BRAUNWALD'S
HEART DISEASE

A TEXTBOOK OF CARDIOVASCULAR MEDICINE

EDITION

12

BRAUNWALD'S
HEART
DISEASE

A TEXTBOOK OF CARDIOVASCULAR MEDICINE

Edited by

PETER LIBBY, MD
Mallinckrodt Professor of Medicine
Harvard Medical School
Brigham and Women's Hospital
Boston, Massachusetts

ROBERT O. BONOW, MD
Max and Lilly Goldberg Distinguished Professor of Cardiology
Department of Medicine
Northwestern University Feinberg School of Medicine
Chicago, Illinois

DOUGLAS L. MANN, MD
Lewin Distinguished Professor of Cardiovascular Disease
Washington University School of Medicine in St. Louis
Saint Louis, Missouri

GORDON F. TOMASELLI, MD
Professor of Medicine (Cardiology)
The Marilyn and Stanley M. Katz Dean
Albert Einstein College of Medicine
Executive Vice President and Chief Academic Officer
Montefiore Medicine
Bronx, New York

DEEPAK L. BHATT, MD, MPH
Executive Director of Interventional Cardiovascular Programs
Brigham and Women's Hospital
Senior Physician
Brigham and Women's Hospital
Professor of Medicine
Harvard Medical School
Boston, Massachusetts

SCOTT D. SOLOMON, MD
The Edward D. Frohlich Distinguished Chair
Professor of Medicine
Harvard Medical School
Senior Physician
Brigham and Women's Hospital
Boston, Massachusetts

Founding Editor and Online Editor

EUGENE BRAUNWALD, MD,
MD(Hon), ScD(Hon), FRCP
Distinguished Hersey Professor of Medicine
Harvard Medical School
Founding Chairman, TIMI Study Group
Brigham and Women's Hospital
Boston, Massachusetts

ELSEVIER

ELSEVIER
1600 John F. Kennedy Blvd.
Ste. 1800
Philadelphia, PA 19103-2899

BRAUNWALD'S HEART DISEASE: A TEXTBOOK OF
CARDIOVASCULAR MEDICINE, TWELFTH EDITION
Copyright © 2022 by Elsevier Inc.

TWO-VOLUME SET ISBN: 978-0-323-72219-3
SINGLE VOLUME ISBN: 978-0-323-82467-5
INTERNATIONAL EDITION ISBN: 978-0-323-82468-2

Notice

Knowledge and best practice in this field are constantly changing. As new research and experience broaden our knowledge, changes in practice, treatment and drug therapy may become necessary or appropriate. Readers are advised to check the most current information provided (i) on procedures featured or (ii) by the manufacturer of each product to be administered, to verify the recommended dose or formula, the method and duration of administration, and contraindications. It is the responsibility of the practitioner, relying on their own experience and knowledge of the patient, to make diagnoses, to determine dosages and the best treatment for each individual patient, and to take all appropriate safety precautions. To the fullest extent of the law, neither the Publisher nor the Authors assume any liability for any injury and/or damage to persons or property arising out of or related to any use of the material contained in this book.

The Publisher

Previous editions copyrighted 2019, 2015, 2012, 2008, 2005, 2001, 1997, 1992, 1988, 1984, 1980 by Elsevier Inc.

Library of Congress Control Number: 2021936447

Executive Content Strategists: Dolores Meloni, Robin Carter
Senior Content Development Specialist: Anne Snyder
Publishing Services Manager: Catherine Jackson
Senior Project Manager: John Casey
Design Direction: Renee Duenow

About the cover:
Professor C. Michael Gibson is well known in interventional cardiology for his many contributions to clinical science. He has had leadership positions in many pivotal clinical trials that have influenced our practice and guidelines. He originated the TIMI myocardial perfusion grade. He currently leads the Baim Institute for Clinical Research, an academic research organization at Boston's Beth Israel Hospital. Beyond his investigative prowess, Professor Gibson is an unusually talented artist. The editor-in-chief was delighted that he agreed to provide art for the cover for this 12th edition of Braunwald's Heart Disease. This addition is particularly appropriate because of Dr. Gibson's long-term association with Dr. Braunwald's research in ischemic heart disease. The editors are proud to have his artistic rendition of the now classic *Heart Disease* logo grace the cover of our book.

Printed in United States of America

9 8 7 6 5 4 3 2 1

To
Beryl, Oliver, and Brigitte
Pat, Rob, Sam, Laura, and Yoko
Benjamin Tan
Charlene, Sarah, Emily, and Matthew
Shanthala, Vinayak, Arjun, Ram, and Raj
Caren, Will and Lyz, Katie and Zach, and Dan

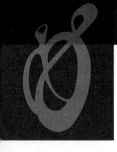

Contributors

Keith D. Aaronson, MD, MS
Bertram Pitt MD Collegiate Professor of Cardiovascular Medicine
Professor of Internal Medicine
Division of Cardiovascular Medicine
University of Michigan
Ann Arbor, Michigan
Chapter 59. Mechanical Circulatory Support

Michael J. Ackerman, MD, PhD
Windland Smith Rice Cardiovascular Genomics Research Professor
Professor of Medicine, Pediatrics, and Pharmacology
Mayo Clinic College of Medicine and Science
Department of Cardiovascular Medicine (Division of Heart Rhythm
    Services and the Windland Smith Rice Genetic Heart Rhythm
    Clinic)
Department of Molecular Pharmacology & Experimental
    Therapeutics (Windland Smith Rice Sudden Death Genomics
    Laboratory)
Department of Pediatric and Adolescent Medicine (Division of
    Pediatric Cardiology)
Mayo Clinic
Rochester, Minnesota
Chapter 63. Genetics of Cardiac Arrhythmias

Philip A. Ades, MD
Endowed Professor of Medicine
Division of Cardiology
University of Vermont College of Medicine
Director, Cardiac Rehabilitation and Prevention
University of Vermont Medical Center
Burlington, Vermont
*Chapter 15. Exercise Physiology and Exercise Electrocardiographic
    Testing*

Christine M. Albert, MD
Chair and Professor of Cardiology
Smidt Heart Institute, Cedars-Sinai Medical Center
Los Angeles, California
Chapter 70. Cardiac Arrest and Sudden Cardiac Death

Michelle A. Albert, MD, MPH
Professor of Medicine
Director, Center for the Study of Adversity and Cardiovascular Disease
    (NURTURE Center)
University of California at San Francisco
San Francisco, California
*Chapter 93. Heart Disease in Racially and Ethnically Diverse
    Populations*

Mark J. Alberts, MD
Chief of Neurology
Hartford Hospital
Hartford, Connecticut;
Co-Physician-in-Chief
Ayer Neuroscience Institute
Hartford HealthCare
Professor of Neurology
University of Connecticut
Storrs, Connecticut
Chapter 45. Prevention and Management of Ischemic Stroke

Sadeer Al-Kindi, MD
Assistant Professor of Medicine
Case Western Reserve University
Harrington Heart and Vascular Institute
University Hospitals Cleveland Medical Center
Cleveland, Ohio
Chapter 3. Impact of the Environment on Cardiovascular Health

Nandan S. Anavekar, MBBCh
Professor of Medicine
Department of Cardiovascular Diseases
Department of Radiology
Mayo Clinic College of Medicine and Science
Rochester, Minnesota
*Chapter 80. Infectious Endocarditis and Infections of Indwelling
    Devices*

Zachi Attia, PhD
Department of Cardiovascular Medicine
Mayo Clinic College of Medicine and Science
Rochester, Minnesota
Chapter 11. Artificial Intelligence in Cardiovascular Medicine

Sonya V. Babu-Narayan, MBBS, BSc, PhD, FRCP
Adult Congenital Heart Disease
Royal Brompton Hospital
Reader, National Heart and Lung Institute
Imperial College London
London, United Kingdom
*Chapter 82. Congenital Heart Disease in the Adolescent and
    Adult*

Larry M. Baddour, MD
Professor of Medicine
Mayo Clinic College of Medicine and Science
Rochester, Minnesota
*Chapter 80. Infectious Endocarditis and Infections of Indwelling
    Devices*

Aaron L. Baggish, MD
Associate Professor of Medicine
Harvard Medical School
Director, Cardiovascular Performance Program
Massachusetts General Hospital
Boston, Massachusetts
Chapter 32. Exercise and Sports Cardiology

C. Noel Bairey Merz, MD
Women's Guild Endowed Chair in Women's Health
Director, Barbra Streisand Women's Heart Center
Erika J. Glazer Women's Heart Research Initiative Director
Director, Linda Joy Pollin Women's Heart Health Program
Barbra Streisand Women's Heart Center
Cedars-Sinai Heart Institute
Los Angeles, California
Chapter 91. Cardiovascular Disease in Women

George L. Bakris, MD, MA
Professor of Medicine
Section of Endocrinology, Diabetes and Metabolism
Director, American Heart Association Comprehensive Hypertension
    Center
UChicago Medicine
Chicago, Illinois
*Chapter 26. Systemic Hypertension: Mechanisms, Diagnosis, and
    Treatment*

Gary J. Balady, MD
Professor of Medicine
Boston University School of Medicine
Director, Non-Invasive Cardiovascular Laboratories
Boston Medical Center
Boston, Massachusetts
*Chapter 15. Exercise Physiology and Exercise Electrocardiographic
    Testing*

David T. Balzer, MD
Professor of Pediatrics
Division of Pediatric Cardiology
Washington University School of Medicine in St. Louis
Saint Louis, Missouri
*Chapter 83. Catheter-Based Treatment of Congenital Heart Disease in
    Adults*

Joshua A. Beckman, MD
Professor of Medicine
Division of Cardiovascular Medicine
Vanderbilt University College of Medicine
Director, Section of Vascular Medicine
Vanderbilt University Medical Center
Nashville, Tennessee
*Chapter 23. Anesthesia and Noncardiac Surgery in Patients with Heart
    Disease*

Donald M. Bers, PhD
Distinguished Professor and Chair
Department of Pharmacology
University of California, Davis
Davis, California
Chapter 46. Mechanisms of Cardiac Contraction and Relaxation

Aruni Bhatnagar, PhD
Professor of Medicine
University of Louisville
Louisville, Kentucky
*Chapter 28. Cardiovascular Disease Risk of Nicotine and Tobacco
    Products*

Deepak L. Bhatt, MD, MPH
Executive Director of Interventional Cardiovascular Programs
Brigham and Women's Hospital
Senior Physician
Brigham and Women's Hospital
Professor of Medicine
Harvard Medical School
Boston, Massachusetts
Chapter 41. Percutaneous Coronary Intervention
Chapter 44. Treatment of Noncoronary Obstructive Vascular Disease

Bernadette Biondi, MD
Professor of Internal Medicine
Department of Clinical Medicine and Surgery
Federico II University
Naples, Italy
Chapter 96. Endocrine Disorders and Cardiovascular Disease

Ron Blankstein, MD
Associate Director, Cardiovascular Imaging Program
Director, Cardiac Computed Tomography
Co-Director, Cardiovascular Imaging Training Program
Brigham and Women's Hospital
Professor of Medicine and Radiology
Harvard Medical School
Boston, Massachusetts
Chapter 20. Cardiac Computed Tomography

Erin A. Bohula, MD, DPhil
TIMI Study Group and Division of Cardiology
Brigham and Women's Hospital
Harvard Medical School
Boston, Massachusetts
Chapter 38. ST-Elevation Myocardial Infarction: Management

Marc P. Bonaca, MD, MPH
Executive Director
CPC Clinical Research
Professor of Medicine
Cardiology and Vascular Medicine
University of Colorado
Aurora, Colorado
Chapter 35. Approach to the Patient with Chest Pain
Chapter 43. Peripheral Artery Diseases

Robert O. Bonow, MD
Max and Lilly Goldberg Distinguished Professor of Cardiology
Department of Medicine
Northwestern University Feinberg School of Medicine
Chicago, Illinois
Chapter 72. Aortic Valve Stenosis
Chapter 73. Aortic Regurgitation
Chapter 76. Mitral Regurgitation

Barry A. Borlaug, MD
Professor of Medicine
Mayo Medical School
Director, Circulatory Failure Research
Consultant, Cardiovascular Diseases
Mayo Clinic College of Medicine and Science
Rochester, Minnesota
Chapter 46. Mechanisms of Cardiac Contraction and Relaxation

Jason S. Bradfield, MD
Associate Professor of Medicine
Director, Specialized Program for Ventricular Tachycardia
UCLA Cardiac Arrhythmia Center
Ronald Reagan UCLA Medical Center
Los Angeles, California
Chapter 102. Cardiovascular Manifestations of Autonomic Disorders

Eugene Braunwald, MD, MD(Hon), ScD(Hon), FRCP
Distinguished Hersey Professor of Medicine
Harvard Medical School
Founding Chairman, TIMI Study Group
Brigham and Women's Hospital
Boston, Massachusetts
Chapter 1. Cardiovascular Disease: Past, Present, and Future
Chapter 39. Non-ST Elevation Acute Coronary Syndromes

Alan C. Braverman, MD
Alumni Endowed Professor in Cardiovascular Diseases
Director, Marfan Syndrome and Aortopathy Clinic
Washington University School of Medicine in St. Louis
Director, Inpatient Cardiology Firm
Barnes-Jewish Hospital
Saint Louis, Missouri
Chapter 42. Diseases of the Aorta

CONTRIBUTORS

John E. Brush Jr., MD
Senior Medical Director
Sentara Health Research Center
Sentara Healthcare
Professor of Medicine
Department of Internal Medicine
Eastern Virginia Medical School
Norfolk, Virginia
Chapter 5. Clinical Decision-Making in Cardiology

Hugh Calkins, MD
Catherine Ellen Poindexter Professor of Cardiology
Professor of Medicine
Director, Cardiac Arrhythmia Service
The Johns Hopkins Medical Institutions
Baltimore, Maryland
Chapter 66. Atrial Fibrillation: Clinical Features, Mechanisms, and Management
Chapter 71. Hypotension and Syncope

John M. Canty Jr., MD
SUNY Distinguished and Albert and Elizabeth Rekate Professor of Medicine
Division of Cardiovascular Medicine
Jacobs School of Medicine and Biomedical Sciences
University at Buffalo
Buffalo, New York
Chapter 36. Coronary Blood Flow and Myocardial Ischemia

Robert M. Carney, PhD
Professor of Psychiatry
Washington University School of Medicine in St. Louis
Saint Louis, Missouri
Chapter 99. Psychiatric and Psychosocial Aspects of Cardiovascular Disease

Y.S. Chandrashekhar, MD
Professor of Medicine
Division of Cardiology
University of Minnesota
Chief of Cardiology
VA Medical Center
Minneapolis, Minnesota
Chapter 75. Mitral Stenosis

Peng-Shen Chen, MD
Cedars-Sinai Medical Center
Los Angeles, California
Chapter 71. Hypotension and Syncope

Mina K. Chung, MD
Professor of Medicine
Cardiovascular and Metabolic Sciences
Lerner Research Institute
Cleveland Clinic Lerner College of Medicine of Case Western Reserve University
Staff, Cardiovascular Medicine
Cleveland Clinic
Cleveland, Ohio
Chapter 69. Pacemakers and Implantable Cardioverter-Defibrillators

Leslie T. Cooper Jr., MD
Professor of Medicine
Chair, Department of Vascular Medicine
Mayo Clinic
Jacksonville, Florida
Chapter 55. Myocarditis

Mark A. Creager, MD
Professor of Medicine and Surgery
Geisel School of Medicine at Dartmouth
Hanover, New Hampshire;
Director, Heart and Vascular Center
Heart and Vascular Center
Dartmouth-Hitchcock Medical Center
Lebanon, New Hampshire
Chapter 43. Peripheral Artery Diseases

Paul C. Cremer, MD
Assistant Professor of Medicine
Cleveland Clinic Lerner College of Medicine of Case Western Reserve University
Associate Director of Cardiovascular Training Program
Cleveland Clinic Foundation
Cleveland Clinic
Cleveland, Ohio
Chapter 86. Pericardial Diseases

Juan A. Crestanello, MD
Professor of Surgery
Mayo Clinic College of Medicine and Science
Rochester, Minnesota
Chapter 80. Infectious Endocarditis and Infections of Indwelling Devices

Anne B. Curtis, MD
Charles and Mary Bauer Professor and Chair
SUNY Distinguished Professor
Department of Medicine
Jacobs School of Medicine and Biomedical Sciences
University at Buffalo
Buffalo, New York
Chapter 61. Approach to the Patient with Cardiac Arrhythmias

George D. Dangas, MD, PhD
Professor of Medicine (Cardiology)
Zena and Michael A Wiener Cardiovascular Institute
Icahn School of Medicine at Mount Sinai
New York, New York
Chapter 21. Coronary Angiography and Intravascular Imaging

James P. Daubert, MD
Professor of Medicine
Cardiology (Electrophysiology)
Duke University Medical Center
Durham, North Carolina
Chapter 69. Pacemakers and Implantable Cardioverter-Defibrillators

James A. de Lemos, MD
Professor of Medicine
Sweetheart Ball-Kern Wildenthal MD PhD Distinguished Chair in Cardiology
UT Southwestern Medical Center
Dallas, Texas
Chapter 40. Stable Ischemic Heart Disease

Jean-Pierre Després, PhD
Professor
Kinesiology Department
Université Laval
Scientific Director
VITAM – Centre de recherche en santé durable
Centre intégré universitaire de santé et de services sociaux de la Capitale-Nationale
Québec City, Québec, Canada
Chapter 30. Obesity: Medical and Surgical Management

Stephen Devries, MD
Executive Director
Gaples Institute for Integrative Cardiology
Deerfield, Illinois;
Division of Cardiology
Northwestern University Feinberg School of Medicine
Chicago, Illinois
Chapter 34. Integrative Approaches to the Management of Patients with Heart Disease

Marcelo F. Di Carli, MD
Seltzer Family Professor of Radiology and Medicine
Harvard Medical School
Executive Director, Cardiovascular Imaging Program
Chief, Division of Nuclear Medicine and Molecular Imaging
Brigham and Women's Hospital
Boston, Massachusetts
Chapter 18. Nuclear Cardiology

Sharmila Dorbala, MD, MPH
Professor of Radiology
Harvard Medical School
Director, Nuclear Cardiology
Division of Nuclear Medicine and Molecular Imaging
Brigham and Women's Hospital
Boston, Massachusetts
Chapter 18. Nuclear Cardiology

Adam L. Dorfman, MD
Professor
Departments of Pediatrics and Radiology
Director, Non-Invasive Imaging, Division of Pediatric Cardiology
University of Michigan Medical School
C.S. Mott Children's Hospital
Ann Arbor, Michigan
Chapter 82. Congenital Heart Disease in the Adolescent and Adult

Dirk J. Duncker, MD, PhD
Professor of Experimental Cardiology
Department of Cardiology
Erasmus MC, University Medical Center Rotterdam
Rotterdam, The Netherlands
Chapter 36. Coronary Blood Flow and Myocardial Ischemia

Kenneth A. Ellenbogen, MD
Martha M. and Harold W. Kimmerling Professor of Cardiology
Director, Electrophysiology and Pacing
Virginia Commonwealth University School of Medicine
Richmond, Virginia
Chapter 64. Therapy for Cardiac Arrhythmias

Thomas H. Everett IV, PhD
Associate Professor of Medicine
The Krannert Institute of Cardiology and Division of Cardiology
Indiana University School of Medicine
Indianapolis, Indiana
Chapter 71. Hypotension and Syncope

James C. Fang, MD
Professor of Medicine
Division of Cardiovascular Medicine
University of Utah
Executive Director, Cardiovascular Service Line
University of Utah Health Sciences
Salt Lake City, Utah
Chapter 13. History and Physical Examination: An Evidence-Based Approach

G. Michael Felker, MD, MHS
Professor of Medicine
Vice Chief for Clinical Research
Division of Cardiology
Duke University School of Medicine
Director, Cardiovascular Research
Duke Clinical Research Institute
Durham, North Carolina
Chapter 49. Diagnosis and Management of Acute Heart Failure

Jerome L. Fleg, MD
Medical Officer
Division of Cardiovascular Sciences
National Heart, Lung, and Blood Institute
Bethesda, Maryland
Chapter 90. Cardiovascular Disease in Older Adults

Lee A. Fleisher, MD
Professor
Anesthesiology and Critical Care
Professor of Medicine
University of Pennsylvania Perelman School of Medicine
Philadelphia, Pennsylvania
Chapter 23. Anesthesia and Noncardiac Surgery in Patients with Heart Disease

Daniel E. Forman, MD
Professor of Medicine
University of Pittsburgh
Chair, Section of Geriatric Cardiology
Divisions of Geriatrics and Cardiology
University of Pittsburgh Medical Center
Director, Cardiac Rehabilitation
VA Pittsburgh Healthcare System
Pittsburgh, Pennsylvania
Chapter 90. Cardiovascular Disease in Older Adults

Kenneth E. Freedland, PhD
Professor of Psychiatry
Washington University School of Medicine in St. Louis
Saint Louis, Missouri
Chapter 99. Psychiatric and Psychosocial Aspects of Cardiovascular Disease

Paul Friedman, MD
Norman Blane & Billie Jean Harty Chair
Mayo Clinic Department of Cardiovascular Medicine Honoring Robert L. Frye, MD
Professor of Medicine
Mayo Clinic College of Medicine and Science
Rochester, Minnesota
Chapter 11. Artificial Intelligence in Cardiovascular Medicine

J. Michael Gaziano, MD, MPH
Professor of Medicine
Harvard Medical School
Chief, Division of Aging
Brigham and Women's Hospital
Director, Preventive Cardiology
VA Boston Healthcare System
Boston, Massachusetts
Chapter 2. Global Burden of Cardiovascular Disease

Thomas A. Gaziano, MD, MSc
Associate Professor
Harvard Medical School
Physician
Cardiovascular Medicine Division
Brigham & Women's Hospital
Boston, Massachusetts
Chapter 2. Global Burden of Cardiovascular Disease

Jacques Genest, MD
Professor of Medicine
Faculty of Medicine
McGill University
Research Institute of the McGill University Health Centre
Montreal, Quebec, Canada
Chapter 27. Lipoprotein Disorders and Cardiovascular Disease

Robert Gerszten, MD
Herman Dana Professor of Medicine
Harvard Medical School
Chief, Division of Cardiovascular Medicine
Beth Israel Deaconess Medical Center
Boston, Massachusetts
Chapter 8. Proteomics and Metabolomics in Cardiovascular Medicine

Linda D. Gillam, MD, MPH
Dorothy and Lloyd Huck Chair
Department of Cardiovascular Medicine
Morristown Medical Center
Morristown, New Jersey;
Professor of Medicine
Thomas Jefferson University
Philadelphia, Pennsylvania
Chapter 16. Echocardiography

John R. Giudicessi, MD, PhD
Assistant Professor of Medicine
Department of Cardiovascular Medicine (Division of Heart Rhythm Services and the Windland Smith Rice Genetic Heart Rhythm Clinic)
Mayo Clinic College of Medicine and Science
Rochester, Minnesota
Chapter 63. Genetics of Cardiac Arrhythmias

Robert P. Giugliano, MD, SM
Staff Physician
Cardiovascular Medicine
Brigham and Women's Hospital
Professor of Medicine
Harvard Medical School
Boston, Massachusetts
Chapter 39. Non-ST Elevation Acute Coronary Syndromes

Ary L. Goldberger, MD
Professor of Medicine
Harvard Medical School
Department of Medicine
Beth Israel Deaconess Medical Center
Boston, Massachusetts
Chapter 14. Electrocardiography

Jeffrey J. Goldberger, MD, MBA
Professor of Medicine
Chief, Cardiovascular Division
University of Miami Miller School of Medicine
Miami, Florida
Chapter 70. Cardiac Arrest and Sudden Cardiac Death

Samuel Z. Goldhaber, MD
Professor of Medicine
Harvard Medical School
Director, Thrombosis Research Group
Associate Chief and Clinical Director
Division of Cardiovascular Medicine
Brigham and Women's Hospital
Boston, Massachusetts
Chapter 87. Pulmonary Embolism and Deep Vein Thrombosis

William J. Groh, MD, MPH
Clinical Professor of Medicine
Medical University of South Carolina
Chief of Medicine
Ralph H. Johnson VAMC
Charleston, South Carolina
Chapter 100. Neuromuscular Disorders and Cardiovascular Disease

Martha Gulati, MD, MS
Chief of Cardiology
Professor of Medicine
University of Arizona–Phoenix
Phoenix, Arizona
Chapter 91. Cardiovascular Disease in Women

Rebecca Tung Hahn, MD
Director of Interventional Echocardiography
Center for Interventional and Vascular Therapy
Columbia University Medical Center
New York, New York
Chapter 76. Mitral Regurgitation

Gerd Hasenfuss, MD
Professor of Medicine
Chair, Department of Cardiology and Pneumology
University of Göttingen Medical Center
Göttingen, Germany
Chapter 47. Pathophysiology of Heart Failure

Howard C. Herrmann, MD
John W. Bryfogle Jr. Professor of Cardiovascular Medicine
Division of Cardiovascular Medicine
University of Pennsylvania Perelman School of Medicine
Health System Director for Interventional Cardiology
Hospital of the University of Pennsylvania
Philadelphia, Pennsylvania
Chapter 78. Transcatheter Therapies for Mitral and Tricuspid Valvular Heart Disease

Joerg Herrmann, MD
Professor of Medicine
Department of Cardiovascular Medicine
Mayo Clinic
Rochester, Minnesota
Chapter 22. Invasive Hemodynamic Diagnosis of Cardiac Disease
Chapter 57. Cardio-Oncology: Approach to the Patient

Ray E. Hershberger, MD
Professor of Internal Medicine
Director, Division of Human Genetics
Division of Cardiovascular Medicine
Section of Heart Failure and Cardiac Transplantation
Dorothy M. Davis Heart and Lung Research Institute
Wexner Medical Center at the Ohio State University
Columbus, Ohio
Chapter 52. The Dilated, Restrictive, and Infiltrative Cardiomyopathies

Carolyn Y. Ho, MD
Associate Professor of Medicine
Cardiovascular Division
Brigham and Women's Hospital
Boston, Massachusetts
Chapter 54. Hypertrophic Cardiomyopathy

Priscilla Y. Hsue, MD
Professor
Department of Medicine
University of California, San Francisco
San Francisco, California
Chapter 85. Cardiovascular Abnormalities in HIV-Infected Individuals

W. Gregory Hundley, MD
Professor of Medicine
Chairman, Cardiology Division
VCU School of Medicine
Director, Pauley Heart Center
Virginia Commonwealth University Health
Richmond, Virginia
Chapter 98. Tumors Affecting the Cardiovascular System

Silvio E. Inzucchi, MD
Professor, Internal Medicine (Endocrinology)
Yale University School of Medicine
Clinical Chief, Endocrinology
Director, Yale Diabetes Center
Yale-New Haven Hospital
New Haven, Connecticut
Chapter 31. Diabetes and the Cardiovascular System

Francine L. Jacobson, MD, MPH
Thoracic Radiologist
Brigham and Women's Hospital
Harvard Medical School
Boston, Massachusetts
Chapter 17. Chest Radiography in Cardiovascular Disease

James L. Januzzi Jr., MD
Physician
Cardiology Division
Massachusetts General Hospital
Hutter Family Professor of Medicine
Harvard Medical School
Boston, Massachusetts
Chapter 48. Approach to the Patient with Heart Failure

Karen E. Joynt Maddox, MD, MPH
Associate Professor of Medicine
Cardiovascular Division
Washington University School of Medicine in St. Louis
Co-Director, Center for Health Economics and Policy
Institute for Public Health at Washington University
Saint Louis, Missouri
Chapter 6. Impact of Health Care Policy on Quality, Outcomes, and Equity in Cardiovascular Disease

Jonathan M. Kalman, MBBS, PhD
Director of Cardiac Electrophysiology
Department of Cardiology
Royal Melbourne Hospital, Melbourne
Professor of Medicine
University of Melbourne
Melbourne, Victoria, Australia
Chapter 65. Supraventricular Tachycardias

Suraj Kapa, MD
Assistant Professor of Medicine
Cardiovascular Diseases
Mayo Clinic College of Medicine and Science
Rochester, Minnesota
Chapter 11. Artificial Intelligence in Cardiovascular Medicine

Morton J. Kern, MD
Professor of Medicine
University California, Irvine
Orange, California;
Chief of Medicine and Cardiology
Veterans Administration Long Beach Healthcare System
Long Beach, California
Chapter 22. Invasive Hemodynamic Diagnosis of Cardiac Disease

Scott Kinlay, MBBS, PhD
Chief, Cardiology (acting)
Director Cardiac Catheterization Laboratory and Vascular Medicine
VA Boston Healthcare System
West Roxbury, Massachusetts
Physician, Cardiovascular Division
Brigham and Women's Hospital
Associate Professor in Medicine
Harvard Medical School
Adjunct Associate Professor in Medicine
Boston University Medical School
Boston, Massachusetts
Chapter 44. Treatment of Noncoronary Obstructive Vascular Disease

Allan L. Klein, MD, FRCP(C)
Professor of Medicine
Cleveland Clinic Lerner College of Medicine of Case Western Reserve University
Director, Center for the Diagnosis and Treatment of Pericardial Diseases
Department of Cardiovascular Medicine
Heart, Vascular and Thoracic Institute
Cleveland Clinic
Cleveland, Ohio
Chapter 86. Pericardial Diseases

Robert A. Kloner, MD, PhD
Professor of Medicine (Clinical Scholar)
Cardiovascular Division
Keck School of Medicine of University of Southern California
Los Angeles, California;
Chief Science Officer
Scientific Director of Cardiovascular Research Institute
Huntington Medical Research Institutes
Pasadena, California
Chapter 84. Cardiomyopathies Induced by Drugs or Toxins

Kirk U. Knowlton, MD
Director of Cardiovascular Research
Intermountain Healthcare Heart Institute
Adjunct Professor
Department of Medicine
University of Utah
Salt Lake City, Utah;
Professor Emeritus of Medicine
University of California, San Diego
La Jolla, California
Chapter 55. Myocarditis

Eric V. Krieger, MD
Professor of Medicine
Division of Cardiology
University of Washington School of Medicine
Director, Adult Congenital Heart Service
University of Washington Medical Center
Seattle Children's Hospital
Seattle, Washington
Chapter 82. Congenital Heart Disease in the Adolescent and Adult

Harlan M. Krumholz, MD, SM
Harold H. Hines, Jr. Professor of Medicine
Section of Cardiovascular Medicine
Department of Medicine
Department of Health Policy and Management
School of Public Health
Yale School of Medicine
Center for Outcomes Research and Evaluation
Yale New Haven Hospital
New Haven, Connecticut
Chapter 5. Clinical Decision-Making in Cardiology

CONTRIBUTORS

Dharam J. Kumbhani, MD, SM
Associate Professor of Medicine
Section Chief, Interventional Cardiology
Department of Internal Medicine
University of Texas Southwestern Medical Center
Dallas, Texas
Chapter 41. Percutaneous Coronary Intervention

Raymond Y. Kwong, MD, MPH
Professor of Medicine
Harvard Medical School
Director of Cardiac Magnetic Resonance Imaging
Cardiovascular Division
Brigham and Women's Hospital
Boston, Massachusetts
Chapter 19. Cardiovascular Magnetic Resonance Imaging

Bonnie Ky, MD, MSCE
Associate Professor of Medicine and Epidemiology
Division of Cardiovascular Medicine
Senior Scholar
Department of Biostatistics, Epidemiology and Informatics
University of Pennsylvania School of Medicine
Philadelphia, Pennsylvania
Chapter 56. Cardio-Oncology: Managing Cardiotoxic Effects of Cancer Therapies

Carolyn S.P. Lam, MBBS, PhD, MRCP, MS
Professor
Cardiovascular Academic Clinical Program
Duke–National University of Singapore
Senior Consultant Cardiologist
National Heart Centre Singapore
Singapore
Chapter 51. Heart Failure with Preserved and Mildly Reduced Ejection Fraction

Eric Larose, DVM, MD, FRCPC
Professor and Head of Cardiology Division
Department of Medicine
Chair of Research & Innovation in Cardiovascular Imaging
Université Laval
Cardiologist, Institut universitaire de cardiologie et de pneumologie de Québec – Université Laval
Quebec City, Quebec, Canada
Chapter 30. Obesity: Medical and Surgical Management

John M. Lasala, MD, PhD
Professor of Medicine
Director, Structural Heart Disease Program
Cardiology Division
Washington University School of Medicine in St. Louis
Saint Louis, Missouri
Chapter 83. Catheter-Based Treatment of Congenital Heart Disease in Adults

Daniel J. Lenihan, MD
President, International Cardio-Oncology Society
Professor of Medicine
Director, Cardio-Oncology Center of Excellence
Cardiovascular Division
Washington University School of Medicine in St. Louis
Saint Louis, Missouri
Chapter 98. Tumors Affecting the Cardiovascular System

Eric J. Lenze, MD
Professor of Psychiatry
Washington University School of Medicine in St. Louis
Saint Louis, Missouri
Chapter 99. Psychiatric and Psychosocial Aspects of Cardiovascular Disease

Martin B. Leon, MD
The Mallah Family Professor of Cardiology
Director, Center for Interventional Vascular Therapy
Columbia University Irving Medical Center
NY Presbyterian Hospital
Founder and Chairman Emeritus
Cardiovascular Research Foundation
New York, New York
Chapter 74. Transcatheter Aortic Valve Replacement

Martin M. LeWinter, MD
Professor Emeritus of Medicine and Molecular Physiology and Biophysics
Larner College of Medicine at the University of Vermont
Attending Cardiologist
University of Vermont Medical Center
Burlington, Vermont
Chapter 86. Pericardial Diseases

Peter Libby, MD
Mallinckrodt Professor of Medicine
Harvard Medical School
Brigham and Women's Hospital
Boston, Massachusetts
Chapter 10. Biomarkers and Use in Precision Medicine
Chapter 24. The Vascular Biology of Atherosclerosis
Chapter 25. Primary Prevention of Cardiovascular Disease
Chapter 27. Lipoprotein Disorders and Cardiovascular Disease
Chapter 37. ST-Elevation Myocardial Infarction: Pathophysiology and Clinical Evolution

JoAnn Lindenfeld, MD
Professor of Medicine
Samuel S Riven MD Directorship in Cardiology
Vanderbilt University Medical Center
Nashville, Tennessee
Chapter 58. Devices for Monitoring and Managing Heart Failure

Brian R. Lindman, MD, MSc
Associate Professor of Medicine
Medical Director, Structural Heart and Valve Center
Cardiovascular Division
Vanderbilt University Medical Center
Nashville, Tennessee
Chapter 72. Aortic Valve Stenosis

Michael J. Mack, MD
Chair, Cardiovascular Service Line
Baylor Scott & White Health
President, Baylor Scott & White Research Institute
Dallas, Texas
Chapter 74. Transcatheter Aortic Valve Replacement

Mohammad Madjid, MD, MS
Associate Professor of Medicine
McGovern Medical School
University of Texas Health Science Center at Houston
Interventional Cardiologist
Heart and Vascular Institute
Memorial Hermann Hospital
Houston, Texas
Chapter 94. Endemic and Pandemic Viral Illnesses and Cardiovascular Disease: Influenza and COVID-19

Douglas L. Mann, MD
Lewin Distinguished Professor of Cardiovascular Disease
Washington University School of Medicine
Saint Louis, Missouri
Chapter 47. Pathophysiology of Heart Failure
Chapter 48. Approach to the Patient With Heart Failure
Chapter 50. Management of Heart Failure Patients with Reduced Ejection Fraction

Bradley A. Maron, MD
Associate Professor of Medicine
Division of Cardiovascular Medicine
Brigham and Women's Hospital
Harvard Medical School
Department of Cardiology
Boston VA Healthcare System
Boston, Massachusetts
Chapter 88. Pulmonary Hypertension

Nikolaus Marx, MD
Professor of Medicine / Cardiology
Head of the Department of Internal Medicine I
University Hospital Aachen
Aachen, Germany
Chapter 31. Diabetes and the Cardiovascular System

Justin C. Mason, PhD, FRCP
Professor of Vascular Rheumatology
Vascular Sciences and Rheumatology
Imperial College London
London, United Kingdom
Chapter 97. Rheumatic Diseases and the Cardiovascular System

Mathew S. Maurer, MD
Arnold and Arlene Goldstein Professor of Cardiology
Professor of Medicine
Columbia University College of Physicians and Surgeons
Center for Advanced Cardiac Care
Columbia University Medical Center
Director, Clinical Cardiovascular Research Laboratory for the Elderly
New York, New York
Chapter 53. Cardiac Amyloidosis

Peter A. McCullough, MD, MPH
Consultant Cardiologist
Clinical Professor of Medicine
Department of Internal Medicine
Texas A&M College of Medicine
Dallas, Texas
Chapter 101. Interface Between Renal Disease and Cardiovascular Illness

Darren K. McGuire, MD, MHSc
Professor, Internal Medicine
Division of Cardiology
University of Texas Southwestern Medical Center
Dallas, Texas
Chapter 31. Diabetes and the Cardiovascular System

John McMurray, OBE BSc (Hons), MB ChB (Hons), MD, FRCP
Professor of Medical Cardiology
Deputy-Director (Clinical), Institute of Cardiovascular and Medical Sciences
BHF Cardiovascular Research Centre
University of Glasgow
Honorary Consultant Cardiologist
Queen Elizabeth University Hospital
Glasgow, Scotland, United Kingdom
Chapter 4. Clinical Trials in Cardiovascular Medicine

Elizabeth M. McNally, MD, PhD
Director, Center for Genetic Medicine
Northwestern University Feinberg School of Medicine
Chicago, Illinois
Chapter 100. Neuromuscular Disorders and Cardiovascular Disease

Roxana Mehran, MD
Professor of Medicine (Cardiology)
Director of Interventional Cardiovascular Research and Clinical Trials
Zena and Michael A. Wiener Cardiovascular Institute
Icahn School of Medicine at Mount Sinai
New York, New York
Chapter 21. Coronary Angiography and Intravascular Imaging

John M. Miller, MD
Professor of Medicine
Indiana University School of Medicine
Director, Cardiac Electrophysiology Services
Indiana University Health
Indianapolis, Indiana
Chapter 64. Therapy for Cardiac Arrhythmias

David M. Mirvis, MD
Professor Emeritus
Preventive Medicine
University of Tennessee College of Medicine
Memphis, Tennessee
Chapter 14. Electrocardiography

Ana Olga Mocumbi, MD, PhD
Associate Professor
Internal Medicine
Universidade Eduardo Mondlane
Head of Division
Non Communicable Diseases
Instituto Nacional de Saúde
Maputo, Mozambique
Chapter 81. Rheumatic Fever

Samia Mora, MD
Associate Professor of Medicine
Harvard Medical School
Associate Physician
Brigham and Women's Hospital
Boston, Massachusetts
Chapter 25. Primary Prevention of Cardiovascular Disease
Chapter 27. Lipoprotein Disorders and Cardiovascular Disease

Fred Morady, MD
McKay Professor of Cardiovascular Disease
Department of Medicine
University of Michigan
Ann Arbor, Michigan
Chapter 66. Atrial Fibrillation: Clinical Features, Mechanisms, and Management

Alanna A. Morris, MD, MSc
Associate Professor of Medicine
Director, Heart Failure Research
Emory University School of Medicine
Atlanta, Georgia
Chapter 93. Heart Disease in Racially and Ethnically Diverse Populations

David A. Morrow, MD, MPH
Professor of Medicine
Harvard Medical School
Boston, Massachusetts
Chapter 37. ST-Elevation Myocardial Infarction: Pathophysiology and Clinical Evolution
Chapter 38. ST-Elevation Myocardial Infarction: Management
Chapter 40. Stable Ischemic Heart Disease

Dariush Mozaffarian, MD, DrPH
Dean, Friedman School of Nutrition Science & Policy
Jean Mayer Professor of Nutrition
Tufts University School of Medicine
Boston, Massachusetts
Chapter 29. Nutrition and Cardiovascular and Metabolic Diseases

xiv

CONTRIBUTORS

Kiran Musunuru, MD, PhD, MPH, ML
Professor of Cardiovascular Medicine and Genetics
Cardiovascular Institute
University of Pennsylvania Perelman School of Medicine
Philadelphia, Pennsylvania
Chapter 7. Applications of Genetics to Cardiovascular Medicine

Robert J. Myerburg, MD
Professor of Medicine and Physiology
Department of Medicine
University of Miami Miller School of Medicine
Miami, Florida
Chapter 70. Cardiac Arrest and Sudden Cardiac Death

Pradeep Natarajan, MD, MMSc
Director of Preventive Cardiology
Massachusetts General Hospital
Assistant Professor of Medicine
Harvard Medical School
Boston, Massachusetts;
Associate Member
Program in Medical and Population Genetics
Broad Institute of Harvard and MIT
Cambridge, Massachusetts
Chapter 7. Applications of Genetics to Cardiovascular Medicine

Stanley Nattel, MDCM
Professor
Department of Medicine
Paul-David Chair in Cardiovascular Electrophysiology
Montreal Heart Institute
University of Montreal
Montreal, Quebec, Canada
Chapter 62. Mechanisms of Cardiac Arrhythmias

Rick A. Nishimura, MD
Judd and Mary Morris Leighton Professor of Cardiovascular Diseases
Department of Cardiovascular Medicine
Mayo Clinic College of Medicine and Science
Rochester, Minnesota
Chapter 73. Aortic Regurgitation

Vuyisile T. Nkomo, MD, MPH
Cardiologist
Professor of Medicine
Department of Cardiovascular Medicine
Mayo Clinic College of Medicine and Science
Rochester, Minnesota
Chapter 77. Tricuspid, Pulmonic, and Multivalvular Disease

Peter Noseworthy, MD
Consultant
Cardiovascular Diseases
Mayo Clinic College of Medicine and Science
Rochester, Minnesota
Chapter 11. Artificial Intelligence in Cardiovascular Medicine

Patrick T. O'Gara, MD
Professor of Medicine
Harvard Medical School
Senior Physician
Cardiovascular Division
Brigham and Women's Hospital
Boston, Massachusetts
Chapter 13. History and Physical Examination: An Evidence-Based Approach
Chapter 79. Prosthetic Heart Valves

Jeffrey E. Olgin, MD
Gallo-Chatterjee Distinguished Professor
Chief, Division of Cardiology
University of California, San Francisco
San Francisco, California
Chapter 68. Bradyarrhythmias and Atrioventricular Block

Steve R. Ommen, MD
Division of Cardiovascular Diseases
Mayo Clinic College of Medicine and Science
Rochester, Minnesota
Chapter 54. Hypertrophic Cardiomyopathy

Catherine M. Otto, MD
Professor of Medicine
J. Ward Kennedy-Hamilton Endowed Chair in Cardiology
Division of Cardiology
University of Washington School of Medicine
Director, Heart Valve Clinic
Associate Director, Echocardiography
University of Washington Medical Center
Seattle, Washington
Chapter 72. Aortic Valve Stenosis

Francis D. Pagani, MD, PhD
Otto Gago MD Endowed Professor of Cardiac Surgery
Department of Cardiac Surgery
University of Michigan
Ann Arbor, Michigan
Chapter 59. Mechanical Circulatory Support

Kristen K. Patton, MD
Professor of Medicine
Division of Cardiology
University of Washington
Seattle, Washington
Chapter 68. Bradyarrhythmias and Atrioventricular Block

Patricia A. Pellikka, MD
The Betty Knight Scripps Professor of Medicine
Mayo Clinic College of Medicine and Science
Vice Chair, Academic Affairs and Faculty Development
Consultant, Department of Cardiovascular Medicine
Director, Ultrasound Research Center
Mayo Clinic
Rochester, Minnesota
Chapter 77. Tricuspid, Pulmonic, and Multivalvular Disease

Gregory Piazza, MD, MS
Staff Physician
Cardiovascular Division
Department of Medicine
Section Head, Vascular Medicine
Brigham and Women's Hospital
Boston, Massachusetts
Chapter 87. Pulmonary Embolism and Deep Vein Thrombosis

Philippe Pibarot, DVM, PhD
Professor
Department of Medicine
Québec Heart & Lung Institute
Université Laval
Québec City, Quebec, Canada
Chapter 79. Prosthetic Heart Valves

Paul Poirier, MD, PhD, FRCPC
Chief, Cardiac Prevention/Rehabilitation
Institut universitaire de cardiologie et de pneumologie de Québec –
    Université Laval
Professor
Faculty of Pharmacy
Université Laval
Quebec City, Quebec, Canada
Chapter 30. Obesity: Medical and Surgical Management

Doiraraj Prabhakaran, MD, DM (Cardiology), MSc, FRCP
Vice President, Research and Policy
Public Health Foundation of India
Executive Director, Centre for Chronic Disease Control
Gurgaon, Haryana, India;
Professor
Department of Epidemiology
London School of Hygiene and Tropical Medicine
London, United Kingdom
Chapter 2. Global Burden of Cardiovascular Disease

Sanjay Rajagopalan, MD
Professor of Medicine
Director, Case Cardiovascular Research Institute
Case Western Reserve University
Chief, Division of Cardiovascular Medicine
Harrington Heart and Vascular Institute
University Hospitals Cleveland Medical Center
Cleveland, Ohio
Chapter 3. Impact of the Environment on Cardiovascular Health

Michael J. Reardon, MD
Professor of Cardiothoracic Surgery
Department of Cardiovascular Surgery
Houston Methodist Hospital
Houston, Texas
*Chapter 78. Transcatheter Therapies for Mitral and Tricuspid Valvular
    Heart Disease*
Chapter 98. Tumors Affecting the Cardiovascular System

Susan Redline, MD, MPH
Peter C. Farrell Professor of Sleep Medicine
Harvard Medical School
Senior Physician
Division of Sleep and Circadian Disorders
Departments of Medicine and Neurology
Brigham and Women's Hospital
Boston, Massachusetts
Chapter 89. Sleep-Disordered Breathing and Cardiac Disease

Shereif Rezkalla, MD
Adjunct Professor of Medicine
University of Wisconsin
Madison, Wisconsin;
Department of Cardiology and Cardiovascular Research
Marshfield Clinic Health System
Marshfield, Wisconsin
Chapter 84. Cardiomyopathies Induced by Drugs or Toxins

Michael W. Rich, MD
Professor of Medicine
Division of Cardiology
Washington University School of Medicine in St. Louis
Saint Louis, Missouri
Chapter 90. Cardiovascular Disease in Older Adults
*Chapter 99. Psychiatric and Psychosocial Aspects of Cardiovascular
    Disease*

Paul M Ridker, MD, MPH
Eugene Braunwald Professor of Medicine
Harvard Medical School
Director, Center for Cardiovascular Disease Prevention
Brigham and Women's Hospital
Boston, Massachusetts
Chapter 10. Biomarkers and Use in Precision Medicine
Chapter 25. Primary Prevention of Cardiovascular Disease

Dan M. Roden, MD
Professor of Medicine, Pharmacology, and Biomedical Informatics
Senior Vice President for Personalized Medicine
Vanderbilt University School of Medicine
Nashville, Tennessee
*Chapter 9. Principles of Drug Therapeutics, Pharmacogenomics, and
    Biologics*

Frederick L. Ruberg, MD
Associate Professor of Medicine
Section of Cardiovascular Medicine
Department of Medicine and Amyloidosis Center
Boston Medical Center
Boston University School of Medicine
Boston, Massachusetts
Chapter 53. Cardiac Amyloidosis

Marc S. Sabatine, MD, MPH
Chair, TIMI Study Group
Lewis Dexter MD Distinguished Chair in Cardiovascular Medicine
Brigham and Women's Hospital
Professor of Medicine
Harvard Medical School
Boston, Massachusetts
Chapter 35. Approach to the Patient with Chest Pain

Prashanthan Sanders, MBBS, PhD
Director, Centre for Heart Rhythm Disorders
School of Medicine
University of Adelaide
Director, Cardiac Electrophysiology and Pacing
Department of Cardiology
Royal Adelaide Hospital
Director, Heart Rhythm Group
Heart Health
South Australian Health and Medical Research Institute
Adelaide, Australia
Chapter 65. Supraventricular Tachycardias

Marc Schermerhorn, MD
George H. A. Clowes Jr. Professor of Surgery
Harvard Medical School
Chief, Division of Vascular and Endovascular Surgery
Beth Israel Deaconess Medical Center
Boston, Massachusetts
Chapter 42. Diseases of the Aorta

Benjamin M. Scirica, MD, MPH
Associate Professor of Medicine
Harvard Medical School
Senior Investigator, TIMI Study Group
Associate Physician, Cardiovascular Division
Brigham and Women's Hospital
Boston, Massachusetts
*Chapter 37. ST-Elevation Myocardial Infarction: Pathophysiology and
    Clinical Evolution*

Arnold H. Seto, MD, MPA
Associate Clinical Professor
University of California, Irvine
Cardiologist
Veterans Administration Long Beach Healthcare System
Long Beach, California
Chapter 22. Invasive Hemodynamic Diagnosis of Cardiac Disease

Sanjiv J. Shah, MD
Neil Stone MD Professor of Medicine
Division of Cardiology
Northwestern University Feinberg School of Medicine
Chicago, Illinois
Chapter 51. Heart Failure with Preserved and Mildly Reduced Ejection Fraction

Shabana Shahanavaz, MBBS
Associate Professor of Pediatrics
Director, Cardiac Catheterization Laboratory
The Heart Institute
Cincinnati Children's Hospital
Cincinnati, Ohio
Chapter 83. Catheter-Based Treatment of Congenital Heart Disease in Adults

Kalyanam Shivkumar, MD, PhD
Professor of Medicine (Cardiology), Radiology, and Bioengineering
Director, UCLA Cardiac Arrhythmia Center and Electrophysiology Programs
Director, Adult Cardiac Catheterization Laboratories
Ronald Reagan UCLA Medical Center
Los Angeles, California
Chapter 102. Cardiovascular Manifestations of Autonomic Disorders

Candice K. Silversides, SM, MD
Professor of Medicine
University of Toronto Pregnancy and Heart Disease Program
Toronto, Ontario, Canada
Chapter 92. Pregnancy and Heart Disease

Samuel C. Siu, MD, SM, MBA
Professor of Medicine
Division of Cardiology
Schulich School of Medicine and Dentistry
Western University
London, Ontario, Canada
Chapter 92. Pregnancy and Heart Disease

Scott D. Solomon, MD
The Edward D. Frohlich Distinguished Chair
Professor of Medicine
Harvard Medical School
Senior Physician
Brigham and Women's Hospital
Boston, Massachusetts
Chapter 4. Clinical Trials in Cardiovascular Medicine
Chapter 16. Echocardiography
Chapter 51. Heart Failure with Preserved and Mildly Reduced Ejection Fraction
Chapter 94. Endemic and Pandemic Viral Illnesses and Cardiovascular Disease: Influenza and COVID-19

Matthew J. Sorrentino, MD
Professor of Medicine
Section of Cardiology
UChicago Medicine
Chicago, Illinois
Chapter 26. Systemic Hypertension: Mechanisms, Diagnosis, and Treatment

Randall C. Starling, MD, MPH
Professor of Medicine
Kaufman Center for Heart Failure
Heart, Thoracic and Vascular Institute
Cleveland Clinic
Cleveland, Ohio
Chapter 60. Cardiac Transplantation

William G. Stevenson, MD
Professor of Medicine
Division of Cardiology
Vanderbilt University Medical Center
Nashville, Tennessee
Chapter 67. Ventricular Arrhythmias

John R. Teerlink, MD, FRCP(UK)
Professor of Medicine
University of California School of Medicine, San Francisco,
    Director, Heart Failure
Director, Echocardiography
Section of Cardiology
San Francisco Veteran Affairs Medical Center
San Francisco, California
Chapter 49. Diagnosis and Management of Acute Heart Failure

David J. Tester, BS
Associate Professor of Medicine
Mayo Clinic College of Medicine and Science
Department of Molecular Pharmacology & Experimental
    Therapeutics (Windland Smith Rice Sudden Death Genomics
    Laboratory)
Mayo Clinic
Rochester, Minnesota
Chapter 63. Genetics of Cardiac Arrhythmias

Randal Jay Thomas, MD, MS
Professor of Medicine
Mayo Clinic Alix School of Medicine
Medical Director, Cardiac Rehabilitation Program
Division of Preventive Cardiology
Department of Cardiovascular Medicine
Mayo Clinic
Rochester, Minnesota
Chapter 33. Comprehensive Cardiac Rehabilitation

Paul D. Thompson, MD
Chief of Cardiology, Emeritus
Hartford Hospital
Hartford, Connecticut
Chapter 32. Exercise and Sports Cardiology

Gordon F. Tomaselli, MD
Professor of Medicine (Cardiology)
The Marilyn and Stanley M. Katz Dean
Albert Einstein College of Medicine
Executive Vice President and Chief Academic Officer
Montefiore Medicine
Bronx, New York
Chapter 61. Approach to the Patient with Cardiac Arrhythmias
Chapter 62. Mechanisms of Cardiac Arrhythmias
Chapter 66. Atrial Fibrillation: Clinical Features, Mechanisms, and Management
Chapter 100. Neuromuscular Disorders and Cardiovascular Disease

Mintu P. Turakhia, MD, MAS
Associate Professor of Medicine (Cardiovascular Medicine)
Executive Director, Center for Digital Health
Stanford University
Stanford, California;
Chief, Cardiac Electrophysiology
VA Palo Alto Health Care System
Palo Alto, California
Chapter 12. Wearable Devices in Cardiovascular Medicine

Anne Marie Valente, MD
Associate Professor
Pediatrics and Internal Medicine
Harvard Medical School
Director, Boston Adult Congenital Heart Program
Children's Hospital Boston
Brigham and Women's Hospital
Boston, Massachusetts
Chapter 82. Congenital Heart Disease in the Adolescent and Adult

Orly Vardeny, PharmD, MS
Associate Professor of Medicine
Center for Care Delivery and Outcomes Research
Minneapolis VA Health Care System and University of Minnesota
Minneapolis, Minnesota
Chapter 94. Endemic and Pandemic Viral Illnesses and Cardiovascular Disease: Influenza and COVID-19

David D. Waters, MD
Professor Emeritus
Department of Medicine
University of California, San Francisco
San Francisco, California
Chapter 85. Cardiovascular Abnormalities in HIV-Infected Individuals

Jeffrey I. Weitz, MD, FRCP(C)
Professor of Medicine and Biochemistry
McMaster University
Executive Director
Thrombosis and Atherosclerosis Research Institute
Hamilton, Ontario, Canada
Chapter 95. Hemostasis, Thrombosis, Fibrinolysis, and Cardiovascular Disease

Nanette Kass Wenger, MD
Professor of Medicine (Cardiology) Emeritus
Emory University School of Medicine
Consultant, Emory Heart and Vascular Center
Atlanta, Georgia
Chapter 90. Cardiovascular Disease in Older Adults

Walter R. Wilson, MD
Professor of Medicine
Mayo Clinic College of Medicine and Science
Rochester, Minnesota
Chapter 80. Infectious Endocarditis and Infections of Indwelling Devices

Justina C. Wu, MD, PhD
Assistant Professor of Medicine
Harvard Medical School
Director of Echocardiography
Brigham and Women's Hospital
Boston, Massachusetts
Chapter 16. Echocardiography

Katja Zeppenfeld, MD, PhD
Professor of Cardiology
Leiden University Medical Centre
Leiden, The Netherlands
Chapter 67. Ventricular Arrhythmias

Michael R. Zile, MD
Charles Ezra Daniels Professor of Medicine
Division of Cardiology
Medical University of South Carolina
Charleston, South Carolina
Chapter 58. Devices for Monitoring and Managing Heart Failure

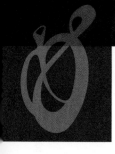

Preface

The knowledge relevant to the practice of cardiology continues to grow by leaps and bounds. Scientific and clinical advances have occurred at such a rapid pace that clinicians often suffer information overload. Communications about advances in cardiovascular medicine inundate practitioners on a seemingly minute-to-minute basis through journals, mailings, text messages, newsletters, social media, webinars, advertisements, and other electronic and print media. How can a practitioner or trainee sift through this cacophony to discern reliable, durable, and important information critical for practice?

This textbook of cardiovascular medicine offers a solution to this quandary. The 12th edition of *Braunwald's Heart Disease* provides a comprehensive, carefully curated, balanced, and unbiased distillation not only of the tried and true, but especially the latest advances in our field. This volume should serve the novice and experienced practitioner alike. Trainees and those preparing for certification or recertification examinations can use this text for an overall review of contemporary cardiovascular medicine. Practitioners confronting a particular clinical problem can consult the appropriate section of the book on an as-needed basis to answer the clinical question at hand to aid on-the-spot clinical decision making. While not a basic science textbook, this volume builds on Dr. Braunwald's founding vision and reviews fundamental pathophysiologic mechanisms to furnish a foundation for informed practice where appropriate.

Cardiovascular medicine has expanded so enormously that few if any individuals can maintain mastery of the entire scope of practice. Sub-specialization and even sub-sub-specialization have increased. Yet, each of us encounters issues within these super-specialized areas when we care for and counsel our own patients. The palette of patients' problems often overlaps the fine divisions our specialty has developed. This book aims to provide a ready reference so that we can update our knowledge with recent and authoritative information in areas of cardiovascular medicine afield from our own primary areas of expertise. The online content of this textbook contains additional new figures and tables, as well as over 200 videos that add to the printed version. Furthermore, through twice monthly online updates by Dr. Braunwald and through Elsevier's ClinicalKey, this textbook undergoes constant updating. Indeed, with the addition of companion volumes, the *Heart Disease* family has become a living learning system and comprehensive reference.

As necessitated by evolution and progress in cardiovascular medicine, in planning this 12th edition the editors have carefully reviewed the content to reflect current knowledge. This edition has 14 totally new chapters. For example, we have added chapters on artificial intelligence in cardiology and on the use of wearables in cardiovascular medicine. These two topics will doubtless change our practices profoundly. We expect that future editions will continue to build on these and other novel areas that will provide us with innovative tools to confront our patients' problems.

We have added a new chapter, "Impact of the Environment on Cardiovascular Health," as we recognize increasingly the clinical importance of this critical interface. Another new chapter, "Cardiovascular Disease Risk of Nicotine and Tobacco Products," highlights the concerning increase in smokeless tobacco use among youth. The burgeoning field of cardio-oncology has expanded coverage in the 12th edition, with two chapters devoted to different aspects of this topic. Expanded coverage of valvular heart disease includes a new chapter on interventions for mitral and tricuspid valvulopathies, which complements an updated chapter on percutaneous interventions for the aortic valve. These additions acknowledge the growing role of structural heart disease interventions in tackling these conditions.

The period of planning and preparation of this 12th edition coincided with the pandemic caused by SARS-CoV-2. We would be remiss not to include an expanded discussion of viral heart diseases in a new chapter, as our specialty needs to prepare for likely future viral pandemics, as well as deal with the potentially long-term cardiovascular consequences of COVID-19. Of course, each and every chapter in the book has undergone extensive updating and revision to reflect advances since the last edition. To this end, a number of chapters are completely written de novo by new authors. Indeed, the 12th edition boasts almost 80 new authors, reflecting our commitment to continuous refreshment and review of the content.

Our field can take considerable pride in the rapid advances in both basic and clinical investigation that this book highlights. Yet, we face a disconnect between these advances and their application to practice. To this end we include a new chapter, "Impact of Health Care Policy on Quality and Outcomes of Cardiovascular Disease," that focuses on practical societal approaches to ensure that our patients can benefit from the clinical and basic scientific advances in our field. Moreover, closing gaps in offering progress in cardiovascular medicine to racially, ethnically, geographically diverse, or underserved populations presents a global challenge. We focus on cardiovascular conditions in particular segments of the population—women, people with diabetes, and those with HIV/AIDS—that may require specialized approaches; each of these and others have been accorded a separate chapter. The global pandemic has placed disparities and inequities in health care in stark relief, locally and globally. To address this problem, a new chapter, "Heart Disease in Racially and Ethnically Diverse Populations," deals with cardiovascular conditions that confront disadvantaged segments of our population.

Finally, the Editors were fortunate to enlist Professor Eugene Braunwald, the founder of this textbook, to contribute an opening chapter, "Cardiovascular Disease: Past, Present, and Future," which shares his vision from his uniquely broad perspective. We have striven to uphold the standards that he set for this textbook from the first five editions that he edited solo. We have aimed to emulate his editorial prowess and example of refreshing every page of this textbook in each edition to maximize its utility for all who care for patients with or at risk of developing cardiovascular disease.

Peter Libby
Robert O. Bonow
Douglas L. Mann
Gordon F. Tomaselli
Deepak L. Bhatt
Scott D. Solomon

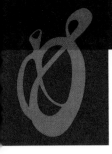

Preface to the First Edition

Cardiovascular disease is the greatest scourge affecting the industrialized nations. As with previous scourges — bubonic plague, yellow fever, and small pox — cardiovascular disease not only strikes down a significant fraction of the population without warning but also causes prolonged suffering and disability in an even larger number. In the United States alone, despite recent encouraging declines, cardiovascular disease is still responsible for almost 1 million fatalities each year and more than half of all deaths; almost 5 million persons afflicted with cardiovascular disease are hospitalized each year. The cost of these diseases in terms of human suffering and material resources is almost incalculable.

Fortunately, research focusing on the prevention, causes, diagnosis, and treatment of heart disease is moving ahead rapidly. Since the early part of the twentieth century, clinical cardiology has had a particularly strong foundation in the basic sciences of physiology and pharmacology. More recently, the disciplines of molecular biology, genetics, developmental biology, biophysics, biochemistry, experimental pathology and bioengineering have also begun to provide critically important information about cardiac function and malfunction.

In the past 25 years, in particular, we have witnessed an explosive expansion of our understanding of the structure and function of the cardiovascular system—both normal and abnormal—and of our ability to evaluate these parameters in the living patient, sometimes by means of techniques that require penetration of the skin but also with increasing accuracy, by noninvasive methods. Simultaneously, remarkable progress has been made in preventing and treating cardiovascular disease by medical and surgical means. Indeed, in the United States, a steady reduction in mortality from cardiovascular disease during the past decade suggests that the effective application of this increased knowledge is beginning to prolong human life span, the most valued resource on earth.

To provide a comprehensive, authoritative text in a field that has become as broad and deep as cardiovascular medicine, I enlisted the aid of a number of able colleagues. However, I hoped that my personal involvement in the writing of about half of the book would make it possible to minimize the fragmentation, gaps, inconsistencies, organizational difficulties, and impersonal tone that sometimes plague multiauthored texts. Although *Heart Disease: A Textbook of Cardiovascular Medicine* is primarily a clinical treatise and not a textbook of fundamental cardiovascular science, an effort has been made to explain, in some detail, the scientific bases of cardiovascular diseases.

To the extent that this book proves useful to those who wish to broaden their knowledge of cardiovascular medicine and thereby aids in the care of patients afflicted with heart disease, credit must be given to the many talented and dedicated persons involved in its preparation. I offer my deepest appreciation to my fellow contributors for their professional expertise, knowledge, and devoted scholarship, which has so enriched this book. I am deeply indebted to them for their cooperation and willingness to deal with a demanding editor.

Eugene Braunwald
1980

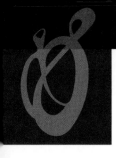

Acknowledgments

The conception and creation of this textbook of over 100 chapters and almost 2000 pages required the expertise, assistance, and skills of many dedicated individuals. We thank the contributors who have authored the chapters that comprise this textbook. We recognize the leadership of Ms. Dolores Meloni, executive content strategist at Elsevier, for her guidance and assistance at all stages of the planning and preparation of this volume. Ms. Anne Snyder, senior content development specialist, provided invaluable and detailed assistance on a daily basis. The editors owe her a great debt of gratitude. Mr. John Casey, senior project manager, cheerfully worked with the authors and the editors in executing the composition and proofing of this tome and accommodating last-minute additions and alterations to make the print edition as accurate and up to date as possible. The editors would not have been able to produce this book and ensure its quality without all of these contributions.

We also thank colleagues the world over who provided suggestions on how to improve *Braunwald's Heart Disease* and identified points that could use clarification. We welcome such input that will enable us to improve this edition in subsequent printings and plan future editions to meet our readers' needs even better.

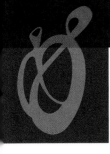

Contents

CONTENTS

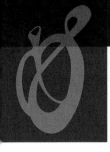

Video Contents

46 Mechanisms of Cardiac Contraction and Relaxation

DONALD M. BERS AND BARRY A. BORLAUG

MICROANATOMY OF CONTRACTILE CELLS AND PROTEINS

Ultrastructure of Contractile Cells

The major function of cardiac muscle cells (*cardiomyocytes or myocytes*) is to execute cardiac excitation-contraction-relaxation that depends on the electrical calcium ion (Ca^{2+}) transport and contractile properties.[1,2] Cardiomyocytes constitute approximately 75% of total ventricular volume and weight, but only one third of the total number of cells there.[1-4] Approximately half of each ventricular myocyte is occupied by myofibrils of the myofibers and 30% by mitochondria (Fig. 46.1 and Table 46.1). A *myofiber* is a group of cardiomyocytes held together by surrounding collagen connective tissue, the latter being a major component of the extracellular matrix. Further strands of collagen connect myofibers to each other.

Ventricular myocytes are roughly brick shaped, typically $150 \times 20 \times 12\ \mu m$ (see Table 46.1), and are connected at the long ends by specialized junctions that mechanically and electrically couple the myocytes with each other. Atrial myocytes are smaller and more spindle shaped ($<10\ \mu m$ in diameter and $<100\ \mu m$ in length). When examined under a light microscope, atrial and ventricular myocytes have cross striations and are often branched. Each myocyte is bounded by a complex cell membrane, the *sarcolemma* (muscle plasma membrane), and is filled with rodlike bundles of *myofibrils* containing the contractile elements. The sarcolemma invaginates to form an extensive transverse tubular network (*transverse tubules* [T tubules]) that extends the extracellular space into the interior of the cell (see Figs. 46.1 and 46.2). Ventricular myocytes are typically binucleate, and these nuclei contain most of the cell's genetic information. Some smaller or more juvenile myocytes have one nucleus and some up to three to four nuclei. Rows of mitochondria are located between the myofibrils and also immediately beneath the sarcolemma. Mitochondria function mainly to generate the energy, in the form of adenosine triphosphate (ATP), that is needed to maintain cardiac contractile function and the associated ion gradients. The *sarcoplasmic reticulum* (SR) is a specialized form of endoplasmic reticulum that is critical for calcium (Ca^{2+}) cycling, which is the on-off switch for contraction. When the wave of electrical excitation reaches the T tubules, voltage-gated Ca^{2+} channels open to provide relatively small entry of Ca^{2+}, which triggers additional release of Ca^{2+} from the SR via closely apposed Ca^{2+} release channels. This is the Ca^{2+} that initiates myocardial contraction. Ca^{2+} sequestration by the SR and extrusion from the myocyte causes relaxation (diastole).

Anatomically, the SR is a lipid membrane–bounded, fine interconnected network spreading throughout the myocytes. The Ca^{2+} release channels (or ryanodine receptors [RyRs]) are concentrated at the part of the SR that is in very close apposition to the T tubular Ca^{2+} channel. These are called terminal cisternae or the junctional sarcoplasmic reticulum (jSR). The second part of the SR, the longitudinal, free, or network SR, consists of ramifying tubules that surround the myofilaments (see Fig. 46.1) that take Ca^{2+} back up into the SR and thus drive relaxation. Such Ca^{2+} uptake is achieved by the ATP-consuming Ca^{2+} pump known as SERCA (sarcoendoplasmic reticulum Ca^{2+}–adenosine triphosphatase, or SR Ca-ATPase). The Ca^{2+} taken up into the SR is then stored at high concentration, in part bound to Ca^{2+}-buffering proteins, including calsequestrin, before being released again in response to the next wave of depolarization. Cytoplasm or sarcoplasm refers to the intracellular fluid and proteins therein, but excludes the contents of organelles such as the mitochondria, nucleus, and SR. The cytoplasm is crowded with myofilaments, but this is the fluid within which the concentration of Ca^{2+} rises and falls to cause cardiac contraction and relaxation.

Subcellular Microarchitecture

There are many microdomains and even nanometer-scale nanodomains involved in molecular signaling that convey messages within

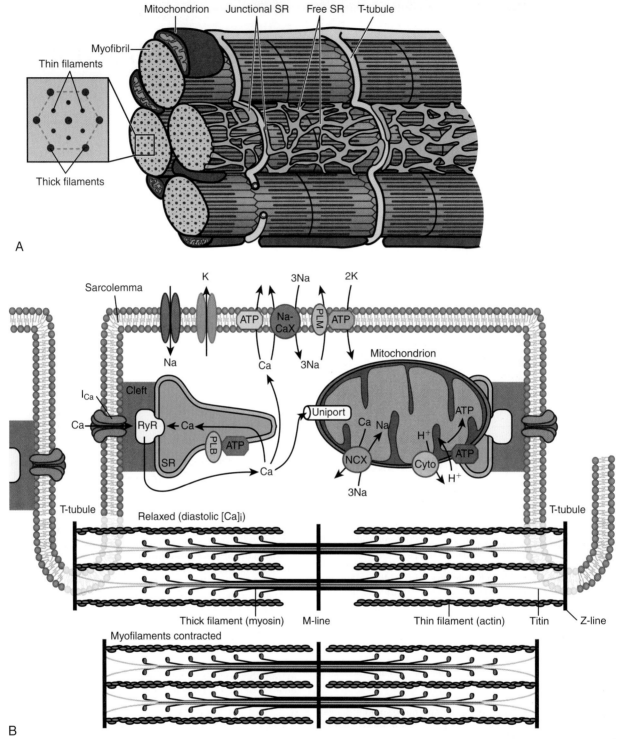

FIGURE 46.1 Ultrastructural components of excitation-contraction coupling in ventricular myocytes, viewed anatomically (**A,** with *inset* showing an end-on view of thick and thin filament organization) and schematically **(B).** The action potential is conducted along the surface sarcolemma and sarcolemma that extends into the T tubules. Ca^{2+} current (I_{Ca}) at sites of junctional SR clefts trigger local Ca^{2+} release, and the Ca^{2+} diffuses throughout the cytosol to activate myofilament contraction. The $[Ca^{2+}]_i$ quickly declines at each beat because of Ca^{2+} uptake via the SR Ca^{2+}-ATPase (ATP/PLB), extrusion via sarcolemmal Na^+/Ca^{2+} exchange (NCX) and Ca^{2+}-ATPase (and mitochondrial Ca^{2+} uniport), allowing relaxation (diastole) to proceed. The myofibrils are bundles of contractile proteins that are organized into a regular sarcomeric array, bounded longitudinally by Z-lines that are immediately adjacent to T tubules that run in parallel. In diastole (*bottom*) the thin filaments (containing mainly actin) create a cage around the thick filaments (containing mainly myosin) that have cross-bridges (myosin heads) that extend toward the thin filament. Myosin molecule tails all face the center of the sarcomere, creating a zone around the M-line devoid of myosin heads. During systole, the myosin cross-bridges pull the thin filament "cage" toward the M-line, thus shortening the sarcomere length (additional details are in subsequent figures). *ATP,* Adenosine triphosphate; *PLB,* phospholamban; *SR,* sarcoplasmic reticulum; *T tubules,* transverse tubules. (**A** Redrawn, based on a classic sketch by Fawcett DW, McNutt NS: The ultrastructure of the cat myocardium: I. Ventricular papillary muscle [*J Cell Biol.* 1969;42:1–45].)

TABLE 46.1 Characteristics of Cardiac Cells, Organelles, and Contractile Proteins

MICROANATOMY OF HEART CELLS			
	VENTRICULAR MYOCYTE	ATRIAL MYO-CYTE	PURKINJE CELLS
Shape	Long and narrow	Elliptical	Long and broad
Length (μm)	75–170	20–100	150–200
Diameter (μm)	15–30	5–6	35–40
Volume (μm³)	15,000–100,000	400–1500	135,000–250,000
T tubules	Plentiful	Rare or none	Absent
Intercalated disc	Prominent end-to-end transmission	Side-to-side as well as end-to-end transmission	Very prominent abundant gap junctions Fast; end-to-end transmission
General appearance	Mitochondria and sarcomeres very abundant Rectangular branching bundles with little interstitial collagen	Bundles of atrial tissue separated by wide areas of collagen	Fewer sarcomeres, paler

COMPOSITION AND FUNCTION OF VENTRICULAR CELL		
ORGANELLE	PERCENTAGE OF CELL VOLUME	FUNCTION
Myofibril	≈50–60	Interaction of thick and thin filaments during contraction cycle
Mitochondria	16 in neonate 33 in adult rat 23 in adult man	Provide ATP chiefly for contraction
T-system	≈1	Transmission of electrical signal from sarcolemma to cell interior
SR	10 in neonate 2–3 in adult	Takes up and releases Ca²⁺ during contraction cycle
SR terminal cisternae	0.33 in adult	Site of calcium storage and release
Rest of network of SR	Rest of volume	Site of calcium uptake en route to cisternae
Sarcolemma	Very low	Control of ionic gradients, channels for ions (action potential), maintenance of cell integrity, receptors for drugs and hormones
Nucleus	≈3	Transcription
Lysosomes	Very low	Intracellular digestion and proteolysis
Sarcoplasm (= cytoplasm) (includes myofibril but not mitochondria or SR)	~60	Cytosolic volume within which [Ca²⁺]ᵢ rises and falls

ATP, Adenosine triphosphate; *SR,* sarcoplasmic reticulum.

myocytes. These include the jSR-T-tubule junctions where T-tubular Ca²⁺ channels are within 10 nm of a cluster of RyR channels in the jSR membrane to produce the synchronous Ca²⁺ transients that control contraction. There are also sarcolemmal receptor complexes, such as beta-adrenergic receptors that have specific molecular partners (more below) that produce second messengers (cyclic nucleotides) that can diffuse to other functional targets in the myocyte. *Caveolae* (small,

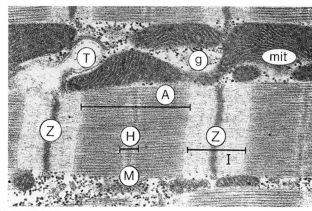

FIGURE 46.2 The sarcomere is the distance between the two Z-lines. Note the presence of numerous mitochondria (*mit*) sandwiched between the myofibrils and the presence of T tubules (*T*), which penetrate into the muscle at the level of the Z-lines. This two-dimensional picture should not disguise the fact that the Z-line is really a "Z-disc," as is the M-line (*M*), also shown in Figure 46.1. *A,* Band of actin-myosin overlap; *g,* glycogen granules; *H,* central clear zone containing only myosin filament bodies and the M-line; *I,* band of actin filaments, titin, and Z-line (rat papillary muscle, 32,000×). (Courtesy Dr. J. Moravec, Dijon, France.)

Mitochondrial Ca and Na Transport: Connection to Metabolism

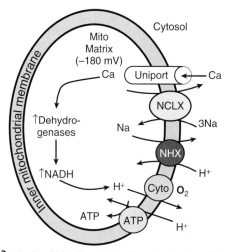

FIGURE 46.3 Mitochondrial Ca²⁺ regulation. The intramitochondrial matrix is very negative with respect to the cytosol (–180 mV). Ca²⁺ enters mitochondria via the Ca²⁺ uniporter in the inner mitochondrial membrane and is extruded by Na⁺/Ca²⁺ exchange (*NCLX*). Na⁺ is extruded via Na⁺/H⁺ exchange (NHX). Protons (H⁺) are pumped out of mitochondria by the cytochrome (*Cyto*) systems, thereby allowing H⁺ to enter via F₀F₁ ATP synthase (*ATP*). When mitochondrial [Ca] is increased, it activates mitochondrial dehydrogenases, which increase NADH levels and provide additional reducing equivalent protons to the electron transport chain. (Modified from Bers DM. *Excitation-Contraction Coupling and Cardiac Contractile Force.* Dordrecht, Netherlands: Kluwer Academic; 2001.)

flask-shaped sarcolemmal invaginations) are also microdomains with key localized signaling cascades. *Scaffolding proteins* such as caveolin, A-kinase anchoring proteins (AKAPs), and the RyR itself bring interacting molecules closely together at these locations. These complexes can also release components that translocate and signal elsewhere in the cell, such as the nucleus, where they can signal for myocyte growth. Another type of subcellular shuttling is involved in transporting the ATP produced in mitochondria to sites where it is used (e.g., myofilaments), which is facilitated by the location of creatine kinase, an enzyme that converts creatine phosphate to ATP.

Mitochondrial Morphology and Function

The typical ventricular myocyte has approximately 8000 mitochondria, each of which is ovate with a long axis measuring 1 to 2 μm and short axis of 300 to 500 nm. Mitochondria have two membranes: outer and inner mitochondrial membranes (OMM and IMM; Figs. 46.1 and 46.3).

The IMM is "crumpled" into folds called cristae, which provide a large surface area within a small volume. The IMM also contains the cytochrome complexes that make up the respiratory chain, including F_0-F_1 ATP synthase. The space within the IMM, the mitochondrial matrix, contains enzymes of the tricarboxylic acid (TCA) cycle and other key metabolic components. These components provide reducing equivalent protons that are pumped out of the matrix by the cytochromes, and it is this proton pumping that creates the very negative voltage with respect to cytosol (ψ_m = −180 mV). The proton pumping out of the matrix also creates a trans-IMM [H^+] gradient, which together with the very negative ψ_m creates a strong electrochemical gradient for protons to enter the matrix. The energy from this "downhill" proton flux is used by the $F_0$$F_1$ ATP synthase to make ATP. However, in the absence of the normal proton and ψ_m, this elegant F_0-F_1 ATP synthase runs backward, consuming ATP. The ATP produced in the matrix is transported across the IMM by an adenine nucleotide transporter that exchanges mitochondrial ATP for cytosolic adenosine diphosphate (ADP). This system is exquisitely regulated to maintain cytosolic [ATP] and [ADP] constant during dramatic changes in cardiac workload.[5] The multiple control mechanisms involved in this process are not fully understood, but one is relevant to excitation-contraction coupling. Increased cardiac work in a physiologic setting is usually driven by higher-amplitude and/or more frequent Ca^{2+} transients. This elevation in average intracellular [Ca^{2+}] ([Ca^{2+}]$_i$) also increases mitochondrial matrix [Ca^{2+}] ([Ca^{2+}]$_m$), which activates key dehydrogenases in the TCA cycle and also pyruvate dehydrogenase to restore levels of reduced nicotinamide adenine dinucleotide (NADH), which drives cytochrome activity and helps restore (ATP) toward normal.

This raises the issue of how mitochondria regulate [Ca^{2+}]$_m$, because there is also a huge electrochemical gradient favoring entry of Ca^{2+} into mitochondria.[2] Indeed, [Ca^{2+}]$_m$ is typically similar to [Ca^{2+}]$_i$ and is kept at that level by a mitochondrial Na/Ca exchanger (NCLX), which uses the also steep Na^+ electrochemical gradient to pump Ca^{2+} out of the mitochondria.[2] However, this would load the mitochondria with Na^+, so Na^+ must also be extruded from the mitochondria. This is accomplished by the mitochondrial Na/H exchanger in the IMM, but a consequence is that this influx of H^+ costs energy. That is, these protons could have entered the mitochondria via the F_0-F_1 ATP synthase making ATP, but instead they were used to extrude Na^+ and Ca^{2+}. Thus in a sense the mitochondrion can make ATP or extrude Ca^{2+}. This becomes important when myocytes (or other cells) experience Ca^{2+} overload. In the short term, mitochondria can take up large amounts of Ca^{2+} to protect the cell from short-term Ca^{2+} overload, but chronic high [Ca^{2+}]$_i$ has dire consequences. First, this Ca^{2+} uptake can diminish ψ_m and occurs at the expense of ATP production (as noted), thus hampering energetic recovery from such stress. Second, elevated [Ca^{2+}]$_i$ and [Ca^{2+}]$_m$ can facilitate opening of the mitochondrial permeability transition pore, which immediately dissipates ψ_m, results in the F_0 F_1 ATP synthase consuming rather than making ATP, and allows the matrix contents to be released to the cytosol. This is usually the death knell for individual mitochondria, as well as the cells that rely on their robust function.

Thus, mitochondria can rapidly become agents of cell death as just described, as well as by producing excessive reactive oxygen species (ROS), which can promote necrotic cell death through the mitochondrial permeability transition pore and release of proapoptotic proteins (see Chapter 47).[6] Mitochondria can also induce mitochondrial

autophagy, or *mitophagy*, which selectively and adaptively clears damaged mitochondria. Increased oxidative stress and apoptotic proteases can inactivate mitophagy and thereby cause cell death.[7] Mitochondria can also undergo fission, sometimes with one daughter mitochondrion being less healthy and targeted for mitophagy. They can also undergo fusion, to merge smaller ones into a larger mitochondrion. Fission, fusion and mitophagy are normal and healthy parts of mitochondrial life, and dysfunction of any of these can have pathologic consequences.

Contractile Proteins

The two chief contractile proteins are the motor protein *myosin* on the thick filament and *actin* on the thin filament (see Figs. 46.1B and 46.2). Ca^{2+} initiates the contraction cycle by binding to the thin filament regulatory protein *troponin C* to relieve the inhibition otherwise exerted by this troponin complex (Fig. 46.4). The thin actin filaments are connected to the *Z-lines* at either end of the *sarcomere*, which is the functional contractile unit that is repeated through the filaments. The sarcomere is limited on either side by a Z-line, which with the thin filaments creates a "cage" around the thick myosin filament that extends from the center of the sarcomere outward toward the Z-line. During contraction, the myosin heads grab onto actin and pull the

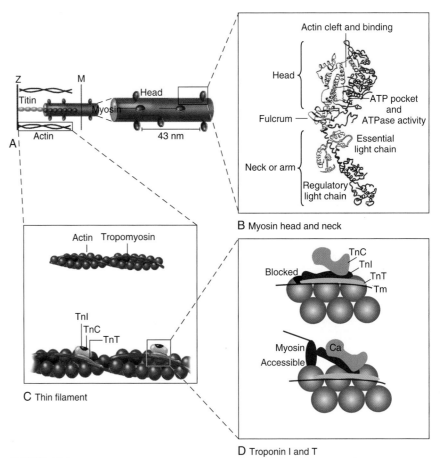

FIGURE 46.4 Key contractile protein interactions. The thin actin filament **(A)** interacts with the myosin head **(B)** when Ca^{2+} ions arrive at troponin C (*TnC*) **(C)**. This causes troponin-tropomyosin shifts to expose the actin site to which a myosin head can attach. **A,** The thin actin filament contains TnC and its Ca^{2+} binding sites. When TnC is not activated by Ca^{2+}, troponin I (*TnI*) stabilizes troponin T (*TnT*) and tropomyosin (*Tm*) along the actin filament to block myosin cross-bridge binding **(D). B,** The molecular structure of the myosin head, based on Rayment and colleagues,[8] is composed of heavy and light chains. The heavy head chain in turn has two major domains: one of 70 kDa (i.e., 70,000 molecular weight) that interacts with actin at the actin cleft and has an ATP binding pocket. The "neck" domain of 20 kDa, also called the "lever," is an elongated alpha helix that extends and bends and has two light chains surrounding it as a collar. The essential light chain is part of the structure. The other regulatory light chain may respond to phosphorylation to influence the extent of the actin-myosin interaction. **C,** TnC with sites in the regulatory domain for activation by calcium and for interaction with TnI. **D,** Binding of calcium to TnC causes TnI to shift binding from TnT to TnC, allowing the TnT-Tm complex to shift deeper into the actin groove and expose the myosin binding domain on actin. (Modified from Opie LH. *Heart Physiology, from Cell to Circulation.* Philadelphia: Lippincott Williams & Wilkins; 2004. Figure copyright L. H. Opie, 2004. **D,** Modified from Solaro RJ, Van Eyk J. Altered interactions among thin filament proteins modulate cardiac function. *J Mol Cell Cardiol.* 1999;28:217.)

actin filaments toward the center of the sarcomere. The thin and thick filaments can thus slide over each other to shorten the sarcomere and cell length, without the individual actin or myosin molecules actually changing length (see Fig. 46.1B). The interaction of the myosin heads with actin filaments that is switched on when Ca^{2+} arrives is called cross-bridge cycling. As the actin filaments move inward toward the center of the sarcomere, they draw the Z-lines closer together so that the sarcomere length shortens. The energy for contraction is provided by breakdown of ATP (myosin is an ATPase).

Titin and Length Sensing

Titin is a giant molecule, the largest protein yet described. It is extraordinarily long, elastic, and slender (Fig. 46.5). Titin extends from the Z-line into the thick filament, approaching the M-line, and connects the thick filament to the Z-line (see Fig. 46.1). Titin has two distinct segments: an inextensible anchoring segment and an extensible elastic segment that stretches as sarcomere length increases. Thus the titin molecule can stretch between 0.6 and 1.2 μm in length and has multiple functions. First, it tethers myosin and thick filaments to the Z-line, thereby stabilizing sarcomeric structure. Second, as it stretches and relaxes, its elasticity contributes to the stress-strain relationship of cardiac and skeletal muscle. At short sarcomere lengths, the elastic domain is coiled up on itself to generate restoring force (see Fig. 46.5), similar to a spring, helping to relengthen the sarcomere and aid early diastolic filling. These changes in titin help explain the *series elastic element* that was inferred from mechanics studies as elasticity in series with the myosin filaments. Third, the increased diastolic stretch of titin as

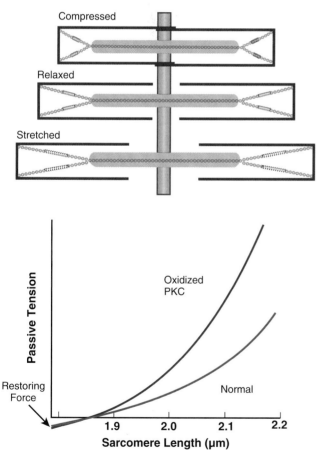

the length of the sarcomere in cardiac muscle is increased causes the enfolded part of the titin molecule to straighten. This stretched molecular spring then limits overstretching of sarcomeres and end-diastolic volume (EDV) and returns some potential energy during systole as the sarcomeres shorten during cardiac ejection.[4] Fourth, titin may transduce mechanical stretch into growth signals. Sustained diastolic stretch, as in volume overload, can cause titin-dependent signaling to muscle LIM protein (MLP) attached to the Z-line end of titin.[8] MLP is proposed to be a stretch sensor that transmits the signals that result in the myocyte growth pattern characteristic of volume overload, and it may be defective in a subset of human dilated cardiomyopathy.[9]

Molecular Basis of Muscular Contraction

Although the molecular level details underlying the cross-bridge cycle are complex, cross bridges appear to exist in either a strong or a weak binding state (but a super-relaxed state also exists).[10] During diastole, myosin heads normally have ATP bound (Fig. 46.6B) and hydrolyzed to ADP plus inorganic phosphate (Pi), although ADP-Pi is not yet released and the energy of ATP is not yet fully consumed (Fig. 46.6C). Thus the cross bridges are poised and ready to bind to actin. This interaction is permitted when Ca^{2+} arrives and binds to troponin C, shifting the position of the troponin-tropomyosin complex on the actin filament (see Fig. 46.4C, D). This enables the poised myosin heads to form strong binding cross bridges with actin molecules (Fig. 46.6D) and use the energy stored in myosin-ADP-P_i to rotate the myosin head while bound to actin in the *power stroke* (and release P_i) while still in the strong binding state (Fig. 46.6D and E). Once a particular cross bridge proceeds through the power stroke (using the energy previously stored in the ATP molecule), it will remain in the strong binding or *rigor* state (Fig. 46.6A) until ATP binds again to myosin, causing a shift back to the weak binding state and allowing cross-bridge detachment and ATP hydrolysis (Fig. 46.6C). As long as $[Ca^{2+}]_i$ and [ATP] remain high, the cycle can continue with myosin-ADP-Pi binding to a new actin molecule. The weak binding state predominates when $[Ca^{2+}]_i$ falls and Ca^{2+} dissociates from troponin C, allowing relaxation during diastole. If intracellular (ATP) declines too far (e.g., during ischemia), ATP cannot bind and disrupt the rigor linkage, leaving cross bridges locked in the strong binding state (as in rigor mortis).

Actin and Troponin Complex

The Ca^{2+} on-switch of cross-bridge cycling is mediated by a series of interactions within the troponin, tropomyosin, and actin complex (see Fig. 46.4C, D). Thin filaments are composed of two helical intertwining actin filaments, with a long tropomyosin molecule that spans seven actin monomers located in the groove between the two actin filaments. Also, at every seventh actin molecule (38.5 nm along this structure) there is a three-protein regulatory *troponin complex:* troponin C (Ca^{2+} binding), I (inhibitory), and T (tropomyosin binding).

When $[Ca^{2+}]_i$ is low, the position of tropomyosin blocks the myosin heads from interacting effectively with actin. As a result, most cross bridges are in the "blocked position," with a few visiting the weak binding state. Ca^{2+} binding with troponin C causes troponin C to bind more tightly to troponin I (see Fig. 46.4D), which allows tropomyosin to roll deeper into the thin filament groove,[1] thereby opening access to allow myosin binding to actin. This allows the cross-bridge cycle to proceed (see Fig. 46.6). As they form, strong cross bridges can nudge tropomyosin deeper into the actin groove, allowing cross-bridge attachment at one site to enhance actin-myosin at its "nearest-neighbor" sites. This cooperatively spreads activation farther along the myofilaments.[1,4]

Myosin Structure and Function

Each myosin head is the terminal part of the myosin heavy chain molecule. The other ends of two myosin molecules (tails) intertwine as a coil that forms the bulk of the thick filament. Also, a short "neck" leads to the myosin head that protrudes out from the filament (see Fig. 46.4). According to the Rayment model, the base of the head and/or neck region changes configuration during the power stroke previously described.[8] Each head has an *ATP-binding pocket* and a narrow cleft that extends from the base of this pocket to the actin-binding face (see Fig. 46.6).[11]

FIGURE 46.5 Titin is a huge elastic elongated protein that connects myosin and the M-line to the Z-line. It is a bidirectional spring that develops passive force in stretched sarcomeres and resting force in shortened sarcomeres. **Upper panel,** As the sarcomere is stretched to its maximum physiologic diastolic length of 2.2 μm, titin stretches and increases passive force generated (contributing to end-diastolic pressure). At short lengths (*top*), which may reflect end-systole, substantial restoring force is generated, shown as negative tension **(lower panel).** Note that oxidation and PKC-dependent phosphorylation increase titin stiffness. (Modified with permission of the American Heart Association, from Lewinter MM, Granzier HL. Titin is a major human disease gene. *Circulation.* 2013;127:938–944.)

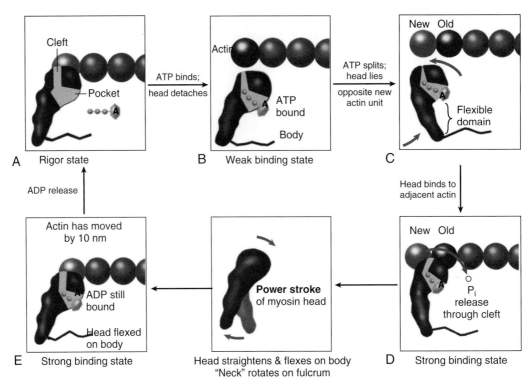

FIGURE 46.6 Cross-bridge cycling molecular model. The cross-bridge (only one myosin head depicted) is pear shaped, and the catalytic motor domain interacts with the actin molecule and is attached to an extended alpha helical "neck region," which acts as a lever arm. The nucleotide pocket that binds adenosine triphosphate (ATP) is in the catalytic domain. The actin binding cleft bisects the catalytic motor domain. Starting with the rigor state **(A)**, binding of ATP to the pocket **(B)** is followed by ATP hydrolysis **(C)**, which alters the actin binding domain, favoring release from actin. The binding to actin is enhanced when phosphate is released, and the myosin head strongly attaches to actin to induce the power stroke **(D and E)**. During the power stroke the head rotates around the head-neck fulcrum. As the head flexes, the actin filament can be displaced by approximately 10 nm **(E)**, causing shortening (although during isometric contraction the neck region stretches and bears force). In this process, ADP is also released, so the binding pocket becomes vacant, resulting in the rigor state again **(A)** until ATP binds to release the cross bridge.

During the power stroke when there is no mechanical load on the muscle, the myosin head flexes and can move the actin filament by approximately 10 nm.[1] When the pocket releases ADP and binds ATP, the cross bridge releases back to an orientation more perpendicular to the direction of the thin and thick filaments. During isometric (or isovolumic) contraction, the cross bridges rotate but cannot fully move the actin filament, and the stretched strong binding cross bridges bear force. During shortening (ejection), the actin filament moves during the power stroke, accompanied by decreases in sarcomere length and ventricular volume.

Note that myosin heads stick out from the thick filament in six directions in an organized array to allow interactions with each of six actin filaments that surround each thick filament (see Fig. 46.1A). The myosin molecules are also oriented in reversed longitudinal directions on either side of the M-line (which itself contains only myosin tails), such that each side is trying to pull the Z-lines toward the center. That is, when cross bridges are in the strong binding or rigor linkages, they form "chevrons" (or *arrows*) pointing toward the Z-line on that side of the M-line.

Each cycle of the cross bridge consumes one molecule of ATP, and this *myosin ATPase activity* is the major site of ATP consumption in the beating heart. Thus, when the heart is more strongly activated, the level of ATP consumption is similarly increased. The two myosin heads that stick out from an intertwined pair of myosin molecules seem to work through a hand-over-hand action such that the myosin dimer never fully releases the thin filament during the activation period.[12] There are also two main myosin isoforms in cardiac myocytes, alpha and beta, which have similar molecular weight but exhibit substantially different cross-bridge cycle and ATPase rates. The beta-myosin heavy chain (β-MHC) isoform exhibits a slower ATPase rate and is the predominant form in adult humans. In small mammals (rats and mice), the faster α-MHC form normally predominates but shifts to the β-MHC pattern during chronic stress and heart failure.[4] β-MHC has been targeted therapeutically using both gain and loss of function approaches. Mavacamten is a novel therapeutic myosin inhibitor that targets the excessive contractility and impaired relaxation, myocardial energetics and compliance in patients with obstructive hypertrophic cardiomyopathy (oHCM). In the

PIONEER clinical trial (NCT03470545), mavacamten improved exercise capacity, left ventricular (LV) outflow tract obstruction, New York Heart Association (NYHA) functional class, and health status in patients with oHCM (see also Chapter 54). Omecamtiv mecarbil is a novel therapeutic that activates myosin ATPase and enhances myosin cross-bridge formation and duration, thereby prolonging myocardial contraction. The GALACTIC-HF trial demonstrated that treatment with the selective cardiac myosin activator omecamtiv mecarbil reduced the incidence of a composite of a heart-failure event or death from cardiovascular causes in patients with heart failure and reduced EF[12a] (see also Chapter 49).

Each myosin molecule neck also has two light chains (see Fig. 46.4A). The *essential myosin light chain* (MLC-1) is more proximal to the myosin head and may limit the contractile process by interaction with actin. The *regulatory myosin light chain* (MLC-2) is a potential site for phosphorylation (e.g., in response to beta-adrenergic stimulation) and may promote cross-bridge cycling.[13] In vascular smooth muscle, which lacks the troponin-tropomyosin complex, contraction is activated by the Ca^{2+}-dependent myosin light chain kinase (MLCK) rather than by Ca^{2+} binding to troponin C (as in striated muscle). Myosin-binding protein C appears to traverse the myosin molecules in the A-band, thereby potentially tethering the myosin molecules and stabilizing the myosin head with respect to the thick and thin filaments. Defects in myosin, myosin-binding protein C, and several other myofilament proteins are genetically linked to familial hypertrophic cardiomyopathy.[14]

Graded Effects of $[Ca^{2+}]_i$ on Cross-Bridge Cycle

The myofilaments are activated in a graded rather than all-or-none manner as a function of $[Ca^{2+}]_i$ (Fig. 46.7), such as at $[Ca^{2+}]_i$ rises force of contraction increases going up the curve. Then as $[Ca^{2+}]_i$ declines relaxation proceeds (back to the diastolic point). The dynamics and regulation of Ca^{2+} transients in cardiac myocytes are discussed in the following section, but a major physiologic mechanism for regulating cardiac contractility (e.g., during sympathetic activity) is to increase peak $[Ca^{2+}]_i$ and more fully activate the myofilaments. The higher the

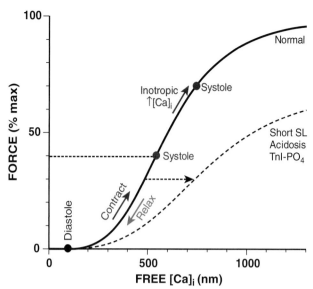

FIGURE 46.7 Myofilament Ca^{2+} sensitivity. Active force development in cardiac muscle depends on the cytosolic free $[Ca]_i$. As $[Ca]_i$ rises during systole, force develops as dictated by the sigmoidal myofilament Ca^{2+} sensitivity curve (*solid curve*; Force = $100/(1+[600\ nm]/[Ca]_i)^4$). As $[Ca]_i$ declines relaxation ensues and force declines. If peak $[Ca]_i$ increases (as in inotropy) the peak force can reach a higher value. At shorter sarcomere length (SL), acidosis, and troponin I (TnI) phosphorylation, the myofilament Ca^{2+} sensitivity is reduced, and the former two also decrease maximal force (*dashed curve*).

$[Ca^{2+}]_i$, the more fully saturated are the Ca^{2+} binding sites on troponin C, and consequently, more sites are available for cross bridges to form. When more cross bridges are working in parallel, the myocyte (and heart) can develop greater force (or ventricular pressure). There is high cooperativity in this process, in large part because of the "nearest-neighbor" effect mentioned earlier. That is, Ca^{2+} bound to a single troponin C molecule encourages local cross-bridge formation, and both Ca^{2+} binding and cross-bridge formation directly enhance the likelihood of cross-bridge formation in the seven actin molecules controlled by one tropomyosin molecule. Furthermore, the openness of that domain directly enhances that of the neighboring domain with respect to both Ca^{2+} binding and cross-bridge formation. This cooperativity means that a small change in $[Ca^{2+}]_i$ can have a great effect on the strength of contraction.

Length-Dependent Activation and the Frank-Starling Effect

Besides $[Ca^{2+}]_i$, the other major factor influencing the strength of contraction is sarcomere length at the end of diastole (preload), just before the onset of systole. Both Otto Frank and Ernest Starling observed that the more the diastolic filling of the heart, the greater the strength of the heartbeat. The increased heart volume translates into increased sarcomere length, which acts by a length-sensing mechanism. A part of this Frank-Starling effect has historically been ascribed to increasingly optimal overlap between the actin and myosin filaments. Clearly, however, there is also a substantial increase in myofilament Ca^{2+} sensitivity with an increase in sarcomere length (see Fig. 46.7).[1] A plausible mechanism for this regulatory change may reside in the decreasing interfilament spacing as heart muscle is stretched. That is, the myocyte is at constant volume (over the cardiac cycle), so as the cell shortens, it must thicken, and conversely, when it is stretched, the cell becomes thinner and filament spacing becomes narrower. This attractive lattice-dependent explanation for the Frank-Starling relationship has been challenged by careful x-ray diffraction studies,[4] which found that reducing sarcomere lattice spacing by osmotic compression failed to influence myofilament Ca^{2+} sensitivity. Although several mechanisms could contribute to myofilament Ca^{2+} sensitization at longer sarcomere length, the issue is unresolved.

When changes in diastolic length (or preload) are the cause of altered contractile strength, it is said to be a Frank-Starling (or Starling) effect. Conditions in which contraction is strengthened independent of sarcomere length (e.g., typically by increased Ca^{2+} transient amplitude) are referred to as positive *inotropic states* or enhanced *contractility*. The distinction between these heterometric (Starling) and homeometric (inotropic) mechanisms of altered cardiac strength is functionally and therapeutically important.

Cross-Bridge Cycling Differs from Cardiac Contraction-Relaxation Cycle

The cardiac cycle of Wiggers (see Fig. 46.16) must be distinguished from the cross-bridge cycle. The cardiac cycle reflects the overall changes in pressure in the left ventricle, whereas the cross-bridge cycle is the repetitive interaction between myosin heads and actin. During isovolumic contraction (before aortic valve opening), the sarcomeres do not shorten appreciably, but cross bridges are developing force, although not all simultaneously. That is, at any given moment, some myosin heads will be flexing or flexed (resulting in force generation), some will be extending or extended, and some will be attached weakly to actin and some detached from actin. Numerous such cross-bridge cycles, each lasting microseconds, are integrated to produce the resulting force (and pressure). When ventricular pressure (sum of cross-bridge forces) reaches aortic pressure (afterload), ejection begins and is associated with the cross bridges actively moving the thin actin filaments toward the center of the sarcomere (M-line), thereby shortening the sarcomere. Note that as ejection proceeds (and sarcomeres shorten), myofilament Ca^{2+} sensitivity declines (see Fig. 46.7). Thus, both $[Ca^{2+}]_i$ decline and shortening cause a progressive decline in the contractile state as systole gives way to diastole. Both the Ca^{2+} transient properties and the myofilament Ca^{2+} sensitivity and cross-bridge cycling rate are altered under physiologic conditions, such as sympathetic stimulation and local acidosis or ischemia, as discussed later.

Force Transmission

Volume and pressure overload may have different effects on myocardial growth because of different patterns of force transmission.[4] Whereas increased diastolic force is transmitted longitudinally by titin to reach MLP, the postulated sensor (see earlier), increased systolic force may be transmitted laterally (i.e., at right angles) by the Z-disc and cytoplasmic actin to reach the cytoskeletal proteins and cell-to-matrix junctions, such as the focal adhesion complex. This mechanical force is translated into signals by the dystrophin and integrin protein complexes that mediate force transmission between the intracellular cytoskeleton, the extracellular matrix, and neighboring cells. These can activate intrinsic short-term adaptive such as the Anrep effect, as well as signaling to the nucleus to activate the growth pathways via altered gene regulation, as addressed in other chapters.

CONTRACTILE PROTEIN DEFECTS AND CARDIOMYOPATHY

Genetic-based hypertrophic and dilated cardiomyopathies not only produce hearts that look and behave very differently but also have diverse molecular causes. These cardiomyopathies in general are linked to mutant genes that cause abnormalities in the force-generating system, such as β-MHC, MLCs, myosin-binding protein C, troponin subunits, and tropomyosin (see Chapter 52). One hypothesis is that mutations that increase myofilament calcium sensitivity, contractility, and energy demand result in concentric hypertrophy,[15] whereas mutations that reduce myofilament calcium sensitivity or force generation or that result in non-force-generating cytoskeletal proteins (e.g., dystrophin, nuclear lamin, cytoplasmic actin, titin) lead to a dilated cardiomyopathy. Although useful, such broad distinction between the two types of cardiomyopathy is oversimplified, with several examples of overlapping mechanisms.

CALCIUM ION FLUXES IN CARDIAC CONTRACTION-RELAXATION CYCLE

Calcium Movements and Excitation-Contraction Coupling

Ca^{2+} is central to cardiac contraction and relaxation, and the associated Ca^{2+} fluxes that link contraction to the wave of excitation (excitation-contraction coupling) are now well understood and accepted.[1,2] Each QRS complex in the electrocardiogram (ECG) represents the synchronization of ventricular myocyte action potentials (APs) that trigger Ca^{2+} transients and consequent contraction-relaxation in each myocyte (Fig. 46.8A). Relatively small amounts of Ca^{2+} (trigger Ca^{2+}) enter and leave the cardiomyocyte during each cardiac cycle, with larger amounts being released and taken back up by the SR (see Fig. 46.8B). Each AP depolarization opens voltage-gated L-type Ca^{2+} channels in the T tubules that are physically near the junctional SR, and that local Ca^{2+} influx activates SR Ca^{2+} release channels (RyRs) to release additional Ca^{2+} which can diffuse to cause a whole-cell Ca^{2+} transient that activates contraction. In this Ca^{2+}-induced Ca^{2+} release mechanism, a smaller amount of Ca^{2+} entering via the calcium current (I_{Ca}) triggers the release of a larger amount of Ca^{2+} into the cytosol.[1,4] In the human ventricle and large mammals, SR Ca^{2+} release is three to four times larger than Ca^{2+} influx by I_{Ca}. In rat and mouse myocytes, however, SR Ca^{2+} cycling is more than 10 times greater than sarcolemmal Ca^{2+} flux.[1] The combined Ca^{2+} release and influx elevates $[Ca^{2+}]_i$ and promotes binding of Ca^{2+} to troponin C and thus contractile activation. Contraction is terminated mainly by Ca^{2+} reuptake into the SR by SERCA and extrusion from the myocyte by Na^+/Ca^{2+} exchange (NCX) which return $[Ca^{2+}]_i$ to the diastolic level.

Calcium Release and Uptake by Sarcoplasmic Reticulum

Sarcoplasmic Reticulum Network and Ca^{2+} Movements

Electron and fluorescence microscopy studies show that the SR is a continuous network surrounding the myofilaments with connections across Z-lines and transversely between myofibrils. Moreover, the lumens of the entire SR network and nuclear envelope are connected in adult cardiac myocytes. This allows relatively rapid diffusion of Ca^{2+} within the SR to balance free $[Ca^{2+}]$ within the SR ($[Ca^{2+}]_{SR}$).[16,17] The total SR Ca^{2+} content is the sum of $[Ca^{2+}]_{SR}$ plus Ca^{2+} bound to intra-SR Ca^{2+} buffers (especially calsequestrin). SR Ca^{2+} content is critical to normal cardiac function and electrophysiology, and its abnormalities contribute to systolic and diastolic dysfunction and arrhythmias. $[Ca^{2+}]_{SR}$ dictates the SR Ca^{2+} content and driving force for Ca^{2+} release and also regulates RyR release channel gating.[17]

Junctional Sarcoplasmic Reticulum and Ryanodine Receptor

The RyR channels that mediate SR Ca^{2+} release are mainly located in the jSR membrane at the junctions with the T tubule.[1] Each junction has 50 to 250 RyR channels on the jSR that are directly under and nearly touching a cluster of 20 to 40 sarcolemmal L-type Ca^{2+} channels across a 15-nm junctional gap (that is crowded with protein). RyR2 (the cardiac isoform) functions both as a Ca^{2+} channel and as a scaffolding protein that localizes numerous key regulatory proteins to the jSR.[1,4] On the large cytosolic side, these include proteins that can stabilize RyR gating (e.g., calmodulin [CaM], FK-506 binding protein [FKBP-12.6]); kinases that can regulate RyR gating by phosphorylation (e.g., protein kinase A [PKA], Ca^{2+}/CaM-dependent protein kinase II [CaMKII]); and the protein phosphatases PP1 and PP2A, which dephosphorylate the RyR. Inside the SR, the RyR also couples to several proteins (e.g., junctin, triadin, and via these, calsequestrin) that similarly regulate RyR gating and, in the case of calsequestrin, provides a local reservoir of buffered Ca^{2+} close to the release channel. The actual RyR channel is made up of a symmetric tetramer of RyR molecules, each of which may have the aforementioned regulatory proteins associated with it. Thus the RyR receptor complex is very large (>7000 kDa; Fig. 46.8).[18] When the T tubule is depolarized, one or more L-type Ca^{2+} channels open, and local cleft $[Ca^{2+}]$ increases sufficiently to activate at least one local jSR RyR (multiple channels here ensure high-fidelity signaling). The Ca^{2+} released from these first openings recruit additional RyRs in the junction through Ca^{2+}-induced Ca^{2+} release to amplify release of Ca^{2+} into the junctional space. The Ca^{2+} diffuses out of this space throughout the sarcomere to activate contraction. Each of the approximately 20,000 jSR regions in the typical ventricular myocyte seems to function independently in response to local activation by I_{Ca}. Thus the global Ca^{2+} transient in the myocyte at each beat is the spatiotemporal summation of SR Ca^{2+} release events from thousands of jSR regions, synchronized by the upstroke of the AP and activation of I_{Ca} at each junction.

Turning Off Ca^{2+} Release: Breaking Positive Feedback

Ca^{2+}-induced Ca^{2+} release is a positive feedback process, but it is now known that SR Ca^{2+} release turns off when $[Ca]_{SR}$ drops by approximately 50% (i.e., from a diastolic value of 1 mM to a nadir of 400 μM).[13] Elegant studies have documented how I_{Ca} is inactivated by high local $[Ca^{2+}]$, and

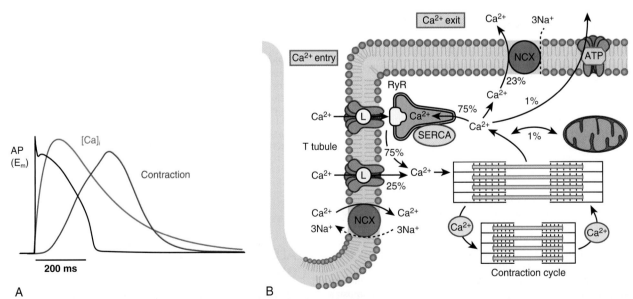

FIGURE 46.8 Myocyte Ca^{2+} fluxes during excitation-contraction (E–C) coupling. Rapid depolarization during the action potential (AP) triggers the Ca^{2+} transient that activates contraction **(A)**. **B,** Crucial features are (1) Ca^{2+} entry via the voltage-activated L-type Ca^{2+} channels, which triggers release of more Ca^{2+} from the SR; (2) a tiny amount of Ca^{2+} may enter via Na^+/Ca^{2+} exchange early in the action potential; and (3) removal of Ca^{2+} ions from the cytosol is mainly via the SR Ca-ATPase (SERCA; 75%) and Na^+/Ca^{2+} exchange (24%), with tiny amounts transported by mitochondrial Ca^{2+} uniport and the sarcolemmal Ca-ATPase (1%). The sodium pump (Na^+/K^+-ATPase) extrudes the Na^+ ions that entered during Na^+ current and Na^+/Ca^{2+} exchange action. Note that extracellular and intra-SR $[Ca^{2+}]$ (1 to 2 mm) is much higher than diastolic $[Ca^{2+}]_i$ (0.10 μm). Mitochondria can act as a buffer against excessive changes in cytosolic Ca^{2+}. (**B** modified from diagram by Bers DM. Cardiac excitation-contraction coupling. *Nature.* 2002;415:198.)

this robust calcium-dependent inactivation is mediated by binding of Ca^{2+} to the CaM that is already associated with that channel. When Ca^{2+} binds to CaM, it alters channel conformation such that I_{Ca} inactivation is favored. I_{Ca} is also subject to voltage-dependent inactivation during the AP plateau, and thus inactivation limits further entry of Ca^{2+} into the cell.

As for Ca^{2+}-dependent RyR activation, several mechanisms may contribute to breaking its inherent positive feedback. Although not necessarily most compelling, one mechanism is analogous to Ca^{2+}/ CaM-dependent inactivation of I_{Ca}. That is, binding of Ca^{2+} to CaM that is prebound to RyR2 favors closure of RyR channels and inhibits reopening (Fig. 46.9).[19] A second mechanism, undoubtedly important, is that RyR2 gating is also sensitive to luminal $[Ca^{2+}]_{SR}$ such that high $[Ca^{2+}]_{SR}$ favors opening and low $[Ca^{2+}]_{SR}$ favors closure.[20] Indeed, release of Ca^{2+} from the SR during normal Ca^{2+} transients is robustly turned off when $[Ca^{2+}]_{SR}$ falls to approximately half its normal value (400 μM, which is still 500 times higher than bulk $[Ca^{2+}]_i$), almost regardless of the rate of SR Ca^{2+} release.[15,16] A third and related mechanism is that as Ca^{2+} release proceeds and $[Ca^{2+}]_{SR}$ declines, Ca^{2+} flux through the RyR falls and junctional $[Ca^{2+}]$ also falls, all of which tend to disrupt the positive feedback. That is, the RyR is less sensitive to activating Ca^{2+} (because $[Ca^{2+}]_{SR}$ is low) and lower $[Ca^{2+}]$ on the cytosolic side also activates more weakly.[21]

CALMODULIN: VERSATILE MEDIATOR OF Ca^{2+} SIGNALING

CaM has four Ca^{2+}-binding sites, resembles troponin C, and participates in many different cellular pathways, from ion channels to transcriptional regulation.[19] In many cases (e.g., L-type Ca^{2+}, Na^+, and some K^+ channels; RyR and inositol 1,4,5-triphosphate receptors), CaM is already prebound or "dedicated" such that elevation of local $[Ca^{2+}]_i$ can rapidly induce Ca^{2+}-CaM effects on their gating (see Fig. 46.9).[22,23] Indeed, more than 90% of the CaM in myocytes is already bound to cellular targets before Ca^{2+} binds to and activates it. Nevertheless, many myocyte CaM targets (e.g., CaMKII, calcineurin, nitric oxide synthase [NOS]) compete for this limited pool of "promiscuous" CaM. Thus, CaM signaling in myocytes is complex and is further complicated by the effects of CaMKII, which influences some of the same targets and processes as CaM itself does.[19,23]

CALCIUM SPARKS AND WAVES

In addition to SR Ca^{2+} release triggered by I_{Ca} during normal excitation-contraction coupling, there is a finite probability that a given RyR will open stochastically. Because of local Ca^{2+}-induced Ca^{2+} release in the junctional cleft, this can lead to spontaneous local SR Ca^{2+} release events known as Ca^{2+} sparks.[21,24] Under normal resting conditions, these Ca^{2+} sparks have a low probability (approximately 10^{-4}), which means that at any moment there might be one or two Ca^{2+} sparks per myocyte. Because local $[Ca^{2+}]_i$ declines rapidly as Ca^{2+} diffuses away from the initiating cleft, the resulting local $[Ca^{2+}]_i$ at the next cleft (1 to 2 μm away) is normally too low to trigger that neighboring site. Thus, Ca^{2+} sparks are very local events (within 2 μm in the cell). However, the probability of Ca^{2+} sparks is greatly enhanced when $[Ca^{2+}]_i$ or $[Ca^{2+}]_{SR}$ is elevated or under conditions in which the RyR is otherwise sensitized (e.g., by oxidation or CaMKII). These conditions can greatly enhance the likelihood that SR Ca^{2+} release from one junction will be sufficient to trigger neighboring junctions 1 to 2 μm away and result in propagating Ca^{2+} waves throughout the whole myocyte. These Ca^{2+} waves can be arrhythmogenic. The Ca^{2+} wave can activate substantial inward current through NCX (see later), which can depolarize the membrane potential and contribute to both early and delayed afterdepolarizations (EADs and DADs) during the AP plateau or during diastole, respectively. EADs result in prolongation of the AP duration, and DADs can initiate premature ventricular complexes (PVCs).

Calcium Uptake into Sarcoplasmic Reticulum by Sarcoendoplasmic Reticulum Ca^{2+}– Adenosine Triphosphatase

Ca^{2+} is transported into the SR by SERCA, which constitutes nearly 90% of the SR protein. Its molecular weight is 115 kDa, with 10 transmembrane domains and large cytosolic and small SR-luminal domains. Three isoforms exist, but in cardiac myocytes the dominant form is SERCA2a. For each molecule of ATP hydrolyzed by this enzyme, two calcium ions are taken up into the SR (Fig. 46.10; see also Fig. 46.9). SR Ca^{2+} uptake is the primary driver of cardiac myocyte relaxation, and reuptake starts as soon as $[Ca^{2+}]_i$ begins to rise. Because Ca^{2+} removal is slower than Ca^{2+} influx and release, a characteristic rise and fall in $[Ca^{2+}]_i$ called the Ca^{2+} transient takes place. As $[Ca^{2+}]_i$ falls, Ca^{2+} dissociates from troponin C, which progressively switches off the myofilaments. A reduction in SERCA expression or function (as seen in heart failure or energetic limitations) can thus directly result in slower rates of cardiac relaxation. In addition, the strength of SR Ca^{2+} uptake directly influences the diastolic SR Ca^{2+} content and $[Ca^{2+}]_{SR}$, which dictates both the sensitivity of the RyR and the flux rate of SR Ca^{2+} release. Thus, SR Ca^{2+} uptake and release are an integrated system.

Phospholamban (PLB) was so named by its discoverers Tada and Katz[25] to mean "phosphate receiver." PLB is a single-transmembrane pass protein that binds directly to SERCA2a. Under basal conditions, this reduces the affinity of SERCA for cytosolic Ca^{2+}, which results in slower SR Ca^{2+} uptake at any given $[Ca^{2+}]_i$. However, when PLB is phosphorylated by either PKA or CaMKII (at Ser16 or Thr17, respectively), the inhibitory effect is relieved, thereby resulting in increased rates of SR Ca^{2+} uptake, cardiac relaxation (lusitropic effect), and increased SR Ca^{2+} content, which drives stronger contraction (inotropic effect; see Fig. 46.10).

The Ca^{2+} taken up into the SR is stored within the SR before the next release. Calsequestrin is a highly charged, low-affinity Ca^{2+} buffer ($K_d = 600$ μM) found primarily inside the jSR, where it enhances the local availability of Ca^{2+} for release through the nearby RyR. Calreticulin is another Ca^{2+}-storing protein that is similar to calsequestrin in structure and function. There is also evidence that calsequestrin and two other proteins located in the SR membrane (junctin and triadin) may regulate the properties of the RyR and be part of the mechanism by which higher $[Ca]_{SR}$ enhances RyR opening.[20] Reuptake by SERCA occurs everywhere

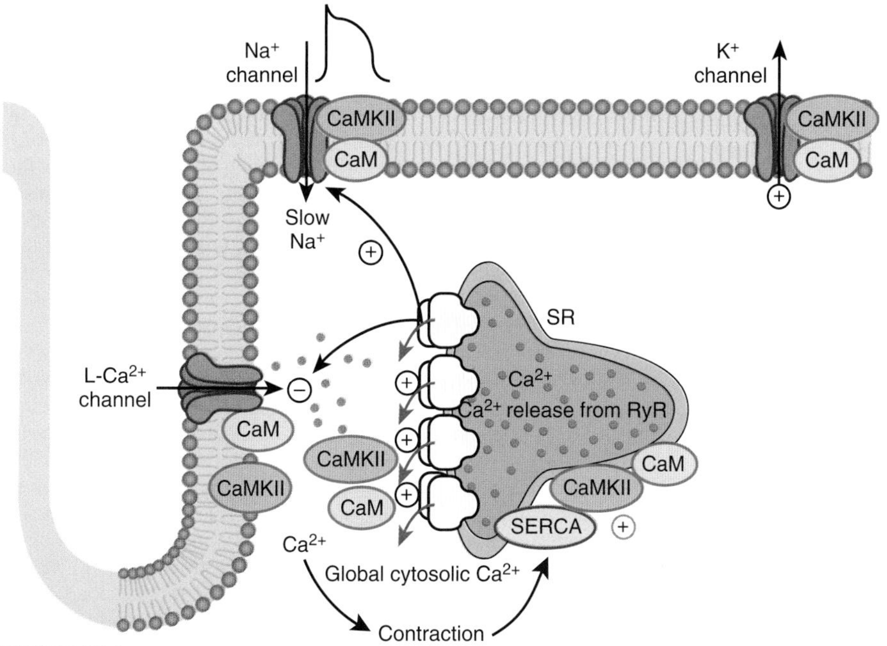

FIGURE 46.9 Role of CaM and CaMKII in regulating intracellular $[Ca^{2+}]$. The rising cytosolic Ca^{2+} concentration in systole activates the Ca^{2+} regulatory system whereby Ca^{2+}-CaM causes inactivation of L-type Ca^{2+} current and RyR release. This negative feedback system limits cellular Ca^{2+} gain. The effects of CaMKII can also modulate these systems.[22] For example, (1) CaMKII limits the extent of Ca^{2+}-dependent inactivation and enhances Ca^{2+} current amplitude, (2) it increases the fraction of SR Ca^{2+} released from the RyR in response to the Ca^{2+} current trigger (which can be arrhythmogenic), (3) it phosphorylates PLB to enhance SR Ca^{2+} uptake by SERCA, and (4) it can modulate Na^+ and K^+ channel gating in ways that are also proarrhythmic.[22,23]

in the SR membrane, including the network SR that surrounds the myofilaments. Diffusion of Ca²⁺ within the SR is relatively fast, which allows restoration of $[Ca^{2+}]_{SR}$ at the jSR to occur quickly after Ca²⁺ is taken back up everywhere.[26] Indeed, during normal Ca²⁺ release, intra-SR Ca²⁺ diffusion is rapid enough to limit Ca²⁺ gradients between SR release sites in the jSR and the Ca²⁺ uptake sites. This diffusion also ensures that $[Ca^{2+}]_{SR}$ is relatively uniform throughout the myocyte, which facilitates the uniformity of SR Ca²⁺ release and myofilament activation throughout the cell.

SARCOLEMMAL CONTROL OF Ca²⁺ AND Na⁺

Calcium and Sodium Channels

Excitation-contraction coupling is initiated by voltage-induced opening of the sarcolemmal L-type Ca²⁺ channels. The channels are pore-forming macromolecular proteins that span the sarcolemmal lipid bilayer to allow a highly selective pathway for transfer of ions into the heart cell when the channel changes from a closed to an open state. Ion channels have two major properties: gating and permeation. Ca²⁺ and Na⁺ channels have two functional "gates," activation and inactivation. At the normal resting membrane potential, the activation gates are closed and the inactivation gate is open, so the channels are available to open on depolarization in their characteristic voltage-gated manner. On activation, the inactivation gate starts to close, and the kinetics of inactivation depends on voltage, time, and local $[Ca^{2+}]_i$. Recovery from inactivation (which makes the channels available for activation again) is also time, voltage, and Ca²⁺ dependent. Thus, after the AP ends, time is required for the Ca²⁺ and Na⁺ channels to recover from inactivation.

Permeation (or conductance) refers to the actual flow of ions or current through the open channel. Ca²⁺ and Na⁺ channels are highly selective for Ca²⁺ and Na⁺, respectively, relative to other physiologic ions. However, nonphysiologic ions can also permeate; barium (Ba²⁺) and strontium (Sr²⁺) readily permeate Ca²⁺ channels, and lithium (Li⁺) permeates Na⁺ channels, and these ions are sometimes used experimentally to study I_{Ca} and I_{Na}. The concentration of the permeant ion influences the conductance, and in simple Ohm's law terms ($I_{Ca} = g_{Ca}[E_m - E_{Ca}]$), current is the product of conductance (g_{Ca}; which depends on gating and permeation) times the electrochemical driving force ($E_m - E_{Ca}$), which is the difference between the membrane potential (E_m) and the potential that exactly counterbalances the transmembrane $[Ca^{2+}]$ gradient (E_{Ca}, typically +120 mV but changes as $[Ca]_i$ changes). Thus, depolarization activates both Ca²⁺ and Na⁺ channels but also decreases the driving force for the currents.

Molecular Structure of Ca²⁺ and Na⁺ Channels

Both Ca²⁺ and Na⁺ channels contain a major alpha subunit with four transmembrane domains (I to IV), each of which has six transmembrane helices (S1 to S6) and a pore loop between S5 and S6. Each channel also has associated auxiliary subunits (α2δ, β, and γ for Ca²⁺ channels) that may influence trafficking and gating.[1] Activation is now understood in molecular terms as outward movement of the charged S4 transmembrane segment (called the *voltage sensor*) in each of the four domains of Na⁺ and Ca²⁺ channels. This S4 voltage dependence differs among channels, and Na⁺ channels are activated at more negative E_m than are Ca²⁺ channels. *Inactivation* is more complex and involves multiple channel domains, and channels accumulate in this state during prolonged depolarization. The open state is typically the last of a sequence of multiple molecular closed conformations. However, there is typically a binary switch between closed and open such that the single-channel conductance is either near zero or at a constant open conductance. This stochastic nature means that it is often better to speak of the *probability of channel opening* for a single channel, while the whole-cell current integrates flux through all the stochastic channels.

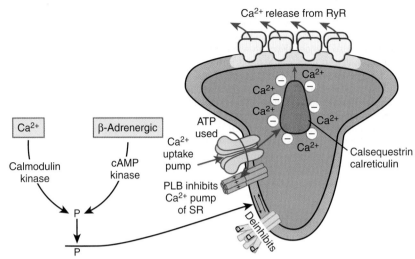

FIGURE 46.10 Ca²⁺ uptake into the SR by SERCA2a. An increased rate of uptake of Ca²⁺ into the SR enhances the rate of relaxation (*lusitropic effect*). PLB, when phosphorylated (*P*), removes the inhibition exerted on the Ca²⁺ pump by its dephosphorylated form. Thereby, Ca²⁺ uptake is increased either in response to enhanced cytosolic $[Ca^{2+}]$ or in response to beta-adrenergic agonists or CaMKII activation (which can be secondary to the beta-adrenergic system).[1,23,32]

T-Versus L-Type Ca²⁺ Channels

The cardiovascular system has two major types of sarcolemmal Ca²⁺ channels, T-type and L-type channels. T (transient)–type channels open at a more negative voltage, have short bursts of opening, and do not interact with conventional Ca²⁺ antagonist drugs.[1] In adult ventricular myocytes, there is normally little T-type I_{Ca} (except under pathophysiologic conditions). Even when expressed in ventricular myocytes, T-type channels do not seem to target the regions where RyRs are, and consequently do not participate in excitation-contraction coupling per se. However, measurable T-type I_{Ca} is present in neonatal ventricular myocytes, Purkinje fibers, and some atrial cells (especially pacemaker cells). In these locations the negative activation voltages may allow T-type I_{Ca} to contribute to pacemaker function. Thus, in ventricular myocytes, L-type currents predominate.

L-Type Ca²⁺ Channel Localization and Regulation

L (long-lasting)–type Ca²⁺ channels are concentrated in the T tubules at jSR sites, where they are positioned for Ca²⁺-induced Ca²⁺ release from the RyR. A fraction of L-type Ca²⁺ channels are also localized in caveolae, where they may participate in local Ca²⁺ signaling, which is distinct from triggering of SR Ca²⁺ release. L-type Ca²⁺ channels are inhibited by Ca²⁺ channel blockers such as verapamil, diltiazem, and the dihydropyridines. I_{Ca} is rapidly activated during the rising phase of the AP, but the combination of Ca²⁺ influx via I_{Ca} itself and local SR Ca²⁺ release causes rapid Ca²⁺-dependent inactivation of I_{Ca}. Voltage-dependent inactivation also contributes to I_{Ca} decline during the AP, but I_{Ca} continues at low levels throughout the AP.[27] Inward I_{Ca} is an important contributor to the plateau phase of the cardiac AP, and excess I_{Ca} or failure of inactivation can prolong the duration of the AP and participate in EADs.

During beta-adrenergic stimulation, cyclic adenosine monophosphate (cAMP) and PKA activity increases and results in phosphorylation of the Ca²⁺ channel and alteration of its gating properties. Notably, most of the molecular components of this beta-adrenergic receptor–cAMP-PKA and phosphatase pathway are localized directly at the L-type Ca²⁺ channel, which facilitates rapid sympathetic activation of I_{Ca}. PKA-dependent phosphorylation of the channel shifts activation (and inactivation) to more negative voltages and increases the open time of the channel. This combination can greatly increase I_{Ca}, which increases both the fraction of SR Ca²⁺ release and the Ca²⁺ load of the cell and SR (to enhance further the Ca²⁺ transient amplitude and inotropic state).

Sodium Channels

Voltage-gated cardiac Na⁺ current is carried mainly by the Nav1.5 *cardiac* isoform, but a minor component is attributed to several other, *neuronal* isoforms. The Nav1.5 channels are especially concentrated at the ends of the myocyte near intercalated discs, but the overall density of I_{Na} is relatively uniform between the T tubule and surface membrane.[28] Depolarization activates I_{Na}, and peak I_{Na} is very large and drives the upstroke of the cardiac AP. Voltage-dependent inactivation of I_{Na} is very rapid, and under normal conditions, Na+ channels inactivate within 4 milliseconds of depolarization. However, a tiny fraction of Na+ channels remain open (or reopen), thereby creating a small but persistent influx of Na+ throughout the plateau of the AP. This so-called late sodium current (I_{NaL}) is characterized by ultraslow, voltage-independent inactivation and reactivation.[29] Although the amplitude of I_{NaL} is small (<1% of peak I_{Na}), because peak I_{Na} is so large, this I_{NaL} still constitutes a significant inward current during the plateau phase of the AP. Under pathophysiologic conditions, the amount of I_{NaL} can increase significantly, which can result in acquired long-QT (LQT) syndrome and also cause Na+ and Ca2+ loading of myocytes, which carries additional arrhythmogenic potential. Thus, I_{NaL} has emerged as a potentially important therapeutic target.[22,30]

Ca²⁺/CALMODULIN-DEPENDENT PROTEIN KINASE II ALTERS GATING OF I_{Na}, I_{Ca}, AND OTHER CHANNELS

CaMKII is known to be upregulated and chronically activated in numerous pathophysiologic conditions (e.g., ischemia-reperfusion, heart failure, ROS). Also, CaMKII-dependent Na+ channel phosphorylation causes increased I_{NaL}, which may produce an acquired form of LQT3 syndrome in patients with genetically normal Na+ channels (see Fig. 46.9).[22,30] At the same time, CaMKII also shifts Na+ channel availability to more negative voltages, enhances intermediate inactivation, and slows recovery from inactivation, all loss-of-function effects that could cause an acquired Brugada syndrome–like condition. Indeed, this can foster both phenotypes, depending on the heart rate (HR): LQT syndrome at a lower HR and Brugada syndrome at a higher HR.[22] CaMKII also modulates Ca2+ and potassium (K+) channel currents, which can further promote arrhythmogenesis through EADs and enhanced transmural dispersion of repolarization.[22]

Ion Exchangers and Pumps

To maintain steady-state Ca2+ and Na+ balance, the amount of Ca2+ and Na+ entering during each AP must be exactly balanced by efflux before the next beat. This is the definition of steady state. For Ca2+, Na+/Ca2+ exchange (NCX) is responsible for extruding most of the Ca2+ that entered by I_{Ca} and NCX, whereas a very small fraction is extruded by the plasma membrane Ca2+-ATPase (PMCA). NCX uses the inward [Na+] electrochemical gradient from 3 Na+ ions to pump each Ca2+ ion into the extracellular space against a large electrochemical gradient (and PMCA uses 1 ATP to pump each Ca2+ ion). The main mechanism for extruding Na+ from the cell is Na+,K+-ATPase, which pumps 3 Na+ ions out for each ATP consumed. Note that NCX also indirectly uses the energy from Na+,K+-ATPase to perform its function.

Sodium-Calcium Exchanger

During relaxation, SR Ca2+-ATPase and NCX compete for the removal of cytosolic Ca2+, with the SR pump normally being dominant.[1,4] NCX is reversible, so the direction of Ca2+ flux depends on the membrane potential and [Na+] and [Ca2+] on both sides of the sarcolemma. The E_m at which the inward electrochemical potential is the same for 3 Na+ ions as for 1 Ca2+ ion to enter is the reversal or equilibrium potential (E_{NCX}, similar to that for ion channels). When E_m is higher than this voltage, entry of Ca2+ is favored, whereas for E_m below E_{NCX}, the Ca2+ efflux mode is thermodynamically favored. During diastole ($E_m = -80$ mV), NCX normally extrudes Ca2+, but because [Ca2+]$_i$ is low during diastole, the Ca2+ flux rate is low (low substrate concentration). As the AP rises to a peak, E_m normally exceeds E_{NCX} and Ca2+ influx is favored, but this occurs only briefly because the high local [Ca2+]$_i$ near the membrane drives NCX back into the Ca2+ extrusion mode. When the AP repolarizes, the negative E_m further enhances the Ca2+ extrusion flux, and at this time, [Ca2+]$_i$ is above the diastolic level, so NCX can transport Ca2+ effectively. Note that if SR Ca2+ release is small and/or I_{Ca} is small or [Na+]$_i$ is abnormally high (as occurs in heart failure), NCX can continue to bring Ca2+ into the cell during much of the AP duration and in that sense can partially compensate for the lack of I_{Ca} or SR Ca2+ release.[1] NCX is also allosterically activated by increasing [Ca2+]$_i$.[31] Although such regulation is time dependent,

it may provide a mechanism to enhance the cell's ability to extrude Ca2+ when [Ca2+]$_i$ is chronically high, as well as to keep NCX from driving [Ca2+]$_i$ and indirectly [Ca2+]$_{SR}$ to inappropriately low levels when cytosolic Ca2+ is in short supply.

Under normal conditions in human or rabbit ventricular myocytes, the steady-state condition occurs when the relative Ca2+ removal from the cytosol by SERCA and NCX is 70% to 75% and 20% to 25%, respectively, with PMCA contributing 1% or less (see Fig. 46.8). In heart failure, in which SERCA is downregulated and NCX may be upregulated, the SERCA and NCX contributions are closer to the same. In the mouse and rat ventricle, the difference is larger (92% SERCA, 7% NCX). This steady state involves all the various Ca2+ transport systems dynamically, but the relative rates of Ca2+ flux by SERCA and NCX at physiologic [Ca2+]$_i$ are useful. These removal fluxes must also pertain to the integrated Ca2+ fluxes into the cytosol. That is, the combination of Ca2+ entry by I_{Ca} and NCX in human and mouse ventricle would be 25% and 8%, respectively. In other words, amplification of the Ca2+ transient by SR Ca2+ release is only approximately fourfold for human or rabbit ventricle (and less in heart failure) but approximately 12-fold for mouse or rat ventricle.

HEART RATE AND Na⁺/Ca²⁺ EXCHANGE

NCX participates in the force-frequency relationship (treppe or Bowditch phenomenon).[1] An increasing HR (independent of sympathetic activation) increases the amount of Na+ and Ca2+ entry per unit time and also diminishes the time available for extrusion of Na+ and Ca2+. This will tend to increase the amount of Ca2+ in the SR simply because of more frequent I_{Ca} pulses and less time for removal of Ca2+ from the cell. However, the same happens for Na+, and the elevation in [Na+]$_i$ also limits the ability of NCX to extrude Ca2+, which further increases the amount of Ca2+ in the myocyte and SR when the cell achieves a new steady state. This NCX effect (once referred to as the "sodium pump lag" hypothesis) thus amplifies the intrinsic inotropic effect of an increase in HR.

Sodium Pump (Na⁺,K⁺–Adenosine Triphosphatase)

During the normal heartbeat, Na+ enters the myocyte mainly by Na+ channels and NCX, with NCX being quantitatively most important.[32] Na+/H+ exchange also mediates significant Na+ influx, particularly when cells are acidotic. In the steady state, this Na+ influx is matched by an equal Na+ efflux, mediated mainly by sarcolemmal Na+,K+-ATPase (the Na+ pump). The Na+ pump is activated by internal Na+ or external K+ and transports 3 Na+ ions out and 2 K+ ions in per ATP molecule used. During this process, one positive charge leaves the cell, and thus Na+,K+-ATPase is electrogenic and carries an outward current.[32] Na+,K+-ATPase in the heart is modulated by the endogenous accessory protein *phospholemman* (PLM), which works in a manner analogous to the PLB-SERCA2a mechanism. That is, at baseline, PLM reduces the intracellular Na+ affinity of Na+,K+-ATPase, but when it is phosphorylated (by either PKA or protein kinase C [PKC]), that inhibitory effect is relieved.[32] Thus, during sympathetic activation, Na+,K+-ATPase activity is increased at any given [Na+]$_i$ to keep up better with the higher rates of Na+ influx that occur under this condition.

Digitalis glycosides inhibit Na+,K+-ATPase and have been used for more than 200 years as a cardiac inotropic drug for the treatment of heart failure, although their use has diminished in recent years (see also Chapter 50). Partial inhibition of Na+,K+-ATPase causes an increase in [Na+]$_i$ in myocytes, which limits the ability of NCX to extrude Ca2+, resulting in enhanced myocyte and SR Ca2+ loading and release. A limitation with this approach is the narrow therapeutic range, and too much inhibition can lead to myocyte Ca2+ overload and trigger arrhythmias. However, this emphasizes the close interrelationship between Na+ and Ca2+ regulation mediated by the powerful NCX present in cardiac myocytes.

ADRENERGIC SIGNALING SYSTEMS

Physiologic Fight-or-Flight Response

During the classic adrenergic fight-or-flight response, cardiac myocyte beta-adrenergic receptors are activated, which leads to increased cAMP production and PKA activation and consequent phosphorylation and altered function of numerous myocyte targets. This results in an increased HR (*positive chronotropy*), increased contractility (*positive inotropy*), faster cardiac relaxation (*positive lusitropy*), and enhanced conduction velocity through the conduction system (*positive dromotropy*). These events enhance cardiac output by enhancing the HR, stroke volume, and diastolic filling. Thus, the adrenergic response is a key physiologic mechanism for increasing cardiac output in response to increased metabolic and hemodynamic demands.

During the adrenergic response, norepinephrine is released by sympathetic neurons at small swellings on small end-branches, or *varicosities*, into the local myocyte environment (Fig. 46.11), analogous to synaptic transmission. Norepinephrine is synthesized in the varicosities from dopa and dopamine and the amino acid tyrosine and stored within the terminals in *storage granules* (or *vesicles*) for release upon adrenergic nervous impulse. Thus, when central stimulation increases during excitement or exercise, an increased number of sympathetic nerve impulses liberate an increased amount of norepinephrine from the terminals into the close vicinity of myocyte surface (akin to neuronal synaptic clefts). Most of the released norepinephrine is taken back up by the nerve terminal varicosities to reenter the storage vesicles or to be metabolized. The released norepinephrine at these *synaptic clefts* interacts with both alpha- and beta-adrenergic receptors on myocytes and also alpha-adrenergic receptors in arterioles (Table 46.2). The beta-adrenergic effects on the sinoatrial (SA) node and conduction system contribute to the chronotropic and dromotropic effects mentioned earlier, whereas those on myocytes are responsible mainly for the inotropic and lusitropic effects. These effects can also be modulated by coactivation of myocyte alpha-adrenergic receptors. Increased alpha-adrenergic activity causes arteriolar constriction and increased vascular impedance, although local metabolic control of arteriolar resistance is strong in the heart and dominates in controlling coronary resistance in arterioles. Parasympathetic (vagal) innervation is strongest in the conduction system, where local release of acetylcholine (ACh) activates muscarinic receptors and tends to slow the HR and conduction velocity (see Fig. 46.11). In these conditions the HR and blood pressure fall. The influence of these main effector pathways is also modulated by numerous other signaling factors, such as local adenosine and nitric oxide (NO) and the powerful neuromodulator angiotensin II, which can also potentiate release of norepinephrine and vasoconstriction. Both alpha- and beta-adrenergic receptors are part of the family of seven–transmembrane domain G protein–coupled receptors (GPCRs).

Beta-Adrenergic Receptor Subtypes

Cardiac beta-adrenergic receptors are chiefly (80%) the beta$_1$ subtype, with 20% being beta$_2$ in the left ventricle. Most noncardiac receptors are beta$_2$. Whereas beta$_1$ receptors are linked to the stimulatory G protein G$_s$, a component of the G protein–adenylyl cyclase system, beta$_2$ receptors are linked to both G$_s$ and the inhibitory protein G$_i$ (Fig. 46.12), so their signaling pathway bifurcates at the first postreceptor step.[4] In humans the main positive inotropic response to adrenergic activation is mediated via beta$_1$ adrenergic receptors. Some beta$_2$ stimulation by salbutamol (albuterol) can appear to be inotropic but may at least in part be through beta$_2$ receptors on the terminal neurons of cardiac sympathetic nerves, thereby causing norepinephrine release which in turn exerts dominant beta$_1$ effects.[4] Indirect evidence suggests that the G$_i$ pathway is relatively augmented in heart failure, whereas the strength of the G$_s$ path is lessened because of uncoupling of G$_s$ from the beta receptor (see Chapter 47). There also appears to be a small

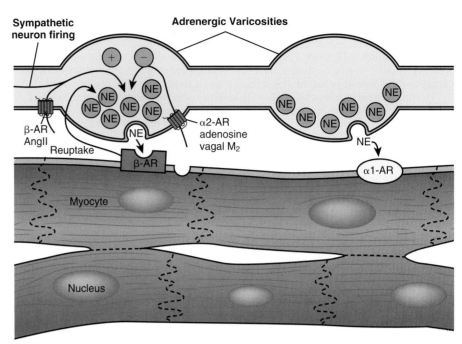

FIGURE 46.11 Norepinephrine (NE) release from sympathetic neurons. NE is released from storage granules in adrenergic varicosities into narrow, synapse-like spaces near its receptors in the sarcolemma of the cardiac and smooth muscle myocytes of the heart and arterial walls. In cardiomyocytes, beta-adrenergic receptor (βAR) activation increases heart rate (chronotropy), contractile force (inotropy) and relaxation (lusitropy), and conduction (dromotropy). However, NE also activates cardiac myocyte alpha$_1$-adrenergic receptors, which can further modulate contractility and myocyte signaling cascades. In arterioles, NE predominantly causes vasoconstriction via postsynaptic alpha$_1$ receptors. NE also stimulates presynaptic alpha$_2$ receptors to invoke feedback inhibition that can limit its own release. Circulating epinephrine stimulates vascular vasodilatory beta$_2$ receptors but also presynaptic receptors on the nerve terminal, which promotes NE release. Angiotensin II (AngII) is also powerfully vasoconstrictive and acts both by stimulation of NE release (presynaptic receptors, as indicated schematically) and directly on arteriolar AngII receptors. M$_2$ is muscarinic receptor, subtype two.

TABLE 46.2 Comparative Cardiovascular Effects of Alpha- and Beta-Adrenergic Receptor Stimulation

	ALPHA1 MEDIATED	BETA MEDIATED
Electrophysiologic effects	±	++
		Conduction
		Pacemaker
		Heart rate
		− AP duration
Myocardial mechanics	±	++
		Contractility, lusitropy
		Stroke volume
		Cardiac output
Myocardial metabolism	±	++
	Glycolysis	O$_2$ uptake ↑
		ATP consumption
Signal systems	GPCR, can activate PKC and MAPK	GPCR, activates cAMP and PKA
Coronary arterioles	++	+ Direct dilation
	Constriction	+++ Indirect dilation (metabolic)
Peripheral arterioles	+++	+
	Constriction	Dilation
	SVR ↑	SVR ↓
	SBP ↑	SBP ↓

AP, Action potential; *cAMP,* cyclic adenosine monophosphate; *GPCR,* G protein–coupled receptor; *MAPK,* mitogen-activated protein kinase; *PK,* protein kinase; *PKC,* protein kinase C; *SBP,* systolic blood pressure; *SVR,* systemic vascular resistance.
Modified from Opie LH. *Heart Physiology, from Cell to Circulation.* 4th ed. Philadelphia: Lippincott, Williams & Wilkins; 2004.

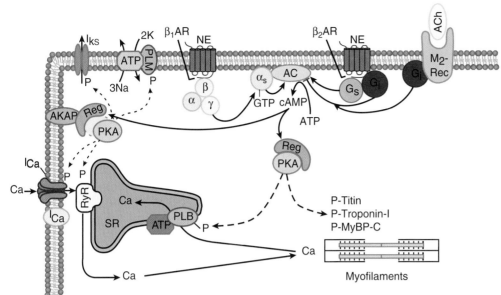

FIGURE 46.12 Beta-adrenergic and muscarinic activation in cardiac myocytes interact. Activation of beta$_1$-adrenergic receptors (β_1AR) activate adenylyl cyclase (*AC*) via G$_s$ (via the activated alpha subunit (α_s) dissociation from the beta and gamma subunits (β and γ). AC produces cAMP, which activates protein kinase A (*PKA*), which phosphorylates (*P*) several key functional targets (*broken arrows*). β$_2$-AR activate both G$_s$ and G$_i$, which activate or inhibit AC, respectively. Activation of muscarinic M$_2$ receptors (*M$_2$-Rec*) by acetylcholine (*ACh*) from parasympathetic neurons inhibits AC via G$_i$.*PLB*, Phospholamban; *PLM*, phospholemman; *Reg*, regulatory subunit of PKA. (Modified from Bers DM. *Excitation-Contraction Coupling and Cardiac Contractile Force*. Dordrecht, Netherlands: Kluwer Academic; 2001.)

number of beta$_3$-adrenergic receptors in cardiac myocytes that seem to produce more G$_i$-mediated negative inotropic signaling, mediated in part by NO, but this pathway is not as well understood. The beta-adrenergic receptor site is highly stereospecific, the best fit among catecholamines being achieved with the synthetic agent isoproterenol rather than with the naturally occurring catecholamines norepinephrine and epinephrine. In the case of beta$_1$ receptors, the order of agonist activity is isoproterenol > epinephrine = norepinephrine, whereas in the case of beta$_2$ receptors, the order is isoproterenol > epinephrine > norepinephrine. Human beta$_1$ and beta$_2$ receptors have been cloned and studied extensively.[4] The transmembrane domains are the site of agonist and antagonist binding, whereas the cytoplasmic domains interact with G proteins.

Alpha-Adrenergic Receptor Subtypes

The two alpha-adrenergic receptor isoforms are alpha$_1$ and alpha$_2$. Those on the sarcolemma of vascular smooth muscle are vasoconstrictor alpha$_1$ receptors, whereas those situated on the terminal varicosities are alpha$_2$-adrenergic receptors that feed back (see Fig. 46.11) to inhibit release of norepinephrine. Pharmacologically, an alpha$_2$-adrenergic receptor mediates a response in which the effects resemble those of the pharmacologic agent phenylephrine. Among catecholamines, the relative potencies of alpha$_1$-agonists are norepinephrine > epinephrine > isoproterenol. Physiologically, norepinephrine liberated from nerve terminals is the chief stimulus to vascular alpha$_1$-adrenergic activity. Both alpha$_1$ and alpha$_2$ receptors are also found in cardiac myocytes, where their activation can fine-tune Ca^{2+} transients, ionic currents, and myofilament properties acutely, but they are also known to be important modulators of cardiac remodeling (in both adaptive and maladaptive contexts).[33]

G Proteins

G proteins are a superfamily of proteins that bind guanine triphosphate (GTP) and other guanine nucleotides. G proteins are crucial in carrying the signal onward from the agonist and its receptor to the activity of the membrane-bound enzyme system that produces the second messenger cAMP (Fig. 46.13; see also Fig. 46.12).[4] Thus the combination of the beta receptor, G protein complex, and adenylyl cyclase is the crux of beta-adrenergic signaling.

THE STIMULATORY G PROTEIN G$_s$

The G protein itself is a heterotrimer composed of G$_\alpha$, G$_\beta$, and G$_\gamma$, which on receptor stimulation splits into the alpha subunit that is bound to GTP and the beta-gamma subunit. Either of these subunits may regulate different effectors such as adenylyl cyclase, phospholipase C, and ion channels. The activity of adenylyl cyclase is controlled by two different G protein complexes, namely, G$_s$, which stimulates, and G$_i$, which inhibits. The alpha subunit of G$_s$ (α_s) combines with GTP and then separates from the other two subunits to enhance the activity of adenylyl cyclase. The beta and gamma subunits (beta-gamma) appear to be linked structurally and functionally.

THE INHIBITORY G PROTEIN G$_i$

In contrast, a second trimeric GTP-binding protein, G$_i$, is responsible for inhibition of adenylyl cyclase.[4] During stimulation of muscarinic and some beta$_2$-adrenergic receptors, GTP binds to the inhibitory alpha subunit α$_i$. The latter then dissociates from the beta-gamma subunits. The beta-gamma subunits act as follows. By stimulating the enzyme guanosine triphosphatase (GTPase), they break down the active α$_s$ subunit (α$_s$-GTP) to limit activation of adenylyl cyclase which occurs in response to G$_s$ stimulation. Furthermore, the beta-gamma subunit activates the K$_{ACh}$ channel, which can slow SA node firing and thereby contribute to the bradycardic effect of cholinergic stimulation. The α$_i$ subunit may also activate another potassium channel (K$_{ATP}$) that stabilizes the diastolic membrane potential. The major physiologic stimulus for G$_i$ is thought to be vagal muscarinic receptor stimulation (although beta$_2$-adrenergic receptors may contribute as well). In addition, adenosine, by interaction with A$_1$ receptors, couples to G$_i$ to inhibit contraction and HR. The adenosine A$_2$ receptor paradoxically increases cAMP. The latter effect, only of ancillary significance in the myocardium, is of major importance in vascular smooth muscle, where it induces vasorelaxation. Pathologically, G$_i$ is increased in experimental postinfarct heart failure[4] and in donor hearts before cardiac transplantation.[4]

A THIRD G PROTEIN, G$_q$

This protein links a group of GPCRs, including the alpha-adrenergic receptor and those for angiotensin II and endothelin-1, to another membrane-associated enzyme, phospholipase C, and then to PKC and PKD (and IP$_3$-induced Ca^{2+} mobilization). G$_q$ has at least four isoforms, two of which have been found in the heart. This G protein, unlike G$_i$, is not susceptible to inhibition by pertussis toxin. Overexpression of G$_q$ in mice induces a dilated cardiomyopathy,[4] which is of interest because angiotensin II and endothelin, which act through G$_q$, are overactive in human heart failure. Conversely, when the activity of G$_q$ is genetically inhibited, the hypertrophic response to pressure overload is attenuated, wall stress increases, but cardiac function is relatively well maintained.

Cyclic Adenosine Monophosphate and Protein Kinase A

Adenylyl Cyclase

Adenylyl cyclase (also called adenylate or adenyl cyclase) catalyzes formation of the second messenger cAMP. Several isoforms exist, but AC5 and AC6 are most prominent in cardiac myocytes, and these isoforms are partially inhibited by high [Ca^{2+}]$_i$. Adenylyl cyclase, when stimulated by G$_s$, produces cAMP, which acts through multiple intracellular signals (including importantly PKA) to mediate the chronotropic, inotropic, lusitropic, and dromotropic effects of cardiac beta-adrenergic agonists. In contrast, cholinergic (and vagal) stimulation can inhibit adenylyl cyclase through G$_i$ to slow HR, but also limit cAMP formation downstream of G$_s$ activation.

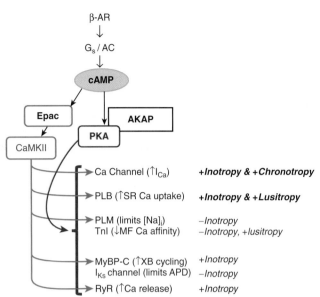

FIGURE 46.13 Key roles of PKA (and CaMKII) in beta-adrenergic responses. Major intracellular effects of beta-agonist catecholamines are via the formation of cyclic adenosine monophosphate (cAMP), which increases the activity of PKA and also Epac (exchange protein activated by cAMP). PKA is localized by A-kinase anchoring proteins (AKAPs) that target PKA function to local nanodomains. Epac also activates CaMKII which can phosphorylate and modulate function of some of the same targets as PKA (often by phosphorylation at different amino acids).

Adenylyl cyclase is the only enzyme that produces cAMP, using low concentrations of Mg^{2+}-ATP as substrate. It is a transmembrane enzyme, with most mass on the cytoplasmic side where G proteins interact. Cyclic guanosine monophosphate (cGMP) is a related second messenger that often antagonizes cAMP effects. cAMP has very rapid turnover as a result of a constant dynamic balance between its formation by adenylyl cyclase and conversion to AMP by phosphodiesterases (PDEs). Several major PDE isoforms have different substrate specificity (cAMP versus cGMP) and are differentially regulated by cyclic nucleotides and Ca^{2+}/calmodulin.[34] In general, directional changes in the tissue content of cAMP can be related to directional changes in cardiac contractile activity, but local subcellular domains may have differential cAMP and PKA regulation that depends in part on PDE isoform localization. For example, while beta-adrenergic stimulation increases both cAMP and PKA target phosphorylation, differences may occur at ion channel and myofilament target sites.[35] *Forskolin* is a potent direct adenylyl cyclase activator, and isobutyl methylxanthine (*IBMX*) is a PDE inhibitor that inhibits all PDE isoforms. These are widely used agents experimentally, but isoform-specific PDE inhibitors are being explored as more targeted therapeutic strategies. A number of hormones or peptides can couple to myocardial adenylyl cyclase independent of the beta-adrenergic receptor. These include glucagon, thyroid hormone, prostacyclin, and calcitonin gene–related peptide.

There is also a GTP *exchange protein* directly *activated* by *cAMP* (*Epac*) that is activated in parallel to cAMP-dependent PKA activation. This allows additional parallel signaling downstream of beta-adrenergic activation. For example, beta-adrenergic activation of SR Ca^{2+} release is mediated by cAMP-Epac–dependent signaling to CaMKII and consequent RyR2 phosphorylation,[36] and not by PKA activation.

Protein Kinase A

PKA occurs in two isoforms, but PKA-II predominates in cardiac cells. It is now clear that many key cAMP effects are mediated by activation of PKA and phosphorylation of key proteins.[37] Each PKA complex is composed of two regulatory (R) and two catalytic (C) subunits, the latter of which transfers the terminal phosphate of ATP to serine and threonine residues of the protein substrates. When cAMP interacts with the inactive protein kinase, it binds to the R subunits, causing partial release and activation of the C subunits. A former dogma was that the C subunits were completely released from the R subunits, but more recent evidence suggests that a loose tethering likely remains when PKA is active. The R subunits are bound to specific AKAPs that target

PKA-dependent phosphorylation at specific subcellular targets.[38] This helps to explain the local compartmentalization of cAMP and PKA signaling. Indeed, there is good evidence that beta-adrenergic receptors, G proteins, adenylyl cyclase, PKA, AKAP, PDE, and phosphatases can all complex at targets such as the L-type Ca^{2+} channel and RyR2 to facilitate local PKA-dependent signaling (see Fig. 46.13).[16,39,40]

Beta$_1$-Adrenergic and Protein Kinase A Signaling in Ventricular Myocytes

The sequence of events for PKA activation is as follows (see Fig. 46.12): catecholamine stimulation → beta receptor → molecular changes → binding of GTP to the α_s subunit of G protein → GTP-α_s subunit stimulating adenylyl cyclase → formation of cAMP from ATP → activation of cAMP-dependent PKA, locally bound by an AKAP → phosphorylation of the target proteins. The L-type Ca^{2+} channel is rapidly phosphorylated by this cascade, which results in both a large increase in the amount of peak I_{Ca} and a shift in the activation voltage to more negative potentials. This increases the amount of Ca^{2+} that enters the cell at each beat and also enhances excitability (including in pacemaker cells). In addition, the higher I_{Ca} triggers more SR Ca^{2+} release, but the higher peak I_{Ca} and SR Ca^{2+} release also enhance Ca-dependent inactivation of I_{Ca}, which limits the total amount of Ca^{2+} entry during the AP. This contributes to an increased Ca^{2+} transient amplitude, the inotropic effect, and also the chronotropic and dromotropic effects of PKA in heart (Figs. 46.12–46.14).

Another major contributor to the inotropic effect of PKA in the heart is phosphorylation of PLB. PLB is associated with SERCA2 and at baseline inhibits the Ca^{2+} pump by reducing its affinity for Ca^{2+}. On phosphorylation of PLB by PKA (or CaMKII), the inhibitory effect is relieved and the Ca^{2+} pumping function greatly enhanced. This allows more Ca^{2+} to accumulate inside the SR during the cardiac cycle, which enhances the amount that can then be released (thereby contributing to inotropy). The faster rate of SR Ca^{2+} uptake is also the major factor in accelerating relaxation, the lusitropic effect of PKA. This occurs because twitch $[Ca^{2+}]_i$ decline is faster, which allows faster Ca^{2+} dissociation from the myofilaments.

Phosphorylation of troponin I by PKA also contributes to the enhanced lusitropic effect of beta-adrenergic agonists (see Fig. 46.13). PKA-dependent troponin I phosphorylation reduces myofilament sensitivity for calcium, which is intrinsically negatively inotropic, but has the benefit of faster dissociation of Ca^{2+} from myofilaments, which hastens relaxation and diastolic filling. In addition, myosin-binding protein C is also a target for PKA, and its phosphorylation appears to be responsible for accelerating the cross-bridge turnover rate. This effect also serves largely to offset the negative inotropic effect of troponin I phosphorylation and also may hasten the rate of sarcomere shortening at a given $[Ca^{2+}]$ and mechanical load, which could enhance stroke volume.[41]

PKA also phosphorylates the RyR, although the impact of this effect is controversial.[42] One group has suggested that this displaces the immunophilin FKBP-12.6 from its binding to RyR2, thereby activating RyR openings, and that this is an important part of the beta-adrenergic inotropy and cardiac dysfunction in heart failure.[43] However, this idea has been strongly challenged by extensive mechanistic experimental data and theoretical arguments from numerous groups worldwide.[42] Although the effects of PKA on the cardiac RyR may enhance the rate of RyR activation during excitation-contraction coupling, it does not seem to increase the amount released (for a given I_{Ca} trigger and SR Ca^{2+} load),[44] nor does it directly enhance the likelihood of spontaneous SR Ca^{2+} release events.[45] Moreover, even when the RyR is sensitized, it causes enhanced SR Ca^{2+} release only for several beats, which then drives greater efflux of Ca^{2+} from the cell (by NCX) and reduces the SR Ca^{2+} content such that it cannot explain the enhanced Ca^{2+} transients during beta-adrenergic activation.[46]

PKA also phosphorylates PLM, a small PLB-like protein that regulates Na^+,K^+-ATPase (see earlier).[32] This is actually a sensible integral part of the fight-or-flight response because the increase in HR incurs more frequent I_{Na} pulses and Ca^{2+} influx (by I_{Ca}) that causes more Na^+ influx by NCX, resulting in a major increase in $[Na^+]_i$. This Na^+,K^+-ATPase activation limits the rise in $[Na^+]_i$ during sympathetic activation and thus allows NCX to remain functional in removing Ca^{2+} from the myocyte.

The increase in Na$^+$,K$^+$-ATPase function thus is somewhat negatively inotropic (by limiting [Na$^+$]$_i$). This is opposite the effect mediated by inhibition of Na$^+$,K$^+$-ATPase by digitalis cardiac glycosides. Notably, digitalis toxicity is associated with cellular Ca^{2+} overload and arrhythmogenesis. Consequently, Na$^+$,K$^+$-ATPase stimulation may limit these arrhythmogenic consequences associated with higher Ca^{2+} loading.

BETA-ADRENERGIC RECEPTOR DESENSITIZATION

There is a potent and rapid feedback mechanism whereby beta-adrenergic receptor stimulation can be muted so that the signal can be turned off (see Fig. 46.14). Physiologically, this mechanism of beta-adrenergic receptor desensitization occurs within minutes. Sustained beta-agonist stimulation recruits a G protein–coupled receptor kinase (GRK2; also called beta-adrenergic receptor kinase 1 [βARK1]). GRK2 phosphorylates a site on the carboxyl-terminal of the beta-adrenergic receptor, which by itself does not switch off signaling. However, GRK2 activity increases beta receptor affinity for arrestins, which uncouple receptor signaling. Beta-arrestin is a scaffolding and signaling protein that links to one of the cytoplasmic loops of the beta-adrenergic receptor and lessens activation of adenylyl cyclase, thereby inhibiting receptor function. Furthermore, beta-arrestin can switch agonist coupling from G$_s$ to G$_i$ and also lead to internalization of the beta-adrenergic receptor.[4] Resensitization of the receptor occurs if the phosphate groups are removed by a phosphatase, and the receptor then more readily linked to G$_s$ (or by recycling the internalized receptor to the surface). Beta-arrestin signaling can also evoke an alternative protective path by activating the epidermal growth factor receptor (EGFR), which leads to the protective extracellular signal–related kinase (ERK)/MAPK pathway (see Fig. 46.14).[47] Although the GRK2-arrestin effects are best described for the beta$_2$ receptor, they also occur with the beta$_1$ receptor. Prolonged beta receptor stimulation, as in hyperadrenergic conditions, is linked to adverse end results in that it both impairs contractile function and enhances adverse signaling. As discussed in Chapter 47, this mechanism also plays a role in long-term desensitization of the beta-adrenergic receptor as in heart failure, and transgenic mice overexpressing GRK2 are protected from heart failure.[48]

Ca^{2+}/Calmodulin-Dependent Protein Kinase II

CaMKII is a serine/threonine-specific protein kinase that is regulated by the Ca^{2+}/CaM complex. CaMKII is involved in many signaling cascades in the heart, and several of the key proteins that are phosphorylated by PKA are also phosphorylated by CaMKII (see Fig. 46.13), typically at different amino acids. Moreover, there is good evidence that CaMKII is activated during beta-adrenergic stimulation.[23] Thus, CaMKII signaling is often coactivated with PKA and can synergize at downstream targets.[23,49] CaMKII activates L-type Ca^{2+} channels (I$_{Ca}$ facilitation), which results in increased peak I$_{Ca}$ and also slows down inactivation, thereby boosting total Ca^{2+} influx by I$_{Ca}$. CaMKII also phosphorylates PLB at Thr17 (vs. at Ser16 by PKA) and, by the same mechanism as for PKA, can enhance SR Ca^{2+} uptake. However, the CaMKII effects on I$_{Ca}$ and SERCA/PLB are typically smaller in magnitude than the effects of PKA activation, so PKA is probably dominant physiologically at these targets. CaMKII can also phosphorylate RyR2 at Ser2814, close to a recognized PKA target site (2808). In contrast to PKA, it is more universally agreed that

CaMKII strongly activates the RyR and that this effect may be important in causing a diastolic SR Ca^{2+} leak, which can both reduce the SR Ca^{2+} content (contributing to both systolic and diastolic dysfunction) and contribute to triggered arrhythmias.[22,23,42] CaMKII can also phosphorylate cardiac Na$^+$ and K$^+$ channels and lead to arrhythmogenic consequences.[22,23] CaMKII-dependent activation of the late Na$^+$ current may also lead to elevated intracellular [Na$^+$] and [Ca^{2+}], which can create Ca^{2+} overload and trigger arrhythmias. Myofilament proteins are also targets for CaMKII (e.g., myosin-binding protein C and titin),[50] but the relative functional importance of this effect is not yet fully resolved. The chronic activation of CaMKII in pathologic states such as heart failure makes these pathways important to keep in mind.

CHOLINERGIC AND NITRIC OXIDE SIGNALING

Cholinergic Signaling

Parasympathetic stimulation reduces the HR and is negatively inotropic. As in adrenergic signaling, there is an extracellular messenger (ACh), a GPCR (the *cholinergic* muscarinic receptor in heart; M$_2$), and a sarcolemmal signaling system (G protein system, specifically G$_i$, see Fig. 46.12). Receptor stimulation produces a negative chronotropic response that is inhibited by atropine. NO, also formed by beta$_3$-adrenergic signaling,[51] facilitates cholinergic signaling at two levels, the nerve terminal and myocyte enzyme system that produces the second messenger cGMP. *Neuregulins* are growth factors that maintain the activity of the muscarinic receptor, thereby indirectly helping to balance the normal parasympathetic modulation of excess beta-adrenergic stimulation.[52,53]

Muscarinic G$_i$ activation also inhibits adenylyl cyclase, which functionally integrates the input from activating G$_s$ (e.g., from beta$_1$-adrenergic and other receptors) and the inhibitory effects of G$_i$ (from M$_2$ muscarinic and other receptors; Fig. 46.12). As a result, vagal stimulation also limits [cAMP] resulting from ambient sympathetic tone. The net effect is slowing of the HR. This is partly because cardiac vagal innervation is highest in the SA and atrioventricular (AV) nodes, with lower density in atrial myocardium and the lowest density in ventricular myocardium. Consequently, vagal activity has less strong effects on atrial or ventricular myocyte electrophysiology, Ca^{2+} transients, or contractility than on conduction system cells, but that is also because these cells lack major pacemaker function and have higher inward rectifier I$_{K1}$ channels that already stabilize diastolic membrane potential at more negative values. Nevertheless, vagal activation can shorten the AP duration in the atria and, to a lesser degree, in the ventricles (primarily by I$_{K(Ach)}$ activation).

CYCLIC GUANOSINE MONOPHOSPHATE SIGNALING IN THE HEART

The second messenger cGMP typically has negative inotropic effects in the heart, in contrast to its cyclic nucleotide cousin cAMP. Cyclic GMP is produced from GTP in cardiac myocytes mainly by soluble and particulate guanylyl cyclases, which are activated downstream of NO and natriuretic peptide receptor activation, respectively (Fig. 46.15), and possibly by cholinergic effects. Local subcellular microdomains in which NO and cGMP signaling take place are also likely to exist.[39] When local [cGMP]

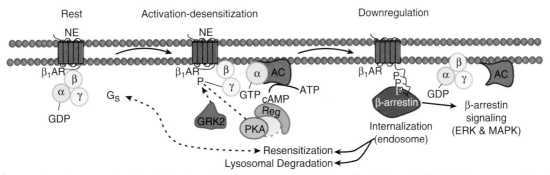

FIGURE 46.14 Beta$_1$-adrenergic receptor (β$_1$AR) activation, desensitization, downregulation, and recycling. Prolonged β$_1$AR activation causes recruitment of a G-protein receptor kinase (GRK2) that phosphorylates the receptor and favors recruitment of beta-arrestin (β-arrestin). β-arrestin promotes its own signaling cascades (e.g. via extracellular receptor and MAP kinase (ERK and MAPK) as well as internalization of the β$_1$AR into endosomes. From there β$_1$AR can either be degraded or recycled to the cell surface. (Modified from Bers DM. *Excitation-Contraction Coupling and Cardiac Contractile Force.* Dordrecht, Netherlands: Kluwer Academic; 2001.)

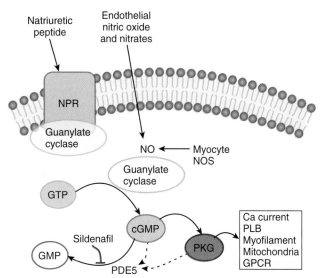

FIGURE 46.15 Nitric oxide (NO) and the natriuretic peptide receptor (NPR) activate guanylate cyclase (via particulate and soluble cyclases, respectively), resulting in production of cyclic guanosine monophosphate (cGMP) and activation of protein kinase G (PKG). PKG can phosphorylate numerous myocyte targets that tend to counteract cyclic adenosine monophosphate (cAMP) and PKA effects at some targets (with some exceptions). Phosphodiesterase 5 (PDE5) breaks down cGMP, and PDE5 inhibitors (e.g., sildenafil) can thus increase cGMP levels. Notably, high cGMP and PKG levels promote vasodilation and negative inotropic effects, and antianginal nitrates promote vasodilation by this mechanism.

is elevated, it can stimulate protein kinase G (PKG), which results in inhibitory cardiac effects such as a decreased HR and negative inotropic response. These effects are largely achieved by modulation of Ca^{2+} entry through L-type Ca^{2+} channels and through alteration of internal Ca^{2+} cycling.[53,54] PKG has also been suggested to be a critical suppressor of pathophysiologic hypertrophy.[55]

cGMP is broken down by PDE, and seven PDE isoforms are expressed in the heart, some of which break down both cAMP and cGMP (PDE1 to PDE3), whereas PDE4 is cAMP specific and PDE5 is cGMP specific.[54] Cell-permeable analogues of cGMP have antiadrenergic effects, potentially by activating PDE2 that also breaks down cAMP. PDE5 has achieved prominence as a result of its inhibition by sildenafil and related compounds that all enhance penile vasodilation. Emerging data show wider therapeutic potential. Thus sildenafil, by accumulation of cGMP, combats the harmful excessive adrenergic stimulation of contractile function. Furthermore, through cGMP, sildenafil can inhibit excess LV growth in response to aortic constriction.[56] Conversely, in human cardiac hypertrophy and heart failure, PDE5 is more highly expressed, which may exacerbate adverse remodeling. The key target of cGMP, PKG, as with its counterpart PKA, colocalizes with its targets to control substrate phosphorylation.[57] The anchoring protein for PKG may be the same AKAP as for PKA, thus allowing tight subcellular colocalization and regulation of the counterposed activities of cAMP and cGMP and of their respective upstream signaling cascades.[54]

Nitric Oxide

The focus of the Nobel Prize Award for 1998, NO is a unique messenger in that it is formed in so many tissues, is a gas, and is a physiologic free radical. NO is generated in the heart by one of three isoenzymes.[53] All three isoforms are present in the heart. NOS1 (nNOS, or neuronal NOS) and NOS3 (eNOS, or endothelial NOS) are always present, whereas NOS2 (iNOS, or inducible NOS) expression is induced in pathological conditions.[58,59] Both NOS1 and NOS3 are activated by local Ca^{2+}-CaM, where relatively low concentrations of Ca^{2+}-CaM suffice to activate NOS activation. In contrast, NOS2 constitutively produces NO, independent of Ca^{2+}-CaM activation. NO can directly activate soluble guanylate cyclase (see Fig. 46.15), feeding into the cGMP signaling system, but many other myocyte proteins are *S*-nitrosylated by NO which can modulate their function, including CaMKII.[59,60]

CONTRACTILE PERFORMANCE OF THE HEART

There are five main determinants of ventricular mechanical performance: preload (or Frank-Starling mechanism), afterload, contractility, lusitropy (diastolic function), and HR. This section describes the cardiac cycle and then the determinants of LV function.

The Cardiac Cycle

The cardiac cycle, fully assembled by Lewis[61] but first conceived by Wiggers,[62] yields important information on the temporal sequence of events (Fig. 46.16). The three basic events with respect to the left ventricle are LV contraction, LV relaxation, and LV filling (Table 46.3). Similar mechanical events occur in the right ventricle.

Left Ventricular Contraction

LV pressure increases as Ca^{2+} arrives at the contractile proteins after cellular depolarization, triggering actin-myosin interaction.[4] This occurs shortly after the upstroke of the ventricular AP, indicated by the QRS complex of the ECG (Fig. 46.16). When LV pressure exceeds pressure in the left atrium (normally 8 to 15 mm Hg), the mitral valve closes, causing the mitral component of the first sound, M_1. Right ventricular (RV) pressure changes are usually slightly delayed because of electrical conduction, such that tricuspid valve closure (T_1), follows M_1. The phase of LV contraction after mitral closure and before aortic opening when the LV volume is fixed is referred to as *isovolumic contraction*. As more myofibers become activated, LV pressure proceeds to increase until it exceeds aortic pressure, causing the aortic valve to open (usually a clinically silent event). Opening of the aortic valve is followed by the phase of *rapid ejection*. The rate of ejection is determined by the pressure gradient across the aortic valve, as well as the elastic properties of the aorta and the arterial tree, which undergo systolic expansion. LV pressure rises to a peak and then starts to fall.

Left Ventricular Relaxation

As myocyte $[Ca^{2+}]_i$ starts to decline because of SR Ca^{2+} uptake, Ca^{2+} dissociates from troponin C, thereby preventing further cross-bridge formation.[4] As this state of relaxation progresses, the rate of LV ejection of blood into the aorta falls (*phase of reduced ejection*). During this phase, blood flow from the left ventricle to the aorta rapidly diminishes but is maintained by aortic recoil—the Windkessel effect.[4] When the pressure in the aorta significantly exceeds the falling LV pressure, the aortic valve closes, which creates the first component of the second sound, A_2 (the second component, P_2, results from closure of the pulmonic valve as pulmonary artery pressure exceeds RV pressure). Thereafter, the ventricle continues to relax. Because the mitral valve is still closed during this phase after aortic closure, LV volume does not change (*isovolumic relaxation*). The rate of pressure decay during isovolumic relaxation is related to the magnitude of systolic shortening in the preceding contraction, similar to a spring compressed below its unstressed slack length.[63] When LV pressure falls to below that in the left atrium, the mitral valve opens (normally silent), and the filling phase of the cardiac cycle restarts (see Fig. 46.16).

Left Ventricular Filling Phases

Following mitral valve opening, the phase of rapid or early filling occurs and accounts for most of the increase in LV volume during diastole.[4] Under normal circumstances, this is caused by a negative pressure gradient from atrium to the LV apex, creating a suction effect, especially during exercise, when LV filling rates must be augmented to increase cardiac output.[63] Such rapid filling may cause the physiologic third heart sound (S_3), when there is a hyperkinetic circulation, or a pathologic S_3 when left atrial (LA) and LV diastolic pressures are elevated in congestive heart failure.[4] As pressures in the atrium and ventricle equalize, LV filling virtually stops (diastasis, separation). Renewed filling requires that atrial pressure exceed LV pressure. This is achieved by atrial systole (or the "LA kick"), which is especially important at a high

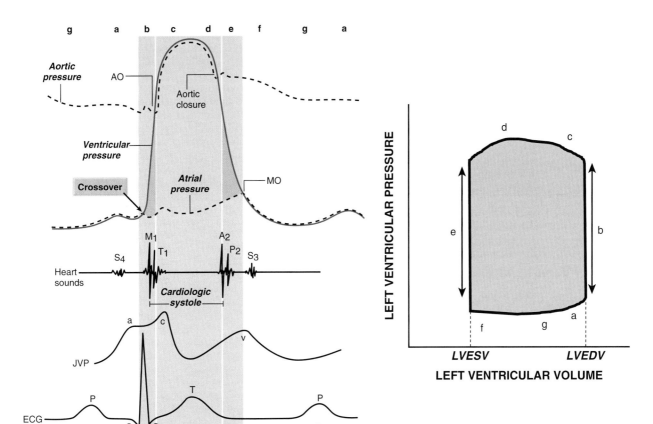

The Lewis or Wiggers Cycle

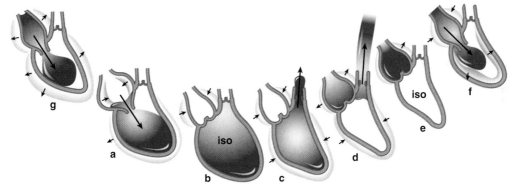

FIGURE 46.16 Mechanical events in the cardiac cycle depicted as pressure versus time **(upper left)** and left ventricular pressure versus volume **(upper right).** The visual phases of the ventricular cycle are shown in the **bottom panel.** For an explanation of phases a to g in upper right and bottom panels, see Table 46.3. *a*, Wave produced by right atrial contraction; *A₂*, aortic valve closure, aortic component of the second sound; *AO*, aortic valve opening, normally inaudible; *c*, carotid wave artifact during the rapid LV ejection phase; *ECG*, electrocardiogram; *JVP*, jugular venous pressure; *LVEDV*, left ventricular end-diastolic volume; *LVESV*, left ventricular end-systolic volume; *M₁*, mitral component of the first sound at the time of mitral valve closure; *MO*, mitral valve opening, may be audible in mitral stenosis as the opening snap; *P₂*, pulmonary component of the second sound, pulmonary valve closure; *S₃*, third heart sound; *S₄*, fourth heart sound; *T₁*, tricuspid valve closure, second component of the first heart sound; *v*, venous return wave, which causes pressure to rise with the tricuspid valve closed. (Modified from Opie LH. *Heart Physiology, from Cell to Circulation*. Philadelphia: Lippincott, Williams & Wilkins; 2004. Figure copyright L.H. Opie, 2004. **Bottom panel** modified from Shepherd JT, Vanhoutte PM. *The Human Cardiovascular System*. New York: Raven Press; 1979:68.)

HR, as during exercise, or when the left ventricle fails to relax normally, as in patients with LV hypertrophy or increased chamber stiffness.[4]

DEFINITIONS OF SYSTOLE AND DIASTOLE

In Greek, systole means "contraction" and diastole means "to send apart." The start of systole can be regarded as the beginning of isovolumic contraction, when LV pressure exceeds the atrial pressure, or as mitral valve closure (M₁). Physiologic systole lasts from the start of isovolumic contraction to the peak of the ejection phase (see Fig. 46.16 and Table 46.3). Physiologic diastole commences as Ca²⁺ is taken back into

the SR, so that myocyte relaxation dominates over contraction, and as the LV pressure starts to fall, as shown on the pressure-volume curve. In contrast, cardiologic systole is longer than physiologic systole and is demarcated by the interval between the first heart sound (M₁) to the closure of the aortic valve (A₂). The remainder of the cardiac cycle automatically becomes cardiologic diastole. For the cardiologist, protodiastole is the early phase of rapid filling, the time when S₃ can be heard (also referred to as a protodiastolic gallop). This sound probably reflects ventricular wall vibrations during rapid filling and becomes audible with an increase in LV diastolic pressure, wall stiffness, or rate of filling.

TABLE 46.3 The Cardiac Cycle

Left Ventricular Contraction
Isovolumic contraction (b)
Maximal ejection (c)
Left Ventricular Relaxation
Start of relaxation and reduced ejection (d)
Isovolumic relaxation (e)
LV filling: rapid phase (f)
Slow LV filling (diastasis) (g)
Atrial systole or kick (a)

The letters a to g refer to the phases of the cardiac cycle shown in Wiggers' diagram (see Fig. 46.16). These letters are arbitrarily allocated so that atrial systole (a) coincides with the A wave and (c) with the C wave of jugular venous pressure.

Contractility Versus Loading Conditions
Contractility
Contractility, or the *inotropic state of the heart,* reflects the inherent capacity of the myocardium to contract independently of changes in preload or afterload.[63] These are key terms in the language of cardiology. At the molecular level, an increased inotropic state is usually explained by either enhanced Ca^{2+} transients or enhanced myofilament Ca^{2+} sensitivity and typically results in a greater rate of contraction to reach a greater peak force. Frequently, increased contractile function is associated with enhanced rates of relaxation, or a lusitropic effect (e.g., as during beta-adrenergic activation). Contractile function is an important regulator of myocardial oxygen (O_2) uptake. Factors that increase contractility include exercise, adrenergic stimulation, digitalis, and other inotropic agents.

Preload
It is important to stress that any change in the contractility should be independent of the loading conditions. An increase in stroke volume that is caused by an increase in preload alone may not reflect an increase in contractility per se. Ventricular preload describes the degree of myocardial stretch or distention before contraction has started and is best represented at the chamber level by the LV EDV. Because volume is difficult to measure accurately and precisely in practice, preload is often estimated by LV end-diastolic pressure (EDP), but it is important to remember that the relationship between EDP and EDV varies between patients, especially when diastolic dysfunction or ventricular interdependence are present. In such patients, a higher EDP is required to achieve a given EDV, meaning that preload may be normal or even low despite elevated intracardiac filling pressures.

Afterload
Afterload refers in a broad sense to the forces opposing LV ejection.[4,63] Afterload is often oversimplified as being equal to aortic blood pressure but is more accurately described as aortic *impedance* or *elastance,* which incorporates steady and oscillatory components of cardiac load. LV afterload can also be expressed by the wall stress that exists during systole. When preload increases, the stroke volume rises according to Starling's law if all other factors are held constant. Conversely, when afterload increases, stroke volume drops.

Starling's Law of the Heart
Venous Filling Pressure and Heart Volume
In 1918, Starling related the venous pressure in the right atrium to the heart volume in a dog heart-lung preparation.[4] He proposed that, within physiologic limits, the larger the volume of the heart, the greater the energy of its contraction and the amount of chemical change at each contraction. Starling did not, however, measure sarcomere length. He could only relate *LV volume* to cardiac output. In practice the LV volume is not often measured, rather making use of a variety of surrogate measures, such as LVEDP or the pulmonary capillary wedge pressure

(PCWP). The relation between LVEDV and LVEDP is curvilinear, with the slope reflecting LV compliance (bottom portion of pressure-volume loop, Fig. 46.16). The venous filling pressure can be measured in humans by cardiac catheterization, as can the stroke volume.

Frank and Isovolumic Contraction
If a larger heart volume increases the initial length of the muscle fiber, to increase stroke volume and thus cardiac output, diastolic stretch of the left ventricle (and increased sarcomere length) increases the force of contraction.[4] In 1895, Otto Frank had already reported that the greater the initial LV volume, the more rapid the rate of rise in pressure, the greater the peak pressure reached, and the faster the rate of relaxation. Thus, he described both a positive *inotropic effect* and an increased lusitropic effect. These complementary findings of Frank and Starling are often combined into the *Frank-Starling law.* Thus an increase in the strength of contraction can generally be categorized as either a *Frank-Starling effect* (increased sarcomere length) or an inotropic effect (altered Ca^{2+} transient or myofilament Ca^{2+} sensitivity), although both effects can occur simultaneously, as with physical exercise, where venous return to the heart is increased while β-1 adrenergic receptors are being activated by catecholamines to augment the Ca^{2+} transient. Being able to parse effects mechanistically in this way can be helpful in selecting therapeutic interventions.

Preload and Afterload Are Interlinked
Although the previous distinctions between preload and afterload are useful, one can influence the other. By the Frank-Starling law, an increased LV volume leads to increased contractile function, which in turn will increase the systolic aortic pressure and thus the afterload in the subsequent contraction cycle. During LV ejection, sarcomere length progressively declines, decreasing both myofilament Ca^{2+} sensitivity and maximal force, which along with progressive $[Ca^{2+}]_i$ decline, reduces contractile force. Afterload also dynamically changes during ejection and declines as ejection wanes.

PRELOAD AND DIASTOLIC PRESSURES MAY BECOME UNCOUPLED IN DISEASED HEARTS
LV pressure and volume are nonlinearly related because of myocardial compliance variations. In patients with reduced diastolic LV compliance, a higher EDP is required to achieve a similar EDV (preload). While the left and right ventricles influence each another in series (right ventricle pumps blood to left ventricle), factors in the right heart and pericardium also may influence LV pressure when there is enhanced ventricular interdependence, for example, with RV dilation from acute infarction or pulmonary embolism, or pericardial restraint caused by fibrotic constrictive pericarditis.[64] In these situations, EDP may be high even when EDV is normal or low, because the right heart and pericardium are applying "external pressure" that uncouples pressure from preload volume.

The true "distending" pressure that determines LV preload volume is referred to as the LV transmural pressure and can be calculated by EDP minus the external pericardial pressure. Pericardial pressure is approximated by right atrial pressure; thus transmural pressure can be estimated by the difference between EDP (or PCWP) and right atrial pressure.[64]

Force-Length Relationships and Ca^{2+} Transients
Acute changes in sarcomere length do not alter the Ca^{2+} transient appreciably. Thus the favored explanation for the steep length-tension relationship of cardiac muscles is enhanced myofilament Ca^{2+} sensitivity as the initial sarcomere length increases (via the Frank-Starling effect) (Fig. 46.17).

Anrep Effect: Abrupt Increase in Afterload
When the aortic pressure is elevated abruptly, ejection is limiting, tending to increase EDV, which acutely increases force and pressure at the next beat by the Frank-Starling effect. However, in a slower adaptation that takes seconds to minutes, the inotropic state of the heart increases (and Ca^{2+} transients are larger). Both phases of this can be readily recapitulated in isolated muscle strips from the heart. This slow force response or adaptation is referred to as the *Anrep effect.* Extensive study has implicated stretch-induced activation of several important

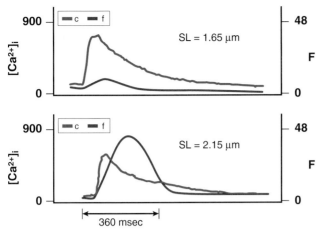

FIGURE 46.17 Length-dependent enhancement of myofilament Ca sensitivity. In the **top panel**, sarcomere length (*SL*) is 1.65 μm, which produces modest developed force (*f*). In the **bottom panel**, at near-maximal sarcomere length (2.15 μm), the Ca²⁺ transient (*c*) is almost unchanged, but causes much greater force development. (Modified from Backx PH, ter Keurs HEDJ. Fluorescent properties of rat cardiac trabeculae microinjected with fura-2 salt. *Am J Physiol.* 1993;264:H1098.)

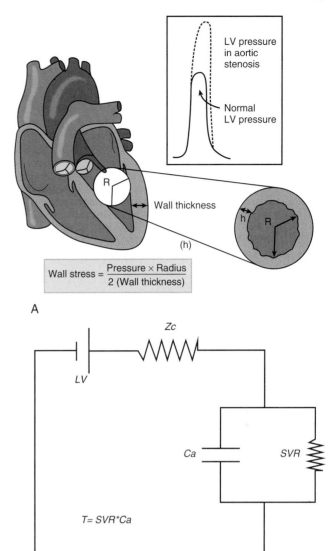

$$\text{Wall stress} = \frac{\text{Pressure} \times \text{Radius}}{2\ (\text{Wall thickness})}$$

A

$$T = SVR * Ca$$

$$Ea = \frac{SVR + Zc}{t_s + T(1-e^{-td/T})} \sim \frac{ESP}{SV}$$

B

FIGURE 46.18 A, Wall stress increases as afterload increases. The formula shown is derived from Laplace's law. The increased left ventricular (LV) pressure in aortic stenosis is compensated for by LV wall hypertrophy, which decreases the denominator on the right side of the equation. **B,** Electrical circuit analog of the arterial system as it relates to LV afterload, based on the three-element Windkessel model. The LV generates current (flow, cardiac output) that is ejected through an upstream impedance in the proximal aorta (characteristic impedance, *Zc*) upstream of total arterial compliance (*Ca*) and systemic vascular resistance (*SVR*) that arranged in parallel. Effective arterial elastance (*Ea*) is a lumped measure of net arterial "stiffness" that is related to each of these components and can be estimated by the ratio of end-systolic LV pressure (*ESP*) to stroke volume (*SV*). Ea (and thus arterial afterload) increases as Zc or SVR increases or as Ca decreases. *R,* Radius. (**A** from Opie LH. *Heart Physiology, from Cell to Circulation.* Philadelphia: Lippincott Williams & Wilkins; 2004. Figure copyright L.H. Opie, 2004; **B** from Borlaug BA, Kass DA. Ventricular-vascular interaction in heart failure. *Heart Fail Clin* 2008; 4:23-36.)

autocrine/paracrine myocyte signaling pathways in this slowly developing inotropic effect. Recent work suggests that increased afterload causes a NOS1- and CaMKII-dependent increase in Ca²⁺ transients to cause this myocyte-intrinsic gradual inotropic effect.[65,66]

Wall Stress

Wall stress develops when tension is applied to a cross-sectional area, and the units are force per unit area (Fig. 46.18). According to Laplace's law, wall stress = (pressure × radius)/(2 × wall thickness). This equation, although an oversimplification, emphasizes two points. First, the larger the LV size and radius, the higher is the wall stress.[4] Second, at any given radius (LV size), the greater the pressure developed by the left ventricle, the greater is the wall stress. An increase in wall stress achieved by either of these two mechanisms (LV size or intraventricular pressure) will increase myocardial O₂ uptake, because a greater rate of ATP use is required for the myofibrils to develop more tension.

In cardiac hypertrophy, Laplace's law explains the effects of changes in wall thickness on wall stress (see Fig. 46.18). The increased wall thickness from hypertrophy balances the increased pressure, and wall stress remains unchanged during the phase of compensatory hypertrophy.[4] The concept that this change is compensatory and beneficial has been challenged by a mouse model in which the process of hypertrophy was genetically inhibited so that wall stress increased in response to a pressure load, yet these mice had better cardiac mechanical function than did the wild-type mice in which compensatory hypertrophy developed.[4] Another clinically useful concept is that in congestive heart failure, the heart dilates so that the increased radius elevates wall stress. Furthermore, because ejection of blood is inadequate, the radius stays too large throughout the contractile cycle, and both end-diastolic and end-systolic wall stress is higher. This decreases LV efficiency, increases myocardial O₂ demand, and augments release of natriuretic peptide levels. The overall reduction in heart size decreases wall stress and improves LV function.[4]

WALL STRESS, PRELOAD, AND AFTERLOAD

This definition brings in both the volume and the fiber length that define the radius.[4] Preload can be defined as the wall stretch at the end of diastole, and therefore at the maximal resting length of the sarcomere (see Fig. 46.18). Measurement of wall stress in vivo is difficult because use of the radius of the left ventricle (see the preceding sections) neglects the confounding influence of the complex LV anatomy. Surrogate preload indices include LVEDP or dimensions (the latter being the major and minor axes of the heart in a two-dimensional echocardiographic view). Afterload, being the load on the contracting myocardium, is also the wall stress during LV ejection. Increased afterload means that increased intraventricular pressure has to be generated first to open the aortic

valve and then during the ejection phase. These increases will translate into increased myocardial wall stress, which can be measured either as an average value or at end-systole.

Peak systolic wall stress reflects the three major components of afterload: peripheral resistance, arterial compliance, and peak intraventricular pressure.[4] Decreased arterial compliance and increased afterload can be anticipated with aortic remodeling and dilation, as in severe systemic hypertension or in older adult patients. The systolic timing of the afterload can also influence LV relaxation. In experimental and human studies, a late systolic load, as when the aorta has stiffened, is associated with impaired LV systolic shortening and diastolic relaxation.[67,68] This is why it is crucial to consider both afterload and preload when evaluating indices of LV function based on the velocity or extent of tissue motion using echocardiography.[68]

Aortic impedance or *elastance* gives another accurate measure of LV afterload (see Fig. 46.18). The advantage of impedance/elastance compared to wall stress is that this measure is totally independent of heart size or wall thickness. The aortic impedance reflects the ratio of aortic pressure to flow across different frequency harmonics. During systole, when the aortic valve is open, an increased afterload will communicate itself to the ventricles by increasing wall stress. In LV failure, aortic impedance is augmented not only by peripheral vasoconstriction (high systemic vascular resistance), but also by decreases in aortic compliance (ability of aorta to "yield" during systole), especially with aging. The problem with the clinical measurement of aortic impedance is that it is expressed in the frequency domain, which is cumbersome to relate to time-domain measures of LV function. An alternative index of LV afterload is the *arterial elastance* (Ea), estimated by the relationship between end-systolic LV pressure and stroke volume (see Fig. 46.18). Ea is derived from the Windkessel model of the arterial system, which includes upstream characteristic impedance (Zc) and a downstream resistance and capacitor that are situated in parallel. Thus, Ea incorporates both mean resistive components of load along with HR and aortic compliance.

Heart Rate and Force-Frequency Relationship
Treppe or Bowditch Effect

An increased HR progressively enhances the force of ventricular muscle contraction, even in isolated papillary muscle preparations and isolated myocytes, the *Bowditch staircase phenomenon.*[4] Alternative names are the *treppe* (German, "steps") phenomenon, positive inotropic effect of activation, or force-frequency relationship (Fig. 46.19A). Conversely, a decreased HR has a negative staircase effect. However, at a very high HR, force progressively decreases. These effects at the myocyte level

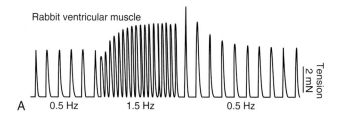

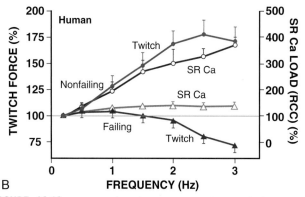

FIGURE 46.19 Heart rate dependence on contraction: Bowditch staircase or *treppe* phenomenon. **A,** An increased stimulation rate increases the force of contraction. The tension developed by rabbit ventricular muscle is shown in mN. During the first shortened diastolic interval the first beat is smaller, an effect caused mainly by refractoriness of the SR Ca^{2+} release channel. As the 1.5-Hz stimulation approaches a steady state, the contraction is progressively increased, an effect attributable to the gain in myocyte Na^+ and Ca^{2+} and enhanced SR Ca^{2+} content. When the diastolic interval is prolonged (first beat at 0.5 Hz), the first beat is especially large because the SR Ca^{2+} load is still elevated and there is more time for the RyR to recover from refractoriness. The larger Ca^{2+} transient then drives higher extrusion of Ca^{2+} from the cell as the initial 0.5-Hz steady state is eventually achieved. **B,** With an increasing heart rate, normal nonfailing ventricular muscle exhibits a progressive increase in SR Ca^{2+} content (*SR Ca*) and a positive force-frequency relationship that peaks at approximately 2.5 Hz. The decline at 3 Hz is caused by reduced fractional SR Ca^{2+} release. In failing human ventricular muscle, the SR fails to increase its Ca^{2+} content appreciably at higher heart rates; this results in a negative force-frequency relationship (which is dominated by the refractoriness, but here is not compensated by increased SR Ca^{2+}). SR Ca^{2+} in these experiments was assessed by rapid-cooling contractures (*RCC*). (From Bers DM. *Excitation-Contraction Coupling and Cardiac Contractile Force.* Dordrecht, Netherlands: Kluwer Academic; 2001.)

are largely attributable to changes in Na^+ and Ca^{2+} in the myocyte. At a higher HR, there is more Na^+ and Ca^{2+} entry per unit time and less time for the cell to extrude these ions, which results in higher $[Na^+]_i$ and cellular and SR Ca^{2+} content.[1] The increase in SR Ca^{2+} content increases the amount of Ca^{2+} released during the AP, the primary cause of the increase in contractility at higher HRs. The elevation in $[Na^+]_i$ also further reduces the efficacy of NCX in extruding Ca^{2+} during the cardiac cycle, thereby leading to further gains in cellular (and SR) Ca^{2+}. A new steady-state Ca^{2+} load will be achieved when the increased Ca^{2+} transients cause Ca^{2+} extrusion by NCX to match the amount of Ca^{2+} influx at each beat (and similarly when Na^+,K^+-ATPase extrudes the amount of Na^+ that enters per beat). This is the definition of steady state, with no net gain or loss of cellular Ca^{2+} (or Na^+) from beat to beat.

To the extent that the SR can take up this extra Ca^{2+} load at a higher HR, diastolic $[Ca^{2+}]_i$ and stiffness remain low. This is helped by an increase in the rate of SR Ca^{2+} uptake at a higher HR (known as "frequency-dependent acceleration of relaxation") mediated by faster SR Ca^{2+} uptake function (although the mechanism is not fully resolved).[1] However, if SR Ca^{2+}-ATPase and NCX are unable to remove Ca^{2+} sufficiently from the cytoplasm during the time between beats, an increase in diastolic $[Ca^{2+}]_i$ and force/stiffness will occur. This is an important contributor to prolongation of relaxation and elevation in cardiac filling pressures as occurs in patients with ventricular hypertrophy or heart failure.[69]

Systolic function is also limited at increasing HRs. The primary reason for this at physiologic HRs is that the SR Ca^{2+} release process has refractoriness that is reminiscent of that seen with voltage-gated Na^+ and Ca^{2+} channels. Thus, at higher HRs, even when a normal AP and Ca^{2+} current signal occurs, the fraction of SR Ca^{2+} released can be reduced (see Fig. 46.19B).[1] In a sense, the resulting Ca^{2+} transient and contraction at increasing HRs can be seen as the product of the increasing SR Ca^{2+} content times the declining fractional SR Ca^{2+} release, with the former factor being dominant (especially at more moderate HR) but the latter being progressively limiting.

In the intact heart this scenario is complicated by alterations in filling time and consequent changes in preload. That is, at higher HRs there will also be a reduced filling time that will limit preload (EDV), and thus a negative Frank-Starling effect will modulate the positive and negative inotropic effects to limit the overall strength of LV contraction. In addition, higher aortic elastance (Ea) at increased HRs will also increase cardiac afterload and limit the ability of the left ventricle to eject blood. Thus, both fundamental myocyte and hemodynamic properties combine to influence net cardiac function at increased HRs.

Premature ventricular complexes (PVCs) or *extrasystoles* can also modulate contraction in understandable ways. When a PVC occurs during the time when SR Ca^{2+} release is partially refractory and the left ventricle has not been refilled, the strength of that PVC will be very weak and may even fail to open the aortic valve. However, because the PVC had low SR Ca^{2+} release, less Ca^{2+} current inactivation and less Ca^{2+} extrusion from the cell occur and result in much higher SR Ca^{2+} release at the next (postextrasystolic) beat following the usual compensatory pause (because of AV node refractoriness during the next sinus node beat). Similarly, by the time the postextrasystolic beat occurs, the much smaller LV ejection and continued LV filling result in greater preload, reduced afterload, and a larger Ca^{2+} transient. These cellular and hemodynamic effects combine to cause an extremely strong, postextrasystolic potentiation beat that a person can often sense as the heart "skipping a beat." Patients with greater postextrasystolic potentiation have increased risk for adverse outcomes, probably because the greater potentiation reflects more severe abnormalities in Ca^{2+} handling within cardiac myocytes in the diseased heart.[70]

Physiologic Force-Frequency Relationship and Optimal Heart Rate

When the HR increases under physiologic conditions, it is usually accompanied and partially mediated by sympathetic beta-adrenergic activation at myocytes throughout the heart. As discussed earlier, this will increase Ca^{2+} current influx, the rate of SR Ca^{2+} uptake, and the amount of SR Ca^{2+} released during the beat, which greatly amplifies the inotropic and lusitropic effects associated with alteration of the HR without sympathetic activation. However, the beta-adrenergic system also enhances Na⁺,K⁺-ATPase activity to limit the rise in $[Na^+]_i$ that occurs at the higher HR, and this would temper the overall inotropic effect. Normally, peak contractile force at a fixed muscle length (isometric contraction) increases, and a peak is reached at about 150 to 180 beats/min (see Fig. 46.19B).[1,4] In situ, the optimal HR is also dependent on the previous hemodynamic factors and a functioning sympathetic system, so the exact value of the HR when cardiac output starts to decrease rather than increase is more difficult to specify and likely varies among people. Pacing rates of up to 150 beats/min can be tolerated, whereas higher rates cannot because of the development of AV block. In contrast, during exercise, indices of LV function still increase up to a maximum HR of about 170 beats/min, presumably because of enhanced contractile function and peripheral vasodilation.[4] The critical HR associated with a fall-off in LV function likely occurs at lower values in diseased hearts, but this is not well understood and likely varies between patients.

Myocardial Oxygen Uptake

Myocardial O_2 demand can be increased by elevations in HR, preload, or afterload (Fig. 46.20), factors that can all precipitate myocardial ischemia in those with coronary artery disease (CAD). Because myocardial O_2 uptake ultimately reflects the rate of mitochondrial metabolism and thus ATP production, any increase in ATP requirement will be reflected in increased O_2 uptake. In general, factors increasing wall stress will increase O_2 uptake. Increased afterload causes increased systolic wall stress, which requires greater O_2 uptake. Increased diastolic wall stress, resulting from increased preload (EDV), will also require more oxygen because the greater stroke volume must be ejected against the afterload. In states of enhanced contractile function, the rate of change in wall stress is increased. Because systolic blood pressure (SBP) is an important correlate of afterload, a practical index of O_2 uptake is SBP × HR, the *double product*. The concept of wall stress in relation to O_2 uptake also explains why heart size is such an important determinant of myocardial O_2 uptake (because a larger radius increases wall stress). In patients with heart failure, the increase in myocardial O_2 demand during exercise outstrips the ability to augment myocardial O_2 supply, contributing to ischemia which is associated with an increase in myocyte injury.[71]

Work of the Heart

External work (pressure × volume) is done by the heart, with stroke volume (or cardiac output) being the volume moved against arterial blood pressure. *Volume work* (associated with increased stroke volume) requires less oxygen than *pressure work* does (increased pressure or HR), and one might suppose that external work is not an important determinant of myocardial O_2 uptake. However, three determinants of myocardial O_2 uptake are involved: preload (because this helps determine stroke volume), afterload (in part determined by blood pressure), and HR. *Minute work* can be defined as the product of SBP, stroke volume, and HR (SBP × SV × HR). Not surprisingly, heart work is related to O_2 uptake. This *pressure-work index* takes into account both the double product (SBP × HR) and HR × SV (i.e., cardiac output). The *pressure-volume area* is another index of cardiac work or O_2 uptake but requires invasive monitoring for accurate measurements (see Fig. 46.18). External cardiac work can account for up to 40% of the total myocardial O_2 uptake.

INTERNAL WORK (POTENTIAL ENERGY)

Total O_2 consumption is related to the total work of the heart (area *abcd* in Fig. 46.21), which means that both external work (area *abce*) and the volume-pressure triangle joining the end-systolic volume-pressure point

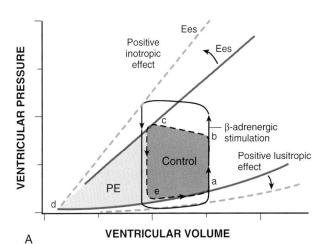

A

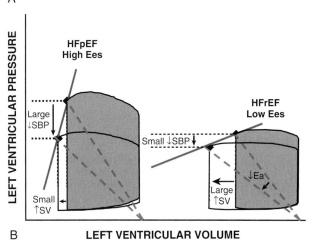

B

FIGURE 46.21 Pressure-volume loop of the left ventricle. **A,** Note the effects of beta-adrenergic catecholamines with both positive inotropic (increased slope of line *Ees*) and increased lusitropic (relaxant) effects. *Ees* is slope of the pressure-volume relationship. The total pressure-volume area (for the control area, see *abcd*) is closely related to myocardial O_2 uptake. The area *cde* is the component of work spent in generating potential energy (*PE*). **B,** Representative left ventricular (LV) pressure-volume loops in a patient with heart failure and preserved ejection fraction (HFpEF, *left*) and heart failure with reduced ejection fraction (HFrEF, *right*) demonstrating the differential effects of vasodilator therapy. In HFpEF, the end-systolic pressure volume relationship is steep, Ees is high, and reductions in arterial afterload or elastance (*Ea*) from acute vasodilator therapy (in this case, nitroprusside infusion) lead to dramatic reductions in systolic blood pressure (*SBP*) and modest increases in stroke volume (*SV*, defined by the width of the pressure-volume loop). In the patient with HFrEF, contractility is depressed, Ees is low, and the end-systolic pressure volume relationship is accordingly shallow. Thus the same degree of vasodilation (reduction in Ea) causes much less reduction in SBP and much more increase in forward SV. (**A** modified from Opie LH. *Heart Physiology, from Cell to Circulation.* Philadelphia: Lippincott, Williams & Wilkins; 2004. Figure copyright L.H. Opie, 2004; **B** modified from Schwartzenberg S, Redfield MM, From AM, Sorajja P, Nishimura RA, Borlaug BA. Effects of vasodilation in heart failure with preserved or reduced ejection fraction implications of distinct pathophysiologies on response to therapy. J Am Coll Cardiol 2012; 59:442-51.)

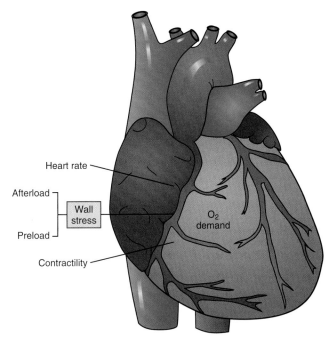

FIGURE 46.20 Major determinants of the O_2 demand of the normal heart: heart rate, wall stress, and contractile function. (Modified with permission from Opie LH. *Heart Physiology, from Cell to Circulation.* Philadelphia: Lippincott Williams & Wilkins; 2004. Figure copyright L.H. Opie, 2004.)

to the origin (area *cde*; marked PE).[72] Although this area has been called internal work, more strictly it should be called the "potential energy" that is generated within each contraction cycle but not converted to external work. Such potential energy at the end of systole (point c) may be likened to the potential energy of a compressed spring.

Efficiency of work is the relationship between the work performed and myocardial O_2 uptake.[4] Metabolically, efficiency is increased by promotion of glucose rather than fatty acids as the major myocardial fuel, as oxidation of glucose produces more ATP relative to O_2 consumed (higher P/O ratio). Conversely, heart failure decreases the efficiency of work, although the basis is not fully understood. Because as little as 12% to 14% of O_2 uptake may be converted to external work,[4] it is probably the "internal work" that becomes less demanding. Ion fluxes ($Na^+/K^+/Ca^{2+}$) account for approximately 20% to 30% of the ATP requirement of the heart, so most ATP is spent on actin-myosin interaction and much of that on the generation of heat rather than on external work. An increased initial muscle length sensitizes the contractile apparatus to Ca^{2+}, thereby theoretically increasing the efficiency of contraction by diminishing the amount of Ca^{2+} flux required.

Measurements of Contractile Function
Force-Velocity Relationship and Maximum Contractile Function in Muscle Models
If contractility is truly independent of load and the HR, unloaded heart muscle stimulated at a fixed rate should have a maximum value of contractile function for any given magnitude of the cytosolic Ca^{2+} transient. This value, the V_{max} of muscle contraction, is defined as the *maximal velocity of contraction* when there is no afterload to prevent maximal rates of cardiac ejection.[4] Beta-adrenergic stimulation increases V_{max}, and converse changes are found in failing myocardium. V_{max} is also termed V_0 (maximum velocity at zero load). As the load increases, the velocity of shortening decreases. A limitation of this relatively simple concept is that V_{max} cannot be measured directly but must be extrapolated from the *force-velocity relationship* to the velocity axis intercept. The other extreme condition is zero muscle shortening, with all the energy going into the development of pressure (P_0) or force (F_0). This situation is an example of *isometric contraction* (with internal cross-bridge stretching).

Isometric Versus Isotonic Contraction
Data for P_0 are obtained under isometric conditions (length unchanged). When muscle is allowed to shorten against a steady load, the conditions are *isotonic* (*tonic*, "contractile force").[4] Thus the force-velocity curve may be a combination of initial isometric conditions followed by isotonic contraction and then abrupt and total unloading to measure V_{max}. Although isometric conditions can be found in the whole heart (e.g., during isovolumic contraction), isotonic conditions are rare because afterload is constantly changing during the ejection period, and complete unloading is impossible. However, as shortening progresses during ejection, the maximal P_0 declines and velocity is lower for any given nonzero load. Therefore the force-velocity relationship is heuristically useful, but measurements in vivo are limited.

Pressure-Volume Loops
Accordingly, measurements of pressure-volume loops are among the best of the current approaches for assessment of the contractile behavior of the intact heart (see Figs. 46.18 and 46.21). A crucial measurement is the *end-systolic elastance* (Ees) from the pressure-volume relationship.[4] When the loading conditions are changed, alterations in the slope of this line joining the different E_s points (the end-systolic pressure-volume relationship [ESPVR]) are generally a good load-independent index of the contractile performance of the heart. In clinical practice, the need to change the loading conditions and the requirement for invasive monitoring for the full pressure-volume loop lessen the usefulness of this index. Measurement of LV volume adequately and continuously throughout the cardiac cycle is not easy. During a positive inotropic intervention, the pressure-volume loop changes in characteristic ways, resulting in a smaller end-systolic volume and a higher end-systolic pressure, so the slope of the pressure-volume relationship (E_s) has moved upward and to the left (see Fig. 46.21A). When the positive inotropic

intervention consists of beta-adrenergic stimulation, the enhanced relaxation (lusitropic effect) may result in a lower pressure-volume curve during ventricular filling.

VENTRICULAR FUNCTION IN HEART FAILURE (SEE ALSO CHAPTER 47)
In patients with heart failure and reduced ejection fraction (HFrEF), the ventricle is dilated, EF is low, and contractility is severely depressed.[73] As such, the pressure-volume loop is shifted to the far right on the volume axis, and the (ESPVR, contractility) is very shallow (see Fig. 46.21B). In this setting, a reduction in arterial afterload (Ea) produces modest reductions in blood pressure despite often dramatic increases in stroke volume. This heightened "afterload dependence" of the LV in HFrEF serves as the hemodynamic basis for aggressive use of vasodilators in this disease. In contrast, patients with heart failure and preserved ejection fraction (HFpEF) display an increased Ees (steep ESPVR). In this patient, the same degree of afterload reduction (decrease in Ea) using a vasodilator causes a much more dramatic drop in blood pressure, with little improvement in forward stroke volume.

Limitations of the Concept of Contractility
Despite all the previous procedures that can be adopted in an attempt to measure true contractility (or the inotropic state), the concept has at least two serious defects: (1) the absence of any noninvasive index that can be measured unequivocally and (2) the impossibility of separating the cellular and chamber-level mechanisms of changes in contractile function from those of load or the HR. Thus an increased HR, by the changes in Na^+ and Ca^{2+} handling noted earlier, gives rise to increased cytosolic Ca^{2+} transients and contraction, which is clearly an inotropic effect. However, the simultaneous changes in preload and afterload also involve Frank-Starling effects, which complicates this picture in the clinical setting. Similarly, increased preload involves increased fiber stretch, which in turn causes enhanced myofilament Ca^{2+} sensitivity, a factor that in a sense is built into the Frank-Starling effect. However, additional changes in myofilament Ca^{2+} sensitivity (e.g., during acidosis or alpha-adrenergic activation) would be attributed to inotropic changes. *So there is a clear overlap between contractility, which should be independent of load or HR, and the effects of load and HR on the cellular mechanisms.*[3,4] Even though this does not undermine the importance of the intrinsic mechanistic distinctions between contractility/inotropy and Frank-Starling mechanisms, the distinction can be blurred by the clinical context and available measurements. For example, in humans with atrial fibrillation and constantly varying ventricular frequency, contractility inferred from pressure-volume loops constantly changes from beat to beat. It is then more difficult to infer a "true" change in LV contractility versus operation of the Frank-Starling mechanism because of varying diastolic filling times.[4]

Left Ventricular Relaxation and Diastolic Dysfunction
Normal diastolic function allows the ventricle to fill adequately during rest and exercise, without an abnormal increase in LA pressure.[63] The phases of diastole are isovolumic pressure decline and filling. The filling phase is divided into early rapid filling, diastasis, and atrial systole. Early rapid filling contributes 70% to 80% of LV filling in normal individuals. Early diastolic filling is driven by the LA-to-LV pressure gradient, which is dependent on a complex interplay of factors, including myocardial relaxation, LV elastic recoil, LV diastolic stiffness, LA pressure, ventricular interaction, pericardial constraint, pulmonary vein properties, and mitral orifice area. Diastasis occurs in mid-diastole when LA and LV pressures equalize and transmitral flow becomes nil. In normal persons, atrial systole contributes 15% to 25% of LV diastolic filling. This contribution depends on the PR interval, atrial inotropic state, atrial preload, atrial afterload, autonomic tone, and HR. In patients with atrial fibrillation this component is lost. Chapter 51 further details the basic mechanisms of LV relaxation, as well as measurements of LV relaxation. In addition to being important in heart failure, abnormalities in diastolic relaxation and stiffness develop as part of normal aging, and this cardiac aging process seems to be accelerated in the presence of obesity.[74]

Right Ventricular Function

Most of the foregoing principles and discussions also apply to the right ventricle, and the differences are not discussed in any detail here. RV myocytes are fundamentally the same as those in the left ventricle, with some minor, mainly quantitative differences in their ion channel, electrophysiology, Ca^{2+} handling, and myofilament properties. The most important functional differences are in the chamber geometry related to Laplace's law and the normal levels of pressure developed (lower pressure in the right ventricle and pulmonary circulation).[75] The right ventricle has a larger radius of curvature, which would tend to increase wall tension, but it normally develops much lower pressure, which greatly reduces wall tension (wall tension = [radius × pressure]/ [2 × thickness]). RV wall thickness is also lower such that the normal characteristics of RV shape and size are functionally matched to the different prevailing conditions on the right ventricle. The right ventricle is poorly suited to eject against high pressures, as in pulmonary hypertension, and this heightened afterload-dependence is further accentuated in patients with heart failure.[76]

Atrial Function

The left atrium has five main functions.[4,77] First and best known, the left atrium functions as a blood-receiving reservoir chamber. Second, it also is a contractile chamber that by presystolic contraction helps complete LV filling with an atrial kick. Third, the left atrium functions as a conduit that empties its contents into the left ventricle down a pressure gradient after the mitral valve opens. Fourth, it is a *blood volume sensor* in the heart and releases atrial natriuretic peptide (ANP) in response to stretch so that ANP-induced diuresis can help restore blood volume to normal. Notably, in congestive heart failure, when the renin-angiotensin system causes fluid retention and exacerbates the elevation in LA pressure and volume, ANP secretion is elevated. Fifth, the left atrium contains receptors for the afferent arms of various reflexes, including mechanoreceptors that increase the sinus discharge rate, thereby contributing to the tachycardia of exercise as venous return increases (Bainbridge reflex).[3,4]

The atrial pressure-volume loop is very different in shape from that of the ventricles in that it resembles a figure 8. The atria have a number of differences in structure and function from the ventricles, including smaller myocytes with fewer T tubules, a shorter AP duration, and more fetal myosin isoforms (both heavy and light chains).[78] The more rapid atrial repolarization is caused by increased outward potassium currents, such as I_{to}, and also has faster Ca^{2+} transient kinetics. In general, these histologic and physiologic changes might be related to the decreased need for the atria to generate high intrachamber pressures, rather than being sensitive to changes in volume while retaining enough contractile action to help with LV filling and to respond to inotropic stimuli. *Atrial remodeling* refers to a variety of ionic, structural, contractile, and metabolic changes that are induced by insults such as chronic atrial tachyarrhythmias, including atrial fibrillation,[78] or by LA stretch and enlargement. Cellular mechanisms include decreased L-type Ca^{2+} channel activity,[78] increased abnormal collagen,[79] and probably adverse stretch-induced signaling. The results include poor contractile performance and increased initiation and perpetuation of atrial fibrillation. Atrial remodeling and deterioration in LA function lead to worsening pulmonary hypertension and secondary RV dysfunction in patients with heart failure.[77,80]

FUTURE PERSPECTIVES

During the last 20 years we have gained tremendous molecular and cellular insight into a much richer, quantitatively detailed understanding of the individual steps in the overall excitation-contraction-relaxation process. In addition, there is a greatly enhanced understanding about how all these processes interact at the cellular and tissue level, how they are regulated by numerous interacting signaling pathways, and what goes wrong during certain cardiac pathologies. This is a very complex system, and diseases such as heart failure are also extremely complex. In the coming 5 years we can expect further clarification of all these systems, likely with a better understanding of signaling in local microdomains and protein complexes. At present, however, we must use this rich mechanistic knowledge to test novel therapeutic strategies for heart failure (e.g., SERCA2 overexpression, RyR inhibitors, GRK2 inhibitors, myofilament enhancers). This work may provide novel effective therapies but will also help us better understand how the fundamental systems impacted by these approaches integrate into the behavior of the whole system. This emphasizes how critical it is to integrate our knowledge of these many systems that dynamically regulate contraction and relaxation over multiple physical scales (molecules to cell to heart to animal) and time scales (milliseconds to seconds, minutes, hours, days, and years), as well as in multiple disciplinary and methodologic perspectives, to help bring the entire system to a higher level of understanding. In this way the therapeutic strategies that we must also continue to test are likely to improve.

ACKNOWLEDGMENT

We honor the memory of Dr. Lionel H. Opie who contributed to previous versions of this chapter over the years.

REFERENCES
Microanatomy of Contractile Cells and Proteins
1. Bers DM. *Excitation-Contraction Coupling and Cardiac Contractile Force.* Dordrecht, Netherlands: Kluwer Academic Press; 2001.
2. Bers DM. Calcium cycling and signaling in cardiac myocytes. *Annu Rev Physiol.* 2008;70:23–49.
3. Opie LH. *Heart Physiology, from Cell to Circulation.* 4th ed. Philadelphia: Lippincott Williams & Wilkins; 2004.
4. Opie LH, Bers DM. Mechanisms of cardiac contraction and relaxation. In: Mann DL, Zipes DP, Libby P, Bonow RO, eds. *Braunwald's Heart Disease: a Textbook of Cardiovascular Medicine.* 10th ed. Philadelphia: Elsevier Saunders; 2015:429–453.
5. Covian R, Balaban RS. Cardiac mitochondrial matrix and respiratory complex protein phosphorylation. *Am J Physiol Heart Circ Physiol.* 2012;303:H940–H966.
6. Dorn GW Jr, Kitsis RN. The mitochondrial dynamism-mitophagy-cell death interactome: multiple roles performed by members of a mitochondrial molecular ensemble. *Circ Res.* 2015;116:167–182.
7. Kubli DA, Gustafsson AB. Mitochondria and mitophagy: the yin and yang of cell death control. *Circ Res.* 2012;111:1208–1221.
8. Rayment I, Holden HM, Whittaker M. Structure of the actin-myosin complex and its implications for muscle contraction. *Science.* 1993;261:58–65.
9. Gigli M, Begay RL, Morea G, et al. A review of the giant protein titin in clinical molecular diagnostics of cardiomyopathies. *Front Cardiovasc Med.* 2016;3:21.
10. Hooijman P, Stewart MA, Cooke R. A new state of cardiac myosin with very slow ATP turnover: a potential cardioprotective mechanism in the heart. *Biophys J.* 2011;100:1969–1976.
11. Knoll R, Hoshijima M, Hoffman HM, et al. The cardiac mechanical stretch sensor machinery involves a Z disc complex that is defective in a subset of human dilated cardiomyopathy. *Cell.* 2002;111:943–955.
12. Beausang JF, Shroder DY, Nelson PC, Goldman YE. Tilting and wobble of myosin V by high-speed single-molecule polarized fluorescence microscopy. *Biophys J.* 2013;104:1263–1273.
12a. Teerlink JR, Diaz R, Felker GM, et al; GALACTIC-HF Investigators. Cardiac myosin activation with omecamtiv mecarbil in systolic heart failure. *N Engl J Med.* 2021;384(2):105–116.
13. Warren SA, Briggs LE, Zeng H, et al. Myosin light chain phosphorylation is critical for adaptation to cardiac stress. *Circulation.* 2012;126:2575–2588.
14. McNally EM, Golbus JR, Puckelwartz MJ. Genetic mutations and mechanisms in dilated cardiomyopathy. *J Clin Invest.* 2013;123:19–26.
15. Bers DM, Shannon TR. Calcium movements inside the sarcoplasmic reticulum of cardiac myocytes. *J Mol Cell Cardiol.* 2013;58:59–66.

Calcium Fluxes in Cardiac Contraction-Relaxation Cycle
16. Zima AV, Picht E, Bers DM, Blatter LA. Termination of cardiac Ca^{2+} sparks: role of intra-SR $[Ca^{2+}]$, release flux, and intra-SR Ca^{2+} diffusion. *Circ Res.* 2008;103:e105–e115.
17. Bers DM. Cardiac sarcoplasmic reticulum calcium leak: basis and roles in cardiac dysfunction. *Annu Rev Physiol.* 2014;76:107–127.
18. Bers DM. Macromolecular complexes regulating cardiac ryanodine receptor function. *J Mol Cell Cardiol.* 2004;37:417–429.
19. Saucerman JJ, Bers DM. Calmodulin binding proteins provide domains of local Ca^{2+} signaling in cardiac myocytes. *J Mol Cell Cardiol.* 2012;52:312–316.
20. Radwanski PB, Belevych AE, Brunello L, et al. Store-dependent deactivation: cooling the chain-reaction of myocardial calcium signaling. *J Mol Cell Cardiol.* 2013;58:77–83.
21. Sato D, Bers DM. How does stochastic ryanodine receptor-mediated Ca leak fail to initiate a Ca spark? *Biophys J.* 2011;101:2370–2379.
22. Bers DM, Grandi E. Calcium/calmodulin-dependent kinase II regulation of cardiac ion channels. *J Cardiovasc Pharmacol.* 2009;54:180–187.
23. Anderson ME, Brown JH, Bers DM. Camkii in myocardial hypertrophy and heart failure. *J Mol Cell Cardiol.* 2011;51:468–473.
24. Cheng H, Lederer WJ. Calcium sparks. *Physiol Rev.* 2008;88:1491–1545.
25. Tada M, Katz AM. Phosphorylation of the sarcoplasmic reticulum and sarcolemma. *Annu Rev Physiol.* 1982;44:401–423.
26. Picht E, Zima AV, Shannon TR, et al. Dynamic calcium movement inside cardiac sarcoplasmic reticulum during release. *Circ Res.* 2011;108:847–856.

Sarcolemmal Control of Ca^{2+} and Na^+
27. Morotti S, Grandi E, Summa A, et al. Theoretical study of L-type Ca^{2+} current inactivation kinetics during action potential repolarization and early afterdepolarizations. *J Physiol.* 2012;590:4465–4481.
28. Orchard C, Brette F. T-tubules and sarcoplasmic reticulum function in cardiac ventricular myocytes. *Cardiovasc Res.* 2008;77:237–244.
29. Maltsev VA, Reznikov V, Undrovinas NA, et al. Modulation of late sodium current by Ca^{2+}, calmodulin, and CaMKII in normal and failing dog cardiomyocytes: similarities and differences. *Am J Physiol Heart Circ Physiol.* 2008;294:H1597–H1608.
30. Wimmer NJ, Stone PH. Anti-anginal and anti-ischemic effects of late sodium current inhibition. *Cardiovasc Drugs Ther.* 2013;27:69–77.

31. Ginsburg KS, Weber CR, Bers DM. Cardiac Na⁺-Ca²⁺ exchanger: dynamics of Ca²⁺-dependent activation and deactivation in intact myocytes. *J Physiol*. 2013;591:2067–2086.
32. Despa S, Bers DM. Na⁺ transport in the normal and failing heart—remember the balance. *J Mol Cell Cardiol*. 2013;61:2–10.

Adrenergic Signaling Systems

33. Woodcock EA, Du XJ, Reichelt ME, Graham RM. Cardiac alpha 1-adrenergic drive in pathological remodelling. *Cardiovasc Res*. 2008;77:452–462.
34. Mika D, Leroy J, Fischmeister R, Vandecasteele G. Role of cyclic nucleotide phosphodiesterases type 3 and 4 in cardiac excitation-contraction coupling and arrhythmias. *Med Sci (Paris)*. 2013;29:617–622.
35. Barbagallo F, Xu B, Reddy GR, et al. Genetically encoded biosensors reveal PKA hyperphosphorylation on the myofilaments in rabbit heart failure. *Circ Res*. 2016;119:931–943.
36. Pereira L, Cheng H, Lao DH, et al. Epac2 mediates cardiac beta1-adrenergic-dependent sarcoplasmic reticulum Ca²⁺ leak and arrhythmia. *Circulation*. 2013;127:913–922.
37. Bers DM. Cardiac excitation-contraction coupling. *Nature*. 2002;415:198–205.
38. Kritzer MD, Li J, Dodge-Kafka K, Kapiloff MS. AKAPs: the architectural underpinnings of local cAMP signaling. *J Mol Cell Cardiol*. 2012;52:351–358.
39. Castro LR, Verde I, Cooper DM, Fischmeister R. Cyclic guanosine monophosphate compartmentation in rat cardiac myocytes. *Circulation*. 2006;113:2221–2228.
40. Harvey RD, Hell JW. Cav1.2 signaling complexes in the heart. *J Mol Cell Cardiol*. 2013;58:143–152.
41. Negroni JA, Morotti S, Lascano EC, et al. Beta-adrenergic effects on cardiac myofilaments and contraction in an integrated rabbit ventricular myocyte model. *J Mol Cell Cardiol*. 2015;81:162–175.
42. Bers DM. Ryanodine receptor S2808 phosphorylation in heart failure: smoking gun or red herring? *Circ Res*. 2012;110:796–799.
43. Marks AR. Calcium cycling proteins and heart failure: mechanisms and therapeutics. *J Clin Invest*. 2013;123:46–52.
44. Ginsburg KS, Bers DM. Modulation of excitation-contraction coupling by isoproterenol in cardiomyocytes with controlled SR Ca²⁺ load and Ca²⁺ current trigger. *J Physiol*. 2004;556:463–480.
45. Valdivia HH, Kaplan JH, Ellis-Davies GC, Lederer WJ. Rapid adaptation of cardiac ryanodine receptors: modulation by Mg²⁺ and phosphorylation. *Science*. 1995;267:1997–2000.
46. Eisner DA, Kashimura T, O'Neill SC, et al. What role does modulation of the ryanodine receptor play in cardiac inotropy and arrhythmogenesis? *J Mol Cell Cardiol*. 2009;46:474–481.
47. Engelhardt S. Alternative signaling: cardiomyocyte beta1-adrenergic receptors signal through EGFRs. *J Clin Invest*. 2007;117:2396–2398.
48. Sato PY, Chuprun JK, Schwartz M, Koch WJ. The evolving impact of G protein-coupled receptor kinases in cardiac health and disease. *Physiol Rev*. 2015;95:377–404.
49. Hegyi B, Bers DM, Bossuyt J. CaMKII signaling in heart diseases: emerging role in diabetic cardiomyopathy. *J Mol Cell Cardiol*. 2019;127:246–259.
50. Bardswell SC, Cuello F, Kentish JC, Avkiran M. CMYBP-C as a promiscuous substrate: phosphorylation by non-PKA kinases and its potential significance. *J Muscle Res Cell Motil*. 2012;33:53–60.

Cholinergic and Nitric Oxide Signaling

51. Niu X, Watts VL, Cingolani OH, et al. Cardioprotective effect of beta-3 adrenergic receptor agonism: role of neuronal nitric oxide synthase. *J Am Coll Cardiol*. 2012;59:1979–1987.
52. Okoshi K, Nakayama M, Yan X, et al. Neuregulins regulate cardiac parasympathetic activity: muscarinic modulation of beta-adrenergic activity in myocytes from mice with neuregulin-1 gene deletion. *Circulation*. 2004;110:713–717.
53. Ziolo MT, Bers DM. The real estate of NOS signaling: location, location, location. *Circ Res*. 2003;92:1279–1281.
54. Takimoto E. Cyclic GMP-dependent signaling in cardiac myocytes. *Circ J*. 2012;76:1819–1825.
55. Zhang M, Takimoto E, Lee DI, et al. Pathological cardiac hypertrophy alters intracellular targeting of phosphodiesterase type 5 from nitric oxide synthase-3 to natriuretic peptide signaling. *Circulation*. 2012;126:942–951.

56. Takimoto E, Champion HC, Li M, et al. Chronic inhibition of cyclic GMP phosphodiesterase 5a prevents and reverses cardiac hypertrophy. *Nat Med*. 2005;11:214–222.
57. Dodge-Kafka KL, Langeberg L, Scott JD. Compartmentation of cyclic nucleotide signaling in the heart: the role of A-kinase anchoring proteins. *Circ Res*. 2006;98:993–1001.
58. Zhang YH, Casadei B. Sub-cellular targeting of constitutive NOS in health and disease. *J Mol Cell Cardiol*. 2012;52:341–350.
59. Murphy E, Kohr M, Menazza S, et al. Signaling by S-nitrosylation in the heart. *J Mol Cell Cardiol*. 2014;73:18–25.
60. Erickson JR, Nichols CB, Uchinoumi H, et al. S-nitrosylation induces both autonomous activation and inhibition of calcium/calmodulin-dependent protein kinase II. *J Biol Chem*. 2015;290:25646–25656.

Contractile Performance of Intact Hearts

61. Lewis T. *The Mechanism and Graphic Registration of the Heart Beat*. London: Shaw & Sons; 1920.
62. Wiggers CJ. *Modern Aspects of Circulation in Health and Disease*. Philadelphia: Lea & Febiger; 1915.
63. Borlaug BA. The pathophysiology of heart failure with preserved ejection fraction. *Nat Rev Cardiol*. 2014;11:507–515.
64. Borlaug BA, Reddy YNV. The role of the pericardium in heart failure: implications for pathophysiology and treatment. *JACC Heart Fail*. 2019:574–585.
65. Konstam MA, Kiernan MS, Bernstein D, et al. Evaluation and management of right-sided heart failure: a scientific statement from the American Heart Association. *Circulation*. 2018;137:e578–e622.
66. Jian Z, Han H, Zhang T, et al. Mechanochemotransduction during cardiomyocyte contraction is mediated by localized nitric oxide signaling. *Sci Signal*. 2014;7:ra27.
67. Chirinos JA, Segers P, Rietzschel ER, et al. Early and late systolic wall stress differentially relate to myocardial contraction and relaxation in middle-aged adults: the ASKLEPIOS study. *Hypertension*. 2013;61:296–303.
68. Borlaug BA, Melenovsky V, Redfield MM, et al. Impact of arterial load and loading sequence on left ventricular tissue velocities in humans. *J Am Coll Cardiol*. 2007;50:1570–1577.
69. Runte KE, Bell SP, Selby DE, et al. Relaxation and the role of calcium in isolated contracting myocardium from patients with hypertensive heart disease and heart failure with preserved ejection fraction. *Circ Heart Fail*. 2017;8:e004311.
70. Sinnecker D, Dirschinger RJ, Barthel P, et al. Postextrasystolic blood pressure potentiation predicts poor outcome of cardiac patients. *J Am Heart Assoc*. 2014;3:e000857.
71. Obokata M, Reddy YNV, Melenovsky V, et al. Myocardial injury and cardiac reserve in patients with heart failure and preserved ejection fraction. *J Am Coll Cardiol*. 2018;72:29–40.
72. Suga H, Hisano R, Hirata S, et al. Mechanism of higher oxygen consumption rate: pressure-loaded vs volume-loaded heart. *Am J Physiol*. 1982;242:H942–H948.
73. Schwartzenberg S, Redfield MM, From AM, et al. Effects of vasodilation in heart failure with preserved or reduced ejection fraction implications of distinct pathophysiologies on response to therapy. *J Am Coll Cardiol*. 2012;59:442–451.
74. Wohlfahrt P, Redfield MM, Lopez-Jimenez F, et al. Impact of general and central adiposity on ventricular-arterial aging in women and men. *JACC Heart Fail*. 2014;2:489–499.
75. Konstam MA, Kiernan MS, Bernstein D, et al. Evaluation and management of right-sided heart failure: a scientific statement from the American Heart Association. *Circulation*. 2018;137:e578–e622.
76. Melenovsky V, Hwang SJ, Lin G, et al. Right heart dysfunction in heart failure with preserved ejection fraction. *Eur Heart J*. 2014;35:3452–3462.
77. Reddy YNV, Obokata M, Verbrugge FH, et al. Atrial dysfunction in patients with heart failure with preserved ejection fraction and atrial fibrillation. *J Am Coll Cardiol*. 2020;76(9):1051–1064.
78. Grandi E, Pandit SV, Voigt N, et al. Human atrial action potential and Ca²⁺ model: sinus rhythm and chronic atrial fibrillation. *Circ Res*. 2011;109:1055–1066.
79. Maillet M, van Berlo JH, Molkentin JD. Molecular basis of physiological heart growth: fundamental concepts and new players. *Nat Rev Mol Cell Biol*. 2013;14:38–48.
80. Melenovsky V, Hwang SJ, Redfield MM, et al. Left atrial remodeling and function in advanced heart failure with preserved or reduced ejection fraction. *Circ Heart Fail*. 2015;8:295–303.

 # 47 Pathophysiology of Heart Failure

GERD HASENFUSS AND DOUGLAS L. MANN

This chapter focuses on the molecular and cellular changes that underlie heart failure with a reduced ejection fraction (HFrEF), with an emphasis on the role of neurohormonal activation and left ventricular (LV) remodeling as the primary determinants for disease progression in HF. The hemodynamic, contractile, and wall motion disorders in HF are discussed in the chapters on cardiac contraction and relaxation (Chapter 46), echocardiography (Chapter 16), cardiac catheterization (Chapter 22), and radionuclide imaging (Chapter 18). The clinical assessment of patients with HF is discussed in Chapter 48, and Chapter 51 discusses the pathogenesis of HF with preserved ejection fraction.

PATHOGENESIS

As shown in Figure 47.1A, HFrEF is initiated after an index event either damages the heart muscle, with a resultant loss of functioning cardiac myocytes or, alternatively, disrupts the ability of the myocardium to generate force, thereby preventing the heart from contracting normally. This index event may have an abrupt onset, as in the case of a myocardial infarction (MI); it may have a gradual or insidious onset, as in the case of hemodynamic pressure or volume overloading; or it may be hereditary, as in the case of many of the genetic cardiomyopathies. Regardless of the nature of the inciting event, the feature that is common to each of these index events is that they all, in some manner, produce a decline in pumping capacity of the heart. The circulatory changes that arise from impaired myocardial pump function are sensed by peripheral arterial baroreceptors as "underfilling" of the circulation. These sensory and other peripheral receptors (e.g., metaboreceptors and ergoreceptors) activate a series of compensatory mechanisms discussed below that lead to changes in heart rate and cardiac contractility, salt and water retention, and constriction of the peripheral blood vessels.[1]

In some patients LV function will recover spontaneously after resolution or removal of the inciting stress that compromised myocardial function; however, in a significant proportion of patients LV function will remain depressed. Some patients with LV dysfunction will remain asymptomatic or minimally symptomatic after the initial decline in pumping capacity of the heart, or symptoms develop only after the dysfunction has been present for some time. The precise reasons why patients with LV dysfunction remain asymptomatic are not known. One potential explanation is that a number of compensatory mechanisms that become activated in the setting of cardiac injury or depressed cardiac output are sufficient to modulate LV function within a physiologic/homeostatic range, such that the patient's functional capacity is preserved or is depressed only minimally. However, sustained activation of neurohormonal systems leads to peripheral vasoconstriction, salt and water retention by the kidney, as well as a series of end-organ changes within the myocardium that contribute to worsening LV dilation (referred to as LV remodeling) and LV dysfunction (Fig. 47.1B). As HF progresses patients undergo the transition from asymptomatic to symptomatic HF.

Neurohormonal Mechanisms

A growing body of experimental and clinical evidence suggests that HF progresses as a result of the overexpression of biologically active molecules that are capable of exerting deleterious effects on the heart and circulation (see Fig. 47.1B).[1] The portfolio of compensatory mechanisms that have been described thus far includes activation of the sympathetic nervous system (SNS) and the renin-angiotensin aldosterone system (RAAS), which are responsible for maintaining cardiac output through increased retention of salt and water; peripheral arterial vasoconstriction and increased contractility; and inflammatory mediators that are responsible for mediating cardiac repair and remodeling. It bears emphasis that *neurohormone* is largely a historical term, reflecting the original observation that many of the molecules that were elaborated in HF were produced by the neuroendocrine system and thus acted on the heart in an endocrine manner. It has since become apparent, however, that a great many of the so-called classic neurohormones such as norepinephrine (NE) and angiotensin II are synthesized directly within the myocardium by myocytes and thus act in an autocrine and paracrine manner. Nonetheless, the important unifying concept that arises from the neurohormonal model is that the overexpression of portfolios of biologically active molecules contributes to disease progression by virtue of the deleterious effects these molecules exert on the heart and circulation.

Activation of Sympathetic Nervous System

The decrease in cardiac output in HF activates a series of compensatory adaptations that are intended to maintain cardiovascular homeostasis. One of the most important adaptations is activation of the sympathetic (adrenergic) nervous system, which occurs early in the course of HF. Activation of the SNS in HF is accompanied by a concomitant withdrawal of parasympathetic tone (**eFig. 47.1**). Although these disturbances in autonomic control initially were attributed to loss of the inhibitory input from arterial or cardiopulmonary baroreceptor reflexes, increasing evidence indicates that excitatory reflexes also may participate in the autonomic imbalance that occurs in HF.[2] In healthy persons, "high-pressure" carotid sinus and aortic arch baroreceptors and "low-pressure" cardiopulmonary mechanoreceptors provide inhibitory signals to the central nervous system (CNS) that repress the sympathetic outflow to the heart and peripheral circulation. Under normal conditions, inhibitory inputs from high-pressure carotid sinus and aortic arch baroreceptors and the low-pressure cardiopulmonary mechanoreceptors are the principal inhibitors of sympathetic outflow, whereas discharge from the nonbaroreflex peripheral chemoreceptors and from muscle *metaboreceptors* are the major excitatory inputs to sympathetic outflow. The vagal limb of the baroreceptor heart rate reflex also is responsive to arterial baroreceptor afferent inhibitory input. Healthy persons display low sympathetic discharge at rest and have a high heart rate variability. In patients with HF, however, inhibitory input from baroreceptors and mechanoreceptors decreases and excitatory input increases, with the net result that there is a generalized increase in sympathetic nerve traffic and blunted parasympathetic nerve traffic, leading to loss of heart rate variability and increased peripheral vascular resistance.[3]

As a result of the increase in sympathetic tone, there is an increase in circulating levels of NE, a potent adrenergic neurotransmitter. The elevated levels of circulating NE result from a combination of increased release of NE from adrenergic nerve endings and its

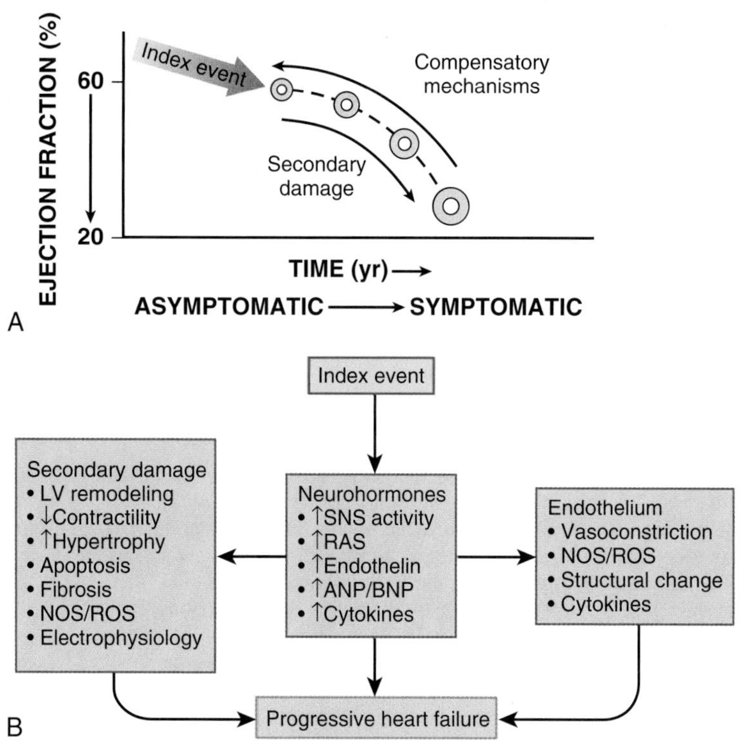

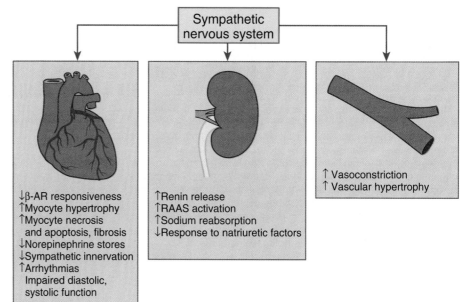

FIGURE 47.1 Pathogenesis of heart failure (HF). **A,** HF begins after a so-called index event produces an initial decline in pumping capacity of the heart. **B,** After this initial decline in pumping capacity, a variety of compensatory mechanisms are activated, including the adrenergic nervous system, the renin-angiotensin system (RAS), and the cytokine systems. In the short term, these systems are able to restore cardiovascular function to a normal homeostatic range, with the result that the patient remains asymptomatic. With time, however, the sustained activation of these systems can lead to secondary end-organ damage within the ventricle, with worsening LV remodeling and subsequent cardiac decompensation. As a result of these changes, patients undergo the transition from asymptomatic to symptomatic HF. *ANP/BNP,* Atrial/brain-type natriuretic peptide; *NOS,* nitric oxide synthase; *ROS,* reactive oxygen species; *SNS,* sympathetic nervous system. (From Mann DL. Mechanisms and models in HF: a combinatorial approach. *Circulation.* 199;100:99; and Kaye DM, Krum H. Drug discovery for heart failure: a new era or the end of the pipeline? *Nat Rev Drug Discov.* 2007;6:127.)

FIGURE 47.2 Activation of the sympathetic nervous system. Increased sympathetic nervous system (SNS) activity may contribute to the pathophysiology of congestive heart failure (HF) by multiple mechanisms involving cardiac, renal, and vascular function. In the heart, increased SNS outflow may lead to desensitization of beta-adrenergic receptors (β-ARs), myocyte hypertrophy, necrosis, apoptosis, and fibrosis. In the kidneys, increased SNS activation induces arterial and venous vasoconstriction, activation of the renin-angiotensin-aldosterone system (RAAS), increase in salt and water retention, and an attenuated response to natriuretic factors. In the peripheral vessels, neurogenic vasoconstriction and vascular hypertrophy are induced by increased SNS activity. (From Nohria A, et al. Neurohormonal, renal and vascular adjustments in heart failure. In Colucci WS, editor. *Atlas of Heart Failure.* 4th ed. Philadelphia: Current Medicine; 2008:106.)

consequent "spillover" into the plasma, as well as reduced uptake of NE by adrenergic nerve endings. In patients with advanced HF, the circulating levels of NE in resting patients are two to three times those found in normal persons. Indeed, plasma levels of NE predict mortality in patients with HF. Whereas the normal heart usually extracts NE from the arterial blood, in patients with moderate HF the coronary sinus NE concentration exceeds the arterial concentration, indicating increased adrenergic stimulation of the heart. However, as HF progresses there is a significant decrease in the myocardial concentration of NE. The mechanism responsible for cardiac NE depletion in severe HF is not clear and may relate to an "exhaustion" phenomenon resulting from the prolonged adrenergic activation of the cardiac adrenergic nerves in HF. In addition, there is decreased activity of myocardial tyrosine hydroxylase, which is the rate-limiting enzyme in the synthesis of NE. In patients with cardiomyopathy, iodine 131 (^{131}I)–labeled metaiodobenzylguanidine (MIBG), a radiopharmaceutical that is taken up by

adrenergic nerve endings, is not taken up normally, suggesting that NE reuptake is also depressed.

Increased sympathetic activation of the beta$_1$-adrenergic receptor results in increased heart rate and force of myocardial contraction, with a resultant increase in cardiac output (see Chapter 46). In addition, the heightened activity of the adrenergic nervous system leads to stimulation of myocardial alpha$_1$-adrenergic receptors, which elicits a modest positive inotropic effect, as well as peripheral arterial vasoconstriction (Fig. 47.2). Although NE enhances both contraction and relaxation and maintains blood pressure, myocardial energy requirements are augmented, which can intensify ischemia when myocardial oxygen (O_2) delivery is restricted. The augmented adrenergic outflow from the CNS also may trigger ventricular tachycardia or even sudden cardiac death, particularly in the presence of myocardial ischemia. Thus, activation of the SNS provides short-term support that has the potential to become maladaptive over the long term. Moreover, increasing evidence suggests

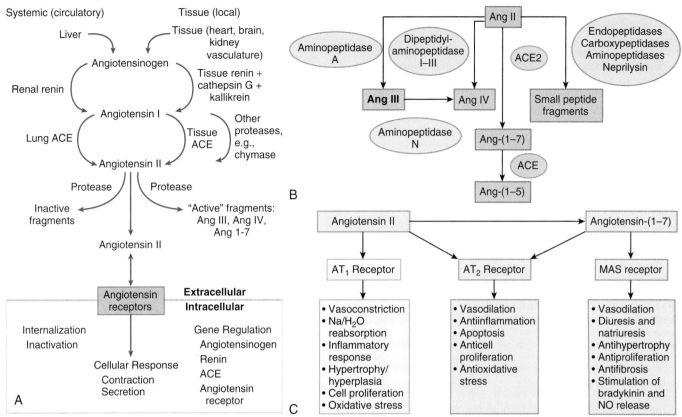

FIGURE 47.3 **A,** The systemic and tissue components of the renin-angiotensin system (RAS). Several tissues, including myocardium, vasculature, kidney, and brain, have the capacity to generate angiotensin II independent of the circulating RAS. Angiotensin II produced at the tissue level may play an important role in the pathophysiology of heart failure (HF). *ACE,* Angiotensin-converting enzyme; *Ang,* angiotensin. **B,** Angiotensin II degradation pathways. Angiotensin II is degraded by angiotensin-converting enzyme 2 (ACE2) to form Ang-(1–7), which subsequently can be degraded by ACE to form Ang-(1–5). Other pathways of angiotensin II degradation include aminopeptidase A to Ang-(2–8), dipeptidyl-aminopeptidase I–III to Ang IV, and neprilysin and various peptidases to other small peptide products. Ang-(2–8) and Ang IV may also be reversibly interchanged via aminopeptidase N. **C,** Action of angiotensin II type 1 (AT$_1$) and type 2 (AT$_2$) receptors and MAS-mediated signaling. *NO,* Nitric oxide. (**A,** Modified from Timmermans PB, Wong PC, Chiu AT, et al. Angiotensin II receptors and angiotensin II receptor antagonists. *Pharmacol Rev.* 1993;45:205; **B,** Modified from Batlle D, Wysocki J, Soler MJ, Ranganath K, et al. Angiotensin-converting enzyme 2: enhancing the degradation of angiotensin II as a potential therapy for diabetic nephropathy. *Kidney Int.* 2012;81:520–528; and **C,** Modified from Iwai M, Horiuchi M. Devil and angel in the renin-angiotensin system. *Hypertens Res.* 2009;32:533–536.)

that apart from the deleterious effects of sympathetic activation, parasympathetic withdrawal also may contribute to the pathogenesis of HF. Withdrawal of parasympathetic nerve stimulation has been associated with decreased nitric oxide (NO) levels, increased inflammation, increased sympathetic activity, and worsening LV remodeling. Several clinical trials with direct vagal nerve stimulation did not meet their primary endpoint but additional studies are ongoing.[4]

Activation of the Renin-Angiotensin System

In contrast with the SNS, the components of the renin-angiotensin system (RAS) are activated comparatively later in HF. The presumptive mechanisms for RAS activation in HF include renal hypoperfusion, decreased filtered sodium reaching the macula densa in the distal tubule, and increased sympathetic stimulation of the kidney, leading to increased renin release from juxtaglomerular apparatus. As shown in Figure 47.3, renin cleaves four amino acids from circulating angiotensinogen, which is synthesized in the liver, to form the biologically inactive decapeptide angiotensin I. Angiotensin-converting enzyme (ACE) cleaves two amino acids from angiotensin I to form the biologically active octapeptide (1 to 8) angiotensin II. Most ACE activity (approaching 90%) in the body is found in tissues; the remaining 10% is found in a soluble (non–membrane-bound) form in the interstitium of the heart and vessel wall. The importance of tissue ACE activity in HF is suggested by the observation that ACE messenger RNA (mRNA) and ACE-binding sites and ACE activity are increased in explanted human hearts.[5] Angiotensin II also can be synthesized using renin-independent pathways through the enzymatic conversion of angiotensinogen to angiotensin I by kallikrein and cathepsin G (Fig. 47.3A). The tissue production of angiotensin II also may occur

along ACE-independent pathways, through the activation of chymase. This latter pathway may be of major importance in the myocardium, particularly when the levels of renin and angiotensin I are increased by the use of ACE inhibitors. Angiotensin II itself can undergo further proteolysis to generate three biologically active fragments: angiotensin III (2 to 8), angiotensin IV (3 to 8), and angiotensin 1 to 7 (Fig. 47.3B). The latter results mainly from angiotensin II cleavage by angiotensin converting enzyme 2 (ACE2), which is a type I transmembrane carboxypeptidase with 40% homology to ACE. ACE2 has also been identified as the cellular receptor of SARS-CoV-2 (see also Chapter 94).[5]

Angiotensin II exerts its effects by binding to two G protein–coupled receptors (GPCRs), the angiotensin type 1 (AT$_1$) and angiotensin type 2 (AT$_2$) receptors. The predominant angiotensin receptor in the vasculature is the AT$_1$ receptor. Although both AT$_1$ and AT$_2$ receptor subtypes are present in human myocardium, the AT$_2$ receptor predominates in a 2:1 molar ratio. Cellular localization of the AT$_1$ receptor in the heart is most abundant in nerves distributed in the myocardium, whereas the AT$_2$ receptor is localized more specifically in fibroblasts and the interstitium. Activation of the AT$_1$ receptor leads to vasoconstriction, cell growth, aldosterone secretion, and catecholamine release, whereas activation of the AT$_2$ receptor leads to vasodilation, inhibition of cell growth, natriuresis, and bradykinin release (Fig. 47.3C). Studies have shown that the AT$_1$ receptor and mRNA levels are downregulated in failing human hearts, whereas AT$_2$ receptor density is increased or unchanged, so that the ratio of AT$_1$ to AT$_2$ receptors decreases. The MAS receptor is a GPCR that is expressed primarily in the brain and testes but also in the heart (see Fig. 47.3C).

Angiotensin II has several important actions that are critical to maintaining short-term circulatory homeostasis. The sustained expression of angiotensin II is maladaptive, however, leading to fibrosis of the heart, kidneys, and other organs. Angiotensin II can also lead to worsening neurohormonal activation by enhancing the release of NE from sympathetic nerve endings, as well as stimulating the zona glomerulosa of the adrenal cortex to produce aldosterone. Analogous to angiotensin II, aldosterone provides short-term support to the circulation by promoting the reabsorption of sodium in exchange for potassium in the distal segments of the nephron. However, the sustained expression of aldosterone may exert harmful effects by provoking hypertrophy and fibrosis within the vasculature and the myocardium, contributing to reduced vascular compliance and increased ventricular stiffness. In addition, aldosterone provokes endothelial cell dysfunction, baroreceptor dysfunction, and inhibition of NE uptake, any of which may lead to worsening HF. The mechanism of action of aldosterone in the cardiovascular system appears to involve oxidative stress, with resultant inflammation in target tissue. Although the exact role of angiotensin III (2 to 8), angiotensin IV (3 to 8), and angiotensin 1 to 7 in HF are not known, experimental studies suggest that angiotensin 1 to 7 counteracts the effects of angiotensin II, and attenuates LV remodeling.[1] In contrast, angiotensin III directly stimulates the zona glomerulosa of the adrenal glands to produce aldosterone,[6] which promotes sodium resorption in the distal collecting duct of the kidney. Angiotensin III also has an important role in vasopressin release in the brain, which controls water retention in the distal collecting duct of the kidney. Angiotensin III in the brain can also modulate cardiac nervous sympathetic hyperactivity, as well as LV remodeling after MI.[1]

OXIDATIVE STRESS

Reactive oxygen species (ROS) are a normal byproduct of aerobic metabolism. In the heart, the potential sources for ROS include the mitochondria, xanthine oxidase, and nicotinamide-adenine dinucleotide phosphate (NADPH) oxidase (Fig. 47.4). ROS can modulate the activity of a variety of intracellular proteins and signaling pathways, including essential proteins involved in myocardial excitation-contraction coupling, such as ion channels, sarcoplasmic reticulum (SR) calcium release channels, and myofilament proteins, as well as signaling pathways that are coupled to myocyte growth.[7] "Oxidative stress" occurs when the production of ROS exceeds the buffering capacity of antioxidant defense systems, leading to an excess of ROS within the cell. Substantial evidence indicates that the level of oxidative stress is increased both systemically and in the myocardium of patients with HF. Oxidative stress in the heart may be caused by reduced antioxidant capacity and increased production of ROS, which may arise secondary to mechanical strain of the myocardium, neurohormonal stimulation (angiotensin

II, alpha-adrenergic agonists, endothelin-1 [ET-1]), or inflammatory cytokines (tumor necrosis factor [TNF], interleukin [IL]-1). Excessive mitochondria-derived ROS in cardiac myocytes have been demonstrated in experimental models of HF and may contribute to contractile dysfunction in advanced HF. Increased xanthine oxidase expression and activity have been reported in canine rapid pacing–induced HF and patients with end-stage HF. Moreover, increased expression and activity of myocardial NADPH oxidases have been demonstrated in both experimental and human HF in cultured cardiac myocytes,[7] ROS stimulate myocyte hypertrophy, reexpression of fetal gene programs, and apoptosis. ROS also can modulate fibroblast proliferation and collagen synthesis and trigger increased matrix metalloproteinase (MMP) abundance and activation. ROS also can affect the peripheral vasculature in HF by decreasing the bioavailability of NO. These and other observations have led to the suggestion that strategies to reduce ROS may be of therapeutic value in patients with HF. However, xanthine oxidase inhibition with allopurinol to reduce oxidative stress in hyperuremic patients with HF did not improve clinical status or cardiac function in a clinical trial.[8]

The importance of aldosterone, independent of angiotensin II, has been demonstrated by clinical trials (see Chapter 50) showing that low-dose spironolactone increased the survival of patients with New York Heart Association (NYHA) class II to IV systolic HF, as well as improved survival after MI, independent of changes in volume or electrolyte status.[9]

Neurohormonal Alterations of Renal Function

One of the signatures of advancing HF is increased salt and water retention by the kidneys. Traditional theories have ascribed this increase to either "forward" failure, which attributes sodium retention to inadequate renal perfusion as a consequence of impaired cardiac output, or "backward" failure, which emphasizes the importance of increased venous pressure in favoring transudation of salt and water from the intravascular to the extracellular compartment. These mechanisms have largely been supplanted by the concept of decreased *effective arterial blood volume*, which postulates that despite blood volume expansion in HF, inadequate cardiac output sensed by baroreceptors in the vascular tree leads to a series of compensatory neurohormonal adaptations that resemble the homeostatic response to acute blood loss.[6] As illustrated in Figure 47.5, a falling cardiac output or redistribution of the circulating blood volume is sensed by baroreceptors in the left ventricle, aortic arch, carotid sinus, and renal afferent arterioles. The loss of inhibitory input from arterial or cardiopulmonary baroreceptor reflexes leads to sustained activation of the SNS and the RAS. An implantable barostimulation device that activates the carotid

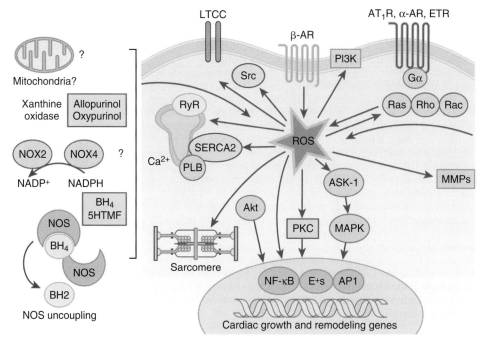

FIGURE 47.4 Cellular sources of reactive oxygen species (ROS) and ROS signaling in cardiac hypertrophy. ROS-generating systems are shown on the *left* and include xanthine oxidase, nicotinamide-adenine dinucleotide phosphate (NADPH) oxidases (NOX2, NOX4), nitric oxide synthase (NOS), and mitochondrial complexes. ROS activation has protean effects on calcium handling, myofilament function, matrix activation, kinase and phosphatase stimulation, and transcriptional regulation of matrix metalloproteinases (MMPs). *Akt*, Protein kinase B; *ASK-1*, apoptosis signal-regulating kinase 1; *ETR*, endothelin receptor; *5HTMF*, 5-hydrotetramethylpholate; *LTCC*, L-type calcium channel; *MAPK*, mitogen-activated protein kinase; *NF-κB*, nuclear factor-kappaB; *PKC*, protein kinase C; *PI3K*, phosphatidylinositol 3-kinase; *PLB*, phospholamban; *RyR*, ryanodine receptor; *SERCA2*, sarcoendoplasmic reticulum Ca²⁺-ATPase. (Modified from McKinsey TA, Kass DA. Small-molecule therapies for cardiac hypertrophy: moving beneath the cell surface. *Nat Rev Drug Discov.* 2007;6:617.)

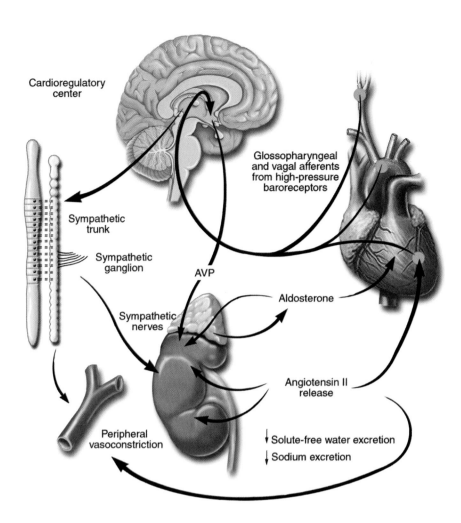

FIGURE 47.5 Unloading of high-pressure barocep-tors (*green circles*) in the left ventricle, carotid sinus, and aortic arch generates afferent signals that stimulate cardioregulatory centers in the brain, resulting in the activation of efferent pathways in the sympathetic nervous system. The sympathetic nervous system (SNS) appears to be the primary integrator of the neurohumoral vasoconstrictor response to arterial underfilling. Activation of renal sympathetic nerves stimulates the release of arginine vasopressin (*AVP*). Sympathetic activation also causes peripheral and renal vasoconstriction, as does angiotensin II. Angiotensin II constricts blood vessels and stimulates the release of aldosterone from the adrenal gland, and it also increases tubular sodium reabsorption and causes remodeling of cardiac myocytes. Aldosterone also may have direct cardiac effects, in addition to increasing the reabsorption of sodium and the secretion of potassium (K^+) and hydrogen (H^+) ions in the collecting duct. The *black arrows* designate circulating hormones. (Modified from Schrier RW, Abraham WT. Hormones and hemodynamics in heart failure. *N Engl J Med*. 1999;341:577.)

baroreceptors to decrease sympathetic activation and increase vagal tone improved quality of life, exercise capacity, and NT-proBNP in patients with symptomatic HF in the BeAT-HF (Barostimulation for Heart Failure).[10]

There is little evidence to suggest that a primary renal abnormality is responsible for the initial sodium retention in the heart; however, there is mounting evidence that secondary changes in the kidney contribute importantly to volume overload as HF progresses. Volume overload in HF is multifactorial and is secondary, at least in part, to several factors that have the potential to cause increased sodium reabsorption, including activation of the SNS, activation of RAS, reduced renal perfusion pressures, and blunting of renal responsiveness to natriuretic peptides. Increased renal sympathetic nerve–mediated vasoconstriction leads to decreased renal blood flow, as well as increased renal tubular sodium and water reabsorption throughout the nephron. Renal sympathetic stimulation also can lead to the nonosmotic release of arginine vasopressin (AVP) from the posterior pituitary, which reduces the excretion of free water and contributes to worsening peripheral vasoconstriction, as well as increased endothelin (ET) production.[1] Increased renal venous pressure can also lead to renal interstitial hypertension, with the development of tubular injury and renal fibrosis.

ARGININE VASOPRESSIN

AVP is a pituitary hormone that plays a central role in the regulation of free water clearance and plasma osmolality (see Fig. 47.5). Under normal circumstances, AVP is released in response to an increase in plasma osmolality, leading to increased retention of water from the collecting duct. Of note, circulating AVP is elevated in many patients with HF, even after correction for plasma osmolality (i.e., nonosmotic release),[1] and may contribute to the hyponatremia that occurs in HF. The cellular effects of AVP are mediated mainly by interactions with

three types of receptors, termed V_1, V_2, and V_3 (previously V_{1b}). The V_1 receptor, the most widespread subtype, is found primarily in vascular smooth muscle cells. The V_3 receptor has a more limited distribution and is located mainly in the CNS. The V_2 receptors are found primarily in the epithelial cells in the renal collecting duct and the thick ascending limb. AVP receptors are members of the GPCRs. The V_1 receptors mediate vasoconstriction, platelet aggregation, and stimulation of myocardial growth factors, whereas V_3 modulates adrenocorticotropic hormone (ACTH) secretion from the anterior pituitary. The V_2 receptor mediates antidiuretic effects by stimulating adenyl cyclase to increase the rate of insertion of water channel–containing vesicles into the apical membrane. Because the vesicles contain preformed functional water channels, termed *aquaporins,* their localization in the apical membranes in response to V_2 stimulation increases the water permeability of the apical membrane, leading to water retention. The "vaptans," vasopressin receptor antagonists with V_1 (relcovaptan) or V_2 (tolvaptan, lixivaptan) selectivity or nonselective V_1/V_2 activity (conivaptan), have been shown to reduce body weight and reduce hyponatremia in clinical trials (see Chapters 49 and 50).

Increased renal sympathetic activity leads to increased renin production by the kidneys, with a resultant sustained activation of RAAS, despite an expanded extracellular volume. Angiotensin II facilitates retention of sodium and water by multiple renal mechanisms, including a direct proximal tubular effect, as well as through activation of aldosterone, which leads to increased sodium resorption in the distal tubule. Angiotensin II also stimulates the thirst center of the brain and provokes the release of AVP and aldosterone, both of which can lead to further dysregulation of salt and water homeostasis.

A number of counterregulatory neurohormonal systems become activated in HF to offset the deleterious effects of the vasoconstricting neurohormones (**eTable 47.1**). Metabolites of vasodilatory prostaglandins, including prostaglandin E_2 (PGE_2) and prostacyclin

(PGI$_2$), are elevated in patients with HF. In addition to being a vasodilator, PGE$_2$ enhances renal sodium excretion and modulates the antidiuretic action of AVP. One class of the most important counterregulatory neurohormonal systems that become activated in HF are the natriuretic peptides, including ANP and brain (B-type) natriuretic peptide (BNP). Under physiologic conditions, ANP and BNP function as natriuretic hormones that are released in response to increases in atrial and myocardial stretch, often secondary to excessive sodium intake. Once released, these cardiac peptides act on the kidney and peripheral circulation to unload the heart, through increased excretion of sodium and water, while inhibiting the release of renin and aldosterone (Fig. 47.6). In the setting of RAAS activation, the release of ANP and BNP may serve as an important counterregulatory mechanism that maintains sodium and water homeostasis. However, for reasons that are not entirely clear, the renal effects of the natriuretic peptides appear to become blunted with advancing HF, leaving the effects of RAAS unopposed.[11] Potential reasons for this blunting include low renal perfusion pressure, relative deficiency or altered molecular forms of the natriuretic peptides, and decreased levels of natriuretic peptide receptors.

NATRIURETIC PEPTIDES

The natriuretic peptide system consists of five structurally similar peptides: ANP, urodilatin (an isoform of ANP), BNP, C-type natriuretic peptide (CNP), and dendroaspis natriuretic peptide (DNP) (Fig. 47.6A).[12] ANP, a 28–amino acid peptide hormone, is produced principally in the cardiac atria, whereas BNP, a 32–amino acid peptide originally isolated from porcine brain, was later identified as a hormone that was primarily produced in the cardiac ventricles. Both ANP and BNP are secreted in response to increasing cardiac wall tension; however, other factors such as neurohormones (e.g., angiotensin II, ET-1, catecholamines) or physiologic factors (e.g., age, gender, renal function) may also play a role in their regulation. The biosynthesis, secretion, and clearance of BNP differs from ANP, suggesting that these two natriuretic peptides have discrete physiologic and pathophysiologic roles. Whereas ANP is secreted in short bursts in response to acute changes in atrial pressure, the activation of BNP is regulated transcriptionally in response to chronic

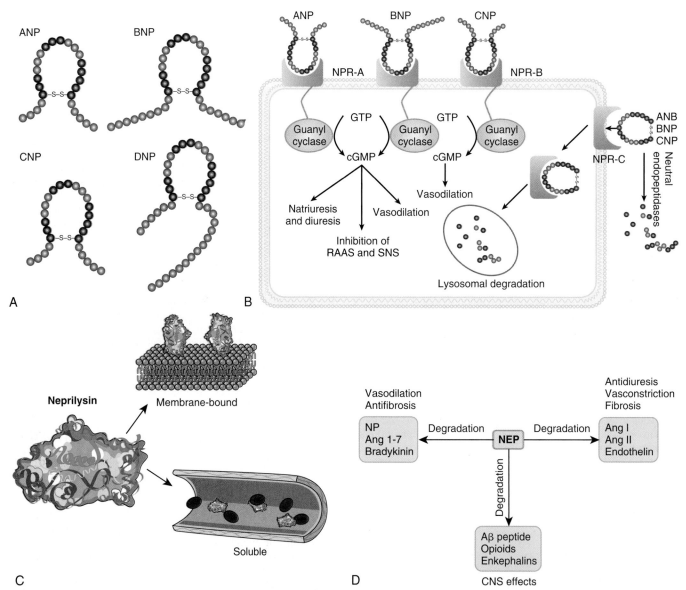

FIGURE 47.6 Natriuretic peptides. **A,** The similar 17–amino acid disulfide ring in natriuretic peptides A, B, C, and D. Identical amino acid sequences are marked in *purple.* **B,** Action and clearance of the natriuretic peptides. **C,** Neprilysin is a membrane-bound enzyme that can be released from the cell surface, producing a soluble form that can be detected in the blood. **D,** Neutral endopeptidases (*NEP*) degrade a variety of different peptides. *NP,* natriuretic peptide. (**B** modified from Gardner RS, Chong KS, McDonagh TA, et al. B-type natriuretic peptides in heart failure. *Biomark Med.* 2007;1:243; **C** modified from Bayes-Genis A, Barallat J, Galán A, et al. Soluble neprilysin is predictive of cardiovascular death and heart failure hospitalizations in heart failure patients. *J Am Coll Cardiol.* 2015;65:657–665; **D** modified from Volpe M, Carnovali M, Mastromarino V. The natriuretic peptides system in the pathophysiology of heart failure: from molecular basis to treatment. *Clin Sci (Lond)* 2016;130:57.)

increases in atrial/ventricular pressure. ANP and BNP initially are synthesized as prohormones that are subsequently proteolytically cleaved, respectively, by corin and furin, to yield large, biologically inactive N-terminal fragments (NT-ANP and NT-BNP) and smaller, biologically active peptides (i.e., ANP and BNP). ANP has a relatively short half-life of approximately 3 minutes, whereas BNP has a plasma half-life of approximately 20 minutes. CNP, which is located primarily in the vasculature, also is released as a prohormone that is cleaved into biologically inactive form (NT-CNP) and a 22–amino acid, biologically active form (i.e., CNP).

Figure 47.6B illustrates the signaling pathway of the natriuretic peptide system. The natriuretic peptides stimulate the production of the intracellular second-messenger cyclic guanosine monophosphate (cGMP), via binding to the natriuretic peptide A receptor (NPR-A), which preferentially binds ANP and BNP, and the natriuretic peptide B receptor (NPR-B), which preferentially binds CNP. Both NPR-A and NPR-B are coupled to particulate guanylate cyclase. Activation of NPR-A and NPR-B results in natriuresis, vasorelaxation, inhibition of renin and aldosterone, inhibition of fibrosis, and increased lusitropy. The natriuretic peptide C receptor (NPR-C) is not linked to cGMP and serves as a clearance receptor for the natriuretic peptides.

All three natriuretic peptides are degraded by two major mechanisms: NPR-C–mediated internalization, followed by lysosomal degradation and enzymatic degradation by neutral endopeptidase (NEP) 24.11 (neprilysin), which is widely expressed in multiple tissues, where it often is colocalized with ACE. Both ACE and NEP are membrane-bound zinc-containing metallopeptidases involved in the metabolism of a variety of biologic peptides.[13]

Neprilysin, like many other membrane-bound metalloproteases, can be released from the cell surface, producing a non–membrane-associated soluble form that retains catalytic activity. NEP preferentially cleaves small peptides on the N-terminal side of hydrophobic residues (Fig. 47.6C). NEP has a wide range of tissue distribution, including vascular endothelium, smooth muscle cells, myocytes, fibroblasts, kidney tubule cells, and nerve cells. NEP degrades multiple peptides, including natriuretic peptides (Fig. 47.6D), angiotensin I, angiotensin II, ET-I, adrenomedullin, opioids, bradykinin, chemotactic peptides, enkephalins, and a[14]myloid-β peptide (Aβ). NEP inhibition of degradation of natriuretic peptides results in vasorelaxation, natriuresis, inhibition of hypertrophy, and fibrosis. On the other hand, inhibition of degradation of other vasoactive peptides, such as angiotensin II, angiotensin 1 to 7, and ET, opposes the vasodilatory effects of natriuretic peptides. Accordingly, NEP inhibition has variable effects on blood pressure. NEP inhibition increases urinary kinin levels, which may contribute to its natriuretic effects. NEP plays an important role in clearance of amyloid peptides in the brain. In particular, NEP is of major relevance for degrading the amyloid-beta peptides (Aβ), which play a significant role in neurotoxicity, and formation of amyloid plaques from Aβ aggregates in complex with other proteins is a hallmark of Alzheimer disease. Overexpression of neprilysin ameliorated the development of Alzheimer disease, and disruption of the neprilysin gene induces cognitive dysfunction in a mouse model of Alzheimer disease. Because of the potentially beneficial effects of natriuretic peptides in HF, NEP inhibition was pursued as a rational approach for HF therapy. The early use of omapatrilat, a dual vasopeptidase inhibitor that inhibits both ACE and NEP, was not shown to be more effective than ACE inhibition alone in HF patients.[14] However, the use of a combined AT₁ receptor antagonist and a neprilysin inhibitor (valsartan/sacubitril, LCZ696) was shown to have a favorable impact on HF outcome, including quality of life, exercise capacity, and more importantly, HF hospitalization and total mortality, in the PARADIGM-HF trial (see Chapter 50).

The biologic importance of the natriuretic peptides in renal sodium handling has been demonstrated in multiple studies using NPR antagonists, as well as overexpression of ANP or BNP. In experimental HF models, either acute blockade of NPR-A and NPR-B or chronic genetic disruption of NPR-A blunts the renal natriuretic response to acute volume expansion, demonstrating the renal protective action of natriuretic peptide activation. The infusion of a recombinant human ANP and BNP exerts beneficial hemodynamic effects, characterized by decreases in arterial and venous pressures, increase in cardiac output, and suppression of neurohormonal activation in humans, resulting in their clinical development as therapeutic agents for human HF (see Chapter 49). In addition to their important biologic role, the natriuretic peptides have provided important diagnostic and prognostic information in HF (see Chapter 48).

Neurohormonal Alterations in the Peripheral Vasculature

In patients with HF, the complex interactions between the autonomic nervous system and local autoregulatory mechanisms tend to preserve circulation to the brain and heart while decreasing blood flow to the skin, skeletal muscles, splanchnic organs, and kidneys. This intense visceral vasoconstriction during exercise helps to divert the limited cardiac output to exercising muscle but contributes to hypoperfusion of the gut and kidneys. The most powerful stimulus for peripheral vasoconstriction is sympathetic activation, which releases the potent vasoconstrictor NE. Other vasoconstrictors that contribute to maintaining circulatory homeostasis include angiotensin II, ET, neuropeptide Y, urotensin II, thromboxane A₂, and AVP (see eTable 47.1). The increased sympathetic adrenergic stimulation of the peripheral arteries and the increased concentrations of circulating vasoconstrictors contribute to the arteriolar vasoconstriction and to the maintenance of arterial pressure. The sympathetic stimulation of the veins contributes to an increase in venous tone, which helps to maintain venous return and ventricular filling and to support cardiac performance by Starling's law of the heart (see Chapter 46). For more information see the online supplement "Vasoconstricting Peptides in Heart Failure."

As noted, the vasoconstricting neurohormones activate counterregulatory vasodilator responses, including release of natriuretic peptides, NO, bradykinin, adrenomedullin, apelin, and vasodilating PGI₂ and PGE₂ (see eTable 47.1). Under normal circumstances, the continuous release of NO (endothelium-derived relaxing factor) from the endothelium counteracts these vasoconstricting factors and allows for appropriate vasodilatory responses during exercise. As HF advances, however, the endothelial cell–mediated vasodilatory responsiveness is lost, which contributes to the excessive peripheral arterial vasoconstriction that is emblematic of advanced HF. Of interest, the vasodilator response can be restored by the administration of L-arginine, a precursor of endothelium-derived NO.

Nitric Oxide

The free radical gas NO is produced by three isoforms of NO synthase (NOS). All three isoforms are present in the heart, including NOS1 (neuronal NOS [nNOS]), NOS2 (inducible NOS [iNOS]) and NOS3 (so-called endothelial-constitutive NOS [eNOS]). NOS1 has been detected in cardiac conduction tissue, in intracardiac neurons, and in the SR of cardiac myocytes. NOS2 is an inducible isoform that is not normally expressed in the myocardium but is synthesized de novo in virtually all cells in the heart in response to inflammatory cytokines. NOS3 is expressed in coronary endothelium and endocardium and in the sarcolemma and transverse (T)-tubule membranes of cardiac myocytes. NOS1 and NOS3 can be activated by calcium or calmodulin, whereas the induction of NOS2 is calcium independent. NO activates soluble guanylate cyclase (**eFig. 47.2A**). Vericiguat, an oral soluble guanylate cyclase stimulator, reduced the composite of death from cardiovascular causes and first HF hospitalization in the VICTORIA (Vericiguat Global Study in Subjects with Heart Failure with Reduced Ejection Fraction) trial (see Chapter 50).[15]

Under normal circumstances, the continuous release of NO (endothelium-derived relaxing factor) from the endothelium counteracts the vasoconstricting factors and allows for appropriate vasodilatory responses during exercise. This activation leads to the production of cGMP, which in turn activates protein kinase G (PKG) and cascade of different signaling events. In normal persons, NO released by endothelial cells mediates vasodilation in the peripheral vasculature through cGMP-mediated relaxation of vascular smooth muscle. In patients with HF, endothelium-dependent NO-mediated dilation of the peripheral vasculature is blunted, which has been attributed to decreased NOS3 expression and activity.

The actions of NO on the myocardium are complex and include both short-term alterations in function and energetics and longer-term effects on structure. NO modulates the activity of several key calcium channels involved in excitation-contraction coupling as well as mitochondrial respiratory complexes. This type of regulation is accomplished by spatial localization of different NOS isoforms in distinct cellular microdomains involved in excitation-contraction coupling. Specifically, NOS1 localizes to the SR in proximity to the ryanodine receptor (RyR) and sarcoendoplasmic reticulum calcium–adenosine triphosphatase (SR Ca²⁺-ATPase, SERCA2a), and NOS3 is found in sarcolemmal caveolae compartmentalized with cell surface receptors and the L-type Ca^{2+} channel (eFig. 47.2B). NO also participates in mitochondrial respiration, the process that fuels excitation-contraction coupling. The different NOS isoforms also may participate in the process of cardiac remodeling. LV remodeling was ameliorated and survival improved after MI in transgenic mice deficient in NOS2. By contrast, overexpression of NOS3 resulted in improved remodeling after MI. These contrasting effects of NOS2 and NOS3 may reflect the differences in amount of NO produced, which is much higher with NOS2. Emerging evidence indicates an imbalance between increasing free radical production and decreased NO generation in HF, which has been termed the "nitroso-redox imbalance." NOS uncoupling secondary to a deficiency of tetrahydrobiopterin may further contribute to the nitroso-redox imbalance.[16] The nitroso-redox imbalance probably contributes to disease progression in HF secondary to increased oxidative stress, as well as loss of the peripheral vasodilatory effects of NO.

BRADYKININ

Kinins are vasodilators that are released from inactive protein precursors (kininogens) through the action of proteolytic enzymes termed *kallikreins.* The biologic actions of the kinins are mediated by binding to B_1 and B_2 receptors. Most cardiovascular actions are initiated by the B_2 receptor, which is distributed widely in tissues, where it binds bradykinin and kallidin. The B_1 receptor binds the metabolites of bradykinin and kallidin. Stimulation of the B_2 receptor leads to vasodilation, which is mediated by the activation of NOS3, phospholipase A_2, and adenylyl cyclase. Studies suggest that bradykinin plays an important role in the regulation of vascular tone in HF.[17] The breakdown of bradykinin is catalyzed by ACE and neprilysin, so these enzymes not only lead to the formation of a potent vasoconstrictor (angiotensin II) but also mediate the breakdown of a vasodilator (bradykinin). The augmentation of bradykinin levels likely contributes to the beneficial actions of ACE inhibitors and NEP inhibitors (see Chapter 50).

ADRENOMEDULLIN

Adrenomedullin is a 52-amino acid vasodilatory peptide that originally was discovered in human pheochromocytoma tissue. Subsequently, high levels of adrenomedullin immunoreactivity were detected in cardiac atrium and adrenal and pituitary glands, with lower levels detected in the ventricle, kidney, and vasculature.[18] Adrenomedullin binds to a number of G-protein coupled receptors (GPRCs) that are present in multiple cell types, including on endothelial and vascular smooth muscle cells. Circulating concentrations of adrenomedullin are elevated in cardiovascular disease and HF in proportion to the severity of cardiac and hemodynamic impairment. Increasing evidence suggests that adrenomedullin may play a compensatory role in HF by offsetting the deleterious effects of excessive peripheral vasoconstriction. For example, the excretion of adrenomedullin that is stimulated by volume overload is thought to be protective by preserving endothelial barrier function. Moreover, adrenomedullin inhibits the renin-angiotensin-aldosterone system. Recently, a new immunoassay that specifically measures the biologically active form of adrenomedullin has been developed and may become a biomarker for tissue congestion.[19]

APELIN

Apelin is a vasoactive peptide that is an endogenous ligand for the GPCR APJ. The *APJ* gene encodes a receptor that most closely resembles the angiotensin receptor AT_1. However, the APJ receptor does not bind angiotensin II. In the cardiovascular system, apelin elicits endothelium-dependent, NO-mediated vasorelaxation and reduces arterial blood pressure. In addition, apelin demonstrates potent inotropic activity without stimulating concomitant cardiac myocyte hypertrophy. Apelin also produces diuresis by inhibition of AVP activity. In experimental animals, apelin concentrations are significantly lower in failing hearts and are increased after treatment with an angiotensin receptor blocking agent. Furthermore, apelin levels are significantly reduced in patients with HF compared with controls and are significantly increased after cardiac resynchronization. The APJ receptor is a bifunctional GPCR that conveys cytoprotective signals after endogenous ligand stimulation and also acts as a mechanosensor to decrease cardiac hypertrophy after hemodynamic pressure overload.[20] Recently, the apelin receptor has been shown to be activated by a novel endogenous peptide ligand referred to as Apela/Elabela/Toddler (ELA).[21] In contrast to apelin, the expression of ELA is mainly enriched in stem cells, the kidney, prostate, and vascular endothelium. ELA exerts similar cardiovascular effects as apelin and may be more potent than apelin. ELA is also downregulated in experimental models

and humans with HF. The ELP-AJP axis is currently being evaluated as a therapeutic target in patients with chronic HF.[21]

ADIPOKINES

Although adipose tissue was once considered a simple storage depot for fat, it is now known to synthesize and secrete a family of proteins collectively referred to as adipokines (see eFig. 47.3). Adipokines include adiponectin, TNF, plasminogen activator inhibitor type 1 (PAI-1), transforming growth factor-β, and resistin. Leptin is a 16-kDa protein hormone that plays a key role in regulating energy intake and energy expenditure. The product of the ob gene, leptin is predominantly synthesized and secreted by adipocytes, although the heart is also a site of leptin synthesis. The initial role of leptin was thought to decrease appetite through hypothalamic stimulation and thus regulation of food intake. However, elevated circulating levels of leptin and soluble leptin receptor, which act via activating a family of receptor (ob.R) isoforms, are markedly elevated in patients with HF.[22] Leptin may affect myocardial function by promoting activation of both the SNS and the RAS. Moreover, leptin can stimulate the secretion of aldosterone.[22] Several studies suggest that leptin directly induces hypertrophy in both human and rodent cardiac myocytes.[23] Leptin resistance may lead to an accumulation of lipids in non-adipose peripheral tissues, resulting in a variety of "lipotoxic" effects, including cardiac myocyte apoptosis.

Adiponectin is a 224–amino acid polypeptide that modulates a number of metabolic processes, including glucose regulation and fatty acid oxidation. Although adiponectin initially was thought to be exclusively produced by adipose tissue, recent studies have demonstrated adiponectin expression in the heart. Studies in adiponectin-deficient mice demonstrated progressive cardiac remodeling after hemodynamic pressure overloading, whereas administration of adiponectin diminished infarct size, apoptosis, and TNF production after myocardial ischemia-reperfusion in both wild-type and adiponectin-deficient mice. Adiponectin inhibits cardiac hypertrophy, inflammation, and fibrosis. Moreover, adiponectin suppresses aldosterone secretion. Thus, adiponectin has been proposed as a potential biomarker of HF, as well as a potential therapeutic target for the treatment of HF.[23]

INFLAMMATORY MEDIATORS

As shown in Figure 47.7 myocardial injury leads to the activation of the innate and adaptive immune systems in the heart. Whereas the innate immune system provides a global, nonspecific defense against tissue injury, the adaptive immune system provides a highly specific response mediated by B cells and T cells.[24] The innate immune system is activated by transmembrane and cytosolic receptors that recognize molecular motifs from endogenous material released by dying or stressed cells (damage-associated molecular patterns [DAMPs]). These receptors, referred to as pattern recognition receptors (PRRs), are expressed by cells residing in the heart, including cardiac myocytes, endothelial cells, and tissue-resident immune cells. PRRs in the heart include Toll-like receptors (TLRs), RIG-I-like receptors (retinoic acid-inducible), NOD-like receptors (NLRs), the NLRP3 inflammasome, pentraxins, and C-type lectin receptors. Transcriptional profiling of human heart samples showed that failing and non-failing hearts have distinct expression profiles of genes related to innate immune responses, and the expression profiles of these genes were different in samples from patients with ischemic and non-ischemic HF.[24] Activation of PRRs by DAMPs initiates downstream signaling cascades that regulate the expression of ensembles of genes encoding pro-inflammatory cytokines, including TNF, IL-1β, and IL-6, as well as chemokines, both of which serve as downstream "effectors" of the innate immune system. Activation of the innate immune system can lead subsequently to the activation of humoral immunity, through recruitment and stimulation of B cells and T cells. Activation of innate and adaptive immune responses provides the heart with a short-term adaptation to increased stress (physiologic inflammation). However, this inflammatory response can become dysregulated and result in chronic inflammation that leads to LV dysfunction and LV remodeling. Circulating levels of proinflammatory cytokines (e.g., CRP, TNF, IL-1β, IL-6) are increased in patients with HF and correlate with adverse patient outcomes.[25] As shown in Table 47.1, the sustained expression of inflammatory mediators is sufficient to recapitulate virtually all aspects of the HF phenotype, by provoking deleterious changes in cardiac myocytes and nonmyocytes, as well as changes in the myocardial extracellular matrix (ECM). The clinical relevance of these findings is suggested by a prespecified analysis of the CANTOS (Cardiovascular Risk Reduction Study) trial, which showed that targeted anti-cytokine therapy with canakinumab (a monoclonal antibody against IL-1β) reduced HF-related hospitalizations and mortality in patients with previous MI. Importantly, canakinumab-treated patients who achieved on-treatment hsCRP

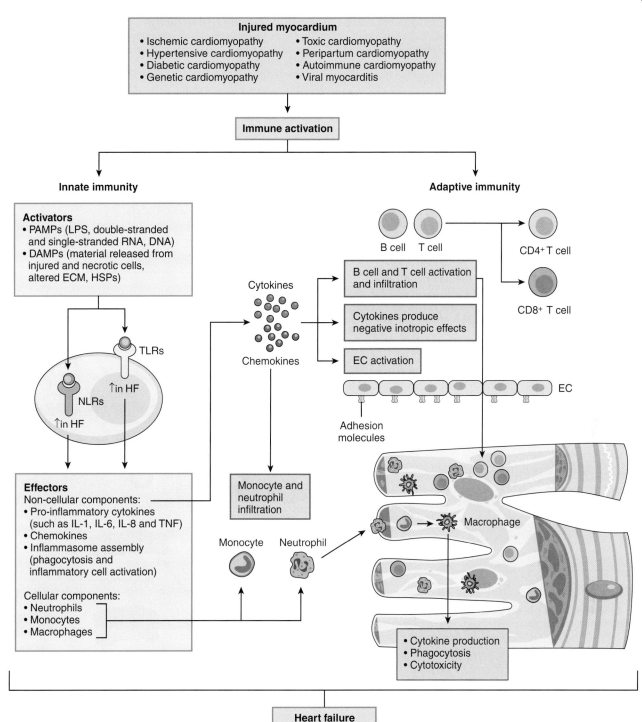

FIGURE 47.7 The innate and adaptive immune systems in heart failure. A variety of cardiac disease states that lead to cardiac injury can activate the innate immune response in the heart through binding of pathogen-associated molecular patterns (PAMPs) or damage-associated molecular patterns (DAMPs) to pattern-recognition receptors (PRRs), such as Toll-like receptors (TLRs) and NOD-like receptors (NLRs), present on cardiomyocytes and tissue-resident immune cells. Activation of PRRs induces a variety of non-cellular effectors in the heart, including pro-inflammatory cytokines and chemokines and activation of the complement system, which lead to endothelial cell (EC) activation and recruitment of monocytes and neutrophils. Activation of the innate immune system triggers the activation of the adaptive immune response through the recruitment of B cells and T cells to the injured myocardium. *ECM*, Extracellular matrix; *HF*, heart failure; *HSP*, heat shock protein; *LPS*, lipopolysaccharide; *TNF*, tumor necrosis factor. (From Adamo L, Rocha-Resende C, Prabhu SD, Mann DL. Reappraising the role of inflammation in heart failure. *Nat Rev Cardiol*. 220;5:269–285.)

concentrations of less than 2 mg/L had significant reductions in the risk of HF related outcomes, including all-cause death when compared with patients receiving placebo, suggesting that inflammation contributes to the progression of HF.[26]

Left Ventricular Remodeling

Although the neurohormonal concept explains many aspects of disease progression in the failing heart, increasing clinical evidence suggests that current neurohormonal models fail to completely explain the basis for this progression. That is, although neurohormonal antagonists stabilize and in some cases reverse certain aspects of the disease process in HF, in the overwhelming majority of patients, it will progress, albeit more slowly. It has been suggested that LV remodeling is directly related to future deterioration in LV performance and a less favorable clinical course in HFrEF patients. LV remodeling is influenced by hemodynamic, neurohormonal, epigenetic, and genetic factors (**eFig. 47.4**),[27] as well as by comorbid conditions. Although the complex changes that occur in the heart during LV remodeling have traditionally been described in anatomic terms, the process of LV remodeling also has an important impact on the biology of the cardiac myocyte, on changes in the volume of myocyte and nonmyocyte components of the myocardium, and on the geometry and architecture of the LV chamber (Table 47.2).

Alterations in Biology of Cardiac Myocyte

Numerous studies have suggested that failing human cardiac myocytes undergo a number of important changes that might be expected to lead to a progressive loss of contractile function. These include decreased alpha-myosin heavy chain gene expression with a concomitant increase in beta-myosin heavy chain expression, progressive loss of myofilaments in cardiac myocytes, alterations in cytoskeletal proteins, and alterations in excitation-contraction coupling and in energy metabolism, as well as desensitization of beta-adrenergic signaling (see Table 47.2).

TABLE 47.1 Effects of Inflammatory Mediators on Left Ventricular Remodeling

Alterations in the Biology of the Myocyte
Myocyte hypertrophy
Fetal gene expression
Negative inotropic effects
Increased oxidative stress
Alterations in the Biology of Nonmyocytes
Conversion of fibroblasts to myofibroblasts
Upregulation of AT_1 receptors on fibroblasts
Increased matrix metalloproteinase secretion by fibroblasts
Alterations in the Extracellular Matrix
Degradation of the matrix
Myocardial fibrosis
Progressive Myocyte Loss
Necrosis
Apoptosis

TABLE 47.2 Overview of Left Ventricular Remodeling

Alterations in Myocyte Biology
Excitation-contraction coupling
Myosin heavy chain (fetal) gene expression
Beta-adrenergic desensitization
Hypertrophy
Myocytolysis
Cytoskeletal proteins
Myocardial Changes
Myocyte loss
Necrosis
Apoptosis
Autosis
Alterations in extracellular matrix
Matrix degradation
Myocardial fibrosis
Alterations in Left Ventricular Chamber Geometry
Left ventricular (LV) dilation
Increased LV sphericity
LV wall thinning
Mitral valve incompetence

Cardiac Myocyte Hypertrophy

Two basic patterns of cardiac hypertrophy occur in response to hemodynamic overload (Fig. 47.8). In pressure overload hypertrophy (e.g., with aortic stenosis or hypertension), increased systolic wall stress leads to the addition of sarcomeres in parallel, an increase in myocyte cross-sectional area, and increased LV wall thickening. This pattern of remodeling has been referred to as "concentric" hypertrophy (Fig. 47.8A) and has been linked with alterations in Ca^{2+}/calmodulin-dependent protein

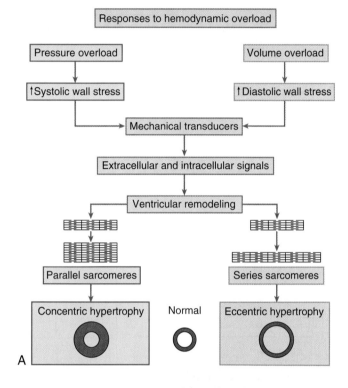

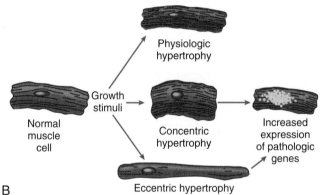

FIGURE 47.8 The pattern of cardiac and cellular remodeling that occurs in response to hemodynamic overloading depends on the nature of the inciting stimulus. **A,** When the overload is predominantly due to an increase in pressure (e.g., with systemic hypertension or aortic stenosis), the increase in systolic wall stress leads to the parallel addition of sarcomeres and widening of the cardiac myocytes, resulting in "concentric" cardiac hypertrophy. When the overload is predominantly due to an increase in ventricular volume, the increase in diastolic wall stress leads to the series addition of sarcomeres, lengthening of cardiac myocytes, and left ventricular (LV) dilation, which is referred to as "eccentric" chamber hypertrophy. **B,** Phenotypically distinct changes occur in the morphology of myocytes in response to the type of hemodynamic overload that is superimposed. When the overload is predominantly due to an increase in pressure, the increase in systolic wall stress leads to the parallel addition of sarcomeres and widening of the cardiac myocytes. When the hemodynamic overload is predominantly due to an increase in ventricular volume, the increase in diastolic wall stress leads to the series addition of sarcomeres with consequent lengthening of cardiac myocytes. The expression of maladaptive genes is increased in both eccentric and concentric hypertrophy, but not in physiologic myocyte hypertrophy as occurs with exercise (see Table 47.2). (**A** from Colucci WS, ed. *Heart Failure: Cardiac Function and Dysfunction.* 2nd ed. Philadelphia: Current Medicine; 1999:4.2. **B** modified from Hunter JJ, Chien KR. Signaling pathways for cardiac hypertrophy and failure. *N Engl J Med.* 1999;341:1276.)

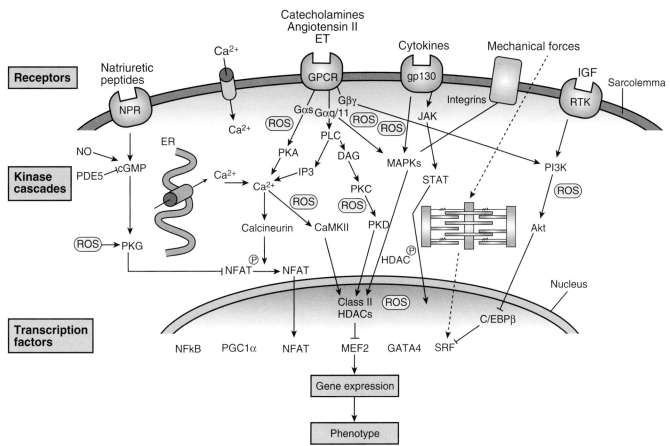

FIGURE 47.9 Cellular signaling pathways in cardiac myocyte hypertrophy. Many signaling pathways have the potential to regulate the growth of cardiac cells acting through an increasingly complex network of intracellular signaling cascades. Agonists for α-adrenergic, angiotensin, and endothelin (*ET*) receptors couple to phospholipase C (*PLC*) and calcium influx channels by way of G proteins. Activation of PLC results in the generation of two second messengers, inositol triphosphate (*IP3*) and diacylglycerol (*DAG*). IP3 causes the release of calcium from intracellular stores, and DAG activates protein kinase C (*PKC*). Changes in intracellular calcium stores can activate Ca²⁺/calmodulin-dependent kinases (*CaMKII*), as well as calcineurin, which can affect gene expression in multiple ways. PKC and G proteins can affect gene expression by activating mitogen-activated protein kinase (*MAPK*) cascades. Histone deacetylase complexes (*HDACs*) are emerging as important negative regulators of genes involved in cardiac hypertrophy. Cytokines and peptide growth factors, such as insulin-like growth factor (*IGF*), can be elaborated by various cells within the heart and may act in an autocrine or paracrine manner. These growth factors activate cellular receptors that usually possess receptor tyrosine kinase (*RTK*) activity and are coupled to a cascade of protein kinase. Mechanical deformation of cardiac myocytes through matrix-integrin interactions can lead to activation or modulation of several signaling pathways, at least in part through autocrine action of released agonists such as angiotensin. Both nitric oxide (NO) and oxidative stress may be induced after stimulation of signaling pathways and modulate the activity of kinase cascades and transcription factors leading to alterations in contractile phenotype, growth, and death in myocytes. *Akt,* Protein kinase B; *C/EBPβ,* CCAAT/enhancer binding protein-β; *ER,* endoplasmic reticulum; *GATA4,* GATA-binding protein; *gp130,* glycoprotein 130; *GPCR,* G protein–coupled receptor; *JAK,* Janus kinase; *MEF2,* myocyte enhancer factor; *NFAT,* nuclear factor of activated T cells; *NFκB,* nuclear factor-kappaB cells; *NPR,* natriuretic peptide receptor; *P,* phosphorylation; *PDE5,* phosphodiesterase type 5; *PGC1α,* peroxisome proliferator–activated receptor gamma, coactivator 1 alpha; *PKA, PKD, PKG,* protein kinases A, D, G; *STAT,* signal transducer and activator of transcription; *SRF,* serum response factor. (From Shah AM, Mann DL. In search of new therapeutic targets and strategies for heart failure: recent advances in basic science. *Lancet.* 2011;378:704.)

kinase II–dependent signaling (Fig. 47.9).²⁸ By contrast, in volume overload hypertrophy (e.g., with aortic and mitral regurgitation), increased diastolic wall stress leads to an increase in myocyte length with the addition of sarcomeres in series, thereby engendering increased LV ventricular dilation. This pattern of remodeling has been referred to as "eccentric" hypertrophy (because of the position of the heart in the chest), or a "dilated" phenotype (see Fig. 47.7A), and has been linked with protein kinase B (Akt) activation (see Fig. 47.8).²⁸ Patients with HF classically present with a dilated left ventricle with or without LV wall thinning. The myocytes from these failing ventricles have an elongated appearance that is characteristic of myocytes obtained from hearts subjected to chronic volume overload.

Cardiac myocyte hypertrophy also leads to changes in the biologic phenotype of the myocyte that are secondary to reactivation of portfolios of genes normally not expressed postnatally. The reactivation of these fetal genes, the so-called fetal gene program, also is accompanied by decreased expression of a number of genes that are normally expressed in the adult heart. As discussed later, activation of the fetal gene program may contribute to the contractile dysfunction that develops in the failing myocyte. As shown in Figure 47.9, the stimuli for the genetic reprogramming of the myocyte include mechanical stretch/strain of the myocyte, neurohormones (e.g., NE, angiotensin II), inflammatory cytokines (e.g., TNF, IL-1β, IL-6), other peptides and growth

factors (e.g., ET), and ROS (e.g., superoxide, NO). These stimuli occur both locally within the myocardium, where they exert autocrine/paracrine effects, and systemically, where they exert endocrine effects.

The early stage of cardiac myocyte hypertrophy is characterized morphologically by increases in the number of myofibrils and mitochondria, as well as enlargement of mitochondria and nuclei. At this stage, the cardiac myocytes are larger than normal, but with preservation of cellular organization. As hypertrophy continues, there is an increase in the number of mitochondria, as well as the addition of new contractile elements in localized areas of the cell. Cells subjected to longstanding hypertrophy show more obvious disruptions in cellular organization, such as extremely enlarged nuclei with highly lobulated membranes, accompanied by the displacement of adjacent myofibrils with loss of the normal registration of the Z-bands. The late stage of hypertrophy is characterized by loss of contractile elements (myocytolysis) with marked disruption of Z-bands and severe disruption of the normal parallel arrangement of the sarcomeres, accompanied by dilation and increased tortuosity of T tubules.

Alterations in Excitation-Contraction Coupling

As discussed in Chapter 46, excitation-contraction coupling refers to the cascade of biologic events that begins with the cardiac action potential and ends with myocyte contraction and relaxation. Impaired

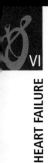

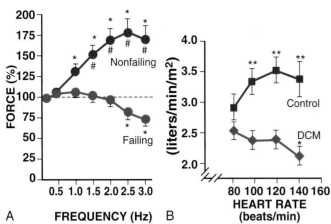

A   FREQUENCY (Hz)   B   HEART RATE (beats/min)

FIGURE 47.10 Relationship between contraction frequency and cardiac performance (force-frequency relation) in heart failure. **A,** Relationship between stimulation frequency and force generation of isolated muscle strip preparations from nonfailing and failing human hearts. In nonfailing myocardium, contractile force increases up to a stimulation rate of approximately 2.5 Hz (150 beats/min), whereas contractile force does not significantly increase in failing myocardium. (*indicates $P < 0.05$ versus 0.25 Hz; # indicates $P < 0.05$ between failing and nonfailing myocardium.) **B,** Cardiac index versus heart rate in patients with and without heart failure (HF). Heart rate was changed by temporary pacing during cardiac catheterization, and cardiac output was measured by thermodilution. In patients without HF, cardiac index increases with higher heart rates up to 120 beats/min, but it declines continuously in patients with HF. (*indicates $P < 0.05$ and **$P < 0.01$ versus lowest pacing rate.) *DCM,* Dilated cardiomyopathy. (**A,** Modified from Pieske B, Maier LS, Bers DM, Hasenfuss G. Ca2+ handling and sarcoplasmic reticulum Ca2+ content in isolated failing and nonfailing human myocardium. *Circ Res.* 1999;85:38; and **B,** modified from Hasenfuss G, Holubarsch C, Hermann HP, et al. Influence of the force-frequency relationship on haemodynamics and left ventricular function in patients with non-failing hearts and in patients with dilated cardiomyopathy. *Eur Heart J.* 1994;15:164.)

contraction and relaxation of the failing heart is most prominent at high heart rates, which results in a depressed force-frequency relationship. This has been demonstrated both in isolated strips of human myocardium and in clinical observations of patients (Fig. 47.10). Normally, higher contraction frequency increases cardiac performance because of a frequency-dependent augmentation of intracellular Ca^{2+} transients. By contrast, in the failing myocardium, a decline in force generation is seen with higher heart rates that is secondary to a decrease in amplitude of intracellular Ca^{2+}, a prolonged decline of the Ca^{2+} transient, and increased levels of diastolic calcium. The reduced intracellular Ca^{2+} transient is secondary to depletion of Ca^{2+} from the SR, the result of three major defects in calcium cycling that occur in the failing heart: (1) increased Ca^{2+} leak through RyRs, (2) impaired SR Ca^{2+} uptake from reduced SERCA2a (SR calcium pump) protein levels and function, and (3) increased expression and function of the sarcolemmal Na^+/Ca^{2+} exchanger (NCX).

Increased Ca^{2+} Leak

Ca^{2+} enters the cell during the action potential through L-type calcium channels and triggers a release of a much larger amount of calcium from the SR through RyRs. Although controversy surrounds the expression levels of RyRs in HF, as well as the coupling of RyRs to L-type Ca^{2+} channels, there is general agreement that the diastolic Ca^{2+} leak in HF is the result of RyR opening during diastole.[29] The resultant release of calcium from the SR event is referred to as a "Ca^{2+}-spark." The pathophysiologic mechanism underlying the diastolic Ca^{2+} leak in HF has been attributed to increased phosphorylation of the RyR by protein kinase A (PKA), Ca^{2+}/calmodulin-dependent protein kinase II (CaMKII), and decreased binding of the RyR stabilizing protein calstabin (FKBP12.6). Experimental studies suggest that PKA-dependent phosphorylation of the RyR may provoke Ca^{2+} leak by destabilizing the association between calstabin and FKB (see Chapter 46). Interestingly, in dogs, beta-adrenergic blockers prevent the development of Ca^{2+} leak by restoring RyR stabilization by FKBP12.6.[29] This observation has led to the suggestion that the increase in contractile function following treatment with beta blockers is secondary to RyR stabilization. The role of excess PKA-dependent RyR phosphorylation in the cause of HF

appears somewhat paradoxical, in that the β-receptor is downregulated in HF. One current proposal is that there are microdomains in close proximity to the RyR where there is increased PKA phosphorylation and more cyclic adenosine monophosphate (cAMP) and decreased activity of the type 4 phosphodiesterase (PDE4D3).[30] In addition to its contribution to reduced SR Ca^{2+} content, increased leak seems to be relevant for arrhythmias in HF. This results from activation of NCX: Ca^{2+} leaking out of the SR activates NCX to remove Ca^{2+} from the cytosol in exchange of Na^+. Because NCX is electrogenic (3 Na^+ versus 1 Ca^{2+}), the increased influx of Na^+ results in a net inward current generating the so-called delayed afterdepolarizations (DADs), which serve as a trigger of arrhythmias. A recent study suggests that the increased leak may have a dominant role for the induction of ventricular arrhythmias and sudden cardiac death rather than for the development of contractile failure.[31]

Sarcoplasmic Reticulum Ca^{2+} Reuptake and Sarcolemmal Ca^{2+} Elimination

Relaxation of the contractile proteins occurs after dissociation of Ca^{2+} from troponin C and Ca^{2+} elimination from the cytosol. In the human heart, there are two main mechanisms responsible for elimination of Ca^{2+} from the cytosol: SR uptake of Ca^{2+} by the SERCA2a Ca^{2+} pump and transsarcolemmal Ca^{2+} elimination through NCX. Under normal conditions, approximately 75% of Ca^{2+} is taken up by the SR and 25% extruded from the cell through NCX. In HF there is decreased uptake of Ca^{2+} by the SR secondary to decreased SERCA2a protein levels and SERCA2a function. In addition, phosphorylation of phospholamban (PLB) is reduced in the failing heart, resulting in increased PLB-dependent inhibition of the SR Ca^{2+} pump.[32] In addition to PLB, the activity of SERCA is inhibited by the binding of small transmembrane micropeptides, myoregulin and dwarf open reading frame (DWORF), which lower the affinity of SERCA for Ca^{2+} and decrease the rate of Ca^{2+} reuptake into the SR.[33] The decrease of SR Ca^{2+} uptake in the failing heart results in a relative increase of transsarcolemmal Ca^{2+} elimination by the NCX, which is most likely secondary to increased expression of NCX protein. Restoring deficient SERCA2a by gene transfer has been shown to improve contractile function and restore electrical stability experimentally. However, the CUPID trial failed to show clinical benefit of SERCA2a gene transfer in patients with HF.[34] Although the increase in NCX activity may result in increased Ca^{2+} elimination from the myocyte, thereby preserving diastolic calcium levels and preventing diastolic dysfunction when SR calcium uptake is reduced, increased NCX activity may further reduce SR Ca^{2+} accumulation/content and may therefore reduce Ca^{2+} activation of contractile proteins. As noted, electrogenic NCX activity induces DADs and arrhythmias.

ALTERATIONS IN T-TUBULES

Cardiac excitation–contraction coupling occurs primarily at the sites of T-tubule/SR junctions (see Chapter 46). Organization of the T-tubule network is essential for coordinated excitation and synchronous activation of Ca^{2+} release from the SR. The L-type Ca^{2+} channels are located mainly on the T-tubule membrane in close proximity to RyRs on the SR. Studies have shown that there is extensive remodeling of the T-tubule system in experimental models of HF, as well as myocardial samples from failing human hearts.[35] T-tubule remodeling within cardiac myocytes leads to loss of coordinated Ca^{2+} release and contraction of ventricular cardiac myocytes, which could contribute to worsening LV dysfunction in HF. Junctophilin-2 (JP2) has been identified as an important protein that serves to bridge the physical gap between T-tubules and the SR, and thus is essential for maintaining EC coupling. Loss of JP2 expression has been demonstrated in failing human hearts and several HF models.[35]

Action Potential Duration and Sodium Handling

Several factors contribute to the prolongation of the action potential duration, which is a ubiquitous finding in failing hearts.[36] The transient outward potassium current (Ito) and the inward rectifier potassium current (Ik1) both are reduced in HF. In addition, the increased inward Na^+ current through the NCX and persistent activity of the sodium channel also may contribute to prolongation of the action potential.

The latter mechanism, also termed the "late sodium current," may be important in the pathogenesis of cardiac arrhythmias in HF. As discussed in Chapter 46, the voltage-gated Na^+ channels are activated on depolarization of the cell membrane, leading to rapid influx of Na^+ that is responsible for the fast upstroke of the action potential (**eFig. 47.5**). Under normal conditions, Na^+ channels inactivate a few milliseconds after depolarization. However, it is now recognized that some Na^+ channels remain open (or reopen), leading to a small but persistent influx of Na^+ throughout the plateau of the action potential, which generates a "late" sodium current (INa).[37] Late INa is sufficient to lead to a substantial influx of Na^+ into the cell in HF, with consequent prolongation of the action potential and early afterdepolarizations (EADs), which may be a significant source of increased arrhythmias in HF. High levels of intracellular Na^+ also may lead to cellular acidosis secondary to increased sodium-proton exchange activity. Increased intracellular Na^+ also influences the electrogenic driving forces for the NCX, thereby reducing Ca^{2+} extrusion through the forward mode of the NCX, which when combined with reduced activity of the SERCA2a pump, may be a cause of the elevated diastolic cytosolic calcium levels and disturbed diastolic function in HF. Inhibition of the late Na^+ current with the inhibitor ranolazine can improve disturbed diastolic function in isolated myocardium from failing human hearts and also may exhibit antiarrhythmic properties.[38] Of note, the different contributions to altered Ca^{2+} handling may vary significantly from patient to patient, which may explain some of the heterogeneity among different HF phenotypes. If SERCA2a expression is decreased and intracellular sodium is high, both systolic and diastolic function will be impaired. By contrast, higher NCX expression with moderately elevated intracellular Na^+ will result in excess transsarcolemmal calcium elimination, and diastolic function will be preserved. However, this may be associated with increased arrhythmias secondary to increased NCX activity.

Abnormalities in Contractile and Regulatory Proteins

Early studies showed that the activity of myofibrillar ATPase was reduced in the hearts of patients who died of HF. Furthermore, reductions in the activity of myofibrillar ATPase, actomyosin ATPase, or myosin ATPase have been demonstrated in several animal models of HF. Subsequent studies showed that these abnormalities in ATPase activity could be explained by a shift to the fetal isoform of myosin heavy chain (MHC) in cardiac hypertrophy and failure. In rodents the predominant MHC is the "fast" V1 isoform (alpha-MHC [MYHC6]), which has high ATPase activity. With pressure-induced hypertrophy or after MI in rodents, re-expression of the "slow" V3 fetal isoform of MHC that has low ATPase activity (beta-MHC [MYHC7]) and decreased expression of the V1 isoform have been observed. Although translating this information to human HF proved to be more challenging, because the predominant MHC isoform in humans is the slower V3 isoform (MYHC7), polymerase chain reaction (PCR) techniques have shown that MYHC6 accounts for approximately 33% of MHC mRNA in normal human myocardium, whereas MYHC6 mRNA abundance decreases to approximately 2% in failing hearts. Furthermore, when myocardial biopsy was performed in patients receiving beta blockers, reciprocal changes were observed in the levels of MYHC6 (increase) and MYHC7 (decrease) mRNA, and an increase in the MYHC6/MYHC7 ratio was noted in those who demonstrated an improvement in LV function. However, these changes in myosin isoform shifts did not occur in HF patients who showed no improvement in LV function with beta blockers. Thus the decreased expression of MYHC6 may play a significant role in the pathophysiology of dilated cardiomyopathy (DCM).

Another important modification of contractile proteins that contributes to contractile dysfunction is proteolysis of the myofilaments themselves (myocytolysis). Myocardial biopsy samples from patients with advanced LV dysfunction show a significant reduction in the volume of myofibrils per cell, which may contribute to the development of cardiac decompensation.

Alterations in the expression and/or activity of myofilament regulatory proteins also have been proposed as a potential mechanism for the decrease in cardiac contractile function in HF (Table 47.3), including the myosin light chains, the troponin-tropomyosin complex, and titin. Changes in myosin light chain isoforms have been observed in the

TABLE 47.3 Changes in the Biology of the Failing Myocyte

PROTEIN	CHANGE IN HUMAN HEART FAILURE
Plasma Membrane	
L-type calcium channels	Decreased*,†
Sodium/calcium exchanger	Increased*,†
Sodium pump	Reexpression of fetal isoforms
Beta₁-adrenergic receptor	Decreased*,†
Beta₂-adrenergic receptor	Increased*
Alpha₁-adrenergic receptor	Increased*
Contractile Proteins	
Myosin heavy chain (MHC)	Reversion to fetal isoform (↓MYHC6/MYHC7)
Myosin light chain (MLC)	Reversion to fetal isoform
Actin	Normal*
Titin	Isoform switch (↑N2BA/N2B), hypophosphorylated
Troponin I	Normal*, hypo- and hyperphosphorylated‡
Troponin T	Isoform switch, hyperphosphorylated‡
Troponin C	Normal*
Tropomyosin	Normal*
Sarcoplasmic Reticulum	
SERCA2a	Decreased*,†
Phospholamban	Hypophosphorylated
Ryanodine receptor	Hyperphosphorylated†
Calsequestrin	Normal*
Calreticulin	Normal*

*Refers to protein level.
†Refers to functional activity.
‡Hyperphosphorylation results in decreased Ca^{2+} sensitivity.
Modified from Katz AM. *Physiology of the Heart*. Philadelphia: Lippincott Williams & Wilkins; 2001.

atria and ventricles of patients whose hearts have been subjected to mechanical overload. Although changes in the abundance and/or isoforms of troponins TnI and TnC have not been reported in HF, isoform shifts have been reported in TnT (see Chapter 46). In normal adult myocardium, TnT is expressed as a single isoform (cTnT3). In myocardium samples from patients with end-stage HF, however, both the fetal cTnT1 and the cTnT4 isoforms are expressed at increased levels, which might be expected to lead to a decrease in maximal active tension. Changes in the titin (*TTN*) isoform from N2B, which is expressed postnatally and is stiffer, to N2BA, the more distensible fetal isoform, have been associated with increased compliance in hearts from patients with HF. As discussed in Chapter 52, truncating variants in *TTN* are common, and are associated with 10% to 20% of cases of DCM depending upon cohort studied (Fig. 52.4).

Abnormalities in Cytoskeletal Proteins

The cytoskeleton of cardiac myocytes consists of actin, the intermediate filament desmin, the sarcomeric protein titin (see Chapter 46), and alpha- and beta-tubulin, which form the microtubules by polymerization. Vinculin, talin, dystrophin, and spectrin constitute a separate group of membrane-associated proteins. In numerous experimental studies, a role for cytoskeletal and membrane-associated proteins has been implicated in the pathogenesis of HF. In patients with DCM, titin is downregulated, and the cytoskeletal proteins desmin and membrane-associated proteins such as vinculin and dystrophin are upregulated. Proteolytic digestion of the dystrophin molecule has been identified as a possible reversible cause of HF. Loss of integrity of the cytoskeleton and its linkage of the sarcomere to the sarcolemma and ECM would be expected to lead to contractile dysfunction at the myocyte level, as well as at the myocardial level.

Beta-Adrenergic Desensitization

Ventricles obtained from HF patients demonstrate a marked reduction in beta-adrenergic receptor density, isoproterenol-mediated adenyl cyclase stimulation, and the contractile response to beta-adrenergic agonists.[39] The downregulation of beta-adrenergic receptors is likely mediated by increased levels of NE in the vicinity of the receptor. In patients with DCM, this reduction in receptor density involves primarily the beta1-receptor protein and mRNA and is proportional to the severity of HF. In contrast, the level of beta2-adrenergic receptor protein and mRNA are unchanged or increased. In addition, there are increases in the expression of beta-adrenergic receptor kinase 1 (βARK1, also called G protein–coupled receptor kinase 2 [GRK2]), a member of the family of GPCR kinases, in failing human hearts. As noted in Chapter 46, βARK phosphorylates the cytoplasmic loops of both beta1- and beta2-adrenergic receptors and increases the affinity of these receptors for a scaffolding protein termed beta-arrestin (see Fig. 46.14). The binding of beta-arrestins to the cytoplasmic tail of the beta receptor not only uncouples the receptor from heterotrimeric G proteins, but also targets the receptor for internalization in clathrin-coated vesicles. Although this internalization fosters receptor dephosphorylation and serves as a prelude to recycling the beta receptor to the surface for reactivation, at some point receptor entry via endocytosis is not followed by recycling, but rather leads to receptor trafficking to lysosomes and receptor degradation. Increased βARK (GRK2) activity may therefore contribute to the desensitization of both beta1 and beta2 receptors in patients with HF. Desensitization of the beta receptors can be both beneficial and deleterious in HF; by reducing LV contractility, desensitization may be deleterious. However, by reducing energy expenditure of the energy-starved myocardium and protecting the myocyte from the deleterious effects of sustained adrenergic stimulation, this adaptive response is beneficial. Interestingly, lymphocyte GRK2 protein levels were shown to be independent predictors of cardiovascular mortality in patients with HF and added prognostic and clinical value over demographic and clinical variables.[40]

Alterations in the Myocardium

The changes that occur in failing myocardium may be categorized broadly into those that occur in the volume of cardiac myocytes and those that occur in the volume and composition of the ECM. For changes in the myocyte component of the myocardium, increasing evidence suggests that progressive myocyte loss, through necrotic, apoptotic, or cell death pathways linked to autophagy, may contribute to progressive cardiac dysfunction and LV remodeling.

NECROSIS

Although necrosis initially was thought to be a "passive" form of cell death, emerging evidence indicates that necrotic cell death also is "regulated."[41] The relative proportion of unregulated versus regulated necrotic death in the heart is not currently known; however, regulated necrosis is an important component of MI, HF, and cerebrovascular accident (stroke). The hallmark features of necrosis are loss of plasma membrane integrity and depletion of cellular adenosine triphosphate (ATP). Dysfunction of the plasma membrane in necrotic cells leads to cell swelling and rupture. There is also swelling of organelles such as the mitochondria. In the heart, increased plasma membrane permeability allows Ca^{2+} to leak into the cell, exposing the contractile proteins to very high concentrations of this activator, which in turn initiates extreme interactions between the myofilaments (contraction bands), further contributing to disruption of the cellular membrane. Necrotic myocyte death occurs in ischemic heart disease, myocardial injury, toxin exposure (e.g., daunorubicin; see Chapter 56), infection, and inflammation. Neurohormonal activation also can lead to necrotic cell death. For example, concentrations of NE available within myocardial tissue, as well as circulating levels in patients with advanced HF, are sufficient to provoke myocyte necrosis in experimental model systems. Moreover, excessive stimulation with angiotensin II, ET, or TNF has been shown to provoke myocyte necrosis in experimental models.

In contrast with apoptosis, the rupture of cell membranes with cell necrosis releases intracellular contents, which include the release of so-called danger-associated molecular patterns (DAMPs) that are sufficient to evoke an intense inflammatory reaction, leading to the influx of granulocytes, macrophages, and collagen-secreting fibroblasts into the area

of injury. The final result is a fibrotic scar, which may alter the structural and functional properties of the myocardium.[42] The regulated cell death pathways that have been studied thus far include TNF signaling through the type 1 TNF receptor (TNFR1) and opening of the mitochondrial permeability transition pore (MPTP) in the inner mitochondrial membrane, resulting in loss of the electrical potential difference (ΔΨm) across the inner mitochondrial membrane, leading to ATP depletion (eFig. 47.6A).

APOPTOSIS

Apoptosis, or programmed cell death, is an evolutionarily conserved process that allows multicellular organisms to selectively remove cells through a highly regulated program of cell suicide. Apoptosis is mediated by two pathways (eFig. 47.6B). The extrinsic pathway uses cell surface receptors, whereas the intrinsic pathway involves the mitochondria and endoplasmic reticulum (ER), and each of these pathways leads to caspase activation. In addition, connections between the pathways amplify signals, increasing the efficiency of killing. The intrinsic pathway is responsible for transducing most apoptotic stimuli, including those caused by inadequate nutrients or survival factors, hypoxia, oxidative stress, nutrient stress, proteotoxic stress, DNA damage, and chemical and physical toxins. These stimuli ultimately converge at the mitochondria to trigger the release of apoptogenic proteins, such as cytochrome c, and at the ER to stimulate the release of luminal Ca^{2+}.[43] Apoptosis plays important roles in development and in postnatal life, when it is critical for tissue homeostasis and surveillance for damaged or transformed cells. However, under pathologic circumstances, such as acute ischemia and in DCM, the apoptotic program can be triggered inappropriately, resulting in inadvertent cell death that can lead to organ failure. In contrast with the cell swelling that characterizes necrosis, during apoptosis the cell shrinks and eventually breaks up into small, membrane-surrounded fragments. The latter often contain bits of condensed chromatin referred to as apoptotic bodies. Maintenance of plasma membrane integrity until late in the apoptotic process allows the dying cell to be engulfed by macrophages, which prevents the release of the reactive intracellular contents, thereby preventing an inflammatory reaction.

Cardiac myocyte apoptosis has been shown to occur in failing human hearts.[44] Indeed, many of the factors implicated in the pathogenesis of HF, including catecholamines acting through beta1-adrenergic receptor, angiotensin II, ROS including NO, inflammatory cytokines (e.g., TNF), and mechanical strain, have been shown to trigger apoptosis in vitro. Moreover, activation of either the extrinsic or the intrinsic cell death pathway provokes progressive LV dilation and decompensation in transgenic mice.[45] Nonetheless, the exact physiologic significance and consequence(s) of apoptosis in human HF have been difficult to determine because of the uncertainty about the actual rate of cardiac myocyte apoptosis in the failing human heart.[44] The aggregate clinical and experimental data, however, suggest that apoptosis is likely to play an important role in HF.

AUTOPHAGY

Autophagy refers to the homeostatic cellular process of sequestering organelles, proteins, and lipids in a double-membrane vesicle inside the cell (autophagosome), where the contents are subsequently delivered to the lysosome for degradation. Unlike necrosis and apoptosis, autophagy is primarily a survival mechanism that regulates the quality and abundance of intracellular proteins and organelles. In mammalian cells, autophagy serves two physiologic purposes: one is to continuously degrade intracellular proteins at low levels, referred to as "basal or constitutive autophagy," which is responsible for clearance of excess or damaged organelles thereby maintaining the quality of essential intracellular components. The second purpose is to supply amino acids that are requisite for cell survival during conditions of environmental stress (e.g., nutrient deprivation), referred to as "adaptive autophagy." Prior studies have established a critical role for basal autophagy in the heart.[46] Accumulation of autophagosomes and autophagic substrates are increased in human HF.[47] Insufficient autophagy in the heart can lead to shortage of properly functioning intracellular organelles; moreover, accumulation of damaged mitochondria and damaged proteins can lead, respectively, to increased oxidative stress and increased ER stress. Autophagy can also induce cell death with distinctive morphologic characteristics and mechanisms of regulation, referred to as autosis.[48] Autosis has several unique morphologic features that differentiate it from necrosis and apoptosis, including increased autophagosomes/autolysosomes, as well as focal swelling of the perinuclear space at late stages. Experimental studies have shown that autosis contributes to cardiac myocyte cell death and increased myocardial injury following ischemia reperfusion injury in the heart.[48] Of note autosis is inhibited by in vitro and in vivo by Na+,K+-ATPase antagonists, such as cardiac glycosides. The role of autosis in the pathogenesis of HF remains to be determined.

Although the distinction between necrosis and apoptosis is apparent in certain circumstances, it often is less clear in the failing heart. Indeed, similar mechanisms can operate in both types of cell death. Thus, instead of the existence of distinct types of cell death in HF, a more likely scenario is a continuum of cell death responses that contribute to progressive myocyte loss and disease progression.

Alterations in the ECM constitute the second important myocardial adaptation that occurs during cardiac remodeling. The myocardial ECM consists of a basement membrane, a fibrillar collagen network that surrounds the myocytes, proteoglycans and glycosaminoglycans, and specialized proteins such as matricellular proteins. The major fibrillar collagens in the heart are types I and III, with a type I/III ratio of approximately 1.3:1 to 1.9:1. The organization of myocardial fibrillar type I and type III collagen ensures the structural integrity of adjoining myocytes and is essential for maintaining alignment of myofibrils within the myocyte through the interaction of collagen and integrins and the cytoskeletal proteins (Fig. 47.11A). *Matricellular proteins* are a class of nonstructural ECM proteins exerting regulatory functions, most likely through their interactions with cell surface receptors, the structural proteins, and soluble extracellular factors such as growth factors and cytokines. *Osteopontin* (OPN [Eta-1]) is a matricellular protein that is expressed in various cell types, including cardiac myocytes and fibroblasts and myofibroblasts (Fig. 47.11B). Because of its localization and molecular properties, OPN is likely to be involved in the communication between the ECM and cardiac myocytes, which implies a role in cardiac remodeling after hemodynamic overloading. OPN is markedly upregulated in animal models of cardiac hypertrophy and failure and myocardial ischemia and in the hearts of patients with DCM. OPN is elevated in the peripheral circulation of patients in direct relation to HF disease severity.[49]

During cardiac remodeling, important alterations in the ECM include changes in fibrillar collagen synthesis and degradation (Fig. 47.12) and in the degree of collagen cross-linking, as well as loss of collagen struts that connect the individual cardiac myocytes. Markers of collagen turnover have been shown to be increased in patients with DCM compared with age-matched controls.[50] In patients with idiopathic or ischemic DCM, serum N-terminal peptide type III collagen propeptide (PIIINP) levels have been shown to be independent predictors of mortality.[51] In the RALES trial (see Chapter 50), serum C-terminal peptide type I collagen propeptide (PIP) and PIIINP were decreased in the spironolactone-treated patients but not in the placebo group, suggesting that aldosterone may play an important role in ECM synthesis. Moreover, it is becoming increasingly apparent that the three-dimensional organization of the ECM plays an important role in regulating cardiac structure and function in HF.

CARDIAC FIBROBLASTS AND MAST CELLS

The cardiac fibroblast, which accounts for almost 90% of nonmyocyte cells in the heart, is the primary cell type that is responsible for the secretion of a majority of ECM components in the heart, such as collagens I, III, and IV and laminin and fibronectin. In response to mechanical stress and neurohormonal activation and inflammation, a subset of fibroblasts undergoes phenotypic conversion to myofibroblasts that are characterized by increased expression of α-smooth muscle actin and enhanced secretory activity. Recent studies have shown that myofibroblasts, which are responsible for the collagen secretion and contraction/realignment of the nascent collagen fibers, arise from tissue-resident fibroblasts that become activated after tissue injury.[52] Myofibroblasts migrate into the area surrounding tissue and play an important role in the final scar formation. Cardiac myofibroblasts also may regulate the phenotype of cardiac myocytes through multiple paracrine signaling pathways (Fig. 47.11B). Several lines of evidence suggest that cardiac fibroblasts and myocytes release proteins that regulate neighboring cells.[53] The proteins that have been implicated thus far include transforming growth factor-β1 (TGF-β1), fibroblast growth factor-2 (FGF2), members of the IL-6 family, and the recently discovered cytokine IL-33. Increasing evidence also suggests that mast cells, which are bone marrow–derived cells that "home" to and reside in the myocardium, also play an important role in remodeling of the

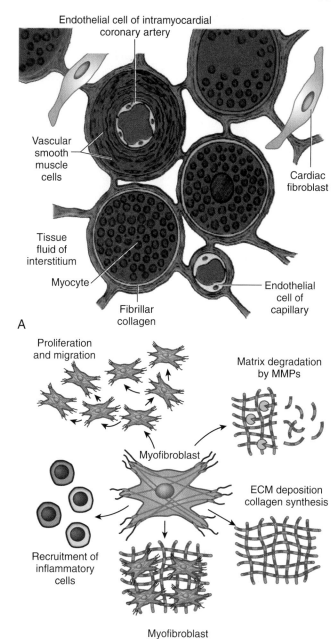

A

B

FIGURE 47.11 Extracellular matrix in heart failure. **A,** Although myocytes are the major components of heart on the basis of mass, they represent only a minority on the basis of number. Nonmyocyte cellular constituents of the myocardium include fibroblasts, smooth muscle cells, and endothelial cells. Myocytes and nonmyocytes are interconnected by a complex of connective tissue and extracellular matrix (ECM). Components of ECM include collagens, proteoglycans, glycoproteins (e.g., fibronectin), several peptide growth factors, and proteases (e.g., plasminogen activators) and collagenases (e.g., matrix metalloproteinases [MMPs]). **B,** Interactions among cardiac fibroblasts, myocytes, and ECM. In response to biomechanical stress, peptide growth factors in ECM and adjacent cardiac fibroblasts release an ensemble of peptide growth factors that activate hypertrophic signaling pathways in cardiac myocytes. Activated cardiac myofibroblasts express elevated levels of various proinflammatory and profibrotic factors that directly contribute to inflammatory cell infiltration and fibroblast proliferation, secrete high levels of MMPs and other ECM-degrading enzymes that facilitate fibroblast migration, and contribute to the deposition of collagen and other ECM proteins, leading to scar formation. (**A** modified from Weber KT, Brilla CG. Pathological hypertrophy and cardiac interstitium. *Circulation.* 1991;83:1849; **B** from Travers JG, Kamal FA, Robbins J, et al. Cardiac fibrosis: the fibroblast awakens. *Circ Res.* 2016;118:1021–1240. Copyright 2016 American Heart Association.)

ECM. Myocardial mast cells are located mainly around blood vessels and between myocytes, where they are capable of releasing profibrotic cytokines and growth factors that influence ECM remodeling. In experimental studies, mast cells that are recruited to the heart during inflammation were responsible for TGF-β1–mediated fibroblast activation, myocardial fibrosis, and LV diastolic dysfunction.[54]

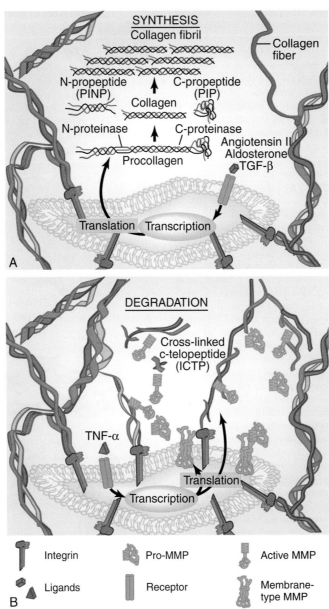

FIGURE 47.12 Collagen synthesis and degradation. **A,** Intracellular signals generated by neurohormonal and/or mechanical stimulation of cardiac fibroblasts results in transcription and translation of nascent collagen proteins containing amino terminal (N-terminal) and carboxyl terminal (C-terminal) propeptides that prevent collagen from assembling into mature fibrils. Once secreted into the interstitium, these propeptides are cleaved by N- and C-proteinases, yielding two procollagen fragments and a mature triple-stranded collagen molecule. In the case of collagen type I, these propeptides are referred to as N-terminal peptide type I collagen propeptide (PINP) and C-terminal peptide type I collagen propeptide (PIP). Removal of the propeptide sequences allows the secreted collagen molecule to integrate into growing collagen fibrils, which can then further assemble into collagen fibers. After the collagen fibrils form in the extracellular space, their tensile strength is greatly strengthened by the formation of covalent cross-links between the lysine residues on the collagen molecules. **B,** The degradation of the collagen matrix within the myocardium entails a number of biochemical events involving several protease systems. Degradation of collagen fibrils occurs through catalytic cleavage of the three collagen alpha chains at a single locus by interstitial collagenase, yielding 36-kDa and 12-kDa collagen telopeptides that maintain their helical structure and thus are resistant to further proteolytic degradation. The large 36-kDa telopeptide spontaneously denatures into nonhelical gelatin derivatives, which in turn are completely degraded by interstitial gelatinases. The small 12-kDa pyridinoline cross-linked C-terminal telopeptide resulting from the cleavage of collagen type I (ICTP) is found intact in blood, where it appears to be derived from tissues, with a stoichiometric ratio of 1:1 between the number of collagen type I molecules degraded and that of ICTP released. (From Deschamps AM, Spinale FG. Extracellular matrix. In: Walsh RA, ed. *Molecular Mechanisms of Cardiac Hypertrophy and Failure.* Boca Raton, FL: Taylor & Francis; 2005:101–116.)

As noted earlier, one of the histologic signatures of advancing HF is the progressive increase in collagen content of the heart (myocardial fibrosis). Studies in failing human myocardium have shown a quantitative increase in collagen types I, III, VI, and IV, along with fibronectin, laminin, and vimentin, and a decrease in the type I/III collagen ratio in patients with ischemic cardiomyopathy. Moreover, clinical studies show a progressive loss of cross-linking of collagen in the failing heart, as well as loss of connectivity of the collagen network with individual myocytes, which would be expected to result in profound alterations in LV structure and function. Furthermore, loss of cross-linking of the fibrillar collagen has been associated with progressive LV dilation after myocardial injury. The accumulation of collagen can occur on a "reactive" basis around intramural coronary arteries and arterioles (perivascular fibrosis) or in the interstitial space (interstitial fibrosis) and does not require myocyte cell death (eFig. 47.7). Alternatively, collagen accumulation can occur as a result of microscopic scarring, which develops in response to cardiac myocyte cell death. This scarring or "replacement fibrosis" is an adaptation to the loss of parenchyma and is therefore critical to preserve the structural integrity of the heart. The increased fibrous tissue would be expected to lead to increased myocardial stiffness, which presumably would result in decreased myocardial shortening for a given degree of afterload. In addition, myocardial fibrosis may provide the structural substrate for atrial and ventricular arrhythmias, thus potentially contributing to inhomogeneous activation, bundle branch block, and dyssynchrony, as well as sudden death (see Chapter 70). Although the full complement of molecules responsible for fibroblast activation is not known, many of the classic neurohormones (e.g., angiotensin II, aldosterone) and cytokines (ET, TGF-β, cardiotrophin-1) that are expressed in HF are sufficient to provoke fibroblast activation. Studies in patients with aortic valve replacement for aortic stenosis have shown that the baseline burden of myocardial fibrosis was associated with worse LV function, a greater degree of pathologic LV remodeling, and more pronounced HF symptoms. Moreover, burden of myocardial fibrosis was an independent predictor of all-cause and cardiovascular mortality after transcatheter aortic valve implantation.[55] Indeed, the use of ACE inhibitors, beta blockers, and aldosterone receptor antagonists has been associated with a decrease in myocardial fibrosis in experimental HF models and in human HF.[56]

Although the fibrillar collagen matrix initially was thought to form a relatively static complex, it is now recognized that these structural proteins can undergo rapid turnover. A major development in understanding the pathogenesis of cardiac remodeling was the discovery that a family of collagenolytic enzymes, the *matrix metalloproteinases*, is activated within the failing myocardium. Conceptually, ECM disruption would be expected to lead to LV dilation and wall thinning as a result of mural realignment of myocyte bundles and within the LV wall, as well as LV dysfunction as a result of dyssynchronous contraction of the left ventricle. Although the precise biochemical triggers responsible for activation of MMPs are not known, TNF and other cytokines and peptide growth factors expressed within the failing myocardium are capable of activating MMPs.

However, the biology of matrix remodeling in HF is likely to be much more complex than the simple presence or absence of MMP activation because degradation of the matrix also is controlled by glycoproteins termed *tissue inhibitors of matrix metalloproteinases (TIMPs)*. TIMPs are

capable of regulating the activation of MMPs by binding to and preventing these enzymes from degrading the collagen matrix of the heart. The TIMP family at present consists of four distinct members, TIMP-1, -2, -3, and -4, each of which is constitutively expressed in the heart by fibroblasts as well as myocytes. TIMPs are secreted proteins that act as the natural inhibitors of active forms of all MMPs, although the efficiency of MMP inhibition varies among the different members. The extant literature suggests that MMP activation can lead to progressive LV dilation, whereas TIMP expression favors progressive myocardial fibrosis. For more information see the online supplement "Matrix Metalloproteinases and Tissue Inhibitors of Metalloproteinases."

NONCODING RNAS

Once considered "transcriptional noise," noncoding RNAs have emerged as potential biomarkers as well as therapeutic targets in HF. The noncoding portion of the genome is actively transcribed, generating thousands of regulatory short and long noncoding RNAs that are capable of regulating gene networks. Noncoding RNAs are classified based on their length. Small noncoding RNAs are less than 200 nucleotides in size and include both small interfering RNAs (siRNAs) and microRNAs (miRNAs). Transcripts larger than 200 nucleotides are called long noncoding RNAs (lncRNAs). MicroRNAs are involved in virtually all cellular processes. The lncRNAs also regulate gene and protein levels but through more complicated and diverse mechanisms.

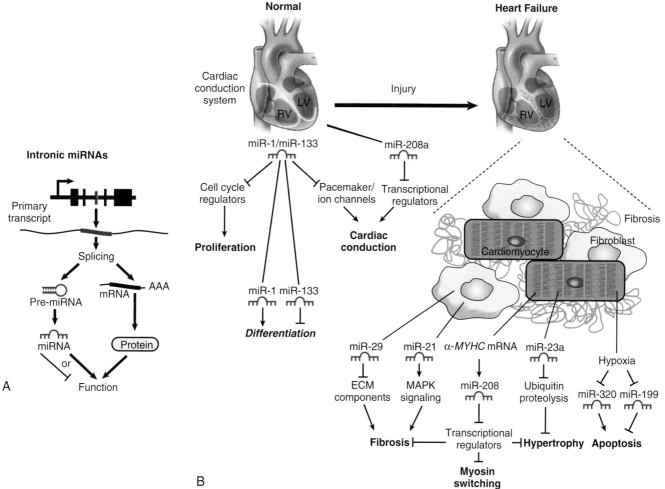

FIGURE 47.13 MicroRNAs (miRNAs) and the heart. **A,** The potential modes of miRNA-based regulation of gene expression are illustrated. Intronic microRNAs are encoded within an intron of a host gene. Messenger RNA splicing generates a protein coding transcript and a microRNA stem-loop. A common mechanism of miRNA function involves the modest repression of several mRNAs in a common biologic process by a single miRNA, most commonly through transcriptional silencing, or through enhanced mRNA degradation. Intronic miRNAs often regulate similar processes to that of the protein encoded by the host gene. *AAA,* Polyadenylated tail of the transcript; pre-miRNA, precursor miRNA. **B,** Functional role of miRNAs in the normal and failing heart. A normal heart and a hypertrophic/failing heart are shown in schematic form, depicting miRNAs that contribute to normal function or pathologic remodeling. All *arrows* denote the normal action of each component or process. The miRNAs miR-1 and miR-133 are involved in the development of a normal heart **(left)** by regulating proliferation, differentiation, and cardiac conduction. After cardiac injury **(right),** various miRNAs contribute to pathologic remodeling and the progression to heart failure: miR-29 blocks fibrosis by inhibiting the expression of extracellular matrix (ECM) components, whereas miR-21 promotes fibrosis; miR-208 controls myosin isoform switching, cardiac hypertrophy, and fibrosis; and miR-23a promotes cardiac hypertrophy by inhibiting ubiquitin proteolysis, which itself inhibits hypertrophy. Hypoxia results in the repression of miR-320 and miR-199, which promote and block apoptosis, respectively. (Modified from Small EM, Olson EN. Pervasive roles of microRNAs in cardiovascular biology. *Nature.* 2011;469:336.)

Experimental studies have shown that microRNAs have a profound effect on cardiac remodeling. MicroRNAs are noncoding RNAs that pair with specific "target" mRNAs and negatively regulate their expression through translational repression or mRNA degradation (gene silencing). The binding specificity of microRNAs depends on complementary base pairing of the approximately 6 nucleotide (nt) region at the 5′ end of the microRNA with the 3′ untranslated region (UTR) of the corresponding mRNA target. As shown in Figure 47.13A, binding of microRNAs to their cognate target mRNAs typically leads to decreased expression of target genes. Individual microRNAs modulate the expression of collections of mRNA targets that often have related functions, thereby governing complex biologic processes. Recent studies have suggested that microRNAs contribute to adverse or pathologic remodeling in experimental HF models.[57] As shown in Figure 47.13B, microRNAs regulate key components of the remodeling process, including cardiac myocyte biology, cell fate, ECM remodeling, and neurohormonal activation. Given that microRNAs are coordinately upregulated in response to stress signals, and that microRNAs regulate the expression levels of gene networks that determine the "heart failure phenotype," it is tempting to speculate that microRNAs, acting singly or in combination, may be responsible for modulating the transition from adaptive to pathologic cardiac remodeling. Moreover, it is possible that certain microRNAs may themselves become therapeutic targets using chemically modified oligonucleotides to target specific microRNAs and disrupt the binding between a specific microRNA and a specific mRNA target[57] Long noncoding RNAs are mechanistically more complex than microRNAs and likely modulate the genome at multiple different levels. For example, lncRNAs may interact with RNAs, proteins, and DNA and can either activate or silence the interaction with other molecules through conformational switching. Recent studies have shown that the profile of myocardial lncRNAs is altered in human HF, and that several lncRNAs are responsible for regulating cardiac structure and function following hemodynamic overload.[58] Inhibition of miR132, a non-coding microRNA that regulates cardiac hypertrophy and autophagy in cardiac myocytes using a synthetic locked nucleic acid antisense oligonucleotide inhibitor (antimiR-132 [CDR132L]), was shown to dose-dependently improve LV function in a large animal model of ischemic injury.[59] CDR132L has been shown to be safe in a phase I safety study in patients with NYHA class I-III HF (NCT04045405), and will be studied in a forthcoming phase II clinical trial in patients with acute myocardial infarction.

Alterations in Left Ventricular Structure

The alterations in the biology of the failing myocyte, as well as in the failing myocardium, are largely responsible for the progressive LV dilation and dysfunction that occur during cardiac remodeling. Many of the structural changes that accompany LV remodeling may contribute to worsening HF (**eTable 47.2**). Indeed, one of the first observations regarding the abnormal geometry of remodeled ventricle was the consistent finding that the remodeled heart was not only larger but also more spherical in shape. An important point in this context is that a change in LV shape from a prolate ellipse to a more spherical shape results in an increase in meridional wall stress of the left ventricle, thereby creating a de novo energetic burden for the failing heart. Because the load on the ventricle at end-diastole contributes importantly to the afterload on the ventricle at the onset of systole, LV dilation itself will increase mechanical energy expenditure of the ventricle, which exacerbates the underlying problems with energy utilization in the failing ventricle (Fig. 47.14).

CARDIAC ENERGETICS AND MITOCHONDRIAL BIOLOGY

Energy transfer in the cardiac myocyte occurs in three stages: uptake and metabolism, energy production through oxidative phosphorylation, and energy transfer by means of the creatine kinase (CK) shuttle (**eFig. 47.8**). Each stage of this process can lead to contractile dysfunction of the heart. Studies in patients with end-stage cardiomyopathy have shown that myocardial ATP concentration, the total adenine nucleotide pool (ATP, ADP, and AMP), CK activity (required for synthesis of ATP), creatine phosphate (CrP) concentration, and CrP/ATP ratio are all decreased in HF. In addition, decreased levels of creatine phosphokinase have been reported, which would slow phosphocreatine shuttle, further exacerbating energy utilization in the failing heart.[60] Thus, in the failing heart, key components of the cardiac energetic system are downregulated. It is unclear at present, however, whether these energetic changes are biomarkers or drivers of LV dysfunction.

Although several mechanisms have been proposed to explain the fall in ATP content in HF, one mechanism that has received considerable attention relates to changes in substrate utilization in HF. Under normal conditions, the adult heart derives most of its energy through oxidation of fatty acids in mitochondria. The genes involved in this key energy

metabolic pathway are transcriptionally regulated by members of the nuclear receptor superfamily, specifically the fatty acid–activated peroxisome proliferator–activated receptors (PPARs) and the nuclear receptor coactivator, PPAR-gamma coactivator-1α (PGC-1α). In experimental HF models, an initial decrease is seen in the oxidation of fatty acids secondary to downregulation of fatty acid–metabolizing genes, with a resultant shift toward glycolytic metabolism. Recent studies indicate that enhanced myocardial ketone use may be adaptive in HF; moreover, provisional studies in experimental models of HF and humans with HF have suggested a role for exogenous ketone therapy.[61] These observations have given rise to the suggestion that metabolic modulation may be beneficial in HF. Trimetazidine, which is a direct inhibitor of myocardial fatty acid oxidation has been approved for human use for the treatment of angina pectoris and myocardial ischemia. Clinical trials and several meta-analyses have shown that when trimetazidine is added to conventional HF therapy, it leads to improvements in NYHA functional class, LV end-systolic volume, and LV ejection fraction.[62] Trimetazidine is recommended in the ESC/HFA 2016 guidelines for the treatment of angina pectoris not responsive to beta blocker in HFrEF patients (class IIb, level of evidence A). There is no recommendation for trimetazidine in the setting of HF alone.[63]

In addition to loss of substrate, ATP generation may be impaired in the failing heart secondary to abnormalities in mitochondrial dynamics.[64] The number of mitochondria are determined through biogenic renewal and by autophagic removal (mitophagy). Studies in yeast have demonstrated that maintaining normal mitochondrial morphology and function depends on the dynamic balance of mitochondrial *fusion* and *fission* (division), collectively called "mitochondrial dynamics." The balance between mitochondrial fusion and fission determines the number, morphology, and activity of mitochondria in the heart. Fusion and fission modulate multiple mitochondrial functions, ranging from energy and ROS production to Ca^{2+} homeostasis and cell death through apoptosis programmed necrosis. Although studies in human HF are limited, data suggest that mitochondrial fusion may be reduced, which would be predicted to lead to reduced O_2 consumption and alterations in mitochondrial metabolism. Of note, abnormally small and fragmented mitochondria have been observed in end-stage DCM, myocardial hibernation, and congenital heart disease, suggesting that mitochondrial fusion/fission becomes dysregulated in cardiac disease. However, the contribution of abnormalities in mitochondrial fission/fusion in HF as a cause versus a consequence of myocardial injury remains unknown. The phase II PROGRESS-HF clinical trial, which was a randomized trial that used a mitochondrial-targeting protein (elamipretide) that enhances mitochondrial ATP synthesis and prevents mitochondrial fragmentation, did not improve LV function at 4 weeks in patients with stable HFrEF when compared with placebo.[65]

LV wall thinning also occurs as the ventricle begins to dilate and remodel. The increase in wall thinning along with the increase in afterload created by LV dilation leads to a functional "afterload mismatch" that may further contribute to a decrease in forward cardiac output. Increased LV wall stress also can lead to sustained expression of stretch-activated genes (angiotensin II, ET, TNF) and stretch activation of hypertrophic signaling pathways. Moreover, the high end-diastolic wall stress might be expected to lead to episodic hypoperfusion of the subendocardium with resultant worsening of LV function, as well as increased oxidative stress, with the resultant activation of gene families that are sensitive to free radical generation (e.g., TNF, IL-1β). Another important mechanical problem from progressive LV dilation is that the papillary muscles are pulled apart, resulting in incompetence of the mitral valve and development of "functional mitral regurgitation." In addition to the loss of forward blood flow, mitral regurgitation results in further hemodynamic volume overloading of the ventricle. Together, the mechanical burdens engendered by LV remodeling might lead to increased LV dilation, decreased forward cardiac output, and increased hemodynamic overloading (see Fig. 47.14), any of which is sufficient to contribute to worsening LV function independent of the patient's neurohormonal status.

REVERSIBILITY OF LEFT VENTRICULAR REMODELING AND RECOVERY OF LEFT VENTRICULAR FUNCTION

Clinical studies have shown that medical and device therapies that reduce HF morbidity and mortality also lead to decreased LV volume and mass and restore a more normal elliptical shape to the ventricle. These salutary changes represent the summation of a series of integrated biologic changes in cardiac myocyte size and function (**eTable 47.3**),

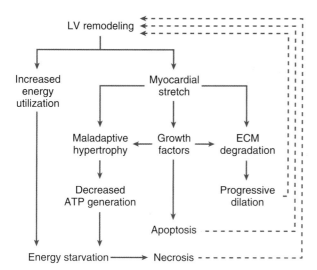

FIGURE 47.14 Self-amplifying nature of left ventricular (LV) remodeling. LV remodeling results in increased afterload on the heart, which increases energy utilization and further stimulates cardiac growth through stretch-mediated activation of growth factors. The former contributes directly to a state of energy starvation, whereas the latter contributes to further cardiac remodeling, including increased myocyte hypertrophy and further matrix remodeling. The sustained activation of growth stimuli also promotes apoptosis and myocardial fibrosis, which contribute to LV dysfunction and LV remodeling. (Modified from Katz AM. *Heart failure.* Philadelphia: Lippincott Williams & Wilkins; 2000.)

as well as modifications in LV structure and organization that are accompanied by shifts of the LV end-diastolic pressure-volume relationship toward normal. For want of better terminology, these changes are collectively referred to as "reverse LV remodeling." In the context of the present discussion, reverse LV remodeling refers to the restoration of more normal cardiac myocyte size and LV chamber geometry, resulting in a leftward shift of the end-diastolic pressure volume relationship toward normal values.[66] Importantly, reverse LV remodeling is associated with improved myocyte contractility and improved LV chamber contractility. It is important to recognize that reverse LV remodeling is associated with fewer HF hospitalizations and decreased cardiovascular mortality, and that there is a direct correlation between the extent of reverse LV remodeling and the improvement in cardiac survival.[66] Insofar as the calculation of LV ejection fraction incorporates LV end-diastolic volume in the denominator of the equation, decreases in LV end-diastolic volume are associated with a reciprocal increase in LV ejection fraction.

Although the biological basis for reverse LV remodeling and recovery of LV function is incompletely understood, several general concepts have emerged. The most prominent theme is that cardiac remodeling is a dynamic process that occurs in a bidirectional manner (i.e. forward and reverse), and that cardiac remodeling involves the coordinated regulation of multiple molecular and cellular changes that contribute to phenotypic changes in the size, shape, and function of the heart. Basic and clinical studies have consistently shown that many of the cellular and anatomic changes that occur during forward LV remodeling revert toward the normal less pathologic phenotype during reverse LV remodeling. Moreover, studies that have examined serial changes in gene expression during reverse LV remodeling have shown the normalization of gene transcription related to myocyte contractility occur before changes in genes related to the ECM, suggesting that return of myocyte function is required for reversal of the changes in LV geometry in the failing heart.[67] In addition to changes in adult cardiac myocytes during reverse LV remodeling, there are a number of important changes that occur within the myocardial ECM.[68] A second important theme, which has direct bearing on the concept of myocardial remission (discussed below), is that many of the multilevel molecular changes that occur during forward LV remodeling remain dysregulated in reverse remodeled hearts, despite improvements in structural and functional abnormalities. Transcriptional profiling of reverse remodeled hearts reveals the emergence of new sets of genes that belong to ontogenies that are not expressed in non-failing hearts.[69] Viewed together, these findings suggest that reverse LV remodeling is not simply a mirror image of the

molecular and cellular pathways that become dysregulated during forward LV remodeling, but rather that reverse LV remodeling represents a coordinated multilevel process that allows the heart to adopt a new, less pathologic steady state that is associated with improved pump function and improved clinical prognosis.

Interestingly, in recognized subsets of patients, the heart undergoes reverse LV remodeling with recovery of LV function either spontaneously or after medical and device therapies or valve replacement. The recognition that LV ejection fraction improves substantially in a subset of HFrEF patients who are treated with evidenced-based medical and device therapies has led to intense interest in their outcomes and clinical management (discussed in Chapter 48).

Importantly, the subsequent clinical course of these patients is associated with fewer future HF events.[66] Recent studies have shown that, even among patients who experience complete normalization of LV function and LV structure after implementation of guideline directed medical therapies, a significant proportion of patients with a recovered LV ejection will develop recurrent LV dysfunction and recurrent HF events. The biological explanation for why some HFrecEF patients become stable clinically for prolonged periods ("myocardial remission"),[66] and why some HFrecEF patients, with similar improvements in LV structure and function "relapse" and redevelop clinical signs and symptoms of HF with recurrent LV dysfunction events is not known, but represents a significant unmet clinical need, as well as significant financial burden for health care systems that have to manage HF readmissions. One plausible explanation for this phenomenon, which is based on the consistent finding that the reverse remodeled heart retains many of the molecular features of the failing heart, is that reverse LV remodeling represents a transition to a new less pathologic steady state that allows the heart to maintain LV pump function under normal conditions, but that this adaptation has less biological and contractile reserve capacity, and is therefore more prone to redevelop LV dysfunction in response to hemodynamic, neurohormonal, or environmental stress.

FUTURE PERSPECTIVES

The clinical syndrome of HF can be considered in terms of several different clinical model systems, including cardiorenal, hemodynamic, and neurohormonal. Each of the models has strengths and weaknesses in explaining the mechanisms responsible for HF, as well as in developing effective new therapies for HF. Nonetheless, current models for explicating the mechanisms for HF are inadequate and do not adequately describe disease progression in HF. Moreover, they do not provide an adequate scaffold for understanding newer device therapies that appear to work through neurohormonally independent mechanisms. This emphasizes the importance of cardiac remodeling as a mechanism of disease progression in HF. Future therapeutic advances are likely to require a more comprehensive understanding and analysis of the pathobiology of HF, particularly cell-cell interactions during LV remodeling, as well as the complex interactions that govern the process of reverse LV remodeling. In this regard, the emerging field of systems biology, which uses network theory to describe how the interrelationships between genes, proteins, and metabolites determine functional changes at the level of the cell, tissue, and organ, may allow investigators to accelerate the pace of novel target identification, as well as improve the likelihood of success in clinical trials.

REFERENCES
Pathogenesis: Neurohormonal Mechanisms
1. Hartupee J, Mann DL. Neurohormonal activation in heart failure with reduced ejection fraction. *Nat Rev Cardiol.* 2017;14(1):30–38.
2. Notarius CF, Millar PJ, Floras JS. Muscle sympathetic activity in resting and exercising humans with and without heart failure. *Appl Physiol Nutr Metab.* 2015;40(11):1107–1115.
3. Floras JS, Ponikowski P. The sympathetic/parasympathetic imbalance in heart failure with reduced ejection fraction. *Eur Heart J.* 2015;36(30):1974-1982.
4. Anand IS, Konstam MA, Klein HU, et al. Comparison of symptomatic and functional responses to vagus nerve stimulation in ANTHEM-HF, INOVATE-HF, and NECTAR-HF *ESC Heart Fail.* 2020;7(1):75–83.
5. Ky B, Mann DL. COVID-19 clinical trials: a primer for the cardiovascular and cardio-oncology communities. *JACC Basic Transl Sci.* 2020;5(5):501–517.

6. Hartupee J, Mann DL. Positioning of inflammatory biomarkers in the heart failure landscape. *J Cardiovasc Transl Res*. 29013;6:485-492.

7. Hafstad AD, Nabeebaccus AA, Shah AM. Novel aspects of ROS signalling in heart failure. *Basic Res Cardiol*. 2013;108(4):359.

8. Givertz MM, Anstrom KJ, Redfield MM, et al. Effects of xanthine oxidase inhibition in hyperuricemic heart failure patients: the EXACT-HF study. *Circulation*. 2015;131:1763–1771.

9. Jennings DL, Kalus JS, O'Dell KM. Aldosterone receptor antagonism in heart failure. *Pharmacotherapy*. 2005;25(8):1126–1133.

10. Zile MR, Lindenfeld J, Weaver FA, et al. Baroreflex activation therapy in patients with heart failure with reduced ejection fraction. *J Am Coll Cardiol*. 2020;76(1):1–13.

11. Lee CY, Burnett JC Jr. Natriuretic peptides and therapeutic applications. *Heart Fail Rev*. 2007;12(2):131–142.

12. Volpe M, Rubattu S, Burnett J Jr. Natriuretic peptides in cardiovascular diseases: current use and perspectives. *Eur Heart J*. 2014;35(7):419–425.

13. Chen Y, Burnett JC Jr. Biochemistry, therapeutics, and biomarker implications of neprilysin in cardiorenal disease. *Clin Chem*. 2017;63(1):108–115.

14. Volpe M, Carnovali M, Mastromarino V. The natriuretic peptides system in the pathophysiology of heart failure: from molecular basis to treatment. *Clin Sci (Lond)*. 2016;130(2):57–77.

15. Armstrong PW, Pieske B, Anstrom KJ, et al. Vericiguat in patients with heart failure and reduced ejection fraction. *N Engl J Med*. 2020;382(20):1883–1893.

16. Carnicer R, Crabtree MJ, Sivakumaran V, et al. Nitric oxide synthases in heart failure. *Antioxid Redox Signal*. 2013;18(9):1078–1099.

17. Su JB. Different cross-talk sites between the renin-angiotensin and the kallikrein-kinin systems. *J Renin Angiotensin Aldosterone Syst*. 2014;15(4):319–328.

18. Yanagawa B, Nagaya N. Adrenomedullin: molecular mechanisms and its role in cardiac disease. *Amino Acids*. 2007;32(1):157–164.

19. Voors AA, Kremer D, Geven C, et al. Adrenomedullin in heart failure: pathophysiology and therapeutic application. *Eur J Heart Fail*. 2019;21(2):163–171.

20. Koguchi W, Kobayashi N, Takeshima H, et al. Cardioprotective effect of apelin-13 on cardiac performance and remodeling in end-stage heart failure. *Circ J*. 2012;76(1):137–144.

21. Ma Z, Song J, Martin S, et al. The Elabela-APJ axis: a promising therapeutic target for heart failure. *Heart Fail Rev*. 2020.

22. Packer M. Leptin-Aldosterone-Neprilysin axis: identification of its distinctive role in the pathogenesis of the three phenotypes of heart failure in people with obesity. *Circulation*. 2018;137(15):1614–1631.

23. Abel ED, Litwin SE, Sweeney G. Cardiac remodeling in obesity. *Physiol Rev*. 2008;88(2):389–419.

24. Adamo L, Rocha-Resende C, Prabhu SD, Mann DL. Reappraising the role of inflammation in heart failure. *Nat Rev Cardiol*. 2020;5(17):269–285.

25. Mann DL. Innate immunity and the failing heart: the cytokine hypothesis revisited. *Circ Res*. 2015;116(7):1254–1268.

26. Everett BM, Cornel J, Lainscak M, et al. Anti-Inflammatory therapy with canakinumab for the prevention of hospitalization for heart failure. *Circulation*. 2019;139:1289–1299.

Pathogenesis: Left Ventricular Remodeling

27. Hershberger RE, Morales A, Siegfried JD. Clinical and genetic issues in dilated cardiomyopathy: a review for genetics professionals. *Genet Med*. 2010;12(11):655–667.

28. Toischer K, Rokita AG, Unsold B, et al. Differential cardiac remodeling in preload versus afterload. *Circulation*. 2010;122(10):993–1003.

29. Dridi H, Kushnir A, Zalk R, et al. Intracellular calcium leak in heart failure and atrial fibrillation: a unifying mechanism and therapeutic target. *Nat Rev Cardiol*. 2020.

30. Lehnart SE, Maier LS, Hasenfuss G. Abnormalities of calcium metabolism and myocardial contractility depression in the failing heart. *Heart Fail Rev*. 2009;14(4):213–224.

31. Mohamed BA, Hartmann N, Tirilomis P, et al. Sarcoplasmic reticulum calcium leak contributes to arrhythmia but not to heart failure progression. *Sci Transl Med*. 2018;10(458):eaan0724.

32. Walweel K, Laver DR. Mechanisms of SR calcium release in healthy and failing human hearts. *Biophys Rev*. 2015;7(1):33–41.

33. Anderson DM, Makarewich CA, Anderson KM, et al. Widespread control of calcium signaling by a family of SERCA-inhibiting micropeptides. *Sci Signal*. 2016;9(457):ra119-.

34. Penny WF, Hammond HK. Randomized clinical trials of gene transfer for heart failure with reduced ejection fraction. *Hum Gene Ther*. 2017;28(5):378–384.

35. Guo A, Zhang C, Wei S, Chen B, Song L-S. Emerging mechanisms of T-tubule remodelling in heart failure. *Cardiovasc Res*. 2013;98(2):204–215.

36. Aiba T, Tomaselli GF. Electrical remodeling in the failing heart. *Curr Opin Cardiol*. 2010;25(1):29–36.

37. Moreno JD, Clancy CE. Pathophysiology of the cardiac late Na current and its potential as a drug target. *J Mol Cell Cardiol*. 2012;52(3):608–619.

38. Sossalla S, Wagner S, Rasenack EC, et al. Ranolazine improves diastolic dysfunction in isolated myocardium from failing human hearts—role of late sodium current and intracellular ion accumulation. *J Mol Cell Cardiol*. 2008;45(1):32–43.

39. Lohse MJ, Engelhardt S, Eschenhagen T. What is the role of beta-adrenergic signaling in heart failure? *Circ Res*. 2003;93(10):896–906.

40. Rengo G, Pagano G, Filardi PP, et al. Prognostic value of lymphocyte G protein-coupled receptor kinase-2 protein levels in patients with heart failure. *Circ Res*. 2016;118(7):1116–1124.

41. Konstantinidis K, Whelan RS, Kitsis RN. Mechanisms of cell death in heart disease. *Arterioscler Thromb Vasc Biol*. 2012;32(7):1552–1562.

42. Zhang W, Lavine KJ, Epelman S, et al. Necrotic myocardial cells release damage-associated molecular patterns that provoke fibroblast activation in vitro and trigger myocardial inflammation and fibrosis in vivo. *J Am Heart Assoc*. 2015;4(6):e001993.

43. Del Re DP, Amgalan D, Linkermann A, et al. Fundamental mechanisms of regulated cell death and implications for heart disease. *Physiol Rev*. 2019;99(4):1765–1817.

44. Abbate A, Narula J. Role of apoptosis in adverse ventricular remodeling. *Heart Fail Clin*. 2012;8(1):79–86.

45. Haudek SB, Taffet GE, Schneider MD, Mann DL. TNF provokes cardiomyocyte apoptosis and cardiac remodeling through activation of multiple cell death pathways. *J Clin Invest*. 2007;117(9):2692–2701.

46. Nakai A, Yamaguchi O, Takeda T, et al. The role of autophagy in cardiomyocytes in the basal state and in response to hemodynamic stress. *Nat Med*. 2007;13(5):619–624.

47. Hartupee J, Szalai GD, Wang W, et al. Impaired protein quality control during left ventricular remodeling in mice with cardiac restricted overexpression of tumor necrosis factor. *Circ Heart Fail*. 2017;10(12).

48. Sciarretta S, Maejima Y, Zablocki D, Sadoshima J. The role of autophagy in the heart. *Annu Rev Physiol*. 2017.

49. Rosenberg M, Meyer FJ, Gruenig E, et al. Osteopontin predicts adverse right ventricular remodelling and dysfunction in pulmonary hypertension. *Eur J Clin Invest*. 2012;42(9):933–942.

50. Spinale FG, Zile MR. Integrating the myocardial matrix into heart failure recognition and management. *Circ Res*. 2013;113(6):725–738.

51. Zannad F, Rossignol P, Iraqi W. Extracellular matrix fibrotic markers in heart failure. *Heart Fail Rev*. 2010;15(4):319–329.

52. Kanisicak O, Khalil H, Ivey MJ, et al. Genetic lineage tracing defines myofibroblast origin and function in the injured heart. *Nat Commun*. 2016;7:12260.

53. Kakkar R, Lee RT. Intramyocardial fibroblast myocyte communication. *Circ Res*. 2010;106(1):47–57.

54. Zhang W, Chancey AL, Tzeng HP, et al. The development of myocardial fibrosis in transgenic mice with targeted overexpression of tumor necrosis factor requires mast cell-fibroblast interactions. *Circulation*. 2011;124:2106–2116.

55. Puls M, Beuthner BE, Topci R, et al. Impact of myocardial fibrosis on left ventricular remodelling, recovery, and outcome after transcatheter aortic valve implantation in different haemodynamic subtypes of severe aortic stenosis. *Eur Heart J*. 2020;41(20):1903–1914.

56. Wilcox JE, Mann DL. Beta-blockers for the treatment of heart failure with a mid-range ejection fraction: deja-vu all over again? *Eur Heart J*. 2018;39(1):36–38.

57. Small EM, Olson EN. Pervasive roles of microRNAs in cardiovascular biology. *Nature*. 2011;469(7330):336–342.

58. Thum T. Facts and updates about cardiovascular non-coding RNAs in heart failure. *ESC Heart Fail*. 2015;2(3):108–111.

59. Foinquinos A, Batkai S, Genschel C, et al. Preclinical development of a miR-132 inhibitor for heart failure treatment. *Nat Commun*. 2020;11(1):633.

60. Neubauer S. The failing heart—an engine out of fuel. *N Engl J Med*. 2007;356(11):1140–1151.

61. Selvaraj S, Kelly DP, Margulies KB. Implications of altered ketone metabolism and therapeutic ketosis in heart failure. *Circulation*. 2020;141(22):1800–1812.

62. Rosano GM, Vitale C. Metabolic modulation of cardiac metabolism in heart failure. *Card Fail Rev*. 2018;4(2):99–103.

63. Ponikowski P, Voors AA, Anker SD, et al. 2016 ESC Guidelines for the diagnosis and treatment of acute and chronic heart failure: the Task Force for the diagnosis and treatment of acute and chronic heart failure of the European Society of Cardiology (ESC) Developed with the special contribution of the Heart Failure Association (HFA) of the ESC. *Eur Heart J*. 2016;37:2129–2200.

64. Murphy E, Ardehali H, Balaban RS, et al. Mitochondrial function, biology, and role in disease: a scientific statement from the American Heart Association. *Circ Res*. 2016;118(12):1960–1991.

65. Butler J, Khan MS, Anker SD, et al. Effects of elamipretide on left ventricular function in patients with heart failure with reduced ejection fraction: the PROGRESS-HF Phase 2 trial. *J Card Fail*. 2020;26(5):429–437.

Reversibility of Heart Failure

66. Wilcox JE, Fang JC, Margulies KB, Mann DL. Heart failure with a recovered ejection fraction. *J Am Coll Cardiol*. 2020;76:719–734.

67. Weinheimer CJ, Kovacs A, Evans S, et al. Load-Dependent changes in left ventricular structure and function in a pathophysiologically relevant murine model of reversible heart failure. *Circ Heart Fail*. 2018;11(5):e004351.

68. Kim GH, Uriel N, Burkhoff D. Reverse remodelling and myocardial recovery in heart failure. *Nat Rev Cardiol*. 2018;15(2):83–96.

69. Margulies KB, Matiwala S, Cornejo C, et al. Mixed messages: transcription patterns in failing and recovering human myocardium. *Circ Res*. 2005;96:592–599.

48 Approach to the Patient with Heart Failure

JAMES L. JANUZZI JR. AND DOUGLAS L. MANN

HEART FAILURE DEFINITION AND EPIDEMIOLOGY

Heart failure (HF) is a complex clinical syndrome resulting from structural and functional impairment of ventricular filling or ejection of blood. While the clinical syndrome of HF may arise due to abnormalities or disorders involving all aspects of cardiac structure and function, most patients have impairment of myocardial function, ranging from normal ventricular size and function to marked dilation and reduced function. While symptoms of HF frequently depend on the presence of elevated left or right heart filling pressures, the term "congestive" HF is no longer preferred, as many patients do not have overt congestion at the time of evaluation, and their symptoms may be due to reduction in cardiac output, for example.

The global incidence and prevalence rates of HF have reached epidemic proportions, as evidenced by the relentless increase in the number of HF hospitalizations, the growing number of HF deaths, and the spiraling costs associated with the care of HF patients. The overall prevalence of HF is increasing in part because our current therapies of cardiac disorders (such as myocardial infarction, valvular heart disease, and arrhythmias) are allowing patients to survive longer. Worldwide, HF affects nearly 23 million people. In the United States, the most recent epidemiologic data suggest that 6.2 million adult Americans have HF, and it is estimated that by 2030 the prevalence will increase 46% from current estimates.[1] Estimates of the prevalence of symptomatic HF in the general European population are similar to that in the United States, and ranges from 0.4% to 2%.[2] The prevalence of HF rises exponentially with age, and affects 4% to 8% of people over the age of 65 years (Fig. 48.1A). Although the relative incidence of HF is lower in women than men for all age groups, women constitute at least half of the cases of HF because of their longer life expectancy and the overall prevalence of HF is greater in women than men ≥80 years of age.[3] The age-adjusted incidence of HF appears greatest in black men, followed by black women, white men, and white women; the higher incidence of HF in blacks was attributed to the greater levels of atherosclerotic risk factors in this population (Fig. 48.1B).[1] In North America and Europe, the lifetime risk of developing HF is approximately one in five for a 40-year-old. Risk factors for HF include ischemic heart disease, incident or prevalent myocardial infarction, myocarditis, valvular heart disease, tachycardia, diabetes mellitus, structural heart disease related to congenital heart disease, sleep apnea, excessive drug or alcohol use, as well as obesity. A significant percentage (approximately 30% to 40%) of nonischemic HF is thought to be due to genetic factors (see Chapter 52).

In addition certain medications may increase the risk for HF, including nonsteroidal antiinflammatory medications and cancer chemotherapy.

The distribution of ejection fraction (EF) across unselected populations of HF patients is bimodal with peaks centered around 35% and 55%.[3] Approximately half of patients have HF with preserved EF (HFpEF [see Chapter 51]), while the balance have HF with reduced EF (HFrEF [see Chapter 50])[3]; HFpEF is generally defined as a left ventricular EF ≥50%, whereas HFrEF is generally defined as an EF less than 40%. Insofar as treatment strategies for treating HF are based on these two categories, these distinctions are critical and consensus is not present regarding this classification or how to consider those with HF and an EF between 40% and 50%[4]; this latter category of patients is often excluded from clinical trials, although recent HFpEF trials have included patients down to an EF of 45%.

The prevalence of HFpEF increases dramatically with age and is much more common in women than in men at any age.[1] The prevalence of HFpEF appears to be increasing, perhaps as a function of the aging population and increased recognition of the diagnosis.

An increasingly important population of patients are those with HF and "recovered" EF (HFrecEF).[5,6] Although increases in left ventricular ejection fraction (LVEF) may occur "spontaneously" in some forms of dilated cardiomyopathy (DCM), the changes generally occur in the setting of the use of guideline-directed medical and device therapy.[6] Moreover, it is usually not possible to clearly discern the "spontaneous" component to the improvement in myocardial function, because most patients are treated with guideline-directed medical therapy (GDMT). It is important to recognize that the subgroup of HFrEF patients with a recovered LVEF are clinically distinct from patients with HF with a preserved EF (HFpEF), who also have an LVEF greater than 50% along with the presence of HF signs and symptoms. Improvements in LVEF with GDMT can lead to a complete normalization of LVEF (i.e., >50%) or a partial normalization of LVEF (40% to 50%) (Fig. 48.2). Estimates of the proportion of patients with improved LVEF range widely (e.g., 10% to 40%) due to variable definitions, and the use of both observational and clinical trial datasets. Patients in this category have somewhat characteristic demographics, in that they are more likely to be younger, female, to have nonischemic HF, shorter duration of HF, and to have less remodeling of their left ventricle at the time of diagnosis. Genetic factors may play a role in recovery of EF, as certain mutations (such as those involving the titin gene) may be associated with more robust improvement in LVEF after therapy. A recent consensus statement suggested that patients

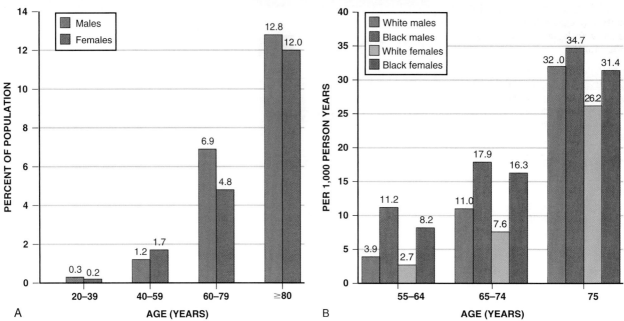

FIGURE 48.1 Prevalence and outcomes of heart failure in the United States. **A,** Prevalence of heart failure by gender and age. **B,** Prevalence of heart failure by age and racial or ethnic group. (From Virani SS, Alonso A, Benjamin EJ, et al. Heart Disease and Stroke Statistics—2020 Update: a report from the American Heart Association. *Circulation.* 2020;141[9]:e139–e596.)

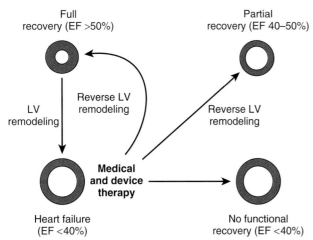

FIGURE 48.2 Changes in left ventricular (LV) ejection fraction (EF) with guideline-directed medical or device therapies (GDMT) in patients with heart failure with a reduced EF (HFrEF). HF and "recovered" EF (HFrecEF) patients treated with GDMT may have a complete recovery of left ventricular (LV) ejection fraction (EF) greater than 50%, partial recovery of LVEF (EF 40% to 50%), or no functional recovery of LVEF (EF <40%). (From Wilcox JE, Fang JC, Margulies KB, Mann DL. Heart failure with a recovered left ventricular ejection fraction. *J Am Coll Cardiol.* 2020;76[6]:719–734.)

with a recovered LVEF should be referred to as HFrecEF, to denote that they were initially HF patients with a remodeled (e.g., dilated) LV. This terminology also avoids confusing these patients with patients with HFpEF who have an LVEF greater than 50%, as well as with patients with an intermediate LVEF (40% to 50%) that may represent HFpEF patients with deteriorating LVEF.

As noted above, one of the major hurdles toward our understanding of this unique group of patients is the lack of standardization with regard to the definition of HFrecEF. A working definition of HFrecEF that is consistent with the majority of studies in the literature includes: (1) documentation of a decreased LVEF less than 40% at baseline, (2) ≥10% absolute improvement in LVEF, and (3) a second measurement of LVEF greater than 40%. These improvements in LVEF are typically accompanied by a reduction in LV volumes.[6]

Patients with HF and improved EF represent a therapeutic conundrum. Although demonstrating improvement in LVEF, many of these patients may have persistent biochemical signs of HF pathophysiology

with abnormal concentrations of natriuretic peptides, and a recent study suggested that discontinuation of GDMT for HF was accompanied by an unacceptably high rate (44%) of recrudescent HFrEF.[7] Further, many patients with HF and improved EF remain at risk of adverse outcomes including return of depressed left ventricular function or hospitalization for HF. Although more studies are needed, the existing data suggest that HFrecEF patients should continue receiving GDMT despite normalization of LVEF, because of the concern for recurrence of HF, as well as the clinical observation that, among patients who experience a relapse and recurrent decline in LVEF, there is a higher likelihood of recurring myocyte injury and a diminished ability to recover LVEF the second time around.[6]

Classification of Heart Failure

Patients with HF are classified according to symptomatology and the stage of the disease. The American College of Cardiology/American Heart Association (ACC/AHA) HF staging approach (Table 48.1) emphasizes the importance of development and progression of disease,[8] whereas the New York Heart Association (NYHA) functional classification focuses more on exercise tolerance in those with established HF (see Table 48.1). While suffering from considerable subjectivity, the NYHA functional classification is widely used. Use of both systems in conjunction provides a reasonable framework for clinician communication and patient prognostication; the NYHA functional classification is also used to determine eligibility for certain therapies, such as mineralocorticoid receptor antagonists, or cardiac resynchronization therapy.

When the diagnosis of HF is suspected, the goals of the clinical assessment are to determine whether HF is present, define the underlying cause and the type of HF (HFrEF vs. HFpEF), assess the severity of HF, as well as identify comorbidities that can influence the clinical course and response to treatment. While the diagnosis of HF can be straightforward when the patient presents with a constellation of the classic signs and symptoms in the appropriate clinical setting (Tables 48.2 and 48.3), no sign or symptom alone can define the presence or severity of HF. Furthermore, detection of diagnostic physical findings of HF is imprecise, often requiring other diagnostic tools. Thus, as depicted in Figure 48.3, the clinical assessment of HF most often depends on information that is gleaned from a variety of sources including the history (both past and present), physical examination, laboratory tests, cardiac imaging, and functional studies.

TABLE 48.1 American College of Cardiology/American Heart Association (ACC/AHA) Stages of Heart Failure (HF) Compared to the New York Heart Association (NYHA) Functional Classification

	ACC/AHA STAGES OF HEART FAILURE	NYHA FUNCTIONAL CLASSIFICATION	
A	At high risk for HF but without structural heart disease or symptoms of heart failure.	None	
B	Structural heart disease but without signs or symptoms of heart failure.	I	No limitation of physical activity. Ordinary physical activity does not cause symptoms of heart failure.
C	Structural heart disease with prior or current symptoms of heart failure.	I	No limitation of physical activity. Ordinary physical activity does not cause symptoms of heart failure.
		II	Slight limitation of physical activity. Comfortable at rest, but ordinary physical activity results in symptoms of heart failure.
		III	Marked limitation of physical activity. Comfortable at rest, but less than ordinary activity causes symptoms of heart failure.
D	Refractory heart failure requiring specialized interventions.	IV	Unable to carry on any physical activity without symptoms of heart failure, or symptoms of heart failure at rest.

HF, Heart failure.

THE MEDICAL HISTORY AND PHYSICAL EXAMINATION

A complete medical history and carefully focused physical examination are the foundation of the assessment in HF patients, providing important information regarding etiology of HF, identifying possible exacerbating factors, and lending pivotal data for proper management (see Chapter 13). The information obtained guides the further direction of the patient's evaluation and enables the clinician to make the most judicious use of additional tests. Further, the history helps to evaluate incongruent results that may emerge during the diagnostic process, and it can obviate the need for needless further testing.

Heart Failure Symptoms and Signs

Patients with HF may complain of a vast array of symptoms, the most common of which are listed in Table 48.2. While none of these are entirely sensitive or specific for identifying the presence of congestion (see Table 48.4), some are more reliable than others for this indication. Importantly, none are specific to HFpEF versus HFrEF. Worsening dyspnea is a cardinal symptom of HF, and is typically related to increases in cardiac filling pressures but also may represent restricted cardiac output.[9] The absence of worsening dyspnea, however, does not necessarily exclude the diagnosis of HF, because patients may accommodate symptoms by substantially modifying their lifestyle. Probing more deeply into the current level of activity may uncover a decline in exercise capacity that is not immediately apparent. Dyspnea at rest is often mentioned by patients hospitalized with HF and has a high-diagnostic sensitivity and significant prognostic ramifications in this population. However, it is also cited by

TABLE 48.2 Using the Medical History to Assess the Heart Failure Patient

Symptoms associated with heart failure include:

1. Fatigue
2. Shortness of breath at rest or during exercise
3. Dyspnea
4. Tachypnea
5. Cough
6. Diminished exercise capacity
7. Orthopnea
8. Paroxysmal nocturnal dyspnea
9. Nocturia
10. Weight gain/Weight loss
11. Edema (of the extremities, scrotum, or elsewhere)
12. Increasing abdominal girth or bloating
13. Abdominal pain (particularly if confined to the right upper quadrant)
14. Loss of appetite or early satiety
15. Cheyne-Stokes respirations (often reported by the family rather than the patient)
16. Somnolence or diminished mental acuity

Historical information that is helpful in determining if symptoms are due to heart failure include:

1. A past history of heart failure
2. Cardiac disease (e.g., coronary artery, valvular or congenital disease, previous myocardial infarction)
3. Risk factors for heart failure (e.g., diabetes, hypertension, obesity)
4. Systemic illnesses that can involve the heart (e.g., amyloidosis, sarcoidosis, inherited neuromuscular diseases)
5. Recent viral illness or history of HIV or Chagas disease
6. Family history of heart failure or sudden cardiac death
7. Environmental and/or medical exposure to cardiotoxic substances
8. Substance abuse
9. Noncardiac illnesses that could affect the heart indirectly (including high output states such as anemia, hyperthyroidism, arteriovenous fistulae)

patients with many other medical conditions, so that the specificity and positive predictive value of dyspnea at rest alone are low. Patients may sleep with their heads elevated to relieve dyspnea while recumbent (orthopnea); additionally, dyspnea while lying on the left side (trepopnea) may occur. Paroxysmal nocturnal dyspnea, shortness of breath developing while recumbent, is one of the most highly reliable indicators of HF. Cheyne-Stokes respiration (also referred to as periodic or cyclic respiration) is common in advanced HF and is usually associated with low cardiac output and sleep-disordered breathing (see also Chapters 50 and 89). The presence of Cheyne-Stokes respiration is generally indicative of an adverse prognosis.[10] Nocturnal cough is a frequently overlooked symptom of HF. These symptoms all typically reflect pulmonary congestion, whereas a history of weight gain, increasing abdominal girth, early satiety, and the onset of edema in dependent organs (extremities or scrotum) indicate right heart congestion; while nonspecific, right upper quadrant pain due to congestion of the liver is common in those with significant right HF, and may be incorrectly attributed to other conditions. Another cardinal symptom of HF is fatigue, generally held to be reflective of reduction in cardiac output as well as abnormal skeletal muscle metabolic responses to exercise.[11] Other causes of fatigue in HF may include major depression, anemia, renal dysfunction, endocrinologic abnormalities, as well as side effects to medications. Unintended weight loss, often leading to cachexia, may be prominent and is a major prognostic indicator.[12]

OTHER HISTORICAL INFORMATION

Information about a patient's past and current medical problems and a multigenerational family history as well as social history provides the background upon which symptoms are interpreted and a management plan is designed.

The presence of hypertension, coronary artery disease, and/or diabetes is particularly helpful because these conditions account for approximately 90% of the population attributable risk for HF in the United States.[13]

TABLE 48.3 Physical Findings of Heart Failure

1. Tachycardia
2. Extra beats or irregular rhythm
3. Narrow pulse pressure or thready pulse*
4. Pulses alternans*
5. Tachypnea
6. Cool and/or mottled extremities*
7. Elevated jugular venous pressure
8. Dullness and diminished breath sounds at one or both lung bases
9. Rales, rhonchi, and/or wheezes
10. Apical impulse displaced leftward and/or inferiorly
11. Sustained apical impulse
12. Parasternal lift
13. S3 and/or S4 (either palpable and/or audible)
14. Tricuspid or mitral regurgitant murmur
15. Hepatomegaly (often accompanied by right upper quadrant discomfort)
16. Ascites
17. Pre-sacral edema
18. Anasarca*
19. Pedal edema
20. Chronic venous stasis changes

*Indicative of more severe disease.

The medical history should also focus on what drugs are taken by the patient; notable agents associated with incident HF include cancer chemotherapy,[14] diabetes drugs (e.g., thiazolidinediones), ergot-based antimigraine drugs, appetite suppressants, certain antidepressants and antipsychotic agents (notably including clozapine), decongestants such as pseudoephedrine (due to its ability to trigger severe hypertension), as well as antiinflammatory agents such as the antimalarial drug hydroxychloroquine (uncommonly associated with an infiltrative cardiomyopathy) or nonsteroidal antiinflammatory drugs. The latter class of agents is well recognized to lead to HF through their ability to worsen renal function, trigger hypertension, and lead to fluid retention, particularly in older adults. A history of use of herbal remedies and dietary supplements should be obtained. Environmental or toxic exposures including alcohol or drug abuse should be carefully sought. A multigenerational family history should be taken for prior HF or sudden cardiac death. Information about the presence of comorbidities (as described later in the chapter) is essential in devising management plans. While most etiologies of HF are cardiac, it is worth remembering that some systemic illnesses (e.g., anemia, hyperthyroidism) can cause this syndrome without direct cardiac involvement (see Chapter 96).

The Physical Examination

The physical findings listed in Table 48.2 complement information from the medical history in defining the presence and severity of HF (see also Chapter 13). The signs of HF have been extensively described, and much as with the history of patients with HF, components of the physical exam have variable sensitivity and specificity for the diagnosis (see Table 48.4),[15] in part due to the subtlety of some physical findings as well as variability in the physical diagnostic skills of the examiner. No physical finding in HF is absolutely pathognomonic for HFpEF versus HFrEF[15]

An evaluation for the presence and severity of HF should include consideration of the patient's general appearance, measurement of vital signs in the seated and standing position, examination of the heart and pulses, and assessment of other organs for evidence of congestion, hypoperfusion, or indications of comorbid conditions. The patient's general appearance conveys vital information. The examiner should assess the patient's body habitus and state of alertness, as well as

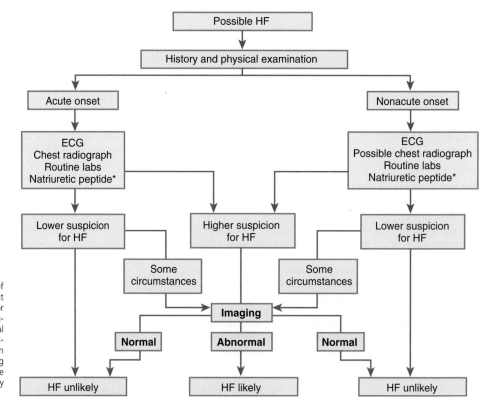

FIGURE 48.3 Flow chart for the evaluation of patients with heart failure (HF). Appropriate cut points for natriuretic peptide testing to identify or exclude HF are discussed in eTable 48.1. The diagnosis of HF is made using a combination of clinical judgment and initial and subsequent testing. Following thorough history and physical examination together with initial diagnostic testing, imaging (such as with echocardiography [ECG]) may still be necessary in ambiguous cases to definitively identify or exclude the diagnosis.

TABLE 48.4 Sensitivity and Specificity of History and Physical Exam Components for the Diagnosis of Elevated Filling Pressures in Patients with Heart Failure

H&P FINDING	FREQUENCY	SENSITIVITY	SPECIFICITY	PREDICTIVE VALUE POSITIVE	PREDICTIVE VALUE NEGATIVE	LR POSITIVE	LR NEGATIVE	OR (95% CI)
Values expressed as percentages unless otherwise indicated. LR indicates likelihood ratio; OR, odds ratio.								
Rales (≥1/3 lung fields)	26/192	15	89	69	38	1.32	1.04	1.4 (0.6, 3.4)
S3	123/192	62	32	61	33	0.92	0.85	0.8 (0.4, 1.5)
Ascites (moderate/massive)	31/192	21	92	81	40	2.44	1.15	2.8 (1.1, 7.3)
Edema (≥2+)	73/192	41	66	67	40	1.20	1.11	1.3 (0.7, 2.5)
Orthopnea (≥2 pillows)	157/192	86	25	66	51	1.15	1.80	2.1 (1, 4.4)
Hepatomegaly (>4 finger breadths)	23/191	15	93	78	39	2.13	1.09	2.3 (0.8, 6.6)
Hepatojugular reflux	147/186	83	27	65	49	1.13	1.54	1.7 (0.9, 3.5)
JVP ≥12 mm Hg	101/186	65	64	75	52	1.79	1.82	3.3 (1.8, 6.1)
JVP <8 mm Hg	18/186	4.3	81	28	33	0.23	0.85	0.2

JVP, Jugular venous pressure.

whether the patient is comfortable, short of breath, coughing, or in pain. The skin exam may show pallor or cyanosis due to under-perfusion, stigmata of alcohol abuse (such as spider angiomata or palmar erythema), erythema nodosum due to sarcoidosis, bronzing due to hemachromatosis, or easy bruising from amyloidosis; additional findings supporting amyloidosis include deltoid muscle infiltration (leading to the "shoulder pad sign"), tongue hypertrophy, and bilateral thenar wasting from carpal tunnel syndrome. The details of inspection and palpation of the heart are discussed in Chapter 13. By observing or palpating the apical impulse, the examiner can rapidly determine heart size and quality of the point of maximal impulse. In cases of severe HF, a palpable impulse corresponding to a third heart sound may be present. Cardiac auscultation (Chapter 13) is a crucial part of HF evaluation.

A characteristic holosystolic murmur of mitral insufficiency is heard in many HF patients. Tricuspid insufficiency, which is also common, can be differentiated from mitral insufficiency by the location of the murmur at the left sternal border, an increased intensity of the murmur during inspiration, and the presence of prominent "V" waves in the jugular venous waveform. Both mitral and tricuspid insufficiency murmurs may become softer as volume overload is treated, and a reduction in ventricular size (with corresponding reduction in annular diameter) improves valve coaptation and competency. Aortic stenosis is an important cause of HF because its presence greatly alters management. The presentation of aortic stenosis may be subtle, however, because the intensity of the murmur depends on blood flow across the valve and this may be reduced as HF develops. The presence of a third heart sound is a crucially important finding and suggests increased ventricular filling volume; while difficult to identify, a third heart sound is highly specific for HF, and carries a substantial prognostic meaning. A fourth heart sound usually indicates reduced ventricular compliance. In advanced HF, the third and fourth heart sounds may be superimposed, resulting in a summation gallop.

A key objective of the examination in HF patients is to detect and quantify the presence of volume retention, with or without pulmonary and/or systemic congestion. As with symptoms, evidence of congestion does not always indicate with certainty that HF is present, nor does absence of manifest congestion definitively exclude the diagnosis. Patients with HFpEF and HFrEF do not generally show significant differences in frequency or significance of the stigmata of volume overload.[16]

The most definitive method for assessing a patient's volume status by physical examination is by the measurement of jugular venous pressure (JVP), which is discussed in detail in Chapter 13. An elevated JVP has good sensitivity (70%) and specificity (79%) for elevated left-sided filling pressure (see Table 48.4).[15] The sensitivity and specificity of the JVP in detecting congestion can be considerably improved by exerting

pressure on the right upper quadrant of the abdomen while assessing venous pulsations in the neck (hepatojugular reflux). Changes in JVP with therapy usually parallel changes in left-sided filling pressure. Limitations of JVP assessment include difficulties in its evaluation due to body habitus as well as significant interobserver variability in its estimation. Increase in the JVP may lag behind left heart filling pressures or may not rise at all if pulmonary artery pressure is increased to the extent that right ventricular failure or tricuspid insufficiency occur. Conversely, the JVP may be elevated without an increase in left ventricular filling pressures in patients with pulmonary arterial hypertension, in those with isolated right ventricular pressure, or when isolated severe tricuspid regurgitation is present.

While pulmonary congestion is exceedingly common in HF, physical findings indicating its presence are variable, and many are nonspecific. Dullness to percussion and diminished breath sounds at one or both lung bases suggests the presence of a pleural effusion. Bilateral pleural effusions are most common but when an effusion is present unilaterally, it is usually right sided with only approximately 10% occurring exclusively on the left side. Leakage of fluid from pulmonary capillaries into the alveoli can be manifest as rales or rhonchi, while wheezing may occur due to reactive bronchoconstriction. Pulmonary rales due to HF are usually fine in nature and extend from the base upward while those due to other causes (e.g., pulmonary fibrosis) tend to be coarser. Importantly, rales or rhonchi may be absent in congested patients with advanced HF; this may reflect compensatory increase in local lymphatic drainage. The occurrence of so-called "cardiac asthma" is due to the physical presence of fluid in the bronchial wall as well as secondary bronchospasm,[17] and can commonly result in an incorrect diagnosis of obstructive airways disease exacerbation, with consequent mis-triage and incorrect therapy with bronchodilators; such incorrect management may be associated with increased risk for mortality.[18]

Lower-extremity edema is a common finding in volume-overloaded HF patients but may commonly be the result of venous insufficiency (particularly after saphenous veins have been harvested for coronary artery bypass grafts) or as a side effect of medications (e.g., calcium channel blockers). Careful inspection of the JVP helps improve the specificity of pedal edema for HF.

Detecting reduced cardiac output and systemic hypoperfusion are key components of the examination. While patients with poor systemic perfusion usually have low systolic and narrow pulse pressures as well as weak and thready pulses, this relationship is not exact. Many patients with systolic blood pressure in the range of 80 mm Hg (or even lower) may have adequate perfusion while others with reduced cardiac output may maintain blood pressure in the normal range at the expense of tissue perfusion by greatly increasing systemic vascular resistance. Findings suggesting reduced cardiac output include poor mentation,

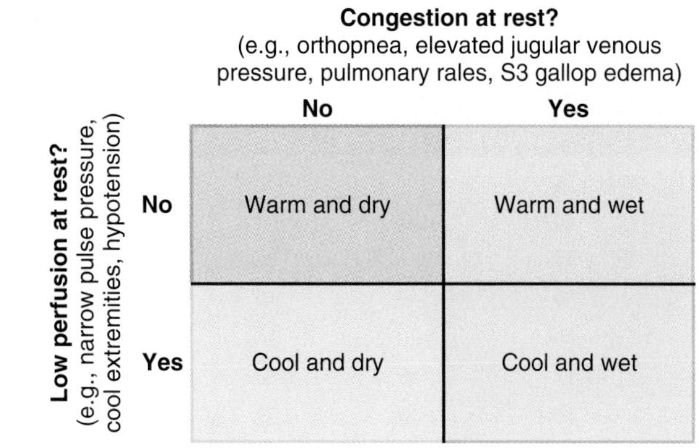

Congestion at rest?
(e.g., orthopnea, elevated jugular venous pressure, pulmonary rales, S3 gallop edema)

FIGURE 48.4 Schema for categorizing patients with heart failure (HF) on the basis of perfusion (warm versus cold) and presence of congestion (dry versus wet). In doing so, four categories may be identified, which have different treatment strategies. The four categories of HF identified in this schema have different treatment strategies. (Based on data from Nohria A, Tsang SW, Fang JC, et al. Clinical assessment identifies hemodynamic profiles that predict outcomes in patients admitted with heart failure. *J Am Coll Cardiol.* 2003;41:1797.)

reduced urine output, mottled skin, and cool extremities. Of these, cool extremities are the most broadly useful.

Assessment for systemic congestion taken together with evaluation for reduced cardiac output may be useful to categorize patients (Fig. 48.4) into "dry/warm" (uncongested with normal perfusion), "wet/warm" (congested with normal perfusion, the most common combination found in decompensated HF), "dry/cold" (uncongested but hypoperfused), and "wet/cold" (cardiogenic shock),[19] as discussed in Chapter 49. These categories are not only prognostic, but also inform treatment decision making.

ROUTINE LABORATORY ASSESSMENT

A suggested algorithm for the diagnostic evaluation of HF is presented in Figure 48.3. The laboratory testing and imaging modalities described below provide important information for the diagnosis and management of patients with suspected or proven HF.

Chest Radiography

Despite advances in other imaging technologies the chest X-ray remains a very useful component of the assessment, particularly when the clinical presentation is ambiguous. Results of chest radiography are additive to clinical variables from history and physical examination, and similarly complement the results of biomarker testing. Accordingly, chest radiography should be a routine part of the early evaluation of patients presenting with symptoms suggestive of acutely decompensated HF (see also Chapter 17).

The classical chest X-ray pattern in patients with pulmonary edema is a "butterfly" pattern of interstitial and alveolar opacities bilaterally fanning out to the periphery of the lungs. Many patients, however, present with more subtle findings, in which increased interstitial markings including Kerley B lines (thin horizontal linear opacities extending to the pleural surface caused by accumulation of fluid in the interstitial space), peri-bronchial cuffing, and evidence of prominent upper lobe vasculature (indicating pulmonary venous hypertension) are the most prominent findings. Pleural effusions and/or fluid in the right minor fissure may also be seen. In many cases, particularly in those with very advanced HF, the chest X-ray may be entirely clear, despite significant symptoms of dyspnea; the negative predictive value of chest radiography is too low to definitively exclude HF.[20]

The Electrocardiogram

The electrocardiogram (ECG) is a standard part of the initial evaluation of a patient with suspected HF, as it may provide important clues regarding incident HF, while also assisting in understanding when

previously diagnosed patients experience an episode of decompensation (see also Chapter 14). In patients with HF, the ECG is infrequently normal, but may only show nonspecific findings; thus, much like the chest radiography, the positive predictive value of ECG far surpasses the negative predictive value in this setting.

Sinus tachycardia due to sympathetic nervous system activation is seen with advanced HF or during episodes of acute decompensation; beside increasing the likelihood for the diagnosis finding of elevated heart rate it is a prognostic finding in HF as well. The presence of atrial arrhythmia on the ECG as well as the ventricular response may provide clues as to the cause of HF, as well as explain why a patient may have developed decompensated symptoms; identifying atrial arrhythmia with a rapid ventricular response also provides a target for therapeutic interventions. Increased ventricular ectopy identifies a patient at risk for sudden death, particularly when the EF is very low (e.g., <30%).

The presence of increased QRS voltage may suggest left ventricular hypertrophy; in the absence of a prior history of hypertension, such a finding might be caused by valvular heart disease or by hypertrophic cardiomyopathy, particularly if bizarre repolarization patterns are noted. If right ventricular hypertrophy is present, primary or secondary pulmonary hypertension should be considered. Low QRS voltage suggests the presence of an infiltrative disease or pericardial effusion. The presence of Q waves suggests that HF may be due to ischemic heart disease, while new or reversible ST changes identify acute coronary ischemia is present even when chest pain is absent. Indeed, as acute coronary ischemia is a leading cause of acutely decompensated HF, a 12-lead ECG should be immediately obtained in this setting, to exclude acute MI.

The intervals on the ECG may provide important information regarding causes of HF, as well as yielding information with respect to treatment strategy. Prolongation of the PR interval is common in patients in this setting, and may be due to intrinsic conduction disease, but may also be seen in patients with infiltrative cardiomyopathy such as amyloidosis. With the advent of cardiac resynchronization therapy (see Chapter 58) evaluation the QRS complex has become a critical part of the clinical assessment, in that it provides important information regarding the cause of HF, as well as providing pivotal information regarding the therapeutic approach. The QT interval is often prolonged in patients with HF, and may be due to electrolyte abnormalities, myocardial disease, or from effects of commonly used drugs, such as antiarrhythmics. A lengthened QT interval may identify patients at risk for torsades de pointes and is thus an important variable to consider when utilizing therapeutic agents with effects on ventricular repolarization.

Measurement of Blood Chemistry and Hematologic Variables

Patients with new-onset HF and those with acute decompensation of chronic HF should have a panel of electrolytes, blood urea nitrogen, serum creatinine, hepatic enzymes, fasting lipid profile, thyroid stimulating hormone, transferrin saturation, uric acid, a complete blood count, and a urinalysis measured. As discussed below, the natriuretic peptides may be useful for diagnosis as well as for prognostication. A test for human immunodeficiency virus or further screening for hemachromatosis is reasonable in selected patients, while diagnostic tests for rheumatologic diseases or pheochromocytoma are reasonable when suspicion exists for these diseases. When the diagnosis of cardiac amyloidosis is entertained (see also Chapter 53), serum-free light chains may be measured to screen for the AL form of the diagnosis, however no reliable blood tests exist for diagnosis of the transthyretin form of cardiac amyloidosis, which typically requires imaging for its evaluation (see also Chapter 53).

Abnormalities of sodium are common in HF patients, particularly during periods of acute decompensation, and have substantial prognostic meaning. Studies have shown that hyponatremia (defined as serum sodium values below 135 mmol/L) may be found in up to 25% of patients with acute HF, and hyponatremia may also be seen in patients with indolently worsening HF without obvious decompensation.[21] Low-sodium concentrations in HF may be due to worsening volume retention or may be related to the use of diuretics, including thiazides. Hyponatremia is associated with impaired cognitive and neuromuscular function, and when present and persistent, low sodium is strongly prognostic for longer hospital stay, as well as a high risk for mortality.[22] Despite this fact, strategies to correct serum-sodium levels have not been shown to clearly improve the clinical course (see Chapter 50).[23] Hypernatremia, although uncommon, is also prognostic for mortality in patients with HF. Hypokalemia occurs commonly in HF patients who are treated with diuretics. Besides increasing the risk of cardiac arrhythmias, low potassium may also lead to leg cramps and muscle weakness. Conversely, hyperkalemia is less common, and most often is due to effects of medications such as angiotensin-converting enzyme inhibitors or mineralocorticoid inhibition.

Abnormalities of renal function are common in patients with HF, and occur due to renal congestion, inadequate cardiac output, or as a consequence of comorbid conditions.[24] In addition, HF therapies such as diuretics and angiotensin-converting enzyme inhibitors or angiotensin receptor blockers can increase blood urea nitrogen and creatinine. In this regard, abnormalities of renal function may have substantial effects on the ability to aggressively treat HF patients. Furthermore, abnormal renal function represents one of the more powerful prognostic variables gleaned from routine laboratory testing in HF. For these reasons, assessment of renal function should be performed as part of the initial evaluation of HF, and then periodically repeated during follow-up.

In patients hospitalized with acutely decompensated HF (see Chapter 49), registry data suggest that 60% to 70% have a reduced estimated glomerular filtration rate[25]; among such patients, the initial blood urea nitrogen and serum creatinine concentrations are both independently predictive of death.[26] Following admission, approximately 30% of patients with acute HF may also develop an increase in serum creatinine by ≥0.3 mg/dL, which is similarly prognostic for mortality.[24,25] The causes of this so-called "cardiorenal" syndrome are complex, but include the severity of right heart congestion, increased intraabdominal pressure, as well as renal hypoperfusion from inadequate cardiac output. On the other hand, worsening renal function may also occur from aggressive decongestion strategies; such decline in renal function has been linked to improved (rather than worse) prognosis, as it presumably indicates a more thorough treatment for congestion, the trigger for acute HF hospitalization.[27] Accordingly, when faced with worsening renal function, the clinician must perform a careful examination to assess volume status and tissue perfusion to decide on appropriate therapies to manage the situation. Lastly, improvement in renal function may follow therapies improving the severity of congestion, although such a finding is still associated with poor long-term prognosis.

Diabetes mellitus is common in HF patients and hyperglycemia has emerged as a possible risk factor for adverse outcome in affected patients. Because diuretics can cause gout, measuring uric acid levels can help in patient management; elevated serum uric acid levels have been noted to be prognostic, and therapies to lower their concentration are now being studied to improve HF outcomes. Abnormalities in aspartate aminotransferase, alanine aminotransferase, alkaline phosphatase, bilirubin, or lactate dehydrogenase may occur in HF patients as a consequence of either hemodynamic derangements leading to hepatic congestion, or may be due to medications, and it is important to follow levels periodically. An unexpected increase in prothrombin time in patients receiving warfarin therapy may be an early harbinger of decompensation as it may reflect impaired synthetic capacity of a congested liver. Albumin levels are an indication of the patient's nutritional status and they may be depressed due to poor appetite or impaired absorption across an engorged bowel wall; hypoalbuminemia is prognostic for mortality in acute and chronic HF.

Hematologic abnormalities are exceedingly common in HF, affecting nearly 40% of affected patients. Low hemoglobin levels have been associated with more severe HF symptoms, reduced exercise capacity and quality of life, and increased mortality.[28] While anemia may be a consequence of chronic disease in HF patients, a low hemoglobin level should trigger an evaluation to detect treatable causes, particularly iron deficiency. Increasing attention has also been given to the red cell distribution width as a prognostic variable in both acutely decompensated and chronic HF.[29] The white blood cell count and differential is helpful in detecting the presence of infection that is responsible for destabilizing a previously well-compensated patient and could provide a clue that HF is due to uncommon cause such as eosinophilic infiltration of the myocardium.

Beyond standard laboratory testing, the measurement of biomarkers has emerged over the past decade as important adjunct to the initial and subsequent evaluation of patients with suspected or proven HF. Biomarkers are now routinely used for distinguishing HF from other conditions and to establish severity of the diagnosis, and also to provide useful prognostic information in HF patients. Lastly,

TABLE 48.5 Biomarkers Used in Assessing Patients with Heart Failure

Inflammation[*,†,‡]

C-reactive protein

Tumor necrosis factor

Fas (APO-1)

Interleukins 1, 6, and 18

Oxidative stress[*,†,§.]

Oxidized low-density lipoproteins

Myeloperoxidase

Urinary biopyrrins

Urinary and plasma isoprostanes

Plasma malondialdehyde

Extracellular-matrix remodeling[*,§]

Matrix metalloproteinases

Tissue inhibitors of metalloproteinases

Collagen propeptides

Propeptide procollagen type I

Plasma procollagen type III

Neurohormones[*,†,§]

Norepinephrine

Renin

Angiotensin II

Aldosterone

Arginine vasopressin

Endothelin

Myocyte injury[*,†,§]

Cardiac-specific troponins I and T

Myosin light-chain kinase I

Heart-type fatty-acid protein

Creatine kinase MB fraction

Myocyte stress[†,‡,§,¶]

B-type natriuretic peptide/N-terminal pro-B type natriuretic peptide

Midregional proadrenomedullin

ST2

New Biomarkers[†]

Chromogranin

Galectin 3

Osteoprotegerin

Adiponectin

Growth differentiation factor 15

Insulin-like growth factor binding protein 7

*Biomarkers in this category aid in elucidating the pathogenesis of heart failure.
†Biomarkers in this category provide prognostic information and enhance risk stratification.
‡Biomarkers in this category can be used to identify subjects at risk for heart failure.
§Biomarkers in this category are potential targets of therapy.
¶Biomarkers in this category are useful in the diagnosis of heart failure and in monitoring therapy.

there is considerable interest in determining the ability of biomarkers to guide therapy both in the acute and chronic settings. As shown in Table 48.5, Braunwald has proposed that HF biomarkers be divided into six distinct categories with an additional one reserved for biomarkers that have not yet been classified (see also Chapter 8 and 10).[30]

As articulated,[31] clinically useful biomarkers of HF should be easily measured with high analytical precision, should reflect important processes involved in HF presence and progression, should not recapitulate clinical information already available at the bedside, and must provide clinically useful information for caregivers to more swiftly and reliably establish/reject a diagnosis, to more accurately estimate prognosis, or to inform more successful therapeutic strategies. Only the natriuretic peptides have met these requirements, although other promising biomarkers exist for use in HF assessment.

Natriuretic Peptides

The natriuretic peptides are useful biomarkers for HF diagnosis, estimation of HF severity and prognosis, and possibly for management of HF as well. The most commonly measured natriuretic peptides are B-type natriuretic peptide (BNP) and its amino-terminal cleavage pro-peptide equivalent, NT-proBNP; these two biomarkers are released from cardiomyocytes in response to stretch, and highly precise assays exist for their detection in blood (see also Chapter 47). Given the preponderance of myocardium in the ventricles, BNP and NT-proBNP mainly reflect ventricular stretch and are synthesized in response to wall stress. Atrial natriuretic peptide (ANP) is another member of the class of natriuretic peptides and is synthesized and secreted from atrial tissue; a mid-regional pro-ANP assay is now available and appears to deliver comparable results to BNP and NT-proBNP when tested in HF patients.[32]

Due to the differences in their clearance BNP and NT-proBNP have considerably different half-lives (BNP: 20 minutes; NT-proBNP: 90 minutes), and thus they circulate with very different concentrations. Both natriuretic peptides have become an important part of the HF assessment, however much like any diagnostic test, clinicians must always remember the broad array of structural and functional reasons for BNP or NT-proBNP release to correctly interpret their values.[33] Natriuretic peptide levels tend to increase progressively with worsening NYHA functional class, and tend to be higher in HFrEF, compared to HFpEF, despite independent contributions of diastolic function to their concentrations. Patients with acute HF most often have higher values for BNP and NT-proBNP, compared to chronic stable patients, however this is by no means a universal finding, and knowledge of an individual's natriuretic peptide value when stable may be useful to better interpret a change when a change in symptoms occurs.

When using BNP or NT-proBNP, the clinician should remember that beyond left ventricular systolic and diastolic dysfunction, concentrations of both peptides are higher in patients with valvular heart disease, pulmonary hypertension, ischemic heart disease, atrial arrhythmias, and even pericardial processes such as constriction.[33] Elevation of BNP or NT-proBNP—often marked—is nearly ubiquitous in infiltrative cardiomyopathies such as cardiac amyloidosis; these elusive diagnoses should be considered in a patient with significant elevation of natriuretic peptide but without obvious congestion. Additionally, numerous relevant medical covariates with effects on natriuretic peptide values must also be kept in mind. For example, both BNP and NT-proBNP concentrations increase with age, thought to identify accumulating structural heart disease in older patients. Both natriuretic peptides are higher in patients with renal failure, partially reflective of slower clearance, but also similarly identifying heart disease in this population of patients with prevalent cardiovascular risk factors. Elevated natriuretic peptide values can also be seen in hyperdynamic states, including sepsis. Patients who have right ventricular dysfunction as a result of pulmonary embolus may have elevated natriuretic peptide concentrations. It is also important to recognize that angiotensin receptor neprilysin inhibitors (ARNIs [see Chapter 50]) may modestly increase levels of BNP, but this finding is not universal and may be transient. As NT-proBNP is not a substrate for neprilysin, its concentrations remain reflective of the clinical picture; in patients under treatment with ARNI, changes in NT-proBNP are associated with LV remodeling parameters (such as change in LVEF)[34] and strongly predict outcomes.[35,36]

Obesity is strongly linked to lower-than-expected BNP or NT-proBNP values, despite comparable or higher wall stress in heavier patients. Given the common effect on BNP, NT-proBNP, and MR-proANP, this is not likely to represent a clearance effect (as each are cleared differently), rather more likely to represent suppression of natriuretic peptide gene expression or post-translational modification.

Results of BNP or NT-proBNP, although useful, should always be interpreted in the context of sound clinical judgment, integrated with results of history, physical examination, and other testing; these important biomarkers strongly supplement clinical judgment, but should not replace it. Keeping this in mind, the natriuretic peptides have been shown to be useful to identify and exclude acute HF in the emergency department, as well as more indolent HF in the outpatient setting. Suggested cutoffs for use of natriuretic peptides are shown in **eTable 48.1**.[37]

> Pivotal data for BNP and NT-proBNP testing to diagnose acute HF came from the Breathing Not Properly and ProBNP Investigation of Dyspnea in the Emergency Department (PRIDE) studies respectively. In the Breathing Not Properly, a BNP concentration of 100 pg/mL was highly accurate for the diagnosis of acutely decompensated HF; in PRIDE, an NT-proBNP cutoff of 900 pg/mL provided comparable performance to a BNP of 100 pg/mL. Subsequently, the International Collaborative of NT-proBNP (ICON) investigators showed that age stratification improved positive predictive value of NT-proBNP in acutely dyspneic patients; as well, an NT-proBNP concentration below 300 pg/mL was useful to exclude acutely decompensated HF.[33] These data were more recently reaffirmed in the ICON: Re-evaluation of Acute Diagnostic Cut-Offs in the Emergency Department study, where performance of NT-proBNP to detect or exclude acute HF remained robust in a more contemporary population of patients with acute dyspnea.[38]
>
> Knowledge of natriuretic peptide levels in the emergency department is associated with more rapid diagnosis, lower admission rate, shorter length of hospital stay, and reduced cost. As clinical uncertainty in acute dyspnea is associated with worse prognosis, it is reassuring to note that natriuretic peptide testing is particularly useful in this complex situation.
>
> For patients with less acute presentations of dyspnea in settings other than the ED, values of BNP or NT-proBNP are most often considerably lower; when used for evaluation of the dyspneic ambulatory patient, therefore, the optimized cutoffs from emergency department studies should not be used: lower values are mandatory, and optimized for their negative predictive value to exclude (rather than identify) HF (see **eTable 48.1**).[37] Age stratification again improves diagnostic accuracy in this setting, as older patients are expected to have generally higher concentrations of BNP or NT-proBNP in the absence of clinical HF. If a patient is found to be above such cutoffs, further diagnostic testing such as echocardiography is likely needed. Causes of falsely low BNP or NT-proBNP in the outpatient setting are comparable to those with acute dyspnea.

Natriuretic peptide levels provide useful prognostic information across all ACC/AHA stages of HF even when adjusted for important variables from history, physical examination, echocardiography, or even cardiopulmonary exercise testing (Fig. 48.5). While one natriuretic peptide measurement is prognostically meaningful, serial follow up measurements add incrementally important prognostic information. For example, in patients with acute HF, those who do not show a robust reduction in BNP or NT-proBNP by the time of hospital discharge tend to have considerably higher rates of morbidity and mortality.[39] It has thus been suggested that a BNP or NT-proBNP decrease of 30% or more by hospital discharge is desirable. Similarly, in ambulatory HF, chronically elevated or rising natriuretic peptide values identify a particularly high-risk patient population. HF therapies may lower concentrations of BNP and NT-proBNP; when this finding occurs, prognosis is improved.

Other Biomarkers

Other promising biomarkers for use in patients with HF have been identified (see Table 48.5), and some are clinically available. In general, newer biomarkers for HF have been developed to supplement the natriuretic peptides for prognostication. While most have not yet achieved the prerequisite data to justify their widespread use, a few promising biomarkers bear mention.

Concentrations of soluble ST2 (a member of the interleukin receptor family) have been shown to be strongly linked to progressive HF and death in patients across the four ACC/AHA stages of HF.[40] Originally identified in a basic science model of mechanotransduction, ST2 plays a pivotal role in the formation of fibrosis in the heart; elevated concentrations of ST2 are thus associated with progressive cardiovascular dysfunction, remodeling, and risk for death. Soluble ST2

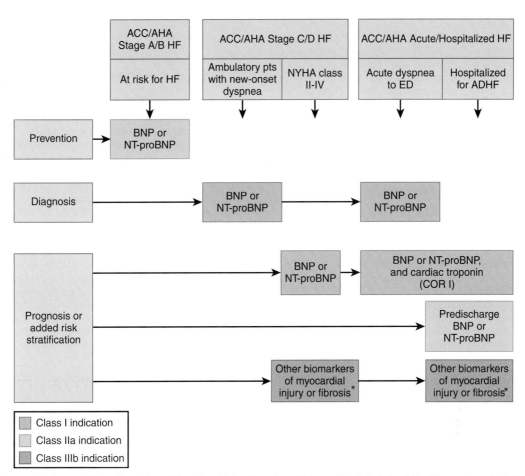

FIGURE 48.5 Indications for the use of biomarkers in heart failure. Key: *Other biomarkers of injury or fibrosis include soluble ST2 receptor, galectin-3, and high-sensitivity troponin. *ACC*, American College of Cardiology; *ADHF*, acute decompensated heart failure; *AHA*, American Heart Association; *BNP*, B-type natriuretic peptide; *COR*, Class of Recommendation; *ED*, emergency department; *HF*, heart failure; *NT-proBNP*, N-terminal pro-B-type natriuretic peptide; *NYHA*, New York Heart Association; *pts*, patients. (Modified from Yancy CW, Jessup M, Bozkurt B, et al. 2017 ACC/AHA/HFSA Focused Update of the 2013 ACCF/AHA Guideline for the Management of Heart Failure: a report of the American College of Cardiology/American Heart Association Task Force on Clinical Practice Guidelines and the Heart Failure Society of America. *J Am Coll Cardiol.* 2017;70[6]:776–803.)

concentrations are additive to natriuretic peptides for prognostication, are useful in both HFrEF and HFpEF, and are similarly dynamic to natriuretic peptides in their changes following HF therapies; in patients with both acutely decompensated and chronic HF, a chronically elevated or rising ST2 value strongly predicts adverse outcome.[41,42] Notably, among apparently normal patients in a population-based analysis, ST2 values predicted future HF beyond other biomarkers such as BNP as well as echocardiographic parameters.[43] This implies the biochemical changes of ventricular remodeling may be detectable well before conventional biomarkers or imaging are abnormal.

The myofibrillar proteins, troponin T and I, are indicators of cardiomyocyte injury and may be elevated in HF patients in the absence of an acute coronary syndrome or even significant coronary artery disease. With the emergence of highly sensitive troponin assays, even more patients may be found to have elevated concentrations of these important predictors of risk.[44] While an elevated troponin value does not specifically identify myocardial necrosis due to coronary artery disease per se, given the importance of acute MI in the triggering of acute HF, a troponin should always be measured in this setting, although interpreted with caution. Elevated troponin concentrations in community-based normal subjects are prognostic for onset of HF (particularly if rising in serial measurement). Troponin is independently predictive of increased mortality risk across the HF spectrum.

Other novel biomarkers are emerging and may have a role in the comprehensive evaluation of the patient with HF; many of these novel markers reflect systemic stress or disarray of organs outside of the heart. For example, the mid-regional fragment of pro-adrenomedullin is a biomarker reflective of vascular and systemic stress and is powerfully prognostic for short-term adverse outcome (see also Chapter 47).[32] In a similar fashion, growth differentiation factor-15, another marker of cardiovascular stress, strongly predicts outcomes not only in established HF, but may also be prognostic for new-onset HF in apparently well subjects.[43] Lastly, novel biomarkers of renal dysfunction are emerging as strong predictors of cardiovascular risk beyond the standard measures of blood urea nitrogen or serum creatinine. Cystatin C (a ubiquitous protein found in all nucleated cells whose clearance is directly related to glomerular filtration) and β trace protein are two renal function markers whose values are tightly related to outcomes in HF, while neutrophil gelatinase-associated lipocalin, N-acetyl-β-D-glucosaminidase, and kidney injury molecule-1 are promising biomarkers of acute renal injury whose values rise well before renal function is perceived to be worsening, and impart important prognostic information in HF patients.[45]

Ultimately, for the comprehensive evaluation of HF, it seems likely that a combination or panel of biomarkers will prove to be the most useful way of assessing prognosis.

RISK SCORING FOR PROGNOSIS

During initial and subsequent evaluation of the patient with HF, the clinician should routinely assess the potential for adverse outcome. Besides biomarker testing, a number of validated methods for risk stratification in HF exist, including a variety of multivariable clinical risk scores for use in both ambulatory and hospitalized patients. One well-validated risk score (the Seattle Heart Failure model) is available in an internet-based application (www.seattleheartfailuremodel.org) and has been shown to provide robust information regarding risk of mortality in ambulatory HF patients.[46] For patients hospitalized with acute symptoms, the model developed by the Acute Decompensated Heart Failure National Registry (ADHERE) incorporates three routinely measured variables upon hospital admission (systolic blood pressure, blood urea nitrogen, and serum creatinine), and partitions subjects into categories with a 10-fold difference in risk (from 2.1% to 21.9%).[46] Importantly, clinical risk scores have not performed as well in estimating risk of hospital readmission. For this purpose, natriuretic peptide results may be of more use, particularly when measured after in-patient treatment, just prior to discharge; a lack of BNP or NT-proBNP reduction by 30% during in-patient treatment may identify those at higher risk for short-term death or rehospitalization.

RIGHT HEART CATHETERIZATION

Measurement of intracardiac pressures and hemodynamics (see also Chapter 22) as part of the diagnostic work-up or for guiding therapy is less commonly performed now than in the past, because biomarkers and noninvasive imaging techniques provide much of the information that was previously available only by heart catheterization. Nonetheless, as right heart catheterization affords unequivocal assessment of hemodynamics and filling pressures, it is particularly useful in cases where there is uncertainty about the cause of a patient's symptoms and in situations where precise measurements are required to guide therapy or decision making (e.g., selection of patients for heart transplantation). In addition, right heart catheterization is of value (and should be considered) in those with HF complicated by clinically significant hypotension, systemic hypoperfusion, dependence on inotropic infusions, or persistently severe symptoms despite adjustment of recommended therapies.

An invasive assessment with right heart catheterization is important to assess the pulmonary vascular resistance, a necessary part of the evaluation for heart transplantation. When pulmonary artery pressures are found to be elevated, response to pulmonary arterial vasodilating agents can be determined in this context, and provides important information determining whether a patient with pulmonary hypertension will be acceptable for cardiac transplantation. In addition, obtaining the pulmonary artery wedge pressure is useful for assessing volume status. The pulmonary artery wedge pressure usually estimates the left ventricular end-diastolic pressure if no obstruction to flow between the left atrium and left ventricle exists. While determination of hemodynamic variables at rest suffices in most patients, there are cases where exercise helps to reveal the presence and/or magnitude of abnormal intracardiac pressures and flow. Pulmonary hypertension, for example, can be highly dynamic and exercise measurements may be needed.

> Use of hemodynamic monitoring to guide therapy was evaluated in patients with advanced HF in the Evaluation Study of Congestive Heart Failure and Pulmonary Artery Catheterization Effectiveness (ESCAPE) trial.[47] The results did not show any clear benefit on morbidity and mortality of pulmonary artery-guided management compared to careful clinical assessment. The failure to affect postdischarge outcomes appears to be related to the fact that the hemodynamic improvements that were affected during hospitalization reverted back toward baseline within a relatively short period of time. Consequently, "tailored therapy" of HF is used less commonly now than in the past, but has a role particularly in patients with HF complicated by hypotension, systemic hypoperfusion, and end-organ dysfunction.

ENDOMYOCARDIAL BIOPSY

The role of endomyocardial biopsy for evaluating patients with HF is also discussed in Chapter 55. In general, biopsy of the myocardium is performed if a disorder with a unique prognosis or one which would benefit from a specific treatment regimen is suspected and the diagnosis cannot be made by conventional methods. The incremental diagnostic, therapeutic, and prognostic benefit offered by the information obtained from a biopsy must be weighed against the risks of the procedure. The sensitivity of endomyocardial biopsy may vary, depending on the cause of HF; for example, sensitivity is higher in more diffuse disease states

such as myocarditis or amyloidosis, while more patchy disease states such as sarcoidosis may be less easily detected using biopsy.

DETECTING COMORBID CONDITIONS

The incidence of HF rises sharply from the sixth decade onward which is coincident with the time when other chronic diseases begin to manifest. In addition, many of the conditions leading to the development of HF (e.g., diabetes, hypertension, atherosclerosis) affect organs other than the heart. Thus, comorbidities are quite common in HF patients, and have a profound effect on the course of affected patients: a substantial percentage of hospitalizations suffered by patients with HF are in fact non-HF related, and not precipitated by a cardiac condition in more than half of cases.[48] Comorbidities not only complicate the course of patients with concomitant HF, but they also have a substantial impact on ability to manage patients with HF; as an example, chronic kidney disease may limit application of agents blocking the renin-angiotensin-aldosterone system. Lastly, the presence of comorbidities reduces the prognostic benefits of GDMT; for example, atrial fibrillation reduces benefit of many therapies, including beta blockers and cardiac resynchronization. With recent data suggesting aggressive management of hypertension and use of sodium-glucose co-transporter 2 inhibitors for diabetes mellitus care both may reduce HF events,[49,50] this illustrates detection and management of comorbidities is a particularly relevant exercise.

ASSESSMENT OF QUALITY OF LIFE

HF has a profound effect on quality of life, and poor health-related quality of life is a powerful predictor of adverse prognosis in HF patients. Change in health-related quality of life is now also considered an approvable endpoint for HF therapies. Determinants of poor quality of life in HF include female gender, younger age, higher body-mass index, worse symptoms, as well as the presence of depression and sleep apnea.[51] Improved quality of life has been reported following standard HF drug treatment intensification, cardiac resynchronization therapy, or in disease management programs. Given its importance, at the initial and subsequent visits, consideration should be given for quality-of-life assessment, whether through standard history or through the use of validated tools for its estimation such as the Kansas City Cardiomyopathy Questionnaire.

CARDIOPULMONARY EXERCISE TESTING

Exercise intolerance is a prime symptom of HF. Despite this fact, quantification of exercise tolerance is imprecise (see also Chapter 15); standard approaches such as the NYHA criteria or the 6-minute walk test are subjective and insensitive measures of functional capacity. Additionally, the 6-minute walk test does not reveal how close the patient may be to their maximal capacity for exercise, does not discriminate between the causes of impaired exercise capacity (e.g., cardiac, pulmonary, orthopedic) or poor motivation, and does not account for the effects of conditioning and/or age; older age may undermine accuracy of the 6-minute walk test. When more precise information is needed, cardiopulmonary exercise testing (CPX) is often used because it allows for identification of causes of exercise intolerance and quantification of exercise capacity, and delivers important physiologic information not routinely available from standard stress testing.[52]

> CPX is performed using treadmill or cycle exercise, continued to symptom limitation. Analysis of gas exchange at rest, during exercise, and in the recovery phase following exertion is performed, and measures of oxygen uptake (V_{O_2}), expiratory ventilation (V_E), and carbon dioxide output (V_{CO_2}) are generated, typically expressed as a ratio of their slope. The maximum V_{O_2} is the standard expression of capacity for endurance, based on the Fick equation, which states that V_{O_2} = cardiac output × [oxygen content$_{arterial}$ − oxygen content$_{venous}$]. Thus, V_{O_2} is a direct function of cardiac output, and indeed very strong associations are established between maximal V_{O_2}, cardiac output, and risk for death. The V_E/V_{CO_2} slope is an expression of efficiency of pulmonary CO_2 clearance

during exercise and has also been suggested to be powerfully prognostic. These variables are often used in conjunction with each other in the assessment of advanced HF.

Use of CPX is a standard part of the routine evaluation prior to heart transplantation; moderate to severely reduced maximal Vo_2 values (e.g., <14 mL $O_2 \cdot kg^{-1} \cdot min^{-1}$) are often used as a prognostic threshold in this setting, while maximal Vo_2 values less than 10 mL $O_2 \cdot kg^{-1} \cdot min^{-1}$ are considered severe, and particularly prognostic when the V_E/Vco_2 slope is ≥45.0. Many evidence-based medical and devices therapies for HF, such as certain drugs, cardiac resynchronization therapy, or exercise may result in improvement in CPX parameters, however this is not universal. For example, beta blockers have significant influence on survival, but do not significantly improve maximal Vo_2. Thus, as beta blockers improve prognosis across all ranges of maximal Vo_2, aggressive use of these agents may necessarily result in a lower optimal cut point than less than 14 mL $O_2 \cdot kg^{-1} \cdot min^{-1}$ for referral for cardiac transplantation. While CPX is most validated in HFrEF, it appears to be of prognostic value in HFpEF, although data are more limited.

USE OF IMAGING MODALITIES IN THE DIAGNOSIS AND MANAGEMENT OF PATIENTS WITH HEART FAILURE

Noninvasive cardiac imaging serves a vital role in the assessment of patients with HF and is essential for determining whether the patient should be classified as HFpEF or HFrEF (see also Chapters 16 to 20). Imaging may help confirm the diagnosis of HF by assessing the presence and severity of structural and functional changes in the heart, provide clues about the etiology of cardiac dysfunction (i.e., congenital heart disease, valvular abnormalities, pericardial disease, coronary artery disease), risk stratify patients, and possibly guide treatment strategies. Imaging modalities can also be used to help assess the efficacy of therapeutic interventions, provide ongoing prognostic information, and further guide treatment. The primary noninvasive cardiac imaging modalities used to evaluate HF patients are echocardiography (Chapter 16), magnetic resonance imaging (MRI; Chapter 19), computed tomography (CT; Chapter 20), and nuclear imaging, including single photon emission computed tomography (SPECT) and positron emission tomography (PET) techniques (Chapter 18). Imaging modalities often provide complementary data and each has the capacity to provide unique information in individual patients. While the initial evaluation of a patient with newly diagnosed HF should include a transthoracic echocardiogram, further imaging with MRI, CT, and/ or nuclear techniques may be considered depending upon the need to further address questions regarding cardiac structure and function, etiology, and issues such as the potential for reversibility of systolic dysfunction with revascularization.

Echocardiography and Lung Ultrasound

Transthoracic echocardiography is an important part of the evaluation of HF,[53] can be performed without risk to the patient, does not involve radiation exposure, and can be performed at the bedside if necessary (see also Chapter 16). Increasing use of handheld echocardiography has facilitated evaluation at the point of care, such as in the emergency department setting in the context of an acute presentation.

Echocardiography is particularly well suited for evaluating the structure and function of both the myocardium and heart valves and providing information about intracardiac pressures and flows. For patients with HFrEF, LV volumes and systolic function can be assessed semi-quantitatively, or quantified using the biplane method and the modified Simpson's rule. Information about the morphology and relative sizes of the cardiac chambers may suggest specific diagnoses. For example, concentric LV hypertrophy with severe bi-atrial enlargement raises the possibility that HF is due to an infiltrative process such as amyloidosis, particularly in the absence of a prior diagnosis of hypertension; in cases such as this, strain imaging may be helpful to evaluate for the characteristic "apical sparing" seen in patients with amyloid cardiomyopathy. Diastolic function is assessed using Doppler measurements, including analyses of the mitral valve inflow pattern (early [E] and atrial [A] waveforms), tissue velocities at the mitral valve annulus, pulmonary vein flow, and the left atrial volume indexed to body surface area (see Chapter 16). Diastolic dysfunction can be further classified as grades I to III based on the above measurements, with incremental prognostic importance in HF as worsening grades of diastolic dysfunction are noted. Ratio of early mitral valve inflow to mitral valve annulus velocity determined using tissue Doppler (E/e′) is particularly helpful to determine presence and severity of diastolic dysfunction; a ratio of 15 or greater is abnormal. Pulmonary hypertension in patients without significant systolic dysfunction or pulmonary disease suggests that diastolic dysfunction may be present. Another advantage of echocardiography is the ability to noninvasively estimate right heart pressures. For example, right atrial pressures are estimated by the inferior vena cava (IVC) diameter and the relative change in diameter upon inspiration. Normal IVC diameter and inspiratory collapse of at least 50% are associated with normal RA pressures, while increased IVC diameter and smaller inspiratory changes indicate elevated RA pressure.

Lung ultrasound (LUS) has become increasingly used to evaluate patients presenting to the emergency department setting; it has been found to be useful to diagnose interstitial pulmonary edema and fluid overload through the detection of vertical reverberation artifacts, known as B-lines. Such B-lines are created at the acoustic interface between two structures with differing acoustic impedances, such as fluid-filled structures and alveolar air. Also known as "comets," in the appropriate setting, such B-lines may be highly sensitive and specific for presence of HF, particularly when incorporated with clinical judgment and other tools such as chest radiography and natriuretic peptide testing.

Magnetic Resonance Imaging

MRI provides high-quality imaging of the heart and involves no radiation, which is a significant advantage over CT (see also Chapter 19). Diagnostic images can be obtained in nearly all patients and unlike echocardiography, images can be obtained in arbitrary tomographic planes. MRI is excellent for evaluating cardiac morphology, chamber sizes, and cardiac function. Using different pulse sequences with and without gadolinium contrast, MRI can characterize myocardial tissue and assess myocardial viability. Cardiac MRI can distinguish ischemic from nonischemic cardiomyopathies based upon the pattern of delayed gadolinium enhancement from T1-weighted images: ischemic cardiomyopathies usually show characteristic sub-endocardial enhancement at the sites of prior infarctions, while nonischemic dilated cardiomyopathies most commonly have either no enhancement, mid-wall enhancement, or other patterns depending upon the cause (Fig. 48.6). Additionally, MRI is extremely useful to identify the presence of myocarditis, and may be similarly helpful in the diagnosis of specific cardiomyopathies such as infiltrative processes or left ventricular noncompaction. Use of MRI-compatible pacemakers and defibrillators has facilitated more widespread use of MRI imaging, however clinicians are advised to confirm device compatibility before imaging.

Cardiac Computed Tomography

The current role of cardiac CT in HF is mainly to help determine whether or not obstructive coronary artery disease is present via the use of CT angiography, an important application particularly for patients with lower likelihood for coronary artery disease (see also Chapter 20). Emerging applications of CT angiography may be to assist in assessment of coronary venous anatomy prior to CRT lead placement. Recent advances in CT technology have led to less radiation exposure, however cardiac CT angiography still involves administering iodinated contrast, a concern in patients who are at risk for developing nephrotoxicity.

Nuclear Imaging

A wide array of nuclear imaging techniques have been developed for the assessment of HF (see also Chapter 18). In particular, SPECT and

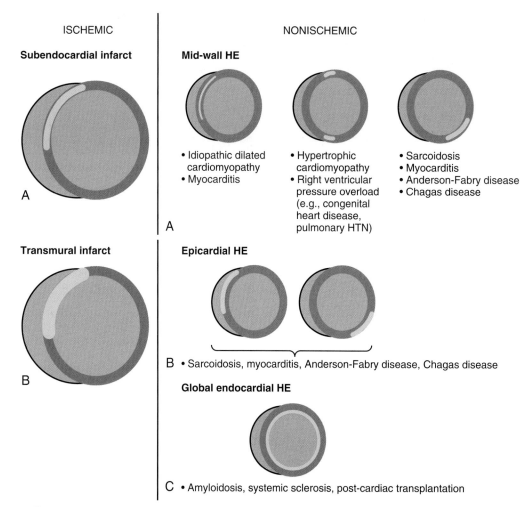

ISCHEMIC

Subendocardial infarct

A

Transmural infarct

B

NONISCHEMIC

Mid-wall HE

- Idiopathic dilated cardiomyopathy
- Myocarditis

A

- Hypertrophic cardiomyopathy
- Right ventricular pressure overload (e.g., congenital heart disease, pulmonary HTN)

- Sarcoidosis
- Myocarditis
- Anderson-Fabry disease
- Chagas disease

Epicardial HE

B • Sarcoidosis, myocarditis, Anderson-Fabry disease, Chagas disease

Global endocardial HE

C • Amyloidosis, systemic sclerosis, post-cardiac transplantation

FIGURE 48.6 Patterns of hyperenhancement (HE) with magnetic resonance imaging (MRI) in various disease states. *HTN*, Hypertension. (Modified from Mahrholdt H, Wagner A, Judd RM, et al. Delayed enhancement cardiovascular magnetic resonance assessment of non-ischaemic cardiomyopathies. *Eur Heart J.* 2005;26:1461.)

PET technologies are well-suited for assessing myocardial ischemia and viability, and for evaluating myocardial function. The use of nuclear imaging to determine myocardial viability is discussed in Chapter 18. ^{18}F-fluorodeoxyglucose (^{18}F-FDG) PET scanning may be particularly helpful for diagnosis prognosis, and management of cardiac sarcoidosis[54]; a characteristic heterogeneous uptake pattern in the myocardium may be seen in patients with cardiac sarcoidosis in contrast to diffuse uptake seen in DCM and normal subjects. Following successful treatment with immunosuppressive medication, ^{18}F-FDG uptake may normalize. ^{99m}Technicium pyrophosphate (^{99m}Tc-PYP) scanning has become a major imaging modality for diagnosing transthyretin amyloidosis (see Chapter 53). Although ^{99m}Tc-PYP scans are more frequently positive in patients with transthyretin amyloidosis, they can also be modestly positive in patients with AL amyloid (see Chapter 53).[55] Lastly, cardiac scans using ^{123}I-metaiodobenzylguanidine (MIBG) may provide objective evaluation of cardiac sympathetic function; this imaging strategy may predict risk for sudden death due to arrhythmia in NYHA class II or III HFrEF when the heart-to-mediastinal ratio of ^{123}I-MIBG is low.[56]

TIMING OF ADVANCED HEART FAILURE REFERRAL

Among patients with advanced HFrEF, early identification and timely referral of select patients to a HF specialist is critical so that those with advanced disease can be considered for heart transplantation or mechanical circulatory support (see also Chapter 50). This window of opportunity is missed if referral is delayed until multiorgan failure develops, as such patients may no longer be candidates for these

therapies. High-risk features include need for intravenous inotropic agents, worsening NYHA symptom severity or congestion refractory to diuretic use, rising natriuretic peptide concentrations, end-organ dysfunction, EF less than 35%, ventricular arrhythmias, recurrent hospitalizations, progressive intolerance to HF therapies, or low blood pressure/high heart rate.

SUMMARY AND FUTURE PERSPECTIVES

As treatment options for HF continue to evolve, there will be increased emphasis on more rapid, accurate, and cost-effective assessment of patients with the goal being to provide unambiguous information about the presence, severity, and cause of HF. New insights into the biology of cardiac dysfunction are likely to lead to the development of therapeutic approaches that are specific to the underlying etiology. Continued advances in the use of biomarkers and imaging techniques to diagnose, stage, and determine etiology of HF will be needed to meet these future demands. Even as these diagnostic modalities increase in their precision and accuracy, the information obtained through the history and physical examination will remain at the core of our ability to understand how to employ these tests most judiciously and to treat patients most effectively.

REFERENCES

Heart Failure Diagnosis and Epidemiology

1. Roger VL. Epidemiology of heart failure. *Circ Res.* 2013;113(6):646–659.
2. Guha K, McDonagh T. Heart failure epidemiology: European perspective. *Curr Cardiol Rev.* 2013;9(2):123–127.
3. Writing Group Members, Mozaffarian D, Benjamin EJ, et al. Executive summary: heart disease and stroke statistics—2016 update: a report from the American Heart Association. *Circulation.* 2016;133(4):447–454.

4. Kapoor JR, Kapoor R, Ju C, et al. Precipitating clinical factors, heart failure characterization, and outcomes in patients hospitalized with heart failure with reduced, borderline, and preserved ejection fraction. *JACC Heart Fail.* 2016;4(6):464–472.
5. Gulati G, Udelson JE. Heart failure with improved ejection fraction: is it possible to escape one's past? *JACC Heart Fail.* 2018;6(9):725–733.
6. Wilcox JE, Fang JC, Margulies KB, Mann DL. Heart failure with recovered left ventricular ejection fraction: JACC Scientific Expert Panel. *J Am Coll Cardiol.* 2020;76(6):719–734.
7. Halliday BP, Wassall R, Lota AS, et al. Withdrawal of pharmacological treatment for heart failure in patients with recovered dilated cardiomyopathy (TRED-HF): an open-label, pilot, randomised trial. *Lancet.* 2019;393(10166):61–73.

The Medical History and Physical Examination

8. Yancy CW, Jessup M, Bozkurt B, et al. 2013 ACCF/AHA guideline for the management of heart failure: a report of the American College of Cardiology Foundation/American Heart Association Task Force on practice guidelines. *J Am Coll Cardiol.* 2013;62(16):e147–239.
9. Solomonica A, Burger AJ, Aronson D. Hemodynamic determinants of dyspnea improvement in acute decompensated heart failure. *Circ Heart Fail.* 2012;6(1):53–60.
10. Damy T, Margarit L, Noroc A, et al. Prognostic impact of sleep-disordered breathing and its treatment with nocturnal ventilation for chronic heart failure. *Eur J Heart Fail.* 2012;14(9):1009–1019.
11. Yu DS, Chan HY, Leung DY, et al. Symptom clusters and quality of life among patients with advanced heart failure. *J Geriatr Cardiol.* 2016;13(5):408–414.
12. Rahman A, Jafry S, Jeejeebhoy K, et al. Malnutrition and cachexia in heart failure. *JPEN J Parenter Enteral Nutr.* 2016;40(4):475–486.
13. Avery CL, Loehr LR, Baggett C, et al. The population burden of heart failure attributable to modifiable risk factors: the ARIC (Atherosclerosis Risk in Communities) study. *J Am Coll Cardiol.* 2012;60(17):1640–1646.
14. Higgins AY, O'Halloran TD, Chang JD. Chemotherapy-induced cardiomyopathy. *Heart Fail Rev.* 2015;20(6):721–730.
15. Kelder JC, Cramer MJ, van Wijngaarden J, et al. The diagnostic value of physical examination and additional testing in primary care patients with suspected heart failure. *Circulation.* 2011;124(25):2865–2873.
16. Ho JE, Gona P, Pencina MJ, et al. Discriminating clinical features of heart failure with preserved vs. reduced ejection fraction in the community. *Eur Heart J.* 2012;33(14):1734–1741.
17. Buckner K. Cardiac asthma. *Immunol Allergy Clin North Am.* 2013;33(1):35–44.
18. Dharmarajan K, Strait KM, Lagu T, et al. Acute decompensated heart failure is routinely treated as a cardiopulmonary syndrome. *PloS One.* 2013;8(10):e78222.
19. Nohria A, Tsang SW, Fang JC, et al. Clinical assessment identifies hemodynamic profiles that predict outcomes in patients admitted with heart failure. *J Am Coll Cardiol.* 2003;41(10):1797–1804.

Routine Laboratory Assessment

20. Sartini S, Frizzi J, Borselli M, et al. Which method is best for an early accurate diagnosis of acute heart failure? Comparison between lung ultrasound, chest X-ray and NT pro-BNP performance: a prospective study. *Intern Emerg Med.* 2016.
21. Urso C, Brucculeri S, Caimi G. Acid-base and electrolyte abnormalities in heart failure: pathophysiology and implications. *Heart Fail Rev.* 2015;20(4):493–503.
22. Mohammed AA, van Kimmenade RR, Richards M, et al. Hyponatremia, natriuretic peptides, and outcomes in acutely decompensated heart failure: results from the International Collaborative of NT-proBNP Study. *Circ Heart Fail.* 2010;3(3):354–361.
23. O'Connell JB, Alemayehu A. Hyponatremia, heart failure, and the role of tolvaptan. *Postgrad Med.* 2012;124(2):29–39.
24. Legrand M, Mebazaa A, Ronco C, Januzzi Jr JL. When cardiac failure, kidney dysfunction, and kidney injury intersect in acute conditions: the case of cardiorenal syndrome. *Crit Care Med.* 2014;42(9):2109–2117.
25. Damman K, Valente MA, Voors AA, et al. Renal impairment, worsening renal function, and outcome in patients with heart failure: an updated meta-analysis. *Eur Heart J.* 2014;35(7):455–469.
26. Fonarow GC, Adams Jr KF, Abraham WT, et al. Risk stratification for in-hospital mortality in acutely decompensated heart failure: classification and regression tree analysis. *J Am Med Assoc.* 2005;293(5):572–580.
27. Lala A, McNulty SE, Mentz RJ, et al. Relief and recurrence of congestion during and after hospitalization for acute heart failure: insights from diuretic optimization strategy evaluation in acute decompensated heart failure (DOSE-AHF) and cardiorenal rescue study in acute decompensated heart failure (CARESS-HF). *Circ Heart Fail.* 2015;8(4):741–748.
28. Cleland JG, Zhang J, Pellicori P, et al. Prevalence and outcomes of anemia and hematinic deficiencies in patients with chronic heart failure. *JAMA Cardiol.* 2016;1(5):539–547.
29. Huang YL, Hu ZD, Liu SJ, et al. Prognostic value of red blood cell distribution width for patients with heart failure: a systematic review and meta-analysis of cohort studies. *PloS One.* 2014;9(8):e104861.
30. Braunwald E. Biomarkers in heart failure. *N Engl J Med.* 2008;358(20):2148–2159.

31. van Kimmenade RR, Januzzi Jr JL. Emerging biomarkers in heart failure. *Clin Chem.* 2011;58(1):127–138.
32. Shah RV, Truong QA, Gaggin HK, et al. Mid-regional pro-atrial natriuretic peptide and pro-adrenomedullin testing for the diagnostic and prognostic evaluation of patients with acute dyspnoea. *Eur Heart J.* 2012;33(17):2197–2205.
33. Ibrahim N, Januzzi JL. The potential role of natriuretic peptides and other biomarkers in heart failure diagnosis, prognosis and management. *Expert Rev Cardiovasc Ther.* 2015;13(9):1017–1030.
34. Januzzi Jr JL, Prescott MF, Butler J, et al. Association of change in N-terminal pro-B-type natriuretic peptide following Initiation of Sacubitril-Valsartan treatment with cardiac structure and function in patients with heart failure with reduced ejection fraction. *J Am Med Assoc.* 2019;1–11.
35. Januzzi Jr JL, Camacho A, Pina IL, et al. Reverse cardiac remodeling and outcome after initiation of sacubitril/valsartan. *Circ Heart Fail.* 2020;13(6):e006946.
36. Zile MR, Claggett BL, Prescott MF, et al. Prognostic implications of changes in N-terminal pro-B-type natriuretic peptide in patients with heart failure. *J Am Coll Cardiol.* 2016;68(22):2425–2436.
37. Kim HN, Januzzi Jr JL. Natriuretic peptide testing in heart failure. *Circulation.* 2011;123(18):2015–2019.
38. Januzzi Jr JL, Chen-Tournoux AA, Christenson RH, et al. N-terminal pro-B-type natriuretic peptide in the emergency department: the ICON-RELOADED study. *J Am Coll Cardiol.* 2018;71(11):1191–1200.
39. Salah K, Kok WE, Eurlings LW, et al. A novel discharge risk model for patients hospitalised for acute decompensated heart failure incorporating N-terminal pro-B-type natriuretic peptide levels: a European coLlaboration on Acute decompeNsated Heart Failure: ELAN-HF Score. *Heart.* 2014;100(2):115–125.
40. Shah RV, Januzzi Jr JL. Soluble ST2 and galectin-3 in heart failure. *Clin Lab Med.* 2014;34(1):87–97 (vi–vii).
41. Aimo A, Vergaro G, Passino C, et al. Prognostic value of soluble suppression of tumorigenicity-2 in chronic heart failure: a meta-analysis. *JACC Heart Fail.* 2017;5(4):280–286.
42. Aimo A, Vergaro G, Ripoli A, et al. Meta-analysis of soluble suppression of tumorigenicity-2 and prognosis in acute heart failure. *JACC Heart Fail.* 2017;5(4):287–296.
43. Wang TJ, Wollert KC, Larson MG, et al. Prognostic utility of novel biomarkers of cardiovascular stress: the Framingham Heart Study. *Circulation.* 2012;126(13):1596–1604.
44. Januzzi Jr JL, Filippatos G, Nieminen M, Gheorghiade M. Troponin elevation in patients with heart failure: on behalf of the third universal definition of myocardial infarction global task force: heart failure section. *Eur Heart J.* 2012;33(18):2265–2271.
45. Metra M, Cotter G, Gheorghiade M, et al. The role of the kidney in heart failure. *Eur Heart J.* 2012;33(17):2135–2142.

Risk Scoring for Prognosis

46. Alba AC, Agoritsas T, Jankowski M, et al. Risk prediction models for mortality in ambulatory patients with heart failure: a systematic review. *Circ Heart Fail.* 2013;6(5):881–889.

Right Heart Catheterization

47. Kahwash R, Leier CV, Miller L. Role of the pulmonary artery catheter in diagnosis and management of heart failure. *Cardiol Clin.* 2011;29(2):281–288.

Detecting Comorbid Conditions

48. van Deursen VM, Damman K, van der Meer P, et al. Co-morbidities in heart failure. *Heart Fail Rev.* 2012.
49. Group SR, Wright Jr JT, Williamson JD, et al. A randomized trial of intensive versus standard blood-pressure control. *N Engl J Med.* 2015;373(22):2103–2116.
50. Zinman B, Wanner C, Lachin JM, et al. Empagliflozin, cardiovascular outcomes, and mortality in type 2 diabetes. *N Engl J Med.* 2015;373(22):2117–2128.

Assessment of Quality of Life

51. Garin O, Herdman M, Vilagut G, et al. Assessing health-related quality of life in patients with heart failure: a systematic, standardized comparison of available measures. *Heart Fail Rev.* 2014;19(3):359–367.

Cardiopulmonary Exercise Testing and Imaging Modalities

52. Malhotra R, Bakken K, D'Elia E, Lewis GD. Cardiopulmonary exercise testing in heart failure. *JACC Heart Fail.* 2016;4(8):607–616.
53. Omar AM, Bansal M, Sengupta PP. Advances in echocardiographic imaging in heart failure with reduced and preserved ejection fraction. *Circ Res.* 2016;119(2):357–374.
54. Aggarwal NR, Snipelisky D, Young PM, et al. Advances in imaging for diagnosis and management of cardiac sarcoidosis. *Eur Heart J Cardiovasc Imaging.* 2015;16(9):949–958.
55. Maurer MS. Noninvasive identification of ATTRwt cardiac amyloid: the Re-emergence of nuclear Cardiology. *Am J Med.* 2015;128(12):1275–1280.
56. Travin MI. Clinical applications of myocardial innervation imaging. *Cardiol Clin.* 2016;34(1):133–147.

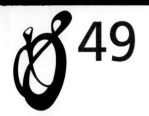 # 49 Diagnosis and Management of Acute Heart Failure

G. MICHAEL FELKER AND JOHN R. TEERLINK

Acute heart failure (AHF) is among the most common causes for hospitalization in patients older than 65 years in the developed world. Increasingly, the spectrum of worsening HF is recognized to encompass not just patients requiring acute hospitalization, but also worsening of HF in outpatient settings and in patients already hospitalized. The prevalence of HF is projected to continue to increase over time due to a convergence of several epidemiologic trends: the aging of the population, given the age-related incidence of HF; the reduction in hypertension-related mortality and the greatly improved survival after myocardial infarction (MI), resulting in more patients living with chronic heart failure (see Chapter 48); and the availability of effective therapy for prevention of sudden death (see Chapters 58 and 70) (Fig. 49.1). AHF is increasingly recognized as a distinct disorder with unique epidemiology, pathophysiology, treatments, and outcomes.

EPIDEMIOLOGY

Nomenclature and Definition

A variety of overlapping terms have been used to characterize AHF in the literature, including "acute heart failure syndromes" (AHFS), "acute decompensated heart failure" (ADHF), "acute decompensation of chronic heart failure" (ADCHF), "worsening heart failure" (WHF), and "hospitalization for heart failure" (HHF). Although none of these is universally accepted, we will use the terminology "acute heart failure" in this chapter for simplicity. Broadly speaking, AHF can be defined as the new onset or recurrence of symptoms and signs of HF requiring urgent or emergent therapy and resulting in unscheduled care or hospitalization. An important source of confusion with this proposed definition is the word "acute"—although this suggests a sudden onset of symptoms, many patients may have a more sub-acute course, with gradual worsening of symptoms that ultimately reaches a level of severity sufficient to seek unscheduled medical care.

Scope of the Problem

In the United States, HF is the primary diagnosis for more than 1 million hospitalized patients annually, and a secondary diagnosis for an additional 3 million hospitalizations.[1] Similar numbers of hospitalizations are reported in Europe.[2] The direct and indirect costs associated with HF approach 40 billion US dollars per year in the United States, and the majority of these expenditures are related to the costs

of hospitalizations.[3,4] As noted earlier, the overall prevalence of chronic heart failure continues to grow. However, recent data suggest that the age-adjusted rate of HHF has begun to decrease, at least for primary heart failure events.[1] To what extent these changes are related to more effective treatments of chronic heart failure or alternatively, changes in care to create alternative care pathways for avoiding hospitalization is unknown. Changes in medical care (especially in the United States) have led to increased efforts to manage milder forms of WHF without hospitalization, utilizing outpatient diuretic clinics and observation units, although available data suggest that even these milder forms of decompensation are still associated with adverse prognosis.[5,6] Despite these potentially encouraging trends, AHF will be a major clinical and economic problem for health care systems for the foreseeable future. An important development in the understanding of the epidemiology, clinical characteristics, and outcomes of patients with AHF has been the development of large, relatively unselected registries of AHF which provide a "real-world" perspective on the epidemiology and outcomes of AHF worldwide (Table 49.1).[7]

Ejection Fraction

On the basis of available registry data, 40% to 50% of patients hospitalized have heart failure with preserved ejection fraction (HFpEF). Important epidemiologic differences exist between heart failure with reduced ejection fraction (HFrEF) and HFpEF (see Chapter 48). The in-hospital mortality of patients with HFpEF appears to be lower compared with that of patients with HFrEF, but post-discharge rehospitalization rates and long-term mortality after hospitalization are similarly high for both groups. Patients with AHF and HFpEF are more likely to be rehospitalized for and to die from non-CV causes than patients with AHF and HFrEF, reflecting their more advanced age and greater burden of comorbidity. More recently, the concept of heart failure with "mid-range ejection fraction" or "mildly reduced ejection fraction," that is, HF-mrEF, has been proposed as an additional refinement of the standard HFrEF vs HFpEF dichotomy, but specific data on AHF outcomes in this group are limited (Fig. 49.2).[8]

Age, Race, and Gender

There are significant differences in the epidemiology of AHF based on age, race, and gender. AHF disproportionally affects older people, with a mean age of 75 years in large registries. AHF affects men and women

Additional content is available online at Elsevier eBooks for Practicing Clinicians

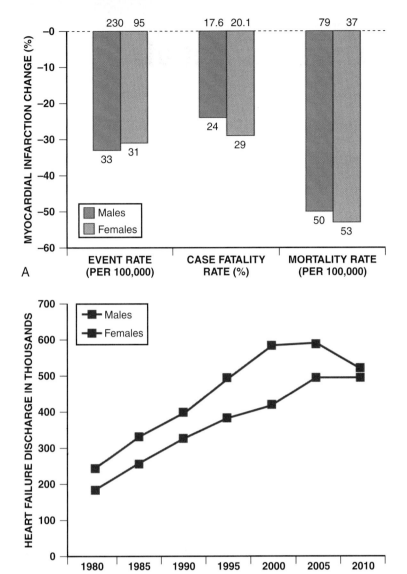

FIGURE 49.1 Reduction in myocardial infarction (MI) and increase in acute heart failure hospitalizations. **A,** Percentage change in MI rates and fatality rates in England from 2002 to 2010. **B,** Hospital discharges for heart failure by gender from 1980 to 2010. (From Braunwald E. The war against heart failure: the Lancet lecture. *Lancet.* 2015;385[9970]:812–824.)

failure, but also can complicate diagnosis and management. Hypertension is the most prevalent concurrent condition, present in approximately two-thirds of the patients (see also Chapter 26), whereas coronary artery disease (CAD) is present in about half and dyslipidemia in over one-third (see Chapters 27 and 40).[11,12] Other conditions that are the result of the vascular injury produced by these diseases, such as stroke, peripheral vascular disease, and chronic kidney disease are also very common in patients with AHF. Diabetes mellitus is present in over 40% of US patients, most likely related to increasing incidence of obesity, and ranges from 27% to 38% in Europe. The interaction between heart failure status and diabetes has been a subject of substantial interest, given the evolving data that some classes of anti-diabetic drugs, specifically the sodium-glucose co-transporter-2 (SGLT-2) inhibitors and glucagon-like peptide-1 (GLP-1) agonists, have a favorable impact on heart failure outcomes (see Chapter 50). Atrial fibrillation can both precipitate AHF and complicate its management.

Global Differences in Acute Heart Failure

Although the majority of data continues to emerge from North America and from Europe, AHF is increasingly recognized as a global issue, and important differences between regions of the world have emerged in terms of epidemiology, therapy, and outcomes.[13] Although there are a variety of country- or region-specific registries (see Table 49.1), to date most available data highlighting these differences have come from large global outcome trials. Although these studies can provide important insight into regional differences, they suffer from inherent selection bias of clinical trials and may not be truly representative of the general population. The recently reported REPORT-HF registry provides a more contemporary assessment of AHF globally (see Table 49.1).[7]

PATHOPHYSIOLOGY

The pathophysiology of AHF is complex and highly variable, with many overlapping pathogenic mechanisms that may be operative to a greater or lesser degree. This fundamental heterogeneity complicates the attempt to create a unified conceptual model. A useful framework for understanding of the pathophysiology of AHF is to consider it as the result of the interaction of underlying substrate, initiating mechanisms or triggers, and amplifying mechanisms, all of which contribute to a common set of clinical signs and symptoms (primarily related to congestion, end-organ dysfunction, or both) that define the clinical picture of AHF (Fig. 49.3). In this context, substrate refers to underlying cardiac structure and function. The underlying substrate may be one of normal ventricular function, for example patients without a prior history of HF who develop AHF because of sudden changes in ventricular function from an acute insult such as MI or acute myocarditis (see Chapter 55). Alternatively, some patients may have no prior history of HF but abnormal substrate (e.g., stage B patients with asymptomatic LV dysfunction) with a first presentation of heart failure (de novo heart failure). Finally, most patients with AHF have a substrate of chronic compensated HF who then decompensate and present with AHF (sometimes termed decompensated chronic heart failure [DCHF]).

Initiating mechanisms vary according to and interact with the underlying substrate and may be cardiac or extra-cardiac. For patients with normal substrate (normal myocardium), a substantial insult to cardiac performance (e.g., acute myocarditis) is generally required to lead to the clinical presentation of AHF. For patients with abnormal substrate at baseline (asymptomatic LV dysfunction), smaller perturbations (e.g., poorly controlled hypertension, atrial fibrillation, or ischemia) may precipitate an AHF episode. For patients with a substrate of compensated or stable chronic HF, medical or dietary nonadherence, drugs

almost equally, but there are important differences by gender. In the ADHERE registry women admitted for AHF were older than men (74 vs. 70 years), and more frequently had preserved systolic function (51% vs. 28%).[9] Differences in ethnic groups have been studied most extensively in the United States and have focused primarily on differences between African American and white patients. In the Organized Program to Initiate Lifesaving Treatment in Hospitalized Patients with Heart Failure (OPTIMIZE-HF) registry, African American patients admitted with AHF were younger (64 vs. 75 years), more likely to have left ventricular (LV) systolic dysfunction (57% vs. 51%) with a lower mean EF (35% vs. 40%), hypertensive cause for heart failure (39% vs. 19%), renal dysfunction, and diabetes compared to the non–African American group.[10] Lower crude mortality rates have been reported for African Americans compared to non–African American patients, but when adjustments are made for these differences in comorbidities and age, mortality rates are similar.

Comorbidities

Concomitant diseases are very common in patients admitted with AHF, reflective of the older population. These comorbidities not only represent diseases that are risk factors for the development of heart

VI

HEART FAILURE

TABLE 49.1 Demographics and Comorbidities of Patients Hospitalized with Acute Heart Failure from Selected Studies

	ADHERE (n = 187,565)	OPTIMIZE-HF (n = 48,612)	PERNA et al. (n = 2974)	EHFS II (n = 3580)	ATTEND (n = 4841)	DAMASCENO (n = 1006)	REPORT-HF (n = 18,102)
Region	US	US	Argentina	Europe	Japan	Africa	Global
Age (years)	75	73	68	70	73	52	67
Male (%)	48	48	59	61	58	49	61
Preserved EF (%)	53	51	26	52	47	25	45
Prior HF (%)	76	88	50	63	36	–	57
Medical History							
Coronary artery disease	57%	50%		54%	N/A		48%
Myocardial infarction	30%	N/A	22%		N/A		N/A
Hypertension	74%	71%	66%	62%	69%	56%	64%
Atrial fibrillation or flutter	31%	31*%	27%	39%	40%	18%	31%
Chronic kidney disease	30%	20%	10%	17%	N/A	8%	20%
Diabetes	44%	42%	23%	33%	34%	11%	37%
COPD/Asthma	31%	34%	15%	19%	12%	N/A	N/A

Data from ADHERE: ADHERE Scientific Advisory Committee. Acute Decompensated Heart Failure National Registry (ADHERE®) Core Module Q1 2006 Final Cumulative National Benchmark Report: Scios, Inc.; July, 2006. OPTIMIZE-HF: Gheorghiade M, Abraham WT, Albert NM, et al. Systolic blood pressure at admission, clinical characteristics, and outcomes in patients hospitalized with acute heart failure. *JAMA.* 2006;296:2217–2226. Argentina: Perna ER, Barbagelata A, Grinfeld L, et al. Overview of acute decompensated heart failure in Argentina: lessons learned from 5 registries during the last decade. *Am Heart J.* 2006;151:84–91. EHFS II: Nieminen MS, Brutsaert D, Dickstein K, et al. EuroHeart Failure Survey II (EHFS II): a survey on hospitalized acute heart failure patients: description of population. *Eur Heart J.* 2006;27:2725–2736. ATTEND: Sato N, Gheorghiade M, Kajimoto K, et al. Hyponatremia and in-hospital mortality in patients admitted for heart failure (from the ATTEND registry). *Am J Cardiol.* 2013;111:1019–25, and Dr Naoki Sato, personal communication. AFRICA: Damasceno A, Mayosi BM, Sani M, et al. The causes, treatment, and outcome of acute heart failure in 1006 Africans from 9 countries: results of the sub-Saharan Africa survey of heart failure. *Arch Intern Med.* 2012;172:1386–94. REPORT-HF: Tromp J, Bamadhaj S, Cleland JGF, et al. Post-discharge prognosis of patients admitted to hospital for heart failure by world region, and national level of income and income disparity (REPORT-HF): a cohort study. *Lancet: Global Health* 2020;8:e411–e422

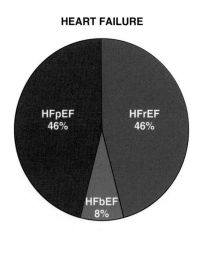

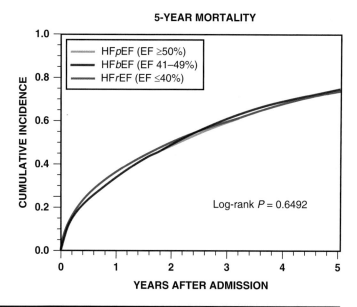

OUTCOMES-5-YEAR EVENT RATES (%)					
	Mortality	Readmission	CV Readmission	HF Readmission	Mortality/Readmission
HFrEF	75.3	82.2	63.9	48.5	96.4
HFbEF	75.7	85.7	63.3	45.2	97.2
HFpEF	75.7	84.0	58.9	40.5	97.3

FIGURE 49.2 Outcomes after acute heart failure (AHF) hospitalization by ejection fraction. *HFbEF,* HF with borderline ejection fraction; *HFpEF,* HF with preserved ejection fraction; *HFrEF,* HF with reduced ejection fraction. (From Shah KS, Xu H, Matsouaka RA, et al. Heart failure with preserved, borderline, and reduced ejection fraction: 5-year outcomes. *JACC.* 2017;70[20]:2476–2486.)

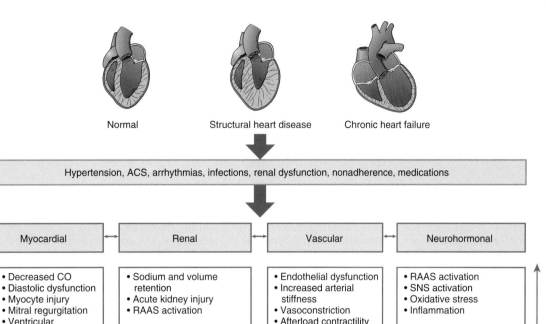

FIGURE 49.3 Schematic of the pathophysiology of acute heart failure.

such as nonsteroidal antiinflammatory agents or thiazolidinediones, and infectious processes are all common triggers for decompensation.

Regardless of the substrate or initiating factors, a variety of "amplifying mechanisms" perpetuate and contribute to the episode of decompensation. These include neurohormonal and inflammatory activation, ongoing myocardial injury with progressive myocardial dysfunction, worsening renal function, and interactions with the peripheral vasculature, all of which may contribute to the propagation and worsening of the AHF episode.

Congestion

Systemic or pulmonary congestion often due to a high ventricular diastolic pressure dominates the clinical presentation of most patients hospitalized for AHF. Congestion can be seen as a final common pathway producing clinical symptoms leading to hospitalization. An oversimplified view of AHF pathophysiology is that gradual increases in intravascular volume lead to symptoms of congestion and clinical presentation, and normalization of volume status with diuretic therapy results in restoration of homeostasis. Although some data suggest that increases in body weight often precede decompensation and hospitalization for HF, careful studies using implantable hemodynamic monitors suggest that increases in invasively measured LV filling pressures can occur without substantial changes in body weight.[14] These observations have led to increasing interest in the concept of volume redistribution and the dynamic role of the vasculature as a contributing mechanism to decompensation in heart failure (discussed in more detail in "Vascular Mechanisms" section below).

One important concept is the distinction between "clinical congestion" and "hemodynamic congestion." Although patients present with signs and symptoms of systemic congestion such as dyspnea, rales, elevated jugular venous pressure (JVP), and edema, this state is often preceded by "hemodynamic congestion," defined as high ventricular

diastolic pressures without overt clinical signs. Similarly, clinical congestion may resolve with treatment but hemodynamic congestion may persist, leading to a high risk of rehospitalization. It has been postulated that hemodynamic congestion may contribute to the progression of HF because it may result in increased wall stress as well as in renin-angiotensin-aldosterone system (RAAS) and sympathetic nervous system (SNS) activation. This may trigger a variety of molecular responses in the myocardium, including myocyte loss and increased fibrosis. The natriuretic peptides (see Chapter 47), which are the intrinsic counter-regulatory hormone in heart failure, may have abnormal processing that leads to diminished biologic activity in patients with advanced heart failure.[15] In addition, elevated diastolic filling pressures may decrease coronary perfusion pressure, resulting in sub-endocardial ischemia that may further exacerbate cardiac dysfunction. Increased LV filling pressures can also lead to acute changes in ventricular architecture (more spherical shape), contributing to worsening mitral regurgitation. These mechanisms also play an important role in pathologic remodeling of the ventricle, a chronic process that may be accelerated by each episode of decompensation. Consistent with this paradigm is the well-established clinical observation that each hospitalization for AHF heralds a substantial worsening of the long-term prognosis, an effect that appears additive with recurrent hospitalizations.[16] Data from studies with implantable hemodynamic monitors have confirmed that chronically elevated filling pressures (i.e., hemodynamic congestion) are associated with increased risk of future events.[17] With the recognition of congestion as the most common aspect of AHF presentation, there has been a formal attempt to better assess and quantitate congestion in heart failure.[18]

Myocardial Function

Although a variety of extra-cardiac factors play important roles in AHF, impairments of cardiac function (systolic, diastolic, or both) remain central to our understanding of this disorder (see also Chapter 46). Changes in systolic function and decreased arterial filling can initiate a cascade of effects that are adaptive in the short term but maladaptive when elevated chronically, including stimulation of the SNS and RAAS. Activation of these neurohormonal axes leads to vasoconstriction, sodium and water retention, volume redistribution from other vascular beds, increases in diastolic filling pressures, and clinical symptoms. In patients with underlying ischemic heart disease, initial defects in systolic function may initiate a vicious cycle of decreasing coronary perfusion, increased myocardial wall stress, and progressively worsening cardiac performance. Increased LV filling pressures and changes in LV geometry can worsen functional mitral regurgitation, further decreasing cardiac output.

Importantly, abnormalities in diastolic function are present in heart failure patients regardless of EF. The impairment of the diastolic phase may be related to passive stiffness, abnormal active relaxation of the left ventricle, or both. Hypertension, tachycardia, and myocardial ischemia (even in the absence of CAD) can further impair diastolic filling. All of these mechanisms contribute to higher LV end-diastolic pressures, which are reflected back to the pulmonary capillary circulation. Diastolic dysfunction alone may be insufficient to lead to AHF, but it serves as the substrate on which other precipitating factors (such as atrial fibrillation, CAD, or hypertension) lead to decompensation. One underappreciated aspect of myocardial function in AHF relates to the interdependence of the left and right ventricles. Because of the constraints of the pericardial space, distention of either ventricle due to increased filling pressures can result in direct impingement of diastolic filling of the other ventricle. This may be particularly operative in clinical scenarios leading to abrupt failure of the right ventricle (such as pulmonary embolism or right ventricular (RV) infarction), resulting in diminished filling of the left ventricle and arterial hypotension.

The availability of increasingly sensitive assays for circulating cardiac troponins has led to evolution of our understanding of the role of myocardial injury in AHF pathophysiology. Data from both registries and clinical trial populations indicate that circulating cardiac troponins are elevated in a large proportion of patients with AHF, even in the absence of clinically overt myocardial ischemia.[19,20] In a representative analysis of data from the RELAX-AHF study using a highly sensitive assay, 90% of patients enrolled had a troponin T level above the 99th percentile upper reference limit at baseline, and troponin elevation was associated with post-discharge outcomes out to 180 days (Fig. 49.4).[21]

The precise mechanisms mediating myocardial injury in AHF are poorly defined, but increased myocardial wall stress, decreased coronary perfusion pressure, increased myocardial oxygen demand, endothelial dysfunction, activation of the neurohormonal and inflammatory pathways, platelet activation, and altered calcium handling may all contribute to myocyte injury even in the absence of epicardial CAD.[19] Specific therapeutic interventions that may increase myocardial oxygen demand (such as positive inotropic agents) or decrease coronary artery perfusion pressure (such as some vasodilators) may exacerbate myocardial injury and further contribute to the cycle of decompensation. Whether avoidance of myocardial injury is a specific target for therapy in AHF remains a subject of active investigation.

Renal Mechanisms

The kidney plays two fundamental roles relative to the pathophysiology of HF: it modulates loading conditions of the heart by controlling intravascular volume and is responsible for neurohormonal outputs (i.e., the RAAS system). Abnormalities of renal function are extremely common in patients with AHF and may be underestimated by creatinine alone.[22] Baseline chronic kidney disease is an established risk factor for poor outcomes in AHF (see Risk Stratification section later), but our understanding of the implications of changes in renal function during AHF treatment has continued to evolve.[23] The term "cardio-renal syndrome" has been increasingly used to describe pathologic interactions between the cardiac and renal axes in the setting of heart failure. Although specific definitions and nomenclature have varied, in the context of AHF the cardio-renal syndrome describes the clinical situation of worsening measures of renal function in the setting of persistent congestion. This clinical scenario has been associated with poor outcomes in a variety of observational studies. Multiple studies have investigated the pathophysiology and risk factors for this phenomenon, which is related to an intricate interplay of patient characteristics (age), comorbidities (baseline renal function as assessed by glomerular filtration rate [GFR], diabetes mellitus, hypertension), neurohormonal activation (especially of RAAS and SNS), and hemodynamic factors (central venous congestion, and less frequently arterial underfilling with renal hypoperfusion), as well as other factors such as activation of inflammatory cascades and oxidative stress.[24] Although often assumed to be related to low cardiac output and renal blood flow, careful hemodynamic studies have repeatedly confirmed that the strongest predictor of worsening renal function in heart failure patients relates to elevated central venous pressure (CVP), which is reflected back to the renal veins and leads directly to changes in GFR.[25] Importantly, recent data have emphasized the importance of evaluating changes in renal function in the context of the overall clinical picture. Worsening renal function in the setting of ongoing clinical improvement is generally reflective of successful decongestion and does not portend a poor prognosis (Fig. 49.5).[26] Although there has been substantial interest in the utility of newer biomarkers to identify episodes of frank kidney injury prior to changes in markers of renal function, the clinical utility of these markers remains uncertain. A detailed

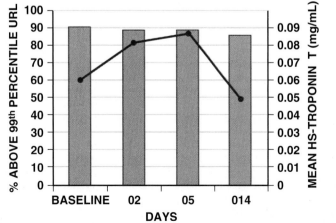
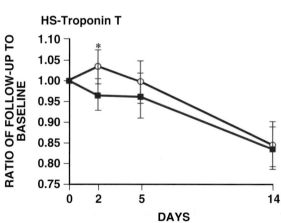

FIGURE 49.4 Incidence of elevated (above the 99th percentile upper reference limit) high-sensitivity troponin T in the RELAX-AHF study and effect of serelaxin therapy on troponin levels. (From Felker GM, Mentz FJ, Teerlink JR, et al. Serial high sensitivity cardiac troponin T measurement in acute heart failure: insights from the RELAX-AHF study. *Eur J Heart Fail*. 2015;17:1262–1270; and Metra M, Cotter G, Davison BA, et al. Effect of serelaxin on cardiac, renal, and hepatic biomarkers in the relaxin in acute heart failure (RELAX-AHF) development program: correlation with outcomes. *J Am Coll Cardiol*. 2013;61:196–206.)

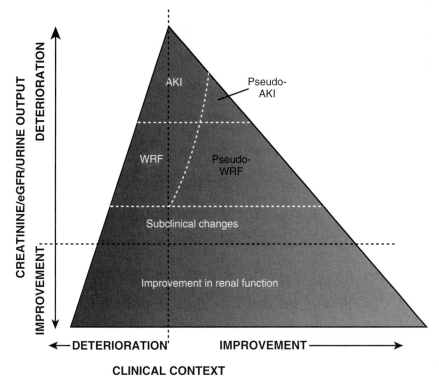

FIGURE 49.5 Schematic of changes in renal function within different clinical context in acute heart failure. AKI, acute kidney injury; WRF, worsened renal function. (From Damman K, Testani JM. The kidney in heart failure: an update. *Eur Heart J.* 2015;36:1437–1444.)

classification system for understanding the interplay between cardiac performance and renal function has been proposed and provides a framework for understanding the complex pathophysiology underlying the cardio-renal syndrome.[24]

Vascular Mechanisms

While abnormalities in cardiac function are central to the pathogenesis of AHF, there is increasing appreciation for the importance of the peripheral vasculature in this disorder. Abnormalities of endothelial function related to nitric oxide dependent regulation of vascular tone are well described in heart failure.[27] Arterial stiffness, which is related to but distinct from blood pressure, increases cardiac loading conditions and is associated with incident heart failure and worse outcomes. Peripheral vasoconstriction in the setting of AHF redistributes blood centrally, increasing pulmonary venous congestion and edema. As noted earlier, elevated CVP reduces renal function, resulting in greater fluid retention, which further elevates venous pressures. Peripheral arterial vasoconstriction increases afterload, LV filling pressures, and post-capillary pulmonary venous pressures, resulting in worsening of pulmonary edema and dyspnea. This increased afterload causes greater ventricular wall stress and increased myocardial ischemia and cardiac arrhythmias. Abnormal vascular compliance also predisposes these patients to marked blood pressure liability with relatively minor changes in intravascular volume, causing precipitous increases in afterload and ultimately in LV filling pressures resulting in pulmonary congestion. The effects of this vascular abnormality are amplified by LV diastolic dysfunction.

The clinical observation that vasodilator treatment can improve dyspnea in many acutely hypertensive patients without significant diuresis has led to the concept that afterload-contractility mismatch can lead to increased diastolic filling pressures in the setting of minimal total body volume changes. Similarly, the recognition of the large capacitance of the venous (in particular the splanchnic circulation) system has led to increased interest in volume shifts from the "venous reservoir" into the effective circulatory volume as a potentially important and under-recognized mechanism in AHF.[28] These shifts can be mediated by SNS activation, and this has been proposed as a potential

explanation between the apparent disconnect between changes in filling pressures and changes in body weight during chronic hemodynamic monitoring. Whether fluid shifts involving this venous reservoir can be modulated therapeutically is a subject of active investigation.[29]

Neurohormonal and Inflammatory Mechanisms

Although elevations of circulating neurohormones are well-documented in patients with AHF, the precise role of neurohormonal activation in the pathophysiology of AHF remains to be fully delineated. Increased plasma concentrations of norepinephrine, plasma renin activity, aldosterone, and endothelin-1 (ET-1) have all been reported in patients with AHF—all of these axes are associated with vasoconstriction and volume retention, which could contribute to myocardial ischemia and congestion, thus exacerbating cardiac decompensation. Inflammatory activation and oxidative stress may also play a role. Pro-inflammatory cytokines such as tumor necrosis factor-alpha and interleukin-6 are elevated in patients with AHF and have direct negative inotropic effects on the myocardium as well as increasing capillary permeability and inducing endothelial dysfunction.[30,31] In addition to direct effects, this activation stimulates the release of other factors, such as the potent pro-coagulant tissue factor and ET-1, which can lead to further myocardial suppression, disruption of the pulmonary alveolar capillary barrier, and increased platelet aggregation and coagulation (potentially worsening ischemia).

EVALUATION OF THE ACUTE HEART FAILURE PATIENT

The initial evaluation of the patient with AHF focuses on the following critical aspects: (1) establishing a definitive diagnosis of AHF as rapidly and efficiently as possible; (2) emergent treatment for potentially life-threatening conditions (e.g., shock, respiratory failure); (3) identifying and addressing any relevant clinical triggers or other condition requiring specific treatment (e.g., acute coronary syndrome [ACS], acute pulmonary embolism, etc.); (4) risk stratification in order to triage patient to appropriate level of care (e.g., intensive care unit [ICU], telemetry unit, observation unit); and (5) defining the clinical profile of the patient (based on blood pressure, volume status, and renal function) in order to rapidly implement the most appropriate therapy. A proposed flow diagram for the initial evaluation of patients with suspected AHF is shown in Figure 49.6.[32]

Classification

The inherent heterogeneity of AHF makes the development of a comprehensive classification scheme difficult, and no single classification system has garnered universal acceptance. There are several relevant domains to consider in classifying patients with AHF (Fig. 49.7). These include underlying **substrate** (i.e., whether there is a prior history of structural heart disease or a background of chronic HF), **severity** (from mild symptoms to cardiogenic shock), **acuity** (gradual onset vs. sudden/acute onset), and **triggers** (which may be readily apparent or unknown). Each of these concepts is discussed briefly below.

Substrate

New-onset or de novo heart failure makes up about 20% of hospitalizations for AHF.[12] These patients may have no prior history of cardiovascular disease or risk factors (e.g., acute myocarditis), but more commonly, they have a background of risk factors for HF (stage A heart failure according to the

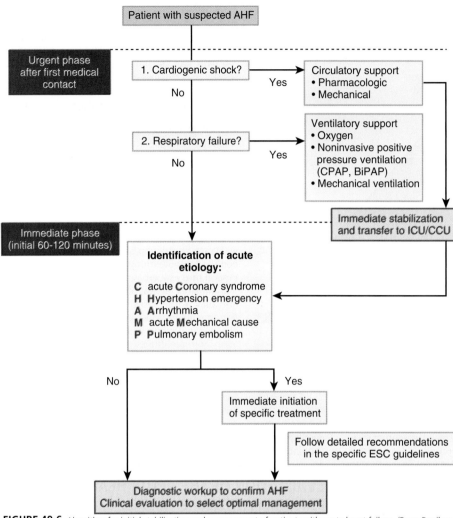

FIGURE 49.6 Algorithm for initial stabilization and management of patients with acute heart failure. (From Ponikowski P, Voors AA, Anker SD, et al. 2016 ESC Guidelines for the diagnosis and treatment of acute and chronic heart failure: the Task Force for the diagnosis and treatment of acute and chronic heart failure of the European Society of Cardiology (ESC) developed with the special contribution of the Heart Failure Association (HFA) of the ESC. *Eur Heart J.* 2016 Jul 14;37[27]:2129–2200.)

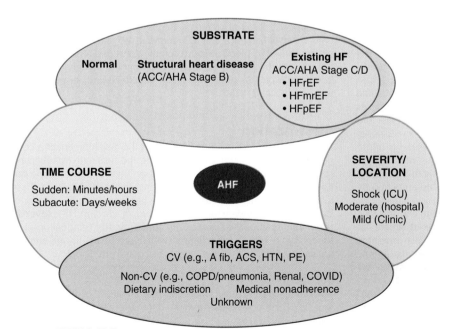

FIGURE 49.7 Systematic approach to classification of patients with acute heart failure.

American College of Cardiology/American Heart Association [ACC/AHA] guidelines) or preexisting structural heart disease (stage B heart failure according to the ACC/AHA guidelines) (see also Chapters 48 and 50). Many of these patients with de novo heart failure develop AHF in the setting of ACS. The majority of AHF patients have a history of preexisting chronic heart failure. These patients often have a less dramatic clinical presentation because the chronic nature of the disorder has allowed for recruitment of compensatory mechanisms and remodeling (e.g., increased pulmonary lymphatic capacity). Additionally, these patients are typically already being treated with neurohormonal antagonists and loop diuretics, such that neurohormonal activation may be less profound but diuretic resistance may be more common. In patients with AHF with a background of chronic HF, these patients can be further sub-classified by ejection fraction (i.e., HFrEF, HFmrEF, HFpEF) or by cause (i.e., ischemic, nonischemic, etc.) although these factors less often impact acute management of the AHF episode.

Severity

Patients with AHF may range from modestly decompensated patients who require intensification of oral diuretics in the outpatient setting to patients with frank cardiogenic shock. Severity of presentation may be disconnected from severity of background HF. Patients with mild hypertensive heart disease may present in profound respiratory distress requiring intubation, whereas patients with very advanced chronic heart failure may present with more subtle symptoms such as fatigue and early satiety. The most severe presentations of cardiogenic shock have signs and symptoms of organ hypoperfusion despite adequate preload. Systolic blood pressure (SBP) is often (although not always) decreased, and evidence of frank or impending end-organ dysfunction (renal, hepatic, CNS) is common. Cardiogenic shock is relatively uncommon (4% of AHFS presentations in EuroHeart Failure Survey II [EHFS II]) in broad community registries but more common in tertiary care settings.

Acuity

The time course of worsening symptoms is a key component of the history for many forms of acute cardiovascular disease and AHF is no exception. Patients may develop symptoms very suddenly (over minutes) or very gradually (over weeks or longer). As noted above, the acuity of symptoms may not be aligned with the severity of heart failure and the long-term prognosis but has clear implications for the immediacy of therapy needed for stabilization. The fact that many patients may have slowly developing symptoms over days to weeks presents the possibility that early intervention with intensified therapy may prevent some hospitalizations.[33]

Triggers

AHF may be triggered by very clear precipitants or alternatively the reason for decompensation may be obscure. In the OPTIMIZE-HF registry, 61% of enrolled subjects had an identifiable clinical precipitant, with pulmonary processes (15%), myocardial ischemia (15%), and arrhythmias (14%) being the most common.[34] More than one precipitant was identified in a substantial minority of the study population. Of the identified triggers, worsening renal function was associated with the highest in-hospital mortality (8%), whereas nonadherence to diet or medication or uncontrolled hypertension had a much better prognosis (<2% in-hospital mortality for each). Infection with the novel coronavirus Sars-CoV-2 is a rapidly evolving trigger of AHF that is discussed in detail elsewhere (see Chapter 94). In patients with a background of HFpEF, acute hypertension is a common trigger for decompensation, and may overlap with the syndrome of hypertensive emergency. Acute hypertension may be triggered by a high sympathetic tone related to dyspnea and accompanying anxiety (reactive hypertension) or acute hypertension with accompanying changes in afterload may be a trigger for decompensation. Both of these mechanisms may be operative in a given patient, and cause and effect relationships may be difficult to discern. Frank pulmonary edema with evident rales and florid congestion on chest x-ray is much more common in this group of patients than in those with more gradual onset of symptoms, likely related to difference in LV compliance, acuity of pressure changes, and pulmonary lymphatic capacity. Although often strikingly ill at the time of initial presentation with hypoxemia and the possible need for noninvasive ventilation (NIV) or even intubation, this group tends to respond well to therapy and have lower in-hospital mortality.[12]

Symptoms of Acute Heart Failure

The most common reasons for patients to seek medical care for AHF are symptoms related to congestion. A list of the most common presenting symptoms is provided in Table 49.2. Dyspnea is the most common symptom and is present in over 90% of patients presenting with AHF. The duration and time course of symptom onset can vary markedly as noted above. The sensation of dyspnea is a complex phenomenon that is influenced by multiple physiologic, psychological, and social factors, and can vary dramatically between patients.[35] Patients may also present with symptoms related to systemic venous congestion, including peripheral edema, weight gain, early satiety, and increasing abdominal girth. Importantly, atypical symptoms can predominate, especially in older patients, where fatigue, depression, altered mental status, and sleep disruptions may be the primary complaints. Bendopnea, or the sensation of dyspnea on bending over, is a commonly reported symptom that has recently been validated experimentally.[36]

Physical Examination

Despite advances in diagnostics technology, biomarkers, and imaging, heart failure remains a clinical diagnosis and the physical examination continues to play a fundamental role (see Chapters 13 and 48). A useful framework in the bedside evaluation of patients with AHF is that developed by Stevenson and colleagues, which focuses on the adequacy of perfusion ("cold" vs. "warm") and congestion at rest ("wet" vs. "dry").[37] While this framework does not completely encompass the heterogeneity of AHF, it does focus the evaluation on two critical aspects that will significantly influence both prognosis and choice of treatments.

Assessing blood pressure is a critical part in the evaluation of patients with AHF; hypotension is one of the strongest predictors of poor outcomes and helps to define appropriate therapeutic interventions. SBP is typically normal or elevated in patients with AHF, with almost 50% presenting with SBP greater than 140 mm Hg. The combination of underlying hypertension and the marked increase in sympathetic stimulation that accompanies AHF can result in elevations of SBP consistent with hypertensive urgencies or emergencies (12% of patients had an SBP over 180 mm Hg on admission). Patients with very low SBP are uncommon, with only 2% of patients in ADHERE presenting with an SBP less than 90 mm Hg. Although blood pressure is generally related to cardiac output and the state of organ perfusion, it

is important to recognize that hypotension and hypoperfusion are not synonymous. Patients with systemic hypoperfusion may present with normal blood pressure, and similarly patients with advanced forms of heart failure may have chronically low blood pressure not associated with acute hypoperfusion. Pulse pressure (the difference between systolic and diastolic blood pressure) is a useful measure that is an indirect marker of cardiac output. A low pulse pressure is a marker of a low cardiac output and confers an increased risk in patients admitted with AHF. A high pulse pressure may alert the physician to a high output state including the possibility of unrecognized thyrotoxicosis, aortic regurgitation, or anemia.

The JVP is a barometer of systemic venous hypertension and is the single most useful physical examination finding in the assessment of patients with AHF. The accurate assessment of the JVP is highly dependent on examiner skill. The JVP reflects the right atrial pressure, which typically (although not always) is an indirect measure of LV filling pressures. JVP may not reflect LV filling pressures in isolated RV failure (e.g., from pulmonary hypertension or RV infarct), and significant tricuspid regurgitation can complicate the assessment of the JVP because the large "CV wave" of tricuspid regurgitation can lead to its overestimation.

Rales or inspiratory crackles are the most common physical examination finding and have been noted in 66% to 87% of patients admitted for AHF. However, rales are often not heard in patients with a background of chronic heart failure and pulmonary venous hypertension, due to increased lymphatic drainage, reinforcing the important clinical pearl that the absence of rales does not necessarily imply normal LV filling pressures. Cool extremities with palpable peripheral pulses suggest decreased peripheral perfusion consistent with a marginal cardiac index, marked vasoconstriction, or both. Of note, the temperature should be assessed at the lower leg as opposed to the foot, and this assessment is relative to the temperature of the examiner's hands.

TABLE 49.2 Common Presenting Symptoms and Signs of Decompensated Heart Failure

SYMPTOMS	SIGNS
Predominantly related to volume overload	
Dyspnea (exertional, paroxysmal nocturnal dyspnea, orthopnea, or at rest); cough; wheezing	Rales, pleural effusion
Foot and leg discomfort	Peripheral edema (legs, sacral)
Abdominal discomfort/bloating; early satiety or anorexia	Ascites/increased abdominal girth; right upper quadrant pain or discomfort; hepatomegaly/splenomegaly; scleral icterus
	Increased weight
	Elevated jugular venous pressure, abdominojugular reflux
	Increasing S_3, accentuated P_2
Predominantly related to Hypoperfusion	
Fatigue	Cool extremities
Altered mental status, daytime drowsiness, confusion, or difficulty concentrating	Pallor, dusky skin discoloration, Hypotension
Dizziness, pre-syncope, or syncope	Pulse pressure (narrow)/proportional pulse pressure (low)
	Pulsus alternans
Other signs and symptoms of AHF	
Depression	Orthostatic hypotension (hypovolemia)
Sleep disturbances	S_4
Palpitations	Systolic and diastolic cardiac murmurs

AHF, Acute heart failure.

Peripheral edema is present in up to 65% of patients admitted with AHF and is less common in patients presenting with predominantly low-output heart failure or cardiogenic shock. As with rales, the presence of edema has a reasonable positive predictive value for AHF but a low sensitivity, so its absence does not exclude that diagnosis. Edema due to AHF is usually dependent, symmetric, and pitting. It is estimated that a minimum of 4 liters of extracellular fluid is accumulated to produce clinically detectable edema.

Other Diagnostic Testing
Biomarkers

The natriuretic peptides are a family of important counter-regulatory hormones in HF with vasodilatory and other effects (see Chapters 47 and 48). In the context of AHF, both brain natriuretic peptide (BNP) and N-terminal pro-BNP (NT-proBNP) have been shown to play an important role in the differential diagnosis of patients presenting in the emergency department with dyspnea, and are now Class I recommendations in clinical guidelines.[38] In diagnostic testing, natriuretic peptides have greater negative predictive value (i.e., the ability to rule out heart failure as a cause of dyspnea) than positive predictive value (i.e., the ability to definitively identify a diagnosis of heart failure as the cause of dyspnea). As with all biomarker testing, false-positives (e.g., due to MI or pulmonary embolism) and false-negatives (primarily due to obesity, which results in lower natriuretic peptide levels for a given degree of heart failure) may occur. Although natriuretic peptide levels tend to be lower in patients with HFpEF than those with reduced systolic function, natriuretic peptide testing cannot reliably distinguish HFpEF from HFrEF in an individual patient. As noted previously, measurement of cardiac troponin is frequently elevated in patients presenting with AHF, and elevated levels are associated with worse in-hospital and post-discharge outcomes. Assessment of cardiac troponin in patients with AHF is now a Class I recommendation in clinical guidelines and serves to both establish prognosis as well as inform the likelihood of concurrent ACS. It is important to note that elevation of troponin in the context of a typical AHF hospitalization without clinical evidence of ACS is not synonymous with a Type II MI based on the updated fourth universal MI definition.[39]

Other Laboratory Testing

Assessment of renal function is a critical component in the management of patients with AHF. Estimated glomerular filtration rates (eGFRs) should be calculated because serum creatinine may underestimate the degree of renal dysfunction, especially in older adults. Blood urea nitrogen (BUN) is more directly related to the severity of AHF than creatinine, as it integrates both renal function and neurohormonal activation in AHF. A wide variety of other biomarkers, including ST2, galectin 3, and GDF15, have been evaluated in patients with AHF, but none are currently recommended for routine use in patients with AHF.[40] In patients in whom the diagnosis of AHF is uncertain, testing to establish alternative causes (e.g., D-dimer to evaluate for pulmonary embolism or procalcitonin to evaluate for evidence of infection) may be useful.

Chest Radiography, Electrocardiogram, and Echocardiogram

Chest radiography is commonly performed at the time of presentation in patients with dyspnea and is a fundamental test in the evaluation of patients with suspected AHF. In the ADHERE registry, 90% of patients underwent chest radiography during hospitalization and there was evidence of congestion in over 80% of these patients. In patients with a background of chronic heart failure and/or slow onset of symptoms, evidence of congestion on chest x-ray may be subtle and frank pulmonary edema is often absent despite substantially elevated filling pressures.

The electrocardiogram (ECG) is another standard diagnostic test that is appropriate in all patients presenting with AHF (see Chapter 14). Careful attention for ECG changes suggestive of ischemia is of importance because troponin elevation is common in AHF regardless of cause. Arrhythmias are also a common trigger for AHF, and atrial fibrillation is present in 20% to 30%.

Utilization of echocardiography (see Chapter 16) is very high in patients with AHF—over 80% of patients in EHFS II had an echocardiogram performed during the index hospitalization.[12] An echocardiogram is generally the single most useful test in evaluating the cause in the patient with AHF. Echocardiography can assess global systolic and diastolic function, regional wall motion abnormalities, valvular function, hemodynamics including estimates of filling pressures and cardiac output, and pericardial disease. The tissue Doppler ratio of peak early diastolic trans-mitral blood flow velocity (E) to the peak early diastolic mitral annular tissue velocity (E_a) (E:E_a ratio) has been shown to be additive to BNP measures in diagnosing AHF patients presenting with dyspnea. An E:E_a ratio of greater than 15 predicts a pulmonary capillary wedge pressure (PCWP) greater than 15 mm Hg and has been demonstrated to be accurate in the emergency room and intensive care settings.

Risk Stratification

Risk stratification can serve as important clinical tools by helping to identify those patients at both ends of the spectrum of risk; patients who are at very high risk may be observed more closely or treated more intensively, whereas patients at low risk may avoid hospitalization altogether or need less rigorous follow-up and monitoring. A variety of predictive models have been developed in AHF, which can generally be divided into two groups: those focused on in-hospital mortality, and those focused on post-discharge events (death or rehospitalization). Commonly used predictive models are summarized in Table 49.3. Although individual models differ, several variables occur repeatedly in risk models in a variety of settings: older age, lower blood pressure, higher heart rate, higher BUN and creatinine, and hyponatremia. In

TABLE 49.3 Selected Risk Prediction Models in Acute Heart Failure

	POPULATION	SAMPLE SIZE	ENDPOINTS	C-INDEX	KEY PREDICTORS
ADHERE[140]	US registry	65275	In-hospital mortality	n/a	↑BUN, ↑Cr, ↓SBP, ↑age
OPTIMIZE in hospital[141]	US registry	48612	In-hospital mortality	0.75	↑age, ↑HR, ↓SBP, ↑Cr, ↓Na
OPTIMIZE post discharge[142]	US registry	4402	60–90-day outcomes	0.72	↑age, ↑Cr, reactive airway dz, liver dz, ↓SBP, ↓Na, depression
PROTECT[143]	Global RCT	2015	In-hospital outcomes	0.67	↑BUN, ↑RR, ↓SBP, ↑HR, ↓albumin
EFFECT[144]	Canadian population data	4031	30-day and 1-year mortality	0.80	↑age, SBP, ↑RR, ↑BUN, ↓Na
OPTIME-CHF[145]	Global RCT	949	60-day mortality	0.77	↑age, ↑BUN, ↓Na, ↓Hb
ESCAPE[146]	US RCT	423	6-month mortality	0.76	↑BNP, ↑age, ↑BUN, Na, mechanical ventilation, ↑diuretic dose

BNP, Brain natriuretic peptide; *BUN,* blood urea nitrogen; *Cr,* creatinine; *Hb,* hemoglobin; *HR,* heart rate; *RCT,* randomized controlled trial; *RR,* respiratory rate; *SBP,* systolic blood pressure settings where natriuretic peptides are available, they are also powerful predictors of long-term risk, although they may be stronger predictors at hospital discharge than on admission.

MANAGEMENT OF THE PATIENT WITH ACUTE HEART FAILURE

Phases of Management

The management of AHF patients may be considered in the context of four phases of treatment with distinct goals. Optimal therapy requires a high level of coordination between the in-hospital and post-discharge caregivers and care plan. Different treatment strategies and a detailed description of various therapies will be presented later.

Phase I: Urgent/Emergent Care

The initial goals in the management of a patient presenting with AHF are to expeditiously establish the diagnosis (as discussed above), treat life-threatening abnormalities, initiate therapies to provide symptom

relief, and identify the cause and precipitating triggers for the episode of AHF.

Initial therapies may follow the algorithm in Fig. 49.8. In patients with hypoxemia ($SaO_2 < 90\%$), oxygen administration is recommended. Although oxygen saturation on presentation is inversely related to short-term mortality, inhaled oxygen ($F_iO_2 \geq 0.4$) may cause detrimental hemodynamic effects (such hyperoxia-induced vasoconstriction) in patients with systolic dysfunction,[41] therefore it is not routinely recommended for patients without hypoxemia.[42] In patients with obstructive pulmonary disease, high concentrations of inhaled oxygen should not be used to avoid the risk of respiratory depression and worsening hypercarbia. Early clinical studies and meta-analyses suggest that in patients with cardiogenic pulmonary edema, treatment with continuous positive airway pressure (CPAP) or noninvasive intermittent positive pressure ventilation (NIPPV) improves symptoms and physiologic variables, and reduces the need for invasive ventilation and mortality.[43] The Three Interventions in Cardiogenic Pulmonary Oedema (3CPO) trial enrolled 1069 patients with pulmonary edema who were randomized to standard oxygen therapy, CPAP, or NIPPV.[44]

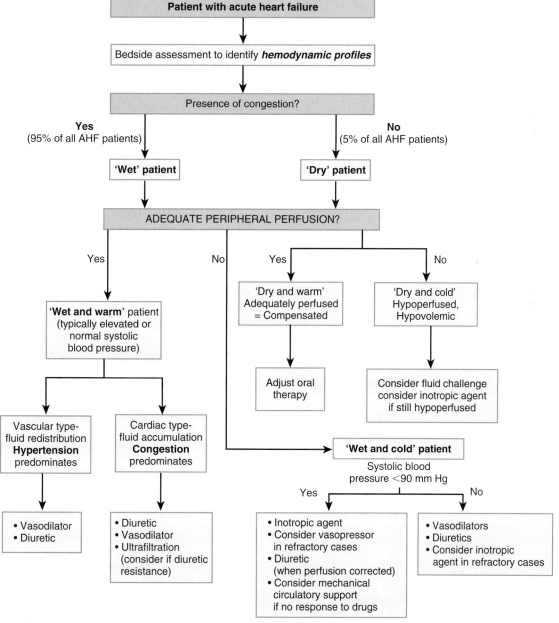

FIGURE 49.8 Algorithm for management of patients admitted with acute heart failure (AHF) based on degree of congestion and perfusion. (From Ponikowski P, Voors AA, Anker SD, et al. 2016 ESC Guidelines for the diagnosis and treatment of acute and chronic heart failure: the Task Force for the diagnosis and treatment of acute and chronic heart failure of the European Society of Cardiology (ESC) developed with the special contribution of the Heart Failure Association (HFA) of the ESC. Eur Heart J. 2016;37:2129–2200.)

NIV with CPAP or NIPPV was associated with greater improvement in patient-reported dyspnea, heart rate, acidosis, and hypercapnea after 1 hour of therapy, although it was not associated with a 7-day mortality benefit nor a decreased need for intubation when compared with standard oxygen therapy. Contraindications to the use of NIV include immediate need for endotracheal intubation (inability to protect the airways, life-threatening hypoxia) and lack of patient cooperation (altered sensorium, unconsciousness, anxiety, inability to tolerate mask). Caution should be used in patients with cardiogenic shock, RV failure, and severe obstructive airway disease. Potential side effects and complications include anxiety, claustrophobia, dry mucous membranes, worsening RV failure, hypercapnea, pneumothorax, and aspiration. Mechanical ventilation with endotracheal intubation is required in about 4% to 5% of all patients.[12,45] Morphine use has been associated with increased likelihood of mechanical ventilation, ICU admission, prolonged hospital stay, and mortality in some retrospective analyses.

Intravenous loop diuretics are the most frequently administered pharmacologic therapy for AHF; over 75% of patients in the emergency department receive intravenous diuretics, with a mean door to first intravenous administration time of 2.2 hours in ADHERE.[45] Whereas some patients with volume redistribution rather than hypervolemia may derive benefit from vasodilators alone, symptomatic patients with objective evidence of congestion consistent with pulmonary or systemic venous hypertension or edema should generally receive urgent diuretic therapy for relief of symptoms related to congestion. Initial therapy is typically a bolus injection with a dose between 1 and 2.5 times the patient's oral loop diuretic dose for patients on chronic diuretic therapy (see section on Diuretics below).[46] In the absence of hypotension, vasodilators may have a role in the initial therapy of patients with pulmonary edema and poor oxygenation. A treatment strategy of early initiation of intravenous nitrate therapy in patients with severe cardiogenic pulmonary edema has been shown to reduce the need for mechanical ventilation and the frequency of MI.[47]

Although low-risk patients may potentially be discharged with careful follow-up, the vast majority of patients who present to the emergency department with AHF are hospitalized.[48] Although fewer than 5% of heart failure patients are initially treated in an emergency department observation unit, these specialized care centers may be effective in decreasing hospitalizations, ICU and critical care unit (CCU) admissions, and related health care costs while maintaining the quality of patient care.[49] In general, hospitalization is recommended for patients with evidence of significant decompensated heart failure, including hypotension, worsening renal function, or altered mentation; significant hypoxemia, hemodynamically significant arrhythmia (most commonly atrial fibrillation either with rapid ventricular response or new onset); and ACS. Hospitalization should be considered in patients with worsened congestion, even in the absence of dyspnea and often reflected by significant weight gain (≥5 kg), other signs or symptoms of pulmonary or systemic congestion, newly diagnosed heart failure, complications of heart failure therapy (such as electrolyte disturbances, frequent implantable cardioverter-defibrillator [ICD] firings), or other associated comorbid conditions.[50]

SPECIFIC CLINICAL PRESENTATIONS
Atrial Fibrillation with Rapid Ventricular Response
Atrial fibrillation (see Chapter 66) with rapid ventricular response is the most common tachyarrhythmia requiring treatment in patients with AHF. It may be difficult to determine with certainty whether the atrial fibrillation was a trigger for AHF or a result of decompensation. Although the ventricular response frequently decreases in parallel with the relief of dyspnea, and consequent decreased sympathetic drive, additional therapy may be required. Immediate cardioversion is generally not indicated except in the unstable patient, as cardioversion while the patient remains significantly decompensated is associated with a high rate of recurrent atrial fibrillation. In patients with systolic dysfunction, intravenous digoxin (in the absence of an accessory pathway), cautious use of beta blocker therapy, or amiodarone may be used. Diltiazem and other agents that suppress ventricular function should be avoided in patients with significant systolic dysfunction but may be effective in patients with preserved function.

Right Ventricular Heart Failure
The most common cause of RV HF in AHF is left-sided failure. Isolated RV HF is relatively rare and is generally due to acute RV infarction, acute pulmonary embolism, or severe pulmonary hypertension. Isolated RV HF caused by an acute RV infarction is best treated with early reperfusion, whereas hemodynamically significant pulmonary embolism may be treated with thrombolytics. Hemodynamic stabilization by optimizing CVPs via carefully monitored fluid loading (target CVP approximately 10 to 12 mm Hg) and increasing RV systolic function with intravenous inotropic support under invasive hemodynamic guidance may also be necessary.[51] Selective pulmonary artery vasodilation by inhaled (nitric oxide, prostacyclin analogs) or intravenous (prostacyclin analogs, sildenafil) agents may improve RV function through decreased afterload. If the patient is mechanically ventilated, normoxia and hypocarbia should be goals using moderate tidal volumes (approximately 8 mL/kg) and as low a PEEP as possible (<12 cm H_2O) to maintain moderate plateau pressures.

Acute Coronary Syndromes (see Chapters 37 and 39)
ACS may be the underlying trigger in patients presenting with AHF, but as noted above, the diagnosis is confounded by the high prevalence of elevated troponins in AHF itself. These patients may present with chest discomfort, electrocardiographic changes consistent with ischemia, and elevated serum troponin. Aggressive therapy for ACS should be rapidly instituted. In the absence of cardiogenic shock, inodilators should be avoided in both patients with ACS and significant asymptomatic coronary disease because experimental data have shown that they can cause necrosis of ischemic and/or hibernating myocardium.

Cardiogenic Shock (see Chapter 38)
Cardiogenic shock is characterized by marked hypotension (SBP <80 mm Hg) lasting more than 30 minutes, associated with severe reduction of cardiac index (usually <1.8 L/min/m²) in spite of adequate LV filling pressure (PCWP >18 mm Hg), resulting in organ hypoperfusion. Cardiogenic shock is an unusual presentation of AHF, occurring in less than 4% of the patients in EHFS II,[12] most of whom had a MI. Mechanical complications of acute myocardial infarction (AMI) such as mitral regurgitation, cardiac rupture with ventricular septal defect or tamponade, and isolated RV infarct may also be causes in this setting. Intravenous inotropes or even vasoconstrictors may be required in these patients, with mechanical circulatory support, such as intra-aortic balloon pump (IABP) or other forms of temporary mechanical support, including ECMO, may be required as a bridge to heart transplant or other mechanical intervention. A variety of evolving approaches to providing hemodynamic support are now available, which may permit temporary stabilization until decisions about the appropriateness of other therapies (such as durable mechanical support or transplantation) can be made (see Chapters 59 and 60).

Phase II: Hospital Care
The goals for the management of a patient with AHF during the hospitalization phase are to complete the diagnostic and acute therapeutic processes that were initiated at the time of initial presentation, to optimize the patient's hemodynamic profile, volume status, and clinical symptoms, and to initiate or optimize chronic heart failure therapy. Monitoring of daily weights, fluid intake and output, and vital signs, including orthostatic blood pressure, as well as a daily assessment of symptoms and signs is crucial. Laboratory monitoring should include daily analysis of electrolytes and renal function. Diagnostic evaluations should include an echocardiogram, if not recently performed. Evaluation for myocardial ischemia may be needed if there is suspicion of ischemia as a trigger of decompensation. Dietary sodium restriction (2 g daily) and fluid restriction (2 liters daily) may be useful to help treat congestion, although the utility of sodium and fluid restriction in this setting has increasingly been called into question.[52] The increased risk of venous thromboembolism in heart failure is exacerbated by the decreased mobility of hospitalized patients with AHF and venous thromboembolism prophylaxis is indicated in all patients unless there is a clear contraindication.

It should be recognized that AHF hospitalization represents an opportunity to review and optimize chronic heart failure therapy. Although changes in renal function may necessitate dose adjustment or temporary discontinuation of RAAS inhibitors (angiotensin-converting enzyme [ACE] inhibitors, angiotensin receptor blocker

[ARB], angiotensin receptor neprilysin inhibitor [ARNI], and/or mineralocorticoid receptor antagonists), in general discontinuation of guideline directed medical therapy should be avoided where possible. Patients admitted on beta blockers have a lower occurrence of ventricular arrhythmias, a shorter length of stay, and reduced 6-month mortality compared to those not receiving them. Patients who had beta blockers withdrawn had significantly lower outpatient use of beta blockers and higher in-hospital mortality, short-term mortality, and combined short-term rehospitalization and mortality, even after adjustments for potential confounders.[53] Therefore, patients should continue beta blocker therapy during the admission for AHF, unless significant hypotension or cardiogenic shock are present. Identification of other untreated targets (e.g., revascularization, consideration of cardiac resynchronization therapy [CRT] in appropriate candidates, etc.) should be performed during the hospitalization. Recent data from the PIONEER trial suggest that hospitalization is an ideal time to transition to sacubitril-valsartan therapy in appropriate patients rather than defer this to the outpatient setting.[54] The hospitalization phase of AHF management is also an opportunity to provide education and behavioral therapies to patients. Patients should receive specific and clear education about heart failure, including indications for specific drugs, outpatient monitoring of fluid status through daily weights, self-adjustment of diuretics, exercise programs, and nutritional counseling, as well as possible consultation with physical and occupational therapy. Comorbidities should be aggressively addressed as these often complicate heart failure management. The hospitalization is also a possible opportunity to enroll the patient in appropriate heart failure disease management programs.

The Cardio-Renal Syndrome in Hospitalized Patients

The *cardio-renal syndrome* (see Chapter 101) represents a significant therapeutic challenge in patients with AHF. Cardio-renal syndrome is often described as the clinical state where the volume overload of heart failure is resistant or refractory to treatment due to progressive renal insufficiency. A commonly used practical definition is an increase in serum creatinine of greater than 0.3 mg/dL (or 25% decreases in GFR) despite evidence of persistent clinical or hemodynamic congestion. Using this definition, the cardio-renal syndrome occurs in approximately 25% to 35% of the patients admitted with AHF, associated with longer lengths of stay and higher post-discharge mortality.[23] This definition of the cardio-renal syndrome emphasizes the importance of persistent congestion, as multiple studies have suggested that changes in renal function during successful decongestion therapy are usually transient and may not be associated with adverse outcomes.[26,55]

Although the diagnosis of the cardio-renal syndrome may be straightforward, the clinical management is a major challenge. Because absolute serum creatinine concentrations can be misleading, eGFR should be calculated in patients with AHF. As noted above, arterial under-filling due to over-diuresis or low cardiac output does not appear to be the most frequent primary cause of worsening renal function, although hypotension can be an important factor.[56] Progressive deterioration of renal function (BUN >80 mg/dL and creatinine >3.0 mg/dL) or hyperkalemia may necessitate discontinuation of RAAS inhibitors, although use of other vasodilators should be considered, either intravenous (i.e., nitroglycerin or nitroprusside) or oral (isosorbide dinitrate and hydralazine). Increasing doses of diuretics are typically required, although diuretic resistance may be profound. The degree of diuretic resistance, sometimes quantified as diuretic efficiency, is known to be associated with increased length of stay and adverse prognosis.[57]

Urine sodium measurements may provide a useful guide to initial diuretic response.[58] Although ultrafiltration is often considered in this scenario, clinical trial data have not supported the efficacy or safety of this approach.[59]

In-Hospital Worsening Heart Failure

Traditional assessments of the inpatient course of patients with AHF have generally lacked granularity and focused primarily on in-hospital mortality. However, there has been increasing emphasis from both a clinical and research perspective on difference in the clinical "trajectory" of patients during inpatient AHF treatment. It is apparent that different patients may have markedly different clinical courses during inpatient therapy for AHF, from relatively uncomplicated courses marked by steady improvement in heart failure status, to those characterized by progressive deterioration in clinical status (Fig. 49.9).[5] Fundamentally, the concept of in-hospital WHF encompasses clinical worsening (as manifest by worsening signs and/or symptoms of heart failure) that necessitates a significant intensification of therapy. Both terminology and specific definitions of WHF have varied between studies, leading to widely varying estimates of prevalence from 5% to 42%. In general, the development of WHF during inpatient AHF therapy is associated with both longer length of inpatient stay (by approximately 5 days in a recent pooled analysis) and adverse post-discharge outcomes (approximately 50% to 100% increase in 30 or 60 day death or HF rehospitalization).[60] As expected, different severity of WHF implies different risk, with WHF treated with increased diuretics alone associated with less increase in baseline risk than WHF requiring IV inotropes or mechanical circulatory or respiratory support. Although there has been substantial interest from researchers and regulators in the concept of WHF as a clinical trial endpoint in recent AHF studies, to date no interventions have provided definitive evidence that they are able to impact this clinical endpoint.

Phase III: Pre-Discharge Planning

The pre-discharge phase focuses on the goals of evaluating readiness for discharge, optimizing chronic oral therapy, minimizing the side effects of treatments, and ultimately preventing early readmission and improving symptoms and survival. Although there may be pressures to rapidly discharge patients, careful optimization of medical regimen prior to discharge may reduce the risk of subsequent readmissions and improve long-term outcomes.[61] Despite the fact that most patients present with congestion, many patients are discharged without significant weight loss. Available data demonstrate that persistent clinical congestion at discharge was associated with a high risk for rehospitalization.[62] Similarly, elevations of discharge BNP level have been shown to be

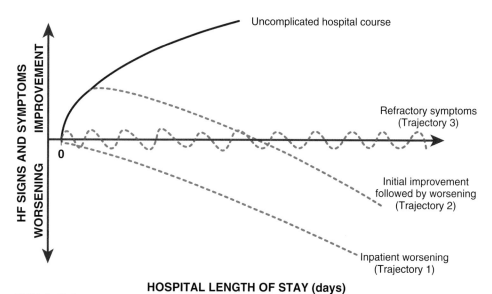

FIGURE 49.9 Various clinical trajectories of patients with acute heart failure during inpatient management. (From Butler J, Gheorghiade M, Kelkar A, et al. In-hospital worsening heart failure. *Eur J Heart Fail*. 2015;17:1104–1113.)

associated with risk for rehospitalization post-discharge.[63] Evaluation of functional capacity with simple maneuvers such as climbing one flight of stairs or walking down the corridor may be a simple and valuable tool to use prior to discharge.

Pharmacologic therapies known to improve long-term outcomes in chronic heart failure, such as beta blockers, ACE inhibitors or ARBs, ARNIs, and mineralocorticoid receptor antagonists, should be initiated as soon as reasonable during the hospitalization and prior to discharge in hemodynamically stable, appropriate patients. In patients already treated chronically with these agents prior to this episode of AHF, they should generally be continued during hospitalization. Clinical practice guidelines provide general criteria for considerations of hospital discharge, although substantial clinical judgment is still required (Table 49.4).[64]

Phase IV: Post-Discharge Management

Early recurrence of signs and symptoms of HF suggestive of worsening volume overload and/or neurohormonal activation are likely to contribute to the high rates of readmission that are observed in AHF.[65] Prompt interventions may therefore allow intervention to prevent the progression of volume overload and new admissions. At least some rehospitalizations for heart failure appear to be preventable.[66] A series of studies have also investigated the benefits of post-discharge support, especially patient-centered discharge instructions, transition coaches, follow-up telephone calls, and early physician follow-up, although results of these studies have been mixed in terms of impact on outcomes.[67,68] A follow-up appointment is optimally scheduled within approximately 7 to 10 days post-discharge, but closer follow-up (in less than a week) should be considered for patients with high-risk features.

General Approaches to Acute Heart Failure Therapy
Targeting Congestion

Treatment strategies for AHF have been largely empiric and limited by an incomplete understanding of its epidemiology and pathophysiology, as well as the relatively blunt nature of the available therapeutic tools.

TABLE 49.4 Considerations Prior to Discharge after Acute Heart Failure Hospitalization

Recommended for all heart failure patients
• Exacerbating factors addressed
• Near-optimal volume status observed
• Transition from intravenous to oral diuretic successfully completed
• Patient and family education completed, including clear discharge instructions
• LVEF documented
• Smoking cessation counseling initiated
• Near-optimal pharmacologic therapy achieved, including ACE inhibitor and beta blocker (for patients with reduced LVEF), or intolerance documented
• Follow-up clinic visit scheduled, usually for 7–10 days
Should be considered for patients with advanced heart failure or recurrent admissions for heart failure
• Oral medication regimen stable for 24 hr
• No intravenous vasodilator or inotropic agent for 24 hr
• Ambulation before discharge to assess functional capacity after therapy
• Plans for post-discharge management (scale present in home, visiting nurse or telephone follow up generally no longer than 3 days after discharge)
• Referral for disease management, if available

ACE, Angiotensin-converting enzyme; *LVEF,* left ventricular ejection fraction.
Adapted from Heart Failure Society of America; Lindenfeld J, Albert NM, et al. HFSA 2010 comprehensive heart failure practice guideline. *J Card Failure.* 2010;16(6):e1–e194.

The current general approach focuses on the successful treatment of clinical and hemodynamic congestion, while limiting untoward effects on myocardial or end-organ function, identifying addressable triggers, and optimizing proven long-term therapies. This approach incorporates information from three main aspects of the patient's clinical presentation: blood pressure, volume status, and renal function.

Blood Pressure

Blood pressure reflects the interaction between vascular tone and myocardial pump function and is one of the most important prognostic indicators in AHF (see above). Most patients present with elevated blood pressures and consequently will benefit from and safely tolerate vasodilator therapy. Vasodilators may decrease preload by reversing venous vasoconstriction and the related central volume redistribution from the peripheral and splanchnic venous systems, and reduce afterload by decreasing arterial vasoconstriction with a resultant improvement in cardiac and renal function. Vasodilators are the primary therapy for AHF with pulmonary edema, and for non-hypotensive patients with low cardiac output (poor peripheral or central perfusion with SBPs above 85 to 100 mm Hg). A systematic review of clinical studies supported the ability of vasodilators to improve short-term symptoms and appear safe to administer, but revealed no data suggesting an impact on mortality.[69] However, in an international registry of 4953 patients admitted for AHF (ALARM-HF; 75% admitted to ICU/CCU care settings), analysis of a propensity-based matched cohort of 1007 matched pairs demonstrated improved in-hospital survival in patients treated with vasodilators and diuretics compared to patients only treated with diuretics with 7.8% compared to 11.0% in-hospital mortality, respectively ($P = 0.016$).[70] Interestingly, this difference in survival was particularly evident in patients with SBP less than 120 mm Hg (Fig. 49.10). The selection of agent depends on the clinical situation, local practice, and availability (see section on Specific Therapies below).

Hypotension (SBP below 85 to 90 mm Hg) or signs of peripheral hypoperfusion are poor prognostic signs in patients with AHF. Treating the potentially reversible, underlying causes, such as ACS, pulmonary embolus, and (rarely) hypovolemia, is essential. Hypovolemic hypotension, usually related to over-diuresis, is unusual in patients presenting with symptomatic AHF, and unappreciated volume overload may be present, especially in obese patients in whom neck veins and ascites are difficult to assess. If there is clear evidence of hypovolemia, carefully monitored "fluid challenges" may be attempted, although rapid intravenous fluid boluses can precipitate congestive symptoms. Asymptomatic hypotension, as an isolated finding in the absence of congestion and poor peripheral or central perfusion, does not require emergent treatment. Inotropic therapy may be indicated for persistent symptomatic hypotension or evidence of hypoperfusion in the setting of advanced systolic dysfunction. An analysis of 954 propensity-matched pairs of patients from the ALARM-HF registry suggested that IV catecholamine use was associated with 1.5-fold increase in in-hospital mortality for dopamine or dobutamine use and a greater than 2.5-fold increase for norepinephrine or epinephrine use.[70] Specific inotropic agents vary by country and local clinical practice (see section on specific agents below). In most patients, invasive pulmonary artery catheter monitoring is not necessary, because the measures of urine output, blood pressure, and end-organ function may be clinically evaluated. The use of vasoconstrictors, such as high-dose dopamine, phenylephrine, epinephrine, and norepinephrine, should generally be avoided unless absolutely necessary for refractory symptomatic hypotension or hypoperfusion. Rarely, over dosage of afterload-reducing agents can precipitate admissions for AHF with a clinical presentation similar to cardiogenic shock or "pseudo-sepsis," in which case careful administration of vasoconstrictors may be indicated.

Volume Status

Most patients with AHF have evidence of volume overload and for patients in whom this is the dominant presenting feature, such as those with significant peripheral edema or ascites, intravenous diuretics remain the foundation of AHF therapy. Patients with clinically evident congestion typically have 4 to 5 liters of excess volume and amounts greater than 10 liters are not uncommon. The choice of diuretic regimen is influenced by the amount and rapidity of the desired fluid removal and the renal function (see below). Diuresis addresses the underlying abnormality and frequently improves symptoms and signs of elevated filling pressures. However, intravenous vasodilator therapy may provide more rapid relief in highly symptomatic patients with evidence of pulmonary congestion. In fact, many patients with hypertensive AHF may require minimal diuretics. Surprisingly, in a study of 131,430 admissions for heart failure, 11% of the patients received a median of 1 liter of intravenous fluids, predominantly normal saline, during the first 2 days of hospitalization. Patients receiving intravenous fluids had increased rates of subsequent critical care admission, intubation, renal replacement therapy, and hospital death compared with those who received only diuretics.[71] Thus, careful attention to volume status is critical, as patients' symptoms of congestion may resolve despite persistent hemodynamic congestion (i.e., elevated filling pressures). Hospital discharge before hemodynamic congestion is fully treated appears to be a common cause of rehospitalization.[72]

Renal Function

Renal function (see Chapter 101) is the third main aspect of a contemporary approach to treatment of the patient with AHF. Treatment of AHF in the presence of normal renal function is generally uncomplicated. Diuretics may be given in standard doses, although renal function, electrolytes, and volume status must be carefully monitored. However, approximately two-thirds of patients present with at least moderate renal insufficiency.[22] This may be from preexisting kidney disease or

may be a manifestation of WHF. Abnormal renal function is typically associated with some degree of diuretic resistance, and higher doses of diuretics or other strategies may be needed (see section on Diuretics below). The important clinical problem of worsening renal function during AHF therapy, the cardio-renal syndrome, is discussed above.

Invasive Hemodynamic Strategy

Invasive hemodynamic management with pulmonary artery catheterization (PAC) may be a useful strategy in the management of some patients with AHF. PAC is an invasive procedure that provides detailed hemodynamic data, including direct assessment of filling pressures and cardiac output, and calculation of pulmonary and systemic vascular resistance. Potential risks of PAC include bleeding, infection, arrhythmias, and rare catastrophic events, such as pulmonary artery rupture or infarction. The use of PAC in the routine management of AHF has been a subject of controversy. The Evaluation Study of Congestive Heart Failure and Pulmonary Artery Catheterization Effectiveness (ESCAPE) was a randomized controlled trial of 433 patients with severe symptomatic heart failure despite recommended therapies randomized to receive therapy guided by clinical assessment and PAC or by clinical assessment alone.[73] In ESCAPE, use of PAC did not significantly affect the days alive and out of hospital during the first 6 months (133 vs. 135 days), mortality (43 vs. 38 deaths), or the number of days hospitalized (8.7 vs. 8.3 days) compared to clinical assessment alone. Based on the results of the ESCAPE trial, the use of PAC in AHF management has declined—in EHFS II, only 5% of patients had a PAC during AHF hospitalization. Importantly, the

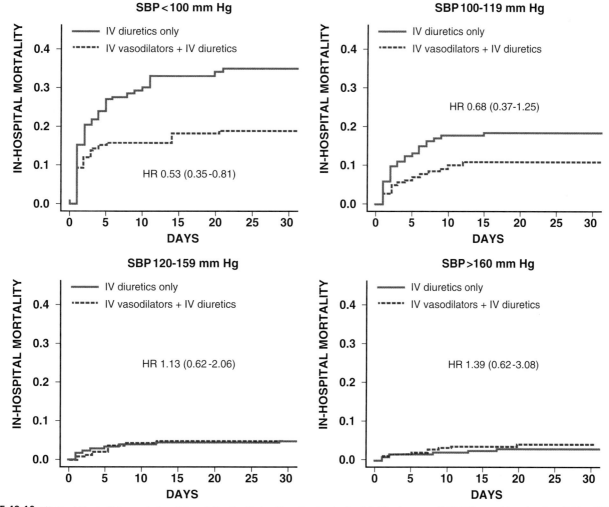

FIGURE 49.10 Effects of IV vasodilators on in-hospital mortality of patients with various levels of systolic blood pressure (SBP). SBP ranged from less than 100 to ≥160 mm Hg. The number of patients is 318, 334, 668, and 694 for SBP less than 100, 100–119, 120–159, and ≥160 mm Hg, respectively. *HR*, Hazard ratio. Value in parenthesis is the 95% confidence interval. (From Mebazaa A, Parissis J, Porcher R, et al. Short-term survival by treatment among patients hospitalized with acute heart failure: the global ALARM-HF registry using propensity scoring methods. *Intensive Care Med*. 2011;37:290–301.)

ESCAPE study excluded patients in whom the treating clinician did not have equipoise about the need for invasive hemodynamic measurement. Invasive hemodynamic assessment with PAC may still play an important role in selected patients, especially those with shock or other severe hemodynamic compromise, with oliguria or anuria, or with unclear hemodynamics and poor response to therapy. In patients with advanced heart failure in whom PAC is used to tailor therapy, an LV filling pressure as approximated by PCWP of less than 16 mm Hg, right atrial pressure less than 8 mm Hg, and a systemic vascular resistance between 1000 and 1200 dynes sec cm^{-5} are useful targets.

Process of Care, Outcomes, and Quality Assessment

The first point of contact at the admitting hospital for most patients (80%) is the emergency department.[74] Many patients with AHF may be effectively managed in and safely discharged from the emergency department and specific algorithms for care and criteria for discharge are evolving.[75] Once the patient with AHF is hospitalized, there appear to be substantial geographic differences in process of care and hospital course worldwide. In the U.S. ADHERE registry, 23% of patients were admitted to an ICU setting, whereas a substantially higher proportion (51%) had an ICU stay in a similar European registry (EHFS II). Median length of stay is also markedly different across geographic regions, with length of stay in the United States of approximately 4 days. Median length of stay is approximately twice as long in Europe (median of 9 days in EHFS II), and even higher in Japan (21 days in ATTEND registry). These differences in length of stay do not appear to be fully explained by differences in case mix or severity of illness. The longer length of stay outside the United States is generally associated with lower rates of short-term

rehospitalization, although a cause-and-effect relationship is not fully established. A focus on reducing length of stay in the United States appears to have been accompanied by an increase in post-discharge events, both mortality and (in particular) rehospitalization.[76] In contrast in the U.S. Veterans Affairs hospitals, heart failure hospitalizations have increased slightly while 30-day mortality has decreased significantly.[77] In general, the natural history of AHF is characterized by relatively low in-hospital mortality but a high rate of recurrent post-discharge events (Table 49.5). Inpatient mortality in AHF ranges between 3% and 7%, with the notable exception of patients in cardiogenic shock, who have a markedly increased in-hospital mortality (40% in EHFS II).[12] Although in-hospital mortality is low, hospitalization for AHF portends a substantial worsening of the clinical course in many patients. In the EVEREST study, despite careful attention to evidence-based care in the context of a large clinical trial, 26% of enrolled patients had died in a median follow-up period of 9.9 months. Of all deaths, 41.0% were due to HF, 26.0% due to sudden cardiac death, 2.6% due to AMI, 2.2% due to stroke, and 13.2% due to non-cardiovascular causes.[78]

The Rehospitalization Problem

The high rates of rehospitalization after discharge from a heart failure hospitalization have become a major focus of clinicians, policy makers, and payers. Claims data using the U.S. Medicare sample suggest a striking rate of rehospitalization in older patients, with a 30-day rehospitalization rate of 27%, although rates are substantially lower in younger non-Medicare cohorts.[79,80] Rates of rehospitalization within 6 months approach 50% in many cohorts, in particular older adults. Of note, approximately half of the rehospitalizations are not heart failure related, which underscores the total burden of comorbidity in heart failure patients as well as the challenges in affecting this event rate with heart failure-focused interventions. In the EVEREST, careful

TABLE 49.5 Outcomes in Acute Heart Failure Patients from Selected Trials and Registries

STUDY	PATIENTS (N)	RE-HOSPITALIZATION	MORTALITY IN-HOSPITAL	MORTALITY POST-DISCHARGE
Trials				
ASCEND-HF	7,141	6% at 30 days		13% at 6 mo
EVEREST	4,133	12% at 30 days	3%	26% at 9.9 mo
RELAX-AHF	1,161	9% at 60 days		9% at 6 mo
RELAX-AHF-2	6,545	19% Hosp for HF or RF at 6 mo		12% at 6 mo
TRUE-HF	2,157	7% HF Hosp at 30 days		21% CV death at 15 mo
Registries				
Lee (Canada)	4,031	N/A	8.7%	10.6% 30 days 31% 1 year
ADHERE (US)	187,565	N/A	3.8%	N/A
OPTIMIZE-HF (US)	41,267	30% at 60–90 days	3.8%	8.0% at 60–90 days
Tavazzi (Italy)	2,807	38.1% at 6 months	7.3%	12.8% at 6 months
EHFS II (EU)	3,580	N/A	6.7%	N/A
ATTEND (Japan)	4,837	N/A	6.3%	N/A
Damasceno (sub-Saharan Africa)	1,006	9% at 60 days (all cause)	4.2%	18% at 6 months

Data from O'Connor CM, Starling RC, Hernandez AF, et al. Effect of nesiritide in patients with acute decompensated heart failure. N Engl J Med. 2011;365:32–43. Konstam MA, Gheorghiade M, Burnett Jr JC, et al. Effects of oral tolvaptan in patients hospitalized for worsening heart failure: the EVEREST outcome trial. JAMA. 2007;297:1319–1331. Teerlink JR, Cotter G, Davison BA, et al. Serelaxin, recombinant human relaxin-2, for treatment of acute heart failure (RELAX-AHF): a randomised, placebo-controlled trial. Lancet. 2013;381:29–39. Teerlink MM, Cotter G, Davison BA, et al. Effects of serelaxin in patients with acute heart failure. N Engl J Med. 2019;381:716–726. Packer M, O'Connor C, McMurray JJV, et al. Effect of ularitide on cardiovascular mortality in acute heart failure. N Engl J Med. 2017;376:1956–1964. Lee DS, Austin PC, Rouleau JL, et al. Predicting mortality among patients hospitalized for heart failure: derivation and validation of a clinical model. JAMA. 2003;290:2581–2587. ADHERE Scientific Advisory Committee Acute Decompensated Heart Failure National Registry (ADHERE®) Core Module Q1 2006 Final Cumulative National Benchmark Report: Scios, Inc.; July, 2006. Gheorghiade M, Abraham WT, Albert NM, et al. Systolic blood pressure at admission, clinical characteristics, and outcomes in patients hospitalized with acute heart failure. JAMA. 2006;296:2217–2226. Tavazzi L, Maggioni AP, Lucci D, et al. Nationwide survey on acute heart failure in cardiology ward services in Italy. Eur Heart J. 2006;27:1207–1215. Nieminen MS, Brutsaert D, Dickstein K, et al. EuroHeart Failure Survey II (EHFS II): a survey on hospitalized acute heart failure patients: description of population. Eur Heart J. 2006;27:2725–2736. Sato N, Gheorghiade M, Kajimoto K, et al. Hyponatremia and in-hospital mortality in patients admitted for heart failure (from the ATTEND registry). Am J Cardiol. 2013;111:1019–1025. Damasceno A, Mayosi BM, Sani M, et al. The causes, treatment, and outcome of acute heart failure in 1006 Africans from 9 countries: results of the sub-Saharan Africa survey of heart failure. Arch Int Med. 2012;172:1386–1394.

adjudication of post-discharge hospitalizations showed that 46% were for heart failure, 15% for other cardiovascular causes, and 39% were for non-cardiovascular causes.[78] These rehospitalizations represent a major driver of health expenditures, accounting for over 39 billion US dollars spent on heart failure care per year in the United States.[4] Although controversial, reducing rehospitalization rates for heart failure has been identified as a major focus of quality improvement and cost containment by payers such as the US Centers for Medicare and Medicaid Services. As a result, a variety of interventions and initiatives related to inpatient management, discharge planning, and transitions of care have been implemented in an attempt to decrease rehospitalization rates for heart failure, although the nature, implementation, and effectiveness of these practices have varied widely across health systems.[81] Despite these significant efforts, recent evidence suggests only a minor impact on rehospitalizations.[82] There is also uncertainty about what proportion of rehospitalizations are avoidable, although a systematic review suggests that a quarter or more may be preventable.[66] To date, only improved utilization of proven evidence-based therapies (such as beta blockers and ACE inhibitors) during acute hospitalization has been shown to improve post-discharge outcomes.[61] Hospital discharge before congestion is adequately treated appears to be a common cause of early readmission.[72] Early post-discharge follow-up has also been associated with lower rehospitalization rates in retrospective registry data.[68] A variety of other interventions centered on telemedicine, disease monitoring, and disease management remain under active investigation.

Specific Therapies
Diuretics

Loop diuretics are the primary pharmacologic treatment for volume overload in patients with AHF, and typically result in rapid symptom relief in most patients.[83] (Diuretics are discussed in detail in Chapter 50.) Loop diuretics (furosemide, torsemide, bumetanide, and ethacrynic acid; Table 49.6) can lead to excretion of up to 25% of the filtered sodium and intravenous administration avoids variable bioavailability and allows for rapid onset of action (typically within 30 to 60 minutes). Preliminary data suggest that genetic variants modulate the response to furosemide in patients with decompensated HF.[84] Based on the results of the DOSE study described below, initial doses of approximately 2.5 times the outpatient dose should be considered for patients on chronic oral diuretic therapy, with underlying renal dysfunction, or with severe volume overload. Given the steep dose-response curve of these agents, titration should be rapid with doubling of the dose until an effective response is noted. If there is significant volume overload (>5 to 10 liters) or diuretic resistance, a continuous intravenous infusion can be considered. Despite their ubiquitous use in AHF, loop diuretics have generally not been tested in rigorously controlled clinical trials. Loop diuretics may lead to neurohormonal activation and electrolyte repletion, and have been associated in observational studies with both increased risk of worsening renal function and decreased survival, although a recent analysis suggested no relationship between diuretic exposure and 30-day all-cause death or HF hospitalization.[85] The DOSE trial was a randomized, double-blind study that prospectively compared diuretic strategies in AHF.[86] Using a 2 × 2 factorial design, 308 patients were randomized to treatment with IV furosemide using either twice-daily bolus dosing or a continuous infusion and to either a low (equivalent to the numerical value of the oral outpatient dose given IV) or high (2.5 times the oral dose given IV) dose strategy. There was no significant difference in either of the co-primary endpoints of global assessment of symptoms or change in creatinine at 72 hours with administration by bolus compared to infusion or with the low- versus high-dose strategy. The high-dose strategy was associated with greater relief of dyspnea and net fluid loss at 72 hours, although more patients in the high-dose group had a transient increase in creatinine greater than 0.3 mg/dL, which resolved by the time

TABLE 49.6 Therapeutic Approaches for Volume Management in Acute Heart Failure

SEVERITY OF VOLUME OVERLOAD	DIURETIC	DOSE (MG)	COMMENTS
Moderate	Furosemide, or	20–40 mg or up to 2.5 times oral dose	Intravenous administration preferable in symptomatic patients
	Bumetanide, or	0.5–1.0	Titrate dose according to clinical response
	Torsemide	10–20	Monitor Na^+, K^+, creatinine, BP
Severe	Furosemide, or	40–160 or 2.5 times oral dose 5–40 mg/hr infusion	Intravenously
	Bumetanide, or	1–4 / 0.5–2 mg/hr infusion (max 2–4 mg/hr, limit 2–4 hr)	Bumetanide and torsemide have higher oral bioavailability than furosemide, but intravenous administration preferable in AHF
	Torsemide	20–100/ 5–20 mg/hr	
	Ultrafiltration	200–500 mL/hr	Adjust ultrafiltration rate to clinical response, monitor for hypotension; consider hematocrit sensor
Refractory to loop diuretics	Add HCTZ, or	25–50 twice daily	Combination with loop diuretic may be better than very high dose of loop diuretics alone
	Metolazone, or	2.5–10 once daily	Metolazone more potent if creatinine clearance <30 mL/min
	Chlorothiazide, or	250–500 mg IV 500–1000 mg po	
	Spironolactone	25–50 once daily	Spironolactone best choice if patient not in renal failure and normal or low serum K^+, although may not be very potent
In case of alkalosis	Acetazolamide	0.5	Intravenously
Refractory to loop diuretic and thiazides	Add dopamine (renal vasodilation), or dobutamine or milrinone (inotropic agent)		
	Ultrafiltration, or hemodialysis if co-existing renal failure		

of hospital discharge (Table e49.1). The significance of this finding is unclear; although there were no apparent differences in hospital length of stay or days alive out of the hospital, the study was not powered for long-term clinical outcomes. Overall, there were no differences in results between the continuous infusion and intermittent bolus strategies in the clinical trial setting of DOSE, suggesting that whichever approach is most likely to reliably produce the desired diuresis in the particular local clinical practice should be used.

In the setting of diuretic resistance, administration of a thiazide-like diuretic that blocks the distal tubule can provide significant augmentation of the diuretic effect.[87] Intravenous chlorothiazide (500 to 1000 mg) or oral metolazone (2.5 to 10 mg) given prior to the loop diuretic are effective agents, although care must be taken to monitor for hypotension, worsening renal function, and electrolyte abnormalities, which may be profound. Nonsteroidal anti-inflammatory drugs can greatly reduce the efficacy of diuretics by reducing renal synthesis of vasodilatory prostaglandins, and these agents should be avoided. If hypokalemia is a persistent problem with replacement requirements, administration of a potassium-sparing diuretic, such as spironolactone or eplerenone, should be considered, and may also provide synergistic diuretic effects, especially at higher doses,[88] as well as long-term beneficial effects on outcomes.

Vasodilators

In the absence of hypotension, vasodilators can be used as first-line therapy in combination with diuretics in the management of AHF patients to improve congestive symptoms (Table 49.7).[89] As noted above, in the ALARM-HF registry using propensity-matching techniques, patients admitted with AHF and treated with diuretics and vasodilators had significantly better in-hospital survival compared to patients treated with diuretics alone or those treated with inotropes,[70] while another more recent analysis of 11,078 patients admitted for AHF demonstrated no mortality benefit at 7, 30, or 365 days[90] consistent with the findings of a systematic review.[69] After extensive review of these and other data, the U.K. National Institute for Health and Care Excellence found no evidence to support the routine use of vasodilators in patients with AHF.[91] However, in practice vasodilators appear to provide symptom relief in these patients. Vasodilators can be classified as: (1) predominantly venous dilators, with consequent reduction in preload; (2) arterial dilators, leading to a decrease in afterload; and (3) balanced vasodilators, with combined action on both the venous and the arterial system. Currently available vasodilators include the organic nitrates (nitroglycerin and isosorbide dinitrate), sodium nitroprusside (SNP), and nesiritide. All of these drugs act by activating soluble guanylate cyclase (sGC) in the smooth muscle cells, leading to higher intracellular concentrations of cGMP and consequent vessel relaxation (see Chapter 47). They should be used with caution in patients who are preload or after-load dependent (e.g., severe diastolic dysfunction, aortic stenosis, and CAD), because they may cause severe hypotension. BP should be monitored frequently and the drug discontinued if symptomatic hypotension develops.

Nitrates

Organic nitrates are one of the oldest therapies for AHF. These agents are potent venodilators, producing rapid decreases in pulmonary venous and ventricular filling pressures and improvement in pulmonary

TABLE 49.7 Intravenous Vasoactive Agents for the Treatment of Acute Heart Failure

INTRAVENOUS MEDICATION	INITIAL DOSE	EFFECTIVE DOSE RANGE*	COMMENTS
Vasodilators			
Nitroglycerin; glyceryl trinitrate	20 µg/min	40–400 µg/min	Hypotension, headache; Tolerance with continuous use after 24 hr
Isosorbide dinitrate	1 mg/hr	2–10 mg/hr	Hypotension, headache; Tolerance with continuous use within 24 hr
Nitroprusside	0.3 µg/kg/min	0.3–5 µg/kg/min (usually <4 µg/kg/min)	Caution in patients with active myocardial ischemia; Hypotension; cyanide side effects (nausea, dysphoria); thiocyanate toxicity; light sensitive
Nesiritide†	2 µg/kg bolus with 0.010–0.030 µg/kg/min infusion‡	0.010–0.030 µg/kg/min	Up-titration: 1 µg/kg bolus, then increase infusion rate by 0.005 µg/kg/min no more frequently than every 3 hr, up to a maximum of 0.03 µg/kg/min)
			Hypotension, headache (less than with organic nitrates)
Inotropes			
Dobutamine	1–2 µg/kg/min	2–20 µg/kg/min	For inotropy and vasodilation; Hypotension, tachycardia, arrhythmias; ?mortality
Dopamine	1–2 µg/kg/min	2–4 µg/kg/min	For inotropy and vasodilation; Hypotension, tachycardia, arrhythmias; ?mortality
	4–5 µg/kg/min	5–20 µg/kg/min	For inotropy and vasoconstriction; Tachycardia, arrhythmias; ?mortality
Milrinone	25–75 µg/kg bolus over 10–20 min‡ followed by infusion	0.10–0.75 µg/kg/min	For vasodilation and inotropy; Hypotension, tachycardia, arrhythmias; Renal excretion; ?mortality
Enoximone†	0.25–0.75 mg/kg	1.25–7.5 µg/kg/min	For vasodilation and inotropy; Hypotension, tachycardia, arrhythmias; ?mortality
Levosimendan†	12-24 µg/kg bolus over 10 min* followed by infusion	0.5–2.0 µg/kg/min	For vasodilation and inotropy; active metabolite present for approximately 84 hr; Hypotension, tachycardia, arrhythmias; ?mortality
Epinephrine		0.05–0.5 µg/kg/min	For vasoconstriction and inotropy; Tachycardia, arrhythmias, end-organ hypoperfusion; ?mortality
Norepinephrine		0.2–1.0 µg/kg/min	For vasoconstriction and inotropy; Tachycardia, arrhythmias, end-organ hypoperfusion; ?mortality

Use higher dose range for chronic diuretic use, renal insufficiency, and severe volume overload. Diuretic naïve patients should receive lower doses, initially.
*In general, titration of medication is accomplished by doubling of dose with careful monitoring for adverse effects.
†Not approved for use in all countries.
‡Some clinicians do not administer a bolus dose, so as to decrease the risk of hypotension. Bolus not recommended in patients with hypotension.

congestion, dyspnea, and myocardial oxygen demand at low doses. At slightly higher doses and in the presence of vasoconstriction, nitrates are also arteriolar vasodilators, reducing afterload and increasing cardiac output. Nitrates are relatively selective for epicardial, compared to intramyocardial, coronary arteries, resulting in increased coronary blood flow and making them useful for patients with concomitant active myocardial ischemia. The starting dose of nitroglycerin is usually 20 μg/min with rapid up-titration occurring every 5 to 15 minutes in either 20 μg/min increments or doubling of the dose. The dose may initially be titrated to the goal of immediate symptom relief, but a blood pressure reduction of at least 10 mm Hg in mean arterial pressure with a SBP greater than 100 mm Hg may be preferable. The nitrate dose may need to be reduced if SBP is 90 to 100 mm Hg and will often need to be discontinued with SBP less than 90 mm Hg. Intravenous nitrate use appears to be more common in Europe than in the United States (38% in EHFS-II but only 9% in ADHERE).[12,45] Organic nitrates may also be administered orally, sublingually, or by spray, allowing for convenient emergent treatment prior to establishing intravenous access.

There is limited clinical trial experience with organic nitrates. Early administration of high-dose intravenous nitrates is beneficial in improving arterial oxygenation and potentially preventing some consequences of AHF (MI, need for mechanical ventilation), compared to furosemide alone[47] or NIV,[92] although these studies were small and not blinded. In a study designed to evaluate nesiritide in patients with dyspnea at rest from decompensated heart failure, nitroglycerin treatment in 143 patients demonstrated nonsignificant, mild decreases in PCWP and no significant improvement in patient-assessed dyspnea within 3 hours, but the dose was remarkably low (42 μg/min).[93] In a small, single-site sub-study[94] where nitroglycerin was aggressively up-titrated to a mean dose of 155 μg/min by 3 hours, there were significant decreases in PCWP (4- to 6-mm Hg decrease from baseline) from 1 to 12 hours, but no difference at 24 hours. The major limitation of organic nitrates is the tolerance that typically develops within 24 hours. Headache is the most common adverse effect (20% within 24 hours[93]). Symptomatic hypotension (5%) may also be noted, but generally resolves when nitrate therapy is discontinued. Given the risk of severe hypotension with potentially catastrophic consequences, the recent use of phosphodiesterase 5 inhibitors (sildenafil, tadalafil, vardenafil, etc.) should be ruled out prior to administration of nitrates.

Sodium Nitroprusside

SNP induces a balanced reduction in afterload and preload that is exquisitely titratable, due to a very short half-life (seconds to a few minutes) and is particularly effective in the setting of markedly elevated afterload (e.g., hypertensive AHF) and moderate-severe mitral regurgitation. Intravenous administration is usually monitored with an indwelling arterial line, although automated blood pressure cuffs are now used in many centers. Titration of the SNP dose to rapidly improve symptoms and/or to achieve an SBP of 90 to 100 mm Hg are typical goals, and invasive pulmonary artery catheters may assist in meeting other hemodynamic goals. Tapering the dose of nitroprusside prior to discontinuation is advised to avoid the possibility of "rebound hypertension." Physician discomfort with the cyanide metabolites and the historical institutional requirements for invasive arterial monitoring has limited the use of this highly effective therapy to fewer than 1% of patients with AHF in Europe and the United States.[12,45]

Nitroprusside, a pro-drug that is rapidly metabolized to nitric oxide and cyanide, has no inherent arrhythmogenic properties, may improve myocardial oxygen demand by reducing afterload and wall stress, creates no significant electrolyte disturbances, and is rarely toxic. Despite its potency, severe hypotension is unusual and rapidly resolves. However, significant vasodilation of the intra-myocardial vasculature has been noted, possibly producing a coronary steal phenomenon, and consequently, nitroprusside is not recommended for patients with active myocardial ischemia. The most common complaints with nitroprusside are related to the cyanide metabolite, including nausea, abdominal discomfort, dissociative feelings, and dysphoria. Cyanide rarely accumulates in patients, but impaired hepatic function and doses of greater than 250 μg/min for over 48 hours increase this risk. The thiocyanate metabolite can accumulate in patients with moderate to severe renal insufficiency when exposed to prolonged infusions of high doses (usually >400 μg/

min) over days and is usually not relevant in the treatment of AHF. Cyanide levels may be measured, but rarely return in a timely fashion to be useful.

There are no randomized studies of nitroprusside in patients with AHF, although multiple studies demonstrated dramatic reduction in PCWP (15 mm Hg) and marked increases in cardiac output, associated with increases in diuresis, natriuresis, and decreased neurohormonal activation. In a contemporary analysis of 175 consecutive patients admitted for AHF, intravenous SNP was associated with greater hemodynamic improvement and lower rates of inotropic support or worsening renal function during hospitalization and with lower rates of all-cause mortality after discharge, despite a worse hemodynamic profile at baseline.[95]

NESIRITIDE

Nesiritide (recombinant human B-type natriuretic peptide) is identical to endogenous BNP and causes potent vasodilation in the venous and arterial vasculatures, resulting in significant reductions in venous and ventricular filling pressures and mild increases in cardiac output. As with other vasodilators, nesiritide may reduce diuretic requirements, but in clinical studies, there is limited evidence for a significant direct "natriuretic" effect. Nesiritide may be used for treatment of patients with acutely decompensated congestive heart failure who have dyspnea at rest or with minimal activity, but it should not be administered for the indication of replacing diuretics, enhancing diuresis, protecting renal function, or improving survival. An optional bolus of 2 μg/kg followed by a 0.01 μg/kg/min infusion is the recommended starting dose for nesiritide. There is limited clinical trial experience with up-titration of the drug, but for patients who remain symptomatic with evidence of volume overload and sufficient blood pressure, up-titration may be considered. Nesiritide has clear effects on hemodynamics and has limited need for frequent dose adjustments and an absence of tolerance, but its high cost and lack of clear clinical benefit beyond other less expensive and more readily titratable agents have limited its use. The Vasodilation in the Management of Acute CHF (VMAC) trial randomized 489 patients with decompensated CHF and dyspnea at rest to placebo, nitroglycerin, or nesiritide.[93] After 3 hours, patients receiving nesiritide had a significantly greater decrease in PCWP compared to both nitroglycerin and placebo, and improvement in dyspnea compared to placebo (no difference from nitroglycerin). A pooled analysis of the randomized, controlled clinical trial data suggested that nesiritide may be associated with an increased risk of worsening renal function as well as increased mortality. To address these issues, the ASCEND-HF trial randomized 7141 patients with AHF to nesiritide or placebo for 24 to 168 hours.[96] At 30 days, there were no difference between patients receiving nesiritide and those receiving placebo with regard to the composite endpoint of death or rehospitalization for heart failure. The clinical effects on dyspnea were relatively modest and have generally not been felt to be clinically important compared to placebo. Use of nesiritide had no impact on worsening renal function but was associated with an increase in the rate of hypotension. Another small study (ROSE-AHF) enrolled 360 patients admitted for AHF to specifically assess the effect of low-dose nesiritide on congestion and renal function.[97] In this study, nesiritide had no beneficial effect on urine output or cystatin-C, nor on any of the other secondary endpoints reflective of decongestion, renal function, or clinical outcomes, although it was associated with more symptomatic hypotension.

Nesiritide exerts its activity via guanylyl cyclase-linked natriuretic peptide receptors (NPR A and B) causing cGMP-mediated vasodilation. Hypotension, at times prolonged (over 2 hours[93]) despite the relatively short (18 minute) half-life of the peptide, is more common in patients with volume depletion and consequently, nesiritide use should be limited to those with congestive signs and symptoms. Headache also occurs, although less frequent than with nitroglycerin. Other actions of nesiritide include neurohormonal antagonism with reduction in vasopressin, aldosterone, and sympathetic tone, and alteration of intra-renal hemodynamics and glomerular filtration. Nesiritide did not improve urine output or renal function in AHF patients with worsening creatinine.[97]

Inotropes and Inodilators

The inotropic drugs and inodilators (inotropic drugs with vasodilatory properties) increase cardiac output through cyclic adenosine monophosphate (cAMP)-mediated inotropy and reduce PCWP through vasodilation (see Table 49.7).[98] However, retrospective data from both registries and trials of AHF patients suggest that even the short-term use (hours to few days) of IV inotropes (except for digoxin) is associated with significant side effects such as hypotension, atrial or ventricular arrhythmias, and an increase in in-hospital[70] and possibly long-term mortality.[99] Patients with CAD may be at higher risk of adverse events due to reduced coronary perfusion and increased myocardial oxygen requirements with possible myocardial ischemia and injury. Therefore, these agents are reserved for use in selected situations of hypoperfusion when other interventions are inappropriate or have failed. The use of these drugs should be limited to patients with reduced EF, who present with low SBP (<90 mm Hg) or low measured cardiac output in the presence of signs of congestion and organ hypoperfusion such as decreased mentation or reduced urine output.[32,50] Despite these recommendations, inotropes are still frequently used in patients with HFpEF in some regions. Inotropic agents for AHF should be used with close hemodynamic and telemetry monitoring and should be stopped as soon as adequate organ perfusion is restored. All of these agents may increase conduction through the atrioventricular node, causing a rapid ventricular response in patients presenting with atrial fibrillation. Additionally, IV inotropes may be used in cardiogenic shock as a temporary therapy to prevent hemodynamic collapse or as a life-sustaining bridge to more definitive therapy for those patients awaiting mechanical circulatory support, ventricular assist devices, or cardiac transplantation. In North American and European registries, approximately 15% and 25% of patients were treated with inotropic agents, although given the minimal supportive clinical evidence, there is marked local variability in the use of these drugs.[100]

Dobutamine

Dobutamine is the most commonly used positive inotrope in Europe and the United States, despite evidence that it increases mortality.[101,102] Dobutamine at doses of 1 to 2 µg/kg/min may improve renal perfusion in patients with cardiogenic shock, although higher doses (5 to 10 µg/kg/min) may be necessary for more profound hypoperfusion. Tachyphylaxis may occur with infusions of over 24 to 48 hours, partially due to receptor desensitization. In general, dobutamine (or dopamine) is the preferred inotrope in patients with significant hypotension and in the setting of significant renal dysfunction, given the renal excretion of milrinone. Concomitant beta blocker therapy will result in competitive antagonism of the effects of dobutamine and higher doses of dobutamine (10 to 20 µg/kg/min) may be required to obtain the desired hemodynamic effects. The lowest effective dose of dobutamine should be used in the context of continuous blood pressure and rhythm monitoring. Dobutamine should be gradually weaned off and clinical status re-evaluated with each dose adjustment. Temporary adjustments to afterload-reducing agents or diuretics may assist in weaning.

As an agonist of both beta$_1$ and beta$_2$ adrenergic receptors (see Chapter 38) with variable effects on the alpha receptors, dobutamine has multiple actions. Beta-receptor stimulation results in increased inotropy and chronotropy through increases in intracellular cAMP and calcium, as well as via direct activation of voltage sensitive calcium channels. At low doses, stimulation of beta$_2$ and alpha receptors causes vasodilation, resulting in decreased aortic impedance and systemic vascular resistance with reduction in afterload and indirect increases in cardiac output. At higher doses, vasoconstriction can ensue with decreased venous capacitance and increased right atrial pressure. Adverse effects of dobutamine include tachycardia, increasing ventricular response to atrial fibrillation, increased atrial and ventricular arrhythmias, myocardial ischemia, and possibly cardiomyocyte necrosis via direct toxic effects and induction of apoptosis.[103]

While the hemodynamic and other effects of dobutamine have been studied, there is only one placebo-controlled, randomized trial in patients with AHF. Although there are some methodologic concerns, the CAlcium Sensitizer or Inotrope or NOne in low output heart failure (CASINO) study demonstrated significantly increased mortality with dobutamine compared to placebo, consistent with the results of other studies of this class of agents.[101]

Dopamine

In both the United States and Europe, dopamine is used as often as dobutamine, presumably as a vasoconstrictor and for its putative effects on renal vasodilation. As a precursor to the synthesis of norepinephrine, an agonist of both adrenergic and dopaminergic receptors, and an inhibitor of norepinephrine uptake, dopamine has complex effects that vary significantly with dose. Initiation of dopamine therapy causes a rapid release of norepinephrine that can precipitate tachycardia, as well as atrial and ventricular arrhythmias. In addition, intermediate to high doses can cause significant vasoconstriction, precipitating heart failure and poor perfusion. Dopamine should be gradually weaned from these doses down to 3 to 5 µg/kg/min and then discontinued to avoid potential hypotensive effects of low-dose dopamine.

Low-dose dopamine (≤2 µg/kg/min) has been proposed to cause specific dilation of renal, splanchnic, and cerebral arteries, potentially increasing renal blood flow in a selective manner, as well as promoting natriuresis through direct distal tubular effects. The DAD-HF study of 60 patients admitted for AHF suggested that a combination of low-dose furosemide and low-dose dopamine resulted in comparable urine output and dyspnea relief, but improved renal function profile and potassium homeostasis compared to high-dose furosemide.[104] However, the DAD-HF II study of 161 patients found no beneficial effect of the addition of low-dose dopamine to furosemide.[105] In the ROSE-AHF study of 360 patients hospitalized with AHF, low-dose dopamine did not increase urine volume during 72 hours, did not improve cystatin C concentrations, but did reduce hypotension and increased tachycardia compared to placebo.[97] Therefore, there does not appear to be an indication for low-dose dopamine therapy to improve renal function.

Intermediate-dose dopamine (2 to 10 µg/kg/min) results in enhanced norepinephrine release, stimulating cardiac receptors with an increase in inotropy and mild stimulation of peripheral vasoconstricting receptors. Because the positive inotropic effect is largely dependent upon myocardial catecholamine stores, which are often depleted in patients with advanced heart failure, dopamine is a poor inotrope in patients with severe systolic dysfunction.

High-dose dopamine (10 to 20 µg/kg/min) causes peripheral and pulmonary artery vasoconstriction, mediated by direct agonist effects on alpha$_1$ adrenergic receptors. These doses pose a significant risk of precipitating limb and end-organ ischemia and should be used cautiously.

Epinephrine

Epinephrine is a full beta-receptor agonist and a potent inotropic agent with balanced vasodilator and vasoconstrictor effects. The direct effect of epinephrine on increasing inotropy independent of myocardial catecholamine stores makes epinephrine a useful agent in the treatment of transplant patients with denervated hearts.

Phosphodiesterase Inhibitors

cAMP is a ubiquitous signaling molecule that increases inotropy, chronotropy, and lusitropy in cardiomyocytes and causes vasorelaxation in vascular smooth muscle (see Chapter 46). Phosphodiesterase IIIa is compartmentalized in the cardiac and vascular smooth muscle, where it terminates the signaling activity of cAMP by degrading it to AMP. Many specific inhibitors of PDE IIIa, such as milrinone and enoximone, have been developed to provide organ-specific improvements in hemodynamics through increasing myocardial and vascular smooth muscle cell cAMP concentrations. In theory, subcellular localization may provide the possibility to stimulate inotropy without increasing heart rate with low doses of highly specific phosphodiesterase inhibitors (PDEI). The independence of the mechanism from adrenergic receptors bypasses receptor down-regulation, desensitization, and antagonism by beta blockers. Although studies have shown improved hemodynamic efficacy with PDEI compared to dobutamine in patients on beta blocker therapy, such limitations of dobutamine's effects are not typically clinically relevant. In addition, this mechanism allows for synergistic effects with beta receptor agonists, such as dobutamine. Such combination therapy may be useful in patients with markedly reduced LV systolic function. PDEI cause significant peripheral and pulmonary vasodilation, reducing afterload and preload, while increasing inotropy. These effects make them well suited for patients with LV dysfunction and pulmonary hypertension or post-transplant patients.

Milrinone is the most commonly used PDEI, but only 3% of patients in ADHERE[45] and less than 1% in EHFS II[12] received it. Milrinone therapy may be initiated with a 25 to 75 µg/kg bolus over 10 to 20 min, although in clinical practice the bolus dose is usually omitted. Infusions are typically started at 0.10 to 0.25 µg/kg/min and may be up-titrated to hemodynamic effect. Given the elimination half-life of 2.5 hours and the pharmacodynamic half-life of over 6 hours, effects from up-titration are delayed by at least 15 minutes after dosage adjustment. Also due to these pharmacodynamics, patients who have had prolonged administration of milrinone may have delayed deterioration, so they should be observed for at least 48 hours after cessation. Milrinone is renally excreted, necessitating dose adjustment in the presence of renal dysfunction or substitution with dobutamine. Milrinone has many side effects, including hypotension and atrial and ventricular arrhythmias. In OPTIME-CHF (Outcomes of a Prospective Trial of Intravenous Milrinone for Exacerbations of Chronic Heart Failure),[106] 951 patients admitted with exacerbation of systolic heart failure not requiring intravenous inotropic support were randomized to milrinone or placebo infusion. There was no difference in the primary endpoint of days hospitalized for cardiovascular causes with 60 days, but significant increases in sustained hypotension and new atrial arrhythmias were noted in the milrinone-treated patients. In addition, a post-hoc sub-group analysis demonstrated increased mortality in patients with an ischemic cause of heart failure who received milrinone.[99] This study reinforces the caution that must be exercised in selecting these agents for the treatment of patients with AHF.

ENOXIMONE

Enoximone is also a PDE IIIa inhibitor that is available in Europe. Dosing is essentially 10 times that of milrinone, with a bolus dose of 0.25 to 0.75 mg/kg bolus over 10 to 20 minutes, followed by an infusion of 1.25 µg/kg/min. It is extensively metabolized by the liver into renally cleared active metabolites, so doses should be reduced in the setting of either renal or hepatic insufficiency. Otherwise, the above comments apply to this PDEI as well.

Levosimendan

Levosimendan is a novel agent that increases myocardial contractility and produces peripheral vasodilation, through cardiac myofilament calcium sensitization by calcium-dependent (systolic) troponin C binding and activation of vascular smooth muscle potassium channels, respectively. Levosimendan also has some PDEI activity, which some contend is responsible for its inotropic activity in patients.[107] Levosimendan was administered to almost 4% of patients in EHFS II[12] and is available in over 40 countries (although not in the United States), where it is used in patients with reduced LV systolic function and hypoperfusion in the absence of severe hypotension. Although it may be given with a bolus of 12 to 24 µg/kg over 10 minutes, many clinicians directly initiate a continuous infusion at a rate of 0.05 to 0.10 µg/kg/min, which may be up-titrated to 0.2 µg/kg/min. In clinical trials, levosimendan has been shown to significantly increase cardiac output, reduce PCWP and afterload, and improve dyspnea. The potent vasodilating effects of levosimendan can cause significant hypotension, the risk of which may be reduced by maintaining filling pressures.[98] Levosimendan has an active, acetylated metabolite with a half-life of over 80 hours, allowing it to have hemodynamic effects days after discontinuation of the infusion.

Initial clinical studies demonstrated reduced arrhythmias and improved survival with levosimendan compared to placebo and dobutamine. REVIVE-II (Randomized multicenter evaluation of intravenous levosimendan efficacy versus placebo in the short term treatment of decompensated heart failure), a recent study of 600 patients, demonstrated significant improvement in the clinical status, serial BNP, and hospital length of stay with levosimendan treatment compared to standard care, but there were also more episodes of hypotension, atrial fibrillation, and ventricular ectopy, as well as a nonsignificant increase in early deaths at 14 to 90 days.[108] SURVIVE (Survival of patients with AHF in need of intravenous inotropic support trial) randomized 1327 patients with systolic dysfunction, evidence of low cardiac output, and dyspnea at rest despite diuretics and vasodilators to either levosimendan or dobutamine. An early reduction in mortality was not sustained through 180 days, but levosimendan was associated with a greater incidence of atrial fibrillation and lower incidence of WHF compared to dobutamine.[109]

Vasopressors

These agents should be reserved for patients with marked hypotension in whom central organ hypoperfusion is evident. Vasopressors will redistribute cardiac output centrally at the expense of peripheral perfusion and increased afterload. *Norepinephrine* is a potent agonist of the beta$_1$ and the alpha$_1$ receptors, but is a weaker agonist of beta$_2$ receptors, resulting in marked vasoconstriction. In general, it is the preferred vasopressor for cardiogenic shock.[32] In the SOAP II trial, 1679 patients with shock were randomized to either dopamine or norepinephrine with a nonstatistical difference increase in mortality with dopamine associated with a significant increase in arrhythmic events.[110] In a subgroup analysis including the 280 patients with cardiogenic shock, norepinephrine had improved survival compared to dopamine. *Phenylephrine* is a selective alpha$_1$ receptor agonist with potent direct arterial vasoconstrictor effects. This agent may be used in case of severe hypotension, particularly when the hypotension is related to systemic vasodilation, rather than to a decrease in cardiac output. As noted above, *dopamine* may also be used for its vasoconstrictor properties. All of these agents may induce end-organ hypoperfusion and tissue necrosis.

OTHER PHARMACOLOGIC THERAPIES
Digoxin

Digoxin rapidly improves hemodynamics without increasing heart rate or decreasing BP and may be considered in patients with a low BP due to a low cardiac output.[111] Digoxin may be used intravenously with an initial bolus of 0.5 mg IV. It should be given slowly because a rapid administration may cause systemic vasoconstriction. The initial bolus should be followed by an oral or IV dose of 0.25 mg at least 12 hours after the initial dose. In patients who continue to have signs and symptoms of HF, digoxin therapy should be continued in addition to other therapies, with a dose resulting in a trough serum concentration of less than 1 ng/mL. Ischemia, hypokalemia, and hypomagnesemia may increase the likelihood of developing digitalis intoxication, even at the therapeutic doses. Digoxin should not be used in patients with moderate to severe renal impairment, ongoing ischemia, or advanced AV block.

Arginine Vasopressin Antagonists

Arginine vasopressin (AVP), also known as antidiuretic hormone, is the main regulator of plasma osmolality. Vasopressin levels are inappropriately high in both acute and chronic HF and are thought to have a major role in the pathophysiology of HF. In particular, vasopressin appears to be the major contributor to the development of the hyponatremia observed in patients with HF. In patients with AHF, volume overload, and persistent hyponatremia at risk for or having active cognitive symptoms, therapy with a vasopressin antagonist for short-term improvement in serum sodium concentration may be considered. Currently available vasopressin antagonists are tolvaptan (an oral, selective V2 receptor antagonist) and conivaptan (a V1$_a$/V2 receptor antagonist for IV use). Although both agents have been approved for the treatment of clinically significant hypervolemic and euvolemic hyponatremia, they have not been shown to improve long-term outcomes in heart failure and are not currently approved for this indication. The Efficacy of Vasopressin Antagonism in Heart Failure Outcome Study with Tolvaptan (EVEREST) was an international trial that evaluated more than 4000 patients admitted with AHF and reduced EF. Tolvaptan added to standard therapy for AHF modestly improved signs and symptoms during hospitalization and modestly reduced body weight without affecting renal function, HR, or BP, but post-discharge survival and readmission rate were not affected by chronic post-discharge therapy with tolvaptan.[112,113] A recent small double blind study of short-term (48 hours) therapy with tolvaptan vs placebo in AHF, the TACTICS study, did not show a clinically important benefit of tolvaptan therapy in this setting.[114] In patients with AHF, the addition of conivaptan to standard therapy increased urine output without a significant improvement in signs or symptoms or decrease in body weight.[115]

Calcium Channel Blockers

Calcium channel blockers (CCBs) without significant myocardial depressant effects, such as nicardipine and clevidipine, may be potentially useful in patients with AHF presenting with severe hypertension refractory to other therapies. In a pilot study of 104 patients with hypertensive AHF who exhibited pulmonary congestion, clevidipine rapidly provided significant blood pressure control associated with improvement in dyspnea compared to standard of care.[116]

Other Nonpharmacologic Therapies
Ultrafiltration

Peripheral ultrafiltration is an available modality to remove sodium and water in hospitalized patients with HF. The theoretical advantage of ultrafiltration is the removal of isotonic fluid, resulting in greater and more reliable salt removal, potentially without the neurohormonal activation seen with diuretics.[83] Potential limitations of ultrafiltration include the need for large-bore venous access, systemic anticoagulation, and increased complexity of nursing care related to management of the device. Although theoretically attractive, the appropriate use of ultrafiltration in AHF remains uncertain.

The Ultrafiltration Versus Intravenous Diuretics for Patients Hospitalized for Acute Decompensated Heart Failure (UNLOAD) trial randomized 200 patients with AHF to veno-venous ultrafiltration or standard of care within 24 hours of initial presentation. Patients receiving ultrafiltration demonstrated a greater reduction in body weight at 48 hours, but no improvements in dyspnea and/or renal function.[117] Intriguingly, there was a reduction in post-discharge events at 90 days with ultrafiltration, although the number of events was small. Other recent studies have raised questions about the optimal use of ultrafiltration in heart failure. In an observational study of 63 patients with persistent congestion refractory to hemodynamically guided intensive medical therapy, slow continuous ultrafiltration resulted in improved hemodynamics, yet was associated with high incidence of subsequent transition to renal replacement therapy and high in-hospital mortality.[118] The Cardiorenal Rescue Study in Acute Decompensated Heart Failure (CARRESS) randomized 188 patients with AHF, worsened renal function, and persistent congestion to a strategy of stepped pharmacologic care (intravenous diuretics dosed by the investigator to maintain urine output of 3 to 5 L/day plus intravenous vasodilators or inotropes if needed to achieve target urine output) or ultrafiltration (fluid removal rate 200 mL/hr).[59] Ultrafiltration resulted in similar weight loss (approximately 12 pounds), but resulted in an increase in creatinine levels, compared to standard care, and was associated with more serious adverse events, especially kidney failure, bleeding complications, and intravenous catheter-related complications.

CARRESS enrolled a high-risk population with a composite rate of death or rehospitalization at 60 days of over 50%. The AVOID-HF study (Aquapheresis Versus Intravenous Diuretics and Hospitalizations for Heart Failure, NCT01474200) was designed as an 810-patient trial that was terminated early after 224 patients were enrolled. Although underpowered, there were trends suggesting longer time to first HF event and fewer HF and cardiovascular events in the adjustable ultrafiltration group compared to those randomized to adjustable intravenous loop diuretics.[119] There was no difference in renal function, but more patients assigned to ultrafiltration experienced adverse events.

HYPERTONIC SALINE

Administration of hypertonic saline (HSS; 3%) along with high-dose furosemide and sodium and fluid restriction may be associated with greater diuretic and clinical response. The SMAC-HF study randomized 1771 patients hospitalized for AHF to a single-blind strategy of hypertonic saline solution (150 mL 3% NS) plus furosemide 250 mg intravenous bolus twice daily and sodium restriction to 120 mmol/day versus furosemide 250 mg intravenous bolus twice daily and sodium restriction to 80 mmol/day; both groups received a fluid intake of 1000 mL/day.[120] After discharge, the HSS group continued with 120 mmol Na/day; the second group continued with 80 mmol Na/day. There was a shorter length of stay, increased creatinine clearance at discharge, reduced readmission rate, and improved survival for patients in the hypertonic saline group. These hypothesis-generating data are intriguing, but they are limited by the unblinded study design and the potential confounding by post-discharge management. Larger, prospective, blinded trials are needed to further evaluate this therapeutic approach prior to adoption for clinical practice.

Potential New Therapies

Most of the large clinical trials of new therapies for AHF have been negative in terms of efficacy and/or safety (Table 49.8). A variety of potential explanations have been proposed including lack of drug efficacy, patient selection, timing of therapy, and endpoints.[121] Nonetheless, given the diverse pathophysiology of AHF, it may be unrealistic to expect that

TABLE 49.8 Selected Clinical Trials for Acute Heart Failure

TRIAL	TREATMENT ARMS	POPULATION	RESULTS
VMAC (2002) $N = 489$	Nesiritide (Nes; 0.01–0.03 µg/kg/min with optional 2 µg/kg bolus; from 24 hr up to 7 days) vs Placebo (Pla; only during first 3 hr) vs Nitroglycerin (NTG; from 24 hr up to 7 days)	Dyspnea at rest / ≥2 signs of HF within 72 hours / CXR with pulmonary edema	Change in PCWP, at 3 h (1°): −5.8 mm Hg Nes, −3.8 mm Hg NTG, −2 mm Hg Placebo ($p < 0.001$); at 24: −8.2 mm Hg Nes, −6.3 mm Hg NTG ($p < 0.04$). / Self-evaluation of dyspnea at 3 h, Likert (1°): Nes vs Pla, $p = 0.03$; Nes vs NTG, $p = 0.56$; a 24 h: NTG vs Nes, $p = 0.13$. / Self-evaluation of global clinical status, at 3 hr: Nes vs Pla, $p = 0.07$; Nes vs NTG, $p = 0.33$; at 24 hr: NTG vs Nes, $p = 0.08$.
OPTIME-HF (2002) $N = 951$	Milrinone (0.5 µg/kg/min, titratable to 0.75) vs Placebo, for 48–72 hr	Presenting within 48 hr / Known systolic HF / LEVF ≤40%	Days with CV hospitalization or dead in 60 days (1°): Milrinone, 12.3 vs Pla 12.5 ($p = 0.71$) / Failure of therapy due to AE within 48 hr: Milrinone 20.6% vs Pla 9.2% ($p < 0.001$). / Excess sustained hypotension ($p = 0.004$), new atrial fibrillation/flutter ($p < 0.001$), VT/VF ($p = 0.06$).
ESCAPE (2005) $N = 433$	Pulmonary artery catheter (PAC)-guided therapy vs clinical assessment (CA)-guided therapy	LVEF ≤30% / SBP ≤125 mm Hg / ≥1 sign and ≥1 symptom of HF / 3 months HF symptoms despite ACEi and diuretics	Days alive out of hospital during 6 months (1°): PAC, 133 days vs CA, 135 (HR 1.00; 95% CI 0.82–1.21; $p = 0.99$). / Greater number of adverse events in PAC group
VERITAS (2007) $N = 1435$	Tezosentan (Tezo; 5 mg/hr for 30 min, followed by 1 mg/hr for 24–72 hr) vs Placebo	Presenting within 24 hr / Persistent dyspnea / Respiratory rate ≥24 bpm / At least two of: elevated BNP/NT-proBNP, clinical pulmonary edema, CXR with congestion, LV systolic dysfunction	Change in dyspnea AUC, 24 hr (1°): VERITAS-1, Tezo −562 vs Pla −550 mm * h ($p = 0.80$); VERITAS-2, Tezo −367 vs Pla −342 ($p = 0.60$) / Death or worsening HF, 7 days: VERITAS-1 + 2, Tezo 26.3% vs. Pla 26.4 ($p = 0.95$)

TABLE 49.8 Selected Clinical Trials for Acute Heart Failure—cont'd

TRIAL	TREATMENT ARMS	POPULATION	RESULTS
SURVIVE (2007) N = 1327	Levosimendan (Levo; loading 12 µg/kg, followed 0.1–0.2 µg/kg/min; for 24 hr) vs Dobutamine (Dob; 5 µg/kg/min, titratable up to 40 µg/kg/min; for at least 24 hr)	LVEF ≤30% Requiring IV inotropic support At least one of following: dyspnea at rest, oliguria, PCWP ≥18 mm Hg or CI ≤V2.2 L/min/m²	All-cause mortality, 180 days (1°): Levo, 26% vs. Dob 28% (HR 0.91; 95% CI 0.74–1.13; p = 0.40) Change in BNP from baseline to 24 hr: Levo, –631 vs. Dob, –397, p < 0.001. No change in dyspnea at 24 hr, days alive out of hospital at 180 days, all-cause mortality at 31 days, CV mortality at 180 days.
EVEREST (2007) N = 4133	Tolvaptan (Tol; 30 mg po qd) vs Placebo, for at least 60 days	Randomized within 48 hr NYHA III–IV symptoms LVEF ≤40% Signs of volume expansion	Composite of changes in global clinical status and body weight, 7 days (1°): p < 0.001, for Tol superiority; no difference in clinical status; Change in body weight, 1 day: Tol, –1.76 kg vs. Pla, –0.97; p < 0.001. All-cause mortality (1°): Tol, 25.9% vs Pla 26.3% (HR 0.98, 95% CI 0.87–1.11, superiority p = 0.68; non-inferiority p < 0.001) CV death or HF hospitalization (1°): Tol, 42.0% vs. Pla 40.2% (HR 1.04, 95% CI 0.95–1.14, superiority p = 0.55)
UNLOAD (2007) N = 200	Ultrafiltration (UF; fluid removal titrated by investigator up to 500 mL/hr) vs Diuretic (titrated by investigator, at least twice daily oral dose), for 48 hr	Randomized within 24 hr ≥2 signs of congestion	Weight loss, 48 hr (1°): UF, –5.0 kg vs Diuretics, –3.1, p = 0.001 Dyspnea score, 48 hr (1°): UF, 6.4 vs Diuretics, 6.1; p = 0.35 HF rehospitalization, 90 days: UF, 0.22 vs Diuretics, 046, p = 0.022; Days rehospitalized: UF, 1.4 days vs Diuretics, 3.8; p = 0.022; Unscheduled HF visits: UF, 21% pts vs Diuretics, 44%, p = 0.009.
3CPO (2008) N = 1069	Noninvasive positive pressure ventilation (NIPPV) vs continuous positive airway pressure (CPAP) vs oxygen therapy (O₂)	Clinical diagnosis of Cardiogenic pulmonary edema CXR with pulmonary edema Respiratory rate >20 bpm Arterial pH <7.35	All-cause mortality, 7 days (1°): NIPPV + CPAP 9.5% vs O₂ 9.8% (OR 0.97, 95% CI 0.63–1.48; p = 0.87) Composite death or intubation, 7 days (1°): NIPPV + CPAP, 11.1% vs O₂ 11.7% (OR 0.94, 95% CI 0.59–1.51; p = 0.81) NIPPV + CPAP better than O₂: Change in arterial pH, 1 hr (p < 0.001); Dyspnea score, 1 hr (p = 0.008)
PROTECT (2010) N = 2033	Rolofylline 30 mg vs. placebo for up to 3 days	Randomized within 24 hr, Persistent dyspnea at rest or with minimal activity, estimated CrCl 20–80 mL/min, BNP ≥500 pg/mL or NT-proBNP ≥2000 pg/mL, IV loop diuretic therapy	Clinical composite (1°): OR for rolofylline 0.92, 95% CI 0.78–1.09, p = 0.35
DOSE (2011) N = 308	Low vs. high dose furosemide Continuous vs intermittent intravenous bolus 1:1:1:1 2×2 factorial design	Randomized within 24 hr, ≥1 sign and ≥1 symptom of HF, history of chronic HF treated with furosemide 80–240 mg/day (or equivalent) for at least 1 month	Global assessment of symptoms (1°): 4236 ± 1440 AUC bolus vs. 4373 ± 1404 AUC cont inf, P = 0.47; 4171 ± 1436 AUC low dose vs 4430 ± 1401 AUC high dose, P = 0.06 Mean change in SCr (1°): 0.05 mg/dL bolus vs. 0.07 mg/dL continuous, P = 0.45; 0.04 mg/dL low dose vs. 0.08 mg/dL high dose, P = 0.21.
ASCEND-HF (2011) N = 7141	Nesiritide (Nes) 0.01 µg/kg/min with optional 2 µg/kg bolus (from 24 hr up to 7 days) vs. Placebo (Pla)	Hospitalized for ADHF, dyspnea at rest or with minimal activity, ≥1 sign and ≥1 objective measure of ADHF, randomized within 24 hr of first IV treatment for ADHF	Self-reported dyspnea moderately or markedly better At 6 hr: 42.1% Pla vs 44.5% Nes, P = 0.03* At 24 hr: 66.1% Pla vs 68.2% Nes, P = 0.007* (*did not meet prespecified US regulatory requirement of significance) Death or rehospitalization for HF at 30 days: 10.1% Pla vs 9.4% Nes (HR 0.93, 95% CI 0.8–1.08, P = 0.31)

Continued

TABLE 49.8 Selected Clinical Trials for Acute Heart Failure—cont'd

TRIAL	TREATMENT ARMS	POPULATION	RESULTS
CARRESS-HF (2012) N = 188	Ultrafiltration (UF) vs stepped pharmacologic care (Pharm)	Develop cardiorenal syndrome before (within 6 weeks) or after (within 7 days from admission) hospitalization.	Change in creatinine level: UF, +0.23 mg/dL vs Pharm, −0.04 ± 0.53 mg/dL in the pharmacologic-therapy group vs in the ultrafiltration group, P = 0.003 Weight loss: 5.5 ± 5.1 kg [12.1 ± 11.3 lb] in the pharmacologic-therapy group vs.5.7 ± 3.9 kg [12.6 ± 8.5 lb] in the ultrafiltration group, P = 0.58 Serious adverse events: 72% in the ultrafiltration group vs. 57% in the pharmacologic-therapy group, P = 0.03
RELAX-AHF (2013) N = 1161	Serelaxin (Ser) 30 µg/kg/day vs. Placebo (Pla) for 48 hr	Patients with dyspnea at rest or on minimal exertion, congestion on chest x-ray, BNP ≥350 ng/L (or NT-proBNP ≥1400 ng/L), eGFR 30–75 mL/min/1.73 m², and SBP > 125 mmHg	Change in dyspnea by VAS AUC to day 5 (1′): 19% improvement by Ser compared to placebo by VAS AUC (448 mm *h, 95% CI 120–775), p = 0.007. Proportion of patients with moderately or markedly improved dyspnea by Likert scale at all 3 early timepoints (6, 12, 24 hr; 1°): Ser 27% vs. Pla 26%, P = 0.70 Days alive out of hospital up to day 60: Ser 48.3 vs. Pla 47.7, p = 0.37 180-day mortality: Pla 65 deaths vs. Ser 42, HR 0.63 (95% CI 0.43–0.93), P = 0.02
REVIVE-2 (2013) N = 600	Levosimendan (Levo; loading 12 µg/kg, followed by 0.1–0.2 µg/kg/min; for 24 h) vs Placebo	Dyspneic at rest LVEF ≤35%	Clinical composite endpoint, 5 d (1°): Levo superior, p = 0.015 More frequent hypotension and cardiac arrhythmias, during the infusion period; numerically higher risk of death, 90 d (REVIVE 1&2: Levo, 49 deaths/350 pts; vs Placebo, 40/ 350, P = 0.29)
ROSE (2013) N = 360	Dopamine (2 µg/kg/min; n = 122) Nesiritide (0.005 µg/kg/min without bolus; n = 119) Pooled placebo group (n = 119)	Acute heart failure Renal dysfunction (eGFR 15–60 mL/min/1.73 m²) Randomized within 24 hr of admission	Compared to placebo: Dopamine: No significant effect on 72-hr cumulative urine volume or on the change in cystatin C level; Increased tachycardia Nesiritide: No significant effect on 72-hr cumulative urine volume or on the change in cystatin C level
DAD-HF II (2014) N = 161	8-hr continuous infusions of: (a) high-dose furosemide (HDF, n = 50, 20 mg/hr), (b) low-dose furosemide and low-dose dopamine (LDFD, n = 56, 5 mg/hr and 5 µg kg⁻¹ min⁻¹, respectively), or (c) low-dose furosemide (LDF, n = 55, furosemide 5 mg/hr).	Dyspnea on minimal exertion or rest dyspnea Oxygen saturation <90% on admission arterial blood gas One or more of the following: (a) signs of congestion, (b) interstitial congestion or pleural effusion on chest x-ray, and (c) elevated serum B-type natriuretic peptide levels	No significant differences in 60-day and one-year all-cause mortality and hospitalization for HF, dyspnea relief (Borg index), worsening renal function, and length of stay
AVOID-HF (2016) N = 224 (810 planned)	Adjustable ultrafiltration (AUF; N = 110) Adjustable intravenous loop diuretics (ALD; N = 114).	Chronic daily oral loop diuretics Fluid overload Received ≤2 iv loop diuretic doses Randomized within 24 hr of admission to hospital	Estimated days to first HF event for the AUF (62) and ALD (34) group (p = 0.106). At 30 days, compared with the ALD group, the AUF group had fewer HF and cardiovascular events Renal function changes were similar More AUF patients with adverse events.
ATOMIC-AHF (2016) N = 606	3 sequential cohorts (approximately 200 patients per cohort): Cohort 1: Omecamtiv mecarbil (OM, target plasma concentration 115 ng/mL) vs. Placebo Cohort 2: OM (target plasma concentration, 230 ng/mL) vs.Placebo Cohort 3: OM (target plasma concentration 310 ng/mL) vs Placebo	LVEF ≤40% Dyspnea at rest or with minimal exertion Elevated natriuretic peptides Randomized within 24 hr of initial IV diuretic.	Dyspnea relief: No significant difference compared to placebo (3 OM dose groups and pooled placebo: placebo, 41%; OM cohort 1, 42%; cohort 2, 47%; cohort 3, 51%; p 0.33); Increased dyspnea relief in Cohort 3 at 48 hr (placebo, 37% vs.OM, 51%; p = 0.034) and through 5 days (p 0.038) Plasma concentration-related increases in LV systolic ejection time (p < 0.0001) and decreases in end-systolic dimension (p < 0.05).

TABLE 49.8 Selected Clinical Trials for Acute Heart Failure—cont'd

TRIAL	TREATMENT ARMS	POPULATION	RESULTS
ATHENA-HF (2017) N = 360	(a) Placebo or 25 mg spironolactone (b) High-dose spironolactone (100 mg) daily for 96 hr	AHF with at least one sign and one symptom of HF NT-proBNP ≥1000 pg/mL or BNP ≥250 pg/mL within 24 hr Potassium ≤5.0 mEq/liter eGFR ≥30 mL/min/1.73m² SBP >90 mm Hg	1° endpoint, Change in NT-proBNP at 96 hr: NS (p = 0.57) All 2° endpoints and day 30 all-cause mortality or heart failure hospitalization: NS
BLAST-AHF (2017) N = 621	(a) Placebo (N = 183) (b) TRV027 1 mg/hr (N = 128) (c) TRV027 5 mg/hr (N = 182) (d) TRV027 25 mg/hr (N = 125)	History of heart failure (HF) Elevated natriuretic peptides ≥2 physical HF signs SBP ≥120 mm Hg and ≤200 mm Hg eGFR (sMDRD) 20–75 mL/min/1.73m² Excluded if use of ARBs 7 days prior, IV inotropes or vasopressors within 2 hr prior, or IV nitrates within 1 hr prior to randomization	1° endpoint (comprised of multiple outcomes, analyzed as a composite z-score), including (1) time from baseline to death through day 30, (2) time from baseline to heart failure rehospitalization through day 30, (3) the first assessment timepoint following worsening heart failure through day 5, (4) change in dyspnea visual analog scale (VAS) score calculated as the area under the curve (AUC) representing the change from baseline over time from baseline through day 5, and (5) length of initial hospital stay (in days) from baseline: No difference in any group.
TACTICS (2017) N = 257	(a) Placebo (N = 128) (b) Tolvaptan (N = 129)	AHF within 24 hr of presentation Elevated natriuretic peptides + 1 additional sign or symptom of congestion Serum sodium ≤140 mmol/L	Dyspnea relief by Likert scale was similar between tolvaptan and placebo at 8 hr (25% moderately or markedly improved for tolvaptan vs 28% placebo, p = 0.59) and at 24 hr (50% tolvaptan vs 47% placebo, p = 0.80). The proportion defined as responders at 24 hr (primary study endpoint) was 16% for tolvaptan and 20% for placebo (p = 0.32). Tolvaptan resulted in greater weight loss and net fluid loss compared to placebo, but tolvaptan-treated patients were more likely to experience worsening renal function during treatment.
SECRET of CHF (2017) N = 250	(a) Placebo (N = 128) (b) Tolvaptan 30 mg/day (N = 122)	AHF within 36 hr Active dyspnea Any of the following: (1) eGFR <60 mL/min/1.73 m²; (2) hyponatremia; or (3) diuretic resistance (urine output #125 mL/hr following intravenous furosemide ≥40 mg)	1° endpoint, 8- and 16-hr dyspnea reduction: NS (p = 0.46; p = 0.78) 2° endpoint: significantly greater weight reduction with tolvaptan (Day 1: −2.4 ± 2.1 kg vs.−0.9 ± 1.8 kg; p < 0.001). 2° endpoint: dyspnea reduction was greater with tolvaptan at Day 3 (p = 0.01).
TRUE-AHF (2017) N = 2157	(a) Placebo (N = 1069) (b) Ularitide (N = 1088)	Men or women, aged 18–85 years Unplanned hospitalization or ED visit for acutely decompensated heart failure Dyspnea at rest, worsened within the past week Evidence of heart failure on chest X-ray BNP >500 pg/mL or NT-pro BNP >2000 pg/mL Persistence of dyspnea at rest despite ≥40 mg of IV furosemide (or equivalent) Systolic BP ≥116 mm Hg and ≤180 mm Hg Start of study drug infusion within 12 hr after initial clinical assessment	1° endpoints, Cardiovascular death: Ularitide 235 deaths, Placebo 225; HR = 1.03 (96% CI:0.85–1.25); p = 0.75 1° endpoints, Hierarchical clinical composite at 48 hr: p = 0.82 2° endpoints, Intensive care LOS during first 120 hr, Hospital length of stay during first 30 days, Episodes of in-hospital WHF during first 120 hr, Proportion with WHF during first 120 hr, Rehospitalization for HF within 30 days of hospital discharge, Duration (hours) of IV therapy for HF during index admission, All-cause mortality or CV hospitalization at 6 months: All NS; Change in NT-proBNP at 48 hr: 47% decrease with ularitide (p < 0.001); Change in serum creatinine during first 72 hr: Increased with ularitide (p = 0.005) Adverse events: Hypotension: Placebo, 10.1% vs. Ularitide, 22.4%. No difference in renal events.

Continued

TABLE 49.8 Selected Clinical Trials for Acute Heart Failure—cont'd

TRIAL	TREATMENT ARMS	POPULATION	RESULTS
RELAX-AHF-2 (2019) N = 6545	(a) Placebo (n = 3271) (b) Serelaxin 30 μg/kg/d (n = 3274)	Presented within 16 hr prior to randomization for AHF. Dyspnea at rest or with minimal exertion, Pulmonary congestion on chest radiograph, BNP ≥500 pg/mL or NT-proBNP ≥2000 pg/mL, SBP ≥125 mm Hg, eGFR ≥25 and ≤75 mL/min/1.73 m², Received at least 40 mg furosemide (or its equivalent) at any time between presentation and the start of screening.	1° endpoint, Cardiovascular death through day 180: Serelaxin, 285 (8.7%) patients vs Placebo, 290 (8.9%); hazard ratio, 0.98; 95% CI, 0.83–1.15; P = 0.77) 1° endpoint, Worsening heart failure through Day 5: Serelaxin, 227 (6.9%) patients vs. Placebo, 252 (7.7%); hazard ratio, 0.89; 95% CI, 0.75–1.07; P = 0.19) 2° endpoints: No significant difference in All-cause death at 180 days, Length of index hospital stay, or Cardiovascular death or rehospitalization for heart failure or renal failure at 180 days.
RELAX-AHF-EU (2019) N = 2666 (3183 planned)	(a) Standard-of-Care (SoC; n = 894) (b) Serelaxin 30 μg/kg/day + SoC (n = 1756)	Presented within 16 hr prior to randomization for AHF. Dyspnea, Pulmonary congestion on chest radiograph, BNP ≥500 pg/mL or NT-proBNP ≥2000 pg/mL), SBP ≥125 mm Hg, eGFR ≥25 and ≤75 mL/min/1.73m² Received at least 40 mg furosemide (or its equivalent) at any time between presentation and the start of screening.	Prospective, randomized, open-label, blinded-endpoint (PROBE) trial 1° endpoint, adjudicated Worsening heart failure/all-cause death through Day 5: significantly reduced in the serelaxin+SoC vs. SoC group (5.0% vs. 6.9%; hazard ratio 0.71; 95% confidence interval 0.51–0.98; P = 0.0172) (absolute risk reduction 1.9%, number needed to treat 53)
GALACTIC (2019) N = 788	(a) Usual care (n = 402) (b) Early intensive and sustained vasodilation therapy throughout the hospitalization (n = 386)	Hospitalized for AHF Dyspnea (NYHA III/IV) BNP ≥500 ng/L or NT-proBNP ≥2000ng/L. SBP ≥100 mm Hg Planned treatment in a general ward	Prospective, randomized, open-label blinded end-point (PROBE) trial 1° endpoint, composite of all-cause mortality or rehospitalization for AHF at 180 days: Vasodilators, 117 patients (30.6%; 55 deaths [14.4%]) vs Usual Care, 111 patients (27.8%; 61 deaths [15.3%]) (absolute difference for the primary end point, 2.8% [95% CI, −3.7%–9.3%]; adjusted hazard ratio, 1.07 [95% CI, 0.83–1.39]; P = .59).

ACEi, Angiotensin-converting enzyme (ACE) inhibitor; AUC, area under the curve; HF, heart failure; LOS, length of stay; NTG, nitroglycerin; PAC, premature atrial complex; PCWP, pulmonary capillary wedge pressure; VAS, visual analogue scale; VMAC, vasodilation in the management of acute CHF; WHF, worsening heart failure.
Data from VMAC Investigators. Intravenous nesiritide vs nitroglycerin for treatment of decompensated congestive heart failure: a randomized controlled trial. JAMA. 2002;287:1531–40. Cuffe MS, Califf RM, Adams KF, et al. Short-term intravenous milrinone for acute exacerbation of chronic heart failure: a randomized controlled trial. JAMA. 2002;287:1541–1547. Binanay C, Califf RM, Hasselblad V, et al. Evaluation study of congestive heart failure and pulmonary artery catheterization effectiveness: the ESCAPE trial. JAMA. 2005;294:1625–1633. McMurray JJ, Teerlink JR, Cotter G, et al. Effects of tezosentan on symptoms and clinical outcomes in patients with acute heart failure: the VERITAS randomized controlled trials. JAMA. 2007;298:2009–2019. Mebazaa A, Nieminen MS, Packer M, et al. Levosimendan vs dobutamine for patients with acute decompensated heart failure: the SURVIVE Randomized Trial. JAMA. 2007;297:1883–1891. Gheorghiade M, Konstam MA, Burnett JC, et al. Short-term clinical effects of tolvaptan, an oral vasopressin antagonist, in patients hospitalized for heart failure: the EVEREST Clinical Status TRIALS. JAMA. 2007;297:1332–1343. Konstam MA, Gheorghiade M, Burnett JC Jr, et al. Effects of oral tolvaptan in patients hospitalized for worsening heart failure: the EVEREST Outcome Trial. JAMA. 2007;297:1319–1331. Costanzo MR, Guglin ME, Saltzberg MT, et al. Ultrafiltration versus intravenous diuretics for patients hospitalized for acute decompensated heart failure. J Am Coll Cardiol. 2007;49:675–683. Gray A, Goodacre S, Newby DE, et al. Noninvasive ventilation in acute cardiogenic pulmonary edema. N Engl J Med. 2008;359:142–151. Giamouzis G, Butler J, Starling RC, et al. Impact of dopamine infusion on renal function in hospitalized heart failure patients: results of the Dopamine in Acute Decompensated Heart Failure (DAD-HF) Trial. J Card Fail. 2010;16:922–930. Massie BM, O'Connor CM, Metra M, et al. Rolofylline, an adenosine A1-receptor antagonist, in acute heart failure. N Engl J Med. 2010;363:1419–28. Felker GM, Lee KL, Bull DA, et al. Diuretic strategies in patients with acute decompensated heart failure. N Engl J Med. 2011;364:797–805. O'Connor CM, Starling RC, Hernandez AF, et al. Effect of nesiritide in patients with acute decompensated heart failure. N Engl J Med. 2011;365:32–43. Bart BA, Goldsmith SR, Lee KL, et al. Ultrafiltration in decompensated heart failure with cardiorenal syndrome. N Engl J Med. 2012;367:2296–2304. Teerlink JR, Cotter G, Davison BA, et al. Serelaxin, recombinant human relaxin-2, for treatment of acute heart failure (RELAX-AHF): a randomised, placebo-controlled trial. Lancet. 2013;381:29–39. Packer M, Colucci WS, Fisher L, et al. Effect of levosimendan on the short-term clinical course of patients with acutely decompensated heart failure. JACC Heart Fail. 2013;1:103–111. Chen HH, Anstrom KJ, Givertz MM, et al. Low-dose dopamine or low-dose nesiritide in acute heart failure with renal dysfunction: the ROSE acute heart failure randomized trial. JAMA. 2013;310:2533–2543. Triposkiadis FK, Butler J, Karayannis G, et al. Efficacy and safety of high dose versus low dose furosemide with or without dopamine infusion: the Dopamine in Acute Decompensated Heart Failure II (DAD-HF II) trial. Int J Cardiol. 2014;172:115–121. Costanzo MR, Negoianu D, Jaski BE, et al. Aquapheresis versus intravenous diuretics and hospitalizations for Heart Failure. JACC Heart Fail. 2016;4:95–105. Teerlink JR, Felker GM, McMurray JJ, et al. Acute treatment with omecamtiv mecarbil to increase contractility in acute heart failure: the ATOMIC-AHF Study. J Am Coll Cardiol. 2016;67:1444–1455. Felker GM, Mentz RJ, Cole R, et al. Efficacy and safety of tolvaptan in patients hospitalized with acute heart failure. J Am Coll Cardiol. 2016; (epub ahead of print).

a single drug would exert beneficial effects in all patients with AHF. There remain areas of significant unmet need in the treatment of AHF, including vasodilators with proven clinical benefits, agents that improve myocardial performance without significant adverse effects, and agents that improve or protect renal function. There are a number of interesting compounds that are undergoing development and/or clinical evaluation.

Vasodilating Agents

A variety of novel molecules with vasodilator properties are in development as therapeutics for AHF.[89]

Serelaxin

Relaxin was first identified as a major hormone of pregnancy with powerful systemic and renal vascular effects, as well as beneficial effects on cardiac preconditioning and ischemia, inflammation, fibrosis, and apoptosis. Serelaxin (recombinant human relaxin-2) demonstrated encouraging effects in a dose-finding pilot study of 234 patients with AHF.[122] The Phase III RELAX-AHF (Efficacy and Safety of Relaxin for the Treatment of Acute Heart Failure) trial enrolled 1161 patients within 16 hours of presentation who had dyspnea, congestion, mild-to-moderate renal insufficiency, and SBP greater than 125 mm Hg and randomized them to standard of care with a 48-hour infusion of either serelaxin (30 μg/kg/day) or placebo.[123] The trial demonstrated efficacy of serelaxin in improving dyspnea as quantified by the area under the curve of the change from baseline dyspnea visual analog scale over 5 days, which was associated with improvements in signs of congestion, decreased in-hospital WHF, shorter length of stay, and both cardiovascular and all-cause mortality at 180 days. There were no significant changes in the dyspnea score as assessed by the 7-level Likert scale over the first 24 hours nor any endpoint related to HF rehospitalizations. Serelaxin treatment was also associated with improved markers of end-organ damage or dysfunction, including cardiac, renal, and hepatic markers.[124] There were no serious adverse events of hypotension or other safety signals in the serelaxin-treated patients. Mechanistic studies have confirmed serelaxin's beneficial effects on hemodynamics[125] and renal function.[126] The RELAX-AHF-2 trial, enrolling over 6600 patients admitted for AHF, evaluated the effects of serelaxin compared to placebo on WHF through 5 days and 180-day cardiovascular mortality and showed no significant benefit (Fig. 49.11).[127]

Natriuretic Peptides

Multiple different natriuretic peptides continue to be developed and investigated for the treatment of AHF, including naturally occurring and alternatively spliced peptides and chimeric designer peptides. Urodilatin, a modified version of pro-ANP, is a 32-amino-acid hormone, synthesized and secreted from the distal tubules of the kidney that regulates renal sodium absorption and water homeostasis via binding to NPR1 receptors and increasing intracellular cGMP levels. Ularitide, a synthetically produced urodilatin, has demonstrated beneficial effects on hemodynamics and symptom relief in two studies of patients with AHF.[128] The TRUE-AHF trial (NCT01661634) enrolled 2157 patients with symptomatic AHF and randomized them to a 48-hour infusion of either ularitide (15 ng/kg/min) or placebo. Ularitide did not significantly improve either primary endpoint of the clinical composite endpoint through 5 days or cardiovascular mortality during the course of the study. Ularitide had no beneficial effect on any secondary endpoint without evidence of end-organ protection and increased creatinine associated with a doubling of hypotension (see Fig. 49.11).[129]

NEUROHORMONAL ANTAGONISTS

Direct renin inhibitors (DRIs) block the first enzymatic step in the RAAS cascade, leading to a profound suppression of this neurohormonal system (see Chapters 47 and 50). Given the role of RAAS in the pathogenesis and complications of HF, as well as the improved survival associated with its inhibition, further blockade of this system may confer additional survival benefits. *Aliskiren* is the first oral DRI on the market and currently approved for the treatment of hypertension. The ASTRONAUT trial enrolled 1639 hemodynamically stable patients a median 5 days after admission for AHF with EF less than 40%, elevated natriuretic peptides, and signs or symptoms of fluid overload who were randomized to daily oral aliskiren or placebo.[130] Aliskiren treatment was associated with higher rates of hyperkalemia, hypotension, and renal impairment/renal failure compared to placebo after a median follow-up of 11.3 months, but there was no difference in cardiovascular death or heart failure rehospitalization at 6 or 12 months. *Endothelin receptor antagonists* block the actions of ET-1, the most powerful endogenous vasoconstrictor that is produced by the vascular endothelial cells. It exerts its effects by binding to two receptors, ET_A and ET_B, located on the vascular smooth muscle cells, resulting in significant systemic arterial vasoconstriction. *Tezosentan*, a nonselective ET_{A-B} antagonist, has been shown to improve hemodynamics in patients with AHF. The Value of Endothelin Receptor Inhibition with Tezosentan in Acute Heart Failure Study (VERITAS) studied more than 1400 patients admitted with AHF in a large, international trial. The addition of IV tezosentan to standard therapy did not improve symptoms nor decrease WHF or mortality at 7 days after randomization.[131] Another approach to neurohormonal antagonism in AHF included the *angiotensin II type I receptor beta-arrestin-biased ligand, TRV027*, which increases signaling of the beta-arrestin mediated pathways stimulating inotropy while simultaneously antagonizing the classic G-protein angiotensin II signaling pathways. The BLAST-AHF study enrolled 621 patients admitted with AHF in a dose-ranging study of a 48 to 96 hour infusion of TRV027 compared to placebo.[132] TRV027 did not confer any benefit over placebo at any dose with regards to the primary composite endpoint or any of the individual components, although there were no significant safety issues.

SOLUBLE GUANYLATE CYCLASE ACTIVATORS AND STIMULATORS

Cinaciguat is the first compound in a new class of vasodilators. Their mechanism of action is similar to that of organic nitrates (and their end product NO) because both classes of drugs activate the sGC in smooth muscle cells, thus leading to the synthesis of cGMP and subsequent

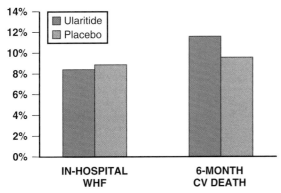

TRUE–HF

	Ularitide	Placebo
Age (years)	68	68
Male sex (%)	66%	66%
NT–proBNP (median, pg/mL)	7156	7121
SBP (mm Hg)	134	135

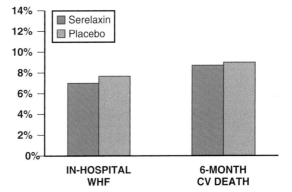

RELAX-AHF-2

	Serelaxin	Placebo
Age (years)	73	73
Male sex (%)	60%	59%
NT–proBNP (median, pg/mL)	6153	6035
SBP (mmHg)	146	146

FIGURE 49.11 Overview of study population and primary results from TRUE-HF (ularitide) and RELAX-AHF-2 (serelaxin) randomized clinical trials. (Adapted from Metra M, Teerlink JR, Cotter G, et al. Effects of serelaxin in patients with acute heart failure. *N Engl J Med.* 2019;381:716–726; Packer M, O'Connor C, McMurray JJV, et al. Effect of ularitide on cardiovascular mortality in acute heart failure. *N Engl J Med.* 2017;376:1956–1964.)

vasodilation. Cinaciguat has been shown to improve hemodynamics in patients with AHF; however, at high doses, it has been associated with significant hypotension, which resulted in the termination of early clinical studies.[133] *Vericiguat* is an oral sGC stimulator that has been studied in patients enrolled in studies within 4 weeks of a WHF event. In the SOCRATES-Reduced study of 456 patients, vericiguat did not significantly improve log transformed NT-proBNP concentrations compared to placebo, but there was a suggestion of a dose response.[134]

INOTROPIC AGENTS
Cardiac Myosin Activators
Cardiac myosin activators represent a new mechanistic class of agents designed to increase myocardial contractility. These agents increase the transition rate from the weakly bound to the strongly bound state necessary for initiation of a force-generating power stroke. Unlike current inotropes, they increase the systolic ejection time without altering the rate of LV pressure development, resulting in increased stroke volume and cardiac output without increases in intracellular cAMP or calcium. *Omecamtiv mecarbil* is the first agent of this class to undergo testing in man. In both healthy volunteers and patients with chronic stable HFrEF, administration of omecamtiv mecarbil produced dose-dependent increases in systolic ejection time, fractional shortening, stroke volume, and ejection fraction and was well-tolerated over a broad range of plasma concentrations.[135] In a phase IIb dose-finding study of 606 patients with AHF (ATOMIC-AHF; NCT01300013), intravenous omecamtiv mecarbil did not meet the primary endpoint of dyspnea improvement compared to the pooled placebo, but it was generally well-tolerated, increased systolic ejection time, and improved dyspnea in the high-dose group.[136]

Istaroxime
Istaroxime, the prototype of a new class of drugs, exerts its actions on the myocyte in two ways: (1) via stimulation of the membrane-bound Na-K/ATPase, and (2) by enhancing the activity of the sarcoendoplasmic reticulum Ca/ATPase type 2a (SERCA-2a). These distinct mechanisms, respectively, result in increased cytosolic calcium accumulation during systole, with positive inotropic effects, and in rapid sequestration of cytosolic calcium into the sarcoplasmic reticulum during diastole, leading to an enhanced lusitropic effect. The HORIZON-HF study evaluated 120 patients admitted with AHF and decreased EF. The addition of istaroxime to standard therapy lowered PCWP and HR and increased SBP. The higher infusion dose increased cardiac index and reduced LVED volume. There were no changes in neurohormones, renal function, or troponin I levels during the short 6-hour infusion.[137,138]

RENOPROTECTIVE AGENTS
Therapeutics to prevent or treat acute kidney injury and maintain or improve renal function in the setting of AHF are an important unmet need. *Adenosine A₁ receptor antagonists* have been developed to increase renal blood flow and enhance diuresis without activating the tubuloglomerular feedback. *Rolofylline* is a highly selective adenosine A₁ receptor antagonist that has been studied in patients with HF. Despite the positive trends seen in the PROTECT-Pilot study, the Phase III PROTECT trial failed to show any clinical benefit, including renal protection,[139] and was associated with more seizure and stroke events when compared to placebo. Given these results, it is doubtful that these agents will undergo further evaluation in AHF.

FUTURE PERSPECTIVES

AHF remains one of the most challenging cardiovascular problems with unacceptably high post-discharge rehospitalization and mortality rates. The development of new therapies has been a persistent challenge over recent decades and most patients are still treated primarily with intravenous loop diuretics. Current management consists primarily of treating the manifestations of the syndrome rather than central pathophysiologic derangements. Improvement in understanding of underlying pathophysiology and better targeting of treatments to specific patient groups most likely to benefit will potentially provide greater success in developing efficacious new therapies for AHF. Given the heterogeneity of the AHF population, it is unlikely that a "one-therapy-fits-all" approach will lead to an improvement in outcomes.

At the same time that new therapies are sought, continued efforts to improve and standardize the use of "best practices" in terms of process of care, transitions of care, and post-discharge follow-up will potentially allow us to better use currently available therapies to improve outcomes from this highly morbid condition.

REFERENCES
Epidemiology
1. Jackson SL, Tong X, King RJ, et al. National burden of heart failure events in the United States, 2006 to 2014. Circ Heart Fail. 2018;11:e004873.
2. Ponikowski P, Anker SD, AlHabib KF, et al. Heart failure: preventing disease and death worldwide. ESC Heart Failure. 2014;1:4–25.
3. Heidenreich PA, Albert NM, Allen LA, et al. Forecasting the impact of heart failure in the United States: a policy statement from the American Heart Association. Circ Heart Fail. 2013;6:606–619.
4. Voigt J, John MS, Taylor A, et al. A reevaluation of the costs of heart failure and its implications for allocation of health resources in the United States. Clin Cardiol. 2014;37:312–321.
5. Butler J, Gheorghiade M, Kelkar A, et al. In-hospital worsening heart failure. Eur J Heart Failure. 2015;17:1104–1113.
6. Okumura N, Jhund PS, Gong J, et al. Importance of clinical worsening of heart failure treated in the outpatient setting: evidence from the Prospective Comparison of ARNI with ACEI to Determine Impact on Global Mortality and Morbidity in Heart Failure trial (PARADIGM-HF). Circulation. 2016;133:2254–2262.
7. Filippatos G, Angermann CE, Cleland JGF, et al. Global differences in characteristics, precipitants, and initial management of patients presenting with acute heart failure. JAMA Cardiol. 2020;5:401–410.
8. Kapoor JR, Kapoor R, Ju C, et al. Precipitating clinical factors, heart failure characterization, and outcomes in patients hospitalized with heart failure with reduced, borderline, and preserved ejection fraction. JACC (J Am Coll Cardiol): Heart Fail. 2016;4:464–472.
9. Galvao M, Kalman J, Demarco T, et al. Gender differences in in-hospital management and outcomes in patients with decompensated heart failure: analysis from the acute decompensated heart failure national registry (ADHERE). J Card Fail. 2006;12:100–107.
10. Yancy CW, Abraham WT, Albert NM, et al. Quality of care of and outcomes for African Americans Hospitalized with heart failure: findings from the OPTIMIZE-HF (Organized Program to Initiate Lifesaving Treatment in Hospitalized Patients with Heart Failure) registry. J Am Coll Cardiol. 2008;51:1675–1684.
11. Adams Jr KF, Fonarow GC, Emerman CL, et al. Characteristics and outcomes of patients hospitalized for heart failure in the united States: rationale, design, and preliminary observations from the first 100,000 cases in the Acute Decompensated Heart Failure National Registry (ADHERE). Am Heart J. 2005;149:209–216.
12. Nieminen MS, Brutsaert D, Dickstein K, et al. EuroHeart Failure Survey II (EHFS II): a survey on hospitalized acute heart failure patients: description of population. Eur Heart J. 2006;27:2725–2736.
13. Metra M, Mentz RJ, Hernandez AF, et al. Geographic differences in patients in a global acute heart failure clinical trial (from the ASCEND-HF trial). Am J Cardiol. 2016;117:1771–1778.

Pathophysiology
14. Zile MR, Bennett TD, S. John Sutton M, et al. Transition from chronic compensated to acute decompensated heart failure: pathophysiological insights obtained from continuous monitoring of intracardiac pressures. Circulation. 2008;118:1433–1441.
15. Dries DL, Ky B, Wu AHB, et al. Simultaneous assessment of unprocessed ProBNP1-108 in addition to processed BNP32 improves identification of high-risk ambulatory patients with heart failure. Circ Heart Fail. 2010;3:220–227.
16. Solomon SD, Dobson J, Pocock S, et al. Influence of nonfatal hospitalization for heart failure on subsequent mortality in patients with chronic heart failure. Circulation. 2007;116:1482–1487.
17. Stevenson LW, Zile M, Bennett TD, et al. Chronic ambulatory intracardiac pressures and future heart failure events. Circ Heart Fail. 2010;3:580–587.
18. Gheorghiade M, Follath F, Ponikowski P, et al. Assessing and grading congestion in acute heart failure: a scientific statement from the acute heart failure committee of the heart failure association of the European Society of Cardiology and Endorsed by the European Society of Intensive Care Medicine. Eur J Heart Fail. 2010;12:423–433.
19. Januzzi JL, Filippatos G, Nieminen M, Gheorghiade M. Troponin elevation in patients with heart failure: on behalf of the third universal definition of myocardial infarction global Task force: heart failure section. Eur Heart J. 2012;33:2265–2271.
20. Kociol RD, Pang PS, Gheorghiade M, et al. Troponin elevation in heart failure prevalence, mechanisms, and clinical implications. J Am Coll Cardiol. 2010;56:1071–1078.
21. Felker GM, Mentz RJ, Teerlink JR, et al. Serial high sensitivity cardiac troponin T measurement in acute heart failure: insights from the RELAX-AHF study. Eur J Heart Fail. 2015;17:1262–1270.
22. Heywood JT, Fonarow GC, Costanzo MR, et al. High prevalence of renal dysfunction and its impact on outcome in 118,465 patients hospitalized with acute decompensated heart failure: a report from the ADHERE database. J Cardiac Fail. 2007;13:422–430.
23. Damman K, Testani JM. The kidney in heart failure: an update. Eur Heart J. 2015;36:1437–1444.
24. Ronco C, Cicoira M, McCullough PA. Cardiorenal syndrome type 1: pathophysiological crosstalk leading to combined heart and kidney dysfunction in the setting of acutely decompensated heart failure. J Am Coll Cardiol. 2012;60:1031–1042.
25. Mullens W, Abrahams Z, Francis GS, et al. Importance of venous congestion for worsening of renal function in advanced decompensated heart failure. J Am Coll Cardiol. 2009;53:589–596.
26. Metra M, Davison B, Bettari L, et al. Is worsening renal function an ominous prognostic sign in patients with acute heart failure? The role of congestion and its interaction with renal function. Circ Heart Fail. 2012;5:54–62.
27. Marti CN, Gheorghiade M, Kalogeropoulos AP, et al. Endothelial dysfunction, arterial stiffness, and heart failure. J Am Coll Cardiol. 2012;60:1455–1469.
28. Fallick C, Sobotka PA, Dunlap ME. Sympathetically mediated changes in capacitance. Circ Heart Fail. 2011;4:669–675.
29. Fudim M, Boortz-Marx RL, Ganesh A, et al. Splanchnic Nerve Block for Chronic Heart Failure. JACC Heart failure; 2020.
30. Milo-Cotter O, Cotter-Davison B, Lombardi C, et al. Neurohormonal activation in acute heart failure: results from VERITAS. Cardiology. 2011;119:96–105.
31. Bozkurt B, Mann DL, Deswal A. Biomarkers of inflammation in heart failure. Heart Failure Reviews. 2010;15:331–341.

Evaluation of the Acute Heart Failure Patient
32. Ponikowski P, Voors AA, Anker SD, et al. ESC Guidelines for the diagnosis and treatment of acute and chronic heart failure: the task force for the diagnosis and treatment of acute and chronic heart failure of the European Society of Cardiology (ESC) developed with the special contribution of the Heart Failure Association (HFA) of the ESC. Eur Heart J. 2016;37:2129–2200.
33. Greene SJ, Mentz RJ, Felker GM. Outpatient worsening heart failure as a target for therapy: a review. JAMA Cardiol. 2018;3:252–259.

34. Fonarow GC, Abraham WT, Albert NM, et al. Factors identified as precipitating hospital admissions for heart failure and clinical outcomes: findings from OPTIMIZE-HF. *Arch Intern Med.* 2008;168:847–854.
35. Pang PS, Cleland JG, Teerlink JR, et al. A proposal to standardize dyspnoea measurement in clinical trials of acute heart failure syndromes: the need for a uniform approach. *Eur Heart J.* 2008;29:816–824.
36. Thibodeau JT, Turer AT, Gualano SK, et al. Characterization of a novel symptom of advanced heart failure: bendopnea. *JACC Heart Fail.* 2014;2:24–31.
37. Nohria A, Tsang SW, Fang JC, et al. Clinical assessment identifies hemodynamic profiles that predict outcomes in patients admitted with heart failure. *J Am Coll Cardiol.* 2003;41:1797–1804.
38. Maisel AS, Krishnaswamy P, Nowak RM, et al. Rapid measurement of B-Type natriuretic peptide in the emergency diagnosis of heart failure. *N Engl J Med.* 2002;347:161–167.
39. Thygesen K, Alpert JS, Jaffe AS, et al. Fourth universal definition of myocardial infarction (2018). *J Am Coll Cardiol.* 2018;72:2231–2264.

Management of the Patient with Acute Heart Failure

40. Chow SL, Maisel AS, Anand I, et al. Role of biomarkers for the prevention, assessment, and management of heart failure: a scientific statement from the American Heart Association. *Circulation.* 2017;135:e1054–e1091.
41. Park JH, Balmain S, Berry C, et al. Potentially detrimental cardiovascular effects of oxygen in patients with chronic left ventricular systolic dysfunction. *Heart.* 2010;96:533–538.
42. Sepehrvand N, Ezekowitz JA. Oxygen therapy in patients with acute heart failure: friend or foe? *JACC Heart Fail.* 2016;4:783–790.
43. Vital FM, Saconato H, Ladeira MT, et al. Non-invasive positive pressure ventilation (CPAP or bilevel NPPV) for cardiogenic pulmonary edema. *Cochrane Database Syst Rev.* 2008:CD005351.
44. Gray A, Goodacre S, Newby DE, et al. Noninvasive ventilation in acute cardiogenic pulmonary edema. *N Engl J Med.* 2008;359:142–151.
45. ADHERE Scientific Advisory Committee. *Acute Decompensated Heart Failure National Registry (ADHERE®) Core Module Q1 2006 Final Cumulative National Benchmark Report.* Scios, Inc.; 2006.
46. Ellison DH, Felker GM. Diuretic treatment in heart failure. *N Engl J Med.* 2018;378:684–685.
47. Cotter G, Metzkor E, Kaluski E, et al. Randomised trial of high-dose isosorbide dinitrate plus low-dose furosemide versus high-dose furosemide plus low-dose isosorbide dinitrate in severe pulmonary oedema. *Lancet.* 1998;351:389–393.
48. Weintraub NL, Collins SP, Pang PS, et al. Acute heart failure syndromes: emergency department presentation, treatment, and disposition: current approaches and future aims: a scientific statement from the American Heart Association. *Circulation.* 2010;122:1975–1996.
49. Collins SP, Pang PS, Fonarow GC, et al. Is hospital admission for heart failure really necessary?: the role of the emergency department and observation unit in preventing hospitalization and rehospitalization. *J Am Coll Cardiol.* 2013;61:121–126.
50. Yancy CW, Jessup M, Bozkurt B, et al. 2013 ACCF/AHA guideline for the management of heart failure: a report of the American College of Cardiology Foundation/American Heart Association Task force on practice guidelines. *J Am Coll Cardiol.* 2013;62:e147–e239.
51. Green EM, Givertz MM. Management of acute right ventricular failure in the intensive care unit. *Curr Heart Fail Rep.* 2012;9:228–235.
52. Aliti G, Rabelo ER, Clausell N, et al. Aggressive fluid and sodium restriction in acute decompensated heart failure: a randomized clinical trial. *JAMA Intern Med.* 2013;173:1058–1064.
53. Prins KW, Neill JM, Tyler JO, et al. Effects of beta-blocker withdrawal in acute decompensated heart failure: a systematic review and meta-analysis. *JACC Heart Fail.* 2015;3:647–653.
54. Velazquez EJ, Morrow DA, DeVore AD, et al. Angiotensin-neprilysin inhibition in acute decompensated heart failure. *N Engl J Med.* 2019;380:539–548.
55. Testani JM, Chen J, McCauley BD, et al. Potential effects of aggressive decongestion during the treatment of decompensated heart failure on renal function and survival. *Circulation.* 2010;122:265–272.
56. Dupont M, Mullens W, Finucan M, et al. Determinants of dynamic changes in serum creatinine in acute decompensated heart failure: the importance of blood pressure reduction during treatment. *Eur J Heart Fail.* 2013;15:433–440.
57. Testani JM, Brisco MA, Turner JM, et al. Loop diuretic efficiency: a metric of diuretic responsiveness with prognostic importance in acute decompensated heart failure. *Circ Heart Fail.* 2014;7:261–270.
58. Felker GM, Ellison DH, Mullens W, et al. Diuretic therapy for patients with heart failure. JACC state-of-the-art review. *J Am Coll Cardiol.* 2020;75:1178–1195.
59. Bart BA, Goldsmith SR, Lee KL, et al. Ultrafiltration in decompensated heart failure with cardiorenal syndrome. *N Engl J Med.* 2012;367:2296–2304.
60. Davison BA, Metra M, Cotter G, et al. Worsening heart failure following admission for acute heart failure: a pooled analysis of the protect and RELAX-AHF studies. *JACC Heart Fail.* 2015;3:395–403.
61. Fonarow GC, Abraham WT, Albert NM, et al. Association between performance measures and clinical outcomes for patients hospitalized with heart failure. *J Am Med Assoc.* 2007;297:61–70.
62. Ambrosy AP, Pang PS, Khan S, et al. Clinical course and predictive value of congestion during hospitalization in patients admitted for worsening signs and symptoms of heart failure with reduced ejection fraction: findings from the EVEREST trial. *Eur Heart J.* 2013;34:835–843.
63. Kociol RD, Horton JR, Fonarow GC, et al. Admission, discharge, or change in B-type natriuretic peptide and long-term outcomes: data from Organized Program to Initiate Lifesaving Treatment in Hospitalized Patients with Heart Failure (OPTIMIZE-HF) linked to Medicare claims. *Circ Heart Fail.* 2011;4:628–636.
64. Yancy CW, Jessup M, Bozkurt B, et al. 2013 ACCF/AHA guideline for the management of heart failure: a report of the American College of cardiology foundation/American heart association Task force on practice guidelines. *J Am Coll Cardiol.* 2013;62:e147–e239.
65. Gheorghiade M, Vaduganathan M, Fonarow GC, et al. Rehospitalization for heart failure: problems and perspectives. *J Am Coll Cardiol.* 2013;61:391–403.
66. van Walraven C, Bennett C, Jennings A, et al. Proportion of hospital readmissions deemed avoidable: a systematic review. *CMAJ (Can Med Assoc J).* 2011;183:E391–E402.
67. Hansen LO, Young RS, Hinami K, et al. Interventions to reduce 30-day rehospitalization: a systematic review. *Ann Intern Med.* 2011;155:520–528.
68. Hernandez AF, Greiner MA, Fonarow GC, et al. Relationship between early physician follow-up and 30-day readmission among Medicare beneficiaries hospitalized for heart failure. *J Am Med Assoc.* 2010;303:1716–1722.
69. Alexander P, Alkhawam L, Curry J, et al. Lack of evidence for intravenous vasodilators in ED patients with acute heart failure: a systematic review. *Am J Emerg Med.* 2015;33:133–141.
70. Mebazaa A, Parissis J, Porcher R, et al. Short-term survival by treatment among patients hospitalized with acute heart failure: the global ALARM-HF registry using propensity scoring methods. *Intensive Care Med.* 2011;37:290–301.
71. Bikdeli B, Strait KM, Dharmarajan K, et al. Intravenous fluids in acute decompensated heart failure. *JACC Heart Fail.* 2015;3:127–133.
72. Blair JE, Khan S, Konstam MA, et al. Weight changes after hospitalization for worsening heart failure and subsequent re-hospitalization and mortality in the EVEREST trial. *Eur Heart J.* 2009;30:1666–1673.
73. Binanay C, Califf RM, Hasselblad V, et al. Evaluation study of congestive heart failure and pulmonary artery catheterization effectiveness: the ESCAPE trial. *J Am Med Assoc.* 2005;294:1625–1633.
74. Collins S, Storrow AB, Albert NM, et al. Early management of patients with acute heart failure: state of the art and future directions. A consensus document from the Society for Academic Emergency Medicine/Heart Failure Society of America Acute Heart Failure working group. *J Cardiac Fail.* 2015;21:27–43.
75. Miro O, Levy PD, Mockel M, et al. Disposition of emergency department patients diagnosed with acute heart failure: an international emergency medicine perspective. *Eur J Emerg Med.* 2017;24:2–12.
76. Bueno H, Ross JS, Wang Y, et al. Trends in length of stay and short-term outcomes among Medicare patients hospitalized for heart failure, 1993-2006. *J Am Med Assoc.* 2010;303:2141–2147.
77. Heidenreich PA, Sahay A, Kapoor JR, et al. Divergent trends in survival and readmission following a hospitalization for heart failure in the Veterans Affairs health care system 2002 to 2006. *J Am Coll Cardiol.* 2010;56:362–368.
78. O'Connor CM, Miller AB, Blair JE, et al. Causes of death and rehospitalization in patients hospitalized with worsening heart failure and reduced left ventricular ejection fraction: results from Efficacy of Vasopressin Antagonism in Heart Failure Outcome Study with Tolvaptan (EVEREST) program. *Am Heart J.* 2010;159:841–849.e1.
79. Allen LA, Tomic KES, Smith DM, et al. Rates and predictors of 30-day readmission among commercially insured and medicaid-enrolled patients hospitalized with systolic heart failure/clinical perspective. *Circ Heart Fail.* 2012;5:672–679.
80. Jencks SF, Williams MV, Coleman EA. Rehospitalizations among patients in the medicare fee-for-service program. *N Engl J Med.* 2009;360:1418–1428.
81. Bradley EH, Curry L, Horwitz LI, et al. Contemporary evidence about hospital strategies for reducing 30-day readmissions: a national study. *J Am Coll Cardiol.* 2012;60:607–614.
82. Bergethon KE, Ju C, DeVore AD, et al. Trends in 30-day readmission rates for patients hospitalized with heart failure: findings from the get with the guidelines-heart failure registry. *Circ Heart Fail.* 2016;9. https://doi.org/10.1161/CIRCHEARTFAILURE.115.002594.
83. Felker GM, Mentz RJ. Diuretics and ultrafiltration in acute decompensated heart failure. *J Am Coll Cardiol.* 2012;59:2145–2153.
84. de Denus S, Rouleau JL, Mann DL, et al. A pharmacogenetic investigation of intravenous furosemide in decompensated heart failure: a meta-analysis of three clinical trials. *Pharmacogenomics J.* 2017;17:192–200.
85. Mecklai A, Subacius H, Konstam MA, et al. In-hospital diuretic agent use and post-discharge clinical outcomes in patients hospitalized for worsening heart failure: insights from the EVEREST trial. *JACC Heart Fail.* 2016;4:580–588.
86. Felker GM, Lee KL, Bull DA, et al. Diuretic strategies in patients with acute decompensated heart failure. *N Engl J Med.* 2011;364:797–805.
87. Jentzer JC, DeWald TA, Hernandez AF. Combination of loop diuretics with thiazide-type diuretics in heart failure. *J Am Coll Cardiol.* 2010;56:1527–1534.
88. Bansal S, Lindenfeld J, Schrier RW. Sodium retention in heart failure and Cirrhosis. *Circ Heart Fail.* 2009;2:370–376.
89. Singh A, Laribi S, Teerlink JR, Mebazaa A. Agents with vasodilator properties in acute heart failure. *Eur Heart J.* 2017;8:317–325.
90. Ho EC, Parker JD, Austin PC, Tu JV, et al. Impact of nitrate use on survival in acute heart failure: a propensity-matched analysis. *J Am Heart Assoc.* 2016;5(2):e002531.
91. National Clinical Guideline Centre. *Acute Heart Failure: Diagnosing and Managing Acute Heart Failure in adults. NICE Clinical Guideline 187 Methods, Evidence and Recommendations.* National Institute for Health and Care Excellence; 2014.
92. Sharon A, Shpirer I, Kaluski E, et al. High-dose intravenous isosorbide-dinitrate is safer and better than Bi-PAP ventilation combined with conventional treatment for severe pulmonary edema. *J Am Coll Cardiol.* 2000;36:832–837.
93. Investigators VMAC. Intravenous nesiritide vs nitroglycerin for treatment of decompensated congestive heart failure: a randomized controlled trial. *J Am Med Assoc.* 2002;287:1531–1540.
94. Elkayam U, Akhter MW, Singh H, et al. Comparison of effects on left ventricular filling pressure of intravenous nesiritide and high-dose nitroglycerin in patients with decompensated heart failure. *Am J Cardiol.* 2004;93:237–240.
95. Mullens W, Abrahams Z, Francis GS, et al. Sodium nitroprusside for advanced low-output heart failure. *J Am Coll Cardiol.* 2008;52:200–207.
96. O'Connor CM, Starling RC, Hernandez AF, et al. Effect of nesiritide in patients with acute decompensated heart failure. *New Engl J Med.* 2011;365:32–43.
97. Chen HH, Anstrom KJ, Givertz MM, et al. Low-dose dopamine or low-dose nesiritide in acute heart failure with renal dysfunction: the ROSE acute heart failure randomized trial. *J Am Med Assoc.* 2013;310:2533–2543.
98. Hasenfuss G, Teerlink JR. Cardiac inotropes: current agents and future directions. *Eur Heart J.* 2011;32:1838–1845.
99. Felker GM, Benza RL, Chandler AB, et al. Heart failure etiology and response to milrinone in decompensated heart failure: results from the OPTIME-CHF study. *J Am Coll Cardiol.* 2003;41:997–1003.
100. Partovian C, Gleim SR, Mody PS, et al. Hospital patterns of use of positive inotropic agents in patients with heart failure. *J Am Coll Cardiol.* 2012;60:1402–1409.
101. Coletta AP, Cleland JG, Freemantle N, Clark AL. Clinical trials update from the European Society of Cardiology heart failure meeting: SHAPE, BRING-UP 2 VAS, COLA II, FOSIDIAL, BETACAR, CASINO and meta-analysis of cardiac resynchronisation therapy. *Eur J Heart Fail.* 2004;6:673–676.
102. Follath F, Cleland JG, Just H, et al. Efficacy and safety of intravenous levosimendan compared with dobutamine in severe low-output heart failure (the LIDO study): a randomised double-blind trial. *Lancet.* 2002;360:196–202.
103. Adamopoulos S, Parissis JT, Iliodromitis EK, et al. Effects of levosimendan versus dobutamine on inflammatory and apoptotic pathways in acutely decompensated chronic heart failure. *Am J Cardiol.* 2006;98:102–106.
104. Giamouzis G, Butler J, Starling RC, et al. Impact of dopamine infusion on renal function in hospitalized heart failure patients: results of the Dopamine in Acute Decompensated Heart Failure (DAD-HF) Trial. *J Cardiac Fail.* 2010;16:922–930.
105. Triposkiadis FK, Butler J, Karayannis G, et al. Efficacy and safety of high dose versus low dose furosemide with or without dopamine infusion: the Dopamine in Acute Decompensated Heart Failure II (DAD-HF II) trial. *Int J Cardiol.* 2014;172:115–121.
106. Cuffe MS, Califf RM, Adams Jr KF, et al. Short-term intravenous milrinone for acute exacerbation of chronic heart failure: a randomized controlled trial. *J Am Med Assoc.* 2002;287:1541–1547.
107. Orstavik O, Ata SH, Riise J, et al. Inhibition of phosphodiesterase-3 by levosimendan is sufficient to account for its inotropic effect in failing human heart. *Br J Pharmacol.* 2014;171:5169–5181.
108. Packer M, Colucci WS, Fisher L, et al. Effect of levosimendan on the short-term clinical course of patients with acutely decompensated heart failure. *JACC Heart Fail.* 2013;1:103–111.
109. Mebazaa A, Nieminen MS, Packer M, et al. Levosimendan vs dobutamine for patients with acute decompensated heart failure: the SURVIVE Randomized Trial. *J Am Med Assoc.* 2007;297:1883–1891.
110. De Backer D, Biston P, Devriendt J, et al. Comparison of dopamine and norepinephrine in the treatment of shock. *N Engl J Med.* 2010;362:779–789.
111. Gheorghiade M, Braunwald E. Reconsidering the role for digoxin in the management of acute heart failure syndromes. *J Am Med Assoc.* 2009;302:2146–2147.
112. Gheorghiade M, Konstam MA, Burnett Jr JC, et al. Short-term clinical effects of tolvaptan, an oral vasopressin antagonist, in patients hospitalized for heart failure: the EVEREST Clinical Status Trials. *J Am Med Assoc.* 2007;297:1332–1343.

113. Konstam MA, Gheorghiade M, Burnett Jr JC, et al. Effects of oral tolvaptan in patients hospitalized for worsening heart failure: the EVEREST Outcome Trial. *J Am Med Assoc.* 2007;297:1319–1331.

114. Felker GM, Mentz RJ, Cole R, et al. Efficacy and safety of tolvaptan in patients hospitalized with acute heart failure. *J Am Coll Cardiol.* 2016;69(11):1399–1406.

115. Goldsmith SR, Elkayam U, Haught WH, et al. Efficacy and safety of the vasopressin V1A/V2-receptor antagonist conivaptan in acute decompensated heart failure: a dose-ranging pilot study. *J Cardiac Fail.* 2008;14:641–647.

116. Peacock WF, Chandra A, Char D, et al. Clevidipine in acute heart failure: results of the a study of blood pressure control in acute heart failure-A pilot study (PRONTO). *Am Heart J.* 2014;167:529–536.

117. Costanzo MR, Guglin ME, Saltzberg MT, et al. Ultrafiltration versus intravenous diuretics for patients hospitalized for acute decompensated heart failure. *J Am Coll Cardiol.* 2007;49:675–683.

118. Patarroyo M, Wehbe E, Hanna M, et al. Cardiorenal outcomes after slow continuous ultrafiltration therapy in refractory patients with advanced decompensated heart failure. *J Am Coll Cardiol.* 2012;60:1906–1912.

119. Costanzo MR, Negoianu D, Jaski BE, et al. Aquapheresis versus intravenous diuretics and hospitalizations for heart failure. *JACC Heart failure.* 2016;4:95–105.

120. Paterna S, Fasullo S, Parrinello G, et al. Short-term effects of hypertonic saline solution in acute heart failure and long-term effects of a moderate sodium restriction in patients with compensated heart failure with New York Heart Association Class III (Class C) (SMAC-HF Study). *Am J Med Sci.* 2011;342:27–37.

121. Felker GM, Pang PS, Adams KF, et al. Clinical trials of pharmacological therapies in acute heart failure syndromes: lessons learned and directions forward. *Circ Heart Fail.* 2010;3:314–325.

122. Teerlink JR, Metra M, Felker GM, et al. Relaxin for the treatment of patients with acute heart failure (Pre-RELAX-AHF): a multicentre, randomised, placebo-controlled, parallel-group, dose-finding phase IIb study. *Lancet.* 2009;373:1429–1439.

123. Teerlink JR, Cotter G, Davison BA, et al. Serelaxin, recombinant human relaxin-2, for treatment of acute heart failure (RELAX-AHF): a randomised, placebo-controlled trial. *Lancet.* 2013;381:29–39.

124. Metra M, Cotter G, Davison BA, et al. Effect of serelaxin on cardiac, renal, and hepatic biomarkers in the Relaxin in Acute Heart Failure (RELAX-AHF) development program: correlation with outcomes. *J Am Coll Cardiol.* 2013;61:196–206.

125. Ponikowski P, Mitrovic V, Ruda M, et al. A randomized, double-blind, placebo-controlled, multicentre study to assess haemodynamic effects of serelaxin in patients with acute heart failure. *Eur Heart J.* 2014;35:431–441.

126. Voors AA, Dahlke M, Meyer S, et al. Renal hemodynamic effects of serelaxin in patients with chronic heart failure: a randomized, placebo-controlled study. *Circ Heart Fail.* 2014;7:994–1002.

127. Metra M, Teerlink JR, Cotter G, et al. Effects of serelaxin in patients with acute heart failure. *N Engl J Med.* 2019;381:716–726.

128. Anker SD, Ponikowski P, Mitrovic V, et al. Ularitide for the treatment of acute decompensated heart failure: from preclinical to clinical studies. *Eur Heart J.* 2015;36:715–723.

129. Packer M, O'Connor C, McMurray JJV, et al. Effect of ularitide on cardiovascular mortality in acute heart failure. *N Engl J Med.* 2017;376:1956–1964.

130. Gheorghiade M, Bohm M, Greene SJ, et al. Effect of aliskiren on postdischarge mortality and heart failure readmissions among patients hospitalized for heart failure: the ASTRONAUT randomized trial. *J Am Med Assoc.* 2013;309:1125–1135.

131. McMurray JJ, Teerlink JR, Cotter G, et al. Effects of tezosentan on symptoms and clinical outcomes in patients with acute heart failure: the VERITAS randomized controlled trials. *J Am Med Assoc.* 2007;298:2009–2019.

132. Felker GM, Butler J, Collins SP, et al. Heart failure therapeutics on the basis of a biased ligand of the angiotensin-2 type 1 receptor: rationale and design of the BLAST-AHF study (Biased Ligand of the Angiotensin Receptor Study in Acute Heart Failure). *JACC Heart Fail.* 2015;3:193–201.

133. Erdmann E, Semigran MJ, Nieminen MS, et al. Cinaciguat, a soluble guanylate cyclase activator, unloads the heart but also causes hypotension in acute decompensated heart failure. *Eur Heart J.* 2013;34:57–67.

134. Gheorghiade M, Greene SJ, Butler J, et al. Effect of vericiguat, a soluble guanylate cyclase stimulator, on natriuretic peptide levels in patients with worsening chronic heart failure and reduced ejection fraction: the SOCRATES-REDUCED randomized trial. *J Am Med Assoc.* 2015;314:2251–2262.

135. Liu LC, Dorhout B, van der Meer P, et al. Omecamtiv mecarbil: a new cardiac myosin activator for the treatment of heart failure. *Expert Opin Investig Drugs.* 2016;25:117–127.

136. Teerlink JR, Felker GM, McMurray JJ, et al. Acute treatment with omecamtiv mecarbil to increase contractility in acute heart failure: the ATOMIC-AHF study. *J Am Coll Cardiol.* 2016;67:1444–1455.

137. Gheorghiade M, Blair JE, Filippatos GS, et al. Hemodynamic, echocardiographic, and neurohormonal effects of istaroxime, a novel intravenous inotropic and lusitropic agent: a randomized controlled trial in patients hospitalized with heart failure. *J Am Coll Cardiol.* 2008;51:2276–2285.

138. Shah SJ, Blair JE, Filippatos GS, et al. Effects of istaroxime on diastolic stiffness in acute heart failure syndromes: results from the hemodynamic, echocardiographic, and neurohormonal effects of istaroxime, a novel intravenous inotropic and lusitropic agent: a randomized controlled trial in patients hospitalized with heart failure (HORIZON-HF) trial. *Am Heart J.* 2009;157:1035–1041.

139. Massie BM, O'Connor CM, Metra M, et al. Rolofylline, an adenosine A1-receptor antagonist, in acute heart failure. *N Engl J Med.* 2010;363:1419–1428.

140. Fonarow GC, Adams Jr KF, Abraham WT, et al. Risk stratification for in-hospital mortality in acutely decompensated heart failure: classification and regression tree analysis. *J Am Med Assoc.* 2005;293:572–580.

141. Abraham WT, Fonarow GC, Albert NM, et al. Predictors of in-hospital mortality in patients hospitalized for heart failure: insights from the Organized Program to Initiate Lifesaving Treatment in Hospitalized Patients with Heart Failure (OPTIMIZE-HF). *J Am Coll Cardiol.* 2008;52:347–356.

142. O'Connor CM, Abraham WT, Albert NM, et al. Predictors of mortality after discharge in patients hospitalized with heart failure: an analysis from the Organized Program to Initiate Lifesaving Treatment in Hospitalized Patients with Heart Failure (OPTIMIZE-HF). *Am Heart J.* 2008;156:662–673.

143. O'Connor CM, Mentz RJ, Cotter G, et al. The PROTECT in-hospital risk model: 7-day outcome in patients hospitalized with acute heart failure and renal dysfunction. *Eur J Heart Fail.* 2012;14:605–612.

144. Lee DS, Stitt A, Austin PC, et al. Prediction of heart failure mortality in emergent care: a cohort study. *Ann Intern Med.* 2012;156:767–775. W-261,W-2.

145. Felker GM, Leimberger JD, Califf RM, et al. Risk stratification after hospitalization for decompensated heart failure. *J Cardiac Fail.* 2004;10:460–466.

146. O'Connor CM, Hasselblad V, Mehta RH, et al. Triage after hospitalization with advanced heart failure: the ESCAPE (Evaluation Study of Congestive Heart Failure and Pulmonary Artery Catheterization Effectiveness) risk model and discharge score. *J Am Coll Cardiol.* 2010;55:872–878.

50 Management of Heart Failure Patients with Reduced Ejection Fraction

DOUGLAS L. MANN

The epidemiology and clinical assessment of patients with heart failure (HF) is reviewed in Chapter 48, whereas the following chapter will focus on the management of patients with a reduced ejection fraction, which is referred to as *HFrEF*. The diagnosis and management of patients with acute HF is discussed in Chapter 49, and the management of patients with an HF with a preserved ejection fraction (HFpEF) is discussed in Chapter 51.

ETIOLOGY

As shown in Table 50.1, any condition that leads to an alteration in left ventricular (LV) structure or function can predispose a patient to developing HF. Although the etiology of HF in patients with HFrEF differs from that of patient with HFpEF (see Chapter 48), there is considerable overlap between the etiologies of these two conditions. In industrialized countries, coronary artery disease (CAD) is the predominant cause in etiology in men and women and is responsible for 60% to 75% of cases of HF. Hypertension contributes to the development of HF in a significant number of patients, including most patients with CAD. Both CAD and hypertension interact to augment the risk of HF. Rheumatic heart disease remains a major cause of HF in Africa and Asia, especially in the young. Hypertension is an important cause of HF in the African and African American population. Chagas disease is still a major cause of HF in South America.[1] As developing nations undergo socioeconomic development, the epidemiology of HF is becoming similar to that of Western Europe and North America, with CAD emerging as the single most common cause of HF.

In 20% to 30% of the cases of HFrEF, the exact etiologic basis is not known. These patients are referred to as having dilated or *idiopathic* cardiomyopathy if the cause is unknown (see Chapter 52). Prior viral infection (Chapter 55) or toxin exposure (e.g., alcohol [Chapter 84] or use of chemotherapeutic agents [Chapters 56 and 57]) may also lead to a dilated cardiomyopathy. Although excessive alcohol consumption can promote cardiomyopathy, alcohol consumption per se is not associated with increased risk for HF, and alcohol may protect against the development of HF when consumed in moderation.[2] It is also becoming increasingly clear that a large number of the cases of dilated cardiomyopathy are secondary to specific genetic defects, most notably those in the cytoskeleton (see Chapter 52). Most of the forms of familial dilated cardiomyopathy are inherited in an autosomal dominant fashion. Mutations of genes encoding cytoskeletal proteins (desmin, cardiac myosin, vinculin) and nuclear membrane proteins (lamin) have been identified thus far. Dilated cardiomyopathy is also associated with Duchenne, Becker, and limb girdle muscular dystrophies (see Chapter 100). Conditions that lead to a high cardiac output (e.g., arteriovenous fistula, anemia) are seldom responsible for the development of HF in a normal heart. However, in the presence of underlying structural heart disease, these conditions often lead to overt congestive failure.

PROGNOSIS

Although several recent reports have suggested that the mortality for HF patients is improving, the overall mortality rate remains higher than for many cancers, including those involving the bladder, breast, uterus, and prostate. In the Framingham Study, the median survival was 1.7 years for men and 3.2 years for women, with only 25% of men and 38% of women surviving 5 years. European studies have confirmed a similar poor long-term prognosis (Fig. 50.1).[3] More recent data from the Framingham Study have examined long-term trends in the survival of patients with HF and shown improved survival in both men and

TABLE 50.1 Risk Factors for Cardiac Failure (Olmstead County)

RISK FACTOR	ODDS RATIO (95% CI)	P VALUE	POPULATION ATTRIBUTABLE RISK (96 = 5% CI)		
			OVERALL	WOMEN	MEN
Coronary heart disease	3.05 (2.36–3.95)	<.001	0.20 (0.16–0.24)	0.16 (0.12–0.20)	0.23 (0.16–0.30)
Hypertension	1.44 (1.18–1.76)	<.001	0.20 (0.10–0.30)	0.28 (0.14–0.42)	0.13 (0.00–0.26)
Diabetes	2.65 (1.98–3.54)	<.001	0.12 (0.09–0.15)	0.10 (0.06–0.14)	0.13 (0.08–0.18)
Obesity	2.00 (1.57–2.55)	<.001	0.12 (0.08–0.16)	0.12 (0.07–0.17)	0.13 (0.07–0.19)
Ever smoker	1.37 (1.13–1.68)	.002	0.14 (0.06–0.22)	0.08 (0.00–0.15)	0.22 (0.07–0.37)

From Dunlay SM, Weston SA, Jacobsen SJ, et al. Risk factors for heart failure: a population-based case-control study. *Am J Med.* 2009;122:1023–1028.

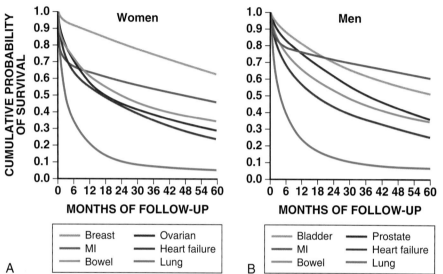

FIGURE 50.1 Survival in heart failure patients compared to cancer. Five-year survival following a first admission to any Scottish hospital in 1991 for heart failure, myocardial infarction, and the four most common sites of cancer specific to women (**A**) and men (**B**). (Modified from Stewart S, MacIntyre K, Hole DJ, et al. More "malignant" than cancer? Five-year survival following a first admission for heart failure. *Eur J Heart Fail.* 2001;3:315–322.)

women, with an overall decline in mortality of approximately 12% per decade from 1950 to 1999. Moreover, recent reports from Scotland, Sweden, and the United Kingdom also suggested that survival rates may be improving following hospital discharge.[3] Of note, the mortality of HF in epidemiologic studies is substantially higher than that reported in clinical HF trials involving drug and/or device therapies, in which the mortality figures are often deceptively low because the patients enrolled in trials are younger, are more stable clinically, and tend to be followed more closely clinically.

The role of gender and HF prognosis remains a controversial issue with respect to HF outcomes. Nonetheless, the aggregate data suggest that women with HF have a better overall prognosis than do men.[4] However, women appear to have a greater degree of functional incapacity for the same degree of LV dysfunction and also have higher prevalence of HF with a normal EF (see Chapter 51). Controversy has also arisen regarding the impact of race on outcome, with higher mortality rates being reported in blacks in some but not all studies. In the United States HF affects approximately 3% of blacks, whereas in the general population, the prevalence is about 2%.[5] Blacks with HF present at an earlier age and have more advanced LV dysfunction and a worse New York Heart Association (NYHA) class at the time of diagnosis. Although the reasons for these differences are not known, as noted above, differences in HF etiology might explain some of these observations. There may also be additional socioeconomic factors that may influence outcomes in black patients, such as geographic location and access to health care. Age is one of the stronger and most consistent predictors of adverse outcome in HF (see Special Populations below).[6]

Many other factors have been associated with increased mortality in HF patients (Table 50.2). Most of the factors listed as outcome predictors have survived, at least, univariate analysis, with many standing out independently when multifactorial analysis techniques are employed. Nonetheless, it is extraordinarily difficult to determine which prognostic variable is most important to predicting individual patient outcome in either clinical trials or, more importantly, during the day-to-day management of an individual patient. To this end several multivariate models for predicting the HF prognosis have been developed and validated. The Seattle Heart Failure Model was derived by retrospectively investigating predictors of survival among HF patients in clinical trials. The Seattle Heart Failure Model provides an accurate estimate of 1-, 2-, and 3-year survival with the use of easily obtained clinical, pharmacologic, device, and laboratory characteristics, and is accessible free of charge to all health care providers as an interactive web-based program (http://depts.washington.edu/shfm).

Biomarkers and Prognosis (see also Chapter 48)

The observation that the renin angiotensin-aldosterone, adrenergic, and inflammatory systems are activated in HF (see Chapter 47) has prompted the examination of the relationships between a variety of biochemical measurements and clinical outcomes (Table 50.3). Strong inverse correlations have been reported between survival and plasma levels of norepinephrine, renin, arginine vasopressin (AVP), aldosterone, atrial and brain natriuretic peptides (BNP and NT-proBNP), endothelin-1, and inflammatory markers such as tumor necrosis factor (TNF), soluble TNF receptors, C reactive protein, galactin-3, pentraxin-3, and soluble ST2. The GUIDE-IT trial (Guiding Evidence Based Therapy Using Biomarker Intensified Treatment in Heart Failure) was designed to prospectively study the relationship between change in natriuretic peptide concentration, cardiac remodeling, and clinical events in HFrEF patients. Although GUIDE-IT was stopped prematurely because biomarker-guided treatment was not more effective than usual care in improving outcomes, the Echocardiographic Substudy showed that lowering NT-proBNP to less than 1000 pg/mL by 12 months was associated with reverse LV remodeling and improved outcomes, regardless of the treatment strategy employed. These findings suggest the response to treatment as assessed by change in NT-proBNP is more important than the treatment strategy. Markers of oxidative stress, such as oxidized low-density lipoprotein and serum uric acid, have also been associated with worsening clinical status and impaired survival in patients with chronic HF. Cardiac troponin T and I, sensitive

TABLE 50.2 Etiology of Chronic Heart Failure

Myocardial Disease

Coronary artery disease
  Myocardial infarction*
  Myocardial ischemia*

Chronic pressure overload
  Hypertension*
  Obstructive valvular disease*

Chronic volume overload
  Regurgitant valvular disease
  Intracardiac (left-to-right) shunting
  Extracardiac shunting

Nonischemic dilated cardiomyopathy
  Familial/genetic disorders
  Infiltrative disorders*
  Toxic/drug-induced damage
  Metabolic disorder*
  Viral or other infectious agents

Disorders of Rate and Rhythm

Chronic bradyarrhythmias

Chronic tachyarrhythmias

Pulmonary Heart Disease

Cor pulmonale

Pulmonary vascular disorders

High-output states

Metabolic Disorders

Thyrotoxicosis

Nutritional disorders (beriberi)

Excessive Blood Flow Requirements

Systemic arteriovenous shunting

Chronic anemia

*Indicates conditions that can also lead to heart failure with a preserved ejection fraction.

TABLE 50.3 Prognostic Variable in Heart Failure Patients

Demographics	**Exercise Testing**
Gender	Metabolic assessment
Race	BP response
Age	Heart rate response
Heart Failure Etiology	6-min walk
CAD	Peak V_{O_2}
IDCM	Anaerobic threshold
Valvular heart disease	VE/V_{CO_2}
Myocarditis	Oxygen uptake slope
Hypertrophy	**Metabolic**
Alcohol	Serum sodium
Anthracyclines	Thyroid dysfunction
Amyloidosis	Anemia
Hemachromatosis	Acidosis/alkalosis
Genetic factors	**Chest X-ray**
Comorbidities	Congestion
Diabetes	Cardiothoracic ratio
Systemic hypertension	**ECG**
Pulmonary hypertension	Rhythm (atrial fibrillation or arrhythmias)
Sleep apnea	
Obesity/cachexia (body mass)	Voltage
Renal insufficiency	QRS width
Hepatic abnormalities	QT interval
COPD	Signal-average EKG (T-wave alternans)
Clinical Assessment	
NYHA class (symptoms)	HR variability
Syncope	**Biomarkers**
Angina pectoris	NE, PRA, AVP, aldosterone
Systolic versus diastolic dysfunction	ANP, BNP, NT-proBNP, endothelin
Hemodynamics	TNF, sTNFR 1,2, galectin-3, pentraxin-3, sST2
LVEF	Cardiac troponins, hematocrit
RVEF	**Endomyocardial Biopsy**
PAP	Inflammatory states
PCWP	Degree of fibrosis
CI	Degree of cellular disarray
PAP-PCWP	Infiltrative processes
Exercise hemodynamics	

BNP, brain natriuretic peptides; *BP*, blood pressure; *CAD*, coronary artery disease; *CI*, cardiac index; *COPD*, chronic obstructive pulmonary disease; *CRP*, C-reactive protein; *ESR*, erythrocyte sedimentation rate; *HR*, hazard ratio; *IDCM*, idiopathic dilated cardiomyopathy; *IL*, interleukin; *LVEF*, left ventricular ejection fraction; *NE*, norepinephrine; *NYHA*, New York Heart Association; *PAP*, pulmonary artery pressure; *PAP-PCWP*, gradient across lung; *PCWP*, pulmonary capillary wedge pressure; *PRA*, plasma renin activity; *RVEF*, right ventricular ejection fraction; *sST2*, soluble suppression of tumorigenesis-2; *TNF*, tumor necrosis factor; *V_{CO_2}*, volume of exhaled carbon dioxide; *VE*, ventilation.

Modified from Young JB. The prognosis of heart failure. In: Mann DL, eds. *Heart Failure: A Companion to Braunwald's Heart Disease.* Philadelphia: Elsevier; 2004:489–506.

markers of myocyte damage, may be elevated in patients with non-ischemic HF and predict adverse cardiac outcomes, as well as the development of incident HF.[7] The association between a low hemoglobin/hematocrit and adverse HF outcomes has also long been recognized, and has garnered considerable recent attention after several reports illustrated the independent prognostic value of anemia in patients with HF with either reduced or normal ejection fraction.[8]

Published estimates of the prevalence of anemia (defined as a hemoglobin concentration of <13 g/dL in men and <12 g/dL in women) in HF patients vary widely, ranging from 4% to 50% depending on the population studied and definition of anemia that is used. In general, anemia is associated with more HF symptoms, worse NYHA functional status, greater risk of HF hospitalization, and reduced survival.[9] However, it is unclear whether anemia is a cause of decreased survival, or simply a marker of more advanced disease. The underlying cause for anemia is likely multifactorial, including reduced sensitivity to erythropoietin receptors, the presence of a hematopoiesis inhibitor, and/or a defective iron supply for erythropoiesis given as possible explanations.

A standard diagnostic workup should be undertaken in anemic HF patients, recognizing that no definite etiology is identified in many of these patients. Correctable causes of anemia should be treated according to practice guidelines. The role for blood transfusions in patients with cardiovascular disease is controversial. Although a "transfusion threshold" for maintaining the hematocrit greater than 30% in patients with cardiovascular disease has been generally been accepted, this clinical practice has been based more on expert opinion rather than on direct evidence that documents the efficacy of this form of therapy. Given the risks and costs of red blood cell transfusion, the evanescent benefits of blood transfusions in patients with chronic anemia, coupled with the unclear benefit in HF patients, the routine use of blood transfusion cannot be recommended for treating the anemia that occurs in stable HF patients. Treatment of anemic HF patients with mild to moderate anemia (hemoglobin level 9.0 to 12.0 g/dL) with the erythropoietin analog darbepoetin alpha was evaluated in the RED-HF (Reduction of Events With Darbepoetin Alfa in Heart Failure) trial. As shown in **eFigure 50.1** there was no significant difference in the primary outcome variable of death from any cause or hospitalization for worsening HF (hazard ratio [HR] in the darbepoetin alfa group, 1.01; 95% confidence interval [CI] 0.90–1.13; P = 0.87), nor the secondary outcome (see eFig. 50.1B) of cardiovascular death or time to first hospitalization for worsening HF (HR in the darbepoetin alfa group 10.01, 95% CI 0.89 to 1.14; P = 0.2). The lack of effect of darbepoetin alfa was consistent across all prespecified subgroups. Importantly, treatment with darbepoetin alfa led to an early (within 1 month) and sustained increase in the hemoglobin level throughout the study.

Iron deficiency is a common comorbidity in patients with HFrEF, and has been associated with increased mortality and a poorer quality of life, regardless of whether there is concomitant anemia.[10] The definition of iron deficiency in HF differs from other conditions of chronic inflammation and is defined as: ferritin less than 100 μg/L or ferritin of 100 to 299 μg/L with a transferrin saturation less than 20%. Correction of iron deficiency in anemic and nonanemic patients with HFrEF (EF <30% to 45%) has been studied in several clinical trials.[11] Two of the three randomized trials conducted thus far have used intravenous ferric carboxymaltose (FCM). Studies with FCM have demonstrated an improvement in symptoms, exercise capacity, and health-related quality of life; however, the effects on major clinical events remain uncertain.[9] The one randomized clinical trial that used an oral iron polysaccharide (Oral Iron Repletion Effects On Oxygen Uptake in Heart Failure [IRONOUT]; NCT02188784), did not show an improvement in peak Vo_2 by cardiopulmonary exercise testing at 16 weeks. Based on the results of the randomized trials with intravenous iron supplementation, the current ACC/AHA/HFSA guidelines recommend (class IIb, LOE B-R) that intravenous iron replacement might be reasonable in patients with NYHA class II and III HF and iron deficiency (ferritin <100 ng/mL or 100 to 300 ng/mL if transferrin saturation is <20%) to improve functional status and quality of life.[12] Although the US guidelines do not recommend any specific formulation, the European guidelines recommend treatment with IV FCM in symptomatic HF patients with iron deficiency to improve HF symptoms and quality of life (class IIa, Level of Evidence A recommendation).[9]

Renal Insufficiency (see also Chapter 101)

Renal insufficiency is associated with poorer outcomes in patients with HF; however, there remains some uncertainty whether renal impairment is a simply a marker for worsening HF or whether renal impairment might be causally linked to worsening HF. Though more common in patients hospitalized for HF, at least some degree of renal impairment is still present in about half of stable HF outpatients. Patients with renal hypoperfusion or intrinsic renal disease show an impaired response to diuretics and angiotensin-converting enzymes inhibitors (ACEIs) and are at increased risk of adverse effects during treatment with digitalis. In a recent meta-analysis the majority of HF patients had some degree of renal impairment. These patients represented a high-risk group with an approximately 50% increased relative mortality risk when compared with patients who had normal renal function.[13] Similar findings were observed in the Acute Decompensated Heart Failure National Registry (ADHERE) (see Chapter 49). In the Second Prospective Randomized Study of Ibopamine on Mortality and Efficacy, impaired renal function was a stronger predictor of mortality than impaired LV function and NYHA class in patients with advanced HF (Fig. 50.2). Thus, renal insufficiency is a strong, independent predictor of adverse outcomes in HF patients. As will be discussed, below, treatment with sodium-glucose transporter-2 (SGLT2) inhibitors stabilizes renal function in patients with HFrEF.[14]

APPROACH TO THE PATIENT

HFrEF should be viewed as continuum that is comprised of four interrelated stages (see Fig. 50.3).[15] Stage A includes patients who are at high risk for developing HF, but without structural heart disease or symptoms of HF (e.g., patients with diabetes or hypertension). Stage B includes patients who have structural heart disease but without symptoms of HF (e.g., patients with a previous myocardial infarction [MI] and asymptomatic LV dysfunction). Stage C includes patients who have structural heart disease who have developed symptoms of HF (e.g., patients with a previous MI with shortness of breath and fatigue). Stage D includes patients who refractory HF requiring special interventions (e.g., patients with refractory HF

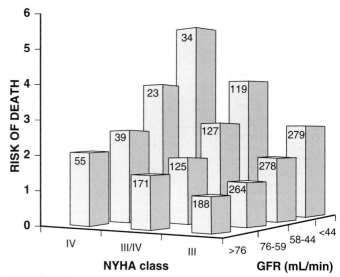

FIGURE 50.2 Effect of renal function on outcomes in heart failure patients. Three-dimensional bar graph showing risk of mortality (vertical axis) in relation to decreasing New York Heart Association (NYHA) class (horizontal axis) and decreasing quartiles of glomerular filtration rate (GFRc; diagonal axis). (From Hillege HL, Girbes AR, de Kam PJ, et al. Renal function, neurohormonal activation, and survival in patients with chronic heart failure. *Circulation.* 2000;102:203–210.)

who are awaiting cardiac transplantation). The clinical assessment of patients with HFrEF is discussed in detail in Chapter 48, and the diagnosis and management of patients with HFpEF is discussed in detail in Chapter 51.

Patients at High Risk for Developing Heart Failure (Stage A)

For patients at high risk of developing HFrEF, every effort should be made to prevent HF, using standard practice guidelines to treat preventable conditions that are known to lead to HF, including hypertension (see Chapter 26), hyperlipidemia (see Chapter 27), and diabetes (see Chapter 31). In this regard, ACEIs are particularly useful in preventing HF in patients who have a history of atherosclerotic vascular disease, diabetes mellitus, or hypertension with associated cardiovascular risk factors.

POPULATION SCREENING

At present there is limited information available to support the screening of broad populations to detect undiagnosed HF and/or asymptomatic LV dysfunction. Although initial studies suggested that determination of BNP or NT-proBNP levels (see also Chapter 48) might be useful for screening, the positive predictive value for these tests in a low-prevalence and asymptomatic population for the purpose of detecting cardiac dysfunction varies among studies, and the possibility of false-positive results has significant cost-effectiveness implications.

Patients who are at very high risk of developing cardiomyopathy (e.g., those with a strong family history of cardiomyopathy or those receiving cardiotoxic interventions [see Chapters 56 and 57]) are appropriate targets for more aggressive screening such as 2-D echocardiography to assess LV function. St Vincent's Screening To Prevent Heart Failure (STOP-HF) showed that, in patients with known cardiovascular risk factors, screening with BNP testing followed by collaborative care between internists and cardiovascular specialists resulted in a significant reduction in LV dysfunction (odds ratio [OR], 0.55; 95% CI, 0.37 to 0.82; P = 0.003). Although there was no significant reduction in clinical HF events, there was a significant decrease in the incidence rates of emergency hospitalization for major cardiovascular events.[16] However, the routine periodic assessment of LV function in low-risk patients is not currently recommended. Several sophisticated clinical scoring systems have been developed to screen for HF in population-based studies, including the Framingham Criteria, which screens for HF on the basis of clinical criteria, and the National Health and Nutrition Survey (NHANES) which uses self-reporting of symptoms to identify HF patients (Table 50.4). However, as discussed in Chapter 48, additional laboratory testing is usually necessary to definitively make the diagnosis of HF when these methodologies are used.

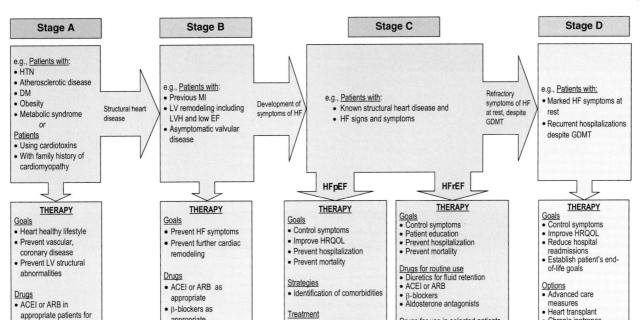

FIGURE 50.3 Stages in the development of heart failure and recommended therapy by stage. *ACEI,* Angiotensin-converting enzyme inhibitor; *AF,* atrial fibrillation; *ARB,* angiotensin-receptor blocker; *CAD,* coronary artery disease; *CRT,* cardiac resynchronization therapy; *DM,* diabetes mellitus; *EF,* ejection fraction; *GDMT,* guideline-directed medical therapy; *HF,* heart failure; *HFpEF,* heart failure with preserved ejection fraction; *HFrEF,* heart failure with reduced ejection fraction; *HRQOL,* health-related quality of life; *HTN,* hypertension; *ICD,* implantable cardioverter-defibrillator; *LV,* left ventricular; *LVH,* left ventricular hypertrophy; *MCS,* mechanical circulatory support; *MI,* myocardial infarction. (Modified from Hunt SA, Abraham WT, Chin MH, et al. 2009 focused update incorporated into the ACC/AHA 2005 Guidelines for the Diagnosis and Management of Heart Failure in Adults: a report of the American College of Cardiology Foundation/American Heart Association Task Force on Practice Guidelines: developed in collaboration with the International Society for Heart and Lung Transplantation. *Circulation.* 2009;119:e391–e479; and Yancy CW, Jessup M, Bozkurt B, et al. 2013 ACCF/AHA Guideline for the Management of Heart Failure: A Report of the American College of Cardiology Foundation/American Heart Association Task Force on Practice Guidelines. Circulation 2013;128(16):e240-327.)

Management of Patients With Symptomatic and Asymptomatic Heart Failure

Transient Left Ventricular Dysfunction

As noted in Chapter 47, the clinical syndrome of HF with reduced EF begins after an initial index event produces a decline in ejection performance of the heart. However, it is important to recognize that LV dysfunction may develop transiently in a variety of different clinical settings that may not invariably lead to the development of the clinical syndrome of HF. Figure 50.4 illustrates the important relationship between LV dysfunction (transient and sustained) and the clinical syndrome of HF (asymptomatic and symptomatic). LV dysfunction with pulmonary edema may develop acutely in patients with previously normal LV structure and function. This occurs most commonly postoperatively following cardiac surgery, or in the setting of severe brain injury, after a systemic infection, or after cessation of tachycardia. The general pathophysiologic mechanism involved is either some form of "stunning" of functional myocardium (see also Chapter 49), or activation of proinflammatory cytokines that are capable of suppressing LV function (see Chapter 47). Emotional stress can also precipitate severe, reversible LV dysfunction that is accompanied by chest pain, pulmonary edema, and cardiogenic shock in patients without coronary disease (Takotsubo syndrome [stress cardiomyopathy]). In this setting LV dysfunction is thought to occur secondary to the deleterious effects of catecholamines following heightened sympathetic stimulation.[17] Microvascular dysfunction has been suggested as an important pathogenetic determinant of myocardial ischemia in Takotsubo syndrome.[17] If LV dysfunction persists following the initial cardiac injury, patients may remain asymptomatic for a period of months to years; however, the weight of epidemiologic and clinical evidence suggests that at some point these patients will undergo the transition to overt symptomatic HF.

Defining the Appropriate Strategy (see Fig. 50.4)

The main goals of treatment are to reduce symptoms, prolong survival, improve quality of life, and prevent disease progression. As will be discussed below, the current pharmacologic device, and surgical therapeutic armamentarium for the management of patients with a reduced EF allows health care providers to achieve each of these goals in the great majority of patients. Once patients have developed structural heart disease (Stage B to D), the choice of therapy for patients with HF with a reduced EF depends on their NYHA functional classification (see Chapter 48, Table 48.1). Although this classification system is notoriously subjective, and has large interobserver variability, it has withstood the test of time and continues to be widely applied to patients with HF. For patients who have developed LV systolic dysfunction, but who remain asymptomatic (class I), the goal should be to slow disease progression by blocking neurohormonal systems that lead to cardiac remodeling (see Chapter 47). For patients who have developed symptoms (class II to IV), the primary goal should be to alleviate fluid retention, lessen disability, and reduce the risk of further disease progression and death. As will be discussed subsequently, these goals generally require a strategy that combines diuretics (to control salt and water retention) with neurohormonal interventions (to minimize cardiac remodeling).

General Measures

Identification and correction of the condition(s) responsible for the cardiac structural and/or functional abnormalities is critical (see Table 50.2), insofar as some of conditions that provoke LV structural and functional abnormalities are potentially treatable and/or reversible. Patients with HF often have multiple comorbid conditions that may interact with the syndrome of HF and or the choice of therapeutics. The 2013 ACC/AHA practice guidelines recognized the importance of comorbidities in HF, including hypertension, anemia, diabetes, arthritis, chronic kidney disease, and depression, but did not provide specific recommendations.

VI

HEART FAILURE

TABLE 50.4 Diagnostic Criteria for Heart Failure in Population-Based Studies

FRAMINGHAM CRITERIA		
MAJOR CRITERIA	**MINOR CRITERIA**	**MAJOR OR MINOR CRITERIA**
Paroxysmal nocturnal dyspnea or orthopnea	Ankle edema	Weight loss >4.5 kg in 5 days in response to treatment
Neck-vein distention	Night cough	
RALES	Dyspnea on exertion	
Cardiomegaly	Hepatomegaly	
Acute pulmonary edema	Pleural effusion	
S3 gallop	Vital capacity decreased one third from maximal capacity	
Increased venous pressure >16 cm H$_2$O	Tachycardia (rate >120/min)	
Hepatojugular reflux		

NHANES CRITERIA		
CATEGORIES	**CRITERIA**	**SCORE**
History	*Dyspnea:*	1
	Do you stop for breath when walking at an ordinary pace?	
	Do you stop for breath after walking for about 100 yards on flat ground?	1
	When hurrying on a hill	2
	When walking at an ordinary pace	2
Physical examination	*Heart rate:*	
	>110 beats/min	1
	91–110 beats/min	2
	Jugular venous pressure (>6 cm H$_2$O):	
	Alone	1
	Plus hepatomegaly or edema	2
	Rales:	
	Basilar crackles	1
	Crackles more than basilar crackles	2
Chest radiography	Upper zone flow redistribution	1
	Interstitial pulmonary edema	2
	Interstitial edema plus pleural fluid	3
	Alveolar fluid plus pleural fluid	3

The diagnosis of HF using the Framingham criteria requires the simultaneous presence of at least two major criteria or one major criterion in conjunction with two minor criteria. Minor criteria are acceptable only if they cannot be attributed to another medical condition (such as pulmonary hypertension, chronic lung disease, cirrhosis, ascites, or the nephrotic syndrome). NHANES-1 criteria: diagnosis of HF is score ≥three points.
NHANES, National Health and Nutrition Survey.
Modified from Ho KK, Pinsky JL, Kannel WB, et al. The epidemiology of heart failure: the Framingham Study. *J Am Coll Cardiol.* 1993;22:6A–13A; and Schocken DD, Arrieta MI, Leaverton PE, et al. Prevalence and mortality rate of congestive heart failure in the United States. *J Am Coll Cardiol.* 1992;20:301–306.

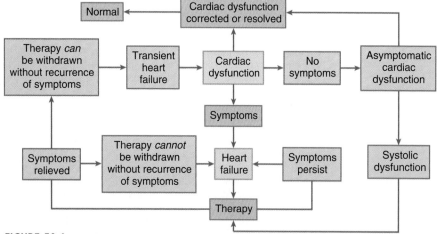

FIGURE 50.4 Relationship between cardiac dysfunction, symptomatic heart failure, and asymptomatic heart failure following appropriate treatment. (From Swedberg K, Cleland J, Dargie H, et al. Guidelines for the diagnosis and treatment of chronic heart failure: executive summary (update 2005): The Task Force for the Diagnosis and Treatment of Chronic Heart Failure of the European Society of Cardiology. *Eur Heart J.* 2005;26:1115–1140.)

However, the 2017 ACC/AHA/HFSA focused guideline update did provide specific recommendations for the treatment of hypertension, anemia, and sleep-disordered breathing.[18] In addition to searching for reversible etiologies and comorbidities that contribute to the development of HF, it is equally important to identify factors that provoke worsening HF in stable patients (Table 50.5). Among the most common causes of acute decompensation in a previously stable patient are dietary indiscretion and inappropriate reduction of HF therapy, either from patient self-discontinuation of medication, or alternatively from physician withdrawal of effective pharmacotherapy (e.g., because of concern over azotemia). HF patients should be advised to stop smoking and to limit alcohol consumption to two standard drinks per day in men or one standard drink per day in women. Patients suspected

TABLE 50.5 Factors That May Precipitate Acute Decompensation in Patients with Chronic Heart Failure

Dietary indiscretion
Inappropriate reduction in HF medications
Myocardial ischemia/infarction
Arrhythmias (tachycardia or bradycardia)
Infection
Anemia

Initiation of medications that worsen the symptoms of HF
  Calcium antagonists (verapamil, diltiazem)
  Beta-blockers
  Nonsteroidal antiinflammatory drugs
  Thiazolidinediones
  Antiarrhythmic agents (all class I agents, sotalol [class III])
  Anti-TNF antibodies

Alcohol consumption
Pregnancy
Worsening hypertension
Acute valvular insufficiency

HF, Heart failure; *TNF,* tumor necrosis factor.
From Mann DL. Heart Failure and Cor Pulmonale. In: Kasper DL, et al., eds. *Harrison's Principles of Internal Medicine.* 17th ed. New York: McGraw-Hill; 2007:1448.

of having an alcohol-induced cardiomyopathy should be advised to abstain from alcohol consumption indefinitely. Excessive temperature extremes and heavy physical exertion should be avoided. Certain drugs are known to make HF worse and should also be avoided. For example, nonsteroidal antiinflammatory drugs (NSAIDs), including cyclooxygenase-2 inhibitors (COX2), are not recommended in patients with chronic HF because the risk of renal failure and fluid retention is markedly increased in the setting of reduced renal function and/or ACEI use. Patients should be advised to weigh themselves on a regular basis to monitor weight gain and alert a health care provider or adjust their diuretic dose in the case of a sudden unexpected weight gain of greater than 3 to 4 pounds over a 3-day period. Although there is no documented evidence of the effects of immunization in HF patients, they are at high risk of developing pneumococcal disease and influenza. Accordingly, clinicians should consider recommending influenza and pneumococcal vaccines to their HF patient to prevent respiratory infections. It is equally important to educate the patient and family about HF, the importance of proper diet, as well the importance of compliance with the medical regimen. Supervision of outpatient care by a specially trained nurse or physician assistant and/or specialized HF clinics have all been found to be helpful, particularly in patients with advanced disease (see Disease Management below).

Activity
Although heavy physical labor is not recommended for patients with HF, routine modest exercise has been shown to be beneficial in selected patients with NYHA class I to III HFrEF. The HF-ACTION trial (Controlled Trial Investigating Outcomes of Exercise Training) was a large multicenter randomized controlled study whose primary endpoint was a composite of all-cause mortality and all-cause hospitalization. Secondary endpoints included all-cause mortality, all-cause hospitalization, and the composite of cardiovascular mortality or HF hospitalization. HF-ACTION failed to show a significant improvement in all-cause mortality or all-cause hospitalization (HR, 0.93; 95% CI 0.84 to 1.02; p = 0.13) in patients who received a 12-week (3 times/wk) exercise training program followed by 25 to 30 minute, 5 days/wk home-based, self-monitored exercise workouts on a treadmill or stationary bicycle (eFig. 50.2A). Moreover, there was no difference in all-cause mortality (HR, 0.96; 95% CI 0.79 to 1.17;

p = 0.70; eFig. 50.2B). However, there was a trend towards decreased cardiovascular mortality or HF hospitalizations (HR, 0.87; 95% CI 0.74 to 0.99 p = 0.06) and quality of life was significantly improved in the exercise group.[19] For euvolemic patients regular isotonic exercise such as walking or riding a stationary-bicycle ergometer may be useful as an adjunct therapy, to improve clinical status after patients have undergone exercise testing to determine suitability for exercise training (ensuring that patient does not develop significant ischemia or arrhythmias). Exercise training is not recommended, however, in HFrEF patients who have had a major cardiovascular event or procedure within the last 6 weeks, in patients receiving cardiac devices that limit the ability to achieve target heart rates, and in patients with significant arrhythmia or ischemia during baseline cardiopulmonary exercise testing.

Diet
Dietary restriction of sodium (2 to 3 g daily) is recommended in all patients with the clinical syndrome of HF and preserved or depressed EF. Further restriction (<2 g daily) may be considered in moderate to severe HF. Fluid restriction is generally unnecessary unless the patient is hyponatremic (<130 mEq/L), which may develop because of activation of the renin angiotensin system, excessive secretion of AVP, or loss of salt in excess of water from prior diuretic use. Fluid restriction (<2 L/day) should be considered in hyponatremic patients (<130 mEq/L), or for those patients whose fluid retention is difficult to control despite high doses of diuretics and sodium restriction. Caloric supplementation is recommended for patients with advanced HF and unintentional weight loss or muscle wasting (cardiac cachexia); however, anabolic steroids are not recommended for these patients because of the potential problems with volume retention. The measurement of nitrogen balance, caloric intake, and prealbumin may be useful in determining appropriate nutritional supplementation. The use of dietary supplements ("nutraceuticals") should be avoided in the management of symptomatic HF because of the lack of proven benefit and the potential for significant interactions with proven HF therapeutics.

MANAGEMENT OF FLUID RETENTION

Many of the clinical manifestations of the syndrome of HF result from excessive salt and water retention that leads to an inappropriate volume expansion of the vascular and extravascular space. The use of implantable devices to monitor HF is discussed in Chapter 58. This chapter will focus on the use of diuretics in chronic HFrEF. Although both digitalis and low doses of ACEIs enhance urinary sodium excretion, few volume-overloaded HF patients can maintain proper sodium balance without the use of diuretic drugs. Indeed, attempts to substitute ACEIs for diuretics have been shown to lead to pulmonary edema and peripheral congestion. As shown in Figure 50.5, diuretic-induced negative sodium and water balance can decrease LV dilation, functional mitral insufficiency, and decrease mitral wall stress and subendocardial ischemia. In short-term clinical trials diuretic therapy has led to a reduction in jugular venous pressures, pulmonary congestion, peripheral edema, and body weight, all of which were observed within days of initiation of therapy. In intermediate-term studies, diuretics have been shown to improve cardiac function, symptoms, and exercise tolerance in HF patients.[20] To date, there have been no long-term studies of diuretic therapy in HF; thus, their effects on morbidity and mortality are not clearly known. Although retrospective analyses of clinical trials suggest that diuretic use is associated with worse clinical outcomes,[20] a meta-analysis (Cochrane Review) suggested that treatment with diuretic therapy produced a significant reduction in mortality (OR 0.24; 95% CI 0.07 to 0.83; p = 0.02) and worsening HF (OR 0.07; 95% CI 0.01 to 0.52; p = 0.01).[20] However, given the retrospective nature of this review, this analysis cannot be used as formal evidence to recommend the use diuretics to reduce HF mortality.

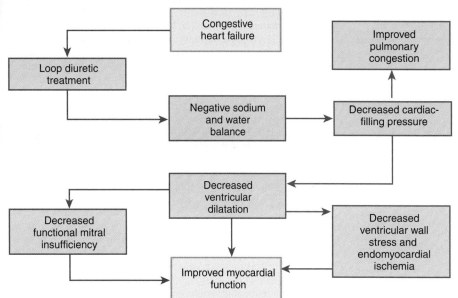

FIGURE 50.5 Potential beneficial effects of diuretics on myocardial function. Diuretic-induced negative sodium and water balance can decrease left ventricular (LV) dilation, functional mitral insufficiency, and decrease mitral wall stress and subendocardial ischemia. However, treatment with diuretics can also lead to deterioration of renal function and worsening neurohormonal activation. (Modified from Schrier RW. Use of diuretics in heart failure and cirrhosis. *Semin Nephrol.* 2011;31:503–512.)

Diuretic Classes

A number of classification schemes have been proposed for diuretics on the basis of their mechanism of action, their anatomical locus of action within the nephron, and the form of diuresis that they elicit (solute versus water diuresis). The most common classification for diuretics employs an admixture of chemical (e.g., thiazide diuretic), site of action (e.g., loop diuretics), or clinical outcomes (e.g., potassium-sparing diuretics). The loop diuretics increase sodium excretion by up to 20% to 25% of the filtered load of sodium, enhance free water clearance, and maintain their efficacy unless renal function is severely impaired. In contrast, the thiazide diuretics increase the fractional excretion of sodium to only 5% to 10% of the filtered load, tend to decrease free water clearance, and lose their effectiveness in patients with impaired renal function (creatinine clearance <40 mL/min). Consequently, the loop diuretics have emerged as the preferred diuretic agents for use in most patients with HF. Diuretics that induce a water diuresis (aquaretics) include demeclocycline, lithium, and vasopressin V2 receptor antagonists, each of which inhibits the action of AVP on the collecting duct through different mechanisms, thereby increasing free water clearance. Drugs that cause solute diuresis are subdivided into two types: osmotic diuretics, which are nonresorbable solutes that osmotically retain water and other solutes in the tubular lumen; and drugs that selectively inhibit ion transport pathways across tubular epithelia, which constitute the majority of potent, clinically useful diuretics. The classes of diuretics and individual class members are listed in Table 50.6 and their renal sites of action are depicted in Figure 50.6.

Loop Diuretics

The agents classified as loop diuretics, including furosemide, bumetanide, and torsemide, act by competing with chloride for binding to the Na^+-K^+-$2Cl^-$ symporter (NKCC2) on the apical membrane of epithelial cells in the thick ascending loop of Henle (site II, Fig. 50.6). Because furosemide, bumetanide, and torsemide are bound to plasma proteins, delivery of these drugs to the tubule by filtration is limited. However, these drugs are secreted efficiently into the tubular lumen by organic anion transporters (OAT1 and OAT2) at the basolateral membrane of proximal convoluted tubule epithelial cells and by multidrug

resistance–associated protein 4 (and others) at the apical membrane or these cells.[21] Thus, the efficacy of loop diuretics is dependent upon sufficient renal plasma blood flow and proximal tubular secretion to deliver these agents to their site of action. Probenecid shifts the plasma concentration-response curve for furosemide to the right by competitively inhibiting furosemide excretion by the organic acid transport system. The bioavailability of furosemide ranges from 40% to 70% of the oral dose. In contrast the oral bioavailability of bumetanide and torsemide exceed 80%. Accordingly, these agents may be more effective in advanced HF or those with right-sided HF, albeit at considerably greater cost. Agents in a second functional class of loop diuretics typified by ethacrynic acid exhibit a slower onset of action and have delayed and only partial reversibility. Ethacrynic acid may be safely used in sulfa-allergic HF patients.

MECHANISMS OF ACTION

Loop diuretics are believed to improve symptoms of congestion by several mechanisms. First, loop diuretics reversibly bind to and reversibly inhibit the action of the Na^+-K^+-$2Cl^-$ cotransporter, thereby preventing salt transport in the thick ascending loop of Henle. Inhibition of this symporter also inhibits Ca^{++} and Mg^{++} resorption by abolishing the transepithelial potential difference that is the driving force for absorption of these cations. By inhibiting the concentration of solute within the medullary interstitium, these drugs also reduce the driving force for water resorption in the collecting duct, even in the presence of AVP (see also Chapter 47). The decreased resorption of water by the collecting duct results in the production of urine that is nearly isotonic with plasma. The increase in delivery of Na^+ and water to the distal nephron segments also markedly enhances K^+ excretion, particularly in the presence of elevated aldosterone levels.

Loop diuretics also exhibit several characteristic effects on intracardiac pressure and systemic hemodynamics. Furosemide acts as a venodilator and reduces right atrial and pulmonary capillary wedge pressure within minutes when given intravenously (0.5 to 1.0 mg/kg). Similar data, although not as extensive, have accumulated for bumetanide and torsemide. This initial improvement in hemodynamics may be secondary to the release of vasodilatory prostaglandins, insofar as studies in animals and humans have demonstrated that the venodilatory actions of furosemide are inhibited by indomethacin. There have also been reports of an acute rise in systemic vascular resistance with in response to loop diuretics, which has been attributed to transient activation of the systemic or intravascular renin-angiotensin system (RAS), which is secondary to loop diuretics directly stimulating renin secretion by macula densa cells.

The potentially deleterious rise in LV afterload reinforces the importance of initiating vasodilator therapy with diuretics in patients with acute pulmonary edema and adequate blood pressure (see Chapter 49).

Thiazide and Thiazide-Like Diuretics

The benzothiadiazides, also known as *thiazide diuretics*, were the initial class of drugs that were synthesized to block the Na^+-Cl^- transporter in the cortical portion of the ascending loop of Henle and the distal convoluted tubule (site III, Fig. 50.6). Subsequently, drugs that share similar pharmacologic properties became known as thiazide-like diuretics, even though they were technically not benzothiadiazine derivatives. Metolazone, a quinazoline sulfonamide, is a thiazide-like diuretic that is used in combination with furosemide, in patients who become resistant to diuretics (see below). Because thiazide and thiazide-like diuretics prevent maximal dilution of urine, they decrease the kidney's ability to increase free water clearance and may therefore contribute to the development of hyponatremia. Thiazides increase Ca^{2+} resorption in the distal nephron (Fig. 50.6)

TABLE 50.6 Diuretics for Treating Fluid Retention in Chronic Heart Failure

DRUG	INITIAL DAILY DOSE(S)	MAXIMUM TOTAL DAILY DOSE	DURATION OF ACTION
Loop Diuretics*			
Bumetanide	0.5–1.0 mg once or twice	10 mg	4–6 hr
Furosemide	20–40 mg once or twice	600 mg	6–8 hr
Torsemide	10–20 mg once	200 mg	12–16 hr
Ethacrynic acid	25–50 mg once or twice	200 mg	6 hr
Thiazide Diuretics**			
Chlorothiazide	250–500 mg once or twice	1000 mg	6–12 hr
Chlorthalidone	25 mg once	100 mg	24–72 hr
Hydrochlorothiazide	25 mg once or twice	200 mg	6–12 hr
Indapamide	2.5 mg once	5 mg	36 hr
Metolazone	2.5–5.0 mg once	5 mg	12–24 hr
Potassium-Sparing Diuretics			
Amiloride	5.0 mg once	20 mg	24 hr
Triamterene	50–100 mg twice	300 mg	7–9 hr
AVP Antagonists			
Satavaptan	25 mg once	50 mg once	NS
Tolvaptan	15 mg once	60 mg once	NS
Lixivaptan	25 mg once	250 mg twice	NS
Conivaptan (IV)	20 mg IV loading dose followed by	100 mg once	7–9 hr
	20 mg continuous IV infusion/day	40 mg IV	
Sequential Nephron Blockade			
Metolazone	2.5–10 mg once plus loop diuretic		
Hydrochlorothiazide	25–100 mg once or twice plus loop diuretic		
Chlorothiazide (IV)	500–1000 mg once plus loop diuretic		

*Equivalent doses: 40 mg furosemide = 1 mg bumetanide = 20 mg torsemide = 50 mg of ethacrynic acid.
**Do not use if estimated glomerular filtration is less than 30 mL/min or with cytochrome 3A4 inhibitors.
Unless indicated, all doses are for oral diuretics.
mg, Milligrams; *IV*, intravenous. *NS*, not specified.
Modified from Hunt SA, et al. ACC/AHA 2005 guideline update for the diagnosis and management of chronic heart failure in the adult: a report of the American College of Cardiology/American Heart Association Task Force on Practice Guidelines. *J Am Coll Cardiol.* 2005;46:e1–e82.

by several mechanisms, occasionally resulting in a small increase in serum Ca^{2+} levels. In contrast, Mg^{2+} resorption is diminished and hypomagnesemia may occur with prolonged use. Increased delivery of NaCl and fluid into the collecting duct directly enhances K^+ and H^+ secretion by this segment of the nephron, which may lead to clinically important hypokalemia.

MECHANISMS OF ACTION
The site of action of these drugs within the distal convoluted tubule has been identified as the Na^+-Cl^- symporter of the distal convoluted tubule. Although this cotransporter shares approximately 50% amino acid homology with the Na^+/K^+/$2Cl^-$ symporter of the ascending limb of the loop of Henle, it is insensitive to the effects of furosemide. This cotransporter (or related isoforms) is also present on cells within the vasculature and many cell types within other organs and tissues and may contribute to some of the other actions of these agents, such as their utility as antihypertensive agents. Similar to the loop diuretics, the efficacy of thiazide diuretics is dependent, at least in part, upon proximal tubular secretion to deliver these agents to their site of action. However, unlike the loop diuretics the plasma protein binding varies considerably among the thiazide diuretics; accordingly, this parameter will determine the contribution that glomerular filtration makes to tubular delivery of a specific diuretic.

Mineralocorticoid Receptor Antagonists
Mineralocorticoids (MRAs) such as aldosterone cause retention of salt and water and increase the excretion of K^+ and H^+ by binding to specific MRA receptors. Spironolactone (first-generation MRA) and eplerenone (second-generation MRA) are synthetic MRA receptors that act on the distal nephron to inhibit Na^+/K^+ exchange at the site of aldosterone action (Site IV, Fig. 50.6).

MECHANISMS OF ACTION
Spironolactone has antiandrogenic and progesterone-like effects, which may cause gynecomastia or impotence in men, and menstrual irregularities in women. To overcome these side effects, eplerenone was developed by replacing the 17 alpha-thioacetyl group of spironolactone with a carbomethoxy group. As a result of this modification, eplerenone has greater selectivity for the MRA receptor than for steroid receptors and has less sex hormone side effects than does spironolactone. Eplerenone is further distinguished from spironolactone by its shorter half-life and the fact that it does not have any active metabolites. Although spironolactone and eplerenone are both weak diuretics, clinical trials have shown that both of these agents have profound effects on cardiovascular morbidity and mortality (Fig. 50.7) by virtue of their ability to antagonize the deleterious effects of aldosterone in the cardiovascular system (see Chapter 47). Hence these agents are used in HF for their ability to antagonize the renin angiotensin aldosterone system (see below), rather than for their diuretic properties. Spironolactone (see Table 50.6) and its active metabolite, canrenone, competitively inhibit the binding of aldosterone to MRA or type I receptors in many tissues, including epithelial cells of the distal convoluted tubule and collecting duct. These cytosolic receptors are ligand-dependent transcription factors, which upon binding of the ligand (e.g., aldosterone), translocate to the nucleus where they bind to hormone response elements present in the promoter of some genes, including several involved in vascular and myocardial fibrosis, inflammation, and calcification.

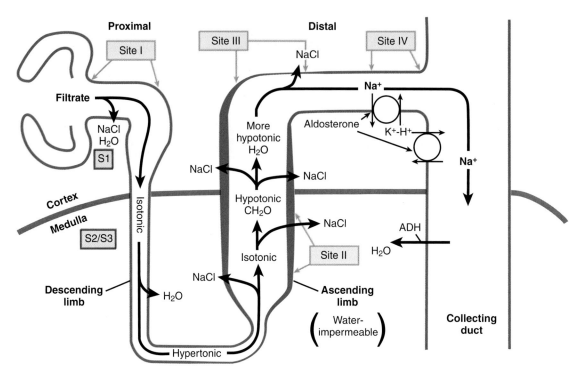

Site I (proximal convoluted tubule): carbonic anhydrase inhibitors, SGLT2 inhibitors
Site II (ascending loop of Henle): loop diuretics
Site III (distal convoluted tubule): thiazide and thiazide-like diuretics
Site IV (late distal tubule and collecting duct): potassium-sparing diuretics, MRAs
S1-S3 segments of proximal convoluted tube

FIGURE 50.6 Sites of action of diuretics in the kidney. (Modified from Wile D. Diuretics: a review. *Ann Clin Biochem.* 2012;49:419–431.)

While first- and second-generation steroid-based MRAs have been shown to reduce HF mortality rates, the broader use of these agents in HF patients has been limited by significant side effects, most notably hyperkalemia. Novel, potent, and selective "third-generation" nonsteroidal MRAs that combine the potency and efficacy of spironolactone with the selectivity of eplerenone, and have less hyperkalemia, have recently entered clinical trials. Finerenone (BAY 94-8862) is a nonsteroidal MRA that was compared to eplerenone in patients with worsening chronic HF and type 2 diabetes mellitus and/or chronic kidney disease in the phase IIb ARTS-HF (MinerAlocorticoid-Receptor antagonist Tolerability Stud) trial.[22] ARTS-HF was a randomized, double-blind, comparator-controlled multicenter trial in 1066 patients with HF (left ventricular ejection fraction [LVEF] ≤40%). The primary endpoint was the percentage of individuals with a decrease of greater than 30% in plasma NT-proBNP from baseline to Day 90. When compared with eplerenone, finerenone was well tolerated and resulted in a 30% or greater decrease in NT-proBNP levels, which was similar to the proportion of patients observed in the eplerenone-treatment group. The composite clinical endpoint of death from any cause, cardiovascular hospitalizations, or emergency presentation for worsening HF until Day 90, which was a prespecified secondary endpoint occurred less frequently in all finerenone-dose groups except for the lowest doses.

Potassium-Sparing Diuretics

Triamterene and amiloride are referred to as *potassium-sparing diuretics.* These agents share the common property of causing a mild increase in NaCl excretion, as well as having antikaluretic properties. Triamterene is a pyrazinoylguanidine derivative, whereas amiloride is a pteridine. Both drugs are organic bases that are transported into the proximal tubule, where they block Na^+ reabsorption in the late distal tubule and collecting duct (site IV, Fig. 50.7). However, since Na^+ retention occurs in more proximal nephron sites in HF, neither amiloride nor triamterene is effective in achieving a net negative Na^+ balance when given alone in HF patients. Both amiloride and triamterene appear to share a similar mechanism of action. Considerable evidence suggests that amiloride blocks Na^+ channels in the luminal membrane of the

principal cells in the late distal tubule and collecting duct, perhaps by competing with Na^+ for negatively charged areas within the pore of the Na^+ channel. Blockade of Na^+ channels leads to hyperpolarization of the luminal membrane of the tubule, which reduces the electrochemical gradient that provides the driving force for K^+ secretion into the lumen. Amiloride and its congeners also inhibit Na^+/H^+ antiporters in renal epithelial cells and in many other cell types, but only at concentrations that are higher than those used clinically.

Carbonic Anhydrase Inhibitors

The zinc metalloenzyme carbonic anhydrase plays an essential role in the $NaHCO_3$ resorption and acid secretion in the proximal tubule (site I, see Fig. 50.6). Although weak diuretics, carbonic anhydrase inhibitors (see Table 50.6) such as acetazolamide, potently inhibit carbonic anhydrase, resulting in near-complete loss of $NaHCO_3$ resorption in the proximal tubule. The use of these agents in patients with HF is confined to temporary administration to correct the metabolic alkalosis that occurs as a "contraction" phenomenon in response to the administration of other diuretics. When used repeatedly, these agents can lead to metabolic acidosis as well as severe hypokalemia.

Sodium-Glucose Transporter-2 Inhibitors

The SGLT2 is a high-capacity, low-affinity transporter that is located in the S1 and S2 segments of the proximal tubule in the kidneys (Site I, Fig. 50.6). SGLT2 accounts for 90% of glucose reabsorption by the kidney, whereas the lower-capacity higher-affinity SGLT1, located in the S3 segment of the proximal tubules, accounts for the remaining 10% of glucose absorption. SGLT2 is also responsible for proximal tubular reabsorption of sodium, and the passive absorption of chloride that is driven by the resulting electrochemical gradient in the proximal tubule lumen. The increased absorption of sodium and chloride in the proximal tubule results in lower chloride concentration delivered to the macula densa, which in turn results in dilation of the afferent arteriole and increased glomerular filtration through "tubulo-glomerular feedback," which preserves renal blood flow and glomerular filtration rate.

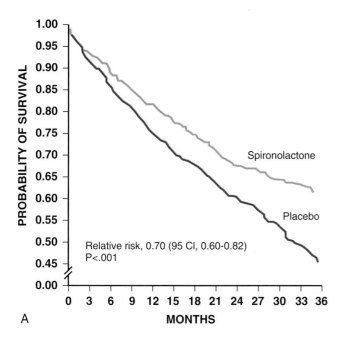

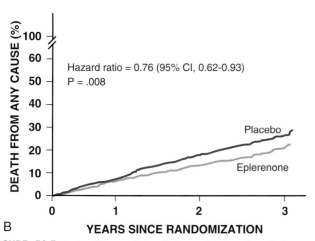

FIGURE 50.7 Kaplan-Meier analysis of the probability of survival among patients in the placebo and treatment groups in the RALES trial (**A**) with spironolactone and the EMPHASIS trial (**B**) using eplerenone. (Modified from Pitt B, Zannad F, Cody R, et al. The effect of spironolactone on morbidity and mortality in patients with severe heart failure. Randomized Aldactone Evaluation Study Investigators. *N Engl J Med.* 1999;341:709–717; and Zannad F, McMurray JJ, Krum H, et al. Eplerenone in patients with systolic heart failure and mild symptoms. *N Engl J Med.* 2011;364:11–21.)

SGLT2 inhibitors result in a 1:1 stoichiometric inhibition of sodium and glucose uptake in the proximal tubule of the kidney. This leads to contraction of the plasma volume and modest lowering of blood pressure, without activation of the sympathetic nervous system. The contraction of plasma volume may contribute to changes in markers of hemoconcentration with SGLT2 inhibitors, including increases in blood urea nitrogen and hematocrit, although the latter may also be on the basis of increased erythropoiesis. In addition, the proximal natriuresis that occurs with SGLT2 inhibition results in afferent arteriole vasoconstriction through tubulo-glomerular feedback, thereby reducing glomerular hyperfiltration (Fig. 50.8). Experimental studies showed that SGLT2 inhibitors reduced hyperfiltration and decreased inflammatory and fibrotic responses of proximal tubular cells.[23] Beyond effects on traditional cardiovascular risk factors such as HbA$_{1c}$ and weight, SGLT2 inhibition also reduces plasma uric acid levels by 10% to 15% by increasing uricosuria via exchange of filtered glucose. Elevated uric acid levels have been implicated in worsening HF because of oxidative stress and inflammation.

Vasopressin Antagonists

As discussed in Chapter 47, increased circulating levels of the pituitary hormone AVP contribute to the increased systemic vascular resistance and positive water balance in HF patients. The cellular effects of AVP are mediated by interactions with three types of receptors, V$_{1a}$, V$_{1b}$, and V$_2$ (see Chapter 47). Selective V$_{1a}$ antagonists block the vasoconstricting effects of AVP in peripheral vascular smooth muscle cells, whereas V$_2$ selective receptor antagonists inhibit recruitment of aquaporin water channels into the apical membranes of collecting duct epithelial cells, thereby reducing the ability of the collecting duct to resorb water. Combined V$_{1a}$/V$_2$ antagonists lead to a decrease in systemic vascular resistance and prevent the dilutional hyponatremia that occurs in HF patients.[24]

The AVP antagonists or "vaptans" (see Table 50.6) were developed to selectively block the V$_2$ receptor (e.g., tolvaptan, lixivaptan, satavaptan) or nonselectively block both the V$_{1a}$/V$_2$ receptors (e.g., conivaptan). All four AVP antagonists increase urine volume, decrease urine osmolarity, and have no effect on 24-hour sodium excretion (see also Chapter 49)[24] Long-term therapy with the V$_2$ selective vasopressin antagonist tolvaptan did not improve mortality but appears to be safe in patients with advanced HF.[25] Currently two vasopressin antagonists are Food and Drug Administration (FDA)-approved (conivaptan and tolvaptan) for the treatment of clinically significant hypervolemic and euvolemic hyponatremia (serum Na$^+$ ≤125) that is symptomatic and which resisted correction with fluid restriction in patients with HF; however, neither of these agents is currently specifically approved for the treatment of HF. Use of these agents is appropriate after traditional measures to treat hyponatremia have been tried, including water restriction and maximization of medical therapies such as ACEIs or angiotensin receptor blockers (ARBs) which block or decrease angiotensin II. The use of vaptans in hospitalized HF patients is discussed in Chapter 49.

Diuretic Treatment of Heart Failure

Patients with evidence of volume overload or a history of fluid retention should be treated with a diuretic to relieve their symptoms. In symptomatic patients, diuretics should be always used in combination with neurohormonal antagonists that are known to prevent disease progression. When patients have moderate to severe symptoms or renal insufficiency, a loop diuretic is generally required. Diuretics should be initiated in low doses (see Table 50.6) and then titrated upward to relieve signs and symptoms of fluid overload. A typical starting dose of furosemide for patients with systolic HF and normal renal function is 40 mg, although doses of 80 to 160 mg are often necessary to achieve adequate diuresis. Loop diuretics have a sigmoidal dose-response curve. Importantly, in both HF and renal insufficiency, the dose response for loop diuretics shifts downward and to the right (Fig. 50.9A). Because of the steep dose-response curve and effective threshold for loop diuretics (see Fig. 50.9B), it is critical to find an adequate dose of loop diuretic that leads to a clear-cut diuretic response. One commonly employed method for finding the appropriate dose is to double the dose until the desired effect is achieved, or the maximal dose of diuretic is reached. Once patients have achieved an adequate diuresis, it is important to document their "dry weight" and make certain that patients weigh themselves daily in order to maintain their dry weight.

Although furosemide is the most commonly used loop diuretic, the oral bioavailability of furosemide is approximately 40% to 79%. Therefore, bumetanide or torsemide may be preferable because of their increased bioavailability. With the exception of torsemide, the commonly used loop diuretics are short-acting (<3 hours). For this reason, loop diuretics usually need to be given at least twice daily. Some patients may develop hypotension or azotemia during diuretic therapy. While the rapidity of diuresis should be slowed in these patients, diuretic therapy should be maintained at a lower level until the patient becomes euvolemic, insofar as persistent volume overload may compromise the effectiveness of some neurohormonal antagonists. Intravenous administration of diuretics may be necessary to relieve congestion acutely (see Fig. 50.9B and Chapter 49), and can be done safely in the outpatient setting. After a diuretic effect is achieved with short-acting loop diuretics, increasing administration frequency to twice or even three

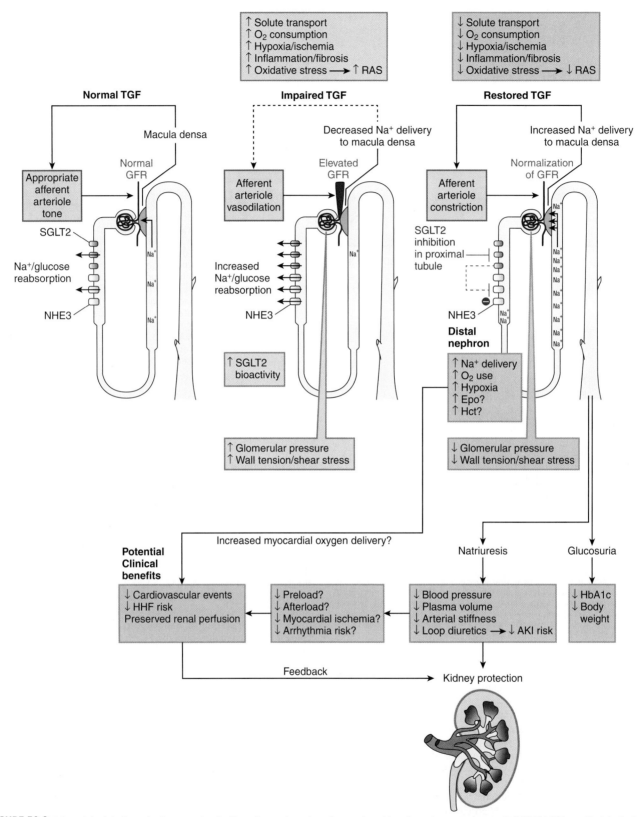

FIGURE 50.8 Selected physiologic mechanisms associated with cardiovascular and renal protection with sodium-glucose transporter-2 (SGLT2) inhibitors. Physiologic changes that occur in the setting of SGLT2 inhibitors, as well as their potential contribution to cardiovascular and renal protection, are depicted. *Red boxes* represent aberrant changes, whereas *yellow boxes* represent protective changes. *Small red circle with a white line* represents inhibition of function. *AKI*, Acute kidney injury; *Epo*, erythropoietin; *GFR*, glomerular filtration rate; *HbA₁c*, glycosylated hemoglobin; *Hct*, hematocrit; *HHF*, hospitalization for heart failure; *Na⁺*, sodium; *NHE3*, sodium–hydrogen antiporter 3; *O₂*, oxygen; *RAS*, renin-angiotensin system; *SGLT2*, sodium-glucose cotransporter-2; *TGF*, tubuloglomerular feedback. (From Cherney DZ, Odutayo A, Aronson R, et al. Sodium Glucose Cotransporter-2 Inhibition and Cardiorenal Protection. *J Am Coll Cardiol.* 2019;74[20]:2511–2524.)

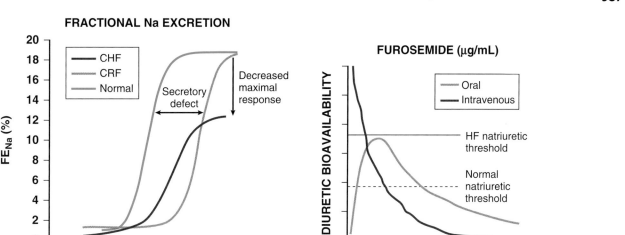

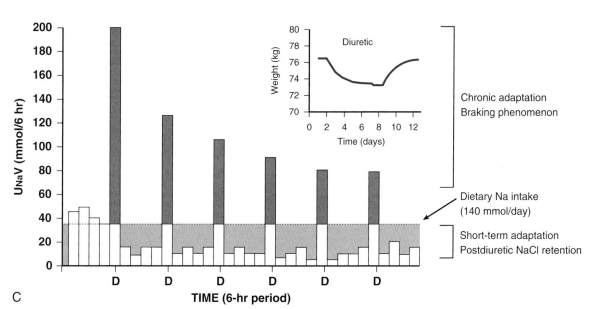

FIGURE 50.9 Pharmacokinetic and pharmacodynamic properties of loop diuretics. **A,** Dose-response curves of loop diuretics in normal patients versus patients with chronic renal failure (CRF) and chronic heart failure. **B,** Comparison of pharmacokinetics of oral versus intravenous loop diuretics *(LD)*. **C,** An example of the braking phenomenon, whereby each additional dose of LD results in progressively less natriuresis. Each period of natriuresis is followed by a period of postdiuretic sodium retention. *ADHF,* Acute decompensated heart failure. **Inset**: effect of a diuretic on body weight, taken as an index of ECF volume. Note that steady state is reached within 6 to 8 days despite continued diuretic administration. (Modified from Ellison DH. Diuretic therapy and resistance in congestive heart failure. *Cardiology.* 2001;96:132-143.)

times per day will provide more diuresis with less physiologic perturbation than larger single doses. Once the congestion has been relieved, treatment with diuretics is continued to prevent the recurrence of salt and water retention in order to maintain the patient's ideal dry weight.

Complications of Diuretic Use

Patients with HF who are receiving diuretics should be monitored for complications of diuretics on a regular basis. The major complications of diuretic use include electrolyte and metabolic disturbances, volume depletion, as well as worsening azotemia. The interval for reassessment should be individualized based on severity of illness and underlying renal function, the use of concomitant medications such as ACEIs, ARBs and aldosterone antagonists, the past history of electrolyte imbalances, and/or need for more aggressive diuresis.

Electrolyte and Metabolic Disturbances

Diuretic use can lead to potassium depletion, which can predispose the patient to significant cardiac arrhythmias. Renal potassium losses from diuretic use can be also exacerbated by the increase in circulating levels of aldosterone observed in patients with advanced HF, as

well by the marked increases in distal nephron Na^+ delivery that follow use of either loop or distal nephron diuretics. The level of dietary salt intake may also contribute to the extent of renal K^+ wasting with diuretics.

In the absence of formal guidelines with respect to the level of maintenance of serum K^+ levels in HF patients, many experienced HF clinicians have advocated that the serum K^+ should be maintained between 4.0 and 5.0 mEq/L because HF patients are often treated with pharmacologic agents that are likely to provoke proarrhythmic effects in the presence of hypokalemia (e.g., digoxin, type III antiarrhythmics, beta-agonists, or phosphodiesterase inhibitors). Hypokalemia can be prevented by increasing the oral intake of KCL. The normal daily dietary K^+ intake is approximately 40 to 80 mEq. Therefore, to increase this by 50% requires an additional 20 to 40 mEq K^+ supplementation daily. However, in the presence of alkalosis, hyperaldosteronism, or Mg^{2+} depletion, hypokalemia is quite unresponsive to increased dietary intake of KCL, and more aggressive replacement is necessary. If supplementation is necessary, oral potassium supplements in the form of KCL extended-release tablets or liquid concentrate should be used whenever possible. Intravenous potassium is potentially hazardous and should be avoided except in emergencies. Where appropriate, the use of an MRA may also prevent the development of hypokalemia.

The use of aldosterone-receptor antagonists is often associated with the development of life-threatening hyperkalemia, particularly when they are combined with ACEIs, ARBs, or angiotensin receptor-neprilysin inhibitors (ARNIs).[26] Potassium supplementation is generally stopped after the initiation of aldosterone antagonists, and patients should be counseled to avoid high potassium–containing foods. The management of acute hyperkalemia (>6.0 mEq/L) may require a short-term cessation of potassium-retaining agents and/or renin-angiotensin-aldosterone system (RAAS) inhibitors; however, RAAS inhibitors should be carefully reintroduced as soon as possible while monitoring potassium levels. Two new potassium binders, patiromer and sodium zirconium cyclosilicate, have been studied in HF patients with hyperkalemia. Patiromer is a nonabsorbed, cation-exchange polymer that contains a calcium-sorbitol counterion, and works by binding potassium in the lumen of the gastrointestinal tract, resulting in a reduction of serum-potassium levels within 7 hours of the first dose. Patiromer is FDA-approved for the treatment of hyperkalemia, but should not be used as an emergency treatment for life-threatening hyperkalemia because of its delayed onset of action. The initial clinical studies in patients with HF have shown that these therapies reduce serum potassium and prevent recurrent hyperkalemia in HF patients with chronic kidney disease who were receiving RAAS inhibitors.[27]

Diuretics may be associated with multiple other metabolic and electrolyte disturbances, including hyponatremia, hypomagnesemia, metabolic alkalosis, hyperglycemia, hyperlipidemia, and hyperuricemia. Hyponatremia is usually observed in HF patients with very high degrees of RAAS activation and/or AVP levels. Aggressive diuretic use can also lead to hyponatremia. Hyponatremia can typically be treated by more stringent water restriction. Both loop and thiazide diuretics can cause hypomagnesemia, which can aggravate muscle weakness and cardiac arrhythmias. Magnesium replacement should be administered for signs or symptoms of hypomagnesemia (arrhythmias, muscle cramps), and can be routinely given (with uncertain benefit) to all subjects receiving large doses of diuretics or requiring large amounts of K+ replacement. The modest hyperglycemia and/or hyperlipidemia produced by thiazide diuretics is not usually clinically important, and blood glucose and lipids are usually easily controlled using standard practice guidelines. Metabolic alkalosis can generally be treated by increasing KCL supplementation, lowering diuretic doses, or transiently using acetazolamide.

Hypotension and Azotemia

The excessive use of diuretics can lead to a decreased blood pressure, decreased exercise tolerance, and increased fatigue, as well as impaired renal function. Hypotensive symptoms usually resolve after a decrease in the dose or frequency of diuretics in patients who are volume depleted. However, in most instances the use of diuretics is associated with decrease in blood pressure and/or mild azotemia that do not lead to patient symptoms. In this instance reductions in the diuretic dose are not necessary, particularly if the patient remains edematous. In some patients with advanced, chronic HF, elevated BUN and creatinine concentrations may be necessary to maintain control of congestive symptoms.

Neurohormonal Activation

Diuretics may increase the activation of endogenous neurohormonal systems in HF patients, which can lead to disease progression unless patients are receiving treatment with a concomitant neurohormonal antagonist (e.g., ACEI or beta-blocker).

Ototoxicity

Ototoxicity, which is more frequent with ethacrynic acid than the other loop diuretics, can manifest as tinnitus, hearing impairment, and deafness. Hearing impairment and deafness are usually, but not invariably, reversible. Ototoxicity occurs most frequently with rapid intravenous injections, and least frequently with oral administration.

Diuretic Resistance and Management

One of the inherent limitations of diuretics is that they achieve water loss via excretion of solute at the expense of glomerular filtration, which in turn activates a set of homeostatic mechanisms that ultimately limit their effectiveness. In normal subjects the magnitude of natriuresis following a given dose of diuretic declines over time as a result of the so-called "braking phenomenon" (see Fig. 50.9C). Studies have shown that the time-dependent decline in natriuresis for a given diuretic dose is critically dependent upon reduction of the extracellular fluid volume, which leads to an increase in solute and fluid reabsorption in the proximal tubule. In addition, contraction of the extracellular volume can lead to stimulation of efferent sympathetic nerves, which reduces urinary Na+ excretion by reducing renal blood flow, stimulating renin (and ultimately aldosterone) release, which in turn stimulates Na+ reabsorption along the nephron (see also Chapter 47). The magnitude of the natriuretic effect of potent loop diuretics may also decline in HF patients, particularly as HF progresses. Although the bioavailability of these diuretics is generally not decreased in HF, the potential delay in their rate of absorption may result in peak drug levels within the tubular lumen in the ascending loop of Henle that are insufficient to induce maximal natriuresis. The use of intravenous formulations may obviate this problem (see Chapter 49). However, even with intravenous dosing, a rightward shift of the dose-response curve is observed between the diuretic concentration in the tubular lumen and its natriuretic effect in HF (see Fig. 50.9A). Moreover, the maximal effect (ceiling) is lower in HF. This rightward shift has been referred to as "diuretic resistance" and is likely due to several factors in addition to the braking phenomenon described above. First, most loop diuretics (with the exception of torsemide) are short-acting drugs. Accordingly, after a period of natriuresis, the diuretic concentration in plasma and tubular fluid declines below the diuretic threshold. In this situation, renal Na+ reabsorption is no longer inhibited and a period of antinatriuresis or postdiuretic NaCl retention ensues. If dietary NaCl intake is moderate to excessive, postdiuretic NaCl retention may overcome the initial natriuresis in patients with excessive activation of the adrenergic nervous system and RAS. This observation forms the rationale for administering short-acting diuretics several times per day to obtain consistent daily salt and water loss. Second, there is a loss of renal responsiveness to endogenous natriuretic peptides as HF advances (see Chapter 47). Third, diuretics increase solute delivery to distal segments of the nephron, causing epithelial cells to undergo both hypertrophy and hyperplasia. Although the diuretic-induced signals that initiate changes in distal nephron structure and function are not well understood, chronic loop diuretic administration increases the Na-K-ATPase activity in the distal collecting duct and cortical collecting tubule, as well as increases the number of thiazide-sensitive Na-Cl cotransporters in the distal nephron, which increases the solute resorptive capacity of the kidney as much as threefold.

In patients with HF an abrupt decline in cardiac and/or renal function or patient noncompliance with their diuretic regimen or diet may lead to diuretic resistance. Apart from these more obvious causes, it is important to query the patient with regard to the concurrent use of drugs that adversely affect renal function, such as NSAIDs and COX-2 inhibitors (see Table 50.5), and certain antibiotics (trimethoprim and gentamicin). The relative risk of increased HF hospitalization varies between individual NSAIDs; including a 1.16 (95% CI 1.07 to 1.27) increase for naproxen, a 1.18 (95% CI 1.12 to 1.23) increase for ibuprofen, a 1.19 (1.15 to 1.24) increase for diclofenac, and a 1.51 (95% 1.33 to 1.71) increase for indomethacin. The use of the COX-2 inhibitors, etoricoxib and rofecoxib, was also associated with increased risk of hospitalization.[28] The insulin-sensitizing thiazolidinediones (TZDs) have also been linked to increased fluid retention in patients with HF, although the clinical significance of this finding is not known. It has been suggested that TZDs activate proliferator-activated receptor-gamma expression in the renal collecting duct, which enhances expression of cell-surface epithelial Na+ channels. Moreover, studies in healthy men have shown that pioglitazone stimulates plasma renin activity that may contribute to increased Na+ retention. Rarely, drugs such as probenecid, or high plasma concentrations of some antibiotics, may compete with the organic ion transporters in the proximal tubule responsible for the transfer of most diuretics from the recirculation into the tubular lumen. The use of increasing doses of vasodilators, with or without a marked decline in intravascular volume as a result of concomitant diuretic therapy, may lower renal perfusion pressure below that necessary to maintain normal autoregulation and glomerular filtration in patients with RAS from atherosclerotic disease. Accordingly, a reduction in renal blood flow may occur despite an increase in cardiac output, thereby leading to a decrease in diuretic effectiveness.

A patient with HF may be considered to be resistant to diuretic drugs when moderate doses of a loop diuretic do not achieve the desired reduction of the extracellular fluid volume. In outpatients, a common and useful method for treating the diuretic-resistant patient is to administer two classes of diuretic concurrently. Adding a proximal tubule diuretic or a distal collecting tubule diuretic to a regimen of loop diuretics is often dramatically effective ("sequential nephron blockade"). As a general rule, when adding a second class of diuretic the dose of loop diuretic should not be altered, because the shape of the dose-response curve for loop diuretics is not affected by the addition of other diuretics, and the loop diuretic must be given at an effective dose for it to be effective. The combination of loop and distal collecting tubule diuretics has been shown to be effective through several mechanisms.[29] One is that distal collecting tubule diuretics have longer half-lives than loop diuretics and may thus prevent or attenuate postdiuretic NaCl retention. A second mechanism by which distal collecting tubule diuretics potentiate the effects of loop diuretics is by inhibiting Na^+ transport along the proximal tubule, insofar as most thiazide diuretics also inhibit carbonic anhydrase. They also inhibit NaCl transport along the distal renal tubule, which may counteract the increased solute resorptive effects of the hypertrophied and hyperplastic distal epithelial cells.

The selection of a distal collecting tubule diuretic to use as second diuretic is a matter of choice. Many clinicians choose metolazone because its half-life is longer than that of some other distal collecting tubule diuretics, and because it has been reported to remain effective even when the glomerular filtration rate is low. However, direct comparisons between metolazone and several traditional thiazides have shown little difference in natriuretic potency when they are included in a regimen with loop diuretics in HF patients.[30] Distal collecting tubule diuretics may be added in full doses (50 to 100 mg/day hydrochlorothiazide or 2.5 to 10 mg/day metolazone; see Table 50.6) when a rapid and robust response is needed. However, such an approach is likely to lead to excessive fluid and electrolyte depletion if patients are not followed up extremely closely. One reasonable approach to combination therapy is to achieve control of fluid overload by initially adding full doses of distal collecting tubule diuretic on a daily basis and then decreasing the dose of this diuretic to three times weekly to avoid excessive diuresis. An alternative strategy in hospitalized patients is to administer the same daily parenteral dose of a loop diuretic by continuous intravenous infusion, which leads to sustained natriuresis because of the continuous presence of high drug levels within the tubular lumen (see also Chapter 49), and avoids postdiuretic ("rebound") resorption of Na^+ (see Fig. 50.9C). This approach requires the use of a constant-infusion pump but permits more precise control of the natriuretic effect achieved over time, particularly in carefully monitored patients. It also diminishes the potential for a too-rapid decline in intravascular volume and hypotension as well as the risk of ototoxicity in patients given large bolus intravenous doses of a loop diuretic. A typical continuous furosemide is initiated with a 20- to 40-mg intravenous loading dose as a bolus injection, followed by a continuous infusion of 5 to 10 mg/hr for a patient who had been receiving 200 mg of oral furosemide per day in divided doses. The Diuretic Optimal Strategy Evaluation in Acute Heart Failure (DOSE) study showed that there was no significant difference in patient symptoms or renal function when patients with acute decompensated HF were treated by an IV bolus of furosemide compared to IV infusion of furosemide (see Chapter 49), suggesting that whichever approach is most likely to reliably produce the desired dieresis should be used.

Another common reason for diuretic resistance in advanced HF is the development of the cardiorenal syndrome (see also Chapters 49 and 101), which is recognized clinically as worsening renal function that limits diuresis in patients with obvious clinical volume overload.[31] In patients with advanced HF the cardiorenal syndrome is frequently present in patients who have repeated HF hospitalizations, and in whom adequate diuresis is difficult to obtain because of worsening indices of renal function. This impairment in renal function often is dismissed as "pre-renal"; however, when measured carefully, neither cardiac output nor renal perfusion pressure have been shown to be reduced in diuretic-treated patients who develop cardiorenal syndrome. Importantly, worsening indices of renal function contribute to longer hospital stays, and predict higher rates of early rehospitalization and death.[32] The mechanisms for and treatment of the cardiorenal syndrome remain poorly understood.

Device-Based Therapies for Management of Fluid Status (See also Chapter 58)

The use of mechanical methods of fluid removal, such as extracorporeal ultrafiltration (UF), may be needed to achieve adequate control of fluid retention, particularly in patients who become resistant and/or refractory to diuretic therapy. Extracorporeal UF removes salt and water isotonically by driving the patient's blood through a highly permeable filter via an extracorporeal circuit in an arteriovenous or venovenous mode. Alternative extracorporeal methods include continuous hemofiltration, continuous hemodialysis, or continuous hemodiafiltration. With slow continuous UF, the patient's intravascular fluid volume remains stable as fluid shifts from the extravascular space into the intravascular space, with the result that there is no deleterious activation of neurohormonal systems. UF has been shown to reduce right atrial and pulmonary artery wedge pressures and increase cardiac output, diuresis, and natriuresis without changes in heart rate, systolic blood pressure, renal function, electrolytes, or intravascular volume.[33]

The Relief for Acutely Fluid-Overloaded Patients With Decompensated Congestive Heart Failure (RAPID-CHF) trial, which was the first randomized controlled trial of UF for acute decompensated HF, enrolled 40 patients who were randomized to receive either usual care (diuretic) or a single 8-hour UF (using a proprietary device) in addition to usual care. The primary endpoint was weight loss 24 hours after enrollment. Fluid removal after 24 hours was approximately twofold greater in the UF group.[33] The Ultrafiltration versus IV Diuretics for Patients Hospitalized for Acute Decompensated Congestive Heart Failure (UNLOAD) compared the long-term safety and efficacy of UF therapy (using a proprietary device) to intravenous diuretics in a multicenter trial involving 200 patients, who were assessed at entry and at intervals out to 90 days. The primary endpoint of the trial was total weight loss during the first 48 hours of randomization and the change in dyspnea score during the first 48 hours of randomization. Although the two treatments were similar in their ability to relieve dyspnea, UF was associated with significantly greater fluid loss over 48 hours and a lower rate of rehospitalization during the next 90 days.[33] The use of UF in high-risk patients who are developing the cardiorenal syndrome was explored in the Cardiorenal Rescue Study in Acute Decompensated HF (CARRESS) trial, which showed that UF resulted in similar weight loss, but resulted in an increase in creatinine levels, compared to standard care, and was associated with more serious adverse events and intravenous catheter-related complications (see Chapter 49).[33]

Given the cost, need for venous access, and the nursing support necessary to implement UF, this intervention will require additional studies to determine its role in the management of volume overload in HF patients. In addition to extracorporeal methods for relieving volume overload, peritoneal dialysis can be used as a viable alternative therapy for the short-term management of refractory congestive symptoms for patients in whom vascular access cannot be obtained, or for whom appropriate extracorporeal therapies are not available.

PREVENTION OF DISEASE PROGRESSION (TABLE 50.7 AND FIG. 50.10)

Drugs that interfere with the excessive activation of renin angiotensin-aldosterone system and the adrenergic nervous system can relieve the symptoms of HFrEF patients by stabilizing and/or reversing LV remodeling (see Chapter 47). In this regard ACEIs/ARBs and beta-blockers have emerged as cornerstones of modern HF therapy for patients with a depressed EF (see Fig. 50.10).

Angiotensin-Converting Enzyme Inhibitors

There is overwhelming evidence that ACEIs should be used in symptomatic and asymptomatic patients with a reduced EF (<40%) (class I indication). ACEIs interfere with the renin angiotensin system by inhibiting the enzyme that is responsible for the conversion of angiotensin I to angiotensin II (see Chapter 47). However, because ACEIs also inhibit kininase II, they may lead to the upregulation of bradykinin, which may further enhance the effects of angiotensin suppression. ACEIs stabilize

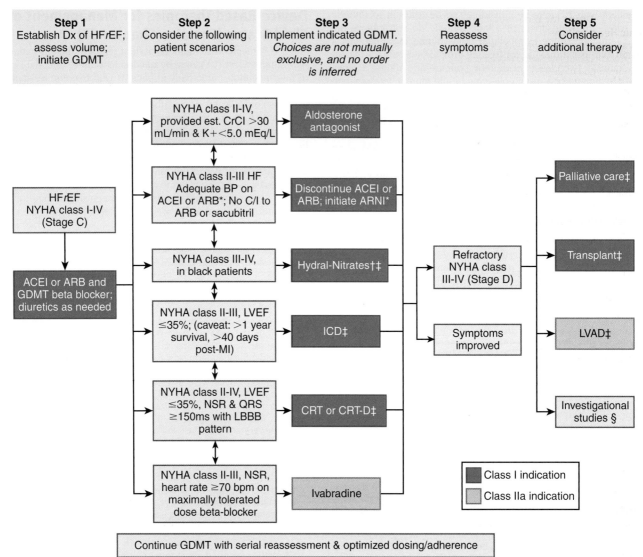

FIGURE 50.10 Treatment algorithm Stage C and D heart failure with a reduced ejection fraction. For all medical therapies, dosing should be optimized and serial assessment exercised. See text for details. (Key: *See text for important treatment directions. †**Hydral-Nitrates green box**: The combination of ISDN/HYD with ARNI has not been robustly tested. BP response should be carefully monitored. ‡See 2013 ACC/AH heart failure guidelines. §Participation in investigational studies is also appropriate for stage C, NYHA class II and III HF. *ACEI*, Angiotensin-converting enzyme inhibitor; *ARB*, angiotensin receptor blocker; *ARNI*, angiotensin receptor neprilysin inhibitor; *BP*, blood pressure; *bpm*, beats per minute; *C/I*, contraindication; *CrCl*, creatinine clearance; *CRT-D*, cardiac resynchronization therapy–device; *Dx*, diagnosis; *GDMT*, guideline-directed management and therapy; *HF*, heart failure; *HFrEF*, heart failure with reduced ejection fraction; *ICD*, implantable cardioverter-defibrillator; *ISDN/HYD*, isosorbide dinitrate hydral-nitrates; *K+*, potassium; *LBBB*, left bundle branch block; *LVAD*, left ventricular assist device; *LVEF*, left ventricular ejection fraction; *MI*, myocardial infarction; *NSR*, normal sinus rhythm; *NYHA*, New York Heart Association. (Modified from Yancy CW, Jessup M, Bozkurt B, et al. 2017 ACC/AHA/HFSA Focused Update of the 2013 ACCF/AHA Guideline for the Management of Heart Failure: A Report of the American College of Cardiology/American Heart Association Task Force on Clinical Practice Guidelines and the Heart Failure Society of America. *J Am Coll Cardiol.* 2017;70:776–803.)

LV remodeling, improve patient symptoms, prevent hospitalization, and prolong life. Because fluid retention can attenuate the effects of ACEIs, it is preferable to optimize the dose of diuretic first, before starting the ACEI. However, it may be necessary to reduce the dose of diuretic during the initiation of an ACEI, in order to prevent symptomatic hypotension. ACEIs should be initiated in low doses, followed by increments in dose if lower doses have been well tolerated. Titration is generally achieved by doubling doses every 3 to 5 days. The dose of ACEI should be increased until the doses used are similar to those that have been shown to be effective in clinical trials (see Table 50.7). Higher doses are more effective than lower doses in preventing hospitalization. For stable patients, it is acceptable to add therapy with beta-blocking agents before full target doses of either ACEIs are reached. Blood pressure (including postural changes), renal function, and potassium should be evaluated within 1 to 2 weeks after initiation of ACEIs, especially in patients with preexisting azotemia, hypotension, hyponatremia, diabetes mellitus, or in those taking potassium supplements. Abrupt withdrawal of treatment with an ACEI may lead to clinical deterioration

and should, therefore, be avoided in the absence of life-threatening complications (e.g., angioedema, hyperkalemia).

The efficacy of ACEIs has been consistently demonstrated in clinical trials with patients with asymptomatic and symptomatic LV dysfunction (Fig. 50.11).[9,15] These trials recruited a broad variety of patients, including women and the elderly, as well as patients with a wide range of causes and severity of LV dysfunction. The consistency of data from the Studies on Left Ventricular Dysfunction (SOLVD) Prevention Study, Survival and Ventricular Enlargement (SAVE), and the Trandolapril Cardiac Evaluation (TRACE) has shown that asymptomatic patients with LV dysfunction will have less development of symptomatic HF and hospitalizations (Table 50.8) when treated with an ACEI. ACEIs have also consistently shown benefit for patients with symptomatic LV dysfunction. As shown in Table 50.8, all placebo-controlled chronic HF trials have demonstrated a reduction in mortality. Further, the absolute benefit is greatest in patients with the most severe HF. Indeed, the patients with NYHA class IV HF in the Cooperative North Scandinavian Enalapril Survival Study (CONSENSUS I) had a much larger effect size than the SOLVD Treatment Trial, which in turn had a larger effect size than the SOLVD Prevention Trial. Although only three placebo-controlled mortality trials

TABLE 50.7 Drugs for the Prevention and Treatment for Chronic Heart Failure

	INITIATING DOSE	MAXIMAL DOSE
Angiotensin-Converting Enzyme Inhibitors		
Captopril	6.25 mg 3 times	50 mg 3 times
Enalapril	2.5 mg twice	10 mg twice
Lisinopril	2.5–5.0 mg once	20 mg once
Ramipril	1.25–2.5 mg once	10 mg once
Fosinopril	5–10 mg once	40 mg once
Quinapril	5 mg twice	40 mg twice
Trandolapril	0.5 mg once	4 mg once
Angiotensin Receptor Blockers		
Valsartan	40 mg twice	160 mg twice
Candesartan	4–8 mg once	32 mg once
Losartan	12.5–25 mg once	50 mg once
Angiotensin Receptor Neprilysin Inhibitor		
Sacubitril/Valsartan	24 mg/26 mg 2 times daily***	97 mg/103 mg 2 times daily***
Beta-Receptor Blockers		
Carvedilol	3.125 mg twice	25 mg twice (50 mg twice if >85 kg)
Carvedilol-CR	10 mg once	80 mg once
Bisoprolol	1.25 mg twice	10 mg once
Metoprolol succinate CR	12.5–25 mg qd	target dose 200 mg qd
Mineralocorticoid Receptor Antagonists		
Spironolactone	12.5–25 mg once	25–50 mg once
Eplerenone	25 mg once	50 mg once
Other Agents		
Combination of hydralazine/isosorbide dinitrate	25 to 50 mg/10 mg 3 times	100 mg/40 mg 3 times
Fixed dose of hydralazine/ isosorbide dinitrate	37.5 mg/20 mg (one tablet) 3 times	75 mg/40 mg (two tablets) 3 times
Digoxin*	0.125 mg qd	≤0.375 mg/day**
Ivabradine	5 mg twice daily	7.5 mg twice daily

*Dosing should be based on ideal body weight, age, and renal function.
**Trough level should be 0.5 to 1 ng/mL though absolute levels have not established.
***(mg sacubitril/mg valsartan).
Modified from Mann DL. Heart Failure and Cor Pulmonale, In: Kasper DL, et al., eds. *Harrison's Principles of Internal Medicine*. 17th ed. New York: McGraw-Hill; 2007:1449.

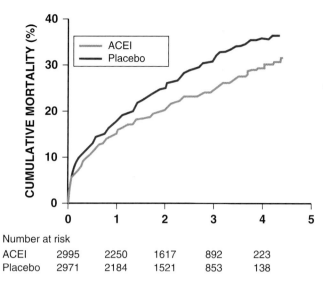

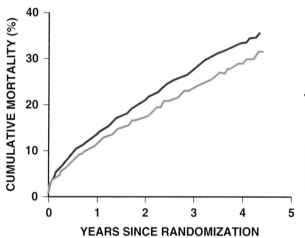

FIGURE 50.11 Meta-analysis of angiotensin-converting enzyme inhibitors (ACEI) in heart failure with reduced ejection fraction (HFrEF). **A,** Kaplan-Meier curves for mortality for patients with HF with a depressed EF treated with an ACEI following acute myocardial infarction (three trials). **B,** Kaplan-Meier curves for mortality for patients with HF with a depressed EF treated with an ACEI in five clinical trials, including post-infarction trials. The benefits of ACEI were observed early and persisted long term. (Modified from Flather MD, Yusuf S, Køber L, et al. Long-term ACE-inhibitor therapy in patients with heart failure or left-ventricular dysfunction: a systematic overview of data from individual patients. ACE-Inhibitor Myocardial Infarction Collaborative Group. *Lancet.* 2000;355:1575–1580.)

have been conducted in patients with chronic HFrEF, the aggregate data suggest that ACEIs reduce mortality in direct relation to the degree of severity of chronic HF. The Vasodilator in Heart Failure II (V-HeFT-II) trial provided evidence that ACEIs improve the natural history of HF through mechanisms other than vasodilation, inasmuch as subjects treated with enalapril had significantly lower mortality than subjects treated with the vasodilatory combination of hydralazine plus isosorbide dinitrate (which does not directly inhibit neurohormonal systems). Although enalapril is the only ACEI that has been used in placebo-controlled mortality trials in chronic HF, as shown in Table 50.8, multiple ACEIs have proven to be more or less equally effective when administered in oral form within the first week of the ischemic event in MI trials. ACEIs markedly enhance

survival in patients with signs or symptoms of HF after MI. In addition to these effects on mortality, ACEIs improve the functional status of patients with HF. In contrast, ACEIs only produce small benefits in exercise capacity. Taken together, these observations support the conclusion that the effects of ACEIs on the natural history of chronic HF, post-MI LV dysfunction, or patients at high risk of developing HF represent a "class effects" of these agents. Nonetheless, it should be emphasized that patients with a low blood pressure (<90 mm Hg systolic), or impaired renal function (serum creatinine >2.5 mg/mL) were not recruited and/or represent a small proportion of patients who participated in these trials. Thus, the efficacy of these agents for these latter patient populations is less well established.

Side Effects of Angiotensin-Converting Enzyme Inhibitor Use

The majority of the adverse effects of ACEIs are related to suppression of the renin angiotensin system. The decreases in blood pressure and mild azotemia often seen during the initiation of therapy are, in general, well tolerated and do not require a decrease in the dose of the ACEI. However, if hypotension is accompanied by dizziness or if the

TABLE 50.8 Mortality Rates in Placebo-Controlled Trials Conducted in Patients with Chronic Heart Failure (EF < 40%) or Patients with Acute Myocardial Infarction or at Risk for Heart Failure

TRIAL NAME	AGENT	NYHA CLASS	NO. OF SUBJECTS ENROLLED	12-MONTH PLACEBO MORTALITY (%)	12-MONTH EFFECT SIZE (%)	P VALUE 12 MONTHS (FULL F/U)
Angiotensin-Converting Enzyme Inhibitors *Heart Failure*						
CONSENSUS-1	Enalapril	IV	253	52	↓31	0.01 (0.0003)
SOLVD-Rx	Enalapril	I-III	2569	15	↓21	0.02 (0.004)
SOLVD-Asx	Enalapril	I, II	4228	5	0	0.82 (0.30)
Post–Myocardial Infarction						
SAVE	Captopril	—	2231	12	↓18	0.11 (0.02)
AIRE	Ramipril	—	1986	20	↓22	0.01 (0.002)
TRACE	Trandolapril	—	1749	26	↓16	0.046 (0.001)
Angiotensin Receptor Blockers *Heart Failure*						
VAL-HeFT	Valsartan	II-IV	5010	9	0	NS (0.80)
CHARM-Alternative	Candesartan	II-IV	2028	NS	NS	NS (0.02)
CHARM-Added	Candesartan	II-IV	2547	NS	NS	NS (0.11)
HEAAL	Losartan	II-IV	3846	NS	NS	NS (0.24)
Post–Myocardial Infarction						
VALIANT	Valsartan	—	14,703	19.5*	NS	NA (0.98)**
Angiotensin Receptor Neprilysin Inhibitors						
PARADIGM	Sacubitril/ Valsartan	II-IV	8442	NS	NS	NS(P < 0.001)
Mineralocorticoid Receptor Antagonists *Heart Failure*						
RALES	Spironolactone	III, IV	1663	24	↓25	NS (<0.001)
EMPHASIS	Eplerenone	II	2737	9	NS	NS (< 0.01)
Post–Myocardial Infarction						
EPHESUS	Eplerenone	I	6632	12	↓15	NS (0.005)
Beta-blockers *Heart Failure*						
CIBIS-I	Bisoprolol	III, IV	641	21	↓20***	NS (0.22)
U.S. Carvedilol	Carvedilol	II, III	1094	8	↓66***	NS (< 0.001)
ANZ—Carvedilol	Carvedilol	I,II,II	415	NS	NS	NS (> 0.1)
CIBIS-II	Bisoprolol	III, IV	2647	12	↓34***	NS (0.001)
MERIT-HF	Metoprolol CR	II-IV	3991	10	↓35***	NS (0.006)
BEST	Bucindolol	III, IV	2708	23	↓10***	NS (0.16)
COPERNICUS	Carvedilol	Severe	2289	28	↓38***	NS (0.0001)
Post–Myocardial Infarction						
CAPRICORN	Carvedilol	I	1959	NS	↓23*	NS (0.03)
BEAT	Bucindolol	I	343		↓12*	NS (0.06)

*In VALIANT the compactor group was enalapril; **Reflects differences between valsartan and enalapril; ***Effect size at the conclusion of the trial.

Note: Twelve-month mortality rates were taken from the survival curves when data were not directly available in published material.

AIRE, Acute Infarction Ramipril Efficacy; *BEAT,* bucindolol evaluation in acute myocardial infarction trial; *BEST,* Beta Blocker Evaluation of Survival Trial; *CAPRICORN,* Carvedilol Post-Infarct Survival Control in Left Ventricular Dysfunction; *CHARM,* candesartan in heart failure-assessment of reduction in mortality and morbidity; *CHF,* congestive heart failure; *CIBIS,* Cardiac Insufficiency Bisoprolol Study; *CONSENSUS,* Cooperative North Scandinavian Enalapril Survival Study; *COPERNICUS,* Carvedilol Prospective Randomized Cumulative Survival; *EPHESUS,* Eplerenone Post-Acute Myocardial Infarction Heart Failure Efficacy and Survival Study; *HEEAL,* Heart Failure Endpoint Evaluation of Angiotensin II Antagonist Losartan; *MERIT-HF,* Metoprolol CR/XL Randomized Interventional Trial in Congestive Heart Failure; *MI,* myocardial infarction; *MRAs,* mineralocorticoid receptor antagonists; *NS,* not specified; *NYHA,* New York Heart Association; *PARADIGM,* Prospective comparison of ARNI with ACEI to Determine Impact on Global Mortality and morbidity in Heart Failure trial; *RALES,* Randomized Aldactone Evaluation Study; *SAVE,* Survival and Ventricular Enlargement; *SOLVD,* Studies of Left Ventricular Dysfunction; *TRACE,* Trandolapril Cardiac Evaluation; *Val-HeFT,* Valsartan Heart Failure Trail; *VALIANT,* Valsartan in Acute Myocardial Infarction Trial.

Modified from Bristow MR, Linas S, Port DJ. Drugs in the treatment of heart failure. In: Zipes DP, et al., eds. *Braunwald's Heart Disease.* 7th ed. Philadelphia: Elsevier, 2004:573.

renal dysfunction becomes severe, it may be necessary to decrease the dose of the diuretic if significant fluid retention is not present, or alternatively decrease the dose of the ACEI if significant fluid retention is present. Potassium retention may also become problematic if the patient is receiving potassium supplements or a potassium-sparing diuretic. Potassium retention that is not responsive to these measures may require a reduction in the dose of ACEI. The side effects of ACEIs that are related to kinin potentiation include a nonproductive cough (10% to 15% of patients) and angioedema (1% of patients). In patients who cannot tolerate ACEIs because of cough or angioedema, ARBs are the next recommended line of therapy. Patients intolerant to ACEIs because of hyperkalemia or renal insufficiency are likely to experience the same side effects with ARBs. The combination of hydralazine and an oral nitrate should be considered for these latter patients (see Table 50.7).

Angiotensin Receptor Blockers

ARBs (see Table 50.7) are well tolerated in patients who are intolerant of ACEIs because of cough, skin rash, and angioedema and should, therefore, be used in symptomatic and asymptomatic patients with an EF less than 40% who are ACE intolerant for reasons other than hyperkalemia or renal insufficiency (class I indication). Although ACEIs and ARBs inhibit RAAS, they do so by a different mechanism. Whereas ACEIs block the enzyme responsible for converting angiotensin I to angiotensin II, ARBs block the effects of angiotensin II on the angiotensin type 1 receptor (see Chapter 47), the receptor subtype that is responsible for virtually all the adverse biological effects relevant to a angiotensin II on cardiac remodeling (see Chapter 47). Multiple ARBs are available to clinicians for the treatment of HFrEF. Three of these, losartan, valsartan, and candesartan, have been extensively evaluated in the setting of HFrEF (see Table 50.7). ARBs should be initiated with the starting doses shown in Table 50.7, which can be up-titrated every 3 to 5 days by doubling the dose of ARB. As with ACEIs, blood pressure, renal function, and potassium should be reassessed within 1 to 2 weeks after initiation and followed closely after changes in dose.

In symptomatic HFrEF patients who were intolerant to ACE inhibitors the aggregate clinical data suggest that ARBs are as effective as ACEIs in reducing HF morbidity and mortality. Candesartan significantly reduced all-cause mortality, cardiovascular death, or hospital admission in the Candesartan Heart Failure: Assessment of Reduction in Mortality and Morbidity trial (CHARM-Alternative Trial) (eFig. 50.3).[9,15] Importantly candesartan reduced all-cause mortality, irrespective of background ACE-inhibitor or beta-blocker therapy. Similar findings were shown with valsartan in the small subgroup of patients not receiving an ACE inhibitor in the Valsartan Heart Failure Trial (Val-Heft). A direct comparison of ACEI and ARBs was assessed in the Losartan Heart Failure Survival Study (ELITE-II), which showed that although losartan did not improve survival in elderly HF patients when compared to captopril, losartan was significantly better tolerated. The question of the impact of high-dose versus low-dose ARB antagonism in ACEI-intolerant patients was evaluated in the Heart Failure Endpoint Evaluation of Angiotensin II Antagonist Losartan (HEAAL) trial.[34] During 4.7 years of follow-up, high-dose losartan (150 mg daily) was superior to low-dose losartan (50 mg daily) for the composite outcome of death or admission for heart failure (HR 0.90; 95% CI 0.82 to 0.99; (p = 0.027). Although there were more side effects with high-dose losartan, these adverse events infrequently led to discontinuation of therapy, suggesting that up-titration of ARBs may confer clinical benefit in HFrEF patients.

One large trial evaluated ARB compared to ACEI in post-MI patients who developed LV dysfunction or signs of HF. The Valsartan in Acute Myocardial Infarction Trial (VALIANT) compared losartan, captopril, and the combination of the two agents on mortality in patients with MI complicated by LV systolic dysfunction, HF or both. During a follow-up period of 24.7 months, there was no significant difference in all-cause mortality in the valsartan group as compared with the captopril group (HR 1.00; 97.5 CI 0.90 to 1.11), nor was there a significant difference in all-cause mortality in the valsartan-captopril group when compared to the captopril group (HR 0.98; 97.5% CI 0.89 to 1.09; P = 0.73). Non-inferiority testing showed that valsartan was noninferior to captopril with respect to mortality (P = 0.004).[9,15] Two large HFrEF trials compared ACEI and ARB versus ACE inhibitor alone. In the CHARM-Added trial, the addition of candesartan to ACE inhibitor led to a reduction

in the primary outcome of CV death or HF hospitalization (HR 0.85; 95% CI: 0.75 to 0.96).[34] However, the addition of candesartan to an ACE inhibitor resulted in an increase in the incidence of hyperkalemia increased from 0.7% to 3.4%. The addition of valsartan to an ACEI had no beneficial effect on mortality in the Valsartan Heart Failure Trial (Val-HeFT) when compared to placebo, whereas the combined endpoint of mortality and morbidity was significantly (13.2%) lower with valsartan than with placebo because of a reduction in the number of patients hospitalized for HF.[34] The interpretation of both of these trials is confounded by the observation that the dose of ACEI in the placebo may have been suboptimal.

Although one meta-analysis suggests that ARBs and ACEIs have similar effects on all-cause mortality and HF hospitalizations,[35] and although ARBs may be considered as initial therapy rather than ACEIs following MI, the ACC/AHA/HFSA guidelines recommend that ACE inhibitors remain first line therapy (class I indication) for the treatment of HFrEF, whereas ARBs were recommended for ACE-intolerant patients (class IIa indication).[9,15] The guidelines also indicate that ARBs may be considered in persistently symptomatic patients with HFrEF who are already being treated with an ACE inhibitor and a beta-blocker in whom an aldosterone antagonist is not indicated or tolerated (class IIb indication).[9]

Side Effects of Angiotensin Receptor Blocker Use

Both ACEIs and ARBs have similar effects on blood pressure, renal function, and potassium. Therefore, the problems of symptomatic hypotension, azotemia, and hyperkalemia will be similar for both of these agents. Although less frequent that with ACEIs, angioedema has also been reported in some patients who receive ARBs. In patients who are intolerant to ACEIs and ARBs, the combined use of hydralazine and isosorbide dinitrate (H-ISDN) may be considered as a therapeutic option in such patients (see Table 50.7). However, compliance with this combination has generally been poor because of the large number of tablets required and the high incidence of adverse reactions.

Angiotensin Receptor Neprilysin Inhibitors

A new therapeutic class of agents that antagonize RAAS and inhibit the neutral endopeptidase system has been developed recently. The first-in-class therapeutic agent is a molecule that combines valsartan (an AT1 receptor antagonist) with sacubitril (a neprilysin inhibitor) in a 1:1 mixture. The combination of an ARNI slows the degradation of natriuretic peptides, bradykinin and adrenomedullin, thereby enhancing diuresis, natriuresis and myocardial relaxation, as well as inhibiting renin and aldosterone secretion., while selectively blocking the AT1-receptor reduces vasoconstriction, sodium, and water retention and myocardial hypertrophy (see Chapter 47).[36] In the Prospective comparison of ARNI with ACEI to Determine Impact on Global Mortality and morbidity in Heart Failure trial (PARADIGM-HF) trial,[37] the use of fixed dose sacubitril/valsartan resulted in striking reductions in all-cause mortality, cardiovascular mortality, and HF hospitalizations when compared with the use of an ACE inhibitor (enalapril) alone in patents with mild to moderate HF (NYHA class II to IV; LVEF ≤35%) (Fig. 50.12) that was characterized by either mildly elevated natriuretic peptide levels (BNP greater than 150 pg/mL or NT-proBNP ≥ 600 pg/mL), or a prior hospitalization in the preceding 12 months and elevated natriuretic peptide levels (BNP ≥100 pg/mL or NT-proBNP ≥400 pg/mL) who were also able to tolerate both a target dose of enalapril (10 mg twice daily) and then subsequently sacubitril/valsartan (200 mg twice daily). ARNIs should be administered in low doses (sacubitril 24 mg/valsartan 26 mg twice daily) in ACEI/ARB naïve patients, or at moderate doses (sacubitril 49 mg/valsartan 51 mg twice daily) in patients who are tolerating ACEIs/ARBs. The target dose of sacubitril/valsartan in PARADIGM-HF was 97/103 mg twice daily. Although the most recent update of the ACC/AHA/HFSA guidelines do not recommend starting HFrEF patients on ARNIs (see Fig. 50.10), in patients with chronic HFrEF NYHA class II or III who are tolerating an ACE inhibitor or an ARB, ARNIs are recommended as a replacement to further reduce morbidity and mortality (class I indication).[12] Given that less than 1% of the patients in the PARADIGM-HF had NYHA class IV HF, ARNIs are not currently recommended for patients with advanced HF symptomatology.

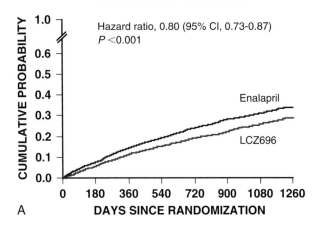

DEATH FROM CARDIOVASCULAR CAUSES OR HOSPITALIZATION FOR HF

Hazard ratio, 0.80 (95% CI, 0.73-0.87)
$P < 0.001$

A

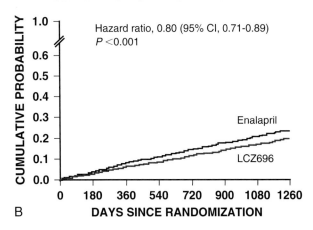

DEATH FROM CARDIOVASCULAR CAUSES

Hazard ratio, 0.80 (95% CI, 0.71-0.89)
$P < 0.001$

B

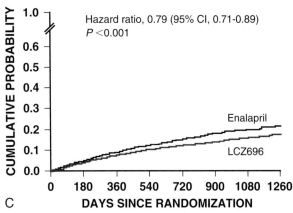

HOSPITALIZATION FOR HEART FAILURE

Hazard ratio, 0.79 (95% CI, 0.71-0.89)
$P < 0.001$

C

FIGURE 50.12 Kaplan-Meier analysis of outcomes in the PARADIGM trial. **A,** Death from cardiovascular causes or hospitalization for heart failure (the primary endpoint). **B,** Death from cardiovascular cause. **C,** Hospitalization for heart failure. (Modifed from McMurray JJ, Packer M, Desai AS, et al. Angiotensin-neprilysin inhibition versus enalapril in heart failure. *N Engl J Med.* 2014;317:993–1004.)

The LIFE trial (NCT02816736), which compared sacubitril/valsartan with valsartan in HFrEF patients with advanced chronic HF and NYHA class IV symptoms in the previous 3 months, showed that sacubitril/valsartan was not superior to valsartan in terms of lowering NT-proBNP.[38] The use of ARNIs in acute HF is discussed in Chapter 49.

Side Effects of Angiotensin Receptor Neprilysin Inhibitors

The use of an ARNI is associated with hypotension (approximately 14%), hyperkalemia (4%), cough (11%), and a very low-frequency incidence of angioedema. Oral neprilysin inhibitors, used in combination with ACE inhibitors, can lead to angioedema; accordingly, the concomitant use of ACEIs and ARNIs is contraindicated (class III recommendation). For patients who are switching from ACEIs to sacubitril/valsartan, the ACEI should be withheld for at least 36 hours before initiating sacubitril/valsartan in order to minimize the risk of angioedema caused by overlapping ACE and neprilysin inhibition. There are additional concerns about the effects of sacubitril/valsartan on the degradation of beta-amyloid peptide in the brain, which could theoretically accelerate amyloid deposition. The optimal titration and tolerability of ARNIs, particularly with regard to blood pressure and the adjustment of concomitant HF medications, will require addition clinical experience.

Beta-Blockers

Beta-blocker therapy represents a major advance in the treatment of HF patients with a depressed EF. Beta-blockers interfere with the harmful effects of sustained activation of the central nervous system, by competitively antagonizing one or more adrenergic receptors (α_1, β_1 and β_2). Although there are a number of potential benefits to blocking all three receptors, most of the deleterious effects of sympathetic activation are mediated by the β_1 adrenergic receptor.

The functional effects of beta-blocker therapy on the failing heart are biphasic. Administration of beta-blockers may be associated with an early, short-term deterioration in cardiac function, consistent with the negative inotropic effects of withdrawing adrenergic drive. However, when given in concert with ACE inhibitors, treatment with beta-blockers is associated with decrease in LV volumes (reverse LV remodeling), favorable changes in LV shape, as well as improved LVEF. From a clinical standpoint, this initial deterioration in LV function is generally not apparent if β-blocker therapy is initiated gradually and slowly up-titrated in patients who are relatively euvolemic. In the long term when given in concert with ACEIs, beta-blockers improve patient symptoms, prevent hospitalization, and prolong life. Therefore beta-blockers are indicated for patients with symptomatic or asymptomatic HF and a depressed EF less than 40% (class I indication). Three beta-blockers have been shown to be effective in reducing the risk of death in patients with chronic HF: bisoprolol and sustained-release metoprolol succinate both competitively block the β1 receptor, and carvedilol competitively blocks the α1, β1, and β2 receptors. Analogous to the use of ACEIs, beta-blockers should be initiated in low doses (see Table 50.7), followed by gradual increments in the dose if lower doses have been well tolerated. The dose of beta-blocker should be increased until the doses used are similar to those that have been reported to be effective in clinical trials (see Table 50.7). However, unlike ACEIs, which may be up-titrated relatively rapidly, the dose titration of beta-blockers should proceed no sooner than two-week intervals, because the initiation and/or increased dosing of these agents may lead to worsening fluid retention because of the abrupt withdrawal of adrenergic support to the heart and the circulation. Therefore, it is important to optimize the dose of diuretic before starting therapy with beta-blockers. If worsening fluid retention does occur, it is likely to occur within 3 to 5 days of initiating therapy, and will be manifest as increase in body weight and/or symptoms of worsening HF. The increased fluid retention can usually be managed by increasing the dose of diuretics. Patients need not be taking high doses of ACEIs before being considered for treatment with a beta-blocker, because most patients enrolled in the beta-blocker trials were not taking high doses of ACEIs. Furthermore, in patients taking a low dose of an ACEI, the addition of a beta-blocker produces a greater improvement in symptoms and reduction in the risk of death than an increase in the dose of the ACEI. Studies have shown that beta-blockers can be safely started before discharge, even in patients hospitalized for HF, provided that the patient is stable and does not require intravenous HF therapy. Contrary to early reports, the aggregate results of clinical trials suggest that beta-blocker therapy is well tolerated by the great majority of HF patients (>85%), including patients with comorbid conditions such as diabetes mellitus, chronic obstructive lung disease, and peripheral vascular disease. Nonetheless, there is a subset of patients (10% to 15%) who remain intolerant to beta-blockers because of worsening fluid retention or symptomatic hypotension.

The first placebo-controlled multicenter trial with a beta-blocking agent was the Metoprolol in Dilated Cardiomyopathy (MDC) trial, which used the shorter-acting tartrate preparation at a target dose of 50 mg three times a day in symptomatic HF patients with idiopathic dilated cardiomyopathy. Metoprolol tartrate at an average dose of 108 mg/day reduced the prevalence of the primary endpoint of death or need for cardiac transplantation by 34%, which did not quite reach statistical significance (p = 0.058). The benefit was due entirely to a reduction by metoprolol in the morbidity component of the primary endpoint, with no favorable trends in the mortality component of the primary endpoint. A more efficacious formulation of metoprolol was subsequently developed, metoprolol (succinate) CR/XL, which has a better pharmacologic profile than metoprolol tartrate because of its controlled-release profile and longer half-life. In the Metoprolol CR/XL Randomized Intervention Trial in Congestive Heart Failure (MERIT-HF), metoprolol CR/XL provided a significant relative risk reduction of 34% reduction in mortality in subjects with mild to moderate HF and moderate to severe systolic dysfunction when compared with the placebo group (Fig. 50.13, top).[9,15] Importantly, metoprolol CR/X reduced mortality from both sudden death and progressive pump failure. Further, mortality was reduced across most demographic groups, including older versus younger subjects, nonischemic versus ischemic etiology, and lower versus higher ejection fractions.

Bisoprolol is a second-generation β_1 receptor-selective blocking agent with approximately 120-fold higher affinity for human $\beta1$ versus $\beta2$ receptors. The first trial performed with bisoprolol was the Cardiac Insufficiency Bisoprolol Study I (CIBIS-I) trial, which examined the effects of bisoprolol on mortality in subjects with symptomatic ischemic or non-ischemic cardiomyopathy. CIBIS-I showed a nonsignificant (p = 0.22) 20% risk reduction for mortality at 2 years follow-up. Because the sample size for CIBIS-I was based on an unrealistically high expected event rate in the control group, a follow-up trial with more conservative effect size estimates and sample size calculations was conducted. In CIBIS-II bisoprolol reduced all-cause mortality by 32% (11.8% versus 17.3%, (p = 0.002), sudden cardiac death by 45% (3.6% versus 6.4%, (p = 0.001), HF hospitalizations by 30% (11.9% bisoprolol versus 17.6% placebo, (p < 0.001), and all-cause hospitalizations by 15% (33.6% versus 39.6%, (p = 0.002) (see Fig. 50.13, middle). The CIBIS-III trial addressed the important question of whether an initial treatment strategy using the beta-blocker bisoprolol was noninferior to a treatment strategy of using an ACEI (enalapril) first, among patients with newly diagnosed mild to moderate HF. The two strategies were compared in a blinded manner with regard to the combined primary endpoint of all-cause mortality or hospitalization, as well as with regard to each of the components of the primary endpoint individually. Although the per-protocol primary endpoint analysis of death or rehospitalization did not meet the prespecified criteria for noninferiority, the intent-to-treat analysis showed that bisoprolol was noninferior to enalapril (HR 0.94, 95% CI 0.77 to 1.16, (p = 0.019 for noninferiority). Although CIBIS-III did not provide clear-cut evidence to justify starting with a beta-blocker first, the overall safety profile of the two strategies was similar. Current guidelines continue to recommend starting with an ACEI first, followed by the addition of a beta-blocker.

Of the three beta-blockers that are approved for the treatment of HF, carvedilol has been studied most extensively (see Table 50.8). The phase III U.S. Trials Program, composed of four individual trials managed by single Steering and Data and Safety Monitoring Committee, was stopped prematurely because of a highly significant (p < 0.0001) 65% reduction in mortality with carvedilol that was observed across all four trials. This was followed by a second study, the Australia-New Zealand Heart Failure Research Collaborative Group Carvedilol Trial (ANZ-Carvedilol), which showed there was a significant improvement in LVEF (p < 0.0001) and a significant (p = 0.0015) reduction in LV end-diastolic volume index in the carvedilol-treated group at 12 months, as well a significant relative risk reduction of 26% in the clinical composite of death or hospitalization for the carvedilol group at 19 months. Rates of hospitalization were also significantly lower for patients treated with carvedilol (48%) compared to placebo (58%). The Carvedilol Prospective Randomized Cumulative Survival (COPERNICUS) study extended these benefits to patients with more advanced HF. In COPERNICUS patients with advanced HF symptoms had to be clinically euvolemic and have an LVEF less than 25%. When compared with placebo, carvedilol reduced the mortality risk at 12 months by 38% (see Table 50.8) and the relative risk of death or HF hospitalization by 31% (see Fig. 50.13, bottom). Carvedilol has also been evaluated in a post-MI trial which enrolled patients with LV dysfunction. The Carvedilol Post-Infarct Survival Controlled Evaluation (CAPRICORN) trial was a randomized, placebo-controlled trial designed to test the long-term efficacy of carvedilol on

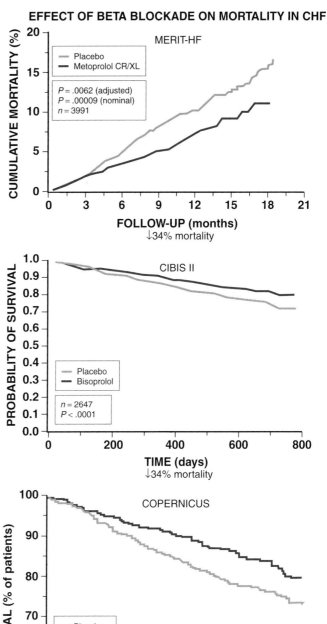

EFFECT OF BETA BLOCKADE ON MORTALITY IN CHF

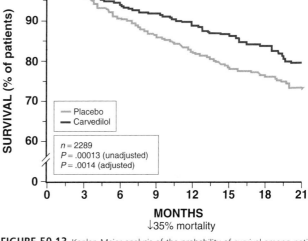

FIGURE 50.13 Kaplan-Meier analysis of the probability of survival among patients in the placebo and beta-blocker groups in the MERIT-HF (top), CIBIS II (middle), and COPERNICUS (bottom) trials. *CHF,* Chronic heart failure; *CI,* confidence interval. (Data from The Cardiac Insufficiency Bisoprolol Study II [CIBIS II]. *Lancet.* 1999;353:9–13; Metoprolol CR/XL randomized intervention trial in congestive heart failure [MERIT-HF]. *Lancet.* 1999;353:2001–2007; and Packer M, Coats AJS, Fowler MB, et al; for The Carvedilol Prospective Randomized Cumulative Survival Study Group. Effect of carvedilol on survival in severe chronic heart failure. *N Engl J Med.* 2001;344:1651–1658.)

morbidity and mortality in patients with LV dysfunction after MI who were already treated with ACEIs. Although carvedilol did not reduce the prespecified primary endpoint of mortality plus cardiovascular hospitalization, it did significantly reduce total mortality by 23% (p = 0.03), cardiovascular mortality by 25 % (p < 0.05), and nonfatal MI by 41% (p = 0.014). Finally, in the Carvedilol or Metoprolol European Trial (COMET) carvedilol (target dose 25 mg twice daily) was compared with immediate-release metoprolol tartrate (target dose 50 mg twice daily) with respect to the primary endpoint of all-cause mortality. In COMET carvedilol was associated with a significant 33% reduction in all-cause mortality when compared with metoprolol tartrate (33.9% versus 39.5%, HR 0.83, 95% CI 0.74 to 0.93, P = 0.0017).[9,15] Based on the results of the COMET trial, short-acting metoprolol tartrate is not recommended for use in the treatment of HF. The results of the COMET trial emphasize the importance of using doses and formulations of beta-blockers that have been shown to be effective in clinical trials. There have been no trials to ascertain whether the survival benefits of carvedilol are greater than those of metoprolol (succinate) CR/XL when both drugs are used at the appropriate target doses.

Not all studies with beta-blockers have been universally successful, suggesting that the effects of beta-blockers should not necessarily be viewed broadly as a class effect. Indeed, early studies with the first generation of nonspecific β_1 and β_2 receptors without ancillary vasodilating properties (e.g., propranolol) resulted in significant worsening of HF and death. The Beta Blocker Evaluation of Survival Trial (BEST) evaluated the third-generation beta-blocking agent bucindolol, which is a completely nonselective β_1 and β_2 blocker with some α_1 receptor blockade properties. Although the BEST trial showed that there was a nonsignificant (p = .10) 10% reduction in total mortality in the bucindolol-treated group, there was a statistically significant (p = 0.01) 19% reduction in mortality in white patients. The differential response of bucindolol in white patients has been suggested to be secondary to a polymorphism (Arginine 389) in the beta$_1$-adrenergic receptor that is more prevalent in white patients **(see the online supplement, Pharmacogenomics)**. Nebivolol is a selective β1 receptor antagonist with ancillary vasodilatory properties that are mediated, at least in part, by nitric oxide (NO). In the Study of Effects of Nebivolol Intervention on Outcomes and Rehospitalization in Seniors with Heart Failure (SENIORS), nebivolol significantly reduced the composite outcome of death or cardiovascular hospitalizations (HR: 0.86; 95% CI 0.74 to 0.99; (p < 0.04), which was the primary endpoint of the trial; however, nebivolol did not reduce mortality significantly. Although approximately 35% of the patients in SENIORS had an LVEF greater than 35%; more than half of these patients had an EF ranging from 35% to 50%, and thus would not be considered as HF with a midrange LVEF or HFpEF patients. Nebivolol is not FDA approved for the treatment of HFrEF.

Side Effects of Beta-Blockers

The adverse effects of beta-blockers are generally related to the predictable complications that arise from interfering with the adrenergic nervous system. These reactions generally occur within several days of initiating therapy, and are generally responsive to adjusting concomitant medications, as described above. Treatment with a beta-blocker can be accompanied by feelings of general fatigue or weakness. In most instances, the increased fatigue spontaneously resolves within several weeks or months; however, in some patients, it may be severe enough to limit the dose of beta-blocker or require the withdrawal or reduction of treatment. Therapy with beta-blockers can lead to bradycardia and/or exacerbate heart block. Moreover, beta-blockers (particularly those that block the α_1 receptor) can lead to vasodilatory side effects. Accordingly, the dose of beta-blockers should be decreased if the heart rate decreases to less than 50 beats/min and/or second- or third-degree heart block develops, or symptomatic hypotension develops. Continuation of beta-blocker treatment during an episode of acute decompensation is safe, although dose reduction may be necessary.[39] Beta-blockers are not recommended for patients with asthma with active bronchospasm.

Mineralocorticoid Receptor Antagonists

Although classified as potassium-sparing diuretics, MRAs that block the effects of aldosterone (e.g., spironolactone) have beneficial effects that are independent of the effects of these agents on sodium balance. Although ACEI may transiently decrease aldosterone secretion, with chronic therapy there is a rapid return of aldosterone to levels similar to those before ACEI, which is referred to as *aldosterone breakthrough.*[40] The administration of an MRA is recommended for patients with NYHA class II to IV HF who have a depressed EF (≤35%), and who are receiving standard therapy including diuretics, ACEIs, and beta-blockers (class I indication) (see Fig. 50.10).[41] The dose of aldosterone antagonist should be increased until the doses used are similar to those that have been shown to be effective in clinical trials (see

Table 50.7). Spironolactone should be initiated at a dose of 12.5 to 25 mg daily, and up-titrated to 50 mg daily, whereas eplerenone should be initiated as doses of 25 mg/day and increased to 50 mg daily (see Table 50.7). As noted above, potassium supplementation is generally stopped after the initiation of aldosterone antagonists, and patients should be counseled to avoid high-potassium foods. Potassium levels and renal function should be rechecked within 3 days and again at 1 week after initiation of an aldosterone antagonist. Subsequent monitoring should be dictated by the general clinical stability of renal function and fluid status but should occur at least monthly for the first 6 months.

The first evidence that MRAs could produce a major clinical benefit in HF was demonstrated by the Randomized Aldactone Evaluation Study (RALES) trial,[9,15] which evaluated spironolactone (25 mg/day initially, titrated to 50 mg/day for signs of worsening HF) versus placebo in NYHA class III or IV HF patients with a LVEF less than 35%, who were being treated with an ACEI, a loop diuretic, and, in most cases, digoxin. As shown in Figure 50.7A, spironolactone led to a 30% reduction in total mortality when compared with placebo (p = 0.001). The frequency of hospitalization for worsening HF was also 35% lower in the spironolactone group than in the placebo group. Although the mechanism for the beneficial effect of spironolactone has not been fully elucidated, prevention of extracellular matrix remodeling (see Chapter 47) and prevention of complications secondary to hypokalemia are plausible mechanisms. Although spironolactone was well tolerated in RALES, gynecomastia was reported in 10% of men who were treated with spironolactone, as compared with 1% of men in the placebo group (P < 0.001). The Eplerenone in Mild Patients Hospitalization and Survival Study in Heart Failure (EMPHASIS-HF) trial, which was performed in patients with NYHA class II HF with an EF less than 30% (or 35% if the QRS width was >130 msec), demonstrated that eplerenone (titrated to 50 mg/day) led to a significant 27% decrease in cardiovascular death or HF hospitalization (HR 0.63; 95% CI 0.54 to 0.74; P < 0.001) (see Fig. 50.7B).[9,15] There were also significant decreases in all-cause death (24%), cardiovascular death (24%), all-cause hospitalization (23%), and HF hospitalizations (43%). Importantly, the effect of eplerenone was consistent across all prespecified subgroups. In contrast to the RALES trial, which was conducted prior to the widespread adoption of beta-blockers, the background therapy for EMPHASIS-HF included ACEIs or ARBs and beta-blockers. The findings in RALES and EMPHASIS-HF are consistent with findings in randomized clinical trials in patients with acute MI and LV dysfunction. The Eplerenone Post-Acute Myocardial Infarction Heart Failure Efficacy and Survival Study (EPHESUS) evaluated the effect of eplerenone (titrated to a maximum of 50 mg/day) on morbidity and mortality among patients with acute MI complicated by LV dysfunction and HF. Treatment with eplerenone led to 15% decrease in all-cause death in the EPHESUS trial (RR 0.85; 95% CI 0.75 to 0.96; P = 0.008). Based on the results of the RALES and EMPHASIS-HF trials,[9,15] aldosterone antagonists are currently recommended for all patients with persistent NYHA class II to IV symptoms and an EF ≤35%, in addition to treatment with an ACEI (or an ARB if an ACEI is not tolerated) and a beta-blocker (class I indication).

Side Effects of Mineralocorticoid Receptor Antagonists

The major problem with the use of aldosterone antagonists is the development of life-threatening hyperkalemia, which is more prone to occur in patients who are receiving potassium supplements, or who have underlying renal insufficiency. Aldosterone antagonists are not recommended when the serum creatinine is greater than 2.5 mg/dL (or creatinine clearance is <30 mL/min) or serum potassium is greater than 5.5 mmol/L. The development of worsening renal function should lead to consideration regarding stopping aldosterone antagonists because of the potential risk of hyperkalemia. Painful gynecomastia may develop in 10% to 15% of patients who use spironolactone, in which case eplerenone may be substituted.

Renin Inhibitors

Aliskiren is an orally active direct renin inhibitor that appears to suppress RAS to a degree similar to ACE inhibitors.[42] Although the benefits of ACEIs and ARBs in HF have been clearly established, these agents provoke a compensatory increase in renin and downstream intermediaries of the renin-angiotensin-aldosterone system, which may attenuate the effects of ACEIs and ARBs ("aldosterone breakthrough"). Aliskiren is

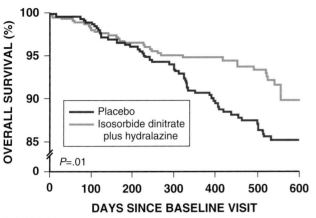

FIGURE 50.14 Kaplan-Meier analysis of the probability of survival among patients in the placebo and isosorbide dinitrate plus hydralazine treatment arms of the A-HeFT study. (Modified from Taylor AL, Ziesche S, Yancy C, et al. Combination of isosorbide dinitrate and hydralazine in blacks with heart failure. *N Engl J Med.* 2004;351:2050–2057.)

a nonpeptide inhibitor that binds to the active site (S1/S3 hydrophobic binding pocket) of renin, thereby preventing the conversion of angiotensinogen to angiotensin I (see Fig. 47.3). In the Aliskiren Observation of Heart Failure Treatment (ALOFT) trial[43] treatment with aliskiren significantly (p < 0.01) decreases NT-proBNP and urinary aldosterone excretion. Based on these promising early results, several large pivotal outcomes trials were initiated to determine whether adding aliskiren to standard HF therapy would improve clinical outcomes. However, both the Aliskiren Trial on Acute Heart Failure Outcomes (ASTRONAUT)[44] and the Efficacy and Safety of Aliskiren and Aliskiren/Enalapril Combination on Morbi-mortality in Patients With Chronic Heart Failure (ATMOSPHERE)[45] clinical trials failed to improve outcomes in HFrEF patients. Aliskiren is not currently recommended as an alternative to an ACEI, ARBs, or in combination with ACEIs for the treatment of HFrEF.

Combination of Hydralazine and Isosorbide Dinitrate

Therapy with the combination of H-ISDN has been shown to reduce all-cause mortality in African Americans. There are two placebo-controlled trials (V-HeFT-I and A-HeFT) and one active-controlled (V-HeFT) randomized trial with H-ISDN in HFrEF patients. In A-HeFT, a total 1050 self-identified African American HFrEF patients with NYHA class III to IV HF who were receiving standard medical therapy for HF were randomized to placebo or fixed dose H-ISDN. The primary endpoint was a weighted composite score of all-cause mortality, first hospitalization for HF, and quality of life. The study was terminated early because of a significantly higher mortality rate (10.2% versus 6.2%, P = 0.02) in the placebo group than in the H-ISDN treatment group (Fig. 50.14). The combination of H-ISDN is recommended (class

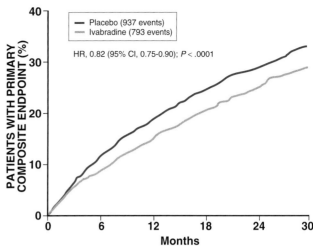

FIGURE 50.15 Kaplan-Meier cumulative event curves for the primary composite endpoint of cardiovascular death or hospitalization for worsening HF in patients treated with ivabradine compared to placebo. (Modified from Swedberg K, Komajda M, Böhm M, et al. Ivabradine and outcomes in chronic heart failure (SHIFT): a randomised placebo-controlled study. *Lancet.* 2010;376:875–885.)

I indication) for African Americans with NYHA class III to IV HFrEF who remain symptomatic despite concomitant use of ACE inhibitors, beta blockers, and aldosterone antagonists (see Fig. 50.10).[46] There is evidence to suggest that the combination of H-ISDN is beneficial as a first line therapy in non-African Americans with HFrEF, although this has never been tested formally in a clinical trial.[15] The combination of H-ISDN is used in patients who are intolerant to ACEI/ARBs/ARNIs (class IIa recommendation).

I_f-Channel Inhibitor

Ivabradine is a heart rate-lowering agent that acts by selectively blocking the cardiac pacemaker I_f ("funny") current that controls the spontaneous diastolic depolarization of the sinoatrial node. Ivabradine blocks I_f channels in a concentration-dependent manner by entering the channel pore from the intracellular side, and thus can only block the channel when it is open. The magnitude of I_f inhibition is directly related to the frequency of channel opening and would therefore be expected to be most effective at higher heart rates. Ivabradine was shown to improve outcomes in the Systolic Heart Failure Treatment with the I_f Inhibitor Ivabradine Trial (SHIFT), which enrolled symptomatic patients with an LVEF ≤35%, who were in sinus rhythm with heart rate ≥70 beats/min and on standard medical therapy for HF (including beta-blockers). In the SHIFT trial ivabradine (up-titrated to a maximal dosage of 7.5 mg twice daily) reduced the primary composite outcome of cardiovascular death or HF hospitalization by 18% (HR 0.82, 95% CI 0.75 to 0.90, (p < 0.0001) (Fig. 50.15). The composite

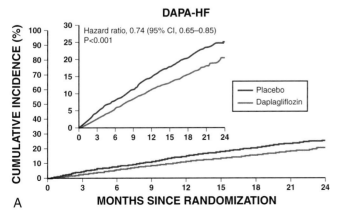

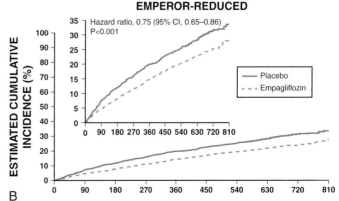

FIGURE 50.16 Kaplan-Meier Analysis of SGLT2 inhibitors in HFrEF patients. **A,** Effect of dapagliflozin on worsening heart failure or cardiovascular death in NYHA class II to IV HF patients with an LVEF of ≤40 in the DAPA-HF trial. **B,** Effect of empagliflozin on CV death or hospitalization for worsening heart failure in NYHA class II to IV HF patients with an LVEF of ≤40 in the EMPEROR-Reduced trial. *HF,* Heart failure; *HfrEF,* heart failure with reduced ejection fraction; *LVEF,* left ventricular ejection fraction; *NYHA,* New York Heart Association; *SGLT2,* sodium-glucose transporter-2. (**A** from McMurray JJV, Solomon SD, Inzucchi SE, et al. Dapagliflozin in Patients with Heart Failure and Reduced Ejection Fraction. *N Engl J Med.* 2019;381[21]:1995–2008; **B** from Packer M, Anker SD, Butler J, et al. Cardiovascular and Renal Outcomes with Empagliflozin in Heart Failure. *N Engl J Med.* 2020;383[15]:1413–1424.)

endpoint was driven primarily by reducing hospital admissions for worsening HF (HR 0.74, CI 0.66 to 0.83; (*p* < 0.0001), insofar as there was no decrease in cardiovascular deaths (HR 0.91; 95% CI 0.80 to 1.03), (*p* = 0.13) or all-cause deaths.[47] Given that ivabradine lowered heart rate by approximately 10 beats/min and that only 26% of the patients in the trial were on optimal doses of beta-blockers, it is possible that titrating beta-blockers to recommended disease may have reduced the HF hospitalizations to a similar degree. Ivabradine is recommended by the ACC/AHA/HFSA guidelines (class IIa recommendation) to reduce HF hospitalization in HFrEF patients in sinus rhythm with a HR greater than 70 beats/min who are receiving guideline-directed medical therapy (GDMT).

Sodium-Glucose Transporter-2 Inhibitors

Medicines in the SGLT2 class of inhibitors include canagliflozin, dapagliflozin, and empagliflozin. The landmark EMPA-REG OUTCOME (Empagliflozin Cardiovascular Outcome Event Trial in Type 2 Diabetes Mellitus Patients) demonstrated that empagliflozin reduced death from CV causes by 38%, hospitalization for HF by 35%, and progression to end-stage kidney disease in patients with type 2 DM and established CV disease (see also Chapter 31).[48] The question of whether SGLT2 inhibitors are beneficial in HFrEF patients without diabetes has been addressed in two large clinical trials, which showed that dapagliflozin (DAPA-HF) and empagliflozin (EMPEROR-Reduced) significantly reduced worsening HF and CV death in NYHA class II to IV HF patients (Fig. 50.16).[49,50]

> In the DAPA-HF trial (Effect of Dapagliflozin on the Incidence of Worsening Heart Failure or Cardiovascular Death in Patients With Chronic Heart Failure), 4744 patients with NYHA class II, III, or IV HF and an LVEF of ≤ 40% were randomized to receive either dapagliflozin (10 mg once daily) or placebo, in addition to GDMT.[49] The primary outcome was a composite of worsening HF (hospitalization or an urgent visit resulting in intravenous therapy for HF) or cardiovascular death. After a follow-up of 18.2 months, dapagliflozin was associated with a 26% reduction in risk (HR, 0.74; 95% CI, 0.59 to 0.83; p = 0.00001) (see Fig. 50.16A). Importantly, event rates for all the components of the composite outcome favored dapagliflozin; hospitalizations for worsening HF were reduced (HR 0.70; 95% CI, 0.59 to 0.83), as well as death from CV cause (HR 0.82; 95% CI 0.69 to 0.98). The outcomes were similar in patients with and without diabetes. Moreover, this benefit was consistent across all subgroups of background therapy and combinations of background therapy analyzed, with HRs ranging from 0.57 to 0.86 and no significant randomized treatment-by-subgroup interaction. There was no difference in a composite of worsening renal function. In the EMPEROR-Reduced (Empagliflozin outcome trial in Patients with Chronic Heart Failure With Reduced Ejection Fraction) trial 3730 patients with NYHA class II, III, or IV HF and an ejection fraction of LVEF of ≤ 40% were randomized to receive empagliflozin (10 mg once daily) or placebo, in addition to standard guideline-directed medical therapy. The primary outcome was a composite of CV death or hospitalization for worsening HF. After a median follow-up of 16 months, empagliflozin was associated with 25% reduction in risk (HR 0.75; 95% CI, 0.65 to 0.86; *P* < 0.001) (see Fig. 50.16B).[50] The primary outcome was similar in patients with or without diabetes. In contrast to DAPA-HF, the primary endpoint in EMPEROR-Reduced was driven by decreased HF hospitalization (HR, 0.70; 95% CI, 0.58 to 0.85); whereas there was no significant difference in CV mortality (HR 0.92; 95% CI, 0.75 to 1.12). Although the reasons for the discrepancy in CV outcomes between these two trials are not known, the patients in EMPEROR-Reduced had on average more severe HF than those in DAPA-HF, raising the possibility that SGLT2 inhibitors are less effective in advanced HF. Another important difference between EMPEROR-Reduced and DAPA-HF is that a composite renal outcome was significantly reduced with the use of empagliflozin, whereas it was not with dapagliflozin. At the time of this writing, neither the ACC/AHA/HFSA guidelines nor the European HF guidelines have provided recommendations with respect to the use of SGLT2 inhibitors in HFrEF. However, the Canadian Cardiovascular Society and the Canadian Heart Failure Society recommend the use of SGLT2 inhibitors in patients with mild or moderate HF who have an LVEF less than 40% or less to improve symptoms and quality of life and to reduce the risk of hospitalization and cardiovascular mortality.[51]

Soluble Guanylate Cyclase Stimulators

As discussed in Chapter 47, in HF there is an imbalance between oxidative stress and NO availability (see Fig. 47.4). The decrease in NO bioavailability contributes to the development of endothelial dysfunction, as well as LV dysfunction. Vericiguat is a novel oral soluble guanylate cyclase (see Fig. 47.6) stimulator that enhances the cyclic guanosine monophosphate (GMP) production pathway, by directly stimulating soluble guanylate cyclase activity, as well as sensitizing soluble guanylate cyclase to endogenous NO.[52] In the Vericiguat Global Study in Subjects with Heart Failure with Reduced Ejection Fraction (VICTORIA) trial, 5050 patients with chronic NYHA class II to IV HF and an LVEF less than 45% were randomized to receive vericiguat (target dose, 10 mg once daily) or placebo, in addition to GDMT.[52] The primary outcome was a composite of CV death or first hospitalization for HF. At 10.8 months of follow-up there were fewer CV death and HF hospitalizations in the vericiguat group than in the placebo group (HR 0.90; 95% CI 0.82 to 0.98; *P* = 0.02). There was, however, no significant difference in CV death in the vericiguat group when compared with the placebo group (HR 0.93; 95% CI 0.81 to 1.06). At the time of this writing, neither the ACC/AHA/HFSA guidelines nor the European HF guidelines have provided recommendations with respect to the use of vericiguat in HFrEF patients.

Myosin Activators

Cardiac myosin activators represent a new mechanistic class of therapeutic agents designed to increase myocardial contractility without increasing intracellular concentrations of cyclic adenosine monophosphate and calcium, and without increasing myocardial oxygen consumption, thus avoiding the major toxic effects of classic inotropic agents (see Chapter 49). Omecamtiv mecarbil is a small-molecule activator of myosin that prolongs myocardial systole by increasing the fraction of sarcomeric myosin molecules that are strongly bound to actin (see Chapter 46), thereby leading to increased myocardial force generation and increased contractility. Administration of omecamtiv mecarbil in patients with HFrEF results in dose-dependent increases in systolic ejection time, fractional shortening, stroke volume, and LVEF. In the Chronic Oral Study of Myosin Activation to Increase Contractility in Heart Failure (COSMIC-HF), a phase 2 trial, 448 patients with HFrEF were randomized to receive placebo or omecamtiv mecarbil (25 mg twice daily with pharmacokinetic-guided dose selection to 50 mg twice daily) for 20 weeks. In patients who received omecamtiv mecarbil, systolic ejection time and stroke volume both increased, while diastolic filing parameters were not worsened.[53] The GALACTIC-HF (Global Approach to Lowering Adverse Cardiac Outcomes Through Improving Contractility in Heart Failure trial [NCT02929329]), which enrolled 8200 patients with HFrEF, showed that treatment with omecamtiv mecarbil significantly reduced the composite of CV death or HF hospitalization and other urgent treatment for HF compared to placebo in patients treated with standard of care (HR 0.92; 95% CI 0.86 to 0.99; (p = 0.025).

MANAGEMENT OF PATIENTS WHO REMAIN SYMPTOMATIC

As noted above an ACEI/ARB or ARNI, a beta-blocker and MRAs should be standard background therapy for patients with HFrEF. However, the addition of an ARB to the combination of ACEI or MRA is not recommended in HFrEF patients because of the risk of hyperkalemia. Moreover, the combination of ARNI with an ACEI is not recommended because of the risk of angioedema. Additional pharmacologic therapy (polypharmacy) or device therapy (see below) should be considered in patients who have persistent symptoms or progressive worsening despite optimized therapy with evidence-based medical and device therapies. Digoxin is recommended for patients with symptomatic HFrEF to reduce hospitalizations despite receiving standard therapy, including ACEIs (or ARBs), ARNIs, beta-blockers, and MRA receptor antagonists (class IIa indication).

Cardiac Glycosides

Digoxin, first described by William Withering in 1775, is by far the oldest drug in the HF armamentarium. Digoxin and digitoxin are the most frequently used cardiac glycosides. Given that digoxin is most commonly used, and is the only glycoside that has been evaluated in placebo-controlled trials, there is little reason to prescribe other cardiac glycosides for the management of patients with chronic HF. Digoxin exerts its effects by inhibiting the sodium potassium adenosine trisphosphate (Na^+-K^+ ATPase) pump in cell membranes, including the sarcolemmal Na^+-K^+ ATPase pump of cardiac myocytes (see Chapters 46 and 47). Inhibition of Na^+-K^+ ATPase pump leads to an increase in intracellular calcium and hence increased cardiac contractility, which led to the suggestion that beneficial effects of digoxin were secondary to its inotropic properties. However, the more likely mechanism of digoxin in HF patients is to sensitize Na^+-K^+ ATPase activity in vagal afferent nerves, leading to an increase in vagal tone that counterbalances the increased activation of the adrenergic system in advanced HF. Digoxin also inhibits Na^+-K^+ ATPase activity in the kidney and may therefore blunt renal tubular resorption of sodium. Therapy with digoxin is commonly initiated and maintained at a dose of 0.125 to 0.25 mg daily. For the great majority of patients the dose should be 0.125 mg daily and the serum digoxin level should be less than 1.0 ng/mL, especially in elderly patients, patients with impaired renal function, and patients with a low lean body mass. Higher doses (e.g., digoxin >0.25 mg daily) are rarely used, and not recommended for the management of HF patients in sinus rhythm or who have atrial fibrillation (AF). Further details about digitalis, including details about mechanism of action, pharmacokinetics, and interaction with other commonly used drugs can be found in **the online supplement, Digoxin**.

Although clinicians have used cardiac glycosides to treat patients with chronic HF for well over 200 years, there is still considerable debate regarding the effectiveness of the cardiac glycosides in HF patients. Whereas small-and medium-sized trials conducted in the 1970s and 1980s yielded equivocal results, two relatively large digoxin withdrawal studies in the early 1990s, the Randomized Assessment of Digoxin and Inhibitors of Angiotensin-Converting Enzyme (RADIANCE) and the Prospective Randomized Study of Ventricular Function and Efficacy of Digoxin (PROVED), provided strong support for clinical benefit from digoxin.[15] In these studies, worsening HF and HF hospitalizations developed in more patients who were withdrawn from digoxin than in patients who were maintained on digoxin. Insofar as withdrawal studies are difficult to interpret with respect to efficacy of a given therapeutic agent, the Digoxin Investigator Group (DIG) trial was a prospective trial conducted to assess the role of digitalis in chronic HF. Although the DIG trial showed that digoxin had a neutral effect on the primary endpoint of mortality, digoxin reduced hospitalizations (including 30-day readmissions for HF),[15] and favorably affected the combined endpoints of death or hospitalization due to worsening HF. Data from the DIG trial indicated a strong trend (p = 0.06) toward a decrease in deaths secondary to progressive pump failure, which was offset by an increase in sudden and other nonpump failure cardiac deaths (p = 0.04). One of the most important findings to emerge from the DIG trial was that mortality was directly related to the digoxin serum level.[15] In men enrolled in the DIG trial, trough levels between 0.6 and 0.8 ng/mL were associated with decreased mortality, suggesting that trough levels of digitalis should be maintained between 0.5 and 1.0 ng/mL. There is also evidence that digoxin may be potentially harmful in women. In a post-hoc multivariable analysis of the DIG trial, digoxin was associated with a significantly higher risk (23%) of death from any cause among women, but not men, possibly because of the relatively lower body weights in women, who were prescribed doses of digoxin the basis of a nomogram rather than trough levels.[15] The DIG trial was conducted prior to the widespread use of β-blockers, and no large trial of digoxin in addition to contemporary GDMT with both ACE inhibitors and β-blockers has been performed.

Complications of Digoxin Use

The principal adverse effects of digoxin are (1) cardiac arrhythmias including heart block (especially in the elderly) and ectopic and reentrant cardiac rhythms, (2) neurologic complaints such as visual disturbances, disorientation, and confusion, and (3) gastrointestinal symptoms such as anorexia, nausea, and vomiting. As noted above, these side effects can generally be minimized by maintaining trough levels of 0.5 to 0.8 ng/mL. In patients with HF, overt digitalis toxicity tends to emerge at serum concentrations that are greater than 2.0 ng/mL; however, digitalis toxicity may occur with lower digoxin levels, particularly if hypokalemia or hypomagnesemia coexist. Oral potassium administration is often useful for atrial, AV junctional, or ventricular ectopic rhythms, even when the

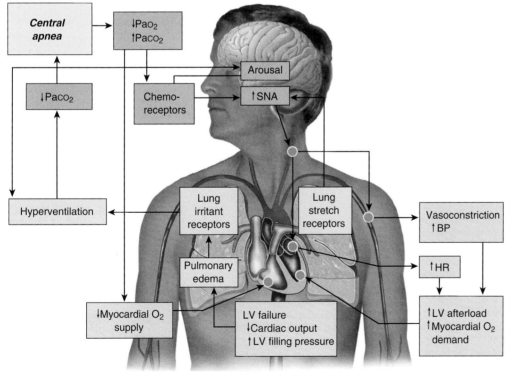

FIGURE 50.17 Pathophysiology of central sleep apnea and Cheyne-Stokes respiration in heart failure (HF). HF leads to increased left ventricular (LV) filling pressure. The resulting pulmonary congestion activates lung vagal irritant receptors, which stimulate hyperventilation and hypocapnia. Superimposed arousals cause further abrupt increases in ventilation and drive the partial pressure of carbon dioxide in arterial blood ($Paco_2$) below the threshold for ventilation, triggering a central apnea. Central sleep apneas are sustained by recurrent arousal resulting from apnea-induced hypoxia and the increased effort to breathe during the ventilatory phase because of pulmonary congestion and reduced lung compliance. Increased sympathetic activity causes increases in blood pressure (BP) and heart rate (HR) and increases myocardial oxygen (O_2) demand in the presence of reduced supply. *SNA*, Sympathetic nervous system activity; *Pao₂*, partial pressure of oxygen in arterial blood. (Redrawn from Bradley TD, Floras JS. Sleep apnea and heart failure. Part II: Central sleep apnea. *Circulation.* 20003;107:1822.)

serum potassium is in the normal range, unless high-grade AV block is also present. However, serum K⁺ levels must be monitored carefully to avoid hyperkalemia, especially in patients with renal failure or taking aldosterone receptor antagonists. Potentially life-threatening digoxin toxicity can be reversed by antidigoxin immunotherapy using purified Fab fragments (see online supplement for details). The concomitant use of quinidine, verapamil, spironolactone, flecainide, propafenone, and amiodarone can increase serum digoxin levels and may increase the risk of adverse reactions (see online supplement). Patients with advanced heart block should not receive digitalis unless a pacemaker is in place.

N-3 Polyunsaturated Fatty Acids

There is a large body of experimental evidence suggesting that n-3 polyunsaturated fatty acids (PUFA) have favorable effects on inflammation, including a reduction of endothelial activation and production of inflammatory cytokines, platelet aggregation, autonomic tone, blood pressure, heart rate, and LV function. The Gruppo Italiano per lo Studio della Sopravvivenza nell'Insufficienza cardiaca-Heart Failure (GISSI-HF) showed that long-term administration of 1 g/day of omega n-3 PUFA resulted in a significant reduction in both all-cause mortality (adjusted HR 0.91; 95.5% CI 0.83 to 0.99; p = 0.041) and all-cause mortality and cardiovascular admissions (adjusted HR 0.92; 99% CI 0.850 to 0.999; p = 0.009), in all the predefined subgroups, including HF patients with nonischemic cardiomyopathy.[54] The most recent ACC/AHA/HFSA and ESC guidelines endorse the use of n-3 PUFAs as adjunctive therapy (class IIa indication) for HFrEF patients who are receiving optimal evidence-based medical therapy.[9]

PHARMACOGENOMICS/PERSONALIZED MEDICINE

As discussed in Chapter 9, *pharmacogenomics* is the study of how genetic variations affect drug response, including genetic variants of enzymes that metabolize drugs, variants in drug receptors or drug transporters, as well as drug targets. These variations can result in gain or loss of therapeutic efficacy, influence optimal drug dosing of a drug, or favor alternative drug treatment. Given the tremendous heterogeneity that exists in HF patients, it is likely that genetic variations play a significant role in determining drug metabolism, disposition, and functional activity in HF patients. Recent advances in the field of pharmacogenetics suggest an analysis of underlying gene polymorphism in disease-causing pathways may one day enable clinicians to develop personalized therapeutic regimens for HF patients. Indeed, polymorphisms have been identified in the genes that appear to influence the therapeutic efficacy of ACEIs, beta-blockers, nitrates, and diuretics. An overview of the major genetic variations in these pathways, and the proposed functional impact of these polymorphisms, is presented in the online supplement, Pharmacogenomics.

Personalized medicine seeks to use genetic information to "personalize" and improve diagnosis, prevention, and therapy. The personalized management of HF involves a large spectrum of potential applications, from diagnosis of monogenic disorders (see Chapters 52 to 54) to prevention and management strategies based on modifier genes, as well as to pharmacogenomics. However, the major challenge in applying pharmacogenomics to everyday clinical practice in patients with HFrEF is the absence of robust clinical data that supports the differential utilization of neurohormonal antagonists in the management of HFrEF patients with specific gene polymorphisms.[55] Indeed, all of the extant pharmacogenomic analyses in HFrEF have come from post-hoc, retrospective analyses of clinical trial data or from observational patient series studies, rather than prospective outcomes studies that have randomized HFrEF patients to a pharmacogenomic-guided therapy versus standard of care. The study Genetically Targeted Therapy for the Prevention of Symptomatic Atrial Fibrillation in Patients With Heart Failure (GENETIC-AF) enrolled patients with paroxysmal or persistent AF, HF, and an LVEF less than 50%.[56] Patients who had a specific genotype for the beta-1 adrenergic receptor (β1389 Arg/Arg genotype) were randomized to bucindolol or metoprolol succinate. The primary endpoint was a composite outcome of all-cause mortality or recurrent AF or atrial flutter at 24 weeks. The trial also incorporated a unique adaptive design that permitted patients to be transitioned into phase III clinical trial, if an interim analysis suggested benefit of bucindolol. At 24 weeks event rates for the bucindolol group (54%) were similar to those of the metoprolol group (53%), with a HR of 1.01 (95% CI: 0.71 to 1.42). However, when GENETIC-AF patients were divided between those with HRrEF (LVEF <40%) and those with HF with a midrange EF (HFmrEF), there was a reduction of approximately 60% in the primary endpoint of recurrent AF/flutter or all-cause mortality for patients with HFmrEF, which was not observed in patients with HFrEF.[56] The PRECISION-HF trial will evaluate the effect of bucindolol in HF patients with a β1389 Arg/Arg genotype and an LVEF ≥40% and ≤55%.

MANAGEMENT OF ATHEROSCLEROTIC DISEASE

The clinical evaluation of atherosclerotic cardiovascular heart disease in HF patients is discussed in Chapter 48. In patients with a prior MI and HF without angina, the use of ACEIs and beta-blockers has been shown to decrease the risk of reinfarction and death. Although the role of aspirin in HF patients of ischemic etiology has not been clearly established in randomized trials, and remains controversial because of the concern that aspirin may attenuate the beneficial effects of ACEI, long-term treatment with an antiplatelet agents, including aspirin (75 to 81 mg), is recommended for patients with HF due to ischemic etiology, regardless of whether they are receiving ACEIs.[57] Alternative antiplatelet agents (e.g., clopidogrel) may not interact adversely with ACEIs and may have superior effects in preventing clinical events; however, their ability to favorably affect outcomes in HF has not been demonstrated. Both beta-blockers and ivabradine (in selected patients) are effective for controlling angina in HFrEF patients.[58]

Although coronary artery bypass grafting (CABG) has not been shown to improve cardiac function or symptoms, or prevent reinfarction or death in HF patients without angina, CABG has been shown to improve symptoms and survival in patients with modestly reduced EF and angina. The Surgical Treatment for Ischemic Heart Failure (STICH) trial showed that CABG did not reduce all-cause death (HR 0.86 [95% CI 90.7 to 1.04]; *P* = .12), which was the primary endpoint of the trial; CABG did, however, reduce the composite endpoint of cardiovascular death, death from any cause, or hospitalization for cardiovascular causes (HR for CABG 0.74 [95% CI, 0.64 to 0.85]; *P* < 0.001), which was a prespecified secondary analysis. The 10-year follow-up to the original STICH trial demonstrated a significantly lower mortality in patients who underwent CABG when compared to medical therapy. The results of STICH suggest that CABG is beneficial in HF patients of ischemic etiology, who are otherwise suitable for surgery. Although the data are less robust, percutaneous coronary intervention (PCI) may be considered as an alternative to CABG in patients unsuitable for surgery. Current ACC/AHA/HFSA guidelines (class I indication) recommend revascularization with CABG or PCI for HFrEF patients on appropriate medical therapy, who have angina and suitable coronary anatomy for revascularization, especially left main stenosis (>50%) or left main equivalent disease.

MANAGEMENT OF VALVULAR DISEASE

Functional mitral regurgitation secondary to LV dysfunction and LV remodeling in HFrEF is powerful predictor of adverse clinical outcomes. Two randomized clinical trials have examined percutaneous mitral valve repair (PMVR) using the MitraClip closure device in addition to GDMT in HFrEF patients with moderate to severe mitral regurgitation. The MitraClip device for Severe Functional/ Secondary Mitral Regurgitation (MITRA-FR) did not demonstrate any improvement in the composite of death from any cause or unplanned hospitalization for HF at 12 months (OR 1.16; 95% CI, 0.73 to 1.84; $P = 0.53$), whereas the Cardiovascular Outcomes Assessment of the Mitra-Clip Percutaneous Therapy for Heart Failure Patients with Functional Mitral Regurgitation (COAPT) trial showed a significant decrease in all hospitalizations for HF (HR 0.53; 95% CI 0.40 to 0.70; $P < 0.001$). In the COAPT trial, death from any cause (prespecified secondary outcome) within 24 months occurred in significantly fewer patients in the device group when compared to the control group (HR 0.62; 95% CI 0.46 to 0.82; $P < 0.001$). Importantly, these two trials differed with respect to patient characteristics and outcome definitions and duration of follow-up. At the time of this writing the ACC/AHA/HFSA and European Society of Cardiology have not provided guidelines for the use of PMVR in HFrEF.

SPECIAL POPULATIONS

Women (see also Chapter 91)

Although women account for a significant proportion of the growing HF epidemic, they have been poorly represented in clinical trials. Women with HF are more likely to be older (see Fig. 48.1), have a preserved ejection fraction (see Chapter 51) and nonischemic etiology for their HF. Although some studies have reported that HF outcomes are worse for women with than for men, the aggregate data suggest that women have a survival advantage when they develop HF. Although the explanation for this observation is unclear, it may be related to gender differences in etiology for HF. Nonetheless, while women appear to have a survival advantage after the diagnosis of HF, they experience increased morbidity, with worse equality of life, and have increased depression. Moreover, women are at increased risk of developing HF following acute MI.[59] Pooled analysis of several large-scale prospective clinical trials with β-blockers and ACEIs suggest that these agents provide similar survival benefits in women with reduced ejection fraction as in men.[59]

Race/Ethnicity

Epidemiologic and clinical trial data have raised awareness of potential areas of concern regarding the evaluation and treatment of HF in specific racial and ethnic groups. The efficacy of pharmacologic treatments in such subgroups is somewhat controversial, because there have been so few randomized clinical trials of HF treatment that have prespecified a subgroup analysis of outcomes stratified by race or ethnicity, that also have sufficient numbers of subjects for meaningful statistical analysis. Several retrospective analyses have highlighted that differences between African American and white populations in response to some standard HF therapies. Unfortunately, few data exist for Hispanic and Asian HF populations. Retrospective analyses from SOLVD and the V-HeFT trials suggested that African Americans do not benefit from ACEIs. In contrast, post-hoc analysis of studies with approved beta-blockers have found that African American patients benefit, although the magnitude of the effect appears to be diminished.[60] As noted above, the use of The H-ISDN was associated with a significant 43% reduction in the rate of death from any cause in the A-HeFT trial (see Fig. 50.14) and a significant 33% relative reduction in the rate of first hospitalization for HF. The mechanism for the beneficial effect of the hydralazine isosorbide regimen may be related to

an improvement in NO bioavailability; however, the combination therapy group also had a small (but significant) effect on blood pressure lowering.

Elderly Persons (see also Chapter 90)

As noted at the outset, the prevalence of HF increases with age (see Fig. 48.1) and is the most common reason for hospitalization in elderly patients. Of note, the presentation of HF may differ in elderly patients with HF. Although they commonly present with the classic symptoms of dyspnea and fatigue, the elderly are more likely than younger patients to present with atypical symptoms such as altered mental status, depression, or poor executive functioning.[6] The therapeutic approach to HF with a reduced EF in the elderly should be, in principal, identical to that in younger patients with respect the choice of pharmacologic therapy. However, altered pharmacokinetic and pharmacodynamic properties of cardiovascular drugs in the elderly may require that these therapies be applied more cautiously, with reductions in drug dosages when appropriate (see also Chapter 90). Other complicating factors may include, blunting of baroreceptor function, and orthostatic dysregulation of blood pressure, which may make it difficult to use target doses of some neurohormonal antagonists. Multidisciplinary HF programs have been successful in decreasing the rate of readmission and associated morbidity in elderly patients (see below).

Patients with Cancer

Patients with cancer are particularly predisposed to the development of HF as a result of the cardiotoxic effects of many cancer chemotherapeutic agents. The management of these patients is discussed in Chapters 56 and 57.

ANTICOAGULATION AND ANTIPLATELET THERAPY

Patients with HF have an increased risk for arterial or venous thromboembolic events. In clinical HF trials the rate of stroke ranges from 1.3% to 2.4%/yr. Depressed LV function is believed to promote relative stasis of blood in dilated cardiac chambers with increased risk of thrombus formation. Thromboembolism prophylaxis in patients with HF and AF should be individualized and based on an assessment of the risk of stroke versus the risk of bleeding on an anticoagulant. In general most patients with HFrEF will have an increased risk of stroke, as assessed by a variety of risk scores (e.g., Cardiac failure, Hypertension, Age ≥75 (Doubled), Diabetes, Stroke (Doubled)-Vascular disease, Age 65 to 74 and Sex category (Female) [CHA2DS2-VASc]). A recent meta-analysis of clinical trials in patients with nonvalvular AF suggests that, when compared to warfarin, novel oral anticoagulants (NOACs) have a favorable risk-benefit profile, with significant reductions in stroke, intracranial hemorrhage, and mortality, and with similar major bleeding as for warfarin, but increased gastrointestinal bleeding.[61] Other studies have suggested comparable efficacy but fewer major bleeding events. On the basis of these studies, the ESC HF guidelines recommend NOACs, recognizing that their safety in older subjects and subjects with impaired renal function is not known.[9] Anticoagulation is also recommended for all patients with a history of systemic or pulmonary emboli, including stroke or transient ischemic attack. Patients with symptomatic or asymptomatic ischemic cardiomyopathy and documented recent large anterior MI or recent MI with documented LV thrombus should be treated with warfarin (goal INR 2.0 to 3.0) for the initial 3 months after MI unless there are contraindications. The question of whether HF patients who are in sinus rhythm should be treated with anticoagulants to reduce stroke was addressed in the Warfarin Versus Aspirin in Reduced Cardiac Ejection Fraction (WARCEF) trial, which showed that treatment with warfarin as compared with aspirin did not reduce the composite outcome of time to ischemic stroke, intracerebral hemorrhage, or death from any cause (HR 0.93; 95% CI, 0.79 to 1.10, P = 0.40).[62] Although treatment with warfarin was associated with a significant reduction in the rate of ischemic stroke (HR 0.52; 95% CI, 0.33 to 82; P = 0.005), this benefit was offset by a significant increase in the rate of major hemorrhage. Interestingly, the rates of intracerebral and intracranial hemorrhage did not differ significantly between the two treatment groups. Based on the results of the WARCEF trial, there is no compelling reason to use warfarin rather than aspirin in HF patients with a reduced LVEF who are in sinus rhythm.

MANAGEMENT OF CARDIAC ARRHYTHMIAS

AF is the most common arrhythmia in HF (see also Chapters 65 and 66), and occurs in 15% to 30% of patients. AF may lead to worsening HF symptoms (see Table 50.5), and increases the risk of thromboembolic complications, particularly stroke. The Atrial Fibrillation and Congestive Heart Failure (AF-CHF) trial tested rate control versus rhythm control in patients with chronic HFrEF (EF <35%) and a history of AF. In AF-CHF a strategy of rhythm control (pharmacologic or electrical cardioversion) was superior to a strategy of controlling ventricular rate with respect to reducing death from cardiovascular causes (HR rhythm-control group 1.06; 95% CI 0.86 to 1.30; P = 0.59).[63] Secondary outcomes were also similar in the rate and rhythm control groups, including death from any cause, stroke, worsening HF, and the composite of death from cardiovascular causes, stroke, or worsening HF.[63] Accordingly, a rhythm-control strategy is best suited for patients with a reversible secondary cause of AF, or in patients who are not amenable to a rate strategy. For control of heart rate in HFrEF patients with AF, beta-blockers are preferred over digoxin, insofar as digoxin does not provide rate control during exercise. Although the effectiveness of beta-blockers in HFrEF patients with coexisting AF was cast in doubt by a patient-level meta-analysis, a recent substudy of the AF-CHF trial showed that the use of beta-blockers was associated with significantly lower mortality, but no difference in CV and non-CV hospitalization in patients with HFrEF and AF. The mortality reduction was not altered by the type of AF (i.e., paroxysmal or persistent) or the proportion of time spent in AF.[64] Importantly, the combination of digoxin and a beta-blocker is more effective than a beta-blocker alone in controlling the ventricular rate at rest. When beta-adrenergic blockers cannot be used, amiodarone has been used by some physicians, but chronic use has potentially significant risks, including thyroid disease and lung toxicity (see below). The short-term intravenous administration of diltiazem or amiodarone has been used for the acute treatment of patients with AF with very rapid ventricular response; however, the negative inotropic effects of nondihydropyridine calcium channel blockers such as diltiazem and verapamil must be considered if these agents are used. The optimum control of ventricular rate in patients with HF and AF is unclear at present. Although a resting ventricular response of 60 to 80 beats/min and a ventricular response between 90 and 115 beats/min during moderate exercise has been suggested by some experts, the RACE II study (Rate Control Efficacy in Permanent Atrial Fibrillation: a Comparison between Lenient versus Strict Rate Control II) did not show a difference in a composite of clinical outcomes when a strategy of strict rate control (<80 beats/min at rest and <110 beats/min during a 6 minute walk) was compared with lenient rate control.[65] Recognizing that sustained tachycardia can lead to a cardiomyopathy, AV node ablation and cardiac resynchronization (CRT) have been suggested for control of ventricular rate (<100 to 110 beats/min) in extreme cases of a rapid ventricular response with AF.[9]

Most antiarrhythmic agents, with the exception of amiodarone and dofetilide, have negative inotropic effects and are proarrhythmic. Amiodarone is a class III antiarrhythmic that has little or no negative inotropic and/or proarrhythmic effects and is effective against most supraventricular arrhythmias (see also Chapter 66). Amiodarone is the preferred drug for restoring and maintaining sinus rhythm and may improve the success of electrical cardioversion in patients with HF. Amiodarone increases the level of phenytoin and digoxin, and will prolong the INR in patients taking warfarin. Therefore it is often necessary to reduce the dose of these drugs by as much as 50% when initiating therapy with amiodarone. The risks of adverse events, such as hyperthyroidism, hypothyroidism, pulmonary fibrosis, and hepatitis are

relatively low, particularly when lower doses of amiodarone are used (100 to 200 mg/day). Dronedarone is a novel antiarrhythmic drug that reduces the incidence of AF and atrial flutter and has electrophysiologic properties that are similar to those of amiodarone, but does not contain iodine, and thus does not cause iodine-related adverse reactions. Although dronedarone was significantly more effective than placebo in maintaining sinus rhythm in several studies, the ANDROMEDA trial (European Trial of Dronedarone in Moderate to Severe Congestive Heart Failure) had to be terminated prematurely because of a twofold increase in mortality (HR 2.13; 95% CI 1.07 to 4.25; P = .167) in the dronedarone-treated HF patients.[66] The excess mortality was predominantly related to worsening of HF. As a result of this study dronedarone is contraindicated in patients with class IV HF, or those with class II or III HF who have had a recent HF decompensation. Because of the risk of proarrhythmic effects of antiarrhythmic agents in patients with LV dysfunction, it is preferable to treat ventricular arrhythmias with implantable cardioverter-defibrillators (ICDs), either alone or in combination with amiodarone (see also Chapter 69).

Two randomized clinical trials in HFrEF patients have demonstrated a reduction in all-cause mortality and hospitalizations with catheter ablation for AF. The AATAC (Ablation versus Amiodarone for Treatment of Atrial Fibrillation in Patients With Congestive Heart Failure and an Implanted ICD/CRTD) trial showed that catheter ablation of AF was superior to amiodarone in terms of achieving freedom from AF at long-term follow-up (primary endpoint) and reducing unplanned hospitalization and mortality (secondary endpoint RR 0.55; 95% CI 0.39 to 0.76).[67] The CASTLE-AF (Catheter Ablation versus Standard Conventional Treatment in Patients with Left Ventricular Dysfunction and Atrial Fibrillation) trial showed that catheter ablation reduced death from any cause or hospitalization for worsening HF (primary endpoint) in NYHA class II to IV HFrEF patients (HR 0.62; 95% CI 0.43 to 0.87; P = 0.007) with symptomatic paroxysmal or persistent AF.[68]

DEVICE THERAPY

Cardiac Resynchronization

CRT is discussed in detail in Chapters 58 and 69. When CRT is added to optimal medical therapy in patients in sinus rhythm there is a significant decrease in patient mortality and hospitalization, a reversal of LV remodeling, as well as improved quality of life and exercise capacity (see Chapter 58).[9,46] CRT should be considered for patients in NYHA class II to IV HF with a depressed EF less than 30% to 35% and a wide QRS who are on GDMT, and may be considered in select patients with NYHA class I HF with a wide QRS. For eligible patients, consideration should be given for implantation of CRT with an ICD (CRT-ICD).

Implantable Cardioverter-Defibrillators

ICDs are discussed in detail in Chapters 58, 69, and 70. Briefly, the prophylactic implantation of ICDs in patients with mild to moderate HF (NYHA class II to III) has been shown to reduce the incidence of sudden cardiac death in patients with ischemic or nonischemic cardiomyopathy (see Chapters 58 and 69). Accordingly, implantation of an ICD should be considered for patients in NYHA class II to III HF with a depressed EF less than 30% to 35%, who are on are on GDMT, and who have a reasonable expectation of survival with a good functional status for more than 1 year (class I indication). CRT-ICD should be considered for NYHA class IV patients.

SLEEP-DISORDERED BREATHING

The general topic of sleep disorders in cardiovascular disease is discussed in detail Chapter 89. HF patients with a reduced EF (<40%) commonly exhibit sleep-disordered breathing: approximately 40% of patients exhibit central sleep apneas (CSA), commonly referred to as Cheyne-Stokes breathing (see also Chapter 48); whereas another 10% exhibit obstructive sleep apneas (OSA). CSA associated with Cheyne-Stokes respiration is a form of periodic breathing in which central apneas and hypopneas alternate with periods of hyperventilation that have a waxing-waning pattern of tidal volume. Risk factors for the development of CSA in an HF patient include male gender, age older than 60 years, the presence of AF, and hypocapnia.[69] Figure 50.17 illustrates the proposed mechanisms that underlie periodic oscillations in ventilation in HF, including heightened sensitivity to arterial partial pressure and long circulation time. The main clinical significance of CSA in HF is its association with increased mortality. Whether this is simply because Cheyne-Stokes respiration with central sleep apnea is a reflection of advanced disease with poor LV function, or whether its presence constitutes a separate and additive adverse influence on outcomes is not clear. This statement notwithstanding, multivariate analyses suggest that central sleep apnea remains an independent risk factor for death or cardiac transplantation, even after controlling for potentially confounding risk factors. The potential mechanism(s) for adverse outcomes in HF patients with CSA may be attributed to marked neurohumoral activation (especially norepinephrine). Studies have suggested that Cheyne-Stokes respirations can resolve with proper treatment of HF. However, if the patient continues to have symptoms related to sleep-disordered breathing for the treatment of nocturnal hypoxemia in OSA, despite optimization of HF therapies, a comprehensive overnight sleep study-polysomnography is indicated.

Although current guidelines recommend that continuous positive airway pressure (CPAP) may be reasonable to improve sleep quality and daytime sleepiness in patients with OSA,[12] there is no consensus as to how CSA should be treated. Insofar as CSA is to some extent a manifestation of advanced HF, the first consideration is to optimize drug therapy, including aggressive diuresis to lower cardiac-filling pressure, along with the use of ACEIs/ARBs, ARNIs, beta-blockers and MRAs, which may lessen the severity of CSA. In some cases, however, metabolic alkalosis arising from diuretic use may predispose to CSA by narrowing the difference between the circulating $Paco_2$ level and the $Paco_2$ threshold that is necessary for apnea to develop. The use of nocturnal oxygen and devices that provide CPAP has been reported to alleviate CSA, abolish apnea-related hypoxia, decrease nocturnal norepinephrine levels, as well as producing symptomatic and functional improvement in HF patients when used in the short term (up to 1 month). However, the effects of supplemental oxygen on cardiovascular endpoints over more prolonged periods have not been assessed. Although there is no direct evidence that treatment of sleep-disturbed breathing prevents the development of HF, treatment with CPAP has been shown to improve LV structure and function in patients with either obstructive or central sleep apnea disturbed-breathing syndrome.[69] Despite these objective measurements of improvement with CPAP, this treatment modality did not lead to a prolongation of life in the Canadian Continuous Positive Airway Pressure for Patients with Central Sleep Apnea and Heart Failure (CANPAP) trial,[69] which was discontinued early after concerns about the early divergence of transplantation-free survival favoring the control group. There was no difference in the primary endpoint of death or transplantation (p = 0.54), nor was there a significant difference in the frequency of hospitalization between groups (0.56 vs. 0.61 hospitalizations per patient year, (p = 0.45). However, a post-hoc analysis of the CANPAP study suggested that adequate suppression of CSA by CPAP was associated with improved heart transplant–free survival.[69] The role of adaptive servo-ventilation (ASV), which alleviates CSA by delivering servo-controlled inspiratory pressure support on top of expiratory positive airway pressure, was evaluated in the SERVE-HF trial (Treatment of Sleep-Disordered Breathing with Predominant Central Sleep Apnea by Adaptive Servo Ventilation in Patients with Heart Failure).[70] In patients with HFrEF (LVEF ≤ 45%) who predominantly had CSA, ASV had no effect on the primary endpoint, which was a time-to-event analysis of the first event of death from any cause, lifesaving cardiovascular intervention (cardiac transplantation, implantation of a ventricular assist device, resuscitation after sudden cardiac arrest, or appropriate lifesaving shock), or unplanned hospitalization for worsening HF. However, all-cause mortality (HR 1.28 [95% CI, 1.06 to 1.55]; P = 0.01) and cardiovascular mortality (HR 1.34 [95% CI, 1.09 to 1.65]; p = 0.006) were significantly higher in the ASV group than in the control group. Therefore, ASV is not recommended in patients with NYHA class II to IV HFrEF and predominantly CSA (Level III: harm[12]). Thus, the data remain unclear whether elimination of apnea will lead to improved clinical outcomes. Other therapies that have been proposed for sleep-disordered breathing in HF include nocturnal oxygen, CO_2 administration (by adding dead space), theophylline, and acetazolamide and diaphragmatic pacing; these have not yet been systematically studied in outcome-based prospective randomized trials (see Chapter 89).

DISEASE MANAGEMENT

Despite the compelling scientific evidence that ACEIs/ARBs, beta-blockers, and aldosterone antagonists reduce hospitalizations and mortality in patients with HF, these life-prolonging therapies continue to be underutilized outside of the highly artificial environment of clinical trials. Indeed, numerous studies in a variety of different clinical settings have documented that a significant proportion of patients with HF are not receiving treatment with guideline-recommended, evidence-based therapies. The failure to deliver optimal medical care to HF patients is almost certainly multifactorial, as it is with other complex chronic conditions that have substantial morbidity and mortality. Further, the elderly nature of many HF patients, who often have a myriad of comorbidities, also presents special challenges to health care providers. Optimal HF care includes a trained network of healthcare providers involved in the delivery of HF management and interventions, including nurses, case managers, physicians, pharmacists, case workers, dietitians, physical therapists, psychologists, and information systems specialists; a method for communicating this knowledge to the patient, including patient education, education of caregivers and family members, medication management, peer support, or some form of post-acute care; and a method of ensuring that the patient has received and understood the knowledge; a system for encouraging adherence to the recommended regimen and monitoring patient compliance (Fig. 50.18). Numerous studies have shown that many of the challenges to delivering optimal care to HF patients can be met through an integrated specialized HF clinic approach that uses nurse and physician extenders to deliver and ensure the implementation of care. Technology-driven strategies that employ low-cost telemonitoring also appear promising in terms of improving HF management and outcomes (see also Chapter 58)[71]; however, the optimum approach to noninvasive remote monitoring is uncertain and the data from randomized clinical trials have been inconsistent, and so these strategies are not recommended by current practice guidelines.

A disease management approach to HF has been shown to reduce hospitalizations and increase the percentage of patients receiving ideal, guideline-recommended therapy. Recent studies demonstrate that disease management programs need not be confined to the outpatient setting and that hospital-based disease management systems can also improve medical care and education of hospitalized HF patients and accelerate use of evidence-based, guideline-recommended therapies by administering them before hospital discharge.[41] Although disease management strategies can lead to improved survival, it is not clear that these strategies are necessarily more cost effective. Accordingly, the biggest challenge to disease management programs will be to determine how to support the additional personnel required in this model of care.

PATIENTS WITH REFRACTORY END-STAGE HEART FAILURE (STAGE D)

Most patients with HFrEF respond well to evidenced-based pharmacologic and nonpharmacologic treatments and enjoy a good quality of life with a meaningful prolongation of life. However, for reasons that are not clear, some patients do not improve or will experience a rapid recurrence of symptoms despite optimal medical and device therapies. These individuals represent the most advanced stage of HF (stage D) and should be considered for specialized treatment strategies, such as mechanical circulatory support (see Chapter 59), continuous intravenous positive inotropic therapy, or referral for cardiac transplantation (see Chapter 60). However, before a patient is considered to have refractory HF, physicians should identify any contributing conditions (see Table 50.5) and ensure that all conventional medical strategies have been optimally employed. When no further therapies are appropriate, the focus of disease management should shift to palliation of symptoms.

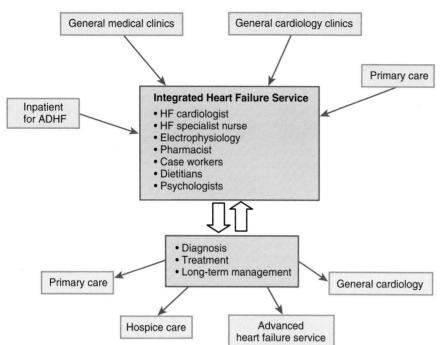

FIGURE 50.18 Integrated disease management program in heart failure. (Modified from McDonagh TA. Lessons from the management of chronic heart failure. *Heart.* 2005;91[suppl 2]:ii24–ii27.)

INTEGRATION OF PALLIATIVE CARE INTO HEART FAILURE CARE

Ideally, patients should continue to be cared for by a team of health care providers with whom they have established a longitudinal relationship, and who apply palliative care principles (Table 50.9). Palliative care is designed to improve quality of life for patients and their families through anticipation of declining health status and major events, clarification of goals of care, relief of physical symptoms, provision of psychosocial and spiritual support, coordination of care, and assistance with bereavement (Fig. 50.19).[72] The high prevalence, morbidity, and lethality of HF creates a substantial need for palliative care at the end of life. However, many providers of cardiovascular care do not distinguish between palliative care and hospice, nor do they understand the indications for these services. Palliative approaches to care should be integrated throughout the care of patients with cardiovascular disease, with intensification during major events and approaching the end of life.

Primary Palliative Care

All clinicians caring for patients with advanced cardiovascular disease play a role in the provision of supportive and palliative interventions. This role is vital insofar as (1) many of the therapies that improve symptoms and quality of life derive from treatment of the underlying cardiovascular disease; (2) prognosis and complex decisions are often best understood by the cardiovascular specialist; (3) integrated care is often preferable to further fragmentation through another consult team; and (4) there are not enough palliative care specialists to provide such services to everyone in need. Provision of supportive care by the usual care team has been designated as "primary" palliative care, to distinguish it from "secondary" or "subspecialty" palliative care.[73] Clinicians supervising inpatient or longitudinal care for patients with cardiovascular disease should regard expertise in providing palliative care as integral to their professional competence.

Hospice

The term *hospice* is used to describe a specific model of palliative care that is offered to patients who are at the end of life with a terminal disease when curative or life-prolonging therapy is no longer a focus of

treatment. Historically, hospice was developed for patients with cancer, but it is increasingly used for patients with cardiovascular disease, with 14.7% of admissions to US hospices in 2014 having a primary diagnosis of heart disease. In the United States, referral is guided by the Centers for Medicare and Medicaid Services (CMS) hospice eligibility guidelines, which require that a physician estimate that life expectancy is 6 months or less.[74] While the 6-month time period is rarely reached, patients who survive beyond it can usually continue to receive hospice benefits if the prognosis remains poor.

Treatment of Symptoms Approaching End of Life

Progressive symptoms are the most common reason for reductions in health status among patients with HF. Indeed, symptom burden at the end of life is often greater than for patients with advanced lung or pancreatic cancer.[75] Accordingly, the design of the cardiovascular regimen and general palliative approaches are critical near the end of life. The best treatment to relieve late-stage cardiac symptoms is often continuation of the regimen that was initiated to decrease progression from earlier stages of disease. The primary treatment of symptomatic congestion remains diuretic therapy. Supplementation with oral, sublingual, or topical nitrates can temporarily help redistribute volume when adequate diuresis cannot be achieved. If symptoms relate to diuretic resistance or hypotension, decrease or discontinuation of neurohormonal antagonists may improve comfort by enhancing diuretic response and

TABLE 50.9 Key Messages for Managing Patients with Cardiovascular Disease Nearing End of Life

1. Worsening disease should trigger preparation with patients and families, but without specifically answering the question of how much time remains, which is usually bounded by wide uncertainty.

2. "What-if" conversations should be standard prior to any major intervention in the setting of advanced cardiac disease or other serious medical conditions, including frailty.

3. Difficult discussions now will simplify difficult decisions in the future.

4. Shared decisions include a broad spectrum of potential interventions beyond those relating to resuscitation preferences.

5. Deactivation of the defibrillation function of ICDs should be explained and offered regularly to patients with poor prognosis and must be done before transition to hospice.

6. Palliative care specialist consultation may be particularly helpful to facilitate decision making within challenging family dynamics and to improve relief of refractory symptoms.

7. Clinicians with existing relationships should shoulder the primary responsibility for presenting an end-of-life plan consistent with values and goals expressed by patient and family.

8. The transition separating "Do Everything" from hospice may be bridged through a phase of "Quality Survival" during which time patients increasingly weigh the benefits, risks, and burdens of initiating or continuing life-sustaining treatments.

9. Revision of the medical regimen for symptom relief and quality of life may involve discontinuation of some recommended therapies and addition of therapies not usually recommended.

10. The end-of-life plan should honor patient preference for site of death as feasible, with agreement upon a "Plan B" if that becomes unsupportable.

From Allen LA, Stevenson LW. Management of patients with cardiovascular disease approaching end of life. In: Zipes DP, Libby P, Bonow RO, et al., eds. *Braunwald's Heart Disease.* 11th ed. Elsevier; 2019:590.

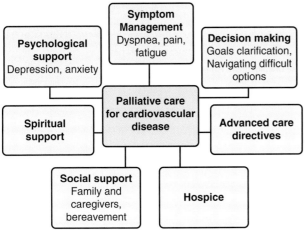

FIGURE 50.19 Components of palliative care for end-stage heart failure. (From Allen LA, Stevenson LW. Management of patients with cardiovascular disease approaching end of life. In: Zipes DP, Libby P, Bonow RO, et al., eds. *Braunwald's Heart Disease.* 11th ed. Elsevier; 2019:590.)

increasing systemic blood pressure **(eTable 50.1)**. Although discontinuation of these agents is associated with worsening HF over time in stable patients, it is unlikely to worsen cardiac function or symptoms in the final days of life. Caution is required in certain situations; for example, withdrawal of beta-blockers may worsen symptom burden in patients with frequent angina or tachyarrhythmias. Relaxation of chronic sodium and fluid restriction often worsens symptoms of congestion; but favorite foods and beverages can be a major factor in quality of life and social interaction for some patients at a time when few other shared pleasures remain. Further discussion of treatment strategies is presented in **the online supplement, End of Life Care.**

FUTURE PERSPECTIVES

As discussed in the foregoing chapter treatment with ACEIs/ARBs, beta-blockers, MRAs, and cardiac devices has substantially improved quality and quantity of life for patients with HFrEF. Moreover, recent success with the use of ARNIs and SGLT2 inhibitors has opened up the possibility of combining traditional neurohormonal approaches with additional drugs, whose mode of action is not completely understood. Ongoing approaches with small molecules that modulate contractility and gene therapy, accompanied by growing appreciation of the role of pharmacogenomics (see Chapter 7), will undoubtedly lead to further advances in the field.

REFERENCES
Etiology and Prognosis
1. Bocchi EA. Heart failure in South America. *Curr Cardiol Rev.* 2013;9(2):147–156.
2. Walsh CR, Larson MG, et al. Alcohol consumption and risk for congestive heart failure in the Framingham Heart Study. *Ann Intern Med.* 2002;136(3):181–191.
3. McMurray JJ, Adamopoulos S, Anker SD, et al. ESC guidelines for the diagnosis and treatment of acute and chronic heart failure 2012: the task force for the diagnosis and treatment of acute and chronic heart failure 2012 of the European Society of Cardiology. Developed in collaboration with the Heart Failure Association (HFA) of the ESC. *Eur Heart J.* 2012;33:1787–1847.
4. Go AS, Mozaffarian D, Roger VL, et al. Heart disease and stroke statistics—2013 update: a report from the American Heart Association. *Circulation.* 2013;127(1):e6–e245.
5. Yancy CW. Heart failure in African Americans. *Am J Cardiol.* 2005;96(7B):3i–12i.
6. Thomas S, Rich MW. Epidemiology, pathophysiology, and prognosis of heart failure in the elderly. *Heart Fail Clin.* 2007;3(4):381–387.
7. Jaffe AS, Miller WL. Meta-analyses and interpretation of troponin values in heart failure. *JACC Heart Fail.* 2018;6(3):198–200.
8. von HS, Anker MS, Jankowska EA, et al. Anemia in chronic heart failure: can we treat? What to treat? *Heart Fail Rev.* 2012;17(2):203–210.
9. Ponikowski P, Voors AA, Anker SD, et al. 2016 ESC Guidelines for the diagnosis and treatment of acute and chronic heart failure: the task force for the diagnosis and treatment of acute and chronic heart failure of the European Society of Cardiology (ESC)Developed with the special contribution of the Heart Failure Association (HFA) of the ESC. *Eur Heart J.* 2016;37:2129–2200.
10. Fitzsimons S, Doughty RN. Iron deficiency in patients with heart failure. *Eur Heart J Cardiovasc Pharmacother.* 2015;1(1):58–64.
11. von Haehling S, Ebner N, Evertz R, et al. Iron deficiency in heart failure. *An Overview.* 2019;7(1):36–46.

Approach to the Patient and Management
12. Yancy CW, Jessup M, Bozkurt B, et al. 2017 ACC/AHA/HFSA focused update of the 2013 ACCF/AHA guideline for the management of heart failure: a report of the American College of Cardiology/American Heart Association Task force on clinical practice guidelines and the Heart Failure Society of America. *Circulation.* 2017;136(6):e137–e161.

13. Cole RT, Masoumi A, Triposkiadis F, et al. Renal dysfunction in heart failure. *Med Clin North Am.* 2012;96(5):955–974.
14. Kelly RB. Microtubules, membrane traffic, and cell organization. *Cell.* 1990;61:5–7.
15. Yancy CW, Jessup M, Bozkurt B, et al. 2013 ACCF/AHA guideline for the management of heart failure: a report of the American College of Cardiology Foundation/American Heart Association Task Force on Practice Guidelines. *Circulation.* 2013;128:e240–e327.
16. Ledwidge M, Gallagher J, Conlon C, et al. Natriuretic peptide-based screening and collaborative care for heart failure: the STOP-HF randomized trial. *J Am Med Assoc.* 2013;310(1):66–74.
17. Dias A, Nunez Gil IJ, Santoro F, et al. Takotsubo syndrome: state-of-the-art review by an expert panel - part 1. *Cardiovasc Revasc Med.* 2019;20(1):70–79.
18. Yancy CW, Jessup M, Bozkurt B, et al. 2017 ACC/AHA/HFSA focused update of the 2013 ACCF/AHA guideline for the management of heart failure: a report of the American College of Cardiology/American Heart Association Task Force on Clinical Practice Guidelines and the Heart Failure Society of America. *J Am Coll Cardiol.* 2017;70(6):776–803.
19. O'Connor CM, Whellan DJ, Lee KL, et al. Efficacy and safety of exercise training in patients with chronic heart failure: HF-ACTION randomized controlled trial. *J Am Med Assoc.* 2009;301(14):1439–1450.
20. Faris RF, Flather M, Purcell H, et al. Diuretics for heart failure. *Cochrane Database Syst Rev.* 2012;2:CD003838.
21. Ellison DH, Felker GM. Diuretic treatment in heart failure. *N Engl J Med.* 2017;377(20):1964–1975.
22. Filippatos G, Anker SD, Bohm M, et al. A randomized controlled study of finerenone vs. eplerenone in patients with worsening chronic heart failure and diabetes mellitus and/or chronic kidney disease. *Eur Heart J.* 2016;37(27):2105–2114.
23. Cherney DZ, Odutayo A, Aronson R, et al. Sodium glucose cotransporter-2 inhibition and cardiorenal protection. *J Amer Coll Cardiol.* 2019;74(20):2511–2524.
24. Finley JJ, Konstam MA, Udelson JE. Arginine vasopressin antagonists for the treatment of heart failure and hyponatremia. *Circulation.* 2008;118(4):410–421.
25. Konstam MA, Gheorghiade M, Burnett Jr JC, et al. Effects of oral tolvaptan in patients hospitalized for worsening heart failure: the EVEREST Outcome Trial. *J Am Med Assoc.* 2007;297(12):1319–1331.
26. Juurlink DN, Mamdani MM, Lee DS, et al. Rates of hyperkalemia after publication of the randomized Aldactone evaluation study. *N Engl J Med.* 2004;351(6):543–551.
27. Pitt B, Bakris GL, Bushinsky DA, et al. Effect of patiromer on reducing serum potassium and preventing recurrent hyperkalaemia in patients with heart failure and chronic kidney disease on RAAS inhibitors. *Eur J Heart Fail.* 2015;17(10):1057–1065.
28. Arfe A, Scotti L, Varas-Lorenzo C, et al. Non-steroidal anti-inflammatory drugs and risk of heart failure in four European countries: nested case-control study. *BMJ.* 2016;354:i4857.
29. Wile D. Diuretics: a review. *Ann Clin Biochem.* 2012;49(Pt 5):419–431.
30. Ellison DH. Diuretic therapy and resistance in congestive heart failure. *Cardiology.* 2001;96(3–4):132–143.
31. Stevenson LW, Nohria A, Mielniczuk L. Torrent or torment from the tubules? challenge of the cardiorenal connections. *J Am Coll Cardiol.* 2005;45(12):2004–2007.
32. Schefold JC, Filippatos G, Hasenfuss G, et al. Heart failure and kidney dysfunction: epidemiology, mechanisms and management. *Nat Rev Nephrol.* 2016;12(10):610–623.
33. Mentz RJ, Kjeldsen K, Rossi GP, et al. Decongestion in acute heart failure. *Eur J Heart Fail.* 2014;16(5):471–482.
34. Leong DP, McMurray JJV, Joseph PG, Yusuf S. From ACE inhibitors/ARBs to ARNIs in coronary artery disease and heart failure (Part 2/5). *J Am Coll Cardiol.* 2019;74(5):683–698.
35. Lee VC, Rhew DC, Dylan M, et al. Meta-analysis: angiotensin-receptor blockers in chronic heart failure and high-risk acute myocardial infarction. *Ann Intern Med.* 2004;141(9):693–704.
36. Braunwald E. The path to an angiotensin receptor antagonist-neprilysin inhibitor in the treatment of heart failure. *J Am Coll Cardiol.* 2015;65(10):1029–1041.
37. Rubio DM, Schoenbaum EE, Lee LS, et al. Defining translational research: implications for training. *Acad Med.* 2010;85(3):470–475.
38. Mann DL, Greene SJ, Givertz MM, et al. Sacubitril/valsartan in advanced heart failure with reduced ejection fraction: rationale and design of the LIFE trial. *JACC Heart Fail.* 2020.
39. Jondeau G, Neuder Y, Eicher JC, et al. B-CONVINCED: beta-blocker CONtinuation Vs. INterruption in patients with Congestive heart failure hospitalized for a decompensation episode. *Eur Heart J.* 2009;30(18):2186–2192.
40. Schrier RW. Aldosterone "escape" vs "breakthrough". *Nat Rev Nephrol.* 2010;6(2):61.
41. Jessup M, Abraham WT, Casey DE, et al. 2009 focused update: ACCF/AHA guidelines for the diagnosis and management of heart failure in adults: a report of the American College of Cardiology Foundation/American Heart Association Task Force on Practice Guidelines: developed in collaboration with the International Society for Heart and Lung Transplantation. *Circulation.* 2009;119(14):1977–2016.
42. Seed A, Gardner R, McMurray J, et al. Neurohumoral effects of the new orally active renin inhibitor, aliskiren, in chronic heart failure. *Eur J Heart Fail.* 2007;9(11):1120–1127.
43. Cleland JG, Abdellah AT, Khaleva O, et al. Clinical trials update from the European Society of Cardiology Congress 2007: 3CPO, ALOFT, PROSPECT and statins for heart failure. *Eur J Heart Fail.* 2007;9(10):1070–1073.
44. Gheorghiade M, Bohm M, Greene SJ, et al. Effect of aliskiren on postdischarge mortality and heart failure readmissions among patients hospitalized for heart failure: the ASTRONAUT randomized trial. *J Am Med Assoc.* 2013;309(11):1125–1135.
45. McMurray JJ, Krum H, Abraham WT, et al. Aliskiren, enalapril, or aliskiren and enalapril in heart failure. *N Engl J Med.* 2016;374(16):1521–1532.
46. Yancy CW, Jessup M, Bozkurt B, et al. 2016 ACC/AHA/HFSA focused update on new pharmacological therapy for heart failure: an update of the 2013 ACCF/AHA guideline for the management of heart failure: a report of the American College of Cardiology/American Heart Association Task Force on Clinical Practice Guidelines and the Heart Failure Society of America. *J Am Coll Cardiol.* 2016.
47. Swedberg K, Komajda M, Bohm M, et al. Ivabradine and outcomes in chronic heart failure (SHIFT): a randomised placebo-controlled study. *Lancet.* 2010;376(9744):875–885.
48. Zinman B, Wanner C, Lachin JM, et al. Empagliflozin, cardiovascular outcomes, and mortality in type 2 diabetes. *N Engl J Med.* 2015;373(22):2117–2128.
49. McMurray JJV, Solomon SD, Inzucchi SE, et al. Dapagliflozin in patients with heart failure and reduced ejection fraction. *N Engl J Med.* 2019.
50. Packer M, Anker SD, Butler J, et al. Cardiovascular and renal outcomes with empagliflozin in heart failure. *N Engl J Med.* 2020.
51. O'Meara E, McDonald M, Chan M, et al. CCS/CHFS heart failure guidelines: clinical trial update on functional mitral regurgitation, SGLT2 inhibitors, ARNI in HFpEF, and Tafamidis in Amyloidosis. *Can J Cardiol.* 2020;36(2):159–169.
52. Armstrong PW, Pieske B, Anstrom KJ, et al. Vericiguat in patients with heart failure and reduced ejection fraction. *N Engl J Med.* 2020;382(20):1883–1893.
53. Teerlink JR, Felker GM, McMurray JJ, et al. Chronic Oral Study of Myosin Activation to Increase Contractility In Heart Failure (COSMIC-HF): a phase 2, pharmacokinetic, randomised, placebo-controlled trial. *Lancet.* 2016;388(10062):2895–2903.
54. GISSI-HF Investigators. Effect of n-3 polyunsaturated fatty acids in patients with chronic heart failure (the GISSI-HF trial): a randomised, double-blind, placebo-controlled trial. *Lancet.* 2008;372:1223–1230.
55. Krittanawong C, Namath A, Lanfear DE, Tang WH. Practical pharmacogenomic approaches to heart failure therapeutics. *Curr Treat Options Cardiovasc Med.* 2016;18(10):60.
56. Piccini JP, Abraham WT, Dufton C, et al. Bucindolol for the maintenance of sinus rhythm in a genotype-defined HF population: the GENETIC-AF trial. *JACC Heart Fail.* 2019;7(7):586–598.

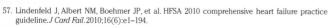

57. Lindenfeld J, Albert NM, Boehmer JP, et al. HFSA 2010 comprehensive heart failure practice guideline. *J Card Fail.* 2010;16(6):e1–194.
58. Borer JS, Swedberg K, Komajda M, et al. Efficacy profile of ivabradine in patients with heart failure plus angina pectoris. *Cardiology.* 2017;136(2):138–144.
59. Dunlay SM, Roger VL. Gender differences in the pathophysiology, clinical presentation, and outcomes of ischemic heart failure. *Curr Heart Fail Rep.* 2012;9(4):267–276.
60. Lanfear DE, Hrobowski TN, Peterson EL, et al. Association of beta-blocker exposure with outcomes in heart failure differs between African American and white patients. *Circ Heart Fail.* 2012;5(2):202–208.
61. Ruff CT, Giugliano RP, Braunwald E, et al. Comparison of the efficacy and safety of new oral anticoagulants with warfarin in patients with atrial fibrillation: a meta-analysis of randomised trials. *Lancet.* 2014;383(9921):955–962.
62. Homma S, Thompson JL, Pullicino PM, et al. Warfarin and aspirin in patients with heart failure and sinus rhythm. *N Engl J Med.* 2012;366(20):1859–1869.
63. Roy D, Talajic M, Nattel S, et al. Rhythm control versus rate control for atrial fibrillation and heart failure. *N Engl J Med.* 2008;358(25):2667–2677.
64. Cadrin-Tourigny J, Shohoudi A, Roy D, et al. Decreased mortality with beta-blockers in patients with heart failure and coexisting atrial fibrillation: an AF-CHF substudy. *JACC Heart Fail.* 2017;5(2):99–106.
65. Van Gelder IC, Groenveld HF, Crijns HJ, et al. Lenient versus strict rate control in patients with atrial fibrillation. *N Engl J Med.* 2010;362(15):1363–1373.
66. Kober L, Torp-Pedersen C, McMurray JJ, et al. Increased mortality after dronedarone therapy for severe heart failure. *N Engl J Med.* 2008;358(25):2678–2687.
67. Di Biase L, Mohanty P, Mohanty S, et al. Ablation versus amiodarone for treatment of persistent atrial fibrillation in patients with congestive heart failure and an implanted device: results from the AATAC multicenter randomized trial. *Circulation.* 2016;133(17):1637–1644.
68. Marrouche NF, Brachmann J, Andresen D, et al. Catheter ablation for atrial fibrillation with heart failure. *N Engl J Med.* 2018;378(5):417–427.
69. Sharma B, McSharry D, Malhotra A. Sleep disordered breathing in patients with heart failure: pathophysiology and management. *Curr Treat Options Cardiovasc Med.* 2011;13(6):506–516.
70. Cowie MR, Woehrle H, Wegscheider K, et al. Adaptive servo-ventilation for central sleep apnea in systolic heart failure. *N Engl J Med.* 2015;373(12):1095–1105.

Disease Management, Patients with End-Stage Heart Failure and Palliative Care

71. Maric B, Kaan A, Ignaszewski A, Lear SA. A systematic review of telemonitoring technologies in heart failure. *Eur J Heart Fail.* 2009;11(5):506–517.
72. Braun LT, Grady KL, Kutner JS, et al. Palliative care and cardiovascular disease and stroke: a policy statement from the American Heart Association/American Stroke Association. *Circulation.* 2016;134(11):e198–e225.
73. World Palliative Care Alliance; WHO. *Global Atlas of Palliative Care at the End of Life. 2014.* Worldwide Palliative Care Alliance; 2014.
74. CMS Services. Medicare benefit policy manual: coverage of hospice services under hospital insurance. In: CMS Services, ed. *Centers for Medicare and Medicaid Services Rev.* 246th ed. Centers for Medicare and Medicaid Services; 2018.
75. Bekelman DB, Rumsfeld JS, Havranek EP, et al. Symptom burden, depression, and spiritual well-being: a comparison of heart failure and advanced cancer patients. *J Gen Intern Med.* 2009;24(5):592–598.

51 Heart Failure with Preserved and Mildly Reduced Ejection Fraction

CAROLYN S.P. LAM, SANJIV J. SHAH, AND SCOTT D. SOLOMON

The pathophysiologic definition of heart failure (HF)—the "inability of the heart to pump blood to the body at a rate commensurate with its needs, or to do so only at the cost of high filling pressures"[1]—is based on the presence of hemodynamic congestion that results in a clinical syndrome characterized by breathlessness, fatigue, and edema but importantly makes no assumption regarding underlying left ventricular (LV) ejection fraction (EF). Yet with the advent of major randomized clinical trials in HF that included an upper LVEF exclusion criterion, the diagnosis of HF became intertwined with ejection fraction. The focus on patients with reduced LVEF has been understandable given their higher mortality rates and the benefit observed in trials of neurohormonal agents. Isolated case reports and small case series in the 1980s served as reminders that HF could occur in the absence of overt reduction in LVEF.[2-4] However, this syndrome received little attention until the more widespread use of noninvasive assessment of LVEF provided robust epidemiologic evidence of the scope of HF in the absence of reduced LVEF. Collectively, these early epidemiologic data showed that approximately half of patients with HF did not have a markedly reduced LVEF and that these patients had a significantly increased risk of death and hospitalization compared with the general population.[5,6]

Although the term HFpEF is nearly universally used currently, there remains debate what LVEF cutoff should be used to define it and indeed what to name this broad syndrome. Whereas some have used the term to define HF with EF above the range generally considered reduced (40% or less), a nomenclature that was first used to distinguish the component of the CHARM program in which patients had HF and LVEF >40%, the most recent guidelines suggest that "HFpEF" be defined using an LVEF cutoff of ≥50%,[7-9] (instead of >40% in CHARM-Preserved). The 2016 European Society of Cardiology HF Guidelines adopted the term "HF with mid-range EF" to refer to patients with LVEF 40% to 50%, while the 2013 American College of Cardiology/American Heart Association HF Guidelines used "borderline" to describe this group. Importantly, this new nomenclature led to an upsurge of publications related to this previously neglected subgroup of HF.[10] More recently, "HF with mid-range EF" has been renamed as "HF with mildly reduced EF."[11,12] Accordingly, this chapter discusses the epidemiology, pathophysiology, diagnosis, and therapy of patients with HFpEF and HF with mildly reduced ejection fraction (HFmrEF). Of note, most epidemiologic and pathophysiologic studies in patients with HF and EF >40% have focused on the subgroup with HFpEF (EF ≥50%), although several completed and ongoing clinical trials have included both types of patients.

EPIDEMIOLOGY

Estimates of the prevalence and incidence of HFpEF and HFmrEF depend on the definition used, method of ascertainment, and population studied. As HF is a clinical syndrome, its ascertainment in epidemiologic studies is challenging, typically relying on hospitalization diagnostic codes with or without additional adjudication using well-accepted clinical criteria such as the Framingham criteria.[13] Furthermore, the determination of LVEF is not always available at the time of HF presentation or using standardized state-of-the-art methods (including echocardiography).

Prevalence

Multiple community-based cohorts have reported on the prevalence of HFpEF in diverse populations across the United States and Europe (eTable 51.1). Together, these studies showed that approximately half the HF population have LVEF >50%. Although the overall prevalence of HF in the community increases with age, the prevalence of HFpEF is higher in women than in men at any given age (eFig. 51.1), although men are more represented at lower ejection fractions.[14]

Estimating temporal trends in the prevalence of HFpEF is challenged by changes in diagnostic criteria and measurement techniques. Early epidemiologic studies did not include echocardiography, but increased awareness, availability, and routine use of both (more advanced) echocardiography and natriuretic peptides may have contributed to a reported increase in the prevalence of HFpEF and HFmrEF in recent years. Nonetheless, large studies of hospitalized HF in the United States consistently show that the proportion of hospitalized HFpEF has increased over time relative to hospitalized HF with reduced EF (HFrEF).[5] Among 110,621 patients hospitalized for HF in 275 U.S. hospitals in Get With the Guidelines-Heart Failure, from 2005 to 2010, the proportion of patients with LVEF ≥40% increased from 48% to 53%, with a projected increase to 65% by 2020.[15,16] The latter study also provided estimates of the proportion of patients with LVEF in the 40% to 50% range, which averaged ~15% and did not change over time. Conversely, the proportion with LVEF ≥50% increased from 33% in 2005 to 39% in 2010, while the proportion with LVEF <40%, decreased from 52% to 47% over the same time frame. Similar observations have been reported in Japan.[17,18] *In summary, the prevalence of HFpEF and HFmrEF is high and increasing over time relative to HFrEF, a phenomenon related to aging of the population,[19] making these the predominant forms of HF in aging societies.*

TABLE 51.1 Risk Factors for Heart Failure

HFpEF	sHR* (95% CI)	P
Age, per 10 years	1.90 (1.74-2.07)	<0.0001
Male sex	0.93 (0.78-1.11)	0.43
Systolic BP, per 20 mm Hg	1.14 (1.05-1.24)	0.003
Body mass index, per 4 kg/m²	1.28 (1.21-1.37)	<0.0001
Antihypertensive treatment	1.42 (1.18-1.71)	0.0002
Previous myocardial infarction	1.48 (1.12-1.96)	0.006

HFrEF	sHR* (95% CI)	P
Age, per 10 years	1.66 (1.52-1.80)	<0.0001
Male sex	1.84 (1.55-2.19)	<0.0001
Systolic BP, per 20 mm Hg	1.20 (1.10-1.30)	<0.0001
Body mass index, per 4 kg/m²	1.19 (1.11-1.28)	<0.0001
Antihypertensive treatment	1.35 (1.13-1.63)	0.001
Diabetes mellitus	1.83 (1.48-2.26)	<0.0001
Current smoker	1.41 (1.14-1.75)	0.0015
Previous myocardial infarction	2.60 (2.08-3.25)	<0.0001
ECG LV hypertrophy	2.12 (1.55-2.90)	<0.0001
Left bundle branch block	3.17 (2.11-4.78)	<0.0001

BP, Blood pressure; *CI*, confidence interval; *sHR*, sub-distribution hazard ratio; *LV*, left ventricular.
Adapted from Ho JE, et al. Predictors of new-onset heart failure: differences in preserved versus reduced ejection fraction. Circ Heart Fail. 2013;6(2):279-286.

Incidence

The reported incidence of HFpEF and HFmrEF in community-based studies has varied, from a 12-year cumulative HF incidence of 4.2% in the Prevention of Renal and Vascular End-Stage Disease (PREVEND) study (36.9% HF with EF >45%) to 13.7% (53.3% HF with EF >45%) in the Cardiovascular Health Study (CHS), with the incidence rate related to the baseline age of the population (lower incidence in younger cohorts).[20,21] The age- and sex-adjusted incidence of HF declined from 3.2 to 2.2 cases per 1000 person-years from 2000 to 2010 in Olmstead County, Minnesota; with a smaller reduction for HFpEF than HFrEF, and more pronounced reduction in women than in men.[22] As a result, HFpEF constituted an increasing proportion of incident HF cases over time (from 47.8% in 2000-2003 to 56.9% in 2004-2007 and 52.3% in 2008-2010).[22]

Risk Factors

Although population-based longitudinal studies have established the well-known clinical risk factors for incident HF, few have taken into account different HF types. In the Framingham Heart Study (FHS),[23] an examination of predictors of 8-year risk of HF patients with LVEF >45% versus those with LVEF ≤45% showed that predictors of all incident HF included older age, male sex, hypertension, higher body mass index (BMI), increasing heart rate, coronary artery disease (CAD), diabetes mellitus, smoking, valve disease, lower HDL cholesterol, atrial fibrillation, and the presence of LV hypertrophy or left bundle branch block. Specifically in those with higher LVEF, risk factors included higher BMI, smoking, and a history of atrial fibrillation. In contrast male sex, hypertension, higher heart rate, prior cardiovascular disease, higher cholesterol level, LV hypertrophy, and left bundle branch block were associated with higher risk of HFrEF. However, older age was associated with a higher risk of HFpEF and HFmrEF whereas male sex and prior myocardial infarction were associated with higher risk of HFrEF (Table 51.1).[23] Of note, the cumulative incidences of HFpEF and HFmrEF in men and women were similar; whereas the cumulative incidence of HFrEF in men was markedly higher than in women.

Pooling individual level data from FHS, PREVEND, and CHS,[20] independent predictors of incident HF with EF >45% included older age,

higher systolic blood pressure, increased BMI, antihypertensive treatment, and previous myocardial infarction. After adjusting for other clinical risk factors, sex was not an independent predictor in the model specific for HF with EF >45%. Instead, male sex was independently associated with significantly higher risk for HFrEF. Left bundle branch block, previous myocardial infarction, smoking, and LV hypertrophy were more strongly associated with HFrEF, whereas older age was more strongly associated with HF with EF >45% (see Table 51.1).[20] In summary, aging is a potent risk factor for heart failure with LVEF >40%. Although women predominate among patients with HFpEF and the prevalence of HFpEF is higher in women than men at any age (see eFig. 51.1), this may be related to aging rather than to an intrinsically higher risk of HFpEF in women versus men, because women outlive men on average (Fig. 51.1).

Atrial Fibrillation

Atrial fibrillation is the most common arrhythmia in patients with HFpEF and HFmrEF, with a prevalence of 20% to 40% at the time of presentation, and occurring in two-thirds of these patients at some point during their course.[24,25] Both atrial fibrillation and HF are age-related conditions that frequently coexist, and share common clinical manifestations (e.g., breathlessness and effort intolerance).[26,27] Furthermore, atrial fibrillation is a potent and independent prognostic factor in patients with HFpEF and HFmrEF.[28-30] In addition, atrial fibrillation can complicate the diagnosis of HF because atrial fibrillation alone increases natriuretic peptides, even in the absence of overt HF.

Prognosis
Mortality

Estimates of mortality in HFpEF and HFmrEF have differed depending on baseline status of the study population (especially hospitalized versus outpatient status), study design (epidemiologic study versus clinical trial), LVEF cutoff level used, and various selection biases (use of natriuretic peptide level for the diagnosis, missing LVEF data, participation bias). In general, mortality rates reported in unselected observational studies are higher than in clinical trial populations, and those in cohorts of hospitalized, acute decompensated HF is higher than in outpatient cohorts of chronic HF.

Epidemiologic reports showed that the high 5-year mortality rates in hospitalized HFpEF were comparable or only slightly lower compared with that in HFrEF (Fig. 51.2),[5,6] with estimates ranging from 53% to 74% and no change over the past decade.[22] The Meta-Analysis Global Group in Chronic Heart Failure (MAGGIC) meta-analysis, inclusive of data from clinical trials, reported that patients with HFpEF had lower risk of death from any cause compared with those with HFrEF independent of age, sex, and etiology.[31] The death rate was 12.1 (95% CI: 11.7, 12.6) per 100 patient-years in HFpEF and 14.1 (95% CI: 13.8, 14.4) per 100 patient-years in HFrEF, with an adjusted hazard ratio (HR) of 0.68 (95% CI: 0.64, 0.71) for HFpEF versus HFrEF (Fig. 51.2, *bottom left panel*); death rates were lower in randomized trials alone, and the lower risk in HFpEF than HFrEF was more prominent in ambulatory versus hospitalized patients.[31] More recently, a prospective multicenter longitudinal study in Singapore and New Zealand, specifically designed to compare outcomes among HF types, found that over 2 years, all-cause death rates were 7.5 (95% CI: 6.0 to 9.3) per 100 patient-years in HFpEF and 10.9 (95% CI: 9.6 to 12.4) per 100 patient-years in HFrEF, thus confirming a lower risk of death in HFpEF (adjusted HR 0.62; 95% CI: 0.46 to 0.85) compared with HFrEF (Fig. 51.2, *right panel*).[32]

Beyond all-cause mortality rates, cause of death differs in HFpEF and HFmrEF compared with HFrEF. As expected with older age and greater prevalence of age-related comorbidities in those with higher LVEF, the proportion of deaths from noncardiovascular causes is generally higher in HFpEF and HFmrEF than in HFrEF, accounting for 32% to 49% of deaths in HFpEF in observational studies[33,34] and 28% to 30% in clinical trials. Importantly, cardiovascular causes still comprise the predominant cause of death even in HF patients with LVEF above 40%

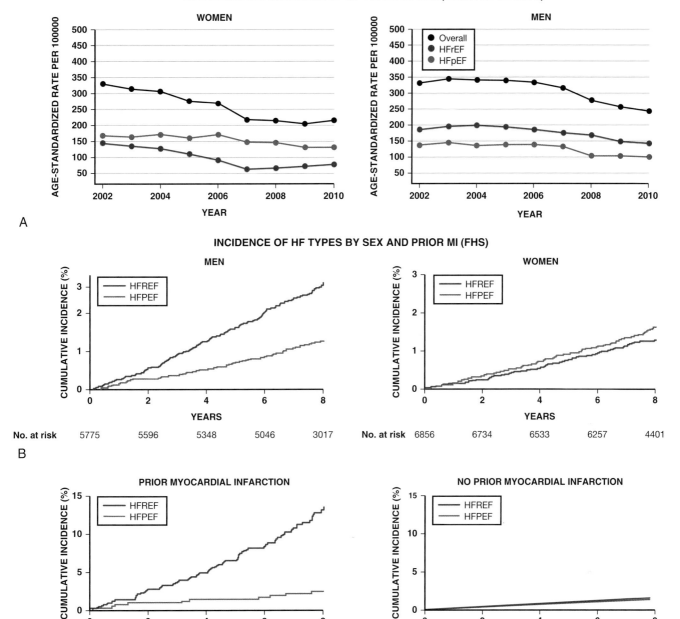

FIGURE 51.1 Prevalence and incidence of HF types by sex. A, Age-adjusted incidence of HF types by sex. **B,** Incidence of HF types by sex. **C,** Incidence of HF types by prior myocardial infarction (from Framingham Heart Study). (**A** adapted from Gerber Y, et al. A contemporary appraisal of the heart failure epidemic in Olmsted County, Minnesota, 2000 to 2010. JAMA Intern Med. 2015;175(6):996-1004. **B, C** modified from Ho JE, et al. Predictors of new-onset heart failure: differences in preserved versus reduced ejection fraction. Circ Heart Fail. 2013;6[2]:279-286.)

(eFig. 51.2).[35] Among cardiovascular causes of death, sudden death accounted for up to 43% of cardiovascular mortality (~25% to 30% of total deaths) in clinical trials that included patients with HF and LVEF >40%, with HF deaths accounting for another 20% to 30% of cardiovascular deaths (eFig. 51.3).[34]

Hospitalization

In contrast to lower death rates compared with HFrEF, the high hospitalization rates in HFpEF and HFmrEF are similar, if not even higher, than in HFrEF.[22,36] Following a new diagnosis of HFpEF, patients were hospitalized an average of 1.39 times per year in Olmsted County,

Minnesota,[22] with hospitalizations for noncardiovascular causes being more common (0.88 per person-year) than cardiovascular hospitalizations (0.46 per person-year). Although total hospitalization rates were similar across the spectrum of LVEF, noncardiovascular hospitalizations were higher in those with HFpEF, whereas cardiovascular hospitalizations were lower, when compared with HFrEF.

Importantly, recurrent hospitalizations are common in HFpEF and HFmrEF and contribute to a high total hospitalization burden.[37] Compared with epidemiologic studies, the proportion of cardiovascular hospitalizations in HFpEF clinical trials was higher: 56% of hospitalizations in the Irbesartan in Heart Failure and Preserved Ejection

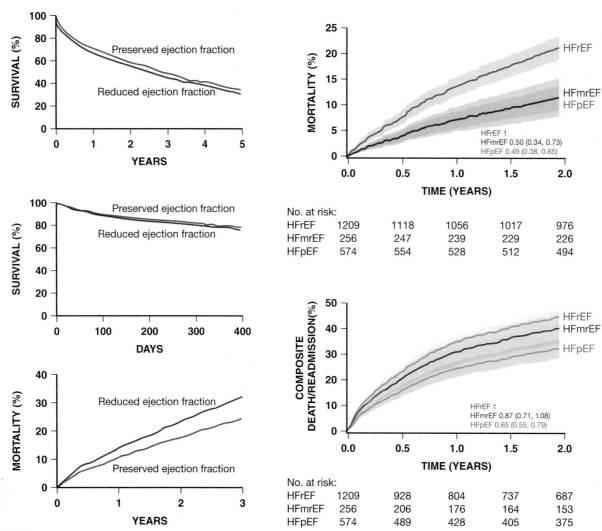

FIGURE 51.2 Survival among patients with heart failure in two epidemiologic studies, an individual patient-level meta-analysis (inclusive of clinical trials), and a prospective dual nation multicenter observational study. (From Owan TE, et al. N Engl J Med. 2006;355:251-259; Bhatia RS, et al, N Engl J Med. 2006;355:260–269; MAGGIC, Eur Heart J. 2012;33:1750-1757; Lam CSP, et al Eur Heart J. 2018;39[20]:1770-1780.)

Fraction (I-PRESERVE) trial[38] and 55% of hospitalizations in CHARM-Preserved.[37] Of note, a prior HF hospitalization heralds a higher risk of death or rehospitalization, with the highest risk close to the time postdischarge and declining over time.[38-40]

Quality of Life

Beyond mortality and hospitalizations, patients with HFpEF also have significantly reduced quality of life, similar to that in HFrEF. Health-related quality of life is often measured in HFpEF clinical trials using either the Kansas City Cardiomyopathy Questionnaire (KCCQ) or the Minnesota Living with Heart Failure Questionnaire (MLHFQ). In the Treatment of Preserved Cardiac Function Heart Failure With an Aldosterone Antagonist (TOPCAT) trial, 43% of participants at baseline had either very low or low KCCQ scores (0 to 50), indicating poor quality of life.[41] In PARAGON-HF, mean KCCQ-overall summary score at randomization was 71, with lowest mean KCCQ score in the symptom stability domain.[42] Low KCCQ scores correlated with worse New York Heart Association functional class, higher NT-proBNP concentration, and more signs and symptoms of HF.

Prior studies have also shown that KCCQ is a valid and reliable measure of health status in HFpEF, has comparable performance in patients with HFpEF and HFrEF,[43] and may be used in serial evaluations to reflect risk of subsequent death and cardiovascular hospitalization in HFpEF and HFrEF.[44-45] Compared with patients with HFrEF in the Prospective Comparison of ARNI with an ACE-Inhibitor to Determine Impact on

Global Mortality and Morbidity in Heart Failure (PARADIGM-HF) trial, those with HFpEF in PARAGON-HF had lower mean scores in nearly all domains, as well as lower mean scores in most physical and social activities (except for intimate or sexual relationships).[42]

DIAGNOSIS

The diagnosis of HFpEF and HFmrEF relies on (1) a clinical diagnosis of HF and (2) evidence of a preserved or only mildly reduced LVEF (LVEF >40%). The former is corroborated by typical signs and symptoms of HF, which are similar across the spectrum of LVEF, including evidence of elevated cardiac filling pressures on physical examination (elevated jugular venous pressure), as well as supportive testing including biomarkers (elevated natriuretic peptides), echocardiography (increased E/e′ ratio, dilated inferior vena cava, or left atrial [LA] enlargement), or invasive hemodynamic testing (elevated pulmonary capillary wedge pressure [PCWP]). The specific LVEF cutoff for HFpEF has been debated and has been different in different contexts, with recent guidelines suggesting that HFpEF should be defined as LVEF ≥50% and HFmrEF defined as LVEF between 40% and 49%.[9] Nevertheless, many clinicians and trials have used the term HFpEF to refer to patients with HF and LVEF as low as 40%.

In patients hospitalized with HF or in outpatients with overt HF and signs of fluid overload (including chest radiographic evidence of pulmonary vascular congestion or pulmonary edema), the diagnosis is

TABLE 51.2 Noncardiac Etiologies That Can Mimic the HFpEF Syndrome

Obesity
Chronic lung disease
Chronic kidney disease with minimal cardiac structural or functional abnormalities
Primary cirrhosis
Extrinsic compression of the LA, LV, or IVC
IVC obstruction
Lymphedema
Anemia

often straightforward. However, the diagnosis can be challenging in patients with dyspnea and exercise intolerance who do not have overt signs of elevated filling pressures and natriuretic peptide levels below typical thresholds used to make the diagnosis of HF, which occurs commonly in some patients (up to 30% to 40%, especially in patients who are obese).[46] In these patients, provocative testing (e.g., exercise) can be useful to make the diagnosis by echocardiography (elevated E/e' ratio at peak exercise) or invasive hemodynamic testing (PCWP ≥25 mm Hg with passive leg raise or during exercise).[47] It is important to proceed with invasive hemodynamic testing (with or without exercise) in any patient with suspected HFpEF or HFmrEF in whom the diagnosis is in question because signs and symptoms of HF can be nonspecific and many of the comorbidities that coexist with HFpEF and HFmrEF can mimic the HF syndrome.

Echocardiographic evidence of LV diastolic dysfunction is challenging and should not be used as the sole criteria for the diagnosis of HFpEF for several reasons: (1) diastolic function on echocardiography may be uninterpretable, equivocal, or misinterpreted; (2) many older patients without the HF syndrome have evidence of diastolic dysfunction; (3) while echocardiography is useful for the diagnosis of impaired relaxation, E/e' ratio (an estimate of LV filling pressures) is often in the indeterminate range (8 to 15), and echocardiography has not proven useful for the assessment of LV chamber compliance in the clinical setting. Thus, while the presence of diastolic dysfunction in the appropriate clinical context is supportive, the absence of significant diastolic dysfunction should not be used to exclude the diagnosis of HFpEF, and further testing with exercise stress or invasive hemodynamics should be considered.

The diagnosis of HFpEF and HFmrEF relies on the exclusion of noncardiac causes of dyspnea, exercise tolerance, or fluid overload. For example, a patient with severe chronic obstructive pulmonary disease on oxygen would likely have symptoms of dyspnea and exercise intolerance and may have signs of central venous congestion due to cor pulmonale with right ventricular hypertrophy. Although the patient has symptoms of "heart failure," the diagnosis is COPD and not HF. Thus, in each patient with suspected HFpEF and HFmrEF, it is important to consider alternate etiologies (Table 51.2).

HFpEF Diagnostic Scores

Two scoring systems have been developed to assist in the diagnosis of HFpEF in patients with dyspnea in whom the diagnosis is in question: the H₂FPEF[48] score and the HFA-PEFF score[49] (Fig. 51.3). Both of these scores offer simple approaches to the diagnosis of HFpEF, and although not specifically designed for HFmrEF, may be helpful in the diagnosis of HFmrEF as well. The H₂FPEF score was systematically derived and validated at a single center (Mayo Clinic, Rochester, MN).[48] HFpEF was diagnosed in patients with PCWP ≥15 mm Hg at rest or ≥25 mm Hg during exercise. The final diagnostic model included the following weighted components: BMI >30 g/m² (2 points), 2 or more antihypertensive medications (1 point), atrial fibrillation (3 points), echocardiographic pulmonary artery (PA) systolic pressure >35 mm Hg (1 point), age >60 years (1 point), and echocardiographic E/e' >9 (1 point). The overall score AUC was 0.84 and the score was found to be superior to other consensus criteria developed for the diagnosis of HFpEF. The score was then validated in a separate test, where it was found to perform well (AUC,

0.89). The authors developed a nomogram that provides the likelihood of the HFpEF diagnosis based on the calculated score in an individual patient (Fig. 51.3A). Given the ease of use of the H₂FPEF score, it may be particularly helpful in the primary care setting where at-risk patients with dyspnea could be screened using the score to help establish the diagnosis.

The HFA-PEFF score was developed by a group of experts convened by the European Society of Cardiology Heart Failure Association.[49] The "PEFF" mnemonic stands for Pre-test assessment; Echocardiography and natriuretic peptide score; Functional testing; and Final etiology. The recommended pretest assessment involves evaluation of HF symptoms and signs, clinical comorbidities typically associated with HFpEF, laboratory tests, electrocardiography, and echocardiography (Fig. 51.3B). The HFA-PEFF score is based on functional and morphologic echocardiographic criteria, and natriuretic peptide criteria. Components of the functional domain include echocardiographic tissue Doppler e' velocities, E/e' ratio, tricuspid regurgitation velocity, and LV global longitudinal strain. Components of the morphologic domain include LA volume index, LV mass index, relative wall thickness, and LV wall thickness. Each domain included major criteria (2 points) or minor criteria (1 point) (Fig. 51.3B). A score of ≥5 points is diagnostic of HFpEF, whereas a score of <2 points excludes HFpEF. In both the H₂FPEF and HFA-PEFF scores have been further assessed for external validation and although not perfect, appear to be clinically useful for making the diagnosis of HFpEF.

KEY TESTS FOR THE EVALUATION OF HFpEF AND HFmrEF
Biomarkers
Natriuretic peptides (NPs; B-type natriuretic peptide [BNP] and N-terminal pro-BNP [NT-proBNP]) are the most widely studied and used diagnostic and prognostic biomarkers in HFpEF and HFmrEF. NPs are secreted by both the ventricular and atrial myocardium in response to increased wall stress, which is directly related to chamber size and inversely related to wall thickness. NP levels are consistently on average higher in patients with HFrEF compared with patients with higher LVEF most likely due to the increased ventricular dilation in lower LVEF patients.[50] In patients with HFrEF, LV dilation is common and wall thickness is frequently normal, whereas in HFpEF, LV volumes are normal or small, and wall thickness can be increased. Thus, for any given rise in LV diastolic pressure elevation, patients with HFpEF or HFmrEF often have lower NP levels compared with HFrEF, and these syndromes have been considered states of relative NP deficiency, which may contribute to the clinical syndrome, including hypertension and fluid retention.

Although an elevated NP level can be helpful to diagnose HF in patients with LVEF >40%, other causes of elevated NP levels such as atrial fibrillation, pulmonary arterial hypertension, primary RV failure, acute pulmonary embolism, and chronic kidney disease must be considered in the differential diagnosis. NP levels should not be used to exclude the diagnosis of HF in patients with intermediate to high pretest probability because 30% to 40% of patients with HFpEF have NP levels below typical diagnostic thresholds, NP levels are lower in HFpEF and HFmrEF than in HFrEF, and morbid obesity is associated with lower NP levels due to NP clearance receptors on adipocytes and lower NP production in obese patients. In these patients, further diagnostic testing should be performed. In patients with prevalent HFpEF and HFmrEF, elevated NP levels are a useful prognostic marker.

High-sensitivity troponin (hsTnT) is also useful in the evaluation of patients with HFpEF and HFmrEF, and elevation in hsTnT can signify a more "myocardial" phenotype of HFpEF, can alert the clinician to the potential presence of an infiltrative cardiomyopathy such as cardiac amyloidosis, and may reflect impaired subendocardial perfusion due to coronary microvascular dysfunction, particularly if measured during or immediately after exercise testing. Moreover, elevated levels portend a worse prognosis.[51,52] In the future, proteomic or metabolomic analysis of the blood may provide additional insight into better diagnostic tests and sub-phenotyping in HFpEF and HFmrEF.

Echocardiography (see Chapter 16)
Comprehensive echocardiography, including Doppler and tissue Doppler imaging, along with speckle-tracking echocardiography for the assessment of cardiac mechanics, should be performed on all patients with suspected or known HFpEF and HFmrEF. Conventional echocardiography provides important diagnostic and etiologic clues in these patients. Importantly, echocardiography is essential to rule out other causes of a patient's signs and symptoms, including other forms of heart disease. Although not all patients with HFpEF or HFmrEF have LV hypertrophy, the majority have concentric LV remodeling, defined by a relative wall thickness (2 × posterior wall thickness/LV end-diastolic dimension) >0.42.[53] Assessment of LV mass index in relation to relative

	Clinical Variable	Values	Points
H₂	**H**eavy	Body mass index > 30 kg/m²	2
	Hypertensive	2 or more antihypertensive medicines	1
F	**A**trial fibrillation	Paroxysmal or persistent	3
P	**P**ulmonary hypertension	Doppler echocardiographic estimated pulmonary artery systolic pressure > 35 mmHg	1
E	**E**lder	Age > 60 years	1
F	**F**illing pressure	Doppler echocardiographic E/e' > 9	1
H₂FPEF score			Sum (0–9)

Total points   0 1 2 3 4 5 6 7 8 9

Probability of HFpEF   0.2 0.3 0.4 0.5 0.6 0.7 0.8   0.9   0.95

A

	Functional	Morphological	Biomarker (SR)	Biomarker (AF)
Major	Septal e' < 7 cm/s or lateral e' < 10 cm/s or Average E/e' ≥ 15 or TR velocity > 2.8 m/s (PASP > 35 mm Hg)	LAVI > 34 mL/m² or LVMI ≥ 149/122 g/m² (m/w) and RWT > 0,42	NT-proBNP > 220 pg/mL or BNP > 80 pg/mL	NT-proBNP > 660 pg/mL or BNP > 240 pg/mL
Minor	Average E/e' 9–14 or GLS < 16%	LAVI 29–34 mL/m² or LVMI > 115/95 g/m² (m/w) or RWT > 0,42 or LV wall thickness ≥ 12 mm	NT-proBNP 125–220 pg/mL or BNP 35–80 pg/mL	NT-proBNP 365–660 pg/mL or BNP 105–240 pg/mL

Major criteria : 2 points	≥ 5 points: HFpEF
Minor criteria : 1 point	2–4 points: Diastolic stress test or invasive hemodynamic measurements

B

FIGURE 51.3 **HFpEF scores. A,** Description of the H₂FPEF score and point allocations for each clinical characteristic (*top*), with associated probability of having heart failure with preserved ejection fraction (HFpEF) based on the total score as estimated from the model (*bottom*). **B,** Calculating and interpreting the HFA-PEFF score. Echocardiographic and natriuretic peptide heart failure with preserved ejection fraction workup and scoring system (diagnostic workup). (**A** from Reddy YNV, et al. A simple, evidence-based approach to help guide diagnosis of heart failure with preserved ejection fraction. Circulation. 2018;138[9]:861-870. **B** from Pieske B, et al. How to diagnose heart failure with preserved ejection fraction: the HFA-PEFF diagnostic algorithm: a consensus recommendation from the Heart Failure Association [HFA] of the European Society of Cardiology [ESC]. Eur Heart J. 2019;40(40):3297-3317.)

wall thickness can also be helpful because it can be used to categorize LV geometry (normal, concentric remodeling, concentric hypertrophy, or eccentric hypertrophy), which can provide clues to the etiology (Fig. 51.4A). LA volume is also very useful for the diagnosis because it provides insight into chronic LA pressure overload. Although maximal LA volume index to body surface area ≥34 mL/m² is the guideline-based cutoff for LA enlargement, it can be challenging to use because of the high prevalence of obesity in these patients, which results in lower values. For these reasons, it is important to examine the LA in relation to the other chambers of the heart. An LA that is as large or larger than the

LV implies that the LA is not emptying properly to adequately fill the LV, which is common in HFpEF. Therefore, LA minimal volume or LA reservoir strain (see later) may be better tools to help diagnose and manage these patients. It is important to note that other conditions can result in LV hypertrophy and/or LA enlargement in the setting of a preserved LVEF. These include athlete's heart, high output states (e.g., cirrhosis), and atrial fibrillation, underscoring the importance of comprehensive echocardiographic assessment in these patients.

Conventional echocardiography is also useful for the assessment of load on the right heart in patients with HFpEF and HFmrEF. Elevated

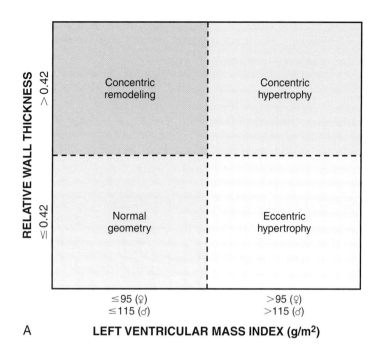

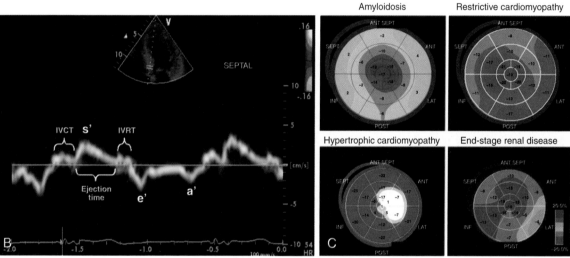

FIGURE 51.4 **A,** Hypertrophy subtypes: comparison of relative wall thickness (RWT). Patients with normal LV mass can have either concentric remodeling (normal LV mass with increased RWT >0.42) or normal geometry (RWT ≤0.42) and normal LV mass. Patients with increased LV mass can have either concentric (RWT >0.42) or eccentric (RWT ≤0.42) hypertrophy. These LV mass measurements are based on linear measurements. **B,** Tissue Doppler imaging can be used to determine the extent of myocardial involvement in HFpEF. Reductions in systolic (s'), early diastolic (e'), and late diastolic (a') velocities, prolongation of isovolumic contraction time (IVCT) and isovolumic relaxation time (IVRT), and reduction in ejection time are all signs of a sick myocardium. **C,** LV global longitudinal strain bullseye maps. The strain maps show particular patterns suggestive of amyloidosis (*upper left*), restrictive cardiomyopathy (*upper right*), apical hypertrophic cardiomyopathy (*lower left*), and end-stage renal disease with a pattern suggestive of Fabry disease (*lower right*). *ANT,* Anterior; *ANT SEPT,* anteroseptal; *INF,* inferior; *LAT,* lateral; *POST,* posterolateral; *SEPT,* septal. (**A** from Lang RM, et al. Recommendations for cardiac chamber quantification by echocardiography in adults: an update from the American Society of Echocardiography and the European Association of Cardiovascular Imaging. Eur Heart J Cardiovasc Imaging. 2015;16[3]:233-270; **B** from Shah SJ. 20th Annual Feigenbaum lecture: echocardiography for precision medicine-digital biopsy to deconstruct biology. J Am Soc Echocardiogr. 2019;32[11]:1379-1395e1372; **C** from Marwick TH, et al. Myocardial strain in the assessment of patients with heart failure: a review. JAMA Cardiol. 2019;4[3]:287-294.)

pulmonary artery systolic pressure (>40 mm Hg) especially when coupled with LA enlargement or dysfunction, is common in HFpEF, and this elevation is considered secondary to left sided heart disease. As HFpEF worsens, RV enlargement and dysfunction often occur in response to chronic elevation in LA and pulmonary venous pressures. Thus, it is important to examine and quantify the right heart on echocardiography in all patients with HFpEF with indices such as RV fractional area change (normal >35%), tricuspid annular plane systolic excursion (normal >1.6 cm), and RV s' velocity (normal >10 cm/sec). The ratio of tricuspid regurgitation velocity (in m/sec) to RV outflow tract velocity time integral (in cm) >0.18 is indicative of elevated total pulmonary resistance and should prompt evaluation of the possibility of pulmonary vascular disease. Assessment of septal flattening during systole and diastole provides insight into RV pressure and volume overload, respectively. Notching of the RV outflow tract pulse wave Doppler velocity

profile is a sign that pulmonary vascular resistance (PVR) is elevated due to interruption of the normal forward RV outflow by the reflected wave from the stiff distal pulmonary vasculature. Finally, assessment of inferior vena cava size and collapsibility, along with hepatic vein flow, can provide valuable information on estimated right atrial pressure and etiologies such as severe tricuspid regurgitation, constrictive pericarditis, and restrictive cardiomyopathy. Assessment of the RV and right atrium on echocardiography is also important for differentiating heart failure from pulmonary arterial hypertension.[54]

Measures of Diastolic Function and Strain. Tissue Doppler imaging (TDI) can be helpful in the assessment of patients with suspected HFpEF or HFmrEF (Fig. 51.4B). The early diastolic (e') velocity is a marker of LV relaxation and is usually reduced in patients with heart failure regardless of LVEF. However, TDI provides additional clues for the diagnosis and management of HFpEF; thus, clinicians should examine the s' and a' velocities along with the ejection time and the isovolumic contraction and relaxation times on the TDI tracing. The s' velocity (a marker of longitudinal motion of the myocardium) is often reduced in HFpEF patients, especially in patients with CAD or infiltrative cardiomyopathy. A reduced a' velocity is reflective of impaired LA contraction and/or reduced LV end-diastolic chamber compliance.

Speckle-tracking echocardiography has emerged as an important diagnostic and prognostic tool in patients with HFpEF and HFmrEF and has provided insights into the pathophysiology.[55] Similar to s' velocity, a reduced absolute LV global longitudinal strain (GLS) value is indicative of reduced longitudinal fiber LV function (a marker of LV subendocardial function, which is often affected by risk factors that lead to HFpEF) even in the setting of a preserved LVEF and is often present in patients with HFpEF.[56] Although values of GLS can vary based on type of echocardiography machine and software used, an absolute GLS value of >18% is considered normal, 16% to 18% borderline, and <16% abnormal (Fig. 51.4C). Polar bullseye maps of the LV longitudinal strain pattern are also useful for determining the potential etiology of HFpEF (Fig. 51.4C) because it can help differentiate patients who have diffuse myocardial fibrosis from those who have cardiac amyloidosis, who would generally have an apical sparing pattern.

Strain measures of the left atrium and right ventricle can also be performed. LA longitudinal strain consists of three components (reservoir, conduit, and booster strains). LA reservoir strain is indicative of the ability of the LA to fill during ventricular systole; when reduced, it is associated with poor prognosis and reflects increased LA pressure and/or reduced compliance of the LA.[57] LA conduit strain reflects the ability of the LA to empty properly during passive filling of the LV in early diastole, and LA booster strain is indicative of the ability of the LA contractile function. When LA strain indices are abnormal out of proportion to the extent of LV dysfunction, a primary LA myopathy as a cause of HFpEF should be considered. Reduced RV free wall strain is often present in HFpEF and is also associated with adverse events; it can be reduced in the setting of elevated pulmonary vascular resistance or a primary myocardial process that is affecting both the LV and the RV and resulting in HFpEF.

Most compensated patients with HFpEF do not have symptoms at rest but become very symptomatic with exertion. Thus, exercise echocardiography can be very useful in the evaluation of HFpEF patients.[58] Despite the routine use of exercise testing in other cardiovascular conditions (especially CAD), exercise testing is still underutilized in the diagnosis and management of HFpEF. Exercise echocardiography can provide an assessment of ischemia (i.e., wall motion abnormalities), LV filling pressures (e.g., E/e' and PA systolic pressure), and can rule out dynamic valvular disease (such as exercise-induced mitral regurgitation). In HFpEF patients, bicycle stress echocardiography is typically easier for patients compared with treadmill testing because HFpEF patients are often older, frail, and debilitated.

Cardiac Magnetic Resonance Imaging (see Chapter 19)

Although echocardiography can provide a wealth of information to assist with the diagnosis and management of HFpEF and HFmrEF, acoustic windows can be challenging in many HFpEF patients because of the high prevalence of obesity and concomitant lung disease. Furthermore, echocardiography is limited in its ability to provide tissue characterization and assessment of extracardiac structures. For these reasons, cardiac magnetic resonance (CMR) imaging can be a very useful diagnostic test in HFpEF and HFmrEF.[59]

CMR is the reference standard for assessment of cardiac structure and global systolic function given its high temporal resolution. Furthermore, late gadolinium enhancement provides assessment of myocardial scar, which may be due to myocardial infarction, myocarditis, or specific cardiomyopathies depending on its distribution. However, some patients with HFpEF and HFmrEF have diffuse myocardial fibrosis which cannot be easily detected on conventional CMR imaging with contrast; instead, T1 mapping with quantitation of the extracellular volume content can be used and when elevated (typically >25%) is indicative of either diffuse myocardial fibrosis or extracellular deposition of proteins as is seen in cardiac amyloidosis (eFig. 51.4A). T2 mapping is also useful for the diagnosis of myocardial edema, which can be present in cases of myocarditis (eFig. 51.4B). In addition, T2* imaging can be useful for the quantitation of myocardial iron content when the diagnosis of hemochromatosis is under consideration. CMR imaging is also useful to detect thickening and/or enhancement of the pericardium (eFig. 51.4C). Dynamic deep breathing cine images can also detect evidence of diastolic septal bounce which reflects ventricular interdependence and can be seen in the setting of constrictive pericarditis. Finally, vasodilator perfusion CMR imaging can be used to detect coronary macrovascular

and microvascular perfusion defects (eFig. 51.4D), the latter of which is indicative of coronary microvascular dysfunction and is present in a large proportion of patients with HFpEF.[60]

Cardiac Catheterization (see Chapter 22)

In patients in whom noninvasive tests are equivocal and the diagnosis of HFpEF is in question, if there is need to differentiate between pulmonary arterial hypertension and HFpEF (i.e., pulmonary venous hypertension), or if there are questions about the physiology or volume status of a patient with known HFpEF, cardiac catheterization remains the reference standard for assessment of invasive hemodynamics.

Important clinical decisions are made on the basis of invasive hemodynamic testing; thus, proper and careful technique is essential. Pressure tracings should be scrutinized not only for the correct measurement of pressure values but also for the clues provided by the pressure waveforms. In general, pressure measurements should be made at end-expiration during normal, free breathing without asking the patient to perform breath hold maneuvers. Respiratory variation in intracardiac pressure measurements is often exaggerated in HFpEF patients because of the frequent presence of concomitant morbid obesity and chronic lung disease (eFig. 51.5). Right atrial pressure and PCWP tracings should be measured mid-A wave or at the base of the A wave in patients in sinus rhythm and at the base of the V wave in patients with atrial arrhythmias in the absence of A waves.

Tall A waves in the RA pressure tracing are indicative of preserved RA contractile function and a stiff RV. Tall V waves in the RA pressure tracing can be seen in severe tricuspid regurgitation or in the presence of a stiff RA (eFig. 51.6A). A rapid X and Y descent can be seen in patients with the HFpEF clinical syndrome who have a restrictive cardiomyopathy (which can be isolated to the RV) or constrictive pericarditis. A rise in RA pressure during inspiration (Kussmaul's sign) can be seen in patients with HFpEF who have a stiff RV, constrictive pericarditis, or significant tricuspid regurgitation (eFig. 51.6B). A high RV nadir pressure can be indicative of significant volume overload, and an exaggerated A wave in the RV pressure tracing can be seen in patients with a stiff RV. A dip-and-plateau (square root sign) morphology of the RV pressure tracing can be seen in restrictive cardiomyopathy or constrictive pericarditis.

Patients with HFpEF and HFmrEF often have elevated PA pressures, which is most commonly due to pulmonary venous hypertension. PA pulse pressure (PA systolic minus PA diastolic pressure) is often elevated in HFpEF and HFmrEF due to proximal PA stiffening. A high PA systolic pressure can also occur because of the reflected wave from the distal pulmonary pressures (often due to a high PCWP), which causes augmentation of the PA pressure waveform in systole. High PA systolic and PA pulse pressures can lead to high mean PA pressures causing the pulmonary vascular resistance (PVR) to be elevated in HFpEF patients. Elevated PVR (>3 Wood units) primarily due to PA systolic pressure elevation can be differentiated from PVR elevation due to concomitant pulmonary arteriopathy and venopathy by examining the diastolic pressure gradient (DPG; PA diastolic pressure minus PCWP) which will be elevated (>5 to 7 mm Hg) in these cases. The ratio of pulmonary to systemic vascular resistance can also be helpful in HFpEF patients; a high ratio is suggestive of the presence of intrinsic pulmonary vascular disease.

By definition, PCWP should be elevated at rest (≥15 mm Hg) or with passive leg raise or exercise (≥25 mm Hg) in patients with HFpEF and HFmrEF (eFig. 51.7A). Tall V waves in the PCWP tracing (eFig. 51.7B) are also often seen either at rest, during exercise, or during intravenous fluid challenge in HFmrEF and HFpEF and typically reflects a stiff LA more commonly than severe mitral regurgitation. Although PCWP and LV end-diastolic pressure (LVEDP) are often thought of as interchangeable, there can be important differences in the PCWP and LVEDP values, which, in turn, can provide insight into cardiovascular physiology.[61] PCWP is an integrated measure of the burden of LA stiffness (and indirectly the LV stiffness) on the pulmonary circulation, while the LVEDP only provides information on LV compliance. Thus, if PCWP can be measured accurately, it is the best measure to use for the calculation of PVR because poor LA compliance (with resultant accentuated LA pressure waves) is what the pulmonary circulation "sees" and what overloads it, not the LVEDP.

Assessment of cardiac output and stroke volume are important to rule out high-output HF, which has specific etiologies and differs from typical HFpEF. Either thermodilution or Fick cardiac output can be used, but the latter can suffer from assumptions made of oxygen consumption, and direct measurement of oxygen consumption is preferred when available. A low stroke volume in the setting of HFpEF is an important sign and should be interrogated further to determine the cause. Restrictive cardiomyopathy, LA failure due to atrial fibrillation or LA myopathy, valvular heart disease, pulmonary vascular disease, and RV failure are all potential causes of a low stroke volume in the setting of elevated cardiac filling pressures.

Dynamic "perturbation" during invasive hemodynamic testing can be very helpful in patients with HFpEF and can be done with passive leg raise, exercise, fluid challenge, and administration of systemic vasodilators. In patients with unexplained dyspnea, a passive leg raise alone can be helpful for making the diagnosis of HFpEF.[62] As mentioned earlier, exercise can be used in equivocal cases, and exercise invasive hemodynamic testing is considered to be the gold standard test for diagnosis. V waves in the PCWP tracing often become exaggerated during exercise because the LA is unable to handle the extra load that occurs due to splanchnic vasoconstriction leading to a large volume shift of blood from the splanchnic circulation and liver to the stiff left heart. Assessment of the relative rise in mean PA pressure and PCWP during exercise can also be helpful. In patients with passive pulmonary venous hypertension, the mean PA pressure and PCWP will rise in parallel with increasing cardiac output during exercise whereas the mean PA pressure will rise more rapidly compared with PCWP in the setting of intrinsic pulmonary vascular disease (Fig. 51.5). A fluid challenge (10 cc/kg of warmed normal saline over a few minutes) can be safely administered to patients with HFpEF who have an RA pressure ≤12 mm Hg. Exaggerated rise in PCWP is indicative of HFpEF; exaggerated rise in PA pressure relative to PCWP is indicative of pulmonary vascular disease; and lack of augmentation (or reduced) cardiac output after fluid challenge can be seen in the setting of constrictive pericarditis, RV failure, or LA dysfunction. In patients with elevated PVR, administration of a systemic vasodilator such as intravenous nitroprusside can be helpful to differentiate pulmonary venous hypertension from intrinsic pulmonary vascular disease. If nitroprusside administration results in reduction in SVR, PCWP, and mean PA pressure, the pulmonary hypertension is likely due to pulmonary venous hypertension. However, if there is a reduction in SVR and PCWP and yet the mean PA pressure remains elevated (in which case the PVR and DPG will also remain elevated), intrinsic pulmonary vascular disease is likely present.

Coronary evaluation is also helpful in patients with suspected HFpEF or HFmrEF. Although most often first examined noninvasively with nuclear or echocardiographic stress testing (or via coronary computed tomography), invasive coronary angiography is helpful when the diagnosis of CAD or ischemia is uncertain. Coronary vasodilator testing with assessment of coronary flow reserve (CFR) and the index of microvascular resistance (IMR) are also helpful in determining whether or not coronary microvascular dysfunction are present.[63] CFR is defined as the ratio of hyperemic coronary flow (in response to adenosine, for example) to resting coronary flow, and can be measured using invasive coronary flow testing, positron emission tomography (PET), CMR, or transthoracic Doppler echocardiography. The cutoff for defining coronary microvascular dysfunction varies by type of study but is generally defined as CFR <2.0 to 2.5. A reduced CFR can be due to intrinsic coronary microvascular dysfunction but can also be present in patients with epicardial CAD, extrinsic compression of the coronary microvasculature (e.g., due to interstitial myocardial fibrosis), coronary microvascular capillary rarefaction (due to severely diseased coronary microvasculature), or elevated cardiac filling pressures. IMR, which is more specific to the coronary microvasculature, may be less susceptible to hemodynamic factors but currently can be measured only with invasive coronary flow

techniques. An IMR ≥23 is abnormal and indicative of coronary microvascular dysfunction. The combination of a reduced CFR and elevated IMR is most specific for coronary microvascular dysfunction and has been associated with a poor prognosis in HFpEF patients.

Endomyocardial Biopsy

Although not routinely indicated, endomyocardial biopsy can be safely performed during right heart catheterization in patients in whom there is a suspicion for infiltrative or toxic cardiomyopathies. In a single-center study of 108 patients with HFpEF who underwent endomyocardial biopsy, myocardial fibrosis and cardiomyocyte hypertrophy were very common (93% and 88%, respectively) but were mild in the majority of cases. In particular, myocardial fibrosis was absent in 7%, mild or patchy in 66%, moderate in 17%, and severe in only 10% of patients. Of the 108 patients examined, 15 (14%) of the patients were found to have cardiac amyloidosis, 50% in whom the diagnosis was unsuspected.[64] Although there was no evidence of overt inflammation in the biopsy samples, evidence of monocyte infiltration was common in HFpEF, with twofold higher CD68+ cells/mm2 compared with controls. Figure 51.6 displays representative histologic findings of myocardial biopsy specimens in HFpEF patients.

Cardiopulmonary Exercise Testing

Cardiopulmonary exercise testing (CPET) is the reference standard test for assessment of exercise intolerance and dyspnea. CPET is especially useful to distinguish heart failure from other causes of dyspnea, including lung disease, anemia, obesity, or deconditioning. In patients in whom the diagnosis of HFpEF has been established, CPET can be useful to pinpoint the source of exercise intolerance, as shown in Table 51.3, and can be used to classify HF into sub-phenotypes based on differential combination of CPET abnormalities.[65] Nevertheless, CPET cannot diagnose all cases of HFpEF. Reduced peak oxygen consumption is reflective of inadequate augmentation of cardiac output and/or peripheral skeletal muscle extraction during exercise, both of which are frequently present in HFpEF. However, some patients, particularly those with early, milder forms of HFpEF, have an isolated problem of elevated LV filling pressures during exercise, and can still augment cardiac output appropriately.[66] Thus, additional testing, such as diastolic stress echocardiography or invasive exercise hemodynamics may be necessary to rule in or rule out heart failure in such patients.

Extracardiac Considerations

Aorta. Increased central aortic stiffness is common in HFpEF and HFmrEF and may be a major driver of its pathogenesis. Reflected waves from a stiff systemic vasculature result in augmentation of aortic pressure, which in turn creates increased load on the LV during ventricular systole and increases systolic LV wall stress.[67] Increased aortic stiffening can also reduce the ability of the aorta to act as a buffer to the pulsatile flow resulting in barotrauma to organs such as the kidney and brain. A variety of techniques are available for the measurement of aortic stiffness, including systemic pulse pressure (systolic minus diastolic blood pressure), arterial tonometry (for measurement of aortic augmentation index and pulse wave velocity), and imaging techniques such as echocardiography and CMR, which can be used to calculate pulse wave velocity.
Lungs. Systematic evaluation of pulmonary function, including chest radiography, pulmonary function tests (PFTs), and computed

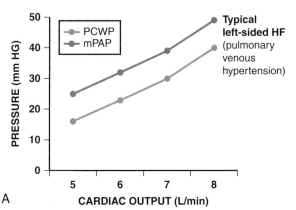

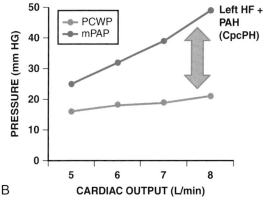

FIGURE 51.5 A, In patients with HFpEF or HFmrEF who develop isolated pulmonary venous hypertension due to left heart disease, the PCWP and mean PA pressure (mPAP) will go up in parallel as cardiac output increases with exercise. **B,** In patients with HFpEF or HFmrEF who develop combined post- and precapillary pulmonary hypertension (CpcPH), mPAP will rise more steeply than the rise in PCWP as cardiac output increases with exercise.

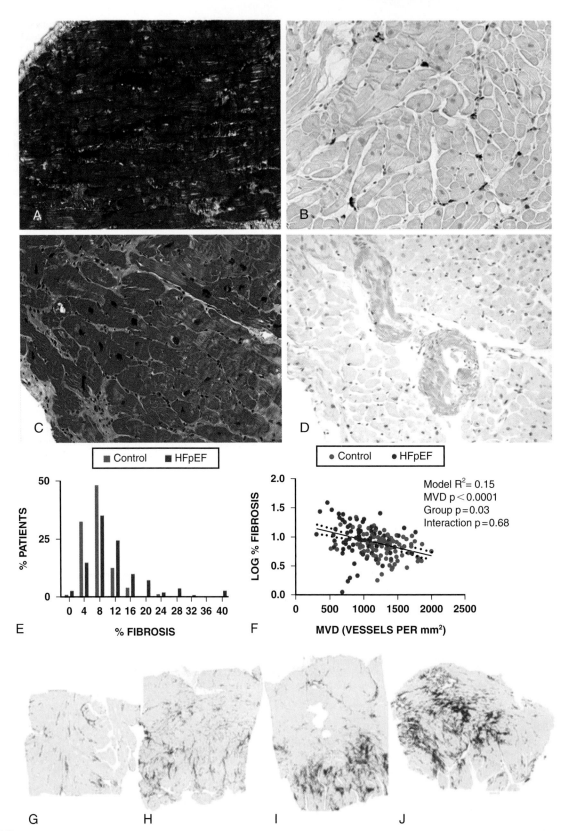

FIGURE 51.6 **A-D,** Endomyocardial biopsy in HFpEF. **A,** Interstitial fibrosis (blue) on Masson's trichrome stain. **B,** CD68+ cells (brown) on immunohistochemistry. **C,** Myocyte hypertrophy on hematoxylin and eosin stain. **D,** Cardiac amyloidosis on Congo Red stain. **E-J,** Cardiac fibrosis in HFpEF and control. **E,** The frequency distribution for percent area fibrosis is shifted upward in HFpEF. **F,** Log-transformed percent area fibrosis increases similarly with decreasing MVD in HFpEF and controls, but it remains higher in HFpEF than in control at any level of MVD. **G-J,** representative examples of SAB stained left ventricular sections with algorithm-defined fibrosis (red), myocardium (*yellow*), and space (*white*) from HFpEF patients with 3% **(G)**, 7% **(H)**, 10% **(I)**, and 21% **(J)** fibrosis. *HFpEF,* heart failure with preserved ejection fraction; *MVD,* microvascular density; *SAB,* sulfated Alcian blue. (**A-D** adapted from Hahn V, et al. Endomyocardial biopsy characterization of heart failure with preserved ejection fraction and prevalence of cardiac amyloidosis. JACC Heart Fail. 2020;8[9]:712-724; **E-J** adapted from Mohammed S, et al. Coronary microvascular rarefaction and myocardial fibrosis in heart failure with preserved ejection fraction. Circulation. 2015;131[6]:550-559.)

TABLE 51.3 Cardiopulmonary Exercise Testing in HFpEF and HFmrEF

CPET PARAMETER	INTERPRETATION
RER <1.05	Submaximal test limited by noncardiopulmonary factor
Peak V_{O_2} < 80% predicted	Indicative of impaired exercise capacity
Discrepancy between unindexed peak V_{O_2} and indexed peak V_{O_2}	In patients with obesity-induced limitation of exercise capacity, unindexed peak V_{O_2} (percent predicted) will be relatively preserved but once indexed to body weight will be much more abnormal
Peak V_E/maximum voluntary V_E <70%	Evaluate for intrinsic pulmonary disease
Reduced O_2 pulse	Look for low stroke volume as a potential cause
Blunted heart rate response	Medication-induced (e.g., beta blocker) versus chronotropic incompetence
Elevated V_E/V_{CO_2}	Can be a sign of elevated PA pressure and PVR; and does not require a maximal test; also a prognostic sign in HFpEF
Exercise oscillatory breathing	Indicative of a worse prognosis in HFpEF

tomography (CT) of the chest is important in patients suspected with HFpEF and HFmrEF to exclude a pulmonary cause of symptoms. Chronic lung diseases, particularly chronic obstructive pulmonary disease (COPD), are often present in patients with HFpEF and HFmrEF and can contribute to its pathogenesis. In patients with COPD with hyperinflation, a chronically underfilled left heart can lead to reduced stroke volume and cardiac output, which triggers neurohormonal activation and can lead to systemic hypertension, which can eventually cause HF. Patients with COPD and chronic bronchitis appear to share risk factors with HFpEF and HFmrEF such as obesity. In patients with either COPD or interstitial lung disease, pulmonary hypertension can result in RV dysfunction, which can further exacerbate HFpEF and right heart failure. Even in the absence of chronic lung disease, HFpEF and HFmrEF patients may have abnormal PFT findings, including reduced forced vital capacity (especially in the setting of obesity) and reduced diffuse capacity of carbon monoxide (COPD) due to pulmonary venous congestion, interstitial edema, alveolar edema, and pulmonary vascular disease.

Central and obstructive sleep apnea (CSA and OSA, respectively) are also common in HFpEF and HFmrEF. CSA can occur in decompensated HF regardless of underlying EF, and increased laryngeal edema and obesity can result in OSA. Thus, overnight polysomnography can be useful in the assessment of HFpEF but should be performed after adequate diuresis to ensure that fluid overload alone is not the cause of either CSA or OSA.[68]

Kidney. Impaired renal function is important in the pathogenesis of HFpEF, often coexists with HFpEF, and can be a major cause of fluid retention. However, because of the crude nature of clinical assessment of renal function (which is reliant on creatinine for estimation of glomerular filtration rate [GFR]), assessment of renal function in HFpEF is often inaccurate and misleading. In patients with overt fluid overload, the serum creatinine level can be hemodiluted, resulting in false reassurance of "normal" renal function. Conversely, diuresis in HFpEF is often halted due to elevation in serum creatinine despite its beneficial effects because clinicians fail to understand the concept of hemoconcentration during diuresis.[69] Several studies have shown that hemoconcentration during diuresis, despite being associated with rising serum creatinine, is associated with improved outcomes in the setting of HF.

Skeletal Muscle. Several studies have demonstrated the concept of sarcopenic obesity in HFpEF.[70] As in other chronic diseases, there is loss of skeletal muscle and increased intramuscular adiposity. Furthermore, there is a transition between type I to type II muscle fibers in HFpEF, which results in impaired exercise tolerance in HFpEF.[71] Patients with HFpEF also have systemic microvascular dysfunction, which, when present in the skeletal muscles, results in decreased oxygen extraction, which has been shown to account for 50% of the reduction in peak V_{O_2} in HFpEF patients. CPET is therefore a useful tool for the assessment of skeletal muscle dysfunction in HFpEF (based on measurement of arteriovenous O_2 difference). Magnetic resonance spectroscopy can also be

utilized to directly examine skeletal muscle energetics and skeletal muscle composition, though such techniques are currently primarily used in the research setting.

Liver. In patients with signs and symptoms of HFpEF, clinical evaluation of the liver is important to exclude primary cirrhosis with high-output heart failure. Nonalcoholic fatty liver disease (NAFLD) is common in morbidly obese patients and is associated with worse LV longitudinal strain, diastolic dysfunction, and higher stroke volume in the general population, all of which can contribute to a HFpEF phenotype.[72] Conversely, severe HFpEF with right heart failure can result in passive congestion of the liver, ultimately leading to cirrhosis. Therefore, liver function tests (particularly bilirubin and alkaline phosphatase as markers of liver congestion) and radiologic assessment of the liver by ultrasound, CT, or MRI can be useful in teasing out the role of the liver in patients with HFpEF.

Adipose Tissue. Increased visceral adiposity is a major contributor to HFpEF pathophysiology and is not always apparent by simply examining the BMI in HFpEF patients.[73] Certain subgroups of patients, especially those of South Asian descent, can have lower BMI but high visceral adiposity. Excessive epicardial adipose tissue may be particularly relevant to the pathophysiology of HFpEF patients.[47,74] Multiple methods for evaluating the presence and extent of visceral adiposity are available, including waist-hip circumference ratio, dual-energy X-ray absorptiometry (DEXA) scanning, and CT or MRI of the chest and abdomen. Several biomarkers, including increased triglyceride/HDL ratio, hyperglycemia with insulin resistance, increased plasminogen activator inhibitor-1 (PAI-1), and reduced vitamin D levels are also indicative of increased visceral adiposity.

PATHOPHYSIOLOGY

Pathophysiology of HFpEF and HFmrEF

From a hemodynamic perspective, the cardinal abnormality in HFpEF patients is LV end-diastolic pressure elevation (with resultant LA pressure elevation) at rest or with exertion. Patients with HFpEF have marked elevation in PCWP with minimal exertion (see eFig. 51.7A). How and why cardiac pressure elevation occurs in HFpEF has been a matter of intense investigation over the past 25 years. In HFrEF, the primary cardiac insult results in myocardial injury (e.g., myocardial infarction, genetic cardiomyopathy, toxins [including chemotherapy], pathogens [e.g., viruses], or other causes), leading to progressive ventricular dysfunction, ventricular dilatation, and elevated filling pressure. Similar mechanisms may be in part responsible for the clinical syndrome in HFmrEF, especially in patients whose LVEF is reduced because of ischemic heart disease. The mechanisms of myocardial dysfunction in HFpEF, where LVEF is normal, remains unclear.

Once HFpEF is clinically overt, a variety of potential pathophysiologic abnormalities can be present (Fig. 51.7).[75] Although the presence of abnormal myocardial relaxation and reduced LV chamber compliance are common in HFpEF and previously thought to be the major pathophysiologic abnormality in HFpEF, it is likely that HFpEF represents a systemic syndrome with multiple cardiac and extracardiac pathophysiologic mechanisms beyond diastolic dysfunction. From a cardiac perspective, LV systolic dysfunction is often impaired despite a preserved LVEF. Longitudinal fiber LV systolic dysfunction (i.e., abnormal LV global longitudinal strain and reduced TDI s' velocities) are often present in HFpEF[57]; furthermore, patients with HFpEF often have impaired LV contractile reserve. LA dysfunction is common in HFpEF, and some patients may have a primary LA myopathy out of proportion to LV dysfunction. Worse LA reservoir function (i.e., impaired ability of the LA to expand during LV systole) promotes chronic increases in pulmonary venous pressure, which can lead to pulmonary hypertension and right-sided heart failure. Atrial dilation in response to the HFpEF syndrome often leads to mitral and tricuspid annular dilation with resultant mitral and tricuspid regurgitation, both of which can exacerbate the HFpEF syndrome. Additional potential mechanisms in HFpEF include abnormal ventricular-arterial coupling and chronotropic incompetence.

Systemic and coronary endothelial dysfunction are common in HFpEF. CFR is reduced in up to 75% of HFpEF patients,[60] and evidence of coronary microvascular disease is present in the majority of HFpEF

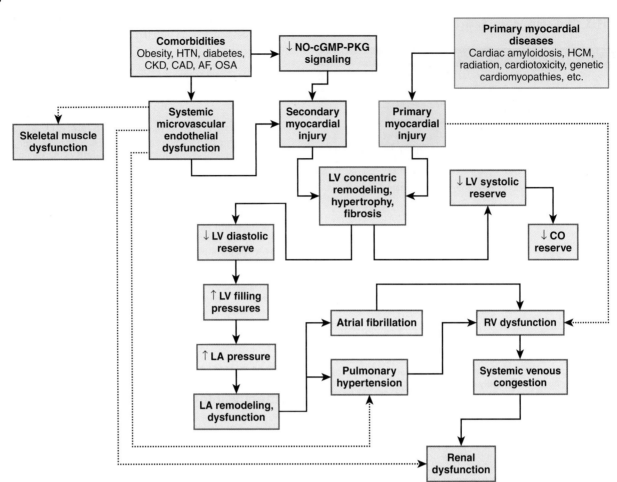

FIGURE 51.7 Etiologic and pathophysiologic model of HFpEF. Etiologic and pathophysiologic model of heart failure with preserved ejection fraction. HFpEF can result from primary or secondary myocardial injury, with the latter being more typical of the syndrome. Comorbidities are thought to lead to systemic inflammation, which is associated with systemic endothelial dysfunction and decreased NO-cGMP-PKG signaling that result in secondary myocardial injury. Other diseases such as cardiac amyloidosis and HCM result in primary myocardial injury. Regardless of the cause, LV concentric remodeling and hypertrophy ensues, which results in a cascade of LV dysfunction, LA dysfunction, and RV dysfunction, ultimately leading to pulmonary and systemic venous congestion. Systemic endothelial dysfunction also likely contributes to skeletal muscle dysfunction and renal dysfunction, both of which are present in the vast majority of HFpEF patients. *AF,* Atrial fibrillation; *CKD,* chronic kidney disease; *CAD,* coronary artery disease; *cGMP,* cyclic guanosine monophosphate; *CO,* cardiac output; *HCM,* hypertrophic cardiomyopathy; *HTN,* hypertension; *LA,* left atrial; *LV,* left ventricular; *NO,* nitric oxide; *OSA,* obstructive sleep apnea; *PKG,* protein kinase G; *RV,* right ventricular. (From Shah SJ. Innovative clinical trial designs for precision medicine in heart failure with preserved ejection fraction. J Cardiovasc Transl Res. 2017;10[3]:322-336.)

patients on autopsy[76] (Fig. 51.8). Reduced CFR is associated with systemic endothelial dysfunction and worse cardiac structure and function in HFpEF and may be a key factor underlying the poor systolic and diastolic reserve present in the setting of HFpEF. In addition, coronary microvascular dysfunction can involve the RV, resulting in impaired RV function independent of RV dysfunction due to increased RV afterload. Systemic endothelial dysfunction can lead to pulmonary, renal, and skeletal muscle dysfunction in HFpEF, all of which likely lead to and exacerbate the HFpEF syndrome.

Less is known about the underlying pathophysiology of HFmrEF due to a general lack of detailed studies in this HF subtype. Because of the mildly reduced LVEF, HFmrEF share some pathophysiologic similarities with patients with HFrEF. Longitudinal systolic dysfunction (i.e., abnormal LV global longitudinal strain) and impaired contractile reserve are more exaggerated in HFmrEF compared with HFpEF. Nevertheless, HFmrEF patients share many of the same comorbidities as HFpEF and may therefore also share some pathophysiologic similarities such as systemic and coronary endothelial dysfunction, abnormal ventricular-arterial coupling, and chronotropic incompetence.

Molecular Mechanisms Underlying HFpEF And HFmrEF
Several molecular mechanisms have been investigated in preclinical studies of HFpEF.[77] Comorbidity-induced systemic inflammation and endothelial dysfunction, cyclic guanosine monophosphate (cGMP)-protein kinase G (PKG) deficiency, interstitial myocardial fibrosis related to hypertension and diabetes, abnormal cardiomyocyte calcium handling,

lipotoxicity, metabolic defects in fuel utilization and efficiency, and loss of cytoprotective signaling are some of the molecular mechanisms thought to be present in common forms of HFpEF, as shown in Figure 51.9.[75] Less is known about the molecular mechanisms of HFmrEF due to the lack of basic science studies of this HF phenotype.

The comorbidity-inflammation-endothelial dysfunction paradigm has garnered recent attention in HFpEF because patients with HFpEF often have multiple comorbidities such as hypertension, obesity, diabetes, chronic kidney disease, CAD, and COPD, and markers of systemic inflammation are more potent risk factors for incident HFpEF compared with incident HFrEF. Comorbidities are thought to result in systemic inflammation leading to endothelial dysfunction in multiple organs throughout the body. Inflammation-induced endothelial dysfunction affects the myocardium, lungs, skeletal muscle, and kidneys leading to diverse HFpEF phenotypes with variable amounts of myocardial remodeling and dysfunction, pulmonary hypertension, renal sodium retention, and deficient skeletal muscle oxygen extraction during exercise. In the heart, inflammation-induced coronary endothelial dysfunction can result in coronary microvascular dysfunction with subendocardial ischemia, particularly during exertion. Endothelial inflammation also causes increased reactive oxygen species, reduced nitric oxide bioavailability, and production of peroxynitrite, resulting in reduced soluble guanylate cyclase activity, lower cGMP content, and reduced PKG. Decreased PKG has protean manifestations germane to HFpEF: increased cardiomyocyte hypertrophy, increased cardiomyocyte stiffness (due to changes in titin phosphorylation), pulmonary vasoconstriction, impaired renal and skeletal muscle function, and increased adiposity. Inflammation also results in increased endothelial expression of adhesion molecules, which attract infiltrating leukocytes that secrete transforming growth factor β

(TGF-β), which converts fibroblasts to myofibroblasts thereby enhancing interstitial collagen deposition and promoting interstitial myocardial fibrosis.[78,79]

Systemic inflammation also leads to the activation of monocytes and macrophages, which release pro-fibrotic cytokines including interleukin-10 and TGF-β, thereby promoting interstitial fibrosis in multiple organs, including the heart.[80] Importantly, collagen cross-linking tends to be higher in HFpEF with increased profibrotic potential in HFpEF compared with HFrEF.[78] Measurement of circulating markers of fibrosis in HFpEF and HFmrEF patients have shown that collagen synthesis is increased, and collagen degradation is decreased. Both mineralocorticoid antagonists and sacubitril/valsartan appear to reverse these

processes resulting in a less pro-fibrotic profile in HFpEF and HFmrEF patients treated with these drugs.[78,81]

Although endothelium-derived NO is reduced in HFpEF, inducible NO synthase (iNOS), which is activated by systemic inflammation, may be upregulated and could be a pathogenic factor leading to HFpEF. In a recent study that utilized a novel 2-hit mouse model of HFpEF leading to hypertension and obesity, NOS was upregulated, which resulted in nitrosative stress of the endonuclease inositol-requiring protein 1α (IRE1α), leading to defective splicing of an unfolded protein response effector (the spliced form of X-box-binding protein 1 [XBP1s]). XBP1s, in turn, was reduced in both the rodent HFpEF model and also in myocardial samples from patients with HFpEF. Defective splicing of XBP1s leads

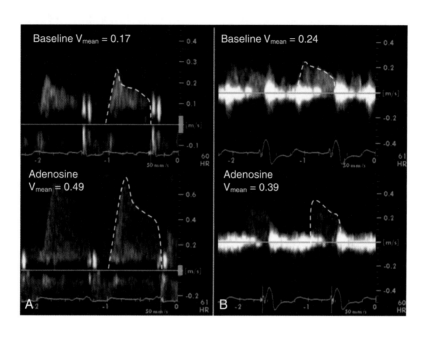

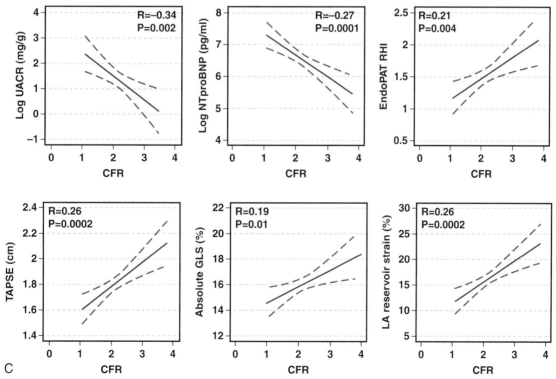

FIGURE 51.8 Coronary microvascular dysfunction in HFpEF and HFmrEF. A and **B,** Examples of transthoracic coronary Doppler echocardiography tracings at rest and with adenosine in a HFpEF patient without coronary microvascular dysfunction **(A)** versus a HFpEF patient with coronary microvascular dysfunction **(B)**. The patient without coronary microvascular dysfunction had a normal coronary flow reserve (2.88), whereas the patient with coronary microvascular dysfunction had a reduced coronary flow reserve (1.63). **C,** Correlations between coronary flow reserve (CFR) and biomarkers, systemic endothelial function, and echocardiographic parameters in the PROMIS-HFpEF study. *EndoPAT,* endothelial peripheral artery tonometry; *GLS,* left ventricular global longitudinal strain; *LA,* left atrial; *NTproBNP,* N-terminal pro-B-type natriuretic peptide; *RHI,* reactive hyperemia index, a marker of systemic endothelial function; *TAPSE,* tricuspid annular plane systolic excursion; *UACR,* urinary albumin-to-creatinine ratio.

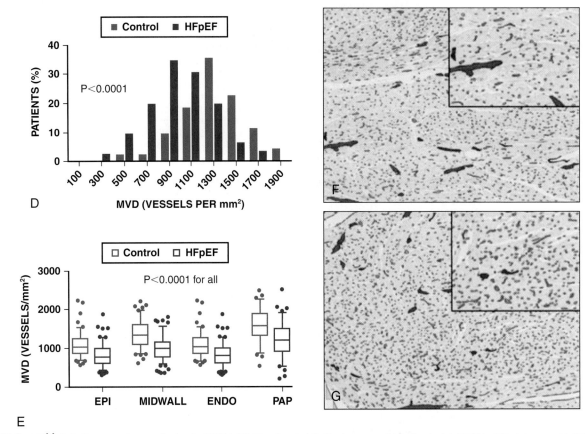

FIGURE 51.8 cont'd D-G, Coronary microvascular density (MVD) in HFpEF and control. **D,** The frequency distribution for total MVD is shifted downward in HFpEF. **E,** Tukey box plots (*box*, median, 75th, and 25th percentiles; *whiskers*, highest value within 75th percentile plus 1.5 × IQR and lowest value within the 25th percentile minus 1.5 × IQR; symbols show outliers if present) of regional MVD demonstrate similar reduction in MVD across the subepicardial (*Epi*), midmyocardial (*Midwall*), subendocardial (*Endo*), and papillary muscle (*Pap*) in HFpEF. Representative examples of antiplatelet endothelial cell adhesion molecule-1/ anti-CD31 stained left ventricular sections with algorithm-defined capillaries (*yellow*), precapillary arterioles (*orange*), and larger intramyocardial arteries (*red*) illustrate **(F)** the lower MVD in HFpEF in comparison with **(G)** control subjects. *CD31,* cluster of differentiation 31; *HFpEF,* heart failure with preserved ejection fraction; *IQR,* interquartile range. (A-C adapted from Shah SJ, et al. Prevalence and correlates of coronary microvascular dysfunction in heart failure with preserved ejection fraction: PROMIS-HFpEF. Eur Heart J. 2018;39[37]:3439-3450; D-G from Mohammed S, et al. Coronary microvascular rarefaction and myocardial fibrosis in heart failure with preserved ejection fraction. Circulation. 2015;131[6]:550-559.)

to increased levels of unfolded proteins within the cardiomyocytes, which are thought to interfere with normal cardiomyocyte function.[82]

Multiple mechanisms present in HFpEF can result in stiffening of titin, the major molecular spring within the cardiomyocyte, thereby leading to increased passive stiffness of cardiomyocytes (with resultant increased LV chamber stiffness). As stated earlier, reduced PKG leads to abnormal phosphorylation of key sites within titin and increases in its stiffness. Other mechanisms of increased stiffness of titin include cardiomyocyte stretch induced ERK-2 signaling, sympathetically mediated PKA stimulation, reactive oxygen species-induced CaMKII abnormalities, and endothelin- and angiotensin-II-mediated increases in PKCα.[75]

Abnormal calcium homeostasis in cardiomyocytes has long been known to be associated with abnormalities in systolic and diastolic function and are likely impaired in HFpEF and HFmrEF patients. T-tubule disruption, increased calcium entry into cardiomyocytes due to enhanced late inward sodium current, defective ryanodine receptor functioning, reduced SERCA2a activity, and abnormal myofilament calcium handling are all potential mechanisms underlying defective cardiomyocyte calcium homeostasis and could represent therapeutic targets in HFpEF and HFmrEF.[75]

Strategies for Phenotypic Subtyping of HFpEF

Because of the heterogeneous nature of the HFpEF syndrome, multiple potential mechanisms, and widespread endothelial dysfunction that can variably affect multiple organs with varying severity, several potential HFpEF sub-phenotypes exist.[83] For these reasons, the creation of a rationale, unified classification system for HFpEF has been challenging. Nevertheless, several ways of classifying HFpEF are available and can assist with clinical management of HFpEF (Table 51.4): (1) clinical subtypes (based on etiologic and echocardiographic features); (2) dominant HFpEF pathophysiology; (3) clinical presentation (exercise-induced LA pressure elevation, overt volume overload, or pulmonary hypertension/RV failure); and (4) extent of cardiac (vs. extracardiac) involvement. While these HFpEF sub-phenotypes are not necessarily mutually exclusive and

may represent different stages of the disease they are nevertheless helpful in the clinical setting and also may explain why HFpEF clinical trials have met with little success. For example, a HFpEF patient with exercise-induced LA pressure elevation with minimal signs of overt fluid overload and a HFpEF patient with significant RV enlargement/dysfunction and pulmonary hypertension may both have elevated natriuretic peptides and LA enlargement and therefore meet inclusion of contemporary HFpEF clinical trials. However, the management of these two types of patients would likely differ dramatically in the clinical setting. The first patient may benefit from structured exercise training whereas the second patient may benefit from implantable hemodynamic monitoring to guide diuresis. Besides pathophysiologic and etiologic sub-phenotypes of HFpEF, it is now also recognized that there are important geographical differences in HFpEF, likely related to different underlying risk factors and genetic backgrounds.[84]

TREATMENT OF HFPEF AND HFMREF

The treatment of HF with a LVEF of 40% or less (HFrEF) has been informed by an abundance of large clinical outcomes trials that have tested several classes of pharmacologic and device therapies and afforded clinicians a full armamentarium of treatments designed to reduce morbidity and mortality (see also Chapter 50). In contrast, there have been limited large clinical outcomes trials to inform therapeutic approaches in patients with HF and LVEF >40%, and treatment of these patients has been mostly empiric. While many of the basic principles of HF management are similar regardless of LVEF, several therapies that have proven beneficial in HFrEF have shown no or limited benefit in patients with HF and higher LVEF (>55% to 60%). Moreover, the treatment of HFpEF and HFmrEF is complicated by the added complexity

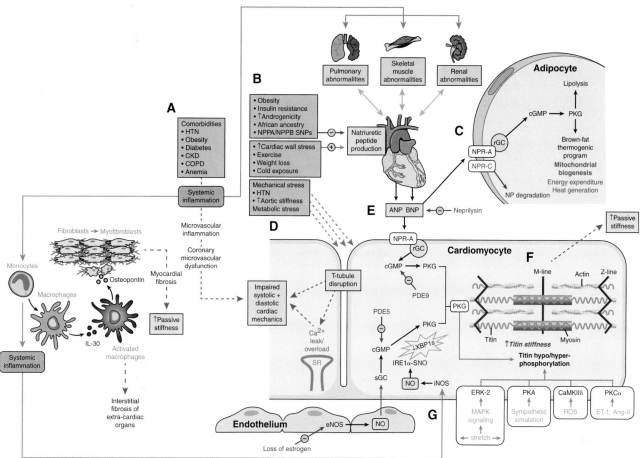

FIGURE 51.9 Proposed molecular mechanisms underlying HFpEF. A, Comorbidities are common in HFpEF and are thought to lead to systemic inflammation, which results in microvascular inflammation, widespread endothelial dysfunction (in multiple organs), and coronary microvascular dysfunction, leading to abnormal systolic and diastolic cardiac mechanics and poor cardiac reserve. Systemic inflammation also leads to the activation of monocytes and macrophages, which release profibrotic cytokines, including IL-10 and transforming growth factor-β, thereby promoting interstitial organ fibrosis, which in the heart increases passive myocardial stiffness. **B,** Several factors promote a relative natriuretic peptide (NP) deficiency state in HFpEF, including obesity, sedentary lifestyle, African ancestry, insulin resistance, increased androgenicity in women, genetic variation in the *NPPA* and *NPPB* genes, and a lower amount of wall stress for the severity of heart failure (compared with heart failure with reduced ejection fraction). **C,** NPs are active in adipose tissue, where the relative ratio of the NP receptor A (*NPRA*) to NP receptor C (*RC*) is important in dictating whether beneficial NP effects are possible. With increased NPRA, there is increased cGMP and protein kinase G (*PKG*) production, leading to lipolysis and the brown-fat thermogenic program. With increased NPRC, these beneficial effects are minimized because there is increased NP breakdown. **D,** Mechanical and metabolic stressors on the cardiomyocyte lead to T-tubule disruption and abnormal calcium handling within the cardiomyocyte, which leads to intracellular calcium overload and inefficient myocardial contraction and relaxation. **E,** NPs act through a receptor guanylate cyclase (rGC) pathway that results in the creation of cGMP and stimulation of PKG, which has a variety of beneficial effects in the heart and multiple other organs. There is also an intracellular, soluble guanylate cyclase that is stimulated by nitric oxide (*NO*), which also leads to increased cGMP and activation of PKG. Phosphodiesterase (*PDE*) 5 results in the breakdown of the NO-based cGMP pool, whereas PDE9 results in the breakdown of the NP-based cGMP pool. **F,** Multiple mechanisms present in HFpEF can result in stiffening of titin, the major molecular spring within the cardiomyocyte, thereby leading to increased cardiomyocyte (and subsequently cardiac chamber) passive stiffness. Because of insufficient NPs and NO, PKG is reduced in HFpEF, which leads to hypophosphorylation of key sites within titin and increases its stiffness. Extracellular signal–regulated kinase 2 (ERK-2; stimulated by increased cardiomyocyte stretch), protein kinase A (PKA; stimulated by sympathetic stimulation), calmodulin-dependent protein kinase II (CaMKII; stimulated by reactive oxygen species [ROS]), and protein kinase Cα (PKCα; stimulated by endothelin-1 [ET-1] and angiotensin-II) all can have deleterious prostiffening effects on titin. **G,** Although endothelium-de-rived NO is reduced in HFpEF, inducible NO synthase (*iNOS*), which is activated by systemic inflammation, is upregulated and could be a pathogenic factor leading to HFpEF. In a recent study that used a novel two-hit mouse model of HFpEF (Nω-nitro-l-arginine methyl ester, which induces hypertension (HTN)]+high-fat diet [obesity]), iNOS was upregulated, which resulted in *S*-nitrosylation (nitrosative stress) of the endonuclease inositol-requiring protein 1α (*IRE1α*), leading to defective splicing of an unfolded protein response effector (the spliced form of X-box-binding protein 1 [*XBP1s*]). XBP1s, in turn, was reduced in both the rodent HFpEF model and in myocardial samples from patients with HFpEF, leading to increased levels of unfolded proteins within the cardiomyocytes, which are thought to interfere in normal cardiomyocyte function. *ANP,* atrial NP; *BNP,* brain NP; *CKD,* chronic kidney disease; *COPD,* chronic obstructive pulmonary disease; *eNOS,* endothelial NO synthase; *IL,* interleukin; *MAPK,* mitogen-activated protein kinase; *SNO,* S-nitrosylation; *SNP,* single nucleotide polymorphism. (From Shah SJ, et al. Research priorities for heart failure with preserved ejection fraction: National Heart, Lung, and Blood Institute Working Group Summary. Circulation. 2020;141[12]:1001-1026.)

of diagnosis in a syndrome in which signs and symptoms overlap with other diseases, and in which clear evidence of cardiac abnormalities are often lacking, a problem that has also confounded the testing of therapies in clinical trials.

General Considerations
Exclusion of Other Causes of Signs/Symptoms

Once the diagnosis of HFpEF or HFmrEF is clear, it is important to recognize that several potential etiologies can result in signs and symptoms of HF, a preserved or mildly reduced LVEF, and elevated cardiac filling pressures (Table 51.5). Because the signs and symptoms associated with HFpEF and HFmrEF are relatively nonspecific, it is necessary that other diseases that can mimic these be considered and ruled out.

Ischemic heart disease resulting in anginal equivalent of shortness of breath can be mistaken for HF. Hypertensive crisis can present with signs and symptoms of HF that can be alleviated with blood pressure control. Both obstructive and interstitial forms of lung disease, as well as pulmonary venoocclusive disease, can mimic the shortness of breath in HF, and elevation in pulmonary pressures can lead to right-sided symptoms and signs, including early satiety, pleural effusions, and edema. All of these conditions have pathophysiologic features that are distinct from HF and can be treated by specific therapies.

Additionally, several distinct disease entities that can present with HF and in which ejection fraction can be relatively preserved should be ruled out, including amyloid heart disease, hypertrophic cardiomyopathy, and constrictive pericarditis (see also Chapters 53, 54, and 86). There are several clinical clues that should alert the clinician to the

TABLE 51.4 Classification Schemes for HFpEF

CLASSIFICATION SCHEME	CATEGORIES OF HFPEF	DESCRIPTION
Clinical classification	"Garden-variety" HFpEF	Hypertension, diabetes, obesity, and/or chronic kidney disease
	CAD-HFpEF	Typically multivessel CAD with prior coronary revascularization
	Right heart failure–HFpEF	Predominant right-sided HF with or without pulmonary hypertension
	Atrial fibrillation–predominant HFpEF	Atrial arrhythmias dominate the clinical presentation
	HCM-like HFpEF	These patients do not have genetic forms of HCM, but their clinical course and echocardiography features are typical of HCM
	High-output HFpEF	Typically due to liver disease and severe anemia
	Valvular HFpEF	Multiple moderate valvular lesions
	Rare causes of HFpEF	For example, infiltrative cardiomyopathies, cardiotoxicities, and genetic cardiomyopathies
Presentation phenotypes	Exercise-induced increase in LA pressure	These patients typically are very breathless with exertion but do not have overt signs of volume overload and typically do not have a history of HF hospitalization
	Volume overload	Signs and symptoms of volume overload: typically have a history of HF hospitalization
	RV failure + pulmonary hypertension	Right heart failure predominates the clinical picture: often pulmonary hypertension is present and systemic blood pressure is reduced
Myocardial phenotypes	Type 1: HCM	Typical genetic forms of HCM
	Type 2: infiltrative	Cardiac amyloidosis and other forms of infiltrative or restrictive cardiomyopathies
	Type 3: non-HTN. non-LVH	No history of hypertension and LV wall thickness <1.2 cm
	Type 4: HTN	Typical, "garden-variety" form of HFpEF with history of HTN
Latent class analysis	A: younger males with CAD, lower LVEF	Based on latent class analysis of the I-PRESERVE and CHARM-Preserved trials. The authors used latent class analysis of 11 clinical features (age, gender, BMI, atrial fibrillation. CAD, diabetes, hyperlipidemia, valvular disease, alcohol use, cGFR, and hematocrit) to find six distinct groups of HFpEF in IPRESERVE and validated these findings in CHARM-Preserved
	B: younger females with lowest NT-proBNP	
	C: obesity, hyperlipidemia, diabetes mellitus, anemia, and renal insufficiency	
	D: obese females	
	E: older males with CAD, lowest LVEF	
	F: female predominance, advanced age, lower BMI, atrial fibrillation, CKD, highest NT-proBNP	
Phenomapping	Pheno-group 1: BNP deficiency syndrome	Based on model-based clustering of 67 continuous variables (phenotypes): physical characteristics, vital signs, ECG data laboratory data, and echocardiography parameters
	Pheno-group 2: obesity–cardiometabolic phenotype	
	Pheno-group 3: RV failure + cardiorenal phenotype	

BMI, Body mass index; *CAD,* coronary artery disease; *CKD,* chronic kidney disease; *HCM,* hypertrophic cardiomyopathy; *HTN,* hypertension; *LVH,* left ventricular hypertrophy; *LVEF,* left ventricular ejection fraction; *NTproBNP,* N-terminal pro-B-type natriuretic peptide; *RV,* right ventricular.
Data from Shah SJ. Precision medicine for heart failure with preserved ejection fraction: an overview. *J Cardiovasc Transl Res.* 2017;10(3):233–244.

TABLE 51.5 Differential Diagnosis of HFpEF

ETIOLOGY	DIAGNOSTIC TOOLS	TREATMENT
Cardiac amyloidosis	Monoclonal proteins, radionuclide scintigraphy, biopsy	Tafamidis (for transthyretin amyloidosis) or chemotherapy (for light-chain amyloidosis); avoid neurohormonal antagonists
Hypertrophic cardiomyopathy	Echocardiography, cardiac MRI	Beta blockers, calcium channel blockers, or septal reduction therapies (for obstructive cardiomyopathy); avoid vasodilators
Cardiac sarcoidosis	Cardiac MRI, FDG-PET, biopsy	Immunosuppressive agents
Constrictive pericarditis	Echocardiography, cardiac MRI or CT imaging, invasive hemodynamic measurements	Pericardiectomy
Valvular heart disease	Echocardiography, invasive hemodynamic measurements with ventriculography	Surgical or percutaneous valve interventions
Coronary artery disease	Invasive coronary angiography, stress imaging[†] or CT imaging	Revascularization, aspirin, statins, beta blockers, and nitrates
High-output heart failure	Evaluate for arteriovenous shunts and liver disease	Treatments directed at the cause of high cardiac output (such as fistula ligation for shunts, liver transplantation for cirrhosis)
Myocarditis	Cardiac MRI, endomyocardial biopsy	Immunosuppressive agents for some types (such as giant cell myocarditis or eosinophilic myocarditis)
Toxins	Assessment of clinical history, blood testing, endomyocardial biopsy	Removal of offending toxin (such as alcohol, cocaine, chemotherapy or radiation therapy, or heavy metals)

possibility of an atypical cause of the syndrome (Table 51.6). While these diseases can overlap with HFpEF and HFmrEF, the specific underlying etiology and pathophysiology are distinct, and targeted treatment options are either available or emerging.

Pathophysiologic Considerations of Therapy

The pathophysiology of HF, regardless of LVEF, is characterized by insufficient cardiac output to meet the body's metabolic needs, elevation in cardiac filling pressures, or both. Despite normal or mildly reduced LVEF, stroke volume (and hence cardiac output) can be low in patients with HFpEF and HFmrEF because of relatively small LV volume and LA failure, resulting in an inability to augment stroke volume during exertion, or to do so only by elevating filling pressure. Thus, while cardiac output may be sufficient at rest, during exertion it may be insufficient, resulting in symptoms. Unlike HFrEF where augmentation of stroke volume can potentially be of value, in HF with higher LVEF, it is not clear that increases in contractile function would be of benefit, as LVEF is already relatively high, even though patients with HFpEF do often have evidence of LV systolic dysfunction and impaired contractile reserve. One situation in which inadequate cardiac output might contribute to a patients' symptoms in HFpEF and HFmrEF is *chronotropic incompetence*, in which patients lack the ability to adequately increase heart rate in the setting of exertion.[85] In cases of true chronotropic incompetence, in which the contribution of medications such as beta blockers or calcium channel blockers has been ruled out, pacemaker therapy may have a role in ensuring adequate cardiac output (see later and Chapters 68 and 69).

LV diastolic dysfunction is present in the majority of patients with HFpEF and HFmrEF, and likely contributes to the pathophysiology of the syndrome. While several lusitropic therapies have been tested in patients with HFpEF and HFmrEF, few therapies other than blood pressure management (see later) have been shown to specifically improve diastolic function.

Mortality Reduction in HFpEF and HFmrEF

The overall goals of HF therapy are to reduce mortality, reduce hospitalization, and improve symptoms and functional capacity. Although mortality is increased in patients with HFpEF and HFmrEF compared with the general population, the absolute incidence of mortality in HF declines as LVEF rises, as does the proportion of deaths attributed to noncardiovascular causes. It has therefore been more difficult to demonstrate mortality benefit in HFpEF and HFmrEF than in HFrEF, both because of the lower event rates, and because therapies that are predominantly aimed at the cardiovascular system will be less able to modify noncardiovascular mortality.[86] Thus, reducing mortality in patients with HFpEF and HFmrEF requires focusing on factors that contribute to known risk factors for death, including treatment of both cardiac and noncardiac comorbidities that increase that risk. Beyond mortality reduction it is important to recognize that reduction in hospitalization and improvement in symptoms and functional capacity are critical patient-centered goals in the management of HFpEF and HFmrEF.

TABLE 51.6 Clues to Atypical Causes of HFpEF

CLUE TO ATYPICAL CAUSE OF HFPEF	NOTES/RATIONALES
HFpEF in a younger patient (age <55 years), especially if conventional HFpEF risk factors are lacking	Patients with common forms of HFpEF are often older and frequently have multiple comorbidities; if these are absent there may be an atypical cause of HFpEF.
Low BP, or LV hypertrophy without hypertension	Hypertension is very common in HFpEF; LV hypertrophy without hypertension is an indicator of an atypical cause of HFpEF.
Definite HFpEF (e.g., documented elevated LV filling pressures, prior HF hospitalization) but low H_2FPEF score	The H_2FPEF score combines common HFpEF risk factors with Doppler echocardiographic evidence of elevated LV filling pressures; if the score is low but definite HF is present, an atypical cause of HFpEF should be excluded.
Kussmaul's sign: ↑JVP with inspiration	Kussmaul's sign can be a sign of constrictive pericarditis, restrictive cardiomyopathy, severe tricuspid regurgitation, or a primary RV cardiomyopathy.
Persistent, low-level troponin elevation	Persistent low-level troponin elevation can be a sign of infiltrative cardiomyopathy such as cardiac amyloidosis.
Low prealbumin (= transthyretin)	Transthyretin (also known as prealbumin) can be measured clinically. A reduced transthyretin level may be indicative of increased propensity for transthyretin cardiac amyloidosis (but is not diagnostic of this disorder, so further testing must be completed).
Restrictive cardiomyopathy	On echocardiography, look for a "sparkling" myocardium, severely reduced tissue Doppler s' and e' velocities, preserved radial function and reduced longitudinal function, and hepatic vein systolic flow reversal during inspiration. On invasive hemodynamics look for concordant LV and RV pressure tracings during respiration.
Constrictive pericarditis	On echocardiography, look for a diastolic septal bounce, preserved e' velocity, septal e' velocity equal to or greater than lateral e' velocity, respiratory variation in mitral inflow, preserved longitudinal function and reduced radial function, and systolic flow reversal during expiration. On invasive hemodynamics, look for discordant LV and RV pressure tracings during respiration.

Empiric Therapy of HFpEF and HFmrEF
Decongestive Therapy with Diuretics

As in all patients with HF, those with HFpEF and HFmrEF typically have some degree of volume overload. Many will have evidence of elevated intracardiac filling pressures, both at rest and during exertion, which contributes to shortness of breath, orthopnea, paroxysmal nocturnal dyspnea, and right-sided symptoms such as lower extremity edema and early satiety. Thus, decongestive therapy with diuretics remains empiric cornerstone therapy for patients with HFpEF and HFmrEF. While diuretic therapy has not been specifically tested in HFpEF and HFmrEF in rigorous clinical trials, there is sufficient empiric evidence and overall collective experience, in addition to evidence from strategy trials using intracardiac monitoring (see later) that most clinicians agree that these patients require and benefit from diuretic therapy. Both the choice of type of diuretic (e.g., loop diuretic versus thiazide diuretic) and the frequency of use are empiric. As with other forms of HF, loop diuretics tend to be more potent than thiazide diuretics, but there are limited data to inform which diuretics are best. Combining loop and thiazide diuretics can be useful in patients in whom volume management is more challenging, or who become refractory to treatment, and empiric use of variable dose and frequency based on careful monitoring of a patient's weight is a commonly utilized strategy. Likewise, combinations of thiazide and potassium sparing diuretics are commonly used empirically in HFpEF and play a role both in decongestion and treatment of hypertension. Mineralocorticoid receptor antagonists (MRAs) are weak diuretics, although their potential benefits in HFpEF may go beyond their diuretic properties (see later), and in the setting of chronic loop diuretic therapy, sodium resorption in other areas of the nephron are heightened; thus, the addition of an MRA to loop diuretic therapy can result in augmented diuresis. As is the case in HFrEF, overdiuresis and volume depletion can predispose patients, especially elderly patients, to hypotension and renal dysfunction, and caution should be taken to avoid overdiuresis in vulnerable patients.

Blood Pressure Management

Although the general principles of blood pressure management (see also Chapter 26) apply to patients with HFpEF and HFmrEF, there may be an additional rationale for lowering blood pressure in these patients. Blood pressure lowering has been shown to improve measures of diastolic function.[87] Although not specifically conducted in patients with HF, several trials of intensive versus standard blood pressure treatment, including HYVET[88] and SPRINT,[89] demonstrated reduction in HF hospitalizations in patients assigned to more intensive blood pressure lowering arms, suggesting that blood pressure reduction may be useful as a means to reduce HF hospitalizations in at-risk patients. Although most of the neurohormonal modulators that have been tested rigorously in HFpEF and HFmrEF are antihypertensive agents, post hoc analyses have suggested that the potential beneficial effects of therapy appeared to be independent of blood pressure reduction,[90] suggesting that the benefits of these agents extend beyond blood pressure lowering.

Atrial Fibrillation

Atrial fibrillation is extremely common in patients with HFpEF and HFmrEF (see earlier), and even patients who have never experienced atrial fibrillation are at markedly increased risk of developing atrial fibrillation. Atrial fibrillation can worsen HF in these patients by reducing the LA contribution to cardiac output and by reducing diastolic filling time when heart rates are rapid. Stroke volume is typically reduced even in patients with atrial fibrillation who have controlled heart rates due to reduced filling and emptying of the LA. Patients with HFpEF who are compensated are more likely to decompensate when they go into atrial fibrillation.[91]

The principles of treatment of atrial fibrillation in patients with HFpEF and HFmrEF are similar to the treatment of atrial fibrillation in general (see Chapter 66), including both rate control and anticoagulation. Beta blockers can be helpful in prevention of atrial fibrillation in those who are in sinus rhythm but have been in atrial fibrillation in the past although the experience in HFpEF and HFmrEF is largely anecdotal. One outstanding question in the treatment of atrial fibrillation in patients with HFpEF and HFmrEF is whether rhythm control rather than just rate control would reduce hospitalizations for HF, and, if so, which rhythm control strategies would be best. Most practitioners agree that patients with HFpEF and HFmrEF who are symptomatic despite empiric therapy and remain in atrial fibrillation deserve a trial of restoration of sinus rhythm, either through electrical or chemical cardioversion or an ablation procedure, although there are no randomized data to support this recommendation. The benefit observed in randomized trials of atrial fibrillation ablation in HFrEF raises the possibility that ablation might be a viable strategy in HFpEF and HFmrEF as well, although there are no rigorous clinical trials. The use of prophylactic rhythm control in patients with paroxysmal atrial fibrillation is also unclear, although beta blockade is often used in these patients empirically. Whether other antiarrhythmic drugs or ablation would reduce the incidence of atrial fibrillation–related hospitalization in these patients remains unknown. Unless contraindicated, anticoagulation with warfarin or a direct-acting oral anticoagulant should be utilized in patients with HFpEF and HFmrEF because of the high risk of thromboembolism in patients with concomitant atrial fibrillation and HF.

Management of Other Comorbidities

Comorbidities such as hypertension, obesity, diabetes, CAD, chronic kidney disease, chronic lung disease, sleep apnea, and anemia are extremely common in patients with HFpEF and HFmrEF. Generally, these comorbidities should be managed according to established guidelines in patients with HFpEF and HFmrEF. Maintaining euvolemia is important in patients with concomitant chronic lung disease and obstructive sleep apnea because elevated pulmonary venous pressure will exacerbate hypoxemia in patients with parenchymal lung disease, and oropharyngeal edema can exacerbate obstructive sleep apnea. Obesity is a very frequent comorbidity in HFpEF, and even when BMI is <30 kg/m^2, significant visceral adiposity is often present in HFpEF. Obesity is also a major determinant of NYHA class and exercise intolerance in HFpEF. Thus, treatment of obesity should be part of the therapeutic plan in HFpEF patients. Lifestyle modifications (see later) can be useful in improving several comorbidities commonly present in patients with HFpEF and HFmrEF.

Specific Pharmacologic Treatment
Calcium Channel Blockers and Beta Blockers

Both nondihydropyridine calcium channel blockers and beta blockers, which have previously been thought to improve myocardial diastolic properties, have been neutral in small trials in HFpEF and HFmrEF. There are virtually no data to support a role for calcium channel blockers in either HFpEF or HFmrEF beyond blood pressure lowering. The SENIORS trial tested the selective beta blocker nebivolol in patients with HF and showed a modest overall reduction in all-cause mortality or cardiovascular hospitalization.[92] That there was no heterogeneity in the treatment response based on ejection fraction has led some to conclude that this beta blocker might be beneficial in patients with HF and higher LVEF, although only 15% of patients in the trial had LVEF >50%. Carvedilol was tested in 245 patients in the J-DHF trial followed for 3.2 years and was not associated with greater reduction in cardiovascular death or HF hospitalization, although the trial was markedly underpowered. Others have suggested that beta blockade might be detrimental in patients with HFpEF,[93] although the data to support harm are likely confounded. The role of beta blockers for rate reduction in patients with atrial fibrillation, or in prevention of atrial fibrillation, is well established, and these benefits likely extend to patients with HFpEF or HFmrEF. Because beta blockers can lower blood pressure, they might limit the use of therapies that also affect blood pressure and for which more data exist. Nevertheless, the proportion of patients with HFpEF and HFmrEF taking beta blockers for hypertension is high, approaching 80% in recent clinical trials. In patients with reduced cardiac output at rest or during exertion, withdrawal of nondihydropyridine calcium channel blockers or beta blockers may be warranted, particularly in those patients with lack of augmentation of stroke volume during exercise. In these patients, improving chronotropic responsiveness may help augment cardiac output during exertion, thereby potentially improving symptoms.

Renin-Angiotensin-Aldosterone System Inhibitors

Neurohormonal modulators, particularly renin-angiotensin-aldosterone (RAAS) inhibitors have been the cornerstone of treatment of HFrEF but have proven less effective in large clinical trials of HFpEF. The postulated effects of RAAS inhibition in HFpEF and HFmrEF include lowering blood pressure, improvement of diastolic function, and reduction of myocardial fibrosis. Overall, there is less activation of the renin-angiotensin system in HF with higher ejection fraction, which might account for the limited therapeutic success of these agents.

Angiotensin Converting Enzyme Inhibitors

The initial CONSENSUS trial compared enalapril versus placebo in NYHA Class IV HF irrespective of ejection fraction, although the majority likely had HFrEF because cardiomegaly was an entry requirement. The ACE inhibitor perindopril was compared with placebo in patients with HF and LVEF >45% in the PEP-CHF trial,[94] an 850-patient trial in which event rates were lower than expected and in which many patients withdrew from therapy after a year (with a high frequency of crossover to ACE inhibitor therapy in the placebo arm). Overall, the hazard ratio for the primary endpoint, a composite of all-cause mortality and unplanned HF hospitalization, was 0.92 (95% CI 0.70 to 1.21), although at 1 year, before a substantial number of dropouts from the ACE inhibitor arm, there was nominal reduction in both the primary endpoint and HF hospitalization, as well as improvement in functional class and 6-minute walk test distance.

Angiotensin Receptor Blockers

Two large outcomes trials with angiotensin receptor blockers have been performed in patients with HF and LVEF >40%: CHARM-Preserved,[95] which compared candesartan to placebo in patients with HF and LVEF >40%, and I-PRESERVE,[96] which compared irbesartan to placebo in patients with HF and LVEF >45%. CHARM-Preserved was a component of the larger CHARM program that enrolled patients with HF across the ejection fraction spectrum; entry criteria for the entire program were similar regardless of ejection fraction. CHARM-Preserved enrolled 3023 patients with HF and LVEF >40%, and the hazard ratio for the primary endpoint of time to first HF hospitalization or cardiovascular

TABLE 51.7 Comparison of HFpEF Trials: Design and Inclusion Criteria

	CHARM-P	PEP-CHF	I-PRESERVE	TOPCAT	PARAGON-HF	EMPEROR-PRESERVED	DELIVER-HF
N	3023	850	4128	3445	4800	5988	6200
Treatment arms	Candesartan vs. placebo	Perindopril vs. placebo	Irbesartan vs. placebo	Spironolactone vs. placebo	Sacubitril/valsartan vs. valsartan	Empagliflozin vs. placebo	Dapagliflozin vs. placebo
Key inclusion criteria	NYHA Class II to IV, prior CV hospitalization	Clinical diagnosis of DHF with ≥ signs/symptoms of HF, ≥2 of the following: LAE/LVH/Impaired LV filling/AFib	NYHA Class II to IV + any corroborating evidence (e.g., HF sign), LVH or LAE considered optional corroborating evidence, HFH required unless in NYHA Class III to IV	≥1 HF symptom + ≥1 HF sign, elevated NP or HFH	NYHA Class II to IV, Elevated NT-proBNP (adjusted for atrial fibrillation and higher if no recent HF hospitalization), structural heart disease (LAE or LVH)	NYHA Class II to IV, elevated NT-proBNP.	NYHA Class II to IV, elevated NT-proBNP (adjusted for atrial fibrillation), structural heart disease (LAE or LVH)
Endpoint	First of either CVD or HFH	First of either all-cause death of HFH	First of either all-cause death or CVH	First of either CVD, HFH, or RSD	CVD and TOTAL HFH (first and recurrent).	CVD or hospitalization for HF	CVD or hospitalization for HF either in the full population or in patients with LVEF <60%

death was 0.89 (95% CI 0.77 to 1.03), $P = 0.12$. This result was stronger in several prespecified and post hoc analyses, including an analysis adjusting for baseline covariates, and in analyses using total number of hospitalization events rather than time to first event.[37] There was no observed effect on mortality. In contrast, the I-PRESERVE trial did not show a benefit comparing irbesartan to placebo in patients with HF and an LVEF above 45%. The primary outcome of all-cause death or cardiovascular hospitalization was similar between treatment groups (HR 0.95, 95% CI 0.86 to 1.05; $P = 0.35$). Each of these trials had slightly different inclusion and exclusion criteria (Table 51.7). More contemporary clinical trials in this population have shown that the majority of patients with HFpEF are treated with ACE inhibitors or angiotensin receptor blockers despite lack of a specific indication for these therapies, suggesting that in the majority of patients being treated, these agents are being used for comorbidities such as hypertension, chronic kidney disease, or diabetes.

Mineralocorticoid Receptor Antagonists

Mineralocorticoid receptor antagonists (MRAs) are potassium-sparing diuretics that have been used as a diuretic and for treatment of hypertension for several decades. Their benefit in HF was first shown in severe HFrEF (see also Chapter 50). Aldosterone is a known contributor to fibrosis in the heart, vasculature, and kidneys, and MRA receptor activation has been implicated in disorders of blood vessels, including hypertension and endothelial dysfunction, and abnormalities of cardiac structure, including myocardial hypertrophy. Moreover, experimental evidence supported a potential role for MRAs in reducing myocardial fibrosis,[97] improving diastolic function,[98] and endothelial vasomotor function.

These data provided the rationale for the TOPCAT trial,[99] which compared spironolactone to placebo in 3445 patients with HFpEF. The entry criteria for TOPCAT required signs and symptoms of HF with either elevation in natriuretic peptides or a history of HF hospitalization within the past year, and only patients with potassium <5.0 mmol/L, serum creatinine <2.5 mg/dL, and estimated glomerular filtration rate ≥30 mL/min/1.73 m² were included. The primary endpoint of the trial was a composite of cardiovascular death, HF hospitalization or aborted cardiac arrest, and the overall results showed an 11% nonsignificant risk reduction (HR 0.89, 95% CI 0.77 to 1.04, $P = 0.14$).[100] The trial enrolled patients from several countries around the world, and following unblinding, it became apparent that patients enrolled in the United States, Canada, Argentina, and Brazil had a nearly fivefold higher event rate than in patients enrolled in Russia and the Republic of Georgia, raising the possibility that patients enrolled in these regions may not have had HF.[101] The treatment effect of spironolactone was similarly attenuated in these regions. These revelations and subsequent

metabolite data showing that a high proportion of sampled patients in Russia and the Republic of Georgia were not taking study drug[102] raised the possibility that in the right patients in whom the therapy was being taken, spironolactone would have shown benefit (Fig. 51.10A).

These data have been used to support incorporation of spironolactone, a generic and inexpensive therapy generic, into several guidelines for potential use in HFpEF (currently listed in the AHA/ACC/HFSA guidelines as a class IIb indication). Because spironolactone is readily available, but can elevate serum potassium, the decision to use it in patients with HFpEF and HFmrEF should be based on individual benefit-risk determination. For example, patients in TOPCAT with evidence of chronic kidney disease demonstrated a reduced benefit-risk ratio compared with those with better renal function,[103] whereas patients with HF with LVEF 45% to 60% appeared to benefit the most from spironolactone in TOPCAT.[104] Based on available data, unless otherwise contraindicated, an MRA should be added to loop diuretic therapy instead of potassium supplementation in patients with HFpEF and HFmrEF. When using an MRA in HFpEF or HFmrEF, potassium and renal function should be closely monitored 1 week and 1 month after initiating MRA therapy, and on a regular basis thereafter. Recently an FDA advisory voted in support of an indication for spironolactone in HFpEF.

Angiotensin Receptor Neprilysin Inhibition

Sacubitril/valsartan in a crystalline compound composed of the angiotensin receptor blocker valsartan and sacubitril, a prodrug neprilysin inhibitor. Neprilysin breaks down several vasoactive peptides, including the biologically active natriuretic factors, ANP, BNP, and CNP; adrenomedullin; endothelin; and angiotensin II; pairing both a neprilysin inhibitor with a renin-angiotensin system (RAS) inhibitor simultaneously blocks the RAS and augments the endogenous vasoactive peptide system.[105] Sacubitril/valsartan reduced cardiovascular mortality, HF hospitalization and all-cause mortality in 8399 patients with HFrEF in the PARADIGM-HF trial.[106] In a phase II trial in patients with HF and LVEF of 45% or greater, sacubitril/valsartan reduced NT-proBNP, a natriuretic peptide marker that is not directly affected by a neprilysin inhibitor, improved NYHA class, and reduced LA size compared with valsartan.[107] Based on these findings, the PARAGON-HF trial tested sacubitril/valsartan compared with valsartan in 4822 patients with NYHA Class II to IV HF, and LVEF ≥45%.[108] In contrast to prior HFpEF trials, patients were required to have elevation in natriuretic peptides and evidence of structural heart disease (see Table 51.7). Moreover, the primary endpoint of PARAGON-HF was a composite of cardiovascular death and total (first and recurrent) HF hospitalizations utilizing a novel recurrent events analysis (see also Chapter 4). PARAGON-HF showed a 13% reduction in total HF hospitalizations and cardiovascular death (rate ratio 0.87, 95% CI 0.75 to 1.01, $P = 0.059$), which just missed statistical significance. Nevertheless, several secondary end-points, including measures of functional status, quality of life, and renal function were strongly suggestive of a true benefit. Moreover, there was evidence of substantial heterogeneity, with a treatment effect that was most pronounced in patients with LVEF that was at or below the median of 57%, and in women, with women appearing to derive greater benefit than men to a higher ejection fraction[109] (Fig. 51.10B). These findings have led to an FDA expanded approval for the use of sacubitril/valsartan in patients with chronic HF, noting that benefit was most evident in those with ejection fraction below normal.

Device Therapy in HFpEF and HFmrEF
Diagnostic Devices
A number of therapeutic and diagnostic devices have been tested, or are currently being tested, in HFpEF and HFmrEF. Several diagnostic devices have been developed to aid physicians in remote

management of patients with HF (see Chapter 58). The CardioMEMS heart sensor is an implantable hemodynamic monitor that is inserted into a pulmonary artery and transmits pulmonary pressures to health-care providers. In the CHAMPION trial,[110] the CardioMEMS sensor was tested in conjunction with a protocol-driven algorithm by which physicians utilized device information to make therapeutic changes. Patients were randomized to either an algorithm-based strategy based on utilizing remote data from the device, or standard medical therapy. Patients in the device-strategy arm demonstrated a significant decrease in pulmonary artery diastolic and systolic pressures, as well as a 52% decrease in HF-related events, an increase in days alive out of hospital and improvement in quality of life. The benefit observed was similar in patients across the spectrum of ejection fraction, suggesting that careful assessment of hemodynamic variables and application of therapeutic algorithms based on these assessments could improve outcomes in patients with HF regardless of ejection fraction. These devices are likely most helpful in HFpEF and HFmrEF patients

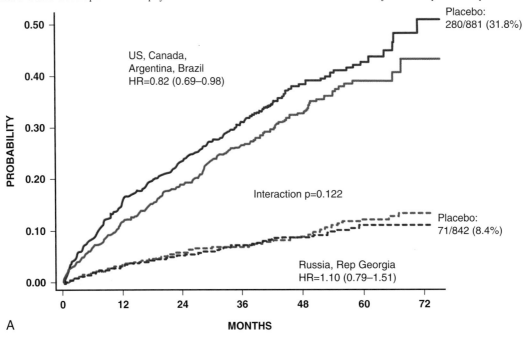

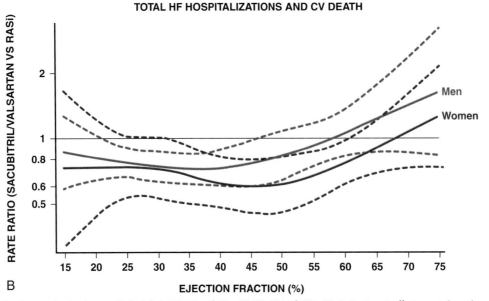

FIGURE 51.10 Phase III randomized controlled trials in HFpEF and HFmrEF. HFpEF and HFmrEF. A, Treatment effect comparing spironolactone and placebo in both the Americas region (United States, Canada, Argentina, Brazil) and in Russia and Republic of Georgia in the TOPCAT trial. The event rate in Russia and Republic of Georgia was approximately fivefold lower than in the Americas. **B,** Treatment effect for sacubitril/valsartan across the spectrum of heart failure from both the PARADIGM-HF and PARAGON-HF trials. The treatment benefit of sacubitril/valsartan declines as ejection fraction rises into the normal range in both men and women, with women deriving greater benefit to a higher ejection fraction than men.

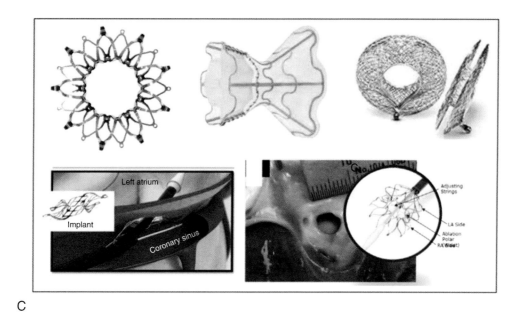

C

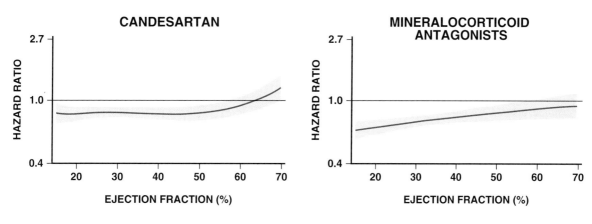

CANDESARTAN

MINERALOCORTICOID ANTAGONISTS

SACUBITRIL/VALSARTAN

D

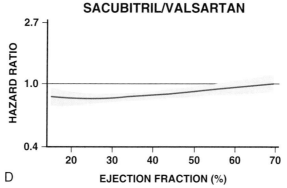

FIGURE 51.10 cont'd C, Interatrial shunt devices designed to lower left atrial pressure in heart failure. **D,** Treatment effect of the ARB candesartan, the MRA spironolactone, and sacubitril/valsartan across the spectrum of ejection fraction showing evidence of benefit for all three therapies in the reduced and mildly reduced ejection fractions. (**A** from Pfeffer MA, et al. Regional variation in patients and outcomes in the Treatment of Preserved Cardiac Function Heart Failure With an Aldosterone Antagonist (TOPCAT) trial. *Circulation.* 2015;131[1]:34-42. **B** from Solomon SD, et al. Sacubitril/valsartan across the spectrum of ejection fraction in heart failure. *Circulation.* 141[5]:352-361. **C** from Griffin JM, et al. Impact of interatrial shunts on invasive hemodynamics and exercise tolerance in patients with heart failure. J Am Heart Assoc. 2020;9[17]:e016760. **D** from Dewan P, et al. Interactions between left ventricular ejection fraction, sex and effect of neurohumoral modulators in heart failure. Eur J Heart Fail. 2020;22[5]:898-901.)

who experience frequent hospitalizations and can be helpful in keeping these patients out of the hospital. Many of these patients have the cardiorenal syndrome; implantable hemodynamic monitoring can be helpful to carefully guide diuresis in order to maintain euvolemia without exacerbating renal dysfunction. Several other diagnostic devices, including those that monitor heart rate and rhythm, impedance, respiration and other parameters are currently being tested in HFpEF and HFmrEF.

Therapeutic Devices

As elevation of LA pressures represents the pathophysiologic sine qua non of HF, another strategy that has been explored is the placement of a shunt device between the left and right atria to lower LA pressures both at rest and on exertion. Interatrial shunt devices have been tested in preliminary trials (Fig.51.10C), which have suggested that this approach is both safe and might improve hemodynamics;[111,112] pivotal data will be forthcoming from ongoing trials.

Neither ICDs nor CRT devices are currently recommended for patients with LVEF above 40%, although some patients with HFpEF and HFmrEF are at risk for sudden death, and dyssynchrony may contribute to worsening hemodynamics in patients with HF regardless of LVEF.[113] Patients with chronotropic incompetence who satisfy other requirements for standard pacemaker placement may benefit from pacemaker therapy. In addition, in patients with HFpEF and HFmrEF who already have pacemakers for other reasons and evidence of low resting cardiac output or inadequate stroke volume increase with exercise, raising the basal pacemaker rate or increasing the rate responsiveness of the pacemaker may improve symptoms and exercise tolerance.

Lifestyle Modification and Exercise Training

Both diet and lifestyle modification may have a role in the treatment of HFpEF and HFmrEF, although neither have been rigorously studied. As with HFrEF, sodium and fluid restriction may be useful in HFpEF, especially in patients with evidence of fluid overload. While strategies meant to treat obesity, including bariatric surgery, have been shown to have a variety of beneficial cardiovascular effects (see also Chapter 30), whether obesity reversal would improve outcomes in HFpEF is unknown. Pharmacologic treatment of obesity is currently being tested in clinical trials in HFpEF and HFmrEF.

In contrast to most pharmacologic intervention trials for HFpEF, exercise-based interventions have consistently demonstrated clinically meaningful improvements in objectively measured exercise capacity (peak oxygen uptake, total exercise time, and 6-minute walk distance), symptoms, and quality of life.[114] The benefits have been ascribed to the effect of exercise on a number of factors that influence exercise tolerance, including general metabolic benefits and effects on skeletal muscle.[115,116] While the majority of exercise trials have tested aerobic (endurance) training, others have incorporated strength training or high-intensity interval training. One of the major factors influencing the success of exercise programs is adherence, which has been only modest in trials.[117] In a randomized trial of patients with obesity and HFpEF, in which both caloric restriction and aerobic exercise were tested in a factorial design, the combination of approaches led to improved exercise capacity, quality of life in conjunction with greater weight loss and improvement in inflammatory biomarkers.[118] A recent multi-center trial of high-intensity interval training versus moderate continuous training versus guideline-based physical activity advice (control) in HFpEF patients showed that the two types of exercise training resulted in some improvement in peak V_{O_2} at 3 months (although not meeting the prespecified minimal clinically important difference of 2.5 mL/kg/min) compared with control during which time exercise training was done in a supervised setting.[119] However, after the initial 3 months, these improvements were attenuated during telehealth exercise over the next 9 months. Results for high intensity interval training and moderate continuous training were similar. Overall, these data suggest that exercise training can be useful to improve exercise tolerance and quality of life in patients with HFpEF and HFmrEF and should be recommended with a specific exercise program prescription in all patients.

Unsuccessful and Potentially Harmful Treatments in HFpEF

Numerous treatments have been tested unsuccessfully in HFpEF. Phosphodiesterase type 5 (PDE5) inhibitors have shown benefit and are currently approved for treatment of pulmonary arterial hypertension, but in several randomized trials in HFpEF, including in HFpEF with known elevation in pulmonary pressures, PDE5 inhibitors failed to show hemodynamic benefits.[120,121] Vericiguat, a soluble guanylate cyclase inhibitor, has been tested in two phase II trials in HFpEF and failed to show hemodynamic benefits or improvement in quality of life.[122,123] Neither organic[124] nor inorganic nitrates[125] have proven beneficial in HFpEF thus far, and isosorbide mononitrate was associated with lower activity levels compared with placebo in HFpEF in the NEAT trial.[124] Ivabradine, a pure heart rate reducing agent, was tested in the EDIFY trial in 179 patients with HFpEF,[126] and failed to show improvement of E/e', 6-minute walk test distance, or NT-proBNP at 6 months.

Emerging Concepts in the Treatment of HFpEF and HFmrEF

Emerging data suggest that patients with HF and LVEF that is above the range generally considered "reduced" but below normal (which overlaps with the HFmrEF category) may be phenotypically intermediate between HFrEF and HFpEF but may respond to therapies that have been proven beneficial in patients with HFrEF. Post hoc analyses from both the CHARM-Preserved and TOPCAT trials suggest greater treatment benefit with either candesartan or spironolactone in patients with LVEFs at the lower end of the spectrum of LVEF enrolled in those trials (Fig. 51.10D), and with treatment responses similar to what was seen in patients with HFrEF for the same therapies.[127] In a prespecified analysis, the PARAGON-HF trial also found significant therapeutic heterogeneity based on LVEF with patients in the lower end of the ejection fraction spectrum studied (LVEF <57%) demonstrating greater benefit from sacubitril/valsartan compared with valsartan.[108] These data collectively suggest that HF patients with mildly reduced ejection fraction may benefit from therapies that benefit HFrEF patients, and this concept is reflected in the recent FDA approval for sacubitril/valsartan.

Ongoing Clinical Trials in HFpEF

Several pharmacologic therapies are currently being tested in large outcomes trials in patients with HF and LVEF >40%. SGLT-2 inhibitors have been shown to reduce morbidity and cardiovascular mortality in HFrEF. In the EMPEROR-Preserved trial empagliflozin compared with placebo reduced first heart failure hospitalization or cardiovascular death in patients with HFpEF. These results were driven by reduction in heart failure hospitalization and the benefit declined with increasing ejection fraction.[128] The DELIVER trial (testing data dapagliflozin compared with placebo) will report in early 2022. Recently, two trials demonstrated marked reduction in HF hospitalization in patients with diabetes and recent hospitalization for HF with the SGLT-1/2 inhibitor sotagliflozin, including in patients with LVEF >40%.[129] Because SGLT-2 inhibitors have been shown to have similar overall effects in patients with and without diabetes in HFrEF, these data are encouraging for the role of these agents in HFpEF and HFmrEF. Another large outcomes trial in HFpEF and HFmrEF is testing the nonsteroidal MRA finerenone, which may have potential advantages over steroidal MRAs such as spironolactone. Spironolactone is also currently being tested in two additional large outcomes trials in HFpEF (SPIRRIT and SPIRIT trials) in an effort to validate the findings in TOPCAT-Americas. Numerous additional trials are currently underway in HFpEF, with the hope that novel treatments beyond diuretics and neurohormonal therapies will begin to demonstrate beneficial results in these patients.

REFERENCES

1. Braunwald E. *Heart Disease: A Textbook of Cardiovascular Medicine*. 4th ed. Philadelphia: Saunders; 1992.
2. Dougherty AH, Naccarelli GV, Gray EL, Hicks CH, Goldstein RA. Congestive heart failure with normal systolic function. *Am J Cardiol*. 1984;54(7):778–782.
3. Topol EJ, Traill TA, Fortuin NJ. Hypertensive hypertrophic cardiomyopathy of the elderly. *N Engl J Med*. 1985;312(5):277–283.
4. Soufer R, Wohlgelernter D, Vita NA, et al. Intact systolic left ventricular function in clinical congestive heart failure. *Am J Cardiol*. 1985;55(8):1032–1036.
5. Owan TE, Hodge DO, Herges RM, et al. Trends in prevalence and outcome of heart failure with preserved ejection fraction. *N Engl J Med*. 2006;355(3):251–259.
6. Bhatia RS, Tu JV, Lee DS, et al. Outcome of heart failure with preserved ejection fraction in a population-based study. *N Engl J Med*. 2006;355(3):260–269.
7. Yancy CW, Jessup M, Bozkurt B, et al. 2017 ACC/AHA/HFSA focused update of the 2013 ACCF/AHA guideline for the management of heart failure: a report of the American College of Cardiology/American Heart Association task force on clinical practice guidelines and the Heart Failure Society of America. *Circulation*. 2017;136(6):e137–e161.
8. Yancy CW, Jessup M, Bozkurt B, et al. 2013 ACCF/AHA guideline for the management of heart failure: executive summary: a report of the American College of Cardiology Foundation/American Heart Association Task Force on practice guidelines. *Circulation*. 2013;128(16):1810–1852.
9. Ponikowski P, Voors AA, Anker SD, et al. 2016 ESC Guidelines for the diagnosis and treatment of acute and chronic heart failure: the task force for the diagnosis and treatment of acute and chronic heart failure of the European Society of Cardiology (ESC) developed with the special contribution of the Heart Failure Association (HFA) of the ESC. *Eur Heart J*. 2016;37(27):2129–2200.
10. Nauta JF, Hummel YM, van Melle JP, et al. What have we learned about heart failure with mid-range ejection fraction one year after its introduction? *Eur J Heart Fail*. 2017;19(12):1569–1573.
11. Bozkurt B, Coats A, Tsutsui H. Universal definition and classification of heart failure. *J Card Fail*. 2021.
12. Lam CSP, Voors AA, Piotr P, et al. Time to rename the middle child of heart failure: heart failure with mildly reduced ejection fraction. *Eur Heart J*. 2020;41(25):2353–2355.
13. McKee PA, Castelli WP, McNamara PM, Kannel WB. The natural history of congestive heart failure: the Framingham study. *N Engl J Med*. 1971;285(26):1441–1446.
14. Ceia F, Fonseca C, Mota T, et al. Prevalence of chronic heart failure in southwestern Europe: the EPICA study. *Eur J Heart Fail*. 2002;4(4):531–539.

15. Steinberg BA, Zhao X, Heidenreich PA, et al. Trends in patients hospitalized with heart failure and preserved left ventricular ejection fraction: prevalence, therapies, and outcomes. *Circulation*. 2012;126(1):65–75.
16. Oktay AA, Rich JD, Shah SJ. The emerging epidemic of heart failure with preserved ejection fraction. *Curr Heart Fail Rep*. 2013;10(4):401–410.
17. Nochioka K, Shiba N, Kohno H, et al. Both high and low body mass indexes are prognostic risks in Japanese patients with chronic heart failure: implications from the CHART study. *J Card Fail*. 2010;16(11):880–887.
18. Shiba N, Nochioka K, Miura M, et al. Trend of westernization of etiology and clinical characteristics of heart failure patients in Japan: first report from the CHART-2 study. *Circ J*. 2011;75(4):823–833.
19. Dunlay SM, Roger VL. Understanding the epidemic of heart failure: past, present, and future. *Curr Heart Fail Rep*. 2014;11(4):404–415.
20. Ho JE, Enserro D, Brouwers FP, et al. Predicting heart failure with preserved and reduced ejection fraction: the International Collaboration on Heart Failure Subtypes. *Circ Heart Fail*. 2016;9(6). https://doi.org/10.1161/CIRCHEARTFAILURE.1115.003116.
21. Dunlay SM, Roger VL, Redfield MM. Epidemiology of heart failure with preserved ejection fraction. *Nat Rev Cardiol*. 2017;14(10):591–602.
22. Gerber Y, Weston SA, Redfield MM, et al. A contemporary appraisal of the heart failure epidemic in Olmsted County, Minnesota, 2000 to 2010. *JAMA Intern Med*. 2015;175(6):996–1004.
23. Ho JE, Lyass A, Lee DS, et al. Predictors of new-onset heart failure: differences in preserved versus reduced ejection fraction. *Circ Heart Fail*. 2013;6(2):279–286.
24. Santhanakrishnan R, Wang N, Larson MG, et al. Atrial fibrillation begets heart failure and vice versa: temporal associations and differences in preserved versus reduced ejection fraction. *Circulation*. 2016;133(5):484–492.
25. Zakeri R, Chamberlain AM, Roger VL, Redfield MM. Temporal relationship and prognostic significance of atrial fibrillation in heart failure patients with preserved ejection fraction: a community-based study. *Circulation*. 2013;128(10):1085–1093.
26. Kotecha D, Lam CS, Van Veldhuisen DJ, et al. Heart failure with preserved ejection fraction and atrial fibrillation: vicious twins. *J Am Coll Cardiol*. 2016;68(20):2217–2228.
27. Lam CS, Rienstra M, Tay WT, et al. Atrial fibrillation in heart failure with preserved ejection fraction: association with exercise capacity, left ventricular filling pressures, natriuretic peptides, and left atrial volume. *JACC Heart Fail*. 2017;5(2):92–98.
28. Kotecha D, Chudasama R, Lane DA, et al. Atrial fibrillation and heart failure due to reduced versus preserved ejection fraction: a systematic review and meta-analysis of death and adverse outcomes. *Int J Cardiol*. 2016;203:660–666.
29. Linssen GC, Rienstra M, Jaarsma T, et al. Clinical and prognostic effects of atrial fibrillation in heart failure patients with reduced and preserved left ventricular ejection fraction. *Eur J Heart Fail*. 2011;13(10):1111–1120.
30. Olsson LG, Swedberg K, Ducharme A, et al. Atrial fibrillation and risk of clinical events in chronic heart failure with and without left ventricular systolic dysfunction: results from the Candesartan in Heart failure-Assessment of Reduction in Mortality and morbidity (CHARM) program. *J Am Coll Cardiol*. 2006;47(10):1997–2004.
31. Meta-analysis Global Group in Chronic Heart Failure (MAGGIC). The survival of patients with heart failure with preserved or reduced left ventricular ejection fraction: an individual patient data meta-analysis. *Eur Heart J*. 2012;33(14):1750–1757.
32. Lam CSP, Gamble GD, Ling LH, et al. Mortality associated with heart failure with preserved vs. reduced ejection fraction in a prospective international multi-ethnic cohort study. *Eur Heart J*. 2018;39(20):1770–1780.
33. Aschauer S, Zotter-Tufaro C, Duca F, et al. Modes of death in patients with heart failure and preserved ejection fraction. *Int J Cardiol*. 2017;228:422–426.
34. Vaduganathan M, Patel RB, Michel A, et al. Mode of death in heart failure with preserved ejection fraction. *J Am Coll Cardiol*. 2017;69(5):556–569.
35. Solomon SD, Anavekar N, Skali H, et al. Influence of ejection fraction on cardiovascular outcomes in a broad spectrum of heart failure patients. *Circulation*. 2005;112(24):3738–3744.
36. Nichols GA, Reynolds K, Kimes TM, et al. Comparison of risk of re-hospitalization, all-cause mortality, and medical care resource utilization in patients with heart failure and preserved versus reduced ejection fraction. *Am J Cardiol*. 2015;116(7):1088–1092.
37. Rogers JK, Pocock SJ, McMurray JJ, et al. Analysing recurrent hospitalizations in heart failure: a review of statistical methodology, with application to CHARM-Preserved. *Eur J Heart Fail*. 2014;16(1):33–40.
38. Carson PE, Anand IS, Win S, et al. The hospitalization burden and post-hospitalization mortality risk in heart failure with preserved ejection fraction: results from the I-PRESERVE trial (Irbesartan in Heart Failure and Preserved Ejection Fraction). *JACC Heart Fail*. 2015;3(6):429–441.
39. Bello NA, Claggett B, Desai AS, et al. Influence of previous heart failure hospitalization on cardiovascular events in patients with reduced and preserved ejection fraction. *Circ Heart Fail*. 2014;7(4):590–595.
40. Vaduganathan M, Claggett BL, Desai AS, et al. Prior heart failure hospitalization, clinical outcomes, and response to sacubitril/valsartan compared with valsartan in HFpEF. *J Am Coll Cardiol*. 2020;75(3):245–254.
41. Lewis EF, Kim HY, Claggett B, et al. Impact of spironolactone on longitudinal changes in health-related quality of life in the treatment of preserved cardiac function heart failure with an aldosterone antagonist trial. *Circ Heart Fail*. 2016;9(3):e001937.
42. Chandra A, Vaduganathan M, Lewis EF, et al. Health-related quality of life in heart failure with preserved ejection fraction: the PARAGON-HF trial. *JACC Heart Fail*. 2019;7(10):862–874.
43. Joseph SM, Novak E, Arnold SV, et al. Comparable performance of the Kansas City Cardiomyopathy Questionnaire in patients with heart failure with preserved and reduced ejection fraction. *Circ Heart Fail*. 2013;6(6):1139–1146.
44. Pokharel Y, Khariton Y, Tang Y, et al. Association of serial Kansas City Cardiomyopathy Questionnaire assessments with death and hospitalization in patients with heart failure with preserved and reduced ejection fraction: a secondary analysis of 2 randomized clinical trials. *JAMA Cardiol*. 2017;2(12):1315–1321.
45. Butler J, Hamo CE, Udelson JE, et al. Exploring new endpoints for patients with heart failure with preserved ejection fraction. *Circ Heart Fail*. 2016;9(11).
46. Anjan VY, Loftus TM, Burke MA, et al. Prevalence, clinical phenotype, and outcomes associated with normal B-type natriuretic peptide levels in heart failure with preserved ejection fraction. *Am J Cardiol*. 2012;110(6):870–876.
47. Obokata M, Reddy YNV, Pislaru SV, et al. Evidence supporting the existence of a distinct obese phenotype of heart failure with preserved ejection fraction. *Circulation*. 2017;136(1):6–19.
48. Reddy YNV, Carter RE, Obokata M, et al. A simple, evidence-based approach to help guide diagnosis of heart failure with preserved ejection fraction. *Circulation*. 2018;138(9):861–870.
49. Pieske B, Tschope C, de Boer RA, et al. How to diagnose heart failure with preserved ejection fraction: the HFA-PEFF diagnostic algorithm: a consensus recommendation from the Heart Failure Association (HFA) of the European Society of Cardiology (ESC). *Eur Heart J*. 2019;40(40):3297–3317.
50. Iwanaga Y, Nishi I, Furuichi S, et al. B-type natriuretic peptide strongly reflects diastolic wall stress in patients with chronic heart failure: comparison between systolic and diastolic heart failure. *J Am Coll Cardiol*. 2006;47(4):742–748.
51. Fudim M, Ambrosy AP, Sun JL, et al. High-sensitivity troponin I in hospitalized and ambulatory patients with heart failure with preserved ejection fraction: insights from the Heart Failure Clinical Research Network. *J Am Heart Assoc*. 2018;7(24):e010364.
52. Obokata M, Reddy YNV, Melenovsky V, et al. Myocardial injury and cardiac reserve in patients with heart failure and preserved ejection fraction. *J Am Coll Cardiol*. 2018;72(1):29–40.
53. Katz DH, Beussink L, Sauer AJ, et al. Prevalence, clinical characteristics, and outcomes associated with eccentric versus concentric left ventricular hypertrophy in heart failure with preserved ejection fraction. *Am J Cardiol*. 2013;112(8):1158–1164.
54. McLaughlin VV, Shah SJ, Souza R, Humbert M. Management of pulmonary arterial hypertension. *J Am Coll Cardiol*. 2015;65(18):1976–1997.
55. Marwick TH, Shah SJ, Thomas JD. Myocardial strain in the assessment of patients with heart failure: a review. *JAMA Cardiol*. 2019;4(3):287–294.
56. Kraigher-Krainer E, Shah AM, Gupta DK, et al. Impaired systolic function by strain imaging in heart failure with preserved ejection fraction. *J Am Coll Cardiol*. 2014;63(5):447–456.
57. Freed BH, Daruwalla V, Cheng JY, et al. Prognostic utility and clinical significance of cardiac mechanics in heart failure with preserved ejection fraction: importance of left atrial strain. *Circ Cardiovasc Imaging*. 2016;9(3).
58. Obokata M, Kane GC, Reddy YN, et al. Role of diastolic stress testing in the evaluation for heart failure with preserved ejection fraction: a simultaneous invasive-echocardiographic study. *Circulation*. 2017;135(9):825–838.
59. Barison A, Aimo A, Todiere G, et al. Cardiovascular magnetic resonance for the diagnosis and management of heart failure with preserved ejection fraction. *Heart Fail Rev*. 2020.
60. Shah SJ, Lam CSP, Svedlund S, et al. Prevalence and correlates of coronary microvascular dysfunction in heart failure with preserved ejection fraction: PROMIS-HFpEF. *Eur Heart J*. 2018;39(37):3439–3450.
61. Reddy YNV, Nishimura RA. Not all secondary mitral regurgitation is the same-potential phenotypes and implications for mitral repair. *JAMA Cardiol*. 2020.
62. Borlaug BA, Nishimura RA, Sorajja P, et al. Exercise hemodynamics enhance diagnosis of early heart failure with preserved ejection fraction. *Circ Heart Fail*. 2010;3(5):588–595.
63. Dryer K, Gajjar M, Narang N, et al. Coronary microvascular dysfunction in patients with heart failure with preserved ejection fraction. *Am J Physiol Heart Circ Physiol*. 2018; 314(5):H1033–H1042.
64. Hahn VS, Yanek LR, Vaishnav J, et al. Endomyocardial biopsy characterization of heart failure with preserved ejection fraction and prevalence of cardiac amyloidosis. *JACC Heart Fail*. 2020;8(9):712–724.
65. Houstis NE, Eisman AS, Pappagianopoulos PP, et al. Exercise intolerance in heart failure with preserved ejection fraction: diagnosing and ranking its causes using personalized O_2 pathway analysis. *Circulation*. 2018;137(2):148–161.
66. Reddy YNV, Olson TP, Obokata M, et al. Hemodynamic correlates and diagnostic role of cardiopulmonary exercise testing in heart failure with preserved ejection fraction. *JACC Heart Fail*. 2018;6(8):665–675.
67. Chirinos JA. Deep phenotyping of systemic arterial hemodynamics in HFpEF (Part 2): clinical and therapeutic considerations. *J Cardiovasc Transl Res*. 2017;10(3):261–274.
68. Sanderson JE, Fang F, Lu M, et al. Obstructive sleep apnoea, intermittent hypoxia and heart failure with a preserved ejection fraction. *Heart*. 2021;107(3):190–194.
69. Griffin M, Rao VS, Fleming J, et al. Effect on survival of concurrent hemoconcentration and increase in creatinine during treatment of acute decompensated heart failure. *Am J Cardiol*. 2019;124(11):1707–1711.
70. Kitzman DW, Haykowsky MJ, Tomczak CR. Making the case for skeletal muscle myopathy and its contribution to exercise intolerance in heart failure with preserved ejection fraction. *Circ Heart Fail*. 2017;10(7).
71. Kitzman DW, Nicklas B, Kraus WE, et al. Skeletal muscle abnormalities and exercise intolerance in older patients with heart failure and preserved ejection fraction. *Am J Physiol Heart Circ Physiol*. 2014;306(9):H1364–H1370.
72. VanWagner LB, Wilcox JE, Colangelo LA, et al. Association of nonalcoholic fatty liver disease with subclinical myocardial remodeling and dysfunction: a population-based study. *Hepatology*. 2015;62(3):773–783.
73. Kitzman DW, Shah SJ. The HFpEF obesity phenotype: the elephant in the room. *J Am Coll Cardiol*. 2016;68(2):200–203.
74. Packer M. Epicardial adipose tissue may mediate deleterious effects of obesity and inflammation on the myocardium. *J Am Coll Cardiol*. 2018;71(20):2360–2372.
75. Shah SJ, Borlaug BA, Kitzman DW, et al. Research priorities for heart failure with preserved ejection fraction: National Heart, Lung, and Blood Institute working group summary. *Circulation*. 2020;141(12):1001–1026.
76. Mohammed SF, Hussain S, Mirzoyev SA, et al. Coronary microvascular rarefaction and myocardial fibrosis in heart failure with preserved ejection fraction. *Circulation*. 2015;131(6):550–559.
77. Mishra S, Kass DA. Cellular and molecular pathobiology of heart failure with preserved ejection fraction. *Nat Rev Cardiol*. 2021.
78. Shah SJ, Kitzman DW, Borlaug BA, et al. Phenotype-specific treatment of heart failure with preserved ejection fraction: a multiorgan roadmap. *Circulation*. 2016;134(1):73–90.
79. Paulus WJ, Tschope C. A novel paradigm for heart failure with preserved ejection fraction: comorbidities drive myocardial dysfunction and remodeling through coronary microvascular endothelial inflammation. *J Am Coll Cardiol*. 2013;62(4):263–271.
80. DeBerge M, Shah SJ, Wilsbacher L, Thorp EB. Macrophages in heart failure with reduced versus preserved ejection fraction. *Trends Mol Med*. 2019;25(4):328–340.
81. Cunningham JW, Claggett BL, O'Meara E, et al. Effect of sacubitril/valsartan on biomarkers of extracellular matrix regulation in patients with HFpEF. *J Am Coll Cardiol*. 2020;76(5):503–514.
82. Schiattarella GG, Altamirano F, Tong D, et al. Nitrosative stress drives heart failure with preserved ejection fraction. *Nature*. 2019;568(7752):351–356.
83. Shah SJ. Precision medicine for heart failure with preserved ejection fraction: an overview. *J Cardiovasc Transl Res*. 2017;10(3):233–244.
84. Tromp J, Ferreira JP, Janwanishstaporn S, et al. Heart failure around the world. *Eur J Heart Fail*. 2019;21(10):1187–1196.
85. Phan TT, Shivu GN, Abozguia K, et al. Impaired heart rate recovery and chronotropic incompetence in patients with heart failure with preserved ejection fraction. *Circ Heart Fail*. 2010;3(1):29–34.
86. Wolsk E, Claggett B, Køber L, et al. Contribution of cardiac and extra-cardiac disease burden to risk of cardiovascular outcomes varies by ejection fraction in heart failure. *Eur J Heart Fail*. 2017;20(3):504–510.
87. Solomon SD, Janardhanan R, Verma A, et al. Effect of angiotensin receptor blockade and antihypertensive drugs on diastolic function in patients with hypertension and diastolic dysfunction: a randomised trial. *Lancet*. 2007;369(9579):2079–2087.
88. Beckett NS, Peters R, Fletcher AE, et al. Treatment of hypertension in patients 80 years of age or older. *New Engl J Med*. 2008;358(18):1887–1898.
89. Group SR, Wright Jr JT, Williamson JD, et al. A randomized trial of intensive versus standard blood-pressure control. *N Engl J Med*. 2015;373(22):2103–2116.
90. Selvaraj S, Claggett B, Shah SJ, et al. Systolic blood pressure and cardiovascular outcomes in heart failure with preserved ejection fraction: an analysis of the TOPCAT trial. *Eur J Heart Fail*. 2017;20(3):483–490.
91. Cikes M, Claggett B, Shah AM, et al. Atrial fibrillation in heart failure with preserved ejection fraction. *JACC Heart Failure*. 2018;6(8):689–697.
92. van Veldhuisen DJ, Cohen-Solal A, Böhm M, et al. Beta-blockade with nebivolol in elderly heart failure patients with impaired and preserved left ventricular ejection fraction. *J Am Coll Cardiol*. 2009;53(23):2150–2158.

93. Silverman DN, Plante TB, Infeld M, et al. Association of β-blocker use with heart failure hospitalizations and cardiovascular disease mortality among patients with heart failure with a preserved ejection fraction. *JAMA Network Open*. 2019;2(12):e1916598.

94. Cleland JG, Tendera M, Adamus J, et al. The perindopril in elderly people with chronic heart failure (PEP-CHF) study. *Eur Heart J*. 2006;27(19):2338–2345.

95. Pfeffer MA, Swedberg K, Granger CB, et al. Effects of candesartan on mortality and morbidity in patients with chronic heart failure: the CHARM-Overall programme. *Lancet*. 2003;362(9386):759–766.

96. Massie BM, Carson PE, McMurray JJ, et al. Irbesartan in patients with heart failure and preserved ejection fraction. *New Engl J Med*. 2008;359(23):2456–2467.

97. Suzuki G, Morita H, Mishima T, et al. Effects of long-term monotherapy with eplerenone, a novel aldosterone blocker, on progression of left ventricular dysfunction and remodeling in dogs with heart failure. *Circulation*. 2002;106(23):2967–2972.

98. Bauersachs J, Heck M, Fraccarollo D, et al. Addition of spironolactone to angiotensin-converting enzyme inhibition in heart failure improves endothelial vasomotor dysfunction. *J Am Coll Cardiol*. 2002;39(2):351–358.

99. Desai AS, Lewis EF, Li R, et al. Rationale and design of the treatment of preserved cardiac function heart failure with an aldosterone antagonist trial: a randomized, controlled study of spironolactone in patients with symptomatic heart failure and preserved ejection fraction. *Am Heart J*. 2011;162(6):966–972.e910.

100. Pitt B, Pfeffer MA, Assmann SF, et al. Spironolactone for heart failure with preserved ejection fraction. *New Engl J Med*. 2014;370(15):1383–1392.

101. Pfeffer MA, Claggett B, Assmann SF, et al. Regional variation in patients and outcomes in the Treatment of Preserved Cardiac Function Heart Failure With an Aldosterone Antagonist (TOPCAT) trial. *Circulation*. 2015;131(1):34–42.

102. de Denus S, O'Meara E, Desai AS, et al. Spironolactone metabolites in TOPCAT — new insights into regional variation. *New Engl J Med*. 2017;376(17):1690–1692.

103. Beldhuis IE, Myhre PL, Claggett B, et al. Efficacy and safety of spironolactone in patients with HFpEF and chronic kidney disease. *JACC Heart Failure*. 2019;7(1):25–32.

104. Solomon SD, Claggett B, Lewis EF, et al. Influence of ejection fraction on outcomes and efficacy of spironolactone in patients with heart failure with preserved ejection fraction. *Eur Heart J*. 2016;37(5):455–462.

105. Vardeny O, Miller R, Solomon SD. Combined neprilysin and renin-angiotensin system inhibition for the treatment of heart failure. *JACC Heart Failure*. 2014;2(6):663–670.

106. McMurray JJV, Packer M, Desai AS, et al. Angiotensin–neprilysin inhibition versus enalapril in heart failure. *New Engl J Med*. 2014;371(11):993–1004.

107. Solomon SD, Zile M, Pieske B, et al. The angiotensin receptor neprilysin inhibitor LCZ696 in heart failure with preserved ejection fraction: a phase 2 double-blind randomised controlled trial. *Lancet*. 2012;380(9851):1387–1395.

108. Solomon SD, McMurray JJV, Anand IS, et al. Angiotensin–neprilysin inhibition in heart failure with preserved ejection fraction. *New Engl J Med*. 2019;381(17):1609–1620.

109. Solomon SD, Vaduganathan M, Claggett B L, et al. Sacubitril/valsartan across the spectrum of ejection fraction in heart failure. *Circulation*. 2020;141(5):352–361.

110. Abraham WT, Adamson PB, Bourge RC, et al. Wireless pulmonary artery haemodynamic monitoring in chronic heart failure: a randomised controlled trial. *Lancet*. 2011;377(9766):658–666.

111. Hasenfuß G, Hayward C, Burkhoff D, et al. A transcatheter intracardiac shunt device for heart failure with preserved ejection fraction (REDUCE LAP-HF): a multicentre, open-label, single-arm, phase 1 trial. *Lancet*. 2016;387(10025):1298–1304.

112. Feldman T, Mauri L, Kahwash R, et al. Transcatheter interatrial shunt device for the treatment of heart failure with preserved ejection fraction (REDUCE LAP-HF I [Reduce Elevated Left Atrial Pressure in Patients with Heart Failure]): a phase 2, randomized, sham-controlled trial. *Circulation*. 2018;137(4):364–375.

113. Santos ABS, Kraigher-Krainer E, Bello N, et al. Left ventricular dyssynchrony in patients with heart failure and preserved ejection fraction. *Eur Heart J*. 2013;35(1):42–47.

114. Pandey A, Parashar A, Kumbhani DJ, et al. Exercise training in patients with heart failure and preserved ejection fraction. *Circ Heart Fail*. 2015;8(1):33–40.

115. Dhakal BP, Malhotra R, Murphy RM, et al. Mechanisms of exercise intolerance in heart failure with preserved ejection fraction. *Circ Heart Fail*. 2015;8(2):286–294.

116. Pandey A, Khera R, Park B, et al. Relative impairments in hemodynamic exercise reserve parameters in heart failure with preserved ejection fraction. *JACC Heart Fail*. 2018;6(2):117–126.

117. Fleg JL, Cooper LS, Borlaug BA, et al. Exercise training as therapy for heart failure. *Circ Heart Fail*. 2015;8(1):209–220.

118. Kitzman DW, Brubaker P, Morgan T, et al. Effect of caloric restriction or aerobic exercise training on peak oxygen consumption and quality of life in obese older patients with heart failure with preserved ejection fraction. *J Am Med Assoc*. 2016;315(1):36.

119. Mueller S, Winzer EB, Duvinage A, et al. Effect of high-intensity interval training, moderate continuous training, or guideline-based physical activity advice on peak oxygen consumption in patients with heart failure with preserved ejection fraction: a randomized clinical trial. *J Am Med Assoc*. 2021;325(6):542–551.

120. Hoendermis ES, Liu LCY, Hummel YM, et al. Effects of sildenafil on invasive haemodynamics and exercise capacity in heart failure patients with preserved ejection fraction and pulmonary hypertension: a randomized controlled trial. *Eur Heart J*. 2015;36(38):2565–2573.

121. Redfield MM, Chen HH, Borlaug BA, et al. Effect of phosphodiesterase-5 inhibition on exercise capacity and clinical status in heart failure with preserved ejection fraction. *J Am Med Assoc*. 2013;309(12):1268.

122. Armstrong PW, Lam CSP, Anstrom KJ, et al. Effect of vericiguat vs placebo on quality of life in patients with heart failure and preserved ejection fraction. *J Am Med Assoc*. 2020;324(15):1512.

123. Pieske B, Maggioni AP, Lam CSP, et al. Vericiguat in patients with worsening chronic heart failure and preserved ejection fraction: results of the SOluble guanylate Cyclase stimulatoR in heArT failurE patientS with PRESERVED EF (SOCRATES-PRESERVED) study. *Eur Heart J*. 2017;38(15):1119–1127.

124. Redfield MM, Anstrom KJ, Levine JA, et al. Isosorbide mononitrate in heart failure with preserved ejection fraction. *New Engl J Med*. 2015;373(24):2314–2324.

125. Borlaug BA, Anstrom KJ, Lewis GD, et al. Effect of inorganic nitrite vs placebo on exercise capacity among patients with heart failure with preserved ejection fraction. *J Am Med Assoc*. 2018;320(17):1764.

126. Komajda M, Isnard R, Cohen-Solal A, et al. Effect of ivabradine in patients with heart failure with preserved ejection fraction: the EDIFY randomized placebo-controlled trial. *Eur J Heart Fail*. 2017;19(11):1495–1503.

127. Dewan P, Jackson A, Lam CSP, et al. Interactions between left ventricular ejection fraction, sex and effect of neurohumoral modulators in heart failure. *Eur J Heart Fail*. 2020;22(5):898–901.

128. Anker SD, Butler J, Filippatos G, et al; EMPEROR-Preserved Trial Investigators. Empagliflozin in heart failure with a preserved ejection fraction. *N Engl J Med*. Aug 27, 2021. https://doi.org/10.1056/NEJMoa2107038.

129. Bhatt DL, Szarek M, Steg PG, et al. Sotagliflozin in patients with diabetes and recent worsening heart failure. *N Engl J Med*. 2021;384(2):117–128.

52 The Dilated, Restrictive, and Infiltrative Cardiomyopathies

RAY E. HERSHBERGER

There remains no satisfying universal definition of cardiomyopathy. Even though it is now agreed that myocardial disease secondary to atherosclerotic coronary artery disease (CAD), valvular disease, congenital heart disease, and systemic hypertension should not be classified as a cardiomyopathy, opinion differs as to whether the condition should be defined on the basis of morphology and whether molecular disturbances such as the channelopathies should be included. An American Heart Association definition[1] described cardiomyopathies as "a heterogeneous group of diseases of the myocardium associated with mechanical and/or electrical dysfunction that usually (but not invariably) exhibit inappropriate ventricular hypertrophy or dilation and are due to a variety of causes and frequently are genetic. Cardiomyopathies either are confined to the heart or are part of a generalized systemic disorder often leading to cardiovascular death or progressive heart failure–related disability." This classification included patients with predominantly electrical dysfunction of the heart, a group not included in a European Working Group definition.[2] Both U.S. and European experts, however, have recognized the growing importance of genetics in patients with cardiomyopathy since these position papers were released.

The ability to combine genetic information with phenotypic information regarding both left ventricular (LV) and right ventricular (RV) structure and function forms the basis of cardiovascular genetic medicine (Fig. 52.1). Clinical genetic testing enhances the care of patients who present with symptoms as well as family members of these patients through proper cascade risk assessment. Despite the expansion of ClinVar, a publicly accessible database of clinically relevant variants, the field still lacks a comprehensive variant- coupled with phenotype-specific database. Nevertheless, as genomic information proliferates, coupled with useful and accurate phenotype information in large, publicly accessible databases, such information will both help predict the natural history and guide therapy.

Clinical genetic testing made feasible by next-generation sequencing over the past decade has rapidly expanded with many commercially available options that are commonly supported by US insurers with appropriate documentation and pre-test genetic counseling. Although this brings opportunities to define a cardiomyopathy by assigning a specific genetic etiology, it also brings new challenges: knowing which tests to order, how to conduct pretest counseling and obtain consent, and how to interpret genetic test results. Table 52.1[3–5] presents an overview of the classification of cardiomyopathies based on key phenotype information. Phenotype information includes key cardiac morphology, physiology, and cellular and molecular pathology data, supported by details of the patient's environment relevant to the specific disease in question.[6]

Despite rapid expansion of genetic knowledge, clinical, or phenotype, information continues to drive the interpretation of genetic information.[4,5] This can be expressed as a phenotype-first (vs. genotype-first) approach to genetic medicine. In short, for the cardiomyopathies, we still rely on phenotype information to identify an individual with a clinical abnormality that fits into one of the conventional categories (dilated cardiomyopathy [DCM], arrhythmogenic right ventricular cardiomyopathy [ARVC], hypertrophic cardiomyopathy [HCM], restrictive cardiomyopathy [RCM]), and we then interpret specific variants in genes having been curated for their relevance by phenotype. It is abundantly clear that nearly all that we think we understand about cardiomyopathy genetics has been gained from a phenotype-first approach. This will remain in the mainstream for the foreseeable future, because when a genotype-first approach is used, we observe differences, sometimes quite dramatic, in variants considered to be highly likely to be pathogenic in individuals who have no evidence of the phenotype of interest, as has recently been shown in a remarkably reduced estimated penetrance of truncating variants in ARVC genes.[7] Thus, phenotype assessment still relies on the most complete and comprehensive information regarding LV and RV chamber size and function, at times also informed by the presence and character of conduction system disease and arrhythmias, as well as cellular and subcellular function. Numerous genes have had rare variants reported in association with one or more of the genetic cardiomyopathies (Fig. 52.2). This observation itself argues that a phenotype-first approach will need to continue until greater mechanistic insights are available to explain how variants in the same gene, perhaps influenced by an individual's specific genetic, epigenetic, or environmental background, or from alternative disease models (e.g., an oligemic model[8]), cause divergent phenotypes.

The enormous progress made to understand the genetic basis of cardiomyopathy has only led to new questions yet to be addressed. Perhaps most important is that of environmental influence on a genetic background predisposing to cardiomyopathy. Hypertension has been postulated as the most prevalent environmental aspect to hasten the emergence of cardiomyopathy. But it is now also clear that given an appropriate genetic background, established myocardial toxins such as alcohol[9] or drugs used to treat cancer[10] can facilitate the development of DCM. The interplay of genetics with environment to influence disease onset and presentation remains as a major incompletely understood aspect of cardiomyopathy.

Moreover, the prevailing and prototypical genetic paradigm has been mendelian for the cardiomyopathies, that is, where one highly penetrant variant in a well-established gene explains the specific cardiomyopathy phenotype in all affected members of a multigenerational pedigree. This view, rightfully so, has been based on the

Phenome ⟷ Genome

FIGURE 52.1 Interaction of genome and phenome. The *arrow* depicts the bimodal interaction between genes and the environment, or the genome and phenome. The goal of human genetic studies has always been to understand genomic variation and its impact on phenotypes, and vice versa. Our ultimate understandings are limited by the depth and integrity of data of both types, and then how well each data type is integrated and leveraged with the other for the greatest insight into health and disease.

very large pedigrees that provided the basis to find the first genes that underlie the cardiomyopathies. While this continues to be the nearly universal paradigm for HCM and the long QT syndrome, a growing body of data, still preliminary, suggests that ARVC and DCM have genetic complexity beyond mendelian in a substantial number of probands and families.[8,11,12]

Finally, although this chapter focuses primarily on nonsyndromic cardiomyopathies, there are multiple syndromes in which a cardiomyopathy develops in concert with multiorgan system involvement. HCM (see Chapter 54) is also mentioned briefly herein because of its significant genetic overlap with DCM (see Fig. 52.2), as is amyloid cardiomyopathy (see Chapter 53) due to its phenotypic presentation as a RCM.

THE DILATED CARDIOMYOPATHIES

DCM is characterized by an enlarged left ventricle with systolic dysfunction that is not caused by ischemic or valvular heart disease. At the outset the DCM nomenclature can be confusing because the DCM term can be applied regardless of etiology, that is, ischemic, valvular, or other causes based only on LV enlargement and reduced function. Thus, a clear grasp of this nomenclature is foundational to navigating the clinical and genetic literature around DCM.[13] Due to the prevalence of ischemic cardiomyopathy, the most common clinical and clinical research approach is to sort DCM into ischemic or nonischemic categories. However, the latter category, having systolic dysfunction and LV enlargement, can include virtually any etiology (except ischemic), including genetic cause. In this category resides those patients diagnosed with "idiopathic" DCM, where other clinically identifiable causes have been excluded. When multiple individuals are identified in a family meeting idiopathic DCM criteria, such families are assigned a *familial* DCM diagnosis.[13] These DCM families provided the initial substrate for the discovery of the first DCM genes. For clinical practice, though, most DCM rigorously classified as idiopathic presents as sporadic, not familial, DCM, even after the clinical screening of first-degree family members. The question, not yet resolved, remains as to whether nonfamilial DCM results principally from underlying rare variant genetic cause. A nearly completed NIH study[12,14] may provide clarity to this fundamental question. A related question applicable to all of the cardiomyopathies is whether cause stems largely from one single highly penetrant rare variant, or is the amalgamation of genetics, both rare, with a possibly substantial oligogenic overlay for some conditions, and common, along with possible epigenetic and environmental impacts.

When investigating a patient with DCM, a full history, including risk factors for CAD, should be acquired.[13] Unless the patient is questioned in detail, the duration of symptoms may be significantly underestimated. Angina may occur, even in the absence of epicardial coronary disease, but symptoms suggestive of angina should raise the possibility of CAD. Patients should be questioned carefully about alcohol consumption (see Chapter 84), both present and past. If a spouse is available, that person's input may be of great value because underreporting of heavy alcohol intake is common. A history to elicit exposure to cardiotoxic drugs, such as anthracyclines or others commonly given for cancer treatment, is also important, although the clinician should be aware that other much less commonly used drugs such as chloroquine or hydroxychloroquine can also underlie cardiomyopathy. Other well-established myocardial toxins, even if rare, such as heavy metal exposure from ingestion or inhalation, should also be ruled out. Finally,

a history directed to finding subtle signs of neuromuscular disease is always indicated, as key proteins of several genes causing cardiomyopathy are also expressed in skeletal muscle.[13]

A family history is essential for all patients with any type of cardiomyopathy. Known diagnoses of cardiomyopathy should be elicited in all first-, second-, and third-degree relatives, as well as any family members who have had history of heart failure or sudden cardiac death. Relevant procedures include family members who have had coronary bypass operations, which implies ischemic etiology. If possible to exclude ischemic etiology, a family history of devices such as pacemakers, implantable cardioverter-defibrillators (ICDs), or ventricular assist devices, or a history of heart transplant, should raise concern for shared genetic risk between family members. Patients will commonly have little medically informed family history information available unless prompted to obtain this either before or following the initial medical interview. Notably, symptoms suggestive of heart failure but also of sudden cardiac death are commonly conflated and reported as the relevant family member having had a "heart attack." Relevant medical records can be invaluable, especially of such close relatives who have recently died of cardiovascular cause.

Findings on clinical examination may reflect the biventricular dysfunction that may present in DCM (see Chapters 13 and 48), although DCM also commonly presents with predominant LV involvement. Electrocardiography frequently reveals LV hypertrophy, nonspecific ST-T wave changes, or bundle branch block (see Chapter 48). Conduction system disease has specific gene associations (e.g., *LMNA* cardiomyopathy). Pathologic Q waves may be present, although their presence should also raise the possibility of advanced atherosclerotic heart disease. In advanced cases with extensive fibrosis, low-voltage limb leads may be seen.

Echocardiography (see also Chapter 16) reveals LV systolic dysfunction (Fig. 52.3) that may also show biventricular dysfunction in at least one third of cases,[15] all of which can range from mild to severe. LV wall thickness is almost always within the normal range, but the LV mass is invariably increased. Most commonly, global LV hypokinesis is present, but regional wall motion abnormalities may also be seen, particularly septal dyskinesis in those with left bundle branch block. Disproportionate thinning of a dyskinetic wall should raise the possibility of CAD rather than primary cardiomyopathy. Mitral and tricuspid regurgitation is frequently present and may be severe, even when the clinical examination does not reveal a loud murmur. Other than impaired leaflet coaptation, the mitral and tricuspid valves appear to be structurally normal, and valvular structural abnormalities suggest primary valvular disease rather than cardiomyopathy. Diastolic function in DCM ranges from normal to restrictive (see also Chapter 51). A restrictive pattern is most commonly seen in patients with volume overload in "decompensated" heart failure and often improves with initiation of diuretic or vasodilator therapy.

Coronary angiography (see Chapter 21) should be considered in all patients who have risk factors for CAD, most importantly cigarette smoking or a prominent family history of early-onset CAD observed in familial hypercholesterolemia, or in those who are of an age where CAD is commonly observed regardless of added risk factors, conventionally above 40 years in males and above 45 years in females. Alternatively, computed tomography (CT) coronary angiography (see Chapter 20) may be used, although it does not allow hemodynamic study, which may be useful in some patients. Because CAD is common, the functional significance of any obstructive coronary lesions found should be carefully evaluated insofar as their presence may be coincidental to DCM.

Cardiac magnetic resonance imaging (CMR) (see also Chapter 19) has become foundational for the evaluation of a patient who presents with a recently diagnosed cardiomyopathy. A pattern of nontransmural delayed gadolinium enhancement in a noncoronary distribution in a dilated left ventricle suggests a nonischemic cause. Certain conditions, such as sarcoidosis, may have a rather typical appearance. CMR is able to evaluate the extent of myocardial fibrosis in DCM and may provide information complementary to that obtained with cardiac biopsy. Unless a specific condition is suspected, cardiac biopsy is often unrewarding in the evaluation of DCM, but it may occasionally provide an

TABLE 52.1 Classification of the Cardiomyopathies by Phenome and Genome

TYPE	PHENOME			SYSTEMIC CONDITIONS, CLINICAL FEATURES, RISK FACTORS	GENOME	
	MORPHOLOGY	PHYSIOLOGY	PATHOLOGY		NONSYNDROMIC, USUALLY SINGLE GENE	SYNDROMIC
Dilated (DCM)	Dilation of LV or LV and RV with minimal or no wall thickening	Reduced contractility is the primary defect; variable degree of diastolic dysfunction	Myocyte hypertrophy; scattered fibrosis	Hypertension; alcohol; thyrotoxicosis, myxedema; persistent tachycardia; toxins (e.g., chemotherapy, especially anthracyclines); radiation	Diverse gene ontology (see Fig. 52.2; Fig. 52.6) with >30 genes implicated (see also **eTable 52.1**)	Diverse array of associated conditions, especially muscular dystrophies: Emery-Dreifuss muscular dystrophy, limb-girdle muscular dystrophy, Duchenne/Becker muscular dystrophy; Laing distal myopathy; Barth syndrome; Kearns-Sayre syndrome; others[3-5]
Restrictive (RCM)	Usually normal chamber sizes; minimal to moderate wall thickening	Contractility normal or near-normal with a marked increase in end-diastolic filling pressure	Specific to type, diagnosis: amyloid, iron, glycogen storage disease, others	Endomyocardial fibrosis, amyloid, sarcoid, scleroderma, Churg-Strauss syndrome, cystinosis, lymphoma, pseudoxanthoma elasticum, hypereosinophilic syndrome, carcinoid	If not associated with systemic genetic disease, genetic cause usually from sarcomeric gene rare variants (see eTable 52.1)	Gaucher disease, hemochromatosis, Fabry disease, familial amyloidosis; mucopolysaccharidoses, Noonan syndrome
Hypertrophic (HCM)	Usually normal or reduced internal chamber dimension; wall thickening pronounced, especially septal hypertrophy	Systolic function increased or normal	Myocyte hypertrophy, classically with disarray	Severe hypertension can confound clinical diagnosis	Rare variants of genes encoding sarcomeric proteins (see Chapter 54; also see eTable 52.1)	Noonan syndrome, LEOPARD syndrome, Danon syndrome, Fabry disease, Wolff-Parkinson-White syndrome, Friedreich ataxia, MERRF, MELAS (see Chapter 100)
Arrhythmogenic right ventricular cardiomyopathy (ARVC)	Scattered fibrofatty infiltration, classically of RV but also of LV; dilation of RV or LV, or both, is common but not universal	Ventricular arrhythmias (VT, VF) early or late, reduced contractility with progressive disease; can mimic DCM	Islands of fatty replacement; fibrosis	Palmoplantar keratoderma, wooly hair in Naxos syndrome	Rare variants of genes encoding proteins of desmosome (see Fig. 52.2; Fig. 52.6, eTable 52.1, and eFig. 52.4)	Naxos syndrome
Inflammatory	Normal or dilated without hypertrophy	Reduced systolic function	Inflammatory infiltrates	Hypereosinophilic syndrome (see text), acute myocarditis (see Chapter 55)		
Ischemic	Normal or dilated without hypertrophy	Reduced systolic function	Areas of infarcted myocardium	Hypercholesterolemia, hypertension, diabetes, cigarette smoking, family history		Familial hypercholesterolemia
Infectious	Normal or dilated without hypertrophy	Reduced systolic function	Specific to infection	Viral (especially acute myocarditis); protozoal (e.g., Chagas disease); bacterial, direct infection (e.g., Lyme disease) or from acute cellular toxicity as result of systemic toxins (e.g., Streptococcus, gram-negative, others) (see Chapter 55)	Genetic predisposition to infection and/or variable response to infective agent	

LV, Left ventricle; MELAS, mitochondrial encephalopathy, lactic acidosis, and strokelike symptoms; MERRF, myoclonic epilepsy associated with ragged-red fibers; RV, right ventricle; VF, ventricular fibrillation; VT, ventricular tachycardia.

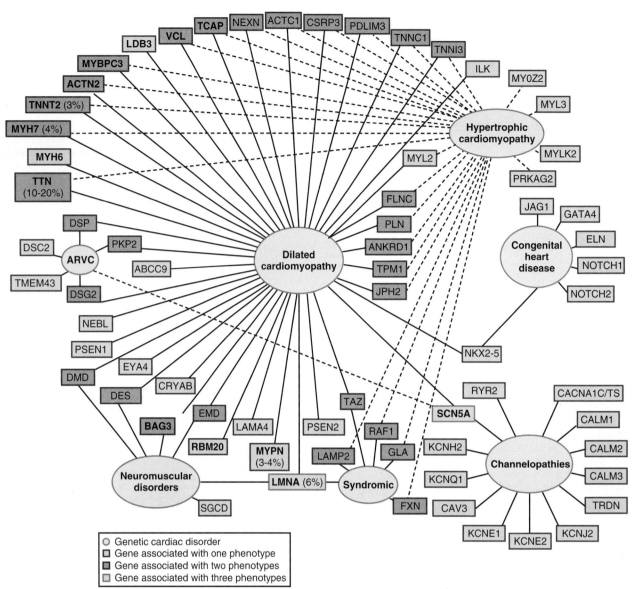

FIGURE 52.2 Relationships of genes implicated in causing cardiovascular and related phenotypes. The gene relationships for several cardiovascular phenotypes are shown, with the principal focus on dilated cardiomyopathy (DCM) genetics. Common cardiac phenotypes are shown in the *purple ovals,* and *lines* connect each phenotype to the gene or genes (shown in a box) of which rare variants have been implicated in causing the phenotype. The gene boxes are color-coded according to the number of phenotypes with which they are associated: *blue* indicates one phenotype, *red* indicates two phenotypes, and *yellow* indicates three phenotypes (as shown in the lower left corner of the figure). For a gene causing 3% or more of familial DCM cases, the frequency is included with its name. Hypertrophic cardiomyopathy (HCM) gene associations are indicated by *dotted lines.* Well-established HCM genes include two sarcomere genes (*MYH7* and *MYBPC3*) that together account for 80% of HCM cases for which a genetic cause can be identified. Three other sarcomere genes (*TNNT2, TNNI3,* and *TPM1*) account for an additional 15% of such cases. The other numerous genes implicated have caused only one or a few reported cases. The evidence in support of rare variants in the genes shown and their relevance for the specified cardiomyopathy varies considerably.

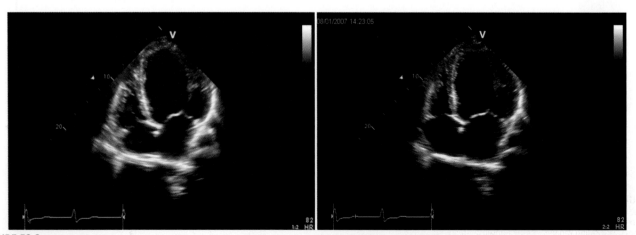

FIGURE 52.3 Echocardiogram in a patient with dilated cardiomyopathy. The end-diastolic frame **(left)** and end-systolic frame **(right)** in a 40-year-old man with severe dilated cardiomyopathy (DCM; ejection fraction <20%) are shown. Note the globular left ventricular (LV) shape, typical of advanced DCM. Despite the severe reduction in LV ejection fraction, he had only mild symptoms, attributable, in part, to preservation of stroke volume because of the marked increase in LV end-diastolic volume.

unexpected diagnosis. Multimodality imaging has become the norm for most cases of DCM.[16]

Once a diagnosis has been established in a patient meeting rigorous clinical criteria for idiopathic DCM, a full genetic evaluation should be initiated.

Genetics of Dilated Cardiomyopathy

In a significant proportion of patients with DCM, no obvious cause can be found even with a comprehensive clinical evaluation; these patients are assigned a diagnosis of *idiopathic DCM*. Family-based studies from the 1990s have shown that if clinical screening with an electrocardiogram (ECG) and/or echocardiogram is conducted in the first-degree family members of patients with DCM, evidence of DCM will be found in 10% to 20% or more,[17] thereby establishing a diagnosis of *familial DCM*. Familial DCM is now known to have a genetic basis of diverse ontology (see Fig. 52.2).[11] Despite the discovery of many genes, plausible genetic cause can only be identified in 25% to 30% of familial cases, with lower sensitivity in sporadic cases of DCM, as more stringent analytical approaches have become the norm.[12] In the largest series to date of 1040 individuals with DCM, with presumed mostly sporadic disease and assuming a mendelian paradigm, sensitivity of testing was approximately 15% when the enrichment of rare variants was assessed compared to population controls.[18] Truncating variants in the giant scaffolding protein titin (*TTN*) have been shown to be the most common, associated with 10% to 20% of cases of DCM depending upon cohort studied (Fig. 52.4).[18–20] Penetrance issues are also highly relevant for *TTN*, also illustrated by genetics-first approaches, with evidence suggesting a marked reduction in penetrance in individuals of African ancestry compared to European ancestry.[21] The proportion of rare variants thought to be causative of DCM attributed to any specific gene is much smaller, usually ranging from less than 1% to 3% (**eTable 52.1**). Even though familial DCM is now considered to have a genetic basis due to the observed heritability, the issue of whether sporadic DCM (that is, where no evidence of familial DCM is apparent after clinical screening of relatives) has a genetic basis has not been

resolved. While some sporadic cases will show pathogenic or likely pathogenic variants, many will only harbor a rare variant of unknown significance or no variants in any known DCM genes.[12]

Patients with DCM typically have an asymptomatic phase for many years before symptomatic heart failure, an arrhythmia, or an embolic event develops later in the course of the disease (Fig. 52.5).[22] Occasionally, asymptomatic but clinically detectable DCM is discovered serendipitously during routine or preprocedural medical screening, usually prompted by subtle abnormalities on an ECG that prompt an echocardiogram. The time span needed for clinical disease to develop illustrates the remarkable ability of the myocardium to maintain normal—or close to normal—cardiac output and filling pressure for years despite clinically detectable asymptomatic DCM. This principle underlies the observation that the family history is much less sensitive than clinical screening by echocardiography in detecting DCM among family members of an individual with a new diagnosis of idiopathic DCM. This also emphasizes the necessity of clinical screening of all first-degree family members when a new diagnosis of any cardiomyopathy has been made.

Genetics of Familial Dilated Cardiomyopathy

The genes shown to cause familial DCM are classified by subcellular location (gene ontology). As shown in Figure 52.2 and **eTable 52.1**, most of the implicated genes encode sarcomere, Z-disc, or cytoskeleton proteins. The broad representation of other genes encoding a wide variety of proteins demonstrates the diverse pathways that can lead to a final phenotype of DCM.[11] Presumably, other yet unknown pathways may also be relevant in the pathogenesis of DCM. More than 30 genes have been identified to cause DCM (referred to as locus heterogeneity) of diverse subcellular localization (Fig. 52.6). The diverse subcellular locations of genes implicated in DCM differentiate this form of cardiomyopathy from HCM (see also Chapter 54) and ARVC, which are caused by variants in genes encoding sarcomeric or desmosomal proteins, respectively (see Fig. 52.2). In addition to locus heterogeneity, the molecular genetics of DCM is also characterized by

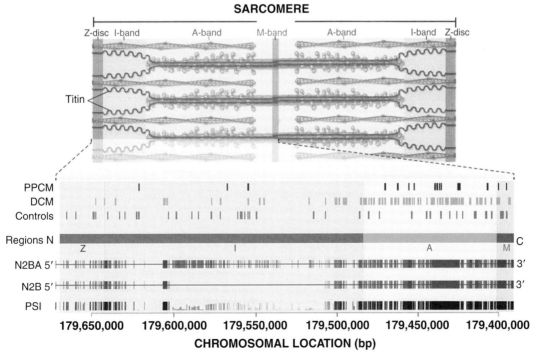

FIGURE 52.4 The giant protein titin and its involvement in dilated cardiomyopathy (DCM). Titin, the largest protein in the body, which is made up of more than 35,000 amino acids, is encoded by *TTN*, which acts as a scaffolding protein for sarcomere assembly. The large size of *TTN* made investigation extremely challenging prior to the development of next-generation sequencing strategies. Recent work has implicated truncating variants of *TTN* in 15% to 25% of familial DCM patients and 10% to 15% of nonfamilial DCM patients. Truncating variants include nonsense, frameshift, splice site, or other variants that cause the protein to be truncated. The upper part of the diagram shows the protein structure, with sarcomeric regions labeled (Z-disc and I, A, and M bands). The lower portion shows the locations of truncating variants in peripartum cardiomyopathy (PPCM), DCM, or controls. The exons of the primary two cardiovascular transcripts expressed (N2BA, N2B) are shown, along with their proportions spliced in (PSI). (From Ware JS, Li J, Mazaika E, et al. Shared genetic predisposition in peripartum and dilated cardiomyopathies. *N Engl J Med.* 2016;374:233–241.)

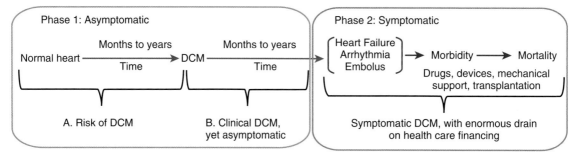

FIGURE 52.5 Asymptomatic and symptomatic phases of dilated cardiomyopathy (DCM). Phase 1 includes two periods, both asymptomatic. In the first period (1A), individuals who harbor one or more rare DCM variants have a risk of developing DCM over time. During this phase, genetic information identifies the individuals who would benefit from periodic clinical screening to detect early clinical disease. In phase 1B, DCM is present but asymptomatic, at times for years, and may evade detection unless periodic clinical cardiovascular imaging efforts detect it. Once disease has been detected, medical therapy can be initiated in an effort to prevent progression to phase 2. In phase 2, disease becomes late-stage and symptomatic with heart failure, arrhythmia, or embolus, the presenting features of DCM. (From Morales A, Hershberger RE. The rationale and timing of molecular genetic testing for dilated cardiomyopathy. *Can J Cardiol*. 2015;31:1309–1312.)

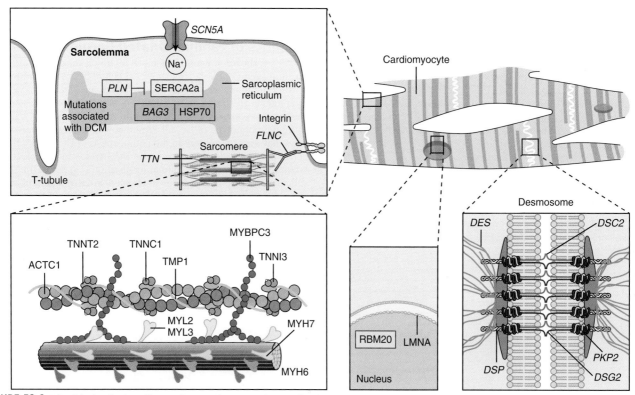

FIGURE 52.6 Subcellular localization of key cardiomyopathy proteins (see text for abbreviations). (Adapted from Schultheiss H-P, Fairweather D, Caforio ALP, et al. Dilated cardiomyopathy. *Nat Rev Dis Primers*. 2019;5:32. https://doi.org/10.1038/s41572-019-0084-1.)

allelic heterogeneity; that is, rare variants commonly occur at many locations in a DCM gene, and many rare variant sites in genes shown to cause both DCM and HCM are specific to that cardiomyopathy (**eFig. 52.1**). So-called overlap phenotypes particularly for sarcomeric genes have occasionally been reported, wherein rare variants that have been shown to cause DCM, HCM, and RCM may be seen in an extended pedigree. One family has been reported showing all three phenotypes (HCM, RCM, DCM) with one *TNNT2* rare variant.[23]

Clinical Genetics of Dilated Cardiomyopathy

DCM is characterized by a relatively unitary final phenotype[11] of "generic" DCM. That is, for almost all genes implicated in DCM, there are no unique or distinguishing clinical features that have been associated with specific gene rare variants. The only general variation in phenotype commonly recognized[17,24] is "DCM with prominent conduction system disease," which has been observed in lamin A/C (*LMNA*) DCM and some cases of sodium channel (*SCN5A*) or desmin (*DES*) DCM (see eTable 52.1). Occasionally, a clinically mild muscular dystrophy phenotype can be identified in patients with *LMNA* cardiomyopathy

and a new diagnosis of DCM. However, if the muscular dystrophy is prominent, in most cases it will have been identified in a neuromuscular clinic with DCM being an incidental finding at the time of evaluation. Regardless of the setting, when a new diagnosis of idiopathic DCM is made, vigilance in detecting syndromic disease is essential, with particular attention being directed to neuromuscular phenotypes.

Most cases of familial DCM are transmitted via autosomal dominant inheritance, with the offspring of a mutation carrier having a 50% chance of inheriting the rare variant (Fig. 52.7). Autosomal recessive disease has been reported, particularly in consanguineous families. X-linked DCM resulting from rare variants in the gene for Duchenne muscular dystrophy (DMD) in patients without any findings of muscular dystrophy has been reported both in males and in carrier females, although the prevalence of DMD-DCM in cohorts of patients with idiopathic DCM has not been studied systematically. Mitochondrial DCM has also been reported, particularly in the setting of syndromic disease.[11]

Familial DCM is characterized by age-dependent penetrance, which means that an individual harboring a DCM-causing allele will manifest

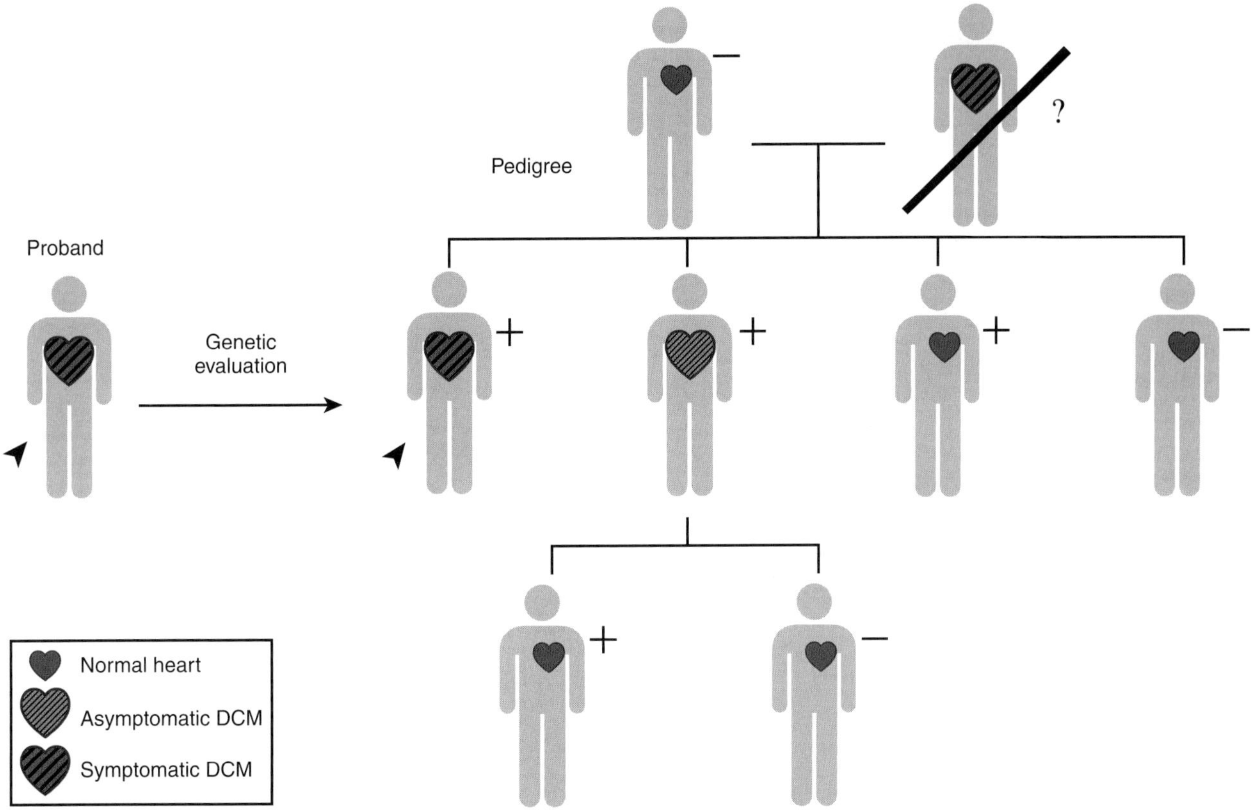

FIGURE 52.7 Genetic evaluation for cardiomyopathy. The goal of a genetic evaluation is to assess genetic risk of the proband and the proband's at-risk family members. The proband is the first patient identified with the trait or disease of interest, here depicted as an individual with dilated cardiomyopathy (DCM) and shown as an enlarged heart. The at-risk relatives can be shown by a pedigree, or a graphical depiction of the family relationships. A genetic evaluation includes a comprehensive family history for three generations or more and genetic and family counseling for all patients and families. In this example, the proband's mother died with a known diagnosis of DCM, but neither a genetic evaluation nor family screening was undertaken. With a new diagnosis of cardiomyopathy, clinical screening of first-degree relatives is indicated. In this example, the proband's three siblings are clinically evaluated. One is found to have asymptomatic DCM; the other two do not have clinical evidence of DCM. Because DCM has been found in one sibling, the sibling's children also have undergone clinical cardiovascular screening. A genetic evaluation is also indicated. In most cases, genetic testing should be undertaken for the one clearly affected person in a family to facilitate family screening and management. In this case, the proband is sequenced first, and a pathogenic rare variant is identified. This permits sequencing of the at-risk family members. The affected sibling is a mutation carrier, as is one unaffected sibling, who will be advised to have ongoing surveillance with clinical screening for early-onset DCM so that treatment can be initiated prior to the development of symptomatic DCM. One sibling is shown to not carry the mutation, so that individual can be released from clinical surveillance. The affected sibling's offspring can now also undergo genetic testing to assess risk. The one who is a mutation carrier will need clinical surveillance for development of DCM, with early intervention to attempt to prevent symptomatic disease. In this pedigree, the negative genetic testing result of the unaffected individual in the first generation indicates that the rare variant, inherited by multiple individuals in the second generation, was transmitted from the affected individual in the first generation. The finding that three affected family members all carried the same rare variant builds the evidence that the variant indeed is the pathogenic variant in this family. The *solid diagonal line* in the first generation represents a deceased individual.

evidence of the DCM phenotype with increasing age.[17,24] Most genetic DCM cases become evident in the fourth to seventh decades, although DCM occurring in adolescence, childhood, or infancy is not uncommon. Variations in the age at onset of DCM are common across families with rare variants in the same DCM gene, at times marked, and even in family members of an extended pedigree with the same rare variant (see Fig. 52.7). Penetrance in familial DCM is commonly incomplete; that is, an individual with a disease-causing allele may not manifest any aspect of the disease phenotype (see Fig. 52.7). Also, expression is variable in that the clinical features and the phenotype can vary significantly between individuals in the same family or between families with the same rare variant. Both incomplete penetrance and variable expressivity confound the assessment of familial DCM in family pedigrees. This is particularly relevant for a newly discovered or novel candidate rare variant in a family because full segregation of the candidate rare variant with the disease phenotype in one or more extended families is one of the most helpful approaches for determining the pathogenicity of such variants.

Incomplete penetrance and variable expressivity at times result in marked phenotypic variability within and between families with DCM, even with the same rare variant. The explanation for this phenomenon is not clear. Both environmental and genetic factors have been postulated and range from intrinsic (e.g., hypertension) and extrinsic phenomic components (e.g., toxins, viruses, adverse or favorable drug exposure) to a combination of various genomic variants resulting in

a different genetic milieu (e.g., a second rare variant in a different disease gene, risk alleles in the same or other relevant DCM pathways, variability in epigenetics or gene expression, and others).

Allelic heterogeneity, in which rare variants in one gene can give rise to different and distinct phenotypes seemingly unrelated to one another (see Fig. 52.2 and eFig. 52.1), is also observed with some DCM genes, and knowledge of these allelic variants can be critical when considering a genetic diagnosis of DCM. One of the most remarkable examples is *LMNA*, which encodes the proteins lamin A and lamin C, key components of the inner nuclear membrane. For example, mutations in *LMNA* cause a distinctive DCM phenotype in which conduction system disease and arrhythmia occur before the onset of DCM. Mutant lamin proteins also cause a variety of syndromic diseases spanning striated muscle, adipose, nerve, and vascular tissues. These phenotypes, collectively termed the *laminopathies*, include skeletal myopathies (autosomal dominant Emery-Dreifuss muscular dystrophy, limb-girdle muscular dystrophy type 1B, and others [see Chapter 100]), lipodystrophy syndromes, peripheral neuropathy, and accelerated aging syndromes, most notably Hutchinson-Gilford progeria.

Approach to Clinical Genetic Evaluation

With a new cardiomyopathy diagnosis a genetic evaluation should be initiated.[4,5] A genetic evaluation precedes genetic testing, and at times may not require genetic testing. Genetic testing (Fig. 52.8) is always

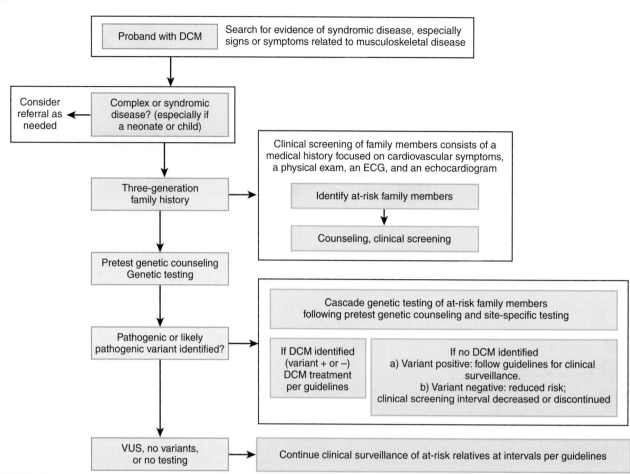

FIGURE 52.8 Flow diagram of clinical genetic testing. The conceptual approach to clinical genetic testing of a proband, the individual first identified in the family of interest, and the proband's at-risk family members, is shown. VUS, variant of unknown significance. Please see Fig. 52.7 for how this could be implemented into a multigenerational family.

TABLE 52.2 Genetic Cardiomyopathy Guidelines*

1	Family history of at least three generations
2	Clinical screening for first-degree relatives
3	Referral for genetic evaluation as needed
4	Genetic testing for DCM, HCM, ARVC, or RCM
5	Genetic counseling for patients and families
6	Cardiovascular evaluation for secondary findings
7 and 8	Therapies based on phenotype are recommended
9	Consider ICD** use before usual criteria are met

ARVC, Arrhythmogenic right ventricular cardiomyopathy; *DCM*, dilated cardiomyopathy; *HCM*, hypertrophic cardiomyopathy; *RCM*, restrictive cardiomyopathy.
*See text for expanded explanation. From the Heart Failure Society of America[4] and the American College of Genetics and Genomics.[5]
***ICD*, Implantable cardioverter-defibrillator.

recommended to be performed as a component of a genetic evaluation.[4,5] Components of a genetic evaluation for a new diagnosis of cardiomyopathy include five key tasks (Table 52.2). This first two are fundamental and will help define the nature and extent of the cardiomyopathy observed in a patient and include (1) a comprehensive family history for at least three generations, and (2) the clinical screening of all first-degree relatives for cardiomyopathy (see Fig. 52.7). Evidence of cardiomyopathy in closely related family members defines familial cardiomyopathy, and this clinical determination is strong evidence for genetic etiology. This information may also aid in the interpretation and inferences drawn from genetic test results. If local evaluative expertise is not available, (3) a referral for expert evaluation is recommended, especially for complex clinical or genetic cases, or infants or children where syndromic and metabolic disease should be considered and

excluded. Then (4) genetic testing (see Fig. 52.8) and (5) genetic counseling should be provided for DCM, ARVC, HCM, and RCM, all of which have been shown to have a genetic basis.[4,5]

The sixth item (see Table 52.2) provides guidance for cardiovascular specialists who are sent individuals who have secondary (sometimes referred to as incidental) genetic findings in genes known to cause cardiovascular disease, such as the cardiomyopathies. In most cases these variants have been observed in clinical exome testing or expanded medically relevant gene panels. In short, a search for the relevant phenotypic features of the condition should be undertaken,[4,5] understanding that penetrance in a "genetics-first" approach rather than a "phenotype-first" approach may give dramatically different penetrance estimates (e.g., for ARVC variants[7]), as noted above. The remaining items (see Table 52.2) reflect current medical or device interventions, including a recommendation for early ICD use as may be indicated by a specific genetic diagnosis that incurs substantial risk of sudden cardiac death before LV systolic dysfunction reaches an ejection fraction less than 35%.

Guidelines for evaluation and clinical genetic testing for DCM, applicable to all cardiomyopathies with a possible genetic cause (see Fig. 52.8), include a comprehensive three- to four-generation search of the family history for any evidence of any type of cardiomyopathy, muscular dystrophy, or other evidence of syndromic disease that may have a cardiomyopathy component. However, as noted earlier, even if it is obtained by a skilled genetics professional, the family history may well be negative because DCM is commonly asymptomatic in family members. Accordingly, cardiovascular clinical screening of all first-degree relatives is essential; history taking, a physical examination, an ECG, and echocardiography should be acquired at a minimum. If evidence of DCM is identified in a relative, screening of that relative's first-degree relatives is indicated (i.e., stepwise or cascade clinical screening).

Genetic testing, within the context of genetic counseling, is indicated with any evidence of familial disease because identification of a disease-associated rare variant (in one or more clearly affected family members) can permit molecular genetic testing of other at-risk family members with preclinical disease and thereby aid in their risk stratification. Those who test negative for the family's disease-associated rare variant should have a significantly reduced risk for the development of DCM; those harboring the family DCM rare variant should undergo enhanced clinical screening to detect early DCM, with the rationale that early drug intervention, for example with an angiotensin-converting enzyme (ACE) inhibitor or a beta blocker, may delay or prevent progression of the disease.

Genetic Testing

Genetic testing (see Fig. 52.8) is now conducted by next-generation sequencing in panels of genes ranging from 50 to 80 or more. In the United States, most insurers pay for genetic testing with appropriate genetic counseling and diagnosis coding. Genetic testing should always be conducted within the context of genetic counseling, the goals of which are to review the genetic inheritance patterns and clinically relevant facts regarding idiopathic and familial DCM and ensure that a comprehensive family history has been completed and properly interpreted, including identification of at-risk relatives. Counseling is also essential to provide information regarding the risks, benefits, and limitations of clinical genetic testing, including the possible consequences of uncertain or inconclusive results or the discovery of heritable disease and its potential psychological implications. These processes are time-consuming and require specialized knowledge; guidelines suggest that referral of patients to individuals or centers with experience should be considered if local resources for completion of the process are not available.

Post-test counseling is indicated regardless of finding a pathogenic or likely pathogenic variant in a relevant cardiomyopathy gene, because the sensitivity of genetic testing, that is, the likelihood that a relevant rare variant will be found, ranges from 20% to 25% for DCM, and 25% to 50% for ARVC and HCM. Sensitivity of testing for RCM is 10%. If testing does not return a pathogenic or likely pathogenic variant, at-risk first-degree family members are counseled to continue with clinical surveillance. If a pathogenic or likely pathogenic variant is identified in the proband, then testing of any other family members who already show evidence of cardiomyopathy builds the case that the identified variant is indeed relevant for disease (see Fig. 52.7). Other at-risk family members who do not yet show a phenotype can be tested to aid in their risk stratification. Those who test negative for the family's disease-associated rare variant should have a significantly reduced risk for the development of cardiomyopathy; those harboring the family rare variant should undergo enhanced clinical screening to detect early disease. The rationale for this for DCM and ARVC is that early drug intervention, for example with an ACE inhibitor, a beta blocker, or an ICD, may delay or prevent progression of the disease or sudden death.

The recommendation for genetic testing recognizes that with the greater number of genes being tested in pan-cardiomyopathy panels, a greater number of variants of uncertain significance may be encountered.[4,5,22] Clinicians ordering clinical genetic testing must understand this concept and be prepared to deal with this reality as the results become available. The emergence of next-generation sequencing of panels of genes has fueled an extremely active period for reevaluation of testing strategies, including approaches to interpreting large numbers of variants. All of this will require careful, comprehensive translational research to understand the optimal testing strategies, including the accumulation of large databases of disease-associated variants.

Therapy for Dilated Cardiomyopathy

Therapy for DCM is similar to that for all types of heart failure with a reduced ejection fraction and is discussed in detail in Chapter 50. Attention should be paid to treatment of atrial arrhythmias (see Tachycardia-Induced Cardiomyopathy, later). In selected patients, cardiac resynchronization therapy should be considered (see Chapter 58),

and/or referral for a ventricular assist device or cardiac transplantation may be also needed (see also Chapters 59 and 60).

Arrhythmogenic Right Ventricular Cardiomyopathy

ARVC is now considered a genetically determined cardiomyopathy that has been historically characterized by lethal arrhythmias in relatively young adults and with fibrofatty replacement of the myocardium, especially of the right ventricle. The ARVC nomenclature is preserved to reflect the current medical literature.[25] Some have proposed to change the nomenclature to the simpler "arrhythmogenic cardiomyopathy" while enlarging the "arrhythmic" phenotypes[26] well beyond the conventional task force-specific ARVC category;[25] but issues have been noted with this approach[27] including an effort to take into account the arrhythmias that occur in cardiomyopathies beyond ARVC. A recognized misnomer in the ARVC term is that biventricular involvement occurs in up to 50% of cases and a small proportion of cases affect predominantly the left ventricle (eFigs. 52.2 and e52.3). Nevertheless, the current approach works well: the applied task force criteria (eTable 52.2) provide a reasonable sensitivity to a specific gene ontology, that is, genes encoding proteins of the desmosome (see Fig. 52.6). The disorder is classically conceptualized as having three stages: an early subclinical phase in which imaging studies are negative but during which sudden cardiac death can still occur; next, a phase in which (usually) RV abnormalities are obvious without any clinical manifestation of RV dysfunction but with the development of a symptomatic ventricular arrhythmia; and, finally, progressive fibrofatty replacement and infiltration of the myocardium leading to severe RV dilation and aneurysm formation and associated right-sided heart failure (see eFig. 52.2). LV dilation and failure may also arise at this stage or may occur later (sometimes referred to as phase 4).[28] Exercise is a key facilitator of arrhythmias at all stages of disease.[25,26,28]

The electrical manifestations of ARVC reflect the pathologic disturbance. In the early stage, slow conduction and electrical uncoupling may lead to a fatal arrhythmia. As the disease progresses, fibrofatty infiltration results in inhomogeneous activation and a further delay in conduction. The predominant site of cardiac involvement, known as the triangle of dysplasia, was believed to involve the RV outflow tract, an area below the tricuspid valve, and the RV apex. However, recent data suggest that the RV apex is only involved in advanced disease and that an area involving the basal inferior and anterior right ventricle and the posterolateral left ventricle may be most commonly involved.[29] Patients with ARVC exhibit a typical monomorphic ventricular tachycardia (VT) characterized by left bundle branch block morphology with a superior axis[30] and typical T wave inversions extending to V_3 or beyond. A classic "epsilon wave" in the right precordial leads is a specific but insensitive finding (Fig. 52.9).

Genomic Cause of Arrhythmogenic Right Ventricular Cardiomyopathy

Unlike genetic DCM, which has extensive locus heterogeneity, ARVC is driven by rare variants in genes encoding proteins that are key for cell-to-cell adhesion (eFig. 52.4).[28] Extensive work over the past decade has implicated genes encoding the desmosome, one of three key components of the intercalated disc, the end-to-end connection between ventricular myocytes,[28,31] in the pathogenesis of ARVC. In addition to desmosomes, the intercalated disc includes gap junctions mediating small-molecule communications. Mechanical coupling is mediated through the desmosome and adherens junctions (see Chapter 46), and disruptions of desmosomal proteins have been associated with ARVC. The classic hallmark of ARVC, fibrofatty replacement, is now understood to be related to aberrant Wnt signaling of desmosomal proteins, as well as direct plakoglobin signaling, which transforms myocytes into adipocytes with disease progression.[28,31]

MOLECULAR GENETICS

When a genetic cause can be identified, rare variants in the genes encoding plakophilin 2 (PKP2), desmoglein 2 (DSG2), and desmoplakin (DSP) account for most genetic causes of ARVC (see eTable 52.1 and Fig. 52.2).

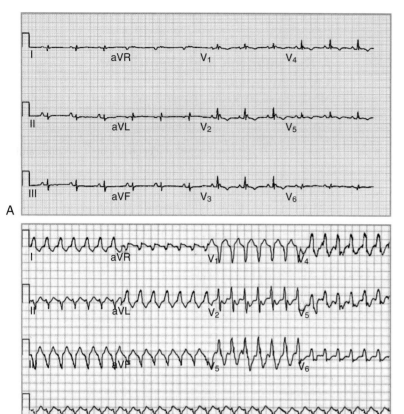

FIGURE 52.9 Arrhythmogenic right ventricular cardiomyopathy (ARVC). **A,** Electrocardiogram (ECG) of a patient with ARVC. A typical ECG shows inverted T waves in the anterior precordial leads and an "epsilon potential" early during ventricular repolarization representing a "late potential" caused by delayed depolarization of an area of the right ventricle. **B,** Ventricular tachycardia in a patient with ARVC. There are left bundle branch block morphologic findings with a leftward axis. (From Hauer RN, Cox MGPJ, Groeneweg JA. Impact of new electrocardiographic criteria in arrhythmogenic cardiomyopathy. *Front Physiol.* 2012;3:352.)

Rare variants in other genes encoding the desmosomal proteins (desmocollin [*DSC2*], junction plakoglobin [*JUP*]) or affecting desmosomal physiology (e.g., transmembrane protein [*TMEM*]) also cause ARVC (see Fig. 52.6; **eTable 52.1**). The ClinGen gene-validity curation for ARVC has found these six genes to have definitive evidence.[32] The degree of locus heterogeneity is similar for HCM and ARVC, in which five or fewer genes contribute to most of the identifiable genetic causes. However, as for DCM and HCM, the genes implicated in ARVC show extensive allelic heterogeneity.

CLINICAL GENETICS

The autosomal recessive syndromic *Naxos disease*, so named because it was discovered on the Greek island of Naxos, is manifested as ARVC cosegregating with palmoplantar keratoderma and wooly hair. Molecular genetic analysis has shown a homozygous two–base pair frameshift deletion of *JUP*, which encodes plakoglobin. This observation first implicated the desmosome in ARVC and prompted the molecular genetic discovery of other desmosomal proteins. Other rare variants in *JUP* have also been associated with cutaneous disease or wooly hair phenotypes, although cardiovascular phenotypes have not been identified in most of these allelic variants.[31] A second autosomal recessive syndromic disease, *Carvajal syndrome*, resembles Naxos disease in that individuals have palmoplantar keratoderma and wooly hair, but individuals with Carvajal syndrome manifest DCM, not ARVC. Carvajal syndrome is caused by a frameshift rare variant in *DSP*, which encodes desmoplakin.[31] Other rare variants in *DSP* have been identified with only ARVC or with only skin or hair manifestations. Even though reduced penetrance and variable expressivity are commonly observed in all genetic cardiomyopathies, these features may be particularly prominent in ARVC, recently highlighted in a genetics first study where penetrance was estimated to be only 6%,[7] in part because of the difficulty of assessing the phenotype and also because the arrhythmia component may be the only feature of the disease in some individuals long before structural changes can be identified. ARVC has also been noted to have highly variable penetrance, in part attributed to an oligogenic basis in some.[27]

Diagnosis

The more advanced the disease, the easier the diagnosis, but recognition of earlier stages, which may be manifested as aborted sudden death without detectable structural abnormalities, can be difficult. In addition, with increasing use of CMR for the diagnosis of cardiac pathology, a trend toward overdiagnosis of ARVC is now being recognized (see also Chapter 19). Although, in experienced hands, CMR is a useful tool for both diagnosis and evaluation of the extent of structural abnormalities in ARVC, early disease may not be apparent despite ventricular arrhythmia,[33] and overdiagnosis of the disease by less-experienced CMR readers has been recognized. Endomyocardial biopsy for ARVC is one of the diagnostic criteria but is rarely undertaken because of the potential for higher complication rates and for false-negative findings.[33] The diagnosis of ARVC currently rests primarily on the combination of clinical, electrocardiographic, and genetic findings, which are divided into major and minor diagnostic criteria as proposed in a 2010 consensus statement (see eTable 52.2).

Approach to Clinical Genetic Evaluation, Including
Clinical Genetic Testing

The general approach to genetic evaluation reviewed above for DCM is fully relevant for ARVC. Current studies estimate that a plausible genetic cause can be identified in approximately half of ARVC cases.[4,34,35] The impact of multiple rare variants in desmosomal genes has been emphasized, as well as the impact of the revised task force clinical criteria, which has increased the sensitivity of molecular genetic testing.[35] A study of 439 index patients and their 562 family members showed an earlier onset of disease in those who were positive for the rare variant, although clinical characteristics were similar for both groups with disease onset.[36] Genetic testing is indicated for ARVC so that cascade testing of at-risk family members can be accomplished. This is particularly relevant for ARVC insofar as arrhythmias, especially sudden cardiac death, can occur before other phenotypic features become evident. Pan-cardiomyopathy testing, especially for a phenotype of prominent VT, ventricular fibrillation, or sudden cardiac death with biventricular dilation and systolic dysfunction of unknown cause otherwise consistent with DCM, may also yield rare variants in the genes associated with ARVC. Even though conventional recommendations currently discourage the use of genetic testing for the diagnosis of ARVC, molecular genetic testing will probably be used more frequently in the near future to assist in making the diagnosis, especially as genetic testing proliferates and is used more commonly for all cardiomyopathies regardless of phenotype.

Differential Diagnosis

The differential diagnosis of ARVC in the early stages (before the onset of visible structural abnormalities) includes idiopathic and RV outflow tract VTs. The morphology of the classic ARVC-related VT differs from these entities, and in the presence of precordial T wave inversion during sinus rhythm, ARVC should be the initial diagnosis. Cardiac sarcoidosis may occasionally mimic ARVC morphologically and be indistinguishable, even with multiple imaging modalities. Cardiac biopsy in patients with sarcoidosis often fails to show the pathognomonic granulomas but may reveal extensive fibrosis, which may also be confused with ARVC.

Treatment

Currently, the mainstay of therapy for ARVC is suppression and prevention of ventricular arrhythmias and the risk for sudden cardiac death, and prevention of disease progression. A systematic review estimated arrhythmic events at approximately 10% per year, with predictors being male gender, syncope, T wave inversions in V_3 to V_6,

RV dysfunction, prior VT or ventricular fibrillation, and exercise.[37] Intense physical exertion is associated with an earlier onset of symptoms and an increased risk of sustained VT, and therefore patients with a diagnosis of ARVC are advised not to participate in athletic activity.[38] The classic monomorphic VT in ARVC with predominant RV involvement is generally well tolerated, even at a rapid rate, possibly because of preserved LV function in most patients. Nevertheless, VT of a different morphology may occur and sudden death is not uncommon. Antiarrhythmic drugs may suppress a symptomatic arrhythmia but have not been shown to prevent sudden death. Beta-blocking agents may suppress catecholamine-triggered arrhythmia and slow progression of ventricular dysfunction and have been recommended as potentially valuable in all patients with ARVC.[38] An ICD is recommended in patients with aborted sudden death, syncope, or decreased LV function and may be considered in other patients (**eFig. 52.5**). Catheter ablation has not been shown to reduce sudden death but is valuable in a patient with an ICD and frequent arrhythmias or in occasional patients with very well-tolerated single-morphology VT. Ablation appears to be most successful when lesions are made in both the epicardial and endocardial surfaces of the heart; it should be performed only at centers experienced in the technique, either as a combined procedure or with epicardial ablation reserved for recurrence after endocardial ablation.[39] Heart failure may occur in advanced ARVC and is treated with standard drugs. Because a history of vigorous sustained exercise among carriers of a pathogenic ARVC desmosome rare variant is associated with an earlier onset of symptoms and a higher prevalence of VT or ventricular fibrillation,[40] there is a task force recommendation that persons with definite or suspected ARVC should not compete in most competitive sports.

Alcoholic and Diabetic Cardiomyopathies

Excessive alcohol intake is cardiotoxic and may be manifested as DCM, and is discussed in detail in Chapter 84.[41] The importance of obtaining as accurate an alcohol history as possible in assessing patients with DCM cannot be overstated. The existence of a specific diabetic cardiomyopathy independent of the effect of diabetes on the vasculature is debated, both in terms of its existence and in the form that it takes. Abnormalities initially in diastolic and then systolic function are prevalent in diabetic patients, but their clinical relevance to the development of overt disease is unclear.[42] Nevertheless, data do support good glycemic control as a preventative against the development of heart failure (see Chapter 31).[43] The addition of SGLT2 inhibitors to the management of diabetic patients with heart failure with reduced ejection fraction is discussed in Chapter 50.

Left Ventricular Noncompaction

In 2006 LVNC was included as a genetic cardiomyopathy in an AHA scientific statement.[1] In 2008, the European Society of Cardiology questioned whether LVNC should be classified as a cardiomyopathy or "merely a congenital or acquired morphologic trait that is shared by many phenotypically distinct cardiomyopathies."[2] Most authorities have suggested that evidence to classify LV noncompaction (LVNC) as a distinct cardiomyopathy is insufficient,[4,44–49] and rather consider LVNC as a morphologic trait that is shared by many cardiomyopathies as well as by other conditions, such as the channelopathies and congenital heart disease. A pattern of LVNC can emerge with intense exercise or pregnancy and resolve with diminished exercise or in the postpartum period, thus suggesting a paradigm of remodeling and reverse remodeling as seen in other conditions affecting LV size or function. Underlying this debate is the lack of adverse outcomes of LVNC itself, as published accounts of adverse events stem from a defined cardiomyopathy or arrhythmia phenotype. Mounting evidence has increased to favor a variant phenotype rather than one inherently pathologic.[46,48] LVNC does not have its own gene ontology but intersects with those of DCM, HCM, and ARVC (see Fig. 52.6; **eTable 52.1**).

Defining the LVNC phenotype has been confounded by various echocardiographic or CMR approaches that have led to an estimate of its frequency in a population-based study of as high as 23%; furthermore, the concordance of three different echocardiographic diagnostic schemata was congruent in only 30% of cases.[45] These diagnostic criteria have been summarized and include four that are echocardiographic-based and two that are cardiac CMR-based (**eTable 52.3**). If LVNC is identified in concert with another cardiomyopathy (DCM, HCM, RCM) the approach to the primary cardiomyopathy will drive the genetic evaluation process, as outlined earlier. It is not clear that any specific management is indicated for LVNC independent of some other cardiovascular diagnosis or complication.

Tachycardia-Induced Cardiomyopathy

Tachycardia for a prolonged period can result in diastolic and systolic ventricular dysfunction, even in the absence of other cardiac diseases. This condition is known as tachycardia-induced cardiomyopathy.[50] It is a diagnosis that can be made only retrospectively when correction of an arrhythmia is associated with improved ventricular function. However, it should be considered in any patient with tachycardia and LV systolic dysfunction who is not in sinus rhythm. The cardiomyopathy may be manifested either as an isolated condition or in association with preexisting cardiac disease. Thus a patient with mild DCM in whom atrial fibrillation develops may have a tendency for the development of decompensated heart failure, not only because of the loss of atrial function but also because the rapid, irregular rate of atrial fibrillation leads to further systolic dysfunction. Hyperthyroidism should be ruled out because it may cause both tachycardia and, rarely, an independent DCM. The "purest" form of tachycardia-induced cardiomyopathy is probably that caused by incessant or extremely frequent atrial tachycardia or permanent reciprocating junctional tachycardia, often in a child or young patient with systolic dysfunction.[51] However, almost any arrhythmia can cause tachycardia-induced cardiomyopathy, including very frequent premature ventricular contractions (PVCs) or recurrent nonsustained VT.[52] Incessant atrial tachycardia causing tachycardia-induced cardiomyopathy may be mistaken for sinus tachycardia. If a previous ECG is available, comparison may be helpful, with specific attention being paid to subtle differences in P-wave morphology.

The duration of the arrhythmia, more than the heart rate, is probably a critical factor in tachycardia-induced cardiomyopathy. Among 30 patients with incessant atrial tachycardia and tachycardia-induced cardiomyopathy, the mean duration of symptoms was 6 years. The mean ventricular response was just 117 beats/min, and rate control (primarily by ablation) was associated with normalization of the ejection fraction in all but one patient.[51] A decreased ejection fraction in the presence of atrial fibrillation may occasionally improve after the restoration of sinus rhythm. If the ventricular rate is well controlled, improvement of LV systolic function in atrial fibrillation with a reduced ejection fraction is uncommon, but it is important to assess ventricular rate control with 24-hour monitoring to confirm control during both exercise and rest. Most patients with PVC-associated tachycardia-induced cardiomyopathy have more than 20,000 PVCs over a 24-hour period, but the condition has also been described with a lesser frequency of arrhythmia.[39] Catheter ablation of PVCs, if possible, is generally associated with improvement in ventricular function in these patients.

Most cases of tachycardia-induced cardiomyopathy improve within 3 to 6 months after correction of the arrhythmia, but occasionally patients have been seen with late improvement, up to 1 year. Because the rapid, irregular ventricular response to atrial fibrillation is associated with marked beat-to-beat variation in the ejection fraction, the most accurate way to determine whether an improvement in systolic function has really occurred is to evaluate the ejection fraction early after restoration of sinus rhythm and then compare it with a reevaluation 3 to 6 months later.

Following restoration of sinus rhythm, subtle abnormalities in LV function may remain, such as mild LV dilation despite normalization of the ejection fraction, and recurrence of arrhythmia can be associated with deterioration of LV function.[53] In an animal model, tachycardia was associated with diastolic dysfunction often before a decrease in systolic function. Tachycardia-induced LV diastolic dysfunction may occur in humans in the presence of a normal ejection fraction. Although poorly studied, it may be responsible for the symptoms of heart failure in some patients with arrhythmia and a preserved LV ejection fraction.[54] Few data on improvement in diastolic dysfunction following correction of arrhythmia are available.

Peripartum Cardiomyopathy

Peripartum cardiomyopathy (PPCM) has been defined as DCM that occurs in a temporal relationship to pregnancy (see also Chapter 92). While PPCM has traditionally been considered etiologically separate from DCM, evidence now clearly indicates that at least a portion of PPCM cases results from genetic risk, at least in part, from genes known to cause DCM. Definitive evidence of this was recently shown,[20] where 172 women with PPCM underwent sequencing for DCM genes, with *TTN* truncating variants (TTNtvs) identified in 26 of the 172 (15%). A similar frequency of TTN truncating mutations in cohorts of patients with DCM is suggestive that at least a portion of PPCM may be DCM occurring during pregnancy. Two earlier studies also observed that in some proportion of cases a rare variant genetic cause, similar to that of DCM, was at play,[55,56] where rare variants in DCM genes were present in 6 of 19 women who had sequence information available.[55] In a second earlier study, among 90 families with DCM, 6% were found to have at least one member with PPCM, and genetic screening of relatives of three patients with PPCM who failed to show complete recovery revealed undiagnosed DCM in all three families.[56] From these studies comes the recommendation that in DCM occurring during or following pregnancy, the same guidelines for DCM presented earlier should be followed, namely, obtaining a comprehensive family history, performing clinical screening of first-degree relatives, and conducting genetic testing.

However, it can also be argued that of the many additional women who harbor TTNtvs only a small fraction develop PPCM, and the additional risk factors, whether genetic, epigenetic, or endogenous environmental factors, may well be at play.[57] Extensive prior studies have implicated risk for DCM during pregnancy that range from autoimmune conditions or nutritional deficiencies to inflammation of the myocardium. Animal models of vascular-hormonal features known to be associated with PPCM, focused primarily on elevated prolactin and its physiology and downstream signaling in late pregnancy and the peripartum period, have contributed to this vascular hypothesis. Bromocriptine, now considered experimental only, had been earlier advocated for treatment based on data from uncontrolled studies, but more recent randomized (without a control group) studies have shown no convincing benefit, and the significant adverse effects of bromocriptine await a properly randomized and controlled trial to show benefit.[57]

Clinical Features

The U.S. incidence is estimated to be between 1 in 1000 and 1 in 4000 live births, with a major risk factor that of African ancestry; significantly higher incidence has been reported in countries with predominant African ancestry. Preeclampsia, older age, and multiple-fetus pregnancies are also risk factors. In patients with PPCM, symptoms and signs of heart failure develop during late pregnancy or after delivery, similar to those of any patient with heart failure caused by LV systolic dysfunction. Most diagnoses are made in the 4 months following delivery; prepartum diagnoses are most commonly made in the last month of pregnancy. However, the disorder has also been described in early pregnancy (pregnancy-associated cardiomyopathy). Because symptoms similar to those of heart failure (dyspnea, fatigue, and edema) may occur in normal pregnancy, it is possible that a proportion of cases have a delayed diagnosis. Furthermore, because spontaneous resolution of LV dysfunction is known to occur, mild cases in the peripartum period may be overlooked. Given the rarity of the disease, it is not possible to precisely determine the incidence of PPCM in subsequent pregnancies of patients who have had a previous episode. However, recurrence appears to be related to the degree of recovery from the initial episode; PPCM seems less likely to recur in women who enter a second pregnancy with a normal ejection fraction than in those with a persistent reduction in the ejection fraction.[58]

In approximately 50% of patients with PPCM who are given standard medical therapy, the LV ejection fraction returns to normal, although the patients may still be at risk for recurrent PPCM. The remainder are often stabilized with medical therapy; however, a proportion of patients may experience progressive heart failure. Following delivery, treatment of PPCM is the same as for other causes of systolic dysfunction. However, if heart failure occurs during pregnancy, ACE inhibitors or angiotensin-receptor blockers are contraindicated because of the risk for fetotoxic effects. Diuretics should be used with caution, and metoprolol should be used rather than carvedilol. Eplerenone should be avoided, but spironolactone can be used cautiously later in pregnancy. Heart transplantation has been performed in patients with severe PPCM. In the United States, approximately 5% of all women undergoing cardiac transplantation have PPCM as their primary indication; it represents the fourth most common cause in women. Post-transplantation outcomes of PPCM are similar to those for other indications.

Takotsubo Cardiomyopathy (see also Chapters 37 and 38)

Takotsubo cardiomyopathy (TC) (referred to as Takotsubo syndrome [TTS] in Europe)[59,60] or stress-induced cardiomyopathy, is an acute, reversible condition first recognized in the 1990s, now with an updated uniform definition (Table 52.3). It is estimated that in 2012, about 5500 patients were admitted to U.S. hospitals with TC, with an even greater number developing the condition while they were in the hospital secondary to a comorbid condition or stress. In an International Takotsubo Registry of 1750 patients, 89.8% were women, the vast majority postmenopausal.[61] Chest pain was the predominant symptom in 76%, dyspnea in 47%, and syncope in 7.7%. A preceding physical trigger occurred in 36% and an emotional trigger in 28%, and troponin values were elevated in 87%, with ST elevation shown on the ECG in almost half of the patients. While men can be affected, women are 10-fold more likely to show TC overall, and women older than 55 years are five times more likely to experience TC compared to those less than 55 years.[59] Of those younger than 50 years, men were more commonly affected with more antecedent neurologic or psychiatric disorders compared to older individuals.[62]

A complete explanation for the pathophysiology of TC remains elusive, but activation of the sympathetic nervous system appears central, with an identifying emotional or physiologic stimulus preceding onset in most cases. Multi-vessel epicardial coronary artery spasm has been postulated as the pathophysiologic pathway due to the generalized myocardial contractile abnormalities that do not follow a specific coronary artery territory, as observed in acute coronary obstruction in atherosclerotic disease. Abnormalities of coronary microcirculation have also been postulated. Familial clustering has only rarely been observed, and genetics, if at play, may be from common variants that facilitate adrenergic signaling or its downstream amplification.

The diagnosis of TC, and in particular, differentiating it from an acute coronary syndrome in the emergency room, has been aided by an algorithm developed by an international Takotsubo task force (Table 52.4).

> The LV contractile abnormalities in TC are prominent, and although they involve the LV apex (resulting in the synonym of "apical ballooning syndrome") in more than 80% of patients (**eFig. 52.6**), regional wall motion abnormalities may be limited to the midventricular wall or other LV walls in a minority of patients. Compensatory hyperdynamic contraction of the basal LV segments with associated apical LV dyskinesis may result in acute LV outflow tract obstruction because of systolic anterior motion of the mitral valve with an associated outflow tract gradient and hypotension. Although the long-term prognosis is good, an in-hospital mortality rate of 4.1% has been reported, primarily because of irreversible cardiogenic shock, LV rupture, or embolization of LV thrombi. Malignant ventricular arrhythmia, particularly torsades de pointes associated with Takotsubo-related QT prolongation, may occur, as (rarely) may complete heart block.[63]

TABLE 52.3 International Takotsubo Diagnostic Criteria (InterTAK Diagnostic Criteria)

1. Patients show transient* left ventricular dysfunction (hypokinesia, akinesia, or dyskinesia) presenting as apical ballooning or midventricular, basal, or focal wall motion abnormalities. Right ventricular involvement can be present. Besides these regional wall motion patterns, transitions between all types can exist. The regional wall motion abnormality usually extends beyond a single epicardial vascular distribution; however, rare cases can exist where the regional wall motion abnormality is present in the subtended myocardial territory of a single coronary artery (focal TTS).**

2. An emotional, physical, or combined trigger can precede the takotsubo syndrome event, but this is not obligatory.

3. Neurologic disorders (e.g., subarachnoid hemorrhage, stroke/transient ischemic attack, or seizures) as well as pheochromocytoma may serve as triggers for takotsubo syndrome.

4. New electrocardiogram (ECG) abnormalities are present (ST-segment elevation, ST-segment depression, T wave inversion, and QTc prolongation); however, rare cases exist without any ECG changes.

5. Levels of cardiac biomarkers (troponin and creatine kinase) are moderately elevated in most cases; significant elevation of brain natriuretic peptide is common.

6. Significant coronary artery disease is not a contradiction in takotsubo syndrome.

7. Patients have no evidence of infectious myocarditis.**

8. Postmenopausal women are predominantly affected.

*Wall motion abnormalities may remain for a prolonged period of time or documentation of recovery may not be possible. For example, death before evidence of recovery is captured.
**Cardiac magnetic resonance imaging is recommended to exclude infectious myocarditis and diagnosis confirmation of takotsubo syndrome.
From Ghadri JR, Wittstein IS, Prasad A, et al. International Expert Consensus Document on Takotsubo Syndrome (Part I): Clinical Characteristics, Diagnostic Criteria, and Pathophysiology. Eur Heart J. 2018;39:2032–2046.

TABLE 52.4 An InterTAK Clinical Score to Differentiate Takotsubo Syndrome from Acute Coronary Syndrome

Female sex 25 points

Emotional stress 24 points

Physical stress 13 points

No ST-segment depression (except aVR) (12 points)

Psychiatric disorders 11 points

Neurologic disorders 9 points

QTc prolongation 6 points

≤70 points, low/intermediate probability of TTS; >70 points, high probability

From Ghadri JR, Cammann VL, Jurisic S, et al. A novel clinical score (InterTAK Diagnostic Score) to differentiate takotsubo syndrome from acute coronary syndrome: results from the International Takotsubo Registry. Eur J Heart Fail. 2017;19:1036–1042.

RESTRICTIVE AND INFILTRATIVE CARDIOMYOPATHIES

The RCMs are a heterogeneous group of diseases characterized by a nondilated left ventricle, often with a normal or near-normal LV ejection fraction. The predominant manifestation is diastolic dysfunction as a result of myocardial disease, and although severe hypertensive disease, aortic stenosis, and some cases of HCM may feature restrictive pathophysiology, these conditions are not classified as RCMs. Some infiltrative cardiac diseases such as amyloidosis (see Chapter 53) produce an RCM, whereas others, such as sarcoidosis, have an infiltrative component but appear as RCM or DCM. Thus, just as DCM is a morphologic condition that encompasses several causes of cardiomyopathy, the terms restrictive cardiomyopathy and infiltrative cardiomyopathy are pathophysiologic and anatomic definitions of cardiomyopathies that have overlaps with several well-defined conditions.

Approach to Identifying a Cause of Restrictive Cardiomyopathy

Because RCM is not always an isolated cardiac disease but may arise secondary to other acquired or genetic diseases, the diagnostic approach is challenging for the cardiovascular specialist (see Table 52.1). Endomyocardial biopsy may be more relevant for the diagnosis of a specific cause in patients with RCM than in those with DCM or HCM insofar as RCM may be caused by an infiltrative cardiac process without systemic involvement or with subclinical involvement of other organs.[64] However, CMR imaging with T1, T2, and extracellular volume mapping has increased the diagnostic yield and thus reduced the need for endomyocardial biopsy. When a cause cannot be identified, the condition is known as idiopathic RCM. Unlike with DCM, familial RCM is distinctly uncommon. Regardless of whether a cause can be found, a comprehensive family history should always be obtained as should clinical screening of first-degree relatives. As noted above, genetic testing is now indicated for any case of RCM where the etiology is uncertain or unknown, even when the family history is negative (see Fig. 52.8).

Clinical and Molecular Genetics of Restrictive Cardiomyopathy

The clinical genetic features of familial RCM are similar to those of DCM in that reduced penetrance and a variable age at onset are commonly observed. Genes with rare variants implicated in the cause of idiopathic and nonsyndromic RCM are in most cases ones that encode sarcomeric proteins (see eTable 52.1).[65,66] Although some locus heterogeneity is apparent, it is much less so than with DCM (see eTable 52.1). Because cardiac hemodynamic findings commonly exhibit restrictive physiology in HCM, the genetic similarity of HCM and RCM suggests that in these cases the RCM phenotype at times may be viewed as a "minimally hypertrophic" HCM phenotype with prominent restrictive physiology. As noted earlier, at times "overlap" or "crossover"

Therapy

TC is a self-limited disorder, usually with rapid resolution of symptoms and LV dysfunction. Classification has been recommended into lower-risk and higher-risk categories, with the latter based on an LV ejection fraction of less than 45%, hypotension and an outflow tract gradient of greater than 40 mm Hg, and/or the presence of an arrhythmia. Use of an ACE inhibitor or a beta blocker, or both, is recommended in the higher-risk groups. Because of the occasional association with acute QT prolongation, care should be taken to avoid using QT-prolonging medications, such as macrolide antibiotics or certain antiarrhythmic agents. In patients with hypotension associated with TC, pressors should be used with caution because LV outflow tract obstruction may be precipitated. Occasionally, thrombus formation may occur in the dyskinetic segment, and anticoagulation is routinely used for this indication. In most cases resolution is complete or nearly complete within days to weeks, although the major adverse events, including cardiogenic shock or death, mandate observation of the acute phase of TC in an intensive care unit (ICU) setting. Major adverse events occur in approximately 5% of individuals, with younger males most at risk. The recurrence risk has been estimated at 5%, usually within the first year. Overall mortality of TC has been estimated to follow that of coronary disease, even though most patients have no demonstrable atherosclerotic plaque. The use of ACE inhibitors long term have been shown to reduce recurrence. In contrast, prophylactic use of beta blockers has not been shown to reduce recurrence, even though attempting to minimize a catecholamine-induced trigger provides a rationale for their use. Likewise, for depression or other psychiatric disorders, treatment has been postulated to possibly reduce recurrence, but evidence is lacking largely due to the difficulty of conducting controlled trials when the recurrence rate is low. Even though a visualized thrombus mandates anticoagulation, long-term anticoagulation has not been recommended.

HEART FAILURE

VI

phenotypes of RCM and HCM have been observed in families with rare variants in sarcomeric genes that demonstrate this principle.[65,66]

Clinical Features of Idiopathic Restrictive Cardiomyopathy

Idiopathic RCM has been described in individuals from infancy to late adulthood; it usually carries a poor prognosis, especially in children.[67] The disease is rare, and the largest adult series contains only 91 cases seen over a 17-year period.[68] In one series of 32 unrelated patients with end-stage disease, RCM was considered to be genetically determined either by the identification of pathogenic rare variants (60%) or by evidence of familial disease without a known pathogenic rare variant (in an additional 5 patients), for a total of 75%.[69] Symptoms of idiopathic RCM are nonspecific and reflect the presence of heart failure. Dyspnea is an initial complaint in most patients; edema occurs in approximately half; and palpitations, fatigue, and orthopnea are reported by 22% to 33%. Physical examination is usually consistent with biventricular heart failure, with jugular venous distention noted in most patients but ascites and significant edema being found in advanced cases. Atrial fibrillation is common, and a third heart sound is heard in one in four patients; murmurs are not a feature. Assuming that amyloidosis has been excluded, the ECG has normal voltage, with only a minority of patients showing intraventricular conduction delay.

Echocardiography reveals a typical pattern of biatrial enlargement and nondilated ventricles with a normal or near normal LV ejection fraction and LV wall thickness (Fig. 52.10). At *cardiac catheterization* RV and LV filling pressures are elevated with a dip-and-plateau tracing often seen; unlike in constrictive pericarditis, however, equalization of diastolic pressures is uncommon. Careful evaluation of simultaneously recorded LV and RV pressures during respiration demonstrates concordant changes in systolic pressures in RCM, rather than a discordance (inspiratory increase in RV systolic pressure with a simultaneous decrease in LV pressure) seen in constrictive pericarditis (**eFig. 52.7**).[70] Endomyocardial biopsy demonstrates nonspecific findings such as myocyte hypertrophy, interstitial fibrosis, and, not uncommonly, endocardial fibrosis. The survival rate is reduced in comparison with that of an age- and sex-matched population; the observed survival rate from the time of diagnosis is 64% at 5 years and 37% at 10 years.[71] Most deaths are associated with cardiac causes, either suddenly or secondary to heart failure, although a third die of noncardiac causes related to progressive age.

The differential diagnosis of idiopathic RCM includes the infiltrative cardiomyopathies, such as amyloidosis, or constrictive pericarditis.[72] Unlike idiopathic RCM, amyloidosis is associated with increased LV wall thickness and subtle abnormalities in LV systolic function, with specific findings on cardiac biopsy; it can also be heritable with variants in *TTR* (see also Chapter 53). Constrictive pericarditis is more difficult to differentiate from RCM because most of the clinical features overlap between the two disorders. A thickened pericardium noted on echocardiography, CT, or CMR in a patient with heart failure and a preserved ejection fraction without wall thickening suggests constrictive pericarditis; however, it bears emphasis that 18% of patients with constrictive pericarditis have normal pericardial thickness.[70] Advanced echocardiographic or CMR-imaging techniques may be of help in distinguishing constrictive pericarditis from RCM (see also Chapters 16 and 19), but endomyocardial biopsy may be required unless an alternative diagnosis is clear. Treatment of idiopathic RCM is generally limited to medical treatment emphasizing judicious use of diuretics, but in selected advanced cases, cardiac transplantation has been performed with similar outcomes as in those with nonrestrictive cardiomyopathy.[68]

Sarcoid Cardiomyopathy

Sarcoidosis is a multisystem disorder of unknown cause characterized histologically by noncaseating granulomas. In the United States the disease is most commonly seen in the black population and is more common in women than in men. Sarcoid has a higher incidence in Scandinavia and Japan. Cardiac involvement takes the form of ventricular dysfunction, heart block, and/or ventricular arrhythmias. Despite

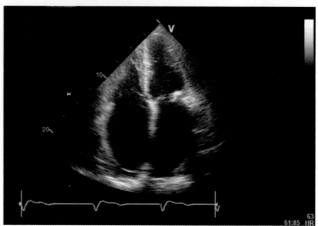

FIGURE 52.10 Echocardiogram showing restrictive cardiomyopathy. An apical four-chamber view is shown in an 80-year-old man with long-standing restrictive cardiomyopathy (RCM). The left ventricular (LV) ejection fraction was normal, with evidence of severe diastolic dysfunction on echocardiography and cardiac catheterization. Note the massive biatrial enlargement and normal LV wall thickness.

frequently being described as an RCM, sarcoid heart disease can also present as a DCM, occasionally with aneurysm formation. Although most patients with sarcoid cardiomyopathy also have evidence of noncardiac disease, particularly lung disease, clinically isolated cardiac sarcoidosis is increasingly being recognized as a cause of heart block and ventricular arrhythmias. Sudden death, presumably from heart block or a ventricular arrhythmia, may be the first manifestation either of sarcoidosis itself or of heart disease in a patient with known pulmonary or systemic sarcoid. The prevalence of cardiac involvement in patients with pulmonary sarcoidosis was previously thought to be no more than 5%, but autopsy studies indicate a much higher prevalence, and recent cardiac imaging studies have demonstrated abnormalities in at least 25% of patients with pulmonary sarcoidosis.[73]

Pathology

The pathology of sarcoid heart disease raises puzzling questions about the cause of the systolic dysfunction, which can be severe. Noncaseating granulomas, the hallmark of the disease, are patchily distributed even in severe disease and thus may not alone account for the severe systolic dysfunction. Granulomatous lesions are associated with edema and inflammation, and widespread myocardial fibrosis is seen late in the disease (Fig. 52.11). The patchy nature of granulomatous infiltration and the sometimes extensive fibrosis render cardiac biopsy a low-yield procedure for detecting diagnostic histology in cardiac sarcoidosis, and finding granulomas may be difficult even at autopsy, because end-stage disease is characterized predominantly by fibrosis.[74] Occasionally, the right ventricle may be severely and predominantly involved. Recently several cases of meeting criteria for ARVC with a typical appearance on multimodality imaging have been described that are later found to show noncaseating granulomas and other signs consistent with sarcoidosis.[75,76] RV function can be impaired in patients with severe pulmonary sarcoidosis and pulmonary hypertension, even in the absence of direct sarcoid involvement of the heart.

Clinical Features

The most common noncardiac site of sarcoid involvement is the lungs, with approximately half of patients having overt parenchymal disease and the remainder having isolated bilateral hilar lymphadenopathy. Other findings, in decreasing order of frequency, are hepatic and gastrointestinal involvement, ocular sarcoidosis, and neurologic sarcoidosis. Skin involvement in sarcoidosis is not uncommon, and lesions appear to have a predilection for scars and tattoos. In patients with established extracardiac sarcoid, LV systolic dysfunction is most commonly due to associated cardiac sarcoidosis.

The most common clinical feature of cardiac sarcoidosis is biventricular heart failure. Mitral regurgitation, often caused by papillary muscle involvement in addition to LV dilation, may be severe.

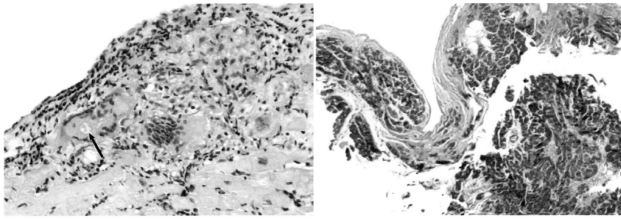

FIGURE 52.11 Myocardial biopsy for sarcoid cardiomyopathy. The **left panel** shows an initial biopsy specimen (hematoxylin-eosin staining) with an inflammatory noncaseating granuloma typical of sarcoid. The *arrow* points to an "asteroid body" in the cytoplasm of the giant cell; this is a common finding in various granulomatous diseases. The **right panel** shows a follow-up biopsy specimen (Masson trichrome stain, initial magnification 100×) in the same patient. No granulomas are present, and there is now extensive interstitial fibrosis (*green-staining area*). This demonstrates how granulomas may be missed on biopsy, particularly in advanced sarcoid cardiomyopathy, when fibrosis is extensive. (From Leone O, Veinot JP, Angelini A, et al. 2011 consensus statement on endomyocardial biopsy from the Association for European Cardiovascular Pathology and the Society for Cardiovascular Pathology. *Cardiovasc Pathol.* 2012;21:245.)

Sarcoid granulomas have a predilection for the cardiac conduction system, and high-degree atrioventricular (AV) block may occur, either as an initial manifestation of cardiac sarcoidosis or later in the disease (Fig. 52.12). Both atrial and ventricular arrhythmias are common, the latter arising from either ventricle. Once causes such as Lyme disease have been ruled out, complete heart block in a young patient suggests sarcoidosis, especially if ventricular arrhythmias are present, and imaging should be pursued in all such cases. Sudden cardiac death is almost always associated with grossly visible scarring and fibrosis at autopsy. A rare manifestation of cardiac sarcoidosis is acute sarcoid myocarditis, characterized by high-degree AV block, malignant ventricular arrhythmia, and heart failure. It may be difficult to distinguish this from giant cell myocarditis unless systemic features of sarcoid are also present.

Diagnosis

Laboratory testing for sarcoidosis is generally unrewarding. An elevated sedimentation rate may be present but is nonspecific, as is a finding of elevated immunoglobulins. Hypercalcemia (believed to be due to activation of vitamin D by macrophages in sarcoid granulomas), although uncommon, is a useful clue. Although elevation of serum ACE may be helpful for diagnosis, there is a wide range in the normal population because of a polymorphism in the *ACE* gene. Normal ACE levels may be seen in patients with untreated sarcoidosis, and serial ACE levels do not appear to correlate with treatment response.

CMR with gadolinium enhancement (see also Chapter 19) is a sensitive test for detecting cardiac abnormalities (Fig. 52.13). Delayed gadolinium enhancement may be found in either a coronary or noncoronary distribution, is usually nontransmural, and has a predilection for the basal and/or midventricular septum.[73] The finding of myocardial late gadolinium enhancement by CMR in a patient with proven extracardiac sarcoidosis is a marker for subsequent major cardiac events, including sudden death, and the risk of major events is proportional to the amount of late gadolinium enhancement.[77] In the acute stage, T2-weighted imaging may show myocardial edema, which is characterized by focal areas of thickening and increased signal intensity on T2-weighted and early gadolinium-enhanced images.[78]

[18]F-fluorodeoxyglucose (FDG) positron emission tomography (PET) scanning (see also Chapter 18, Figs. 18.2, 18.36, 18.37, and 18.39) is complementary to CMR in patients with sarcoidosis; it reveals areas of inflammation in active disease, permits serial evaluation of response to therapy, and is becoming an important tool for the diagnosis and management of cardiac disease.[79] An example of a combined PET-CT scan in a patient with cardiac amyloidosis is shown in Figure 52.14.

TISSUE BIOPSY

A positive cardiac biopsy showing noncaseating granulomas is diagnostic of cardiac sarcoidosis if giant cell myocarditis is ruled out. However, the patchy nature of the granulomatous infiltration results in a low yield of positive biopsies. Targeted biopsy of another organ, such as enlarged hilar lymph nodes, may give a higher yield, or alternatively, biopsy of an area of definite abnormality seen on PET or CMR may be valuable. Although the 2006 recommendations of the Japanese Society of Sarcoidosis and of the Granulomatous Disorders suggest diagnosis by a combination of major and minor criteria, including myocardial biopsy, PET-CT and CMR are more sensitive and are playing an increasing role. An algorithm for the diagnosis of cardiac sarcoidosis is presented in **eFigure 52.8**.

Treatment

No randomized clinical trials of the treatment of cardiac sarcoidosis have been completed, although the design of a Canadian study where patients will be randomized to prednisone or prednisone plus methotrexate has been published.[80] Standard heart failure therapy should be instituted if heart failure is present, but in addition, steroid therapy is often given, particularly in patients with newly diagnosed sarcoidosis and systolic dysfunction. Steroids are frequently effective in noncardiac sarcoidosis, and nonrandomized data suggest a benefit in patients with cardiac sarcoid complicated by heart failure, particularly early in the disease when irreversible fibrosis has not yet developed. Prednisone is generally initiated in doses between 1 mg/kg and 40 mg daily and tapered gradually over a period of several months with careful monitoring.[81] Methotrexate is often used as a second agent if steroid therapy is unsuccessful,[82] and several recent case reports have shown promising responses to anti-tumor necrosis factor (anti-TNF) monoclonal antibodies.

Management of arrhythmia often requires a pacemaker and/or ICD. On the assumption that high-degree AV block in systemic sarcoidosis is a marker of associated myocardial sarcoidosis, use of a pacemaker-ICD has been recommended for any patient with sarcoidosis who requires pacing. Prophylactic use of an ICD based on a reduced ejection fraction, similar to other patients with heart failure with a depressed ejection fraction, is also appropriate (see also Chapter 58), but the role of an ICD in a patient with sarcoidosis and mild cardiac disease but no high-degree AV block or frequent ventricular arrhythmia is less clear.[83] The 2014 Heart Rhythm Society Consensus Recommendations for ICD implantation in patients with cardiac sarcoidosis are a useful guide, and suggest incorporation of advanced imaging and possible electrophysiologic study in such patients (**eTable 52.4**).[84] A recent meta-analysis of 585 patients from 10 studies showed substantial benefit of ICD placement, with 39% receiving appropriate therapy over a mean follow-up period of 25 months.[85] Cardiac transplantation may be undertaken in patients with severe cardiac sarcoidosis after careful evaluation for noncardiac involvement. Less than 0.2% of transplants in the United States are performed for cardiac sarcoidosis; outcomes are at least equivalent to those of other cardiac transplant patients.[85]

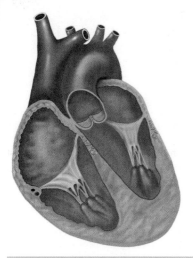

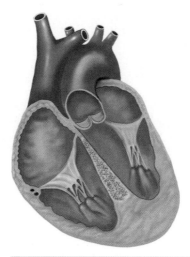

Small patches of basal involvement, usually clinically silent

Large area of septal involvement, often clinically manifest as heart block

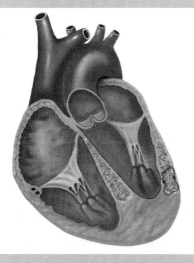

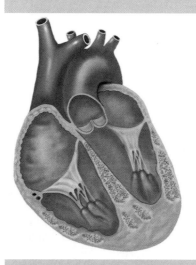

Re-entrant circuit involving area of granuloma/fibrosis leading to VT

Extensive areas of LV and RV involvement, often clinically manifest as heart failure +/− heart block +/− VT

FIGURE 52.12 Illustrative examples of the extent of cardiac sarcoid pathologic changes in relation to clinical manifestations of the disease. (From Birnie DH, Nery PB, Ha AC, Beanlands RSB. Cardiac sarcoidosis. *J Am Coll Cardiol.* 2016;68:411–421.)

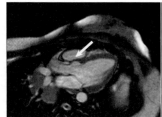

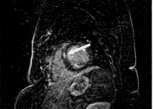

FIGURE 52.13 Cardiac MRI in a patient with sarcoidosis. Heart failure developed late in pregnancy and was initially diagnosed as peripartum cardiomyopathy (PPCM). Echocardiography revealed a reduced ejection fraction with the basal septal thinning typical of sarcoidosis. The appearance was confirmed on MRI (**left panel**, *arrow*). Delayed gadolinium uptake showed midmyocardial gadolinium uptake (**right panel**, *arrow*) consistent with sarcoidosis, which was subsequently confirmed on a biopsy specimen.

Fabry Disease

Fabry disease is caused by progressive lysosomal accumulation of neutral glycosphingolipids, primarily globotriaosylceramide; it results from deficiency of the enzyme alpha-galactosidase A, which is encoded by *GLA* on the X chromosome.[86] As an X-linked condition, most disease occurs in males with transmission by female carriers, although significant disease in later years can also be seen in women.[86–88] The disease phenotype encompasses diverse signs and symptoms with the following major manifestations: angiokeratomas, acroparesthesias, anhidrosis, ocular changes, and eventually cardiovascular, cerebrovascular, and renal disease, all largely related to the central pathophysiology of small-vessel vascular disease from the deposition of glycosphingolipid and consequent vascular insufficiency. The hallmark of the classic early-onset disease in males in childhood is episodic crises of severe pain in the extremities (acroparesthesias), characterized by burning pain in the distal end of the extremities, triggered by a variety of stressors, and resulting in ischemia of peripheral nerves from small-vessel disease. Angiokeratomas, red and purple punctate dermal lesions involving the lower midsection, buttocks, thighs, and upper part of the legs, may be one of the earliest signs of the disease and accumulate progressively with age. Anhidrosis is also an early finding in most cases. A survey of the phenotypic characteristics derived from a Fabry registry[87] showed that the age at onset and phenotypic variability were related to the degree of alpha-galactosidase A deficiency, with less than 1% of the activity associated with the earliest and most aggressive disease (**eTable 52.5**).[86–88]

Most morbid and mortal manifestations of Fabry disease are related to cardiovascular, cerebrovascular, and renal disease and occur in men in midlife who have had the classic phenotype and onset in early life, although the age at onset of advanced disease is variable and in some cases it may occur in the second and third decades. Cerebrovascular issues related to small-vessel disease include transient ischemic attacks and thrombosis resulting in stroke in up to a quarter of patients in a variety of locations, most commonly the posterior circulation. Cardiovascular involvement is not usually clinically apparent until the third or fourth decade, but eventually some manifestation of cardiovascular disease occurs in most patients. The most common finding is LV hypertrophy on echocardiography, although the degree of hypertrophy is mild in many cases in the third decade but is progressive with age. Worsening LV hypertrophy is associated with angina that occurs consequent to small-vessel disease, and epicardial coronary disease is uncommon. Findings on the ECG initially include a short PR interval and LV hypertrophy, with later evidence of heart block. Nonspecific intraventricular conduction delays are also seen. Bradycardia is common and a few patients will require pacemakers. Nonspecific ST-T changes are also common. Echocardiographic features range from mild to severe LV hypertrophy, the latter being more common in older patients, and mild to significant diastolic dysfunction. In most cases systolic function is normal, although heart failure has been reported with advanced disease. Palpitations and arrhythmia also occur.

Atypical phenotypes of Fabry disease have been categorized as cardiac or renal variants. Although most classic Fabry disease

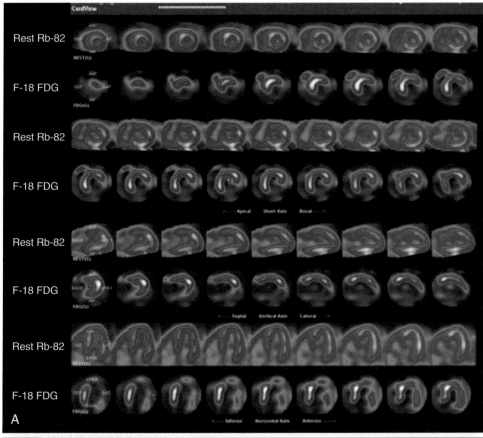

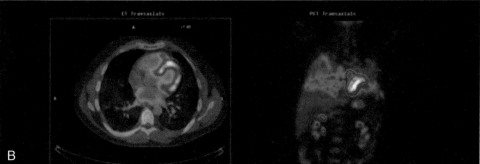

FIGURE 52.14 Positron emission tomography (PET) scan in a patient with sarcoidosis. A combined resting PET scan using rubidium-82 and ¹⁸F-FDG (a glucose analogue) is shown for a 53-year-old man with a history of pulmonary sarcoidosis who had palpitations and atrial flutter. **A,** From the top, each pair of images represents the rubidium-82 scan and, underneath it, the corresponding ¹⁸F-FDG image. The scans show a basal and midanteroseptal perfusion defect with intense FDG uptake in these regions suggestive of myocardial inflammation. Normal myocardium does not exhibit any FDG uptake because it is using free fatty acids. **B,** Combined CT-PET images in the same patient demonstrating the intense cardiac uptake. (Courtesy of Dr. Sharmila Dorbala, Brigham and Women's Hospital, Boston. From Dubrey SW, Falk RH. Diagnosis and management of cardiac sarcoidosis. *Prog Cardiovasc Dis.* 2010;52:336.)

individuals (0.5%) were identified, four of the seven being women 45 to 72 years of age, all with significant LV hypertrophy (ranging from 15 to 22 mm). Only three had other signs of Fabry disease, most commonly angiokeratomas. Exclusion of rare variants in other genes encoding sarcomeric proteins known to cause HCM was not reported in this study, but comprehensive molecular (panel) testing for HCM would now identify sarcomeric variants, as well as *GLA* variants. Fabry disease has also been found in unexplained cardiomyopathy cases with gadolinium uptake where all other usual genetic causes have been excluded.[90]

The diagnosis of Fabry disease rests on showing reduced alpha-galactosidase A activity and molecular genetic testing for rare variants in *GLA*. An endomyocardial biopsy alpha-galactosidase A specimen showing inclusions in vascular endothelial cytoplasm on light or electron microscopy can also lead to the diagnosis (**eFig. 52.9**). Because the cardiovascular findings in adults with Fabry disease usually include LV hypertrophy, in many cases a diagnosis of HCM is considered. Genetic testing with gene panels now includes *GLA* to ensure that atypical cases of Fabry disease will not be missed.

Importantly, treatment of Fabry disease is available as intravenous enzyme replacement therapy (ERT), which can arrest the deposition of globotriaosylceramide and in some cases reverse the disease phenotype, ameliorate symptoms, and restore organ function. For this reason, the diagnosis of Fabry disease is important, even though rarely encountered by most physicians.

Another commercially approved treatment for Fabry disease in an oral chaperone therapy called migalastat is a pharmacologic chaperone that reversibly binds to the active site of the alpha-galactosidase and stabilizes the protein, which allows it to be trafficked from the endoplasmic reticulum into

is syndromic, as noted earlier, and in the vast majority of cases a diagnosis of Fabry disease will be established before referral for cardiovascular or renal consultation, occasionally patients will be referred to cardiovascular or renal specialists for organ-specific disease before the diagnosis of Fabry disease is made. The atypical cardiac variant phenotype has few or none of the classic signs and symptoms but rather may be manifested as unexplained LV hypertrophy in the sixth to eighth decades, at times accompanied by cardiomyopathy, mitral insufficiency, and mild proteinuria but minimal or no renal dysfunction. Because of its protean manifestations, the frequency of Fabry disease in patients who have unexplained LV hypertrophy consistent with a diagnosis of HCM has been investigated. In a study of 1386 patients at 13 European centers that included men and women older than 35 and 40 years, respectively, all with diagnoses of HCM, systematic screening for Fabry disease was performed by searching for *GLA* rare variants, and when identified, it was confirmed by alpha-galactosidase A levels.[89] Seven

the lysosome where it exerts its action. Migalastat is only approved for use in Fabry disease patients who have GLA variants that result in abnormally folded, less stable forms of the alpha-galactosidase A, so-called amenable variants. Newer approaches, including periodic administration of mRNA encoding human α-Gal A, are now in preclinical studies,[91] which if successful could expand therapeutic options.

Gaucher Disease and Glycogen Storage Diseases

Gaucher disease is an autosomal recessive glycogen storage disease that results from deficient beta-glucocerebrosidase enzyme activity caused by homozygous or compound heterozygous rare variants in *GBA*.[92] The clinical spectrum of disease varies greatly and ranges from a lethal acute perinatal form and a subacute juvenile form, both of which share major central nervous system disease, to a mostly asymptomatic adult form; all forms share splenomegaly, hepatomegaly, cytopenia, and pulmonary disease because of deposition of glucosylceramide in reticuloendothelial cells, including peripheral blood leukocytes. Cardiac involvement is uncommon to rare but has been reported in patients with allelic variants, with mitral and aortic valve calcification leading to valvular insufficiency and stenosis in the setting of corneal opacification and splenomegaly. Recurrent pericarditis resulting in constriction, as well as DCM with systolic dysfunction, has also been reported. ERT is now available, and in most cases will stabilize or reverse the disease process, thus accentuating the relevance of identifying Gaucher disease.

Hemochromatosis

Hemochromatosis is a disease caused by iron overload in which iron infiltrates major organs, especially the liver, heart, thyroid, gonads, skin, and pancreatic islet cells, to give the characteristic clinical findings of advanced disease that include cirrhosis, cardiomyopathy, diabetes, and endocrine disease. Hemochromatosis is categorized as hereditary (or primary) when arising from genetic disease or as secondary when caused by increased absorption associated with the thalassemias, sickle cell disease, or the sideroblastic anemias, or when related to excess blood transfusions for myelodysplasia or aplastic anemia. The content and distribution of iron are tightly regulated because of its toxicity and the inability of the body to excrete iron. Recent progress has been made in further understanding the molecular mechanisms of iron adsorption, use, storage, and recycling.[93]

HFE (hemochromatosis gene)-associated hereditary hemochromatosis is an autosomal recessive disease that in almost all cases results from the homozygous rare variant Cys282Tyr, although 3% to 8% of cases are compound heterozygotes for Cys282Tyr and His63Asp. The carrier frequency of the Cys282Tyr variant ranges as high as 11% in individuals of European descent, although the disease is twice as likely to develop in women and penetrance varies even with Cys282Tyr homozygotes.[94] A recent study with homozygous His63Asp showed only hypertension with minimal cardiac hypertrophy but without other adverse events.[95] The onset of clinical disease from iron overload is insidious, and signs and symptoms are insensitive and nonspecific. Screening tests include serum ferritin and percent transferrin saturation, with the accepted level being 200 ng/mL in women and 300 ng/mL in men or 45% in women and 50% in men. If both tests are negative, iron overload is effectively excluded. With elevated transferrin saturation, molecular genetic testing for *HFE* is indicated. With elevated transferrin saturation and ferritin levels higher than 1000, iron removal, usually by phlebotomy, is indicated, and evaluation of liver and cardiac function is indicated.

The cardiovascular findings of hemochromatosis, regardless of cause, are similar and may bring the patient to medical attention before diagnosis because of other organ system involvement in a minority of cases, so clinicians always need to consider hemochromatosis in the differential diagnosis of a nondilated cardiomyopathy with mild to moderate systolic dysfunction. Cardiovascular dysfunction begins with a restrictive nondilated phenotype that with advancing disease progresses to systolic dysfunction, mild to moderate LV dilation consistent with DCM, and then advanced disease and eventual heart failure.[96] In most cases, arrhythmias and conduction system disease accompany the progressive myocardial dysfunction and include AV and bundle branch blocks and bradyarrhythmias and tachyarrhythmias, some of which may result in syncope and sudden cardiac death. CMR has evolved to become a sensitive noninvasive diagnostic modality. A definitive tissue-based diagnosis of iron overload causing cardiac dysfunction can also be made by endomyocardial biopsy, which may be particularly useful if other testing is inconclusive or the degree of cardiovascular involvement by hemochromatosis is confounded by other cardiovascular disease (e.g., coronary disease). Definitive treatment is centered on iron removal, usually by phlebotomy in *HFE*-associated hereditary hemochromatosis, and as iron stores are depleted, cardiac function will improve in most cases, sometimes to a dramatic degree. Cardiac transplantation can be avoided in most patients with timely diagnosis and phlebotomy.

Endomyocardial Disease

The endomyocardial diseases, another cause of RCM, are unified by the finding of endocardial fibrosis. Several conditions share the pathologic end phenotype of fibrosis of the endocardium, but no unifying hypothesis for this pathology has emerged, and each condition may have its own distinctive cause. *Endomyocardial fibrosis* (EMF), a disease first described in Uganda in 1948 (initially termed tropical endocardial disease or endocardial fibroelastosis [EFE]), may well be the most common cause of RCM worldwide.[97] Although only rarely observed in North America, related conditions that pathologically resemble EMF include Löffler endocarditis, usually observed in adults, or the distinctly different onset of *neonatal endocardial fibroelastosis* associated with hypoplastic left-heart syndrome and other congenital heart disease or in utero mumps infection. EFE, recently recapitulated in a model system,[98] can be differentiated from EMF by its epidemiology and more diffuse involvement of the left ventricle, whereas endocardial fibrosis more involves the RV and LV apices and subvalvular apparatus. Neonatal EFE has been observed in a few families, and a genetic cause has been considered (see Online Mendelian Inheritance in Man [OMIM] 226000), and the X-linked *Barth syndrome* (see OMIM 302060) is categorized as a DCM with associated EFE, a proximal skeletal myopathy, and growth retardation.

Carcinoid Heart Disease

Carcinoid heart disease is a rare condition that occurs as part of carcinoid syndrome, a systemic disorder mediated by elevated circulating levels of vasoactive substances, including serotonin (5-hydroxytryptamine [5-HT]), 5-hydroxytryptophan, histamine, bradykinin, tachykinins, and prostaglandins produced by a rare metastatic neuroendocrine malignancy, carcinoid.[99] *Carcinoid syndrome* is characterized by a triad of symptoms—flushing, diarrhea, and bronchospasm—that occur in association with hepatic metastases. The metastases produce high levels of these vasoactive substances, particularly 5-HT, which reaches the systemic circulation via the hepatic vein. High levels in the right side of the heart cause progressive fibrotic endocardial plaque (eFig. 52.10).[100] Inactivation in the lung to hydroxyindoleacetic acid (5-HIAA) generally protects the left-sided heart structures, but these structures may become involved if levels are very high or if a patent foramen ovale allows right-to-left shunting.[101] Carcinoid heart disease has also very rarely been described in association with nonmetastatic ovarian cancer.

The characteristic pathologic features of carcinoid heart disease are right-sided valve thickening and retraction resulting from myofibroblast proliferation along with deposition of collagen and smooth muscle cells. Tricuspid annular and subvalvar involvement and pulmonary root constriction also occur, thereby adding to the valvular dysfunction. Very rarely the heart is involved directly by carcinoid metastases.[99] Physical examination reveals evidence of RV volume and pressure overload with murmurs of tricuspid and pulmonary regurgitation and stenosis. In the late stage of the disease, peripheral edema and ascites with low cardiac output occur, although the valvular disease may be hemodynamically severe before significant clinical deterioration takes place. Symptoms of right-sided heart failure in the setting of known carcinoid syndrome are highly suggestive of carcinoid heart disease, but cardiac involvement may occasionally be the initial feature of carcinoid syndrome. Chest radiography and electrocardiography are generally unrevealing in carcinoid heart disease. Elevation of urinary 5-HIAA levels is highly specific and moderately sensitive for the diagnosis of carcinoid syndrome, and the echocardiographic and CMR features of thickened immobile tricuspid and pulmonary valves with combined stenosis and regurgitant lesions are highly suggestive of carcinoid heart disease (eFig. 52.11).[102]

Untreated patients with carcinoid syndrome have a median survival time of 3 to 4 years, and the presence of carcinoid heart disease shortens this to less than 1 year.[99] Therapy is not generally curative and includes debulking the hepatic metastases by embolization or partial hepatic resection and by the use of octreotide, a somatostatin analogue that binds to somatostatin receptors on the surface of carcinoid tumor cells and inhibits the secretion of vasoactive substances. Newer treatment includes radiation therapy delivered by peptide receptor-linked radiotherapy.[103] Although the development and progression of carcinoid heart disease are associated with increasing 5-HIAA levels,[104,105] a decrease in 5-HIAA levels afterward does not appear to cause a change in the cardiac valvular lesions, and they may even progress. Valve replacement in carcinoid heart disease can be performed successfully[101] but carries unique challenges, such as the development of an *acute carcinoid crisis* characterized by profound hypotension, severe flushing bronchoconstriction, and arrhythmias. Thus a surgical and anesthetic team knowledgeable about the condition and working with an endocrinologist, both intraoperatively and perioperatively, is of critical importance. Once advanced carcinoid valve disease is recognized on echocardiography, surgery is recommended even in the absence of significant right-sided heart dysfunction; patients who have undergone surgery are believed to be likely to have a more favorable outcome.[99]

Löffler (Eosinophilic) Endocarditis

Löffler endocarditis occurs within the spectrum of the hypereosinophilic conditions in which increased numbers of eosinophils invade and damage tissues in a variety of organs, including the endocardium and myocardium, by releasing highly active biologic substances. The cause of the eosinophilia in Löffler endocarditis includes known and idiopathic causes, such as a broad spectrum of helminthic or other parasitic infections, malignancy including carcinoma or eosinophilic leukemia, and allergy including drug reactions, all of which may have associated hypereosinophilia, as well as idiopathic hypereosinophilia syndrome. Hypereosinophilia has been defined as either a chronic absolute eosinophil count higher than 1500 cells/mL for at least 1 month, although hypereosinophilia persisting for 6 months or longer is common, or pathologic evidence of hypereosinophilic tissue invasion. One family has been reported with autosomal dominant transmission linked to 5q31-q33, and more recently, hypereosinophilia syndrome in the setting of myeloproliferative disease has responded to tyrosine kinase inhibitors, but a unifying genetic or environmental hypothesis is not yet available.

Hypereosinophilic syndromes affecting the heart, although rare, when present cause considerable morbidity and mortality. Some cases of myocardial hypereosinophilic disease may be identified at endomyocardial biopsy during evaluation for idiopathic RCM, and in such situations a thorough evaluation for an underlying cause should be completed. Regardless of cause, eosinophilic-mediated cardiac disease has been categorized into three stages: acute, intermediate, and fibrotic. In the acute phase, usually characterized by few or no signs or symptoms, eosinophils invade the myocardium, degranulate, and aided by lymphocytes, cause intense myocardial inflammation and eventually myocardial necrosis. Even though findings on echocardiography may be normal during this phase, contrast-enhanced CMR can detect disease,[106,107] and myocardial biomarkers may be elevated to variable degrees. In the second stage, thrombus favoring the apices covers the affected endocardium. Symptoms include chest pain or dyspnea. Other evidence of disease includes mitral or tricuspid valvular regurgitation, cardiomegaly, and heart failure. Embolism of endocardial thrombus to the brain or other organs is common and may be the initial feature of the disease. The ECG may show T wave inversions, and imaging studies will reveal mural thrombus in affected areas, at times so extensive that large portions of the myocardial chamber are obliterated with clot. The third fibrotic phase progresses with diffuse scarring that results in endocardial fibrosis and RCM. The scar process commonly involves the mitral and tricuspid subvalvular structures; it impairs their mobility and leads to valvular regurgitation. Valve leaflet scarring can also occur. If disease can be identified in the first stage, therapy is focused on treatment of the underlying condition. Corticosteroids and cytolytic therapies have been used with some response. The fibrotic stage needs to be addressed surgically by valve release, repair, or replacement and by resection of the endocardial scar to mitigate the restrictive nature of the endocardial fibrosis.

Endomyocardial Fibrosis

EMF, an unusual disease in North America but common in Africa, is characterized by fibrosis of the LV and RV apical endocardium causing an RCM.[97] First reported in Uganda, it has been found in tropical regions of Africa, the south Asian subcontinent, and Brazil, although it is also found in subtropical Africa and some cases occur rarely in moderate climates, including North America. A population prevalence of approximately 20% in rural Mozambique has been reported,[108] with more males affected than females (23% vs. 17%). In addition, family clustering was identified in this study, although whether this was related to environmental exposure common to the family units selected for study, to a genetic predisposition, or to both was not addressed. A bimodal peak in age has been noted in several studies, with onset in the first decade and a second peak occurring in the second to fourth decades of life.

The cause of EMF remains unknown, but its pathology resembles that of other conditions in North America that are more commonly encountered, such as eosinophilic cardiomyopathy or hypereosinophilic syndrome, discussed earlier. However, elevated eosinophil counts in peripheral blood or cardiac tissue from endomyocardial biopsy have seldom been observed in EMF. Although one or more infectious agents could be causal, no consistent unifying infectious cause has been established. Environmental exposure to cerium, a rare element present in affected areas, has also been considered. Family-based disease has been observed in several reports, but whether familial predisposition is related to environmental or genetic causes, or to both, remains unknown.

In most cases heart failure symptoms from left or right restrictive physiology predominate the clinical findings and include dyspnea on exertion, paroxysmal nocturnal dyspnea, and edema. Ascites, at times a prominent feature, is common to all the endomyocardial diseases. Cardiovascular imaging shows restrictive filling with apical fibrosis that commonly involves the mitral and tricuspid subvalvular apparatus, accompanied by atrial enlargement. As noted earlier, successful surgical resection of the endocardial fibrosis with valve repair or replacement can have a dramatic effect on symptoms and survival, although the operation itself is associated with a significant risk for morbidity and mortality.

FUTURE PERSPECTIVES

Enormous progress has recently been made in understanding the genetic basis of cardiomyopathy, accelerated in large part by large panel and genome-wide next-generation sequencing strategies. The genomic information reviewed herein, limited in most cases by numbers of well-phenotyped individuals with rare variant surveys of only a few known genes, will give way to comprehensive genome-wide strategies to identify and understand rare and common variants relevant to disease susceptibility and cause, including structural and other nonprotein coding genomic variants, in much larger populations. This will enable a more comprehensive and insightful understanding of the genomic basis of human disease. Our present rudimentary understandings of "mendelian genetics," likely an oversimplified concept of "single-gene" genetics for many of the cases of DCM and ARVC, in the next few years will evolve into greater insight to the complexity that likely underlies the cardiomyopathies.

REFERENCES
The Dilated Cardiomyopathies

1. Maron BJ, Towbin JA, Thiene G, et al. Contemporary definitions and classification of the cardiomyopathies: an American Heart Association scientific statement from the council on clinical cardiology, heart failure and transplantation committee; quality of care and outcomes research and functional genomics and translational biology interdisciplinary working groups; and council on epidemiology and prevention. *Circulation*. 2006;113:1807–1816.
2. Elliott P, Andersson B, Arbustini E, et al. Classification of the cardiomyopathies: a position statement from the European Society of Cardiology working group on myocardial and pericardial diseases. *Eur Heart J*. 2008;29:270–276.
3. Hershberger RE, Cowan J, Morales A, Siegfried JD. Progress with genetic cardiomyopathies: screening, counseling, and testing in dilated, hypertrophic, and arrhythmogenic right ventricular dysplasia/cardiomyopathy. *Circ Heart Fail*. 2009;2:253–261.
4. Hershberger RE, Givertz M, Ho CY, et al. Genetic evaluation of cardiomyopathy—a heart failure society of America practice guideline. *J Card Fail*. 2018;24(5):281–302.
5. Hershberger RE, Givertz MM, Ho CY, et al. Genetic evaluation of cardiomyopathy: a clinical practice resource of the American College of Medical Genetics and Genomics (ACMG). *Genet Med*. 2018;20:899–909.
6. Piran S, Liu P, Morales A, Hershberger RE. Where genome meets phenome: rationale for integrating genetic and protein biomarkers in the diagnosis and management of dilated cardiomyopathy and heart failure. *J Am Coll Cardiol*. 2012;60:283–289.
7. Carruth ED, Young W, Beer D, et al. Prevalence and electronic health record-based phenotype of loss-of-function genetic variants in arrhythmogenic right ventricular cardiomyopathy-associated genes. *Circ Genom Precis Med*. 2019;12:e002579.

8. Cowan JR, Kinnamon DD, Morales A, et al. Multigenic disease and bilineal inheritance in dilated cardiomyopathy is illustrated in nonsegregating LMNA pedigrees. *Circ Genom Precis Med.* 2018;11:e002038.

9. Ware JS, Amor-Salamanca A, Tayal U, et al. Genetic etiology for alcohol-induced cardiac toxicity. *J Am Coll Cardiol.* 2018;71:2293–2302.

10. Garcia-Pavia P, Kim Y, Restrepo-Cordoba MA, et al. Genetic variants associated with cancer therapy-induced cardiomyopathy. *Circulation.* 2019;140:31–41.

11. Hershberger RE, Hedges DJ, Morales A. Dilated cardiomyopathy: the complexity of a diverse genetic architecture. *Nat Rev Cardiol.* 2013;10:531–547.

12. Morales A, Kinnamon DD, Jordan E, et al. Variant interpretation for dilated cardiomyopathy: refinement of the American College of Medical Genetics and Genomics/ClinGen guidelines for the DCM precision medicine study. *Circ Genom Precis Med.* 2020;13:e002480.

13. Hershberger RE, Morales A, Siegfried JD. Clinical and genetic issues in dilated cardiomyopathy: a review for genetics professionals. *Genet Med.* 2010;12:655–667.

14. Kinnamon DD, Morales A, Bowen DJ, et al. Toward genetics-driven early intervention in dilated cardiomyopathy: design and implementation of the DCM precision medicine study. *Circ Cardiovasc Genet.* 2017;10:e001826.

15. Gulati A, Ismail TF, Jabbour A, et al. The prevalence and prognostic significance of right ventricular systolic dysfunction in nonischemic dilated cardiomyopathy. *Circulation.* 2013;128:1623–1633.

16. Donal E, Delgado V, Bucciarelli-Ducci C, et al. Multimodality imaging in the diagnosis, risk stratification, and management of patients with dilated cardiomyopathies: an expert consensus document from the European Association of Cardiovascular Imaging. *Eur Heart J Cardiovasc Imaging.* 2019;20:1075–1093.

17. Burkett EL, Hershberger RE. Clinical and genetic issues in familial dilated cardiomyopathy. *J Am Coll Cardiol.* 2005;45:969–981.

18. Mazzarotto F, Tayal U, Buchan RJ, et al. Reevaluating the genetic contribution of monogenic dilated cardiomyopathy. *Circulation.* 2020;141:387–398.

19. Herman DS, Lam L, Taylor MR, et al. Truncations of titin causing dilated cardiomyopathy. *N Engl J Med.* 2012;366:619–628.

20. Ware JS, Li J, Mazaika E, et al. Shared genetic predisposition in peripartum and dilated cardiomyopathies. *N Engl J Med.* 2016;374:233–241.

21. Haggerty CM, Damrauer SM, Levin MG, et al. Genomics-first evaluation of heart disease associated with titin-truncating variants. *Circulation.* 2019;140:42–54.

22. Morales A, Hershberger RE. The rationale and timing of molecular genetic testing for dilated cardiomyopathy. *Can J Cardiol.* 2015;31:1309–1312.

23. Menon S, Michels V, Pellikka P, et al. Cardiac troponin T mutation in familial cardiomyopathy with variable remodeling and restrictive physiology. *Clin Genet.* 2008;74:445–454.

24. Hershberger RE, Siegfried JD. State of the Art Review. Update 2011: clinical and genetic issues in familial dilated cardiomyopathy. *J Am Coll Cardiol.* 2011;57:1641–1649.

25. James CA, Calkins H. Arrhythmogenic right ventricular cardiomyopathy: progress toward personalized management. *Annu Rev Med.* 2019;70:1–18.

26. Towbin JA, McKenna WJ, Abrams DJ, et al. 2019 HRS expert consensus statement on evaluation, risk stratification, and management of arrhythmogenic cardiomyopathy. *Heart Rhythm.* 2019;16:e301–e372.

27. Elliott PM, Anastasakis A, Asimaki A, et al. Definition and treatment of arrhythmogenic cardiomyopathy: an updated expert panel report. *Eur J Heart Fail.* 2019;21:955–964.

28. Corrado D, Basso C, Judge DP. Arrhythmogenic cardiomyopathy. *Circ Res.* 2017;121:784–802.

29. Te Riele AS, James CA, Philips B, et al. Mutation-positive arrhythmogenic right ventricular dysplasia/cardiomyopathy: the triangle of dysplasia displaced. *J Cardiovasc Electrophysiol.* 2013;24:1311–1320.

30. Hauer RN, Cox MG, Groeneweg JA. Impact of new electrocardiographic criteria in arrhythmogenic cardiomyopathy. *Front Physiol.* 2012;3:352.

31. Swope D, Li J, Radice GL. Beyond cell adhesion: the role of armadillo proteins in the heart. *Cell Signal.* 2013;25:93–100.

32. ClinGen Cardiovascular Domain Working Group.

33. te Riele AS, James CA, Rastegar N, et al. Yield of serial evaluation in at-risk family members of patients with ARVD/C. *J Am Coll Cardiol.* 2014;64:293–301.

34. den Haan AD, Tan BY, Zikusoka MN, et al. Comprehensive desmosome mutation analysis in North Americans with arrhythmogenic right ventricular dysplasia/cardiomyopathy. *Circ Cardiovasc Genet.* 2009;2:428–435.

35. Quarta G, Muir A, Pantazis A, et al. Familial evaluation in arrhythmogenic right ventricular cardiomyopathy: impact of genetics and revised task force criteria. *Circulation.* 2011;123:2701–2709.

36. Groeneweg JA, Bhonsale A, James CA, et al. Clinical presentation, long-term follow-up, and outcomes of 1001 arrhythmogenic right ventricular dysplasia/cardiomyopathy patients and family members. *Circ Cardiovasc Genet.* 2015;8:437–446.

37. Bosman LP, Sammani A, James CA, et al. Predicting arrhythmic risk in arrhythmogenic right ventricular cardiomyopathy: a systematic review and meta-analysis. *Heart Rhythm.* 2018;15:1097–1107.

38. Corrado D, Wichter T, Link MS, et al. Treatment of arrhythmogenic right ventricular cardiomyopathy/dysplasia: an international task force consensus statement. *Circulation.* 2015;132:441–453.

39. Santangeli P, Zado ES, Supple GE, et al. Long-term outcome with catheter ablation of ventricular tachycardia in patients with arrhythmogenic right ventricular cardiomyopathy. *Circ Arrhythm Electrophysiol.* 2015;8:1413–1421.

40. James CA, Bhonsale A, Tichnell C, et al. Exercise increases age-related penetrance and arrhythmic risk in arrhythmogenic right ventricular dysplasia/cardiomyopathy-associated desmosomal mutation carriers. *J Am Coll Cardiol.* 2013;62:1290–1297.

41. Guzzo-Merello G, Segovia J, Dominguez F, et al. Natural history and prognostic factors in alcoholic cardiomyopathy. *JACC Heart Fail.* 2015;3:78–86.

42. Jia G, Hill MA, Sowers JR. Diabetic cardiomyopathy: an update of mechanisms contributing to this clinical entity. *Circ Res.* 2018;122:624–638.

43. Fitchett D, Zinman B, Wanner C, et al. Heart failure outcomes with empagliflozin in patients with type 2 diabetes at high cardiovascular risk: results of the EMPA-REG OUTCOME(R) trial. *Eur Heart J.* 2016;37:1526–1534.

44. Sen-Chowdhry S, McKenna WJ. Left ventricular noncompaction and cardiomyopathy: cause, contributor, or epiphenomenon? *Curr Opin Cardiol.* 2008;23:171–175.

45. Kohli SK, Pantazis AA, Shah JS, et al. Diagnosis of left-ventricular non-compaction in patients with left-ventricular systolic dysfunction: time for a reappraisal of diagnostic criteria? *Eur Heart J.* 2008;29:89–95.

46. Arbustini E, Weidemann F, Hall JL. Left ventricular noncompaction: a distinct cardiomyopathy or a trait shared by different cardiac diseases? *J Am Coll Cardiol.* 2014;64:1840–1850.

47. Anderson RH, Jensen B, Mohun TJ, et al. Key questions relating to left ventricular noncompaction cardiomyopathy: is the emperor still wearing any clothes? *Can J Cardiol.* 2017;33:747–757.

48. Hershberger RE, Morales A, Cowan J. Is left ventricular noncompaction a trait, phenotype, or disease? The evidence points to phenotype. *Circ Cardiovasc Genet.* 2017;10.

49. Ross SB, Jones K, Blanch B, et al. A systematic review and meta-analysis of the prevalence of left ventricular non-compaction in adults. *Eur Heart J.* 2020;41:1428–1436.

50. Gopinathannair R, Etheridge SP, Marchlinski FE, et al. Arrhythmia-induced cardiomyopathies: mechanisms, recognition, and management. *J Am Coll Cardiol.* 2015;66:1714–1728.

51. Medi C, Kalman JM, Haqqani H, et al. Tachycardia-mediated cardiomyopathy secondary to focal atrial tachycardia: long-term outcome after catheter ablation. *J Am Coll Cardiol.* 2009;53:1791–1797.

52. Hasdemir C, Ulucan C, Yavuzgil O, et al. Tachycardia-induced cardiomyopathy in patients with idiopathic ventricular arrhythmias: the incidence, clinical and electrophysiologic characteristics, and the predictors. *J Cardiovasc Electrophysiol.* 2011;22:663–668.

53. Dandamudi G, Rampurwala AY, Mahenthiran J, et al. Persistent left ventricular dilatation in tachycardia-induced cardiomyopathy patients after appropriate treatment and normalization of ejection fraction. *Heart Rhythm.* 2008;5:1111–1114.

54. Selby DE, Palmer BM, LeWinter MM, Meyer M. Tachycardia-induced diastolic dysfunction and resting tone in myocardium from patients with a normal ejection fraction. *J Am Coll Cardiol.* 2011;58:147–154.

55. Morales A, Painter T, Li R, et al. Rare variant mutations in pregnancy-associated or peripartum cardiomyopathy. *Circulation.* 2010;121:2176–2182.

56. van Spaendonck-Zwarts KY, van Tintelen JP, van Veldhuisen DJ, et al. Peripartum cardiomyopathy as a part of familial dilated cardiomyopathy. *Circulation.* 2010;121:2169–2175.

57. Davis MB, Arany Z, McNamara DM, et al. Peripartum cardiomyopathy: JACC state-of-the-art review. *J Am Coll Cardiol.* 2020;75:207–221.

58. Elkayam U, Tummala PP, Rao K, et al. Maternal and fetal outcomes of subsequent pregnancies in women with peripartum cardiomyopathy. *N Engl J Med.* 2001;344:1567–1571.

59. Ghadri JR, Wittstein IS, Prasad A, et al. International expert consensus document on takotsubo syndrome (Part I): clinical characteristics, diagnostic criteria, and pathophysiology. *Eur Heart J.* 2018;39:2032–2046.

60. Ghadri JR, Wittstein IS, Prasad A, et al. International expert consensus document on takotsubo syndrome (Part II): diagnostic workup, outcome, and management. *Eur Heart J.* 2018;39:2047–2062.

61. Templin C, Ghadri JR, Diekmann J, et al. Clinical features and outcomes of takotsubo (stress) cardiomyopathy. *N Engl J Med.* 2015;373:929–938.

62. Cammann VL, Szawan KA, Stahli BE, et al. Age-related variations in takotsubo syndrome. *J Am Coll Cardiol.* 2020;75:1869–1877.

63. Syed FF, Asirvatham SJ, Francis J. Arrhythmia occurrence with takotsubo cardiomyopathy: a literature review. *Europace.* 2011;13:780–788.

Restrictive Cardiomyopathies

64. Stollberger C, Finsterer J. Extracardiac medical and neuromuscular implications in restrictive cardiomyopathy. *Clin Cardiol.* 2007;30:375–380.

65. Kaski JP, Syrris P, Burch M, et al. Idiopathic restrictive cardiomyopathy in children is caused by mutations in cardiac sarcomere protein genes. *Heart.* 2008;94:1478–1484.

66. Caleshu C, Sakhuja R, Nussbaum RL, et al. Furthering the link between the sarcomere and primary cardiomyopathies: restrictive cardiomyopathy associated with multiple mutations in genes previously associated with hypertrophic or dilated cardiomyopathy. *Am J Med Genet.* 2011;155A:2229–2235.

67. Webber SA, Lipshultz SE, Sleeper LA, et al. Outcomes of restrictive cardiomyopathy in childhood and the influence of phenotype: a report from the Pediatric Cardiomyopathy Registry. *Circulation.* 2012;126:1237–1244.

68. Depasquale EC, Nasir K, Jacoby DL. Outcomes of adults with restrictive cardiomyopathy after heart transplantation. *J Heart Lung Transplant.* 2012;31:1269–1275.

69. Gallego-Delgado M, Delgado JF, Brossa-Loidi V, et al. Idiopathic restrictive cardiomyopathy is primarily a genetic disease. *J Am Coll Cardiol.* 2016;67:3021–3023.

70. Talreja DR, Edwards WD, Danielson GK, et al. Constrictive pericarditis in 26 patients with histologically normal pericardial thickness. *Circulation.* 2003;108:1852–1857.

71. Ammash NM, Seward JB, Bailey KR, et al. Clinical profile and outcome of idiopathic restrictive cardiomyopathy. *Circulation.* 2000;101:2490–2496.

72. Pereira NL, Grogan M, Dec GW. Spectrum of restrictive and infiltrative cardiomyopathies: Part 1 of a 2-part series. *J Am Coll Cardiol.* 2018;71:1130–1148.

73. Patel MR, Cawley PJ, Heitner JF, et al. Detection of myocardial damage in patients with sarcoidosis. *Circulation.* 2009;120:1969–1977.

74. Bagwan IN, Hooper LV, Sheppard MN. Cardiac sarcoidosis and sudden death. The heart may look normal or mimic other cardiomyopathies. *Virchows Arch.* 2011;458:671–678.

75. Vasaiwala SC, Finn C, Delpriore J, et al. Prospective study of cardiac sarcoid mimicking arrhythmogenic right ventricular dysplasia. *J Cardiovasc Electrophysiol.* 2009;20:473–476.

76. Kerkar A, Hazard F, Caleshu C, et al. Pathological overlap of arrhythmogenic right ventricular cardiomyopathy and cardiac sarcoidosis. *Circ Genom Precis Med.* 2019;12:452–454.

77. Murtagh G, Laffin LJ, Beshai JF, et al. Prognosis of myocardial damage in sarcoidosis patients with preserved left ventricular ejection fraction: risk stratification using cardiovascular magnetic resonance. *Circ Cardiovasc Imaging.* 2016;9:e003738.

78. Gupta A, Singh Gulati G, Seth S, Sharma S. Cardiac MRI in restrictive cardiomyopathy. *Clin Radiol.* 2012;67:95–105.

79. Ramirez R, Trivieri M, Fayad ZA, et al. Advanced imaging in cardiac sarcoidosis. *J Nucl Med.* 2019;60:892–898.

80. Birnie D, Beanlands RSB, Nery P, et al. Cardiac sarcoidosis multi-center randomized controlled trial (CHASM CS- RCT). *Am Heart J.* 2020;220:246–252.

81. Sadek MM, Yung D, Birnie DH, et al. Corticosteroid therapy for cardiac sarcoidosis: a systematic review. *Can J Cardiol.* 2013;29:1034–1041.

82. Cremers JP, Drent M, Bast A, et al. Multinational evidence-based World Association of Sarcoidosis and Other Granulomatous Disorders recommendations for the use of methotrexate in sarcoidosis: integrating systematic literature research and expert opinion of sarcoidologists worldwide. *Curr Opin Pulm Med.* 2013;19:545–561.

83. Birnie DH, Nery PB, Ha AC, Beanlands RS. Cardiac sarcoidosis. *J Am Coll Cardiol.* 2016;68:411–421.

84. Perkel D, Czer LS, Morrissey RP, et al. Heart transplantation for end-stage heart failure due to cardiac sarcoidosis. *Transplant Proc.* 2013;45:2384–2386.

85. Halawa A, Jain R, Turagam MK, et al. Outcome of implantable cardioverter defibrillator in cardiac sarcoidosis: a systematic review and meta-analysis. *J Interv Card Electrophysiol.* 2020.

86. Mehta A, Hughes DA. Fabry Disease. 1993.

87. Eng CM, Fletcher J, Wilcox WR, et al. Fabry disease: baseline medical characteristics of a cohort of 1765 males and females in the Fabry Registry. *J Inherit Metab Dis.* 2007;30:184–192.

88. Wilcox WR, Oliveira JP, Hopkin RJ, et al. Females with Fabry disease frequently have major organ involvement: lessons from the Fabry Registry. *Mol Genet Metab.* 2008;93:112–128.

89. Elliott P, Baker R, Pasquale F, et al. Prevalence of Anderson-Fabry disease in patients with hypertrophic cardiomyopathy: the European Anderson-Fabry Disease survey. *Heart.* 2011;97:1957–1960.

90. Moonen A, Lal S, Ingles J, et al. Prevalence of Anderson-Fabry disease in a cohort with unexplained late gadolinium enhancement on cardiac MRI. *Int J Cardiol.* 2020;304:122–124.

91. Zhu X, Yin L, Theisen M, et al. Systemic mRNA therapy for the treatment of Fabry disease: preclinical studies in wild-type mice, fabry mouse model, and wild-type non-human primates. *Am J Hum Genet.* 2019;104:625–637.

92. Pastores GM, Hughes DA. Gaucher Disease. 1993.

93. Fleming RE, Ponka P. Iron overload in human disease. *N Engl J Med.* 2012;366:348–359.

94. Barton JC, Edwards CQ. *HFE Hemochromatosis. GeneReviews(R)*; 2000. Apr 3 [Updated 2018 Dec 6].
95. Selvaraj S, Seidelmann S, Silvestre OM, et al. HFE H63D polymorphism and the risk for systemic hypertension, myocardial remodeling, and adverse cardiovascular events in the ARIC study. *Hypertension*. 2019;73:68–74.
96. Murphy CJ, Oudit GY. Iron-overload cardiomyopathy: pathophysiology, diagnosis, and treatment. *J Card Fail*. 2010;16:888–900.
97. Bhattacharyya S, Correia-de-Sa P, Yacoub M. Endomyocardial fibrosis: an update after 70 years. *Curr Cardiol Rep*. 2019;21:148.
98. Friehs I, Illigens B, Melnychenko I, et al. An animal model of endocardial fibroelastosis. *J Surg Res*. 2012.
99. Davar J, Connolly HM, Caplin ME, et al. Diagnosing and managing carcinoid heart disease in patients with neuroendocrine tumors: an expert statement. *J Am Coll Cardiol*. 2017;69:1288–1304.
100. Bhattacharyya S, Davar J, Dreyfus G, Caplin ME. Carcinoid heart disease. *Circulation*. 2007;116:2860–2865.
101. Castillo JG, Silvay G, Solis J. Current concepts in diagnosis and perioperative management of carcinoid heart disease. *Semin CardioThorac Vasc Anesth*. 2012.
102. Agha AM, Lopez-Mattei J, Donisan T, et al. Multimodality imaging in carcinoid heart disease. *Open Heart*. 2019;6:e001060.
103. Davis LM, Nicou N, Martin W, et al. Timing of peptide receptor radiotargeted therapy in relation to cardiac valve surgery for carcinoid heart disease in patients with neuroendocrine metastases and cardiac syndrome. A single-centre study from a centre of excellence. *Nucl Med Commun*. 2020;41:575–581.
104. Bhattacharyya S, Toumpanakis C, Chilkunda D, et al. Risk factors for the development and progression of carcinoid heart disease. *Am J Cardiol*. 2011;107:1221–1226.
105. Buchanan-Hughes A, Pashley A, Feuilly M, et al. Carcinoid heart disease: prognostic value of 5-hydroxyindoleacetic acid levels and impact on survival—a systematic literature review. *Neuroendocrinology*. 2021;111:1–15.
106. Debl K, Djavidani B, Buchner S, et al. Time course of eosinophilic myocarditis visualized by CMR. *J Cardiovasc Magn Reson*. 2008;10:21.
107. Qureshi N, Amin F, Chatterjee D, et al. MR imaging of endomyocardial fibrosis (EMF). *Int J Cardiol*. 2011;149:e36–e37.
108. Mocumbi AO, Ferreira MB, Sidi D, Yacoub MH. A population study of endomyocardial fibrosis in a rural area of Mozambique. *N Engl J Med*. 2008;359:43–49.

The Dilated, Restrictive, and Infiltrative Cardiomyopathies

53 Cardiac Amyloidosis

FREDERICK L. RUBERG AND MATHEW S. MAURER

The systemic amyloidoses are a group of diseases characterized by the extracellular deposition of insoluble, misfolded fibrillar proteins in the form of β-pleated sheets, resulting in organ dysfunction. First applied to human disease by Rudolph Virchow in 1854, amyloid derives its name from the Latin amylum or starch, because amyloid was initially and erroneously thought to be composed of cellulose owing to a positive iodine-staining reaction. Amyloid deposits evaluated by electron microscopy demonstrated that amyloid fibrils are nonbranching protein structures, 80 to 100 Angstroms in width and of variable length. They are resistant to proteolysis. Amyloid fibrils avidly bind to the histologic stain Congo red imparting a hyaline pink appearance under light microscopy, while under polarized light, fibrils reflect a characteristic apple-green birefringence.[1] Precursor protein identification is essential to define the type of amyloidosis, inform prognosis, and guide therapy. The taxonomy is defined by abbreviating the type with an A (for amyloid) followed by a protein abbreviation.[2] The two most common types of amyloidosis that affect the heart are light chain (AL) amyloidosis and transthyretin (ATTR) amyloidosis. ATTR amyloidosis is further subclassified by the sequence of the *TTR* gene, which resides on chromosome 18. Hereditary or variant transthyretin amyloidosis (hATTR or ATTRv) results from single nucleotide polymorphisms of the *TTR* gene and are inherited in an autosomal dominant fashion. In ATTRv, amino acid substitution results in a destabilization and misfolding process that leads to amyloidogenesis. Historical nomenclature places a one- or three-letter abbreviation for the normal amino acid at the position of substitution in the protein followed by the substituted amino acid (e.g., ATTR Val122Ile signifies isoleucine replacing valine at position 122 in the TTR amino acid sequence). More contemporary nomenclature includes the 20-amino acid signal peptide sequence in the count of residues such that pVal142Ile (or pV142I) refers to the same variant as Val122Ile. In contrast, wild-type transthyretin amyloidosis (ATTRwt) is a sporadic disease characterized by a normal *TTR* genetic sequence, with unclear causes of TTR misfolding. Secondary amyloidosis (AA), composed of serum amyloid A protein, can result from intense and persistent systemic inflammation but rarely affects the heart. Finally, uncommon genetic variants also known to affect the heart include atrial natriuretic peptide (ANP), apolipoprotein A1 (ApoA1), fibrinogen (Afib), and gelsolin (Agel). This chapter will focus attention on AL and ATTR amyloidosis, by far the most relevant types for the practicing clinician.

EPIDEMIOLOGY

Light Chain Amyloidosis

Epidemiologic studies suggest that AL amyloidosis is a rare disease with an annual incidence of approximately 1 per 100,000 individuals, accounting for approximately 5000 new annual cases in the United States. Cardiac involvement can be demonstrated in up to 70% of cases of AL amyloidosis. Although AL amyloidosis can affect individuals from the fourth decade of life onward, the prevalence of AL amyloidosis increases with age, with a median age of diagnosis at 63 years, and slight male predominance (between 55% and 65%). The current estimated prevalence is 40 to 58 cases per million persons. AL amyloidosis is related to, but distinct from, multiple myeloma and monoclonal gammopathy of unknown significance (MGUS) (other clonal plasma cell disorders). Among patients with MGUS, only a small percentage will develop AL amyloidosis (1% overall, relative risk 8.8). Although most patients with AL amyloidosis do not have multiple myeloma, up to 10% to 15% of patients with multiple myeloma have coexisting AL amyloidosis.[3]

Transthyretin Amyloidosis

The epidemiology ATTR amyloidosis varies by type (ATTRwt and ATTRv) and by specific variant, but conclusive data regarding population incidence and prevalence are lacking. Autopsy studies have demonstrated that up to 25% of decedents older than age 85 years have demonstrable myocardial TTR amyloid deposits, with a prevalence that increases with age, male sex, and is associated with a clinical diagnosis of heart failure.[4] Contemporary imaging suggests that of older (>60 year) patients hospitalized with heart failure and preserved ejection fraction with an increased left ventricular wall thickness, between 10% and 15% of patients may have ATTRwt amyloidosis. Other studies of older individuals with severe aortic stenosis demonstrate similar prevalence and male predilection for ATTRwt amyloidosis.[5] Larger-scale epidemiology studies designed to assess the prevalence of ATTRwt amyloidosis are presently underway.

In contrast to ATTRwt, hATTR or ATTRv is caused by a genetic mutation in the TTR gene. The TTR gene is composed of 4 exons (127 amino acids) in which more than 100 mutations have been described that can cause hereditary amyloidosis. Linked to a genetic founder, each variant is endemic to a particular geographic region or follows population migration patterns. Disease expression manifests as a polyneuropathy or cardiomyopathy (previously termed familial amyloidogenic polyneuropathy [FAP] or cardiomyopathy [FAC]). Phenotypic penetrance varies widely by mutation and increases with age (Table 53.1). The most common variant observed outside of the United States is pVal50Met (Val30Met), endemic to Portugal, northern Sweden, Japan, and Brazil. This variant causes predominantly a polyneuropathy phenotype, but at a later age of onset causes amyloid cardiomyopathy. The pThr80Ala (Thr60Ala) variant first identified in a northern region of the Republic of Ireland, causes both cardiomyopathy and polyneuropathy. Prevalence can approach 1% in endemic areas but is very uncommon elsewhere in the world. By far the most common *TTR* variant is pVal142Ile (Val122Ile), which has been reproducibly identified in approximately 3.5% of self-identified Black persons in the United States.[6] As a cause of ATTR cardiomyopathy, this allele frequency translates into more than 1.6 million persons in the United States as carriers and therefore at risk

Additional content is available online at Elsevier eBooks for Practicing Clinicians

TABLE 53.1 Comparison of the Most Common Types of Cardiac Amyloidosis

FEATURES	AL	ATTR					
PRECURSOR PROTEIN	LIGHT CHAIN—KAPPA OR LAMBDA	VARIANT TTR					
		CARDIOGENIC			NEUROPATHIC/MIXED		
SPECIFIC MUTATION		VAL122ILE (pV142I)	LEU111MET (pL131M)	ILE68LEU (pI88L)	THR60ALA (pT80A)	VAL30MET (pV50M)	WILD-TYPE TTR
Average age (range)	63 (30–80)	72 (47–90)	48 (35–60)	71 (40–80)	66 (41–82)	Early onset (30–50) Endemic, neuropathic Late onset (>50)—nonendemic, mixed phenotype	75 (50–>100)
Gender (% male)	55%–60%	70%	64%	78%	60%	50%	90%
Race/ethnicity	Not specific	Black/Afro-Caribbean	Danish	Italian	Irish	Portuguese, Swedish, Japanese	Not specific
Cardiac involvement (%)	~70%	100%	100%	96%	100%	More common in late onset	100%
Fat pad biopsy	70%–80%*	<50%	<50%	<50%	<50%	<50%	<20%
Primary referral route	Hematology, cardiology, nephrology, dermatology	Cardiology	Cardiology	Cardiology	Neurology and cardiology	Neurology and cardiology	Cardiology
Extracardiac manifestations	Nephrotic syndrome/renal failure Autonomic dysfunction Purpura Macroglossia Carpal tunnel syndrome	Autonomic dysfunction Carpal tunnel Lumbar spinal stenosis	Carpal tunnel syndrome	Polyneuropathy (rare) Carpal tunnel syndrome	Polyneuropathy Autonomic dysfunction Carpal tunnel syndrome	Polyneuropathy Autonomic dysfunction GI motility disorder Carpal tunnel syndrome	Carpal tunnel syndrome Lumbar spinal stenosis Biceps Tendon Rupture
Median survival/stage	1: Not reached (at 12 years) 2: 9.4 years 3: 4.3 years 3b: 1 year	1: 54 months 2: 28.8 months 3: 17.7 months	NR	Median overall survival of 36 months	1: 77 months 2: 54 months 3: 21 months	Survival usually >10 years and improved with liver transplant and tafamidis	1: 75 months 2: 46 months 3: 20 months

AL, light chain amyloidosis; *ATTR*, transthyretin amyloidosis; *NAC*, National Amyloidosis Centre, London, UK; *NR*, not reported.
*Dependent on extent of amyloid.

for ATTR cardiomyopathy. In addition, individuals of Hispanic/Latino ancestry may also harbor this mutation which increases the risk of developing heart failure nearly 50%. Unfortunately, among the vast majority of allele carriers with heart failure, the diagnosis is delayed or missed.[7] That stated, the phenotypic penetrance of ATTR cardiomyopathy is unclear and depends upon the age of ascertainment, with increasing penetrance with advancing age. Other *TTR* variants seen worldwide that predominantly result in ATTR cardiac amyloidosis include pIle88Leu (Ile68Leu, Italy) and pLeu131Met (Leu111Met, Denmark).[8]

PATHOPHYSIOLOGY

In AL amyloidosis, a dysregulated plasma cell clone produces kappa or lambda immunoglobulin light chain fragments that have a propensity to misfold, aggregate, and deposit in the myocardial interstitium. Lambda light chain amyloidosis is more common than kappa, and organ systems affected include the heart, kidneys, liver, nervous system (including autonomic nervous system), gastrointestinal tract, and soft tissues. The titer of light chain does not predict the site of target organ deposition. Cardiac AL amyloidosis is viewed as a "toxic-infiltrative" cardiomyopathy involving two mechanisms: (1) interstitial and/or

perivascular amyloid fibril deposition leading to disruption of tissue architecture, microvascular dysfunction with angina/ischemia, and inhibition of contractile/relaxation functions and (2) direct toxicity to cardiomyocytes through, in part, p38 mitogen-activated protein kinase (MAPK) signaling. Interstitial deposition results in a restrictive cardiomyopathy and heart failure, and direct cellular toxicity is thought to occur through induction of reactive oxygen species and apoptosis in cardiomyocytes.[3]

Transthyretin, also known as prealbumin, is a tetrameric protein consisting of four identical subunits, synthesized in the liver, but also by the choroid plexus and retinal pigmented epithelial cells. TTR derives its name from its function as a circulating transporter of thyroid hormone and retinol (vitamin A). In hATTR, amino acid substitutions alter the properties of the protein favoring tetramer dissociation which is the rate-limiting step in amyloid fibril formation. Monomers then misfold and aggregate into amyloid fibrils that deposit in body tissues with specific organ tropism. Precisely why native (i.e., genetically normal), wild-type TTR becomes kinetically unstable and aggregates is unclear, but the process definitively occurs with advancing age (typically older than 60 years). Disease expression may also be influenced by age-related degradation in cellular systems that manage misfolded proteins. ATTR amyloidosis results in progressive myocardial deposition (infiltrating between myocytes) and restrictive cardiomyopathy and/or a small fiber, length-dependent peripheral and autonomic neuropathy. Tissue tropism or organ system involvement in ATTR amyloidosis is incompletely understood; however, there is developing evidence that the amyloid fibril composition may play a role. Amyloid deposits composed of TTR fragments (type A fibrils) are associated with later-onset disease with cardiac involvement in ATTRv and with ATTRwt, whereas full-length TTR fibrils (type B fibrils) in amyloid deposits correlate with earlier-onset disease without a strong cardiac phenotype.[9]

CLINICAL FEATURES AND PROGNOSIS

There are various impediments that hinder the recognition of cardiac amyloidosis by the cardiovascular clinician. First, the disease is generally perceived to be rare and presents with clinical and imaging features associated with more common conditions. Second, cardiac amyloidosis was, until recently, an untreatable disease with extremely poor prognosis lending credence to therapeutic nihilism. Third and finally, the diagnostic approach required endomyocardial biopsy, a procedure not appropriate in a scenario of low-pretest likelihood or for widespread screening. Recent discoveries in epidemiology, advancements in diagnostic imaging, and the development of novel therapeutics have rendered each of these conceptions invalid. Nevertheless, significant delays in disease recognition persist. Among patients with ATTR amyloidosis, data demonstrate increasing frequency of hospitalizations and visits for heart failure without disease recognition in the 3 years preceding ultimate diagnosis.[10]

Although differing by precursor protein, the final common pathophysiologic pathway of cardiac amyloidosis is one of myocardial infiltration and progressive impairment in diastolic and systolic function that elicits symptoms of congestive heart failure. Left ventricular ejection fraction (LVEF) is preserved in early stages of the disease, while longitudinal contraction is impaired. Progressive infiltration and/or direct myocyte toxicity subsequently results in decrement in global left and right ventricular systolic function. Signs of heart failure in more advanced disease become predominantly right-sided, with lower extremity edema, ascites, and hepatic enlargement. For this reason, the disease, particularly in early stages, is misrecognized for more common wall-thickening processes such as hypertensive remodeling or hypertrophic cardiomyopathy (HCM). The electrocardiogram (ECG) classically demonstrates a low-voltage pattern in approximately 50% of patients with AL cardiac amyloidosis, while inferior or anterior pseudoinfarcts are seen in greater than 70% of AL cases. Low voltage is seen in only 25% to 40% of patients with ATTR, while up to 15% can show evidence of left ventricular hypertrophy. Conduction disease progressing to heart block is more commonly a feature of ATTR amyloidosis. Atrial dysrhythmias, particular atrial fibrillation (AF) and flutter, are seen in up to 40% to 60% of patients with wtATTR amyloidosis at diagnosis and in up to 90% over time. The risk of intracardiac thrombus is increased in all patients with cardiac amyloidosis, even those in sinus rhythm, with stroke or systemic embolization occurring in some patients. Although a low-voltage pattern itself can be attributable to other causes (pericardial effusion, lung hyper-expansion), integration of increased wall thickness seen by echocardiography in the setting of a low-voltage pattern (the mass to voltage ratio), increases diagnostic accuracy.

One strategy to increase recognition involves identification of other, noncardiac features of AL or ATTR amyloidosis in the context of heart failure. Clinical features of AL amyloidosis are myriad and follow organ system infiltration including renal (proteinuria, often nephrotic range), soft tissue (macroglossia, carpal tunnel syndrome), gastrointestinal (bleeding), or neurologic (peripheral or autonomic neuropathy). Periorbital ecchymosis resulting from capillary fragility is considered a pathognomonic feature of AL amyloidosis and is not seen in ATTR amyloidosis. Hereditary ATTR amyloidosis presents as a small fiber, length-dependent peripheral neuropathy manifesting as parenthesis, pain, or sensory loss on the hands and feet. However, autonomic neuropathy, most commonly manifesting as abnormal sweating, orthostatic hypotension, gastrointestinal dysmotility, and erectile dysfunction, can also be observed in AL or ATTR. As noted previously, different TTR variants present with either cardiomyopathy or neuropathy symptoms, or both. For example, the pVal50Met variant causes predominantly neuropathy in early-onset disease (third or fourth decade) but cardiomyopathy and neuropathy in later onset (sixth or seventh decade of life). The pThr80Ala variant causes either cardiomyopathy or neuropathy, or both, with onset in the fifth decade. The common variant pVal142Ile affects individuals of West African origin generally in the seventh decade of life, but nearly exclusively causes cardiomyopathy. Rare ATTRv manifestations resulting from leptomeningeal involvement include hydrocephalus and vitreous opacities. Wild-type ATTR was previously held to be principally a cardiac-restricted disease, although soft tissue deposition manifesting as carpal tunnel syndrome, lumbar spinal stenosis (ligamentum flavum thickening), and spontaneous tendon ruptures (biceps in particular) is now widely recognized. It is held that the orthopedic/soft tissue manifestations of ATTRwt amyloidosis precede the cardiac, often by many years. The presence of neuropathy in ATTRwt is often difficult to disentangle for other age-associated neuropathies or comorbidities (including diabetes mellitus or alcohol intake).

Prognosis

The prognosis of AL cardiac amyloidosis varies greatly depending upon two important contingencies: the stage of disease upon diagnosis and, importantly, the response to chemotherapy directed against the affected plasma cell clone. Prognosis is assessed by a combination of biomarker risk assessment models and cardiac imaging. Biomarker testing (Mayo or Boston University scoring systems) involves measurement of brain natriuretic peptides (NT-pro-BNP or BNP), cardiac troponin I or T, and direct measurement of lambda and kappa light chain.[11,12] Patients are classified into stages depending upon the values of these biomarkers. Recent data demonstrate that median survival for stage 2 patients (with either troponin or BNP above threshold) is approximately 9.5 years, whereas for those with advanced disease (stage 3b), median survival remains approximately 1 year. Imaging studies demonstrate that poor prognosis is also associated with lower echocardiographic stroke volume, increasing impairment global longitudinal strain, increasingly severe cardiac magnetic resonance imaging (CMR) late gadolinium enhancement (LGE), and increasing CMR extracellular volume fraction (ECV).[13] Each of these imaging features is a marker of more advanced disease and is strongly associated with cardiac biomarkers. Hematologic response status and change in cardiac biomarkers with treatment also predict prognosis. The attainment of a complete hematologic response is the goal of all therapy and is strongly associated with improved survival. A reduction in BNP or NT-pro BNP of greater than 30% from baseline is also indicative of a cardiac response and is associated with improved prognosis.

The prognosis of ATTR amyloidosis differs between hereditary and wild-type genotype. Similar to AL amyloidosis, staging systems using cardiac biomarkers and renal function have been developed to inform prognosis. Despite the larger population of affected patients as compared with AL, data limited to case series estimate median survival in ATTRwt amyloidosis to be approximately 3.5 years and for ATTRv amyloidosis pVal142Ile to be approximately 2.5 years from diagnosis. However, as in AL, prognosis depends upon stage of disease at diagnosis. Using a combination of NT-proBNP and troponin T (Mayo system) or NT-proBNP and estimated glomerular filtration rate (eGFR, National Amyloidosis Centre system), data demonstrate that for ATTRwt median survival following diagnosis ranges from 5 to 7 years for stage 1 (early stage) to 2 to 3 years for stage 3 (advanced stage).[14,15] It is important to emphasize that the natural history studies currently available do not account for contemporary TTR-specific therapies which can extend survival. Like AL, imaging also informs prognosis with increasing CMR LGE and ECV and worsening global longitudinal strain associated with impaired survival.

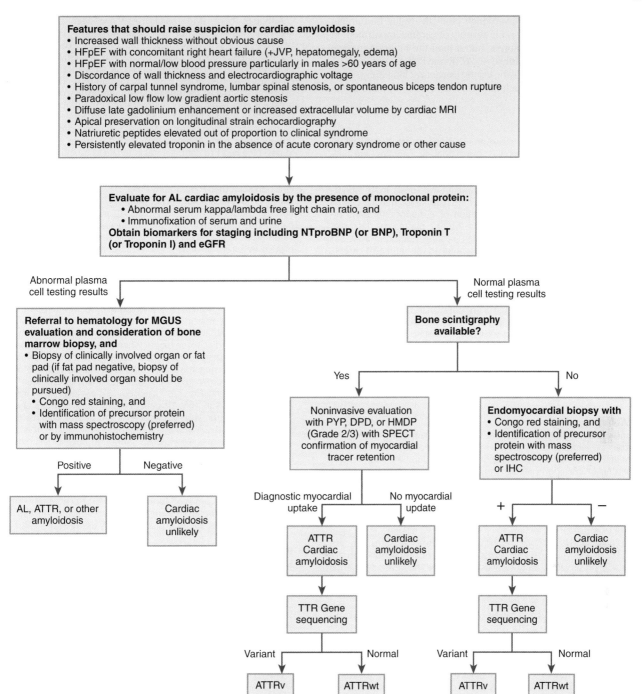

FIGURE 53.1 Algorithm for cardiac amyloidosis diagnosis. Accurate diagnosis of cardiac amyloidosis can be made by tissue biopsy or by noninvasive methods (bone-seeking nuclear tracers) following exclusion of monoclonal protein. Note appropriate testing for monoclonal protein involves serum-free light chain assay and serum and urine immunofixation electrophoresis (not serum protein electrophoresis). Nuclear imaging with bone-seeking radiotracers (PYP, DPD, or HMDP) can be performed concurrent to monoclonal protein assessment to afford additional information. *DPD,* 99mTc-3,3-diphosphono-1,2-propanedicarboxylic acid; *HMDP,* 99mTc-hydhydroxyl-methylene-diphosphonate; *MGUS,* monoclonal gammmopathy of unknown significance; *PYP,* 99mTc-pyrophosphate.

DIAGNOSIS

The critical step to enable a diagnosis of cardiac amyloidosis is clinical suspicion forged, in part, by attention to associated signs/symptoms and reassessment of changes in clinical features previously attributed to other processes. Examples of the latter point include intolerance to beta blockade (a feature of restrictive filling), intolerance to angiotensin-converting enzyme (ACE) inhibitors, angiotensin receptor blockers (ARBs), or angiotensin receptor/neprilysin inhibitors (ARNIs), or a reduced requirement for antihypertensives. Heightened awareness in specific affected populations is also essential, such as severe aortic stenosis, particularly the low-flow, low-gradient phenotype. In addition,

several "red flag" features have been proposed including extreme left ventricle (LV) wall thickening (>15 mm), discordant ECG voltage as predicted from wall thickness, orthopedic/soft tissue manifestations, and characteristic patterns on imaging testing.[16] A clinical algorithm to guide the approach toward accurate diagnosis of cardiac amyloidosis can be found in Figure 53.1.

Diagnosis of amyloidosis classically requires tissue biopsy with Congo red (or Thioflavin) staining and precursor protein identification by immunohistochemistry and/or mass spectrometry. In the case of AL amyloidosis, a tissue biopsy is required to establish the diagnosis. Establishment of cardiac amyloidosis, however, does not require an endomyocardial biopsy, as supportive evidence from imaging and biomarker testing afford a very high predictive value for cardiac involvement.[17] Furthermore, it is the severity of cardiac impairment in AL that defines treatment regimens, rather than the binary adjudication of cardiac involvement. Unlike AL, ATTR amyloidosis can now be accurately diagnosed with imaging testing (nuclear scintigraphy) combined with testing for light chain amyloidosis, when performed in the proper clinical context.

BIOMARKERS

Persistent and unexplained elevation in cardiac biomarkers, including the aforementioned troponins and natriuretic peptides, are hallmark features of cardiac amyloidosis but are nonspecific. Although candidates have been proposed, there are no specific biomarkers yet reported that can definitively identify cardiac amyloidosis. In AL, abnormal increase in either lambda (more common) or kappa free light chain with abnormal ratio, and/or identification of a monoclonal band on immunofixation electrophoresis is indicative of a plasma cell dyscrasia. In the proper context, these findings can increase suspicion for AL but are not diagnostic. Furthermore, it is common in the setting of chronic kidney disease to observe a kappa predominance with abnormal free light chain ratio, confusing interpretation. In addition, MGUS incidence increases with age and plasma cell testing abnormalities can be seen in up to 40% to 50% of patients with ATTR amyloidosis.[18] Thus hematologic consultation is indispensable in unclear scenarios. A serum protein electrophoresis (SPEP) is insensitive for identifying AL amyloidosis and should not be obtained without subsequent immunofixation. Emerging data suggest that lower prealbumin (TTR) concentration may identify patients with ATTRv amyloidosis and can inform prognosis in ATTRwt. Similarly, the TTR ligand retinol-binding protein 4 (RBP4), also appears to identify ATTRv pVal142Ile amyloidosis, although its capacity to predict prognosis has not been well explored.[19]

IMAGING

Cardiac imaging plays an essential role in the diagnostic pathway for cardiac amyloidosis identification (Table 53.2). Recently published multisocietal consensus recommendations for the acquisition, analysis, and reporting of imaging in cardiac amyloidosis have conferred important standardization.[20,21] Echocardiography is indispensable (see also Chapter 16). Findings include increased biventricular thickening (above the upper limit of normal for age and sex but often ≥12 mm for the LV), dilated atria, interatrial septal thickening, valvular thickening, evidence of right ventricular thickening, pericardial effusion, dilated inferior vena cava, diastolic dysfunction, and increased left atrial pressures (see also Fig. 16.31 and Video 16.28). Global measures of systolic function are generally preserved in early to midstage disease; however, segmental variation in systolic function is evident early. Global longitudinal strain is often reduced and in specific, basal segments often are hypokinetic relative to apical segments. This distinctive pattern is described as "apical sparing" (Fig. 53. 2) and can be quantified with longitudinal systolic strain deformational imaging with an approximate apical/basal ratio of greater than 2 or apical/basal+mid strain greater than 0.7 (relative apical sparing). Increased LVEF/global longitudinal strain ratio greater than 4 is also suggestive of amyloid cardiomyopathy.[22] Echocardiographic features, although raising suspicion of amyloid cardiomyopathy, are not in themselves diagnostic. Another echocardiographic parameter that has utility in identifying cardiac amyloidosis and predicting clinical outcomes is the myocardial contraction fraction (MCF, ratio of LV stroke volume to myocardial wall volume).

CMR imaging (see Chapter 19) with LGE affords the capacity to visualize the extracellular space expansion that results from amyloid fibril deposition.[23] As in echocardiography, AL and ATTR patterns overlap; thus, although useful for adjudication of amyloid from nonamyloid, the specific type cannot be reliably identified. Cardiac amyloidosis demonstrates diffuse enhancement throughout the myocardial segments, either in a global subendocardial or transmural pattern, often with atrial involvement. The inability to suppress ("null") the myocardium in cine-inversion recovery (Look-Locker) sequences is a common feature. LGE CMR is approximately 85% to 90% sensitive and specific for identification of amyloid cardiomyopathy in patients with clinically suspected disease. As extracellular amyloid fibril deposition increases, the interstitial space between myocytes expands. Parametric T1 mapping demonstrates increased native (noncontrast) T1 and ECV is typically greater than 0.40. One distinct advantage of CMR over other imaging modalities is its capacity to differentiate other diseases that may mimic the amyloid cardiomyopathy phenotype (e.g., HCM, Fabry disease).

Although bone avid radiotracers have been used for myocardial infarction imaging for more than 40 years, it is now recognized that the tracers ^{99m}Tc-pyrophosphate (PYP), ^{99m}Tc-3,3-diphosphono-1,2-propanedicarboxylic acid (DPD), and ^{99m}Tc-hydroxyl-methylenediphosphonate (HMDP) can detect cardiac amyloidosis and differentiate ATTR from AL (see Figs. 18.34, 18.35, and eFig. 18.7). Using a simple semiquantitative methodology (the Perugini score), cardiac tracer uptake is compared with rib with grade 0 (no uptake) to grade 3 (cardiac uptake greater than rib) and determined either after 1 or 3 hours of tracer incubation. Alternatively, ATTR cardiac amyloidosis can be differentiated from AL using ^{99m}Tc PYP (the tracer available in United States) by a heart to contralateral lung (H/CL) quantitative uptake ratio of greater than 1.5 from a region of interest drawn over the heart and contralateral chest after a 1 hour of tracer incubation. Single-photon emission computed tomography (SPECT) is required to confirm myocardial (and not blood pool) tracer uptake. A large international collaboration using a cohort of biopsy-proven AL and ATTR cardiac amyloidosis patients demonstrated that nuclear tracers provided 100% specificity when grade 2 or 3 uptake was seen in the absence of a monoclonal protein by serum or urine in individuals with heart failure and typical echocardiographic or CMR features of amyloidosis.[24] In addition, a multicenter study validated these results with ^{99m}Tc-PYP and additionally showed H/CL ratio greater than 1.6 conferred worse survival.[25] It is essential that lab testing excludes evidence of a monoclonal gammopathy in conjunction with nuclear imaging to properly interpret the testing results. For these reasons, ATTR cardiac amyloidosis can now be diagnosed using bone avid tracers and blood testing without the need for confirmatory cardiac tissue biopsy when properly applied. It is appropriate to note that there remains some disagreement in the optimal timing of imaging following tracer injection. That stated, with the adoption, awareness, and growing availability of this imaging technique, recognition of ATTR amyloidosis has increased. Nuclear techniques have noted ATTR amyloidosis in 16% of patients with aortic stenosis undergoing transcatheter aortic valve replacement and 5% of patients with presumed HCM, with 26% of those referred for HCM older than 80 years of age having cardiac amyloidosis. Although nuclear techniques hold great promise as a means to screen for ATTR amyloidosis when applied in the proper clinical context, endomyocardial biopsy remains necessary in cases of demonstrated monoclonal gammopathy or in cases of equivocal tracer uptake and high clinical suspicion. Although not widely available, positron emission tomography (PET) tracers specific for amyloid deposits (florbetapir, florbetaben, 11C-Pittsburgh-B) also identify cardiac amyloidosis and may prove clinically useful in the future.

BIOPSY

Endomyocardial biopsy remains the "gold standard" for diagnosis of cardiac amyloidosis and is considered 100% sensitive and specific if biopsy specimens are collected from multiple sites (four or more are recommended). Definitive typing for the precursor protein must be determined by immunohistochemistry or via the more preferred, laser dissection with tandem mass spectrometry (LC MS/MS) analysis. Endomyocardial biopsy carries a small but notable risk of perforation, tamponade, or access site complications and as such is reserved for confirmatory testing in suspected cases wherein imaging testing is inconclusive (or isolated AL cardiac amyloidosis). Abdominal fat aspirate with Congo red staining can be helpful; however, sensitivity for ATTRwt is low (only approximately 20%) and a negative result should not dissuade continued evaluation.[26] Biopsies of other sites (e.g., gastrointestinal), have widely reported sensitivities/specificities, and as with fat aspirate, a negative result should not dissuade further testing in scenarios of high clinical suspicion.

GENOTYPING

Genotyping of TTR is a final critical step in the ATTR amyloidosis diagnostic algorithm because it has implications for treatment as well as raises the possibility of gene inheritance for first-degree relatives. One approach proposed as means to achieve amyloidosis screening involves widespread genotyping. Such an approach can accurately identify known variants associated with ATTR amyloidosis, although it is important to note that clinical penetrance is unclear and varies with age and family history. This has been most widely explored for the pVal142Ile genotype. Although data clearly demonstrate that the inheritance of the pVal142Ile allele increases the risk of heart failure,[7] evidence from other studies suggest that the allele does not necessarily result in imaging evidence of ATTR amyloidosis.[27] Furthermore, a genotyping-only approach will fail to identify ATTRwt, the most common type of cardiac amyloidosis. Although rare, the possibility of non-TTR variants including gelsolin, AApoA1, A2, and AFib (fibrinogen) should be considered in the presence of defined cardiac amyloidosis and a strong family history with normal TTR gene sequence.

TABLE 53.2 Comparison of Diagnostic Imaging Modalities in Cardiac Amyloidosis

FEATURE	ECHOCARDIOGRAPHY	MRI	BONE SCINTIGRAPHY
Clinical clues	Pericardial or pleural effusions, thick right ventricle, small LV cavity, intra-atrial septal thickening, and impaired global longitudinal strain characteristically with sparing of the apex	Elevated native T1, increased extracellular volume fraction, late gadolinium enhancement in any pattern, abnormal gadolinium kinetics	Diagnostic for transthyretin amyloid cardiomyopathy (ATTR-CM) if normal light chain assays and grade 2/3 cardiac uptake with confirmation of myocardial retention by SPECT False positives due to AL cardiac amyloidosis, previous myocardial infarction, diffuse myocardial scarring, overlying previous rib fracture, blood pool, hydroxychloroquine toxicity, and unusual forms of cardiac amyloidosis (ApoA1)
Relative cost	$	$$	$
Specialized expertise required for interpretation	No	Yes	No
Exposure to ionizing radiation	No	No	Yes
Cardiac devices affect image quality	No	Yes	No
Can identify nonamyloid causes of LV thickening	Yes (valvular disease, HCM, diastolic function) though amyloid CM may also be present	Yes (infiltrative disease, HCM)	No
Distinguish AL and ATTR	No	No	Yes*
Markers of worse prognosis	Lower stroke volume, greater regional variation in global longitudinal strain, worse global longitudinal strain, lower MCF, low EF (late phase)	Late gadolinium enhancement, higher extracellular volume fraction, higher native T1	H/CL ratio ≥1.6 at 1 hr

AL, Amyloidogenic light chain; *ApoA1*, apolipoprotein A1; *EF*, ejection fraction; *H/CL*, heart to contralateral lung; *HCM*, hypertrophic cardiomyopathy; *LV*, left ventricle; *MCF*, myocardial contraction fraction; *SPECT*, Single-photon emission computed tomography.
*In the context of normal serum and urine immunofixation electrophoresis and serum kappa/lambda ratio.

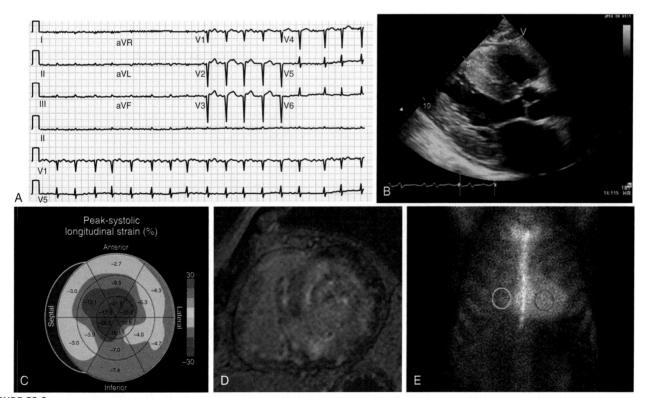

FIGURE 53.2 Electrocardiographic and imaging findings in cardiac amyloidosis. A 77-year-old male with dyspnea and palpitations presents for evaluation. **A,** Electrocardiogram (ECG) demonstrates atrial fibrillation, with low voltage in the limb leads and a pseudoinfarct pattern in the anterior leads. **B,** Still-frame image from parasternal long-axis echocardiogram illustrating severely increased wall thickness (19 mm) discordant from ECG low-voltage findings. **C,** Echocardiographic global longitudinal strain polar map showing apical-sparing pattern. **D,** Cardiac MR with phase-sensitive inversion recovery late gadolinium enhancement (PSIR-LGE) imaging demonstrating diffuse subendocardial and transmural enhancement. **E,** Planar Tc99m pyrophosphate (PYP) image showing grade 3 tracer uptake, confirmed by single-photon emission computed tomography (SPECT), with a heart to contralateral chest ratio of 1.7. Endomyocardial biopsy confirmed ATTRwt amyloidosis.

CLINICAL MANAGEMENT

Supportive Non–Disease-Modifying Therapies

In contrast to other etiologies of heart failure, the evidence basis underlying clinical management in cardiac amyloidosis, although increasing, remains sparse. As such, management strategies are largely drawn from smaller, nonrandomized, observational case series. That being stated, aforementioned consensus recommendations for imaging and a recently reported AHA Scientific Statement distilled available evidence into coherent recommendations to guide clinical management.[28] In general, the approach to a patient with cardiac amyloidosis involves treatment of the underlying cause (chemotherapy for AL, TTR-directed therapies for ATTR) and concurrent management of heart failure, arrhythmia, and concomitant symptoms. As such, the general principles underlying non–disease-modifying therapy for cardiac amyloidosis include symptom management, maintenance of euvolemia, avoidance of polypharmacy (particularly in elderly patients), avoidance of medications that may cause symptomatic hypotension, implantation of electrical devices (pacemakers, defibrillators), and consideration of advanced circulatory support/transplant for refractory heart failure in a minority of patients.

MANAGEMENT OF HEART FAILURE

Maintenance of euvolemia and optimization of perfusion in patients with cardiac amyloidosis can be a distinct challenge. Perturbations of filling hemodynamics from diastolic dysfunction with impairment of stroke volume (restriction), renal dysfunction from intrinsic renal disease, poor perfusion, or the cardiorenal syndrome, and in some individuals, concurrent autonomic dysfunction from amyloid neuropathy renders a very narrow range of tolerable circulating volume. Bioavailable loop diuretics and aldosterone antagonists are the preferred first-line agents with frequent dose adjustments to address changes in volume status that may result from concomitant chemotherapies for AL amyloidosis, such as steroids. Patients with orthostasis from poor vascular tone owing to impaired autonomic function may require the alpha-agonist midodrine to maintain adequate systolic blood pressure.

Evidence-based therapies that have proven beneficial in other causes of heart failure including ACE inhibitors, ARBs, ARNIs, and beta blockers are generally poorly tolerated in patients with advanced cardiac amyloidosis owing to fixed stroke volume and impaired hemodynamic compensatory mechanisms. Lower doses are often useful to manage hypertension or AF heart rate in earlier stage patients. Non-dihydropyridine calcium channel blockers (CCBs) are generally contraindicated in cardiac amyloidosis because they can bind amyloid fibrils (demonstrated in AL only), and worsen heart failure through heart-rate slowing, negative inotropy, and potentiation of conduction block. Interestingly, the affinity of TTR amyloid fibrils for various bone-seeking radiotracers is thought to be calcium related, thereby suggesting a potential mechanism for increased binding of CCBs to amyloid fibrils. Dihydropyridine CCBs may be useful as adjunctive agents for blood pressure management, particularly in the context of renal dysfunction, although potentiation of lower-extremity edema may limit application. Although an in vitro study demonstrated that isolated AL amyloid fibrils bind digoxin with high affinity, digoxin has been recently reconsidered if used cautiously as adjunctive management in AF rate control.[29]

ARRHYTHMIA MANAGEMENT

Atrial dysrhythmias, particularly AF and atrial flutter, are extremely common in ATTR amyloidosis and less commonly seen in AL amyloidosis. Management involves anticoagulation to prevent thromboembolism and rate control, and if exacerbating symptoms of heart failure, rhythm control is also appropriate. As with maintenance of euvolemia, heart rate control can also be challenging to optimize because both tachycardia and bradycardia are poorly tolerated, resulting from restrictive hemodynamics. Maintaining sinus rhythm and the atrial contribution to ventricular filling in cardiac amyloidosis may be less important because many patients have significantly reduced atrial mechanical function, reducing the atrial contribution to ventricular filling. Regularization and slowing of heart rate likely provide equal or greater benefit. The stroke risk among patients with AF and cardiac amyloidosis is exceedingly high because of blood stasis and elevated pressures, and atrial amyloid deposition may potentiate thrombosis. Left atrial appendage thrombosis has been observed in the context of normal sinus rhythm

and after therapeutic anticoagulation, underscoring the imperative to perform transesophageal echocardiography prior to attempts at restoration of sinus rhythm by cardioversion.[30] Heparins, vitamin K antagonists, or direct-acting oral anticoagulants are all effective in reducing thromboembolic risk and should be considered as indefinite therapy with minimal interruption. As specified in recent American College of Cardiology/American Heart Association/Heart Rhythm Society (ACC/AHA/HRS) recommendations, agents that may be used for rhythm control include amiodarone (most commonly) and dofetilide.[29] Data supporting the use of catheter ablation in cardiac amyloidosis are limited. In early-stage patients, cavotricuspid isthmus ablation may help to maintain sinus rhythm in the setting of atrial flutter, while pulmonary venous isolation procedures are generally less effective at controlling AF than in nonamyloid populations.

In ATTR in particular, deposits of amyloid fibrils infiltrate the conduction system, with a significant percentage of patients requiring permanent pacing. Pacing following AV junctional ablation for refractory AF management can also be considered. Biventricular pacing can be considered for patients with preexisting reduced LVEF. The routine use of automatic implantable cardioverter-defibrillators (ICDs) in patients with cardiac amyloidosis is debatable as sudden cardiac death related to ventricular tachycardia (VT) or ventricular fibrillation (VF) is relatively uncommon and mortality typically results from pulseless electrical activity. If anticipated survival is less than 1 year, then practice guidelines do not recommend ICD placement for the primary prevention of sudden cardiac death.[29] Device implantation for primary prevention is debatable, although ICD placement after aborted sudden death or sustained VT/VF is less controversial provided survival is expected to exceed 1 year.

ADVANCED CIRCULATORY SUPPORT AND ORGAN TRANSPLANTATION

Selected patients with advanced heart failure may qualify for orthotopic heart transplantation (OHT) and/or mechanical circulatory support (MCS) after careful assessment for the extent of systemic involvement. Acceptable outcomes have been reported in small series of carefully selected patients with AL that underwent OHT followed by treatment for AL (typically stem cell transplant–based regimens but more recently targeted anti-plasma cell therapy alone). Similarly, outcomes after OHT in ATTR patients with wild-type or cardiac-restricted variant disease (typically pVal142Ile) do not differ from those transplanted for other nonamyloid indications. Patients with ATTRv can be treated with OHT followed by TTR-specific pharmacotherapies to slow allograft TTR deposition. MCS with left ventricular assist devices (LVADs) or total artificial heart has been reported as a bridge to transplant in a small number of highly selected patients, but outcomes are worse in part because of small ventricular chamber size leading to suction events and, in the case of LVAD, concomitant right heart failure.

The majority of circulating TTR protein (95%) is produced by the liver. Orthotopic liver transplantation (OLT) replaces amyloidogenic mutant TTR with wild-type TTR and theoretically arrests amyloid formation. Prior to contemporary pharmaceutical therapies, OLT was the only available TTR-specific treatment for ATTRv amyloidosis. The treatment is largely effective among patients without demonstrable cardiac involvement; however, among those with cardiac amyloidosis, there is still a risk of progressive cardiac deposition after isolated OLT owing to continued wild-type TTR deposition upon the template of previous amyloid deposits. Combined OHT and OLT was formerly a strategy in ATTRv disease with a neuropathic *TTR* variant but has been largely rendered obsolete by contemporary therapies.[28]

Disease-Targeted Therapeutics
Light Chain Amyloidosis

The ultimate goal of chemotherapy for AL amyloidosis is elimination of the plasma cell clone that produces the amyloidogenic light chain. Arresting amyloid production reverses disease progression, preserves organ function, and enhances survival. Chemotherapeutics are drawn from the armamentarium of agents developed for multiple myeloma. The objective is attainment of a complete hematologic response (CR) defined as normalization of the involved free light chain and light chain ratio, elimination of a monoclonal band by immunofixation electrophoresis, and normalization of the bone marrow plasma cell population. Degrees of hematologic response are defined by the proportion of light chain reduction from complete, very good partial,

TABLE 53.3 Therapies for Amyloidogenic Transthyretin Amyloidosis

DRUG NAME	MECHANISM OF ACTION	INDICATION	ROUTE	DOSE	COMMON, SERIOUS OR POTENTIAL SIDE EFFECTS	CONCOMITANT THERAPY	MONITORING	COST
Patisiran	Silencer	Neuropathy	IV	0.3 mg/kg q3 weeks up to 30 mg	Infusion-related reactions Vitamin A deficiency	With IV infusion: • IV steroids • Acetaminophen • IV H1 blocker • IV H2 blocker • Daily vitamin A supplements	None	$450,000 annual list price $345,000 average effective net annual price
Inotersen	Silencer	Neuropathy	SQ	284 mg weekly	Thrombocytopenia/ glomerulonephritis, requiring testing before treatment and monitoring during therapy Infusion-site reactions, fever Vitamin A deficiency	Daily vitamin A supplements	Weekly platelet counts. Every 2 weeks measures of serum creatinine, eGFR urinalysis, and urine protein to creatinine ratio	$450,000 annual list price $345,000 average effective net annual price
Tafamidis meglumine	Stabilizer	Neuropathy/ Cardio-myopathy	Oral	20 mg once a day 80 mg once a day	Side effects were less common than with placebo in cardiomyopathy	None	None	€100,000 per year $225,000 per year
Tafamidis free salt	Stabilizer	Cardio-myopathy	Oral	61 mg once a day	Unknown	None	None	$225,000 per year
Diflunisal	Stabilizer	Neuropathy/ Cardio-myopathy	Oral	250 mg PO twice a day	Related to NSAID properties: • Bleeding • Hypertension • Fluid retention • Renal dysfunction	Proton pump inhibitor	Monitor renal function, platelet count, hemoglobin 1–2 weeks after initiation and then every 3 months	$300-500 per year

eGFR, Estimated glomerular filtration rate; *hATTR*, Hereditary transthyretin amyloidosis; *NSAID*, nonsteroidal antiinflammatory drug.

partial, and no response. As noted earlier, the biomarker scoring systems developed for prognosis are also used to follow response to treatment. First-line strategies vary by institutional experience and must be individualized to a particular patient. In appropriately selected patients managed at highly specialized referral centers with extensive experience, high-dose melphalan-based chemotherapy coupled with autologous stem cell transplant (HDM/SCT) can be applied as a means to rapidly reduce the light chain concentration. In such centers, a complete or very good partial response can be induced in approximately 60% of patients with a peritransplant mortality less than 2% while durable, long-term complete response (>15 years) can be achieved.[31] Eligibility for HDM/SCT is defined by various clinical parameters including (but not limited to) LVEF, pulmonary function, blood pressure, and performance status.[32] For those not eligible for HDM/SCT, contemporary advances in chemotherapy offer many alternative and highly effective options. Regimens include combinations of drugs such as proteasome inhibitors, immune modulators, and most recently, monoclonal antibodies. In specific, a monoclonal antibody targeting the CD38-receptor (daratumumab), developed for the treatment of patients with relapsed multiple myeloma, has produced a rapid and profound hematologic response with minimal toxicity.[33] This agent, which can be delivered subcutaneously, results in robust hematologic and organ responses with an acceptable safety profile.[34] Daratumumab is the first and only agent specifically approved by FDA for AL amyloidosis and is now

considered first line therapy in combination with cytoxan, bortizimib, and dexamthasone.

Transthyretin Amyloidosis

There are numerous pharmacologic strategies developed to ameliorate ATTR amyloidosis, including TTR silencing or knockdown, TTR stabilization, and TTR amyloid fibril disruption/extraction (Table 53.3). Presently, there are three U.S. Food and Drug Administration (FDA)-approved therapies for ATTR amyloidosis including the TTR silencers patisiran and inotersen, and the TTR stabilizer tafamidis, with additional novel agents in clinical trials. In addition, the FDA-approved nonsteroidal antiinflammatory drug (NSAID) diflunisal has been repurposed for ATTR amyloidosis treatment and demonstrated efficacy in smaller, nonrandomized, retrospective studies.

TTR Stabilizers

As a therapeutic class, TTR stabilizers are orally available small molecules that bind to TTR and inhibit its dissociation and subsequent amyloid fibril formation. Tafamidis is a benzoxazole derivative lacking NSAID activity specifically engineered to bind to the thyroxine-binding sites of TTR with high affinity and selectivity, stabilizing the tetramer and slowing dissociation and subsequent aggregation. The efficacy of tafamidis in ATTR cardiac amyloidosis was demonstrated in the phase III clinical study Amyloid Transthyretin

Amyloidosis Cardiomyopathy Trial (ATTR-ACT), where treatment resulted in lower all-cause mortality and reduction in cardiovascular hospitalizations.[35] Treatment also resulted in a lower rate of decline in distance for the 6-minute walk test and in the Kansas City Cardiomyopathy Questionnaire (KCCQ-OS) as compared with controls. Tafamidis was approved in May of 2019 as the only therapeutic approved for ATTRwt cardiac amyloidosis. Given its extremely high initial cost, the cost-effectiveness of the therapy was deemed poor despite the efficacy.[36]

Diflunisal is an NSAID that, like tafamidis, binds to the TTR tetramer at the thyroxine-binding site, kinetically stabilizing it from dissociation. Used off-label in a phase III study of patients with ATTRv amyloidosis, diflunisal at a reduced dose of 250 mg twice daily improved symptoms of amyloid polyneuropathy.[37] Retrospective studies have demonstrated the safety of diflunisal in selected patients with eGFR greater than 45 mL/min and efficacy as determined by improved echocardiographic markers of decline with increased survival in treated patients. Diflunisal has emerged as a cost-effective alternative therapy in selected patients with careful monitoring of volume status and renal function.[4] An additional stabilizer with a separate molecular TTR-binding site (acoramidis, or AG10) is currently in a phase III clinical trial with promising preliminary results from smaller phase II studies.[38]

TTR Silencers

TTR protein silencers hold great promise to halt or even reverse ATTR cardiac amyloidosis by significantly reducing circulating TTR. Patisiran is a small interfering RNA (siRNA) delivered intravenously that specifically targets hepatic TTR messenger RNA (mRNA) to elicit degradation and subsequent inhibition of TTR protein translation. Administered every 3 weeks, the drug reduces circulating TTR protein levels by approximately 90%. Patisiran must be co-administered with corticosteroids and histamine receptor blockers to blunt immune/histamine response. Efficacy of patisiran in ATTRv amyloidosis with polyneuropathy was demonstrated in the phase III APOLLO trial, where patients randomized to active drug experienced improved neuropathy (as measured by the modified neuropathy impairment score, mNIS+7) and quality of life.[39] More than 50% of patients in APOLLO had cardiac amyloid involvement, and in a cardiac subgroup analysis with wall thickness greater than 13 mm, patisiran resulted in significant improvements in NT-proBNP, LV wall thickness, global longitudinal strain, and gait speed compared with placebo.[40] Patisiran was approved by the FDA for ATTRv amyloidosis and polyneuropathy, with or without cardiomyopathy. Patisiran and another RNA interfering therapeutic, vutrisiran (delivered subcutaneously every 3 months) are presently being evaluated in phase III trials of cardiac amyloidosis patients that includes those with ATTRwt.

The 2′-O-methoxyethyl–modified antisense oligonucleotide inotersen is a short synthetic RNA that binds and inhibits translation of target hepatic *TTR* mRNA, thereby suppressing expression. Efficacy of inotersen in ATTRv amyloidosis in ameliorating clinically assessed polyneuropathy and quality of life was demonstrated in the NEURO-TTR study.[41] Inotersen received FDA approval for ATTRv amyloid polyneuropathy with or without cardiomyopathy (as in patisiran). Both agents were deemed not cost-effective in cost-effective analyses based on current U.S. prices.[42] Given observed toxicities of thrombocytopenia and glomerulonephritis (both 3%), inotersen was approved with a Risk Evaluation and Mitigation Strategy (REMS) that includes weekly monitoring of platelet counts and every 2-week monitoring of renal function and urinary protein. A small, open-label study of inotersen in patients with ATTR cardiomyopathy demonstrated stabilization of LV wall thickness, mass, global longitudinal strain, and functional capacity.[43] Ongoing clinical trials of inotersen and the related ligand-conjugated antisense oligonucleotide (LICA, trial CADRIO-TTRansform) in ATTR cardiac amyloidosis, including ATTRwt, are ongoing. A promising, early-stage report of a clustered regularly interspaced short palindromic repeats and associated Cas9 endonuclease (CRISPR-Cas9) based therapeutic (NTLA-2001) affords the potential for permanent silencing of TTR expression.[44]

CONCLUSION

The diagnostic and therapeutic landscape for cardiac amyloidosis has dramatically changed over the recent past. A disease that formerly was conceived as uncommon and untreatable is now increasingly recognized with available therapies that dramatically extend survival and mitigate symptoms. Advances in noninvasive diagnosis coupled with concurrent demonstration of efficacy and approval of specific therapies has shifted cardiac amyloidosis from a rarely encountered and untreatable "zebra," to a condition that cardiovascular clinicians should consider in daily practice.

REFERENCES

Etiologies

1. Sipe JD, Cohen AS. Review: history of the amyloid fibril. *J Struct Biol*. 2000;130:88–98.
2. Wechalekar AD, Gillmore JD, Hawkins PN. Systemic amyloidosis. *Lancet*. 2016;387:2641–2654.
3. Merlini G, Dispenzieri A, Sanchorawala V, et al. Systemic immunoglobulin light chain amyloidosis. *Nat Rev Dis Primers*. 2018;4:38.
4. Ruberg FL, Grogan M, Hanna M, et al. Transthyretin amyloid cardiomyopathy: JACC state-of-the-art review. *J Am Coll Cardiol*. 2019;73:2872–2891.
5. Castano A, Narotsky DL, Hamid N, et al. Unveiling transthyretin cardiac amyloidosis and its predictors among elderly patients with severe aortic stenosis undergoing transcatheter aortic valve replacement. *Eur Heart J*. 2017;38:2879–2887.
6. Buxbaum JN, Ruberg FL. Transthyretin V122I (pV142I)* cardiac amyloidosis: an age-dependent autosomal dominant cardiomyopathy too common to be overlooked as a cause of significant heart disease in elderly African Americans. *Genet Med*. 2017;19:733–742.
7. Damrauer SM, Chaudhary K, Cho JH, et al. Association of the V122I hereditary transthyretin amyloidosis genetic variant with heart failure among individuals of African or Hispanic/Latino ancestry. *J Am Med Assoc*. 2019;322:2191–2202.
8. Maurer MS, Hanna M, Grogan M, et al. Genotype and phenotype of transthyretin cardiac amyloidosis: THAOS (transthyretin amyloid outcome survey). *J Am Coll Cardiol*. 2016;68:161–172.
9. Suhr OB, Lundgren E, Westermark P. One mutation, two distinct disease variants: unravelling the impact of transthyretin amyloid fibril composition. *J Intern Med*. 2017;281:337–347.
10. Lane T, Fontana M, Martinez-Naharro A, et al. Natural history, quality of life, and outcome in cardiac transthyretin amyloidosis. *Circulation*. 2019;140:16–26.

Diagnosis

11. Kumar S, Dispenzieri A, Lacy MQ, et al. Revised prognostic staging system for light chain amyloidosis incorporating cardiac biomarkers and serum free light chain measurements. *J Clin Oncol*. 2012;30:989–995.
12. Lilleness B, Ruberg FL, Mussinelli R, et al. Development and validation of a survival staging system incorporating BNP in patients with light chain amyloidosis. *Blood*. 2019;133:215–223.
13. Falk RH, Quarta CC, Dorbala S. How to image cardiac amyloidosis. *Circ Cardiovasc Imaging*. 2014;7:552–562.
14. Gillmore JD, Damy T, Fontana M, et al. A new staging system for cardiac transthyretin amyloidosis. *Eur Heart J*. 2018;39:2799–2806.
15. Grogan M, Scott CG, Kyle RA, et al. Natural history of wild-type transthyretin cardiac amyloidosis and risk stratification using a novel staging system. *J Am Coll Cardiol*. 2016;68:1014–1020.
16. Witteles RM, Bokhari S, Damy T, et al. Screening for transthyretin amyloid cardiomyopathy in everyday practice. *JACC Heart Failure*. 2019;7:709–716.
17. Aljama MA, Sidiqi MH, Dispenzieri A, et al. Comparison of different techniques to identify cardiac involvement in immunoglobulin light chain (AL) amyloidosis. *Blood Adv*. 2019;3:1226–1229.
18. Phull P, Sanchorawala V, Connors LH, et al. Monoclonal gammopathy of undetermined significance in systemic transthyretin amyloidosis (ATTR). *Amyloid*. 2018;25:62–67.
19. Arvanitis M, Simon S, Chan G, et al. Retinol binding protein 4 (RBP4) concentration identifies V122I transthyretin cardiac amyloidosis. *Amyloid*. 2017;24:120–121.
20. Dorbala S, Ando Y, Bokhari S, et al. ASNC/AHA/ASE/EANM/HFSA/ISA/SCMR/SNMMI expert consensus recommendations for multimodality imaging in cardiac amyloidosis: Part 1 of 2-evidence base and standardized methods of imaging. *J Card Fail*. 2019;25:e1–e39.
21. Dorbala S, Ando Y, Bokhari S, et al. ASNC/AHA/ASE/EANM/HFSA/ISA/SCMR/SNMMI expert consensus recommendations for multimodality imaging in cardiac amyloidosis: Part 2 of 2-diagnostic criteria and appropriate utilization. *J Card Fail*. 2019;25:854–865.
22. Pagourelias ED, Mirea O, Duchenne J, et al. Echo parameters for differential diagnosis in cardiac amyloidosis: a head-to-head Comparison of deformation and nondeformation parameters. *Circ Cardiovasc Imaging*. 2017;10:e005588.
23. Martinez-Naharro A, Baksi AJ, Hawkins PN, Fontana M. Diagnostic imaging of cardiac amyloidosis. *Nat Rev Cardiol*. 2020;17:413–426.
24. Gillmore JD, Maurer MS, Falk RH, et al. Nonbiopsy diagnosis of cardiac transthyretin amyloidosis. *Circulation*. 2016;133:2404-2012.
25. Castano A, Haq M, Narotsky DL, et al. Multicenter study of planar technetium 99m pyrophosphate cardiac imaging: predicting survival for patients with ATTR cardiac amyloidosis. *JAMA Cardiol*. 2016;1:880–889.
26. Quarta CC, Gonzalez-Lopez E, Gilbertson JA, et al. Diagnostic sensitivity of abdominal fat aspiration in cardiac amyloidosis. *Eur Heart J*. 2017;38:1905–1908.
27. Quarta CC, Buxbaum JN, Shah AM, et al. The amyloidogenic V122I transthyretin variant in elderly black Americans. *N Engl J Med*. 2015;372:21–29.

Management

28. Kittleson MM, Maurer MS, Ambardekar AV, et al. Cardiac amyloidosis: evolving diagnosis and management: a scientific statement from the American heart association. *Circulation*. 2020;142:e7–e22.
29. Towbin JA, McKenna WJ, Abrams DJ, et al. 2019 HRS expert consensus statement on evaluation, risk stratification, and management of arrhythmogenic cardiomyopathy. *Heart Rhythm*. 2019;16:e301–e372.
30. El-Am EA, Dispenzieri A, Melduni RM, et al. Direct current cardioversion of atrial arrhythmias in adults with cardiac amyloidosis. *J Am Coll Cardiol*. 2019;73:589–597.
31. Muchtar E, Gertz MA, Kumar SK, et al. Improved outcomes for newly diagnosed AL amyloidosis over the years 2000–2014: cracking the glass ceiling of early death. *Blood*. 2017;129:2111–2119.
32. Varga C, Comenzo RL. High-dose melphalan and stem cell transplantation in systemic AL amyloidosis in the era of novel anti-plasma cell therapy: a comprehensive review. *Bone Marrow Transplant*. 2019;54:508–518.
33. Sanchorawala V, Sarosiek S, Schulman A, et al. Safety, tolerability, and response rates of daratumumab in relapsed AL amyloidosis: results of a phase 2 study. *Blood*. 2020;135:1541–1547.

34. Palladini G, Kastritis E, Maurer MS, et al. Daratumumab plus CyBorD for patients with newly diagnosed AL amyloidosis: safety run-in results of ANDROMEDA. *Blood.* 2020;136:71–80.

35. Maurer MS, Schwartz JH, Gundapaneni B, et al. Tafamidis treatment for patients with transthyretin amyloid cardiomyopathy. *N Engl J Med.* 2018;379:1007–1016.

36. Kazi DS, Bellows BK, Baron SJ, et al. Cost-effectiveness of tafamidis therapy for transthyretin amyloid cardiomyopathy. *Circulation.* 2020;141:1214–1224.

37. Berk JL, Suhr OB, Obici L, et al. Repurposing diflunisal for familial amyloid polyneuropathy a randomized clinical trial. *J Am Med Assoc.* 2013;310:2658–2667.

38. Judge DP, Falk RH, Maurer MS, et al. Transthyretin stabilization by AG10 in symptomatic transthyretin amyloid cardiomyopathy. *J Am Coll Cardiol.* 2019.

39. Adams D, Gonzalez-Duarte A, O'Riordan WD, et al. Patisiran, an RNAi therapeutic, for hereditary transthyretin amyloidosis. *N Engl J Med.* 2018;379:11–21.

40. Scott D, Solomon DA, Kristen A, et al. Effects of patisiran, an RNA interference therapeutic, on cardiac parameters in patients with hereditary transthyretin-mediated amyloidosis: an analysis of the APOLLO study. *Circulation.* 2019;139(4):431–443.

41. Benson MD, Waddington-Cruz M, Berk JL, et al. Inotersen treatment for patients with hereditary transthyretin amyloidosis. *N Eng J Med.* 2018;379:22–31.

42. Inotersen and Patisiran for Hereditary Transthyretin Amyloidosis. *Effectiveness and Value Evidence Report.* Institute for Clinical and Economic Review (ICER); 2018.

43. Dasgupta NR, Benson MD. Treatment of ATTR cardiomyopathy with a TTR specific antisense oligonucleotide, inotersen. *Amyloid.* 2019;26:20–21.

44. Gillmore JD, Gane E, Taubel J, et al. CRISPR-Cas9 in vivo gene editing for transthyretin amyloidosis. *N Engl J Med* 2021;385:493–502.

54 Hypertrophic Cardiomyopathy

CAROLYN Y. HO AND STEVE R. OMMEN

Hypertrophic cardiomyopathy (HCM) is a primary disorder of the myocardium. It is defined by the presence of unexplained left ventricular hypertrophy (LVH), occurring in the absence of identifiable factors that may account for increased left ventricular wall thickness, including pressure overload and infiltrative or storage disorders. Classically, myocyte hypertrophy, disarray, and myocardial fibrosis are present histologically. The prevalence has been estimated to be 1 in 500 in the general population. Familial disease is well characterized, and pathogenic variants in the genes encoding the cardiac sarcomere are the most common etiology of HCM. Pathogenic sarcomeric variants are present in more than 60% of patients with a family history of HCM, but are also seen in individuals with sporadic disease. However, the cause of disease cannot be easily identified in many patients. Additionally, there is substantial heterogeneity in cardiac morphology and disease course, ranging from low symptom burden and relatively normal longevity to marked functional limitations, advanced heart failure, and sudden cardiac death. Clinical management requires assessment of the individual patient's pathophysiology and symptoms, as well as systematic evaluation of family members. This chapter describes the diagnosis, natural history, and management of HCM.

DIAGNOSIS, MORPHOLOGY, AND ETIOLOGY OF HYPERTROPHIC CARDIOMYOPATHY

Diagnosis and Morphology

Hypertrophic cardiomyopathy (HCM) is a highly complex disorder with a myriad of effects on the heart. Historically and currently the diagnosis of HCM has relied solely on the most overt feature: left ventricular hypertrophy that has developed in the absence of an obvious cause. In many ways this remains a diagnosis of exclusion. A maximum left ventricular wall thickness of ≥15 mm has been the standard threshold to diagnose disease in adults, although a threshold of ≥13 mm is recommended if there is a family history of HCM or if the individual in question carries a disease-causing (pathogenic) sarcomeric gene variant.[1] Standards for diagnosing pediatric-onset HCM have been more variable but typically require a left ventricular wall thickness at least two standard deviations greater than the body surface area–corrected population mean (z score ≥2.5).[2,3]

At the histopathologic level, HCM is characterized by myocyte hypertrophy, disarray, and fibrosis (Fig. 54.1). These intrinsic tissue abnormalities, particularly myocyte hypertrophy and myocardial fibrosis, likely contribute to clinical manifestations of heart failure (systolic and diastolic) and to the genesis of arrhythmias (ventricular and atrial). Notably, these histologic changes are not uniformly distributed and affect deeper layers of the myocardium; therefore endocardial biopsy is generally not useful in yielding a tissue diagnosis of HCM.

The location and degree of hypertrophy are variable, and ventricular volumes are typically small. Although asymmetric septal hypertrophy resulting in reversed septal curvature is the classic and most common morphologic subtype of HCM, hypertrophy can involve any left ventricular (LV) segment and may be focal or concentric (Fig. 54.2). Apical HCM is a well-described morphologic variant in which hypertrophy involves the distal LV, below the level of the papillary muscles. As such, apical HCM is not associated with left ventricular outflow tract obstruction (LVOTO). Apical HCM was first reported in Japan[4] and is more prevalent in individuals of Japanese versus European descent (13% to 25% vs. 1% to 2%).[5] Although early studies suggested a more benign prognosis for apical HCM, a broad spectrum of clinical outcomes has been described.[6]

Septal morphology and location of hypertrophy are moderately predictive of genetic background. Patients with classic reversed septal curvature are most likely to have pathogenic sarcomeric gene variants whereas patients with a sigmoidal septum (discrete upper septal thickening) or apical hypertrophy are least likely to have sarcomeric disease.[7,8] This latter pattern of hypertrophic remodeling is relatively common in older adults with hypertension and thus nonspecific. However, even within families with HCM who share the same underlying pathogenic sarcomeric variant, both the degree and morphology of hypertrophy are often varied.[9]

The differential diagnosis for HCM includes other conditions that may also result in increased left ventricular wall thickness, including syndromic, metabolic, storage, or infiltrative disorders (e.g., Noonan syndrome/RASopathies, Fabry disease, Pompe disease, cardiac amyloidosis, mitochondrial disease) and compensatory or secondary hypertrophic heart disease attributed to pressure overload (hypertension) or intense athletic training. These disorders are genocopies—phenotypically similar but genetically different—that mimic HCM as they share a common feature of cardiac hypertrophy. However, they are distinct from HCM and have different underlying pathobiology and natural history (Table 54.1). For HCM to be diagnosed with confidence, these conditions should be excluded. Age of presentation can be informative. Family history should be carefully ascertained to determine if disease is genetic, and if so, the pattern of inheritance can provide valuable information. Clinical features and physical examination should focus on identifying key extracardiac features, such as bilateral carpal tunnel

Additional content is available online at Elsevier eBooks for Practicing Clinicians

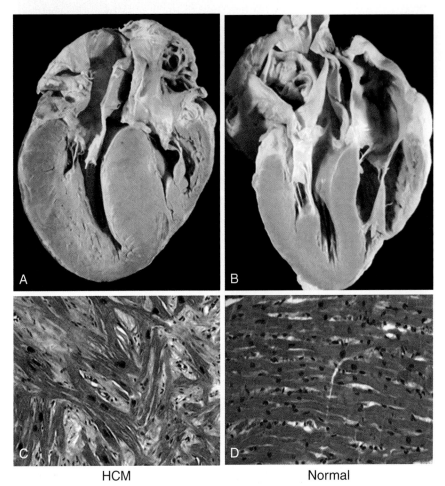

HCM   Normal

FIGURE 54.1 Gross and microscopic appearance of hypertrophic cardiomyopathy (HCM). **A** and **C,** HCM characterized by left ventricular hypertrophy, myocyte disarray, and myocardial fibrosis. **B**and **D,** Normal heart.

disease. The cause of HCM in patients who do not carry sarcomere variants (non-sarcomeric HCM) remains largely unknown but likely reflects more complex interactions between genetic background and environment.

The sarcomere (Fig. 54.4) is the fundamental unit of contraction of all muscle cells. Cardiac sarcomeric proteins are organized into thick (myosin heavy and light chains, myosin binding protein C) and thin (actin, the troponin complex, and α-tropomyosin) filaments that interdigitate with muscle fiber shortening and lengthening. Excitation-contraction coupling relies on highly coordinated alterations in protein confirmation and calcium flux to drive thick and thin filament interaction and cardiac contraction and relaxation.[15] Membrane depolarization by the action potential elicits calcium influx through L-type calcium channels on the cardiomyocyte membrane. Ryanodine receptors on the sarcoplasmic reticulum (SR) are then activated to trigger calcium-induced calcium release. With the resultant increase in intracellular Ca^{2+} concentration, calcium binds to troponin C, leading to conformational changes in troponins I and T that release steric hindrance of tropomyosin from actin, permitting actin-myosin cross-bridge formation. Adenosine triphosphate (ATP) is then hydrolyzed to allow actin-myosin detachment and reuptake of calcium into the SR through the sarcoplasmic reticulum calcium-ATPase (SERCA) to complete the heart's chemomechanical cycle.

The exact mechanisms by which sarcomeric gene variants lead to the complex phenotype of HCM are not completely understood and likely involve multiple underlying pathways. Most pathogenic variants that cause HCM appear to act in a dominant negative or poison peptide fashion whereby mutant proteins are incorporated into the sarcomere and alter contractile performance.[16,17] *MYBPC3* is an exception in that the majority of pathogenic variants in *MYBPC3* result in premature termination codons and haploinsufficiency appears to be the predominant mechanism of disease.[18–20] Animal and basic science models have identified increased force generation, increased calcium sensitivity, impaired and disordered relaxation, and abnormal myocardial energetics, including increased energy consumption, as fundamental abnormalities associated with sarcomeric variants and HCM.[18,21–25]

Some of these fundamental findings have been corroborated by investigating individuals who carry pathogenic sarcomeric gene variants but have not yet developed a clinically overt phenotype of HCM. Studying these at-risk preclinical or subclinical variant carriers allows interrogation of the early manifestations of sarcomeric variants without confounding effects created by pathophysiologic abnormalities that accompany cardiac remodeling and disease development. Abnormalities in myocardial structure, function, and biochemistry are identifiable prior to the development of LVH. Decreased LV cavity size,[26] impaired LV relaxation, increased LV ejection fraction (LVEF),[27,28] altered myocardial energetics,[22,29] electrocardiographic abnormalities,[30] increased mitral valve leaflet length,[31,32] and evidence of a profibrotic state[33,34] can be identified in sarcomeric variant carriers when left ventricular wall thickness is normal. These findings also emphasize that although LVH is the most obvious manifestation, it is not an absolute marker of HCM. Further investigation is needed to characterize the entire spectrum of disease.

syndrome, biceps tendon rupture, skin changes (suggesting amyloidosis, particularly transthyretin [ATTR] amyloidosis), plasma cell dyscrasias (suggesting light chain (AL) amyloidosis), skin, neurologic and renal involvement (suggesting Fabry disease), and syndromic features (suggesting Noonan syndrome and mitochondrial disease). Cardiac magnetic resonance imaging (CMR) can help characterize myocardial tissue composition, identifying evidence of fibrosis or other infiltrative processes; however, biopsy (myocardial or of another affected site) is sometimes warranted to obtain a tissue diagnosis. Genetic testing can also provide key information to differentiate HCM from genocopies that also result in increased LV wall thickness (see Genetic Testing section later).

Etiology and Genetic Basis of Hypertrophic Cardiomyopathy

HCM was the first genetic cardiomyopathy to be characterized at the molecular level. Seminal genetic studies performed on families with HCM in the 1980s to 1990s established that HCM is a disease of the sarcomere—most frequently caused by pathogenic variation in genes encoding cardiac-specific sarcomeric proteins (Table 54.2), particularly myosin binding protein C (*MYBPC3*), myosin heavy chain (*MYH7*), troponin T (*TNNT2*), troponin I (*TNNI3*), myosin light chains (*MYL2* and *MYL3*), alpha-tropomyosin (*TPM1*), and actin (*ACTC*).[10–13] Sarcomeric variants are found in approximately 30% of HCM patients with apparently sporadic disease and over 60% of patients with a family history of HCM[14] or among those diagnosed in childhood. Variants in MYBPC3 and *MYH7* are most common; collectively responsible for over 80% of sarcomeric HCM (caused by pathogenic sarcomeric variants identified by genetic testing) (Fig. 54.3). The population prevalence of HCM is approximately 1:500,[1] making it the most common monogenic heart

PATHOPHYSIOLOGY

The clinical manifestations of HCM can be tied to a complex interplay of cellular abnormalities, impaired myocardial function, and anatomic changes that alter hemodynamics, and may predispose to

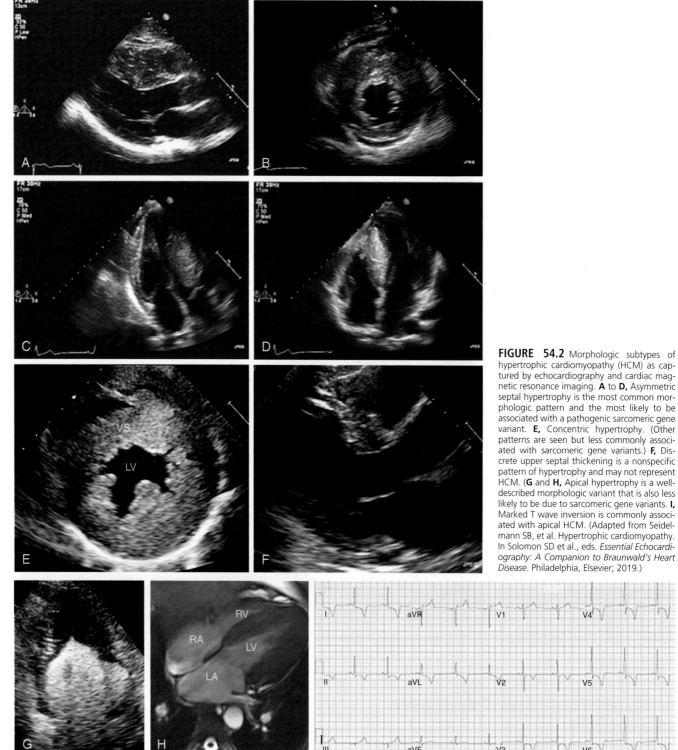

FIGURE 54.2 Morphologic subtypes of hypertrophic cardiomyopathy (HCM) as captured by echocardiography and cardiac magnetic resonance imaging. **A** to **D,** Asymmetric septal hypertrophy is the most common morphologic pattern and the most likely to be associated with a pathogenic sarcomeric gene variant. **E,** Concentric hypertrophy. (Other patterns are seen but less commonly associated with sarcomeric gene variants.) **F,** Discrete upper septal thickening is a nonspecific pattern of hypertrophy and may not represent HCM. (**G** and **H,** Apical hypertrophy is a well-described morphologic variant that is also less likely to be due to sarcomeric gene variants. **I,** Marked T wave inversion is commonly associated with apical HCM. (Adapted from Seidelmann SB, et al. Hypertrophic cardiomyopathy. In Solomon SD et al., eds. *Essential Echocardiography: A Companion to Braunwald's Heart Disease.* Philadelphia, Elsevier; 2019.)

development of arrhythmias. At the cellular level, abnormal calcium handling and altered interaction between actin-myosin has been identified, leading to abnormal contraction and relaxation. Coupled with the inherent stiffness of the hypertrophied left ventricle, some degree of diastolic dysfunction is present in nearly all patients with HCM.[35–37] Early diastolic tissue Doppler velocities are reduced in most patients with HCM, and abnormalities can be identified before the development of overt LVH in individuals who carry pathogenic sarcomeric variants.[38,39] Because the capillary network is less dense in HCM, subendocardial ischemia is readily manifest and can further worsen diastolic

function. Delayed relaxation impacts the entire left ventricle at the macroscopic and myofilament level and also has carry-over effects on systolic function. However, contractile function has been more difficult to characterize. Animal, tissue, and cellular models of HCM have generally, but not universally, suggested increased contractility. There is some evidence suggesting that individuals who carry pathogenic sarcomeric variants but have not yet developed HCM (preclinical HCM) have preserved or slightly increased systolic strain by echo.[27,40] However, echocardiographic and CMR-derived systolic strain are abnormal in most patients with clinically overt HCM, potentially as a result of developing

TABLE 54.1 Genocopies of Hypertrophic Cardiomyopathy and Differentiating Features

ETIOLOGIES	TYPICAL AGE AT PRESENTATION	SYSTEMIC FEATURES	DIAGNOSTIC CONSIDERATIONS
RASopathies	Infants (0–12 months) and toddlers	Dysmorphic features	Geneticist assessment and genetic testing
Glycogen storage diseases, other metabolic or mitochondrial diseases		Failure to thrive	
		Metabolic acidosis	Newborn metabolic screening and additional metabolic assessment
RASopathies	Early childhood	Dysmorphic features	Biochemical screening
Mitochondrial diseases		Delayed or abnormal cognitive development	Genetic testing
		Visual or hearing impairment	
Friedrich ataxia	School age and adolescence	Skeletal muscle weakness or movement disorder	Biochemical screening
Danon disease			Neuromuscular assessment
Mitochondrial disease			Genetic testing
Friedrich ataxia	Late adolescence and adulthood	Movement disorder	Biochemical screening
Glycogen storage disorder (e.g., Fabry disease)		Peripheral or autonomic neuropathy	Neuromuscular assessment
Infiltrative disorders (e.g., light chain (AL) or transthyretin (ATTR) cardiac amyloidosis)		Renal dysfunction	Genetic testing
		Skin involvement	Biopsy
		Plasma cell dyscrasia	
		Bilateral carpal tunnel syndrome, biceps tendon rupture	

Adapted from Ommen SR, Mital S, Burke MA, et al. AHA/ACC guideline for the diagnosis and treatment of patients with hypertrophic cardiomyopathy: a report of the American College of Cardiology/American Heart Association Joint Committee on Clinical Practice Guidelines. *J Am Coll Cardiol.* 2020;76(25):e159–e240.

TABLE 54.2 Major Genes Associated with Hypertrophic Cardiomyopathy and Genocopies

CORE SARCOMERIC GENES	PROTEIN ENCODED	% HCM ATTRIBUTABLE[4]
MYBPC3	Cardiac myosin-binding protein C	~50%
MYH7	Cardiac β myosin heavy chain	30%–35%
TNNI3	Cardiac troponin I	~5%
TNNT2	Cardiac troponin T	~5%
TPM1	α-tropomyosin	<3%
MYL2	Myosin regulatory light chain	<3%
MYL3	Myosin essential light chain	<3%
ACTC1	α-cardiac actin	~1%
Other HCM-Associated Genes		
CSRP3	Muscle LIM protein	<1%
TNNC1	Cardiac troponin C	<1%
ACTN2	α-actinin	<1%
JPH2	Junctophilin-2	Rare
Genocopies		
Storage Diseases		
LAMP2 (Danon disease)	Lysosome-associated membrane protein 2 (X chromosome)	
PRKAG2 (Glycogen storage disease)	Protein Kinase AMP-Activated Non-Catalytic Subunit Gamma 2	
GLA (Fabry disease)	α-galactosidase (X chromosome)	
Infiltrative Disease		
TTR (familial amyloidosis)	Transthyretin	
Noonan syndrome/RASopathies		
PTPN11 (Noonan syndrome)	Protein tyrosine phosphatase non-receptor type 11	
RAF1	Raf-1 Proto-Oncogene	

HCM, Hypertrophic cardiomyopathy.

myocardial abnormalities (fibrosis, disarray, hypertrophy) that accompany clinically overt disease. Moreover, calculated LVEF may not be a reliable measure of overall systolic function in HCM as the small LV cavity size associated with HCM is in the denominator of the formula and may artificially elevate ejection fraction. Accordingly, patients with HCM are considered to have significantly impaired systolic function if the ejection fraction less than 50%.

The most clinically apparent, and treatable, pathophysiologic mechanism in HCM is that of LVOTO.[41–43] Obstruction is present at rest or with physiologic provocation in up to two-thirds of patients with HCM and occurs as the hypertrophied septum redirects flow across, rather than along the mitral valve, which causes systolic anterior motion (SAM), further narrowing the outflow tract. The mitral valve itself is often elongated and positioned more anteriorly, which amplifies this effect.[44,45] The anterior mitral leaflet, rather than closing normally, is pushed further into the outflow tract, narrowing the latter and interfering with coaptation. Together, this results in increased LV systolic pressure and obstruction to outflow, particularly in late systole, increased myocardial oxygen demand, and posteriorly directed mitral regurgitation (Fig. 54.5). Patients are considered to have obstructive physiology if they have maximum instantaneous gradients across the outflow tract of at least 30 mm Hg. Resting or provoked gradients exceeding 40 to 50 mm Hg are considered capable of causing limiting symptoms. Patients with effort-related symptoms and resting LVOT gradients less than 40 mm Hg should have provocative maneuvers included with noninvasive evaluation. Bedside maneuvers such as Valsalva or squat-to-stand can be helpful in identifying latent outflow obstruction.[46] Provocation with exercise (e.g., exercise echocardiography) is a highly relevant and physiologic method to assess effort intolerance and should be considered in patients with symptoms whose resting gradients are not sufficiently high to account for their symptoms.[47,48] Symptom management is discussed under "Clinical Management," later.

Atrial fibrillation (AF) is a common arrhythmia in patients with HCM and is associated with decreased quality of life and a relatively high risk for systemic thromboembolism.[49–51] The loss of atrial contribution to LV filling, and the compromised diastolic filling period with rapid heart rates can result in decreased LV preload and thereby increased LVOT gradient. Aggressive rate control or restoration of sinus rhythm, both in combination with oral anticoagulation are felt to be important for patients with HCM (see Clinical Management, Management of Atrial Fibrillation, later).

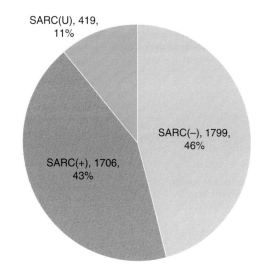

SARC(U), 419, 11%

SARC(−), 1799, 46%

SARC(+), 1706, 43%

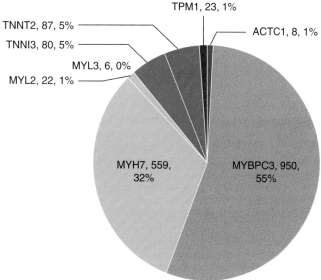

TPM1, 23, 1%

TNNT2, 87, 5%

TNNI3, 80, 5%

MYL3, 6, 0%

MYL2, 22, 1%

ACTC1, 8, 1%

MYH7, 559, 32%

MYBPC3, 950, 55%

FIGURE 54.3 Top, Prevalence of sarcomeric versus nonsarcomeric hypertrophic cardiomyopathy (HCM). Examining 3924 HCM probands who had genetic testing and are cared for at high-volume HCM centers participating in the multicenter Sarcomeric Human Cardiomyopathy Registry (SHaRe),[49] 43% had pathogenic or likely pathogenic sarcomeric variants (SARC(+)), 46% did not have clinically significant variants identified (SARC(−)), and 11% had sarcomeric variants of unknown significance (SARC(U)). **Bottom,** Distribution of sarcomeric genes in HCM. Focusing on patients with sarcomeric HCM, myosin heavy chain and myosin binding protein C are most commonly implicated, collectively accounting for over 80% of HCM with an identified genetic etiology. *MYH7,* Myosin heavy chain; *MYBPC3,* myosin binding protein C; *MYL2/MYL3,* myosin essential and regulatory light chain; *TNNI3,* troponin I; *TNNT2,* troponin T; *TPM1,* alpha-tropomyosin; *ACTC1,* actin.

Ventricular arrhythmias are also an important cause for concern in HCM.[52] Sudden cardiac arrest occurs in just less than 1% of patients with HCM each year necessitating periodic risk assessment to identify patients with features that suggest higher risk and who may benefit from implantable cardioverter-defibrillator (ICD) placement (see Clinical Management, Sudden Cardiac Death Risk Stratification later). Nonfatal ventricular arrhythmias can also be problematic for some patients. This is often felt to result from intramyocardial scar and/or apical LV aneurysm.

NATURAL HISTORY

Natural history has been difficult to study and accurately characterize because disease course is highly variable. Many patients experience relatively normal longevity and modest symptom burden, whereas many others experience adverse clinical outcomes including heart failure, arrhythmias, and sudden cardiac death. Several large, multicenter HCM registries have recently been developed to better characterize clinical

outcomes and their predictors.[49,53–55] Overall morbidity in HCM is dominated by heart failure and atrial fibrillation. Similarly, mortality is driven by complications of heart failure and noncardiac death, both of which are more common than lethal arrhythmias. Genotype is associated with clinical outcomes. Patients with sarcomeric HCM are diagnosed at an earlier age and had a greater burden and earlier onset of HCM-related complications than patients with nonsarcomeric HCM.[49,56–58] Sex also impacts the clinical course in HCM. Females are typically diagnosed at an older age and typically have more symptomatic heart failure and higher mortality.[59,60]

The lifetime cumulative burden of HCM was shown to be greatest in patients diagnosed earlier in life, and those with sarcomere mutations.[49] While the incidence of malignant ventricular arrhythmias and risk for sudden cardiac death decline with age, the risk for heart failure and atrial fibrillation increases. The majority of these HCM-related complications occur later in life, becoming most prevalent by middle to late adulthood, even in patients diagnosed before age 40 years (Fig. 54.6). These observations underscore the need for lifelong surveillance and for developing effective strategies to attenuate progressive disease burden.

Approximately 8% of patients with HCM experience more advanced cardiac remodeling marked by a decrease in LV systolic function.[61] Because HCM is characteristically associated with increased LVEF, an LVEF of 50% or less is abnormal and has traditionally defined HCM with LV systolic dysfunction (HCM-LVSD). Risk predictors for incident development of systolic dysfunction included the presence of pathogenic sarcomeric variants, particularly in thin filament genes, increased left ventricular wall thickness, left ventricular dilation, and borderline low ejection fraction (50% to 59%). The natural history of HCM-LVSD is variable; however, the majority of patients experience adverse events. Approximately one-third of patients died or required cardiac transplantation or durable mechanical support within a decade of developing systolic dysfunction.[61] Risk predictors of poor prognosis for patients with HCM-LVSD are multiple pathogenic/likely pathogenic sarcomeric variants, atrial fibrillation, and LVEF less than 35%.[61] Management is discussed later under "Clinical Management."

GENETIC TESTING AND FAMILY MANAGEMENT

Genetic Testing

The goals of genetic testing are to provide a definitive diagnosis in patients with known or suspected HCM and to guide management of at-risk or undiagnosed relatives.[62] There are two major types of genetic testing: diagnostic and predictive/variant confirmation testing in families. *Diagnostic genetic testing* is performed on an individual with unexplained LVH or a clinical diagnosis of HCM, typically using multigene panels specifically tailored for HCM that include at least the core sarcomeric genes (*MYH7, MYBPC3, TNNT2, TNNC1, TNNI3, TPM1, MYL2, MYL3, ACTC1*), as well as genes associated with other conditions that result in increased LV wall thickness, including glycogen storage disease and lysosome storage diseases (*LAMP2, PRKAG2, GLA* [Fabry disease], *GAA* [Pompe disease]), metabolic and mitochondrial disease, hereditary amyloidosis (*TTR*), and other genetic syndromes such as Noonan syndrome (involving genes in the Ras/MAP kinase pathway) (see Table 54.2). As such, diagnostic genetic testing can clarify diagnosis and identify the underlying disease process, including differentiating HCM from these genocopies. Accurately making these distinctions will critically impact clinical management.

One of the greatest challenges for genetic testing is determining whether an identified sequence variant is the cause of disease. In contrast to typical laboratory testing, genetic testing is probabilistic and classifies variants along a continuum that reflects the estimated likelihood that a variant is disease causing, based on current evidence. The American College of Medical Genetics and Genomics and the Association for Molecular Pathology developed guidelines for variant interpretation, proposing five tiers of classification: pathogenic, likely pathogenic, uncertain significance, likely benign, and benign, drawing upon a variety of evidence, including population, functional, computational, and segregation data to determine classification.[63] Variants classified as pathogenic and likely pathogenic are generally considered

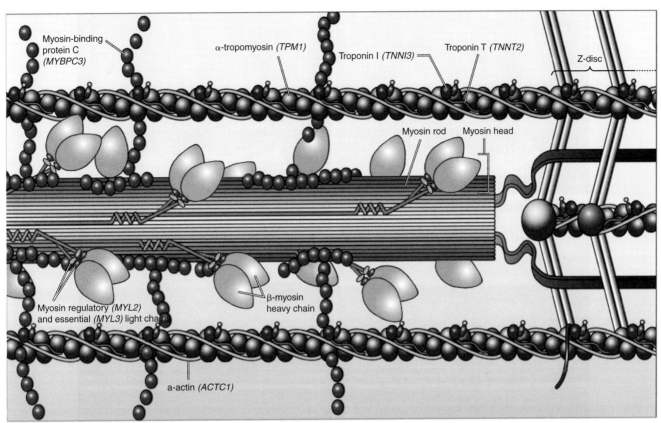

FIGURE 54.4 Cardiac sarcomere. The sarcomere is the fundamental unit of contraction for cardiac myocytes. Pathogenic variants in the genes that encode the different elements of the sarcomere are the most common genetic cause of hypertrophic cardiomyopathy. (Adapted from Seidelmann SB, et al. Hypertrophic cardiomyopathy. In Solomon SD et al., eds. *Essential Echocardiography: A Companion to Braunwald's Heart Disease*. Philadelphia, Elsevier; 2019.)

"positive" genetic testing results, meaning there is reasonable to high confidence that they are the genetic etiology of disease. These results may be considered for clinical decision making, including predictive genetic testing. A classification of a variant of uncertain significance (VUS) is an indeterminate result that does not provide a definitive genetic etiology and should not be used for clinical decision making or predicting risk in unaffected relatives. Negative results should be considered cautiously because this does not imply that genetic disease is excluded but rather indicates that a causative variant was not identified with available technology and knowledge. Clinical evaluation of at-risk healthy relatives is often still advisable. Additional genetic testing may be considered in the future if there are important advances in knowledge and technology. Furthermore, variants of uncertain significance should be reassessed periodically to determine if new data have emerged that allows reclassification into a more definitive category.

Family Management

Because HCM is often genetic, management extends beyond the individual patient to also include their family. The goals of family screening are to provide timely cardiac evaluation and initiate early treatment that may help mitigate adverse outcomes, particularly sudden death and symptomatic heart failure. The initial step is to obtain a multigenerational family history, ideally in pedigree format, to capture family structure, medical diagnoses and events, and ages and causes of death. This type of structured review assists in determining if familial disease is present, establish the inheritance pattern, and identify relatives at risk for developing disease. If familial disease is confirmed or cannot be excluded, clinical screening is performed to identify affected relatives and to follow currently unaffected relatives who are at risk for developing clinical disease.

The systematic process of evaluating relatives at risk for a genetic condition is termed cascade testing and may incorporate both clinical screening and genetic testing (Figs. 54.7 and 54.8). If genetic etiology has not been established in the family or if relatives do not wish to pursue genetic testing, the family evaluation relies on clinical screening

(physical examination, electrocardiogram, echocardiogram) for first-degree relatives of an individual with HCM. If HCM is diagnosed in relatives during screening, their first-degree relatives are evaluated, and so forth. Due to the variable penetrance and expressivity of HCM, symptoms or signs may not develop until early or middle adulthood; thus longitudinal clinical screening is recommended for at-risk relatives.

The overall strategy for family screening is summarized in Figure 54.8. Initiation and repetition of clinical screening (echocardiography and ECG) varies by age. For adult and adolescent first-degree relatives of patients with HCM, screening is recommended to commence at the time of diagnosis in the proband and repeated at regular intervals (late childhood through adolescence every 1 to 2 years, and every 5 years through adulthood). For younger children, clinical screening can commence at any time but no later than the onset of puberty. Earlier initiation of screening can be considered if there is a family history of early-onset HCM, a particularly malignant history of HCM-related adverse outcomes, and/or heightened parental concern. For children and adolescents, once clinical screening is initiated, the repeat surveillance interval is every 1 to 2 years.[3]

If a definitively pathogenic variant is identified by diagnostic genetic testing on an affected family member, focused *predictive or variant confirmation genetic testing* can be offered to relatives to determine whether the variant has been inherited in other relatives. Relatives found to carry the pathogenic variant are at risk of developing disease. They should undergo serial clinical evaluation and be informed of the risk of transmission to offspring (see Figs. 54.7 and 54.8). However, the penetrance (the likelihood that an individual who carries a variant develops disease) of pathogenic variants is variable and cannot be predicted prospectively. In addition to not being able to accurately predict when or if HCM will develop, we currently are not able to predict how severe manifestations will be (expressivity). Therefore, broad longitudinal clinical follow-up of all at-risk relatives is currently recommended. In contrast, relatives who have negative predictive genetic testing and do not carry their family's pathogenic variant can generally be reassured that they neither they nor their children are at increased risk for developing HCM. They can be dismissed from longitudinal screening, although they should undergo prompt

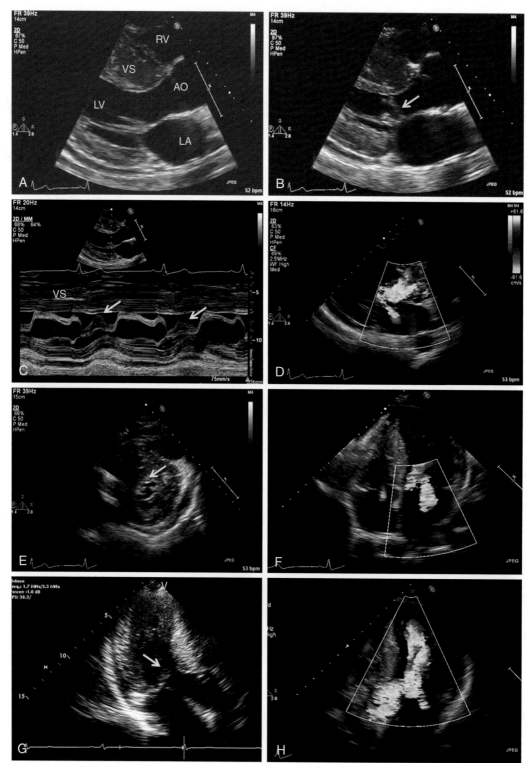

FIGURE 54.5 Systolic anterior motion of the mitral valve and left ventricular outflow tract obstruction. Still-frame images illustrate typical systolic anterior motion (SAM), showing the anterior mitral leaflet as it makes septal contact, producing mechanical impedance to LV outflow and mitral regurgitation. **A,** Parasternal long axis view in diastole. **B,** Parasternal long axis view in midsystole showing typical SAM in which the anterior mitral leaflet bends acutely (*arrows*), becoming almost perpendicular to the LV outflow tract in systole, resulting in focal septal contact and obstruction to flow (Video 54.1). **C,** M-mode depiction of mitral valve motion demonstrating anterior motion of the mitral valve and septal contact in midsystole (*arrows*). The degree and duration of SAM-septal contact relates directly to the magnitude of the outflow gradient. **D,** Parasternal long axis image in midsystole with color Doppler demonstrating turbulent flow in the LV outflow tract due to systolic anterior motion and posteriorly directed mitral regurgitation (Video 54.2). **E,** Parasternal short axis image in midsystole showing that the typical anterior motion of the mitral valve occurs in the center of the anterior mitral valve leaflet (*arrow* demonstrates septal contact). **F,** Apical four-chamber view in midsystole with color Doppler demonstrating turbulent flow in the LV outflow tract and mitral regurgitation. **G** and **H,** Apical three- and five-chamber view in midsystole demonstrating elongated mitral leaflets, particularly the anterior leaflet (AML), producing LV outflow obstruction from SAM (*arrow*) as shown by the accompanying color Doppler image. *AO,* Aorta; *LA,* left atrium; *LV,* left ventricle; *RV,* right ventricle; *VS,* ventricular septum. (From Seidelmann SB, et al. Hypertrophic cardiomyopathy. In: Solomon SD et al., eds. *Essential Echocardiography: A Companion to Braunwald's Heart Disease.* Philadelphia, Elsevier; 2019.)

evaluation in response to clinical changes. In cases where diagnostic genetic testing is not performed or a causal variant is not identified (diagnostic genetic testing was negative or identified variants were not definitively pathogenic), predictive genetic testing for healthy, at risk relatives is not an option and serial clinical evaluation is the default strategy, typically starting with first-degree relatives of affected individuals and expanding as new diagnoses are made.

Predictive genetic testing can also be used for reproductive planning either with prenatal testing (using amniocentesis or chorionic villus sampling) during an ongoing pregnancy to determine whether

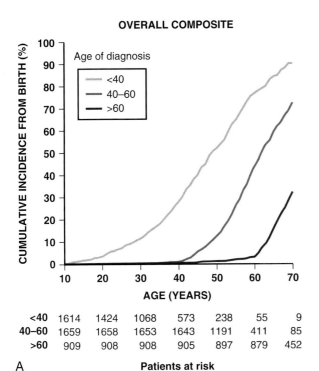

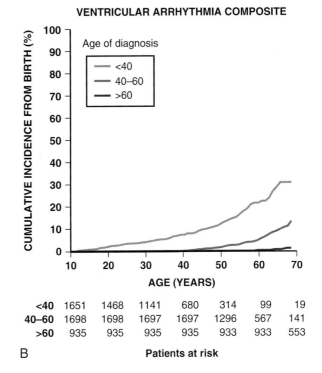

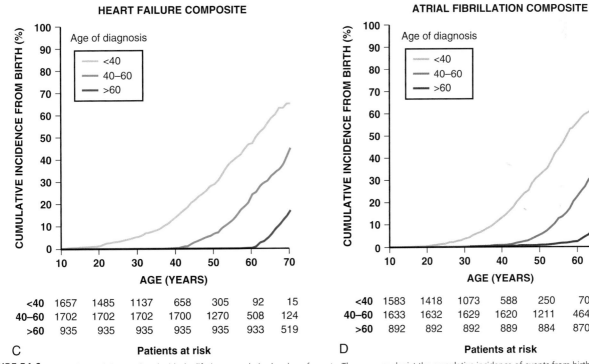

FIGURE 54.6 Age at diagnosis is associated with the lifetime cumulative burden of events. These curves depict the cumulative incidence of events from birth for outcomes of interest, stratified by age at diagnosis <40, 40 to 60, and >60 years. Earlier age at diagnosis is associated with a higher burden of adverse events. **A,** Overall composite outcome (first occurrence of all-cause mortality, sudden cardiac death, resuscitated cardiac arrest, appropriate implantable cardioverter-defibrillator therapy, cardiac transplantation, LV assist device implantation, New York Heart Association class III/IV symptoms, atrial fibrillation). **B,** Ventricular arrhythmia composite (first occurrence of sudden cardiac death, resuscitated cardiac arrest, or appropriate implantable cardioverter-defibrillator therapy). **C,** Heart failure composite (first occurrence of cardiac transplantation, LV assist device implantation, LVEF <35%, or New York Heart Association class III/IV symptoms). **D,** Atrial fibrillation. (From Ho CY, Day SM, Ashley EA, et al. Genotype and lifetime burden of disease in hypertrophic cardiomyopathy: insights from the sarcomeric human cardiomyopathy registry (SHaRe). *Circulation.* 2018;138:1387–1398.)

or not the fetus inherited the causal variant or through preimplantation genetic diagnosis (PGD). With PGD, genetic testing is performed on a single cell from embryos created using in vitro fertilization. Only embryos without evidence for the family's pathogenic variant are used for implantation, with a goal of achieving pregnancy without transmitting the genetic susceptibility for HCM.

CLINICAL MANAGEMENT

Sudden Cardiac Death Risk Stratification

The approach to the patient with HCM involves advice about family screening/surveillance (discussed earlier), risk stratification for SCD, and management of symptoms. As mentioned earlier, SCD occurs in

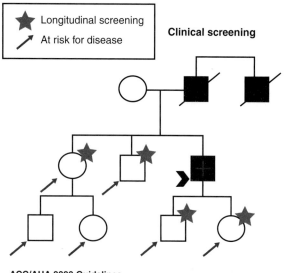

Clinical screening

Predictive genetic testing

Longitudinal screening

At risk for disease

No planned
follow-up
needed

Clinical
management
for HCM

No planned
follow-up
needed

Not at risk;
genotyping not
performed

Longitudinal
screening
required

ACC/AHA 2020 Guidelines:

Children and Adolescents from genotype-positive family and/or family with early onset HCM: Initiate screening at the time of family diagnosis; repeat evaluation every 1 to 2 years.

All other children and adolescents: Initiate screening following family diagnosis and no later than puberty; repeat evaluation every 2 to 3 years.

Adults: Initiate screening at the time of family diagnosis; repeat evaluation every 3 to 5 years.

ESC 2014 Guidelines:

10–20 years: every 1–2 years
>20 years: every 2–5 years

A

B

FIGURE 54.7 Family screening strategies using **(A)** clinical evaluation or **(B)** genetic testing. **A,** Clinical screening: All family members are at risk for developing hypertrophic cardiomyopathy (HCM) (*red arrows*). Guidelines recommend that all first-degree relatives (*blue stars*) of an affected individual undergo serial, longitudinal clinical screening to monitor for disease development. If found to have HCM (or develop HCM during follow-up), their first-degree relatives should be screened; a process referred to as *cascade screening*. The frequency of longitudinal screening varies by age and clinical status and is outlined in the 2020 ACC/AHA and 2014 ESC guidelines.[1,3] **B,** Predictive genetic testing is recommended for all members of families in whom a pathogenic variant has been identified. This allow unambiguous identification of relatives who are and are not at risk for developing HCM. With these results, family screening can evolve from broad, longitudinal screening of all potentially at-risk relatives **(A)** to focused longitudinal screening of relatives who are definitively at risk for disease by virtue of having inherited the family's pathogenic variant (*red plus signs and arrows* in **B**). Relatives who have not inherited the family's pathogenic variant (*red minus sign*) and their children are not at risk of developing HCM. Longitudinal follow-up is not required unless there is a clinical change in these patients. *Black arrowheads* indicate family proband. *Squares* indicate males and *circles* indicate females. *Solid black squares* indicate relatives diagnosed with HCM, and *open circles and squares* denote clinically unaffected relatives. (Adapted from Ahluwalia M, Ho CY. Heart 2021;107:183–189.)

just less than 1% of patients with HCM each year, and the appropriate utilization of ICDs has resulted in significantly improved outcomes. Patients who have previously experienced cardiac arrest or sustained ventricular arrhythmias have class 1 indications for ICD placement as secondary prevention.[1,3] Risk assessment and advice regarding primary-prevention ICDs remains a blend of science and clinical judgement (Fig. 54.9). Several clinical features have been associated with SCD, but the importance of the risk factors varies with age (i.e., some risk markers carry more weight in children than adults, and vice versa), and the overall risk appears to diminish with advanced age.[64–66] Although there are numerous exceptions, generally, the more severe the phenotypic expression of HCM, the higher the risk for SCD. Massive LV wall thickness (either as a binary variable or as a continuous variable), syncope felt to be arrhythmogenic, family history of SCD, overt systolic dysfunction, LV apical aneurysm, nonsustained ventricular tachycardia (NSVT), and extensive intramyocardial scarring (as assessed with CMR) have all been identified as being associated with SCD. Severe LVOTO has also been shown to be associated with SCD, but the effect size is modest and given the inherently dynamic nature of obstruction, this metric can be problematic to use in practice. Left atrial size, as a surrogate for phenotypic severity, has also been incorporated into risk calculators.[67] These tools can be useful to help patients with one or more of the SCD risk markers understand the magnitude of that risk.

In adult patients, the risk markers that appear to carry the most significance are massive hypertrophy (wall thickness approaching or exceeding 30 mm), family history of SCD in first-degree relatives younger than the age of 40 to 50 (or potentially multiple second-degree

relatives), arrhythmogenic syncope, LV systolic dysfunction, and LV apical aneurysm. NSVT appears to be more important for younger patients or when the runs of NSVT are frequent, longer, and/or faster.[3,68] Extensive late gadolinium enhancement (LGE) on CMR indicates scarring in the LV wall which has also been shown to be associated with adverse outcomes including heart failure and ventricular arrhythmias.[69]

For children with HCM, massive hypertrophy (defined as z score approaching 20), arrhythmogenic syncope, and NSVT appear to be the most prominent risk predictors of SCD.[64] There are discordant data regarding family history of SCD, but a family event may be most useful if the event occurred in very young family members, or if it has occurred in multiple family members. Systolic dysfunction, apical aneurysm, and extensive LGE have not widely studied in children with HCM, but if present would seem important to consider as representing a particularly severe phenotype. The decision to proceed with ICD placement in children also must consider the complexity of placement, the need to account for somatic growth, and the greater number of years a device will be present.[70]

Management of Symptoms

Apart from SCD risk stratification, management of patients with HCM has traditionally focused on symptom management. Although clinical trial evidence is relatively scant, no pharmacologic agent has been shown to improve survival, and no invasive therapy has been shown to alter mortality in asymptomatic patients. This means that asymptomatic patients do not require initiation of therapy. Advice on health lifestyle, family evaluation, and management of other health concerns

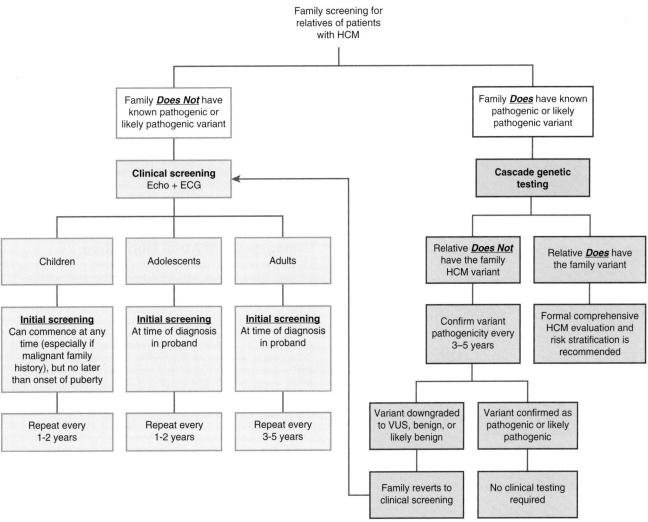

FIGURE 54.8 Strategy for family screening. Current recommendations suggest that clinical screening be repeated every 1 to 2 years during late childhood to early adulthood and every 5 years throughout adulthood. (From Ahluwalia M, Ho CY. Cardiovascular genetics: the role of genetic testing in diagnosis and management of patients with hypertrophic cardiomyopathy. *Heart*. 2021;107[3]:183–189.)

are the focus for these patients. For patients who have exertional dyspnea, angina, or syncope/presyncope, it is useful to base treatment on whether the symptoms are driven by obstructive physiology, nonobstructive disease, arrhythmia, or other processes (Fig. 54.10).

PATIENTS WITH OBSTRUCTIVE HYPERTROPHIC CARDIOMYOPATHY

Dyspnea, chest pain/pressure, and/or presyncope that vary from day to day are the hallmark symptoms attributable to LVOTO. Because gradient is highly dependent on loading conditions, anything that causes systemic vasodilation (e.g., ambient temperature, postprandial state, alcohol consumption) or volume depletion may exacerbate symptoms. Symptoms are most dramatically promoted by physical effort as systemic vascular resistance drops and contractility is augmented. Patients are rarely symptomatic at rest unless there is another disease state (e.g., sepsis) that alters loading conditions dramatically. Although randomized clinical trials have not been performed, the general approach for symptomatic patients with obstructive physiology is to optimize volume status (encourage vigorous hydration), eliminate or reduce any vasodilator therapies, and empirically start beta blockers, verapamil, or diltiazem because these agents have negative chronotropic effects which help maximize preload by increasing the diastolic filling interval, and negative inotropic effects.[3] Therapeutic efficacy is guided by the symptomatic response of the patient, not changes in gradient. If patients remain symptomatic after maximizing one of these

agents, then switching to one of the other agents is the usual next step in care. Persistent symptoms beyond this prompts consideration of advanced options including disopyramide (added to one of the other agents).[71] Novel agents that directly target the enhanced actin-myosin interaction of HCM are in trials at this time (see Clinical Trials and Emerging Therapy, later).[72]

Although medical therapies are used to target myocardial function and/or loading conditions to indirectly improve obstruction, septal reduction therapy (surgical septal myectomy or alcohol septal ablation) directly addresses the anatomic cause of obstruction. Septal myectomy has evolved since its introduction over 60 years ago.[73] Performed via an aortotomy, muscle resection is now extended and involves a larger surface area of the septum down to the level of the papillary muscles. Some operators also include plication or other manipulation of the anterior mitral leaflet, particularly if mitral regurgitation or mitral valve pathology is thought to contribute importantly to pathophysiology.[74–76] Successful myectomy normalizes the flow pattern in the ventricle such that the mitral valve can coapt normally and outflow tract gradient is substantially reduced or abolished (Fig. 54.11). Muscle does not "regrow" at the myectomy site; therefore results are durable (recurrent or residual obstruction likely results from inadequate initial resection). In experienced centers, operative (30-day) mortality is less than 1% with a 90% to 95% success rate.[77,78]

Septal ablation is a percutaneous procedure during which alcohol is infused into the septal perforator artery that supplies the obstructive hypertrophied septum. This results in a scar which causes retraction of the septum as the myocardium remodels post infarct (Fig. 54.12).

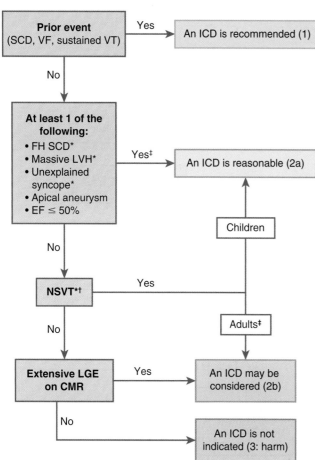

FIGURE 54.9 Patient selection for ICD placement. *ICD decisions in pediatric patients with HCM are based on ≥1 of these major risk factors: family history of HCM SCD, NSVT on ambulatory monitor, massive LVH, and unexplained syncope. †It would seem most appropriate to place greater weight on frequent, longer, and faster runs of NSVT. ‡In patients >16 years of age, 5-year risk estimates can be considered to fully inform patients during shared decision-making discussions. *CMR,* Cardiovascular magnetic resonance; *EF,* ejection fraction; *FH,* family history; *HCM,* hypertrophic cardiomyopathy; *ICD,* implantable cardioverter-defibrillator; *LGE,* late gadolinium enhancement; *LVH,* left ventricular hypertrophy; *NSVT,* nonsustained ventricular tachycardia; *SCD,* sudden cardiac death; *VF,* ventricular fibrillation; *VT,* ventricular tachycardia. (Adapted from Ommen SR, Mital S, Burke MA, et al. AHA/ACC guideline for the diagnosis and treatment of patients with hypertrophic cardiomyopathy: a report of the American College of Cardiology/American Heart Association Joint Committee on Clinical Practice Guidelines. *J Am Coll Cardiol.* 2020;76[25]:e159–e240.)

Patients who respond to ablation have similar symptomatic improvements as patients treated with septal myectomy, and long-term survival is similar.[79,80] However, there is a higher need for reintervention following ablation, and higher rate of heart block requiring permanent pacemaker placement. Clinical decision making to determine whether to pursue myectomy versus ablation can be complex and considers factors including access to experienced operators, a comprehensive discussion of the benefits and risks of both procedures, and patient-specific features that may make one option more appropriate, including septal morphology and suitable coronary artery anatomy. Patients who have other cardiovascular disease requiring surgical intervention are usually treated with surgical myectomy. Younger patients, patients with more severe LVH (>18 mm), and patients with severe resting gradients (>100 mm Hg) appear to have better outcomes with surgery.[81] Patients who are frail or have significant comorbidity that makes a surgical approach riskier are better candidates for septal ablation.

PATIENTS WITH NONOBSTRUCTIVE HYPERTROPHIC CARDIOMYOPATHY

Patients who do not have obstructive physiology can also have symptoms of angina or dyspnea. The former is likely due to subendocardial ischemia, and the latter falls into a spectrum of heart failure with preserved ejection fraction. Empiric treatment also uses beta blockers, verapamil, or diltiazem as first agents. Diuretics are used for patients with persistent dyspnea and/or signs of congestion. Nonobstructive patients with preserved systolic function (i.e., LVEF >50%) and severe symptoms that do not respond to these therapies are often considered for advanced heart failure options (medical therapy and advanced therapies) in accordance with the heart failure guidelines (see Fig. 54.10).[82] Cardiac transplantation is typically pursued as mechanical circulatory support has not been widely successful, particularly if LV cavity size is small.

As described previously under Natural History, specific to patients with HCM, systolic dysfunction is believed to be present when LVEF falls below 50% (as compared with ejection fraction <40%) with most other forms of cardiomyopathy guideline-directed management for systolic heart failure should be applied when appropriate.[3]

Management of Atrial Fibrillation

It has been estimated that up to half of patients with HCM may experience atrial fibrillation, with prevalence increasing with age.[49] Similar to other patients, this may be asymptomatic. However, patients with HCM, particularly those with obstructive physiology, are prone to develop symptoms when preload is decreased. The onset of atrial fibrillation can substantially reduce preload through loss of atrial contribution to LV filling, and as heart rates increase, the diastolic filling period is truncated. Slowing the heart rate and restoring sinus rhythm are important targets for therapy. Beta blockers, verapamil, and diltiazem can be helpful for rate control, and amiodarone, dofetilide, sotalol, and disopyramide have all be used for rhythm control.[3] The potential for proarrhythmia needs consideration in HCM, particularly in patients who do not have an ICD. Catheter ablation is considered a reasonable option for patients whose AF is not well controlled with medications. Similarly, for patients with HCM and AF who are referred for surgical myectomy, intraoperative AF ablation techniques can be added.

The risk of thromboembolism in patients with HCM and AF is higher than in patients without structural heart disease.[83] As such, risk-scoring systems (e.g., CHADs2VASc) are not used in patients with HCM, but rather oral anticoagulation is considered appropriate in all patients with both HCM and AF. Direct oral anticoagulants or warfarin are considered as viable options in patients with HCM. As with other patients with AF lasting more than 24 hours, the recommendation for oral anticoagulation is clear. For AF episodes less than 24 hours, the choice to initiate anticoagulation would need to be individualized accounting for bleeding risk, total AF burden, and other risk factors for thromboembolism.

Exercise and Sports Participation

The benefits of a healthy lifestyle that includes regular light to moderate physical activity appear to extend to patients with HCM.[84,85] The challenge is that among competitive athletes who have had cardiac arrest, HCM is overrepresented as an underlying diagnosis. This fact led to a generalized exclusion of individuals with HCM from participation in competitive athletics regardless of their clinical status.[86] The increasing societal interest in higher-intensity exercise led to renewed studies to determine for patients with HCM if there was a safe intensity level. These investigations, starting from the population of patients with HCM rather than from patients with cardiac arrest, have not shown increased adverse event rates with increasing effort intensity or participation in sports.[87,88] Taken together, these seemingly disparate results likely reflect that the highest level of physical activity (competitive sports) does represent a level of increased risk for cardiac arrest, but that the incremental relative risk of participation compared with nonparticipation is so small that the most recent studies are underpowered to detect that risk. From a practical standpoint, each person with HCM who is interested in higher-intensity training must be informed of this risk, the inability to accurately estimate the risk, and determine his or her own level of tolerance for the unknown risk.[3]

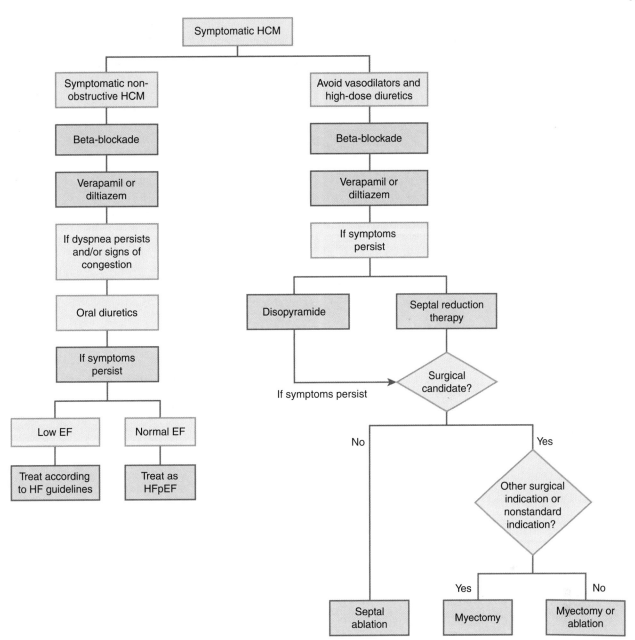

FIGURE 54.10 Management of symptoms in patients with hypertrophic cardiomyopathy.

CLINICAL TRIALS AND EMERGING THERAPIES

Owing to its relative rarity and heterogeneous disease expression, very few robust, prospective, appropriately controlled trials have been performed in HCM. To date, fewer than 100 trials have been published, the vast majority studying fewer than 50 patients and lacking randomization, blinding, or comparison with placebo.[89,90] Historically and currently, treatment has relied on off-label use of available medications (beta blockers, L-type calcium channel blockers, and disopyramide) to mitigate symptoms by leveraging nonspecific pharmacologic properties. These limitations have been well recognized and, in concert with growing understanding of underlying disease pathways, there has been renewed interest in developing more mechanistically driven therapies. However, small trials of potentially promising therapeutic targets in obstructive and nonobstructive HCM have failed to demonstrate efficacy. These include attempts to modulate myocardial energetics using perhexiline and trimetazidine,[91,92] to inhibit the late-sodium channel using ranolazine and eleclazine,[93,94] and to decrease fibrosis using spironolactone, valsartan, and losartan.[95–98]

Newer treatments and concepts in development include disease-modifying and prevention strategies, targeting sarcomeric variant carriers prior to development of clinically overt HCM, myosin inhibitors, and gene-based therapies. No treatments have been proven to alter the natural history of disease or to be beneficial for either sarcomeric variant carriers with normal LV wall thickness or for asymptomatic patients with HCM. However, with improved understanding of how sarcomere variants cause HCM, treatments are being pursued attempting to target early, disease-initiating pathways. The goal of these therapies would be to attenuate disease progression and, ultimately, disease emergence. Studies in mouse models of sarcomeric HCM have demonstrated that treatment with agents, including diltiazem, losartan, and mavacamten (see later), was able to attenuate disease development if given early in life, prior to the development of diagnostic features of disease.[99–101] Pilot efforts at translation to human disease are being attempted, but further investigation and experience are required.[102,103]

Novel, oral selective allosteric inhibitors of cardiac myosin ATPase have recently been developed to address fundamental abnormalities associated with HCM, namely increased contractile force. The first such agent, mavacamten, reduces actin-myosin cross-bridge formation, thereby reducing myocardial contractility and improving myocardial energetics.[104] Animal studies demonstrated that mavacamten reduces

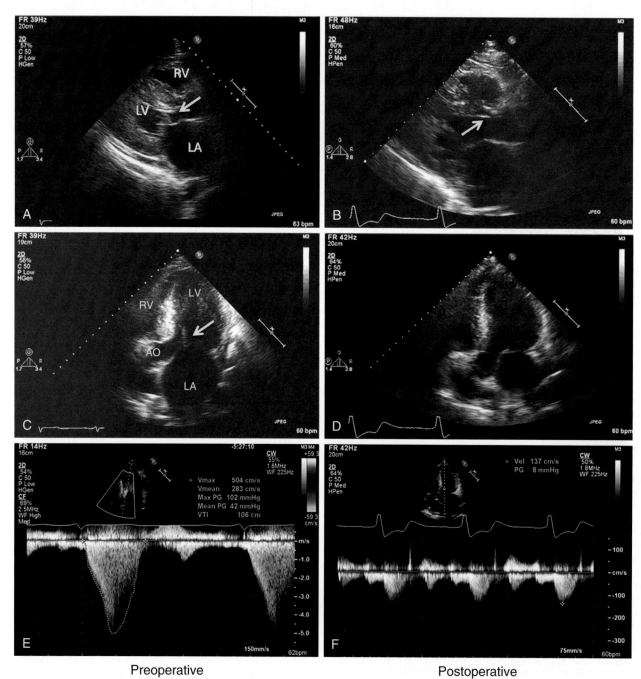

FIGURE 54.11 Surgical myectomy to manage symptomatic obstructive hypertrophic cardiomyopathy (HCM). **A,** Preoperative: Parasternal long axis view shows marked hypertrophy of the septum and systolic anterior motion of the mitral valve (SAM) (*arrow*). **B,** Postoperative: Parasternal long axis view shows a myectomy "trough" (*arrow*) representative of the portion of the upper septum that was resected, resulting in an increase of the cross-sectional area of the LV outflow tract, ultimately, eliminating SAM and LVOT obstruction. **C,** Preoperative: Apical five-chamber view showing hypertrophy of the ventricular septum and SAM (*arrow*). **D,** Postoperative: Apical five-chamber view showing resection of the basal ventricular septum and resolution of SAM. **E,** Preoperative: Apical five-chamber view with continuous wave Doppler showing a peak velocity of 5.0 m/sec. **F,** Postoperative: Apical five-chamber view with continuous wave Doppler showing a reduction in peak velocity to 1.4 m/sec post resection. *AO,* Aorta; *LA,* left atrium; *LV,* Left ventricle; *RV,* right ventricle; *VS,* ventricular septum. (From Seidelmann SB, et al. Hypertrophic cardiomyopathy. In: Solomon SD, et al., eds. *Essential Echocardiography: A Companion to Braunwald's Heart Disease.* Philadelphia, Elsevier; 2019.)

myocardial contraction in a dose-dependent manner and relieves left ventricular outflow obstruction.[101,105] A phase III clinical trial of mavacamten versus placebo in patients with symptomatic obstructive HCM demonstrated that treatment with mavacamten significantly improved exercise capacity, LVOT obstruction, symptoms, and health status.[72] Substantial reduction in outflow tract gradients were achieved with only modest reduction in LVEF; however, careful dose titration and monitoring are required given that the mechanism of action is to decrease contractility. Furthermore, although initial experience with myosin inhibitors targeted patients with obstructive HCM and focused on reducing contractility and obstruction, there is also potential mechanistic rationale that myosin inhibitors may improve relaxation

abnormalities and impaired myocardial energetics associated with disease.[104,106] A phase II study of mavacamten versus placebo in patients with symptomatic nonobstructive HCM demonstrated that treatment with mavacamten was associated with a significant reduction in N-terminal propeptide of B-type natriuretic peptide.[107] Although this initial experience has been promising, further investigation is needed to determine long-term safety and benefit over standard therapy.

Gene-based therapy is also emerging as a potential strategy, including genome editing, exon skipping, allele-specific silencing, spliceosome-mediated RNA trans-splicing, and gene replacement.[108,109] The therapeutic goal is to replace, remove, or mitigate the effect of the germline genetic defect. Technologies are being developed and tested

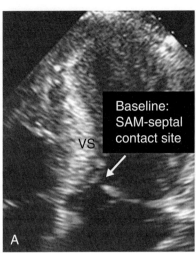 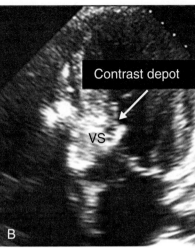 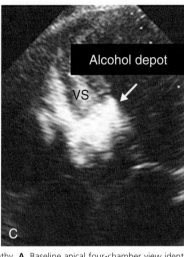

FIGURE 54.12 Alcohol septal ablation for management of symptomatic obstructive hypertrophic cardiomyopathy. **A,** Baseline apical four-chamber view identifies the area of maximal systolic anterior motion (SAM)-septal contact to target for ablation (*arrow*). **B,** Intracoronary injection of echocardiographic contrast is used to verify that the identified septal perforator branch supplies the target area of the ventricular septum, at the site of maximal SAM-septal contact. The region supplied by the injected septal branch is highlighted by the contrast agent manifest as an echogenic signal created by the accumulation of contrast within the myocardium (*arrow*). Contrast defines the site of potential ablation and determines if infarction size will be too large or involve unintended structures such as the right ventricle. **C,** After defining the site of potential ablation, alcohol is injected into the selected septal perforator branch, targeting the region of the septum that is highlighted by intracoronary contrast and seen as an intensely echobright signal from the alcohol collection within the myocardium (*arrow*). (From Seidelmann SB, et al. Hypertrophic cardiomyopathy. In: Solomon SD, et al., eds. *Essential Echocardiography: A Companion to Braunwald's Heart Disease*. Philadelphia, Elsevier; 2019.)

in animal and human-induced pluripotent stem cell models of HCM. Genetic variants resulting in haploinsufficiency as the mechanism of disease, such as most HCM caused by *MYBPC3* variants, may be most amenable to gene therapy.

SUMMARY

HCM is a primary myocardial disorder defined by otherwise unexplained left ventricular hypertrophy. As an intriguing and complex clinical entity and the first cardiomyopathy to be explained at the molecular genetic level, HCM has been the focus of intense clinical and basic science investigation for decades. Optimal clinical management requires thoughtful assessment of an individual patient's pathophysiology, as well as systematic care of their family. Further studies to better understand the relationships between genotype, phenotype, and outcomes over a lifetime are critical to improve risk stratification and to guide patient management. These insights will also support development of targeted therapies intended to modify disease progression and prevent adverse sequelae.

REFERENCES

1. Elliott PM, Anastasakis A, Borger MA, et al. 2014 ESC guidelines on diagnosis and management of hypertrophic cardiomyopathy: the task force for the diagnosis and management of hypertrophic cardiomyopathy of the European Society of Cardiology (ESC). *Eur Heart J.* 2014;35:2733–2779.
2. Norrish G, Field E, McLeod K, et al. Clinical presentation and survival of childhood hypertrophic cardiomyopathy: a retrospective study in United Kingdom. *Eur Heart J.* 2019;40:986–993.
3. Ommen SR, Mital S, Burke MA, et al. 2020 AHA/ACC guideline for the diagnosis and treatment of patients with hypertrophic cardiomyopathy: a report of the American College of Cardiology/American Heart Association Joint Committee on Clinical Practice Guidelines. *J Am Coll Cardiol.* 2020;76:e159–e240.
4. Yamaguchi H, Ishimura T, Nishiyama S, et al. Hypertrophic nonobstructive cardiomyopathy with giant negative T waves (apical hypertrophy): ventriculographic and echocardiographic features in 30 patients. *Am J Cardiol.* 1979;44:401–412.
5. Kitaoka H, Doi Y, Casey SA, et al. Comparison of prevalence of apical hypertrophic cardiomyopathy in Japan and the United States. *Am J Cardiol.* 2003;92:1183–1186.
6. Hughes RK, Knott KD, Malcolmson J, et al. Apical hypertrophic cardiomyopathy: the variant less known. *J Am Heart Assoc.* 2020;9:e015294.
7. Bos JM, Will ML, Gersh BJ, et al. Characterization of a phenotype-based genetic test prediction score for unrelated patients with hypertrophic cardiomyopathy. *Mayo Clin Proc.* 2014;89:727–737.
8. Gruner C, Ivanov J, Care M, et al. Toronto hypertrophic cardiomyopathy genotype score for prediction of a positive genotype in hypertrophic cardiomyopathy. *Circ Cardiovasc Genet.* 2013;6:19–26.
9. Arad M, Penas-Lado M, Monserrat L, et al. Gene mutations in apical hypertrophic cardiomyopathy. *Circulation.* 2005;112:2805–2811.
10. Geisterfer-Lowrance AA, Kass S, Tanigawa G, et al. A molecular basis for familial hypertrophic cardiomyopathy: a beta cardiac myosin heavy chain gene missense mutation. *Cell.* 1990;62:999–1006.
11. Georgakopoulos D, Christe ME, Giewat M, et al. The pathogenesis of familial hypertrophic cardiomyopathy: early and evolving effects from an alpha-cardiac myosin heavy chain missense mutation [see comments]. *Nat Med.* 1999;5:327–330.
12. Seidman CE, Seidman JG. Identifying sarcomere gene mutations in hypertrophic cardiomyopathy: a personal history. *Circ Res.* 2011;108:743–750.
13. Watkins H, McKenna WJ, Thierfelder L, et al. Mutations in the genes for cardiac troponin T and alpha-tropomyosin in hypertrophic cardiomyopathy. *N Engl J Med.* 1995;332:1058–1064.
14. Alfares AA, Kelly MA, McDermott G, et al. Results of clinical genetic testing of 2,912 probands with hypertrophic cardiomyopathy: expanded panels offer limited additional sensitivity. *Genet Med.* 2015;17:880–888.
15. Eisner DA, Caldwell JL, Kistamas K, Trafford AW. Calcium and excitation-contraction coupling in the heart. *Circ Res.* 2017;121:181–195.
16. Bottinelli R, Coviello DA, Redwood CS, et al. A mutant tropomyosin that causes hypertrophic cardiomyopathy is expressed in vivo and associated with an increased calcium sensitivity. *Circ Res.* 1998;82:106–115.
17. Cuda G, Fananapazir L, Epstein ND, Sellers JR. The in vitro motility activity of beta-cardiac myosin depends on the nature of the beta-myosin heavy chain gene mutation in hypertrophic cardiomyopathy. *J Muscle Res Cell Motil.* 1997;18:275–283.
18. van Dijk SJ, Dooijes D, dos Remedios C, et al. Cardiac myosin-binding protein C mutations and hypertrophic cardiomyopathy: haploinsufficiency, deranged phosphorylation, and cardiomyocyte dysfunction. *Circulation.* 2009;119:1473–1483.
19. Helms AS, Tang VT, O'Leary TS, et al. Effects of MYBPC3 loss-of-function mutations preceding hypertrophic cardiomyopathy. *JCI Insight.* 2020;5.
20. Helms AS, Thompson AD, Glazier AA, et al. Spatial and functional distribution of MYBPC3 pathogenic variants and clinical outcomes in patients with hypertrophic cardiomyopathy. *Circ Cardiovasc Genet.* 2020;13(5):396–405.
21. Sequeira V, Wijnker PJ, Nijenkamp LL, et al. Perturbed length-dependent activation in human hypertrophic cardiomyopathy with missense sarcomeric gene mutations. *Circ Res.* 2013;112:1491–1505.
22. Witjas-Paalberends ER, Guclu A, Germans T, et al. Gene-specific increase in the energetic cost of contraction in hypertrophic cardiomyopathy caused by thick filament mutations. *Cardiovasc Res.* 2014;103:248–257.
23. Marian AJ, Braunwald E. Hypertrophic cardiomyopathy: genetics, pathogenesis, clinical manifestations, diagnosis, and therapy. *Circ Res.* 2017;121:749–770.
24. Alamo L, Ware JS, Pinto A, et al. Effects of myosin variants on interacting-heads motif explain distinct hypertrophic and dilated cardiomyopathy phenotypes. *eLife.* 2017;6.
25. Toepfer CN, Garfinkel AC, Venturini G, et al. Myosin sequestration regulates sarcomere function, cardiomyocyte energetics, and metabolism, informing the pathogenesis of hypertrophic cardiomyopathy. *Circulation.* 2020;141:828–842.
26. Ho CY, Day SM, Colan SD, et al. The burden of early phenotypes and the influence of wall thickness in hypertrophic cardiomyopathy mutation carriers: findings from the HCMNet study. *JAMA Cardiol.* 2017;2:419–428.
27. Ho CY, Carlsen C, Thune JJ, et al. Echocardiographic strain imaging to assess early and late consequences of sarcomere mutations in hypertrophic cardiomyopathy. *Circ Cardiovasc Genet.* 2009;2:314–321.
28. Ho CY, Cirino AL, Lakdawala NK, et al. Evolution of hypertrophic cardiomyopathy in sarcomere mutation carriers. *Heart.* 2016.
29. Crilley JG, Boehm EA, Blair E, et al. Hypertrophic cardiomyopathy due to sarcomeric gene mutations is characterized by impaired energy metabolism irrespective of the degree of hypertrophy. *J Am Coll Cardiol.* 2003;41:1776–1782.
30. Lakdawala NK, Thune JJ, Maron BJ, et al. Electrocardiographic features of sarcomere mutation carriers with and without clinically overt hypertrophic cardiomyopathy. *Am J Cardiol.* 2011;108:1606–1613.
31. Captur G, Lopes LR, Mohun TJ, et al. Prediction of sarcomere mutations in subclinical hypertrophic cardiomyopathy. *Circ Cardiovasc Imaging.* 2014;7:863–871.
32. Groarke JD, Galazka PZ, Cirino AL, et al. Intrinsic mitral valve alterations in hypertrophic cardiomyopathy sarcomere mutation carriers. *Eur Heart J Cardiovascular Imaging.* 2018;19:1109–1116.
33. Ho CY, Lopez B, Coelho-Filho OR, et al. Myocardial fibrosis as an early manifestation of hypertrophic cardiomyopathy. *N Engl J Med.* 2010;363:552–563.
34. Ho CY, Abbasi SA, Neilan TG, et al. T1 measurements identify extracellular volume expansion in hypertrophic cardiomyopathy sarcomere mutation carriers with and without left ventricular hypertrophy. *Circ Cardiovasc Imaging.* 2013;6:415–422.
35. Paulus WJ, Lorell BH, Craig WE, et al. Comparison of the effects of nitroprusside and nifedipine on diastolic properties in patients with hypertrophic cardiomyopathy: altered left ventricular loading or improved muscle inactivation? *J Am Coll Cardiol.* 1983;2:879–886.
36. Soullier C, Obert P, Doucende G, et al. Exercise response in hypertrophic cardiomyopathy: blunted left ventricular deformational and twisting reserve with altered systolic-diastolic coupling. *Circ Cardiovasc Imaging.* 2012;5:324–332.

37. Villemain O, Correia M, Khraiche D, et al. Myocardial stiffness assessment using Shear wave imaging in pediatric hypertrophic cardiomyopathy. *JACC Cardiovasc Imaging.* 2018;11:779–781.

38. Ho CY, Sweitzer NK, McDonough B, et al. Assessment of diastolic function with Doppler tissue imaging to predict genotype in preclinical hypertrophic cardiomyopathy. *Circulation.* 2002;105:2992–2997.

39. Nagueh SF, McFalls J, Meyer D, et al. Tissue doppler imaging predicts the development of hypertrophic cardiomyopathy in subjects with subclinical disease. *Circulation.* 2003;108:395–398.

40. Williams LK, Misurka J, Ho CY, et al. Multilayer myocardial mechanics in genotype-positive left ventricular hypertrophy-negative patients with hypertrophic cardiomyopathy. *Am J Cardiol.* 2018;122:1754–1760.

41. Maron MS, Olivotto I, Betocchi S, et al. Effect of left ventricular outflow tract obstruction on clinical outcome in hypertrophic cardiomyopathy. *N Engl J Med.* 2003;348:295–303.

42. Maron MS, Olivotto I, Zenovich AG, et al. Hypertrophic cardiomyopathy is predominantly a disease of left ventricular outflow tract obstruction. *Circulation.* 2006;114:2232–2239.

43. Sorajja P, Nishimura RA, Gersh BJ, et al. Outcome of mildly symptomatic or asymptomatic obstructive hypertrophic cardiomyopathy: a long-term follow-up study. *J Am Coll Cardiol.* 2009;54:234–241.

44. Numata S, Yaku H, Doi K, et al. Excess anterior mitral leaflet in a patient with hypertrophic obstructive cardiomyopathy and systolic anterior motion. *Circulation.* 2015;131:1605–1607.

45. Sherrid MV, Gunsburg DZ, Moldenhauer S, Pearle G. Systolic anterior motion begins at low left ventricular outflow tract velocity in obstructive hypertrophic cardiomyopathy. *J Am Coll Cardiol.* 2000;36:1344–1354.

46. Ayoub C, Geske JB, Larsen CM, et al. Comparison of valsalva maneuver, amyl nitrite, and exercise echocardiography to demonstrate latent left ventricular outflow obstruction in hypertrophic cardiomyopathy. *Am J Cardiol.* 2017;120:2265–2271.

47. Joshi S, Patel UK, Yao SS, et al. Standing and exercise doppler echocardiography in obstructive hypertrophic cardiomyopathy: the range of gradients with upright activity. *J Am Soc Echocardiogr.* 2011;24:75–82.

48. Reant P, Dufour M, Peyrou J, et al. Upright treadmill vs. semi-supine bicycle exercise echocardiography to provoke obstruction in symptomatic hypertrophic cardiomyopathy: a pilot study. *Eur Heart J Cardiovasc Imaging.* 2018;19:31–38.

49. Ho CY, Day SM, Ashley EA, et al. Genotype and lifetime burden of disease in hypertrophic cardiomyopathy: insights from the Sarcomeric Human Cardiomyopathy Registry (SHaRe). *Circulation.* 2018;138:1387–1398.

50. Olivotto I, Cecchi F, Casey SA, et al. Impact of atrial fibrillation on the clinical course of hypertrophic cardiomyopathy. *Circulation.* 2001;104:2517–2524.

51. Rowin EJ, Orfanos A, Estes NAM, et al. Occurrence and natural history of clinically silent episodes of atrial fibrillation in hypertrophic cardiomyopathy. *Am J Cardiol.* 2017;119:1862–1865.

52. Link MS, Bockstall K, Weinstock J, et al. Ventricular tachyarrhythmias in patients with hypertrophic cardiomyopathy and defibrillators: triggers, treatment, and implications. *J Cardiovasc Electrophysiol.* 2017;28:531–537.

53. Elliott P, Charron P, Blanes JR, et al. European cardiomyopathy pilot registry: EURObservational Research Programme of the European society of Cardiology. *Eur Heart J.* 2016;37:164–173.

54. Charron P, Elliott PM, Gimeno JR, et al. The Cardiomyopathy Registry of the EURObservational Research Programme of the European Society of Cardiology: baseline data and contemporary management of adult patients with cardiomyopathies. *Eur Heart J.* 2018;39:1784–1793.

55. Neubauer S, Kolm P, Ho CY, et al. Distinct subgroups in hypertrophic cardiomyopathy in the NHLBI HCM registry. *J Am Coll Cardiol.* 2019;74:2333–2345.

56. Sedaghat-Hamedani F, Kayvanpour E, Tugrul OF, et al. Clinical outcomes associated with sarcomere mutations in hypertrophic cardiomyopathy: a meta-analysis on 7675 individuals. *Clin Res Cardiol.* 2018;107:30–41.

57. Ingles J, Burns C, Bagnall RD, et al. Nonfamilial hypertrophic cardiomyopathy: prevalence, natural history, and clinical implications. *Cir Cardiovasc Genet.* 2017;10.

58. Li Q, Gruner C, Chan RH, et al. Genotype-positive status in patients with hypertrophic cardiomyopathy is associated with higher rates of heart failure events. *Cir Cardiovasc Genet.* 2014;7:416–422.

59. Olivotto I, Maron MS, Adabag AS, et al. Gender-related differences in the clinical presentation and outcome of hypertrophic cardiomyopathy. *J Am Coll Cardiol.* 2005;46:480–487.

60. Geske JB, Ong KC, Siontis KC, et al. Women with hypertrophic cardiomyopathy have worse survival. *Eur Heart J.* 2017;38:3434–3440.

61. Marstrand P, Han L, Day SM, et al. Hypertrophic cardiomyopathy with left ventricular systolic dysfunction: insights from the SHaRe registry. *Circulation.* 2020;141:1371–1383.

62. Cirino AL, Harris S, Lakdawala NK, et al. Role of genetic testing in inherited cardiovascular disease: a review. *JAMA Cardiol.* 2017;2:1153–1160.

63. Richards S, Aziz N, Bale S, et al. Standards and guidelines for the interpretation of sequence variants: a joint consensus recommendation of the American College of Medical Genetics and Genomics and the Association for Molecular Pathology. *Genet Med.* 2015;17:405–424.

64. Miron A, Lafreniere-Roula M, Steve Fan CP, et al. A validated model for sudden cardiac death risk prediction in pediatric hypertrophic cardiomyopathy. *Circulation.* 2020;142:217–229.

65. Norrish G, Cantarutti N, Pissaridou E, et al. Risk factors for sudden cardiac death in childhood hypertrophic cardiomyopathy: a systematic review and meta-analysis. *Eur J Prev Cardiol.* 2017;24:1220–1230.

66. Rowin EJ, Sridharan A, Madias C, et al. Prediction and prevention of sudden death in young patients (<20 years) with hypertrophic cardiomyopathy. *Am J Cardiol.* 2020;128:75–83.

67. O'Mahony C, Jichi F, Pavlou M, et al. A novel clinical risk prediction model for sudden cardiac death in hypertrophic cardiomyopathy (HCM risk-SCD). *Eur Heart J.* 2014;35:2010–2020.

68. Monserrat L, Elliott PM, Gimeno JR, et al. Non-sustained ventricular tachycardia in hypertrophic cardiomyopathy: an independent marker of sudden death risk in young patients. *J Am Coll Cardiol.* 2003;42:873–879.

69. Weng Z, Yao J, Chan RH, et al. Prognostic Value of LGE-CMR in HCM: a meta-analysis. *JACC Cardiovasc Imaging.* 2016;9:1392–1402.

70. Maron BJ, Spirito P, Ackerman MJ, et al. Prevention of sudden cardiac death with implantable cardioverter-defibrillators in children and adolescents with hypertrophic cardiomyopathy. *J Am Coll Cardiol.* 2013;61:1527–1535.

71. Sherrid MV, Barac I, McKenna WJ, et al. Multicenter study of the efficacy and safety of disopyramide in obstructive hypertrophic cardiomyopathy. *J Am Coll Cardiol.* 2005;45:1251–1258.

72. Olivotto I, Oreziak A, Barriales-Villa R, et al. Mavacamten for treatment of symptomatic obstructive hypertrophic cardiomyopathy (EXPLORER-HCM): a randomised, double-blind, placebo-controlled, phase 3 trial. *Lancet.* 2020.

73. Nguyen A, Schaff HV. Surgical myectomy: subaortic, midventricular, and apical. *Cardiol Clin.* 2019;37:95–104.

74. Balaram SK, Ross RE, Sherrid MV, et al. Role of mitral valve plication in the surgical management of hypertrophic cardiomyopathy. *Ann Thorac Surg.* 2012;94:1990–1997; discussion 1997-8.

75. Hong JH, Schaff HV, Nishimura RA, et al. Mitral regurgitation in patients with hypertrophic obstructive cardiomyopathy: implications for concomitant valve procedures. *J Am Coll Cardiol.* 2016;68:1497–1504.

76. Schoendube FA, Klues HG, Reith S, et al. Long-term clinical and echocardiographic follow-up after surgical correction of hypertrophic obstructive cardiomyopathy with extended myectomy and reconstruction of the subvalvular mitral apparatus. *Circulation.* 1995;92:II122–II127.

77. McLeod CJ, Ommen SR, Ackerman MJ, et al. Surgical septal myectomy decreases the risk for appropriate implantable cardioverter defibrillator discharge in obstructive hypertrophic cardiomyopathy. *Eur Heart J.* 2007;28:2583–2588.

78. Ommen SR, Maron BJ, Olivotto I, et al. Long-term effects of surgical septal myectomy on survival in patients with obstructive hypertrophic cardiomyopathy. *J Am Coll Cardiol.* 2005;46:470–476.

79. Batzner A, Pfeiffer B, Neugebauer A, et al. Survival after alcohol septal ablation in patients with hypertrophic obstructive cardiomyopathy. *J Am Coll Cardiol.* 2018;72:3087–3094.

80. Nguyen A, Schaff HV, Hang D, et al. Surgical myectomy versus alcohol septal ablation for obstructive hypertrophic cardiomyopathy: a propensity score-matched cohort. *J Thorac Cardiovasc Surg.* 2019;157:306–315 e3.

81. Sorajja P, Binder J, Nishimura RA, et al. Predictors of an optimal clinical outcome with alcohol septal ablation for obstructive hypertrophic cardiomyopathy. *Catheter Cardiovasc Interv.* 2013;81:E58–E67.

82. Yancy CW, Jessup M, Bozkurt B, et al. 2017 ACC/AHA/HFSA focused update of the 2013 ACCF/AHA guideline for the management of heart failure: a report of the American College of Cardiology/American Heart Association Task Force on Clinical Practice Guidelines and the Heart Failure Society of America. *Circulation.* 2017;136:e137–e161.

83. Guttmann OP, Rahman MS, O'Mahony C, et al. Atrial fibrillation and thromboembolism in patients with hypertrophic cardiomyopathy: systematic review. *Heart.* 2014;100:465–472.

84. Saberi S, Wheeler M, Bragg-Gresham J, et al. Effect of moderate-intensity exercise training on peak oxygen consumption in patients with hypertrophic cardiomyopathy: a randomized clinical trial. *J Am Med Assoc.* 2017;317:1349–1357.

85. Piercy KL, Troiano RP, Ballard RM, et al. The physical activity guidelines for Americans. *J Am Med Assoc.* 2018;320:2020–2028.

86. Maron BJ, Levine BD, Washington RL, et al. Eligibility and disqualification recommendations for competitive athletes with cardiovascular abnormalities: task force 2: preparticipation screening for cardiovascular disease in competitive athletes: a scientific statement from the American Heart Association and American College of Cardiology. *Circulation.* 2015;132:e267–e272.

87. Harmon KG, Asif IM, Klossner D, Drezner JA. Incidence of sudden cardiac death in National Collegiate Athletic Association athletes. *Circulation.* 2011;123:1594–1600.

88. Ullal AJ, Abdelfattah RS, Ashley EA, Froelicher VF. Hypertrophic cardiomyopathy as a cause of sudden cardiac death in the young: a meta-analysis. *Am J Med.* 2016;129:486–496 e2.

89. Ammirati E, Contri R, Coppini R, et al. Pharmacological treatment of hypertrophic cardiomyopathy: current practice and novel perspectives. *Eur J Heart Fail.* 2016;18:1106–1118.

90. Wong TC, Martinez M. Novel pharmacotherapy for hypertrophic cardiomyopathy. *Cardiol Clin.* 2019;37:113–117.

91. Abozguia K, Elliott P, McKenna W, et al. Metabolic modulator perhexiline corrects energy deficiency and improves exercise capacity in symptomatic hypertrophic cardiomyopathy. *Circulation.* 2010;122:1562–1569.

92. Coats CJ, Pavlou M, Watkinson OT, et al. Effect of trimetazidine dihydrochloride therapy on exercise capacity in patients with nonobstructive hypertrophic cardiomyopathy: a randomized clinical trial. *JAMA Cardiol.* 2019;4:230–235.

93. Olivotto I, Camici PG, Merlini PA, et al. Efficacy of ranolazine in patients with symptomatic hypertrophic cardiomyopathy: the RESTYLE-HCM randomized, double-blind, placebo-controlled study. *Circ Heart Fail.* 2018;11:e004124.

94. Olivotto I, Hellawell JL, Farzaneh-Far R, et al. Novel approach targeting the complex pathophysiology of hypertrophic cardiomyopathy: the impact of late sodium current inhibition on exercise capacity in subjects with symptomatic hypertrophic cardiomyopathy (LIBERTY-HCM) trial. *Circ Heart Fail.* 2016;9:e002764.

95. Kawano H, Toda G, Nakamizo R, et al. Valsartan decreases type I collagen synthesis in patients with hypertrophic cardiomyopathy. *Circ J.* 2005;69:1244–1248.

96. Penicka M, Gregor P, Kerekes R, et al. The effects of candesartan on left ventricular hypertrophy and function in nonobstructive hypertrophic cardiomyopathy: a pilot, randomized study. *J Mol Diagn.* 2009;11:35–41.

97. Axelsson A, Iversen K, Vejlstrup N, et al. Efficacy and safety of the angiotensin II receptor blocker losartan for hypertrophic cardiomyopathy: the INHERIT randomised, double-blind, placebo-controlled trial. *Lancet Diabetes Endocrinol.* 2015;3:123–131.

98. Maron MS, Chan RH, Kapur NK, et al. Effect of spironolactone on myocardial fibrosis and other clinical variables in patients with hypertrophic cardiomyopathy. *Am J Med.* 2018;131:837–841.

99. Semsarian C, Ahmad I, Giewat M, et al. The L-type calcium channel inhibitor diltiazem prevents cardiomyopathy in a mouse model. *J Clin Invest.* 2002;109:1013–1020.

100. Teekakirikul P, Eminaga S, Toka O, et al. Cardiac fibrosis in mice with hypertrophic cardiomyopathy is mediated by non-myocyte proliferation and requires Tgf-beta. *J Clin Invest.* 2010;120:3520–3529.

101. Green EM, Wakimoto H, Anderson RL, et al. A small-molecule inhibitor of sarcomere contractility suppresses hypertrophic cardiomyopathy in mice. *Science.* 2016;351:617–621.

102. Ho CY, Lakdawala NK, Cirino AL, et al. Diltiazem treatment for pre-clinical hypertrophic cardiomyopathy sarcomere mutation carriers: a pilot randomized trial to modify disease expression. *JACC Heart Fail.* 2015;3:180–188.

103. Ho CY, McMurray JJV, Cirino AL, et al. The Design of The Valsartan for Attenuating Disease Evolution in Early Sarcomeric Hypertrophic Cardiomyopathy (VANISH) trial. *Am Heart J.* 2017;187:145–155.

104. Kawas RF, Anderson RL, Ingle SRB, et al. A small-molecule modulator of cardiac myosin acts on multiple stages of the myosin chemomechanical cycle. *J Biol Chem.* 2017;292:16571–16577.

105. Stern JA, Markova S, Ueda Y, et al. A small molecule inhibitor of sarcomere contractility acutely relieves left ventricular outflow tract obstruction in feline hypertrophic cardiomyopathy. *PloS One.* 2016;11:e0168407.

106. Mamidi R, Li J, Doh CY, et al. Impact of the myosin modulator mavacamten on force generation and cross-bridge behavior in a murine model of hypercontractility. *J Am Heart Assoc.* 2018;7:e009627.

107. Ho CY, Mealiffe ME, Bach RG, et al. Evaluation of mavacamten in symptomatic patients with nonobstructive hypertrophic cardiomyopathy. *J Am Coll Cardiol.* 2020;75:2649–2660.

108. Prondzynski M, Mearini G, Carrier L. Gene therapy strategies in the treatment of hypertrophic cardiomyopathy. *Pflugers Arch.* 2019;471:807–815.

109. Ma H, Marti-Gutierrez N, Park SW, et al. Correction of a pathogenic gene mutation in human embryos. *Nature.* 2017;548:413–419.

55 Myocarditis

LESLIE T. COOPER JR. AND KIRK U. KNOWLTON

OVERVIEW AND DEFINITION

In its broadest sense, *myocarditis* refers to any inflammation of the myocardium. Inflammation can be found after any form of injury to the heart, including ischemic damage, mechanical trauma, and genetic cardiomyopathies. More specifically, however, *classic myocarditis* refers to inflammation of the heart muscle occurring as a result of exposure to either discrete external antigens, such as viruses, bacteria, parasites, toxins, or drugs, or internal triggers, such as autoimmune activation against self-antigens. Although viral infection remains the most commonly identified cause of myocarditis, drug hypersensitivity and toxic drug reactions, other infections, and peripartum cardiomyopathy also can lead to myocarditis.

The pathogenesis of myocarditis is a classic paradigm of cardiac injury followed by immunologic response from the host resulting in cardiac inflammation. The relative incidence of viral causes is continually evolving as new diagnostic tools based on molecular epidemiology become available. Indeed, more than 20 viruses have been associated with myocarditis, and the most frequent are currently parvovirus B19 (B19V) and human herpesvirus 6.[1] Enteroviruses such as coxsackievirus B continue to be commonly identified pathogens, and strains of enterovirus remain widely used in mouse models of the disease.[2] If the host immune response is overwhelming or inappropriate, the inflammation may destroy the heart tissue acutely or may linger, producing cardiac remodeling that leads to dilated cardiomyopathy (DCM), heart failure, or death. Fortunately for most patients, clinical myocarditis often is self-limited if proper support and follow-up care are available. In many cases the virus is cleared successfully, and the immune response is downmodulated. In some patients, however, an autoimmune reaction to endogenous antigens lingers beyond this phase and can cause persistent cardiac dysfunction. Sometimes viral genomes persist in the heart with or without acute inflammation.[3] Viral genomes commonly are detected in endomyocardial biopsy (EMB) specimens from patients with DCM and may signal a disease-related infection. As discussed in this chapter, with new insights into the understanding of the pathophysiology of myocarditis and new therapies for this condition, the outlook for affected patients is continuing to improve.

EPIDEMIOLOGY

As estimated in the 2019 Global Burden of Disease study the prevalence of myocarditis in 2019 was 712,780 (612,466 to 817,245, 95% uncertainty interval [UI]) or a prevalence rate of 9.21 per 100,000 (7.92 to 10.56, 95% UI).[4] This rate increased from 8.04 (6.85 to 9.19, 95% UI) in 1990. Disability from myocarditis is largely due to heart failure.

The age standardized, global disability-adjusted life years (DALYs) rate per 100,000 due to myocarditis in 2019 was 977,238 (803,762 to 1,126,804, 95% UI). There were an estimated 32,449 (23,164 to 37,087, 95% UI) deaths or 0.42 (0.30 to 0.48, 95% UI) deaths per 100,000 due to myocarditis.[4]

The death rate from myocarditis is higher in the first year of life than between ages 1 and 14 years for both males and females. After age 15 years, DALYs, number of deaths, and death rate due to myocarditis are higher in males than females.[4]

The rates of myocarditis vary by region with higher rates seen in parts of Southeast Asia, East Asia, Oceania, Central Europe, Eastern Europe, and Central Asia (Table 55.1). Myocarditis can be difficult to distinguish from other forms of cardiomyopathy in areas that rely on clinical presentation and echocardiography for diagnosis, suggesting imprecision in diagnosis within the larger category of cardiomyopathy. Myocarditis is responsible for sudden cardiovascular death in approximately 2% of infants, 5% of children, and 5% to 14% of young athletes.[4–6]

Myocarditis is responsible for a substantial minority of DCM cases (see also Chapters 48 and 52). In a review of DCM case series from 1978 to 1995 in which EMB was performed, the incidence of biopsy-proven myocarditis varied widely, ranging from 0.5% to 67%, with an average of 10.3%. Data from the U.S. Pediatric Cardiomyopathy Registry, in which 46% (222/485) of children with an identified cause of DCM had myocarditis, are illustrative of recent reports. As in most DCM case series, only a minority of children in this series, 34% of 1426, had a specific cause of DCM identified.[7] The differing histologic criteria used to define myocarditis are responsible for some of the variation in the reported prevalence of myocarditis. The standard Dallas criteria define idiopathic myocarditis as an inflammatory infiltrate of the myocardium with necrosis and/or degeneration of adjacent myocytes not typical of the ischemic damage associated with coronary artery disease (Fig. 55.1A and Table 55.2).[8] These criteria have been criticized because of interreader variability in interpretation, lack of prognostic value, and low sensitivity due in part to sampling error. Specific immunohistochemical stains that detect cellular antigens, such as anti-CD3 (T lymphocytes), anti-CD68 (macrophages), and class I and II human leukocyte antigens (see Fig. 55.1B), may have greater sensitivity for small infiltrates than that of hematoxylin-eosin stain. Markers of complement activity such as C4d also are commonly found in native cardiomyopathic hearts. Newer immunohistochemical stains have a greater predictive value for cardiovascular events than the Dallas criteria.[9]

The presence of viral genomes in heart tissue may indicate an active infectious myocarditis. In the posttransplantation setting, the presence of viral genomes in myocardial biopsy material predicts future rejection episodes and graft loss in children.[10] Viruses for which testing is commonly done in the setting of suspected myocarditis are B19V, adenovirus, cytomegalovirus, enterovirus, Epstein-Barr virus, hepatitis

3 20

C virus, herpes simplex viruses 1, 2, and 6, and influenza viruses A and B. New diagnostic criteria that rely on higher B19V copy numbers or evidence of active viral replication have been proposed.[2] For epidemiologic studies in which universal EMB is not feasible, diagnostic classifications that rely on clinical syndromes, biomarkers, and/or imaging abnormalities have been used (Table 55.3).[11]

SPECIFIC ETIOLOGIC AGENTS

In most cases, myocarditis is triggered by an inciting event, such as infection or exposure to a drug or toxin that activates the immune response. A subset of cases is due to primary immunologic abnormalities in the affected patient. Advanced techniques in virology, immunology, and molecular biology have demonstrated that there are many potential causes of myocarditis. Almost any infectious agent has been associated with myocarditis. In clinical practice, however, it is often difficult to identify a specific etiologic agent.

Viruses

Viral infection has been implicated as one of the most common infectious causes of myocarditis (Table 55.4). The earliest evidence of virus infection and its association with myocarditis and pericarditis was acquired during outbreaks of influenza, poliomyelitis, measles, and mumps, and in cases of pleurodynia associated with enterovirus infection.[12] Modern virologic and molecular techniques have demonstrated that adenoviruses, enteroviruses, and parvovirus are among the most commonly identified infectious agents in myocarditis. Although SARS-CoV-2 viral genomes and proteins have been identified in the heart tissue, the presence of SARS-CoV-2 viral genomes in the heart is generally not accompanied by a classic lymphocytic myocarditis (see also Chapter 94).

The precise incidence of myocarditis caused by these infectious agents varies geographically and temporally (Fig. 55.2). Nevertheless, in meta-analyses, polymerase chain reaction (PCR) studies in patients with clinically suspected myocarditis or cardiomyopathy who subsequently underwent heart biopsy demonstrated that virus could be identified 3.8 times more frequently in patients with myocarditis than in control subjects. Additional evidence indicates that persistence of the viral genome in patients with cardiomyopathy is associated

TABLE 55.1 Deaths from Myocarditis by Geographic Regions (Global Burden of Disease Study 2019)

GEOGRAPHIC REGION	DEATHS PER 100,000	95% UNCERTAINTY INDEX
Southeast Asia, East Asia, and Oceania	0.76	0.46–0.93
Central Europe, Eastern Europe, and Central Asia	0.79	0.57–0.93
High-income regions*	0.29	0.18–0.30
Latin America and Caribbean	0.22	0.18–0.35
North Africa and Middle East	0.36	0.26–0.65
South Asia	0.21	0.15–0.29
Sub-Saharan Africa	0.20	0.13–0.33

*High income regions are defined as Southern Latin America, Western Europe, High Income North America, Australasia, and High Income Asia Pacific.
From Roth GA, Mensah GA, Johnson CO, et al. Global burden of cardiovascular diseases and risk factors, 1990 to 2019: update from the global burden of disease 2019. *J Am Coll Cardiol.* 2020;76:2982–3021. Epublished DOI: 10.1016/j.jacc.2020.11.010.

TABLE 55.2 Endomyocardial Biopsy Diagnosis of Myocarditis: The Dallas Criteria

Definition
Idiopathic *myocarditis*: "an inflammatory infiltrate of the myocardium with necrosis and/or degeneration of adjacent myocytes not typical of the ischemic damage associated with coronary artery disease"

Classification

First biopsy
- Myocarditis with or without fibrosis
- Borderline myocarditis (repeat biopsy may be indicated)
- No myocarditis

Subsequent biopsy
- Ongoing (persistent) myocarditis with or without fibrosis
- Resolving (healing) myocarditis with or without fibrosis
- Resolved (healed) myocarditis with or without fibrosis

	DESCRIPTORS	
	INFLAMMATORY INFILTRATE	FIBROSIS
Distribution	Focal, confluent, diffuse	Endocardial, interstitial
Extent	Mild, moderate, severe	Mild, moderate, severe
Type	Lymphocytic, eosinophilic, granulomatous, giant cell, neutrophilic, mixed	Perivascular, replacement

Modified from Leone O, Veinot JP, Angelini A, et al. 2011 consensus statement on endomyocardial biopsy from the Association for European Cardiovascular Pathology and the Society for Cardiovascular Pathology. *Cardiovasc Pathol.* 2012;21:245.

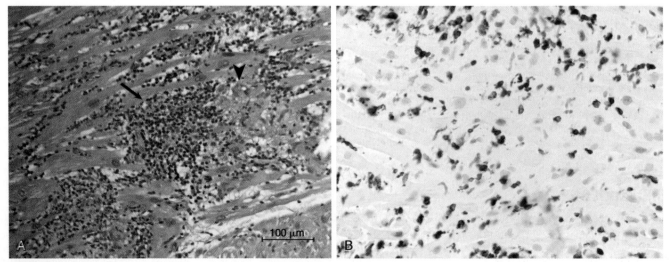

FIGURE 55.1 A, Acute myocarditis with widespread lymphocytic and histiocytic infiltrate *(arrow)* and associated myocyte damage *(arrowhead).* **B,** CD3 immunostaining of T lymphocytes in a patient with acute myocarditis. (Courtesy of Dylan Miller, MD. From Cooper LT. Myocarditis. *N Engl J Med.* 2009;360:1526.)

TABLE 55.3 Three-Tiered Clinical Classification for Diagnosis of Myocarditis by Level of Diagnostic Certainty

DIAGNOSTIC CATEGORY	CRITERIA	HISTOLOGIC CONFIRMATION	BIOMARKER, ECG, OR IMAGING ABNORMALITIES CONSISTENT WITH MYOCARDITIS	TREATMENT NEEDED
Possible subclinical acute myocarditis	In the clinical context of possible myocardial injury *without* cardiovascular symptoms but with at least one of the following: Biomarkers of cardiac injury raised / ECG findings suggestive of cardiac injury / Abnormal cardiac function on echocardiogram or CMR	Absent	Required	Not known
Probable acute myocarditis	In clinical context of possible myocardial injury *with* cardiovascular symptoms and at least one of the following: Biomarkers of cardiac injury raised / ECG findings suggestive of cardiac injury / Abnormal cardiac function on echocardiogram or CMR	Absent	Required	Per clinical syndrome
Definite myocarditis	Histologic or immunohistologic evidence of myocarditis	Present	Not required	Tailored to specific cause

CMR, Cardiac magnetic resonance imaging; *ECG,* electrocardiogram.
Modified from Sagar S, Liu PP, Cooper LT, Jr. Myocarditis. *Lancet.* 2012;379:738.

TABLE 55.4 Causes of Myocarditis

VIRUSES AND VIRAL DISORDERS	BACTERIA AND BACTERIAL DISORDERS	CARDIOTOXINS	HYPERSENSITIVITY MEDIATORS AND FACTORS
Adenovirus*	*Chlamydia*	Anthracycline drugs*	Cephalosporins
B19V	Cholera	Arsenic	Clozapine
Coxsackievirus B*	Leptospirosis	Carbon monoxide	Diuretics
Cytomegalovirus*	Lyme disease	Catecholamines	Hypereosinophilia
Epstein-Barr virus	*Mycoplasma*	Chagas disease	Insect bites
Hepatitis C virus	*Neisseria*	Cocaine*	Kawasaki disease
Herpes simplex virus	Relapsing fever	Copper	Lithium
HIV*	*Salmonella*	Ethanol*	Sarcoidosis
Influenza virus	Spirochete	Heavy metals	Snake bites
Mumps	*Staphylococcus*	Lead	Sulfonamides
Poliovirus	*Streptococcus*	Leishmaniasis	Systemic disorders
Rabies	Syphilis	Malaria	Tetanus toxoid
Rubella	Tetanus	Mercury	Tetracycline
SARS-CoV-2	Tuberculosis	Protozoa	Wegener granulomatosis
Varicella-zoster virus			
Yellow fever			

*Frequent cause of myocarditis.
HIV, Human immunodeficiency virus.
Modified from Elamm C, Fairweather D, Cooper LT. Pathogenesis and diagnosis of myocarditis. *Heart J.* 2012;98:835.

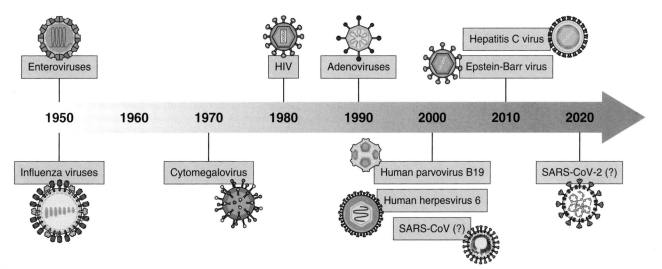

FIGURE 55.2 Prominent viruses associated with inflammatory cardiomyopathy over time. Over the years, the number of recognized viruses associated with inflammatory cardiomyopathy has grown. This evolution is partly influenced by the intentional detection of a broader repertoire of viruses over time as well as by the occurrence of novel viruses or virus genotypes in the heart. The association between severe acute respiratory syndrome coronavirus (SARS-CoV) and SARS-CoV-2 and inflammatory cardiomyopathy is not yet clear. "(?)" denotes unclear, needing further investigation; HIV, human immunodeficiency virus. (Adapted from Tschope C, Ammirati E, Bozkurt B, et al. Myocarditis and inflammatory cardiomyopathy: current evidence and future directions. *Nat Rev Cardiol.* 2020;Oct 12:1–25. https://doi.org/10.1038/s41569-020-00435-x.)

with increased ventricular dysfunction and worse outcome during follow-up.

Enteroviruses, Including Coxsackieviruses. Coxsackievirus is a member of the Enterovirus genus, Picornaviridae family. It is a nonenveloped lytic virus. Its capsid proteins harbor a single, positive-strand RNA genome of 7.4 Kb. Throughout the history of studies that address the causes of myocarditis, enteroviruses such as coxsackievirus B3 or echovirus are commonly identified in a subset of patients at a higher frequency than in control subjects. Using molecular techniques such as PCR and in situ hybridization, the enterovirus genome has been identified in the heart of 15% to 30% of patients with myocarditis and 7% to 30% of specimens with DCM, although the incidence in different studies varies considerably. Coxsackievirus infection meets the criteria of Koch's postulates as a cause of myocarditis in humans: It can be regularly found in the lesions of the disease; it has been isolated in pure culture from patients with myocarditis; and when inoculated into a mouse it can recapitulate the disease, after which the virus can be recovered from the heart of the infected mouse.

Coxsackievirus is a close relative of the poliovirus and rhinovirus, viruses that have been studied extensively. Although the disease phenotypes are different, the many similarities in viral replication cycles have facilitated an understanding of the mechanisms by which coxsackievirus can cause disease. Coxsackievirus typically enters the host through the gastrointestinal or respiratory system. It uses the coxsackievirus-adenovirus receptor (CAR), a transmembrane adhesion protein, as its primary receptor for cell entry. It can cause a broad range of clinical syndromes, including meningitis, skin rashes, acute respiratory illness, skeletal myositis, and myocarditis. Most recently, evaluation of patients with myocarditis has demonstrated a decrease in the prevalence of enteroviruses in the myocardium. This is particularly evident in Western Europe. The reason for this decrease is not clear but may be related to a herd immunity that occurs after a period of prolonged exposure to the virus. The lower incidence may also be confounded by seasonal outbreaks of enterovirus infections, thereby making the exact incidence dependent on the outbreaks.

Adenovirus. Adenoviruses are nonenveloped DNA viruses that also use CAR (adenovirus types 2 and 5), as well as integrins, as receptors for entry into the target cell. The adenovirus capsid harbors a double-stranded DNA genome. Adenoviruses commonly infect mucosal surfaces. The adenovirus genome is consistently identified in a subset of patients with myocarditis. The incidence in myocarditis patients has been recorded to be as high as 23% and as low as less than 2%.[13] Although mechanisms of adenoviral infection have been studied in considerable detail in cell culture and other diseases, it has been challenging to study adenovirus-mediated myocarditis, in the face of difficulties identifying an appropriate mouse model using the same adenoviruses that affect humans.

Parvovirus. The role of parvovirus B19 (B19V) of the genus Erythrovirus in the pathogenesis of myocarditis has been identified as a potentially important contributor to myocarditis because of the high prevalence of B19V DNA in hearts of patients with myocarditis. Parvovirus is a nonenveloped, nonlytic virus with a single-strand, positive-strand DNA genome of approximately 5.6 Kb. Humans are the only known host for B19V, making it challenging to study in animal models, but examples of myocarditis in mice stimulated with the capsid protein VP1 or antibodies against VP1 have been reported.[14] Its primary receptor is globoside, also known as group P antigen. This antigen is found primarily on erythroid progenitors, erythroblasts, and megakaryocytes. It also has been shown to be expressed on endothelial cells. This finding may be important for its role in the pathogenesis of myocarditis. The infection is thought generally to be spread by the respiratory route. The incidence of infection in the general population is also high, with evidence of B19V infection demonstrated in approximately 50% of children at age 15 years, and detectable IgG directed against B19V found in as many as 80% of older adult patients. With PCR studies, the PVB genome has been identified in 11% to 56% of patients with myocarditis and in 10% to 51% of patients with DCM.[14]

In keeping with the high prevalence of B19V in the general population, the pathogenic role of B19V continues to be clarified. In one study, B19V was assessed by immunohistochemistry and PCR assay. The investigators found that B19V was detectable by immunohistologic analysis in 65% of patients with myocarditis, 35% of patients with DCM, and 8% of noninflamed control hearts. The viral load was assessed by genome copy numbers in the samples that were positive for B19V on immunohistologic analysis. The viral load was significantly higher in patients with acute myocarditis, followed by those with DCM, and it

was lowest in the patients with normal hearts without inflammation. In addition, viral RNA replicative intermediates were detected only in patients with inflamed hearts. It has also been determined that evidence of viral transcription is associated with an anomalous host myocardial transcriptome.[15,16] These findings indicate that the amount of B19V viral DNA is associated with the disease phenotype. Of importance, the virus was found in endothelial cells and not myocardial cells. Other studies have suggested a bystander role for B19V in adult myocarditis, with persistence of low-level B19V titers a frequent finding, but unrelated to ongoing myocardial injury. Additional experimentation is needed to determine mechanisms by which B19V could contribute to myocarditis and cardiomyopathy.

Human Immunodeficiency Virus. The improved survival rate of patients with human immunodeficiency virus (HIV) infection has affected the incidence of heart disease in this population (see also Chapter 85). Myocarditis with lymphocytic infiltration has been reported in 40% to 52% of patients who die of acquired immunodeficiency syndrome (AIDS). The incidence of myocardial disease, however, appears to have decreased with increased antiretroviral therapy. For more information see the online supplement, "Human Immunodeficiency Virus."

Hepatitis C Virus. Hepatitis C virus infection appears to be mainly associated with cardiomyopathy in Asian countries such as Japan. A low incidence of hepatitis C virus antibodies (4.4%) was identified in patients who were studied in the Myocarditis Treatment Trial. This occurrence rate was nevertheless higher than that (1.8%) in the general U.S. population. Perhaps the higher incidence of hepatitis C virus infection in DCM is related to the overall higher incidence of this infection in Asia. Myocardial biopsy samples from patients with cardiomyopathy have demonstrated the presence of the hepatitis C viral genome, and a rise in serum antibody titers has been documented in patients so affected. The phenotype associated with hepatitis C virus also has been reported to include hypertrophic cardiomyopathy, suggesting that hepatitis C may have a direct effect on growth and hypertrophy of the myocardial cells. Symptomatic myocarditis generally is observed in the first to third weeks of illness. It has been reported that heart function can return to normal with clearance of the virus.

Influenza Virus. Influenza A virus infection is a well-recognized cause of myocarditis, and this association should be kept in mind during periodic outbreaks of influenza A. The exact incidence of myocarditis with influenza A outbreaks is not known, but it generally is considered to be in the 5% range. During pandemics such as the 2009 H1N1 pandemic, myocarditis was reported in 5% to 15% of cases as diagnosed by changes on the electrocardiogram (ECG) and the presence of cardiac symptoms. Some cases manifested with fulminant myocarditis. Histopathologic examination usually demonstrates the presence of the inflammatory infiltrate that is typical of myocarditis (see also Chapter 94).

Coronavirus. As the world has turned its attention to the COVID-19 pandemic, it became clear during the early stages of the disease that patients who were admitted to the hospital for COVID-19 had a 20% to 35% incidence of myocardial injury manifested by an increase in troponin and type B natriuretic factor. It was also clear that the extent of myocardial injury correlated directly with a worsening prognosis of intubation and death. It was assumed initially that this myocardial injury was secondary to a classical form of myocarditis precipitated by infection of cardiac cells by SARS-CoV-2. Case reports from some of the most severely affected areas supported that hypothesis. However, diagnoses were often made by clinical findings and evidence of myocarditis on cardiac magnetic resonance (cMR) imaging. Subsequent reports of myocarditis have been varied, which may be related to definitions that used to define myocarditis.[17] An autopsy report from a young person with sudden death found to have COVID-19 demonstrated that SARS-CoV-2 could be identified within isolated, but adjacent myocytes. Correlative experiments in human IPS-derived cardiomyocytes (hiPS-CMs) demonstrate that hiPS-CMs can be infected by SARS-CoV-2 and that cell fusion can be mediated by proteolytically activated SPIKE protein.[18] The pathogenesis of cardiac injury in COVID-19 is complex with mechanisms that include viral mediated injury, microvascular dysfunction/thrombosis, cytokines, and type II myocardial infarctions. The histological features seen at autopsy include increased macrophages and cytokine elevation. Classic lymphocytic myocarditis is relatively uncommon in COVID-19 patients.[19,20] Additional research will be needed to clearly define mechanisms of cardiac injury following SARS-CoV2 infection. The cause of injury is likely multifactorial with evidence of inflammation as manifest by macrophage infiltration and less commonly a typical lymphocytic myocarditis.

Attention has turned to whether myocarditis or cardiac injury might be identified by cardiac MR after patients recover from COVID-19. Myocarditis identified by MR after SARS-CoV-2 infection varies widely, from

0.6% in young athletes to 32% in older patients with elevated troponin.[21] COVID-19 in children and young adults <21 years of age was associated with a multisystem inflammatory syndrome (MIS-C). A total of 36/99 (36%) of the patients were diagnosed with Kawasaki disease or atypical (or incomplete) Kawasaki disease, whereas 52/99 (53%) had clinical evidence of myocarditis (see also Chapter 94).[17] COVID vaccines have been highly successful at reducing the risk of illness and hospitalization from SARS-CoV-2 infection. A small increase in the rate of myocarditis and pericarditis has been observed following mRNA vaccines. The rate of myocarditis and pericarditis has been reported as 1.0 per 100,000 and 1.8 per 100,000, respectively. None of the patients that had myocarditis or pericarditis died following vaccination. Additional studies are needed to confirm these findings. In addition, the incidence and severity of vaccine-associated myocarditis and pericarditis is much less than the devastating effects of COVID-19 infection.[21a]

Bacteria

Nonviral pathogens such as bacteria and parasites can affect the heart and, in some cases, activate an immune reaction in the heart. Virtually any bacterial agent can cause myocardial dysfunction, but it does not necessarily mean that the bacterium has infected the myocardium. In the case of sepsis or other severe bacterial infections, the myocardial dysfunction generally is attributed to activation of inflammatory mediators (see Chapter 47). Of note, however, bloodstream infection by virtually any bacterial infection can result in metastatic foci in the myocardium. This finding is most commonly associated with bacterial endocarditis. Some bacterial infections are well known to have specific effects on the heart that can be mediated by direct infection or activation of inflammatory mechanisms. The most common of these include diphtheria, rheumatic heart disease, and streptococcal infections.

Corynebacterium Infection. Myocardial involvement with *Corynebacterium diphtheriae* is a serious complication and is the most common cause of death in diphtheria. In up to one half of fatal cases, evidence of cardiac involvement can be found. Studies from the last decade indicate that there is evidence of myocardial involvement in 22% to 28% of patients. The overall incidence has decreased in developed countries because of vaccination, but recently there have been a growing number of unprotected individuals in developed countries as well. This may be related to vaccine avoidance. *C. diphtheriae* produces an exotoxin that severely damages the myocardium and the cardiac conduction system. Cardiac damage is due to the liberation of this exotoxin, which inhibits protein synthesis by interfering with host translational mechanisms. The toxin appears to have an affinity for the cardiac conduction system. Both antitoxin therapy and antibiotics are important in the treatment of diphtheria.

Streptococcal Infection. The most commonly detected cardiac complication after beta-hemolytic streptococcal infection is acute rheumatic fever, which is followed by rheumatic valve disease in approximately 60% of affected patients. Rarely, involvement of the heart by the streptococcus may produce a nonrheumatic myocarditis distinct from acute rheumatic carditis (see also Chapter 97). This clinical entity is characterized by the presence of an interstitial infiltrate composed of mononuclear cells with occasional polymorphonuclear leukocytes, which may be focal or diffuse. In contrast with rheumatic heart disease, streptococcal myocarditis usually occurs coincident with the acute infection or within a few days of the pharyngitis. Electrocardiographic abnormalities, including ST elevation and prolongation of the PR and QT intervals, are common. Rare sequelae may include sudden death, conduction disturbances, and arrhythmias.

Tuberculosis. Involvement of the myocardium by Mycobacterium tuberculosis (not tuberculous pericarditis) is rare. Tuberculous involvement of the myocardium occurs by means of hematogenous or lymphatic spread or may arise directly from contiguous structures and may cause nodular, miliary, or diffuse infiltrative disease. On occasion, it may lead to arrhythmias, including atrial fibrillation and ventricular tachycardia, complete atrioventricular block, heart failure, left ventricular aneurysms, and sudden death.

Whipple Disease. Although overt involvement is rare, intestinal lipodystrophy, or Whipple disease, is not uncommonly associated with cardiac involvement. Periodic acid–Schiff–positive macrophages can be found in the myocardium, pericardium, coronary arteries, and heart valves of patients with this disorder. Electron microscopy has demonstrated rod-shaped structures in the myocardium similar to those found in the small intestine, representing the causative agent of the disease, Tropheryma whipplei, a gram-negative bacillus related to the actinomycetes. An inflammatory infiltrate and foci of fibrosis also may be present. The valvular fibrosis may be severe enough to result in aortic regurgitation and mitral stenosis. Although it usually is asymptomatic, nonspecific electrocardiographic changes are most common; systolic murmurs, pericarditis, complete heart block, and even overt congestive heart failure may occur. Antibiotic therapy appears to be effective in treatment of the basic disease, but relapses can occur, often more than 2 years after the initial diagnosis.

Lyme Carditis. Lyme disease is caused by a tick-borne spirochete (*Borrelia burgdorferi*). It usually begins during the summer months with a characteristic rash (erythema chronicum migrans), followed by acute neurologic, joint, or cardiac involvement, usually with few long-term sequelae. Early studies indicated that up to 10% of untreated patients with Lyme disease demonstrated evidence of transient cardiac involvement, the most common manifestation being atrioventricular block of variable degree. With the early use of antibiotics, however, Lyme carditis is now considered to be a rare manifestation.[22] Of patients with Lyme disease reported to the Centers for Disease Control (CDC), only 1.1% were identified as having Lyme carditis.[23] Syncope due to complete heart block is frequent with cardiac involvement because of the commonly associated depression of ventricular escape rhythms. Diffuse ST-segment and T wave abnormalities are transient and usually asymptomatic. An abnormal gallium scan is compatible with cardiac involvement, and the demonstration of spirochetes in myocardial biopsy specimens of patients with Lyme carditis suggests a direct cardiac effect. Patients with second-degree or complete heart block should be hospitalized and undergo continuous electrocardiographic monitoring. Temporary transvenous pacing may be required for a week or longer in patients with a high-grade block. It is thought that antibiotics can prevent subsequent complications and may shorten the duration of the disease; therefore, they are used routinely in patients with Lyme carditis. Intravenous antibiotics are suggested, although oral antibiotics can be used when only mild cardiac involvement is present. Corticosteroids may reduce myocardial inflammation and edema, which in turn can shorten the duration of the heart block. It is thought that treatment of the early manifestations of the disease will prevent development of late complications.

Protozoa

Chagas disease is one of the major causes of nonischemic cardiomyopathy throughout the world, although the incidence is changing. In a remarkable tale of discovery at the beginning of the 20th century, Carlos Chagas almost single-handedly identified the parasite, *Trypanosoma cruzi*, which causes the entity now known as Chagas disease. He also elucidated the relatively complex life cycle of the parasite in poor, rural areas of Brazil. The parasite resides in and replicates in an infected host such as an armadillo or a domestic cat. The parasite then infects triatomine insects, including the hematophagous reduviid bug that feeds on the blood of infected vertebrate carriers. The triatomine acts as the vector of infection when it bites a human, depositing the parasite in its feces in the area of the bite wound, conjunctiva, or other mucous membranes. Transmission can also occur through blood transfusions, organ transplantation, consumption of food or beverages that have been contaminated by the vector or vector feces, as well as *in utero* from mother to fetus. Once within the now-infected individual, the parasite replicates and infects target organs such as the heart. Parasitic infection of cardiac myocytes and activation of the associated immune function damage the heart and other organs and lead to the clinical manifestations of Chagas disease; Fig. 55.3 shows the life cycle.[24]

Chagas disease is endemic in poor, rural areas of Central and South America (eFig. 55.1). The distribution of Chagas disease is changing to include more urban and traditionally nonendemic areas because of migration of infected individuals from the rural to urban areas. Vector control initiatives in the endemic areas and aggressive screening of the blood supply has reduced the overall incidence of Chagas disease. In the 1980s, 17.4 million people were infected in 18 endemic countries.[25] By 2010, it was estimated that the number of infected persons had dropped to nearly 5.7 million. In 1990, it was

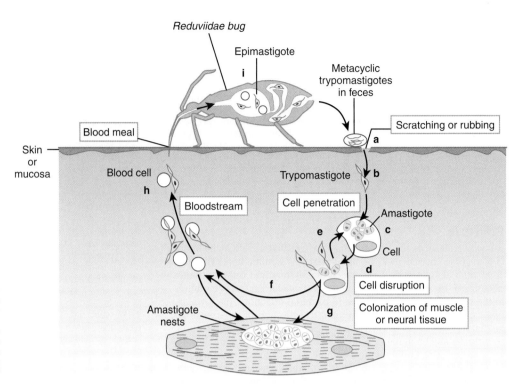

FIGURE 55.3 The life cycle of *Trypanosoma cruzi*. Reduviidae bugs transmit *T. cruzi*. While partaking of a blood meal *(a)*, the insect defecates on the host's skin, releasing the infective trypomastigote form of the parasite. The trypomastigotes penetrate the host's skin or mucous membrane through abrasions caused by scratching or rubbing the bitten area *(b)*. Trypomastigotes can infect host cardiac, skeletal, smooth muscle, or neural cells, subsequently giving rise to the round amastigote form that can replicate intracellularly *(c)*. Amastigotes can give rise to trypomastigotes that can lyse cells *(d)*. Amastigotes and trypomastigotes released from dying cells can propagate the infection or reenter the circulation *(e-g)*. Insects can pick up the parasite when consuming a blood meal *(h)*; it develops into the epimastigote form that replicates in the insect gut *(i)*. (From Macedo AM, Oliveira RP, Pena SDJ. Chagas' disease: role of parasite genetic variation in pathogenesis. *Expert Rev Mol Med.* 2002;4:1.)

estimated that 700,000 new cases were diagnosed each year. In 2010, that number had decreased to 29,925. Similarly, the number of annual deaths from Chagas disease has decreased, from 50,000 per year in 1990 to approximately 12,500 per year.[26] However, at the same time that Chagas disease is decreasing worldwide, the incidence in the developed world is increasing because of immigration from endemic areas. It is currently estimated that 240,000 to 350,000 people in the United States are infected with *T. cruzi*.[26] This has important implications in relation to blood transfusion and organ donation, because the infectious agent can be transferred from donor to recipient; this is a particularly important consideration in the immunocompromised transplant recipient.

Symptoms from *T. cruzi* infection typically begin 1 to 2 weeks after a bite from an infected triatomine, or can occur up to a few months after transfusion of infected blood. The parasite load can affect the severity of clinical presentation. The initial acute phase of the disease begins 1 to 2 weeks after infection and lasts for up to 4 to 8 weeks. In the acute phase, the most sensitive diagnostic test is the identification of *T. cruzi* genetic material in the blood using PCR assay. During the acute phase of parasite infection, most affected patients are either asymptomatic or have a mild, subacute febrile illness. Other potential manifestations include adenopathy, hepatomegaly, myocarditis, and meningoencephalitis. Cardiovascular abnormalities during the acute phase might include nonspecific ECG changes, first-degree atrioventricular block, and cardiomegaly on chest x-ray examination. Death occurs from myocarditis or meningoencephalitis in less than 5% to 10% of symptomatic patients. In up to 90% of patients, the symptoms of disease resolve spontaneously, even without therapeutic intervention. Of these, approximately 60% to 70% develop an intermediate form of the disease that is characterized by the absence of signs or symptoms of cardiac or gastrointestinal involvement. Although these patients will remain seropositive throughout life, there are no other laboratory findings of Chagas disease. The prognosis is excellent for this form of the disease.

The other 30% to 40% of patients will develop manifestations of the chronic Chagas disease 5 to 15 years after the acute phases of the disease. Cardiac involvement in the chronic form of Chagas is characterized by myocardial fibrosis, destruction of the conduction system, ventricular dilation, thinning of the apex of the heart, and formation of a thrombus in the apex of the heart. These changes lead to DCM, symptomatic heart failure, arrhythmias, atrioventricular and bundle branch block, and possible thromboembolism. The Latin American guidelines for the diagnosis and treatment of cardiovascular involvement in Chagas disease define

5 different stages of Chagas heart disease based on the presence or absence of ECG changes, LV dysfunction, and development of symptoms of heart failure.[27] Gastrointestinal disturbances also can be a prominent part of the presentation. Congenital transmission of the parasite to a fetus from the mother is another important mechanism of transmission of the parasite. Conversely, the parasite can be passed from the mother to the infant at the time of birth. *T. cruzi* also has been shown to infect the placenta and subsequently infect the fetus in utero. Congenital transmission occurs in 1% to 5% of pregnancies when the mother has chronic Chagas disease. Congenital transmission of this disease results in spontaneous abortion, premature birth, or infection of organs in the fetus.[26]

Benznidazole and nifurtimox, which both inhibit *T. cruzi* DNA replication, and are effective against the trypomastigote and amastigote forms of the parasite, are currently the only treatments for treating Chagas disease. Benznidazole is considered to be the first line of therapy because of its better tolerability; however, both drugs produce significant side effects. Current treatment recommendations are based on the phase of the disease and age of the patient. The cure rates for treating congenital cases (96%) and children in the acute (76%) early chronic phase (62%) are well established. However, the cure rates for adults with chronic disease are less well established.[28] Treatment with benznidazole is recommended for children in acute and congenital cases, reactivations, and in the chronic indeterminate phase. The therapy of adult patients with intermediate or established Chagas cardiomyopathy remains controversial. The BENEFIT trial was a prospective study of 2854 patients with Chagas cardiomyopathy randomized to receive benznidazole or placebo for up to 80 days. The primary outcome variable was a clinical composite of death, resuscitated cardiac arrest, sustained ventricular tachycardia, insertion of a pacemaker or implantable cardioverter-defibrillator, cardiac transplantation, new heart failure, stroke, or other thromboembolic event. BENEFIT showed that although benznidazole significantly reduced the detection of parasite in the serum, it had no effect on the primary outcome (adjusted HR, 0.92; 95% CI, 0.81 to 1.06; p = 0.26).[29] Current guidelines recommend that adults ≤50 years of age in the indeterminate phase with minimal cardiac involvement should be offered treatment.[28] However, there is insufficient evidence supporting effectiveness of treatment in older adults and adults with cardiomyopathy. Nonetheless, given that it is not currently possible to predict which asymptomatic adult patients > 50 years of age will progress to the chronic form of the disease, it may be reasonable to also consider therapy for this group of patients on a case-by-case basis, because treatment remains the best way to prevent morbidity and mortality in Chagas disease.[28]

Helminths

Infection by a wide variety of helminth parasites, commonly *Trichinella* and *Echinococcus*, can result in myocardial injury ultimately progressing to cardiomyopathy. For more information see the online supplement, "Helminths."

Physical Agents, Including Adverse Drug Effects

A wide variety of substances other than infectious agents can act on the heart and damage the myocardium. In some cases, the damage is acute, transient, and associated with evidence of an inflammatory myocardial infiltrate with myocyte necrosis (e.g., with the arsenicals and lithium). Other agents that damage the myocardium can lead to chronic changes with resulting histologic evidence of fibrosis and a clinical picture of a dilated or restrictive cardiomyopathy. Numerous chemicals and drugs (both industrial and therapeutic) can lead to cardiac damage and dysfunction. Several other physical agents (e.g., radiation, excessive heat, hypothermia) also can contribute directly to myocardial damage. For more information see the online supplement, "Additional Physical Agents That Cause Myocarditis."

Drugs. Drug-induced hypersensitivity syndrome may involve the heart and be associated with myocarditis. The syndrome usually emerges within 8 weeks of the initiation of a new drug but can occur at any time after drug consumption. Common agents include antiepileptics, antimicrobials, allopurinol, and sulfa-based drugs. Dobutamine, often used for hemodynamic support in patients with failing hearts, may be associated with eosinophilic myocarditis, and the drug should be stopped when eosinophilia appears or when an unexpected decline in left ventricular function is noted. Presenting characteristics may include a rash (unless the patient is immunologically compromised), fever, and multiorgan dysfunction (including hepatitis, nephritis, and myocarditis). Diffuse myocardial involvement may result in systemic hypotension and thromboembolic events. CMR imaging and measurement of cardiac biomarkers may help identify patients with cardiac involvement. EMB may demonstrate eosinophils, histiocytes, lymphocytes, myocardial necrosis, and occasionally granuloma and vasculitis. Myocardial involvement is patchy, so a definitive diagnosis is made only when the biopsy findings are positive. Corticosteroids and drug withdrawal usually resolve this syndrome; however, some patients may display a prolonged and relapsing course.

Clozapine is an effective antipsychotic medication that is used to treat severe, refractory schizophrenia. Myocarditis is a rarely reported side effect of clozapine therapy, with the initial incidence reported at between 0.01% and 0.001%. More recent observations, however, have found an incidence of myocarditis in 1% to 10% of patients. Perhaps the increased incidence is related to an increased awareness of the risk. Myocarditis can develop at any time during treatment but occurs most frequently within the first 4 days to 22 weeks after initiation of clozapine. The peak incidence is at around 19 to 21 days. Clozapine-related myocarditis probably is the result of a hypersensitivity reaction. It may be accompanied by eosinophilia, with eosinophilic infiltration seen in myocardial biopsy material. Clozapine also is a potent anticholinergic compound, and high levels associated with altered metabolism from CYP450 enzymes also could contribute to the cardiac effects. With clear evidence of myocarditis in a patient taking this drug, immediate discontinuation is indicated.[30]

Vaccination for smallpox among uniformed service members has been demonstrated to be associated with myopericarditis. In a prospective assessment of myocarditis following smallpox vaccination, clinical myopericarditis and subclinical myocarditis were noted at an incidence of 463 and 2868 per 100,000 subjects, respectively (in a healthy cohort the incidence was 2.2 clinical myopericarditis patients per 100,000). There were no cases of clinical myopericarditis or subclinical myocarditis in a control group that received trivalent influenza vaccination.[31]

As new chemotherapeutic agents are developed to target specific pathways in the heart, it is becoming increasingly apparent that cancer chemotherapy can induce cardiomyopathy that may be associated with myocarditis (see also Chapters 56 and 57). Antibodies against programmed cell death-1 (PD-1) (nivolumab, pembrolizumab, cemiplimab), T-lymphocyte-associated protein-4 (CTLA-4) (ipilimumab), and programmed cell death ligand 1 (PD-L1) (atezolizumab, avelumab, durvalumab)—termed "immune checkpoint inhibitors" (ICIs)—have revolutionized cancer treatment by increasing native immune activation and enhancing tumor antigen expression. As an unwanted consequence of immune activation, self-antigens (once regulated by checkpoint receptors) are recognized as foreign and result in autoimmunity including myocarditis in 0.3% to 1.0%. Fulminant myocarditis has been treated with high-dose corticosteroids and sometimes alemtuzumab or abatacept, T cell inhibitors.[32]

PATHOGENESIS OF VIRAL MYOCARDITIS

Much of the current understanding of the pathogenesis of myocarditis is derived from mouse models of enteroviral infection, particularly coxsackievirus B3, and rodent models of autoimmune myocarditis. The principles derived from these models have been applied to human myocarditis of different causes.[2] The description of the pathogenesis draws from cellular animal and human data. The pathogenesis of viral myocarditis can be divided into three major components: viral infection and replication, immunologic response (innate and adaptive immune response), and, ultimately, a phase of chronic cardiac remodeling (Fig. 55.4). MicroRNAs have also been shown to have a role in myocarditis. (For more information see the online supplement, "MicroRNAs in Myocarditis.")

Viral Infection

Viruses enter the host through a variety of locations, including the gastrointestinal system and respiratory system. The virus may undergo initial replication in the host in organs such as the liver, spleen, and pancreas. Ultimately, the virus reaches the heart via dissemination through the blood or lymphatic vessels. The steps include attachment of the virus to its receptor, entry of the virus into the cell, replication of the virus within the affected cell in the heart, and for lytic viruses, exit of the virus from the cell to allow infection of other cardiac cells. In the case of coxsackievirus, the virus infects the cardiac myocyte. In addition, however, other viruses may infect other cells in the heart, such as B19V that has been demonstrated to infect the cardiac endothelial cell and is not found in the cardiac myocyte.[16]

Initially, the virus binds to a viral receptor, ultimately resulting in internalization of the virus (eFig. 55.2). This process includes entry of the viral capsid proteins and the viral genome. In the case of coxsackieviruses and adenoviruses, the receptor is a transmembrane molecule, CAR, named for these two viruses, which are known to use it as a receptor.[33] Genetic deletion of CAR in the cardiac myocyte markedly inhibits infection of the heart and development of myocarditis.[34] In addition to CAR, coxsackievirus infection can be facilitated by interaction with the decay-accelerating factor (DAF), or CD55. CAR acts as a receptor in both human and mouse cells. CAR is a tight junction protein in noncardiac cells and is expressed at high levels in the intercalated disc of myocardial cells. Entry of the virus through the receptor activates a signaling complex that includes p56^{lck}, Abl, and Fyn kinase.[33]

On entry of the enterovirus into the cell, the positive, single-strand RNA is released from the icosahedral capsid and translated using host translational mechanisms. The viral RNA is translated as a single, monocistronic polyprotein, which is cleaved into its separate peptides by the viral proteases 2A and 3C; through an autocatalytic cleavage process, VP0 is cleaved into VP2 and VP4. This results in generation of capsid and nonstructural proteins, including an RNA-dependent RNA polymerase that is required for replication of the viral genome. The other nonstructural proteins also are required for replication of the positive-strand RNA through a negative-strand intermediate. Once the numbers of viral capsid proteins have been amplified and the positive-strand RNA has replicated, the positive-strand RNA is encapsidated into the newly formed viral capsid proteins VP1, VP2, VP3, and VP4. The encapsidated coxsackievirus RNA is released from the myocardial cell through a process of cell lysis and disruption of the sarcolemmal membrane.

Several mechanisms are recognized to affect membrane integrity, thus affecting in turn release of the replicated virus. Muscle cells rely on the subsarcolemmal protein dystrophin and the associated proteins in the dystrophin-glycoprotein complex to maintain the integrity of the sarcolemmal membrane. Hereditary absence of dystrophin in Duchenne muscular dystrophy, for example, causes cardiac and skeletal muscle dysfunction (see Chapter 100). In enterovirus-induced murine myocarditis, it has been demonstrated that one of the nonstructural proteins, protease 2A, is able to directly cleave dystrophin, thus disrupting the dystrophin-glycoprotein complex. This decreases the sarcolemmal

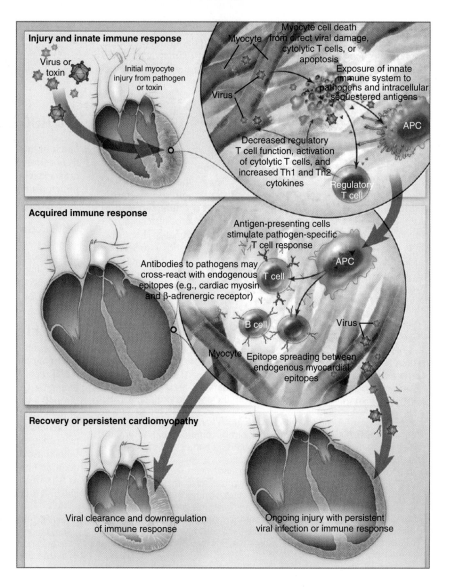

FIGURE 55.4 Pathogenesis of myocarditis. The current understanding of the cellular and molecular pathogenesis of postviral and autoimmune myocarditis is based solely on animal models. In these models, the progression from acute injury to chronic dilated cardiomyopathy may be simplified into a three-stage process. Acute injury leads to cardiac damage, exposure of intracellular antigens such as cardiac myosin, and activation of the innate immune system. Over weeks, specific immunity that is mediated by T lymphocytes and antibodies directed against pathogens and similar endogenous heart epitopes causes robust inflammation. In most patients, the pathogen is cleared and the immune reaction is downregulated, with few sequelae. In other patients, however, the virus is not cleared, and it causes continued myocyte damage; heart-specific inflammation may persist because of mistaken recognition of endogenous heart antigens as pathogenic entities. *APC,* antigen-presenting cell. (From Cooper LT. Myocarditis. *N Engl J Med.* 2009;360:1526.)

membrane integrity and facilitates the release of the virus from the myocardial cell. When dystrophin is not present in the mouse heart, as occurs in Duchenne muscular dystrophy, coxsackievirus is released more efficiently from the myocyte to infect adjacent cells.[35] However, when a dystrophin protein is expressed that cannot be cleaved by protease 2A, viral replication and the extent of myocardial damage is decreased.[35] Proteases 2A and 3C can cleave other host proteins that are involved in the maintenance of membrane integrity, initiation of translation of host proteins, regulation of apoptosis, innate immune response, and serum response factor.[3]

As genetic profiles have been assessed in patients, especially children with myocarditis, there is a growing body of literature that supports the concept that abnormalities in the cytoskeletal proteins occur more frequently in patients with myocarditis than in control populations. One study demonstrates that, in patients with acute myocarditis, there is an increase in the percentage who have homozygous or compound heterozygous variants in genes that have been associated with DCM. Interestingly, they found that potentially pathogenic variants occurred in the genes DSP, PKP2, and TNNI3 that code for the cytoskeletal and contractile proteins desmoplakin, plakophilin-2, and troponin I type 3. In addition, there were alterations in BAG3, which encodes BCL2-associated athanogene 3, which is an important mediator of apoptosis. Other genes that were abnormal in acute myocarditis included SCN5A, which encodes the sarcolemmal sodium channel, voltage-gated type V alpha subunit, which has been associated with the dystrophin-glycoprotein complex. Finally, RYR2, which encodes the ryanodine receptor 2, was mutated.[36] Additional evidence for an interaction between myocarditis and cytoskeletal abnormalities has been demonstrated in other case reports including one in monozygotic twins with a desmoplakin gene

variant.[37] Desmoplakin cardiomyopathy has been shown to have an inflammatory component as well.[38]

Generally, the activation of the innate and adaptive, antigen-specific immune response eliminates or greatly reduces the replication of the virus within the host cell. In some cases, however, the virus can persist within the myocardium. In keeping with the presence of the enteroviral genome in a subset of patients with DCM, it is thought that persistence of the enteroviral genome could contribute to the ongoing remodeling that occurs with DCM. The feasibility of this concept has been shown in a mouse model, in which low-level, cardiac-specific expression of a replication-defective enteroviral genome can cause cardiomyopathy. However, the proportion of patients in whom the enteroviral genome can be identified with reverse transcriptase PCR (rtPCR) or in situ hybridization techniques generally is less than 10%. The early phases of enteroviral infection and intramyocardial innate immunity can now be studied in human-induced pluripotent stem cells that are differentiated to cardiac myocytes.[39]

Other types of viruses also have been detected in cardiac biopsy specimens from patients with DCM. These viruses include B19V, herpesvirus, cytomegalovirus, hepatitis C virus, and others. Distinguishing whether the presence of a viral genome in each patient is causative or an incidental finding in cardiomyopathy has not been trivial. For example, the B19V viral genome can be detected in a high percentage of patients independent of whether they have cardiomyopathy. It has been demonstrated that only 15.9% of patients that have evidence of

B19V DNA on EMB have evidence of B19V mRNA. Interestingly, there is a significant difference in expression profiling in the biopsies that show transcriptionally active B19V, suggesting that transcriptional activity of the B19V may have a role in the pathogenesis.[16]

enterovirus-positive patients, IFN-β may improve survival rates.[41] For more information see the online supplement, "The Role of Innate Immunity in Myocarditis."

Innate Immunity

Innate immunity is effective during the earliest stages of virus infection. It is an antigen-independent defense mechanism that protects the host from a broad range of microbial pathogens. Innate immunity is initiated in the first days of enteroviral infection and is the major immune mechanism responsible for inhibiting viral infection and replication during the first 4 to 5 days after infection (Fig. 55.5). In addition to innate immune mechanisms in noncardiac organs, important innate immune responses also are activated in the cardiac myocyte.[40] One of the classic and best-characterized examples of innate immunity is the activation of interferon (IFN) signaling that occurs with viral infection. The two broad classes of IFNs use different receptors: Type I IFNs bind to the IFN-α receptor and include IFN-α and IFN-β, whereas IFN-γ is the sole type II IFN member. Both types I and II IFNs are effective at limiting viral replication when added to infected cells or when administered to a coxsackievirus-infected mouse.[40] The absence of type I IFN receptors or IFN-β in mice is associated with a marked increase in mortality rates but has less effect on early viral replication in the heart. In a phase II clinical trial, it has been demonstrated that administration of IFN-β to virus-positive patients with symptoms of heart failure caused significant clearance or reduction of the virus load and improvement in the New York Heart Association (NYHA) functional class and quality of life. In

Acquired Immunity

Acquired immunity becomes a prominent manifestation of viral myocarditis beginning approximately 4 to 5 days after the viral infection, although the peak and pattern of activation are variable. The acquired immune response is an antigen-specific response that is directed to a single antigen and is mediated by T and B cells. T cells are targeted to infected cells and attempt to limit infection by destroying the host cell through secretion of cytokines or perforins. These can contribute to the death of the infected cell through necrotic and/or apoptotic mechanisms. Thus, although T cell–mediated immune mechanisms are important for controlling and limiting viral replication, they also can have detrimental effects on the infected organ by stimulating cell death mechanisms in the infected host. Appropriately limiting the T cell and B cell immune mechanisms could limit damage to the heart, but such inhibition needs to be balanced by the need to inhibit viral replication.[42]

The acquired immune process is initiated when the variable region of the T cell receptor binds to peptides with specific amino acid sequences that are recognized as foreign to the host. When CD4+ T cells interact with antigen-presenting cells such as dendritic cells, the CD4+ cells can differentiate into different effector cell subsets, such as the classic Th1 and Th2 cell subtypes, namely Th17 and T regulatory (Treg) cells. Cytokines in the cellular microenvironment can control how the cells differentiate. The precise cellular signaling cascades and pattern

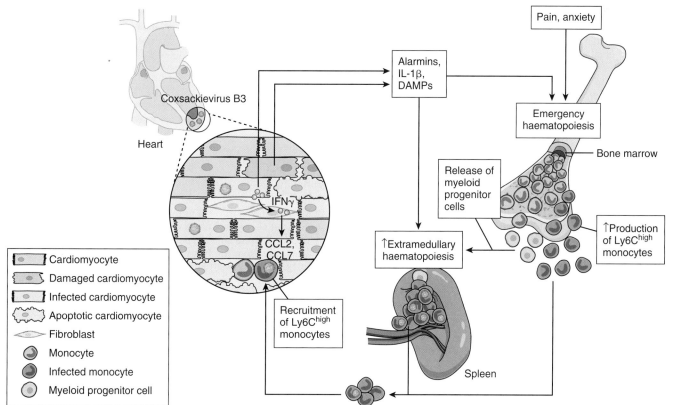

FIGURE 55.5 Cardiosplenic axis in coxsackievirus B3-induced myocarditis. In the heart, coxsackievirus B3 infection of cardiomyocytes leads to cell damage and death and the release of IL-1β and damage-associated molecular patterns (DAMPs), which trigger the recruitment and activation of cells from the innate immune system. Pain, anxiety, and the release of danger signals into the systemic circulation trigger emergency hematopoiesis in the bone marrow, leading to medullary monocytopoiesis as well as release of myeloid progenitor cells into the circulation. Myeloid progenitor cells then migrate to the spleen, where extramedullary monocytopoiesis takes place to replenish the pool of proinflammatory Ly6C^high monocytes, which can be rapidly mobilized to the damaged heart. In the heart, interferon γ (IFNγ) released by infected cardiomyocytes boosts the production by fibroblasts of the pro-inflammatory C-C motif chemokines CCL2 and CCL7, which promote the homing of Ly6C^high monocytes to the heart. Given that the spleen is a target organ of coxsackievirus B3 and monocytes target cells of coxsackievirus B3, the recruited Ly6C^high monocytes might be infected with coxsackievirus B3 and thereby transport the virus into the heart, further contributing to the viral infection. Activation of the innate immune system in the heart is beneficial for its antiviral effects but excessive or persistent activation can lead to exaggerated and/or chronic inflammation that triggers myocardial destruction and remodeling, culminating in cardiac dysfunction. (Adapted from Tschope, C, Ammirati E, Bozkurt B, et al. Myocarditis and inflammatory cardiomyopathy: current evidence and future directions. *Nat Rev Cardiol.* 2020;Oct 12:1–25. https://doi.org/10.1038/s41569-020-00435-x.)

of cytokine production that are associated with differentiation of these distinct T cell subtypes has been reviewed elsewhere.[42,43] Appropriate regulation of effector T cells is needed to control infections and at the same time avoid inappropriate immunologic destruction of host tissue such as myocardial cells. Activation of T cells also leads to B cell activation, which results in secretion of antigen-specific antibodies directed against the invading pathogen. After initial activation, the immune cells undergo clonal expansion to attack the source of antigen, which could include a viral coat protein or, in some cases, proteins in the cardiac myocyte such as myosin. There is evidence that cross reaction with the host may occur because of "molecular mimicry" between the virus and the host. Treg cells have important functions for the suppression of Th1-cell and Th2-cell immune responses and were previously identified as T-helper cells. They are characterized by the expression of the forkhead transcription factor, Foxp3, and are defined as $CD4^+CD25^+Foxp3^+$. The classic model held that commitment of $CD4^+$ cells to the different effector lineages involved stable programs of gene expression and that once differentiated, they maintained that effector phenotype even as changes in the microenvironment occurred. This model, however, has evolved, because of evidence that $CD4^+$ T cells have an element of plasticity in that they can alter their functional programs and in this way change the balance between Treg cells and cytokine-producing T cells and the type of cytokines that they produce.[42] This plasticity may be important as new therapeutic strategies are developed. The activation of T cells is highly dependent on an interaction with the innate immune-signaling cascade. For example, signaling through the T cell receptor uses p56lck. It is interesting that p56lck also has been shown to bind to the CAR-DAF receptor complex and that it is involved in viral entry. When p56lck is genetically deleted from the mouse, typical myocarditis is almost eliminated, with no significant mortality rates after infection.[44]

Alterations in any of the pathogenic mechanisms just described could, theoretically, affect the susceptibility to viral infection. For example, alterations in the mechanism of viral entry and replication, innate or acquired immune-signaling mechanisms, or the integrity of the sarcolemmal membrane could affect the susceptibility to develop myocarditis on exposure to a given virus. Nutrition is also likely to influence the susceptibility to viral infection. It is thought that a deficiency of selenium can increase the risk of myocarditis, as has been described in the Keshan province in China. When selenium deficiency was prevented, the incidence of myocarditis and DCM decreased. Furthermore, selenium deficiency in mice also increased the susceptibility to enteroviral myocarditis. The number of mechanisms known to affect the susceptibility to myocarditis in humans is far from complete.

Cardiac Remodeling

Remodeling of the heart after cardiac injury (see also Chapter 47) can significantly affect cardiac structure and function, and the degree of such remodeling may mean the difference between appropriate healing and the development of DCM. The virus can directly enter the endothelial cells and myocytes and effect changes that lead to direct cell death or hypertrophy. The virus also can modify the myocyte cytoskeleton, as mentioned earlier, leading to DCM. The inflammatory process outlined earlier for both innate and acquired immunity can lead to cytokine release and activation of matrix metalloproteinases that digest the interstitial collagen and elastin framework of the heart (see Chapter 47).

CLINICAL SYNDROMES

Myocarditis has a wide-ranging array of potential clinical presentations, a feature that contributes to the difficulties in diagnosis and classification. The clinical picture may be one of asymptomatic electrocardiographic or echocardiographic abnormalities or may include signs and symptoms of chest pain, cardiac dysfunction, arrhythmias or heart failure, and/or hemodynamic collapse. Transient electrocardiographic or echocardiographic abnormalities have been observed frequently during community viral outbreaks or influenza epidemics,

but most patients remain asymptomatic from a cardiac standpoint and have few long-term sequelae. Chest pain from myocarditis may resemble typical angina and be accompanied by ECG changes, including ST-segment elevation. Coronary vasospasm, demonstrated using intracoronary acetylcholine infusion, is one cause for chest pain in patients with clinical signs of myocarditis in the absence of significant coronary atherosclerosis. Chest pain also may mimic that in pericarditis, suggesting epicardial inflammation with adjacent pericardial involvement. The outcome of myopericarditis generally is good, with only two sudden deaths reported from four published case series ($N = 128$). For more information see the online supplement, "Specific Clinical Presentations of Myocarditis."

Myocarditis typically has a bimodal distribution in terms of age in the population, with the acute or fulminant presentation more commonly seen in young children and teenagers. By contrast, the presenting symptoms are more subtle and insidious, often with DCM and heart failure, in the older adult population. The difference in presentation probably is related to the maturity of the immune system, whereby the young tend to mount an exuberant response to the initial exposure of a provocative antigen. By contrast, older persons would have developed a greater degree of tolerance and show a chronic inflammatory response only to the chronic presence of a foreign antigen or with a dysregulated immune system that predisposes to autoimmunity. Myocarditis probably is responsible for 10% to 50% of new-onset cases of idiopathic DCM, a rate that varies depending on the criteria used for diagnosis. Viral myocarditis has been associated with heart failure from both systolic and isolated diastolic dysfunction.[45]

The presentation of myocarditis varies by cause. For example, B19V frequently causes chest pain from endothelial dysfunction, whereas ventricular arrhythmias and heart block are more common in giant cell myocarditis (GCM).[45] Associated physical examination findings point to specific causes for myocarditis. Enlarged lymph nodes with hilar adenopathy on the chest radiograph may suggest systemic sarcoidosis. A pruritic, maculopapular rash with an elevated eosinophil count suggests a hypersensitivity reaction to a drug or toxin. Patients who present with DCM complicated by sustained or symptomatic ventricular tachycardia or high-grade heart block are at high risk for having GCM or cardiac sarcoidosis. A study of 72 young Finnish patients with initially unexplained atrioventricular block revealed that 25% had either cardiac sarcoidosis (19%) or GCM (6%). Of these 18 patients, 7 (39%) experienced sustained ventricular tachycardia or cardiac death or required transplantation over an average follow-up period of 48 months (Fig. 55.6).[46] A prospective study of 12 patients with biopsy-proven GCM revealed that 25% of patients with a cardiomyopathy of less than 6 months' duration that failed to respond to usual care or was complicated by ventricular tachycardia or high-grade heart block had GCM.[47] In patients who fail to recover from an acute episode of myocarditis, the persistence of left ventricular dysfunction can sometimes be due to ongoing immune activation or chronic myocarditis. Failure to clear virus from the heart has been postulated to underlie some cases of persistent heart failure. Recognition of endogenous proteins, such as cardiac myosin, as "foreign" may contribute to ongoing inflammation even after successful viral clearance.[4,48] In clinical practice, the distinction between a noninflammatory DCM and a chronic inflammatory DCM with or without viral infection requires EMB. As discussed below, the lack of positive large-scale trial data supporting either immunosuppression or antiviral therapy currently limits the application of EMB in this setting.

DIAGNOSTIC APPROACHES

The diagnosis of myocarditis traditionally has required a histologic diagnosis according to the classic Dallas criteria. However, because of low sensitivity due to the patchy nature of the inflammatory infiltrates in the myocardium and the reluctance of clinicians to perform an invasive diagnostic procedure, myocarditis is severely underdiagnosed. Because the incidence of the disease is likely to be much higher than is appreciated, a high level of clinical suspicion, together with hybrid clinical and laboratory criteria and new imaging modalities, may help

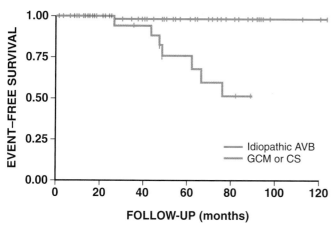

FIGURE 55.6 Kaplan-Meier curves for survival free of major adverse cardiac events (cardiac death, cardiac transplantation, ventricular fibrillation, or treated sustained ventricular tachycardia) in patients with pacemaker implantation for atrioventricular block (AVB) that remained idiopathic or AVB due to cardiac sarcoidosis (CS) or giant cell myocarditis (GCM). (From Kandolin R, Lehtonen J, Kupari M. Cardiac sarcoidosis and giant cell myocarditis as causes of atrioventricular block in young and middle-aged adults. *Circ Arrhythm Electrophysiol.* 2011;4:303.)

secure the diagnosis without necessarily resorting to biopsy in all cases (see Table 55.3).[2] Although clinical and imaging criteria have been used to estimate the myocarditis prevalence in various cohorts without EMB confirmation, such criteria probably sacrifice diagnostic specificity.

Laboratory Testing

The role of cardiac injury biomarkers in screening for myocarditis in patients with acute viral illness has been investigated in accordance with the hypothesis that a diagnosis of heart damage in this setting may indicate a greater risk of arrhythmias or cardiomyopathy. In this regard, elevated cardiac troponin values help to confirm cases of suspected myocarditis. Whereas older studies suggested that the sensitivity of troponins for myocarditis was low, more recent studies using more sensitive assays in less chronic disease support the value of troponin. For example, troponin levels predicted the severity of myocarditis and short-term prognosis in a case series of 65 children with recent-onset myocarditis. Fulminant myocarditis was associated with higher levels of cardiac troponins I and T (cTnI and cTnT) than acute myocarditis, and a higher cardiac troponin level was associated with a lower left ventricular ejection fraction.[49] In a case series of adults hospitalized with acute or fulminant myocarditis, creatine kinase–MB concentrations of greater than 29.5 ng/mL predicted in-hospital death with a sensitivity of 83% and a specificity of 73%. A growing literature also supports a role for TnI as an autoantigen as well as a biomarker for diagnosis.[50]

Renko and associates prospectively measured cTnI levels in 1009 children to determine the incidence of myocarditis in children hospitalized for an acute infection. TnI levels exceeded the screening limit (0.06 μg/L) in only six children, none of whom had electrocardiographic or echocardiographic abnormalities. Thus, the incidence of acute myocarditis during childhood viral infections appears to be low, so routine TnI screening for asymptomatic myocarditis in unselected children without cardiac symptoms probably is not indicated.[51] The rate of asymptomatic increases in troponin after smallpox vaccination is as high as 28.7 per 1000.[32] The risk of acute cardiomyopathy appears low in the first year after smallpox vaccination, but the longer-term significance of a troponin rise in this setting is not known.

A variety of other biomarkers have demonstrated prognostic value in acute myocarditis. In children with fulminant myocarditis, higher serum creatinine, lactate, and aspartate transaminase (AST) levels are associated with increased in-hospital mortality rates.[52] N-terminal pro–B type (brain) natriuretic peptide (NT-pro-BNP) is predictably elevated in children with acute DCM due to myocarditis and generally declines rapidly in children who recover left ventricular function.[53] In

adults, higher interleukin-10 and soluble Fas concentrations are associated with an increased risk of death. Anti–heart antibodies have been reported to predict an increased risk of death or need for transplantation. However, few anti–heart antibody tests are standardized or available in clinical laboratories. Nonspecific biomarkers of inflammation, such as the leukocyte count, C-reactive protein, and erythrocyte sedimentation rate, have low specificity. Circulating viral antibody titers do not correlate with tissue viral genomes and are rarely of diagnostic use in clinical practice.[54]

Pathognomonic ECG findings are lacking in acute myocarditis, but nonspecific repolarization changes and sinus tachycardia are common (see also Chapter 14). PR-segment depression and diffuse ST-segment elevation may accompany a clinical presentation of myopericarditis. The presence of a QRS width greater than 120 milliseconds in duration and Q waves is associated with a great risk of cardiac death or need for heart transplantation.[55]

Cardiac Imaging

An assessment of left ventricular function by means of cardiac imaging (see also Chapters 16 to 19) is essential in all cases of suspected myocarditis. Echocardiography is an excellent choice for imaging, although there are no specific echocardiographic features of myocarditis. In patients who have an acute cardiomyopathy, the most common pattern is a dilated, spherical ventricle with reduced systolic function. Patients with heart failure due to fulminant myocarditis typically present with small cardiac chambers and mild and reversible ventricular hypertrophy from inflammation. Right ventricular dysfunction is less common and heralds a poor prognosis. Of interest, segmental wall motion abnormalities often are present early and may mimic the regional changes seen in a myocardial infarction. A pericardial effusion usually signifies myopericarditis.

CMR (see Chapter 19) has become the primary noninvasive imaging modality for assessment of myocardial inflammation in patients with suspected myocarditis. Certain patterns of signal abnormality on CMR are strongly suggestive of acute myocarditis (eFig. 55.3).[56] Myocardial necrosis can be detected by late gadolinium enhancement (LGE). The T1-weighted, myocardial-delayed enhancement technique can quantitate regions of damage and possibly predict the risk of cardiovascular death and ventricular arrhythmias after myocarditis.[57] T2-weighted imaging can be used to detect myocardial edema. However, the T2-weighted, short tau inversion recovery (STIR) and T1-weighted-delayed postcontrast signal abnormalities seen in acute myocarditis usually decrease with time. The sensitivity and specificity of CMR in suspected myocarditis more than 14 days after symptom onset were poor (sensitivity, 63%; specificity, 40%).[58] Thus, CMR performs best in the setting of acute cardiomyopathy or chest pain with elevated troponin. Both T1- and T2-weighted sequences should be used, to optimize the sensitivity and specificity.[59] An anteroseptal pattern of delayed enhancement is associated with greater risk of MACE as is an increase in DGE on follow-up CMR 6 months after presentation. A decrease in LGE on follow-up CMR is associated with a low risk of MACE.[57] Because of the absence of large-scale multicenter data with CMR in myocarditis, current recommendations with respect to the CMR diagnosis of myocarditis are based on expert opinion, rather than rigorous data of pulse sequences that have been evaluated against myocardial biopsy in clearly defined clinical subsets of patients. The "Lake Louise Criteria" (eTable 55.1) is a consensus document that provides suggested CMR criteria for diagnosing myocardial inflammation in patients with suspected myocarditis. The diagnostic accuracy of the Lake Louise Criteria ranges from 68% to 78%, depending on the number of tissue markers used in CMR studies.[60]

Although most nuclear imaging techniques are ancillary in the evaluation of suspected myocarditis, positron emission tomography (PET) imaging remains useful for diagnosing cardiac sarcoidosis.[61] Isiguzo and colleagues recently showed a significant association of metabolism-perfusion mismatch by rubidium-fluorodeoxyglucose (FDG) PET with clinically active disease in cardiac sarcoidosis patients.[62] Case control series suggest that patients with cardiomyopathy or ventricular arrhythmias due to cardiac sarcoidosis may benefit from steroid therapy.

Endomyocardial Biopsy

EMB remains essential for the diagnosis of specific forms of myocarditis.[63] The rate of major complications with EMB is less than 1 in 1000 when the procedure is done by experienced operators. In children with suspected myocarditis, EMB demonstrating myocarditis can identify responders to medical treatment. Because myocarditis may only involve regions of one ventricle, several large-volume cardiac centers are routinely performing left as well as right ventricular biopsy. In these centers, the safety of left ventricular biopsy is equivalent to that of right ventricular biopsy, and the diagnostic yield is greater.[64,65]

The clinical scenarios in which EMB is most useful are suspected GCM and fulminant lymphocytic myocarditis in the setting of an acute cardiomyopathy (Fig. 55.7).[66,67] GCM should be considered in acute DCM that fails to respond to usual care or is complicated by high-grade heart block or sustained ventricular tachycardia. The use of immunosuppressive therapy that includes cyclosporine probably increases the transplant-free survival rate in patients with GCM whose symptoms are of less than 6 months' duration.[47,68] Histologically, GCM is defined by a diffuse or multifocal inflammatory infiltrate of lymphocytes and multinucleated giant cells in the absence of granuloma. In contrast with cardiac sarcoidosis, in which the giant cells are located within the granuloma, the giant cells often are located at the edges of the inflammation, where myocyte damage is present. Eosinophils are significantly more common in GCM, whereas fibrosis is significantly more common in cardiac sarcoidosis. Immunohistochemistry may be beneficial in differentiating GCM from cardiac sarcoidosis.

PROGNOSIS

The prognosis for patients with acute myocarditis varies in relation to the clinical scenario and degree of left ventricular dysfunction at presentation.[69] Patients who present with myopericarditis or chest pain suggestive of an acute coronary syndrome usually do well if their left ventricular function is normal or near normal.[70] However, approximately 15% of patients with myopericarditis may develop recurrent myopericarditis. In acute DCM, the risk of death or need for cardiac transplantation is increased in those myocarditis patients with lower left ventricular function, lower right ventricular function, and higher pulmonary artery pressures. In children, the time course of left ventricular functional recovery extends to at least 8 years, and the overall risk of death or requirement for transplantation approaches 30% (Fig. 55.8).[71,72] In patients with a recent onset of DCM who were bridged to recovery with a left ventricular assist device, myocardial inflammation was present but fibrosis was less evident.[73] There is a risk of late heart failure due to diastolic dysfunction years after the apparent resolution of acute myocarditis.[45]

In chronic DCM, the presence of inflammatory cells on EMB may define a subset of patients who will improve with a short course of immunosuppression. Some investigators have demonstrated that the presence of active myocarditis defined by immunohistology, but not conventional Dallas criteria, predicts the risk of death or need for transplantation. The presence of viral genomes on EMB may portend a poor outcome. Older clinical data for enteroviruses in acute cardiomyopathy were mostly consistent with this conclusion, but in recent years, the impact of viral genomes on the outcome has been questioned. Possibly the variable findings with respect to viral genomes may be due to a changing spectrum of viruses, from enteroviruses to B19V and human herpesvirus 6. In addition, genetic background differences in study populations, and possibly unmeasured environmental toxins or nutritional deficiencies, may account for differences in study outcomes. Studies that have evaluated the impact of CMR imaging–associated delayed gadolinium enhancement on the cardiovascular risk following acute myocarditis generally support an association between delayed gadolinium enhancement and subsequent arrhythmic events.[59]

TREATMENT

The first-line therapy for all patients with myocarditis and heart failure is supportive care (see Chapter 50). A small proportion of patients will require hemodynamic support that ranges from vasopressors (see Chapter 49) to intraaortic balloon pump and ventricular assist devices (see Chapter 59) (Fig. 55.9). Guidelines for myocarditis management have been published by the American Heart Association (AHA),[74] Japanese Circulatory Society, and European Society of Cardiology (ESC) working group on myocarditis and pericarditis.[63] In patients who present with an acute DCM and a syndrome of heart failure, the current American College of Cardiology (ACC)/AHA guidelines for heart failure care should be followed.[45] Clinical experience suggests that standard pharmacotherapy is effective in myocarditis, although trials of heart failure management in myocarditis have not been done.

Routine treatment of mild to moderately severe acute myocarditis with immunosuppressive drugs is not recommended for adults.

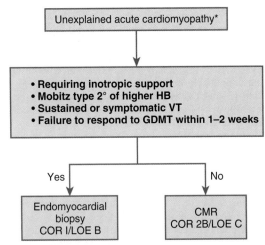

FIGURE 55.7 Algorithm for the evaluation of suspected myocarditis in the setting of unexplained acute cardiomyopathy. Unexplained acute cardiomyopathy will usually present as a dilated cardiomyopathy. However, patients with fulminant myocarditis may have normal end-diastolic diameter with mildly increased left ventricular wall thickness. It is also important to exclude ischemic, hemodynamic (valvular, hypertensive), metabolic, and toxic causes of acute cardiomyopathy, as indicated clinically. *CMR*, Cardiac magnetic resonance imaging; *COR*, class of recommendation; *LOE*, level of evidence. (From Bozkurt B, Colvin M, Cook J, et al; American Heart Association Committee on Heart Failure and Transplantation of the Council on Clinical Cardiology; Council on Cardiovascular Disease in the Young; Council on Cardiovascular and Stroke Nursing; Council on Epidemiology and Prevention; and Council on Quality of Care and Outcomes Research. Current Diagnostic and Treatment Strategies for Specific Dilated Cardiomyopathies: A Scientific Statement From the American Heart Association. *Circulation*. 2016;134:e579-e646.)

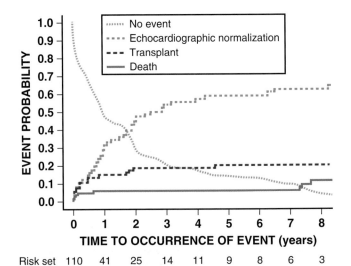

FIGURE 55.8 Crude cumulative incidence rates of echocardiographic normalization, cardiac transplantation, and death among children with biopsy-confirmed myocarditis. (From Foerster SR, Canter CE, Cinar A, et al. Ventricular remodeling and survival are more favorable for myocarditis than for idiopathic dilated cardiomyopathy in childhood: an outcomes study from the Pediatric Cardiomyopathy Registry. *Circ Heart Fail*. 2010;3:689.)

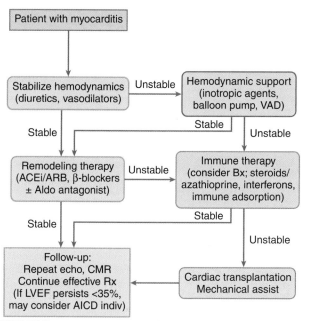

FIGURE 55.9 Treatment algorithms for patients with myocarditis, depending on hemodynamic stability and response to general supportive and remodeling treatment regimen at each step. All patients require aggressive support and appropriate follow-up. Immune therapy at present is still indicated mainly to support those who have failed to improve spontaneously. *ACEi,* Angiotensin-converting enzyme inhibitor; *AICD,* automatic implantable cardioverter-defibrillator; *Aldo,* aldosterone; *ARB,* angiotensin receptor blocker; *Bx,* biopsy; *CMR,* cardiac magnetic resonance; *echo,* echocardiography; *indiv,* based on individual assessment of risk versus benefit; *LVEF,* left ventricular ejection fraction; *VAD,* ventricular assist device.

These data are based on the U.S. Myocarditis Treatment Trial, in which immunosuppression with prednisone and either azathioprine or cyclosporine effected similar changes in the left ventricular ejection fraction and transplant-free survival rates compared with placebo. Significant exceptions are recognized, including those of patients with GCM, cardiac sarcoidosis, eosinophilic myocarditis, and myocarditis associated with inflammatory connective tissue disorders. Also, the data from case-controlled series regarding the use of intravenous immunoglobulin (IVIG) and immunosuppressive drugs are neutral to favorable in the pediatric literature. Treatment of viral infection may be helpful in the management of posttransplantation viral heart disease in children.[10] However, in adult patients with chronic DCM and viral genomes detected by PCR in heart biopsy tissues, one trial series suggests that 6 mIU of IFN-β three times per week improves enteroviral or adenoviral heart infection.[41] There may be a role for a short course of immunosuppression in patients with chronic DCM who fail to respond to guideline-based heart failure management. In the Tailored Immunosuppression in Inflammatory Cardiomyopathy (TIMIC) trial, 85 patients with chronic inflammatory cardiomyopathy without persistent viral infection were randomly assigned to receive either prednisone and azathioprine or placebo. Immunosuppressive treatment was associated with an increase in the left ventricular ejection fraction from 26% to 46% and an improved quality of life, whereas none of the patients in the placebo arm improved their left ventricular ejection fraction.[75] Larger, multicenter trials are needed to assess whether immunosuppression will affect clinically meaningful end points such as the risk of death or admission to hospital in this population.

Patients with ventricular arrhythmias or heart block due to acute myocarditis should be hospitalized for electrocardiographic monitoring. Arrhythmias usually resolve after several weeks. The ACC/AHA/ESC guidelines for the management of arrhythmias recommended that acute arrhythmia emergencies be managed conventionally in the setting of myocarditis. Generally, the indications for an implantable cardiac defibrillator (ICD) are the same as with nonischemic DCM. In the setting of GCM or cardiac sarcoidosis, the high rate of ventricular arrhythmias may warrant early consideration for an ICD. In patients

with suspected lymphocytic myocarditis and nonsustained ventricular tachycardia, a temporary external defibrillator vest may be used while it is determined whether the arrhythmias will persist after the acute inflammatory phase.

Mechanical circulatory support (see also Chapter 59) or extracorporeal membrane oxygenation may allow a bridge to transplantation or recovery in patients with cardiogenic shock despite optimal medical care. In those patients who recover, the time to recovery in acute myocarditis varies, ranging from a few weeks to a few months. Transplantation also is an effective therapy for patients with myocarditis who have refractory heart failure despite optimal medical therapy and mechanical circulatory support. Survival rates after transplantation for myocarditis are similar to survival rates for other causes of cardiac transplantation. However, the risk of graft loss may be greater in children who undergo transplantation.

FUTURE PERSPECTIVES

One of the major gaps in the management of myocarditis is the lack of a sensitive and specific noninvasive test. In this regard, diagnostic techniques are evolving to identify novel blood-based biomarkers reflecting cardiac inflammation through microarray and proteomic analysis of tissues from both laboratory models and patient samples.[3] Moreover, with improved understanding of pathophysiologic mechanisms, new therapies also are being developed and evaluated in clinical trials. These new treatments, including cell-based therapies that selectively inhibit T cell responses, induce apoptosis of activated T cells, and increase Treg cells, will be evaluated in planned clinical trials. Such prospective investigations should be designed specifically to establish efficacy in women. Translational studies focused on genomic markers in biopsy samples and peripheral blood should help refine risk assessments and target therapies to the populations at highest need.

REFERENCES
Definition and Epidemiology
1. Schultheiss HP, Kuhl U, Cooper LT. The management of myocarditis. *Eur Heart J.* 2011;32:2616–2625.
2. Heymans S, Eriksson U, Lehtonen J, Cooper LT. The quest for new approaches in myocarditis and inflammatory cardiomyopathy. *J Am Coll Cardiol.* 2016;68:2348–2364.
3. Fung G, Luo H, Qiu Y, et al. Myocarditis. *Circulation Res.* 2016;118:496–514.
4. Mensah GA, Roth GA, Fuster V. The global burden of cardiovascular diseases and risk factors. *J Am Coll Cardiol.* 2019;74:2529–2532.
5. Maron BJ, Udelson JE, Bonow RO, et al. Eligibility and disqualification recommendations for competitive athletes with cardiovascular abnormalities: Task Force 3: hypertrophic cardiomyopathy, arrhythmogenic right ventricular cardiomyopathy and other cardiomyopathies, and myocarditis. *Circulation.* 2015;132.
6. Harmon KG, Asif IM, Maleszewski JJ, et al. Incidence and etiology of sudden cardiac arrest and death in high school athletes in the United States. *Mayo Clin Proc.* 2016;91:1493–1502.
7. Towbin JA, Lowe AM, Colan SD, et al. Incidence, causes, and outcomes of dilated cardiomyopathy in children. *J Am Med Assoc.* 2006;296:1867.
8. Leone O, Veinot JP, Angelini A, et al. 2011 consensus statement on endomyocardial biopsy from the association for European Cardiovascular Pathology and the Society for Cardiovascular Pathology. *Cardiovasc Pathol.* 2012;21:245–274.
9. She RC, Hammond EH. Utility of immunofluorescence and electron microscopy in endomyocardial biopsies from patients with unexplained heart failure. *Cardiovasc Pathol.* 2010;19:e99–e105.
10. Moulik M, Breinholt JP, Dreyer WJ, et al. Viral endomyocardial infection is an independent predictor and potentially treatable risk factor for graft loss and coronary vasculopathy in pediatric cardiac transplant recipients. *J Am Coll Cardiol.* 2010;56:582–592.
11. Nunes MCP, Beaton A, Acquatella H, et al. Chagas cardiomyopathy: an update of current clinical knowledge and management: a scientific statement from the American Heart Association. *Circulation.* 2018;138.

Specific Etiologic Agents
12. Knowlton KU, Anderson JL, Savoia MC, Oxman MN. Myocarditis and pericarditis. *Mandell, Douglas, and Bennett's Principles and Practice of Infectious Diseases.* 9th ed. Philadelphia: Elsevier; 2019:1151–1164.
13. Manga P, McCutcheon K, Tsabedze N, et al. HIV and nonischemic heart disease. *J Am Coll Cardiol.* 2017;69:83–91.
14. Verdonschot J, Hazebroek M, Merken J, et al. Relevance of cardiac parvovirus B19 in myocarditis and dilated cardiomyopathy: review of the literature. *Eur J Heart Fail.* 2016;18:1430–1441.
15. Ammirati E, Frigerio M, Adler ED, et al. Management of acute myocarditis and chronic inflammatory cardiomyopathy: an expert consensus document. *Circ Heart Fail.* 2020;13:e007405.
16. Kuhl U, Lassner D, Dorner A, et al. A distinct subgroup of cardiomyopathy patients characterized by transcriptionally active cardiotropic erythrovirus and altered cardiac gene expression. *Basic Res Cardiol.* 2013;108.
17. Knowlton KU. Pathogenesis of SARS-CoV-2 induced cardiac injury from the perspective of the virus. *J Mol Cell Cardiol.* 2020;147:12–17.
18. Jay S, David P, Chanakha N, et al. SARS-CoV-2 direct cardiac damage through spike-mediated cardiomyocyte fusion. *Nat Res.* 2020.
19. Basso C, Leone O, Rizzo S, et al. Pathological features of COVID-19-associated myocardial injury: a multicentre cardiovascular pathology study. *Eur Heart J.* 2020;41:3827–3835.
20. Haluschka MK, Vander Heide RS. Myocarditis is rare in COVID-19 autopsies: cardiovascular findings across 277 postmortem examinations. *Cardiovasc Pathol.* 2020;50:107300.

21. Martinez MW, Tucker AM, Bloom OJ, et al. Prevalence of inflammatory heart disease among professional athletes with prior COVID-19 infection who received systematic return-to-play cardiac screening. *JAMA Cardiol.* 2021;6(7):745–752.
21a. Diaz GA, Parsons GT, Gering SK, et al. Myocarditis and pericarditis after vaccination for COVID-19. *JAMA.* Published online August 4, 2021. doi:10.1001/jama.2021.13443.
22. Krause PJ, Bockenstedt LK. Lyme disease and the heart. *Circulation.* 2013;127.
23. Forrester JD, Meiman J, Mullins J, et al. Notes from the field: update on Lyme carditis, groups at high risk, and frequency of associated sudden cardiac death—United States. *MMWR Morb Mortal Wkly Rep.* 2014;63:982–983.
24. Lidani KCF, Andrade FA, Bavia L, et al. Chagas disease: from discovery to a worldwide health problem. *Front Public Health.* 2019;7:166.
25. Moncayo Á, Silveira AC. Current epidemiological trends for Chagas disease in Latin America and future challenges in epidemiology, surveillance and health policy. *Mem Inst Oswaldo Cruz.* 2009;104:17–30.
26. Bern C, Messenger LA, Whitman JD, Maguire JH. Chagas disease in the United States: a public health approach. *Clin Microbiol Rev.* 2019;33.
27. Santos E, Menezes Falcao L. Chagas cardiomyopathy and heart failure: from epidemiology to treatment. *Rev Port Cardiol.* 2020;39:279–289.
28. Meymandi S, Hernandez S, Park S, et al. Treatment of Chagas disease in the United States. *Curr Treat Options Infect Dis.* 2018;10:373–388.
29. Morillo CA, Marin-Neto JA, Avezum A, et al. Randomized trial of benznidazole for chronic Chagas' cardiomyopathy. *N Engl J Med.* 2015;373:1295–1306.
30. De Berardis D, Serroni N, Campanella D, et al. Update on the adverse effects of clozapine: focus on myocarditis. *Curr Drug Safety.* 2012;7:55–62.
31. Engler RJM, Nelson MR, Collins Jr LC, et al. A prospective study of the incidence of myocarditis/pericarditis and new onset cardiac symptoms following smallpox and influenza vaccination. *PloS One.* 2015;10:e0118283–e.
32. Bonaca MP, Olenchock BA, Salem J-E, et al. Myocarditis in the setting of cancer therapeutics: proposed case definitions for emerging clinical syndromes in Cardio-Oncology. *Circulation.* 2019;140:80–91.

Pathogenesis

33. Coyne CB, Bergelson JM. Virus-induced Abl and Fyn kinase signals permit coxsackievirus entry through Epithelial tight junctions. *Cell.* 2006;124:119–131.
34. Shi Y, Chen C, Lisewski U, et al. Cardiac deletion of the coxsackievirus-adenovirus receptor Abolishes coxsackievirus B3 infection and prevents myocarditis in vivo. *J Am Coll Cardiol.* 2009;53:1219–1226.
35. Lim B-K, Peter AK, Xiong D, et al. Inhibition of Coxsackievirus-associated dystrophin cleavage prevents cardiomyopathy. *J Clini Invest.* 2013;123:5146–5151.
36. Belkaya S, Kontorovich AR, Byun M, et al. Autosomal recessive cardiomyopathy presenting as acute myocarditis. *J Am Coll Cardiol.* 2017;69:1653–1665.
37. Kissopoulou A, Fernlund E, Holmgren C, et al. Monozygotic twins with myocarditis and a novel likely pathogenic desmoplakin gene variant. *ESC Heart Fail.* 2020;7:1210–1216.
38. Smith ED, Lakdawala NK, Papoutsidakis N, et al. Desmoplakin cardiomyopathy, a fibrotic and inflammatory form of cardiomyopathy distinct from typical dilated or Arrhythmogenic right ventricular cardiomyopathy. *Circulation.* 2020;141:1872–1884.
39. Bouin A, Gretteau P-A, Wehbe M, et al. Enterovirus persistence in cardiac cells of patients with idiopathic dilated cardiomyopathy is linked to 5' terminal genomic RNA-deleted viral populations with viral-encoded proteinase activities. *Circulation.* 2019;139:2326–2338.
40. Yajima T, Knowlton KU. Viral myocarditis. *Circulation.* 2009;119:2615–2624.
41. Schultheiss H-P, Piper C, Sowade O, et al. Betaferon in chronic viral cardiomyopathy (BICC) trial: effects of interferon-β treatment in patients with chronic viral cardiomyopathy. *Clini Res Cardiol.* 2016;105:763–773.
42. Zhou L, Chong MMW, Littman DR. Plasticity of CD4+ T cell lineage differentiation. *Immunity.* 2009;30:646–655.
43. Huber SA. Viral myocarditis and dilated cardiomyopathy: etiology and pathogenesis. *Curr Pharm Des.* 2016;22:408–426.
44. Liu P, Aitken K, Kong Y-Y, et al. The tyrosine kinase p56lck is essential in coxsackievirus B3-mediated heart disease. *Nat Med.* 2000;6:429–434.
45. Kociol RD, Cooper LT, Fang JC, et al. Recognition and initial management of fulminant myocarditis. *Circulation.* 2020;141.
46. Kandolin R, Lehtonen J, Kupari M. Cardiac sarcoidosis and giant cell myocarditis as causes of atrioventricular block in young and middle-aged adults. *Circ Arrhythm Electrophysiol.* 2011;4:303–309.
47. Kandolin R, Lehtonen J, Salmenkivi K, et al. Diagnosis, treatment, and outcome of giant-cell myocarditis in the era of combined immunosuppression. *Circ Heart Fail.* 2013;6:15–22.
48. Ammirati E, Veronese G, Brambatti M, et al. Fulminant versus acute nonfulminant myocarditis in patients with left ventricular systolic dysfunction. *J Am Coll Cardiol.* 2019;74:299–311.

Diagnostic Approaches

49. Al-Biltagi M, Issa M, Hagar HA, et al. Circulating cardiac troponin levels and cardiac dysfunction in children with acute and fulminant viral myocarditis. *Acta Paediatr.* 2010;99:1510–1516.
50. Kaya Z, Katus HA, Rose NR. Cardiac troponins and autoimmunity: their role in the pathogenesis of myocarditis and of heart failure. *Clini Immunol (Orlando, Fla).* 2010;134:80–88.
51. Renko M, Leskinen M, Kontiokari T, et al. Cardiac troponin-I as a screening tool for myocarditis in children hospitalized for viral infection. *Acta Paediatr.* 2009.
52. Younis A, Matetzky S, Mulla W, et al. Epidemiology characteristics and outcome of patients with clinically diagnosed acute myocarditis. *Am J Med.* 2020;133:492–499.
53. Mlczoch E, Darbandi-Mesri F, Luckner D, et al. NT-pro BNP in acute childhood myocarditis. *J Pediatr.* 2012;160:178–179.
54. Mahfoud F, Gartner B, Kindermann M, et al. Virus serology in patients with suspected myocarditis: utility or futility? *Eur Heart J.* 2011;32:897–903.
55. Ukena C, Mahfoud F, Kindermann I, et al. Prognostic electrocardiographic parameters in patients with suspected myocarditis. *Eur J Heart Fail.* 2011;13:398–405.
56. Gräni C, Eichhorn C, Bière L, et al. Prognostic value of cardiac magnetic resonance tissue characterization in risk stratifying patients with suspected myocarditis. *J Am Coll Cardiol.* 2017;70:1964–1976.
57. Aquaro GD, Ghebru Habtemicael Y, Camastra G, et al. Prognostic value of repeating cardiac magnetic resonance in patients with acute myocarditis. *J Am Coll Cardiol.* 2019;74:2439–2448.
58. Lurz P, Luecke C, Eitel I, et al. Comprehensive cardiac magnetic resonance imaging in patients with suspected myocarditis. *J Am Coll Cardiol.* 2016;67:1800–1811.
59. Ferreira VM, Schulz-Menger J, Holmvang G, et al. Cardiovascular magnetic resonance in non-ischemic myocardial inflammation. *J Am Coll Cardiol.* 2018;72:3158–3176.
60. Friedrich MG, Sechtem U, Schulz-Menger J, et al. Cardiovascular magnetic resonance in myocarditis: A JACC White Paper. *J Am Coll Cardiol.* 2009;53:1475–1487.
61. Blankstein R, Osborne M, Naya M, et al. Cardiac positron emission tomography enhances prognostic assessments of patients with suspected cardiac sarcoidosis. *J Am Coll Cardiol.* 2014;63:329–336.
62. Isiguzo M, Brunken R, Tchou P, et al. Metabolism-perfusion imaging to predict disease activity in cardiac sarcoidosis. *Sarcoidosis Vasc Diffuse Lung Dis.* 2011;28:50–55.
63. Caforio ALP, Pankuweit S, Arbustini E, et al. Current state of knowledge on aetiology, diagnosis, management, and therapy of myocarditis: a position statement of the European Society of Cardiology Working Group on Myocardial and Pericardial Diseases. *Eur Heart J.* 2013;34:2636–2648.
64. Yilmaz A, Kindermann I, Kindermann M, et al. Comparative evaluation of left and right ventricular endomyocardial biopsy. *Circulation.* 2010;122:900–909.
65. Chimenti C, Frustaci A. Contribution and risks of left ventricular endomyocardial biopsy in patients with cardiomyopathies. *Circulation.* 2013;128:1531–1541.
66. Cooper LT, Baughman KL, Feldman AM, et al. The role of endomyocardial biopsy in the management of cardiovascular disease. *Circulation.* 2007;116:2216–2233.
67. Bennett MK, Gilotra NA, Harrington C, et al. Evaluation of the role of endomyocardial biopsy in 851 patients with unexplained heart failure from 2000–2009. *Circ Heart Fail.* 2013;6:676–684.
68. Maleszewski JJ, Orellana VM, Hodge DO, et al. Long-term risk of recurrence, morbidity and mortality in giant cell myocarditis. *Am J Cardiol.* 2015;115:1733–1738.

Prognosis and Treatment

69. Gilotra NA, Bennett MK, Shpigel A, et al. Outcomes and predictors of recovery in acute-onset cardiomyopathy: a single-center experience of patients undergoing endomyocardial biopsy for new heart failure. *Am Heart J.* 2016;179:116–126.
70. Imazio M, Brucato A, Barbieri A, et al. Good prognosis for pericarditis with and without myocardial involvement. *Circulation.* 2013;128:42–49.
71. Foerster SR, Canter CE, Cinar A, et al. Ventricular remodeling and survival are more favorable for myocarditis than for idiopathic dilated cardiomyopathy in childhood. *Circ Heart Fail.* 2010;3:689–697.
72. Alvarez JA, Orav EJ, Wilkinson JD, et al. Competing risks for death and cardiac transplantation in children with dilated cardiomyopathy: results from the pediatric cardiomyopathy registry. *Circulation.* 2011;124:814–823.
73. Boehmer JP, Starling RC, Cooper LT, et al. Left ventricular assist device support and myocardial recovery in recent onset cardiomyopathy. *J Cardiac Fail.* 2012;18:755–761.
74. Bozkurt B, Colvin M, Cook J, et al. Current diagnostic and treatment strategies for specific dilated cardiomyopathies: a scientific statement from the American Heart Association. *Circulation.* 2016;134.
75. Seferović PM, Polovina M, Bauersachs J, et al. Heart failure in cardiomyopathies: a position paper from the heart failure association of the European Society of Cardiology. *Eur J Heart Fail.* 2019;21:553–576.

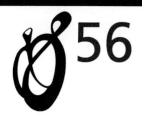# 56 Cardio-Oncology: Managing Cardiotoxic Effects of Cancer Therapies

BONNIE KY

Cardiovascular (CV) disease and cancer are highly prevalent and two major causes of mortality worldwide, resulting in a substantial public health burden. Global estimates suggest 422 million prevalent cases of CV disease.[1] Each year, there are an estimated 17 million incident cases of cancer.[2] CV disease accounts for an estimated 17.9 million deaths and cancer 9.6 million deaths worldwide each year.[3] The overlap in the epidemiology of these two diseases, as well as the shared biologic mechanisms of both CV disease and cancer have led to the birth and maturation of the field of cardio-oncology.

Cardio-oncology is a multidisciplinary field that encompasses the following broad clinical areas: (1) the care of patients with pre-existing CV risk factors or disease who develop cancer; (2) cancer patients and survivors who are at greater propensity for the development of CV risk factors or disease secondary to cancer or cancer therapy; and (3) patients with active or a prior history of cancer who subsequently develop overt CV risk factors or disease. Incident CV disease related to cancer therapy is often termed *cardiotoxicity*. The diseases encompassed by the term include not only heart failure (HF) (see Chapters 49–51), cardiomyopathy (CM), and left ventricular (LV) dysfunction (often referred to as cancer therapeutics related cardiac dysfunction, or CTRCD), but also a broad range of CV disease states, including hypertension (HTN) (see Chapter 26), coronary disease and myocardial ischemia (see Chapters 37, 38, 40), arrhythmia (see Chapters 65–68), pulmonary HTN (see Chapter 88), pericardial disease (see Chapter 86), valvular disease (see Chapters 72–76), myocarditis (see Chapter 55), peripheral arterial disease (PAD; see Chapter 43), and venous and arterial thrombosis.

Both the incidence and significance of cardiotoxicity with cancer therapy are believed to be growing. There are several potential reasons for this. First, survival rates among cancer patients are increasing, potentially related to early detection and more effective treatment regimens, and as a result, the observed "late effects" of cancer therapies are becoming more evident. Second, cancer therapies are rapidly evolving, and while many conventional chemotherapies are still being used, new drug development has led to the development of "targeted" strategies, many of which can also affect fundamental signaling pathways that are necessary for cardiomyocyte and endothelial cell function and homeostasis. This chapter reviews the epidemiology, clinical manifestations, and pathophysiology of CV disease with commonly used chemotherapeutic agents, targeted therapies, immune therapies, hormonal therapy, and radiation therapy (RT) (Table 56.1, Fig. 56.1). Care of the CV patient prior to, during, and after therapy and strategies to mitigate cardiotoxicity are discussed in Chapter 57.

EPIDEMIOLOGY, CLINICAL MANIFESTATIONS, AND PATHOPHYSIOLOGY OF CANCER THERAPY CARDIOTOXICITY

Traditional Chemotherapeutic Agents
Anthracyclines
The American College of Cardiology and American Heart Association HF Guidelines classify exposure to cardiotoxic therapies, such as anthracyclines, as stage A HF.[4] Reports of the incidence of anthracycline-associated cardiotoxicity have varied widely in the literature, in part, secondary to the variability in the definition of CV outcomes across retrospective analyses and the lack of systematic and rigorously ascertained longitudinal follow-up data, particularly in adults. Historically, cardiotoxicity has been classified as acute, subacute, or chronic although recent studies have substantially challenged this paradigm.

A study of 2625 patients treated with anthracyclines, primarily for breast cancer and hematologic disease, followed over a median of 5.2 years (interquartile range [IQR] 2.6 to 8.0) with serial echocardiography monitoring noted an overall incidence of cardiotoxicity of 9%.[5] Cardiotoxicity was defined as a decrease in the LV ejection fraction (LVEF) of more than 10% from baseline to less than an absolute value of 50%. In 98% of cases, cardiotoxicity was detected within the first year after chemotherapy had been completed, with a median time between the last dose of anthracyclines and the development of cardiotoxicity of 3.5 months (IQR, 3 to 6). In five patients, cardiotoxicity was detected after 5.5 years. The LVEF at the completion of chemotherapy and the cumulative anthracycline dose were independently associated with cardiotoxicity risk. A very small number of patients were hospitalized; the majority were managed as outpatients. HF therapy was initiated in all patients who developed cardiotoxicity, and 82% of the patients recovered their LVEF, either fully or partially. Data from a carefully phenotyped, prospective observational cohort study of breast cancer patients treated with standard dosages of anthracyclines, doxorubicin 240 mg/m², also support the observation that modest declines in quantitative LVEF, on the order of 3% to 4%, occur and are detectable during the 1 to 2 years after the initiation of anthracycline chemotherapy.[6] Altogether, these findings suggest that declines in cardiac function, which may be subclinical, can occur relatively early after chemotherapy completion; these data also challenge the notion of irreversible LVEF declines.

Anthracyclines are a mainstay of therapy in childhood cancers. Cardiotoxicity, when carefully evaluated, is also observed in patients early after exposure to anthracyclines. In clinical trial participants

TABLE 56.1 Cardiotoxic Effects of Cancer Therapies

AGENT	REPORTED CARDIOTOXIC EFFECTS	COMMENTS
Anthracyclines		
Doxorubicin, daunorubicin, epirubicin, idarubicin, mitoxantrone	Cardiac arrhythmias, CM, HF	Risk factors include cumulative dose, although genetic variation may confer increased risk at lower dosages; conventional CV risk factors and disease; age; gender; additional cardiotoxic therapies, including RT or trastuzumab
Anti-Microtubule Therapies—Taxanes (See Supplement)		
Paclitaxel, docetaxel	Arrhythmia, myocardial ischemia	May exacerbate risk of anthracycline cardiotoxicity secondary to pharmacokinetic effects
Alkylating and Alkylating-Like Agents (See Supplement)		
Cyclophosphamide	Myopericarditis, arrhythmias	Rare; CV complications reported primarily at high dosages; emerging data in the transplant setting may suggest increased CV risk.
Cisplatin, carboplatin, oxaliplatin	Vasculotoxicity, including endothelial dysfunction, arterial vasospasm, HTN	Small studies suggest acute vasculotoxic effects; relationship to long-term events unknown.
Antimetabolites (See Supplement)		
5-Fluorouracil, capecitabine	Coronary vasospasm, myocardial ischemia, infarction, arrhythmias, ECG changes, sudden death	May be related to endothelial injury, vasoconstriction, and vasospasm; typically managed with nitrates and calcium channel blockers
Monoclonal Antibody Tyrosine Kinase Inhibitors		
Bevacizumab	HTN, CM, HF, thrombosis	Low risk of CM or HF
Trastuzumab	CM, HF	Increased risk of CM and HF with anthracyclines; HTN, obesity, and borderline normal baseline LVEF are also established risk factors; many LVEF declines are reversible, but as noted in clinical trial data, in approximately 20% of patients, reversibility is not seen
Pertuzumab	CM, HF	Risk of CM and HF remains incompletely defined, but thus far, it has been modest
Proteasome Inhibitors		
Bortezomib and carfilzomib	CM, HF, edema, HTN, acute coronary syndrome, pulmonary hypertension, arrhythmia	Bortezomib is a reversible proteasome inhibitor; carfilzomib is an irreversible proteasome inhibitor; cardiotoxicity rates greater
Small-Molecule Tyrosine Kinase Inhibitors		
Sunitinib	HTN, CM, HF, ischemia, thrombosis	Risk of HTN that tends to occur early; relationship between afterload and CM risk remains to be determined
Sorafenib	HTN, CM, ischemia, thrombosis	Risk of HTN; also associated with ischemia
Imatinib	Edema, pericardial effusion	Very low risk of CM
Nilotinib	Peripheral vascular disease, ischemic heart disease, QT prolongation, cardiometabolic effects	Multi-targeted oral tyrosine kinase inhibitor; cardiometabolic effects include hyperglycemia and hyperlipidemia
Ponatinib	Peripheral vascular disease, ischemic heart disease, HTN, HF	Multi-targeted oral tyrosine kinase inhibitor
Dasatinib	Pulmonary HTN, pericardial effusion	Cardiopulmonary status should be evaluated prior to and during therapy
Ibrutinib	HTN, atrial fibrillation, ventricular arrhythmias, HF, bleeding	Bruton's tyrosine kinase inhibitor
Immune-Modulating Agents		
Immune checkpoint inhibitors	Myocarditis	Myocarditis is very rare but can be fulminant; worse with combination therapy; typically occurs earlier in course of therapy but can occur at any time
CAR T cell therapy	Cytokine release syndrome associated adverse CV events (hypotension, arrhythmia)	Treatment for cytokine release syndrome includes tocilizumab
Androgen-Deprivation Therapy		
Leuprolide, goserelin, triptorelin, degarelix, flutamide, bicalutamide	Metabolic syndrome, ischemia, coronary artery disease, HTN	Mixed data regarding an increased risk of adverse CV events with mechanisms of CV disease unclear; patients with pre-existing CV disease may be at a more substantially increased risk
Estrogen-Receptor Modulators		
Tamoxifen	Thrombosis	Favorable effects on lipids
Aromatase inhibitors (anastrozole, letrozole, exemestane)	Hypercholesterolemia, HTN, HF, combined endpoint of dysrhythmia, valvular disease, and pericarditis	Studies evaluated aromatase inhibitors in comparison to tamoxifen and demonstrated worse CV effects
Radiation Therapy	Valvular disease, pericardial disease, vascular disease, ischemia, coronary artery disease, CM, HF	Major CV events tend to occur late, although early abnormalities in cardiac function and perfusion are observed; mean heart dose associated with mortality

CM, Cardiomyopathy; *CV,* cardiovascular; *ECG,* electrocardiogram; *HF,* heart failure; *HTN,* hypertension; *RT,* radiation therapy.

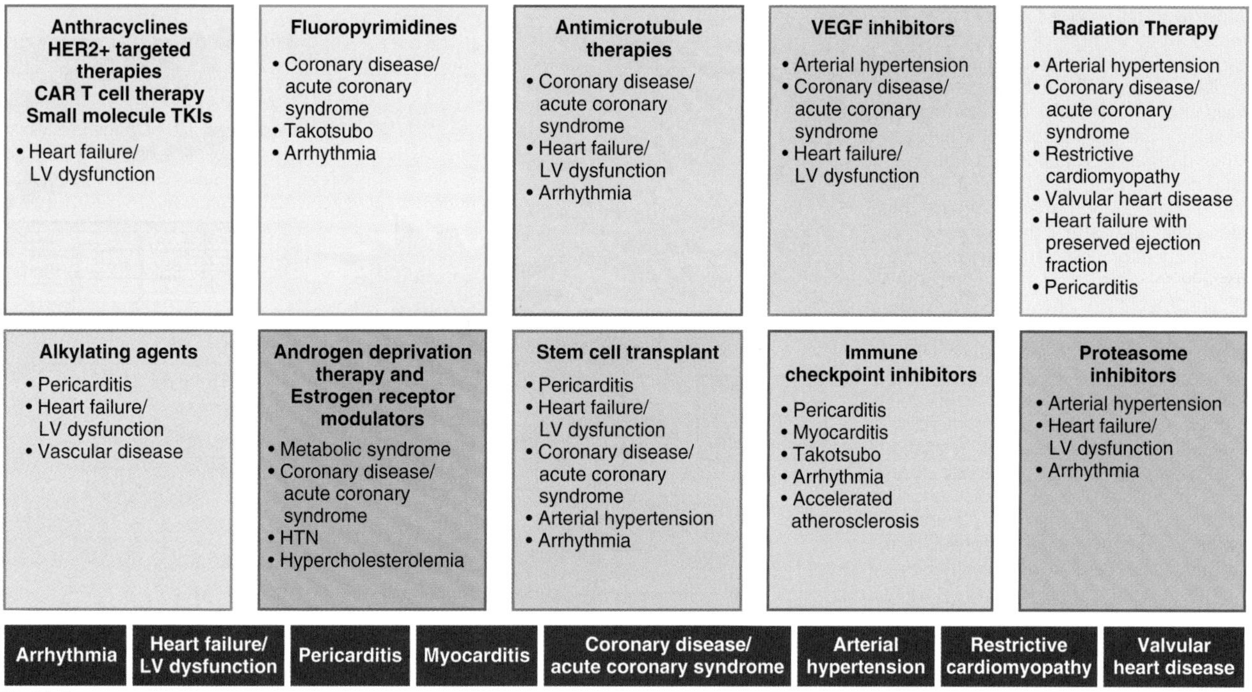

Anthracyclines HER2+ targeted therapies CAR T cell therapy Small molecule TKIs	Fluoropyrimidines	Antimicrotubule therapies	VEGF inhibitors	Radiation Therapy
• Heart failure/ LV dysfunction	• Coronary disease/ acute coronary syndrome • Takotsubo • Arrhythmia	• Coronary disease/ acute coronary syndrome • Heart failure/ LV dysfunction • Arrhythmia	• Arterial hypertension • Coronary disease/ acute coronary syndrome • Heart failure/ LV dysfunction	• Arterial hypertension • Coronary disease/ acute coronary syndrome • Restrictive cardiomyopathy • Valvular heart disease • Heart failure with preserved ejection fraction • Pericarditis

Alkylating agents	Androgen deprivation therapy and Estrogen receptor modulators	Stem cell transplant	Immune checkpoint inhibitors	Proteasome inhibitors
• Pericarditis • Heart failure/ LV dysfunction • Vascular disease	• Metabolic syndrome • Coronary disease/ acute coronary syndrome • HTN • Hypercholesterolemia	• Pericarditis • Heart failure/ LV dysfunction • Coronary disease/ acute coronary syndrome • Arterial hypertension • Arrhythmia	• Pericarditis • Myocarditis • Takotsubo • Arrhythmia • Accelerated atherosclerosis	• Arterial hypertension • Heart failure/ LV dysfunction • Arrhythmia

Arrhythmia	Heart failure/ LV dysfunction	Pericarditis	Myocarditis	Coronary disease/ acute coronary syndrome	Arterial hypertension	Restrictive cardiomyopathy	Valvular heart disease

FIGURE 56.1 Cardiotoxicities of common cancer therapies. This figure demonstrates commonly used cancer therapies and the associated potential cardiovascular risk factors and diseases. *CAR*, Chimeric antigen receptor; *HER2*, human epidermal growth factor receptor 2; *LV*, left ventricular; *TKI*, tyrosine kinase inhibitor; *VEGF*, vascular endothelial growth factor (Adapted from Harries I, Liang K, Williams M, et al. Magnetic resonance imaging to detect cardiovascular effects of cancer therapy. *JACC Cardio Oncl.* 2020;2(2):270–292.)

younger than 30 years of age receiving frontline treatment for acute myelogenous leukemia, the cumulative incidence of cardiotoxicity, as defined by National Cancer Institute Common Terminology Criteria for Adverse Events (version 3.0) grade 2 or worse LV systolic dysfunction, was 12%.[7] The standard induction and intensification treatment protocol included daunorubicin and mitoxantrone. In this study, 25% of the cardiotoxicity events were infection associated and 70% of these occurred early, with a median time to cardiotoxicity of 4.3 months (IQR, 3.1 to 5.9) after chemotherapy initiation. Both 5-year event free and overall survival were significantly worsened in patients who suffered from cardiotoxicity. These findings not only indicate an early cardiotoxicity onset, but also suggest treatment-related cardiotoxicity in children results in worse overall outcomes.

Clinical risk factors for anthracycline-induced cardiotoxicity include age of exposure, traditional, modifiable CV risk factors (HTN, diabetes, obesity, and hyperlipidemia), prior chest RT, anthracycline dose, genetic factors, and pre-existing CV disease. In adult survivors of childhood cancer, the prevalence of CM is 4.7% to 10.7%, and increases with age, with an adjusted odds of CM development 2.7 (95% CI 1.1 to 6.9) fold greater compared to patients not exposed to anthracyclines.[8] More recent studies also suggest that the association between anthracycline dose and HF is modified by age of treatment, with a greater relative risk (RR) of CV disease among those who received high-dose anthracycline chemotherapy (≥250 mg/m²) at ≤13 years of age, as compared to children older than 13 years.[9] Here, children that were ≤13 years at diagnosis had a RR of 2.4 to 4.0 fold of any CV disease compared to those older than 13 years. In addition to modifiable CV risk factors and age at anthracycline exposure, concomitant treatment exposures such as RT (>15 Gy) are associated with an increased risk of CV disease. In 1820 adult survivors of childhood cancer treated with anthracyclines, chest-directed RT, or both, there was a high prevalence of subclinical dysfunction in those with an LVEF ≥50%, with abnormal GLS in 28% and diastolic dysfunction in 8.7%,[10] greatest in those who received both anthracyclines and RT.

While multiple studies document a dose-dependent relationship between anthracycline exposure and risk of HF and CM, it is recognized that anthracycline cardiotoxicity can occur at any dose. Older retrospective analyses suggest an incidence of HF, as defined by

clinical signs and symptoms, of 1.7% at a cumulative dose of 300 mg/m², 4.7% at 400 mg/m², 15.7% at 500 mg/m², and 48% at 650 mg/m².[5] It is notable that standard errors for many of these estimates are large, given the small sample sizes. Moreover, with respect to dose, emerging data suggest that the equivalency ratios for mitoxantrone relative to doxorubicin is 10.5 (95% CI 6.2 to 19.1), much greater than previously published (0.6 (95% CI 0.4 to 1.0) for daunorubicin, 0.8 (95% CI 0.5 to 2.8) for epirubicin).[11] Data from childhood cancer survivors also indicate that genetic variations in single-nucleotide polymorphisms modify the association between the anthracycline dose and CM risk and confer an increased risk of cardiotoxicity at lower dosages.[12] The genetic determinants of anthracycline cardiotoxicity is an active area of research, with ongoing studies in candidate genes and genome-wide association studies. Additional content on this topic is presented in an online supplement, "Genetics of Anthracycline Cardiotoxicity."

Several basic mechanisms have been proposed to explain anthracycline-induced cardiotoxicity. The first is formation of reactive oxygen species (ROS) and increased oxidative stress via redox cycling of the quinone moiety of doxorubicin, formation of anthracycline-iron complexes, and topoisomerase-2β (Top2β) inhibition (Fig. 56.2).[13] Furthermore, anthracyclines have shown to cause impaired calcium signaling and intracellular sequestration affecting myocardial relaxation, a decrease in cardiac progenitor cells, and alterations in neuregulin (NRG)/ErbB signaling.[13,14] Recent data also suggest a role for phosphoinositide 3-kinase γ (PI3Kγ) in the pathophysiology of anthracycline cardiotoxicity, perhaps related to the release of mitochondrial DNA by injured organelles and contained autolysosomes.[15] The most widely cited and unifying mechanism is the formation of ROS, leading to oxidative stress and subsequent injury to cardiac myocytes and endothelial cells.[13,14] The quinone moiety of the anthracycline enters cells and undergoes redox cycling, generating free radicals via both an enzymatic pathway involving the mitochondrial respiratory chain and also via a nonenzymatic pathway involving direct interactions between anthracyclines and intracellular iron. Toxic hydroxyl radicals from anthracycline-iron complexes act as cytotoxic messengers. This results in impaired mitochondrial function, cellular membrane damage, and cytotoxicity. Nitric oxide synthase (NOS) also contributes to the generation of anthracycline-mediated reactive nitrogen species, worsening nitrosative stress. The formation of ROS may occur via the isozyme Top2, and, more specifically, Top2β,

1094

in cardiomyocytes.[13] Mice lacking Top2β are protected from anthracycline-induced DNA damage, cardiomyocyte death, and declines in cardiac function. These findings need to be validated. Interestingly, dexrazoxane, an iron chelator and cardioprotectant, binds to Top2β and results in Top2βdegradation.

Data derived from in vitro and in vivo animal models support the hypothesis that anthracyclines also affect the population of cardiac progenitor cells. Anthracycline chemotherapy may also render cardiomyocytes more susceptible to alterations in NRG-1 and ErbB signaling and downstream pro-survival pathways.[13,14] In vitro studies have demonstrated an inhibitory effect of doxorubicin on hypoxia-inducible factor (HIF) and downstream pathways. Anthracyclines also result in impaired diastolic relaxation via calpain-dependent titin proteolysis. More recent studies have used human induced pluripotent stem cell–derived cardiomyocytes (hiPSC-CMs) to model the predilection to anthracycline cardiotoxicity in patients, and corroborated decreased cell viability, impaired mitochondrial and metabolic function, impaired calcium handling, decreased antioxidant pathway activity, and increased ROS production as mechanisms of toxicity.[16]

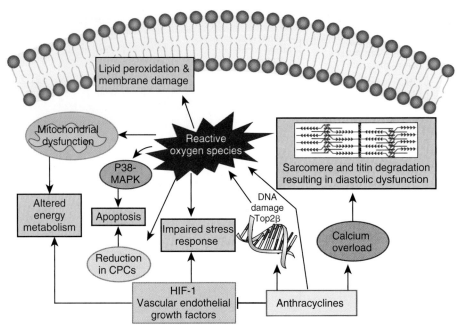

FIGURE 56.2 Proposed mechanisms of anthracycline cardiotoxicity. Using anthracyclines results in the generation of reactive oxygen species (ROS), potentially via topoisomerase 2β inhibition, as well as calcium overload, reduction in cardiac progenitor cells (CPCs), and hypoxia-inducible factor (HIF) inhibition.

Several other traditional chemotherapeutic agents, including taxanes, alkylating and alkylating-like agents, and antimetabolites can also lead to cardiotoxicity (see online supplement "Cardiotoxicity of Traditional Chemotherapeutic Agents").

Additional Cancer Therapies
Proteasome Inhibitors

Proteasome inhibitors, including bortezomib and carfilzomib, are used in the treatment of relapsed or refractory and newly diagnosed cases of multiple myeloma. Bortezomib is a reversible nonselective inhibitor of proteasomes that blocks chymotrypsin-like activity at the 26S proteasome; carfilzomib is an irreversible selective inhibitor of proteasomes that blocks chymotrypsin activity of the 20S proteasome.

The reported incidence of all-grade and grade 3 and higher adverse CV events with these proteasome inhibitors from a meta-analysis of Phase 1 to 3 clinical trials was 18.1% and 8.2%, respectively.[17] HF (4.1%) and HTN (12.2%) were the most common adverse CV events, followed by arrhythmias (2.4%) and ischemia (1.8%). In a multi-center, longitudinal prospective cohort study of 95 patients, the rates of adverse CV events were much greater, occurring in 50.7% in patients receiving carfilzomib and 16.7% receiving bortezomib.[18] Most occurred during carfilzomib therapy; HF and HTN were similarly noted as most common, with grade 3 and 4 HF and HTN events occurring in 20% and 23%, respectively. Arrhythmia, acute coronary syndrome, and pulmonary HTN were also noted. In case series, both HF with preserved and reduced ejection fraction have been reported. Predictors of adverse CV events with carfilzomib include a history of HF, baseline diastolic dysfunction, higher doses of carfilzomib, and abnormal NT-proBNP levels at baseline or during therapy. It is postulated that proteasome inhibitors alter protein homeostasis[19] and reduce phosphorylation of AMPKalpha and downstream autophagy related proteins, such as Raptor.[20]

IMMUNOTHERAPY
Immune Checkpoint Inhibitors

Immune checkpoint inhibitors have become the standard of care in the treatment of a variety of solid and liquid tumors, revolutionizing cancer care, replacing cytotoxic therapies for many malignancies.

These monoclonal antibodies, which target cytotoxic T lymphocyte-associated antigen 4 (CTLA-4) and the programmed death receptor (PD-1) and its ligand PD-L1, are associated with a risk of immune-related adverse events. In a retrospective analysis of 448 patients with advanced melanoma treated in Phase I-III trials, 94.9% of treated patients experienced adverse events over a median follow-up of 13.2 months, with 55.4% being grade 3 to 4. Dermatologic, gastrointestinal, endocrine, hepatic, and pulmonary adverse events are most common. Myocarditis, however, occurs much less frequently, on the order of 0.06% to 1%,[21,22] but is notable given its potential morbidity and mortality.

The data related to immunotherapy cardiotoxicity are still emerging. Many published studies are derived from retrospective cohort studies or case series. These suggest that myocarditis typically occurs early, at a median time of 34 to 65 days, but over a broad range as there are also published reports of late myocarditis. Additional clinical manifestations include dyspnea, palpitations, and HF. Biomarkers, including troponin and natriuretic peptides have been studied as diagnostic and prognostic tools, as have imaging markers including global longitudinal strain, with associations with adverse cardiac events in small studies.[23–25]

Combination therapies have been noted to be associated with an approximate twofold increased risk of myocarditis compared to monotherapy. Myositis has also been reported to be common in patients who develop myocarditis. The relevance of other autoimmune diseases or CV disease or risk factors in the development of myocarditis remains incompletely defined. Other toxicities have been reported with immunotherapy, including arrhythmias, pericardial effusions, and CM. Whether these are completely distinct entities from myocarditis is not clear. Moreover, there are emerging data regarding potential associations with accelerated atherosclerosis.

Chimeric Antigen Receptor T Cell Therapies

Chimeric antigen receptor (CAR) T cells targeting CD19 are a newer class of therapies that have shown to be highly effective in the treatment of refractory and relapsing hematologic malignancies, including pediatric acute lymphoblastic leukemia and adult large B-cell lymphoma.[26] Toxicities associated with CAR T cell therapy include cytokine release syndrome, a multi-organ system toxicity that occurs with widespread release of inflammatory cytokines and chemokines, including interleukin (IL)-2, soluble IL-2Ra, interferon gamma, IL-6, soluble IL-6R, and granulocyte-macrophage colony-stimulating factor. Adverse CV events most commonly occur with cytokine release syndrome, and include hypotension, arrhythmia, HF, and potentially cardiac death. Treatment for cytokine release syndrome includes tocilizumab.

TARGETED THERAPY

The treatment of a number of malignant neoplasms has changed dramatically with the advent of targeted therapies. As opposed to traditional chemotherapeutics which target basic cellular processes present in most cells, these therapies target pathways that are dysregulated in cancerous cells. It was hoped that this approach would reduce toxicities typical of conventional chemotherapeutics and be more effective at treating the cancer. However, concerns about cardiotoxicity have surfaced for several agents, likely given the mechanistic commonalities to both CV disease and cancer.

ErbB Antagonists (Trastuzumab, Pertuzumab)

Trastuzumab is a humanized monoclonal antibody that binds subdomain IV of human epidermal growth factor receptor 2 (HER2)/neu, also known as ErbB2. Trastuzumab exerts its antitumor effects by blocking HER2 cleavage, resulting in antibody-dependent, cell-mediated cytotoxicity and inhibition of ligand-independent, HER2-mediated signaling affecting the following downstream pathways: PI3K, serine/threonine-specific protein kinase Akt, mitogen-activated protein kinase (MAPK), extracellular-signal–regulated kinase 1/2 (ERK1/2), and the mechanistic target of rapamycin (mTOR).[13] Trastuzumab also exerts antiangiogenic effects. First approved by the Food and Drug Administration (FDA) in 1998 for metastatic disease, it received indications for early-stage HER2+ breast cancer in 2007.

Phase III clinical trials with trastuzumab suggest that the risk of severe HF is low, on the order of 1.7% to 4.1%, but the risk of LVEF declines is greater, on the order of 7.1% to 18.6%.[5,27] Compared to retrospective and prospective cohort studies, these rates are lower. This may be secondary to the lack of generalizability of the clinical trial population given stringent exclusion/inclusion criteria. Retrospective analyses from various large data sources, including the Surveillance, Epidemiology, and End Results (SEER) Program, the Cancer Research Network, and the Canadian health care system database, indicate a higher incidence of HF and CM.[5] SEER analyses suggested an HF incidence of 41.9% at 3 years following combination therapy with anthracyclines and trastuzumab; however, these data are also subject to limitations including potential misclassification. In the Cancer Research Network, there was a 20.1% incidence of HF and/or CM with combination therapy. Ontario Cancer Registry data suggested an estimated cumulative 5-year incidence of HF of 5.2% with trastuzumab regimens, with a HF risk that was greatest in the first 1.5 years of cancer therapy.[28] In this analysis, patients treated with sequential anthracyclines and trastuzumab therapy had a cumulative incidence of 6.6% for major cardiac events at 3 years. The adjusted risk of major cardiac events was higher with sequential therapy (HR 3.96, 95% CI 3.01 to 5.22) and trastuzumab without anthracyclines (HR 1.76, 95% CI 1.19 to 2.60) compared with other chemotherapy. There are clear data that indicate the risk of HF and CM with trastuzumab therapy is increased in the setting of sequential anthracycline and trastuzumab exposure. Additional risk factors for trastuzumab cardiotoxicity include obesity, a lower baseline LVEF, HTN, or diabetes; non-Caucasian race; and older age.

Importantly, LVEF declines with trastuzumab are largely reversible and typically occur during therapy. As a consequence, trastuzumab-associated cardiotoxicity was initially termed type II dysfunction, to distinguish it from anthracycline-associated cardiotoxicity, termed type I dysfunction.[5] This classification has largely fallen out of favor

secondary to its oversimplification and because of the lack of strong evidence that the biologic underpinnings and clinical manifestations of anthracycline and trastuzumab cardiotoxicity are fundamentally distinct without overlap. Moreover, the reversibility of LVEF declines with trastuzumab is not universally observed. In the HERceptin Adjuvant (HERA) Trial, a phase III randomized trial of trastuzumab, approximately 20% to 30% of patients did not demonstrate LVEF recovery, and some patients suffered a subsequent decline in LVEF even after an initial recovery was noted. Conversely, as noted above, LVEF recovery is observed with anthracyclines.[29] There are also data to suggest that there are longer-term consequences and a risk of late HF with trastuzumab.[30]

Dose delays and interruptions have also been shown to be associated with worse overall survival rates, emphasizing the importance of safe cancer therapy delivery. The clinical determinants of LV recovery, as defined by an improvement in LVEF, have not been rigorously defined with trastuzumab, but observations suggest that temporary cessation of therapy and/or institution of cardiac medications (e.g., angiotensin-converting enzyme [ACE] inhibitors and beta blockers) are associated with recovery. Very small studies have also suggested that trastuzumab can be continued in the setting of modest LVEF declines, of 40% or greater.[31] Longitudinal data defining the changes in cardiac size and function over time suggest that measures of LV size (primarily end-systolic volumes), contractility (longitudinal and circumferential strain), and ventricular-arterial coupling (afterload) are independently associated with LVEF decline and recovery.[6]

It is widely speculated that the cardiac dysfunction observed with trastuzumab is a direct consequence of ErbB2 inhibition in cardiomyocytes, but this remains to be definitively proven.[13,14] Basic studies have been limited, in part, by the lack of robust systems to directly study the in vitro and in vivo effects of trastuzumab. The NRG/ErbB system functions as a paracrine and juxtacrine system between microvascular endothelial cells and cardiomyocytes. NRG-1 is expressed in vascular endothelial cells, and ErbB2 and ErbB4 are expressed in cardiomyocytes and endothelial cells. Recombinant NRG-1β activates ErbB2 and ErbB4 receptor phosphorylation in cardiomyocytes in vitro. Important downstream mediators, as noted above, include PI3K/Akt, MAPK/ERK, steroid receptor activator (Src)/focal adhesion kinase, and NOS. All of these pathways are fundamental for cardiac homeostasis, cell survival, mitochondrial function, cell growth, and focal adhesion formation. Mice with a cardiac-specific deletion of ErbB2 develop dilated CM and demonstrate exaggerated systolic dysfunction after pressure overload compared with wild-type mice. ErbB2 and ErbB4 expression is preserved during compensated hypertrophy, but it declines in the early stages of systolic dysfunction in mice subjected to pressure overload. Overall, these findings suggest that perturbations in ErbB receptor signaling are important in the maintenance of cardiac function. Data also suggest that disruption of ErbB2 signaling results in endothelial dysfunction and an altered vascular phenotype, potentially contributing to the cardiomyopathic phenotype.

There are a number of newer ErbB antagonists, including pertuzumab, ado-trastuzumab Emtansine (T-DM1), and tucatinib. Pertuzumab is a humanized monoclonal antibody that binds HER2 at subdomain II of the HER2 extracellular domain; it is administered in conjunction with trastuzumab for high-risk and metastatic HER2+ breast cancer.[32] Pertuzumab also stimulates antibody-dependent, cell-mediated cytotoxicity, and prevents dimerization to other ligand-activated HER receptors, especially HER3. Although the CV effects are still being elucidated, Phase III trial data have not demonstrated a substantial cardiotoxic signal with pertuzumab and trastuzumab, T-DM1, or tucatinib that is greater than trastuzumab alone.[32] However, the external validity of these findings remains a question, as the epidemiology of LVEF declines and recovery have not completely been defined in the non-clinical trial setting.

Tyrosine Kinase Inhibitors and Monoclonal Antibodies

Many of the targeted cancer therapeutics inhibit the activity of tyrosine kinases (TKs). TKs attach phosphate groups to tyrosine residues of other proteins, thereby changing the activity, subcellular localization, and rate of degradation of the proteins. In the normal cell, these wild-type (i.e., normal) TKs play many roles in regulating basic cellular functions. However, in leukemias and cancers, the gene encoding the causal (or contributory) TKs is amplified (leading to overexpression) or mutated, leading to a constitutively activated state that drives proliferation of the cancerous clonal cells or blocks their normal death.

Vascular Endothelial Growth Factor Signaling Pathway Inhibitors

Vascular endothelial growth factor receptor (VEGFR) signaling pathway inhibitors are used in the treatment of metastatic renal cell cancers; gastrointestinal stromal tumors; and thyroid, hepatocellular, and colon cancers. Bevacizumab is a humanized recombinant anti-VEGF antibody. The CV risks associated with bevacizumab include HTN, a low incidence of HF (1.6%, but with a RR of 4.7 compared with placebo), and arterial thromboembolic events (7.1% with bevacizumab versus 2.5% with chemotherapy alone).

Sorafenib, sunitinib, axitinib, pazopanib, lenvatinib, cabozantinib, and vandetanib are other small-molecule tyrosine kinase inhibitors (TKIs) that inhibit multiple TKs, in addition to the VEGFR signaling pathway.,[13,33] These antiangiogenic TKIs have been associated with HTN, CM and HF, cardiac ischemia, and arterial thrombotic events. Of these agents, we focus on describing the epidemiology and basic mechanisms of sunitinib, because it is one of the most well studied agents to date. This discussion is relevant to other TKIs that have primarily off-target effects on VEGFR and PDGFR.

> Sunitinib results in HTN, as well as declines in LVEF. In phase III trials and subsequent clinical experience, the incidence of HTN ranges from 5% to 47% and the incidence of significant LVEF declines is estimated to be on the order of 10%.[14] HTN secondary to sunitinib tends to occur early, with the median time to HTN (defined as a systolic blood pressure of ≥140 mm Hg or diastolic blood pressure of ≥90 mm Hg) occurring within 1 to 20 days of the first two cycles of sunitinib therapy. The incidence of systolic HTN in one pooled analysis was 58% by the end of cycle 1 and 80% by the end of cycle 2. Increases in blood pressure tend to be greater in those with a history of HTN. Additional single center retrospective data suggest that average systolic blood pressure increases of 8.5 mm Hg and diastolic blood pressure increases of 6.7 mm Hg occur with any TKI therapy, greatest with axitinib.[34]
>
> Prospective observational data suggest that the rate of LV dysfunction in the metastatic renal cell cancer population, as defined by declines in LVEF, is on the order of 9.7%. Most of these events occur early after the initiation of therapy, primarily within the first 3 months. LVEF declines have also been observed to be reversible and manageable, although predictors of recovery remain to be defined. The mechanisms of sunitinib cardiotoxicity are believed to be secondary to the inhibition of signaling pathways critical to CV homeostasis, energy compromise, and increased afterload.[14]

Bcr-Abl Targeted Therapies

Imatinib, the first targeted small-molecule TK inhibitor of the fusion protein Bcr-Abl, which arises from the chromosomal translocation that creates the Philadelphia chromosome, revolutionized the treatment of chronic myeloid leukemia.[35] However, clinically, imatinib may be associated with a very low incidence of HF, with admittedly conflicting data. Newer generation Bcr-Abl TKIs have raised more substantive concerns. Dasatinib, with more potent activity than imatinib against Bcr-Abl, has been associated with significant pulmonary HTN that is observed to be largely reversible with cessation of the drug. This finding prompted the FDA to recommend that patients be evaluated for cardiopulmonary disease prior to and during dasatinib treatment. Nilotinib and ponatinib have both been associated with PVD and ischemic heart disease. Moreover, nilotinib has been associated with cardiometabolic effects, including hyperglycemia and hyperlipidemia, and QT prolongation. The incidence of PVD has been reported to be 1.3% to 6.2%, and the incidence of combined CV events, including ischemic heart disease, cerebrovascular disease, and PVD, is on the order of 10% to 15.9%.[35] Ponatinib has been associated with HTN, ischemic events, and HF, potentially related to VEGFR1-3 inhibition. In the Ponatinib Ph-Positive Acute Lymphoblastic Leukemia and CML Evaluation (PACE)

trial, 6% of patients experienced CV events, 3% experienced cerebrovascular events, and 4% experienced PAD at 12 months.[36] At a median follow-up of 24 months, the cumulative incidences increased to 10%, 7%, and 7%, respectively. The biologic mechanisms of cardiotoxicity remain unknown, but again are likely related to their multi-targeted kinase inhibition. Comprehensively deciphering the mechanisms of these kinase inhibitors remains challenging given their nonselectivity; as they typically affect more than 30 different kinases. Ibrutinib is a small molecule Bruton's TKI that is used in the treatment of chronic lymphocytic leukemia, Waldenstrom macroglobulinemia, mantle cell lymphoma, marginal zone lymphoma, and chronic graft versus host disease. CV toxicities include HTN, atrial fibrillation and supraventricular arrhythmias, ventricular arrhythmias, HF, and bleeding. One pharmacovigilance database study indicated an elevated reporting odds ratio (ROR) for each of these, that occurred soon after the first dose.[37] For HTN, the ROR was 1.7 (95% CI 1.5 to 1.9); supraventricular arrhythmias (largely atrial fibrillation) 23.1 (95% CI 21.6 to 24.7); ventricular arrhythmias 4.7 (95% CI 3.7 to 5.9); HF 3.5 (95% CI 3.1 to 3.8); and central nervous system bleeding 3.7 (3.4 to 4.1). These were each associated with an increased risk of death, except HTN.

HORMONAL THERAPY

Androgen Deprivation Therapies

In prostate cancer, androgen deprivation therapy (ADT) is used to reduce levels of androgens in the circulation and decrease prostate cell growth. ADT includes gonadotropin-releasing hormone (GnRH) agonists, such as leuprolide, goserelin, and triptorelin; GnRH antagonists (Degarelix); and antiandrogens, such as flutamide and bicalutamide. These therapies have adverse cardiometabolic effects, and low testosterone is also implicated in metabolic syndrome. Studies suggest that they result in increased body weight (particularly visceral adiposity), decreased insulin sensitivity, and dyslipidemia (increased low-density lipoprotein [LDL] and triglycerides). Changes in body composition occur early, within the first few months of therapy. Multiple cohort studies indicate an increased risk of CV events in men with prostate cancer. Moreover, treatment with ADT has also been associated with adverse CV events, including coronary disease, myocardial infarction, HF, sudden cardiac death, or death due to CV disease. Not all studies corroborate this effect, however, including a meta-analyses of 4141 patients from 8 randomized trials. It may also be that these effects are worsened in patients with preexisting CV disease, and new CV events have been reported within the first 6 months of initiation of therapy.[38] CV risk in patients treated with ADT may vary according to severity of comorbidities, with ADT reported as having a greater and worse impact on CV survival in patients who have greater baseline CV risk and worse overall comorbidities.

Selective Estrogen Receptor Modulators and Aromatase Inhibitors

Tamoxifen is a selective estrogen receptor modulator widely used in adjuvant therapy for estrogen receptor–positive breast cancer. Data regarding the cardioprotective effect of tamoxifen have been conflicting. Tamoxifen does exert a favorable effect on lipids, with a reduction in total cholesterol and LDL levels. Some studies demonstrate a potential effect on decreasing the ischemic heart disease incidence, with a RR of 0.76 (95% CI, 0.60 to 0.95; $P = 0.02$), although other studies demonstrate no significant effect.[39] An increased risk of thromboembolic events, however, is well established; they occur largely during the first 2 years of exposure and in older women. A meta-analysis from the Early Breast Cancer Trialists' Collaborative Group confirmed a significant, but small, increased risk in venous thromboembolism with tamoxifen.

Aromatase inhibitors (e.g., anastrozole, letrozole, exemestane) block the conversion of androgens to estrogen. The two major classes that are currently in use differ according to their ability to bind reversibly versus irreversibly to aromatase. Data regarding the potential CV effects of aromatase inhibitors have been conflicting, but it is hypothesized that these agents inhibit the beneficial effects of estrogen related to the regulation of lipids, coagulation, antioxidant systems, and nitric oxide production. Aromatase inhibitors are associated with worse hypercholesterolemia and HTN, and a longer duration of exposure is reportedly associated with an increased risk of CV disease. Pooled data analyses from multiple large cohort studies suggest that there is a modestly increased risk of CV disease, as defined by myocardial infarction, angina, or HF with aromatase inhibitors compared with tamoxifen (odds ratio [OR], 1.26; 95% CI, 1.10 to 1.43; p < 0.001).[40] Another large retrospective analysis determined that compared with tamoxifen, aromatase inhibitors were not associated with an increased risk of CV ischemia or stroke, or HF/CM, but were associated with a combined outcome of dysrhythmia, valvular dysfunction, and pericarditis.[41] A population-based, retrospective cohort study suggested that in 23,525 women newly diagnosed with breast cancer, of which 17,922 initiated treatment with an aromatase inhibitor (n = 8139) or tamoxifen (n = 9783), aromatase inhibitors were associated with an increased risk of HF (incidence rate, 5.4 versus 1.8 per 1000 person-years; HR 1.86 95% CI 1.14 to 3.03) and CV mortality (incidence rate, 9.5 versus 4.7 per 1000 person-years; HR 1.50, 95% CI 1.11 to 2.04) compared with tamoxifen.[42]

RADIATION THERAPY

RT has been critical for improved cancer control and survival rates. Despite these gains, incidental irradiation to cardiac structures results in an increased risk of CV morbidity and mortality.[43] The clinical manifestations of RT cardiotoxicity include coronary disease, CM and HF, valvular disease, arrhythmia, and pericardial disease. Increasing data suggest that early subclinical changes, including cardiac perfusion defects and longitudinal strain abnormalities, can occur earlier, within 6 months of RT, even with the use of current techniques.

In a meta-analysis of over 23,000 women with breast cancer, there was an excess of deaths not resulting from breast cancer as early as 5 years following RT, principally due to CV disease and lung cancer. Subsequent studies support these results. In one study of women treated from 1954 to 1984 evaluated approximately 28 years after cancer therapy, RT was associated with a 1.76-fold increased risk of cardiac mortality and a 1.33-fold increased risk of vascular mortality. Patients with left-sided disease had a 1.56-fold increased risk of cardiac mortality compared with right-sided disease. Moreover, a study of women treated for breast cancer between 1958 and 2001 suggested that major CV events increased by 7.4% for each Gy increase in mean heart dose.[44]

Studies in lymphoma survivors corroborate an association between RT dose to the heart and a progressive risk of CV disease, with a CV complications risk three- to five-fold greater than the general population. Relative to healthy age-matched controls, the standard incidence ratio was 3.19 for coronary artery bypass surgery, 1.55 for revascularization, 9.19 for valve surgery, 12.91 for pericardial stripping or pericardiocentesis, and 1.9 for defibrillator or pacemaker placement.

Most recently, data from the lung cancer population have also suggested an increased CV risk. In RTOG 0617, a randomized trial of standard versus high-dose RT in locally advanced lung cancer, high-dose RT was associated with a 38% increased risk of all-cause mortality,[45] and RT dose to the heart specifically was associated with worse overall survival. A single-center retrospective analysis of 748 non-small cell lung cancer patients treated with RT (median age 65 years, IQR 57 to 73 years), of whom 35.8% had pre-existing coronary disease, noted that coronary disease, HF, or cardiac death occurred in 10.3%.[46]

In addition to the RT dose delivered (total and mean heart dose), which is a critical determinant of the development of cardiac disease, additional risk factors include the radiation field, younger age, higher number of fractions, concomitant chemotherapy (anthracyclines), CV risk factors (diabetes, tobacco use, obesity, HTN, hypercholesterolemia), and CV disease.

Irradiation also results in valvular disease with leaflet thickening, fibrosis, and calcification. Left-sided valves are more commonly affected, particularly the aortic valve, followed by the mitral and tricuspid valves. Fibrosis and calcification of the aortic root, aortic valve annulus, aortic valve leaflets, aortic-mitral intervalvular fibrosa, mitral valve annulus, and the base and mid portions of the mitral valve leaflets typically occur. Sparing of the mitral valve tips and commissures has been noted as a distinguishing feature. Regurgitation is more common than stenosis, with the exception of the aortic valve. The reported incidence of significant valve disease is 1% at 10 years, 5% at 15 years, and 6% at 20 years, with the incidence increasing significantly after 20 years and related to dose. The pathophysiology of radiation-induced heart disease may be related to an increase in TGF-β and osteogenic factors, including bone morphogenetic protein 2, osteopontin, and alkaline phosphatase.

RT is also associated with the development of HF and CM. Diffuse myocardial fibrosis and microvascular and macrovascular injury result in systolic and diastolic dysfunction, and can manifest as a restrictive CM phenotype. RT has also been associated with an increased risk of HF with preserved ejection fraction. On a microvascular level, irradiation results in endothelial cell loss and dysfunction, increased inflammation, and decreased capillary density. On a macrovascular level, there is proximal (ostial) involvement of coronary arteries, and lesions can be fibrous, fibrocalcific, fibrofatty, and laden with cholesterol and lipid. Irradiation also results in autonomic dysfunction, defined by an elevated resting heart rate and abnormal heart rate recovery. Finally, radiation-induced pericardial disease can occur acutely, as pericarditis and pericardial effusions. Pericardial thickening and constrictive pericarditis have also been noted, and can be delayed several weeks to years after RT.

STEM CELL TRANSPLANTATION

Advances in hematopoietic stem cell transplantation (HCT) for hematologic malignancies have led to improvements in transplant outcomes resulting in a growing survivor population. However, CV disease is a competing risk and a major cause of morbidity and mortality in this population. Compared with the general population, there is a markedly increased rate of CV death, HF/CM, and ischemic heart disease, with incidence rate differences on the order of 3.6 (1.7 to 5.5), 8.8 (5.7 to 11.8), and 3.3 (0.7 to 5.9), respectively.[47] These effects are worsened in younger survivors less than 60 years of age. Moreover, there is a significantly increased hazard of CV death (HR 2.3, 95% CI 1.1 to 48) and HF/CM (HR 1.9, 95% 1.1 to 3.3). Highly prevalent, modifiable CV risk factors in the HCT survivor population contribute significantly to CV disease. The burden of modifiable CV risk factors after HCT in this population is substantial. At 1-year post transplant, HCT survivors (median age 44 years) have a cumulative incidence of HTN of 28.4%; dyslipidemia 33.6%, diabetes 10.8%, and multiple CV risk factors 16.1%.[47] These numbers increase substantially over time, and at 10 years, 37.7% suffer from HTN, 46.7% from dyslipidemia, 18.1% diabetes, and 31.4% multiple CV risk factors.

MECHANISTIC OVERLAP BETWEEN CARDIOVASCULAR DISEASE AND CANCER

An emerging area in the field of cardio-oncology research that links both cancer-associated mutations and CV disease is clonal hematopoiesis. (Additional content on this topic is presented in an online supplement "Mechanistic Overlap Between CV Disease and Cancer"; see also Chapter 24)

FUTURE PERSPECTIVES

The field of cardio-oncology continues to evolve. The need for the dedicated CV care of cancer patients will continue to grow as both cancer and CV disease remain highly prevalent; as there is a growing population of survivors; and as newer cancer therapies affect fundamental CV signaling pathways, resulting in both subclinical and overt cardiotoxic effects. With this growth comes a call to: (1) advance our understanding of the basic pathophysiologic mechanisms; (2) translate these findings to improve upon cancer therapeutics and cardioprotective strategies; (3) understand the epidemiology and natural history of cardiotoxicity and CV remodeling with cancer therapies; (4) develop robust mechanisms to identify high-risk CV patients; and (5) personalize the delivery of therapy to maximize its oncologic effectiveness and minimize its cardiotoxic potential. There is a great need for continued clinical and research education and expertise and collaborative efforts among cardiologists, oncologists, industry partners, patient advocates, and the National Institutes of Health and FDA, as well as analogous global organizations, so that a framework can be built to address gaps in knowledge and personalize care through evidence-based medicine.[48]

REFERENCES

Epidemiology, Clinical Manifestations, and Pathophysiology of Cancer Therapy Cardiotoxicity

1. Roth GA, Johnson C, Abajobir A, et al. Global, regional, and national burden of cardiovascular diseases for 10 causes, 1990 to 2015. *J Am Coll Cardiol.* 2017;70(1):1–25.
2. American Cancer Society. *Global Cancer Facts & Figures.* 4th ed. Atlanta: American Cancer Society; 2018.
3. Roth GA, Abate D, Abate KH, et al. Global, regional, and national age-sex-specific mortality for 282 causes of death in 195 countries and territories, 1980–2017: a systematic analysis for the Global Burden of Disease Study 2017. *Lancet.* 2018;392(10159):1736–1788.

Traditional Chemotherapeutic Agents

4. Yancy CW, Jessup M, Bozkurt B, et al. 2013 ACCF/AHA guideline for the management of heart failure: a report of the American College of Cardiology Foundation/American Heart Association Task Force on practice guidelines. *Circulation.* 2013;128(16):e240–e327.
5. Bloom MW, Hamo CE, Cardinale D, et al. Cancer therapy-related cardiac dysfunction and heart failure: Part 1: definitions, pathophysiology, risk factors, and imaging. *Circ Heart Fail.* 2016;9(1):e002661.
6. Narayan HK, Finkelman B, French B, et al. Detailed echocardiographic phenotyping in breast cancer patients: associations with ejection fraction decline, recovery, and heart failure symptoms over 3 years of follow-up. *Circulation.* 2017;135(15):1397–1412.
7. Getz KD, Sung L, Ky B, et al. Occurrence of treatment-related cardiotoxicity and its impact on outcomes among children treated in the AAML0531 clinical trial: a report from the Children's Oncology Group. *J Clin Oncol.* 2019;37(1):12–21.
8. Mulrooney DA, Armstrong GT, Huang S, et al. Cardiac outcomes in adult survivors of childhood cancer exposed to cardiotoxic therapy: a cross-sectional study. *Ann Intern Med.* 2016;164(2):93–101.
9. Bates JE, Howell RM, Liu Q, et al. Therapy-related cardiac risk in childhood cancer survivors: an analysis of the childhood cancer survivor study. *J Clin Oncol.* 2019;37(13):1090–1101.
10. Armstrong GT, Joshi VM, Ness KK, et al. Comprehensive echocardiographic detection of treatment-related cardiac dysfunction in adult survivors of childhood cancer: results from the St. Jude lifetime cohort study. *J Am Coll Cardiol.* 2015;65(23):2511–2522.
11. Feijen EAM, Leisenring WM, Stratton KL, et al. Derivation of anthracycline and anthraquinone equivalence ratios to doxorubicin for late-onset cardiotoxicity. *JAMA Oncol.* 2019;5(6):864–871.
12. Zamorano JL, Lancellotti P, Rodriguez Muñoz D, et al. 2016 ESC Position Paper on cancer treatments and cardiovascular toxicity developed under the auspices of the ESC Committee for Practice guidelines: the task force for cancer treatments and cardiovascular toxicity of the European Society of Cardiology (ESC). *Eur Heart J.* 2016;37(36):2768–2801.
13. Ky B, Vejpongsa P, Yeh ET, et al. Emerging paradigms in cardiomyopathies associated with cancer therapies. *Circ Res.* 2013;113(6):754–764.
14. Hahn VS, Lenihan DJ, Ky B. Cancer therapy-induced cardiotoxicity: basic mechanisms and potential cardioprotective therapies. *J Am Heart Assoc.* 2014;3(2):e000665.
15. Li M, Sala V, De Santis MC, et al. Phosphoinositide 3-kinase gamma inhibition protects from anthracycline cardiotoxicity and reduces tumor growth. *Circulation.* 2018;138(7):696–711.
16. Burridge PW, Li YF, Matsa E, et al. Human induced pluripotent stem cell-derived cardiomyocytes recapitulate the predilection of breast cancer patients to doxorubicin-induced cardiotoxicity. *Nat Med.* 2016;22(5):547–556.

Additional Cancer Therapies

17. Waxman AJ, Clasen S, Hwang WT, et al. Carfilzomib-associated cardiovascular adverse events: a systematic review and meta-analysis. *JAMA Oncol.* 2018;4(3):e174519.
18. Cornell RF, Ky B, Weiss BM, et al. Prospective study of cardiac events during proteasome inhibitor therapy for relapsed multiple myeloma. *J Clin Oncol.* 2019;37(22):1946–1955.
19. Willis MS, Patterson C. Proteotoxicity and cardiac dysfunction–Alzheimer's disease of the heart? *N Engl J Med.* 2013;368(5):455–464.
20. Efentakis P, Kremastiotis G, Varela A, et al. Molecular mechanisms of carfilzomib-induced cardiotoxicity in mice and the emerging cardioprotective role of metformin. *Blood.* 2019;133(7):710–723.

Immunotherapy

21. Johnson DB, Balko JM, Compton ML, et al. Fulminant myocarditis with combination immune checkpoint blockade. *N Engl J Med.* 2016;375(18):1749–1755.
22. Mahmood SS, Fradley MG, Cohen JV, et al. Myocarditis in patients treated with immune checkpoint inhibitors. *J Am Coll Cardiol.* 2018;71(16):1755–1764.
23. Awadalla M, Mahmood SS, Groarke JD, et al. Global longitudinal strain and cardiac events in patients with immune checkpoint inhibitor-related myocarditis. *J Am Coll Cardiol.* 2020;75(5):467–478.
24. Zhang L, Awadalla M, Mahmood SS, et al. Cardiovascular magnetic resonance in immune checkpoint inhibitor-associated myocarditis. *Eur Heart J.* 2020;41(18):1733–1743.
25. Chitturi KR, Xu J, Araujo-Gutierrez R, et al. Immune checkpoint inhibitor-related adverse cardiovascular events in patients with lung cancer. *JACC (J Am Coll Cardiol): CardioOncol.* 2019;1(2):182–192.
26. Ghosh AK, Chen DH, Guha A, et al. CAR T cell therapy–related cardiovascular outcomes and management. *JACC (J Am Coll Cardiol): CardioOncol.* 2020;2(1):97–109.

Targeted Therapies

27. Advani PP, Ballman KV, Dockter TJ, et al. Long-term cardiac safety analysis of NCCTG N9831 (Alliance) adjuvant trastuzumab trial. *J Clin Oncol.* 2016;34(6):581–587.
28. Goldhar HA, Yan AT, Ko DT, et al. The temporal risk of heart failure associated with adjuvant trastuzumab in breast cancer patients: a population study. *J Natl Cancer Inst.* 2016;108(1).
29. Cardinale D, Colombo A, Bacchiani G, et al. Early detection of anthracycline cardiotoxicity and improvement with heart failure therapy. *Circulation.* 2015;131(22):1981–1988.
30. Banke A, Fosbøl EL, Ewertz M, et al. Long-term risk of heart failure in breast cancer patients after adjuvant chemotherapy with or without trastuzumab. *JACC Heart Fail.* 2019;7(3):217–224.
31. Leong DP, Cosman T, Alhussein MM, et al. Safety of continuing trastuzumab despite mild cardiotoxicity. *JACC (J Am Coll Cardiol): CardioOncol.* 2019;1(1):1–10.
32. Jerusalem G, Lancellotti P, Kim SB. HER2+ breast cancer treatment and cardiotoxicity: monitoring and management. *Breast Cancer Res Treat.* 2019;177(2):237–250. https://doi.org/10.1007/s10549-019-05303-y.
33. Haas NB, Manola J, Ky B, et al. Effects of adjuvant sorafenib and sunitinib on cardiac function in renal cell carcinoma patients without overt metastases: results from ASSURE, ECOG 2805. *Clin Cancer Res.* 2015;21(18):4048–4054.
34. Waliany S, Sainani KL, Park LS, et al. Increase in blood pressure associated with tyrosine kinase inhibitors targeting vascular endothelial growth factor. *JACC (J Am Coll Cardiol): CardioOncology.* 2019;1(1):24–36.
35. Moslehi JJ, Deininger M. Tyrosine kinase inhibitor-associated cardiovascular toxicity in chronic myeloid leukemia. *J Clin Oncol.* 2015;33(35):4210–4218.
36. Cortes JE, Kim DW, Pinilla-Ibarz J, et al. A phase 2 trial of ponatinib in Philadelphia chromosome-positive leukemias. *N Engl J Med.* 2013;369(19):1783–1796.
37. Salem JE, Manouchehri A, Bretagne M, et al. Cardiovascular toxicities associated with ibrutinib. *J Am Coll Cardiol.* 2019;74(13):1667–1678.

Hormonal Therapy

38. O'Farrell S, Garmo H, Holmberg L, et al. Risk and timing of cardiovascular disease after androgen-deprivation therapy in men with prostate cancer. *J Clin Oncol.* 2015;33(11):1243–1251.
39. Davies C, Pan H, Godwin J, et al. Long-term effects of continuing adjuvant tamoxifen to 10 years versus stopping at 5 years after diagnosis of oestrogen receptor-positive breast cancer: ATLAS, a randomised trial. *Lancet.* 2013;381(9869):805–816.
40. Amir E, Seruga B, Niraula S, et al. Toxicity of adjuvant endocrine therapy in postmenopausal breast cancer patients: a systematic review and meta-analysis. *J Natl Cancer Inst.* 2011;103(17):1299–1309.
41. Haque R, Shi J, Schottinger JE, et al. Cardiovascular disease after aromatase inhibitor use. *JAMA Oncol.* 2016;2(12):1590–1597.
42. Khosrow-Khavar F, Filion KB, Bouganim N, et al. Aromatase inhibitors and the risk of cardiovascular outcomes in women with breast cancer: a population-based cohort study. *Circulation.* 2020;141(7):549–559.

Radiation Therapy

43. Early Breast Cancer Trialists' Collaborative G, Darby S, McGale P, et al. Effect of radiotherapy after breast-conserving surgery on 10-year recurrence and 15-year breast cancer death: meta-analysis of individual patient data for 10,801 women in 17 randomised trials. *Lancet.* 2011;378(9804):1707–1716.
44. Darby SC, Ewertz M, McGale P, et al. Risk of ischemic heart disease in women after radiotherapy for breast cancer. *N Engl J Med.* 2013;368(11):987–998.
45. Bradley JD, Paulus R, Komaki R, et al. Standard-dose versus high-dose conformal radiotherapy with concurrent and consolidation carboplatin plus paclitaxel with or without cetuximab for patients with stage IIIA or IIIB non-small-cell lung cancer (RTOG 0617): a randomised, two-by-two factorial phase 3 study. *Lancet Oncol.* 2015;16(2):187–199.
46. Atkins KM, Rawal B, Chaunzwa TL, et al. Cardiac radiation dose, cardiac disease, and mortality in patients with lung cancer. *J Am Coll Cardiol.* 2019;73(23):2976–2987.

Stem Cell Transplantation

47. Armenian SH, Ryan TD, Khouri MG. Cardiac dysfunction and heart failure in hematopoietic cell transplantation survivors: emerging paradigms in pathophysiology, screening, and prevention. *Heart Fail Clin.* 2017;13(2):337–345.

Future Directions

48. Minasian LM, Dimond E, Davis M, et al. The evolving design of NIH-funded cardio-oncology studies to address cancer treatment-related cardiovascular toxicity. *JACC (J Am Coll Cardiol): CardioOncol.* 2019;1(1):105–113.

57 Cardio-Oncology: Approach to the Patient

JOERG HERRMANN

Never in history have there been more cancer survivors than presently, and thus, never have the chances been greater for a cardiologist to treat a patient with a cancer diagnosis. The latter conclusion holds true even more so in view of the general aging of the population and the fact that aging is a risk factor for both cancer and cardiovascular diseases (CVD).[1,2] The same applies to obesity, and a sedentary lifestyle and smoking add to the list of factors that increase the risk not only for CVD but also cancer. Thus, the cancer patient of today often presents with cardiovascular (CV) risk factors and diseases that require optimal management, in particular as they can complicate cancer care. Furthermore, cancer therapy can cause CVD, as outlined in **Chapter 56**, with significant implications for morbidity and mortality. Indeed, cancer patients with CVD, either present before or developing during cancer therapy, have worse overall survival, emphasizing the call for the optimal management of both.[3] This call extends to all cardiologists, who need to have a basic understanding of how to approach CVD in the cancer patient, as well as those who specialize in this area that has become known as cardio-oncology.

One intuitive and practical approach to the cancer patient with CVD can be summarized under the acronym SCI-FI (CV **S**ubject, Oncology **C**ontext, Cardio-Oncology **I**nteraction, and **F**ollow-up on **I**ntervention, Fig. 57.1). It begins with the CV issue in question, then takes the oncology/hematology context into consideration, and finally integrates these entities. The three CVD groups to be attentive to in particular are cardiomyopathy/heart failure (HF), vascular disease, and arrhythmias. These compose most of the referrals and can lead to fatal outcomes if not recognized and managed appropriately. Last but not least, the specific management aspects of these CVD vary by stage of presentation in the continuum of cancer care: before, during, or after cancer therapy (Fig. 57.2). This chapter will follow this framework.

APPROACH TO THE CANCER PATIENT AT RISK OF OR WITH CARDIOVASCULAR DISEASES BEFORE CANCER THERAPY

Patients who were diagnosed with cancer and are about to undergo oncological or hematological treatment are referred for a cardiology consultation most commonly out of concern that the presence or risk of CVD could pose a threat to the completion of cancer therapy and the patient. A comprehensive understanding of CVD, as well as cancer, its treatment, and how it affects the CV system is needed to address such referrals. A conceptual model that provides a useful foundation and can almost universally be applied is the multiple-hit model (Fig.

57.3).[4] The key concept is that injuries from cancer therapies add to any pre-existing impairment of CV function decreasing the CV reserve to the point of its exhaustion and eventually the clinical appearance of disease states. Very pertinent questions for any patient who is to undergo cancer therapy with concerns for CVD are: how much of the CV reserve is left, what is the margin for toxicities, and what is to be expected? Aligned with this basic concept, applicable consensus documents and guidelines are in general agreement that all cancer patients who are about to start any (potentially) cardiotoxic therapy should have a baseline assessment of cardiac function, with echocardiography as the preferred imaging modality, an assessment of any potential CVD and CV risk factors, and optimal control of any of the CV abnormalities identified.[5]

Cardiomyopathy/Heart Failure Considerations

Cardiotoxicity has historically received the greatest interest and over the years has been defined by many different criteria (see also Chapter 56). Moreso, two subtypes had been proposed on the basis of the cardiotoxicity reversibility pattern (irreversible cardiac injury, or type 1, and reversible cardiac dysfunction, or type 2), and the 2014 American Society of Echocardiography (ASE)/European Association of Cardiovascular Imaging (EACI) consensus document assigned all (potentially) cardiotoxic medication to one of these two groups.[5] This model even set the tone for pre-, on-, and posttreatment evaluations. However, recent data have challenged this concept and indicate that breast cancer patients who experienced trastuzumab cardiotoxicity have an impaired CV function even years later.[6] Furthermore, improvement in cardiac function may be seen even in patients with anthracycline cardiotoxicity.[7,8] Alternative classification systems have been proposed, and in the general approach to cancer patients at risk of cardiac dysfunction it might be useful to consider the mechanisms that can account for the decrease in cardiac function: (1) directly harmful effects on the myocardium, (2) indirectly harmful effects on the myocardium, for example, via progression of coronary artery disease (CAD), ischemia, metabolic derangement, and (3) mediated by inflammation (Table 57.1).[9] Such an approach directs to optimal treatment strategies, for example, neurohormonal blockade in case of cardiomyopathy versus improvement in coronary blood flow in case of CAD or coronary vasospasm versus antiinflammatory in case of myocarditis. For preventive efforts and screening recommendations for cardiomyopathy see supplementary text online.

Radiation-induced heart disease involves every structure of the heart and can lead to restrictive cardiomyopathy, constrictive pericarditis, valvular heart disease, and conduction and autonomic function

General Cardio-Oncology Approach (SCI-FI)

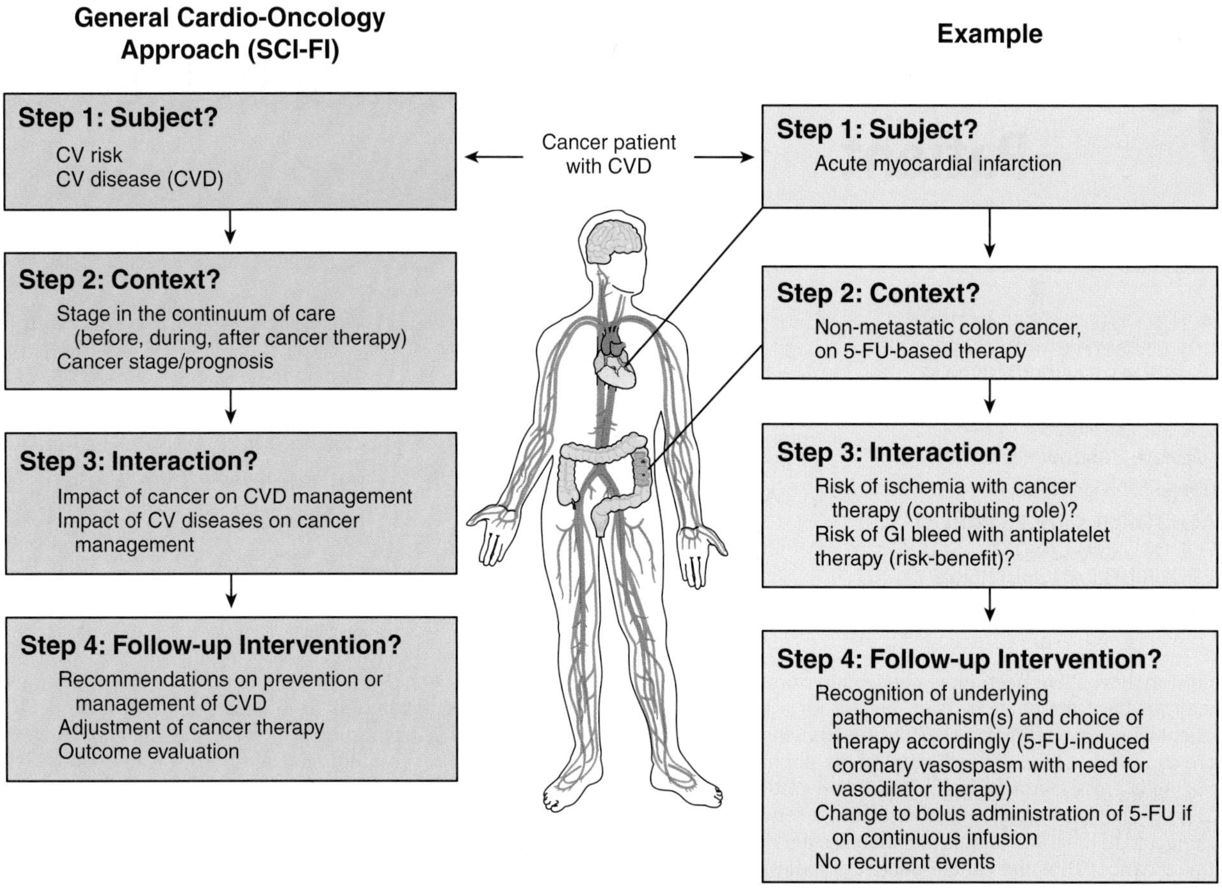

Step 1: Subject?

CV risk
CV disease (CVD)

↓

Step 2: Context?

Stage in the continuum of care
(before, during, after cancer therapy)
Cancer stage/prognosis

↓

Step 3: Interaction?

Impact of cancer on CVD management
Impact of CV diseases on cancer
management

↓

Step 4: Follow-up Intervention?

Recommendations on prevention or
management of CVD
Adjustment of cancer therapy
Outcome evaluation

← Cancer patient with CVD →

Example

Step 1: Subject?

Acute myocardial infarction

↓

Step 2: Context?

Non-metastatic colon cancer,
on 5-FU-based therapy

↓

Step 3: Interaction?

Risk of ischemia with cancer
therapy (contributing role)?
Risk of GI bleed with antiplatelet
therapy (risk-benefit)?

↓

Step 4: Follow-up Intervention?

Recognition of underlying
pathomechanism(s) and choice of
therapy accordingly (5-FU-induced
coronary vasospasm with need for
vasodilator therapy)
Change to bolus administration of 5-FU if
on continuous infusion
No recurrent events

FIGURE 57.1 Approach to the cancer patient at risk of or with cardiovascular disease (CVD). The basic approach starts with defining the CVD problem in the context of the patient's malignancy and its treatment. This interplay is evaluated further to reach a conclusion on the management of both CVD and the malignancy. Follow-up assessment allows for the adjustment of recommendations and the successful management of the patient. *5-FU,* 5-fluorouracil; *GI,* gastrointestinal.

abnormalities (see also Chapter 56).[10,11] Every patient undergoing chest and/or neck radiation therapy should therefore be carefully counseled. Patients with a history of CAD and myocardial infarction (MI) in particular should be informed about the risks and benefits of undergoing chest radiation therapy. An increased risk of acute coronary events was seen in particular in this subgroup of women who underwent radiation therapy for breast cancer.[12] The risk of these events is not immediate but within the timeline of years. Time to onset of cardiomyopathy is usually beyond 10 years and classically presents as restrictive cardiomyopathy and HF with preserved ejection fraction.[13] Reduction of dose exposure is the best preventive strategy and several techniques are available. Anti-inflammatory and antioxidant therapies including statins and angiotensin converting enzyme (ACE) inhibitors are theoretically attractive but have not been proven beneficial in clinical practice.

Vascular Disease Considerations

In addition to the historically well-known increased risk of venous thromboembolism (VTE), cancer patients can present with typical and atypical chest pain episodes, MI, transient ischemic attack, stroke, claudication, critical limb ischemia, and Raynaud's.[14] Based on pathophysiology, one may propose three main vascular toxicity types: acute thrombosis, acute vasospasm, and accelerated atherosclerosis (Table 57.2).[15]

The risk of venous thrombosis in cancer patients relates not to a single but several factors (patient-, cancer-, and treatment-related). These are captured in risk prediction models such as the most widely used Khorana risk score.[16] Based on data indicating a 60% reduction in VTE and/or VTE-related deaths, practice guidelines of various societies suggest the use of direct oral anticoagulants (DOACs) as primary thromboprophylaxis in ambulatory cancer patients who are about to start chemotherapy and have a Khorana score ≥2, if there are no drug-drug interactions and no high-risk scenario for bleeding.[16]

Low-molecular-weight heparin (LMWH) remains an option for outpatient thromboprophylaxis in high-risk patients. For patients with multiple myeloma receiving "IMiD"-based combination therapy, current guidelines recommend aspirin 81 to 325 mg daily if none or only one individual/myeloma risk factor, otherwise LMWH equivalent to 40 mg enoxaparin daily or full-dose warfarin. In hospitalized patients with major surgery or acute medical illness, thromboprophylaxis with heparin or LMWH is recommended per standard recommendations with consideration for 4 weeks extension in high-risk postoperative patients in the setting of abdominal and pelvic surgery for malignancy.

Regarding arterial thromboembolic events (ATEs), the highest risk period is within 1 month before and after cancer diagnosis, thereafter declining by persisting for at least 12 months.[17,18] Advanced (stage 3 and 4) cancers and those of the gastrointestinal tract and the lung pose the highest malignancy-related risk categories for ATEs, similar to VTE.[18] A therapy-related risk of ATEs is seen in particular with vascular endothelial growth factor (VEGF) inhibitors and platinum drugs.

Acute vasospasm should be anticipated for patients to be started on 5-fluorouracil (5-FU), capecitabine, paclitaxel, cisplatin, bleomycin, VEGF inhibitors such as sorafenib, and Bcr-Abl inhibitors such as dasatinib.[15] Risk factors for 5-FU cardiotoxicity have variably been described but likely a history of cardiac disease (in particular ischemic heart disease [IHD]) and especially MI is relevant. Furthermore, smoking is likely of significance for peripheral vasoconstriction.[19] Accelerated atherosclerosis in cancer patients is most commonly associated with radiation therapy but has received attention with the use of Bcr-Abl inhibitors such as nilotinib and ponatinib in recent years; it may also be seen with VEGF inhibitors and cisplatin.[15] For preventive efforts and screening recommendations for cardiovascular disease see supplementary text online.

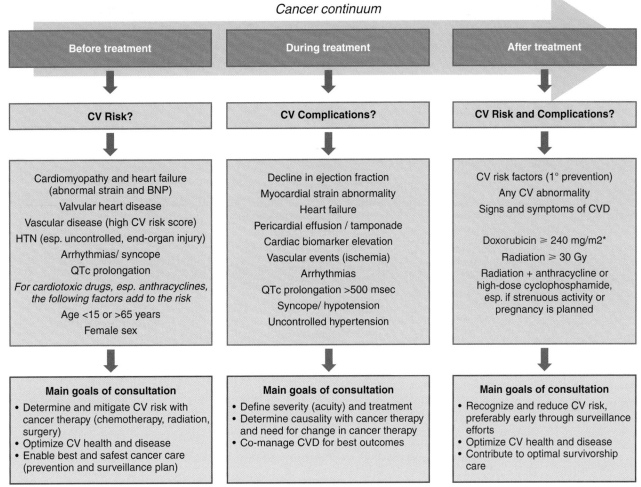

Cancer continuum

| Before treatment | During treatment | After treatment |

CV Risk? / **CV Complications?** / **CV Risk and Complications?**

CV Risk?

Cardiomyopathy and heart failure
(abnormal strain and BNP)

Valvular heart disease

Vascular disease (high CV risk score)

HTN (esp. uncontrolled, end-organ injury)

Arrhythmias/ syncope

QTc prolongation

*For cardiotoxic drugs, esp. anthracyclines,
the following factors add to the risk*

Age <15 or >65 years

Female sex

CV Complications?

Decline in ejection fraction

Myocardial strain abnormality

Heart failure

Pericardial effusion / tamponade

Cardiac biomarker elevation

Vascular events (ischemia)

Arrhythmias

QTc prolongation >500 msec

Syncope/ hypotension

Uncontrolled hypertension

CV Risk and Complications?

CV risk factors (1° prevention)

Any CV abnormality

Signs and symptoms of CVD

Doxorubicin ≥ 240 mg/m2*

Radiation ≥ 30 Gy

Radiation + anthracycline or
high-dose cyclophosphamide,
esp. if strenuous activity or
pregnancy is planned

Main goals of consultation
- Determine and mitigate CV risk with cancer therapy (chemotherapy, radiation, surgery)
- Optimize CV health and disease
- Enable best and safest cancer care (prevention and surveillance plan)

Main goals of consultation
- Define severity (acuity) and treatment
- Determine causality with cancer therapy and need for change in cancer therapy
- Co-manage CVD for best outcomes

Main goals of consultation
- Recognize and reduce CV risk, preferably early through surveillance efforts
- Optimize CV health and disease
- Contribute to optimal survivorship care

FIGURE 57.2 Cardiovascular disease management aspects across the cancer continuum. The needs of cancer patients vary based on their stand relative to treatment and so do the goals of the cardio-oncology consultation. Orienting oneself to this grid serves well in a practice that aims to cover the vast scope of cardiology and oncology/hematology.

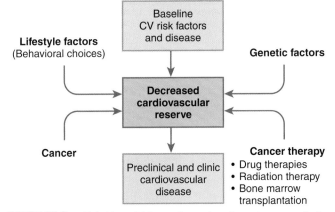

FIGURE 57.3 Multiple-hit model for cardio-oncology. In most cancer patients a number of factors (or "hits") lead to the clinical emergence of cardiovascular disease (CVD). Many patients already have cardiovascular risk factors or (subclinical) CVD that lower the reserve to tolerate additional stressors such as cancer and cancer therapy. Lifestyle factors and genetics further influence the equation.

Arrhythmia Considerations

Patients with cancer who have electrocardiogram (ECG) abnormalities, impaired exercise capacity, or CVD at baseline should be assumed to be more susceptible to cancer therapy-induced arrhythmias, as are those undergoing treatment regimens with known cardiotoxicity potential. Therefore, as a general rule, comorbidities that could represent a possible arrhythmogenic substrate should be identified and treated aggressively before and during cancer therapy. Early identification and appropriate management of cardiac ischemia, dysfunction, and remodeling is also likely to be the best strategy to modulate the arrhythmogenic substrate and improve outcomes in patients with cancer therapy-induced arrhythmias. These recommendations hold true for QTc prolongation and related ventricular arrhythmias.[9]

Crizotinib, dasatinib, lapatinib, nilotinib, pazopanib, sorafenib, sunitinib, vandetanib, and vemurafenib should be administered with caution in patients with pre-existing QTc prolongation or QTc-prolongation-related risk factors. As illustrated for several tyrosine kinase inhibitors (TKIs), such as vandetanib, electrolytes should be corrected before initiation of cancer therapy (goal value for serum K+ levels ≥4 mEq/L and for magnesium and calcium within normal limits) and monitored along with ECGs, as outlined above (at baseline, at 2 to 4 weeks, at 8 to 12 weeks, and every 3 months thereafter). The common cutoffs for the QTc interval are 450 msec before and 500 msec during therapy (the one exception being nilotinib 480 msec). Full-dose therapy can be given if the QTc is less than 450 msec, half-dose if between 450 and upper limit, no dose if above the upper limit.[9]

The other common reason for referral is atrial fibrillation (AF), more commonly pre-existing though some cancer populations and therapeutics have been recognized as being more predisposed. The impact in terms of morbidity and mortality is the same and the approach to these patients should be the same as in the general population.[9] For additional discussion on the management of AF see supplemental text online.

TABLE 57.1 Overview of the Three Principal Presentations of Cardiotoxicity with Cancer Therapy

	CATEGORIES OF CANCER THERAPY-RELATED CARDIOTOXICITIES		
	Direct Impairing Effect on the Myocardium	Indirect Impairing Effect on the Myocardium	Impairing Effect Owing to Myocarditis
Risk with Cancer Therapy			
Doxorubicin	+	+	+ (toxic or reactive)
Cyclophosphamide	+	+	+ (toxic or reactive)
5-Fluorouracil	+	+	NR
HER2 inhibitors	+	Inconclusive findings	NR
VEGF inhibitors	+ (TKIs)	+	NR
Immune checkpoint inhibitors	Inconclusive findings	+	+ (immune-mediated)
Radiation therapy	+ (at high dose)	+	+ (toxic or reactive)
Diagnosis			
Imaging	• Echocardiogram • Cardiac MRI • MUGA scan	• (Stress) echocardiogram • (Stress) cardiac MRI • Stress Sestamibi–PET • CT coronary angiogram • Vasoreactivity studies	• Cardiac MRI • PET • Echocardiogram
Biomarkers	• Cardiac troponins • Natriuretic peptides (especially chronically)	• Thyroid function studies • Cytokines • Catecholamines	• Cardiac troponins • Natriuretic peptides
Management			
Treatment	• Stop cancer therapy • Beta-blocker (carvedilol and nebivolol) • ACE inhibitor • ARB • Spironolactone	• Stop cancer therapy • Therapy directed to the underlying cause (e.g., correction of myocardial ischemia or valve disease)	• Stop cancer therapy • For ICI: anti-inflammatory or immunosuppressive therapy, supportive care (e.g., ECMO)
Prevention	• Screening for comorbidities • For anthracyclines: cardiovascular medications (as above) • Exercise	• Screening for predisposing conditions • For radiation therapy: dose reduction, for example by shielding, positioning or proton beam • Dose and type of administration of cancer therapeutics	• Screening for comorbidities (efficacy not proven) • Early detection with biomarkers and/or ECG changes (heart blocks, ventricular arrhythmias including ectopy and tachycardia, atrial fibrillation)

ACE, Angiotensin converting enzyme; *ARB*, angiotensin receptor blocker; *CT*, computed tomography; *ECMO*, extracorporeal membrane oxygenation; *ICI*, immune checkpoint inhibitor; *MRI*, magnetic resonance imaging; *MUGA*, multigated acquisition scan; *NR*, not reported; *PET*, positron emission tomography; *TKI*, tyrosine kinase inhibitors; *VEGF*, vascular endothelial growth factor.
From Herrmann J. Adverse cardiac effects of cancer therapies: cardiotoxicity and arrhythmia. *Nat Rev Cardiol*. 2020;17:474–502.

TABLE 57.2 Overview of the Three Principal Presentations of Arterial Vascular Toxicity with Cancer Therapy

PRESENTATION	ACUTE VASOSPASM	ACUTE THROMBOSIS	ACCELERATED ATHEROSCLEROSIS
Onset after cancer therapy	Days to weeks	Weeks to months	Months to years
Reversibility	Very likely	Likely	Very unlikely
Examples of cancer therapeutics	5-fluorouracil, capecitabine, platinum drugs, VEGF inhibitors	Platinum drugs, bleomycin, vinca alkaloids, VEGF inhibitors, ICIs	Nilotinib, ponatinib, cisplatin, VEGF inhibitors
Treatment	Nitrates, calcium-channel blocker (CCB)	Thrombectomy with/without PTCA, stent, DAPT, statin therapy	Revascularization, aspirin, statin, amlodipine, ACE-inhibitor, exercise
On-therapy screening	Signs and symptoms	Signs and symptoms	Signs and symptoms
Prevention	Vasoreactivity studies, ECG (ST-segment elevation monitoring	vWF levels, circulating endothelial cell and/or endothelial progenitor cell levels	Ankle–brachial index, cardiac stress test, coronary CT angiography

ACE, angiotensin-converting enzyme; *ASCDV*, atherosclerotic cardiovascular disease; *CCB*, calcium channel blockers; *CT*, computed tomography; *CVD*, cardiovascular disease; *DAPT*, dual antiplatelet therapy; *ECG*, electrocardiogram; *ICI*, immune checkpoint inhibitor; *PTCA*, percutaneous transluminal coronary angioplasty; *VEGF*, vascular endothelial growth factor; *vWF*, von Willebrand factor.
From Herrmann J. Vascular toxic effects of cancer therapies. *Nat Rev Cardiol*. 2020;17:503–522.

APPROACH TO THE CANCER PATIENT AT RISK OF OR WITH CARDIOVASCULAR DISEASES DURING CANCER THERAPY

Patients are referred for a cardiology evaluation during active cancer treatment most commonly to seek guidance on how a noted CVD issue could be managed, its causal relationship with cancer therapy, and its overall impact on the patient's cancer treatment plan. Such management decisions and judgment calls are among the most challenging given the unique characteristics and comorbidities of patients with active cancer, demanding a broader knowledge and experience with their trajectory. Standard practice guidelines written for the general population may need to be modified, although for the most part these should be followed and translate into better clinical outcomes. Pertinent societal recommendations and considerations for cancer patients with CVD presentations are covered elsewhere.[9,15] The 2020 European Society of Medicine Oncology (ESMO) recommendations for management of cardiac disease in cancer patients are outlined in **eTable 57.1**.[20]

Cardiomyopathy/Heart Failure Management

Cardiotoxicity is commonly used as an umbrella term for any cardiac abnormality encountered with cancer therapy. The first step is therefore to define the abnormality, its causes, and implications. Of the advocated cardiac surveillance parameters, left ventricular ejection fraction (LVEF) is most commonly reported and reacted to. That being said, various consensus documents have forwarded different definitions of cardiotoxicity,

and the consensus definition that emerges is a drop of greater than 10% to below the lower limit of normal, which is set at 53% in the ASE/EACI consensus and at 50% in the ESMO consensus.[5,20] The cutoff to stop cancer therapy is not universally defined but most would agree with an LVEF of 40% as originally outlined for trastuzumab therapy for cessation of therapy and as outlined in the most recent ESMO document.[20] Cancer therapy of any type is to be discontinued in any patient who develops HF. These patients as well as those with an EF less than 50% should receive neurohormonal therapy in accordance with the American Heart Association (AHA)/American College of Cardiology (ACC) HF guidelines (Chapter 50).[21] For global longitudinal strain (GLS), a 15% relative change (confirmed within 2 to 3 weeks upon repeat assessment) is considered to represent subclinical left ventricular dysfunction and is predictive of a more evident future decline in LVEF. At present, however, there is no clear guidance how to react to such changes.[5] The same holds true for cTn elevations, though it has been used as a trigger to start ACE inhibitor therapy. For both parameters, the main merit is in the high negative predictive value.

As outlined above, it is important not to default to the assumption that a decline in cardiac function is always due to the cancer therapy, and even when it is, that is always due to a direct (toxic) effect on the cardiomyocytes. Some cancer therapeutics affect the vasculature more so than the myocardium and a decline in cardiac function is seen because of a reduction in blood supply. This would be even more so in the case in patients with CAD and other CVD conditions. The pre-therapy evaluation therefore serves a very important role as does an evaluation for any additional contributing factor during therapy should complications arise. Very important in view of the increasing use and the potential fatal implications is the recognition of ICI myocarditis (Fig. 57.4). For further

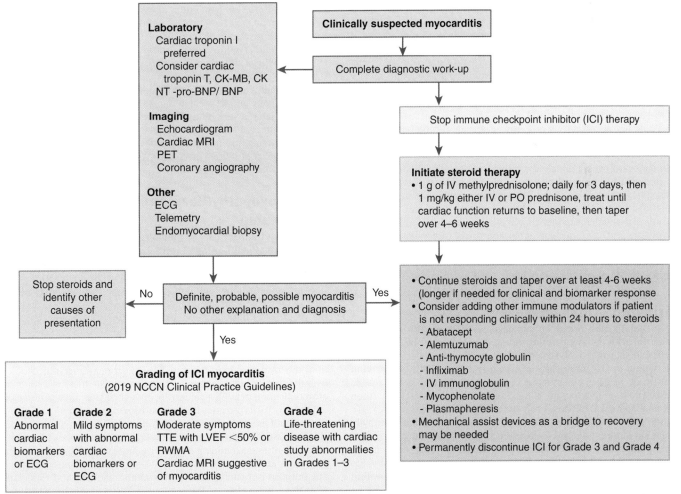

FIGURE 57.4 Outline of the approach to immune checkpoint inhibitor (ICI) myocarditis. Some patients on ICI therapy may undergo routine, serial (e.g., every 4 weeks) testing with biomarkers (cardiac troponin and natriuretic peptides) and electrocardiograms (ECG), while others present with symptoms that raise concerns for myocarditis. The work-up includes cardiac imaging studies, coronary angiography, and endomyocardial biopsy as prompted clinically. ICI therapy is to be stopped and steroids are to be started already at this stage. Once a diagnosis of myocarditis is substantiated, steroids are continued with additional immunosuppressive therapies as needed. Depending on the grade/severity of myocarditis, ICI is not to be resumed. *CK,* creatine kinase; *BNP,* brain natriuretic peptide; *ECG,* electrocardiogram; *LVEF,* left ventricular ejection fraction; *MRI,* magnetic resonance imaging; *PET,* positron emission tomography; *TTE,* transthoracic echocardiogram; *RWMA,* regional wall motion abnormalities.

discussion on cardiomyopathy management see the supplemental text online.

Vascular Disease Management

Management of VTE in cancer patients is challenging because of their predisposition to both thrombosis and bleeding. Recurrence of VTE despite anticoagulation (so-called anticoagulation failure) is seen in 15% of patients on warfarin (rate of 2.5% per month).[22] LMWH has superior efficacy in this regard at similar major bleeding rates than warfarin. Compared with LMWH, DOACs have similar (edoxaban) or improved (rivaroxaban, apixaban) efficacy rates but higher bleeding rates, especially gastrointestinal (GI) bleeding rates.[23] Patients with mucosal tumors (GI/GU malignancy) should receive anticoagulation other than with DOACs. Treatment should continue for as long as the cancer disease process is deemed active, and at a minimum for 3 to 6 months.

As outlined above, cancer patients are also at risk of ATEs,[17] and presentations range from unstable angina to MI with and without arrhythmias (polymorphic ventricular tachycardia [VT] or heart block) in the coronary circulation, from transient ischemic attack to stroke in the carotid/cerebral circulation, and bowel ischemia, acute renal failure, and critical limb ischemia in the peripheral circulation. Treatment is in agreement with current practice guidelines and is outlined in Chapters 43 and 45. Antiplatelet therapy is a key element and based on current ACC/AHA guidelines, dual antiplatelet therapy (DAPT) should be continued for 1 year in patients with ACS, thereafter guided by risk calculators such as the DAPT score (see also Chapters 37 and 40).[24] These, however, do not take malignancy into consideration. Similar to VTE recommendations, one might argue for the continuation of DAPT as long as active cancer is present; however, there are no data for such a recommendation yet. Moreover, all of these interventions need to be balanced with the bleeding risk. In this context thrombocytopenia is an important factor to consider and the Society for Cardiovascular Angiography and Interventions (SCAI) recommendations for platelet cutoffs are as following: for surgical interventions platelet counts greater than 50K are recommended, for percutaneous coronary intervention (PCI) with DAPT platelet counts greater than 30K, and for angiography platelet counts greater than 10K.[25]

While acute coronary vasospasm, especially if profound and prolonged, can lead to MI, VT/ventricular fibrillation to the point of sudden cardiac death (SCD), and cardiac dysfunction, even Takotsubo's, HF, and cardiogenic shock, the typical presentation is angina with concomitant ST-segment elevation on ECG, resolving promptly with vasodilator therapy. In case of 5-FU, the presentation can be so typical that treatment with vasodilator therapy is both diagnostic and therapeutic. For patients experiencing acute vasospasm, vasodilators such as nitrates and calcium channel blockers (CCBs) are mainstay therapy and have been used even in combination. For further discussion on management of acute vasospasm as well as accelerated atherosclerosis see the supplemental text online.

Arrhythmia Management

QTc prolongation noted on surveillance ECGs should prompt the adjustment of therapy. For most drugs, therapy should be held if the QTc interval exceeds 500 msec and resumed at a reduced dose upon resolution of QTc prolongation. With nilotinib, any QTc greater than 480 msec requires cessation of therapy until the QTc is 450 to 480 msec (then resume therapy at half dose) or less than 450 msec (then resume therapy at full dose). Any grade 4 (that is, life-threatening) QTc event also precludes any further cancer therapy. Ventricular arrhythmias should be managed as usual according to clinical guidelines.[26] Important to address in cancer patients on multiple other medications are drug-drug interactions and electrolyte abnormalities (goal value for serum K^+ levels ≥ 4 mEq/L and for calcium and magnesium within normal limits).

The principles and goals of the management of AF in patients with cancer are generally the same as those in the general population, albeit with some important nuances. The first is a more lenient heart rate goal (<115 beats/min [bpm]) with the use of beta-blockers, CCBs, and digoxin. The second is the potential for drug-drug interactions, especially with antiarrhythmic drugs, which are indicated if patients remain symptomatic. An illustrating example is ibrutinib as outlined in the extended online content.

Anticoagulation in patients with cancer can be problematic in general and especially in patients receiving ibrutinib because of a predisposition to bleeding.[27] Ibrutinib has a unique antiplatelet effect, inhibiting mainly von Willebrand factor (vWF) and collagen-mediated platelet activation (in addition to fibrinogen-activated platelet activation).[28] Importantly, these activation pathways are distinct from those inhibited by aspirin (cyclooxygenase) and thienopyridines adenosine diphosphate ((ADP) receptor), and combination therapy would lead to a profoundly additive effect and bleeding risk; therefore, this strategy is not recommended. Anticoagulation strategies in cancer patients are outlined above. For further discussion on management of arrhythmias see the supplemental text online.

APPROACH TO THE CANCER PATIENT AT RISK OF OR WITH CARDIOVASCULAR DISEASES AFTER CANCER THERAPY

Patients who have completed their cancer therapy and are cured of their disease (survivors) remain at risk of secondary malignancies as well as long-term consequences and complications of their malignancy and its treatment. These patients are referred to see a cardiologist to discuss long-term risk and preventive strategies. Often though, cardiologists may encounter these patients presenting with CVD, which can be due to (a) the continuum of vascular disease that was present even before the cancer treatment, and/or (b) the new development of vascular disease during or after completion of cancer therapy. Whereas the first scenario requires follow-up and treatment in keeping with published guidelines, the second scenario has to take into account the uniqueness of the cancer therapy the patient has received. Some cancer therapeutics affect the CV system only for the time of therapy, and especially if any impact is ruled out at the time, any newly developing CVD years later is very difficult to causally link to it. The situation is different with cancer therapies that have a prolonged effect and late onset. Cultivating an understanding of the most likely clinical course and potential contributing mechanisms is again the most recommendable approach.

Cardiomyopathy/Heart Failure in Cancer Survivorship

The profound impact cancer therapies can have on the CV system has been very well illustrated in cardiopulmonary exercise studies outlining a drop in peak VO_2 (**eFig. 57.1**).[29] A sharp decline in exercise capacity is seen after cancer therapy, which, however, may not become evident at the time. It may, and likely will with additional risk factors, progress to the symptomatic stage. This matches conceptually the progression through the AHA HF stages. Patients after exposure to cardiotoxic therapy are considered to be in Stage A HF just like patients with hypertension, diabetes, and other well-known risk predisposition. How to best follow these patients and when to act and in which format is not well defined. Serial echocardiographic studies over the first 3 years after cancer therapy indicate that the main negative deflection in LVEF is occurring in the first year after start of cancer therapy.[30] This provides the rationale for current American Society of Clinical Oncology (ASCO) and National Comprehensive Cancer Network (NCCN) follow-up recommendations (see below). However, several studies do outline a cumulative increase in HF presentations over time and not only in patients after anthracycline-based therapy, but also in patients after trastuzumab treatment and especially after the combination of these agents.[31,32] Reportedly, breast cancer patients who underwent chemotherapy also have an increased risk of late (10+ years) CV mortality. The sequence and causal link of reduction of cardiac function, HF, and mortality in these patients is yet to be proven though, as is the mantra of early detection and intervention.[33] Following radiation therapy, an increase in HF rates is seen after 15 years in breast cancer patients and an exponential increase in CV events follow the same timeline in lymphoma patients after chest radiation.[34] The effects of anthracycline exposure and radiation therapy are additive. While anthracycline therapy in adults leads to a dilative cardiomyopathy and HF with reduced LVEF, radiation therapy classically leads to a restrictive cardiomyopathy and HF with preserved LVEF. As HF can be the final common pathway of the various elements in the spectrum of radiation-induced heart disease, all contributing factors need to be evaluated, including ischemic and structural heart disease. Otherwise, treatment recommendations follow the ACC/AHA HF guidelines for the various stages of HF. Exercise is to be encouraged and cardio-oncology rehabilitation programs have emerged.[35] For further discussion on cardiomyopathy/HF in cancer survivorship see the supplemental text online.

Vascular Disease in Cancer Survivorship

Cancer patients have a sixfold higher risk of VTE recurrence with an annual rate as high as 30% in the absence of anticoagulation and as high as 20% even within the initial 6 months on anticoagulation therapy. The rate of VTE recurrence differs significantly by cancer type, stage of disease, and progression over time; specific risk factors include brain, lung, pancreatic, or ovarian cancer; myeloproliferative or myelodysplastic disorders; stage IV cancer; cancer stage progression; or leg paresis.[22] The original and modified Ottawa prediction scores were developed to risk stratify for recurrent VTE; among the variables included in the score, female gender and lung cancer increase the risk, whereas breast cancer and stage I (/II) decrease the risk.[36] If outlined risk factors are present, it is likely best to continue anticoagulation (premature discontinuation of anticoagulation should be avoided). Importantly, the risk for VTE remains increased in cancer survivors, especially in childhood cancer survivors who face a 25-fold higher risk than their non-diseased siblings.[37,38]

> In terms of VTE, most cancer therapies do not pose a long-term risk though exceptions need to be recognized. The first is cisplatin, and its circulating levels can remain detectable for decades after completion of cancer therapy. The second is Bcr-Abl TKIs, especially nilotinib and ponatinib, though ischemic events may not relate to thrombosis (alone); the same holds true for radiation therapy.[12] Proactive screening for thrombosis is usually not done; the evaluation is driven by signs and symptoms. In these patients it remains important to consider embolic thrombotic events (VTE with patent foramen ovale, marantic endocarditis, AF, atrial or ventricular thrombus) as well as plaque rupture or erosion with subsequent in situ thrombosis. Treatment is directed toward the underlying etiology and per guidelines with options including anticoagulation, fibrinolysis, antiplatelet therapy, and revascularization.[39,40] Preventive efforts are mainly secondary prevention efforts and are directed toward improving endothelial health and reducing the risk of thrombus formation. For the long-term (>1 year past event) use of DAPT, the presumed anti-ischemic benefit must be weighed against the bleeding risk. Calculators to estimate these risks are available but need to be validated in cancer patients and the long-term dynamics of thrombotic risk in these patients remain to be defined.[24,41]

For many years after completion of therapy, cancer patients can experience an altered vasoreactivity profile, which can present as typical and atypical angina, microvascular angina, cardiac syndrome X, and Raynaud's. CCBs are usually first-line therapy for patients with Raynaud's, especially slow-release/long-acting dihydropyridine CCB such as nifedipine XL. They may also be more effective than nitrates in cases of microcirculatory involvement (microvascular angina).

Accelerated atherosclerosis is the leading entity in terms of vascular risk after completion of cancer therapy. The risk is particularly high in patients who received Bcr-Abl inhibitors or radiation therapy, and also after allogenic bone marrow transplantation. These patients may benefit from preemptive screening of vascular territories most likely to be involved, including ankle-brachial index (ABI), carotid ultrasound and noninvasive coronary imaging, and stress tests. Following chest radiation therapy, consensus guidelines recommend a cardiac stress test every 5 years in patients with defined high-risk features. As the increase in risk with the combination of radiation therapy and CV risk factors is profound, regular screening for these is recommended.[11] For patients who present with accelerated atherosclerosis (progressive arterial occlusive disease), treatment is in keeping with societal guidelines. For further discussion on vascular disease in cancer survivorship see the supplemental text online.

Arrhythmias in Cancer Survivorship

Arrhythmias in cancer survivors are most commonly expected after radiation therapy to the chest and therapies that exerted a lasting negative effect on cardiac function. This includes patients who sustained a MI as a consequence of cancer therapy with subsequent scar formation. Patients after anthracycline therapy may have such poor heart function that they are at risk of malignant arrhythmias and SCD. Indeed, current literature is supportive of the fact that among patients with a LVEF less than 35% and meeting qualifications for an ICD/cardiac resynchronization therapy-defibrillator (CRT-D) the risk of VT and ventricular fibrillation and the benefit from device therapy is the same for anthracycline and dilated/ischemic cardiomyopathy. Device therapy should therefore not be withheld for cancer survivors. AF can be seen in those with cardiomyopathy or valvular heart disease, especially after radiation therapy. Management follows standard guidelines. Heart block can be seen after radiation therapy. Sinus tachycardia is by far the most common rhythm abnormality in cancer patients, even as a reflection of autonomic dysfunction, after radiation as well as after anthracycline therapy.

CARDIO-ONCOLOGY CARE TEAM AND CLINICS

Cardio-oncology allows for further specialization and dedicated care of cancer patients with CVD. A multidisciplinary team is at the core of the cardio-oncology clinic and expands to a larger network that includes general practitioners and other subspecialties as patients are undergoing long-term comprehensive care (Fig. 57.5). Three milestones can be distinguished toward establishing a cardio-onco-hematology clinic (vision, institutional support and organization, and implementation and operation). The structure and scope of the cardio-onco-hematology clinic needs to be individualized for the specific practice environment it is to successfully operate in and will require reevaluation and re-adjustment based on outcome measures and developments in the field.[42] The overreaching goal of the clinic and the outlined approach in this chapter is to enable cancer patients to receive the best possible cancer therapy at the lowest possible CV risk.

FUTURE PERSPECTIVES

It is the expectation that in the years to come the demands for cardio-oncology will grow and with it the need for education (including core knowledge and competencies), best practice recommendations (including practice guidelines and quality metrics), and research (providing the much-needed evidence base). These currently ongoing developments will refine the approach to the cancer patient at risk of or with evident CVD or CV toxicity. In addition, emerging trends will shape the cardio-oncology practice including ongoing advances in cancer therapies, artificial intelligence innovations, and changing health care environments such as those imposed by viral pandemics.

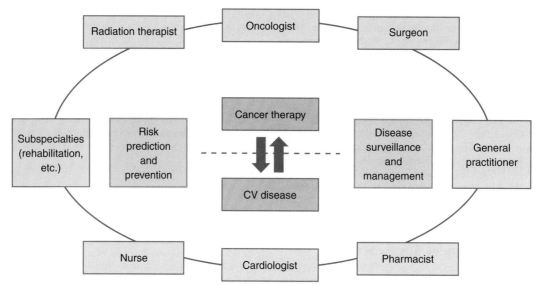

FIGURE 57.5 The cardio-oncology network. The cardio-oncology approach is multidisciplinary in nature. It requires the expertise and interaction of multiple providers to most optimally follow and treat the cancer patient through their continuum of care.

REFERENCES

Approach to the Cancer Patient at Risk of or with Cardiovascular Diseases Before Cancer Therapy

1. Herrmann J. Adverse cardiac effects of cancer therapies: cardiotoxicity and arrhythmia. *Nat Rev Cardiol.* 2020;17(8):474–502.
2. Herrmann J. Vascular toxic effects of cancer therapies. *Nat Rev Cardiol.* 2020;17(8):503–522.
3. Youn JC, et al. Cardiovascular disease burden in adult patients with cancer: an 11-year nation-wide population-based cohort study. *Int J Cardiol.* 2020;317:167–173.
4. Jones LW, et al. Early breast cancer therapy and cardiovascular injury. *J Am Coll Cardiol.* 2007;50(15):1435–1441.
5. Plana JC, et al. Expert consensus for multimodality imaging evaluation of adult patients during and after cancer therapy: a report from the American Society of Echocardiography and the European Association of Cardiovascular Imaging. *J Am Soc Echocardiogr.* 2014;27(9):911–939.
6. Yu AF, et al. Long-term cardiopulmonary consequences of treatment-induced cardiotoxicity in survivors of ERBB2-positive breast cancer. *JAMA Cardiol.* 2020.
7. Cardinale D, et al. Early detection of anthracycline cardiotoxicity and improvement with heart failure therapy. *Circulation.* 2015;131(22):1981–1988.
8. Mazur M, et al. Burden of cardiac arrhythmias in patients with anthracycline-related cardiomyopathy. *JACC Clin Electrophysiol.* 2017;3(2):139–150.
9. Herrmann J. Adverse cardiac effects of cancer therapies: cardiotoxicity and arrhythmia. *Nat Rev Cardiol.* 2020.
10. Lancellotti P, et al. Expert consensus for multi-modality imaging evaluation of cardiovascular complications of radiotherapy in adults: a report from the European Association of Cardiovascular Imaging and the American Society of Echocardiography. *J Am Soc Echocardiogr.* 2013;26(9):1013–1032.
11. Iliescu C, et al. SCAI expert consensus statement: evaluation, management, and special considerations of cardio-oncology patients in the cardiac catheterization laboratory (Endorsed by the Cardiological Society of India, and Sociedad Latino Americana De Cardiologia Intervencionista). *Catheter Cardiovasc Interv.* 2016;87(5):895–899.
12. Darby SC, et al. Risk of ischemic heart disease in women after radiotherapy for breast cancer. *N Engl J Med.* 2013;368(11):987–998.
13. Saiki H, et al. Risk of heart failure with preserved ejection fraction in older women after contemporary radiotherapy for breast cancer. *Circulation.* 2017;135(15):1388–1396.
14. Herrmann J, et al. Vascular toxicities of cancer therapies: the old and the new—an evolving avenue. *Circulation.* 2016;133(13):1272–1289.
15. Herrmann J. Vascular toxic effects of cancer therapies. *Nat Rev Cardiol.* 2020.
16. Key NS, et al. Venous thromboembolism prophylaxis and treatment in patients with cancer: ASCO clinical practice guideline update. *J Clin Oncol.* 2020;38(5):496–520.
17. Oren O, Herrmann J. Arterial events in cancer patients-the case of acute coronary thrombosis. *J Thorac Dis.* 2018;10(suppl 35):S4367–S4385.
18. Navi BB, et al. Risk of arterial thromboembolism in patients with cancer. *J Am Coll Cardiol.* 2017;70(8):926–938.
19. Wigley FM, Flavahan NA. Raynaud's phenomenon. *N Engl J Med.* 2016;375(6):556–565.

Approach to the Cancer Patient at Risk of or with Cardiovascular Diseases During Cancer Therapy

20. Curigliano G, et al. Management of cardiac disease in cancer patients throughout oncological treatment: ESMO consensus recommendations. *Ann Oncol.* 2020;31(2):171–190.
21. Yancy CW, et al. ACC/AHA/HFSA focused update of the 2013 ACCF/AHA guideline for the management of heart failure: a report of the American College of Cardiology/American Heart Association task force on clinical practice guidelines and the Heart Failure Society of America. *J Am Coll Cardiol.* 2017.
22. Chee CE, et al. Predictors of venous thromboembolism recurrence and bleeding among active cancer patients: a population-based cohort study. *Blood.* 2014;123(25):3972–3978.
23. Li A, et al. Direct oral anticoagulant (DOAC) versus low-molecular-weight heparin (LMWH) for treatment of cancer associated thrombosis (CAT): a systematic review and meta-analysis. *Thromb Res.* 2019;173:158–163.

24. Yeh RW, et al. Development and validation of a prediction rule for benefit and harm of dual antiplatelet therapy beyond 1 year after percutaneous coronary intervention. *J Am Med Assoc.* 2016;315(16):1735–1749.
25. Iliescu CA, et al. SCAI expert consensus statement: evaluation, management, and special considerations of cardio-oncology patients in the cardiac catheterization laboratory (endorsed by the Cardiological Society of India, and Sociedad Latino Americana De Cardiologia Intervencionista). *Catheter Cardiovasc Interv.* 2016;87(5):E202–E223.
26. Al-Khatib SM, et al. AHA/ACC/HRS guideline for management of patients with ventricular arrhythmias and the prevention of sudden cardiac death: a report of the American College of Cardiology/American Heart Association task force on clinical practice guidelines and the Heart Rhythm Society. *J Am Coll Cardiol.* 2018;72(14):e91–e220.
27. Aguilar C. Ibrutinib-related bleeding: pathogenesis, clinical implications and management. *Blood Coagul Fibrinolysis.* 2018;29(6):481–487.
28. Shatzel JJ, et al. Ibrutinib-associated bleeding: pathogenesis, management and risk reduction strategies. *J Thromb Haemost.* 2017;15(5):835–847.

Approach to the Cancer Patient at Risk of or with Cardiovascular Diseases After Cancer Therapy

29. Koelwyn GJ, et al. Running on empty: cardiovascular reserve capacity and late effects of therapy in cancer survivorship. *J Clin Oncol.* 2012;30(36):4458–4461.
30. Narayan HK, et al. Detailed echocardiographic phenotyping in breast cancer patients: associations with ejection fraction decline, recovery, and heart failure symptoms over 3 years of follow-up. *Circulation.* 2017;135(15):1397–1412.
31. Chen J, et al. Incidence of heart failure or cardiomyopathy after adjuvant trastuzumab therapy for breast cancer. *J Am Coll Cardiol.* 2012;60(24):2504–2512.
32. Bowles EJ, et al. Risk of heart failure in breast cancer patients after anthracycline and trastuzumab treatment: a retrospective cohort study. *J Natl Cancer Inst.* 2012;104(17):1293–1305.
33. Bradshaw PT, et al. Cardiovascular disease mortality among breast cancer survivors. *Epidemiology.* 2016;27(1):6–13.
34. Lee CK, Aeppli D, Nierengarten ME. The need for long-term surveillance for patients treated with curative radiotherapy for Hodgkin's disease: University of Minnesota experience. *Int J Radiat Oncol Biol Phys.* 2000;48(1):169–179.
35. Gilchrist SC, et al. Cardio-oncology rehabilitation to manage cardiovascular outcomes in cancer patients and survivors: a scientific statement from the American Heart Association. *Circulation.* 2019;139(21):e997-e1012.
36. Delluc A, et al. Accuracy of the Ottawa score in risk stratification of recurrent venous thromboembolism in patients with cancer-associated venous thromboembolism: a systematic review and meta-analysis. *Haematologica.* 2020;105(5):1436–1442.
37. Madenci AL, et al. Long-term risk of venous thromboembolism in survivors of childhood cancer: a report from the childhood cancer survivor study. *J Clin Oncol.* 2018;JCO2018784595.
38. Faber J, et al. Burden of cardiovascular risk factors and cardiovascular disease in childhood cancer survivors: data from the German CVSS-study. *Eur Heart J.* 2018;39(17):1555–1562.
39. O'Gara PT, et al. ACCF/AHA guideline for the management of ST-elevation myocardial infarction: a report of the American College of Cardiology Foundation/American Heart Association task force on practice guidelines. *J Am Coll Cardiol.* 2013;61(4):e78–e140.
40. Amsterdam EA, et al. AHA/ACC guideline for the management of patients with non-ST-elevation acute coronary syndromes: a report of the American College of Cardiology/American Heart Association task force on practice guidelines. *J Am Coll Cardiol.* 2014;64(24):e139–e228.
41. Costa F, et al. Derivation and validation of the predicting bleeding complications in patients undergoing stent implantation and subsequent dual antiplatelet therapy (PRECISE-DAPT) score: a pooled analysis of individual-patient datasets from clinical trials. *Lancet.* 2017;389(10073):1025–1034.
42. Herrmann J, Loprinzi C, Ruddy K. Building a cardio-onco-hematology program. *Curr Oncol Rep.* 2018;20(10):81.

58 Devices for Monitoring and Managing Heart Failure

JOANN LINDENFELD AND MICHAEL R. ZILE

While implantable cardioverter defibrillators (ICDs) were first approved by the U.S. Food and Drug Administration (FDA) for the secondary prevention of sudden cardiac death (SCD) in 1985, the advent of device-based therapy for the management of heart failure (HF) did not begin until 2001 when the FDA approved cardiac resynchronization therapy (CRT) to reduce the symptoms of moderate to severe HF. In 2003, the Center for Medicaid Services (CMS) issued the first coverage decision for the use of ICDs for the primary prevention of SCD in patients with HF and reduced ejection fraction (HFrEF) post–myocardial infarction (post-MI) followed later by more expansive coverage to include nonischemic HFrEF patients. After a hiatus of nearly two decades, several new therapeutic devices that target central sleep apnea (CSA), secondary mitral regurgitation (SMR), abnormal myocardial contractility, and autonomic imbalance have been approved by the FDA for the treatment of patients with HF. Devices have also been developed to monitor and transmit physiologic data that provide important information about the events preceding HF exacerbations, allowing testing of treatment strategies based on remotely monitored data to avert HF exacerbations, reduce HF hospitalizations (HFHs), and reduce mortality. This chapter reviews the use of CRT, ICDs, and newer approved devices for management of HF and discusses the ability of monitoring devices to provide data to improve symptoms and reduce HF exacerbations. Medical management of HF is discussed in Chapters 48 to 51.

VENTRICULAR DYSSYNCHRONY: THE TARGET OF CARDIAC RESYNCHRONIZATION THERAPY

Intraventricular conduction abnormalities are common in patients with chronic HF and are associated with increased morbidity and mortality.[1] Conduction delay resulting in a QRS duration greater than 120 msec on the surface electrocardiogram has been termed electrical dyssynchrony. The difference in the timing of mechanical contraction or relaxation between different segments of the left ventricle that results from electrical dyssynchrony has been termed mechanical dyssynchrony and can result in suboptimal ventricular filling, a reduction in left ventricular (LV) contractility, greater degree and prolonged duration of mitral regurgitation (MR), and paradoxical septal wall motion.[2] Using this definition of a QRS duration of greater than 120 milliseconds, about one-third of patients with HFrEF have ventricular dyssynchrony.[2] CRT improves

ventricular dyssynchrony with implantation of pacing leads to pace both the right and left ventricles. Optimal placement of two leads, one on the right ventricular septum and a second in the coronary sinus at the site of latest LV activation allows for simultaneous or near simultaneous activation of both ventricles and improves inter- and intra-ventricular synchrony. Early studies demonstrated a benefit of CRT in patients with HFrEF and ventricular dyssynchrony on hemodynamics, functional outcomes and quality of life (QoL) leading to the initial indications for this therapy.[3] These results led to large-scale randomized controlled trials (RCTs) confirming the beneficial effects of CRT on functional status and demonstrating an important morbidity and mortality benefit.

Randomized Controlled Trials of Cardiac Resynchronization Therapy in New York Heart Association Class III and IV HFrEF Patients (Table 58.1)

The following RCTs are considered among the most important studies of CRT in the severe HFrEF patient population: the Multisite Stimulation in Cardiomyopathy (MUSTIC) study,[4] the Multicenter InSync Randomized Clinical Evaluation (MIRACLE) trial,[5] the MIRACLE ICD trial,[6] the CONTAK CD trial,[7] the Comparison of Medical Therapy, Pacing and Defibrillation in Heart Failure (COMPANION),[8] and the Cardiac Resynchronization in Heart Failure (CARE HF) trial.[9] To understand and compare the size and design, clinical benefits, baseline medical therapy, and limitations of CRT with or without an ICD, these studies are described in Table 58.1 with specific comments in the text that follows.

Multisite Stimulation in Cardiomyopathy (MUSTIC) Trial. The MUSTIC trial was a single-blind randomized controlled crossover study of CRT that enrolled 67 patients with enrollment criteria outlined in Table 58.1.[4] The CRT device was implanted in all patients and after a run-in period, patients were randomized to either VVI pacing at a fixed rate of 40 beats/min ("inactive pacing") or atrio-biventricular pacing ("active pacing") for 12 weeks followed by a crossover to the alternate treatment assignment. Forty-eight patients completed the study. The primary endpoint of peak exercise oxygen consumption (Vo_2) improved with CRT vs. no CRT as did all the secondary endpoints. The blinded crossover design of this trial suggested substantial improvements in

TABLE 58.1 Pivotal Trials for Cardiac Resynchronization Therapy

TRIAL (YEAR PUBLISHED)	N	INCLUSION CRITERIA	STUDY DESIGN	MEAN FOLLOW-UP	PRIMARY ENDPOINT	SECONDARY ENDPOINTS	MEDICAL THERAPY*
MUSTIC (2001)	67	• QRS >150 msec • NYHA Classes III and IV • LVEF<35% • Sinus rhythm	Single-blind, crossover RCT CRT on vs. CRT off	24 wk	CRT on vs. CRT off 6MHWD (active vs. inactive pacing) 399 ± 100 m vs. 326 ± 134 m (p ≤ 0.001)	CRT on vs. CRT off QoL 29.6 ± 21.3 vs. 43.2 ± 22.8 (p < 0.001) Vo₂ 16.2 ± 4.7 vs. 15 ± 4.9 mL/kg/min (p < 0.029)	ACEI/ARB 96% BB 28% MRA 22% Diuretics† 94% Digoxin 48%
MIRACLE (2002)	453	• QRS ≥130 msec • NYHA III, IV • LVEF ≤35%	Double-blind prospective RCT CRT on vs. CRT off	6 mo	CRT on vs. CRT off 6MWHD + 39 vs. +10 M (p = 0.001) QoL −18 vs. −9 points (p < 0.001) NYHA Improved (p < 0.001)	CRT on vs. CRT off Measures of exercise performance (Vo₂) and total exercise time, LVEF, area of MR jet, QRS duration—all improved (p < 0.001)	ACEI/ARB 93% BB 62% MRA NR Diuretics† 94% Digoxin 78%
MIRACLE-ICD (2003)	369	• QRS ≥130 msec • NYHA Classes III, IV • LVEF ≤35% • Indication for secondary prevention • ICD or history of inducible sustained ventricular tachycardia	Double-blind, prospective RCT CRT-ICD implanted in all with CRT off in control group	6 mo	CRT on vs. off 6MWHD +55 CI = 44-79] vs. +53 m [CI = 43-75] (p = 0.36) QoL −17.5 [CI = −21 to −14] vs. −11.0 [CI = −16 to −7] m (p = 0.02) NYHA Improved (p = 0.007)	CRT on vs. off No significant differences in changes in left ventricular size or function, overall HF status, survival, and rates of hospitalization	ACEI/ARB 93% BB 62% MRA NR Diuretics† 93%
CONTAK CD (2003)	490	• QRS ≥120 msec • NYHA Classes II-IV • LVEF ≤35% • Indication for primary prevention ICD	Single-blind, prospective RCT parallel-controlled CRT-ICD implanted with CRT off in control group	6 mo	CRT vs. no CRT Progression of HF, defined as ACM, hospitalization for HF, and VT/VF requiring device intervention 15% reduction in HF progression with CRT vs. no CRT (p = 0.35)	CRT vs. no CRT Vo₂ 0.8 mL/kg/min vs. 0.0 mL/kg/min (p = 0.03) 6MHWD 35 m vs. 15 m (p = 0.043) QoL (p = NS)	ACEI/ARB 81% BB 45% MRA NR Diuretics† 92% Digoxin 72%
COMPANION (2004)	1520	• QRS ≥120 msec • NYHA Classes III-IV • LVEF ≤35%	Prospective RCT Randomized 1:2:2 to OPT (optimal medical therapy) vs. CRT-D (CRT+ICD) vs. CRT-P (CRT alone)	NR	Time to ACM or hospitalization for any cause CRT-P vs. OPT (HR= 0.81; p = 0.014) CRT-D vs. OPT (HR, 0.80; P = 0.01)	ACM CRT-P vs. OPT (reduced by 24%, p = 0.059) CRT-D vs. OPT (reduced 36%, p = 0.003) 6MWD OPT vs. CRT-P vs. CRT-I 1 ± 93 vs. 40 ± 96 (p < 0.001) vs. 46 ± 98 (p < 0.001) QoL OPT vs. CRT-P vs. CRT-D −12 ± 23 vs. −25 ± 26 (p < 0.001) vs. −26 ±28 (p < 0.001)	ACEI/ARB 89% BB 68% MRA 53% Loop diuretics 94%
CARE HF (2005)	813	• QRS≥150 msec or 120-150 msec with echocardiographic dyssynchrony • NYHA Classes III-IV • LVEF ≤35%	Unblinded, prospective RCT CRT vs. no CRT	29.4 mo	CRT vs. no CRT Time to ACM or unplanned cardiovascular hospitalization HR = 0.63; 95% CI = 0.51-0.77; P < 0.001	CRT vs. no CRT ACM (HR= 0.64; 95% CI 0.48-0.85; P < 0.002) QoL difference (mean ± SD) at 90 −10 (−8 to −12) (p < 0.001)	ACEI/ARB 95% BB 70% MRA 54% Loop diuretics 44% Digoxin 40%

TABLE 58.1 Pivotal Trials for Cardiac Resynchronization Therapy—cont'd

TRIAL (YEAR PUBLISHED)	N	INCLUSION CRITERIA	STUDY DESIGN	MEAN FOLLOW-UP	PRIMARY ENDPOINT	SECONDARY ENDPOINTS	MEDICAL THERAPY*
REVERSE (2008)	610	• QRS ≥120 msec • NYHA Classes I-II • LVEF ≤40%	Double-blind, prospective RCT CRT on vs. off	12 mo	CRT on vs. off Clinical composite response (improved, unchanged or worsened) CRT on vs. off 16% vs. 21% worsened (p = 0.19)	CRT on vs. off LVESVI −18.4 ± 29.5 vs. −1.3 ± 23.4 mL/m² (p < 0.0001)	ACE/ARB 96% BB 96% MRA NR Diuretics NR
MADIT-CRT (2009)	1820	• QRS ≥130 msec • NYHA Classes I-II • LVEF ≤30% • Candidate for primary prevention ICD	Unblinded, prospective double-blind CRT-ICD vs. ICD	2.4 yr	CRT-ICD vs. ICD ACM or HF event CRT-ICD 17.2% vs. ICD 25.3% (HR = 0.66, CI = 0.52-0.84, p = 0.001)	CRT-ICD vs. ICD ACM 6.8% vs. 7.3% (p = 0.99) HF events CRT-ICD 13.9% vs. 22.8% (p < 0.001)	ACEI 77% ARB 21% BB 93% MRA 32% Diuretics† 76%
RAFT (2010)	1798	• QRS ≥120 msec or ≥200 msec if paced • NYHA Classes II-III • LVEF ≤30%	Double-blind, prospective RCT ICD-CRT vs. ICD alone	40 mo	ICD-CRT vs. ICD ACM or HFH HR 0.75, CI 0.64-0.87 (p < 0.0001)	ICD-CRT vs. ICD ACM HR 0.75, CI 0.62-0.91 (p < 0.0001) AE double in ICD-CRT compared with ICD at 30 days	ACEI/ARB 96% BB 90% MRA 42% Diuretics† 85% Digoxin 34%
ECHO-CRT (2012)	809	• QRS ≤130 msec • NYHA Classes III-IV • LVEF ≤30% and echo evidence of LV dyssynchrony	Prospective RCT CRT vs. control	19.4 mo	CRT vs. control ACM or first HFH HR 1.20, CI = 0.92-1.57, p = 0.15	CRT vs. control ACM HR 1.81, CI, 1.11-2.93 (p = 0.02)	ACEI/ARB 95% BB 96% MRA 61% Diuretics 86%
BLOCK-HF (2013)	691	• Indications for pacing with AV block • NYHA Classes I-III • LVEF ≤50% • Patients with standard indication for CRT excluded	Prospective RCT CRT vs. RV pacing	37 mo	CRT vs. RV pacing Time to ACM or urgent HF visit or a 15% increase in LVESVI HR, 0.74; CI, 0.60-0.90	CRT vs. RV pacing ACM + urgent HF care HR 0.73, CI 0.56-0.94 ACM + HFH HR 0.77, CI 0.58-1.00 ACM HR 0.83, CI 0.59-1.17 HFH HR 0.68 (049-0.94)	NR

*All medical therapy for CRT group.
†All diuretic types.
ACEI, Angiotensin converting enzyme inhibitors; *ACM*, all-cause mortality; *AE*, adverse events; *ARB*, angiotensin receptor blockers; *BB*, beta blockers; *CI*, confidence intervals; *HF*, heart failure; *HFH*, heart failure hospitalization; *HR*, hazard ratio; *LVEF*, left ventricular ejection fraction; *MRA*, mineralocorticoid receptor antagonists; *NR*, not reported; *NYHA*, New York Heart Association Classification; *QoL*, quality of life (Minnesota Living with Heart Failure for all studies); *RCT*, randomized controlled trial; *RV*, right ventricular; *6MHWD*, 6-minute hall walk distance; *Vo₂*, peak exercise oxygen consumption.

functional capacity and QoL with CRT that were dependent on ongoing pacing.

Multicenter InSync Randomized Clinical Evaluation (MIRACLE). MIRACLE was the first prospective RCT designed to evaluate the benefits of CRT in patients with the inclusion criteria outlined in Table 58.1.[5] Patients assigned to CRT experienced an improvement in each of the primary endpoints at 6 months: 6MHWD, NYHA functional class, and QoL. The trial also provided evidence of substantial LV reverse remodeling with CRT as outlined in Table 58.1. The results of this trial led to FDA approval of the InSync system in 2001, the first approved CRT system in the United States.

Multicenter Insync–Implantable Cardioverter-Defibrillator Randomized Clinical Evaluation. MIRACLE ICD was a prospective RCT designed to evaluate the benefits of an implantable cardiac defibrillator (ICD) + CRT vs. ICD alone.[6] The inclusion criteria and primary endpoints were the same as in MIRACLE with the additional requirement that subjects have an indication for a secondary prevention ICD or have a history of inducible sustained ventricular tachycardia. With CRT, the improvements in QoL and (NYHA) classification were similar to those in

MIRACLE but there was no difference in 6MHWD. However, Vo₂ and total exercise time were improved. The ventricular remodeling benefits seen with CRT in MIRACLE were not reproduced in MIRACLE ICD. The combined CRT-ICD device used in this study was approved by the FDA in June 2002 for use in NYHA Class III and IV HFrEF patients with ventricular dyssynchrony and an ICD indication.

CONTAK CD. CONTAK CD was similar to MIRACLE ICD except NYHA Class II patients were enrolled.[7] Both the study design (crossover) and primary endpoint (Vo₂) were changed during the study to a parallel design and a composite HF progression endpoint. The 15% reduction in HF progression was not significant but Vo₂ and 6MWHD were improved. Significant reductions in ventricular dimensions and improvement in left ventricular ejection fraction (LVEF) similar to those seen in MIRACLE were demonstrated with CRT.

Comparison of Medical Therapy, Pacing, and Defibrillation in Heart Failure (COMPANION). COMPANION randomized patients to optimal medical therapy (OPT), CRT-P (CRT alone), and CRT-D (CRT+ICD) and was the first reported large RCT to include mortality in the primary endpoint.[8] COMPANION confirmed the results of earlier CRT trials in improving symptoms, exercise tolerance, and QoL for HF patients with electrical dyssynchrony. COMPANION was also the first large RCT to demonstrate the impact of CRT-D in reducing all-cause mortality (ACM) and suggested incremental benefit from combined ICD and CRT therapies.

Mean systolic blood pressure was significantly higher in both the CRT-P and CRT-D groups compared to the OPT group at 3, 6, and 12 months (Fig. 58.1). This improvement in systolic blood pressure following CRT may allow uptitration of guideline-directed medical therapy (GDMT), further improving morbidity and mortality.

Cardiac Resynchronization in Heart Failure Trial. The CARE-HF trial convincingly demonstrated the benefits of CRT+ medical therapy vs. medical therapy alone on morbidity and mortality in patients with NYHA Class III or IV HF and ventricular dyssynchrony[9] (Fig. 58.2). CRT also led to a significant reduction in MR area by echocardiography and significant myocardial reverse remodeling and reduced N-terminal pro B-type natriuretic peptide (NT-proBNP) at 18 months. These benefits were achieved irrespective of the use of beta blockers, mineralocorticoid receptor antagonists (MRAs), or digoxin. In addition, the mean systolic blood pressure was 5.8 mm Hg (CI, 3.5 to 8.2, p = 0.001) higher in the CRT group than in the control group at 3 months; this difference was maintained at 18 months, confirming the blood pressure improvements in COMPANION.

Randomized Controlled Trials of Cardiac Resynchronization Therapy in NYHA Class I and II Patients (Table 58.1)

CRT studies described earlier in this chapter focused specifically on patients with HFrEF and NYHA Classes III and IV. These studies also provided preliminary data that informed the design of studies that allowed expanded indications to patients with an LVEF between 30% and 35% and NYHA Class I and II HFrEF patients.

The echo data from MIRACLE-ICD suggested a significant improvement in LV remodeling with CRT even in the small cohort of NYHA Class II patients enrolled similar to that seen in the more symptomatic patients in CARE-HF[10] This finding led to three important trials with CRT in patients with mild HF including the Resynchronization Reverses Remodeling in Systolic Left Ventricular Dysfunction (REVERSE) trial,[11] Multicenter Automatic Defibrillator Implantation Trial with Cardiac Resynchronization Therapy (MADIT-CRT),[12] and Resynchronization/defibrillation for Ambulatory Heart Failure Trial (RAFT).[13]

Resynchronization Reverses Remodeling in Systolic Left Ventricular Dysfunction Trial. The primary endpoint (an HF composite) in REVERSE was not significantly changed but the CRT-on vs. CRT-off group had a greater improvement in measures of LV remodeling.[11] As noted in CARE-HF, the benefits of CRT on remodeling were present irrespective of the presence or dose of beta blockers. Despite the negative primary endpoint, this trial suggested a benefit of CRT on ventricular remodeling in mildly symptomatic HFrEF patients.

Multicenter Automatic Defibrillator Implantation Trial With Cardiac Resynchronization Therapy. The MADIT-CRT trial was an unblinded RCT designed to determine if CRT + primary prevention ICD vs. primary prevention ICD alone reduced the risk of ACM and nonfatal HF events in HFrEF patients with NYHA Class I (ischemic etiology) and NYHA Class II (ischemic or nonischemic etiology) symptoms.[12] The significant reduction in the primary endpoint was due to a reduction in HF events in both the ischemic and nonischemic groups. A subsequent

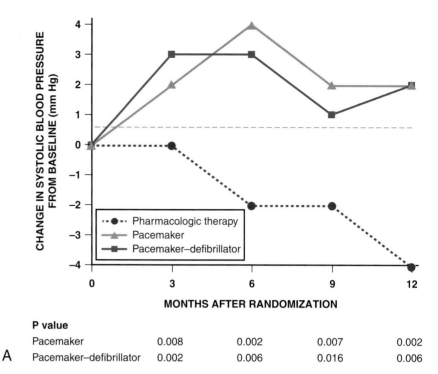

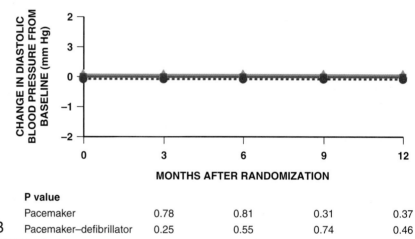

	P value			
A Pacemaker	0.008	0.002	0.007	0.002
Pacemaker–defibrillator	0.002	0.006	0.016	0.006

	P value			
B Pacemaker	0.78	0.81	0.31	0.37
Pacemaker–defibrillator	0.25	0.55	0.74	0.46

FIGURE 58.1 Median change from baseline in systolic **(A)** and diastolic **(B)** blood pressure at 3, 6, 9, and 12 months in the COMPANION trial. *P* values are for the comparison with optimal pharmacologic therapy. (Modified from Bristow MR, et al. Cardiac-resynchronization therapy with or without an implantable defibrillator in advanced chronic heart failure. *N Engl J Med.* 2004;350:2140-2150.)

analysis demonstrated that the benefit of CRT was seen only in those with a left bundle branch block (LBBB).[14] A larger benefit of CRT was noted for women (HR = 0.37, CI 0.22 to 0.62) than men (HR = 0.76, CI 0.59 to 0.97, p = 0.01 for interaction) and in patients with a QRS of 150 milliseconds or longer. The MADIT-CRT trial led the FDA to expand the indication for CRT to NYHA Class II or ischemic Class I patients, with LVEF less than 30%, QRS duration longer than 130 milliseconds, and LBBB. MADIT-CRT also demonstrated substantial improvement in ventricular size and function in patients randomized to CRT, with the outcomes benefit directly related to the degree of reverse remodeling.[15]

Initially the RAFT trial included patients in NYHA Class II and III but when the CARE HF trial showed a reduction in mortality for NYHA Class III patients, the protocol was revised to include only patients in Class II.[13] The RAFT trial was the first to show a mortality benefit of combined CRT-ICD over an ICD alone, and a mortality reduction with the addition of CRT in patients in NYHA Class II HF. *The results of REVERSE, MADIT-CRT, and RAFT resulted in the FDA expanding the indication CRT to include patients with mildly symptomatic HF.*

Cardiac Resynchronization Therapy in Patients With Narrow QRS Complex and Mechanical Dyssynchrony. Patients with HFrEF and a

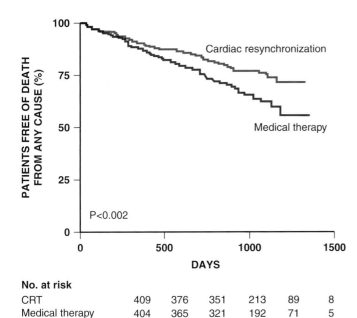

FIGURE 58.2 Kaplan-Meier estimates of survival in patients randomized to cardiac resynchronization therapy (CRT) compared to conventional medical therapy in the CARE-HF trial. (Modified from Cleland JGF, et al. The effect of cardiac resynchronization on morbidity and mortality in heart failure. *N Engl J Med.* 2005;352:1539-1549.)

No. at risk

CRT	409	376	351	213	89	8
Medical therapy	404	365	321	192	71	5

narrow QRS complex may demonstrate mechanical dyssynchrony using imaging techniques such as echocardiography. Small trials suggested a benefit in these patients but a larger trial, Echocardiography Guided Cardiac Resynchronization Therapy (EchoCRT), did not confirm these benefits.[16] The primary endpoint was not significant, but the secondary endpoint of ACM was higher in the CRT group than in the control group (Table 58.3), demonstrating the potential for harm in using CRT in narrow-QRS patients. Thus CRT is considered contraindicated in these patients.

Patients Requiring Right Ventricular pacing. Early studies of CRT specifically excluded patients with high degrees of atrioventricular block to avoid the confounding effects of right ventricular (RV) pacing with its potential to cause ventricular dyssynchrony.[3] To determine whether CRT might reduce mortality, morbidity, and adverse LV remodeling in patients requiring RV pacing, the Biventricular vs. Right Ventricular Pacing in Heart Failure Patients with Atrioventricular Block (BLOCK HF) study was designed.[17] Patients with standard guideline indications for CRT were excluded. Patients received a CRT and ICD (ICD if the patient had an indication for ICD therapy) and were assigned to standard RV pacing or CRT. Patients randomly assigned to CRT had a significantly lower incidence of the primary outcome than did those assigned to RV pacing (Table 58.2) This led to a guideline recommendation to consider CRT in patients with and LVEF of ≤50% who require RV pacing.

Indications for Cardiac Resynchronization Therapy in Patients with Heart Failure

Although electrical and mechanical dyssynchrony often coexist, CRT guideline recommendations are based on electrical dyssynchrony alone. This recommendation is due to the volume of clinical trial data using QRS duration as an enrollment criterion and the results of the Predictors of Response to CRT (PROSPECT) study.[18] The PROSPECT trial was designed to find echocardiographic or tissue Doppler measures of dyssynchrony that predicted a positive response to CRT by improvement in a clinical composite score or a ≥15% reduction in left ventricular end-systolic volume (LVESV) at 6 months in patients with standard CRT indications. No single measure had adequate sensitivity or specificity to improve patient selection for CRT beyond the current QRS guidelines.

Limitations of Cardiac Resynchronization Therapy

While, overall, RCTs have shown that HFrEF patients derive substantial benefits from CRT, some patients are "nonresponders" and do not have reductions in symptoms or HF hospitalizations and do not

achieve LV reverse remodeling. Factors reported to contribute to the nonresponder rate include suboptimal LV lead placement, suboptimal atrioventricular (AV) and ventricular-ventricular (VV) timing, ventricular scar, and HF disease progression.[3] Factors associated with a particularly beneficial (super) response include LBBB, longer QRS duration, female sex, lack of prior myocardial infarction, and smaller left atrial volume.[19] Patients may have a wide range of responses to CRT (or any medical or device therapy) as outlined in Fig. 58.3. Super responders show a large benefit—some as "super" as normalization of ventricular function. Some patients (nonprogressors) do not show a measurable benefit of CRT, but also do not have the predicted worsening HF over time as do nonresponders. Negative responders are those who have clinical worsening of their disease after CRT implantation. A number of advances in CRT pacing are being developed to address the nonresponder rate, including biomarker-guided selection, optimal AV and VV timing, and the use of epicardial and endocardial LV pacing leads.[3]

CRT has been standard therapy for HFrEF for nearly two decades but there are a number of clinical situations for which more data would be valuable. Perhaps the most important of these is the benefit of CRT in patients with atrial fibrillation (AF). Patients with AF were excluded from most of the pivotal trials of CRT but the prevalence of AF is as high as 40% in some HFrEF studies. Because of the lack of strong clinical trial data, the recommendations for CRT in patients with persistent AF with or without AV nodal ablation and RV pacing are weaker than those for similar patients with sinus rhythm. In patients with AF, adequate rate control or AV ablation to allow consistent pacing is important to achieve a response[20] Another gap in knowledge for CRT is in patients with HF and preserved or mid-range ejection fraction in whom mechanical and electrical dyssynchrony may be present, but no large studies have yet addressed the benefits of CRT in these patients.[21]

SUDDEN CARDIAC DEATH IN CHRONIC HEART FAILURE

Sudden cardiac death (SCD) is a leading cause of mortality in patients with HFrEF and occurs at a rate severalfold higher than in the general population (see also Chapter 70). Given this high rate of SCD, the use of prophylactic ICDs was hypothesized to reduce total mortality in HFrEF. A series of studies performed more than two decades ago have provided proof of this hypothesis.

Randomized Controlled Trials of Implantable-Cardioverter Defibrillators for Primary Prevention of SCD in HFrEF

The most important trials establishing a role for ICDs as primary prevention of mortality in HFrEF patients are the Multicenter Automatic Defibrillator Implantation II Trial (MADIT II),[22] Prophylactic Defibrillator Implantation in Patients with Nonischemic Dilated Cardiomyopathy (DEFINITE),[23] and the Sudden Cardiac Death–Heart Failure Trial (SCD-HeFT).[24] A more recent study, the Danish Study to Assess the Efficacy of ICDs in Patients with Non-ischemic Systolic Heart Failure on Mortality (DANISH) trial, has raised questions regarding the efficacy of prophylactic ICD use in nonischemic HF patients.[25] To allow comparison of these studies their size and design, clinical benefits, baseline medical therapy, and limitations are outlined in Table 58.2, with specific comments in the text that follows.

Multicenter Automatic Defibrillator Implantation II Trial. MADIT II was designed and powered to assess the survival benefit of ICDs in post-MI patients with reduced EF (<30%).[22] The trial was stopped early because of a marked benefit of ICD therapy. Survival benefits of ICD therapy were present in all age groups and NYHA classes.

Prophylactic Defibrillator Implantation in Patients With Nonischemic Dilated Cardiomyopathy Trial. The DEFINITE trial was the first RCT evaluating an ICD for primary prevention of ACM in patients with nonischemic cardiomyopathy.[23] At the time the trial was conducted there were inadequate data regarding the benefit of an ICD in nonischemic HF patients and previous observations had suggested that prophylactic amiodarone might reduce the risk of SCD in these patients. Although the primary endpoint of ACM was not reduced with an ICD, a post hoc analysis suggested a highly significant reduction in SCD with an ICD. This result was based on SCD in 3 patients in the ICD group and 14 in the control group. The mortality in DEFINITE was lower than in MADIT II, perhaps in part, due to the higher use of angiotensin-converting enzyme inhibitors (ACEIs) and beta blockers. The study was underpowered for ACM but did suggest a strong trend toward a survival advantage based on the expected reduction in SCD for patients receiving an ICD.

Sudden Cardiac Death: Heart Failure Trial. The results of the SCD-HeFT trial have had a substantial impact on current practice guidelines for ICDs.[24] SCD-HeFT randomized patients to three arms—comparing an ICD to amiodarone and placebo in patients with both ischemic and nonischemic causes of HFrEF (Fig. 58.4). Similar degrees of benefit on ACM with an ICD were noted in patients with ischemic and nonischemic HFrEF, confirming the findings of MADIT II and DEFINITE. The neutral results on ACM with amiodarone effectively ended its routine use for primary prevention of SCD in HFrEF. The SCD-HeFT trial provided

the most robust evidence to date supporting the prophylactic use of an ICD in patients with NYHA Class II and III HFrEF irrespective of etiology. **Danish Study to Assess the Efficacy of ICDs in Patients with Nonischemic Systolic Heart Failure on Mortality.** With improvements in medical therapy that reduce both SCD and death from progressive HF the value of primary prevention ICDs in patients with nonischemic HF has been questioned. The DANISH trial randomized patients with non-ischemic HFrEF to usual clinical care vs. usual care plus an ICD. Fifty-eight percent of patients in each group received CRT.[25] There was no benefit of primary prevention ICD implantation on ACM in this patient group. However, the secondary endpoint of SCD was significantly reduced in patients in the ICD group. While the results questioned the use of prophylactic ICDs in a nonischemic HFrEF population who had appropriate CRT use, the substantial reduction in SCD, overall, and the decrease in ACM in younger patients have left considerable uncertainty about ICD use in patients with nonischemic HFrEF.

Using older trials for guideline recommendations is increasingly problematic as new medical therapies continue to reduce the risk of both progressive HF death and SCD in HFrEF, potentially reducing the

TABLE 58.2 Pivotal Trials for ICDs for Primary Prevention of SCD

TRIAL (YEAR PUBLISHED)	N	INCLUSION CRITERIA	STUDY DESIGN	% ISCHEMIC	MEAN FOLLOW-UP	PRIMARY ENDPOINT	MORTALITY/ YEAR	MEDICAL THERAPY*
MADIT II (2002)	1232	• LVEF ≤30% • Prior MI • ≥1 month post-MI	RCT 3:2 ICD + medical therapy vs. medical therapy	100%	20 mo	ICD + MT vs. MT ACM HR = 0.69 (95% CI, 0.51-0.93; P = 0.016)	ICD 8.5% Control 11.9%	ACEI 68% ARB NR BB 70% MRA NR Dig 57% Diuretics† 72%
DEFINITE (2004)	458	• Nonischemic • LVEF <36% • PVCs or NSVT	RCT ICD + MT vs. MT	0%	29 mo	ICD + MT vs. MT ACMHR = 0.65 (95% CI, 0.40-1.06; P = 0.08) Post hoc analysis of SCD HR = 0.20 (95% CI, 0.06-0.71; P = 0.006) (no. of events = 17)	ICD 3.9% Control 7.0%	ACEI 84% ARB 14% BB 86% MRA NR Dig 42% Diuretics† 87%
SCD-HeFT (2005)	2521	• LVEF ≤35% • NYHA Classes II-II • >3 mo post-HF onset	RCT ICD + MT vs. amiodarone + MT vs. MT	52%	45.5 mo	ACM ICD vs. MT HR = 0.77 (97.5% CI, 0.62-0.96, p = 0.007) Amiodarone + MT vs. MT HR = 0.77 (97.5% CI, 0.86-1.3, P = 0.53)	ICD 5.8% Control 7.6%	ACEI/ ARB 94% BB 69% MRA 20%‡+ Dig 67% Loop diuretics 82%
DANISH (2016)	1116	• LVEF ≤35% • NYHA Classes II-II (or IV if CRT planned) • NT-proBNP >200 pg/mL • Nonischemic	RCT ICD + MT vs. MT	0%	67.6 mo	ICD + MT vs. MT ACM HR = 0.87 (95% CI, 0.68-1.12; P = 0.28) Other endpoints CV death HR = 0.77 (95% CI, 0.57-1.05; P = 0.10) SCD HR = 0.50 (95% CI, 0.31-0.82; P = 0.005)	ICD 4.4% Control 5.0%	ACEI/ ARB 96% BB 92% MRA 59% Dig NR Loop diuretics NR CRT 58%

*All medical therapy for CRT group.
†All diuretic types.
‡potassium-sparing diuretics (unknown % of MRA)

Abbreviations as for Table 58.1. *ACM*, All-cause mortality; *ACMHR*, all-cause mortality hazard ratio; *ARB*, angiotensin receptor blockers; *BB*, beta blockers; *CRT*, cardiac resynchronization therapy; *CV*, cardiovascular; *HR*, hazard ratio; *ICD*, implantable cardiac defibrillator; *LVEF*, left ventricular ejection fraction; *MI*, myocardial infarction; *MRA*, mineralocorticoid receptor antagonists; *MT*, medical therapy; *NR*, not reported; *NSVT*, nonsustained ventricular tachycardia; *NYHA*, New York Heart Association; *PVCs*, premature ventricular contractions; *RCT*, randomized controlled trial; *SCD*, sudden cardiac death.

absolute benefit of ICDs.[26] While the absolute rate of both SCD and progressive HF increase as NYHA symptom class worsens, the relative risk of SCD is higher in less symptomatic patients. Thus, by improving symptom class, improved medical therapy for HFrEF may shift the relative percentage of deaths to more SCD increasing the potential benefit of ICDs.[3] Indeed recent meta-analyses support the efficacy of ICD use for nonischemic cardiomyopathy, despite the results of the DANISH trial.[27] Furthermore, in a recent analysis of the Prospective Comparison of ARNI (Angiotensin Receptor–Neprilysin Inhibitor) with ACEI (Angiotensin-Converting–Enzyme Inhibitor) to Determine Impact on Global Mortality and Morbidity in HF Trial (PARADIGM-HF), ICD use was associated with lower rates of SCD, regardless of HFrEF etiology.[28] Thus it is unlikely that current guideline recommendations for ICDs will change, despite the results of the DANISH trial.

GUIDELINES FOR CARDIAC RESYNCHRONIZATION AND IMPLANTABLE CARDIOVERTER-DEFIBRILLATORS IN HEART FAILURE WITH A REDUCED EJECTION FRACTION

The American College of Cardiology, American Heart Association, and Heart Rhythm Society (ACC/AHA/HRS) 2012 guidelines for device-based therapy of cardiac rhythm abnormalities,[29] and 2017 guidelines for management of patients with ventricular arrhythmias and the prevention of sudden cardiac death,[30] and the 2017 AHA/ACC/HFSA Heart Failure Guidelines[31] provide the most recent recommendations for CRT and ICD therapies. The only Class I recommendation for CRT is for patients with LVEF ≤35%, LBBB with QRS duration of ≥150 msec, sinus rhythm, NYHA Class II, III, or ambulatory Class IV, and receiving GDMT. The only Class I indication for primary prevention ICD is for patients with HFrEF at least 40 days post-MI with LVEF <35%, NYHA Class II or II, and receiving GDMT. There are a number of Class II recommendations.[29-31]

NEW IMPLANTABLE THERAPEUTIC DEVICES FOR HEART FAILURE (TABLE 58.3)

Abnormal myocardial contractility often leads to HF resulting in a number of secondary manifestations including neurohormonal activation, autonomic imbalance, arrhythmias, ventricular dyssynchrony, myocardial remodeling, secondary mitral regurgitation (SMR), and sleep disordered breathing. These manifestations generally become more common and more severe as HF progresses. Device therapy has been instrumental in filling gaps in treatment for some of these manifestations that were only partially addressed or not addressed at all with medical therapy. For example, CRT improves myocardial dyssynchrony still present after GDMT and ICDs treat the ventricular arrhythmias that still occur despite GDMT in HFrEF patients. More recently, devices have been developed to reduce episodes of central sleep

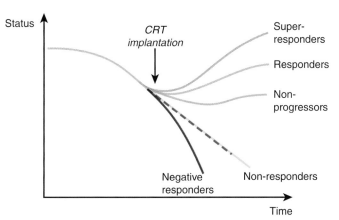

FIGURE 58.3 Possible clinical courses after CRT implantation. Responders show a measurable effect, whereas superresponders show excellent response up to normalization after CRT implantation. Nonprogressors do not show a benefit of CRT, but also do not follow their predicted natural course of deterioration as a result of chronic heart failure (*dashed line*) like nonresponders. Negative responders demonstrate clinical worsening of their disease after CRT implantation.*CRT*, cardiac resynchronization therapy. (From Steffel J, Ruschitzka F. Superresponse to cardiac resynchronization therapy. Circulation. 2014;130:87-90.)

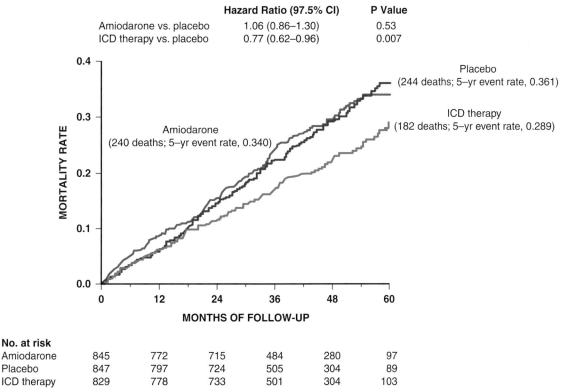

	Hazard Ratio (97.5% CI)	P Value
Amiodarone vs. placebo	1.06 (0.86–1.30)	0.53
ICD therapy vs. placebo	0.77 (0.62–0.96)	0.007

No. at risk						
Amiodarone	845	772	715	484	280	97
Placebo	847	797	724	505	304	89
ICD therapy	829	778	733	501	304	103

FIGURE 58.4 Kaplan-Meier estimates of survival in patients randomized to an ICD compared to conventional medical therapy or conventional medical therapy plus amiodarone in the SCD-HeFT trial. (Modified from Bardy GH, et al. Amiodarone or an implantable cardioverter-defibrillator for congestive heart failure. *N Engl J Med.* 2005;352:225-237.)

apnea, reduce SMR, improve myocardial contractility, and restore autonomic imbalance in HFrEF patients. The pivotal clinical trials for new approved therapeutic devices for HFrEF include the Remede System Pivotal Study,[32] the Cardiovascular Outcomes Assessment of the Mitra-Clip Percutaneous Therapy for Heart Failure Patients with Functional Mitral Regurgitation (COAPT) trial,[33] the Evaluate Safety and Efficacy of the OPTIMIZER System in Subjects with Moderate-to Severe Heart Failure (FIX-HF-5C),[34] and the BAROSTIM NEO-Baroreceptor Activation Therapy for Heart Failure (BEAT-HF) trial.[35]

Central Sleep Apnea

Both obstructive sleep apnea and CSA are common even in optimally medically managed patients with HFrEF and are associated with worse symptoms and increased mortality.[36] The Remede system was designed to avert episodes of CSA by direct stimulation of the phrenic nerve via a transvenous lead in either the left pericardiophrenic or right brachiocephalic vein connected to a pulse generator. The device is programmed to deliver stimulation during sleep, thereby preventing episodes of CSA. The Remede System Pivotal Study enrolled 151 subjects, 96 of whom had NYHA Class I-IV HF.[32] At 6 months, the device "on" group was more likely to have a ≥50% reduction in Apnea-Hypopnea Index (AHI) from baseline (51% vs. 11%). The Remede system (Respicardia, Minnetonka, MN) was FDA approved in 2017 for the treatment of moderate to severe CSA in adult patients. The device does not have a specific guideline indication for HF and it remains uncertain if CSA should be routinely treated in patients with HFrEF because of concern generated by the Adaptive Servo-Ventilation for Central Sleep Apnea in Systolic HF (SERVE-HF) trial.[37] The SERVE-HF trial randomized 1625 subjects with HFrEF and predominantly CSA to adaptive servo-ventilation (ASV) or control. ASV had no significant effect on the primary endpoint, time to the first event of death from any cause, lifesaving cardiovascular intervention, or unplanned hospitalization for worsening HF, but all-cause and cardiovascular mortality were both increased with ASV. The increase in mortality was due to an increase in cardiovascular death without a preceding hospitalization for worsening HF.[38] Thus additional data are necessary to determine if the excess mortality seen in SERVE-HF in patients with HFrEF and CSA was due to the treatment modality (ASV) or the reduction in CSA.

Transcatheter Mitral Valve Repair Secondary (Functional) Mitral Regurgitation

SMR is associated with a poor prognosis in patients with HFrEF.[39] Two recent trials, Cardiovascular Outcomes Assessment of the MitraClip Percutaneous Therapy for HF Patients with Functional Mitral Regurgitation (COAPT)[33] and Percutaneous Repair with the MitraClip Device for Severe Functional/Secondary Mitral Regurgitation (MITRA-FR)[40] evaluated the role of transcatheter edge to edge repair (TEER) of the mitral valve in patients with HFrEF and moderately severe to severe SMR and demonstrated markedly differently results, with COAPT demonstrating a large benefit on HFH and ACM and MITRA-FR demonstrating no benefit. (See also Chapter 78.) The explanation for these disparate results remains a source of considerable discussion. However, in 2019, the FDA approved the MitraClip (Abbott, Menlo Park, CA) device for repair of moderately severe to severe SMR in patients with symptomatic HF and an LVEF of 20% to 50% despite optimally titrated (GDMT based on the results of the COAPT trial). The 2020 ACC/AHA Valvular Heart Disease Guidelines have a new IIa recommendation for TEER of the mitral valve in patients with chronic severe secondary MR related to LV systolic dysfunction and symptomatic HF who meet the inclusion criteria of the COAPT trial.[41]

Cardiac Contractility Modulation

Myocardial contractility is impaired in patients with HFrEF despite optimal GDMT. Cardiac contractility modulation (CCM) uses the Optimizer Smart System (Impulse Dynamics, Stuttgart, Germany), which includes an implantable pulse generator (IPG), one atrial and two ventricular leads, a programmer, and a transcutaneous charger.[42] The

IPG stimulates the ventricular myocardium with high-voltage, nonexcitatory (does not stimulate contraction) impulses to improve myocardial contractility.[42] The precise molecular mechanism by which CCM improves contractility is uncertain but does appear to be associated with improved myocardial calcium handling.[42] The FIX-HF-5C trial combined patients from a similar previous trial (FIX-HF-5) and 160 new subjects with an LVEF ≥25% and ≤45%, NYHA Class III or IV symptoms, QRS duration <130 msec, and normal sinus rhythm with[34,43] (Table 58.3). The difference in peak VO2 favored the CCM group, as did all the secondary endpoints (Table 58.3). The FDA approved the Optimizer Smart System) in with the indications outlined in Table 58.3. There are no current guideline recommendations for CCM.

Baroreflex Activation Therapy

HF is associated with autonomic imbalance—enhanced activation of the sympathetic nervous system and decreased parasympathetic activity—that results in increased heart rate and blood pressure, myocardial remodeling, decreased diuresis and enhanced renin secretion as well as increased morbidity and mortality.[44] Baroreflex activation therapy (BAT) is designed to restore this autonomic imbalance by inhibiting the sympathetic system and activating the parasympathetic system by electrically stimulating the baroreceptors in the carotid sinus.

The BAROSTIM NEO system (CVRx, Inc., Minneapolis, MN), consists of a pulse generator and a carotid sinus lead implanted surgically to deliver BAT. In a randomized, open-label phase II trial of 146 subjects with NYHA Class III and an LVEF of ≤35% comparing GDMT alone to GDMT + BAT, each of the three primary endpoints—6MHWD, QoL, and NT-pro BNP—was improved in the BAT group.[45] The benefits were most prominent in the subgroup of patients without CRT.[46] Thus CRT was an exclusion in the subsequent phase III BEAT-HF trial. Initial results demonstrated significant improvements in QoL and 6MHW distance but not NT pro-BNP at 6 months.[35] However, patients with an NT-proBNP <1600 pg/mL benefitted significantly from BAT. Thus, an additional cohort of patients enrolled concurrently, with the same inclusion criteria, and a requirement for an NT-proBNP <1600 pg/mL were analyzed. Combining this cohort with the subjects in the early cohort with NT-proBNP <1600 pg/mL (*n* = 246 patients) resulted in a highly statistically significant benefit of BAT for all three endpoints (Table 58.3). These beneficial changes occurred despite a disproportionately increased use of ACEI/ARB, beta blockers, and MRAs during the 6-month study period in the GDMT alone group.[35] Based on the totality of data, BAT was approved by the FDA on August 16, 2019. The BEAT-HF trial was the first trial designed under the FDA expedited access pathway for premarket approval of devices and has a planned postmarket phase (now fully enrolled) to expand the indication to reduction of HF hospitalizations and cardiovascular mortality.[47]

IMPLANTABLE DEVICES TO MONITOR HEART FAILURE

Device-Based Heart Failure Diagnostics

Despite advances in medical and device therapy for HFrEF, HFH and mortality remain high. In addition, no therapies have been developed for HFpEF that have been shown to definitely reduce HFH and mortality.[48] The cost of care for HF in the United States is expected to double by 2030, with HFH accounting for 80% of the costs, thus there is intense interest in reducing HFH to both reduce societal costs of HF and improve QoL for patients.[48] Studies using changes in heart rate, blood pressure, body weight, and symptoms or any combination of these parameters to predict an HF exacerbation and guide therapies that prevent HFH have had inconsistent success. There are several potential reasons for these disappointing results. Some of these metrics are relatively insensitive in predicting an HF exacerbation, some become abnormal only late in the course of HF decompensation, and some are difficult to assess in a continuous and remote fashion.[49] These issues led to the search for physiologic parameters that might be more sensitive and specific in predicting HFH. Many implantable CRT, ICD, and pacemaker devices can now record and transmit individual

TABLE 58.3 Pivotal Trials of New Therapeutic Devices for Heart Failure

TRIAL (YEAR PUBLISHED)	N	THERAPEUTIC TARGET	INCLUSION CRITERIA	STUDY DESIGN	PRIMARY ENDPOINT	FDA APPROVAL DATE AND INDICATION	MEDICAL THERAPY[†]
Remede System Pivotal Study (2016)	151 (96 with HF)	Central sleep apnea	AHI of ≥ 20 central sleep apnea events per hour with central sleep apneas ≥ 50% of all apneas	RCT Neurostimulation vs. no neurostimulation	% of patients with a reduction in AHI of ≥50% from baseline to 6 mo Neurostimulation vs. no neurostimulation 51 vs. 11% (CI = 25-54, p < 0.001)	10.6.2017 Remede System Indicated for the treatment of moderate to severe central sleep apnea in adult patients	NR
COAPT (2018)	614	Secondary mitral regurgitation	• LVEF 20%-50% • 3-4 + MR • NYHA Class II-IVa • LVESD ≤70 mm	RCT MitraClip + optimal GDMT vs. optimal GDMT alone	Freedom from all HFH for 24 mo HR = 0.53 (95% CI = 0.40-0.70, p < 0.001)	3.14.2019 MitraClip NT and NTR/XTR Delivery System: for the treatment of symptomatic, moderate-to-severe secondary MR in patients with LVEF 20%-50% and LVESD ≤70 mm	ACEI/ARB/ARNI 72% BB 91% MRA 51% Diuretics 89%
FIX-HF-5C (2018)	160*	Myocardial contractility	• LVEF 25%-45% • NYHA Classes III-IV • NSR • QRS<130 msec • No CRT indication	RCT Cardiac contractility modulation (CCM) vs. control	CCM vs. control Peak Vo$_2$ +0.84 mL O$_2$/kg/min (0.12-1.55) (posterior probability of 0.989) Secondary endpoint of 6MHWD and QoL also improved	3.21.2019 Optimizer Smart system: to improve 6MHWD, QoL, and functional status of NYHA Class III HF patients who remain symptomatic despite GDMT, are in normal sinus rhythm, and not indicated for CRT and have an LVEF of 25%-45%	NR
BEAT-HF (2020)	408	Autonomic imbalance	• LVEF ≤35% • NYHA Class III or II (if recent III) • QRS<130 msec • No CRT indication	RCT Baroreflex activation therapy (BAT) vs. control	BAT vs. control All three of following must be significant: QoL −14.1 (95% CI = −19 to −9, p < 0.001) 6MHWD +60 m (95% CI = 40-80 m, p < 0.001) NT-proBNP −25% (95% CI = −38 to −9, p = 0.004)	8.16.2019 BAROSTIM NEO system: For the improvement of symptoms of HF-QoL, 6MHWD, and functional status (NYHA) for patients who are in NYHA Class III or Class II (if recent Class III) have an LVEF ≤35%, an NT-proBNP < 1600 pg/mL, and no indication for CRT	ACEI/ARB/ARNI 88% BB 95% MRA 48% Diuretics 85%

*30% borrowing from FIX-HF-5.
†All diuretic types.
ACEI, Angiotensin converting enzyme inhibitors; *ARB*, angiotensin receptor blockers; *BB*, beta blockers; *HF*, heart failure; *CCM*, cardiac contractility modulation; *GDMT*, guideline-directed medical therapy; *HFH*, heart failure hospitalization; *HR*, hazard ratio; *LVEF*, left ventricular ejection fraction; *LVESD*, left ventricular end systolic diameter; *MRA*, mineralocorticoid receptor antagonists; *NT-proBNP*, brain natriuretic peptide; *NYHA*, New York Heart Association; *QoL*, quality of life; *RCT*, randomized controlled trial.

physiologic parameters including atrial and ventricular heart rate and rhythm, patient activity level, heart rate variability, and intrathoracic impedance, a measure of lung water. Some devices also record measurements of respiratory activity such as rapid shallow breathing, respiratory rate, and tidal volume as well as the presence and intensity of third and fourth heart sounds.[50] Some of these metrics, alone or combined in a predictive model, change in the days to weeks prior to an HFH and predict the likelihood of an impending HFH allowing time for an intervention to reverse the decompensation and prevent an HFH.[49-51] In addition to monitoring individual device-based HF diagnostic parameters, algorithms based on combined parameters can stratify patients into subgroups of high risk, medium risk, and low risk for HFH.[50] These metrics can be measured remotely and be transmitted to secure networks for monitoring by providers. Several of these multisensor, multiparameter, integrated, diagnostic risk scores have been validated and approved by the FDA including HeartLogic (Boston Scientific) and TriageHF (Medtronic). However, to date, randomized trials in which providers use individual monitoring parameters or algorithms combining multiple parameters to guide therapy have not consistently led to a reduction in HFH or mortality.[52-54]

Ventricular Filling Pressures as a Target for Monitoring

Data using an implantable right ventricular pressure monitor that provides an estimate of diastolic pulmonary artery pressure (PAP) has shown that one of the earliest and most consistent changes prior to an HF exacerbation is an increase in estimated diastolic PAP that closely reflects the increase in pulmonary capillary wedge pressure (PCWP).[55] Estimated diastolic PAP most often rises gradually, generally preceding symptoms and HFH by days to weeks[55] (Fig. 58.5A). While these changes in PAP are generally small, they are accurately measured by implantable devices, are similar in patients with HFrEF and HFpEF, and are not consistently associated with changes in body weight.[55] Algorithms based on multisensors have demonstrated a similar timeline prior to an HF exacerbation (Fig. 58.5B).[50] Both high baseline estimated diastolic PAP and an increase in estimated diastolic PAP are associated with increased HFH and increased mortality.[56] These data stimulated the development of implantable devices to directly measure PAP and the design of a large RCT using direct PAP monitoring.

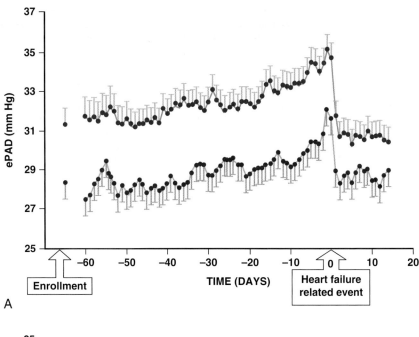

A

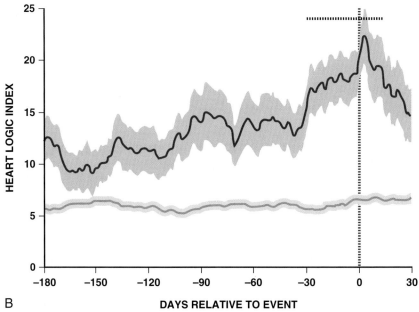

B

FIGURE 58.5 A, Daily median implantable hemodynamic monitor (IHM)-derived pressures (ePAD) in patients who experienced a heart failure related event (HFRE). Trends in daily median estimated pulmonary artery diastolic pressures (ePAD) are shown beginning 60 days before a hypervolemic HFRE and continuing for 14 days after the event. Systolic HF patients are represented by blue circles and diastolic HF patients by red circles. **B,** Temporal profile of HeartLogic index trends in patients with and without heart failure events. Data are displayed as mean ± SEM. The shaded regions represent the SEM. HeartLogic index in patients with usable HFE (*blue line*) aligned by the date of the HFE (*vertical line*) at day 0; HeartLogic index in patients without HFE (*black line*) aligned by the last available HeartLogic index date for each patient (day 30). (**A** from Zile MR, et al. Transition from chronic compensated to acute decompensated heart failure: pathophysiological insights obtained from continuous monitoring of intracardiac pressures. *Circulation.* 2008;118:1433-1441; **B** from Boehmer JP, et al. A multisensor algorithm predicts heart failure events in patients with implanted devices: results from the MultiSENSE study. *JACC Heart Fail.* 2017;5:216-225.)

Implantable Hemodynamic Monitors

The CardioMEMS Heart Sensor Allows Monitoring of Pressure to Improve Outcomes in NYHA Class III Heart Failure Patients (CHAMPION) trial evaluated the use of the CardioMEMs heart sensor—a device implanted in a small pulmonary artery that records high-fidelity pulmonary artery pressures that are downloaded and transmitted intermittently. The CHAMPION trial randomized HF patients with the implanted device, regardless of LVEF, to two groups: one in which clinicians were able to view PAP and respond according to a

suggested algorithm or to standard of care alone without access to PAP.[57] The CHAMPION trial differed from prior studies of implantable hemodynamic monitors in that specific pressure targets and treatment algorithms were suggested by protocol to ensure adequate testing of the hypothesis. The primary endpoint of the trial was the rate of HFH over 6 months, and long-term outcomes were also prospectively evaluated. Over a 6-month period, significantly fewer HFH occurred in the treatment group (83) than in the control group (120). During the entire single-blinded follow-up averaging 15 months, the treatment group had a 37% RRR in HF hospitalizations compared with the control group

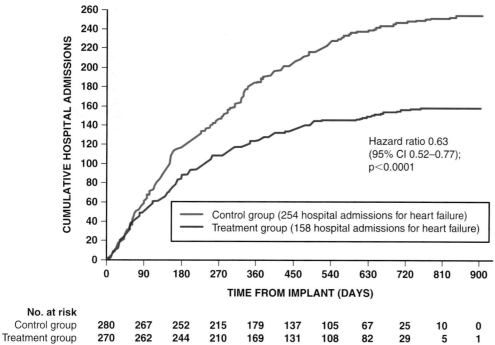

FIGURE 58.6 Primary (6-month) and extended results of the CHAMPION trial for the primary endpoint of heart failure (HF) hospitalization rate. (Modified from Abraham WT, et al. Wireless pulmonary artery haemodynamic monitoring in chronic heart failure: a randomised controlled trial. *Lancet.* 2011;377:658-666.)

(p < 0.001) (Fig. 58.6). Twice as many medication changes occurred in the actively monitored group and two-thirds of these changes were increases in medication doses while one-third were decreases.[58] The majority of pressure-based medication changes (≈75%), as expected, were diuretics. All four prespecified secondary endpoints were met favoring the treatment group, including PAP reduction, proportion of patients hospitalized for HF, days alive and out of the hospital for HF, and QoL score. Importantly, all results mentioned above were statistically significant in both the HFrEF and HFpEF patients; in fact, the highest reduction in HFH (52%) occurred in the HFpEF subgroup, which composed 22% of the patients studied.

The results of the CHAMPION trial led to FDA approval of the first implantable hemodynamic monitoring system in 2014, for use in HFrEF and HFpEF patients with NYHA Class III symptoms and a history of HF hospitalization within the previous year. The CHAMPION trial confirmed previous data that higher baseline estimated diastolic PAP predicts mortality and increases in PAP from baseline in PAP are also associated with increased mortality.[55]

Building on the results of this trial, the Hemodynamic-GUIDEd Management of Heart Failure (GUIDE-HF) Trial was designed. GUIDE-HF is a multicenter, trial consisting of a fully enrolled, double-blind, randomized arm (*n* = 1000) and a larger unblinded, unrandomized arm that is still enrolling.[59] In the randomized arm, patients with both NYHA Class II to IV, HFrEF or HFpEF and either or both a previous HFH or elevated BNP or NT-proBNP level underwent device implantation and then were randomized 1:1 to either PAP-guided therapy vs. no PAP guided therapy (control) for 12 months. The primary endpoint is ACM + HFH and is scheduled to be reported in 2021. Other implantable hemodynamic monitors are currently in development. Current AHA/ACC/HFSA guidelines do not include a recommendation for PAP monitoring.

INTERPLAY BETWEEN DRUGS AND DEVICES

As new medical and device therapies for HF are developed it will be important to refine and standardize definitions of response in order to initiate or continue therapies in likely "responders" (see Fig. 58.3). As HFrEF is generally a progressive disease, nonprogression may be a favorable response in some patients.[19] Further, it will be necessary to understand the interplay and potential synergies of drugs and devices. For example, CRT raises the systolic blood pressure, creating opportunity to either maintain or further uptitrate medical therapies that were limited by hypotension pre-CRT[8,9,60] (see Fig. 58.1). In the MADIT-CRT trial the greater degree of myocardial remodeling in the CRT group the more likely it was for patients to remain on either an ACEI or angiotensin receptor blocker (ARB) and/or to reduce diuretic doses or avoid diuretics entirely.[61] The ability to continue ACEI/ARBs and/or avoid diuretic escalation with CRT were both associated with a lower risk of ACM + HFH.[61] Furthermore, in a study of 650 patients who were on maximally tolerated GDMT prior to CRT, post-CRT uptitration of ACEI/ARB and beta blockers was possible in 45% and 57%, respectively.[62] Successful uptitration of either therapy was associated with a large reduction in ACM + HFH, a finding confirmed in another large observational trial.[63] It is, however, possible that the ability to uptitrate medical therapy following CRT is a marker of a group with better outcomes rather than the result of uptitration of medical therapy.

There is also an intriguing possibility that medical therapy may enhance the response to device therapies. A retrospective analysis of the COMPANION trial suggested that the relative benefit of CRT was larger with the addition of each of three classes of neurohormonal antagonists (ACEI/ARB, beta blockers, and MRA).[60] A similar result was suggested from a recent analysis of a CRT registry.[64] Further studies are required to determine whether this is a synergistic effect of CRT and medical therapies or if the ability to add or uptitrate medical therapy is a marker for patients who are more responsive to CRT.

Finally, it is important to remember that devices must be monitored to ensure proper functioning. CRT becomes less beneficial and perhaps ineffective as the percentage of pacing falls below 95%.[65] Patients with HFrEF may develop indications for device therapies over time so that candidacy for devices should be reconsidered at intervals, especially if HF worsens. LBBB appears in about 2.4% of HFrEF patients per year[1] and moderately severe or severe MR in about 3% to 4% per year in HFrEF patients on maximally tolerated GDMT.[36] The development of LBBB and/or significant SMR provides opportunities for CRT and TMVr, respectively, and should be considered in any HFrEF patient, especially in those who have progression of HF.

CONCLUSIONS

Implantable devices for monitoring and managing HF, particularly HFrEF, have become an integral part of standard therapy. Recently, several therapeutic devices have been developed and approved to address important pathophysiologic mechanisms often incompletely addressed by medical therapy. Additional data will inform the most beneficial use of these devices and their potential synergies with medical therapy.

REFERENCES

Dyssynchrony

1. Kristensen SL, Castagno D, Shen L, et al. Prevalence and incidence of intraventricular conduction delays and outcomes in patients with heart failure and reduced ejection fraction: insights from PARADIGM-HF and ATMOSPHERE [published online ahead of print, 2020 Jul 28]. *Eur J Heart Fail.* 2020.
2. Kirk JA, Kass DA. Cellular and molecular aspects of dyssynchrony and resynchronization. *Card Electrophysiol Clin.* 2015:585–597.
3. Hussein AA, Wilkoff BL. Cardiac implantable electronic device therapy in heart failure. *Circ Res.* 2019;124:1584–1597.

Randomized Controlled Trials of Cardiac Resynchronization Therapy

4. Cazeau S, Leclercq C, Lavergne T, et al. Effects of multisite biventricular pacing in patients with heart failure and intraventricular conduction delay. *N Engl J Med.* 2001;344(12):873–880.
5. Abraham WT, Fisher WG, Smith AL, MIRACLE Study Group, et al. Multicenter InSync randomized clinical evaluation. Cardiac resynchronization in chronic heart failure. *N Engl J Med.* 2002;346:1845–1853.
6. Young JB, Abraham WT, Smith AL, et al. Combined cardiac resynchronization and implantable cardioversion defibrillation in advanced chronic heart failure: the MIRACLE ICD Trial. *J Am Med Assoc.* 2003;289:2685–2694.
7. Higgins SL, Hummel JD, Niazi IK, et al. Cardiac resynchronization therapy for the treatment of heart failure in patients with intraventricular conduction delay and malignant ventricular tachyarrhythmias. *J Am Coll Cardiol.* 2003;42:1454–1459.
8. Bristow MR, Saxon LA, Boehmer J, et al. Cardiac-resynchronization therapy with or without an implantable defibrillator in advanced chronic heart failure. *N Engl J Med.* 2004;350:2140–2150.
9. Cleland JG, Daubert JC, Erdmann E, et al. The effect of cardiac resynchronization on morbidity and mortality in heart failure. *N Engl J Med.* 2005;352:1539–1549.
10. Abraham WT, Young JB, León AR, et al. Effects of cardiac resynchronization on disease progression in patients with left ventricular systolic dysfunction, an indication for an implantable cardioverter-defibrillator, and mildly symptomatic chronic heart failure. *Circulation.* 2004;110:2864–2868.
11. Linde C, Abraham WT, Gold MR, et al. Randomized trial of cardiac resynchronization in mildly symptomatic heart failure patients and in asymptomatic patients with left ventricular dysfunction and previous heart failure symptoms. *J Am Coll Cardiol.* 2008;52:1834–1843.
12. Moss AJ, Hall WJ, Cannom DS, et al. Cardiac-resynchronization therapy for the prevention of heart-failure events. *N Engl J Med.* 2009;361:1329–1338.
13. Tang AS, Wells GA, Talajic M, et al. Cardiac-resynchronization therapy for mild-to-moderate heart failure. *N Engl J Med.* 2010;363:2385–2395.
14. Zareba W, Klein H, Cygankiewicz I, et al. Effectiveness of cardiac resynchronization therapy by QRS morphology in the Multicenter Automatic Defibrillator Implantation Trial-Cardiac Resynchronization Therapy (MADIT-CRT). *Circulation.* 2011;123:1061–1072.
15. Solomon SD, Foster E, Bourgoun M, et al. Effect of cardiac resynchronization therapy on reverse remodeling and relation to outcome: multicenter automatic defibrillator implantation trial: cardiac resynchronization therapy. *Circulation.* 2010;122:985–992.
16. Ruschitzka F, Abraham WT, Singh JP, et al. Cardiac-resynchronization therapy in heart failure with a narrow QRS complex. *N Engl J Med.* 2013;369:1395–1405.
17. Curtis AB, Worley SJ, Adamson PB, Biventricular vs. Right Ventricular Pacing in Heart Failure Patients with Atrioventricular Block (BLOCK HF) Trial Investigators, et al. Biventricular pacing for atrioventricular block and systolic dysfunction. *N Engl J Med.* 2013;368:1585–1593.
18. Chung ES, Leon AR, Tavazzi L, et al. Results of the predictors of response to CRT (PROSPECT) trial. *Circulation.* 2008;117:2608–2616.
19. Steffel J, Ruschitzka F. Superresponse to cardiac resynchronization therapy. *Circulation.* 2014;130(1):87–90.
20. Ruwald MH, Mittal S, Ruwald AC, et al. Association between frequency of atrial and ventricular ectopic beats and biventricular pacing percentage and outcomes in patients with cardiac resynchronization therapy. *J Am Coll Cardiol.* 2014;64:971–981.
21. Friedman DJ, Emerek K, Kisslo J, et al. Left bundle-branch block is associated with asimilar dyssynchronous phenotype in heart failure patients with normal and reduced ejection fractions. *Am Heart J.* 2020;231:45–55.

Primary Prevention of Sudden Cardiac Death

22. Moss AJ, Zareba W, Hall WJ, et al. Prophylactic implantation of a defibrillator in patients with myocardial infarction and reduced ejection fraction. *N Engl J Med.* 2002;346:877–883.
23. Kadish A, Dyer A, Daubert JP, et al. Prophylactic defibrillator implantation in patients with nonischemic dilated cardiomyopathy. *N Engl J Med.* 2004;350:2151–2158.
24. Bardy GH, Lee KL, Mark DB, Sudden Cardiac Death in Heart Failure Trial (SCD-HeFT) Investigators, et al. Amiodarone or an implantable cardioverter-defibrillator for congestive heart failure. *N Engl J Med.* 2005;352:225–237.
25. Køber L, Thune JJ, Nielsen JC, DANISH Investigators, et al. Defibrillator implantation in patients with nonischemic systolic heart failure. *N Engl J Med.* 2016;375:1221–1230.
26. Shen L, Jhund PS, Petrie MC, et al. Declining risk of sudden death in heart failure. *N Engl J Med.* 2017;377:41–51.
27. Shun-Shin MJ, Zheng SL, Cole GD, et al. Implantable cardioverter defibrillators for primary prevention of death in left ventricular dysfunction with and without ischaemic heart disease: a meta-analysis of 8567 patients in the 11 trials. *Eur Heart J.* 2017;38:1738–1746.
28. Rohde LE, Chatterjee NA, Vaduganathan M, et al. Sacubitril/valsartan and sudden cardiac death according to implantable cardioverter-defibrillator use and heart failure cause: a PARADIGM-HF analysis. *JACC Heart Fail.* 2020;8:844–855.

Guidelines

29. Tracy CM, Epstein AE, Darbar D, et al. 2012 ACCF/AHA/HRS focused update of the 2008 guidelines for device-based therapy of cardiac rhythm abnormalities: a report of the American College of Cardiology Foundation/American Heart Association Task Force on Practice Guidelines and the Heart Rhythm Society [corrected]. *Circulation.* 2012;126:1784–1800.
30. Al-Khatib SM, Stevenson WG, Ackerman MJ, et al. 2017 AHA/ACC/HRS guideline for management of patients with ventricular arrhythmias and the prevention of sudden cardiac death: executive summary: a report of the American College of Cardiology/American Heart Association Task Force on Clinical Practice Guidelines and the Heart Rhythm Society. *Heart Rhythm.* 2018;15:e190–e252.
31. Yancy CW, Jessup M, Bozkurt B, et al. 2017 ACC/AHA/HFSA focused update of the 2013 ACCF/AHA guideline for the management of heart failure: a report of the American College of Cardiology/American Heart Association Task Force on Clinical Practice Guidelines and the Heart Failure Society of America. *Circulation.* 2017;136(6):e137–e161.

New Therapeutic Devices for Heart Failure

32. Costanzo MR, Ponikowski P, Javaheri S, et al. Transvenous neurostimulation for central sleep apnoea: a randomised controlled trial. *Lancet.* 2016;388:974–982.
33. Stone GW, Lindenfeld J, Abraham WT, et al. Transcatheter mitral-valve repair in patients with heart failure. *N Engl J Med.* 2018;379:2307–2318.
34. Abraham WT, Kuck KH, Goldsmith RL, et al. A randomized controlled trial to evaluate the safety and efficacy of cardiac contractility modulation. *JACC Heart Fail.* 2018;6(10):874–883.
35. Zile MR, Lindenfeld J, Weaver FA, et al. Baroreflex activation therapy in patients with heart failure with reduced ejection fraction. *J Am Coll Cardiol.* 2020;76(1):1–13.
36. Coats AJS. Monitoring for sleep-disordered breathing in heart failure. *Eur Heart J Suppl.* 2019;21(suppl M):M36–M39.
37. Cowie MR, Woehrle H, Wegscheider K, et al. Adaptive servo–ventilation for central sleep apnea in systolic heart failure. *N Engl J Med.* 2015;373:1095–1105.
38. Eulenburg C, Wegscheider K, Woehrle H, et al. Mechanisms underlying increased mortality risk in patients with heart failure and reduced ejection fraction randomly assigned to adaptive servoventilation in the SERVE-HF study: results of a secondary multistate modelling analysis. *Lancet Respir Med.* 2016;4:873–881.
39. Nasser R, Van Assche L, Vorlat A, et al. Evolution of functional mitral regurgitation and prognosis in medically managed heart failure patients with reduced ejection fraction. *JACC Heart Fail.* 2017;5:652–659.
40. Obadia JF, Messika-Zeitoun D, Leurent G, et al. Percutaneous repair or medical treatment for secondary mitral regurgitation. *N Engl J Med.* 2018;379(24):2297–2306.
41. Otto CM, Nishimura RA, Bonow RO, et al. 2020 ACC/AHA guideline for the management of patients with valvular heart disease: a report of the American College of Cardiology/American Heart Association Joint Committee on Clinical Practice Guidelines. *J Am Coll Cardiol.* 2020;80:S0735–S1097.
42. Campbell CM, Kahwash R, Abraham WT. Optimizer Smart in the treatment of moderate-to-severe chronic heart failure. *Future Cardiol.* 2020;16:13–25.
43. Wiegn P, Chan R, Jost C, et al. Safety, Performance, and efficacy of cardiac contractility modulation delivered by the 2-lead optimizer Smart system: the FIX-HF-5C2 Study. *Circ Heart Fail.* 2020;13.
44. Sobowale CO, Hori Y, Ajijola OA. Neuromodulation therapy in heart failure: combined use of drugs and devices. *J Innov Card Rhythm Manag.* 2020;11(7):4151–4159.
45. Abraham WT, Zile MR, Weaver FA, et al. Baroreflex activation therapy for the treatment of heart failure with a reduced ejection fraction. *JACC Heart Fail.* 2015;3(6):487–496.
46. Zile MR, Abraham WT, Weaver FA, et al. Baroreflex activation therapy for the treatment of heart failure with a reduced ejection fraction: safety and efficacy in patients with and without cardiac resynchronization therapy. *Eur J Heart Fail.* 2015;17:1066–1074.
47. Zile MR, Abraham WT, Lindenfeld J, et al. First granted example of novel FDA trial design under expedited access pathway for premarket approval: BeAT-HF. *Am Heart J.* 2018;204:139–150.

Implantable Devices to Monitor Heart Failure

48. Jackson SL, Tong X, King RJ, et al. National burden of heart failure events in the United States, 2006 to 2014. *Circ Heart Fail.* 2018;11(12):e004873.
49. Abraham WT, Perl L. Implantable hemodynamic monitoring for heart failure patients. *J Am Coll Cardiol.* 2017;70:389–398.
50. Boehmer JP, Hariharan R, Devecchi FG, et al. A multisensor algorithm predicts heart failure events in patients with implanted devices: results from the MultiSENSE study. *JACC Heart Fail.* 2017;5:216–225.
51. Ali O, Hajduczok AG, Boehmer JP. Remote physiologic monitoring for heart failure. *Curr Cardiol Rep.* 2020;22:68.
52. Heist EK, Herre JM, Binkley PF, et al. Analysis of different device-based intrathoracic impedance vectors for detection of heart failure events (from the Detect Fluid Early from Intrathoracic Impedance Monitoring study). *Am J Cardiol.* 2014;114:1249–1256.
53. Morgan JM, Kitt S, Gill J, et al. Remote management of heart failure using implantable electronic devices. *Eur Heart J.* 2017;38(30):2352–2360.
54. Hindricks G, Taborsky M, Glikson M, et al. Implant-based multiparameter telemonitoring of patients with heart failure (IN-TIME): a randomised controlled trial. *Lancet.* 2014;384:583–590.
55. Zile MR, Bennett TD, St John Sutton M, et al. Transition from chronic compensated to acute decompensated heart failure: pathophysiological insights obtained from continuous monitoring of intracardiac pressures. *Circulation.* 2008;118:1433–1441.
56. Zile MR, Bennett TD, El Hajj S, et al. Intracardiac pressures measured using an implantable hemodynamic monitor: relationship to mortality in patients with chronic heart failure. *Circ Heart Fail.* 2017;10:1–9.
57. Abraham WT, Adamson PB, Bourge RC, et al. Wireless pulmonary artery haemodynamic monitoring in chronic heart failure: a randomised controlled trial. *Lancet.* 2011;377:658–666.
58. Costanzo MR, Stevenson LW, Adamson PB, et al. Interventions linked to decreased heart failure hospitalizations during ambulatory pulmonary artery pressure monitoring. *JACC Heart Fail.* 2016;4:333–344.
59. Lindenfeld J, Abraham WT, Maisel A, et al. Hemodynamic-GUIDEd management of Heart Failure (GUIDE-HF). *Am Heart J.* 2019;214:18–27.

Interplay Between Drugs and Devices

60. Bristow MR, Saxon LA, Feldman AM, et al. Lessons learned and insights gained in the design, analysis, and outcomes of the COMPANION trial. *JACC Heart Fail.* 2016;4:521–535.
61. Penn J, Goldenberg I, McNitt S, et al. Changes in drug utilization and outcome with cardiac resynchronization therapy: a MADIT-CRT substudy. *J Card Fail.* 2015l;21:541–547.
62. Martens P, Verbrugge FH, Nijst P, et al. Feasibility and association of neurohumoral blocker uptitration after cardiac resynchronization therapy. *J Card Fail.* 2017;23:597–605.
63. Witt CT, Kronborg MB, Nohr EA, et al. Optimization of heart failure medication after cardiac resynchronization therapy and the impact on long-term survival. *Eur Heart J Cardiovasc Pharmacother.* 2015;1:182–188.
64. Schmidt S, Hürlimann D, Starck CT, et al. Treatment with higher dosages of heart failure medication is associated with improved outcome following cardiac resynchronization therapy. *Eur Heart J.* 2014;35:1051–1060.
65. Ruwald MH, Mittal S, Ruwald AC, et al. Association between frequency of atrial and ventricular ectopic beats and biventricular pacing percentage and outcomes in patients with cardiac resynchronization therapy. *J Am Coll Cardiol.* 2014;64(10):971–981.

59 Mechanical Circulatory Support

KEITH D. AARONSON AND FRANCIS D. PAGANI

Mechanical circulatory support (MCS) devices are mechanical pumps designed to assist or replace the function of the left and/or right ventricle(s) of the heart. Important features that characterize MCS devices include: (1) location of the pumping chamber; (2) ventricle(s) supported by the pump; (3) pumping mechanism; and (4) intended use and duration of support (Table 59.1). Typically, temporary MCS devices, used for days or weeks of support, are *extracorporeal* (or *paracorporeal*) pumps (pump located outside the body), whereas durable devices, used for months to years of support, are implantable (*intracorporeal*) systems.

INDICATIONS, STRATEGIES, AND DEVICE SELECTION

MCS devices are indicated to provide hemodynamic support to patients with cardiogenic shock or symptomatic advanced heart failure (HF) refractory to guideline-directed medical care. The goal of MCS therapy is to provide hemodynamic support to the patient in one of three clinical scenarios: (1) patients with severe but potentially reversible heart dysfunction until native heart function sufficiently recovers to have the MCS device successfully withdrawn for anticipated long-term survival without MCS (i.e., bridge to recovery, BTR); (2) patients with severe and irreversible heart dysfunction who are failing medical therapy, to allow sufficient time for allocation and transplantation of a donor heart (i.e., bridge to heart transplantation, BTT); or (3) patients with severe and irreversible heart dysfunction who are failing medical therapy but not eligible for heart transplantation, for permanent support (i.e., destination therapy [DT]). Candid discussion with each patient about which ventricular assist device (VAD) treatment strategy is being used is both legally and morally essential, allays unreasonable expectations, and improves patient satisfaction. However, that discussion should include the understanding that recipients often move between strategies as their clinical circumstances evolve. The decision to initiate MCS must include an analysis of the intended use and clinical setting, patient variables and conditions, the type of MCS devices available for the selected indication, medical society guidelines for use of the device, and financial considerations.

Bridge to Recovery

BTR refers to the use of MCS devices in patients with acute cardiogenic shock or acute decompensated HF that is refractory to guideline-directed medical therapy. In these clinical scenarios, there is a reasonable expectation that the myocardial injury is reversible and that myocardial function will recover during a short period of temporary MCS; this is generally the default strategy when applying temporary

MCS. The use of MCS for BTR is the most common application of MCS in the United States.[1] Examples of reversible forms of myocardial injury are acute myocardial infarction (AMI), acute myocarditis, and postcardiotomy cardiogenic shock resulting from ischemic myocardial stunning. Several types of MCS devices can provide temporary circulatory support in these circumstances, including intra-aortic balloon pumps (IABP) (Fig. 59.1), surgically or percutaneously placed extracorporeal/paracorporeal VADs (Figs. 59.2 to 59.4), and systems for extracorporeal life support (ECLS; Fig. 59.5) (or extracorporeal membrane oxygenation [ECMO]), which can provide both cardiac and pulmonary support. Typically, temporary MCS devices such as the IABP, Impella VAD (Abiomed, Inc., Danvers, MA), or TandemHeart VAD (TandemLife, Inc., Pittsburgh, PA) are placed percutaneously to enable rapid initiation of cardiac support and subsequent ease of removal when cardiac function recovers. Some types of extracorporeal VAD systems (i.e., CentriMag VAD; Abbott Labs, Chicago, IL) require major operative procedures with sternotomy or less-invasive thoracotomy incisions for access and placement of the outflow and inflow cannulas, and more frequently are initiated in the operating room for postcardiotomy HF following failure to wean from cardiopulmonary bypass (CPB; see Fig. 59.2).

The assumption that myocardial injury is reversible may not be accurate, and this may be especially so when the patient presents with significant hemodynamic compromise and significant organ injury. Temporary MCS may be instituted with the expectation of clinical improvement, but the subsequent recognition that myocardial recovery has not occurred and is unlikely to occur despite an extended period of hemodynamic support requires strategic adjustment. In such situations, temporary MCS can be continued as a bridge to placement of a durable, implantable VAD or total artificial heart (TAH; *bridge to bridge* [BTB] application), or continued as a bridge to heart transplantation.[2] The use of temporary MCS devices in this way is not an approved indication for these devices but occasionally may be appropriate because of the inherent difficulties in accurately assessing the potential for myocardial recovery in all clinical settings. Historically, durable, implantable VADs have been the most common form of MCS to provide BTT support. However, recent changes to the United States heart transplant allocation system have given greater relative priority to patients supported with temporary MCS devices, including ECMO, compared to durable, implantable VADs.[2] As a result, there has been a significant change in clinical practice patterns with more patients being bridged to heart transplantation with temporary MCS devices, particularly with IABP counterpulsation support.[2]

As a rule, patients should be excluded from consideration for temporary MCS if myocardial recovery is unlikely and the option of heart transplantation or implantation of a long-term, durable VAD is not feasible. In these clinical scenarios, MCS should not be instituted and is considered futile.

Bridge to Transplantation

The second indication for MCS applies to patients presenting with cardiogenic shock or decompensated advanced HF refractory to guideline directed medical management in whom myocardial function is

TABLE 59.1 Terminology Describing Characteristics of Mechanical Circulatory Support Devices

Pump Location
Extracorporeal: Pump located outside the body
Paracorporeal: Pump located outside but adjacent to the body
Intracorporeal: Pump implanted within the body
Orthotopic: In the normal position of the heart (TAH)

Ventricle Supported
LV support (LVAD)
RV support (RVAD)
Biventricular support (BiVAD)
Biventricular replacement (TAH)

Intended Use
Short-term: Days to weeks (BTR indication)
1. Patient remains hospitalized
2. Patient tethered to pump
Long-term: Months to years (BTT or DT indication)
1. Patient discharged with untethered, "hands-free" mobility

Pump Mechanism[6,7]
Pulsatile flow, volume displacement with:
1. Pneumatic actuation, *or*
2. Electrical actuation
Continuous-flow rotary pump with *axial design* (flow of blood is along axis of symmetry of pump) *and*
1. Bearing support of impeller (mechanical pivot), *or*
2. Magnetic or hydrodynamic levitation of impeller (bearingless design)
Continuous-flow rotary pump with *centrifugal design* (flow of blood from center to periphery of pump) *and*
1. Bearing support of impeller, *or*
2. Magnetic or hydrodynamic levitation of impeller (bearingless design)

BiVAD, Biventricular assist device; *BTR,* bridge to recovery; *BTT,* bridge to transplantation; *DT,* destination therapy; *LVAD,* left ventricular assist device; *RVAD,* right ventricular assist device; *TAH,* total artificial heart.

unlikely to recover (e.g., longstanding ischemic, valvular, or idiopathic cardiomyopathy; severe AMI or myocarditis), and who are considered eligible for heart transplantation. Durable, implantable MCS devices designed for long-term use (months to years) permit untethered patient mobility and discharge from the hospital and are appropriate devices for BTT indication (Figs. 59.6 to 59.8). A major operative procedure, including CPB, is generally required for placement in most patients, although newer, smaller device designs permit less-invasive implant techniques without CPB.[3] These devices are ideally placed in patients with significant symptoms of HF who are either receiving intravenous (IV) inotropes or who are not on inotropes but have limiting symptoms at rest or with minimal activity, and in whom hemodynamics are stable and end-organ function is preserved or slowly deteriorating. Select patients with acutely unstable hemodynamics and compromised organ function may be better served by a bridge to decision (BTD) strategy consisting of temporary MCS, followed by placement of a durable MCS device only for those who respond with improvements in hemodynamics and organ function. Although durable, implantable MCS devices (VADs) are most frequently used in situations of chronic irreversible cardiac dysfunction, recovery of myocardial function may also occur to such a degree to permit removal of the durable MCS device.[4,5] Patients thought to have irreversible dysfunction, but who demonstrate sufficient recovery of cardiac function to permit explant of durable, implantable VADs, are most commonly young patients with short durations of HF and with a nonischemic cause of the HF.[4,5]

Recently, clinical trials evaluating newer durable, implantable MCS devices (left ventricular assist devices [LVADs]) have developed alternative terminology for durable, implantable MCS device use and have used the terms "short-term" support to refer to clinical situations where patients are receiving durable VADs as BTT therapy or BTR and "long-term" support to refer to clinical situations where patients are receiving durable VADs as BTT or DT.[6,7] Although confusing to use the term "short-term support" to refer to an indication for temporary and durable devices, the important message is that the ultimate indication for durable VAD implantation in a significant proportion of patients is unknown at the time of implant and patients may transition to either heart transplantation or DT depending on the clinical course following device implantation. Importantly, the initial intent—BTT or DT—does not appear to have a significant impact on long-term survival with durable VAD therapy.[7]

Destination Therapy

The feasibility of durable, implantable MCS devices to provide long-term support demonstrated through the BTT experience prompted further expansion of indications for durable, implantable MCS devices as a permanent alternative to heart transplantation. DT is the application of durable, implanted MCS in patients with chronic refractory symptoms of advanced HF that result from irreversible forms of either nonischemic or ischemic cardiomyopathy and who are ineligible for heart transplantation. Use of durable, implantable devices that permit

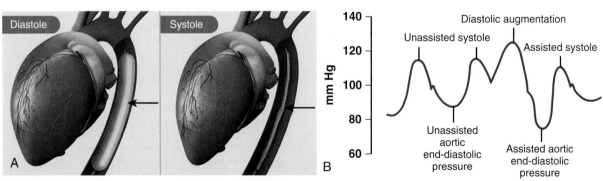

FIGURE 59.1 A, Intra-aortic balloon pump (IABP) positioned in descending aorta and inflated during diastole (increasing diastolic blood pressure and coronary perfusion) and deflated during systole (reducing ventricular afterload). **B,** Aortic pressure tracing during IABP support. Balloon counterpulsation is occurring after every other heartbeat (1:2 counterpulsation). With correct timing, balloon inflation begins immediately after aortic valve closure, signaled by the dicrotic notch of the arterial waveform. Compared with unassisted ejection, the pump augments diastolic blood flow by increasing peak aortic pressure during diastole. Balloon deflation before systole decreases ventricular afterload, with lower aortic end-diastolic pressure and lower peak systolic pressure.

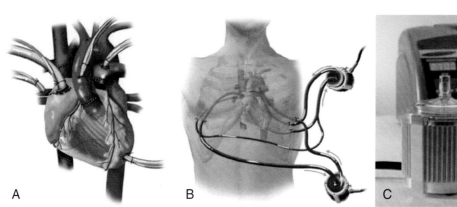

FIGURE 59.2 Temporary extracorporeal mechanical circulatory support: CentriMag Ventricular Assist System (Abbott Labs, Chicago, IL). **A,** Surgically implanted cannula for biventricular support configuration. *Left ventricular support*: A cannula is positioned in the right superior pulmonary vein (cannula depicted on the far left of the picture) and drains blood from the left atrium and pumps it back to the aorta. (Alternative cannula configuration includes a cannula inserted into the left ventricular apex (far bottom right of the figure) draining the left ventricle and returning blood to the cannula positioned in the ascending aorta). *Right ventricular support*: A cannula positioned in the right atrial appendage (second from left) drains blood from the right atrium and pumps it to the main pulmonary artery (cannula in the upper right corner of the figure). **B,** Cannula connected to external blood pumps (extracorporeal pumps) supporting right and left ventricles. **C,** The CentriMag is a continuous-flow rotary pump with centrifugal design and full magnetic levitation of the internal rotor.

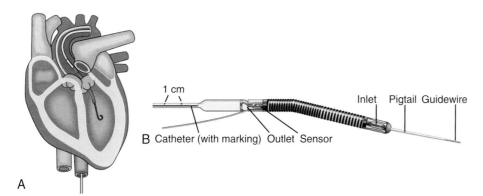

FIGURE 59.3 Temporary mechanical circulatory support: Impella (Abiomed, Inc., Danvers, MA). **A,** The Impella is a continuous-flow, microaxial pump designed to propel blood from the left ventricle into the ascending aorta, in series with the left ventricle. The tip is positioned within the left ventricle, and blood is pumped from the left ventricle into the ascending aorta. **B,** The tip of the catheter is a flexible pigtail loop that stabilizes the device within the left ventricle. The catheter connects to a cannula that contains the pump inlet and outlet areas, motor housing, and pump-pressure monitor. The proximal end of the catheter is connected to the external pump. (From Thunberg CA, Gaitan BD, Arabia FA, et al. Ventricular assist devices today and tomorrow. *J Cardiothorac Vasc Anesth.* 2010;24:656.)

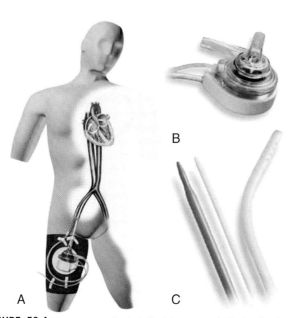

FIGURE 59.4 Temporary mechanical circulatory support: TandemHeart percutaneous ventricular assist device (pVAD) (TandemLife, Inc., Pittsburgh, PA). **A,** The TandemHeart pVAD has four components: a centrifugal pump with hydrodynamic levitation of the internal rotor positioned on the right thigh **(B)**, a 21F transseptal cannula **(C)**, a femoral arterial cannula, and a control console.

untethered "hands-free" patient mobility at home is appropriate in this clinical situation. A major operative procedure is required for placement of these implantable pumps, which, as in the setting of BTT, are ideally used in patients with significant symptoms of advanced HF

with stable hemodynamics and without manifestations of significant organ injury, irreversible frailty, or cachexia. The benefits of MCS for DT, in terms of survival, function, and quality of life, for the treatment of chronic advanced HF were first established in a prospective, randomized trial known as REMATCH (Randomized Evaluation of Mechanical Assistance in the Treatment of Congestive Heart Failure).[8] REMATCH evaluated the use of a durable, implantable LVAD compared with optimal medical management (OMM) for refractory chronic advanced HF. LVAD therapy halved (relative risk [RR], 0.52; 95% confidence interval [CI] 0.34 to 0.78) the mortality seen in the control population (92% at 2 years) treated with OMM. Despite serious adverse events (e.g., stroke, infection, bleeding, and device malfunction) attributable to MCS, LVAD recipients experienced a better quality of life than those in the OMM group.

Patients evaluated for DT must meet specific criteria for reimbursement from CMS that include: (1) ineligibility for heart transplantation; (2) significant functional limitations consistent with New York Heart Association (NYHA) Class IIIB or IV symptoms for 45 of the preceding 60 days, despite the use of maximally tolerated doses of drugs outlined in guidelines for HF treatment; (3) left ventricular ejection fraction (LVEF) less than 25%; and (4) a peak exercise oxygen consumption (peak VO_2) of 14 mL/kg/min or less, unless the patient is dependent on IV inotropes for 14 days or IABP for 7 days.[9] Although the current reimbursement framework requires determination of DT or BTT status, it is often not possible when assessing VAD candidacy to accurately determine future transplant eligibility. Many patients present with hemodynamic compromise, significant pulmonary hypertension, organ injury, cachexia, or debilitation, all of which represent relative contraindications to heart transplantation but may be reversible with a period of MCS.

The terms *bridge to candidacy* (BTC) and *bridge to decision* reflect the unknown efficacy of MCS therapy to reverse the clinical conditions that represent relative barriers to heart transplantation. In a similar vein, patients receiving MCS for BTT indication may experience significant

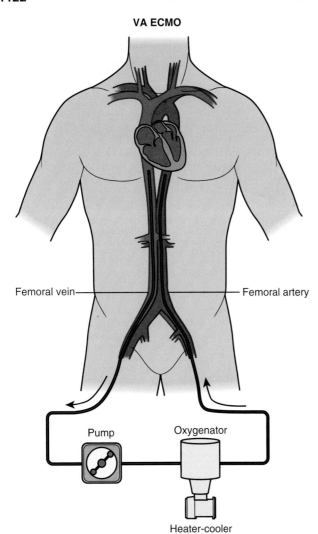

VA ECMO

Femoral vein

Femoral artery

Pump

Oxygenator

Heater-cooler

FIGURE 59.5 Extracorporeal life support (ECLS) or extracorporeal membrane oxygenation (ECMO) circuit. The ECMO circuit is used to establish rapid initiation of mechanical circulatory support. The circuit consists of a pump (typically a centrifugal pump system), oxygenator, and heater-cooler element. A typical configuration for emergent application of ECMO is percutaneous placement of cannulas in the femoral vein and femoral artery.

complications after implantation of an MCS device that could adversely affect transplantation candidate status. Recent clinical trials investigating new devices for durable VAD therapy have attempted to reframe VAD candidacy without reference to transplant candidacy by using patient characteristics and physiologic parameters to define an indication for "long-term support."[6,7,10] In the future, this unifying indication of long-term support with coverage determination likely will encompass MCS therapy with durable devices for long-term support independent of transplant eligibility.

DESIGN OF VENTRICULAR ASSIST DEVICES

An MCS pump or pumps may be positioned extracorporeally (outside the body) (see Figs. 59.1 through 59.5) or intracorporeally (contained within the body) (see Figs. 59.6 through 59.9) as a biventricular assist device (BiVAD), a right ventricular assist device (RVAD), or more often as an LVAD. The pump's flow characteristic further classifies pump type as *pulsatile flow* or *continuous flow*. The older generation, pulsatile flow, volume displacement pumps, such as the HeartMate XVE and Novacor LVAS, were large, had limited durability, and are now of only historical interest.[11] Newer-generation continuous-flow pumps are smaller, capable of a similar degree of pumping support (6 to 10 liters per minute [L/min]), more durable, and functionally dependent on both preload and afterload. These include the HeartMate 3 (HM3)

(see Fig. 59.6), the HeartMate II (HMII) (see Fig. 59.7), and HeartWare ventricular assist device (HVAD) (see Fig. 59.8).[6,7,10,12–16] For more information see the online supplement "Engineering Designs of Ventricular Assist Devices." The improvements in design attributes of the newest continuous-flow pump (HM3) with centrifugal design, including complete magnetic levitation of the internal rotor, decreased mechanical wear, operation at low flow, and improved potential for hemocompatibility were recently studied in the MOMENTUM 3 (Multi-center Study of MagLev Technology in Patients Undergoing MCS Therapy with Heart-Mate 3) clinical trial.[6,7,10,16]

PATIENT SELECTION, COMORBIDITY, AND TIMING OF INTERVENTION

Appropriately timing the initiation of MCS is crucial to obtaining satisfactory patient outcomes. There are no absolute hemodynamic criteria to meet to initiate MCS for any indication. Generally, patients presenting with acute forms of myocardial injury exhibit recognizable changes in hemodynamics. A cardiac index less than 1.8 to 2.2 L/min/m², systolic blood pressure less than 90 mm Hg, pulmonary capillary wedge pressure (PCWP) greater than 20 mm Hg, and evidence of poor tissue perfusion, reflected by oliguria, rising serum creatinine, arterial lactate, and liver transaminases, mental status changes, or cool extremities, despite the use of guideline directed medical therapy, constitute general indications for initiation of MCS.[17–19] Patient history and overall clinical setting also need to be considered in the decision. When the patient's clinical status reaches this degree of hemodynamic compromise, the risk of death is substantial, exceeding more than 50% at 30 days, despite the availability of OMM, invasive circulatory monitoring, thrombolysis, and IABP support.[17–19]

More subtle indications to initiate MCS may be present, particularly in patients with chronic advanced HF who are being evaluated for BTT or DT. These indications include resting tachycardia, progressive organ dysfunction, and persistent significant HF symptoms resulting in limited functional capacity and poor quality of life despite guideline directed medical therapy, with or without inotrope use.[20,21] In chronic HF patients who had previously maintained good end-organ function and functional performance despite substantially compromised hemodynamics, deterioration in end-organ function or progressive decline in functional performance may occur in the absence of any significant change in hemodynamic parameters.[22] Ambulatory patients with NYHA Class IIIB or IV symptoms who do not tolerate guideline directed medical therapy for advanced HF, or who experience renal insufficiency or hypotension with optimal dosages of angiotensin-converting enzyme (ACE) inhibitors or beta blockers, may need evaluation for MCS therapy.[22] Patients who require inotrope therapy or who do not tolerate inotrope therapy as a result of refractory ventricular arrhythmias, or those who have life-threatening coronary anatomy and unstable angina not amenable to revascularization and are at risk of imminent death (hours, days, or weeks), may be considered for MCS without necessarily meeting hemodynamic criteria.

Renal Function

Renal dysfunction has consistently been one of the greatest risks for morbidity and mortality with the use of MCS.[23] Renal dysfunction may be secondary to decreased perfusion of the kidney in cardiogenic shock or advanced HF, but elevated central venous pressure is the hemodynamic abnormality most closely associated with worsening renal function during in-hospital diuresis. Kidney dysfunction may result from intrarenal hemodynamic derangements reflecting overactivity of the renin-angiotensin-aldosterone (RAAS) and sympathetic nervous systems in advanced HF as well as from the effects of guideline directed medical therapy blocking these systems (although renal deterioration resulting from the latter should generally not limit their use) and immune-mediated nephrotoxicity or complications of noncardiac comorbidity. In patients with shock or advanced HF, it is difficult to assess the reversibility of renal dysfunction. Acute onset of renal failure requiring renal replacement therapy is not necessarily a contraindication to initiate short-term MCS but may be a greater obstacle to successful long-term support with implantable devices for BTT and in particular, DT. In the setting of cardiogenic shock with acute renal failure, establishing normal hemodynamics with MCS may resolve the renal failure in a relatively short period. However, a preimplant creatinine clearance of less than 30 mL/min/m² is associated with a 22% 3-month mortality in recipients of a continuous-flow LVAD, and this constitutes a relative contraindication to durable LVAD implantation at most centers.[23] Thus the degree and duration of cardiogenic shock, along with the patient's baseline renal function, must be considered in estimating the probability of recovery of renal function.

Pulmonary Function and Pulmonary Hypertension (see Chapter 88)

HF may be associated with a restrictive pattern on pulmonary function testing. However, this often improves with removal of interstitial fluid and pleural effusions after placement of an MCS device and resolution of lung congestion. Patients with a long history of smoking or a history of other intrinsic lung disease with significant abnormalities on pulmonary function testing—for example, less than 50% of predicted normal value for forced vital capacity (FVC), forced expiratory volume at 1 second (FEV₁), or diffusion capacity for carbon monoxide (DLco)—should undergo high-resolution computed tomography (CT). Patients with low oxygen saturation (<92%) on room air also require evaluation with echocardiography to rule out a right-to-left shunt from an atrial septal defect or patent foramen ovale. If results are negative, spiral (helical) CT or radionuclide scanning (in patients without pulmonary abnormalities on chest radiography) is warranted to rule out thromboembolic disease. Patients with severe pulmonary disease and HF patients with chronically elevated pulmonary venous pressures may have an elevated pulmonary vascular resistance (PVR) that is fixed (not responsive to pulmonary artery vasodilators). High fixed PVR (thresholds vary from 3 to 6 Wood units) represents a contraindication to heart transplantation and consequently to use of LVAD for BTT indication. Moderate elevations in PVR can be encountered in patients with cardiogenic shock and especially in those with long-established HF and does not preclude successful use of LVAD, if lowering of PVR (reversibility) is achieved with inotropes or pulmonary vasodilators. PVR frequently declines a few months after LVAD implantation, so patients deemed not transplantable because of elevated PVR at the time of implant may later become eligible. Perioperative hypoxia secondary to significant underlying lung disease may contribute to pulmonary vasoconstriction, leading to right ventricular (RV) failure after institution of VAD support. Sleep apnea is present in a significant number of patients with HF, which may contribute to pulmonary hypertension.

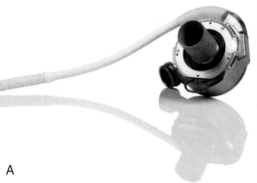 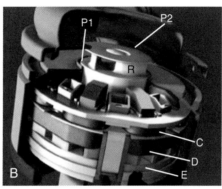

FIGURE 59.6 Implantable durable left ventricular assist device—HeartMate 3 (HM3, Abbott Labs, Chicago, IL). **A,** The HM3 left ventricular assist device (LVAD) is a continuous-flow rotary pump with centrifugal design and complete magnetic levitation of the internal rotor. The blood pump is positioned within the pericardial space, with its integral inflow conduit in the left ventricle and outflow graft (*not shown*) attached to the ascending aorta. The percutaneous power cable is tunneled through the abdominal wall and is attached to the system controller that receives power from two lithium-ion batteries. The implanted components include the inflow cannula, pump housing, motor, control electronics, outflow graft and bend relief, and percutaneous driveline. The HM3 uses a centrifugal flow pump that has a capacity to pump blood up to 10 L/min. Left ventricular (LV) blood is drawn into the inflow cannula along a central axis and is expelled at right angles by and between the impeller blades of a rotor rotating about the central axis. Blood is angularly accelerated and travels around a volute before it is diffused to a desired pressure and flow rate by being directed tangentially into the outflow graft. The pump rotor is fully supported by magnetic levitation, obviating mechanical or fluid bearings and essentially eliminating mechanical wear as a reliability factor. Both drive (i.e., rotation) and levitation of the rotor is accomplished using a single stator comprising iron pole pieces, a back-iron, copper coils, and position sensors. Measuring the position of a permanent magnet in the rotor and controlling the current in the drive and levitation coils enables active control of the radial position and rotational speed of the rotor. Because the permanent magnet is attracted to the iron pole pieces, the rotor passively resists excursion in the axial direction, whether translating or tilting. The electronics and software necessary to control motor drive and levitation are integrated into the lower housing with the stator; these components plus the rotor comprise the motor. **B,** Cross section of an implantable durable continuous-flow rotary pump with centrifugal design and complete magnetic levitation of the internal rotor. The rotor (*R*) is magnetically levitated by electromagnetic coils (*C*) and rotated by motor drive coils (*D*). The levitated rotor produces wide recirculation passages radially (*P1*) and axially (*P2*). A second axial passage beneath the rotor is hidden in this view. Motor electronics (*E*) are incorporated into the implantable pump. (From Heatley G, Sood P, Goldstein D, et al. Clinical trial design and rationale of the Multicenter Study of MagLev Technology in Patients Undergoing Mechanical Circulatory Support Therapy with HeartMate 3 (MOMENTUM 3) investigational device exemption clinical study protocol. *J Heart Lung Transplant.* 2016;35:528.)

Hepatic Function

Preoperative total bilirubin level (in the absence of Gilbert syndrome) and transaminase levels more than three times normal are independent risk factors for RV failure and reduced survival following LVAD implantation. The cause of the hyperbilirubinemia may be multifactorial, including congestive hepatopathy, cirrhosis, or a combination of causative disorders. Abnormal liver function often is associated with abnormal coagulation factors, as well as low serum albumin. Attempts should be made to normalize all indices of liver function and the cause(s) of any abnormalities preoperatively. The presence of portal hypertension with liver cirrhosis is a contraindication to initiating MCS support. A history of significant alcohol use should be ruled out in

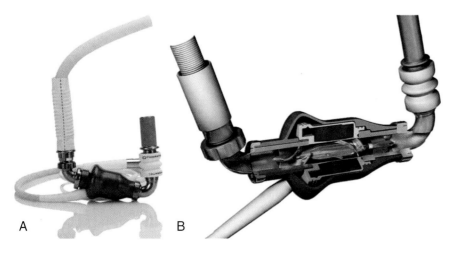

FIGURE 59.7 Implantable durable left ventricular assist device—HeartMate II (HMII; Abbott Labs, Chicago, IL). **A,** The HMII left ventricular assist device (LVAD) is a continuous-flow rotary pump with axial design and mechanical support of the internal rotor. The device is positioned outside the pericardial space in a preperitoneal pump pocket. The inlet cannula is inserted into the apex of the left ventricle, and the outflow graft is attached to the ascending aorta. **B,** Internal view of the HMII device demonstrating blood flow path with internal rotor containing a magnet suspended by mechanical pivots (stators) and external wiring (coils), creating a rotating magnetic field that spins the rotor (and internal magnet).

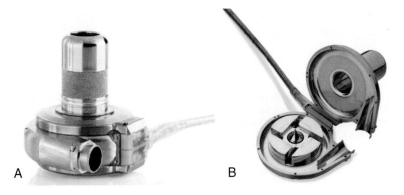

FIGURE 59.8 Implantable durable left ventricular assist device (LVAD)—HeartWare ventricular assist device (HVAD; Medtronic, Inc., Minneapolis, MN). **A,** The HVAD LVAD is a continuous-flow rotary pump with centrifugal design and hydrodynamic and magnetic levitation of the internal rotor. The pump is positioned within the pericardial space with the integrated inlet cannula positioned within the apex of the left ventricle and the outflow graft (*not shown*) sewn to the ascending aorta. The percutaneous driveline traverses the skin and attaches to an external controller and power source (batteries). **B,** Internal view of the pump demonstrating internal rotor that is levitated by magnets (passive magnetic field) positioned in the impeller and central post. Hydrodynamic forces generated by the top surface of the impeller stabilize impeller position.

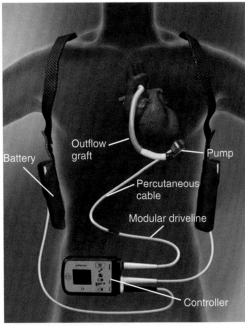

FIGURE 59.9 Typical configuration for a wearable durable left ventricular assist device (LVAD). The pump is attached to the apex of the left ventricle, and the outflow graft is attached to the ascending aorta. The power supply for implantable pumps is delivered through a percutaneous lead (also referred to as driveline) that traverses the skin and connects the external power system (batteries or stationary power unit) with the internal pump. The external components of an implantable system generally consist of a power source (i.e., batteries or an alternating-current [AC] power unit) and a small, portable computer (controller) that controls device speed and monitors device function.

all potential candidates for MCS therapy, especially those with abnormal liver function. Patients also should be tested for previous infection with hepatitis A, B, and C viruses. Ultrasound visualization of the liver is a good screening test in patients with significant hepatomegaly to rule out infiltrative disease, mass, or other pathologic condition that may warrant biopsy. Decrease in hepatic congestion and recovery of synthetic function can occur with institution of MCS.

Right Ventricular Function

Patients with advanced HF frequently have coexisting RV failure, a major contributor to morbidity and mortality after initiation of MCS.[24–26] RV failure is most commonly a result of LV failure. Compared to patients with HF resulting from coronary artery disease, patients with a non-ischemic cause are more likely to develop significant RV failure and have a three- to fourfold greater risk of requiring both LV and RV support. Patients who require BiVAD support have significantly higher preoperative creatinine and total bilirubin levels and a greater need for mechanical ventilation before MCS device insertion than patients requiring LVAD support only. The need for BiVAD support is associated with substantially worse survival with both short-term and long-term MCS devices because of a greater degree of compromised preoperative organ function.[24] RV failure is a prominent factor leading to renal dysfunction after LVAD implantation, because significantly elevated

right atrial (RA) pressures lead to changes in glomerular filtration from cortical to medullary nephrons, with secondary reduction in urine output and resistance to diuretic therapy. Preoperative optimization of RV function with a goal RA pressure ideally at 10 to 12 mm Hg is important in reducing the need for postoperative RV support. The higher the left atrial (LA) pressure or PCWP at device implantation, the greater is the benefit to the right ventricle and pulmonary artery pressure when the left ventricle is totally unloaded and LA pressure falls. Postoperative recovery of RV function, however, may lag for several days, because total decompression of the left ventricle allows a significant shift of the interventricular septum toward the left ventricle, with further distention and dysfunction of the RV.[25–30]

Coagulation (see Chapter 95)

Coagulopathy is a significant risk factor and a common abnormality noted in patients with refractory HF. An abnormal international normalized ratio (INR) in the absence of warfarin use is of added concern because it may reflect chronically high RA pressures, leading to hepatic congestion and, ultimately, to hepatic fibrosis and cirrhosis. Prolonged abnormal INR and low platelet count combined with use of anticoagulation or antiplatelet therapy are associated with significant perioperative bleeding, requiring multiple transfusions, leading to increased PVR, RV failure, decline in renal function, hemodynamic instability, and multiple-organ failure. In addition, patients with severe HF typically have a nutritional basis for abnormal coagulation because of depletion of several specific coagulation factors, such as factor VII. The minimum preoperative screen for coagulation abnormalities should include INR, platelet count, and in view of the high likelihood of previous heparin exposure, a heparin-induced thrombocytopenia (HIT) assay. The presence or development of HIT is associated with a high risk of bleeding, as well as thrombosis of MCS devices.

Other Medical Considerations

Other important medical considerations in instituting MCS include the presence or absence of significant aortic, mitral, or tricuspid valve disease, coronary artery disease, and atrial and ventricular arrhythmias, as well as intracardiac shunts. For more information see the online supplement "Patient Selection, Comorbidity, and Timing of Intervention."

PATIENT OUTCOMES

Temporary Mechanical Circulatory Support

Temporary MCS is indicated in patients with cardiogenic shock refractory to medical therapy when *rapidly achieved* augmentation of cardiac output and reduction of ventricular filling pressures are required to sustain life.[1] When used in the setting of medically refractory myocarditis or Takotsubo cardiomyopathy, temporary MCS may provide time for spontaneous recovery and discontinuation of MCS. When cardiogenic shock complicates longstanding HF, temporary MCS can provide the time needed for patients, family members, and physicians to make critical decisions about long-term MCS and heart transplantation. Patients with HF severe enough to warrant long-term MCS but with reversible clinical characteristics (e.g., coagulopathy from hepatic congestion, acute renal failure from low cardiac output and high RA pressure, hypoalbuminemia resulting from cardiac cachexia and bowel edema) that put them at high risk for perioperative death with a long-term device may benefit from temporary MCS, if their risk profile could be substantially improved with temporary MCS to the extent that they would become good candidates for a durable MCS device. The clinical evaluation of temporary MCS devices for treatment of cardiogenic shock generally has not involved randomized clinical trials but rather has relied on the use of prospective, single-arm observation studies to validate device design, safety, and efficacy. Table 59.2 summarizes extracorporeal assist devices and their characteristics.

Intra-Aortic Balloon Pump (see Chapter 38)

The IABP pump remains the most commonly used MCS device (see Fig. 59.1). The IABP consists of a balloon catheter and a pump console to control the timing of balloon inflation and deflation. The catheter is a double-lumen, 7.5- to 8.0-French (F) catheter with a polyethylene balloon attached at its distal end, with one lumen of the catheter attached to the pump and used to inflate the balloon with gas. Helium is used because its low viscosity facilitates rapid transfer in and out of the balloon, and because it absorbs very rapidly in blood if the balloon ruptures. Timing of balloon inflation and deflation is based on electrocardiogram (ECG) or pressure triggers. The balloon inflates with the onset of diastole, which roughly corresponds with electrophysiologic repolarization or the middle of the T wave on the surface ECG, or just after the dicrotic notch on the aortic pressure tracing. Following diastole, the balloon rapidly deflates at the onset of LV systole, which is timed electrocardiographically to the peak of the R wave on the surface ECG. The IABP increases diastolic blood pressure, decreases afterload, decreases myocardial oxygen consumption, increases coronary artery perfusion, and modestly enhances cardiac output. The IABP provides modest ventricular unloading but does increase mean arterial pressure and coronary blood flow. Patients must have some level of LV function and electrical stability for an IABP to be effective because any increase in cardiac output depends on the work of the heart itself. Optimal hemodynamic effect from the IABP depends on several factors, including the balloon's position in the aorta, the blood displacement volume, the balloon diameter in relation to aortic diameter, the timing of balloon inflation in diastole and deflation in systole, and the patient's own heart rate, blood pressure, and vascular resistance.

The efficacy of IABP counterpulsation was recently evaluated in the SHOCK II clinical trial (Randomized Clinical Study of Intra-aortic Balloon Pump Use in Cardiogenic Shock Complicating Acute Myocardial Infarction), a randomized, prospective, open-label, multicenter trial comparing IABP therapy with best available medical therapy for treatment of acute myocardial infraction (AMI) complicated by cardiogenic shock.[31] All patients were expected to undergo early revascularization (by means of percutaneous coronary intervention or bypass surgery). At 30 days, 119 patients in the IABP group (39.7%) and 123 patients in the control group (41.3%) had died (RR with IABP, 0.96; 95% CI 0.79 to 1.17; $P = 0.69$). No significant differences were found in secondary endpoints or in process-of-care measures, including the time to hemodynamic stabilization, the length of stay in the intensive care unit,

TABLE 59.2 Temporary Mechanical Circulatory Support Devices*

DEVICE	PUMP MECHANISM	PUMP ENERGY SOURCE	METHOD OF PLACEMENT	VENTRICLE SUPPORTED	DEGREE OF SUPPORT[†]
Intra-aortic balloon pump (IABP) (several manufacturers)	Counterpulsation	Pneumatic	Percutaneous placement via femoral artery or operative placement in ascending aorta or axillary artery	Principal effect: reduction of left ventricular (LV) afterload and increase in coronary perfusion	Partial-support device
Extracorporeal life support (ECLS) (several manufacturers depending on pump selected)	Continuous-flow rotary pump with centrifugal design	Variable; depends on pump used for ECLS circuit (most frequently a continuous-flow rotary pump with centrifugal design)	Percutaneous or operative placement	Venous-arterial configuration. Partial unloading of right and left ventricles by reduction in preload with oxygenation of blood	Full-support device (4–6 L/min)
CentriMag VAD (Abbott Labs, Chicago, IL)	Continuous-flow rotary pump with centrifugal design (magnetic levitation; no bearing)	Electric motor	Operative placement	Right, left, or biventricular support	Full-support device (4–6 L/min)
TandemHeart pVAD (TandemLife, Inc., Pittsburgh, PA)	Continuous-flow rotary pump with centrifugal design (hydrodynamic support of impeller)	Electric motor	Percutaneous placement. Requires transseptal placement of cannula for left atrial drainage. Arterial return to femoral artery	LV support[‡]	Partial-support device (2–4 L/min)
Impella 2.5, CP, 5.0, or RP (Abiomed Inc., Danvers, MA)	Continuous-flow rotary pump with microaxial design (bearing support of impeller)	Electric motor	Percutaneous via femoral artery (Impella 2.5, CP, or 5.0) or operative placement via aorta or axillary artery depending on device size (Impella 5.0, CP). Placement across aortic valve (Impella 5.0, CP). Inflow from left ventricle and outflow in ascending aorta	LV support or right ventricular (RV) support (Impella RP)[‡]	Partial-support device 1–3 L/min for Impella 2.5 or full-support device 3.5–4 L/min for Impella CP 5 L/min for Impella 5.0

*The table includes representative mechanical circulatory support devices and is not meant to be an exhaustive listing of all devices currently available in the United States or internationally.
[†]Values of cardiac support represent approximate ranges and capabilities of the device.
[‡]Impella RP designed specifically for right ventricular support. Provides 4 liters or greater of flow.

serum lactate levels, dose and duration of catecholamine therapy, and renal function. The use of IABP counterpulsation did not significantly reduce 30-day mortality in patients with AMI complicated by cardiogenic shock for whom an early revascularization strategy was planned. There have not been adequately powered randomized clinical trials of IABP therapy to assess for a mortality benefit in cardiogenic shock occurring outside the context of an AMI.

IABP placement via the left axillary artery is increasingly being used for advanced HF patients who require short-term hemodynamic support as a bridge to transplantation. In part, this is the result of the October 2018 revision to the UNOS Heart Allocation Policy that prioritizes heart donor allocation to patients receiving temporary MCS over those receiving durable MCS. Moreover, in patients for whom the degree of hemodynamic support afforded by an IABP is adequate for successful bridging, major surgery and the associated prolonged recovery is avoided, as is the forced immobility and resulting further deconditioning associated with transfemoral insertion. In the largest single center published experience, 133 of 195 patients (68%) receiving an axillary IABP were successfully bridged to transplant (120 patients) or durable implanted LVAD (13 patients).[32] Sixteen patients died while on IABP and 18 needed additional circulatory support. Forty-nine percent (49%) needed bedside repositioning of the IABP, 37% required fluoroscopic exchange or repositioning, and IABP removal occurred in 14%. Unique complications of axillary IABP are folding of the balloon within the aorta or entry of the catheter tip into a branch of the abdominal aorta (Fig. 59.10). Kinking of the balloon may occur without eliciting system alarms so serial surveillance x-rays to confirm positioning are essential. Other complications included bacteremia requiring antibiotic treatment (9.2%), left arm ischemia (3.5%), mesenteric ischemia (3%), and stroke (2.6%). A fully ambulatory counterpulsation device intended for more prolonged hemodynamic support in the outpatient setting, potentially in less advanced HF patients, is under investigation (Fig. 59.11).[33]

Extracorporeal Life Support and Extracorporeal Membrane Oxygenation

ECMO provides cardiopulmonary support for patients whose heart and/or lungs can no longer provide adequate physiologic support (see Fig. 59.5).[34,35] ECMO can be configured for respiratory support (venovenous [VV-ECMO]) or for respiratory and circulatory support (venoarterial [VA-ECMO]). In cases of biventricular failure, VA-ECMO is the MCS device of choice for patients in cardiogenic shock and impaired oxygenation, because it provides full cardiopulmonary support. ECMO may be placed at the bedside without fluoroscopic guidance. ECMO is similar to a CPB circuit used in cardiac surgery with some modifications. VA-ECMO involves a circuit composed of a continuous-flow centrifugal pump for blood propulsion (most commonly) and a membrane oxygenator for gas exchange. A venous cannula drains deoxygenated blood into a membrane oxygenator for gas exchange, and oxygenated blood is subsequently infused into the patient through an arterial cannula. VA-ECMO provides systemic circulatory support with

flow capabilities approximating 4 to 6 L/min depending on cannula size. Because of the increase in systemic afterload, however, VA-ECMO alone may not significantly reduce ventricular wall stress and may result in LV distension in cases where residual LV function is inadequate to eject against the increase in systemic afterload.[36] This may result in high myocardial oxygen demand (secondary to high filling pressures and volume). This may have negative consequences on myocardial recovery unless the LV is unloaded by concomitant IABP, an LV vent, atrial septostomy, or use of a percutaneous LV-to-aorta VAD. Inadequate LV unloading may also result in pulmonary hemorrhage.

Numerous large clinical series have reported successful use of ECLS for cardiac and respiratory support in adult, pediatric, and neonatal patients.[34,35,37–41] Reports of contemporary survival outcomes are significantly impacted by adult or pediatric application, cause of the cardiac

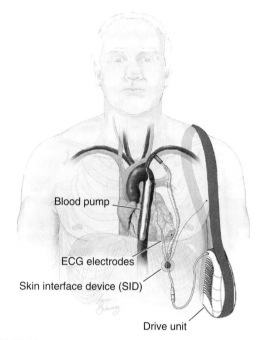

FIGURE 59.11 The iVAS is an external heart assist device that has several components. The intravascular component is a 50-cc displacement pump (similar to an intra-aortic balloon) placed in the descending aorta. The skin interface device (SID) is an electromechanical and pneumatic conduit with a chimney that allows for shuttling of air between the pump and external driver and communication of the captured electrocardiogram (ECG) signals that are transmitted to the driver from 3 subcutaneous electrodes. The SID is placed onto the lower chest cage and connects a driver to an external driveline. An external and wearable drive unit provides compressed ambient air to inflate and deflate the pump. (From Jeevanandam V, Song T, Onsager D, et al. The first-in-human experience with a minimally invasive, ambulatory, counterpulsation heart assist system for advanced congestive heart failure. *J Heart Lung Transplant.* 2018;37(1):1–6.)

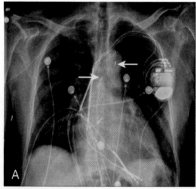 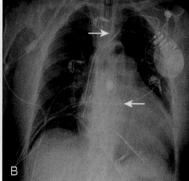 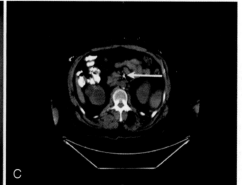

FIGURE 59.10 Images depicting complications unique to axillary intra-aortic balloon pumps (IABP). **A,** Chest radiograph of IABP folded into the aortic arch with the distal marker at the aortic knob and the proximal marker in the ascending aorta (*arrows*). **B,** Chest radiograph of IABP partially folded into the ascending aorta. The distal marker is pulled up into the thoracic aorta whereas the proximal marker remains close to ideal position (*arrows*). **C,** Abdominal computed tomography of the metallic tip of the IABP projecting into a branch of the abdominal aorta (*arrow*). (From Bhimaraj A, Agrawal T, Duran A, et al. Percutaneous left axillary artery placement of intra-aortic balloon pump in advanced heart failure patients. *JACC Heart Fail.* 2020;8(4):313–323.)

and/or respiratory failure, and heterogeneity of the patient population and mode of presentation.[34,35,37–41]

Left Atrium to Aorta Assist Device

The TandemHeart percutaneous ventricular assist device (pVAD) is a paracorporeal device inserted as a LA–aorta assist device that pumps blood from the left atrium to the femoral artery through a transseptal positioned LA cannula, thereby entirely bypassing the LV (see Fig. 59.4). The TandemHeart system includes a 21F transseptal cannula, a centrifugal pump, a femoral arterial cannula, and a control console. The TandemHeart is approved by FDA to incorporate an oxygenator to the circuit, allowing for concomitant LV unloading and oxygenation. The centrifugal blood pump contains a hydrodynamic bearing that supports a spinning impeller. The impeller is powered by a brushless direct-current (DC) electromagnetic motor, rotating between 3000 and 7500 rpm. The external console controls the pump and provides battery backup in case of power failure. A continuous infusion of heparinized saline flows into the lower chamber of the pump, which provides lubrication and cooling, and prevents thrombus formation. The redirection of blood from the left atrium reduces LV preload, LV workload, filling pressures, wall stress, and myocardial oxygen demand. The increase in arterial blood pressure and cardiac output supports systemic perfusion.[36] The flow through the TandemHeart is additive to LV output through the aortic valve (parallel circulation). However, the contribution from the native heart is typically reduced as MCS support is increased due to changes in LV loading conditions (i.e., decrease in preload and increase in afterload). Coronary flow is driven by the perfusion pressure (diastolic pressure–RA pressure). With a parallel circulation, the aorta is perfused and pressured by both the left ventricle and the TandemHeart. Not infrequently, LV contraction (native heart output) may be negligible, and systemic perfusion is pump dependent, with a flat mean arterial pressure curve. This situation can result in stasis of blood within the aortic root, resulting in thrombus formation and stroke.

In a randomized comparison of the IABP with the TandemHeart, the TandemHeart provided more effective improvement in cardiac power index as well as other hemodynamic and metabolic variables compared to the IABP.[42,43] Moreover, complications, such as severe bleeding and limb ischemia, were encountered more frequently after TandemHeart VAD support. Thirty-day mortality rates were similar between the groups, but the study was underpowered to compare mortality between groups.

Left Ventricle to Aorta Assist Device

The Impella is a continuous flow microaxial pump designed to pump blood from the LV into the ascending aorta, in series with the LV (see Fig. 59.3). Several versions of the pump are available, including the Impella 2.5, Impella CP, Impella CP with SmartAssist, Impella 5.0, Impella LD, and Impella 5.5 with SmartAssist. The pumps are U.S. FDA-approved to treat patients with cardiogenic shock. A pump specifically designed to support the right ventricle, the Impella RP is U.S. FDA-approved to treat right HF or decompensation following left VAD implantation, myocardial infarction, heart transplant, or postcardiotomy failure to wean from CPB. The SmartAssist technology uses optical sensors to assess aortic pressure. The devices for LV assist are designed to be placed via the femoral artery, either percutaneously (Impella 2.5 and CP) or with a surgical cutdown (Impella 5.0 and 5.5). Alternate access sites such as the subclavian artery have also been described. The Impella pumps blood from the LV into the ascending aorta, thereby unloading the LV and increasing forward flow. It reduces myocardial oxygen consumption, increases coronary perfusion, improves mean arterial pressure, and reduces PCWP.[36] The Impella 2.5 provides a greater increase in cardiac output than the IABP but less than the TandemHeart device. The more powerful Impella CP and 5.0 devices are comparable to the TandemHeart device in terms of support. Similar to the TandemHeart, adequate RV function or concomitant RVAD is necessary to maintain LV preload and hemodynamic support during biventricular failure or unstable ventricular arrhythmias.

In a prospective, randomized clinical trial comparing the Impella 2.5 to the IABP, cardiac index was significantly increased in patients with the Impella 2.5 compared with patients supported with an IABP.[44]

Overall mortality rates at 30 days were similar in both groups, but the study was not adequately powered to assess for a mortality difference.[44]

Despite the absence of suitably powered randomized clinical trials demonstrating a mortality benefit over IABP therapy (which itself has no proven mortality benefit), the use of temporary MCS devices in patients with cardiogenic shock is likely to continue. In comparison with an IABP, these devices provide a much larger increment in cardiac output and superior LV unloading.[44,45]

Devices Intended for Long-Term Mechanical Circulatory Support

The introduction of continuous-flow technology into clinical practice was a milestone in the field of MCS therapy and led to significant improvements in survival and reduction of serious major adverse events, especially in the area of device malfunction. Compared with pulsatile-flow devices, continuous-flow technology provides functionally equivalent hemodynamic support improvement of kidney and liver function. Long-term survival with continuous-flow technology is significantly better with half the rate of stroke and infection and one-third the rate of device malfunction compared to pulsatile-flow technology. Table 59.3 summarizes the characteristics of durable MCS devices intended for long-term use.

Durable Implantable Left Ventricular Assist Devices

HeartMate 3

The HM3 is FDA-approved for both short-term (BTR or BTT indication) and long-term (BTT, BTC, or DT indication) support of patients with advanced HF (see Fig. 59.6). The HM3 recently completed clinical evaluation in the MOMENTUM 3 clinical trial. MOMENTUM 3 was a multicenter randomized clinical trial evaluating the HM3 to the HMII pump.[6,10] The final analysis included 1028 enrolled patients: 516 in the HM3 group and 512 in the HMII group. In the final analysis of the primary endpoint, 397 patients (76.9%) in the HM3 group, as compared with 332 (64.8%) in the HMII group, remained alive and free of disabling stroke or reoperation to replace or remove a malfunctioning device at 2 years (RR, 0.84; 95% CI, 0.78 to 0.91; P < 0.001 for superiority). There was no difference in deaths alone. Pump replacement was less common in the HM3 group than in the HMII group (12 patients [2.3%] vs. 57 patients [11.3%]; RR, 0.21; 95% CI, 0.11 to 0.38; P < 0.001). The numbers of events per patient-year for stroke of any severity, major bleeding, and gastrointestinal hemorrhage were lower in the HM3 group than in the HMII group (Table 59.4 and **eTable 59.1**).

HeartMate II

The HMII (see Fig. 59.7) is intended for long-term support of patients with advanced HF and is the most evaluated MCS device to date, with more than 20,000 implantations worldwide. Patient outcomes after implantation of the HMII have been extensively evaluated in five major scientific reports on its use for BTT and DT indications within the context of pre- and post-approval clinical trials (see Table 59.4 and eTable 59.1).[12,44–47] For more information see the online supplement the online supplement "Patient Outcomes."

HeartWare Ventricular Assist Device

[NOTE: On June 3, 2021, worldwide sales and distribution of the HVAD was discontinued by the manufacturer. This was in response to a study showing poorer survival at 1 year with the HVAD than with the HM3, with a hazard ratio ~ 3.[49a] At the time of this publication, previously implanted patients continue to be supported by this device, and it is recommended that the HVAD not be prophylactically exchanged for an alternative LVAD.[49b]]

The HVAD has undergone clinical evaluation in the United States for BTT indication in a prospective, nonrandomized clinical trial, ADVANCE (see Table 59.4 and eTable 59.1).[50,51] The unique feature of ADVANCE was the use of a contemporaneous, observational control arm derived from registrants entered into Interagency Registry for Mechanically Assisted Circulatory Support (INTERMACS). The primary outcome in ADVANCE was success defined as survival on the originally implanted device, transplantation, or explantation for ventricular recovery at

TABLE 59.3 Long-term Durable Mechanical Circulatory Support Devices*

DEVICE	PUMP MECHANISM	PUMP ENERGY SOURCE	METHOD OF PLACEMENT	VENTRICLE SUPPORTED	INDICATION
HeartMate 3 (Abbott Labs, Chicago, IL)	Continuous-flow rotary pump with centrifugal design and magnetic levitation of internal impeller	Electric motor Power to pump delivered via percutaneous lead with external power source and computer controller	Operative	Left ventricle Implantable pump with intrapericardial placement	Approved for "Short-term" and "Long-term" support (intended for BTT, BTC, or DT indication)
HeartMate II (Abbott Labs, Chicago, IL)	Continuous flow rotary pump with axial design with mechanical pivot support of internal impeller	Electric motor Power to pump delivered via percutaneous lead with external power source and computer controller	Operative	Left ventricle Implantable pump requiring preperitoneal pocket	BTT, DT
HVAD (Medtronic, Minneapolis, MN)	Continuous-flow rotary pump with centrifugal design with magnetic and hydrodynamic levitation of internal impeller	Electric motor Power to pump delivered via percutaneous lead with external power source and computer controller	Operative	Left ventricle Implantable pump with intrapericardial placement No preperitoneal pocket required	BTT, DT
SynCardia TAH-t (SynCardia Systems, Tucson, AZ)	Pulsatile, volume displacement (50-cc and 70-cc displacement devices)	Pneumatic Patient tethered to portable drive unit	Operative	Biventricular support Orthotopic placement with removal of both ventricles	BTT DT[†]

*The table includes representative mechanical circulatory support devices and is not meant to be an exhaustive list of all devices currently available in the United States or internationally.
[†]Currently under clinical evaluation for DT indication.
BTC, Bridge to candidacy; BTT, Bridge to transplantation; DT, destination therapy.

TABLE 59.4 Clinical Trials of Durable, Implantable Continuous-Flow Rotary Devices for Mechanical Circulatory Support in United States

CLINICAL TRIAL	PATIENTS (n)	FOLLOW-UP DURATION	STUDY DEVICE SURVIVAL (6 MONTHS/1 YEAR/2 YEARS)	COMPARATOR GROUP (PATIENTS, DEVICE USED)	TRIAL DESIGN	COMPARATOR GROUP SURVIVAL (6 MONTHS/1 YEAR/2 YEARS)
HeartMate II Pivotal BTT trial[12]	133	Median duration of support: 126 days	75%/68%/—	None	Observational Single arm	N/A
HeartMate II Pivotal BTT trial and CAP[46]	281	Median duration of support: 155 days	82%/73%/72% (18 months)	None	Observational Single arm	N/A
HVAD Pivotal BTT trial[50]	140	Duration of follow-up: 89.1 patient-years	94%/86%/—	499 Commercially implanted devices for BTT (INTERMACS)	Observational Contemporaneous control group	90%/85%/—
HVAD Pivotal BTT trial and CAP[51]	332	—	91%/84%/—	None	Observational Single arm	N/A
HeartMate II Post-approval BTT study[49]	169	Median duration of support: 386 days	90%/85%/—	169 HeartMate XVE or Thoratec pVAD or IVAD (INTERMACS)	Observational Contemporaneous control group	79%/70%/—
HeartMate II Pivotal DT trial—original cohort[47]	134	Median duration of support: 1.7 years	—/68%/58%	66 HeartMate XVE	Randomized clinical trial	—/55%/24%
HeartMate II Pivotal DT trial—CAP[48]	281	Median duration of support: 1.7 years	—/73%/63%	None	Observational Single arm	N/A
HVAD DT Pivotal Trial[52]	297	Complete follow-up to 24 months	(—/—/60%)	148 HeartMate II	Randomized	(—/—/68%)
HeartMate 3 Pivotal trial[6]	516	Complete follow-up to 24 months	90%/86.6%/79%	512 HeartMate II	Randomized clinical trial	89%/84%/77%

CAP, Continued access protocol; N/A, not applicable.

180 days and was evaluated for both noninferiority and superiority. A total of 140 patients received the investigational pump, and 499 patients received a commercially available pump (the HMII in at least 95% of cases) implanted contemporaneously. Success was achieved in 90.7% of patients on the investigational pump and in 90.1% of controls, establishing the noninferiority of the investigational pump (P < 0.001; 15% noninferiority margin). At 6 months, median 6-minute walk distance increased by 128.5 meters, and both disease-specific and global quality-of-life scores improved significantly. The HVAD was approved for use in the United States for the BTT indication in 2012. The HVAD underwent clinical evaluation in the United States for DT indication in the ENDURANCE and ENDURANCE Supplemental Trials (A Clinical Trial to Evaluate the HeartWare Ventricular Assist System).[52,53] In the ENDURANCE trial, 297 participants were assigned to the HVAD and 148 participants assigned to the control device, the HMII. The primary endpoint, defined as survival at 2 years free from disabling stroke or device removal for malfunction or failure, was achieved in 164 patients in the HVAD group and 85 patients in the HMII group.[52] The analysis of the primary endpoint showed noninferiority of the HVAD relative to the HMII device (estimated success rates, 55.4% and 59.1%, respectively, calculated by the Weibull model; absolute difference, 3.7 percentage points; 95% upper confidence limit, 12.56 percentage points; P = 0.01 for noninferiority). More patients in the HMII group than in the study group had device malfunction or device failure requiring replacement (16.2% vs. 8.8%), and more patients in the HVAD group had strokes (29.7% vs. 12.1%). Quality of life and functional capacity improved to a similar degree in the two groups. Due to the high rate of stroke in the HVAD device in ENDURANCE, a supplemental clinical trial was performed to investigate the effect of an improved blood pressure control management algorithm on incidence of stroke associated with HVAD support.[53] The primary endpoint for the trial was the 12-month incidence of transient ischemic attack or stroke with residual deficit 24 weeks post-event. The ENDURANCE Supplemental trial demonstrated that an enhanced blood pressure protocol significantly reduced mean arterial blood pressure. However, the primary endpoint was not achieved (14.7% with HVAD vs. 12.1% with the HMII, noninferiority [margin 6%] P = 0.14). However, a post-hoc analysis of a secondary composite endpoint, consisting of freedom from death, disabling stroke, or need for device replacement or urgent transplantation, demonstrated superiority of HVAD (76.1%) versus the HMII (66.9%) (P = 0.04). The incidence of stroke in HVAD subjects was reduced 24.2% in ENDURANCE Supplemental compared with ENDURANCE (P = 0.10), and hemorrhagic cerebrovascular accident was reduced by 50.5% (P = 0.02).

Total Artificial Heart
SynCardia Total Artificial Heart–Temporary
Another option for MCS is the TAH. The 70-mL stroke volume version of the SynCardia CardioWest Total Artificial Heart–Temporary (TAH-t; Fig. 59.12) was evaluated in a large, prospective, nonrandomized trial conducted in five centers for BTT indication in 81 patients at risk for imminent death from irreversible biventricular cardiac failure.[54] The study cohort was compared with a nonrandomized, observational control cohort of 35 patients. The primary study endpoints included the rates of survival to heart transplantation and survival after transplantation. The rate of survival to transplantation was 79% (95% CI 68% to 87%). Of the 35 patients in the control cohort who met the same entry criteria but did not receive the TAH-t, 16 (46%) survived to transplantation (P < 0.001). Overall, the 1-year survival rate among the patients who received the TAH was 70%, compared with 31% among the controls (P < 0.001). After transplantation, 1-year and 5-year survival rates among patients who had received the TAH were 86% and 64%.[54] The SynCardia TAH-t was approved by the FDA for BTT in 2007. The TAH-t is currently being evaluated in the United States for DT indication. A smaller version of the device (50-cc ventricle) is also available.

INTERAGENCY REGISTRY OF MECHANICALLY ASSISTED CIRCULATORY SUPPORT

An important milestone in the advance of MCS therapy has been the development of the INTERMACS. INTERMACS is a national registry

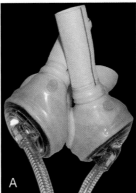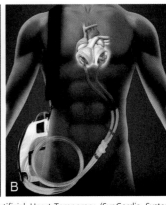

FIGURE 59.12 SynCardia Total Artificial Heart–Temporary (SynCardia Systems, Tucson, Arizona). **A,** The TAH-t consists of a right and left prosthetic ventricle. The prosthetic ventricles, made of biocompatible polyurethane, have a capacity of 70 mL. A 50-cc prosthetic ventricle is also available for use in patients with small body habitus. The ventricles are pneumatically driven with four flexible polyurethane diaphragms positioned between the blood surface and the air sac. When compressed air is forced into the air sacs simultaneously, compression is affected onto the blood sac and ejection occurs in simulation of cardiac systole. Cardiac ejection in the TAH-t thus occurs in parallel from the left and right sides. As the air sac is deflated, the blood sac is filled passively from the atrial connection. Two mechanical valves are situated along the prosthetic ventricle to provide unidirectional inflow and outflow. The prosthetic ventricles are connected by quick-connect silicone cuffs to two atrial connectors on the cuffs (not shown), and two connectors on the end of the grafts are sewn to the aorta and pulmonary artery. The compressed air is delivered by an external console (not shown) through two separate air tubes connected to the right and left prosthetic ventricles. The console has two independent controllers that allow redundancy for emergency backup. Compressed air cylinders inside the console can be used to mobilize the patient. **B,** Portable drive unit to permit hospital discharge and improve patient mobility is also available.

currently administered by The Society of Thoracic Surgeons, and is the largest available data repository for the study of durable MCS outcomes.[55] INTERMACS was formerly a collaboration between National Heart, Lung and Blood Institute (NHLBI), FDA, Centers for Medicare and Medicaid Services (CMS), device manufacturers, and the professional community and began prospective patient enrollment and data collection in June 2006. In March 2009, CMS and the U.S. Department of Health and Human Services mandated that all U.S. hospitals approved for use of MCS for DT enter MCS patient data into INTERMACS for all non-investigative MCS devices approved by FDA. Although mandated data entry was discontinued by CMS in October 2013, the number of DT implants entered annually into INTERMACS has increased. Since the inception of INTERMACS, the ongoing evolution of strategies for device application and the types of available devices has continued to refine the landscape of MCS. A major limitation of INTERMACS is the inability to enter patient information on investigative devices currently in evaluation in the United States, which represents a barrier for capture of all patients receiving durable, implantable MCS therapy. To date, data on more than 22,000 patients receiving durable MCS therapy have been reported to INTERMACS.[55] The overall survival rate for all patients undergoing primary implantation of a durable MCS device is approximately 82% at 1 year and 72% at 2 years (Fig. 59.13).[55] A competing outcomes analysis demonstrates that at 5 years, 23% of patients remain alive on support, 34% have undergone heart transplantation, 39% have died, and 4% underwent device explantation for myocardial recovery.[55]

One of the most important contributions to the MCS field has been the development of a subjective classification system based on severity of illness, termed "INTERMACS Patient Profiles," which range from Profile 1 (critical cardiogenic shock) to Profile 7 (advanced NYHA Class III HF) (Table 59.5).[56] This classification system has added enhanced resolution of patient outcomes in the advanced stages of HF or cardiogenic shock beyond that offered by the NYHA classification system. INTERMACS patient profiles are associated with short-term survival following LVAD implantation and are used to inform appropriate timing of intervention with durable, implantable MCS devices. Patients undergoing implantation of an MCS device who have critical cardiogenic shock (INTERMACS Patient Profile 1) have worse long-term outcomes than patients with more stable forms of advanced HF (INTERMACS Patient Profile levels 2 through 7).[57] Patients with significant organ dysfunction at MCS device implantation, accompanied

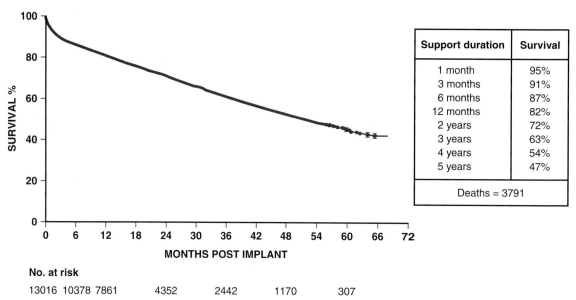

Support duration	Survival
1 month	95%
3 months	91%
6 months	87%
12 months	82%
2 years	72%
3 years	63%
4 years	54%
5 years	47%
Deaths = 3791	

No. at risk

13016 10378 7861   4352   2442   1170   307

FIGURE 59.13 Actuarial survival after implantation of primary continuous-flow left ventricular assist devices without concomitant right ventricular assist device (RVAD) support. The *curve* displays the Kaplan-Meier survival estimates over time. (Data from Teuteberg JJ, Cleveland JC Jr, Cowger J, et al. The Society of Thoracic Surgeons Intermacs 2019 Annual Report: The changing landscape of devices and indications. *Ann Thorac Surg.* 2020;109:649–660.)

TABLE 59.5 INTERMACS Patient Profiles

PROFILE	DEFINITION	DESCRIPTION
1	"Crashing and burning"	Life-threatening hypotension and rapidly escalating inotropic pressor support, with critical organ hypoperfusion confirmed by worsening acidosis and lactate levels.
2	"Inotrope dependent and worsening"	Shows signs of continuing deterioration in nutrition, renal function, fluid retention, or other major status indicator *or* refractory volume overload, ± evidence of impaired perfusion, with inotropic infusion intolerance due to tachyarrhythmias, clinical ischemia, or other.
3	"Stable on inotropes"	Clinically stable on mild-moderate doses of IV inotropes (or has a temporary MCSD) after repeated failures to wean without symptomatic hypotension, worsening symptoms, or progressive organ dysfunction. May be either at home or in the hospital.
4	"Frequent flyer/resting symptoms"	At home on oral therapy but frequently has symptoms of congestion at rest or with ADLs. May have orthopnea, SOB during ADLs, GI symptoms, disabling ascites, or severe lower extremity edema.
5	"Exercise intolerant"	Comfortable at rest but unable to engage in any activity, living predominantly within the house or housebound. No congestive symptoms, but may have chronically elevated volume status, frequently with renal dysfunction, and may be characterized as exercise intolerant.
6	"Walking wounded"	Comfortable at rest without evidence of fluid overload, but able to do some mild activity. ADLs are comfortable and minor activities outside the home can be performed, but fatigue results within a few minutes of any meaningful physical exertion. Occasional episodes of worsening symptoms; likely to have had a hospitalization for heart failure within the past year.
7	"Advanced NYHA Class III"	Clinically stable with a reasonable level of comfortable activity, despite history of previous decompensation that is not recent. Usually able to walk more than a block. Any decompensation requiring IV diuretics or hospitalization within the previous month should make this person a Patient Profile 6 or lower.

ADLs, Activities of daily living; *GI,* gastrointestinal; *IV,* intravenous; *MCSD,* mechanical circulatory support device; *NYHA,* New York Heart Association; *SOB,* shortness of breath.
From Stevenson LW, Pagani FD, Young JB, et al. INTERMACS profiles of advanced heart failure: the current picture. *J Heart Lung Transplant.* 2009;28:535–541.

by a greater degree of hemodynamic compromise, are significantly more likely to require BiVAD support and are at higher risk for major adverse events and at significantly higher risk for death during use of MCS devices.

FUTURE PERSPECTIVES

Recent rapid technological advancements and successful clinical application of MCS have provided a major impetus to extending the use of this modality. Important initiatives that will contribute significantly to future directions in MCS therapy include (1) introduction of new MCS devices that focus on miniaturization and biventricular support applications; (2) implementation of partial-support MCS devices and management paradigms to enhance long-term myocardial recovery; (3) design of fully implantable MCS devices, with elimination of the percutaneous lead and introduction of wireless energy transfer; (4) specific developments in the field of pediatric MCS, including appropriately designed MCS devices, clinical trials, and national registry development;

(5) evaluation of MCS therapy in patients with less advanced HF; and (6) harmonization of the global MCS experience through international registry initiatives.

The percutaneous lead has been a significant source of morbidity and adversely influences quality of life for patients on MCS support.[58] The introduction of wireless energy transfer will allow MCS systems to receive energy transcutaneously without the need for the percutaneous lead.[59] The entire MCS system will be implantable, with an internal power source providing short periods of support, allowing the patient to pursue activities that are restricted with current technology, such as swimming and bathing. The incorporation of this type of technology, if successful, can be expected to increase patient satisfaction and quality of life significantly.

Important developments in the pediatric field include the PumpKIN Trial (Pumps in Kids, Infants and Neonates).[60] PumpKIN is an NHLBI initiative to investigate the use of several novel pump designs and ECLS systems for pediatric MCS application. The trial is investigating an implantable pump design based on the Jarvik 2000 VAD.[61] The initiative is a collaboration between industry, clinical centers, and the New England Research Institutes (NERI), designated as the data-coordinating center for the trial.

Widespread interest in MCS therapies has resulted in global adoption and clinical application of this technology. An understanding of international outcomes based on uniform definitions of outcomes and adverse events is essential to the sustainability of MCS therapy and to foster efficient device development and clinical evaluation. IMACS is an international registry collaboration supported by the International Society of Heart and Lung Transplantation and INTERMACS that was initiated to achieve international cooperation on reporting of MCS outcomes.[62] Efforts to create uniform registration and reporting requirements worldwide constitute an important initiative of the FDA to facilitate clinical device evaluation in the United States.[63]

REFERENCES

Indications and Device Selection

1. Rihal CS, Naidu SS, Givertz MM, et al. 2015 SCAI/ACC/HFSA/STS clinical expert consensus statement on the use of percutaneous mechanical circulatory support devices in cardiovascular care: endorsed by the American Heart Association, the Cardiological Society of India, and Sociedad Latino Americana de Cardiologia Intervencion; Affirmation of Value by the Canadian Association of Interventional Cardiology-Association Canadienne de Cardiologie d'intervention. *J Am Coll Cardiol.* 2015;65:e7–e26.
2. Hanff TC, Harhay MO, Kimmel SE, et al. Trends in mechanical support use as a bridge to adult heart transplant under new allocation rules. *JAMA Cardiol.* 2020:e200667.
3. McGee Jr E, Danter M, Strueber M, et al. Evaluation of a lateral thoracotomy implant approach for a centrifugal-flow left ventricular assist device: the lateral clinical trial. *J Heart Lung Transplant.* 2019;38:344–351.
4. Wever-Pinzon O, Drakos SG, McKellar SH, et al. Cardiac recovery during long-term left ventricular assist device support. *J Am Coll Cardiol.* 2016;68:1540–1553.
5. Topkara VK, Garan AR, Fine B, et al. Myocardial recovery in patients receiving contemporary left ventricular assist devices: results from the Interagency Registry for Mechanically Assisted Circulatory Support (INTERMACS). *Circ Heart Fail.* 2016;9(7). https://doi.org/10.1161/CIRCHEARTFAILURE.116.003157 e003157.
6. Mehra MR, Uriel N, Naka Y, et al. A fully magnetically levitated left ventricular assist device—final report. *N Engl J Med.* 2019;380:1618–1627.
7. Goldstein DJ, Naka Y, Horstmanshof D, et al. Association of clinical outcomes with left ventricular assist device use by bridge to transplant or destination therapy intent: the multicenter study of Maglev Technology in Patients Undergoing Mechanical Circulatory Support Therapy with Heartmate 3 (MOMENTUM 3) randomized clinical trial. *JAMA Cardiol.* 2020;5:411–419.
8. Rose EA, Gelijns AC, Moskowitz AJ, et al. Long-term mechanical left ventricular assistance for end-stage heart failure. *N Engl J Med.* 2001;345:1435.
9. Centers for Medicare & Medicaid Services. Decision Memo for ventricular assist devices as destination therapy (CAG-00119R). Assessed June 1, 2020 https://www.cms.gov/medicare-coverage-database/details/nca-decision-memo.aspx?NCAId=268.
10. Heatley G, Sood P, Goldstein D, MOMENTUM 3 Investigators, et al. Clinical trial design and rationale of the multicenter study of Maglev Technology in Patients Undergoing Mechanical Circulatory Support Therapy with Heartmate 3 (MOMENTUM 3) investigational device exemption clinical study protocol. *J Heart Lung Transplant.* 2016;35:528–536.

Design of Ventricular Assist Devices

11. Frazier OH, Rose EA, Oz MC, et al. Multicenter clinical evaluation of the HeartMate vented electric left ventricular assist system in patients awaiting heart transplantation. *J Thorac Cardiovasc Surg.* 2001;122:1186.
12. Miller LW, Pagani FD, Russell SD, et al. Use of a continuous-flow device in patients awaiting heart transplantation. *N Engl J Med.* 2007;357:885.
13. Pagani FD. Continuous flow rotary left ventricular assist devices with "3rd generation" design. *Semin Thorac Cardiovasc Surg.* 2008;20:255.
14. Moazami N, Fukamachi K, Kobayashi M, et al. Axial and centrifugal continuous flow rotary pumps: a translation from pump mechanics to clinical practice. *J Heart Lung Transplant.* 2013;32:1.
15. Netuka I, Sood P, Pya Y, et al. Fully magnetically levitated left ventricular assist system for treating advanced heart failure: a multicenter study. *J Am Coll Cardiol.* 2015;66:2579–2589.
16. Mehra MR, Naka Y, Uriel N, et al. A fully magnetically levitated circulatory pump for advanced heart failure. *N Engl J Med.* 2017;376:440–450.

Patient Selection, Comorbidities, and Timing of Intervention

17. Reynolds HR, Hochman JS. Cardiogenic shock: current concepts and improving outcomes. *Circulation.* 2008;117:686–697.
18. Hochman JS, Sleeper LA, Webb JG, et al. Early revascularization in acute myocardial infarction complicated by cardiogenic shock. *N Engl J Med.* 1999;341:625.
19. Vahdatpour C, Collins D, Goldberg S. Cardiogenic shock. *J Am Heart Assoc.* 2019;8(8):e011991.
20. Yancy CW, Jessup M, Januzzi JL. 2017 ACC expert consensus decision pathway for optimization of heart failure treatment: answers to 10 pivotal issues about heart failure with reduced ejection fraction. *J Am Coll Cardiol.* 2018;71:201–230.
21. Yancy CW, Jessup M, Bozkurt B, et al. 2017 ACC/AHA/HFSA focused Update of the 2013 ACCF/AHA guideline for the management of heart failure: a report of the American College of Cardiology/American Heart Association Task Force on clinical practice guidelines and the Heart Failure Society of America. *Circulation.* 2017;136:e137–e161.
22. Guglin M, Zucker MJ, Borlaug BA. Evaluation for heart transplantation and LVAD implantation. *J Am Coll Cardiol.* 2020;75:1471–1487.
23. Kirklin JK, Naftel DC, Kormos RL, et al. Quantifying the effect of cardiorenal syndrome on mortality after left ventricular assist device implant. *J Heart Lung Transplant.* 2013;32:1205–1213.
24. Kormos RL, Teuteberg JJ, Pagani FD, et al. Right ventricular failure in patients with the HeartMate II continuous-flow left ventricular assist device: incidence, risk factors, and effect on outcomes. *J Thorac Cardiovasc Surg.* 2010;139:1316.
25. Kiernan MS, Grandin EW, Brinkley Jr M, et al. Early right ventricular assist device use in patients undergoing continuous-flow left ventricular assist device implantation: incidence and risk factors from the Interagency registry for mechanically assisted circulatory support. *Circ Heart Fail.* 2017;10(10):e003863.
26. Cleveland JC, Naftel DC, Reece TB, et al. Survival after biventricular assist device implantation: an analysis of the Interagency registry for mechanically assisted circulatory support database. *J Heart Lung Transplant.* 2011;30:862.
27. Kukucka M, Potapov E, Stepanenko A, et al. Acute impact of left ventricular unloading by left ventricular assist device on the right ventricle geometry and function: effect of nitric oxide inhalation. *J Thorac Cardiovasc Surg.* 2011;141:1009.

28. Santamore WP, Gray LA. Left ventricular contributions to right ventricular systolic function during LVAD support. *Ann Thorac Surg.* 1996;61:350.
29. Pavie A, Leger P. Physiology of univentricular versus biventricular support. *Ann Thorac Surg.* 1996;61:347.
30. Mandarino WA, Winowich S, Gorcsan J, et al. Right ventricular performance and left ventricular assist device filling. *Ann Thorac Surg.* 1997;63:1044.

Patient Outcomes

31. Thiele H, Zeymer U, Neumann FJ, et al. Intraaortic balloon support for myocardial infarction with cardiogenic shock. *N Engl J Med.* 2012;367:1287.
32. Bhimaraj A, Agrawal T, Duran A, et al. Percutaneous left axillary artery placement of intra-aortic balloon pump in advanced heart failure patients. *JACC Heart Fail.* 2020;8(4):313–323.
33. Jeevanandam V, Song T, Onsager D, et al. The first-in-human experience with a minimally invasive, ambulatory, counterpulsation heart assist system for advanced congestive heart failure. *J Heart Lung Transplant.* 2018;37(1):1–6.
34. Rao P, Khalpey Z, Smith R, et al. Venoarterial extracorporeal membrane oxygenation for cardiogenic shock and cardiac arrest. *Circ Heart Fail.* 2018;11(9):e004905.
35. Guglin M, Zucker MJ, Bazan VM, et al. Venoarterial ECMO for adults: JACC scientific expert panel. *J Am Coll Cardiol.* 2019;73:698–716.
36. Burkhoff D, Sayer G, Doshi D, Uriel N. Hemodynamics of mechanical circulatory support. *J Am Coll Cardiol.* 2015;66:2663–2674.
37. Squiers JJ, Lima B, DiMaio JM. Contemporary extracorporeal membrane oxygenation therapy in adults: fundamental principles and systematic review of the evidence. *J Thorac Cardiovasc Surg.* 2016;152(1):20–32.
38. Rastan AJ, Dege A, Mohr M, et al. Early and late outcomes of 517 consecutive adult patients treated with extracorporeal membrane oxygenation for refractory postcardiotomy cardiogenic shock. *J Thorac Cardiovasc Surg.* 2010;139:302–311.e1.
39. Bartlett RH, Roloff DW, Custer JR, et al. Extracorporeal life support: the University of Michigan experience. *J Am Med Assoc.* 2000;283:904.
40. Aubin H, Petrov G, Dalyanoglu H, et al. A supra-institutional network for remote extracorporeal life support: a retrospective cohort study. *JACC Heart Fail.* 2016;4:698–708.
41. Eckman PM, Katz JN, El Banayosy A, et al. Veno-arterial extracorporeal membrane oxygenation for cardiogenic shock: an introduction for the busy clinician. *Circulation.* 2019;140:2019–2037.
42. Thiele H, Sick P, Boudriot E, et al. Randomized comparison of intra-aortic balloon support with a percutaneous left ventricular assist device in patients with revascularized acute myocardial infarction complicated by cardiogenic shock. *Eur Heart J.* 2005;26:1276.
43. Burkhoff D, Cohen H, Brunckhorst C, et al. TandemHeart Investigators Group. A randomized multicenter clinical study to evaluate the safety and efficacy of the TandemHeart percutaneous ventricular assist device versus conventional therapy with intraaortic balloon pumping for treatment of cardiogenic shock. *Am Heart J.* 2006;152.469.e1-469.e4698.
44. Seyfarth M, Sibbing D, Bauer I, et al. A randomized clinical trial to evaluate the safety and efficacy of a percutaneous left ventricular assist device versus intra-aortic balloon pumping for treatment of cardiogenic shock caused by myocardial infarction. *J Am Coll Cardiol.* 2008;52:1584.
45. Werdan K, Gielen S, Ebelt H, Hochman JS. Mechanical circulatory support in cardiogenic shock. *Eur Heart J.* 2014;35:156–167.
46. Pagani FD, Miller LW, Russell SD, et al. Extended mechanical circulatory support with a continuous flow rotary left ventricular assist device. *J Am Coll Cardiol.* 2009;54:312.
47. Slaughter MS, Rogers JG, Milano CA, et al. Advanced heart failure treated with continuous-flow left ventricular assist device. *N Engl J Med.* 2009;361:2241.
48. Park SJ, Tector A, Piccioni W, et al. Left ventricular assist devices as destination therapy: a new look at survival. *J Thorac Cardiovasc Surg.* 2005;129(9):2005; erratum 129:1464.
49. Starling RC, Naka Y, Boyle AJ, et al. Results of the post–U.S. Food and Drug Administration–approval study with a continuous flow left ventricular assist device as a bridge to heart transplantation: a prospective study using the INTERMACS (Interagency Registry for Mechanically Assisted Circulatory Support). *J Am Coll Cardiol.* 2011;57:1890.
49a. Pagani FD, Cantor R, Cowger J, et al. Concordance of treatment effect: an analysis of The Society of Thoracic Surgeons Intermacs Database [published online ahead of print, 2021 Jun 1]. *Ann Thorac Surg.* 2021;S0003-4975(21)00929-2. https://doi.org/10.1016/j.athoracsur.2021.05.017.
49b. Medtronic Recalls HVAD Pump Implant Kits Due to Delayed or Failed Restart After the Pump is Stopped. U.S. Food and Drug Administration Website. https://www.fda.gov/medical-devices/medical-device-recalls/medtronic-recalls-hvad-pump-implant-kits-due-delayed-or-failed-restart-after-pump-stopped. Accessed July 7, 2021.
50. Aaronson KD, Slaughter MS, Miller LW, et al. Use of an intrapericardial, continuous-flow, centrifugal pump in patients awaiting heart transplantation. *Circulation.* 2012;125:3191.
51. Slaughter MS, Pagani FD, McGee EC, et al. HeartWare ventricular assist system for bridge to transplant: combined results of the bridge to transplant and continued access protocol trial. *J Heart Lung Transplant.* 2013;32:675.
52. Rogers JG, Pagani FD, Tatooles AJ, et al. Intrapericardial left ventricular assist device for advanced heart failure. *N Engl J Med.* 2017;376:451–460.
53. Milano CA, Rogers JG, Tatooles AJ, et al. HVAD: the ENDURANCE supplemental trial. *JACC Heart Fail.* 2018;6:792–802.
54. Copeland JG, Smith RG, Arabia FA, et al. Cardiac replacement with a total artificial heart as a bridge to transplantation. *N Engl J Med.* 2004;351:859.

Interagency Registry of Mechanically Assisted Circulatory Support

55. Teuteberg JJ, Cleveland Jr JC, Cowger J, et al. The Society of Thoracic Surgeons INTERMACS 2019 annual report: the changing landscape of devices and indications. *Ann Thorac Surg.* 2020;109:649–660.
56. Stevenson LW, Pagani FD, Young JB, et al. INTERMACS profiles of advanced heart failure: the current picture. *J Heart Lung Transplant.* 2009;28:535–541.
57. Kormos RL, Cowger J, Pagani FD, et al. The Society of Thoracic Surgeons Intermacs database annual report: evolving indications, outcomes, and scientific partnerships. *J Heart Lung Transplant.* 2019;38:114–126.

Future Perspectives

58. Goldstein DJ, Naftel D, Holman W, et al. Continuous-flow devices and percutaneous site infections: clinical outcomes. *J Heart Lung Transplant.* 2012;31:1151.
59. Pya Y, Maly J, Bekbossynova M, et al. First human use of a wireless coplanar energy transfer coupled with a continuous-flow left ventricular assist device. *J Heart Lung Transplant.* 2019;38:339–343.
60. Baldwin JT, Borovetz HS, Duncan BW, et al. The national, heart, lung, and blood institute pediatric circulatory support program: a summary of the 5-year experience. *Circulation.* 2011;123:1233.
61. Adachi I. Current status and future perspectives of the PumpKIN trial. *Transl Pediatr.* 2018;7:162–168.
62. Kirklin JK, Mehra MR. The dawn of the ISHLT Mechanical Assisted Circulatory Support (IMACS) registry: fulfilling our mission. *J Heart Lung Transplant.* 2012;31:115.
63. US Food and Drug Administration Center for Devices and Radiological Health. Japan–U.S. "Harmonization by doing" HBD Pilot Program initiative; 2010. http://www.fda.gov/MedicalDevices/DeviceRegulationandGuidance/InternationalInformation/ucm053067.htm.

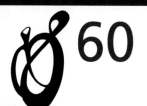

60 Cardiac Transplantation

RANDALL C. STARLING

HISTORICAL ASPECTS

Cardiac transplantation in humans began over 50 years ago in Cape Town, South Africa.[1] After rapid initial growth in the United States, transplantation stopped because of poor outcomes. The initial 1-year survival was only approximately 20%, and most centers ceased cardiac transplantation programs. In 1984 with the approval of cyclosporine, there was a proliferation of heart transplant centers in the United States as the survival improved significantly. Currently, there are over 140 active heart transplant centers in the United States. The valiant efforts of pioneering heart surgeons, cardiologists, pathologists, and immunologists have all contributed to the ongoing improvements in the technical and management aspects of cardiac transplantation now achieving outstanding short- and long-term outcomes.

EPIDEMIOLOGY OF HEART TRANSPLANTATION

Heart transplantation is performed internationally, as well as at over 140 centers in the United States. The International Society of Heart and Lung Transplantation (ISHLT; https://ishlt.org/research-data/registries/ttx-registry) maintains an international registry that contains in excess of 140,000 heart transplants, reported from 390 international centers. The Scientific Registry of Transplant Recipients (https://www.srtr.org/transplant-centers/?organ=heart) is a USA-based registry of heart transplant recipients and provides program specific outcomes. The United Network of Organ Sharing (UNOS; https://unos.org/) also provides extensive information for heart transplant centers and outcomes. In 2019 a record number of 3552 heart transplants were performed in the United States, representing a 4.2% increase over the 3408 transplants performed in 2018. Over the past decade the number of heart transplants has continuously grown; in 2010 2332 heart transplants were performed compared with 3552 heart transplants in 2019, representing a 34% increase in 9 years in heart transplant volume. There were 669 heart transplants performed in Europe in 2019 (https://www.eurotransplant.org/organs/heart/).

The tremendous growth in transplant volume has been attributed to successful treatment of hepatitis C and expansion of the donor pool.[2] Secondly, the opiate crisis in the United States and Europe has increased the numbers of suitable donors secondary to drug overdoses.[3,4] Based on early and emerging outcomes data, the results are equivalent using these donors. Combined heart-lung, heart-liver, and heart-kidney transplantation can be performed with excellent results, but the numbers are very limited.

EVALUATION OF THE POTENTIAL RECIPIENT

Medical Issues

The benchmark for the consideration of cardiac transplantation is marked reduction in functional capacity despite implementation of all conventional therapies (see also Chapters 50 and 59). The advanced heart failure specialist must consider and exhaust all treatment options before recommending transplantation. Figure 60.1 summarizes the details of testing and evaluation for patients undergoing an evaluation for cardiac transplantation. The convention is to measure exercise capacity objectively with cardiopulmonary exercise testing or a 6-minute walk test. A peak oxygen consumption ($\dot{V}o_2$) less than 50% of age and gender predicted is considered a marked functional limitation. In general, a peak $\dot{V}o_2$ of less than 10 mL-kg-minute is considered as an indication for cardiac transplantation, and a peak $\dot{V}o_2$ less than 14 mL/kg/min is considered a poor prognosis. A 6-minute walk of less than 300 m is considered a marked impairment. Additional testing is required for a full review of all organ systems, with a goal to ensure there are no life-threatening comorbidities and or conditions that would complicate the ability to survive heart transplant surgery or limit life span for noncardiac reasons. Most malignancies in remission and/or with a disease-free interval for 5 years or longer will not preclude cardiac transplantation. Concomitant severe renal, pulmonary, or hepatic disease may indicate a need for the consideration of dual organ transplantation. The details of full evaluation for heart transplantation in the patient with advanced heart failure are described in detail in a recent American College of Cardiology report.[5] Figure 60.2 provides an algorithm for the consideration of heart transplantation and left ventricular assist device (LVAD) (see also Chapter 59). Evaluation of the pulmonary artery pressures and pulmonary vascular resistance (PVR) is essential. Patients with World Health Organization (WHO) group 2 pulmonary artery hypertension (see also Chapter 88) generally respond well to diuresis and pharmacologic or mechanical unloading with acceptable PVR. Patients with elevation of the PVR and transpulmonic gradient refractory to treatment may require consideration of heart and lung transplantation. Many patients listed for cardiac transplantation will require support with LVAD while awaiting a donor heart. In the United States, almost

Additional content is available online at Elsevier eBooks for Practicing Clinicians

Evaluation of the Heart Transplant Candidate

- Clinical history and physical examination
- Laboratory evaluation: Complete blood count, basic metabolic panel, liver function tests, urinalysis, coagulation studies, thyroid evaluation, urine drug screen, alcohol level, HIV testing, hepatitis testing, tuberculosis screening, CMV IgG and IgM, RPR/VDRL, panel reactive antibodies, ABO and Rh blood type, lipids, hemoglobin A1c
- Chest x-ray, pulmonary function testing
- ECG
- Right and left heart catheterization
- Cardiopulmonary exercise testing
- Age- appropriate malignancy screening
- Psychosocial evaluation (including substance abuse history, mental health, and social support)
- Financial screening

FIGURE 60.1 Evaluation of the heart transplant candidate. (From Guglin M, Zucker MJ, Borlaug BA, et al. ACC Heart Failure and Transplant Member Section and Leadership Council. Evaluation for Heart Transplantation and LVAD Implantation: JACC Council perspectives. *J Am Coll Cardiol.* 2020;75:1471–1487.)

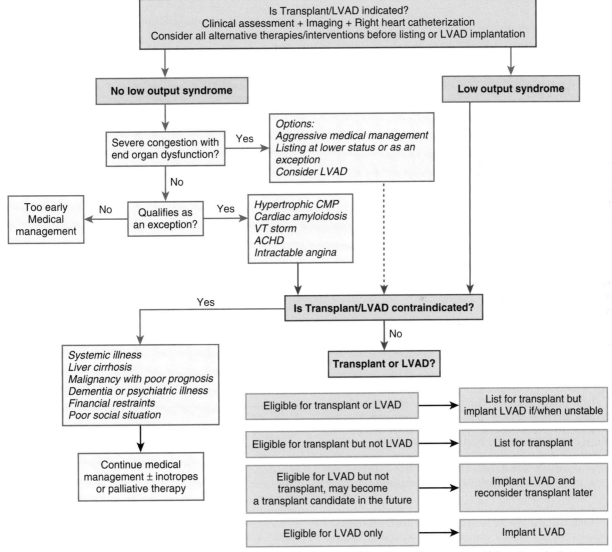

FIGURE 60.2 Algorithm for choosing cardiac transplantation or left ventricular assist device (LVAD) in patients with advanced heart failure. The evaluation process within the advanced heart failure center consists of three main parts: identification of indications for heart transplantation and/or LVAD implantation, ruling out contraindications, and deciding on the strategy: proceed with listing, proceed with LVAD placement, continue management, or administer palliative care. In the latter two scenarios, the patient may be sent back to the referring center or co-managed by both teams. *ACHD,* Adult congenital heart disease; *CMP,* cardiomyopathy; *VT,* ventricular tachycardia. (From Guglin M, Zucker MJ, Borlaug BA, et al. Evaluation for heart transplantation and LVAD implantation. *J Am Coll Cardiol.* 2020;75[12]:1471–1487.)

half of those transplanted are on LVAD historically. Transplant outcomes are essentially equivalent with LVAD support when compared with those not supported with LVAD. A decision to support with LVAD prior to transplant is made by the local transplant team and relates to waiting time, severity of illness, and decisions related to best strategy to achieve a successful heart transplant.

Age is a variable that generates robust discussion. There is a "U-" shaped relationship historically regarding mortality post heart transplant, with increased mortality in those younger than 18 years of age and those older than 65 years of age. There are numerous isolated reports of excellent survival in recipients older than age 65 to 70 years from individual centers. The registry data clearly demonstrate reduced survival that increases by decade of age older than 60 years. Individual centers generally have established algorithms for patient treatment with LVAD and heart transplantation related to recipient age. Some centers have adopted an approach of using donors that would be otherwise discarded (e.g., donor age older than 55 years) as "extended donors" for potential recipients that exceed local established upper limits of age. The ethics of transplantation and allocation of a "scarce" resource is often discussed when evaluating which patient groups will be most likely to have successful outcomes with heart transplantation.

Psychosocial Evaluation

The Stanford Integrated Psychosocial Assessment for Transplantation (SIPAT) is used by most U.S. heart transplant centers to quantify a candidate's psychosocial milieu and determine compliance and social support.[6] It has been well established that lack of a support structure and noncompliance portend poor outcomes after cardiac transplantation. The SIPAT is an objective tool that quantifies and scores each candidate and has been linked to survival post transplantation. The ISHLT has published guidelines for the psychosocial evaluation of adult heart transplant recipients.[7] The psychosocial evaluation is an integral and essential component of a heart transplant evaluation. The social worker is an active, important member of every heart transplant team.

Substance Abuse

Most U.S. programs will not consider an active user of a tobacco product for transplant and require cessation for a minimum of 6 months before listing for transplant. Substance abuse is considered a contraindication to heart transplantation. A patient with an active opiate addiction will not be considered for heart transplantation and will be referred to an addiction specialist for recommendations for recovery. The use of cannabis is generally considered a contraindication, but there are statewide variations. Most heart failure centers will offer LVAD to patients with advanced heart failure and active addiction; hence providing a lifesaving device to enable the patient an opportunity to embark upon a recovery program with the hope for potential transplant listing in the future.

DONOR ALLOCATION SYSTEM

Allocation of donor hearts in the United States is based upon a new algorithm developed by the United Network for Organ Sharing that was implemented October 2018. In contrast to the prior donor allocation system which categorized patients as status 1A, 1B, and 2, there are now six categories that were designated, based upon severity of illness, diagnosis, and risk factors felt to be associated with wait list mortality (Table 60.1).[8] When an offer is made, the center has 30 minutes to respond and must decide based upon recipient condition and donor variables to accept or decline the donor offer. The changes were designed to reduce the waiting list mortality and reduce waiting times, while maintaining excellent outcomes. Early indicators suggest that there is an evolving shift from durable LVAD support to short-term support devices, including an intra-aortic balloon pump and percutaneous LVAD (see also Chapter 59).

The short-term survival of recipients listed and receiving a transplant under the old and new allocation systems has been observed to be comparable. The modification to the allocation system has resulted in several changes to the clinical management of patients undergoing heart transplantation. The implications of these practice changes should be closely monitored to ensure, at minimum, equivalent outcomes. The impact of the revised allocation system has shown a marked increase in the use of the intra-aortic balloon pump pretransplant with the Scientific Registry for Transplant Recipients (SRTR) registry report demonstrating an increase from 7.6% to 28.3% after the allocation revision. There is variability across UNOS regions in the proportion of patients undergoing heart transplantation at the most urgent listing statuses,[1–3] ranging from 29% in region six (Pacific Northwest) to 63% in region eight (Central Plains). Clinicians may

TABLE 60.1 Adult Heart Allocation Criteria for Medical Urgency Status

Tier		
1.	i.	VA ECMO (up to 7 days)
	ii.	Nondischargeable BIVAD
	iii.	Mechanical circulatory support with life-threatening ventricular arrhythmia
2.	i.	Intra-aortic balloon pump (up to 14 days)
	ii.	Acute percutaneous endovascular circulatory support (up to 14 days of support)
	iii.	Ventricular tachycardia/ventricular fibrillation; mechanical circulatory support not required
	iv.	Mechanical circulatory support with device malfunction/device failure
	v.	Total artificial heart
	vi.	Dischargeable BIVAD or RVAD
3.	i.	LVAD for up to 30 days
	ii.	Multiple inotropes of single high-dose inotrope with continuous hemodynamic monitoring
	iii.	Mechanical circulatory support with device infection
	iv.	Mechanical circulatory support with thromboembolism
	v.	Mechanical circulatory support with device-related complications other than infection, thromboembolism, device
4.	i.	Diagnosis of congenital heart disease (CHO) with:
		a. Unrepaired/incompletely repaired complex CHO, usually with cyanosis
		b. Repaired CHD with two ventricles
		c. Single ventricle repaired with Fontan or modifications
	ii.	Diagnosis of ischemic heart disease with intractable angina
	iii.	Diagnosis of hypertrophic cardiomyopathy
	iv.	Diagnosis of restrictive cardiomyopathy
	v.	Stable LVAD patient after 30 days
	vi.	Inotropes without hemodynamic monitoring
	vii.	Diagnosis of amyloidosis
	viii.	Retransplant
5.	i.	Approved combined organ-transplants: heart-lung, heart-liver, heart-kidney
6.	i.	All remaining active candidates
7.	i.	Inactive/not transplantable

BIVAD, biventricular assist device; *LVAD,* left ventricular assist device; *RVAD,* right ventricular assist device; *VA ECMO,* venoarterial extracorporeal membrane oxygenation.

recommend placement of a balloon pump or extracorporeal membrane oxygenation to sustain life and hence expedite transplantation, which might potentially expose patients to higher daily risks of device complications. In some geographic regions, waiting times appear to be shorter for those in urgent need. The use of durable LVAD as bridge to transplant (BTT) has declined. Meanwhile, among patients with a durable LVAD listed for transplant, transplantation rates are low, and these patients are listed as status 4. When a specified device-related complication occurs, it may permit escalation to status 2 or 3, hence hopefully facilitating a shorter waiting time.

THE CARDIAC DONOR

Donor Evaluation

In light of an inadequate number and increasing organ demand, efficacious donor management and selection are crucial in maintaining excellent transplant volumes and outcomes. Obviously, it is critical

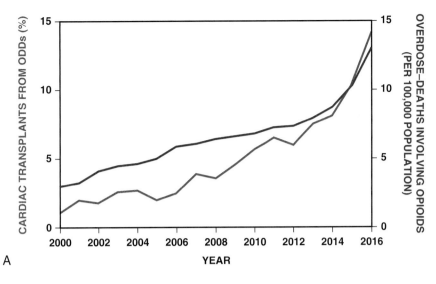

A

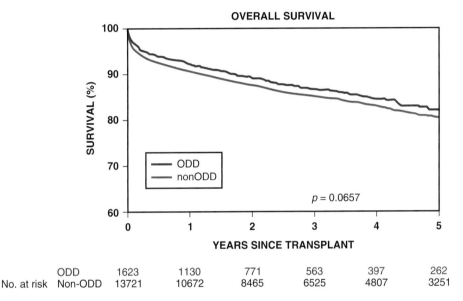

	ODD	1623	1130	771	563	397	262
No. at risk	Non-ODD	13721	10672	8465	6525	4807	3251

B

FIGURE 60.3 Impact of the opioid epidemic on heart transplantation. **A,** National average percentage of cardiac transplants from overdose-death donors (ODD) compared with overdose deaths involving opioids per 100,000 population. **B,** Kaplan-Meier analysis for survival on the basis of ODD status. *blue line,* Non-ODD; *No.,* number; *Red line,* ODD. (From Phillips KG, Ranganath NK, Malas J, et al. Impact of the opioid epidemic on heart transplantation: donor characteristics and organ discard. *Ann Thorac Surg.* 2019;108[4]:1133–1139.)

risk factors. The final decision to accept a heart for transplantation is made at the time of harvesting, after direct examination of the heart for coronary calcification, as well as left ventricular hypertrophy or dilation. Many regions have instituted a process of systematically reviewing donor turndown events to reduce variability and increase confidence in expanded criteria for donors. These outcome reviews have resulted in improved donor organ utilization and transplant volumes.[10]

Hepatitis C and Drug Overdose Cause of Death

Over the past 5 years it has become more common to accept donor organs that are hepatitis C–positive donors or donors when the cause of death is related to overdose. As shown in Figure 60.3A the percent of overdose-death donors was 1.1% in 2000 and rose to 14.2% in 2017.[11]

Registry data indicate that survival with overdose-death donors is equivalent to non–overdose-death donors (see Fig. 60.3B). The advent of antiviral agents now permits use of use of hepatitis C–positive donors and subsequent cure if seroconversion occurs.[2] Prolonged follow-up will provide important information as to the suitability of these donor organs. An early report suggests that hepatitis C–positive donor recipients may experience a higher frequency of acute allograft rejection.[12] Although this report was in a limited cohort of 22 viremic recipients, it will be imperative to track the outcomes of these patients carefully. Any systemic viral infection that involves the endothelium could, in theory, accelerate coronary vascular disease. At present this expanded donor pool will save lives at minimum with excellent short-term survival.

Donation After Circulatory Determined Death Donors

This form of organ donation is now beginning to advance in the United States in efforts to expand the donor pool. Donation after circulatory determined death (DCD) involves donors with devastating brain injury who depend on life support but do not meet the legal criteria for brain death. After the withdrawal of life support, death is declared on the basis of cardiac arrest and organ harvest ensues thereafter. If widely adopted, DCD has the estimated potential to increase overall heart transplant volume by more than 20%. A report from the United Kingdom over a 5-year period from 2015 to 2020 at a single transplant center demonstrated a 48% increase in transplantation with similar 30-day and 1-year survival between DCD and standard donors.[13] The history, techniques, and role for the future is explained in detail regarding the potential to expand the donor pool.[14]

to obtain a complete medical history for the donor, including any relevant cardiovascular disorders before brain death. All donors are screened for communicable diseases, including viral disorders such as hepatitis and HIV infection. Specific information that is relevant for the assessment of cardiac donor suitability also includes the presence or absence of thoracic trauma, disseminated cancer, donor hemodynamic stability, pressor and inotropic requirements, duration of cardiac arrest, and need for cardiopulmonary resuscitation. In some cardiac donors, hemodynamic deterioration may be caused by brain death. Cardiac echocardiography is required on all donors, and coronary arteriography is required to evaluate the presence of coronary artery disease in donors older than 45 to 50 years, depending on other risk factors.

The acceptable cold ischemia time for cardiac transplantation is approximately 4 to 5 hours; systems of ex vivo heart perfusion of human heart donors are under investigation.[9] Prolonged ischemic time has been shown to be a significant risk factor for death after cardiac transplantation, especially when it is coupled with other risk factors, such as older donor age. Donors up to the age of 60 to 65 years are currently considered, depending on transport distance and other donor

SURGICAL CONSIDERATIONS

The two most common surgical approaches for the implantation of the donor heart are the biatrial and the bicaval anastomoses. The bicaval anastomosis technique was introduced with the intention to reduce right atrial size, to minimize distortion of the recipient heart, to preserve atrial conduction pathways, and to decrease tricuspid regurgitation. This alternative procedure entails five anastomoses: left atrium, pulmonary artery, aorta, inferior vena cava, and superior vena cava. Although no prospective trial has been conducted to establish the superiority of either technique, the bicaval technique is now being done most often in the United States, primarily because it appears to decrease the need for permanent pacemakers in transplant recipients.[15] Most important, the number of patients coming to transplantation with ventricular assist devices in place has steadily increased, so that transplant procedures are riskier and result in more device-related complications. Each prior sternotomy increases risk; it is now commonplace for the heart transplant recipient to have undergone one or more prior sternotomies, and this should not be considered as a contraindication.

The most common reason for failure to wean a heart transplant recipient from cardiopulmonary bypass is right-sided heart failure, evidenced by a low cardiac output despite a rising central venous pressure. The right side of the heart can be seen in the surgical field to dilate and to contract poorly. Intraoperative transesophageal echocardiography shows a dilated, poorly contracting right ventricle and an underfilled, vigorously contracting left ventricle. Right ventricular function may be enhanced with inotropes and pulmonary vasodilators, but the prognostic importance of preoperative PVR becomes obvious in these first few hours after surgery.[16] A most important and essential element of assessing suitability for cardiac transplantation is to measure the PVR. Often a challenge with vasodilator therapy and adjunctive measures to improve left heart function and reduce pulmonary capillary wedge pressure are necessary to determine reversibility of WHO group 2 pulmonary hypertension. Patients receiving LVAD as BTT with pulmonary hypertension often normalize after unloading with LVAD, and serial measures with right heart catheterization are often required to document reversal.

IMMUNOSUPPRESSION

Immunosuppressive regimens begin with the simultaneous use of three classes of drugs: glucocorticoids, calcineurin inhibitors (CNIs), and antiproliferative agents.[17] In the immediate postoperative period, immunosuppressive agents are given parenterally with a quick transition to oral formulations. In a subset of patients, transplant teams use a variety of drugs for "induction therapy" to rapidly enhance immune tolerance. This practice was based upon the prior experiences in renal transplantation. Over the past 30 years there has been a vast experience with different agents.[18] Globally, transplant centers are divided, and approximately half use induction therapy.[19] The arguments in favor of induction are to minimize the risk of rejection and to minimize steroid use. The downsides include infection, malignancy, and the potential for mortality as a consequence. The two most commonly used agents are basiliximab and T cell cytolytic agents. Basiliximab is a chimeric mouse-human monoclonal antibody to the α chain (CD25) of the interleukin-2 (IL-2) receptor of T cells. Antithymocyte globulins (ATGs) are the T cell cytolytic agents. A large registry analysis compared recipients receiving no induction versus basiliximab or ATGs.[20] Survival was equivalent with no induction or ATGs and reduced with basiliximab. More deaths attributable to malignancy were seen in the ATG group. Another common practice is to delay the introduction of a CNI early after transplant, to avoid the potential associated nephrotoxicity. A "renal sparing" approach without a CNI and use of an induction agent in theory may prevent early post-transplant acute kidney injury.

The mainstay of chronic immunotherapy is corticosteroids. Steroids are given intravenously (IV) preoperatively and postoperatively and are rapidly converted to oral therapy. There is tremendous variability regarding steroid dosing, and most centers aim to remove steroids after the first year if it is feasible. Corticosteroids are nonspecific

antiinflammatory agents that work primarily by lymphocyte depletion. Side effects are common and include cushingoid appearance, fluid retention, hypertension, dyslipidemia, weight gain with central obesity, gastrointestinal bleeding, pancreatitis, cataract formation, hyperglycemia, and osteoporosis with avascular necrosis of bone. Bone densitometry monitoring and treatment with vitamin D and calcium supplements are often necessary.

The advent of the CNI cyclosporine, approved for use in the United States in 1984, was a pivotal landmark that changed heart transplantation in the United States. The introduction of cyclosporine, the first in class CNI led to improved survival, fewer infections, and the ability to minimize steroid use. There are two CNIs, cyclosporine and tacrolimus, commonly in use. Nephrotoxicity and hypertension are common adverse events. Tacrolimus was subsequently developed with the hope for superior efficacy and fewer adverse events. Their primary mechanism of action involves binding to specific proteins (cyclophilin or FK-binding protein) to form complexes that block the action of calcineurin, a key participant in T cell activation. They suppress the immune system by blocking T cell proliferation through the inhibition of its key signaling phosphatase calcineurin, thus called CNIs. The CNIs serve to block the signal transduction pathways responsible for T cell and B cell activation.

Tacrolimus is the CNI currently used and may be administered IV, orally, or sublingually. Tacrolimus is given twice a day, and the dosing is based upon monitoring 12-hour trough levels. Target trough levels tend to decrease after the first year. The most common patient-centered adverse events are tremor and hypertension. Acute nephrotoxicity, usually reversible, can be seen and is potentiated by the concurrent use of nonsteroid antiinflammatory agents, which should be strictly avoided. Chronic nephrotoxicity is a late consequence of CNI use and may be definitively diagnosed only by renal biopsy and pathology. Hirsutism, gingival hyperplasia, hyperlipidemia, and neuropathy may also occur.

Antiproliferative agents work to either directly or indirectly inhibit the expansion of activated T cell and B cell clones after antigen presentation. Historically, azathioprine was the first agent used in this class and served as the mainstay of immunosuppression with steroids before the routine use of cyclosporine. Mycophenolate mofetil (MMF) has replaced azathioprine as the first-line antiproliferative agent based upon clinical trials demonstrating superiority and a reduction in rejection with hemodynamic compromise.[21] MMF is hydrolyzed to mycophenolic acid, which inhibits de novo purine synthesis. Both azathioprine and MMF cause leukopenia as their major adverse effect; the use of MMF can be limited by diarrhea and nausea and may be associated with a form of colitis. MMF is given IV or orally twice a day. There is an enteric coated, long-acting once-a-day form of the drug. There is also concern that viral infections, primarily cytomegalovirus (CMV), may be more prevalent in the presence of MMF.

Mammalian target of rapamycin (mTOR) are immunosuppressive drugs that inhibit the mTOR, which is a serine/threonine-specific protein kinase. Rapamycin inhibits cellular proliferation and cell cycle progression, and it was discovered to have immunosuppressive properties in the 1980s. Sirolimus (often called rapamycin) and everolimus are two mTOR inhibitors that block activation of T cells after autocrine stimulation by IL-2. They also are known to inhibit proliferation of endothelial cells and fibroblasts. Originally, it was hoped that mTOR inhibitors might have unique characteristics to reduce the scourge of cardiac transplantation, cardiac allograft vasculopathy (CAV). A clinical trial published in 2003 provided optimism for the role of this class of immunosuppressive drugs, showing a reduction in CAV.[22] Their action is complementary to that of CNIs, and both sirolimus and everolimus have been used as maintenance immunosuppression, as alternatives to standard immunosuppression, and as rescue drugs for rejection. The mTOR inhibitors have been shown to slow progression of CAV in patients with established disease and to reduce development of de novo CAV.[23,24] The use of sirolimus as a primary immunosuppressive agent has been observed to reduce CAV and improve survival, but definitive data from randomized clinical trials do not exist.[25] The drugs inhibit the proliferation of fibroblasts and may theoretically cause delayed wound healing although this was not observed with everolimus in the randomized trial with de novo use. Finally, reduced

TABLE 60.2 ISHLT Standardized Cardiac Biopsy Grading Compared with an Earlier System

2004 SYSTEM		1990 SYSTEM	
GRADE 0 R	**NO REJECTION**	**GRADE 0**	**NO REJECTION**
Grade 1 R, mild	Interstitial and/or perivascular infiltrate with up to one focus of myocyte damage	Grade 1, mild	
		A—focal	Focal perivascular and/or interstitial infiltrate without myocyte damage
		B—diffuse	Diffuse infiltrate without myocyte damage
Grade 2 R, moderate	Two or more foci of infiltrate with associated myocyte damage	Grade 2, moderate (focal)	One focus of infiltrate with associated myocyte damage
Grade 3 R, severe	Diffuse infiltrate with multifocal myocyte damage ± edema, ± hemorrhage, ± vasculitis	Grade 3, moderate	
		A—focal	Multifocal infiltrate with myocyte damage
		B—diffuse	Diffuse infiltrate with myocyte damage
		Grade 4, severe	Diffuse, polymorphous infiltrate with extensive myocyte damage ± hemorrhage ± vasculitis

ISHLT, International Society of Heart and Lung Transplantation.
Modified from Stewart S, Winters GL, Fishbein MC, et al. Revision of the 1990 working formulation for the standardization of nomenclature in the diagnosis of heart rejection. *J Heart Lung Transplant.* 2005;24:1710.

occurrence of CMV viremia and infection has been observed with everolimus-based regimens and forms the basis for use in some recipients with recurrent CMV disease. Despite the accumulated efficacy data with everolimus, it has not been approved by the FDA for the indication of cardiac transplantation and its use is "off label" in the United States. The main concern of the FDA was related to worse renal outcomes observed in the two large, randomized trials performed in the United States.[22,26–28] The withdrawal of CNI and replacement with mTOR should be considered with caution and careful observation if implemented.

REJECTION

Rejection, which once limited the effectiveness of cardiac transplantation, has become a much less common occurrence in the current era. Rejection has been primarily an asymptomatic diagnosis based upon surveillance endomyocardial biopsy and pathologic examination of the specimens. Although heart biopsy has been considered the "gold standard," it is well established that there may be significant variability between pathologists with concordance studies showing up to 25% of biopsies receiving different pathologic grades. This has created variability among centers and the requirement for external pathology panels is a necessity in clinical trials. Over the past decade, noninvasive and laboratory-based assays have become available, challenging the need for routine, frequent surveillance endomyocardial biopsies.

From the beginning, rejection has referred to the infiltration of lymphocytes within the myocardium. The intensity of the lymphocytic infiltration and the degree of myocyte injury and necrosis determines the pathologic grade of rejection. Heart biopsies are graded by a standardized international grading system developed by the International Society for Heart and Lung Transplantation shown in Table 60.2.[29] Rejection is subdivided as cellular and antibody mediated.

Cellular Rejection

Cellular rejection has been the basis of surveillance endomyocardial biopsy justification. Early reports indicated up to 50% of patient demonstrating moderate forms of rejection in the first 6 months; currently the rates observed have decreased to approximately 10%. Factors contributing to the reduced rates are related to improved donor-recipient matching with improvements in organ matching based upon "virtual" crossmatching and improvements in immunosuppressive regimens. Virtual crossmatch uses solid phase assays to detect anti-HLA antibodies in the recipient and allows exclusion of donors with unacceptable HLA antigens. The previous mandate for a negative prospective crossmatch has been largely eliminated based upon the use of virtual

crossmatches and high concordance with final crossmatches when lymphoid tissue from the donor becomes available.

In most cases of cellular rejection diagnosed from a surveillance endomyocardial biopsy, the patient is asymptomatic and will have no evidence of cardiac allograft dysfunction. This explains why imaging of the functioning allograft with echo is insensitive to detect cellular rejection, which most often is a pathologic diagnosis without changes in heart function or physiology. Most often, cellular rejection is treated by steroid augmentation or adjustment of baseline immunosuppressive medications. Heart biopsies that are triggered by patient symptoms, or a decline in graft function that demonstrates moderate to severe cellular rejection require hospitalization, IV steroids, and other adjunctive therapies often including antithymocyte globulin. Some patients will require hemodynamic monitoring or inotropic or mechanical support; fortunately for most patients, graft dysfunction from cellular rejection is reversible with treatment and full recovery is expected. Numerous other techniques, including cardiac MRI (see also Chapter 19), have been studied, with varying degrees of effectiveness, but none have replaced the endomyocardial biopsy.[30]

The advent of gene expression profiling assays has proliferated over the past decade and become mainstream to monitor the cardiac allograft. A commercially available test, the AlloMap, is based upon a validated 11 gene panel to diagnosis cellular rejection. The panel of 11 informative genes and 9 controlled genes detects changes in gene expression associated with acute rejection and provides an actionable score. The usefulness of this test was studied in a multicenter study over a decade ago; however, the uptake of the blood test to replace endomyocardial biopsy has been gradual.[31] Most recently an ancillary blood test measuring donor-derived cell-free DNA has been developed, envisioned to be combined with gene expression profiling to monitor the cardiac allograft.[32]

Antibody-Mediated Rejection

Antibody-mediated rejection (AMR) was formally defined based on the 2005 ISHLT publication revising the pathologic standards for rejection. Prior to this formulation, it was recognized that heart transplant recipients would present with graft dysfunction and hemodynamic compromise and only mild cellular rejection present on heart biopsy. Eventually, it was observed that most of these patients had developed donor-specific antibodies to HLA loci. Subsequently with the advent of staining for complement, the observation of complement deposition in the heart biopsies of patients with hemodynamic compromise led to the terminology of "humoral rejection with hemodynamic compromise." Hence the terminology of AMR was formally defined and subsequently refined in 2011.[33] AMR remains a challenge; there is variability in monitoring, and currently there is not a validated noninvasive or blood test. Most often, HLA antibody in the form of donor-specific assays are present, but it is also known that non-HLA antibody may be implicated in AMR. Heart biopsy and the presence of complement with adjunctive histologic criteria are the basis of the pathologic diagnosis. The treatment is less standardized but most often includes cytolytic agents, antibody depletion, and specific therapies directed at B cell lymphocytes.[34] AMR can present early or late post transplant, and the most vulnerable patients are those with positive crossmatch, elevated preformed antibody levels, and demographically multiparous female recipients. AMR is often associated with graft dysfunction and hemodynamic compromise. Treatment may require prolonged antibody depletion with plasmapheresis, and protocols with photopheresis have been described.

Recently a tissue-based molecular diagnostic system has been developed aimed to increase the accuracy of both T cell–mediated cellular rejection and AMR.[35] RNA is extracted from endomyocardial biopsy specimens, and analyses are performed to detect rejection-associated transcripts associated with known profiles from renal transplant T cell–mediated and AMR. The hope is that this modality will provide a new tool to improve the accuracy of diagnosis and calibration of histology interpretations.

OUTCOMES AFTER HEART TRANSPLANTATION

Surveillance for Rejection and Coronary Artery Vasculopathy

The conventions for performing heart biopsy and coronary angiography were established decades ago by the original U.S. heart transplant programs. Endomyocardial biopsies were performed 12 to 15 times the first year post transplant and gradually reduced in frequency after year 1. Many programs continued surveillance heart biopsies twice a year indefinitely. Much variation exists throughout the United States now, with some programs stopping endomyocardial biopsy after the first year and using laboratory and imaging techniques and only a clinical event-driven approach to heart biopsy. The majority of U.S. programs perform routine surveillance heart biopsies at minimum for the first year post transplant. As was discussed, the endomyocardial biopsy is the only technique that can diagnose both cellular and AMR. AMR can be diagnosed by light microscopy on the basis of histology and either immunohistochemistry or immunofluorescence. The limitation of the gene expression profiling assay (AlloMap) is that it is validated only for cellular rejection. Most heart transplant programs follow their recipients long term and continue routine testing and clinic visits designed to diagnose asymptomatic rejection or coronary disease before a clinical manifestation occurs.

The convention for surveillance coronary angiography is yearly for the lifetime of the transplant recipient. Coronary artery vasculopathy (CAV) is common and can occur within the first year after transplant or much later after the first decade. Monitoring techniques have included coronary angiography, intravascular ultrasound (IVUS), and coronary optical coherence tomography. The latter two procedures are primarily investigational, although IVUS is used in conjunction with percutaneous coronary interventions (PCIs) routinely. Based on evidence obtained from clinical trials, it was felt that IVUS determined findings of coronary changes even without the concurrent demonstration of angiographic disease were important and predictive of the development of angiographic disease. Insurers typically will not reimburse for IVUS studies, and its use for surveillance has waned recently. Many patients with high-grade, epicardial coronary obstructions may be asymptomatic when referred for surveillance cardiac cath. Most patients are treated with drug-eluting stents, even if asymptomatic. The dogma has been that denervated heart transplant recipients do not always exhibit typical angina. Most noninvasive techniques have been studied for CAV surveillance; however, they lack the necessary sensitivity and specificity to replace the routine use of coronary angiography. Perhaps the most promising noninvasive strategy for coronary surveillance is the use of PET imaging.[36] At present, coronary angiography yearly or less frequently and supplemented with yearly noninvasive stress imaging is the basis for CAV surveillance. It is believed that aspirin and statin use should be routine in heart transplant recipients even

without elevation of low-density lipoprotein (LDL). Lipid abnormalities should be aggressively treated.

Survival

Patients with stage D heart failure are estimated to have a mortality of 50% at 6 months and nearly 100% at 1 year. These projections are based on reported mortality for patients deemed to be inotrope dependent. When listing a patient for transplant, most often the decision is based upon reduced quality of life and poor functional capacity. Advances in medical and device therapies for heart failure have markedly reduced mortality; hence a patient listed for transplant may have an estimated 1-year mortality of 20% to 30% or less depending on the clinical situation. Acknowledging the potential "survival benefit" is important when recommending cardiac transplantation. From a long-term perspective the survival advantage for transplantation becomes very clear when looking at survival projections at 10 years and beyond. Thus two common situations exist; the hospitalized patient in extremis related to an acute event or chronic decompensation and the "walking wounded" patient with chronic heart failure being managed as an outpatient with poor quality of life and reduced exercise tolerance. LVADs have played a role in the management of patients in both scenarios and provided both improved survival and quality of life while waiting for a donor heart; it is referred to as the "bridge to transplant" strategy for LVAD therapy (see also Chapter 59).

The major source of information for heart transplantation survival is based upon the ISHLT registry that contains data on over 146,000 transplants. The registry is updated yearly and provides detailed information related to demographics, era, and immunosuppression. The 2019 registry report shows survival related to era of transplantation: the median survival from 1992 to 2001 was 10.5 years and increased to 12.5 years in the era 2002 to 2009 (Fig. 60.4).[37] Survival, activity, and outcome metrics for all U.S. heart transplant programs can be viewed in detail on the Health Resources and Services Administration (HRSA) website *The Scientific Registry for Transplant Recipients* (https://srtr.transplant.hrsa.gov /).[38] Many successful U.S. heart transplant programs report 1-year survival greater than 90% and 3-year survival greater than 85%. There are over 140 active heart transplant programs in the United States, with volumes varying from fewer than 10 to more than 100 transplants each year. Data from the SRTR show the common causes of mortality in the first 5 years after transplant (Fig. 60.5), including graft failure, infection, coronary artery disease, and malignancy. A feared and fortunately uncommon complication is primary graft failure (PGF). PGF typically occurs in the early post-transplant period and can manifest as profound allograft dysfunction and cardiogenic shock without evidence of acute rejection or any specific etiology. PGF is felt to be related to ischemic time, age of the donor, preservation, and surgical factors that are poorly understood. Patients require support often with extracorporeal membrane oxygenation, and many will fully recover; however, the 30-day mortality rate is 30%.[39] Numerous factors related to the donor including age, mechanism of brain death, and gender may all influence early and late outcomes.[40] Over the past decade the donor pool has been expanded by using organs that in the past would have been discarded, yet outstanding outcomes have been maintained or improved.

As noted earlier, the allocation system for heart donors changed in October 2018. The changes were designed to reduce the waiting list mortality and reduce waiting times, while maintaining excellent outcomes. Early indicators suggest that there is an evolving shift from durable LVAD support to short-term support devices, including an intra-aortic balloon pump and percutaneous LVAD. The argument has been made that LVAD will provide equivalent survival to transplantation and lengthen the overall life span for an individual, acknowledging the median survival post heart transplant is limited to approximately 12 years. Contemporary data (Fig. 60.6) suggest that the 1- and 5-year survival for heart transplant (with or without BTT LVAD support) is superior when compared with outcomes of patients receiving a chronic or destination (DT) LVAD.[40] Overall 1-year survival was 87.7% in those wait-listed for heart transplant compared with 76.4% in the DT LVAD group, whereas the 5-year

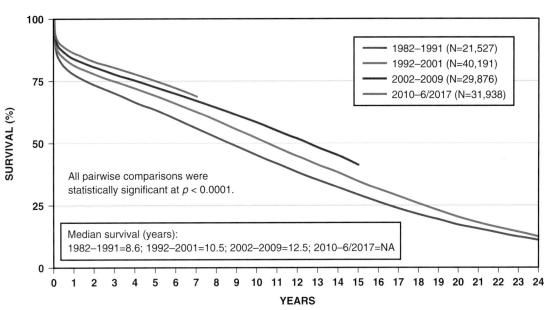

FIGURE 60.4 Kaplan-Meier survival estimates for adult heart transplant patients by era. (From Khush KK, Cherikh WS, Chambers DC, et al. International Society for Heart and Lung Transplantation. The International Thoracic Organ Transplant Registry of the International Society for Heart and Lung Transplantation: Thirty-sixth adult heart transplantation report—2019; focus theme: Donor and recipient size match. *J Heart Lung Transplant.* 2019;38[10]:1056–1066. doi: 10.1016/j.healun.2019.08.004. Epub 2019 Aug 10. Erratum in: *J Heart Lung Transplant.* 2020;39:91. https://ishltregistries.org/registries/slides.asp?yearToDisplay=2020.)

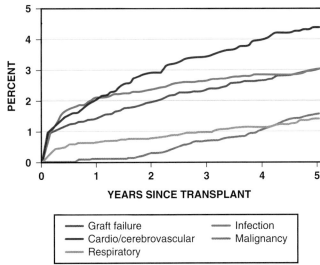

FIGURE 60.5 Five-year cumulative incidence of death by cause among adult heart transplant recipients, 2012–2013. Primary causes of death are as reported on the Organ Procurement Transplant Network Transplant Recipient Registration and Follow-up Forms. Other causes of death include hemorrhage, trauma, nonadherence, unspecified other, unknown, etc. Cumulative incidence is estimated using Kaplan-Meier competing risk methods. (From https://srtr.transplant.hrsa.gov/annual_reports/2018/Heart.aspx)

survival was 72.1% in the heart transplant group versus 36.1% in the DT LVAD group.[41] The improvement in survival was primarily related to whether or not the patient underwent heart transplantation. Given that there may have been medical reasons why certain patients were deemed DT versus BTT, a randomized clinical trial to definitively address is required. The clinical data that are available suggest that clinical outcomes with cardiac transplantation are superior to those of DT LVAD therapy.[40]

Functional Outcomes

Cardiac transplantation dramatically improves quality of life and functional capacity. The improvement is referenced based upon the pretransplant degree of impairment. A normal heart transplant recipient's exercise capacity is below that of an age-matched control, normal individual but much improved compared with pretransplant. A recent

report showed that peak $\dot{V}O_2$ of less than or equal to 60% and VE/VCO_2 greater than or equal to 34 with exercise were associated with a high hazard for CAV in heart transplant recipients at 1 year after transplant.[42] Cardiac rehabilitation is routinely recommended for all heart transplant recipients to optimize their recovery potential.[43] The Karnofsky Index, which is routinely reported after cardiac transplantation, provides an objective measure of functional capacity. Most heart transplant recipients reach near-normal function based on their Karnofsky grade, and over 90% are physically fit to return to most all occupations with excellent cardiopulmonary function. A typical heart transplant recipient should expect to regain full activity and be able to return to usual social and employment activities within 6 to 12 months after transplantation.

INFECTION

A successful result after cardiac transplantation is a balance between preventing rejection and overzealous use of immunosuppression. The incidence of rejection has decreased, but opportunistic infection remains an important risk due to immunosuppression. Infections cause approximately 20% of deaths within the first year after transplantation and continue to be a common contributing factor in morbidity and mortality throughout the recipient's life. The most common infections are bacterial and viral, specifically CMV. The recipient and the donor are assessed for prior CMV infection with IgG antibody titers.[44] The highest risk for CMV infection is from a CMV-positive donor in a negative CMV recipient. Standard prophylaxis for CMV infection with valganciclovir for 3 to 6 months post transplant reduces the burden of disease. Routinely patients are monitored for CMV DNA, which may become seropositive in the absence of a clinical infection. The spectrum of disease may vary from asymptomatic viremia to a serious, tissue-invasive infection, for example CMV pneumonitis. The use of an mTOR inhibitor (everolimus) may be considered in a high-risk patient with recurrent CMV infection concurrent with the elimination of mycophenolic acid mofetil to mitigate the risk of future active CMV infection. Mortality is highest for fungal infections, followed by protozoal, bacterial, and viral infections. Aspergillosis and candidiasis are the most common fungal infections after heart transplantation. *Pneumocystis jirovecii* and herpes simplex virus infections and oral candidiasis, require prophylactic regimens to be used during the first 6 to 12 months after transplantation. Prophylactic IV ganciclovir or oral valganciclovir generally is given for variable periods

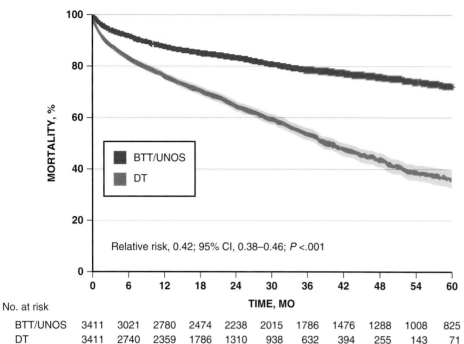

No. at risk											
BTT/UNOS	3411	3021	2780	2474	2238	2015	1786	1476	1288	1008	825
DT	3411	2740	2359	1786	1310	938	632	394	255	143	71

FIGURE 60.6 Survival curves comparing strategies of wait-listing for heart transplant, with or without left ventricular assist device (LVAD) when compared with LVAD destination therapy (DT). The strategy of wait-listing for heart transplant (with or without LVAD) was associated with a superior outcome at 5 years (relative risk [RR], 0.42; 95% CI, 0.38–0.46) after adjusting for select clinical factors. These survival curves accounted for waiting-list mortality with or without bridge to transplant (BTT) LVAD. (From Lala A, Rowland JC, Ferket BC, et al. Strategies of wait-listing for heart transplant vs durable mechanical circulatory support alone for patients with advanced heart failure. *JAMA Cardiol.* 2020;5:652–659.)

in CMV-seronegative recipients of a transplant from a CMV-positive donor. Patients who undergo transplantation with infected LVAD represent a unique and high-risk group for infectious complications post heart transplantation. Surgical management with irrigation and infection control at the time of transplant and prolonged postoperative antibiotics are necessary.

MEDICAL COMPLICATIONS AND COMORBID CONDITIONS

The complications that follow heart transplantation reflect, in part, the premorbid status of a majority of transplant recipients, who have vascular disease and other significant medical conditions.[45] After 5 years, more than 90% of recipients have hypertension, at least 80% have hyperlipidemia, and more than 30% have diabetes, as shown in Table 60.3. Each year after transplantation, clinically significant CAV—which is the major limitation to long life after transplantation—will develop in a larger number of patients. By 5 years, almost 30% of recipients will have CAV, and at least half will be so afflicted at 10 years. It is the most common reason why retransplant is undertaken in the United States (Fig. 60.7). Likewise, progressive renal insufficiency is an insidious problem that is only recently being addressed by substitution protocols to limit the administration of CNIs. Safety and efficacy remain devoid of evidence for the use of mTOR inhibitors as a replacement for CNIs.

Malignancy

Patients are generally considered for transplantation if they have at least a 5-year disease-free interval regarding a preexisting malignancy such as breast, lung, or colon cancer. Malignancy after cardiac transplant is related to a number of risk factors, including age, race, cigarette use, and others (Table 60.4). Most U.S. transplant centers require a cigarette-free interval of a minimum of 6 months before permitting active listing for transplant. More than 10% of adult heart transplant recipients may develop de novo malignancy between years 1 and 5 after transplantation, which is accompanied by increased mortality.[46] Lymphoma and lung cancer are the most common malignancies, with reduced 5-year survival rates of 32% and 21%, respectively, after

the time of diagnosis.[47] A dialogue between the transplant cardiologist and the treating oncologist is necessary (see also Chapters 56 and 57) both to discuss the advantage of immunosuppression reduction, as well as monitoring for cardiotoxicity with specific agents with known cardiotoxicity, such as anthracyclines, immune checkpoint inhibitors, and tyrosine kinase inhibitors. Sirolimus, which is uncommonly used as a chronic maintenance immunosuppressive drug, has been associated with reduced occurrences of malignancies in a single center study.[48] Specific to transplant is a malignancy known as post-transplant lymphoproliferative disorder (PTLD). There are known risk factors for PTLD, including an Epstein-Barr virus (EBV)-negative recipient of an EBV+ donor and the use of induction immunotherapy, and others risks that are less well established.[49] Specific treatment often includes immunosuppression reduction, rituximab, and close follow-up monitoring. Skin malignancies are common in all solid organ recipients, and prophylaxis includes limiting exposure to ultraviolet light and liberal use of sunscreen and barrier protection.

Diabetes

Patients in whom new-onset diabetes mellitus develops after transplantation are at increased risk for morbidity and mortality. Accumulating evidence suggests that long-term outcomes, including patient survival and graft survival, may be adversely affected. Much of the diabetes that occurs is attributed to the high-dose corticosteroids used early after transplant surgery, but it is now appreciated that the CNIs play an important role as well. Impaired B cell function appears to be the primary mechanism of CNI-induced new-onset diabetes.

The risk factors for the development of diabetes after transplantation include obesity, increased age, family history of diabetes, abnormal glucose tolerance, and African American or Hispanic descent. Changing trends in the demographics of transplant patients, such as increased age and increased body mass index (BMI), suggest that these patients may now be at a greater risk for new-onset diabetes than in the past. Increased BMI increases risk of insulin resistance, and corticosteroids can cause glucose intolerance, insulin resistance, and frank hyperglycemia. African Americans are more likely to develop new-onset diabetes mellitus regardless of the immunosuppression used but are particularly susceptible after treatment with tacrolimus.

Hypertension

Hypertension is prevalent in heart transplant recipients and associated with the use of CNIs.[50] The control of hypertension and achieving a target blood pressure can be challenging and often require multiple agents (see also Chapter 26). Calcium channel blockers and ACE inhibitors are commonly used. Long-term use of CNIs may lead to the development of chronic kidney disease and refractory hypertension. It is recommended to aggressively treat all cardiac risk factors, including optimal blood pressure control in heart transplant recipients.

Renal Insufficiency

The development of chronic kidney disease is a concern and potentially avoidable after cardiac transplant. A major contributor to the risk of renal disease is CNI nephrotoxicity. The cumulative incidence of chronic renal failure (defined as a glomerular filtration rate of 29 mL/min per 1.73 m² of body-surface area or less or the development of end-stage renal disease [ESRD]) 5 years after cardiac transplant is

TABLE 60.3 Cumulative Post–Heart Transplant Morbidity Rates for Adult Patients

OUTCOME	WITHIN 5 YEARS (%)	TOTAL NO. OF PATIENTS WITH KNOWN RESPONSE	WITHIN 10 YEARS	TOTAL NO. OF PATIENTS WITH KNOWN RESPONSE
Hypertension	92	13,023	Not available	Not available
Renal dysfunction	52	15,769	68%	5428
Abnormal creatinine <2.5 mg/dL	33		39%	
Creatinine >2.5 mg/dL	15		20%	
Chronic dialysis	2.9		6.0%	
Renal transplantation	1.1		3.6%	
Hyperlipidemia	88	14,372	Not available	Not available
Diabetes	38	15,458	Not available	Not available
Cardiac allograft vasculopathy	30	11,511	50%	3146

Cumulative prevalence in survivors at 5 and 10 years after transplantation (January 1995 to June 2013).
Adapted from Lund LH, Edwards LB, Kucheryavaya AY, et al. The registry of the International Society for Heart and Lung Transplantation: thirty-first official adult heart transplant report—2014; focus theme: retransplantation. *J Heart Lung Transplant*. 2014;33:996–1008.

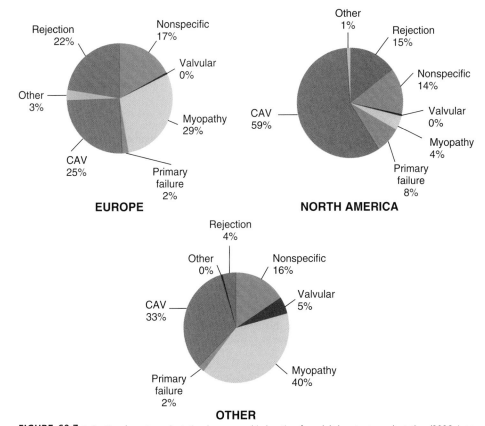

FIGURE 60.7 Indication for retransplantation by geographic location for adult heart retransplantation (2006–June 2013). *CAV*, Coronary allograft vasculopathy. (From Lund LH, Edwards LB, Kucheryavaya AY, et al. The registry of the International Society for Heart and Lung Transplantation: thirty-first official adult heart transplant report—2014; focus theme: retransplantation. *J Heart Lung Transplant*. 2014;33[10]:996–1008.)

10.9%.[51] Known contributing risk factors include age, gender, diabetes mellitus, hypertension, and hepatitis C infection. The high mortality associated with ESRD post heart transplant can be significantly mitigated with renal transplantation (see also Chapter 101).

Hyperlipidemia

Hyperlipidemia is common after transplantation, as it is in the general population. The concern has been that many studies have demonstrated an association of hyperlipidemia with the development of CAV and cerebrovascular and peripheral vascular disease, with the attendant morbidity and mortality of these vascular disorders. Typically, total cholesterol, LDL cholesterol, and triglycerides increase by 3 months after transplantation and then generally fall somewhat after the first year. A number of drugs commonly used after transplantation contribute to the hyperlipidemia observed. Corticosteroids may lead to

insulin resistance, increased free fatty acid synthesis, and increased very-LDL production. Cyclosporine increases serum LDL cholesterol and binds to the LDL receptor, decreasing its availability to absorb cholesterol from the bloodstream; tacrolimus probably causes less hyperlipidemia. Sirolimus and MMF also have unfavorable effects on lipids. Sirolimus in escalating doses has been shown to result in prominent elevation of triglyceride levels.

Lipid-lowering therapy with any statin, or HMG-CoA reductase inhibitor, was strongly associated with a marked improvement in 1-year survival in the Heart Transplant Lipid registry. In heart transplant recipients, pravastatin and simvastatin have been associated with outcome benefits in survival, severity of rejection, incidence of CAV, and even malignancies.[52]

Cardiac Allograft Vasculopathy

The development of coronary artery vasculopathy (CAV) is a well-known limitation of cardiac transplantation. CAV may occur in young or older recipients, and its prevalence increases with older donor age. CAV remains the most prominent long-term complication of heart transplantation, with an annual incidence rate of 5% to 10%. CAV is detected angiographically in up to 20% of transplant hearts at 1 year and in 40% to 50% at 5 years. CAV occurring early is predominantly an immune-mediated phenomena with myointimal proliferative lesions characterized by intense cellular infiltration. CAV occurring after the first decade and beyond is similar in its pathologic characteristics as native coronary artery disease. There is evidence to implicate donor-specific antibody production, and AMR with accelerated CAV. CAV angiographically is graded by the ISHLT grading system (Table 60.5) and characterized by diffuse disease and the distal obliteration or "pruning" of the coronary arteries (Fig. 60.8).[53] ISHLT CAV grade 3 represents the most extensive degree of coronary disease based upon angiographic assessment. A single center experience has observed worsening severity of CAV was associated with progressively worse long-term survival. Among patients with CAV, long-term survival in those with CAV amenable to PCI was greater than that in those with severe CAV not treatable with PCI.[54] There is evidence that statin therapy improves outcomes for heart transplant recipients, and statin use is advised in all patients irrespective of lipid levels. The

TABLE 60.4 Multivariable Risk Model for First Invasive Malignancy

LATE PHASE VARIABLE	RELATIVE RISK	P-VALUE
Older age (60 vs. 45 years)	2.1	<0.0001
Black male recipient	1.4	0.04
History of cigarette use	1.2	0.05
History of invasive malignancy	1.6	0.02
Earlier date of transplant (1995 vs. 2005)	2.1	<0.0001

TABLE 60.5 Recommended Nomenclature for Cardiac Allograft Vasculopathy

ISHLT CAV$_0$	(Not significant): No detectable angiographic lesion
ISHLT CAV$_1$	(Mild): Angiographic left main (LM) <50%, or primary vessel with maximum lesion of <70%, or any branch stenosis <70% (including diffuse narrowing) without allograft dysfunction
ISHLT CAV$_2$	(Moderate): Angiographic LM <50%; a single primary vessel >70%, or isolated branch stenosis >70% in branches of 2 systems, without allograft dysfunction
ISHLT CAV$_3$	(Severe): Angiographic LM >50%, or two or more primary vessels >70% stenosis, or isolated branch stenosis >70% in all 3 systems; or ISHLT CAV$_1$ or CAV$_2$ with allograft dysfunction (defined as LVEF <45% usually in the presence of regional wall motion abnormalities) or evidence of significant restrictive physiology (which is common but not specific; see text for definitions)

Definitions	
	a. A primary vessel denotes the proximal and middle 33% of the left anterior descending artery, the left circumflex, the ramus and the dominant or co-dominant right coronary artery with the posterior descending and posterolateral branches.
	b. A secondary branch vessel includes the distal 33% of the primary vessels or any segment within a large septal perforator, diagonals and obtuse marginal branches or any portion of a nondominant right coronary artery.
	c. Restrictive cardiac allograft physiology is defined as symptomatic heart failure with echocardiographic E to A velocity ratio >2 (>1.5 in children), shortened isovolumetric relaxation time (<60 msec), shortened deceleration time (<150 msec), or restrictive hemodynamic values (right atrial pressure >12 mm Hg, pulmonary capillary wedge pressure >25 mm Hg, cardiac index <2 L/min/m^2).

CAV, Coronary artery vasculopathy; *ISHLT,* International Society of Heart and Lung Transplantation; *LVEF,* left ventricular ejection fraction.
From Mehra MR, Crespo-Leiro MG, Dipchand A, et al. International Society for Heart and Lung Transplantation working formulation of a standardized nomenclature for cardiac allograft vasculopathy—2010. *J Heart Lung Transplant.* 2010;29(7):717–727.

use of low-dose aspirin (81 mg) is also recommended substantiated by isolated reports demonstrating improved survival with aspirin use.[55] Ultimately the only treatment for extensive CAV may be retransplantation. Patients with extensive CAV and no other risk factors experience improved long-term survival with retransplantation; however, medical management in the absence of systolic dysfunction should be considered.[56,57] Lack of donor organs creates an ethical discussion when considering the option of retransplantation. The option of using an mTOR inhibitor (everolimus, sirolimus) as part of the immunosuppressive regimen in patients with established CAV has been advocated.[58] The strategy for heart transplant recipients for the longitudinal surveillance, and follow-up of established CAV varies widely across centers. Although yearly coronary angiography was the initial standard, followed by the use of IVUS in conjunction with angiography, more centers now are using various noninvasive testing protocols. CAV remains an area in dire need of continued research to establish best practices for primary and secondary prevention.

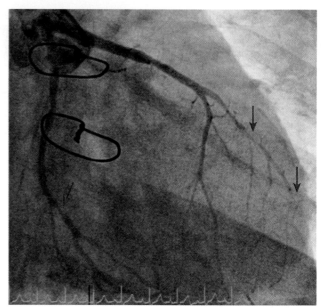

FIGURE 60.8 Coronary artery angiogram showing coronary artery vasculopathy in a heart transplant patient. *Arrows* indicate distal obliteration or "pruning" of the right and left coronary arteries.

FUTURE PERSPECTIVES

The 50th anniversary of cardiac transplantation was recently celebrated and provided the opportunity to reflect upon the tremendous progress that has occurred over the past 5 decades. Successful transplantation requires excellence in multiple facets including organ harvesting and preservation, surgical implantation, immunosuppression, and post-transplant surveillance, and multi-disciplinary care. Clearly over the past 2 decades a shift has occurred with greater care pre- and post-transplant provided by cardiologists. Importantly, the discipline of transplant cardiology emerged in 2010 with the opportunity for board certification in the United States. Organ preservation systems have been developed for longer ischemic times with good organ function. Surgical techniques have been refined. The standard approach to monitor for rejection with histology is now moving toward molecular diagnostics and fewer invasive endomyocardial biopsies. The emergence of effective treatment for hepatitis C and the knowledge that donor death related to opiate overdose is not a contraindication to heart transplant donation have resulted in an expanding donor pool and a greater number of heart transplants. The challenges that will need to be addressed in the future include personalizing, minimizing, and improving immunosuppression and overall protocols. The prospect of immune tolerance does not appear to be a near-term reality; hence we must continue to immunosuppress our patients. Our goal must be to determine the least amount of immunosuppression necessary to avoid the adverse impact of immunotherapy while maintaining graft survival. Mechanical circulatory support has also advanced tremendously over the past 25 years (see Chapter 59) but still cannot match the outcomes with cardiac transplantation. CAV remains a devastating problem limiting the long-term success of cardiac transplantation and should remain an active area of research to advance the field. The mechanisms of early coronary vasculopathy are certainly primarily immune mediated and will be overcome only if we understand and develop treatments to prevent and/or mitigate. Evidence is required to improve outcomes, which is challenging in heart transplantation with limited patient numbers.[59] Risk factor modification is imperative in this patient population at high risk for vascular complications. The future may find that sodium-glucose cotransporter inhibitors have an important role to mitigate adverse events, but well-designed randomized clinical trials must be conducted to advance our knowledge. For now, cardiac transplantation unquestionably remains the best treatment option for eligible potential recipients with stage D, advanced heart failure.

ACKNOWLEDGMENTS

The author gratefully acknowledges Drs. Mariell Jessup, Pavan Alturi, and Michael A. Acker, whose chapter on this topic in the prior edition of *Braunwald's Heart Disease: A Textbook of Cardiovascular Medicine* served as the partial basis for the current chapter.

This chapter is dedicated in memory of the late David O. Taylor, MD, and the advanced heart failure and cardiac transplant medicine fellows that have trained at the Cleveland Clinic.

REFERENCES

History, Epidemiology and Evaluation of the Recipient

1. Stehlik J, Kobashigawa J, Hunt SA, et al. Honoring 50 years of clinical heart transplantation in *Circulation*: in-depth State-of-the-Art review. *Circulation*. 2018;137(1):71–87.
2. Woolley AE, Singh SK, Goldberg HJ, et al. Heart and lung transplants from HCV-infected donors to uninfected recipients. *N Engl J Med*. 2019;380(17):1606–1617.
3. Vaduganathan M, Machado SR, DeFilippis EM, et al. Organ donation and drug intoxication-related deaths in the United States. *N Engl J Med*. 2019;380(6):597–599.
4. Mehra MR, Jarcho JA, Cherikh W, et al. The drug-Intoxication epidemic and solid-organ transplantation. *N Engl J Med*. 2018;378(20):1943–1945.
5. Guglin M, Zucker MJ, Borlaug BA, et al. Evaluation for heart transplantation and LVAD implantation: JACC Council perspectives. *J Am Coll Cardiol*. 2020;75(12):1471–1487.

Donor and Surgery Considerations, Allocation, Immunosuppression

6. Maldonado JR, Sher Y, Lolak S, et al. The Stanford Integrated psychosocial assessment for transplantation: a prospective study of medical and psychosocial outcomes. *Psychosom Med*. 2015;77(9):1018–1030.
7. Dew MA, DiMartini AF, Dobbels F, et al. The 2018 ISHLT/APM/AST/ICCAC/STSW recommendations for the psychosocial evaluation of adult cardiothoracic transplant candidates and candidates for long-term mechanical circulatory support. *J Heart Lung Transplant*. 2018;37(7):803–823.
8. Truby LK, Rogers JG. Advanced heart failure: epidemiology, diagnosis, and therapeutic approaches. *JACC Heart Fail*. 2020;8(7):523–536.
9. Ardehali A, Esmailian F, Deng M, et al. Ex-vivo perfusion of donor hearts for human heart transplantation (PROCEED II): a prospective, open-label, multicentre, randomised non-inferiority trial. *Lancet*. 2015;385:2577–2584.
10. Smith JW, O'Brien KD, Dardas T, et al. Systematic donor selection review process improves cardiac transplant volumes and outcomes. *J Thorac Cardiovasc Surg*. 2016;151:238–243.
11. Phillips KG, Ranganath NK, Malas J, et al. Impact of the opioid epidemic on heart transplantation: donor characteristics and organ discard. *Ann Thorac Surg*. 2019;108(4):1133–1139.
12. Gidea CG, Narula N, Reyentovich A, et al. Increased early acute cellular rejection events in hepatitis C-positive heart transplantation. *J Heart Lung Transplant*. 2020;S1053–2498(20)31624-7.
13. Messer S, Cernic S, Page A, et al. 5-Year single Centre early experience of heart transplantation from Donation After Circulatory Determined death (DCD) donors. *J Heart Lung Trans*. 2020;S1053–2498(20):31765-4.
14. Rajab TK, Jaggers J, Campbell DN. Heart transplantation following donation after cardiac death: history, current techniques, and future. *J Thorac Cardiovasc Surg*. 2020;S0022-5223(20)30529-8.
15. Davies RR, Russo MJ, Morgan JA, et al. Standard versus bicaval techniques for orthotopic heart transplantation: an analysis of the United Network for Organ Sharing database. *J Thorac Cardiovasc Surg*. 2010:700–708, 8 e1–2.
16. Bermudez CA, Rame JE. Reversible but risky: pulmonary hypertension in advanced heart failure is the Achilles' heel of cardiac transplantation. *J Thorac Cardiovasc Surg*. 2015;150:1362–1363.
17. Soderlund C, Radegran G. Immunosuppressive therapies after heart transplantation—the balance between under- and over-immunosuppression. *Transplant Rev (Orlando)*. 2015;29:181–189.
18. Whitson BA, Kilic A, Lehman A, et al. Impact of induction immunosuppression on survival in heart transplant recipients: a contemporary analysis of agents. *Clin Transplant*. 2015;29:9–17.
19. Khush KK, Potena L, Cherikh WS, et al. The international thoracic organ transplant registry of the international Society for heart and lung transplantation: 37th adult heart transplantation report-2020; focus on deceased donor characteristics. *J Heart Lung Transplant*. 2020;S1053–2498(20):31660-0.
20. Nozohoor S, Stehlik J, Lund LH, et al. Induction immunosuppression strategies and long-term outcomes after heart transplantation. *Clin Transplant*. 2020;34:e13871.
21. Kobashigawa JA, Meiser BM. Review of major clinical trials with mycophenolate mofetil in cardiac transplantation. *Transplantation*. 2005;80(suppl 2):S235–S243.
22. Eisen HJ, Tuzcu EM, Dorent R, et al. Everolimus for the prevention of allograft rejection and vasculopathy in cardiac-transplant recipients. *N Engl J Med*. 2003;349(9):847–858.
23. Topilsky Y, Hasin T, Raichlin E, et al. Sirolimus as primary immunosuppression attenuates allograft vasculopathy with improved late survival and decreased cardiac events after cardiac transplantation. *Circulation*. 2012;125(5):708–720.
24. Kobashigawa JA, Pauly DF, Starling RC, et al. Cardiac allograft vasculopathy by intravascular ultrasound in heart transplant patients: substudy from the everolimus versus mycophenolate mofetil randomized, multicenter trial. *JACC Heart Fail*. 2013;1(5):389–399.
25. Asleh R, Briasoulis A, Kremers WK, et al. Long-term sirolimus for primary immunosuppression in heart transplant recipients. *J Am Coll Cardiol*. 2018;71(6):636–650.
26. Eisen HJ. CAVEAT mTOR: You've heard about the benefits of using mTOR inhibitors, here are some of the risks. *Am J Transplant*. 2020;21:449–450.
27. Tsay AJ, Eisen HJ. mTOR inhibitors vs calcineurin inhibitors: a Catch-22-preventing nephrotoxicity or acute allograft rejection after heart transplantation. *Am J Transplant*. 2019;19(11):2967–2968.
28. Eisen HJ, Kobashigawa J, Starling RC, et al. Everolimus versus mycophenolate mofetil in heart transplantation: a randomized, multicenter trial. *Am J Transplant*. 2013;13(5):1203–1216.

Rejection, Outcomes, Infection

29. Stewart S, Winters GL, Fishbein MC, et al. Revision of the 1990 working formulation for the standardization of nomenclature in the diagnosis of heart rejection. *J Heart Lung Transplant*. 2005;24(11):1710–1720.
30. Estep JD, Shah DJ, Nagueh SF, et al. The role of multimodality cardiac imaging in the transplanted heart. *JACC Cardiovasc Imaging*. 2009;2(9):1126–1140.
31. Pham MX, Teuteberg JJ, Kfoury AG, et al. Gene-expression profiling for rejection surveillance after cardiac transplantation. *N Engl J Med*. 2010;362(20):1890–1900.
32. Khush KK, Patel J, Pinney S, et al. Noninvasive detection of graft injury after heart transplant using donor-derived cell-free DNA: a prospective multicenter study. *Am J Transplant*. 2019;19(10):2889–2899.
33. Berry GJ, Angelini A, Burke MM, et al. The ISHLT working formulation for pathologic diagnosis of antibody-mediated rejection in heart transplantation: evolution and current status (2005–2011). *J Heart Lung Transplant*. 2011;30(6):601–611.
34. Colvin MM, Cook JL, Chang P, et al. Antibody-mediated rejection in cardiac transplantation: emerging knowledge in diagnosis and management: a scientific statement from the American Heart Association. *Circulation*. 2015;131(18):1608–1639.
35. Halloran PF, Potena L, Van Huyen JD, et al. Building a tissue-based molecular diagnostic system in heart transplant rejection: the heart Molecular Microscope Diagnostic (MMDx) System. *J Heart Lung Transplant*. 2017;36(11):1192–1200.
36. Chih S, Chong AY, Erthal F, et al. PET assessment of epicardial intimal disease and Microvascular dysfunction in cardiac allograft vasculopathy. *J Am Coll Cardiol*. 2018;71(13):1444–1456.
37. ISHLT registry. www. https://ishltregistries.org/registries/slides.asp.
38. Scientific registry of transplant recipients. https://www.srtr.org/transplant-centers/?organ=heart&recipientType=adult&query=.
39. Kittleson MM, Kobashigawa JA. Cardiac transplantation: current outcomes and contemporary controversies. *JACC Heart Fail*. 2017;5(12):857–868.
40. Khush KK, Potena L, Cherikh WS, et al. The international thoracic organ transplant registry of the international society for heart and lung transplantation: 37th adult heart transplantation report-2020; focus on deceased donor characteristics. *J Heart Lung Transplant*. 2020;39(10):1003–1015.
41. Lala A, Rowland JC, Ferket BS, et al. Strategies of wait-listing for heart transplant vs durable mechanical circulatory support alone for patients with advanced heart failure. *JAMA Cardiol*. 2020;5(6):652–659.
42. Mingxi DY, Liebo MJ, Lundgren S, et al. Impaired exercise tolerance early after heart transplantation is associated with development of cardiac allograft vasculopathy. *Transplantation*. 2020;104(10):2196–2203.
43. Kobashigawa JA, Leaf DA, Lee N, et al. A controlled trial of exercise rehabilitation after heart transplantation. *N Engl J Med*. 1999;340(4):272–277.
44. Kotton CN, Kumar D, Caliendo AM, et al. The Third international Consensus guidelines on the management of cytomegalovirus in solid-organ transplantation. *Transplantation*. 2018;102(6): 900–931.

Medical Complications, Comorbidities, and Future Perspective

45. Singh TP, Milliren CE, Almond CS, Graham D. Survival benefit from transplantation in patients listed for heart transplantation in the United States. *J Am Coll Cardiol*. 2014;63:1169–1178.
46. Youn JC, Stehlik J, Wilk AR, et al. Temporal trends of de novo malignancy development after heart transplantation. *J Am Coll Cardiol*. 2018;71(1):40–49.
47. Higgins RS, Brown RN, Chang PP, et al. A multi-institutional study of malignancies after heart transplantation and a comparison with the general United States population. *J Heart Lung Transplant*. 2014;33(5):478–485.
48. Asleh R, Clavell AL, Pereira NL, et al. Incidence of malignancies in patients treated with sirolimus following heart transplantation. *J Am Coll Cardiol*. 2019;73(21):2676–2688.
49. Dierickx D, Habermann TM. Post-transplantation lymphoproliferative disorders in adults. *N Engl J Med*. 2018;378(6):549–562.
50. Campbell PT, Krim SR. Hypertension in cardiac transplant recipients: tackling a new face of an old foe. *Curr Opin Cardiol*. 2020;35(4):368–375.
51. Ojo AO, Held PJ, Port FK, et al. Chronic renal failure after transplantation of a nonrenal organ. *N Engl J Med*. 2003;349(10):931–940.
52. Frohlich GM, Rufibach K, Enseleit F, et al. Statins and the risk of cancer after heart transplantation. *Circulation*. 2012;126:440–447.
53. Mehra MR, Crespo-Leiro MG, Dipchand A, et al. International Society for Heart and Lung Transplantation working formulation of a standardized nomenclature for cardiac allograft vasculopathy-2010. *J Heart Lung Transplant*. 2010;29(7):717–727. Erratum in: J Heart Lung Transplant. 2011 Mar;30(3):360. PMID: 20620917.
54. Agarwal S, Parashar A, Kapadia SR, et al. Long-term mortality after cardiac allograft vasculopathy: implications of percutaneous intervention. *JACC Heart Fail*. 2014;2(3):281–288.
55. Kim M, Bergmark BA, Zelniker TA, et al. Early aspirin use and the development of cardiac allograft vasculopathy. *J Heart Lung Transplant*. 2017;36(12):1344–1349.
56. Goldraich LA, Stehlik J, Kucheryavaya AY, et al. Retransplant and medical therapy for cardiac allograft vasculopathy: international Society for heart and lung transplantation registry analysis. *Am J Transplant*. 2016;16(1):301–309.
57. Barghash MH, Pinney SP. Heart retransplantation: Candidacy, outcomes, and management. *Curr Transplant Rep*. 2020;7(1):12–17.
58. Asleh R, Alnsasra H, Lerman A, et al. Effects of mTOR inhibitor-related proteinuria on progression of cardiac allograft vasculopathy and outcomes among heart transplant recipients. *Am J Transplant*. 2021;21:626–635.
59. Shah MR, Starling RC, Schwartz Longacre L, et al. Heart transplantation research in the next decade–a goal to achieving evidence-based outcomes: National Heart, Lung, and Blood Institute Working Group. *J Am Coll Cardiol*. 2012;59(14):1263–1269.

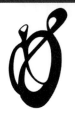

61 Approach to the Patient with Cardiac Arrhythmias

ANNE B. CURTIS AND GORDON F. TOMASELLI

The evaluation of patients with suspected cardiac arrhythmias is highly individualized and must include a comprehensive assessment of the patient. Evaluation of the patient begins with a careful history and physical examination and should usually progress from the simplest to the most complex diagnostic test, from the least invasive and safest to the most invasive and risky, and from the least expensive out-of-hospital evaluations to those that require hospitalization and sophisticated, costly, and potentially risky procedures. However, two key features—the history and the electrocardiogram (ECG)—are pivotal in directing the diagnostic evaluation and treatment. The physical examination is focused on determining whether there is cardiopulmonary disease that is associated with specific cardiac arrhythmias. The absence of significant cardiopulmonary disease often, but not always, suggests a benign cause of a cardiac rhythm disturbance. The judicious use of noninvasive diagnostic tests is an important element in the evaluation of patients with arrhythmias, and the most important is the ECG, particularly if recorded at the time of symptoms.

An evidence-based approach to the history and physical examination for patients with suspected cardiovascular (CV) disease is presented in Chapter 13. This chapter focuses on features most germane to the patient with cardiac rhythm disturbances. However, it is essential to understand that the general medical condition of the patient may profoundly influence the presentation of any cardiac arrhythmia. This chapter discusses the approach to and diagnostic evaluation of the patient with a suspected arrhythmia, keeping in mind that arrhythmia management has two goals: addressing the patient's symptoms as well as whatever risks the arrhythmia poses to the individual.

GENERAL APPROACH TO THE HISTORY AND PHYSICAL EXAM

History

Patients with cardiac arrhythmias exhibit a wide spectrum of clinical presentations, ranging from asymptomatic incidental ECG abnormalities to survival from sudden cardiac arrest (SCA). The presenting features may vary with circumstances, and arrhythmias are common in the setting of CV and medical diseases, leading to overlap of symptoms and signs. The history is key to directing the evaluation of patients. In general, the more severe the presenting symptoms, the more aggressive are the evaluation and treatment. The presence of structural heart disease and prior myocardial infarction (MI) often dictates a change in

the approach to the management of syncope or a presumed cardiac arrhythmia.

In assessing a patient with a known or suspected arrhythmia, several key pieces of information should be obtained that can help determine a diagnosis or guide further diagnostic testing. The mode of onset of an episode can provide clues about the type of arrhythmia or preferred treatment option. For example, palpitations that occur in the setting of exercise, fright, or anger are often caused by catecholamine-sensitive automatic or triggered tachycardias that may respond to adrenergic blocking agents. Palpitations that occur at rest or that awaken the patient can be caused by enhanced vagal tone; an example of such an arrhythmia is atrial fibrillation (AF). Lightheadedness or syncope occurring in the setting of a tightly fitting collar or turning the head suggests carotid sinus hypersensitivity. The triggering event may help establish the presence of an inherited ion channel abnormality such as the long-QT syndrome (LQTS) (see Chapter 63). The mode of termination of episodes can also be helpful: palpitations that are reliably terminated by breath-holding or by Valsalva or other vagal maneuvers probably involve the atrioventricular (AV) node as an integral part of a tachycardia circuit. On occasion, focal atrial tachycardia (AT) or ventricular tachycardia (VT) can be terminated with vagal maneuvers, as can VT originating in the right ventricular outflow tract. Patients should be asked about the frequency and duration of episodes and the severity of symptoms. These features help guide how aggressively and quickly the physician needs to pursue a diagnostic or therapeutic plan (a patient with daily episodes associated with near-syncope or severe dyspnea warrants a more expeditious evaluation than does one with infrequent episodes of mild palpitations and no other symptoms). Patients should be encouraged to report their heart rate during an episode (either rapid or slow, regular or irregular) by counting the pulse directly or by using a blood pressure or heart rate monitor, wearable, or smart phone application. Devices recording an ECG waveform provide the most reliable data.

A careful drug and dietary history should also be sought; some nasal decongestants can provoke tachycardia episodes, whereas beta-adrenergic receptor-blocking eye drops for the treatment of glaucoma can drain into tear ducts, be absorbed systemically, and precipitate syncope secondary to bradycardia. Dietary supplements, particularly those containing stimulants, can cause arrhythmias. A growing list of drugs can directly or indirectly affect ventricular repolarization and produce or exacerbate long-QT interval–related tachyarrhythmias (see Chapter 9). The patient should be questioned about the presence of systemic

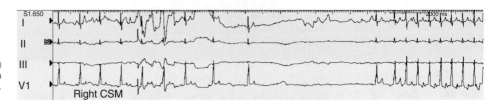

FIGURE 61.1 Right carotid sinus massage (CSM) produces sinus arrest and a 7.2-second pause in a patient with episodic dizziness. (Image courtesy Dr. Joseph Marine.)

illnesses that may be associated with arrhythmias, such as chronic obstructive pulmonary disease, thyrotoxicosis (see Chapter 94), pericarditis (Chapter 86), and chronic heart failure (Chapters 49 and 50), as well as previous chest injury, surgery, radiation therapy, or chemotherapy.

A family history of a significant cardiac arrhythmia may not directly inform the prognosis of a patient, but it should alert the practitioner to the possibility of a heritable trait such as a channelopathy (Chapter 63), cardiomyopathy (Chapters 52 and 54) or neuromuscular disease (Chapter 100) that may increase susceptibility to development of an arrhythmia.

Physical Examination

In the absence of symptoms, the physical examination is focused on determining whether CV or general medical disease is present. The lack of significant cardiopulmonary disease often, but not always, suggests benignity of a rhythm disturbance. Conversely, palpitations, syncope, or near-syncope in the setting of significant heart or lung disease have a more ominous prognosis. In addition, the physical examination may reveal the presence of a persistent arrhythmia such as AF. The detailed approach to the CV physical examination is outlined in Chapter 13 and may suggest the presence of structural heart disease (and thus generally a clinically more serious situation with a worse overall prognosis), even in the absence of an arrhythmia episode. For example, a laterally displaced or dyskinetic apical impulse, a regurgitant or stenotic murmur, or a third heart sound in an older adult can denote significant myocardial or valvular dysfunction or damage.

The general physical examination is also important and can identify medical conditions associated with cardiac manifestations and arrhythmias. Inspection of the skin may reveal erythema chronicum migrans, the rash associated with Lyme disease; hair loss and exophthalmos may reflect the presence of thyroid disease; and ptosis, cataracts, and skeletal muscle wasting or myotonia may indicate the presence of neuromuscular disease (see Chapter 100). Even facial features may suggest an associated rhythm disorder (e.g., cataracts and early balding with myotonic dystrophy, micrognathia, and low-set ears in Andersen-Tawil syndrome).

If tachycardia is present, the priorities are evaluation of the heart rate and blood pressure, and to obtain a 12-lead ECG if the patient is hemodynamically stable. If it is not possible to obtain an ECG, several clues on the physical examination can help to make a diagnosis. The presence of regular cannon A waves in the jugular venous pulse would be consistent with 1:1 retrograde ventriculoatrial activation, as in tachycardias such as atrioventricular reentrant tachycardia (AVRT), atrioventricular nodal reentrant tachycardia (AVNRT), and some junctional tachycardias and VTs. In contrast, patients may have physical examination features of AV dissociation, such as intermittent "cannon" A waves, indicative of right atrial contraction against a closed tricuspid valve, variable intensity of the first heart sound, and variable peak systolic blood pressure, consistent with arrhythmias, including VT and nonparoxysmal AV junctional tachycardia, without retrograde capture of the atria (see Chapter 13).

The Valsalva maneuver and carotid sinus massage (CSM) during the physical examination can be useful to interrupt arrhythmias sensitive to autonomic tone or identify the patient with a hypersensitive carotid sinus reflex. CSM is performed with the patient supine and comfortable and the head turned slightly away from the side being stimulated. The examiner first needs to listen carefully over both carotid arteries to be certain that no bruit is present. The area of the carotid sinus, at the artery's bifurcation, is palpated lightly at the angle of the jaw until a good pulse is felt. Even this minimal amount of pressure can induce a hypersensitive response in susceptible individuals. If no initial effect

is noted, a side-to-side or rotating motion of the fingers over the site is performed for up to 5 seconds. Lack of effect on the ECG after 5 seconds of pressure adequate to cause mild discomfort is considered a negative response. Because responses to carotid massage may differ on the two sides, the maneuver can be repeated on the opposite side; however, both sides should never be stimulated simultaneously. Findings may not be readily reproducible, even within minutes of a prior attempt. Gentle massage is usually sufficient to terminate a sensitive tachycardia or produce significant periods of sinus arrest or AV block in susceptible patients. The most definitive responses to CSM are tachycardia termination, as may be observed in AVRT, AVNRT, sinus node reentry, adenosine-sensitive AT, and idiopathic right ventricular outflow tract tachycardia. CSM can gradually slow a sinus tachycardia without termination and decrease the ventricular response to AT, atrial flutter, and AF without termination, allowing examination of atrial activity. CSM transiently terminates the permanent form of AV junctional reciprocating tachycardia, which then restarts when carotid massage ceases. CSM generally does not affect reentrant ventricular or junctional tachycardias (Fig. 61.1). During wide-QRS tachycardias with a 1:1 relationship between the P waves and QRS complexes, vagal influence can terminate or slow a supraventricular tachycardia (SVT) that depends on the AV node for perpetuation; on the other hand, vagal effects on the AV node can transiently block retrograde conduction and thus establish the diagnosis of VT by demonstrating AV dissociation (Fig. 61.2). Because the effect of either of these physical maneuvers typically lasts only seconds, clinicians must be ready to observe or record any changes in rhythm on an ECG when the maneuver is performed.

SIGNS AND SYMPTOMS

Palpitations

Palpitations are the awareness of the heartbeat that may be caused by a rapid heart rate, irregularities in heart rhythm, or an increase in the force of cardiac contraction, as occurs with a post–extrasystolic beat; however, this perception can also exist in the setting of a completely normal cardiac rhythm. Patients who complain of palpitations describe the sensation of an unpleasant awareness of a forceful, irregular, or rapid beating of the heart. Many patients are acutely aware of any cardiac irregularity, whereas others are oblivious, even to long runs of a rapid VT or AF with a rapid ventricular rate. The latter is particularly noteworthy because if untreated, it may be associated with stroke or may produce a tachycardia-induced cardiomyopathy. Patients may use terms such as a "pounding" or "flipping" sensation in the chest; a fullness or pounding in the throat, neck, or chest; or a pause in the heartbeat, or "skipped beat." The skip often results from the pause after a premature ventricular complex (PVC) or the resetting of sinus rhythm after a premature atrial complex (PAC). Usually, the premature beat, particularly if it is a ventricular extrasystole, occurs too early to permit sufficient ventricular filling to cause a sensation when the ventricle contracts. The ventricular systole that ends the compensatory pause is often responsible for the actual palpitation, the result of a more forceful contraction from prolonged ventricular filling or increased motion of the heart in the chest.

Anxiety over such symptoms is usually the complaint that brings the patient to the physician's attention. Premature atrial or ventricular complexes constitute the most common causes of palpitations. If the premature complexes are frequent, or particularly if a sustained tachycardia is present, patients are more likely to have additional symptoms, such as lightheadedness, syncope or near-syncope, chest discomfort, fatigue, or shortness of breath. The context and symptoms associated

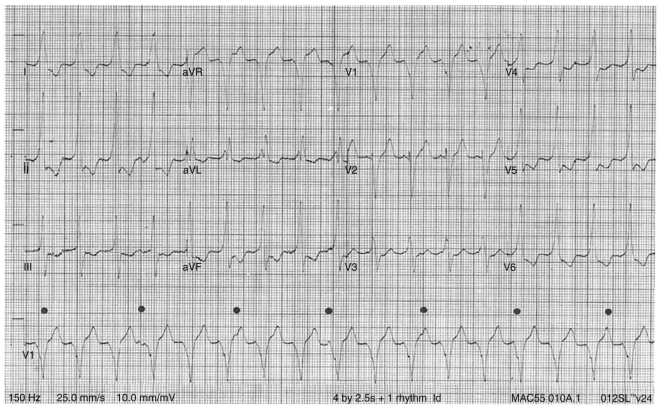

FIGURE 61.2 Wide complex tachycardia with AV dissociation establishing the diagnosis of ventricular tachycardia. P waves are dissociated from the QRS complexes and are indicated by the red dots; the sinus rate is approximately 40 beats/min.

with palpitations can be diagnostically and prognostically informative. Low-risk features include isolated palpitations not induced by exercise, the absence of structural heart disease or symptoms such as syncope or chest pain, no family history of sudden cardiac death (SCD), and a normal 12-lead ECG. Associated symptoms, such as syncope or chest pain, the presence of structural heart disease or a documented arrhythmia, and family history of SCD may be associated with a more ominous cause of palpitations.[1]

The differential diagnosis of palpitations is broad. The age of the patient and the presence of associated CV problems influence the nature of the symptoms. For example, an SVT at a rate of 180 beats/min can provoke chest pain in a patient with coronary artery disease (CAD) or syncope in a patient with aortic stenosis but may result in mild breathlessness in an otherwise healthy young person. The onset and offset of palpitations can suggest the etiology of the arrhythmia. A sudden, abrupt onset, "like a light switch turning on," is consistent with a paroxysmal tachycardia such as AVNRT (see Chapter 65), whereas gradual speeding and slowing are more consistent with atrial or sinus tachycardia. However, even tachycardias that start abruptly can begin and end with extra beats appearing to have a more gradual onset and offset. Termination by Valsalva maneuver or CSM suggests a tachycardia incorporating nodal tissue in the reentrant pathway, such as sinus node reentry, AVRT, or AVNRT (see Chapters 62 and 65).

The rate of an untreated tachycardia often narrows diagnostic possibilities, and patients should be taught to count their radial or carotid pulse rate, noting whether it is regular or irregular. Ventricular rates of 150 beats/min should always suggest the diagnosis of atrial flutter with 2:1 AV block (see Chapter 65), whereas most SVTs, such as those caused by AVNRT or AVRT, usually occur at rates exceeding 150 beats/min. The rates of VTs overlap with those of SVTs. Patients with bradyarrhythmias may have symptoms of low cardiac output, including fatigue, weakness, dizziness, dyspnea, and syncope (see Chapter 68). Palpitations can result from an increased force of contraction associated with longer ventricular filling times and may be prominent symptoms in bradycardias.

Syncope, Presyncope, and Altered Level of Consciousness

Syncope, commonly referred to as "fainting" or "passing out," is a transient, self-limited loss of consciousness and posture resulting from a drop in blood pressure with cerebral hypoperfusion and should always prompt a search for a cause (see Chapter 71). It is important to distinguish syncope from other causes of transient loss of consciousness, such as seizures, metabolic disorders (hypoglycemia, hypoxia [e.g., airline decompression]), intoxication, cataplexy, and pseudosyncope. The etiologies of true syncope are varied with similarly diverse prognoses. The unheralded loss of consciousness in any patient, even if benign from the cardiac perspective, can be dangerous depending on the circumstances (e.g., while driving a vehicle, or standing at the top of a flight of stairs). However, because syncope can be a harbinger of SCD, it is important to identify cardiac from more benign causes of syncope (eTable 61.1).[2–4] When caused by a cardiac arrhythmia, the onset of syncope is rapid and the duration is usually brief, with or without a preceding aura, and it is not typically followed by a postictal confusional state. It can be associated with bodily injury if the patient falls while unconscious. Palpitations preceding a syncope may support an arrhythmic cause of syncope but are often absent if the loss of consciousness is rapid. Seizure activity is uncommon and occurs mostly after prolonged asystole or a rapid ventricular arrhythmia. Therefore, the seizure does not begin with or anticipate the syncope, whereas in epileptic seizures, convulsive movements start within seconds of the onset of syncope. Tongue biting or incontinence is also uncommon in cardiac syncope. In summary, syncope with early seizure activity is frequently caused by epilepsy, whereas later seizure activity is more likely caused by a cardiac arrhythmia with cerebral hypoperfusion.

The history of syncope should be elicited and interpreted carefully, because older people who have fallen might deny loss of consciousness during the event because of retrograde amnesia. Common arrhythmic causes of syncope include bradyarrhythmias caused by sinus node dysfunction or AV block and tachyarrhythmias, most often ventricular, but on occasion supraventricular. Bradycardia can follow tachycardia in patients with the bradycardia-tachycardia syndrome, and treatment of both may be necessary. Of the reflex syncopes—neurocardiogenic, carotid hypersensitivity, and situational—neurocardiogenic is the most common. It should be differentiated from syncope caused by orthostasis, which may be seen in autonomic failure (e.g., due to diabetes).[5] Vasodepressor and cardioinhibitory syncope usually unfold more slowly and can be preceded by manifestations of autonomic hyperactivity such as nausea, abdominal cramping, diarrhea, sweating, or yawning. In fact, palpitations are common in this setting. On recovery, the patient may be bradycardic, pale, sweaty, and fatigued, unlike the patient recovering from a Stokes-Adams attack or an episode of VT, who may be flushed and may have a sinus tachycardia, usually without persistent mental confusion. Palpitations and presyncope on standing can be symptoms of postural orthostatic tachycardia syndrome (POTS).[6] Drug-induced (orthostatic hypotension, bradyarrhythmia) and nonarrhythmic cardiac causes of syncope such as aortic stenosis, hypertrophic cardiomyopathy, pulmonary stenosis, pulmonary hypertension, and acute MI can be excluded by the history, physical examination, ECG, echocardiography, and other laboratory tests. Noncardiac causes of syncope, such as hypoglycemia, transient ischemic attack, and psychogenic causes, can often be excluded by a careful history (see Chapter 71).

Sudden Cardiac Arrest and Aborted Sudden Cardiac Death

SCD is common, although estimates of the incidence are confounded by inadequate case identification and secular trends that have influenced both the rates and the etiologies of sudden death (see Chapter 70).[7] SCD caused by cardiac arrhythmias is most often the result of VT or ventricular fibrillation (VF); however, it can result from profound bradycardia, as might be observed in complete heart block or asystole. A variety of noncardiac conditions may be associated with life-threatening arrhythmias, including neurologic diseases (stroke, intracranial hemorrhage, epilepsy, neuromuscular disease, and Parkinson disease), diabetes, obesity, cirrhosis, anorexia, and bulimia. In well-adjudicated cases, coronary heart disease (CHD) is the most common finding in SCD and can be the first and last manifestation. Up to 80% of cases of SCD occur in patients with some form of structural heart disease, such as CHD, cardiomyopathy, or congenital heart disease. Other cardiac causes of SCD, referred to as "autopsy negative," include primary electrical diseases such as LQTS, Brugada syndrome, catecholaminergic polymorphic ventricular tachycardia (CPVT), idiopathic ventricular fibrillation (IVF), and under some circumstances, Wolff-Parkinson-White (WPW) syndrome (see Chapters 63 and 65). The remaining sudden deaths are usually not cardiac in etiology.

For the purposes of evaluation, SCA should be considered as SCD that someone has survived. It is essential that patients who have SCA undergo a comprehensive evaluation to identify the cause and proper treatment. A history of cardiac disease is critically important in directing the evaluation and management, as is a family history of SCD or significant cardiac arrhythmias. The circumstances at the time of SCA are often informative. Cardiac symptoms that predate the SCD suggest preexisting structural heart disease. A variety of precipitating factors can provide clues to the etiology of SCA. Exercise, emotional upset, or stress may precipitate cardiac arrest in the setting of a variety of structural heart diseases, arrhythmogenic cardiomyopathy (arrhythmogenic right ventricular cardiomyopathy/dysplasia, ARVC/D), and primary electrical diseases such as LQTS (types 1 and 2) and CPVT. SCD in LQTS3 or Brugada syndrome is more likely to occur at rest or with sleep. Fever is a common precipitant of the characteristic ECG abnormality (Fig. 61.3) and arrhythmias in Brugada syndrome.

Medications and recreational drugs can increase the risk of lethal arrhythmias; patients should be asked about the use of antiarrhythmic drugs, stimulants, decongestants, psychotropics, antibiotics, alcohol, amphetamines, cocaine, and supplements, especially those used for weight loss and energy enhancement. Patients with LQTS and Brugada syndrome should be cautioned about the use of medications that may increase risk of arrhythmias. Drugs that should be avoided are listed on https://www.crediblemeds.org/ and http://www.brugadadrugs.org/, respectively. Structural heart diseases, such as dilated (DCM) or hypertrophic (HCM) cardiomyopathy (HCM SCD risk calculator https://doc-2do.com/hcm/webHCM.html) are associated with delayed ventricular repolarization, an acquired form of LQTS, and the same drugs can produce life-threatening arrhythmias in these patients.

The presence of a family history of serious ventricular arrhythmias, premature sudden death, stillbirths, sudden infant death syndrome (SIDS), unexplained motor vehicle and other accidents, and relatives with permanent pacemakers or implantable cardioverter-defibrillators (ICDs) may be relevant and will influence the evaluation of presumed heritable arrhythmias. If available, biologic materials from related decedents may be suitable for genetic testing or a molecular autopsy in suspected cases of heritable causes of SCD.

CLINICAL AND LABORATORY TESTING

The history, physical examination, and ECG are of paramount importance in the evaluation of patients with a suspected arrhythmia. A number of other studies, alone or in combination, may assist in the diagnosis and management of patients with cardiac arrhythmias.

Resting Electrocardiogram

The judicious use of noninvasive diagnostic tests is an important element in the evaluation of patients with arrhythmias, and there is no test more important than the ECG (see Chapter 14). Uncommon but

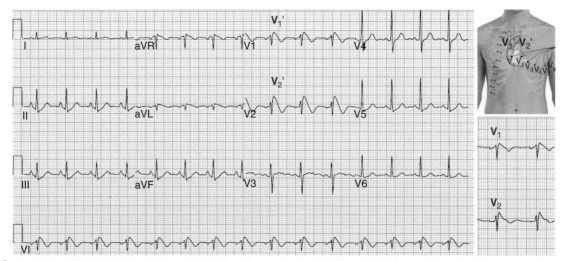

FIGURE 61.3 12-Lead electrocardiogram from a patient with Brugada syndrome with V_1' and V_2' recorded in the second intercostal space, as shown on the torso. *Inset,* Appearance of leads V1 and V2 in the standard positions in this patient.

diagnostically important signatures of electrophysiologic disturbances may be unearthed on the resting ECG, such as delta waves in WPW syndrome, prolongation or shortening of the QT interval, right precordial ST-segment abnormalities characteristic of Brugada syndrome, and epsilon waves in ARVC/D (Fig. 61.4).

During an arrhythmia, the ECG is the primary tool for diagnosis; an electrophysiologic study (EPS), in which intracardiac electrode catheters are used to record activity from several regions of the heart at one time, is more definitive but infrequently available immediately. A 12-lead ECG in addition to a long continuous recording with the use of a lead that shows distinct P waves is often helpful for closer analysis; typically, this is one of the inferior leads (II, III, and aVF), V₁, or aVR. The ECG obtained during an arrhythmia may be diagnostic by itself and obviate the need for further diagnostic testing.

Fig. 61.5 depicts an algorithm for the diagnosis of specific tachyarrhythmias from the 12-lead ECG (see Chapters 65 and 67). A major branch point in the differential diagnosis concerns the QRS duration: wide-QRS (>0.12 second) tachycardias are often VTs, and narrow-QRS (≤0.12 second) tachycardias are almost always SVTs, but there is some overlap (Table 61.1). Next, the most important questions to answer, regardless of QRS width, concern the characteristics of P waves. If P waves are not clearly visible on the regular ECG, atrial activity can occasionally be discerned by placing the right and left arm leads in various anterior chest positions (so-called Lewis leads), by recording atrial electrograms using intracardiac right atrial recordings (via permanent or temporary transvenous pacing leads), or by using esophageal electrodes or an echocardiogram. The last three methods are not readily available in most clinical situations and consume valuable time when dealing with a sick patient. A long rhythm strip can usually be obtained and can yield important clues by revealing P waves if perturbations occur during the arrhythmia (e.g., changes in rate, premature complexes, sudden termination, and the effect of physical maneuvers, as noted earlier). In a stable patient, if P waves are not clearly visible, the administration of adenosine by rapid intravenous bolus (6 mg followed by 12 mg if no response to the first dose) while running a rhythm strip may cause transient AV block and either terminate the tachycardia or allow discernment of P waves and diagnosis of the arrhythmia (Fig. 61.6).

Each arrhythmia should be approached in a systematic manner to answer several key questions; as suggested earlier, many of these questions relate to P wave characteristics and underscore the importance of assessing the ECG carefully for them. If P waves are visible, are the atrial and ventricular rates identical? Are the P-P and R-R intervals regular or irregular? If irregular, is it a consistent, repeating irregularity? Is there a P wave related to each QRS complex? Does the P wave seem to precede (long RP interval) or follow (short RP interval) the QRS complex (Fig. 61.7)? Are the resultant RP and PR intervals constant?

Are all P waves and QRS complexes identical? Is the P wave vector normal or abnormal? Are P, PR, QRS, and QT durations normal? Once these questions have been addressed, the clinician needs to assess the significance of the arrhythmia in view of the clinical setting. Should it be treated, and if so, how? For SVTs with a normal QRS complex, a branching decision tree such as that shown in Fig. 61.5 may be useful.

The Ladder Diagram: A ladder diagram, derived from the ECG, is used to depict depolarization and conduction schematically to aid in understanding the rhythm (Fig. 61.8). Because the ECG and therefore the ladder diagram represent electrical activity as a function of time along the x-axis, conduction is indicated by the lines of the ladder diagram sloping in a left-to-right direction. Activity originating in an ectopic site such as the ventricle is indicated by lines emanating from that tier. Sinus nodal discharge and conduction and, under certain circumstances, AV junctional discharge and conduction can only be inferred; their activity is not directly recorded on the ECG.

Cardiac Imaging

The prognostic implications of a cardiac arrhythmia depend on context, most importantly the presence of structural heart disease. The presence of structural heart disease may be apparent from the history and physical examination, chest radiograph, and ECG itself. Cardiac imaging plays an important role in the detection and characterization of myocardial structural abnormalities that can render the heart more susceptible to arrhythmias. Ventricular tachyarrhythmias, for instance, occur more frequently in patients with ventricular systolic dysfunction and chamber dilation, in HCM, and in the setting of infiltrative diseases such as sarcoidosis. Supraventricular arrhythmias may be associated with particular congenital conditions, including AV reentry in the setting of Ebstein anomaly (see Chapter 82). Echocardiography (Chapter 16) is frequently employed to screen for disorders of cardiac structure and function. Increasingly, magnetic resonance imaging (MRI) of the myocardium (Chapter 19) is being used to screen for scar burden, fibrofatty infiltration of the myocardium as seen in ARVC, and other structural changes that affect arrhythmia susceptibility. Both contrast-enhanced MRI and 18F-fluorodeoxyglucose positron emission tomography with computed tomographic transmission (18F-FDG PET/CT) have been used in the diagnosis, management, and response to treatment of cardiac sarcoidosis (Fig. 61.9) (see Chapter 18).

Stress Electrocardiography

Exercise electrocardiographic stress testing may be particularly useful in the evaluation of patients who experience symptoms with exertion (Chapter 15). Exercise stress testing is important in determining the

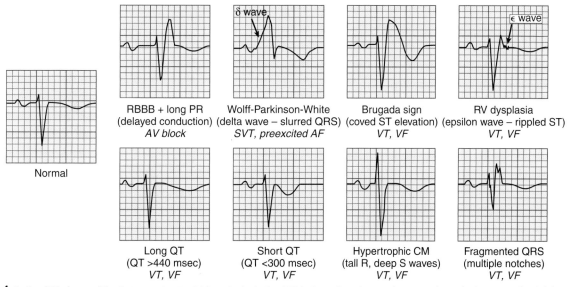

FIGURE 61.4 Resting QRS abnormalities that suggest potential for arrhythmia. Lead V1 is shown in each example; a normal complex is presented at *left* for reference. *CM,* Cardiomyopathy; *RBBB,* right bundle branch block; *RV,* right ventricular.

presence of myocardial demand ischemia and other arrhythmic substrates, such as alterations in repolarization and the dynamic behavior of the QT interval (see Chapter 63). Microscopic alterations in the T wave (T wave alternans, see below) at low heart rates may identify patients at risk for ventricular arrhythmias. Altered heart rate recovery may indicate autonomic dysfunction associated with heightened arrhythmic risk. A persistent elevation in heart rate after the end of exercise (delay in return to baseline) is associated with a worse CV prognosis, as is a rapid resting heart rate.

It is important to recognize that not all arrhythmias induced by exercise have an ominous prognosis. Approximately one third of individuals without heart disease will have ventricular ectopy associated with exercise. Typically, this manifests as occasional uniform PVCs, more likely to occur at faster heart rates, and not reproducible from one test to the next. Three to six beats of nonsustained VT can occur in normal subjects, especially elderly persons, and its occurrence neither implicates ischemia or other forms of heart disease nor predicts

increased CV morbidity or mortality. However, multiform PVCs and VT are an infrequent response to exercise in healthy individuals; thus, the development of more complex ventricular arrhythmias during exercise testing should prompt a search for underlying structural heart disease.[8,9] Ventricular ectopy occurs in about half of patients with CAD, generally appearing more reproducibly and at lower heart rates (<130 beats/min) than in healthy individuals and often in the early recovery period. Frequent PVCs (>10 per minute), polymorphic PVCs, and VT are more likely to occur in patients with CAD. PVCs at rest can be suppressed by exercise in patients with CAD; therefore, this observation does not necessarily imply a benign prognosis or absence of underlying structural heart disease.

Patients who have symptoms consistent with an arrhythmia induced by exercise (e.g., syncope, sustained palpitations) should be considered for stress testing. Stress testing may be indicated to provoke supraventricular and ventricular arrhythmias, to determine the relationship of the arrhythmia to activity, to aid in choosing antiarrhythmic therapy

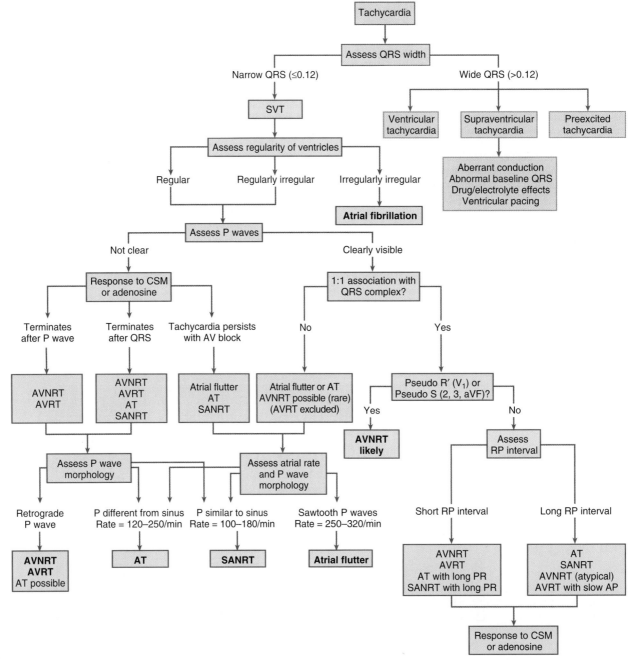

FIGURE 61.5 Stepwise approach to diagnosis of the type of tachycardia based on a 12-lead electrocardiogram during the episode. The initial step is to determine whether the tachycardia has a wide or narrow QRS complex. For wide-complex tachycardia, see Table 61.1; the remainder of the algorithm is helpful in diagnosis of the type of narrow-complex tachycardia. *AP,* Accessory pathway; *AT,* atrial tachycardia; *AVNRT,* atrioventricular nodal reentrant tachycardia; *AVRT,* atrioventricular reciprocating tachycardia; *CSM,* carotid sinus massage; *SANRT,* sinoatrial nodal reentry tachycardia.

TABLE 61.1 Electrocardiographic Distinctions for Diagnosis of Wide–QRS Complex Tachycardia

FAVOR SUPRAVENTRICULAR TACHYCARDIA	FAVOR VENTRICULAR TACHYCARDIA
Initiation with a premature P wave	Initiation with a premature QRS complex
Tachycardia complexes identical to those in resting rhythm	Tachycardia beats identical to PVCs during sinus rhythm
"Long-short" sequence preceding initiation	"Short-long" sequence preceding initiation
Changes in the P-P interval preceding changes in the R-R interval	Changes in the R-R interval preceding changes in the P-P interval
QRS contours consistent with aberrant conduction (V_1, V_6)	QRS contours inconsistent with aberrant conduction (V_1, V_6)
Slowing or termination with vagal maneuvers	AV dissociation or other non-1:1 AV relationship
Onset of the QRS to its peak (positive or negative) <50 msec	Onset of the QRS to its peak (positive or negative) ≥50 msec
	Fusion beats, capture beats
QRS duration ≤0.14 sec	QRS duration >0.14 sec
Normal QRS axis (0–+90 degrees)	Left-axis deviation (especially –90–180 degrees)
	Concordant R-wave progression pattern
	Contralateral bundle branch block pattern from the resting rhythm
	Initial R, q, or r >40 msec or notched Q in aVR
	Absence of an "rS" complex in any precordial lead

AV, Atrioventricular; *PVC,* premature ventricular complexes.

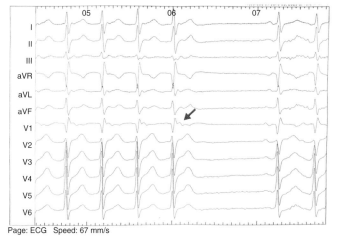

Page: ECG   Speed: 67 mm/s

FIGURE 61.6 Supraventricular tachycardia, typical AV reentry tachycardia terminated by 6 mg of IV adenosine. The tachycardia terminates with a retrograde P wave *(arrow).* After the pause, the temporal relationship of the P wave to the QRS changes indicating conversion to sinus rhythm.

and uncovering proarrhythmic responses, and to provide some insight into the mechanism of the tachycardia.

Exercise testing has diagnostic or prognostic value in patients with primary electrical abnormalities such as LQTS, CPVT, and Brugada syndrome (see Chapter 63). Since the QT interval can be normal in up to one quarter of patients with genetically proven LQTS, exercise testing can stress repolarizing reserves and can be useful to expose ECG abnormalities in these patients. An abnormal response of the QT interval to the heart rate acceleration produced by standing is seen in patients with LQTS compared with normal patients. Exercise testing can unmask polymorphic PVCs and VT in patients with CPVT (Fig. 61.10).[10] In patients with Brugada syndrome, significant ST-segment

elevation with coving of the ST segment during the recovery phase predicts arrhythmic events during follow-up.[11]

Long-Term Electrocardiogram Recording: Holter Monitoring, Event Recording, and Insertable Loop Recorders

The fundamental diagnostic principle in managing patients with an undocumented cardiac rhythm disturbance is to record the ECG during a symptomatic episode and establish a causal relation between the arrhythmia and symptoms. As importantly, recording normal sinus rhythm during a patient's typical symptomatic episode effectively excludes cardiac arrhythmia as a cause. In patients not suspected of having a life-threatening arrhythmia, Holter monitoring and event recording, continuously or intermittently, record the ECG over longer periods, enhancing the possibility of observing the cardiac rhythm during symptoms (eTable 61.2). The type and duration of ECG monitoring depend on the frequency of symptoms. Most continuous recording systems are equipped with patient-triggered recording to enable correlation of the ECG with symptoms. Continuous recording systems do not require patient recognition of an arrhythmia but some do allow for patient-activated ECG data transmission.

In Hospital Electrocardiographic Recording

ECG monitoring systems are used in increasing proportions of inpatients regardless of history or suspicion of arrhythmias. These systems can provide valuable information about rhythm abnormalities, including mode of onset and termination, and allow prompt acquisition of a full 12-lead ECG for more detail. Telemetry can disclose intermittent heart block in a patient with presyncope that may warrant consideration of pacemaker implantation or reveal nonsustained VT in a patient with previous MI and left ventricular dysfunction and prompt an EPS for further assessment of risk. Although telemetry is helpful in many cases, it can be misleading: artifacts can simulate VT or VF, heart block, or asystole. Careful scrutiny is necessary to avoid unnecessary tests and procedures in patients with these artefactual arrhythmias (Fig. 61.11).

Ambulatory Electrocardiographic (Holter) Recording

Continuous electrocardiographic recorders include the traditional Holter monitor and digitally record three or more electrocardiographic channels for 24 to 48 hours. Computers scan the recording, with human oversight, to provide a report with snapshot recordings of symptomatic events and other important findings such as asymptomatic arrhythmias or ST-segment changes. Holter monitoring is most useful in patients with frequent (daily or more often) symptoms. From 25% to 50% of patients experience a symptom during a 24-hour recording; in 2% to 15% the complaint is caused by an arrhythmia (Fig. 61.12). The ability to correlate symptoms temporally with abnormalities on the ECG is one of the strengths of this technique. Guidelines for the use of ambulatory electrocardiographic recording for diagnosis, risk assessment, efficacy of antiarrhythmic drug therapy, assessment of cardiac rhythm device management, and monitoring for myocardial ischemia is summarized in the Guidelines section of the online chapter and eTable 61G.1 through eTable 61G.3. This section addresses the requirement for maintenance of clinical competence in ambulatory electrocardiography.

Significant rhythm disturbances are uncommon in healthy young persons. Sinus bradycardia with heart rates of 35 to 40 beats/min, sinus arrhythmia with pauses exceeding 3 seconds, sinoatrial exit block, type I (Wenckebach) second-degree AV block (often during sleep), wandering atrial pacemaker, junctional escape complexes, and PACs and PVCs can be observed and are not necessarily abnormal. Frequent and complex atrial and ventricular rhythm disturbances are less frequently observed, however, and type II second-degree AV conduction disturbances (see Chapter 68) are not recorded in normal patients. Elderly patients have a higher prevalence of arrhythmias, some of which may be responsible for neurologic symptoms (Fig. 61.13, see Chapter 90).

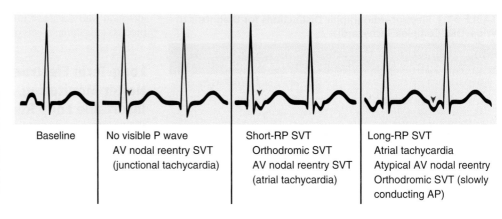

FIGURE 61.7 Differential diagnosis of types of supraventricular tachycardia based on timing of atrial activity (RP and PR intervals). **Left,** Normal beat. The types of tachycardia are listed below the representative electrocardiographic patterns that they can produce, as categorized by P wave position relative to the QRS complex. An *arrowhead* shows the location of the P wave in each example. Diagnoses in parentheses are rare causes of the noted findings. *AP,* Accessory pathway.

Baseline

No visible P wave
AV nodal reentry SVT
(junctional tachycardia)

Short-RP SVT
Orthodromic SVT
AV nodal reentry SVT
(atrial tachycardia)

Long-RP SVT
Atrial tachycardia
Atypical AV nodal reentry
Orthodromic SVT (slowly conducting AP)

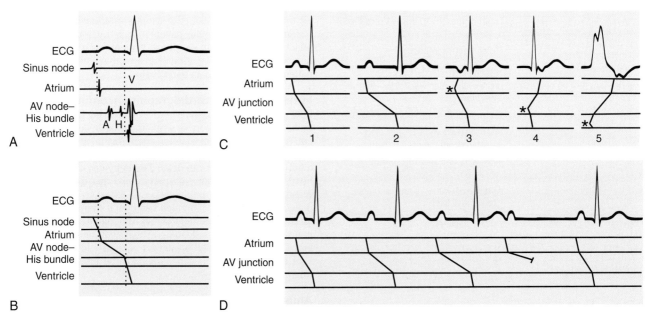

FIGURE 61.8 Intracardiac signals and ladder diagrams. **A,** A single beat is shown with accompanying intracardiac signals from the sinus node, right atrium, atrioventricular (AV) nodal and His bundle regions, and right ventricle. **B,** The same beat is shown with the accompanying ladder diagram below. Cardiac regions have been divided into tiers separated by horizontal lines. Vertical *dotted lines* denote onset of the P wave and QRS complexes. The relatively steep lines indicate rapid conduction through the atrium, His bundle, and ventricular muscle and more gently sloping lines the slower conduction in the sinus and AV nodes. **C,** Different situations with accompanying explanatory ladder diagrams. Beat 1 is normal, as in **B**; beat 2 shows first-degree AV delay, with the more gradual slope than normal in the AV nodal tier signifying very slow conduction in this region. In beat 3 an atrial premature complex is shown (starting in the atrial tier at the *asterisk*) and is producing an inverted P wave on the ECG. In beat 4 an ectopic impulse arises in the His bundle *(asterisk)* and propagates to the ventricle, as well as retrogradely through the AV node to the atrium. In beat 5 a ventricular ectopic complex *(asterisk)* conducts retrogradely through the His bundle and AV node and eventually to the atrium. **D,** Wenckebach AV cycle (type I second-degree block). As the PR interval progressively increases from left to right in the figure, the slope of the line in the AV nodal region flattens until it fails to propagate at all after the fourth P wave (small line perpendicular to the sloping AV nodal conduction line), after which the cycle repeats. *A,* Atrial recording; *H,* His recording; *V,* ventricular recording.

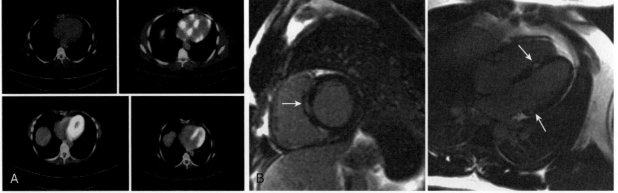

FIGURE 61.9 Sarcoidosis **A,** Four images show the pattern of 18F-fluorodeoxyglucose uptake on positron emission tomography (PET) scan. **B,** Two cardiac magnetic resonance images show evidence of delayed gadolinium enhancement in the midwall of the left ventricle *(arrows)*. (Modified from Hamzeh N, Steckman DA, Sauer WH, et al. Pathophysiology and clinical management of cardiac sarcoidosis. *Nat Rev Cardiol.* 2015;12:278.)

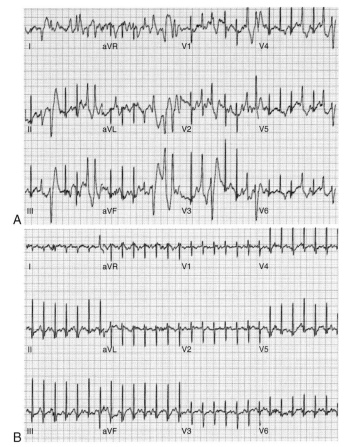

FIGURE 61.10 Exercise-induced polymorphic premature ventricular complexes and ventricular tachycardia (VT) in a young woman with dizziness; palpitations caused by a ryanodine receptor (RyR2) mutation producing catecholaminergic polymorphic VT (CPVT). **A,** ECG at peak exercise before treatment. **B,** ECG while receiving treatment with nadolol and flecainide.

It is worth repeating that the long-term prognosis of even frequent and complex PVCs in asymptomatic healthy patients is very good, without an increased risk of mortality. However, frequent PVCs (>15% of the total) have been shown to produce a cardiomyopathy and heart failure in some people, which can be reversed following elimination of the PVCs. Most patients with ischemic heart disease, particularly after MI (see Chapters 37 to 39), exhibit PVCs when they are monitored for 24 hours. The frequency of PVCs progressively increases during the first several weeks and then decreases at about 6 months after infarction. Frequent and complex PVCs are associated with a two- to five-fold increased risk for cardiac or sudden death in patients after MI, but treating these PVCs may not improve the prognosis. Recent data indicate that ablation of PVCs after MI may improve previously depressed ventricular function.[12]

Long-term recording of the ECG has also exposed potentially serious arrhythmias and complex ventricular ectopy in patients with left ventricular hypertrophy, as well as in those with hypertrophic, dilated, and ischemic cardiomyopathy; in those with mitral valve prolapse (see Chapter 76); in those with otherwise unexplained syncope (Chapter 71) or transient vague cerebrovascular symptoms or stroke; and in those with conduction disturbances, sinus node dysfunction, bradycardia-tachycardia syndrome, WPW syndrome (Chapter 65), and pacemaker malfunction (Chapter 69). It has been shown that asymptomatic AF occurs far more often than symptomatic episodes in patients with AF.

Variations of Holter recording have been used for particular applications. Some monitoring systems are able to reconstruct a full 12-lead ECG from a seven-electrode recording system. This is especially useful in trying to document the ECG morphology of VT before an ablation procedure or a consistent morphology of PVCs that may arise from an ablatable focus of VT or VF. Most Holter recording and analysis systems can place a clearly recognizable deflection on the recording when a pacemaker stimulus is detected, facilitating diagnosis of potential pacemaker malfunction. On occasion, artifacts on the ECG can mimic bradycardias or tachycardias and lead to erroneous therapy. Finally, most systems can also provide heart rate variability and QT data (see below). Use of these systems for detection of myocardial ischemia (ST-segment analysis) has yielded mixed results for both specificity and sensitivity.

Event Recording
In many patients, the 24- or 48-hour snapshot provided by the Holter recording is insufficient to document the cause of the patient's symptoms. Event recorders are indicated when symptoms occur less frequently (e.g., several episodes per month), and because the monitors are typically patient activated, and well-suited for correlating symptoms with rhythm disturbances. These devices come in various forms and are kept by the patient for an extended time, often up to 30 days. Event recorders can be continuous with auto-triggered or patient-activated recording (**eFig. 61.1**). Discontinuous transtelephonic monitoring systems without looping memory require patient activation. When being worn by the patient, digital recordings can be made during symptomatic episodes and can be transmitted to a receiving station by telephone at the patient's convenience (see Fig. 61.13). Some of these recorders store more than 30 seconds of the ECG before the patient activates the recording. These loop recorders record continuously, but only a small window of time is present in memory at any moment. When the patient presses the event button, the current window is frozen while the device continues recording for another 30 to 60 seconds, depending on how it is configured. Event recorders are highly effective in documenting infrequent events, but the quality of the recordings is more subject to motion artifact than with Holter monitors, and usually only one channel can be recorded. With most systems, the device automatically begins recording the rhythm when the heart rate increases or decreases outside preset parameters. Some systems incorporate cell phone technology that automatically notifies a central monitoring facility when certain conditions are met (e.g., extreme bradycardia or tachycardia). This can significantly shorten the time between occurrence and effective treatment of serious arrhythmias.

The use of wearables for cardiac monitoring has enabled detection of abnormalities in heart rate and rhythm on a much broader basis than physician-prescribed monitoring.[13] Fitness bands and other wearables may have accelerometers that detect movement during exercise and other daily activities and correlate it with heart rate. There are a number of other devices that are accurate and easy to use, including smartphones and watches that use camera-based plethysmography to assess heart rate and rhythm. Algorithms have been developed to detect irregularity of the heart rate and notify a patient of "possible AF." Although heart rate measurements tend to be fairly accurate, subsequent cardiac monitoring to confirm AF in patients alerted to a possible arrhythmia has shown confirmation of AF in less than half of the patients.[14] Both iPhones and Android phones have applications for real-time ECG monitoring. They are useful for on-demand arrhythmia diagnosis and monitoring arrhythmia burden and are being used as a phenotyping platform in population studies (**eFig. 61.2**).[15–17] A small, lightweight device is available that has two electrodes on which the fingers of the left and right hands are placed to record a lead I ECG rhythm strip for 30 seconds. More recently, a third electrode has been added that allows for all six limb leads to be recorded. These rhythm strips can be uploaded to the cloud and downloaded to a physician's office for subsequent verification of the rhythm. The latest versions of smartwatches can also record a single-lead rhythm strip by opening an app and placing the fingers of the hand opposite to the watch on the crown of the watch for 30 seconds.

Most currently available pacemakers and ICDs can provide Holter-like data when premature beats or tachycardia episodes occur and can store electrograms of these events from the implanted leads (Fig. 61.14). Dual-chamber devices can record atrial and ventricular high-rate episodes that can be correlated with the electrograms during such events (see Chapter 69). The device can then be interrogated and the electrograms printed for analysis. Many implanted device systems incorporate remote monitoring so that if symptoms develop, the information can be transmitted via the Internet to the physician's office, thus enabling more prompt diagnosis and treatment than if the patient had to schedule an outpatient visit. For serious rhythm disturbances, such as sustained VT, this information can lead to timely changes in therapy; in other cases, such as incidentally discovered AF, therapeutic implications (e.g., initiation of anticoagulation) are less clear. Implantable monitors or insertable loop recorders (ILRs) are typically used for the evaluation of suspected serious arrhythmias that occur infrequently and cannot be provoked at diagnostic EPS. An ILR, a single-lead ECG monitoring device placed subcutaneously at approximately the level of the anterior second rib, monitors the cardiac rhythm for as long as 24 to 36 months. Both P waves and QRS complexes can be recorded by an ILR. These devices have both auto-triggered and patient-activated arrhythmia-recording capabilities (**eFig. 61.3**). Use of such devices has been successful in recording tachyarrhythmias and, more often, bradyarrhythmias. The devices can be configured to store patient-activated episodes, automatically activated recordings (heart rate outside preset parameters), or a combination of these. ECG recordings can be sent to an analyzing center transtelephonically and then to physicians via the Internet. Interrogation of ILRs can also be performed remotely over a landline telephone. Technologic advances have resulted in further reduction in size and ease of implantation of ILRs, which has led to increased clinical deployment of these devices. ILRs have primarily been used in the evaluation of syncope, but their use is increasing in monitoring arrhythmia density, especially AF.[18]

ELECTROCARDIOGRAM DYNAMICS/ANALYTICS

Various methods for evaluating components of the ECG and heart rate have been developed, mainly for the purpose of enhancing SCD risk stratification of patients. Few of them are used routinely today because of suboptimal sensitivity and specificity. **Heart rate variability** is used to evaluate vagal and sympathetic influences on the sinus node (inferring that the same activity is also occurring in the ventricles) and to identify patients at risk for a CV event or death. R-R variability predicts all-cause mortality after MI, as does left ventricular ejection fraction or nonsustained VT.[19,20] Similar results have been obtained in patients with dilated cardiomyopathy (see Chapters 50 and 52).

Heart rate turbulence is a measure of reflex vagal control of the heart. Abnormal heart rate turbulence is a strong independent predictor of mortality in patients with CAD and dilated cardiomyopathy. **QRS and QT dispersion and T wave**

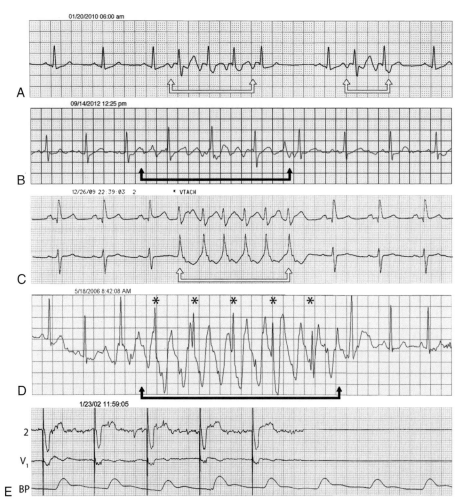

FIGURE 61.11 Electrocardiographic events and artifacts. **A,** Sinus rhythm punctuated by short episodes of atrial tachycardia with a more rapid rate (between the *white arrows*). **B,** Pseudo–atrial arrhythmia. Sinus rhythm is present throughout (no variation in the R-R interval) despite the appearance of an artifact that mimics short episode of atrial flutter or fibrillation (between the *black arrows*). **C,** Nonsustained VT (between the *white arrows*) with wide rapid QRS complexes not preceded by a P wave and seen in two monitor leads. **D,** Pseudo-VT. Despite the appearance of VT (between the *black arrows*), sinus rhythm is present throughout (including complexes indicated by *asterisks*). **E,** Pseudo–pacemaker failure. After the first five paced complexes, the ECG is flat in *both* monitor leads, thus suggesting failure of pacemaker output; however, the pulse contour on the blood pressure (BP) tracing indicates that the heart is still contracting and the pacemaker is still working whereas the ECG monitor is not.

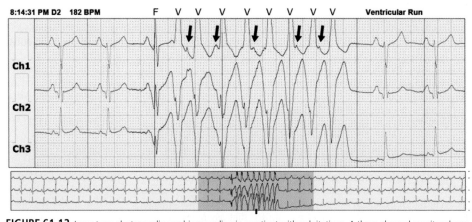

FIGURE 61.12 Long-term electrocardiographic recording in a patient with palpitations. A three-channel monitor shows sinus rhythm followed by nine wide QRS complexes of VT (labeled "V"); the complex that precedes these is a fusion between the normal complex and wide ("F"). *Arrows* indicate retrograde P waves during tachycardia. The presence of fewer P waves than QRS complexes and a fusion complex at the outset confirm the diagnosis of VT (which correlated with the patient's palpitations).

abnormalities are a reflection of heterogeneity in refractoriness and conduction velocity, which is a hallmark of reentrant arrhythmias. Dispersion indices usually measure the maximum difference (shortest to longest) in the intervals of interest. Abnormally high QRS and QT dispersion have been correlated with risk for overall mortality and arrhythmic death in patients with various disorders. **Signal-averaged electrocardiography and late potentials** Signal averaging is a method that improves the signal-to-noise ratio when signals are recurrent and noise is random. Signal averaging can detect late ventricular potentials of 1 to 25 μV that correspond to the delayed and fragmented conduction in the ventricles recorded with direct mapping techniques in patients with VT (**eFig. 61.4**). In specific situations, it can be helpful, as in a patient suspected of having ARVC. **T wave alternans** is beat-to-beat alternation in the amplitude or morphology of the ECG recording of ventricular repolarization, the ST segment, and the T wave. It has been found in conditions favoring the development of ventricular tachyarrhythmias, such as ischemia and LQTS, and in patients with ventricular arrhythmias. A positive T wave alternans test result has been associated with a worse arrhythmic prognosis in various disorders, including ischemic heart disease and nonischemic cardiomyopathy. **Body surface mapping** is used to provide a complete picture of the effects of currents from the heart on the body surface. The potential distributions are represented by contour lines of equal potential, and each distribution is displayed instant by instant throughout activation, recovery, or both. **Electrocardiographic imaging** is a method for recording cardiac electrical activity at the skin surface and spatially integrating it with imaging data (currently, cardiac CT scanning). Using complex mathematical processing of electrical data collected from 224 electrodes on the skin surface, this technique can plot or project atrial and ventricular electrical activity on an epicardial "shell" of the patient's own heart and thereby follow the course of activation or repolarization during sinus rhythm or an arrhythmia (**eFig 61.5**).[21]

HEAD UP TILT

Tilt-table testing (TTT) is useful in the evaluation of patients without structural heart disease and recurrent syncope in whom there is a suspicion that exaggerated vagal tone producing cardioinhibitory and/or vasodepressor responses may play a causal role (**eFig. 61.6**). In patients with structural heart disease, TTT may be indicated in those with syncope in whom other causes (e.g., asystole, tachyarrhythmias) have been excluded. TTT has been suggested as a useful tool in the diagnosis of and therapy for recurrent idiopathic vertigo, chronic fatigue syndrome, recurrent transient ischemic attacks, and repeated falls of unknown etiology in elderly patients without much evidence. Importantly, TTT is relatively contraindicated in the presence of severe CAD with proximal coronary stenoses, known severe cerebrovascular disease, severe mitral stenosis, and obstruction to left ventricular outflow (e.g., aortic stenosis).

Patients are placed on a tilt table in the supine position and tilted upright to a maximum of 60 to 80 degrees for 20 to 45 minutes or longer if necessary. Isoproterenol, administered as a bolus or infusion, may provoke syncope in patients whose initial upright TTT result shows no abnormalities or, after a few minutes of tilt, may shorten the time needed to produce a positive response on the test. An initial intravenous isoproterenol dose of 1 μg/min can be increased in 0.5-μg/min steps until symptoms occur or a maximum of 4 μg/min is given. Isoproterenol induces a vasodepressor response in upright susceptible patients (decrease in heart rate and blood pressure along with near-syncope or syncope). Tilt-table test (TTT) results are positive in two-thirds to three-fourths of patients susceptible to neurally mediated syncope. They are reproducible in approximately 80% of patients but have a 10% to 15% false-positive response rate. A positive test result is more meaningful when it reproduces symptoms that have occurred spontaneously.

The physiologic response to TTT is incompletely understood; however, redistribution of blood volume and increased ventricular contractility occur consistently. Exaggerated activation of a central reflex in response to TTT produces a stereotypic response of an initial increase in heart rate, followed by drop in blood pressure and then a reduction in heart rate characteristic of neurally-mediated hypotension (see eFig. 61.6). Positive responses can be divided into cardioinhibitory, vasodepressor, and mixed categories (**eFig. 61.7**). In patients with orthostatic hypotension and autonomic insufficiency, blood pressure will drop with only a minimal increase in heart rate. Patients with neurocardiogenic syncope or near syncope have been treated with beta blockers, disopyramide, theophylline, selective serotonin reuptake inhibitors, midodrine, fludrocortisone, salt loading, tilt-training, and thigh-high support stockings, alone or in combination. However, none of these treatments is reliably effective in most patients.

POTS is another aberrant variant of a neurocardiogenic reflex characterized

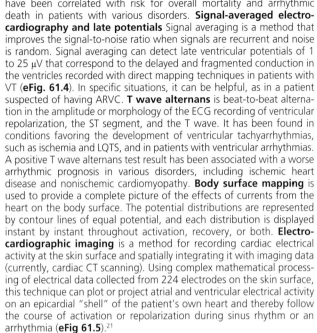

6/25/2003 8:01:15 PM[M]   Speed: 25 mm/s Gain: 10 mm/mV High-pass filter: none Low-pass filter: 40Hz
0h02m01s85 ... 0h02m09s98
Event 2 continued   CH1

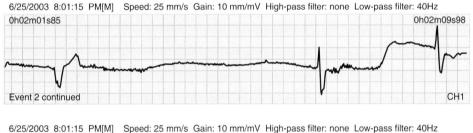

6/25/2003 8:01:15 PM[M]   Speed: 25 mm/s Gain: 10 mm/mV High-pass filter: none Low-pass filter: 40Hz
0h02m09s88 ... 0h02m18s01
CH1

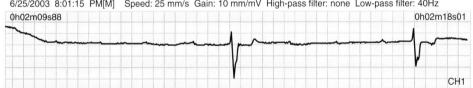

FIGURE 61.13 Continuous electrocardiographic recording from a patient-activated event monitor during an episode of lightheadedness. Sinus rhythm at 75 beats/min with sudden AV block is present with pauses of longer than 4 seconds, and in the *bottom strip* there is an effective heart rate of approximately 8 beats/min.

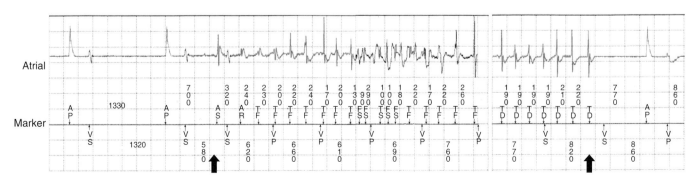

FIGURE 61.14 Recordings from a pacemaker log showing an episode of atrial fibrillation (AF) at its onset *(left arrow)* and termination *(right arrow)*, more than four days later. Two atrial paced complexes (AP) are followed by an episode of AF characterized by rapid erratic deflections. When the episode ends, atrial pacing resumes. The patient was unaware of the episode, but when discovered at a routine office follow-up visit, this information prompted initiation of anticoagulation in light of an elevated stroke risk and newly discovered AF.

by the inability to tolerate the upright posture and a dramatic increase (>30 beats/min) in heart rate (>120 beats/min) within 10 minutes of assuming an upright posture. A wide array of symptoms complicates the diagnosis of POTS, which is often confused with anxiety disorder, inappropriate sinus tachycardia, chronic fatigue syndrome, and fibromyalgia.[22,23] Data from an international registry suggest that endurance- and strength-training programs may be useful in managing POTS.[24]

Invasive Electrophysiologic Testing

The EPS is central to the understanding and treatment of many cardiac arrhythmias. The indications for EPS fall into several broad categories: to define the mechanism of an arrhythmia, to deliver catheter-based ablative treatment, and to determine the etiology of symptoms that may be caused by an arrhythmia (e.g., syncope, palpitations). An invasive EPS involves introducing multipolar electrode catheters into the venous or arterial system and positioning them at various intracardiac sites or percutaneously into the pericardium to record or stimulate cardiac electrical activity. The positioning of these catheters is guided by complementary imaging modalities including fluoroscopy, intracardiac echocardiography (ICE) and electroanatomic mapping (EAM), often using MRI and CT to merge cardiac images with the EAM information. Guidelines for the use of electrophysiological procedures for diagnosis and therapeutic intervention are summarized in the Guidelines section of the online chapter and eTables 61G.4 and 61G.5. This section addresses the requirement for maintenance of clinical competence in electrophysiological procedures including electrophysiological studies, catheter ablation, and cardiac rhythm device implantation and management.

The components of the EPS are baseline measurements of conduction under resting and stressed (rate or pharmacologic) conditions and maneuvers, both pacing and pharmacologic, to induce arrhythmias. Assessment of AV conduction at rest is done by positioning electrodes along the septal leaflet of the tricuspid valve and measuring the atrial-His interval (an estimate of AV nodal conduction time; normally, 60 to 125 milliseconds) and the His-ventricular (H-V) interval (a measure of infranodal conduction; normally, 35 to 55 milliseconds). The heart is stimulated from portions of the atria or ventricles and from the region of the His bundle, bundle branches, accessory pathways, and other structures. EP studies are performed *diagnostically* to provide information about the type of clinical rhythm disturbance and insight into its electrophysiologic mechanism. EPS are used *therapeutically* to terminate a tachycardia by electrical stimulation or electroshock, to evaluate the effects of therapy by determining whether a particular intervention modifies or prevents electrical induction of a tachycardia or whether an electrical device properly senses and terminates an induced tachyarrhythmia, and to ablate myocardium involved in the tachycardia and prevent further episodes. EPS have also been used prognostically to identify patients at risk for SCD. The study can be helpful in patients with AV block, intraventricular conduction disturbance, sinus node dysfunction, tachycardia, and unexplained syncope or palpitations (see Chapter 71).

An EPS is usually effective at initiating VT and SVT when these tachyarrhythmias have occurred spontaneously. Particularly for VT, programmed stimulation is used in a systematic attempt to induce the arrhythmia. Short bursts of fixed rate ventricular pacing (e.g., eight beats at 100 to 150 beats/min, corresponding to a pacing cycle length of 600 to 400 msec) are followed by single ventricular extrastimuli at varying coupling intervals, and eventually two or three extrastimuli are added. The ability to induce an arrhythmia using such stimulation techniques before an intervention (e.g., drug therapy or catheter or surgical ablation) allows one to assess the efficacy of treatment afterward by using the same stimulation techniques and demonstrating noninducibility. However, false-negative responses (not finding a particular electrical abnormality known to be present) and false-positive responses (induction of a nonclinical arrhythmia) may complicate interpretation of the results because many lack reproducibility. Altered autonomic tone in a supine patient undergoing EPS, hemodynamic or ischemic influences,

changing anatomy (e.g., new infarction) after the study, day-to-day variability, and the use of an artificial trigger (electrical stimulation) to induce the arrhythmia are several of many factors that can explain the occasional disparity between test results and spontaneous occurrence of arrhythmia. Overall, the diagnostic validity and reproducibility of these studies are good, and they are safe when performed by skilled clinical electrophysiologists.

ATRIOVENTRICULAR BLOCK

In patients with AV block, the site of block usually dictates the clinical course of the patient and whether a pacemaker is needed (see Chapter 68). In general, the site of AV block can be determined from analysis of the surface ECG. When the site of block cannot be determined from such an analysis and when knowing the site of block is imperative for management of the patient, an invasive EPS is indicated. Candidates include symptomatic patients in whom His-Purkinje block is suspected but not established, patients with second- or third-degree AV block, for whom information about the site of block or its mechanism may help direct therapy or assess prognosis, and patients suspected of having concealed His bundle extrasystoles. Patients with block in the His-Purkinje system become symptomatic because of periods of bradycardia or asystole and require pacemaker implantation more often than do patients who have AV nodal block. Type I (Wenckebach) AV block in older patients can have clinical implications similar to those for type II AV block. However, the results of EPS for evaluating the conduction system must be interpreted with caution. In rare cases, the process of recording conduction intervals alters their values. For example, catheter pressure on the AV node or His bundle can cause prolongation of the atrial-His or H-V interval and could lead to erroneous diagnosis and therapy. Finally, patients with AV block treated with a pacemaker who continue to be symptomatic and in whom a causal ventricular tachyarrhythmia is suspected are also candidates for EPS.

INTRAVENTRICULAR CONDUCTION DISTURBANCE

For patients with an intraventricular conduction disturbance, an EPS provides information about the duration of the H-V interval, which can be prolonged with a normal PR interval, or normal with a prolonged PR interval. A prolonged H-V interval (>55 msec) is associated with a greater likelihood of the development of a complete AV block (but typically the rate of progression is slow, 2% to 3% annually) and for having structural heart disease and a higher mortality.[25] The finding of very long H-V intervals (>80 to 90 msec) identifies patients at increased risk for the development of AV block. The H-V interval has high specificity (approximately 80%) but low sensitivity (66%) for predicting the development of complete AV block. During an EPS, atrial pacing is used to uncover abnormal His-Purkinje conduction. A positive response is provocation of distal His block during 1:1 AV nodal conduction at rates of 135 beats/min or less. Again, sensitivity is low but specificity is high. Drug infusion, such as with procainamide or ajmaline (not available in the United States), sometimes exposes abnormal His-Purkinje conduction (Fig. 61.15). An EPS is indicated in patients with an intraventricular conduction disturbance with symptoms (syncope or presyncope) that appear to be related to a bradyarrhythmia when no other cause of symptoms is identified, including with prolonged ECG monitoring. However, for many of these patients, ventricular tachyarrhythmias rather than AV block can be the cause of their symptoms, with obvious therapeutic implications. Consequently, programmed stimulation to see if ventricular tachyarrhythmias can be provoked is a standard part of the evaluation of such patients with EPS.

SINUS NODE DYSFUNCTION

Demonstration of slow sinus rates, sinus exit block, or sinus pauses on an ECG temporally related to symptoms suggests a causal relationship and usually obviates the need for further diagnostic studies (see Chapters 65 and 68). Carotid sinus pressure that results in several seconds of complete asystole or AV block and reproduces the patient's usual symptoms exposes the presence of a hypersensitive carotid sinus reflex. CSM must be done cautiously; rarely, it can precipitate a stroke. Neurohumoral agents, adenosine, or stress testing can be used to evaluate the effects of autonomic tone on sinus node automaticity and sinoatrial conduction time (SACT).

Sinus Node Recovery Time

Sinus node recovery time (SNRT) is a technique that can be useful for evaluating sinus node function. Atrial pacing is initiated at a fixed rate faster than the sinus rate for 30 to 60 seconds, after which is it abruptly terminated. The interval between the last paced high right atrial response and the first spontaneous (sinus) high right atrial response after termination of pacing is measured to determine SNRT. Because the spontaneous sinus rate influences SNRT, the value is corrected by subtracting the spontaneous sinus node cycle length (before pacing) from the SNRT (Fig. 61.16). This value, the corrected SNRT (CSNRT), is generally shorter than 525 milliseconds. A prolonged CSNRT has been found in patients suspected of having sinus node dysfunction. After cessation of pacing, the first return sinus cycle can be normal but can be followed by secondary pauses (a strong indicator of sinus node dysfunction). It is important to evaluate AV node and His-Purkinje function in patients with sinus node dysfunction because many also exhibit impaired AV conduction.

Sinoatrial Conduction Time

SACT can be estimated by simple pacing techniques based on the assumptions that (1) conduction times into and out of the sinus node are equal, (2) no depression of sinus node automaticity occurs, and (3) the pacemaker site does not shift after premature stimulation. These assumptions can be erroneous, particularly in patients with sinus node dysfunction. The sensitivity of the SACT and SNRT tests is only approximately 50% for each test alone and 65% when combined. The specificity, combined, is approximately 88%, with a low predictive value. Thus, if these test results are abnormal, the likelihood of the patient having sinus node dysfunction is great. However, normal results do not exclude the possibility of sinus node disease. Candidates for invasive EPS to evaluate sinus node function are symptomatic patients in whom sinus node dysfunction is suspected but has not yet been established as a cause of the symptoms. In patients with suspected clinical sinus node dysfunction, EPS is also important in excluding other causes of symptoms (e.g., tachyarrhythmias).

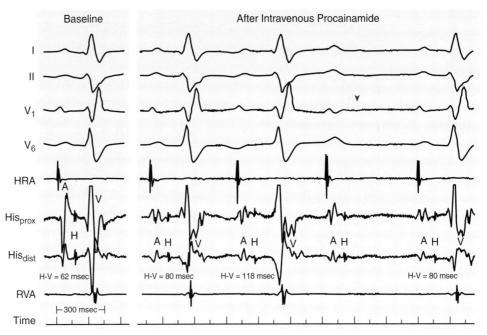

FIGURE 61.15 Testing the His-Purkinje system. A 43-year-old woman with sarcoidosis underwent EPS after a syncopal episode. Surface leads I, II, V₁, and V₆ are shown, with intracardiac recordings from catheters in the high right atrium *(HRA)*, the proximal *(His$_{prox}$)*, and distal *(His$_{dist}$)* electrode pairs of a catheter at the AV junction to record the His potential, and right ventricular apex *(RVA)*. During baseline recording, the H-V interval is only slightly prolonged (62 msec). After infusion of intravenous procainamide, the H-V interval is longer and infra-His Wenckebach block is present. *Arrowhead* denotes the missing QRS complex caused by infra-His block. A, Atrial electrogram; H, His potential; V, ventricular electrogram.

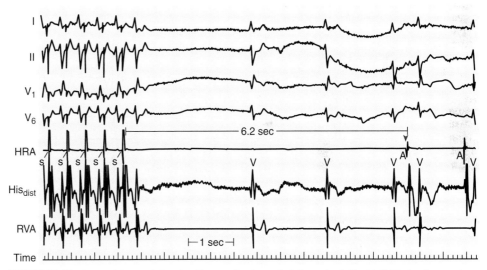

FIGURE 61.16 Abnormal sinus node function. The recording format is similar to that in Fig. 61.15. The last five complexes of a 1-minute burst of atrial pacing *(S)* at a cycle length of 400 msec are shown, after which pacing is stopped. The sinus node does not spontaneously discharge (sinus node recovery time (SNRT)) until 6.2 seconds later *(arrowhead)*. Three junctional escape beats occurred before this time. His$_{dist}$, Distal electrode pair; HRA, high right atrium; RVA, right ventricular apex.

TACHYCARDIA

In patients with tachycardias, an EPS can be used to diagnose the arrhythmia, to determine and deliver therapy, to establish the anatomic sites involved in the tachycardia, to identify patients at high risk for the development of serious arrhythmias, and to gain insight into the mechanisms responsible for the arrhythmia (see Chapters 65 and 67). The study can differentiate aberrant supraventricular conduction from ventricular tachyarrhythmias when standard electrocardiographic criteria are equivocal. An SVT is recognized electrophysiologically by an H-V interval equaling or exceeding that recorded during a normal sinus rhythm (Fig. 61.17). In contrast, during VT, the H-V interval is shorter than normal, or the His deflection cannot be recorded clearly because of superimposition of the larger ventricular electrogram. Only two situations exist in which a consistently short H-V interval occurs: during retrograde activation of the His bundle from activation originating in the ventricle (i.e., PVC, ventricular pacing, or VT) and during AV conduction over an accessory pathway (preexcitation syndrome). Atrial pacing at rates exceeding the tachycardia

rate can demonstrate the ventricular origin of a wide-QRS tachycardia by producing fusion and capture beats and normalization of the H-V interval. The only VT that exhibits an H-V interval equal to or slightly exceeding the normal sinus H-V interval is bundle branch reentry, but His activation will be in the retrograde direction.

An EPS should be considered for the following circumstances: (1) in patients who have symptomatic, recurrent, or drug-resistant supraventricular or ventricular tachyarrhythmias to help select optimal therapy; (2) in patients with tachyarrhythmias occurring too infrequently to permit adequate diagnostic or therapeutic assessment; (3) for differentiation of SVT and aberrant conduction from VT; (4) whenever nonpharmacologic therapy, such as the use of electrical devices, catheter ablation, or surgery, is contemplated; (5) in patients surviving an episode of cardiac arrest occurring more than 48 hours after acute MI or without evidence of an acute Q wave MI in an effort to establish a mechanism; and (6) for assessment of the risk for sustained VT in

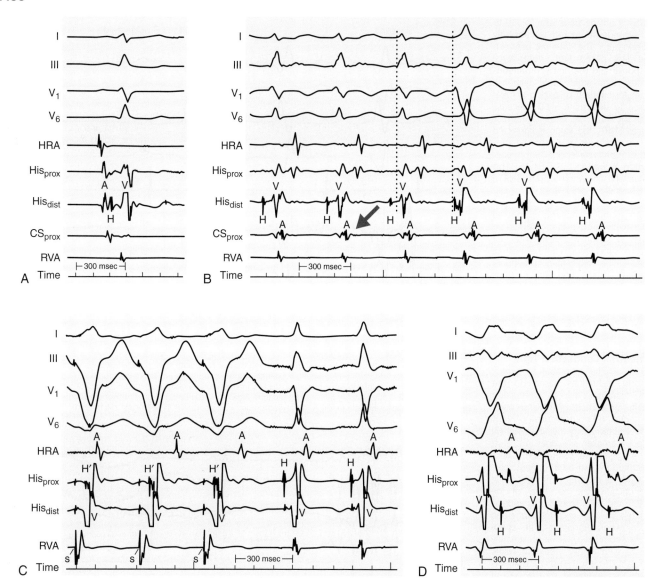

FIGURE 61.17 Bundle of His recordings in a format similar to that in Figs. 61.14 and 61.15. **A,** Baseline sinus rhythm with normal AV conduction. **B,** Orthodromic supraventricular tachycardia (SVT) with retrograde conduction over a left-sided accessory pathway throughout the tracing (earliest atrial activation in CS_{prox}, *arrow*). The first three beats have a narrow QRS complex with a normal H-V interval; the last three QRS complexes represent a fusion of conduction over the AV node–His bundle and a slowly conducting right-sided accessory pathway (left bundle aberrant conduction is a clue). The His potential occurs after onset of the wide QRS complex *(dashed lines)*. **C,** Three paced ventricular beats are shown with a retrograde His potential (H′), followed by initiation of AV node reentrant SVT (atrial depolarization near the end of the QRS complex, as seen in the HRA tracing). **D,** VT with delayed activation of the His potential and complete retrograde AV node block (dissociated atrial complexes). CS_{prox}, Proximal coronary sinus; His_{dist}, distal electrode pair; His_{prox}, proximal electrode pair; *HRA,* high right atrium; *RVA,* right ventricular apex.

patients with a previous MI, ejection fraction of 0.3 to 0.4, no evidence of heart failure, and nonsustained VT on an ECG. In general, EPS is not indicated in patients with LQTS and torsades de pointes.

The process of initiation and termination of SVT or VT with programmed electrical stimulation to establish precise diagnoses and help select sites for catheter ablation is the most common application of EPS in patients with tachycardia. Noninvasive stimulation from an implanted pacemaker or defibrillator can be used to test the effects of drug therapy given in an attempt to decrease the frequency of arrhythmias, as well as to test the ICD's ability to detect and treat VT that has been slowed or otherwise altered by drug effect.

UNEXPLAINED SYNCOPE

The three common arrhythmic causes of syncope are sinus node dysfunction, AV block, and tachyarrhythmias. Of the three, tachyarrhythmias are most reliably evaluated in the electrophysiology laboratory, followed by sinus node abnormalities and His-Purkinje block. Patients with a single episode of syncope and no evidence of structural heart disease, as well as those with a nondiagnostic EPS, have a low incidence of sudden death and an 80% remission rate over the ensuing 10 years. In those with recurrent syncope, the test is falsely negative

in 20%, usually because of failure to find an AV block or sinus node dysfunction. Conversely, in many patients with structural heart disease, several abnormalities may be present that could account for syncope and can be diagnosed at EPS. Deciding which among these abnormalities is responsible for syncope and therefore requires therapy, and of what type, can be difficult (Fig. 61.18). Mortality and the incidence of SCD are determined mainly by the presence of underlying heart disease (see Chapter 70).

Syncopal patients considered for an EPS are those whose spells remain undiagnosed despite general, neurologic, and noninvasive cardiac evaluation, particularly if the patient has structural heart disease. The diagnostic yield is approximately 70% in that group but only 12% in patients without structural heart disease. Therapy for a putative cause found during EPS prevents recurrence of syncope in approximately 80% of patients. Among arrhythmic causes of syncope, intermittent conduction disturbances are the most difficult to diagnose. EPS are poor in establishing this diagnosis despite an array of provocative tests that can be used. When tachyarrhythmias have been thoroughly sought and excluded and clinical suspicion for intermittent heart block is high (e.g., bundle branch block or long H-V interval), empiric permanent pacing may be justified.

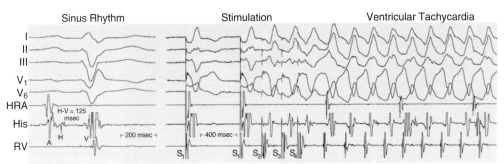

FIGURE 61.18 Surface ECG and intracardiac recordings in a patient with prior myocardial infarction and syncope. The format is similar to previous figures. In **left panel,** a sinus rhythm complex shows a right bundle branch block and left axis deviation, with a very prolonged H-V interval of 125 milliseconds (normal, 35 to 55); thus heart block could have caused syncope. However, in **right panel,** ventricular stimulation with three extrastimuli (S2, S3, S4) induces sustained VT, another potential cause of syncope (note the different time scales in the two panels).

PALPITATIONS

An EPS is indicated in patients with palpitations who have had a pulse documented by medical personnel to be inappropriately rapid or slow without an electrocardiographic recording and in those suspected of having clinically significant arrhythmias without electrocardiographic documentation. In patients with syncope or palpitations, the sensitivity of EPS may be low but can be increased at the expense of specificity. For example, more aggressive pacing techniques (e.g., use of three or four premature stimuli), administration of drugs (e.g., isoproterenol), or left ventricular pacing can increase the likelihood of induction of ventricular arrhythmias by precipitating nonclinical ventricular tachyarrhythmias, such as nonsustained polymorphic VT or VF. Similarly, aggressive techniques during atrial pacing can induce nonspecific episodes of atrial flutter (AF). A diagnostic dilemma arises when the patient's clinical, symptom-producing arrhythmia is one of these nonspecific arrhythmias that can be produced in a normal patient who has no arrhythmia. In most patients, these arrhythmias are regarded as *nonclinical* (i.e., nonspecific responses to intense stimulation). In other patients, such as those with hypertrophic or dilated nonischemic cardiomyopathy, they may be clinically relevant arrhythmias. However, induction of sustained SVT (e.g., AVNRT, AVRT) or monomorphic VT is almost never an artifact of stimulation, no matter how intense. Initiation of these arrhythmias in patients who have not had known spontaneous episodes of these tachycardias is uncommon and provides important information; for example, the induced tachyarrhythmia may be clinically significant and responsible for the patient's symptoms. In addition, inducible SVT episodes can have important implications for patients with ICDs that may deliver inappropriate therapy for such arrhythmias. In general, other abnormalities, such as prolonged sinus pauses after overdrive atrial pacing or His-Purkinje block, are not induced in patients who do not or may not spontaneously experience these abnormalities.

Complications of Electrophysiologic Studies

The risks associated with undergoing only an EPS are small. Myocardial perforation with cardiac tamponade, pseudoaneurysms at arterial access sites, and provocation of nonclinical arrhythmias can occur, each with less than a 1/500 incidence; the addition of therapeutic maneuvers (e.g., ablation) to the procedure increases the incidence of complications. In many centers, diagnostic EPS and even ablation procedures are performed on an outpatient basis (i.e., same-day discharge). With the increasing use of extensive ablation in the left atrium to treat AF, an increase in systemic thromboembolic complications has been observed, as have pericardial effusion and tamponade, valve damage, and phrenic nerve injury (see Chapter 66).[26–29] In addition pericardial approaches (subxyphoid and anterior) to epicardial VT ablation can rarely be associated with pericardial bleeding, RV puncture, and very rarely the need for cardiac surgery.[30]

DIRECT CARDIAC MAPPING: RECORDING POTENTIALS DIRECTLY FROM THE HEART

Cardiac mapping is a method whereby potentials recorded directly from the heart are spatially depicted as a function of time in an integrated manner. The location of recording electrodes (e.g., epicardial, intramural, or endocardial) and the recording mode used (unipolar vs. bipolar), as well as the method of display (isopotential, isochronal, unipolar, or bipolar voltage maps), depend on the problem under consideration. Direct cardiac mapping by catheter electrodes or less frequently at cardiac surgery can be used to identify and localize the areas responsible for rhythm disturbances in patients with supraventricular and ventricular tachyarrhythmias for catheter or surgical ablation, isolation, or resection. Conditions amenable to this approach include accessory pathways associated with WPW syndrome, the slow or fast pathways in AVNRT, AV node–His bundle ablation, sites of origin of focal AT and VTs, isolated pathways essential for the maintenance of reentrant ATs or VTs, and various substrates responsible for episodes of AF (**Videos 61.1 and 61.2**) (see Chapter 66). Mapping can also be used to delineate the anatomic course of the His bundle and phrenic nerve to avoid injury during catheter ablation or open heart surgery for repair of congenital heart disease.

Specialized mapping systems use computers to log not only the activation times and electrogram amplitude (voltage) at various points in the heart, but also the physical locations from which they were obtained. The mapping information acquired in this way can be displayed on a screen to show relative activation times in a color-coded sequence. Using such systems, dozens or even hundreds of sites can be sampled relatively quickly, thereby leading to a clear picture of cardiac activation and potential target sites for ablation (Figs. 61.19 and 61.20). These systems can also record the signal amplitude at each site sampled to allow differentiation of normal from scarred myocardium, which can help in planning ablation strategies (Fig. 61.21). Other mapping systems can acquire data from several thousand points simultaneously by using a multipolar electrode array. This may be useful for hemodynamically unstable tachycardias or those that terminate spontaneously within seconds, which precludes detailed point-to-point mapping.

Pace mapping is a technique in which pacing is performed at putative sites from which arrhythmias arise (a focus) or exit (reentrant circuit). The greater the degree of "match" in QRS complexes (for VT) or intracardiac activation sequences (for ATs), the more likely that the paced site may be an appropriate site for ablation. Software has been developed to calculate the fidelity of match of the paced complexes to the target arrhythmia; ideally, this should approach 100% (see Chapter 64, and Figs. 64.17 and 64.19). Other algorithms have been developed to analyze propagation patterns during complex arrhythmias such as AF by recording signals from multielectrode "basket" catheters in the atrium (Fig. 61.22). This has resolved many cases of an apparently chaotic rhythm to one in which erratic patterns of propagation emanate from a stable rapid source (either rotor or focus). Ablation at these source sites can eliminate AF in some cases. Lastly, although computerized mapping systems acquire activation time and voltage at given sites in the heart, these features have been displayed separately. Current mapping systems have the ability to integrate previous imaging studies (CT, MRI) into the procedure for additional anatomic reference and to derive anatomic information by moving a catheter throughout a cardiac chamber to develop a contour of its inner surface, on which activation or voltage data can be plotted.

GUIDELINES

See the online chapter for Guidelines.

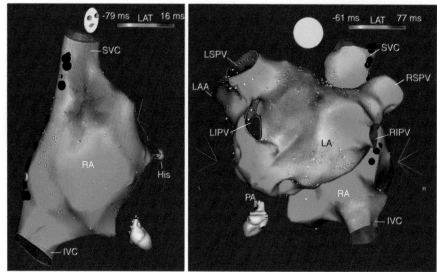

FIGURE 61.19 Electroanatomic maps of focal atrial tachycardias. **Left,** A focal right atrial tachycardia is shown from a right lateral view. A color-coded time scale of activation is shown at the top right; *red* indicates earliest activation and *purple,* latest. This atrial tachycardia arose in the anterolateral right atrium *(RA),* slightly anterior to where the sinus node resides; ablation here eliminated tachycardia while leaving sinus node function unaffected. **Right,** Activation map of a left atrial focal tachycardia with a posterior view of both RA and left atrium *(LA).* The tachycardia arose from the region of the *small red spot* at top center of the LA, with all other areas activated centrifugally. Ablation at this site eliminated the tachycardia. *SVC,* Superior vena cava; *IVC,* inferior vena cava; *His,* His bundle area *(orange dots); LIPV,* left inferior pulmonary vein *(PV); LSPV,* left superior PV; *RIPV,* right inferior PV; *RSPV,* right superior PV.

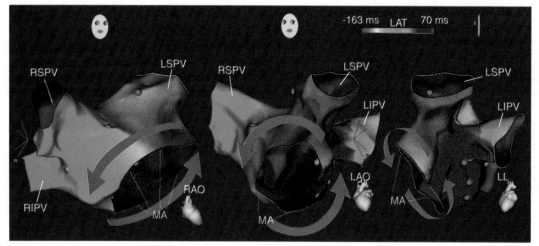

FIGURE 61.20 Electroanatomic activation map of "perimitral" reentrant atrial flutter. Three views of the left atrium are shown: right anterior oblique *(RAO),* left anterior oblique *(LAO),* and left lateral *(LL).* The wave front propagates around the mitral annulus *(MA)* in a "counterclockwise" direction as indicated by *orange arrows;* in this complete circuit, early activation *(red)* abuts late activation *(purple)* at the lateral mitral annulus. The cycle length of the tachycardia was 235 msec, almost completely described by the points shown in the figure (from −163 to +70 msec, a total of 233 msec; time scale at *top*). Abbreviations as in Fig. 61.19.

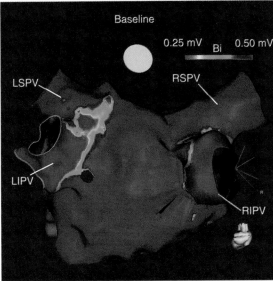

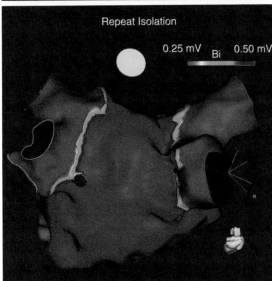

FIGURE 61.21 Electroanatomic left atrial voltage maps during sinus rhythm in a patient with recurrent atrial fibrillation after prior pulmonary vein (PV) isolation. **Top,** Posterior view of the left atrium at baseline, showing low voltage (*red,* tantamount to electrical isolation) in the left *(LIPV)* and right *(RIPV)* inferior PVs, but high residual voltage *(purple)* in the left *(LSPV)* and right *(RSPV)* superior PVs. **Bottom,** After repeat ablation around the PVs, the superior veins now have no residual voltage *(red)*; all four PVs are now isolated. The patient has had no recurrence of symptoms. Voltage scales are shown at *top right* of each panel.

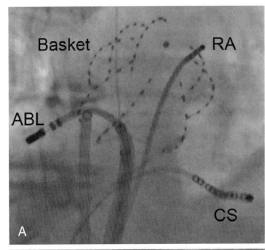

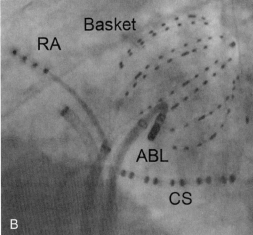

FIGURE 61.22 Basket catheter for mapping atrial fibrillation. Right **(A)** and left **(B)** anterior oblique fluoroscopic views of an eight-spline, eight electrodes per spline (64 total electrodes) "basket" catheter in the left atrium; other catheters are right atrial *(RA)*, coronary sinus *(CS)*, and an ablation catheter *(ABL)* in the right inferior pulmonary vein.

REFERENCES

Signs and Symptoms

1. Giada F, Raviele A. Clinical approach to patients with palpitations. *Card Electrophysiol Clin.* 2018;10:387–396.
2. Goldberger ZD, Petek BJ, Brignole M, et al. ACC/AHA/HRS versus ESC guidelines for the diagnosis and management of syncope: JACC guideline comparison. *J Am Coll Cardiol.* 2019;74:2410–2423.
3. Puppala VK, Akkaya M, Dickinson O, et al. Risk stratification of patients presenting with transient loss of consciousness. *Cardiol Clin.* 2015;33:387–396.
4. Albassam OT, Redelmeier RJ, Shadowitz S, et al. Did this patient have cardiac syncope?: the rational clinical examination systematic review. *J Am Med Assoc.* 2019;321:2448–2457.
5. Novak P. Autonomic disorders. *Am J Med.* 2019;132:420–436.
6. Bryarly M, Phillips LT, Fu Q, et al. Postural orthostatic tachycardia syndrome: JACC focus seminar. *J Am Coll Cardiol.* 2019;73:1207–1228.
7. Wong CX, Brown A, Lau DH, et al. Epidemiology of sudden cardiac death: global and regional perspectives. *Heart Lung Circ.* 2019;28:6–14.
8. Jeserich M, Merkely B, Olschewski M, et al. Patients with exercise-associated ventricular ectopy present evidence of myocarditis. *J Cardiovasc Magn Reson.* 2015;17:100.

Clinical and Laboratory Testing

9. Kim J, Kwon M, Chang J, et al. Meta-analysis of prognostic implications of exercise-induced ventricular premature complexes in the general population. *Am J Cardiol.* 2016;118:725–732.
10. Skinner JR, Winbo A, Abrams D, et al. Channelopathies that lead to sudden cardiac death: clinical and genetic aspects. *Heart Lung Circ.* 2019;28:22–30.
11. Subramanian M, Prabhu MA, Harikrishnan MS, et al. The utility of exercise testing in risk stratification of asymptomatic patients with type 1 brugada pattern. *J Cardiovasc Electrophysiol.* 2017;28:677–683.
12. Marcus GM. Evaluation and management of premature ventricular complexes. *Circulation.* 2020;141:1404–1418.
13. Sana F, Isselbacher EM, Singh JP, et al. Wearable devices for ambulatory cardiac monitoring: JACC state-of-the-art review. *J Am Coll Cardiol.* 2020;75:1582–1592.
14. Perez MV, Mahaffey KW, Hedlin H, et al. Large-scale assessment of a smartwatch to identify atrial fibrillation. *N Engl J Med.* 2019;381:1909–1917.
15. Wasserlauf J, You C, Patel R, et al. Smartwatch performance for the detection and quantification of atrial fibrillation. *Circ Arrhythm Electrophysiol.* 2019;12:e006834.
16. Turakhia MP, Desai M, Hedlin H, et al. Rationale and design of a large-scale, app-based study to identify cardiac arrhythmias using a smartwatch: the apple heart study. *Am Heart J.* 2019;207:66–75.
17. Godin R, Yeung C, Baranchuk A, et al. Screening for atrial fibrillation using a mobile, single-lead electrocardiogram in Canadian primary care clinics. *Can J Cardiol.* 2019;35:840–845.
18. Giancaterino S, Lupercio F, Nishimura M, et al. Current and future use of insertable cardiac monitors. *JACC Clin Electrophysiol.* 2018;4:1383–1396.
19. Melillo P, Izzo R, Orrico A, et al. Automatic prediction of cardiovascular and cerebrovascular events using heart rate variability analysis. *PloS One.* 2015;10:e0118504.
20. Al-Zaiti SS, Pietrasik G, Carey MG, et al. The role of heart rate variability, heart rate turbulence, and deceleration capacity in predicting cause-specific mortality in chronic heart failure. *J Electrocardiol.* 2019;52:70–74.
21. Rudy Y. Noninvasive ECG imaging (ECGI): mapping the arrhythmic substrate of the human heart. *Int J Cardiol.* 2017;237:13–14.

1162

ARRHYTHMIAS, SUDDEN DEATH, AND SYNCOPE   VII

22. Sheldon RS, Grubb 2nd BP, Olshansky B, et al. 2015 heart rhythm society expert consensus statement on the diagnosis and treatment of postural tachycardia syndrome, inappropriate sinus tachycardia, and vasovagal syncope. *Heart Rhythm.* 2015;12:e41–e63.
23. Raj SR, Guzman JC, Harvey P, et al. Canadian cardiovascular society position statement on postural orthostatic tachycardia syndrome (POTS) and related disorders of chronic orthostatic intolerance. *Can J Cardiol.* 2020;36:357–372.
24. George SA, Bivens TB, Howden EJ, et al. The international pots registry: evaluating the efficacy of an exercise training intervention in a community setting. *Heart Rhythm.* 2016;13:943–950.

Invasive EP Testing

25. Boule S, Ouadah A, Langlois C, et al. Predictors of advanced his-purkinje conduction disturbances in patients with unexplained syncope and bundle branch block. *Can J Cardiol.* 2014;30:606–611.
26. Voskoboinik A, Sparks PB, Morton JB, et al. Low rates of major complications for radiofrequency ablation of atrial fibrillation maintained over 14 years: a single centre experience of 2750 consecutive cases. *Heart Lung Circ.* 2018;27:976–983.
27. Peichl P, Wichterle D, Pavlu L, et al. Complications of catheter ablation of ventricular tachycardia: a single-center experience. *Circ Arrhythm Electrophysiol.* 2014;7:684–690.
28. Dukkipati SR, Choudry S, Koruth JS, et al. Catheter ablation of ventricular tachycardia in structurally normal hearts: indications, strategies, and outcomes-part i. *J Am Coll Cardiol.* 2017;70:2909–2923.
29. Shivkumar K. Catheter ablation of ventricular arrhythmias. *N Engl J Med.* 2019;380:1555–1564.
30. Keramati AR, DeMazumder D, Misra S, et al. Anterior pericardial access to facilitate electrophysiology study and catheter ablation of ventricular arrhythmias: a single tertiary center experience. *J Cardiovasc Electrophysiol.* 2017;28:1189–1195.

Guidelines

31. Crawford MH, Bernstein SJ, Deedwania PC, et al. ACC/AHA guidelines for ambulatory electrocardiography. A report of the American College of Cardiology/American Heart Association task force on practice guidelines (committee to revise the guidelines for ambulatory electrocardiography). Developed in collaboration with the North American Society for Pacing and Electrophysiology. *J Am Coll Cardiol.* 1999;34:912–948.
32. Kadish AH, Buxton AE, Kennedy HL, et al. ACC/AHA clinical competence statement on electrocardiography and ambulatory electrocardiography: a report of the ACC/AHA/ACP-ASIM task force on clinical competence (ACC/AHA Committee to develop a clinical competence statement on electrocardiography and ambulatory electrocardiography) endorsed by the International Society for Holter and Noninvasive Electrocardiology. *Circulation.* 2001;104:3169–3178.
33. Zipes DP, Calkins H, Daubert JP, et al. 2015 ACC/AHA/HRS advanced training statement on clinical cardiac electrophysiology (a revision of the ACC/AHA 2006 update of the clinical competence statement on invasive electrophysiology studies, catheter ablation, and cardioversion). *J Am Coll Cardiol.* 2015;66:2767–2802.
34. Zipes DP, DiMarco JP, Gillette PC, et al. Guidelines for clinical intracardiac electrophysiological and catheter ablation procedures. A report of the American College of Cardiology/American Heart Association task force on practice guidelines (committee on clinical intracardiac electrophysiologic and catheter ablation procedures), developed in collaboration with the North American Society of Pacing and Electrophysiology. *J Am Coll Cardiol.* 1995;26:555–573.
35. Shen WK, Sheldon RS, Benditt DG, et al. 2017 ACC/AHA/HRS guideline for the evaluation and management of patients with syncope: a report of the American College of Cardiology/American Heart Association task force on clinical practice guidelines and the Heart Rhythm Society. *J Am Coll Cardiol.* 2017;70:e39–e110.
36. Aliot EM, Stevenson WG, Almendral-Garrote JM, et al. EHRA/HRS expert consensus on catheter ablation of ventricular arrhythmias: developed in a partnership with the European Heart Rhythm Association (EHRA), a registered branch of the European Society of Cardiology (ESC), and the Heart Rhythm Society (HRS); in collaboration with the American College of cardiology (ACC) and the American Heart Association (AHA). *Heart Rhythm.* 2009;6:886–933.

# 62 Mechanisms of Cardiac Arrhythmias

STANLEY NATTEL AND GORDON F. TOMASELLI

FOUNDATIONS OF CARDIAC ELECTROPHYSIOLOGY

The Functions of the Cardiac Electrical System

While this might come as a surprise to some electrophysiologists, the role of the electrical system of the heart is not to generate nice-looking action potentials (APs) and conduction patterns. Its role is to subserve and control the mechanical function of the heart appropriately. The key elements of this function are illustrated in Figure 62.1A. The electrical system must initiate contraction at a rate and rhythm that is appropriate to the body's moment-to-moment needs for blood supply to various organs. Appropriate timing of the contraction of different parts of each cardiac chamber (atria and ventricles) needs to be ensured, as does the relative timing of the atria versus the ventricles. The atria serve a primer-pump role and need to contract before the ventricles with an appropriate delay to allow optimal ventricular filling (which is a key determinant of cardiac contractility via the Frank-Starling principle). Finally, excessively rapid and excessively slow rates must be prevented, as these can have disastrous effects on cardiac function.

As illustrated by the schematic diagram of the relationship between heart rate and cardiac output in Figure 62.1B, cardiac output is more or less a linear function of the heart rate between about 50 and 150 beats/min (consistent with the relationship cardiac output = heart rate × stroke volume, as long as stroke volume is fairly constant). At heart rates below or above this range, cardiac output can fall precipitously. The key properties underlying the functions listed in Figure 62.1A are automaticity, conduction, electromechanical coupling, and refractoriness. The central cellular characteristic that underlies these properties and cardiac electrical function is the cardiac action potential.

The Cardiac Action Potential

The cardiac action potential (AP) is illustrated in Figure 62.2. The AP is a graph of the voltage difference between the inside of a cardiac cell and the outside of the cell (as seen from the inside, for example by a fine-tipped electrode placed inside the cell, eFig. 62.1), as a function of time. Cardiac cells normally have a negative intracellular resting potential, which for most of the heart (working atrial and ventricular muscle, specialized His-Purkinje conducting system) is about −80 to −90 mV. The exceptions are the sinoatrial (SA) and central atrioventricular (AV) node regions, which have resting potentials between about −50 and −65 mV. The cardiac AP is by convention divided into four phases, the AP-upstroke (phase 0), which depolarizes the cell from its negative resting potential to a potential positive to 0 mV; the initial rapid repolarization phase (phase 1); the so-called plateau (phase 2) in which the AP voltage changes relatively slowly; and the final (phase 3) rapid repolarization phase, which brings the cell back to its resting potential (referred to as phase 4).

During phase 0, there is a rapid inrush of positively charged Na^+ ions that mediate depolarization and carry a large inward current (the direction of current is by convention defined by the movement of positive ions), which provides the energy for electrical conduction. Phase 1 sets the voltage level for the subsequent critical phase 2. Phase 2 is the portion of the AP during which Ca^{2+} enters the cell and causes a large secondary release of Ca^{2+} from the sarcoplasmic reticulum (SR), the main cellular Ca^{2+}-storage organelle. The SR Ca^{2+}-release rapidly increases free intracellular $[Ca^{2+}]$, which causes cellular contraction and mediates electromechanical coupling. Finally, phase 3 (carried by a rapid egress of K^+) brings the cell back to its negative resting potential. Because the cell cannot be activated by normal means at voltages positive to −60 mV, from when the cell reaches −60 mV during phase 0 until the time that it repolarizes to −60 mV during phase 3 the cell cannot be fired and is "refractory" to activation. Thus, the timing of phase 3 sets the refractory period (RP). The mechanisms by which the crucial AP properties are set depend critically on the function of ion channels, which is discussed in detail below.

Physiology of Ion Channels

Electrical signaling in the heart involves the passage of ions through ionic channels. The sodium, potassium, calcium, and chloride (Na^+, K^+, Ca^{2+}, and Cl^-) ions are the major charge carriers, and their movement across the cell membrane through channel pores creates a flow of current that generates excitation and signals in cardiac myocytes (Table 62.1).

When a semipermeable membrane allows an ion to cross, and the concentration of the ion is different on the two sides of the membrane, a small number of ions will move across the membrane and create an electrical field. For example, consider the case of K^+ and the cardiac cell membrane. The concentration of K^+ is maintained (by a complex set of pumps and transporters) at about 150 mM inside the cardiac cell and is about 4 mM outside (eTable 62.1). Cardiac cell membranes are highly permeable to K^+ at rest, largely because of a specific ion channel, the inward-rectifier K^+ channel (carrying the current I_{K1}). K^+ tends to leave the cell, down its chemical gradient. However, each K^+ ion that leaves the cell (unaccompanied by a negative ion, because the cell membrane

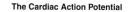

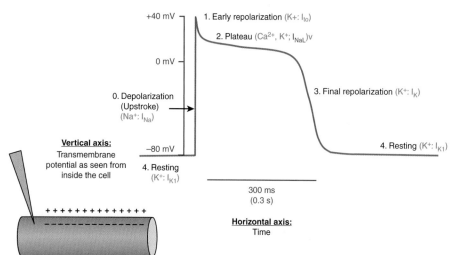

is largely impermeable to them at rest) leaves the interior of the cell with a slightly negative charge relative to the outside. Equilibrium is created when the chemical force tending to push K^+ out of the cell is balanced by an equal and opposite electrical force created by the net intracellular negative charge tending to pull the K^+ back into the cell. The voltage at which these forces balance is called the "equilibrium potential." In the case of K^+, the equilibrium potential is given by the Nernst equation ($E = RT/F \cdot \ln([K^+_o]/[K^+_i])$, where R is the universal gas constant, T = absolute temperature, F = Faraday's constant, and $[K^+_o]$, $[K^+_i]$ = extracellular and intracellular K^+ concentration, respectively. This value, designated "E_K," for K^+ equilibrium potential, is about −95 mV. Thus, at rest the high permeability to K^+ results in a resting potential of about −90 mV (see Fig. 62.2), close to the K^+ equilibrium potential.

As shown in Figure 62.2, membrane voltages during a cardiac AP vary over the range of approximately −90 to +30 mV. Each phase of the cardiac AP is characterized by its dominant ionic permeabilities (shown in green in Fig. 62.2), which determine the direction in which the transmembrane potential moves during that phase. Phase 0 happens when there is a rapid increase in membrane permeability to Na^+, and K^+ permeability falls, making Na^+ the dominant conductance. At the peak of phase 0 (the "overshoot"), the cell moves close to the Na^+ equilibrium potential, which is quite positive because in contrast to K^+, Na^+ is more concentrated outside the cell than inside and the Na^+ chemical force makes it move into the cell, making the interior more positive. Phase 1 is carried by a transient, rapid exit of K^+ from the cell. Because the calculated reversal potential of a cardiac Ca^{2+} channel is +64 mV (assuming $P_K/P_{Ca} = 1/3000$, $Ca_i = 100$ nM, and $Ca_o = 2$ mM), passive Ca^{2+} flux is into the cell. During phase 2, the transmembrane potential is governed by balanced permeabilities to Ca^{2+} and K^+, while during phase 3 a rapid increase in K^+ permeability offsets the decreasing Ca^{2+} conductance and repolarizes the cell. In some cardiac cells (notably His-Purkinje cells) a late Na^+ current (I_{NaL}) contributes inward current during the phase 2 plateau.

The changes in ionic permeabilities during the AP are determined by the opening and closing of ion channels. The opening of ion channels allows selected ions to flow passively down the electrochemical activity gradient at a very high rate (>10^6 ions per second). The high transfer rates and restriction to "downhill" fluxes not stoichiometrically coupled to the hydrolysis of energy-rich phosphates distinguish ion channel mechanisms from other ion-transporting structures (pumps and exchangers), such as the sarcolemmal Na^+,K^+–adenosine triphosphatase (Na^+,K^+–ATPase, which largely maintains the physiological Na^+ and K^+ concentrations inside the cell), sarcoendoplasmic reticulum (SR) Ca^{2+}-ATPase (SERCA, the SR Ca^{2+}-uptake mechanism), or the Na^+/Ca^{2+} exchanger (NCX, which removes from the cell interior the extra Ca^{2+} that has entered during phase 2). Ion channels may be induced to open or close (gated) by extracellular and intracellular receptor-ligands, changes in transmembrane voltage ("voltage-gated"), or mechanical stress (see Table 62.1). The most important ion channels in generating the AP are voltage-gated. Ion currents and gating of single ion channels can best be studied by means of the "patch-clamp" technique, in which a glass microelectrode tip is attached to the cell membrane (to record single channel opening), and in some cases a small patch of membrane is torn away to allow electrical continuity between the inside of the cell and the contents of the microelectrode (to measure transmembrane currents). The microelectrode is filled with an electrically conducting fluid that is connected to an amplifier that measures the potential difference between the microelectrode and a reference electrode, generally located in the extracellular fluid.

The *permeability ratio* is commonly used to define a channel's ionic selectivity, defined as the ratio of the permeability of one ion type to that of the main permeant ion type. Permeability ratios of voltage-gated K^+ and Na^+ channels for other monovalent and divalent (e.g., Ca^{2+})

Functions of the Cardiac Electrical System

• To initiate rhythmic contraction at a rate appropriate to the needs of the body.
• To ensure appropriate timing of contraction for each cardiac chamber.
• To prevent heart rates that are excessively slow or rapid for the body's needs.

A

B

FIGURE 62.1 A, Functions of the cardiac electrical system. **B,** Plot of the cardiac output as a function of heart rate.

The Cardiac Action Potential

FIGURE 62.2 A representative ventricular action potential, with phases numbered 0 to 4. The major ionic currents active during each phase are shown in green type. The late Na current I_{NaL} is augmented in some forms of heritable and acquired heart disease. The drawing at lower left of the figure depicts cardiac muscle impaled with an electrode. The resting membrane potential of the inside of the cell is negative with respect to the outside.

TABLE 62.1 Synopsis of Transsarcolemmal Ionic Currents in Mammalian Cardiac Myocytes

CURRENT	SUBUNIT	FUNCTIONAL PROPERTIES
A. Sodium Currents		
I_{Na}	Nav1.5, Nav1.1, Nav1.3, Nav1.6, Nav1.8 (alpha subunits)	TTX-resistant (Nav1.5, Nav1.8) and TTX-sensitive (Nav1.1, Nav1.3, Nav1.6) voltage-gated currents; Nav1.5 is the major cardiac isoform; neuronal Na^+ channel isoforms contribute to SA node pacemaking and ventricular repolarization
B. Calcium Currents		
$I_{Ca.L}$	Cav1.2 (alpha subunit)	L-type (*l*ong lasting, *l*arge conductance) Ca^{2+} currents through voltage-gated Ca^{2+} (Cav) channels blocked by dihydropyridine antagonists (e.g., nifedipine), phenylalkylamines (e.g., verapamil), benzodiazepines (e.g., diltiazem), and various divalent ions (e.g., Cd^{2+}); activated by dihydropyridine agonists (e.g., Bay K 8644); responsible for phase 0 depolarization and propagation in SA and AV nodal tissue and contributing to the plateau of atrial, His-Purkinje, and ventricular cells; main trigger of Ca^{2+} release from the sarcoplasmic reticulum (Ca^{2+}-induced Ca^{2+} release); the noninactivating or "window" component underlies EADs
$I_{Ca.T}$	Cav3.1/alpha$_{1G}$ (alpha subunit)	T-type (*t*ransient current, *t*iny conductance) Ca^{2+} currents through Cav channels blocked by mibefradil and efonidipine but insensitive to dihydropyridines; may contribute an inward current to the later phase of phase 4 depolarization in pacemaker cells and action potential propagation in AV nodal cells; role in triggering Ca^{2+}-induced Ca^{2+} release uncertain
I_f	HCN4 (alpha subunit)	Hyperpolarization-activated "funny" current carried by Na^+ and K^+ in SA and AV nodal cells and His-Purkinje cells; involved in generating phase 4 depolarization; increases the rate of impulse initiation in pacemaker cells
C. Potassium Currents		
I_{K1}	Kir2.1 (alpha subunit)	K^+ current through inwardly rectifying K^+ (Kir) channels, voltage-dependent block by Ba^{2+} at micromolar concentrations; responsible for maintaining resting the membrane potential in atrial, His-Purkinje, and ventricular cells; channel activity is a function of both membrane potential and $[K^+]_o$; inward rectification appears to result from depolarization-induced internal block by Mg^{2+} and neutral or positively charged amino acid residues in the cytoplasmic channel pore
$I_{K.G}$ ($I_{K.ACh}$, $I_{K.Ade}$)	Kir3.1/Kir3.4 (alpha subunit)	Inwardly rectifying K^+ current activated by muscarinic (M_2) and purinergic (type 1) receptor stimulation via GTP regulatory (G) protein signal transduction; expressed in SA and AV nodal cells and atrial cells, where it causes hyperpolarization and action potential shortening; activation causes negative chronotropic and dromotropic effects
I_{Ks}	KvLQT1, Kv7.1 (alpha subunit)/ minK (beta subunit)	K^+ current carried by a voltage-gated K^+ (Kv) channel (delayed rectifier K^+ channel); plays a major role in determining phase 3 of the action potential
I_{Kr}	hERG, Kv11.1 (alpha subunit)/ MiRP1 (beta subunit)	Rapidly activating component of delayed rectifier K^+ current; I_{Kr} specifically blocked by dofetilide and sotalol in a reverse use–dependent manner; inward rectification of I_{Kr} results from depolarization-induced fast inactivation; plays a major role in determining the APD
I_{Kur}	Kv1.5 (alpha subunit)	K^+ current through a Kv channel with ultrarapid activation but ultraslow inactivation kinetics; expressed in atrial myocytes; determines the APD
$I_{K.Ca}$	SK1-3 (alpha subunit)	K^+ current through small-conductance Ca^{2+}-activated channels; blocked by apamin and expressed in human atrial and ventricular myocytes; determines the APD; upregulated in failing cardiomyocytes
I_{to} (I_{to1}, I_A)	Kv4.3 (alpha subunit)/KChIP2 (beta subunit)	Transient outward K^+ current through voltage-gated (Kv) channels; exhibits fast activation and inactivation and recovery kinetics; blocked by 4-aminopyridine in a reverse use–dependent manner; contributes to the time course of phase 1 repolarization; transmural differences in I_{to} properties contribute to regional differences in early repolarization
D. Chloride Currents		
$I_{Cl.Ca}$ (I_{to2})	?	4-Aminopyridine–resistant transient outward current carried by Cl^- ions; activated by an increase in intracellular calcium level; blocked by stilbene derivatives (SITS, DIDS); contributes to the time course of phase 1 repolarization; may underlie spontaneous transient inward currents under conditions of Ca^{2+} overload; molecular correlate uncertain
$I_{Cl.cAMP}$	?	Time-independent chloride current regulated by the cAMP/adenylate cyclase pathway; slightly depolarizes resting membrane potential and significantly shortens the APD; antagonizes action potential prolongation associated with beta-adrenergic stimulation of $I_{Ca.L}$
$I_{Cl.swell}$ or $I_{Cl.vol}$	?	Outwardly rectifying, swelling-activated Cl^- current; inhibited by 9-anthracene carboxylic acid; activation causes resting membrane depolarization and action potential shortening
$I_{K.ATP}$	Kir6.2 (alpha subunit)/SUR	Time-independent K^+ current through Kir channels activated by a fall in intracellular ATP concentration; inhibited by sulfonylurea drugs, such as glibenclamide; activated by pinacidil, nicorandil, cromakalim; causes shortening of the APD during myocardial ischemia or hypoxia
$I_{Cir.swell}$	?	Inwardly rectifying, swelling-activated cation current; permeable to Na^+ and K^+; inhibited by Gd^{3+}; depolarizes resting membrane potential and prolongs terminal (phase 3) repolarization
E. Electrogenic Pumps and Exchangers		
$I_{Na/Ca}$	NCX1.1	Current carried by Na^+/Ca^{2+} exchanger; causes net Na^+ outward current and Ca^{2+} inward current (reverse mode) or net Na^+ inward and Ca^{2+} outward current (3 Na^+ for 1 Ca^{2+}); direction of Na^+ flux depends on membrane potential and intracellular and extracellular concentrations of Na^+ and Ca^{2+}; Ca^{2+} influx mediated by $I_{Na/Ca}$ can trigger SR Ca^{2+} release; underlies I_{ti} (transient inward current) under conditions of intracellular Ca^{2+} overload

Continued

TABLE 62.1 Synopsis of Transsarcolemmal Ionic Currents in Mammalian Cardiac Myocytes—cont'd

CURRENT	SUBUNIT	FUNCTIONAL PROPERTIES
$I_{Na/K}$	Alpha subunit/beta subunit	Na⁺ outward current generated by Na⁺,K⁺-ATPase (stoichiometry: 3 Na⁺ leave and 2 K⁺ enter); inhibited by digitalis
I_{ti}	?	Transient inward current activated by Ca²⁺ waves; I_{ti} possibly reflects 3 Ca²⁺-dependent components: I_{NCX}, $I_{Cl,Ca}$, and a *TRPM4* (transient receptor potential cation channel, member 4 gene)–mediated current
F. Electroneutral Ion-Exchanging Proteins		
Ca²⁺-ATPase	SERCA2	Extrudes cytosolic calcium
Na/H	Cardiac myocytes express isoform NHE1	Exchanges intracellular H⁺ for extracellular Na⁺; specifically inhibited by the benzoylguanidine derivatives HOE 694 and HOE 642; inhibition causes intracellular acidification
Cl⁻-HCO₃⁻		Exchanges intracellular HCO₃⁻ for external Cl⁻; inhibited by SITS
Na⁺-K⁺-2Cl⁻	Na-K-Cl NKCC1	Cotransporter blocked by amiloride

APD, Action potential duration; *AV,* atrioventricular; *DIDS,* 4,4′-diisothiocyanatostilbene-2,2′-disulfonic acid; *EADs,* early afterdepolarizations; *GTP,* guanosine triphosphate; *SA,* sinoatrial; *SITS,* 4-acetamido-4′-isothiocyanatostilbene-2,2′-disulfonic acid; *TTX,* tetrodotoxin.

cations (cations are positively charged ions, so called because they are attracted to a "cathode" or negative electrode) versus their permeant ion are usually less than 1:10. Voltage-gated Ca²⁺ channels exhibit a more than 1000-fold discrimination against Na⁺ and K⁺ ions (e.g., P_K/P_{Ca} = 1/3000) and all of these are impermeable to anions (negatively charged ions like Cl⁻, attracted to an "anode").

Because ions are charged, net ionic flux through an open channel is determined by both the concentration and the electrical gradients across the membrane (electrodiffusion). As discussed above, the potential at which the passive flux of ions resulting from the chemical driving force is exactly balanced by the electrical driving force is called the *equilibrium* or *reversal potential* of the channel. In a channel that is perfectly selective for one ion species, the reversal potential equals the thermodynamic equilibrium potential of that ion, E_S, which is given by an equation of the form:

$$E_S = (RT/zF) \ln([S_o]/[S_i])$$

where $[S_i]$ and $[S_o]$ are the intracellular and extracellular concentrations of the permeant ion, respectively, z is the valence of the ion, R is the gas constant, F is the Faraday constant, T is the absolute temperature (kelvin), and ln is the natural logarithm (the Nernst equation is this equation applied to K⁺). If the current through an open channel is carried by more than one permeant ion, the reversal potential becomes a weighted mean of all the equilibrium potentials.

ION FLUX THROUGH VOLTAGE-GATED CHANNELS

The activation of voltage-dependent cardiac channels generally increases with membrane depolarization. Channels do not have a sharp voltage threshold for opening. Rather, the dependence of channel activation on membrane potential is a continuous function of voltage and follows a sigmoidal curve (Fig. 62.3A, *blue curve*). The potential at which activation is half-maximal and the steepness of the activation curve govern channel permeability changes in response to changes in membrane potential. Some channels (like Na⁺, L-type Ca²⁺ and transient-outward K⁺ channels) also show inactivation, with a voltage dependence qualitatively similar to activation but generally occurring at more negative voltages (Fig. 62.3A, *gold curve*). Both channel activation and inactivation are time-dependent, with a change in voltage causing a progressive change in gating toward the steady-state values shown in Figure 62.3A. The time constant of a gating process indicates the time required to get to about 63% of steady state, and ranges from about 1 msec (msec, 1/1000 second) for Na⁺ channel activation to about 5 to 10 msec for L-type Ca²⁺ channels to 100 msec for delayed-rectifier K⁺ channels. Inactivation is generally about an order of magnitude slower than activation.

Activation occurs rapidly on membrane depolarization, causing channel opening. Inactivation proceeds with a slight delay because of its slower kinetics, allowing for a substantial number of channels to open and carry current before inactivation occurs. If membrane depolarization persists, the channel remains inactivated and cannot reopen. Inactivation curves of the various cardiac voltage-gated ion channels differ in their voltage dependence. For example, sustained membrane depolarization to −50 mV (as may occur in acutely ischemic myocardium) causes almost complete inactivation of the Na⁺ channel, whereas the L-type Ca²⁺ channel (see Voltage-Gated Ca²⁺ Channels) exhibits little inactivation at this membrane potential. Activation and inactivation

curves can overlap over a voltage range with finite steady-state conductance (hatched area in Fig. 62.3A), in which case a steady-state non-inactivating inward current can flow, potentially causing spontaneous depolarization. L-type Ca²⁺ channel and Na⁺ channel window currents have been implicated in the genesis of triggered activity arising from early afterdepolarizations (EADs).[1]

Channels recover from inactivation and then enter the closed state, from which they can be reactivated and open again (Fig. 62.3B). Rates of recovery from inactivation vary among the different types of voltage-dependent channels and usually follow monoexponential or multiexponential time courses, with time constants ranging from a few milliseconds for Na⁺ current to several seconds for some subtypes of K⁺ currents.

PRINCIPLES OF IONIC CURRENT MODULATION

The whole-cell current amplitude I is the product of the number of functional channels in the membrane available for opening (N), the probability that a channel will open (P_o), and the single-channel current amplitude (i) (Fig. 62.3C), or $I = N \cdot P_o \cdot i$. Changes in total current therefore result from alterations in N, P_o, i, or any combination of these factors. Changes in the number of available channels in the cell membrane result from up- or down-regulation of the expression of ion channel–encoding genes. The magnitude of the single-channel current amplitude depends in part on the ionic concentration gradient across the membrane. Changes in channel activation (i.e., P_o) can result from phosphorylation or dephosphorylation of the channel protein, or from gene mutations that alter channel gating or conductivity properties.

Phases of the Cardiac Action Potential

As discussed above, the cardiac AP consists of five phases: *phase 0,* upstroke or rapid depolarization; *phase 1,* early rapid repolarization; *phase 2,* plateau; *phase 3,* final rapid repolarization; and *phase 4,* resting membrane potential and diastolic depolarization (see Fig. 62.2 and eFig. 62.1). These phases are the result of passive ion fluxes moving down their electrochemical gradients established by active ion pumps and exchange mechanisms. Each ion moves primarily through its own ion-specific channel. Different regions in the heart have different AP morphologies. However, two specific regions have quite distinct APs from the rest of the heart: the SA and AV nodes. Unlike the APs shown in Figure 62.2, these areas have APs with much less negative resting potentials and much slower phase-0 upstrokes (Fig. 62.4), often referred to as "slow-response APs." The following discussion explains the detailed electrogenesis of each of these phases and how it can be altered.

RESTING MEMBRANE POTENTIAL

The intracellular potential during electrical quiescence in diastole is −50 to −95 mV, depending on the type of cell (Table 62.2 and Figure 62.4).

Outward potassium current through open, inwardly rectifying K⁺ channels (I_{K1}) under normal conditions determines the resting membrane potential in atrial and ventricular myocytes, as well as in the specialized conducting cells of the His-Purkinje system. Slow-response tissues have a less negative resting potential because they have much

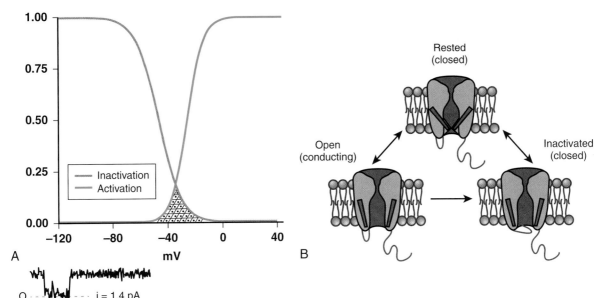

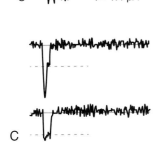

O ---- i = 1.4 pA

C

FIGURE 62.3 A, Curves that describe the voltage dependence of channel opening or the transition from the rested, closed to the open, conducting state (activation curve, *teal*) and channel availability (inactivation, *gold*). The inactivation or availability curve describes the voltage dependence of the occupancy of the inactivated state, and channels may transition to the inactivated state by way of the open or the rested, closed state. Generally, an inactivated channel must first return to the closed state to be available to open again. The crosshatched area indicates voltages at which there is steady-state opening of the channels because there is finite activation and inactivation is incomplete. In this overlap region, steady-state "window current" flows and can cause excessive action-potential depolarization and/or arrhythmogenic afterdepolarizations. **B,** Principal conformations of voltage-dependent channels. The position of the activation gate changes with the transition from closed to open, and the transition to the inactivated state is determined by the position of the inactivation gate. **C,** Single-channel current recordings showing the opening of sodium (Na) channels in response to a step change in voltage. The *middle tracing* reflects the activity of two channels, each with a single-channel amplitude of 1.4 pA.

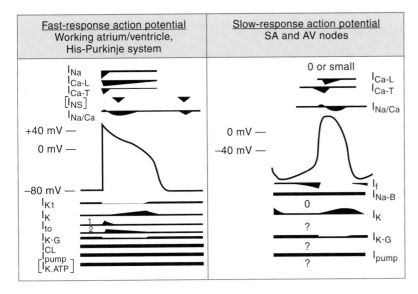

FIGURE 62.4 Currents and channels involved in generating resting membrane and action potentials. The time course of a stylized action potential of atrial and ventricular cells is shown on the **left** and that of sinoatrial (SA) node cells is on the **right.** Above and below are the various channels and pumps that contribute the currents underlying the electrical events. (See Table 62.1 for identification of the symbols and description of the channels or currents.) Where possible, the approximate time courses of the currents associated with the channels or pumps are shown symbolically, without trying to represent their magnitudes relative to each other. I_K incorporates at least two currents, I_{Kr} and I_{Ks}. There appears to be an ultrarapid component as well, designated I_{Kur}. The *heavy bars* for I_{CL}, I_{pump}, and $I_{K.ATP}$ indicate only the presence of these channels or pump, without implying magnitude of currents, because the magnitude would vary with physiologic and pathophysiologic conditions. The channels identified by *brackets* (I_{NS} and $I_{K.ATP}$) are active only under pathologic conditions. I_{NS} may represent a swelling-activated cation current. For the SA node cells, I_{NS} and I_{K1} are small or absent. *Question marks* indicate that experimental evidence is not yet available to determine the presence of these channels in SA node cell membranes. Although it is likely that other ionic current mechanisms exist, they are not shown here because their roles in electrogenesis are not sufficiently well defined.

lower I_{K1} channel-density in their membranes than other parts of the heart.

The intracellular ion concentrations that govern the AP are set by a group of ion pumps and exchangers that transport ions more slowly than open ion channels, but are active continuously throughout the cardiac cycle. The most important pump in establishing the transmembrane ionic distribution gradient is the Na-K pump, which pumps Na+ out of the cell and simultaneously pumps K+ into the cell against their respective chemical gradients, keeping the intracellular K+ concentration high and the intracellular Na+ concentration low. The Na-K pump is

"electrogenic": each cycle of the pump carries 3 Na+ ions out for every 2 K+ ions pumped in, leaving a net negative intracellular charge. The rate of Na+-K+ pumping must increase as the heart rate increases to maintain the same ionic gradients, because the cell gains a small amount of Na+ and loses a small amount of K+ with each depolarization. Rapid cardiac activation makes the resting potential more negative because of the electrogenic properties of the activated Na-K pump. The energy for the Na-K pump is generated by its catalytic activity that breaks high-energy phosphate bonds in adenosine triphosphate (ATP), so it is often called the "Na+,K+-ATPase." Excess inhibition of Na+,K+-ATPase function (e.g.,

TABLE 62.2 Properties of Transmembrane Potentials in Heart Cells

PROPERTY	SA NODAL CELL	ATRIAL MYOCYTE	AV NODAL CELL	HIS PURKINJE CELL	VENTRICULAR MYOCYTE
Resting potential (mV)	−50 to −60	−80 to −90	−60 to −70	−90 to −95	−80 to −90
Action Potential Features					
Amplitude (mV)	60–70	110–120	70–80	120	110–120
Overshoot (mV)	0–10	30	5–15	30	30
Duration (msec)	100–300	100–300	100–300	300–500	200–300
V̇max (V/sec)	1–10	100–200	5–15	500–700	100–200
Propagation velocity (m/sec)	<0.05	0.3–0.4	0.1	2–3	0.3–0.4
Fiber diameter (μm)	5–10	10–15	1–10	100	10–15

AV, Atrioventricular; *SA*, sinoatrial; *V̇max*, maximal rise of membrane potential.
Modified from Sperelakis N. Origin of the cardiac resting potential. In: Berne RM et al., eds. *Handbook of Physiology: The Cardiovascular System*. Bethesda, MD: American Physiological Society; 1979:190.

by digitalis glycoside toxicity) can cause substantial cardiac-cell depolarization and seriously impair cardiac electrical function, leading to conduction block and arrhythmias.

The resting potential can be made more negative by interventions that increase the K^+ permeability; for example, both adenosine and acetylcholine (ACh) activate a G-protein coupled K^+ channel ($I_{K.G}$, Table 62.1) and increase resting K^+ conductance. In fast-response tissues, the normal resting K^+ conductance is high and $I_{K.G}$ activation produces small changes in resting potential. However, in SA and AV nodes, with very limited baseline K^+ conductance, $I_{K.G}$ activation substantially increases resting K^+ conductance and can have a major hyperpolarizing effect that slows automaticity and conduction.

PHASE 0: UPSTROKE (RAPID DEPOLARIZATION)

Cardiac activation normally proceeds from the SA node pacemaker and is conducted throughout the heart. Electrical changes in the AP follow a relatively fixed time and voltage relationship that differs according to specific cell types (Fig. 62.5). The AP can also be initiated by an electrical stimulus, as is induced by an artificial pacemaker. Normally, the AP morphology is independent of the size of the depolarizing stimulus, provided that the pulse exceeds a threshold value. Small, subthreshold depolarizing stimuli depolarize the membrane in proportion to the strength of the stimulus, but fail to elicit an AP. When the stimulus is sufficiently intense to depolarize membrane potential to a threshold value in the range of about −70 to −65 mV (for normal fast-response tissues), an "all-or-none" response results.

The upstroke of the cardiac AP in fast-response tissues results from a rapid increase in membrane conductance for Na^+. Rapid depolarization opens Na^+ channels before they have a chance to close via inactivation. When the depolarization is sufficiently rapid, Na^+ channel opening allows Na^+ ions to enter the cell, depolarizing it rapidly and causing more channels to open, producing further depolarization in a self-sustaining process (the "all-or-none" phase 0 depolarization). This process stops when Na^+ channels inactivate to a significant degree (within 1 to 2 msec), allowing the membrane to reach a voltage of about +40 mV, near the Na^+ equilibrium potential (+60 mV).

The rate at which depolarization occurs during phase 0, that is, the maximum rate of change in voltage over time, is indicated by the expression dV/dt_{max} or $\dot{V}max$ (see Table 62.2). $\dot{V}max$ (dV/dt_{max}) is an indicator of the rate and magnitude of phase 0 Na^+ entry into the cell, which is a determinant of tissue conduction velocity (CV). Depolarization must be rapid in order to initiate a fast-response AP. A slow depolarization allows Na^+ channels to inactivate, reducing the maximal conductance they can achieve when activated from that depolarized potential. Thus, clinical processes like hyperkalemia, which slowly depolarize the cell (by reducing the transmembrane K^+ concentration gradient and consequently the K^+ equilibrium potential) result in reduced phase 0 Na^+ current and can produce important conduction slowing.

In cardiac Purkinje fibers, the SA node region, and to a lesser extent, ventricular muscle, different populations of Na^+ channels exist. By far the most common is the tetrodotoxin (TTX)-resistant Nav1.5 isoform (encoded by the *SCN5A* gene). The Nav1.8 TTX-resistant isoform (*SCN10a*) contributes little to peak I_{Na}, but plays an important role in the late Na^+ current (I_{NaL}) that contributes importantly to the prolongation of AP-duration (APD) with cardiac disease or ion-channel mutations.

TTX-sensitive Na^+ channels may also participate in I_{NaL}, although the precise contribution remains to be better defined.[2]

Normal fast-response APs have phase 0 dV/dt_{max} values of the order of 200 to 1000 mV/msec. Slow-response APs in the SA and AV nodes have much slower upstrokes (of the order of 4 to 20 mV/msec) because of the slower activation of Ca^{2+} channels compared to Na^+ channels (see Figs. 62.4 and 62.5). The slow phase 0 upstroke is associated with much slower conduction in slow versus fast response tissues. Slow conduction through the AV node is responsible for creating a delay between atrial and ventricular activation, helping to ensure optimal efficiency of the atrial "primer pump" function to optimize ventricular filling just before ventricular contraction. Under certain circumstances, diseased working myocardial cells can have slow-response type cells (see Fig. 62.5F).

The threshold for activation of $I_{Ca.L}$ is about −30 to −40 mV. In fibers of the fast-response type, $I_{Ca.L}$ is normally activated during phase 0 caused by the fast I_{Na}. Current flows through both fast and slow channels during the latter part of the AP upstroke. However, $I_{Ca.L}$ is much smaller than the peak I_{Na} and therefore contributes little to the AP until the fast I_{Na} is inactivated after completion of phase 0. Thus, $I_{Ca.L}$ affects mainly the plateau of APs recorded in atrial and ventricular muscle and His-Purkinje fibers. $I_{Ca.L}$ may play a prominent role in depolarized fast-response cells in which I_{Na} has been inactivated, if conditions are appropriate for slow-channel activation. Although T-type Cav channels have not been directly recorded in human myocardium, the corresponding genes have been cloned from human hearts, and experimental evidence in animals has suggested that these channels might play an important role in determining SA node automaticity and AV nodal conduction.[3]

PHASE 1: EARLY RAPID REPOLARIZATION

Following phase 0, the membrane repolarizes rapidly and transiently to almost 0 mV (early notch), partly because of inactivation of I_{Na} and concomitant activation of several outward currents. The most important of these in the human heart is the 4-aminopyridine–sensitive transient outward K^+ current, commonly termed I_{to} (or I_{to1}), which is activated rapidly by depolarization and then rapidly inactivates. Both the density and the recovery of I_{to} from inactivation exhibit transmural gradients in the left and right ventricular (RV) free wall, with the density decreasing and reactivation becoming progressively prolonged from epicardium to endocardium. Transmural differences in the expression of KChIP2, the auxiliary subunit that forms the I_{to} channel in working atrial and ventricular muscle along with Kv4.3 pore-forming alpha subunits, contributes to the transmural gradient in I_{to} properties and densities.[4] This gradient gives rise to regional differences in AP shape, with increasingly slower phase 1 restitution kinetics and diminution of the notch along the transmural axis (**eFig. 62.2**). These regional differences create transmural voltage gradients, thereby increasing dispersion of repolarization and allowing for arrhythmogenic transmural current flow, contributing to arrhythmogenesis in Brugada syndrome (see Chapters 63 and 67). Downregulation of I_{to} is at least partially responsible for slowing of phase 1 repolarization in failing human cardiomyocytes.

Studies have demonstrated that these changes in the phase 1 notch of the cardiac AP cause a reduction in the kinetics and peak amplitude of the AP–evoked intracellular Ca^{2+} transient because of failed recruitment and synchronization of SR Ca^{2+} release through $I_{Ca.L}$ (**eFig. 62.3**). Thus, modulation of I_{to} appears to play a physiologic role in controlling cardiac excitation-contraction coupling. It remains to be determined whether transmural differences in phase 1 repolarization translate into similar differences in regional contractility that are important for overall contractile function.

The 4-aminopyridine–resistant, Ca^{2+}-activated chloride current $I_{Cl.Ca}$ (or I_{to2}) might also contribute to outward current during phase 1 repolarization.[1] This current is activated by the AP–evoked intracellular Ca^{2+} transient. Other chloride currents may also play a role in early repolarization, such as the cyclic adenosine monophosphate (cAMP)- or swelling-activated chloride conductances $I_{Cl.cAMP}$ and $I_{Cl.swell}$.

PHASE 2: PLATEAU

During the plateau phase, which may last several hundred milliseconds, membrane conductance of all ions falls to rather low values. Accordingly, smaller changes in current are needed to produce changes in transmembrane potential than near the resting potential. This phenomenon makes the plateau a vulnerable time for the generation of arrhythmogenic afterdepolarizations (see discussion of EADs below). The plateau is maintained by competition between the outward current carried by K^+ and the inward current carried by Ca^{2+} moving through $I_{Ca,L}$ and Na^+ being exchanged for internal Ca^{2+} by the NCX. After depolarization, I_{K1} conductance falls to low levels during the plateau as a result of inward rectification, despite the large electrochemical driving force on K^+ ions.

The plateau is a critical time for Ca^{2+} entry through activated L-type Ca^{2+} channels. The entry of Ca^{2+}, principally during the plateau, triggers a much larger secondary release of Ca^{2+} from SR stores and is an essential component of cardiac excitation-contraction coupling (see Chapter 46).

Several potassium currents are open during the plateau phase, including the rapid (I_{Kr}) and slow (I_{Ks}) components of the delayed rectifier current I_K (see Voltage-Gated K^+ Channels). "Delayed rectification" refers to the time-dependent opening of the I_K channel. In addition, I_{Kr} shows a phenomenon called "inward rectification," which involves a decrease in channel opening at more positive potentials. Inward rectification is a prominent feature of the background I_{K1} channel, whose conductance drops dramatically at positive potentials to prevent wasteful excess loss of K^+ and allow efficient phase 0 depolarization. I_{Kr} also shows prominent inward rectification, due to extremely rapid inactivation that occurs during depolarization. This fast inactivation mechanism is sensitive to changes in extracellular K^+, with the degree of inactivation being accentuated at low extracellular K^+ concentrations, explaining how hypokalemia can prolong APD (by decreasing I_{Kr}).

I_{Ks} also contributes to plateau duration. Mutations in the KvLQT1 subunit, which in combination with the I_{Ks} ancillary (beta) subunit (KCNE1, encoding a protein also called minK) carries I_{Ks}, are associated with abnormally prolonged ventricular repolarization (long-QT syndrome [LQTS] type 1; see Chapters 63 and 67). Although I_{Ks} activates slowly compared to the APD, it is only slowly inactivated. Therefore, increases in heart rate cause I_{Ks} activation to accumulate, contributing to APD abbreviation at higher heart rates.

In conditions of reduced intracellular ATP concentration (e.g., hypoxia, acute ischemia), K^+ efflux through activated I_{KATP} channels reduces APD and increases K^+ concentration in the extracellular space, which in turn decreases the K driving force, I_{K1} amplitude, and cell resting potential. Other ionic mechanisms that control plateau duration include I_{CaL} inactivation and steady-state (window-current) components of both I_{Na} and $I_{Ca.L}$.

PHASE 3: FINAL RAPID REPOLARIZATION

Repolarization of the terminal portion of the AP proceeds rapidly largely because of changes in two currents: time-dependent inactivation of I_{CaL}, with a decrease in the inward movement of positive charges, and activation of repolarizing K^+ currents, particularly I_{Kr} and I_{Ks}, which increase the movement of positive charges out of the cell. As the cell repolarizes, the transmembrane potential moves to voltages at which the inward rectification of I_{K1} is removed, so I_{K1} contributes substantially to the terminal part of phase 4. A small-conductance Ca^{2+}-activated K^+ current, I_{KCa}, expressed in human atrial myocytes, may also contribute to phase 3 repolarization.[5]

Loss-of-function mutations in the human ether-a-go-go–related or hERG gene (KCNH2), which encodes the pore-forming (α) subunit of I_{Kr}, delay phase 3 repolarization and predispose to the development arrhythmias associated with LQTS. A wide range of non-cardiac drugs, such as erythromycin, many antipsychotics, antimalarial/anti-inflammatory drugs like hydroxychloroquine, and antifungal drugs such as ketoconazole, inhibit I_{Kr} and can cause acquired forms of LQTS (see Chapters 63 and 67). A decrease in I_{K1} function, as occurs in heart failure or mutations in the associated KCNJ2 gene, prolong APD and reduce resting membrane potential.

PHASE 4: DIASTOLIC DEPOLARIZATION

Normally, the membrane potential of atrial and ventricular muscle cells remains steady throughout diastole. In specialized conducting cells of the His-Purkinje system and in the SA and AV nodes, the resting membrane potential does not remain constant in diastole but gradually depolarizes (see Figs. 62.4 and 62.5). The property possessed by spontaneously automatic cells is called spontaneous phase 4 diastolic depolarization. When spontaneous phase 4 depolarization reaches a

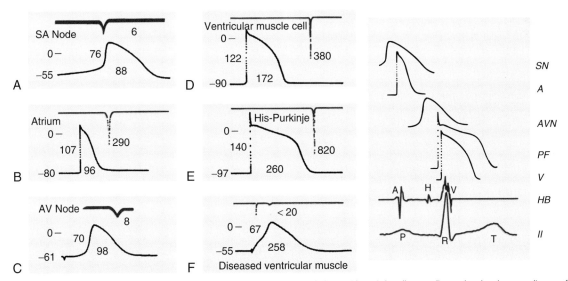

FIGURE 62.5 Action potentials recorded from different tissues in the heart **(left)** remounted along with a His bundle recording and scalar electrocardiogram from a patient **(right)** to illustrate the timing during a single cardiac cycle. **A** to **F,** Top tracing is dV/dt of phase 0, and the second tracing is the action potential. For each panel, the numbers (from *left to right*) indicate maximum diastolic potential (mV), action potential amplitude (mV), action potential duration at 90% of repolarization (milliseconds), and rate of depolarization of phase 0 (V/sec). Zero potential is indicated by the *short horizontal line* next to the zero on the upper left of each action potential. **A,** Rabbit sinoatrial node. **B,** Canine atrial muscle. **C,** Rabbit AV node. **D,** Canine ventricular muscle. **E,** Canine Purkinje fiber. **F,** Diseased human ventricle. Note that the action potentials recorded in **A, C,** and **F** have reduced resting membrane potentials and amplitudes relative to the other action potentials. In the right panel, *A,* Atrial muscle potential; *AVN,* atrioventricular nodal potential; *HB,* His bundle recording; *II,* lead II; *PF,* Purkinje fiber potential; *SN,* sinus nodal potential; *V,* ventricular muscle potential. Horizontal calibration on the left: 50 milliseconds for **A** and **C,** 100 milliseconds for **B, D, E,** and **F;** 200 milliseconds on the right. Vertical calibration on the left: 50 mV; horizontal calibration on the right: 200 milliseconds. (Modified from Gilmour RF Jr, Zipes DP. Basic electrophysiology of the slow inward current. In: Antman E, Stone PH, eds. *Calcium blocking agents in the treatment of cardiovascular disorders.* Mount Kisco, NY: Futura; 1983:1–37.)

voltage at which a sufficient number of phase 0 inward current channels (Na+ channels in His-Purkinje system, Ca2+ channels in SA and AV nodes) open, spontaneous cell-firing occurs. The voltage at which an AP is generated is called the "threshold potential." The time from the maximum (most negative) diastolic potential (MDP) at the end of phase 3 to the arrival at threshold potential determines the "intrinsic" spontaneous cycle length of the tissue. The intrinsic rate of SA node automaticity normally exceeds the intrinsic rate of other potentially automatic pacemaker sites; thus the SA mode maintains dominance of the cardiac rhythm. The SA node is heavily innervated by the parasympathetic and sympathetic nervous systems. Parasympathetic activation slows SA node automaticity and sympathetic activation accelerates it. This dual control allows for very fine regulation of SA node rate in relation to the body's needs, with heart rate being the most important single determinant of cardiac output (see Fig. 62.1). Enhanced or abnormal automaticity at other sites (as well as other arrhythmia mechanisms, see below) can cause them to discharge at rates faster than the SA node and usurp control of cardiac rhythm for one or many cycles (see Chapter 65). The intrinsic pacemaking ability of other tissues produces important "escape" rhythms should the sinus node fail or should conduction between the atria and ventricles be blocked because of disease in the AV node or specialized His-Purkinje ventricular conducting system.

Normal Automaticity

Two models of contributors to SA node pacemaking have been proposed.[3] In the "membrane clock" model, HCN channels (see Cardiac Pacemaker Channels and Table 62.1) are activated by repolarization from the plateau to normal diastolic membrane potentials. HCN channels carry a current called I_f ("funny current"), often called the "pacemaker current," with the unusual feature of time-dependent activation at negative potentials (unlike all other voltage-dependent cardiac channels). During the diastolic interval between consecutive APs, the probability of HCN channels being open increases. Open HCN channels conduct both Na+ and K+, but at these negative membrane potentials at which the driving force for Na+ is high and for K+ is low, Na+ entry predominates. The inward Na+ current through HCN channels depolarizes pacemaker cells to threshold, repetitively triggering APs to generate a periodically firing pacemaker.[1,3]

In the "Ca2+ clock" model, periodic increases in [Ca2+]i serve as an internal generator of rhythmic signals that are transformed into changes in membrane voltage via modulation of calcium-sensitive ion channels and transporters in the cell membrane. This concept is illustrated in Figure 62.6, in which simultaneous [Ca2+]i and voltage measurements in isolated SA node myocytes are used as an example. Local submembrane increases in [Ca2+]i (denoted by the white *arrows* in Fig. 62.6B) occurring during the latter part of the spontaneous diastolic depolarization (transmembrane APs are shown in blue) precede the rapid upstroke of the AP. SR Ca2+-release activates the Na+/Ca2+ exchange inward (i.e., depolarizing) current (I_{NCX}), which then results in membrane depolarization, which activates membrane L-type Ca2+ channels to initiate the AP phase-0 upstroke. Thus, the NCX plays an essential role in converting the driver intracellular Ca2+ signals into membrane (i.e., voltage) signals. Once an AP has been initiated, two highly interacting, concurrent series of events proceed (Fig. 62.6C). In a surface membrane delimited series of events, depolarization-induced activation of I_K leads to membrane repolarization, which is followed by slow diastolic depolarization via a number of inward currents, particularly I_f and I_{CaT} (see Table 62.1). In a second, parallel cycle of events, AP–induced SR Ca2+ release is followed by Ca2+ reuptake into the SR, giving rise to spontaneous Ca2+-release and subsequent inward I_{NCX}.

In reality, the calcium and membrane clock systems function together, to ensure that the important SA node pacemaking function is protected by system redundancy, somewhat like dual computers producing a fail-safe system controlling key aircraft guidance functions.

The rate of SA node discharge is regulated by autonomic and other influences. Alterations in the slope of diastolic depolarization, MDP, or threshold potential can alter the discharge rate. For example, if the slope of diastolic depolarization steepens, the discharge rate increases (e.g., Fig. 62.6A, dashed line). The molecular mechanisms that mediate acceleration of the SA node discharge rate in response to adrenergic stimulation are complex. Adrenergic stimulation increases inward HCN current, mainly by virtue of cyclic AMP shifting the HCN channel activation curve to more depolarized

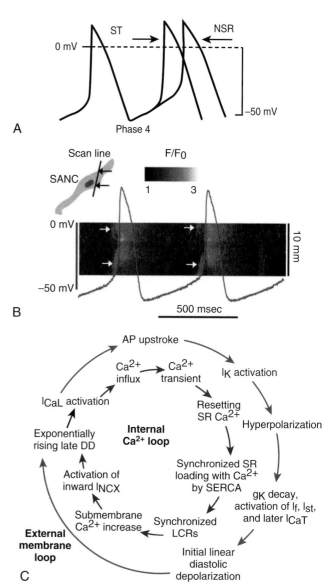

FIGURE 62.6 A, Sympathetic stimulation of heart rate in the sinoatrial node (SAN). Simulated SAN action potentials during baseline *(NSR)* and sympathetic stimulation *(ST [sinus tachycardia]).* Sympathetic stimulation increases the rate of diastolic depolarization *(not shown)* and shifts the maximum diastolic potential to a less negative value, thereby accelerating action potential firing. **B** and **C,** Spontaneous sarcoplasmic reticulum (SR) Ca2+-release events trigger membrane excitation in SAN myocytes. **B,** Confocal line scan images of Ca2+ signals measured in spontaneously beating rabbit sinoatrial node cells (SANC) with simultaneous recording *(blue lines)* of transmembrane action potentials; the orientation of the scan line is shown in the inset. *Arrows* in the confocal image show the local Ca2+ release in the submembrane space during late diastolic depolarization that precedes the rapid upstroke of the action potential. **C,** Model of sinoatrial node cell pacemaking, as suggested by Maltsev and coworkers. I_{NCX}, Na+/Ca2+ exchange current; *DD,* diastolic depolarization; *LCR,* local Ca2+ release; *SERCA,* sarcoendoplasmic reticulum Ca2+-ATPase. (**B** and **C** from Maltsev VA, Vinogradovad TM, Lakatta EG. The emergence of a general theory of the initiation and strength of the heartbeat. *J Pharmacol Sci.* 2006;100:338.)

potentials.[1] In addition, cAMP-activation of protein kinase A (PKA) increases phosphorylation of key Ca2+-handling proteins like the cardiac ryanodine-receptor (RyR2), phospholamban (see Chapter 46), SERCA, and voltage-gated Ca2+ channels. Phosphorylation of these proteins increases the rate of spontaneous SR Ca2+ release and SR Ca2+ uptake via synergistic activation of these proteins. ACh shifts the MDP to more negative values, moving it further away from threshold and slowing the spontaneous firing rate.

PASSIVE MEMBRANE ELECTRICAL PROPERTIES
In addition to the active electrical properties that govern APs, cardiac electrical function is also determined by passive electrical properties. When a cell membrane depolarizes, the Na+ that rushes in changes the

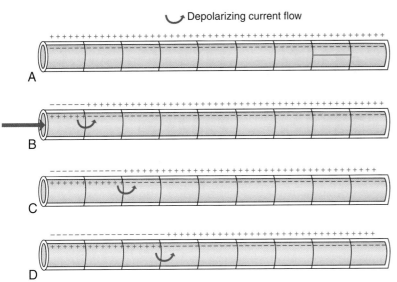

↪ Depolarizing current flow

FIGURE 62.7 Schematic of an electrical impulse traversing a cardiac fiber bundle. The bundle is comprised of electrically coupled cardiomyocytes simulating a continuous cable. **A**, A resting bundle, with a negative *(inside)* transmembrane potential. **B**, Activation of the bundle from the left; the first cardiomyocyte in the bundle is depolarized, initiating an action potential and cell-to-cell current flow *(curved arrow)* and causing progressive depolarization of cells in the fiber (**C** and **D**).

local transmembrane potential quite strongly. Figure 62.7 illustrates how an electrical impulse travels along a cardiac fiber bundle composed of multiple cardiac cells (cardiomyocytes). Cardiomyocytes are electrically coupled to each other by low-resistance "gap junctions" (see below), making a bundle of cardiac fibers behave like a continuous cable. Panel A represents the resting bundle, with cardiomyocytes having a transmembrane potential of −80 mV due to more negative charges on the internal side of the membrane. Panel B illustrates what happens when an impulse arrives from an activated cell to the left, depolarizing the first cardiomyocyte in the bundle. The cell membrane, depolarized to threshold, undergoes phase 0 and changes rapidly from being relatively negative internally (−80 mV transmembrane potential) to becoming positive (+40 mV). A flow of electrical current (by definition, movement of positive ions) ensues as illustrated by the curved arrow in B, depolarizes adjacent membrane to threshold and causes cellular activation, as shown in C. The impulse then spreads further as shown in D, and eventually makes its way to the end of the bundle. One major determinant of impulse spread is how fast depolarizing current flow spreads from the activated region to the region that is not yet activated. When a depolarizing current is passed across an electrical resistor (like the lipid cell membrane), the voltage change produced depends on the resistance (by virtue of Ohm's law, $E = IR$, where E = voltage change, I = current, R = resistance). Thus, membrane resistance is an important factor governing conduction speed in the heart. The resting fast-response cardiac cell membrane has a relatively low resistance because of the high K^+ conductance through I_{K1}; rapid conduction therefore requires a very large current flow (ensured by large phase 0 Na^+ current). Slow-channel tissue has a much higher resistance because of lack of I_{K1}, allowing the relatively small I_{CaL} to produce conduction, albeit much more slowly than in fast-response tissue. Membrane resistance is a very important "passive" membrane property, as opposed to active membrane functions mediated by ion channels.

Molecular Structure of Key Cardiac Ion Channels and Transporters

The changes in membrane permeability that mediate the phases of the cardiac AP are largely produced by the time- and voltage-dependent function of cardiac ion channels, the building blocks of biologic electricity in the heart, brain, skeletal muscle, and other excitable tissues. Specialized transmembrane glycoproteins form ion channels: ion-selective pores in cell membranes that open and close *(gating)* in response to an appropriate biologic signal. The

ion channels most centrally involved in controlling cardiac AP gate in response to changes in transmembrane voltage ("voltage-gated channels"). Other physiologically important channels respond to chemical ligands such as ACh, ATP, and Ca^{2+}. Electrophysiologic studies have detailed the functional properties of Na^+, Ca^{2+}, and K^+ currents in cardiomyocytes, and molecular cloning has revealed a large number of pore-forming (α) and auxiliary (β, γ, and δ) subunits that form ion channels. Mutations in the genes encoding cardiac ion channel subunits are responsible for many forms of inherited cardiac arrhythmias (see Chapter 63). The expression and functional properties of myocardial ion channels also change in a number of acquired disease states, and these alterations can predispose to cardiac arrhythmias.[6]

VOLTAGE-GATED NA+ CHANNELS

Voltage-gated Na^+ (Nav) channel pore-forming (α) subunits have four homologous domains (I to IV), each of which contains six-transmembrane–spanning regions (designated S1 to S6), and these four domains come together to form the Na^+-permeable pore (Fig. 62.8A).[7] Among the multiple Nav α subunits, Nav1.5 (which is encoded by the *SCN5A* gene) is the most strongly expressed in mammalian myocardium. The name of the voltage-gated sodium channel protein consists of the chemical symbol of the principal permeating ion (Na^+) and v, which indicates its principal physiologic regulator (voltage). The number following v indicates the gene subfamily (Nav1), and the number following the decimal point identifies the specific channel isoform (e.g., Nav1.1). An identical nomenclature applies to voltage-gated calcium and potassium channels. Mutations in *SCN5A*, which are associated with LQT3 syndrome, disrupt Nav channel inactivation and thereby give rise to a sustained inward Na^+ current during the plateau phase of the AP and to APD prolongation. Mutations in *SCN5A* are also linked to Brugada syndrome. Brugada syndrome mutations result in reduced I_{Na} amplitude, which leads to slowing of the phase 0 AP upstroke, reduced AP amplitude, and altered phase 1 early repolarization.

Nav1.5 pore-forming α subunits coassemble with one to two auxiliary Nav β subunits to form functional cell-surface Na^+ channels in cardiomyocytes.[8] Nav β subunits appear to play an important role in anchoring ion channel proteins to the cell membrane. Subpopulations of Nav1.5 channels are present in different subcellular regions, such as the intercalated disc and T-tubular membranes. As with many other ion channels, Nav1.5 channels are part of macromolecular complexes including both channel and regulatory proteins.[8,9]

VOLTAGE-GATED Ca2+ CHANNELS

As with Nav channels, cardiac voltage-gated Ca^{2+} (Cav) channels are assemblies of a pore-forming $α_1$ subunits and auxiliary Cav β or Cav $α_2$−δ subunits (see Fig. 62.8C). Among the various Cav channels, Cav1.2, also known as $α_{1C}$ encoded by the *CACNA1C* gene, is the prominent Cav $α_1$ subunit expressed in mammalian myocardium. Cav1.2 channels exhibit many of the time- and voltage-dependent properties and pharmacologic sensitivities of cardiac L-type Ca^{2+} currents (see Table 62.1). Cav1.3 channel subunits may also form L-type Ca^{2+} channels, particularly in the SA node and atria. Accessory subunits modulate the functional properties of Cav channels.[10]

Cav3.1/$α_1$ G alpha subunits form a Ca^{2+}-selective channel with time- and voltage-dependent characteristics and pharmacologic sensitivities that resemble those of the low-voltage activated T-type Ca^{2+} channel. Disruption of the gene encoding Cav3.1 subunits *(CACNA1G)* in mice slows the sinus node rate and AV conduction, and reduces the heart-rate response to adrenergic stimulation, consistent with a role in SA and AV node function.[11]

VOLTAGE-GATED K+ CHANNELS

Voltage-gated K^+ channels (Kv) are the most diverse family of voltage-dependent channels in the heart. Kv channels are composed of four separate pore-forming (α) subunits, each containing six-membrane–spanning domains (S_1 through S_6)[12] (see Fig. 62.8B). Kvα subunits expressed in the human heart include members of the Kv1, Kv4, hERG

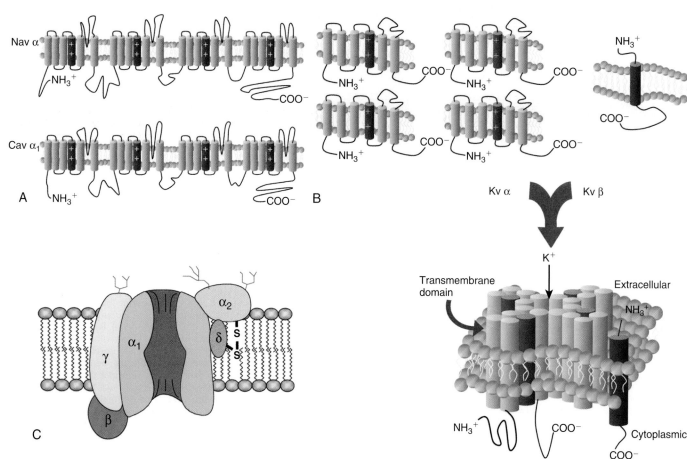

FIGURE 62.8 Transmembrane topology and schematic of the structure of ion channels. **A,** Voltage-gated Na+ and Ca2+ channels are composed of a single tetramer consisting of four covalently linked repeats of the six-transmembrane–spanning motifs. **B,** Voltage-gated K+ channels are composed of four separate subunits, each containing a single six-transmembrane–spanning motif. Inwardly rectifying K+ channels are formed by inward rectifier K+ channel pore-forming (alpha) subunits (Kir). In contrast to voltage-gated K+ channel alpha subunits, the Kir alpha subunits have only two (not six) transmembrane domains. **C,** All ion channels are multisubunit proteins, as exemplified by the schematic subunit structure of L-type Ca channels.

(Kv7), and KvLQT (Kv11) subfamilies. In addition, Kv channel α subunit proteins interact with Kv channel accessory subunits, including minK, KChIP2, and MiRP1 (see Table 62.1), to form functional cell surface channels with distinct time- and voltage-dependent properties. Co-assembly of the Kv4.3 α subunits and the accessory subunit KChIP2 gives rise to the cardiac transient outward Kv channel I_{to} (see Phase 1: Early Rapid Repolarization). hERG α subunits, possibly together with MiRP1 accessory subunits, form functional cardiac I_{Kr} channels. Mutations in the gene encoding hERG *(KCNH2)* have been shown to underlie congenital LQT2 syndrome. These LQT2 mutations are loss-of-function mutations that lead to reduced functional I_{Kr} channel expression or to alterations in channel processing or trafficking (see Chapter 63).

KvLQT1 α subunits associate with minK (encoded by *KCNE1*) accessory subunits to form channels that carry slowly activating, noninactivating K+ currents, identified with I_{Ks} in human myocardium. Mutations in the gene encoding KvLQT1 α subunits, *KCNQ1*, are linked to LQT1 syndrome. Mutations in the minK-encoding gene *KCNE1* are associated with LQT5 syndrome. These mutations are all loss-of-function mutations that reduce expression of functional I_{Ks} channels in the cell membrane.

Kv1.5 α subunits contribute to K+-selective channels with time- and voltage-dependent characteristics that underlie the rapidly activating and slowly inactivating I_{Kur} in human atrial myocytes.[13] I_{Kur} is downregulated in the atria of patients with chronic AF.

Small-conductance, Ca2+-sensitive K+ channels are tetrameric assemblies of SK α subunits (encoded by *KCNN1-3*) and underlie a Ca2+-activated K+ current, I_{KCa}, in human cardiomyocytes.[5] Common variants in *KCNN3* discovered in genome-wide analyses have been associated with AF.[14]

INWARDLY RECTIFYING CARDIAC K+ CHANNELS

Kir channels in cardiac myocytes, as in other cells, conduct inward current at membrane potentials negative to E_K (see earlier, Physiology of Ion Channels) and smaller outward currents (due to inward rectification) at membrane potentials positive to E_K. The current through Kir channels is a function of both the membrane potential and the extracellular K+ concentration ($[K^+]_o$) and is the major determinant of the resting membrane potential in working myocardium and the specialized ventricular conducting system. When $[K^+]_o$ increases, the E_K moves to more positive values and the cell depolarizes.

Inward rectification reduces the permeability of K+ channels at depolarized voltages to prevent too much K+ leaving the cell. Mechanisms include channel block by binding of magnesium and positively charged organic ions to the channel (for I_{K1}) and extremely rapid inactivation (for I_{Kr}).[15] In contrast to Kv α subunits, Kir α subunits have only two (not six) transmembrane domains. The α subunits Kir2.1 and Kir2.2 encoded by *KCNJ2* and *KCNJ3*, respectively, are the main subunits underlying the I_{K1} inwardly rectifying current in cardiomyocytes.

The K+-selective sarcolemmal $I_{K.ATP}$ channel is formed by the association of pore-forming Kir6 α subunits and sulfonylurea receptor (SUR) subunits. In cardiomyocytes, Kir6.2 α subunits (encoded by *KCNJ11*) assemble with SUR1 and SUR2 subunits encoded by *ABCC8* and *ABCC9,* respectively, to carry $I_{K.ATP}$. Different anatomic regions of the heart may express $I_{K.ATP}$ comprised of differing channel and SUR subunits. $I_{K.ATP}$ channels play a pivotal role in myocardial ischemia and preconditioning, by reducing APD and myocardial metabolic demands when cellular ATP content goes down. Opening of cardiac sarcolemmal $I_{K.ATP}$ channels underlies ST-segment elevation during acute myocardial ischemia. $I_{K.ATP}$ is an important regulator of the function of multiple tissues. For example, in blood vessels, $I_{K.ATP}$ leads to vasodilation and in the pancreas, $I_{K.ATP}$ inhibits insulin secretion. Drugs like nicorandil and diazoxide open ATP-sensitive K+ channels, whereas sulfonylurea compounds (e.g., glibenclamide) inhibit $I_{K.ATP}$. In addition to the sarcolemmal $I_{K.ATP}$ channel an ATP-sensitive potassium conductance in mitochondria (mitoK[ATP]) is involved in cardioprotection and arrhythmias. The molecular composition of this channel is uncertain but likely involves another type of inwardly rectifying K+ channel.[16]

The ACh-activated K+ channel $I_{K.ACh}$ is a heteromultimer of two inwardly rectifying potassium channel subunits, Kir3.1 and Kir3.4.[12,15] Stimulation of $I_{K.ACh}$ by vagally secreted ACh hyperpolarizes SA and AV node cells, decreases the slope of spontaneous depolarization in the SA node, slowing heart rate, and slows conduction in the AV node. Adenosine, through type 1 purinergic receptor–mediated G-protein activation, opens the $I_{K.ACh}$ channel (in this context carrying a current referred to as $I_{K.Ado}$) in atrial, SA node, and AV node cells. Adenosine and vagal-enhancement maneuvers are useful for the acute termination of arrhythmias involving the AV node as part of the reentry circuit, such as atrioventricular reentrant (AVRT) and atrioventricular nodal reentrant tachycardias (AVNRT) (see later, Mechanisms of Arrhythmogenesis).

CARDIAC PACEMAKER CHANNELS

The I_f pacemaker current prominently contributes to diastolic depolarization in all tissues with spontaneous automaticity. I_f activates slowly at negative potentials and deactivates rapidly with depolarization, carrying a mixed monovalent cation (Na+ and K+) current. I_f is highly regulated; beta-adrenergic stimulation increases the probability of channel opening by shifting the channel's activation curve to more positive potentials, accelerating diastolic depolarization. The HCN channels underlying I_f are topologically similar to voltage-dependent K+ channels and related to cyclic nucleotide–gated channels in photoreceptors in the retina. Of the four known HCN pore-forming α subunits, HCN4 is the most highly expressed in the mammalian myocardium. Mutations in the human *HCN4* gene have been linked to familial sinus bradycardia and inappropriate sinus tachycardia.[17] I_f-blocking drugs have been approved for the treatment of angina and are under investigation for the treatment of various forms of heart failure and arrhythmias.[18]

ELECTROGENIC TRANSPORTERS
Na+/Ca2+ Exchanger

The NCX is an ion transporter that exchanges three Na+ ions for one Ca2+ and is very strongly expressed in the mammalian heart. With each cycle, NCX exchanges three positive charges (Na+ ions) for every Ca2+ ion (two positive charges) that it handles, producing a net current in the direction of Na+ movement (its function is therefore "electrogenic"). NCX almost always functions to extrude Ca2+, resulting in a net inward current. The cardiac NCX is a transmembrane glycoprotein proposed to have nine-transmembrane repeats based on hydropathy analysis (Fig. 62.9A,B). The intracellular loop contains domains that bind Ca2+ (CBD 1 and 2) and the endogenous NCX inhibitory domain, XIP.

Ion exchange through NCX can occur in either direction. With each heartbeat, the phase-2 entry of Ca2+ triggers a large cytosolic Ca2+ release from SR stores through the release-channel RyR2. Intracellular [Ca2+] then increases from the resting level of less than 100 nM to approximately 1 μM. Outward Ca2+ flux through the NCX (in exchange for Na+, generating an inward current) along with Ca2+ reuptake into the SR by the SR Ca2+-ATPase (SERCA) remove cytosolic Ca2+ during diastole, restoring diastolic [Ca2+] to its resting level. NCX current is time-independent and largely reflects changes in intracellular [Ca2+] during the AP. Thus, NCX can contribute to determining the transmembrane voltage. At depolarized potentials, reverse-mode Na+/Ca2+ exchange (Ca2+ influx, net outward current) can occur; however, the role of reverse-mode exchange in initiating SR Ca2+ release and contraction is uncertain.

NCX current is an important component of the inward current that underlies delayed afterdepolarizations (DADs). DADs are spontaneous membrane depolarizations after complete repolarization of the AP. They generally result from spontaneous diastolic SR Ca2+ release events under pathologic conditions. The cytosolic Ca2+ transient resulting from Ca2+ release causes Ca2+ to be extruded via NCX in exchange for extracellular Na+ release, producing a depolarizing inward current. When the resulting membrane depolarization reaches threshold it initiates an ectopic AP; repeated DADs can cause or trigger tachyarrhythmias.[19]

Na+,K+-ATPase

Also called the Na+ pump, Na+,K+-ATPase maintains the high intracellular K+ and low intracellular Na+ concentration of cardiomyocytes. The Na+ pump belongs to the widely distributed class of P-type ATPases cation transporters. The P-type designation refers to the formation of a phosphorylated aspartyl intermediate during the catalytic cycle. The Na+,K+-ATPase hydrolyzes a molecule of ATP to transport two K+ into the cell and three Na+ out and thus is electrogenic, generating a time-independent hyperpolarizing outward current. The Na+,K+-ATPase is oligomeric, consisting of α and β subunits and a tissue-specific regulator protein called phospholemman (PLM). PLM belongs to a family of single-membrane–spanning proteins called FXYD proteins, which share a characteristic 35-amino acid sequence including a PFXYD (proline-phenylalanine-X-tyrosine-aspartic acid) sequence in their extracellular domain. PLM (FXYD1) is expressed in heart and skeletal muscle, which binds to and inhibits Na+,K+-ATPase, acting as an important endogenous regulator.[20]

Na+,K+-ATPase isoforms are diverse and exhibit tissue-specific distributions. The structural diversity of the Na+,K+-ATPase comes from variations in α and β genes, splice variants of the α subunits and promiscuity of subunit associations. The α subunit is catalytic and binds digitalis glycosides in the extracellular linker between the first and second membrane-spanning region (Fig. 62.9C and D).

Gap Junction Channels and Intercalated Discs

Another family of ion channel proteins critical to cardiac electrophysiology forms gap junctional channels. These dodecameric channels are found in the intercalated discs between adjacent cells (Fig. 62.10A,B). Three types of specialized junctions make up each intercalated disc. The macula adherens (or "desmosome") and the fascia adherens form areas of strong adhesion between cells that provide linkage for the transfer of mechanical energy from one cell to the next. The *nexus*, also called the tight or gap junction (Fig. 62.10C–E), is a region of functional intercellular contact in the intercalated disc. Membranes at these junctions are separated by only about 10 to 20 Å and are connected by hexagonally packed subunit bridges (or "gap junction channels"). These specialized channels provide biochemical and low-resistance electrical coupling between adjacent cells, by establishing aqueous pores that directly link their cytoplasm. Gap junctions allow the movement of ions (e.g., Na+, Cl−, K+, Ca2+) and small molecules (e.g., cAMP, cGMP,inositol 1,4,5-triphosphate [IP_3]) between adjacent cells, thereby linking their interiors.

Gap junctions permit a multicellular structure such as the heart to function electrically as an orderly, synchronized, interconnected unit. Gap junctions are mostly located at cell ends. Thus, the anatomic and biophysical properties of cardiac muscle bundles vary according to the direction in which they are measured, a property called "anisotropy." CV is generally two to three times faster longitudinally, in the direction of the long axis of the fiber, than it is transversely, perpendicular to this long axis. Resistivity (the inverse of permeability) is lower longitudinally than transversely. Cardiac conduction is discontinuous because of resistive discontinuities created by the gap junctions. The *safety factor for conduction*, the energy for normal conduction relative to the minimum energy that propagates, determines the success of AP propagation. Interestingly, the *safety factor for propagation* is greater transversely than horizontally. Conduction delay or block thus occurs more easily in the longitudinal direction than it does transversely.

Gap junctions also provide "biochemical coupling," which permits cell-to-cell movement of ATP (or other high-energy phosphates), cyclic nucleotides, and IP_3, the activator of the IP_3-sensitive SR Ca2+-release channel. Diffusion of second-messenger substances through gap junctional channels enables coordinated responses of the myocardial syncytium to physiologic stimuli.[21]

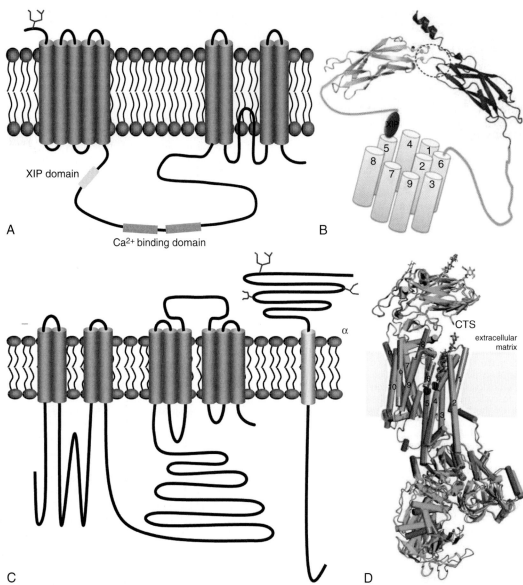

FIGURE 62.9 Transmembrane topology and predicted structures of Na$^+$/Ca^{2+} exchanger (NCX) and the Na$^+$,K$^+$-ATPase (Na pump). **A,** Predicted topology of NCX, the cytoplasmic segment includes an autoinhibitory domain (XIP) and two Ca^{2+}-binding domains. **B,** Predicted structure; the cytoplasmic surface is on top. **C,** Topologic structure of the α and β subunits of Na$^+$,K$^+$-ATPase. **D,** Overlapping structures of the Na pump bound to three different cardiotonic steroids. *CTS,* Cardiotonic steroid. (**B** from Khaninshvilli D. The SLC8 gene family of sodium-calcium exchangers (NCX)—structure, function, and regulation in health and disease. *Mol Aspects Med.* 2013;34:220–235. **D** from Laursen M, Gregersen JL, Yatime L, et al. Structures and characterization of digoxin- and bufalin-bound Na+,K+-ATPase compared with the ouabain-bound complex. *Proc Natl Acad Sci U S A.* 2015;112:1755–1760.)

Gap junction function is dynamic. When the intracellular calcium level rises, as in myocardial infarction (MI), gap junctions close to seal off injured from noninjured cells. Acidosis increases, and alkalosis decreases, gap junctional resistance. Increased gap junctional resistance slows the rate of AP propagation, leading to conduction delay or block. The small number of transverse gap junctions means that inactivation of gap junctions impairs transverse conduction to a greater degree than longitudinal, resulting in increased anisotropy.

Connexins are the proteins that form the intercellular channels of gap junctions. Six connexin proteins assemble to form a *"connexon,"* a hemichannel that connects to a complementary connexon hemichannel in an adjacent cell to create a permeable channel connecting the cells. Each connexon is formed by six integral membrane connexin subunits, which surround an aqueous pore and thereby create a low-resistance connection (Fig. 62.10A). *Connexin 43,* a 43-kDa polypeptide, is the most abundant cardiac connexin in heart cells, with connexins 40 and 45 being found in smaller amounts. Ventricular muscle expresses connexins 43 and 45, whereas atrial muscle and the specialized conduction system express connexins 43, 45, and 40.

The various connexin types form gap junctional channels with characteristic unitary conductances, voltage sensitivities, and permeabilities. Tissue-specific connexin expression and the spatial distribution of gap junctions contribute to distinct conduction properties of cardiac tissues. The functional diversity of cardiac gap junctions is further enhanced by the ability of different connexin isoforms to form hybrid gap junctional channels with unique electrophysiologic properties (Fig. 62.10B). These channel chimeras appear to have a major function in controlling impulse transmission at the SA node–atrium border, the atrium–AV node transitional zone, and the Purkinje-myocyte border.[1,22]

Alterations in the distribution and function of cardiac gap junctions are associated with increased susceptibility to arrhythmias. Conduction slowing and arrhythmogenesis have been associated with redistribution of connexin 43 (Cx43) gap junctions from the end of cardiomyocytes to the lateral borders and with decreased phosphorylation of Cx43 in a dog model of nonischemic dilated cardiomyopathy (Fig. 62.10C–E). Adult mice genetically engineered to lack cardiac Cx43 exhibited increased susceptibility to the induction

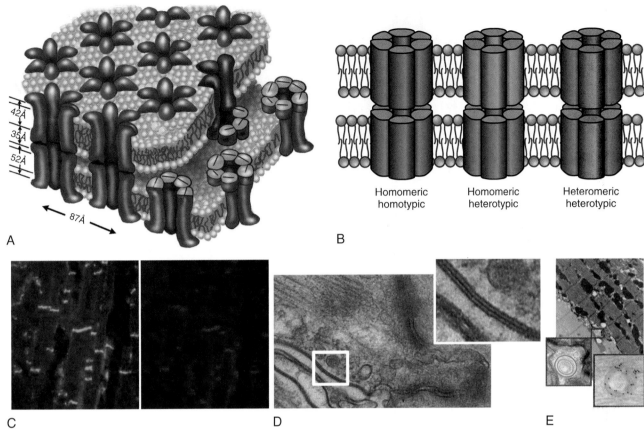

FIGURE 62.10 A, Model of the structure of a gap junction based on the results of x-ray diffraction studies. Individual channels are composed of paired hexamers in the membranes of adjacent cells and adjoin in the extracellular gap to form an aqueous pore that provides continuity of the cytoplasm of the two cells; Å, ångstroms. **B,** Mixing of connexin subunits to form gap junction channels may occur at interfaces between tissue types in the heart. Homomeric, homotypic channels contain a single connexin isoform; homomeric, heterotypic channels are composed of connexons (hemichannels) comprising a single connexin isoform; and heteromeric, heterotypic channels are made from connexons containing more than one connexin isoform. **C,** Connexin 43 (Cx43) is concentrated at the intercalated discs at cell ends in ventricular myocardium *(green)* and colocalizes with junctional proteins such as N-cadherin *(red)*. **D,** Electron microscopic view of an intercalated from normal ventricular myocardium reveals a pentalaminar membrane *(inset)* characteristic of gap junctions. **E,** Remodeling of gap junctions in the failing heart. Immunoreactive Cx43 is increased along lateral cell borders, and annular gap junctions that label with anti-Cx43 immunogold antibodies *(insets)* can be observed. (**A** from Saffitz JE. Cell-to-cell communication in the heart. *Cardiol Rev.* 1995;3:86; **C** and **E** modified from Hesketh GA, Shah MH, Halperin VL, et al. Ultrastructure and regulation of lateralized connexin43 in the failing heart. *Circ Res.* 2010;106:1153–1163.)

of fatal tachyarrhythmias. Side-to-side electrical coupling between cardiomyocytes is reduced following acute MI, exaggerating anisotropy and facilitating reentrant activity. Lastly, mutations in the atrial-specific connexin 40 gene have been associated with AF.[23] Normal electrical coupling of cardiomyocytes through gap junctions depends on cell-to-cell mechanical coupling through adhesion junctions. Defects in cell-cell adhesion prevent normal localization of connexins in gap junctions, potentially causing lethal tachyarrhythmias. Mutations in *desmoplakin,* a protein that links desmosomal adhesion molecules to *desmin,* a filament protein of the cardiomyocyte cytoskeleton, and *plakoglobin,* a protein that connects N-cadherins to actin and desmosomal cadherins to desmin, produce autosomal recessive variants of arrhythmogenic RV cardiomyopathy (ARVC), Carvajal disease, and Naxos disease, respectively (see Chapter 52).[24] Notably, restoring plakoglobin (*JUP* gene) levels in a mouse model of Naxos disease caused by a truncation of plakoglobin prevented cardiac dysfunction, consistent with a loss of function defect of the truncated protein. Loss of N-cadherin expression in mouse hearts decreases Cx43 expression in gap junctions, impairs and promotes arrhythmias.

STRUCTURE AND FUNCTION OF THE CARDIAC ELECTRICAL NETWORK

Sinoatrial Node

The SA node is a spindle-shaped structure composed of a fibrous tissue matrix containing closely packed cells. In man, it is 10 to 20 mm long

and 2 to 3 mm wide, narrowing caudally toward the inferior vena cava (IVC). The SA node is superficial, lying less than 1 mm from the epicardial surface, laterally in the right atrial sulcus terminalis at the junction of the superior vena cava (SVC) and right atrium. The proximity to the right phrenic nerve is an important consideration when catheter ablation or modification of the sinoatrial node (SAN) is contemplated (Fig. 62.11). The artery supplying the SAN branches from the right (55% to 60% of the time) or the left (40% to 45%) circumflex coronary artery and approaches the node around the junction of the SVC and right atrium (**eFigs. 62.4** and **62.5**).

Atrioventricular Junctional Area and Intraventricular Conduction System
Atrioventricular Node

Based on histology and immunolabeling, the normal AV junctional area is composed of multiple distinct structures, including transitional tissue, inferior nodal extension (INE), compact portion, penetrating bundle, His bundle, atrial and ventricular muscle, central fibrous body, tendon of Todaro, and valves (Fig. 62.12A and **eFig. 62.7**).[26] The properties of AV node cells are diverse, with the compact AV node populated by relatively depolarized cells displaying slow response APs and cells more like working atrium in other sections.[27]

At the level of the AV junction, the tract of nodal tissue is divided into two major components, the INE and the penetrating bundle.[26,28]

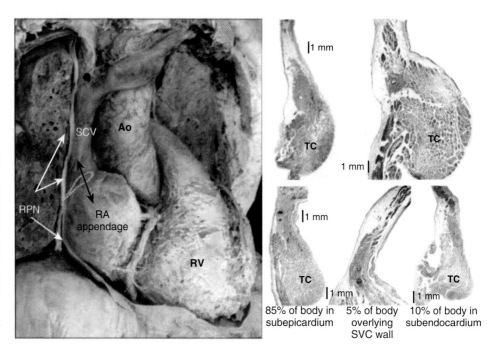

FIGURE 62.11 Left, Anterior view of the heart in a cadaver that has been dissected to show the course of the right phrenic nerve *(RPN)* relative to the right atrium *(RA)*. The anticipated location of the sinus node outlined with the *dots*. The *double-headed arrow* represents the sectioning plane used for making the cross sections through the sinus node and the terminal crest *(TC)* shown in the histologic sections. *Ao,* Aorta; *RV,* right ventricle; *SCV,* superior caval vein. The histologic sections in the two **upper right panels** show variations in sizes of the sinus node cross section and the TC. With this stain (Masson trichrome), the node is recognizable by its fibrous matrix *(green)* and its artery. Two **lower right panels** show variations in nodal location relative to the epicardial and endocardial surfaces and to the SCV. *SVC,* Superior vena cava. (From Ho SY, Sanchez-Quintana D. Anatomy and pathology of the sinus node. *J Interv Card Electrophysiol.* 2016;46:3–8.)

The INE is located between the coronary sinus and the tricuspid valve, and the end of the INE is covered by transitional tissue (Fig. 62.12D). The small myocytes in the INE are dispersed among connective tissue and do not express connexin 43, whereas myocytes in the transitional zone do express Cx43; however, unlike the Cx43-positive atrial myocytes in the working myocardium, they are loosely packed between collagen septa (Fig. 62.12B, C). The INE is continuous with the penetrating bundle, which penetrates the fibrous tissue separating the atria and ventricles and emerges in the ventricles as the bundle of His. Both structures are covered by connective tissue and are therefore enclosed. Myocytes in the *penetrating bundle* express Cx43 and are dispersed among connective tissue. A tract of Cx43-positive nodal tissue projects into the Cx43-negative INE.

The compact portion of the AV node (Fig. 62.12A) is a superficial structure lying just beneath the right atrial endocardium, anterior to the ostium of the coronary sinus, and directly above the insertion of the septal leaflet of the tricuspid valve. It is at the apex of a triangle formed by the tricuspid annulus and the *tendon of Todaro* (Fig. 62.12), which originates in the central fibrous body and passes posteriorly through the atrial septum to continue with the Eustachian valve. The term *triangle of Koch*, however, has to be used with caution because histologic studies of anatomically normal adult hearts have demonstrated that the tendon of Todaro, which forms one side of the triangle of Koch, is absent in about two thirds of hearts. The compact node is located at the junction where the Cx43-negative nodal tissue meets the Cx43-positive nodal tissue (see Fig. 62.12B–D).

In 85% to 90% of human hearts, the arterial supply to the AV node is derived from a branch of the right coronary artery that originates at the posterior intersection of the AV and interventricular grooves (crux). A branch of the circumflex coronary artery provides the arterial supply to the AV node in the remaining hearts (**eFig. 62.8**).

During normal anterograde AV conduction, the AP propagates from the SAN through atrial working myocardium (while the involvement of specialized internodal conduction pathways has been suggested, their existence remains controversial) and enters the tract of nodal tissue at two points (see Fig. 62.12D; see also **Video 62.1**). The first point is at the end of the INE (next to the penetrating bundle) via transitional tissue. This conduction pathway most likely corresponds to the fast-pathway route. Second, the AP enters near the atrial origin of the INE. This conduction pathway probably constitutes the slow-pathway route. The AP cannot enter nodal tissue at other tissue points, because of separation by a vein and connective tissue. From the two entry points, the APs propagating anterogradely and retrogradely along the INE usually

annihilate each other, whereas the APs entering the nodal tract via the transitional zone propagate into the compact node and then reach the His bundle to enter the left and right bundle branches.

Transmembrane APs recorded from cardiomyocytes in situ at various locations within the nodal tract exhibit distinct shapes and time courses. Cells from the compact AV node are depolarized and have much slower phase 0 upstrokes due to the relatively small underlying Ca^{2+} current.[27] This smaller rate of depolarization, along with more limited electrical coupling, results in slowing of conduction across the compact portion and penetrating bundle (CV <10 cm/sec versus 35 cm/sec in atrial working myocardium), thereby giving rise to the AV conduction delay. APs from extranodal atrial tissue and the His bundle have more negative diastolic potentials and faster upstrokes than myocytes in the transitional zone and penetrating bundle.

Bundle of His (Penetrating Portion of Atrioventricular Bundle)

This structure is the continuation of the penetrating bundle on the ventricular side of the AV junction before it divides to form the left and right bundles. Myocytes in the His bundle are small and Cx43 positive (see Fig. 62.12). Large, well-formed fasciculoventricular connections between the penetrating portion of the AV bundle and the ventricular septal crest are occasionally found in adult hearts, possibly underlying preexcitation. Branches from the anterior and posterior descending coronary arteries supply the upper muscular interventricular septum with blood, which makes the conduction system at this site more impervious to ischemic damage unless the ischemia is extensive.

Bundle Branches (Branching Portion of Atrioventricular Bundle)

The bundle branches begin at the superior margin of the muscular interventricular septum, immediately beneath the membranous septum, with cells of the left bundle branch (LBB) cascading downward as a continuous sheet onto the septum beneath the noncoronary aortic cusp (Fig. 62.13A). The AV bundle may then give off other discrete bundle tracts. Sometimes these constitute a true bifascicular system with an anterosuperior branch and an inferoposterior system, constituting (when damaged) the anatomical basis of electrocardiographic left anterior and left posterior hemiblock respectively. In other cases, the AV bundle may give rise to a group of central fibers, and in still others, the offshoots appear as a network without clear division into a fascicular system (Fig. 62.13B,C). The right bundle branch continues intramyocardially as an unbranched extension of the AV bundle down the right side of the interventricular septum to the apex of the right ventricle

Purkinje fibers penetrate only the inner third of the endocardium, whereas in pigs, they almost reach to the epicardium. These differences influence changes produced by myocardial ischemia, because Purkinje fibers are more resistant to ischemia than ordinary myocardial fibers. Purkinje myocytes are found in the His bundle and bundle branches, and cover most of the endocardium of both ventricles (see Fig. 62.13B); they align to form multicellular bundles in longitudinal strands separated by collagen. Although conduction of cardiac impulses is their principal function, large free-running Purkinje fibers composed of many Purkinje cells, often called *false tendons*, are capable of contraction. APs propagate within the thin Purkinje fiber bundles from the base to the apex before activating surrounding myocytes. Purkinje myocytes have less well-developed transverse tubules (**eFig. 62.9**), which reduces membrane capacitance and thus accelerates AP propagation. Purkinje fiber coupling relies on connexins 40 and 45. The molecular identity of the connexin type at the Purkinje fiber–myocyte junction (PMJ) is unclear. Purkinje cells have markedly longer repolarization times than surrounding myocytes (see Fig. 62.5E) and may be preferential sites of afterdepolarization generation.

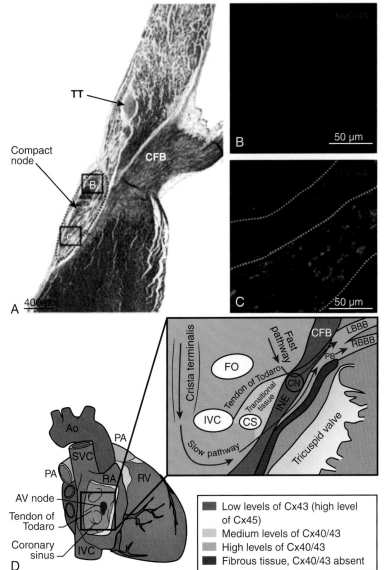

FIGURE 62.12 **A,** Masson's trichrome–stained section through the compact node of the rabbit heart (*red,* myocytes; *blue,* connective tissue). The compact node is enclosed with a *dashed line.* **B** and **C,** High-magnification images of boxed regions in **A** (**B** is the compact node; **C** is the lower nodal bundle) showing Cx43 expression (immunofluorescence, *bright-green* punctate spots). **C,** *Dotted yellow lines* divide tissue into Cx43-negative (*top*) and Cx43-positive (*bottom*) regions. (Modified from Dobrzynski H, Nikolski VP, Sambelashvili AT, et al. Site of origin and molecular substrate of atrioventricular junctional rhythm in the rabbit heart. *Circ Res.* 2003;93:1102–1110.) *CFB,* Central fibrous body; *TT,* tendon of Todaro. **D,** Color-coded map of the distribution of connexins (Cx) in the atrioventricular (AV) junction. *Ao,* Aorta; *CN,* compact AV node; *CS,* coronary sinus; *FO,* foramen ovale; *INE,* inferior nodal extension; *IVC,* inferior vena cava; *LBBB,* left bundle branch block; *PA,* pulmonary artery; *PB,* penetrating bundle; *RA,* right atrium; *RBBB,* right bundle branch block; *RV,* right ventricle. (From Temple IP, Inada S, Dobrzynski H, et al. Connexins and the atrioventricular node. *Heart Rhythm.* 2010;10:297.)

and base of the anterior papillary muscle. In some human hearts, the His bundle traverses the right interventricular crest and gives rise to a right-sided narrow stem origin of the LBB. The anatomy of the LBB system can be variable and may not conform to a constant bifascicular division. However, the concept of a trifascicular system remains useful to both electrocardiographers and clinicians (see Chapter 14).

Terminal Purkinje Fibers
The Purkinje fibers connect with the ends of the bundle branches to form interweaving networks on the endocardial surface of both ventricles and transmit the cardiac impulse almost simultaneously to the right and left ventricular endocardium. Purkinje fibers tend to be less concentrated at the base of the ventricle and at the papillary muscle tips. They penetrate the myocardium transmurally from the endocardium for varying distances, depending on the species. In humans,

Innervation of Atrioventricular Node, His Bundle, and Ventricular Myocardium
Pathways of Innervation
The AV node and His bundle region are richly innervated by cholinergic and adrenergic fibers with densities exceeding the ventricular myocardium.[1] Innervation density is variable in the AV junctional area. For example, the INE has a higher density of cholinergic and adrenergic nerves than working atrial myocardium; the opposite is true for the compact node. Ganglia, nerve fibers, and nerve nets lie close to the AV node.

In general, autonomic neural input to the heart exhibits some degree of "sidedness," with the right sympathetic and vagal nerves affecting the SA node more than the AV node and the left sympathetic and vagal nerves affecting the AV node more than the SA node. The distribution of neural input to the SA and AV nodes is complex because of substantial overlapping innervation. Despite the overlap, specific branches of the vagal and sympathetic nerves can be shown to innervate certain regions preferentially. Stimulation of the right stellate ganglion produces sinus tachycardia with less effect on AV nodal conduction, whereas stimulation of the left stellate ganglion generally shifts the sinus pacemaker to an ectopic site and consistently shortens AV nodal conduction time and refractoriness. Left stellate stimulation produces variable and usually smaller degrees of SAN acceleration. Stimulation of the right cervical vagus nerve primarily slows the SA nodal discharge rate, whereas stimulation of the left vagus primarily prolongs AV nodal conduction time and refractoriness. Neither sympathetic nor vagal stimulation affects normal conduction in the His bundle. The negative dromotropic response of the heart to vagal stimulation is mediated by the activation of $I_{K,ACh}$, which hyperpolarizes AV nodal cells, making them harder to activate.

Most efferent sympathetic impulses reach the canine ventricles over the ansae subclavia, branches from the stellate ganglia. Sympathetic nerves then synapse primarily in the caudal cervical ganglia and form individual cardiac nerves that innervate relatively localized parts of the ventricles. The major route to the heart is the recurrent cardiac nerve on the right side and the ventrolateral cardiac nerve on the left. In general, the right sympathetic chain shortens refractoriness primarily of the anterior portion of the ventricles, and the left affects primarily the posterior surface of the ventricles, although overlapping areas of distribution occur. Asymmetrical sympathetic activation may be associated with arrhythmogenesis and stellate ganglion block is sometimes used to treat certain refractory ventricular arrhythmia syndromes.

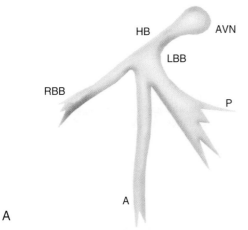

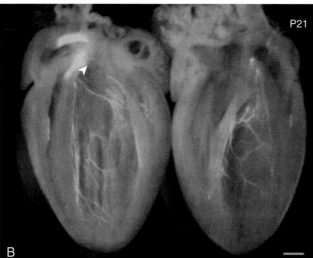

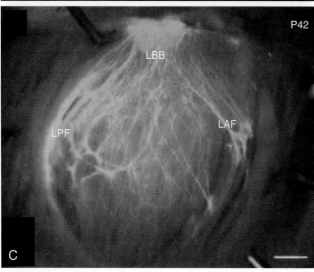

FIGURE 62.13 A, Schematic representation of the trifascicular bundle branch conduction system. **B** and **C,** Whole mount of murine hearts expressing contactin-2 eGFP reporter gene (Cntn2EGFP) demonstrate the presence of Cntn2 throughout the cardiac conduction system. The hearts are from mice **(B)** 21 days (P21) and **(C)** 42 days (P42) postpartum. There is robust expression of Cntn2 within the atrioventricular node *(AVN) (arrowhead)* His bundle *(HB),* bundle branches, and Purkinje network. Scale bars = 500 μm. *LAF,* Left anterior fascicle; *LBB,* left bundle branch; *LPF,* left posterior fascicle; *RBB,* right bundle branch. (**A** modified from Rosenbaum MB et al. *The Hemiblocks.* Oldsmar, FL: Tampa Tracings; 1970, cover illustration; **B** and **C** from Maass K, Shekhar A, Lu J, et al. Isolation and characterization of embryonic stem cell–derived cardiac Purkinje cells. *Stem Cells.* 2015;33:1102–1112.)

The intraventricular route of sympathetic nerves generally follows the coronary arteries. Afferent and efferent sympathetic nerves travel in the superficial layers of the epicardium and dive to innervate the endocardium. Vagal fibers travel intramurally or subendocardially and travel to the epicardium at the AV groove (Fig. 62.14A). Sympathetic nerve density in the left ventricle is higher in the epicardial than endocardium, which at least in part results from transmural gradients in cytokines during cardiac development that influence sympathetic nerve growth (Fig. 62.14B).[1,29]

Effects of Vagal Stimulation

The principal effects of vagus nerve activation are due to opening of $I_{K,ACh}$ channels. In addition, vagal discharge modulates cardiac sympathetic activity at prejunctional and postjunctional sites by regulating the amount of norepinephrine released and by inhibiting cAMP-induced phosphorylation of cardiac proteins, including ion channels and calcium pumps. Tonic vagal stimulation thus produces a greater absolute reduction in the SAN rate in the presence of tonic background sympathetic stimulation, a sympathetic-parasympathetic interaction termed *accentuated antagonism.* In contrast, changes in AV conduction during concomitant sympathetic and vagal stimulation are essentially the algebraic sum of the individual AV conduction responses to tonic vagal and sympathetic stimulation alone. Cardiac responses to brief vagal bursts begin and dissipate quickly; in contrast, cardiac responses to sympathetic stimulation commence and dissipate more slowly. Periodic *vagal bursting,* as may occur each time that a systolic pressure wave arrives at the baroreceptor regions in the aortic and carotid sinuses, induces phasic changes in sinus cycle length and can entrain the sinus node to discharge faster or slower at periods identical to those of the vagal burst. In a similar phasic manner, vagal bursts prolong AV nodal conduction time and are influenced by background levels of sympathetic tone. Because the peak vagal effects on sinus rate and AV nodal conduction occur at different times in the cardiac cycle, a brief vagal burst can slow the sinus rate without affecting AV nodal conduction or can prolong AV nodal conduction time and not slow the sinus rate.

Effects of Sympathetic Stimulation

Nonuniform distribution of sympathetic nerves—and thus norepinephrine levels—may produce nonuniform electrophysiologic effects during sympathetic activation because the ventricular content of norepinephrine is greater at the base than at the apex of the heart. In humans, both direct and reflex sympathetic stimulation increases regional differences in cardiac repolarization. The dispersion of repolarization is significantly enhanced in patients with ischemic cardiomyopathy.[1] Afferent vagal activity is higher in the posterior ventricular myocardium, which may account for the vagomimetic effects of inferior MI.

The vagi exert very small effects on ventricular tissue; decreased contractility and prolonged refractoriness are demonstrable under careful experimental observation. In addition, the vagus can exert indirect effects by modulating sympathetic influences.

Beyond the beat-to-beat regulation of rate and contractile force, sympathetic input to the heart, through both translational and posttranslational modifications, exerts long-term regulation of adrenergic receptor sensitivity and ion channels. These long-term changes in autonomic responsiveness and cardiac electrical properties appear to be mediated, at least in part, by highly localized signaling cascades involving neurally released molecules such as NPY.[1] In addition, adrenergic neurotransmitters (both released in the heart and in circulating forms) have major neurohumoral effects and promote cellular and structural remodeling that contribute to heart failure and arrhythmias.

Arrhythmias and the Autonomic Nervous System

Alterations in vagal and sympathetic innervation (autonomic remodeling) can influence the development of arrhythmias and contribute to sudden cardiac death (SCD) from ventricular tachyarrhythmias.[30] Damage to nerves extrinsic to the heart, such as the stellate ganglia,

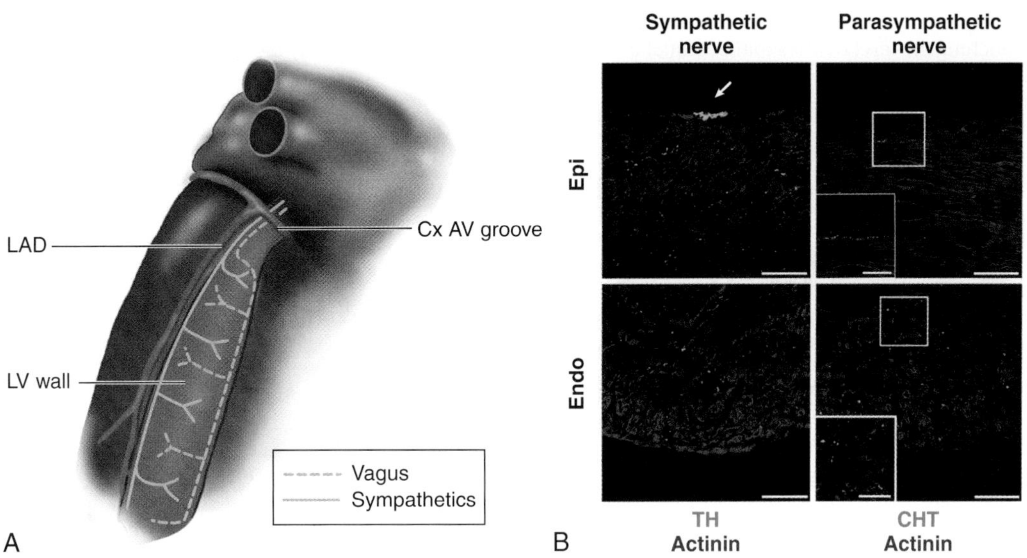

FIGURE 62.14 **A,** Intraventricular route of the sympathetic and vagal nerves to the left ventricle (*LV*); *LAD,* left anterior descending artery. **B,** Distribution of sympathetic and parasympathetic nerves in the mammalian heart. Immunofluorescence staining for the sympathetic and parasympathetic nerve markers tyrosine hydroxylase (*TH*) and choline transporter (*CHT*) is shown in the LV of a rat heart (*green,* nerves; *red,* alpha-actinin, a cardiomyocyte marker). TH-positive nerves are more abundant in the subepicardial (Epi) layer than in the subendocardial (Endo) layer. *Arrow* indicates sympathetic nerves at the epicardial surface. No CHT-positive nerves are present at the epicardial surface, and CHT-positive nerves are more abundant in the subendocardial layer. Higher magnification views of the boxed regions are shown in the *insets.* Scale bars = 100 μm. (**A** from Ito M, Zipes DP. Efferent sympathetic and vagal innervation of the canine right ventricle. *Circulation.* 1994;90:1459. By permission of the American Heart Association; **B** from Kanazawa H, Ieda M, Kimura K, et al. Heart failure causes cholinergic transdifferentiation of cardiac sympathetic nerves via gp130-signaling cytokines in rodents. *J Clin Invest.* 2010;120:408.)

and to intrinsic cardiac nerves from diseases that may affect primarily nerves, such as viral infections, or from diseases that secondarily cause cardiac damage may produce cardioneuropathy. Although the mechanisms by which altered sympathetic innervation modulates cardiac electrical properties are largely unknown, spatially heterogeneous sympathetic hyperinnervation could result in enhanced dispersion of myocardial excitability and refractoriness through patchy adrenergic stimulation of ionic currents, including $I_{Ca,L}$, I_{Ks}, and I_{Cl} (see Table 62.1). Sympathetic hypoinnervation has been shown to increase the sensitivity of adrenergic receptors to activation by circulating catecholamines (*denervation supersensitivity*) (**eFig. 62.10**).

Numerous studies have suggested an important role of altered cardiac sympathetic innervation in arrhythmogenesis. Nerve growth factor (NGF) infusion into the left stellate ganglion in dogs with chronic MI causes spatially heterogeneous sympathetic cardiac hyperinnervation (nerve sprouting) and dramatically increases the incidence of SCD from ventricular tachyarrhythmias. Malignant ventricular arrhythmias are preceded by increased neuronal discharge. Explanted human hearts from transplant recipients with a history of arrhythmias exhibit greater and more heterogeneous expression of sympathetic nerve fibers versus patients without arrhythmias. In a canine model of heart failure with dyssynchronous ventricular contraction, cardiac resynchronization therapy (CRT) restored sympathovagal balance and reduced arrhythmogenic afterdepolarizations. In patients with congestive heart failure, sympathetic neural tone is upregulated, leading to adverse myocardial effects, including depletion of cardiac norepinephrine content, adverse cellular remodeling, tissue fibrosis and lethal arrhythmias, and arrhythmogenesis.[31] Neurotransmitter switching and transdifferentiation from catecholaminergic into cholinergic neurons occurs in the chronically failing heart.

The junctions between PVs and the left atrium are highly innervated. Sympathetic and parasympathetic nerves are colocalized and concentrated in "ganglionated plexuses" around the PVs. Selective ablation of ganglionated plexuses, as well as regional ablation targeting anatomic areas containing ganglionated plexuses, has been shown to prevent paroxysmal AF in some but not all clinical and experimental studies (**eFig. 62.11**).[32] Mutations in genes encoding cardiac ion channel subunits also affect channel function in the central and peripheral autonomic nervous system and thereby result in abnormal firing properties of affected neurons.[1] This observation may partially explain the clinical finding that SCD in some variants of LQTS (see Chapters 63 and 67)

is typically preceded by sympathetic arousal. Also, the antiarrhythmic efficacy of surgical left cardiac sympathetic denervation has previously been demonstrated in young patients with catecholaminergic polymorphic ventricular tachycardia (CPVT, see later). Thus the cardiac sympathetic nervous system provides a potentially useful target for treating patients at risk for clinical arrhythmias.[29] Overall, while there are some established indications for targeted autonomic-nerve manipulation in cardiac arrhythmias, the clear indications are limited and this is still an evolving area.

MECHANISMS OF ARRHYTHMOGENESIS

The mechanisms responsible for cardiac arrhythmias are generally divided into disorders of impulse formation, disorders of impulse conduction, or combinations of both (Table 62.3). In many cases, currently available diagnostic tools do not permit unequivocal determination of the electrophysiologic mechanisms responsible for many clinical arrhythmias. It is clinically difficult to separate microanatomic reentry from automaticity, and often one is left with the consideration that a particular arrhythmia is "most consistent with" or "best explained by" one or the other electrophysiologic mechanism. Some tachyarrhythmias can be started by one mechanism and perpetuated by another. This is particularly true of reentrant arrhythmias, which often require an initiating premature activation resulting from some type of abnormal impulse generation. Entrainment and the response to the creation of critical lines of block by ablation (e.g., for AV reentrant arrhythmias, atrial flutter, critical conduction channels for ventricular tachyarrhythmias) can identify arrhythmias caused by macroreentry (see later and Chapter 65).

Disorders of Impulse Formation

Disorders of impulse formation are characterized by an inappropriate discharge rate of the normal pacemaker, the SA node (e.g., sinus rates too fast or too slow for physiologic needs of patient), or discharge of an ectopic pacemaker that then controls the atrial or ventricular rhythm, either as an escape rhythm or accelerated automaticity. Pacemaker discharges from ectopic sites, often called *latent* or *subsidiary* pacemakers, can occur in fibers located in several parts of the atria, coronary sinus and PVs, AV valves, portions of the AV junction, and His-Purkinje system. Usually kept from reaching the level of threshold potential because of overdrive suppression by the more rapidly firing sinus node, ectopic pacemaker activity at one of these latent sites manifests when the SAN rate slows or block occurs between the SA node and the ectopic pacemaker site, permitting *escape* of the latent pacemaker at the latter's normal discharge rate. A clinical example would be sinus bradycardia to a rate of 45 beats/min that permits an AV junctional escape complex to occur at a rate of 50 beats/min.

The discharge rate of a latent pacemaker can accelerate inappropriately and usurp control of cardiac rhythm from the SA node, as may occur with a premature ventricular complex (PVC) or a burst of ventricular tachycardia (VT). Such disorders of impulse formation can be caused by alteration in a *normal* pacemaker mechanism (e.g., phase 4 diastolic depolarization that is physiologically normal for SA node or for ectopic site such as a Purkinje fiber, but occurs inappropriately fast or slow) or by a physiologically *abnormal* pacemaker mechanism.

A patient with persistent sinus tachycardia at rest or sinus bradycardia during exertion exhibits inappropriate SAN rates, but the underlying ionic mechanisms responsible can still be basically normal, with changes in the kinetics or magnitude of relevant currents underlying the abnormal rate. Conversely, when a patient experiences VT during acute MI, myocardial ischemia and infarction can depolarize normally non-automatic myocardial cells to membrane potentials at which inactivation of K^+-currents and activation of I_{CaL} cause automatic discharge.

Abnormal Automaticity

The mechanisms responsible for normal automaticity are described earlier (Phase 4: Diastolic Depolarization). Abnormal automaticity can arise from cells that have reduced maximum diastolic potentials, often at membrane potentials positive to –50 mV, in the activation range of both I_K and I_{CaL}. Automaticity at membrane potentials more negative than –70 mV may be caused by I_f. Electrotonic effects from surrounding normally polarized or more depolarized myocardium influence the development of automaticity.

Partial depolarization and failure to reach normal maximal diastolic potential can induce automatic discharges in most if not all cardiac fibers. Although this type of spontaneous automatic activity has been found in human atrial and ventricular fibers, its relationship

to the genesis of clinical arrhythmias has not been established. Abnormal automaticity in Purkinje cells can be caused by spontaneous, submembrane Ca^{2+} elevations through activation of calcium-sensitive membrane conductances, similar to processes identified in SA node myocytes. Rhythms resulting from abnormal automaticity may be slow atrial, junctional, or ventricular escape rhythms; certain types of atrial tachycardias (ATs) (e.g., those produced by digitalis or perhaps those coming from PVs); accelerated junctional (nonparoxysmal junctional tachycardia) and idioventricular rhythms (see Chapters 65 and 67).

Triggered Activity

Triggered activity is initiated by *afterdepolarizations*, which are depolarizing oscillations in membrane voltage induced by one or more preceding APs. Thus, triggered activity is related to *the consequences of a preceding impulse or series of impulses*, without which electrical quiescence occurs (Figs. 62.15 and 62.16). This triggering activity is not caused by an automatic self-generating mechanism, and the term "triggered automaticity" is therefore contradictory. Afterdepolarizations can occur before or after full repolarization of the fiber, termed *early afterdepolarizations* when they arise before full repolarization of the AP (Fig. 62.15C) or *delayed afterdepolarizations* (see Fig. 62.15B) when they occur after completion of repolarization (phase 4), at more negative membrane potentials than EADs. Not all afterdepolarizations reach the threshold potential, but those that do can trigger another afterdepolarization and thus self-perpetuate.

Delayed Afterdepolarizations

DADs and triggered activity have been demonstrated in Purkinje fibers, atrial and ventricular muscle cells in a wide range of experimental and clinical contexts (see Fig. 62.16). When fibers in the rabbit, canine, simian, and human mitral valves and in the canine tricuspid valve and coronary sinus are superfused with norepinephrine, they exhibit the capability for sustained, triggered rhythmic activity that may correspond to some forms of clinical tachyarrhythmia.

In vivo, atrial and ventricular arrhythmias caused by triggered activity have been reported in experimental models and in humans. Clinical arrhythmias likely due to DADs include some arrhythmias precipitated by digitalis, spontaneous atrial ectopic beats, and some cases of AF

TABLE 62.3 Mechanisms of Arrhythmias

DISORDER	EXPERIMENTAL EXAMPLES	CLINICAL EXAMPLES
Disorders of Impulse Formation		
Automaticity		
Normal automaticity	Normal in vivo or in vitro in SA nodal, AV nodal, and Purkinje cells	Sinus tachycardia or bradycardia inappropriate for the clinical situation; possibly ventricular parasystole
Abnormal automaticity	Depolarization-induced automaticity in Purkinje myocytes	Accelerated ventricular rhythms after myocardial infarction
Triggered Activity		
EADs	Drugs (sotalol, *N*-acetylprocainamide, terfenadine, erythromycin), cesium, barium, low $[K^+]_o$	Acquired LQTS and associated ventricular arrhythmias
DADs	Gain-of-function mutations in the gene encoding RyR2	Catecholaminergic polymorphic ventricular tachycardia; atrial ectopic beats
Disorders of Impulse Conduction		
Block and Reentry		
Bidirectional or unidirectional without reentry	SA, AV, bundle branch, Purkinje muscle	Sinoatrial, AV, bundle branch block
Unidirectional block with reentry	AV node, Purkinje-muscle junction, infarcted myocardium	Reciprocating tachycardia in Wolff-Parkinson-White syndrome, AV nodal reentry tachycardia, ventricular tachycardia caused by bundle branch reentry
Combined Disorders		
Interactions between automatic foci	Depolarizing or hyperpolarizing subthreshold stimuli speed or slow the automatic discharge rate	Modulated parasystole
Interactions between automaticity and conduction	Deceleration-dependent block, overdrive suppression of conduction, entrance and exit block	Similar to experimental

AV, Atrioventricular; *DADs,* delayed afterdepolarizations; *EADs,* early afterdepolarizations; *LQTS,* long-QT syndrome; *SA,* sinoatrial.

arising from DADs in PVs and arrhythmias caused by certain congenital arrhythmia syndromes (e.g., CPVT). The accelerated idioventricular rhythm and VTs 1 day after experimental canine MI may be caused by DADs, and certain specific VTs, such as those arising in the RV outflow tract, may be caused by DADs, whereas other data suggest that EADs are responsible.

Major Role of Intracellular Ca²⁺-Handling Abnormalities in Delayed Afterdepolarization Generation

It is well-recognized that DADs result from the activation of a calcium-sensitive inward current elicited by spontaneous increases in intracellular free calcium concentration due to aberrant diastolic Ca²⁺ release (see Fig. 62.16). Acquired or inherited abnormalities in the properties and/or function of the SR RyR2 calcium-release channels or SR calcium-binding proteins underlie spontaneous calcium-release events.

As discussed above, rapid mobilization of Ca²⁺ from the SR into the cytosol is mediated by the synchronous opening of RyRs. The cardiac RyR is composed of four equivalent subunits (homotetramer), each encoded by the *RYR2* gene. During cardiac systole, the small influx of calcium ions through L-type Cav channels triggers a massive release of Ca²⁺ from the SR via synchronous opening of RyR2 channels, a process called Ca²⁺-induced Ca²⁺ release (see Chapter 46). During diastole, RyR2 channels close and Ca²⁺ is recycled into the SR via calcium pumps, thereby refilling SR Ca²⁺ stores for the next release cycle. The duration and amplitude of Ca²⁺ efflux from the SR are therefore tightly controlled by the gating of RyR2 channels. RyR2 interacts with a number of accessory proteins to form a macromolecular Ca²⁺-release complex (**eFig. 62.12**). Proteins interact with RyR2 at multiple sites within the cytosolic domains of RyR2 and in the SR (e.g., calsequestrin, the major calcium-binding protein in the SR lumen). Among the cytosolic ligands, FKBP-12.6 (calstabin 2) has been implicated in stabilizing the closed state of the RyR2 channel and thus preventing diastolic Ca²⁺ leakage.[1]

Mutations in the human *RYR2* gene and in *CASQ2*, which encodes calsequestrin, have been linked to CPVT. Experimental studies have revealed that the *RYR2* and *CASQ2* mutations that underlie CPVT increase the sensitivity of the RyR2 channel to luminal Ca²⁺ activation.

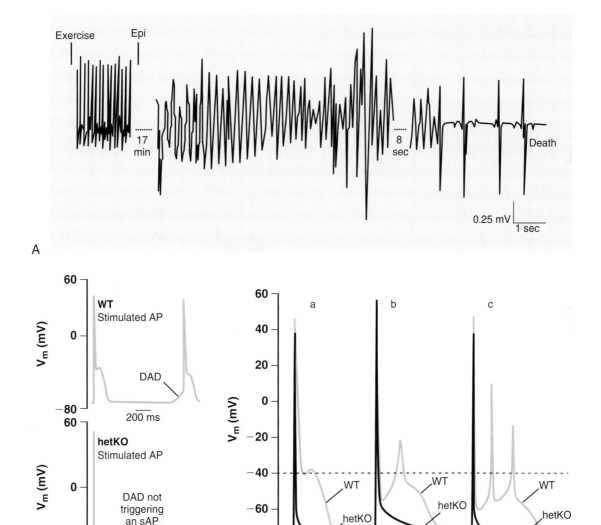

FIGURE 62.15 A, Electrocardiogram after exercise and administration of epinephrine in a mouse heterozygous for a loss-of-function mutation in the gene encoding ankyrin-B (AnkB⁻/⁺). Polymorphic ventricular tachycardia (torsades de pointes) occurred within about 17 minutes of epinephrine administration, followed by marked bradycardia and death 2 minutes after the arrhythmia. **B,** Impaired translation of delayed afterdepolarizations (DADs) into spontaneous action potentials (APs) in heterozygous knockout of Na⁺/Ca²⁺ exchanger (hetKO) versus wild-type (WT) exposed to isoproterenol and an arrhythmogenic pacing protocol. The first AP is initiated by current injection. The second AP in the **upper panel** is triggered by a DAD in the WT; it fails to generate an AP in the hetKO. **C,** Early afterdepolarizations (EADs) in WT and heterozygous knockout of Na⁺/Ca²⁺ exchanger. The EAD shape varied between low-amplitude, slow-transient membrane fluctuations (a), spike-like depolarizations (b), and steep upstrokes (c). (**A** from Mohler PJ, Schott JJ, Gramolini AO, et al. Ankyrin-B mutation causes type 4 long-QT cardiac arrhythmia and sudden cardiac death. *Nature.* 2003;421:634; **B** and **C** from American Heart Association; Bögeholz N, Pauls P, Bauer BK, et al. Suppression of early and late afterdepolarizations by heterozygous knockout of the Na⁺/Ca²⁺ exchanger in a murine model. *Circ Arrhythm Electrophysiol.* 2015;8:1210.)

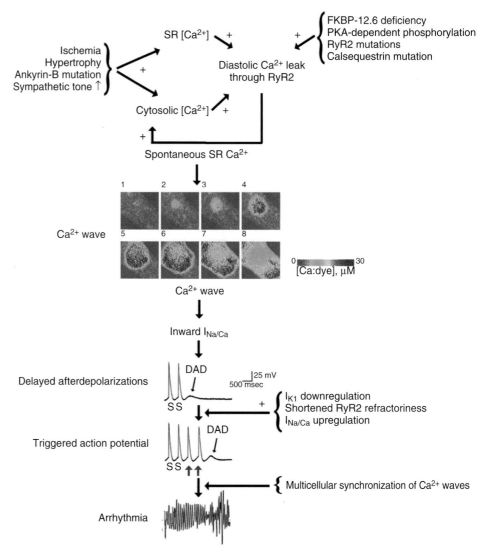

FIGURE 62.16 Proposed sequence of events leading to delayed afterdepolarizations (DADs) and triggered tachyarrhythmia. **Top panel,** Congenital (e.g., gain-of-function mutations in the *RYR2* or *CASQ2* genes) or acquired (e.g., ischemia, hypertrophy, increased sympathetic tone, heart failure) factors will cause a diastolic Ca^{2+} leak through RyR2 that results in localized and transient increases in [Ca^{2+}]$_i$ in cardiomyocytes. **Middle panel,** Representative series of images showing changes in [Ca^{2+}]$_i$ during a Ca^{2+} wave in a single cardiomyocyte loaded with a Ca^{2+}-sensitive fluorescent dye. Images were obtained at 117-msec intervals. Focally elevated Ca^{2+} (*frame 2*) diffuses to the adjacent junctional sarcoplasmic reticulum (SR), where it initiates more Ca^{2+} release events that result in a propagating Ca^{2+} wave (*frames 3 to 8*). **Bottom panel,** The Ca^{2+} wave, through activation of inward I$_{Na/Ca}$, will depolarize the cardiomyocyte (DAD). If of sufficient magnitude to overcome the source-sink mismatch, the DAD will depolarize the cardiomyocyte above threshold and result in a single or repetitive premature activations (*red arrows*), which can trigger an arrhythmia. Downregulation of the inwardly rectifying potassium current (I$_{K1}$), upregulation of I$_{Na/Ca}$, and shortened Ca^{2+} signaling refractoriness because of ryanodine receptor phosphorylation and/or oxidation can promote the generation of DAD-triggered action potentials. *S*, Stimulus. (Modified from Rubart M, Zipes DP. Mechanisms of sudden cardiac death. *J Clin Invest.* 2005;115:2305. With permission from the Journal of Clinical Investigation.)

Thus, increased catecholamine release due to adrenergic stimulation (e.g., from emotional or physical stress), which increases SR Ca^{2+} stores and phosphorylates RyR2 (increasing its Ca^{2+} sensitivity further), enhances the propensity for spontaneous, diastolic SR Ca^{2+} release and DAD-triggered arrhythmias (accounting for the "C" in CPVT). The regulatory protein FKBP-12.6 appears to inhibit RyR2 sensitivity and Ca^{2+} release. Reduced FKBP-12.6 binding caused by PKA–mediated RyR2 hyperphosphorylation has been implicated in cardiac arrhythmogenesis associated with heart failure. Polymorphic VT, as well as inducible AF, develop in FKBP-12.6–deficient mice on adrenergic stimulation. Treatment with the 1,4-benzothiazepine derivatives JTV519 and S107, which restore FKBP-12.6 affinity for RyR2, has been shown to suppress CPVT in FKBP-12.6–deficient mice, although these agents also have other potential antiarrhythmic actions.[1] Purkinje myocytes isolated from mice heterozygous for a CPVT-causing mutation in *RyR2* are more susceptible to arrhythmogenic Ca^{2+}-handling abnormalities than nonmutant cardiomyocytes, and Purkinje cells appear to be more prone to developing arrhythmogenic afterdepolarizations than working ventricular myocytes.[33]

The IP$_3$ receptor (IP3R) is another Ca^{2+}-release channel in cardiomyocytes that is activated by binding of the second messenger IP$_3$ and cytosolic Ca^{2+}. The IP3R exists as a homotetramer or heterotetramer, each subunit encoded by the *ITPR1*, *ITPR2*, or *ITPR3* gene (**eFig. 62.13**). The type 2 IP3R is the predominant subtype in atrial myocytes, where they are located near RyR2 channels at the SR Ca^{2+}-release sites and contribute to altered excitation-contraction coupling and arrhythmogenesis in the atria. In Purkinje myocytes, type 1 IP3Rs colocalize with type 3 RyR in the subsarcolemmal space to form a functional dyad that regulates electrical excitability. IP$_3$-dependent Ca signaling has been implicated in cardiac arrhythmias due to ischemia and reperfusion injury,

inflammation, and cardiac failure. IP3Rs are upregulated in heart failure and AF.[1] In atrial and Purkinje myocytes, IP$_3$ causes spontaneous [Ca^{2+}]$_i$ transients, Ca^{2+} waves, and Ca^{2+} alternans and facilitates the generation of afterdepolarizations. Recent work suggests that perinuclear IP$_3$R upregulation in AF may enhance nuclear Ca^{2+} load and contribute the gene-reprogramming associated with AF-related remodeling.[34]

The cascade of events linking cellular Ca^{2+}-handling abnormalities to cardiac arrhythmias is illustrated in Figure 62.16. Ca^{2+} leak via RyR2 during diastole gives rise to localized increases in cytosolic calcium concentrations in single cardiomyocytes. Since RyR2 release occurs in response to a critical level of Ca^{2+}, RyR2 leak may occur because of increased RyR2 sensitivity or increased Ca^{2+} load. When large enough, the focally elevated Ca^{2+} resulting from RyR2 release causes a propagating Ca^{2+} wave that depolarizes the cardiomyocyte membrane and triggers a DAD through activation of the inward Na$^+$/Ca^{2+} exchange current (I$_{Na/Ca}$) which handles the increased Ca^{2+}. Calmodulin kinase type-II (CaMKII) is a key player in promoting DADs, via phosphorylation of multiple membrane proteins, in particular RyR2 which, when CaMKII-phosphorylated shows enhanced sensitivity to Ca^{2+}. CaMKII inhibition suppresses arrhythmogenic DADs and may provide a strategy for new therapeutic development.[35,36] Because intracellular Na$^+$ is exchanged for Ca^{2+}, drugs that reduce I$_{Na}$ suppress Na$^+$ load and, indirectly, Ca^{2+} load, NCX current, and DADs. DADs likely play a causative role in arrhythmogenesis in the failing heart, where enhanced CaMKII activity, upregulation of I$_{Na/Ca}$, and downregulation of the inward rectifier K$^+$ current I$_{K1}$, facilitate DAD generation.[37]

Short coupling intervals and pacing at rates more rapid than the triggered activity rate (*overdrive pacing*) increase the amplitude and shorten the cycle length of DADs after cessation of pacing (*overdrive acceleration*), because they enhance cellular Ca^{2+} loading. The clinical implication is that tachyarrhythmias caused by DAD-triggered activity may not be suppressed easily or indeed may be precipitated by rapid rates, either spontaneously, as with sinus tachycardia, or induced by pacing. Because a single premature stimulus can theoretically both initiate and terminate triggered activity, differentiation from reentry (see later) becomes difficult.

Early Afterdepolarizations

Various interventions can cause EADs, with most of them delaying repolarization. The sentinel finding in clinically identifiable EAD-associated syndromes is thus prolongation of the electrocardiographic QT interval, the macroscopic manifestation of cellular APD prolongation. EADs almost certainly play a central role in the tachyarrhythmias seen in the acquired and congenital forms of LQTS (see Fig. 62.15 and Chapters 63 and 67).

Long-QT Syndrome

Patients with heritable LQTS have an abnormally prolonged ventricular APD and are at increased risk of SCD from ventricular tachyarrhythmias (see Chapters 63 and 67). When the AP is excessively prolonged, the membrane potential remains at levels that allow recovery of enough steady-state Ca^{2+} (particularly during phase 2) or Na^+ (during phase 3) current to depolarize the cell, producing an EAD. It appears that, because of their longer APD and unique Ca^{2+} handling properties, Purkinje cells are particularly sensitive to EAD-inducing interventions.[33,38] Purkinje cell EADs raise to threshold adjacent ventricular muscle cells that have already repolarized, producing an unstimulated extrasystole. This activation can initiate tachyarrhythmias either by the induction of unstable transmural reentry or via repetitive rapid EADs inducing repetitive ventricular beats in rapid succession. Transmural variation in APD can produce substantial repolarization gradients, particularly under EAD-promoting conditions, creating favorable conditions for reentry in which functional conduction block within the ventricular wall plays an important role.

While DADs and EADs clearly have different features and occur under different conditions, both centrally involve cell Ca^{2+} homeostasis and abnormal Ca^{2+} dynamics are central to both. APD is a major determinant of Ca^{2+} entry; EAD-associated APD prolongation increases Ca^{2+} influx through L-type Ca^{2+} channels and produces Ca^{2+} loading in the SR, thus increasing the likelihood of DAD generation. Thus, EADs and DADs may occur together with common initiating conditions.[39]

Genetically modified mice have been used extensively to model congenital arrhythmogenic disorders, including LQTS. While for some LQTS forms the ionic derangements show similar physiology in mice and men (e.g., I_{Na} inactivation deficiencies responsible for LQT3), for others (particularly delayed-rectifier K^+ channel abnormalities), the mouse APD does not share the same determinants with human. The ability to generate patient-specific human iPSCs offers a new paradigm for modeling human disease. These have been used extensively to model and study mechanisms of LQTS.[40] For example, a Medline search with the term "iPSC cardiomyocytes long QT syndrome" identified 169 papers (as of April 2021). Cardiomyocytes differentiated from iPSC cells of LQTS patients recapitulate the disease phenotype in vitro, including marked APD prolongation and increased susceptibility to spontaneous or pharmacologically induced triggered activity. A study of cardiomyocytes derived from LQTS patient–specific iPSCs is summarized in **eFigure 62.14**. Large-scale production of human iPSC–derived cardiomyocytes has made it possible to generate sufficient numbers of uniform cardiac monolayers and higher-order three-dimensional models that can be used for the study of arrhythmia mechanisms in vitro.[41] Collectively, pluripotent stem cell technology now offers a unique platform to evaluate patient-specific arrhythmia mechanisms, to evaluate and optimize patient therapy and for high-throughput screens for drug proarrhythmic effects.[42]

Experimental observations have also suggested an important role of transmural or longitudinal heterogeneity of repolarization. Marked transmural dispersion of repolarization can create a vulnerable window for the development of reentry. Direct experimental evidence of the existence of transmural dispersion in the AP has been provided for the human heart. Normal hearts showed midmyocardial islands of cells that had distinctly long APDs with steep local APD gradients. In contrast, failing hearts were observed to have significantly reduced transmural repolarization gradients and to lack islands of cells with delayed repolarization. The ionic mechanisms underlying transmural dispersion of repolarization in the human heart likely include spatial variations in expression of the transient outward potassium current I_{to} and the delayed rectifier potassium current I_{Ks} (see Table 62.1).[1,43]

Sympathetic stimulation can increase EAD amplitude to provoke ventricular tachyarrhythmias. Beta-adrenergic stimulation produces a balanced increase in inward (especially $I_{Ca,L}$) and outward (I_{Ks}) currents. In LQT1, the I_{Ks} alpha subunit is defective and adrenergic stimulation causes an unopposed increase in depolarizing current, potentially producing important APD prolongation and EADs. LQT1 patients are particularly prone to adrenergic provocation of ventricular arrhythmias and tend to respond well to beta-adrenoceptor blockers.

Acquired LQTS and torsades de pointes from class III antiarrhythmic drugs like quinidine, sotalol, or dofetilide and a host of non-cardiac agents like cisapride, erythromycin, moxifloxacin, and psychoactive drugs, likely mediated by EADs (see Chapters 9 and 64).[44] Almost all of these drugs block I_{Kr} - the hERG alpha-subunit that has a large inner vestibule which easily accommodates many drugs that have HERG-block as an off-target effect.[45] Screening for hERG block and potential QT - prolongation are thus now an important part of the preclinical toxicology screen for most new drugs.[46] The problem is compounded by the idiosyncratic nature of the proarrhythmic effect, related in large measure to genetically determined "repolarization reserve." In addition, drugs may additively prolong APD and provoke EADs/torsades de pointes. In addition, drug interactions at the level of hepatic metabolism or (less commonly) renal excretion may increase the concentration of an at-risk compound.[47]

Disorders of Impulse Conduction

Conduction delay and block can result in bradyarrhythmias or tachyarrhythmias. Bradyarrhythmias occur when the propagating impulse is blocked and is followed by asystole or a slower escape rhythm; tachyarrhythmias occur when the delay and block produce reentrant excitation (see later, Reentry). Various factors involving both active and passive membrane properties determine the CV and successful propagation of an impulse. These factors include the stimulating efficacy of the propagating impulse, which is related to the amplitude and rate of rise of phase 0 (an indicator of the size of the activating phase 0 inward current); the excitability of the tissue into which the impulse is conducted; and the geometry of the tissue.

DECELERATION-DEPENDENT BLOCK
Diastolic depolarization has been suggested as a cause of conduction block at slow rates, so-called bradycardia- or deceleration-dependent block (see Chapter 68). However, excitability and the speed of impulse propagation increase as the membrane depolarizes until approximately −70 mV despite a reduction in AP amplitude (supernormal conduction). This type of block has also been referred to as "phase 4 block," but experiments in Purkinje fiber bundles have demonstrated that diastolic (phase 4) depolarization is not a necessary condition for the occurrence of deceleration-dependent block. Evidently, depolarization-induced inactivation of fast Na^+ channels is offset by other factors, such as a reduction in the difference between membrane potential and threshold potential and an increase in membrane excitability.

TACHYCARDIA-DEPENDENT BLOCK
More often, impulses are blocked at rapid rates or short cycle lengths as a result of incomplete recovery of refractoriness (postrepolarization refractoriness) caused by incomplete time- or voltage-dependent recovery of excitability. For example, such incomplete recovery is the usual mechanism responsible for a nonconducted premature P wave or one that conducts with a functional bundle branch block.

DECREMENTAL CONDUCTION
"Decremental conduction" refers to the phenomenon whereby an impulse with a low safety factor loses activation effectiveness as it spreads anterogradely. This property is most typically seen in the AV node, in relation to the relatively small amplitude of phase 0 Ca^{2+}

FIGURE 62.17 **Reentry and entrainment. A** to **E,** Criteria for entrainment exemplified in a case of postinfarction ventricular tachycardia (VT). **A,** *left,* Two leads of the ECG of a VT and intracardiac recordings from a mapping catheter (Map) at a left ventricular site critical for VT continuation, as well as from the right ventricular apex (RV). Note the diastolic potential *(red arrowhead)* during VT. Recordings are similarly arranged in all subsequent panels. **A,** *right,* RV pacing in the setting of sinus rhythm. **B,** RV pacing at a cycle length (CL) slightly shorter than VT produces a QRS complex that is a blend between fully VT and fully paced ("fusion") complexes. All recordings are accelerated to the paced CL, and after pacing ceases, the same VT resumes. Each fused QRS complex is identical, and the last beat is entrained, but surface fusion is absent. **C** and **D,** The same phenomena, but at shorter-paced CLs. Note that the fused QRS complex appears to be more similar to pacing than to VT as the pacing CL shortens. **B** to **D,** Progressive degrees of fusion on ECG. Map recording of **B, C,** and **D** also shows a progression of fusion, with both the morphology and timing of a portion of the electrogram changing with faster pacing. **E,** Finally, an even shorter-paced CL results in a sudden change in both map electrogram (block in small diastolic potential, *red arrowhead)* and surface ECG, which is now fully paced. When pacing ceases, VT has been interrupted. **F,** Diagrammatic representation of the reentrant circuit during spontaneous atrial flutter (AFL) and transient entrainment of the AFL. **Left,** Reentrant circuit during spontaneous type I AFL; *f* = circulating wavefront of the AFL. **Center,** Introduction of the first pacing impulse (X) during rapid pacing from a high atrial site during AFL. The *black arrowhead* indicates entry of the pacing impulse into the reentrant circuit, where it is conducted orthodromically (Ortho) and antidromically (Anti). The antidromic wavefront of the pacing impulse (X) collides with the previous beat, in this case the circulating wavefront of the spontaneous AFL *(f),* which results in an atrial fusion beat and, in effect, terminates the AFL. However, the orthodromic wavefront from the pacing impulse (X) continues the tachycardia and resets it to the pacing rate. **Right,** Introduction of the next pacing impulse (X + 1) during rapid pacing from the same high atrial site. The *black arrowhead* again indicates entry of the pacing impulse into the reentrant circuit, where it is conducted orthodromically and antidromically. Once again, the antidromic wavefront from the pacing impulse (X + 1) collides with the orthodromic wavefront of the previous beat. In this case, it is the orthodromic wavefront of the previous paced beat (X), and an atrial fusion beat results. The orthodromic wavefront from the pacing impulse (X + 1) continues the tachycardia and resets it to the pacing rate. In all three parts, *arrows* indicate the direction of spread of the impulses; the *serpentine line* indicates slow conduction through a presumed area of slow conduction *(stippled region)* in the reentrant circuit. (**A** to **E** from Zipes DP. A century of cardiac arrhythmia: in search of Jason's golden fleece. *J Am Coll Cardiol.* 1999;34:959; **F** from Waldo AL. Atrial flutter: entrainment characteristics. *J Cardiovasc Electrophysiol.* 1997;8:337.)

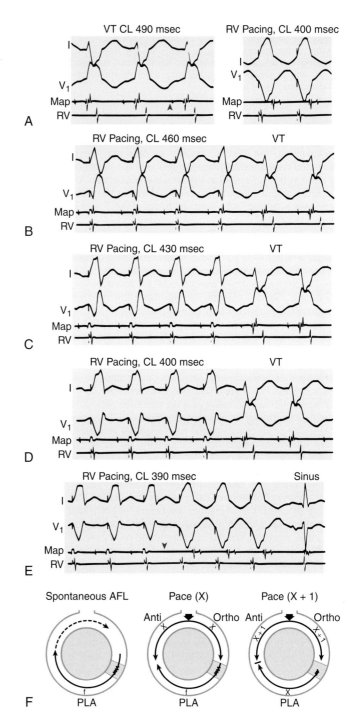

current in slow channel tissue, especially at fast rates and in the presence of disease. It is also a feature of diseased tissue with conduction impairment due to cell death, fibrosis, and/or reduced phase 0 activating current. Decremental conduction is associated with increased risk of conduction block.

REENTRY

During the normal cardiac cycle, activation begins in the SAN pacemaker and continues until the entire heart has been activated. The cardiac impulse stops propagating when all fibers have been discharged and are completely refractory. During this absolute RP, the cardiac impulse has "no place to go." Activation is then reinitiated by the next sinus impulse. If, however, a group of fibers not activated during the initial wave of depolarization recovers excitability in time to be reactivated before the impulse dies out, the fibers may serve as a link to reexcite areas that were just discharged and have now recovered from the initial depolarization. Such a process has been given various names—reentry, reentrant excitation, circus movement, reciprocal or echo beat, and reciprocating tachycardia—and all have approximately the same meaning.

ENTRAINMENT

Entraining a tachycardia (i.e., increasing the rate of the tachycardia through capture of the reentry circuit by pacing),[48] with resumption of the intrinsic rate of the tachycardia when pacing is stopped, is a clinically accessible way to establish the presence of reentry (Fig. 62.17A). Entrainment represents capture or continuous resetting of the tachycardia by the pacing-induced activation. Each pacing stimulus creates a wavefront that travels in an anterograde direction (orthodromic) and resets the tachycardia to the pacing rate. A wavefront propagating retrogradely in the opposite direction (antidromic) collides with the orthodromic wavefront of the previous beat. In the clinical example shown in Figure 62.17, as the RV pacing rate is increased, the paced QRS morphology (Fig. 62.17B–D) changes, the result of more of the tachycardia circuit being captured by the anterograde activation wave, yet when pacing is stopped, the tachycardia is still present; this is referred to as *progressive fusion*. These wavefront interactions create electrocardiographic and electrophysiologic features that can be explained only by reentry. Therefore, the demonstration of

entrainment can be used to prove the reentrant mechanism of a clinical tachycardia and form the basis for localizing the pathway traveled by the tachycardia wavefront. Such localization can be useful to guide ablation therapy.

Anatomic Reentry

Anatomic reentry inspired the first conceptual models of reentry.[48] In anatomic reentry, there is a discrete anatomical barrier separating alternate conduction pathways, and allowing reentry to be initiated and maintained. A conceptual model presented as a schematic of the occurrence of anatomic reentry with the required conditions is shown in Figure 62.18. In many individuals, the AV node behaves as if there are two functionally independent pathways with common connections at top and bottom, but longitudinally dissociated in between. Typically, the pathway with the faster conduction has a longer RP. Both pathways have RPs much shorter than the SAN cycle

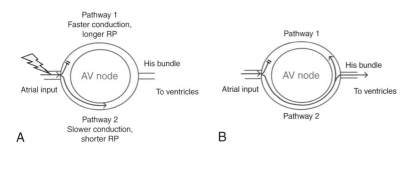

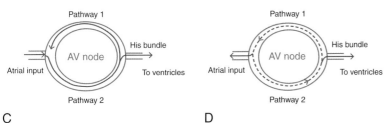

FIGURE 62.18 Schematic of reentry in the AV node (AVN). Differences in conduction and refractoriness in the fast (1) and slow (2) pathways permit reentry to occur. **A,** Activation of the AVN from the atrium with block in the fast, longer refractory period pathway with conduction down the slow pathway. **B,** Activation of the His bundle and ventricle from the slow pathway with the activation wave retrogradely activating the fast pathway. **C,** Atrial activation from the AVN over the fast pathway with a short time from ventricular (QRS) to atrial (retrograde P) activation. **D,** Typical AV node reentry tachycardia circuit.

length, so a premature beat is required in order to engage the AV node during the RP of either pathway. Figure 62.18A illustrates a premature beat arriving during the RP of the fast pathway (here designated Pathway 1) but after the shorter-RP pathway (Pathway 2) has recovered excitability. The impulse then travels antegradely down Pathway 2 to the His bundle entrance, conducting via the His bundle to the ventricles (Fig. 62.18B). If the distal end of Pathway 1 has now had time to recover, the impulse will propagate retrogradely up Pathway 1 (Fig 62.18C). If the circuit time (the time to leave each point in the circuit and get back to the initial point of reference) is longer than the RP of Pathway 2, it will now be reexcited in the antegrade direction and the process can continue indefinitely (Fig 62.18D) if the conditions are right. The key determinants are: (1) alternative conducting pathways separated longitudinally but with connections at each end; (2) different RPs of the alternate pathways allowing for block of a premature beat in one pathway; and (3) a circuit time longer than the longest RO in the pathway.

A realistic example of AV nodal reentry using different pathways is illustrated in Figure 62.19. Because the two pathways have different electrophysiologic properties (e.g., shorter RP and slower conduction in one pathway versus a longer RP and faster conduction in the other), the impulse is first blocked anterogradely in the fast pathway with the longer RP and then propagates slowly in the adjacent slow pathway, whose RP is shorter (Fig. 62.19A). If conduction in this alternative route is sufficiently slow, the propagating impulse finds tissue that has recovered from refractoriness throughout its circuit, exciting tissue beyond the blocked pathway and returning in the reverse direction along the pathway initially blocked (Fig. 62.19B). A clinical arrhythmia caused by anatomic reentry is most likely to have a monomorphic morphology on ECG (**Video 62.2**). For anatomic reentry to occur, the time for conduction within the depressed but unblocked area and for excitation of the distal segments must exceed the RP of the initially blocked pathway and the tissue proximal to the site of block.

CONDITIONS FOR ANATOMIC REENTRY
The length of the pathway is fixed and determined by the anatomy. Conditions that depress CV or abbreviate the RP promote the development of reentry in this model, whereas prolonging refractoriness and

speeding CV hinder it. The maintenance of anatomic reentry requires the existence of an "excitable gap," a region ahead of the reentrant wavefront that has recovered excitability and is available for re-excitation. Conceptually, the distance traveled by the impulse in one RP is the minimum distance that can support reentry with anatomical reentry. This distance, termed the reentrant wavelength (λ) is equal to the minimum circuit time (the RP) multiplied by the mean CV. The actual length of the pathway minus λ gives the length of the excitable gap.

In reentrant circuits with an excitable gap, CV determines the revolution time of the impulse around the circuit and therefore the rate of the tachycardia. Prolongation of refractoriness does not influence the revolution time around the circuit or the rate of the tachycardia, with the rare exception when the revolution exactly equals the RP and makes the impulse propagate in relatively refractory tissue. Anatomic reentry occurs in patients with Wolff-Parkinson-White (WPW) syndrome (Fig. 62.20), in AV nodal reentry, in some atrial flutters, and in some VTs.

Functional Reentry
Functional reentry lacks confining anatomic boundaries and can occur in contiguous fibers that exhibit functionally different electrophysiologic properties caused by local differences in transmembrane AP, APD, or other determinants of excitability. Dispersion of excitability, refractoriness, or both, as well as anisotropic distributions of intercellular resistance, permit initiation and maintenance of reentry. Functional heterogeneities in the electrophysiologic properties of the myocardium have been shown to contribute to the generation and maintenance of tachycardia and fibrillation. These heterogeneities can be fixed, as in the case of spatial redistribution of gap junctions in the failing heart or infarct border zone, or with spatial gradients in the magnitude of the background K+ current I_{K1}. They can also change dynamically, as in an acutely ischemic myocardium or in the presence of dynamic autonomic tone changes that influence RP in a spatially heterogeneous way (e.g., vagal AF).

An important concept in understanding functional reentry is that of a spiral wave rotor.[49] The development of functional block along a line of tissue causes the impulse to circulate around the initial zone of block. The pattern of propagation is often represented as a circle or ellipse, but its shape depends on underlying tissue properties, anisotropy, and heterogeneity. A schematic of such a system is shown in Figure 62.21A. The reentrant wavefront (shown by a solid red curve) has a curvature that is greatest near the center of the wave, and gradually decreases at portions of the front progressively further from the core. Behind the propagating wavefront, there is a zone of refractory tissue that ends at the dashed red curve, with the tissue inside the dashed border having recovered excitability. Where the curvature is relatively flat (see brown box and insert), the propagating wavefront stimulates a region of tissue in front of it that is about the same size as the wavefront. As the curvature increases (black box), the emanating wavefront has to activate much larger regions of tissue relative to the source wavefront. At the center of the spiral is a zone where the curvature is so great that the source-sink mismatch causes failure of activation. This zone creates a "core" of excitable but non-excited tissue. If the properties of the tissue are such that the recirculating "rotor" can continue uninterrupted, the resulting stable rotor will cause a sustained tachycardia. An example of such a reentrant wave in simulated 2-dimensional tissue is shown in Figure 62.21B. If there are multiple unsynchronized rotors, or a single rotor with a variable tissue response with irregular propagation patterns, fibrillation results. Fibrillatory activity can be maintained by highly unstable rotors, providing their rate of formation is greater or equal to their rate of destruction.

The detection of rotors in tissue can be facilitated by the use of "phase mapping," which defines the activation at each point in space relative to the phase in an activation cycle in which it occurs.[49] At the inner tip of the activation wavefront, there is a location at which all phases meet, called a "phase singularity" (PS). Identifying and following the PS trajectory over time is useful to keep track

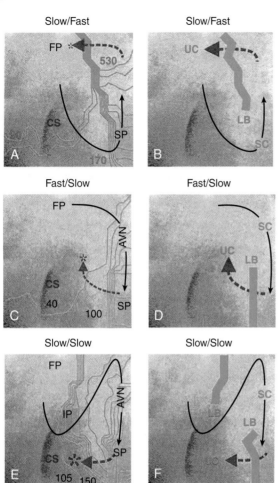

FIGURE 62.19 Reentrant circuits of different types of atrioventricular nodal reentrant tachycardia (AVNRT). Pictures of the optical activation maps of A₂ stimuli obtained from three different experiments at A₂ coupling intervals of 190, 220, and 190 milliseconds, respectively, were merged with the pictures of the mapping area to show the initiation of echo beats in **A** (Slow/Fast), **C** (Fast/Slow), and **E** (Slow/Slow) circuits. The numbers on the maps indicate the activation times in reference to the A₂ stimulus. The *black arrow* indicates anterograde conduction, and the *asterisk* and the *dashed red arrow* represent the site of earliest retrograde atrial activation. The corresponding locations of the lines of block (LB, *green*), slow anterograde conduction (SC, *black arrow*), and unidirectional conduction (UC, *red*) are shown in **B, D,** and **F,** respectively. CS, Coronary sinus; FP, fast pathway; IP, intermediate pathway; SP, slow pathway. (From Wu J, Zipes DP. Mechanisms underlying atrioventricular nodal conduction and the reentrant circuit of atrioventricular nodal reentrant tachycardia using optical mapping. *J Cardiovasc Electrophysiol.* 2002;13:831.)

of complex, often short-lived rotors. Sophisticated mapping studies have revealed reentrant rotors in a wide range of experimental and clinical arrhythmias, including VT and atrial and ventricular fibrillation.[50]

Specific Arrhythmias Illustrating Mechanistic Principles

Other chapters in this book deal with various forms of specific arrhythmias including supraventricular and VTs, flutter, and fibrillation (see Chapters 65 and 67). We will discuss a variety of arrhythmias here focused on their mechanistic properties to illustrate the basic principles of electrophysiology and arrhythmogenesis discussed in the present chapter.

Atrial Flutter

Reentry is the most likely cause of the usual form of atrial flutter, with the reentrant circuit being confined to the right atrium in typical atrial flutter, where it usually travels counterclockwise in a caudocranial direction in the interatrial septum and in a craniocaudal

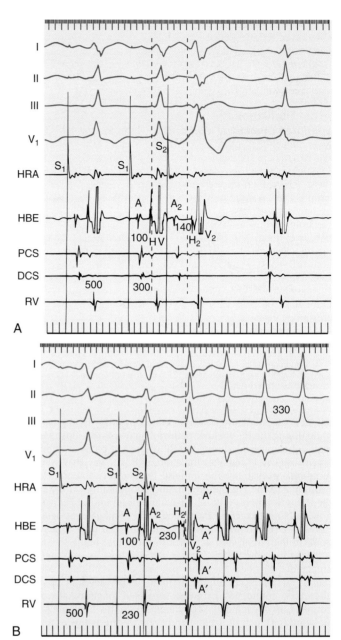

FIGURE 62.20 A, Wolff-Parkinson-White syndrome. Following high right atrial pacing at a cycle length of 500 milliseconds (S₁–S₁), premature stimulation at a coupling interval of 300 milliseconds (S₁–S₂) produces physiologic delay in AV nodal conduction, which results in an increase in the A-H interval from 100 to 140 milliseconds but no delay in the AV interval. Consequently, activation of the His bundle follows activation of the QRS complex (*second interrupted line*), and the QRS complex becomes more anomalous in appearance because of increased ventricular activation over the accessory pathway. **B,** Induction of reciprocating AV tachycardia. Premature stimulation at a coupling interval of 230 milliseconds prolongs the A₂–H₂ interval to 230 milliseconds and results in anterograde block in the accessory pathway and normalization of the QRS complex (a slight functional aberrancy in the nature of incomplete right bundle branch block occurs). Note that H₂ precedes onset of the QRS complex (*interrupted line*). Following V₂, the atria are excited retrogradely (A′) beginning in the distal coronary sinus, followed by atrial activation in leads recording from the proximal coronary sinus, His bundle, and high right atrium. A supraventricular tachycardia is initiated at a cycle length of 330 milliseconds. I, II, III, and V₁ indicate scalar electrocardiographic leads. A, H–V, atrial, His bundle, and ventricular activation during the drive train; A₂, H₂,V₂, atrial, His bundle, and ventricular activation during the premature stimulus; DCS, distal coronary sinus electrogram; HBE, His bundle electrogram; HRA, high right atrium; PCS, proximal coronary sinus electrogram; RV, right ventricular electrogram. Timelines are in 50- and 10-millisecond intervals. S₁, Stimulus of the drive train; S₂, premature stimulus. (From Zipes DP, Mahomed Y, King RD, et al. Wolff-Parkinson-White syndrome: cryosurgical treatment. *Indiana Med.* 1986;89:432.)

direction in the right atrial free wall. An area of slow conduction is present in the posterolateral to posteromedial inferior area of the right atrium, along with a central area of block that can include an anatomic (IVC) and functional component. This area of slow conduction is rather constant and represents the site of successful ablation of typical atrial flutter. Ablation results are consistent with a macroreentry circuit.

Different reentrant circuits exist in patients with other types of atrial flutter, such as those that occur after surgery or ablation or that are associated with an atrial septal defect (see Chapter 82).

Atrial Fibrillation
Spatiotemporal Organization and Focal Discharge
AF is characterized by rapid irregular atrial activity. The classical theory is that of multiple disorganized reentrant waves, encapsulated by Moe's "multiple-wavelet hypothesis," but a variety of competing theories and ideas of AF pathophysiology have emerged (see Chapter 66).[49,51] While atrial activation during AF appears to be random, there is in fact an underlying organization, likely related to both discrete determining electrophysiological characteristics and non-random sources. The activity of underlying sources may be reflected in dominant frequencies of activation in spectral analyses of recordings of atrial electrical activity. The notion that a single or small number of underlying focal or rotor sources underlie AF and may be susceptible to targeted ablation is a very attractive idea. There is extensive evidence that the PVs are particularly prone to host both focal and reentrant sources, and PV ablation is the single most effective procedure for AF management.[52] The localization of sources in other regions, which seem to be increasingly important as AF becomes more persistent and enduring, has proved difficult and is the object of extensive ongoing technological, scientific, and clinical investigation.[53]

Several experimental models have been used to study the structural and basic electrophysiologic properties of PVs that are thought to play a role in initiation and maintenance of AF. Morphologic studies have demonstrated the presence of complex anatomic structures and phenotypically different cardiomyocytes in PVs.[1,54] Electrophysiologic studies have shown that both reentrant and nonreentrant mechanisms (automaticity and triggered activity) may underlie initiation of AF from the PVs.

ION CHANNEL ABNORMALITIES IN ATRIAL FIBRILLATION
Monogenic (Familial) Atrial Fibrillation
Although familial forms of AF are relatively rare, identification of mutations in AF kindreds has provided valuable insight into the molecular pathways underlying the arrhythmia. Most mutations linked to familial AF have been located in genes that encode sodium or potassium channel subunits. Functional analyses of these mutations have revealed either gain-of-function or loss-of-function effects. Mutations in genes encoding pore-forming alpha or auxiliary beta subunits of the delayed rectifier potassium channel and the voltage-gated sodium channel (I_{Ks} and I_{Na}, respectively; see Table 62.1) have been reported in familial AF. The mechanisms by which these mutations cause AF are not fully understood. Gain-of-function mutations in I_{Ks} give rise to increased repolarizing currents, which then shorten the APD and atrial refractoriness, thereby facilitating fibrillatory activity. An augmented inward sodium current can increase excitability and promote triggered activity. Conversely, a reduced inward sodium current might promote reentry by favoring block and the initiation of reentry. Other potassium channel mutations in the KCNJ2 and KCNA5 genes, which encode the inward rectifier and ultrarapid delayed rectifier potassium current, respectively, have been associated with AF (see Table 62.1). Finally, mutations in the GJA5 gene, which encodes the gap junction channel subunit connexin 40, have been linked to familial AF. Abnormal intercellular electrical coupling can produce conduction heterogeneity, localized block, and facilitated reentry.

Polygenic Factors in Atrial Fibrillation
A significant portion of AF risk is heritable. Genome-wide association studies (GWAS) have identified variations in multiple genomic regions that are associated with lone AF. These regions encode ion channels (e.g., calcium-activated potassium channel gene KCNN3, HCN channel gene HCN4), transcription factors related to cardiopulmonary development (e.g., homeodomain transcription factor PRRX1), and cell-signaling molecules (e.g., CAV1, a cellular membrane protein involved in signal transduction). The mechanistic links between these genetic variations and susceptibility to AF remain to be determined.[55] Only a small percentage of the AF risk can be attributed to known gene polymorphisms; a

more expansive approach combining GWAS, whole blood epigenome-wide association, and transcriptome-wide association reveals almost 2000 genes linked to AF and accounts for about three times as much (about 10% vs. 3%) of the AF risk.[56] Nevertheless, there are still major risk determinants outside present genetically identified factors. With the rapid technologic development of genetic approaches and the creation of ever-larger merged databases, the identification of genetic factors underlying AF will certainly progress; however, since genetics account for only a portion of AF risk and disease factors like hypertension, heart disease, diabetes, and toxins (cigarette smoke, environmental pollution, etc.) are also major determinants there will likely be a limit to how much insight into AF risk genetic studies can provide.

A number of studies have probed the primary role of abnormalities in ion channel expression or related properties in causing AF. In human tissue studies, diastolic Ca^{2+} leak and associated triggered activity in right atrial appendage myocytes are associated with paroxysmal and persistent AF, as well as post-operative AF (**eFig. 62.15**).[57] Conduction abnormalities are frequently found in AF patients and are likely related to reentry-promoting tissue fibrosis[58,59] and disturbances in connexin expression and/or function.[21,58]

Remodeling of the Atria
Remodeling of atrial structure and/or electrical function occurs as a result of risk factors, heart disease, and AF itself, and appears to be a key determinant of AF occurrence, persistence, and resistance to therapy. Prolonged rapid atrial rates cause electrophysiologic alterations in the atria, including shortening and loss of the physiologic rate adaptation of refractoriness and a decrease in CV. The ionic mechanisms underlying shortening of the RP and slowing of conduction includes downregulation of L-type Ca^{2+} and Na^+ currents, upregulation of I_{K1}, and disturbances in connexin expression and distribution.[57] In addition, remodeling of autonomic innervation and function appears to play an important role in both triggering and maintaining AF.[60] Rapid rates and a variety of underlying conditions promote the development of atrial fibrosis, which favors AF progression. Finally, there is extensive emerging evidence that inflammatory signaling plays a central role in AF pathophysiology, contributing to the ion channel/transporter and structural changes that underlie the AF substrate.[61,62]

Sinus Node Reentry
The SA node shares with the AV node electrophysiologic features like the potential for dissociation of conduction; that is, an impulse can be conducted in some nodal fibers but not in others, permitting reentry to occur (see Chapter 65). The reentrant circuit can be located entirely within the SA node or may involve both the SA node and atrium. Supraventricular tachycardias caused by sinus node reentry are generally less symptomatic than other SVTs because of slower rates. Ablation of the SA node may occasionally be necessary for refractory tachycardia.

Atrial Reentry
Reentry within the atrium, unrelated to the SA node, can be a cause of SVT in humans. Distinguishing AT caused by automaticity or afterdepolarizations from AT sustained by reentry over small areas (i.e., microanatomic reentry) is difficult.

Atrioventricular Nodal Reentry
The mechanisms underlying AV node reentry are discussed in detail above. For further information, see Chapter 65.

Preexcitation Syndrome
Preexcitation results from fibers that bypass the AV node and allow for more rapid communication between atria and ventricles than is normally permitted by the AV node. These connections can produce the substrate for anatomical reentry involving the atria, AV node, ventricles, and bypass tract, generally referred to as "*atrioventricular reciprocating tachycardia*" (AVRT). In most patients who have reciprocating tachycardias associated with WPW syndrome, the accessory pathway conducts more rapidly than the normal AV node but takes a longer time to recover excitability; that is, the anterograde RP of the accessory pathway exceeds that of the AV node. Consequently, a premature

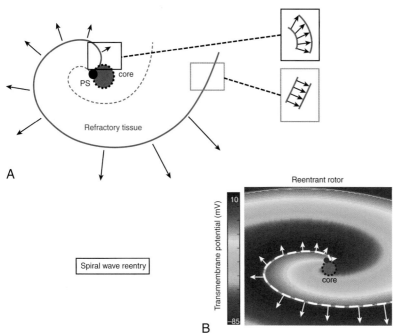

FIGURE 62.21 Spiral wave reentry due to functional block generating a rotor. **A,** Reentrant wavefront (*solid red curve*) with greatest curvature near the center of the wave. Tissue behind the wavefront (ending at the *dashed red curve*), with the tissue inside the dashed border having recovered excitability. The core is characterized by a high degree of curvature causing inexcitability due to source-sink mismatch. **B,** An example of a reentrant wave in simulated 2-dimensional tissue.

atrial complex that occurs sufficiently early is blocked anterogradely in the accessory pathway and continues to the ventricle over the normal AV node and His bundle. After the ventricles have been excited, the impulse is able to enter the accessory pathway retrogradely and return to the atrium. A continuous conduction loop of this type establishes the circuit for the tachycardia. The usual (orthodromic) activation wave during such a reciprocating tachycardia in a patient with an accessory pathway occurs anterogradely over the normal AV node–His-Purkinje system and retrogradely over the accessory pathway, which results in a normal-duration QRS complex (see Fig. 62.20). Occasionally, the activation wave travels in a reverse (antidromic) direction to the ventricles over the accessory pathway and to the atria retrogradely up the AV node. Two accessory pathways can form the circuit in some patients with antidromic AVRT. In some patients, the accessory pathway may be capable of only retrograde conduction ("concealed"), but the circuit and mechanism of AVRT remain the same. Less frequently, the accessory pathway can conduct only anterogradely. The pathway can be localized by ECG analysis. Developmental studies in mice have demonstrated that myocardium-specific inactivation of T-box 2 (Tbx2), a transcription factor essential for AV canal patterning, leads to the formation of fast-conducting accessory pathways, malformation of the annulus fibrosus, and ventricular preexcitation in mice.[63]

Ventricular Tachycardia Caused by Reentry
Reentry in the ventricle, both anatomic and functional, as a cause of sustained VT has been supported by many animal and clinical studies (see Chapter 67). Reentry in ventricular muscle, with or without contributions from specialized tissue, is responsible for many or most VTs in patients with ischemic heart disease. The area of microreentry appears to be small, and less often a macroreentry circuit is found around the infarct scar. Surviving myocardial tissue separated by connective tissue provides serpentine routes of activation traversing infarcted areas that can establish reentry pathways. Bundle branch reentry, macroreentry using the specialized conduction system, can cause sustained VT, particularly in patients with dilated cardiomyopathy.

Both figure-of-eight and single-circle reentrant loops have been described as circulating around an area of functional block or as conducting slowly across an apparent area of block created by anisotropy. When intramural myocardium survives, it can form part of the reentrant loop. Structural discontinuities that separate muscle bundles—as

a result of the naturally occurring myocardial fiber orientation and anisotropic conduction, as well as collagen matrices formed from the fibrosis after MI—establish the basis for slowed conduction and fragmented electrograms, which can lead to reentry. After MI, the surviving epicardial border zone undergoes substantial electrical remodeling, including reduced CV and increased anisotropy associated with the occurrence of reentrant circuits and VT. Slowing of conduction arises from alterations in the spatial distribution and electrophysiologic properties of connexin 43 gap junctions, as well as from reduced voltage-gated sodium current. It has been speculated that myocyte depolarization secondary to electrotonic coupling to adjacent myofibroblasts (which typically have a much more depolarized potential) plays a role in electrical dysfunction in postinfarction border-zone myocardium. While sophisticated studies using advanced microscopy techniques suggest that such coupling is possible,[64] their actual role in clinically relevant arrhythmogenesis and potential for therapeutic targeting are still uncertain. During acute ischemia, various factors, including elevated $[K^+]_o$ and reduced pH, combine to create depressed APs in ischemic cells that impede conduction and can lead to reentry. A great deal of effort has gone into defining the ionic basis of these changes; however, efforts to apply this knowledge to provide viable clinical therapeutics have largely failed and interest has shifted to primary prevention against the atherosclerosis leading to MI and prevention of myocardial damage by rapid reperfusion of acutely ischemic tissue via interventional procedures.

Brugada Syndrome
Brugada syndrome is a congenital sudden death syndrome involving characteristic electrocardiographic abnormalities. These typically include ST-segment elevation (unrelated to ischemia, electrolyte abnormalities, or structural heart disease) in the right precordial (V_1 to V_3) leads of the ECG, often but not always accompanied by an apparent right bundle branch block (see Fig. 61.3). Early repolarization in localized myocardial regions is often a central factor, although conduction abnormalities have also been observed, and the relative role of repolarization versus depolarization abnormalities remains controversial. The hereditary nature of the syndrome is well established; however, a wide variety of genes and ion-channel abnormalities have been associated and it is apparent that simple mendelian transmission does not explain the phenotypic expression in many cases.[65] The single most common genetic abnormalities in Brugada syndrome are loss-of-function mutations in *SCN5A* (Table 62.1), which encodes the pore-forming cardiac sodium channel alpha subunit Nav1.5, and mutations in *SCN1B*, *SCN2B*, and *SCN3B*, which encode the function-modifying sodium channel beta subunits (see Chapter 63). However, mutations in the α and β subunits of the Ca^{2+} channel and several potassium channel genes have been found in some patients with Brugada syndrome, as have mutations in the glycerol-3-phosphate dehydrogenase 1–like *(GPD1L)* and other genes that encode proteins that regulate the functional expression of the Na^+ current I_{Na}. Brugada syndrome–associated gene defects cause a reduction or loss of sodium or calcium current in combination with altered functional properties of voltage-gated sodium channels.[65] While the apparent localization of Brugada syndrome substrates points to the potential applicability of catheter ablation, results to date have been mixed and improvement is needed before ablation becomes an effective and widely applicable therapy.[66]

Catecholaminergic Polymorphic Ventricular Tachycardia
CPVT is an inherited arrhythmogenic syndrome characterized by stress-induced, adrenergically mediated polymorphic VT occurring in structurally normal hearts. The common mechanism underlying RyR2-associated CPVT is spontaneous diastolic Ca^{2+} leak from the SR via RyR2, leading to intracellular Ca^{2+} waves and triggered activity. While RyR2 mutations are responsible for about 95% of cases, CPVT can also

occur because of mutations in genes encoding calsequestrin, calmodulin, and triadin, all proteins that interact with RyR2 and regulate its function.[67] Beta-adrenergic tone resulting from stimulation by catecholamines has a central role in modulating RyR2 function, both by increasing RyR2-sensitivity to Ca^{2+} by enhancing PKA and CaMKII-mediated phosphorylation, and by increasing SR Ca^{2+}-loading through increased $I_{Ca,L}$ and SERCA activity, effects that largely account for the "C" in CPVT. Thus, beta-adrenergic receptor blockade is the mainstay of CPVT therapy. For patients that are not adequately controlled by beta-blockers, flecainide is a safe and largely effective therapy,[68] acting by directly inhibiting RyR2 Ca^{2+}-release and/or by inhibiting I_{Na} to decrease cellular excitability and cellular Ca^{2+}-loading through the reduced phase-0 Na^+-influx and subsequent exchange for extracellular Ca^{2+} via NCX.

Arrhythmogenic Right Ventricular Cardiomyopathy

ARVC is an inherited myopathy characterized by sustained monomorphic VT and sudden death (see Chapter 52). At least 16 genes have been associated with ARVC-causing mutations.[69] The majority are mutations in genes encoding proteins of the cardiac desmosome, a component of the intercalated disc essential for mechanical coupling between cardiomyocytes. Mutations in the desmosomal proteins, intercalated disk proteins, nuclear envelope proteins, along with desmin, titin, phospholamban, channel proteins, and growth factors have been identified in patients with ARVC. Approximately 20% to 45% of the pathogenic mutations linked to ARVC are in the gene encoding plakophilin 2 (*PKP2*), which interacts with other cytoskeletal proteins to stabilize the desmosome. Loss of *PKP2* expression reduces the voltage-gated sodium current and connexin 43 expression at the intercalated disc and thus results in slowed AP propagation. Shared phenotypic, genetic, and functional features suggest pathogenic links between ARVC and Brugada syndrome.[69] The pathophysiology of ARVC illustrates the interrelatedness of tissue mechanical integrity and cardiac bioelectricity, as well as the critical role of the intercalated disk in electrophysiological function.

Ventricular Fibrillation: Fibrillation Initiation and Maintenance

Previous experimental and simulation investigations point to reentry as the central mechanism underlying VF (see Chapter 67). While the reentry underlying VF was classically thought to be randomly maintained by wandering wavelets of activation, more recent investigations have suggested underlying spatiotemporal organization and pointed to the role of spiral-wave reentry in maintaining VF. Important roles have been identified for both focal activity in initiating reentry and rotor sources maintaining VF.[70] These have been translated into promising ablation approaches for patients with recurrent VF episodes.[71] For a demonstration of wavefront dynamics during fibrillation, see **Video 62.3**.

The hallmark of cardiac fibrillation is ongoing wave break (or wave splitting). Wave break is caused by conduction block occurring at a specific site along the wavefront while the remaining portions of the front continue to propagate. This localized block, wave break, causes splitting of a primary spiral wavefront into two daughter wavelets. The daughter wavefronts can collide and annihilate each other, or can form independent reentry-supporting spiral-wave generators.[49,70] Two hypotheses exist regarding the genesis of wave breaks during fibrillation. The "mother rotor" hypothesis states that VF is maintained by a single, stationary, intramural stable reentrant circuit (i.e., the mother rotor) in a dominant domain, which has the shortest RP from which activations propagate into the more slowly activating domains with longer RPs. In this case, the fastest activating (i.e., dominating) rotor rather than ongoing wave break is the engine driving cardiac fibrillation, and wave break occurs only secondarily. High-resolution electrical mapping has suggested that fast activation during VF is driven by Purkinje fibers. Spatial heterogeneity in the magnitude of ionic currents has been implicated in the generation of spatial gradients in activation rates and in maintaining rotor stability in the fastest activating regions. For example, the magnitude of the inward rectifying K^+ current I_{K1} (see Table 62.1) is a critical determinant of rotor frequency and sustainability.[49]

The involvement of rotors in cardiac fibrillation does not require the presence of a single or small number of dominant rotors. As long as the destruction and creation rate of rotors are such that a critical number of rotor generators are present at all times, fibrillation will sustain itself indefinitely. A major determinant of the dynamically induced component of heterogeneity leading to reentry has been identified as electrical restitution, or variation of the AP duration and CV with the diastolic interval. For example, it has been proposed that the breakup of periodic waves is precipitated by APD alternans sufficiently large to cause conduction block along the spiral wavefront. Simulations have shown that a reentrant rotor becomes unstable and breaks down into multiple rotors when the slope of the restitution curve for the APD versus the diastolic interval is greater than 1. At the cellular level, the steepness of the APD restitution curve and intracellular calcium level ($[Ca^{2+}]_i$) dynamics cause the APD and $[Ca^{2+}]_i$ transient to alternate. Given the bidirectional coupling between changes in $[Ca^{2+}]_i$ and membrane potential—for example, the membrane potential determines the activity of L-type Ca channels, and conversely, the $[Ca^{2+}]_i$ transient amplitude strongly modulates the APD through its effects on Ca^{2+}-sensitive currents (e.g., $I_{Na/Ca}$ and I_{Ca}) during the AP plateau—an alternation in $[Ca^{2+}]_i$ transient amplitude causes a secondary alternation in the APD. Recent work has shown that AF-induced Ca^{2+}-handling remodeling promotes aberrant RyR2 Ca^{2+}-releases associated with enhanced Ca^{2+} and APD alternans, leading to a vulnerability spatially discordant alternans that initiates and stabilizes AF.[72] Manipulations that alter cellular Ca^{2+}-handling in a way that decreases alternans might provide novel approaches to prevent fibrillation.

REFERENCES

1. Tomaselli GF, Rubart M, Zipes DP. Mechanisms of cardiac arrhythmias. In: Zipes DP, Libby P, Bonow RO, Mann DL, Tomaselli GF, eds. *Braunwald's Heart Disease, a Textbook of Cardiovascular Medicine*. 11th ed. Philadelphia, PA: Elsevier; 2016.
2. Bengel P, Ahmad S, Tirilomis P, et al. Contribution of the neuronal sodium channel Nav1.8 to sodium- and calcium-dependent cellular proarrhythmia. *J Mol Cell Cardiol*. 2020;144:35–46.
3. Carmeliet E. Pacemaking in cardiac tissue. From Ik2 to a coupled-clock system. *Physiol Rep*. 2019;7:e13862.
4. Yang KC, Nerbonne JM. Mechanisms contributing to myocardial potassium channel diversity, regulation and remodeling. *Trends Cardiovasc Med*. 2016;26:209–218.
5. Shamsaldeen YA, Culliford L, Clout M, et al. Role of SK channel activation in determining the action potential configuration in freshly isolated human atrial myocytes from the SKArF study. *Biochem Biophys Res Commun*. 2019;512:684–690.
6. Rahm AK, Lugenbiel P, Schweizer PA, et al. Role of ion channels in heart failure and channelopathies. *Biophys Rev*. 2018;10:1097–1106.
7. Jiang D, Shi H, Tonggu L, et al. Structure of the cardiac sodium channel. *Cell*. 2020;180:122–134 e110.
8. Ahern CA, Payandeh J, Bosmans F, et al. The hitchhiker's guide to the voltage-gated sodium channel galaxy. *J Gen Physiol*. 2016;147:1–24.
9. Balse E, Eichel C. The cardiac sodium channel and its protein partners. *Handb Exp Pharmacol*. 2018;246:73–99.
10. Briot J, Tetreault MP, Bourdin B, et al. Inherited ventricular arrhythmias: the role of the multi-subunit structure of the L-type calcium channel complex. *Adv Exp Med Biol*. 2017;966:55–64.
11. Li Y, Zhang X, Zhang C, et al. Increasing t-type calcium channel activity by beta-adrenergic stimulation contributes to beta-adrenergic regulation of heart rates. *J Physiol*. 2018;596:1137–1151.
12. Nerbonne JM. Molecular basis of functional myocardial potassium channel diversity. *Card Electrophysiol Clin*. 2016;8:257–273.
13. Jeevaratnam K, Chadda KR, Huang CL, et al. Cardiac potassium channels: physiological insights for targeted therapy. *J Cardiovasc Pharmacol Ther*. 2018;23:119–129.
14. Tucker NR, Clauss S, Ellinor PT. Common variation in atrial fibrillation: navigating the path from genetic association to mechanism. *Cardiovasc Res*. 2016;109:493–501.
15. Grandi E, Sanguinetti MC, Bartos DC, et al. Potassium channels in the heart: structure, function and regulation. *J Physiol*. 2017;595:2209–2228.
16. Papanicolaou KN, Ashok D, Liu T, et al. Global knockout of ROMK potassium channel worsens cardiac ischemia-reperfusion injury but cardiomyocyte-specific knockout does not: implications for the identity of mitoKATP. *J Mol Cell Cardiol*. 2020;139:176–189.
17. Baruscotti M, Bucchi A, Milanesi R, et al. A gain-of-function mutation in the cardiac pacemaker HCN_4 channel increasing cAMP sensitivity is associated with familial inappropriate sinus tachycardia. *Eur Heart J*. 2017;38:280–288.
18. Ide T, Ohtani K, Higo T, et al. Ivabradine for the treatment of cardiovascular diseases. *Circ J*. 2019;83:252–260.
19. Kistamas K, Veress R, Horvath B, et al. Calcium handling defects and cardiac arrhythmia syndromes. *Front Pharmacol*. 2020;11:72.
20. Himes RD, Smolin N, Kukol A, et al. L30A mutation of phospholemman mimics effects of cardiac glycosides in isolated cardiomyocytes. *Biochemistry*. 2016;55:6196–6204.
21. Delmar M, Laird DW, Naus CC, et al. Connexins and disease. *Cold Spring Harb Perspect Biol*. 2018;10.
22. Hoagland DT, Santos W, Poelzing S, et al. The role of the gap junction perinexus in cardiac conduction: potential as a novel anti-arrhythmic drug target. *Prog Biophys Mol Biol*. 2019;144:41–50.
23. Noureldin M, Chen H, Bai D. Functional characterization of novel atrial fibrillation-linked GJA5 (Cx40) mutants. *Int J Mol Sci*. 2018;19.
24. Vimalanathan AK, Ehler E, Gehmlich K. Genetics of and pathogenic mechanisms in arrhythmogenic right ventricular cardiomyopathy. *Biophys Rev*. 2018;10:973–982.
25. Eckhardt LL, Kalscheur MM. Replacing hardware with "viralware". *J Am Coll Cardiol*. 2019;73:1688–1690.
26. Markowitz SM, Lerman BB. A contemporary view of atrioventricular nodal physiology. *J Interv Card Electrophysiol*. 2018;52:271–279.
27. Billette J, Tadros R. An integrated overview of AV node physiology. *Pacing Clin Electrophysiol*. 2019;42:805–820.
28. George SA, Faye NR, Murillo-Berlioz A, et al. At the atrioventricular crossroads: dual pathway electrophysiology in the atrioventricular node and its underlying heterogeneities. *Arrhythm Electrophysiol Rev*. 2017;6:179–185.
29. Fukuda K, Kanazawa H, Aizawa Y, et al. Cardiac innervation and sudden cardiac death. *Circ Res*. 2015;116:2005–2019.

30. Manolis AA, Manolis TA, Apostolopoulos EJ, et al. The role of the autonomic nervous system in cardiac arrhythmias: the neuro-cardiac axis, more foe than friend? *Trends Cardiovasc Med*. 2020.
31. Bencivenga L, Liccardo D, Napolitano C, et al. Beta-adrenergic receptor signaling and heart failure: from bench to bedside. *Heart Fail Clin*. 2019;15:409–419.
32. Stavrakis S, Kulkarni K, Singh JP, et al. Autonomic modulation of cardiac arrhythmias: methods to assess treatment and outcomes. *JACC Clin Electrophysiol*. 2020;6:467–483.
33. Boyden PA, Dun W, Robinson RB. Cardiac Purkinje fibers and arrhythmias; the GK Moe award Lecture 2015. *Heart Rhythm*. 2016;13:1172–1181.
34. Qi XY, Vahdahi Hassani F, Hoffmann D, et al. Inositol trisphosphater receptors and nuclear calcium in atrial fibrillation. *Circ Res*. 2021;128:619–635.
35. Nassal D, Gratz D, Hund TJ. Challenges and opportunities for therapeutic targeting of calmodulin kinase II in heart. *Front Pharmacol*. 2020;11:35.
36. Sufu-Shimizu Y, Okuda S, Kato T, et al. Stabilizing cardiac ryanodine receptor prevents the development of cardiac dysfunction and lethal arrhythmia in ca(2+)/calmodulin-dependent protein kinase IIδc transgenic mice. *Biochem Biophys Res Commun*. 2020;524:431–438.
37. Hegyi B, Morotti S, Liu C, et al. Enhanced depolarization drive in failing rabbit ventricular myocytes: calcium-dependent and beta-adrenergic effects on late sodium, l-type calcium, and sodium-calcium exchange currents. *Circ Arrhythm Electrophysiol*. 2019;12:e007061.
38. Iyer V, Roman-Campos D, Sampson KJ, et al. Purkinje cells as sources of arrhythmias in long QT syndrome type 3. *Sci Rep*. 2015;5:13287.
39. Koleske M, Bonilla I, Thomas J, et al. Tetrodotoxin-sensitive Na$_v$s contribute to early and delayed afterdepolarizations in long QT arrhythmia models. *J Gen Physiol*. 2018;150:991–1002.
40. Sala L, Gnecchi M, Schwartz PJ. Long QT syndrome modelling with cardiomyocytes derived from human-induced pluripotent stem cells. *Arrhythm Electrophysiol Rev*. 2019;8:105–110.
41. van Gorp PRR, Trines SA, Pijnappels DA, et al. Multicellular in vitro models of cardiac arrhythmias: focus on atrial fibrillation. *Front Cardiovasc Med*. 2020;7:43.
42. da Rocha AM, Campbell K, Mironov S, et al. hiPSC-CM monolayer maturation state determines drug responsiveness in high throughput pro-arrhythmia screen. *Sci Rep*. 2017;7:13834.
43. Priori SG, Napolitano C. J-wave syndromes: electrocardiographic and clinical aspects. *Card Electrophysiol Clin*. 2018;10:355–369.
44. Woosley RL, Black K, Heise CW, et al. CredibleMeds.org: what does it offer? *Trends Cardiovasc Med*. 2018;28:94–99.
45. Butler A, Helliwell MV, Zhang Y, et al. An update on the structure of hERG. *Front Pharmacol*. 2019;10:1572.
46. Wallis R, Benson C, Darpo B, et al. CiPA challenges and opportunities from a non-clinical, clinical and regulatory perspectives. An overview of the safety pharmacology scientific discussion. *J Pharmacol Toxicol Methods*. 2018;93:15–25.
47. Etchegoyen CV, Keller GA, Mrad S, et al. Drug-induced QT interval prolongation in the intensive care unit. *Curr Clin Pharmacol*. 2017;12:210–222.
48. Aguilar M, Nattel S. The pioneering work of George Mines on cardiac arrhythmias: groundbreaking ideas that remain influential in contemporary cardiac electrophysiology. *J Physiol*. 2016;594:2377–2386.
49. Nattel S, Xiong F, Aguilar M. Demystifying rotors and their place in clinical translation of atrial fibrillation mechanisms. *Nat Rev Cardiol*. 2017;14:509–520.
50. Hansen BJ, Zhao J, Li N, et al. Human atrial fibrillation drivers resolved with integrated functional and structural imaging to benefit clinical mapping. *JACC Clin Electrophysiol*. 2018;4:1501–1515.
51. Dharmaprani D, Schopp M, Kuklik P, et al. Renewal theory as a universal quantitative framework to characterize phase singularity regeneration in mammalian cardiac fibrillation. *Circ Arrhythm Electrophysiol*. 2019;12:e007569.
52. Terricabras M, Verma A. Is pulmonary vein isolation enough for persistent atrial fibrillation? *J Cardiovasc Electrophysiol*. 2020.
53. Hyman MC, Marchlinski FE. Persistent atrial fibrillation: when the pulmonary veins are no longer the answer. *J Cardiovasc Electrophysiol*. 2020;31:1861–1863.
54. Bond RC, Choisy SC, Bryant SM, et al. Ion currents, action potentials, and noradrenergic responses in rat pulmonary vein and left atrial cardiomyocytes. *Physiol Rep*. 2020;8:e14432.
55. Choi SH, Jurgens SJ, Weng LC, et al. Monogenic and polygenic contributions to atrial fibrillation risk: results from a national biobank. *Circ Res*. 2020;126:200–209.
56. Wang B, Lunetta KL, Dupuis J, et al. Integrative omics approach to identifying genes associated with atrial fibrillation. *Circ Res*. 2020;126:350–360.
57. Nattel S, Heijman J, Zhou L, et al. Molecular basis of atrial fibrillation pathophysiology and therapy: a translational perspective. *Circ Res*. 2020;127:51–72.
58. Callegari S, Macchi E, Monaco R, et al. A clinico-pathological "bird's-eye" view of left atrial myocardial fibrosis in 121 patients with persistent atrial fibrillation: developing architecture and main cellular players. *Circ Arrhythm Electrophysiol*. 2020.
59. Nattel S. Molecular and cellular mechanisms of atrial fibrosis in atrial fibrillation. *JACC Clin Electrophysiol*. 2017;3:425–435.
60. Gussak G, Pfenniger A, Wren L, et al. Region-specific parasympathetic nerve remodeling in the left atrium contributes to creation of a vulnerable substrate for atrial fibrillation. *JCI Insight*. 2019;4.
61. Hiram R, Xiong F, Naud P, et al. The inflammation-resolution promoting molecule resolvin-d1 prevents atrial proarrhythmic remodeling in experimental right heart disease. *Cardiovasc Res*. 2021;117:1776–1789.
62. Yao C, Veleva T, Scott Jr L, et al. Enhanced cardiomyocyte nlrp3 inflammasome signaling promotes atrial fibrillation. *Circulation*. 2018;138:2227–2242.
63. Meyers JD, Jay PY, Rentschler S. Reprogramming the conduction system: onward toward a biological pacemaker. *Trends Cardiovasc Med*. 2016;26:14–20.
64. Schultz F, Swiatlowska P, Alvarez-Laviada A, et al. Cardiomyocyte-myofibroblast contact dynamism is modulated by connexin-43. *FASEB J*. 2019;33:10453–10468.
65. Cerrone M. Controversies in Brugada syndrome. *Trends Cardiovasc Med*. 2018;28:284–292.
66. Rizzo A, de Asmundis C, Brugada P, et al. Ablation for the treatment of Brugada syndrome: current status and future prospects. *Expert Rev Med Devices*. 2020;17:123–130.
67. Wleklinski MJ, Kannankeril PJ, Knollmann BC. Molecular and tissue mechanisms of catecholaminergic polymorphic ventricular tachycardia. *J Physiol*. 2020;598:2817–2834.
68. Wang G, Zhao N, Zhong S, et al. Safety and efficacy of flecainide for patients with catecholaminergic polymorphic ventricular tachycardia: a systematic review and meta-analysis. *Medicine (Baltim)*. 2019;98:e16961.
69. Gandjbakhch E, Redheuil A, Pousset F, et al. Clinical diagnosis, imaging, and genetics of arrhythmogenic right ventricular cardiomyopathy/dysplasia: JACC state-of-the-art review. *J Am Coll Cardiol*. 2018;72:784–804.
70. Aras KK, Kay MW, Efimov IR. Ventricular fibrillation: rotors or foci? Both! *Circ Arrhythm Electrophysiol*. 2017;10.
71. Singh P, Noheria A. Ablation approaches for ventricular fibrillation. *Curr Treat Options Cardiovasc Med*. 2018;20:21.
72. Liu T, Xiong F, Qi XY, et al. Altered calcium handling produces reentry-promoting action potential alternans in atrial fibrillation-remodeled hearts. *JCI Insight*. 2020;5.

# 63 Genetics of Cardiac Arrhythmias

JOHN R. GIUDICESSI, DAVID J. TESTER, AND MICHAEL J. ACKERMAN

Cardiac arrhythmias encompass a large and heterogenous group of electrical abnormalities of the heart with or without underlying structural heart disease. Cardiac arrhythmias can be innocuous, can predispose to the development of potentially lethal stroke or embolus, or can present emergently with a life-threatening condition that may result in sudden cardiac death (SCD), one of the most common causes of death in the developed countries. In the United States, for example, an estimated 300,000 to 400,000 individuals die suddenly each year, with the vast majority involving the elderly; 80% are caused by ventricular fibrillation (VF) in the context of ischemic heart disease. In comparison, SCD in the young is relatively uncommon, with an incidence between 1.3 and 8.5 per 100,000 patient-years.[1] However, tragically, thousands of otherwise healthy individuals under the age of 40 years die suddenly each year without warning signs. Most SCD in the young can be attributed to structural cardiovascular anomalies identifiable at autopsy. However, 30% to 50% of sudden death in the young remains unexplained following a complete autopsy and medicolegal investigation (see Chapter 70).

Potentially lethal and inheritable arrhythmia syndromes—classified under "the cardiac channelopathies" including congenital long QT syndrome (LQTS), Brugada syndrome (BrS), catecholaminergic polymorphic ventricular tachycardia (CPVT), and related disorders—involve electrical disturbances with the propensity to cause fatal arrhythmias in the setting of a structurally normal heart. These often unassuming electrical abnormalities have the capacity to cause the heart of an unsuspecting individual to develop a potentially lethal arrhythmia, leading to a sudden and early demise of an otherwise healthy individual. In fact, it is now recognized that nearly a third of autopsy-negative sudden unexplained death (SUD) in the young and approximately 10% of sudden infant death syndrome (SIDS) stem from these inherited cardiac channelopathies.[1]

Through molecular advances in the field of cardiovascular genetics, the underlying bases responsible for many inherited cardiac arrhythmia syndromes have been identified, while other underlying genetic substrates are on the cusp of discovery. Over the past two decades, a set of themes including extreme genetic heterogeneity, reduced/incomplete penetrance, and variable expressivity have proven to be central themes among the cardiac channelopathies. However, for some disorders, important genotype-phenotype correlations have been recognized and have provided diagnostic, prognostic, and therapeutic impact.

Given the potentially devastating impact that these disorders can have on a family and their communities, we sought to illustrate the clinical description, genetic basis, and the genotype-phenotype correlations associated with these inherited arrhythmia syndromes.

Specifically, this chapter will discuss cardiac channelopathies, focusing on the subset of QT-opathies [LQTS including calmodulinopathic LQTS, triadin knockout (TKO) syndrome, Timothy syndrome (TS), cardiac-only Timothy syndrome (COTS), short QT syndrome (SQTS), and drug-induced torsade de pointes (DI-TdP)] and other channelopathies [Andersen-Tawil syndrome (ATS), ankyrin-B syndrome (ABS), BrS, CPVT, early repolarization syndrome (ERS), familial atrial fibrillation (FAF), idiopathic ventricular fibrillation (IVF), multifocal ectopic Purkinje-related premature contractions (MEPPC), progressive cardiac conduction defect (PCCD), and sick sinus syndrome (SSS)].

THE QT-OPATHIES

Long QT Syndrome
Clinical Description and Manifestations of Long QT Syndrome
Congenital LQTS comprises a distinct group of cardiac channelopathies characterized by delayed repolarization of the myocardium resulting in heart rate-corrected QT prolongation (QTc >480 msec as the 50th percentile among individuals with genetically confirmed LQTS; Fig. 63.1A) and an increased risk of syncope, seizures, and SCD in the setting of a structurally normal heart. The incidence of LQTS may exceed 1 in 2500 persons. However, individuals with LQTS may not manifest QT prolongation on a resting 12-lead surface electrocardiogram (ECG). This repolarization abnormality almost always is without consequence; however, it is rarely triggered by exertion, swimming, emotion, auditory stimuli such as an alarm clock, or the postpartum period, which can cause the heart to become electrically unstable and develop a life-threatening and sometimes lethal arrhythmia, torsade de pointes (TdP) (see Chapter 70). Though the cardiac rhythm often returns to normal spontaneously, resulting in only transient syncope, 5% of untreated and unassuming LQTS individuals succumb to a fatal arrhythmia as their sentinel event. However, it is estimated that nearly half of individuals experiencing SCD, stemming from this very treatable arrhythmogenic disorder, may have exhibited prior warning signs (i.e., exertional syncope, family history of premature sudden death) that went unrecognized. LQTS may explain approximately 20% of autopsy-negative SUD in the young and 10% of SIDS.[1]

GENETIC BASIS FOR LONG QT SYNDROME
LQTS is a genetically heterogeneous disorder of cardiac repolarization inherited predominantly in an autosomal dominant pattern (formerly referred to as Romano-Ward syndrome). It is rarely inherited in a recessive pattern as illustrated by Jervell and Lange-Nielsen Syndrome (JLNS),

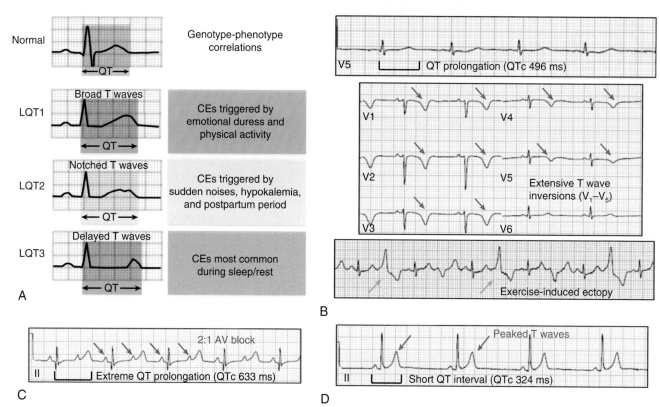

FIGURE 63.1 Notable electrocardiographic findings in the QT-opathies. **A,** Canonical (i.e., LQT1-3) long QT syndrome genotype-specific electrocardiogram patterns and clinically relevant genotype-phenotype correlations. **B,** QTc prolongation (top panel, *black bracket*), extensive precordial T wave inversions (middle panel, *blue arrows*), and exercise-induced ventricular ectopy (bottom panel, *orange arrows*) observed in a triadin knockout syndrome patient homozygous for p.D18fs*13-TRDN. **C,** Rhythm strip from a Timothy syndrome patient harboring p.G406R-CACNA1C that displays extreme QTc prolongation (*black bracket*) and 2:1 atrioventricular block (*blue arrows*). **D,** Rhythm strip from a patient with short QT syndrome displaying characteristic QTc shortening (*black bracket*) and peaked T waves (*blue arrows*). *AV,* Atrioventricular; *CEs,* cardiac events; *QTc,* heart rate-corrected QT interval.

characterized by extreme QTc prolongation, high risk of SCD, and sensorineural hearing loss. Spontaneous/sporadic germline mutations can account for nearly 5% to 10% of LQTS. To date, hundreds of mutations have now been identified in LQTS-susceptibility genes responsible for a nonsyndromic "classical" LQTS phenotype. In addition, three extremely rare, multisystem disorders (ATS formerly referred to as LQT7; ABS formerly referred to as LQT4; and TS formerly referred to as LQT8) associated with marked QTc prolongation and an array of extra-cardiac manifestations have also been described and are detailed in the later sections of this chapter.

Approximately 75% of patients with a clinically robust diagnosis of LQTS host either loss-of-function or gain-of-function pathogenic/likely pathogenic variants in one of these three major/canonical LQTS genes (eTable 63.1)—KCNQ1-encoded I_{Ks} (K_v7.1) potassium channel (LQT1, approximately 35%, loss-of-function); KCNH2-encoded I_{Kr} (K_v11.1) potassium channel (LQT2, approximately 30%, loss-of-function); and SCN5A-encoded I_{Na} (Na_v1.5) sodium channel (LQT3, approximately 10%, gain-of-function)—which are responsible for the inscription of the cardiac action potential (Fig. 63.2). Approximately 5% to 10% of patients have multiple mutations and such patients present at a younger age and with greater expressivity.[1]

Following the discovery of the canonical LQTS-susceptibility genes in 1995 and 1996, rapid advances in deoxyribonucleic acid (DNA) sequencing technology has facilitated the discovery of new disease-susceptibility genes in scenarios (i.e., singletons and small pedigrees) not feasible with classical linkage analysis.[2] As a result, the last two decades have seen a rapid explosion in the number of new disease-susceptibility genes, which includes the 14 minor LQTS-susceptibility genes that may underlie an additional 5% to 10% of LQTS cases (eTable 63.1).

However, many of the minor LQTS-susceptibility genes (e.g., AKAP9, ANK2, CAV3, KCNE1, KCNE2, SCN4B, and SNTA1; eTable 63.1) were discovered using hypothesis-driven, candidate-based analysis of

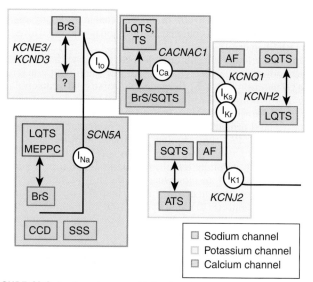

FIGURE 63.2 Cardiac action potential disorders. Illustrated are the key ion currents (*white circles*) along the ventricular cardiomyocyte's action potential that are associated with potentially lethal cardiac arrhythmia disorders. Disorders resulting in gain-of-function mutations are shown in *green rectangles* and those with loss-of-function mutations shown in *blue rectangles*. For example, while gain-of-function mutations in the SCN5A encoding cardiac sodium channel responsible for INa, lead to LQTS, loss-of-function SCN5A mutations result in BrS, CCD, and SSS. *AF,* Atrial fibrillation; *ATS,* Andersen-Tawil syndrome; *BrS,* Brugada syndrome; *CCD,* cardiac conduction disease; *LQTS,* long QT syndrome; *MEPPC,* multifocal ectopic Purkinje-related premature contractions; *SSS,* sick sinus syndrome; *SQTS,* short QT syndrome; *TS,* Timothy syndrome.

biologically plausible genes rather than unbiased approaches (linkage analysis, next-generation sequencing-based trio/pedigree analysis, etc.).[2,3] Furthermore, many putative disease-causative variants used to establish these minor LQTS disease-gene associations (GDAs) were discovered before the true background rate of rare and presumably innocuous amino acid-altering variants was illuminated by large-scale sequencing projects such as the Genome Aggregation Database (gnomAD).[4] Therefore, it comes as little surprise that some putative LQTS-causative nonsynonymous variants are observed at frequencies in public exomes/genomes that far exceed the anticipated contribution of the minor LQTS-susceptibility gene in which it resides (i.e., 1:250,000 or 0.0004% for a ≤1% contributor) or in some cases the estimated prevalence of LQTS as a whole (i.e., 1:2500 or 0.04%).[3,5]

As a result, the strength of many minor LQTS GDAs is rightfully in question. To this end, the Clinical Genome Resource (ClinGen) Clinical Domain Channelopathy Working Group recently released a semiquantitative, evidence-based assessment of the GDA strength for the 17 putative LQTS-susceptibility genes.[6,7] However, the canonical LQTS-susceptibility genes (*KCNQ1*/LQT1, *KCNH2*/LQT2, and *SCN5A*/LQT3) and redundant genes (*CALM1-3*) responsible for calmodulinopathic LQTS received "definitive" evidence designations, and the majority of the remaining LQTS-susceptibility genes received a "limited" or "disputed" evidence designation (see eTable 63.1).[6,7] As a result, the majority (9/17; 53%) of alleged LQTS-susceptibility genes have now been demoted to so-called gene of uncertain significance (GUS) status.[6]

Unfortunately, owing to the limited number of sentinel variants used to establish initial GDAs, nearly all novel, nonsynonymous variants identified in a minor LQTS-GUS are destined to receive, at best, an ambiguous variant of uncertain significance (VUS) designation in accordance with the current American College of Medical Genetics and Genomics (ACMG) guidelines.[8,9] Therefore, the continued inclusion of GUS on gene panels likely elevates the signal-to-noise ratio associated with LQTS genetic testing as well as the risk of genetic testing misinterpretation, and subsequent diagnostic miscues.[8,9]

However, in light of (1) the increasing contribution of common genetic variants (oligogenic/polygenic basis) to the genetic architecture of LQTS, particularly in the approximately 10% to 20% of individuals that remain genotype-negative,[10,11] (2) clear role of rare and common variants in some GUS, most notably the *KCNE1*-encoded MiRP1 β-subunit,[8,12–14] in low penetrant and acquired/drug-induced forms of LQTS, and (3) potential that new evidence could elevate the ClinGen designation of a minor LQTS GUS, it is difficult to argue for the blanket removal of all limited- and disputed-evidence genes from commercial LQTS genetic testing panels at this time.

As minor LQTS GUS are likely to remain on LQTS genetic testing panels for the foreseeable future, ordering health care professionals should prioritize clinically actionable (ACMG pathogenic/likely pathogenic) variants identified in ClinGen definitive (*KCNQ1*, *KCNH2*, *SCN5A*, and *CALM1-3*), strong (*TRDN*), and moderate (*CACNA1C*) evidence genes and approach any variant (ACMG pathogenic, likely pathogenic, or VUS) identified in a ClinGen limited/disputed evidence gene with caution, as detailed in Figure 63.3. Importantly, if any doubt exists in regards to the clinical implications of variants labeled, currently or previously, as pathogenic/likely pathogenic in a GUS or VUS in definitive, strong, or moderate-evidence LQTS-susceptibility genes, strong consideration should be given to referring the patient to a dedicated Cardiovascular Genomics Clinic with the suitable infrastructure and expertise needed to carefully interpret, continually reappraise, and if needed act on these genetic findings (see Fig. 63.3).[2]

Phenotypic Correlates for the Three Canonical Long QT Syndrome Genotypes

Specific genotype/phenotype associations in LQTS have emerged, suggesting relatively gene-specific triggers, ECG patterns, and response to therapy (see Fig. 63.1A). Swimming and exertion-induced cardiac events are strongly associated with mutations in *KCNQ1* (LQT1), whereas auditory triggers and events occurring during the postpartum period most often occur in patients with LQT2. While exertion- or emotional stress-induced events are most common in LQT1, events occurring during periods of sleep/rest are most common in LQT3. In a study of 721 LQT1 and 634 LQT2 genetically confirmed patients from the U.S. portion of the international LQTS registry, a multivariate analysis was used to assess the independent contribution of clinical and mutation-specific factors in the occurrence of a first triggered event associated with exercise, arousal, or sleep/rest.[1] Among the 221 symptomatic

LQT1 patients, their first cardiac event was most often associated with exercise (55%) followed by sleep/rest (21%), arousal (14%), and non-specific (10%) triggers, whereas the 204 symptomatic LQT2 patients most often had their first event associated with either arousal triggers (44%) or nonexercise/nonarousal triggers (43%), and only 13% of the symptomatic LQT2 patients had an exercise-induced triggered first event. For LQT2 patients, the rate of arousal-triggered events was similar between male and female children, whereas there was a significantly higher rate of arousal-triggered events in women than men (26% vs. 6%, at age 40 years) following the onset of adolescence. Characteristic gene-suggestive ECG patterns have been described previously. LQT1 is associated with a broad-based T wave, LQT2 with a low amplitude notched or biphasic T wave, and LQT3 with a long isoelectric segment followed by a narrow-based T wave (see Fig. 63.1A).

However, exceptions to these relatively gene-specific T wave patterns exist, and due caution must be exercised with making a pre-genetic test prediction of the particular LQTS subtype involved, as the most common clinical mimicker of the LQT3-looking ECG is seen among patients with LQT1. This is key because the underlying genetic basis heavily influences the response to standard LQTS pharmacotherapy where beta blockers are extremely protective in LQT1 patients and moderately protective in patients with LQT2 and LQT3. Additionally, targeting the pathologic, LQT3-associated late sodium current with agents such as mexiletine, flecainide, or ranolazine represents a gene-specific therapeutic option for LQT3. Attenuation in repolarization with clinically apparent shortening in the QTc has been demonstrated with such a strategy and recently, a reduction in LQT3-triggered events using this strategy has been demonstrated. While the generalization that beta-blocker efficacy is genotype-type dependent has been well accepted, the effectiveness of beta-blocker therapy may be largely trigger-specific, rather than dependent on genotype. For both LQT1 and LQT2 patients, beta-blockade was associated with a pronounced 71% (LQT2 patients) to 78% (LQT1 patients) reduction in the risk for exercise-triggered cardiac events, but had no statistically significant effect on the apparent risk for arousal- or sleep/rest-triggered events.[1] However, it should be noted that many symptomatic LQT1 and LQT2 patients experience a subsequent cardiac event associated with a different trigger. For example, an LQT2 patient first presenting with an arousal event or event during sleep may present subsequently with an exercise-triggered event. Therefore, beta-blocker therapy remains first-line therapy even for patients experiencing a non-exercise-associated first event.

In addition, intra-genotype risk stratification has been realized for the two most common subtypes of LQTS based on mutation type, mutation location, and cellular function. Patients with LQT1 secondary to *Kv7.1* missense mutations localizing to the transmembrane-spanning domains clinically have a twofold greater risk of a LQT1-triggered cardiac event than LQT1 patients with mutations localizing to the C-terminal region. In addition, missense mutations localizing to the so-called cytoplasmic loops (C-loops) within the transmembrane-spanning domains, an area of the protein involved in adrenergic channel regulation, are associated with the highest rate of both exercise- and arousal-triggered events, but were not associated with an increase rate of sleep/rest associated events.[1] C-loop $K_v7.1$ missense mutations were consistently associated with a sixfold increase in risk for exercise-triggered events compared to non-missense mutations, and a nearly threefold increase compared to N- and C-terminal missense mutations.[1]

Patients with mutations resulting in a greater degree of $K_v7.1$ loss-of-function at the cellular in vitro level (dominant negative) have a twofold greater clinical risk compared to mutations that damaged the biology of the $K_v7.1$ channel less severely (haploinsufficiency). Adding to the traditional clinical risk factors, molecular location and cellular function are independent risk factors used in the evaluation of patients with LQTS.

Akin to molecular risk stratification in LQT1, patients with LQT2 secondary to $K_v11.1$ pore-region mutations have a longer QTc, a more severe clinical manifestation of the disorder, and experience significantly more arrhythmia-related cardiac events occurring at a younger age than those LQT2 patients with non-pore mutations in $K_v11.1$.[1] Similarly, in a Japanese cohort of LQT2 patients, those with

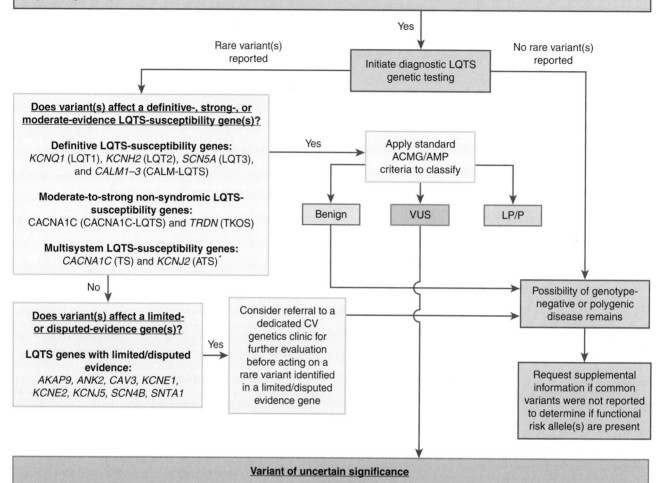

FIGURE 63.3 A rational approach to long QT syndrome genetic testing initiation and interpretation. *Blue boxes* denote basic considerations pertaining to the initiation of long QT syndrome genetic testing. *Light yellow boxes* denote a tiered approach to the assessment of rare variants in long QT syndrome-susceptibility genes with variable gene-disease association evidence strength. *Orange boxes* denote basic considerations pertaining to the identification of rare variants of uncertain significance in self-sufficient long QT syndrome-susceptibility genes that currently lack sufficient evidence to classify as either benign or pathogenic/likely pathogenic. *Due to the lack of a true QT prolongation phenotype, the authors recommend against the routine inclusion of *KCNJ2* on diagnostic LQTS testing panels. *ACMG*, American College of Medical Genetics and Genomics; *AMP*, Association for Molecular Pathology; *LP*, likely pathogenic; *LQTS*, long QT syndrome; *P*, pathogenic; *TKOS*, triadin knockout syndrome; *TS*, Timothy syndrome; *GUS*, gene of uncertain significance; *VUS*, variant of uncertain significance. (Adapted from Giudicessi JR, et al. *Trends Cardiovasc Med.* 2018;28[7]:453–464.)

pore mutations had a longer QTc, though not significant among probands, non-probands with pore mutations experienced their first cardiac event at an earlier age than those with a non-pore mutation. Most recently, additional information has been gleaned suggesting that LQT2 patients with mutations involving the transmembrane pore region had the greatest risk for cardiac events, those with frame-shift/nonsense mutations in any region had an intermediate risk, and those with missense mutations in the C-terminus had the lowest risk for cardiac events. Interestingly, LQT2 patients with mutations in the pore-loop region of the $K_v11.1$ channel have a greater than twofold increased risk for arousal-triggered events, and LQT2 patients with non-pore loop TM region mutations have a nearly sevenfold increase in the risk for exercise-triggered cardiac events compared with patients with N-terminal/C-terminal mutations.[1]

Incomplete penetrance and variable expressivity are clinical hallmark features of LQTS, and it has been long thought that co-inheritance

of a true disease-causing mutation and either a common or rare channel genetic variant may determine the expressed severity of the disorder. For example, the co-existence of the common *K897T-KCNH2* polymorphism and the *A1116V-KCNH2* mutation (on opposite alleles) led to a more severe clinical course in a single Italian LQTS family. The *A1116V* mutation by itself produced a sub-clinical phenotype of mild QT prolongation and an asymptomatic course, while the proband hosting both variants had clinically overt disease consisting of a diagnostic QT prolongation, presyncopal episodes, and cardiac arrest. Besides cardiac ion channels, single nucleotide polymorphisms (SNPs) of non-ion channel genes like *NOS1AP* (the gene encoding the nitric oxide synthase 1 adapter protein), *ADRA2C* (alpha-2C adrenergic receptor), and *ADRB1* (beta-1 adrenergic receptor) can modify disease severity in LQTS.[1]

There is compelling evidence for a strong disease modifying effect of a 3′ untranslated region (3′UTR) *KCNQ1* allele-specific haplotype in LQT1 mutation positive pedigrees; the magnitude of the effect on the QTc and symptomology go well beyond any other currently described genetic modifiers.[1] The *KCNQ1* gene encodes a single $K_v7.1$ ion channel alpha subunit that assemble to create a pore-forming $K_v7.1$ tetrameric channel. Therefore, if a patient had a heterozygous *KCNQ1* mutation (i.e., one normal *KCNQ1* gene allele and one mutant allele), one would expect that if both the normal and mutant gene alleles were expressed in equal amounts, then 1/16 of the $K_v7.1$ channels would be a normal homomeric tetramer and 1/16 of the $K_v7.1$ channels would be a mutant homomeric tetramer. The remaining channels would be hybrids containing both normal and mutant alpha-subunits. If expression of the normal *KCNQ1* gene allele was somehow suppressed, then there would be relatively more *KCNQ1* mutant alpha-subunits translated and ultimately assembled to provide more dysfunctional $K_v7.1$ channels, thus leading to a more severe manifestation of the disorder (see eFig. 63.1). The opposite would be true if the mutation containing the *KCNQ1* allele was suppressed.

Most genes have a 3'UTR that generates an mRNA transcript containing regions of cis-regulatory binding sites for small noncoding microRNAs (miRNAs) that bind to the transcript and ultimately inhibit that gene's expression. Naturally occurring genetic variation within these 3'UTRs (miR-SNPs) can either abolish existing or creating new miRNA binding sites. SNPs in the *KCNQ1* 3'UTR create a "suppressive" haplotype by generating new miRNA binding sites that suppress the expression of the *KCNQ1* allele in which they reside. Inheritance of the "suppressive" haplotype residing on the normal "healthy" allele produced a more severe LQT1 phenotype, whereas the inheritance of the "suppressive" haplotype residing on the same allele as the *KCNQ1* mutation gave a less severe LQT1 phenotype (shorter QTc and fewer symptoms).[1] This intriguing discovery both explains a significant component of reduced penetrance and variable expressivity that is a common feature of arrhythmia syndromes, and also represents a paradigm shift in our thinking about disease-modifying genetic-drivers of mendelian disorders (as one of the most important genetic determinants of disease severity in LQT1 appears to be the 3'UTR *KCNQ1* haplotype on the allele inherited from the unaffected "non-LQTS" parent).

In line with the concept that common variants within noncoding regions of the human genome may impact the penetrance and expressivity (a.k.a. clinical variability) of rare LQTS pathogenic/likely pathogenic variants, recent studies have demonstrated that an aggregate polygenic risk score (PRS) comprised of common variants that influence QTc duration at the level of population[15-17] can explain 2% to 15% of the clinical variability observed among LQTS patients.[10,18] Although the clinical utility of these PRSs in the management of genotype-positive LQTS patients remains unclear, they do provide intriguing and potentially clinically relevant insights into the genetic architecture of the 10% to 20% of LQTS patients that remain genotype-negative for monogenic LQTS.

Of note, the recent rare disease genome-wide association study (GWAS) by Lahrouchi et al.[10] provided compelling evidence, by way of a 68 SNP/common variant–weighted PRS, that genotype-negative LQTS likely represents a polygenic subtype that arises secondary to the accumulation of multiple QTc-prolonging common genetic variants. Interestingly, in comparison to patients with canonical LQTS (i.e., LQT1-LQT3), these genotype-negative patients had longer aggregate QTc intervals and a similar rate of event-free survival.[10] These observations are in line with those from other genetic heart diseases considered, at least initially, to be predominantly mendelian/monogenic such as familial hypercholesterolemia and BrS.[19]

LQTS, like many cardiovascular disorders, appears to have a more complex genetic architecture than anticipated initially that likely includes monogenic, oligogenic, and polygenic subtypes (Fig. 63.4).[2] As our understanding of the genetic architecture underlying LQTS continues to grow, it appears increasingly likely that commercial gene panel-based LQTS genetic tests in use today require an overhaul to better accommodate assessment of the 10% to 20% of patients that have oligogenic/polygenic subtypes, and the genetic background that influences the penetrance and expressivity of canonical LQTS-causative variants.

Calmodulinopathic Long QT Syndrome

In the early 2010s, three independent, unbiased exome sequencing studies implicated heterozygous sporadic/de novo pathogenic variants in the biologically redundant *CALM1*, *CALM2*, and *CALM3* genes that collectively encode calmodulin (an ubiquitously expressed and essential calcium-handling protein) in infants/young children with extreme QT prolongation (i.e., >600 msec) and adrenergic-triggered life-threatening ventricular arrhythmias.[20] Subsequently, pathogenic variants in *CALM1-3* have also been identified in patients with *CPVT*, *IVF*, and *CPVT/LQTS* overlap phenotypes. However, recent data from the multicenter International Calmodulinopathy Registry indicate that LQTS (49%) and CPVT (28%) phenotypes predominate.[20]

From a pathophysiological perspective, it is interesting to note that all LQTS-causative *CALM1-3* mutations described to date localize within or proximal to calcium-coordinating residues of the C-terminal lobe (C-lobe) of calmodulin and impart a marked reduction in calcium-binding affinity.[20,21] Although calmodulin is known to regulate a number of cardiac ion channels, the predominant effect of LQTS pathogenic/likely pathogenic *CALM1-3* variants appears to be loss of calcium-dependent inactivation (CDI) of the L-type calcium channel (LTCC) resulting in unrestrained calcium influx (i.e., $LTCC/I_{CaL}$ gain-of-function).[21] In contrast, CPVT pathogenic/likely pathogenic variants in *CALM1-3* localized at the N-terminal (N-lobe) and C-lobe increase RyR2-binding affinity/single channel open probability and spontaneous calcium release from the sarcoplasmic reticulum rather than calcium-binding affinity.[21]

Unfortunately, the calmodulinopathies (such as CALM-LQTS and CALM-CPVT) are frequently refractory to conventional LQTS- and CPVT-directed therapies (beta-blockers).[20] At present, it is not known whether the varying levels of neurodevelopmental delay observed in a minority of patients with a calmodulinopathy (17%) are secondary to anoxic brain injury in the setting of recurrent cardiac arrhythmias or are related to developmental effects of perturbed calcium-handling in the central nervous system.[20] Regardless, a combination of pharmacologic, sympathectomy, and device-related therapies is typically required and even then is often inadequate. As such, the calmodulinopathies represent an important target for gene-therapy and other targeted precision medicine approaches.

Triadin Knockout Syndrome

In 2015, Altmann et al. described a rare autosomal recessive form of LQTS characterized by transient/consistent QT prolongation with extensive precordial (V_1–V_4) T wave inversions (see Fig. 63.1B), severe and often refractory exercise-induced ventricular arrhythmias during childhood. In addition, they described mild-to-moderate proximal skeletal myopathy secondarily due to either homozygous (p.D18fs*13-TRDN and p.K147fs0*-TRDN) or compound heterozygous (p.N9fs*5-TRDN and p.K147fs*0-TRDN) frame-shift/null pathogenic/likely pathogenic variants in *TRDN*-encoded triadin (a key structural component of the cardiac release unit [CRU]).[21,22] Interestingly, some of the same TRDN null variants (p.D18fs*13-TRDN and p.N9fs*5-TRDN) were implicated previously in recessively inherited CPVT,[21] suggesting that Triadin knockout syndrome (TKOS) may represent a unique clinical entity with clinical characteristics of both LQTS and CPVT.

To this end, a recent study from the International TKOS Registry attempted to clarify the phenotype observed in individuals with homozygous/compound heterozygous TRDN null variants.[23] Whereas the mean QTc observed in TKOS patients was 472 ± 34 msec, exercise-induced ectopy was observed in 89%.[23] Furthermore, 90% of TKOS patients experienced SCA/SCD, and 74% suffered breakthrough cardiac events despite a myriad of medical, surgical (sympathectomy), and device therapy highlighting the malignant nature of the distinct TKOS clinical phenotype.[23]

Like calmodulinopathies, TKOS is primarily a disorder of calcium-handling. Although the TKOS patient-specific human induced pluripotent stem cell-derived cardiomyocytes (iPSC-CM) have yet to be characterized, insights gleaned from ventricular arrhythmia-prone *TRDN* null mice suggest that complete ablation of triadin, as would be expected in TKOS patients, disrupts the approximation of the

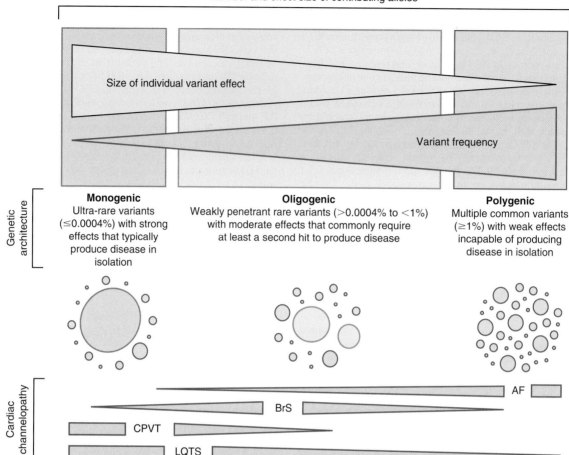

FIGURE 63.4 The spectrum of genetic variation underlying the heritable component of select cardiac channelopathies. At the severe (*red*) end of the spectrum are ultra-rare disease-causative pathogenic variants with strong effects on gene function that typically result in monogenic disorders. In the middle of the spectrum (*yellow*) are weakly penetrant and comparably more common rare variants with moderate effects on gene function that rarely produce disease in isolation, but in the presence of one or more second hits result in so-called oligogenic disease. At the benign (*green*) end of the spectrum are common variants with weak effects on gene function, largely discovered through large genome-wide association studies, that are incapable of producing disease in isolation, but may confer disease risk when multiple risk-associated common variants are present within the genome of an individual exposed to environmental risk factors, resulting in so-called polygenic disease. In recognition that the genetic architecture of most cardiac channelopathies is variable, *blue triangles* denote the spectrum of genetic variation shown to contribute to genetic basis of select cardiac channelopathies. *AF,* Atrial fibrillation; *BrS,* Brugada syndrome; *CPVT,* catecholaminergic polymorphic ventricular tachycardia; *LQTS,* long QT syndrome. (Adapted from Giudicessi JR, Ackerman MJ. *Transl Res.* 2013;161[1]:1–14.)

T-tubule and junctional sarcoplasmic reticulum within the cardiac dyad and reduces the expression of key proteins such as RyR2, calsequestrin2, and junctin reducing the co-localization of the LTCC/RyR2 and RyR2/Calsequestrin2 in the CRU.[21] The resulting remodeling of the CRU leads to reduced sarcoplasmic reticulum calcium release and impaired LTCC CDI that ultimately leads to calcium overload in the sarcoplasmic reticulum.[21] These molecular events likely contribute to an underlying proarrhythmic electrophysiological substrate capable of triggering delayed afterdepolarization- and/or early afterdepolarization-mediated ventricular arrhythmias. This explains the distinct and particularly malignant clinical phenotype, with elements of LQTS and CPVT, observed in TKOS patients.[21,23]

Timothy Syndrome
Clinical Description and Manifestations of Timothy Syndrome

Timothy syndrome (TS) is an extremely rare (<30 patients described worldwide) multisystem, highly lethal arrhythmia disorder, associated with both cardiac and extracardiac abnormalities. The typical cardiac manifestation of TS includes fetal bradycardia, extreme prolongation of the QT interval (QTc >500 msec) often with macroscopic T wave alternans and 2:1 atrioventricular block at birth (see Fig. 63.1C). These abnormalities often coincide with congenital heart defects or cardiomyopathies. Extracardiac abnormalities often consist of simple syndactyly

(webbing of the toes and fingers), dysmorphic facial features, abnormal dentition, immune deficiency, severe hypoglycemia, and developmental delay (including autism). Currently, most TS patients die before reaching puberty. While the majority of TS has been described as sporadic/de novo occurrences, few cases with somatic mosaicism associated with a less severe phenotype have recently been described. For example, the *CACNA1C* mutation may be present in the patient's skeletal muscle, but could only be present in traces or even completely absent in other cell types of the human body (i.e., absent in heart, blood lymphocytes), where the patient may present with simple syndactyly.

GENETIC BASIS FOR TIMOTHY SYNDROME

In 2004, Splawski et al. identified the molecular basis for this highly lethal arrhythmia and named it *Timothy syndrome* (TS) after Katherine Timothy, Drs. Keating's and Splawski's study coordinator who meticulously phenotyped these cases.[1] Remarkably, in all 13 unrelated patients where DNA was available, Splawski identified the same recurrent sporadic de novo missense mutation, p.G406R-CACNA1C, in the alternatively spliced exon 8A of the *CACNA1C*-encoded cardiac LTCC (Ca$_v$1.2), which is important for excitation-contraction coupling in the heart and mediates an inward depolarizing current in cardiomyocytes (see eTable 63.1, Fig. 63.2) similar to the cardiac sodium channel Na$_v$1.5. Through alternative splicing, the human L-type Ca channel consists of two mutually exclusive isoforms: one containing exon 8A and the other with exon 8. A year later, they described two cases of atypical TS with similar features of TS yet without syndactyly. As with other TS cases, these two atypical cases were identified as having sporadic de novo *CACNA1C* mutations in exon 8. One case hosted a mutation analogous to the classic TS mutation, *p.G406R-CACNA1C*, whereas the other case hosted a *p.G402R-CACNA1C* missense mutation. All three mutations confer gain-of-function to the LTCC/Ca$_v$1.2 channels through impaired channel inactivation and reside very near the end of the S6 transmembrane segment of domain 1 in the beginning of the intracellular loop between domain I and II of the Ca$_v$1.2 alpha subunit.

In 2011, Gillis et al. identified a novel *CACNA1C* mutation, *p.A1473G-CACNA1C*, in a single patient with a prolonged QT interval, dysmorphic facial features, syndactyly, and joint contractures consistent with TS.[1] In 2015, Boczek et al. identified a novel *CACNA1C* mutation, *p.I1166T-CACNA1C*, in a patient exhibiting a TS phenotype with QT prolongation, patent ductus arteriosus, seizures, facial dysmorphism, joint hypermobility, hypotonia, hand anomalies, intellectual impairment, and tooth decay.[24] Patch-clamp analysis of *p.I1166T-CACNA1C* demonstrated a novel electrophysiological phenotype distinct from the loss of inactivation seen with the previously established TS mutations. Instead, p.I1166T-CACNA1C electrophysiological studies illustrated a loss of current density and a gain-of-function shift in activation, leading to an increase in window current.[24] Interestingly, both p.I1166T-CACNA1C's and p.A1473G-CACNA1C's topological position (a few amino acids away from the S6 transmembrane segment of the domain III and IV, respectively) in the channel architecture is very similar to the position of the three original TS mutations (S6 segment of domain I).

Cardiac-Only Timothy Syndrome

In 2015, Boczek et al. used exome sequencing to identify a novel *CACNA1C* mutation p.R518C-CACNA1C that was most likely responsible for the observed phenotype in a large pedigree with concomitant LQTS, hypertrophic cardiomyopathy (HCM), congenital heart defects, and sudden cardiac death.[25] None of the patients had extracardiac phenotypes, such as those observed with TS. A subsequent *CACNA1C* exon 12 specific analysis in 5 additional unrelated index cases with a similar phenotype of LQTS and a personal/family history of HCM identified 2 additional pedigrees with mutations at the same amino acid position; either p.R518C-CACNA1C or p.R518H-CACNA1C. Patch-clamp studies on both revealed a complex Ca$_v$1.2 electrophysiological phenotype consisting of loss of current density and inactivation in combination with increased window and late current. All three pedigrees hosting p.R518C-CACNA1C/p.R518H-CACNA1C presented with this unique and atypical phenotypic sequela consistent with cardiac-only Timothy syndrome (COTS).[25]

The spectrum of QT-opathies associated with LTCC/Ca$_v$1.2 gain-of-function currently encompasses nonsyndromic LQTS (i.e., CACNA1C-LQTS/LQT8), COTS, and TS.[21] The electrophysiological mechanisms and clinical phenotypes that differentiate this spectrum of LTCC/Ca$_v$1.2-mediated disorders are detailed in Figure 63.5 and are the focus of several recent comprehensive reviews.[21,26]

Short QT Syndrome
Clinical Description and Manifestations of Short QT Syndrome

Short QT syndrome (SQTS), first described in 2000 by Gussak et al., is associated with a short QT-interval (usually ≤320 msec) on a 12-lead ECG (Fig. 63.1D), paroxysmal atrial fibrillation (AF), syncope, and an increased risk for SCD. Giustetto et al. analyzed the clinical presentation of 53 patients with SQTS from 29 families (the largest cohort studied to date). They found that 62% of the patients were symptomatic, with cardiac arrest being the most common symptom (31% of patients) and frequently the first manifestation of the disorder. A fourth of the patients had a history of syncope, and nearly 30% had a family history of SCD. Symptoms including syncope or cardiac arrest most often occurred during periods of rest or sleep. Nearly one-third presented with AF. SCD was observed during infancy, suggesting the potential role for SQTS as a rare pathogenic basis for some cases of SIDS.[1]

GENETIC BASIS FOR SHORT QT SYNDROME
SQTS is most often inherited in an autosomal dominant manner; however, some de novo sporadic cases have been described. To date, mutations in six genes (see eTable 63.1) have been implicated in the pathogenesis of SQTS, including gain-of-function mutations in the potassium channel encoding genes *KCNH2* (SQT1), *KCNQ1* (SQT2), and *KCNJ2* (SQT3) and loss-of-function mutations in *CACNA1C* (SQT4), *CACNB2b* (SQT5), and *CACNA2D1* (SQT6) encoding for LTCC alpha, beta, and delta subunits, respectively (see eTable 63.1, Fig. 63.2).[1] However, despite the identification of these SQTS-susceptibility genes, the proportion of SQTS expected to be SQT1-6 genotype positive and that awaiting genetic elucidation are unknown. It is estimated that over 75% of SQTS remains elusive genetically.

Genotype-Phenotype Correlates in Short QT Syndrome
While there are insufficient data to clearly define genotype-phenotype correlations in SQTS (probably fewer than 60 cases have been described in the literature to date), gene-specific ECG patterns are beginning to emerge. The typical ECG pattern consists of a QT-interval of ≤320 msec (QTc ≤340 msec) and tall, peaked T waves in the precordial leads with either a short ST segment present or no ST-segment at all. The T waves tend to be symmetrical in SQT1 but asymmetrical in SQT2-4. In SQT2, inverted T waves can be observed. In SQT5, a BrS-like ST elevation in the right precordial lead could be observed as well.[1]

Owing to the prematurely small sample size, a recent report revealed that SQTS patients with *KCNH2* mutations have a shorter QT and a greater response to hydroquinidine therapy than patients with a non-KCNH2 mediated SQTS.[1] Based on a clinical variable analysis of 65 mutation-positive SQTS patients among 132 SQTS cases previously reported in the literature, Harrell et al. indicated that patients with *KCNH2*-mediated SQTS (SQT1) exhibit a later age of onset of manifestation, whereas patients with *KCNQ1*-mediated SQTS (SQT2) have a higher prevalence of bradyarrhythmias and AF.[27]

Drug-Induced Torsade de Pointes (see Chapter 9)
Clinical Description and Manifestations of Drug-Induced Torsade de Pointes

Drug-induced long QT syndrome (DI-LQTS) and torsades de pointes is a multifactorial clinical entity that tends to surface in the setting of multiple modifiable (electrolyte abnormalities such as hypokalemia, co-administration of multiple QT-prolonging drugs, drug accumulation due to renal/hepatic impairment or inhibition of cytochrome P450 metabolism) and non-modifiable (female sex, underlying genetic disposition, structural heart disease, and diabetes) risk factors (see Chapters 9 and 64). The estimated incidence of DI-LQTS/DI-TdP is drug-dependent, while class III anti-arrhythmic agents range between 1% and 8% depending on the drug and dose. DI-TdP and subsequent sudden death are rare events; however, the list of potential "QT-liability" or "torsadegenic" drugs is extensive and includes both anti-arrhythmic drugs (quinidine, sotalol and dofetilide) and many noncardiac medications (antipsychotics, methadone, antimicrobials, antihistamines, and the gastrointestinal stimulant cisapride [see https://www.crediblemeds.org for a comprehensive list]).[1]

hERG/K$_v$11.1 Channel Blockade and Cardiac Repolarization Reserve

In addition to their intended function/mechanism of action, the vast majority of drugs associated with DI-LQTS and DI-TdP also cause unwanted, intracellular drug-induced blockade of the rapidly activating component of phase 3 delayed rectifier K$^+$ current (I$_{Kr}$) conducted by *KCNH2*-encoded hERG/K$_v$11.1 K$^+$ channels. In effect, QT-prolonging drugs create a "LQT2-like" phenotype through reduced repolarization efficiency, lengthening and exaggerated spatial dispersion of the cardiac action potential. However, I$_{Kr}$ drug blockade alone does not appear sufficient to provide the potentially lethal TdP substrate. One particular thesis centers on the observation that cardiac repolarization relies on the interaction of several ion currents that provide some level of redundancy in order to protect against extreme QT prolongation by "QT-liability" drugs. This so-called repolarization reserve may be reduced through anomalies in the repolarization machinery as a result of common or rare genetic variants in critical ion channels that produce a subclinical loss

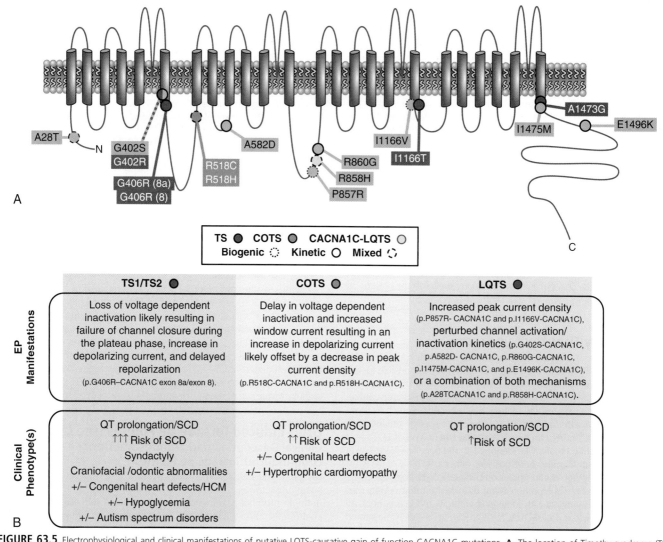

FIGURE 63.5 Electrophysiological and clinical manifestations of putative LQTS-causative gain-of-function CACNA1C mutations. **A,** The location of Timothy syndrome (TS; *red circles*)-, cardiac-only Timothy syndrome (COTS; *orange circles*)-, and LQTS (CACNA1C-LQTS; *green circles*)-causative CACNA1C pathogenic variants are depicted on the Cav1.2 linear protein topology. Biogenic (*small dashed outline*), biophysical/kinetic (*solid outline*), and mixed (*large dashed outline*) electrophysiologic manifestations of individual CACNA1C pathogenic variants are indicated by the contrasting circle outlines. **B,** Summary of the electrophysiological and clinical manifestations of TS, COTS, and LQTS. *EP,* Electrophysiologic; *HCM,* hypertrophic cardiomyopathy; *SCD,* sudden cardiac death. (Adapted from Giudicessi JR, et al. *Circ Arrhythm Electrophysiol.* 2016;9[7]:e002480.)

of the repolarizing I_{Ks} and I_{Kr} currents.[1] Prior studies have demonstrated that (1) 10% to 15% of patients with DI-TdP host rare ion channel mutations,[1] and (2) weighted-effect PRSs, designed to measure the aggregate effect of QTc-influencing common genetic variants identified previously in the general population[9,17] can identify those at greatest risk of developing an exaggerated QTc response/TdP following exposure to known QT prolonging drugs.[28] As a result, these studies provide further credence to the concept that multiple genetic and environmental hits to the "repolarization reserve" are involved in the pathogenesis of DI-LQTS/DI-TdP.

Furthermore, emerging evidence suggests that drug-induced blockade of hERG/K_v11.1 channels is not the only mechanism involved in the pathogenesis of DI-LQTS/DI-TdP. Over the last several years, inhibition of phosphoinositide 3-kinase (PI3K) signaling and its downstream effect on multiple depolarizing and repolarizing currents [primarily reduced I_{Kr} and increased late/sustained Na$^+$ (I_{NaL}) currents] has emerged as another important mechanism underling DI-LQTS/DI-TdP risk.[28] Interestingly, drugs such as dofetilide, sotalol, and azithromycin that also inhibit PI3K and increase I_{NaL} current appear to be more torsadogenic than those that only cause hERG/K_v11.1 blockade. Therefore, in vitro markers of DI-LQTS risk, most notably the hERG/K_v11.1 half-maximal inhibitory concentration (IC_{50}), which is used currently for pre-clinical drug screening,

may underestimate the true DI-LQTS/DI-TdP liability of some pharmacologic agents.[28]

Common Ion Channel Polymorphisms and DI-TdP Risk
(see Chapter 9).

Among the common polymorphisms of the *KCNH2*-encoding I_{Kr} potassium channel, the p.K897T-KCNH2 and p.R1047L-KCNH2 polymorphisms have gained the most attention. Paavonen et al. observed that p.T897-KCNH2 channels exhibit slower activation kinetics with a higher degree of inactivation, an alteration expected to decrease channel function and perhaps alter drug sensitivity since several commonly used drugs inhibiting I_{Kr} channel function bind preferentially to the inactivated state of the channel. This finding reveals that p.T897T-KCNH2 may genetically "reduce repolarization reserve" and facilitate a pro-arrhythmic response that may be enhanced in the setting of I_{Kr} channel blocking drugs. In fact, p.K897T-KCNH2 appears to affect the QTc response to ibutilide in a gender-specific manner. In one study, among 105 AF patients treated with dofetilide, p.R1047L-KCNH2 was over-represented among those patients who developed DI-TdP. Besides these common potassium channel alpha-subunit polymorphisms, three common polymorphisms (p.D85N-KCNE1, p.T8A-KCNE2, and p.Q9E-KCNE2) involving auxiliary beta subunits have been implicated in drug-induced arrhythmia susceptibility.[1]

Of note, there is particularly strong epidemiological (DI-LQTS odds ratio of 9.0 [3.5 to 22.9]) and functional (decreased I_{Ks} and I_{Kr} secondary to altered activation/inactivation kinetics) evidence to support a role for p.D85N-KCNE1, a common variant observed in approximately 1% of individuals of European-descent, in DI-LQTS/DI-TdP risk.[29] In addition, p.D85N-KCNE1 may cause transient QTc prolongation in isolation[8,14] and influence QTc duration in both the general population[8] and congenital LQTS patients.[10] Nevertheless, owing to its common nature, some commercial genetic testing companies continue to relegate reporting of p.D85N-KCNE1 and other clinically relevant common variants (p.K897T-KCNH2, p.S1103Y-SCN5A, etc.) to supplemental reports that must be requested by the ordering health care professional.[8]

In addition to common genetic variants that affect the KVLQT1/K_v7.1 (I_{Ks}) and hERG/K_v11.1 (I_{Kr}) potassium channels, common variants in the *SCN5A*-encoded Na_v1.5 cardiac sodium channel that increase late sodium current may also serve as potentially pro-arrhythmic genetic substrate in patients exposed to QT-prolonging drugs. Of note, the p.S1103Y-SCN5A common variant observed in approximately 8% to 10% of individuals of African descent has been associated with baseline QT prolongation and a small persistent risk of arrhythmia/SCD across the age spectrum (DI-LQTS odds ratio of 8.7 [3.2 to 23.9]).[8] Interestingly, in heterologous expression systems the very subtle biophysical alterations imparted by p.S1103Y-SCN5A do not appear to alter action potential duration (APD). However, in the setting of a "second hit" such as hERG/K_v11.1 block or intracellular acidosis, the modest increase in late sodium current generated by p.S1103Y-SCN5A significantly prolongs the APD in in vitro and in silico models.[8]

Recent GWAS have associated common variants of the *NOS1AP*-encoded nitric oxide synthase 1 adapter protein (NOS1AP) with QT interval duration. NOS1AP is a regulator of the neuronal nitric oxide synthase (nNOS), which regulates intracellular calcium levels and myocyte contraction through its effect on the LTCCs. Common SNPs in *NOS1AP* are associated with drug-induced QT prolongation and ventricular arrhythmia.[1] This association was most pronounced among those patients using amiodarone, one of the most common antiarrhythmic drugs. It has been hypothesized that individuals hosting genetic variants in *NOS1AP* that suppress the gene's expression may in turn result in increased LTCC currents and subsequently QT prolongation and such individuals may be at increased arrhythmogenic risk while on amiodarone.[1] However, although QT prolongation is observed routinely with amiodarone, DI-TdP attributed to amiodarone is exceedingly rare.

Additionally, genetic variation or individual differences in drug elimination or metabolism may contribute to individual risk for drug DI-TdP. For example, patients with genetically mediated reduction in CYP3A enzymatic activity could be vulnerable to DI-TdP in the setting of I_{Kr} blockers that depend on the cytochrome P450 enzyme CYP3A for its metabolism.[1]

THE OTHER CHANNELOPATHIES

Andersen-Tawil Syndrome

Clinical Description and Manifestations of Andersen-Tawil Syndrome

ATS, first described in 1971 in a case report by Andersen and later described by Tawil in 1994, is now recognized as a rare (≤1:1,000,000) autosomal-dominant cardiac channelopathy characterized clinically by the triad of periodic paralysis, frequent ventricular ectopy/arrhythmia (Fig. 63.6A), and variable developmental abnormalities.[1]

Initially, ATS was classified erroneously as a multisystem form of LQTS (and called LQT7) due to the inclusion of prominent U-waves that result in substantial prolongation of the QT-U interval (see Fig. 63.6A).[2] However, once the U-waves are excluded properly, the QTc values of ATS patients are typically within the normal range (i.e., <440 msec).[2] Furthermore, the burden and nature of the electrocardiographic abnormalities (mostly ventricular bigeminy, polymorphic VT, and in rare circumstances bi-directional VT) observed in ATS is reminiscent of the electrocardiographic hallmarks of CPVT and can lead to misdiagnosis. However, the presence of these findings at rest as well

as the variable presence of micrognathia, low-set ears, widely spaced eyes, and clinodactyly helps differentiate ATS from CPVT. Correctly distinguishing between true ATS and CPVT is critical as the treatment strategies are quite different.

Of note, despite an often-alarming burden of ventricular ectopy, the long-term prognosis in ATS has generally been considered favorable. However, in the largest multicenter registry of ATS patients assembled to date, Mazzanti et al. demonstrated recently that the rate of SCA/SCD in ATS (9.3%)[30] was much higher than reported previously (2.7%) and similar to the lifetime SCA/SCD observed in other cardiac channelopathies such as LQTS (~13%). As such, the natural history of ATS could be more malignant than anticipated previously and the efficacy of conventional pharmacotherapies in terms of SCA/SCD prevention (i.e., nadolol plus flecainide, amiodarone) remains currently in question.[30]

GENETIC BASIS FOR ANDERSEN-TAWIL SYNDROME

To date, more than 40 unique mutations in *KCNJ2* have been described as causative for ATS1. Mutations in *KCNJ2* account for approximately two-thirds of ATS, while the molecular basis of the residual third of ATS cases remains genetically and mechanistically elusive. However, the prevalence of *KCNJ2* mutations may be as high as 75% to 80% for patients with at least two ATS phenotypic features (i.e., typical ATS).[1] Most ATS-associated mutations in *KCNJ2* are inherited in an autosomal dominant inheritance pattern, however as much as one-third of mutations in *KCNJ2* could be sporadic de novo occurrences. In addition, somatic mosaicism has also been described in at least one *KCNJ2*-associated ATS family. Localized to chromosome 17q23, *KCNJ2* encodes for Kir2.1, a two-membrane spanning repeat potassium channel alpha subunit expressed in brain, skeletal muscle, and heart that is critically responsible for the inward rectifying cardiac I_{K1} current (see eTable 63.1, Fig. 63.2). In the heart, I_{K1} plays an important role in setting the heart's resting membrane potential, buffering extracellular potassium, and modulating the action potential waveform. Most *KCNJ2* mutations described in ATS are missense mutations that cause a loss-of-function of I_{K1} either through a dominant negative effect on Kir2.1 subunit assembly or through haploinsufficiency as a result of protein trafficking defects.[1]

Phenotypic Correlates in *KCNJ2*-Mediated Andersen-Tawil Syndrome (ATS1)

Genotype-specific electrocardiographic features of ATS are beginning to emerge. Zhang et al. examined ECG T-U morphology and found that 91% of *KCNJ2* mutation positive ATS1 patients had characteristic T-U-wave patterns (including prolonged terminal T wave down-slope, a wide T-U junction, and biphasic and enlarged U-waves) compared to none of the 61 unaffected family members or 29 genotype-negative ATS patients. In a subsequent study, 88% of *KCNJ2* mutation positive ATS patients had an abnormal U-wave. Additionally, while the U-wave is markedly abnormal in ATS1, it is typically normal in LQTS. Consequently, this *KCNJ2* gene-specific T-U morphology can be very useful in differentiating ATS1 patients from *KCNJ2* mutation-negative ATS and LQT1-3 patients. This could facilitate a cost-effective approach towards genetic testing of the appropriate disorder. Interestingly, topological location of *KCNJ2* mutations may influence the phenotypic expression of ATS features. The vast majority (approximately 90%) of *KCNJ2* mutations reside either in the N- or C-terminus of this two-transmembrane single pore channel. C-terminal mutations appear to be more often associated with typical ATS (>2 ATS features), dysmorphism, and periodic paralysis. Meanwhile, N-terminal mutations were more often observed in atypical ATS (only 1 ATS feature, predominately a cardiac phenotype only) cases.[1]

Ankyrin-B Syndrome

The *ANK2* gene encodes for ankyrin B protein, a member of large family of proteins that anchor various integral membrane proteins to the spectrin-based cytoskeleton. Specifically, ankyrin B is involved in anchoring the Na/K-ATPase, Na/Ca exchanger, and InsP3 receptor to specialized microdomains in the cardiomyocyte transverse tubules. In murine models, *ANK2* haploinsufficiency results in altered calcium handling and a complex cardiac phenotype consisting of atrial arrhythmias, sinus bradycardia, modest heart rate-corrected QT

1200

ARRHYTHMIAS, SUDDEN DEATH, AND SYNCOPE

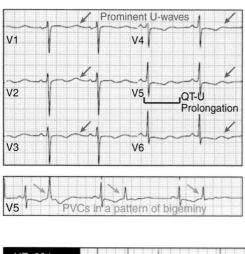

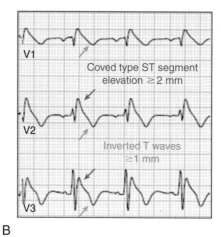

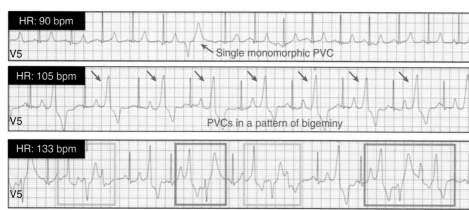

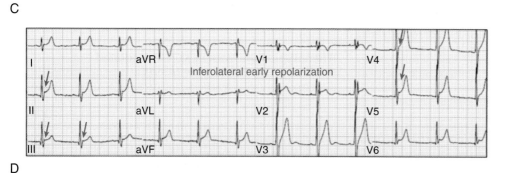

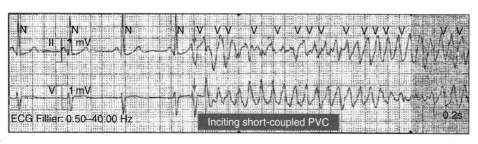

interval prolongation, catecholamine-induced ventricular arrhythmias, and a propensity for SCD.[31] In humans, loss-of-function variants in *ANK2* were shown to cause a dominantly inherited cardiac arrhythmia with an increased risk for SCD in the setting of overt QTc prolongation. As a result, *ANK2* was subsequently assigned the label of type 4 LQTS (LQT4). However, subsequent studies have demonstrated that baseline QTc prolongation is inconsistently observed in ankyrin B syndrome (ABS). Similar to ATS, this initial discrepancy appears to have been caused partly by the erroneous inclusion of prominent U-waves/sinusoidal T-U abnormalities in QTc calculations. As a result, the QT-U interval may appear markedly prolonged in ABS, but true QTc values typically reside in the normal-to-borderline range as commonly reported. As a result, this disorder has been renamed SSS with bradycardia or the ABS.[1]

Of note, the first human *ANK2* mutation (*p.E1425G-ANK2*) was identified in a large multi-generational French kindred presenting with "atypical LQTS" displaying a phenotype of prolonged QT-interval, severe sinus bradycardia, polyphasic T waves and AF.[1] Following this sentinel discovery, significant loss-of-function ankyrin B variants of differing degrees of functionality have now been identified in patients with a wide array of arrhythmia including bradycardia, sinus node dysfunction (SND), delayed cardiac conduction/conduction block, IVF, AF, DI-LQTS, exercise-induced VT, and even BrS and CPVT phenotypes.

However, it is important to note that 2% to 4% of ostensibly healthy white and 8% to 10% of black subjects (including the most common "black" specific variant *p.L1622I-ANK2*) also host rare variants in *ANK2*, making it difficult to distinguish ABS-causative variants from background genetic noise (i.e., VUS). Furthermore, the majority of alleged ABS-causative loss-of-function variants, including *p.E1424G-ANK2*, used to establish the initial GDA between *ANK2* and ABS have now been observed with perplexingly high frequency in public exomes/genomes (i.e., >100 individuals). This revealed that the genetic basis of ABS may be substantially more complex than initially anticipated.[5]

Brugada Syndrome
Clinical Description and Manifestations of Brugada Syndrome

Brugada syndrome (BrS) is a heritable arrhythmia syndrome characterized clinically by spontaneous or

FIGURE 63.6 Select electrocardiographic findings in the non-QT-opathies. **A,** Prominent U-waves (*blue arrows*), QT-U interval prolongation (*black bracket*), and frequent ventricular ectopy (*orange arrows*) in a p.R82W-KCNJ2–positive Andersen-Tawil syndrome patient. After exclusion of the U-wave in the top panel, the patient's QT interval (443 msec) is within normal limits. **B,** A spontaneous type 1 Brugada syndrome pattern (coved/downsloping ST elevation ≥2 mm [*blue arrows*] with T wave inversions ≥1 mm [*orange arrows*] in the right precordial leads) in a genotype-negative patient with Brugada syndrome and easily inducible ventricular fibrillation from the right ventricular outflow tract on electrophysiology study. **C,** The progression of exercise-induced ventricular ectopy in a p.N98S-CALM1-positive catecholaminergic polymorphic ventricular tachycardia patient. During the early stages of exercise (*top panel*), occasional premature ventricular contractions (*blue arrow*) are observed. With increasing workloads (*middle panel*), more complex patterns of ventricular ectopy, most notable premature ventricular contractions in a pattern of bigeminy (*blue arrows*), is observed. At peak exercise (*bottom panel*), untreated or sub-optimally treated patients' manifest findings such as bi-directional couplets (*orange box*) and triplets (*gold boxes*) and bidirectional ventricular tachycardia (nonsustained in this case; *blue box*). **D,** Early repolarization in the inferior and lateral leads observed in a genotype-negative patient who presented with a sentinel cardiac arrest and has suffered appropriate implantable cardioverter defibrillator shocks. **E,** Telemetry rhythm strip demonstrating so-called short coupled torsades de pointes (premature ventricular contraction with a coupling interval of approximately 300 msec is indicated by *blue arrows*) in a genotype-negative patient who presented with a sentinel out-of-hospital cardiac arrest.

class I antiarrhythmic-provoked coved type ST-segment elevation (≥2 mm) followed by a negative T wave in ≥1 mm right precordial leads (V$_1$ or V$_2$, often referred to as a type 1 Brugada ECG pattern; Fig. 63.6B) on ECG and an increased risk of SCD during rest, sleep, or febrile episodes.[1] Although initially thought to disproportionately affect males with structurally normal hearts, recent imaging,[32,33] post-mortem necropsy, and concomitant electroanatomic mapping/targeted endomyocardial biopsy[34] studies have provided evidence that BrS is defined by electroanatomic and structural abnormalities involving the right ventricular outflow tract (RVOT) epicardium. As a result, BrS is best classified as a focal epicardial arrhythmogenic cardiomyopathy rather than a true cardiac channelopathy.

GENETIC BASIS OF BRUGADA SYNDROME

Classically, BrS is considered a mendelian/monogenic disorder inherited in an autosomal dominant fashion. However, many BrS cases arise sporadically, and marked incomplete penetrance and variable expressivity is a hallmark of the disorder. Therefore, the use of unbiased gene-discovery techniques (i.e., linkage analysis and trio/pedigree-based exome sequencing) to identify monogenic causes of BrS have largely proven unsuccessful.

At present, loss-of-function pathogenic/likely pathogenic variants in the SCN5A-encoded Na$_v$1.5 cardiac sodium channel underlie approximately 20% to 30% of BrS cases and constitute Brugada syndrome type 1 (BrS1). Interestingly, the yield of mutation detection may be significantly higher among familial forms than in sporadic cases. In one study, SCN5A mutations were identified in 38% of familial BrS cases compared to none in 27 sporadic cases (p = 0.001). The majority of the mutations were missense (66%), followed by frameshift (13%), nonsense, (11%), splice-site (7%), and in-frame deletions/insertions (3%) mutations. Approximately 3% of the genotype-positive patients host multiple putative pathogenic SCN5A mutations. Similar to the genotype-phenotype observations in LQTS, patients hosting multiple SCN5A mutations tend to be younger at diagnosis (29.7 ± 16 years) than those having a single mutation (39.2 ± 14.4 years).[1] Similar to LQT3, there is no particular mutational "hotspot," as nearly 80% of the BrS related SCN5A mutations occur as "private" single family mutations.

However, nearly 10% of the 438 unrelated putative disease-causative SCN5A variant-positive patients hosted one of the following four mutations: p.E1784K-SCN5A (14 patients), p.F861Wfs*90-SCN5A (11 patients), p.D356N-SCN5A (8 patients), and p.G1408R-SCN5A (7 patients). Interestingly, the most common occurring BrS1 mutation (p.E1784K-SCN5A) has also been reported as the most commonly seen LQT3-associated SCN5A mutation, illustrating how the same exact DNA alteration in a given gene can lead to two distinct cardiac arrhythmia syndromes. This is most likely a result of other environmental or genetic modifying factors. In fact, p.E1784K-SCN5A represents the quintessential example of a cardiac sodium channel mutation with the capacity to provide for a mixed clinical phenotype of LQT3, BrS, and conduction disorders.[1]

Besides ultra-rare pathogenic/likely pathogenic variants, common genetic variants in SCN5A (and other genes) also contribute a substantive role in the pathogenesis of BrS. In particular, a rare disease GWAS identified and validated the association of three genetic loci [SCN5A (rs11708996) SCN10A (rs10428132) on chromosome 3 and HEY2 (rs9388451) on chromosome 6] in BrS patients of European descent. Interestingly, the likelihood of manifesting a type 1 BrS ECG pattern rose substantially as individuals accumulated risk alleles within these genetic loci (two risk alleles conferred an odds ratio of 1.9 whereas greater than four risk alleles conferred an odds ratio of 21.5). Importantly, this simple "PRS" has now been validated independently in Japanese and Taiwanese cohorts.[19,35] However, approximately 1.5% of individuals of European-descent possess greater than 4 risk alleles in the aforementioned BrS-associated genetic loci identified by Bezzina et al.[19] Therefore, it is highly unlikely that these common genetic loci are sufficient to cause BrS, a disorder with an estimated prevalence less than 1:5000 (0.02%).[19,36]

In addition to putative BrS-causative SCN5A rare variants and the polygenic cocktail of common variants in SCN5A, SCN10A, and HEY2, alleged BrS-susceptibility variants have now been described in greater than 20 additional BrS-susceptibility genes (see eTable 63.1). Mechanistically, many of the "minor" BrS-susceptibility genes encode components of the Na$_v$1.5 macromolecular complex and have been shown to perturb Na$_v$1.5 trafficking in vitro (GPD1L, RANGRF [aka MOG1], PKP2, SLMAP, and the more recently described RRAD)[1,37] or gating/conduction

(SCN1B, SCN2B, and SCN3B) and decrease I$_{Na}$ in a manner analogous to BrS-causative variants in SCN5A. The vast majority of the remaining minor BrS-susceptibility genes encode pore-forming α- and accessory β-subunits that impart either a loss-of-function to the depolarizing L-type calcium current (I$_{Ca,L}$; CACNA1C, CACNA2D1, and CACNB2) or a gain-of-function to repolarizing transient outward (I$_{to}$; KCND3, KCNE3, and KCNE5) and ATP-sensitive potassium (I$_{KATP}$; ABCC9 and KCNJ8) currents.[1]

However, with the notable exception of the p.A280V-GPD1L variant in the GPD1L-encoded glycerol-3-phosphate dehydrogenase 1-like protein (discovered using linkage analysis)[1] and the recently described p.R211H-RRAD variant in RRAD-encoded Ras-Related Associated with Diabetes GTPase discovered by exome sequencing,[37] the remaining minor BrS-susceptibility genes were largely discovered using hypothesis-driven candidate gene approaches. Unfortunately, the only BrS-susceptibility gene where rare variants are statistically over-represented in BrS cases versus controls is SCN5A.[38]

In this context, it is surprising that SCN5A is the only BrS-susceptibility gene to receive a ClinGen "definitive" evidence designation.[39] Although some of the more recently described BrS-susceptibility genes (RRAD, SEMA3A) were not assessed, the 20 BrS-susceptibility genes that were evaluated by the ClinGen Channelopathy Working Group all received "disputed" evidence designations demoting them to ambiguous GUS status.[39] As a result, extreme caution should be used when interpreting any rare variant identified in alleged minor BrS-susceptibility gene and the identification of such a variant should **never** be used as the sole means of diagnosing a BrS.[40,41] Ultimately, the (1) the probable demise of most alleged minor BrS-susceptibility genes,[39] (2) large number of BrS cases that remain genetically elusive, and (3) low penetrance and variable expressivity associated with many BrS-causative SCN5A pathogenic variants determines whether the majority of BrS is a genetically heterogeneous monogenic disorder or an admixture of monogenic, oligogenic/polygenic, and nongenetic etiologies that through developmental- and/or immune-mediated mechanisms result in a shared final common pathway of epicardial RVOT inflammation, fibrosis, and conduction disorders (Fig. 63.7).

Phenotypic Correlates of SCN5A-Mediated Brugada Syndrome

As the majority of BrS cases remain elusive genetically, genotype-phenotype correlations in BrS have not been analyzed to the same degree as in LQTS. SCN5A mutations are associated with a higher incidence of conduction abnormalities in BrS patients, and the presence of a long PQ interval may be indicative of SCN5A-mediated BrS1. In fact, Crotti et al., reported that compared to a less than 10% yield for a positive SCN5A genetic test for those with a PQ less than 200 msec, the yield was almost 40% among those with a PQ interval ≥200 msec. Interestingly, young BrS males (<20 years, 83%) had a significantly higher SCN5A pathogenic/likely pathogenic variant detection rate than males aged 20 to 40 years (21%) and those over 40 years (11%, P < 0.0001). In addition, BrS1, patients with non-sense, frameshift, and premature truncation causing mutations exhibit a more severe phenotype. Unlike LQTS genetic testing where the triad of diagnostic, prognostic, and therapeutic impact has been fulfilled, BrS genetic testing is currently limited by its lower yield (25% for BrS versus 75% for LQTS) and relative absence of a therapeutic contribution from knowing the genotype.[1] As a result, the clinical utility of BrS genetic testing is limited largely to SCN5A-specific genetic testing in order to facilitate the cascade screening of potentially at-risk relatives.[42-44]

Catecholaminergic Polymorphic Ventricular Tachycardia

Clinical Description and Manifestations of Catecholaminergic Polymorphic Ventricular Tachycardia

Catecholaminergic polymorphic ventricular tachycardia (CPVT) is a heritable arrhythmia syndrome that affects an estimated 1 in 10,000 individuals, and manifests clinically with exercise-induced syncope or sudden death in individuals with otherwise structurally normal hearts. Similar to LQT1, swimming is a potentially lethal arrhythmia-precipitating trigger in CPVT. In fact, both LQT1 and CPVT have been shown to underlie several cases of unexplained drowning or near-drowning in the young healthy swimmer. However, aside from

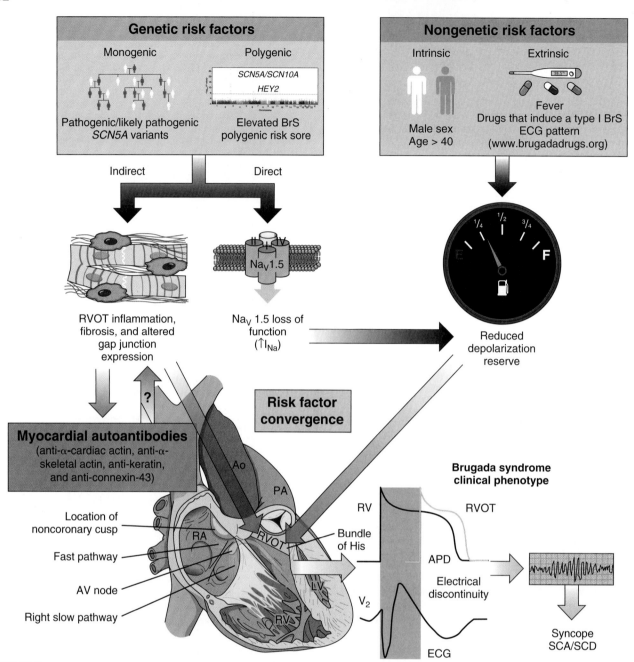

FIGURE 63.7 The evolving genetic architecture and pathophysiology of Brugada syndrome. The contribution of genetic (*blue box*) and nongenetic (*gray box*) risk factors to Brugada syndrome pathogenesis. *Black arrows* denote the potential myocardial and electrophysiological effect(s) of known genetic and nongenetic risk factors. *Blue arrows* demonstrate the recent identification of myocardial autoantibodies sensitive and specific for Brugada syndrome, as well as their potential role in disease pathogenesis. *Gray arrows* demonstrate the convergence of myocardial and electrophysiological effects in the right ventricular outflow tract resulting in a localized delay in depolarization/conduction. *Yellow arrows* demonstrate how electrical discontinuity between the right ventricular (black tracing) and right ventricular outflow tract (yellow tracing) are capable of generating the classic electrocardiogram findings observed in Brugada syndrome as well as an increased risk of syncope and/or sudden cardiac arrest/death secondary to sustained ventricular arrhythmias. *AP*, Action potential; *BrS*, Brugada syndrome; *ECG*, electrocardiogram; I_{Na}, RV, right ventricle; *RVOT*, right ventricular outflow tract; *SCA*, sudden cardiac arrest; *SCD*, sudden cardiac death.

nonspecific findings such as bradycardia and subtle U-waves, the resting 12-lead ECG in CPVT is completely normal. As a result, the use of exercise stress testing (EST), or catecholamine provocation testing (CPT), is needed to unearth the adrenergically induced ventricular ectopy/arrhythmias (Fig. 63.6C), including the pathognomonic finding of bidirectional VT (Fig. 63.6C), that serve as the electrocardiographic hallmarks of CPVT.[1]

Clinically, a presentation of exercise-induced syncope or cardiac arrest in the setting of a QTc less than 460 msec should always prompt first consideration of CPVT rather than so-called "concealed" or "normal QT interval" LQT1. Furthermore, exercise-induced premature ventricular complexes occurring in a pattern of bigeminy is a far

more likely observation than the more specific but less sensitive finding of bidirectional VT. Unfortunately, failure to perform an EST/CPT or the misinterpretation of appropriately obtained EST/CPT results represents a common reason for a delayed or missed CPVT diagnosis.[45] As a result, the 2017 ACC/AHA/HRS guidelines have called for the inclusion of an EST (or CPT for those unable to exercise) in the primary evaluation of all patients presenting with arrhythmic symptoms occurring during exertion or emotion.[42] However, as over a quarter of CPVT patients in the Pediatric and Congenital Electrophysiology Society multicenter CPVT registry that experienced a prior SCA did so during non-exertional wakeful activities (i.e., rest and playing a musical instrument),[46] the argument could be made to extend the inclusion of an EST/CPT in the work-up of all unexplained SCA survivors.

Once thought to manifest only during childhood, recent studies have suggested that the age of first presentation can range from infancy to 40 years of age. CPVT's potential lethality is illustrated by mortality rates of 30% to 50% by 35 years of age and the presence of a positive family history of young (<40 years) SCD for more than a third of CPVT individuals and in as many as 60% of families hosting RyR2 mutations. Moreover, approximately 15% of autopsy negative SUD in the young and some cases of SIDS have been attributed to CPVT.[1]

GENETIC BASIS OF CATECHOLAMINERGIC POLYMORPHIC VENTRICULAR TACHYCARDIA

Perturbations in key components of intracellular calcium-induced calcium release from the sarcoplasmic reticulum serve as the pathogenic basis for CPVT (see Chapter 62). Inherited in an autosomal dominant fashion, mutations in the *RYR2*-encoded cardiac ryanodine receptor/calcium release channel represent the most common genetic subtype of CPVT (CPVT1), accounting for 60% of clinically "strong" cases of CPVT (eTable 63.1 and Fig. 63.8). Gain-of-function mutations in RyR2 produce leaky calcium release channels leading to excessive calcium release, particularly during sympathetic stimulation that can precipitate calcium overload, delayed depolarizations (DADs), and ventricular arrhythmias. Again, most unrelated CPVT families are identified with their own unique *RYR2* mutation and about 5% of unrelated mutation-positive patients host multiple putative pathogenic mutations.

RYR2 is one of the largest genes in the human genome with 105 exons that transcribe/translate one of the largest cardiac ion channel proteins comprising 4967 amino acid residues. While there appears to be no specific mutation "hot-spots," there are three regional "hotspots" or "domains" where unique mutations reside (see Fig. 63.8). Greater than 90% of *RYR2* mutations discovered to date represent

missense mutations; however, as much as 5% of unrelated CPVT patients host large gene rearrangements consistent with large whole exon deletions, similar to findings with LQTS. While to date genotype-phenotype correlations are very limited, a recent publication revealed that family members hosting C-terminal (ion channel-forming domain) RyR2 mutations may have a higher burden of nonsustained ventricular tachycardia (NSVT) than those hosting N-terminal or central domain RyR2 localizing mutations.[1]

Strikingly, nearly a third of "possible/atypical" LQTS (QTc <480 msec) cases with exertion-induced syncope have also been identified as *RYR2* mutation positive. In fact, it has been reported that nearly 30% of patients with CPVT have been misdiagnosed as "LQTS with normal QT-intervals" or "concealed LQTS," indicating the critical importance of properly distinguishing between CPVT and LQTS at the clinical level, as risk assessments and treatment strategies of these unique disorders may vary. Similarly, loss-of-function variants in the *KCNJ2*-encoded $K_{ir}2.1$ potassium channel (the same gene/mechanism that causes ATS) have also been observed in patients diagnosed with CPVT who experience exercise-induced bi-directional VT. Although a distinct electrophysiological phenotype (protein kinase A-dependent I_{K1} reduction) has been elucidated for the type 3 CPVT (CPVT3)-causative *KCNJ2* variant (p.Val227Phe-KCNJ2),[1] it is unclear if ATS and CPVT3 represent a disease continuum or separate entities differentiated by distinct electrophysiological/pathophysiological mechanisms.[1]

In addition to *KCNJ2*, pathogenic/likely pathogenic variants in three additional genes (*CASQ2*-encoded calequestrin-2, *TRDN*-encoded triadin, and *CALM1*- and *CALM3*-encoded calmodulin) also have been implicated in the pathogenesis of CPVT (see eTable 63.1). Whereas *CASQ2* and *TRDN* were associated with autosomal recessive forms of CPVT, *CALM1/CALM3*, like *RYR2* and *KCNJ2*, is associated with an autosomal dominant form (see eTable 63.1). However, the recent realization that some CASQ2-CPVT-causative variants are capable of generating a CPVT phenotype in heterozygous individuals has re-defined the heritability of this minor CPVT subtype (i.e., both an autosomal dominant and recessive disorder).[47]

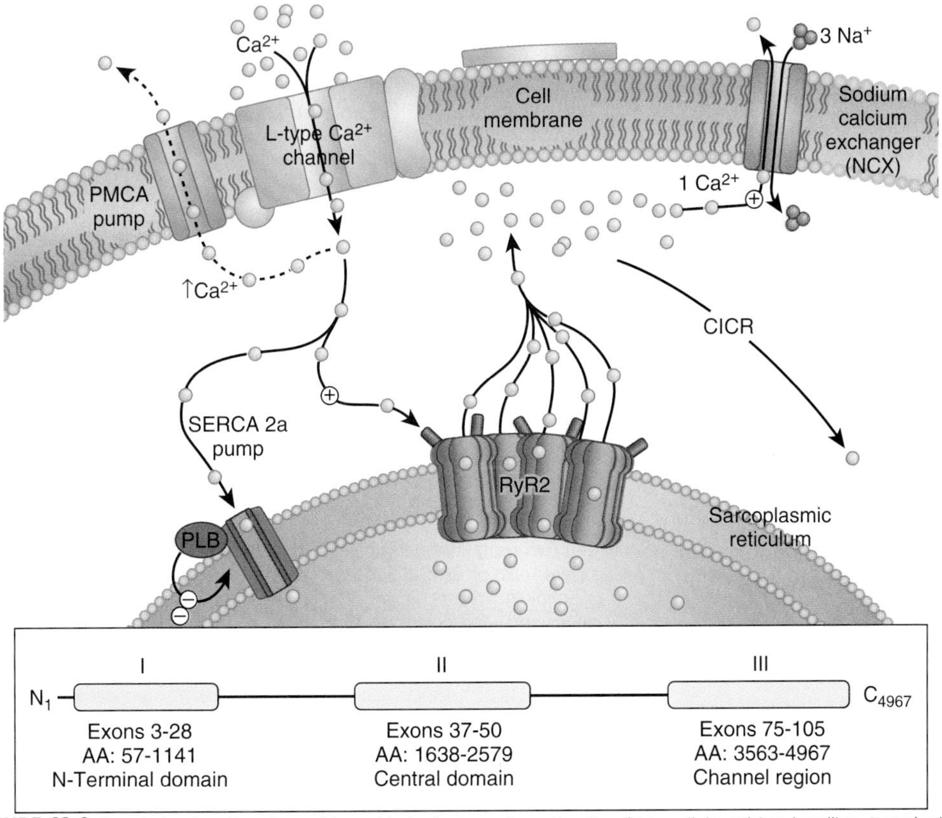

Calcium Release Channel Deficiency Syndrome

In early 2020, Tester et al. described two seemingly unrelated, multigenerational Amish families with multiple recessively inherited and exercise-associated youthful SUDs. Interestingly, exome sequencing and subsequent analysis using an autosomal recessive model failed to identify any homozygous or compound heterozygous nonsynonymous variants within a candidate gene(s).[48] However, copy number variant analysis identified a homozygous tandem duplication involving the 5′ untranslated/promoter regions and the first four exons of *RYR2* in all affected individuals (i.e., youthful SCA/SCD) with available genetic material. Unlike CPVT1, patients with this new disorder termed "calcium release channel deficiency syndrome" or CRC deficiency syndrome display relatively nonspecific ECG findings (i.e., intermittent QTc prolongation with U-waves) and modest or no ventricular ectopy during EST/CPT or prolonged ambulatory Holter monitoring.[48]

Mechanistically, CRC deficiency syndrome patient-specific

FIGURE 63.8 Catecholaminergic polymorphic ventricular tachycardia: a disorder of intracellular calcium handling. Perturbations in key components of the calcium-induced calcium release (CICR) mechanism responsible for cardiac excitation-contraction coupling is the pathogenic basis for CPVT. At the center of this mechanism is the *RYR2*-encoded cardiac ryanodine receptor/calcium release channel located in sarcoplasmic reticulum membrane. Mutations in RyR2 are clustered and distributed in three "hot-spot" regions of this 4967 amino acid (AA) protein; Domain I or N-terminal Domain (AA 57-1141), Domain II or the Central Domain (AA 1638-2579), and Domain III or Channel Region (AA 3563-4967).

iPSC-CM display a profound reduction in the transcription and translation of RyR2, and loss of calcium responsiveness to isoproterenol and caffeine. Therefore, unlike the RyR2 gain-of-function (i.e., hyperactive/hyperreactive "leaky" channels) observed in CPVT1, CRC deficiency syndrome appears to result in RyR2 loss-of-function that nearly ablates calcium-induced calcium release in response to catecholamine infusion.[49]

Interestingly, RyR2 loss-of-function variants (e.g., p.A4860G-RYR, and p.S4938F-RYR2) have also been observed in patients with so-called short-coupled TdP/PVC-triggered VF and unremarkable ESTs diagnosed with either atypical CPVT or IVF.[50] As such, these studies provide compelling evidence that genetic defects in RyR2 likely increase SCA/SCD risk through a variety of electrophysiologic mechanisms, which may have both risk-stratification and management implications in the future.

Early Repolarization Syndrome
Clinical Description and Manifestations of Early Repolarization Syndrome
The early repolarization (ER) pattern is characterized by the elevation (≥1 mm above baseline) of the QRS-ST junction (the so-called J-point) manifesting as either QRS slurring (at the transition of the QRS to the ST-segment) or notching (a positive deflection inscribed on terminal S wave), ST-segment elevation with upper concavity and prominent T waves in ≥2 contiguous leads (Fig. 63.6D). The prevalence of the ER pattern in the general population has been reported to range from less than 1% to 13%, depending on age, sex, race, and the criteria for J-point elevation. This electrocardiographic phenomenon has long been considered an innocuous variant among healthy individuals. However, Haissaguerre et al. have noted that J-point elevation (≥1 mm above baseline) on inferolateral ECG leads was over represented significantly (31%) and was greater in magnitude among 206 case subjects who experienced cardiac arrest due to IVF compared to 412 (5%, p < 0.001) age, sex, race, and level of physical activity matched controls. Those patients with ER were more often males and have a personal history of syncope or cardiac arrest during sleep than those without ER pattern. Other studies have observed an over representation of J-point elevation in IVF patients compared to controls, with the same male predominance among those with ER.[1]

In a community-based general population of 10,864 middle-aged (30 to 59 years of age, 52% male) Finnish subjects, Tikkanen et al. identified 630 subjects overall (5.8%) with J-point elevation of at least 0.1 mV; J-point elevation. This overall prevalence of ER pattern was reduced to only 0.33% when considering a J-point elevation of ≥0.2 mV. Following a 30-year follow-up with the end point being cardiac death, Tikkanen et al. noted that compared to subjects without a J-point elevation, subjects with ER (J-point ≥0.1 mV) in the inferior leads had both an increased risk of cardiac death (adjusted relative risk [ARR] = 1.28, 95% confidence interval [CI] = 1.04 to 1.59; P = 0.03) and arrhythmias (ARR = 1.43, 95% CI = 1.06 to 1.94, p = 0.03) and this risk was further elevated (cardiac death, ARR = 2.98, 95% CI = 1.85 to 4.92, p < 0.001; arrhythmia, ARR = 2.92; 95% CI = 1.45 to 5.89, p < 0.001) with increasing elevation (≥0.2 mV) of the J-point. However, ER pattern localizing to only the lateral leads did not show a statistically significant association with increased risk for arrhythmic cardiac death.[1] Obviously, the vexing clinical conundrum with respect to this Inferolateral Early Repolarization syndrome is distinguishing the potentially lethal ERS from the all too often observed juvenile ER pattern seen in healthy individuals, particularly athletes.

GENETIC BASIS FOR EARLY REPOLARIZATION SYNDROME
The inclination for a genetic basis for ERS stems from Haissaguerre's observation that 16% of their IVF patients with an ER pattern had a family history of unexplained sudden death. The first gene to be implicated in ERS was described by Haissaguere et al., who reported finding a rare, functionally uncharacterized, missense mutation (p.S422L-KCNJ8) in the KCNJ8-encoding pore-forming subunit Kir6.1 of the ATP-sensitive potassium channel in a 14-year-old female with IVF. Since then, this same mutation has been described now in additional cases of BrS and ERS and has been shown to have a gain-of-function in

electrophysiological phenotype. However despite its abnormal in vitro functional phenotype, it is now appreciated that p.S422L-KCNJ8 is far more common than once thought, thus questioning its pathophysiological role. In fact, since its implication in disease, p.S422L-KCNJ8 is now known to have heterozygous frequency of 0.5% (168/33,363) among European Caucasians in the exome aggregation consortium (ExAC) and as high as 4% among the Ashkenazi Jewish population. Thus, these findings reveal that this variant may be a functional common variant that contributes to disease phenotype rather than a monogenic disease-causative pathogenic mutation.[1] In addition, gain-of-function variants in ABBC9, a component of the hetero-octameric $K_{ir}6.1$ ATP-sensitive potassium channels, and the KCND3-encoded $K_v4.3$ voltage-gated potassium channel as well as loss-of-function variants in the LTCC (CACNA1C, CACNB2b, and CACNA2D1) and $Na_v1.5$ (SCN5A and SCN10A) macromolecular complex constituents have been linked to ERS.[36] However, not all of these genetic variants have been characterized functionally, while p.S422L-KCNJ8 could appear to be over-represented in public exomes/genomes.

As such, no definitive evidence exists to show that ERS has a mendelian/monogenic (i.e., single gene) basis. Although initial ER pattern GWAS studies were inconclusive, a recent larger GWAS study identified a statistical association between a locus in KCND3 and an ER pattern (not ERS).[51] In light of the clinical similarities between the so-called J-wave syndromes (i.e., ERS and BrS) and the emerging polygenic genetic architecture of BrS, it stands to reason that the bulk of ERS may also have a oligogenic/polygenic basis driven by relatively common functional risk alleles such as p.S422L-KCNJ8.

Familial Atrial Fibrillation (see Chapter 66)
Clinical Description and Manifestations of Familial Atrial Fibrillation
AF is the most common cardiac arrhythmia with a prevalence of about 1% in the general population and 6% in people over the age of 65 years. Most often AF is associated with underlying cardiac pathology, including cardiomyopathy, valvular disease, hypertension, and atherosclerotic cardiovascular disease and is responsible for over a third of cardioembolic episodes. However, AF can present even at an early age without any identifiable cardiac anomalies and is termed lone AF, accounting for 2% to 16% of all AF cases. Further, approximately one-third of lone AF patients have a family history of AF suggesting familial forms of the disease.[1]

GENETIC BASIS FOR FAMILIAL ATRIAL FIBRILLATION
While the majority of FAF remains genetically elusive, several genetic loci and causative genes have been described in recent decades. In 1996, Brugada et al. identified three families with autosomal dominant arterial fibrillation (AF). The age of onset ranged from in utero to 45 years. Genetic linkage analysis of these families revealed a novel locus for AF on chromosome 10 (10q22). In 2003, a second locus at 6q14-16, again associated with autosomal dominant inheritance, was identified. To date, the underlying causative genes for both loci remain unknown.

However, in 2003 an AF-associated locus on chromosome 11 in a large four-generation family and subsequent identification of a SQTS-like gain-of-function variant, p.S140G-KCNQ1, in $K_v7.1$ (I_{Ks}) was identified, thus providing a causal link between a cardiac potassium ion channel mutation and FAF for the first time. Interestingly, a second de novo mutation involving KCNQ1 was identified in a patient with a severe form of AF and SQTS presenting in utero.[1]

Following these discoveries, gain-of-function variants a number of genes encoding potassium channel α- [KCNH2 ($K_v11.1$), KCNJ2 ($K_{ir}2.1$), KCND3 (I_{to}), and KCNJ8 ($K_{ir}6.1$) and accessory β-subunits (KCNE1, KCNE2, KCNE3, KCNE4, and KCNE5) have been linked to familial AF. In addition, loss-of-function variants in genes encoding potassium channel α-subunits [KCNJ5 (I_{KACh}), KCNA5 (I_{Kur}), and hyperpolarization-activated cyclic nucleotide gated channel 4 (HCN4) (I_f)] have also been described.[52]

Besides these potassium channels, $Na_v1.5$ has also been implicated in lone and familial AF. In fact, AF is a fairly common arrhythmia among patients with loss-of-function sodium cardiac channelopathies (up to 15% to 20% of BrS cases developing AF). In 2008, a novel SCN5A mutation (p.M1875T-SCN5A) in a family characterized with juvenile onset of atrial arrhythmias that progressed to AF in the absence of structural heart disease or ventricular arrhythmias was described. Functional studies of this mutant channel produced an increased peak current density and a depolarizing shift of activation (gain-of-function). *SCN5A* channel mutations have been identified in approximately 3% of AF cases.[1] Moreover, putative AF-causative variants have also been described in Na$_v$1.5 accessory β-subunits (*SCN1B*, *SCN2B*, *SCN3B*, *SCN4B*, and *SCN1Bb*) as well as the *SCN10A*-encoded Na$_v$1.8 sodium channel through a modulatory effect on late sodium current.[52]

In addition, non-ion channel genes have been implicated in familial and lone AF. Hodgson-Zingman et al. identified a frameshift mutation in the *NPPA* gene in a large pedigree with FAF. *NPPA* encodes for the atrial natriuretic peptide which modulates ionic currents in myocardial cells and may shorten atrial conduction time. The clinical phenotype of neonatal onset of AF, with an autosomal recessive inheritance pattern, was recently linked to a mutation in *NUP155*, which encodes for a member of the nucleoporins family of proteins. Gollob et al. identified 4 heterozygote *GJA5* missense mutations in 4 of 15 patients with early onset idiopathic AF. Most interestingly, three of the four mutations were shown to be in cardiac tissue only (somatic) and not germline in origin. *GJA5* encodes for the cardiac gap-junction protein connexin 40 that is predominantly expressed in atrial myocytes and mediates the finely orchestrated electrical activation of the atria. Yang et al. have identified either *GATA4* (*p.S70T-GATA4* and *p.S160T-GATA4*), or *GATA5* (*p. G184V-GATA5*, *p.K218T-GATA5* and *p.A266P-GATA5*) missense mutations in 5/130 (3.8%) unrelated Han Chinese individuals with familial AF.[1] *GATA4* and *GATA5* belong to a family of cardiac transcription factors critical for cardiogenesis.

Importantly, the overall fraction of AF cases that have a mendelian/monogenic (i.e., single gene) basis is exceedingly small and the clinical utility of genetic testing in familial/lone AF-susceptibility is limited. Rather, as demonstrated by recent AF GWAS, the heritable component for the vast majority of AF patients is likely polygenic in nature and arises secondary to the contribution of a number of relatively common variants residing in genes that encode ion channel macromolecular complexes (e.g., *CAV1*, *KCNN3*, *KCND3*), structural proteins (i.e., *NEBL*, *TTN*, *SYNE2*), transcription factors (e.g., *PITX2*, *TBX5*, *ZFHX3*), and those with a myriad of other functions.[52] Although recent GWAS meta-analyses have demonstrated that the collective contribution of AF-associated loci explain approximately 11% of AF heritability,[53] the translation of these findings into clinically meaningful PRSs capable of enhancing AF risk prediction independent of or in concert with traditional risk factors has been slow.[54]

Idiopathic Ventricular Fibrillation
Clinical Description and Manifestations of Idiopathic Ventricular Fibrillation

VF is a major cause of SCD and often is the "final common arrhythmic pathway" for all the aforementioned channelopathies. In the absence of an identifiable cardiac (structural and genetic), respiratory, metabolic, or toxicological cause, resuscitated cardiac arrest victims in which VF is documented are termed "idiopathic" ventricular fibrillation (IVF).[43] In essence, like SIDS, IVF is a diagnosis of exclusion and can stem from several underlying mechanisms. It accounts for as much as 10% of sudden deaths, especially in the young. About 30% of IVF-labeled individuals will have recurrent episodes of VF. In 20% of such cases, there is a family history of sudden death or IVF, suggesting a hereditary component in some cases. Unfortunately, the vast majority of IVF patients are diagnosed only after experiencing a sentinel out-of-hospital cardiac arrest.

GENETIC BASIS FOR IDIOPATHIC VENTRICULAR FIBRILLATION

At present, pathogenic/likely pathogenic variants in *CALM1-3*-encoded calmodulin, the *IRX3*-encoded Iroquois homeobox gene family transcription factor, *RYR2*-encoded RyR2 calcium release channel, and a promoter haplotype in the *DPP6* gene locus on chromosome 7q36 have been found to be linked to IVF.[1,55] However, many patients with IVF-causative variants in these genes have documented evidence of short-coupled TdP/PVC-triggered VT/VF (Fig. 63.6e), which is often considered to be synonymous with IVF but could represent a distinct clinical entity/phenotype.

Despite the identification of these IVF-susceptibility genes, the current ACC/AHA and EHRA/HRS guideline-endorsed role for genetic testing in individuals with IVF is to provide further evidence of a specific underlying SCD-predisposing genetic heart disease (i.e., a cardiomyopathy in a pre-cardiomyopathic electrical state or cardiac channelopathy) when there is reasonable clinical suspicion.[42] However, given the likelihood of unearthing ≥1 ambiguous VUS in a strong evidence channelopathy- or cardiomyopathy-susceptibility gene, the 2013 HRS/EHRA guidelines discouraged the use of large gene panels as seen in pan-arrhythmia, pan-cardiac, and exome-based genetic testing in individuals with a diagnosis of IVF.

Even with this guidance, several referral centers have published their experience with genetic testing in IVF, most using large commercial gene panels (i.e., pan-arrhythmia or pan-cardiac genetic testing) and/or exome sequencing.[29,56–58] Of note, within the slate of SCD-predisposing channelopathy- and cardiomyopathy-susceptibility genes tested variably in each study, the yield of ambiguous VUS (range 15% to 26%) far exceeded that of clinically-actionable pathogenic/likely pathogenic variants (range 2% to 17%; eFig. 63.2).[29,56–58] As such, the decision to pursue any form of genetic testing in IVF should not be taken lightly and should be performed in a dedicated cardiovascular genetics clinic.

Multifocal Ectopic Purkinje-Related Premature Contractions

In addition to AF, LQTS, BrS, and progressive cardiac conduction disease (PCCD), pathogenic/likely pathogenic genetic variants in the *SCN5A*-encoded Na$_v$1.5 cardiac sodium channel have been linked to MEPPC. This rare condition results in a high burden of narrow complex, polymorphic ventricular ectopy of fascicular/Purkinje origin, increased risk of sudden death, and in some cases, a reversible and likely PVC-mediated dilated cardiomyopathy.[59,60]

Initially, MEPPC was thought to arise secondary to a specific gain-of-function variant (*p.R222Q-SCN5A*) observed in several unrelated families. However, additional variants within (*p.G213N-SCN5A*, *p.R225P-SCN5A*, and *p.L828F-SCN5A*) or in close proximity (*p.I141V-SCN5A* and *p.M1851V-SCN5A*) to the S4 transmembrane segments that play a critical role in Na$_v$1.5 voltage-sensing have been observed in patients with a MEPPC-like phenotype with time.[60] Furthermore, it appears that some LQT3-causative variants (voltage-sensing domain variants such as *p.N1325S-SCN5A* and *p.R1623Q-SCN5A*) are capable of causing a LQT3-MEPPC overlap syndrome consisting of QTc prolongation and frequent narrow complex PVCs/short-coupled ventricular arrhythmias that is associated with a higher risk of VF (SCA and appropriate ICD shocks) when present.[61]

Mechanistically, the majority of MEPPC-causative *SCN5A* variants result in the generation of increased "window current" that arise secondary to hyperpolarizing shifts in Nav1.5 voltage-dependent activation and inactivation.[59,62] Interestingly, despite possessing *SCN5A* variants that cause a LQT3-like Na$_v$1.5 gain-of-function, patients with MEPPC have normal QTc values suggesting that cardiac APD is not prolonged globally. Recent evidence from a *p.R222Q-SCN5A* knock-in murine cardiomyocyte/Purkinje cell model suggest that this phenomenon is due to the generation of an APD-shortening outward gating-pore current conducted through alternative cation permeation pathways adjacent to the S4 transmembrane.[63,64] Therefore, the absence of QTc prolongation in MEPPC may be explained by the offsetting effects of increased Na$_v$1.5 window current amplitude (APD-prolonging) and the generation of a distinct outward gating-pore current (APD-shortening) on cardiac repolarization.

Progressive Cardiac Conduction Disease
Clinical Description and Manifestations of Progressive Cardiac Conduction Defect

Cardiac conduction disease (CCD) causes a potentially life-threatening alteration in normal impulse propagation through the cardiac conduction system. CCD can be a result of several physiologic mechanisms, acquired or congenital, in the presence or absence of structural heart disease. PCCD, also known as Lev-Lenègre disease, is one of the most common cardiac conduction disturbances in the absence of structural heart disease and is characterized by progressive (age-related) impairment of impulse propagation through the His-Purkinje system, with right or left bundle branch block and widening of the QRS complex. This leads to a complete AV block, syncope, and occasionally sudden death.

ARRHYTHMIAS, SUDDEN DEATH, AND SYNCOPE

VII

GENETIC BASIS FOR PROGRESSIVE CARDIAC CONDUCTION DISEASE

In 1999, Schott et al. further expanded the spectrum of loss-of-function *SCN5A* disease with the inclusion of familial PCCD. They identified a splice-site *SCN5A* mutation (c.3963+2 T>C) associated with an autosomal dominant inheritance pattern in a large French family. Since then, investigators have identified over 30 PCCD-associated mutations in *SCN5A*. In addition to *SCN5A*, mutations in *SCN1B* can cause BrS with conduction disease. These mutations present with a loss-of-function phenotype through reduced current density and enhanced slow inactivation of the channel. As with most loss-of-function *SCN5A*-mediated disorders, the phenotypic expression of PCCD can be complex and is often present with a concomitant BrS or BrS-like phenotype. In fact, PCCD is the prevailing phenotype in BrS-associated *SCN5A* pathogenic/likely pathogenic variant carriers, where the penetrance of conduction defects can be as high as 76%.[1]

In 2009, Meregalli et al. demonstrated that *SCN5A* variant type can have a profound effect on the severity of PCCD and BrS. Studying 147 individuals hosting one of 32 different *SCN5A* variants, Meregalli found that patients with either a premature truncation mutation (i.e., nonsense or frameshift) or a severe loss-of-function missense mutation (>90% reduction in peak I_{Na}) had a significantly longer PR interval compared with those patients with missense variants having less impairment to the sodium current (≤90% reduction). Furthermore, these patients had significantly more episodes of syncope than those with an "active" variant.[1] These findings suggest that those mutations with a more deleterious loss of sodium current produce a more severe phenotype of syncope and conduction defect, providing the first evidence for intra-genotype risk stratification associated with *SCN5A* loss-of-function disease.

Gain-of-function variants (*p.E7K-TRPM4, p.R164W-TRPM4, p.A432T-TRPM4,* and *p.G844D-TRPM4*) in the *TRPM4*-encoded transient receptor potential melastatin type 4 ion channel have been identified as a cause of autosomal dominant isolated cardiac conduction disorder and progressive familial heart block. This is possible by classical linkage analysis and subsequent mutational analysis of *TRPM4* in four different large multi-generational pedigrees. As such, the calcium-activated nonselective cation channel contributes importantly to the cardiac conduction system.[1]

Sick Sinus Syndrome

Clinical Description and Manifestations of Sick Sinus Syndrome

SND or "sick sinus syndrome" (SSS) manifesting as inappropriate sinus bradycardia, sinus arrest, atrial standstill, tachycardia-bradycardia syndrome, or chronotropic incompetence is the leading diagnosis for pacemaker implantation (see Chapter 68). SSS commonly occurs in the elderly (1 in 600 cardiac patients >65 years of age) with acquired cardiac conditions including cardiomyopathy, congestive heart failure, ischemic heart disease, or metabolic diseases. However, there are no identifiable cardiac anomalies or conditions underlying sinus node dysfunction ("idiopathic SND"), which can occur at any age including in utero in a significant number of cases. Additionally, familial forms of idiopathic SND consistent with autosomal dominant inheritance with reduced penetrance and recessive forms with complete penetrance have been reported.[1]

GENETIC BASIS OF SICK SINUS SYNDROME

Mutational analysis of small cohorts and case reports of patients with idiopathic SSS have so far implicated four genes: *SCN5A, HCN4, ANK2,* and *MYH6* (see eTable 63.1). To date, 15 putative SSS-causative variants have been reported in *SCN5A*. These variants either produced nonfunctional sodium channels through loss of expression or channels with mild to severe loss-of-function through altered biophysical properties of the channel. In 2003, based on prior observations of arrhythmias and conduction disturbances, *SCN5A* was identified as a gene for congenital SSS diagnosed in the first decade of life. Compound heterozygote variants (p.T220I-SCN5A + p.R1623X-SCN5A, p.P1298L-SCN5A + p.G1408R-SCN5A, and p.delF1617-SCN5A + p.R1632H-SCN5A) implicated *SCN5A* in autosomal recessive SSS.[1] Moreover, many of the *SCN5A* positive patients displayed a mixed phenotype consisting of SSS, BrS and/or CCD. The expressivity of the mixture can be highly variable within affected families, and the environmental and/or genetic modifiers responsible for this

phenomenon are poorly understood. A patient with SSS, CCD, and recurrent VT was described with an *p.L1821fsX10-SCN5A* frameshift variant that exhibited a 90% reduction in current density (consistent with BrS/SSS/CCD), and an increase in late sodium current (consistent with LQT3) for those channels that are expressed. The absence of symptoms in a number of other family members highlights the incomplete or low penetrance of this *SCN5A*-mediated disorder.

Two loss-of-function variants in *HCN4*, have been identified in idiopathic SND. The *HCN4* gene encodes the so-called I_f "funny" or pacemaker current and plays a key role in the automaticity of the sinus node. In one study, a frameshift variant (*p.P544fsX30-HCN4*) was identified in a patient with idiopathic SND. In another study, a patient with idiopathic SND had a missense variant (*p.D553N-HCN4*) that resulted in abnormal trafficking of the pacemaker channel. Interestingly, while the frameshift mutation identified in a 66-year-old woman produced a mild phenotype associated with sinus rhythm during exercise, the *p.D553N-HCN4* missense mutation identified in a 43-year-old woman was associated with severe bradycardia, recurrent syncope, QT prolongation, and polymorphic ventricular tachycardia (TdP), suggesting the potential for lethality in *HCN4*-mediated disease.[1] Further studies (larger cohorts) are required to determine if the preliminary 10% to 15% yield for defective *HCN4*-encoded pacemaker channels in idiopathic SND (derived from the two small cohorts) is durable.

Genetic dysfunction in *ANK2*-encoded ankyrin B has been reported in two large families with high penetrant and severe SND. Ankyrin B is essential for normal membrane organization of ion channels and transporters in the cardiomyocytes within the SA node and is required for proper physiological cardiac pacing. Dysfunction of ankyrin B-based trafficking pathway causes abnormal electrical activity in the SA node and SND. Like the $Na_v1.5$ sodium channel, variants in *ANK2* have been associated with a variety of cardiac dysfunctions.

In a GWAS in the Icelandic population including 792 individuals with SSS and 37,592 controls, a rare missense variant (c.2161C>T, *p.R721W-MYH6*) in *MYH6*-encoded alpha heavy chain 6 subunit of cardiac myosin was significantly associated with SSS. Moreover, the lifetime risk of being diagnosed with SSS was only 6% for non-carriers of c.2161C>T compared to 50% for carriers of the *MYH6* variant. Ishikawa et al. identified a 3 bp in-frame deletion resulting in a single amino acid deletion (*p.delE933-MYH6*) in a genotype-negative proband with SSS. The mutant slowed down action potential propagation when heterologously expressed in HL-1 atrial myocytes. Moreover, morpholino knockdown of *MYH6* in zebrafish led to a reduced heart rate that could be restored when co-expressed with wild-type *MYH6*, but not when co-expressed with *dE933-MYH6*.[1]

CONCLUSIONS

This novel discipline of genetic cardiology has grown substantially over the past two decades. The pathogenic insights into the molecular underpinnings for nearly all these syndromes have matured through the entire continuum of research from discovery, translation, incorporation into routine clinical practice. This bench-to-bedside maturation now requires the learned interpretation of the available genetic tests for these syndromes with a clear understanding of the diagnostic, prognostic, and therapeutic implications associated with genetic testing of these channelopathies.

FUTURE PERSPECTIVES

As illustrated by LQTS, genetic testing in the cardiac channelopathies has the potential to substantially impact the diagnosis, risk-stratification, and clinical management of patients with these potentially lethal but highly treatable genetic heart disorders. However, the full promise of precision genomic medicine is far from being completely realized. As such, over the next decade, well-designed and adequately powered studies as well as educational efforts are needed to:

1. Better define the genetic architecture of the cardiac channelopathies (Fig. 63.4), particularly in regards to the role of limited- and disputed-evidence disease-susceptibility genes (also known as GUSs), the ability of common genetic variants/PRSs to explain genotype-negative disease, and the marked incomplete penetrance and variable expressivity observed in these putative mendelian/monogenic disorders.

1206

2. Enhance our ability to distinguish pathogenic/likely pathogenic variants from rare and likely innocuous background genetic noise in definitive/strong evidence cardiac channelopathy-susceptibility genes.

3. Strengthen the genetics/genomics literacy of all cardiovascular health care providers and improve access to dedicated cardiovascular genetics clinics/cardiovascular-specific genetic counseling.

4. Use our ever-expanding understanding of the genetic and electrophysiological basis of cardiac channelopathies to develop new and targeted therapies, particularly for disorders (e.g., TS, TKOS, CASQ2-CPVT/CPVT2) that are often refractory to available medical, surgical, and device therapies.

These efforts will allow cardiovascular health care providers to fully capitalize on the promise of precision genomic medicine and deliver genetics- and genomics-guided care to an increasing number of patients with monogenic- and polygenic-driven cardiac arrhythmias.

REFERENCES

QT-opathies

1. Tester DJAM. Genetics of cardiac arrhythmias. In: Zipes D, Mann DL, Libby P, Bonow RO, Tomaselli GF, eds. *Braunwald's Heart Disease: A Textbook of Cardiovascular Medicine*. Elsevier; 2019:604–618.
2. Giudicessi JR, Wilde AAM, Ackerman MJ. The genetic architecture of long QT syndrome: a critical reappraisal. *Trends Cardiovasc Med*. 2018;28(7):453–464.
3. Giudicessi JR, et al. Variant frequency and clinical phenotype call into question the nature of minor, nonsyndromic long-QT syndrome-susceptibility gene-disease associations. *Circulation*. 2020;141(6):495–497.
4. Karczewski KJ, et al. The mutational constraint spectrum quantified from variation in 141,456 humans. *Nature*. 2020;581(7809):434–443.
5. Giudicessi JR, Ackerman MJ. Established loss-of-function variants in ANK2-encoded ankyrin-B rarely cause a concerning cardiac phenotype in humans. *Circ Genom Precis Med*. 2020;13(2):e002851.
6. Adler A, et al. An international, multicentered, evidence-based reappraisal of genes reported to cause congenital long QT syndrome. *Circulation*. 2020;141(6):418–428.
7. Strande NT, et al. Evaluating the clinical validity of gene-disease associations: an evidence-based framework developed by the clinical genome Resource. *Am J Hum Genet*. 2017;100(6):895–906.
8. Giudicessi JR, et al. Classification and reporting of potentially proarrhythmic common genetic variation in long QT syndrome genetic testing. *Circulation*. 2018;137(6):619–630.
9. Giudicessi JR, Kullo IJ, Ackerman MJ. Precision cardiovascular medicine: state of genetic testing. *Mayo Clin Proc*. 2017;92(4):642–662.
10. Lahrouchi N, et al. Transethnic genome-wide association study provides insights in the genetic architecture and heritability of long QT syndrome. *Circulation*. 2020;142(4):324–338.
11. Turkowski KL, et al. The QTc-polygenic risk score (QTc-PRS) and its contribution to type 1, type 2, and type 3 long QT syndrome in probands and genotype-positive family members. *Circ Genom Precis Med*. 2020.
12. Roberts JD, et al. An international multicenter evaluation of type 5 long QT syndrome: a low penetrant primary arrhythmic condition. *Circulation*. 2020;141(6):429–439.
13. Garmany R, et al. Clinical and functional reappraisal of alleged type 5 long QT syndrome: causative genetic variants in the KCNE1-encoded minK beta-subunit. *Heart Rhythm*. 2020;17(6):937–944.
14. Lane CM, et al. Long QT syndrome type 5-Lite: defining the clinical phenotype associated with the potentially proarrhythmic p.Asp85Asn-KCNE1 common genetic variant. *Heart Rhythm*. 2018;15(8):1223–1230.
15. Pfeufer A, et al. Common variants at ten loci modulate the QT interval duration in the QTSCD Study. *Nat Genet*. 2009;41(4):407–414.
16. Newton-Cheh C, et al. Common variants at ten loci influence QT interval duration in the QTGEN Study. *Nat Genet*. 2009;41(4):399–406.
17. Arking DE, et al. Genetic association study of QT interval highlights role for calcium signaling pathways in myocardial repolarization. *Nat Genet*. 2014;46(8):826–836.
18. Turkowski KL, et al. Corrected QT interval-polygenic risk score and its contribution to type 1, type 2, and type 3 long QT syndrome in probands and genotype-positive family members. *Circ Genom Precis Med*. 2020;13(4):e002922.
19. Bezzina CR, et al. Common variants at SCN5A-SCN10A and HEY2 are associated with Brugada syndrome, a rare disease with high risk of sudden cardiac death. *Nat Genet*. 2013;45(9):1044–1049.
20. Crotti L, et al. Calmodulin mutations and life-threatening cardiac arrhythmias: insights from the International Calmodulinopathy Registry. *Eur Heart J*. 2019;40(35):2964–2975.
21. Giudicessi JR, Ackerman MJ. Calcium revisited: new insights into the molecular basis of long-QT syndrome. *Circ Arrhythm Electrophysiol*. 2016;9(7).
22. Altmann HM, et al. Homozygous/compound heterozygous triadin mutations associated with autosomal-recessive long-QT syndrome and pediatric sudden cardiac arrest: elucidation of the triadin knockout syndrome. *Circulation*. 2015;131(23):2051–2060.
23. Clemens DJ, et al. International triadin knockout syndrome registry. *Circ Genom Precis Med*. 2019;12(2):e002419.
24. Boczek NJ, et al. Novel Timothy syndrome mutation leading to increase in CACNA1C window current. *Heart Rhythm*. 2015;12:211–219.
25. Boczek NJ, et al. Identification and functional characterization of a novel CACNA1C-mediated cardiac disorder characterized by prolonged QT intervals with hypertrophic cardiomyopathy, congenital heart defects, and sudden cardiac death. *Circulation*. 2015;8(5):1122–1132.
26. Landstrom AP, Dobrev D, Wehrens XHT. Calcium signaling and cardiac arrhythmias. *Circ Res*. 2017;120(12):1969–1993.
27. Harrell DT, et al. Genotype-dependent differences in age of manifestation and arrhythmia complications in short QT syndrome. *Int J Cardiol*. 2015;190:393–402.
28. Giudicessi JR, Ackerman MJ, Camilleri M. Cardiovascular safety of prokinetic agents: a focus on drug-induced arrhythmias. *Neuro Gastroenterol Motil*. 2018;30(6):e13302.
29. Giudicessi JR, Ackerman MJ. Role of genetic heart disease in sentinel sudden cardiac arrest survivors across the age spectrum. *Int J Cardiol*. 2018;270:214–220.

Other Channelopathies

30. Mazzanti A, et al. Natural history and risk stratification in andersen-tawil syndrome type 1. *J Am Coll Cardiol*. 2020;75(15):1772–1784.
31. Koenig SN, Mohler PJ. The evolving role of ankyrin-B in cardiovascular disease. *Heart Rhythm*. 2017;14(12):1884–1889.
32. Bastiaenen R, et al. Late gadolinium enhancement in Brugada syndrome: a marker for subtle underlying cardiomyopathy? *Heart Rhythm*. 2017;14(4):583–589.
33. Gray B, et al. Relations between right ventricular morphology and clinical, electrical and genetic parameters in Brugada Syndrome. *PloS One*. 2018;13(4):e0195594.
34. Pieroni M, et al. Electroanatomic and pathologic right ventricular outflow tract abnormalities in patients with Brugada syndrome. *J Am Coll Cardiol*. 2018;72(22):2747–2757.
35. Juang JJ, et al. Validation and disease risk assessment of previously reported genome-wide genetic variants associated with Brugada syndrome: SADS-TW BrS registry. *Circ Genom Precis Med*. 2020.
36. Antzelevitch C, et al. J-Wave syndromes expert consensus conference report: emerging concepts and gaps in knowledge. *Heart Rhythm*. 2016;13(10):e295–324.
37. Belbachir N, et al. RRAD mutation causes electrical and cytoskeletal defects in cardiomyocytes derived from a familial case of Brugada syndrome. *Eur Heart J*. 2019;40(37):3081–3094.
38. Le Scouarnec S, et al. Testing the burden of rare variation in arrhythmia-susceptibility genes provides new insights into molecular diagnosis for Brugada syndrome. *Hum Mol Genet*. 2015;24(10):2757–2763.
39. Hosseini SM, et al. Reappraisal of reported genes for sudden arrhythmic death. *Circulation*. 2018;138(12):1195–1205.
40. Behr ER, et al. Role of common and rare variants in SCN10A: results from the Brugada syndrome QRS locus gene discovery collaborative study. *Cardiovasc Res*. 2015;106(3):520–9.
41. Le Scouarnec S, et al. Testing the burden of rare variation in arrhythmia-susceptibility genes provides new insights into molecular diagnosis for Brugada syndrome. *Hum Mol Genet*. 2015;24(10):2757–63.
42. Al-Khatib SM, et al. 2017 AHA/ACC/HRS guideline for management of patients with ventricular arrhythmias and the prevention of sudden cardiac death: a report of the American College of Cardiology/American Heart Association task force on clinical practice guidelines and the Heart Rhythm Society. *Circulation*. 2018;138(13):e272–e391.
43. Priori SG, et al. HRS/EHRA/APHRS expert consensus statement on the diagnosis and management of patients with inherited primary arrhythmia syndromes: document endorsed by HRS, EHRA, and APHRS in May 2013 and by ACCF, AHA, PACES, and AEPC in June 2013. *Heart Rhythm*. 2013;10(12):1932–1963.
44. Priori SG, et al. 2015 ESC guidelines for the management of patients with ventricular arrhythmias and the prevention of sudden cardiac death: the task force for the management of patients with ventricular arrhythmias and the prevention of sudden cardiac death of the European Cociety of Cardiology (ESC). Endorsed by: Association for European Paediatric and Congenital Cardiology (AEPC). *Eur Heart J*. 2015;36(41):2793–2867.
45. Giudicessi JR, Ackerman MJ. Exercise testing oversights underlie missed and delayed diagnosis of catecholaminergic polymorphic ventricular tachycardia in young sudden cardiac arrest survivors. *Heart Rhythm*. 2019;16(8):1232–1239.
46. Roston TM, et al. The clinical and genetic spectrum of catecholaminergic polymorphic ventricular tachycardia: findings from an international multicentre registry. *Europace*. 2018;20(3):541–547.
47. Ng K, et al. An international multi-center evaluation of inheritance patterns, arrhythmic risks, and underlying mechanisms of CASQ2-catecholaminergic polymorphic ventricular tachycardia. *Circulation*. 2020;142(10):932–947.
48. Tester DJ, et al. Identification of a novel homozygous multi-exon duplication in RYR2 among children with exertion-related unexplained sudden deaths in the Amish community. *JAMA Cardiol*. 2020;5(3):13–18.
49. Tester DJ, et al. Molecular characterization of the calcium release channel deficiency syndrome. *JCI Insight*. 2020;5(15).
50. Fujii Y, et al. A type 2 ryanodine receptor variant associated with reduced Ca(2+) release and short-coupled torsades de pointes ventricular arrhythmia. *Heart Rhythm*. 2017;14(1):98–107.
51. Teumer A, et al. KCND3 potassium channel gene variant confers susceptibility to electrocardiographic early repolarization pattern. *JCI Insight*. 2019;4(23).
52. Feghaly J, et al. Genetics of atrial fibrillation. *J Am Heart Assoc*. 2018;7(20):e009884.
53. Nielsen JB, et al. Biobank-driven genomic discovery yields new insight into atrial fibrillation biology. *Nat Genet*. 2018;50(9):1234–1239.
54. Weng LC, et al. Genetic predisposition, clinical risk factor burden, and lifetime risk of atrial fibrillation. *Circulation*. 2018;137(10):1027–1038.
55. Koizumi A, et al. Genetic defects in a His-Purkinje system transcription factor, IRX3, cause lethal cardiac arrhythmias. *Eur Heart J*. 2016;37(18):1469–1475.
56. Leinonen JT, et al. The genetics underlying idiopathic ventricular fibrillation: a special role for catecholaminergic polymorphic ventricular tachycardia? *Int J Cardiol*. 2018;250:139–145.
57. Mellor G, et al. Genetic testing in the evaluation of unexplained cardiac arrest: from the CASPER (cardiac arrest survivors with preserved ejection fraction registry). *Circ Cardiovasc Genet*. 2017;10(3).
58. Visser M, et al. Next-generation sequencing of a large gene panel in patients initially diagnosed with idiopathic ventricular fibrillation. *Heart Rhythm*. 2017;14(7):1035–1040.
59. Laurent G, et al. Multifocal ectopic Purkinje-related premature contractions: a new SCN5A-related cardiac channelopathy. *J Am Coll Cardiol*. 2012;60(2):144–156.
60. Wilde AAM, Amin AS. Clinical spectrum of SCN5A mutations: long QT syndrome, Brugada syndrome, and cardiomyopathy. *JACC Clin Electrophysiol*. 2018;4(5):569–579.
61. Barake W, et al. Purkinje system hyperexcitability and ventricular arrhythmia risk in type 3 long QT syndrome. *Heart Rhythm*. 2020;17(10):1768–1776.
62. Ter Bekke RMA, et al. Beauty and the beat: a complicated case of multifocal ectopic Purkinje-related premature contractions. *HeartRhythm Case Rep*. 2018;4(9):429–433.
63. Daniel LL, et al. SCN5A variant R222Q generated abnormal changes in cardiac sodium current and action potentials in murine myocytes and Purkinje cells. *Heart Rhythm*. 2019;16(11):1676–1685.
64. Moreau A, et al. Gating pore currents are defects in common with two Nav1.5 mutations in patients with mixed arrhythmias and dilated cardiomyopathy. *J Gen Physiol*. 2015;145(2):93–106.

64 Therapy for Cardiac Arrhythmias

JOHN M. MILLER AND KENNETH A. ELLENBOGEN

It is estimated that almost a third of people will have a problematic tachyarrhythmia, most often atrial fibrillation (AF), at some point during a normal life span. Thus, most clinicians will need to manage their patients' rhythm problems, or those treatments may impact or may be impacted by treatment of the patient's other disorders. Treatment of patients with tachyarrhythmias has evolved dramatically over the last 40 years and has become more complex and specialized. A few, relatively ineffective antiarrhythmic drugs (AADs) were the only therapeutic option until the late 1960s, when surgical therapy to cure (not just suppress) tachyarrhythmias was developed. This mode in turn was replaced by catheter ablation for better control or even cure of many types of supraventricular tachycardias (SVTs) and ventricular tachycardias (VTs) in the absence of structural heart disease starting in the 1980s. The implantable cardioverter-defibrillator (ICD) was introduced in the early 1980s and has become standard therapy for patients with serious ventricular arrhythmias in the presence of structural heart disease. Some patients require a combination of treatments, such as an ICD and AADs or surgery and an ICD; drug therapy can also affect ICD function, positively or negatively. Drug therapy for arrhythmias, at one time the only option, has largely been replaced as the mainstay of therapy by ablation or implanted devices. In most patients, however, tachyarrhythmias are initially treated with AADs, and thus these agents continue to have a significant role in management of patients with a variety of arrhythmias.

PHARMACOLOGIC THERAPY

The principles of clinical pharmacokinetics and pharmacodynamics are discussed in Chapter 9.

General Considerations Regarding Antiarrhythmic Drugs

Most of the AADs currently available can be classified according to whether they exert blocking actions predominantly on sodium (Na$^+$), potassium (K$^+$), or calcium (Ca^{2+}) channels and/or what receptors they block (Table 64.1). The commonly used classification (Vaughan Williams) is still a useful framework for categorizing drug action but is limited because it is based on the electrophysiologic effects exerted by an arbitrary concentration of the drug, generally on a laboratory preparation of normal cardiac tissue.

In practice, the actions of these drugs are complex and depend on tissue type, degree of acute or chronic damage, heart rate, membrane potential, ionic composition of the extracellular milieu, autonomic influences (see Chapter 102), genetics (see Chapter 63), age (Chapter 90), and other factors (see Table 64.1). Many drugs exert more than one type of electrophysiologic effect or operate indirectly, such as by altering hemodynamics, myocardial metabolism, or autonomic neural transmission. Therefore, it is more appropriate to think of classes of

action rather than classes of drugs, although the major classification schemes categorize drugs by their predominant action. Some drugs have active metabolites that exert effects different from those of the parent compound. Not all drugs in the same class have identical effects (e.g., amiodarone, sotalol, and ibutilide). Whereas all class III agents are dramatically different, some drugs in different classes have overlapping actions (e.g., class IA and class IC drugs). Thus, in vitro studies on healthy myocardium usually establish the idealized properties of AADs rather than their actual antiarrhythmic properties in vivo. Since many AADs affect ventricular repolarization and thus have the potential for producing lethal ventricular arrhythmias, development and approval of new agents is uncommon (no new agents in the United States since dronedarone in 2009).[1]

Despite its limitations, the Vaughan Williams classification is widely known and provides a useful communication shorthand, but the reader is cautioned that drug actions are more complex than those depicted by the classification. A more realistic but not widely used framework regarding AADs is provided by the "Sicilian Gambit." This approach to drug classification is an attempt to identify the mechanisms of a particular arrhythmia, to determine the vulnerable parameter of the arrhythmia most susceptible to modification, to define the target most likely to affect the vulnerable parameter, and then to select a drug that will modify the target (Table 64.2; also see Table 64.1).[2] More recently, a modified Vaughan Williams classification has been proposed that takes into account additional drug targets, including effects on connexins, molecules underlying longer-term signaling processes, and mechanically sensitive ion channels (Fig. 64.1).[3] This revised classification, incorporating advances in both basic and clinical sciences, also emphasizes that most AADs affect multiple targets and can be used to facilitate decisions about drug choices in specific clinical settings. Classes 0-VII have been described; currently available agents are limited to Classes 0-IV and several unclassified drugs.

Drug Classification
Class 0
This class includes drugs that block the HCN channel mediated pacemaker current (I_f). Inhibition of the I_f channel (or "funny" current) reduces the depolarization rate of the sinus node pacemaker cells and reduces heart rate.

According to the Vaughan Williams classification, class I drugs predominantly block the voltage gated fast sodium channel (I_{Na}). These in turn are divided into four subgroups, classes IA, IB, IC and ID (eTable 64.1). Some also block potassium channels at pharmacologically relevant concentrations.

Class IA
This class includes drugs that reduce $\dot{V}_{max}$ (rate of rise in action potential upstroke [phase 0]) and prolong the action potential duration (APD; see Chapter 62)—quinidine, procainamide, and disopyramide. The kinetics of onset and offset of class IA drugs blocking the Na$^+$

Additional content is available online at Elsevier eBooks for Practicing Clinicians

TABLE 64.1 Actions of Drugs Used in Treatment of Arrhythmias

	CHANNELS							RECEPTORS				PUMPS	PREDOMINANT CLINICAL EFFECTS		
	NA*														
DRUG	FAST	MED	SLOW	CA	K_R	K_S	HCN	α	β	M₂	P	NA-K ATPASE	LV FUNCTION	SINUS RATE	EXTRACARDIAC
Quinidine		●A			◉			O	O				—	↑	◉
Procainamide		●I			◉								↓	—	◉
Disopyramide		●A			◉				O				↓	var	●
Ajmaline		●A											—	—↓	O
Lidocaine	O												—	—↓	O
Mexiletine	O												—	—	O
Phenytoin	O												—	—	◉
Flecainide			●A		O								↓	—	O
Propafenone		●A			O				◉				↓	↓	O
Propranolol	O								●				↓	↓	O
Nadolol									●				↓	↓	O
Amiodarone	O			◉	●	◉	◉	◉	◉				—	↓	●
Dronedarone	O			◉	●	◉		◉	◉				—	↓	O
Sotalol					●				●				↓	↓	O
Ibutilide	activator				O								—	↓	O
Dofetilide					●								—	—	O
Verapamil	O			●			◉						↓	↓	O
Diltiazem				◉									↓	↓	O
Adenosine											□		—	↓	◉
Digoxin										O		●	↑	↓	◉
Atropine										●			—	↑	◉
Ranolazine	O				O								—	—	O
Ivabradine							●						O	↓	O

*Fast, med (medium), and slow refer to kinetics of recovery from sodium (Na) channel blockade.
Relative potency of blockade or extracardiac side effect: O, low; ◉, moderate; ●, high; □, agonist; A, activated state blocker; I = inactivated state blocker.
—, minimal effect; ↑, increase; ↓, decrease; var, variable effects.
Ca, calcium channel; HCN, hyperpolarization-activated cyclic nucleotide-gated channel; K_R, Rapid component of delayed rectifier K⁺ current; K_s, slow component of delayed rectifier K⁺ current; LV, left ventricular; M₂, muscarinic receptor subtype 2; Na, sodium channel; NaK- ATPase, sodium pump; P, A₁ purinergic receptor;.
Modified from Schwartz PJ, Zaza A. Haemodynamic effects of a new multifactorial antihypertensive drug. *Eur Heart J.* 1992;13:26.

channel is of intermediate rapidity (<5 seconds) when compared with class IB and class IC agents.

Class IB
This class of drugs does not reduce $\dot{V}_{max}$ and shortens the APD—mexiletine, phenytoin, and lidocaine. The kinetics of onset and offset of these drugs in blocking the sodium channel is rapid (<500 milliseconds).

Class IC
This class of drugs, including flecainide and propafenone, can reduce $\dot{V}_{max}$ slow conduction velocity, and prolong refractoriness minimally. These drugs have slow onset and offset kinetics (10 to 20 seconds).

Class ID
This class of drugs includes ranolazine, which preferentially inhibits the late Na⁺ current affecting APD and recovery and increases refractoriness and repolarization reserve. Class ID drugs cause a reduction in early afterdepolarization-induced triggered activity.

Class II
These drugs block beta-adrenergic receptors and include propranolol, metoprolol, nadolol, carvedilol, nebivolol, and timolol.

Class III
This class of drugs predominantly blocks potassium channels (e.g., I_{Kr}) and prolongs repolarization. Included are sotalol, amiodarone,

dronedarone, and ibutilide. Although these drugs are all classified as class III, they differ significantly in their effects on additional ion channels. For example, amiodarone is a nonselective K⁺ channel blocker while the other agents primarily block I_{Kr}.

Class IV
This class of drugs predominantly blocks the L-type or slow calcium channel ($I_{Ca.L}$)—verapamil, diltiazem, nifedipine, and others (felodipine blocks $I_{Ca.T}$).

Antiarrhythmic agents appear to cross the cell membrane and interact with receptors in the membrane channels when the channels are in the resting, activated, or inactivated state (see Table 64.1 and Chapter 62), and each of these interactions is characterized by different association and dissociation rate constants of a drug from its receptor. Such interactions depend on voltage and time. Transitions among resting, activated, and inactivated states are time- and voltage-dependent. When the drug is bound (associated) to a receptor site at or close to the channel pore (the drug may not actually "plug" the channel), the channel cannot conduct, even in the activated state.

USE DEPENDENCE
Some drugs exert greater inhibitory effects on the upstroke of the action potential at more rapid rates of stimulation and after longer periods of stimulation, a characteristic called *use dependence*. Drugs with this property depress V_{max} to a greater extent after the channel has been "used" (i.e., after action potential depolarization rather than after a rest period). Agents with class IB action exhibit rapid binding and unbinding from their receptor site on the channel protein, or exhibit

TABLE 64.2 Classification of Drug Actions on Arrhythmias Based on Modification of Vulnerable Parameter

MECHANISM	ARRHYTHMIA	VULNERABLE PARAMETER (EFFECT)	DRUGS (EFFECT)
Automaticity			
Enhanced normal	Inappropriate sinus tachycardia	Phase 4 β-adrenergic induced rate acceleration and I_f block	β-Adrenergic blocking agents and I_f blockers
Abnormal	Atrial tachycardia	Maximum diastolic potential (hyperpolarization)	M_2 agonist
		Phase 4 depolarization (decrease)	Ca^{2+} or Na^+ channel blocking agents
			M_2 agonist
	Accelerated idioventricular rhythms	Phase 4 depolarization (decrease)	Ca^{2+} or Na^+ channel blocking agents
Triggered Activity			
EAD	Torsades de pointes	Action potential duration (shorten)	β-adrenergic agonists; vagolytic agents (increase rate)
		EAD (suppress)	Ca^{2+} channel blocking agents; Mg^{2+}; β-adrenergic blocking agents; ranolazine
DAD	Digitalis-induced arrhythmias	Calcium overload (unload)	Ca^{2+} channel blocking agents
		DAD (suppress)	Na^+ channel blocking agents
	RV outflow tract ventricular tachycardia	Calcium overload (unload)	β-adrenergic blocking agents
		DAD (suppress)	Ca^{2+} channel blocking agents; adenosine
Reentry—Na^+ Channel Dependent			
Long excitable gap	Typical atrial flutter	Conduction and excitability (depress)	Type IA, IC Na^+ channel blocking agents
	Circus movement tachycardia in WPW	Conduction and excitability (depress)	Type IA, IC Na^+ channel blocking agents
	Sustained uniform ventricular tachycardia	Conduction and excitability (depress)	Na^+ channel blocking agents
Short excitable gap	Atypical atrial flutter	Refractory period (prolong)	K^+ channel blocking agents
	Atrial fibrillation	Refractory period (prolong)	K^+ channel blocking agents
	Circus movement tachycardia in WPW	Refractory period (prolong)	Amiodarone, sotalol
	Polymorphic and uniform ventricular tachycardia	Refractory period (prolong)	Type IA Na^+ channel blocking agents
	Bundle branch reentry	Refractory period (prolong)	Type IA Na^+ channel blocking agents; amiodarone
	Ventricular fibrillation	Refractory period (prolong)	
Reentry—Ca^{2+} Channel Dependent			
	AV nodal reentrant tachycardia	Conduction and excitability (depress)	Ca^{2+} channel blocking agents
	Circus movement tachycardia in WPW	Conduction and excitability (depress)	Ca^{2+} channel blocking agents
	Verapamil-sensitive ventricular tachycardia	Conduction and excitability (depress)	Ca^{2+} channel blocking agents

AV, Atrioventricular; *DAD,* delayed afterdepolarization; *EAD,* early afterdepolarization; *RV,* right ventricular; *WPW,* Wolff-Parkinson-White syndrome.
Modified from Task Force of the Working Group on Arrhythmias of the European Society of Cardiology. The Sicilian gambit: a new approach to the classification of antiarrhythmic drugs based on their actions on arrhythmogenic mechanisms. *Circulation.* 1991;84:1831. Copyright 1991, American Heart Association.

use-dependent block of the fast channel at fast rates. Class IC drugs have slow kinetics, and class IA drugs are intermediate. With increased time spent in diastole (slower rate), a greater proportion of receptors unbind drug, and the drug exerts less effect. The clinical consequence is that these drugs with slower kinetics have greater electrophysiologic effects at more rapid heart rates. For example, a class IC drug would cause more Na^+ channel blockade at more rapid heart rates, and this translates into greater QRS widening with faster heart rates. Unhealthy cells with reduced (i.e., abnormal) membrane potentials recover more slowly from drug actions than do healthier cells with more negative (i.e., normal) membrane potentials. This is referred to as *voltage dependence of block.*

REVERSE USE DEPENDENCE
Some drugs exert greater effects at slow rates than at fast rates, a property known as *reverse use dependence.* This is particularly true for drugs that lengthen repolarization; in the ventricle the QT interval becomes more prolonged at slow rather than at fast rates. This effect is not an ideal antiarrhythmic property, because prolongation of refractoriness should be increased at fast rates to interrupt or prevent a tachycardia and should be minimal at slow rates to avoid precipitation of torsades de pointes (TdP).

MECHANISMS OF ARRHYTHMIA SUPPRESSION
Given that enhanced automaticity, triggered activity, or reentry can cause cardiac arrhythmias (see Chapter 62), *mechanisms* by which AADs suppress arrhythmias in general can only be postulated (see Table 64.2) as some arrhythmias may encompass multiple mechanisms. AADs can slow the spontaneous discharge frequency of an automatic pacemaker by depressing the slope of diastolic depolarization, shifting the threshold voltage toward zero, or hyperpolarizing the resting membrane potential. In general, most AADs at therapeutic concentrations depress the automatic firing rate of spontaneously discharging ectopic sites while minimally affecting the discharge rate of the normal sinus node. Other agents act directly on the sinus node to slow heart rate, whereas drugs that exert vagolytic effects, such as disopyramide and quinidine, can increase the sinus rate. Drugs that suppress early (early afterdepolarization [EAD]) or delayed (delayed afterdepolarization [DAD]) afterdepolarizations can eliminate triggered arrhythmias based on these mechanisms.

Reentry depends critically on the interrelationships between refractoriness and conduction velocity, the presence of unidirectional block in one of the pathways, and other factors that influence refractoriness and conduction, such as excitability (see Chapter 62). An antiarrhythmic agent can stop ongoing reentry that is already present or

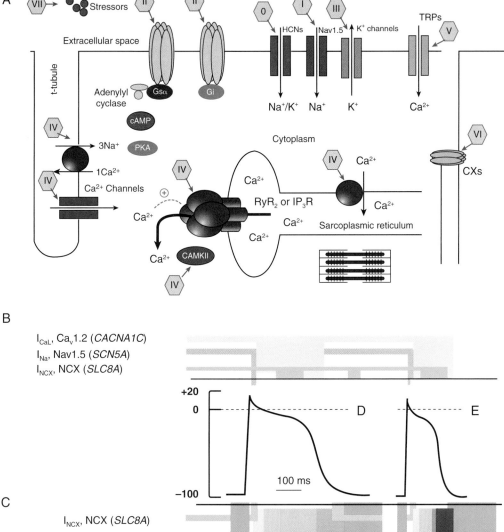

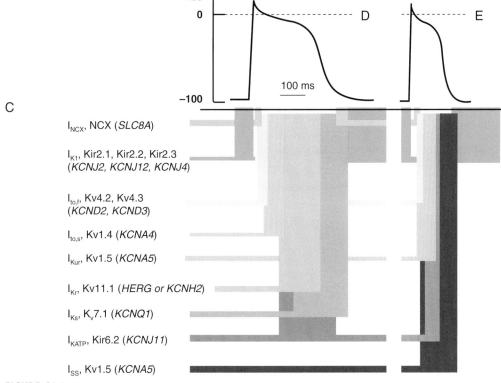

FIGURE 64.1 A, Surface and intracellular membrane ion channels, ion exchangers, transporters, and ionic pumps involved in cardiomyocyte electrophysiological excitation and activation; Roman numerals in blue hexagons refer to classes (*0*, HCN channel blockers; *I*, voltage-gated sodium channel blockers; *II*, autonomic inhibitors/activators; *III*, potassium channel blockers/openers; *IV*, calcium channel modulators; *V*, mechanosensitive channel blockers; *VI*, gap junction channel blockers; *VII*, upstream target modulators). **B** to **E,** Activation and inactivation of ion channels, currents, underlying proteins, and encoding genes and their contributions to (**B**) inward depolarizing and (**C**) outward repolarizing currents inscribing cardiac action potentials (APs). Ventricular (**D**) and atrial (**E**) APs comprise rapid depolarizing (phase 0), early repolarizing (phase 1), brief (atrial) or prolonged (ventricular) phase 2 plateaus (phase 2), phase 3 repolarization, and phase 4 electric diastole. In these, inward Na+ or Ca2+ currents drive phase 0 depolarization and Ca2+ current maintains the phase 2 plateau (**B**), and a range of outward K+ currents (**C**) drive phase 1 and phase 3 repolarization. Phase 4 resting potential restoration is accompanied by a refractory period required for Na+ channel recovery. The resulting wave of electric activity and refractoriness is propagated through successive sino-atrial node, atrial, atrioventricular, Purkinje, and endocardial and epicardial ventricular cardiomyocytes. *CaMKII* indicates calcium/calmodulin kinase II; *Cx*, connexin; *Gi*, inhibitory G protein; *Gs*, stimulatory G-protein; *HCN*, hyperpolarization-activated cyclic nucleotide-gated channel; *Nav1.5*, cardiac Na+ channel protein; *PKA*, protein kinase A; *RyR2*, cardiac ryanodine receptor type 2; *TRP*, transient receptor potential channel. (Adapted from Lei M, Wu L, Terrar DA, et al. Modernized classification of cardiac antiarrhythmic drugs. *Circulation.* 2018;138:1879–1896 with permission. Copyright (c) 2018, American Heart Association.)

can prevent it from starting if the drug depresses or, alternately, improves conduction. For example, improving conduction can (1) eliminate unidirectional block so that reentry cannot begin or (2) facilitate conduction in the reentrant loop so that the returning wavefront reenters too quickly, encounters cells that are still refractory, and is extinguished. A drug that depresses conduction can transform unidirectional block into bidirectional block and thus terminate reentry or prevent it from starting by creating an area of complete block in the reentrant pathway. Conversely, a drug that slows conduction without producing block or significantly lengthening refractoriness can actually promote reentry. Lastly, most AADs share the ability to prolong refractoriness relative to their effects on APD; that is, the ratio of the effective refractory period (ERP) to APD exceeds 1.0. If a drug prolongs the refractoriness of fibers in the reentrant pathway, the pathway may not recover excitability in time to be depolarized by the reentering impulse, and reentrant propagation ceases. Different types of reentry influence the effectiveness of a drug.

In considering the properties of a drug, it is important to define carefully the situation or model from which conclusions are drawn. Electrophysiologic, hemodynamic, autonomic, pharmacokinetic, and adverse effects can all differ in normal individuals compared with patients, in normal versus abnormal tissue, in cardiac muscle compared with specialized conduction fibers, and in atrial versus ventricular muscle (eTable 64.2).

DRUG METABOLITES

Drug metabolites can add to or alter the effects of the parent compound by exerting similar actions, competing with the parent compound, or mediating drug toxicity. Quinidine has at least four active metabolites, but none with a potency exceeding that of the parent drug, and none implicated in causing TdP. About 50% of procainamide is metabolized to *N*-acetylprocainamide (NAPA), which prolongs repolarization and is a less effective sodium channel blocker but competes with procainamide for renal excretion and can increase the parent drug's elimination half-life. A lidocaine metabolite can compete with the parent drug for sodium channels and partially antagonize its blocking effect.

PHARMACOGENETICS

Genetically determined metabolic pathways account for many of the differences in patients' responses to some drugs (see Chapter 9).[4]

The superfamily of cytochrome P-450 (CYP450) enzymes metabolize propafenone, hydroxylate several beta blockers, and biotransform flecainide. The CYP4502D6 exhibits extensive genetic and functional heterogeneity. Lack of this enzyme (in approximately 7% of white patients and 5% of Blacks) reduces metabolism of the parent compound and thereby leads to increased plasma concentrations of the parent drug and reduced concentrations of metabolites. Propafenone is metabolized by CYP450 to a compound with slightly less antiarrhythmic and beta-adrenergic blocking effects, as well as fewer central nervous system (CNS) side effects. Thus, poor metabolizers may experience more heart rate slowing and neurotoxicity than extensive metabolizers do.

Drugs such as rifampin, phenobarbital, and phenytoin induce the synthesis of larger amounts of various CYP450 isoforms, which leads to lower concentrations of the parent drugs because of extensive metabolism, whereas erythromycin, clarithromycin, fluoxetine, and grapefruit juice inhibit enzyme activity, which leads to accumulation of the parent compound. Therefore, clinicians caring for patients who take AADs should be sensitive to the effects of non-cardiac medications and supplements on AAD metabolism and elimination and drug-drug interactions. Over-the-counter (OTC) drugs such as proton pump inhibitors can promote hypokalemia and hypomagnesemia and interact with a simple antibiotic such as ceftriaxone to cause TdP.[5,6] Many astute clinicians use, and refer their patients to, websites such as Crediblemeds.org, where updated information on drug interactions of this type is available. A list of drugs that prolong the QT interval can also be found at www.sads.org.

Clinical Use

In treating cardiac rhythm disorders, most drugs are given on a daily basis (in one to three doses) to prevent episodes from occurring or, in some cases of AF, to control the ventricular rate. Efficacy can be judged in various ways, depending on the clinical circumstances. Symptom reduction (in the case of benign arrhythmias, such as most premature ventricular complexes [PVCs]) and electrocardiographic monitoring (long-term or event; see Chapter 61) are useful; electrophysiologic study (EPS) has been used in the past, with suppression of electrical induction of arrhythmia being the goal, but is rarely used for this purpose currently. Interrogation of implanted devices can also provide an indicator of the success of drug therapy by providing PVC counts and burden of atrial arrhythmias.

In some patients, tachycardia episodes are infrequent enough (months between occurrences) and symptoms mild enough that reactive drug administration is more reasonable than chronic daily dosing. The patient takes a medication only after an episode has started, in the hope that the tachycardia can be terminated and a visit to a physician's office or emergency department avoided. This "pill in the pocket" strategy has worked well for some patients with AF, who have been given one of various medications orally in a monitored setting to ensure safety as well as efficacy before allowing self-medication at home or elsewhere.

Adverse Effects

AADs produce one group of adverse effects related to excessive dosage and plasma concentrations that result in both non-cardiac (e.g., neurologic defects) and cardiac (e.g., heart failure, some arrhythmias) toxicity. Another group of side effects unrelated to plasma concentrations is termed *idiosyncratic*; examples include amiodarone-induced pulmonary fibrosis and some arrhythmias, such as quinidine-induced TdP, which can occur in individuals with a forme fruste of long-QT syndrome (i.e., marked prolongation of normal QT interval in the presence of certain medications; see Chapters 9 and 63). Genetic variants can underlie susceptibility to idiosyncratic reactions.

The U.S. Food and Drug Administration (FDA) has recently determined that the risk of adverse events during pregnancy and lactation (previously categorized as A, B, C, D, and X; see Table 64.3) should be modified (the Pregnancy and Lactation Labeling rule of 2015). The old classification scheme was confusing and did not accurately differentiate the risks to the fetus. This rule applies to all new prescription drugs after June 2015 and is being phased in gradually for drugs approved between 2001 and 2015. This process is underway but until completed, adverse event risk in this setting is characterized using the previous classification.[7] We have attempted to summarize some information about AAD safety during pregnancy in Table 64.4.

Proarrhythmia

Drug-induced or drug-exacerbated cardiac arrhythmias (proarrhythmia) constitute a major clinical problem.[1,8] Proarrhythmia can manifest as an increase in frequency of a preexisting arrhythmia, sustaining of a previously non-sustained arrhythmia (even making it incessant), or development of arrhythmias that the patient has not previously experienced. Electrophysiologic mechanisms are probably related to prolongation of repolarization or an increase in transmural dispersion, development of EADs with resultant TdP, and alterations in reentry pathways to initiate or sustain tachyarrhythmias. Proarrhythmic events can occur in as many as 5% to 10% of patients receiving antiarrhythmic agents; heart failure increases this risk. Reduced left ventricular function, treatment with digitalis and diuretics, bradycardia and a longer pretreatment QT interval identify patients who experience AAD-induced ventricular fibrillation (VF). The more commonly known proarrhythmic events occur within several days of

TABLE 64.3 Antiarrhythmic Drug Use During Pregnancy

Considered Safe
Adenosine (C)
Propranolol (C)
Metoprolol (C)
Lidocaine (B)
Digoxin* (C)
Sotalol (B)
Verapamil (C)
Limited Data; Recommend Use With Caution
Adenosine (C)
Propranolol (C)
Metoprolol (C)
Carvedilol (C)
Propafenone (C)
Flecainide* (C)
Propafenone (C)
Sotalol* (B)
Diltiazem (C)
Verapamil (C)
Ivabradine (D)
Contraindicated
Amiodarone (D)
Dronedarone (X)

A, No demonstrated risk to the fetus based on well-controlled human studies; *B*, No demonstrated risk to the fetus based on animal studies; *C*, Animal studies have demonstrated fetal adverse events, but no human study data; *D*, Demonstrated high human fetal risk, and X: demonstrated high risk for human fetal abnormalities and should not be used.

*Digoxin, flecainide, and sotalol have been used to treat fetal arrhythmias during pregnancy.

Adapted from Regitz-Zagrosek V, Ross-Hesselink JW, Bauersachs J, et al. 2018 ESC guidelines for the management of cardiovascular diseases during pregnancy. *Eur Heart J.* 2018;39:3165–3241.

beginning drug therapy or changing dosage and are represented by such developments as incessant VT and long-QT–related TdP. In the Cardiac Arrhythmia Suppression Trial (CAST), however, researchers found that encainide and flecainide reduced spontaneous ventricular arrhythmias but were associated with a total mortality of 7.7%, versus 3.0% in the placebo group. Deaths were equally distributed throughout the treatment period, indicating that another type of proarrhythmic response can occur sometime after the beginning of drug therapy. Such late proarrhythmic effects may be related to drug-induced exacerbation of the regional myocardial conduction delay caused by ischemia and to heterogeneous drug concentrations that can promote reentry. In the future, a candidate antiarrhythmic compound's potential for proarrhythmia may be modeled computationally and tested in stem cells.

The availability of catheter ablation (see later) and implantable devices (pacemakers and ICDs; see Chapter 69) to treat a wide variety of arrhythmias has largely relegated drug therapy to a secondary role in the treatment of serious arrhythmias. Drugs are still useful to prevent or to decrease the frequency of recurrences in patients who have relatively infrequent episodes of benign tachycardias, as well as in those who have had incomplete success with catheter ablation procedures and in patients with an ICD, to decrease the frequency of shocks because of supraventricular or ventricular arrhythmias.

Antiarrhythmic Agents
Class IA Agents
Quinidine

Quinidine and quinine are isomeric alkaloids isolated from cinchona bark. Although quinidine shares the antimalarial, antipyretic, and vagolytic actions of quinine, only quinidine has direct cellular electrophysiologic effects. It blocks several channels, including the rapid inward sodium channel (I_{Na}), I_{Kr}, I_{to}, and to a lesser extent the slow inward calcium channel, I_{Ks}, and the adenosine triphosphate (ATP)–sensitive potassium current (K_{ATP}). Quinidine causes alpha-adrenergic and cholinergic blockade. The ultimate biologic effect of the drug in a given patient depends on heart rate, drug concentration, and which channels are more prominently affected. Because of decreased demand for quinidine, manufacturing had ceased for a time, with little remaining supply in many countries, but recent renewed demand for its use in patients with Brugada syndrome and idiopathic VF have resulted in quinidine becoming more readily available.

ELECTROPHYSIOLOGIC ACTIONS

Quinidine exerts little effect on automaticity of the normal sinus node but suppresses automaticity in normal Purkinje fibers (see eTable 64.2; see also Tables 64.1, 64.2, and eTable 64.1). In patients with sinus node dysfunction, quinidine can further depress sinus node automaticity. Quinidine lengthens the QT interval in part via formation of EADs in experimental preparations and in humans, which appears to be responsible for TdP. Because of its significant anticholinergic effect and the reflex sympathetic stimulation resulting from alpha-adrenergic blockade, which causes peripheral vasodilation, quinidine can cause a reflex increase in the sinus node discharge rate and improve atrioventricular (AV) nodal conduction. Quinidine prolongs repolarization, an effect that is more prominent at slow heart rates (reverse use dependence) because of block of I_{Kr} (as well as enhancing the late inward Na⁺ current at low concentrations). Faster rates result in more block of sodium channels and less unblocking because a smaller percentage of time is spent in the rested state (use dependence). Isoproterenol can modulate the effects of quinidine on reentrant circuits in humans. Quinidine at higher doses inhibits the late inward Na⁺ current. As noted, quinidine blocks the transient outward current I_{to}, which probably explains its efficacy in suppressing ventricular arrhythmias in Brugada syndrome and patients with idiopathic VF (see Chapter 63).

HEMODYNAMIC EFFECTS

Quinidine induces vasodilation by blocking alpha-adrenergic receptors and can cause significant hypotension. It does not cause significant direct myocardial depression.

PHARMACOKINETICS

Plasma quinidine concentrations peak at approximately 1.5 to 3 hours after an oral dose of a quinidine gluconate preparation (see Table

64.4). Approximately 80% of plasma quinidine is protein bound, especially to α₁-acid glycoprotein. Both the liver and the kidneys remove quinidine; dose adjustments may be made to achieve appropriate serum concentrations. Its elimination half-life is 8 to 9 hours after oral administration.

DOSAGE AND ADMINISTRATION. The usual oral dose of quinidine sulfate for an adult is 300 to 600 mg four times daily, which results in a steady-state level within about 24 hours (see Table 64.4). A loading dose of 600 to 800 mg produces an earlier effective concentration. Oral doses of the gluconate are about 30% higher than those of the sulfate form. Important interactions with other drugs occur.

INDICATIONS. Quinidine is a versatile AAD that was used previously to treat premature supraventricular and ventricular complexes and sustained tachyarrhythmias. However, because of its side effect profile and potential for causing TdP, as well as its limited usefulness in preventing VT and VF in most applications, its use has decreased greatly. In recent years, however, interest has increased in quinidine for treating primary (idiopathic) VF, ventricular arrhythmias in patients with Brugada syndrome (see Chapter 63),[9] and short-QT syndrome. Quinidine crosses the placenta so it can be used to treat fetal arrhythmias.

ADVERSE EFFECTS. The most common adverse effects of chronic oral quinidine therapy are gastrointestinal (GI) and include nausea, vomiting, diarrhea, abdominal pain, and anorexia (milder with the gluconate form). CNS toxicity includes tinnitus, hearing loss, visual disturbances, confusion, delirium, and psychosis (cinchonism). Allergic reactions include rash, fever, immune-mediated thrombocytopenia, hemolytic anemia, and rarely, anaphylaxis. Side effects may preclude long-term administration of quinidine in 30% to 40% of patients.

Quinidine can slow cardiac conduction, sometimes to the point of block, which is manifested as prolongation of the QRS duration or as sinoatrial (SA) or AV nodal conduction disturbances. Quinidine can produce syncope in 0.5% to 2.0% of patients, most often the result of a self-terminating episode of TdP. Quinidine prolongs the QT interval in most patients (not dose related), regardless of whether ventricular arrhythmias occur, but significant QT prolongation (QT interval of 500 to 600 milliseconds) is often a characteristic of patients with quinidine-related syncope, who may have a genetic predisposition underlying such a response (see Chapter 9). Many of these patients are also receiving digitalis or diuretics or have hypokalemia; women are more susceptible than men. Importantly, syncope is unrelated to plasma concentrations of quinidine or the duration of therapy, although most episodes occur within the first 2 to 4 days of therapy initiation, often after conversion of AF to sinus rhythm. This proarrhythmic effect during initiation of treatment is reproducible and because of this, the drug should not be taken on an intermittent basis. Therapy of proarrhythmia requires immediate discontinuation of use of the drug; magnesium given intravenously (2 g over 1 to 2 minutes, followed by an infusion of 3 to 20 mg/min) is the initial drug treatment of choice. Atrial or ventricular pacing can be used to suppress the ventricular tachyarrhythmia, perhaps by suppressing EADs. When pacing is not available, isoproterenol can be given with caution. The arrhythmia gradually dissipates as quinidine is cleared and the QT interval returns to baseline. Affected patients should not use quinidine thereafter and also should avoid other drugs that prolong the QT interval (see Crediblemeds.org).

Drugs that induce hepatic enzyme production, such as phenobarbital and phenytoin, can shorten the duration of action of quinidine by increasing its rate of elimination. Quinidine can increase plasma concentrations of flecainide by inhibiting the CYP450 enzyme system. Quinidine can elevate serum digoxin concentrations by decreasing its clearance and volume of distribution and the affinity of tissue receptors.

Procainamide

ELECTROPHYSIOLOGIC ACTIONS

The cardiac actions of procainamide on automaticity, conduction, excitability, and membrane responsiveness resemble those of quinidine (see

TABLE 64.4 Dosage and Other Information for Clinical Use of Common Antiarrhythmic Agents

DRUG	USUAL DOSAGE RANGES — INTRAVENOUS (MG) LOADING	INTRAVENOUS (MG) MAINTENANCE	ORAL (MG) LOADING	ORAL (MG) MAINTENANCE	TIME TO PEAK PLASMA CONCENTRATION (ORAL) (HR)	EFFECTIVE SERUM OR PLASMA CONCENTRATION (MCG/ML)	HALF-LIFE (HR)	BIOAVAILABILITY (%)	MAJOR ROUTE OF ELIMINATION	PREGNANCY CLASS
Quinidine	6–10 mg/kg at 0.3–0.5 mg/kg/min	—	800–1000	300–600 q6h	1.5–3.0	3–6	5–9	60–80	Liver > kidneys	C
Procainamide	6–13 mg/kg at 0.2–0.5 mg/kg/min	2–6 mg/min	500–1000	250–1000 q4–6h	1	4–10	3–5	70–85	Kidneys > liver	C
Disopyramide	1–2 mg/kg over 15–45 min*	1 mg/kg/hr*	N/A	100–300 q6-8h	1–2	2–5	4–10	80–90	Kidneys	C
Lidocaine	1–2 mg/kg at 20–50 mg/min	1–4 mg/min	N/A	N/A	N/A	1–5	1–2	N/A	Liver	B
Mexiletine	500 mg*	0.5–1.0 g/24 hr*	400–600	150–300 q8-12h	2–4	0.75–2.0	10–17	80–90	Liver	C
Phenytoin	100 mg q5min for ≤1000mg	N/A	1000	100–400 q12-24h	8–12	10–20	18–36	50–70	Liver	D
Flecainide	2 mg/kg*	100–200 q12h*	N/A	50–200 q12h	3–4	0.2–1.0	20	95	Kidneys	C
Propafenone	1–2 mg/kg*	N/A	600–900	150–300 q8-12h	1–3	0.5–2.0	2–10 (extensive metabolizers); 10-32 (poor metabolizers)	3–25	Liver	C
Propranolol	0.25–0.5 mg q5min to ≤0.20 mg/kg	N/A	N/A	10–200 q6-8h	4	0.02–0.2	3–6	35–65	Liver	C
Amiodarone	15 mg/min for 10 min; 1 mg/min for 6 hr; 0.5 mg/min thereafter	0.5 mg/min	400 to 800 mg/day for 7-14 days	200–600 qd	Variable	0.5–1.5	56 days	25	Liver	D
Dronedarone	N/A	N/A	N/A	400 mg q12h	3–4	0.3–0.6	13–19	70–90	Liver	X
Sotalol	60–112.5 mg over 1 h	75–112.5 mg over 5 h	N/A	80–160 q12h	2.5–4	2.5	10–20	90–100	Kidneys	B
Ibutilide	1 mg over 10 min	N/A	N/A	N/A	N/A	N/A	2–12		Kidneys	C
Dofetilide	N/A	N/A	N/A	0.125–0.5 q12h	N/A	N/A	7–13	90	Kidneys	C
Verapamil	5–10 mg over 1–2 min	0.005 mg/kg/min	N/A	80–120 q6-8h	1–2	0.10–0.15	3–8	20–35	Liver, kidneys	C
Adenosine	6–18 mg (rapidly)	N/A	N/A	N/A	N/A	N/A	Seconds	100	Blood cells	C
Digoxin	0.5–1.0 mg	0.125–0.25 qd	0.5–1.0	0.125–0.25 qd	2–6	0.0008–0.002	36–48	60–80	Kidneys	C
Ranolazine	N/A	N/A	N/A	500–1000 bid	4–6	N/A	7	60–75	Kidneys > liver	C
Ivabradine	N/A	N/A	N/A	2.5–7.5 mg bid	1	N/A	6	40%	Gut and liver	D

Pill in the Pocket Approach

1. Chronic oral beta blocker therapy or diltiazem or verapamil
2. If NOT on chronic beta blocker therapy, rapid acting beta blockers such as metoprolol 25–50 mg, propranolol 20–80 mg, diltiazem 30–90 mg or verapamil 30–60 mg at least 30 min prior to antiarrhythmic drug therapy
3. Flecainide as single dose of 200–300 mg; 200 mg if weight <70 kg

OR

Propafenone as single dose of 450–600 mg; 450 mg if weight <70 kg

Recommended that the first dose of a class IC agent or first trial of pill in the pocket consideration should be given to have it administered under monitored therapy

*Intravenous use investigational or unavailable in United States.

N/A, not applicable; q4-6h, every 4 to 6 hours; qd, every day; bid, twice daily.

Results presented may vary according to doses, disease state, and IV or oral administration.

Pregnancy Class: A, controlled studies show no fetal risk; B, no controlled studies, but no evidence of fetal risk; C, fetal risk cannot be excluded; fetal harm unlikely; D, positive fetal risk; drug should be avoided unless in a life-threatening situation or safer alternatives do not exist; X, contraindicated in pregnancy. Categorization of safety during pregnancy and lactation is currently undergoing revision.

Tables 64.1, 64.2, and eTables 64.1, 64.2). Procainamide predominantly blocks the inactivated state of I_{Na}. It also blocks I_{Kr}, I_{K1}, and $I_{K,ATP}$. Like quinidine, procainamide usually prolongs the ERP more than it prolongs the APD and thus may prevent reentry. Procainamide exerts the least anticholinergic effects among type IA drugs. High levels of NAPA, such as in patients with renal disease, can produce EADs, triggered activity, and TdP. Because of decreased demand, availability of intravenous (IV) and oral procainamide is greatly limited.

HEMODYNAMIC EFFECTS
Procainamide can depress myocardial contractility in high concentrations. It does not produce alpha blockade but can result in peripheral vasodilation, possibly through antisympathetic effects on the brain or spinal cord, which can impair cardiovascular reflexes (e.g., provoking orthostatic symptoms).

PHARMACOKINETICS
Oral administration produces a peak plasma concentration in approximately 1 hour. Approximately 80% of oral procainamide is bioavailable; the overall elimination half-life of procainamide is 3 to 5 hours, with 50% to 60% of the drug eliminated by the kidneys and 10% to 30% metabolized by the liver (see Table 64.4). The drug is acetylated to NAPA, which is excreted almost exclusively by the kidneys. As renal function decreases and in patients with heart failure, NAPA levels increase and, because of the risk for serious cardiotoxicity, need to be carefully monitored in these situations. NAPA has an elimination half-life of 7 to 8 hours, but the half-life exceeds 10 hours if high doses of procainamide are used. Increased age, congestive heart failure, and reduced creatinine clearance lower the clearance of procainamide and necessitate a reduced dosage.

DOSAGE AND ADMINISTRATION. Procainamide can be given by the oral, IV, or intramuscular (IM) route to achieve plasma concentrations in the range of 4 to 10 μg/mL and produce an antiarrhythmic effect (see Table 64.4). Several IV regimens have been used to administer procainamide, but usually doses of 10 to 15 mg/kg are used at a rate of up to 50 mg/min until the arrhythmia has been controlled, hypotension results, or the QRS complex is prolonged more than 50%. With this method, the plasma concentration falls rapidly during the first 15 minutes after the loading dose, with parallel effects on refractoriness and conduction. A constant-rate IV infusion of procainamide can be given at a dosage of 2 to 6 mg/min, depending on the patient's response.

Oral administration of procainamide requires a 3- to 4-hour dosing interval at a total daily dose of 2 to 6 g, with a steady-state concentration being reached within 1 day. When a loading dose is used, it should be twice the maintenance dose. Frequent dosing is required because of its short elimination half-life in normal persons. For the extended-release forms of procainamide, dosing is at 6- to 12-hour intervals. Procainamide by IM injection is almost 100% bioavailable.

INDICATIONS. Procainamide is used to treat both supraventricular and ventricular arrhythmias in a manner comparable to that of quinidine. Although both drugs have similar electrophysiologic actions, either drug can effectively suppress a supraventricular or ventricular arrhythmia that is resistant to the other drug. Procainamide can be used to convert recent-onset AF to sinus rhythm. As with quinidine, prior treatment with beta or calcium channel blockers is recommended to prevent acceleration of the ventricular response during atrial flutter or fibrillation after procainamide therapy. Procainamide can block conduction in the accessory pathway of patients with Wolff-Parkinson-White (WPW) syndrome and can be used in patients with AF and a rapid ventricular response related to conduction over the accessory pathway. It can produce His-Purkinje block and is sometimes administered during an EPS to stress the His-Purkinje system and evaluate the need for a pacemaker (see Fig. 61.15). However, it should be used with caution in patients with evidence of His-Purkinje disease (bundle branch block) for whom a ventricular pacemaker is not readily available.

Procainamide is more effective than lidocaine in acutely terminating sustained VT. IV procainamide is recommended along with IV amiodarone and IV sotalol in the Advanced Cardiac Life Support (ACLS) Guidelines for the treatment of stable wide QRS tachycardia presumed to be VT. Most consistently, procainamide slows the VT rate, a change correlated with the increase in QRS duration. The drug also has diagnostic applications when given intravenously (10 mg/kg over 5 to 10 minutes). In patients with suspected Brugada syndrome who have a normal resting electrocardiogram (ECG), drug infusion can result in the characteristic "Brugada sign," whereas in patients with WPW syndrome, the drug can cause sudden loss of preexcitation.

ADVERSE EFFECTS. Noncardiac adverse effects from administration of procainamide include rash, myalgia, digital vasculitis, and Raynaud phenomenon. Fever and agranulocytosis may be the result of hypersensitivity reactions, and a complete blood count should be assessed at regular intervals. GI side effects are less frequent than with quinidine, and adverse CNS side effects are less frequent than with lidocaine. Toxic concentrations of procainamide can diminish myocardial performance and promote hypotension. Various conduction disturbances or ventricular tachyarrhythmias can occur, similar to those produced by quinidine. NAPA can cause QT prolongation and TdP. In the absence of sinus node disease, procainamide does not adversely affect sinus node function. In patients with sinus node dysfunction, however, procainamide can prolong sinus node recovery time and worsen symptoms in some patients with bradycardia-tachycardia syndrome.

Arthralgia, fever, pleuropericarditis, hepatomegaly, and hemorrhagic pericardial effusion with tamponade have been described in a systemic lupus erythematosus (SLE)-like syndrome related to procainamide administration. The syndrome occurs more frequently and earlier in patients who are slow acetylators of procainamide and is genetically influenced (see Chapter 9). Acetylation of procainamide to form NAPA appears to block the SLE-inducing effect. In 60% to 70% of patients receiving long-term procainamide therapy, anti-nuclear antibodies (ANAs) develop, with clinical symptoms occurring in 20% to 30%; this is reversible when procainamide is stopped. Positive serologic test results are not necessarily a reason to discontinue drug therapy; however, the development of symptoms with a positive anti-DNA antibody generally indicates that drug therapy should be discontinued. Corticosteroid administration in these patients may eliminate the symptoms. In this syndrome, in contrast to naturally occurring SLE, the brain and kidneys are typically spared, and there is no predilection for women.

Disopyramide
Disopyramide has been approved in the United States for oral administration to treat patients with ventricular and supraventricular arrhythmias.

ELECTROPHYSIOLOGIC ACTIONS
Disopyramide produces electrophysiologic effects similar to those of quinidine and procainamide, causing use-dependent block of I_{Na} and non–use-dependent block of I_{Kr} (see Tables 64.1, 64.2, and eTables 64.1, 64.2).

Disopyramide is a muscarinic blocker and can increase the sinus node discharge rate and shorten AV nodal conduction time and refractoriness when the nodes are under cholinergic (vagal) influence. It exerts greater anticholinergic effects than quinidine and does not appear to affect alpha or beta adrenoceptors. The drug prolongs atrial and ventricular refractory periods, but its effect on AV nodal conduction and refractoriness is not consistent. Disopyramide prolongs His-Purkinje conduction time, but infra-His block rarely occurs. It can be administered safely to patients who have first-degree AV delay and narrow QRS complexes.

HEMODYNAMIC EFFECTS
Disopyramide suppresses ventricular systolic performance and is a mild arterial vasodilator. The drug should generally be avoided in patients with reduced left ventricular systolic function because they tolerate its negative inotropic effects poorly.

PHARMACOKINETICS

Oral disopyramide is 80% to 90% absorbed, with a mean elimination half-life of 8 to 9 hours in healthy volunteers but almost 10 hours in patients with heart failure (see Table 64.4). Renal insufficiency prolongs its elimination time. Thus, in patients with renal, hepatic, or cardiac insufficiency, loading and maintenance doses need to be reduced. Peak blood levels after oral administration occur in 1 to 2 hours. Approximately 50% of an oral dose is excreted unchanged in urine, with 30% occurring as the mono-N-dealkylated metabolite. The metabolites appear to exert less effect than the parent compound. As with other class IA antiarrhythmic drugs, macrolide antibiotics inhibit its metabolism.

DOSAGE AND ADMINISTRATION. Doses are generally 100 to 300 mg orally every 6 hours, with a range of 400 to 1200 mg/day (see Table 64.4). A controlled-release preparation can be given as 200 to 300 mg every 12 hours.

INDICATIONS. Disopyramide appears to be comparable to quinidine and procainamide in reducing the frequency of PVCs and effectively preventing recurrence of VT in selected patients. Disopyramide has been combined with other drugs, such as mexiletine, to treat patients who do not respond or respond only partially to one drug.

Although rarely used for this, disopyramide helps prevent recurrence of AF after successful cardioversion as effectively as quinidine and may terminate atrial flutter. In treating patients with AF, particularly atrial flutter, the ventricular rate must be controlled before disopyramide is administered, or the combination of a decrease in atrial rate with vagolytic effects on the AV node can result in 1:1 AV conduction during atrial flutter (see Chapter 66). It has been used in patients with hypertrophic cardiomyopathy for both AF therapy and its negative inotropic effect.

ADVERSE EFFECTS. Three types of adverse effects follow disopyramide administration. The most common effects are related to the drug's potent parasympatholytic properties and include urinary hesitancy or retention, constipation, blurred vision, closed-angle glaucoma, and dry mouth. Symptoms are less with the sustained-release form. Second, disopyramide can produce ventricular tachyarrhythmias frequently associated with QT prolongation and TdP. Cross-sensitization to both quinidine and disopyramide occurs in some patients, and TdP can develop while receiving either drug. When drug-induced torsades de pointes (DI-TdP) occurs, agents that prolong the QT interval should be used cautiously or not at all. Lastly, disopyramide can reduce contractility of the normal ventricle, but the depression of ventricular function is much more pronounced in patients with preexisting ventricular failure. Rarely, cardiovascular collapse can result.

Ajmaline

Ajmaline, a rauwolfia derivative, has been used extensively to treat patients with ventricular and supraventricular arrhythmias in Europe and Asia but is not available in the United States.

ELECTROPHYSIOLOGIC ACTIONS

As with other class IA drugs, ajmaline produces use-dependent block of INa; it also weakly blocks IKr. The drug has mild anticholinergic activity (see Tables 64.1, 64.2, and eTables 64.1, 64.2).

HEMODYNAMIC EFFECTS

Ajmaline mildly suppresses ventricular systolic performance but does not affect peripheral resistance. It also inhibits platelet activity more potently than aspirin does.

PHARMACOKINETICS, DOSAGE, AND ADMINISTRATION

Ajmaline is well absorbed with a mean elimination half-life of 13 minutes in most patients, thus making it poorly suited to long-term oral use. The dose for termination of acute arrhythmia is generally 50 mg intravenously infused over 1 to 2 minutes.

INDICATIONS

Although it is useful for terminating SVTs by IV infusion, other medications have largely supplanted ajmaline for this purpose and its use

has evolved to that of a diagnostic tool. When administered intravenously at doses of 50 mg over a 3-minute period, or 10 mg/min, to a total dose of 1 mg/kg, ajmaline can have the following effects: (1) delta wave disappearance in patients with WPW syndrome (indicating an accessory pathway anterograde ERP longer than 250 milliseconds); (2) ST-T abnormalities and interventricular conduction block in patients with occult Chagasic cardiomyopathy; (3) heart block in patients with bundle branch block and syncope, but in whom no rhythm disturbance had been discovered; and (4) right precordial ST elevation in patients with suspected Brugada syndrome in whom findings on the resting ECG are normal. It is in this last setting that ajmaline is used most frequently.

ADVERSE EFFECTS

Ajmaline can produce mild anticholinergic side effects, as well as mild depression of left ventricular systolic function, and can worsen AV conduction in patients with His-Purkinje disease. Rare occurrences of TdP have been reported. Ajmaline can increase the defibrillation threshold.

Class IB Agents
Lidocaine

ELECTROPHYSIOLOGIC ACTIONS

Lidocaine blocks I_{Na}, predominantly in the open or inactivated state. It has rapid onset and offset kinetics and does not affect normal sinus node automaticity in usual doses but does depress other normal and abnormal forms of automaticity, as well as EADs and DADs in Purkinje fibers in vitro (see Tables 64.1, 64.2, and eTables 64.1, 64.2). Lidocaine has only a modest depressant effect on $\dot{V}_{max}$; however, faster rates of stimulation, acidosis, increased extracellular K^+ concentration, and reduced membrane potential (changes that can result from ischemia) increase the ability of lidocaine to block I_{Na}. Lidocaine can convert areas of unidirectional block into bidirectional block during ischemia and inhibit the development of VF by preventing fragmentation of organized large wavefronts into heterogeneous wavelets.

Except in very high concentrations, lidocaine does not affect slow-Ca channel–dependent action potentials despite its moderate suppression of the Ca current. Lidocaine has minimal effect on atrial fibers and does not affect conduction in accessory pathways. Depressed automaticity or conduction can develop in patients with preexisting sinus node dysfunction, abnormal His-Purkinje conduction, or junctional or ventricular escape rhythms. Part of lidocaine's effects may involve inhibition of cardiac sympathetic nerve activity.

HEMODYNAMIC EFFECTS

Clinically significant adverse hemodynamic effects are rarely noted with lidocaine at the usual drug concentrations unless left ventricular function is severely impaired.

PHARMACOKINETICS

Lidocaine is used only parenterally because oral administration results in extensive first-pass hepatic metabolism and unpredictably low plasma levels, as well as excessive metabolites that can produce toxicity (see Table 64.4). Hepatic metabolism of lidocaine depends on hepatic blood flow; severe hepatic disease or reduced hepatic blood flow, as in heart failure or shock, can greatly decrease the rate of lidocaine metabolism. Beta-adrenoceptor blockers can decrease hepatic blood flow and increase the serum concentration of lidocaine. Prolonged infusion can reduce lidocaine clearance. Its elimination half-life averages 1 to 2 hours in normal individuals, longer than 4 hours in patients after uncomplicated myocardial infarction (MI), longer than 10 hours in patients after MI complicated by heart failure, and even longer in the presence of cardiogenic shock. Maintenance doses should be reduced by one third to one half in patients with low cardiac output.

DOSAGE AND ADMINISTRATION. Although lidocaine can be given intramuscularly, the IV route is most often used, with an initial bolus of 1 to 2 mg/kg body weight at a rate of 20 to 50 mg/min and a second injection of half the initial dose 20 to 40 minutes later to maintain the therapeutic concentration (see Table 64.4).

If the initial bolus of lidocaine is ineffective, up to two more boluses of 1 mg/kg may be administered at 5-minute intervals. Patients who require more than one bolus to achieve a therapeutic effect generally need a higher maintenance dose to sustain these higher concentrations, with infusion rates in the range of 1 to 4 mg/min to produce steady-state plasma levels of 1 to 5 mg/mL in patients with uncomplicated MI. These rates must be reduced during heart failure or shock because of the concomitant reduced hepatic blood flow. Higher doses and concentrations are unlikely to provide additional benefit but do increase the risk for toxicity.

INDICATIONS. Lidocaine has moderate efficacy against ventricular arrhythmias of diverse causes; it is generally ineffective against supraventricular arrhythmias and rarely terminates monomorphic VT. Although once used in an attempt to prevent VF in the first 2 days after acute MI, its efficacy was marginal, and because it can produce side effects such use is now not recommended.

ADVERSE EFFECTS. The most frequently reported adverse effects of lidocaine are dose-related manifestations of CNS toxicity: dizziness, paresthesias, confusion, delirium, stupor, coma, and seizures. Occasional sinus node depression and His-Purkinje block have been reported. Rarely, lidocaine can cause malignant hyperthermia.

Mexiletine

Mexiletine, a local anesthetic congener of lidocaine with anticonvulsant properties, is used for the oral treatment of patients with symptomatic ventricular arrhythmias. It is rarely used as a single agent for the treatment of ventricular arrhythmias.

ELECTROPHYSIOLOGIC ACTIONS

Mexiletine is similar to lidocaine in many of its electrophysiologic actions. In vitro, mexiletine shortens the APD and ERP of Purkinje fibers and, to a lesser extent, ventricular muscle. It depresses the V_{max} of phase 0 by blocking I_{Na}, especially at faster rates, and depresses the automaticity of Purkinje fibers but not of the normal sinus node. Its onset and offset kinetics are rapid. Hypoxia or ischemia can increase its effects (see Tables 64.1, 64.2, and eTables 64.1, 64.2).

Mexiletine can result in severe bradycardia and abnormal sinus node recovery time in patients with sinus node disease, but not in those with a normal sinus node. It does not affect AV nodal conduction and can depress His-Purkinje conduction, but not greatly, unless conduction was abnormal initially. Mexiletine does not appear to affect human atrial muscle. It does not affect the QT interval. It has been used in treating a variety of other disorders, including erythromelalgia (red, painful extremities) in children and myotonia.

HEMODYNAMIC EFFECTS

Mexiletine exerts no major hemodynamic effects on ventricular contractile performance or peripheral resistance.

PHARMACOKINETICS

Mexiletine is rapidly and almost completely absorbed after oral ingestion by volunteers, with peak plasma concentrations being attained in 2 to 4 hours (see Table 64.4). Its elimination half-life is approximately 10 hours in healthy individuals but 17 hours in post-MI patients. Therapeutic plasma levels of 0.5 to 2 mcg/mL are maintained by oral doses of 200 to 300 mg every 6 to 8 hours. Absorption with less than a 10% first-pass hepatic effect occurs in the upper part of the small intestine and is delayed and incomplete in patients receiving narcotics or antacids. Approximately 70% of the drug is protein bound; the apparent volume of distribution is large because of extensive tissue uptake. Normally, mexiletine is eliminated metabolically by the liver, with less than 10% being excreted unchanged in urine. Doses should be reduced in patients with cirrhosis or left ventricular failure. Renal clearance of mexiletine decreases as urinary pH increases. Its known metabolites exert no electrophysiologic effects. Metabolism can be increased by phenytoin, phenobarbital, and rifampin and can be reduced by cimetidine.

DOSAGE AND ADMINISTRATION. The recommended starting dose is 200 mg orally every 8 hours when rapid arrhythmia control is not essential (see Table 64.4). Doses may be increased or decreased by 50 to 100 mg every 2 to 3 days and are better tolerated when given with food. The total daily dose should generally not exceed 1200 mg. In some patients, administration every 12 hours can be effective.

INDICATIONS. Mexiletine is a moderately effective antiarrhythmic agent for the treatment of acute and chronic ventricular tachyarrhythmias, but not SVTs. Success rates vary from 6% to 60% and can be increased in some patients if mexiletine is combined with other drugs such as procainamide, beta blockers, quinidine, disopyramide, propafenone, or amiodarone. Most studies show no clear superiority of mexiletine over other class I agents. Mexiletine may be very useful in children with congenital heart disease and serious ventricular arrhythmias. In treating patients with a long QT interval, mexiletine may be safer than drugs that increase the QT interval further, such as quinidine. Limited experience in treating subsets of patients with long-QT syndrome (LQT3, which is related to the *SCN5A* gene for the cardiac sodium channel) suggests a beneficial role (see Chapter 63). Mexiletine has also been used to treat myotonia in patients with neuromuscular diseases such as myotonic dystrophy. Involvement of the conduction system in these diseases can predispose these patients to advanced life-threatening heart rate slowing, mandating mexiletine be used with caution or backup pacing in this situation (Chapter 100).

ADVERSE EFFECTS. Up to 40% of patients may require a change in dose or discontinuation of mexiletine therapy as a result of adverse effects, including tremor, dysarthria, dizziness, paresthesia, diplopia, nystagmus, confusion, nausea, vomiting, and dyspepsia. Cardiovascular side effects are rare but include hypotension, bradycardia, and exacerbation of arrhythmia. The adverse effects of mexiletine appear to be dose related, and toxic effects can occur at plasma concentrations that are sub-therapeutic or only slightly higher than therapeutic levels. Therefore, its effective use requires careful titration of dose and monitoring for adverse effects and possibly plasma concentration. Lidocaine use as an AAD should be avoided in patients receiving mexiletine.

Phenytoin

Phenytoin was used originally to treat seizure disorders. Its value as an AAD is limited to rare cases of digitalis-toxic atrial and ventricular tachyarrhythmias (for which more rapid and effective control can be achieved with digitalis-specific antibodies) and occasional cases of ventricular arrhythmias when used in combination with other agents (see Tables 64.1, 64.2, 64.4 and eTables 64.1, 64.2).

Class IC Agents

Flecainide

Flecainide is approved by the FDA to treat patients with life-threatening ventricular arrhythmias, as well as various supraventricular arrhythmias.

ELECTROPHYSIOLOGIC ACTIONS

Flecainide exhibits marked use-dependent depressant effects on the rapid sodium channel by decreasing V_{max} and has slow onset and offset kinetics (see Tables 64.1, 64.2, and eTables 64.1, 64.2). Drug dissociation from the sodium channel is slow, with time constants of 10 to 30 seconds (versus 4 to 8 seconds for quinidine and <1 second for lidocaine). Thus, marked drug effects can occur at physiologic heart rates. Flecainide shortens the duration of the Purkinje fiber action potential but prolongs it in ventricular muscle, actions that, depending on the circumstances, could enhance or reduce electrical heterogeneity and create or suppress arrhythmias. Flecainide profoundly slows conduction in all cardiac fibers and, in high concentrations, inhibits the slow Ca^{2+} channel (see Chapter 62). Conduction time in the atria, ventricles, AV node, and His-Purkinje system is prolonged. Minimal increases in atrial or ventricular refractoriness or in the QT interval result. Anterograde and retrograde refractoriness in accessory pathways can increase significantly in a use-dependent manner. Sinus node function remains unchanged in normal individuals but may be depressed in patients with sinus node dysfunction. Flecainide can facilitate or inhibit reentry and may transform AF to flutter. Pacing and defibrillation thresholds are characteristically slightly to significantly increased.

HEMODYNAMIC EFFECTS

Flecainide depresses cardiac performance, particularly in patients with compromised ventricular systolic function, and should be used cautiously or not at all in those with moderate or severe ventricular systolic dysfunction.

PHARMACOKINETICS

Flecainide is at least 90% absorbed, with peak plasma concentrations achieved in 3 to 4 hours. Its elimination half-life in patients with ventricular arrhythmias is 20 hours, with 85% of the drug excreted unchanged or as an inactive metabolite in urine (see Table 64.4). Its two major metabolites have less potency than the parent drug. Elimination is slower in patients with renal disease and heart failure, and doses should be reduced in these situations. Therapeutic plasma concentrations range from 0.2 to 1.0 mcg/mL. Approximately 40% of the drug is protein bound. Increases in serum concentrations of digoxin (15% to 25%) and propranolol (30%) result during co-administration with flecainide. Propranolol, quinidine, and amiodarone may increase flecainide serum concentrations. Five to 7 days of dosing may be required to reach a steady-state concentration in some patients.

DOSAGE AND ADMINISTRATION. The starting dose is 100 mg every 12 hours, increased in increments of 50 mg twice daily, no sooner than every 3 to 4 days, until efficacy is achieved or an adverse effect is noted, or to a maximum of 400 mg/day (see Table 64.4). Cardiac rhythm and QRS duration should be monitored after changes in dose.

INDICATIONS. Flecainide is indicated for the treatment of life-threatening ventricular tachyarrhythmias, SVTs, and paroxysmal AF. Encouraging experimental and early clinical data support its use for catecholaminergic polymorphic VT (see Chapter 63). The dosage is adjusted to achieve the desired effect, but the serum concentration should not exceed 1.0 µg/mL. Flecainide is particularly effective in suppressing PVCs and short runs of non-sustained VT. As with other class I AADs, no data from controlled studies indicate that the drug favorably affects survival or sudden cardiac death, and data from CAST indicate increased mortality in patients with coronary artery disease (CAD). Flecainide produces a use-dependent prolongation of VT cycle length, which can improve hemodynamic tolerance. Flecainide is also useful for various SVTs, such as atrial tachycardia (AT), atrial flutter, and AF (including oral loading to terminate episodes acutely). Flecainide and propafenone may both be used in combination with beta or calcium channel blockers as a "pill in the pocket" approach to terminate AF as an outpatient (Table 64.4). When flecainide toxicity occurs, isoproterenol can reverse some of its electrophysiologic effects. It is important to slow the ventricular rate before treatment of AF with flecainide (e.g., with beta blockers or verapamil or diltiazem) to avoid the 1:1 AV conduction of slowed atrial flutter that may result from the effect of flecainide on fibrillation. Flecainide has been used to treat fetal arrhythmias and arrhythmias in children. Flecainide administration can produce ST elevation in lead V_1, characteristic of Brugada syndrome, in susceptible patients (see Chapter 63) and has been used as a diagnostic tool in persons suspected of having this disorder.

ADVERSE EFFECTS. Proarrhythmic effects are some of the most important adverse effects of flecainide. Its marked slowing of conduction precludes its use in patients with second-degree AV block without a pacemaker and warrants cautious administration in patients with intraventricular conduction disorders. Worsening of existing ventricular arrhythmias or the onset of new ventricular arrhythmias can occur in 5% to 30% of patients, especially in those with preexisting sustained VT, cardiac decompensation, and higher doses of the drug. Failure of the flecainide-related arrhythmia to respond to therapy, including electrical cardioversion-defibrillation, may result in mortality as high as 10% in patients in whom proarrhythmic events develop. Negative inotropic effects can precipitate or worsen heart failure episodes. Patients with sinus node dysfunction may experience sinus arrest, and an increase in the pacing and defibrillation thresholds may develop in those with pacemakers and ICDs, respectively. In CAST, patients treated with flecainide had higher mortality or nonfatal cardiac arrest compared to the placebo group, possibly related to an interaction between the drug and myocardial ischemia. Exercise can amplify the conduction slowing in the ventricle produced by flecainide and in some cases can precipitate a proarrhythmic response. Therefore, exercise testing has been recommended to screen for proarrhythmia (as well as occult ischemia) before and periodically during treatment. CNS complaints, including confusion and irritability, represent the most frequent noncardiac adverse effects. The safety of flecainide during pregnancy has not been determined, although as noted previously, it is occasionally used to treat fetal arrhythmias. It is concentrated in breast milk to a level 2.5- to 4-fold higher than in plasma. High doses of class IC agents can result in a markedly prolonged QRS duration, bundle branch block and wide and bizarre QRS morphologies during tachycardia.

Propafenone

Propafenone has been approved by the FDA for the treatment of patients with life-threatening ventricular tachyarrhythmias, as well as AF.

ELECTROPHYSIOLOGIC ACTIONS

Propafenone blocks the fast sodium current in a use-dependent manner in Purkinje fibers and to a lesser degree in ventricular muscle (see Tables 64.1, 64.2, and eTables 64.1, 64.2). Its use-dependent effects contribute to its ability to terminate AF. Its dissociation constant from the receptor is slow, similar to that of flecainide. Effects are greater in ischemic than in normal tissue and with reduced membrane potentials. Propafenone decreases excitability and suppresses spontaneous automaticity and triggered activity. The drug is a weak blocker of I_{Kr} and beta-adrenergic receptors. Although ventricular refractoriness increases, slowing of conduction is the major effect. Propafenone has several active metabolites that exert electrophysiologic effects. It depresses sinus node automaticity, and the A-H, H-V, PR, and QRS intervals increase, as do the refractory periods of all tissues. The QT interval increases only as a function of increased QRS duration.

HEMODYNAMIC EFFECTS

Propafenone and 5-hydroxypropafenone exhibit negative inotropic properties at high concentrations. In patients with left ventricular ejection fraction (EF) exceeding 40%, the negative inotropic effects are well tolerated, but patients with preexisting left ventricular dysfunction and congestive heart failure may exhibit worsening of their symptoms.

PHARMACOKINETICS

With more than 95% of the drug absorbed, the maximum plasma concentration of propafenone is achieved in 1 to 3 hours (see Table 64.4). Systemic bioavailability is dose dependent and ranges from 3% to 40% because of variable presystemic clearance. Bioavailability increases as the dose increases, and the plasma concentration is therefore not linearly related to dose. A threefold increase in dosage (300 to 900 mg/day) results in a 10-fold increase in plasma concentration, presumably because of saturation of hepatic metabolic mechanisms. Propafenone is 97% bound to alpha$_1$-acid glycoprotein, with an elimination half-life of 5 to 8 hours. Maximum therapeutic effects occur at serum concentrations of 0.2 to 1.5 µg/mL. The marked interpatient variability in pharmacokinetics and pharmacodynamics may be the result of genetically determined differences in metabolism (see Chapter 9). Approximately 7% of the white population are poor metabolizers and have an elimination half-life of 15 to 20 hours for the parent compound. The (+)-enantiomer provides nonspecific beta-adrenergic receptor blockade with 2.5% to 5% of the potency of propranolol, but because plasma propafenone concentrations may be 50 or more times higher than propranolol levels, these beta-blocking properties may be relevant. Poor metabolizers have a greater beta receptor–blocking effect than extensive metabolizers.

DOSAGE AND ADMINISTRATION

Most patients respond to oral propafenone doses of 150 to 300 mg every 8 hours, not to exceed 1200 mg/day (see Table 64.4). Doses are similar for patients of both metabolizing phenotypes. A sustained-release form is available for the treatment of AF; dosing is 225 to 425 mg twice daily. Concomitant food administration increases its bioavailability, as does hepatic dysfunction. No good correlation between the plasma propafenone concentration and suppression of arrhythmia has been shown. Doses should not be increased more often than every 3 to 4 days. Propafenone increases plasma concentrations of warfarin, digoxin, and metoprolol.

INDICATIONS. Propafenone is indicated for the treatment of paroxysmal SVT, AF, and life-threatening ventricular tachyarrhythmias, and effectively suppresses spontaneous PVCs and nonsustained and sustained VT. Acute termination of AF episodes occurred with a single 600-mg oral dose of propafenone in 76% of patients given the drug (twice the rate of those given placebo). It has been used effectively in the pediatric age group. Propafenone increases the pacing threshold but minimally affects the defibrillation threshold. The beta blocking effect contributes to a reduction in the sinus rate during exercise.

ADVERSE EFFECTS. Minor noncardiac effects occur in approximately 15% of patients, with dizziness, disturbances in taste, and blurred vision being the most common and GI side effects next. Exacerbation of bronchospastic lung disease can occur because of mild beta-blocking effects. Cardiovascular side effects develop in 10% to 15% of patients, including AV block, sinus node depression, and worsening of heart failure. Proarrhythmic responses, which occur more often in patients with a history of sustained VT and decreased EF, appear less often than with flecainide. Applicability of data from CAST about flecainide to propafenone is not clear but limiting the use of propafenone in a manner similar to that of other class IC drugs seems prudent; however, its beta-blocking actions may make it different. The safety of propafenone administration during pregnancy has not been established (class C).

Class II Agents
Beta Adrenoceptor–Blocking Agents
Although many beta adrenoceptor–blocking drugs have been approved for use in the United States, metoprolol, carvedilol, atenolol, propranolol, and esmolol have been most widely used to treat supraventricular and ventricular arrhythmias. Acebutolol, nadolol, timolol, betaxolol, pindolol, and bisoprolol have been used less extensively for the treatment of arrhythmias. Metoprolol, atenolol, carvedilol, timolol, and propranolol decrease overall mortality and sudden death after MI (see Chapter 70). It is generally thought that beta blockers possess class effects, and that when titrated to the proper dose, all can be used effectively to treat cardiac arrhythmias, hypertension, or other disorders. However, differences in pharmacokinetic or pharmacodynamic properties that confer safety, reduce adverse effects, or affect dosing intervals or drug interactions influence the choice of agent. For example, nadolol may be particularly effective in patients with long-QT syndrome (see Chapter 63). Also, some beta blockers, such as sotalol, pindolol, and carvedilol, exert unique actions in addition to beta receptor blockade.

Beta receptors can be separated into those that affect predominantly the heart (β_1) and those that affect predominantly blood vessels and the bronchi (β_2). In low doses, selective beta blockers can block β_1 receptors more than they block β_2 receptors and might be preferable for the treatment of patients with pulmonary or peripheral vascular disease. In high doses, the "selective" β_1 blockers also block β_2 receptors. Carvedilol also exerts alpha-blocking effects and is used primarily in patients with heart failure (see Chapters 49 and 50). It is a relatively poor agent for rate control in AF because of the alpha-blocking–induced hypotension that accompanies doses large enough to block the AV node adequately.

Some beta blockers exert intrinsic sympathomimetic activity; that is, they slightly activate the beta receptor. These drugs appear to be as efficacious as beta blockers without intrinsic sympathomimetic actions and may cause less slowing of the heart rate at rest and less prolongation of AV nodal conduction time. They have been shown to induce less depression of left ventricular function than do beta blockers without intrinsic sympathomimetic activity. Beta blockers without intrinsic sympathomimetic activity have been shown to reduce mortality in patients after MI, with nonselective agents possibly conferring slightly greater benefit (see Chapters 37 and 38).

The following discussion focuses on the use of propranolol as a prototypic antiarrhythmic agent but is generally applicable to other beta blockers.

ELECTROPHYSIOLOGIC ACTIONS
Beta blockers exert an electrophysiologic action by competitively inhibiting binding of catecholamines at beta adrenoceptor sites (see Tables 64.1, 64.2, and eTables 64.1, 64.2). Thus, beta blockers exert their major effects in cells most actively stimulated by adrenergic actions. At a beta-blocking concentration, propranolol slows spontaneous automaticity in the sinus node or in Purkinje fibers that are being stimulated by adrenergic tone and produces an I_f block (see Chapter 62). Beta blockers also block the $I_{Ca,L}$ stimulated by beta agonists. In the absence of adrenergic stimulation, only high concentrations of propranolol slow normal automaticity in Purkinje fibers, probably by a direct membrane (ion channel blocking) action.

Concentrations that cause beta receptor blockade, but no local anesthetic effects, do not alter the normal resting membrane potential, maximum diastolic potential amplitude, V_{max}, repolarization, or refractoriness of atrial, Purkinje, or ventricular muscle cells in the absence of catecholamine stimulation. However, in the presence of isoproterenol, a relatively pure beta receptor stimulator, beta blockers reverse isoproterenol's accelerating effects on repolarization. Propranolol reduces

the amplitude of digitalis-induced DADs and suppresses triggered activity in Purkinje fibers.

Propranolol slows the sinus discharge rate in humans by 10% to 20%, although severe bradycardia occasionally results if the heart is particularly dependent on sympathetic tone or if sinus node dysfunction is present. The PR interval lengthens, as do AV nodal conduction time and AV nodal effective and functional refractory periods (at a constant heart rate), but refractoriness and conduction in the normal His-Purkinje system remain unchanged, even after high doses of propranolol. Beta blockers do not affect conduction or repolarization in normal ventricular muscle, as evidenced by their lack of effect on the QRS complex and QT interval, respectively.

Because administration of beta blockers that do not have direct membrane action prevents many arrhythmias resulting from activation of the autonomic nervous system, it is thought that the beta-blocking action is responsible for their antiarrhythmic effects. Nevertheless, the possible importance of the direct membrane effect of some of these drugs cannot be discounted totally, because beta blockers with direct membrane actions can affect the transmembrane potentials of diseased cardiac fibers at much lower concentrations than are needed to affect normal fibers directly. However, indirect actions on the arrhythmogenic effects of ischemia are probably the most important.

HEMODYNAMIC EFFECTS
Beta blockers exert negative inotropic effects and can precipitate or worsen heart failure. However, beta blockers clearly improve survival in patients with heart failure (see Chapter 50). By blocking β receptors, these drugs may allow unopposed alpha-adrenergic effects to produce peripheral vasoconstriction and exacerbate coronary artery spasm or pain from peripheral vascular disease in some patients.

Pharmacokinetics
Although various types of beta blockers exert similar pharmacologic effects, their pharmacokinetics differ substantially. Propranolol is almost 100% absorbed, but the effects of first-pass hepatic metabolism reduce its bioavailability to approximately 30% and produce significant interpatient variability in plasma concentration with a given dose (see Table 64.4). Reduced hepatic blood flow, as in patients with heart failure, decreases the hepatic extraction of propranolol; in these patients, propranolol may further decrease its own elimination rate by reducing cardiac output and hepatic blood flow. Beta blockers eliminated by the kidneys tend to have longer half-lives and exhibit less interpatient variability in drug concentration than do beta blockers metabolized by the liver.

DOSAGE AND ADMINISTRATION. The appropriate dose of propranolol is best determined by a measure of the patient's physiologic response, such as changes in resting heart rate or prevention of exercise-induced sinus tachycardia, because wide individual differences exist between the observed physiologic effect and plasma concentration. For example, IV dosing is best achieved by titration of the dose to clinical effect, beginning with doses of 0.25 to 0.50 mg, increasing to 1.0 mg if necessary, and administering doses every 5 minutes until either a desired effect or toxicity is produced or a total of 0.15 to 0.20 mg/kg has been given. In many cases, the short-acting effects of esmolol are preferred. Orally, propranolol is given in four divided doses, usually ranging from 40 to 160 mg/day up to no more than 640 mg/day (see Table 64.4). Some beta blockers, such as carvedilol and pindolol, need to be given twice daily; many are also available as once-daily long-acting preparations. In general, if one agent in adequate doses does not produce the desired effect, other beta blockers will also be ineffective. Conversely, if one agent produces the desired physiologic effect but a side effect develops, another beta blocker can often be substituted successfully.

INDICATIONS. Arrhythmias associated with thyrotoxicosis or pheochromocytoma and arrhythmias largely related to excessive cardiac adrenergic stimulation, such as those initiated by exercise or emotion, often respond to beta-blocker therapy. Beta-blocking drugs do not usually convert chronic atrial flutter or AF to normal sinus rhythm but may do so if the arrhythmia is of recent onset and in patients who have recently undergone cardiac surgery. The atrial rate during atrial flutter or fibrillation is not changed, but the ventricular response decreases because beta blockade prolongs AV nodal conduction time and refractoriness. Esmolol can be used intravenously for rapid control of the heart rate. For reentrant SVTs using the AV node as one of the reentrant pathways, such as AV nodal reentrant tachycardia (AVNRT) and orthodromic reciprocating tachycardia in WPW syndrome or inappropriate sinus tachycardia, or for AT, beta blockers can slow or terminate the tachycardia and can be used prophylactically to prevent a recurrence (see Chapters 65 and 66). Combining beta blockers with digitalis, quinidine, or various other agents can be effective when the beta blocker as a single agent fails.

Beta blockers can be effective for digitalis-induced arrhythmias such as AT, nonparoxysmal AV junctional tachycardia, PVCs, or VT. If a significant degree of AV block is present during digitalis-induced arrhythmia, lidocaine or phenytoin may be preferable to propranolol. Beta blockers can also be useful to treat ventricular arrhythmias associated with prolonged–QT interval syndrome (see Chapter 63) and with mitral valve prolapse (see Chapter 76). For patients with ischemic heart disease, beta blockers do not generally prevent the episodes of recurrent monomorphic VT that occur in the absence of acute ischemia. It is well accepted that several beta blockers reduce the incidence of both total and sudden death after MI (see Chapters 37 and 38). The mechanism of this reduction in mortality is not entirely clear and may be related to reduction of the extent of ischemic damage, autonomic effects, a direct antiarrhythmic effect, or combinations of these factors. Beta blockers may have been protective against proarrhythmic responses in CAST.

ADVERSE EFFECTS. Adverse cardiovascular effects from beta blockers include unacceptable hypotension, bradycardia, and congestive heart failure. The bradycardia can be caused by sinus slowing or AV block. Sudden withdrawal of propranolol in patients with angina pectoris can precipitate or worsen angina and cardiac arrhythmias and cause acute MI, possibly as a result of the heightened sensitivity to beta agonists caused by previous beta blockade (receptor upregulation). Heightened sensitivity may begin several days after cessation of beta-blocker therapy and can last 5 or 6 days. Other adverse effects of beta blockers include worsening of asthma or chronic obstructive pulmonary disease, intermittent claudication, Raynaud phenomenon, mental depression, increased risk for hypoglycemia in insulin-dependent diabetic patients, easy fatigability, disturbingly vivid dreams or insomnia, and impaired sexual function. Many of these side effects were noted less frequently with the use of β_1-selective agents, but even so-called cardioselective beta blockers can exacerbate asthma or diabetic control in individual patients.

Class III Agents
Amiodarone
Amiodarone is an iodinated benzofuran derivative approved by the FDA for the treatment of patients with life-threatening ventricular tachyarrhythmias when other drugs are ineffective or not tolerated.

ELECTROPHYSIOLOGIC ACTIONS
With long-term oral administration, amiodarone prolongs the APD and refractoriness of all cardiac fibers without affecting resting membrane potential (see Tables 64.1, 64.2, and eTables 64.1, 64.2 and Chapter 62). When acute effects are evaluated, amiodarone and its metabolite desethylamiodarone prolong the APD of ventricular muscle but shorten the APD of Purkinje fibers. It depresses V_{max} in ventricular muscle in a rate- or use-dependent manner by blocking inactivated sodium channels, an effect that is accentuated by depolarized and reduced by hyperpolarized membrane potentials. Amiodarone depresses conduction at fast rates more than at slow rates (use dependence). It does not prolong repolarization more at slow than at fast rates (i.e., does not demonstrate reverse use dependence) but does exert time-dependent effects on refractoriness, which may in part explain its high antiarrhythmic efficacy and low incidence of TdP.

Desethylamiodarone has relatively greater effects on fast-channel tissue, which probably contributes to its antiarrhythmic efficacy. The delay in building up adequate concentrations of this metabolite may in part explain the delay in amiodarone's antiarrhythmic action.

Amiodarone noncompetitively antagonizes alpha and beta receptors and blocks conversion of thyroxine (T_4) to triiodothyronine (T_3), which may account for some of its electrophysiologic effects. Amiodarone exhibits slow channel–blocking effects; with oral administration, it slows the sinus rate by 20% to 30% and prolongs the QT interval, at times changing the contour of the T wave and producing U waves.

The ERP of all cardiac tissues is prolonged. The H-V interval increases, and the QRS duration lengthens, especially at fast rates. Amiodarone given intravenously modestly prolongs the refractory period of atrial and ventricular muscle. The PR interval and AV nodal conduction time lengthen. The duration of the QRS complex lengthens at increased rates but less than after oral amiodarone. Thus the increase in prolongation of conduction time (except for AV node), duration of repolarization, and refractoriness is much less with IV administration than after the oral route. Considering these actions, it is clear that amiodarone has class I (blocks I_{Na}), class II (antiadrenergic), and class IV (blocks $I_{Ca,L}$) actions in addition to its class III effects (blocks I_K). Amiodarone's actions approximate those of a theoretically ideal drug that exhibits use-dependent Na$^+$ channel blockade with fast diastolic recovery from block and use-dependent prolongation of the APD. It does not increase and may decrease QT dispersion. Catecholamines can partially reverse some of the effects of amiodarone.

HEMODYNAMIC EFFECTS
Amiodarone is a peripheral and coronary vasodilator. When administered intravenously (150 mg over 10 minutes, then a 1-mg/min infusion), amiodarone decreases the heart rate, systemic vascular resistance, and left ventricular dP/dt. Oral doses of amiodarone sufficient to control cardiac arrhythmias do not depress the left ventricular EF, even in patients with reduced EF. However, because of the antiadrenergic actions of amiodarone, it should be given cautiously, particularly intravenously, to patients with marginal cardiac compensation.

PHARMACOKINETICS
Amiodarone is slowly, variably, and incompletely absorbed, with a systemic bioavailability of 25% to 65% (see Table 64.4). Plasma concentrations peak 3 to 6 hours after a single oral dose. There is a minimal first-pass effect, indicating minimal hepatic extraction. Elimination is by hepatic excretion into bile with some enterohepatic recirculation. Extensive hepatic metabolism occurs, with desethylamiodarone being a major metabolite. Both accumulate extensively in the liver, lung, fat, "blue" skin, and other tissues. The concentration in myocardium is 10 to 50 times that found in plasma. Plasma clearance of amiodarone is low, and renal excretion is negligible. Doses do not need to be reduced in patients with renal disease. Amiodarone and desethylamiodarone are not dialyzable. The volume of distribution is large but variable, with an average of 60 L/kg. Amiodarone is highly protein bound (96%), crosses the placenta (10% to 50%), and is found in breast milk.

The onset of action after IV administration generally occurs within 1 to 2 hours. After oral administration, the onset of action may require 2 to 3 days, often 1 to 3 weeks, and on occasion even longer. Loading doses reduce this time interval. Plasma concentrations relate well to oral doses during chronic treatment and average approximately 0.5 mg/L (0.5 µg/mL) for each 100 mg/day at doses between 100 and 600 mg/day. Amiodarone's elimination half-life is multiphasic, with an initial 50% reduction in plasma concentration 3 to 10 days after cessation of drug ingestion (probably representing elimination from well-perfused tissues), followed by a terminal half-life of 26 to 107 days (mean, 53 days), with most patients in the 40- to 55-day range. To achieve a steady-state concentration without a loading dose takes about 265 days. Interpatient variability in these pharmacokinetic parameters mandates close monitoring of the patient. Therapeutic serum concentrations range from 0.5 to 1.5 µg/mL. Greater suppression of arrhythmias may occur with up to 3.5 µg/mL, but the risk for side effects increases.

DOSAGE AND ADMINISTRATION. There is no standard dosing schedule for amiodarone applicable to all patients. One recommended approach is to treat with 800 to 1200 mg/day for 1 to 3 weeks, 400 to 800 mg/day for 1 to 2 weeks, and finally after 2 to 3 months of treatment, a maintenance dose of 200 mg per day (see Table 64.4). Maintenance drug can be given once or twice daily and should be titrated to the lowest effective dose to minimize the occurrence of side effects; in general, the earlier during drug loading that arrhythmia control is achieved, the lower the maintenance dose can be. Doses as low as 100 mg every other day can be effective in some patients. Regimens must be individualized for a given patient and clinical situation. To achieve more rapid loading and effect in emergencies, amiodarone can be administered intravenously at initial doses of 15 mg/min for 10 minutes, followed by 1 mg/min for 6 hours and then 0.5 mg/min for the remaining 18 hours and the next several days as necessary. Supplemental infusions of 150 mg over a 10-minute period can be used for breakthrough VT or VF. Intravenous infusions can be continued safely for 2 to 3 weeks. IV amiodarone is generally well tolerated, even in patients with left ventricular dysfunction. Patients with depressed EF should receive IV amiodarone with great caution because of hypotension. High-dose oral loading (800 to 2000 mg/day to maintain trough serum concentrations of 2 to 3 μg/mL) may suppress ventricular arrhythmias in 5 to 7 days.

INDICATIONS. Amiodarone has been used to suppress a wide spectrum of supraventricular and ventricular tachyarrhythmias in utero, in adults, and in children, including AV node and AV reentry, junctional tachycardia, atrial flutter and fibrillation, VT and VF associated with CAD, and hypertrophic cardiomyopathy. Success rates vary widely, depending on the population of patients, arrhythmia, underlying heart disease, length of follow-up, definition and determination of success, and other factors. In general, however, the efficacy of amiodarone equals or exceeds that of all other AADs and may be in the range of 60% to 80% for most supraventricular tachyarrhythmias and 40% to 60% for ventricular tachyarrhythmias. IV amiodarone is recommended in the 2015 ACLS algorithm for treatment of a shockable rhythm during the cardiac arrest VF/pulseless VT/cardiac arrest asystole/pulseless electrical activity (PEA) algorithm. Amiodarone may be useful in improving outcomes in patients with ventricular tachyarrhythmia during and after resuscitation from cardiac arrest. Amiodarone given before open heart surgery, as well as postoperatively, has been shown to decrease the incidence of postoperative AF. Amiodarone is superior to class I AADs and sotalol in maintaining sinus rhythm in patients with recurrent AF.

Patients who have an ICD receive fewer shocks if they are treated with amiodarone than if treated with conventional drugs. Amiodarone has little effect on the pacing threshold but typically increases the electrical defibrillation threshold modestly and slows the rate of VT (sometimes below the ICD's detection rate).

Several prospective, randomized controlled trials and meta-analyses have demonstrated improved survival with amiodarone therapy versus placebo. However, amiodarone has been shown to result in inferior survival compared with ICD therapy, and in the SCD-HeFT population (New York Heart Association [NYHA] class II or III heart failure; EF, 35%), survival of amiodarone-treated patients was no different than for the placebo group. The drug may still be used adjunctively in ICD-treated patients to decrease the frequency of shocks from VT and VF episodes or to control supraventricular tachyarrhythmias that elicit device therapy (see Chapter 65). As noted, the drug can slow the ventricular rate during spontaneous VT episodes beneath the detection rate of the device; careful patient assessment and, occasionally, device reprogramming and testing are necessary. It also can be used to slow the ventricular rate during AF and atrial flutter.

Because of the serious nature of the arrhythmias being treated, the unusual pharmacokinetics of the drug, and its adverse effects, consideration should be given to starting amiodarone therapy with the patient hospitalized and monitored for at least several days. Combining other AADs with amiodarone may improve efficacy in some patients.

ADVERSE EFFECTS. Adverse effects are reported by about 75% of patients treated with amiodarone for 5 years, and these effects compel stopping the drug in 18% to 37%. The most frequent side effects requiring drug discontinuation involve pulmonary and GI complaints or abnormal test results. Most adverse effects are reversible with dose reduction or cessation of treatment. Adverse effects are more common when therapy is continued in the long term and at higher doses. Of the non-cardiac adverse reactions, pulmonary toxicity is the most serious[10]; in one study, it occurred in 33 of 573 patients between 6 days and 60 months of treatment, with three deaths. The mechanism is unclear but may involve a hypersensitivity reaction, widespread phospholipidosis, or both. Dyspnea and nonproductive cough are the most common symptoms, along with fine crackles on examination, hypoxia, abnormal gallium scan results, reduced carbon monoxide diffusion capacity (D_{LCO}), and radiographic evidence of pulmonary infiltrates. Amiodarone must be immediately discontinued if such pulmonary changes occur. Corticosteroids can be tried, but no controlled studies have been done to support their use. Up to 10% mortality results in patients with pulmonary inflammatory changes, often in those with unrecognized pulmonary involvement that is attributed to other

causes and is thus allowed to progress. Chest radiography and pulmonary function testing, including D_{LCO}, is recommended at baseline and then yearly chest radiographs are recommended. At maintenance doses lower than 200 mg/day, pulmonary toxicity is uncommon but can still occur. Advanced age, high maintenance doses, and reduced predrug D_{LCO} are risk factors for the development of pulmonary toxicity. An unchanged D_{LCO} on therapy may be a negative predictor of pulmonary toxicity.

Although asymptomatic elevations in liver enzyme levels are found in most patients, amiodarone is not stopped unless values exceed two or three times the upper limit of normal in a patient with initially normal values. Cirrhosis occurs infrequently but may be fatal.[11] Neurologic dysfunction, photosensitivity (perhaps minimized by sunscreens), bluish skin discoloration, GI disturbances, and hyperthyroidism (1% to 2%) or hypothyroidism (2% to 4%) can occur. Because amiodarone appears to inhibit the peripheral conversion of T_4 to T_3, chemical changes result and are characterized by a slight increase in T_4, reverse T_3, and thyroid-stimulating hormone (TSH) and a slight decrease in T_3 levels. The reverse T_3 concentration has been used as an index of drug effect. During hypothyroidism the TSH level increases greatly, whereas the level of T_3 increases in hyperthyroidism. Thyroid function tests should be performed approximately every 3 months for the first year while amiodarone is being taken and once or twice yearly thereafter, or sooner if symptoms develop that are consistent with thyroid dysfunction. Corneal microdeposits occur in almost 100% of adults receiving the drug longer than 6 months. More serious ocular reactions, including optic neuritis and atrophy with visual loss, have been reported but are rare, and causation by amiodarone has not been firmly established.[12] Among the most common side effects limiting long-term drug use are neurologic, and these side effects are both dose and duration related as well as idiosyncratic. Lowering the dose of amiodarone frequently decreases the severity of the side effect. A wide variety of neurologic toxicities have been described including tremor, ataxia, peripheral neuropathy, and rarely myopathy and encephalopathy. Some general guidelines for monitoring outpatients taking amiodarone are seen in Table 64.5.

Cardiac side effects include symptomatic bradycardias in approximately 2% of patients; and the rare development of TdP in 1% to 2%. Despite QT prolongation, amiodarone causes TdP rarely presumably due to the inhibition of multiple K channels and L-type Ca channels.

In general, the lowest possible maintenance dose of amiodarone that is still effective should be used to avoid significant adverse effects. Many supraventricular arrhythmias can be managed successfully with daily dosages of 200 mg or less, whereas ventricular arrhythmias generally require higher doses. Adverse effects are less common at dosages of 200 mg/day or less but can still occur. Monitoring of patients on this agent at any dose is critical.[13]

TABLE 64.5 Recommended Follow-up for Amiodarone

ECG at routine clinic follow ups, and at least every 12 months
Liver function tests at baseline and every 6 months or if patient presents with clinical features of liver disease
Thyroid function test (thyroid stimulating hormone) at baseline and every 4–6 months or if patient presents with clinical features suggestive of thyroid disease
Chest radiography at baseline and every year or for new and changing symptoms
Pulmonary function tests at baseline (including D_{LCO}) and if symptoms develop, especially in patients with underlying lung disease or abnormalities on chest radiography
Skin examination at routine follow-up every 6–12 months
Neurologic examination at routine follow-up. Note side effects are dose- and duration-related. Reduced dose should ameliorate symptoms.
Ophthalmologic examination at baseline if there is visual impairment and yearly or for any change in vision
Be aware of numerous drug interactions and drugs contraindicated with concomitant use of amiodarone, especially drugs that prolong QT interval or interact with amiodarone metabolism

Important interactions with other drugs occur, and when given concomitantly with amiodarone, the doses of warfarin, digoxin, and other AADs should be reduced by one third to one half and the patient observed closely. Drugs with synergistic actions, such as beta blockers or calcium channel blockers, must be given cautiously. The safety of amiodarone during pregnancy is controversial but categorized currently as class D. It should be used in pregnant patients only if no alternatives exist but should be avoided during breastfeeding.

Dronedarone

Dronedarone is approved by the FDA to facilitate maintenance of sinus rhythm in patients with atrial flutter and AF.

ELECTROPHYSIOLOGIC ACTIONS

As with amiodarone, dronedarone alters the activity of multiple cardiac ion channels (see Tables 64.1, 64.2, and eTables 64.1, 64.2). It is a more potent blocker of I_{Na} than amiodarone and exhibits similar effects on the L-type calcium current. Blockade of both I_{Kr} and I_{Ks} by dronedarone is also similar to that by amiodarone, whereas its effect on atrial $I_{K.Ach}$ and antiadrenergic effects (via noncompetitive binding) are significantly more potent than for amiodarone. Sinus node function is depressed to a minor degree. Pacing and defibrillation thresholds are slightly increased.

HEMODYNAMIC EFFECTS

Dronedarone has minimal effect on cardiac performance except in patients with compromised ventricular systolic function and should not be used in those with clinical signs of heart failure.

PHARMACOKINETICS

Dronedarone is 70% to 90% absorbed after oral administration, with peak plasma concentrations achieved in 3 to 4 hours; absorption is enhanced by food (see Table 64.4). Unlike the very long half-life of amiodarone, the elimination half-life of dronedarone is 13 to 19 hours, with 85% of the drug being excreted unchanged in feces and the remainder in urine. Dronedarone is metabolized by and slightly inhibits the activity of CYP3A4 (as well as CYP2D6) and should not be used in conjunction with other agents that strongly inhibit these enzyme systems. There is minimal warfarin interaction, but dronedarone increases serum levels of dabigatran.

DOSAGE AND ADMINISTRATION. The standard recommended dose of dronedarone is 400 mg every 12 hours with food (see Table 64.4). No parenteral form is currently available.

INDICATIONS. Dronedarone is indicated to facilitate cardioversion of atrial flutter or AF or to maintain sinus rhythm after restoration of sinus rhythm. It is slightly less effective than amiodarone and type IC drugs in this regard.[14] In the ANDROMEDA (Antiarrhythmic Trial with Dronedarone in Moderate-to-Severe Congestive Heart Failure Evaluating Morbidity Decrease) study, dronedarone-treated patients had a mortality rate more than twice that of the placebo group (8.1% vs. 3.8%). Similarly, in the PALLAS (Permanent Atrial Fibrillation Outcome Study Using Dronedarone on Top of Standard Therapy) trial, patients with permanent AF who were taking dronedarone had a greater than twofold higher risk for death, stroke, systemic embolism, or MI than did control patients. Thus, the medication should not be used in patients with current or recent episodes of clinical heart failure or those with permanent AF (as a rate control agent). Patients taking dronedarone should be evaluated periodically to ensure that permanent AF or heart failure has not developed.[15]

ADVERSE EFFECTS. A transient, predictable increase in serum creatinine, without adversely affecting actual glomerular filtration or other measures of renal function, occurs with standard dosing and is not a reason to alter the dose or to discontinue use of dronedarone. As noted, patients with NYHA class III or IV heart failure, as well as those with permanent AF, should not be given the drug because these patients have higher mortality. Patients with severe liver dysfunction should not generally receive dronedarone. The QT interval is predictably prolonged, but proarrhythmic effects from this or other mechanisms are rare (although sinus bradycardia is sometimes seen). Rash, photosensitivity, nausea, diarrhea, dyspepsia, headache, and asthenia have occurred in treated patients at higher frequency than in controls.

Absence of the iodine appears to account for the lower prevalence of lung and thyroid toxicity in dronedarone-treated patients than in those taking amiodarone. Dronedarone should not be used during pregnancy (category X, evidence or risk of fetal harm) and is possibly unsafe during breastfeeding.

Sotalol

Sotalol is a nonspecific beta adrenoceptor blocker without intrinsic sympathomimetic activity that prolongs repolarization. It is approved by the FDA to treat patients with life-threatening ventricular tachyarrhythmias and those with AF.[16]

ELECTROPHYSIOLOGIC ACTIONS

Both the d- and l-isomers have similar effects on prolonging repolarization, whereas the l-isomer is responsible for almost all the beta-blocking activity (see Tables 64.1, 64.2, and eTables 64.1, 64.2). Sotalol does not block alpha adrenoceptors and does not block I_{Na} (no membrane-stabilizing effects) but does prolong atrial and ventricular repolarization times by reducing I_{Kr}, thus prolonging the plateau of the action potential. Action potential prolongation is greater at slower rates (reverse use dependence). Resting membrane potential, action potential amplitude, and $\dot{V}_{max}$ are not significantly altered. Sotalol prolongs atrial and ventricular refractoriness, A-H and QT intervals, and sinus cycle length (see Chapter 65).

HEMODYNAMICS

Sotalol exerts a negative inotropic effect only through its beta-blocking action. Although it can slightly increase the strength of contraction by prolonging repolarization, which occurs maximally at slow heart rates, the negative inotropic effects predominate. In patients with reduced cardiac function, sotalol can decrease the cardiac index, increase filling pressure, and precipitate overt heart failure. Therefore, it must be used cautiously in patients with marginal cardiac compensation but is well tolerated in those with normal cardiac function.

PHARMACOKINETICS

Sotalol is completely absorbed and not metabolized, thus making it 90% to 100% bioavailable. It is not bound to plasma proteins, is excreted unchanged primarily by the kidneys, and has an elimination half-life of 10 to 15 hours (see Table 64.4). Peak plasma concentrations occur 2.5 to 4 hours after oral ingestion. Over the dose range of 160 to 640 mg, sotalol displays dose proportionality with plasma concentration (usually in the range of 2.5 μg/mL). The dose must be reduced in patients with renal disease. The beta-blocking effect is half-maximal at 80 mg/day and maximal at 320 mg/day.

DOSAGE. The typical oral dose is 80 to 160 mg every 12 hours, with 2 to 3 days between dose adjustments to attain a steady-state concentration and to monitor the ECG for arrhythmias and QT prolongation (see Table 64.4). Doses exceeding 320 mg/day can be used in patients when the potential benefits outweigh the risk for proarrhythmia. Because of its ability to prolong significantly the QT interval in some patients and cause TdP or provoke severe bradycardia, consideration should be given to inpatient initiation of the drug, especially in those with AF (in whom conversion to sinus bradycardia may cause syncope and/or further QT prolongation at slow rates, as well as in women (with longer baseline QT intervals). Intravenous sotalol has been approved for use in the United States; loading doses of 60 to 112.5 mg (depending on creatinine clearance) can be given over 1 hour, monitoring the QTc interval.

INDICATIONS. Approved by the FDA to treat patients with ventricular tachyarrhythmias and AF, sotalol is also useful to prevent recurrence of a wide variety of SVTs, including atrial flutter, AT, AV node reentry, and AV reentry (see Chapter 65). It slows the ventricular response to atrial tachyarrhythmias, but rarely causes conversion to sinus rhythm. Sotalol appears to be more effective than conventional AADs and may be comparable to amiodarone in the treatment of patients with ventricular tachyarrhythmias, as well as in prevention of recurrences of AF after cardioversion. Sotalol has been used successfully to decrease the incidence of AF after cardiac surgery. It may be effective in fetal and pediatric patients and young adults with congenital heart disease. Unlike most other AADs, sotalol may decrease the frequency of ICD discharges and reduce the defibrillation threshold but typically does not slow VT rates.

ADVERSE EFFECTS. Proarrhythmia is the most serious adverse effect. Overall, new or worsened ventricular tachyarrhythmias occur in approximately 4% of patients taking sotalol; this response is the result of TdP in approximately 2.5% but increases to 4% in patients with a history of sustained VT and is dose related (only 1.6% at 320 mg/day but 4.4% at 480 mg/day). This proarrhythmic effect was probably the cause of excess mortality in patients given *d*-sotalol (the enantiomer lacking a beta-blocking effect) after acute MI in the SWORD (Survival With Oral *d*-Sotalol) trial. Other adverse effects typically seen with other beta blockers also apply to sotalol. Sotalol should be used with caution or not at all in combination with other drugs that prolong the QT interval. However, such combinations have occasionally been used successfully.

Ibutilide

Ibutilide is an agent released for acute termination of episodes of atrial flutter and AF (see Chapter 66). Ibutilide also blocks accessory pathway conduction.

ELECTROPHYSIOLOGIC ACTIONS

As with other class III agents, ibutilide prolongs repolarization (see Tables 64.1, 64.2, and eTables 64.1, 64.2). Although similar to other class III agents that block outward potassium currents, such as I_{Kr}, ibutilide is unique in that it also activates a slow inward sodium current. IV ibutilide has minimal effects on AV conduction or QRS duration, but the QT interval is characteristically prolonged. Ibutilide has no significant effect on hemodynamics.

PHARMACOKINETICS

Ibutilide is administered intravenously and has a large volume of distribution (see Table 64.4). Clearance is predominantly renal, with a drug half-life averaging 6 hours, but with considerable interpatient variability. Protein binding is approximately 40%. One of the drug's metabolites has weak class III effects.

DOSAGE AND ADMINISTRATION. Ibutilide is given as an IV infusion of 1 mg over 10 minutes (see Table 64.4). It should not be given in the presence of a QTc interval longer than 440 milliseconds or other drugs that prolong the QT interval or in patients with uncorrected hypokalemia, hypomagnesemia, or bradycardia. A second 1-mg dose may be given after the first dose is finished if the arrhythmia persists. Patients must have continuous electrocardiographic monitoring throughout the dosing period and for up to 4 hours thereafter because of the risk for ventricular arrhythmias. Pretreatment with IV magnesium may decrease the risk for ventricular arrhythmias and enhance efficacy in treating some atrial arrhythmias. Up to 60% of patients with AF and 70% of those with atrial flutter convert to sinus rhythm after 2 mg of ibutilide has been administered.[17]

INDICATIONS. Ibutilide is indicated for termination of an established episode of atrial flutter or AF. It should not be used in patients with frequent short paroxysms of AF because it merely terminates episodes and is not useful for long-term prevention. Patients whose condition is hemodynamically unstable should proceed to direct-current (DC) cardioversion. Ibutilide has been used safely and effectively in patients who were already taking amiodarone or propafenone, but should be used with caution in these patients. Ibutilide has been administered at transthoracic electrical cardioversion to increase the likelihood of termination of AF. In one study, all 50 patients given ibutilide before attempted electrical cardioversion achieved sinus rhythm, whereas only 34 of 50 who did not receive the drug converted to sinus rhythm. Of note, all 16 patients who did not respond to electrical cardioversion without ibutilide were successfully electrically cardioverted to sinus rhythm when a second attempt was made after ibutilide pretreatment.

Ibutilide prolongs accessory pathway refractoriness and can temporarily slow the ventricular rate during preexcited AF. The drug can rarely terminate episodes of organized AT, as well as sustained, uniform-morphology VT.

ADVERSE EFFECTS. The most significant adverse effect of ibutilide is QT prolongation–related TdP, which occurs in approximately 2% of patients given the drug (twice as often in women as in men). This effect develops within the first 4 hours of dosing or until the QTc has returned to baseline, after which the risk is negligible. Thus, patients must undergo electrocardiographic monitoring for up to 4 hours after dosing (or longer, until QTc returns to baseline). This requirement makes using ibutilide in emergency departments or private offices problematic. The safety of ibutilide during pregnancy has not been well studied, and its use in pregnant women should be restricted to those in whom no safer alternative exists.

Dofetilide

Dofetilide is approved for the acute conversion of AF to sinus rhythm, as well as for chronic suppression of recurrent AF.

ELECTROPHYSIOLOGIC ACTIONS

The sole electrophysiologic effect of dofetilide is block of the rapid component of the delayed rectifier potassium current (I_{Kr}), important in repolarization (see Tables 64.1, 64.2, and eTables 64.1, 64.2). This effect is more prominent in the atria than in the ventricles—30% increase in the atrial refractory period versus 20% in the ventricle. The effect of dofetilide on I_{Kr} is prolongation of refractoriness without slowing conduction, which is believed to be largely responsible for its antiarrhythmic effect. It is also responsible for prolongation of the QT interval on the ECG, which averages 11% but can be much greater. This effect on the QT interval is dose dependent and linear. No other important electrocardiographic changes are observed with the drug. It has no significant hemodynamic effects. Dofetilide is more effective than quinidine at converting AF to sinus rhythm. Its long-term efficacy is similar to that of other agents.[18]

PHARMACOKINETICS

Oral dofetilide is absorbed well, and more than 90% is bioavailable. Its mean elimination half-life is 7 to 13 hours, with 50% to 60% excreted unchanged in urine (see Table 64.4). The remainder of the drug undergoes hepatic metabolism to inert compounds. Significant drug-drug interactions have been reported in patients taking dofetilide; cimetidine, verapamil, ketoconazole, and trimethoprim, alone or in combination with sulfamethoxazole, cause a significant elevation in the dofetilide serum concentration and should not be used with this drug.

DOSAGE AND ADMINISTRATION. Dofetilide is available only as an oral preparation. Dosing is from 0.125 to 0.5 mg twice daily and must be initiated in a hospital setting with continuous electrocardiographic monitoring to ensure that excessive QT prolongation and TdP do not develop (see Table 64.4). Physicians must be specially certified to prescribe the drug. Its dosage must be decreased in the presence of impaired renal function or an increase in the QT interval of more than 15%, or 500 milliseconds. Dofetilide should not be given to patients with a creatinine clearance lower than 20 mL/min or a baseline QTc interval longer than 440 milliseconds.

INDICATIONS. Oral dofetilide is indicated for prevention of episodes of supraventricular tachyarrhythmias, particularly atrial flutter and fibrillation. The role of dofetilide in the treatment of ventricular arrhythmias is less clear; it has been shown to decrease the defibrillation threshold in patients with an ICD, as well as to decrease the frequency of ICD therapies for ventricular arrhythmias.

ADVERSE EFFECTS. The most significant adverse effect of dofetilide is QT interval prolongation–related TdP, which occurs in 2% to 4% of patients. Risk is highest in patients with a baseline prolonged QT interval, in those who are hypokalemic, in those taking some other agent that prolongs repolarization, and after conversion from AF to sinus rhythm. Because the risk for TdP is highest at drug initiation, it should be used continuously and not as intermittent outpatient dosing. The drug is otherwise well tolerated, with few side effects. Its use in pregnancy has not been studied extensively, and it should probably be avoided in pregnant women if possible.

Class IV Agents
Calcium Channel Antagonists: Verapamil and Diltiazem

Verapamil, a synthetic papaverine derivative, is the prototype of a class of drugs that block the slow calcium channel and reduce $I_{Ca,L}$ in cardiac muscle (see Chapter 46). Diltiazem has electrophysiologic actions similar to those of verapamil. Nifedipine and other dihydropyridine agents exhibit minimal electrophysiologic effects at clinically used doses; these drugs are not discussed here.

ELECTROPHYSIOLOGIC ACTIONS

By blocking $I_{Ca,L}$ in all cardiac fibers, verapamil reduces the plateau height of the action potential, slightly shortens muscle action potential at pharmacologic concentrations, and slightly prolongs Purkinje fiber action potential (see Tables 64.1, 64.2, and eTables 64.1, 64.2). It does not appreciably affect the action potential amplitude, V_{max} of phase 0, or resting membrane voltage in cells that have fast-response characteristics related to I_{Na} (e.g., atrial and ventricular muscle, His-Purkinje system). Verapamil suppresses slow responses elicited by various experimental methods, as well as sustained triggered activity and EADs and DADs. Verapamil and diltiazem suppress electrical activity in the normal sinus and AV nodes. Verapamil depresses the slope of diastolic depolarization in sinus node cells, V_{max} of phase 0, and maximum diastolic potential and prolongs conduction time and refractory periods of the AV node. The AV node–blocking effects of verapamil and diltiazem are more apparent at faster rates of stimulation (use dependence) and in depolarized fibers (voltage dependence). Verapamil slows activation of the slow channel and delays its recovery from inactivation.

Verapamil does exert some local anesthetic activity because the *d*-isomer of the clinically used racemic mixture exerts slight blocking effects on I_{Na}. The *l*-isomer blocks the slow inward current carried by calcium, as well as other ions, traveling through the slow channel. Verapamil does not affect calcium-activated adenosine triphosphatase (ATPase), nor does it block beta receptors, but it may block alpha receptors and potentiate vagal effects on the AV node. Verapamil can also cause other effects that indirectly alter cardiac electrophysiology, such as decreasing platelet adhesiveness or reducing the extent of myocardial ischemia.

In humans, verapamil prolongs conduction time through the AV node (the A-H interval) and lengthens AV nodal anterograde and retrograde refractory periods without affecting the P wave or QRS duration or the H-V interval. The spontaneous sinus rate may decrease slightly, an effect only partially reversed by atropine. More often, the sinus rate does not change significantly because verapamil causes peripheral vasodilation, transient hypotension, and reflex sympathetic stimulation, which mitigates any direct slowing effect that verapamil exerts on the sinus node. If verapamil is given to a patient who is also receiving a beta blocker, the sinus node discharge rate may slow because reflex sympathetic stimulation is blocked. Verapamil does not exert a significant direct effect on atrial or ventricular refractoriness or on the anterograde or retrograde properties of accessory pathways. However, reflex sympathetic stimulation after IV verapamil administration may increase the ventricular response over the accessory pathway during AF in patients with WPW syndrome, sometimes dangerously so.

HEMODYNAMIC EFFECTS

Because verapamil interferes with excitation-contraction coupling, it inhibits vascular smooth muscle contraction and causes marked vasodilation in coronary and other peripheral vascular beds. The reflex sympathetic effects of verapamil may reduce its marked negative inotropic action on isolated cardiac muscle, but the direct myocardial depressant effects of verapamil may predominate when the drug is given in high doses. In patients with well-preserved left ventricular function, combined therapy with propranolol and verapamil appears to be well tolerated, but in some cases, beta blockade can accentuate the hemodynamic depressant effects produced by oral verapamil. Patients with reduced left ventricular function may not tolerate the combined blockade of beta receptors and calcium channels; thus, in these patients, verapamil and a beta blocker should be used in combination either cautiously or not at all. Verapamil reduces myocardial oxygen demand while decreasing coronary vascular resistance. Such changes may be indirectly antiarrhythmic.

Peak alterations in hemodynamic variables occur 3 to 5 minutes after completion of a verapamil injection, with the major effects dissipating within 10 minutes. Systemic resistance and mean arterial pressure decrease, as does left ventricular dP/dt_{max}, and left ventricular end-diastolic pressure increases. Heart rate, cardiac index, and mean pulmonary artery pressure do not change significantly in individuals with normal resting left ventricular systolic function. Thus the afterload reduction produced by verapamil significantly counterbalances its negative inotropic action, so the cardiac index may not be reduced. In addition, when verapamil slows the ventricular rate in a patient with tachycardia, hemodynamics may also improve. Nevertheless, caution should be exercised in giving verapamil to patients with myocardial depression or those receiving beta blockers or disopyramide because hemodynamic deterioration may progress in some patients.

PHARMACOKINETICS

After single oral doses of verapamil, measurable prolongation of AV nodal conduction time occurs in 30 minutes and lasts 4 to 6 hours (see Table 64.4). After IV administration, AV nodal conduction delay occurs within 1 to 2 minutes and A-H interval prolongation is still detectable after 6 hours. After oral administration, absorption is almost complete, but its overall bioavailability of 20% to 35% suggests substantial first-pass metabolism in the liver, particularly of the *l*-isomer. Verapamil's elimination half-life is 3 to 8 hours, with up to 70% of the drug excreted by the kidneys. Norverapamil is a major metabolite that may contribute to the electrophysiologic actions of verapamil. Serum protein binding is approximately 90%. With diltiazem, the percentage of heart rate reduction in AF is related to its plasma concentration.

DOSAGE AND ADMINISTRATION. For acute termination of SVT or rapid achievement of ventricular rate control during AF, the most common IV dose of verapamil is up to 10 mg infused over 1 to 2 minutes while cardiac rhythm and blood pressure are monitored (see Table 64.4). A second injection of an equal dose may be given 30 minutes later. The initial effect achieved with the first bolus injection, such as slowing of the ventricular response during AF, can be maintained by continuous infusion of the drug at a rate of 0.005 mg/kg/min. The oral dose is 240 to 480 mg/day in divided doses. Diltiazem is given intravenously at a dose of 0.25 mg/kg as a bolus over 2 minutes, with a second dose in 15 minutes if necessary. Because it is generally better tolerated (less hypotension) with long-term administration, such as for control of the ventricular rate during AF, diltiazem is preferred over verapamil in this setting. Significant hypotension resulting from IV diltiazem can be countered by volume expansion or judicious use of a pure vasoconstrictor agent such as phenylephrine. Orally, doses must be adjusted to the patient's needs, with a 120- to 360-mg range. Various long-acting preparations (once daily) are available for verapamil and diltiazem.

INDICATIONS. After simple vagal maneuvers have been tried and adenosine has been given, IV verapamil or diltiazem is the next treatment of choice for termination of sustained AV node reentry or orthodromic AV reciprocating tachycardia associated with an accessory pathway (see Chapter 65). Verapamil is as effective as adenosine for termination of these arrhythmias. Assuming that the patient is stable, verapamil should definitely be tried before termination is attempted by digitalis administration, pacing, electrical DC cardioversion, or acute blood pressure elevation with vasopressors. Verapamil and diltiazem terminate 60% to 90% or more episodes of paroxysmal SVT within several minutes. Verapamil may also be of use in some fetal SVTs. Although IV verapamil has been given along with IV propranolol, this combination should be used only with great caution because of combined adverse hemodynamic effects.

Verapamil and diltiazem decrease the ventricular response over the AV node during AF or atrial flutter, possibly converting a small number of episodes to sinus rhythm, particularly if the atrial flutter or AF is of recent onset. AF can occur in some patients with atrial flutter after verapamil administration. As noted earlier, in patients with preexcited ventricular complexes during AF associated with WPW syndrome, IV verapamil may accelerate the ventricular response; therefore, the IV route is contraindicated in this situation. Verapamil can terminate some ATs. Even though verapamil can often terminate an idiopathic left septal VT, hemodynamic collapse can occur if IV verapamil is given to patients with the more common forms of VT because these generally occur in the setting of decreased left ventricular systolic function. A general rule for avoiding complications, however, is not to administer verapamil intravenously to any patient with wide-QRS tachycardia unless one is certain of the nature of the tachycardia and its probable response to verapamil.

Orally, verapamil or diltiazem can prevent the recurrence of AV node reentrant and orthodromic AV reciprocating tachycardias associated with an accessory pathway, as well as help maintain a decreased ventricular response during atrial flutter or AF in patients without an accessory pathway. Verapamil has not generally been effective in treating patients who have recurrent ventricular tachyarrhythmias, although it may suppress some forms of VT, such as left septal VT (noted earlier). It can also be useful in patients with ventricular arrhythmias related to coronary artery spasm. Calcium channel blockers have not been shown to reduce mortality or to prevent sudden cardiac death in patients after acute MI, except for diltiazem in those with non–ST-segment elevation infarctions (see Chapter 39).

ADVERSE EFFECTS. Verapamil must be used cautiously in patients with significant hemodynamic impairment or in those receiving beta blockers, as noted earlier. Hypotension, bradycardia, AV block, and asystole are more likely to occur when the drug is given to patients who are already receiving beta-blocking agents. Hemodynamic collapse has been noted in infants, and verapamil should be used cautiously in children younger than 1 year. Verapamil should also be used with caution in patients with sinus node abnormalities because marked depression of sinus node function or asystole can result in some of these patients. IV isoproterenol, calcium, glucagon, dopamine, or atropine, which may be only partially effective, or temporary pacing may be necessary to counteract some of the adverse effects of verapamil. Isoproterenol may be more effective for the treatment of bradyarrhythmias, and calcium may be used for the treatment of hemodynamic dysfunction secondary to verapamil. AV node depression is common in overdoses. Contraindications to the use of verapamil and diltiazem include the presence of advanced heart failure, second- or third-degree AV block without a pacemaker in place, AF and anterograde conduction over an accessory pathway, significant sinus node dysfunction, most VTs, cardiogenic shock, and other hypotensive states. Although these drugs should probably not be used in patients with overt heart failure, if it is caused by one of the supraventricular tachyarrhythmias noted earlier, verapamil or diltiazem may restore sinus rhythm or significantly decrease the ventricular rate and thereby lead to hemodynamic improvement. Also, verapamil can decrease the excretion of digoxin by approximately 30%. Hepatotoxicity may occur on occasion. Verapamil crosses the placental barrier; its use in pregnancy has been associated with impaired uterine contraction, fetal bradycardia, and possibly fetal digital defects. It should therefore be used only if no effective alternatives exist.

Other Antiarrhythmic Agents
Adenosine
Adenosine is an endogenous nucleoside present throughout the body and has been approved by the FDA to treat patients with SVTs.

ELECTROPHYSIOLOGIC ACTIONS
Adenosine interacts with G-protein coupled A_1 receptors present on the extracellular surface of cardiac cells and activates K+ channels ($I_{K.Ach}$, $I_{K.Ado}$) in a manner similar to that produced by acetylcholine (see Tables 64.1, 64.2, and eTables 64.1, 64.2). The increase in K+ conductance shortens the atrial APD, hyperpolarizes the membrane potential, and decreases atrial contractility. Similar changes occur in the sinus and AV nodes. In contrast to these direct effects mediated through the guanine nucleotide regulatory proteins G_i and G_o, adenosine antagonizes catecholamine-stimulated adenylate cyclase to decrease accumulation of cyclic adenosine monophosphate (AMP) and to decrease $I_{Ca.L}$ and the pacemaker current I_f in sinus node cells along with a decrease in V_{max}. Shifts in the pacemaker site within the sinus node and sinus exit block may occur. Adenosine slows the sinus rate in humans, followed within seconds by a reflex increase in the sinus rate. In the AV node, adenosine produces transient prolongation of the A-H interval, often with transient first-, second-, or third-degree AV node block lasting up to a few seconds. The delay in AV nodal conduction is rate dependent. His-Purkinje conduction is not generally affected directly. Adenosine does not affect conduction in normal accessory pathways. Conduction may be blocked in unusual accessory pathways that have long conduction times or decremental conduction properties. Patients with heart transplants exhibit a supersensitive response to adenosine.

PHARMACOKINETICS
Adenosine is removed from the extracellular space by washout, enzymatically by degradation to inosine, by phosphorylation to AMP, or by reuptake into cells through a nucleoside transport system (see Table 64.4). The vascular endothelium and erythrocytes contain these elimination systems, which result in very rapid clearance of adenosine from the circulation. Its elimination half-life is 1 to 6 seconds. Most of adenosine's effects are produced during its first passage through the circulation. Important drug interactions occur; methylxanthines are competitive antagonists, and therapeutic concentrations of theophylline totally block the exogenous effects of adenosine. Dipyridamole is a nucleoside transport blocker that blocks reuptake of adenosine, thus delaying its clearance from the circulation or interstitial space and potentiating its

effect. Smaller adenosine doses should be used in patients receiving dipyridamole and in heart transplant patients where denervation makes the sinus and AV node supersensitive.

DOSAGE AND ADMINISTRATION. To terminate tachycardia, a bolus of adenosine is rapidly injected intravenously at doses of 6 to 12 mg, followed by a flush (see Table 64.4). Pediatric (<50 kg) dosing should be 0.05 to 0.3 mg/kg. When it is injected into a central vein and in patients after heart transplantation or those receiving dipyridamole, the initial dose should be reduced to 3 mg. Transient sinus slowing or AV node block results but lasts less than 5 seconds. Doses higher than 18 mg are unlikely to revert a tachycardia and should not be used.

INDICATIONS. Adenosine has become the drug of first choice to terminate an SVT acutely, such as AV node or AV reentry (see Chapter 65), and is useful in pediatric patients. Adenosine can produce AV nodal block or terminate ATs and sinus node reentry. It results in only transient AV block during atrial flutter or fibrillation and is thus useful only for diagnosis, not therapy. Adenosine terminates a group of VTs whose maintenance depends on adrenergic drive, which is most often located in the right ventricular outflow tract but can be found at other sites as well; however, idiopathic left septal VT rarely responds. When properly administered, adenosine usually causes transient hypotension, chest discomfort, and dyspnea; if tachycardia persists in the absence of these effects, the drug may not have been given correctly. Adenosine has less potential than verapamil for producing prolonged hypotension, should tachycardia persist after injection.

Doses as low as 2.5 mg terminate some tachycardias; doses of 12 mg or less terminate 92% of SVTs, usually within 30 seconds. Successful termination rates with adenosine are comparable to those achieved with verapamil. Because of its effectiveness and extremely short duration of action, adenosine is preferable to verapamil in most cases, particularly in patients who have previously received IV beta adrenoceptor blockers, in those with poorly compensated heart failure or severe hypotension, and in neonates. Verapamil might be chosen first in patients receiving drugs such as theophylline (which is known to interfere with adenosine's actions or metabolism), in patients with active bronchoconstriction, and in those with inadequate venous access.

Adenosine may be useful to help differentiate among causes of wide-QRS tachycardias because it terminates many SVTs with aberrancy or reveals the underlying atrial mechanism and does not block conduction over an accessory pathway or terminate most VTs. In rare cases, however, adenosine terminates some VTs, characteristically those of right ventricular outflow tract origin as noted earlier, and therefore tachycardia termination is not completely diagnostic of an SVT. This agent may predispose to the development of AF and might transiently increase the ventricular response in patients with AF conducting over an accessory pathway. Adenosine may also be useful in differentiating conduction over the AV node from that over an accessory pathway during ablative procedures designed to interrupt the accessory pathway. However, this distinction is not absolute because adenosine can block conduction in slowly conducting accessory pathways and does not always produce block in the AV node.

ADVERSE EFFECTS. Transient side effects occur in almost 40% of patients with SVT given adenosine and usually consist of flushing, dyspnea, and chest pressure. These symptoms are fleeting, lasting less than 1 minute, and are well tolerated. PVCs, transient sinus bradycardia, sinus arrest, and AV block are common when an SVT is terminated abruptly. AF is occasionally observed (12% in one study) with adenosine administration, perhaps because of the drug's effect in shortening atrial refractoriness. Induction of AF can be problematic in patients with WPW syndrome and rapid AV conduction over the accessory pathway.

Digoxin
Cardiac actions of digitalis glycosides have been recognized for several centuries. In adults, digoxin is used mainly for control of the ventricular rate during AF, whereas its use in pediatrics is in a broader range of arrhythmias. Use of digoxin has decreased because of the availability of agents with greater and more reliable efficacy and a

wider therapeutic to toxic drug concentration range. Its use is generally discouraged in adults.

ELECTROPHYSIOLOGIC ACTIONS

Digoxin acts mainly through the autonomic nervous system, in particular by enhancing both central and peripheral vagal tone. These actions are confined largely to slowing of the sinus node discharge rate, shortening of atrial refractoriness, and prolongation of AV nodal refractoriness (see Tables 64.1, 64.2, and eTables 64.1, 64.2). Electrophysiologic effects on the His-Purkinje system and ventricular muscle are minimal, except with toxic concentrations. In studies of denervated hearts, digoxin has relatively little effect on the AV node and causes a mild increase in atrial refractoriness.

The sinus rate and P wave duration are minimally changed in most patients taking digoxin. The sinus rate may decrease in patients with heart failure whose left ventricular performance is improved by the drug; individuals with significant underlying sinus node disease also have slower sinus rates or even sinus arrest. Similarly, the PR interval is generally unchanged, except in patients with underlying AV node disease. The QRS and QT intervals are unaffected. The characteristic ST and T wave abnormalities seen with use of digoxin do not represent toxicity.

PHARMACOKINETICS

IV digoxin yields some electrophysiologic effect within minutes, with a peak effect occurring after 1.5 to 3 hours (see Table 64.4). After oral dosing, the peak effect occurs in 4 to 6 hours. The extent of digoxin absorption after oral administration varies according to the preparation; tablet forms are 60% to 75% absorbed, whereas encapsulated gel forms are almost completely absorbed. Ingestion of cholestyramine or an antacid preparation at the same time as digoxin ingestion decreases its absorption. The serum half-life of digoxin is 36 to 48 hours, and the drug is excreted unchanged by the kidneys.

DOSAGE AND ADMINISTRATION. In acute loading doses of 0.5 to 1.0 mg, digoxin can be given orally or intravenously (see Table 64.4). Chronic daily oral dosing should be adjusted on the basis of clinical indications and the extent of renal dysfunction. Most patients require 0.125 to 0.25 mg/day as a single dose. However, some patients undergoing renal dialysis need as little as 0.125 mg every other day, whereas young patients may require as much as 0.5 mg/day. Serum digoxin levels may be used to monitor compliance with therapy, as well as to determine whether digitalis toxicity is the cause of new symptoms compatible with the diagnosis. However, routine monitoring of digoxin levels is not warranted in patients whose ventricular rate is controlled during AF and who have no symptoms of toxicity.

INDICATIONS. Digoxin can be used intravenously to slow the ventricular rate during AF and atrial flutter; it was formerly used in an attempt to convert SVTs to sinus rhythm, but its onset of action is much slower and its success rate less than that of adenosine, verapamil, or beta blockers. Thus, it is now rarely used in this fashion. Digoxin is more often used orally to control the ventricular rate in permanent ("chronic") AF. When a patient with AF is at rest and vagal tone predominates, the ventricular rate can be maintained between 60 and 100 beats/min in 40% to 60% of cases. However, when the patient begins to exercise, the decrease in vagal tone and increase in adrenergic tone combine to diminish the beneficial effects of digoxin on AV nodal conduction. Patients can experience a marked increase in ventricular rate with even mild exertion. Digoxin is therefore rarely used as a single agent to control the ventricular rate in AF. The drug has little ability to prevent episodes of paroxysmal AF or to control the ventricular rate during episodes and may even provoke episodes in patients with so-called vagal AF. Furthermore, digoxin is not more effective than placebo in terminating episodes of acute- or recent-onset AF.

ADVERSE EFFECTS. The use of digoxin has decreased because of is its potential for serious adverse effects, the narrow window between therapeutic and toxic concentrations and extensive drug-drug interactions. Digitalis toxicity produces various symptoms and signs, including headache, nausea and vomiting, altered color perception, halo vision, and generalized malaise. Less common but more serious than these are digitalis-related arrhythmias, which include bradycardias related to a greatly enhanced vagal effect (e.g., sinus bradycardia or arrest, AV node block) and tachyarrhythmias that may be caused by DAD-mediated triggered activity (e.g., junctional, and fascicular or VT). Worsening renal function, advanced age, hypokalemia, chronic lung

disease, hypothyroidism, and amyloidosis increase a patient's sensitivity to digitalis-related arrhythmias. The diagnosis of toxicity can be confirmed by determination of the serum digoxin level. Therapy for most bradycardias consists of withdrawal of digoxin; atropine or temporary pacing may be needed in symptomatic patients. Phenytoin can be used to control atrial tachyarrhythmias, whereas lidocaine has been successful in treating infranodal tachycardias. Life-threatening arrhythmias can be treated with digoxin-specific antibody fragments. Electrical DC cardioversion should be performed only when absolutely necessary in a digitalis-toxic patient because life-threatening VT or VF can result and can be difficult to control. Some data incriminate digoxin in increasing mortality in patients with AF.[19]

Ranolazine

Ranolazine, approved by the FDA for the treatment of chronic angina, has significant electrophysiologic properties. It has been shown to decrease the incidence of AF, SVT, and ventricular arrhythmias relative to controls in trials of the drug's antianginal effects.

ELECTROPHYSIOLOGIC ACTIONS

Ranolazine blocks I_{Kr}, as well as the late Na current; at higher concentrations, the L-type Ca current is mildly affected (see Tables 64.1, 64.2, and eTables 64.1, 64.2). The drug prolongs atrial and ventricular refractoriness and induces postrepolarization refractoriness; the P wave, PR interval, and QRS are unaffected, but the QT interval is mildly prolonged. Unlike other I_{Kr}-blocking drugs, ranolazine does not induce EADs. Its effects are more pronounced on atrial than on ventricular myocardium, and the drug shows promise for the treatment of AF, particularly when combined with dronedarone.[20]

HEMODYNAMIC EFFECTS

Ranolazine has no important hemodynamic effects; it does not appear to produce meaningful changes in contractility or vascular resistance.

PHARMACOKINETICS

Absorption of oral ranolazine is mediated in part by the P-glycoprotein system, modulators of which may increase or decrease drug exposure. About 75% of a dose is bioavailable, with peak levels reached in 2 to 5 hours (see Table 64.4). Absorption is not affected by food. Its half-life is approximately 7 hours; hepatic metabolism to minimally or wholly inactive products occurs via the CYP3A and, to a lesser extent, the CYP2D6 pathways. Approximately 75% of the drug is excreted in urine, the remainder in feces.

DOSAGE AND ADMINISTRATION. The typical oral dose of ranolazine is 500 mg twice daily, to a maximum of 1000 mg twice daily. The dose should be decreased in the setting of moderate liver disease. It should not be used in conjunction with strong inhibitors of CYP3A, which could increase the drug's serum concentration threefold.

ADVERSE EFFECTS. The most widely known potential adverse effect of ranolazine is QTc prolongation, which averages 6 to 15 milliseconds (sometimes more in patients with severe liver failure), because of inhibition of I_{Kr}. Despite this effect on the QT interval, TdP is rare, probably in part because of only modest QT prolongation combined with the drug's inhibition of the late inward Na current, which mitigates the QT effect. As noted, ranolazine does not cause EADs or increases in transmural dispersion of refractoriness, which are believed to be prerequisites for torsades. Ranolazine produces a mild elevation in measured serum creatinine (0.1 mg/dL) without changing the actual glomerular filtration rate. The drug is pregnancy category C; its concentration in breast milk is unknown.

Ivabradine

Ivabradine is approved by the FDA for reducing the risk of hospitalization for worsening heart failure in patients with stable, symptomatic heart failure and a reduced EF in sinus rhythm with a resting heart rate ≥70 beats/min and taking maximally tolerated doses of beta blockers. Ivabradine has been used to treat inappropriate sinus tachycardia.

ELECTROPHYSIOLOGIC ACTIONS

Ivabradine blocks the pacemaker or "funny" current (I_f), the current responsible for generating spontaneous depolarization in the sinus node. The funny current is a mixed Na$^+$-K$^+$ inward current activated by hyperpolarization. Ivabradine blocks the intracellular portion of the transmembrane ion pore and inhibits cation movement with a high degree of selectivity leading to a reduction in the slope of diastolic depolarization. Ivabradine causes a dose-dependent reduction in heart rate. It has been used to treat inappropriate sinus tachycardia, especially when beta blockers and calcium channel blockers have failed or are poorly tolerated. Little long-term data exists on its efficacy.[21]

HEMODYNAMIC EFFECTS

There are no hemodynamic effects or alterations of cardiac contractility caused by ivabradine.

PHARMACOKINETICS

The drug undergoes extensive first-pass hepatic metabolism and is metabolized by CYP3A4. The dose needs to be adjusted for severe hepatic or renal impairment. The pharmacokinetics properties appear to be linear with respect to dosing.

DOSAGE AND ADMINISTRATION. Ivabradine is typically started at a dose of 5 mg twice per day (2.5 mg bid if the resting heart rate is <60 beats/min) and may be increased to 7.5 mg twice daily to increase its effects. The dosage may be lowered if excessive bradycardia is encountered. The dose is typically titrated after 2 weeks.

SIDE EFFECTS. The drug may cause excessive sinus slowing or AV nodal block, and caution should be exercised when given to patients with sinus bradycardia or first-degree AV block. The most common non-cardiac side effect is visual disturbances, specifically transient flashes of brightness in the visual field. When ivabradine is used in combination with other QT prolonging drugs it may increase the risk of TdP. There may be an increased incidence of AF with this agent. Ivabradine is contraindicated in pregnant mothers due to possible fetal toxicity.

Antiarrhythmic Effects of Nonantiarrhythmic Drugs

Several medications commonly used for other indications also have some degree of antiarrhythmic effect. In some cases, physicians can use these drugs for their standard indications and achieve additional, although often small, amounts of benefit in treating the patient's rhythm disturbance. These drugs include angiotensin-converting enzyme (ACE) inhibitors and angiotensin receptor–blocking agents; aldosterone antagonists such as eplerenone, statins, and omega-3 fatty acids (prevention of sudden death); and these same classes of drugs with the addition of non-dihydropyridine calcium channel blockers and ranolazine (less AF and perhaps VF). The mechanisms whereby these drugs exert their attenuating effect on arrhythmias is not clear in most cases, and they should not be relied on as the sole form of antiarrhythmic therapy. In patients who have arrhythmias, as well as another disorder that requires drug therapy (hypertension, heart failure), one of these medications may be preferable to agents that treat the primary disorder but do not possess antiarrhythmic effects. There are a number of drugs used for other indications that have been considered for repurposed use in the treatment of arrhythmias. Prominent are drugs used to treat neurological disorders such gabapentins, flunarizine, and riluzole which have ion channel blocking effects and vanoxerine a dopamine reuptake inhibitor. It is imperative to remember that all drugs that have effects on electrical properties of the heart can also produce proarrhythmic effects.

New Antiarrhythmic Agents

VERNAKALANT

Vernakalant is a mixed potassium and sodium channel blocker used intravenously for conversion of AF to sinus rhythm. The drug, currently available in Europe, is a use-dependent inhibitor of I_{Na} and blocks the atrial-specific potassium current I_{Kur} as well as $I_{K.ACh}$ and I_{to}. Vernakalant prolongs atrial APD and refractoriness. The safety for IV conversion of AF (initial dose of 3 mg/kg over 10 minutes followed by 2 mg/kg over 15 minutes for persistent arrhythmia) have been demonstrated in the Atrial Arrhythmia Conversion Trials 1 and 3 (ACT1, ACT3). The drug was well tolerated in these studies, with minimal side effects and no TdP episodes. Transient hypotension and bradycardia were observed in 5% to 10% of patients.

ELECTROTHERAPY FOR CARDIAC ARRHYTHMIAS

Direct-Current Electrical Cardioversion

Cardioversion is a general term used to indicate the termination of an arrhythmia, usually a tachyarrhythmia, by various means, including electrical, pharmacologic, or manual/surgical. *Electrical cardioversion* refers to the delivery of an electrical shock to the heart to terminate a tachycardia, flutter, or fibrillation and includes the technique of both synchronous cardioversion (see below) and defibrillation. It offers obvious advantages over drug therapy because under conditions optimal for close supervision and monitoring, a precisely regulated "dose" of electricity can restore sinus rhythm immediately and safely. The distinction between supraventricular and ventricular tachyarrhythmias, crucial to the proper medical management of arrhythmias, becomes less significant, and the time-consuming titration of drugs with potential side effects is obviated.

MECHANISMS

Electrical cardioversion is most effective in terminating tachycardias related to reentry, such as atrial flutter and many cases of AF, AV node reentry, reciprocating tachycardias associated with WPW syndrome, most forms of VT, ventricular flutter, and VF. The electrical shock, by depolarizing all excitable myocardium and possibly by prolonging refractoriness, interrupts reentrant circuits and establishes electrical homogeneity, which terminates reentry. The mechanism by which a shock successfully terminates VF has not been completely explained. If the precipitating factors are no longer present, interruption of the tachyarrhythmia for only the brief time produced by the shock may prevent its return for long periods, even though the anatomic and electrophysiologic substrates required for the tachycardia are still present.

Tachycardias thought to be caused by disorders of impulse formation (automaticity) include parasystole, some forms of AT, junctional tachycardia (with or without digitalis toxicity), accelerated idioventricular rhythm, and relatively uncommon forms of VT (see Chapters 62 and 67). An attempt to cardiovert these tachycardias electrically is not indicated in most cases because they typically recur within seconds after the shock, and release of endogenous catecholamines consequent to the shock can perpetuate the arrhythmia. It has not been established whether cardioversion can terminate tachycardias caused by enhanced automaticity or triggered activity.

Technique

Synchronous cardioversion refers to a specific technique of delivering an electrical shock, usually of lower energy and timed to the QRS complex ("R wave"), to avoid the vulnerable period of the T wave. Before elective synchronous cardioversion, careful physical examination should be performed, including palpation of limb pulses and inspection of the chest wall and airway. A 12-lead ECG is usually obtained before and after cardioversion, as well as a rhythm strip during the shock delivery. The patient, who should be informed completely about what to expect, is in a fasting state and respiratory function and electrolyte values should be normal, with no evidence of drug toxicity. Withholding of digitalis for several days before elective cardioversion in patients without clinical evidence of digitalis toxicity is not necessary, although patients in whom digitalis toxicity is suspected should not be electrically cardioverted until this situation has been corrected. Administration of maintenance AADs 1 to 2 days before planned electrical cardioversion of patients with AF can revert some patients to sinus rhythm, help prevent recurrence of AF once sinus rhythm is restored, and assist in determining the patient's tolerance of the drug for long-term use.[14] There is also evidence that statin drugs, as well as ACE inhibitors and angiotensin receptor blockers, may help prevent recurrence of AF, especially in patients with ventricular dysfunction.[22]

Self-adhesive patches applied in the standard apicoanterior or anteroposterior paddle positions have transthoracic impedances similar to those of paddles and are useful in elective synchronous cardioversions or other situations in which time is available for their application. Patches 12 to 13 cm in diameter can be used to deliver maximum current to the heart, but the benefits of these patches versus patches 8 to 9 cm in diameter have not been clearly established. Larger

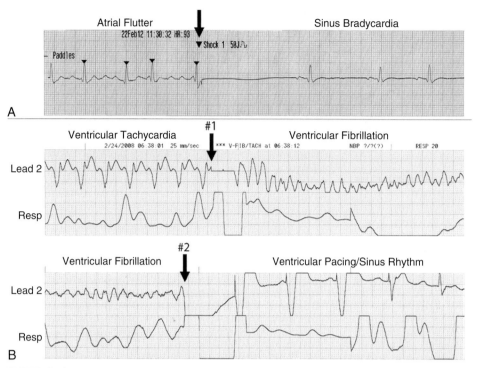

FIGURE 64.2 Cardioversions. **A,** Synchronized shock (note the synchronization mark in the apex of the QRS complex, *arrowhead*) during atrial flutter is followed by sinus bradycardia. **B** *(top),* Shock (*#1*) is delivered during ventricular tachycardia but asynchronously (on the T wave); this results in ventricular fibrillation, which is then treated with a second, asynchronous shock (*#2*) that results in sinus rhythm with tracked ventricular pacing. *Resp,* Respirations.

patches may distribute the intracardiac current over a wider area and reduce the possibility of shock-induced myocardial injury.

A synchronized shock (i.e., one delivered during the QRS complex; Fig. 64.2) is used for all cardioversions except for very rapid ventricular tachyarrhythmias, such as ventricular flutter or VF. For defibrillation of the latter, energies greater than those for synchronous cardioversion are required, and synchronization is not necessary because there is no vulnerable period of the T wave to avoid. Although generally minimal, shock-related myocardial damage increases directly with increases in applied energy, and thus the minimum effective shock should be used. Therefore, shocks are "titrated" when the clinical situation permits. Except for AF, shocks in the range of 25 to 50 joules (J) successfully terminate most SVTs and should be tried initially. If the shock is unsuccessful, a second shock of higher energy can be delivered. The starting level to terminate AF with older monophasic machines should be no less than 100 J, but with newer biphasic systems, a shock as low as 25 J may succeed. Delivered energy can be increased in stepwise fashion; up to 360 J can be used safely. It is critical to remember to resynchronize the defibrillator to the QRS complex after an unsuccessful shock before delivery of another shock to avoid initiation of VF (machines typically revert to the asynchronous mode after each shock). Anteroposterior patches may have a higher efficacy rate by placing more of the atrial mass in the shock vector than is the case with apicoanterior patches. If a shock of 360 J fails to convert the rhythm, 1 or 2 additional shocks at the same energy may still succeed by decreasing chest wall impedance; reversing patch polarity can occasionally help as well. Administration of ibutilide has been shown to facilitate electrical cardioversion of AF to sinus rhythm. Intracardiac or transesophageal defibrillation can be tried if all attempts at external cardioversion fail. For patients with stable VT, starting levels in the range of 25 to 50 J can be used. If there is some urgency to terminate the tachyarrhythmia, the clinician can begin with higher energies. To terminate VF, a biphasic 100 to 200 J shock (200 to 360 J with monophasic machines) is generally used, although much lower energies (<50 J) terminate VF when the shock is delivered soon after onset of the arrhythmia, for example, using previously placed adhesive patches in the electrophysiology laboratory.

During elective cardioversion, a short-acting barbiturate such as methohexital, a sedative such as propofol, or an amnesic such as diazepam or midazolam can be used. A physician skilled in airway management should be in attendance; an IV route should be established; and pulse oximetry, the ECG, and blood pressure should be monitored. All equipment necessary for emergency resuscitation should be immediately accessible. Before cardioversion, 100% oxygen may be administered for 5 to 15 minutes by nasal cannula or facemask and is continued throughout the procedure. Manual ventilation of the patient may be necessary to avoid hypoxia during periods of deepest sedation. Adequate sedation of the patient undergoing even urgent cardioversion is essential.

In up to 5% of patients with AF, sinus rhythm cannot be restored by external countershock despite all the preceding measures, including ibutilide pretreatment and biphasic shocks. It is important to distinguish between inability to *attain* sinus rhythm, indicating failure of the shock to convert the arrhythmia, and inability to *maintain* sinus rhythm after transient termination of fibrillation; the latter condition (early re-initiation of AF) does not respond to higher-energy shocks because fibrillation has already been terminated but quickly recurs. Pretreatment with an AAD may help maintain sinus rhythm after subsequent shocks. Patients in whom AF simply cannot be terminated with an external shock tend to be very obese or have severe obstructive lung disease. In such patients, internal cardioversion can be performed with the use of specially configured catheters that have multiple large electrodes covering several centimeters of the distal portion of the catheter for distributing the shock energy. Internal shocks of 2 to 15 J can terminate AF in more than 90% of patients whose arrhythmia was refractory to transthoracic shock. Esophageal cardioversion has also been reported. Rarely, simultaneous shocks from two defibrillators have been reported to terminate refractory AF or VF.

Indications

As a general rule, any non-sinus tachycardia that produces hypotension, congestive heart failure, mental status changes, or angina and does not respond promptly to medical management should be terminated electrically. Very rapid ventricular rates in patients with AF and WPW syndrome are often best treated by electrical cardioversion. In almost all cases, the patient's hemodynamic status improves after cardioversion. Rarely, a patient may experience hypotension, reduced cardiac output, or congestive heart failure after the shock. This problem may be related to complications of the cardioversion, such as embolic events, myocardial depression resulting from the anesthetic agent or the shock itself, hypoxia, lack of restoration of left atrial contraction despite return of electrical atrial systole, or post-shock arrhythmias. DC countershock of digitalis-induced tachyarrhythmias is contraindicated (see earlier).

Favorable candidates for electrical cardioversion of AF include patients who (1) have symptomatic AF of less than 12 months' duration, (2) continue to have AF after the precipitating cause has been removed (e.g., after treatment of thyrotoxicosis), (3) have a rapid ventricular rate that is difficult to slow, or (4) have symptoms of decreased cardiac output (e.g., fatigue, lightheadedness, dyspnea) attributable to lack of atrial contraction's contribution to ventricular filling. In patients who have indications for chronic anticoagulants to prevent stroke, the hope of avoiding these medications by restoring sinus rhythm is not a reason to attempt cardioversion, because these patients are still at increased risk for thromboembolic events. Several large trials have shown that maintenance of sinus rhythm confers no survival advantage over rate control and anticoagulation; thus, not all patients with newly discovered AF warrant an attempt at restoration of sinus rhythm. Treatment must be determined individually (see Chapter 66). In a recently published study, early cardioversion was not superior at restoring sinus rhythm at 4 weeks compared to a wait-and-see approach with delayed cardioversion.[23]

Unfavorable candidates include patients with (1) digitalis toxicity, (2) no symptoms and a well-controlled ventricular rate without therapy, (3) sinus node dysfunction and various unstable supraventricular tachyarrhythmias or bradyarrhythmias—often bradycardia-tachycardia syndrome—in whom AF finally develops and is maintained, which in essence represents a cure for sick sinus syndrome, (4) little or no symptomatic improvement with normal sinus rhythm, (5) prompt reversion to AF after cardioversion despite drug therapy, (6) a large (>5 cm) left atrium and longstanding AF, (7) episodes of AF that revert spontaneously to sinus rhythm, (8) no mechanical atrial systole after the return of electrical atrial systole, (9) AF and advanced heart block, (10) cardiac surgery planned in the near future, and (11) AAD intolerance. AF is more likely to recur after cardioversion in patients who have significant chronic obstructive lung disease, congestive heart failure, mitral valve disease (particularly mitral regurgitation), AF present longer than 1 year, and an enlarged left atrium (echocardiographic diameter >5.5 cm).

In patients with atrial flutter, slowing the ventricular rate by administration of beta or calcium channel blockers or terminating the flutter with an antiarrhythmic agent may be difficult, and electrical cardioversion is often the initial treatment of choice. For patients with other types of SVT, electrical cardioversion may be used when (1) vagal maneuvers or simple medical management (e.g., IV adenosine and verapamil) has failed to terminate the tachycardia and (2) the clinical setting dictates prompt restoration of sinus rhythm because of hemodynamic decompensation or other clinical consequences of the tachycardia. Similarly, in patients with VT, the hemodynamic and electrophysiologic consequences of the arrhythmias determine the need for and urgency of DC cardioversion. Electrical countershock is the initial treatment of choice for ventricular flutter or VF. Speed is essential (see Chapter 70).

If reversion of the arrhythmia to sinus rhythm does not occur after the first shock, a higher energy level should be tried. When transient ventricular arrhythmias result after an unsuccessful shock, a bolus of lidocaine can be given before delivery of a shock at the next energy level. If sinus rhythm returns only transiently and is promptly supplanted by the tachycardia, a repeated shock can be tried, depending on the tachyarrhythmia being treated and its consequences. Administration of an AAD intravenously may be useful before delivery of the next cardioversion shock (e.g., ibutilide for resistant AF). After cardioversion, the patient should be monitored, at least until full consciousness has been restored and preferably for 1 hour or more thereafter, depending on the duration of recovery from the particular form of sedation or anesthesia used. If ibutilide has been given, the ECG should be monitored for up to 4 hours because TdP can develop in the first few hours after administration.

Results
Electrical cardioversion restores sinus rhythm in up to 95% of patients, depending on the type of tachyarrhythmia. However, sinus rhythm remains after 12 months in less than one third to one half of patients with longstanding persistent AF. Thus, maintenance of sinus rhythm, once established, is the difficult problem, not immediate termination of the tachyarrhythmia. The likelihood of maintaining sinus rhythm depends on the particular arrhythmia, the presence of underlying heart disease, and the response to AAD therapy. Atrial size often decreases after termination of AF and restoration of sinus rhythm, and functional capacity improves.

Complications
Arrhythmias induced by electrical cardioversion are generally caused by inadequate synchronization, with the shock occurring during the ST segment or T wave (see Fig. 64.2). On occasion, even a properly synchronized shock can produce VF. Post-shock arrhythmias are usually transient and do not require therapy. Asystole is rare and typically lasts no more than a few seconds before a sinus or junctional rhythm ensues; most defibrillators are also capable of transcutaneous pacing if needed. Embolic episodes are reported to occur in 1% to 3% of patients converted from AF to sinus rhythm. Prior therapeutic anticoagulation with warfarin (international normalized ratio [INR], 2.0 to 3.0) or newer agents such as dabigatran, rivaroxaban, apixaban or edoxaban, should be used consistently for at least 3 weeks by patients who have no contraindication to such therapy and have had AF for longer than 2 days or of indeterminate duration. It is important to note that 3 weeks of therapeutic anticoagulation is not the same as simply administering warfarin for 3 weeks, because the warfarin dose may not achieve a therapeutic INR. However, the newer agents confer almost immediate anticoagulation, such that 3 weeks of treatment equals 3 weeks of anticoagulation. Anticoagulation for at least 4 weeks afterward is recommended because restoration of atrial mechanical function lags behind that of electrical systolic function, and thrombi can still form due to delayed mechanical recovery, although the atria are electrocardiographically in sinus rhythm. Exclusion of left atrial thrombi by transesophageal echocardiography immediately before cardioversion may not always preclude embolism days or weeks after cardioversion of AF. Atrial thrombi can be present in patients with non–fibrillation-related atrial tachyarrhythmias, such as atrial flutter and AT in patients with congenital heart disease. The same precardioversion and postcardioversion anticoagulation recommendations apply to these patients as to those with AF. Although DC shock has been demonstrated in animals to cause myocardial injury, studies in humans have indicated that elevations in myocardial enzymes after cardioversion are not common. ST-segment elevation, sometimes dramatic, can occur immediately after elective DC cardioversion and can last for up to 1 to 2 minutes, although cardiac enzymes and myocardial scintigraphy may be unremarkable. ST elevation lasting longer than 2 minutes usually indicates myocardial injury unrelated to the shock. A decrease in serum K^+ and Mg^{2+} levels can occur after cardioversion of VT.

Cardioversion of VT can also be achieved by a chest thump. Its mechanism of termination is probably related to a mechanically induced PVC that interrupts a tachycardia circuit and may be related to commotio cordis. The thump cannot be timed accurately and is probably effective only when delivered during a nonrefractory part of the cardiac cycle. The thump can alter a VT and possibly induce ventricular flutter or VF if it occurs during the vulnerable period of the T wave. Because there may be a slightly greater likelihood of converting a stable VT to VF than of terminating VT to sinus rhythm, chest thump cardioversion should not be attempted unless a defibrillator is unavailable.

Implantable Electrical Devices for Treatment of Cardiac Arrhythmias
Implantable devices that monitor the cardiac rhythm and can deliver competing pacing stimuli and low- and high-energy shocks have been used effectively in selected patients (see Chapter 69).

Ablation Therapy for Cardiac Arrhythmias
The purpose of catheter ablation is to destroy myocardial tissue by delivery of energy, generally electrical energy or cryoenergy, through electrodes on a catheter placed next to an area of the myocardium integrally related to onset or maintenance of the arrhythmia. For tachycardias with an apparent focal origin (e.g., automatic, triggered activity, microreentry), the focus itself (<5 mm in diameter) is targeted. In macroreentrant AT and VT, inexcitable scar tissue typically separates strands of surviving myocardium, and wavefronts propagate around these scars. The target for ablation is a narrow portion of myocardium between inexcitable areas (e.g., scar, valve annulus; Fig. 64.3). The first catheter ablation procedures were performed with DC shocks, but this energy source has been supplanted by radiofrequency (RF) energy, which is delivered from an external generator and destroys tissue by controlled heat production.

ARRHYTHMIAS, SUDDEN DEATH, AND SYNCOPE

VII

Lasers and microwave energy sources have been used, but not frequently; cryothermal catheter ablation has been approved for use in humans. When a target tissue has been identified by EPS, the tip of the ablation catheter is maneuvered into apposition with this tissue. After stable catheter position and recordings have been ensured, RF energy is delivered between the catheter tip and an indifferent electrode, usually an electrocautery-type grounding pad on the skin of the patient's thigh. Because energies in the RF portion of the electromagnetic spectrum are poorly conducted by cardiac tissue, RF energy instead causes resistive heating in the cells close to the tip of the catheter (i.e., these cells transduce the electrical energy into thermal energy). When tissue temperature exceeds 50°C, irreversible cellular damage and tissue death occur. An expanding front of conducted heat emanates from the region of

resistive heating while RF delivery continues over the next 30 seconds and results in the production of a homogeneous, roughly hemispheric lesion of coagulative necrosis 3 to 5 mm in diameter (Fig. 64.4A). RF-induced heating of tissue that has inherent automaticity (e.g., His bundle, foci of automatic tachycardias) results in initial acceleration of a rhythm, whereas RF delivery during a reentrant arrhythmia typically causes slowing and termination of the arrhythmia. In most cases, RF delivery is painless, although ablation of atrial or right ventricular tissue can be uncomfortable for some patients.

Cooled-Tip Radiofrequency Ablation

In some situations, the catheter can be delivered to the correct location, but conventional RF energy delivery cannot eliminate the tachycardia. In some of these cases the amount of damage—depth or breadth—caused by standard RF energy is inadequate. With the use of standard RF energy, power delivery is usually regulated to maintain a preset catheter tip temperature (typically, 55°C to 70°C). Tip temperatures higher than 90°C are associated with coagulation of blood elements on the electrode, which precludes further energy delivery and could also cause this material to become detached and embolize. Cooling of the catheter tip by internal circulation of liquid or continuous fluid infusion through small holes in the tip electrode can prevent excessive heating of the tip and allow delivery of higher power, thus producing a larger lesion (see Fig. 64.4B) and potentially enhancing efficacy.[24] Cooled-tip ablation has been used to good advantage in cases in which standard (4-mm tip) catheter ablation has failed, as well as for primary therapy for atrial flutter and fibrillation and VT associated with structural heart disease, in which additional damage to already-diseased areas is not harmful and may be required to achieve the desired result.

Catheter-delivered cryoablation causes tissue damage by freezing cellular structures. Nitrous oxide is delivered to the tip of the catheter, where it is allowed to internally boil and cool the tip electrode, after which the gas is circulated back to the delivery console. Catheter tip temperature can be regulated, with cooling to as low as −80°C. Cooling to 0°C causes reversible loss of function and can be used as a diagnostic test (i.e., termination of a tachycardia when the catheter is in contact with a group of cells critical to its perpetuation, or determining its effect on normal conduction when close to the AV node). The catheter tip can then be cooled more deeply to produce permanent damage and thus cure of the arrhythmia. Cryoablation has been used for pulmonary vein isolation to treat paroxysmal AF by situating a collapsed balloon at the end of a catheter near a pulmonary vein ostium and inflating the balloon with nitrous oxide at −80°C. During cryoballoon occlusion of the vein for 3 to 4 minutes at a time, pulmonary vein isolation can usually be effected with one or two applications.[25] Real-time recordings can be done simultaneously to monitor conduction. Cryoablation appears to cause less endocardial damage than RF energy does and may thus engender less risk for thromboemboli after ablation, as well as less chance of esophageal injury with ablation of AF (although it is not eliminated). However, balloon cryotherapy to isolate right pulmonary veins for the treatment of AF has resulted in phrenic nerve injury, and care must be taken to establish the location of the phrenic nerve. Larger balloon sizes, with more proximal zones of cryoablation, and monitoring

ABLATION FOR FOCAL ARRHYTHMIA

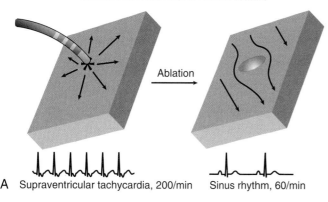

A   Supraventricular tachycardia, 200/min   Sinus rhythm, 60/min

ABLATION FOR REENTRANT ARRHYTHMIA

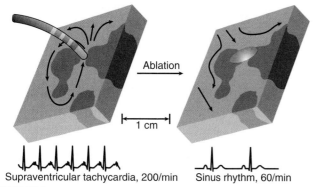

B   Supraventricular tachycardia, 200/min   Sinus rhythm, 60/min

FIGURE 64.3 Strategies for catheter ablation. **A,** Focal tachycardia. *Left,* SVT is caused by an atrial focus, with activation emanating in all directions. *Right,* Ablation of the focus eliminates the arrhythmia with minimal disruption of normal activation. **B,** Macroreentrant SVT in setting of previous atrial damage resulting in scar formation. *Left,* During SVT, a wavefront circulates around a scarred area and through a narrow isthmus between this and another area of scar. *Right,* Ablation at this critical site prevents further reentry.

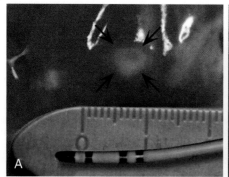
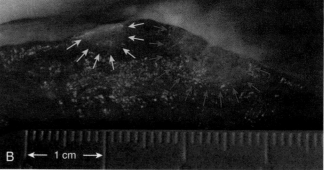

FIGURE 64.4 Radiofrequency lesion in human ventricular myocardium (explanted heart at transplantation). **A,** Energy was applied for 30 seconds at the location denoted by arrows, with the tip of the catheter shown. The lesion is 5 mm in diameter and has a well-demarcated border. A central depression in the lesion results from partial desiccation of tissue. **B,** Extent of radiofrequency lesions (cut surface of specimen in **A**). The lesion outlined by *yellow arrows* was made with a standard electrode (15 W for 30 sec); the lesion outlined by *blue arrows* was made with an irrigated catheter, cooling the tip to allow more power delivery (50 W for 30 sec). The lesion made by the irrigated catheter is more than twice the diameter and 12 times the volume of the standard catheter lesion.

diaphragmatic contraction during transvenous phrenic nerve pacing, have markedly decreased the risk of phrenic damage.

OTHER FORMS OF ABLATION

Laser energy has been used for pulmonary vein isolation and in VT; the wavelengths used cannot penetrate blood and thus the energy must be delivered through a water-filled balloon that is in direct contact with tissue, or blood must be flushed from the endocardial target tissue with saline. Laser energy can be very effective in these applications but the equipment is expensive and remains cumbersome. Pulsed field ablation, in which high energy current is delivered through a variety of electrode designs, can result in irreversible electroporation of target cardiac tissue. This promising technique appears to be capable of causing very focused myocardial damage, destroying heart muscle relatively selectively while almost entirely sparing vascular, esophageal and nerve tissue.[26]

Radiofrequency Catheter Ablation of Accessory Pathways

Location of Pathways

The safety, efficacy, and cost-effectiveness of RF catheter ablation of an accessory AV pathway have made ablation the treatment of choice in most adult and many pediatric patients who have AV reentrant tachycardia (AVRT) or atrial flutter or fibrillation associated with a rapid ventricular response over the accessory pathway (see Chapter 65). When RF energy is delivered to an immature heart, the lesion size can increase as the heart grows; however, this has not been shown to cause problems later in life.

An EPS is performed initially to determine that the accessory pathway is part of the tachycardia circuit or capable of rapid AV conduction during AF and to localize the accessory pathway (the optimal site for ablation). Pathways can exist in the right or left free wall or the septum of the heart (Fig. 64.5). Septal accessory pathways are further classified as superoparaseptal, midseptal, and posterior paraseptal. Pathways classified as posterior paraseptal are posterior to the central fibrous body within the so-called pyramidal space, which is bounded by the posterosuperior process of the left ventricle and the inferomedial aspects of both atria and is behind (posterior to) the true atrial septum. Superoparaseptal pathways are found near the His bundle, and an accessory pathway activation potential as well as a His bundle potential can be recorded simultaneously from a catheter placed at the His bundle region. Midseptal pathways are close to the AV node and can usually be ablated from a right-sided approach; rarely, a left atrial approach is needed. Right posterior paraseptal pathways insert along the tricuspid ring in the vicinity of the coronary sinus ostium, whereas left posterior paraseptal pathways are further into the coronary sinus and may be located at a subepicardial site around the proximal coronary sinus, within a middle cardiac vein or coronary sinus diverticulum, or subendocardially along the ventricular aspect of the mitral annulus.

Pathways at all locations and in all age groups can be ablated successfully. Multiple pathways are present in about 5% of patients. Occasional pathways with epicardial locations may be more easily approached from within the coronary sinus. Rarely, pathways can connect an atrial appendage with adjacent ventricular epicardium, 2 cm or more from the AV groove.

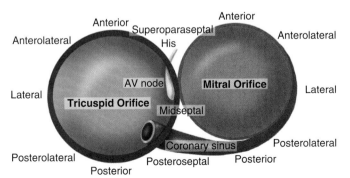

FIGURE 64.5 Locations of accessory pathways by anatomic region. The tricuspid and mitral valve annuli are depicted in a left anterior oblique view. Locations of the coronary sinus, atrioventricular node, and bundle of His are shown. Accessory pathways may connect the atrial to the ventricular myocardium in any of the regions shown.

ABLATION SITE

The optimal ablation site can be found by direct recordings of the accessory pathway (Fig. 64.6), although deflections that mimic accessory pathway potentials can be recorded at other sites. The ventricular insertion site can be determined by finding the site of the earliest onset of the ventricular electrogram in relation to the onset of the delta wave. Other helpful guidelines include unfiltered unipolar recordings that register a QS wave and an accessory pathway signal during preexcitation. A major ventricular potential synchronous with onset of the delta wave can be a target site in left-sided preexcitation, whereas earlier ventricular excitation in relation to the delta wave can be found for right-sided preexcitation. The atrial insertion site of manifest or concealed pathways (i.e., delta wave present or absent, respectively) can be found by locating the site showing the earliest atrial activation during retrograde conduction over

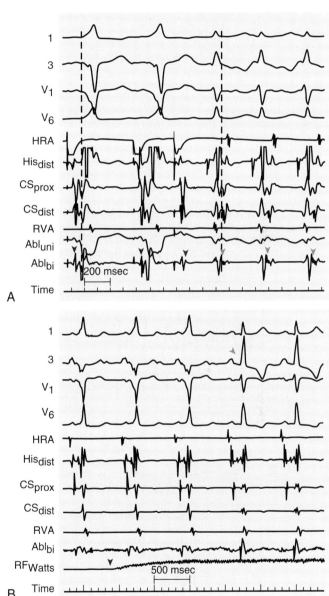

FIGURE 64.6 Wolff-Parkinson-White syndrome. Surface ECG leads 1, 3, V$_1$, and V$_6$ are shown, with intracardiac recordings from high right atrium (HRA), distal His (His$_{dist}$) bundle region, proximal (CS$_{prox}$) and distal (CS$_{dist}$) coronary sinus, right ventricular apex (RVA), and unipolar (Abl$_{uni}$) and bipolar (Abl$_{bi}$) tip electrodes of the ablation catheter. RF power in watts (RF$_{Watts}$) is also shown. **A,** Two beats of atrial pacing are conducted over the accessory pathway (*blue arrowheads* in the Abl$_{bi}$ recording from the site of the accessory pathway) and resulted in a delta wave on the ECG. A premature atrial stimulus *(center)* encounters accessory pathway refractoriness *(red arrowhead)* and instead is conducted over the AV node and bundle of His and resulted in a narrow QRS complex and started an episode of AVRT. After each narrow QRS complex is an atrial deflection, the earliest portion of which is recorded at the ablation site *(green arrowheads)*. **B,** Ablation of this pathway by delivery of RF energy from the ablation catheter tip. The *blue arrowhead* denotes the onset of delivery of RF energy; two QRS complexes later, the delta wave is abruptly lost *(green arrowhead in lead 3)* because of elimination of conduction over the accessory pathway.

the pathway. Reproducible mechanical inhibition of accessory pathway conduction during catheter manipulation and subthreshold stimulation has also been used to determine the optimal site. Accidental catheter trauma should be avoided, however, because it can hide the target for prolonged periods. Right free wall and superoparaseptal pathways are particularly susceptible to catheter trauma.

Left-sided accessory pathways typically cross the mitral annulus obliquely. Consequently, the earliest site of retrograde atrial activation and the earliest site of anterograde ventricular activation are not directly across the AV groove from each other (i.e., ventricular insertion closer to coronary sinus ostium). Identification of the earliest site of atrial activation is usually performed during orthodromic AVRT or relatively rapid ventricular pacing so that retrograde conduction using the AV node does not confuse assessment of the location of the earliest atrial activation.

Successful ablation sites should exhibit anatomic/fluoroscopic stability and consistent electrical characteristics. During sinus rhythm, local ventricular activation at the successful ablation site precedes onset of the delta wave on the ECG by 10 to 35 milliseconds; during orthodromic AVRT, the interval between onset of ventricular activation in any lead and local atrial activation is usually 70 to 90 milliseconds (see Fig. 64.6). When temperature-measuring ablation catheters are used, a stable rise in catheter tip temperature is a helpful indicator of catheter stability and adequate contact between the electrode and tissue. In such a case, tip temperature generally exceeds 50°C. The retrograde transaortic and transseptal approaches have been used with equal success to ablate accessory pathways located along the mitral annulus. Routine performance of an EPS weeks after the ablation procedure is not generally indicated but may be considered in patients who have a recurrent delta wave or symptoms of tachycardia. Catheter-delivered cryoablation can be useful in patients with

septal accessory pathways (located near AV node or His bundle). With use of this system, the catheter tip and adjacent tissue can be reversibly cooled to test a potential site. If accessory pathway conduction fails while normal AV conduction is preserved, deeper cooling can be performed at the site to complete the ablation. If, however, normal AV conduction is worsened, permanent damage is almost always averted by allowing the catheter tip to rewarm quickly.

Atriofascicular accessory pathways have connections consisting of a proximal, AV node–like portion on the atrial side of the annulus, which is responsible for conduction delay and decremental conduction properties, and a long distal segment crossing the annulus and extending along the endocardial surface of the right ventricular free wall, which has electrophysiologic properties similar to those of the right bundle branch. The distal end of the right atriofascicular accessory pathway can insert into the apical region of the right ventricular free wall, close to the distal right bundle branch, or can actually fuse with the latter. Right atriofascicular accessory pathways might represent a duplication of the AV conduction system and can be localized for ablation by recording potentials from the rapidly conducting distal component, which crosses the tricuspid annulus (analogous to the His bundle) and extends to the apical region of the right ventricular free wall. Ablation at such a site on the annulus is usually successful; these pathways are very sensitive to catheter trauma, and the operator must use great care to avoid such trauma (that may eliminate pathway conduction for minutes or hours).

Indications

Ablation of accessory pathways is indicated in patients who have symptomatic AVRT that is drug resistant or who are drug intolerant or do not desire long-term drug therapy. It is also indicated in patients who have AF or other atrial tachyarrhythmias and a rapid ventricular response, by means of an accessory pathway when the tachycardia is drug resistant, or in those who are drug intolerant or do not desire long-term drug therapy. Other potential candidates with an accessory pathway include the following: (1) patients with AVRT or AF with rapid ventricular rates identified during an EPS for another arrhythmia; (2) asymptomatic patients with ventricular preexcitation whose livelihood, profession, important activities, insurability, or mental well-being and the public safety would be affected by spontaneous tachyarrhythmias or by the presence of the electrocardiographic abnormality; (3) patients with AF and a controlled ventricular response by means of the accessory pathway; and (4) patients with asymptomatic preexcitation and a family history of sudden cardiac death. Controversy remains whether all patients with accessory pathways (even those without symptoms) need treatment; however, ablation has such a high success rate and low complication rate that in most centers, patients who need any form of therapy are referred for catheter ablation.

Results

Currently, in the hands of an experienced operator, the success rate for accessory pathway ablation is greater than 95% (slightly less for right free wall pathways, in which stable catheter-tissue contact is more problematic), with a 2% recurrence rate after an apparently successful procedure. There is a 1% to 2% complication rate, including bleeding, vascular damage, myocardial perforation with cardiac tamponade, valve damage, stroke, and MI. Heart block occurs in less than 3% of septal pathways. Procedure-related death is very rare.

Radiofrequency Catheter Modification of AV Node for AV Nodal Reentrant Tachycardias

AV node reentry is a common cause of SVT episodes (see Chapters 62 and 65). Although controversy still exists about the exact nature of the tachycardia circuit, abundant evidence has indicated that two pathways in the region of the AV node participate, one with relatively fast conduction but long refractoriness and the other with shorter refractoriness but slower conduction. Premature atrial complexes can encounter refractoriness in the fast pathway, conduct over the slow pathway, and reenter the fast pathway retrogradely, thereby initiating AV nodal reentrant SVT (Fig. 64.7). Although this is the most common manifestation of

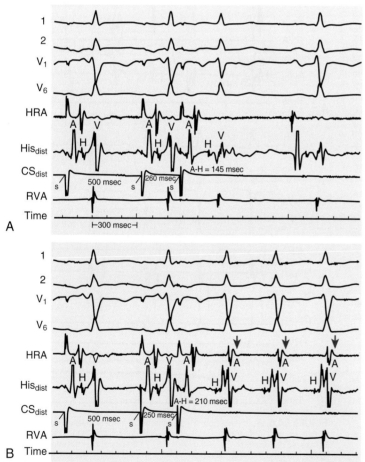

FIGURE 64.7 Atrioventricular node reentry. **A,** Two atrial paced complexes from the coronary sinus (CS) are followed by an atrial premature stimulus at a coupling interval of 260 milliseconds and resulted in an A-H interval of 145 milliseconds. **B,** The same atrial drive train is followed by an atrial extrastimulus 10 milliseconds earlier than before (250 milliseconds). This resulted in a marked increase in the A-H interval to 210 milliseconds, after which atrioventricular (AV) nodal reentrant tachycardia ensues because the extrastimulus encounters block in a "fast" AV node pathway, conducts down a "slow" pathway, and then conducts back up the fast pathway in a repeating fashion. *Red arrowheads* denote atrial electrograms coincident with QRS complexes, characteristic of the most common type of AV node reentry. Recording was done as in the previous figure.

AV node reentry, some patients have what appears to be propagation in the opposite direction in this circuit (anterograde fast, retrograde slow), as well as a "slow-slow" variant. Other, much less common types have been described. Two or more of these variants can exist in the same patient (Fig. 64.8).

FAST PATHWAY ABLATION
Ablation can be performed to eliminate conduction in the fast pathway or the slow pathway. Currently, fast pathway ablation is rarely performed because it is associated with a prolonged PR interval, a higher recurrence rate (10% to 15%), and a slightly higher risk for complete

AV block (2% to 5%) than with slow pathway ablation. One uncommon situation in which fast pathway ablation may be preferred is for patients who have a greatly prolonged PR interval at rest and no evidence of anterograde fast pathway conduction. In such patients, ablation of the anterograde slow pathway may produce complete AV block, whereas retrograde fast pathway ablation can eliminate SVT without altering AV conduction.

SLOW PATHWAY ABLATION
The slow pathway can be located by mapping along the posteromedial tricuspid annulus close to the coronary sinus os. Electrographic recordings are obtained with an atrial-to-ventricular electrogram ratio of less than 0.5 and either a multicomponent atrial electrogram or a recording consistent with a possible slow pathway potential. In the anatomic approach, target sites are selected fluoroscopically. A single RF application eliminates slow pathway conduction in many cases, but in others, serial RF applications may be needed, starting at the most posterior site (near the coronary sinus os) and progressing along the tricuspid annulus more anteriorly. An accelerated junctional rhythm usually occurs when RF energy is applied at a site that will result in successful elimination of SVT (Fig. 64.9). The success rate is equivalent with the anatomic and electrographic mapping approaches, and most often, combinations of both are used and yield success rates of greater than 95%, with less than a 1% chance of complete heart block.[27] Catheter-delivered cryoablation has been used for the treatment of AVNRT with excellent results and is considered by some to be safer than RF (less chance of permanent AV block) but in most series has a somewhat higher rate of SVT recurrence after apparent successful ablation.

Patients in whom slow pathway conduction is completely eliminated almost never have recurrent SVT episodes. Approximately 40% of patients can have evidence of residual slow pathway function after successful elimination of sustained AVNRT, usually manifested as persistent dual AV node physiology and single AV node echoes during atrial extrastimulation. The surest endpoint for slow pathway ablation is elimination of sustained AVNRT, with and without an infusion of isoproterenol or epinephrine.

AVNRT recurs in approximately 5% of patients after slow pathway ablation; repeat ablation is almost always successful. In some patients the ERP of the fast pathway decreases after slow pathway ablation, possibly because of eliminating electrotonic interaction between the two pathways. Atypical forms of reentry can result after ablation, as can apparent parasympathetic denervation, and result in inappropriate sinus tachycardia. This usually resolves within 3 months after ablation.

At present, the slow pathway approach is the preferred method for ablation of typical AVNRT. Ablation of the slow pathway is also a safe and effective means for the treatment of atypical forms of AVNRT. In patients with AVNRT undergoing slow pathway ablation, junctional ectopy during application of the RF energy is a sensitive but nonspecific marker of successful ablation; it occurs in longer bursts at effective than at ineffective target sites. Ventriculoatrial conduction should be expected during the junctional ectopy, and poor ventriculoatrial conduction or actual block may herald subsequent anterograde AV block. Junctional ectopic rhythm is caused by heating of the AV node and does not occur with cryoablation.

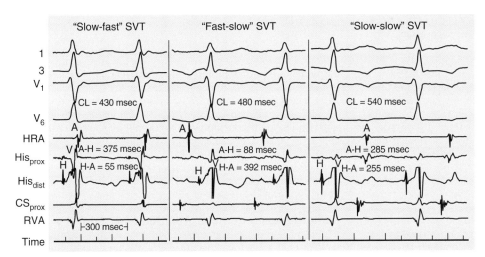

FIGURE 64.8 Three variants of atrioventricular (AV) node reentrant supraventricular tachycardia (SVT) in the same patient. **Left,** Most common type of AV node SVT (anterograde slow pathway, retrograde fast). Atrial activation is coincident with ventricular activation. **Center,** "Atypical" AV node reentry with anterograde fast pathway conduction and retrograde conduction over a slow pathway. **Right,** A rare variety is shown that consists of anterograde conduction over a slow pathway and retrograde conduction over a second slow pathway. Note the similar atrial activation sequences in the last two (coronary sinus before the right atrium), as distinct from that of slow-fast AV node reentry (coronary sinus and right atrial activation almost simultaneous). Note also the different P-QRS relationships, from simultaneous activation (left, short RP interval) to P in front of the QRS (middle, long RP interval) and P midway in the cardiac cycle (right). Recording was done as in previous figures. *CL,* Cycle length.

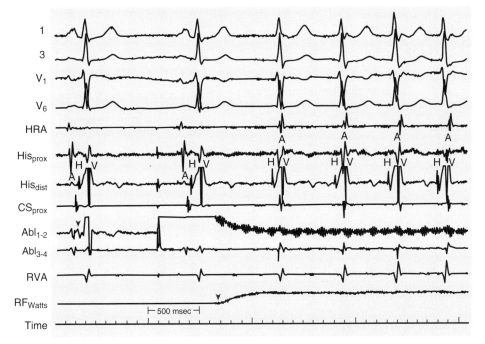

FIGURE 64.9 Atrioventricular node slow pathway modification for cure of atrioventricular (AV) node reentrant supraventricular tachycardia. The ablation recording (*arrowhead* in Abl$_{1-2}$) shows a slurred deflection between the atrial and ventricular electrogram components; this may represent the AV node slow pathway deflection (but it is not the bundle of His deflection, which is instead recorded from a separate catheter 15 mm away). Shortly after the onset of radiofrequency delivery (*arrowhead* in RF$_{Watts}$), an accelerated junctional rhythm begins and gradually speeds up further. Retrograde conduction is present during the junctional rhythm. *Abl$_{3-4}$,* Proximal electrode recording from ablation catheter.

Indications

RF catheter ablation for AVNRT can be considered in patients with recurrent, symptomatic, sustained AVNRT that is drug resistant or who are drug intolerant or do not desire long-term drug treatment. The procedure can also be considered for patients with sustained AVNRT identified during EPS or catheter ablation of another arrhythmia, or when EPS reveals dual–AV node pathway physiology and atrial echoes but without AVNRT in patients with suspected AVNRT clinically.

Results

Most centers currently use slow pathway ablation, which results in a procedural success rate of 98%, a recurrence rate of less than 5%, and an incidence of heart block requiring permanent pacing of 1% or less. Late development of heart block (months to years later) is rare.

Junctional Tachycardia

Junctional tachycardia, often called ectopic junctional tachycardia (although if the location is junctional, by definition it is ectopic) is a rare form of SVT in which the ECG resembles that in AVNRT but is distinct in that (1) the mechanism is automatic, not reentrant, and (2) the atrium is clearly not involved in the tachycardia. This disorder is most often observed in young healthy individuals, in women more often than in men, and is usually catecholamine dependent. Ablation must be carried out close to the His bundle, and the risk for heart block requiring pacemaker insertion exceeds 5%.

Radiofrequency Catheter Ablation of Arrhythmias Related to the Sinus Node

Inappropriate sinus tachycardia is a syndrome characterized by high sinus rates with exercise and at rest. Patients complain of palpitations at all times of day that correlate with inappropriately high sinus rates. They may not respond well to beta-blocker therapy because of lack of desired effect or occurrence of side effects. Ivabradine, which blocks I_f (principal pacemaker current in sinus node) is indicated for treatment of heart failure but has been used with some success in patients with inappropriate sinus tachycardia.[28] When the sinus node area is to be ablated because of drug-refractory symptoms, it can be identified anatomically and electrophysiologically, and ablative lesions are usually placed between the superior vena cava and crista terminalis at sites of early atrial activation. Intracardiac echocardiography can help in defining the anatomy and in positioning the ablation catheter. Isoproterenol may be helpful in "forcing" the site of impulse formation to cells with the most rapid discharge rate. Care must be taken to apply RF energy at the most cephalad sites

first; initial ablation performed farther down the crista terminalis does not alter the atrial rate at the time but can damage any subsidiary pacemaker regions that may be needed after the sinus node has eventually been ablated.

Indications

Patients with *persistent* inappropriate sinus tachycardia should be considered for ablation only after clear failure of medical therapy, because the results of ablation are often less than completely satisfactory. Whenever ablation is performed in the region of the sinus node, the patient should be apprised of the chance of needing a pacemaker after the procedure. Phrenic nerve damage and superior vena caval stenosis are also possibilities.

Results

Although a good technical result may be obtained at the time of the procedure for inappropriate sinus tachycardia, symptoms often persist because of recurrence of rapid sinus rates (at or near preablation rates) or for nonarrhythmic reasons. In some, after the atrial rate decreases, an inappropriately rapid junctional rhythm (80 to 90/min) is present; this may indicate an overall increased sensitivity of cells with pacemaker capacity to catecholamines in these patients. Multiple ablation sessions are needed in some patients, and approximately 20% eventually undergo pacemaker implantation; however, not all these patients have relief of symptoms, including palpitations, despite a normal heart rate.

Radiofrequency Catheter Ablation of Atrial Tachycardia

ATs are a heterogeneous group of disorders; causative factors include rapid discharge of a focus (focal tachycardia) and reentry. The former can occur in anyone, regardless of the presence of structural abnormalities of the atria, whereas reentrant ATs almost always occur in the setting of structurally damaged atria. Symptoms vary from none, with relatively infrequent or slow ATs in patients without heart disease, to syncope (rapid AT with compromised cardiac function) or heart failure (incessant AT over weeks or months). All forms of AT are amenable to catheter ablation (see Chapter 65).

FOCAL ATRIAL TACHYCARDIA

In focal ATs (automatic or triggered foci or microreentry), activation mapping is used to determine the source of the AT by recording the earliest onset of local activation. These tachycardias can behave capriciously and can be practically noninducible during EPS despite the patient complaining of multiple daily episodes before the EPS. Approximately 10% of patients can have multiple atrial foci. Sites tend to cluster near the pulmonary veins in the left atrium and the mouths of the atrial appendages and along the right atrial crista terminalis (Figs. 64.10A, 64.11, and 64.12). Activation times at these sites typically occur only 15 to 40 milliseconds before onset of the P wave on the ECG. Care must be taken to avoid inadvertent damage to the phrenic nerve (see Fig. 64.12); its location can be determined by pacing at high current at a candidate site of ablation while observing for diaphragmatic contraction. Ablation should not be performed at a site at which this is seen, if at all possible.

REENTRANT ATRIAL TACHYCARDIA

As noted, these ATs usually occur in the setting of structural heart disease, especially after previous surgery involving an atrial incision (repair of congenital heart disease such as an atrial septal defect, Mustard or Senning repair of transposed great vessels, or one of a variety of Fontan repairs for tricuspid atresia and other disorders), or previous atrial ablation (e.g., for AF). The region of slow conduction is typically related to an end of an atriotomy or previous ablation scar, the location of

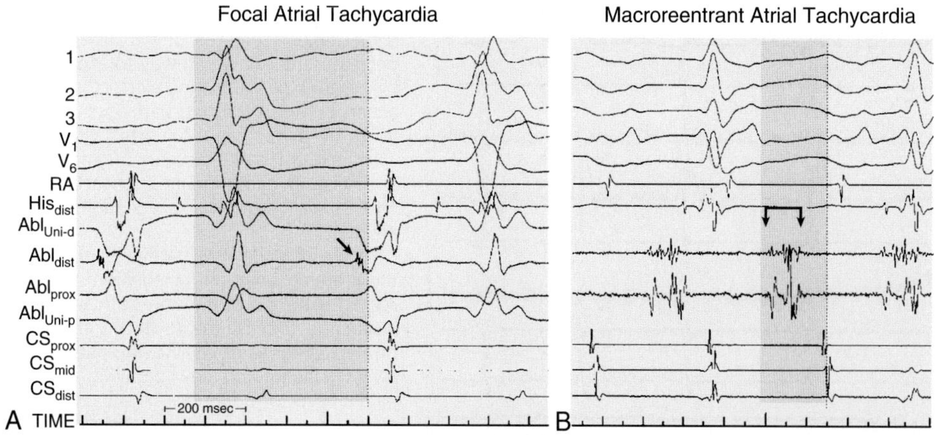

Focal Atrial Tachycardia   Macroreentrant Atrial Tachycardia

FIGURE 64.10 Atrial tachycardia. In both panels the interval from the end of one P wave to the beginning of the next (atrial diastole) is in *gray*. A *dashed line* denotes onset of the P wave during tachycardia. **A,** Focal atrial tachycardia (AT) arising in the right atrium. Two tachycardia complexes are shown; the earliest site found (Abl$_{dist}$, at which ablation eliminated the tachycardia) is shown as a multicomponent recording that starts only approximately 40 milliseconds before onset of the P wave. The unipolar recording (Abl$_{Uni-d}$) has a deep negative deflection (indicating propagation away from the electrode). The activation sequence of recordings is very different from that during sinus rhythm, in which the right atrial (RA) recording is at the onset of the P wave. **B,** Macroreentrant AT in a patient who had undergone repair of an atrial septal defect years earlier. The ablation catheter is in the posterior right atrium, where a fragmented signal (between *arrows*) is recorded that almost fills atrial diastole. Ablation at this site terminated the tachycardia.

which varies from patient to patient. Therefore, preprocedural review of operative and ablation procedure reports and careful electrophysiologic mapping are essential. Because reentry within a complete circuit is occurring, activation can be recorded throughout the entire cardiac cycle. The ablation strategy is to identify regions with mid-diastolic atrial activation during tachycardia (see Fig. 64.10B) that can be proved by pacing techniques to be integral to the tachycardia. Such sites are attractive ablation targets because they are composed of relatively few cells—thus electrical silence on the surface ECG in atrial diastole—and so are more easily eliminated by the small amount of damage effected by a typical application of RF energy. Focal ablation of these sites can then be performed, but often tachycardia can still be initiated (usually at a slower rate) or recurs after the procedure. Because these sites are typically located at a relatively narrow zone between the ends of previous scars, surgical incisions, or ablation lines and another nonconducting barrier (e.g., another scar, caval orifice, valve annulus), a line of ablative lesions is generally made from the end of the scar to the nearest electrical barrier; thus reentry can be prevented (Video 64.1). This technique is analogous to that used in curing atrial flutter (see later). Because these patients frequently have extensive atrial disease with islands of scar that could serve as barriers for additional ATs, specialized mapping techniques may be needed to locate these regions and preemptively connect them with ablative lesions to prevent future AT episodes.

Indications

Catheter ablation for ATs should be considered in patients who have recurrent episodes of symptomatic sustained ATs that are drug resistant, or who are drug intolerant or do not desire long-term drug treatment.

Results

Success rates for ablation of focal AT range from 80% to 95%, largely depending on the ability to induce episodes at EPS. When episodes can be initiated with pacing, isoproterenol, or other means, the AT can usually be ablated. Reentrant ATs, although more readily induced by an EPS, are often more difficult to eliminate completely; initial success rates are high (90%), but recurrences are seen in up to 20% of patients and necessitate drug therapy or another ablation procedure. Complications, which occur in 1% to 2% of patients, include phrenic nerve damage, cardiac tamponade, and heart block (with rare perinodal ATs).

Radiofrequency Catheter Ablation of Atrial Flutter

Atrial flutter can be defined electrocardiographically (most typically, negative sawtooth waves in leads II, III, and aVF at a rate of approximately 300 beats/min) or electrophysiologically (rapid, organized macroreentrant AT, the circuit for which is anatomically determined). Understanding of the reentrant pathway in all forms of atrial flutter is essential for development of an ablation strategy (see Chapter 65).

Reentry in the right atrium, with the left atrium passively activated, constitutes the mechanism of the typical electrocardiographic variety of atrial flutter, with caudocranial activation along the right atrial septum and craniocaudal activation of the right atrial free wall (Fig. 64.13A). Ablating tissue in a line between any two anatomic barriers that transects a portion of the circuit necessary for perpetuation of reentry can be curative. Typically, this is across the isthmus of atrial tissue between the inferior vena caval orifice and the tricuspid annulus (the cavotricuspid isthmus), a relatively narrow point in the circuit. Locations for RF delivery can be guided anatomically or electrophysiologically. Less frequently, the direction of wavefront propagation in this large right atrial circuit is reversed ("clockwise" flutter proceeding cephalad up the right atrial free wall and caudad down the septum, with upright flutter waves in the inferior leads; Fig. 64.13A, left panel). These two arrhythmias constitute cavotricuspid isthmus–dependent flutter, that can be ablated by cavotricuspid isthmus interruption, and are distinct from other rapid atrial arrhythmias that may have a similar appearance on the ECG but use different (and often multiple) circuits in other parts of the right or left atrium. Ablation can be more difficult in these cases, which often occur in the setting of advanced lung disease or previous cardiac surgery or ablation. A common theme in these complex reentrant arrhythmias is the presence of an anatomically determined zone of

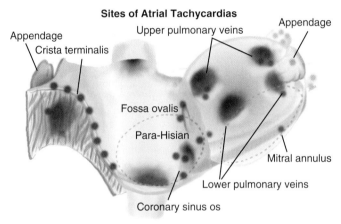

Sites of Atrial Tachycardias

FIGURE 64.11 Locations of origins of focal atrial tachycardias. The atria are viewed from the front with the right atrial free wall retracted to show the interior. Structures are labeled as shown; right atrial foci appear in shades of *blue*, left atrial foci in shades of *red*.

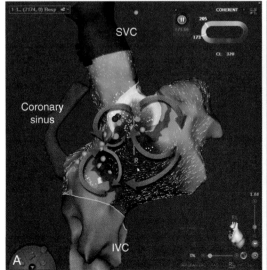
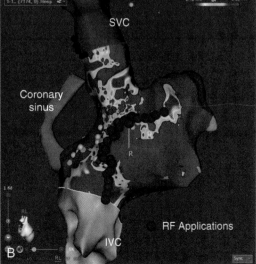

FIGURE 64.12 Reentrant atrial tachycardia. **A,** Electroanatomic activation map of the right atrium is shown in a patient with a previous right atrial incision for closure of an atrial septal defect. *Orange arrows* depict a complex double loop of reentry around presumed scars with a common diastolic pathway between scars. *Small white arrows* depict the vectoral direction of activation during tachycardia. The *color bar* shows progression of activation times during AT (from *red* through *green*, *blue*, and *purple*). The tachycardia cycle length (320 msec) is entirely represented in the range of colors. **B,** *Red dots* denote ablation sites connecting scars (transecting diastolic pathway) and connecting one scar to the *IVC* to preclude reentry around all barriers. *SVC*, superior vena cava; *IVC*, inferior vena cava.

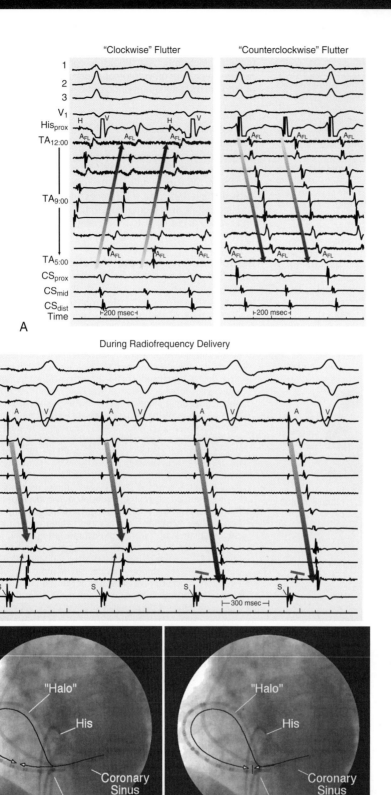

FIGURE 64.13 A, Two forms of atrial flutter in the same patient are shown. A halo catheter with 10 electrode pairs is situated on the atrial side of the tricuspid annulus *(TA),* with recording sites displayed from the top of the annulus (12:00) to the inferomedial aspect (5:00), as shown in the fluoroscopic views in **B.** *Left,* the wavefront of atrial activation proceeds in a clockwise fashion *(arrows)* along the annulus. *Right,* the direction of propagation is the reverse. **B,** Ablation of the isthmus of atrial tissue between the tricuspid annulus and the inferior vena caval orifice for cure of atrial flutter. Recordings are displayed from the multipolar catheter around much of the circumference of the tricuspid annulus (see the left anterior oblique fluoroscopic images). Ablation of this isthmus is performed during coronary sinus pacing. In the two beats on the **left,** atrial conduction proceeds in two directions around the tricuspid annulus, as indicated by arrows and recorded along the halo catheter. In the two beats on the **right,** ablation has interrupted conduction in the floor of the right atrium, thereby eliminating one path for transmission along the tricuspid annulus. The halo catheter now records conduction, proceeding all the way around the annulus. This finding demonstrates a unidirectional block in the isthmus; block in the other direction may be demonstrated by pacing from one of the halo electrodes and observing a similar lack of isthmus conduction. The bundle of His recording in **A** *(right panel)* is lost because of catheter movement.

inexcitability around which an electrical wavefront can circulate. Specialized mapping tools and skills are necessary to achieve successful ablation in these cases.

In patients with AF, an AAD can slow intraatrial conduction to such an extent that atrial flutter results and fibrillation is no longer observed. In some of these patients, ablation of atrial flutter and continued AAD therapy can prevent recurrences of these atrial arrhythmias.

The endpoint of atrial flutter ablation procedures was initially termination of atrial flutter with RF application, accompanied by noninducibility of the arrhythmia. However, with use of these criteria, up to 30% of patients had recurrent flutter because of lack of complete and permanent conduction block in the cavotricuspid isthmus. Thus, the current endpoint of ablation has changed to ensuring a line of bidirectional block is present in this region, usually by pacing from opposite sides of the isthmus (see Fig. 64.13B). With use of these criteria, recurrence rates have fallen to less than 5%.

Indications

Candidates for RF catheter ablation include patients with recurrent episodes of atrial flutter that are drug resistant, those who are drug intolerant, and those who do not desire long-term drug therapy. Many patients who undergo AF ablation (see Chapter 66) also have episodes of flutter during the procedure that can be treated by ablation of the cavotricuspid isthmus at the same setting.

Results

Regardless of circuit location, atrial flutter can be ablated successfully in more than 90% of cases, although patients with complex right or left atrial flutter require more extensive and complex procedures. Recurrence rates are less than 5% except in patients with extensive atrial disease, in whom new circuits can develop over time as new areas of conduction delay and block form. Complications are rare and include inadvertent heart block and phrenic nerve paralysis.

Ablation and Modification of Atrioventricular Conduction for Atrial Tachyarrhythmias

In some patients who have rapid ventricular rates despite optimal drug therapy during complex atrial tachyarrhythmias that are less amenable to ablation, RF ablation can be used to eliminate or modify AV conduction and control the ventricular rates.

To achieve this, a catheter is placed across the tricuspid valve and positioned to record a small His bundle electrogram associated with a large atrial electrogram. RF energy is applied until complete AV block has been achieved and is continued for an additional 30 to 60 seconds (Fig. 64.14). If no change in AV conduction is observed after 15 seconds of RF ablation despite good contact, the catheter is repositioned and the attempt repeated. In occasional patients, attempts at RF ablation via this right-sided approach fail to achieve heart block. These patients can undergo an attempt from

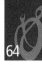

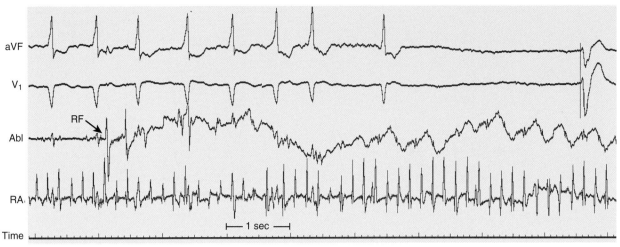

FIGURE 64.14 Atrioventricular nodal ablation for rate control of atrial fibrillation (AF). The ECG shows rapidly conducted AF; application of radiofrequency *(RF)* energy *(arrow)* results in complete AV block within seconds, followed by a ventricular paced complex.

the left ventricle with a catheter positioned along the interventricular septum, just beneath the aortic valve, to record a large His bundle electrogram. Success rates currently approach 100%, with AV conduction recurring in less than 5% of cases. Improved left ventricular function can result from control of the ventricular rate during AF and withdrawal of rate-controlling medications that have negative inotropic action. Permanent right, His bundle or biventricular pacing is typically required after ablation. With continuing advances in direct ablation of complex atrial arrhythmias, AV nodal ablation is less often used currently except in elderly patients. Whereas in some cases the AV junction can be modified to slow the ventricular rate without producing complete AV block by ablation in the region of the slow pathway (as described with AV node modification for AV node reentry), this strategy has been almost entirely abandoned due to poor predictability of long-term outcome despite good acute results.

Indications

Ablation and modification of AV conduction can be considered in the following cases: (1) patients with symptomatic atrial tachyarrhythmias who have inadequately controlled ventricular rates, unless primary ablation of the atrial tachyarrhythmia is possible (especially when a permanent pacemaker is already present for treatment of bradycardia-tachycardia syndrome); (2) similar patients when drugs are not tolerated or patients do not choose to take them, even though the ventricular rate can be controlled; (3) patients with symptomatic, nonparoxysmal junctional tachycardia that is drug resistant or in whom drugs are not tolerated or are not desired; (4) patients resuscitated from sudden cardiac death related to atrial flutter or AF with a rapid ventricular response in the absence of an accessory pathway; and (5) patients with a dual-chamber pacemaker and pacemaker-mediated tachycardia that cannot be treated effectively by drugs or reprogramming of the pacemaker. The last three situations are rarely encountered.

Results

As previously noted, successful interruption of AV conduction can be achieved in almost all cases; recurrent conduction is observed in less than 5%. Significant complications occur in 1% to 2%. In early studies, up to 4% of patients had an episode of sudden death after AV junction ablation despite adequate pacemaker function, presumably because of relative bradycardia after long periods of rapid ventricular rates serving as the setting for repolarization-related ventricular arrhythmias. Since then, backup pacing rates are set to 80 to 90/min for the first 1 to 3 months after ablation in most cases, which has almost entirely eliminated this problem. Improvements in quality-of-life indices, as well as in cost-effectiveness, have been demonstrated for this procedure.

Radiofrequency Catheter Ablation of Atrial Fibrillation
See Chapters 65 and 66.

Radiofrequency Catheter Ablation of Ventricular Arrhythmias (see Chapter 67)

In general, the success rate for ablation of VTs is lower than that for AV node reentry or AV reentry because of the heterogeneity of substrates and presentations. In the ideal case, induction of the VT must be reproducible, with uniform QRS morphology from beat to beat, and VT must be sustained and hemodynamically stable so that the patient can tolerate the VT long enough during the procedure to undergo the extensive mapping necessary to localize optimal ablation target sites. These conditions are often not met. Patients with several electrocardiographically distinct, uniform morphologies of VT can still be candidates for ablation, because in many cases a common reentrant pathway is shared by two or more VT morphologies. Also, the target for ablation must be fairly circumscribed and preferably endocardially situated, although catheter mapping and ablation from the epicardial surface after percutaneous pericardial access is performed in many centers. Very rapid VT, polymorphic VT, and infrequent, nonsustained VT can be addressed with catheter ablation using different strategies.

LOCATION AND ABLATION

RF catheter ablation of VT can be divided into idiopathic VT, which occurs in patients with essentially structurally normal hearts and includes patients with isolated PVCs; VT that occurs in various disease settings but without CAD; and VT in patients with CAD and usually previous MI. In the first group, VTs/PVCs can arise in either ventricle. Right VTs most frequently originate in the outflow tract and have a characteristic left bundle branch block–like, inferior axis morphology (see Chapter 67); less often, VTs/PVCs arise in the inflow tract or free wall. Initiation of tachycardia can often be facilitated by catecholamines. Most left VTs in structurally normal hearts are septal in origin and have a characteristic QRS configuration (i.e., right bundle branch block, superior axis). Other VTs/PVCs also occur and arise from different areas of the left ventricle, including the left ventricular outflow region and the aortic sinuses of Valsalva, and are similar in electrocardiographic appearance and clinical behavior to those arising in the right ventricular outflow tract. VTs in abnormal hearts without CAD can be the result of either intramyocardial or bundle branch reentry, most often observed in patients with dilated cardiomyopathy, or as a focal process. Epicardial foci and circuits are more common in this than in other groups. In patients with bundle branch reentry, ablation of the right bundle branch eliminates the tachycardia. VT can occur in patients with right ventricular dysplasia (see Chapter 63), sarcoidosis, Chagas disease, hypertrophic cardiomyopathy (see Chapters 52 to 54), and a host of other noncoronary disease states.

Activation mapping and pace mapping are effective in patients with idiopathic VTs/PVCs to locate the site of origin of the VT. In *activation mapping* the timing of endocardial electrograms sampled by the mapping catheter as it is moved around the chamber is compared with the onset of the surface QRS complex. Sites that are activated 20 to 40 milliseconds before onset of the surface QRS are near the origin of the arrhythmia. In idiopathic VT/PVCs, ablation at a site at which the unipolar

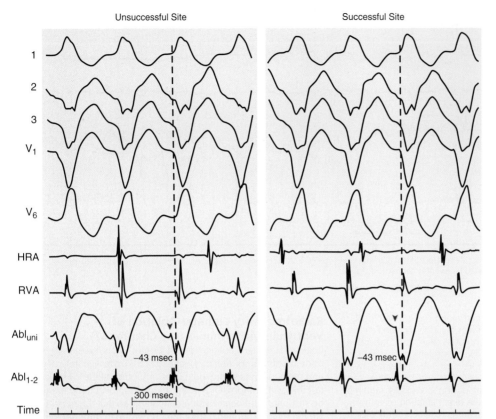

FIGURE 64.15 Recordings from unsuccessful and successful ablation sites in a patient with idiopathic ventricular tachycardia arising in the inferior right ventricular wall. In the recordings from the unsuccessful ablation site, the unipolar signal (*arrowhead*) has a small r wave, which indicates that a portion of the wavefront from the focus of tachycardia is approaching the site from elsewhere. At the successful site, the unipolar recording has a QS configuration, thus indicating that all depolarization is emanating from this site. In each site the bipolar recording (Abl$_{1-2}$) occurs an identical 43 milliseconds before onset of the QRS (*dashed lines*).

electrogram shows a QS complex may yield greater success than if an rS potential is observed (Fig. 64.15). *Pace mapping* involves stimulation of various ventricular sites to produce a QRS contour that duplicates the QRS contour of the spontaneous VT or PVC, thus establishing the apparent site of origin of the arrhythmia (Fig. 64.16). This technique is limited by several methodologic problems but may be useful when the arrhythmia cannot be initiated and when a 12-lead ECG has been obtained during spontaneous episodes. Presystolic Purkinje potentials, as well as very-low-amplitude mid-diastolic signals, can be recorded during VT from sites at which ablation cures VT in most patients with left ventricular VTs that have a right bundle branch block superior axis; this VT characteristically terminates with IV verapamil and is the only significant idiopathic VT with a reentrant basis. Localization of optimal ablation sites for VT in patients with CAD and previous MI can be more challenging than in patients with structurally normal hearts because of the altered anatomy and electrophysiology. Pace mapping has a lower sensitivity and specificity than for idiopathic VT. Furthermore, reentry circuits can sometimes be large and resistant to the relatively small lesions produced by RF catheter ablation in scarred endocardium.

In scar-based VT (e.g., after MI, cardiomyopathies), finding a protected region of diastolic activation used as a critical part of the reentrant circuit is desirable because ablation at this site has a good chance of eliminating the tachycardia (Fig. 64.17). As a result of the extensive derangement in electrophysiology caused by the previous damage (e.g., infarct, myopathy), many areas of the ventricle may have diastolic activation but may not be relevant to perpetuation of the VT. These "bystander sites" make activation mapping more difficult. Pacing techniques such as entrainment can be used to test whether a site is actually part of a circuit or is a bystander. *Entrainment* involves pacing for several complexes during a tachycardia at a rate slightly faster than the VT rate; after pacing is stopped and the same tachycardia resumes, the timing of the first complex relative to the last paced beat is an indicator of how close the pacing site is to a part of the VT circuit (Fig. 64.18). During entrainment, part of the ventricle is activated by the paced wavefront and part by the VT wavefront being forced to exit earlier than it normally would, thereby resulting in a fusion complex on the ECG. Pacing

from within a critical portion of the circuit itself produces an exact QRS match with the VT; fusion occurs only within the circuit and is "concealed" (not evident on the surface ECG). Sites with a low-amplitude, isolated, mid-diastolic potential that cannot be dissociated from the tachycardia by pacing perturbations, at which entrainment with concealed fusion can be demonstrated, are highly likely to be successful ablation sites.

In a significant proportion of patients with VT and structural heart disease, activation mapping and entrainment cannot be performed because of poor hemodynamic tolerance of the arrhythmia or inability to initiate sustained tachycardia during an EPS. In these situations, additional methods can be used that are categorized as *substrate mapping,* in which areas of low electrical voltage or from which very delayed potentials are recorded during sinus rhythm, or at which pacing closely replicates a known VT 12-lead ECG morphology (pace mapping) are targeted for ablation without needing any mapping during VT (Fig. 64.19). Other strategies include searching for and eliminating possible conduction channels within scar tissue, homogenization of scar tissue, or surrounding the arrhythmogenic zone with RF applications to isolate this "core." These methods, usually requiring very extensive ablation in diseased areas, have yielded very good results in many cases. In other patients, hemodynamic support in the form of catecholamine infusion, intra-aortic balloon counterpulsation, or a percutaneous temporary ventricular assist device or extracorporeal membrane oxygenation has been used to facilitate activation mapping during VT.

In patients without structural heart disease, only a single VT is usually present, and catheter ablation of that VT is most often curative. In patients with extensive structural heart disease, multiple VTs are usually present. Most of these patients already have, or soon will have, an ICD; ablation can be used to decrease the frequency of ICD therapies but is generally not intended to cure the patient of all ventricular arrhythmias. Catheter ablation of a single VT in such patients may be only palliative and may not eliminate the need for further AAD or device therapy, but can improve quality of life by decreasing ICD shocks. The genesis of multiple tachycardia morphologies is not clear, although in some cases they are merely different manifestations of one circuit (e.g., different directions of wavefront propagation or exit to the ventricle as a whole), and ablation of one may prevent recurrence of others. The presence of multiple VT morphologies contributes to the difficulties in mapping and ablation of VT in these patients, because pacing techniques used to validate recordings at potential sites of ablation may result in a change in morphology to another VT that may not arise in the same region.

After ablation of VT, ventricular stimulation is repeated to assess efficacy. In some cases, rapid polymorphic VT or VF is initiated. The clinical significance of these arrhythmias is unclear, but some evidence has suggested that they have a low likelihood of spontaneous occurrence during follow-up.

As noted earlier, most cases of polymorphic VT and VF are not currently amenable to standard ablation methods because of hemodynamic instability and beat-to-beat changes in activation sequence. However, some cases appear to have a focal source (similar to the focal sources of AF), and if the focus can be identified and ablated, further arrhythmia episodes can be prevented. In such cases, repeated episodes of arrhythmia have constant electrocardiographic features of the initiating beat or beats, thus suggesting a consistent source, which may be in either ventricle. The electrogram at sites of successful ablation often has very sharp presystolic potentials reminiscent of Purkinje potentials, with a 50- to 100-millisecond delay until onset of the QRS (Fig. 64.20).[29] In some cases of VF, "rotors" (sites of rapid circulation within a small region)

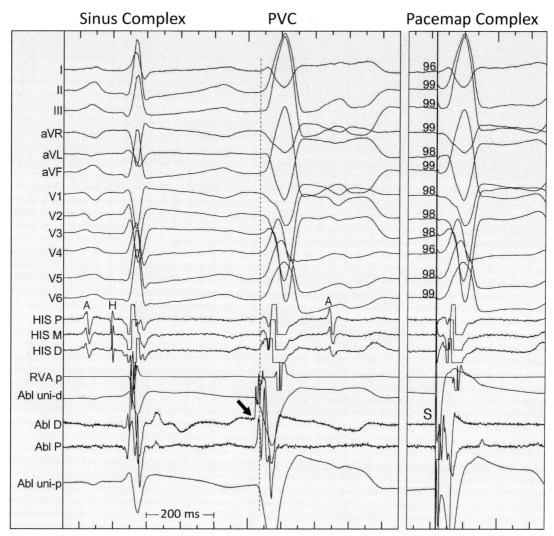

FIGURE 64.16 Premature ventricular complex (PVC) and pace mapping. All 12 surface ECG leads are shown, along with intracardiac recordings in sinus rhythm, a spontaneous PVC, and pacing (S) at the site of Abl D (distal recordings of ablation catheter). The Abl D recording shows a sharp deflection *(arrow)* occurring about 25 milliseconds before onset of the QRS *(dashed line)*. In the **right panel,** pacing is performed from this site. This produces an identical QRS complex in each lead, with a short stimulus–QRS interval; numbers indicate percentage of "match" between PVC and paced QRS complexes using an algorithm in the recording system. Ablation at this site eliminated VT in 2 seconds. *uni*, Unipolar recording; *A*, atrial electrogram; *H*, His electrogram.

have been reported, ablation of which has prevented recurrences (similar to the case with AF). This work is promising but preliminary.

Indications

Patients considered for RF catheter ablation of VT in the absence of structural heart disease are those with symptomatic, sustained monomorphic VT when the tachycardia is drug resistant, when the patient is drug intolerant, or when the patient does not desire long-term drug therapy. Patients with structural heart disease who are candidates for ablation include those with bundle branch reentrant VT and those with sustained monomorphic VT and an ICD who are receiving multiple shocks not manageable by reprogramming or concomitant drug therapy. In some patients (usually without structural heart disease, but also in patients with diseased ventricles), nonsustained VT or even severely symptomatic PVCs warrant RF catheter ablation. In some of these patients, in whom the ventricular ectopy occurs frequently, significant left ventricular systolic dysfunction has occurred (presumably similar to tachycardia-related cardiomyopathy). After successful ablation, ventricular function may improve significantly or even normalize.

Results

In patients with structurally normal hearts, the success rate of VT or PVC ablation is approximately 85%.[30] In patients with postinfarction VT, more than 70% no longer have recurrences of VT after the ablation procedure

despite inducibility of rapid VT or VF; only approximately 30% of patients will have no inducible ventricular arrhythmia of any type and no spontaneous recurrences. As noted earlier, most of these patients already have, or will have, an ICD as backup. Significant complications occur in up to 3%, including vascular damage, heart block, worsening of heart failure, cardiac tamponade, stroke, and valve damage. Death is rare but can occur in patients with severe CAD and/or systolic dysfunction.

NEW MAPPING AND ABLATION TECHNOLOGIES
Multielectrode Mapping Systems

Some of the limitations of ablation are related to inadequate mapping. These problems include having only isolated premature complexes during the EPS instead of sustained tachycardias (in idiopathic AT and VT), nonsustained episodes of VT, poor hemodynamic tolerance of VT, and multiple VT morphologies. Standard mapping techniques sample single sites sequentially and are poorly suited to these situations. New mapping systems are available that enable sampling of many sites simultaneously and incorporate sophisticated computer algorithms for analysis and display of global maps. These mapping systems use various technologies ranging from multiple electrodes situated on each of several splines of a basket catheter, to the use of low-intensity electrical or magnetic fields to localize the tip of the catheter in the heart and record and plot activation times on a contour map of the chamber, to the use of complex mathematics to compute "virtual" electrograms recorded from a mesh electrode situated in the middle of a chamber cavity or on the body surface. Some of these systems are capable of generating activation maps of an entire chamber by using only one

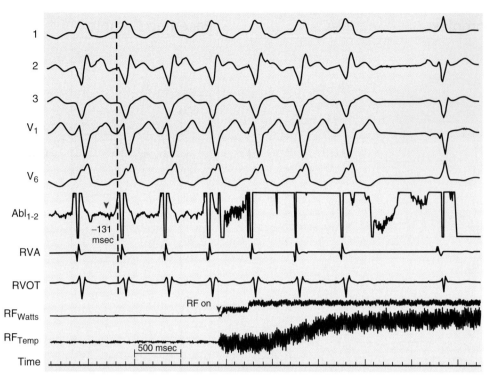

FIGURE 64.17 Radiofrequency ablation of postinfarction ventricular tachycardia. The electrogram in the ablation recording (Abl$_{1-2}$, *arrowhead*) precedes onset of the QRS *(dashed line)* by 131 msec. Ablation here (RF on) results in slight deceleration of VT before termination in 1.3 seconds. Temperature monitored from the catheter tip had just peaked (≈70°C) at the time that VT terminated.

cardiac complex, an obvious advantage in patients with only rare premature complexes, nonsustained arrhythmias, or poor hemodynamic tolerance of sustained arrhythmias.

Epicardial Catheter Mapping

Although most VTs can be ablated from the endocardium, occasional cases are resistant to this therapy. In many of these cases, epicardial ablation may be successful. It is often needed in VT attributable to cardiomyopathy but less frequently in postinfarction patients and those without structural heart disease.

For gaining access to the pericardial space for epicardial mapping and ablation, a long spinal anesthesia needle is introduced from a subxiphoid approach under fluoroscopic guidance. As the pericardium is approached, a small amount of radiocontrast agent is injected. If the tip of the needle is still outside the pericardium, the dye stays where it is injected; when the pericardial space has been entered, the dye disperses and outlines the heart. A guidewire is introduced through the needle and a standard vascular introducer sheath exchanged over the wire. The pericardial space is then accessible for a mapping/ablation catheter, and standard mapping techniques can then

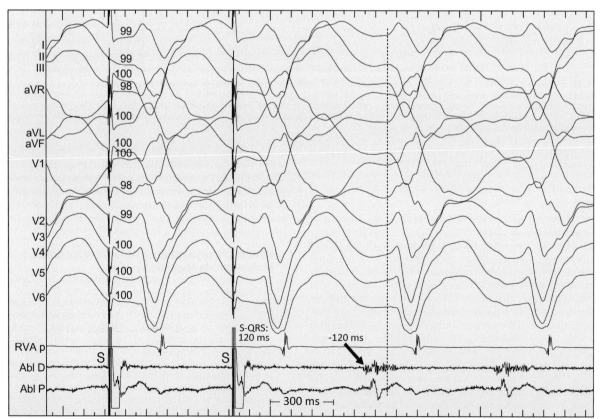

FIGURE 64.18 Concealed" entrainment of postinfarction ventricular tachycardia. The two complexes on the *left* are pacing during VT, with a stimulus *(S)*-QRS interval 120 milliseconds; after pacing ends, VT resumes. The electrogram *(arrow)* in Abl D (distal electrode pair of the ablation catheter) is 120 milliseconds before QRS onset *(dotted line)*. The paced and VT QRS complexes are almost identical (numbers above paced complexes indicate algorithmic "match" assessed by recording system). Ablation at this site quickly terminated VT. *RVA p,* Right ventricular apex; *Abl P,* recording from proximal electrodes on ablation catheter.

be applied. When a site is selected for possible ablation, coronary arteriography is usually warranted to avoid delivery of RF energy near a coronary artery. This is less important in cases of postinfarction VT because the VT substrate is typically in a region of previous transmural infarction. For left ventricular sites, high-output pacing should be performed to assess proximity to the left phrenic nerve; if captured, another ablation site may be sought at which phrenic capture is absent, or a balloon can be placed in the pericardial space (or air or fluid instilled) to physically displace and thus protect the nerve from damage during ablation. Treatment of ventricular arrhythmias in some right ventricular pathologies, such as arrhythmogenic right ventricular cardiomyopathy and Brugada syndrome, often require epicardial mapping and ablation. Epicardial mapping can be used for patients who have previously undergone cardiac surgery, although adhesions may obliterate portions of the pericardial space; on occasion, a small subxiphoid incision is needed for better access and visualization of the space. The most frequent complication of epicardial mapping is pericarditis related to the ablation; cardiac tamponade is rare.

Chemical Ablation

Chemical ablation of an area of myocardium can be used for treatment of VT refractory to drug and standard catheter ablation. Using this specialized technique, an angioplasty catheter is maneuvered into an arterial (or venous) branch in the region of the VT (determined by mapping). After verifying the correct vessel by injecting iced saline into it and observing transient slowing or termination of VT, the angioplasty balloon is inflated (to prevent spillage of alcohol) and 100% ethanol is injected into the vessel. This generally terminates VT and kills the cells responsible for its continuation. Recurrences of tachycardia several days after apparently successful ablation are possible. Excessive myocardial necrosis is the major complication, and alcohol ablation should be considered only when other ablative approaches fail or cannot be done.

Several other mapping/imaging techniques have been developed recently, including integration of a previously obtained computed tomography or magnetic resonance study into computerized mapping systems and use of intracardiac ultrasound to construct a facsimile of the intracardiac anatomy in any chamber during ablation procedures, to guide placement of anatomic ablation and reduce fluoroscopic exposure. Other techniques include use of algorithms to select complex fractionated atrial electrograms for ablation in patients with AF and algorithms to assess the fidelity of pace maps with native tachycardia complexes. Cryoablation, high-frequency focused ultrasound, laser energy, and delivery of RF energy between two catheters on opposite sides of a ventricular wall, or through a needle electrode inserted into myocardium, have had some success in select patients.

Non-Invasive Radioablation

Recently, external radiation has been used to treat VT refractory to medication and catheter ablation strategies.[31] With this method, once a target area in the ventricles has been precisely designated, one of a variety of sources of radiation is focused at these specific coordinates from different angles in order to minimize collateral damage to skin and normal tissue near the ablation target. This technique requires expertise coordinated among many disciplines (electrophysiology, nuclear medicine, radiation physics) and is not widely available; preliminary results are promising.

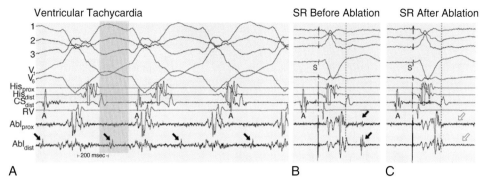

FIGURE 64.19 Mid-diastolic potentials during ventricular tachycardia correlating with late potentials in sinus rhythm (SR). **A,** Ventricular tachycardia (VT); diastole (from the end of one QRS complex to the beginning of the next) is shaded in gray. In the Abl$_{dist}$ recording, a small, sharp signal is seen in mid-diastole that corresponds to a protected corridor of propagation. **B,** After termination of VT with pacing, recording at the same location shows a delayed ("late") potential in SR that tracked ventricular pacing (black arrows; the dashed line denotes the end of the QRS complex). **C,** Ablation here eliminated the late potential (clear arrows), as well as inducible VT. A, Atrial recording; S, stimulus artifact.

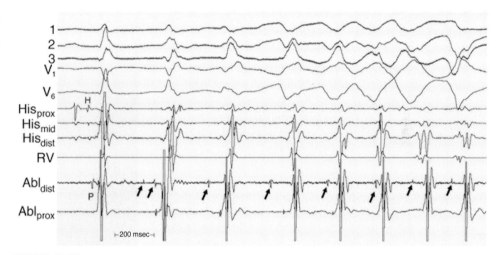

FIGURE 64.20 "Focal ventricular fibrillation." Recordings are shown from a patient with multiple episodes of VF in a day. A sinus rhythm complex, during which a Purkinje potential (P) is recorded from the ablation (Abl) electrode, is followed by a premature complex from this site that is preceded by sharp Purkinje spikes (arrows) that continue to precede subsequent complexes of polymorphic ventricular tachycardia that degenerated to ventricular fibrillation (VF). Ablation at this site eliminated recurrent episodes of VF.

SURGICAL THERAPY FOR TACHYARRHYTHMIAS

The objectives of a surgical approach to treatment of a tachycardia are to excise, isolate, or interrupt tissue in the heart critical for initiation, maintenance, or propagation of the tachycardia while preserving or even improving myocardial function. In addition to a direct surgical approach to the arrhythmia, indirect approaches such as aneurysmectomy, coronary artery bypass grafting, and relief of valvular regurgitation or stenosis can be useful in select patients by improving cardiac hemodynamics and myocardial blood supply. Cardiac sympathectomy (stellate ganglionectomy) alters adrenergic influences on the heart and has been effective in some patients, particularly those who have recurrent VT with long-QT syndrome despite beta blockade, and catecholaminergic polymorphic VT.

Supraventricular Tachycardias

Surgical procedures exist for patients (adults and children) with AT, atrial flutter and fibrillation, AV node reentry, and AV reentry (Fig. 64.21). RF catheter ablation adequately treats most of these patients and thus has replaced direct surgical intervention, except for the occasional patient in whom RF catheter ablation fails or who is

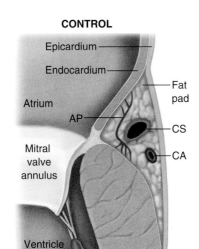
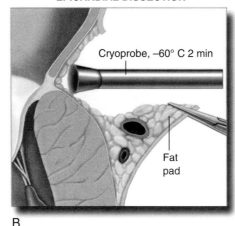
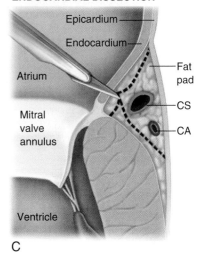

A   B   C

FIGURE 64.21 Schematic diagram showing the two approaches for surgical interruption of an accessory pathway. **A,** Left atrioventricular groove and its vascular contents the coronary sinus *(CS)* and circumflex coronary artery *(CA)*. Multiple accessory pathways *(AP)* course through the fat pad. **B,** Approach for epicardial dissection. **C,** Endocardial dissection. Both approaches clear out the fat pad and interrupt any accessory pathways. (From Zipes DP. Cardiac electrophysiology: promises and contributions. *J Am Coll Cardiol.* 1989;13:1329. Reprinted by permission of the American College of Cardiology.)

undergoing concomitant cardiovascular surgery. In some cases, a prior attempt at RF catheter ablation complicates surgery by obliterating the normal tissue planes that exist in the AV groove or by rendering tissues friable. On occasion, patients with ATs have multiple foci that require surgical intervention. Several surgical procedures have been developed to treat AF and are reviewed in Chapter 66.

Ventricular Tachycardia

In contrast to patients with supraventricular arrhythmias, candidates for surgical therapy for ventricular arrhythmias often have severe left ventricular dysfunction, generally the result of CAD. The cause of the underlying heart disease influences the type of surgery performed. Candidates are patients with drug-resistant, symptomatic, recurrent ventricular tachyarrhythmias who ideally have a segmental wall motion abnormality (scar or aneurysm) with preserved residual left ventricular function, have not benefited from previous attempts at catheter ablation, or are not candidates for catheter ablation because of hemodynamic instability during VT or the presence of left ventricular thrombi (precluding endocardial catheter ablation).

Idiopathic Ventricular Tachycardia/Premature Ventricular Complexes and Nonischemic Cardiomyopathy

Patients with VT or PVCs in the absence of structural heart disease or with nonischemic cardiomyopathy who have undergone unsuccessful drug and catheter ablation therapy for their arrhythmias are candidates for surgical therapy.

The procedure is usually performed through a limited thoracotomy, exposing only the area of the ventricles believed responsible for the arrhythmia. In idiopathic VT/PVC cases, this is often at the basal aspect of the anterior left ventricle, an area where epicardial catheter ablation is difficult because of thick epicardial fat and proximity to major coronary arteries. After exposing the area of the ventricular epicardial surface of interest, mapping is done to confirm the source of the arrhythmia, after which cryoablation is usually performed (Fig. 64.22). This typically results in cessation of the arrhythmia. Extensive ablation is often needed in patients with nonischemic cardiomyopathy, in whom epicardial and intramural scarring in the basal left and right ventricles is a common substrate for ventricular arrhythmias.

Ischemic Heart Disease

In almost all patients who have VT associated with ischemic heart disease, the arrhythmia, regardless of its configuration on the surface ECG, arises in the left ventricle or on the left ventricular side of the interventricular

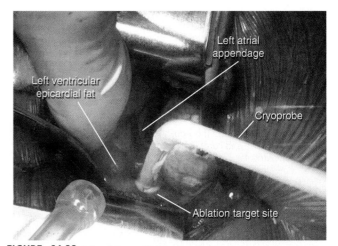

FIGURE 64.22 Epicardial cryoablation for treatment of symptomatic, drug-refractory premature ventricular complexes (PVCs) that could not be ablated from an endo- or epicardial catheter approach. The left ventricular base is exposed through a limited left thoracotomy; after mapping to pinpoint the sites of origin of PVCs, a cryoprobe is used to freeze the area.

septum. The electrocardiographic contour of the VT can change from a right bundle branch block to a left bundle branch block pattern without a change in the site of earliest diastolic activation, thus suggesting that the location of the circuit within the left ventricle remains the same, often near the septum, but that its exit pathway is altered.

Indirect surgical approaches, including coronary artery revascularization, and ventricular aneurysm or infarct resection with or without coronary artery bypass grafting, have been successful in no more than 20% to 30% of VT cases. Coronary artery bypass grafting as a primary therapeutic approach has generally been successful only in patients who experience rapid VT because of severe ischemia, as well as in patients with ischemia-related VF, but it can sometimes be useful in patients with coronary disease resuscitated from sudden death who have no inducible arrhythmias at EPS. These patients generally show a clear relationship between episodes of ventricular arrhythmia and immediately antecedent severe ischemia and have no evidence of infarction or minimal wall motion abnormalities but have preserved overall left ventricular function. Patients with sustained monomorphic VT or only polymorphic VT rarely have their arrhythmias affected by coronary bypass surgery, although it can reduce the frequency of the arrhythmic episodes in some patients and prevent new ischemic events. Percutaneous (temporary) stellate ganglion blockade, or left or bilateral cardiac sympathectomy, has been shown to be effective in controlling refractory VT and VF in many cases.

SURGICAL TECHNIQUES

In general, two types of direct surgical procedures are used, resection and ablation (Fig. 64.23). The first direct surgical approach to VT was encircling endocardial ventriculotomy, which entails performing a transmural ventriculotomy to isolate areas of endocardial fibrosis that were recognized visually; this procedure is rarely used now. Another procedure, subendocardial resection, is based on data indicating that arrhythmias after MI arise mostly at the subendocardial borders between normal and infarcted tissue. Subendocardial resection involves peeling off a 1- to 3-mm-thick layer of endocardium, often near the rim of an aneurysm, that has been demonstrated by mapping procedures to contain sites of mid-diastolic activation recorded during VT. Tachycardias arising from near the base of the papillary muscles are treated with a cryoprobe cooled to −70°C. Cryoablation can also be used to isolate areas of the ventricle that cannot be resected and is often combined with resection. Lasers have also been used with good success, but the equipment is expensive and cumbersome.

For ventricular tachyarrhythmias, operative mortality ranges from 5% to 10%, related to poor LV function and comorbidities extant prior to surgery. Success, defined as the absence of recurrence of spontaneous ventricular arrhythmias, is achieved in 59% to 98% of patients. In experienced centers, operative mortality can be as low as 5% in stable patients undergoing elective procedures, with 85% to 95% of survivors being free of inducible or spontaneous ventricular tachyarrhythmias. Long-term recurrence rates range from 2% to 15% and correlate with results of the patient's postoperative electrophysiologic stimulation study. Operative survival is strongly influenced by the degree of left ventricular dysfunction.

ELECTROPHYSIOLOGIC STUDIES
Preoperative Electrophysiologic Study
In patients for whom direct surgical therapy for VT is planned, a preoperative EPS is usually warranted. This study involves initiation of the VT and electrophysiologic mapping to localize the area to be resected, as is done with catheter ablation. Preoperative catheter mapping is contraindicated in patients with known left ventricular thrombi that might be dislodged by the mapping catheter.

Intraoperative Ventricular Mapping
Electrophysiologic mapping is also performed at surgery, with the surgeon using a handheld probe or an electrode array coupled with computer techniques that instantaneously provide an overall activation map, cycle by cycle. The sequence of activation during VT can be plotted and the area of earliest activation determined. Resection or cryoablation of tissue from which these recordings are made usually cures the VT, thus indicating that they represent a critical portion of the reentrant circuit. When the earliest recordable endocardial electrical activity occurs less than 30 milliseconds before onset of the QRS complex, the critical portions of the circuit may be in the interventricular septum or near the epicardium of the free wall. In some patients, intramural mapping using a plunge needle electrode can be useful. Most centers have used a strategy of "sequential" subendocardial resection in which VT is initiated, mapped, and ablated (resected or cryoablated) while the heart is warm and beating, and stimulation is repeated immediately. If VT can

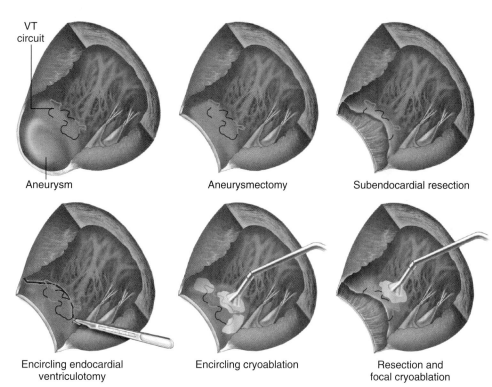

Aneurysm   Aneurysmectomy   Subendocardial resection

Encircling endocardial ventriculotomy   Encircling cryoablation   Resection and focal cryoablation

FIGURE 64.23 Schematic diagram showing surgical procedures for the treatment of postinfarction ventricular tachycardia with a left ventricular aneurysm. A damaged left ventricle is depicted as opened along the lateral wall and showing the septum and papillary muscles. The tachycardia circuit *(upper left)* takes a meandering course near the point where the aneurysm meets normal myocardium and at times is superficial *(purple lines)* and at other times is coursing deeper *(green lines)*. Simple aneurysmectomy that leaves a portion of the aneurysm for suturing often misses the circuit and thus does not cure the arrhythmia. By subendocardial resection, a layer of endocardium and subjacent tissue is removed, including at least some of the tachycardia circuit. Such resection results in elimination of the tachycardia. Encircling endocardial ventriculotomy attempts to isolate the circuit electrically without removal of tissue, but it probably actually works by incising portions of the circuit. Cryoablation can be used to encircle the infarct zone, alone or in combination with resection of damaged tissue too deep in the wall to be resected safely.

still be initiated, mapping and resection are also repeated until VT can no longer be initiated. Reentry around an inferior scar, with a critical diastolic pathway confined to an isthmus of ventricular muscle between the scar and mitral valve annulus, can be cured by cryoablation of this isthmus. Cure rates in this situation exceed 93%, although risk of late exacerbation of heart failure remains a concern.

REFERENCES
Pharmacologic Therapy
1. Lester RM, Olbertz J. Early drug development: assessment of proarrhythmic risk and cardiovascular safety. *Expert Rev Clin Pharmacol.* 2016;9:1611–1618.
2. Rosen MR, Janse MJ. Concept of the vulnerable parameter: the Sicilian Gambit revisited. *J Cardiovasc Pharmacol.* 2010;55:428–437.
3. Lei M, Wu L, Terrar DA, et al. Modernized classification of cardiac antiarrhythmic drugs. *Circulation.* 2018;138:1879–1896.
4. Zaiou M, El Amri H. Cardiovascular pharmacogenetics: a promise for genomically-guided therapy and personalized medicine. *Clin Genet.* 2017;91:355–370.
5. Tomaselli Muensterman E, Tisdale JE. Predictive analytics for identification of patients at risk for QT interval prolongation: a systematic review. *Pharmacotherapy.* 2018;38:813–821.
6. Lorberbaum T, Sampson KJ, Woosley RL, et al. An integrative data science pipeline to identify novel drug interactions that prolong the QT interval. *Drug Saf.* 2016;39:433–441.
7. Wright JM, Page RL, Field ME. Antiarrhythmic drugs in pregnancy. *Expert Rev Cardiovasc Ther.* 2015;13:1433–1444.
8. Li Z, Ridder BJ, Han X, et al. Assessment of an in silico mechanistic model for proarrhythmia risk prediction under the CiPA initiative. *Clin Pharmacol Ther.* 2019;105:466–475.
9. Brodie OT, Michowitz Y, Belhassen B. Pharmacological therapy in Brugada syndrome. *Arrhythm Electrophysiol Rev.* 2018;7:135–142.
10. Mankikian J, Favelle O, Guillon A, et al. Initial characteristics and outcome of hospitalized patients with amiodarone pulmonary toxicity. *Respir Med.* 2014;108:638–646.
11. Hussain N, Bhattacharyya A, Prueksaritanond S. Amiodarone-induced cirrhosis of liver: what predicts mortality? *ISRN Cardiol.* 2013;617943.
12. Wang AG, Cheng HC. Amiodarone-associated optic neuropathy: clinical review. *Neuro Ophthalmol.* 2017;41:55–58.
13. Epstein AE, Olshansky B, Naccarelli GV, et al. Practical management guide for clinicians who treat patients with amiodarone. *Am J Med.* 2016;129:468–475.
14. Valembois L, Audureau E, Takeda A, et al. Antiarrhythmics for maintaining sinus rhythm after cardioversion of atrial fibrillation. *Cochrane Database Syst Rev.* 2019;9:CD005049.
15. De Vecchis R, Ariano C. Effects of dronedarone on all-cause mortality and on cardiovascular events in patients treated for atrial fibrillation: a meta-analysis of RCTs. *Minerva Cardioangiol.* 2019;67:163–171.
16. Kpaeyeh JA, Wharton JM. Sotalol. *Card Electrophysiol Clin.* 2016;8:437–452.
17. Vinson DR, Lugovskaya N, Warton EM, et al. Ibutilide effectiveness and safety in the cardioversion of atrial fibrillation and flutter in the community emergency department. *Ann Emerg Med.* 2018;71:96–108.e2.

18. Naksuk N, Sugrue AM, Padmanabhan D, et al. Potentially modifiable factors of dofetilide-associated risk of torsades de pointes among hospitalized patients with atrial fibrillation. *J Interv Card Electrophysiol.* 2019;54:189–196.
19. Erath JW, Vamos M, Hohnloser SH. Effects of digitalis on mortality in a large cohort of implantable cardioverter defibrillator recipients: results of a long-term follow-up study in 1020 patients. *Eur Heart J Cardiovasc Pharmacother.* 2016;2:168–174.
20. Guerra F, Romandini A, Barbarossa A, et al. Ranolazine for rhythm control in atrial fibrillation: a systematic review and meta-analysis. *Int J Cardiol.* 2017;227:284–291.
21. Koruth JS, Lala A, Pinney S, et al. The clinical use of ivabradine. *J Am Coll Cardiol.* 2017;70:1777–1784.
22. Sanders P, Elliott AD, Linz D. Upstream targets to treat atrial fibrillation. *J Am Coll Cardiol.* 2017;70:2906–2908.

Electrotherapy

23. Pluymaekers N, Dudink E, Luermans J, et al. Early or delayed cardioversion in recent-onset atrial fibrillation. *N Engl J Med.* 2019;380:1499–1508.
24. Houmsse M, Daoud EG. Biophysics and clinical utility of irrigated-tip radiofrequency catheter ablation. *Expert Rev Med Devices.* 2012;9:59–70.

25. Andrade JG, Dubuc M, Guerra PG, et al. The biophysics and biomechanics of cryoballoon ablation. *Pacing Clin Electrophysiol.* 2012;35:1162–1168.
26. Reddy VY, Neuzil P, Koruth JS, et al. Pulsed field ablation for pulmonary vein isolation in atrial fibrillation. *J Am Coll Cardiol.* 2019;74:315–326.
27. Katritsis DG, Zografos T, Siontis KC, et al. Endpoints for successful slow pathway catheter ablation in typical and atypical atrioventricular nodal re-entrant tachycardia: a contemporary, multicenter study. *JACC Clin Electrophysiol.* 2019;5:113–119.
28. Reissmann B, Fink T, Schluter M, et al. Catheter ablation for inappropriate sinus tachycardia: clinical outcomes of sinus node ablation. *HeartRhythm Case Rep.* 2020;6:81–85.
29. Cheniti G, Vlachos K, Meo M, et al. Mapping and ablation of idiopathic ventricular fibrillation. *Front Cardiovasc Med.* 2018;5:123.
30. Marchlinski FE, Haffajee CI, Beshai JF, et al. Long-term success of irrigated radiofrequency catheter ablation of sustained ventricular tachycardia: post-approval THERMOCOOL VT trial. *J Am Coll Cardiol.* 2016;67:674–683.
31. Cuculich PS, Schill MR, Kashani R, et al. Noninvasive cardiac radiation for ablation of ventricular tachycardia. *N Engl J Med.* 2017;377:2325–2336.

# 65 Supraventricular Tachycardias

JONATHAN M. KALMAN AND PRASHANTHAN SANDERS

DEFINITIONS

The 2015 American College of Cardiology/American Heart Association/Heart Rhythm Society (ACC/AHA/HRS) guidelines[1] defined supraventricular tachycardia (SVT) as:

> An umbrella term used to describe tachycardias (atrial and/or ventricular rates in excess of 100 bpm at rest), the mechanism of which involves tissue from the His bundle or above. These SVTs include inappropriate sinus tachycardia, atrial tachycardia (including focal and multifocal AT), macroreentrant AT (including typical atrial flutter), junctional tachycardia, atrioventricular nodal reentrant tachycardia (AVNRT), and various forms of accessory pathway-mediated reentrant tachycardias (AVRT).

They further define paroxysmal SVT (PSVT) as: "A clinical syndrome characterized by the presence of a regular and rapid tachycardia of abrupt onset and termination. These features are characteristic of AVNRT or AVRT, and, less frequently, AT. PSVT represents a subset of SVT."

ASSESSMENT OF THE PATIENT WITH PALPITATIONS

When a patient complains of palpitations, this can reflect a broad range of differing symptoms that will frequently point to the correct diagnosis. For example, some patients may simply develop a subjective awareness of their heartbeat, which is often described as a slow forceful beating. Frequently these symptoms will be most obvious at night and will often be reported while lying on the left-hand side presumably as the cardiac apex is felt more clearly against the chest wall.

Symptoms of ectopic beats are most usually reported as a skipped beat associated with a strange sensation in the throat or an impulse to cough. This may be repetitive, and patients can often describe the frequency of these (every third beat, etc.). The symptoms may occasionally be associated with transient light-headedness and shortness of breath, although these are usually mild and momentary. If repetitive, the symptoms may be described as lasting for hours and it is important to ascertain whether this is a continuous rapid arrhythmia lasting for hours or alternately intermittent symptoms coming and going over hours. Many patients with ectopic beats, including high-burden ectopy, are completely asymptomatic, and the reason for this symptom variance remains unclear.

Symptomatic sinus tachycardia produces regular palpitations with heart rate generally in the range of 120 to 130 bpm, although it can be much faster depending on the underlying cause. Onset of symptoms in inappropriate sinus tachycardia (IAST) may be gradual or sudden as patients may become aware of sinus tachycardia only when a particular heart rate is reached. Termination is gradual usually over many minutes, and episodes can last for hours. Patients may feel breathless on minor exertion, mildly light-headed, and fatigued. Symptoms can overlap with those of SVT.

SVT is usually described as sudden in onset with rapid racing (often too fast to count) with a sensation that the heart is trying to beat out of the chest. The episodes may be triggered by sudden movements such as sudden running for the bus or by bending and standing up. Episodes may last continuously from minutes to hours and terminate suddenly. They may respond to vagal maneuvers. SVT may be associated with transient light-headedness at onset, which is occasionally severe and resulting in presyncope, although syncope is unusual. Accompanying symptoms include anxiety as a secondary phenomenon, although some patients (particularly women) have been given an erroneous diagnosis of panic attacks or primary anxiety disorder. Patients may also become breathless and develop chest discomfort during prolonged episodes. Polyuria may be reported during and early after SVT episodes due to release of atrial natriuretic peptide at these elevated rates. Symptoms are generally more severe in older age-groups, although rate is also an important determinant of symptom severity. Recurrent short bursts (seconds to minutes) of rapid palpitations with normal rhythm interspersed suggests an automatic focal AT. Prolonged irregularly irregular racing points to atrial fibrillation (AF). Sudden syncope is rarely associated with SVT and when arrhythmic in origin generally suggests ventricular tachycardia (VT) or a significant pause as a result of sinus arrest or atrioventricular (AV) block.

The physical examination may be helpful in demonstrating findings associated with valvular pathology, cardiac failure, or thyrotoxicosis or when an incessant or persistent arrhythmia is present. Investigations include a 12-lead electrocardiogram (ECG) in sinus rhythm. This will determine whether preexcitation is present and identify P wave abnormalities and bundle branch block patterns.

Routine blood tests include biochemistry and thyroid function tests. When patients present to an emergency department with tachyarrhythmias, troponin will often be elevated. In this setting, this is a nonspecific response frequently secondary to the tachycardia and not necessarily indicative of obstructive coronary artery disease.[2] An echocardiogram is usually performed to evaluate ventricular function and atrial size and to rule out significant valvular pathology.

Most important is documentation of the tachycardia. This may involve finding ambulance traces or emergency department ECGs. For patients without documented arrhythmias, a range of monitoring strategies are available and may be chosen according to symptom frequency and patient preference. When symptoms occur daily, simple 24-hour Holter monitoring will obtain the diagnosis. Documentation of onset and termination of the arrhythmia may add important diagnostic information. For example, an IAST may have gradual increase in rate over 30 seconds to several minutes, whereas a focal AT usually has sudden onset with a "warm-up" over several beats. For less frequent episodic events, a range of wearable technologies or devices used with a smart phone are now available and this has greatly facilitated documentation of the arrhythmia (see Chapter 61). Alternative approaches include more prolonged monitoring of up to 30 days with a variety of different devices of variable patient tolerability. An implanted loop recorder may be considered in the unusual event that documentation cannot be obtained with simpler monitoring approaches. Finally, in patients with classic symptoms of sudden onset and offset tachycardia highly suggestive of SVT, documentation is not essential and an initial approach of a diagnostic electrophysiologic study (EPS) with a view to catheter ablation may be considered.

SUPRAVENTRICULAR ARRHYTHMIA TYPES

Atrial Premature Complexes or Ectopic Beats

Atrial premature complexes are very common in the general population. In an unselected population over the age of 50, the average frequency was approximately 1 or 2 per hour and increased with each decade of life.[3] Increase in atrial ectopy occurred not only in relation to advancing age but also in association with other cardiovascular disease. Regular physical exercise was protective. Transient increase in atrial ectopics may occur in response to intercurrent illness, in stress and anxiety, and in response to alcohol and caffeine.

Usually ectopic beats are asymptomatic but may be associated with a range of sensations, including a heightened awareness of the heart beating, the sensation that the heart has given an extra beat or missed a beat, a fluttering sensation in the chest or throat, and occasionally a momentary feeling of faintness or dizziness.

A diagnosis is generally made with ECG monitoring with documentation that symptoms occur corresponding with atrial ectopic events.

Although in the vast majority of patients atrial premature complexes are benign, the seminal paper by Haissaguerre et al. described the

triggering of AF by focal atrial ectopics originating from sleeves of myocardium within the pulmonary veins.[4] Subsequent studies showed that patients with both paroxysmal and persistent forms of AF demonstrate an increased atrial ectopic burden when compared with a control population. Furthermore, increased premature atrial complex (PAC) burden is associated with incident AF risk both in the general population and in patients with cryptogenic stroke. Longitudinal studies have described an association between excess PACs (>30/hour or runs of nonsustained AT >20 beats) and the outcomes of incident AF, stroke, and death. In 15-year follow-up, patients with excess PACS and a CHADs-VASc score of 2 or greater demonstrated an annual stroke risk comparable to that of patients with AF.[5] A number of opinions have suggested that atrial ectopy and AF may be markers of an underlying atrial myopathy that is the primary determinant of stroke risk and adverse outcomes.[6,7] Isolated case reports have indicated that frequent PACs (20% to 40% daily burden) also may be associated with development of a reversible cardiomyopathy.[8]

Despite the association of frequent atrial ectopy with potential for adverse events, to date there is no evidence that treatment of isolated atrial ectopy reduces risk or improves long-term outcomes. Therefore, the only indication for treatment of PACs is when they are sufficiently symptomatic. The vast majority of patients with atrial ectopics will not require any treatment other than reassurance. In those with severe symptoms, treatment would initially involve a beta blocker or calcium channel antagonist. Occasionally it might be appropriate to prescribe an antiarrhythmic medication such as flecainide. In highly symptomatic patients unresponsive to or intolerant of medication, catheter ablation may be considered when the ectopic burden is high and the atrial ectopic is unifocal in origin.

The appearance of an atrial ectopic on an ECG is characterized by an early atrial beat with a P wave morphology different from that of the sinus beat. However, the P wave is frequently inscribed within the preceding T wave and the morphology therefore unclear (Fig. 65.1). An atrial ectopic may be conducted normally, with prolongation of the PR interval and possibly aberrancy or widening of the QRS but also may be nonconducted. A nonconducted or blocked atrial ectopic is one of the most common causes of an unexpected pause on an ECG (Fig. 65.1A,

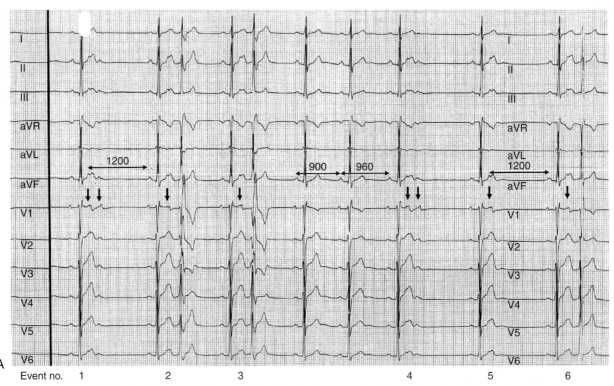

FIGURE 65.1 A, Continuous 12-lead ECG with frequent atrial ectopics. Events 1 and 4 demonstrate 2 atrial ectopic beats in quick succession; the first is inscribed within the initial component of the T wave and the P wave morphology is obscured. The second occurs immediately after the T wave, and the morphology is very different from the sinus morphology. This is particularly evident in lead III and V₁. Neither of these two ectopics in event 1 or 4 are conducted, creating the appearance of an unexpected sinus pause. Similarly, event 5 has a single ectopic beat inscribed within the T wave, which is nonconducted and also creates an apparently unexpected pause. Close inspection of the T wave immediately before the pause clearly demonstrates the mechanism. The pause duration from ectopic to next sinus beat (1200 msec) is longer than a single sinus interval (900 msec). This longer interval includes the conduction time into the node, depolarization and reset of the node possibly with overdrive suppression, and then conduction out from the node (sinoatrial conduction time). Note that in event 1 the pause from first ectopic to the following sinus beat is also 1200 msec, indicating that the second ectopic beat has not resulted in further sinus node reset. This is presumably because the perinodal region was refractory as a result of the immediately preceding ectopic. In events 2, 3, and 6, the ectopic is conducted with a prolonged PR interval as the early ectopic is conducted to the AV node while still relatively refractory and therefore decremental or slow conduction occurs. The QRS complex in these conducted beats demonstrates right bundle branch block aberrancy. The long preceding interval produced by the pause is followed by a short interval, which renders the right bundle branch refractory at that moment. Note that the right bundle branch has a longer refractory period than that of the left bundle branch.

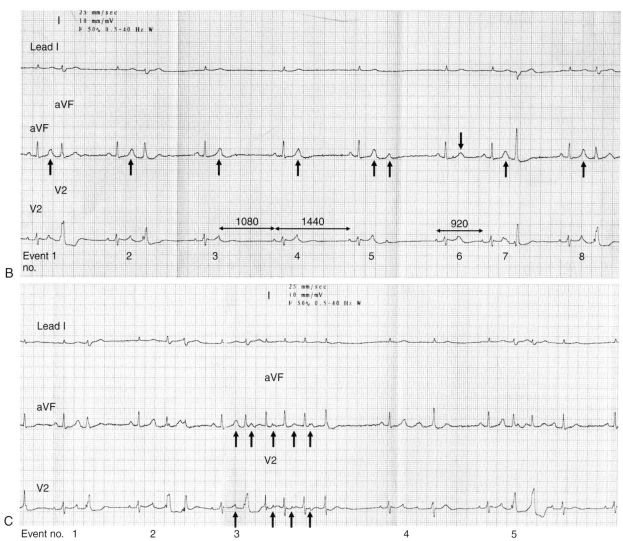

FIGURE 65.1–cont'd B, Continuous 3-lead rhythm strip with high burden of atrial ectopics. In events 1, 2, 7, and 8, the ectopic beat is conducted with a long PR interval and right bundle branch aberrancy. In events 3, 4, and 5 there is a nonconducted atrial ectopic beat occurring within the T wave, creating a pause. The bigeminal pattern of atrial ectopy therefore creates the impression of a marked sinus bradycardia with apparent sinus interval of 1440 msec. In event 5, a second atrial premature beat occurs immediately after the T wave and the visible morphology indicates that this is different from the sinus morphology (best appreciated in aVF). Event 6 is the only normal T wave appearance because there is no inscribed atrial ectopic (*downward pointing arrow*). The sinus interval following the absence of an atrial premature beat is 920 msec rather than the apparent interval of 1440 msec. The interval between the nonconducted atrial premature beat and the following sinus beat (1080 msec) is longer than the sinus interval of 920 msec. **C,** Continuous three-lead ECG in event 1, an atrial premature beat that conducts with a long PR interval and right bundle branch block (RBBB) aberrancy. In events 2, 3, 4, and 5 there are short (variable duration) runs of nonsustained atrial tachycardia. Again we see conduction with a long PR interval and some beats showing RBBB aberrancy. In event 3 the P wave preceding each QRS complex can be clearly seen when examining both aVF and V₂ (*arrows*). This constellation of arrhythmias is frequently observed on monitoring in patients with paroxysmal atrial fibrillation.

B). Nonconducted ectopics in a bigeminal pattern may create the appearance of marked sinus bradycardia (see Fig. 65.1B). Frequent atrial ectopics accompanied by recurrent bursts of nonsustained AT indicates a very active focal trigger or triggers and is a pattern commonly seen in patients who also demonstrate paroxysms of AF (Fig. 65.1C). This is usually because of activity originating in the pulmonary vein sleeves.

Atrial Tachycardias

The term *atrial tachycardia* encompasses a range of different tachycardias that originate in the atria and do not require the participation of the AV node for maintenance of the arrhythmia.[9] These tachycardias have differing arrhythmia mechanisms and are often related to anatomic structures.[9,10] Broadly AT can be considered to be in one of two major categories: focal or macroreentry. Focal AT has been defined as atrial activation starting rhythmically at a small area (focus) from which it spreads out centrifugally.[11] Impulses occur with a given periodicity separated by a quiescent interval recorded on the surface ECG as an isoelectric period. The main tenet of this definition is that, in contrast to activation seen in macroreentrant AT (also termed *atrial flutter* [AFL]), atrial activity originates from a focal location. In macroreentry,

activation occurs around a large central obstacle, such as an anatomic structure or region of scarring; electrical activity can be recorded throughout the *entire* atrial cycle length. These include typical AFL and other well-characterized macroreentrant circuits in the right and left atrium, which are also frequently referred to as types of "atypical AFL." More recently a third category of AT has been described although not routinely included in all classifications. These have been termed "small circuit" or "localized" reentry (see later).[12]

Focal Atrial Tachycardia

Focal AT is a form of SVT characterized by regular, organized atrial activity with discrete P waves and typically an isoelectric segment between P waves (Fig. 65.2, *left*). However, when focal AT rate is particularly rapid, an isoelectric interval may not be apparent (Fig. 65.2, *right*). Focal AT may display some irregularity particularly at onset ("warm-up") and termination ("cool-down"),[1] usually occurring over several beats. Atrial mapping reveals a focal point of origin. Mechanisms of focal AT include abnormal or enhanced automaticity (abnormal impulse initiation in an individual or cluster of myocytes),

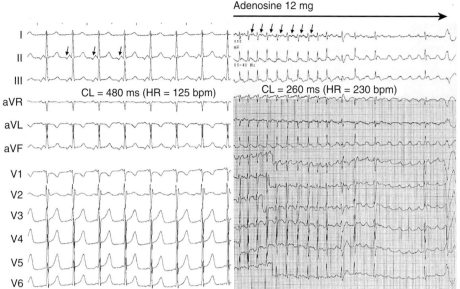

FIGURE 65.2 Focal atrial tachycardia. *Left,* Heart rate is 125 bpm and there is a P wave easily visible before each QRS preceded by a clear isoelectric interval. The P wave morphology is unusual, most notably in the inferior leads, where the pattern demonstrates a biphasic negative-positive appearance incompatible with a sinus origin. This patient (a 22-year-old woman) had an incessant tachycardia originating in the left septal region. This tachycardia falls into the group of long RP tachycardia. *Right,* Rapid tachycardia (heart rate 230 bpm) treated with adenosine. During 1:1 conduction to the ventricle, the P wave appears within the initial part of the T wave, which is deformed (*arrows* on lead I). This is therefore a short R-P tachycardia. The rapid rate coupled with delayed atrioventricular (AV) conduction at this rate is responsible for the position of the P wave within the preceding T wave. After administration of adenosine, AV conduction is blocked but the tachycardia continues uninterrupted. At this rapid rate, there appears to be almost continuous undulation (V₁ and inferior leads) resembling macroreentry. This was a focal atrial tachycardia originating in the left superior pulmonary vein. *CL,* cycle length

tachycardias, rates during sleep may be up to 40 bpm less than those during waking hours.

Patients experience a variety of symptoms, including palpitations, dizziness, chest pain, dyspnea, fatigue, and presyncope.[9] Syncope is unusual unless tachycardia rates are extremely rapid or there is associated underlying structural heart disease.

Tachycardia-mediated cardiomyopathy (TMC) has been reported to occur in a small percentage of patients with incessant ATs. In a large series of patients with focal AT, the incidence of TMC was 10%. TMC occurred exclusively in the context of incessant or very frequent (almost incessant) paroxysmal tachycardia. Patients with TMC were younger, were more frequently male, and had slower tachycardias (mean rate 117 bpm). Incessant tachycardias arise from specific anatomic locations, including the right atrial (RA) and left atrial (LA) appendages (Fig. 65.5) and from the pulmonary venous ostia. Importantly, after successful ablation, left ventricular (LV) function normalizes in virtually all patients.

Embolic events and stroke have rarely been reported in patients with AT, and treatment with anticoagulation is generally not indicated.[1,13] Spontaneous remission of focal AT has been reported in both adults and children after cessation of medical therapy. In fact, the AT disappeared in 55% of patients under the age of 25, compared with just 14% of patients aged 26 or older.

triggered activity (abnormal impulse initiation due to oscillations of membrane potential, termed early or delayed after-depolarizations) and reentry (when myocardial regions activated later in propagation reexcite regions that have already recovered excitability).[13] In practice, there is considerable overlap in electrophysiologic properties, and it is not always possible to be certain of the underlying mechanism during a clinical EPS. For example, tachycardias due either to reentry or to triggered activity may be initiated and terminated with programmed electrical stimulation during an EPS. Tachycardias due to enhanced automaticity and triggered activity may initiate in response to isoprenaline infusion or adrenergic stimulation and may demonstrate multiple spontaneous onsets and terminations (Fig. 65.3). The arrhythmia may also demonstrate cycle length variability (see Fig. 65.3). Finally, focal AT due to either microreentry or triggered activity may be terminated with adenosine.[10]

Epidemiology. Focal AT is the least common mechanism of PSVT, accounting for approximately 10% to 20% of patients with PSVT.[14] Focal AT has a slight preponderance in women, although this has not been a consistent finding in all studies. AT can occur across the age spectrum but gradually increases in prevalence with age and peaking between the age of 40 and 60 years.[15] Automatic AT tends to be more common in younger populations, whereas focal AT due to microreentry is more common in older populations, although many exceptions to this generalization occur. Older patients are more likely to have right-sided AT and multiple ATs.[16] The majority of patients with focal AT do not have underlying structural heart disease or atrial abnormalities, but focal AT may also occur in this context.

Clinical Features. Focal AT is usually manifested by atrial rates between 130 and 250 bpm but may be as low as 100 bpm or as high as 300 bpm[9] (see Fig. 65.2). In general, younger patients tend to have faster AT, with rates up to 340 bpm observed in infants. The P wave morphology is usually different from that of sinus rhythm (see Fig. 65.2), but foci arising from the region of the crista terminalis (particularly the superior crista) may have morphology consistent with a sinus origin (Fig. 65.4). The properties of the atrial focus may be similar to that of the sinus node in that they are responsive to changes in activity and autonomic tone, with the rate varying according to activity. In incessant

Diagnosis and Differential Diagnosis

Detection of AT is usually straightforward. Most patients can be diagnosed by a routine ECG during sustained tachycardia (see Fig. 65.2). However, those with self-reverting paroxysmal AT may require monitoring for diagnosis. If symptoms are frequent, this may require a 24-hour Holter monitor and, if infrequent, various wearable monitoring technologies are available to facilitate ECG documentation if only on a single lead. It should be noted that brief (3 to 10 beats) nonsustained AT is a common finding on routine Holter recordings and is seldom associated with symptoms. Occasionally the ECG differentiation of focal AT from other forms of SVT or from macroreentrant AT may be more challenging.

Inappropriate Sinus Tachycardia versus AT

Differentiating AT from IAST on the ECG alone can at times be difficult, particularly for tachycardias originating at the superior crista terminalis. Although the P wave in AT usually has a morphology different from that of the sinus P wave (see Fig. 65.2), in which case the diagnosis will be clear, when AT arises from the superior crista terminalis these differences may be subtle (see Fig. 65.4). AT usually demonstrates an abrupt onset and termination or may warm up and cool down over 3 or 4 beats. In contrast, IAST gradually increases in rate over approximately 30 seconds to several minutes. In addition, demonstration that onset occurs with a tightly coupled P wave, particularly located in the preceding T wave, is virtually diagnostic of AT (see Fig. 65.3 and eFig. 65.1).

AT versus AVNRT/AVRT

The most important differentiating factor on ECG between AT and AVNRT and AVRT is the R-P relationship. Both typical AVNRT and AVRT have a short R-P interval that does not vary (the former superimposed on the QRS and the latter in the ST segment), and the P wave morphology usually cannot be clearly discerned. Although most commonly associated with a long R-P interval, AT can occur with either a short R-P interval or a long R-P interval depending on the tachycardia rate and the speed of AV nodal conduction. It can therefore mimic either AVNRT or AVRT. The ability to demonstrate "unlinking" or variability of the R to P relationship invariably indicates AT. In AT

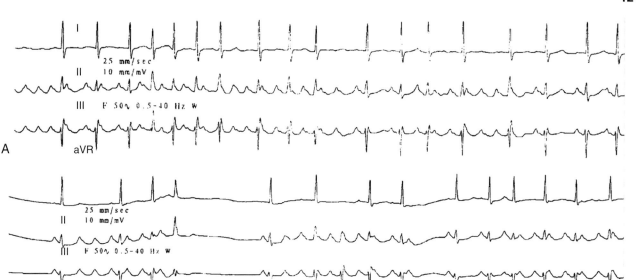

FIGURE 65.3 A, This rhythm strip resembles atrial flutter with continuous P wave undulation. However, on closer inspection, there is marked cycle length variability indicating that this is not macroreentry but rather likely to be focal. **B,** Spontaneous initiations and terminations of the arrhythmia confirming a focal mechanism related either to abnormal automaticity or triggered automaticity. This pattern is incompatible with a reentrant arrhythmia.

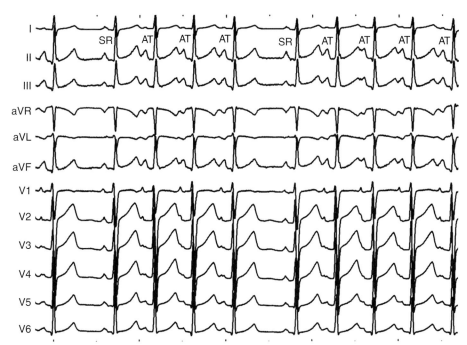

FIGURE 65.4 Continuous 12-lead ECG indicating short bursts of atrial tachycardia from the region of the superior crista terminalis. Note that the P wave morphology of the tachycardia beats (atrial tachycardia [AT]) is very similar to the morphology of the sinus beats (SR).

there may be no isoelectric baseline and the appearance may mimic that of macroreentrant AT (see Fig. 65.2, *right*). Conversely, although macroreentrant AT (including typical AFL) frequently demonstrates a continuous undulation without an isoelectric period on the ECG, patterns resembling focal AT (with an isoelectric period) also have been described. Variation in the tachycardia rate with spontaneous termination and then reinitiation is diagnostic of a focal AT, usually the result of enhanced automaticity or triggered activity (see Fig. 65.3). Spontaneous bursts of tachycardia do not occur with macroreentrant tachycardias.

The rate of the tachycardia does not help discriminate between focal and macroreentrant AT as the rate ranges of both focal AT and macroreentrant AT are too wide to be reliably used for determination of arrhythmia mechanism. The rate range of focal AT is usually between 130 and 250 bpm but may be as low as 100 bpm or as high as 300 bpm. Similarly, although macroreentrant atrial arrhythmias usually have a rate between 240 and 310 bpm, conduction delays within the circuit either due to atrial pathology or use of conduction slowing antiarrhythmics can slow the rate to less than 150 bpm.

Focal AT versus Multifocal AT versus AF

True multifocal AT is a relatively uncommon arrhythmia that occurs in the context of underlying conditions, including pulmonary disease, pulmonary hypertension, coronary disease, and valvular heart disease. However, bursts of focal AT may masquerade as multifocal AT because of the variable P wave appearance when there are varying degrees of fusion with the preceding T wave or QRS complex. Indeed, during rapid focal AT it may be quite difficult to discern a clear P wave morphology because the majority of beats are at least partially obscured by the T waves and QRS complexes unless higher grades of AV conduction block are present (Fig. 65.6). Similarly, when focal AT is fast, it has some P wave interval irregularity in cycle length, and there is varying AV conduction, the trace may superficially resemble AF, particularly if there is only a single monitor lead. A careful appraisal of the trace will generally indicate a P wave fused with the T wave visible before most conducted beats (see Fig. 65.6).

the R-P relationship is incidental and hence possibly variable. In AVRT and AVNRT this relationship will be constant because it is integral to the tachycardia mechanism. Another clue to the diagnosis is the presence of an inferior P wave axis. This excludes AVRT or AVNRT because it suggests an origin high in the atrium. A superiorly directed P wave vector may indicate AVRT or AVNRT or an AT focus originating from the coronary sinus ostium or annular structures. Of note, atypical AVNRT and a concealed accessory pathway with slow retrograde conduction may have long R-P intervals but have constant R-P intervals and a superior P wave axis. Automatic AT may also manifest with recurrent self-limiting bursts of tachycardia that can exhibit warm-up and cool-down phases.

Focal AT versus Macroreentrant AT

In most cases of focal AT it is possible to observe a discrete P wave with an intervening isoelectric interval (see Fig. 65.2A). However, when the atrial rate is very rapid and, if atrial conduction slowing is present,

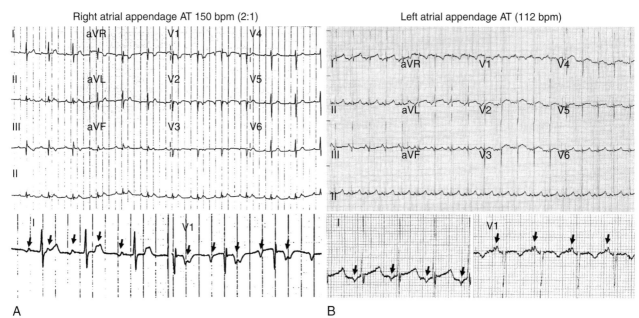

FIGURE 65.5 A, A 12-lead ECG of an incessant tachycardia originating in the right atrial appendage. The atrial rate is 150 bpm, and there is 2:1 conduction to the ventricle. The P wave is deeply inverted from V₁ to V₃ consistent with an origin in the right atrial appendage (anterior location), and lead I has an unusual biphasic negative-positive appearance inconsistent with a sinus origin. **B,** A 12-lead ECG of an incessant tachycardia originating in the left atrial appendage. The P wave morphology is characteristic, showing a broad upright and notched appearance in V₁, a similar pattern in inferior leads (especially well seen in aVF) and a deeply inverted pattern in lead I (characteristic for a left appendage origin). The incessant tachycardia at 112 bpm did not produce symptomatic palpitations, but the patient presented with heart failure due to tachycardia-mediated cardiomyopathy that was reversed after successful ablation.

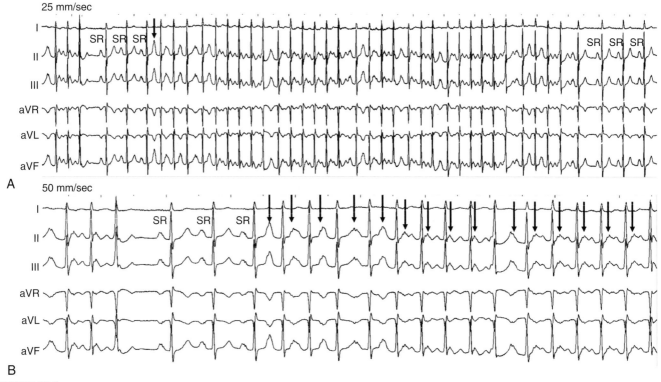

FIGURE 65.6 A, Continuous ECG at a sweep speed of 25 mm/sec; on the left there is termination of an arrhythmia followed by 3 sinus beats (SR) before onset of a rapid irregular tachycardia with a P wave on the peak of the T wave (*arrow*). At first glance this trace suggests atrial fibrillation. The arrhythmia terminates spontaneously on the right of the trace. **B,** The tachycardia initiation is shown at a faster sweep speed (50 mm/sec). It is now possible to see the P wave deforming the T wave and the tail end of the QRS throughout the burst of tachycardia ruling out atrial fibrillation. Because the P wave shows variable fusion with the T wave it is possible to think there is variation in morphology that would suggest a multifocal atrial tachycardia. In fact this was a single-focus atrial tachycardia arising in the left atrial roof.

Anatomic Distribution

Focal ATs do not occur randomly throughout the atria but rather have a characteristic anatomic distribution (Fig. 65.7). In the right atrium they tend to cluster around the crista terminalis,[17] coronary sinus ostium (CS os), para-Hisian or perinodal region, tricuspid annulus (TA), and RA appendage. In the left atrium, the majority originate from the pulmonary veins, with the mitral annulus, LA appendage, and left septum being less common. More recently, focal AT has been described originating from the noncoronary cusp of the aortic valve.[18] The specific reasons for this anatomic distribution remain speculative. For example, the crista terminalis is an area of marked anisotropy with poor transverse but rapid linear

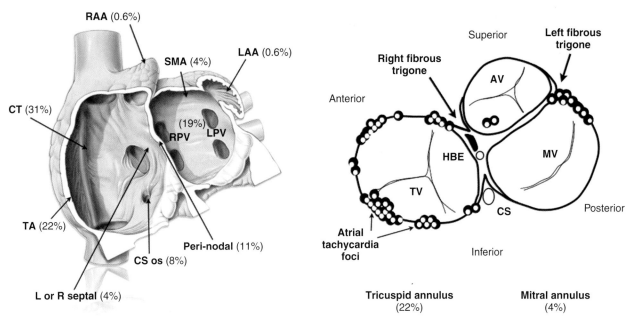

FIGURE 65.7 Anatomic distribution of focal atrial tachycardias. Approximately 75% of atrial tachycardias originate in the right atrium, with the most common locations being the crista terminalis (CT), the tricuspid annulus (TA), the coronary sinus ostium (CS os), and the perinodal region. In the left atrium, the most common location is the ostium of the pulmonary veins and the superior mitral annulus (SMA). Less common locations include the left atrial (LAA) and right atrial appendages (RAA). Tachycardias originating near the midline can sometimes be safely and successfully ablated from within the noncoronary cusp. (From Kistler PM, et al. P-Wave morphology in focal atrial tachycardia: development of an algorithm to predict the anatomic site of origin. J Am Coll Cardiol 2006;48:1010-1017.)

conduction, creating a potential substrate for reentry. In addition, the sinus node complex is located along the crista terminalis, and the presence of automatic tissue with anisotropy may favor abnormal automaticity.

In the context of this classic anatomic distribution, the P wave morphology can provide a reliable and relatively specific guide as to the likely anatomic site of focal AT origin and a number of different P wave algorithms have been proposed.[19] The important caveat is that no significant structural atrial disease is present and the patient has not had prior catheter ablation, because either of these factors may fundamentally change the shape of the P wave. In general, an upright P wave in V_1 suggests LA origin whereas a negative P wave in V1 suggests RA origin.

Sinus Node Reentry
Although the sinus node reentry arrhythmia remains as a separate entity in recent guidelines documents,[1,13] there has been some debate as to whether tachycardias due to reentry within the sinus node truly exist.[11] Sinus node reentry is clinically defined as a tachycardia that can be induced and terminated with programmed stimulation and has a P wave morphology identical or similar to that of the sinus P wave. It is now well recognized that the sinus node is not a discrete structure but rather a diffuse pacemaker complex located along the long axis of the crista terminalis. AT has been described arising from sites along the length of this structure, and it may be best to define these simply as crista terminalis AT.[11]

Management of Focal AT
Acute Management of Focal AT. Initial management of a focal AT in the emergency department might involve administration of adenosine as for other mechanisms of SVT (6 to 12 mg intravenously). For focal AT, the arrhythmia may either terminate, transiently slow, and then return to the pre-adenosine rate or continue with AV block and unmasked P waves (see Fig. 65.2). If unsuccessful, intravenous beta blockers or calcium channel blockers (verapamil or diltiazem) may be effective in hemodynamically stable patients. If ineffective, antiarrhythmic agents such as flecainide, ibutilide, or amiodarone may be considered. Alternatively, if drug treatment is unsuccessful or the patient is hemodynamically unstable, synchronized DC cardioversion may be used. This would be inappropriate for automatic forms of tachycardia with recurrent bursts of tachycardia separated by 1 or more sinus beats. Similarly, for

incessant automatic tachycardias, there is a high probability of recurrence of the arrhythmia after cardioversion.
Chronic Management. Catheter ablation is recommended as a first-line therapy in patients with symptomatic focal AT as an alternative to pharmacologic therapy (class 1).[1,13] Catheter ablation for the most part involves the use of a three-dimensional mapping system to identify the earliest site of atrial activation (Fig. 65.8). Mapping will generally indicate a site from which there is centrifugal spread of activation away from that site. Contemporary ablation series indicate a high procedural success rate in excess of 85% with a very low risk of major complications. The caveat is that for some automatic or triggered forms of focal AT, on occasion all attempts at inducing the arrhythmia may be unsuccessful rendering mapping and ablation impossible on that day.

When catheter ablation is not preferred or not appropriate, pharmacologic management may be considered. However, there are no long-term, randomized, placebo-controlled studies on the use of antiarrhythmic therapy in focal AT. The available studies are observational, with small numbers and mostly conducted over a decade ago. There is widespread agreement that antiarrhythmic agents have low efficacy in the treatment of focal AT.

When drug therapy is preferred, beta blockers or non-dihydropyridine calcium channel blockers (verapamil or diltiazem) may be considered. In patients without structural or ischemic heart disease, propafenone or flecainide also may be considered. Less commonly, agents such as sotalol, amiodarone, or ivabradine have been used.

Inappropriate Sinus Tachycardia
IAST is defined as an elevated heart rate of greater than 100 bpm at rest or on minimal exertion out of keeping with the level of activity or stress.[20,21] The mean 24-hour heart rate is above 90 bpm. The diagnosis can be made when there are accompanying symptoms attributable to the elevated heart rate such as palpitations, breathlessness on minor activity, light-headedness, chest pain, and fatigue. The impact on quality of life can be substantial and is frequently associated with significant psychosocial distress.[20,21] Overwhelmingly the condition manifests in young women. Other than the symptoms that may be debilitating, IAST does not have adverse prognostic significance and reports of tachycardia-induced cardiomyopathy are extremely rare. It is important to rule out secondary causes as a critical part of the initial evaluation before the diagnosis may be considered. A broad range of secondary causes of sinus tachycardia, including anxiety, anemia,

ARRHYTHMIAS, SUDDEN DEATH, AND SYNCOPE

VII

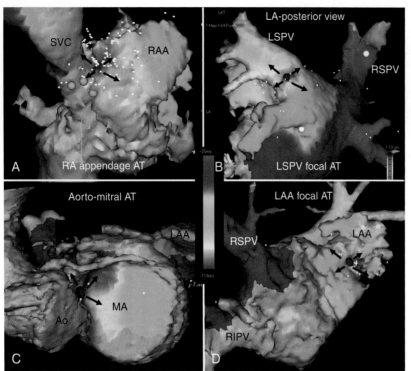

FIGURE 65.8 Three-dimensional electroanatomic maps of focal atrial tachycardia originating from four different anatomic locations. The earliest site of activation is represented by *red*, with *yellow, green, light blue, dark blue,* and *purple* representing progressively later activation. The *black arrows* indicate centrifugal spread away from the site of focal origin where ablation was successful in eliminating the tachycardia. **A,** Origin at the superior base of the right atrial appendage (RAA). **B,** Origin from the posterior inferior ostium of the left superior pulmonary vein. **C,** Origin from the aortomitral continuity. **D,** Origin from the anterior base of the left atrial appendage (LAA). *Ao,* Aortic root; *LA,* left atrium; *LSPV,* left superior pulmonary vein; *MA,* mitral annulus; *RIPV,* right inferior pulmonary vein; *RSPV,* right superior pulmonary vein; *SVC,* superior vena cava.

volume depletion, thyrotoxicosis, fever, pulmonary embolus, cardiac failure, sepsis, stimulants, and drug withdrawal must first be excluded. The heart rate in IAST is not necessarily persistently elevated, and considerable fluctuation is often present. Resting heart rates are frequently in the normal range, and diurnal variation is generally preserved. However, significant rate increases occur with minor activity and positional changes and at other times may be unexplained.[20] Heart rate increases generally occur gradually over 30 seconds to several minutes in contrast to onset of focal AT, which demonstrates sudden onset with a tightly coupled initiating beat and perhaps "warm-up" phenomenon over 2 to 3 beats. The P wave morphology of IAST reflects an origin in the region of the superior crista terminalis in the right atrium with a biphasic positive-negative appearance in V_1 and upright P waves in inferior leads and lead I. This resembles the morphology of a focal AT originating in the same anatomic region. The differential diagnosis also includes both postural orthostatic tachycardia syndrome (POTS) and physical deconditioning, which may have many overlapping features.

The mechanism of IAST is not well understood, and both intrinsic (sinus node hyperactivity) and extrinsic (related to dysautonomia or neurohormonal dysregulation) mechanisms have been suggested. A number of recent reports have described the development of inappropriate sinus tachycardia with elevated mean heart rates and reduced heart rate variability as a manifestation of post COVID-19 syndrome.[21a]

Treatment requires effective communication, support, and reassurance, which may improve outcomes. Lifestyle interventions such as exercise training and volume expansion may be helpful. Ivabradine, a selective blocker of the pacemaker current (I_f) has been found to be safe and effective in several small trials.[1,13] Addition of beta blockade to ivabradine therapy or the use of beta blockers alone may also be useful. However, beta blockers may increase postural dizziness and fatigue. Sinus node modification (catheter ablation) and surgical ablation are not recommended as a part of routine care for patients with IAST. Although these may have early effect and most patients have recurrent symptoms and even with complete surgical removal of the sinus pacemaker complex, fast rates are often generated from the junctional region and left atrium.

Atrial Flutter or Macroreentrant Atrial Tachycardia
Epidemiology

Data indicate that AFL is one of the most common cardiac arrhythmias in humans, with an estimated prevalence of 190,000 people in the United States in 2005. Similar to predictions for AF (Chapter 66), its prevalence is expected to increase to 440,000 by 2050 owing to the increasing aging of the population.[22] AFL often occurs in the context of structural heart disease (e.g., valvular, ischemic heart disease, cardiomyopathy) but may also manifest during an acute disease process (e.g., sepsis, myocardial infarction).

Relationship Between Atrial flutter and Atrial Fibrillation. AFL and AF have been described as two sides of the same coin.[23,24] The two arrhythmias frequently coexist clinically with documented AF in up to 75% of AFL patients. In both animal and human studies, the onset of AFL is usually preceded by a transitional period of AF. When AFL terminates it is also generally via transitional AF (Fig. 65.9). It appears that AF provides both the necessary trigger and electrophysiologic preconditions to initiate and sustain AFL. Furthermore, existing atrial remodeling, which underlies the development of AF, also promotes maintenance of AFL and development of sinus node dysfunction. In addition, antiarrhythmic agents such as flecainide, propafenone, and amiodarone, which slow atrial conduction, promote the conversion of AF to AFL. These agents slow both atrial and ventricular conduction. The atrial rate may slow to 200 to 230 bpm, potentially facilitating 1:1 AV conduction. At these rates, class 1C agents may result in slowed ventricular conduction with the appearance of a very-wide-complex tachycardia resembling VT (Fig. 65.10). It is for this reason that guidelines recommend addition of an AV nodal blocking drug when treating AF with a class 1C agent. An example of AFL with an atrial rate slowed to 230 bpm with amiodarone therapy is shown in Fig. 65.11A. The three panels of Fig. 65.11 show 1:1 conduction resembling a rapid SVT in panel A, the classic 2:1 conduction of typical flutter in panel B, and variable Wenckebach conduction in panel C.

The risk of developing AF late after a flutter ablation is high and increases with both intensity of monitoring and duration of follow-up. In some studies the likelihood of detecting AF during 2 years of follow-up reaches 50%.[25] Risk factors for developing AF after ablation of AFL include previously documented AF, impaired LV function, ischemic and other structural heart disease, and LA enlargement.

Symptoms in patients with AFL resemble those of AF, with palpitations, breathlessness, and reduction in exercise tolerance. A minority of patients with AFL may be minimally symptomatic. In the setting of 1:1 flutter, patients may experience presyncope or syncope. In addition, in the presence of persistent rapid ventricular response rates of 2:1 flutter, patients may develop a decline in LV ejection fraction due to development of a TCM. This is usually fully reversible within approximately 3 months of resumption of sinus rhythm.

Patients with AFL (whether or not AF has also been documented) are considered to have a similar thromboembolic risk to patients with AF. Therefore, recommendation regarding anticoagulation of patients with AFL reflect those for AF both in long-term management and at the time of reversion (pharmacologic, electrical, or with catheter ablation).[1,13]

Classification of Atrial Flutter

The terms *atrial flutter* and *atrial macroreentry* continue to be used interchangeably, with the use of the historical term *atrial flutter* remaining predominant. A suggested AFL classification is shown in Table 65.1, with broad division into those that are dependent on the cavo-tricuspid isthmus (CTI-dependent or typical AFL) and those that are not ("atypical" or non-CTI dependent) (Fig. 65.12). These arrhythmias classically involve reentry around a central obstacle (which may be an anatomic structure or a region of scarring) and the presence of slow conduction to facilitate perpetuation of the arrhythmia.

Atrial flutter: Onset/termination via transitional fibrillation

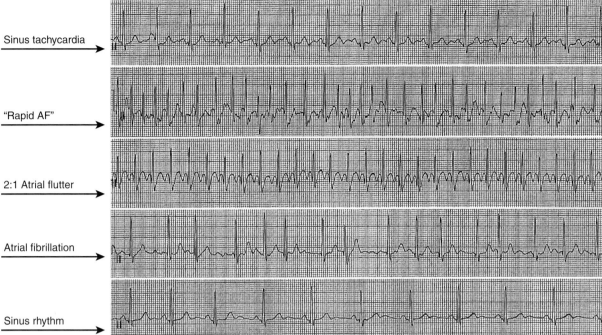

Exercise stress test

Sinus tachycardia →

"Rapid AF" →

2:1 Atrial flutter →

Atrial fibrillation →

Sinus rhythm →

FIGURE 65.9 Exercise stress test indicating progressively: sinus tachycardia, followed by onset of atrial fibrillation (AF) with rapid ventricular response rate, followed by organization into atrial flutter with 2:1 conduction, followed by degeneration back to AF during the recovery phase, and finally termination to sinus rhythm. The example highlights the fact that AF acts as the critical initiator of atrial flutter, establishing regions of functional block and the critical unidirectional block in the flutter circuit required for initiation of the arrhythmia.

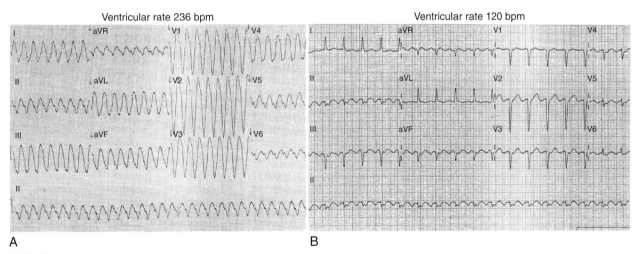

Ventricular rate 236 bpm | Ventricular rate 120 bpm

A | B

FIGURE 65.10 A patient treated with flecainide for atrial fibrillation presents with a wide-complex tachycardia at 236 bpm **(A)** and profound hemodynamic compromise. The patient spontaneously reverted to atrial flutter (AF) with 2:1 conduction with a ventricular rate almost exactly half that of the wide-complex tachycardia **B,** This provides strong evidence that the initial presenting arrhythmia was AF with 1:1 conduction to the ventricle. The profound use-dependent conduction slowing effect of flecainide in the ventricle is responsible for the extremely broad QRS complexes at this rate. This is a potentially life-threatening arrhythmia because of the risk of degeneration into sine wave ventricular tachycardia and asystole. Flecainide was discontinued, and the patient underwent ablation of the atrial flutter.

The term *atypical AFL* denotes a heterogeneous group of macroreentrant circuits that may occur in either atrium or involve both chambers and a range of anatomic boundaries (see Fig. 65.12). These circuits do not involve the CTI. Broadly, atypical AFL may occur in the context of previous atrial surgery (congenital, valvular heart disease, Maze procedures), after catheter ablation for AF (the ablation areas creating scar around which reentry occurs), cardiac transplantation, or in the absence of previous atrial surgery.

Cavo-Tricuspid Isthmus Dependent Flutter. The circuit of (typical) CTI-dependent flutter has been extensively described.[26] Typical flutter is as a macroreentrant circuit within the right atrium. It can be considered to be a broad activation wavefront rotating between the tricuspid

annulus (TA) anteriorly and the crista terminalis-eustachian ridge/inferior vena cava (IVC) posteriorly (Fig. 65.12A). More recently, it is recognized that the posterior barrier may be a line of block running between the superior and IVCs.[26] The CTI is the narrowest anatomic segment of the circuit. In the most common form (approximately 90%) the circuit rotates in a counterclockwise direction when viewed in the frontal plane. In 10%, rotation is clockwise. Numerous variations of this classic circuit have been described,[26] with the most common being lower loop reentry (Fig. 65.12B) where the activation wavefront crosses the posterior line of block. Other less common variations include upper loop reentry and intra-isthmus reentry.

The ECG of typical counterclockwise AFL is characterized by the classic inferior lead flutter wave appearance ("saw-tooth" pattern) demonstrating an initial gradual downsloping segment followed by a deeply inverted component with a terminal positive component (Fig. 65.13A).

TABLE 65.1 Classification of Supraventricular Tachycardias

Atrial arrhythmias
Atrial premature beats
Sinus tachycardias
• Physiologic sinus tachycardia
• Inappropriate sinus tachycardia
• Postural orthostatic tachycardia syndrome (POTS)
• Sinus node reentry (a subset of focal AT)
Focal AT
Multifocal AT
Atrial flutter or macroreentrant atrial tachycardia (MRAT)
• Cavo-tricuspid isthmus-dependent flutter
• Typical atrial flutter—counterclockwise
• Typical atrial flutter—clockwise
• Lower loop reentry
• Intra-isthmus reentry
• Non–cavo-tricuspid isthmus-dependent macroreentry (atypical flutter)
• Right atrial atypical flutter
• Left atrial atypical flutter
Small circuit/localized atrial tachycardia
AV junctional tachycardias
Atrioventricular nodal reentrant tachycardia (AVNRT)
• Typical
• Atypical
Nonreentrant junctional tachycardia
• JET (junctional ectopic or focal junctional tachycardia)
• Other nonreentrant variants
Atrioventricular reentrant tachycardia (AVRT)
• Orthodromic (including PJRT)
• Antidromic (with retrograde conduction through the AVN or, rarely, over another pathway; includes atriofascicular pathways)
Preexcited atrial fibrillation

AT, Atrial tachycardia; *AVN,* atrioventricular node; *JET,* junctional ectopic tachycardia; *PJRT,* permanent junctional reciprocating tachycardia.

In the precordial leads, V_1 classically demonstrates an initial isoelectric component followed by an upright component. With progression across the precordial leads, the initial component becomes inverted and the second component isoelectric such that V_5 and V_6 demonstrate an inverted flutter wave. Lead I is low amplitude/isoelectric and aVL usually upright (see Fig. 65.13A). Unusual flutter wave morphologies may be seen with counterclockwise AFL and a left AFL may occasionally mimic the counterclockwise AFL appearance.[27]

It has long been recognized that typical flutter has a characteristic rate of 300 bpm. With 2:1 conduction, this equates to a ventricular rate of 150 bpm. Both the stereotypical morphology and cycle length reflect the RA anatomy that defines the circuit. However, multiple factors can significantly slow this rate and it is not unusual to see atrial rates as slow as 200 bpm for typical flutter in certain circumstances. Marked RA enlargement, atrial remodeling with significant conduction slowing, and antiarrhythmic agents which slow atrial conduction are associated with slower flutter rates.

In clockwise AFL, although the anatomic boundaries are identical to those of counterclockwise AFL, the wavefront is reversed and there is more variability in the ECG appearance. Nevertheless, characteristic features appear in the inferior leads where a broad and notched upright component is preceded by an inverted segment. V_1 is characterized by a broad negative and usually notched deflection with transition to an upright deflection in V_6 (Fig. 65.13B).

Non Cavo-Tricuspid Isthmus–Dependent Flutter (Atypical Atrial Flutter). Atypical AFL encompasses a range of macroreentrant atrial arrhythmias that are not dependent on the CTI. They have markedly varied ECG characteristics (Fig. 65.13C), and the flutter wave morphology

is generally not particularly useful for determining the circuit location, although some broad generalizations can be made. Atypical flutter may occur primarily in the right or the left atrium. When the V_1 flutter wave is deeply inverted, this is highly likely to represent a right atrial circuit. Conversely, when the V_1 flutter wave is upright, this generally indicates an LA circuit. However, many variations exist and these findings lack sensitivity and specificity. Occasionally, atypical flutter may present ECG characteristics suggesting an isthmus-dependent mechanism. Similarly, the atrial rate in atypical flutter has wide limits (120 to 300 bpm) depending on the underlying circuit and pathology).

AFL is classically described as showing a continuously undulating appearance of the flutter wave on the 12-lead ECG, reflecting continuous atrial activation. This distinguishes macroreentry from focal AT, which typically demonstrates discrete P waves separated by an isoelectric interval. Although this is generally true of CTI-dependent flutter, in patients with atypical flutter, extensive atrial scarring may result in extremely low-amplitude flutter morphology and the appearance of either discrete P waves or very-low-amplitude P waves. Conversely, when focal AT is very rapid (e.g., >250 bpm), the P waves may appear to show continuous undulation.

The pathology underlying atypical flutter is highly variable, and these circuits may occur in the context of (1) prior corrective atrial surgery (congenital heart disease [CHD], valvular heart disease, after a Maze procedure or cardiac transplantation),[28] (2) previous AF ablation, (3) advanced atrial disease associated with atrial enlargement (these patients frequently have underlying pathologies such as heart failure [systolic or diastolic] or unoperated valvular heart disease such as severe mitral regurgitation[29]), or (4) in patients with normal atrial size and without an obvious underlying pathologic condition. In these patients, spontaneous scarring of unknown cause may be found at the time of atrial mapping. These circuits have particularly been described in the RA free wall.[30]

The circuits involved in atypical (non–isthmus dependent) AFL are highly variable and involve a range of anatomic boundaries. These might be anatomic structures, surgical scars, or regions of low voltage and slowed conduction. Stereotypical anatomic locations associated with certain underlying pathologic conditions or procedures have been defined. These include surgical repair of complex CHD such as Mustard or Senning repair, Fontan repair, or simpler atrial surgeries such as atrial septal defect (ASD) repair (Fig. 65.12E). Mitral valve surgery (repair or replacement) has been associated with a high late incidence of both typical and atypical flutter.[31] In patients with prior atrial surgery, circuits particularly involve atriotomy scars and it is important to review operative reports to ascertain the nature of atrial access incisions. The circuits associated with different access incisions vary accordingly. In patients with prior LA ablation, circuits may be around the pulmonary veins (roof dependent) or around the mitral annulus (mitral isthmus dependent). Frequently both circuits may occur in an individual patient (Fig. 65.14). Dual-loop or figure-of-8 reentry has been described when there are two simultaneous circuits. This may occur in either the left atrium (Fig. 65.15) or the right atrium (Fig. 65.16) and is not uncommon in the context of prior AF ablation or prior atrial surgery.[29,30]

Small Circuit Reentry. As noted earlier, a third category of AT termed *small circuit reentry* has been increasing recognized in the era of high-density three-dimensional mapping. These reentrant circuits occur in a localized region with a diameter of 1 to 2 cm; the hallmark is that the entire circuit can be recorded on a single catheter with a high density of electrodes in this specific region (Fig. 65.17). These circuits generally occur in the context of advanced atrial remodeling, and although they have been recognized across a range of pathologies they are most commonly observed in patients with a history of persistent AF, atrial enlargement, and prior AF ablation. It is important to recognize that these circuits are not necessarily due to proarrhythmia created by prior ablation but rather reflect regions of advanced atrial remodeling with markedly slowed conduction, which is a necessary prerequisite to stabilize these small circuits.[12,32]

Treatment

Acute Management. For patients who are hemodynamically unstable, synchronized cardioversion is indicated. For hemodynamically stable patients, DC cardioversion is also preferred if trained personnel are available. Alternatively, intravenous ibutilide or oral dofetilide may be trialed. These should be administered in hospital with careful monitoring for the potential risk of ventricular proarrhythmia. This risk is increased in patients with impaired LV function.

For patients with implanted dual-chamber devices (pacemaker or defibrillator) attempts at high-rate atrial overdrive pacing may be considered if appropriate expertise is available.

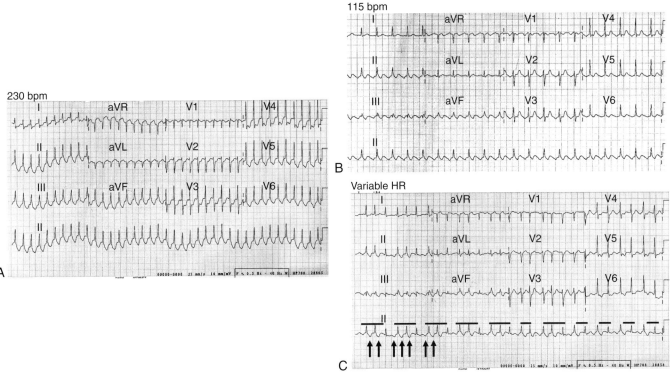

FIGURE 65.11 **A,** Atrial flutter (AF) with 1:1 conduction. Atrial rate is slowed due to amiodarone facilitating 1:1 atrioventricular nodal conduction with a narrow QRS. **B,** Typical AF with 2:1 conduction. **C,** Typical AF with variable Wenckebach-type conduction. The *horizontal lines* highlight the grouped beating of Wenckebach conduction. The *arrows* indicate the flutter waves.

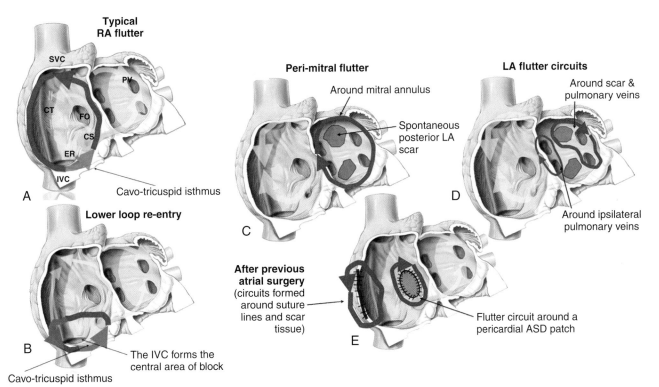

FIGURE 65.12 **Examples of different types of atrial macroreentry or atrial flutter (AF).** **A,** Typical counterclockwise AF confined within the right atrium. *Blue arrow* indicates conduction through the cavo-tricuspid isthmus and the *red arrow* completion of the circuit around the right atrium. The wavefront is constrained between the tricuspid annulus anteriorly (*cutaway* in this image), the posterior line of block formed by the crista terminalis (CT), and the continuation into the eustachian ridge (ER). The left atrium and the posterior right atrium are passively activated (*yellow arrows*) and do not form part of the circuit. **B,** Lower loop reentry with the circuit cutting across the posterior line of block to complete the circuit (*gray arrow*). **C,** Perimitral valve flutter with a region of posterior spontaneous scarring. **D,** Examples of other left atrial macroreentrant circuit with one around the left-sided pulmonary veins and an area of scarring in the posterior left atrium. The other is around the right-sided pulmonary veins. This may occur in an atrium with significant remodeling and conduction slowing or may occur as a result of prior ablation. **E,** Circuits after prior atrial surgery. Most macroreentrant circuits late after atrial septal defect (ASD) repair are typical cavo-tricuspid isthmus–dependent flutter or occur around the atrial incision in the free wall. Circuits around a septal patch are less common. In the current era, most ASDs are closed with a percutaneously placed closure device. *CS,* Coronary sinus ostium; *FO,* fossa ovalis; *IVC,* inferior vena cava; *PV,* pulmonary veins; *SVC,* superior vena cava. (From Lee G, et al. Catheter ablation of atrial arrhythmias: state of the art. Lancet 2012;380(9852):1509-1519.)

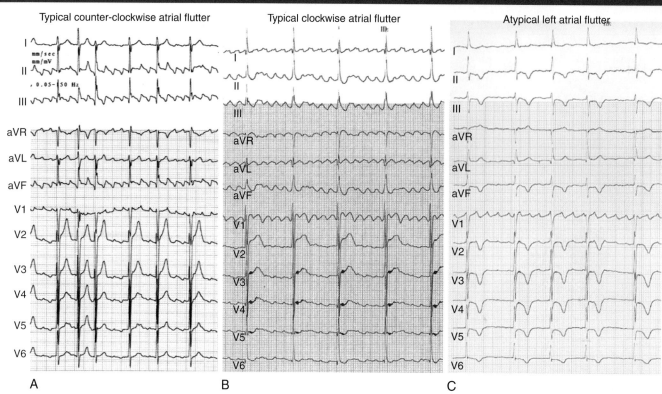

Typical counter-clockwise atrial flutter   Typical clockwise atrial flutter   Atypical left atrial flutter

A   B   C

FIGURE 65.13 Variants of atrial flutter. **A,** ECG of typical counterclockwise atrial flutter (AFL). **B,** ECG of typical clockwise AFL. **C,** ECG of an atypical left AFL.

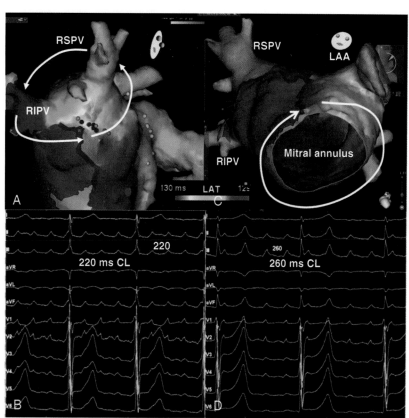

FIGURE 65.14 Patient with a prior history of persistent atrial flutter and previous catheter abla-tion. Three-dimensional color-coded activation maps and corresponding ECGs are shown. Activation timing is earliest in *red* through *yellow, green, light blue,* and *dark blue,* with the latest area activated in *purple.* The *deep red line* where purple meets red is the region of "head meets tail" of a reentrant circuit. **A,** Circuit rotating around the right-sided pulmonary veins in a counterclockwise direction is shown. This is considered a "roof-dependent" flutter. **B,** The corresponding ECG indicates an atypical flutter with upright morphology in V₁ and precordial leads and also upright in inferior leads and a cycle length of 220 msec. An ablation line was created across the atrial roof between the right superior (RSPV) and left superior (LSPV) pulmonary veins. **C,** A remap indicated that the circuit had changed and was now rotating around the mitral annulus in a counterclockwise direction. This may be termed a *mitral isthmus-dependent flutter.* The absence of change in the flutter wave morphology reflects the poor sensitivity and specificity of the flutter morphology for localization of atypical flutter circuits. This is particularly the case in the context of structural heart disease and prior ablation. **D,** With completion of the ablation line there was a sudden increase in cycle length to 260 msec without any apparent change in the flutter wave morphology.

Rate control with oral or intravenous beta block-ers or non-dihydropyridine calcium channel blockers (verapamil or diltiazem) may be used for rate control. Class 1C agents should not be used in patients with AFL because of the risk of slowing atrial rate and facil-itating 1:1 AV conduction with concomitant profound conduction slowing in the ventricle (see Fig. 65.10).

Chronic Therapy. Catheter ablation now represents the cornerstone management strategy in patients with AFL. It may be considered after a first episode or in patients with recurrent or persistent episodes. It is particularly indicated in patients who develop TMC. These recommendations apply to both CTI-dependent (typical) AFL and non–isthmus-dependent (atypical) flutters.

In CTI-dependent flutter, ablation is across the CTI from the annulus to the eustachian ridge at the ante-rior margin of the IVC. The end point is the demon-stration of bidirectional conduction block across this line using standard electrophysiology mapping tech-niques. The acute success rate is in excess of 97%, and the recurrence rate is now approximately 5% to 10%.[1,13] The procedural risk of serious adverse events is under 1%.[33]

In patients with atypical flutter or non–CTI-dependent flutter, the success rate is much more variable and depends on the nature of the underlying cardiac disease. For example, in patients with simple forms of scar-related flutter such as after ASD repair or mitral valve repair, success rates are similarly high, approaching 90%.[30,34] However, the requirement for multiple procedures is more common than for CTI-dependent flutter (>20% to 30%) because the frequent presence of multiple circuits and the late incidence of AF is high (>30% at 2 years). In patients with more advanced forms of surgically repaired CHD such as Fontan repair for univentricular physiology or Mustard/Senning repair for D-transposition of the great arteries (D-TGA), acute success rates are lower, the need for multiple procedures is higher, and long-term recurrences are common.[28,35] Patients generally have multiple different circuits due to the extensive atrial surgery performed and the underlying anatomic abnormalities. Nevertheless, ablation can represent an effective palliative procedure as part of a more

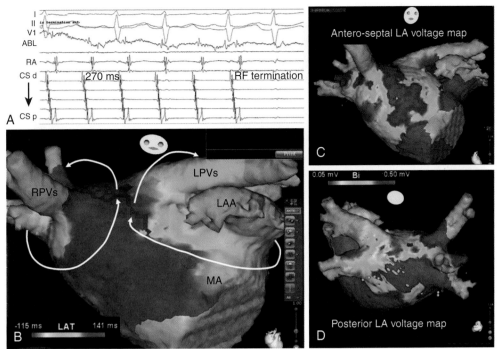

FIGURE 65.15 Example of dual-loop reentry in a patient with prior persistent atrial fibrillation (AF), advanced atrial remodeling, and prior AF ablation. A, Demonstration of ECG recordings and simultaneous intracardiac recordings from the ablation catheter (ABL), the right atrium (RA), and the coronary sinus (CS, distal to proximal) during a radiofrequency application that terminated the flutter. **B,** Electroanatomic color-coded activation map with colors superimposed on the left atrial CT scan, with the earliest activation indicated in *red* through *yellow, green, light blue, dark blue, and purple*. The *deep red line* where purple meets red is the region of "head meets tail" of both simultaneous reentrant circuits. The simultaneous circuits are indicated by the *white arrows* with one rotating around the right pulmonary veins (RPVs) and the other around the left pulmonary veins (LPVs) and the left atrial appendage (LAA). Both circuits are "roof-dependent." Linear ablation through the LA roof from the superior RPV to the superior LPV terminated the flutter as shown in **A**. **C** and **D,** The nature of advanced remodeling in this atrium. The colors in these images indicate atrial voltage with normal amplitudes represented by *purple* and *blue;* and abnormally low voltages by *red* and *yellow*. There are extensive low-voltage regions, indicative of fibrosis and associated with slow conduction in this atrium both anteriorly and septally (**C**) and posteriorly (**D**).

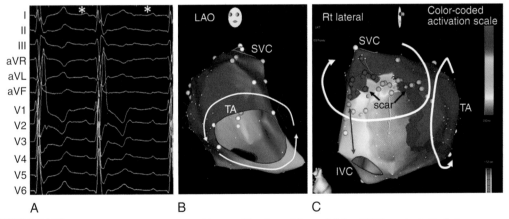

FIGURE 65.16 Dual-loop reentry in a 52-year-old man with prior atrial septal defect (ASD) repair. A, The flutter wave morphology *(asterisks)* is very unusual across all ECG leads. **B,** The three-dimensional electroanatomic map with a counterclockwise circuit around the tricuspid annulus (TA) in the right atrium in the left anterior oblique (LAO) view. Progression of activation is according to the color code at *right*. The activation is characteristic of typical counterclockwise atrial flutter, but the ECG is inconsistent with this. **C,** The right lateral view of the right atrium demonstrates that there are two simultaneous loops of activation. One is around the TA, but the other is around the region of the superior vena cava and an area of scar *(gray patch and blue dots arrowed)*. This is presumed to be the region of the atriotomy scar required for access to repair the ASD. This latter circuit alone would be termed *upper loop reentry*. Ablation in the cavo-tricuspid isthmus interrupted the circuit around the TA without any change in the cycle length due to the ongoing upper loop circuit. Ablation from the scar to the inferior vena cava *(red double-headed arrow)* terminated this second circuit.

general strategy that includes careful attention to structural and hemodynamic issues.[36]

A common form of atypical flutter in the era of AF ablation is due to circuits occurring after AF ablation procedures. These may occur in up to 20% of patients and are more common in those who have undergone persistent AF ablation, particularly when extensive or linear ablation has been performed or in those with more advanced atrial remodeling. Patients may have multiple circuits and the need for multiple procedures

is common.[37,38] Nevertheless, when control can be achieved, the long-term freedom from AF is high.

For patients in whom catheter ablation is contraindicated (e.g., advanced age, comorbidities, patient preference) or is not feasible (e.g., presence of mechanical valves, multiple unstable circuits, previously failed) a number of antiarrhythmic agents may be considered for maintenance of sinus rhythm. These include sotalol, dofetilide, or amiodarone depending on efficacy, tolerability, and nature of comorbidities (e.g., amiodarone preferred in the presence of significant LV dysfunction).

For patients in whom a rhythm control strategy is unsuccessful or not preferred, a rate control strategy may be adopted. This might be with a beta blocker or a nondihydropyridine calcium channel blocker (verapamil or diltiazem). If drug therapy is unsuccessful or poorly tolerated and ventricular response rates remain high, pacing (usually biventricular or His bundle pacing) followed by AV node ablation may be considered.

Due to the frequent coexistence of AF and AFL, anticoagulant management of patients with AFL generally follows the same recommendations as for AF both at the time of reversion and during chronic management, in which decisions should be dictated by the $CHADS_2-VA_2Sc$ score rather than apparent rhythm control.[1,13]

Paroxysmal Supraventricular Tachycardia
ECG Characteristics and ECG Classification of PSVT

SVT is most classically a regular narrow-complex tachycardia with a wide rate range from just in excess of 100 bpm to over 250 bpm in some patients (Fig. 65.18). In some patients bundle branch aberrancy may be present during tachycardia. This is more commonly right bundle aberrancy due to the longer refractory period of the right bundle compared with the left bundle (Fig 65.18A). Occasionally, patients with SVT may have a preexisting bundle branch block even in sinus rhythm, resulting in a wide complex tachycardia that nevertheless has a typical bundle branch block appearance (Fig. 65.19). In cases of aberrancy, the differential diagnosis may include some forms of VT such as a fascicular VT (Fig. 65.20).

The ECG of PSVT can be classified according to the VA relationship (Fig. 65.21). When there are more atrial than ventricular complexes

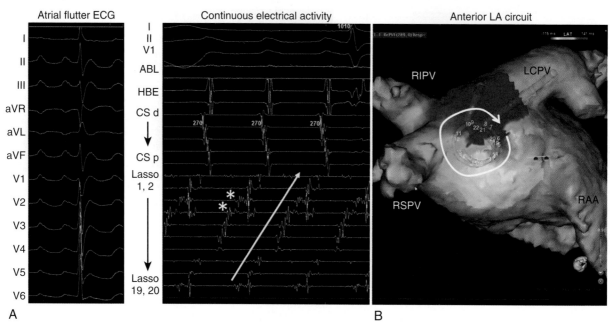

FIGURE 65.17 **Atypical atrial flutter due to small circuit reentry in a patient with a history of persistent atrial fibrillation. A,** Flutter wave morphology, which is upright in V₁ (indicating a probable left atrial origin) and upright in inferior leads (indicating a probable superior origin). The signals in the *middle panel* recorded by a lasso catheter in the anterior left atrium show activation spanning the entire cycle length. The *asterisks* indicate long fractionated multicomponent electrograms that span almost half the tachycardia cycle length and indicate a region of markedly slowed conduction necessary to maintain these small reentrant circuits. These signals reflect advanced atrial remodeling. **B,** An anatomic view of the left atrium viewed from superior aspect. The lasso catheter is shown in the anterior LA roof. The activation sequence goes from *red* through *yellow, green, light blue, dark blue,* and *purple.* Where purple meets red is the "head meets tail" location of the reentrant circuit (*arrow*). This circuit was interrupted by ablation at the site of the fractionated electrograms.

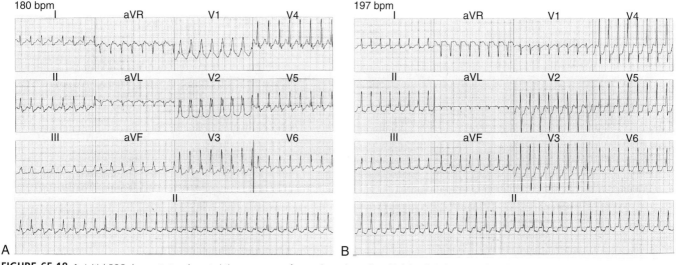

FIGURE 65.18 **A,** Initial ECG demonstrates characteristic appearance of a regular tachycardia, which is relatively narrow but displays a typical right bundle branch block (RBBB) morphology at a heart rate of 180 bpm. The RBBB occurs at initiation when a "long-short" onset sequence finds the right bundle refractory. The RBBB persists due to transeptal concealed conduction (linking). Activation over the left bundle then crosses the septum and invades the right bundle retrogradely maintaining the block to antegrade conduction. **B,** Minutes later, the bundle branch block normalized spontaneously. Two possible mechanisms for this spontaneous resolution are either "accommodation," in which the antegrade refractory period of the right bundle gradually shortens or, alternatively, distal migration of the site of collision between antegrade activation of the RBBB and transeptal retrograde penetration. This resolution despite the higher heart rate confirms that the block was functional. Note also the widespread ST segment depression, which usually does not imply the presence of myocardial ischemia.

the possibilities include focal AT (see Fig. 65.5), AV node reentry with block (Fig. 65.22) or AFL (see Fig. 65.11B, C). When there are fewer atrial than ventricular complexes during a narrow-complex tachycardia, the differential diagnosis includes only quite rare entities, including junctional ectopic tachycardia (JET), a concealed nodofascicular pathway and high septal fascicular VT (see Fig. 65.21). Most commonly, when the atrial and ventricular complexes occur 1:1, the tachycardia can be further defined in terms of whether the P wave falls in the first half of the R-R interval (short RP tachycardia) or the second half of the R-R interval (long RP tachycardia). Short RP tachycardias can be further

divided into those in which the P wave falls largely within the QRS when it may not be visible (RP <70 msec) or after the QRS within the T wave (RP >70 msec) (see Fig. 65.21).

Clinical Presentation

As described in the introduction, PSVT may be viewed as a subset of SVT and involves a classic clinical picture characterized by sudden onset and termination of rapid palpitations documented as a regular narrow-complex tachycardia. This clinical picture implies the presence of AVNRT, AVRT, or less frequently AT.

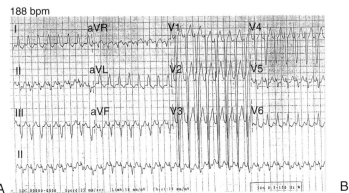

188 bpm

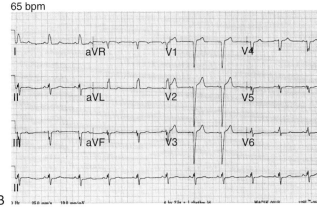

65 bpm

FIGURE 65.19 A, Left bundle branch block and left axis tachycardia at 188 bpm. The appearance is of a typical left bundle with a deep S wave in right precordial leads and in inferior leads and loss of the septal Q wave in the lateral precordial leads. **B,** In sinus rhythm at 65 bpm the identical QRS morphology is present indicating that the ECG is highly likely to represent SVT. The rhythm was proven to be atrioventricular nodal reentrant tachycardia.

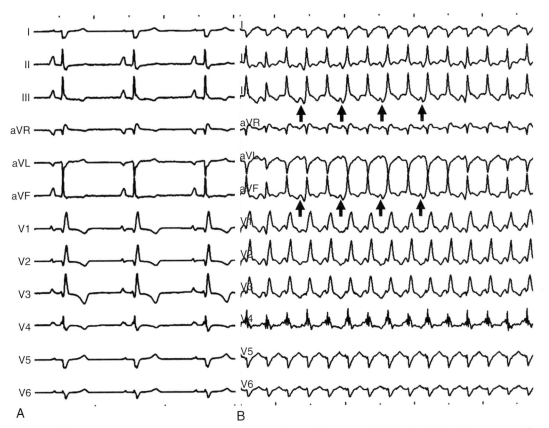

FIGURE 65.20 A, Sinus rhythm ECG demonstrating a right bundle branch block pattern with right axis deviation due to presence of a left posterior hemiblock. **B,** Tachycardia with the identical QRS morphology suggests that this is likely to be a supraventricular tachycardia. However, there is VA dissociation (P waves indicated by the *solid arrows* seen best in lead III and aVF. The mechanism of the arrhythmia was a form of bundle branch reentry with the antegrade limb being the left posterior hemifascicle (hence the same morphology as sinus rhythm) and the retrograde limb being the right bundle, which had slow conduction. *VA,* ventriculoatrial.

rapid rates.[10] In adults with PSVT, asymptomatic episodes are quite uncommon. AF may develop in up to 12% of patients diagnosed with PSVT during follow-up.

Episodes of PSVT are usually initiated by atrial or ventricular ectopic beats or couplets. Patients frequently describe classic triggers such as sudden movements, bending over, or exercise, although a wide range of triggers with variable frequency have been reported.

A description of multiple stop-start episodes in succession usually indicates a focal AT, whereas a single prolonged episode is more common with AVRT or AVNRT. Adults with a long history of episodes that began in childhood and teenage years are more likely to have AVNRT or AVRT rather than AT.

Patients with PSVT may have been diagnosed and treated as having anxiety and panic attacks, a misdiagnosis more commonly observed in women.[10]

Typically, rapid palpitations may be accompanied by light-headedness, chest discomfort, and dyspnea, but the severity of these symptoms varies considerably. Very rapid and more prolonged episodes particularly in older patients are more likely to be associated with severe symptoms. Conversely, younger patients will frequently have no symptoms other than an awareness of rapid palpitations. Intense light-headedness or occasionally presyncope may be reported at onset of the tachycardia and may be perceived immediately before awareness of rapid palpitations. However, syncope is rare in SVT. Patients will often describe fatigue, which may persist for 24 hours after an event. Polyuria is occasionally described as a feature and is presumed to be the result of atrial natriuretic peptide release at

Epidemiology. AV node reentry (AVNRT) is the most common documented mechanism of PSVT in patients undergoing catheter ablation.[15] After the age of 20, AVNRT accounts for the largest number of ablations in each age group. There is a consistent 2:1 female-to-male predominance observed in multiple series. AVRT is the most common mechanism of SVT in the first decade of life, accounting for 55% to 60% of PSVT cases.[15] Thereafter there is a progressive decline that continues through each decade of life such that beyond 60 years of age AVRT represents under 10% of SVT cases. In contrast, the prevalence of AT is low in the first decades of life (<10%), slowly increasing with age to represent over 20% of cases beyond age 60.

AVNRT: Anatomy, Physiology and ECG Characteristics. The AVNRT circuit most probably involves the compact AV node, perinodal transitional inputs to the node, which may be left or right sided (fast and slow pathways), and the perinodal atrial region. However, it must be emphasized that the precise anatomic location of the entire circuit is unknown. The critical components of the circuit are located within the anatomic triangle of Koch bounded anteriorly by the TA, posteriorly by the tendon of Todaro, superiorly by the membranous septum and the penetrating bundle of His, and inferiorly by the ostium of the coronary sinus. At the apex of the triangle is the compact node. The fast AV nodal pathway approaches the compact node at the superior aspect of the triangle, and the slow pathway approaches the node from the inferior aspect of the triangle and the CS os region. In addition, there are both anterior and posterior inputs to the AV node from the left side of the septum, which may participate in tachycardia. A proposed schema for the different forms of AVNRT from the work of Katritsis and Becker is shown in Fig. 65.23.[39] The theoretical possibilities include a right-sided circuit, a left-sided circuit, simultaneous right and left circuits, and figure-of-8 reentry.

Typical AVNRT

The typical form of AVNRT involves antegrade conduction over the slow pathway and retrograde activation via the fast pathway. Retrograde activation to the atrium via the fast pathway occurs synchronously with antegrade activation over the His Purkinje system to the ventricle resulting in simultaneous atrial and ventricular activation. In approximately 50% of cases, the P wave is not visible because it is occurs completely within the QRS. In 45% of cases, the final component of the P wave occurs at the tail end of the QRS, producing a pseudo right bundle appearance in V_1 and a pseudo S wave pattern in the inferior leads (Fig. 65.22A). This appearance has been reported to indicate typical AVNRT with an accuracy of 100%.[40] Occasionally the tachycardia exhibits 2:1 conduction to the ventricle (Fig. 65.22B). This generally occurs early after onset of the arrhythmia and is characterized by the appearance of a P wave exactly in the middle of two consecutive QRS complexes (Fig. 65.22B and eFig. 65.2). The usual site of block is within or below the bundle of His (Fig. 65.22C), and

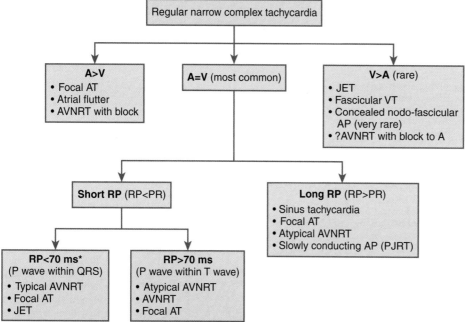

FIGURE 65.21 Algorithm for evaluation of narrow-complex tachycardia. The P wave is either not visible or visible as a pseudo R prime in V_1. The interval of 70 msec is derived from the VA time on the His bundle electrogram during electrophysiologic study. When using the onset of the surface QRS to onset of the visible P wave the intervals used are less than 90 msec and greater than 90 msec. *A,* Atrium; *AP,* accessory pathway; *AT,* atrial tachycardia; *AVNRT,* atrioventricular nodal reentrant tachycardia; *JET,* junctional ectopic tachycardia; *PJRT,* permanent junctional reciprocating tachycardia; *V,* ventricle; *VT,* ventricular tachycardia. (Modified from Brugada J, et al. 2019 ESC guidelines for the management of patients with supraventricular tachycardia the task force for the management of patients with supraventricular tachycardia of the European Society of Cardiology (ESC): developed in collaboration with the Association for European Paediatric and Congenital Cardiology (AEPC). Eur Heart J 2020;41:655-720.)

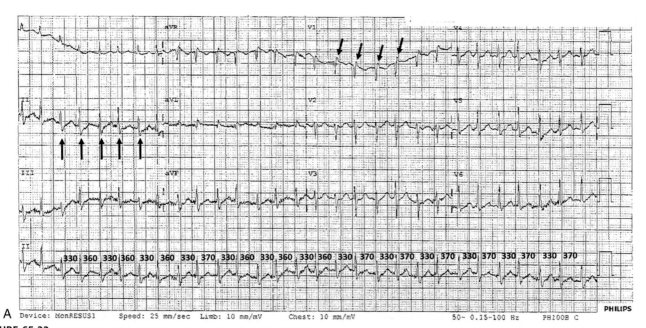

FIGURE 65.22 A, 1:1 atrioventricular nodal reentrant tachycardia (AVNRT). Note the presence of the pseudo R prime in V_1 (*downward arrows*) and the pseudo S wave in inferior leads (*upward arrows*) due to the retrograde P wave. Note also the presence of cycle length alternans varying between 330 and 360/370 msec on alternate beats. This suggests the presence of two antegrade slow pathways. Despite this cycle length alternans, the position of the retrograde P wave remains fixed at the same location in the final component of the QRS as indicated by the *arrows*. This fixed VA time despite cycle length variation rules out focal atrial tachycardia and confirms the presence of typical AVNRT. *VA,* ventriculoatrial.

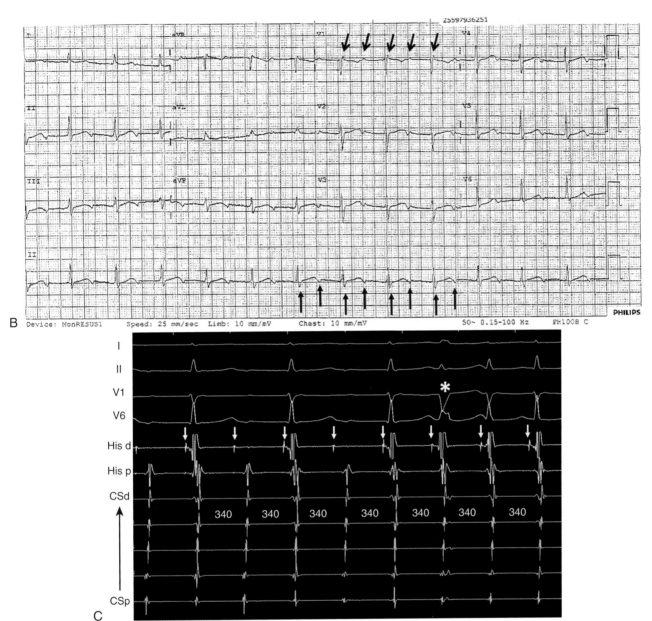

FIGURE 65.22–cont'd **B,** 2:1 AVNRT in the same patient; note that there is a P wave (inverted in inferior leads; upright in V₁) precisely located in the middle between two QRS complexes. In V₁ there is a pseudo R prime at the tail end of the QRS (pseudo partial RBBB) and indicated by the *downward arrows,* which corresponds to the final component of the P wave. This can be readily appreciated by viewing the identical appearance of the P wave located between the two QRS complexes. Similarly, in inferior leads, the pseudo S wave appearance (*upward arrows*) is due to the P wave occurring in the final component of the QRS. Again, this can be appreciated by noting the P wave located between the QRS complexes that has the identical morphology to the pseudo S wave. **C,** Four ECG leads and intracardiac recordings from a His bundle catheter (distal and proximal) and from a coronary sinus catheter (CS) with recordings displayed from proximal at the *bottom* to distal at the *top.* The panel shows 2:1 AVNRT, which changes to 1:1 spontaneously during an electrophysiology study and ablation procedure. The cycle length is 340 msec (176 bpm). On the *left* of the panel, every other His spike (*white arrows*) is not followed by a QRS complex. Thus, there is 2:1 "infra-Hisian" block. This is not pathologic but rather reflects functional block. On the *right* of the screen, the tachycardia spontaneously goes 1:1, with the first beat showing only left bundle aberrancy (*asterisk*) before the tachycardia then becomes 1:1 with narrow complexes (final 2 beats).

although block occurring in a lower final common AV nodal pathway above the His bundle has previously been proposed, definitive evidence for this is lacking.[40] Several ECG features may allow differentiation of *typical* AVNRT from a focal AT:

1. When onset of the tachycardia is recorded, an early atrial ectopic that blocks in the fast pathway (due to the relatively longer refractory period of the fast pathway) conducts down the slow pathway with a long PR interval is highly suggestive of AVNRT. Activity then travels retrogradely via the fast pathway, which has now recovered excitability, and the tachycardia is initiated. Onset of focal AT is also generally with a tightly coupled atrial premature beat, but it will not necessarily be conducted with a long PR interval over a slow pathway.
2. When cycle length variability occurs during the tachycardia, the presence of a fixed ventriculoatrial (VA) relationship (reflecting

fast pathway conduction) provides strong evidence in favor of AVNRT rather than AT, in which this relationship is incidental (see Fig. 65.22A).
3. When termination of the tachycardia is documented, spontaneous termination with a P wave as the final event also provides strong evidence against AT and therefore in favor of AVNRT.

Atypical AVNRT
Atypical AVNRT may be fast-slow or slow-slow, the latter indicating the presence of more than one slow pathway. Fast-slow AVNRT is a long RP tachycardia usually with a PR interval of less than 200 msec (Fig. 65.24).[40] In fast-slow AVNRT the distance from the atrium to His recording (the AH interval) is shorter than the subsequent HA interval. The inferior leads characteristically show inverted P waves due to the

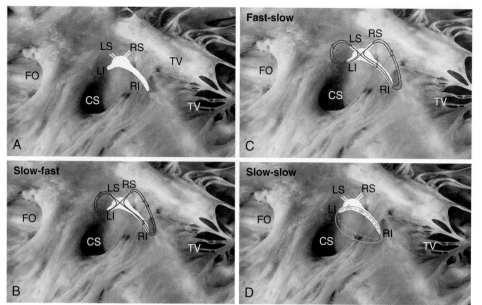

retrograde slow pathway exit that is frequently in the vicinity of the CS os. Slow-slow AVNRT is diagnosed when the VA interval is >70 msec, but the AH interval is longer than the HA interval.

Treatment of AVNRT

ACUTE MANAGEMENT. Patients should be educated in vagal maneuvers to be performed in the supine position with leg elevation.[41] When performed under instruction in the emergency department this may be effective in 40% to 50% of patients.

In patients who fail vagal maneuvers, adenosine 6 to 12 mg intravenous bolus is the treatment of choice. Care must be taken to warn the patient that they may feel chest tightness and a transient sense of impending doom. In patients who fail adenosine reversion, intravenous verapamil or diltiazem or alternatively an intravenous beta blocker (metoprolol or esmolol) may be considered.

DC cardioversion is appropriate in hemodynamically unstable patients or when all other measures fail but is rarely required.

FIGURE 65.23 A proposed schema for the different forms of atrioventricular nodal reentry tachycardia (AVNRT). The theoretical possibilities include a right-sided circuit, a left-sided circuit, simultaneous right and left circuits, and figure-of-8 reentry. **A,** Schema of the anatomy of the atrioventricular nodal region showing the coronary sinus ostium (CS), the tricuspid valve (TV), and the fossa ovalis (FO). The compact node is shown with right inferior (RI), left inferior (LI), right superior (RS), and left superior (LS) inputs to the node. **B,** Slow-fast typical AVNRT circuits. The most common form approaches the node from the RI input and exits from the RS input. A small region of perinodal atrium completes the circuit. The circuit also may be localized to the left-sided inputs. **C,** Fast-slow AVNRT with activation in the reverse direction with input to the node over the RS or LS and exits from wither the RI or LI pathways. **D,** Slow-slow AVNRT uses the two inferior inputs to the node as entrance and exit. As in all forms of AVNRT, perinodal atrium completes the circuit. (From Katritsis DG, Becker A. The atrioventricular nodal reentrant tachycardia circuit: a proposal. Heart Rhythm 2007;4:1354-1360.)

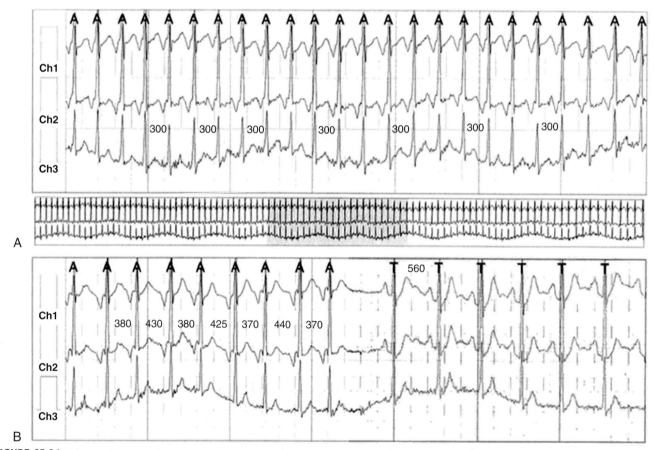

FIGURE 65.24 Holter monitor trace of a long R-P tachycardia with inverted P waves in Ch1 and Ch2 indicative of a superiorly directed axis. The differential diagnosis includes focal atrial tachycardia, atypical atrioventricular nodal reentrant tachycardia (AVNRT), or permanent junctional reciprocating tachycardia (slowly conducting retrograde pathway). **A,** The tachycardia cycle length is relatively fixed at approximately 300 msec (200 bpm). **B,** Immediately before termination the tachycardia cycle length has prolonged and is varying by up to 70 msec (cycle length approximately 400 msec equivalent to heart rate of 150 bpm). Note that even with marked variability the PR interval remains fixed (150 msec), indicating that the variation is in the VA interval. This "unhooking of the VA" favors a diagnosis of focal atrial tachycardia but does not on its own eliminate the other two diagnoses as variable retrograde conduction over a slow atrioventricular nodal pathway or a slowly conducting accessory pathway could produce a similar pattern. Termination with the last complex being ventricular (QRS) is also consistent with all three diagnoses. Indeed, at electrophysiologic study the arrhythmia was proven to be atypical fast-slow AVNRT with variable conduction in the retrograde slow pathway. VA, ventriculoatrial

CHRONIC MANAGEMENT. Patients with infrequent episodes associated with mild symptoms and that are responsive to vagal maneuvers may elect no treatment.

However, for more frequent episodes, unpredictable episodes, or episodes with severe symptoms, the treatment of choice is catheter ablation targeting the slow pathway region.[1,13] Numerous observational trials have documented both the efficacy and safety of catheter ablation for AVNRT. In addition, a recent randomized trial comparing catheter ablation versus antiarrhythmics confirmed the superiority of ablation and the relative long-term inefficacy of medical therapy. At 5 years of follow up none of the ablation patients had a recurrence necessitating hospital presentation compared with over 75% in the medical arm by 2 years.[42] Large series have confirmed the efficacy and safety of catheter ablation for both typical and atypical forms of AVNRT.[43] Long-term success rates in excess of 95% are generally reported. In addition, large contemporary series have reported an incidence of AV block between 0.1% and 0.4% and no mortality.[42,44,45] In the pediatric age group there is a preference toward using cryoablation because some studies have suggested a lower rate of inadvertent AV block, but the recurrence rate is higher.[46,47] However, in the adult population no consistent benefit has been demonstrated with cryoablation.[48] Catheter ablation has been shown to improve quality of life and reduce ongoing costs.

In patients who prefer medical therapy, the first-line long-term treatment options are either a non-dihydropyridine calcium channel blocker (verapamil or diltiazem) or a beta blocker. These may reduce the frequency and duration of events but rarely abolish the tachycardia. In addition, 20% to 50% of patients will discontinue therapy for reasons including inefficacy or intolerance.[40]

Junctional Ectopic Tachycardia (Nonreentrant Junctional Tachycardia). JET is a rare arrhythmia that occurs in several specific clinical contexts:

1. It may occur early after surgical repair of CHD with an incidence of 1% to 5%.[49,50]
2. As a congenital arrhythmia presenting in the first 6 months of life, in which it has been associated with a high morbidity and mortality.[51] In this age group the arrhythmia is more likely to be incessant and has higher rates.
3. In the pediatric age group beyond the age of 6 months. For management, a wide range of antiarrhythmic medications have been trialed and the majority of patients require combination therapy.[52] Complete suppression of the arrhythmia is rare; more frequently the rate and frequency of episodes is decreased. In up to 20% of cases, antiarrhythmics are completely ineffective. The agent with highest reported efficacy is amiodarone. Catheter ablation is playing an increasing role using either radiofrequency or

cryoablation approaches. In the largest study published to date, these modalities had comparable acute efficacy (82% to 85%) and recurrence rates (13% to 14%). Inadvertent permanent third-degree AV block occurred in 3 of 17 (18%) patients who underwent radiofrequency ablation and in none of the cryoablation patients.[53]

4. Rarely, this arrhythmia may manifest in adults.[54] In a small ablation series of JET in adults (mean age 58), recurrence rates (37%), requirement for multiple procedures, and risk of AV block (20%) were high.

The ECG characteristics of JET are those of a narrow-complex tachycardia resembling typical AVNRT with a P wave at the terminal end of the QRS (Fig. 65.25) or with VA dissociation when conduction block is present between the junctional focus and the surrounding atrium. On monitoring, the arrhythmia demonstrates multiple spontaneous (not ectopic induced) onsets and terminations and rates may occur in excess of 250 bpm.

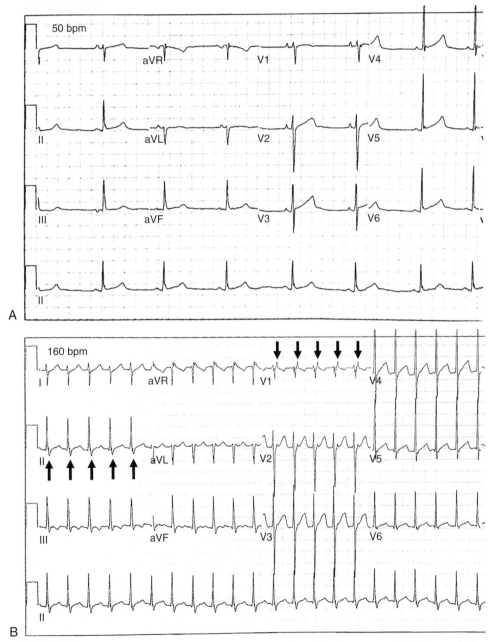

FIGURE 65.25 ECGs recorded in a 12-yr-old boy with incessant tachycardia refractory to medical therapy. **A,** Sinus rhythm at 50 bpm. **B,** Junctional tachycardia at 160 bpm (on Holter monitoring rates would frequently reach 240 bpm during minor activity). Note the presence of the P wave visible after the tail end of the QRS in V₁ as a sharp pseudo R prime (*downward arrows*) and in the inferior leads as a sharp pseudo S wave (*upward arrows* in lead II). On a snapshot ECG, the arrhythmia is indistinguishable from typical atrioventricular reentrant tachycardia. Holter monitoring revealed repeated onsets and terminations with a junctional beat (no preceding P wave).

Tachycardias due to an Accessory Pathway

Accessory Pathway Epidemiology

The prevalence of a Wolff-Parkinson-White (WPW) pattern on a sinus rhythm ECG in the general population has been estimated at between 0.15% and 0.25%. Although not classically considered to be an inherited disorder, the prevalence does increase significantly among first-degree relatives of patients with WPW to 0.55%.[55] However, in many patients, WPW is intermittent and not all with the ECG pattern will develop tachyarrhythmias.

Accessory pathways may occur in the context of the *PRKAG2* gene variant cardiac glycogenosis, which causes a syndrome characterized by cardiomyopathy with increased ventricular wall thickness, conduction disease and AV block, and ventricular preexcitation.[56]

Accessory pathways are classically recognized in patients with Ebstein anomaly, occurring in approximately 25% of this population.[57] They occur in relation to the tricuspid valve malformation and are therefore invariably right sided; frequently there may be multiple pathways, the majority of which are manifest (Fig. 65.26). It is important to recognize that in addition to AVRT, patients with Ebstein anomaly may sustain a wide range of arrhythmias, including typical and atypical AFL, focal AT, AF, and ventricular arrhythmias.

Accessory Pathway Anatomic Considerations. The musculature of the atrium and ventricles is normally separated by the electrically inert fibrous skeleton of the heart, with the only connection being the bundle of His. This electrical conducting bundle penetrates through the central fibrous body of the heart and then divides into the bundle branch system, which directs the impulse to the right and left ventricles. An accessory pathway represents a congenital persistence of bridging AV working myocardium in the form of a muscle bundle. Another form of accessory pathway involves a muscular bridge from the sleeve of myocardium investing the coronary sinus and its branches and the epicardial myocardium of the left ventricle most usually in the posteroseptal region.

Anatomically, accessory pathways are most commonly located along the mitral annulus and termed *left free wall pathways* (60%); approximately 25% are in the septal region of the tricuspid or mitral annulus, and a minority (15%) are on the right free wall.[10]

Concealed vs. Manifest Accessory Pathways. An accessory pathway may conduct in the antegrade direction (termed *manifest* due to the characteristic ECG appearance), the retrograde direction, or both. When an accessory pathway conducts only in the retrograde direction it is termed *concealed* and the surface ECG is normal. On occasion, manifest accessory pathways conduct in the antegrade direction only (these represent only approximately 10% of all accessory pathways).

The WPW ECG

The sinus rhythm 12-lead ECG of WPW classically exhibits a short PR interval (rapid conduction over the accessory pathway) and a slurred QRS onset (delta wave) (Fig. 65.27 and eFig. 65.3). The QRS complex represents a fusion beat between conduction over the accessory pathway and conduction over the AV node. The normal AV node has slow and decremental conduction that accounts for the normal PR interval. *Decrement* refers to the fact that conduction in the AV node slows further for an abnormally fast input such as an AT or AF. In contrast, an accessory pathway generally has rapid antegrade conduction such that there is a very short PR interval and the P wave is followed immediately by the QRS without an isoelectric interval.

Because initial ventricular activation occurs via the accessory pathway inserting directly into ventricular myocardium, the initial appearance of the QRS is a slurred onset and the beginnings of a wide QRS (due to relatively slow ventricular conduction). However, shortly after this onset, activation over the AV node is complete and the remainder of ventricular activation then occurs rapidly over the His-Purkinje fibers. This creates an inflection point in the QRS between the slow delta wave due to ventricular myocardial conduction and the subsequent rapid His-Purkinje upstroke (Fig. 65.28 and Fig. 65.29). The extent of ventricular preexcitation depends on a number of factors, including the anatomic location of the pathway and the relative speed of conduction over the accessory pathway compared with the node. For example, a left lateral accessory pathway may demonstrate minimal preexcitation because by the time atrial activation has spread from the sinus node in the high right atrium over to a left lateral location, antegrade conduction though the AV node may have already occurred. In

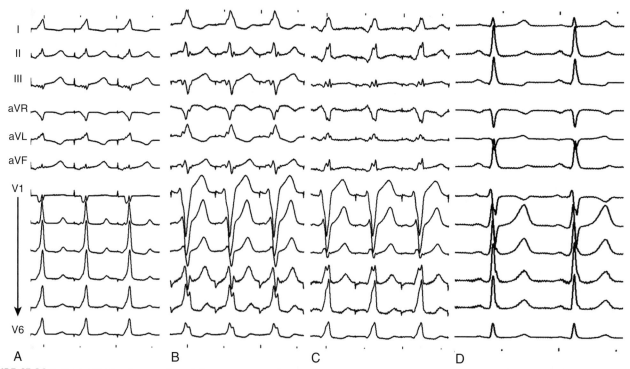

FIGURE 65.26 Patient with Ebstein anomaly and three accessory pathways around the tricuspid annulus. The ECGs were performed during an electrophysiologic study, and pacing is from the atrium near the accessory pathway insertion site in order to maximize the preexcitation. **A,** An accessory pathway located in a midseptal location. The precordial transition is between V₁ and V₂ localizing the pathway to the septum. Leads II and III are isoelectric with a small positive delta wave in lead II. This pattern is consistent with a midseptal location (deeply negative delta waves would suggest a posteroseptal location and steeply positive delta wave in the inferior leads would suggest an anteroseptal location). **B,** A second accessory pathway with a precordial transition occurs after V₃, putting this pathway on the right free wall. The pathway was right lateral. **C,** A third right-sided accessory pathway with another differing delta wave vector. The precordial transition after V₃ indicating right free wall and a more inferiorly directed delta wave axis (upright in lead II and aVF). The pathway was right anterolateral. **D,** After catheter ablation of all three pathways, the QRS morphology normalized.

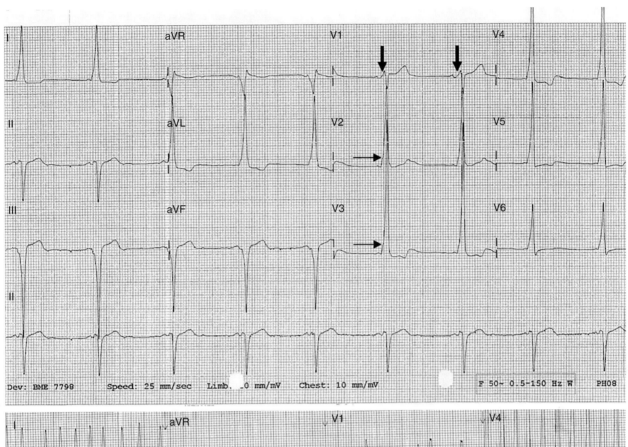

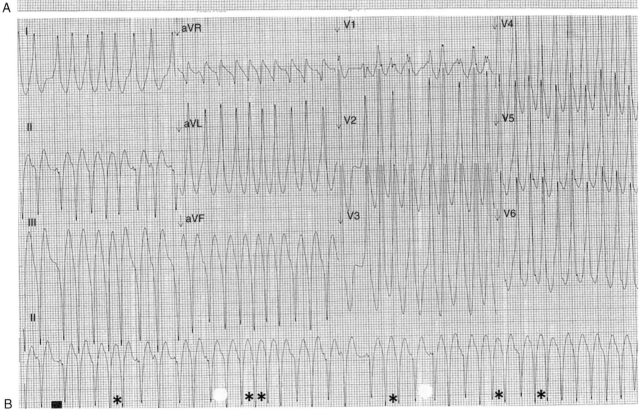

FIGURE 65.27 **A,** Sinus rhythm ECG showing a short PR interval and delta wave classic for Wolf-Parkinson-White syndrome (WPW). The delta wave vector is upright in V₁ (*downward arrows*) and across the precordium and negative in the inferior leads, consistent with a left posterior accessory pathway location. The inflection point between slow ventricular myocardial activation from the delta wave insertion into ventricular myocardium and rapid activation over the His-Purkinje tissue once slower conduction over the atrioventricular node has occurred is well seen in V₂ and V₃ (*horizontal arrows*). **B,** Preexcited atrial fibrillation, the hallmark of which is an irregularly irregular wide-complex tachycardia that appears largely monomorphic (some variability may occur due to capture and fusion). The delta wave morphology is upright in V₁ during maximal preexcitation. There are some very short R-R intervals of 200 msec or less (*asterisks*) equivalent to a heart rate of over 300 bpm. In general, a shortest preexcited R-R interval of less than 250 msec is a risk factor for progression to ventricular fibrillation and sudden death.

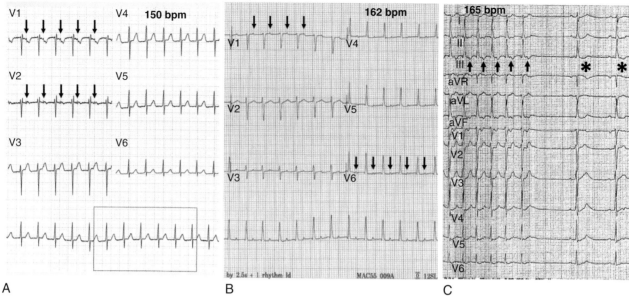

FIGURE 65.28 A, Precordial leads showing atrioventricular reentrant tachycardia (AVRT) with the retrograde P wave clearly observed deforming the T wave in V₁ and in V₂ (*arrows*). The patient had a concealed anteroseptal accessory pathway. **B,** Precordial leads of atrial tachycardia originating from the anteroseptal tricuspid annulus. (The P wave morphology cannot be clearly identified within the T wave). The P wave occupies the same position deforming the T wave as in the AVRT example in panel A. However, the arrhythmia is a focal atrial tachycardia. At this heart rate, there is slow conduction over the AV node to the ventricle such that the P wave is inscribed within the preceding T wave (*arrows*). The arrhythmia is independent of AV nodal conduction, and the position of the P wave is therefore incidental. Nevertheless, on the ECG alone, the two mechanisms cannot be distinguished. **C,** On the left of this continuous 12-lead trace is a regular narrow-complex tachycardia at 165 bpm with the retrograde P wave observed within the T wave (*upward arrows*). There is spontaneous termination with the final activation being the retrograde P wave. This essentially rules out an atrial tachycardia as it would be highly unlikely for the tachycardia to terminate at the precise moment when there was coincidental AV block. This implies antegrade block in the AV node, which must form part of the circuit being either AVRT or atypical atrioventricular nodal reentrant tachycardia. In this case, the arrhythmia was AVRT due to a concealed right posteroseptal accessory pathway. Note that the final 2 sinus beats are not preexcited. The *asterisks* highlight the absence of the retrograde P waves during sinus rhythm.

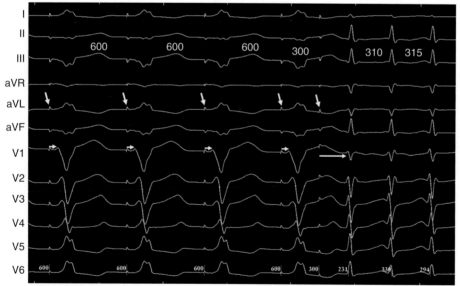

FIGURE 65.29 Continuous 12-lead ECG during atrial programmed stimulation at electrophysiology study. The patient has a right free wall accessory pathway (late precordial transition at V₄). An atrial pacing drive train is being delivered at cycle length of 600 msec (pacing artefact—*downward arrows*). There is a short PR interval, and the QRS morphology is maximally preexcited due to pacing close to the accessory pathway location. An atrial extra-stimulus is introduced at a coupling interval of 300 msec. There is antegrade block in the accessory pathway with a much longer PR interval due to antegrade conduction over the AV node. The QRS of this beat is narrow because preexcitation is no longer present, and all activation occurred over the AV node and His-Purkinje system. Tachycardia is initiated as the accessory pathway–recovered excitability in the retrograde direction setting up the reentrant loop. In this case, the retrograde P waves during these initial tachycardia beats (cycle length 310/315 msec) cannot be clearly detected.

Accessory Pathway Localization. A variety of ECG algorithms to predict the likely anatomic location of the accessory pathway are based on the delta wave vector.[10] Broadly, a positive delta wave in V₁ indicates a left-sided accessory pathway (see Fig. 65.28), a negative delta wave in V₁ with early precordial transition to upright in V₂ usually indicates a right septal accessory pathway (see Fig. 65.29), and later transition of the precordial delta wave at or after V₃ most usually a right free wall accessory pathway (see Fig. 65.27). The pattern in the limb leads aids with localization to relatively more superior or inferior sites or more septal or lateral sites. These algorithms are most specific when there is significant or maximal preexcitation, which can be achieved during EPS by pacing close to the accessory pathway site.[58]

Arrhythmias Associated with Accessory Pathways

ORTHODROMIC AVRT. The most common form of tachycardia associated with an accessory pathway is orthodromic AVRT. In patients with a manifest pathway, this accounts for 90% to 95% of AVRT episodes. This circuit involves antegrade conduction over the AV node and His-Purkinje system and is therefore classically a regular narrow-complex tachycardia. Retrograde conduction occurs over the accessory pathway after ventricular activation. Therefore, the retrograde P wave occurs after ventricular activation and generally creates a visible sharp deflection deforming the T wave most usually best seen in V₁ (see Fig. 65.28). Note that this location of the P wave is not specific to AVRT and may also occur in AT (see Fig. 65.28B) and in atypical AVNRT.

contrast, right free wall pathways, being very close to the AV node, may demonstrate marked preexcitation in sinus rhythm due to the proximity of the accessory pathway to sinus node activation (see Fig. 65.29). An accessory pathway with slow conduction such as an atriofascicular pathway may show no preexcitation because AV nodal conduction is more rapid.

In sinus rhythm, although the accessory pathway conducts more rapidly than the AV node, the refractory period of the accessory pathway (time taken to recover excitability) is usually longer than AV nodal refractory period. This is particularly true in sinus rhythm when the cycle length is long compared with that in tachycardia. Thus, a tight-coupled atrial premature complex can find the accessory pathway refractory but conduct slowly antegradely down the AV node (see Fig. 65.29). Conduction time down the node and His-Purkinje and across the ventricle allows recovery of accessory pathway excitability in the retrograde direction and AV reentry is initiated. When block in the accessory pathway occurs with antegrade conduction over the AV node, preexcitation is lost and the QRS normalizes because all ventricular activation is over the His-Purkinje system.

ANTIDROMIC AVRT. Antidromic AVRT is a regular wide-complex arrhythmia in which antegrade conduction occurs over the accessory pathway (fully preexcited), with retrograde activation occurring over the AV node or over a second accessory pathway present in 30% to 60% of patients with spontaneous antidromic AVRT[13] (Fig. 65.30). The P wave is inscribed within the broad QRS and is usually not visible. It accounts for only approximately 5% of AVRT episodes.

PREEXCITED TACHYCARDIA. In preexcited tachycardia, the arrhythmia originates in the atrium and is conducted passively to the ventricle over the accessory pathway, which acts as a bystander. Examples of this include AT (Fig. 65.31) or AV node reentry with passive conduction over the accessory pathway. A rapidly conducting accessory pathway does not exhibit any decremental conduction in response to a rapid input such as an AT or AF. The development of AF in the presence of an accessory pathway with a short antegrade refractory period (<250 msec) and a shortest R-R interval during AF of less than 250 msec can result in ventricular response rates of up to 300 bpm with the potential to trigger ventricular fibrillation (VF) and sudden death. The characteristic ECG is a wide-complex tachycardia (maximal preexcitation) with an irregularly irregular ventricular rhythm (see Fig. 65.28B and Fig. 65.29B).

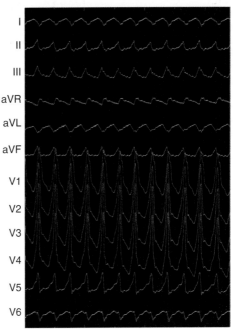

FIGURE 65.30 Antidromic tachycardia recorded during a catheter ablation procedure. The tachycardia is a regular monomorphic wide-complex tachycardia with antegrade conduction over the accessory pathway and retrograde conduction over the atrioventricular node. All ventricular myocardium is depolarized from the accessory pathway insertion point with slow conduction over ventricular myocardium producing maximal preexcitation. The delta wave vector is markedly upright in V_1 (left-sided), upright in inferior leads (anteriorly located) and negative in leads I and aVL (far left lateral) consistent with a left anterolateral pathway. The arrhythmia was proven at electrophysiologic study to be antidromic tachycardia, but the differential diagnosis of this wide-complex regular tachyarrhythmia includes ventricular tachycardia and other forms of preexcited tachycardia.

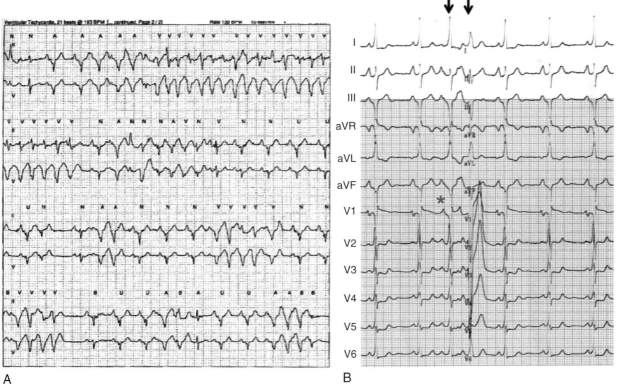

A   B

FIGURE 65.31 A 57-year-old man with recurrent palpitations and presyncope. **A,** Holter monitor trace showing bursts of wide-complex tachycardia. Analysis of the sinus beats suggests the presence of preexcitation. There are bursts of atrial tachycardia with increasing preexcitation. **B,** Continuous 12-lead ECG showing sinus rhythm with an atrial couplet from the atrial tachycardia focus. The first 2 sinus beats are preexcited with a pattern consistent with a right posteroseptal accessory pathway (precordial transition between V_1 and V_2; superiorly directed delta wave axis). There are then two atrial ectopics (*downward arrows*) with an increase in QRS duration due to increasing preexcitation. This occurs due to the decremental conduction properties of the AV node, whereas the accessory pathway demonstrates no such decrement. The atrial ectopic focus P wave is upright in V_1 and upright in inferior leads and was successfully ablated at the ostium of the left superior pulmonary vein.

Treatment of AVRT

As with any regular narrow-complex SVT, initial management may include vagal maneuvers best performed in the supine position with leg elevation.[41]

In patients who fail vagal maneuvers, adenosine 6- to 12-mg intravenous bolus is the treatment of choice but must be used with caution in AVRT due to the potential for induction of AF with rapid antegrade conduction over the accessory pathway. Electrical cardioversion must be available. In patients who fail adenosine reversion, drugs that act on the AV nodal limb of the circuit, including intravenous verapamil or diltiazem or a beta blocker (metoprolol or esmolol), may be considered. Alternatively, drugs acting on the accessory pathway such as ibutilide, procainamide, or a class 1C agent (flecainide or propafenone) may be used. In antidromic tachycardia, drugs active on the accessory pathway are preferred because when multiple accessory pathways are present they may form both limbs of the circuit. DC cardioversion is appropriate in hemodynamically unstable patients or when antiarrhythmic medications fail.

ACUTE TREATMENT OF PREEXCITED AF.
Acute treatment of preexcited AF when the patient is hemodynamically unstable is DC cardioversion. When hemodynamically stable, drugs acting on the accessory pathway such as ibutilide, procainamide, or a class 1C agent (flecainide or propafenone) may be used. Amiodarone should be avoided because enhanced AV nodal conduction and VF have been described in a number of reports. Similarly, AV nodal–blocking drugs should not be used because they may also contribute to a risk of VF.

CHRONIC THERAPY IN AVRT.
Catheter ablation is the treatment of choice for patients with symptoms associated with recurrent AVRT or who have sustained preexcited AF.[1,13]

Contemporary ablation success rates are in the vicinity of 95%, and complications rates are under 1% in experienced centers. In a large series of 11,601 accessory pathway catheter ablations performed between 1998 and 2011 there was a zero mortality.[59]

Beta blockers or non-dihydropyridine calcium channel blockers (verapamil or diltiazem) should be considered for concealed accessory pathway AVRT (no preexcitation on sinus rhythm ECG) when ablation is not preferred or is unsuccessful. Class 1C agents (propafenone or flecainide) may be considered for AVRT with a manifest or concealed accessory pathway when ablation is not preferred or has been unsuccessful and when no other contraindications are present (ischemic heart disease, impaired LV function etc.).[13]

ASYMPTOMATIC WPW.
When WPW is found incidentally on a routine ECG or an ECG performed for a nonarrhythmic indication, it raises the question as to whether the patient is at risk of sudden death and what the most appropriate approach is. This remains a controversial area of electrophysiology. Of patients with asymptomatic WPW, 80% will go through life without arrhythmic events. In the 20% who do develop arrhythmias, the most common is AVRT in 80%. Preexcited AF may develop in 20% to 30%, with the small associated risk of sudden death estimated at 2.4 per 100 person-years in patients with asymptomatic WPW.[13] The risk estimates associated with asymptomatic preexcitation vary widely and depend on the population being considered. Preexcitation has been estimated to cause sudden death in only 3.6 per 10 million person-years in the general population.[60]

There are advocates for invasive testing and ablation if the accessory pathway has a short effective refractory period (ERP),[13,61] whereas others point out that the risk of an adverse outcome is so low that intervention is not warranted as a routine approach.[60,62,63] This exceedingly low risk must be balanced against the small procedural risk and the possibility of accessory pathway recurrence after an initially successful ablation. Nevertheless, the 2019 European Society of Cardiology guidelines provide a Class 1 recommendation of catheter ablation in asymptomatic patients who have an accessory pathway with high-risk properties at EPS. To emphasize the controversy, however, the 2015 ACC/AHA/HRS guidelines provide a class 2A recommendation for diagnostic EPS with a view to catheter ablation of high-risk pathways or alternatively an identical 2A recommendation for observation without further evaluation or treatment.[1] This decision in general involves a detailed discussion and must take into account patient preferences. Patients in high-risk occupations (e.g., pilots) may require catheter ablation to allow maintenance of licensing. Low-risk features of WPW include intermittent loss of preexcitation on ECG, Holter monitoring, or exercise stress test. High-risk features include the presence of multiple accessory pathways, a short antegrade refractory period of the accessory pathway, young age (the risk of sudden cardiac death associated with WPW is highest in the first two decades of life), and symptomatic AVRT episodes. In addition, because children may not describe classic symptoms associated with SVT, the threshold for electrophysiologic evaluation will be considerably lower.

Unusual Forms of Accessory Pathway. Permanent junctional reciprocating tachycardia (PJRT) is an unusual type of long RP SVT that occurs predominantly in infants and children.[64] The arrhythmia is due to a concealed accessory pathway with slow, decremental retrograde conduction. The accessory pathway is most commonly located in the right posteroseptal region but has also been described in the left posteroseptal area, the right free wall, and the left free wall. The tachycardia is incessant in over 50% of patients and not uncommonly results in a TMC. This is generally fully reversible on resumption of persistent sinus rhythm. In a recent large multicenter series of 194 patients with PJRT, the median age at diagnosis was 3.2 months, with the majority being diagnosed before age 1. However, there were patients diagnosed throughout childhood years and into early teenage years. The tachycardia manifests as a long RP rhythm (eFig. 65.4) with spontaneous initiation classically heralded by a slight shortening of the sinus cycle length (Fig. 65.32). Medical therapy is frequently ineffective, and the majority of patients will eventually undergo catheter ablation with a success rate in excess of 90% and low complication rate.[64]

Atriofascicular Pathways and Variants. The original description by Mahaim was of an anatomic connection between the AV node and the right ventricle.[65] Subsequent work describing the electrophysiologic properties of pathways with antegrade only and decremental conduction assumed that this was associated with these previously characterized anatomic connections. However, surgical mapping demonstrated that the majority of these pathways consisted of an accessory AV node and His-Purkinje system with origin from the right atrium with a distal insertion either into the distal right bundle branch (atriofascicular) or into right ventricular myocardium (AV). The most common anatomic location for these atrio-connections is at the anterior lateral TA, but they also may occur at other sites around the tricuspid ring. Because of the antegrade decremental properties of the pathway, patients will usually not have any evidence of preexcitation on a resting 12-lead ECG or minimal preexcitation only because activation occurs first over the AV node (Fig. 65.33A). Tachycardia is an antidromic arrhythmia with antegrade conduction over the pathway and retrograde conduction over the right bundle followed by bundle of His and then AV node (Fig. 65.33B). Less commonly, retrograde conduction occurs over a second accessory pathway. During tachycardia, due to the insertion near the RV apex, the QRS morphology is classically of left bundle branch appearance with a late precordial transition and a superior axis. Atriofascicular pathways have been described in association with Ebstein anomaly, in which accessory pathway conduction can mask the underlying right bundle branch block (Fig. 65.33C). Catheter ablation is the treatment of choice in patients with an atriofascicular pathway. After proving the presence of an atriofascicular pathway responsible for tachycardia, mapping is performed along the lateral tricuspid ring looking for a typical M potential. This is the equivalent of the His bundle potential being a sharp deflection located between the atrial and ventricular signals. Ablation can be technically challenging because of the common difficulty of stabilizing the ablation catheter on the TA, but success can be achieved in over 90% of cases.

Manifest antegrade only nodofascicular and nodoventricular pathways do occur but are rare. The pathway extends from the AV node to the right bundle or RV myocardium. The clinical characteristics appear very similar to those of an atriofascicular pathway (no preexcitation at baseline, with a tachycardia demonstrating left bundle branch block morphology. The distinction is made during a detailed EPS and, in the majority, ablation can be successfully achieved in the slow pathway region.

Rarely a nodofascicular pathway may be concealed, demonstrating retrograde conduction only. These very rare pathways are associated with a narrow-complex tachycardia with antegrade conduction over the AV node and His-Purkinje system and retrograde conduction over the concealed nodofascicular pathway. These pathways are most frequently right sided. The retrograde P wave may be concealed within the QRS,

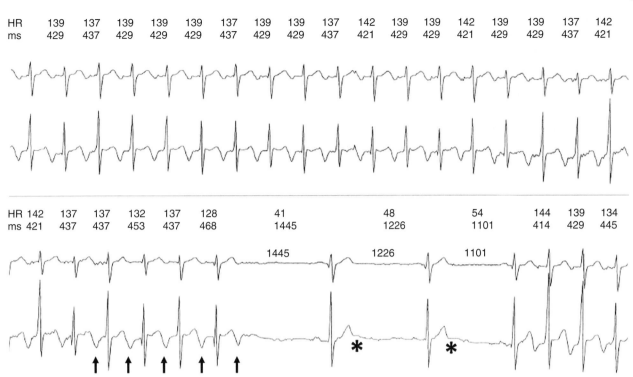

| HR | 139 | 137 | 139 | 139 | 139 | 137 | 139 | 139 | 137 | 142 | 139 | 139 | 142 | 139 | 139 | 137 | 142 |
| ms | 429 | 437 | 429 | 429 | 429 | 437 | 429 | 429 | 437 | 421 | 429 | 429 | 421 | 429 | 429 | 437 | 421 |

| HR | 142 | 137 | 137 | 132 | 137 | 128 | 41 | 48 | 54 | 144 | 139 | 134 |
| ms | 421 | 437 | 437 | 453 | 437 | 468 | 1445 | 1226 | 1101 | 414 | 429 | 445 |

FIGURE 65.32 Holter monitor trace showing a spontaneous termination and then reinitiation of a long-RP tachycardia. Note the inverted P waves closer to the following QRS (*upward arrows*). There is spontaneous termination with the last recording being a retrograde P wave (*final upward arrow*). This effectively rules out an atrial tachycardia. Note that there are then 3 sinus beats (*asterisks* indicating absence of a retrograde P wave) before the tachycardia then reinitiates spontaneously. This spontaneous reinitiation is proceeded by a shortening of the sinus cycle length. This sinus cycle length shortening classically proceeds tachycardia onset in permanent junctional reciprocating tachycardia. This mechanism was confirmed at electrophysiology study.

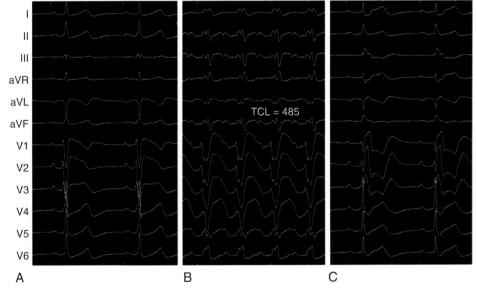

FIGURE 65.33 Recordings made during electrophysiology study and ablation procedure for patient with Ebstein anomaly and atriofascicular pathway. The pathway represents an accessory atrioventricular (AV) node, His-Purkinje system originating on the lateral tricuspid annulus and inserting into the apical region of the right bundle branch. The pathway conducts in the antegrade direction only and shows decremental properties. **A,** Baseline sinus rhythm ECG. The PR interval is normal, and there is only a hint of slurring in the initial portion of the QRS seen particularly in V_4-V_6. **B,** During antidromic preexcited tachycardia (rate 125 bpm) the QRS is broad with an LBBB morphology, late precordial transition after V_4 and a superiorly directed axis. This pattern is characteristic of tachycardia due to antegrade conduction over an atriofascicular pathway with retrograde conduction over the AV node. **C,** After successful ablation of the atriofascicular pathway the underlying first-degree AV block and right bundle branch block pattern characteristic of Ebstein anomaly is now manifest. Before ablation, this pattern had been obscured by the presence of an accessory atriofascicular pathway.

thereby mimicking typical AVNRT, or there may be retrograde block to the atrium in which case there will be VA dissociation during the narrow-complex tachycardia.[66,67]

Supraventricular Tachycardia in Adults Late after Surgical Repair of Congenital Heart Disease. Supraventricular arrhythmias are particularly common in adults late after repair of CHD. The most common mechanism is macroreentrant AT (atypical flutter) due to circuits around scars and prosthetic material. They are most common in patients with more complex forms of CHD such as Fontan repair for single ventricular physiology or Mustard or Senning repair for D-TGA.[68] However, these circuits are also common in less complex forms of CHD such as tetralogy of Fallot and simple forms such as ostium secundum ASD. In patients with complex CHD, the combination of atrial enlargement, atrial surgical scarring, and extensive remodeling often results in the presence of multiple different tachycardia circuits (Fig. 65.34).

Patients with CHD may also develop focal AT or either AVNRT or AVRT.

It is important to be aware that atrial arrhythmias in patients with complex CHD can be life-threatening. Patients often have little hemodynamic reserve, and rapid arrhythmias can lead to cardiac arrest. An arrhythmia that causes stable symptoms with 2:1 conduction may cause hemodynamic collapse if 1:1 conduction develops. This is a significant risk due to the relatively long cycle length of the arrhythmia in many cases.

Medical therapy is commonly with beta blockers for rate control. The threshold for amiodarone use in this population is relatively low because most other antiarrhythmics such as sotalol and class 1C drugs are contraindicated. Bradyarrhythmias are also common and pacing may be required. Catheter ablation is a therapeutic option to control recurrent arrhythmias. In view of extensive atrial scarring, the

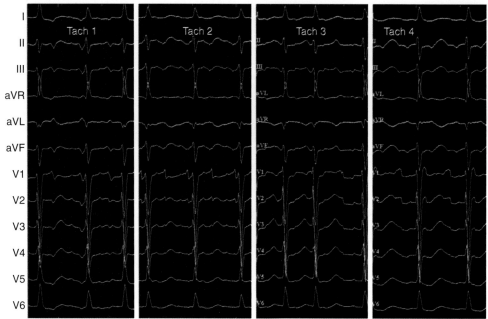

FIGURE 65.34 A 37-year-old man with prior atriopulmonary Fontan due to single ventricular physiology. Four different tachycardia morphologies recorded during an electrophysiology study. These patients frequently have profound right atrial enlargement together with extensive surgical scarring and atrial remodeling, which together create the possibility for numerous different circuits.

QRS (initial RS interval shorter in SVT with aberrancy), (5) chest lead concordance, with negative or positive being highly specific for VT but relatively insensitive; (6) QRS axis (e.g., northwest axis rarely seen in SVT with aberrancy), (7) when available, comparison with the baseline ECG may provide important clues; (8) onsets, terminations, and transitions may provide diagnostic information. For example, transition from wide to narrow complex or the reverse at a similar rate is highly suggestive of SVT with aberrancy; and (9) beyond the ECG alone, the clinical context can provide critically important information. Knowledge of a prior myocardial infarct with persistent scar would point strongly toward VT. Alternatively, a history of paroxysmal AF treated with a class 1C agent such as flecainide suggests atrial flutter with ventricular conduction slowing.

TABLE 65.2 Regular Wide-Complex Tachycardia

Ventricular tachycardia
Fascicular tachycardia

SVT with bundle branch aberrancy
  Rate-related
  Preexisting
  Antiarrhythmic induced (e.g., flecainide)
  Metabolic derangement (e.g., hyperkalemia)

Accessory pathway related
  Antidromic tachycardia
  Preexcited tachycardia (atrial tachycardia or AVNRT with bystander
    accessory pathway)

Rapid ventricular pacing

AVNRT, Atrioventricular nodal reentrant tachycardia; *SVT,* supraventricular tachycardia.

procedure is generally not curative but excellent palliative results can be obtained. Management of adults late after surgical repair of CHD should be undertaken only in specialist units where CHD physicians and electrophysiologists experienced in complex arrhythmia ablation work closely together.

Patients with atrial arrhythmias and CHD generally warrant anticoagulation with an oral anticoagulant.

DIFFERENTIAL DIAGNOSIS OF WIDE COMPLEX TACHYCARDIA

The differential diagnosis of wide-complex tachycardia is considered in Table 65.2. The differentiation of VT from supraventricular tachyarrhythmias associated with broad QRS complexes can be a diagnostic challenge with important clinical implications. A range of different stepwise, points-based, and single criteria methods have been devised that largely are focused on the same key criteria.[69] These have included (1) the AV relationship and specifically whether AV dissociation is present, (2) morphologic QRS criteria asking the question of whether this is a typical left or right bundle branch block pattern; (3) QRS duration (broader in VT), (4) activation velocity of the initial and terminal components of the

REFERENCES
General Considerations

1. Page RL, Joglar JA, Caldwell MA, et al. ACC/AHA/HRS guideline for the management of adult patients with supraventricular tachycardia: a report of the American College of Cardiology/American Heart Association task force on clinical practice guidelines and the Heart Rhythm Society. *J Am Coll Cardiol.* 2016;67:e27–e115.
2. Murer M, Cuculi F, Toggweiler S, et al. Elevated high-sensitivity troponin does not indicate the presence of coronary artery disease in patients presenting with supraventricular tachycardia. *Cardiol J.* 2017;24:642–648.
3. Conen D, Adam M, Roche F, et al. Premature atrial contractions in the general population: frequency and risk factors. *Circulation.* 2012;126:2302–2308.
4. Haissaguerre M, Jais P, Shah DC, et al. Spontaneous initiation of atrial fibrillation by ectopic beats originating in the pulmonary veins. *N Engl J Med.* 1998;339:659–666.
5. Larsen BS, Kumarathurai P, Falkenberg J, et al. Excessive atrial ectopy and short atrial runs increase the risk of stroke beyond incident atrial fibrillation. *J Am Coll Cardiol.* 2015;66:232–241.
6. Marcus GM, Dewland TA. Premature atrial contractions: a wolf in sheep's clothing? *J Am Coll Cardiol.* 2015;66:242–244.
7. Sajeev JK, Koshy AN, Dewey H, et al. Association between excessive premature atrial complexes and cryptogenic stroke: results of a case-control study. *BMJ Open.* 2019;9:e029164.
8. Liuba I, Schaller RD, Frankel DS. Premature atrial complex-induced cardiomyopathy: case report and literature review. *Heart Rhythm Case Rep.* 2020;6:191–193.
9. Roberts-Thomson KC, Kistler PM, Kalman JM. Atrial tachycardia: mechanisms, diagnosis, and management. *Curr Probl Cardiol.* 2005;30:529–573.
10. Olgin JE, Zipes DP. Supraventricular arrhythmias. In: Zipes DP, et al., ed. *Braunwald's Heart Disease, a Textbook of Cardiovascular Medicine.* 11th ed. Philadelphia, PA: Elsevier; 2016.
11. Saoudi N, Cosio F, Waldo A, et al. A classification of atrial flutter and regular atrial tachycardia according to electrophysiological mechanisms and anatomical bases; a statement from a joint expert group from the working group of arrhythmias of the European Society of Cardiology and the North American Society of Pacing and Electrophysiology. *Eur Heart J.* 2001;22:1162–1182.
12. Frontera A, Takigawa M, Haissaguerre M, et al. High-density characterization of a localized reentry circuit occurred after AF ablation. *Pacing Clin Electrophysiol.* 2019;42:111–112.
13. Brugada J, Katritsis DG, Arbelo E, et al. 2019 ESC guidelines for the management of patients with supraventricular tachycardia: the task force for the management of patients with supraventricular tachycardia of the European Society of Cardiology (ESC). *Eur Heart J.* 2020;41:655–720.
14. Poutiainen AM, Koistinen MJ, Airaksinen KE, et al. Prevalence and natural course of ectopic atrial tachycardia. *Eur Heart J.* 1999;20:694–700.
15. Porter MJ, Morton JB, Denman R, et al. Influence of age and gender on the mechanism of supraventricular tachycardia. *Heart Rhythm.* 2004;1:393–396.
16. Hillock RJ, Kalman JM, Roberts-Thomson KC, et al. Multiple focal atrial tachycardias in a healthy adult population: characterization and description of successful radiofrequency ablation. *Heart Rhythm.* 2007;4:435–438.

Supraventricular Arrhythmic Types

17. Morris GM, Segan L, Wong G, et al. Atrial tachycardia arising from the crista terminalis, detailed electrophysiological features and long-term ablation outcomes. *JACC Clin Electrophysiol.* 2019;5:448–458.
18. Beukema RJ, Smit JJ, Adiyaman A, et al. Ablation of focal atrial tachycardia from the non-coronary aortic cusp: case series and review of the literature. *Europace.* 2015;17:953–961.
19. Kistler PM, Roberts-Thomson KC, Haqqani HM, et al. P-wave morphology in focal atrial tachycardia: development of an algorithm to predict the anatomic site of origin. *J Am Coll Cardiol.* 2006;48:1010–1017.
20. Olshansky B, Sullivan RM. Inappropriate sinus tachycardia. *Europace.* 2019;21:194–207.
21. Sheldon RS, Grubb 2nd BP, Olshansky B, et al. 2015 Heart Rhythm Society expert consensus statement on the diagnosis and treatment of postural tachycardia syndrome, inappropriate sinus tachycardia, and vasovagal syncope. *Heart Rhythm.* 2015;12:e41–63.
21a. Arano Llach J, Bazan V, Llados G, et al. Inappropriate sinus tachycardia in post-Covid-19 syndrome. *Europace.* 2021;23(suppl 3):euab116.114.
22. Benjamin EJ, Muntner P, Alonso A, et al. Heart disease and stroke statistics-2019 update: a report from the American Heart Association. *Circulation.* 2019;139:e56–e528.

23. Kumar S, Michaud GF. Atrial fibrillation: mechanisms, clinical features and management. In: Zipes DP, et al., ed. *Cardiac Electrophysiology: From Cell to Bedside*. 7th ed. Philadelphia, PA: Elsevier; 2018.

24. Waldo AL. Atrial fibrillation and atrial flutter: two sides of the same coin!. *Int J Cardiol*. 2017;240:251–252.

25. Maskoun W, Pino MI, Ayoub K, et al. Incidence of atrial fibrillation after atrial flutter ablation. *JACC Clin Electrophysiol*. 2016;2:682–690.

26. Pathik B, Lee G, Sacher F, et al. New insights into an old arrhythmia: high-resolution mapping demonstrates conduction and substrate variability in right atrial macro-re-entrant tachycardia. *JACC Clin Electrophysiol*. 2017;3:971–986.

27. Medi C, Kalman JM. Prediction of the atrial flutter circuit location from the surface electrocardiogram. *Europace*. 2008;10:786–796.

28. Moore BM, Anderson R, Nisbet AM, et al. Ablation of atrial arrhythmias after the atriopulmonary Fontan procedure: mechanisms of arrhythmia and outcomes. *JACC Clin Electrophysiol*. 2018;4:1338–1346.

29. Derval N, Takigawa M, Frontera A, et al. Characterization of complex atrial tachycardia in patients with previous atrial interventions using high-resolution mapping. *JACC Clin Electrophysiol*. 2020;6:815–826.

Management Strategies

30. Markowitz SM, Thomas G, Liu CF, et al. Atrial tachycardias and atypical atrial flutters: mechanisms and approaches to ablation. *Arrhythm Electrophysiol Rev*. 2019;8:131–137.

31. Enriquez A, Santangeli P, Zado ES, et al. Postoperative atrial tachycardias after mitral valve surgery: mechanisms and outcomes of catheter ablation. *Heart Rhythm*. 2017;14:520–526.

32. Luther V, Sikkel M, Bennett N, et al. Visualizing localized reentry with ultra-high density mapping in iatrogenic atrial tachycardia: beware pseudo-reentry. *Circ Arrhythm Electrophysiol*. 2017;10.

33. Holmqvist F, Kesek M, Englund A, et al. A decade of catheter ablation of cardiac arrhythmias in Sweden: ablation practices and outcomes. *Eur Heart J*. 2019;40:820–830.

34. Wang H, Wang C, Chen J, et al. Long-term outcome of catheter ablation for atrial tachyarrhythmias in patients with atrial septal defect. *J Interv Card Electrophysiol*. 2019;54:217–224.

35. Anguera I, Dallaglio P, Macias R, et al. Long-term outcome after ablation of right atrial tachyarrhythmias after the surgical repair of congenital and acquired heart disease. *Am J Cardiol*. 2015;115:1705–1713.

36. Saul JP, Kanter RJ, Writing Commitee, et al. PACES/HRS expert consensus statement on the use of catheter ablation in children and patients with congenital heart disease: developed in partnership with the Pediatric and Congenital Electrophysiology Society (PACES) and the Heart Rhythm Society (HRS). Endorsed by the governing bodies of PACES, HRS, the American Academy of Pediatrics (AAP), the American Heart Association (AHA), and the Association for European Pediatric and Congenital Cardiology (AEPC). *Heart Rhythm*. 2016;13:e251–289.

37. Gopinathannair R, Mar PL, Afzal MR, et al. Atrial tachycardias after surgical atrial fibrillation ablation: clinical characteristics, electrophysiological mechanisms, and ablation outcomes from a large, multicenter study. *JACC Clin Electrophysiol*. 2017;3:865–874.

38. Gucuk Ipek E, Marine J, Yang E, et al. Predictors and incidence of atrial flutter after catheter ablation of atrial fibrillation. *Am J Cardiol*. 2019;124:1690–1696.

39. Katritsis DG, Becker A. The atrioventricular nodal reentrant tachycardia circuit: a proposal. *Heart Rhythm*. 2007;4:1354–1360.

40. Katritsis DG, Josephson ME. Classification, electrophysiological features and therapy of atrioventricular nodal reentrant tachycardia. *Arrhythm Electrophysiol Rev*. 2016;5:130–135.

41. Appelboam A, Reuben A, Mann C, et al. Postural modification to the standard Valsalva manoeuvre for emergency treatment of supraventricular tachycardias (revert): a randomised controlled trial. *Lancet*. 2015;386:1747–1753.

42. Katritsis DG, Zografos T, Katritsis GD, et al. Catheter ablation vs. Antiarrhythmic drug therapy in patients with symptomatic atrioventricular nodal re-entrant tachycardia: a randomized, controlled trial. *Europace*. 2017;19:602–606.

43. Feldman A, Voskoboinik A, Kumar S, et al. Predictors of acute and long-term success of slow pathway ablation for atrioventricular nodal reentrant tachycardia: a single center series of 1,419 consecutive patients. *Pacing Clin Electrophysiol*. 2011;34:927–933.

44. Chrispin J, Misra S, Marine JE, et al. Current management and clinical outcomes for catheter ablation of atrioventricular nodal re-entrant tachycardia. *Europace*. 2018;20:e51–e59.

45. Katritsis DG, Zografos T, Siontis KC, et al. Endpoints for successful slow pathway catheter ablation in typical and atypical atrioventricular nodal re-entrant tachycardia: a contemporary, multicenter study. *JACC Clin Electrophysiol*. 2019;5:113–119.

46. Insulander P, Bastani H, Braunschweig F, et al. Cryoablation of atrioventricular nodal re-entrant tachycardia: 7-year follow-up in 515 patients-confirmed safety but very late recurrences occur. *Europace*. 2017;19:1038–1042.

47. Karacan M, Celik N, Akdeniz C, et al. Long-term outcomes following cryoablation of atrioventricular nodal reentrant tachycardia in children. *Pacing Clin Electrophysiol*. 2018;41:255–260.

48. Chan NY, Mok NS, Yuen HC, et al. Cryoablation with an 8-mm tip catheter in the treatment of atrioventricular nodal re-entrant tachycardia: results from a randomized controlled trial (cryoablate). *Europace*. 2019;21:662–669.

49. Makhoul M, Oster M, Fischbach P, et al. Junctional ectopic tachycardia after congenital heart surgery in the current surgical era. *Pediatr Cardiol*. 2013;34:370–374.

50. El Amrousy DM, Elshmaa NS, El-Kashlan M, et al. Efficacy of prophylactic dexmedetomidine in preventing postoperative junctional ectopic tachycardia after pediatric cardiac surgery. *J Am Heart Assoc*. 2017;6:e004780.

51. Kylat RI, Samson RA. Junctional ectopic tachycardia in infants and children. *J Arrhythm*. 2020;36:59–66.

52. Ergul Y, Ozturk E, Ozgur S, et al. Ivabradine is an effective antiarrhythmic therapy for congenital junctional ectopic tachycardia-induced cardiomyopathy during infancy: case studies. *Pacing Clin Electrophysiol*. 2018;41:1372–1377.

53. Collins KK, Van Hare GF, Kertesz NJ, et al. Pediatric nonpost-operative junctional ectopic tachycardia medical management and interventional therapies. *J Am Coll Cardiol*. 2009;53:690–697.

54. Dar T, Turagam MK, Yarlagadda B, et al. Outcomes of junctional ectopic tachycardia ablation in adult population-a multicenter experience. *J Interv Card Electrophysiol*. 2020.

55. Vidaillet Jr HJ, Pressley JC, Henke E, et al. Familial occurrence of accessory atrioventricular pathways (preexcitation syndrome). *N Engl J Med*. 1987;317:65–69.

56. Lopez-Sainz A, Dominguez F, Lopes LR, et al. Clinical features and natural history of PRKAG2 variant cardiac glycogenosis. *J Am Coll Cardiol*. 2020;76:186–197.

57. Wei W, Zhan X, Xue Y, et al. Features of accessory pathways in adult Ebstein's anomaly. *Europace*. 2014;16:1619–1625.

58. Pambrun T, El Bouazzaoui R, Combes N, et al. Maximal pre-excitation based algorithm for localization of manifest accessory pathways in adults. *JACC Clin Electrophysiol*. 2018;4:1052–1061.

59. Garg J, Shah N, Krishnamoorthy P, et al. Catheter ablation of accessory pathway: 14-year trends in utilization and complications in adults in the United States. *Int J Cardiol*. 2017;248:196–200.

60. Obeyesekere MN, Klein GJ. Application of the 2015 ACC/AHA/HRS guidelines for risk stratification for sudden death in adult patients with asymptomatic pre-excitation. *J Cardiovasc Electrophysiol*. 2017;28:841–848.

61. Pappone C, Santinelli V. Electrophysiology testing and catheter ablation are helpful when evaluating asymptomatic patients with Wolff-Parkinson-White pattern: the pro perspective. *Card Electrophysiol Clin*. 2015;7:371–376.

62. Obeyesekere MN, Klein GJ. Preventing sudden death in asymptomatic Wolf-Parkinson-White patients. *JACC Clin Electrophysiol*. 2018;4:445–447.

63. Skanes AC, Obeyesekere M, Klein GJ. Electrophysiology testing and catheter ablation are helpful when evaluating asymptomatic patients with Wolff-Parkinson-White pattern: the con perspective. *Card Electrophysiol Clin*. 2015;7:377–383.

64. Kang KT, Potts JE, Radbill AE, et al. Permanent junctional reciprocating tachycardia in children: a multicenter experience. *Heart Rhythm*. 2014;11:1426–1432.

65. Hoffmayer KS, Han FT, Singh D, et al. Variants of accessory pathways. *Pacing Clin Electrophysiol*. 2020;43:21–29.

66. Soares Correa F, Lokhandwala Y, Cruz Filho F, et al. Part II: clinical presentation, electrophysiologic characteristics, and when and how to ablate atriofascicular pathways and long and short decrementally conducting accessory pathways. *J Cardiovasc Electrophysiol*. 2019;30:3079–3096.

67. Anderson RH, Sanchez-Quintana D, Mori S, et al. Unusual variants of pre-excitation: from anatomy to ablation: Part I—Understanding the anatomy of the variants of ventricular pre-excitation. *J Cardiovasc Electrophysiol*. 2019;30:2170–2180.

68. Khairy P, Van Hare GF, Balaji S, et al. PACES/HRS expert consensus statement on the recognition and management of arrhythmias in adult congenital heart disease: developed in partnership between the Pediatric And Congenital Electrophysiology Society (PACES) and the Heart Rhythm Society (HRS). Endorsed by the governing bodies of PACES, HRS, the American College of Cardiology (ACC), the American Heart Association (AHA), the European Heart Rhythm Association (EHRA), the Canadian Heart Rhythm Society (CHRS), and the International Society for Adult Congenital Heart Disease (ISACHD). *Can J Cardiol*. 2014;30:e1–e63.

69. Kashou AH, Noseworthy PA, DeSimone CV, et al. Wide complex tachycardia differentiation: a reappraisal of the state-of-the-art. *J Am Heart Assoc*. 2020;9:e016598.

66 Atrial Fibrillation: Clinical Features, Mechanisms, and Management

HUGH CALKINS, GORDON F. TOMASELLI, AND FRED MORADY

ELECTROCARDIOGRAPHIC FEATURES

Atrial fibrillation (AF) is a supraventricular arrhythmia characterized electrocardiographically by low-amplitude baseline oscillations (fibrillatory or f waves from the fibrillating atria) and an irregularly irregular ventricular rhythm. The f waves, 300 to 600 beats/min, are variable in amplitude, shape, and timing. Atrial flutter waves have a rate of 250 to 350 beats/min and are constant in timing and morphology (Fig. 66.1). In lead V_1, f waves sometimes appear uniform and can mimic flutter waves (Fig. 66.2). In some patients, f waves are very small and not perceptible on the electrocardiogram, and the diagnosis of AF is based on the irregularly irregular ventricular rhythm (Fig. 66.3).

The ventricular rate during untreated AF typically is 100 to 160 beats/min. Patients with the Wolff-Parkinson-White (WPW) syndrome can experience ventricular rates during AF exceeding 250 beats/min because of conduction over the accessory pathway (see Chapter 65). The ventricular rate during AF can appear more regular when the rate is extremely rapid (>170 beats/min) (Fig. 66.4), when a junctional tachycardia independently controls the ventricles, when there is high-degree atrioventricular (AV) block with a regular escape rhythm (Fig. 66.5), or when the QRS complexes all are paced. In these cases the diagnosis of AF is based on the presence of f waves. Infrequently, a junctional tachycardia can exhibit Wenckebach exit block (often during digitalis toxicity) and cause a regularly irregular ventricular rate.

CLASSIFICATION OF ATRIAL FIBRILLATION

Atrial fibrillation that terminates spontaneously within 7 days is termed *paroxysmal*, and AF present continuously for more than 7 days is called *persistent*. AF that persists for longer than 1 year is termed *longstanding persistent*. The term *permanent AF* is used when the patient and clinician jointly decide to abandon further attempts at restoring and/or maintaining sinus rhythm.[1] This "acceptance of AF" represents a therapeutic attitude rather than a pathophysiologic characteristic of the AF and should not be taken literally. Some patients with paroxysmal AF occasionally can have episodes that are persistent and vice versa. The predominant form of AF determines how it should be categorized.

A confounding factor in the classification of AF is cardioversion and antiarrhythmic drug (AAD) therapy. For example, if a patient undergoes transthoracic cardioversion 24 hours after AF onset, it is unknown whether the AF would have persisted for more than 7 days. Furthermore, AAD therapy can change persistent AF into paroxysmal AF. The classification of AF should not be altered on the basis of the effects of electrical cardioversion or AAD therapy.

Lone atrial fibrillation refers to AF that occurs in patients younger than 60 years who do not have hypertension or any evidence of structural heart disease. This designation is a historical descriptor that has been variably applied to different low-risk subsets of AF patients. Because the definitions have not been consistent, and the potentially confusing definitions of this term, this designation should be abandoned.

Paroxysmal AF also can be classified clinically on the basis of the autonomic setting in which it most often occurs. Approximately 25% of patients with paroxysmal AF have *vagotonic* AF, in which AF is initiated in the setting of high vagal tone, typically in the evening when the patient is relaxing or during sleep. Drugs exerting a vagotonic effect (e.g., digitalis) can aggravate vagotonic AF, and drugs with a vagolytic effect (e.g., disopyramide) may be particularly appropriate for prophylactic therapy. Adrenergic AF occurs in approximately 10% to 15% of patients with paroxysmal AF in the setting of high sympathetic tone, as during strenuous exertion. In patients with adrenergic AF, beta blockers not only provide rate control but may prevent episodes of AF. Most patients have a mixed or random form of paroxysmal AF, with no consistent pattern of onset. In some, alcohol can be a precipitant.[2,3]

EPIDEMIOLOGY OF ATRIAL FIBRILLATION

Atrial fibrillation is the most common arrhythmia treated in clinical practice and the most common arrhythmia for which patients are hospitalized; approximately 33% of arrhythmia-related hospitalizations are for AF. In 2010 the prevalence of AF was estimated to be between 2.1 and 6.1 million persons. This is predicted to increase to 12.1 million persons by 2030.[4] AF is associated with approximately a fivefold increase in the risk of cerebrovascular accident (stroke), a twofold

Additional content is available online at Elsevier eBooks for Practicing Clinicians

increase in the risk of all-cause mortality, and a twofold increase in cognitive dysfunction.[4] AF also is associated with the development of heart failure and has been linked to sudden death.

The incidence of AF is related to age and sex, ranging from 0.1% per year before age 40 to more than 1.5% per year in women and more than 2% per year in men older than 80. Advanced age, congestive heart failure, male sex, tall stature, a family history of AF at less than 50 years of age, left atrial enlargement, and hypertension are independent risk factors for the development of AF, as are obesity and obstructive sleep apnea. AF is less common in African Americans.[1]

MECHANISMS OF ATRIAL FIBRILLATION

The mechanisms responsible for AF are complex and incompletely understood. The three main mechanistic concepts that have emerged over time consist of multiple reentrant wavelets, rapidly discharging autonomic foci, and a single reentrant circuit with fibrillatory conduction. Considerable progress has been made in defining the mechanisms underlying initiation, perpetuation, and progression of AF.[5-8] A key breakthrough that had an immediate therapeutic impact was the recognition that in many patients, AF is triggered and/or maintained by rapidly firing foci in the pulmonary veins.[7] It is now well accepted the focal firing is the key mechanism underlying initiation and perpetuation of paroxysmal AF. In contrast, the mechanisms that underlie maintenance of persistent AF appear far more complex. In persistent AF, changes in the atrial substrate, including interstitial fibrosis that

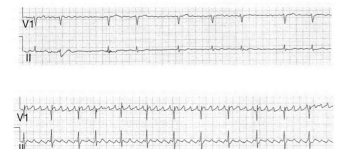

FIGURE 66.1 Comparison between the f waves of AF **(top panel)** and the flutter waves of atrial flutter **(bottom panel).** Note that f waves are variable in rate, shape, and amplitude, whereas flutter waves are constant in rate and morphology. Shown are leads V$_1$ and II.

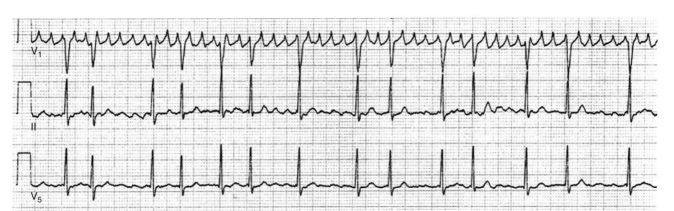

FIGURE 66.2 An example of AF with prominent f waves in V$_1$ that mimic atrial flutter waves. Note that typical f waves are present in leads II and V$_5$, establishing the diagnosis of AF.

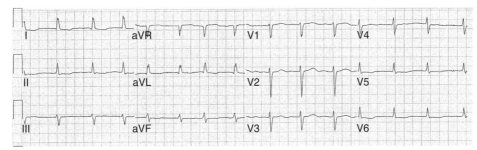

FIGURE 66.3 A 12-lead electrocardiogram of AF in which f waves are not discernible. The irregularly irregular ventricular rate indicates that this is AF.

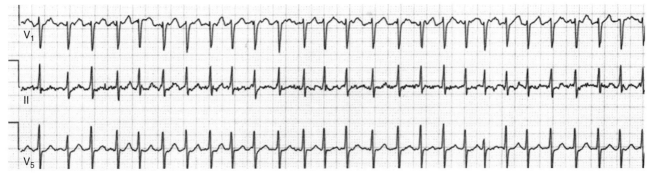

FIGURE 66.4 A recording of AF with a rapid ventricular rate of 160 beats/min. Shown are leads V$_1$, II, and V$_5$. On quick review, there may appear to be a regular rate consistent with paroxysmal supraventricular tachycardia. On closer inspection, it is clear that the rate is irregularly irregular.

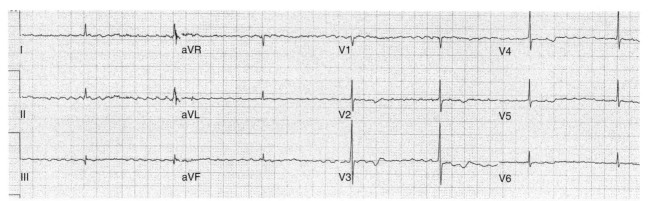

FIGURE 66.5 A 12-lead electrocardiogram of AF and a regular junctional rhythm at a rate of 43 beats/min. There is either underlying third-degree AV block or second-degree AV block with extremely slow atrioventricular conduction allowing a junctional escape rhythm to become manifest.

contributes to slow, discontinuous, and anisotropic conduction, may give rise to wandering or stationary reentry. It is for this reason that the outcomes of AF ablation targeted at the pulmonary veins (PVs) alone results in lower efficacy than in patients with paroxysmal AF.

GENETIC FACTORS

It is now well established that susceptibility to AF is heritable.[9,10] Individuals who have a first-degree relative with AF have a 40% increased risk of developing AF. In the last decade, considerable progress has been made in identifying the genetic determinants of AF. Population-based studies have been used to identify many AF risk loci. A recent study tested the association between AF genetic susceptibility and recurrence of AF after AF ablation using a polygenic risk score. A higher AF genetic susceptibility was associated with younger age and fewer clinical risk factors, but not AF recurrence.[10] Although progress has been made, studies continue to better define the link between genetic factors and AF and how these genetic factors impact the response to therapy.

CAUSES OF ATRIAL FIBRILLATION

The majority of patients with AF have hypertension (usually with left ventricular hypertrophy; Chapter 26) or some other form of structural heart disease. In addition to hypertensive heart disease, the most common cardiac abnormalities associated with AF are ischemic heart disease (Chapters 37 to 40), mitral valve disease (Chapters 75 and 76), hypertrophic cardiomyopathy (Chapter 54), and dilated cardiomyopathy (Chapter 52). Less common causes of AF are restrictive cardiomyopathies such as amyloidosis (Chapter 53), constrictive pericarditis (Chapter 86), and cardiac tumors (see Chapter 98). Severe pulmonary hypertension often is associated with AF (Chapter 88).

Obstructive sleep apnea and obesity are associated with each other, and both independently increase the risk of AF (see Chapter 89).[11] The possible mechanisms of AF in patients with sleep apnea include hypoxia, surges in autonomic tone, and hypertension. Available data suggest that atrial dilation and an increase in local and systemic inflammatory factors are responsible for the relationship between obesity and AF. Obesity is associated with increased deposits of epicardial fat (see Chapter 30). A growing body of data has demonstrated that epicardial fat is strongly associated with the presence, severity, and recurrence of AF in many clinical settings. The most likely arrhythmogenic mechanisms by which epicardial fat predisposes to AF include adipocyte infiltration, profibrotic effects, proinflammatory effects.[12] The LEGACY study demonstrated that sustained weight loss and exercise can reduce the AF burden.[13]

AF is sometimes caused by tachycardia. Patients with tachycardia-induced AF most often have AV nodal reentrant tachycardia or a tachycardia related to WPW syndrome that degenerates into AF. AF in a patient with a history of rapid and regular palpitations before the onset

of irregular palpitations or with a WPW electrocardiographic pattern suggest that the patient may have tachycardia-induced AF. Treatment of the tachycardia that triggers the AF often (but not always) prevents recurrences of AF.

CLINICAL FEATURES

The symptoms of AF range from none to severe and functionally disabling. The most common symptoms are palpitations, fatigue, dyspnea, effort intolerance, and lightheadedness. Polyuria can occur because of release of atrial natriuretic peptide. Many patients with symptomatic paroxysmal AF also have asymptomatic episodes, and some patients with persistent AF have symptoms only intermittently, making it difficult to assess accurately the frequency and duration of AF on the basis of symptoms.

An estimated 25% of patients with AF are asymptomatic, more often elderly patients and patients with persistent AF. Such patients sometimes are erroneously classified as being "asymptomatic" despite having symptoms of fatigue or effort intolerance. Because fatigue is a nonspecific symptom, it may not be clear that the cause is persistent AF. Many elderly patients incorrectly assume that their effort intolerance is attributable to aging. A "diagnostic cardioversion" may be helpful by maintaining sinus rhythm for at least a few days to determine whether a patient feels better in sinus rhythm. This strategy is especially valuable in a patient under the age of 80 years who presents for a routine physical examination and is found to be in AF. Rather than quickly declaring the patient "asymptomatic," many experienced clinicians will restore sinus rhythm with a cardioversion to evaluate symptomatic improvement. This strategy also is useful in patients with newly diagnosed persistent AF as the longer a patient is in continuous AF, the more difficult it is to restore and maintain sinus rhythm. This approach can provide a basis to pursue a rhythm-control versus rate-control strategy.

Syncope, an uncommon symptom of AF, can be caused by a long sinus pause on termination of AF in a patient with the sick sinus syndrome. Syncope also can occur during AF with a rapid ventricular rate because of neurocardiogenic (vasodepressor) syncope triggered by the tachycardia or because of a severe drop in blood pressure caused by a reduction in cardiac output.

Asymptomatic or minimally symptomatic AF patients are not prompted to seek medical care and can present with a thromboembolic complication such as stroke or the insidious onset of heart failure symptoms, eventually presenting in florid congestive heart failure caused by tachycardia-induced cardiomyopathy.

The hallmark of AF on physical examination is an irregularly irregular pulse. Short R-R intervals during AF do not allow adequate time for left ventricular diastolic filling, resulting in a low stroke volume and the absence of palpable peripheral pulse. This results in a "pulse deficit," during which the peripheral pulse is not as rapid as the apical rate. Other manifestations of AF on the physical examination are irregular jugular venous pulsations and variable intensity of the first heart sound.

DIAGNOSTIC EVALUATION

The history should be directed at determination of the type and severity of symptoms, the first onset of AF, whether the AF is paroxysmal or persistent, the triggers of AF, whether the episodes are random or occur at particular times (e.g., during sleep), and the frequency and duration of episodes. When it is unclear from the history, 2 to 4 weeks of continuous or autotrigger ambulatory monitoring, or by mobile cardiac outpatient telemetry, is useful to determine whether AF is paroxysmal or persistent and to quantitate the AF burden in patients with paroxysmal AF. The history also should be directed at identification of potentially correctable causes (e.g., hyperthyroidism, excessive alcohol intake), structural heart disease, and comorbidities.

In a patient who describes irregular or rapid palpitations suggestive of paroxysmal AF, ambulatory monitoring is useful to document whether AF is responsible for the symptoms. If the symptoms occur on a daily basis, a 24-hour Holter recording is appropriate. However, extended monitoring for 2 to 4 weeks with an event monitor or continuous rhythm monitor or by mobile cardiac outpatient telemetry is appropriate for patients whose symptoms are sporadic (see Chapter 61).[14] Another option is an insertable monitor, which is placed subcutaneously and has a battery life of approximately 3 years.[15] A recent trial demonstrated that among patients with a cryptogenic stroke and no AF seen on a 24-hour Holter monitor, AF was detected in 8.9% of patients who had an implantable cardiac monitor within 6 months.[15] One of the most important benefits of a continuous monitor over weeks to years is that the burden of AF can be precisely defined.

Laboratory testing should include thyroid, liver, and renal function blood tests. Echocardiography always is appropriate to evaluate atrial size and left ventricular function and to look for left ventricular hypertrophy, congenital heart disease (see Chapter 82), and valvular heart disease (Chapters 72 to 77). Chest radiography is appropriate if the history or physical examination is suggestive of pulmonary disease (Chapter 17). A stress test is appropriate for evaluation of ischemic heart disease in at-risk patients (Chapter 15).

PREVENTION OF THROMBOEMBOLIC COMPLICATIONS

Risk Stratification

The most important therapeutic goal in AF patients is to prevent thromboembolic complications, especially stroke.[16,17] Anticoagulants (warfarin or one of the direct oral anticoagulants) are far more effective than antiplatelet agents (e.g., aspirin or clopidogrel) for prevention of thromboembolic complications.[16,17] However, because of the risk of hemorrhage from anticoagulants, their use should be limited to patients whose risk of thromboembolic complications is greater than the risk of hemorrhage. Therefore, it is useful to risk stratify patients with AF to identify appropriate candidates for anticoagulation. The guidelines for use of anticoagulants to prevent thromboembolism are outlined in eTable 66.G1 and eTable 66.G2 (see Chapter 95).

The strongest predictors of ischemic stroke and systemic thromboembolism are a history of stroke or transient ischemic episode and mitral stenosis. When patients with AF and a prior ischemic stroke are treated with aspirin, the risk of another stroke is very high, in the range of 10% to 12% per year. At the other end of the risk spectrum are younger patients with AF and no comorbidities whose cumulative 15-year risk of stroke is in the range of 1% to 2%. Aside from prior stroke, the best-established risk factors for stroke in patients with nonvalvular AF are diabetes (relative risk [RR], 1.7), hypertension (RR, 1.6), heart failure (RR, 1.4), and age 70 or older (RR, 1.4 per decade).[1,17,18]

Renal failure also is an independent risk factor for stroke in patients with AF.[19] The RR of a thromboembolic event in the absence of anticoagulation was 1.4 in patients with non–end-stage chronic kidney disease and 1.8 in patients requiring hemodialysis or a renal transplant. The predictive strength of chronic kidney disease for a thromboembolic event appears to be equivalent to that of heart failure and advanced age. Therefore, it may be appropriate to take into account chronic kidney disease when evaluating the risk profile of a patient with AF.

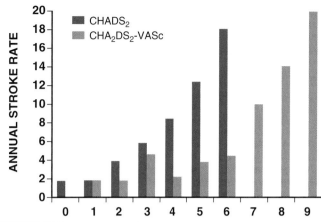

FIGURE 66.6 The annual risk of stroke (percent risk/year) based on the CHADS$_2$ and CHA$_2$DS$_2$-VASc scores. (From Lip GY. Implications of the CHA(2)DS(2)-VASc and HAS-BLED Scores for thromboprophylaxis in atrial fibrillation. Am J Med 2011;124:111-114.)

At present the CHA$_2$DS$_2$-VASc score is recommended for estimation of stroke risk (cardiac failure, hypertension, age >75 years; diabetes, stroke, or transient ischemic attack (TIA), age 65 to 74 years, vascular disease, female sex category).[18,20] Each risk factor counts as 1 point, with the exception of prior stroke or transient ischemic events and age ≥75 years, which count for 2 points. Correction for the inclusion of female sex is accomplished in the updated 2019 AF Guidelines by specifying a higher CHA$_2$DS$_2$-VASc score in women than in men (i.e., ≥3 in women and ≥2 in men to achieve a class I recommendation for anticoagulation) for each anticoagulation cutoff.[18] When considering the CHA$_2$DS$_2$-VASc score, it is important to recognize that there are risk factors for stroke that are not included in the CHA$_2$DS$_2$-VASc score. These include left atrial size, mitral annular calcification, and AF burden (see eTable 66G.1).

The clinical value of the CHA$_2$DS$_2$-VASc score lies in its simplicity and predictive value. There is a direct relationship between the CHA$_2$DS$_2$-VASc score and the annual risk of stroke in the absence of aspirin or anticoagulant therapy. The annual risk of stroke is zero or close to zero when the CHA$_2$DS$_2$-VASc score is 0, compared with approximately 3% when the CHA$_2$DS$_2$-VASc score is 3 (Fig. 66.6).[17] Other risk scores that incorporate other metrics include biomarkers that have been developed and calibrated and may improve risk benefit assessment in AF patients that are candidates for anticoagulation.[21]

The AF burden in persistent AF is 100% and always higher than in patients with paroxysmal AF. It may seem reasonable to assume that the risk of stroke is higher in patients with persistent AF. This recently has been confirmed by several studies, which reported a higher stroke risk in patients with persistent than paroxysmal AF.[17,22] Despite the results of these recent studies, neither the CHA$_2$DS$_2$-VASc score nor the current United States and European AF management guidelines have incorporated AF burden as a risk factor for stroke or into anticoagulation recommendations.[18,23]

Pacemakers and implantable cardioverter-defibrillators (ICDs) that incorporate an atrial lead are capable of detecting short episodes of asymptomatic AF that are subclinical. Subclinical atrial tachyarrhythmias were independently associated with a 2.5-fold increase in the risk of stroke. Long-term intracardiac monitoring in patients with recently implanted pacemakers or ICDs has detected subclinical AF (SCAF) in up to 50% of patients. In a multicenter prospective study, electrocardiographic monitors were implanted in patients ≥65 years of age with left atrium (LA) enlargement or elevated pro-BNP but no history of AF with either CHA$_2$DS$_2$-VASc ≥2, sleep apnea or body mass index (BMI) >30 kg/m^2. About half of the patients had a history of stroke or TIA. SCAF (>5 minutes duration) was detected in 40% of patients who suffered a stroke or TIA and 30% of those who did not over 16 months of follow-up.[24] SCAF is common in older adults and more frequently detected due to the widespread use of implanted electrocardiographic monitoring devices. However, whether anticoagulation lowers stroke risk in this subset of AF patients currently is unknown; SCAF may be a risk marker, not a cause of stroke. The 2019 AHA/ACC/HRS AF Guidelines provides a class I level of evidence (LOE) B recommendation that the presence of recorded atrial high rate episodes on an implanted device should prompt further evaluation to document clinically relevant AF to guide treatment decisions (see eTable 66G.6).[18] It is important to recognize that not all mode switch events that are classified as AF by an implanted device are truly AF. In the absence of data from clinical trials, most clinicians today would advise anticoagulation for patients with device-detected AF who have episodes of at least 5 hours in duration and have an elevated stroke risk profile.

An important consideration in patients treated with an oral anticoagulant is the risk of bleeding. Several risk-scoring systems have been developed to assess a patient's susceptibility to hemorrhagic complications. The scoring system with the best balance of simplicity and accuracy is the HAS-BLED score.[25] The components of this score are hypertension, abnormal renal or liver function, stroke, bleeding history or predisposition, labile international normalized ratio (INR), older adults (>75 years), and concomitant drug (antiplatelet agent or nonsteroidal anti-inflammatory drug) or alcohol use. Each of these components is 1 point. As the score increases from 0 to the maximum of 9, there is a stepwise increase in the risk of bleeding in patients treated with warfarin. While these scores may be helpful in identifying patients at elevated breeding risk, their clinical utility was deemed insufficient to be included as a formal recommendation in the 2014 ACC/AHA/HRS AF Guidelines.[1,18]

The 2019 AHA/ACC/HRS AF Guidelines give a class I LOE A recommendation for anticoagulation of men with a CHA_2DS_2-VASc score of 2 or higher and women with a CHA_2DS_2-VASc score of 3 or higher.[18] For men with a CHA_2DS_2-VASc score of 1 and women with a CHA_2DS_2-VASc score of 2, anticoagulation should be considered (class IIa, LOE A). While the CHA_2DS_2-VASc score provides a valuable guideline for anticoagulation, other factors should be considered, including patient preference. Some patients may prefer to accept an increased risk of stroke instead of long-term anticoagulation. Other patients with a low CHA_2DS_2-VASc score of 0 to 1 may prefer to take an anticoagulant to protect against even the small risk of a stroke (see eTable 66G.1).

Aspirin

Aspirin is not effective for preventing thromboembolic complications in patients with AF. In a meta-analysis of five randomized clinical trials, aspirin did not significantly reduce the risk of stroke compared with placebo in patients with AF.[26] In a large cohort study of patients with nonvalvular AF, aspirin had no therapeutic efficacy for preventing strokes.[1] In several network meta-analyses, the variable and modest reduction in stroke risk with aspirin is not greater than that expected for reduction of risk for vascular stroke. It is notable that a major update of the 2019 ACC/AHA/HRS AF Guidelines, as compared with the 2014 AHA/ACC/HRS AF Guidelines, is that aspirin is no longer recommended for stroke prevention in AF patients.[1,18] In patients with a low CHA_2DS_2-VASc score, the recommended options for stroke prevention are now an anticoagulant versus no therapy (see eTable 66G.1).

Warfarin

A meta-analysis of the major randomized clinical trials that compared warfarin with placebo for prevention of thromboembolism in patients with AF demonstrated that warfarin reduced the risk of all strokes (ischemic and hemorrhagic) by approximately 60%.[26,27] The target INR should be 2.0 to 3.0. This range of INRs provides the best balance between stroke prevention and hemorrhagic complications. In clinical practice, maintenance of the INR in therapeutic range has been challenging, and a large proportion of patients often have an INR of less than 2.0. A large prospective study of community-based practices demonstrated that the mean time in therapeutic range (TTR) in patients treated with warfarin was only 66% and that the TTR was less than 60% in 34% of patients.[28] Even in clinical trials there are significant lapses in maintaining warfarin TTR. Maintaining the INR at a level of 2.0 or higher is important because even a relatively small decrease in INR from 2.0 to 1.7 more than doubles the risk of stroke.

The annual risk of a major hemorrhagic complication during anticoagulation with warfarin is in the range of 1% to 2%, and a strong predictor of major bleeding events is an INR greater than 3.0. For example, the risk of intracranial bleeding is approximately twice as high at an INR of 4.0 than 3.0. This emphasizes the importance of maintaining the INR in the range of 2.0 to 3.0.

Some studies have indicated that advanced age can be a risk factor for intracranial hemorrhage in patients with AF treated with warfarin. However, the available data indicate that warfarin and the direct-acting oral anticoagulants (DOACs) have a favorable risk-to-benefit ratio even in patients older than 75.[29]

Direct-Acting Oral Anticoagulants

Direct thrombin inhibitors and factor Xa inhibitors have several advantages over vitamin K antagonists such as warfarin: (1) a fixed dosing regimen that eliminates the need for monitoring the INR, (2) rapid onset and offset, (3) equal or greater efficacy for stroke prevention, (4) a lower risk of intracranial hemorrhage, (5) no interactions with dietary factors such as alcohol or vitamin-K containing foods, and (6) far fewer drug interactions.[30]

Dabigatran, an oral direct thrombin inhibitor, and rivaroxaban, apixaban, and edoxaban, which are factor Xa inhibitors, are approved by the U.S. Food and Drug Administration (FDA) for prevention of stroke/embolism in patients with nonvalvular AF. Randomized clinical trials demonstrated that each of these four DOACs is noninferior or superior to warfarin in efficacy and safety in patients with nonvalvular AF who had risk factors for stroke.[30] One of the most serious risks of anticoagulation is intracranial hemorrhage. The trials, which were performed for FDA approval of each of these NOACs, revealed that the risk of intracranial hemorrhage is about 50% lower with DOACs compared with warfarin.

Because of these major advantages, the 2019 ACC/AHA/HRS AF Guidelines recommend the use of DOACs over warfarin for prevention of thromboembolic complications in patients with AF (see eTable 66G.1).[18]

DOACs also have some disadvantages compared with warfarin: higher cost, more gastrointestinal side effects in the case of dabigatran, twice-daily dosing for dabigatran and apixaban, the absence of a readily available laboratory test to verify compliance, and restricted use in patients with prosthetic valves. Furthermore, use of these agents requires great care in patients with severe renal disease. The pharmacokinetics of apixaban suggest it could be used in severe renal disease and recent studies have demonstrated safety/efficacy,[31] but randomized controlled trials are needed.

Until recently another limitation of DOACs was that there were no specific reversal agents. However, reversal agents now are available for all DOACs.[30,32-34] The first reversal agent to receive FDA approval, both for uncontrolled bleeding and the need for urgent surgery, was idarucizumab, an antibody fragment that reverses the anticoagulant effects of dabigatran within minutes.[30,34] Since that time andexanet alfa has been approved for acute major bleeding in patients taking a factor Xa inhibitor.[32] A limitation of andexanet alfa is high cost compared with a prothrombin concentrate.

When a reversal agent is not available or not desired, administration of prothrombin complex concentrate can reverse the anticoagulant effect of the DOACs (see eTable 66G.2).

Older studies demonstrated the frequent underutilization of warfarin in patients with AF and risk factors for stroke. The inconvenience and potential risks of warfarin likely contributed to its underutilization. However, the underutilization of and low adherence to oral anticoagulant use in patients with AF has continued to be the case even with the advent of DOACs.[35]

The major professional societies have incorporated recommendations regarding the use of the factor Xa- and direct thrombin-inhibitors into their most recent guidelines for the management of AF.[18,23] As noted above, the ACC/AHA/HRS AF guidelines recommend DOACs over warfarin for prevention of stroke and systemic embolism in patients with nonvalvular paroxysmal or persistent AF and risk factors for stroke. This recommendation is limited to patients without valvular AF. Valvular AF is defined as AF in patients with a prosthetic valve or with moderate to severe mitral stenosis. Based on recent data, the 2019 ACC/AHA/HRS AF Guidelines provide a 2B recommendation for reduced-dose DOAC therapy in patients with moderate to severe kidney disease.[18] These guidelines also state that dabigatran, rivaroxaban, and edoxaban are not recommended in patients with end-stage kidney disease or patients on dialysis. Recent studies indicate the apixaban may be safe to use in such patients.[31]

The results of a large number of clinical trials have indicated that the DOACs are as effective as warfarin for prevention of thromboembolic complications associated with cardioversion.[36] This is the case regardless of whether or not a transesophageal echocardiogram is performed before cardioversion to look for left atrial thrombus.

The onset of action of the DOACs is approximately 1.5 to 2 hours after a dose. Their half-life is approximately 12 hours. The rapid onset of action and washout eliminates the need for bridging therapy with heparin when treatment with one of the DOACs is interrupted for a surgical or invasive medical procedure. Recent data indicate that the risk of major periprocedural complications does not differ significantly between patients who undergo radiofrequency catheter ablation of AF during uninterrupted therapy with warfarin and patients anticoagulated with an uninterrupted DOAC.[30,37]

Low-Molecular-Weight Heparin

Low-molecular-weight heparin (LMWH) has a longer half-life than unfractionated heparin and a predictable antithrombotic effect that is attained with a fixed dosage administered subcutaneously twice daily. Because LMWH can be self-injected outside the hospital, it is a practical alternative to unfractionated heparin for initiation of anticoagulation with warfarin in patients with AF. Bridging therapy with LMWH should be continued until the INR is 2.0 or higher.

Because of its high cost, LMWH rarely is used in clinical practice as a substitute for long-term conventional anticoagulation. In the past, LMWH typically was used as a temporary bridge to therapeutic anticoagulation when therapy with warfarin was initiated or in high-risk patients for a few days before and after a medical or dental procedure when anticoagulation with warfarin was been suspended. In contemporary practice, the use of DOACs has greatly limited the need for LMWH in patients with nonvalvular AF.

Excision or Closure of the Left Atrial Appendage

Approximately 90% of left atrial thrombi form in the left atrial appendage (LAA), and therefore successful excision or closure of the LAA should greatly reduce the risk of thromboembolic complications in patients with AF. Surgical techniques consist of either excision or closure by suturing or stapling. The efficacy of these techniques is variable and probably dependent on both the technique and the operator. Transesophageal echocardiography (TEE) should be performed after surgical closure of the LAA to confirm successful closure before discontinuation of anticoagulation.

In recent years, several percutaneous LAA occlusion and ligation devices have been developed as alternatives to surgical closure techniques. These devices have their greatest utility in high-risk AF patients who cannot tolerate or who refuse to take an oral anticoagulant.

The only percutaneous occlusion device approved by the FDA specifically for stroke prevention as an alternative to warfarin is the WATCHMAN (Boston Scientific, Marlborough, Massachusetts).[38] This nitinol plug covered with fenestrated fabric became widely available for clinical use after FDA approval in 2015 (Fig. 66.7). After implantation of the WATCHMAN using femoral vein access and transeptal catheterization, anticoagulation with warfarin is recommended for at least 45 days, at which time anticoagulation can be discontinued if there is no TEE evidence of peridevice flow.[39] Since initial release of this device, considerable evidence has demonstrated that DOACs can be used instead of warfarin.[40,41]

Another device used in the United States for LAA occlusion is the LARIAT (Sentreheart, Redwood City, California). This device has FDA

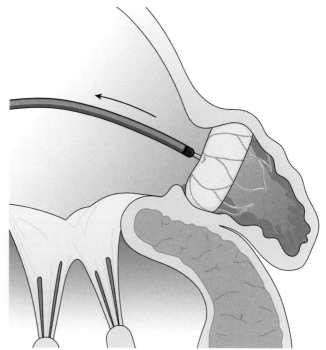

FIGURE 66.7 WATCHMAN device positioned in the left atrial appendage. The delivery sheath is removed once the device is well seated.

approval for soft tissue approximation (not stroke prevention) and has been used off-label in clinical practice in the United States and elsewhere for LAA occlusion. A guidewire with a magnetic tip is inserted into the left atrium after transseptal catheterization and is positioned at the tip of the LAA. It functions as a rail for an epicardial snare. Entry into the pericardial space is attained using a percutaneous approach. A snare with a pretied suture is inserted into the pericardial space and guided toward the LAA (Fig. 66.8). The pretied suture then is tightened to occlude the LAA. In a large multicenter registry, complete LAA closure was achieved in 94% of 712 patients. There was one procedure-related death, and cardiac perforation occurred in 3.4% of patients, with open heart surgery required to repair the perforation in 1.4% of patients.[42] Clinical trial data establishing the efficacy of the LARIAT for stroke prevention are lacking. At present, this device is being used in the AMAZE clinical trial, which is seeking to determine whether PV isolation plus appendage ligation with the LARIAT device is superior to PV isolation alone in patients with persistent AF. The study has completed enrollment and the results should be available in 2021. Percutaneous or surgical LAA occlusion are considered class IIa and IIb recommendations, respectively, in situations where anticoagulation is contraindicated or the patient is undergoing cardiac surgery (see eTable 66G.2).

ACUTE MANAGEMENT OF ATRIAL FIBRILLATION

Patients who present to the emergency department because of AF often have a rapid ventricular rate, and control of the ventricular rate is most rapidly achieved with intravenous diltiazem or esmolol (eTable 66G.3). If the patient is hemodynamically unstable, immediate transthoracic cardioversion may be appropriate. Cardioversion should ideally be preceded by TEE to rule out a left atrial thrombus if the AF has been present for longer than 48 hours or if the duration is unclear and the patient is not already anticoagulated. However, if the patient has marked hemodynamic compromise, immediate cardioversion without a TEE is advised.

If the patient is hemodynamically stable, the decision to restore sinus rhythm by cardioversion is based on several factors, including symptoms, prior AF episodes, age, left atrial size, and current AAD therapy. For example, in an elderly patient whose symptoms resolve once

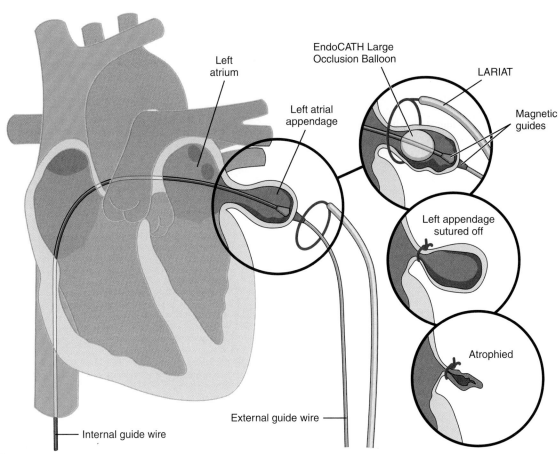

FIGURE 66.8 Steps involved in deploying the LARIAT catheter for occlusion of the left atrial appendage.

the ventricular rate is controlled and who already has had early recurrences of AF despite rhythm-control drug therapy, further attempts at cardioversion usually are not appropriate. On the other hand, cardioversion usually is appropriate for patients with symptomatic AF who present with a first episode of AF or who have had long intervals of sinus rhythm between prior episodes.

If cardioversion is decided upon for a hemodynamically stable patient who presents with AF that does not appear to be self-limited, two management decisions must be made: early versus delayed cardioversion and pharmacologic versus electrical cardioversion.

The advantages of early cardioversion are rapid relief of symptoms, avoidance of the need for TEE or therapeutic anticoagulation for 3 to 4 weeks before cardioversion if cardioversion is performed within 48 hours of AF onset, and possibly a lower risk of early AF recurrence because of less atrial remodeling (see Chapter 64). A reason to defer cardioversion is the unavailability of TEE in a patient who has not been anticoagulated with AF of unclear duration or duration more than 48 hours. Other reasons include a left atrial thrombus by TEE (see Chapter 16), a suspicion (based on prior AF episodes) that AF will convert spontaneously within a few days, or in rare cases, a correctable cause of AF such as hyperthyroidism.

When cardioversion is performed early in the course of an episode of AF, there is the option of either pharmacologic or electrical cardioversion. Pharmacologic cardioversion has the advantage of not requiring general anesthesia or deep sedation. In addition, the probability of an immediate recurrence of AF is lower with pharmacologic cardioversion than with electrical cardioversion. However, pharmacologic cardioversion is associated with the risk of adverse drug effects and is not as effective as electrical cardioversion. Pharmacologic cardioversion is unlikely to be effective if the duration of AF is longer than 7 days.

Drugs that can be administered intravenously for cardioversion of AF consist of ibutilide, procainamide, and amiodarone. For AF episodes fewer than 2 to 3 days in duration, efficacy is approximately 60% to 70% for ibutilide, 40% to 50% for amiodarone, and 30% to 40% for

procainamide. To minimize the risk of QT prolongation and polymorphic ventricular tachycardia (torsades de pointes; see Chapter 67), the use of ibutilide should be limited to patients with an ejection fraction greater than 35%.

Acute pharmacologic cardioversion of AF also can be attempted with oral drugs in patients without structural heart disease. The most common oral agents for acute conversion of AF are propafenone (300 to 600 mg) and flecainide (100 to 200 mg). When flecainide is used, patients generally take a beta blocker on AF onset and then take the flecainide one or more hours later. It is recommended that these drugs be administered under surveillance upon first use, as patients may have a pronounced postconversion pause. If no adverse drug effects are observed, the patient may then be an appropriate candidate for episodic, self-administered AAD therapy on an outpatient basis (the "pill-in-the-pocket" approach).

The efficacy of transthoracic cardioversion exceeds 95%. Biphasic waveform shocks convert AF more effectively than monophasic waveform shocks and allow the use of lower energy shocks, resulting in less skin irritation. An appropriate first-shock strength using a biphasic waveform is 150 to 200 J, followed by higher output shocks if needed. If a 360-J biphasic shock is unsuccessful, ibutilide should be infused before another shock is delivered because it lowers the defibrillation energy requirement and improves the success rate of transthoracic cardioversion.

Transthoracic cardioversion can fail to restore sinus rhythm. An increase in shock strength, an infusion of ibutilide, or repeat CV with greater pressure applied to the defibrillation patches, often results in successful repeat cardioversion. The second type of failure is an immediate recurrence of AF within a few seconds of successful conversion to sinus rhythm. This occurs in approximately 25% of AF episodes less than 24 hours in duration and 10% of episodes more than 24 hours in duration. For this type of cardioversion failure, an increase in shock strength is of no value. If the patient has not been receiving an oral rhythm-control agent, infusion of ibutilide may be helpful to prevent an immediate recurrence of AF.

Regardless of whether cardioversion is performed pharmacologically or electrically, *therapeutic* anticoagulation is necessary for 3 weeks or more before cardioversion to prevent thromboembolic complications if the AF has been ongoing for more than 48 hours. If the time of onset of AF is unclear, for the sake of safety, the AF duration should be assumed to be more than 48 hours. These patients should be therapeutically anticoagulated for 4 weeks after cardioversion to prevent thromboembolic complications that may occur because of atrial stunning. If the patient's stroke risk profile is elevated, anticoagulation should be continued indefinitely. If the duration of AF is known to be less than 48 hours, cardioversion can be performed without anticoagulation. However, if the patient's stroke risk profile is elevated and long-term anticoagulation is advised, immediate initiation of anticoagulation with a DOAC is recommended.[42]

When AF duration exceeds 48 hours or is unclear, an alternative to 3 weeks of therapeutic anticoagulation before cardioversion is anticoagulation with heparin and a TEE to check for a left atrial thrombus. If no thrombi are seen, the patient can be cardioverted safely but still requires 4 weeks of therapeutic anticoagulation after cardioversion to prevent thromboembolism related to atrial stunning. The major clinical benefit of the TEE-guided approach over the conventional approach is that sinus rhythm is restored several weeks sooner. Compared with the conventional approach, the TEE approach has not been found to reduce the risk of stroke or major bleeding or to affect the proportion of patients still in sinus rhythm at 8 weeks after cardioversion. The guidelines for pharmacologic and electrical cardioversion, pharmacologic enhancement of direct current cardioversion of AF and prevention of thromboembolism with acute cardioversion are summarized in eTable 66G.4.[18]

LONG-TERM MANAGEMENT OF ATRIAL FIBRILLATION

Pharmacologic Rate Control Versus Rhythm Control

Several randomized studies have compared a rate-control strategy with a rhythm-control strategy in patients with AF. Overall, these studies have demonstrated a significantly lower rate of rehospitalization with a rate-control strategy but no significant differences in other major outcomes, such as all-cause mortality, strokes, bleeding events, worsening heart failure, or quality of life.[43]

The results of these randomized studies should not be applied systematically to all patients with AF. It is important to note that many patients in the rhythm-control arms of these studies continued to have AF, and that the possible beneficial effects of sinus rhythm over AF could have been negated by adverse effects of the AADs. Furthermore, most patients enrolled in these studies were elderly and had few AF symptoms, and the duration of follow-up was several years. It remains uncertain what the implications are of decades of continuous AF in terms of the risks of stroke, heart failure, dementia, and death.

The decision to pursue a rhythm-control strategy versus a rate-control strategy should be individualized based on several factors. These include the nature, frequency, and severity of symptoms; the length of time that AF has been present continuously in patients with persistent AF; left atrial size; comorbidities; the response to prior cardioversions; age; the side effects and efficacy of the AADs already used to treat the patient; patient age and activity level; and the patient's preference.

The duration of continuous AF is a predictor of the ability to restore and maintain sinus rhythm. The chance of successful AF rhythm control is higher in patients with paroxysmal or early persistent AF (<6 months) than for patients who have been in continuous AF for one or more years. This is an important consideration when faced with asymptomatic or minimally symptomatic patients with newly diagnosed persistent AF. It is well established that the presence of AF is associated with a higher risk of stroke risk, heart failure risk, cognitive dysfunction, and mortality. Recent studies indicate that the stroke risk is higher in a patient with continuous AF than paroxysmal AF.[17,22] While no study has shown that restoration of sinus rhythm with AF ablation impacts any of these complications of AF, it may. Of particular note is the CABANA trial.[44] This prospective randomized clinical trial randomized 2204 patients with AF to catheter ablation or medical therapy. The primary endpoint was a composite of death, disabling stroke, serious bleeding, or cardiac arrest. No difference in the primary endpoint was present after a median follow-up of 48.5 months. But the secondary endpoint of death or cardiovascular hospitalizations was significantly lower in the ablation arm than in the medical therapy arm (51.7% vs. 58.1%, p = 0.001). For this reason, the 2017 HRS/EHRA/ECAS Consensus Document on AF ablation provides a class IIb recommendation for catheter ablation of AF in patients who are asymptomatic.[8]

Pharmacologic Rate Control

An excessively rapid ventricular rate during AF often results in uncomfortable symptoms and decreased effort tolerance and can cause a tachycardia-induced cardiomyopathy if it is sustained for several weeks to months. Optimal heart rates during AF vary with age and should be similar to the heart rates that a patient would have at a particular degree of exertion during sinus rhythm. Heart rate control must be assessed both at rest and during exertion. The 2014 and 2019 ACC/AHA/HRS AF Guidelines advise that the optimal metric for rate control is a resting heart rate <80 beats/min.[1,18] Based on a single European clinical trial, a more lenient rate control metric of <110 beats/min is provided with a class IIb recommendation.[1,18] Assessment of the degree of heart rate control can be obtained with a 24-hour Holter monitor. A 12-lead ECG provides an indication of the resting ventricular rate but fails to provide information on the ventricular rate during a patient's daily activities.

Oral agents available for long-term heart rate control in patients with AF are digitalis, beta blockers, calcium channel antagonists, and amiodarone[1] (see Chapter 64). The first-line agents for rate control are beta blockers and the calcium channel antagonists verapamil and diltiazem. A combination is often used to improve efficacy or to limit side effects by allowing the use of smaller dosages of the individual drugs. In patients with sinus node dysfunction and tachycardia-bradycardia syndrome, the use of a beta blocker with intrinsic sympathomimetic activity (pindolol, acebutolol) may provide rate control without aggravating sinus bradycardia.

Digitalis may adequately control the rate at rest but often does not provide adequate rate control during exertion as it works mainly by increasing vagal tone. Digitalis is no longer recommended for rate control except in patients with heart failure because digitalis has been shown to increase the risk of all-cause mortality, particularly among patients with AF. The 2014 and 2019 AHA/ACC/HRS Guidelines recommend digoxin for rate control only in patients with heart failure (see eTable 66G.3).[1,18]

Amiodarone is much less frequently used for rate control than the other negative dromotropic agents because of the risk of organ toxicity associated with long-term therapy. Amiodarone can be an appropriate choice for rate control if the other agents are not tolerated or are ineffective. For example, amiodarone would be an appropriate choice for a patient with persistent AF, heart failure, and reactive airway disease who cannot tolerate either a calcium channel antagonist or a beta blocker and who has a rapid ventricular rate despite treatment with digitalis. Amiodarone as a rate-control medication is provided with a class IIb recommendation in the 2014 ACC/AHA/HRS AF Guidelines.[1,18]

Pharmacologic Rhythm Control

The results of studies on the efficacy of AADs for suppression of AF suggest that all the available drugs except amiodarone have similar efficacy and are associated with a 40% to 60% reduction in the odds of recurrent AF during 1 year of treatment (see Chapter 64). The one drug that stands out as having higher efficacy than the others is amiodarone. In studies that directly compared amiodarone with sotalol or class I drugs, amiodarone was 60% to 70% more effective in suppressing AF. However, because of the risk of organ toxicity, amiodarone is not appropriate first-line drug therapy for most patients with AF. The 2014 and

2019 AHA/ACC/HRS AF Guidelines[1,18] recommend that amiodarone be used as first-line antiarrhythmic medication only in patients with heart failure.[1,18] In all other subsets of patients, amiodarone should only be used after a less toxic AAD has proven ineffective or poorly tolerated. Because the efficacy of rhythm-control agents other than amiodarone is in the same general range, the selection of a particular AAD to prevent AF often is dictated by the issues of safety and side effects (eTable 66G.5).

Ventricular proarrhythmia from class Ia agents (quinidine, procainamide, disopyramide) and class III agents (sotalol, dofetilide, dronedarone, amiodarone) is manifested as QT prolongation and polymorphic ventricular tachycardia (torsades de pointes). Risk factors for this type of proarrhythmia include female sex, left ventricular dysfunction, hypokalemia, and concomitant use of another QT-prolonging drug. The risk of torsades de pointes appears to be much lower with dronedarone and amiodarone than with the other class III drugs. The ventricular proarrhythmia from class Ic agents (flecainide and propafenone) manifests as monomorphic ventricular tachycardia, sometimes associated with widening of the QRS complex during sinus rhythm, but not QT prolongation. They also increase the propensity for ventricular fibrillation in the setting of myocardial ischemia or infarction (see Chapters 9 and 64). For this reason, class Ic agents are not recommended in patients with established coronary artery disease (CAD).[1,18]

Adverse drug events or side effects resulting in discontinuation of drug therapy are fairly common with rhythm-control drugs, with discontinuation rates reported to be as high as 40%.[45]

The best options for drug therapy to suppress AF depend on the patient's comorbidities. In patients with AF in the setting of a structurally normal heart, flecainide, propafenone, sotalol, dofetilide, and dronedarone are all reasonable first-line drugs. Amiodarone can be considered if the first-line agents are ineffective or not tolerated, especially if AF ablation is not preferred by the patient. As noted above, in patients with CAD, class Ic drugs have been found to increase the risk of death, and the safest first-line options are dofetilide, sotalol, or dronedarone, with amiodarone reserved for use as a second-line agent. In patients with heart failure, several AADs have been associated with increased mortality, and the only two drugs known to have a neutral effect on survival are amiodarone and dofetilide (see Chapter 64).

Dronedarone should not be used as a rate-control agent in patients with persistent AF. At the time of FDA approval, it was not known that dronedarone increased mortality in New York Heart Association (NYHA) Class IV heart failure or patients with a recent episode of decompensated heart failure. After a higher mortality risk was demonstrated in a subsequent randomized clinical trial,[46] dronedarone was labeled as being contraindicated when used as a rate-control agent and also in patients with decompensated heart failure.

Rhythm Control with Agents Other Than Antiarrhythmic Drugs

Experimental studies have indicated that angiotensin-converting enzyme (ACE) inhibitors and angiotensin receptor blockers (ARBs) have favorable effects on electrical and structural remodeling (see Chapters 62 and 64). This explains why some studies have shown that ACE inhibitors and ARBs prevent AF. However, other studies have demonstrated that these agents do not prevent AF. At present, there is insufficient evidence to support the use of ACE inhibitors and ARBs for the sole purpose of preventing AF. Available data also do not support the use of statins or omega-3 polyunsaturated fatty acids (PUFAs) for the prevention of AF.[18]

NONPHARMACOLOGIC MANAGEMENT OF ATRIAL FIBRILLATION

Risk Factor Modification

An important development in AF management in the past decade has been the recognition of the importance of risk factor management in the treatment of patients with AF.[11] Historically, the three pillars of AF

management have been stroke prevention, rate control, and rhythm control. There is now is strong evidence that risk factor management should be considered the fourth pillar of AF management. The modifiable AF risk factors consist of obesity, hypertension, diabetes, sleep apnea, CAD, heart failure, lack of cardiovascular fitness, and tobacco and alcohol use.

An overview of risk factor management in patients with AF is provided in this chapter. More detailed information is provided in the recently published AHA Scientific Statement on Lifestyle and Risk Factor Modification for Reduction in Atrial Fibrillation.[47]

Obesity is closely linked to the development of AF. The risk of developing AF increases 29% with every 5-point increase in BMI. The scientific basis for this link between obesity and AF has been studied extensively in animal models. Several clinical studies have demonstrated that weight loss combined with comprehensive risk factor management reduces AF and also improves the efficacy of catheter ablation.[11,47,48] This has also been shown recently to be a cost-effective treatment strategy.[49]

Hypertension is a modifiable risk factor for AF. Hypertension causes ventricular hypertrophy and atrial enlargement, as well as activation of the renin-angiotensin system.[1,50] One small study enrolling 76 patients with severe resistant hypertension, demonstrated that renal denervation was associated with a significant reduction in both BP and AF burden at 12 months' follow-up.[51] There also is a strong association between diabetes and AF, probably because of fibrotic changes in the atria and downregulation of connexin-43 and associated abnormalities of conduction in the atrium.[52]

Cigarette smoking augments the risk of AF by causing an increase in sympathetic tone, inflammation, endothelial dysfunction, atrial fibrosis, and oxidative stress. Alcohol use has also been linked to development of AF.[2,3] This link results from direct cellular effects of alcohol on atrial myocytes with acute oxidative stress and also from activation of the sympathetic nervous system. A recent study demonstrated that abstinence from alcohol results in a reduction in AF burden.[2]

Physical inactivity is another modifiable AF risk factor. Physical activity has been demonstrated to reduce the incidence of cardiovascular disease. Sedentary lifestyles have also been shown to be other risk factors for AF, particularly obesity. Cardiovascular fitness has been found to reduce the AF burden independent of weight loss.

Another modifiable risk factor to consider is sleep apnea. Sleep apnea is common among AF patients. A number of studies have shown that sleep apnea increases the risk of new-onset AF. Treatment of sleep apnea has been shown to reduce the probability of recurrent AF after cardioversion and AF catheter ablation.

Based on the growing body of literature linking AF development to the presence of modifiable risk factors, especially obesity, the AHA/ACC/HRS 2019 AF Guideline provides a class I LOE B recommendation that overweight and obese patients with AF should lose weight as part of a risk factor modification program.[18] The goal of weight loss ideally should be a BMI of ≤27 kg/m^2 (eTable 66G.6).

Pacing to Prevent Atrial Fibrillation

Multiple studies have been performed to determine whether various atrial pacing strategies can prevent or terminate AF. Overall, there has been no convincing evidence that any atrial pacing strategy is effective in preventing or terminating episodes of AF, and therefore atrial pacing is not indicated for prevention of AF in patients without bradycardia or AV block.

Catheter Ablation of Atrial Fibrillation

Catheter ablation reliably and permanently eliminates several types of arrhythmias, such as AV nodal reentrant tachycardia (AVNRT) and accessory pathway–mediated tachycardias (see Chapters 64 and 65). Success rates greater than 95% are attainable when the arrhythmia substrate is well defined, localized, and temporally stable. In contrast, the arrhythmia substrate of AF is not completely understood, is usually widespread, is variable between patients, and is often progressive. Furthermore, several factors that promote AF cannot be addressed simply by catheter ablation, including comorbidities (e.g., hypertension, obesity, obstructive sleep apnea), structural remodeling of the atria, systemic inflammatory factors, and genetic factors (see Chapter 7). Therefore, whereas late recurrences of AVNRT or accessory pathway conduction are very rare, AF can recur after an initially successful ablation procedure. For this reason, AF ablation should not be considered a "cure" for AF but rather a palliative measure to keep the patient in sinus rhythm for as long as possible.[8] This section of the chapter provides an overview of the techniques and outcomes of catheter ablation of AF.

Catheter Ablation Technique and Outcomes of AF Ablation

Cox and colleagues developed and demonstrated the efficacy of surgical AF ablation in the early 1990s. Although a large number of investigators attempted to replicate the surgical maze procedure with catheter ablation techniques, these clinical trials reported limited success. A major step forward occurred in 1998 when Haissaguerre et al. identified the PVs as the most common site of focal triggers that initiate AF.[7] After an initial approach of focal RF ablation within the PVs, it was quickly recognized that electrical isolation of the PVs is the optimal technique for eliminating triggers and drivers arising in the PVs. This is true for ablation of paroxysmal and persistent AF. Electrical isolation of the PVs can be achieved by focal PV ostial ablation, circumferential ostial ablation, or circumferential ablation in the antral areas of the PVs, 1 to 2 cm from the ostium. Circumferential antral isolation of the PVs results in 1 year of freedom from AF of between 60% and 80% in patients with paroxysmal AF, 40% to 60% in patients with persistent AF, and 20% to 40% in patients with longstanding persistent AF.[8] Because of the lower success rate of antral PV isolation in patients with the persistent forms of AF, a number of strategies have been developed to improve outcomes in this cohort of patients. These techniques include linear ablation to isolate the left atrial posterior wall, linear ablation in other regions of the left atrium and right atrium, ablation of complex fractionated electrograms, ablation of nonpulmonary vein triggers, isolation of the LAA, focal impulse and rotor modulation ablation, ablation of atrial scar identified by MRI or voltage mapping, and electrical isolation of the superior vena cava. Despite single-center cohort studies that reported promising results, none of the adjunctive approaches has been shown to be superior in efficacy compared with the others when subjected to a prospective, randomized clinical trial.[8,53] This remains an active area of clinical investigation and a number of prospective randomized clinical trials are underway.

The efficacy of AF ablation is closely linked with how success is defined and the intensity of ECG monitoring postablation.[54,55] In general, the more monitoring performed, the lower the success rate. The CIRCA-DoSE trial recently examined this relationship closely.[54] In this trial, 346 patients with paroxysmal AF were randomized to catheter ablation with the cryoballoon or with RF energy. An implantable rhythm monitor was implanted at least 1 month before ablation in all patients. The success of AF ablation was approximately 55% at 1 year if the definition of success was defined as freedom from a 30 second or longer episode of an atrial arrhythmia after the 3-month blanking period. The success rate increased to approximately 80% if the definition of success was freedom from a symptomatic atrial arrhythmia. Importantly, AF burden was reduced by approximately 98%. The outcomes of AF ablation were similar in the cryoballoon and RF arms of the study. These results have been reproduced in a more recent trial.[55]

The two most common ablation energy sources are radiofrequency energy and cryoenergy. Radiofrequency energy applied on a point-by-point basis was the first method that became widely adapted for AF ablation. In contemporary practice, radiofrequency ablation typically is performed in association with a three-dimensional electroanatomic mapping system as a nonfluoroscopic navigation guide and to create a visual record of the sites that already have been ablated (Fig. 66.9). To improve anatomic accuracy, the electroanatomic map of the left atrium can be merged with a computed tomography scan or magnetic resonance image of the left atrium and PVs or with an ultrasound image generated by intracardiac echocardiography. An important determinant of lesion depth and durability is *contact force,* and the newest

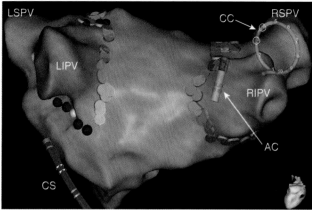

FIGURE 66.9 An electroanatomic map of the left atrium. Icons representing the distal portion of the ablation catheter *(AC)*, circular catheter *(CC)* in the right superior pulmonary vein *(RSPV)*, and a catheter positioned within the coronary sinus *(CS)* are visualized in real time. Circumferential antral ablation was performed around the left and right pulmonary veins. Each one of the *pink, red,* and *yellow* tags represents a site at which radiofrequency energy was delivered. *LIPV,* Left inferior pulmonary vein; *LSPV,* left superior pulmonary vein; *RIPV,* right inferior pulmonary vein.

generation of RF ablation catheters provides the operator with immediate feedback on contact force.

In 2010 a cryoballoon catheter designed to isolate PVs became widely available for use in the United States. In contrast to point-by-point RF ablation around the PVs, the cryoballoon was designed to fit into the antrum of a PV and to create a circumferential ablation lesion using cryoenergy. Cryoenergy is delivered through the entire distal half of the second-generation cryoballoon catheter currently in clinical use. Complete occlusion of the PV by the inflated balloon is essential for reliable PV isolation (Fig. 66.10). Various strategies are used to deliver the cryoenergy, ranging from one or two applications of 3 to 4 minutes to applications of variable duration based on specific freezing parameters[56] (Fig. 66.11).

Avoidance of entry of the cryoballoon into the luminal portion of a PV is important to avoid PV stenosis. The most commonly used cryoballoon catheter has a 28-mm diameter when the balloon is fully inflated. The relatively large size of the balloon typically allows occlusion of a PV from the antrum. A multielectrode catheter inserted through a central lumen of the cryoballoon catheter often allows recording of PV potentials during an application of cryoenergy. The endpoint of the cryoballoon ablation procedure is electrical isolation of all PVs. Disappearance or dissociation of PV potentials within the first minute of a cryoenergy application is a strong independent predictor of durable PV isolation (Fig. 66.12). Other independent predictors are a temperature recorded by a thermocouple proximal to the balloon of at least −40°C within 60 seconds of an application of cryoenergy and an interval thaw time to 0°C of >10 seconds upon completion of a cryoenergy application. In addition to the cryoballoon, a visually-guided laser balloon (VGLB) system now also is available for clinical use.[57] A randomized clinical trial demonstrated that the VGLB was noninferior to radiofrequency catheter ablation in regards to efficacy.[58]

There have been a number of head-to-head comparisons of the safety and efficacy of radiofrequency ablation versus cryoballoon ablation.[54,59] These studies have reported remarkably similar outcomes. The cryoballoon procedures are generally shorter, require more fluoroscopy, and have a higher risk of phrenic nerve injury and a lower risk of pericardial tamponade.[55] The tool an operator chooses is largely based on his or her own personal training and experience. Some operators have great skill with point-by-point RF ablation and rarely if ever use the cryoballoon system. Other operators use the cryoballoon system for 100% of first-time ablation procedures and reserve the RF approach for complete isolation of PVs that cannot be successfully isolated with the cryoballoon catheter, for repeat ablation procedures, and also in patients in whom the operator wishes to ablate sites outside the PVs. RF ablation also may be needed to ablate typical or atypical atrial flutter.

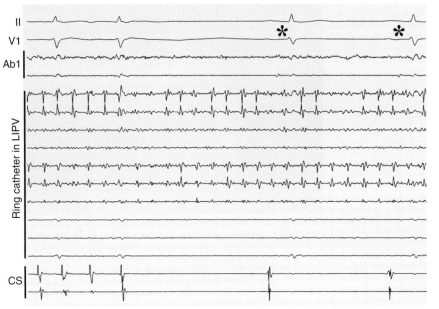

FIGURE 66.10 A tachycardia with a cycle length of 80 milliseconds arising in a left inferior pulmonary vein (LIPV) during AF. AF converted to sinus rhythm (asterisks) during radiofrequency ablation when the LIPV was electrically isolated. The pulmonary vein tachycardia persisted inside the vein. Conversion to sinus rhythm on electrical isolation of the LIPV is strong evidence that the tachycardia arising in the muscle sleeve of this pulmonary vein was the driver of AF in this patient. Shown are leads II and V₁, the electrograms recorded by the ablation catheter (Abl), by a ring catheter in the LIPV, and in the coronary sinus (CS).

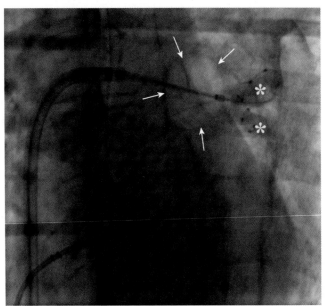

FIGURE 66.11 A right anterior oblique fluoroscopic image of the heart showing a cryoballoon catheter positioned in the antrum of the left inferior pulmonary vein. The 28-mm balloon (arrows) is inflated, and there is no leakage of contrast injected through the lumen of the cryoballoon catheter into the vein (asterisks). This indicates complete occlusion of the vein, a necessary requirement for durable pulmonary vein isolation. A diagnostic ring catheter is positioned within the vein.

When performed by experienced operators, catheter ablation of AF has a major complication rate of 1% to 3%.[8] The potential complications include stroke (0.5%), cardiac tamponade (0.5% to 1.5%), phrenic nerve injury (0.2%), femoral vein-related complications (1%), pulmonary vein stenosis (0.5%), and death (0.1%).

The most feared complication of AF ablation is an atrial esophageal fistula. The risk of esophageal perforation is reported to be in the range of 0.01% to 0.02%.[60] Despite its rarity, this complication is of great concern because it often is lethal. Patients typically present 3 to 14 days after ablation with one or more of the following: dysphagia,

odynophagia, fever, leukocytosis, bacteremia, and stroke. Computed tomography of the chest with intravenous contrast is the diagnostic test of choice. The presence of contrast in the esophagus or air in the mediastinum or cardiac chambers is indicative of an esophageal perforation or fistula formation. Instrumentation of the esophagus should be avoided.

Monitoring of the position of the esophagus and intraluminal esophageal temperature monitoring have been used to prevent esophageal injury during ablation along the posterior wall. Although these maneuvers may reduce the risk, they clearly do not prevent all cases of esophageal injury, since 90% of patients with an esophageal perforation had undergone monitoring of the esophageal position or temperature.[60] There is evidence that limiting the power of RF energy applications to 20 to 25 watts for less than 30 seconds when ablating along the posterior left atrial wall and the use of periprocedural proton pump inhibitors reduce the risk of esophageal injury.[61]

Based on the results of a recent global survey, 72% of patients with an esophageal perforation had evidence of an atrial-esophageal fistula, and mortality among these patients was 79%. In contrast, among the 28% of patients with an esophageal perforation who did not have an atrial-esophageal fistula, mortality was 13%.[60] This highlights the importance of early diagnosis and treatment of esophageal perforations. Early surgical intervention is appropriate regardless of whether an atrial-esophageal fistula is present.

Most published series have reported a small or zero mortality risk.[8,44] However, two recent studies examined the mortality of AF ablation in large claims databases. One study examined the major complication rate and mortality among 190,398 patients in the Nationwide Inpatient Sample.[62] The complication rate was 7.21% and the mortality rate was 0.24%. The complication and mortality rates were more than twice that of patients undergoing ablation for supraventricular tachycardia (SVT). The complication rate was about 30% lower but the in-hospital mortality rate was only 13% of that of patients undergoing ablation for VT.[62] A lower operator- and center-procedure-volume were associated with a higher complication rate. A second recent study reported a similar mortality rate of 0.46%, half of which occurred during an early readmission following the index procedure.[63] These studies serve as a sober reminder that AF ablation can be risky and that both operator experience and center procedure volume are important factors that influence risk.

Indications for Ablation and Selection of Patients

The indications for catheter ablation of AF reflect the safety and efficacy of the procedure.[8,18,23] Various documents have been published that provide specific indications for AF ablation. The most widely recognized management guidelines are the 2014 and 2019 AHA/ACC/HRS AF Guidelines, the 2016 ESC AF Guidelines (see eTable 66G.5), and the 2017 HRS/EHRA/ECAS Consensus Document on AF Ablation. The 2017 HRS/EHRA/ECAS Consensus Document provides the most detailed recommendations.[8] In this section, the appropriate indications for catheter ablation of AF are reviewed.

Several principles should be considered when selecting patients who are appropriate candidates for AF ablation. First, the only proven benefit of AF ablation is an improvement in quality of life. While cohort studies have provided evidence suggesting that AF ablation may reduce stroke risk, heart failure risk, cognitive dysfunction risk, and mortality, none of these benefits have been conclusively proven in randomized clinical trials. As noted earlier, the CABANA trial randomized 2204 patients to ablation or medical therapy. No difference was seen in the composite primary endpoint of death, disabling stroke, serious

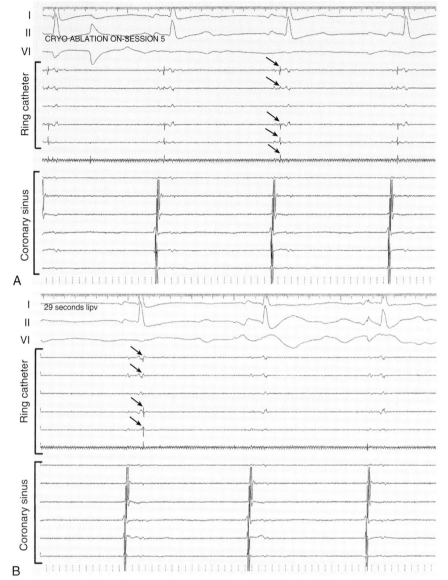

FIGURE 66.12 A, Pulmonary vein potentials *(arrows)* recorded from within the left inferior pulmonary vein at the onset of an application of cryoenergy during sinus rhythm at a rate of 54 beats/min. **B,** At 29 seconds into an application of cryoenergy, there is a conduction delay in the pulmonary vein potentials *(arrows)* followed by their complete disappearance, indicating isolation of the left inferior pulmonary vein *(lipv).* The application of cryoenergy was continued for a total of 4 minutes.

performed as first-line treatment, in preference to an antiarrhythmic medication. Catheter ablation in medication-naïve patients is a class II indication. Similarly, the recommendation for AF ablation in patients with persistent or longstanding persistent AF is weaker than for patients with paroxysmal AF (see eTable 66G.5). This reflects the fact that most trials have primarily enrolled patients with paroxysmal AF and because outcomes after catheter ablation are less satisfactory in patients with the persistent forms of AF.

Surgical Ablation of Atrial Fibrillation

The maze procedure was developed and first reported by Cox et al. in 1987.[1,8] The operation initially required a sternotomy and cardiopulmonary bypass and consisted of multiple atrial incisions to create lines of block and compartmentalize the left atrium and right atrium. In addition, the left and right atrial appendages were excised. Although this procedure had a high success rate, it was technically challenging and the risks were considerable. For this reason, this "cut-and-sew" approach is rarely if ever still performed.

The current iteration of the procedure is the Cox maze 4.[8] This procedure has a similar lesion set, but various tools are used to create the lines of block instead of surgical incisions. These tools include a bipolar clamp RF ablation tool to electrically isolate the PVs. Cryoablation energy delivered with a handheld probe is used to create linear lesions. A bipolar RF clamp is used to electrically isolate the LAA. AF ablation using this open-chest approach is performed in conjunction with open-chest heart surgical procedures such as mitral valve repair or replacement or coronary artery bypass grafting.

Stand-alone surgical AF ablation is performed using a minimally invasive approach referred to as the "mini maze." This procedure involves recreating the maze lesion set using a thorascopic approach with ablation tools specifically designed for percutaneous use.

A single randomized clinical trial[65] and a review of cohort studies[66] have indicated that surgical ablation has greater efficacy than catheter ablation but that it is associated with a higher rate of complications including the need for a permanent pacemaker.[65,66] In many centers this procedure is reserved for AF patients who are poor candidates for catheter ablation, often due to the presence of longstanding persistent AF with severe left atrial dilation, or inefficacy of catheter ablation procedures.

An evolving surgical ablation strategy is a hybrid AF ablation approach in which cardiac surgeons and electrophysiologists participate. Hybrid AF ablation can be performed sequentially during a single ablation session. Some centers prefer a staged approach in which the surgical portion of the procedure is performed first followed by catheter ablation at a separate session, usually several weeks later. The choice of a single combined procedure versus a staged procedure is largely based on operator preference.

Ablation of the Atrioventricular Node

Radiofrequency catheter ablation of the AV node results in complete AV nodal block and substitutes a regular, paced rhythm for an irregular and rapid native rhythm. It is a useful strategy in patients who are symptomatic from AF because of a rapid ventricular rate that cannot be adequately controlled pharmacologically by medications and who either are not good candidates for AF ablation or have already undergone

bleeding, or cardiac arrest.[44] It is notable, however, that a secondary treatment analysis revealed that catheter ablation was associated with a lower mortality than medical therapy. The CASTLE AF study is also important to consider. This trial randomized 363 patients with AF heart failure, each of whom had an ICD, to catheter ablation or medical therapy. After a median follow-up of 37.8 months, the primary composite endpoint of death from any cause or hospitalization for worsening heart failure was lower in the ablation arm.[64]

Because of the absence of strong data demonstrating a survival benefit of AF ablation in the absence of heart failure, this procedure is most commonly performed to improve quality of life in patients with symptomatic AF. Other factors to consider when recommending catheter ablation include the type of AF (paroxysmal, persistent, or longstanding persistent), duration of continuous AF, severity of symptoms and quality of life, age, left atrial size, response to rate- and rhythm-control medications, response to cardioversion, and patient preference.

The optimal patients for AF ablation, for which the guidelines provide a class I indication, are patients with symptomatic paroxysmal AF who have not responded well to least one antiarrhythmic medication.[8,18,23] Because of patient preference, ablation sometimes is unsuccessful attempts at ablation. AV node ablation also can be help-ful in patients with heart failure and AF to maximize the benefits of cardiac resynchronization therapy (CRT) if there already is not 100% ventricular pacing.

In patients with AF and an uncontrolled ventricular rate, AV node ablation improves the left ventricular ejection fraction (EF) if there is a tachycardia-induced cardiomyopathy. AV node ablation also has been shown to improve symptoms, quality of life, and functional capacity and to reduce the use of health care resources.[67-69]

The disadvantages of AV node ablation are that it creates a life-long need for ventricular pacing and does not restore AV synchrony. Although symptoms and functional capacity typically improve after AV node ablation in patients with AF and an uncontrolled ventricular rate, some patients may not feel as well as during sinus rhythm.

Atrioventricular node ablation is a technically simple procedure with an acute and long-term success rate of 98% or higher and a very low risk of complications. In patients with persistent AF, a ventricular pacemaker is implanted. A dual-chamber pacemaker is appropriate if the AF is par-oxysmal. Most patients have a good clinical outcome with right ventricu-lar pacing, but in patients with left ventricular dysfunction, biventricular pacing for CRT is appropriate.[67,69] In some cases, rate-responsive pacing may improve exercise capacity after AV node ablation.[70] In patients with an ischemic or nonischemic cardiomyopathy and EF of 30% to 35% or lower, an ICD may be appropriate for primary prevention of sud-den death. However, a pacemaker without the ICD often is adequate for patients with a borderline EF (30% to 35%) and a rapid ventricular rate because the EF typically improves after the ventricular rate has been controlled by AV node ablation. In patients without a bundle branch block, His bundle pacing is optimal because it avoids the dyssynchrony associated with right ventricular pacing and eliminates the need for a lead in the coronary sinus that is required for biventricular pacing.[71,72]

SPECIFIC CLINICAL SYNDROMES

Postoperative Atrial Fibrillation

Atrial fibrillation is common after open heart surgery, occurring in 25% to 40% of patients who undergo coronary artery bypass graft (CABG) surgery or valve replacement. AF in this setting is associated with a twofold increase in the risk of postoperative stroke and is the most common reason for prolonged hospitalization. The incidence of AF peaks on the second postoperative day. The pathogenesis of postoper-ative AF is multifactorial and probably involves various combinations of adrenergic activation, inflammation, atrial ischemia, electrolyte dis-turbances, and genetic factors.[73] Several risk factors for AF after open heart surgery have been identified, including age over 70 years, history of prior AF, male sex, left ventricular dysfunction, left atrial enlargement, chronic lung disease, diabetes, and obesity.

The incidence of AF after open heart surgery can be significantly reduced by prophylactic treatment with amiodarone,[74] sotalol, or beta blockers (see eTable 66G.6).[75] Hypomagnesemia is common after open heart surgery and can heighten the risk of AF. Magnesium admin-istration has been reported to decrease the risk of postoperative AF. Right atrial or biatrial pacing using temporary electrodes has been reported to reduce the risk of postoperative AF.[76]

A number of other interventions have been assessed for their effi-cacy in reducing the incidence of AF after cardiac surgery, typically not in large randomized clinical trials. The use of colchicine,[77] statins,[78] and steroids[79] to address postoperative inflammation have produced variable results in reducing AF burden. These agents should be used with caution since the impact on postoperative AF may not be a class effect[80] and other adverse effects have been reported.[79] Omega-3 PUFAs also have an anti-inflammatory effect, but randomized studies on their efficacy for preventing postoperative AF have reported con-flicting results.[81]

Another approach to the prevention of AF after cardiac surgery is injection of botulinum toxin into the four major epicardial fat pads at operation. This causes temporary autonomic blockade and has been shown to reduce the incidence of AF after CABG to less than 10% and reduced the AF burden for up three years after surgery.[82]

Patients who develop postoperative AF can be managed using a rate- or rhythm-control strategy. In a randomized comparison of rate- and rhythm-control strategies in patients with AF after cardiac surgery, there were no significant differences between the two strategies in the number of days of hospitalization, mortality, or adverse events.[83] The decision regarding which type of strategy to employ in these patients should be based on the severity of symptoms, hemodynamic effects of the AF, and the patient-specific risk of side effects or adverse reactions to the various rate- and rhythm-control drugs.

AF that occurs after cardiac surgery often resolves within 3 months. In a randomized comparison of rate control versus rhythm control in patients with new-onset AF after cardiac surgery, approximately 95% of patients in both groups were in sinus rhythm at 60 days and had not experienced AF during the prior 30 days.[83] Treatment with an oral anti-coagulant should be continued after discharge. Because new-onset AF after cardiac surgery often does not recur after 60 to 90 days, rhythm-control medications can be discontinued at that time, and if there is no subsequent evidence of symptomatic or asymptomatic AF, as confirmed by monitoring (e.g., 3- to 4-week autotrigger event monitor), anticoagu-lation can be safely discontinued unless needed for another indication.

New-onset AF occurs postoperatively in less than 5% of patients undergoing major noncardiac surgery. Some of the possible mech-anisms of postoperative AF after cardiac surgery (e.g., sympathetic activation, electrolyte abnormalities, hypoxia) most likely also play a role in AF after noncardiac surgery. Beta blockers have been shown to significantly reduce the risk of AF after major noncardiac surgery,[84] but one must be vigilant for the development of bradycardia and hypotension.[85]

Wolff-Parkinson-White Syndrome

Patients with the WPW syndrome and an accessory pathway with a short refractory period can experience a very rapid ventricular rate during AF (see Chapters 64 and 65). Ventricular rates greater than 250 to 300 beats/min can result in loss of consciousness or precipitate ven-tricular fibrillation and a cardiac arrest. Patients with WPW syndrome who present in AF with a rapid ventricular rate should undergo trans-thoracic cardioversion if there is hemodynamic instability. If the patient is hemodynamically stable, intravenous procainamide or ibutilide can be used for pharmacologic cardioversion. Procainamide may be preferable to ibutilide because it blocks accessory pathway conduc-tion and slows the ventricular rate before AF has converted to sinus rhythm. Digitalis and calcium channel antagonists are contraindicated in patients with WPW syndrome and AF. These agents selectively block conduction in the AV node and can result in acceleration of conduc-tion through the accessory pathway.

The preferred therapy for patients with WPW syndrome and AF with a rapid ventricular rate is catheter ablation of the accessory pathway. When performed by experienced operators, the efficacy of catheter ablation is 95% or higher for most types of accessory pathways, and the risk of a major complication is very low. AF typically no longer recurs after successful accessory pathway ablation, probably because AF in the WPW syndrome often is induced by AV reciprocating tachycardia that degenerates into AF (see eTable 66G.6).

Congestive Heart Failure

Atrial fibrillation is a common arrhythmia in patients with heart failure, with a prevalence ranging from 10% in patients with NYHA functional Class I up to 50% in Class IV patients (see Chapters 48 and 49). AF may be the cause of heart failure in patients who present with a nonisch-emic cardiomyopathy and AF with a rapid ventricular rate. It now is recognized that AF can cause left ventricular dysfunction and heart failure even when the ventricular rate is not rapid. In patients with structural heart disease and preexisting left ventricular dysfunction, AF often worsens the heart failure. The deleterious hemodynamic effects of AF are mediated by a rapid and/or irregular ventricular rate and loss of AV synchrony.

The most appropriate rate-control drugs in patients with systolic heart failure are beta blockers and digitalis. If necessary, amiodarone also can be used for rate control. In patients with diastolic heart failure, nondihydropyridine calcium antagonists can be used safely for rate control. Amiodarone and dofetilide are the only two rhythm-control drugs that are not associated with an increased risk of death in patients with heart failure. AV node ablation is appropriate for patients when the ventricular rate during AF is not adequately controlled by drug therapy. Because left ventricular dysfunction and heart failure can be aggravated by right ventricular pacing, biventricular pacing should be instituted after AV node ablation. The decision to implant a biventricular pacemaker versus a biventricular ICD is based on clinical judgment. If it seems likely that the EF will remain less than 30% to 35% after optimal heart rate control, a biventricular ICD is appropriate for primary prevention of sudden cardiac death. It may take 2 to 3 months to evaluate the response of the LVEF to restoration of sinus rhythm. The decision on an ICD can be safely deferred by use of a wearable defibrillator pending reevaluation of the LVEF.

In patients with heart failure who undergo CRT, AF often results in intrinsic and/or fused QRS complexes even when the rate is considered to be adequately controlled. This can limit the extent of biventricular capture, which undermines the maximum therapeutic effect of CRT. If this is the case in a patient with heart failure and AF, AV node ablation is appropriate to maximize the benefit of CRT by allowing 100% biventricular capture.

A large number of trials have been performed to evaluate the safety and efficacy of AF catheter ablation in patients with heart failure.[8,64,86] Meta-analysis of these trials concluded that catheter ablation of AF in patients with heart failure was associated with a greater improvement in LVEF, greater increase in 6-minute walk distance, improved quality of life, and a significantly reduced mortality. Another more recent meta-analysis concluded that AF ablation reduces the risk of death, stroke, and hospitalization compared with medical therapy in heart failure patients.[87] The CASTLE AF trial randomized 363 heart failure patients, each of whom had an ICD in place, to AF catheter ablation or medical therapy. After a median follow-up of 37.8 months, the primary composite endpoint of death from any cause or hospitalization for worsening heart failure was lower in the ablation arm.[64] While these studies strongly suggest that AF ablation should be considered in patients with heart failure, it is important to recognize that these trials were limited by small numbers of highly selected patients. It is for this reason that the 2019 AHA/ACC/HRS AF Guidelines provides only a class IIb recommendation for AF ablation in patients with heart failure.[18]

As in other patients with AF, the decision to pursue a rate-control or a rhythm-control strategy in patients with heart failure should be individualized. But it is important to recognize that sinus rhythm is the best type of rate control. It is also important to recognize that AF can cause or aggravate left ventricular dysfunction and heart failure despite adequate heart rate control. Because of this, a reasonable approach is to first use a rhythm-control strategy in patients with newly diagnosed AF associated with heart failure. Amiodarone or dofetilide can be used to help maintain sinus rhythm after sinus rhythm is restored by cardioversion. If a patient does not want to be on these AADs long term or if these AADs do not prevent early recurrences of AF, catheter ablation of the AF or rate-control alone should be considered.

A rate-control strategy is appropriate for patients who do not respond adequately to amiodarone or dofetilide and either are not suitable candidates for catheter ablation of the AF or have had an unsuccessful outcome from ablation.

Hypertrophic Cardiomyopathy (see Chapter 54)

Atrial fibrillation occurs in approximately 25% of patients with hypertrophic cardiomyopathy (HCM) and can cause severe hemodynamic impairment because of an inadequate diastolic filling time and loss of atrial-ventricular synchrony. Because of a high risk of thromboembolic complications, anticoagulation is indicated in AF patients with HCM, independent of the CHA_2DS_2-VASc score.[1,18]

Severe left ventricular hypertrophy increases the risk of drug-induced torsade de pointes as a complication of AAD therapy. Catheter ablation of AF also is an option. A large number of studies have

reported that catheter ablation in AF is associated with an acceptable efficacy and safety profile.[8]

Pregnancy (see Chapter 92)

The prevalence of AF during pregnancy is very low, approximately 60/100,000 pregnancies. When it occurs, there often is underlying congenital or valvular heart disease, thyrotoxicosis, or electrolyte abnormalities. Pregnancy is associated with a hypercoagulable state, but there are no data indicating that pregnancy increases the risk of thromboembolic complications related to AF. In women with paroxysmal AF before pregnancy, the frequency of episodes may or may not increase during pregnancy.

The decision to anticoagulate a pregnant woman with AF should be made using the same criteria as in nonpregnant women. If anticoagulation is deemed necessary, warfarin (not a DOAC) is recommended from the second trimester until 1 month before the due date, and subcutaneous LMWH is recommended during the first trimester and during the final month of pregnancy.

Transthoracic cardioversion is considered safe at all stages of pregnancy. The recommended pharmacologic agents for acute management of AF consist of intravenous metoprolol for rate control and flecainide or sotalol for conversion to sinus rhythm. If ongoing therapy is deemed necessary, the recommended rate-control drug is digoxin. If ineffective, a beta blocker can be used, but only after the first trimester. If there is no structural heart disease, flecainide and sotalol are recommended for long-term rhythm control.[88] In the patient with structural heart disease, amiodarone is recommended for rhythm control.

FUTURE PERSPECTIVES

The past few years have witnessed significant progress in the field of catheter ablation of AF, but there is room for further improvement and limited data on the durability of rhythm control.[89] The failure to create permanent pulmonary vein isolation often accounts for recurrences of AF after both radiofrequency catheter ablation and cryoballoon ablation. The development of new ablation tools that improve the ability to safely create transmural lesions could reduce the need for redo ablation procedures. At present, several studies are underway to determine whether electroporation, also known as pulse field ablation, may be a more effective and safer energy source than either RF or cryoablation. Early data suggest that this energy source results in a high rate of permanent PV isolation and also reduces the risk of injury to surrounding structures such as the phrenic nerve and esophagus.[90,91]

AF is a progressive condition that results in atrial remodeling. In patients with persistent AF, a better understanding of AF mechanisms could result in more efficient and successful ablation strategies. The best chance for treating AF is early in the course of the disease. New trials are underway to examine the outcomes of early AF ablation even if episodes of paroxysmal or persistent AF are infrequent.

Perhaps most pressing, as the population ages, the incidence of chronic disease and AF will continue to rise. This will create a public health challenge that is linked to other preventable diseases that share modifiable risk factors. This underscores the need for primordial prevention strategies that delay the onset of AF by minimizing risk factors and behaviors and optimizing the management of predisposing diseases.[92]

GUIDELINES

The guidelines on atrial fibrillation are presented in the online chapter.

REFERENCES
Epidemiology
1. Morady F, Zipes DP. Atrial fibrillation: clinical features, mechanisms, and management. In: Zipes DP, et al., ed. *Braunwald's heart disease, a textbook of cardiovascular medicine.* 11 ed. Philadelphia, PA: Elsevier; 2016.
2. Voskoboinik A, Kalman JM, De Silva A, et al. Alcohol abstinence in drinkers with atrial fibrillation. *N Engl J Med.* 2020;382:20–28.

3. Johansson C, Lind MM, Eriksson M, et al. Alcohol consumption and risk of incident atrial fibrillation: a population-based cohort study. *Eur J Intern Med*. 2020;76:50–57.
4. Benjamin EJ, Virani SS, Callaway CW, et al. Heart disease and stroke statistics-2018 update: a report from the American Heart Association. *Circulation*. 2018;137:e67–e492.

Mechanisms

5. Nattel S. Molecular and cellular mechanisms of atrial fibrosis in atrial fibrillation. *JACC Clin Electrophysiol*. 2017;3:425–435.
6. Lee S, Sahadevan J, Khrestian CM, et al. Characterization of foci and breakthrough sites during persistent and long-standing persistent atrial fibrillation in patients: studies using high-density (510-512 electrodes) biatrial epicardial mapping. *J Am Heart Assoc*. 2017;6:e005274.
7. Haissaguerre M, Jais P, Shah DC, et al. Spontaneous initiation of atrial fibrillation by ectopic beats originating in the pulmonary veins. *N Engl J Med*. 1998;339:659–666.
8. Calkins H, Hindricks G, Cappato R, et al. HRS/EHRA/ECAS/APHRS/SOLAECE expert consensus statement on catheter and surgical ablation of atrial fibrillation. *Europace*. 2017;20:e1–e160. 2018.
9. Shoemaker MB, Husser D, Roselli C, et al. Genetic susceptibility for atrial fibrillation in patients undergoing atrial fibrillation ablation. *Circ Arrhythm Electrophysiol*. 2020;13:e007676.
10. Roselli C, Chaffin MD, Weng LC, et al. Multi-ethnic genome-wide association study for atrial fibrillation. *Nat Genet*. 2018;50:1225–1233.
11. Miller JD, Aronis KN, Chrispin J, et al. Obesity, exercise, obstructive sleep apnea, and modifiable atherosclerotic cardiovascular disease risk factors in atrial fibrillation. *J Am Coll Cardiol*. 2015;66:2899–2906.
12. Wong CX, Ganesan AN, Selvanayagam JB. Epicardial fat and atrial fibrillation: current evidence, potential mechanisms, clinical implications, and future directions. *Eur Heart J*. 2017;38:1294–1302.
13. Pathak RK, Middeldorp ME, Meredith M, et al. Long-term effect of goal-directed weight management in an atrial fibrillation cohort: A long-term follow-up study (legacy). *J Am Coll Cardiol*. 2015;65:2159–2169.
14. Tung CE, Su D, Turakhia MP, et al. Diagnostic yield of extended cardiac patch monitoring in patients with stroke or tia. *Front Neurol*. 2014;5:266.
15. Brachmann J, Morillo CA, Sanna T, et al. Uncovering atrial fibrillation beyond short-term monitoring in cryptogenic stroke patients: Three-year results from the cryptogenic stroke and underlying atrial fibrillation trial. *Circ Arrhythm Electrophysiol*. 2016;9:e003333.

Management

16. Sun Q, Chang S, Lu S, et al. The efficacy and safety of 3 types of interventions for stroke prevention in patients with cardiovascular and cerebrovascular diseases: a network meta-analysis. *Clin Ther*. 2017;39:1291. 1312 e1298.
17. Link MS, Giugliano RP, Ruff CT, et al. Stroke and mortality risk in patients with various patterns of atrial fibrillation: results from the ENGAGE AF-TIMI 48 trial (effective anticoagulation with factor Xa next generation in atrial fibrillation-thrombolysis in myocardial infarction 48). *Circ Arrhythm Electrophysiol*. 2017;10:e004267.
18. January CT, Wann LS, Calkins H, et al. AHA/ACC/HRS focused update of the 2014 AHA/ACC/HRS guideline for the management of patients with atrial fibrillation: a report of the American College of Cardiology/American Heart Association task force on clinical practice guidelines and the heart rhythm society. *J Am Coll Cardiol*. 2019;74:104–132. 2019.
19. Bonde AN, Lip GY, Kamper AL, et al. Renal function and the risk of stroke and bleeding in patients with atrial fibrillation: an observational cohort study. *Stroke*. 2016;47:2707–2713.
20. Freedman B, Camm J, Calkins H, et al. Screening for atrial fibrillation: a report of the af-screen international collaboration. *Circulation*. 2017;135:1851–1867.
21. Berg DD, Ruff CT, Jarolim P, et al. Performance of the abc scores for assessing the risk of stroke or systemic embolism and bleeding in patients with atrial fibrillation in engage af-timi 48. *Circulation*. 2019;139:760–771.
22. Takabayashi K, Hamatani Y, Yamashita Y, et al. Incidence of stroke or systemic embolism in paroxysmal versus sustained atrial fibrillation: the Fushimi atrial fibrillation registry. *Stroke*. 2015;46:3354–3361.
23. Kirchhof P, Benussi S, Kotecha D, et al. 2016 ESC guidelines for the management of atrial fibrillation developed in collaboration with EACTS. *Eur Heart J*. 2016;37:2893–2962.
24. Healey JS, Alings M, Ha A, et al. Subclinical atrial fibrillation in older patients. *Circulation*. 2017;136:1276–1283.
25. Proietti M, Rivera-Caravaca JM, Esteve-Pastor MA, et al. Predicting bleeding events in anticoagulated patients with atrial fibrillation: a comparison between the HAS-BLED and GARFIELD-AF bleeding scores. *J Am Heart Assoc*. 2018;7:e009766.
26. Assiri A, Al-Majzoub O, Kanaan AO, et al. Mixed treatment comparison meta-analysis of aspirin, warfarin, and new anticoagulants for stroke prevention in patients with nonvalvular atrial fibrillation. *Clin Ther*. 2013;35:967–984 e962.
27. Tereshchenko LG, Henrikson CA, Cigarroa J, et al. Comparative effectiveness of interventions for stroke prevention in atrial fibrillation: a network meta-analysis. *J Am Heart Assoc*. 2016;5:e003206.
28. Pokorney SD, Simon DN, Thomas L, et al. Patients' time in therapeutic range on warfarin among us patients with atrial fibrillation: results from orbit-af registry. *Am Heart J*. 2015;170:141–148. 148 e141.
29. Shah SJ, Singer DE, Fang MC, et al. Net clinical benefit of oral anticoagulation among older adults with atrial fibrillation. *Circ Cardiovasc Qual Outcomes*. 2019;12:e006212.
30. Steffel J, Verhamme P, Potpara TS, et al. The 2018 European heart rhythm association practical guide on the use of non-vitamin k antagonist oral anticoagulants in patients with atrial fibrillation. *Eur Heart J*. 2018;39:1330–1393.
31. Stanifer JW, Pokorney SD, Chertow GM, et al. Apixaban versus warfarin in patients with atrial fibrillation and advanced chronic kidney disease. *Circulation*. 2020;141:1384–1392.
32. Connolly SJ, Crowther M, Eikelboom JW, et al. Full study report of andexanet alfa for bleeding associated with factor Xa inhibitors. *N Engl J Med*. 2019;380:1326–1335.
33. Tomaselli GF, Mahaffey KW, Cuker A, et al. acc expert consensus decision pathway on management of bleeding in patients on oral anticoagulants: a report of the American College of Cardiology solution set oversight committee. *J Am Coll Cardiol*. 2020;76:594–622.
34. Pollack CV Jr, Reilly PA, Eikelboom J, et al. Idarucizumab for dabigatran reversal. *N Engl J Med*. 2015;373:511–520.
35. Ozaki AF, Choi AS, Le QT, et al. Real-world adherence and persistence to direct oral anticoagulants in patients with atrial fibrillation: a systematic review and meta-analysis. *Circ Cardiovasc Qual Outcomes*. 2020;13:e005969.
36. Gibson CM, Basto AN, Howard ML. Direct oral anticoagulants in cardioversion: a review of current evidence. *Ann Pharmacother*. 2018;52:277–284.
37. Cardoso R, Willems S, Gerstenfeld EP, et al. Uninterrupted anticoagulation with non-vitamin K antagonist oral anticoagulants in atrial fibrillation catheter ablation: lessons learned from randomized trials. *Clin Cardiol*. 2019;42:198–205.
38. Freeman JV, Varosy P, Price MJ, et al. The ncdr left atrial appendage occlusion registry. *J Am Coll Cardiol*. 2020;75:1503–1518.
39. Brouwer TF, Whang W, Kuroki K, et al. Net clinical benefit of left atrial appendage closure versus warfarin in patients with atrial fibrillation: a pooled analysis of the randomized protect-af and prevail studies. *J Am Heart Assoc*. 2019;8:e013525.
40. Boersma LV, Ince H, Kische S, et al. Evaluating real-world clinical outcomes in atrial fibrillation patients receiving the watchman left atrial appendage closure technology: final 2-year outcome data of the Evolution trial focusing on history of stroke and hemorrhage. *Circ Arrhythm Electrophysiol*. 2019;12:e006841.

41. Sondergaard L, Wong YH, Reddy VY, et al. Propensity-matched comparison of oral anticoagulation versus antiplatelet therapy after left atrial appendage closure with watchman. *JACC Cardiovasc Interv*. 2019;12:1055–1063.
42. Lakkireddy D, Afzal MR, Lee RJ, et al. Short and long-term outcomes of percutaneous left atrial appendage suture ligation: results from a us multicenter evaluation. *Heart Rhythm*. 2016;13:1030–1036.
43. Sethi NJ, Feinberg J, Nielsen EE, et al. The effects of rhythm control strategies versus rate control strategies for atrial fibrillation and atrial flutter: a systematic review with meta-analysis and trial sequential analysis. *PLoS One*. 2017;12:e0186856.

Ablation

44. Packer DL, Mark DB, Robb RA, et al. Effect of catheter ablation vs antiarrhythmic drug therapy on mortality, stroke, bleeding, and cardiac arrest among patients with atrial fibrillation: the cabana randomized clinical trial. *JAMA*. 2019;321:1261–1274.
45. Allen LaPointe NM, Dai D, Thomas L, et al. Antiarrhythmic drug use in patients <65 years with atrial fibrillation and without structural heart disease. *Am J Cardiol*. 2015;115:316–322.
46. Boriani G, Blomstrom-Lundqvist C, Hohnloser SH, et al. Safety and efficacy of dronedarone from clinical trials to real-world evidence: implications for its use in atrial fibrillation. *Europace*. 2019;21:1764–1775.
47. Chung MK, Eckhardt LL, Chen LY, et al. Lifestyle and risk factor modification for reduction of atrial fibrillation: a scientific statement from the American Heart Association. *Circulation*. 2020;141:e750–e772.
48. Middeldorp ME, Pathak RK, Meredith M, et al. PREVEntion and regReSsive effect of weight-loss and risk factor modification on atrial fibrillation: the REVERSE-AF study. *Europace*. 2018;20:1929–1935.
49. Pathak RK, Evans M, Middeldorp ME, et al. Cost-effectiveness and clinical effectiveness of the risk factor management clinic in atrial fibrillation: the CENT study. *JACC Clin Electrophysiol*. 2017;3:436–447.
50. Cipollini F, Arcangeli E, Seghieri G. Left atrial dimension is related to blood pressure variability in newly diagnosed untreated hypertensive patients. *Hypertens Res*. 2016;39:583–587.
51. Romanov A, Pokushalov E, Ponomarev D, et al. Pulmonary vein isolation with concomitant renal artery denervation is associated with reduction in both arterial blood pressure and atrial fibrillation burden: data from implantable cardiac monitor. *Cardiovasc Ther*. 2017;35. https://doi.org/10.1111/1755-5922.12264.
52. Fatemi O, Yuriditsky E, Tsioufis C, et al. Impact of intensive glycemic control on the incidence of atrial fibrillation and associated cardiovascular outcomes in patients with type 2 diabetes mellitus (from the action to control cardiovascular risk in diabetes study). *Am J Cardiol*. 2014;114:1217–1222.
53. Verma A, Jiang CY, Betts TR, et al. Approaches to catheter ablation for persistent atrial fibrillation. *N Engl J Med*. 2015;372:1812–1822.
54. Andrade JG, Champagne J, Dubuc M, et al. Cryoballoon or radiofrequency ablation for atrial fibrillation assessed by continuous monitoring: a randomized clinical trial. *Circulation*. 2019;140:1779–1788.
55. Duytschaever M, De Pooter J, Demolder A, et al. Long-term impact of catheter ablation on arrhythmia burden in low-risk patients with paroxysmal atrial fibrillation: the close to cure study. *Heart Rhythm*. 2020;17:535–543.
56. Aryana A, Braegelmann KM, Lim HW, et al. Cryoballoon ablation dosing: from the bench to the bedside and back. *Heart Rhythm*. 2020;17:1185–1192.
57. Tohoku S, Bordignon S, Chen S, et al. From point by point to single shot: evolution of visually guided pulmonary vein isolation using the third-generation laser balloon catheter. *J Cardiovasc Electrophysiol*. Apr 22 2020.
58. Dukkipati SR, Cuoco F, Kutinsky I, et al. Pulmonary vein isolation using the visually guided laser balloon: A prospective, multicenter, and randomized comparison to standard radiofrequency ablation. *J Am Coll Cardiol*. 2015;66:1350–1360.
59. Kuck KH, Furnkranz A, Chun KR, et al. Cryoballoon or radiofrequency ablation for symptomatic paroxysmal atrial fibrillation: reintervention, rehospitalization, and quality-of-life outcomes in the fire and ice trial. *Eur Heart J*. 2016;37:2858–2865.
60. Barbhaiya CR, Kumar S, Guo Y, et al. Global survey of esophageal injury in atrial fibrillation ablation: characteristics and outcomes of esophageal perforation and fistula. *JACC Clin Electrophysiol*. 2016;2:143–150.
61. Kapur S, Barbhaiya C, Deneke T, et al. Esophageal injury and atrioesophageal fistula caused by ablation for atrial fibrillation. *Circulation*. 2017;136:1247–1255.
62. Hosseini SM, Rozen G, Saleh A, et al. Catheter ablation for cardiac arrhythmias: utilization and in-hospital complications, 2000 to 2013. *JACC Clin Electrophysiol*. 2017;3:1240–1248.
63. Cheng EP, Liu CF, Yeo I, et al. Risk of mortality following catheter ablation of atrial fibrillation. *J Am Coll Cardiol*. 2019;74:2254–2264.
64. Marrouche NF, Brachmann J, Andresen D, et al. Catheter ablation for atrial fibrillation with heart failure. *N Engl J Med*. 2018;378:417–427.
65. Boersma LV, Castella M, van Boven W, et al. Atrial fibrillation catheter ablation versus surgical ablation treatment (fast): a 2-center randomized clinical trial. *Circulation*. 2012;125:23–30.
66. Kearney K, Stephenson R, Phan K, et al. A systematic review of surgical ablation versus catheter ablation for atrial fibrillation. *Ann Cardiothorac Surg*. 2014;3:15–29.
67. Mittal S, Musat DL, Hoskins MH, et al. Clinical outcomes after ablation of the AV junction in patients with atrial fibrillation: impact of cardiac resynchronization therapy. *J Am Heart Assoc*. 2017;6:e007270.
68. Garcia B, Clementy N, Benhenda N, et al. Mortality after atrioventricular nodal radiofrequency catheter ablation with permanent ventricular pacing in atrial fibrillation: outcomes from a controlled nonrandomized study. *Circ Arrhythm Electrophysiol Jul*. 2016;9:e003993.
69. Brignole M, Pokushalov E, Pentimalli F, et al. A randomized controlled trial of atrioventricular junction ablation and cardiac resynchronization therapy in patients with permanent atrial fibrillation and narrow qrs. *Eur Heart J*. 2018;39:3999–4008.
70. Palmisano P, Aspromonte V, Ammendola E, et al. Effect of fixed-rate vs. rate-responsive pacing on exercise capacity in patients with permanent, refractory atrial fibrillation and left ventricular dysfunction treated with atrioventricular junction ablation and biventricular pacing (responsible): a prospective, multicentre, randomized, single-blind study. *Europace*. 2017;19:414–420.
71. Vijayaraman P, Subzposh FA, Naperkowski A. Atrioventricular node ablation and His bundle pacing. *Europace*. 2017;19:iv10–iv16.
72. Huang W, Su L, Wu S, et al. Benefits of permanent His bundle pacing combined with atrioventricular node ablation in atrial fibrillation patients with heart failure with both preserved and reduced left ventricular ejection fraction. *J Am Heart Assoc*. 2017;6:e005309.

Postoperative Atrial Fibrillation

73. Dobrev D, Aguilar M, Heijman J, et al. Postoperative atrial fibrillation: mechanisms, manifestations and management. *Nat Rev Cardiol*. 2019;16:417–436.
74. Atreya AR, Priya A, Pack QR, et al. Use and outcomes associated with perioperative amiodarone in cardiac surgery. *J Am Heart Assoc*. 2019;8:e009892.
75. Blessberger H, Lewis SR, Pritchard MW, et al. Perioperative beta-blockers for preventing surgery-related mortality and morbidity in adults undergoing cardiac surgery. *Cochrane Database Syst Rev*. 2019;9:CD013435.
76. Ruan Y, Robinson NB, Naik A, et al. Effect of atrial pacing on post-operative atrial fibrillation following coronary artery bypass grafting: pairwise and network meta-analyses. *Int J Cardiol*. 2020;302:103–107.

77. Lee JZ, Singh N, Howe CL, et al. Colchicine for prevention of post-operative atrial fibrillation: a meta-analysis. *JACC Clin Electrophysiol.* 2016;2:78–85.

78. Zhen-Han L, Rui S, Dan C, et al. Perioperative statin administration with decreased risk of postoperative atrial fibrillation, but not acute kidney injury or myocardial infarction: a meta-analysis. *Sci Rep.* 2017;7:10091.

79. Dvirnik N, Belley-Cote EP, Hanif H, et al. Steroids in cardiac surgery: a systematic review and meta-analysis. *Br J Anaesth.* 2018;120:657–667.

80. Yuan X, Du J, Liu Q, et al. Defining the role of perioperative statin treatment in patients after cardiac surgery: a meta-analysis and systematic review of 20 randomized controlled trials. *Int J Cardiol.* 2017;228:958–966.

81. Wang H, Chen J, Zhao L. N-3 polyunsaturated fatty acids for prevention of postoperative atrial fibrillation: updated meta-analysis and systematic review. *J Interv Card Electrophysiol.* 2018;51:105–115.

82. Romanov A, Pokushalov E, Ponomarev D, et al. Long-term suppression of atrial fibrillation by botulinum toxin injection into epicardial fat pads in patients undergoing cardiac surgery: three-year follow-up of a randomized study. *Heart Rhythm.* 2019;16:172–177.

83. Gillinov AM, Bagiella E, Moskowitz AJ, et al. Rate control versus rhythm control for atrial fibrillation after cardiac surgery. *N Engl J Med.* 2016;374:1911–1921.

84. Bessissow A, Khan J, Devereaux PJ, et al. Postoperative atrial fibrillation in non-cardiac and cardiac surgery: an overview. *J Thromb Haemost.* 2015;13(suppl 1):S304–312.

85. Blessberger H, Lewis SR, Pritchard MW, et al. Perioperative beta-blockers for preventing surgery-related mortality and morbidity in adults undergoing non-cardiac surgery. *Cochrane Database Syst Rev.* 2019;9:CD013438.

Perspectives

86. Ganesan AN, Nandal S, Luker J, et al. Catheter ablation of atrial fibrillation in patients with concomitant left ventricular impairment: a systematic review of efficacy and effect on ejection fraction. *Heart Lung Circ.* 2015;24:270–280.

87. Saglietto A, De Ponti R, Di Biase L, et al. Impact of atrial fibrillation catheter ablation on mortality, stroke, and heart failure hospitalizations: a meta-analysis. *J Cardiovasc Electrophysiol.* 2020;31:1040–1047.

88. Wright JM, Page RL, Field ME. Antiarrhythmic drugs in pregnancy. *Expert Rev Cardiovasc Ther.* 2015;13:1433–1444.

89. Gaita F, Scaglione M, Battaglia A, et al. Very long-term outcome following transcatheter ablation of atrial fibrillation. Are results maintained after 10 years of follow up? *Europace.* 2018;20:443–450.

90. Koruth JS, Kuroki K, Kawamura I, et al. Pulsed field ablation versus radiofrequency ablation: esophageal injury in a novel porcine model. *Circ Arrhythm Electrophysiol.* 2020;13:e008303.

91. Bradley CJ, Haines DE. Pulsed field ablation for pulmonary vein isolation in the treatment of atrial fibrillation. *J Cardiovasc Electrophysiol.* 2020;31(8):2136–2147.

92. Kornej J, Borschel CS, Benjamin EJ, et al. Epidemiology of atrial fibrillation in the 21st century: novel methods and new insights. *Circ Res.* 2020;127:4–20.

67 Ventricular Arrhythmias

WILLIAM G. STEVENSON AND KATJA ZEPPENFELD

Ventricular arrhythmias originate in the ventricular myocardium or His-Purkinje system. These include premature ventricular complexes (PVCs), nonsustained and sustained ventricular tachycardias (VT), and ventricular fibrillation (VF). They can occur in all forms of structural heart disease that involve the ventricles and can be the initial presentation of disease. Sustained arrhythmias are an important cause of sudden death. Some genetic abnormalities of cardiac ion channels can cause sudden death from ventricular arrhythmias despite the absence of structural heart disease. Ventricular arrhythmias that occur in the absence of structural heart disease and a defined ion channel abnormality are referred to as idiopathic and are usually benign. Evaluation and management are guided by symptoms, underlying heart disease, and the risk of arrhythmic sudden death. Because of the differences in prognosis and treatment, proper diagnosis is critical.

PREMATURE VENTRICULAR COMPLEXES, NONSUSTAINED VENTRICULAR TACHYCARDIAS, COUPLETS

Electrocardiographic Recognition

PVCs are due to abnormal impulse formation (automaticity, triggered activity) or reentry (Chapter 62) in the ventricular myocardium or Purkinje system, producing a depolarization wavefront that propagates through the ventricles independent of activation from the atrium and AV node. The mechanism cannot usually be determined with certainty. A PVC is characterized by the premature occurrence of an abnormal QRS complex that usually has a duration exceeding 120 msec. The corresponding T wave is typically broad and in the opposite direction of the major QRS deflection. It is typically not preceded by a P-wave. Premature atrial or junctional beats that conduct with bundle branch block can mimic PVCs.

The timing of the PVC and its interaction with the conduction system determine the effect on rhythm (Fig. 67.1). Often the PVC excitation wavefront propagates retrogradely in the His Purkinje system. It may block in the conduction system or collide in the AV node with the sinus impulse. In either case it fails to reach the atrium and has no effect on sinus node automaticity. The next sinus beat is on time, resulting in a compensatory pause with the R – R interval from the sinus beat preceding the PVC to the one following the PVC equal to twice the sinus cycle length. If the PVC conducts to the atrium, the retrograde

P-wave is usually visible at the end of its QRS. The retrograde P-wave can then reset the sinus node, advancing its next spontaneous depolarization and producing an incomplete compensatory pause (see Fig. 67.1C), which is more commonly associated with premature atrial beats. PVCs can also fall between sinus beats without disturbing AV conduction and without producing a pause, defined as interpolated PVCs (see Fig. 67.1D). If PVCs are relatively late in the cardiac cycle the PVC activation wavefront may collide with a sinus wavefront that has already reached the ventricles, producing fusion beats.

The QRS morphology of the PVC reflects its origin within the ventricles. The wide QRS is due to the initial activation of the ventricles by wavefronts propagating through ventricular myocardium or part of the Purkinje system rather than simultaneously through right and left bundle branches. The ventricular activation sequence is largely determined by the site of initial ventricular activation and hence the QRS morphology is an indication of the location of the ventricular arrhythmia origin (Fig. 67.2). Those that have a dominant S wave in V1 are termed left bundle branch block (LBBB)—like and generally originate in the right ventricular (RV) or interventricular septum. Those with a dominant R wave in V1 are termed right bundle branch block (RBBB)—like and generally originate in the left ventricle (LV) in the morphologically normal heart. Analysis of the frontal plane axis and precordial lead patterns further refine prediction of the likely origin. Initial depolarization of the inferior wall produces a superior frontal plane axis, and depolarization of the anterior wall produces an inferiorly directed frontal plane axis. Exceptions occur and predicting the arrhythmia origin from the QRS morphology is less reliable when structural heart disease with scar that changes ventricular activation is present.

PVCs with a single QRS morphology are referred to as unifocal (see Fig. 67.1E, *beats 3, 5, 7*). The presence of PVCs with different QRS morphologies (see Fig. 67.1D) is referred to as multifocal or multiform and usually indicates more than one PVC focus, although variable conduction away from a single focus is also a possible cause. Frequent multifocal PVCs are more often associated with structural heart disease.

PVCs may occur in repetitive patterns. Every conducted sinus beat followed by a PVC is bigeminy (Fig. 67.2, sites 1, 3, and 4 and Fig. 67.3B). Every two sinus beats followed by a PVC is trigeminy (see Fig. 67.2, site 6). The coupling interval between the sinus beat and PVC may be fixed or variable. A fixed coupling interval is consistent with reentry or triggered activity as the mechanism (Chapter 62). Variable coupling with a common interval between PVCs suggests abnormal automaticity from a parasystolic focus that is relatively protected from ventricular activation from conducted sinus beats.

Additional content is available online at Elsevier eBooks for Practicing Clinicians

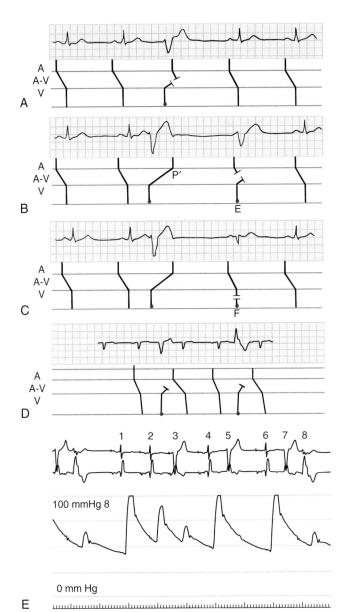

FIGURE 67.1 Premature ventricular complexes (PVCs). **A,** Late PVC results in a compensatory pause. **B,** Slower sinus rate and slightly earlier PVC result in retrograde atrial excitation (P′). The sinus node is reset, followed by a noncompensatory pause. Before the sinus-initiated P wave that follows the retrograde P wave can conduct to the ventricle, a ventricular escape beat (*E*) occurs. **C,** A PVC with a noncompensatory pause similar to **B** except that a ventricular fusion beat (*F*) results after the PVC because of a slightly faster sinus rate. **D,** Interpolated multifocal PVCs are followed by slightly prolonged PR interval of the sinus-initiated beat due to concealed conduction from the PVC into the AV node. **E,** Hemodynamic effect of PVCs. The ECG shows PVCs (beats 3, 5, 7, and 8). The femoral arterial tracing shows a small or absent pressure contour following the PVCs, producing an effective heart rate slower than 30 beats/min.

Two consecutive PVCs are referred to as a PVC couplet (Fig. 67.4C). Three consecutive beats is a triplet. Nonsustained VT is defined as a run of consecutive ventricular beats persisting for 3 beats to 30 seconds (Fig. 67.5A). VT is also characterized by its QRS morphology. Monomorphic VT has the same QRS morphology from beat to beat (see Fig. 67.5A), consistent with a single origin for each beat. Polymorphic VT (see Figs. 67.4B and D and 67.5B) has a continually changing QRS morphology. The initial beats of a run of monomorphic VT may have a variable QRS morphology.

Clinical Features

PVCs occur in apparently healthy individuals but can also be a marker for underlying disease. PVC frequency is associated with mortality and heart failure during long-term follow-up. PVCs are identified on a standard ECG in fewer than 1% of individuals younger than 20 years of age, increasing with age to more than 2% of those older than 50 years.[1] On ambulatory monitoring PVCs increase with age and cardiovascular risk factors including hypertension and smoking.[2] Of 1139 subjects older than 65 years who had normal LV systolic function and no heart failure, the median PVC frequency at baseline was 0.01% (approximately 10 PVCs per day).[3] The 15-year risk of heart failure increased from 19.3% for those with 0.01% PVCs/day to 30.8% for those who had 1% (approximately 1000 PVCs) per day at baseline.

Couplets and nonsustained VTs are less common than PVCs but are often present in patients who have frequent PVCs and increase with underlying disease severity. Runs of VT that are polymorphic, faster than 220 beats/min, or that start near the peak of the T-wave of the preceding sinus beat (see Figs. 67.4 and 67.5B) raise concern for risk of rapid sustained arrhythmias causing syncope or sudden death.[4]

During exercise testing 7 or more PVCs/minute occur at some stage (before, during exertion, or during recovery) in fewer than 10% of patients without a history of heart disease. PVCs may emerge during exertion, then suppress with elevation of sinus rate and reemerge in recovery as the sinus rate slows. Nonsustained VT occurs in fewer than 5%, is typically 5 beats in duration or shorter, and slower than 200 beats/minute. Benign idiopathic arrhythmias often originate from the right ventricular outflow tract (see Fig. 67.5A). Exercise-induced arrhythmias can also be associated with underlying structural heart disease, or be a manifestation of rare genetic arrhythmia syndromes, particularly catecholaminergic polymorphic VT (see Fig. 67.5C) or early arrhythmogenic RV cardiomyopathy. Exercise-induced PVCs and non-sustained VT (NSVT) have been associated with increased mortality during long-term follow-up in some studies, but generally not after adjusting for associated disease and ventricular dysfunction. In competitive athletes without evidence of heart disease, 7% have PVCs during exercise testing, usually fewer than 10, and these were associated with a benign prognosis in one study.[5]

PVCs can be produced by direct mechanical, electrical, or chemical stimulation of the myocardium and are often noted during acute coronary syndromes (see Fig. 67.4C,D), myocarditis,[6] hypoxia, and electrolyte abnormalities, particularly hypokalemia. Management is directed at correcting the underlying illness.

PVCs are commonly asymptomatic. Symptoms include palpitations, lightheadedness, weakness, and fatigue. They are often responsive to sympathetic stimulation, increasing with emotion or exertion. Palpitations are often perceived as a "thump" or strong beat from the sinus beat terminating a longer period of ventricular filling after the PVC (see Fig. 67.1E). When a PVC conducts retrogradely to the atrium, the atria contract against a closed tricuspid valve. These atrial pressure waves may elicit a vagal reflex sensation, similar to pacemaker syndrome.

Physical examination reveals pauses that are often compensatory and do not disturb the expected cadence of the pulse. Although the stroke volume of the PVC is often insufficient to produce a palpable pulse, premature heart sounds are commonly audible. Frequent PVCs may effectively produce bradycardia (see Fig. 67.1E). Cannon A waves may be present in the venous pulse when the atria contract during ventricular systole of the PVC.

Management

The importance of PVCs depends on the clinical setting. Initial evaluation focuses on determining whether PVCs are an indication of underlying structural or electrical heart disease (Table 67.1). Symptoms of syncope, near syncope, anginal chest pain, and dyspnea warrant careful evaluation and can be due to episodes of ventricular tachycardia or other underlying heart disease. Physical examination focuses on signs of underlying heart disease. A 12-lead ECG of the arrhythmia should be obtained whenever possible to confirm the diagnosis and assess its likely origin, which is often a clue to underlying heart disease. Any ECG abnormality warrants further investigation including assessment of biventricular function for cardiomyopathies, and assessment for coronary artery disease in those at risk. Consideration of genetic ion channel abnormalities is also important (see Table 67.1).

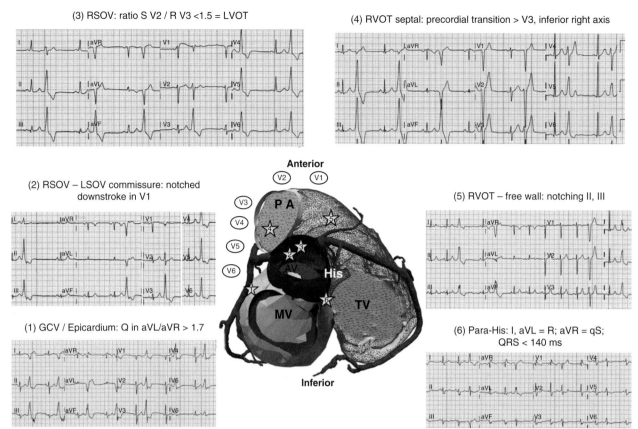

(3) RSOV: ratio S V2 / R V3 <1.5 = LVOT

(4) RVOT septal: precordial transition > V3, inferior right axis

(2) RSOV – LSOV commissure: notched downstroke in V1

(5) RVOT – free wall: notching II, III

(1) GCV / Epicardium: Q in aVL/aVR > 1.7

(6) Para-His: I, aVL = R; aVR = qS; QRS < 140 ms

Anterior

Inferior

FIGURE 67.2 Premature ventricular complexes (PVCs) from the outflow tracts and tricuspid annulus. At the center, the heart is viewed from the base. Sites are indicated by stars with numbers corresponding to the ECG. Depolarization at the RVOT (sites 4, 5) and LVOT/Aorta (sites 2, 3) generates inferiorly directed ventricular activation producing dominant monophasic R waves in II, III, aVF. The RVOT and pulmonary artery sites are anterior to the aorta such that depolarization of the RVOT (sites 4 and 5) produces activation that moves away from the anterior chest wall, producing a qS or minimal initial r in V1, V2. Activation at the LVOT produces initial activation toward V1/V2 such that r/S ratio increases as the PVC originates from progressively more posterior sites (LSOV, GCV). The leftward aspect of the RVOT is left of the aorta, such that PVCs from this location can have a right inferior axis (site 4), whereas PVCs from the aortic valve ring (sites 2, 3) have a left inferior axis, as do PVCs from the rightward aspect of the RVOT and tricuspid annulus. Sites on the tricuspid annulus and those adjacent to the His bundle are lower than the RVOT, and have a more horizontal frontal plane axis. Distinguishing ECG features of these locations are noted. *GCV,* Great cardiac vein; *His,* His bundle; *LSOV,* left sinus of Valsalva; *LVOT,* left ventricular outflow tract; *MV,* mitral valve; *PA,* pulmonary artery; *RSOV,* right sinus of Valsalva; *RVOT,* right ventricular outflow tract; *TA,* tricuspid annulus; *TV,* tricuspid valve.

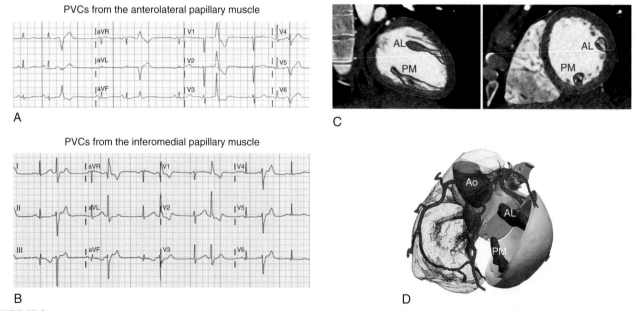

PVCs from the anterolateral papillary muscle

A

PVCs from the inferomedial papillary muscle

B

C

D

FIGURE 67.3 Premature ventricular complexes (PVCs) from the anterior lateral **(A)** and inferior medial **(B)** LV papillary muscles. The LV papillary muscles are mid-cavity structures and produce a right bundle branch block like-configuration with an rS configuration in leads V3, V4 and inferiorly directed axis (anterolateral) or superiorly directed axis (inferomedial papillary muscle). **C,** MR images of the LV with the papillary muscles in long axis *(left)* and short axis *(right)* views. **D,** Left anterior oblique view of the 3-dimensional reconstruction of the LV *(gray)* with overlying RV *(blue)*, aorta *(Ao)*, and coronary arteries *(red)*. The papillary muscles are shown in red. *AL,* Anterolateral papillary muscle; *PM,* posteromedial papillary muscle.

Idiopathic VF

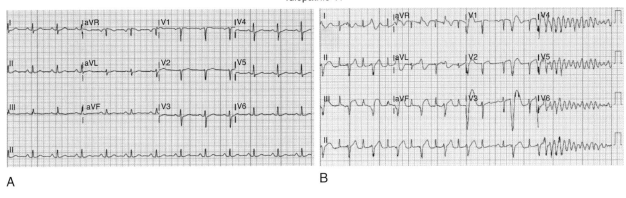

A   B

Acute coronary syndrome

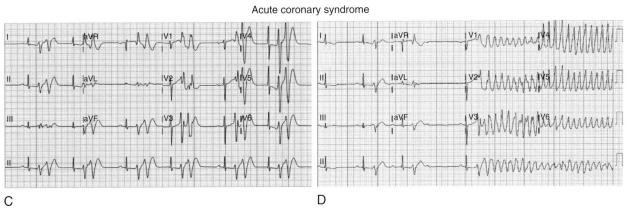

C   D

FIGURE 67.4 Polymorphic ventricular tachycardias (VTs). 12—lead ECG and continuous lead II are shown. **A** and **B**, ECGs from a patient with idiopathic VF. **A**, Normal ECG with normal repolarization, QT. **B**, Ventricular bigeminy with short coupled premature ventricular complexes interrupting the T-wave of the preceding sinus beat initiate polymorphic VT degenerating to ventricular fibrillation. **C** and **D**, During acute myocardial ischemia ventricular couplets with close coupling to the preceding sinus beat. **D**, Closely coupled PVCs are present and initiate polymorphic VT.

Idiopathic Premature Ventricular Complexes/NSVT with No Structural or Electrical Heart Disease

Idiopathic PVCs most often originate from a single site in the right or left ventricular outflow tracts, along the valve annuli, or from a papillary muscle (see Figs. 67.2 and 67.3). Multifocal PVCs are more often associated with underlying structural heart disease. In the absence of associated structural or electrical disease PVCs are benign. Some patients with idiopathic PVCs also have nonsustained or sustained VT from the same focus. Very rarely closely coupled PVCs that start near the peak of the T wave of the preceding sinus beat initiate rapid polymorphic VT/VF that causes cardiac arrest (see Fig. 67.4B).

Asymptomatic PVCs do not require therapy unless they are occurring with sufficient frequency to depress ventricular function. Symptoms often wax and wane over long periods of time and may resolve in over a third of patients.[7] Mild symptoms are often sufficiently managed by reassurance. Removal of provocative factors, such as caffeine, is reasonable. If treatment is required, chronic administration of a beta-blocker is a reasonable first therapy, particularly if PVCs are increased with activity or emotion. Efficacy is relatively low, but symptoms can be improved despite lack of a major impact on PVC frequency. Non-dihydropyridine calcium channel blockers, verapamil or diltiazem, are sometimes effective. Class IC antiarrhythmic drugs flecainide and propafenone can also be effective. Amiodarone can be effective but is avoided due to long-term toxicities.

Catheter ablation should be considered when therapy is warranted and beta-blockers are ineffective or not desired, particularly when a single dominant PVC morphology is identified.[1] The likelihood of successful ablation depends on whether the PVCs are present at the time of the procedure to allow localization of its origin, and whether the focus is accessible. Success rates are greatest for the RV outflow tract, lower for papillary muscles and those that arise from the basal LV septum. A randomized trial found that catheter ablation effectively reduced RV outflow tract PVCs in 81% of patients and was more effective than chronic metoprolol or propafenone therapy.[8] Serious complications are uncommon but femoral bleeding, pseudoaneurysm, cardiac perforation, tamponade, coronary injury, and heart block can occur.

Premature Ventricular Complexes in Structural Heart Disease

In the absence of evidence that PVCs are depressing ventricular function, suppression of PVCs with antiarrhythmic medications has not generally been shown to improve outcomes. Treatment with the Class IC drug flecainide and the Class III drug D-sotalol increased mortality in post-infarct patients, possibly due to proarrhythmic effects.[1] PVCs that are symptomatic or sufficiently frequent to contribute to ventricular dysfunction warrant consideration of therapy. In patients with depressed ventricular function, amiodarone is a therapeutic option, but long-term toxicities are an important consideration (see Chapters 9 and 64). Catheter ablation can be considered if a dominant PVC morphology is present that can be targeted for ablation. During acute myocardial infarction, routine attempts to suppress PVCs with antiarrhythmic medications do not improve outcome and are not warranted. PVCs that trigger recurrent episodes of VF (see Fig. 67.4B) may respond to quinidine.[9]

Premature Ventricular Complex Induced Cardiomyopathy

Very frequent PVCs can cause reversible depression of ventricular function.[10–12] The mechanism is uncertain. Patients may be asymptomatic, or have fatigue, exertional limitation, or heart failure. Most have more than 15% PVCs as assessed from at least 24 hours of ambulatory recording, but PVC frequency during any 24-hour period can vary substantially and ventricular dysfunction has been seen in patients with

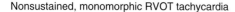

Nonsustained, monomorphic RVOT tachycardia

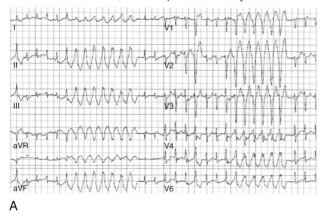

A

Nonsustained, polymorphic VT

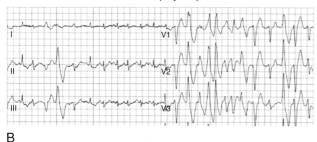

B

Bi-directional VT

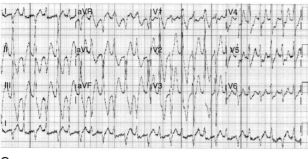

C

FIGURE 67.5 Exercise induced ventricular tachycardias. **A,** Nonsustained monomorphic ventricular tachycardias (VT) occurring in repetitive bursts. VT has a left bundle branch block configuration in V1 with transition after V3 and monophasic R waves in II, III, aVF consistent with origin in the RVOT. **B,** Polymorphic VT. **C,** Bidirectional ventricular tachycardia during exercise in a patient with catecholaminergic polymorphic VT.

only 5% PVCs during a single monitoring period. Multiday ECG monitoring may provide a better assessment of PVC burden.

When depressed ventricular function is encountered in a patient with frequent PVCs there are four major possibilities: (1) cardiac contractility may be normal, but the frequent PVCs are impairing measurement of ventricular function; (2) PVCs are depressing cardiac contractility; (3) an underlying cardiomyopathic process is present and causing the PVCs; and (4) An underlying cardiomyopathy is present and the PVCs are further depressing ventricular function. Sinus QRS duration greater than 130 msec, a PVC burden less than 17%, substantial LV dilation, multifocal PVCs, and areas of late gadolinium enhancement on MR imaging suggest underlying cardiomyopathy.[13] If PVCs are suspected to cause or contribute to cardiomyopathy, suppression of PVCs and reassessment of ventricular function is warranted. Beta-adrenergic blockers and amiodarone are the major pharmacologic options. Catheter ablation is recommended if there is a dominant PVC morphology that can be targeted and antiarrhythmic drug therapy is ineffective, not tolerated, or not preferred for long-term therapy.[1,14]

Patients who have frequent PVCs but normal ventricular function at presentation have a low risk of developing ventricular dysfunction. In a cohort of 100 subjects with greater than 5% PVCs/24 hours and normal LV ejection fraction followed for more than 4 years, PVCs spontaneously decreased to less than 1% in 44%, although they increased again in 9%.[7] Only 4% of patients developed LV ejection fraction less than 50%, all of whom had persistently frequent PVCs. Patients with very frequent PVCs and normal ventricular function warrant follow-up. Optimal risk assessment and surveillance is not defined but annual ambulatory recording and echocardiogram is reasonable for subjects with more than 15% to 20% PVCs.

In patients for whom cardiac resynchronization pacing has improved ventricular function, frequent PVCs can interfere with pacing and impair cardiac function, which may improve following PVC suppression.

ACCELERATED IDIOVENTRICULAR RHYTHM

Electrocardiographic Recognition

The ventricular rate is typically 60 to 100 beats/minute, often only slightly exceeding the sinus rate, producing interference AV dissociation (Fig. 67.6). Conduction of sinus beats to the ventricle producing fusion beats and capture beats is common. The mechanism is likely automaticity. This arrhythmia is usually seen in patients with structural heart disease, particularly during reperfusion of acute myocardial infarction and in myocarditis. It lasts for seconds to minutes and does not usually have an important hemodynamic effect.

Management

Suppressive therapy is rarely necessary but may be needed if loss of AV synchrony and acceleration of heart rate produces symptoms or a fall in blood pressure in a compromised patient. Accelerating the atrial rate with administration of atropine or atrial pacing can suppress the rhythm.

SUSTAINED VENTRICULAR TACHYCARDIA

Ventricular tachycardia can be due to reentry, triggered activity, or automaticity. The management and prognosis depend on the specific type of VT and underlying heart disease.

Monomorphic Ventricular Tachycardia
Electrocardiographic Recognition
Monomorphic VT is a wide QRS tachycardia that has the same QRS configuration from beat to beat indicating a stable ventricular depolarization sequence for each beat (Fig. 67.7). The QRS duration typically exceeds 120 msec, but is occasionally shorter for VTs originating in the septum or that utilize a portion of the Purkinje system. It is usually regular, but 20 msec variation in cycle length is not uncommon, and occasionally marked cycle length variation is encountered in the presence of antiarrhythmic medications, or at the onset and prior to spontaneous termination. Rates can range from slower than 100/min to faster than 270/min.

Monomorphic VT has to be distinguished from other causes of uniform wide QRS tachycardias including supraventricular tachycardia with bundle branch block aberrancy, supraventricular tachycardias conducted to the ventricles over an accessory pathway (preexcited tachycardias **eFig. 67.1**–67.3) (see Chapter 65), and rapid cardiac pacing if a pacemaker or implanted defibrillator is present. Rapid pacing is usually evident from pacing artifacts prior to the QRS. The rate will be at or below the maximum programmed pacing rate and the QRS morphology is the same as that during pacing at slow rates. Interrogation of the pacing device may be needed for confirmation. Preexcited tachycardias are uncommon, can be indistinguishable from monomorphic VT, and should be managed as monomorphic VT when the diagnosis is not certain.

TABLE 67.1 Etiologic Considerations

MONOMORPHIC VT	CARDIAC STRUCTURE	SINUS ECG	FH/GENETICS	VT FEATURES	USUAL INITIAL MANAGEMENT
Coronary disease	Old infarction	Abnormal	CAD+	Multiple morphologies	ICD
NICM	Fibrosis, often in the basal LV	Usually abnormal	40%—LMNA, TTN, PLM, desmosomal	Multiple morphologies	ICD
Post-viral	Fibrosis after healing			Lateral subepicardial LV origin most common	ICD
ARVC	RV fibrosis starts epicardial, LV involvement in some	Abnormal, PVCs	>60% desmosomal mutations	LBBB, multiple morphologies	ICD
Sarcoidosis	LV, RV fibrosis. + FDG PET if active inflammation	AV conduction impairment common, PVCs		RBBB or LBBB, endocardial and epicardial	ICD
Repaired TOF, VSD	Ventricular fibrosis, patch material	RBBB common		LBBB	Dependent on biventricular function
Idiopathic outflow VT	Normal	Normal, PVCs		Single monomorphic VT, PVCs often present	Beta-blocker
Idiopathic LV fascicular reentrant VT	Normal	Normal		Single RBBB monomorphic VT	Beta-blocker, verapamil
Polymorphic VT/VF					
Coronary disease	Acute ischemia	Abnormal	CAD+	Variable initiation	Reperfusion, CAD management
LV failure/hypertrophy from any cause	LVH, fibrosis, dilation	Abnormal			ICD
Acquired LQTS	Normal or any disease	QTc usually >0.48 sec, but can be short	Occasional	Pause dependent PMVT/torsade de pointes	Mg, removal of inciting factors
Idiopathic VF	Normal	Normal or early repolarization	Occasional	PMVT	ICD, quinidine, ablation
Congenital LQTS	Normal	QT prolongation, but variable	Mutations in ion channel genes	PMVT/torsade de pointes	Beta-blocker
Catecholaminergic polymorphic VT	Normal	Normal, PVCs on exertion	Mutation in RyR2, Calsequestrin	Exertion, stress induced polymorphic PVCs, VT	Beta-blocker, flecainide
Brugada syndrome	Normal	Normal or ST elevation V1—2	20%–30% SCN5A, others	Nocturnal cardiac arrest	ICD
Early repolarization	Normal, small epicardial scars?	J-point elevation	Occasional	PMVT/VF	ICD quinidine
Short QT syndrome	Normal	QTc <0.34 – 0.36s	Yes	AF, PMVT	ICD, quinidine

AF, atrial fibrillation; *ARVC,* arrhythmogenic right ventricular cardiomyopathy; *CAD,* coronary artery disease; *FDG PET,* fluorodeoxyglucose positron emission tomography; *FH,* family history; *ICD,* implantable cardioverter defibrillator; *LBBB,* left bundle branch block; *LMNA,* Lamin A/C; *LQTS,* long QT syndrome; *LVH,* left ventricular hypertrophy; *NCIM,* nonischemic cardiomyopathy; *NICM,* non-ischemic cardiomyopathy; *PMVT,* polymorphic ventricular tachycardia; *PVC,* premature ventricular contraction; *RBBB,* right bundle branch block; *RyR2,* type 2 ryanodine receptor; *SCN5A,* cardiac sodium channel gene; *TOF,* tetralogy of Fallot; *TTN,* titin; *PLM,* phospholamban; *VSD,* ventricular septal defect.

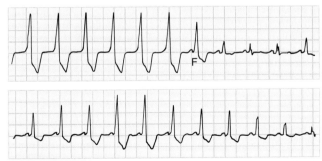

FIGURE 67.6 Accelerated idioventricular rhythm. In this continuous monitor lead recording, an accelerated idioventricular rhythm competes with the sinus rhythm. Wide QRS complexes at a rate of 110 beats/min fuse (*F*) with the sinus rhythm, which takes control briefly, generates the narrow QRS complexes, and then yields once again to the accelerated idioventricular rhythm as the P waves move "in and out" of the QRS complex. This example of isorhythmic AV dissociation may be caused by hemodynamic modulation of the sinus rate via the autonomic nervous system.

Ventricular Tachycardias Versus Supraventricular Tachycardia with Aberrancy

Sustained monomorphic VT is usually regular. The atrium is not involved in the tachycardia. The presence of dissociation between ventricular and atrial activity strongly favors VT over supraventricular tachycardia, the exception being junctional ectopic tachycardia with aberrancy, which is rare in adults, and some rare forms of AV nodal reentry (Chapter 65). Although P waves are often difficult to perceive, AV dissociation may be evident as subtle deflections superimposed on QRS and ST-T waves (Fig. 67.8). AV dissociation may be evident from the presence of fusion beats or capture beats. Vagotonic maneuvers or administration of adenosine may increase AV block exposing a supraventricular arrhythmia with aberration (see eFig. 67.1), or if 1:1 VA conduction is present in VT, may cause transient VA dissociation, confirming VT. It is important to recognize that a 1:1 relation between atrium and ventricle does not exclude VT because retrograde VA conduction may occur such that each QRS is followed by a retrograde p-wave (**eFig. 67.4**). In many cases P-waves are difficult to discern and the relation between P-waves and QRS complexes cannot be determined with certainty.

Comparison of the QRS morphology during tachycardia with that during sinus rhythm can be helpful. The same wide QRS morphology during sinus rhythm and the tachycardia suggests supraventricular tachycardia with aberrancy; this can also occur, however, in patients with bundle branch reentry VT (see below). A number of QRS morphology criteria help distinguish VT from SVT with aberrancy (see

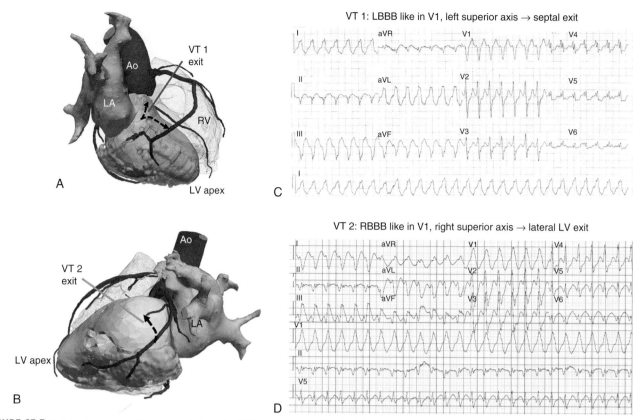

FIGURE 67.7 Sustained monomorphic ventricular tachycardias (VTs) from a patient with prior inferior myocardial infarction. Reconstructed images from segmented magnetic resonance and multidetector computed tomography imaging that shows the coronary arteries (**A,** right inferior projection; **B,** left lateral projection) demonstrate a large area of late gadolinium enhancement (LGE) in the LV consistent with a large inferior wall infarction (*yellow*). Two different VTs originated from this infarct. **C** and **D** show the 12-lead ECGs with a continuous lead I (**C**) or V1, II and V5 (**D**) at bottom. The VT morphologies are defined by the locations of the reentry circuit exits (black arrows) along the infarct margins. **C,** VT is LBBB-like in V1, consistent with a septal exit from a reentry circuit; with a superiorly directed axis, consistent with its location in the inferior LV. **D,** VT is RBBB-like in V1 with a dominant R, and axis directed rightward, consistent with activation preceding from a reentry circuit exit in the lateral wall scar margin. *Ao,* Aorta; *LA,* left atrium; *LV,* left ventricle; *LBBB,* left bundle branch block; *RV,* right ventricle.

Fig. 67.8). None are completely reliable, particularly in advanced heart disease, where the sinus rhythm QRS can be very abnormal (see eFig. 67.3). In structurally normal hearts, VTs that arise from the Purkinje system are more likely to fail to meet QRS criteria for VT.

Mechanisms and Clinical Correlations
Scar—Related Ventricular Tachycardia

The majority of sustained monomorphic VT associated with structural heart disease are due to reentry (Fig. 67.9) through regions of myocardial scar, consisting of fibrosis and surviving myocyte bundles. Diminished coupling between myocyte bundles and complex anatomic arrangement of the bundles contributes to slow conduction and facilitates conduction block needed for reentry. The slow conduction occurs during propagation through the scar, which is typically a small mass of myocardium that does not contribute to the surface ECG. The QRS is inscribed when the VT wavefront reaches the border of the scar and propagates across the ventricles. The QRS configuration reflects the "exit" of the reentry circuit from the scar (see Fig. 67.7). Hence the location of the scar can often be inferred from the VT QRS morphology, which is then an indication of the infarct or scar location. Cardiac imaging will often show the area of scar as a region of late gadolinium enhancement, absence of perfusion, or abnormal wall motion. Small areas of scar, however, particularly in the RV may escape detection with imaging. In the electrophysiology laboratory scars are evident as areas of low electrogram voltage due to replacement of myocardium by fibrosis (see Fig. 67.9A) and abnormal electrograms.

Scars causing VT are often able to support more than one reentry circuit. Hence, patients may have more than one QRS morphology of monomorphic VT (see Fig. 67.7). This is often seen when attempts to

terminate VT by rapid pacing from an ICD initiates a new morphology of VT. Scar is a persistent electrophysiologic substrate such that episodes of VT may recur with variable frequency extending over years, often despite antiarrhythmic drug therapy.

Bundle Branch Reentry and Other Purkinje System—Related Ventricular Tachycardias

In the presence of disease of the Purkinje system and surrounding myocardium VT can be due to reentry circuits that utilize the bundle branches or fascicles. The VT has a QRS morphology consistent with activation of the ventricles from the Purkinje system, resembling bundle branch block. These VTs are uncommon, occurring in fewer than 10% of patients with recurrent VT referred for catheter ablation, but are important to recognize because they can mimic supraventricular tachycardia with aberrancy and most are well treated with ablation.

Bundle branch reentry is the most common form (Fig. 67.10). The circulating wavefront usually propagates down the right bundle branch, through the septum and up the left bundle branch to complete the circuit. VT has a typical LBBB configuration. Rarely the circuit revolves in the reverse direction giving rise to an RBBB configuration. The VT is often rapid, faster than 200/min. It is associated with disease of the Purkinje system and often with severe LV dysfunction. Most patients have an interventricular conduction delay or even a pattern of complete LBBB during sinus rhythm, despite the ability of the left bundle to sustain repetitive retrograde conduction during VT. Catheter ablation of the right bundle branch is curative, but anterograde His Purkinje conduction is often poor, warranting back-up bradycardia pacing. Most patients have other, scar-related VTs that warrant an ICD.

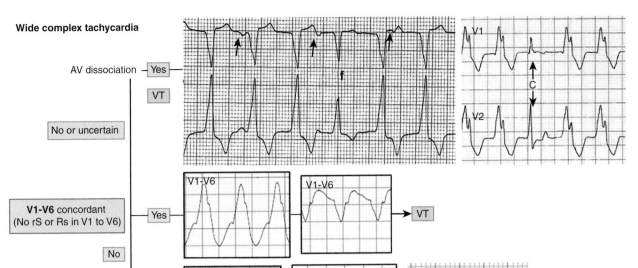

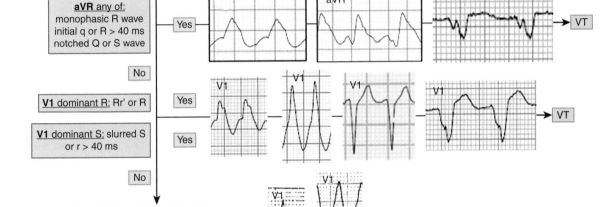

Wide complex tachycardia

AV dissociation — Yes → VT

No or uncertain

V1-V6 concordant (No rS or Rs in V1 to V6) — Yes → VT

No

aVR any of: monophasic R wave initial q or R > 40 ms notched Q or S wave — Yes → VT

No

V1 dominant R: Rr' or R — Yes

V1 dominant S: slurred S or r > 40 ms — Yes → VT

No

V1: typical for RBBB or LBBB r'R or rsR rS with sharp r and S downstroke — Yes → Supraventricular

FIGURE 67.8 Flow diagram for distinguishing VT from SVT with aberrancy. Top ECG panels show AV dissociation *(arrows)* with a fusion beat (f) and capture beat (C). *LBBB,* Left bundle branch block; *RBBB,* right bundle branch block. (From Kindwall KE, Brown J, Josephson ME. Electrocardiographic criteria for ventricular tachycardia in wide complex left bundle branch block morphology tachycardias. *Am J Cardiol.* 1988;61:1279; Wellens HJ, Bär FW, Lie KI. The value of the electrocardiogram in the differential diagnosis of a tachycardia with a widened QRS complex. *Am J Med.* 1978;64:27; Brugada P, Brugada J, Mont L, et al. A new approach to the differential diagnosis of a regular tachycardia with a wide QRS complex. *Circulation.* 1991;83:1649; and Vereckei A, Duray G, Szénási G, et al. New algorithm using only lead aVR for differential diagnosis of wide QRS complex tachycardia. *Heart Rhythm.* 2008;5:89.)

The Purkinje system is also involved in idiopathic LV fascicular tachycardia that is due to reentry involving a portion of the LV Purkinje fascicles for part of the circuit (Fig. 67.11).

Automaticity in the Purkinje system can give rise to fascicular origin tachycardias that have a QRS morphology similar to supraventricular tachycardias with aberrancy.

Purkinje fibers can also be involved in rare malignant arrhythmias.[15] PVCs originating from the RV or LV Purkinje network can initiate rapid polymorphic VT in idiopathic VF. Multifocal ectopic Purkinje-related PVCs due to an *SCN5A* mutation can present with dilated cardiomyopathy that is responsive to arrythmia suppression with quinidine or flecainide.[16]

Focal Origin Ventricular Tachycardias

VT can originate from a small focus of triggered activity or reentry. The mechanism can usually not be established with certainty. These are most often encountered in patients who do not have structural heart disease, often associated with PVCs of the same QRS morphology. Common locations of origin are in the outflow tracts (see Fig. 67.2), including sleeves of myocardium that extend along the aorta or pulmonary artery, along valve annuli and in the papillary muscles. The Purkinje system also gives rise to some focal tachycardias, particularly from the

septum, papillary muscles, and occasionally in infarcts. Focal VTs tend to be enhanced by beta-adrenergic stimulation. The QRS morphology is an excellent guide to their location. Beta-blockers can be helpful and catheter ablation is usually an option when therapy is warranted.

Clinical Features

The clinical presentation of monomorphic VT varies depending on the rate and duration of the arrhythmia, underlying cardiac function, and autonomic adaptations in response to the arrhythmia. Patients may present with palpitations, dyspnea, chest pain, or may be asymptomatic. Rapid VT, faster than 200 beats/min, usually causes hypotension that may present as syncope, or cardiac arrest. VT can degenerate to VF, which may then be the initial rhythm detected by emergency medical responders; this is rare in patients without structural heart disease. Hemodynamic stability during the arrhythmia does not exclude VT.

Acute Management of Sustained Monomorphic Ventricular Tachycardia

Acute management of ongoing VT (Fig. 67.12) follows Advanced Cardiac Life Support guidelines. The patient should be immediately connected to an external defibrillator with ECG monitoring as hypotension

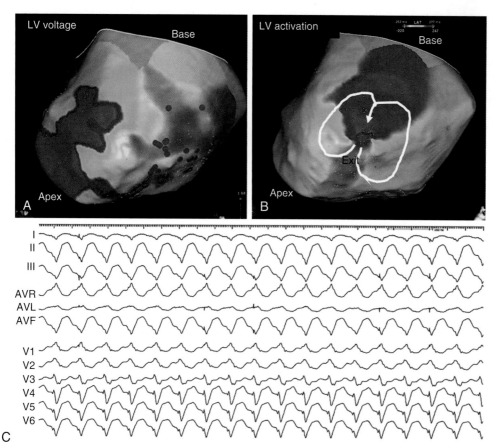

C

FIGURE 67.9 Nonischemic dilated cardiomyopathy with subepicardial scar-related ventricular tachycardias (VT). **A** and **B,** Maps of the epicardial LV viewed from the lateral aspect of the LV. **A,** Voltage map shows an extensive region of low voltage (*red, yellow, green, blue*) over the lateral LV from base to near the apex. **B** and **C** show one of the inducible VTs. In **B,** the activation emerges at the mid-lateral LV (*red,* and propagates clockwise and counterclockwise around the region, returning to the very low voltage region forming a figure-of-eight type of reentry circuit. **C,** ECG of the VT shows an RBBB-like superior rightward axis consistent with the reentry circuit exit in the inferolateral left ventricle. Dissociated atrial pacing spikes are also seen, indicating AV dissociation. The red dots in **A** are ablation sites for this VT, as well as others that were induced. *RBBB,* Right bundle branch block.

or degeneration to VF can occur at any time and may be precipitated by drug administration for attempted termination. QRS synchronous electrical cardioversion should be performed in case of impaired consciousness, hypotension, or pulmonary edema, after sedation if possible if the patient is conscious. For hemodynamically stable wide QRS tachycardia a 12-lead ECG should be obtained. If the diagnosis is uncertain, an intravenous bolus of adenosine may be administered during ECG monitoring, as this may transiently interrupt AV or VA conduction, clarifying the diagnosis (see eFig. 67.1). For acute pharmacologic termination, intravenous procainamide was more effective for termination than amiodarone in one trial.[17] Both are vasodilators that induce hypotension in up to 30% of patients. Procainamide should not be given to patients with end-stage renal disease due to the risks of accumulation of its metabolite n-acetylprocainamide that can cause QT prolongation and polymorphic VT. Intravenous lidocaine is less effective than amiodarone. Intravenous sotalol is available, but experience is limited.

If the patient is known to have an idiopathic VT without structural heart disease, acute management is dependent on the specific VT. Intravenous administration of beta-blockers can often terminate these VTs. If the diagnosis of idiopathic left ventricular fascicular reentrant tachycardia is certain, intravenous verapamil or diltiazem will usually terminate the arrhythmia. Administration of calcium channel blockers is contraindicated for acute management of other sustained VTs due to the risk of inducing hemodynamic instability.

Reversible conditions contributing to the initiation and perpetuation of VT should be sought and corrected including factors that increase sympathetic tone, often related to other acute illness,

hypokalemia, hypoxia, and acidosis. Assessment for evidence of acute MI from ECG and cardiac biomarkers is appropriate, but acute MI is rarely a cause of sustained monomorphic VT. Elevations in cardiac enzymes are more likely to indicate injury secondary to hypotension and ischemia from the VT. Subsequent management is determined by the underlying heart disease and frequency of VT.

Electrical Storm

Sustained monomorphic VT usually occurs as an isolated episode. VT that occurs 3 or more times within 24 hours has been defined as an "electrical storm" and is associated with difficult to control VT and increased mortality.[18,19] Ongoing electrical storm with VT that recurs frequently after cardioversion or is incessant despite termination attempts is a life-threatening emergency. Precipitating factors, most commonly elevated sympathetic tone, should be addressed (eTable 67.1). Very wide sinusoidal tachycardia (see below) should prompt immediate consideration and treatment for hyperkalemia. Intravenous amiodarone and measures to reduce sympathetic tone should be initiated. The nonselective beta-blocker propranolol was more effective than metoprolol in one study, suggesting a role for potent nonselective beta-blockade.[20] Sedation escalating to general anesthesia is often effective. Other means of reducing cardiac sympathetic stimulation include percutaneous stellate ganglion block and high thoracic epidural anesthesia.[21] Patients with electrical storm from monomorphic VT often have a history of VT, have an ICD and are already receiving antiarrhythmic drugs. Assessment of appropriate ICD function and possible proarrhythmic effects from antiarrhythmic medications should be considered. If initial measures are ineffective, emergent catheter ablation should be considered.[1,14,22]

Evaluation and Long-Term Management

After the initial presentation of sustained VT, underlying heart disease should be characterized (see Table 67.1) and consideration given to therapy to reduce the risk of arrhythmia recurrence and sudden death. Most patients will be found to have an area of ventricular scar as the cause, most commonly prior myocardial infarction. The sinus rhythm ECG often suggests the possible underlying disease, with evidence of prior myocardial infarction, or abnormalities suggesting a cardiomyopathic process. An assessment of left and right ventricular function with echocardiography or cardiac MR imaging should be obtained. Evidence of scar or ventricular dysfunction that is not due to coronary artery disease warrants further investigation. Approximately 40% of nonischemic cardiomyopathies are genetic in origin and their detection has prognostic and family screening implications. Arrhythmogenic right ventricular cardiomyopathy (ARVC) and cardiac sarcoidosis (see below) are especially important considerations for patients with RV origin VTs. Other important causes include prior myocarditis, and ventricular scars from prior cardiac surgery, such as repaired tetralogy of

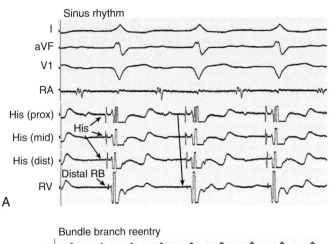

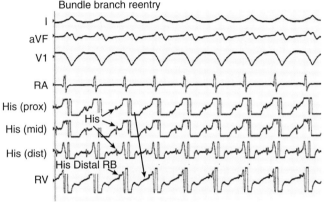

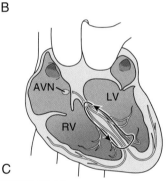

FIGURE 67.10 Surface and intracardiac recordings in a patient with inducible bundle branch reentry ventricular tachycardias. Catheter recording sites are labeled on the left. The His catheter is somewhat distal in its recording position, and the RV catheter is positioned in the right ventricle to record a distal right bundle potential. **A,** His bundle recordings and distal right bundle branch recording (on the RV catheter) during sinus rhythm. Notice that the right bundle potential (*RB*) is normally activated after the His bundle. **B,** Bundle branch reentry induced with the S_1-S_2. The distal His bundle and right bundle are activated anterogradely, and the H-V interval during bundle branch reentry is slightly longer than in sinus rhythm **(A). C,** Schematic of the reentry circuit. The circulating wavefront propagates down the right bundle branch, through the septum and up the left bundle branch to complete the circuit. *prox,* Proximal; *dist,* distal; *RA,* right atrium; *RV,* right ventricle.

Fallot. In the absence of structural heart disease VT is referred to as idiopathic.

Long-Term Therapy

Patients with scar-related sustained monomorphic VT are at risk for cardiac arrest from VT recurrence, which varies with the type and severity of the underlying disease. Placement of an ICD that will terminate VT should it recur is usually warranted provided the patient has a reasonable expectation for survival with acceptable quality of life for the next year and desires the protection of the ICD. ICDs reduce arrhythmic death in patients with depressed ventricular function who have had sustained hypotensive or syncopal VT that is not related to a

reversible cause (secondary prevention), and also in patients who are at increased risk for a first episode of sustained VT (primary prevention of sudden death).[1,23]

ICDs terminate VT by antitachycardia pacing (ATP) or delivery of a cardioversion shock if ATP is not effective (Fig. 67.13), but do not prevent VT occurrences. Of patients who receive an ICD for primary or secondary prevention, 20% to 70% will have spontaneous VT terminated by the device within 3 years depending on the type of disease and presentation. The significance of the recurrences varies. Some are asymptomatic, terminated promptly by ATP, and infrequent such that additional therapy is not required. Others are symptomatic with syncope, or patients remain conscious and experience painful ICD shocks for VT termination. ICD shocks often cause post-traumatic stress disorder and even "mild" recurrences with palpitations and tachycardia termination by pacing may elicit substantial anxiety. VT recurrences are also associated with increased mortality over the following months for several potential reasons.[24] VT may be a marker for more severe disease and disease progression. VT episodes and ICD shocks may elicit detrimental increases in sympathetic tone and lead to implementation or escalation of therapies that have toxicities and potential adverse effects. Following a VT recurrence potential precipitating factors should be sought and addressed. The recurrence may be an indication of deteriorating cardiac function and warrant an assessment of heart failure therapies. Antiarrhythmic drug therapy or catheter ablation to prevent or reduce VT recurrences is often needed (Table 67.2).[25] Early catheter ablation after initial presentation does reduce future VT recurrences but has not been shown to reduce mortality and does expose patients who would not recur to procedure risks.[14,26] The risks and efficacy of catheter ablation varies with the underlying heart disease. Treatment is therefore individualized.

Idiopathic VT in the absence of structural heart disease rarely causes sudden death and an ICD is not usually warranted. Beta-adrenergic blockers or catheter ablation are often effective.

Specific Ventricular Tachycardias
Ischemic Cardiomyopathy

Sustained monomorphic VT may present any time after myocardial infarction, but often more than 10 years after the acute infarction. Remodeling of the infarct scar with fibrosis that promotes slow conduction is likely a factor in the late emergence of scar-related reentrant VT. Most patients have LV ejection fraction of less than 40%. Wide complex tachycardia, syncope, and cardiac arrest are common presentations. Multiple QRS morphologies of VT are common due to multiple potential reentry circuits within the infarct scar (see Fig. 67.7). The QRS morphology reflects the infarct scar location and its border zone with healthy myocardium. Inferior wall infarcts often give rise to VTs that have a superiorly directed frontal plane axis. Anteroseptal infarcts often give rise to LBBB-like VTs when the exit is on the septum and RBBB-like VTs when the VT exit is at the lateral infarct border. Myocardial ischemia is not required, and when present is more often secondary to hemodynamic consequences of VT, rather than primary. Myocardial revascularization does not adequately reduce the risk of recurrent VT.

An episode of sustained VT late after myocardial infarction usually warrants placement of an ICD (Chapters 69 and 70).[1] Recurrent VT terminated by the ICD is detected in up to 70% of patients over the following 2 to 3 years.[14,26] ICDs are also recommended for infarct survivors who are at risk for a first episode of VT based on LV ejection fraction of 35% or less with symptoms of heart failure or less than 30% even in the absence of symptoms provided that they are: (1) at least 40 days from acute infarction and (2) are more than 90 days from a revascularization procedure. These criteria were adopted after trials showed a mortality benefit in those groups. ICDs are also recommended for those with inducible sustained VT at electrophysiology study. ICDs have been shown to reduce mortality in both secondary and primary prevention patients.[1] This benefit, however, is limited for patients with serious comorbidities that limit survival and an ICD should not be implanted

ARRHYTHMIAS, SUDDEN DEATH, AND SYNCOPE

VII

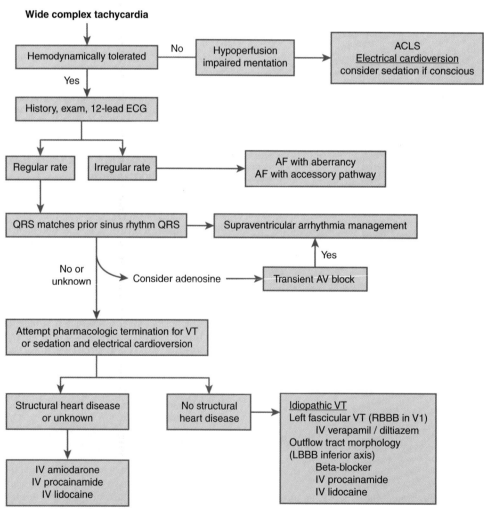

I   aVR   V₁   V₄

II   aVL   V₂   V₅

III   aVF   V₃   V₆

Speed: 25 mm/sec   10 mm/mV   12 Lead ECG   I.U. Medical Center EP Lab

FIGURE 67.11 Left fascicular reentrant ventricular tachycardias. This tachycardia is characterized by a right bundle branch block contour with relatively narrow QRS, typically less than 150 msec. In this instance the axis was superior rightward, consistent with exit from a reentry circuit involving the posterior fascicles of the left bundle branch.

Wide complex tachycardia

Hemodynamically tolerated → No → Hypoperfusion impaired mentation → ACLS / Electrical cardioversion / consider sedation if conscious

↓ Yes

History, exam, 12-lead ECG

Regular rate | Irregular rate → AF with aberrancy / AF with accessory pathway

QRS matches prior sinus rhythm QRS → Supraventricular arrhythmia management

No or unknown → Consider adenosine → Transient AV block → Yes → (Supraventricular arrhythmia management)

Attempt pharmacologic termination for VT or sedation and electrical cardioversion

Structural heart disease or unknown | No structural heart disease → Idiopathic VT
Left fascicular VT (RBBB in V1)
    IV verapamil / diltiazem
Outflow tract morphology
(LBBB inferior axis)
    Beta-blocker
    IV procainamide
    IV lidocaine

IV amiodarone
IV procainamide
IV lidocaine

FIGURE 67.12 Management of the patient with a wide QRS tachycardia.

if the patient does not have a reasonable expectation for survival with acceptable quality of life over the following year.[23]

Over a third of patients will have recurrent VT which often warrants treatment with medications or catheter ablation to reduce recurrences (see Table 67.2). Amiodarone is more effective than sotalol for VT

prevention, but long-term toxicities are of concern.[27] If VT recurs despite amiodarone, outcomes with catheter ablation are more favorable than escalating drug therapy by increasing amiodarone dose or adding mexiletine to amiodarone.[25] During the catheter ablation the infarct containing the VT substrate is usually identifiable as a region of low voltage, abnormal

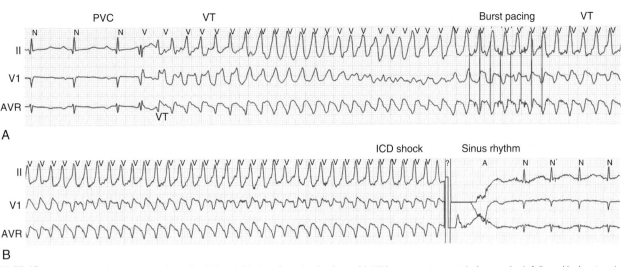

FIGURE 67.13 ICD treatment of ventricular tachycardias (VT). **A,** Initiation of sustained polymorphic VT by a premature ventricular complex is followed by burst pacing from an implanted defibrillation, which fails to terminate the VT, although the QRS becomes more organized. **B,** VT continues and the ICD delivers a shock that converts the rhythm to sinus.

electrograms that can be targeted for ablation without necessarily needing to induce VT.[14] Catheter ablation abolishes VT in about 50% of patients, and reduces the frequency of recurrences in an additional 20% to 30%.[25,28] Procedure-related mortality is 1% to 3% with patients who have severe ventricular dysfunction and comorbidities at greatest risk.[14] Complications occur in 5% to 8%, most commonly femoral bleeding, but stroke, tamponade, and vascular injury can occur. Recurrent VT after catheter ablation is a marker for increased long-term mortality.[28]

Nonischemic Dilated Cardiomyopathy

Areas of late gadolinium enhancement consistent with ventricular scar are detected by cardiac MR imaging in approximately a third of patients with nonischemic dilated cardiomyopathy (NICM) and are associated with increased risk of sudden death. A genetic mutation is identifiable in approximately 40% of patients and is associated with worse long-term mortality, occurrence of VT, and sudden death than those without an identifiable genetic cause of cardiomyopathy.[29] Sustained monomorphic VT occurs in approximately 2% to 3% of patients per year, and polymorphic VT/VF occurs with similar frequency.[29] Sustained monomorphic VT is most commonly due to reentry in regions of scar often near the base of the heart (Figs. 67.9 and 67.14).[30]

Presentation and management are similar to that for VT in ischemic heart disease.[1] An ICD is usually warranted and is also recommended for patients who have had syncope that could be due to VT. Primary prevention ICDs are also recommended for patients who have LV ejection fraction of 35% or less despite medical therapy for ventricular dysfunction and for patients with high-risk genetic cardiomyopathies, including many with lamin A/C mutations.[1,31,32] The benefit of ICDs is greater in patients younger than 60 years of age and is limited in older patients who have other diseases likely to limit survival.

Recurrent episodes of VT requiring suppressive therapy are treated with antiarrhythmic drug therapy or catheter ablation. Catheter ablation is less often successful in NICM compared to coronary disease.[33,34] The VT substrate can be intramural and epicardial (see Fig. 67.9) and more difficult to approach with catheter ablation. Percutaneous pericardial access is more often required to address subepicardial substrate and is associated with a greater risk of bleeding compared to endocardial ablation.[35] Heart block from ablation of VT originating from the basal septum can occur and warrants biventricular pacing.[36]

Arrhythmogenic Right Ventricular Cardiomyopathy

ARVC is an inherited disorder characterized by fibrofatty replacement of the right ventricular free wall that typically extends from the tricuspid annulus and RV outflow region toward the apex creating the substrate for PVCs and sustained monomorphic VT and less commonly polymorphic VT/VF. Other regions of the RV and LV can also be involved. Approximately half of the patients have an identifiable mutation involving a desmosomal protein, most commonly plakophilin-2, desmoplakin, and desmoglein, followed by other desmosomal and non-desmosomal proteins. Inheritance is autosomal dominant for most. Approximately half of patients have a family history of sudden death. LV involvement is not uncommon and may predominate, which has led to use of the term arrhythmogenic cardiomyopathy (AMC). Patients present with palpitations, syncope, or cardiac arrest most commonly in their third or fourth decade. Penetrance is quite variable. Prolonged chronic exercise increases the disease expression and progression and athletes are likely to present earlier than less active individuals. A common presentation is sustained monomorphic VT with an LBBB configuration in V1 (Fig. 67.15). The distinction of ARVC, which has a risk of sudden death from idiopathic VT, which is benign, is extremely important and can be difficult. Task force criteria have been developed for establishing the diagnosis.[37] Both ARVC and idiopathic VT can cause RVOT origin VTs that have an LBBB inferior axis VT. LBBB VT with a superior axis or multiple VTs favors ARVC. The sinus rhythm ECG is normal in idiopathic VT, but commonly shows T wave inversions in V1 to V3 or beyond, which is abnormal in individuals older than 14 years of age (see Fig. 67.15B). A prolonged terminal activation duration (nadir of the S wave to QRS offset >55 msec in V1), or less commonly epsilon waves are found in ARVC. Early in the course of ARVC cardiac imaging may be normal, but more commonly echocardiography shows some degree of RV enlargement. Cardiac MRI may show RV enlargement and areas of late gadolinium enhancement in ARVC. Electrophysiology study can be helpful. Multiple morphologies of inducible VT and isoproterenol induced multiple morphologies of PVCs are common in ARVC and rare in idiopathic VT. RV epicardial and endocardial mapping reveals areas of low amplitude abnormal electrograms in ARVC that are rare in idiopathic VT.[38] Cardiac sarcoid can be indistinguishable from ARVC, sometimes only identified at heart transplantation. AV conduction delay, evidence of septal scar, and evidence of extracardiac sarcoidosis favor sarcoid as the diagnosis (see Fig. 67.15D).

Arrhythmias are commonly provoked by exertion. Chronic therapy with a beta-blocker is recommended.[1] An ICD is recommended for those who have had sustained arrhythmias, syncope, or RV or LV dysfunction with ejection fraction of 35% or less, and is considered for patients with less severe manifestations of disease because the initial symptomatic event can be sudden death. With avoidance of exercise unaffected gene carriers appear to have an excellent outcome without therapy. If VT recurrences require suppression, sotalol, amiodarone, and

ARRHYTHMIAS, SUDDEN DEATH, AND SYNCOPE

VII

TABLE 67.2 Clinical Trials on Treatment to Reduce Ventricular Tachycardia Recurrences in Patients with ICDs

STUDY	PATIENT INCLUSION	ENDPOINTS	TREATMENT ARMS	KEY RESULTS
Antiarrhythmic Drug Trials				
RAID (Zareba 2018)	ICD for primary or secondary prevention. 54% CAD N = 1012	Death + VT/VF	Ranolazine Placebo	No difference in primary outcome
OPTIC (Connolly 2006)	VT or VF receiving an ICD 80% prior MI N = 412	ICD shock for any reason	Randomized to BB, sotalol, or amiodarone + BB	Annual rate of VT treated with ATP or shocks: Amiodarone + BB most effective 13% vs. 39% for sotalol and 45% for BB. Adverse thyroid and pulmonary effects more common with amiodarone
ALPHEE (Kowey 2011)	ICD and VT/VF 75% CAD	Sudden death or appropriate ICD therapy	Amiodarone Placebo	Amiodarone improved primary endpoint: 45.3% vs. 61.5%
(Pacifico 1999)	ICD for VT/VF 70% CAD	Death or ICD shock	Sotalol Placebo	Improved freedom from death or ICD shock in sotalol group (66% vs. 46% at 1 year)
CASCADE substudy (Dolack 1994)	VF out of hospital, CAD, ICD N = 88	ICD shocks	Amiodarone Other AADs	Improved 2 years free survival without ICD shocks for amiodarone vs. other AADs; 77% vs. 42%
Kettering 2002	ICD	VT/VF recurrence	Sotalol Metoprolol	VT/VF recurred in 63% of pts with no difference between groups
QUIDAM (Andorin 2017)	Brugada syndrome	Appropriate ICD shock	Hydroquinidine Placebo 18 months crossover. 50 patients total	2 VF events during placebo treatment. No VF during hydroquinidine treatment, but stopped for side effects in 26%
Catheter Ablation Trials				
VANISH (Sapp 2016)	CAD with SMVT despite AAD therapy N = 259	Death, VT Storm or ICD shock	CA Escalation of AAD	CA Improved outcome overall (59.1% vs. 68.5%); In subanalysis CA similar to switching from sotalol to amiodarone; CA superior to escalating amiodarone
SMS (Kuch 2017)	Unstable VT or cardiac arrest CAD LVEF ≤40% N = 111	Time to first recurrence VT/VF	CA before ICD implant ICD implant with no CA	No difference with recurrent VT in 49% vs. 52.4% at 2 years
VTACH (Kuch 2010)	Hemodynamically tolerated SMVT CAD LVEF ≤50% N = 107	Time to first recurrence VT/VF	CA No CA	CA prolonged time to recurrent VT to 18.6 months vs. 5.6 months
BERLIN VT (Willems 2020)	SMVT, CAD LVEF 30%–50% N = 159	Death or unplanned hospitalization	CA No CA	Terminated for futility. Trends for CA to reduce VT but with more hospitalizations
SMASH-VT (Reddy 2017)	ICD for unstable VT/VF syncope CAD N = 128	Survival free from appropriate ICD therapy	CA No CA	CA reduced ICD therapy to 12% vs. 33%
CALYPSO (AL-Khatib)	CAD with SMVT despite AAD	Feasibility	Ablation AAD	27 enrolled of 243 screened

AAD, Antiarrhythmic drug; *ATP,* antitachycardia pacing; *BB,* beta blocker; *CA,* catheter ablation; *ICD,* implantable cardioverter defibrillator; *SMVT,* sustained monomorphic VT.
Zareba W, Daubert JP, Beck CA, et al. Ranolazine in high-risk patients with implanted cardioverter-defibrillators: the RAID Trial. *J Am Coll Cardiol.* 2018;72:636–645.
Connolly SJ, Dorian P, Roberts RS, et al. Comparison of beta-blockers, amiodarone plus beta-blockers, or sotalol for prevention of shocks from implantable cardioverter defibrillators: the OPTIC Study: a randomized trial. *JAMA.* 2006;295:165–171.
Kowey PR, Crijns HJ, Aliot EM, et al. Efficacy and safety of celivarone, with amiodarone as calibrator, in patients with an implantable cardioverter-defibrillator for prevention of implantable cardioverter-defibrillator interventions or death: the ALPHEE study. *Circulation.* 2011;124:2649–2660.

Continued

Pacifico A, Hohnloser SH, Williams JH, et al. Prevention of implantable-defibrillator shocks by treatment with sotalol. d,l-Sotalol Implantable Cardioverter-Defibrillator Study Group. *N Engl J Med*. 1999;340:1855–1862.

Dolack GL. Clinical predictors of implantable cardioverter-defibrillator shocks (results of the CASCADE trial). Cardiac Arrest in Seattle, Conventional versus Amiodarone Drug Evaluation. *Am J Cardiol*. 1994;73:237–241.

Kettering K, Mewis C, Dornberger V, et al. Efficacy of metoprolol and sotalol in the prevention of recurrences of sustained ventricular tachyarrhythmias in patients with an implantable cardioverter defibrillator. *Pacing Clin Electrophysiol*. 2002;25:1571–1576.

Andorin A, Gourraud JB, Mansourati J, et al. The QUIDAM study: Hydroquinidine therapy for the management of Brugada syndrome patients at high arrhythmic risk. *Heart Rhythm*. 2017;14:1147–1154.

Sapp JL, Wells GA, Parkash R, et al. Ventricular tachycardia ablation versus escalation of antiarrhythmic drugs. *N Engl J Med*. 2016;375:111–121.

Kuck KH, Tilz RR, Deneke T, et al. Impact of substrate modification by catheter ablation on implantable cardioverter-defibrillator interventions in patients with unstable ventricular arrhythmias and coronary artery disease: results from the multicenter randomized controlled SMS (Substrate Modification Study). *Circ Arrhythm Electrophysiol*. 2017;10:e004422.

Kuck KH, Schaumann A, Eckardt L, et al. Catheter ablation of stable ventricular tachycardia before defibrillator implantation in patients with coronary heart disease (VTACH): a multicentre randomised controlled trial. *Lancet*. 2010;375:31–40.

Willems S, Tilz RR, Steven D, et al. Preventive or deferred ablation of ventricular tachycardia in patients with ischemic cardiomyopathy and implantable defibrillator (BERLIN VT): a multicenter randomized trial. *Circulation*. 2020;141:1057–1067.

Reddy VY, Reynolds MR, Neuzil P, et al. Prophylactic catheter ablation for the prevention of defibrillator therapy. *N Engl J Med*. 2007;357:2657–2665.

Al-Khatib SM, Daubert JP, Anstrom KJ, et al. Catheter ablation for ventricular tachycardia in patients with an implantable cardioverter defibrillator (CALYPSO) pilot trial. *J Cardiovasc Electrophysiol*. 2015;26:151–157.

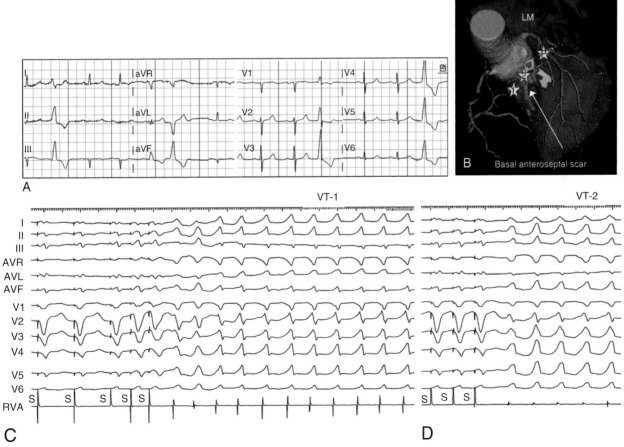

FIGURE 67.14 Arrhythmias in a patient with genetic cardiomyopathy due to a titin (*TTN*) mutation. Frequent PVCs were recognized as a young adult. Several decades later the patient presented with syncope due to ventricular tachycardias (VT) and LV ejection fraction of approximately 40%. **A,** Resting ECG shows sinus rhythm with unifocal PVCs that have an RBBB inferior right axis configuration and dominant R waves from V3 to V6 consistent with activation from a focus at the aortic mitral continuity area (site *P* in **B**). **B,** The voltage map of the LV merged with CT scan and the segmented magnetic resonance–derived scar (in *yellow*) is viewed from the superior aspect. An area of low voltage (*red, green*) consistent with scar is present at the basal LV septum. Purple is greater than 1.5 mV. Ablation areas for the PVCs (site *P*) and VTs (sites *1* and *2*) are shown (*stars*). **C,** During programmed stimulation two extrastimuli following a pacing train at 150 beats/min (*S*) induced sustained monomorphic VT that has a left bundle branch block configuration in V1, dominant R in V2 and axis of + 30 degrees, consistent with activation from site 1 at the LV basal septum. **D,** A burst of rapid pacing was performed during VT-1 (last three stimuli shown) converted VT-1 to VT-2 that has an axis of + 60 degrees, consistent with an exit at site 2. Multiple monomorphic VTs are common in scar-related VT.

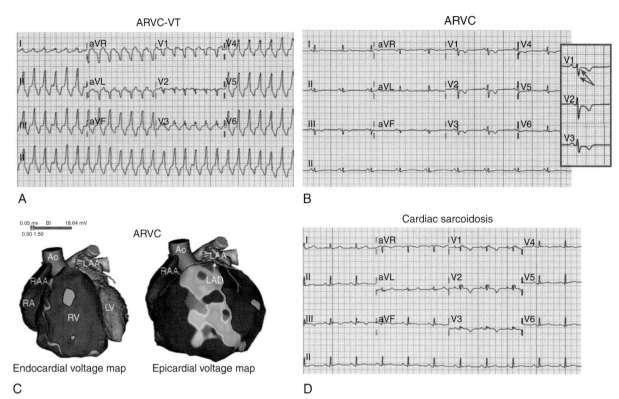

FIGURE 67.15 Arrhythmogenic RV cardiomyopathy (ARVC) (**A** to **C**) can be mimicked by sarcoidosis (**D**). **A,** sustained monomorphic VT has a left bundle branch block–like configuration in V1 and inferior axis consistent with an RVOT origin. **B,** Following conversion to sinus rhythm the ECG shows T wave inversions in V1 to V4 with a delayed S nadir to J point in V1 of greater than 50 msec consistent with an RV abnormality (*arrows* in enlargement at right). **C** and **D** Bipolar voltage maps viewed from an anterior projection. The endocardial bipolar voltage map (*left*) shows a small area of low voltage (*red*) along the tricuspid annulus. The epicardial voltage map (*right*) shows extensive low voltage (*red, yellow, green*) over the entire free wall of the RV. **D,** A 12-lead ECG from a patient with sarcoidosis involving the RV. T wave inversions in V1–V3 can occur in ARVC or sarcoidosis. PR interval prolongation (>0.2 s) favors sarcoidosis over ARVC.

flecainide have been used. Catheter ablation, which often requires an epicardial approach, reduces episodes.[14]

Congenital Heart Disease

The incidence of serious ventricular arrhythmias in the population of adults with congenital heart disease (CHD) is relatively low (<0.1% per year).[39,40] Approximately 10% of deaths, however, are sudden. The risk varies with the specific lesion and increases with severity of heart disease. In patients with progressive failure of the systemic or subpulmonary ventricle polymorphic VT and VF can occur independent of surgical scars. In contrast, sustained monomorphic VT is usually due to reentry facilitated by scar areas that are often associated with prior surgical repair, most commonly in tetralogy of Fallot (Fig. 67.16).[41–43] The substrate for these often-fast VTs has been well characterized. Areas of dense fibrosis owing to surgical incisions, patch material, and the valve annuli form regions of conduction block that define reentry circuit borders and create anatomically defined isthmuses with slow conduction that allow macroreentrant VTs. These isthmuses can be identified during stable rhythm and be ablated with very low rates of VT recurrence if conduction block in the isthmus can be achieved. Catheter ablation is generally considered an adjunct to an ICD, but has been used as an alternative to an ICD in selected patients.[41] VT may be associated with pulmonary regurgitation and RV enlargement late after repair such that percutaneous or surgical pulmonary valve replacement is warranted. It is important to consider ablation for VT prior to or combined with these procedures as placement of a valved conduit does not abolish VT and may prevent future access to the isthmus causing VT.

Hypertrophic Cardiomyopathy

Sudden death occurs at a rate of 1% per year in patients with genetic hypertrophic cardiomyopathy (Chapter 54).[1] Polymorphic VT (PMVT) and VF are the most common rhythms identified at sudden death. These can be precipitated by rapid rates during sinus tachycardia or atrial

fibrillation. Ventricular myocyte disarray, interstitial fibrosis, and susceptibility to myocardial ischemia are likely arrhythmogenic factors. Sustained monomorphic VT is uncommon but can occur due to scar-related reentry, most commonly in patients who have a fibrotic apical aneurysm, which occurs in fewer than 5% of patients.[44,45] An ICD is recommended for survivors of cardiac arrest or sustained VT, or who have had recent unexplained syncope or other markers of sudden death risk (Chapter 70). Nonsustained VT occurs in 20% to 30% of patients on ambulatory monitoring and its relation to risk of sudden death remains controversial, although it is associated with increased risk of spontaneous VT in patients who have received an ICD.[46] Symptomatic PVCs and recurrent VT may respond to therapy with beta-blockers or amiodarone. Catheter ablation can be successful for scar-related sustained monomorphic VT.

Inflammatory Heart Disease
Cardiac Sarcoidosis

Sarcoidosis is characterized by noncaseating granulomas that can involve any organ.[47] Cardiac involvement can cause atrial and ventricular arrhythmias, heart block, and heart failure. VT is the presenting event in one-third of patients.[48] The granulomas heal, leaving areas of fibrosis that can be the substrate for scar-related reentrant sustained monomorphic VT that persists after active inflammation resolves. Purkinje-related arrhythmias also occur. Ventricular scar can occur anywhere in the left or right ventricles. When involvement is confined to the right ventricle the clinical findings can be indistinguishable from arrhythmogenic RV cardiomyopathy.

Cardiac sarcoidosis should be suspected for any patient presenting with ventricular arrhythmias associated with areas of unexplained ventricular scar, but establishing the diagnosis is often difficult. Biopsy of involved noncardiac tissue should be obtained if identified. If involvement is confined to the heart, cardiac biopsy is an option but is unrevealing in the majority of cases due to the often patchy nature of cardiac involvement. Cardiac positron emission tomography with fluorodeoxyglucose (FDG-PET) after a carbohydrate-free diet is helpful

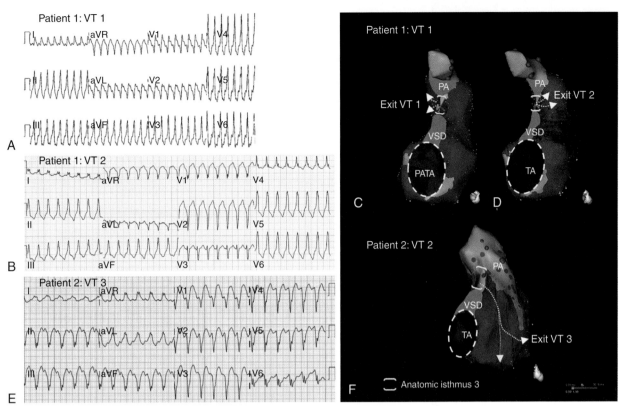

FIGURE 67.16 Tetralogy of Fallot. Ventricular tachycardia (VT) morphology depends on the location of the exit from anatomically defined isthmuses and the extension of surgical incisions. ECGs of VT (**A** and **B**) and RV voltage maps viewed from the posterior projection (**C** and **D**) from patient 1. **A,** VT1 has an RBBB-like V1 with inferior axis due to a leftward exit from the infundibular RVOT isthmus between the pulmonary artery (PA) and VSD patch (**C**). **B,** VT2 has an LBBB configuration with inferior axis, due to exit from the rightward side of the same isthmus as for VT1 (**D**). **E** and **F,** VT from patient 2 has an LBBB, superior axis configuration. This VT also uses an infundibular isthmus, but there is extensive free wall RV scar, so the apparent exit is in the inferior RV, producing the superior axis. This anatomic isthmus bordered by the PA and the VSD patch is the most common isthmus causing VT in repaired tetralogy of Fallot. (From Brouwer C, Kapel GFL, Jongbloed MRM, et al. Noninvasive identification of ventricular tachycardia-related anatomical isthmuses in repaired tetralogy of Fallot: what is the role of the 12-lead ventricular tachycardia electrocardiogram. *JACC Clin Electrophysiol.* 2018;4:1308–1318.)

in revealing active inflammation that supports the diagnosis (Chapter 18). Cardiac MR imaging may show a nonspecific pattern of fibrosis in a distribution that does not follow coronary anatomy (Chapter 19). Management is as for VT in NICM. Sustained VT or syncope warrants placement of an ICD.[1] Sustained VT is usually, but not always, associated with depressed ventricular function. ICDs are also considered for primary prevention of sudden death, particularly if there is evidence of depressed LV function, scar on cardiac MR imaging, or inducible VT at electrophysiologic testing. Immunosuppressive therapy may prevent or slow active disease progression and may improve AV block and PVCs but is unlikely to prevent recurrences of sustained VT once the fibrotic substrate is present. Recurrent episodes of VT are treated with antiarrhythmic drug therapy or catheter ablation. Catheter ablation is often challenging due to the varied scar locations and potential disease progression and recurrence rates exceed 50%.[34]

Myocarditis
Acute myocarditis from viral, autoimmune disease, or toxins can cause arrhythmias and sudden death. Active inflammation associated with myocarditis can cause multifocal PVCs, nonsustained VT, accelerated idioventricular rhythms, and polymorphic VT/VF.[6] In a series of patients with lymphocytic myocarditis, PVCs and nonsustained VT often originated from the inferior LV giving rise to RBBB superior axis QRS morphologies. With healing, myocarditis may leave areas of scar detectable as late gadolinium enhancement on MR imaging that can be a persistent substrate for reentrant sustained monomorphic VT and PVCs. Some patients presenting with PVCs and depressed ventricular function show cardiac inflammation on FDG-PET consistent with myocarditis as a cause of PVCs that sometimes resolves over time.[49,50]

Chagas Disease
Chagas disease is due to infection with the parasite *Trypanosoma cruzi* that is endemic to Latin America, where it is estimated that 6 million

people are infected.[51] As a consequence of migration it is occasionally encountered outside the Western Hemisphere, and in the United States alone an estimated 300,000 people are infected. The acute infection is often unrecognized, but occasionally causes severe myocarditis. The disease then enters a chronic phase with seropositivity and no evidence of heart disease. Over years to decades 20% to 30% of patients develop cardiac disease of varying severity that appears to be due to persistent cardiac inflammation with a low level of parasite present. RBBB, left anterior hemiblock, and PVCs can be early manifestations followed over years by ventricular dysfunction, often with aneurysms, and VT. Sudden death can be the first clinical manifestation of disease and can be from ventricular arrhythmias or heart block. Sustained monomorphic VT is due to scar-related reentry, most commonly from the inferolateral left ventricle giving rise to VT that has an RBBB right axis QRS configuration.

Idiopathic Ventricular Tachycardias
Idiopathic VT is defined as monomorphic VT in patients who do not have structural heart disease Most have a single origin that is indicated by the QRS morphology. PVCs from the same focus are often present. The presence of more than one morphology of monomorphic VT, or VT with different morphologies of PVCs increases concern for underlying heart disease. The prognosis of idiopathic VT is good. The arrhythmia may be controlled by beta-blockers, verapamil or diltiazem as well as antiarrhythmic drugs such as flecainide and propafenone. Most originate from locations amenable to catheter ablation.

Outflow Tract Arrhythmias
The right and left ventricular outflow regions are the most common locations for idiopathic VT as well as PVCs (see Fig. 67.2). These most frequently arise in tissue along the pulmonary or aortic valve rings.

This tissue can extend above the valve ring giving rise to supravalvular foci that require ablation from within the pulmonary artery or aorta. The initiating mechanism is likely triggered activity. VT can be paroxysmal or exercise induced. It may occur as repetitive monomorphic VT with bursts of tachycardia separated by a variable number of sinus beats (see Fig. 67.5A). The QRS morphology of the VT has an inferiorly directed frontal plane axis, with tall monophasic R waves in leads II, III, AVF.[52]

For many patients these arrhythmias are provoked by exertion, stress, isoproterenol infusion, or rapid pacing. Termination with vagal maneuvers can occur. Suppression can often be achieved with beta-blockers or verapamil or diltiazem. Flecainide and propafenone have also been used for chronic therapy. When drug therapy is ineffective, not tolerated, or not desired by the patient, catheter ablation is a useful option. Efficacy varies for specific origins and generally exceeds 80%. Failure of ablation is often due to inability to initiate the arrhythmia to allow mapping in the electrophysiology laboratory, or origin from an inaccessible location that may be deep in the interventricular septum or subepicardial adjacent to a coronary artery where ablation is not performed. Serious complications are uncommon, but can include cardiac perforation, coronary injury, and femoral access site bleeding.

Annular Arrhythmias

Ventricular arrhythmias that arise adjacent to the tricuspid or mitral annuli have clinical characteristics similar to outflow tract arrhythmias with characteristic QRS morphologies that suggest the origin (see Fig. 67.2). Most are amenable to ablation. For those that originate close to the His bundle ablation has a risk of heart block.

Crux Arrhythmias

The crux of the heart encompasses the tissue in the inferior portion of the septum extending from the basal inferior septum near the coronary sinus apically and inferiorly.[53] The QRS shows a left superior frontal plane axis with QS complexes in II, III, and an LBBB or RBBB morphology, often with a prominent R in V2 (see eFig. 67.4). The focus can be subepicardial, and approachable from within the middle cardiac vein or pericardial space for ablation but can also be protected by overlying posterior descending coronary artery and epicardial fat making ablation difficult.

Papillary Muscle Arrhythmias

PVCs, nonsustained VT, and occasionally sustained VT can originate from a focal source within the papillary muscles of the left or right ventricle. From the left ventricular papillary muscles the QRS has an RBBB configuration with either superior axis and S waves in V4 to V6 (posteromedial papillary muscle origin) or inferior rightward axis (anterolateral papillary muscle origin) (see eFig. 67.3).[54] These arrhythmias can be associated with mitral valve prolapse. Most are benign, but very frequent arrhythmias may depress ventricular function and rare cases of papillary muscle PVC-induced VF occur. The presence of mitral annular disjunction (Chapter 76) and myocardial fibrosis in the adjacent LV wall has been associated with more severe arrhythmias.[55] The papillary muscles can also be sources for arrhythmias in cardiomyopathies and coronary artery disease.

Left Fascicular Reentrant Tachycardia

Left fascicular reentrant tachycardia, also known as verapamil-sensitive fascicular tachycardia is due to reentry involving one or more of the left ventricular fascicles and adjacent ventricular tissue in the septum or papillary muscles.[14] Patients are most commonly young adults. There is a male predominance. Tachycardia is sustained, often exercise induced, and hemodynamically tolerated. The most common form involves the LV posterior fascicle giving rise to an RBBB – like tachycardia with a superior left axis (see Fig. 67.11). Less common forms have a right inferior axis, or rarely, a narrow QRS. It can often be terminated by intravenous administration of verapamil, while intravenous administration of class I agents such as procainamide slow the tachycardia without termination. Chronic oral verapamil and beta-blockers have

variable efficacy for preventing episodes. Catheter ablation of the common form is highly effective.

Polymorphic Ventricular Tachycardia
Electrocardiographic and Clinical Features

Polymorphic VT is characterized by a continually changing QRS morphology that indicates the changing ventricular activation sequence (Figs. 67.5, 67.17, and 67.18). Torsade de pointes is a specific type of polymorphic VT that has a waxing and waning QRS amplitude and is often associated with QT prolongation prior to initiation (see Fig. 67.17). The tachycardia is unstable and either terminates spontaneously or degenerates to VF. The distinction of where polymorphic VT ends and VF begins is often not clear. Polymorphic VT presents with light-headedness, syncope, or cardiac arrest. Polymorphic VT can be associated with myocardial ischemia (see Fig. 67.4D), left ventricular hypertrophy, or scar, but also occurs in structurally normal hearts in a number of genetic sudden death syndromes (long QT, short QT, early repolarization [ER], Brugada, catecholaminergic polymorphic VT) as well as digoxin toxicity. The mechanism may be reentry with continually changing reentry paths and has been associated with marked dispersion of ventricular repolarization. In CPVT and digoxin toxicity it is likely due to multiple competing foci of triggered activity. Unlike sustained monomorphic VT it is less likely to be associated with areas of ventricular scar, although scar is occasionally the arrhythmia substrate.[30]

Management

Sustained episodes causing hemodynamic collapse require immediate cardioversion. Following cardioversion further treatment is guided by the likely cause. Possible myocardial ischemia versus prolonged ventricular repolarization as causes should be immediately considered. In patients with coronary artery disease and electrocardiographic evidence of ischemia or ongoing infarction, emergent coronary angiography is often warranted. For torsade de pointes associated with QT prolongation intravenous administration of magnesium sulfate and removal of precipitating factors are first steps.

Specific Disorders with Polymorphic Ventricular Tachycardias
Acute Myocardial Infarction and Ischemia

Polymorphic VT degenerating to VF associated with acute ischemia or infarction is a common cause of out of hospital sudden death in Western societies. Evidence of acute infarction is found in approximately half of out of hospital VF survivors. Polymorphic VT degenerating to VF occurs within the first 24 to 48 hours in up to 10% of patients under care for acute type I myocardial infarction and may occur before, during, or after reperfusion.[1] It also occurs in up to 8% of non-ST elevation infarctions (see Fig. 67.4D). It is associated with a larger infarct territory, worse ventricular function, current smoking, and in some studies, the presence additional comorbidities. The electrocardiographic characteristics of the onset are variable. It may initiate with early or late coupled PVCs, during tachycardia or bradycardia, and with or without a preceding long R to R cycle (pause). With prompt defibrillation it is usually an isolated event. Recurrent episodes suggest ongoing ischemia warranting angiography for consideration of further intervention. Rarely recurrent episodes are due to automaticity from damaged cells in the infarct border region.[22] Amiodarone or quinidine suppress the arrhythmia in some.[9] Episodes usually resolve within days, but catheter ablation is occasionally required.

PMVT/VF during hospitalization for acute myocardial infarction is associated with greater in-hospital mortality, likely related to larger infarct size and comorbidities.[56] Mortality is greater for those with arrhythmia that occurs more than 48 hours after infarction. Although PMVT/VF within the first 48 hours of infarction is associated with greater in-hospital mortality, it is not associated with increased risk of sudden death over the following 5 years for those surviving to hospital discharge, and is not an indication for an ICD.[56]

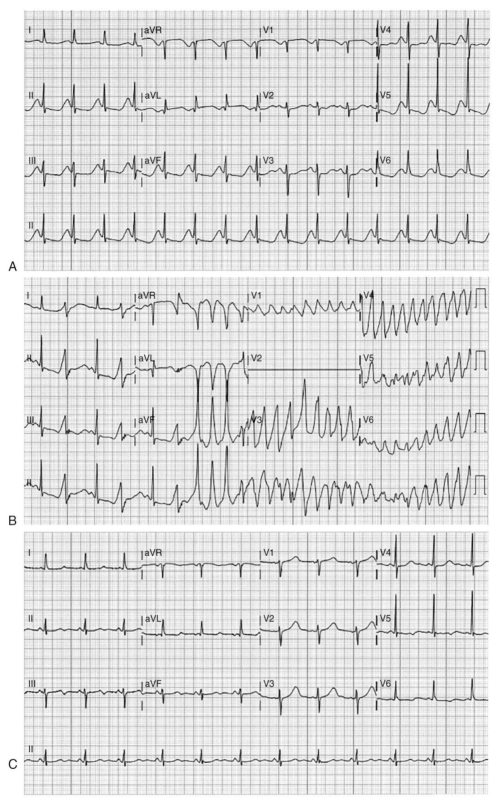

FIGURE 67.17 Long QT syndrome. **A-C** Long QT syndrome type 1. **A,** During hypokalemia there is marked QT prolongation with broad-based T waves. **B,** PVCs with initiation of the polymorphic VT torsade de pointes. **C,** After restoration of potassium, QT interval has shortened markedly. **D-F** Long QT syndrome type 2.

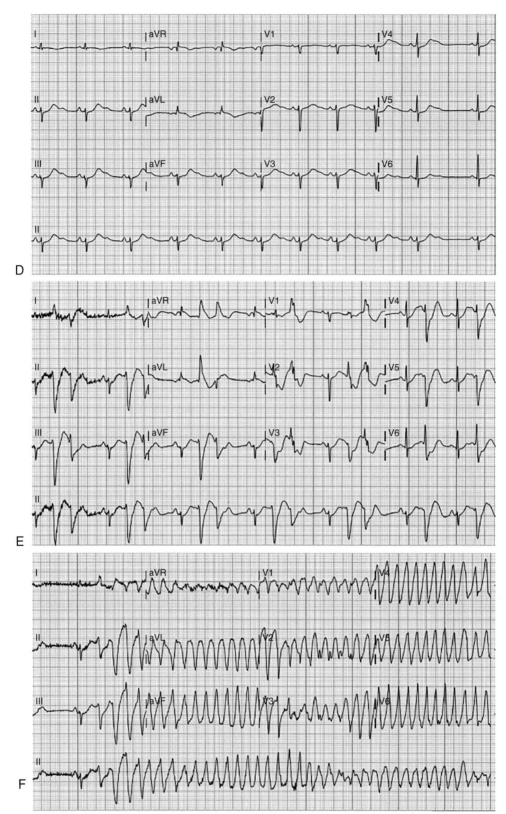

FIGURE 67.17—Cont'd D, QT prolongation with notched T-waves. **E,** PVCs and couplets. **F,** A pause initiates torsade de pointes.

Acquired Long QT Syndrome and Torsade de Pointes

The polymorphic VT torsade de pointes associated with QT interval prolongation is due to prolonged repolarization that allows recovery of time-dependent inward currents with creation of early afterpolarizations that cause PVCs as well as repolarization heterogeneity facilitating reentry. Episodes are usually initiated by heart rate slowing or a PVC-induced pause. PVCs and runs of nonsustained VT are common.

Sustained episodes may degenerate to VF. Prior to VT, the QTc interval is typically prolonged greater than 0.48 sec. Following defibrillation, the QT may be shorter in response to tachycardia and catecholamine administration, obfuscating the initial cause.

Any cause of QT prolongation can cause torsade de pointes. Drugs that block the repolarizing potassium current IKr are the most common offenders (dofetilide, ibutilide, sotalol, quinidine). Amiodarone also

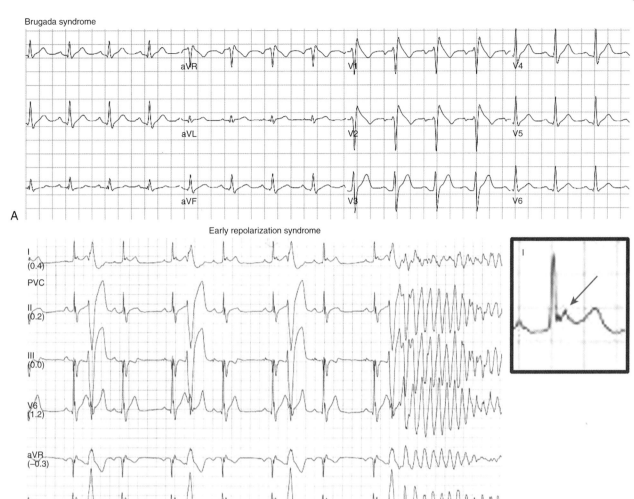

FIGURE 67.18 A, Type 1 ECG pattern of Brugada syndrome with J-point elevation greater than 2 mm in V1, V2. **B,** Early repolarization syndrome. Marked J-point elevation is present in lead I (arrow in *inset*); trigeminal short-coupled PVCs are present, interrupting the T wave of the preceding sinus beat, followed by initiation of polymorphic VT.

prolongs the QT interval, but rarely causes torsade de pointes. Many non-antiarrhythmic drugs also have IKr blocking capability (including a number of psychiatric and antibiotic medications). An updated list is maintained at www.crediblemeds.org. Bradycardia and hypokalemia are also important causes. Women are more susceptible than men, likely due to their sex-related longer QTc. In many cases a combination of factors is responsible. With genetic testing some patients are found to have inherited long QT syndrome.[57] Various combinations of single nucleotide polymorphisms that influence repolarization are genetic factors in determining risk, and have yet to be clarified sufficiently for clinical applications.[58] Drug interactions that increase concentrations of an offending agent or metabolite are also important causes.

Sustained episodes require immediate defibrillation. Recurrent episodes can usually be suppressed by 1 to 2 g of magnesium sulfate administered by rapid intravenous infusion and repeated as needed to suppress PVCs and NSVT. Bradycardia should be corrected by isoproterenol infusion or implementation of pacing at a rate that suppresses PVCs and nonsustained PMVT. Provocative drugs should be stopped and electrolyte abnormalities corrected. Shortening of the QT interval may lag excretion of the drug by several days. Patients who have had torsade de pointes should be viewed as having a susceptibility that warrants avoidance of all medications that can prolong the QT interval.

Inherited Long QT syndrome

The inherited long QT syndrome (LQTS) is due to genetic mutations that impair ventricular repolarization and prolong the QT interval

(Chapter 63).[1,59] The incidence is approximately 1 in 2500. Most are autosomal dominant with variable penetrance. Although many individuals remain asymptomatic, others present with palpitations, syncope, or cardiac arrest due to torsade de pointes that can degenerate to VF (see Fig. 67.17). Episodes can present in childhood and may be misdiagnosed as seizures or benign syncope. A family history of sudden death may be present. The QTc interval is prolonged greater than 0.48 in most symptomatic individuals but can vary over time (see Fig. 67.17A, C) and can be normal on any individual ECG. Risk increases with the degree of QTc prolongation. Some phenotype correlations with genotype are described including classic triggers for arrhythmia episodes and sex differences in risk and timing of presentation and efficacy of therapies (Chapter 63).

Type 1 (LQTS1) causes over a third of congenital LQTS. It is due to a mutation that decreases the repolarizing current IKs. Episodes of syncope are classically triggered by exertion, including swimming, or emotional stress. The ECG typically shows broad symmetric T-wave (see Fig. 67.17A). Chronic therapy with beta-adrenergic blockers is highly effective in preventing episodes.

Type 2 (LQTS2) is due to a mutation that decreases the repolarizing current IKr, which is the same current that is most commonly blocked by agents causing acquired LQTS. Episodes of arrhythmia are classically provoked by emotional stress or surprise, such as sudden noises and are pause dependent. The risk is increased for women during the 9-month post-partum period. The ECG classically shows notched or humped appearing T waves (see Fig. 67.17D), similar to those often observed in acquired LQTS. Chronic therapy with beta-adrenergic blockers is protective.

Type 3 (LQTS3) is due to a mutation in *SCN5A* that increases inward Na current (INa). Episodes of arrhythmia or sudden death tend to occur during sleep and slow heart rates. The ECG typically shows a flat ST segment with a peaked T-wave. Therapy with beta-blockers is recommended. The sodium channel blocker mexiletine significantly shortens the QT interval in some individuals.

Many other mutations have been described that can cause LQTS, including ones with noncardiac features (Timothy Syndrome, Andersen-Tawil Syndrome) and a recessive form accompanied by congenital deafness (Jervell Lange-Nielsen Syndrome) (see Chapter 63).

Management

Management of recurrent acute episodes of polymorphic VT includes intravenous administration of magnesium sulfate and overdrive pacing to shorten the QT interval. Long term, avoidance of QT prolonging medications is critical. Asymptomatic individuals with mild QTc prolongation may not warrant additional therapy.[60] Chronic beta-blocker therapy with propranolol or nadolol is often sufficient, particularly for type 1 and 2 LQTS; metoprolol is less effective.[1] ICDs are considered in patients who have had cardiac arrest or who continue to have symptoms despite therapy. Specific therapeutic strategies for the type of LQTS are emerging, including potassium supplementation for type 2 and sodium channel blockers for type 3 LQTS. Surgical cardiac sympathectomy is an option when these therapies fail. When a proband is discovered, cascade genetic screening for other affected family members is important.

Inherited Short QT Syndrome

The short QT syndrome is characterized by polymorphic VT and atrial fibrillation in patients with a structurally normal heart and a QTc ≤340 to 360 milliseconds.[61] It is rare and caused by mutations that result in gain of function in repolarizing potassium channels (IKr and IKs) or loss of function in the L-type calcium current channel. Patients present with atrial fibrillation or palpitations, syncope, or cardiac arrest from polymorphic VT. Cardiac arrest is the initial manifestation in up to 40% of patients. Symptoms may occur at rest, with routine activity, or with exertion. A family history of sudden death is common. Most patients present with arrhythmias before 40 years of age. There is a male predominance. An ICD is recommended for patients who have had symptomatic arrhythmias. Quinidine may be helpful in diminishing episodes of VT.

J Wave Syndromes: Brugada and Early Repolarization Syndromes

Brugada Syndrome

Brugada syndrome (BrS) is characterized by transient or persistent coved type ST-segment elevation in at least one right pre-cordial ECG lead (see Fig. 67.18A).[62] BrS is associated with syncope and sudden death due to ventricular arrhythmias (see Chapter 63). Approximately 25% to 30% of affected patients have a mutation in the *SCN5A* gene. *SCN5A* mutations may also produce other phenotypes including AV conduction delay, sinus node dysfunction, and atrial fibrillation, features that can occur in BrS, or may occur isolated or in combinations in other family members.[63] Phenotypic manifestations can also overlap with ARVC.[62] Arrhythmic sudden death due to polymorphic VT/VF is the first manifestation in 4% of BrS patients, usually occurring at rest or during sleep. The average age at presentation is 40 years. There is approximately an 8 to 1 male dominance. The arrhythmia mechanisms are debated. There is evidence for both, abnormalities of repolarization with heterogeneously shortened action potentials, as well as abnormal conduction in regions of fibrosis in the subepicardial free wall of the RVOT tract. Rapid monomorphic VT (average cycle length of 298 ± 45 milliseconds) occurs in up to 4.2% of patients with BrS who have received an ICD and is the arrhythmia detected in 31% of those that have an appropriate ICD therapy.[64]

A type-1 ECG—consisting of a coved ST elevation ≥2 mm followed by a descending negative T wave in at least one right precordial lead, with the electrodes positioned in the 2nd, 3rd, or 4th intercostal space that is present either spontaneously or after provocative drug test with

intravenous administration of sodium-channel blockers—is required for diagnosis of BrS. The ECG pattern can vary markedly and be normal at times. Enhanced vagal tone, fever, and several drugs (particularly sodium channel blocking antiarrhythmic and psychotropic drugs) can unmask the BrS pattern in some subjects who otherwise have a normal ECG. The type-2 and type-3 ECGs, defined by a saddleback pattern with broad R' followed by ST elevation ≥2 mm (type-2) or less than 2 mm (type 3) in the anterior precordial leads are not diagnostic and not, by themselves, associated with increased risk for sudden cardiac death (SCD).

The absolute risk of developing VF among asymptomatic patients with a type-1 ECG is lower than initially estimated and the majority of patients are likely to remain asymptomatic. Risk stratification in asymptomatic patients remains controversial and challenging.

Management

The ICD is the only established therapy to protect against SCD and is recommended for patients with a history of cardiac arrest or syncope consistent with an arrhythmia who have a type-1 ECG. In asymptomatic patients, the prognostic value of inducible PMVT at electrophysiology study and a family history of sudden death are less well defined. Lifestyle changes, including avoidance of drugs and intoxicating amounts of alcohol and immediate treatment of fever are important.

For patients with recurrent arrhythmias hydroquinidine or quinidine can reduce or prevent recurrences, but long-term treatment is hampered by side effects. Catheter ablation targeting areas of abnormal electrocardiograms in the subepicardial RVOT can normalize the ECG and prevent PMVT recurrences.[15]

Early Repolarization and J Wave Syndromes

Early repolarization (ER) *syndrome* is diagnosed in (1) a patient with an ER pattern who has been resuscitated from otherwise unexplained VF; or (2) in an SCD victim with a negative autopsy and a previous ECG with the ER pattern. An ER *pattern* is defined as a J-point elevation (or a J-wave producing slurring of the terminal QRS) ≥1 mm in at least 2 contiguous inferior and/or lateral leads of the 12-lead ECG and a QRS duration less than 120 milliseconds in leads without J waves (see Fig. 67.18B). The prevalence of ER varies between 1% and 24% in the general population and is particularly common in young men, athletes, and African Americans. Although the absolute arrhythmia risk is estimated to be very low (0.07%), ER patterns have been associated with VF initiated by Purkinje or myocardial triggers and sudden cardiac death. The ER pattern has also been associated with an increased incidence of ventricular arrythmias during myocardial ischemia and in dilated or hypertrophic cardiomyopathies. The pathophysiology is uncertain.[15,62] Heterogeneity of the transmural voltage gradient across the ventricular wall due to abnormal rapid repolarization or delayed depolarization have been suggested. In contrast to BrS, the abnormal areas may more commonly involve the inferior aspects of the ventricles. Some have been associated with areas of subepicardial fibrosis over the inferior RV or LV that may facilitate reentry, similar to BrS.

There is currently no reliable risk stratification strategy to identify the small subset of patients at high risk among the large number of individuals with an ER pattern. Suspected arrhythmogenic syncope, in particular with a dynamic and high J wave amplitude recorded immediately after the event, J waves greater than 2.0 mm in inferior leads with horizontal/descending ST segment (≤0.1 mV 100 msec after J-point), J waves in several leads, a family history of SCD or ERS, and coexistence of other ECG abnormalities (LQT, short QT, Brugada) appear to be associated with a higher risk.

Management

An ICD is recommended for patients resuscitated from VT or VF or who have had syncope attributable to VT. Oral quinidine therapy can suppress recurrent episodes. Ablation of areas with delayed abnormal fractionated electrograms involving particularly the RV epicardium appears to reduce VF recurrence in highly symptomatic patients and can abolish the ER pattern.[15] In patients with VF storm administration of isoproterenol or quinidine can often suppress the arrhythmia. Ablation targeting the abnormal epicardial substrate or PVC triggers (Figs. 67.4B and 67.18B) can be lifesaving.

Catecholaminergic Polymorphic Ventricular Tachycardias

Catecholaminergic polymorphic VT (CPVT) is a rare disorder characterized by exercise- or stress-induced ventricular arrhythmias including PVCs, bidirectional VT (see Fig. 67.5C), and polymorphic VT/VF (see Chapter 63). These arrhythmias are due to abnormal calcium handling with increased intracellular calcium during sympathetic stimulation causing delayed afterdepolarizations and triggered activity. Mutations in the gene coding for the cardiac ryanodine receptor (*RYR2*) cause an autosomal dominant form. Mutations in the genes coding for calsequestrin, calmodulin, Kir2.1, and triadin cause very rare forms. Patients typically present in childhood with palpitations, syncope, or cardiac arrest during exertion or stress, although a quarter of patients have events during wakeful activity at rest.[65] The resting 12-lead ECG is normal. Exercise stress testing should be performed in suspected cases.[66] Monomorphic PVCs consistent with an outflow-tract origin in ≈60% typically occur at HR of ≈100 bpm, progressing to bigeminy, polymorphic PVCs, and VT or VF at higher rates. Bidirectional VT, although not common, is considered pathognomonic in young individuals without structural heart disease. Bidirectional VT is also seen in digoxin toxicity, myocarditis, and Anderson-Tawil syndrome.

Chronic therapy with beta-adrenergic blockers and limiting exercise are first-line treatments.[1] The addition of flecainide, propafenone, or verapamil suppresses arrhythmias in some patients. Those who continue to have symptoms often benefit from cardiac surgical left sympathectomy. Implantable defibrillators are avoided if possible. Shocks from the device, including inappropriate shocks for supraventricular tachycardia, can elicit sympathetic activation and VT storms.[67]

VENTRICULAR FIBRILLATION

Electrocardiographic Recognition

VF is a terminal arrhythmia followed by death or severe brain injury from lack of perfusion if not corrected within 3 to 5 minutes. It is characterized by irregular undulations of varying contour and amplitude without distinct QRS complexes (Fig. 67.19C).

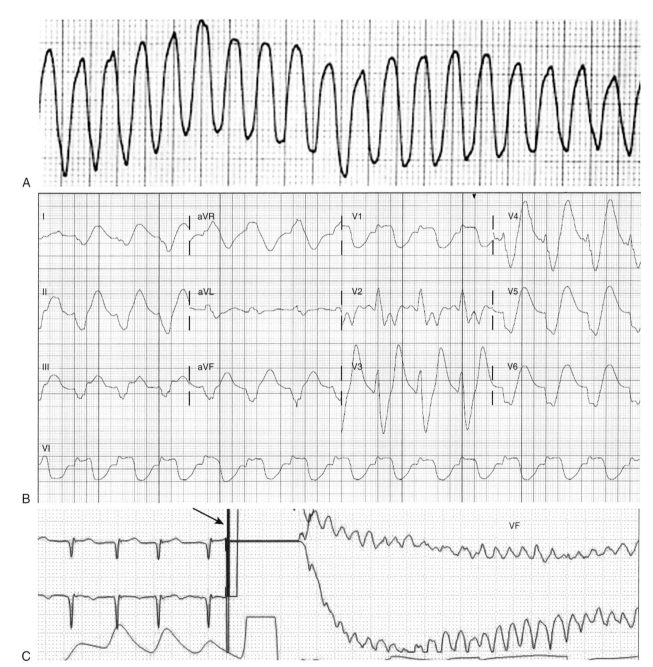

FIGURE 67.19 A, Rapid ventricular flutter. **B,** Slow sinusoidal rhythm with markedly wide QRS complexes due to severe hyperkalemia. **C,** Initiation of ventricular fibrillation by an external cardioversion shock *(arrow)* that fell during the T wave.

Clinical Features

VF and rapid ventricular flutter are most commonly encountered in coronary artery disease with ongoing myocardial ischemia and can follow from polymorphic VT or monomorphic VT of any cause. In structurally normal hearts VF can be elicited by electrical shock (see Fig. 67.19C) or a precordial impact that causes cardiac depolarization during the T-wave (commotio cordis). It can also be caused by very rapid ventricular rates during atrial fibrillation in patients with an accessory pathway in the Wolff-Parkinson-White syndrome or by early PVCs or unusually rapid idiopathic VT to cause idiopathic VF. There is no coordinated cardiac contraction, no detectable blood pressure, and absence of heart sounds. Eventually electrical activity of the heart ceases.

Management

Management should follow basic life support and advanced cardiac life support guidelines. Asynchronous DC cardioversion using 200 J to 400 J is mandatory therapy for VF, ventricular flutter, and pulseless VT. Cardiopulmonary resuscitation is performed until cardioversion can be performed and resumed immediately after each shock. If the first shock is ineffective subsequent shocks should be delivered at maximum defibrillator output. A bolus of intravenous amiodarone of 300 mg can be administered if initial shocks are unsuccessful while cardiopulmonary resuscitation is continued. Recurrent fibrillation is common after an initially successful shock. Close monitoring should be continued with immediate ability to defibrillate again as further evaluation seeks to identify and treat the underlying cause.

VENTRICULAR FLUTTER

Ventricular flutter (see Fig. 67.19A) is a sinusoidal tachycardia during which it is not possible to separate the QRS from the ST-T wave with certainty. Rapid ventricular flutter has rates faster than 280 beats/minute and can be a rapid monomorphic VT for which the etiologies are the same as for slower monomorphic VT, but can also occur during acute myocardial infarction or severe metabolic derangements. It usually produces hemodynamic collapse and degenerates to VF. Immediate electrical cardioversion or defibrillation is required. Correct synchronization of the defibrillator shock to the QRS, rather than T-wave, is not possible and an asynchronous shock should be used, always being prepared to apply a following shock for VF.

Relatively slow ventricular flutter is a wide QRS tachycardia due to slow conduction through the myocardium that can be due to hyperkalemia, drug toxicity, particularly cardiac sodium channel blocking drugs, severe global ischemia, and severe metabolic derangements (see Fig. 67.19B). It is usually associated with hypotension or hemodynamic collapse warranting cardioversion. For suspected hyperkalemia administration of intravenous calcium followed separately by sodium bicarbonate is warranted, followed by measures to lower serum potassium. Toxicity from a sodium channel blocking antiarrhythmic drug including flecainide, propafenone, and procainamide may respond to administration of hypertonic saline, which can be in the form of sodium bicarbonate.[68] Tachycardia increases sodium channel blockade by these drugs. Measures to slow the underlying sinus rate are helpful.

REFERENCES

1. Al-Khatib SM, Stevenson WG, Ackerman MJ, et al. 2017 AHA/ACC/HRS guideline for management of patients with ventricular arrhythmias and the prevention of sudden cardiac death: a report of the American college of cardiology/American heart association task force on clinical practice guidelines and the heart rhythm society. *Circulation*. 2018;138:e272–e391.
2. Kerola T, Dewland TA, Vittinghoff E, et al. Modifiable predictors of ventricular ectopy in the community. *J Am Heart Assoc*. 2018;7:e010078.
3. Dukes JW, Dewland TA, Vittinghoff E, et al. Ventricular ectopy as a predictor of heart failure and death. *J Am Coll Cardiol*. 2015;66:101–109.
4. Kim YR, Nam GB, Kwon CH, et al. Second coupling interval of nonsustained ventricular tachycardia to distinguish malignant from benign outflow tract ventricular tachycardias. *Heart Rhythm*. 2014;11:2222–2230.
5. Verdile L, Maron BJ, Pelliccia A, et al. Clinical significance of exercise-induced ventricular tachyarrhythmias in trained athletes without cardiovascular abnormalities. *Heart Rhythm*. 2015;12:78–85.
6. Peretto G, Sala S, Rizzo S, et al. Ventricular arrhythmias in myocarditis: characterization and relationships with myocardial inflammation. *J Am Coll Cardiol*. 2020;75:1046–1057.
7. Lee AKY, Andrade J, Hawkins NM, et al. Outcomes of untreated frequent premature ventricular complexes with normal left ventricular function. *Heart*. 2019;105:1408–1413.
8. Ling Z, Liu Z, Su L, et al. Radiofrequency ablation versus antiarrhythmic medication for treatment of ventricular premature beats from the right ventricular outflow tract: prospective randomized study. *Circ Arrhythm Electrophysiol*. 2014;7:237–243.
9. Viskin S, Chorin E, Viskin D, et al. Quinidine-responsive polymorphic ventricular tachycardia in patients with coronary heart disease. *Circulation*. 2019;139:2304–2314.
10. Latchamsetty R, Bogun F. Premature ventricular complex-induced cardiomyopathy. *JACC Clin Electrophysiol*. 2019;5:537–550.
11. Huizar JF, Ellenbogen KA, Tan AY, et al. Arrhythmia-induced cardiomyopathy: JACC state-of-the-art review. *J Am Coll Cardiol*. 2019;73:2328–2344.
12. Berruezo A, Penela D, Jauregui B, et al. Mortality and morbidity reduction after frequent premature ventricular complexes ablation in patients with left ventricular systolic dysfunction. *Europace*. 2019;21:1079–1087.
13. Penela D, Fernandez-Armenta J, Aguinaga L, et al. Clinical recognition of pure premature ventricular complex-induced cardiomyopathy at presentation. *Heart Rhythm*. 2017;14:1864–1870.
14. Cronin EM, Bogun FM, Maury P, et al. 2019 HRS/EHRA/APHRS/LAHRS expert consensus statement on catheter ablation of ventricular arrhythmias. *Heart Rhythm*. 2020;17:e2–e154.
15. Nademanee K, Haissaguerre M, Hocini M, et al. Mapping and ablation of ventricular fibrillation associated with early repolarization syndrome. *Circulation*. 2019;140:1477–1490.
16. Doisne N, Waldmann V, Redheuil A, et al. A novel gain-of-function mutation in SCN5A responsible for multifocal ectopic Purkinje-related premature contractions. *Hum Mutat*. 2020;41:850–859.
17. Ortiz M, Martin A, Arribas F, et al. Randomized comparison of intravenous procainamide vs. intravenous amiodarone for the acute treatment of tolerated wide QRS tachycardia: the PROCAMIO study. *Eur Heart J*. 2017;38:1329–1335.
18. Vergara P, Tzou WS, Tung R, et al. Predictive score for identifying survival and recurrence risk profiles in patients undergoing ventricular tachycardia ablation: the I-VT score. *Circ Arrhythm Electrophysiol*. 2018;11:e006730.
19. Vergara P, Tung R, Vaseghi M, et al. Successful ventricular tachycardia ablation in patients with electrical storm reduces recurrences and improves survival. *Heart Rhythm*. 2018;15:48–55.
20. Chatzidou S, Kontogiannis C, Tsilimigras DI, et al. Propranolol versus metoprolol for treatment of electrical storm in patients with implantable cardioverter-defibrillator. *J Am Coll Cardiol*. 2018;71:1897–1906.
21. Meng L, Tseng CH, Shivkumar K, et al. Efficacy of stellate ganglion blockade in managing electrical storm: a systematic review. *JACC Clin Electrophysiol*. 2017;3:942–949.
22. Komatsu Y, Hocini M, Nogami A, et al. Catheter ablation of refractory ventricular fibrillation storm after myocardial infarction. *Circulation*. 2019;139:2315–2325.
23. Beggs SAS, Gardner RS, McMurray JJV. Who benefits from a defibrillator-balancing the risk of sudden versus non-sudden death. *Curr Heart Fail Rep*. 2018;15:376–389.
24. Almehmadi F, Porta-Sanchez A, Ha ACT, et al. Mortality implications of appropriate implantable cardioverter defibrillator therapy in secondary prevention patients: contrasting mortality in primary prevention patients from a prospective population-based registry. *J Am Heart Assoc*. 2017;6.
25. Sapp JL, Wells GA, Parkash R, et al. Ventricular tachycardia ablation versus escalation of antiarrhythmic drugs. *N Engl J Med*. 2016;375:111–121.
26. Willems S, Tilz RR, Steven D, et al. Preventive or deferred ablation of ventricular tachycardia in patients with ischemic cardiomyopathy and implantable defibrillator (BERLIN VT): a multicenter randomized trial. *Circulation*. 2020;141:1057–1067.
27. Kheiri B, Barbarawi M, Zayed Y, et al. Antiarrhythmic drugs or catheter ablation in the management of ventricular tachyarrhythmias in patients with implantable cardioverter-defibrillators: a systematic review and meta-analysis of randomized controlled trials. *Circ Arrhythm Electrophysiol*. 2019;12:e007600.
28. Tung R, Vaseghi M, Frankel DS, et al. Freedom from recurrent ventricular tachycardia after catheter ablation is associated with improved survival in patients with structural heart disease: an International VT Ablation Center Collaborative Group study. *Heart Rhythm*. 2015;12:1997–2007.
29. Gigli M, Merlo M, Graw SL, et al. Genetic risk of arrhythmic phenotypes in patients with dilated cardiomyopathy. *J Am Coll Cardiol*. 2019;74:1480–1490.
30. Piers SR, Everaerts K, van der Geest RJ, et al. Myocardial scar predicts monomorphic ventricular tachycardia but not polymorphic ventricular tachycardia or ventricular fibrillation in nonischemic dilated cardiomyopathy. *Heart Rhythm*. 2015;12:2106–2114.
31. El Moheb M, Nicolas J, Khamis AM, et al. Implantable cardiac defibrillators for people with non-ischaemic cardiomyopathy. *Cochrane Database Syst Rev*. 2018;12:CD012738.
32. Wahbi K, Ben Yaou R, Gandjbakhch E, et al. Development and validation of a new risk prediction score for life-threatening ventricular tachyarrhythmias in laminopathies. *Circulation*. 2019;140:293–302.
33. Zeppenfeld K. Ventricular tachycardia ablation in nonischemic cardiomyopathy. *JACC Clin Electrophysiol*. 2018;4:1123–1140.
34. Vaseghi M, Hu TY, Tung R, et al. Outcomes of catheter ablation of ventricular tachycardia based on etiology in nonischemic heart disease: an international ventricular tachycardia ablation center collaborative study. *JACC Clin Electrophysiol*. 2018;4:1141–1150.
35. Aryana A, Tung R, d'Avila A. Percutaneous epicardial approach to catheter ablation of cardiac arrhythmias. *JACC Clin Electrophysiol*. 2020;6:1–20.
36. Nakamura T, Narui R, Zheng Q, et al. Atrioventricular block during catheter ablation for ventricular arrhythmias. *JACC Clin Electrophysiol*. 2019;5:104–112.
37. Bosman LP, Cadrin-Tourigny J, Bourfiss M, et al. Diagnosing arrhythmogenic right ventricular cardiomyopathy by 2010 Task Force Criteria: clinical performance and simplified practical implementation. *Europace*. 2020;22:787–796.
38. Venlet J, Piers SR, Jongbloed JD, et al. Isolated subepicardial right ventricular outflow tract scar in athletes with ventricular tachycardia. *J Am Coll Cardiol*. 2017;69:497–507.
39. Koyak Z, de Groot JR, Bouma BJ, et al. Sudden cardiac death in adult congenital heart disease: can the unpredictable be foreseen? *Europace*. 2017;19(3):401–406.
40. Wu MH, Lu CW, Chen HC, et al. Adult congenital heart disease in a nationwide population 2000-2014: epidemiological trends, arrhythmia, and standardized mortality ratio. *J Am Heart Assoc*. 2018;7.
41. Kapel GF, Reichlin T, Wijnmaalen AP, et al. Re-entry using anatomically determined isthmuses: a curable ventricular tachycardia in repaired congenital heart disease. *Circ Arrhythm Electrophysiol*. 2015;8:102–109.
42. Brouwer C, Kapel GFL, Jongbloed MRM, et al. Noninvasive identification of ventricular tachycardia-related anatomical isthmuses in repaired tetralogy of Fallot: what is the role of the 12-lead ventricular tachycardia electrocardiogram. *JACC Clin Electrophysiol*. 2018;4:1308–1318.
43. Kapel GF, Sacher F, Dekkers OM, et al. Arrhythmogenic anatomical isthmuses identified by electroanatomical mapping are the substrate for ventricular tachycardia in repaired tetralogy of Fallot. *Eur Heart J*. 2017;38:268–276.
44. Rowin EJ, Maron BJ, Chokshi A, et al. Left ventricular apical aneurysm in hypertrophic cardiomyopathy as a risk factor for sudden death at any age. *Pacing Clin Electrophysiol*. 2018.
45. Igarashi M, Nogami A, Kurosaki K, et al. Radiofrequency catheter ablation of ventricular tachycardia in patients with hypertrophic cardiomyopathy and apical aneurysm. *JACC Clin Electrophysiol*. 2018;4:339–350.
46. Wang W, Lian Z, Rowin EJ, et al. Prognostic implications of nonsustained ventricular tachycardia in high-risk patients with hypertrophic cardiomyopathy. *Circ Arrhythm Electrophysiol*. 2017;10.

47. Birnie DH, Sauer WH, Bogun F, et al. HRS expert consensus statement on the diagnosis and management of arrhythmias associated with cardiac sarcoidosis. *Heart Rhythm*. 2014;11:1305–1323.

48. Kandolin R, Lehtonen J, Airaksinen J, et al. Cardiac sarcoidosis: epidemiology, characteristics, and outcome over 25 years in a nationwide study. *Circulation*. 2015;131:624–632.

49. Ammirati E, Cipriani M, Moro C, et al. Clinical presentation and outcome in a contemporary cohort of patients with acute myocarditis: multicenter Lombardy registry. *Circulation*. 2018;138:1088–1099.

50. Lakkireddy D, Turagam MK, Yarlagadda B, et al. Myocarditis causing premature ventricular contractions: insights from the MAVERIC registry. *Circ Arrhythm Electrophysiol*. 2019;12:e007520.

51. Nunes MCP, Beaton A, Acquatella H, et al. Chagas cardiomyopathy: an update of current clinical knowledge and management: a scientific statement from the American Heart Association. *Circulation*. 2018;138:e169–e209.

52. Anderson RD, Kumar S, Parameswaran R, et al. Differentiating right- and left-sided outflow tract ventricular arrhythmias: classical ECG signatures and prediction algorithms. *Circ Arrhythm Electrophysiol*. 2019;12:e007392.

53. Kawamura M, Gerstenfeld EP, Vedantham V, et al. Idiopathic ventricular arrhythmia originating from the cardiac crux or inferior septum: epicardial idiopathic ventricular arrhythmia. *Circ Arrhythm Electrophysiol*. 2014;7:1152–1158.

54. Al'Aref SJ, Ip JE, Markowitz SM, et al. Differentiation of papillary muscle from fascicular and mitral annular ventricular arrhythmias in patients with and without structural heart disease. *Circ Arrhythm Electrophysiol*. 2015;8:616–624.

55. Dejgaard LA, Skjolsvik ET, Lie OH, et al. The mitral annulus disjunction arrhythmic syndrome. *J Am Coll Cardiol*. 2018;72:1600–1609.

56. Bougouin W, Marijon E, Puymirat E, et al. Incidence of sudden cardiac death after ventricular fibrillation complicating acute myocardial infarction: a 5-year cause-of-death analysis of the FAST-MI 2005 registry. *Eur Heart J*. 2014;35:116–122.

57. Itoh H, Crotti L, Aiba T, et al. The genetics underlying acquired long QT syndrome: impact for genetic screening. *Eur Heart J*. 2016;37:1456–1464.

58. Strauss DG, Vicente J, Johannesen L, et al. Common genetic variant risk score is associated with drug-induced QT prolongation and torsade de pointes risk: a pilot study. *Circulation*. 2017;135:1300–1310.

59. Mazzanti A, Maragna R, Vacanti G, et al. Interplay between genetic substrate, QTc duration, and arrhythmia risk in patients with long QT syndrome. *J Am Coll Cardiol*. 2018;71:1663–1671.

60. MacIntyre CJ, Rohatgi RK, Sugrue AM, et al. Intentional nontherapy in long QT syndrome. *Heart Rhythm*. 2020;17:1147–1150.

61. El-Battrawy I, Besler J, Liebe V, et al. Long-term follow-up of patients with short QT syndrome: clinical profile and outcome. *J Am Heart Assoc*. 2018;7:e010073.

62. Antzelevitch C, Yan GX, Ackerman MJ, et al. J-Wave syndromes expert consensus conference report: emerging concepts and gaps in knowledge. *Europace*. 2017;19:665–694.

63. Wilde AAM, Amin AS. Clinical spectrum of SCN5A mutations: long QT syndrome, Brugada syndrome, and cardiomyopathy. *JACC Clin Electrophysiol*. 2018;4:569–579.

64. Rodriguez-Manero M, Sacher F, de Asmundis C, et al. Monomorphic ventricular tachycardia in patients with Brugada syndrome: a multicenter retrospective study. *Heart Rhythm*. 2016;13:669–682.

65. Roston TM, Yuchi Z, Kannankeril PJ, et al. The clinical and genetic spectrum of catecholaminergic polymorphic ventricular tachycardia: findings from an international multicentre registry. *Europace*. 2018;20:541–547.

66. Giudicessi JR, Ackerman MJ. Exercise testing oversights underlie missed and delayed diagnosis of catecholaminergic polymorphic ventricular tachycardia in young sudden cardiac arrest survivors. *Heart Rhythm*. 2019;16:1232–1239.

67. Roston TM, Jones K, Hawkins NM, et al. Implantable cardioverter-defibrillator use in catecholaminergic polymorphic ventricular tachycardia: a systematic review. *Heart Rhythm*. 2018;15:1791–1799.

68. Brumfield E, Bernard KR, Kabrhel C. Life-threatening flecainide overdose treated with intralipid and extracorporeal membrane oxygenation. *Am J Emerg Med*. 2015;33:1840.e3–1845.

68 Bradyarrhythmias and Atrioventricular Block

KRISTEN K. PATTON AND JEFFREY E. OLGIN

BRADYARRHYTHMIAS

Based on large population studies of healthy individuals, the lower limit of normal resting heart rate is defined as 50 beats/min.[1,2] Frequently, bradyarrhythmias are physiologic, as in well-conditioned athletes with low resting heart rates or in type I atrioventricular (AV) block during sleep. In other cases, bradyarrhythmias can be pathologic. Similar to tachyarrhythmias, bradyarrhythmias can be categorized on the basis of the level of disturbance in the hierarchy of the normal impulse generation and conduction system (from sinus node to AV node to His-Purkinje system) (see Chapter 65 and Table 65.1).

Sinus Bradycardia

Electrocardiographic Recognition

Sinus bradycardia is diagnosed in an adult when the sinus node discharges at a rate less than 50 beats/min (Fig. 68.1A). P waves have a normal contour, and are usually upright in leads I, II, and aVF, and occur before each QRS complex, usually with a constant PR interval longer than 120 msec. Sinus arrhythmia often coexists.

Clinical Features

Sinus bradycardia can result from excessive vagal or decreased sympathetic tone, as an effect of medications, or from anatomic changes in the sinus node. In most cases, symptomatic sinus bradycardia is caused or worsened by the effects of medication. Asymptomatic sinus bradycardia frequently occurs in healthy young adults, particularly well-trained athletes, and decreases in prevalence with advancing age. During sleep, the normal heart rate can fall to 35 to 40 beats/min, especially in adolescents and young adults, with marked sinus arrhythmia sometimes producing pauses of 2 seconds or longer. Eye surgery, coronary arteriography, meningitis, intracranial tumors, increased intracranial pressure, cervical and mediastinal tumors, and certain disease states (e.g., severe hypoxia, myxedema, hypothermia, fibrodegenerative changes, convalescence from some infections, gram-negative sepsis, mental depression) can produce sinus bradycardia. Sinus bradycardia also occurs during vomiting or vasovagal syncope[3,4] (see Chapter 71) and can be produced by carotid sinus stimulation or by the administration of parasympathomimetic drugs, lithium, amiodarone, beta adrenoceptor–blocking drugs, clonidine, propafenone, ivabradine (a specific I_f pacemaker current blocker; see Chapter 62), or calcium antagonists. Conjunctival instillation of beta blockers for glaucoma can produce sinus or AV nodal abnormalities, especially in elderly patients.

In most cases, sinus bradycardia is a benign arrhythmia that can actually be beneficial by producing a longer period of diastole and increasing ventricular filling time, especially in heart failure patients. Conversely, it can be associated with syncope caused by an abnormal autonomic reflex (cardioinhibitory; see Chapter 71). Sinus bradycardia occurs in 10% to 15% of patients with acute myocardial infarction (MI) and may be even more prevalent when patients are seen in the early hours of infarction. Unless it is accompanied by hemodynamic decompensation or arrhythmias, sinus bradycardia is generally associated with a more favorable outcome after MI than sinus tachycardia. It is usually transient and occurs more commonly during inferior than during anterior MI; sinus bradycardia has also been noted during reperfusion with thrombolytic agents (see Chapter 38). Bradycardia that follows resuscitation from cardiac arrest is associated with a poor prognosis.

Management

Treatment of sinus bradycardia is not usually necessary unless cardiac output is inadequate or arrhythmias result from the slow rate. Atropine (0.5 mg intravenously as an initial dose, repeated if necessary) is generally acutely effective; lower doses, particularly given subcutaneously or intramuscularly, can exert an initial parasympathomimetic effect, possibly by a central action. For recurrent symptomatic episodes, temporary or permanent pacing may be needed (see Chapters 64 and 69). Although theophylline and terbutaline can be used to increase the sinus rate, as a general rule, no drugs are available that increase the heart rate reliably and safely during long periods without undesirable side effects.

Sinus Arrhythmia

Sinus arrhythmia is characterized by a phasic variation in sinus cycle length during which the maximum sinus cycle length minus the minimum sinus cycle length exceeds 120 msec or the maximum sinus cycle length minus the minimum sinus cycle length divided by the minimum sinus cycle length exceeds 10% (Fig. 68.1B). It is the most frequent form of arrhythmia and is physiologically normal. P wave morphology does not usually vary, and the PR interval exceeds 120 msec and remains unchanged because the focus of discharge remains relatively fixed within the sinus node. On occasion, the pacemaker focus can wander within the sinus node, or its exit to the atrium may change and produce P waves of a slightly different contour (although not retrograde) and a slightly changing PR interval that exceeds 120 msec.

> Sinus arrhythmia usually occurs in the young, especially those with slower heart rates or with enhanced vagal tone, for example, following the administration of digitalis or morphine, or due to athletic training. The prevalence of sinus arrhythmia decreases with age or with autonomic dysfunction, such as in diabetic neuropathy. Sinus arrhythmia appears in two basic forms. In the respiratory form, the P-P interval cyclically shortens during inspiration, primarily as a result of reflex inhibition of vagal tone, and slows during expiration; breath-holding eliminates the variation in cycle length (see Chapter 61). Nonrespiratory sinus arrhythmia is characterized by a phasic variation in the P-P interval unrelated to the respiratory cycle and can be the result of digitalis intoxication. Loss of sinus rhythm variability is a risk factor for sudden cardiac death (see Chapter 70).

Additional content is available online at Elsevier eBooks for Practicing Clinicians

Symptoms produced by sinus arrhythmia are uncommon, but on occasion, if the pauses are excessively long, palpitations or dizziness can result. Marked sinus arrhythmia can produce a sinus pause sufficiently long to cause syncope if it is not accompanied by an escape rhythm. Treatment is usually unnecessary. Increasing the heart rate by exercise or drugs generally abolishes sinus arrhythmia. Symptomatic individuals may experience relief from palpitations with sedatives, tranquilizers, atropine, ephedrine, or isoproterenol administration, as for the treatment of sinus bradycardia.

VENTRICULOPHASIC SINUS ARRHYTHMIA

The most common example of ventriculophasic sinus arrhythmia occurs during complete AV block and a slow ventricular rate, when P-P cycles that contain a QRS complex are shorter than P-P cycles without a QRS complex. Similar lengthening can be present in the P-P cycle that follows a premature ventricular complex (PVC) with a compensatory pause. Alterations in the P-P interval are probably caused by the influence of the autonomic nervous system responding to changes in ventricular stroke volume.

SINUS PAUSE OR SINUS ARREST

Sinus pause or sinus arrest is recognized by a pause in the sinus rhythm (eFig. 68.1). The P-P interval delimiting the pause does not equal a multiple of the basic P-P interval. Differentiation of sinus arrest, which is thought to be caused by slowing or cessation of spontaneous sinus node automaticity, and therefore is a disorder of impulse formation, from sinoatrial (SA) exit block in patients with sinus arrhythmia can be difficult without direct recordings of sinus node discharge. Failure of sinus nodal discharge results in the absence of atrial depolarization and can also result in ventricular asystole if escape beats initiated by latent pacemakers do not occur (see eFig. 68.1). Involvement of the sinus node by acute MI, degenerative fibrotic changes, digitalis toxicity, stroke, or excessive vagal tone can produce sinus arrest. Transient sinus arrest (especially while sleeping) may have no clinical significance by itself if latent pacemakers promptly escape to prevent ventricular asystole or the genesis of other arrhythmias precipitated by slow rates. Sinus arrest and AV block have been demonstrated in many patients with sleep apnea (see Chapter 89).

Treatment is as outlined earlier for sinus bradycardia. In patients who have a chronic form of sinus node disease characterized by marked

sinus bradycardia or sinus arrest, permanent pacing is often necessary. However, as a general rule, chronic pacing for sinus bradycardia is indicated only in symptomatic patients.

SINOATRIAL EXIT BLOCK

SA exit block is an arrhythmia that is recognized electrocardiographically by a pause resulting from absence of the normally expected P wave (eFig. 68.2). The duration of the pause is a multiple of the basic P-P interval. SA exit block is caused by a conduction disturbance during which an impulse formed within the sinus node fails to depolarize the atria or does so with delay (eFig. 68.3). An interval without P waves that equals approximately two, three, or four times the normal P-P cycle characterizes type II second-degree SA exit block. During type I (Wenckebach) second-degree SA exit block, the P-P interval progressively shortens before the pause, and the duration of the pause is less than two P-P cycles. (See Chapter 14 for further discussion of Wenckebach intervals.) First-degree SA exit block cannot be recognized on the electrocardiogram (ECG) because SA nodal discharge is not recorded. Third-degree SA exit block can be manifested as a complete absence of P waves and is difficult to diagnose with certainty without sinus node electrograms.

Excessive vagal stimulation, acute myocarditis, MI, or fibrosis involving the atrium, as well as drugs such as quinidine, procainamide, flecainide, and digitalis, can produce SA exit block. SA exit block is usually transient. It may be of no clinical importance except to prompt a search for the underlying cause. On occasion, syncope can result if the SA block is prolonged and unaccompanied by an escape rhythm. SA exit block can occur in well-trained athletes. Therapy for patients who have symptomatic SA exit block is as outlined earlier for sinus bradycardia.

Sick Sinus Syndrome
Electrocardiographic Recognition

Sick sinus syndrome is a term applied to a syndrome encompassing several sinus nodal abnormalities, including (1) persistent spontaneous sinus bradycardia inappropriate for the physiologic circumstance, (2) sinus arrest or exit block (Fig. 68.2), (3) combinations of SA and AV conduction disturbances, and often, (4) alternation of paroxysms of rapid regular or irregular atrial tachyarrhythmias and periods of slow atrial and ventricular rates (bradycardia-tachycardia syndrome; Fig. 68.3). More than one of these conditions can be seen in the same patient on different occasions, and their mechanisms are often causally interrelated and combined with an abnormal state of AV conduction or automaticity.

Patients with sinus node disease can be categorized as having intrinsic

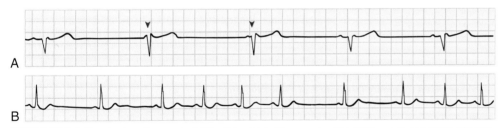

FIGURE 68.1 **A,** Sinus bradycardia at a rate of 40 to 48 beats/min. The second and third QRS complexes *(arrowheads)* represent junctional escape beats. Note the P waves at the onset of the QRS complex. **B,** Nonrespiratory sinus arrhythmia occurring as a consequence of digitalis toxicity. Monitor leads were used.

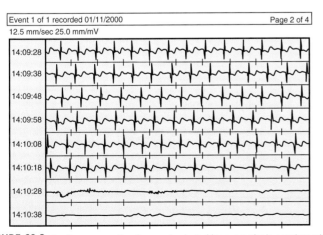

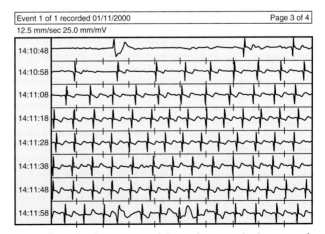

FIGURE 68.2 Continuous recording from an implanted loop recorder in a patient with syncope. The tracing shows paroxysmal sinus node arrest and a sinus pause of nearly 30 seconds. The preceding sinus cycle length appears to lengthen just before the pause, which suggests an autonomic component of the pause. There is also a single ventricular escape complex at 14:10:48.

disease unrelated to autonomic abnormalities or as exhibiting combinations of intrinsic and autonomic abnormalities. Symptomatic patients with sinus pauses or SA exit block frequently show abnormal responses on electrophysiologic testing and can have a relatively high incidence of atrial fibrillation. In children, sinus node dysfunction most frequently occurs in those with congenital or acquired heart disease, particularly after corrective cardiac surgery. Sick sinus syndrome can occur in the absence of other cardiac abnormalities. The course of the disease is frequently intermittent and unpredictable because it is influenced by the severity of the underlying heart disease. Excessive physical training can heighten vagal tone and produce syncope related to sinus bradycardia or AV conduction abnormalities in otherwise normal individuals.

The anatomic basis of sick sinus syndrome can involve total or subtotal destruction of the sinus node, areas of nodal-atrial discontinuity, inflammatory or degenerative changes in the nerves and ganglia surrounding the node, and pathologic changes in the atrial wall. Fibrosis and fatty infiltration occur, and the sclerodegenerative processes generally involve the sinus node and the AV node or the bundle of His and its branches or distal subdivisions. Occlusion of the sinus node artery can cause sinus node dysfunction.

Chronotropic Incompetence

Chronotropic incompetence (CI) is diagnosed when the heart rate does not increase appropriately in the setting of increased physiologic demand (Fig. 68.4). Although many studies use a definition of failure to obtain 80% or 85% of either maximal expected heart rate, or of inadequate heart rate reserve (the difference between resting

heart rate and age predicted maximal heart rate),[2] the variance in individual heart rate range can require meticulous clinical assessment. If required, a reliable technique using ventilatory expired gas analysis during exercise to calculate the chronotropic index allows for an objective calculation of the relationship between metabolic reserve and heart rate reserve adjusted for age and functional capacity (see Chapter 15).[5]

The normal heart rate increase with exercise and rapid decline with cessation of activity results from an exquisite balance of inputs from the sympathetic and parasympathetic nervous system to the sinus node. Increase in heart rate due to physiologic demand is the principal determinant of rate of oxygen consumption (Vo_2) and exercise capacity. The fourfold increase in Vo_2 during exercise is largely due to a 2.2-fold increase in heart rate. Genome-wide association studies have confirmed heritability of heart rate increase with exercise and heart rate recovery. Candidate genes are related to the central nervous system, cardiac development, and cardiac ion channels.[6] Aging alone can confer CI; the age-related decline in heart rate response to exercise is inevitable even in healthy older athletes.

Symptomatic CI is common, and frequently associated with SA node disease, atrial fibrillation, coronary artery disease (CAD), and heart failure.[7] Symptoms are grounded in intolerance of exertion, and often include dyspnea, lightheadedness, and overall limited exercise capacity. Interestingly, beta-blocker therapy is not universally associated with CI in either the CAD or heart failure populations. Similar to sinus bradycardia treatment is based on symptoms. Despite the clear association between CI and mortality, the evidence supporting atrial-based rate responsive pacing therapy and improvement in mortality risk is scant, but promising.

Tachycardia-Bradycardia Syndrome

Tachycardia-bradycardia syndrome (TBS) occurs when a patient has tachyarrhythmias and bradyarrhythmias closely associated in time. That can occur when a tachyarrhythmia, typically atrial fibrillation or atrial flutter terminates, with a resultant excessive post-conversion pause (Fig. 68.5). TBS can also occur during atrial fibrillation when periods of atrial fibrillation with rapid ventricular rates alternate with periods of excessive bradycardia (due to high-grade AV block) during atrial fibrillation. While TBS can occur without medication, it typically occurs as a result of treatment with beta blockers or calcium channel blockers.

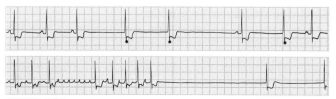

FIGURE 68.3 Sick sinus syndrome with bradycardia-tachycardia in a continuous monitor lead recording. **Top,** Intermittent sinus arrest is apparent with junctional escape beats at irregular intervals *(red circles)*. **Bottom,** A short episode of atrial flutter is followed by almost 5 seconds of asystole before a junctional escape rhythm resumes. The patient became presyncopal at this point.

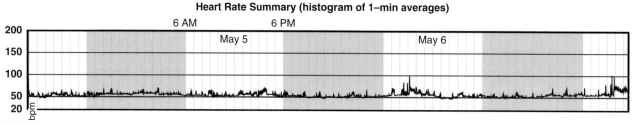

FIGURE 68.4 Three-day monitor revealing markedly suppressed heart rate histogram curve, showing a heart rate range between 55 and 91 beats/min, with an average of 45 beats/min. Correlation of symptoms and rate remain essential.

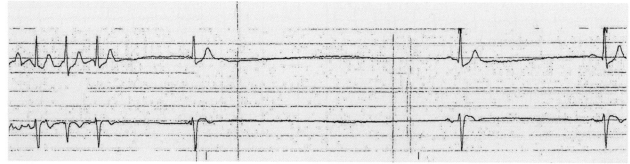

FIGURE 68.5 Telemetry monitor example of atrial fibrillation with rapid ventricular response with termination followed by a sinus pause with a junctional escape beat, and a second, longer sinus pause.

Management

For patients with sick sinus syndrome, treatment depends on the basic rhythm problem but usually involves permanent pacemaker implantation when symptoms are manifest (see Chapter 69). Pacing for bradycardia, combined with drug therapy to treat the tachycardia, is required in those with bradycardia-tachycardia syndrome.

ATRIOVENTRICULAR BLOCK (HEART BLOCK)

Heart block is a disturbance of impulse conduction that can be permanent or transient, depending on the anatomic or functional impairment. It must be distinguished from *interference*, a normal phenomenon that is a disturbance of impulse conduction caused by physiologic refractoriness resulting from inexcitability secondary to a preceding impulse. Interference or block can occur at any site where impulses are conducted, but they are recognized most often between the sinus node and atrium (SA block), between the atria and ventricles (AV block), within the atria (intra-atrial block), or within the ventricles (intraventricular block). SA exit block was discussed earlier (see Sinus Bradycardia). AV block exists if the atrial impulse is conducted with delay or is not conducted at all to the ventricle when the AV junction is not physiologically refractory. During AV block, the site of block can be in the AV node, His bundle, or bundle branches. In some cases of bundle branch block (BBB), the impulse may only be delayed and not completely blocked in the bundle branch, yet the resulting QRS complex may be indistinguishable from a QRS complex generated by a complete BBB.

AV block is classified by severity into three categories. During first-degree heart block, conduction time is prolonged but all impulses are conducted. Second-degree heart block occurs in two forms, Mobitz type I (Wenckebach) and type II. Type I heart block is characterized by progressive lengthening of the conduction time until an impulse is not conducted. Type II heart block denotes an occasional or repetitive sudden block of conduction of an impulse, without prior measurable lengthening of conduction time. When no impulses are conducted, complete or third-degree block is present. The degree of block may depend in part on the direction of impulse propagation. For unknown reasons, retrograde conduction can still occur in the presence of advanced anterograde AV block. The reverse can also occur. Some electrocardiographers use the term *advanced* or *high-grade heart block* to indicate blockage of two or more consecutive impulses.

First-Degree Atrioventricular Block

During first-degree AV block, every atrial impulse is conducted to the ventricles and a regular ventricular rate is produced, but the PR interval exceeds 0.20 second in adults. PR intervals as long as 1.0 second have been noted and can at times exceed the P-P interval, a phenomenon known as *skipped P waves*. Clinically important PR interval prolongation can result from a conduction delay in the AV node (A-H interval), in the His-Purkinje system (H-V interval), or at both sites. Equally delayed conduction over both bundle branches can infrequently produce PR prolongation without significant QRS complex widening. On occasion, intra-atrial conduction delay can result in PR prolongation. If the QRS complex on the ECG is normal in contour and duration, the AV delay almost always resides in the AV node and rarely within the His bundle itself. If the QRS complex shows a BBB pattern, the conduction delay may be within the AV node or the His-Purkinje system (Fig. 68.6). In the latter case, a His bundle electrogram is necessary to localize the site of conduction delay. Acceleration of the atrial rate or enhancement of vagal tone by carotid massage can cause first-degree AV nodal block to progress to type I second-degree AV block. Conversely, type I second-degree AV nodal block can revert to a first-degree block with deceleration of the sinus rate.

Second-Degree Atrioventricular Block

Blocking of some atrial impulses conducted to the ventricle at a time when physiologic interference is not involved defines second-degree AV block (Figs. 68.7 to 68.9; eFig. 68.4). The nonconducted

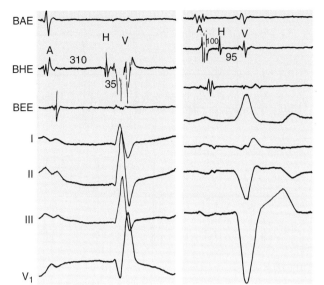

FIGURE 68.6 First-degree atrioventricular (AV) block. One complex during sinus rhythm is shown. **Left,** The PR interval measured 370 msec (PA = 25 msec; A-H = 310 msec; H-V = 39 msec) during a right bundle branch block. Conduction delay in the AV node causes the first-degree AV block. **Right,** The PR interval is 230 msec (PA = 39 msec; A-H = 100msec; H-V = 95 msec) during a left bundle branch block. The conduction delay in the His-Purkinje system is causing the first-degree AV block. *BAE,* Bipolar atrial electrogram; *BEE,* bipolar esophageal electrogram; *BHE,* bipolar His electrogram.

Ladder diagram of typical 4:3 atrioventricular Wenckebach cycle

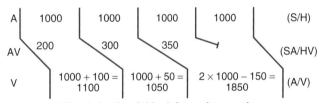

Wenckebach exit block from sinus node

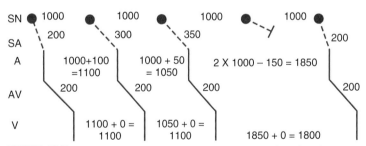

FIGURE 68.7 A, Ladder diagram of typical 4:3 atrioventricular Wenckebach cycle. P waves (A tier) occur at a cycle length of 1000 msec. The PR interval (AV tier) is 200 msec for the first beat and generates a ventricular response (V tier). The PR interval increases by 100 msec in the next complex, which results in an R-R interval of 1100 msec (1000 + 100). The increment in the PR interval is only 50 msec for the third cycle, and the PR interval becomes 350 msec. The R-R interval shortens to 1050 msec (1000 + 50). The next P wave is blocked, and an R-R interval is created that is less than twice the P-P interval by an amount equal to the increments in the PR interval. Thus the Wenckebach features explained in the text can be found in this diagram. If the increment in the PR interval of the last conducted complex increased rather than decreased (e.g., 150 msec rather than 50 msec), the last R-R interval before the block would increase (1150 msec) rather than decrease and thus become an example of an atypical Wenckebach cycle (see Fig. 68.8). **B,** If this were a Wenckebach exit block from the sinus node to the atrium, the sinus node cycle length (S) would be 1000 msec, and the SA interval would increase from 200 to 300 to 350 msec and culminate in a block. These events would not be apparent on a scalar electrocardiogram (ECG). However, the P-P interval on the ECG would shorten from 1100 to 1050 msec, and finally, there would be a pause of 1850 msec (A). If this rhythm were a junctional rhythm arising from the His bundle and conducting to the ventricle, the junctional rhythm cycle length would be 1000 msec (H) and the H-V interval would progressively lengthen from 200 to 300 to 350 msec, whereas the R-R interval would decrease from 1100 to 1050 msec and then increase to 1850 msec (V). The only clue to the Wenckebach exit block would be the changes in cycle length in the ventricular rhythm.

ARRHYTHMIAS, SUDDEN DEATH, AND SYNCOPE

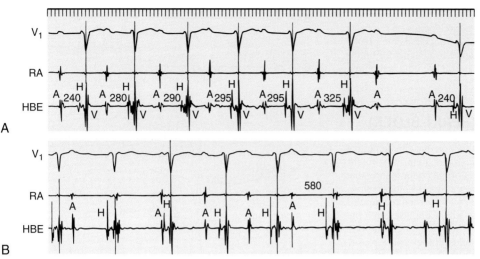

FIGURE 68.8 A, Type I (Wenckebach) atrioventricular (AV) nodal block. During spontaneous sinus rhythm, progressive PR prolongation occurs and culminates in a nonconducted P wave. From the His bundle recording (HBE), it is apparent that the conduction delay and subsequent block occur within the AV node (prolongation of the AH interval). Because the increment in conduction delay does not consistently decrease, the R-R intervals do not reflect the classic Wenckebach structure. **B,** Recorded 5 minutes after the intravenous administration of atropine, 0.5 mg. Atropine has had its predominant effect on sinus and junctional automaticity by this time, with little improvement in AV conduction. Consequently, more P waves are blocked and AV dissociation is present, caused by a combination of AV block and an enhanced junctional discharge rate. When atropine finally improved AV conduction (not shown), 1:1 AV conduction occurred. *RA,* Right atrium.

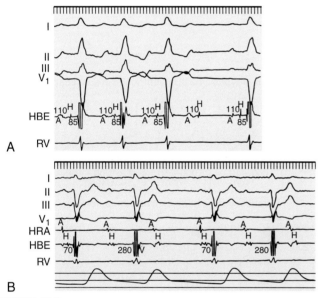

FIGURE 68.9 Type II atrioventricular (AV) block. **A,** The sudden development of His-Purkinje block is apparent. The A-H and H-V intervals remain constant, as does the PR interval. A left bundle branch block is present. **B,** Wenckebach AV block in the His-Purkinje system. The QRS complex exhibits a right bundle branch block morphology. However, note that the second QRS complex in the 3:2 conduction exhibits a slightly different contour from the first QRS complex, particularly in leads III and V$_1$. This finding is the clue that the Wenckebach AV block might be in the His-Purkinje system. The H-V interval increases from 70 to 280 msec, and then a block distal to the His bundle results. *HBE,* His bundle electrogram; *HRA,* high right atrium; *RV,* right ventricle.

P wave can be intermittent or frequent, can occur at regular or irregular intervals, and may be preceded by fixed or lengthening PR intervals. A distinguishing feature is that conducted P waves relate to the QRS complex with recurring PR intervals; that is, the association of P with QRS is not random. Electrocardiographically, typical type I second-degree AV block is characterized by progressive PR prolongation culminating in a nonconducted P wave (Figs. 68.8 and 68.9B), whereas in type II second-degree AV block, the PR interval remains constant before the blocked P wave (Fig. 68.9A). In both cases, the AV block is intermittent and generally repetitive. Frequently, the eponyms Mobitz type I and Mobitz type II are applied to the two types of block, whereas Wenckebach block refers to type I block only. Although Wenckebach

block in the His-Purkinje system in a patient with a BBB can closely resemble an AV nodal Wenckebach block, the site of Wenchekbach block most commonly occurs in the AV node (Fig. 68.9B).[8]

Certain features of type I second-degree block deserve special emphasis because when actual conduction times are not apparent on the ECG—for example, during SA, junctional, or ventricular exit block (see Fig. 68.7)—a type I conduction disturbance can be difficult to recognize. During a typical type I block, the increment in conduction time is greatest in the second beat of the Wenckebach group, and the absolute increase in conduction time decreases progressively over subsequent beats. These two features serve to establish the characteristics of classic Wenckebach group beats: (1) the interval between successive beats progressively decreases, although the conduction time increases (but by a decreasing function); (2) the duration of the pause produced by the nonconducted impulse is less than twice the interval preceding the blocked impulse (which is usually the shortest interval); and (3) the cycle that follows the nonconducted beat (beginning the Wenckebach group) is longer than the cycle preceding the blocked impulse. Although much emphasis has been placed on this characteristic grouping of cycles, primarily to be able to diagnose a Wenckebach exit block, this typical grouping occurs in fewer than 50% of patients with a type I Wenckebach AV nodal block.

Differences in these cycle-length patterns can result from changes in sinus pacemaker rate (e.g., sinus arrhythmia), neurogenic control of conduction, and in the increment of conduction delay. For example, if the PR increment in the last cycle increases, the R-R cycle of the last conducted beat can lengthen rather than shorten. In addition, because the last conducted beat is often at a critical state of conduction, it can become blocked and produce a 5:3 or 3:1 conduction ratio instead of a 5:4 or 3:2 ratio. During a 3:2 Wenckebach structure, the duration of the cycle that follows the nonconducted beat will be the same as the duration of the cycle that precedes the nonconducted beat.

Although it has been suggested that type I and type II AV block are different manifestations of the same electrophysiologic mechanism that differ only quantitatively in the size of the increments, clinical separation of second-degree AV block into types I and II serves a useful function, and in most cases the differentiation can be made easily and reliably from the surface ECG. Type II AV block often antedates the development of Adams-Stokes syncope[3] and complete AV block, whereas type I AV block with a normal QRS complex is generally more benign and does not progress to more advanced forms of AV conduction disturbance. In older people, type I AV block with or without BBB has been associated with a clinical picture similar to that seen in type II AV block.

In a patient with an acute MI, type I AV block usually accompanies inferior infarction (perhaps more often if a right ventricular infarction also occurs), is transient, and does not require temporary pacing, whereas type II AV block occurs in the setting of acute anterior MI, can require temporary or permanent pacing, and is associated with high mortality, generally as a result of pump failure. A high degree of AV block can occur in patients with acute inferior MI and is associated with more myocardial damage and a higher mortality rate than in those without AV block.

Although type I conduction disturbance is ubiquitous and can occur in any cardiac tissue in vivo as well as in vitro, the site of block for the usual forms of second-degree AV block can generally be determined from the surface ECG with sufficient reliability to permit clinical decisions without an invasive electrophysiologic study (EPS). Type I AV block with a normal QRS complex almost always takes place at the level of the AV node, proximal to the His bundle. An exception is the uncommon patient with type I intrahisian block. Type II AV block, particularly in association with a BBB, is localized to the His-Purkinje system. Type I AV block in a patient with a BBB can be caused by a block in the AV node or in the His-Purkinje system. Type II AV block in a patient with a normal QRS complex can be caused by an intrahisian AV block, but the block is likely to be a type I AV nodal block, which exhibits small increments in AV conduction time.

DIFFERENTIATION OF TYPE I FROM TYPE II SECOND-DEGREE ATRIOVENTRICULAR BLOCK

The preceding generalizations encompass most patients with second-degree AV block. However, certain caveats must be heeded to avoid misdiagnosis because of subtle electrocardiographic changes or exceptions.

1. 2:1 AV block can be a form of type I or type II AV block (Fig. 68.10). If the QRS complex is narrow, the block is more likely to be type I and located in the AV node, and one should search for transition of the 2:1 block to a 3:2 block, during which the PR interval lengthens in the second cardiac cycle. If BBB is present, the block can be located in the AV node or His-Purkinje system.
2. AV block can occur simultaneously at two or more levels and cause difficulty in distinguishing between types I and II.
3. If the atrial rate varies, it can alter conduction times and cause type I AV block to stimulate type II block or change type II AV block into type I. For example, if the shortest atrial cycle length that has just achieved 1:1 AV nodal conduction at a constant PR interval is decreased by only 10 or 20 msec, the P wave of the shortened cycle can block conduction at the level of the AV node without an apparent increase in the antecedent PR interval. An apparent type II AV block in the His-Purkinje system can be converted to type I in the His-Purkinje system in some patients by increasing the atrial rate.
4. Concealed premature His depolarizations can create electrocardiographic patterns that simulate type I or II AV block.
5. Abrupt transient alterations in autonomic tone can cause sudden block of one or more P waves without altering the PR interval of the conducted P wave before or after the block. Thus, an apparent type II AV block would be produced at the AV node. Clinically, a burst of vagal tone usually lengthens the P-P interval, as well as produces AV block.
6. The response of the AV block to autonomic changes, either spontaneous or induced, to distinguish type I from type II AV block can be misleading. Although vagal stimulation generally increases and vagolytic agents decrease the extent of type I AV block, such conclusions are based on the assumption that the intervention acts primarily on the AV node and fail to consider rate changes. For example, atropine can minimally improve conduction in the AV node and greatly increase the sinus rate, which results in an increase in AV nodal conduction time and the degree of AV block as a result of the faster atrial rate (see Fig. 68.8B). Conversely, if an increase in vagal

tone minimally prolongs AV conduction time but greatly slows the heart rate, the net effect on type I AV block may be to improve conduction. In general, however, carotid sinus massage improves and atropine worsens AV conduction in patients with His-Purkinje block, whereas the opposite results are to be expected in patients with AV nodal block. Similarly, exercise or isoproterenol is likely to increase the sinus rate and improve AV nodal block but worsen His-Purkinje block. These interventions can help differentiate the site of block without invasive study, although damaged His-Purkinje tissue may be variably influenced by changes in autonomic tone.

7. During type I AV block with high ratios of conducted beats, the increment in PR interval can be quite small and can suggest type II AV block if only the last few PR intervals before the blocked P wave are measured. Comparing the PR interval of the first beat in the long Wenckebach cycle with that of the beats immediately preceding the blocked P wave readily reveals the increment in AV conduction time.
8. The classic AV Wenckebach structure depends on a stable atrial rate and a maximal increment in AV conduction time for the second PR interval of the Wenckebach cycle along with a progressive decrease in PR lengthening in subsequent beats. Unstable or unusual alterations in the increment of AV conduction time or in the atrial rate, often seen with long Wenckebach cycles, result in atypical forms of type I AV block in which the last R-R interval can lengthen because the PR increment increases; such alterations are common.
9. Finally, the PR interval on the ECG consists of conduction through the atrium, AV node, and His-Purkinje system. An increment in H-V conduction, for example, can be masked on the ECG by a reduction in the A-H interval, and the resulting PR interval will not reflect the entire increment in His-Purkinje conduction time. Very long PR intervals (200 msec) are more likely to result from AV nodal conduction delay (and block), with or without concomitant His-Purkinje conduction delay, although an H-V interval of 390 msec is possible. The above discussion highlights the importance of measuring all intervals in an AV block series.

First-degree and type I second-degree AV block can occur in normal healthy children, and Wenckebach AV block can be a normal phenomenon in well-trained athletes, as noted earlier, probably related to an increase in resting vagal tone. On occasion, progressive worsening of the Wenckebach AV conduction disorder can result, and the athlete becomes symptomatic and needs to decondition. In patients who have chronic second-degree AV nodal block (proximal to the His bundle) without structural heart disease, the course is generally benign (except in older age groups), whereas in those with structural heart disease, the prognosis is poor and related to the type and severity of the underlying heart disease.

High-Grade Atrioventricular Block

High-grade, or "advanced," AV block is differentiated from complete AV block by an intermittent relationship between atrial and ventricular activity, yet conduction that is more impaired than in second-degree AV block. Some studies define high-grade AV block as Mobitz type II second-degree or third-degree AV block. The ventricular rhythm will not be regular since the diagnosis of high-grade AV block requires demonstration of intermittent AV conduction. Commonly, two or more consecutive non-conducted P waves are noted on ECG (Fig. 68.11). Etiologies include acute coronary syndromes, rheumatic heart disease, autoimmune disorders, myocarditis, and infiltrative cardiomyopathies.[8] The clinical presentation, symptoms, and outcomes are indistinguishable from third-degree AV block.

Third-Degree (Complete) Atrioventricular Block

Third-degree or complete AV block occurs when no atrial activity is conducted to the ventricles and therefore the atria and ventricles are controlled by independent pacemakers. Thus, complete AV block is one type of complete AV dissociation. The atrial pacemaker can be sinus or ectopic

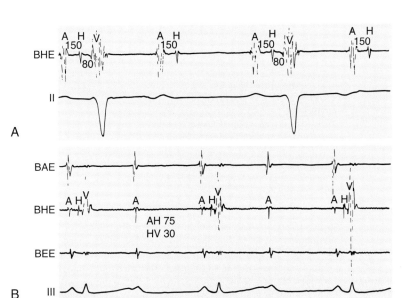

FIGURE 68.10 2:1 atrioventricular (AV) block proximal and distal to the His bundle deflection in two different patients. **A,** 2:1 AV block seen on the scalar electrocardiogram occurs distal to the His bundle recording site in a patient with a right bundle branch block and anterior hemiblock. The A-H interval (150 msec) and H-V interval (80 msec) are both prolonged. **B,** 2:1 AV block proximal to the bundle of His in a patient with a normal QRS complex. The A-H interval (75 msec) and the H-V interval (30 msec) remain constant and normal. *BAE,* Bipolar atrial electrogram; *BEE,* bipolar esophageal electrogram; *BHE,* bipolar His electrogram.

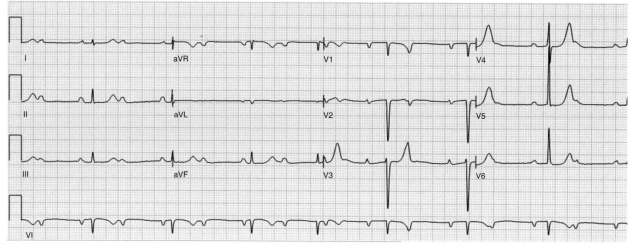

FIGURE 68.11 Electrocardiogram showing high-grade heart block. Sinus rate is 82 beats/min. The RR intervals are variable, indicating intermittent conduction and not complete heart block (QRS #4 and #5 have shorter preceding RR intervals compared with the others).

(tachycardia, flutter, or fibrillation) or can result from an AV junctional focus occurring above the level of block with retrograde atrial conduction. The ventricular focus is usually located just below the region of the block, which can be above or below the His bundle bifurcation. Sites of ventricular pacemaker activity that are in or closer to the His bundle appear to be more stable and can produce a faster escape rate than those located more distally in the ventricular conduction system. The ventricular rate in acquired complete heart block is less than 40 beats/min but can be faster with congenital complete AV block. The ventricular rhythm, usually regular, can vary in response to PVCs, a shift in the pacemaker site, an irregularly discharging pacemaker focus, or autonomic influences.[8]

Complete AV block can result from a block at the level of the AV node (usually congenital; Fig. 68.12), within the bundle of His, or distal to the His in the Purkinje system (usually acquired; eFig. 68.5).[8] Block proximal to the His bundle generally exhibits normal QRS complexes and rates of 40 to 60 beats/min because the escape focus that controls the ventricle arises in or near the His bundle. In complete AV nodal block, the P wave is not followed by a His deflection, but each ventricular complex is preceded by a His deflection (Fig. 68.12). His bundle recording can be useful to differentiate AV nodal from intrahisian block because the intrahisian may carry a more serious prognosis than the AV nodal block. Intrahisian block is recognized infrequently without invasive studies. In patients with AV nodal block, atropine generally speeds both the atrial and the ventricular rate. Exercise can reduce the extent of AV nodal block. Acquired complete AV block occurs most often distal to the bundle of His because of trifascicular conduction disturbance. Each P wave is followed by a His deflection, and the ventricular escape complexes are not preceded by a His deflection (see eFig. 68.5). The QRS complex is abnormal, and the ventricular rate is generally less than 40 beats/min. A hereditary form of conduction block caused by degeneration of the His bundle and bundle branches has been linked to the *SCN5A* gene, which is also responsible for LQT3 (see Chapter 63).

Paroxysmal AV block in some cases can be caused by exaggerated responsiveness of the AV node to vagotonic reflexes.[9] Surgery, electrolyte disturbances, myoendocarditis, tumors, Chagas disease, rheumatoid nodules, calcific aortic stenosis, myxedema, polymyositis, infiltrative processes (e.g., amyloidosis, sarcoidosis, scleroderma), and an almost endless assortment of common and unusual conditions can produce complete AV block. In adults, rapid rates may be followed by block (called *tachycardia-dependent* AV block), which is thought to result from phase 3 block (block caused by incomplete action potential recovery), postrepolarization refractoriness, and concealed conduction in the AV node. Less common than tachycardia-dependent AV block, *pause-dependent paroxysmal* AV block can also occur; it results in AV block after a pause or during relative bradycardia and thus can be difficult to distinguish from vagal AV block. This form of AV block is often referred to as a *phase 4 block* because it is thought that

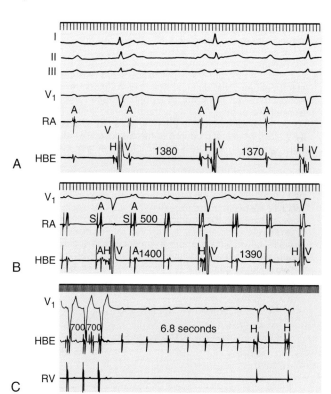

FIGURE 68.12 Congenital third-degree atrioventricular (AV) block. **A,** Complete AV nodal block is apparent. No P wave is followed by a His bundle potential, whereas each ventricular depolarization is preceded by a His bundle potential. **B,** Atrial pacing (cycle length of 500 msec) fails to alter the cycle length of the junctional rhythm. Still, no P wave is followed by a His bundle potential. **C,** After 30 seconds of ventricular pacing (cycle length of 700 msec), suppression of the junctional focus results for almost 7 seconds (overdrive suppression of automaticity). *HBE,* His bundle electrogram; *RA,* right atrium; *RV,* right ventricle.

spontaneous depolarizations during the resting phase of the action potential result in an inability to depolarize, although other mechanisms may also play a role.

In children, the most common cause of AV block is congenital (see Chapter 82). In such circumstances, the AV block can be an isolated finding or associated with other lesions. Neonatal autoimmune disease, from maternal antibodies crossing the placenta, accounts for most cases of heart block in utero or in the immediate neonatal period but only for rare cases of congenital heart block occurring after this period. Anatomic disruption between the atrial musculature and peripheral parts of the conduction system and nodoventricular discontinuity are two common histologic findings. Children are most often asymptomatic; however, in some children, symptoms requiring pacemaker implantation develop. Mortality from congenital AV block is highest in the neonatal period, is much lower during childhood and adolescence, and increases slowly later in life. Adams-Stokes attacks can occur in patients with congenital heart block at any age. It is difficult to predict the prognosis in an individual patient. A persistent heart rate at rest of 50 beats/min or less correlates with the incidence of syncope, and extreme bradycardia can contribute to the frequency of Adams-Stokes attacks in children with congenital complete AV block. The site of block may not distinguish symptomatic children who have congenital or surgically induced complete heart block from those without symptoms. Prolonged recovery times of escape foci after rapid pacing (see Fig. 68.12C), slow heart rates on 24-hour electrocardiographic recordings, and the occurrence of paroxysmal tachycardias may be factors predisposing to the development of symptoms.

Clinical Features

Many of the signs of AV block are evident at the bedside. First-degree AV block can be recognized by a long *a* to *c* wave interval in the jugular venous pulse and by diminished intensity of the first heart sound (S₁) as the PR interval lengthens (see Chapter 13). In type I second-degree AV block, the heart rate may increase imperceptibly with gradually diminishing intensity of S₁; widening of the *a* to *c* interval, terminated by a pause; and an *a* wave not followed by a *v* wave. Intermittent ventricular pauses and *a* waves in the neck not followed by *v* waves characterize type II AV block. S₁ maintains a constant intensity. In complete AV block, the findings are the same as those in AV dissociation (see later).

Significant clinical manifestations of first- and second-degree AV block usually consist of palpitations or subjective feelings of the heart "missing a beat." Persistent 2:1 AV block can produce symptoms of chronic bradycardia. Complete AV block can be accompanied by signs and symptoms of reduced cardiac output, syncope or presyncope, angina, or palpitations from ventricular tachyarrhythmias.

Management

For patients with transient or paroxysmal AV block and presyncope or syncope, the diagnosis can be elusive. Ambulatory monitoring (Holter or external loop recorders) can be useful, but monitoring for longer periods may be necessary, with extended (>3 weeks) Holter or external loop recorders being required. Longer periods of recording require an implantable loop recorder to establish the diagnosis. In patients with presyncope or syncope, one should suspect intermittent infrahisian block in those with BBB or an intraventricular conduction defect. An EPS to evaluate AV conduction thoroughly (including infusion of isoproterenol and/or procainamide) may be warranted to make the diagnosis, particularly in those with severe symptoms (see Chapter 61).

Drugs cannot be relied on to increase the heart rate for more than several hours to several days in patients with symptomatic heart block without producing significant side effects. Therefore, temporary or permanent pacemaker insertion is indicated for patients with symptomatic bradyarrhythmias. For short-term therapy, when the block is likely to be evanescent but still requires treatment or until adequate pacing therapy can be established, vagolytic agents such as atropine are useful for patients who have AV nodal disturbances, whereas catecholamines such as isoproterenol can be used transiently to treat patients who have heart block at any site (see earlier, Sinus Bradycardia). Isoproterenol should be used with extreme caution or not at all in patients with acute MI. The use of transcutaneous or temporary transvenous pacing is preferable. For symptomatic AV block or high-grade AV block (e.g., infrahisian, type II AV block, third-degree heart block not caused by congenital AV block), permanent pacemaker placement is the treatment of choice.[2,9] There is growing evidence that some patients with AV block, especially those with preexisting left ventricle dysfunction, may benefit from biventricular pacing rather than right ventricle–only pacing to prevent the development or progression of symptoms caused by heart failure.[10]

ATRIOVENTRICULAR DISSOCIATION

As the term indicates, *dissociated* or *independent* beating of the atria and ventricles defines AV dissociation. AV dissociation is never a primary disturbance of rhythm but rather is a "symptom" of an underlying rhythm disturbance produced by one of three causes or a combination of causes that prevents the normal transmission of impulses from atrium to ventricle. See the online supplement for content on AV dissociation (eFig. 68.6).

CLASSIFICATION

1. Slowing of the dominant pacemaker of the heart (usually the sinus node), which allows escape of a subsidiary or latent pacemaker. AV dissociation by default of the primary pacemaker to a subsidiary one in this manner is often a normal phenomenon. It may occur during sinus arrhythmia or sinus bradycardia and permit an independent AV junction rhythm to arise (see Fig. 68.1A).
2. Acceleration of a latent pacemaker, for example, a tachycardia in which the atria are not required and that usurps control of the ventricles. An abnormally enhanced discharge rate of a usually slower subsidiary pacemaker is pathologic and typically occurs during nonparoxysmal AV junctional tachycardia or VT without retrograde atrial capture (eFig. 68.7).
3. A block, generally at the AV junction, that prevents impulses formed at a normal rate in a dominant pacemaker from reaching the ventricles and allows the ventricles to beat under the control of a subsidiary pacemaker. Junctional or ventricular escape rhythm during AV block, without retrograde atrial capture, is a common example in which block gives rise to AV dissociation. Complete AV block is not synonymous with complete AV dissociation. Patients who have complete AV block have complete AV dissociation, but patients who have complete AV dissociation may or may not have complete AV block (see Fig. 68.11 and eFig. 68.5).
4. A combination of causes, as when excess digitalis results in the production of nonparoxysmal AV junctional tachycardia associated with SA or AV block.

MECHANISMS

With this classification in mind, it is important to emphasize that AV dissociation is not a diagnosis but a finding and is used in a manner similar to jaundice or fever. One must state that "AV dissociation is present and is caused by…" and then give the cause. An accelerated rate of a slower, normally subsidiary pacemaker and a slower rate of a faster, normally dominant pacemaker that prevents conduction because of physiologic collision and mutual extinction of opposing wavefronts (interference) or the manifestations of AV block are the basic disturbances producing AV dissociation. The atria in all these cases beat independently from the ventricles, under control of the sinus node or ectopic atrial or AV junctional pacemakers, and can exhibit any type of supraventricular rhythm. If a single pacemaker establishes control of both the atria and the ventricles for one beat (capture) or a series of beats (e.g., sinus rhythm, AV junctional rhythm with retrograde atrial capture [see eFigs. 68.4 and 68.5], ventricular tachycardia [VT] with retrograde atrial capture), AV dissociation is abolished for that period. Conversely, whenever the atria and ventricles fail to respond to a single impulse for one beat (PVC without retrograde capture of the atrium) or a series of beats (VT without retrograde atrial capture), AV dissociation exists for that period. Interruption of AV dissociation by one or a series of beats under the control of one pacemaker, anterogradely or retrogradely, indicates that the AV dissociation is incomplete. Complete or incomplete dissociation can also occur in association with all forms of AV block. Usually, when AV dissociation results from AV block, the atrial rate exceeds the ventricular rate. For example, a subsidiary pacemaker with a rate of 40 beats/min can escape in the presence of a 2:1 AV block when the atrial rate is 78 beats/min. If the AV block is bidirectional, AV dissociation results.

Electrocardiographic and Clinical Features

The ECG demonstrates the independence of P waves and QRS complexes. P wave morphology depends on the rhythm controlling the atria—sinus, atrial tachycardia, junctional, flutter, or fibrillation. During complete AV dissociation, both the QRS complex and the P waves appear to be regularly spaced without a fixed temporal relationship to each other. When the dissociation is incomplete, a QRS complex with a supraventricular contour occurs early and is preceded by a P wave at a PR interval exceeding 0.12 second and within a conductible range. This combination indicates ventricular capture by the supraventricular focus. Similarly, a premature P wave with retrograde morphology and a conductible RP interval may indicate retrograde atrial capture by the subsidiary focus.

Physical findings include a variable intensity of the first heart sound as the PR interval changes, atrial sounds, and *a* waves in the jugular venous pulse lacking a consistent relationship to ventricular contraction. Intermittent large (cannon) *a* waves may be seen in the jugular venous pulse when atrial and ventricular contractions occur simultaneously. The second heart sound can split normally or paradoxically, depending on the manner of ventricular activation. A premature beat representing ventricular capture can interrupt a regular heart rhythm. When the ventricular rate exceeds the atrial rate, a cyclic increase in intensity of the first heart sound is produced as the PR interval shortens, climaxed by a very loud sound (bruit de canon). This intense sound is followed by a sudden reduction in intensity of the first heart sound and the appearance of giant *a* waves as the PR interval shortens and P waves "march through" the cardiac cycle.

Management

Management is directed toward the underlying heart disease and precipitating cause. The individual components producing the AV dissociation, not the AV dissociation per se, determine the specific type of therapeutic, antiarrhythmic approach.

Autonomic/Neurally Mediated Bradycardia

Since the sinus node and AV node are richly innervated by the autonomic nervous system, both sinus bradyarrhythmias (sinus pauses, sinus arrest, and sinus arrhythmia) and AV block (typically type I AV block, or intermittent complete block) can be caused by autonomic influences without any underlying conduction system disease.[3] Increases in parasympathetic (vagal) tone can be triggered by a variety of events that can result in bradyarrhythmias and include hypersensitive carotid sinus syndrome, vasovagal syncope, cough syncope, stimulation of the Bezold-Jarisch receptors during an inferior MI, autonomic dysfunction, and others (see Chapter 71).[3]

Electrocardiographic Recognition

Neurally-mediated bradyarrhythmias are characterized most frequently by ventricular asystole caused by cessation of atrial activity as a result of sinus arrest or SA exit block (see Fig. 68.2). AV block is observed less frequently, probably in part because the absence of atrial activity from sinus arrest precludes the manifestations of AV block. However, if an atrial pacemaker maintained an atrial rhythm during the episodes, a higher prevalence of AV block would probably be noted. In symptomatic patients, AV junctional or ventricular escapes generally do not occur or are present at very slow rates, suggesting that heightened vagal tone and sympathetic withdrawal can suppress subsidiary pacemakers located in the ventricles, as well as in supraventricular structures.

Clinical Features

There are generally two types of neutrally mediated responses, and frequently both occur in the same patient to varying degrees. A *cardioinhibitory* response is generally defined as ventricular asystole exceeding 3 seconds, although normal limits have not been definitively established. In fact, asystole exceeding 3 seconds during carotid sinus massage is not common but can occur in asymptomatic subjects (see Fig. 68.2). A *vasodepressor* response is usually defined as a decrease in systolic blood pressure (SBP) of 50 mm Hg or more without associated cardiac slowing or a decrease in SBP exceeding 30 mm Hg when the patient's symptoms are reproduced.

Management

Atropine acutely abolishes cardioinhibitory responses to neurally mediated bradyarrhythmias. However, symptomatic patients with a cardioinhibitory response may benefit from pacemaker implantation. Because AV block can occur with a cardioinhibitory response, some form of ventricular pacing, with or without atrial pacing, is generally required. Atropine and pacing do not prevent the SBP decrease in the vasodepressor response, which may result from inhibition of sympathetic vasoconstrictor nerves and possibly from activation of cholinergic sympathetic vasodilator fibers. Combinations of vasodepressor and cardioinhibitory responses can occur, and vasodepression can account for syncope after pacemaker implantation in some patients. Patients who have neurally mediated bradyarrhythmias that do not cause symptoms require no treatment. Drugs such as digitalis, methyldopa, clonidine, and propranolol can enhance neurally mediated bradyarrhythmias and be responsible for symptoms in some patients. Elastic support hose and sodium-retaining drugs may be helpful in patients with vasodepressor responses.

REFERENCES

1. Rijnbeek PR, van Herpen G, Bots ML, et al. Normal values of the electrocardiogram for ages 16–90 years. *J Electrocardiol*. 2014;47:914–921.
2. Kusumoto FM, Schoenfeld MH, Barrett C, et al. 2018 ACC/AHA/HRS guideline on the evaluation and management of patients with bradycardia and cardiac conduction delay: a report of the American College of Cardiology/American Heart Association task force on clinical practice guidelines and the heart rhythm society. *Circulation*. 2019;140:e382–e482.
3. Bennett MT, Leader N, Krahn AD. Recurrent syncope: differential diagnosis and management. *Heart*. 2015;101:1591–1599.
4. Goldberger ZD, Petek BJ, Brignole M, et al. ACC/AHA/HRS versus ESC guidelines for the diagnosis and management of syncope: JACC guideline comparison. *J Am Coll Cardiol*. 2019;74:2410–2423.
5. Wilkoff BL, Miller RE. Exercise testing for chronotropic assessment. *Cardiol Clin*. 1992;10:705–717.
6. van de Vegte YJ, Tegegne BS, Verweij N, et al. Genetics and the heart rate response to exercise. *Cell Mol Life Sci*. 2019;76:2391–2409.
7. Brubaker PH, Kitzman DW. Chronotropic incompetence: causes, consequences, and management. *Circulation*. 2011;123:1010–1020.
8. Barra SNC, Providencia R, Paiva L, et al. A review on advanced atrioventricular block in young or middle-aged adults. *Pacing Clin Electrophysiol*. 2012;35:1395–1405.
9. Aste M, Brignole M. Syncope and paroxysmal atrioventricular block. *J Arrhythm*. 2017;33:562–567.
10. Tanawuttiwat T, Cheng A. Which patients with AV block should receive CRT pacing? *Curr Treat Options Cardiovasc Med*. 2014;16:291.

# 69 Pacemakers and Implantable Cardioverter-Defibrillators

MINA K. CHUNG AND JAMES P. DAUBERT

Cardiac implantable electrical devices (CIEDs) refer to implanted devices that deliver therapeutic electrical stimuli and include permanent pacemakers and implantable cardioverter-defibrillators (ICDs).

TYPES OF DEVICES

Electrical therapy for cardiac arrhythmias includes low-voltage (typically 1 to 5 V) pacing stimuli (pulses) and high-voltage (typically 500 to 1400 V) stimuli (shocks). Pacemakers deliver pacing pulses to treat bradycardia. ICDs deliver shocks to defibrillate ventricular fibrillation (VF) or to cardiovert ventricular tachycardia (VT). ICDs also have antibradycardia pacing functions that can deliver pacing pulses to treat bradycardia, as well as antitachycardia pacing functions that can deliver sequences of rapid pacing pulses to treat ventricular or atrial tachyarrhythmias. Cardiac resynchronization therapy (CRT) pacemakers (CRT-P) or ICDs (CRT-D) also provide electrical therapy for heart failure in the form of pacing pulses that resynchronize the ventricular contraction sequence. This chapter covers antiarrhythmic electrical therapy delivered by CIEDs. See Chapters 50 and 58 for CRT in the treatment of heart failure and devices for hemodynamic monitoring, and see Chapter 61 for devices implanted for rhythm monitoring.

DEVICE RADIOGRAPHY

Chest and occasionally abdominal radiography can help to identify the type, manufacturer, and integrity of implanted devices. Transvenous system pulse generators are typically located subcutaneously in the upper chest, though in pediatric patients, some older larger devices, or devices with leads inserted via the femoral vein or epicardially, the pulse generator may be in the abdomen. Pacemaker pulse generators are smaller than ICD devices (Figs. 69.1 and 69.2 and eFig. 69.1). Transvenous pacemaker leads are typically implanted with lead tips in the right ventricle and right atrium. Epicardial leads may be tunneled to the devices. ICDs are readily identified by the presence of defibrillation

coils on the leads (see Fig. 69.2). For CRT, leads may be placed in a left ventricular branch of the coronary sinus (Fig. 69.3) or on the LV epicardium. Some pacing leads are now being placed at the His bundle or deep septally from the right ventricle to capture the subendocardial left bundle branch conduction system (Fig. 69.4). Subcutaneous ICDs are typically placed subcutaneously in the left chest along the axillary line with leads tunneled subcutaneously (Fig. 69.5). Leadless devices can also be visualized radiographically (Fig. 69.6B).

TYPES OF PACEMAKERS

Conventional pacemaker components include a pulse generator (PG) that contains the battery and circuitry and the lead system. The lead system consists of one to three leads that are connected to the pacemaker PG via the lead pin. The lead body includes conducting wires that are surrounded by insulating material and connected to sensing and stimulating electrodes. The tip of the leads connect to the heart via an active (screw) or passive (e.g., tine) fixation mechanisms (Fig. 69.7). Conventional single-chamber systems have one lead that usually connect to the right ventricular (RV) endocardium or in some cases to the right atrium (RA). Dual-chamber systems usually have leads that connect to the right ventricle and RA (see Fig. 69.1). Cardiac resynchronization devices have a third lead that is placed to pace the left ventricle (LV) via a lead in a branch of the coronary sinus or implanted on the LV epicardial surface (see Fig. 69.3). (See Chapter 50.) Newer pacemaker configurations include leads intended to pace the cardiac conduction system, using leads placed at the His bundle or into the interventricular septum to capture the left bundle branch (see Fig. 69.4). Leadless pacemakers are also commercially available and include self-contained devices implanted via a catheter to the right ventricle (Fig. 69.6B). These provide single chamber pacing; algorithms that are designed to detect atrial contraction may be able to provide atrial synchronous pacing as well. Investigational leadless devices include right atrial or left ventricular components.

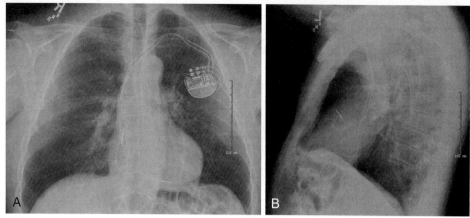

FIGURE 69.1 Chest radiograph of a dual-chamber pacemaker system. Posteroanterior (**A**) and lateral (**B**) projections demonstrate leads extending from the prepectoral pacemaker pulse generator to the right atrium and right ventricular apex.

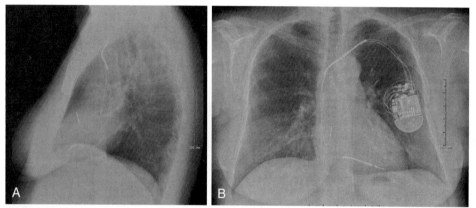

FIGURE 69.2 Chest radiograph of a dual-chamber implantable cardioverter-defibrillator (ICD) system. Lateral (**A**) and posteroanterior (**B**) projections demonstrate the ICD pulse generator in the left prepectoral region with a pacing lead extending to the right atrium and a pace/sense, dual coil defibrillation lead extending to the right ventricular apex. Defibrillation coils are evident in the brachiocephalic-superior vena cava and in the RV portions of the defibrillation lead.

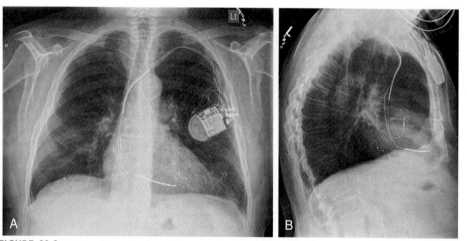

FIGURE 69.3 Chest radiograph of a cardiac resynchronization therapy defibrillator (CRT-D) system. Posteroanterior (**A**) and lateral (**B**) projections demonstrate the CRT-D ICD pulse generator in the left prepectoral region with a pacing lead extending to the right atrium, a pace/sense, dual coil defibrillation lead extending to the right ventricular apex, and a bipolar pacing lead extending to a left ventricular branch of the coronary sinus.

INDICATIONS FOR PACEMAKERS

Simply put, pacemakers are indicated for symptomatic bradycardia.[1] In the early pacemaker era such patients mainly had complete AV block with resultant intermittent asystole known as Stokes-Adams attacks.[2] In higher income countries, more pacemakers are implanted at present

for symptomatic sinus node dysfunction. Patients at high risk of complete atrioventricular (AV) block due to advanced, infranodal conduction system disease may also receive a pacemaker prophylactically.[3] There is a marked age-related pacemaker indication and implantation rate with an overall prevalence of pacemakers of 500/100,000 in the U.S. Medicare population (>65) but 40/100,000 for ages 18 to 64 and 2600/100,000 for age >75.[4]

PACEMAKER LEAD AND GENERATOR DESIGN

Transvenous pacing leads are insulated wires 6 to 8F (2.0 to 2.67 mm) in diameter that carry electrical signals between a pacemaker generator, usually in the prepectoral area (superficial to the pectoralis muscle) and the endocardial surface of the heart (see Fig. 69.7). Bipolar leads have a 1 to 2 mm metallic electrode tip and a slightly larger ring electrode situated about 10 to 15 mm proximally. The electrodes are made of polished titanium and platinum alloys. Unipolar leads, now used much less commonly, though occasionally used in coronary sinus or epicardial placement, have only the tip electrode and use the metallic pacemaker generator surface as the return electrode. The tip is secured to the myocardium with passive fixation (2 to 3 mm flexible polyurethane tines that embed in trabeculated myocardium) or active fixation (via a ~1 mm screw that secures) to the endomyocardium (Fig. 69.7A). Epicardial leads are used primarily in patients with congenital heart disease, tricuspid valve replacement, endocarditis, or in the pediatric age range (Fig. 69.7C). They either screw into or are sewn onto the epicardial surface; the generator resides in the abdominal wall or pectoral region. Ventricular leads comprise RV and coronary sinus LV leads. Epicardial leads can be used on any chamber's epicardial aspect. Leads are insulated with silicone and/or polyurethane and more recently polytetrafluoroethylene. Silicone is soft and flexible but needs to be thicker, has relatively high frictional surface resistance, and is prone to abrasions. Polyurethane is stiffer, more slippery, more durable, and can be made thinner but is prone to two forms of degradation, including environmental stress cracking (ESC) and metal ion oxidation (MIO).[2] Nearly all transvenous leads have a hollow lumen for a thin malleable stylet or wire to shape or advance the lead for implantation. In cross section the lead design can be coaxial with the wire to the tip electrode in the center surrounded by insulation then the ring electrode surrounded by additional insulation or co-radial with the two different (insulated) coils wound together around the central lumen (Fig. 69.7B). Passive fixation leads are generally placed in the RV apex. Active fixation leads can be secured anywhere in the RV or in the RA. Passive fixation atrial leads have a J shape and are placed in the RA appendage, with the tines intended to secure to the trabeculated myocardium there. The connection between the lead and the generator is via a terminal pin that usually conforms to the 3.2 mm diameter IS-1 standard at present, but other size and configurations still exist.[2] Attention to these details is critical when reoperating on patients with very old leads.

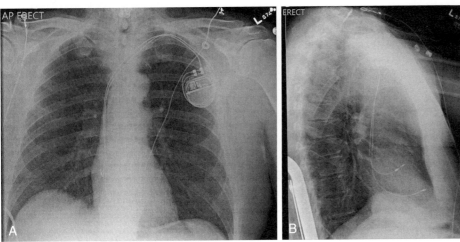

FIGURE 69.4 Chest radiograph of a dual-chamber pacemaker system with ventricular lead placed for left bundle branch pacing. Posteroanterior (**A**) and lateral (**B**) projections demonstrate pacing leads extending from the prepectoral pacemaker pulse generator to the right atrium and right ventricle with the tip inserted septally to achieve left bundle branch pacing.

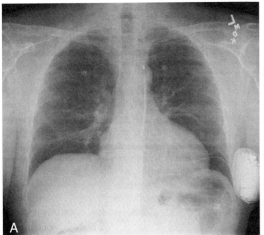

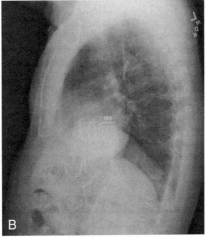

FIGURE 69.5 Chest radiograph of a subcutaneous implantable cardioverter-defibrillator (S-ICD) system. Posteroanterior (**A**) and lateral (**B**) projections demonstrate the ICD pulse generator in the left axillary region with a defibrillation lead tunneled subcutaneously to the left parasternal region.

Pacemaker generators are hermetically sealed titanium casings of varying shapes with a volume of ~10 to 15 cc housing the battery (typically lithium-iodine), sensing circuitry, activity sensors, hybrid circuit RF communication antenna, and logic boards (see eFig. 69.1). Glued to the generator is a clear epoxy header into which the leads are placed and secured using set screws.

CAPTURE AND SENSING

Capture and Stimulation

Modern cardiac pacemakers perform a number of functions, but their most critical two actions remain pacing and sensing. Pacing means delivering a small (compared with a defibrillation shock) electrical stimulus of ~1 to 5 V that captures a small myocardial region adjacent to the pacing electrode yielding a propagating wavefront in the chambers of interest (i.e., the atria or ventricles) (eFig. 69.2).

A pacing stimulus that fails to capture is subthreshold (eFig. 69.3). A stronger stimulus is required during the relative refractory period compared with electrically recovered tissue; cathodal versus anodal stimuli exhibit different characteristics, too.[5] Events leading to capture are complex when the three-dimensional structure and fiber orientation is taken into account with some stimuli leading to hyperpolarization versus depolarization occurring in adjacent regions.[2] Determinants of the threshold for a given pacing lead, above which "capture" occurs, include the stimulus strength (in voltage or current) and the pulse duration. An important relationship is Ohm's law ($V = IR$, where V is voltage, I is current, and R is resistance).

The strength-duration curve describes the relationship between pulse strength (usually voltage) and duration and whether capture occurs or not (Fig. 69.8). At an infinitely long pulse duration, practically estimated as about 1.5 to 2.0 msec, a minimal pulse strength (in V) eliciting capture is known as the rheobase. With shorter pulse durations, the threshold voltage (i.e., that required to capture) gradually and then abruptly increases at very short pulse durations (about 0.1 to 0.2 msec). The pulse duration at which the voltage threshold is twice the rheobase voltage is defined as the chronaxie. These concepts are important to understand threshold measurements, defining a safe margin for capture and optimizing battery longevity. Energy usage by pacing pulses are described by $J = VIt = V^2t(1/R)$ (where J is energy, V = voltage, I = current, t = pulse duration, and R = impedance). Monophasic pulses are used for pacing, whereas biphasic ones have advantages for defibrillation. Cathodal stimulation is used in pacing, so the distal electrode is the cathode. Pacing stimuli can be unipolar, wherein the return pole is the pacemaker generator housing or bipolar with an anodal ring electrode. Under certain circumstances, capture may occur at both sites (i.e., "anodal capture"). Of note, the capacitor-generated pulse declines over the course of the stimulus from a leading to a trailing edge voltage (see eFig. 69.2).

As illustrated in Figure 69.8, increasing the pulse width beyond about 1 msec provides little safety margin. Similarly, increasing the voltage at very short pulse durations (0.1 to 0.15 msec) is ineffective due to the steep ascent of the curve. Examining the energy curve (see Fig. 69.8) illustrates that the optimal combination of safety margin, and efficiency usually is found near the chronaxie.[2] Thresholds can be measured manually by reducing the voltage while maintaining the pulse width constant (or vice versa). A reliable electrocardiogram (ECG) is required to avoid prolonged loss of capture in device-dependent patients and correctly interpret the results for safety and battery longevity.

Thresholds are also measured automatically by most devices, in some or all chambers, usually by assessing for an evoked response indicating tissue capture, as distinguished from electrode polarization right after the pacing pulse (eFig. 69.3). The device can be programmed to adjust the pacing output to achieve a desired safety margin automatically. In some devices, capture is confirmed on a beat-to-beat basis and using a pacing output only slightly (0.125 to 0.5 V) above threshold. In other devices and/or chambers, once the threshold is measured, pacing is set at a programmable amount, often two times the threshold, and the threshold is measured one or more times a day. In the latter scenario, beat-to-beat capture, using an evoked response, is not determined. For some devices, when AV conduction is present, atrial threshold is measured automatically by ascertaining a conducted ventricular event. Alternatively, the native atrial response to a premature atrial test pulse can determine whether capture occurs. LV threshold can be measured by evaluating whether an RV event is sensed after an LV pacing test pulse.

Pacing thresholds frequently vary over time early after implantation. For active fixation leads, transient myocardial injury elicited by securing them produces an elevated threshold for minutes to hours.

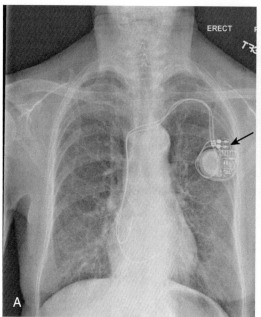
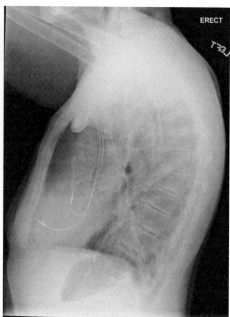
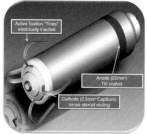
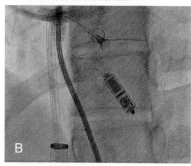
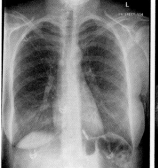
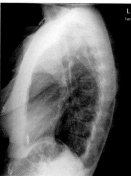

FIGURE 69.6 Transvenous and leadless pacemakers. A, Dual-chamber pacing system with bipolar right atrial active fixation and bipolar right ventricular active fixation leads with PA (*left*) and lateral (*right*) projections. The patient is post-TAVR, which resulted in complete heart block. Note the lead terminal pins (*arrow*) inserted into the pacemaker header and secured with set screws. Terminal pins have had several formats, but IS-1 is used predominantly for pacing leads now. **B,** Leadless cardiac pacemaker (*upper left panel*). *Lower left,* Insertion catheter has been decoupled from the leadless cardiac pacemaker after implantation and is being removed. An angiogram is usually performed through the catheter before implantation. *Right,* leadless cardiac pacemaker in PA and lateral projections in the right ventricular apex. *TAVR,* transcutaneous aortic valve replacement.

Inflammation at the electrode tissue interface leads to a subacute threshold rise resolving in about 6 weeks. However, the magnitude of this rise has been minimized with corticosteroid-eluting leads. Nevertheless, even with such leads, a fibrous capsule develops around the implanted electrode. Smaller electrodes display a higher impedance thus favorably reducing current drain (Ohm's law). However, they are more prone to threshold elevation and exit block due to the reactive fibrous cap. Electrode porosity, a fractal design in effect increasing the surface area, avoiding corrosion, and chemical composition are other important aspects of pacing electrode design.

Drugs, electrolyte perturbations, and metabolic changes also affect pacing thresholds (eTable 69.1). Severe hyperkalemia results in an elevation of pacing thresholds; significant hyperglycemia, severe hypothyroidism, and also acidosis or alkalosis can elevate thresholds. Some studies, but not all, have found that sodium channel blocking drugs (flecainide, propafenone, and others, as well as amiodarone) may elevate the pacing threshold as well. Acute ischemia and chronic infarction may also result in loss of capture.

Electrograms and Sensing Function in Pacemakers

Apart from pacemakers functioning in the asynchronous modes (VOO, DOO; see Table 69.1), pacemakers need to accurately detect underlying atrial and/or ventricular native signals in order to know whether to and when to deliver a pacing stimulus. A stable position abutting viable myocardial tissue makes this possible, but numerous challenges exist. Sensing is dependent on the electrogram (EGM) characteristics, including amplitude and frequency content, but also filtering within the device.

The EGM derives from the temporal change in the local voltage between the two electrodes (for a bipolar lead or between the tip electrode and the generator for a unipolar sensing circuit) as the activation wavefront travels toward and then away from the electrode(s).[6,7] For a unipolar lead, as the wavefront moves toward the electrode, a positive EGM is inscribed and crosses baseline when it reaches the electrode; a negative

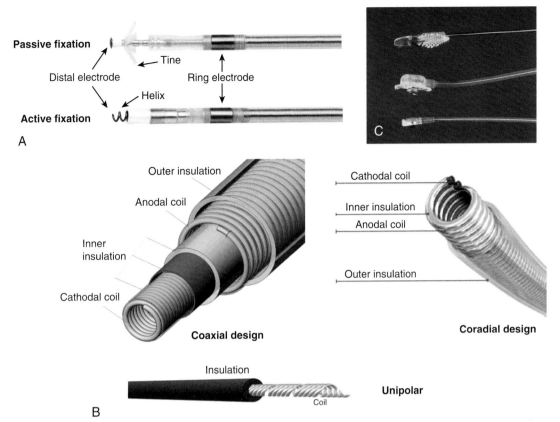

FIGURE 69.7 **Pacing lead design. A,** Lead fixation types. *Top,* Passive fixation (tined design) bipolar lead. *Bottom,* Active fixation bipolar lead with helical screw serving as distal electrode. Active fixation leads may have either extendable-retractable or fixed screws that are covered with mannitol that dissolves after several minutes in the bloodstream. **B,** Lead design types. *Left,* Coaxial leads have the distal or tip electrode (cathodal) coil on the inside with one or more layers of polyurethane or silicone insulation around the coil, the ring or proximal (anodal) electrode's coil wound around that inner insulation, and then another layer (or more) of outer insulation. *Right,* Coradial leads have the distal electrode and proximal electrode's coils individually insulated adjacent to each other and surrounded by one (or more) layers of outer insulation. *Bottom,* Unipolar leads are simple with the single electrode surrounded by insulation. **C,** Epicardial leads, which have puncture, screw-in, or sew-on fixation and contact mechanisms. They are used when endocardial leads are not feasible in certain types of congenital heart disease, young children, and after endocarditis or tricuspid valve replacement.

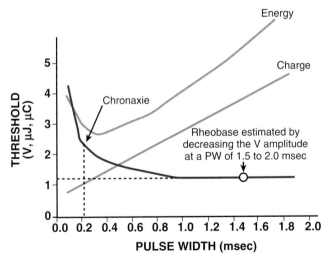

FIGURE 69.8 Strength-duration curve. The red curve displays the chronic, pacing threshold in volts (V), on the y-axis, from a canine at specific pulse durations (x-axis), known as the strength-duration curve. Capture occurs above and to the right of this curve. Also plotted are charge (μC), and energy (μJ) for the combination of voltage and pulse duration. Rheobase is the threshold at an infinitely long pulse width (PW) duration. Chronaxie is the pulse duration at twice the rheobase. (From Stokes K, Bornzin G. The electrode-biointerface stimulation. In Barold SS, editor: Modern Cardiac Pacing. Mount Kisco, NY: Futura; 1985, pp 33-77.)

TABLE 69.1 NASPE/BPEG Generic Code for Bradycardia Pacing

	POSITION			
	I	II	III	IV
Category	Chamber(s) paced	Chamber(s) sensed	Response to sensing	Rate modulation
	O = None	O = None	O = None	O = None
	A = Atrium	A = Atrium	T = Triggered	R = Rate modulation
	V = Ventricle	V = Ventricle	I = Inhibited	
	D = Dual (A + V)	D = Dual (A + V)	D = Dual (T + I)	
Manufacturers' designation only	S = Single (A or V)	S = Single (A or V)		

See text for explanation of use of the code.
BPEG, British Pacing and Electrophysiology Group; *NASPE,* North American Society of Pacing and Electrophysiology.
(Modified from Bernstein AD, et al. The revised NASPE/BPEG generic code for antibradycardia, adaptive-rate, and multisite pacing. Pacing Clin Electrophysiol 2002;25:260.)

signal is inscribed as the waveform moves away. With a bipolar lead the EGM is the difference between the two unipolar electrodes. Thus, the direction of the activation wavefront with respect to the bipolar pair influences the EGM size and shape, too. Bipolar leads in the ventricle sense the activation wavefront (commonly called the local R wave) but may also sense the repolarization signal (local T wave), and rarely the atrial activation event (e.g., if placed basally near the tricuspid annulus). Sensed signals vary in their timing, amplitude, and frequency content (eFig. 69.4). Thus, bandpass filters are used to reduce the likelihood of sensing the wrong electrical events. Sensing of T waves can to some degree be avoided with a high pass filter above about 15 Hz (i.e., excludes lower frequencies). Local atrial and ventricular signals exhibit frequencies in the 5 to 50 Hz range, and T waves and far-field R waves exhibit frequencies in the 1 to 10 Hz range (see eFig. 69.4). The timing of events can also be used to exclude certain signals and thereby avoid inappropriate sensing, for example, the ventricular blanking and refractory periods and the postventricular atrial blanking and postventricular atrial refractory period (eFig. 69.5). The signal from the lead undergoes amplification, filtering, and rectification and is then evaluated for whether it meets the sensing level programmed (see eFig. 69.5). Sensing in the atrial signals is more challenging due to the presence of large far-field ventricular signals. These far-field R waves exhibit a lower frequency range than the local atrial signal, as noted above. At implantation, P waves of about 1.5 mv or greater and R waves of 5 mv or greater are sought. Sensing thresholds for P waves thus are usually set at between 0.25 and 1.0 mv, and in the ventricle at about 2.0 mv. Setting the sensing threshold to a lower number *increases* the sensitivity reducing the chance of undersensing (but increasing the chance of oversensing). With unipolar leads, oversensing of pectoral myopotentials from the generator is a concern; in the ventricle this could lead to asystole in a pacemaker-dependent patient.

Hemodynamic Aspects of Pacing

Severe bradycardia and/or complete heart block with a junctional or ventricular escape adversely affects cardiac output. Instituting ventricular pacing at normal rates dramatically improves cardiac output by 25% to 30%. Restoring AV synchrony augments cardiac output still more by about 20%.[2] Studies in the 1980s demonstrated that chronotropic response was dominant in improving exercise capacity over AV synchrony.

Nevertheless, there are additional advantages of maintaining the AV relationship. When patients were randomized to different rate responsive modes, most preferred a mode that maintained AV synchrony (i.e., DDDR rather than VVIR).[2] Moreover, pacemaker syndrome occurs in 3% to 30% of patients who have ongoing sinus activity (i.e., not atrial fibrillation) when subjected to ventricular pacing. Its manifestations include fatigue, dyspnea, dizziness, neck pulsations, chest pain, and hypotension. It is most common when a fixed VA relationship is present, wherein the atrial contractions encounter closed AV valves. Dual-chamber as compared with single-chamber pacing leads to reduced occurrence of atrial fibrillation and of stroke and better quality of life in follow-up.[2]

For dual-chamber pacing the AV interval is of importance. Pacemaker syndrome can occur with a severely prolonged PR interval analogously to the problem with VA conduction alluded to above. On the other hand, too short of an AV interval or a marked interatrial conduction delay adversely affects performance. A hemodynamically optimal AV interval is typically about 150 msec at rest and somewhat less with exertion.[2]

The potential deleterious effects of RV pacing were initially obscured by the advantages of (1) any pacing over severe bradycardia, (2) AV sequential pacing over ventricular-only pacing, and (3) rate-responsive pacing over fixed-rate pacing. Although slightly reduced LV function occurs acutely, even in patients with normal ventricular function, RV pacing rarely exhibits clinically obvious adverse effects in the short term in such patients.[2] Elegant studies of direct His bundle stimulation clearly identified that both the contribution of atrial systole (by varying PR interval) and ventricular activation sequence (by comparing atrial-His bundle with atrial-RV) influenced ventricular function.

Clinicians became much more aware of the adverse effects of (right) ventricular stimulation on ventricular function, especially over the long term in the early 2000s. The ameliorative role of biventricular pacing (CRT) in treating LBBB-related ventricular dysfunction cemented this observation since conduction with LBBB resembles RV apical pacing. Studies comparing ventricular pacing to native ventricular activation, especially in those with LV systolic dysfunction, demonstrated significantly increased heart failure events.[2] The magnitude of the detriment with RV pacing worsened with greater QRS prolongation and worse baseline LV function.[2]

The adverse effects of RV pacing were initially attributed to the RV apex in particular. However, targeting alternative sites such as the septum actually proved somewhat elusive and led to minimal advantages.[8] Thus, algorithms emerged to limit RV pacing in dual-chamber pacemakers (as discussed later).[2] These algorithms sometimes fostered very prolonged AV intervals, however, with potential hemodynamic consequences akin to pacemaker syndrome and an increased tendency toward atrial fibrillation and pause-dependent arrhythmias.[2]

When ventricular pacing was unavoidable, as in AV block, achieving more physiologic ventricular activation has become important using either biventricular or His bundle or LBB-area pacing.[2,9,10,11]

His Bundle and Left Bundle Branch Area Pacing

Permanent His bundle pacing was reported in a small cohort in 2000. However, owing to the perceived technical difficulty, rudimentary tools, and frequently elevated thresholds, uptake was modest. The field has exploded since 2014 when a cohort study reported high procedural success rates and better outcomes than with conventional DDD pacing.[12] Dedicated sheaths and leads have eventually emerged and more improvements are expected.[9,13] An example is shown in eFigure 69.6. His bundle capture can be selective (see eFig. 69.6) or nonselective wherein local ventricular tissue is captured in addition to the His bundle.[14] The electrocardiography of His bundle pacing has been reviewed.[14] His bundle pacing is being used in advanced AV block but also when atrial pacing is needed with marked first-degree AV block to avoid worsening AV dyssynchrony. In addition, it has been used to correct LBBB leading to corroboration of concepts that BBB could be very proximal or even within the His bundle.[15] Elevated thresholds especially for correcting LBBB but even for His bundle capture in follow-up, and the potential for distal conduction system progression, have led to an iterative approach of targeting the LBBB, its fascicles, or the immediate region (eFig. 69.7).[16]

PACING MODE AND TIMING CYCLES

Definitions

The current convention for naming pacemaker modes stems from 2001 consensus between the North American Society for Pacing and Electrophysiology (NASPE) and the British Pacing and Electrophysiology Groups (see Table 69.1). This convention specifies that five positions describe the functionality of pacemakers. The first position lists the chambers paced (A, V, or both, D). The second similarly describes the chambers sensed. The third letter specifies the device's response(s) to sensed events. Position or letter IV specifies the presence or absence of rate response. Position V specifies the location or absence of multisite pacing (i.e., biatrial or biventricular pacing with at least two stimulation sites in each case).

Timing cycles, usually in msec, characterize the function of a pacemaker in different modes. Various periods, like a clock, run sequentially or simultaneously and specify what the pacemaker will do at the end of the period or during the period if another event occurs.

Common Pacing Modes

VOO is the simplest mode (Fig. 69.9A). From the first through third letter, respectively, the mode paces only in the ventricle, does not sense the atrium or ventricle (O), and behaves asynchronously (O). There is one timing clock, the ventricular escape interval. For example, for VOO 60 bpm, the ventricular escape interval is 1000 msec (60,000 msec/min/60/min = 1000 msec) (see eTable 69.2) Thus every 1000 msec the pacemaker delivers a ventricular pacing pulse (even if a native ventricular beat has occurred).

VVI implies pacing in the ventricle (V) and sensing in the ventricle (V), and if a sensed event occurs, the next scheduled pacing pulse is inhibited (I) (Fig. 69.9B). The sensed event resets the ventricular escape interval. This mode adds a ventricular refractory period, during which sensed events are ignored. This prevents double counting ventricular events or local T waves and falsely inhibiting pacing.

In most pacemakers, applying a magnet converts the function from VVI to VOO. Depending upon the manufacturer, model, and

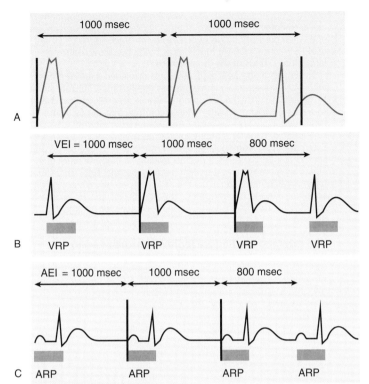

FIGURE 69.9 **Single chamber modes.** **A,** VOO mode. The device does not sense; it paces at a fixed rate even if intrinsic beats occur (third complex). **B,** VVI mode. The VVI timing cycle consists of a defined lower rate limit and a ventricular refractory period (VRP, *gray rectangles*). When the ventricular escape interval (VEI) from the ventricular sensed event of 1000 msec is completed, a paced event occurs. Because no ventricular sensed event occurs within 1000 msec after the paced event, a second ventricular paced event occurs. Because a ventricular sensed event occurs 800 msec later, a ventricular paced event does not occur. A VRP begins with any sensed or paced ventricular activity. **C,** AAI mode. The AAI timing cycle consists of a defined lower rate limit and an atrial refractory period (ARP, *gray rectangles*). When the atrial escape interval (AEI) from the atrial sensed event of 1000 msec is completed, a paced event occurs. Analogous to VVI mode.

programming magnet application may also change the pacing rate and/or initiate other temporary behavior (e.g., performing a pacing threshold test). The VOO mode is useful when oversensing is present as in a lead fracture or is anticipated due to electrocautery or other electromagnetic interference (EMI).

With respect to single chamber atrial pacing, AOO is analogous to VOO and AAI resembles VVI. In AAI, the device paces only in the atrium and senses in the atrium (Fig. 69.9C). In response to a sensed event, the next scheduled pacing pulse is inhibited, resetting the atrial escape interval. This mode, like VVI, has a refractory period, the atrial refractory period, during which sensed events are ignored. This prevents double counting atrial signals, or inappropriate sensing of far-field ventricular events that would falsely inhibit pacing. This mode is infrequently used due to the absence of ventricular support in the event of AV block.

Dual-chamber modes more than double the complexity. In DDD, the most commonly used one, pacing as well as sensing may occur in both the atrium and ventricle, as is evident from the first two letters (Fig. 69.10). The third letter indicates that both inhibition and triggered events occur depending upon the circumstances. DDD preserves AV synchrony where possible. Unlike VVI or AAI there is an upper rate limit in addition to a lower rate limit. The occurrence of pacing versus native activity in the atrium and in the ventricle depends on the programmed rate and AV interval compared with the native sinus rate and AV conduction characteristics. Timing can be based on either the atrium or the ventricle. The AV interval may be different for sensed atrial versus paced atrial events and may shorten with faster rates.

An atrial paced atrial event initiates a post-atrial ventricular blanking period to minimize the chance of the ventricular channel sensing the atrial pacing spike, also called crosstalk, and inappropriately inhibiting resulting in ventricular asystole in the setting of complete AV block. Since crosstalk may even occur after the 40 to 60 msec post-atrial

ventricular blanking period, DDD timing features a ventricular safety pacing interval (ending at about 100 to 110 msec after the atrial pacing spike). Should ventricular sensing occur between the end of the post-atrial ventricular blanking period and the end of the ventricular safety pacing interval (due to crosstalk, a premature ventricular complex [PVC], or very rapid native conduction), the device will V pace using an abbreviated AV interval (~100 to 110 msec). If the sensing in this interval was due to crosstalk, asystole is prevented. If the sensing was due to a PVC, the abbreviated AV interval seeks to pace early enough after a PVC to avoid an R-on-T event (eFig. 69.9). The post-atrial ventricular blanking tries to prevent crosstalk, while the safety pacing interval and function prevents asystole if crosstalk occurs. These blanking and safety pacing intervals don't exist after atrial sensed events. The chance for crosstalk can be reduced by using bipolar rather than unipolar atrial pacing, reducing the atrial output to an appropriate safety margin, using bipolar ventricular (rather than unipolar) sensing, decreasing the ventricular sensitivity (increasing the numerical value), and increasing the post-atrial ventricular blanking period duration.

The ventricular sensed or paced event initiates an atrial refractory period, the postventricular atrial refractory period (PVARP). PVARP seeks to prevent the atrial channel from sensing either the far-field ventricular event or retrograde atrial events initiated by the ventricular event or atrial tachyarrhythmias. As in VVI, a ventricular refractory period is present as well to prevent double counting.

The DDI mode is used much less often (eFig. 69.8). Unlike DDD, it does not exhibit atrial tracking. Thus, it can be useful in the setting of atrial oversensing to avoid inappropriate ventricular pacing. Another use of DDI is when there is intermittent atrial fibrillation but suboptimal atrial sensing prevents mode switching (in DDD); tracking of the AF is avoided in DDI. Operationally, in DDI, if the sinus rate is below the lower rate limit (LRL) the device will atrial pace at the LRL and then either native ventricular conduction will occur or the device will pace the ventricle at the conclusion of the AV delay. If the sinus rate is above the LRL the device will inhibit in the atrium; if AV conduction is absent it will pace the ventricle at the LRL (at a different rate than the atrium is firing, thus losing AV synchrony).

The VDD mode is adequate for patients with intact sinus node function but with AV block (see eFig. 69.8). However, should sinus bradycardia below the LRL develop, the device will pace the ventricle (only, as the initial letter implies) at the LRL losing AV synchrony.

Rate Responsive Pacing

Each of the aforementioned modes can function in a rate responsive fashion as well, provided the pacemaker generator has a sensor (or sensors) for rate adaptive pacing. As discussed above, the most important mechanism for increasing cardiac output with exercise is the capacity to double or triple the heart rate since stroke volume can only be increased slightly compared with rest. Most sensors attempt to detect motion by the patient, such as walking, via an accelerometer.

Limitations to the effectiveness of a motion-based sensor include the potential for a car passenger on a bumpy road or a patient with a tremor to experience a rate increase (worse with vibration sensors), or conversely, for a rock climber or cyclist (whose torso is moving little) to undergo negligible rate augmentation (e.g., with accelerometers). Consequently, numerous modalities have been attempted to detect the need for increased rate including respiratory volume change, catecholamine-induced increased myocardial contractility, the QT interval, pH, dP/dt, central venous temperature, oxygen saturation, peak endocardial acceleration as a measure of myocardial contractility, and RV lead impedance (correlated with contractility or inotropy). Of these, accelerometers are most widely used, with minute ventilation and RV lead impedance also in use.

For the single chamber modes (VOO, VVI, AAI, AOO), which do not have an upper rate limit and only an LRL, their rate-responsive forms (VOOR, VVIR, AAIR, AOOR) now add an upper rate limit. When the patient is at rest, the device paces at the LRL. Otherwise the pacing rate

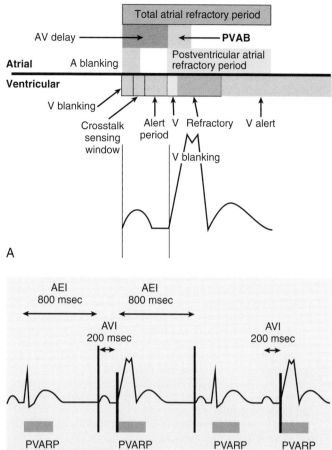

FIGURE 69.10 Basic DDD timing cycle and operation. A, The timing cycle in DDD. *Top,* Atrial channel. *Bottom,* Ventricular channel. Total atrial refractory period (TARP) is the sum of the AV delay and the postventricular atrial refractory period (PVARP). Postventricular atrial blanking (PVAB) is the time that the atrial channel is blanked after a ventricular event. "A blanking" is the atrial blanking period, representing the blanking period after an atrial event. There are two ventricular blanking periods, one after the atrial paced event, which prevents atrial paced events from being sensed on the ventricular channel, and one after the ventricular event. A ventricular sensed event in the crosstalk sensing window will result in safety pacing. There are two ventricular alert periods, one at the end of the AV delay and one after the ventricular refractory period. **B,** Operation of DDD mode. Because an intrinsic atrial event occurs and is followed by an intrinsic ventricular event within the AV interval, no ventricular pacing occurs in the first beat. In ventricular-based timing, the time from a ventricular paced or sensed event to the next atrial paced event is called the atrial escape interval (AEI), which is the lower rate limit interval minus the AV interval. Because no intrinsic atrial event occurs before the AEI times out, a paced atrial event occurs in the second beat. Since no intrinsic ventricular event occurs within the AV interval after this atrial paced event, a ventricular paced event occurs. Following this ventricular paced event an atrial paced event is delivered when the AEI times out 800 msec later to initiate the third beat. Since AV conduction follows this atrial paced event, ventricular pacing is inhibited. The fourth beat begins with an intrinsic atrial event that is not followed by an intrinsic ventricular event within the AV interval. Hence the intrinsic atrial event is "tracked" and followed by a paced ventricular event. See eFigure 69.8 for other timing cycles in DDD. The AV delay may vary for an atrial sensed or atrial paced event, at different rates (rate responsive AV delay), and to minimize RV pacing.

is determined by the sensor. The goal is the gradual increase in rate to match the activity and after return to rest a gradual (not immediate) decrease in rate to baseline. Sensor gain or function can be calibrated to the patient's specific physiology and activities with thresholds and response curves and other adjustments. Devices with dual sensor can use one to cross check the other or to blend the input from the two. For dual-chamber modes, already featuring an upper (tracking) rate limit, a second upper rate limit is defined for the sensor as well as the one for the maximum rate allowed in tracking the atrial rhythm.

Enhancements to the DDD Pacing Mode

Response to Atrial Tachyarrhythmias. When first devised, the DDD mode was highly problematic for patients with atrial tachyarrhythmias because atrial fibrillation would cause the device to abruptly pace at or

near the upper rate limit. This problem led to the development of an ability to detect the presence of atrial fibrillation (flutter or tachycardia) and when present "mode switch" to a non-tracking mode, DDI(R) (Fig. 69.11). Practically DDI(R) functions as VVI(R) but allows ongoing surveillance of the status of the atrial arrhythmia.

To achieve mode switching, atrial events needed to be identified even within certain refractory zones such as the PVARP. A minimal atrial rate to define the arrhythmia is programmable. The device switches back to tracking (DDD or DDDR) when it confirms that the tachyarrhythmia has ended.

A related issue is nonphysiologic noise detection and response. External electromagnetic interference, such as electrocautery, could be sensed as intrinsic cardiac rhythm leading to inappropriate inhibition, and in the pacemaker-dependent patient, asystole. Noise detection and rejection algorithms can allow the device to pace asynchronously in this scenario; if noise is anticipated, the pacemaker can be programmed to an asynchronous mode (DOO, VOO, or AOO) or a magnet could be applied.

The ADI Mode to Reduce Right Ventricular Pacing

While dual-chamber pacing restores AV synchrony, it exhibits the disadvantage of a tendency to pace the right ventricle, even in the absence of complete AV block. As compared with native sinus rhythm, when the atrium is paced, intraatrial conduction is prolonged, and at faster rates AV nodal conduction may be prolonged. These two factors tend to result in ventricular pacing, unless the AV delay is set to a nonphysiologic long setting. Lengthening the AV delay also compromises the upper tracking rate. The heightened focus on the detrimental effect of RV pacing led to the development of modes or algorithms to reduce RV pacing for patients with generally intact AV conduction. Initially, these algorithms consisted of a programmable increase in AV interval. When conduction is lost, pacing occurs at a shorter, more physiologic AV interval, and periodic testing for AV conduction occurs by lengthening the AV delay. However, these proved only moderately effective at reducing RV pacing. Instead new modes that functioned essentially as single chamber atrial pacing (AAI/AAIR) but with backup ventricular pacing in the event of temporary AV block were devised. These can be described in the BPEG naming convention as ADI/ADIR (Fig. 69.12). When persistent AV block develops, the device switches to DDD/DDDR. Some variation of their function among the different manufacturers exists.[17]

Choosing a Single- or Dual-Chamber Pacing Device

Randomized trials have established that dual-chamber pacing is superior in reducing the occurrence of atrial fibrillation and possibly stroke, though a reduction in mortality has not been proven.[2] Consequently a dual-chamber device is favored except when permanent atrial fibrillation is present. The recent availability of single chamber (ventricular) leadless pacemakers has led to a greater usage of these single chamber systems in some patients who would traditionally receive a dual-chamber device. Optimal leadless pacemaker candidates include those with increased infection risk, with limited vascular access, and who are expected to have a low (ventricular) pacing burden, as well as patients with minimal benefit from dual-chamber pacing due to advanced comorbidities or reduced activity.[18] In addition, leadless devices with some atrial tracking capability have been developed, although atrial pacing is not available yet.

Pacemaker Troubleshooting

With growing complexity of pacemaker systems, many suspected pacing abnormalities are eventually deemed normal function after evaluation. Nevertheless, device dysfunction does occur and can result in serious consequence. Potential malfunction should be evaluated thoroughly via a multimodality approach harnessing all potential resources, such as telemetry, multichannel electrocardiography, the device programmer, and knowledge of the programmed parameters including active device algorithms. Moreover, it is important to take into account the patient's location and potential external environment (EMI), radiography, stored device data, and provocative investigation such as pocket manipulation or arm movement. The most frequent

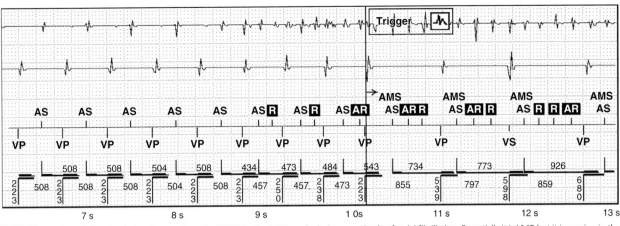

FIGURE 69.11 Mode switch. The device changes from the DDDR to the DDIR mode during an episode of atrial fibrillation. Essentially it is VVIR but it is sensing in the atrium to detect termination of the atrial arrhythmia. This mode prevents tracking an atrial arrhythmia at or near the upper rate. The top channel is the atrial electrogram. The second channel is the ventricular electrogram. The third channel is the marker channel. At the bottom the AA and VV intervals are shown horizontally and the AV intervals displayed vertically. The first five atrial events (AS) are sinus beats tracked with the programmed interval for atrial sensing (AS) and ventricular pacing (VP). Atrial fibrillation begins after the fifth atrial event with AS and AR (atrial refractory) events. Automatic mode switch (AMS) occurs when the number of rapid intervals is met. After AMS, in the DDIR mode, A events are not tracked, and the device exhibits VP or VS (ventricular sensed) events depending upon the conduction rate in atrial fibrillation and patient activity (for rate responsive pacing). When atrial fibrillation ceases, the device resumes atrial tracking (not shown).

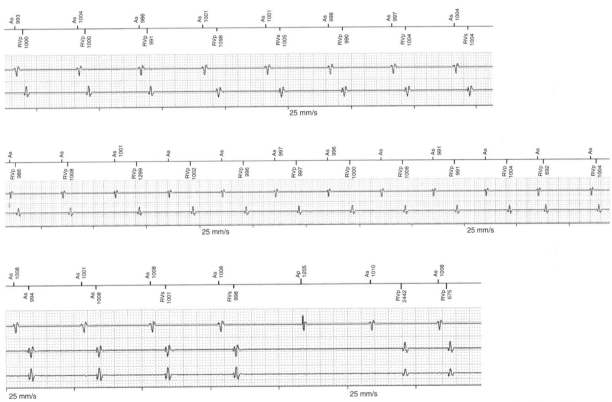

FIGURE 69.12 ADI mode or RV pacing minimization strategy. Marker channel, atrial, and ventricular electrograms from top to bottom in each panel. **Top panel,** AS-RVP (atrial sense-RV paced) occurs; the AV delay is lengthened automatically to try to allow native AV conduction and is successful in transitioning to AS-RVS (RV sensed) rhythm. **Middle panel,** AS-RVP rhythm is present; the AV delay is lengthened automatically to try to allow native AV conduction but is unsuccessful, so the AV delay shortens to the programmed interval for the DDD/DDDR mode in the last two beats. **Bottom panel,** Termination of ADI mode. AS-RVS rhythm is present but the native atrial event does not occur resulting in an AP (atrial paced event). AV conduction does not occur either, possibly due to increased vagal tone; after the next atrial event RVP occurs at the maximal allowed AV delay or maximal V-V interval depending upon the specific mode characteristics. In the last beat, there is resumption of DDD/DDDR mode with the programmed AV delay for that mode. After a programmable time interval, the device will attempt to search for native AV conduction again (as in top panel) by lengthening the AV delay (not shown).

issues are undersensing (eFig. 69.9), failure to capture, failure to pace, and pacing at an unexpected rate (Table 69.2).

Failure to Capture

Especially in the acute period after implantation, pacing lead dislodgement or elevation of threshold (to a value greater than the programmed value) will cause failure to capture (Fig. 69.13). Threshold elevation sometimes is mitigated by device-automated threshold determination and programmed output alteration. Lead fracture or other failure can cause loss of capture. Lead connection issues at the generator's header are also important to consider. Pathologic capture failure must be distinguished from physiologic capture failure that occurs when a pacing impulse falls in the refractory period, sometimes due to undersensing.

Failure to Pace

The flipside of failure to capture is failure to pace. Either can result in ventricular asystole. Failure to pace usually stems from oversensing, either of physiologic signals (P, R, or T waves), of noncardiac or external noise (EMI), of lead fracture, or from a loose header connection (Fig. 69.14). Advanced battery depletion or catastrophic device failure can cause loss of output, too. A special case of failure to pace, called cross-talk, is only possible in dual-chamber devices and is discussed above (eFig. 69.10).

TABLE 69.2 Common Causes of Pacemaker Problems

Failure to Capture
Pacing output below threshold
Changes at electrode-myocardial interface
Output programmed below threshold
Lead dislodgement
Lead insulation failure or conductor fracture
Connection problem between header and lead
Functional failure to capture (undersensing or asynchronous pacing)

Failure to Pace
Corrected by magnet or programming to asynchronous mode
Oversensing of physiologic or nonphysiologic signals
Not corrected by magnet or programming to asynchronous mode
Failure in the pulse generator
Lead conductor fracture
Connection problem between header and lead

Pacing at a Rate Not Consistent with Programmed Rate
Shorter-than-expected escape interval: undersensing
Longer-than-expected escape interval: oversensing
Battery depletion

Unanticipated Rapid Pacing
Pacemaker-mediated tachycardia
Inappropriate ventricular tracking of rapid sensed atrial rates, electromagnetic interference, or myopotentials
Sensor-driven pacing unrelated to patient activity

Unexpected Pacing at or Near the Upper Rate

Several conditions are prominent causes of pacing at or near the upper rate limit (eTable 69.3). One should recall that atrial fibrillation with a rapid, natively conducted ventricular response can result in rapid rates just as in patients without pacemakers. For rate responsive devices, unexpected activation of an accelerometer sensor can occur due to vibratory movement (e.g., transportation) or hyperventilation for minute ventilation devices. In dual-chamber devices, tracking nonphysiologic atrial arrhythmias, atrial lead noise (fracture or EMI), or pacemaker-mediated tachycardia are causes of unexpectedly rapid (ventricular) pacing. Tracking an atrial tachyarrhythmia may occur if mode switch is not programmed on, if the atrial arrhythmia is below the mode switch rate, or if the atrial arrhythmia is undersensed. A special example of the latter is when every other atrial flutter beat falls in the postventricular atrial blanking period. Rapid nonphysiologic signals due to atrial lead fracture can lead to tracking near the upper rate. Similarly, external electromagnetic noise detected by the atrial lead can produce rapid ventricular pacing.

Pacemaker-mediated tachycardia (PMT), or endless loop tachycardia, originates with a ventricular impulse (especially a PVC) that conducts retrogradely to the atrium, where it is sensed and thus triggers a paced ventricular beat at the expiration of the AV delay (eFig. 69.11). Subsequently, that ventricular-paced beat may again conduct retrogradely to the atrium and the "reentrant loop" continues. The ECG shows ventricular pacing at or near the upper rate limit, and retrograde P waves. PMT can be prevented by programming the PVARP to an interval longer than the observed VA conduction interval; in addition, PVARP extension can be programmed to occur for PVCs. Once begun, PMT termination algorithms function by omitting tracking for one atrial event. Applying a magnet will terminate it as well. PMT will not

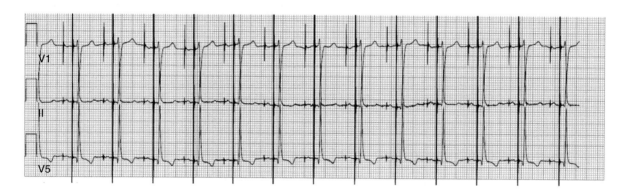

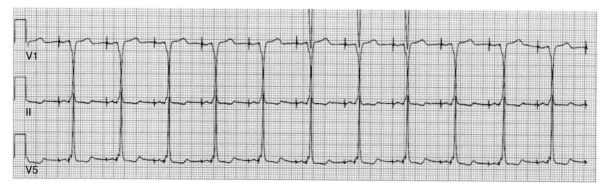

FIGURE 69.13 Failure to capture. Top panel, Unipolar atrial and ventricular pacing via epicardial temporary wires. There is atrial capture (P wave evident after first spike of each beat) but there is an isoelectric interval after the second spike followed by a native (narrow) QRS complex due to intrinsic AV conduction. The device was determined to be delivering ventricular stimuli below the capture threshold. **Bottom panel,** Atrial and ventricular capture after insertion of a permanent pacemaker (with bipolar pacing, note smaller stimulus artifact).

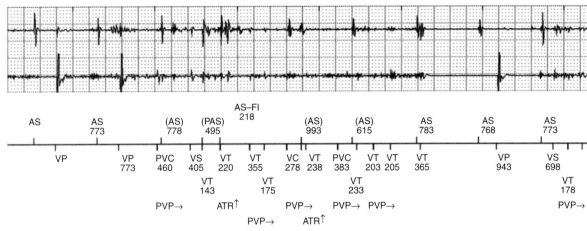

FIGURE 69.14 Failure to pace. The atrial electrogram is on top, ventricular electrogram below, and at the bottom is marker channel. AV block is present. The first two beats are atrial sensed (AS) and ventricular paced (VP). Noise is present on the atrial and ventricular electrograms due to electromagnetic interference or failure of both leads. The ventricular noise is sensed as VT inhibiting pacing output leading to a pause.

occur in the DDI mode since it is dependent upon atrial tracking, but it can occur in VDD, as well as DDD.

Non-reentrant ventricular-atrial synchrony, similar to PMT, also starts most commonly with a PVC that conducts retrogradely. However, due to timing and programming particulars, it falls in the PVARP. Atrial pacing then occurs at the LRL (or at the sensor indicated rate). However, in this scenario the atrial pacing pulse does not capture due to functional refractoriness from the preceding retrograde atrial activation. The sequence then repeats. It can be prevented by shortening the AV delay, reducing the PVARP and/or by reducing the lower rate, such as by inactivating rate-response pacing.[19]

Unexpected Drop in Pacing Rate
If the sinus rate exceeds the upper tracking rate in the setting of AV block, the pacing rate will fall. Dependent upon certain timing relationships (upper tracking rate [UTR], atrioventricular interval [AVI], PVARP), a phenomenon resembling AV Wenckebach or of 2:1 AV block can occur. Ideally, the UTR should be programmed high enough to avoid a drop in pacing rate with exercise. See Figure 69.15 for details.

Pacing-Induced Proarrhythmia
Pacing-induced proarrhythmia includes several subtypes (eFig. 69.12). The simplest form is an R-on-T ventricular pacing in the VOO mode triggering VT or VF. Any form of ventricular or atrial undersensing may allow pacing to trigger an arrhythmia. Even ventricular escape pacing at a low rate can rarely trigger ventricular tachyarrhythmias. A pause in pacing due to loss of capture during a threshold test or an RV pacing-minimization algorithm can initiate VT or VF by a short-long-short sequence. A pacing lead may mechanically trigger ectopic impulses, too. Competitive atrial pacing can trigger atrial tachyarrhythmias. Some manufacturers enable programming of a noncompetitive atrial pacing interval to minimize such events.

Pseudo-Malfunction
Numerous forms of pacemaker function can appear abnormal depending upon the type and amount of ECG data available, the presence or absence of marker channels, and the type of algorithms and programming in effect. ECG records may either suggest a pacing pulse is not present or fail to disclose one (bipolar pacing, dependent on lead vector, etc.). In-person threshold tests with loss of capture or change in rate may be noted on later review of telemetry as a possible abnormality. Similarly, automatic pacing thresholds or AV search algorithms may prompt concern when seen on a monitor strip.

IMPLANTABLE CARDIOVERTER-DEFIBRILLATORS
Types of ICDs
Like implanted pacemakers, conventional ICD components include a PG that contains the battery and circuitry, and a lead system. The PG is larger than those for pacemakers, as the device must contain a larger battery and capacitors capable of generating higher voltage shocks. Transvenous ICDs incorporate fully functional antibradycardic pacing. The lead system consists of at least one lead that has one or two defibrillating coils along with pace/sense electrodes, typically placed at the RV apex (Figs. 69.2 and 69.16). Dual-chamber ICDs include a pace/sense port that is usually connected to a lead placed in the RA, thus providing along with the RV lead, dual-chamber pacing capabilities. A third port for CRT can be connected to a pacing lead placed to pace the LV via a lead in a branch of the coronary sinus or implanted on the LV epicardial surface (see Fig. 69.3). Like pacing systems, newer pacemaker configurations may include a lead intended to pace the cardiac conduction system, using a lead placed at the His bundle or deep into the interventricular septum to capture the left bundle branch. Subcutaneous ICDs are also commercially available and consist of a PG typically placed subcutaneously in the left lateral chest connected to a subcutaneously tunneled sensing and defibrillation lead (Fig. 69.5).

Indications for ICDs
ICDs are indicated for prevention of sudden death from VT/VF, either as *secondary prevention* in patients who have been resuscitated from VT/VF or *primary prevention* in patients who have not had VT/VF but are at sufficiently high risk to warrant protection with an ICD.

Secondary Prevention
ICDs are the treatment of choice for secondary prevention of VT/VF, providing patients remain at risk for recurrence of VT/VF and have sufficient life expectancy and quality of life to justify implantation. The strong consensus for secondary prevention ICDs is based on randomized trials comparing ICD implantation to medical therapy for patients who survived cardiac arrest or hemodynamically significant sustained ventricular arrhythmias (Table 69.3). The largest trial, Antiarrhythmics Versus Implantable Defibrillators (AVID),[20] randomized 1016 patients who were resuscitated from near-fatal VF, sustained VT with syncope, or sustained VT with left ventricular

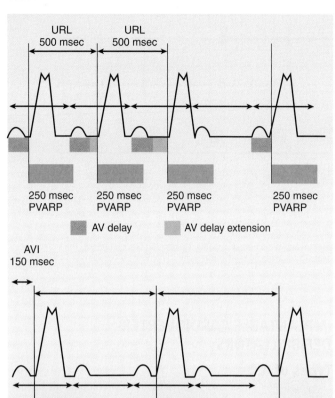

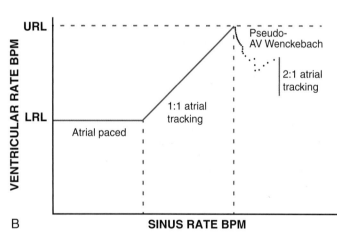

FIGURE 69.15 Upper rate limit behavior of dual-chamber pacemaker. A, *Top,* Pseudo-Wenckebach behavior occurs when the sinus rate exceeds the programmed maximum tracking rate but the P-P interval is longer than the total atrial refractory period (TARP, sum of atrioventricular interval [AVI] and postventricular atrial refractory period [PVARP]). *Bottom,* When the P-P interval is less than the TARP, every other P falls within the PVARP and therefore cannot be tracked. Thus the ventricular rate falls to half the atrial rate (2:1 atrial tracking). **B,** Response of DDD pacemaker *(ordinate)* as sinus rate *(abscissa)* increases. *BPM,* Beats per minute; *LRL,* programmed lower rate limit; *URL,* programmed upper rate limit.

ejection fraction (LVEF) of ≤40% and symptoms suggesting severe hemodynamic compromise due to an arrhythmia to ICD implantation or antiarrhythmic drugs (mostly amiodarone). Overall survival was significantly greater in the ICD group ($p < 0.02$).[20] The 2017 AHA/ACC/HRS Guideline for Management of Patients with Ventricular Arrhythmias and the Prevention of Sudden Cardiac Death[21] recommends ICD implantation in patients who survive sudden cardiac arrest due to VT/VF, hemodynamically unstable VT, stable sustained VT not due to reversible causes, or unexplained syncope with inducible sustained VT on electrophysiologic study, if meaningful

TABLE 69.3 Major ICD Trials for Secondary Prevention of Sudden Cardiac Death

TRIAL	YEAR	TOTAL N	RANDOMIZATION	MORTALITY OUTCOME WITH ICD
AVID (AVID Investigators)	1997	1016	ICD, Class III AAD (mostly amiodarone)	HR 0.62 ($p < 0.02$)
CASH (Kuck et al.)	2000	288	ICD, amiodarone, propafenone, metoprolol	HR 0.766 ($P = 0.081$)
CIDS (Connolly et al.)	2000	659	ICD, amiodarone	RRR 19.7% ($p = 0.142$)

AAD, Antiarrhythmic drug; *HR,* hazard ratio; *ICD,* implantable cardioverter-defibrillator; *RRR,* relative risk ratio.
See reference[20] for individual trials.

survival greater than 1 year is expected (Class I recommendation). An algorithm for secondary prevention of sudden cardiac death in ischemic heart disease is shown in Figure 69.17 and for nonischemic cardiomyopathy in Figure 69.18.

Primary Prevention
Several randomized clinical trials have provided indications for ICD implantation for primary prevention of sudden cardiac death (Table 69.4).[20] Clinical decisions for ICD implantation in ischemic or nonischemic cardiomyopathy are largely informed by three randomized clinical trials. The MADIT II trial of patients with ischemic cardiomyopathy and LVEF of 30% or less demonstrated significant survival benefit of an ICD[20] with survival benefit evident through 8 years of follow-up.[22] The SCD-HeFT trial of patients with LVEF of 35% or less and ischemic or nonischemic cardiomyopathy with NYHA functional Class II or III heart failure found that ICDs reduced total mortality.[20] MUSTT randomized patients with CAD and LVEF 40% or less with asymptomatic nonsustained VT to electrophysiology-guided therapy with antiarrhythmic drugs or ICD implantation versus no antiarrhythmic treatment; patients who received an ICD experienced reduced mortality.[20] However, retrospective analyses suggest that ICDs may not prolong life in identifiable subgroups with extensive comorbidities, including advanced heart failure and renal failure. Further, these trials were performed before present pharmacologic therapy and CRT for HF. A subsequent randomized controlled trial of patients with nonischemic cardiomyopathy and LVEF of 35% or less (DANISH trial) found that ICDs did not reduce total mortality in patients who received guideline-directed medical therapy (GDMT) and indicated CRT pacemakers, though sudden cardiac death mortality was reduced.[20]

Clinical trials do not support ICD implantation in low-LVEF patients within 40 days of myocardial infarction (MI) or 90 days of surgical revascularization; low-LVEF patients with recent percutaneous revascularization are not well represented in clinical trials.[20] With few exceptions,[23] ICD implantation in these patients is not indicated. Algorithms for primary prevention of sudden cardiac death in nonischemic and ischemic heart disease are shown in Figure 69.18 and Figure 69.19.

Expert consensus statements provide recommendations for ICD implantation in patients under specific circumstances not covered in clinical trials[23] and clinical scenarios not addressed by guidelines.[24] These include high-risk patients with less common diseases, including specific cardiomyopathies (e.g., hypertrophic cardiomyopathy; Chapter 54), ion channelopathies (Chapter 63), and certain forms of congenital heart disease (Chapter 82).

ICD LEADS AND GENERATORS
Defibrillation Leads
An ICD system comprises the generator and at least one defibrillation lead. Usually, the generator is implanted pectorally, and a single, transvenous defibrillation lead is implanted in the right ventricle (analogous to a ventricular pacemaker lead) (Fig. 69.20A, *left panel*). Dual-chamber

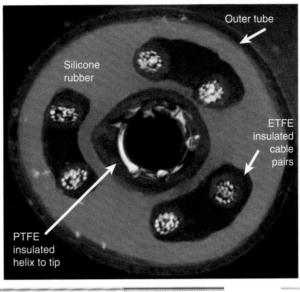

DF4 Dual Coil

B

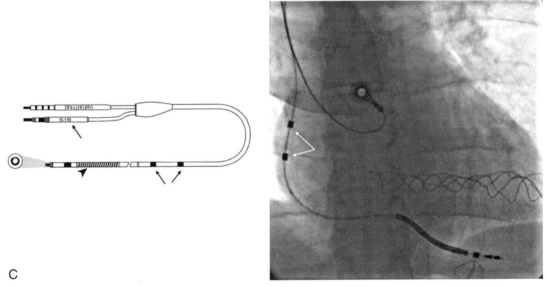

C

FIGURE 69.16 ICD leads. A, Cross section of transvenous ICD lead. *ETFE,* Ethyltetrafluoroethylene; *PTFE,* polytetrafluoroethylene. **B,** Dual coil lead *(arrows* to coils) with in-line modern DF4 header connection. **C,** RV lead with atrial sensing electrodes *(arrows)* and single defibrillation coil *(arrow head).*

ICDs incorporate a bipolar atrial pace-sense lead to provide dual-chamber bradycardia pacing and dual-chamber algorithms that discriminate supraventricular tachycardia (SVT) from VT. CRT-Ds incorporate an LV pacing lead (see Chapter 58). The totally subcutaneous[25] ICD system consists of a defibrillation lead implanted parallel to the sternum and tunneled to the ICD generator located near the left anterior axillary line (see Fig. 69.20B).

ICD Generators
ICD generators include a clear-plastic header that connects to the lead(s) and a titanium can that houses high-voltage electronics, in addition to the battery and other low-voltage components found in pacemakers (see eFig. 69.1B).

Unlike pacemakers, ICDs must deliver high-voltage shocks in addition to low-voltage pacing pulses. However, low-voltage batteries have approximately 1000 times the energy density of high-voltage capacitors. Thus, ICDs require a high-voltage transformer and charging circuit to convert electrochemical energy stored in an electrochemical cell (about 3 V) to the high voltage needed for defibrillation shocks (750

to 900 V for transvenous ICDs; 1400 V for subcutaneous ICDs). Unlike pacemaker batteries, ICD batteries must be able to deliver high current (up to 3 A) and high power (up to 10 W) to provide high-voltage electricity for shocks. The charging circuit requires 6 to 15 seconds for transvenous ICDs and 15 to 25 seconds for subcutaneous ICDs. During charging, high-voltage electricity is stored in a high-voltage capacitor. To deliver the shock, the high-voltage capacitor is disconnected from the charging circuit and connected to the shock electrodes.

ICD SYSTEM SELECTION

Dual- versus Single-Chamber Transvenous ICDs
In addition to providing dual-chamber bradycardia pacing, dual-chamber ICDs provide atrial EGMs that enhance physician interpretation of stored EGMs and permit both diagnostics for AF and dual-chamber algorithms to discriminate SVT from VT. The present

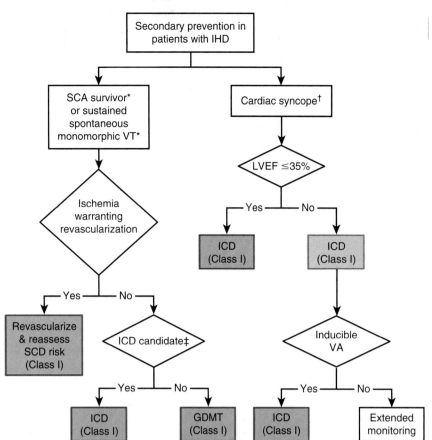

FIGURE 69.17 Secondary prevention of SCD in patients with ischemic heart disease. From 2017 AHA/ACC/ HRS Guideline for Management of Patients With Ventricular Arrhythmias and the Prevention of Sudden Cardiac Death: A Report of the American College of Cardiology/American Heart Association Task Force on Clinical Practice Guidelines and the Heart Rhythm Society. Colors correspond to class of recommendation per reference 21. *Exclude reversible causes. †History consistent with an arrhythmic etiology for syncope. ‡ICD candidacy as determined by functional status, life expectancy, or patient preference. *GDMT,* guideline-directed management and therapy; *ICD,* implantable cardioverter-defibrillator; *IHD,* ischemic heart disease; *LVEF,* left ventricular ejection fraction; *SCA,* sudden cardiac arrest; *SCD,* sudden cardiac death; *VT,* ventricular tachycardia.

consensus recommends reserving dual-chamber ICDs for patients who need dual-chamber pacing or have SVT and monomorphic VT at overlapping ventricular rates.[23]

Transvenous versus Subcutaneous ICD Systems

The subcutaneous ICD[25] eliminates morbidity associated with transvenous lead insertion, lead-related complications during MRI scans, and the hazards of transvenous extraction when lead removal is required. Candidates for a subcutaneous ICD undergo screening using surface ECG electrodes to assess the risk of T wave oversensing or R wave double-counting; 7% to 10% of candidates fail screening. Despite this, inappropriate shocks caused by oversensing are more common in subcutaneous ICDs than in modern transvenous ICDs (5% to 10% versus <2% in the first year).[25-27] Subcutaneous ICDs cannot perform ATP, resynchronization, or long-term bradycardia pacing. However, future models are expected to communicate with leadless capsule pacemakers. eTable 69.4 compares transvenous and subcutaneous ICDs.

TRANSVENOUS DEFIBRILLATION LEADS
Dual Versus Single Coil
Dual-coil leads improved defibrillation efficacy of early ICDs but do not provide a clinically significant advantage for left pectoral implants in present ICDs.[28]

They provide better defibrillation for some right-sided implants as well as reliable atrial cardioversion and alternate EGMs for diagnostic interpretation. However, the proximal coil often adheres to

the superior vena cava. If lead extraction is required, this increases procedural difficulty and may increase risk. Thus, single-coil leads usually are preferred for left pectoral implants in younger patients, but dual coils may be preferable for patients expected to have high defibrillation thresholds (e.g., patients with severe ventricular dysfunction or enlargement), although prediction of high defibrillation thresholds remains suboptimal.

Integrated Versus Dedicated Sensing Bipoles
Compared with dedicated bipolar leads, the integrated bipolar design simplifies the lead by reducing the number of conductors. However, reliable leads have been developed with both designs. Integrated bipolar EGMs have a wider field of view than dedicated bipolar EGMs and are thus more likely to oversense nonphysiologic signals or physiologic signals (such as myopotentials from the chest wall or diaphragm) that do not reflect local myocardial depolarization.[29]

ICD SENSING AND DETECTION
Sensing in ICDs is more challenging than for pacemakers given the top priority of treating lethal arrhythmias, especially VF, and thus needing to sense VF reliably. As discussed under pacemakers, simply increasing the sensitivity level (by decreasing the numerical value) poses a high risk of oversensing other signals, especially T waves. To meet both the goal of sensing potentially small and variable signals in VF along with avoiding sensing normal non–R wave signals (especially T waves), sensing is dynamically adjusted rather than using a constant level as in pacemakers (Fig. 69.21). After a sensed event, the sensitivity becomes greater until the next signal is sensed. The magnitude of the starting mV sensitivity level, after the absolute refractory period, varies on the basis of the most recent native signals but is often 50% to 75% of that value and declines, linearly, exponentially or in steps down to a programmed maximal sensitivity level, usually 0.3 to 0.5 mv. Sensing after pacing in some devices has a longer blanking period but then starts from a lower value to avoid undersensing.

The maximal sensitivity is programmable to various levels in different ICDs. In addition, some manufacturers offer other variations to enhance the ability to detect VF (such as a lower starting level or shorter initial sensing level or blanking period). Conversely, if oversensing of T waves is noted, a higher high-pass filter, longer period before sensing becomes more sensitive, or reduced maximal sensitivity are possible programming options that vary by manufacturer. One manufacturer uses a specific algorithm set that compares the differential of the filtered EGM, which magnifies the difference between R waves and T waves due to a higher slew rate (dv/dt) for R waves to allow pattern recognition of T wave oversensing that can inhibit therapy. Other algorithms try to recognize baseline noise and when noted, adjust the sensing floor to a less sensitive value to avoid myopotential oversensing. Any change in sensing function or decline in native signals can make underdetection of VF possible and consideration should be given to testing for sensing of induced VF.

Building on how a single signal is sensed, the detection of VT and VF can be described (Table 69.5 and Fig. 69.22). One or more zones of detection and therapy are programmable (eFig. 69.13). Within a zone, a rate range or cycle length range is defined. In addition a duration is programmed so as not to treat a nonsustained arrhythmia. All manufacturers use some form of probabilistic detection algorithm in the VF zone, since the marked variability in signal size and coupling interval often leads to some underdetection with some intervals thus falling out of the VF zone. The number of intervals is often specified as X of

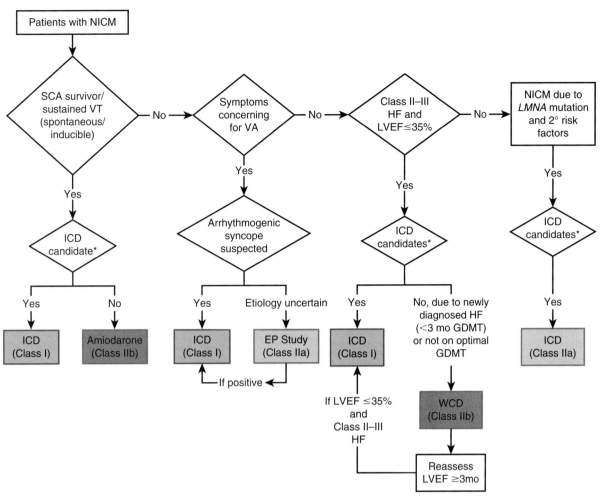

FIGURE 69.18 Secondary and primary prevention of SCD in patients with NICM. Colors correspond to class of recommendation per reference 21. *ICD candidacy as determined by functional status, life expectancy, or patient preference. 2° indicates secondary. *VA*, Ventricular arrhythmia; *WCD*, wearable cardiac defibrillator.

Y, for example 8 of 10 or 30 of 40 intervals for detection. This may or may not be programmable. One manufacturer requires a continuous string of fast beats in a VT zone; others use counters that increment or decrement if slower beats are detected. Each type of zone has its own strengths and weaknesses, requiring a sophisticated knowledge of the device and the patient's possible or likely arrhythmia characteristics. Once VT or VF detection criteria is satisfied, then therapy (ATP or charging for a shock) proceeds.

After the therapy is delivered, the device attempts to detect whether VT or VF is still present or if sinus rhythm has been restored (eFig. 69.14). Because the hemodynamic state deteriorates with longer VT or especially VF, and signals may become more attenuated, redetection criteria are usually a shorter number of intervals, and shocks may be committed to avoid inappropriately aborting therapy for VF.

In addition to rate-based (plus duration) detection criteria, other measures are possible for confirming the presence of VT or VF and differentiating it from SVT, AF, or abnormal sensing (eTable 69.5). These discriminators are considered in VT zones or sometimes in the slower portion of a VF zone but not for the fastest arrhythmias so as to avoid inappropriate withholding of therapy (eFigs. 69.15 and 69.16). In single-chamber devices, available criteria include EGM morphology, sudden onset, and regularity. Morphology criteria compare a previously obtained template of either the rate sensing or shock EGM to the tachycardia under consideration for therapy. If it is deemed to differ by programmable criteria, VT is declared or vice versa. Pitfalls can include aberration, noise on the morphology channel (from exercise for example), or suboptimal template capture. Sudden onset attempts to distinguish sinus tachycardia, which develops gradually, from VT that typically occurs abruptly. Drawbacks with this criterion include a VT that starts slower than the detection rate but then gradually accelerates to the detection rate and thus falsely being declared as SVT (sinus tachycardia). Regularity or stability seeks to identify atrial fibrillation as opposed to

most monomorphic VTs, which display regularity. Obviously polymorphic VT is also irregular, so this criterion should be disabled for fast arrhythmias.

In dual-chamber ICDs the atrial lead can be used to help diagnose the arrhythmia. First, atrial fibrillation can be diagnosed by rate-based criteria. Second, the rate in the ventricle and atria can be compared; if the former is faster, VT is diagnosed and treated. However, there can be undersensing in the atria due to blanking of atrial events during or after ventricular ones. VT, however, can exhibit a constant 1:1 retrograde conduction. The pattern or relationship between the A and V is used in some of these algorithms. The chamber initiating the tachycardia is a powerful diagnostic modality used in one family of devices.

Inappropriate shocks are painful, may lead to myocardial injury and hemodynamic effects, impair patient quality of life, and increase health care costs; when repetitive they may engender a posttraumatic distress syndrome. Rarely, inappropriate therapy can trigger VT or VF. Some but not all studies have identified a mortality signal associated with them. These facts led to research studies focusing on primary prevention patients comparing standard programming with novel programming using faster rate detection criteria and/or longer detection durations before therapy. These studies confirmed the benefit in reducing inappropriate therapy, the safety in doing so (lack of increase in mortality or syncope), and some found a reduction in mortality with the novel programming. Nevertheless, it is undoubtedly true that some patients may present with hemodynamically unstable or otherwise dangerous VT just below the cutoff zone, although such cases are relatively uncommon. Undersensing as well as the unintended function of some algorithms may impair VF sensing and detection that may be fatal. In programming tachycardia detection in

TABLE 69.4 Major ICD Trials for Primary Prevention of Sudden Cardiac Death

TRIAL (FIRST AUTHOR)	YEAR	N	DESIGN	POPULATION	TIMING	MORTALITY, HAZARD RATIO ICD
MADIT (Moss et al.)	1996	196	ICD versus conventional medical therapy	Prior MI; LVEF ≤35%; NSVT; inducible nonsuppressible sustained VT/VF at EPS	>3 wk post MI / >2 mo post CABG / >3 mo post PTCA	0.46 (p = 0.009)
MUSTT (Buxton et al.)	1999	704	Electrophysiology-guided therapy with antiarrhythmic drugs or ICD versus no antiarrhythmic treatment	CAD; LVEF≤40%; asymptomatic NSVT; Inducible sustained ventricular tachyarrhythmia	≥4 d post MI or revascularization	0.40 (p < 0.001)
MADIT II (Moss et al.)	2002	1232	3:2 ICD versus medical therapy	Prior MI LVEF ≤30%	>1 mo post MI / >3 mo post revasc	0.69 (P = 0.016)
SCDHeFT (Bardy et al.)	2005	2521	ICD versus amiodarone versus placebo	Ischemic or nonischemic cardiomyopathy, LVEF ≤35% NYHA FC II or III		0.77 (p = 0.007)
DINAMIT (Hohnloser et al.)	2004	674	ICD versus no ICD	Recent MI, LVEF ≤35%; ↓HRV or average HR ≥80 bpm	6-40 d post MI	1.08 (p = 0.66) Arrhythmic death 0.42 (p= 0.009)
IRIS (Steinbeck et al.)	2009	898	ICD versus no ICD	Recent MI, LVEF ≤40%, HR ≥90 bpm or NSVT	5-31 d post MI	1.04 (p = 0.78) SCD 0.55 (p = 0.049)
CABGPatch (Bigger et al.)	1997	900	Epicardial ICD versus no ICD with CABG	CABG, LVEF ≤35%, abnormal SAECG	At time of CABG	1.07 (NS)
CAT (Bansch et al.)	2002	104	ICD versus no ICD	Nonischemic, recent onset dilated cardiomyopathy	≤9 mo	NS
DEFINITE (Kadish et al.)	2004	458	Single chamber ICD versus medical therapy	Non-ischemic dilated cardiomyopathy, LVEF <36%, and PVCs or NSVT	-	0.65 (p = 0.08)
AMIOVERT (Strickberger et al.)	2003	103	ICD versus amiodarone	Nonischemic dilated cardiomyopathy, LVEF ≤35%, NSVT	-	NS
COMPANION (Bristow et al.)	2004	1520	1:2:2 optimal medical therapy, CRT-P, CRT-D	Ischemic or nonischemic cardiomyopathy, NYHA FC III or IV heart failure, QRS ≥120 msec, PR150 msec	HF hospitalization in preceding 12 mo	0.64 (p = 0.003) CRT-D versus medical therapy
DANISH (Kober et al.)	2016	556	ICD versus usual clinical care; 58% received CRT in both groups	Nonischemic cardiomyopathy LVEF ≤35%		0.87 (p = 0.28); SCD 0.50 (p = 0.005)

See reference[20] for individual trials.
CABG, Coronary artery bypass graft surgery; *CAD,* coronary artery disease; *CRT,* cardiac resynchronization therapy; *EPS,* electrophysiologic study; *HR,* heart rate; *HRV,* heart rate variability; *ICD,* implantable cardioverter defibrillator; *LVEF,* left ventricular ejection fraction; *MI,* myocardial infarction; *NS,* nonsignificant, *NSVT,* nonsustained ventricular tachycardia; *NYHA FC,* New York Heart Association functional class; *PVCs,* premature ventricular complexes; *SAECG,* signal-averaged electrocardiogram; *SCD,* sudden cardiac death; *VF,* ventricular fibrillation; *VT,* ventricular tachycardia.

ICDs, tachyarrhythmia duration detection criteria is recommended to allow the tachycardia to continue at least 6 to 12 seconds, or 30 intervals, to reduce therapies for both primary and secondary prevention ICD patients. Discrimination algorithms (see eFigs. 69.15 and 69.16) to distinguish SVT from VT are also recommended to include rates faster than 200 bpm and potentially up to 230 bpm unless contraindicated, to reduce inappropriate therapies. Furthermore, activation of lead failure alerts are recommended to detect possible lead problems.[30]

ICD THERAPY

General Considerations

Modern ICDs terminate ventricular arrhythmias by antitachycardia pacing and/or by one or more shocks. Except for VF, ATP is often used first, and if unsuccessful shocks are applied (up to five to eight before therapy is ceased). ATP is used preferentially because of the adverse effects of shocks discussed above. As discussed above, zones of therapy for detection are sometimes used (see eFig. 69.13), allowing differentiation of the degree of aggressiveness in diagnosis (longer or shorter detection) and in therapy (none, some to extensive attempts at ATP versus shocks only). Previously, low-energy shocks were used more often, but these result in a similar degree of discomfort and may have a higher propensity at inducing atrial arrhythmias, as well as being unsuccessful for VT or VF and thus requiring more than one shock. Smaller shocks do require a shorter time for charging, but this is infrequently a substantial concern with normal, modern ICD function. In single zone configurations, commonly called a VF zone, many of the actual arrhythmias treated are rapid monomorphic VTs that are amenable to ATP.

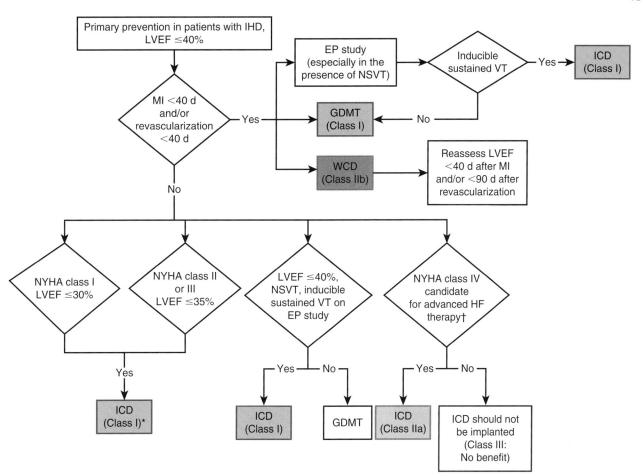

FIGURE 69.19 Primary prevention of SCD in patients with ischemic heart disease and LVEF ≤40%. Colors correspond to class of recommendation per reference 21. *Advanced HF therapy includes CRT, cardiac transplant, and LVAD. †Scenarios exist for early ICD placement in select circumstances such as patients with a pacing indication or syncope thought due to VT. These are detailed elsewhere in an HRS/ACC/AHA expert consensus statement. *MI,* myocardial infarction; *NSVT,* nonsustained ventricular tachycardia; *NYHA,* New York Heart Association. Other abbreviations are as in Fig. 69.17.

Antitachycardia Pacing

Antitachycardia pacing (ATP) differs from bradycardia pacing by the rate at which it is delivered and other aspects (Fig. 69.23). The underpinnings were established by Waldo and colleagues studying the interruption of atrial flutter using epicardial pacing wires after cardiac surgery.[2] To capture locally, at a rate even faster than the tachycardia (leading to relative refractoriness) as well as to penetrate the reentrant circuit, a higher output near the maximal pacing output is used (5 to 8 V), and a train of stimuli (usually 6 to 10) is used to progressively shorten the refractory period and allow access to the circuit. When effective, the ATP impulses enter the reentry circuit, travel in the antidromic direction, and collide with the previous impulse; meanwhile, the ATP impulse conducts in the orthodromic direction (same as during the tachycardia) but blocks due to greater refractoriness because the pacing rate is faster than the tachycardia. In addition to termination, the ATP could have no effect, accelerate the VT, or terminate and reinduce it. Thus, more than one sequence is often used, and if significant acceleration occurs, shocks are used. Two different protocols are commonly used, burst (having a constant cycle length within the train) and ramp (featuring a decrement in cycle length from beginning to end). Some studies have found ramp more effective but more prone to acceleration, and others found burst more effective. Programming more than two sequences has limited yield and delays definitive shock therapy. In single zone programming, only one ATP sequence is used.

For slower VTs, ATP is reportedly effective in 80% to 90% of events, with acceleration occurring 2% to 4% of the time. When applied to faster VTs (188 to 250 bpm), ATP has been reported to be successful for 70% to 80% of events with 2% acceleration. Prior studies had shown lower success rates and higher acceleration occurrences.[2] These success rates need to be interpreted in light of the VT duration before intervention since some VTs will self-terminate. In the MADIT-RIT study, treated VT above 200 bpm occurred half as often in the long duration arm than the conventional arm, implying self-termination occurred in many in the conventional arm, and for the episodes that persisted, the success of ATP appeared lower (58% versus 76%).[31]

In primary prevention, a single zone or two zones beginning at between 185 and 200 bpm is appropriate. A single ATP sequence is now often used to treat rapid MMVT (not VF) in single zone or in the VF zone. Current ATP programming recommendations are that for all patients with structural heart disease and ATP-capable ICDs, ATP should be active for all detection zones, including arrhythmias up to 230 bpm, with one ATP attempt, except when ATP has been documented to be ineffective or proarrhythmic.[30] Burst ATP is preferred to ramp ATP to improve termination rates of VT. For *secondary prevention* patients, when MMVT has been noted, two sequences of ATP may have added value in the fast VT zone, and two to three sequences in a slow VT zone for three-zone programming.[30]

Defibrillation and Cardioversion Shock Therapy

Although the risk of a shock inducing VF has been known since the 1700s and 1800s, the termination of VF by an electric shock was noted incidentally in the late 1800s and established in the 1930s by Wiggers and others.[32] Background work, by Gurvich in the USSR in 1939, established the supremacy of direct current (DC) shock over alternating current (AC) for terminating VF. It was appreciated in the West about 15 years later. Size constraints for implantable defibrillators led to use of a capacitor, and the high incidence of the tail end of the waveform reinducing VF led to truncation of the shock, based on work by John Schuder.

The mechanism of defibrillation has been debated since its demonstration, and theories have included transient incapacitation of the myocardium, halting the fibrillation in a critical mass of the myocardium (not necessarily the entire musculature), and termination of the reentrant rotors plus avoiding triggering new activation wavefronts leading to VF recurrence (Fig. 69.24).[33] Biphasic waveforms with a smaller or shorter second phase have supplanted monophasic waveforms due to lower defibrillation thresholds.[32,34]

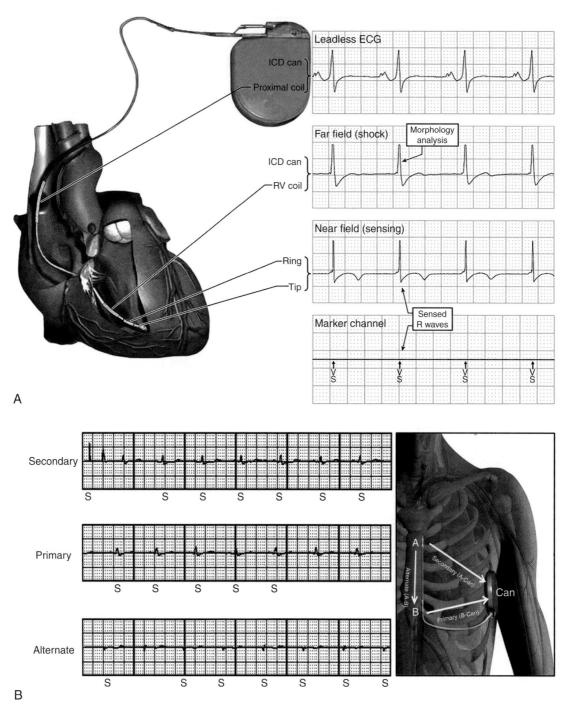

FIGURE 69.20 Implantable cardioverter-defibrillators and electrograms (EGMs). A, *Left,* Single-chamber ICD system, including left pectoral active can and right ventricle (RV) lead. *Right,* Telemetered EGM recorded between proximal coil and can ("leadless ECG"), high-voltage (shock) far-field EGM, and sensing near-field EGM, with annotated markers. The dual-coil lead uses true bipolar sensing between tip and ring electrodes. Marker channel denotes timing of sensed R waves from the near-field EGM *(arrows)* and ICD's classification of each ventricular event by letter symbols. "VS" denotes sensed ventricular events in the sinus rate zone. Sensing is accurate because there is a 1:1 correspondence between ventricular EGMs and markers. Morphology of shock EGMs stored during detected tachycardias is useful for distinguishing ventricular tachycardia from supraventricular tachycardia. Leadless electrocardiograms (ECGs) provide a signal with an identifiable atrial EGM with a single-chamber ICD if a dual-coil lead is used. **B,** Subcutaneous ICD records subcutaneous EGMs from one of three vectors. The amplitude of the alternate vector is smallest (as in this tracing) because it often overlies atrial tissue and the sternum. The secondary vector is prone to myopotential artifact because it usually overlies the pectoralis muscles. *S,* sensed ventricular events in the sinus rate zone. (From Swerdlow CD, Friedman P. Implantable cardioverter-defibrillator: clinical aspects. In Zipes D, Jalife J, editors: Cardiac Electrophysiology: From Cell to Bedside. 7th ed. Philadelphia: Saunders Elsevier; 2018.)

Defibrillation success rates with respect to shock size exhibit a probabilistic relationship with a sigmoidal shape, rather than a distinct threshold like myocardial capture with pacing (Fig. 69.25). Thus testing whether a given implanted lead and device would succeed in terminating VF at a given energy has proved challenging. In early decades, one or more tests involving induction and termination of VF were deemed mandatory to establish a margin of successful defibrillation. But to accurately understand the defibrillation success curve, multiple inductions are needed. Unfortunately, multiple conversions increase the risk of nonconversion, myocardial stunning, and embolization. Shortcuts with one or two inductions at levels sufficiently below the maximum output are moderately predictive of shock success for spontaneous events. An alternative or complementary approach to defibrillation threshold (DFT) testing is upper limit of vulnerability testing (eFig. 69.17). As leads, devices, and waveforms have improved, the likelihood of true defibrillation incapability for a transvenous system, especially left pectoral, is low. Consequently, studies were therefore performed to assess whether not testing after implantation would have inferior or similar outcomes to a limited confirmation of defibrillation efficacy. These studies have shown similar outcomes.[35] Currently, defibrillation testing is recommended in all patients undergoing an S-ICD implant, as DFTs are higher. Defibrillation testing may be reasonable to omit in patients undergoing left pectoral transvenous ICD implantation where appropriate sensing, pacing, and impedance values and well-positioned leads are confirmed by fluoroscopy.[30] For the patient at higher risk for elevated defibrillation, such as with a right pectoral implant or patients undergoing ICD replacements, particularly with older components, testing is reasonable.

In terms of shock energy, lower energies require slightly less charge time but result in similar degree of patient discomfort, so using a maximum energy shock as the first shock is reasonable and minimizes the duration of an episode and the need for more than one (painful) shock. Particularly with evidence that for most patients testing DFTs does not improve outcomes this approach has become more common. Devices can deliver five or more shocks in a given zone for a given episode, after which point more shocks offer negligible benefit. With biphasic shocks the order of the polarity can have some bearing on success, with the RV coil being the anode for the first phase tending to be superior in some studies. For one or more of subsequent shocks, that would only be given in the event of failure of prior shocks, it is typical to try a reversed polarity sequence. Defibrillation success is also influenced by metabolic and drug effects, as well as ischemia and hemodynamic decompensation.

ICD TROUBLESHOOTING

Ventricular Oversensing

In early ICDs, ventricular oversensing of rapid signals usually presented as inappropriate detection of VT/VF with delivered therapy or aborted shocks. In modern ICDs with enhanced sensing features, oversensing typically presents as oversensing alerts.

Oversensing can be classified by EGM morphology, temporal pattern (cyclic versus noncyclic), source type (physiologic versus nonphysiologic), and source location (intracardiac versus extracardiac) (eFig. 69.18). Signals that vary with the cardiac cycle (cyclic signals) indicate an intracardiac source. Nonphysiologic sources usually are extracardiac (e.g., EMI), except for those generated by intracardiac lead failures. Physiologic signals can be intracardiac (P, R, or T waves that cause one oversensed signal per cardiac cycle) or extracardiac (myopotentials). Specific sources can generate oversensed signals with characteristic features that differ from true cardiac EGMs in frequency content and amplitude.[29]

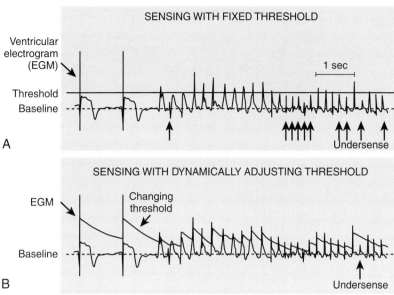

FIGURE 69.21 Fixed versus dynamic sensing threshold in VF. A, Fixed sensitivity requires that the sensed potential exceed a fixed threshold. Because of the highly variable amplitude during VF, undersensing occurs (arrows). If the threshold is lowered, T wave oversensing may occur. Note that the threshold is just above the T wave amplitude during sinus rhythm, first two complexes. B, Dynamic adjustment of sensitivity. At the end of the blanking period after each sensed (or paced) event, the sensing threshold is set to a high value. It then decreases with time until a minimum value is reached. Undersensing is diminished while still retaining a safety margin to prevent T wave oversensing. (Modified from Olson WH. Tachyarrhythmia sensing and detection. In Singer I, editor. Implantable Cardioverter-Defibrillator. Armonk, NY: Futura; 1994, pp 71-107.)

TABLE 69.5 Strategic Programming Principles for Shock Reduction*

PRINCIPLE	RATIONALE
Sufficiently long detection time	Do not treat self-terminating VT. AF with rapid ventricular rate is less likely to exceed the rate threshold for a longer detection time.
Fast VT detection rate in primary prevention patients and secondary-prevention survivors of VF	Do not treat slower tachycardias, which are more likely to be SVT.
SVT-VT discrimination	Do not treat SVT.
ATP in all VT/VF detection zones	ATP is painless. Even in the "VF" zone, most rhythms are monomorphic VT; many can be terminated by ATP.
Maximum shock strength†	Minimize unsuccessful shocks for VT, VF, or AF with rapid ventricular rate.
Enhanced sensing features	Minimize shocks for oversensing.

*Providing AV conduction is normal and discriminator is reliable.
†Adult patients.
AF, Atrial fibrillation; ATP, antitachycardia pacing; SVT, supraventricular tachycardia; VT, ventricular tachycardia.

Shocks: Diagnosis and Management

Minimizing shocks requires strategic programming, use of patient alerts, and remote monitoring. Once shocks occur, diagnosis and management tools include clinical data (history, chest radiograph), ICD diagnostics (e.g., lead impedance trends), and stored EGMs (Fig. 69.26).

Approach to the Patient with Shocks

Figure 69.27 summarizes a three-step approach to the patient who presents with a shock. First, analyze stored EGMs to determine if it was delivered in response to a tachycardia or oversensing. Second, if the shock responded to a tachycardia, determine if

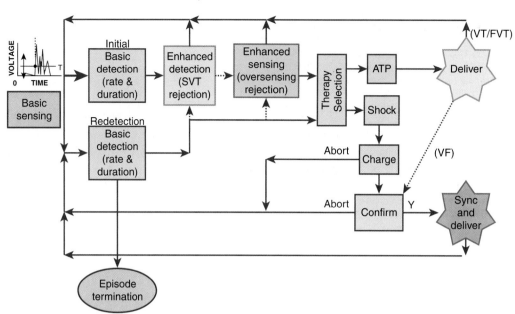

FIGURE 69.22 Overview of ICD detection algorithm. After initial basic (rate and duration) criteria are fulfilled, algorithms apply enhanced detection comprising supraventricular tachycardia–ventricular tachycardia (SVT-VT) discrimination, enhanced sensing features to detect and redetect VT, fast ventricular tachycardia (FVT), and ventricular fibrillation (VF). Enhanced sensing features may be applied either before intervals are counted or (as shown) after rate and duration are fulfilled. In the first case, oversensed signals are rejected, and only validated intervals contribute to the count. In the second case, episodes are classified specifically as oversensing events. Next, SVT-VT discriminators may classify the tachycardia as SVT; otherwise it is classified as VT/VF. When VT/VF is detected, antitachycardia pacing (ATP) is delivered immediately, but shocks require capacitor charging, which takes 6 to 15 seconds for maximum-energy. After charging is completed, ICDs perform a brief *confirmation* or *reconfirmation* process to determine if VT/VF is still present. The shock is delivered if VT/VF is reconfirmed; otherwise it is aborted. After therapy, ICDs monitor the rhythm for persistence of VT/VF or return to baseline. *Redetection* is the process by which ICDs determine whether VT/VF persists; typically it is less strict than initial detection. If VT/VF is redetected, the next programmed therapy is delivered. Simultaneously, ICDs monitor for a sufficient duration of slow intervals to fulfill the *episode termination* criterion, returning to the initial detection criteria. The VT/VF episode continues until either the ICD redetects VT or declares *episode termination*. *Y,* Yes. (Modified from Swerdlow C, et al. Sensing and detection with cardiac implantable electronic devices. In Ellenbogen KA, et al., editors. Clinical Cardiac Pacing, Defibrillation and Resynchronization Therapy. 5th ed. Philadelphia: Saunders; 2017.)

the rhythm is VT or SVT using established principles of ECG and EGM analysis. Third, determine whether an appropriate shock for VT/VF could have been avoided by either strategic programming (see Table 69.5 and eTable 69.6) or nondevice interventions (eTable 69.7).

Because shocks for VT/VF or rapidly conducted AF are associated with increased mortality over subsequent weeks to months,[2] the clinician should not only diagnose and treat the immediate precipitant of shocks but also consider treatments to reduce delayed mortality, including reassessment for HF and ischemia.

The approach to shocks delivered for oversensing is guided by the cause of oversensing. T wave oversensing was once a common cause of inappropriate shocks in transvenous ICDs (Fig. 69.28), but its frequency has been reduced by multiple sensing enhancements and programming options.[29] However, in subcutaneous ICDs, despite electrocardiographic prescreening, it remains the most common cause of oversensing, although a new filtering algorithm has reduced these events.[26,27] Shocks for SVT may be corrected by reprogramming (rate zones or SVT-VT discriminators) and treatment with beta blockers, antiarrhythmic drugs, or ablation. Most avoidable shocks for self-terminating VT may be prevented by strategic programming.

A patient with a *single shock* can be evaluated in person or by remote monitoring within 24 to 48 hours. In contrast, *repetitive shocks* constitute an emergency (see Fig. 69.27). The cause must be determined, and VT/VF detection may be disabled using a programmer or magnet. Repetitive shocks for VT/VF may be caused by multiple unsuccessful shocks for a single episode or recurrent VT/VF after successful shock termination ("VT storm"). Multiple or inappropriate shocks for AF or SVT with rapid rates, or detection of noise, requires prompt intervention for the underlying arrhythmia or malfunction and generally require emergent reprogramming of detection criteria or disabling of detection and hospitalization.

Treatment of VT storm includes reversal of precipitating events, beta blockers, and/or pharmacologic or ablative antiarrhythmic therapy. Neuraxial interventions may also be useful.[36] Causes include acute ischemia, exacerbation of HF, metabolic abnormalities (e.g., hypokalemia, amiodarone-induced hyperthyroidism), and drug proarrhythmia or noncompliance.

Unsuccessful Shocks

Table 69.6 summarizes causes of unsuccessful shocks. If an ICD classifies a shock for VT/VF as unsuccessful, stored EGMs should be reviewed to determine if the shock truly failed to terminate VT/VF or if the ICD misclassified effective therapy as ineffective (e.g., due to immediate arrhythmia recurrence). Because defibrillation success is probabilistic, occasionally shocks fail, but failure of two maximum-output shocks is rare if the safety margin is adequate. Shocks from chronic ICD systems may fail to terminate true VT/VF because of both patient-related and ICD system–related causes. Many patient-related causes can be reversed, but system-related causes usually require operative intervention. ICD data should be reviewed for clues to system-related causes, including excessive detection or charge times, evidence of lead or connection failure, mismatch between programmed and delivered shock strength, and out-of-range high-voltage impedance, suggesting a failure in lead components of the shock circuit. In the absence of a diagnosis, defibrillation testing should be performed.

Failure to Deliver Therapy or Delayed Therapy

Delayed therapy or failure to deliver therapy can be caused by sensing problems, programmed detection parameters, or ICD system malfunction. In modern ICDs, clinically significant undersensing of VF is rare but may be caused by low-amplitude EGMs, rapidly varying EGM amplitudes (see Fig. 69.28C), drug effects, post-shock tissue changes, and device-device or intradevice interactions.[29] Rarely, enhanced

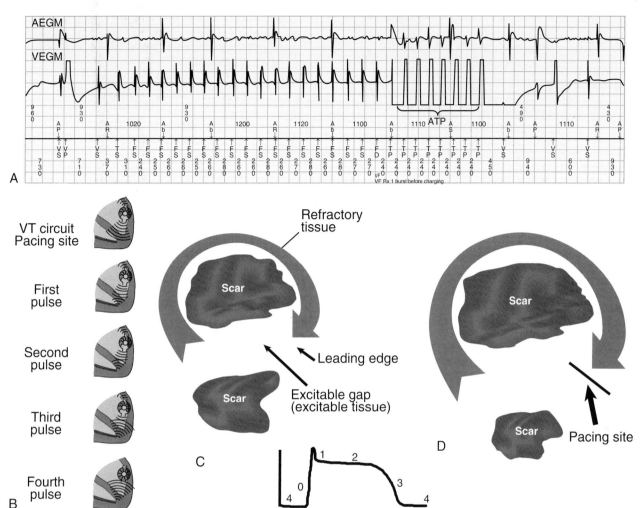

FIGURE 69.23 **Antitachycardia pacing (ATP) for monomorphic ventricular tachycardia (VT). A,** Stored atrial (AEGM) and ventricular (VEGM) electrograms and atrial and ventricular marker channels from an episode of rapid monomorphic VT (cycle length, 240 to 270 msec; rate, 220 to 250 beats/min). VT with AV dissociation begins with the second VEGM. After 18 intervals shorter than the programmed ventricular fibrillation (VF) detection interval of 320 msec, an adaptive train of eight ATP pulses is delivered at a cycle length of 240 msec, 88% of the VT cycle length, to terminate the VT. On the marker channel, VS, TS, and FS indicate intervals classified in the sinus, VT, and VF rate zones, respectively. FD, Detection of VF; TP, ATP. Note that a burst of ATP is delivered even though the intervals are in the VF zone. AP, Atrial paced events. "Ab" and "AR" indicate atrial intervals in the postventricular atrial blanking and refractory periods, respectively. **B,** Vertical panels show a conceptual model of why multiple ATP pulses are required in a train. *Top image* shows that during VT the region between the pacing lead in the right ventricular apex and the VT reentry circuit in the left ventricle is activated by the circuit. Subsequent images represent conditions after the first, second, third, and fourth ATP pulses. After each successive pulse, ATP propagates to more of the region before colliding with the VT wavefront. **C** and **D,** a conceptual model of the interaction between ATP pulses and the VT circuit. **C,** The circuit around a fixed scar is depicted by the *large curved arrow.* The head of the arrow depicts the leading edge of the wavefront, and the body of the arrow back to the tail (*gray*) represents depolarized tissue that is refractory because the wavefront has just propagated through it. The repolarized tissue between the tip and the tail of the arrow is excitable ("excitable gap"). For the head of the arrow to continue around the scar, an excitable gap must be present; if the wavefront encounters refractory tissue, it cannot proceed. **D,** A wavefront generated by an ATP pulse enters the excitable gap and terminates the VT. Tachycardias with a small excitable gap (i.e., the head of the arrow follows the tail very closely so that only a small "moving rim" of excitable tissue is in the circuit) are less likely to be terminated with ATP. (**B-D** from Hayes DL, Friedman PA, editors. Cardiac Pacing and Defibrillation: A Clinical Approach. 2nd ed. West Sussex, UK: Wiley-Blackwell; 2008.)

sensing features may classify VF as oversensing and withhold therapy. VF may be underdetected despite adequate sensing due to device inactivation or programming (sensitivity, rate, duration, SVT-VT discriminators). Lead, connector, or generator malfunction can also prevent shock delivery.

ICD Lead Failure: Presentation and Management

The serious consequences of ICD lead failure combined with reliability concerns for specific lead models have focused efforts on early diagnosis.[37] Excluding leads with known high failure rates, the overall incidence of clinical failure is about 1.3/100 lead-years.[38,2]

Clinical Presentations

Pace-sense malfunctions account for most failures. Oversensing is the most common initial electrical abnormality with either conductor

fracture or insulation breach.[37] Conductor fractures usually cause a characteristic pattern of oversensing[2] (Fig. 69.29). Unlike conductor fractures, insulation breaches themselves do not generate abnormal signals. Instead, oversensing occurs because external signals enter the conductor at the breach; EGM patterns vary, reflecting the source signal (see eFig. 69.18C and F). Several enhanced sensing features incorporate specific features of lead-related oversensing to alert patients and physicians and, in some cases, withhold inappropriate shocks[29,37] (see Fig. 69.28B).

Pacemakers and ICDs periodically measure DC electrical resistance ("impedance") of the pacing circuit. Usually, pacing impedance is in the normal range when oversensing occurs. Pace-sense malfunctions can also present with pacing impedance changes, loss of capture, or abrupt decrease in R wave amplitude. Pacemaker lead failures present identically to failures of ICD pace-sense components, except that oversensing causes only inhibition of pacing, not inappropriate therapy for VF.

Shock-component malfunction presents with shock-impedance changes, abnormal signals on shock EGMs, or failed defibrillation

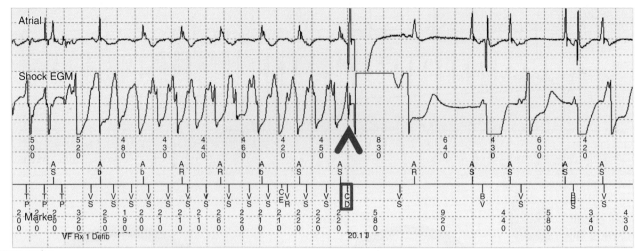

FIGURE 69.24 Dual-chamber EGM showing polymorphic VT with AV dissociation treated with shock. The atrial EGM, high-voltage ("shock") EGM, and dual-chamber marker channel are shown. The red arrowhead denotes shock, designated by *CD* (charge delivered) on the marker channel. After the shock, the atrial rhythm is sinus with premature atrial complexes; the ventricular rhythm is biventricular (BV) paced with premature ventricular complexes (PVCs) in the sinus rate zone (VS). The second BV beat (BV/VS) has a slightly shorter paced AV delay (110 versus 130 msec) than first BV beat because a PVC occurs during the AV delay and triggers "safety pacing," a feature that reduces crosstalk inhibition.

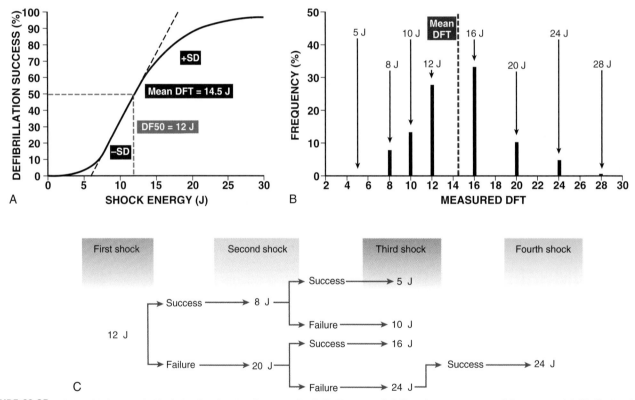

FIGURE 69.25 Relationship in an individual, simulated patient between the defibrillation probability-of-success curve and the measured defibrillation threshold (DFT) using a binary search protocol. A, Patient's defibrillation probability-of-success curve. **B,** Plot showing frequency of individual measured DFT values during repeated testing. **C,** Binary search sequence of three or four test shocks used to measure each DFT, starting at 12 J, the shock strength with a 50% probability of success (DF50). The process defined by the binary search protocol results in a single value, which the clinician records as the patient's "DFT." (Modified from Smits K, Virag N. Impact of defibrillation test protocol and test repetition on the probability of meeting implant criteria. Pacing Clin Electrophysiol 2011;34:1515.)

shocks. Insulation breaches that cause high-voltage short circuits may also cause ICD generator failure.

Impedance and Impedance Trends in Diagnosis of Lead Failure

Conductor fractures may cause abrupt increases in impedance; conversely, insulation breaches may cause abrupt decreases in impedance. eFigure 69.19 shows examples of pace-sense impedance trends in various conditions. Oversensing usually precedes impedance changes in pace-sense component failures, but impedance changes occur before or concurrently with oversensing in a minority of cases. When the cause of oversensing is in doubt, impedance abnormalities confirm the diagnosis of lead failure.

Fractures of high-voltage conductors can present as abrupt increases in shock impedance. Low shock impedance occurs in some high-voltage insulation breaches. However, diagnosing high-voltage insulation breaches by painless measurements of shock impedance is challenging because high-voltage shocks above the insulating material's dielectric breakdown voltage can cause catastrophic short circuits even if low-voltage test pulses encounter intact insulation.

Imaging

The chest x-ray film is unrevealing in most cases of lead failure, but it should be inspected for lead conductor discontinuity, kinks, or acute angles that identify stress points and twisting that suggests "twiddler's syndrome." It is important for excluding alternative causes of oversensing, such as lead dislodgement, abandoned leads, or lead fragments that cause a lead-lead interaction, and incomplete insertion of DF-1 pins into the header (eFig. 69.20A). Cinefluoroscopy in multiple views is more sensitive than chest radiography for identifying "inside-out" insulation breaches that cause cable conductors to protrude outside the outer insulation (externalized cables; eFig. 69.20B,D).[39,40,41]

Approach to the Patient

Figure 69.30 summarizes the approach to patients with findings suggestive of lead failure. All lead-failure diagnostics have false-positives, and the diagnosis of lead failure must be confirmed before surgical intervention to remove a failed lead.[37] Connection problems between the lead and header must be excluded (see eFig. 69.20A). System revision involves either abandoning or extracting the failed lead and inserting a replacement lead. Usually, lead abandonment is associated with lower procedural risk, and lead extraction with fewer long-term problems. The trade-offs depend on multiple factors related to the patient, expertise of the operator/institution, specific lead model, and patient preference.[37,39,40,41]

COMPLICATIONS

Complications can be broken down temporally into acute perioperative and delayed ones (eTable 69.8). Pacemaker and ICD complications are essentially the same with the exception of shock-related issues discussed above under ICD troubleshooting. Some complications are common to all CIED devices while others are unique to transvenous, leadless, or subcutaneous-type devices. While awareness and recognition of complications should be broadly known, techniques and knowledge for the minimization and avoidance of complications, equally important, are available elsewhere.[42,43]

Vascular Access Complications

Common vascular access complications for transvenous devices include pneumothorax, hemothorax, pocket hematoma, and more rarely inadvertent arterial access.[44,45] Pneumothorax occurs in about 1% of implants, is avoidable with the cephalic vein access approach, is minimized with the extrathoracic approach, is diagnosed with chest x-ray, and if large or symptomatic, is treated with a chest tube. Venous injury or other access site bleeding, including arterial cannulation or injury can cause a pocket hematoma or hemothorax. Inadvertent placement of the lead via the subclavian vein or via a patent foramen ovale (PFO) into the left cardiac chambers can lead to stroke. The lateral view on a post-implant chest x-ray is vital to exclude this complication. Acute or subacute subclavian vein thrombosis may lead to ipsilateral upper extremity swelling; it should be managed with elevation and anticoagulation.

Lead Placement Complications

Important complications related to lead placement include cardiac perforation, dislodgement, extracardiac stimulation, and lead terminal pin to header connection problems (see eTable 69.8). Cardiac perforation may present acutely or subacutely; likewise the manifestations may range from overt cardiac tamponade to pericarditis-related pain with a small effusion. Some perforations are only recognized years later having been seemingly occult, in which case the main problem is if extraction is needed for infection. Inadvertent nonmyocardial

stimulation can include the right phrenic nerve from a lateral RA lead, the left phrenic nerve from an LV lead, the diaphragm itself directly from an RV lead (usually perforated but rarely at high output without perforation), and the chest wall including intercostal muscles from possible perforation. Connection issues can present with unexpected pacing observations (such as ventricle first for lead connection reversal), abnormal impedances, noise and oversensing, and loss of capture. They unfortunately require repeat operation to rectify.

Pocket Hematoma and CIED Infections

Device infections include pocket infections and/or systemic presentations (including bacteremia, lead-associated endocarditis, and valvular endocarditis). Presentations of pocket infection vary considerably, including acute pain with pocket swelling due to inflammation and contained pus, subacute pain and inflammatory signs, chronic pain and induration, and generator (or lead) erosion. Infections may present from days to years after implant. Coagulase positive or negative staphylococci are the most common pathogens. Immediate preoperative antibiotics are considered mandatory as they have been shown to reduce infections. Pocket hematomas and repeat operation (such as for hematoma or other complication) markedly increase the risk of infection. Avoiding perioperative heparin, for example, by using uninterrupted warfarin or uninterrupted (or minimally interrupted) direct oral anticoagulant (DOAC) as opposed to heparin bridging reduces the risk of hematoma.[45,46] The management of either pocket infection or systemic infection requires full system removal, including lead extraction (eFig. 69.21).[41,40] Although bacteremia can occur without incurring lead-associated endocarditis, the latter is more common with staphylococci[47] or if vegetations are identified. Recently, an antibiotic-impregnated, dissolvable envelope was found to reduce the risk of device infection, whereas a trial evaluating pocket instilled and additional antibiotics was not superior to a single preoperative antibiotic dose.[48,49]

Subcutaneous ICD Complications

Vascular access complications (pneumothorax, cardiac perforation, etc.) do not pertain to subcutaneous ICDs.[25] Pocket infection occurred in 1.1% of implants in a large series,[26] but systemic infections have not been reported. A trend toward lower total infections was seen in the Praetorian trial compared with transvenous ICDs.[27] Inappropriate shocks have been reduced with new sensing algorithms but still run higher than for transvenous ICDs.[26,27]

Leadless Pacemaker Complications

Leadless pacemaker implantation is not associated with pocket complications or pneumothorax, but can result in femoral access-related complications or cardiac perforation.[50] Initial studies found a higher rate of pericardial complications with leadless (1.0% to 1.5%) than transvenous pacemakers, but one study has shown a decline in such events possibly due to increased operator experience.[50,51] Tricuspid valve injury or regurgitation can occur especially for more basal insertions or from device removal.[52] Device dislodgement and embolization has occurred in 0% to 1.1% of implants. Pocket infection is of course eliminated, and intravascular infection appears to be much less likely even in cases of documented bacteremia, but one case has been reported.[50]

FOLLOW-UP AND MANAGEMENT

Remote Monitoring

The convergence of internet technology, improved telemetry, and enhanced CIED diagnostics permits remote monitoring of multiple device functions and improves patient management[53] (eFig. 69.22). Currently, most ICDs and many pacemakers use "wireless telemetry" to transmit data automatically to a home monitor, which then relays the data to a server via an Internet connection. Smartphone-based

ARRHYTHMIAS, SUDDEN DEATH, AND SYNCOPE

VII

1344

applications are also coming into use for implanted devices. By convention, *remote interrogation* refers to scheduled, routine device interrogation at a distance, corresponding to in-clinic interrogation; *remote monitoring* refers to automatic data transmission based on device-generated alerts.[53] Colloquially, "remote monitoring" includes both. Routine, scheduled transmissions include battery status, pacing and sensing thresholds, lead impedances, and detected arrhythmias. Patients can also initiate transmissions in response to symptoms. Health care providers log into a Web server to review alerts and transmitted data. ICDs and some pacemakers provide programmable alerts for system malfunction (e.g., suspected lead failure), potential programming errors (e.g., VF detection or therapy "off"), or high-risk arrhythmias. Alerts may be transmitted daily or even immediately. Alerts may also notify the patient through audible tones or generator vibration. A "lead integrity alert" reduces inappropriate shocks caused by lead failure.[37]

CIED Diagnostics for Atrial Fibrillation

Remote monitoring can be used to monitor comorbidities if relevant data are stored in the device or input into the local hub from another source. AF is an important comorbidity that can be monitored reliably by CIEDs with an atrial lead. ICD patients with rapidly conducted AF have an increased risk of inappropriate shocks, and early diagnosis may permit treatment or reprogramming to prevent inappropriate therapy. Early treatment of new-onset, persistent AF may reduce exacerbations of HF. Alerts for AF facilitate early anticoagulation and adjustment of rate and rhythm control medications.[53] In CIED patients, asymptomatic AF episodes as short as 5 minutes are associated with an increased rate of stroke, although it is not clear if AF is causal. Present data are insufficient to determine if continuous device monitoring of patients with infrequent paroxysmal AF might permit safe withdrawal of anticoagulation or intermittent use of short-acting anticoagulants.

Device Clinic Follow-Up

Despite the ability to track device and patient status using remote monitoring, in-person follow-up remains helpful, particularly if troubleshooting, reprogramming, or optimization of device therapy is needed. Adjustments in pacing output may help to extend device longevity or maintain a capture safety margin. Inspection of rate histograms and atrial and ventricular pacing trends may indicate a need for sensor or AV delay programming optimization that can enhance exertional tolerance or reduce unnecessary ventricular pacing, respectively. Programming changes can be evaluated and, if needed, changed iteratively using in clinic walk testing. Typical in-person follow-up intervals for patients on remote monitoring are yearly for pacemakers and ICDs. More frequent in-person follow-up is advisable for patients not on remote monitoring (e.g., every 3 to 6 months) or those who are pacemaker-dependent (e.g., every 6 months). In-person follow-up remains necessary for reprogramming or evaluation of suspected malfunction.

Electromagnetic Interference

Ubiquitous electromagnetic waves sometimes interfere with CIEDs, potentially causing temporary or permanent inactivation, inappropriate

FIGURE 69.26 Differential diagnosis of ICD shocks. See text for details.

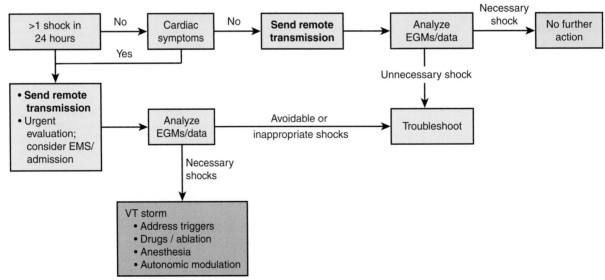

FIGURE 69.27 Approach to the patient with ICD shocks at home. Remote monitoring facilitates care of patients who receive shocks. In the absence of ongoing cardiac symptoms, a single appropriate shock (reviewed remotely) does not require further intervention. Multiple shocks or ongoing symptoms require urgent action to treat VT storm, treat SVT, or troubleshoot to prevent oversensing. (From Swerdlow CD, Friedman P. Implantable cardioverter-defibrillator: clinical aspects. In Zipes D, Jalife J, editors. Cardiac Electrophysiology: From Cell to Bedside. 7th ed. Philadelphia: Elsevier; 2018.)

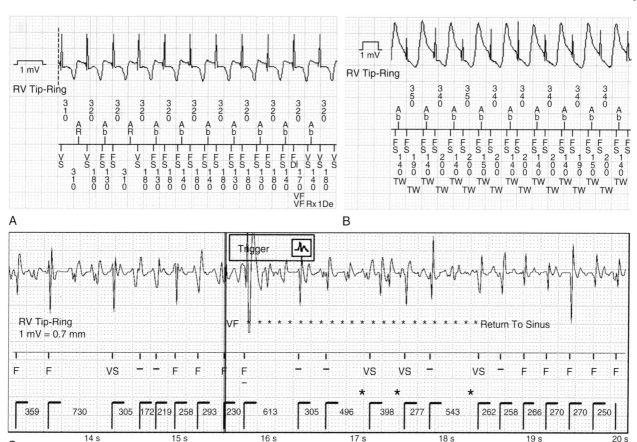

FIGURE 69.28 Abnormal sensing. Wide-band dedicated bipolar RV EGMs during sinus tachycardia with dual-chamber markers. Each EGM shows the characteristic pattern of alternating high-frequency and low-frequency sensed events, with two ventricular events for each atrial event. One millivolt (mV) calibration markers are shown at *left*. **A,** Oversensing of T waves causes inappropriate detection of ventricular fibrillation (VF). High-amplitude T waves cause intermittent oversensing despite adequate (10 mV base to peak) R waves. "VF Rx [Therapy] 1 De" at *lower right* denotes inappropriate detection of VF. **B,** Enhanced sensing algorithm identifies the pattern of T wave oversensing therapy (TW markers) and prevents inappropriate detection of VF despite consistent T wave oversensing. Low-amplitude (1.5 to 4.0 mV) R waves are the root cause of this T wave oversensing. **C,** Undersensing. Dedicated bipolar, filtered EGM is shown during ongoing VF. Between 15 and 18 seconds (s), there are fewer markers than true EGMs indicating undersensing. The single-zone VF detection interval is 360 msec and programmed minimum sensitivity 0.3 mV. Undersensing occurs primarily from amplitude of EGMs changing faster than dynamic sensitivity can adjust despite EGM amplitudes that exceed the minimum sensitivity. Shortly after detection of VF at vertical line (Trigger, VF), three consecutive classified intervals (separated by one unclassified interval) are classified in the sinus zone (VS, *asterisks*). This results in clinically incorrect termination of the device-defined VF episode (Return to Sinus) despite ongoing VF. The ICD subsequently performed a second initial detection of VF and delivered a successful shock. (From Swerdlow CD, Friedman P. Implantable cardioverter-defibrillator: clinical aspects. In Zipes D, Jalife J, editors. Cardiac Electrophysiology: From Cell to Bedside. 7th ed. Philadelphia: Elsevier; 2018.)

TABLE 69.6 Causes of Unsuccessful ICD Shocks

Successful Termination of VT/VF Misclassified by the ICD

VT/VF recurs before the device determines the VT/VF episode has terminated.
Failure to terminate SVT (e.g., sinus tachycardia)
Postshock rhythm is SVT in the VT rate zone.

Patient-Related Factors

Metabolic (hyperkalemia)
Ischemia
Progression of heart failure
Some antiarrhythmic drugs (e.g., amiodarone, type IC)
Pleural or pericardial effusions

Device System–Related Reasons

Insufficient programmed shock strength
Battery depletion
Failure of generator component or lead
Device-lead connection problem
Lead dislodgement
Delayed detection resulting in a prolonged VT/VF that increases required shock strength

ICD, Implantable cardioverter-defibrillator; *SVT,* supraventricular tachycardia; *VF,* ventricular fibrillation; *VT,* ventricular tachycardia.

pacing or inhibition of pacing or shocks, and inappropriate detection of VT/VF.[2]

Nonmedical Sources. Clinically significant EMI is extremely rare for household appliances. Although the risk is very low, patients should hold activated digital cellular phones to the contralateral ear and should avoid carrying phones in the ipsilateral breast pocket. CIED patients may walk through airport metal detectors and electronic article surveillance devices at a normal pace. Prolonged exposure can inhibit pacing and detection of VT/VF, cause inappropriate detection of VT/VF, or (rarely) program VT/VF detection "off."

Medical Sources. Medical sources of EMI are most frequently associated with electrosurgery (electrocautery) or MRI.

Perioperative Management of CIED Patients. A consensus statement requires preoperative determination of pacemaker dependency, device model, type of lead, and plans to use electrocautery to inform management[54] (eTable 69.9). The arterial pulse must be monitored intraoperatively. Intraoperative management strategies may include magnet application or perioperative reprogramming. When a magnet is placed over a pacemaker, it paces asynchronously. In contrast, a magnet placed over an ICD disables detection of VT/VF but does not alter pacing mode.

The risk of oversensing is greatest for monopolar electrocautery delivered between a pen and a remote dispersive ground electrode, especially when the surgical site is in proximity to the device or sensing electrodes.[54] If the surgical incision and dispersive ground pad are both

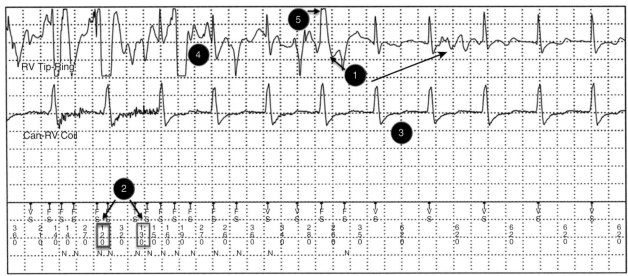

FIGURE 69.29 **EGM conductor fracture or connection problem between DF1 lead and header.** Characteristic features include (1) intermittent nonphysiologic signals, (2) "nonphysiologic" intervals too short to correspond to successive ventricular depolarizations, (3) no abnormal signals on shock channel of dedicated sensing bipole, (4) variable amplitude, morphology, and frequency, and (5) may saturate sensing amplifier. Enhanced sensing feature (lead noise algorithm) prevents inappropriate detection of VF, classifying intervals as "N" (noise) on marker channel. High-frequency signal superimposed on shock channel probably is caused by pectoral myopotentials, which are a normal finding on EGMs, including the can (see eFig. 69.18EF). (From Swerdlow CD, Friedman P. Implantable cardioverter-defibrillator: clinical aspects. In Zipes D, Jalife J, editors. Cardiac Electrophysiology: From Cell to Bedside. 7th ed. Philadelphia: Elsevier; 2018.)

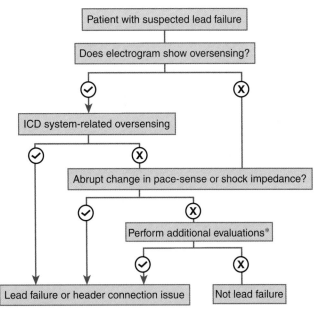

FIGURE 69.30 **Deductive approach to suspected ICD lead failure.** See text for details. *Additional evaluations include real-time, pace-sense electrograms with muscle exercise and pocket manipulation; shock EGMs; differential EGMs; and pacing and sensing thresholds. (From Swerdlow CD, et al. Implantable cardiac defibrillator lead failure and management. J Am Coll Cardiol 2016;67(11):1358-1368.)

below the umbilicus, the risk of EMI is low. Rate-adaptive sensors should be disabled.

Magnetic Resonance Imaging. MRI exposes CIED patients to risks resulting from mechanical forces generated by the static magnetic field, heat and current flow in the leads induced by the radiofrequency fields, and current induced by gradient magnetic fields. MRI-conditional pacemaker and ICD systems employ PGs and leads designed to permit safe imaging under specific MRI conditions when programmed to fixed rate (VOO, DOO) or nonpacing (ODO) modes.[55] MRI of patients with standard CIEDs may be performed safely by implementing rigorous risk mitigation strategies.[2]

Other Medical Procedures and Devices. When external cardioversion is required, defibrillation pads should be placed at least 8 inches (20 cm) from the PG. In ICD patients, cardioversion of AF can be attempted through the device. Ionizing radiation therapy can damage CIED circuitry, and CIEDs should be shielded or if necessary moved to the contralateral side when necessary (e.g., when exposure to the CIED device

will exceed 5 Gy). Left ventricular assist devices (LVADs) cause specific forms of EMI.[2,56] Dialysis procedures pose potential infection risks, particularly if performed ipsilateral to an implanted CIED. If feasible, at implant, contralateral transvenous placement or subcutaneous ICD devices may be considered.

DEVICE LONGEVITY AND REPLACEMENT CONSIDERATIONS
Improvements in battery longevity have led to devices that can last 10 years or longer, depending on pacing use, shocks, and threshold requirements. Device indicators of battery depletion include measures of battery voltage. Devices can be programmed to issue a tone or vibration when elective replacement indicators are reached. Remote monitoring facilitates detection of these indicators. Generally several months of function remain when elective replacement indicators are reached, allowing a margin of time from detection to replacement.

Before device replacement, evaluation should include assessment of lead function to anticipate need for lead extraction, revision or replacement, and ventricular dysfunction that may indicate need for upgrade to an ICD or CRT device. In the event that addition of a lead is planned, venography may be needed. Another consideration is improvement in ventricular function in patients who had implanted ICDs for primary prevention of SCD due to ventricular dysfunction but who have had improvement in ventricular function. However, studies report that although arrhythmic events are reduced when ventricular function improves, risk for arrhythmic events is not entirely mitigated by improvements in ventricular function.[57] Thus, unless there is patient preference otherwise, ICDs are usually replaced with another ICD at time of battery depletion.

Common Clinical Issues in CIED Patients
Psychosocial Issues
ICD patients may experience anxiety about shocks, but they may also feel protected from the risk of sudden death. ICD recipients may benefit from interventions such as counseling, education, and support groups.[58] It is important to provide patients with a plan for what to do when a shock occurs. eTable 69.10 summarizes an approach consistent with the clinical approach in Figure 69.27, which emphasizes that patient-initiated remote transmission is the most rapid and efficient approach to transfer information required for medical decision making to the clinician. ICD patients benefit from counseling after shocks occur.[2] This includes reviewing what triggered the shock and what intervention has been taken to mitigate the trigger, estimating the likelihood of future shocks after this intervention, explaining that shocks are one of multiple challenges of living with heart disease, and usually emphasizing the value of returning to normal activity.

A consensus statement addresses legal and ethical issues related to withdrawal of CIED therapy to reduce suffering at the end of a patient's life.[2,59] This is important because 20% of ICD patients receive painful shocks in their last weeks of life. A patient (or legally defined surrogate decision maker) has the right to request withdrawal of any medical therapy, including CIED therapy, even if such withdrawal allows the patient to die naturally from an underlying disease.

Lifestyle Issues

Driving

Pacemaker patients are not restricted from driving after the perioperative period. Guidelines for ICD patients recommend that patients refrain from driving for 6 months after each shock for VT/VF and for 6 months after ICD implant for secondary prevention.[2] Primary prevention patients are not restricted from driving personal cars (versus commercial vehicles).

Participation in Sports

Exercise improves health and quality of life but may induce VT/VF in patients with specific diseases.[60] Decisions regarding sports participation should be based on the patient's underlying disease, indication for ICD therapy (e.g., primary versus secondary prevention, risk of exercise-induced VT/VF), and risks of specific sports (e.g., ICD system damage in contact sports, risk of trauma with transient loss of consciousness).[60] Athletes with ICDs experience shocks for both VT/VF and SVT more frequently during sports than at rest, but the risk of injury or failure to terminate VT/VF is low.[2] Swimming presents the risk of drowning even if VT/VF is treated promptly.

Drug Interactions

Antiarrhythmic drugs are used in pacemaker patients to prevent AF and in ICD patients to prevent both AF and VT/VF. RCTs report reduction in VT/VF using either sotalol or the combination of amiodarone and beta blockers. However, antiarrhythmic and other drugs have important interactions with devices (see eTable 69.1). Certain antiarrhythmic drugs (e.g., amiodarone, 1C agents) may increase pacing or DFTs. Beta blockers and other drugs that prolong AV conduction may increase RV pacing burden and thereby exacerbate HF. Antiarrhythmic drugs prescribed for VT/VF or AF (e.g., amiodarone) may slow the rate of VT and thus require decreasing the rate threshold to ensure that VT is detected.

REFERENCES

General Considerations

1. Kusumoto FM, Schoenfeld MH, Barrett C, et al. 2018 ACC/AHA/HRS guideline on the evaluation and management of patients with bradycardia and cardiac conduction delay. *J Am College Cardiol.* 2018.
2. Swerdlow CD, Wang PJ, Zipes DP. *Pacemakers and Implantable Cardioverter-Defibrillators. Braunwald's Heart Disease: A Textbook of Cardiovascular Medicine.* Mosby; 2018.
3. Roca-Luque I, Francisco-Pasqual J, Oristrell G, et al. Flecainide versus procainamide in electrophysiological study in patients with syncope and wide QRS duration. *JACC Clin Electrophysiol.* 2019;5:212–219.
4. Bradshaw PJ, Stobie P, Knuiman MW, et al. Trends in the incidence and prevalence of cardiac pacemaker insertions in an ageing population. *Open Heart.* 2014;1:e000177.
5. Galappaththige SK, Gray RA, Roth BJ. Cardiac strength-interval curves calculated using a bidomain tissue with a parsimonious ionic current. *PloS One.* 2017;12:e0171144.

Types of Pacemakers

6. Gaeta S, Bahnson TD, Henriquez C. Mechanism and magnitude of bipolar electrogram directional sensitivity: characterizing underlying determinants of bipolar amplitude. *Heart Rhythm.* 2020;17:777–785.
7. Josephson ME, Anter E. Substrate mapping for ventricular tachycardia: assumptions and misconceptions. *JACC Clin Electrophysiol.* 2015;1:341–352.
8. Worsnick SA, Sharma PS, Vijayaraman P. Right ventricular septal pacing: a paradigm shift. *J Innov Card Rhythm Manag.* 2018;9:3137–3146.
9. Vijayaraman P, Chung MK, Dandamudi G, et al. His bundle pacing. *J Am Coll Cardiol.* 2018;72:927–947.
10. Merchant FM, Mittal S. Pacing-induced cardiomyopathy. *Card Electrophysiol Clin.* 2018;10:437–445.
11. Vijayaraman P, Herweg B, Dandamudi G, et al. Outcomes of His-bundle pacing upgrade after long-term right ventricular pacing and/or pacing-induced cardiomyopathy: insights into disease progression. *Heart Rhythm.* 2019;16:1554–1561.
12. Sharma PS, Dandamudi G, Naperkowski A, et al. Permanent His-bundle pacing is feasible, safe, and superior to right ventricular pacing in routine clinical practice. *Heart Rhythm.* 2015;12:305–312.
13. Vijayaraman P, Naperkowski A, Subzposh FA, et al. Permanent His-bundle pacing: long-term lead performance and clinical outcomes. *Heart Rhythm.* 2018;15:696–702.
14. Burri H, Jastrzebski M, Vijayaraman P. Electrocardiographic analysis for His bundle pacing at implantation and follow-up. *JACC Clin Electrophysiol.* 2020;6:883–900.

Pacing Mode and Timing Cycles

15. Upadhyay GA, Cherian T, Shatz DY, et al. Intracardiac delineation of septal conduction in left bundle-branch block patterns. *Circulation.* 2019;139:1876–1888.
16. Vijayaraman P, Subzposh FA, Naperkowski A, et al. Prospective evaluation of feasibility and electrophysiologic and echocardiographic characteristics of left bundle branch area pacing. *Heart Rhythm.* 2019;16:1774–1782.
17. Auricchio A, Ellenbogen KA. Reducing ventricular pacing frequency in patients with atrioventricular block: is it time to change the current pacing paradigm? *Circ Arrhythm Electrophysiol.* 2016;9:e004404.
18. Tjong FV, Reddy VY. Permanent leadless cardiac pacemaker therapy: a comprehensive review. *Circulation.* 2017;135:1458–1470.
19. Wass SY, Kanj M, Mayuga K, et al. Proarrhythmic effects from competitive atrial pacing and potential programming solutions. *Pacing Clin Electrophysiol.* 2020;43:720–729.
20. Hussein AA, Wilkoff BL. Cardiac implantable electronic device therapy in heart failure. *Circ Res.* 2019;124:1584–1597.
21. Al-Khatib SM, Stevenson WG, Ackerman MJ, et al. AHA/ACC/HRS guideline for management of patients with ventricular arrhythmias and the prevention of sudden cardiac death: executive summary: a report of the American College of Cardiology/American Heart Association Task Force on Clinical Practice Guidelines and the Heart Rhythm Society. *J Am Coll Cardiol.* 2017.

Implantable Cardioverter-Defibrillators

22. Goldenberg I, Gillespie J, Moss AJ, et al. Long-term benefit of primary prevention with an implantable cardioverter-defibrillator: an extended 8-year follow-up study of the multicenter automatic defibrillator implantation trial II. *Circulation.* 2010;122:1265–1271.
23. Kusumoto FM, Calkins H, Boehmer J, et al. HRS/ACC/AHA expert consensus statement on the use of implantable cardioverter-defibrillator therapy in patients who are not included or not well represented in clinical trials. *J Am Coll Cardiol.* 2014.
24. Russo AM, Stainback RF, Bailey SR, et al. ACCF/HRS/AHA/ASE/HFSA/SCAI/SCCT/SCMR 2013 appropriate use criteria for implantable cardioverter-defibrillators and cardiac resynchronization therapy: a report of the American College of Cardiology Foundation Appropriate Use Criteria Task Force, Heart Rhythm Society, American Heart Association, American Society of Echocardiography, Heart Failure Society of America, Society for Cardiovascular Angiography and Interventions, Society of Cardiovascular Computed Tomography, and Society for Cardiovascular Magnetic Resonance. *J Am Coll Cardiol.* 2013.
25. Lewis GF, Gold MR. Safety and efficacy of the subcutaneous implantable defibrillator. *J Am Coll Cardiol.* 2016;67:445–454.
26. Gold MR, Lambiase PD, El-Chami MF, et al. Primary results from the understanding outcomes with the S-ICD in primary prevention patients with low ejection fraction (UNTOUCHED) trial. *Circulation.* 2021;143:7–17.
27. Knops RE, Olde Nordkamp LRA, Delnoy PHM, et al. Subcutaneous or transvenous defibrillator therapy. *N Engl J Med.* 2020;383:526–536.
28. Baccillieri MS, Gasparini G, Benacchio L, et al. Multicentre comparison of shock efficacy using single-vs. dual-coil lead systems and anodal vs. cathodaL polarITY defibrillation in patients undergoing transvenous cardioverter-defibrillator implantation. The MODALITY study. *J Interv Card Electrophysiol.* 2015;43:45–54.
29. Swerdlow CD, Asirvatham SJ, Ellenbogen KA, Friedman PA. Troubleshooting implanted cardioverter defibrillator sensing problems I. *Circ Arrhythm Electrophysiol.* 2014;7:1237–1261.
30. Wilkoff BL, Fauchier L, Stiles MK, et al. 2015 HRS/EHRA/APHRS/SOLAECE expert consensus statement on optimal implantable cardioverter-defibrillator programming and testing. *Heart Rhythm.* 2016;13:e50–86.
31. Schuger C, Daubert JP, Zareba W, et al. Reassessing the role of antitachycardia pacing in fast ventricular arrhythmias in primary prevention implantable cardioverter-defibrillator recipients: results from MADIT-RIT. *Heart Rhythm.* 2020.
32. Cakulev I, Efimov IR, Waldo AL. Cardioversion: past, present, and future. *Circulation.* 2009;120:1623–1632.
33. Chen PS, Shibata N, Dixon EG, et al. Comparison of the defibrillation threshold and the upper limit of ventricular vulnerability. *Circulation.* 1986;73:1022–1028.
34. Dixon EG, Tang AS, Wolf PD, et al. Improved defibrillation thresholds with large contoured epicardial electrodes and biphasic waveforms. *Circulation.* 1987;76:1176–1184.
35. Healey JS, Hohnloser SH, Glikson M, et al. Cardioverter defibrillator implantation without induction of ventricular fibrillation: a single-blind, non-inferiority, randomised controlled trial (SIMPLE). *Lancet.* 2015;385:785–791.
36. Tung R, Shivkumar K. Neuraxial modulation for treatment of VT storm. *J Biomed Res.* 2015;29:56–60.

Complications

37. Swerdlow CD, Kalahasty G, Ellenbogen KA. Implantable cardiac defibrillator lead failure and management. *J Am Coll Cardiol.* 2016;67:1358–1368.
38. Resnic FS, Majithia A, Dhruva SS, et al. Active surveillance of the implantable cardioverter-defibrillator registry for defibrillator lead failures. *Circ Cardiovasc Qual Outcomes.* 2020;13:e006105.
39. Pokorney SD, Mi X, Lewis RK, et al. Outcomes associated with extraction versus capping and abandoning pacing and defibrillator leads. *Circulation.* 2017.
40. Lewis RK, Pokorney SD, Hegland DD, Piccini JP. Hands on: how to approach patients undergoing lead extraction. *J Cardiovasc Electrophysiol.* 2020;31:1801–1808.
41. Kusumoto FM, Schoenfeld MH, Wilkoff BL, et al. 2017 HRS expert consensus statement on cardiovascular implantable electronic device lead management and extraction. *Heart Rhythm.* 2017.
42. Blomström-Lundqvist C, Traykov V, Erba PA, et al. European Heart Rhythm Association (EHRA) international consensus document on how to prevent, diagnose, and treat cardiac implantable electronic device infections-endorsed by the Heart Rhythm Society (HRS), the Asia Pacific Heart Rhythm Society (APHRS), the Latin American Heart Rhythm Society (LAHRS), International Society for Cardiovascular Infectious Diseases (ISCVID), and the European Society of Clinical Microbiology and Infectious Diseases (ESCMID) in collaboration with the European Association for Cardio-Thoracic Surgery (EACTS). *Eur Heart J.* 2020.
43. Carrillo R, Healy C. Clinical cardiac pacing, defibrillation and resynchronization therapy E-book. In: Ellenbogen KA, et al., eds. Elsevier; 2016: 1200.
44. Timmers L, Van Heuverswyn F, De Wilde H, Jordaens L. Evaluating current implantable cardioverter defibrillator implantation procedures: can common complications be minimised. *Expert Rev Cardiovasc Ther.* 2016;14:579–589.
45. Essebag V, Verma A, Healey JS, et al. Clinically significant pocket hematoma increases long-term risk of device infection: BRUISE CONTROL INFECTION study. *J Am Coll Cardiol.* 2016;67:1300–1308.
46. Birnie DH, Healey JS, Wells GA et al. Continued vs. interrupted direct oral anticoagulants at the time of device surgery, in patients with moderate to high risk of arterial thrombo-embolic events (BRUISE CONTROL-2). *Euro Heart J.* 2018ehy413-ehy413.
47. Maskarinec SA, Thaden JT, Cyr DD, et al. The risk of cardiac device-related infection in bacteremic patients is species specific: results of a 12-year prospective cohort. *Open Forum Infect Dis.* 2017;4:ofx132.
48. Tarakji KG, Mittal S, Kennergren C, et al. Antibacterial envelope to prevent cardiac implantable device infection. *N Engl J Med.* 2019;380:1895–1905.
49. Krahn AD, Longtin Y, Philippon F, et al. Prevention of arrhythmia device infection trial: the PADIT trial. *J Am Coll Cardiol.* 2018;72:3098–3109.
50. Lee JZ, Mulpuru SK, Shen WK. Leadless pacemaker: performance and complications. *Trends Cardiovasc Med.* 2018;28:130–141.

51. Roberts PR, Clementy N, Al Samadi F, et al. A leadless pacemaker in the real-world setting: the micra transcatheter pacing system post-approval registry. *Heart Rhythm*. 2017;14:1375–1379.

52. Beurskens NEG, Tjong FVY, de Bruin-Bon RHA, et al. Impact of leadless pacemaker therapy on cardiac and atrioventricular valve function through 12 Months of follow-up. *Circ Arrhythm Electrophysiol*. 2019;12:e007124.

Follow-up and Management

53. Slotwiner D, Varma N, Akar JG, et al. HRS Expert Consensus Statement on remote interrogation and monitoring for cardiovascular implantable electronic devices. *Heart Rhythm*. 2015;12:e69–e100.

54. Crossley GH, Poole JE, Rozner MA, et al. The Heart Rhythm Society (HRS)/American Society of Anesthesiologists (ASA) Expert Consensus Statement on the perioperative management of patients with implantable defibrillators, pacemakers and arrhythmia monitors: facilities and patient management this document was developed as a joint project with the American Society of Anesthesiologists (ASA), and in collaboration with the American Heart Association (AHA), and the Society of Thoracic Surgeons (STS). *Heart Rhythm*. 2011;8:1114–1154.

55. Indik JH, Gimbel JR, Abe H, et al. 2017 HRS expert consensus statement on magnetic resonance imaging and radiation exposure in patients with cardiovascular implantable electronic devices. *Heart Rhythm*. 2017.

56. Yalcin YC, Kooij C, Theuns DAMJ, et al. Emerging electromagnetic interferences between implantable cardioverter-defibrillators and left ventricular assist devices. *Europace*. 2020;22:584–587.

57. Yuyun M, Erqou S, Peralta A, et al. Ongoing risk of ventricular arrhythmias and all-cause mortality at implantable cardioverter defibrillator generator change: a systematic review and meta-analysis. *Circep*. 2021 (in press).

58. Lampert R. Managing with pacemakers and implantable cardioverter defibrillators. *Circulation*. 2013;128:1576–1585.

59. Lampert R, Hayes DL, Annas GJ, et al. HRS expert consensus statement on the management of Cardiovascular Implantable Electronic Devices (CIEDs) in patients nearing end of life or requesting withdrawal of therapy. This document was developed in collaboration and endorsed by the American College of Cardiology (ACC), the American Geriatrics Society (AGS), the American Academy of Hospice and Palliative Medicine (AAHPM); the American Heart Association (AHA), the European Heart Rhythm Association (EHRA), and the Hospice and Palliative Nurses Association (HPNA). *Heart Rhythm*. 2010;7:1008–1026.

60. Zipes DP, Link MS, Ackerman MJ, et al. Eligibility and disqualification recommendations for competitive athletes with cardiovascular abnormalities: Task force 9: arrhythmias and conduction defects: a scientific statement from the American Heart Association and American College of Cardiology. *Circulation*. 2015;132:e315–e325.

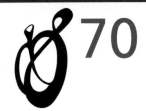

70 Cardiac Arrest and Sudden Cardiac Death

JEFFREY J. GOLDBERGER, CHRISTINE M. ALBERT, AND ROBERT J. MYERBURG

PERSPECTIVE

Sudden cardiac arrest (SCA), and its common consequence sudden cardiac death (SCD), is the common cardiac pathway for death. There are a diverse array of cardiac and noncardiac causes and mechanisms underlying the development of SCA and SCD. While SCA and SCD are most likely deterministic processes rather than true stochastic processes, the inability to delineate these processes presents a challenge in addressing this major public health problem. Current estimates for out-of-hospital SCDs are still in the range of 380,000/year in the United States alone,[1,2] with an additional 200,000 in-hospital cardiac arrests.[3] Generally, its impact is defined by the "rule of 50s": SCD accounts for 50% of all cardiovascular deaths, approximately 50% of all SCDs are unexpected first expressions of a cardiac disorder, and it often strikes during the victim's productive years, accounting for up to 50% of years of potential life lost due to heart disease.[4] Despite recognition of an association between forewarning symptoms of syncope and SCD dating to Hippocrates around 400 BC, advances in prediction, prevention, and management of unexpected SCA and SCD did not begin to emerge until approximately 50 years ago. It is anticipated that the major insights into causes, pathophysiology, and preventive and management strategies developed during the past few decades will continue to evolve.

DEFINITIONS

SCD is not a uniform entity resulting from a single precipitating diagnosis. SCD is natural death from cardiac causes heralded by abrupt loss of consciousness within 1 hour of the onset of an acute change in cardiovascular status. As such detailed information is often lacking, various definitions of SCD include up to a 24 hour period and death during sleep. Moreover, at least half of SCDs are unwitnessed, providing substantial uncertainty to the terminal events. Preexisting heart disease may or may not have been known to be present, but the time and mode of death are unexpected. This definition incorporates the key elements of natural, rapid, and most importantly unexpected death by a cardiac cause or mechanism. It consolidates previous definitions that

have conflicted, mainly because the most useful operational definition of SCD in the past differed for clinicians, cardiovascular epidemiologists, pathologists, and scientists attempting to define pathophysiologic mechanisms. As the epidemiology, clinical expression, causes, and mechanisms began to be understood, these differences merged.

To satisfy clinical, scientific, legal, and social considerations, four temporal elements must be considered: (1) prodromes, (2) onset, (3) cardiac arrest, and (4) biologic death (Fig. 70.1). Because the proximate cause of SCA is an abrupt disturbance in cardiovascular function resulting in loss of consciousness due to cessation of cerebral blood flow, any definition must recognize the brief time interval between onset of the mechanism *directly* responsible for cardiac arrest and the consequent loss of blood flow. The 1-hour definition primarily refers to the duration of the "terminal event," which defines the interval between the onset of symptoms signaling the pathophysiologic disturbance leading to cardiac arrest and the onset of the cardiac arrest itself. Based on human centrifuge studies carried out during the early years of the space program, the time between abrupt cessation of cerebral blood flow and loss of consciousness can be 10 seconds or less.

Prodromes, occurring weeks or months before an event, are generally predictors of an impending cardiac event, but not specific for SCA itself. The same premonitory signs and symptoms may be more specific for imminent cardiac arrest when they begin abruptly. Sudden onset of chest pain, dyspnea, or palpitations and other symptoms of arrhythmias often precede the onset of cardiac arrest and define the onset of the 1-hour terminal event period that brackets the cardiac arrest. The fourth element, biologic death, is an immediate consequence of cardiac arrest, unless there is a successful intervention, and usually occurs within minutes. The generally accepted clinical-pathophysiologic definition of up to 1 hour between onset of the terminal event and biologic death requires qualifications for specific circumstances. For example, since the development of community-based interventions and life support systems, patients may now remain biologically alive for a long period after the onset of a pathophysiologic process that has caused irreversible damage and will ultimately lead to death. In this circumstance, the causative pathophysiologic and clinical event is the cardiac arrest itself rather than the factors responsible for the delayed biologic death. Thus death remains defined biologically, legally, and literally as an absolute and irreversible event timed to cessation of all biologic functions, but most studies link the definition of SCD to the cardiac arrest rather than to a biologic death that occurs during hospitalization after cardiac arrest or within 30 days. Finally, forensic pathologists studying unwitnessed deaths continue to use the definition of sudden death for a person known to be alive and functioning normally 24 hours before, and this remains appropriate within obvious limits. Among the precautions is the recognition that not all sudden deaths are cardiac in origin.[5]

EPIDEMIOLOGY

Epidemiologic Overview

Epidemiologic studies of SCD are difficult to interpret for both theoretical and practical reasons. There are persisting inconsistencies about the definition and challenges in accessing data and adjudicating individual cases in data sets, in determining pathophysiologic mechanisms, and in making distinctions between population risk and individual risk.[6] In addition, the fact that SCA leading to SCD has short-term dynamics superimposed on a long-term static or dynamic substrate introduces unusual epidemiologic complexities, including long-term risk prediction based on the evolution of atherogenesis, myocardial hypertrophy, and ventricular muscle dysfunction over time and modulation by transient (short-term) variables such as ischemia, hemodynamic shifts, atherosclerotic plaque disruption and thrombosis, and autonomic variations. The differences between chronic disease evolution and transient events call for different forms of epidemiologic modeling (Table 70.1A). Furthermore, the emerging field of genetic epidemiology adds another dimension for consideration, and there is a need to focus on

interventional epidemiology, a term coined to define the population dynamics of therapeutic outcomes.

In reference to risk for SCD from coronary heart disease, clinical categories ranging from general population risk to personalized risk profiling are paralleled by the partition of risk predictors into the pathophysiologic categories of substrate-based risk and expression-based risk (Table 70.1B). Substrate-based risk refers to prediction of the evolution or identification of vascular or myocardial substrates that establish risk for SCD (i.e., atherogenesis, scar patterns, remodeling) and to quantification of these risks. It should not be perceived as limited to anatomic features because risk substrates may exist at a molecular level, such as those characterized by the ion channelopathies that are associated with SCD. In contrast, expression-based risk refers to the identification of mechanisms and pathways that contribute to the clinical manifestation of the risk established by the substrate. This category includes plaque transition and acute coronary syndromes

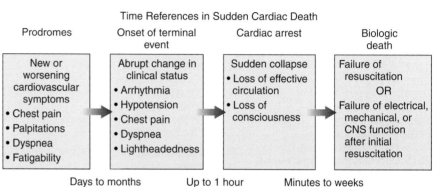

FIGURE 70.1 Sudden cardiac death viewed from four temporal perspectives: (1) prodromes, (2) onset of the terminal event, (3) cardiac arrest, and (4) progression to biologic death. Individual variability of the components influences clinical expression. Some victims experience no prodromes, with onset leading almost instantaneously to cardiac arrest; others may have an onset that lasts up to 1 hour before clinical arrest. Other patients may live days to weeks after the cardiac arrest before biologic death, often because of irreversible brain damage and dependence on life support. These factors influence interpretation of the 1-hour definition. The two most relevant clinical factors are onset of the terminal event and the clinical cardiac arrest itself; legal and social considerations focus on the time of biologic death. CNS, central nervous system.

TABLE 70.1 Pathophysiologic Epidemiology and Utility for Indicators of Risk for Sudden Cardiac Arrest

A. UTILITY FOR RISK PREDICTION			
STRATEGY	EXAMPLES	MEASURES	UTILITY
Conventional risk factors	Framingham risk index	Prediction of evolution of disease	High for the population / Low for the individual
Anatomic disease screening	Coronary calcium score and CT angiography	Identification of abnormal coronary arteries	High for anatomic identification / Low for individual event prediction
Clinical risk profiling	Ejection fraction, stress testing, imaging techniques	Extent of disease	High for small, high-risk subgroups / Low for large, low-risk subgroups
Transient risk predictors	Inflammatory markers; thrombotic cascade	Prediction of unstable plaques; acute changes in vascular status	Uncertain feasibility
Personalized risk predictors	Familial/genetic profiles	Individual SCD expression	Improved clinical precision
B. PATHOPHYSIOLOGIC EPIDEMIOLOGY			
Substrate-based risk	Coronary heart disease		
	State of epicardial and intramyocardial vessels		
	Myocardial infarction		
	Myopathy, infiltration, inflammation, valvulopathy		
	Hypertrophy; myocardial fibrosis		
Expression-based risk	Left ventricular dysfunction and heart failure		
	Metabolic abnormalities		
	Autonomic dysfunction		
Mechanism-based causes	VF/pulseless VT		
	PEA		
	Asystole		

(plaque disruption and thrombogenesis) and their potential for specific expression as an arrhythmic event in susceptible individuals.

Incidence and the Population Burden of Sudden Cardiac Death

The worldwide incidence of out of hospital cardiac arrest (OHCA) leading to SCD is variable[7] and difficult to estimate because numbers vary as a function of reporting practices and the prevalence of coronary heart disease in different countries (see Chapter 2). The annual number of out-of-hospital SCDs in the United States is derived from multiple sources, such as retrospective death certificate data, American Heart Association (AHA) statistical updates based on data from the National Center for Health Statistics,[2] and extrapolations from population-based surveillance. Data from large surveillance studies, such as the Resuscitation Outcomes Consortium (ROC), have contributed additional insight into the subtleties of data collection and interpretation.

Statistical analyses from the same death certificate data sources have ranged from fewer than 250,000 SCDs annually when the etiologic definition is limited to coronary heart disease (International Classification of Diseases, ninth edition [ICD-9], classifications 410-414) to more than 460,000 SCDs/year when all causes are included.[8] Extrapolations from community-based sources set nationwide figures at fewer than 200,000,000 SCDs annually. Because these broad ranges and the reported regional differences in incidence and outcomes of cardiac arrest suggest that an accurate number can be found only by performing carefully designed prospective epidemiologic surveillance studies, the most widely cited estimates remain in the range of 380,000 SCDs annually, as suggested in the 2020 AHA statistical update.[9] These figures suggest an overall incidence of between one and two deaths/1000 persons in the general population. The annual number of emergency rescue (EMS) assessed OHCAs in people of any age in the United States in 2015 was 356,000.[2]

The temporal definition of sudden death strongly influences epidemiologic data. Retrospective death certificate studies have demonstrated that a temporal definition of sudden death of less than 2 hours after the onset of symptoms results in 12% to 15% of all natural deaths being defined as "sudden" and almost 90% of all natural sudden deaths having cardiac causes. In contrast, application of a 24-hour definition of sudden death increases the fraction of all natural deaths falling into the sudden category to more than 30% but reduces the proportion of all sudden natural deaths resulting from cardiac causes to 75%.

Prospective studies have demonstrated that approximately 50% of all deaths caused by coronary heart disease are sudden and unexpected and occur shortly (instantaneous to 1 hour) after the onset of symptoms. Because coronary heart disease is the dominant cause of both sudden and non-SCDs in the United States, the fraction of total cardiac deaths that are sudden is similar to the fraction of deaths from coronary heart disease that are sudden, although there does appear to be geographic variation in the fraction of coronary deaths that are sudden.[3,4] It is also of interest that the age-adjusted decline in mortality from coronary heart disease in the United States during the past half-century has not changed the fraction of coronary deaths that are sudden and unexpected.[4,10] Furthermore, the decreasing age-adjusted mortality does not imply a decrease in absolute numbers of cardiac or sudden deaths because of the growth and aging of the U.S. population and the increasing prevalence of chronic heart disease,[4] including heart failure. Yet a substantial 44% decline in the SCD rate in patients with heart failure and reduced ejection fraction enrolled in clinical trials from 1995 to 2014 has been observed.[11] It does not appear that the cumulative SCD burden in absolute numbers is tracking the age-adjusted decrease in cardiac deaths that has been evolving during the past 40 to 50 years.[12] In a prospective study of SCD victims in Finland undergoing autopsy between 1998 and 2012, while the proportion of SCDs resulting from coronary heart disease decreased, the concomitant increase in SCDs attributable to nonischemic causes maintained a relatively stable rate of SCD.[13] The landscape of SCD over time is further complicated by the suggested shift of mechanisms of out-of-hospital SCA from ventricular tachyarrhythmias to pulseless electrical activity/asystole, in part as a consequence of ICD efficacy.[4]

Population Pools, Risk Gradients, and Time Dependence of Risk

Three factors are of primary importance for identification of populations at risk and consideration of strategies for prevention of SCD: (1) the absolute numbers and event rates (incidence) among population subgroups (Fig. 70.2A), (2) the clinical subgroups in which SCDs occur (Fig. 70.2B), (3) competing risks, and (4) the time dependence of risk.

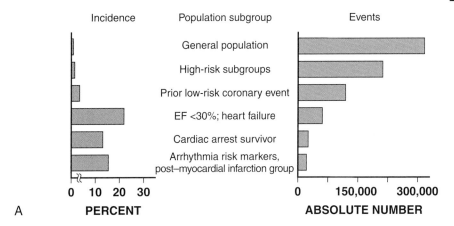

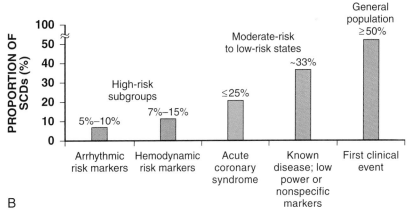

FIGURE 70.2 **Impact of population subgroups and time from events on the clinical epidemiology of sudden cardiac death. A,** Estimates of incidence (percent per year) and the total number of events per year for the general adult population in the United States and for increasingly high-risk subgroups. The overall adult population has an estimated incidence of sudden death of 0.1% to 0.2%/year, which accounts for a total of more than 300,000 events per year. With the identification of increasingly powerful risk factors, the incidence increases progressively, but this is accompanied by a progressive decrease in the total number of events represented by each group. The inverse relationship between incidence and the total number of events is due to the progressively smaller denominator pool in the highest subgroup categories. Successful interventions in larger population subgroups require identification of specific markers to increase the ability to identify specific patients who are at particularly high risk for a future event. (Note: The horizontal axis for the incidence figures is not linear and should be interpreted accordingly.) **B,** Distribution of the clinical status of victims at the time of SCD. Approximately 50% of all cardiac arrests caused by coronary heart disease occur as the first clinical event, and up to an additional 30% occur in the clinical setting of known disease in the absence of strong risk predictors. Less than 25% of victims have high-risk markers based on arrhythmic or hemodynamic parameters. *EF,* Ejection fraction. (**A** modified from Myerburg RJ, et al. Sudden cardiac death: structure, function, and time-dependence of risk. Circulation 1992;85(Suppl I):I2; **B** modified from Myerburg RJ: Sudden cardiac death: exploring the limits of our knowledge. J Cardiovasc Electrophysiol 2001;12:369.)

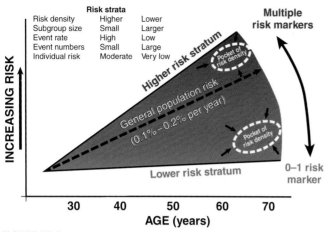

FIGURE 70.3 Stratification of risk as a continuum across the population as a function of age. The mean risk in the general population is demonstrated as a continuum across four decades. The mean risk of approximately 0.1% to 0.2%/year is bracketed by extremes of higher and lower risk strata, with the larger absolute numbers accumulated in the lower-risk strata. The ability to identify high–risk density subgroups within the general population would contribute to better individual risk prediction. (Modified from Myerburg RJ, Junttila MJ. Sudden cardiac death caused by coronary heart disease. Circulation 2012;125:1043.)

Population and Subgroup Risk Versus Individual Risk Assessment

When the estimated 380,000 SCDs that occur annually in the United States are viewed as a global figure for an unselected adult population 35 years and older, the overall incidence is calculated to be in the range of 0.1% to 0.2%/year (1 to 2/1000 population; Fig. 70.2A). This general population includes the large proportion of SCDs that occur as a first clinical manifestation of previously unrecognized heart disease, as well as SCDs that can be predicted with somewhat greater accuracy in higher risk subgroups (Fig. 70.2B), as it is impractical to plan an intervention designed for the general population that would be applied to the 999/1000 who do not have an event to reach and possibly influence the 1/1000 who will experience an event. Figure 70.2A highlights this problem by expressing the incidence (percent per year) of SCD among various subgroups and comparing the incidence figures with the total number of events that occur annually in each subgroup. Thus, despite the large absolute number at risk in the general population and the impact of preventive interventions on population risk for coronary artery disease, the precise ability to identify these individuals for targeted therapy for SCD prevention is an unmet challenge. The cost and risk-to-benefit uncertainties limit the nature of such broad-based interventions and demand a higher resolution of risk identification.[14] Two fundamental approaches for attacking this challenge can be followed: a general population strategy targeting prevention of acquired risk factors such as obesity (primordial prevention) and primary prevention by control of manifest risk factors and a more focused individual risk strategy based on identification and intervention in small subsets of the general population with a high density of risk (Fig. 70.3). Several population-based risk scores have been reported that provide an initial attempt to identify subsets within the general population who have heightened risk of SCD.[15,16] Based on data from the Atherosclerosis Risk in Communities (ARIC) Study, a race-adjusted risk score incorporating readily available variables from the medical record—age, sex, total cholesterol, lipid-lowering and hypertension medication use, blood pressure, smoking status, diabetes, and body mass index—provided good internal discrimination, which held up with external validation in the Framingham study.[17]

On moving from the total adult population to a subgroup at higher risk because of the presence of selected coronary risk factors, there may be a 10-fold or greater increase in the annual incidence of events, with the magnitude being dependent on the number and types of risk factors operating in specific subgroups. Higher resolution is desirable and can be achieved by identification of more specific subgroups. However, the corresponding absolute number of deaths may become progressively smaller as the subgroups become more focused (Fig. 70.2A),

unless the gradients of risk are steep. Applying the ARIC-based risk score[17] to the U.S. National Health and Nutrition Examination Survey, it was noted that there is an exponential rise in calculated risk by decile with a 10-fold gradient in risk between the highest and lowest decile.[18] Up to half of all SCDs attributable to coronary heart disease are first clinical events, and another 20% to 30% occur in subgroups of patients with known coronary heart disease who are profiled to be at relatively low risk for SCD on the basis of current clinically available markers (Fig. 70.2B). It is notable that when the ARIC-based risk score[17] was applied to a general population,[18] those in the highest risk deciles had a very high burden of risk factors. Moreover, these patients may have occult heart disease, providing an opportunity for early detection and treatment.[19] The principle of a high proportion of SCDs occurring as first events or in previously asymptomatic individuals with a high burden of risk factors also applies to SCD in the young (under age 35 years).[20]

Biologic and Clinical Time-Dependent Risk

Temporal elements in risk for SCD have been analyzed in the context of both biologic and clinical chronology. In the former, epidemiologic analyses of risk for SCD in populations have identified three patterns: diurnal, day of the week, and seasonal. General patterns of heightened risk during the morning hours, on Mondays, and during the winter months have been described.[12,21] An exception to the diurnal risk pattern is SCD in sleep apnea, in which the risk tends to be nocturnal.

Ambient temperature is an environmental factor associated with risk for SCD.[22,23] Both excessive cold and excessive heat have been linked to risk for cardiac arrest, although the studies did not determine whether temperature extremes are associated with ventricular tachyarrhythmias versus other mechanisms of cardiac arrest. However, significant cooling of the core temperature can lengthen the time course of repolarization of ventricular myocardium and prolong the QT interval, while sweating associated with increases in core temperature can alter electrolyte balance. Elevated temperature is a risk for SCA in patients with Brugada syndrome[24] (see Chapters 63 and 67). Another environmental variable, short-term ambient air pollution conditions, has been associated with increased risk of OHCA, but not consistently.[12,25,26] In patients with an implantable defibrillator, exposure to fine particulate material correlated significantly to episodes of ventricular tachycardia and fibrillation.[27] A sympathetically mediated mechanism has been postulated.

In the longer term, risk for SCD is not linear as a function of time after changes in cardiovascular status. Survival curves after major cardiovascular events, which identify risk for both SCD and total cardiac death, usually demonstrate that the most rapid rate of attrition occurs during the first 6 to 18 months after an index event. Thus, there is a time dependence of risk that focuses the potential opportunity for maximum efficacy of an intervention during the early period after a cardiovascular event. Even though the rate of attrition decreases after the early spike in mortality, a secondary delayed increase in risk occurs in post–myocardial infarction (MI) patients 2 to 5 years after an index event, probably related to ventricular remodeling and heart failure.

Age, Race, Sex, and Heredity
Age
The incidence of sudden death has two peak ages: within the first year of life (including sudden infant death syndrome [SIDS]; see Chapter 82) and between 45 and 75 years of age. Among the general populations of infants younger than 1 year and middle-aged or older adults, the incidence is surprisingly similar.[28] In adults older than 35 years, the incidence of SCD is in the range of 1/1000 persons/year (Fig. 70.4A), with an age-related increase in risk over time as the prevalence of coronary heart disease increases in parallel with advancing age.

The incidence in infants is 73/100,000 person-years and is most commonly associated with complex congenital heart disease, and the incidence in children and adolescents is approximately 4 to 6/100,000 person-years versus 125/100,000 person-years in adults (Fig. 70.4A).[28] One study demonstrated that approximately 40% of SCDs in this age category were unexplained, based on the absence of an autopsy or premortem clinical diagnosis, but postmortem genetic studies identified a likely cause in 27% of such cases that underwent studies.[29]

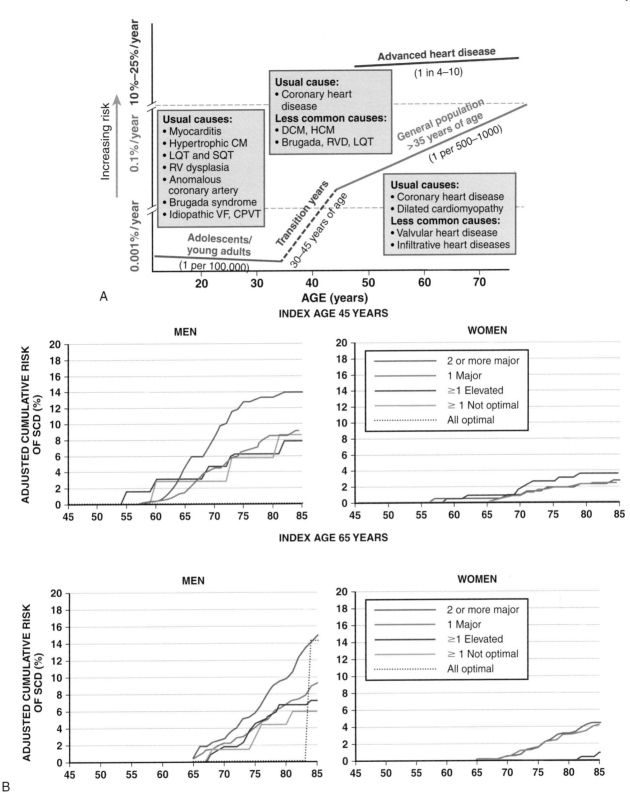

FIGURE 70.4 Age- and sex-specific risks for SCD. A, Age-related and disease-specific risk for SCD. For the general population 35 years and older, the risk for SCD is 0.1% to 0.2%/year (1/500 to 1000 population), with a wide spread in subgroup risk based on the number and power of individual risk factors. Causes are dominated by coronary heart disease and, to a lesser extent, nonischemic cardiomyopathy in this age range. The risk for SCD increases dramatically beyond the age of 35 years and continues to increase past the age of 70 years. In patients older than 30 years with advanced structural heart disease and markers of high risk for cardiac arrest, the event rate may exceed 25%/year, and the age-related risk is attenuated. In adolescents and adults younger than 30 years, the overall risk for SCD is 1/100,000 population or 0.001%/year, with a variety of causes such as inherited structural and electrical disorders, developmental defects, and myocarditis dominating. In adolescents and young adults at risk for SCD from specific identified causes, it is difficult to ascertain the risk in individual patients because of variable expression of the disease state (see text for details). In the transition range from 30 to 45 years of age, the relative frequency of the uncommon disease yields to the dominance of coronary heart disease and nonischemic cardiomyopathy, but both groups of potential causes must be entertained because many of the rare disorders are expressed in that age range. **B,** Lifetime risk for SCD risk as a function of index age (shown for age 45 and 65 years), sex, and risk factor burden derived from the Framingham Heart Study. Boxes show risk factors burden strata coded by colors. *CA,* cardiac arrest; *CM,* cardiomyopathy; *CPVT,* catecholaminergic polymorphic VT; *DCM,* dilated CM; *HCM,* hypertrophic CM; *LQT,* long-QT; *RV,* right ventricular; *RVD,* RV dysplasia; *SQT,* short QT; *VF,* ventricular fibrillation. (**B** from Bogle BM, et al. Lifetime risk for sudden cardiac death in the community. J Am Heart Assoc 2016;5(7):e002398.)

In contrast to incidence, however, the proportion of deaths caused by coronary heart diseases that are sudden and unexpected decreases with advancing age. In the 20- to 39-year age group, approximately 75% of the deaths attributable to coronary heart disease in men are sudden and unexpected, with the proportion falling to approximately 60% in the 45- to 54-year age group and hovering close to 50% thereafter. Age also influences the proportion of any cardiovascular cause among all causes of natural sudden death in that the proportion of coronary deaths and of all cardiac causes of death that are sudden is highest in the younger age groups whereas the fraction of total sudden natural deaths that result from any cardiovascular cause is higher in the older age groups. At the other end of the age range, only 19% of sudden natural deaths in children between 1 and 13 years of age have cardiac causes; the proportion increases to 30% in the 14- to 21-year age group.

In the transition age range between adolescence and young adulthood (to the age of 25 years) and in the middle and older ages (beginning at 35 years of age), coronary heart disease emerges to its position as the dominant cause of SCD. However, rare disorders, such as hypertrophic cardiomyopathy (HCM), Brugada syndrome, long-QT syndrome, right ventricular dysplasia, and idiopathic myocardial fibrosis, are significant contributors to the distribution of causes of SCD in this age group.

Race

A number of studies comparing racial differences in the relative risk for SCD in white and Black with coronary heart disease in the United States had yielded conflicting and inconclusive data. More recent studies demonstrate a higher risk for cardiac arrest and SCD in Blacks than in whites. Data from the ARIC and REGARD studies show that Blacks had an adjusted hazard ratio for SCD of 1.38 to 1.97 compared with whites.[30,31] SCD rates in Hispanic populations have been less well studied but do not appear to show increased risk (see Chapter 93).

Sex

SCD syndrome has a large preponderance in men relative to women during the young adult and early middle-age years because of the protection that women enjoy from coronary atherosclerosis before menopause (Fig. 70.4B). There is at least a threefold increase lifetime risk for SCD among men aged 45 to 65 years compared with women, with only mild attenuation of this accentuated risk at age 75 years.[32] Even though the overall risk for SCD is much lower in younger women, coronary artery disease is the most common cause of SCD in women older than 40 years, and the classic coronary risk factors, including cigarette smoking, diabetes, use of oral contraceptives, and hyperlipidemia, all influence risk in women (see Chapter 91).[4] In an autopsy study, the profile of women experiencing SCD differed significantly from men; women were older (70 versus 64 years), more commonly had nonischemic causes (28% versus 24%) and primary myocardial fibrosis (5.2% versus 2.6%), and more commonly had ECG evidence of left ventricular (LV) hypertrophy with or without repolarization abnormalities.[33]

Heredity

Familial patterns of risk for SCD, which result from known or suspected genetic variations, are emerging as important factors for risk profiling. This concept is generally applicable to both disease development and SCD expression in the common acquired disorders and in a specific sense to inherited arrhythmogenic conditions associated with SCD.[34] The various genetic associations can be separated into four categories (Table 70.2): uncommon inherited primary arrhythmic syndromes (e.g., long-QT syndromes, Brugada syndrome, catecholaminergic polymorphic ventricular tachycardia or fibrillation; see Chapter 63), uncommon inherited structural diseases associated with risk for SCD (e.g., HCM, right ventricular dysplasia; see Chapters 52 and 54), "acquired" or induced risk for arrhythmias (e.g., drug-induced long-QT interval or proarrhythmia, electrolyte disturbances), and common acquired diseases associated with risk for SCD (e.g., coronary heart disease, nonischemic cardiomyopathies; see Chapters 38, 39, and 50). Genetic variants mapped to loci on many chromosomes are being defined as the molecular bases for these entities and associations.

TABLE 70.2 Genetic Contributors to Risk for Sudden Cardiac Death

Genetically Based Primary Arrhythmia Disorders
Congenital long-QT syndrome, short-QT syndrome
Brugada syndrome
Catecholaminergic polymorphic VT/VF
J wave syndromes
Nonsyndromic VT/VF
Inherited Structural Disorders with Risk for Arrhythmic SCD
Hypertrophic cardiomyopathy
Right ventricular dysplasia/cardiomyopathy
Genetic Predisposition to Induced Arrhythmias and SCD
Drug-induced "acquired" long-QT syndrome (drugs, electrolytes)
Electrolyte and metabolic arrhythmogenic effects
Genetic Modulation of Complex Acquired Diseases
Coronary artery disease, acute coronary syndromes
Congestive heart failure, dilated cardiomyopathies

The multiple specific mutations at gene loci-encoding ion channel proteins associated with the various inherited arrhythmia syndromes (see Chapter 63) represent a major advance in the understanding of a genetic and pathophysiologic basis for these causes of sudden death. In addition, the role of modifier genes and mutation specificity in the severity of clinical phenotypes in long–QT interval syndromes (LQTS)[35] and structural diseases such as HCM is of increasing interest. These observations may provide screening tools for individuals at risk, as well as the potential to devise specific therapeutic strategies. In a study of screening ECGs for long-QT in children entering first grade and those in the seventh grade, and subsequent genetic testing in those children who were positive, there was a suggestion that the incidence of inherited LQT was considerably higher (~1/1000) at the age of 12 years (seventh graders) than earlier estimates from studies based on diagnoses from general clinical expressions.[36] Moreover, the cumulative risk of SCA among those with unrecognized or untreated LQTS was reported to be 13% before the age of 40 years.[37] In addition, gene loci identified by genome-wide association studies may also serve as candidates for investigation of the role of low-penetrance mutations or polymorphisms in SCD caused by more common conditions, such as coronary heart disease.[38]

To the extent that SCD is an expression of underlying coronary heart disease, hereditary factors that contribute to risk for coronary heart disease operate nonspecifically for the SCD syndrome. Various studies have identified mutations and relevant polymorphisms along multiple steps of the cascade, from atherogenesis to plaque destabilization, thrombosis, and arrhythmogenesis, each of which is associated with increased risk for a coronary event (Fig. 70.5). Several studies have suggested that SCD as the initial expression of coronary heart disease demonstrates familial clustering, including general population surveillance studies, family histories of cardiac arrest survivors in the community, studies of ventricular fibrillation (VF) during acute MI, and postmortem evaluation of SCD cases (eTable 70.1).

Risk Factors for Sudden Cardiac Death
General Profile of Risk for Sudden Cardiac Death

Risk prediction for SCD is far more challenging than simply profiling risk for coronary artery disease by means of the conventional risk factors for coronary atherogenesis (see Chapters 33 and 34). While the latter is useful for identifying levels of population risk and some aspects of individual risk, it is not sufficient for distinguishing individual patients at risk for SCD from those at risk for other manifestations of coronary heart disease (see Chapters 35 to 40).[6]

Multivariate analyses of selected risk factors (e.g., age, sex, diabetes mellitus, blood pressure/hypertension, current smoking, body mass index, lipid lowering medication use) have demonstrated that the majority of all SCDs occur in the upper deciles of risk (Fig. 70.6). It is likely that the interactions of multiple risk factors potentiates the sum of the individual risks. Comparison of risk factors in victims of SCD with those in people with any manifestation of coronary artery disease does not provide useful patterns to distinguish victims of SCD from the overall pool. However, a history of diabetes mellitus and a tendency to longer QTc intervals on random ECGs are suggested as potential markers of interest for prediction of SCD. ECG analyses by artificial intelligence merits investigation for SCD risk stratification (see Chapter 11). Familial clustering of SCD as a specific

manifestation of the disease may lead to the identification of specific genetic abnormalities that predispose to SCD.[4]

Hypertension is a clearly established risk factor for coronary heart disease and also emerges as a highly significant risk factor in the incidence of SCD (see Chapter 26). However, there is no influence of increasing systolic blood pressure levels on the ratio of sudden deaths to total coronary heart disease deaths. No relationship has been observed between cholesterol concentration and the proportion of coronary deaths that were sudden. Neither the electrocardiographic pattern of LV hypertrophy nor nonspecific ST-T wave abnormalities influence the proportion of total coronary deaths that are sudden and unexpected; only intraventricular conduction abnormalities are suggestive of a disproportionate number of SCDs, an old observation reinforced by data from some device trials that suggest the importance of QRS duration as a risk marker, but one with low individual predictive ability.

The conventional risk factors used in early studies of SCD are risk factors for the evolution of coronary artery disease. The rationale is based on two facts: (1) Coronary disease has been considered the structural basis for 80% of SCDs in the United States, and (2) coronary risk factors are easy to identify because they tend to be present continuously over time (see Fig. 70.5). However, there is evolving evidence that the anatomic consequences of coronary artery disease may not account for as large a proportion of SCDs in adults as previously estimated, with hypertension, LV hypertrophy, and myocardial fibrosis being identified as dominant anatomic/pathophysiologic factors. In a Finnish autopsy study of SCD victims, there was a decline in coronary artery disease with an increase in hypertensive heart disease with LV hypertrophy (and no coronary artery disease).[13] A 10-year longitudinal study of clinical associations identified in hospitalized OHCA victims demonstrated a trend toward decreasing structural heart disease associations, paralleled by an increasing dominance of dynamic, transient pathophysiologic events.[4] Transient

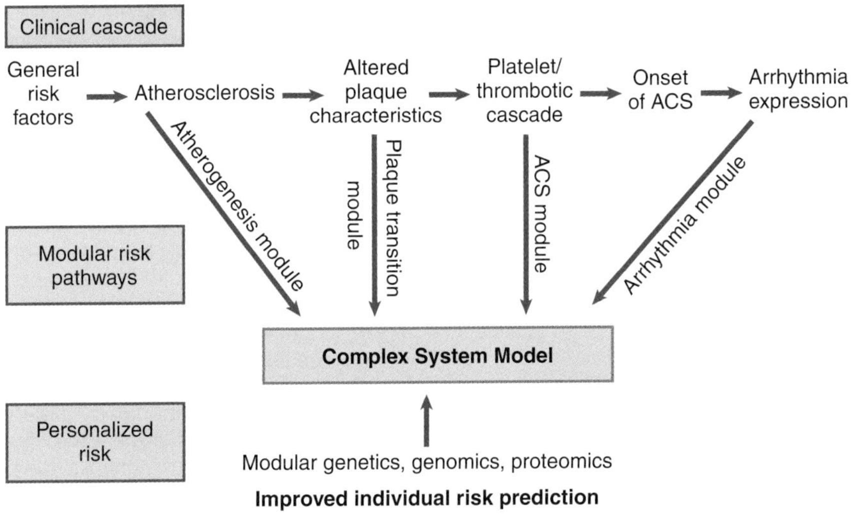

FIGURE 70.5 Coronary atherosclerosis cascade and genetic imprints on the progression to SCD. The cascade from conventional risk factors for coronary atherosclerosis to arrhythmogenesis in SCD related to coronary heart disease includes initiation and development, progression to an active state, initiation of acute coronary syndromes (ACSs), and finally, progression to the specific expression of life-threatening arrhythmias. Multiple factors enter at each level, including specific risk based on the genetic profiles of individual patients. Individual risk based on genetic profiles has been identified for atherogenesis, plaque evolution, the thrombotic cascade, and arrhythmia expression. Stepwise integration of these characteristics may lead to higher single-patient probabilities for individual SCD risk prediction. See text for details. (Modified from Myerburg RJ, Junttila MJ: Sudden cardiac death caused by coronary heart disease. Circulation 2012;125:1043.)

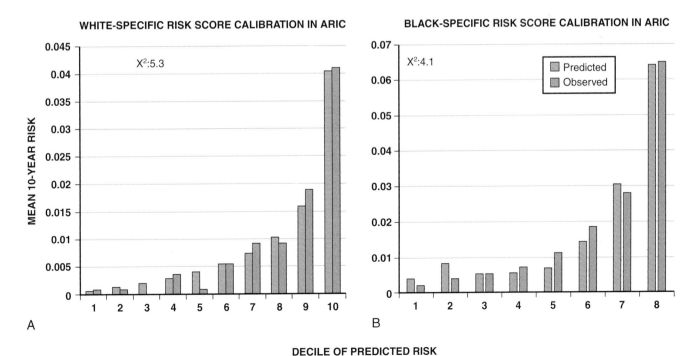

FIGURE 70.6 Risk for sudden death by decile of a multivariate risk score derived in the Framingham Heart Study and calibrated for white (**A**) and Black (**B**) Atherosclerosis Risk in Communities (ARIC) participants. Observed (*red*) and predicted (*blue*) mean 10-year risk of SCD are shown. (From Bogle BM, et al. A simple community-based risk-prediction score for sudden cardiac death. Am J Med 2018;131:532-539.)

pathophysiologic events are being modeled epidemiologically in an attempt to express and use them as clinical risk factors for both profiling and intervention. Nonetheless, data suggest that longitudinal and transient risk predictors may have their power blunted by clinical interventions, such as percutaneous coronary intervention during acute coronary syndromes and post-MI beta blocker therapy.

Identification of specific clinical markers of risk for SCD as a specific expression of both coronary heart disease and other cardiovascular disorders has been a goal for many years. LV ejection fraction has been the most popular of such markers for clinical trials but with limited sensitivity, encouraging investigators to seek additional markers. These additional markers are quite variable, depend on the underlying structural heart disease, and likely reflect the multifactorial basis for SCD.[39-42] Functional metrics such as LV size, strain, and functional status all have demonstrated prognostic significance. Electrical abnormalities in depolarization (QRS duration, fragmented QRS, late potentials) and repolarization, including QT interval, dispersion, and dynamicity, also have prognostic significance. Noninvasive measures of autonomic abnormalities have also demonstrated prognostic significance. Finally, imaging evidence of fibrosis/scarring and autonomic denervation have also demonstrated prognostic significance. Emerging data on the role of biomarkers and genetics may also provide important prognostication. It is notable that no single parameter has adequate predictive power to impact clinical decisions on an individual level.

The general framework for considering SCD risk is to consider the underlying substrate, potential triggers, and other modulating factors. The substrate may represent an anatomical or molecular (e.g., ion channel) abnormality. Common triggers include ventricular ectopic activity and exercise or other conditions of sympathoexcitation. While ventricular ectopic activity was once thought to represent a treatment target for prevention of SCD, the Cardiac Arrhythmia Suppression Trial (CAST) dispelled this notion. Exercise is a well known trigger for SCD, but it must be emphasized that habitual exercise dramatically lowers the risk. Nevertheless, many markers related to exercise have been found to be related to risk of SCD including the acceleration and deceleration of heart rate with and after exercise and exercise repolarization dynamics.[4]

Functional Capacity and Sudden Death

The Framingham Study demonstrated a striking relationship between functional classification and death during a 2-year follow-up period. However, the proportion of deaths that were sudden did not vary with the functional classification, including those free of clinical heart disease and those in functional class IV. Generally, it has been shown that mortality increases with functional class. Competing risk of death from heart failure and other causes does diminish the proportional risk of SCD.[43]

Lifestyle and Psychosocial Factors

A strong association has been found between cigarette smoking and all manifestations of coronary heart disease (see Chapter 28). The Framingham Study demonstrated that cigarette smokers have a two- to threefold increase in risk for sudden death in each decade of life at entry between 30 and 59 years and that this is one of the few risk factors in which the proportion of deaths attributable to coronary heart disease that are sudden increases in association with the risk factor. Importantly, smoking cessation can reverse the excess risk associated with smoking. In support of a direct effect of smoking on arrhythmogenesis, survivors of out-of-hospital cardiac arrest who continued to smoke had a higher recurrence of cardiac arrest than those who stopped.[4]

Alcohol has complex effects on the heart. Light to moderate alcohol consumption was associated with a reduced risk for SCD in the Physicians' Health Study, but there was no reduction in those consuming two or more drinks per day. Alcohol abuse is associated with increased risk of atrial fibrillation, MI, and congestive heart failure,[44] conditions associated with SCD. It is likely that there is a U-shaped relationship between alcohol consumption and SCD (see Chapter 84).

Obesity also influences the proportion of coronary deaths that occur suddenly. With increasing relative weight, the percentage of coronary heart disease deaths that were sudden and total coronary heart disease mortality in the Framingham Study increased linearly. In the

ARIC study, obesity was associated with increased risk of SCD but only in nonsmokers (see Chapter 30).[45]

Associations between levels of physical activity and SCD have been studied with variable results. Epidemiologic observations have suggested a relationship between low levels of physical activity and increased risk for death from coronary heart disease. The Framingham Study, however, showed an insignificant relationship between low levels of physical activity and the incidence of sudden death but a high proportion of sudden to total cardiac deaths with higher levels of physical activity. An association between acute physical exertion and the onset of MI and SCD has been suggested, particularly in individuals who are habitually physically inactive. Analysis from the Physicians' Health Study demonstrated a 17-fold relative increase in SCD associated with vigorous exertion and the 30 minute postexertion period compared with periods of lower level activity or inactive states. However, the absolute risk for events was very low (one event/1.5 million exercise sessions). Habitual vigorous exercise markedly attenuated risk. A clue that intensity of exercise may play a role in SCA risk comes from an observation in college athletes, suggesting that division 1 basketball players are at higher risk than division 2 and division 3 athletes.[46] Information about physical activity relationships in various clinical settings, such as overt and silent disease states, is still lacking (see Chapter 32).

The role of social determinants of health on cardiac risk factors and mortality are well recognized, but no data specifically links this to SCD. There is an association with significant elevations in life change scores during the 6 months before a coronary event, and the association is particularly striking in victims of SCD. In women, it has been reported that those who die suddenly were less often married, had fewer children, and had greater educational discrepancies with their spouses than did age-related control subjects living in the same neighborhood. A history of psychiatric treatment, including phobic anxieties, cigarette smoking, and greater quantities of alcohol consumption than in control subjects also characterized the sudden death group. Behavioral changes (e.g., inactivity) secondary to depression appeared to relate more closely to event rates than did depression itself. Acute psychosocial stressors have been associated with a higher risk for cardiovascular events, including SCD. The risk appears to cluster around the time of the stress in victims with preexisting risk, with the stressor simply advancing the time of an impending event. Natural disasters, such as earthquakes and tsunamis, may be associated with a transient increase in SCD, though specific aggravation of ventricular tachyarrhythmias in patients with implantable defibrillators may not be noted.[47] The possibility of physical stress–induced coronary plaque disruption has been suggested.

Left Ventricular Ejection Fraction in Chronic Ischemic Heart Disease

A marked reduction in the LV ejection fraction is the most powerful of the known predictors of total mortality and SCD in patients with chronic ischemic heart disease, as well as in those at risk for SCD from other causes (see later). Increased mortality, independent of other risk factors, is measurable with ejection fractions higher than 40%, but the greatest rate of change in mortality occurs at levels between 30% and 40%. An ejection fraction of 30% or lower is the single most powerful independent predictor of SCD but has low sensitivity and specificity. Notably, relying on a low ejection fraction as the sole risk-stratifier misses a large number of SCDs that occur at lower incidence rates among the very large subset of patients with normal or moderately reduced ejection fractions and unrecognized disease.[48] Generally, ejection fraction measurements are highly variable, among imaging techniques and even in a given patient depending on loading conditions. Contractility is a major factor determining the ejection fraction and its role in SCD risk may be related to quantifying the extent of scar or myopathy. There are emerging data that LV fibrosis may be a better predictor of cardiac events than ejection fraction alone.[49-51]

Ventricular Arrhythmias in Chronic Ischemic Heart Disease

Most forms of ambient ventricular ectopic activity (premature ventricular complexes [PVCs] and short runs of nonsustained ventricular tachycardia [VT]) have a benign prognosis in the absence of structural heart disease (see Chapters 67 and 40). An exception is the polymorphic forms of nonsustained VT that occur in patients without structural heart disease but can have a molecular, functional, drug-related, or electrolyte-related basis for high-risk arrhythmias. When present in coronary disease-prone age groups, PVCs select a subgroup with a higher probability of coronary artery disease and SCD. Exercise-induced PVCs and short runs of nonsustained VT indicate some level of risk for SCD, even in the absence of recognizable structural heart disease. However, the data available to support this hypothesis are conflicting, with the possible exception of polymorphic runs of nonsustained VT. Additional data suggest that PVCs and nonsustained VT during both the exercise and recovery phases of a stress test predict increased risk. Arrhythmias in the recovery phase, previously thought to be benign, appear to predict higher risk than do arrhythmias in the exercise phase, and there is a gradient of risk with increasing severity of arrhythmias.

The occurrence of PVCs in survivors of MI, particularly if frequent and having complex forms such as repetitive PVCs, predicts an increased risk for SCD and total mortality during long-term follow-up. Data are conflicting on the role of measures of frequency and forms of ventricular ectopic activity as discriminators of risk, but most studies have cited a frequency cutoff of 10 PVCs/hour as a threshold level for increased risk. Several investigators have emphasized that the most powerful predictors among the various forms of PVCs are runs of nonsustained VT, although this relationship is now questioned. It is important to note that much of the foundational data that demonstrated the important prognostic role of ejection fraction after MI also demonstrated the similarly important role of PVC frequency.

While both ejection fraction and PVC frequency were shown to be important prognostic markers after MI, only PVCs were considered to be modifiable with antiarrhythmic drugs. The results of CAST (Cardiac Arrhythmia Suppression Trial; see Chapter 64), which was designed to test the hypothesis that suppression of PVCs by antiarrhythmic drugs alters the risk for SCD after MI, were surprising for two reasons. First, the death rate in the randomized placebo group was lower than expected, and second, the death rate among patients in the encainide and flecainide arms exceeded control rates by more than threefold. The excess death rates may be accounted for by drug-induced proarrhythmia during ischemic events. The SWORD (Survival with Oral d-Sotalol) study, a comparison of d-sotalol with placebo in a post-MI population with a low mortality rate, also demonstrated excess risk in the drug treated group. Whether the conclusions from CAST, CAST II, and SWORD extend beyond the drug studies or to other diseases remains to be learned. What is clear is that markers of risk for SCD do not necessarily represent appropriate treatment targets.

LV dysfunction is the major modulator of risk associated with chronic PVCs after MI. The risk for death predicted by post-MI PVCs is enhanced by the presence of LV dysfunction, which appears to exert its influence most strongly in the first 6 months after infarction. Delayed deterioration of LV function, probably because of remodeling after MI, may increase the risk further.

Emerging Markers of Risk for Sudden Cardiac Death

Decades of evaluations of ECG-based testing for abnormalities in depolarization, repolarization, and cardiac autonomic function provide consistent data linking these markers to mortality and/or SCD risk in populations but with little utility for individual risk prediction and clinical decision making. Emerging tests such as contrast-enhanced magnetic resonance imaging of the infarction, as well as noninfarct patterns of fibrosis seen on MRI delayed hyperenhancement, and sympathetic imaging with 11C-hydroxyephedrine or I-m-iodobenzylguanidine (MIBG) require further evaluation to assess utility for individual risk prediction (see Chapter 18). The potential of genetic risk profiling based on studies of familial clustering of SCD also requires further evaluation.[6]

CAUSES OF SUDDEN CARDIAC DEATH

Coronary Artery Abnormalities

Diseases of the coronary arteries and their consequences have been estimated to account for at least 80% of SCDs in Western countries, but

recent observations suggest that the magnitude of this excess burden may be decreasing.[13] Coronary artery disease is also the most common cause in many areas of the world in which the prevalence of atherosclerosis is lower. As developing nations improve access to health care for communicable disease in the earlier years of life, coronary atherosclerosis and its consequences may emerge as a larger problem.[52] Continued focus on control of underlying risk factors will be key to prevention of SCD.

Despite the established dominant relationship between coronary atherosclerosis and SCD, complete understanding of SCD requires recognition that less common and often rare coronary vascular disorders (Table 70.3) may be identifiable before death and have therapeutic implications. Many of these entities are relatively more common causes of SCD in adolescents and young adults, in whom the prevalence of coronary heart disease-related SCDs is much lower before the age of 30 years[29] (see Fig. 70.4A).

Atherosclerotic Coronary Artery Disease

The structural and functional abnormalities of the coronary vasculature as a result of coronary atherosclerosis interact with the electrophysiologic alterations that result from the myocardial impact of an ischemic burden (see Chapters 37 to 40). The relationship between the vascular and myocardial components of this pathophysiologic model, as well as its modulation by hemodynamic, autonomic, genetic, and other influences, establishes multiple patterns of risk derived from the fundamental disease state (Fig. 70.7). Risk is modulated by multiple factors that can be either transient or persistent, and transient modulations may interact with persistent changes. The myocardial component of this pathophysiologic model is not static over time, and the term persistent must be viewed with caution because of the gradual effects of remodeling after an initial ischemic event and the effects of recurrent ischemic episodes. SCA and SCD resulting from transient ischemia or acute MI differ in physiology and prognosis from the risk for SCA implied by a previous MI with or without subsequent ischemic cardiomyopathy. In general, the short-term risk for life-threatening events is associated more closely with acute ischemia or the acute phase of MI, and longer-term risk is associated more with transient ischemia, myocardial scarring, remodeling, ischemic cardiomyopathy, alterations in autonomic modulation, and heart failure.

Nonatherosclerotic Coronary Artery Abnormalities

Nonatherosclerotic coronary artery abnormalities include congenital lesions, coronary artery embolism, coronary arteritis, and mechanical abnormalities of the coronary arteries. Among the congenital lesions, anomalous origin of a left coronary artery from the pulmonary artery (see Chapters 21 and 82) is relatively common and associated with an increased death rate in infancy and early childhood without surgical treatment. The early risk for SCD is not excessively high, but patients who survive to adolescence and young adulthood without surgical intervention are at risk for SCD. Other forms of coronary arteriovenous fistulas are much less frequent and associated with a low incidence of SCD.

Anomalous Origin of Coronary Arteries from the Wrong Sinus of Valsalva

These anatomic variants are associated with an increased risk for SCD, particularly during exercise. When the anomalous artery passes between the aortic and the pulmonary artery root, the takeoff angle of the anomalous ostium creates a slitlike opening of the vessel that reduces the effective cross-sectional area for blood flow. The less common origin of the left coronary artery from the right sinus of Valsalva is a higher risk variant, but the origin of the right coronary artery from the left sinus of Valsalva, while lower risk, accounts for a proportion of SCDs that should not be ignored, based on the incidence of this anomaly.[53] Congenitally hypoplastic, stenotic, or atretic left coronary arteries are uncommon abnormalities associated with a risk for MI in the young, but not for SCD.

TABLE 70.3 Causes of and Contributing Factors in Sudden Cardiac Death

I. **Coronary artery abnormalities**
- A. Coronary atherosclerosis
  1. Chronic coronary atherosclerosis with acute or transient myocardial ischemia—thrombosis, spasm, physical stress
  2. Acute myocardial infarction, onset and early phase
  3. Chronic atherosclerosis with a change in myocardial substrate, including previous myocardial infarction
- B. Congenital abnormalities of coronary arteries
  1. Anomalous origin from the pulmonary artery
  2. Other coronary arteriovenous fistula
  3. Origin of a left coronary artery from the right or noncoronary sinus of Valsalva (lower incidence; higher risk)
  4. Origin of the right coronary artery from the left sinus of Valsalva (higher incidence; lower risk)
  5. Hypoplastic or aplastic coronary arteries
  6. Coronary-intracardiac shunt
- C. Coronary artery embolism
  1. Aortic or mitral endocarditis
  2. Prosthetic aortic or mitral valves
  3. Abnormal native valves or left ventricular mural thrombus
  4. Platelet embolism
- D. Coronary arteritis
  1. Polyarteritis nodosa, progressive systemic sclerosis, giant cell arteritis
  2. Mucocutaneous lymph node syndrome (Kawasaki disease)
  3. Syphilitic coronary ostial stenosis
- E. Miscellaneous mechanical obstruction of the coronary arteries
  1. Coronary artery dissection in Marfan syndrome
  2. Coronary artery dissection in pregnancy (primarily labor/delivery)
  3. Prolapse of aortic valve myxomatous polyps into the coronary ostia
  4. Dissection or rupture of the sinus of Valsalva
- F. Functional obstruction of the coronary arteries
  1. Coronary artery spasm with or without atherosclerosis
  2. Myocardial bridges

II. **Hypertrophy of the ventricular myocardium**
- A. Left ventricular hypertrophy associated with coronary heart disease
- B. Hypertensive heart disease without significant coronary atherosclerosis
- C. Hypertrophic myocardium secondary to valvular heart disease
- D. Hypertrophic cardiomyopathy
  1. Obstructive
  2. Nonobstructive
- E. Primary or secondary pulmonary hypertension
  1. Advanced chronic right ventricular overload
  2. Pulmonary hypertension in pregnancy (highest risk peripartum)

III. **Myocardial diseases and dysfunction, with or without heart failure**
- A. Chronic congestive heart failure
  1. Ischemic cardiomyopathy
  2. Idiopathic dilated cardiomyopathy, acquired
  3. Hereditary dilated cardiomyopathy
  4. Alcoholic cardiomyopathy
  5. Hypertensive cardiomyopathy
  6. Postmyocarditis cardiomyopathy
  7. Peripartum cardiomyopathy
  8. Idiopathic fibrosis
- B. Acute and subacute cardiac failure
  1. Large acute myocardial infarction
  2. Myocarditis, acute or fulminant
  3. Acute alcoholic cardiac dysfunction
  4. Takotsubo syndrome (uncertain risk for sudden death)
  5. Ball valve embolism in aortic stenosis or prosthesis
  6. Mechanical disruptions of cardiac structures
     - a. Rupture of the ventricular free wall
     - b. Disruption of the mitral apparatus
        (1). Papillary muscle
        (2). Chordae tendineae
        (3). Leaflet
     - c. Rupture of the interventricular septum
        (1). Acute pulmonary edema in noncompliant ventricles

IV. **Inflammatory, infiltrative, neoplastic, and degenerative processes**
- A. Viral myocarditis, with or without ventricular dysfunction
  1. Acute phase
  2. Postmyocarditis interstitial fibrosis
- B. Myocarditis associated with the vasculitides
- C. Sarcoidosis
- D. Progressive systemic sclerosis
- E. Amyloidosis
- F. Hemochromatosis
- G. Idiopathic giant cell myocarditis
- H. Chagas disease
- I. Cardiac ganglionitis
- J. Arrhythmogenic right ventricular dysplasia, right ventricular cardiomyopathy
- K. Neuromuscular diseases (e.g., muscular dystrophy, Friedreich ataxia, myotonic dystrophy)
- L. Intramural tumors
  1. Primary
  2. Metastatic
- M. Obstructive intracavitary tumors
  1. Neoplastic
  2. Thrombotic

V. **Diseases of the cardiac valves**
- A. Valvular aortic stenosis/insufficiency
- B. Mitral valve disruption
- C. Mitral valve prolapse
- D. Endocarditis
- E. Prosthetic valve dysfunction

VI. **Congenital heart disease**
- A. Congenital aortic (potentially high risk) or pulmonic (low risk) valve stenosis
- B. Congenital septal defects with Eisenmenger physiology
  1. Advanced disease
  2. During labor and delivery
- C. Late after surgical repair of congenital lesions (e.g., tetralogy of Fallot)

VII. **Electrophysiologic abnormalities**
- A. Abnormalities of the conducting system
  1. Fibrosis of the His-Purkinje system
     - a. Primary degeneration (Lenègre disease)
     - b. Secondary to fibrosis and calcification of the cardiac skeleton (Lev disease)
     - c. Postviral conducting system fibrosis
     - d. Hereditary conducting system disease
  2. Anomalous pathways of conduction (Wolff-Parkinson-White syndrome, short refractory period bypass tract)
- B. Abnormalities of repolarization
  1. Congenital abnormalities in duration of the QT interval
     - a. Congenital abnormalities in duration of the QT interval
        (1). Romano-Ward syndrome (without deafness)
        (2). Jervell and Lange-Nielsen syndrome (with deafness)
  2. Congenital short QT interval syndrome
  3. Acquired (or provoked) long-QT interval syndromes
     - a. Drug effect (enhanced by predisposition)
        (1). Cardiac, antiarrhythmic
        (2). Noncardiac
        (3). Drug interactions
     - b. Electrolyte abnormality (response modified by genetic predisposition)
     - c. Toxic substances
     - d. Hypothermia
     - e. Central nervous system injury, subarachnoid hemorrhage
  4. Brugada syndrome—right bundle branch block pattern and ST segment elevation in the absence of ischemia
  5. Early repolarization syndrome
- C. Ventricular fibrillation of unknown or uncertain cause
  1. Absence of identifiable structural or functional causes
     - a. Idiopathic ventricular fibrillation
     - b. Short-coupled torsades de pointes, polymorphic ventricular tachycardia
     - c. Nonspecific fibrofatty infiltration in a previously healthy victim (variation of right ventricular dysplasia?)
  2. Sleep-death in Southeast Asians (Brugada syndrome)
     - a. Bangungut
     - b. Pokkuri
     - c. Lai-tai

VIII. **Electrical instability related to neurohumoral and central nervous system influences**
- A. Catecholaminergic polymorphic ventricular tachycardia
- B. Other catecholamine-dependent arrhythmias
- C. Central nervous system related
  1. Psychic stress, emotional extremes (Takotsubo syndrome)
  2. Auditory related
  3. "Voodoo death" in primitive cultures
  4. Diseases of the cardiac nerves
  5. Arrhythmia expression in congenital long-QT syndrome

IX. **Sudden cardiac death in the young**
- A. Sudden cardiac death in newborns
  1. Complex congenital heart disease
  2. Neonatal myocarditis
- B. Sudden infant death syndrome
  1. Immature respiratory control function
  2. Long-QT syndrome
  3. Congenital heart disease
  4. Myocarditis
- C. Sudden death in children
  1. Eisenmenger syndrome, aortic stenosis, hypertrophic cardiomyopathy, pulmonary atresia
  2. After corrective surgery for congenital heart disease
  3. Myocarditis
  4. Genetic disorders of electrical function (e.g., long-QT syndrome)
  5. No identified structural or functional cause

X. **Miscellaneous**
- A. Sudden death during extreme physical activity (seek predisposing causes)
- B. Commotio cordis—blunt chest trauma
- C. Mechanical interference with venous return
  1. Acute cardiac tamponade
  2. Massive pulmonary embolism
  3. Acute intracardiac thrombosis
- D. Cardiorespiratory arrest secondary to mechanical asphyxia
- E. Dissecting aneurysm of the aorta
- F. Toxic and metabolic disturbances (other than the QT interval effects listed above)
  1. Electrolyte disturbances
  2. Metabolic disturbances
  3. Proarrhythmic effects of antiarrhythmic drugs
  4. Proarrhythmic effects of noncardiac drugs
- G. Mimics sudden cardiac death
  1. "Café coronary"
  2. Acute alcoholic states ("holiday heart")
  3. Acute asthmatic attacks
  4. Air or amniotic fluid embolism

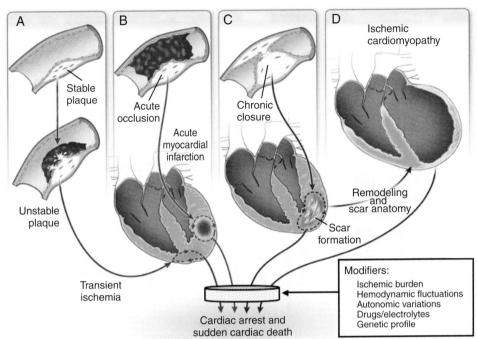

FIGURE 70.7 **Pathophysiology of ventricular tachyarrhythmias in coronary heart disease.** The short- and long-term risks for the development of VT or VF and recurrent events are related to the presence of transient or persistent physiologic factors. VT/VF caused by transient ischemia **(A)** and the acute phase (24 to 48 hours) of myocardial infarction **(B)** are not predictive of recurrent events if the recurrent ischemia is preventable. In contrast, VT/VF associated with healed myocardial infarction, with or without acute transient ischemia **(C)**, is associated with risk for recurrence. Longstanding ischemic cardiomyopathy **(D)**, especially when accompanied by heart failure, establishes a substrate associated with risk for VT/VF and recurrences over time. A series of modifying influences contribute to individual expression. (Modified from Myerburg RJ: Implantable cardioverter-defibrillators after myocardial infarction. N Engl J Med 2008;359:2245.)

Ventricular Hypertrophy and Hypertrophic Cardiomyopathy

LV hypertrophy, an independent risk factor for SCD, is associated with many causes of SCD and may be a physiologic contributor to mechanisms of potentially lethal arrhythmias.[54] Underlying states resulting in LV hypertrophy include hypertensive heart disease with or without atherosclerosis, valvular heart disease, obstructive and nonobstructive HCM (see Chapter 54), primary pulmonary hypertension with right ventricular hypertrophy, and advanced right ventricular overload secondary to congenital heart disease. Each of these conditions is associated with risk for SCD, and it has been suggested that patients with severely hypertrophic ventricles are particularly susceptible to arrhythmic death.

Risk for SCD in patients with obstructive and nonobstructive HCM was identified in the early clinical and hemodynamic descriptions of this entity.[42,55] In patients who have the obstructive form, a majority of all deaths are sudden. However, survivors of cardiac arrest in this group may have a better long-term outcome than might survivors with other causes, and reports have suggested that the risk for primary cardiac arrest and SCD in those with HCM is lower than previously thought. It is suggested that it is now less than 1%/year, perhaps related to risk stratification based therapies such as the implantable cardioverter defibrillator.[42] Yet this is a significant cause for SCD in the young.[56,57]

A substantial proportion of patients with obstructive and nonobstructive HCM have a family history of affected relatives with premature SCDs of unknown cause. Genetic studies have confirmed autosomal dominant inheritance patterns, but with significant allelic and phenotypic heterogeneity. Most of the mutations are at loci that encode elements in the contractile protein complex, the most common being myosin binding protein C and beta-myosin heavy chain, which together account for more than half of identified abnormalities. The genetics of HCM is characterized by a large number of private mutations with variable expression. Possible interaction with modifier genes may account for variable expression among carriers of a specific variant, but there is also a possibility that a number of HCM variants thought to be disease-causing in the Black population are actually benign variants unique

to the Black population that are missed because of underrepresentation in control populations.[58]

Specific clinical markers have not been especially predictive of SCD in individual patients, although young age at onset, a strong family history of SCD in a first-degree relative, magnitude of the LV mass, wall thickness >3 cm, unexplained syncope, nonsustained VT, LV apical aneurysm, and LV systolic dysfunction appear to indicate higher risk. Both a substantial provocable gradient, regardless of the resting gradient, and a high resting gradient alone identify high risk for SCD.[59] The mechanism of SCD in patients with HCM was initially thought to involve outflow tract obstruction, possibly as a consequence of catecholamine stimulation, but later data have focused on lethal arrhythmias as the common mechanism of sudden death in this disease.

The pathogenesis of the arrhythmias in HCM is discussed in Chapter 54. The observation that patients with nonobstructive HCM, such as the diffuse, midcavitary, and to a lesser extent the apical variety, are also at risk for SCD suggests that an electrophysiologic mechanism secondary to the hypertrophied muscle itself plays a major role. In athletes younger than 35 years, HCM is the most common cause of SCD, in contrast to athletes older than 35 years, in whom coronary heart disease is the most common cause.

Cardiomyopathy and Systolic and Diastolic Heart Failure

The advent of therapeutic interventions that provide better control of congestive heart failure has improved the long-term survival of these patients (see Chapters 50 to 52). However, the proportion of patients with heart failure who die suddenly is substantial, especially among those who appear clinically stable (i.e., functional class I or II). The mechanism of SCD may be tachyarrhythmic (VT or VF) or nonshockable bradyarrhythmias or asystole. The absolute risk for SCD increases with deteriorating LV function, but the ratio of sudden to nonsudden deaths is inversely related to the extent of functional impairment. In patients with cardiomyopathy who have good functional capacity (classes I and II), total mortality risk is considerably lower than in those with functional classes III and IV, but the probability that a death will be sudden is higher (Fig. 70.8). Unexplained syncope has been observed to be a powerful predictor of SCD in patients who have functional class III or IV symptoms, regardless of the cause of cardiomyopathy.

Heart failure with preserved ejection fraction (HFpEF) has a risk for mortality over time similar to that of heart failure with reduced ejection fraction (see Chapter 51). In a summary[60] of the cause specific mortality in HFpEF from the I-Preserve, CHARM-Preserved, and TOPCAT trials, 68% were cardiovascular. SCD accounted for approximately 40% of the cardiovascular deaths (27% of all deaths). The precise etiology remains unknown with both VT and bradyarrhythmias recorded in these patients.[61] To date, there have been no targeted interventions that have successfully reduced the risk of SCD in this population.

Ischemic cardiomyopathy provides the strongest association between chronic heart failure and SCD. The prevalence of ischemic cardiomyopathy had been increasing because of better acute MI survival statistics coupled with late remodeling. Other causes include "idiopathic" fibrosis, alcoholic and postmyocarditis cardiomyopathies, peripartum cardiomyopathy (see Chapter 92), and the familial pattern of dilated cardiomyopathy, many of the latter being associated with lamin A/C mutations.[62] Other gene loci have also been implicated. A residual group of undefined causes have been classified as idiopathic cardiomyopathy.

Acute Heart Failure

All causes of acute cardiac failure (see Chapters 47-49), in the absence of prompt interventions, can result in SCD as a result of the circulatory failure itself or secondary arrhythmias. The electrophysiologic mechanisms involved have been proposed to be caused by acute stretching of ventricular myocardial fibers or the His-Purkinje system on the basis of its experimentally demonstrated arrhythmogenic effects. However, the roles of neurohumoral mechanisms and acute electrolyte shifts have not been fully evaluated. Among the causes of acute cardiac failure associated with SCD are massive acute MI, acute myocarditis, acute alcoholic cardiac dysfunction, acute pulmonary edema in any form of advanced heart disease, and a number of mechanical causes of heart failure, such as massive pulmonary embolism, mechanical disruption of intracardiac structures secondary to infarction or infection, and ball valve embolism in aortic or mitral stenosis (see Table 70.3).

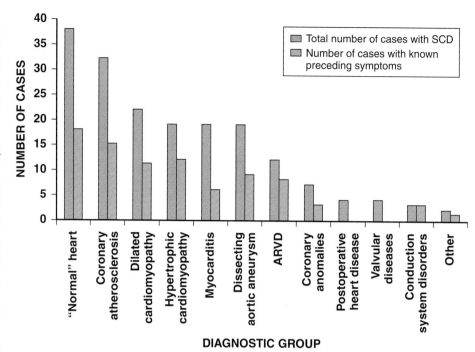

FIGURE 70.8 SCD in adolescents and young adults in Sweden. The frequency of preceding symptoms in 181 cases of SCD in persons 15 to 35 years old is shown by diagnostic group. *ARVD,* Arrhythmogenic right ventricular dysplasia. (Modified from Wisten A, et al. Sudden cardiac death in 15-35-year-olds in Sweden during 1992-99. J Intern Med 2002;252:529.)

Inflammatory, Infiltrative, Neoplastic, and Degenerative Diseases of the Heart. Almost all diseases in this category have been associated with SCD, with or without concomitant cardiac failure. Acute viral myocarditis with LV dysfunction (see Chapters 52 and 55) is commonly associated with cardiac arrhythmias, including potentially lethal arrhythmias. Serious ventricular arrhythmias or SCD can occur in patients with myocarditis, even in the absence of clinical evidence of LV dysfunction. This has most recently been reported following SARS-CoV-2 infection during the COVID-19 pandemic.[63-67] In autopsy series of young people presenting with SCD, myocarditis may be found in up to 10%.[68] As noted during the COVID-19 pandemic, many individuals with myocarditis have no to minimal symptoms (Fig. 70.8). Most data available suggest a bias toward victims younger than 35 years. Focal myocarditis can be associated with SCD and may be missed on autopsy depending on the extent of the cardiac evaluation. Giant cell myocarditis and acute necrotizing eosinophilic myocarditis are particularly virulent for both myocardial damage and arrhythmias. Viral myocarditis can also cause damage isolated to the specialized conducting system and result in a propensity to arrhythmias; the rare association of this process with SCD has been reported. Varicella in adults is a rare cause of striking conduction system disorders, largely involving the intraventricular specialized conducting tissue with very prolonged QRS complexes. LV function is usually preserved, and its relationship to SCD is unclear.

Myocardial involvement in collagen-vascular disorders, tumors, chronic granulomatous diseases, infiltrative disorders, and protozoan infestations varies widely, but SCD can be the initial or terminal manifestation of the disease process in all cases. Among the granulomatous diseases, cardiac sarcoidosis stands out because of the frequency of associated SCD.[69] Clinical cardiac involvement in patients with sarcoidosis is approximately 5% with another 20% to 25% having asymptomatic involvement.[70] The risk for SCD has been related to the extent of cardiac involvement, but ambient arrhythmias, such as nonsustained VT, may indicate risk in such patients with lesser degrees of cardiac involvement. In a report of the pathologic findings in nine patients who died of progressive systemic sclerosis, eight who died suddenly had evidence of transient ischemia and reperfusion histologically, thus suggesting that this might represent spasm of the coronary vessels. Amyloidosis of the heart (see Chapter 53) can also cause sudden death. An incidence of 30% has been reported, and diffuse involvement of ventricular muscle or the specialized conducting system may be associated with SCD. Cardiac involvement can occur in both light chain (AL) and transthyretin (ATTR) amyloid. TTR-associated cardiac amyloid tends to express later in life, almost always after the age of 50 years, and observed in up to 4% of the Black population, with or without the disease. Despite a high incidence of treatment for VT/fibrillation, the role of the implantable defibrillator in improving survival has not been established.[71]

Arrhythmogenic Right Ventricular Dysplasia or Right Ventricular Cardiomyopathy. This condition with a prevalence ranging between 1/1000 and 1/5000[72] is associated with a high incidence of ventricular arrhythmias, including polymorphic nonsustained VT and VF and recurrent sustained monomorphic VT (see Chapters 63 and 67). Importantly, this is a significant underlying etiology for SCD in young people, likely accounting for 10% to 20% of cases.[73] Importantly, in a high proportion of victims, perhaps as many as 80%, the first manifestation of arrhythmogenic right ventricular dysplasia or right ventricular cardiomyopathy (ARVD/C) is "unexplained" syncope or SCD. With more widespread screening and evaluation for ARVD/C, this is being identified among family members of probands who also have substantial risk for VT, but the clinical characteristics suggest a more aggressive course in the subset who present with SCD—occurring at a younger age, in a higher percent of males, and during high levels of exertion.[74]

SCD is often exercise related, and in some areas of the world where screening for HCM has excluded affected athletes from competition, ARVD/C has emerged as the most common cause of sports-related SCD. High-level competitive sports participation is not recommended for those with a confirmed diagnosis.[75] Although it is generally considered a right ventricular abnormality, with possible late involvement of the left ventricle in advanced cases, a left ventricle–dominant pattern has also been described.

ARVD/C is predominantly an inherited disorder in which the variants cause or predispose to the disease, interacting with high right ventricular strain during exercise. In addition, there is some basis for considering that RV arrhythmogenic responses may be caused by very high-intensity athletic activity as a result of repeated RV strain exposures.[76] The inheritance pattern is autosomal dominant, except in one geographically isolated cluster in which it is autosomal recessive (Naxos disease, plakoglobin locus on chromosome 17). Four loci-encoding components of the desmosome (plakoglobin, desmoplakin, plakophilin 2, and desmoglein 2) are collectively the most common known mutations associated with right ventricular dysplasia.[77] Autosomal dominant mutations have also been identified in the ryanodine receptor locus on chromosome 1 (1q42) (see Chapter 63).

Valvular Heart Disease

Before the advent of surgery for valvular heart disease, severe aortic stenosis was associated with high risk for mortality (see Chapter 72). Approximately 70% of deaths were sudden and accounted for an absolute SCD mortality rate of 15% to 20% among all affected patients. In the Contemporary Outcomes After Surgery and Medical Treatment in Patients With Severe Aortic Stenosis (CURRENT AS) registry,[78] the annual rate of SCD was 1.6%/year and 1.1%/year with and without censoring for surgical or transcatheter valve replacement. Even asymptomatic patients experienced a 1.4%/year rate of SCD. In patients with mild to moderate AS, a 0.39%/year rate of SCD has been reported.[79]

The advent of aortic valve replacement has reduced the incidence of SCD, but patients with prosthetic or heterograft aortic valve replacements remain at some risk for SCD caused by arrhythmias, prosthetic valve dysfunction, or coexistent coronary heart disease. The incidence peaks 3 weeks after surgery and then levels off after 8 months. A high incidence of ventricular arrhythmia has been observed during the follow-up of patients with valve replacement, especially those who had aortic stenosis, multiple valve surgery, or cardiomegaly. Among 3726 patients who underwent transcatheter aortic valve replacement, 5.6% were reported to have SCD at average 22 month follow-up.[80] New-onset left bundle branch block was a significant predictor of SCD, but not in those who received a pacemaker, suggesting that AV block may be a significant etiology for SCD in these patients. Similar observations have been made following surgical aortic valve replacement. An association between stenotic lesions of other valves and SCD has not been demonstrated.

Mitral valve prolapse has been associated with SCD. While mitral valve prolapse is common, the risk for SCD is extremely low. There may be a subset of patients with mitral valve prolapse that are particularly susceptible to ventricular arrhythmias and SCD. The estimated incidence of SCD is 0.2% to 0.4% per year.[81] Fibrosis of the papillary muscles and inferobasal left ventricle is noted in these patients. Mapping studies show a papillary muscle origin for ventricular ectopy in patients with mitral valve prolapse and evidence of late gadolinium enhancement in the papillary muscle,[82] though other LV origins for ventricular ectopy have also been noted. SCD is associated with marked redundancy of mitral leaflets, in conjunction with nonspecific ST-T wave changes in inferior leads.

Regurgitant lesions, particularly chronic aortic regurgitation and acute mitral regurgitation, may cause SCD, but the risk is lower than with aortic stenosis. Limited data suggest that inducibility of VT with programmed ventricular stimulation is a significant predictor of arrhythmic events.

Endocarditis of the Aortic and Mitral Valves. This condition may be associated with rapid death resulting from acute disruption of the valvular apparatus (see Chapter 80), coronary embolism, or abscesses of valvular rings or the septum; however, such deaths are rarely true sudden deaths because conventionally defined tachyarrhythmic mechanisms are uncommon. Coronary embolism from valvular vegetations can trigger fatal ischemic arrhythmia on rare occasion.

Congenital Heart Disease. The congenital lesions most commonly associated with SCD are aortic stenosis (see Chapter 82) and communications between the left and right sides of the heart with Eisenmenger physiology. In the latter, the risk for SCD is a function of the severity of pulmonary vascular disease; also, pregnant patients with Eisenmenger syndrome have an extraordinarily high risk for maternal mortality during labor and delivery (see Chapter 92). Potentially lethal arrhythmias and SCD have been described as late complications after surgical repair of complex congenital lesions, particularly tetralogy of Fallot, transposition of the great arteries, and atrioventricular (AV) canal defects. These patients should be observed closely and treated aggressively when cardiac arrhythmias are identified, although the late risk for SCD may not be as high as previously thought.

Electrophysiologic Abnormalities

Acquired disease of the AV node and His-Purkinje system and the presence of accessory AV pathways (see Chapter 68) may be associated with SCD. Clinical surveillance and follow-up studies have suggested that intraventricular conduction disturbances in coronary heart disease are one of the few factors that can increase the proportion of SCD in patients with coronary heart disease. Early studies demonstrated a very high risk for total mortality and SCD during the late in-hospital course and the first few months after hospital discharge in patients with anterior MIs and right bundle branch or bifascicular block. In a later study evaluating the impact of thrombolytic therapy versus the pre–thrombolytic era experience, the incidence of pure right bundle branch block was higher but that of bifascicular block was lower, as were late complications and mortality.

Primary fibrosis (Lenègre disease) or injury secondary to other disorders (Lev disease) of the His-Purkinje system is commonly associated with intraventricular conduction abnormalities and symptomatic AV block and less commonly with SCD. Identification of those at risk and the efficacy of pacemakers for prevention of SCD, rather than only amelioration of symptoms, have been subjects of debate. However, survival appears to depend more on the nature and extent of the underlying disease than on the conduction disturbance itself.

Patients with congenital AV block (see Chapter 68) or nonprogressive congenital intraventricular block, in the absence of structural cardiac abnormalities and with a stable heart rate and rhythm, have been characterized as being at low risk for SCD in the past. Later data have suggested that patients with the patterns of congenital AV block previously thought to be benign are at risk for dilated cardiomyopathy, and routine pacemaker implantation in patients older than 15 years, if not indicated sooner based on symptoms, has been suggested by at least one group. Confirmation from clinical trial data is not available. Hereditary forms of AV block have also been reported in association with a familial propensity to SCD. Sodium channel gene mutations have been associated with progressive conduction system disturbances and variants of Brugada syndrome (see Chapter 63). External ophthalmoplegia and retinal pigmentation with progressive conduction system disease (Kearns-Sayre syndrome), which is associated with mitochondrial DNA variants, may lead to high-grade heart block and pacemaker dependence.

The anomalous pathways of conduction in Wolff-Parkinson-White syndrome are commonly associated with nonlethal arrhythmias. However, when the anomalous pathways of conduction have short anterograde refractory periods, the occurrence of atrial fibrillation may allow the initiation of VF during very rapid conduction across the accessory pathway (see Chapter 65). Patients who have multiple pathways appear to be at higher risk for SCD, as do patients with a familial pattern of anomalous pathways and premature SCD.

Long-QT Syndromes

Congenital long-QT syndrome is a functional abnormality usually caused by mutations affecting ion channel proteins and is associated with environmental or neurogenic triggers that can initiate symptomatic or lethal arrhythmias (see Chapters 63 and 67).[83] Such mutations may occur de novo or more commonly may be transmitted from an apparently normal parent. Syncope is the most common manifestation in symptomatic patients. SCD is less common, although data are limited by the absence of information on undiagnosed carriers in whom fatal cardiac arrest is the first clinical event. For example, the prevalence of long-QT variants in the population is generally cited to be in the range of 1/2000 to 1/2500, but a study from Japan reporting on routine ECG screening among first- and seventh-grade school children provides an estimated prevalence of 1/988, more than double the generally accepted figure from referral populations.[36] Some patients have prolonged QT intervals throughout life without any manifest arrhythmias, whereas others are highly susceptible to symptomatic and potentially fatal ventricular arrhythmias. The concept of modifier genes interacting with the primary defect or physiologic contributors to expression is an area of active investigation.[84]

Higher levels of risk are associated with female sex, greater degrees of QT prolongation or QT alternans, unexplained syncope, family history of premature SCD, and documented torsades de pointes or previous VF. Patients with the syndrome require avoidance of drugs that are associated with QT lengthening and careful medical management, which may include implantable defibrillators. Moreover, it is important to identify and to manage relatives medically who carry the mutation and may be at risk (see Chapters 63, 64, and 67). While abnormalities in genes coding for ion channels are the most frequent causes of long-QT syndrome, there are now multiple LQT types coding for other proteins that are responsible for this syndrome (see Chapter 63).

Even in the absence of manifest long-QT syndrome, from an epidemiologic perspective, there is interest in whether QT interval abnormalities or the propensity thereto, interacting with acquired diseases, predisposes to SCD as a specific clinical expression. In many studies, QT prolongation has been associated with increased SCD, but it is interesting to note that individual components of the QT interval may bear more predictive utility.[85] The hypothesis that common genetic variants may modulate QTc in unselected populations has stimulated interest in the relationship to selective risk for SCD in individuals with acquired diseases. However, a number of rare variants may be even more important.

The acquired form of prolonged–QT interval syndrome refers to excessive lengthening of the QT interval and the potential for the development of torsades de pointes (TdP) in response to environmental influences. As with congenital LQTS, it is more common in women. The syndrome may be caused by drug effects or an individual patient's idiosyncrasies (particularly related to class IA or III antiarrhythmic drugs and psychotropic drugs; see Chapters 9 and 99), electrolyte abnormalities, hypothermia, toxic substances, bradyarrhythmia-induced QT adjustments, and central nervous system injury (most commonly subarachnoid hemorrhage). It had also been reported in intensive weight reduction programs that involved the use of certain liquid protein diets and in patients with anorexia nervosa. Lithium carbonate can prolong the QT interval and unmask Brugada syndrome and has been reported to be associated with an increased incidence of SCD in cancer patients with preexisting heart disease. Drug interactions have been recognized as a mechanism of prolongation of the QT interval and TDP. Inherited polymorphisms or mutations with low penetrance involving the same gene loci associated with phenotypically expressed long-QT syndrome may underlie the acquired form, in many cases. In acquired prolonged-QT syndrome, as in the congenital form, torsades de pointes is commonly the specific arrhythmia that triggers or degenerates into VF.

Short-QT Syndrome. A familial pattern of risk for SCD has been associated with abnormally short QT intervals, defined as a QTc shorter than 300 milliseconds (QT <280 milliseconds). Short-QT syndrome is much less common than long-QT syndrome, and there is little to guide risk profiling other than documented life-threatening arrhythmias and familial clustering of SCD. Several ion channel gene loci variants have been identified, but they account for a minority of cases (see Chapter 63).

Brugada Syndrome

This disorder, now considered part of the J wave syndromes, is characterized by an atypical right bundle branch block pattern and unusual forms of nonischemic ST-T wave elevations in the anterior precordial leads (Fig. 70.9). It is a familial disorder associated with risk for SCD and occurs most commonly in young and middle-aged men (see Chapters 63 and 67). Mutations involving the cardiac Na+ channel gene (*SCN5A*) are the most commonly observed variants but are identified in only a minority of cases, and a number of other ion channel defects have been associated with the syndrome. A variant in *SCN10A* has been observed in more than 16% of affected individuals. The right bundle branch block and ST-T wave changes may be intermittent and evoked or exaggerated by Na+ channel blockers (e.g., ajmaline, flecainide, procainamide). Individual risk for SCD is difficult to predict. Persistent type I electrocardiographic patterns, syncope, sex, and life-threatening arrhythmias, in various combinations, are thought to be the best predictors.[86] Though the role of programmed ventricular stimulation to identify patients at high risk for SCD is debated, a pooled analysis of eight studies incorporating 1312 patients found a hazard ratio of 2.66 (95% confidence interval [CI], 1.44 to 4.92) for inducible sustained or hemodynamically significant polymorphic VT or fibrillation.[4]

Early Repolarization and Sudden Cardiac Death

An association between the electrocardiographic pattern of early repolarization (ER) and risk for idiopathic VF has been described (J wave syndrome; see Chapter 67). ER was limited to the inferior and lateral leads, in contrast to the anterior leads, which associated with the conventional definition of benign ER. The magnitude of J point elevation was significantly greater in cardiac arrest survivors than in controls with ER. It has been estimated that ER accounts for an increase of 139.6 cardiac arrests per 100,000 subjects per year.[87]

The observation that excess risk is expressed later in life suggests a possible interaction between the physiology of ER and structural heart disease, such as coronary heart disease. An association between ER and a higher mortality during acute MI has been reported.[88]

Catecholaminergic Polymorphic Ventricular Tachycardia. Catecholaminergic polymorphic ventricular tachycardia (CPVT) is an inherited syndrome associated with catecholamine-dependent lethal arrhythmias in the absence of forewarning electrocardiographic abnormalities and with at least partial control by beta adrenoceptor-blocking agents (see Chapters 63 and 67). An autosomal dominant pattern involving the ryanodine receptor locus (RyR2) was initially described predominantly in younger patients, with bidirectional or polymorphic VT associated with risk for SCD. Another variant involving autosomal recessive inheritance of calsequestrin loci (*CASQ2*) is observed in approximately

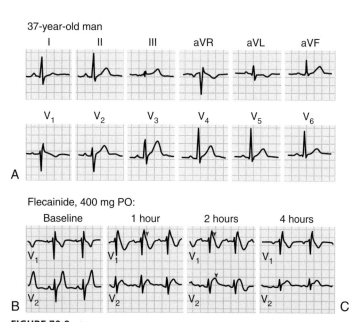

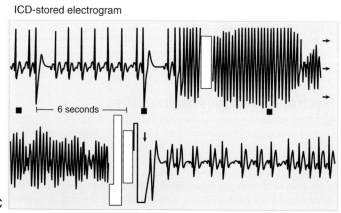

FIGURE 70.9 Electrocardiographic and clinical findings in a 37-year-old man with Brugada syndrome. The patient was resuscitated after out-of-hospital VF. No structural disease was identified. **A,** The 12-lead ECG shows an incomplete right bundle branch block pattern, which is not typical of Brugada syndrome. **B,** The typical repolarization changes associated with Brugada syndrome (*red arrowheads*) were elicited by a single oral dose of flecainide, 400 mg. The patient received an ICD and 6 months later had an appropriate shock (*arrow,* **C**), as shown on the accompanying electrogram stored in the device.

10% of genotyped cases and relatives. Overall incidence has been estimated at 1 in 10,000 with a high mortality in untreated patients.[83]

Electrical Instability Resulting from Neurohumoral and Central Nervous System Influences. The central nervous system can adversely effect cardiac electrophysiology to produce SCD (see Chapters 62 and 102). Epidemiologic data have also suggested an association between behavioral abnormalities and risk for SCD. Psychological stress and emotional extremes have been suggested for many years to be triggering mechanisms for advanced arrhythmias and SCD, but only limited, largely observational data support such associations (see Chapter 99). Takotsubo cardiomyopathy is a catecholamine-mediated condition with a generally good long-term prognosis, but the short-term risk for SCD during the acute phase remains uncertain and can be associated with QT prolongation. The possibility that it contributed to unexplained SCD in the young and middle aged population should be explored.

Stress-induced arrhythmias are better supported than stress-induced risk for mortality, which requires further study. Data from the 1994 Los Angeles earthquake identified an increased rate of fatal cardiac events on that day, but the event rate was reduced during the ensuing 2 weeks, thus suggesting triggering of events about to happen rather than independent causation. Other natural disasters have been associated with a transient increase in SCD.[4,47] Associations between auditory stimulation and auditory auras and SCD have been reported. Auditory abnormalities in some forms of congenital QT prolongation have also been observed.

A variant of TDP characterized by short coupling intervals between a normal impulse and the initiating impulse has been described (eFig. 70.1). It appears to have familial trends and to be related to alterations in autonomic nervous system activity. The 12-lead ECG demonstrates normal QT intervals, but VF and sudden death are common (see Chapters 63 and 67).

The phenomenon of so-called voodoo death has been studied in pockets of isolation in underdeveloped countries. There appears to be an association between isolation from the tribe, a sense of hopelessness, severe bradyarrhythmias, and sudden death. Limited clinical observations and experimental data modeling voodoo death have suggested a mechanism related to parasympathetic overactivity, as opposed to the evidence of an adrenergic basis for syndromes related to acute emotional stress.

Sudden Infant Death Syndrome and Sudden Cardiac Death in Children

SIDS occurs between birth and 6 months of age, is more common in male infants, and had an incidence of 1.2 deaths per 1000 live births before widespread publication of appropriate sleep positions in at-risk infants. In 1992, the American Academy of Pediatrics recommended that infants be placed to sleep in a nonprone position to reduce the risk of SIDS. The SIDS rate dropped from 120 per 100,000 live births in 1992 to 56 per 100,000 live births in 2001.[89] This supports a major role for obstructive sleep apnea as a mechanism. Vulnerability as a result of various mechanisms of dysfunctional central respiratory control, both inherent and related to prematurity, is likely to interact with sleep position as a multicomponent mechanism.

Because of its abrupt nature, a primary cardiac mechanism had been suspected in some cases, and a large study of ECGs of infants suggested prolonged QT intervals associated with risk for SIDS. A near-miss survivor with a de novo mutation of the cardiac Na+ channel gene (SCN5A) provided proof of concept that a long-QT may be a mechanism of SIDS. Subsequent data have supported the notion that as many as 15% of cases of SIDS may occur by this mechanism. Other very rare potential cardiac associations, such as accessory pathways and dispersed or immature AV nodal or bundle branch cells in the annulus, have also been described.

Sudden death in children beyond the SIDS age group and in adolescents and young adults is associated with structural heart disease in most cases. Approximately 25% of cases of SCDs in children occur in those who have undergone previous surgery for congenital cardiac disease. Of the remaining 75%, more than half occur in children who have one of four lesions: congenital aortic stenosis, Eisenmenger syndrome, pulmonary stenosis or atresia, or obstructive HCM (see Chapter 82). Other common causes included myocarditis, hypertrophic and dilated cardiomyopathy, congenital heart disease, and aortic dissection.

Sudden Cardiac Death in Competitive and Recreational Athletes and During Intense Exercise

SCD can occur during or after extreme physical activity in competing athletes or under special circumstances in the general population (see Chapter 32). Examples of the latter include intense conditioning exercise and basic military training. Among adolescent and young adult competitive athletes, the incidence was estimated to be in the range of 1/75,000 annually in Italy, as opposed to less than 1/125,000 for the general nonathlete population in the same age group. A more recent report from Italy revealed a rate of 1/100,000 among competitive athletes and 0.32/100,000 among those involved only in recreational or leisure activity.[90] In the National Collegiate Athletic Association (NCAA) database, there was 1 SCD per 53,703 athlete-years, with increased rates for males and Black athletes.[46] Differences by sport and NCAA division have been reported. The US National Registry similarly reports male predominance and higher prevalence in Blacks.[91]

While regular physical activity is associated with improved survival, there is an incremental risk related to the time period bounded by the exertion and its recovery period compared with other times—the "exercise paradox" for SCD. Overall, the risk is low, <20 per million per year,[46,92] with lower rates in women than men. Most athletes and nonathletes have a previously known or unrecognized cardiac abnormality. In middle-aged and older adults, in whom coronary disease dominates as the cause of SCD, exercise-related deaths appear to be associated with acute plaque disruption. Whether exercise contributed to the initiation of plaque disruption or preexisting disruption simply set the stage for the fatal response during exercise remains unclear. Among adolescent and young adult athletes, HCM with or without obstruction and occult congenital or acquired coronary artery disease are the most common causes identified after death,[59,91] with myocarditis contributing a significant minority. Other causes, such as ARVD/C, mitral valve prolapse, and dilated cardiomyopathy, were less common. In a report of a cohort of U.S. Air Force recruits, a surprisingly large fraction of those who died suddenly during exertion had unsuspected myocarditis. There is therefore general consensus that athletes with myocarditis should be restricted from exercise for 3 to 6 months.[93] With the advent of the COVID-19 pandemic, screening athletes for myocarditis to prevent exercise-induced SCD was widely undertaken. A study of SCA risk in marathon and half-marathon runners suggested that the overall incidence did not appear to be higher than that for the general population in the age group of participants (see Chapter 32).

Diseases attributed to molecular abnormalities, such as long-QT syndrome and right ventricular dysplasia, are increasingly being recognized as causes of SCD in athletes and exercising nonathletes. Blunt chest wall trauma by sports objects, such as baseballs and hockey pucks, can initiate lethal arrhythmias, a syndrome known as commotio cordis.[94]

Sudden death from true cardiac causes in athletes should not be confused with precipitous death related to noncardiac causes, such as acute stroke,[95] heat stroke, or malignant hyperthermia. In the latter, the victim has usually exercised excessively in hot weather, often with athletic gear that impairs heat dissipation and sometimes in association with the use of substances such as ephedrine that may cause vasoconstriction impairing heat exchange. This leads to collapse with markedly elevated core body temperatures and, ultimately, irreversible organ system damage. As a result, the U.S. Food and Drug Administration (FDA) has banned marketing of these substances for enhancement of athletic performance or weight loss.

Other Causes and Circumstances Associated with Sudden Death

A small group of victims has neither previously determined functional abnormality nor identifiable structural abnormalities at postmortem examination. Such events or deaths, when they are associated with documented VF, are classified as idiopathic. Although long-term survival after an idiopathic, potentially fatal event is still unclear, some degree of risk appears to remain. The idiopathic category is decreasing as the molecular causes become better defined, including recognition by postmortem genetic studies. Limited data suggest that higher risk persists primarily in patients with subtle cardiac structural abnormalities, in contrast to patients who are truly normal.

A number of noncardiac-related conditions can also cause or mimic SCD. Sleep apnea is associated with increased risk of SCD,[96] particularly nocturnal death, including deaths attributable to cardiac causes (see Chapter 89). The risk for death peaks during the night rather than in the early morning hours. Another respiratory system–based cause of sudden death is the so-called café coronary, in which food lodges in the oropharynx and causes an abrupt obstruction at the glottis. The holiday heart syndrome is characterized by cardiac arrhythmias, most commonly atrial fibrillation, as well as other cardiac abnormalities associated with alcohol consumption. It has not been determined whether potentially lethal arrhythmias occurring in such settings account for the reported sudden deaths associated with acute alcoholic states. Massive pulmonary embolism (see Chapter 87) can cause acute cardiovascular collapse and sudden death; sudden death in severe acute asthmatic attacks, without prolonged deterioration of the patient's condition, is well recognized. Air or amniotic fluid embolism at the time of labor and delivery may cause sudden death on rare occasion, with the clinical picture mimicking that of SCD.

Finally, a number of abnormalities that do not directly involve the heart may cause sudden deaths that mimic SCD. Such abnormalities include aortic dissection (see Chapter 42), acute cardiac tamponade (see Chapter 86), and rapid exsanguination. The electrical mechanism associated with these deaths is most commonly severe bradyarrhythmias, pulseless electrical activity (PEA), or asystole rather than VT or fibrillation.

Pathology and Pathophysiology. Protocols and observations from postmortem studies of SCD victims have changed in recent years. It is now recommended that cases of SCD that do not have obvious causes identified on routine postmortem studies or available clinical information, have post mortem examinations performed by specialized cardiac pathology centers. This is particularly important for younger populations with unexplained SCA. In a series of autopsy cases referred by a pathologist to an expert cardiac pathologist, there was divergence in final diagnoses. Notably, there was a tendency for the routine autopsy to overdiagnose cardiomyopathy as a cause of death, and CAD was less common than in other studies. However, the study was limited to some extent by being skewed to a younger population, limiting extrapolation of this observation to the overall population.[4] In addition, a number of studies now support the notion that postmortem genetic studies are useful for increasing the probability of identifying a cause that is unexplained based on anatomical findings.[29,97,98]

Earlier pathologic studies in SCD victims across a broad age range reflected the epidemiologic and clinical observations that coronary atherosclerosis is the major predisposing cause. All other causes of SCD (see Table 70.3) collectively account for no more than 20% of cases. In the Postmortem Systematic Investigation of SCD (POST SCD) study,[5] 55.8% of cases with World Health Organization defined SCD were determined to have sudden arrhythmic death. Coronary artery disease accounted for only 32% of all cases, with evidence of acute coronary syndrome in one-third. Noncardiac causes included occult overdose and neurologic causes. Cardiomyopathy and hypertrophy were other significant cardiac causes. The decline in the proportion of SCDs attributed to coronary artery disease, with a concomitant increase in hypertensive cardiomyopathy

and idiopathic myocardial fibrosis has been demonstrated in a longitudinal autopsy series from Finland.[13] Continued attention to the postmortem evaluation of cases labelled as SCD is clearly needed to help guide further attempts at prevention.

Pathology of Sudden Death Caused by Coronary Artery Abnormalities

Coronary Arteries. Extensive atherosclerosis has long been recognized as the most common pathologic finding in the coronary arteries of victims of SCD. The combined results of a number of studies have suggested a general pattern of at least two coronary arteries with 75% or greater narrowing in more than 75% of the victims. Several studies have demonstrated no specific pattern of distribution of coronary artery lesions that preselect for SCD, but the extent of coronary artery narrowing at postmortem examination was greater in SCD victims than in control subjects.

The role of active coronary artery lesions, characterized by plaque fissuring, plaque erosion or rupture, platelet aggregation, and thrombosis, as a major pathophysiologic mechanism of the onset of cardiac arrest has emerged (see Chapters 24 and 37). Disruption, platelet aggregation, and thrombosis are associated with markers of inflammation and various conventional risk factors for coronary atherosclerosis, such as cigarette smoking and hyperlipidemia.

Some of the less common, nonatherosclerotic coronary artery abnormalities have specific pathologic features as well. Coronary artery spasm, an established cause of acute ischemia and SCD, is commonly associated with nonobstructive plaque (Fig. 70.10), and the consequences of spasm/reperfusion has been recognized at postmortem examination. When deep myocardial bridges are identified in association with SCD, patchy fibrosis in areas subserved by the affected vessel

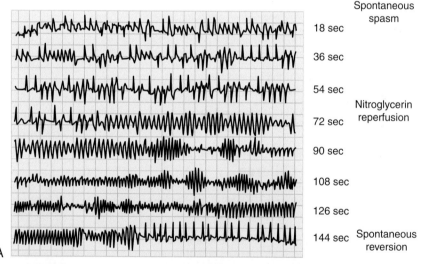

18 sec	Spontaneous spasm
36 sec	
54 sec	
72 sec	Nitroglycerin reperfusion
90 sec	
108 sec	
126 sec	
144 sec	Spontaneous reversion

A

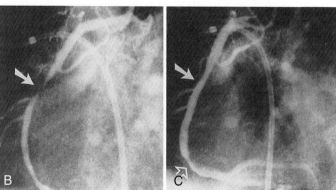

B   C

FIGURE 70.10 Life-threatening ventricular arrhythmias associated with acute myocardial ischemia related to coronary artery spasm and with reperfusion. **A,** Continuous lead II electrocardiographic monitor recording during ischemia (time, 0 to 55 seconds) caused by spasm of the right coronary artery **(B)**. Following the administration of nitroglycerin at approximately 55 seconds, an abrupt transition from repetitive ventricular ectopy to a rapid polymorphic, prefibrillatory tachyarrhythmia occurs (time, 80 to 130 seconds) in association with reversal of the spasm **(C)**. *Closed arrow* indicates the site of spasm before and after nitroglycerin; the *open arrow* indicates a lower grade distal lesion. (Modified from Myerburg RJ, et al: Life-threatening ventricular arrhythmias in patients with silent myocardial ischemia due to coronary artery spasm. N Engl J Med 1992;326:1451.)

is commonly seen at postmortem examination. Coronary vasculitis in association with various autoimmune disorders may cause diffuse myocardial abnormalities, but asymptomatic cardiac involvement or global myocardial dysfunction is more common than SCD.

Myocardium. Myocardial injury in SCD caused by coronary heart disease reflects the extensive atherosclerosis usually present. Studies of victims of out-of-hospital SCD have indicated that healed MI is a common finding in SCD victims, with most investigators reporting frequencies ranging from 40% to more than 70%. The incidence of acute MI is considerably lower, with cytopathologic evidence of recent MI found in approximately 20% of individuals. This estimate corresponds well with the frequency of new MI in of out-of-hospital cardiac arrest survivors. The POST SCD study noted that only one third of the cases attributed to coronary artery disease had evidence of acute coronary syndrome.[5] These pathologic observations do not provide insight into the likely possibility that many SCDs occur as a result of acute coronary syndrome mechanisms and progress from ischemia to fatal arrhythmias without time for structural markers to become visible. Since elevations in troponin levels occur during chest pain syndromes and also in a substantial proportion of cardiac arrest survivors, the determination whether myocardial injury preceded or resulted from the cardiac arrest is difficult to resolve in individual cases.

Ventricular Hypertrophy. Myocardial hypertrophy can coexist and interact with acute or chronic ischemia but appears to confer an independent risk for mortality. No close correlation has been found between increased heart weight and the severity of coronary heart disease in SCD victims; however, heart weight is higher in SCD victims than in those whose death is not sudden despite a similar prevalence of a history of hypertension before death. Risk for hypertrophy-associated mortality is also independent of LV function and the extent of coronary artery disease, and LV hypertrophy itself may predispose to SCD. Experimental data have also suggested increased susceptibility to potentially lethal ventricular arrhythmias in patients with LV hypertrophy and ischemia and reperfusion.

Specialized Conducting System in Sudden Cardiac Death. Fibrosis of the specialized conducting system may be observed in SCD victims. Although this process is associated with AV block or intraventricular conduction abnormalities, its role in SCD is uncertain. Lev disease, Lenègre disease, ischemic injury caused by small-vessel disease, and numerous infiltrative or inflammatory processes can result in such changes. In addition, active inflammatory processes such as myocarditis and infiltrative processes such as amyloidosis, scleroderma, hemochromatosis, and morbid obesity may damage or destroy the AV node, bundle of His, or both and result in AV block.[4]

Focal diseases such as sarcoidosis, rheumatoid arthritis, fibrotic or fatty infiltration of the AV node or His-Purkinje system with apparent discontinuities, Lyme disease, and very rarely Whipple disease (infection with *Tropheryma whipplei*), can also involve the conducting system (see Chapter 68). These various categories of conducting system disease have been considered possible pathologic substrates for SCD that might be overlooked because of the difficulty of performing careful postmortem examinations of the conducting system routinely; careful studies of the conducting system are necessary to identify up to 22% of otherwise unexplained SCDs under the age of 40 years.[99] Focal involvement of conducting tissue by tumors (especially mesothelioma of the AV node but also lymphoma, carcinoma, rhabdomyoma, and fibroma) has also been reported, and rare cases of SCD have been associated with these lesions. It has been suggested that abnormal postnatal morphogenesis of the specialized conducting system may be a significant factor in some cases of SCD in infants and children.

Cardiac Nerves and Sudden Cardiac Death. Intrinsic and extrinsic autonomic dysfunction mediated by altered cardiac innervation and/or neuro-cardiac interactions have a role in SCD (see Chapter 102).[100] Neural involvement can be the result of damage to neural elements within the myocardium (i.e., concomitant with MI leading to a secondary cardioneuropathy) or may be primary, as in diabetic cardiac autonomic neuropathy, which is associated with a 3.5-fold increased risk of SCD, or rarely a selective autonomic neuropathy. Alterations in autonomic function as a compensatory mechanism for cardiac disease, such as heart failure, is well described. Generally, sympathoexcitation, which can be noted with multiple techniques ranging from heart rate variability analysis, catecholamine levels, and direct neural recordings, is associated with poor prognosis and increased risk for ventricular tachyarrhythmias leading to SCD. The role of anatomic changes in neural innervation is also significant. Myocardial infarction has been shown to lead to areas of sympathetic denervation. These may contribute to arrhythmogenesis by a mechanism of denervation supersensitivity to catecholamines causing increased dispersion of refractoriness. Nerve

sprouting due to released nerve growth factors after MI may be important[101,102] in determining changes in cardiac innervation in response to injury. Clinical techniques for sympathetic imaging suggest a changing pattern over time after MI.[103]

Mechanisms and Pathophysiology

Electrical mechanisms of cardiac arrest are divided into tachyarrhythmic and bradyarrhythmic-asystolic events, or conversely shockable versus nonshockable. The tachyarrhythmias include VF and pulseless sustained VT, in which a perceptible pulse may not be present (<60 mm Hg), and adequate blood flow is not maintained. Bradyarrhythmic-asystolic events include severe bradyarrhythmias, PEA (formerly called *electromechanical dissociation* [EMD]), and inability to generate a mechanical event because of complete absence of electrical activity (asystole). To qualify as a mechanism of cardiac arrest, severe bradyarrhythmias must be slow enough to result in an inability to adequately perfuse and maintain consciousness, which usually requires a heart rate of less than 20 beats/min. In PEA, the electrical rate can be considerably faster, but in general much slower than true pulseless VT, with either a narrow or wide QRS complex. The important distinction between PEA and pulseless VT is that pulseless VT is a shockable rhythm. Included in the classification of PEA are the slow agonal rhythms heralding death (random irregular depolarizations that do not generate a pulse), narrow and wide QRS rhythms at rates from 40 to >100 without a pulse. In PEA, there is no perfusion because of absent mechanical activity or mechanical obstruction to blood flow, as in massive pulmonary embolism. However, echocardiographic imaging during PEA has suggested that residual LV wall motion may persist but not be adequate for generating a pulse, as in pulseless VT. This phenomenon has implications for exploring new therapeutic approaches for PEA. Data from the Resuscitation Outcomes Consortium show that PEA accounts for approximately 20% of initial rhythms.[104] Asystole is the most common initial rhythm, though it is likely that many victims found to be asystolic at contact were initially in VF or VT. After a variable time, fibrillation may cease and asystole or less commonly PEA emerges. In contrast to earlier data, the most common initial recording documented in recent years is asystole or PEA.

The occurrence of potentially lethal tachyarrhythmias or severe bradyarrhythmia or asystole is the end of a cascade of pathophysiologic abnormalities that result from complex interactions between coronary vascular events, myocardial injury, variations in autonomic tone, and the metabolic and electrolyte state of the myocardium (see Fig. 70.5). There is no uniform hypothesis of mechanisms by which these elements interact to lead to the final pathway of lethal arrhythmias. However, Figure 70.7 shows models of the pathophysiologic process of SCD that include vascular, myocardial, and functional components. The risk for cardiac arrest is conditioned by the presence of structural abnormalities and modulated by functional variations.

Pathophysiologic Mechanisms of Lethal Tachyarrhythmias
Coronary Artery Structure and Function

Among the large fraction of SCDs associated with coronary atherosclerosis, an extensive distribution of chronic arterial narrowing has been well defined by pathologic studies. However, the specific mechanisms by which these lesions lead to potentially lethal disturbances in electrical stability are not simply the consequence of steady-state reductions in regional myocardial blood flow in association with variable demands (see Chapter 36). A simple increase in myocardial oxygen demand, in the presence of a fixed supply, may be a mechanism of exercise-induced arrhythmias and sudden death during intense physical activity. It is notable that asymptomatic ST depression during exercise testing in men without prevalent coronary artery disease is associated with a doubling of risk of SCD. Yet, the overall risk of SCD during exercise and/or exercise testing even with induced ischemia is extremely low, supporting recommendations for continued exercise in most patients with angina and/or provokable ischemia on stress testing.[105] However, the dynamic nature of the pathophysiologic mechanism of acute coronary events creates a setting in which alterations in the metabolic or electrolyte state of the myocardium may lead to disturbed electrical stability. Active vascular events resulting in an acute or transient reduction in regional myocardial blood flow in the presence of a normal or previously compromised circulation constitute a common mechanism of ischemia, angina pectoris, arrhythmias, and SCD. Coronary artery spasm or modulation of coronary collateral flow, predisposed to by local endothelial dysfunction, further exposes the myocardium to the double hazard of transient ischemia and reperfusion[106] (see Fig. 70.10). Neurogenic influences may also be contributory. Vessel susceptibility and humoral factors, particularly those related to platelet activation and aggregation, also appear to be important mechanisms.

Transition of stable atherosclerotic plaque to an "active" state because of plaque fissuring leading to platelet activation and aggregation followed by thrombosis, is a mechanism that appears to be present in many SCDs related to coronary heart disease (see Chapters 24 and 37). Inflammatory responses in atherosclerotic plaque are now viewed as the condition leading to lesion progression, including erosion, disruption, platelet activation, and thrombosis. In addition to causing a subacute or acute critical reduction in regional blood flow, these mechanisms produce a series of biochemical alterations that may enhance or retard susceptibility to VF by means of vasomotor modulation.

The step in the cascade of coronary artery pathophysiology leading to ischemia-induced arrhythmias that follows conversion to an active plaque involves the thrombotic module of platelet aggregation and thrombosis (see Figs. 70.5 and 70.7; see Chapter 24). However, there is a discrepancy between the relatively high incidence of platelet aggregation or acute thrombi in postmortem studies and the low incidence of evolution of new MI in survivors of out-of-hospital VF. The rapid initiation of lethal arrhythmias, the spontaneous thrombolysis, a dominant role of spasm induced by platelet products, or a combination of these factors may explain this observation.

Acute Ischemia and Initiation of Lethal Arrhythmias

The onset of acute ischemia produces immediate electrical, mechanical, and biochemical dysfunction of cardiac muscle. The specialized conducting tissue is more resistant to acute ischemia than working myocardium, and therefore the electrophysiologic consequences are less intense and delayed in onset in specialized conduction tissue. In addition to the direct effect of ischemia on normal or previously abnormal tissue, reperfusion after transient ischemia can cause lethal arrhythmias (see Fig. 70.10). Reperfusion of ischemic areas can occur by three mechanisms: (1) spontaneous thrombolysis, (2) recruitment of collateral vessels from other vascular beds in response to local ischemia, and (3) reversal of vasospasm. Some mechanisms of reperfusion-induced arrhythmogenesis appear to be related to the duration of ischemia before reperfusion. An array of pathophysiologic changes resulting in intracellular calcium overload is likely the underlying mechanism.[106]

Electrophysiologic Effects of Acute Ischemia. Within the first minutes after experimental coronary ligation, there is a propensity to ventricular arrhythmias that abates after 30 minutes and reappears after several hours (Chapter 62). The initial 30 minutes of arrhythmias is divided into two periods, the first of which lasts for approximately 10 minutes and is presumably directly related to the initial ischemic injury. The second period (20 to 30 minutes) may be related either to reperfusion of ischemic areas or to the evolution of different injury patterns in epicardial and endocardial muscle. Multiple mechanisms of reperfusion arrhythmias have been observed experimentally, including slow conduction and reentry and afterdepolarizations and triggered activity.

At the level of the myocyte, the immediate consequences of ischemia of particular interest are the possible continued influx of Ca^{2+}, which may produce electrical instability; responses to alpha or beta adrenoceptor stimulation, or both; and afterdepolarizations as triggering responses for Ca^{2+}-dependent arrhythmias. Other possible mechanisms studied experimentally include the formation of superoxide radicals in reperfusion arrhythmias and differential responses of endocardial and epicardial muscle activation times and refractory periods during ischemia or reperfusion. The adenosine triphosphate–dependent K^+ current

($I_{K,ATP}$), which is inactive during normal conditions, is activated during ischemia. Its activation results in a strong efflux of K^+ ions from myocytes and markedly shortening of the time course of repolarization, which leads to slow conduction and ultimately to inexcitability. The fact that this response is more marked in epicardium than in endocardium leads to a prominent dispersion of repolarization across the myocardium during transmural ischemia. At an intercellular level, ischemia alters the distribution of connexin-43, the primary gap junction protein between myocytes. This alteration results in uncoupling of myocytes, a factor that is arrhythmogenic because of altered patterns of excitation and regional changes in conduction velocity.

The state of the myocardium at the time of onset of ischemia is important. Tissue healed after previous injury appears to be more susceptible to the electrical destabilizing effects of acute ischemia, as is chronically hypertrophied muscle. Remodeling-induced local stretch, regional hypertrophy, or intrinsic cellular alteration may contribute to this vulnerability. Of more direct clinical relevance is the suggestion that potassium depletion by diuretics and clinical hypokalemia may make ventricular myocardium more susceptible to potentially lethal arrhythmias, in part by its effect on repolarization (QT) duration.

The association of metabolic and electrolyte abnormalities and neurophysiologic and neurohumoral changes with lethal arrhythmias emphasizes the importance of integrating changes in the myocardial substrate with systemic influences. Most direct among myocardial metabolic changes in response to ischemia are local acute increase in interstitial K^+ levels to values exceeding 15 mM, decrease in tissue pH to below 6.0, changes in adrenoceptor activity, and alterations in autonomic nerve traffic, all of which tend to create and maintain electrical instability, especially if it is regional in distribution. Other metabolic changes, such as elevation of cyclic adenosine monophosphate levels, accumulation of free fatty acids and their metabolites, formation of lysophosphoglycerides, and impaired myocardial glycolysis, have also been suggested as myocardial-destabilizing influences. These local myocardial changes integrate with systemic patterns of autonomic fluctuation that can be observed as patterns of altered heart rate variability and fractal dynamics, thus potentially identifying subsets of patients at higher risk for SCD during an acute ischemic event.[4]

Transition from Myocardial Instability to Lethal Arrhythmias

The combination of a triggering event and a susceptible myocardium is a fundamental electrophysiologic concept for the mechanism of initiation of potentially lethal arrhythmias (see Figs. 70.5 and 70.7). The triggering event for VT or VF can be electrophysiologic, ischemic, metabolic, or hemodynamic. For VF, the endpoint of their interaction is disorganization of patterns of myocardial activation into multiple uncoordinated reentrant pathways. Clinical, experimental, and pharmacologic data have suggested that triggering events in the absence of myocardial instability are unlikely to initiate lethal arrhythmias.

Bradyarrhythmias and Asystolic Arrest

The basic electrophysiologic mechanism in this form of arrest is failure of normal subordinate automatic activity to assume the pacing function of the heart in the absence of normal function of the sinus node, AV junction, or both. Asystolic arrest is more common in severely diseased hearts and in patients with a number of end-stage disorders, cardiac and noncardiac. These mechanisms may result, in part, from diffuse involvement of subendocardial Purkinje fibers in advanced heart disease.

Pulseless Electrical Activity

PEA is separated into primary and secondary forms. No one unifying definition for PEA, mechanistically or clinically, is recognized. The common denominator in both is the presence of organized cardiac electrical activity in the absence of effective mechanical function. The absence of rapid return of spontaneous circulation (ROSC) is important in that it excludes transient losses of cerebral blood flow, such as the various patterns of vasovagal reflex syncope, which have different clinical implications. The secondary form of PEA results from an abrupt cessation of cardiac venous return, such as massive pulmonary embolism, acute malfunction of prosthetic valves, exsanguination, and cardiac tamponade from hemopericardium. The primary form is the more familiar; in this form none of these obvious mechanical factors is present, but ventricular muscle fails to produce an effective contraction despite continued electrical activity. It usually occurs as an end-stage event in advanced heart disease, but it can occur in patients with acute ischemic events or, more commonly, after electrical resuscitation from prolonged cardiac arrest. Although it is not thoroughly understood, it appears that diffuse disease, metabolic abnormalities, or global ischemia provides the pathophysiologic substrate. The proximate mechanism for failure of electromechanical coupling may be abnormal intracellular Ca^{2+} metabolism, intracellular acidosis, or perhaps depletion of ATP.

CLINICAL FEATURES OF PATIENTS WITH CARDIAC ARREST

Although the pathologic anatomy associated with SCD caused by coronary artery disease often reflects the changes associated with acute myocardial injury, <20% of survivors of OHCA have clinical evidence of a new transmural MI. Nonetheless, many have elevations in enzyme levels along with nonspecific electrocardiographic changes suggesting myocardial damage, which may be caused by transient ischemia as a triggering event or a consequence of the loss of myocardial perfusion during the cardiac arrest. The recurrence rate is low in survivors of OHCA caused by transmural MI. In contrast, early studies demonstrated a 30% recurrence rate at 1 year and 45% at 2 years in the survivors who did not have a new transmural MI. Recurrence rates decreased subsequently, probably in part due to the result of long-term interventions.

Prodromal Symptoms

Patients at risk for SCD can have prodromes such as chest pain, dyspnea, weakness or fatigue, palpitations, syncope, and a number of nonspecific complaints. Several epidemiologic and clinical studies have demonstrated that such symptoms can presage coronary events, particularly MI and SCD, and result in contact with the medical system weeks to months before SCD.

Attempts to identify early prodromal symptoms specific for SCD risk have not been successful. Although several studies have reported that 12% to 46% of fatalities occur in patients who had seen a physician 1 to 6 months before death, such visits are more likely to presage MI or nonsudden death, and most complaints responsible for these visits are not heart related. However, patients who have chest pain as a prodrome to SCD appear to have a higher probability of intraluminal coronary thrombosis at postmortem examination. Fatigue has been a particularly common symptom in the days or weeks before SCD in a number of studies, but this symptom is nonspecific. The symptoms that occur within the last hours or minutes before cardiac arrest are more specific for heart disease and may include symptoms of arrhythmias, ischemia, and heart failure.

Onset of the Terminal Event

Ambulatory recordings fortuitously obtained during the onset of an unexpected cardiac arrest have indicated dynamic changes in cardiac electrical activity during the minutes or hours before the event. Increasing heart rate and advancing grades of ventricular ectopy are common antecedents of VF. Alterations in autonomic nervous system activity may also contribute to onset of the event. Studies of short-term variations in heart rate variability or related measures have identified changes that correlate with the occurrence of ventricular arrhythmias. Although these physiologic properties may be associated with transient electrophysiologic destabilization of the myocardium, the extent to which they are paralleled by clinical symptoms or events has been less well documented.

Cardiac Arrest

Cardiac arrest is characterized by abrupt loss of consciousness caused by lack of adequate cerebral blood flow as a result of failure of cardiac pump function. In contrast to previous data, the most common electrical mechanism of OHCA currently identified by Emergency Rescue Systems is asystole (50%), with VF/pulseless VT and PEA each estimated in the range of 20% to 25%.[104] The extent to which these proportions of first recorded rhythms reflect the rhythms that trigger the onset of SCA remains unknown because of the lag between onset and EMS arrival. Mechanical causes include rupture of the ventricle, cardiac tamponade, acute obstruction to flow, and acute disruption of a major blood vessel, each of which is more likely to present with PEA or asystole.

Among elderly persons, outcomes after community-based responses to OHCA are not as good as for younger victims. In one study comparing persons younger than 80 years (mean age, 64 years) with those in their 80s and 90s, the survival rate to hospital discharge in the younger group was 19.4% as opposed to 9.4% for octogenarians and 4.4% for nonagenarians. However, when the groups were analyzed according to markers favoring survival (e.g., VF, pulseless VT), the incremental benefit was even better for the elderly than for the younger patients (36%, 24%, and 17%, respectively), but the frequency of ventricular tachyarrhythmias versus nonshockable rhythms was lower in elderly persons. Overall, advanced age is only a weak predictor of an adverse outcome and should not be used in isolation as a reason to not resuscitate.[107] Long-term neurologic status and length of hospitalization were similar in older and younger surviving patients.

The potential for successful resuscitation is a function of the setting in which the cardiac arrest occurs, the mechanism of the arrest, and the underlying clinical status of the victim. The decision whether to attempt to resuscitate is closely related to the potential for success.[108]

At present, there are fewer low-risk patients with otherwise uncomplicated MIs accounting for in-hospital cardiac arrest (IHCA) than previously reported. Patients with IHCA associated with acute MI (AMI), typically had a history of congestive heart failure, and commonly had experienced previous cardiac arrests. Noncardiac-related clinical diagnoses were dominated by renal failure, pneumonia, sepsis, diabetes, and a history of cancer. The strong male preponderance consistently reported in out-of-hospital cardiac arrest studies is not present in in-hospital patients, but the better prognosis of VT or VF mechanisms than PEA or asystolic mechanisms persists (27% versus 8% survival rate). However, the proportion of arrests caused by in-hospital VT or VF is considerably less (33%), with the combination of respiratory arrest, asystole, and PEA dominating the statistics (61%). Similar findings were reported from China.[109] One year survival after IHCA is also influenced by age, sex, race, and presenting rhythm. Strategic factors affecting survival after IHCA include the location in the hospital, the type of hospital, daytime and evening events versus night and weekend events, and a rapid time to performance of defibrillation.[4,110]

A multihospital study of outcomes after IHCA in pediatric patients demonstrated a major improvement in survival to hospital discharge between 2000 and 2009, with a risk-adjusted improvement from 14.3% in 2000 to 43.4% in 2009. There was neither improvement nor worsening of the proportion with residual neurologic deficits. The proportion with VF or pulseless VT decreased from 22% in 2000 to 2003 to 9.7% in 2007 to 2009, and those with asystole decreased from 51.4% to 20%. In contrast, PEA increased from 26.6% to 70.3%. The reason for the dramatic increase in the proportion of PEA events is not clear because respiratory insufficiency as an initial condition increased only modestly, but may be related to the increased proportion of patients maintained on mechanical ventilators at the time of arrest.[4]

Important risk factors for death after in-hospital CPR are listed in eTable 70.2. Survival after IHCA is lower for events that occur during weeknights and weekends than during the daytime and evening hours during the week and more rapid times to defibrillation are advantageous. Such data suggest the need for additional strategies for uniformly rapid in-hospital responses, as well as for the limitations reported for in-hospital early warning systems.

Progression to Biologic Death

The time course for progression from cardiac arrest to biologic death is related to the mechanism of the cardiac arrest, the nature of the underlying disease process, and the delay between onset and resuscitative efforts. The onset of irreversible brain damage usually begins within 4 to 6 minutes after loss of cerebral circulation, and biologic death follows quickly in unattended cardiac arrest. In large series, however, it has been demonstrated that a limited number of victims can remain biologically alive for longer periods and may be resuscitated after delays in excess of 8 minutes before beginning basic life support and in excess of 16 minutes before advanced life support. Despite these exceptions, it is clear that the probability of a favorable outcome—survival neurologically intact—deteriorates *rapidly* as a function of time after cardiac arrest. Younger patients with less severe cardiac disease and the absence of coexistent multisystem disease have a higher probability of a favorable outcome after such delays.

Irreversible injury to the central nervous system usually occurs before biologic death, and the interval may extend days to weeks and occasionally result in very prolonged persistent vegetative states in patients who are resuscitated during the temporal gap between brain damage and biologic death. IHCA caused by VF is less likely to have a protracted course between the arrest and biologic death, with patients surviving after a prompt intervention or succumbing rapidly because of inability to stabilize their cardiac and/or medical conditions. Overall, patients who have ROSC with persistent severe cerebral performance disability or who remain comatose (CPC-3 or -4) have a very low survival rate, both in-hospital and at 6 months postarrest.

Patients whose cardiac arrest is caused by sustained VT with cardiac output inadequate to maintain consciousness can remain in VT for considerably longer periods with blood flow that is marginally sufficient to maintain viability. Thus there is a longer interval between the onset of cardiac arrest and the end of the period that allows successful resuscitation. The lives of such patients usually end in VF or an asystolic event (PEA or asystole) if the VT is not reverted.

The progression in patients with asystole or PEA as the initiating event is more rapid. Such patients, whether in-hospital or out-of-hospital, have a poor prognosis because of advanced heart disease or coexistent multisystem disease. They tend to respond poorly to interventions, even if the heart is successfully paced. Although there has been an increase in survival from PEA in recent years, it is generally limited to the small subgroup of patients with reversible conditions (e.g., respiratory, electrolyte imbalances) that respond well to interventions, and most progress rapidly to biologic death. Cardiac arrests caused by mechanical factors such as tamponade, structural disruption, and impedance to flow by major thromboembolic obstructions to right or LV outflow are reversible only in patients in whom the mechanism is recognized and an intervention is feasible.

Survivors of Cardiac Arrest

Hospital Course

Cardiac arrests during the acute phase of MI may be primarily related to an electrical event, or secondarily to LV dysfunction or cardiogenic shock. Patients who are resuscitated immediately from primary VF associated with ST elevation MI usually stabilize promptly, and no long-term arrhythmia management is recommended based on the early arrhythmia (see Chapters 28 and 37). However, there are data linking early primary VF to heightened short- and long-term mortality.[111,112] The mechanism for excess mortality is not well delineated. Management after secondary cardiac arrest in patients with MI is dominated by the hemodynamic status of the patient.

Survivors of out-of-hospital cardiac arrest may have repetitive ventricular arrhythmias during the initial 24 to 48 hours of hospitalization. These arrhythmias have variable responses to antiarrhythmic therapy, depending on hemodynamic status. The overall rate of recurrent cardiac arrest is low, 10% to 20%, but the mortality rate in patients who have recurrent cardiac arrests is approximately 50%. Only 5% to 10% of in-hospital deaths after out-of-hospital resuscitation are caused by recurrent cardiac arrhythmias. Patients with recurrent cardiac arrest have a high incidence of new or preexisting AV or intraventricular conduction abnormalities.

The most common causes of death in hospitalized survivors of out-of-hospital cardiac arrest are noncardiac events related to central nervous system injury, including anoxic encephalopathy and sepsis related to prolonged intubation and hemodynamic monitoring lines. Approximately 40% of those who arrive at the hospital in coma never awaken after admission to the hospital and die after a median survival of 3.5 days. Two-thirds of those who regain consciousness have no gross deficits, and an additional 20% have persisting cognitive deficits only. Of the patients who do awaken, 25% do so by admission, 71% by the first hospital day, and 92% by the third day. A small number of patients have awakened after prolonged hospitalization. Among those who die in the hospital, 80% do not awaken before death. Therapeutic hypothermia in patients with postcardiac arrest coma is beneficial,[113] even for those with nonshockable rhythms[114] (see next section).

Cardiac causes of delayed death during hospitalization after out-of-hospital cardiac arrest are most commonly related to hemodynamic deterioration, which accounts for about a third of deaths in hospitals. Among all deaths, those that occurred within the first 48 hours of hospitalization were usually caused by hemodynamic deterioration or arrhythmias regardless of neurologic status; later deaths were dominated by neurologic complications. Admission characteristics most predictive of subsequent awakening included motor response, pupillary light response, spontaneous eye movement, and blood glucose level below 300 mg/dL.

Clinical Profile of Survivors of Out-of-Hospital Cardiac Arrest

The clinical features of survivors of out-of-hospital cardiac arrest are heavily influenced by the type and extent of the underlying disease associated with the event. Causation is dominated by coronary heart disease and cardiomyopathies. All other structural heart diseases plus functional abnormalities and toxic or environmental causes are responsible for the remainder.

In a study of 375 survivors of cardiac arrest with normal ejection fractions and no obvious heart disease, genetic testing was performed in 174 patients.[115] Pathogenic variants were identified in 17% of cases for long-QT syndrome, catecholaminergic polymorphic VT, right ventricular dysplasia, idiopathic VF, Brugada syndrome (9%), and HCM. A substantial number of variants of uncertain significance were identified. This highlights the role of genetic testing in the evaluation of the etiology of OHCA in those without structural heart disease.

Postresuscitation Electrocardiographic Changes

Among survivors of OHCA, the 12-lead ECG has proved to be of value only for discriminating risk for recurrence in those whose cardiac arrest was associated with new transmural MI. Patients in whom documented new Q waves develop in association with a clinical picture that supports acute ST-segment elevation MI as the mechanism of cardiac arrest itself are at lower risk for recurrence, unless they develop criteria for postinfarct primary prevention of SCD, such as EF <30% to 40%. In contrast, nonspecific electrocardiographic markers of ischemia, associated with elevation of troponin or creatine kinase MB levels, indicate higher risk for recurrence. Nonspecific repolarization abnormalities (e.g., ST-segment depression, flat T waves) are commonly present, often transiently, after a cardiac arrest. Transient prolongation of the QT interval, often associated with postresuscitation hypokalemia, can follow CPR, and associate with risk of recurrent arrhythmias. A prolonged QRS duration in association with a markedly reduced ejection fraction portends increased risk for mortality.

Left Ventricular Function

LV function is abnormal in most survivors of out-of-hospital cardiac arrest, often severely abnormal, but there is wide variation ranging from severe dysfunction to normal or almost normal function. The severity of myocardial dysfunction estimated shortly after cardiac arrest is due to a combination of myocardial stunning consequent to the cardiac arrest itself and the extent of preexisting dysfunction. Stunning commonly improves within the first 24 to 48 hours,[116] and the residual is assumed to be due to preexisting disease or to the acute injury leading to the cardiac arrest. Reliance on postarrest troponin elevations alone to determine whether MI caused a cardiac arrest can be treacherous because cardiac arrest and even nonlife-threatening sustained arrhythmias, as well as ICD shocks, can be associated with transient elevations. Moreover, troponin levels do not improve risk prediction beyond standard clinical variables. If the ejection fraction is severely reduced initially, failure to begin improvement within the first 48 hours is an adverse short-term prognostic sign. In the CREST model, ejection fraction <30% at the time of admission was a multivariate predictor of a circulatory etiology death.[117] Among survivors to hospital discharge, a reduced ejection fraction is an adverse long-term prognostic sign.

Coronary Angiography

Coronary angiography is performed with increasing frequency during initial hospitalization after OHCA. In a recent report based on data from the National Inpatient Sample, patients, 143,607 of 407,974 survivors (35.2%), underwent coronary angiography, increasing from 27.2% in 2000 to 43.9% 2012, and percutaneous coronary intervention increased from 9.5% in 2000 to 24.1% in 2012.[118] Survivors of OHCA tend to have extensive coronary disease but no specific pattern of abnormalities. Acute coronary lesions, often multifocal, are present in many survivors. Significant lesions in two or more vessels are present in at least 70% of patients who have any coronary lesion. In patients who have recurrent cardiac arrests, the incidence of triple-vessel disease is higher than in those who do not. However, the frequency of moderate to severe stenosis of the left main coronary artery does not differ between cardiac arrest survivors and the overall population of patients with symptomatic coronary heart disease.

Blood Chemistry

Lower serum potassium levels are observed in survivors of cardiac arrest than in patients with AMI or stable coronary heart disease. This finding is often a consequence of resuscitation interventions rather than a preexisting hypokalemic state because of chronic diuretic use or other causes. However, severe preexisting hypokalemia may aggravate the risk for VF and recurrent VF.[119] Among survivors who are hypokalemic during the first 12 to 24 hours after SCA, serum K^+ levels following stabilization should be checked to exclude a chronic potassium-wasting state. Low ionized calcium levels with normal total calcium levels were also observed during resuscitation from out-of-hospital cardiac arrest. Higher resting lactate levels have been reported in out-of-hospital cardiac arrest survivors than in normal subjects. Lactate levels correlated inversely with ejection fractions and directly with PVC frequency and complexity.

Long-Term Prognosis

Studies from Miami and Seattle in the early 1970s had indicated that the risk for recurrent cardiac arrest in the first year after survival of an initial VT/VF event was approximately 30% and at 2 years was 45%. Total mortality at 2 years was approximately 60% in both studies. More recent mortality data, including those from the control groups of secondary prevention ICD trials, have demonstrated improved survival.[120] The Israel ICD registry demonstrated one- and two-year mortality rates of 8% and 11%, respectively,[121] and a European cohort of patients with secondary prevention ICDs for ischemic or dilated cardiomyopathy had 5- and 10-year mortalities of 24% and 51%, respectively.[122] The apparent improved outcomes, independent of the benefit provided by ICD therapy, are probably attributable to the current interventions used in survivors, such as beta adrenoceptor blockers, statins and angiotensin converting enzyme inhibitor (ACEI)/angiotensin receptor blocker (ARBs), anti-ischemic procedures, and heart failure therapies that were not available or in general use at the earlier time. The risk for recurrent cardiac arrest and all-cause mortality is higher during the first 12 to 24 months after the index event and relates best to the ejection fraction during the first 6 months.

MANAGEMENT OF CARDIAC ARREST

The response to cardiac arrest is driven by two principles: (1) maintenance of continuous cardiopulmonary support until ROSC has been

achieved and (2) achieve ROSC as quickly as possible. To achieve these goals, the management strategy is divided into five elements: (1) initial assessment by a witness/bystander and summoning of an emergency response team, (2) basic life support BLS, (3) early defibrillation by a first responder (if available), (4) advanced life support, and (5) postcardiac arrest care. If successful, the algorithm is followed by a sixth element, long-term management. The initial elements can be applied by physicians and nurses, EMTs or paramedics, lay people trained in bystander interventions, and untrained bystanders prompted in CPR by 911 telecommunicators who are trained to prompt callers in BLS technique. Emerging data suggest that telephone prompts by 911 operators can improve survival with preserved neurologic status.[123] Further enhancements may include drones for deployment of automated external defibrillators (AEDs), mobile technology/social media to alert nearby potential responders, and specialized applications.[124-126] Requirements for specialized knowledge and skills increase progressively as the patient is moved through postcardiac arrest management into long-term follow-up care. These emergency response principles are intended for both in-hospital and community-based responses.

In-Hospital Interventions

Development of the coronary care unit resulted in an immediate reduction of in-hospital mortality risk during AMI from 30% to 15% based almost entirely on the reduction of cardiac arrests. Other specialized monitoring and intensive care units demonstrated various levels of benefit as well, but the impact has been less in general care hospital units and for cardiac arrests associated with complex comorbid states or occurring during off-hours.[127] A registry study in the decade from 2000 to 2009 provided trends for risk-adjusted rates of survival to discharge after cardiac arrest in monitored units and general hospital units. Among 84,625 subjects, 20.7% had VF or pulseless VT as the initial rhythm and 79.3% had asystole or PEA, with the proportion of cardiac arrests attributable to asystole/PEA increasing over time ($P < 0.001$). The overall survival rate to discharge increased from 13.7% in 2000 to 22.3% in 2009 ($P < 0.001$), with improvement in both the VT/VF and the PEA/asystole subsets (Fig. 70.11A). Absolute rates of survival to discharge remained higher for the VT/VF group, whereas improvement in survival occurred in the two rhythm groups. The improvement in survival appeared to be due to both improved acute resuscitation actions and postresuscitation care. A small decrease in rates of clinically significant neurologic disability in survivors occurred over time.

Community-Based Interventions

The initial out-of-hospital intervention experience in Miami and Seattle yielded only 14% and 11% rates of survival to discharge, respectively. Subsequent improvements correlated with the addition of emergency medical technicians as another tier of responders to provide CPR and earlier defibrillation. In general, rural areas have lower success rates, and the U.S. national success rate remains approximately 10%.[9] Regional variability is highlighted by a county level analysis from the CARES Surveillance Group and the HeartRescue Project demonstrating survival to discharge rates from 3.4% to 20.1%.[128] A large portion of this variability is explained by rates of bystander CPR, median age, and median household income. Rates of bystander CPR have been shown to increase with a mobile phone technology to alert nearby lay volunteers trained in CPR that there is a nearby OHCA.[124,126]

Reports from different areas in the United States show marked variations in outcomes.[129] Older data from Chicago and New York City provided disturbing outcome data. A study from Chicago reported that only 9% of out-of-hospital cardiac arrest victims survive to be hospitalized and only 2% are discharged alive. Moreover, outcomes in Blacks are worse than those in whites (0.8% versus 2.6%). The fact that a large majority had bradyarrhythmias, asystole, or PEA on initial contact with emergency medical services suggests prolonged times between collapse and arrival of the emergency medical service, absent or ineffective bystander interventions, or both. The New York City report indicated a survival to hospital discharge rate of only 1.4%. Among those who undergo bystander CPR, the rate increases to 2.9%, and bystander

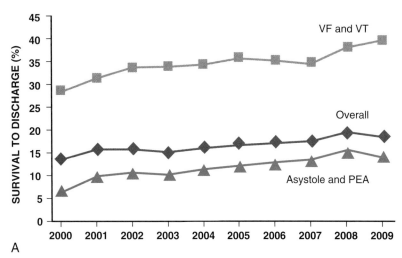

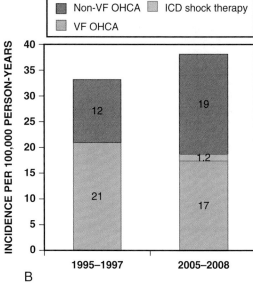

FIGURE 70.11 **Changing incidence of shockable and nonshockable rhythms. A,** Survival to discharge for VF and pulseless VT versus asystole and PEA between 2000 and 2009 (*P* < 0.001 for trend in each survival curve). **B,** In Holland, there was a decrease in the VF event rate with a concomitant increase in non-VF rhythms. Thus, the proportion of events with VF at initial contact is decreasing, as observed in several other studies. (**A** from Girotra S, et al. Trends in survival after in-hospital cardiac arrest. N Engl J Med 2012;367:1912-1920. **B** from Hulleman M, et al. Implantable cardioverter defibrillators have reduced the incidence of resuscitation for out of hospital cardiac arrest caused by lethal arrhythmias. Circulation 2012;126:815-821.)

CPR plus VF as the initial rhythm yields a further increase to 5.3%. Finally, for those whose arrests occurred after the arrival of emergency medical services, the success rate increases further to 8.5%. These trends support the concept that delays and breaks in the in the "chain of survival" have a major negative impact on the results of emergency medical services in densely populated areas. Cardiac arrest data from the COVID-19 pandemic support this observation. The rate of OHCA was substantially increased during comparable time periods before and during the pandemic, with increased mortality perhaps linked to increased time to EMS arrival and reduced frequency of bystander CPR, among other factors.[130] Even communities with low rates of infection demonstrated this pattern.[131] Both bystander CPR and EMS arrival time have been shown to influence survival,[132] providing support for the importance of these community interventions.

There are circumstances in which resuscitative effort in the out-of-hospital setting is deemed futile. A victim found unconscious after an unwitnessed collapse, reasonably assumed to be found after a prolonged interval (e.g., cool skin, rigor mortis), obviously fulfills this classification. However, studies have provided markers of futility under less stark circumstances. In a study involving trained responders with AEDs, only 0.5% of victims survived if (1) the arrest was not witnessed by emergency medical service personnel, (2) there was no ROSC, and (3) no shocks were delivered per protocol. Adding a response time longer than 8 minutes reduced the survival rate to 0.3%, and events unwitnessed by a bystander yielded no survivors.

Impact of Tiered Response Systems

Improvements in both out-of-hospital care and in-hospital technology and practices can contribute to better outcomes, as described in the chain-of-survival concept.[1] Of these two general factors, the influence of out-of-hospital care has been studied in more detail. The importance of early defibrillation for improving outcome has been supported by many studies. These observations have motivated a search for strategies that shorten response times, largely by the development of two-tiered systems in which nonconventional first responders, such as police, firefighters, security guards, and lay bystanders, deploy AEDs that are now commonly available in public places. Available data suggest that this strategy may improve outcome, primarily in public locations (see eFig. 70.2).[133]

In rural communities, earlier defibrillation by ambulance technicians yielded a 19% survival rate versus only 3% for standard CPR. In another report, an analysis of the relationship between response delay and survival to hospital discharge revealed a 48% survival rate

for response times of 2 minutes or less and less than a 10% survival rate when responses were longer than 10 minutes (eFig. 70.2). Another study showed survival decline by 5.2%/min for EMS arrival between 5 and 10 minutes and a further decline of 1.9%/min for arrival between 11 and 15 minutes after collapse.

A second element in out-of-hospital care that contributes to outcome is the role of bystander CPR by laypeople awaiting the arrival of EMS personnel.[134] It has been reported that although there was no significant difference in the percentage of patients successfully resuscitated and admitted to the hospital alive with (67%) or without (61%) bystander intervention, almost twice as many OHCA victims were ultimately discharged alive when they had undergone bystander CPR (43%) than when such support was not provided (22%). Central nervous system protection, expressed as early regaining of consciousness, is the major protective element of bystander CPR. It has been reported that more than 40% of victims whose defibrillation and other advanced life support activities were instituted more than 8 minutes after collapse survived if basic CPR had been initiated less than 2 minutes after onset of the arrest. While it has been suggested that a period of CPR before defibrillation may also be helpful, particularly if the time to defibrillation exceeds 4 minutes from the onset of arrest, the data are unclear.

Importance of Electrical Mechanisms. Several sources have identified a changing distribution of initial rhythms recorded by EMS personnel. When compared with data from the 1970s and 1980s, there has been a decrease in the number of events in which ventricular tachyarrhythmias are the initial rhythm recorded, with a consequent reduction in the proportion of victims who have rhythms amenable to cardioversion-defibrillation (see Fig. 70.11B). Similar observations have been reported in in-hospital settings. Some studies have now suggested that less than 50% of victims have shockable rhythms at initial contact. This could contribute to a reduction in cumulative survival probability with community-based interventions.[129] It is likely that pre-911 delays in recognition of and reaction to an event may be playing a role, in conjunction with longer response times based on geographic considerations. This suggests a need for more extensive public education programs. Thus response times may not accurately reflect true downtimes, and consequently the potential for success is impaired. The 4- to 6-minute time for a desirable response is not optimal. By 4 minutes, significant circulatory and ischemic changes have taken place, and conditions worsen rapidly beyond that time.

The electrical mechanism of out-of-hospital cardiac arrest, as defined by the initial rhythm recorded by EMS personnel, has a powerful impact

TABLE 70.4 Tachyarrhythmic and Nontachyarrhythmic Cardiac Arrest

PRIMARY ARRHYTHMIAS	ELECTRICAL MECHANISMS	MECHANICAL MECHANISMS
Tachyarrhythmic Cardiac Arrest		
Ventricular fibrillation	Absence of organized ventricular depolarization	Absence of LVWM
Pulseless ventricular tachycardia	Organized ventricular pattern; rapid rate	Absent LVWM or LVWM insufficient for organ perfusion
Secondary Arrhythmias		
Sinus tachycardia; other	Sinus or other supraventricular rhythm; narrow QRS	Obstruction to cardiac blood flow; hypovolemia
Nontachyarrhythmic Cardiac Arrest		
PEA, Primary (Initial Rhythm)		
With residual LV contraction	Organized QRS complexes, usually wide	LVWM insufficient for organ perfusion
Without LV contraction	Organized QRS complexes, usually wide	Absence of LVWM
PEA, Secondary		
Postshock	Regular or irregular QRS complexes, usually wide	Absent LVWM or LVWM insufficient for organ perfusion
Primary noncardiac	Regular or irregular QRS complexes, usually wide	Usually LVWM insufficient for organ perfusion; LVWM may be absent
Agonal PEA	Slow, usually irregular, wide QRS	Absence of LVWM
Ventricular asystole	Absent ventricular electrical activity; exclude fine ventricular fibrillation	Absence of LVWM

LV, Left ventricular; *LVWM,* left ventricular wall motion; *PEA,* pulseless electrical activity.
Modified from Myerburg RJ, et al. Pulseless electrical activity: definition, causes, mechanisms, management, and research priorities for the next decade. Report from a National Heart, Lung, and Blood Institute Workshop. Circulation 2013;128:2532.

on outcome. They are generally categorized as shockable (VF, and pulseless VT [pVT]) and nonshockable (PEA, asystole) rhythms (Table 70.4). The distinction between pVT and PEA is sometimes confused and has relevance because it impacts response strategies. The subgroup of patients who are in pVT at the time of first contact, although small, has the best outcome. Eighty-eight percent of patients in cardiac arrest related to VT were successfully resuscitated and admitted to the hospital alive, and 67% were ultimately discharged alive. However, this relatively low-risk group represents less than 10% of all cardiac arrests. Because of the inherent time lag between collapse and initial recordings, it is likely that many more cardiac arrests begin as rapid sustained VT and degenerate into VF before the arrival of rescue personnel.

Patients with a bradyarrhythmia or with asystole or PEA at initial contact have the worst prognosis; only 9% of such patients in the Miami study were admitted to the hospital alive, and none were discharged. In a later experience, some improvement in outcome was noted, although the improvement was limited to patients in whom the initial bradyarrhythmia recorded was an idioventricular rhythm that responded promptly to chronotropic agents in the field. In a large prospective observational in-hospital study of cardiac arrests in children and adults, children had a higher probability of asystole or PEA as the initial documented rhythm but had a better overall survival rate because they had better outcomes of interventions for these rhythms than adults did. Overall survival after PEA appears to be better in recent years, and may be somewhat better than for asystole.[135] Moreover, for patients with an initial nonshockable rhythm that converts to a shockable rhythm, there may also be improved outcomes, but this may depend on how early this conversion occurs and whether the initial rhythm was asystole or PEA.[136]

Bradyarrhythmias also have adverse prognostic implications after defibrillation from VF in the field. Patients with a heart rate lower than 60 beats/min after defibrillation, regardless of the specific bradyarrhythmic mechanism, had a poor prognosis, with 95% of such patients dying before hospitalization or in the hospital. The outcome in the group of patients in whom VF is the initial rhythm recorded is intermediate between the outcomes associated with sustained VT and with bradyarrhythmia and asystole. The proportion of each of the electrophysiologic mechanisms responsible for cardiac arrest varied among the earlier reports, with VF ranging from 65% to more than 90% of the study populations and bradyarrhythmia and asystole ranging from 10% to 30%. However, in reports from densely populated metropolitan areas, the ratios of tachyarrhythmic to bradyarrhythmic or pulseless activity events were reversed, and outcomes were far worse.

Initial Assessment and Basic Life Support

Activities at initial contact with the unconscious victim include diagnostic maneuvers and basic cardiopulmonary support interventions. The first action must be confirmation that collapse is the result of a cardiac arrest. A few seconds of evaluation for response to voice, observation for respiratory movements and skin color, and simultaneous palpation of major arteries for the presence or absence of a pulse yields sufficient information to determine whether a life-threatening incident is in progress. Once a life-threatening incident has been suspected or confirmed, contact with an available emergency medical rescue system (911) for out-of-hospital settings or a "code" team in the hospital should be an immediate priority.

The absence of a carotid or femoral pulse detected by a medical professional, particularly if it is confirmed by the absence of an audible heartbeat, is a primary diagnostic criterion. For lay responders, the pulse check is no longer recommended.[108] Skin color may be pale or intensely cyanotic. Absence of respiratory effort or the presence of only agonal respiratory effort in conjunction with an absent pulse is diagnostic of cardiac arrest; however, respiratory effort can persist for 1 minute or longer after onset of the arrest. In contrast, absence of respiratory effort or the presence of severe stridor with persistence of a pulse suggests a primary respiratory arrest that will lead to cardiac arrest in a short time. In the latter circumstance, initial efforts should include exploration of the oropharynx in search for a foreign body and performance of the Heimlich maneuver, particularly if the incident occurs in a setting in which aspiration is likely (e.g., restaurant death or café coronary).

Chest Thump

A blow to the chest (precordial thump, "thumpversion") may be attempted by a properly trained rescuer. It has been recommended that it be reserved as an advanced life support activity. Precordial thumps will rarely revert apparent VF, VT, and asystole. The use of the precordial thump does not impact ROSC or overall survival. The technique is considered optional for responding to a pulseless cardiac arrest in the absence of monitoring when a defibrillator is not immediately available. It should not be used unmonitored in a patient with a rapid tachycardia without complete loss of consciousness. The thumpversion technique involves one or two blows delivered firmly to the junction of the middle and lower thirds of the sternum from a height of 8 to 10 inches. The effort should be abandoned if a spontaneous pulse does not develop immediately. Another mechanical method, which requires that the patient still be conscious, is so-called cough-induced cardiac compression. It is a conscious act of forceful coughing by the patient that may support forward flow by cyclical increases in intrathoracic pressure during VF or may cause conversion of sustained VT. Available data supporting its successful use are limited; it is not an alternative to conventional techniques.

Basic Life Support—The Initial Steps in Cardiopulmonary Resuscitation

The goal of BLS is to maintain viability of the central nervous system, heart, and other vital organs until definitive ROSC can be achieved. BLS encompasses both the initial responses outlined earlier and their natural flow into establishing perfusion and ventilation. This range of activities can be carried out not only by professional and paraprofessional personnel but also by trained emergency technicians and laypeople. There should be minimal delay between diagnosis and preparatory effort in the initial response and institution of BLS. The first steps are to verify the environmental safety of the site and confirm that the victim is unresponsive. The responder should call for nearby help, activate an emergency response system (via mobile device, if appropriate), and send for an AED.

These principles have measurable impact for both OHCA and IHCA. The survival rate to discharge for IHCA, considering all causes and mechanisms, was reported to be 33% when CPR was initiated within the first minute versus 14% when the time was longer than 1 minute. When VF was the initial rhythm, the corresponding figures were 50% and 32%, respectively. In the out-of-hospital setting, if only one witness is present, notification of emergency personnel (calling 911) is the only activity that should precede BLS. The previous sequence of the "ABC" of BLS—airway, breathing, compression—has been changed to "CAB"—compression, airway, breathing—based on the recognition that compression alone is the better strategy because it minimizes interruptions in perfusion and avoids excessive ventilation.

Circulation

This element of BLS is intended to maintain blood flow (i.e., circulation) until definitive steps can be taken. The rationale is based on the hypothesis that chest compression allows the heart to maintain an externally driven pump function by sequential emptying and filling of its chambers, with competent valves favoring forward direction of flow. In fact, application of this technique has proved successful when it is used as recommended. The palm of one hand is placed over the lower half of the sternum and the heel of the other rests on the dorsum of the lower part of the hand. The sternum is then depressed, with the resuscitator's arms straight at the elbows to provide a less tiring and more forceful fulcrum at the junction of the shoulders and back. By use of this technique, sufficient force is applied to depress the sternum at least 2 inches (>5 cm). Compression is followed by abrupt relaxation, and the cycle is carried out at a rate of about 100 compressions/min.

Techniques of CPR based on the hypothesis that increased intrathoracic pressure is the prime mover of blood, rather than cardiac compression itself, have been evaluated, and the guidelines for conventional CPR ventilatory techniques were modified in 2005. For single responders to victims from infancy (excluding newborns) through adulthood, and for adults responded to by two rescuers, a compression-ventilation ratio of 30:2 is now recommended. For two-rescuer CPR in infants and children, the former compression-ventilation ratio of 15:2 is retained. A more recent modification intended to encourage more bystander participation in CPR and to allay concerns about mouth-to-mouth ventilation of unknown victims is the "hands-only" (compression-only) technique. This technique is particularly important for untrained or remotely trained bystanders who are not confident in their ability to perform compression-ventilation sequences. The 2005 changes in CPR recommendations, in which the number of successive shocks and pulse checks during initial responses is reduced (Electrotherapy for Cardiac Arrhythmias, Chapter 67), are retained in the current recommendations.[4] This is intended in part to increase the cumulative time of circulatory support during CPR before restoration of a spontaneous pulse.

Concept of Cardiocerebral Resuscitation

This concept, also referred to as minimally interrupted cardiac resuscitation, is based on the hypothesis that the primary benefit of CPR is its pumping action rather than the combination of compression and ventilation. It challenges the general guidelines, which assume a benefit of interrupting compression to provide ventilation and that an initial phase of ventilation before initial defibrillation improves outcomes when response times are longer than 4 or 5 minutes. Cardiocerebral resuscitation[137] emphasizes continuous chest compressions, interrupted primarily for single shocks and evaluation of responses to shocks and deferring and limiting ventilatory and certain pharmacologic actions. Despite interesting preliminary data, it is generally agreed that a randomized trial is needed before the minimal interruption concept can replace the current guidelines.

Even though conventional techniques produce measurable carotid artery flow with a record of successful resuscitations, the absence of a pressure gradient across the heart in the presence of an extrathoracic arteriovenous pressure gradient has led to the concept that it is not cardiac compression per se but rather a pumping action produced by changes in pressure in the entire thoracic cavity that optimizes systemic blood flow during resuscitation. Experimental work in which the chest is compressed during ventilations rather than between them (simultaneous compression-ventilation) has demonstrated better extra-thoracic arterial flow. However, increased carotid artery flow does not necessarily equate with improved cerebral perfusion, and the reduction in coronary blood flow caused by elevated intrathoracic pressure with the use of certain techniques may be too high a price for the improved peripheral flow. In addition, a high thoracoabdominal gradient has been demonstrated during experimental simultaneous compression-ventilation, which could divert flow from the brain in the absence of concomitant abdominal binding. On the basis of these observations, new mechanically assisted techniques, including an active decompression phase (i.e., active compression-decompression), have been evaluated for improved circulation during CPR.[138] An impedance threshold device for ventilation has also been developed that in combination with active compression-decompression enhances venous return to the heart. The combination of these two technologies has demonstrated improved survival. Further addition of a "head-up/torso-up" position improves cerebral perfusion and has been reported to almost double resuscitation rates in a community-based study.[139]

Airway

Clearing of the airway is a critical step in preparing for successful resuscitation. This process includes tilting the head backward and lifting the chin, in addition to exploring the airway for foreign bodies, including dentures, and removing them. The Heimlich maneuver should be performed if there is reason to suspect that a foreign body is lodged in the oropharynx. This maneuver entails wrapping the arms around the victim from the back and delivering a sharp thrust to the upper part of the abdomen with a closed fist. If it is not possible for the person in attendance to carry out the maneuver because of insufficient physical strength, mechanical dislodgment of the foreign body can sometimes be achieved by abdominal thrusts with the unconscious patient in a supine position. The Heimlich maneuver is not entirely benign; ruptured abdominal viscera in the victim have been reported, as has a case in which the rescuer disrupted his own aortic root and died. If there is strong suspicion that respiratory arrest precipitated cardiac arrest, particularly in the presence of a mechanical airway obstruction, a second precordial thump should be delivered after the airway has been cleared.

Breathing

With the head placed properly and the oropharynx clear, mouth-to-mouth resuscitation can be initiated if no specific rescue equipment is available. To a large extent the procedure used to establish ventilation depends on the site at which the cardiac arrest occurs. Various devices are available, including plastic oropharyngeal airways, esophageal obturators, masked Ambu bags, and endotracheal tubes. Intubation is the preferred procedure, but time should not be sacrificed, even in the in-hospital setting, while awaiting an endotracheal tube or a person trained to insert it quickly and properly. Thus, in the in-hospital setting, temporary support with Ambu bag ventilation is the usual method until endotracheal intubation can be carried out, and in the out-of-hospital setting, mouth-to-mouth resuscitation is used while awaiting EMS personnel. The effect of various infectious diseases, such as acquired immunodeficiency syndrome, hepatitis B, and SARS-CoV-2, on attitudes about mouth-to-mouth resuscitation by bystanders and even professional personnel in hospitals is an area of concern, likely impacting its use.

Early Defibrillation by First Responders

The time from the onset of cardiac arrest to advanced life support (ACLS) influences outcome. Both early neurologic status and survival are better in patients defibrillated by first responders than if one awaits the assistance of more highly trained paramedics. The term *first responder* refers to the person on scene providing initial CPR and has emerged from minimally trained emergency technicians allowed to carry out defibrillation in conjunction with BLS to nonconventional responders, such as trained security guards and police, and subsequently to lay bystanders knowledgeable in CPR with access to AEDs. Because the time to defibrillation plays a central role in determining outcome in cardiac arrest caused by VF, the development and deployment of AEDs (see Chapter 67) in public locations has had impact on outcomes. This technology is potentially applicable to a number of different strategic models, each with its own benefits and limitations.

Overall, AED use is associated with improved outcomes but the quality of the cumulative evidence had been low to very low.[140] Data from the Resuscitation Outcomes Consortium showed that patients shocked by an AED by a bystander were more likely to survive to discharge (66.5% versus 43.0%) than patients initially shocked by EMS with better functional outcome.[141] Among the strategies that have yielded various levels of identifiable survival benefit to date are deployment in police vehicles, airliners and airports, casinos, and more general community-based sites. Police AED deployment data have been inconsistent in various studies, possibly because of appropriateness for various types of communities and the specific deployment strategies used, but data suggest that it is beneficial in large metropolitan areas. Initial airline data were similarly uncertain, but a more recent report on data from a large airline with a well-organized system has suggested benefit (eFig. 70.3). Similar encouraging results have been reported with the deployment of AEDs in the Chicago airport system. Finally, the special circumstance of casinos, in which continuous television monitoring alerts security officers to medical problems immediately, has yielded impressive survival rates (Fig. 70.12). However, there appears to be a great deal of variability in efficiency on the basis of expected event rates at different types of community sites, and deployment strategies have been suggested on the basis of projected event rates at various locations. Deployment in schools, accompanied by comprehensive response planning, is associated with good outcomes, even with relatively low event rates. A study of the deployment of AEDs in the homes of patients who recently had MIs and were not candidates for implantable defibrillators did not demonstrate benefit. Because the home is the most common site of cardiac arrest and survival rates are lower

than those in public sites, additional strategies for both AEDs and other technologies should be tested. Further research on effective strategies is needed because most community-based cardiac arrests occur in the home. Novel approaches such as the use of drones to deploy AEDs where needed and mobile applications that can locate the nearest AED may alleviate some of these issues.[142]

As is the case with any medical device, malfunctions of AEDs may occur infrequently because of design or manufacturing defects or failure to adhere to manufacturers' recommendations for replacement of batteries and leads. It is an obligation of those responsible for maintaining AEDs to remain cognizant of FDA safety alerts and recalls and the shelf-lives of batteries and leads.

Advanced Life Support

This next step in the resuscitative sequence is designed to achieve stable ROSC and hemodynamic stabilization.[108] Implementation of advanced life support (ACLS) is not intended to suggest an abrupt cessation of BLS activities, but rather a transition from one level of activity to the next. In the past, ACLS required judgments and technical skills that removed it from the realm of activity of lay bystanders and even emergency medical technicians, instead limiting these activities to specifically trained paramedical personnel, nurses, and physicians. With further education of emergency technicians, most community-based CPR programs now permit them to carry out ACLS activities. However, some studies suggest that the addition of ACLS to an otherwise optimized out-of-hospital response system (i.e., bystander CPR and early defibrillation) does not improve survival. In this regard, the development and testing of AEDs that have the ability to sense and analyze cardiac electrical activity and to prompt the user to deliver definitive electrical intervention provide a role for rapid defibrillation by less highly trained rescue personnel (i.e., police, ambulance drivers) and even minimally trained lay bystanders.

The general goals of ACLS are to restore cardiac rhythm to one that is hemodynamically effective, to optimize ventilation, and to maintain and support the restored circulation. Thus, during advanced life support, the patient's cardiac rhythm is promptly cardioverted or defibrillated as the first priority, if appropriate equipment is immediately available. Although a short period of closed-chest cardiac compression immediately before defibrillation has been reported to enhance the probability of survival, especially if circulation has been absent for 4 to 5 or more minutes, the data are unclear. After the initial attempt to restore a hemodynamically effective rhythm, the patient is intubated and oxygenated, if needed, and the heart is paced if bradyarrhythmia or asystole occurs. An intravenous line is established to deliver medications. After intubation, the goal of ventilation is to reverse the hypoxemia and not merely to achieve high alveolar oxygen pressure (po_2). Thus oxygen rather than room air should be used to ventilate the patient; if possible, arterial Po_2 should be monitored. Respiratory support in the hospital by means of an endotracheal tube and Ambu bag—or facemasks in the out-of-hospital setting—is generally used.

Successful ROSC after IHCA is associated with a shorter median duration of resuscitation than is the case in nonsurvivors (12 minutes, interquartile range [IQR] of 6 to 21, versus 20 minutes, IQR of 14 to 30). Nonetheless, hospitals that habitually ran the longest maximum code runs (the median value in the longest quartile was 25 versus 16) generated a higher likelihood of ROSC and survival to discharge. This observation supports longer attempts at resuscitation in patients without do-not-resuscitate orders or futile medical status.

Defibrillation-Cardioversion

Rapid conversion to an effective cardiac electrical mechanism is a key step in successful resuscitation. Delay should be minimal, even when conditions for CPR are optimal. When VF or VT that is pulseless and/or accompanied by loss of consciousness is recognized on a monitor or by telemetry, defibrillation should be carried out immediately. An initial shock of 120 to 200 J by biphasic devices, with the energy level depending on the recommendations for the individual biphasic devices, should be delivered. Energies delivered through AEDs are generally preprogrammed and vary among the devices available. Failure

Casino AED Project: Witnessed Response Times and Outcomes

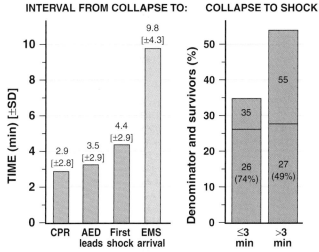

FIGURE 70.12 Results of AED deployment in the controlled environment of casinos. Because the onset of cardiac arrest can frequently be witnessed, short intervals from the onset of collapse to CPR and AED shocks were achieved. Response times were reduced by more than 50% in comparison to the standard emergency medical system (EMS). For those found in VT/VF, the survival rate approached 60% for VT/VF with a witnessed onset. When response time was less than 3 minutes, the survival rate after VT/VF was greater than 70%. (Modified from Valenzuela TD, et al: Outcomes of rapid defibrillation by security officers after cardiac arrest in casinos. N Engl J Med 2000;343:1206.)

VII

of the initial shock to provide an effective rhythm is a poor prognostic sign. Failure of a single adequate shock to restore a pulse should be followed by continued CPR and a second shock delivered after five cycles of CPR. This supersedes the previous strategy of three successive shocks before resuming CPR. The intent is to maximize circulatory time by chest compressions until a pulse has been restored.

If cardiac arrest still persists, the patient is intubated and intravenous access achieved. Epinephrine is administered and followed by repeated defibrillation attempts at maximal output. Although its efficacy is not established, double sequential defibrillation—delivering shocks from two different defibrillators almost simultaneously—may be considered for patients who are refractory to defibrillation.[108] Epinephrine may be repeated at 3- to 5-minute intervals with a defibrillator shock in between. Vasopressin is an effective alternative to epinephrine. However, studies of the value of high-dose versus standard-dose epinephrine and epinephrine versus vasopressin have not demonstrated superiority of one strategy for survival to discharge or neurologic outcome, though some differences in ROSC were noted. In a placebo controlled trial from the United Kingdom, there was improved 30-day survival with epinephrine (3.2% versus 2.4%) but no difference in neurologic outcome as more patients in the epinephrine group had neurologic impairment.[143]

Simultaneously, the rescuer should focus on ventilation to improve oxygenation, reversal of acidosis, and improvement of the underlying electrophysiologic condition to make the heart more likely to reestablish a stable rhythm. Although adequate oxygenation of the blood is crucial in immediate management of the metabolic acidosis of cardiac arrest, additional correction by intravenous administration of sodium bicarbonate has been used. In a small study patients randomized to intravenous sodium bicarbonate or saline for patients undergoing CPR with pH <7.1 or bicarbonate <10 mEq/L, there was no improvement in ROSC or good neurologic survival at one month.[144] Sodium bicarbonate is generally not recommended except in certain conditions such as hyperkalemia and drug overdose.[145]

Pharmacotherapy

For patients who have persistent or recurrent VT or VF despite direct-current cardioversion after epinephrine, intravenous administration of antiarrhythmic agents has been recommended (Chapter 64) during continued resuscitative efforts. Based on a single controlled trial with a survival to hospital admission endpoint, intravenous amiodarone emerged as the initial treatment of choice. Bolus therapy (150 mg), followed by a maintenance dose during the next 18 hours and for several days if necessary, was recommended, depending on response. A bolus of lidocaine (60 to 100 mg) may be given intravenously and the dose repeated in 2 minutes for patients in whom amiodarone is unsuccessful and possibly for those who have an acute transmural MI as the triggering mechanism for the cardiac arrest. In a randomized, placebo controlled, double blind trial, the Resuscitation Outcomes Consortium compared intravenous amiodarone (150 mg, followed by a second bolus if necessary) or lidocaine (60 mg) against placebo. There was no difference between either drug or placebo for survival to discharge outcomes or survival with favorable neurologic status.[146] However, survival to hospital admission was significantly better with both active drugs compared with placebo. In addition, survival to discharge was improved with both drugs among the subgroup with bystander-witnessed arrest, but neither active drug was superior to the other. In another placebo controlled trial, the Resuscitation Outcomes Consortium compared intravenous and intraosseous administration of amiodarone and lidocaine and found that only intravenous administration improved outcomes.[147] Intravenous procainamide is rarely used in this setting any longer, but it may be tried for persisting, hemodynamically stable arrhythmias.

For patients in whom acute hyperkalemia is associated with resistant VF or for those who have hypocalcemia or are toxic from Ca^{2+} entry–blocking drugs, 10% calcium gluconate may be helpful. Calcium should not be used routinely during resuscitation, even though ionized calcium levels may be low during resuscitation from cardiac arrest. Some resistant forms of polymorphic VT or torsades de pointes, rapid monomorphic VT or ventricular flutter (rate ≥260/min), or resistant

VF may respond to intravenous beta blocker therapy or intravenous magnesium sulfate. For patients with acute ventricular arrhythmias or VT storm associated with long-QT syndrome, intravenous magnesium sulfate is often an effective antiarrhythmic, even if it has no effect on QT duration.[145]

Bradyarrhythmic and Asystolic Arrest; Pulseless Electrical Activity

The approach to patients with bradyarrhythmic or asystolic arrest or with PEA differs from the approach to those with a tachyarrhythmic event. When this form of cardiac arrest is recognized, effort should focus first on establishing control of cardiorespiratory status (i.e., continue CPR, intubate, and establish intravenous access), reconfirming the rhythm (in two leads if possible), and finally taking action that favors the emergence of a stable spontaneous rhythm or attempt to pace the heart. Possible reversible causes, particularly for bradyarrhythmia and asystole, should be considered and excluded (or treated) promptly. Such causes include hypovolemia, hypoxia, cardiac tamponade, tension pneumothorax, preexisting acidosis, drug overdose, hypothermia, and hyperkalemia. Epinephrine is commonly used in an attempt to elicit spontaneous electrical activity or to increase the rate of a bradycardia. It has had only limited success, as has intravenous isoproterenol infusions in doses of up to 15 to 20 µg/min. In the absence of an intravenous line, epinephrine 1 mg (10 mL of a 1:10,000 solution) may be given by the intracardiac or intraosseous route, but there is danger of coronary or myocardial laceration with the former. Endotracheal delivery can be used if neither IV or IO can be achieved. The added value of high-dose epinephrine is unclear, as in the case of resistant VF. Atropine is no longer considered of value for PEA or asystole, although it may be of benefit for other bradyarrhythmic mechanisms.

Pacing of a bradyarrhythmic or asystolic heart has been limited in the past by the unavailability of personnel capable of carrying out such procedures at the scene of cardiac arrest. With the development of more effective external pacing systems, the role of pacing and its influence on outcome must now be reevaluated. Unfortunately, to date, no clear benefit to transcutaneous pacing has been established.[145]

The published standards for CPR and emergency cardiac care include a series of teaching algorithms to be used as guides to appropriate care. These general guides are not to be interpreted as inclusive of all possible approaches or contingencies. CPR in pregnant women requires attention to the influence of the gravid uterus on the mechanics of CPR. The pregnant patient should be placed in a left lateral decubitus position with left uterine displacement during CPR to relieve aorto-caval compression,[148] and standard defibrillation has no risk for the fetus. Acute antiarrhythmic drug therapy during ACLS is generally safe, although long-term amiodarone therapy raises concern for potential fetal organ toxicity.

Stabilization of Cardiac Rhythm after Initial Return of Spontaneous Circulation

If frequent PVCs and runs of nonsustained VT persist after restoration of a sinus mechanism, continuous infusion of an effective antiarrhythmic drug may be used, but this is based on the clinical situation and clinical judgement of the provider. Intravenous amiodarone is the preferred agent, but lidocaine is an option for arrhythmias caused by acute ischemic events. On occasion, continuous infusion of propranolol or esmolol is used, sometimes in conjunction with magnesium sulfate, especially for recurrent episodes of polymorphic VT or VT storm unresponsive to amiodarone.

Catecholamines are used for cardiac arrest not only in an attempt to achieve better electrical stability (e.g., conversion from fine to coarse VF or increasing the rate of spontaneous contraction during bradyarrhythmias) but also for their inotropic and peripheral vascular effects. Epinephrine is the first choice among the catecholamines for use in cardiac arrest because it increases myocardial contractility, elevates perfusion pressure, may convert electromechanical dissociation to electromechanical coupling, and improves the chances for successful defibrillation. Because of its adverse effects on renal and mesenteric flow, norepinephrine is a less desirable agent despite its inotropic effects. When the chronotropic effect of epinephrine is undesirable, dopamine or dobutamine is preferable to norepinephrine for inotropic effect. Isoproterenol may be used for the treatment of primary or postdefibrillation bradycardia when heart rate control is the primary goal of therapy intended to improve cardiac output. Calcium chloride is sometimes used in patients with PEA that persists after the administration of catecholamines. The efficacy of this intervention is uncertain. Stimulation of alpha adrenoceptors may be important during definitive resuscitative efforts. For example, the alpha adrenoceptor–stimulating effects of epinephrine and higher dosages of dopamine, which elevate aortic diastolic pressure by peripheral vasoconstriction with increased cerebral and myocardial flow, have been reemphasized.

Postcardiac Arrest Care and Postcardiac Arrest Syndrome

After return of spontaneous or stable assisted circulation, focus shifts to the diagnostic and therapeutic elements of postcardiac arrest syndrome, a field of pathophysiology and clinical intervention that emerged from the recognition that the various elements of injury following cardiac arrest should be organized into a multidisciplinary continuum. The four elements of postcardiac arrest syndrome include brain injury, myocardial dysfunction, systemic ischemia/reperfusion responses, and control of persistent precipitating factors. The therapeutic goal is to achieve and maintain stable electrical, hemodynamic, and central nervous system (CNS) status, based on complex algorithms. The specialized and multidisciplinary nature of postcardiac arrest care have led to the proposal and preliminary data supporting the concept of specialized cardiac centers for postcardiac arrest patients, analogous to trauma or stroke centers. When transporting the hemodynamically unstable or comatose patient, EMS responders would selectively bypass the nearest hospital, in favor of the closest facility having facilities and staff sufficient to manage postcardiac arrest complexities, assuming an added transport time of no more than 15 minutes. The profile of the patient ready for transport is matched to the capabilities of the institution to which the victim is transported, as outlined in Figure 70.13.

For successfully resuscitated cardiac arrest victims, whether the event occurred in or out of the hospital, postcardiac arrest care includes admission to an intensive care unit and continuous monitoring for a

minimum of 48 to 72 hours. Some elements of postcardiac arrest syndrome are common to all resuscitated patients, but the prognosis and certain details of management are specific for the clinical setting in which the cardiac arrest occurred. The major management categories include (1) primary cardiac arrest in patients with AMI; (2) secondary cardiac arrest in patients with AMI; (3) cardiac arrest associated with noncardiac-related diseases, drug effects, or electrolyte disorders; and (4) survival after out-of-hospital cardiac arrest.

Cardiac Arrest in Patients with Hemodynamically Stable Acute Myocardial Infarction

VF in patients with AMI free of concomitant hemodynamic complications (i.e., primary VF; see Chapter 38) is now less common in hospitalized patients compared with the 15% to 20% incidence noted before the availability of cardiac care units. The events that do occur are almost always reverted successfully by prompt interventions in properly equipped emergency departments or cardiac care units. If ventricular arrhythmias persist after successful resuscitation, a lidocaine or amiodarone infusion is used. Antiarrhythmic drugs are generally discontinued after 24 hours if sustained arrhythmias do not recur. The occurrence of VF during the early phase of AMI (i.e., first 24 to 48 hours) does not identify long-term arrhythmic risk and is not an indication for long-term antiarrhythmic or device therapy. Polymorphic VT has similar implications.

Monomorphic VT, which may lead to cardiac arrest in AMI, has different implications as it may be due to the presence of a substrate that has long-term implications or transient electrophysiologic changes due to the acute ischemia and infarction. VF within 48 hours of MI was shown to be associated with a better prognosis than VT. Of those with VT who received an ICD, there was a high rate of appropriate ICD therapy in follow-up. Though monomorphic VT is uncommon in the setting of acute coronary syndromes, it has been shown to be an independent predictor of long-term survival, whereas nonmonomorphic VT was not.[149]

Cardiac arrest caused by bradyarrhythmias or asystole in acute *inferior* wall MI, in the absence of primary hemodynamic deterioration, is uncommon and may respond to atropine or pacing. The prognosis is good, with no special long-term care required in most cases. Persistent

Level	Patient Status	Hospital Resource Minimums
Level 1	Failure to restore circulation; ROSC without regaining consciousness ± hemodynamic instability ± acute coronary syndrome; ± recurrent arrhythmias	Local or regional facility capable of providing highest level of neurological, cardiovascular, and intensive care support 24/7 (ICU/CCU/NICU)
Level 2	ROSC with restoration of consciousness; Persistent hemodynamic instability ± acute coronary syndrome; ± recurrent arrhythmias	Nearest facility capable of providing high level cardiovascular and intensive care support 24/7; cardiac catheterization laboratory capable of providing PCI within 90 minutes
Level 3	ROSC with restoration of consciousness; hemodynamically stable. Evidence of acute coronary syndrome; ± recurrent arrhythmias	Nearest facility with cardiac catheterization laboratory capable of providing PCI within 90 minutes - 24/7
Level 4	ROSC with restoration of consciousness; hemodynamically stable; no evidence of acute coronary syndrome ± recurrent arrhythmias	Nearest facility capable of providing standard ED, ICU/CCU; cardiac catheterization desirable with PCI capability within 24 hours

FIGURE 70.13 A four-tiered EMS bypass model aligning immediate postcardiac arrest status and level of required care is illustrated to reflect a priority-based hospital bypass system. The Copenhagen model provides a foundation for this additional level of coordination. Patients can be transported to the closest facility appropriate to the optimal or minimal care requirements. *CCU,* coronary care unit; *ED,* emergency department; *ICU,* intensive care unit; *NICU,* neurologic intensive care unit; *PCI,* percutaneous coronary intervention; *ROSC,* return of spontaneous circulation. (Modified from Myerburg RJ: Initiatives for improving out-of-hospital cardiac arrest outcomes. Circulation 2014;30:1840-1843.)

symptomatic bradyarrhythmias requiring permanent pacemakers rarely occur in such patients. In contrast, bradyarrhythmic cardiac arrest associated with large *anterior* wall infarctions (and AV or intraventricular block) has a poor prognosis.

Cardiac Arrest in Patients with Hemodynamically Unstable Acute Myocardial Infarction

Cardiac arrest occurring in association with, or as a result of, hemodynamic or mechanical dysfunction during the acute phase of MI has an immediate mortality rate ranging from 59% to 89%, depending on the severity of the hemodynamic abnormalities and size of the MI. Resuscitative efforts commonly fail in such patients, and when they are successful, postcardiac arrest management is often difficult. When secondary cardiac arrest occurs by the mechanisms of VT or VF in this setting, aggressive postresuscitation hemodynamic or anti-ischemic measures may help achieve rhythm stability. Intravenous amiodarone has emerged as the antiarrhythmic therapy of choice. Lidocaine may also be tried if the mechanism appears to be ischemic but is less likely to be successful in this setting than in primary VF. The success of interventions and prevention of recurrent cardiac arrest are closely related to the success in managing the patient's hemodynamic status. The proportion of cardiac arrests caused by bradyarrhythmias or asystole or by PEA is higher in hemodynamically unstable patients with AMI. Such patients usually have large MIs and major hemodynamic abnormalities and may be acidotic and hypoxemic. Even with aggressive therapy, the prognosis after asystolic arrest in such patients is poor, and they are resuscitated only rarely from PEA.

> **Cardiac Arrest Among In-Hospital Patients With Noncardiac Abnormalities.** These patients fall into two major categories: (1) those with life-limiting diseases, such as malignant neoplasms, sepsis, organ failure, end-stage pulmonary disease, and advanced CNS disease, and (2) those with acute toxic or proarrhythmic states that are potentially reversible. In the former category, the ratio of tachyarrhythmic to bradyarrhythmic cardiac arrest is low, and the prognosis for survival of cardiac arrest is poor. Although the data may be somewhat skewed by the practice of assigning "do-not-resuscitate" orders to patients with end-stage disease, the data available for attempted resuscitations show poor outcomes. For the few successfully resuscitated patients in these categories, postarrest management is dictated by the underlying precipitating factors.

Risk Identification by QT Interval Prolongation after Cardiac Arrest

The initial management of survivors of OHCA centers on stabilizing cardiac electrical status, supporting hemodynamics, and providing supportive care for reversal of any organ damage that has occurred as a consequence of the cardiac arrest. The in-hospital risk for recurrent cardiac arrest is relatively low, and arrhythmias account for only 10% of in-hospital deaths after successful out-of-hospital resuscitation. However, the mortality rate during the index hospitalization is 50%, thus indicating that nonarrhythmic mortality dominates the mechanisms of early postresuscitation deaths (30% hemodynamic, 60% CNS related). Antiarrhythmic therapy, usually intravenous amiodarone, is used in an attempt to prevent recurrent cardiac arrest in patients who demonstrate recurrent arrhythmia during the first 48 hours of postarrest hospitalization. Patients who have preexisting or new AV or intraventricular conduction disturbances are at particularly high risk for recurrent cardiac arrest. The routine use of temporary pacemakers has been evaluated in such patients but has not been found to be helpful for prevention of early recurrent cardiac arrest. Invasive techniques for hemodynamic monitoring are used in patients whose condition is unstable but are not used routinely in those whose condition is stable on admission.

Anoxic encephalopathy is a strong predictor of in-hospital death or death within 6 months postdischarge. The induction of therapeutic hypothermia to reduce metabolic demands and cerebral edema should be applied promptly to a postarrest survivor who remains unconscious on hospital admission. A randomized study of prehospital intravenous hypothermia demonstrated a small reduction in ROSC

and no benefit for survival to hospital discharge.[150] The initial temperature target was 32 to 34°C, but subsequent data suggest that a target of 36°C is equally effective and easier to achieve.

During the later convalescent period, continued attention to CNS status, including physical rehabilitation, is of primary importance for an optimal outcome. Respiratory support by conventional methods is used as necessary. Management of other organ system injury (e.g., renal, hepatic), as well as early recognition and treatment of infectious complications, also contributes to ultimate survival.

Long-Term Management of Survivors of Out-of-Hospital Cardiac Arrest

When a survivor of out-of-hospital cardiac arrest has awakened and achieved electrical and hemodynamic stability, usually within a few days if it is to occur at all, decisions must be made about the nature and extent of the workup required to establish a long-term management strategy. The goals of the workup are to identify the specific causative and triggering factors of the cardiac arrest, to clarify the functional status of the patient's cardiovascular system, and to establish long-term therapeutic strategies. Patients who have limited return of CNS function usually do not undergo extensive workups, and patients whose cardiac arrests were triggered by an acute transmural AMI have workups similar to those for other patients with AMI (see Chapter 38).

Survivors of OHCA not associated with AMI who have good return of neurologic function appear to have a long-term survival probability commensurate with their age, sex, and extent of disease when they are treated according to existing guidelines.[151] These patients should undergo diagnostic workups to define the cause of the cardiac arrest and to tailor long-term therapy, the latter targeted to the underlying disease and strategies for prevention of recurrent cardiac arrest or SCD. The workup includes cardiac catheterization with coronary angiography if coronary atherosclerosis is known or considered to be the possible cause of the event, evaluation of the functional significance of coronary lesions by stress imaging techniques if indicated, determination of functional and hemodynamic status, and assessment of whether the life-threatening arrhythmic event was caused by a transient risk associated with AMI or there is persisting risk based on clinical characteristics.

General Care

The general management of survivors of cardiac arrest is determined by the specific cause and the underlying pathophysiologic process. For patients with ischemic heart disease, interventions to prevent myocardial ischemia, optimization of therapy for LV function, and attention to general medical status are all addressed. Although limited data suggest that revascularization procedures may improve the recurrence rate and total mortality rates after survival from OHCA, no properly controlled prospective studies have validated this impression for bypass surgery or percutaneous interventions. The indications for revascularization after cardiac arrest are limited to those who have a generally accepted indication for angioplasty or surgery, including a documented ischemic mechanism of the cardiac arrest.

Although no data from placebo-controlled trials are available to define a benefit of various anti-ischemic strategies (including beta blockers or other medical anti-ischemic therapy) for long-term management after OHCA, medical, catheter interventional, or surgical anti-ischemic therapy, rather than antiarrhythmic drug therapy, is generally considered the primary approach to long-term management of the subgroup of prehospital cardiac arrest survivors in whom transient myocardial ischemia was the inciting factor. Moreover, in an uncontrolled observation comparing cardiac arrest survivors who had ever received beta blockers after the index event with those who had not, a significant improvement in long-term outcome with beta blocker therapy was noted. Further evaluation of the specific role of revascularization procedures and anti-ischemic medical therapy after OHCA is needed.

Whether the various pharmacologic strategies (e.g., angiotensin-converting enzyme inhibitors, carvedilol and other beta-adrenergic blocking agents, and spironolactone) that have been shown to provide a clinical and mortality benefit in patients with LV dysfunction provide a specific SCD benefit separate from a total mortality benefit remains uncertain.

PREVENTION OF CARDIAC ARREST AND SUDDEN CARDIAC DEATH

Prevention of SCA can be classified into five clinical subgroup categories: (1) prevention of recurrent events in survivors of cardiac arrest (secondary prevention) (see Table 69.3); (2) prevention of an initial event in patients at high risk because of advanced heart disease, such as those with low ejection fractions and other markers of risk (primary prevention) (see Table 69.4); (3) primary prevention in patients with less advanced common or uncommon structural heart diseases; (4) primary prevention in patients with structurally normal hearts, subtle or minor structural abnormalities, or genetically based molecular disorders (Table 70.5); and (5) primary prevention in the general population. The last category includes the substantial proportion of SCDs that occur as a first cardiac event in victims previously free of known disease. While all-encompassing preventive strategies have been difficult to establish, the potential public health impact of prevention in the context of limited postcardiac arrest survival suggests that this needs to be incorporated into the global strategy for prevention of SCD (Fig. 70.14).

Four general antiarrhythmic strategies, which are not mutually exclusive, can be contemplated for patients at high risk for cardiac arrest: implantable defibrillators, antiarrhythmic drugs, catheter ablation, and antiarrhythmic surgery. While the mainstay of therapy for the highest risk patients is the implantable defibrillator, there are a variety of nontraditional antiarrhythmic medications that have shown survival benefit. These include beta blockers, angiotensin-converting enzyme (ACE) inhibitors, angiotensin receptor blockers, aldosterone receptor antagonists, combined angiotensin-neprilysin inhibitors, statins, polyunsaturated fatty acids, and SGLT2 inhibitors, among others.[152] The role of antiarrhythmic drug therapy (class I and class III) for secondary prevention of subsequent SCD, as opposed to adjunctive therapy, has not been established, though there is some supportive evidence for the use of amiodarone.[153]

The choice of a therapy, or combinations of therapies, is based on estimation of risk determined by evaluation of the individual patient by various risk-profiling techniques, coupled with available efficacy and safety data.

Methods to Estimate Risk for Sudden Cardiac Death
General Medical and Cardiovascular Risk Markers
The presence and severity of acquired medical disorders (such as coronary atherosclerosis and associated myocardial ischemia or magnetic resonance imaging–defined scar patterns, LV dysfunction and ventricular volume, and heart failure) and general medical conditions (such as hypertension, diabetes, dyslipidemias, chronic renal failure, and cigarette smoking) are integral to estimation of risk for SCD. Although lacking the specificity of individual SCD risk prediction, they provide general indicators of risk and data supporting the benefit of therapies, such as beta blockers, ACE inhibitors and receptor blockers, and statins, in appropriate subgroups of patients. In several recent reports, a series of easily identified markers was used to generate a risk score for SCD among subjects in two long-term population studies

TABLE 70.5 Selected Indications for Implantable Cardioverter-Defibrillators in Genetic Disorders Associated with Risk for Sudden Cardiac Death (Refer to Most Recent Guidelines)

DIAGNOSIS	ICD INDICATION	PRIMARY SOURCE OF DATA	RISK INDICATORS	GUIDELINES CLASSIFICATION	EVIDENCE
HCM	Secondary SCA protection	Registries, cohorts	Previous SCA, sustained VT	Class I	Level B
	Primary SCA protection	Registries, cohorts	For adults ≥1 major risk factor: family history of SCD, Left ventricular thickness ≥30 mm, syncope suspected to be arrhythmic, apical aneurysm, ejection fraction <50%	Class IIa	Level B
ARVD/RVCM	Secondary SCA protection	Registry, case series	Previous SCA, hemodynamically unstable sustained VT	Class I	Level B
			Hemodynamically stable sustained VT	Class IIa	Level B
			Unexplained syncope	Class IIa	Level B
	Primary SCA protection	Registry, case series	Three major, two major and two minor, or one major and four minor risk factors for ventricular arrhythmia*	Class IIa	Level B
				Class IIb	Level B
			Two major, one major and two minor, or four minor risk factors for ventricular arrhythmia*		
Congenital LQT	Secondary SCA protection	Registry, cohorts	Previous SCA	Class I	Level B
	Primary SCA protection	Registry, cohorts	Beta blocker ineffective/not tolerated (intensification is recommended—ICD is an option)	Class 1	Level B
				Class IIb	Level B
			QTc >500 msec on beta blocker (intensification may be considered—ICD is an option)		
Brugada syndrome	Secondary SCA protection	Case cohorts	SCA, sustained VT, recent syncope suspected to be arrhythmic	Class I	Level B
	Primary SCA protection	Case cohorts	Positive electrophysiology study (1-2 extra stimuli)	Class IIb	Level B
CPVT/F	Secondary SCA protection	Small case series	Previous SCA	Class I	Level B
	Primary SCA protection	Small case series	Syncope or VT while taking beta blockers, family history of premature SCA (?)	Class I	Level B

ARVD/RVCM, Arrhythmogenic right ventricular dysplasia/cardiomyopathy; *CPVT/F*, catecholaminergic polymorphic ventricular tachycardia/"idiopathic" ventricular fibrillation; *HCM*, hypertrophic cardiomyopathy; *LQT*, long-QT syndrome; *N-S*, nonsustained; *PVT*, polymorphic ventricular tachycardia; *SQT*, short-QT syndrome; *VA*, ventricular arrhythmia; *(?)*, uncertain.
*Major criteria: nonsustained ventricular tachycardia (NSVT), inducible VT, LVEF ≤49%. Minor criteria: male sex, >1000 premature ventricular complexes (PVCs)/24 hours, RV dysfunction, proband status, two or more desmosomal variants. If both NSVT and PVC criteria are present, then only NSVT can be used.

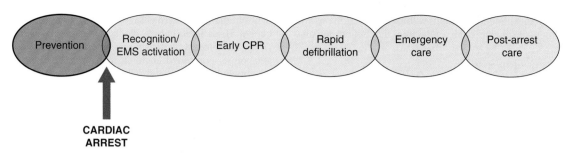

FIGURE 70.14 Prevention of cardiac arrest is an important element of addressing the public health burden of sudden cardiac death. On a case-by-case basis, prevention may be even more effective to improve survival than the well described import and impact of the postcardiac arrest chain of survival. *CPR,* Cardiopulmonary resuscitation; *EMS,* emergency medical services. (From Mitrani RD, Goldberger JJ. Cardiac arrests during the COVID-19 pandemic: the perfect storm. JACC: Clinical Electrophysiology 2021;7:12-15.)

without a history of cardiovascular disease.[16,17] Bogle et al. used only clinical information that is widely available in the electronic health record including age, sex, cholesterol, blood pressure, lipid and blood pressure medication use, diabetes, current smoking, and body mass index. The model demonstrated large, nonlinear, gradients of risk, with the major impact in the highest 1 to 2 deciles. The score yielded very good internal discrimination and very good external discrimination among Framingham participants. This type of model moves in the right direction for individual risk prediction, but it is limited by its effect sizes—approximately a 4% SCD risk over 10 years in the highest decile. This magnitude of risk is not sufficient to justify certain interventions and further risk stratification will be needed to identify even higher risk subgroups at sufficient risk to merit advanced therapies.

In patients with known or suspected coronary heart disease or nonischemic cardiomyopathy, other noninvasive markers of risk are being employed and/or explored, including ejection fraction and measures reflecting autonomic function, depolarization and repolarization abnormalities, and genetic influences on risk for SCD (see Risk Factors for Sudden Cardiac Death). While ejection fraction is the most widely studied and most widely used clinical measure to assess risk for SCD, it is now well appreciated that it lacks sensitivity and specificity. Electrocardiographic based tests for abnormal depolarization and repolarization have enjoyed tremendous enthusiasm and have been evaluated extensively. Abnormal depolarization provides information about conduction; areas of slow or delayed conduction are critical for reentrant tachyarrhythmias. While evaluations of QRS duration, late potentials on signal averaged electrocardiography, and fragmented QRS all show prognostic value, the individual predictive value is not high enough to be used clinically and these are not incorporated in the guidelines. Similarly, abnormal repolarization indices may indicate heterogeneities in repolarization and/or refractoriness that may also be a key requirement for the pathogenesis of reentrant tachyarrhythmias. While evaluations of QT interval duration, QT dispersion, QT alternans, and QT variability, among others, all show prognostic value, the individual predictive value is not high enough to be used clinically and these are not incorporated in the guidelines. Recent data suggest that scores composed of combinations of novel and/or standard ECG markers might add to SCD risk prediction in the general population and in patients with established coronary heart disease.

The role of the autonomic nervous system in the pathogenesis of ventricular tachyarrhythmias and SCD is well appreciated. ECG-based analyses of heart rate variability—time domain, frequency domain, and nonlinear techniques—and heart rate changes with exercise provide prognostic information, but the individual predictive value is not high enough to be used clinically. The only testing/findings currently included in the guidelines[151] are low ejection fraction, nonsustained VT, inducible ventricular tachycardia, and MRI findings of scar (discussed below). It should be noted that although several clinical trials incorporating the ECG-based markers have been negative, dampening enthusiasm for the clinical use of these techniques, these trials also typically incorporated a low ejection fraction which remains a clinically used technique. It may be that risk stratification strategies can be applied that utilize these methods in a strategic fashion.[154]

The potential importance of proper timing for evaluation of risk markers has been explored. There is a well-known time-dependence to risk of SCD following MI.[155] Overlaid on this is a changing proportion of presumed arrhythmic and mechanical causes for SCD, as noted in the VALIANT study.[4] It is therefore not surprising that there is time-dependence to risk stratification. The REFINE study suggested greater risk predictive power for post-MI adverse events when markers were evaluated after 8 weeks versus closer to the index event. Another study of a cohort of 231 patients with acute MI and an initial EF ≤35% reported that the distribution of EFs on echocardiograms at 90 days of follow-up remained at 35% or less in 43%, increased to 36% to 49% in 31%, and increased to 50% or more in 26%.[156] How this impacts future SCD risk remains to be determined.

Ambulatory Monitoring. Although ambulatory monitoring is not routinely recommended as a screening tool, it is used for profiling the risk for development of life-threatening sustained arrhythmias in individuals with certain forms of structural or electrophysiologic disease who are considered to be at high risk (Chapter 61). Notably, nonsustained VT is an actionable finding in certain conditions such as HCM[42,151] and ischemic cardiomyopathy with LV ejection fraction ≤40%.[151] Technologic advances making very long-term monitoring easier allows identification of episodic arrhythmias as causes of relevant symptoms, such as near-syncope and syncope. In addition to the common disorders associated with SCA, loop recorders may be useful for selected individuals with disorders such as HCM, long-QT syndrome, and right ventricular dysplasia and in patients with dilated cardiomyopathy or heart failure.

Programmed Electrical Stimulation for Risk Profiling. Despite a large, albeit somewhat conflicting data base on the role of electrophysiologic testing for risk profiling,[157] particularly in patients with advanced heart disease, its use is currently more limited than in the past. In primary prevention trials such as MADIT and MUSTT, programmed electrical stimulation studies were used to profile risk and suggested large benefits. MADIT II, subsequently enrolled patients with lower ejection fractions than did MADIT or MUSTT and did not use programmed stimulation or other arrhythmia markers; this study demonstrated a survival benefit of ICD therapy without the need for incorporating results of electrophysiologic testing in the treatment decision. This led to a dramatic decline in its use. Nevertheless, based on the criteria in MUSTT, it is currently included in the guidelines.[151] It is the most direct test to evaluate for the presence of substrate for monomorphic VT, but its utility to predict VF is more limited. The question of whether electrophysiologic testing is generally useful has yet to be fully resolved, although it appears to have a role in selected patients and clinical circumstances. Of interest, a follow-up study of patients in MADIT II suggested inducibility was associated with a higher incidence of VT and noninducibility was associated with a higher incidence of VF. The utility of programmed ventricular stimulation to assess for inducible VT was shown in the PRESERVE EF study.[154] In post-MI patients with LV ejection fraction ≥40%, programmed ventricular stimulation was performed if one noninvasive risk factor derived from the signal-averaged ECG and ambulatory 24-hour monitoring was positive. Patients with a positive noninvasive risk factor and inducible VT comprised approximately 7% of the population and experienced approximately an 8% annual rate of major arrhythmic events. The Programmed Ventricular Stimulation to Risk Stratify for Early Cardioverter-Defibrillator Implantation to Prevent Tachyarrhythmias following Acute Myocardial Infarction (PROTECT-ICD) is testing whether programmed ventricular stimulation in patients with LV ejection fraction ≤40% 2 to 40 days after AMI can identify patients who benefit from an ICD.[158] Finally, in patients with nonischemic dilated cardiomyopathy, the accumulated evidence is that programmed ventricular stimulation does provide moderate risk stratification with an approximate doubling of relative risk for those with inducible ventricular tachyarrhythmias.

The secondary prevention trials of cardiac arrest survivors did not seek to determine whether routine electrophysiologic testing offered predictive value. It is not a necessary component of the evaluation unless there is no structural heart disease or a suspicion for a supraventricular tachycardia as the initiating rhythm for cardiac arrest. In the latter patients, treatment targeting the supraventricular tachycardia should be pursued rather than ICD therapy. For the evaluation of precipitating ventricular arrhythmias, most previous studies had demonstrated limitations because of the relatively small fraction of cardiac arrest survivors (an average of less than 50% on the basis of multiple studies) who had inducible ventricular arrhythmias. Under conditions in which a potentially reversible trigger for cardiac arrest can be identified and perhaps in some cardiac arrest survivors in whom transient ischemia was the initiating mechanism and the ejection fraction is normal or near-normal, there might be a persistent limited role for electrophysiologic testing as a guide to therapy.

Cardiac MRI. Cardiac MRI has the ability to define reactive/interstitial fibrosis and replacement fibrosis with T1 mapping/extracellular volume fraction and delayed enhancement.[40] Many studies have related the findings of dense scar and "border zone" to arrhythmic outcomes in patients with ischemic heart disease. The rationale is that the infarct topology and/or size provides the anatomic platform or substrate for reentrant ventricular tachyarrhythmias. While infarct size is correlated with LV ejection fraction, the strength of the correlation is not high . The accumulated evidence over many studies is that late gadolinium enhancement is a strong predictor of arrhythmic events. In a meta-analysis,[50] the hazard ratio for ventricular arrhythmias and SCD associated with late gadolinium enhancement in ischemic cardiomyopathy was 3.87 and in nonischemic cardiomyopathy was 4.32. Importantly, LV ejection fraction above or below 35% did not significantly modulate this risk (hazard ratio 3.72 and 3.53, respectively). The CMR-Guide study is currently under way to assess whether late gadolinium enhancement in patients with ischemic or nonischemic cardiomyopathies with LV ejection fractions between 36% and 50% can be used to stratify arrhythmic risk and demonstrate utility of an ICD.[159]

The utility of substrate delineation in nonischemic and HCM has also been demonstrated. In a study of 339 patients with nonischemic dilated cardiomyopathy and ejection fraction ≥40% followed for a median of 4.6 years, 18% of those with late gadolinium enhancement experienced SCD or aborted SCD compared with 2% without late gadolinium enhancement.[51] After adjusting for age, New York Heart Association class, and ejection fraction, the hazard ratio was 9.2. The cumulative data from many studies is strongly supportive of the role of late gadolinium enhancement in nonischemic, dilated cardiomyopathy, even among those with better ejection fractions (e.g., between 35%-43%).[160] Annual rates for arrhythmic events for those with late gadolinium enhancement was over 6% regardless of ejection fraction and below 2% for those without late gadolinium enhancement. Newer methods for analysis of the substrate—for example the area of interface between scar and surviving myocardium—may also provide more direct pathophysiologic correlation to ventricular tachyarrhythmias.[161] Observational studies also support the value of late gadolinium enhancement in patients with HCM.[162] In a meta-analysis including almost 3000 patients, late gadolinium enhancement was associated with an odds ratio (OR) of 3.41 for SCD.[163] The extent of late gadolinium enhancement was also an important predictor. The guidelines currently do include the use of MRI in patients with nonischemic dilated cardiomyopathy and HCM for assessment of SCD risk but do not provide a recommendation on how to specifically use this information.

Novel Proteomic and Genomic Markers of Risk for Sudden Cardiac Death. Biomarkers released in the setting of inflammation, myocardial stretch, ischemia, hyperglycemia, and renal dysfunction have been associated with SCD in the general population as well as in selected subsets of high-risk patients with heart failure or coronary heart disease.[164] Several of these biologic markers have also been documented to be associated with ICD therapies for ventricular arrhythmias. Individual associations tend to be modest; and thus, biomarkers have yet to be used clinically for SCD risk prediction. However, elevations in these biomarkers may be useful for identifying individuals with undiagnosed coronary or structural heart disease and prompting further diagnostic evaluation and initiation of standard preventive therapies, which would be expected to impact SCD risk. Recent data suggest that individuals with high levels of several of these markers (TC:HDL, hsTnI, NT-proBNP, and hsCRP) in combination are at marked increased risk (HR = 6.9); however, the number of individuals at such high risk is quite small.[165] In addition to standard cardiac and renal biomarkers, levels of very long chain n-3 fatty acid, eicosapentaenoic acid (EPA) and docosahexaenoic acid (DHA), have also been associated with elevated risks of SCD. In four studies within the general population, levels of EPA and DHA have been associated with markedly lower risks of SCD (risk reduction [RR]

= 0.20 to 0.50 for those in the highest versus lowest quartile/tertile).[166] Relationships with SCD appear to be stronger than those observed for other forms of cardiac death, and thus these fatty acids may be able to discriminate risk for SCD from that for other cardiovascular causes.

The genetic basis of SCD in the general population is poorly understood. Several studies have demonstrated a familial predisposition to SCD.[8,167] Three case-control studies demonstrate that a history of SCD among a first-degree relative is an independent risk factor for VF or SCD (e.g., reference[168]) in the setting of acute MI. Two large-scale genome-wide association studies[33,34] and several single candidate gene studies have identified several potential genetic variants associated with SCD risk,[35-42] but these results have not been replicated in larger studies.[169] Data are beginning to accumulate in support of utilizing combinations of genetic variants in the form of genetic risk scores (GRS) to advance SCD risk prediction in the general population[170] and in patients with coronary heart disease (CHD).[171] A GRS composed of 153 genetic variants associated with CHD at genome-wide significance was found to associate with SCD in the setting of CHD in three separate cohorts (OR 1.045 per SD of CHD risk score, $P = 1.7 \times 10^{-7}$] and to predict the occurrence of SCD in patients undergoing stress test, with an improvement in the net reclassification index (NRI) over standard risk factors.[171] In the largest genome-wide association study of SCD published to date, GRS for CHD, BMI, and QT interval were all associated with SCD, suggesting that these risk factors are causally associated with SCD.[169] Despite these promising data, the current role for genetic testing for SCD risk stratification is confined to select patients and families with suspected inherited arrhythmias such as LQTS, Brugada, and CPVT, and cardiomyopathies, such as ARVC, HCM, and DCM.

Strategies to Reduce Risk for Sudden Cardiac Death

Antiarrhythmic Drugs

Historically, the earliest approach to management of risk for out-of-hospital cardiac arrest and VT with hemodynamic compromise was the use of membrane-active antiarrhythmic agents. This approach was based initially on the assumption that a high frequency of ambient ventricular arrhythmias constituted a triggering mechanism for potentially lethal arrhythmias and that their suppression by antiarrhythmic drugs was protective. It was also assumed that electrophysiologic instability of the myocardium, likely associated with regional disease associated changes in refractory periods and conduction velocities, predisposed to potentially lethal arrhythmias and could be positively modified by these drugs. Suppression of inducibility of VT or VF during programmed electrical stimulation studies likely reflected this effect as well and had been a widespread strategy, particularly before the advent of the ICD. Suppression of ambient arrhythmias was demonstrated by the empiric use of amiodarone, beta-adrenergic–blocking agents, or membrane-active antiarrhythmic drugs, but scientifically valid demonstration of a survival benefit was lacking. The discrepancy between ambient arrhythmia suppression and survival benefit was clarified by the results of CAST, which showed that certain class I antiarrhythmic drugs increased mortality despite suppression of ambient ventricular ectopy. In contrast, beta blocker therapy might have some benefit in such patients, and amiodarone might also be effective for some patients, although it did not perform better than the control group in the heart failure patients studied in SCD-HeFT (Sudden Cardiac Death–Heart Failure Trial). A subgroup analysis of patients in AVID suggested that cardiac arrest survivors with EF >35% had identical outcomes with ICDs and amiodarone, but there was no untreated control group to determine both were beneficial versus ineffective. In summary, ambient arrhythmia suppression and empiric antiarrhythmic drug therapy enjoyed a short period of popularity as a strategy for reduction of risk in VT/VF survivors and in high-risk primary prevention candidates, but in time were shown to be ineffective for this purpose.

Surgical Intervention Strategies

Coronary artery bypass surgery can be an effective approach for prevention of SCD in patients with clear acute ischemia induced SCD due to critical coronary artery disease, but for most patients this is not effective as an isolated strategy. The previously popular antiarrhythmic surgical techniques now have limited applications. Intraoperative map-guided cryoablation may be used for patients who have inducible, hemodynamically stable, sustained monomorphic VT during electrophysiologic testing and ventricular and coronary artery anatomy amenable to catheter ablation. However, it has little applicability to survivors of OHCA because the type of arrhythmia favoring this surgical approach is infrequently observed in cardiac arrest survivors. It can be used as adjunctive therapy for ICD recipients whose arrhythmia burden requires frequent shocks.

Catheter Ablation Therapy

The use of catheter ablation techniques to prevent ventricular tachyarrhythmias has been most successful for benign focal tachycardias that may originate from preferential locations in the right or left ventricle (see Chapter 67) and for some reentrant VTs. With rare exceptions, catheter ablation techniques are not used for the treatment of higher risk ventricular tachyarrhythmias or for definitive therapy in patients at risk for progression of the arrhythmic substrate. For VT caused by bundle branch reentrant mechanisms, which occur in cardiomyopathies, as well as in other structural cardiac disorders, ablation of the right bundle branch to interrupt the reentrant cycle has been successful. However, this has limited applicability to the large number of patients with structural heart disease who are at risk for SCD or those who have survived a cardiac arrest. Nonetheless, catheter ablation is an appropriate adjunctive treatment strategy for patients with ICDs who are having multiple tachyarrhythmic events. Catheter-based substrate modification/ablation has been demonstrated to be useful in ICD recipients receiving multiple therapies and performed somewhat better than escalation of antiarrhythmic therapy.[172] Presently, this benefit is limited to reducing the number of patients receiving ICD therapies; further studies are needed to determine whether it has an expanded role for survival. Catheter ablation may have a role in prevention of cardiac arrest in patients with consistent premature ventricular beats that trigger VF, such as may be seen in a wide variety of conditions including idiopathic VF, acute ischemia, and Brugada syndrome. The Purkinje system is frequently a triggering source.[173-175]

Implantable Cardioverter Defibrillators

Development of the implantable cardioverter defibrillator (ICD) added a new dimension to the management of patients at high risk for cardiac arrest (see Chapter 69). After the initial reports of small case series of very high-risk patients in the early 1980s, a number of observational studies confirmed that ICDs can achieve rates of sudden death consistently

less than 5% at 1 year and total death rates in the 10% to 20% range in populations at high risk for mortality, as predicted by mortality surrogates such as historical controls or time to the first delivered appropriate therapy. However, determination of the survival benefit of ICDs remained uncertain and was debated. More than 16 years elapsed between the first clinical use of an implanted defibrillator and publication of the first major randomized clinical trial comparing implantable defibrillator therapy with antiarrhythmic drug therapy. During that period, reports had documented the ability of ICDs to revert potentially fatal arrhythmias but could not identify a valid relative or absolute mortality benefit because of confounding factors, such as competing risks for sudden and nonsudden death and determination of whether appropriate shocks represented the interruption of an event that would have been fatal.

MADIT provided the first randomized trial data on the relative benefit of defibrillators over antiarrhythmic drug therapy (largely amiodarone) for primary prevention of SCD in a high-risk population. The outcome demonstrated a 59% reduction in the relative risk for total mortality at 2 years of follow-up (54% cumulative) and a 19% reduction in the absolute risk of dying at 2 years of follow-up. It was followed over a period of less than 10 years by a series of randomized trial reports evaluating ICD therapy for primary and secondary prevention of SCD in patients with previous MI, previous cardiac arrests, and heart failure.

Although these studies documented the ability of ICDs to revert potentially fatal arrhythmias and showed a relative benefit over amiodarone in some groups of patients, the absence of placebo-controlled trials still prevents quantitation of the true magnitude of any mortality benefit because of the inability of positive-controlled trials to identify the absolute benefit of an intervention. Despite these limitations, an ICD is now the preferred therapy for survivors of cardiac arrest at risk for recurrences and for primary prevention in patients in a number of high-risk categories.

Application of Therapeutic Strategies to Specific Groups of Patients
Secondary Prevention of Sudden Cardiac Death after Survival from Cardiac Arrest

As populations of OHCA survivors began to accumulate from community-based EMS activities, the development of therapeutic strategies intended to improve long-term survival emerged as a mandate for clinical investigators. This mandate is complicated by the inability to do randomized controlled trials and the confounding influence of specific cardiovascular therapies that may also improve survival. Early approaches to long-term therapy centered on the use of antiarrhythmic drugs, largely guided by the results of electrophysiologic testing or the empiric use of antiarrhythmic drugs, particularly amiodarone. Various observational and positive-controlled studies had suggested that suppression of inducible ventricular arrhythmias yielded a better outcome than did failure of suppression and that amiodarone was better than class I antiarrhythmic drugs. This approach is no longer widely used. The first adequately powered secondary prevention trial of ICDs versus antiarrhythmic drugs was published in 1997.[176] This study, the AVID Trial, demonstrated a 27% reduction in the relative risk for total mortality at 2 years of follow-up, with an absolute risk reduction of 7% (Fig. 70.15). It was followed shortly thereafter by reports of two other studies, CIDS (Canadian Implantable Defibrillator Study) and CASH (Cardiac Arrest Study Hamburg), both limited by their enrollment numbers but suggesting trends toward similar benefits (see Table 69.3). A meta-analysis of these data confirmed the benefit of ICDs for secondary prevention,

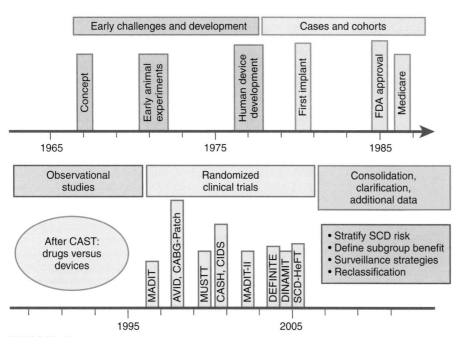

FIGURE 70.15 The concept of an ICD originated in the late 1960s, and development of the technology and proof of concept leading to the first clinical implant extended to 1980. From 1980 until late 1996, data supporting the benefit of ICDs were largely observational or based on small high-risk cohorts or case-control studies. All the major trials for both primary and secondary indications were published during an interval of 10 years between late 1996 and early 2005. Additional studies since then have aided in interpretation of the outcomes from the clinical trials, but there remains a need for consolidation and clarification and for additional data to better define the efficiency of therapy and targeted selection of individual candidates who have a high likelihood of benefit. (Modified from Myerburg RJ, et al. Indications for implantable cardioverter-defibrillators based on evidence and judgment. J Am Clin Cardiol 2009;54:747.)

although only AVID demonstrated a statistically significant survival benefit of an ICD over antiarrhythmic therapy, usually amiodarone. A retrospective subgroup analysis of AVID has also suggested that ICDs had no advantage over antiarrhythmic drugs for VT/VF survivors with ejection fractions >35%. Currently, despite these limitations, ICDs have emerged as the preferred therapy for survivors of OHCA or hemodynamically significant VT, regardless of the ejection fraction, in the absence of identifiable and correctable transient causes of cardiac arrest. The National Cardiovascular Data Registry (NCDR) ICD Registry provides a contemporary report on the outcomes of patients treated with ICD for secondary prevention of SCD.[177] Among 36,434 patients (mean age 65 years, ejection fraction 36%) who received a secondary prevention ICD, 65% for cardiac arrest, the 1- and 2-year mortalities were 10.9% and 16.5%, reflecting better overall survival than the antiarrhythmic drug therapy group in AVID, though this observation should be tempered by many factors including the dramatic change in medical and interventional therapies that have ensued between these reports.

Primary Prevention of Sudden Cardiac Death in Patients with Advanced Heart Disease

After the disturbing outcome of CAST and suggestions of a lack of efficacy or adverse effects of the class I antiarrhythmic drugs in general when used for primary or secondary prevention of SCD, interest shifted to the use of amiodarone and the ICD. Two major trials of amiodarone in post-MI patients, EMIAT and CAMIAT, one of which required ejection fractions lower than 40%, demonstrated no total mortality benefit, even though both trials demonstrated antiarrhythmic benefit, expressed as a reduction in arrhythmic deaths or resuscitated VF. Subgroup analyses have suggested that the concomitant use of beta blockers does confer a mortality benefit.

In parallel with the amiodarone trials, the first randomized controlled trial comparing antiarrhythmic therapy (primarily amiodarone) with ICD therapy (MADIT) was carried out (see Table 69.4). The randomly assigned patients had ejection fractions lower than 35%, nonsustained VT during ambulatory recording, and inducible VT that was not suppressible by procainamide. This very high-risk group demonstrated a 54% reduction in total mortality with ICD therapy versus drug therapy. At the same time, a trial comparing ICD implantation with no specific therapies for arrhythmias in patients with ejection fractions lower than 36% who were undergoing coronary bypass surgery (CABG Patch trial) demonstrated no benefit of defibrillators on total mortality. The only markers for arrhythmic risk required for entry into the study were a low EF and a positive signal-averaged ECG. A third trial, MUSTT, was a complex study designed to determine whether electrophysiologically guided therapy would lead to an improved outcome in patients with ambient nonsustained VT, inducible VT, history of previous MI, and ejection fraction lower than 40%. The results demonstrated that although a statistically significant beneficial effect on total mortality was achieved by guiding therapy according to the results of electrophysiologic testing, when compared with patients with inducible tachycardia who did not receive therapy, the subgroup of patients who received ICDs because they failed to respond to drug therapy accounted for all the benefit. MADIT II was next among the post-MI primary prevention trials, and demonstrated that ICD therapy provided a mortality benefit over conventional therapy in patients with previous MI and ejection fractions lower than 30%, with a relative risk reduction of 28% and an absolute risk reduction of 6% (22% versus 16%) at 2 years (see Fig. 70.15). During long-term follow-up, a constant annualized risk of approximately 8.5% was estimated in survivors, with the most powerful risk predictors being age greater than 65 years, class III or IV heart failure, diabetes, non–sinus rhythm, and elevated blood urea nitrogen levels.

MADIT and MADIT II had set entry requirements of >3 weeks and >1 month after the qualifying infarction, but the actual enrollment in these studies and MUSTT was considerably longer on average. Because both old and recent data suggested higher risk for SCD early after MIs, DINAMIT (Defibrillator in Acute Myocardial Infarction Trial) was designed to evaluate any possible benefit of ICD implantation early after MI in patients with ejection fractions of 35% or lower and other markers of risk. DINAMIT demonstrated no survival benefit attributable to early

implantation of ICDs in patients randomly assigned at 6 to 40 days after MI (mean, 18 days) despite reduced arrhythmic mortality (see Table 69.4). There was also an unexplained increase in nonarrhythmic mortality over conventional therapy that needs to be explored in future studies. The IRIS (Immediate Risk Stratification Improves Survival) trial also evaluated ICD implantation early after a MI (entry criteria for days from infarct to randomization = 5 to 31; mean to randomization = 13 ± 7 days) in patients with either ejection fractions of 40% or lower and other markers of risk or nonsustained VT. No survival benefit was noted with ICD therapy. These data suggest that either some SCDs in the early post-MI period are due to a nonarrhythmic mechanism or that different risk predictors are required in this setting. Indeed, there are limited data supporting both of these possibilities. The VALIANT investigators evaluated autopsy findings in patients considered to be SCD and identified that approximately half of the SCDs in the early post-MI period were due to mechanical complications, with a large proportion of these being recurrent MI and ruptured ventricular aneurysms. Observational data from Australia support the potential for this approach to identifying risk for SCD in the early postinfarction period, and support the rationale for the ongoing PROTECT-ICD trial.[158] Further efforts to properly address SCD risk prediction in this critical time period are necessary.

The promise of early ICD benefit from the intervention studies cited above were all reported between 1996 and 2005 and had been designed and executed beginning in the early 1990s and extending to 2004. Modern day optimized therapy during and after MI, with "optimized" being defined as revascularization and the use of beta blockers, acetylsalicylic acid, statins, and ACE inhibitors, may beneficially influence risk for SCD during long-term follow-up after the event. Moreover, thrombolytic therapy and percutaneous coronary intervention during AMI and other changes in therapy that have occurred between 1995 and 2010 have improved 30-day mortality.

A 2009 to 2011 randomized trial, MADIT-RIT was designed to evaluate ICD therapy programming strategies on delivered shocks and mortality. Higher detection rates and longer detection times were associated with fewer shocks and improved survival compared with conventional programming. Interestingly, cumulative mortality at 24 months in the conventional programming group was 10% versus 16% in the original MADIT II cohort (1997 to 2001), thus suggesting beneficial influences other than ICDs on outcomes. More recent data also demonstrate dramatically lower rates of appropriate ICD therapy than were noted in the primary prevention randomized clinical trials. In the MADIT-RIT study of patients with reduced ejection fraction (mean 26%) who were all treated with an ICD, the incidence of appropriate ICD therapy in the optimally programmed group was 6% at a mean follow-up of 1.4 years. In the PROSE-ICD registry, there were 143 ICD shocks for adjudicated ventricular arrhythmias among 1177 patients (mean ejection fraction 23%) over a 59-month follow-up period (annualized 2.5%/year). The low rate of appropriate ICD shocks supports reconsideration of deployment strategies for ICDs. While the initial randomized clinical trials were critical in establishing the efficacy of the ICD for primary prevention of SCD, they were certainly not designed to ensure that the utilized strategy was optimal. Indeed, it has been demonstrated that within the currently indicated population for primary prevention ICD, there is likely a low-risk subgroup whose risk is low enough that there is no ICD benefit. Similarly, there is a high risk subgroup in whom the competing risks of death are high enough that there is also no clinical benefit to the ICD.[43,178-180] There is substantial opportunity to optimize data and clinical approaches to primary prevention of SCD.

In patients with nonischemic cardiomyopathy, the data for primary prevention are more variable. The DEFINITE study enrolled patients with a history of heart failure, ejection fractions of 35% or lower, and PVCs or nonsustained VT. The statistical significance for the outcome of survival benefit was not established ($P = 0.08$), but the study may have been underpowered. However, the reported results demonstrated a strong trend toward benefit, with a 35% reduction in relative risk and a 6% reduction in absolute risk during 2 years of follow-up. Subgroups with prolonged QRS durations, ejection fractions higher than 20%, and class III heart failure performed better than did the overall cohort data. SCD-HeFT was designed to test the potential benefit of

ICDs versus amiodarone and placebo in patients with functional class II or III congestive heart failure and ejection fractions lower than 35%. Nonischemic cardiomyopathy and ischemic cardiomyopathy were almost equally represented, with 85% of the patients with ischemic cardiomyopathy having a history of MI. The results of this study demonstrated a 23% reduction in relative risk and a 7% reduction in absolute risk during 5 years (Fig. 70.16). Amiodarone provided no added benefit over conventional therapy. In contrast to DEFINITE, the class II patients in SCD-HeFT had better outcomes than did the class III patients. In the Danish Study to Assess the Efficacy of ICDs in Patients with Non-ischaemic Heart Failure on Mortality (DANISH) trial, patients were randomized to receive an ICD or not.[181] Notably 58% of patients in both groups were treated with cardiac resynchronization therapy. No survival benefit was noted with an ICD. The cumulative data do support the efficacy of the ICD in this patient population.[182] However, demonstration of efficacy is not the same as demonstration that a strategy is optimal or efficient.

Primary Prevention in Patients With Less Advanced Common Heart Diseases or Uncommon Diseases. Primary prevention trials have been designed to enroll populations of patients with advanced heart disease who were estimated to be at very high risk for SCD and total mortality as a consequence of the severity of the underlying disease. Most clinical trials testing the question of the relative efficacy of

antiarrhythmic versus ICD therapy have used the ejection fraction as the marker for advanced disease, with the upper limits of qualifying ejection fractions being between 30% and 40% and the majority set at 35%. The mean or median values of those actually enrolled ranged from 21% to 30%, and subgroups with ejection fractions higher than 30%, particularly those in the range of 35% to 40%, had lower if any benefit.

Although the risk for SCD and total mortality is highest in patients with advanced structural heart disease, characterized by low ejection fractions, impaired functional capacity, or both, a substantial proportion of the total SCD burden occurs in patients with coronary heart disease or the various nonischemic cardiomyopathies with ejection fractions between 35% and 40% and higher.[48] In the Pre-DETERMINE cohort of patients with established coronary artery disease without an indication for ICD, adjudicated sudden or arrhythmic death accounted for 56% of all cardiac deaths, with a 4-year cumulative incidence of 2.1%. Moderately reduced ejection fraction, heart failure severity, and age distinguished sudden arrhythmic death from nonsudden arrhythmic death. Clinical subgroups could be identified with differing profiles of total and proportional risk for sudden arrhythmic death which could be used as a guide for future risk profiling and intervention. In addition, in patients with heart failure related to various forms of cardiomyopathy, even though the total mortality risk is considerably lower in patients with functional class I or early class II than in those with late class III or class IV status, the probability of a death being sudden is higher in the former group. Despite this observation, no data are available to guide therapy for primary prevention of cardiac arrest in such patients. This limitation is confounded by the fact that patients in these categories generally have low event rates but cumulatively account for large numbers of SCD (see Fig. 70.2A and B). In addition, certain other structural entities associated with some elevation in risk for SCD in the absence of a severely reduced ejection fraction, such as some patterns of viral myocarditis, HCM, right ventricular dysplasia, and sarcoidosis, are managed without the benefit of clinical trials to guide therapeutic decisions (see Table 69.4). Patients with symptomatic ventricular arrhythmias related to structural disorders such as right ventricular dysplasia, in which most of the mortality risk is arrhythmic, are often advised to have an ICD, even in the absence of a previous cardiac arrest or hemodynamically significant VT. Whether antiarrhythmic therapy would be just as effective remains unknown, but the judgement of using defibrillators in patients with a disorder whose fatal expression is primarily arrhythmic carries the strength of logic, often supported by risk profiling based on observational data of clinical markers. Among the entities in which the family history is helpful in defining risk, clinical judgment is made easier in patients with a strong family history of SCD. Specific support for this approach is derived from genetic studies of individuals with HCM. In addition, clinical observational data have supported the use of ICDs in high-risk subsets of patients with HCM.

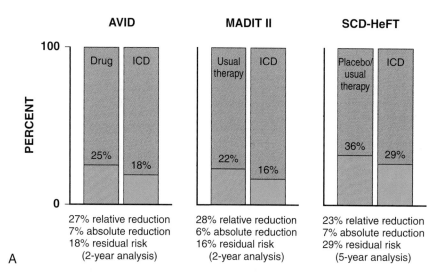

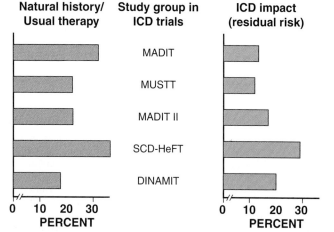

FIGURE 70.16 A, Relative and absolute benefits of ICDs in three ICD trials: a secondary prevention study (AVID) trial, a primary prevention trial (MADIT II), and a heart failure sudden death trial (SCD-HeFT); see text for definitions and trial descriptions. Relative risk reductions indicate proportional differences in outcomes between test and control populations, absolute reductions indicate proportional benefits for individuals, and residual risks indicate mortality remaining after accounting for ICD benefits. **B,** Residual risk after accounting for ICD-associated survival benefit in five major primary prevention ICD clinical trials. (**A** modified from Myerburg RJ, et al. Interpretation of outcomes of antiarrhythmic clinical trials: design features and population impact. Circulation 1998;97:1514.)

Primary Prevention in Patients with Structurally Normal Hearts or Molecular Disorders of Cardiac Electrical Activity

Clinically subtle or unapparent structural disorders and entities with pure electrophysiologic expression, such as the congenital long-QT syndromes, Brugada syndrome, and idiopathic VF, are receiving increasing attention with regard to preventive activities (see Chapter 63).[83] No randomized clinical trials evaluating the utility of ICDs in these patients have been performed, but there is some evidence of efficacy.[183]

The decision-making process for cardiac arrest or symptomatic VT survivors with long-QT syndrome is similar to that for other entities in that those who have survived a potentially fatal arrhythmia are generally treated with ICDs (see Table 70.5). In contrast, individuals who express the electrocardiographic phenotype of long-QT syndrome in the absence of symptomatic arrhythmias are generally treated with beta blocker therapy. Beta blockers are also considered useful for affected family members who have not had an event and for subgroups of long-QT patients with syncope of undocumented mechanism. Between these extremes are asymptomatic affected family members of patients with symptomatic long-QT syndrome. The threshold for consideration of ICD therapy is decreasing, primarily among carriers who breakthrough with symptoms while on beta blocker therapy. Currently, many such clinical therapeutic decisions remain based on judgment rather than driven by data (see Chapter 63). QTc intervals ≥550 msec and syncope while on beta blocker therapy have been shown to be predictors of appropriate ICD shocks.[184]

Among the other molecular arrhythmia syndromes, Brugada syndrome is one for which management strategies remain problematic and debated.[83,86] An ICD is accepted as the secondary prevention strategy in SCA survivors and primary prevention therapy in symptomatic patients with type I Brugada patterns, even though it is based largely on observational data. Studies have suggested that syncope associated with electrocardiographic changes suggestive of the disorder at baseline is a marker of risk sufficient to warrant ICD therapy and that baseline electrocardiographic changes associated with inducibility of ventricular tachyarrhythmias during electrophysiologic testing may also be a marker of risk in some subgroups, although this remains debated. However, a family history of SCD is often considered in judgment-based decisions. Similar arguments, but supported by even fewer data, apply to affected family members of patients with right ventricular dysplasia.

Prediction and Primary Prevention in the General Population

Because SCD is frequently the first clinical expression of underlying structural heart disease or occurs in identified patients profiled to be at low risk (see Fig. 70.2B), there has been longstanding interest in risk profiling and therapeutic strategies targeted to primary prevention. To have a major impact on the problem of SCD in the general population, including adolescents and young adults, we need to move beyond the identification of high-risk patients who have specific clinical entities, advanced or subtle, that predict high risk for SCD. Rather, it is necessary to find small subgroups of patients in the general population at specific risk for SCD as a manifestation of underlying heart disease, if and when that disease becomes manifested. As an example, studies that have demonstrated familial clustering of SCD as the first expression of underlying coronary artery disease and thus suggesting a genetic or behavioral predisposition may provide some help for the future. If highly specific markers related to electrophysiologic properties or along multiple points in the cascade of coronary events (see Fig. 70.5) can be found, preventive therapy before the first expression of an underlying disease may have a major effect on the population burden of SCD. Short of that, successes will be limited to community-based intervention and to subgroups that are easier to identify and in whom it is more justifiable to use prophylactic interventional therapy on the basis of population size and magnitude of risk.

The clinical risk score developed in ARIC and validated in the Framingham study[17] has been implemented in the electronic health record to evaluate risk of SCD among 36,885 primary care patients. Those in the low SCD risk category (deciles 1 to 4) had a mean age of 55.3 ± 11.3 years, 65% were female, 35% were Hispanic, 60% had hypertension, and 65% had diabetes. Those in deciles 9 to 10 (highest risk) were 71.0 ± 9.8 years of age, 91% male, 32% Hispanic, 88% had hypertension, and 91% had diabetes. Among the 7256 patients who were classified in the highest SCD risk category (deciles 9 to 10), these patients were seen frequently by a primary care physician (82%), but only 35% were seen by a cardiologist, 36% had an echocardiogram, and 18% had a stress test. It is interesting to note that patients at the highest risk of SCD without known heart disease actually have a significant burden of occult heart disease, including late gadolinium enhancement, abnormal heart rate recovery after exercise, and pathogenic SNPs related to cardiomyopathy and/or arrhythmias.[19] This presents a potential pathway to identify high risk subgroups that may benefit from some intervention.

Adolescents and young adults, including athletes (see Chapter 32), constitute a group for special consideration. Risk for SCD in these groups is approximately 1% of the risk in the general adult population older than 35 years (see Fig. 70.3).[57] However, most causes of SCD in these populations are not characterized by advanced life-limiting structural heart disease, and therefore surviving cardiac arrest victims can, with appropriate long-term therapy, be expected to have significant extensions of life. Because most deaths are arrhythmic, the ability to identify individuals at risk in advance of a life-threatening arrhythmic event offers more long-term impact than in older populations. For both the general young population and athletes, identification of individuals at risk may lead to prevention of events triggered by physical activity. One study has demonstrated a reduction in SCDs in athletes with the use of widespread electrocardiographic screening. In the United States, strategies for screening of adolescents, young adults, and athletes to identify entities that create risk have largely been limited to medical and family histories and physical examination, although a consensus statement spearheaded by the NCAA has taken a more permissive position on ECG screening.[185] The European and the International Olympic Committee recommendations add electrocardiographic screening for athletes, which continues to be debated in the United States despite data indicating both feasibility and suggestions of cost-effectiveness. Electrocardiographic screening of the general adolescent population, including athletes, can identify many of those at potential risk because of congenital long-QT syndrome, HCM, right ventricular dysplasia, and Brugada syndrome. In Japan, where ECG screening of first and seventh grade school children is routine, the apparent incidence of LQT is considerably higher than recognized in the United States and Europe—1/3298 first graders and 1/988 by the seventh grade versus 1/2000 to 2500 in the general population elsewhere.[36] Although electrocardiographic screening in the adolescent and athletic subgroups is imperfect and usually accompanied by depolarization and repolarization patterns that may be difficult to interpret, this strategy can lead to further testing in appropriate individuals. Echocardiography has also been suggested as a screening method, but it is more expensive and less cost-efficient and does not recognize conditions such as long-QT syndrome and Brugada syndrome.

Risk for SCD must be evaluated in competitive athletes with previously known cardiovascular disorders or those discovered during preparticipation screening, as well as in those with known disorders who wish to participate in recreational sports. Recommendations for competitive athletes, based on the intensity of exercise,[186] the nature of the diseases,[75,187] response strategies,[188] and legal considerations,[189] are available; issues for recreational athletes are more complex because of absence of organizational infrastructures in most instances.

SUDDEN DEATH AND PUBLIC SAFETY

The unexpectedness of SCD has raised questions concerning secondary risk to the public created by people in the throes of cardiac arrest. No data from controlled studies are available to guide public policy regarding people at high risk for potentially lethal arrhythmias and for abrupt incapacitation. In a report of observations on 1348 sudden deaths caused by coronary heart disease in people 65 years or younger during a 7-year period in Dade County, FL, 101 (7.5%) of the deaths occurred in people who were engaged in activities at the time of death that were potentially hazardous to the public (e.g., driving a motor vehicle, working at altitude, piloting aircraft), and 122 (9.1%) of the victims had occupations that could create potential hazards to others if an abrupt loss of consciousness had occurred while they were at work. No catastrophic events occurred as a result of these cardiac arrests.

In specific reference to private automobiles, a study from Seattle identified 33 SCDs per year while driving the estimated 1.32 million vehicles in the community. An analysis of recurrent events in cardiac arrest survivors has suggested limitation of driving privileges for the first 8 months after the index event on the basis of the clustering of recurrent event rates early after the index event. Therefore, although there are likely to be isolated cases in which cardiac arrest causes public hazards, the risk appears to be small, and because it is difficult to identify specific individuals at risk, sweeping restrictions to avoid such risks appear to be unwarranted. The exceptions are people with multisystem disease, particularly senility, and individual circumstances that require specific consideration, such as patients with documented or substantial risk for loss of consciousness associated with the onset of arrhythmias and high-risk patients who have special responsibilities—school bus drivers, aircraft pilots, train operators, and truck drivers.

Among patients with primary prevention ICD implants, it was originally suggested that driving be avoided for 6 months postimplant, but a revision of the recommendations had reduced that to 1 week or more, depending on individual circumstances. Once a therapy has been delivered, the posttherapy guideline of up to 6 months still prevails, again with modification based on individual circumstances and preshock symptoms. Studies of temporal patterns of recurrent ICD shock therapies identified an acceleration of time to recurrent events after a first event has occurred, but with an overall low rate, an observation that may have implications for driving depending on associated symptoms in individual patients.[190,191]

REFERENCES

Perspectives/Definition

1. Berg KM, Cheng A, Panchal AR, et al. Part 7: systems of care: 2020 American Heart Association guidelines for cardiopulmonary resuscitation and emergency cardiovascular care. *Circulation*. 2020;142:S580–S604.
2. Virani SS, Alonso A, Benjamin EJ, et al. Heart disease and stroke statistics-2020 update: a report from the American Heart Association. *Circulation*. 2020;141:e139–e596.
3. Kolte D, Khera S, Aronow WS, et al. Regional variation in the incidence and outcomes of in-hospital cardiac arrest in the United States. *Circulation*. 2015;131:1415–1425.
4. Myerburg RJ, Goldberg JJ. Cardiac arrest and sudden cardiac death. In: Zipes DP, et al., ed. *Braunwald's Heart Disease*. 11 ed. Philadelphia: Elsevier; 2019.
5. Tseng ZH, Olgin JE, Vittinghoff E, et al. Prospective countywide surveillance and autopsy characterization of sudden cardiac death: post scd study. *Circulation*. 2018;137:2689–2700.

Epidemiology

6. Myerburg RJ, Goldberger JJ. Sudden cardiac arrest risk assessment: population science and the individual risk mandate. *JAMA Cardiol*. 2017;2:689–694.
7. Wong CX, Brown A, Lau DH, et al. Epidemiology of sudden cardiac death: global and regional perspectives. *Heart Lung Circ*. 2019;28:6–14.
8. Myerburg RJ, GJJ. Sudden cardiac arrest/death in adults. In: Zipes DP, Jalife J, Stevenson WG, eds. *Cardiac Electrophysiology: from Cell to Bedside*. 7th ed. Philadelphia, PA: Elsevier; 2018:937–948.
9. Virani SS, Alonso A, Aparicio HJ, et al. Heart disease and stroke statistics-2021 update: a report from the American Heart Association. *Circulation*. 2021;143:e254–e743.
10. Huikuri HV, Castellanos A, Myerburg RJ. Sudden death due to cardiac arrhythmias. *N Engl J Med*. 2001;345:1473–1482.
11. Shen L, Jhund PS, Petrie MC, et al. Declining risk of sudden death in heart failure. *N Engl J Med*. 2017;377:41–51.
12. Hayashi M, Shimizu W, Albert CM. The spectrum of epidemiology underlying sudden cardiac death. *Circ Res*. 2015;116:1887–1906.
13. Junttila MJ, Hookana E, Kaikkonen KS, et al. Temporal trends in the clinical and pathological characteristics of victims of sudden cardiac death in the absence of previously identified heart disease. *Circ Arrhythm Electrophysiol*. 2016;9.
14. Myerburg RJ, Ullmann SG. Alternative research funding to improve clinical outcomes: model of prediction and prevention of sudden cardiac death. *Circ Arrhythm Electrophysiol*. 2015;8:492–498.
15. Aro AL, Reinier K, Rusinaru C, et al. Electrical risk score beyond the left ventricular ejection fraction: prediction of sudden cardiac death in the Oregon sudden unexpected death study and the atherosclerosis risk in communities study. *Eur Heart J*. 2017;38:3017–3025.
16. Deo R, Norby FL, Katz R, et al. Development and validation of a sudden cardiac death prediction model for the general population. *Circulation*. 2016;134:806–816.
17. Bogle BM, Ning H, Goldberger JJ, et al. A simple community-based risk-prediction score for sudden cardiac death. *Am J Med*. 2018;131:532-539.e535.
18. Olson KA, Patel RB, Ahmad FS, et al. Sudden cardiac death risk distribution in the United States population (from nhanes, 2005 to 2012). *Am J Cardiol*. 2019;123:1249–1254.
19. Tamariz L, Palacio A, Myerburg R, et al. Asymptomatic patients without known heart disease have markers of occult heart disease. *Am J Cardiol*. 2020;125:1449–1450.
20. Jayaraman R, Reinier K, Nair S, et al. Risk factors of sudden cardiac death in the young: multiple-year community-wide assessment. *Circulation*. 2018;137:1561–1570.
21. Farioli A, Christophi CA, Quarta CC, et al. Incidence of sudden cardiac death in a young active population. *J Am Heart Assoc*. 2015;4:e001818.
22. Kang SH, Oh IY, Heo J, et al. Heat, heat waves, and out-of-hospital cardiac arrest. *Int J Cardiol*. 2016;221:232–237.
23. Onozuka D, Hagihara A. Extreme temperature and out-of-hospital cardiac arrest in Japan: a nationwide, retrospective, observational study. *Sci Total Environ*. 2017;575:258–264.
24. Abdelsayed M, Peters CH, Ruben PC. Differential thermosensitivity in mixed syndrome cardiac sodium channel mutants. *J Physiol*. 2015;593:4201–4223.
25. Dai J, Chen R, Meng X, et al. Ambient air pollution, temperature and out-of-hospital coronary deaths in Shanghai, China. *Environ Pollut*. 2015;203:116–121.
26. Zhao R, Chen S, Wang W, et al. The impact of short-term exposure to air pollutants on the onset of out-of-hospital cardiac arrest: a systematic review and meta-analysis. *Int J Cardiol*. 2017;226:110–117.
27. Folino F, Buja G, Zanotto G, et al. Association between air pollution and ventricular arrhythmias in high-risk patients (aria study): a multicentre longitudinal study. *Lancet Planet Health*. 2017;1:e58–e64.
28. Holmberg MJ, Ross CE, Fitzmaurice GM, et al. Annual incidence of adult and pediatric in-hospital cardiac arrest in the United States. *Circ Cardiovasc Qual Outcomes*. 2019;12:e005580.
29. Bagnall RD, Weintraub RG, Ingles J, et al. A prospective study of sudden cardiac death among children and young adults. *N Engl J Med*. 2016;374:2441–2452.
30. Deo R, Safford MM, Khodneva YA, et al. Differences in risk of sudden cardiac death between blacks and whites. *J Am Coll Cardiol*. 2018;72:2431–2439.
31. Zhao D, Post WS, Blasco-Colmenares E, et al. Racial differences in sudden cardiac death. *Circulation*. 2019;139:1688–1697.
32. Bogle BM, Ning H, Mehrotra S, et al. Lifetime risk for sudden cardiac death in the community. *J Am Heart Assoc*. 2016;5.
33. Haukilahti MAE, Holmstrom L, Vahatalo J, et al. Sudden cardiac death in women. *Circulation*. 2019;139:1012–1021.
34. Bezzina CR, Lahrouchi N, Priori SG. Genetics of sudden cardiac death. *Circ Res*. 2015;116:1919–1936.
35. Schwartz PJ, Crotti L, George Jr AL. Modifier genes for sudden cardiac death. *Eur Heart J*. 2018;39:3925–3931.
36. Yoshinaga M, Kucho Y, Nishibatake M, et al. Probability of diagnosing long QT syndrome in children and adolescents according to the criteria of the HRS/EHRA/APHRS expert consensus statement. *Eur Heart J*. 2016;37:2490–2497.
37. Myerburg RJ. Electrocardiographic screening of children and adolescents: the search for hidden risk. *Eur Heart J*. 2016;37:2498–2501.
38. Tamariz L, Balda J, Pareja D, et al. Usefulness of single nucleotide polymorphisms as predictors of sudden cardiac death. *Am J Cardiol*. 2019;123:1900–1905.
39. Deyell MW, Krahn AD, Goldberger JJ. Sudden cardiac death risk stratification. *Circ Res*. 2015;116:1907–1918.
40. Grani C, Benz DC, Gupta S, et al. Sudden cardiac death in ischemic heart disease: from imaging arrhythmogenic substrate to guiding therapies. *JACC Cardiovasc Imaging*. 2020;13:2223–2238.
41. Halliday BP, Cleland JGF, Goldberger JJ, et al. Personalizing risk stratification for sudden death in dilated cardiomyopathy: the past, present, and future. *Circulation*. 2017;136:215–231.
42. Ommen SR, Mital S, Burke MA, et al. 2020 AHA/ACC guideline for the diagnosis and treatment of patients with hypertrophic cardiomyopathy: a report of the American College of Cardiology/American Heart Association joint committee on clinical practice guidelines. *J Am Coll Cardiol*. 2020;76:e159–e240.
43. Bilchick KC, Wang Y, Cheng A, et al. Seattle heart failure and proportional risk models predict benefit from implantable cardioverter-defibrillators. *J Am Coll Cardiol*. 2017;69:2606–2618.
44. Whitman IR, Agarwal V, Nah G, et al. Alcohol abuse and cardiac disease. *J Am Coll Cardiol*. 2017;69:13–24.
45. Adabag S, Huxley RR, Lopez FL, et al. Obesity related risk of sudden cardiac death in the atherosclerosis risk in communities study. *Heart*. 2015;101:215–221.
46. Harmon KG, Asif IM, Maleszewski JJ, et al. Incidence, cause, and comparative frequency of sudden cardiac death in national collegiate athletic association athletes: a decade in review. *Circulation*. 2015;132:10–19.
47. Chan C, Daly M, Melton I, et al. Two major earthquakes in Christchurch were not associated with increased ventricular arrhythmias: analysis of implanted defibrillator diagnostics. *PloS One*. 2019;14:e0216521.
48. Chatterjee NA, Moorthy MV, Pester J, et al. Sudden death in patients with coronary heart disease without severe systolic dysfunction. *JAMA Cardiol*. 2018;3:591–600.
49. Disertori M, Rigoni M, Pace N, et al. Myocardial fibrosis assessment by lge is a powerful predictor of ventricular tachyarrhythmias in ischemic and nonischemic LV dysfunction: a meta-analysis. *JACC Cardiovasc Imaging*. 2016;9:1046–1055.
50. Ganesan AN, Gunton J, Nucifora G, et al. Impact of late gadolinium enhancement on mortality, sudden death and major adverse cardiovascular events in ischemic and nonischemic cardiomyopathy: a systematic review and meta-analysis. *Int J Cardiol*. 2018;254:230–237.
51. Halliday BP, Gulati A, Ali A, et al. Association between midwall late gadolinium enhancement and sudden cardiac death in patients with dilated cardiomyopathy and mild and moderate left ventricular systolic dysfunction. *Circulation*. 2017;135:2106–2115.

Causes of Sudden Death

52. Herrington W, Lacey B, Sherliker P, et al. Epidemiology of atherosclerosis and the potential to reduce the global burden of atherothrombotic disease. *Circ Res*. 2016;118:535–546.
53. Brothers JA, Frommelt MA, Jaquiss RDB, et al. Expert consensus guidelines: anomalous aortic origin of a coronary artery. *J Thorac Cardiovasc Surg*. 2017;153:1440–1457.
54. Shenasa M, Shenasa H. Hypertension, left ventricular hypertrophy, and sudden cardiac death. *Int J Cardiol*. 2017;237:60–63.
55. Adamczak DM, Oko-Sarnowska Z. Sudden cardiac death in hypertrophic cardiomyopathy. *Cardiol Rev*. 2018;26:145–151.
56. Ha FJ, Han HC, Sanders P, et al. Sudden cardiac death in the young: incidence, trends, and risk factors in a nationwide study. *Circ Cardiovasc Qual Outcomes*. 2020;13:e006470.
57. Ackerman M, Atkins DL, Triedman JK. Sudden cardiac death in the young. *Circulation*. 2016;133:1006–1026.
58. Manrai AK, Funke BH, Rehm HL, et al. Genetic misdiagnoses and the potential for health disparities. *N Engl J Med*. 2016;375:655–665.
59. Maron BJ, Maron MS. Contemporary strategies for risk stratification and prevention of sudden death with the implantable defibrillator in hypertrophic cardiomyopathy. *Heart Rhythm*. 2016;13:1155–1165.
60. Vaduganathan M, Patel RB, Michel A, et al. Mode of death in heart failure with preserved ejection fraction. *J Am Coll Cardiol*. 2017;69:556–569.
61. van Veldhuisen DJ, van Woerden G, Gorter TM, et al. Ventricular tachyarrhythmia detection by implantable loop recording in patients with heart failure and preserved ejection fraction: the VIP-HF study. *Eur J Heart Fail*. 2020;22:1923–1929.
62. Wahbi K, Ben Yaou R, Gandjbakhch E, et al. Development and validation of a new risk prediction score for life-threatening ventricular tachyarrhythmias in laminopathies. *Circulation*. 2019;140:293–302.
63. Clark DE, Parikh A, Dendy JM, et al. COVID-19 myocardial pathology evaluation in athletes with cardiac magnetic resonance (compete cmr). *Circulation*. 2021;143:609–612.
64. Martinez MW, Tucker AM, Bloom OJ, et al. Prevalence of inflammatory heart disease among professional athletes with prior COVID-19 infection who received systematic return-to-play cardiac screening. *JAMA Cardiol*. 2021.
65. Puntmann VO, Carerj ML, Wieters I, et al. Outcomes of cardiovascular magnetic resonance imaging in patients recently recovered from coronavirus disease 2019 (covid-19). *JAMA Cardiol*. 2020;5:1265–1273.
66. Rajpal S, Tong MS, Borchers J, et al. Cardiovascular magnetic resonance findings in competitive athletes recovering from COVID-19 infection. *JAMA Cardiol*. 2021;6:116–118.
67. Starekova J, Bluemke DA, Bradham WS, et al. Evaluation for myocarditis in competitive student athletes recovering from coronavirus disease 2019 with cardiac magnetic resonance imaging. *JAMA Cardiol*. 2021.
68. Ammirati E, Frigerio M, Adler ED, et al. Management of acute myocarditis and chronic inflammatory cardiomyopathy: an expert consensus document. *Circ Heart Fail*. 2020;13:e007405.
69. Ekstrom K, Lehtonen J, Nordenswan HK, et al. Sudden death in cardiac sarcoidosis: an analysis of nationwide clinical and cause-of-death registries. *Eur Heart J*. 2019;40:3121–3128.
70. Birnie D, Ha A, Kron J. Which patients with cardiac sarcoidosis should receive implantable cardioverter-defibrillators: some answers but many questions remain. *Circ Arrhythm Electrophysiol*. 2018;11:e006685.
71. Kim EJ, Holmes BB, Huang S, et al. Outcomes in patients with cardiac amyloidosis and implantable cardioverter-defibrillator. *Europace*. 2020;22:1216–1223.
72. Calkins H, Corrado D, Marcus F. Risk stratification in arrhythmogenic right ventricular cardiomyopathy. *Circulation*. 2017;136:2068–2082.
73. Finocchiaro G, Papadakis M, Robertus JL, et al. Etiology of sudden death in sports: insights from a United Kingdom regional registry. *J Am Coll Cardiol*. 2016;67:2108–2115.

74. Gupta R, Tichnell C, Murray B, et al. Comparison of features of fatal versus nonfatal cardiac arrest in patients with arrhythmogenic right ventricular dysplasia/cardiomyopathy. *Am J Cardiol.* 2017;120:111–117.
75. Zipes DP, Link MS, Ackerman MJ, et al. Eligibility and disqualification recommendations for competitive athletes with cardiovascular abnormalities: task force 9: arrhythmias and conduction defects: a scientific statement from the American Heart Association and American College of Cardiology. *Circulation.* 2015;132. e315-325.
76. La Gerche A, Claessen G, Dymarkowski S, et al. Exercise-induced right ventricular dysfunction is associated with ventricular arrhythmias in endurance athletes. *Eur Heart J.* 2015;36:1998–2010.
77. Bhonsale A, Groeneweg JA, James CA, et al. Impact of genotype on clinical course in arrhythmogenic right ventricular dysplasia/cardiomyopathy-associated mutation carriers. *Eur Heart J.* 2015;36:847–855.
78. Taniguchi T, Morimoto T, Shiomi H, et al. Sudden death in patients with severe aortic stenosis: observations from the current as registry. *J Am Heart Assoc.* 2018;7:e008397.
79. Minners J, Rossebo A, Chambers JB, et al. Sudden cardiac death in asymptomatic patients with aortic stenosis. *Heart.* 2020;106:1646–1650.
80. Urena M, Webb JG, Eltchaninoff H, et al. Late cardiac death in patients undergoing transcatheter aortic valve replacement: incidence and predictors of advanced heart failure and sudden cardiac death. *J Am Coll Cardiol.* 2015;65:437–448.
81. Basso C, Iliceto S, Thiene G, et al. Mitral valve prolapse, ventricular arrhythmias, and sudden death. *Circulation.* 2019;140:952–964.
82. Fulton BL, Liang JJ, Enriquez A, et al. Imaging characteristics of papillary muscle site of origin of ventricular arrhythmias in patients with mitral valve prolapse. *J Cardiovasc Electrophysiol.* 2018;29:146–153.
83. Singh M, Morin DP, Link MS. Sudden cardiac death in long QT syndrome (LQTS), Brugada syndrome, and catecholaminergic polymorphic ventricular tachycardia (CPVT). *Prog Cardiovasc Dis.* 2019;62:227–234.
84. Myerburg RJ. Physiological variations, environmental factors, and genetic modifications in inherited LQT syndromes. *J Am Coll Cardiol.* 2015;65:375–377.
85. O'Neal WT, Singleton MJ, Roberts JD, et al. Association between QT-interval components and sudden cardiac death: the aric study (atherosclerosis risk in communities). *Circ Arrhythm Electrophysiol.* 2017;10.
86. Adler A, Rosso R, Chorin E, et al. Risk stratification in Brugada syndrome: clinical characteristics, electrocardiographic parameters, and auxiliary testing. *Heart Rhythm.* 2016;13:299–310.
87. Cheng YJ, Lin XX, Ji CC, et al. Role of early repolarization pattern in increasing risk of death. *J Am Heart Assoc.* 2016;5.
88. Fan J, Yao FJ, Cheng YJ, et al. Early repolarization pattern associated with coronary artery disease and increased the risk of cardiac death in acute myocardium infarction. *Ann Noninvasive Electrocardiol.* 2020;25:e12768.
89. Moon RY, Task Force On Sudden Infant Death S. SIDS and other sleep-related infant deaths: evidence base for 2016 updated recommendations for a safe infant sleeping environment. *Pediatrics.* 2016;138.
90. Sollazzo F, Palmieri V, Gervasi SF, et al. Sudden cardiac death in athletes in Italy during 2019: Internet-based epidemiological research. *Medicina (Kaunas).* 2021;57.
91. Maron BJ, Haas TS, Ahluwalia A, et al. Demographics and epidemiology of sudden deaths in young competitive athletes: from the United States National Registry. *Am J Med.* 2016;129:1170–1177.
92. Marijon E, Uy-Evanado A, Reinier K, et al. Sudden cardiac arrest during sports activity in middle age. *Circulation.* 2015;131:1384–1391.
93. Pelliccia A, Solberg EE, Papadakis M, et al. Recommendations for participation in competitive and leisure time sport in athletes with cardiomyopathies, myocarditis, and pericarditis: position statement of the sport cardiology section of the European Association of Preventive Cardiology (EAPC). *Eur Heart J.* 2019;40:19–33.
94. Link MS, Estes 3rd NAM, Maron BJ. Eligibility and disqualification recommendations for competitive athletes with cardiovascular abnormalities: task force 13: commotio cordis: a scientific statement from the American Heart Association and American College of Cardiology. *J Am Coll Cardiol.* 2015;66:2439–2443.
95. Kim AS, Moffatt E, Ursell PC, et al. Sudden neurologic death masquerading as out-of-hospital sudden cardiac death. *Neurology.* 2016;87:1669–1673.
96. Heilbrunn E, Ssentongo P, Chinchilli VM, et al. Sudden death in individuals with obstructive sleep apnoea: protocol for a systematic review and meta-analysis. *BMJ Open.* 2020;10:e039774.

Pathology and Pathophysiology

97. Anderson JH, Tester DJ, Will ML, et al. Whole-exome molecular autopsy after exertion-related sudden unexplained death in the young. *Circ Cardiovasc Genet.* 2016;9:259–265.
98. Quenin P, Kyndt F, Mabo P, et al. Clinical yield of familial screening after sudden death in young subjects: the French experience. *Circ Arrhythm Electrophysiol.* 2017;10.
99. Vassalini M, Verzeletti A, Restori M, et al. An autopsy study of sudden cardiac death in persons aged 1-40 years in Brescia (Italy). *J Cardiovasc Med.* 2016;17:446–453.
100. Goldberger JJ, Arora R, Buckley U, et al. Autonomic nervous system dysfunction: JACC focus seminar. *J Am Coll Cardiol.* 2019;73:1189–1206.
101. Huang WA, Boyle NG, Vaseghi M. Cardiac innervation and the autonomic nervous system in sudden cardiac death. *Card Electrophysiol Clin.* 2017;9:665–679.
102. Li CY, Li YG. Cardiac sympathetic nerve sprouting and susceptibility to ventricular arrhythmias after myocardial infarction. *Cardiol Res Pract.* 2015;2015:698368.
103. Gardner RT, Ripplinger CM, Myles RC, et al. Molecular mechanisms of sympathetic remodeling and arrhythmias. *Circ Arrhythm Electrophysiol.* 2016;9:e001359.
104. Kurz MC, Schmicker RH, Leroux B, et al. Advanced vs. Basic life support in the treatment of out-of-hospital cardiopulmonary arrest in the resuscitation outcomes consortium. *Resuscitation.* 2018;128:132–137.
105. Pelliccia A, Sharma S, Gati S, et al. 2020 ESC guidelines on sports cardiology and exercise in patients with cardiovascular disease. *Eur Heart J.* 2021;42:17–96.
106. van der Weg K, Prinzen FW, Gorgels AP. Editor's choice- reperfusion cardiac arrhythmias and their relation to reperfusion-induced cell death. *Eur Heart J Acute Cardiovasc Care.* 2019;8:142–152.

Clinical Features of Patients With Cardiac Arrest

107. Chan PS, McNally B, Nallamothu BK, et al. Long-term outcomes among elderly survivors of out-of-hospital cardiac arrest. *J Am Heart Assoc.* 2016;5:e002924.
108. Merchant RM, Topjian AA, Panchal AR, et al. Part 1: executive summary: 2020 American Heart Association guidelines for cardiopulmonary resuscitation and emergency cardiovascular care. *Circulation.* 2020;142:S337–S357.
109. Shao F, Li CS, Liang LR, et al. Incidence and outcome of adult in-hospital cardiac arrest in Beijing, China. *Resuscitation.* 2016;102:51–56.
110. Hirlekar G, Karlsson T, Aune S, et al. Survival and neurological outcome in the elderly after in-hospital cardiac arrest. *Resuscitation.* 2017;118:101–106.
111. Kosmidou I, Embacher M, McAndrew T, et al. Early ventricular tachycardia or fibrillation in patients with ST elevation myocardial infarction undergoing primary percutaneous coronary intervention and impact on mortality and stent thrombosis (from the harmonizing outcomes with revascularization and stents in acute myocardial infarction trial). *Am J Cardiol.* 2017;120:1755–1760.
112. Takada T, Shishido K, Hayashi T, et al. Impact of late ventricular arrhythmias on cardiac mortality in patients with acute myocardial infarction. *J Interv Cardiol.* 2019;2019:5345178.
113. Nolan JP, Soar J, Cariou A, et al. European resuscitation council and European society of intensive care medicine guidelines for post-resuscitation care 2015: section 5 of the European resuscitation council guidelines for resuscitation 2015. *Resuscitation.* 2015;95:202–222.
114. Lascarrou JB, Merdji H, Le Gouge A, et al. Targeted temperature management for cardiac arrest with nonshockable rhythm. *N Engl J Med.* 2019;381:2327–2337.
115. Mellor G, Laksman ZWM, Tadros R, et al. Genetic testing in the evaluation of unexplained cardiac arrest: from the CASPER (cardiac arrest survivors with preserved ejection fraction registry). *Circ Cardiovasc Genet.* 2017;10.
116. Jozwiak M, Bougouin W, Geri G, et al. Post-resuscitation shock: recent advances in pathophysiology and treatment. *Ann Intensive Care.* 2020;10:170.
117. Bascom KE, Dziodzio J, Vasaiwala S, et al. Derivation and validation of the crest model for very early prediction of circulatory etiology death in patients without ST-segment-elevation myocardial infarction after cardiac arrest. *Circulation.* 2018;137:273–282.
118. Patel N, Patel NJ, Macon CJ, et al. Trends and outcomes of coronary angiography and percutaneous coronary intervention after out-of-hospital cardiac arrest associated with ventricular fibrillation or pulseless ventricular tachycardia. *JAMA Cardiol.* 2016;1:890–899.
119. Rodriguez AP, Badiye A, Lambrakos LK, et al. Refractory ventricular tachycardia storm associated with severe hypokalemia in fanconi syndrome. *Heart Rhythm Case Rep.* 2019;5:374–378.
120. Sawyer KN, Camp-Rogers TR, Kotini-Shah P, et al. Sudden cardiac arrest survivorship: a scientific statement from the American Heart Association. *Circulation.* 2020;141:e654–e685.
121. Sabbag A, Suleiman M, Laish-Farkash A, et al. Contemporary rates of appropriate shock therapy in patients who receive implantable device therapy in a real-world setting: from the Israeli ICD registry. *Heart Rhythm.* 2015;12:2426–2433.
122. Schaer B, Kuhne M, Reichlin T, et al. Incidence of and predictors for appropriate implantable cardioverter-defibrillator therapy in patients with a secondary preventive implantable cardioverter-defibrillator indication. *Europace.* 2016;18:227–231.

Management of Cardiac Arrest

123. Bobrow BJ, Spaite DW, Vadeboncoeur TF, et al. Implementation of a regional telephone cardiopulmonary resuscitation program and outcomes after out-of-hospital cardiac arrest. *JAMA Cardiol.* 2016;1:294–302.
124. Andelius L, Malta Hansen C, Lippert FK, et al. Smartphone activation of citizen responders to facilitate defibrillation in out-of-hospital cardiac arrest. *J Am Coll Cardiol.* 2020;76:43–53.
125. Cheng A, Nadkarni VM, Mancini MB, et al. Resuscitation education science: educational strategies to improve outcomes from cardiac arrest: a scientific statement from the American Heart Association. *Circulation.* 2018;138:e82–e122.
126. Ringh M, Rosenqvist M, Hollenberg J, et al. Mobile-phone dispatch of laypersons for CPR in out-of-hospital cardiac arrest. *N Engl J Med.* 2015;372:2316–2325.
127. Ofoma UR, Basnet S, Berger A, et al. Trends in survival after in-hospital cardiac arrest during nights and weekends. *J Am Coll Cardiol.* 2018;71:402–411.
128. Girotra S, van Diepen S, Nallamothu BK, et al. Regional variation in out-of-hospital cardiac arrest survival in the United States. *Circulation.* 2016;133:2159–2168.
129. van Diepen S, Girotra S, Abella BS, et al. Multistate 5-year initiative to improve care for out-of-hospital cardiac arrest: primary results from the Heart Rescue Project. *J Am Heart Assoc.* 2017;6.
130. Lim ZJ, Ponnapa Reddy M, Afroz A, et al. Incidence and outcome of out-of-hospital cardiac arrests in the COVID-19 era: a systematic review and meta-analysis. *Resuscitation.* 2020;157:248–258.
131. Uy-Evanado A, Chugh HS, Sargsyan A, et al. Out-of-hospital cardiac arrest response and outcomes during the COVID-19 pandemic. *JACC Clin Electrophysiol.* 2021;7:6–11.
132. Mitrani RD, Goldberger JJ. Cardiac arrests during the COVID-19 pandemic: the perfect storm. *JACC Clin Electrophysiol.* 2021;7:12–15.
133. Malta Hansen C, Kragholm K, Pearson DA, et al. Association of bystander and first-responder intervention with survival after out-of-hospital cardiac arrest in North Carolina, 2010-2013. *J Am Med Assoc.* 2015;314:255–264.
134. Nakahara S, Tomio J, Ichikawa M, et al. Association of bystander interventions with neurologically intact survival among patients with bystander-witnessed out-of-hospital cardiac arrest in Japan. *J Am Med Assoc.* 2015;314:247–254.
135. Fukuda T, Ohashi-Fukuda N, Matsubara T, et al. Association of initial rhythm with neurologically favorable survival in non-shockable out-of-hospital cardiac arrest without a bystander witness or bystander cardiopulmonary resuscitation. *Eur J Intern Med.* 2016;30:61–67.
136. Luo S, Zhang Y, Zhang W, et al. Prognostic significance of spontaneous shockable rhythm conversion in adult out-of-hospital cardiac arrest patients with initial non-shockable heart rhythms: a systematic review and meta-analysis. *Resuscitation.* 2017;121:1–8.
137. Ewy GA. Cardiocerebral and cardiopulmonary resuscitation - 2017 update. *Acute Med Surg.* 2017;4:227–234.
138. Riess ML. New developments in cardiac arrest management. *Adv Anesth.* 2016;34:29–46.
139. Pepe PE, Scheppke KA, Antevy PM, et al. Confirming the clinical safety and feasibility of a bundled methodology to improve cardiopulmonary resuscitation involving a head-up/torso-up chest compression technique. *Crit Care Med.* 2019;47:449–455.
140. Holmberg MJ, Vognsen M, Andersen MS, et al. Bystander automated external defibrillator use and clinical outcomes after out-of-hospital cardiac arrest: a systematic review and meta-analysis. *Resuscitation.* 2017;120:77–87.
141. Pollack RA, Brown SP, Rea T, et al. Impact of bystander automated external defibrillator use on survival and functional outcomes in shockable observed public cardiac arrests. *Circulation.* 2018;137:2104–2113.
142. Delhomme C, Njeim M, Varlet E, et al. Automated external defibrillator use in out-of-hospital cardiac arrest: current limitations and solutions. *Arch Cardiovasc Dis.* 2019;112:217–222.
143. Perkins GD, Ji C, Deakin CD, et al. A randomized trial of epinephrine in out-of-hospital cardiac arrest. *N Engl J Med.* 2018;379:711–721.
144. Ahn S, Kim YJ, Sohn CH, et al. Sodium bicarbonate on severe metabolic acidosis during prolonged cardiopulmonary resuscitation: a double-blind, randomized, placebo-controlled pilot study. *J Thorac Dis.* 2018;10:2295–2302.
145. Panchal AR, Bartos JA, Cabanas JG, et al. Part 3: adult basic and advanced life support: 2020 American Heart Association guidelines for cardiopulmonary resuscitation and emergency cardiovascular care. *Circulation.* 2020;142:S366-S468.
146. Kudenchuk PJ, Brown SP, Daya M, et al. Amiodarone, lidocaine, or placebo in out-of-hospital cardiac arrest. *N Engl J Med.* 2016;374:1711–1722.
147. Daya MR, Leroux BG, Dorian P, et al. Survival after intravenous versus intraosseous amiodarone, lidocaine, or placebo in out-of-hospital shock-refractory cardiac arrest. *Circulation.* 2020;141:188–198.
148. Jeejeebhoy FM, Zelop CM, Lipman S, et al. Cardiac arrest in pregnancy: a scientific statement from the American Heart Association. *Circulation.* 2015;132:1747–1773.
149. Hai JJ, Un KC, Wong CK, et al. Prognostic implications of early monomorphic and non-monomorphic tachyarrhythmias in patients discharged with acute coronary syndrome. *Heart Rhythm.* 2018;15:822–829.
150. Bernard SA, Smith K, Finn J, et al. Induction of therapeutic hypothermia during out-of-hospital cardiac arrest using a rapid infusion of cold saline: the rinse trial (rapid infusion of cold normal saline). *Circulation.* 2016;134:797–805.

151. Al-Khatib SM, Stevenson WG, Ackerman MJ, et al. 2017 AHA/ACC/HRS guideline for management of patients with ventricular arrhythmias and the prevention of sudden cardiac death: executive summary: a report of the American College of Cardiology/American Heart Association task force on clinical practice guidelines and the heart rhythm society. *Circulation.* 2018;138:e210–e271.

Prevention of Cardiac Arrest and Sudden Cardiac Death

152. Fernandes GC, Fernandes A, Cardoso R, et al. Association of SGLT2 inhibitors with arrhythmias and sudden cardiac death in patients with type 2 diabetes or heart failure: a meta-analysis of 34 randomized controlled trials. *Heart Rhythm.* 2021.
153. Claro JC, Candia R, Rada G, et al. Amiodarone versus other pharmacological interventions for prevention of sudden cardiac death. *Cochrane Database Syst Rev.* 2015:CD008093.
154. Gatzoulis KA, Tsiachris D, Arsenos P, et al. Arrhythmic risk stratification in post-myocardial infarction patients with preserved ejection fraction: the preserve ef study. *Eur Heart J.* 2019;40:2940–2949.
155. Bui AH, Waks JW. Risk stratification of sudden cardiac death after acute myocardial infarction. *J Innov Card Rhythm Manag.* 2018;9:3035–3049.
156. Brooks GC, Lee BK, Rao R, et al. Predicting persistent left ventricular dysfunction following myocardial infarction: the predicts study. *J Am Coll Cardiol.* 2016;67:1186–1196.
157. Katritsis DG, Zografos T, Hindricks G. Electrophysiology testing for risk stratification of patients with ischaemic cardiomyopathy: a call for action. *Europace.* 2018;20:f148–f152.
158. Zaman S, Taylor AJ, Stiles M, et al. Programmed ventricular stimulation to risk stratify for early cardioverter-defibrillator implantation to prevent tachyarrhythmias following acute myocardial infarction (protect-icd): trial protocol, background and significance. *Heart Lung Circ.* 2016;25:1055–1062.
159. Selvanayagam JB, Hartshorne T, Billot L, et al. Cardiovascular magnetic resonance-guided management of mild to moderate left ventricular systolic dysfunction (CMR guide): study protocol for a randomized controlled trial. *Ann Noninvasive Electrocardiol.* 2017;22.
160. Di Marco A, Anguera I, Schmitt M, et al. Late gadolinium enhancement and the risk for ventricular arrhythmias or sudden death in dilated cardiomyopathy: systematic review and meta-analysis. *JACC Heart Fail.* 2017;5:28–38.
161. Balaban G, Halliday BP, Porter B, et al. Late-gadolinium enhancement interface area and electrophysiological simulations predict arrhythmic events in patients with nonischemic dilated cardiomyopathy. *JACC Clin Electrophysiol.* 2021;7:238–249.
162. Freitas P, Ferreira AM, Arteaga-Fernandez E, et al. The amount of late gadolinium enhancement outperforms current guideline-recommended criteria in the identification of patients with hypertrophic cardiomyopathy at risk of sudden cardiac death. *J Cardiovasc Magn Reson.* 2019;21:50.
163. Weng Z, Yao J, Chan RH, et al. Prognostic value of LGE-CMR in HCM: a meta-analysis. *JACC Cardiovasc Imaging.* 2016;9:1392–1402.
164. Dhindsa DS, Khambhati J, Sandesara PB, et al. Biomarkers to predict cardiovascular death. *Card Electrophysiol Clin.* 2017;9:651–664.
165. Everett BM, Moorthy MV, Tikkanen JT, et al. Markers of myocardial stress, myocardial injury, and subclinical inflammation and the risk of sudden death. *Circulation.* 2020;142:1148–1158.
166. Elagizi A, Lavie CJ, Marshall K, et al. Omega-3 polyunsaturated fatty acids and cardiovascular health: a comprehensive review. *Prog Cardiovasc Dis.* 2018;61:76–85.
167. Kaab S. Genetics of sudden cardiac death - an epidemiologic perspective. *Int J Cardiol.* 2017;237:42–44.
168. Jabbari R, Engstrom T, Glinge C, et al. Incidence and risk factors of ventricular fibrillation before primary angioplasty in patients with first ST-elevation myocardial infarction: a nationwide study in Denmark. *J Am Heart Assoc.* 2015;4:e001399.
169. Ashar FN, Mitchell RN, Albert CM, et al. A comprehensive evaluation of the genetic architecture of sudden cardiac arrest. *Eur Heart J.* 2018;39:3961–3969.
170. Huertas-Vazquez A, Nelson CP, Sinsheimer JS, et al. Cumulative effects of common genetic variants on risk of sudden cardiac death. *Int J Cardiol Heart Vasc.* 2015;7:88–91.
171. Hernesniemi JA, Lyytikainen LP, Oksala N, et al. Predicting sudden cardiac death using common genetic risk variants for coronary artery disease. *Eur Heart J.* 2015;36:1669–1675.
172. Sapp JL, Wells GA, Parkash R, et al. Ventricular tachycardia ablation versus escalation of antiarrhythmic drugs. *N Engl J Med.* 2016;375:111–121.
173. Gianni C, Burkhardt JD, Trivedi C, et al. The role of the purkinje network in premature ventricular complex-triggered ventricular fibrillation. *J Interv Card Electrophysiol.* 2018;52:375–383.
174. Haissaguerre M, Duchateau J, Dubois R, et al. Idiopathic ventricular fibrillation: role of purkinje system and microstructural myocardial abnormalities. *JACC Clin Electrophysiol.* 2020;6:591–608.
175. Nogami A. Mapping and ablating ventricular premature contractions that trigger ventricular fibrillation: trigger elimination and substrate modification. *J Cardiovasc Electrophysiol.* 2015;26:110–115.
176. Borne RT, Katz D, Betz J, et al. Implantable cardioverter-defibrillators for secondary prevention of sudden cardiac death: a review. *J Am Heart Assoc.* 2017;6.
177. Katz DF, Peterson P, Borne RT, et al. Survival after secondary prevention implantable cardioverter-defibrillator placement: an analysis from the NCDR ICD registry. *JACC Clin Electrophysiol.* 2017;3:20–28.
178. Lee DS, Hardy J, Yee R, et al. Clinical risk stratification for primary prevention implantable cardioverter defibrillators. *Circ Heart Fail.* 2015;8:927–937.
179. Merchant FM, Levy WC, Kramer DB. Time to shock the system: moving beyond the current paradigm for primary prevention implantable cardioverter-defibrillator use. *J Am Heart Assoc.* 2020;9:e015139.
180. Younis A, Goldberger JJ, Kutyifa V, et al. Predicted benefit of an implantable cardioverter-defibrillator: the MADIT-ICD benefit score. *Eur Heart J.* 2021;42:1676–1684.
181. Kober L, Thune JJ, Nielsen JC, et al. Defibrillator implantation in patients with nonischemic systolic heart failure. *N Engl J Med.* 2016;375:1221–1230.
182. Pathak RK, Sanders P, Deo R. Primary prevention implantable cardioverter-defibrillator and opportunities for sudden cardiac death risk assessment in non-ischaemic cardiomyopathy. *Eur Heart J.* 2018;39:2859–2866.
183. McNamara DA, Goldberger JJ, Berendsen MA, et al. Implantable defibrillators versus medical therapy for cardiac channelopathies. *Cochrane Database Syst Rev.* 2015:CD011168.
184. Biton Y, Rosero S, Moss AJ, et al. Primary prevention with the implantable cardioverter-defibrillator in high-risk long-QT syndrome patients. *Europace.* 2019;21:339–346.
185. Hainline B, Drezner JA, Baggish A, et al. Interassociation consensus statement on cardiovascular care of college student-athletes. *J Am Coll Cardiol.* 2016;67:2981–2995.
186. Levine BD, Baggish AL, Kovacs RJ, et al. Eligibility and disqualification recommendations for competitive athletes with cardiovascular abnormalities: task force 1: classification of sports: dynamic, static, and impact: a scientific statement from the American Heart Association and American College of Cardiology. *Circulation.* 2015;132. e262-266.
187. Maron BJ, Zipes DP, Kovacs RJ, et al. Eligibility and disqualification recommendations for competitive athletes with cardiovascular abnormalities: preamble, principles, and general considerations: a scientific statement from the American Heart Association and American College of Cardiology. *Circulation.* 2015;132:e256–261.
188. Link MS, Myerburg RJ, Estes 3rd NA, et al. Eligibility and disqualification recommendations for competitive athletes with cardiovascular abnormalities: task force 12: emergency action plans, resuscitation, cardiopulmonary resuscitation, and automated external defibrillators: a scientific statement from the American Heart Association and American College of Cardiology. *Circulation.* 2015;132:e334–338.
189. Mitten MJ, Zipes DP, Maron BJ, et al. Eligibility and disqualification recommendations for competitive athletes with cardiovascular abnormalities: task force 15: legal aspects of medical eligibility and disqualification recommendations: a scientific statement from the American Heart Association and American College of Cardiology. *Circulation.* 2015;132:e346–349.

Sudden Death and Public Safety

190. Kim MH, Zhang Y, Sakaguchi S, et al. Time course of appropriate implantable cardioverter-defibrillator therapy and implications for guideline-based driving restrictions. *Heart Rhythm.* 2015;12:1728–1736.
191. Merchant FM, Hoskins MH, Benser ME, et al. Time course of subsequent shocks after initial implantable cardioverter-defibrillator discharge and implications for driving restrictions. *JAMA Cardiol.* 2016;1:181–188.

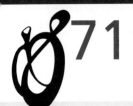

71 Hypotension and Syncope

HUGH CALKINS, THOMAS H. EVERETT IV, AND PENG-SHENG CHEN

DEFINITION

Syncope is a symptom that presents with abrupt, transient, complete loss of consciousness (LOC) associated with the inability to maintain postural tone, with rapid and spontaneous recovery. The presumed mechanism of syncope is cerebral hypoperfusion.[1,2] The metabolism of the brain, in contrast to that of many other organs, is exquisitely dependent on perfusion. Consequently, cessation of cerebral blood flow leads to LOC within approximately 10 seconds. Restoration of appropriate behavior and orientation after a syncopal episode is usually immediate. Retrograde amnesia, although uncommon, can be present in older adults. It is important to recognize that syncope, as previously defined, represents a subset of a much wider spectrum of conditions that can result in transient LOC, including conditions such as cerebrovascular accident (stroke) and epileptic seizures. Nonsyncopal causes of transient LOC differ in their mechanism and duration.[1,2]

Syncope is an important clinical problem because it is common, costly, and often disabling; can cause injury; and can be the only warning sign before sudden cardiac death (SCD) (see Chapter 70).[1-3] Patients with syncope account for 1% of hospital admissions and 3% of emergency department (ED) visits. Up to 50% of young adults report a previous episode of LOC, mostly isolated events that never come to medical attention. The prevalence of a first episode of syncope is particularly high between the ages 10 and 20, with additional peaks at approximately 60 and 80 years.[4] Patients who experience syncope also report greatly reduced quality of life; syncope can result in traumatic injury.

The prognosis of patients with syncope varies greatly with the diagnosis. Patients with syncope in the setting of structural heart disease or primary electrical disease have an increased incidence of SCD and overall mortality. Syncope caused by orthostatic hypotension is associated with a twofold increase in mortality, which reflects the presence of multiple comorbid conditions in this patient group. In contrast, young patients with neurally mediated syncope (NMS) have an excellent prognosis.

CLASSIFICATION

Tables 71.1 and 71.2 present the diagnostic considerations in patients with real or apparent transient LOC and in those with syncope, respectively. Syncope can be distinguished from most other causes of transient LOC by asking whether the LOC was transient, of rapid onset, of short duration, and followed by spontaneous recovery. If the answer to each of these questions is yes and the transient LOC did not result

from head trauma, the diagnostic considerations include true syncope in which the mechanism of transient LOC is global cerebral hypoperfusion, epileptic seizures, psychogenic syncope, and other rare causes. It is important to consider nonsyncopal conditions when evaluating a patient with transient LOC, such as metabolic disorders, epilepsy, or alcohol, as well as conditions in which consciousness is only apparently lost (i.e., conversion reaction). These psychogenic causes of syncope, being recognized with increased frequency, are typically diagnosed in patients 40 years or younger and especially in those with a history of psychiatric disease.[1,5]

The differential diagnosis of syncope (see Table 71.2) most often involves vascular causes, followed by cardiac causes, most frequently arrhythmias. Although knowledge of the common conditions that can cause syncope is essential and allows the clinician to arrive at a probable cause of the syncope in most patients, it is equally important to be aware of several less common but potentially lethal causes of syncope, such as long-QT syndrome, arrhythmogenic right ventricular dysplasia, Brugada syndrome, hypertrophic cardiomyopathy, idiopathic ventricular fibrillation (VF), catecholaminergic polymorphic ventricular tachycardia (VT), short-QT syndrome, and pulmonary emboli (see Chapters 63 and 67).[1,6-11]

It is important to recognize that the distribution of causes of syncope varies both with patient age and with the clinical setting in which the patient is evaluated. NMS and other causes of reflex-mediated syncope are the most frequent causes of syncope at any age and in any setting. Cardiac causes of syncope, especially cardiac tachyarrhythmias and bradyarrhythmias, are the second most common causes of syncope. The incidence of cardiac causes of syncope is higher in older adults and in patients evaluated in the ED. Orthostatic hypotension is extremely uncommon in patients younger than 40 years but is common in much older adults (see Chapter 90).

VASCULAR CAUSES OF SYNCOPE

Vascular causes of syncope, particularly reflex-mediated syncope and orthostatic hypotension, are by far the most common causes and account for at least one third of all syncopal episodes.[12,13] In contrast, vascular steal syndromes are exceedingly uncommon causes of syncope.

Orthostatic Hypotension

Standing upright displaces 500 to 800 mL of blood to the abdomen and lower extremities, thereby resulting in an abrupt drop in venous return

TABLE 71.1 Causes of Real or Apparent Transient Loss of Consciousness

Syncope (see Table 71.2)

Neurologic or cerebrovascular disease
    Epilepsy
    Vertebrobasilar transient ischemic attack

Metabolic syndromes and coma
    Hyperventilation with hypocapnia
    Hypoglycemia
    Hypoxemia
    Intoxication with drugs or alcohol
    Coma

Psychogenic syncope
    Anxiety, panic disorder
    Somatization disorders

TABLE 71.2 Causes of Syncope

Vascular Causes
Anatomic
Vascular steal syndromes (subclavian steal syndrome)
Orthostatic
Autonomic insufficiency
Idiopathic
Volume depletion
Drug and alcohol induced
Reflex Mediated
Carotid sinus hypersensitivity
Neurally mediated syncope (common faint, vasodepressor, neurocardiogenic, vasovagal)
Glossopharyngeal syncope
Situational (acute hemorrhage, cough, defecation, laugh, micturition, sneeze, swallow, postprandial)
Cardiac Causes
Anatomic
Obstructive cardiac valve disease
Aortic dissection
Atrial myxoma
Pericardial disease, tamponade
Hypertrophic obstructive cardiomyopathy
Myocardial ischemia, infarction
Pulmonary embolism
Pulmonary hypertension
Arrhythmias

Bradyarrhythmias
   Atrioventricular block
   Sinus node dysfunction, bradycardia

Tachyarrhythmias
   Supraventricular tachycardia
      Atrial fibrillation
      Paroxysmal supraventricular tachycardia (AVNRT, WPW)
      Other
   Ventricular tachycardia
      Structural heart disease
      Inherited syndromes (ARVD, HCM, Brugada syndrome, long-QT syndrome)
   Drug-induced proarrhythmia
   Implanted pacemaker or ICD malfunction

Syncope of Unknown Origin

ARVD, Arrhythmogenic right ventricular dysplasia; *AVNRT,* atrioventricular nodal reentrant tachycardia; *HCM,* hypertrophic cardiomyopathy; *ICD,* implantable cardioverter-defibrillator; *WPW,* Wolff-Parkinson-White syndrome.

to the heart. This drop leads to a decrease in cardiac output and stimulation of aortic, carotid, and cardiopulmonary baroreceptors, which triggers a reflex increase in sympathetic outflow. As a result, heart rate, cardiac contractility, and vascular resistance increase to maintain stable systemic blood pressure (BP) on standing. *Orthostatic intolerance* is a term used to refer to the signs and symptoms of an abnormality in any portion of this BP control system. Orthostatic hypotension is defined as a 20-mm Hg drop in systolic BP or a 10-mm Hg drop in diastolic BP within 3 minutes of standing. Orthostatic hypotension can be asymptomatic or associated with syncope, lightheadedness/presyncope, tremulousness, weakness, fatigue, palpitations, diaphoresis, and blurred or tunnel vision. Many patients with orthostatic hypotension are asymptomatic despite substantial falls in systolic BP and low upright BPs.[14] These symptoms are often worse immediately on arising in the morning or after meals or exercise. Initial orthostatic hypotension is defined as less than a 40-mm Hg decrease in BP immediately on standing with rapid (<30 seconds) return to normal.[1,2,12] In contrast, *delayed progressive* orthostatic hypotension is characterized by a slow progressive decrease in systolic BP on standing. Syncope that occurs after meals, particularly in older adults, can result from a redistribution of blood to the gut. A decline in systolic BP of approximately 20 mm Hg approximately 1 hour after eating has been reported in up to one third of older adult nursing home residents. Although usually asymptomatic, it can result in lightheadedness or syncope.

Drugs that either cause volume depletion or result in vasodilation are the most common causes of orthostatic hypotension (Table 71.3). Older adult patients are particularly susceptible to the hypotensive effects of drugs because of reduced baroreceptor sensitivity, decreased cerebral blood flow, renal sodium wasting, and an impaired thirst mechanism that develops with aging (see Chapter 90). Orthostatic hypotension can also result from neurogenic causes, which can be subclassified into primary and secondary *autonomic failure* (see Chapter 102). Primary causes are generally idiopathic, whereas secondary causes are associated with a known biochemical or structural anomaly or are seen as part of a particular disease or syndrome.

There are three types of primary autonomic failure. *Pure autonomic failure* (Bradbury-Eggleston syndrome) is an idiopathic sporadic disorder characterized by orthostatic hypotension, usually in conjunction with evidence of more widespread autonomic failure, such as disturbances in bowel, bladder, thermoregulatory, and sexual function. Patients with pure autonomic failure have reduced supine plasma norepinephrine levels. *Multisystem atrophy* (Shy-Drager syndrome) is a sporadic, progressive, adult-onset disorder characterized by autonomic dysfunction, parkinsonism, and ataxia in any combination. The third type of primary autonomic failure is *Parkinson disease* with autonomic failure. A small subset of patients with Parkinson disease may also experience autonomic failure, including orthostatic hypotension. In addition to these forms of chronic autonomic failure is a rare, acute *panautonomic neuropathy.* This neuropathy generally occurs in young people and results in severe, widespread sympathetic and parasympathetic failure with orthostatic hypotension, loss of sweating, disruption of bladder and bowel function, fixed heart rate, and fixed dilated pupils.

Postural orthostatic tachycardia syndrome (POTS) is a clinical syndrome characterized by frequent symptoms that occur with standing (e.g., lightheadedness, palpitations, tremulousness, generalized weakness, blurred vision, exercise intolerance, fatigue), an increase in heart rate of 30 beats/min or more on standing (or ≥40 beats/min in those 12 to 19 years of age), and absence of a more than 20-mm Hg reduction in systolic BP.[1,2,13] The precise pathophysiologic basis for POTS has not been well defined. Some patients have both POTS and NMS.

Reflex-Mediated Syncope

Reflex-mediated, or *situational,* causes of syncope are listed in Table 71.2. In this group of conditions, the cardiovascular reflexes that control the circulation become inappropriate in response to a trigger, which results in vasodilation with or without bradycardia and a drop in BP and global cerebral hypoperfusion. In each case the reflex is composed of a trigger (the afferent limb) and a response (the efferent limb). This group of reflex-mediated

TABLE 71.3 Causes of Orthostatic Hypotension

Drugs

Diuretics

Alpha-adrenergic blocking drugs
  Terazosin (Hytrin), labetalol

Adrenergic neuron-blocking drugs
  Guanethidine

Angiotensin-converting enzyme inhibitors

Antidepressants
  Monoamine oxidase inhibitors

Alcohol

Ganglion-blocking drugs
  Hexamethonium, mecamylamine

Tranquilizers
  Phenothiazines, barbiturates

Vasodilators
  Prazosin, hydralazine, calcium channel blockers

Centrally acting hypotensive drugs
  Methyldopa, clonidine

Primary Disorders of Autonomic Failure

Pure autonomic failure (Bradbury-Eggleston syndrome)

Multisystem atrophy (Shy-Drager syndrome)

Parkinson disease with autonomic failure

Secondary Neurogenic Causes

Aging

Autoimmune disease
  Guillain-Barré syndrome, mixed connective tissue disease, rheumatoid arthritis
  Eaton-Lambert syndrome, systemic lupus erythematosus

Carcinomatosis autonomic neuropathy

Central brain lesions
  Multiple sclerosis, Wernicke encephalopathy
  Vascular lesions or tumors involving hypothalamus and midbrain

Dopamine beta-hydroxylase deficiency

Familial hyperbradykininism

General medical disorders
  Diabetes, amyloid, alcoholism, renal failure

Hereditary sensory neuropathies, dominant or recessive

Infections of the nervous system
  Human immunodeficiency virus infection, Chagas disease, botulism, syphilis

Metabolic disease
  Vitamin B_{12} deficiency, porphyria, Fabry disease, Tangier disease

Spinal cord lesions

Modified from Bannister SR, ed. *Autonomic Failure*. 2nd ed. Oxford: Oxford University Press; 1988:8.

syncopal syndromes has in common the response limb of the reflex, which consists of increased vagal tone and withdrawal of peripheral sympathetic tone and leads to bradycardia, vasodilation, and ultimately, hypotension, presyncope, or syncope. If hypotension secondary to peripheral vasodilation predominates, it is classified as a *vasodepressor-type* reflex response; if bradycardia or asystole predominates, it is classified as a *cardioinhibitory* response; and when both vasodilation and bradycardia play a role, it is classified as a *mixed* response. Specific triggers distinguish these causes of syncope. For example, micturition-induced syncope results from activation of mechanoreceptors in the bladder, defecation-induced syncope results from neural input from gut wall tension receptors, and swallowing-induced syncope results from afferent neural impulses arising from the upper gastrointestinal tract. The two most common types of reflex-mediated syncope, carotid sinus

hypersensitivity and neurally mediated hypotension, are discussed later. Identification of the trigger is of importance because of its therapeutic implications, with avoidance of the trigger, where possible, preventing further syncopal episodes.

Neurally Mediated Hypotension or Syncope (Vasovagal Syncope)

The term *neurally mediated hypotension* or *syncope* (also known as neurocardiogenic, vasodepressor, and vasovagal syncope and "fainting") has been used to describe a common abnormality in regulation of BP characterized by an abrupt onset of hypotension with or without bradycardia. Triggers associated with the development of NMS include orthostatic stress, such as can occur with prolonged standing or a hot shower, and emotional stress, such as can result from the sight of blood.[1,2,13] Neurally mediated hypotension has shown to run in families and three genes have been associated.[15] While our understanding of the genetic basis for neurally mediated hypotension is in its early stages, this is an active area of research. A large proportion of patients with NMS may have minor psychiatric disorders. Patients with syncope caused by neurally mediated hypotension may also have psychogenic pseudosyncope.[5] It has been proposed that NMS results from a paradoxical reflex that is initiated when ventricular preload is reduced by venous pooling. This reduction leads to a decrease in cardiac output and BP, which is sensed by arterial baroreceptors. The resultant increased catecholamine levels, combined with reduced venous filling, leads to a vigorously contracting, volume-depleted ventricle. The heart itself is involved in this reflex by virtue of the presence of mechanoreceptors, or C fibers, consisting of nonmyelinated fibers found in the atria, ventricles, and pulmonary artery. It has been proposed that vigorous contraction of a volume-depleted ventricle leads to activation of these receptors in susceptible individuals. These afferent C fibers project centrally to the dorsal vagal nucleus of the medulla and can result in "paradoxical" withdrawal of peripheral sympathetic tone and an increase in vagal tone, which in turn causes vasodilation and bradycardia. The ultimate clinical consequence is syncope or presyncope. It has been speculated that the fall in BP seen during neurally mediated hypotension mimics a "fictitious hemorrhage." To protect against this fictitious hemorrhage, the brainstem triggers cardioinhibition as protection against the hypothetical loss of blood simulated by the reduction in venous return. The most effective solution to stopping blood loss is to stop the heart.[16] A recent study has shown that in patients who experienced a syncopal episode during a tilt-table test there was sympathetic activation before a syncopal event followed by sympathetic withdrawal and parasympathetic activation.[17] Not all NMS, however, results from activation of mechanoreceptors. In humans the sight of blood or extreme emotion can trigger syncope, thus suggesting that higher neural centers can also participate in the pathophysiology of vasovagal syncope. In addition, central mechanisms can contribute to the production of NMS.

Carotid Sinus Hypersensitivity

Syncope caused by carotid sinus hypersensitivity results from stimulation of carotid sinus baroreceptors located in the internal carotid artery above the bifurcation of the common carotid artery. It is diagnosed by the reproduction of clinical syncope during carotid sinus massage, with a cardioinhibitory response if asystole is longer than 3 seconds or AV block occurs; or a significant vasodepressor response if there is a more than 50-mm Hg drop in systolic BP; or a mixed cardioinhibitory and vasodepressor response.[1] Carotid sinus hypersensitivity is detected in approximately one third of older adult patients evaluated for syncope or falls.[2] It is important, however, to recognize that carotid sinus hypersensitivity is also frequently observed in asymptomatic older adult patients. Thus the diagnosis of carotid sinus hypersensitivity should be approached cautiously after excluding alternative causes of the syncope. Once diagnosed, dual-chamber pacemaker implantation is recommended for patients with recurrent syncope or falls resulting from carotid sinus hypersensitivity that is cardioinhibitory or mixed (class 2A/IIa, level of evidence [LOE] B-R).[1,2,18]

CARDIAC CAUSES OF SYNCOPE

Cardiac causes of syncope, particularly tachyarrhythmias and brad-yarrhythmias, are the second most common cause of syncope and account for 10% to 20% of syncopal episodes (see Table 71.2 and Chapters 65 and 67).VT is the most common tachyarrhythmia that can cause syncope. Supraventricular tachycardia (SVT) can also cause syncope, although the great majority of patients with supraventricular arrhythmias have less severe symptoms, such as palpitations, dyspnea, and lightheadedness. Bradyarrhythmias that can result in syncope include sick sinus syndrome and atrioventricular (AV) block. Anatomic causes of syncope include obstruction to blood flow, such as massive pulmonary embolism (see Chapter 87), atrial myxoma (Chapter 98), or aortic stenosis (Chapter 72).

NEUROLOGIC CAUSES OF TRANSIENT LOSS OF CONSCIOUSNESS

Neurologic causes of transient LOC, including migraines, seizures, Arnold-Chiari malformations, and transient ischemic attacks, are surprisingly uncommon and account for less than 10% of all cases of syncope (see Chapters 45 and 100). Most patients in whom a "neurologic" cause of transient LOC is established are in fact found to have had a seizure rather than true syncope.

METABOLIC CAUSES OF TRANSIENT LOSS OF CONSCIOUSNESS

Metabolic causes of transient LOC are rare and account for less than 5% of syncopal episodes. The most common metabolic causes of syncope are hypoglycemia (see Chapter 31), hypoxia, and hyperventilation. Establishing hypoglycemia as the cause of apparent LOC requires demonstration of hypoglycemia during the syncopal episode. Although hyperventilation-induced syncope has generally been considered to result from a reduction in cerebral blood flow, one study demonstrated that hyperventilation alone was not sufficient to cause syncope. This observation suggests that hyperventilation-induced syncope may also have a psychological component. Psychiatric disorders can also cause syncope. Up to one fourth of patients with syncope of unknown origin may have psychiatric disorders for which apparent syncope is one of the initial symptoms (see Chapter 99).[1]

DIAGNOSTIC TESTS

Identification of the precise cause of the syncope is often challenging. Because syncope usually occurs sporadically and infrequently, it is extremely difficult to examine a patient or obtain an electrocardiogram (ECG) during an episode of syncope. For this reason, the primary goal in the evaluation of a patient with syncope is to arrive at a presumptive determination of the cause of the syncope.

History, Physical Examination, and Carotid Sinus Massage

The history and physical examination are by far the most important components of the evaluation of a patient with transient LOC and syncope and can be used to identify the cause in more than 25% of patients.[1,2,13,19–21] The 2017 ACC/AHA/HRS syncope guidelines provide a class I (LOE B-NR) recommendation for performing a detailed history and physical examination in patients with syncope.[1] Maximal information can be obtained from the clinical history when it is approached in a systematic and detailed manner. Initial evaluation should begin by determining whether the patient did in fact experience a syncopal episode by asking the following: (1) Did the patient experience complete LOC? (2) Was the LOC transient with a rapid onset and short duration? (3) Did the patient recover spontaneously, completely, and without

sequelae? and (4) Did the patient lose postural tone? If the answer to one or more of these questions is negative, other nonsyncopal causes of transient LOC should be suspected. Although falls can be differentiated from syncope by the absence of LOC, an overlap between symptoms of falls and syncope has been reported,[2,22] because older adults may experience amnesia for the LOC episode. When evaluating a patient with syncope, particular attention should then be focused on (1) determining whether the patient has a history of cardiac disease or metabolic disease (i.e., diabetes) or a family history of cardiac disease, syncope, or sudden death; (2) identifying medications that may have played a role in syncope, especially those that may cause hypotension, bradycardia/heart block, or a proarrhythmic response (antiarrhythmics); (3) quantifying the number and chronicity of previous syncopal and presyncopal episodes; (4) identifying precipitating factors, including body position and activity immediately before syncope; and (5) quantifying the type and duration of prodromal and recovery symptoms. It is also useful to obtain careful accounts from witnesses to provide a detailed description of the episode, including how the patient collapsed and the patient's skin color and breathing pattern, duration of unconsciousness, and movements during the episode of unconsciousness. Table 71.4 summarizes features of the clinical history most helpful in differentiating neurally mediated hypotension, arrhythmia, seizures, and psychogenic syncope.

The clinical histories obtained from patients with syncope related to AV block and VT are similar. In each case, syncope typically occurs with less than 5 seconds of warning and few if any prodromal and recovery symptoms. Demographic features suggesting that the syncope results from an arrhythmia such as VT or AV block include male sex, fewer than three previous episodes of syncope, and increased age. Features of the clinical history that point toward a diagnosis of NMS include palpitations, blurred vision, nausea, warmth, diaphoresis, or lightheadedness before syncope and the presence of nausea, warmth, diaphoresis, or fatigue after syncope.

Features of the clinical history useful in distinguishing seizures from syncope include orientation following an event, a blue face or not becoming pale during the event, frothing at the mouth, aching muscles, feeling sleepy after the event, time of seizure relative to onset of syncope—early points to neurologic whereas late suggests arrhythmic cause—and a duration of unconsciousness of longer than 5 minutes.[20] Tongue biting strongly points toward a seizure rather than syncope as the cause of LOC. One recent study reported that a history of tongue biting during an episode of LOC had 33% sensitivity and 96% specificity in predicting a seizure as the cause of the LOC.[21] Other findings suggestive of a seizure as a cause of the syncopal episode include (1) an aura before the episode, (2) horizontal eye deviation during the episode, (3) elevated BP and pulse during the episode, and (4) a headache following the event. Urinary or fecal incontinence can be observed with either a seizure or a syncopal episode but occurs more often with a seizure. Grand mal seizures are usually associated with tonic-clonic movements. It is important to note that syncope caused by cerebral ischemia can result in decorticate rigidity with clonic movements of the arms. Akinetic or petit mal seizures can be recognized by the patient's lack of responsiveness in the absence of loss of postural tone. Temporal lobe seizures last several minutes and are characterized by confusion, changes in level of consciousness, and autonomic signs such as flushing. Vertebral basilar insufficiency should be considered as the cause of the syncope if it occurs in association with other symptoms of brainstem ischemia (i.e., diplopia, tinnitus, focal weakness or sensory loss, vertigo, or dysarthria). Migraine-mediated syncope is often associated with a throbbing unilateral headache, scintillating scotomata, and nausea.

Physical Examination

In addition to a complete cardiac examination, particular attention should be focused on whether structural heart disease is present, defining the patient's level of hydration, and detecting the presence of significant neurologic abnormalities suggestive of dysautonomia or a cerebrovascular accident. Orthostatic vital signs are a critical component of the evaluation. The patient's BP and heart rate should be determined while supine and then repeated each minute for approximately

TABLE 71.4 Differentiation of Syncope Caused by Neurally Mediated Hypotension, Arrhythmias, Seizures, and Psychogenic Causes

	NEURALLY MEDIATED HYPOTENSION	ARRHYTHMIAS	SEIZURES	PSYCHOGENIC
Demographics and clinical setting	Female > male sex Younger age (<55 years) More episodes (>2) Standing, warm room, emotional upset	Male > female sex Older age (>54 years) Fewer episodes (<3) During exertion or supine Family history of sudden death	Younger age (<45 years) Any setting	Female > male sex Occurs in presence of others Younger age (<40 years) Many episodes (often many episodes in a day) No identifiable trigger
Premonitory symptoms	Longer duration (>5 sec) Palpitations Blurred vision Nausea Warmth Diaphoresis Lightheadedness	Shorter duration (<6 sec) Palpitations less common	Sudden onset or brief aura (déjà vu, olfactory, gustatory, visual)	Usually absent
Observations during the event	Pallor Diaphoresis Dilated pupils Slow pulse, low BP Incontinence may occur Brief clonic movements may occur	Blue, not pale Incontinence may occur Brief clonic movements may occur	Blue face, no pallor Frothing at the mouth Prolonged syncope (duration > 5 min) Tongue biting Horizontal eye deviation Elevated pulse and BP Incontinence more likely* Tonic-clonic movements if grand mal	Normal color Not diaphoretic Eyes closed Normal pulse and BP No incontinence Prolonged duration (minutes) common
Residual symptoms	Residual symptoms common Prolonged fatigue common (>90%) Oriented	Residual symptoms uncommon (unless prolonged unconsciousness) Oriented	Residual symptoms common Aching muscles Disoriented Fatigue Headache Slow recovery	Residual symptoms uncommon Oriented

*May be observed with any of these causes of syncope but more common with seizures.
BP, Blood pressure.

3 minutes while standing. The two abnormalities that should be sought are (1) early orthostatic hypotension, defined as a 20-mm Hg drop in systolic BP or a 10-mm Hg drop in diastolic BP within 3 minutes of standing, and (2) POTS, an increase in heart rate of 30 beats/min or more on standing (or ≥40 beats/min in those 12 to 19 years of age), and absence of a more than 20-mm Hg reduction in systolic BP.[1,2,13] The significance of POTS lies in its close overlap with NMS.

Carotid Sinus Massage

Carotid sinus massage should be performed after checking for bruits by applying *gentle* pressure over the carotid pulsation, first one side and then the other, just below the angle of the jaw where the carotid bifurcation is located. Pressure should be applied for 5 to 10 seconds in both the supine and the upright position because an abnormal response to carotid sinus massage is present only in the upright position in up to one third of patients. Since the main complications associated with performing carotid sinus massage are neurologic, it should be avoided in patients with previous transient ischemic attacks, strokes within the past 3 months, and carotid bruits, except if significant stenosis has been excluded by carotid Doppler studies. A normal response to carotid sinus massage is a transient decrease in the sinus rate, prolongation of AV conduction, or both. Carotid sinus hypersensitivity is diagnosed by the reproduction of clinical syncope during carotid sinus massage and the responses previously noted.[1] Diagnosis of carotid sinus hypersensitivity as the cause of the syncope requires reproduction of the patient's symptoms during carotid sinus massage.

Laboratory Testing: Blood Tests

Routine use of blood tests, such as serum electrolytes, cardiac enzymes, glucose, and hematocrit levels, is of low diagnostic value in syncopal patients and therefore not recommended routinely. The 2017 ACC/AHA/HRS syncope guidelines state that targeted blood tests are reasonable in the evaluation of selected patients with syncope identified based on clinical assessment from history, physical examination, and ECG (class IIa, LOE B-NR).[1]

Tilt-Table Test

The tilt-table test is a valuable diagnostic test for evaluating patients with syncope,[1,2,13] with a positive response indicating susceptibility to NMS. The 2017 ACC/AHA/HRS syncope guidelines state that tilt-table testing can be useful for patients with suspected vasovagal syncope if the diagnosis is unclear after initial evaluation (class IIa, LOE B-NR).[1] Upright tilt testing is generally performed for 30 to 45 minutes following a 20-minute horizontal pretilt stabilization phase at an angle between 60 and 80 degrees (with 70 degrees being most common). The sensitivity of the test can be increased, along with an associated fall in specificity, by the use of longer tilt durations, steeper tilt angles, and provocative agents such as isoproterenol or nitroglycerin. When isoproterenol is used, it is recommended that the infusion rate be increased incrementally from 1 to 3 µg/min to increase the heart rate 25% greater than baseline. When nitroglycerin is used, a fixed dose of 300 to 400 µg of nitroglycerin spray should be administered sublingually after a 20-minute unmedicated phase with the patient in the upright position. These two provocative approaches are equivalent in diagnostic accuracy. In the absence of pharmacologic provocation, the specificity of the test has been estimated to be 90%; when provocative agents are used, specificity decreases significantly.

The main indication for upright tilt testing is to confirm a diagnosis of NMS when the initial evaluation was insufficient to establish this diagnosis. Tilt-table testing is also of value in diagnosing psychogenic pseudosyncope.[5] Upright tilt testing is not generally recommended in patients in whom the diagnosis can be established from the initial history and physical examination. However, for some patients, confirmation of the diagnosis with a positive response to upright tilt testing is very reassuring. Induction of reflex hypotension/bradycardia without reproduction of the syncope points toward a diagnosis of NMS but is a less specific response. If a patient has structural heart disease, other cardiovascular causes of syncope should be excluded before considering a positive response to upright tilt testing to be diagnostic of NMS. Upright tilt testing is also indicated in the evaluation of patients for whom the cause of the syncope has been determined (i.e., asystole), but the presence of NMS on upright tilt would influence treatment. Upright tilt testing has also been shown to be of value in patients with psychogenic causes of syncope in that it may trigger LOC in association with a normal BP and heart rate. Induction of LOC with no change in vital signs points strongly toward a diagnosis of psychogenic pseudosyncope. Upright tilt testing has no value in assessing the efficacy of treatment of NMS.

Cardiac Imaging

Echocardiograms are frequently used to evaluate patients with syncope (see Chapter 16), but current guidelines suggest that an echocardiogram should be performed only in patients suspected of having structural heart disease.[1,2] The 2017 ACC/AHA/HRS syncope guidelines state that echocardiography can be useful in selected patients presenting with syncope if structural heart disease is suspected (class IIa, LOE B-NR).[1] The guidelines also state that routine cardiac imaging is not useful in the evaluation of patients with syncope unless cardiac etiology is suspected on the basis of an initial evaluation including history, physical examination, or ECG (class 3/III, LOE B-NR).[1] These guidelines also recommend that computed tomography (CT) or magnetic resonance imaging (MRI) may be useful in selected patients presenting with syncope of suspected cardiac etiology (class IIb, LOE B-NR).[1] Studies have shown that the diagnostic yield of an echocardiogram in a syncope patient with a normal ECG and physical examination is extremely low. Therefore, routine echocardiograms are not advised in this setting. For example, an echocardiogram should be obtained in patients who have clinical features suggestive of a cardiac cause of the syncope, such as syncope with exertion or while supine, a family history of sudden death, or syncope of abrupt onset. Echocardiographic findings considered diagnostic of the cause of syncope include severe aortic stenosis, pericardial tamponade, aortic dissection, congenital abnormalities of the coronary arteries, and obstructive atrial myxomas or thrombi. Findings of impaired right or left ventricular function, evidence of right ventricular overload or pulmonary hypertension (pulmonary emboli), or the presence of hypertrophic cardiomyopathy (see Chapter 54) are of prognostic importance and justify additional diagnostic testing.

Stress Tests and Cardiac Catheterization

Myocardial ischemia is an unlikely cause of syncope and, when present, is usually accompanied by angina (see Chapters 35 and 40). The use of stress tests (see Chapter 15) is best reserved for patients in whom syncope or presyncope occurred during or immediately after exertion in association with chest pain or in a patient at high risk for coronary artery disease.[1,2] The 2017 ACC/AHA/HRS syncope guidelines state exercise stress testing can be useful to establish the cause of syncope in selected patients who experience syncope or presyncope during exertion (class IIa, LOE C-LD).[1] Syncope occurring during exercise is suggestive of a cardiac cause. In contrast, syncope following exercise is usually caused by NMS. Even in patients with syncope during exertion,

exercise stress testing is highly unlikely to trigger another event. Coronary angiography is recommended in patients with syncope suspected to result, directly or indirectly, from myocardial ischemia.

Electrocardiography

The 12-lead ECG is another important component in the workup of a patient with syncope (see Chapter 14). The 2017 ACC/AHA/HRS syncope guidelines provide a class I (LOE B-NR) recommendation for performing an ECG in patients with syncope.[1] The initial ECG results in establishment of a diagnosis in approximately 5% of patients and suggests a diagnosis in another 5% of patients. Specific findings that can identify the probable cause of the syncope include QT prolongation (long-QT syndrome), the presence of a short PR interval and a delta wave (Wolff-Parkinson-White syndrome), the presence of a right bundle branch block pattern with ST-segment elevation (Brugada syndrome), or evidence of acute myocardial infarction, high-grade AV block, or T wave inversion in the right precordial leads (arrhythmogenic right ventricular dysplasia) (see Chapters 63, 65 and 67). Any abnormal finding on the baseline ECG is an independent predictor of cardiac syncope or increased mortality and suggests the need to pursue evaluation of cardiac causes of syncope.[1] Most patients with syncope have normal findings on ECGs, which is useful because it suggests a low likelihood of a cardiac cause of the syncope and is associated with an excellent prognosis, particularly when observed in a young patient with syncope. Despite the low diagnostic yield of electrocardiography, the test is inexpensive and risk free and is considered a standard part of the evaluation of virtually all patients with syncope.[1]

Cardiac Monitoring

Continuous ECG monitoring via telemetry or Holter monitoring is frequently performed in patients with syncope but is unlikely to identify the cause of the syncope (see Chapter 61). Over the past 5 years, patch monitoring and mobile cardiac telemetry have been developed to allow long-term continuous recording of heart rhythm. The mobile cardiac telemetry transmits real-time ECG recordings to a service center. The prescribing physicians are alerted when serious arrhythmias occur. The patch monitoring stores heart rhythm over a 1- to 2-week period for later off-line analyses but does not transmit data real time. Both types of devices may result in higher diagnostic yield in patients with syncope or presyncope than do the conventional event monitors just described. The information provided by ECG monitoring at the time of syncope is extremely valuable in that it allows an arrhythmic cause of syncope to be established or excluded. Another clinically useful finding is detection of symptoms in the absence of an arrhythmia, which is observed in up to 15% of patients undergoing continuous ECG monitoring. It is important to emphasize that the absence of an arrhythmia and symptoms during continuous ECG monitoring may not exclude an arrhythmia as the cause of the syncope. In patients suspected of having an arrhythmia as the cause of the syncope, additional evaluation, such as electrophysiologic (EP) testing or event monitoring, should be considered. Inpatient telemetry monitoring or continuous ECG monitoring is recommended for patients who have clinical or ECG features suggesting an arrhythmic syncope or a history of recurrent syncope with injury. Continuous ECG monitoring and inpatient telemetry monitoring are most likely to be diagnostic when used for the occasional patient with frequent (i.e., daily) episodes of syncope or presyncope.

In patients with extremely infrequent episodes of syncope (e.g., once or twice a year), a traditional non-invasive monitoring device is unlikely to record an event. Implantable event recorders address this problem by triggering automatically on the basis of programmed detection criteria, as well as with a handheld activator, and storing the ECG signal in a circular buffer (see Chapter 61). These devices, with battery lives up to 3 years, store data that can be also be downloaded with remote telemetry. They can be implanted with a minimally procedure in the outpatient clinic or in a procedure room. The main disadvantage of these devices is their cost. Implantable loop recorders have also been shown to improve the diagnostic yield in patients with syncope.[23] However, a Cochrane meta-analysis showed no impact of implantable loop recorders on mortality.[23]

TABLE 71.5 Indications for and Diagnostic Findings of Electrophysiologic Testing in Evaluation of Patients with Syncope

INDICATIONS/DIAGNOSTIC CRITERIA	CLASS	LEVEL OF EVIDENCE
Indications		
In patients with ischemic heart disease when the initial evaluation suggests an arrhythmic cause and there is no established indication for an ICD.	I	B
In patients with BBB, EPS should be considered when noninvasive tests do not establish a diagnosis.	IIa	B
In patients with syncope preceded by sudden and brief palpitations when noninvasive tests do not establish a diagnosis	IIb	B
In patients with syncope and Brugada syndrome, ARVD, or hypertrophic cardiomyopathy, EPS is appropriate in selected cases.	IIb	C
In patients with high-risk occupations, in whom every effort to exclude a cardiovascular cause of syncope is warranted	IIb	C
EPS is not recommended in syncopal patients with normal findings on an ECG, no structural heart disease, and no palpitations.	III	B
Diagnostic Criteria		
EPS is diagnostic and no additional tests are required in the following situations:		
Sinus bradycardia and a prolonged CSNRT (>525 msec)	I	B
BBB and either a baseline H-V interval ≥100 msec or second- or third-degree His-Purkinje block during incremental atrial pacing or with pharmacologic challenge	I	B
Induction of sustained monomorphic VT in patients with a previous myocardial infarction	I	B
Induction of SVT with reproduction of the hypotensive or spontaneous symptoms	I	B
H-V interval between 70 and 100 msec should be considered diagnostic.	IIa	B
Induction of polymorphic VT or VF in patients with Brugada syndrome, patients with ARVD, or patients resuscitated from cardiac arrest	IIb	B
Induction of polymorphic VT or VF in patients with ischemic disease or DCM should not be considered a diagnostic finding.	III	B

ARVD, Arrhythmogenic right ventricular dysplasia; *BBB,* bundle branch block; *CSNRT,* corrected sinus node recovery time; *DCM,* dilated cardiomyopathy; *ECG,* electrocardiogram; *EPS,* electrophysiologic study; *H-V,* His-ventricular; *ICD,* implantable cardioverter-defibrillator; *SVT,* supraventricular tachycardia; *VF,* ventricular fibrillation; *VT,* ventricular tachycardia.
Modified from Moya A, Sutton R, Ammirati R, et al. Guidelines for the diagnosis and management of syncope 2009. *Eur Heart J.* 2009;30:2631.

The 2017 ACC/AHA/HRS syncope guidelines state that the choice of a specific cardiac monitor should be determined on the basis of the frequency and nature of the syncope events (class I, LOE C-EO). The guidelines also state that each of the monitors previously discussed can be useful to evaluate selected ambulatory patients with syncope of suspected arrhythmic etiology (class IIa, LOE B-NR).[1]

Electrophysiologic Testing

EP testing can provide important diagnostic information in patients with syncope by establishing a diagnosis of sick sinus syndrome, carotid sinus hypersensitivity, heart block, SVT, and VT (see Chapter 61). Table 71.5 presents indications for EP testing and diagnostic findings in the evaluation of patients with syncope.[2] The 2017 ACC/AHA/HRS syncope guidelines state that an electrophysiologic study (EPS) can be useful for evaluation of select patients with syncope of suspected arrhythmic etiology (class IIa, LOE B-NR). These guidelines further note that EPS is not recommended for syncope evaluation in patients with a normal ECG and normal cardiac structure and function, unless an arrhythmic etiology is suspected (class III, LOE B-NR).[1] It is generally agreed that EP testing should be performed in patients when the initial evaluation suggests an arrhythmic cause of the syncope,[2] such as those with abnormal findings on an ECG or structural heart disease, those whose clinical history suggests an arrhythmic cause of the syncope, and those with a family history of sudden death. EP testing should not be performed in patients with normal findings on an ECG and no heart disease and in whom the clinical history does not suggest an arrhythmic cause of the syncope. The class II indications for performing EPS are shown in Table 71.5, which indicates that EP testing is appropriate when the results may have an impact on treatment and also in patients with "high-risk" occupations, in whom every effort should be expended to determine the probable cause of the syncope. EP testing is no longer indicated for patients with a severely depressed ejection fraction, because in this setting an implantable cardioverter-defibrillator (ICD) is indicated regardless of the presence or mechanism of the syncope.[1,2]

Electrophysiologic Testing Protocol

A comprehensive EP evaluation should be performed in patients with syncope, including evaluation of sinus node function by measuring the sinus node recovery time (SNRT) and evaluation of AV conduction by measuring the His-ventricular (H-V) interval at baseline, with atrial pacing, and following pharmacologic challenge with intravenous procainamide. In addition, programmed electrical stimulation using standard techniques should be performed to evaluate the inducibility of ventricular and supraventricular arrhythmias. Although the minimal suggested EP protocol includes only double extra stimuli and two basic drive train cycle lengths, it is common practice in the United States to include triple extra stimuli and three basic drive train cycle lengths. It is also common practice to limit the shortest coupling interval to 200 milliseconds. In select patients in whom suspicion for ventricular arrhythmia is high, EP testing with atrial and ventricular programmed stimulation may be repeated following an infusion of isoproterenol, which is of particular importance for patients suspected of having a supraventricular arrhythmia, such as AV nodal reentrant tachycardia or orthodromic AV reciprocating tachycardia, as the cause of the syncope.

Sinus node function is evaluated during EP testing primarily by determining the SNRT. Identification of sinus node dysfunction as the cause of syncope is uncommon during EP tests (<5%). The sensitivity of an abnormal SNRT or corrected SNRT (CSNRT) is approximately 50% to 80%. The specificity of an abnormal SNRT or CSNRT is less than 95%. It is important to note that the absence of evidence of sinus node dysfunction during EP testing does not exclude a bradyarrhythmia as the cause of the syncope (see Chapter 68).

During EP testing, AV conduction is assessed by measuring the AV nodal–to–His bundle conduction time (A-H interval) and the His bundle–to–ventricular conduction time (H-V interval) and also by determining the response of AV conduction to incremental atrial pacing and atrial premature stimuli. If the results of an initial assessment of AV conduction in the baseline state are inconclusive, procainamide (10 mg/kg) can be administered intravenously and atrial pacing and programmed stimulation repeated. Findings on EPS that allow heart block to be established as the probable cause of the syncope are bundle branch block and a baseline H-V interval of 100 milliseconds or longer, or demonstration of second- or third-degree His-Purkinje block during incremental atrial pacing or provoked by an infusion of procainamide (see Table 71.5). An H-V interval of 70 to 100 milliseconds is of less certain diagnostic value. In studies of EP testing to evaluate patients with syncope, AV block was identified as the probable cause of syncope in approximately 10% to 15% of patients.

Although it is uncommon for SVT to result in syncope, this is an important diagnosis to establish because most types of supraventricular arrhythmias can be cured with catheter ablation (see Chapters 64 and 65). The usual setting in which SVT causes syncope is in a patient with underlying heart disease and/or limited cardiovascular reserve, a patient with SVT of abrupt onset and with an extremely rapid rate, or a patient who has a propensity for the development of NMS. The typical pattern is the development of syncope or near-syncope at the onset of the SVT because of an initial drop in BP. The patient often regains consciousness despite continuation of the arrhythmia as a result of activation of a compensatory mechanism. Completion of a standard EP test allows accurate identification of most types of supraventricular arrhythmias that may have caused the syncope, and it should be repeated during an isoproterenol infusion to increase the sensitivity of the study, particularly for detecting AV nodal reentrant tachycardia in a patient with dual–AV node physiology or catecholamine-sensitive atrial fibrillation. An EPS is considered diagnostic of SVT as the cause of syncope when induction of a rapid supraventricular arrhythmia reproduces the hypotensive or spontaneous symptoms (see Table 71.5). A supraventricular arrhythmia is diagnosed as the probable cause of syncope in fewer than 5% of patients who undergo EP testing for evaluation of syncope of unknown origin, but the probability is increased in patients who report a history of palpitations ("heart racing") before syncope.

VT is the most common abnormality uncovered during EP testing in patients with syncope and was identified as the probable cause in approximately 20% of patients (see Chapter 67). In general, an EP test is interpreted as positive for VT when sustained monomorphic VT is induced. Induction of polymorphic VT and VF may represent a non-specific response to EP testing. The diagnostic and prognostic importance of induction of polymorphic VT or VF remains uncertain. An EPS is considered diagnostic of VT as the cause of the syncope when sustained monomorphic VT is induced (see Table 71.5),[2] with less certain diagnostic value with induction of polymorphic VT or VF in patients with Brugada syndrome or arrhythmogenic right ventricular dysplasia and in patients resuscitated from cardiac arrest. The role of EP testing and pharmacologic challenge with procainamide in syncope patients with suspected Brugada syndrome is controversial.[24]

Overall, approximately one third of patients with syncope referred for diagnostic EP testing have a presumptive diagnosis established.

Test to Screen for Neurologic Causes of Syncope

Syncope as an isolated symptom rarely has a neurologic cause. As a result, widespread use of tests to screen for neurologic conditions is rarely diagnostic.[1,2] In many institutions, CT scans, electroencephalograms (EEGs), and carotid duplex scans are overused; these are obtained in more than 50% of patients with syncope. A diagnosis is almost never uncovered that was not first suspected on the basis of a careful history and neurologic examination. A recent systematic review of CT imaging in patients who present with syncope found that more than half of syncope patients had a head CT performed and the diagnostic yield was 1.1% to 3.8%.[25] Transient ischemic attacks that result from carotid disease are not accompanied by LOC. No studies have suggested that carotid Doppler ultrasonography is beneficial in patients with syncope. EEGs should be obtained only in patients with a relatively high likelihood of epilepsy. CT and MRI should be avoided in patients with uncomplicated syncope (see Chapters 19 and 20). Although the low diagnostic yield of screening "neurologic tests" has been recognized for more than a decade, they continue to be overused and result in a dramatic increase in costs.

The 2017 ACC/AHA/HRS syncope guidelines state that MRI and CT of the head are not recommended in the routine evaluation of patients with syncope in the absence of focal neurologic findings or

head injury that support further evaluation (class III, LOE B-NR). The guidelines also provide a class III recommendation for the routine use of carotid artery imaging and EEG in the evaluation of patients with syncope.[1]

APPROACH TO THE EVALUATION OF PATIENTS WITH SYNCOPE

Figure 71.1 outlines the approach to the diagnostic evaluation of a patient with syncope proposed by the 2017 ACC/AHA/HRS Syncope Guidelines.[1] This is consistent with the approach also recommended in the 2018 ESC guidelines.[2] The first step is to take a careful history, perform a physical examination, and obtain an ECG. In some patients the diagnosis can be established based on this limited evaluation. For most patients, the diagnosis is unclear and additional evaluation will be needed as outlined in the Figure 71.1.

The initial evaluation begins with a careful history, physical examination, supine and upright BP, and a 12-lead ECG, followed by additional testing in select patient subgroups, including carotid sinus massage, echocardiography, cardiac ECG monitoring, and tilt-table testing, as discussed earlier. The various types of neurologic testing are generally of little or no value except in the case of head trauma and when nonsyncopal causes of transient LOC such as epilepsy are suspected.

The European and ACC/AHA/HRS guidelines on management of syncope have called attention to the importance of a structured care pathway in the evaluation of patients with syncope.[1,2,26,27] Other studies have reported favorable outcomes when a syncope evaluation unit or standardized approach to the evaluation of syncope is used.[27,28]

MANAGEMENT OF PATIENTS WITH SYNCOPE

Treatment of a patient with syncope has three goals: (1) prolong survival, (2) prevent traumatic injuries, and (3) prevent recurrences of syncope. The approach to treatment of a patient with syncope depends largely on the cause and mechanism of the syncope. For example, the appropriate treatment of a patient with syncope related to AV block would be a pacemaker in most situations. However, a patient with syncope secondary to heart block in the setting of an inferior wall myocardial infarction will not usually require a permanent pacemaker because the heart block usually resolves spontaneously. Similarly, heart block resulting from NMS does not generally require pacemaker implantation. Treatment of a patient with syncope related to Wolff-Parkinson-White syndrome typically involves catheter ablation, and treatment of a patient with syncope related to VT or in the setting of ischemic or nonischemic cardiomyopathy would probably involve placement of an implantable defibrillator (see Chapter 69). However, ICD implantation may not be required for patients with VT/VF occurring within 48 hours of an acute myocardial infarction. For other types of syncope, optimal management may involve discontinuation of an offending pharmacologic agent, an increase in salt intake, or education of the patient.[29]

Other issues that need to be considered include the indication for hospitalization of a patient with syncope and the duration of driving restrictions. Current guidelines recommend that patients with syncope be hospitalized when there is known or suspected heart disease, ECG abnormalities suggestive of arrhythmic syncope, syncope with severe injury or during exercise, and syncope in patients with a family history of sudden death (Table 71.6).[1]

Physicians who care for patients with syncope are often asked to address the issue of driving risk. Patients who experience syncope while driving pose a risk both to themselves and to others. One study has reported that a prior hospitalization for syncope was associated with a small increase in the risk of a motor vehicle accident during follow-up.[30] Although some would argue that all patients with syncope should never drive again because of the theoretical possibility of recurrence, this is an impractical solution that would be ignored by many patients. Factors that should be considered when making a recommendation for a particular patient include: (1) the potential for

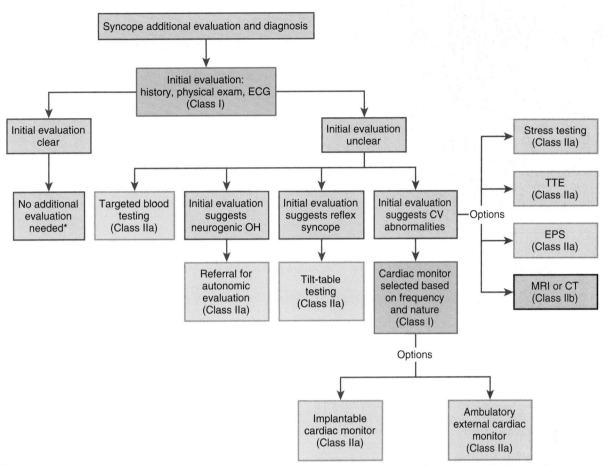

FIGURE 71.1 Diagnostic approach to the evaluation of patients with syncope. *Applies to patients with a normal evaluation, no significant cardiovascular morbidity, or significant injuries with syncope. The recommendation in the yellow boxes are for selected patients; see text for details (Adapted from Writing Committee Members; Shen WK, Sheldon RS, Benditt DG, et al. 2017 ACC/AHA/HRS guideline for the evaluation and management of patients with syncope: A report of the American College of Cardiology/American Heart Association Task Force on Clinical Practice Guidelines and the Heart Rhythm Society. J Am Coll Cardiol 70(5):e39-110.)

TABLE 71.6 Clinical Variables for Identification of High-Risk Syncope Patients Who May Benefit from Hospitalization or an Accelerated Outpatient Evaluation

Severe structural heart disease (low ejection fraction, previous myocardial infarction, heart failure)

Clinical or ECG features suggesting arrhythmic syncope
 Syncope during exertion or while supine
 Palpitations at the time of syncope
 Family history of sudden death
 Nonsustained ventricular tachycardia
 Bifascicular block or QRS >120 msec
 Severe sinus bradycardia (<50 beats/min) in the absence of medications
  or physical training
 Preexcitation
 Prolonged or very short QT interval
 Brugada ECG pattern (right bundle branch block with ST elevation in
  leads V_1–V_3)
 Arrhythmogenic right ventricular dysplasia ECG pattern (T wave inversion
  in leads V_1–V_3 with or without epsilon waves)
 ECG suggestive of hypertrophic dilated cardiomyopathy
 Clinical evidence or suspicion of a pulmonary embolus (clinical setting,
  sinus tachycardia, shortness of breath)
 Severe anemia

Important comorbid conditions
 Significant electrolyte abnormalities
 Severe anemia

ECG, Electrocardiogram.

recurrent syncope, (2) the presence and duration of warning symptoms, (3) whether syncope occurs while seated or only when standing, (4) how often and in what capacity the patient drives, and (5) whether any state laws may be applicable.

When considering these issues, physicians should note that acute illnesses, including syncope, are unlikely to cause a motor vehicle accident. The American Heart Association and the Canadian Cardiovascular Society have published guidelines concerning this issue. For noncommercial drivers, it is generally recommended that driving be restricted for several months. If the patient remains asymptomatic for several months, driving can then be resumed.

Neurally Mediated Syncope

Because NMS and reflex syncope are so common, treatment options are reviewed (Table 71.7).[1,2,13] Treatment of syncope resulting from neurally mediated hypotension begins with a careful history with particular attention on identifying precipitating factors, quantifying the degree of salt intake and current medication use, and determining whether the patient has a previous history of peripheral edema, hypertension, asthma, or other conditions that may alter the approach used for treatment. For most patients with NMS, particularly those with infrequent episodes associated with an identifiable precipitant, education plus reassurance is sufficient. Patients should be educated about common precipitating factors, such as dehydration, prolonged standing, alcohol, and medications (e.g., diuretics, vasodilators). Patients should also be taught to sit or lie down at the onset of symptoms and to initiate physical counterpressure

TABLE 71.7 Treatment of Neurally Mediated and Reflex-Mediated Syncope

TREATMENT	CLASS	LEVEL OF EVIDENCE
Patient education on diagnosis and prognosis	I	C-EO
Physical counterpressure maneuvers can be useful in patients with vasovagal syncope (VVS) who have a sufficiently long prodromal period.	IIa	B-R
Midodrine is reasonable in patients with recurrent VVS with no history of hypertension, heart failure, or urinary retention. Cardiac pacing should be considered with frequent recurrent reflex syncope, age >40 years, and documented spontaneous cardioinhibitory response during monitoring of recurrent syncope.	IIa	B-R
The use of orthostatic training is uncertain in patients with frequent VVS. Midodrine may be indicated in patients with neurally mediated syncope refractory to conservative treatment approaches.	IIb	B-R
Dual-chamber pacing might be reasonable in a select population of patients age 40 or older with recurrent VVS and prolonged spontaneous pauses.	IIb	B-R
Fludrocortisone might be reasonable for patients with recurrent VVS and inadequate response to salt and fluid intake, unless contraindicated.	IIb	B-R
Beta blockers might be reasonable in patients age 42 or older with recurrent VVS.	IIb	B-NR
Encouraging increased salt and fluid intake may be reasonable in select patients with VVS, unless contraindicated.	IIb	C-LD
In select patients with VVS, it may be reasonable to reduce or withdraw medications that can cause hypotension when appropriate.	IIb	C-LD
In select patients with VVS, a selective serotonin reuptake inhibitor might be considered.	IIb	C-LD
Beta blockers are not indicated in pediatric patients with VVS.	IIb	C-LD

Modified from Shen WK, Sheldon RS, Benditt DG, et al. 2017 ACC/AHA/HRS Guideline for the Evaluation and Management of Patients With Syncope: A Report of the American College of Cardiology/American Heart Association Task Force on Clinical Practice Guidelines and the Heart Rhythm Society. *J Am Coll Cardiol.* 2017;70:e39–e110.

maneuvers. One recent study reported that a standardized education protocol significantly reduced traumatic injuries and recurrence of syncope.[29] In this trial the syncope burden was reduced from 0.35 ± 0.3 at initial evaluation to 0.08 ± 0.02 during follow-up. Volume expansion by salt supplementation is also frequently recommended. Ingestion of approximately 500 mL of water acutely improves orthostatic tolerance to tilt in healthy persons and may be of value as prophylaxis for syncope in blood donors. The effectiveness of water ingestion alone in the management of patients with recurrent NMS has not been well studied.

A recent important shift in the approach used for the treatment of NMS has resulted from the effectiveness of "physical" measures and maneuvers in the treatment of patients with this condition.[1] Isometric physical counterpressure maneuvers such as leg crossing or handgrip with arm tensing can prevent syncope in many patients with neurally mediated hypotension. The 2017 ACC/AHA/HRS guidelines on management of syncope identify the following physical measures as class IIA treatments of NMS.[1] It has been reported that 2 minutes of an isometric handgrip maneuver initiated at the onset of symptoms during tilt testing rendered two thirds of patients asymptomatic. Other studies have demonstrated that tilt (standing) training is effective in the treatment of NMS. Standing training involves leaning against a wall with the heel 10 inches (25 cm) from the wall for progressively longer periods for 2 to 3 months. Standing time should initially be 5 minutes two times per day with a progressive increase to 40 minutes twice daily. Although the results of nonrandomized studies of standing training have been positive, the results of randomized trials suggest that standing training may have only limited effectiveness.

In contrast to these effective physical maneuvers, the value of pharmacologic agents is less certain. Medications that are generally relied on to treat NMS include beta blockers, fludrocortisone, serotonin reuptake inhibitors, and midodrine. Despite the widespread use of these agents, the quality and quantity supporting these medications in the treatment of NMS are limited. Table 71.7 shows the recommendation class for each of these medications based on the 2017 ACC/AHA/HRS syncope guidelines.[1] Even though beta blockers were previously considered by many to be first-line therapy, recent studies have reported that the beta blockers metoprolol, propranolol, and nadolol are no more effective than placebo.[13] A recent subanalysis of data from a randomized prospective study evaluating the effectiveness of fludrocortisone (Florinef) reported weak evidence that fludrocortisone may be of therapeutic value despite missing its primary endpoint.[31]

Even though pacemakers have also been found to be valuable in the treatment of some patients with NMS in nonrandomized and nonblinded clinical trials, blinded randomized clinical trials have shown that pacemakers have no benefit.[32-34] In contrast, one recent randomized trial demonstrated the benefit of implanted pacemakers in a select population of patients with NMS.[35] This double-blind placebo-controlled clinical trial randomly assigned 77 patients 40 years or older with recurrent NMS, documented by implantable loop monitor as associated with 3 seconds or longer of asystole or a 6-second or greater pause without syncope, to dual-chamber pacing with rate-drop hysteresis or to sensing only. The 2-year estimated syncope recurrence rate was 57% with pacing off and 25% with pacing on. Overall, the risk for recurrent syncope was reduced by 57% with pacing. The most recent study to examine PPM in neurally mediated syncope was the SPAIN study.[36] Forty-six patients older than 40 years of age with recurrent syncope due to neurally mediated hypotension and a tilt test demonstrating bradycardia less than 40 beats/min for 10 seconds or more than 3 seconds of asystole underwent placement of a dual-chamber pacemaker with closed-loop stimulation. Patients were randomized to DDD pacing with closed loop stimulation or DDI pacing at 30 beats/min for 12 months at a time. The study was positive and revealed that DDD pacing with closed-loop stimulation reduced the syncope burden and prolonged the time to first recurrence of syncope sevenfold. Critics of the study argue that it was not perfectly blinded as patients could sense the activation of the pacing algorithm. Based on the available literature and clinical experience the 2017 ACC/AHA/HRS syncope guidelines provide a class IIb indication for pacing in a specific subgroup of patients with neurally mediated syncope over 40 years of age (see Table 71.7).[1] When considering pacemaker implantation for patients with NMS, pacemakers that provide specialized pacing algorithms are often selected. These include rate-drop hysteresis or closed-loop stimulation[33,34] and closed-loop stimulation which is a form of rate-adaptive pacing that responds to myocardial contraction dynamics by measuring variations in right ventricular intracardiac impedance. When an incipient, neurally mediated syncopal episode is detected, the pacing rate is increased. The SPAIN trial provides important data to demonstrate the potential value of close loop stimulation.[36]

CARDIONEUROABLATION FOR TREATMENT OF NEURALLY MEDIATED SYNCOPE

In 2005 a paper was published describing a new treatment for NMS, referred to as "cardioneuroablation."[37] This report included six patients with NMS. RF ablation was used to ablate the three main cardiac ganglia. All patients responded to this treatment with a mean follow-up duration of 9 months.[37] Several years later this group published an expanded report, also with encouraging results.[38] A slightly different approach based on ablation of the typical autonomic ganglia that have been identified in patients with AF was published by a Chinese team.[39] Among 10 patients with NMS, all were free of recurrent syncope. This group has subsequently published an expanded series, also with excellent results.[40,41] The most recent report describes using the cryoballoon system to accomplish neuromodulation by targeting the four PVs, using a protocol identical to what would be used to ablate AF.[42] Among 26 patients, some of whom also had AF, 84% were free of recurrent NMS during follow-up.[42] A recent editorial has drawn attention to this new treatment strategy.[16] A major limitation of all available data is that no prospective randomized clinical trials have been performed. Clearly this is the next step before "cardioneuroablation" becomes a reality.

FUTURE PERSPECTIVES

As the US population ages and the prevalence of cardiac disease increases, it is inevitable that syncope will become an increasingly common and important problem that physicians of all types will need to address. The 2017 ACC/AHA/HRS syncope guidelines provide a timely, comprehensive update on syncope and also emphasize that further research is needed. A new generation of experts in syncope must help develop further knowledge regarding the diagnosis and management of patients with syncope. A particularly challenging problem is the management of patients with various types of orthostatic hypotension. One of the most exciting developments in this field is the potential that "cardioneuroablation" will emerge as a safe and effective treatment strategy.

REFERENCES

1. Shen WK, Sheldon RS, Benditt DG, et al. 2017 ACC/AHA/HRS guideline for the evaluation and management of patients with syncope. *Circulation*. 2017;136(5):e60–e122.
2. Brignole M, Moya A, de Lange FJ, et al. Guidelines for the diagnosis and management of syncope 2009. *Eur Heart J*. 2018;30:2631.
3. Sutton R, Benditt DG. Epidemiology and economic impact of cardiac syncope in western countries. *Future Cardiol*. 2012;8:467.
4. Ruwald MH, Hansen ML, Lamberts M, et al. The relation between age, sex, comorbidity, and pharmacotherapy and the risk of syncope: a Danish nationwide study. *Europace*. 2012;14:1506.
5. Blad H, Lamberts RJ, van Dijk GJ, Thijs RD. Tilt-induced vasovagal syncope and psychogenic pseudosyncope: overlapping clinical entities. *Neurology*. 2015;85(23):2006–2010.
6. Lieve KV, van der Werf C, Wilde AA. Catecholaminergic polymorphic ventricular tachycardia. *Arrhythm Electrophysiol Rev*. 2016;5(1):45–49.
7. Maron BJ, Rowin EJ, Casey SA, Maron MS. How hypertrophic cardiomyopathy became a contemporary treatable genetic disease with low mortality: shaped by 50 years of clinical research and practice. *JAMA Cardiol*. 2016;1(1):98–105.
8. Calkins H. Arrhythmogenic right ventricular dysplasia/cardiomyopathy: three decades of progress. *Circ J*. 2015;79(5):901–913.
9. Mizusawa Y, Wilde AA. Brugada syndrome. *Circ Arrhythm Electrophysiol*. 2012;5:606.
10. Napolitano C, Bloise R, Monteforte N, Priori SG. Sudden cardiac death and genetic ion channelopathies: long QT, Brugada, short QT, catecholaminergic polymorphic ventricular tachycardia, and idiopathic ventricular fibrillation. *Circulation*. 2012;125:2027.
11. Keller K, Beule J, Balzer JO, Dippold W. Syncope and collapse in acute pulmonary embolism. *Am J Emerg Med*. 2016;34(7):1251–1257.
12. Chisholm P, Anpalahan M. Orthostatic hypotension: pathophysiology, assessment, treatment, and the paradox of supine hypertension—a review. *Intern Med J*. 2017;47(4):370–379.
13. Sheldon RS, Grubb 2nd BP, Olshansky B. 2015 Heart Rhythm Society expert consensus statement on the diagnosis and treatment of postural tachycardia syndrome, inappropriate sinus tachycardia, and vasovagal syncope. *Heart Rhythm*. 2015;12(6):e41–e63.
14. Freeman R, Illigens BMW, Lapusca R, et al. Symptom recognition is impaired in patients with orthostatic hypotension. *Hypertension*. 2020;75(5):1325–1332.
15. Sheldon R, Sandhu R. The search for the genes of vasovagal syncope. *Front Cardiovasc Med*. 2019;6:175.
16. Pachon-M JC. Neurocardiogenic syncope: pacemaker or cardioneuroablation? *Heart Rhythm*. 2020;S1547–5271(20)30177-6.
17. Kumar A, Wright K, Uceda DE, et al. Skin sympathetic nerve activity as a biomarker for syncopal episodes during a tilt table test. *Heart Rhythm*. 2020 (in press).
18. Lopes R, Gonçalves A, Campos J, et al. The role of pacemaker in hypersensitive carotid sinus syndrome. *Europace*. 2011;13:572.
19. Sheldon R, Hersi A, Ritchie D, et al. Syncope and structural heart disease: historical criteria for vasovagal syncope and ventricular tachycardia. *J Cardiovasc Electrophysiol*. 2010;21:1358.
20. Sheldon R. How to differentiate syncope from seizure. *Cardiol Clin*. 2015;33(3):377–385.
21. Brigo F, Nardone R, Bongiovanni LG. Value of tongue biting in the differential diagnosis between epileptic seizures and syncope. *Seizure*. 2012;21:568.
22. Ungar A, Mussi C, Ceccofiglio A, et al. Etiology of syncope and unexplained falls in elderly adults with dementia: Syncope and Dementia (SYD) Study. *J Am Geriatr Soc*. 2016;64(8):1567–1573.
23. Solbiati M, Costantino G, Casazza G, et al. Implantable loop recorder versus conventional diagnostic workup for unexplained recurrent syncope. *Cochrane Database Syst Rev*. 2016;4:CD011637.
24. Myerburg RJ, Marchlinski FE, Scheinman MM. Controversy on electrophysiology testing in patients with Brugada syndrome. *Heart Rhythm*. 2011;8:1972.
25. Viau JA, Chaudry H, Hannigan A, et al. The yield of computed tomography of the head among patients presenting with syncope: a systematic review. *Acad Emerg Med*. 2019;26(5):479–490.
26. Costantino G, Sun BC, Barbic F, et al. Syncope clinical management in the emergency department: a consensus from the first international workshop on syncope risk stratification in the emergency department. *Eur Heart J*. 2016;37(19):1493–1498.
27. Brignole M, Ungar A, Casagranda I, et al. Syncope Unit Project (SUP) investigators. Prospective multicentre systematic guideline-based management of patients referred to the syncope units of general hospitals. *Europace*. 2010;12(1):109–118.
28. Sanders NA, Jetter TL, Brignole M, Hamdan MH. Standardized care pathway versus conventional approach in the management of patients presenting with faint at the University of Utah. *Pacing Clin Electrophysiol*. 2013;36:152.
29. Aydin MA, Mortensen K, Salukhe TV, et al. A standardized education protocol significantly reduces traumatic injuries and syncope recurrence: an observational study in 316 patients with vasovagal syncope. *Europace*. 2012;14:410.
30. Numé AK, Gislason G, Christiansen CB, et al. Syncope and motor vehicle crash risk: a Danish nationwide study. *JAMA Intern Med*. 2016;176(4):503–510.
31. Sheldon R, Raj SR, Rose MS, et al. Fludrocortisone for the prevention of vasovagal syncope: a randomized, placebo-controlled trial. *J Am Coll Cardiol*. 2016;68(1):1–9.
32. Connolly SJ, Sheldon R, Thorpe KE, et al. Pacemaker therapy for prevention of syncope in patients with recurrent severe vasovagal syncope: Second Vasovagal Pacemaker Study (VPS II): a randomized trial. *J Am Med Assoc*. 2003;289(17):2224–2229.
33. Sutton R, de Jong JSY, Stewart JM, et al. Pacing in vasovagal syncope: physiology, pacemaker sensors, and recent clinical trials-precise patient selection and measurable benefit. *Heart Rhythm*. 2020;S1547–5271(20)30084–9.
34. de Jong JSY, Jardine DL, Lenders JWM, Wieling W. Pacing in vasovagal syncope: a physiological paradox?. *Heart Rhythm*. 2019 Sep 24:S1547–5271(19)30855-0.
35. Brignole M, Menozzi C, Moya A, et al. Pacemaker therapy in patients with neurally mediated syncope and documented asystole. Third International Study on Syncope of Uncertain Etiology (ISSUE-3): a randomized trial. *Circulation*. 2012;125(21):2566–2571.
36. Baron-Esquivias G, Morillo CA, Moya-Mitjans A, et al. Dual-chamber pacing with closed loop stimulation in recurrent reflex vasovagal syncope: the Spain study. *J Am Coll Cardiol*. 2017;70(14):1720–1728.
37. Pachon JC, Pachon EI, Pachon JC, et al. Cardioneuroablation"—new treatment for neurocardiogenic syncope, functional AV block and sinus dysfunction using catheter RF-ablation. *Europace*. 2005;7(1):1–13.
38. Pachon JC, Pachon EI, Cunha Pachon MZ, et al. Catheter ablation of severe neurally mediated reflex (neurocardiogenic or vasovagal) syncope: cardioneuroablation long-term results. *Europace*. 2011;13(9):1231–1242.
39. Yao Y, Shi R, Wong T, et al. Endocardial autonomic denervation of the left atrium to treat vasovagal syncope: an early experience in humans. *Circ Arrhythm Electrophysiol*. 2012;5(2):279–286.
40. Sun W, Zheng L, Qiao Y, et al. Catheter ablation as a treatment for vasovagal syncope: long-term outcome of endocardial autonomic modification of the left atrium. *J Am Heart Assoc*. 2016;5(7):e003471.
41. Hu F, Zheng L, Liang E, et al. Right anterior ganglionated plexus: the primary target of cardioneuroablation? *Heart Rhythm*. 2019;16(10):1545–1551.
42. Maj R, Borio G, Osório TG, et al. Conversion of atrial fibrillation to sinus rhythm during cryoballoon ablation: a favorable and not unusual phenomenon during second-generation cryoballoon pulmonary vein isolation. *J Arrhythm*. 2020;36(2):319–327.

72 Aortic Valve Stenosis

BRIAN R. LINDMAN, ROBERT O. BONOW, AND CATHERINE M. OTTO

EPIDEMIOLOGY

In population-based echocardiographic studies, 1% to 2% of persons aged 65 or older and 12% of persons 75 or older had calcific aortic stenosis (AS)[1-3] (see Chapter 90). Among those older than 75, 3.4% (95% confidence interval [CI] 1.1% to 5.7%) have severe AS.[2] The prevalence of aortic valve sclerosis without stenosis, defined as irregular thickening or calcification of the aortic valve leaflets, increases with age and ranges from 9% in populations with a mean age of 54 years to 42% in populations with a mean age of 81 years.[4] The rate of progression from aortic sclerosis to stenosis is 1.8% to 1.9% per year. With the aging of the population, the number of individuals with AS is expected to increase twofold to threefold in developed countries in the coming decades.[3]

CAUSES AND ETIOLOGY

Valvular AS has three principal causes: a congenital bicuspid valve with superimposed calcification, calcification of a normal trileaflet valve, and rheumatic disease (Fig. 72.1). In a U.S. series of 933 patients undergoing aortic valve replacement (AVR) for AS, a bicuspid valve was present in more than 50%, including two thirds of those younger than 70 years and 40% of those older than 70 (see Classic References, Roberts and Ko).

In addition, AS may result from a congenital valve stenosis manifesting in infancy or childhood. Rarely, AS is caused by severe atherosclerosis of the aorta and aortic valve; this form of AS occurs most frequently in patients with severe hypercholesterolemia and is observed in children with homozygous type II hyperlipoproteinemia. Rheumatoid involvement of the valve is a rare cause of AS and results in nodular thickening of the valve leaflets and involvement of the proximal portion of the aorta. Ochronosis with alkaptonuria is another rare cause of AS.

Fixed obstruction to left ventricular (LV) outflow also may occur above the valve (supravalvular stenosis) or below the valve (discrete subvalvular stenosis) (see Fig. 16.41). Dynamic subaortic obstruction may be caused by hypertrophic cardiomyopathy (see Chapter 54).

Calcific Aortic Valve Disease

Calcific (formerly "senile" or "degenerative") aortic valve disease affecting a congenital bicuspid or normal trileaflet valve is now the most common cause of AS in adults. Aortic sclerosis, identified by either echocardiography or computed tomography (CT), is the initial stage of calcific valve disease and, even in the absence of valve obstruction or known cardiovascular disease, is associated with an increased risk of myocardial infarction (MI) and cardiovascular and all-cause mortality.[4] Epidemiologic associations have been documented between cardiovascular risk factors and calcific aortic valve disease, suggesting that treating or preventing these risk factors may lessen the risk of developing AS (Table 72.1).[1,5] Whether better control of modifiable risk factors may slow progression of AS is unknown.[6]

Bicuspid Aortic Valve Disease

Congenital malformations of the aortic valve may be unicuspid, bicuspid, or quadricuspid, or the anomaly may manifest as a dome-shaped diaphragm (see Chapter 82). Unicuspid valves typically produce severe obstruction in infancy and are the most common malformations found in fatal valvular AS in children younger than 1 year but also may be seen in young adults with an anatomy that mimics bicuspid valve disease. A congenital bicuspid aortic valve (BAV) is present in approximately 1% to 2% of the population, with a male predominance of approximately 3:1. Reflecting an underlying but complex genetic basis, a 9% prevalence of BAV has been reported in first-degree relatives of individuals with a BAV.

A BAV may be an isolated abnormality (approximately 50% of the time) or occur in the context of a genetic syndrome (e.g., Turner syndrome), alongside other congenital heart defects (e.g., hypoplastic left heart, coarctation of the aorta), or with a thoracic aortic aneurysm (most common nonvalvular manifestation).[7] The genetic etiologies of BAV are complicated and incompletely understood; several genes appear to play a role with different patterns of inheritance. Familial inheritance is complex and increased when nonvalvular abnormalities accompany a BAV.

The most prevalent anatomy for a bicuspid valve is two cusps with a right-left systolic opening, consistent with congenital fusion of the right and left coronary cusps, seen in 70% to 80% of patients (Fig. 72.2). An anterior-posterior orientation, with fusion of the right and noncoronary cusps, is less common, seen in approximately 20% to 30% of patients. Fusion of the left and noncoronary cusps is rarely seen. A prominent ridge of tissue or raphe may be present in the larger of the two cusps so that the closed valve in diastole may mimic a trileaflet valve. Echocardiographic diagnosis relies on imaging the systolic leaflet opening with only two aortic commissures, but CT is now commonly used to identify or confirm the bicuspid morphology of the valve (Fig. 72.3).

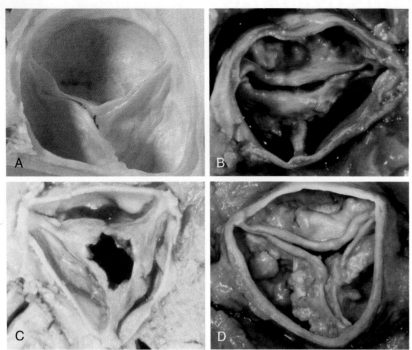

FIGURE 72.1 Major types of aortic valve stenosis. A, Normal aortic valve. **B,** Congenital bicuspid aortic stenosis. A false raphe is present at 6 o'clock. **C,** Rheumatic aortic stenosis. The commissures are fused with a fixed central orifice. **D,** Calcific aortic stenosis. (**A** from Manabe H, Yutani C, editors. *Atlas of Valvular Heart Disease.* Singapore: Churchill Livingstone; 1998:6, 131; **B-D** courtesy Dr. William C. Roberts, Baylor University Medical Center, Dallas, Tex.)

underlying aortopathy (dissection).[8] Often, the diagnosis is unknown until the physical examination reveals manifestations of valve dysfunction or the patient develops symptoms. The risk of aortic dissection in patients with BAV is five to nine times higher than in the general population, but the absolute risk is still quite low (see Chapter 42).[9,10]

Most bicuspid valves function normally until late in life, although a subset of patients present in childhood or adolescence with valve dysfunction. Overall, survival is no different from population estimates.[9,11] Patients with BAV also are at increased risk for endocarditis (0.4 per 100,000), accounting for approximately 1200 deaths per year in the United States. However, the most common cardiac event is need for AVR,[9] and most patients with BAV develop calcific valve stenosis later in life, typically presenting with severe AS after the age of 50 years. Although the histopathologic features of calcific stenosis of a BAV are no different from those of a trileaflet valve, the turbulent flow and increased leaflet stress caused by the abnormal architecture are postulated to result in accelerated valve changes, explaining the earlier average age at presentation in patients with a bicuspid, compared with trileaflet, stenotic valve. BAV disease accounts for greater than 50% of AVRs in the United States and is a common cause of calcific AS, even in older persons. The aortopathy associated with BAV disease often results in aortic dilation and carries an increased risk of aortic dissection. The magnitude of risk appears to vary depending on valve and aortic morphology and on a family history of aortic involvement.[12,13]

Rheumatic Aortic Stenosis

Rheumatic AS results from adhesions and fusions of the commissures and cusps and vascularization of the leaflets of the valve ring, leading to retraction and stiffening of the free borders of the cusps. Calcific nodules develop on both surfaces, and the orifice is reduced to a small, round or triangular opening (see Fig. 72.1C). As a consequence, the rheumatic valve often is regurgitant as well as stenotic. Patients with rheumatic AS invariably have rheumatic involvement of the mitral valve (see Chapter 81). With the decline in rheumatic fever in developed nations, rheumatic AS is decreasing in frequency, although it continues to be a major problem on a worldwide basis.

PATHOPHYSIOLOGY
Valve Calcification and Obstruction

Although calcific AS once was considered to represent the result of years of normal mechanical stress on an otherwise normal valve ("wear and tear"), it is now clear that active biological processes underlies the initiation and progression of calcific aortic valve disease (Fig. 72.4).[1,14-16] Differences in the biology driving the early versus later stages of calcific aortic valve disease could have important implications for medical therapies aimed at preventing, slowing, or reversing the path from aortic sclerosis to severe stenosis, both in terms of which pathways are relevant to target and when along the disease spectrum drugs targeting them are most likely to be effective.[15-17]

Normal valve leaflets comprise the fibrosa (facing the aorta), ventricularis (facing the ventricle), and spongiosa (located between the fibrosa and ventricularis). *Valve interstitial cells* (VICs) are the most predominant cell type; endothelial and smooth muscle cells are also present. Through a complex interplay of molecular events, the pliable, flexible valve becomes stiff and immobile, characterized grossly by fibrosis and calcification. The process is initiated by lipid infiltration and oxidative stress, which attract and activate inflammatory cells and promote the elaboration of cytokines (Fig. 72.5).[1] VICs undergo osteogenic reprogramming that promotes the mineralization of the extracellular matrix and the progression of fibrocalcific remodeling of the valve.

In addition to the genetic underpinnings of BAV, there is evidence indicating a genetic predisposition to valve calcification.[18] Genetic polymorphisms have been linked to the presence of calcific AS, including

TABLE 72.1 Strength of Associations in Observational and Epidemiologic Studies of Clinical Risk Factors and Calcific Aortic Valve Disease (CAVD)

	CAVD ANALYSIS		
RISK FACTOR	CROSS-SECTIONAL	INCIDENT	PROGRESSION
Age	+++	+++	+++
Male sex	++/−	++	0
Height	++	++	0
Body mass index	++	++	0
Hypertension	++	++	0
Diabetes	+++	+++	0
Metabolic syndrome	++	++	+
Dyslipidemia	++	++	0
Smoking	++	++	+
Renal dysfunction	+	0	0
Inflammatory markers	+	0	0
Phosphorus levels	++	0	N/A
Calcium levels	0	0	N/A
Baseline calcium score	N/A	N/A	+++

+, Weak positive association; ++, modest positive association; +++, strong positive association; −, weak negative association; 0, no association seen; N/A, no/insufficient data available.
From Thanassoulis G. Clinical and genetic risk factors for calcific valve disease. In Otto CM, Bonow RO, editors. *Valvular Heart Disease: A Companion to Braunwald's Heart Disease.* 5th ed. Philadelphia: Saunders; 2021;66-78.

Unicuspid valves are distinguished from a bicuspid valve by having only one aortic commissure.

The clinical manifestations of a BAV tend to relate to the function of the aortic valve (stenosis or regurgitation), infection of the aortic valve (endocarditis), or damage to a dilated aorta related to an

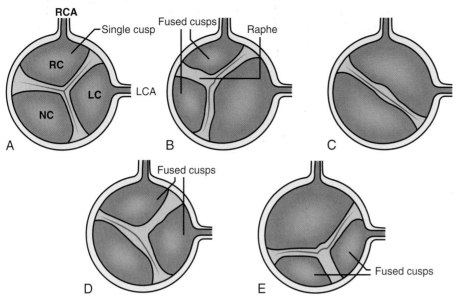

FIGURE 72.2 Comparison of tricuspid and bicuspid aortic valve structures. A, Schematic representation of a normal tricuspid aortic valve with the three cusps. *LC,* Left coronary; *LCA,* left coronary artery; *NC,* noncoronary; *RC,* right coronary; *RCA,* right coronary artery. **B,** Bicuspid valve with right noncoronary cusp fusion and one raphe (the line of union between the fused cusps). **C,** Bicuspid valve with fusion of the right and left coronary cusps and no raphe. **D,** Bicuspid valve with right-left coronary cusp fusion and one raphe. **E,** Bicuspid valve with fusion of the left and noncoronary cusps and one raphe. (From Lindman BR, et al. Calcific aortic stenosis. *Nat Rev Dis Primers.* 2016;2:16006.)

Hypertrophic Myocardial Remodeling. Maintenance of cardiac output in the face of an obstructed aortic valve imposes a chronic increase in LV pressure. In response, the ventricle typically undergoes hypertrophic remodeling characterized by myocyte hypertrophy and increased wall thickness (Fig. 72.6). LV remodeling may manifest as concentric remodeling, concentric hypertrophy, or eccentric hypertrophy. Based on the LaPlace law, LV remodeling reduces wall stress (afterload) and is considered one of the important compensatory mechanisms to maintain LV ejection performance, which is directly affected by afterload (see Classic References, Grossman).

Cardiac hypertrophy in response to pressure overload involves both adaptive and maladaptive processes.[36] Hypertrophic remodeling is not simply related to increased valvular afterload; several factors other than the severity of valve obstruction influence it, including sex, genetics, vascular load, and metabolic abnormalities.[37,38] Additionally, the degree to which LV hypertrophic remodeling is maladaptive versus adaptive and the resulting functional and clinical effects are not simply an issue of total LV mass and geometry; composition and energetics of the myocardium also are important.[36] Preclinical studies have demonstrated that blocking the hypertrophic response to pressure overload did not have deleterious effects on LV performance despite increased wall stress (see Classic References, Hill).

In patients with AS, several studies have now documented that increased LV hypertrophic remodeling is associated with more severe ventricular dysfunction and heart failure (HF) symptoms, as well as higher mortality.[39] In a recent study combining the largest patient numbers with the longest clinical follow-up to date, increased LV mass index before transcatheter aortic valve replacement (TAVR), particularly severe LV hypertrophy (LVH) was associated with increased mortality and rehospitalization over 5 years after the procedure.[40] Related to this, among patients with moderate or severe LVH treated with TAVR, greater LV mass index regression at 1 year is independently associated with lower death and rehospitalization rates out to 5 years.[41] Among those with moderate or severe LVH before TAVR, 39% still had severe LVH at 1 year and this degree of residual LVH was associated with a marked increase in subsequent mortality and rehospitalization rates.[41] Thus, although it may reduce wall stress, LV hypertrophic remodeling also may have longer-term deleterious effects that translate into impaired ventricular performance and worse clinical outcomes.

Myocardial Fibrosis. Although not routinely assessed in clinical practice, myocardial fibrosis is now well established as a risk factor for adverse clinical outcomes in patients with AS.[34,42-44] As a part of the hypertrophic remodeling process, diffuse and replacement myocardial fibrosis (not fibrosis from prior MI) may develop (see Chapter 19), although the incidence and extent of fibrosis are variable and unpredictable and the underlying biologic mechanisms not yet clarified (Fig. 72.7; see also Fig 72.6).[42,43,45] Diffuse fibrosis tends to regress after AVR, whereas replacement fibrosis does not.[34,45-47] Both the amount of diffuse fibrosis and the presence of replacement fibrosis are associated with subsequent mortality (Fig. 72.8).[34,42-44] Importantly, patients with severe fibrosis, despite a normal LV ejection fraction (LVEF), are more likely to have worse preoperative HF symptoms and less likely to experience improvement in symptoms midterm after AVR, compared to those with no or minimal fibrosis before valve replacement.[48]

Myocardial Ischemia. In patients with AS, the hypertrophied left ventricle, increased systolic pressure, and prolongation of ejection all elevate myocardial oxygen (O_2) consumption.[49] At the same time, even in the absence of epicardial coronary artery disease (CAD), decreased myocardial capillary density in the hypertrophied ventricle, endothelial cell loss, increased LV end-diastolic pressure (LVEDP), and a shortened diastole all serve to decrease the coronary perfusion pressure gradient and myocardial blood flow (see Chapter 36). Together, these conditions create an imbalance between myocardial O_2 supply and demand, yielding ischemia. Impaired myocardial flow reserve underlies symptoms of angina in patients with AS that is often indistinguishable from that caused by epicardial coronary obstruction.[50] Exercise or other states of increased O_2 demand may exacerbate this ischemic imbalance and

those involving the vitamin D receptor, interleukin (IL)-10 alleles, estrogen receptor, transforming growth factor (TGF)-β receptor, and the apolipoprotein E4 allele.[18] The most consistently observed genetic association is for lipoprotein(a) (Lp(a)). In a genome-wide association study (GWAS) based on a meta-analysis of data on nearly 7000 patients from three population-based cohorts, a single-nucleotide polymorphism (SNP) in Lp(a) was associated with aortic valve calcification, serum Lp(a) levels, and incident AS (hazard ratio [HR], 1.68; CI 1.32 to 2.15).[19] This association has been confirmed in several other cohorts.[20-22] Recent evidence suggests a potential link between Lp(a) and AS through lipoprotein-associated phospholipase A_2 (Lp-PLA$_2$) and ectonucleotide pyrophosphatase/phosphodiesterase family member 2 (ENPP2), also known as *autotaxin*.[23-27] Lp(a) transports both Lp-PLA$_2$ and autotaxin, and each of these is found in increased abundance in stenotic aortic valves.[25,26] Lp-PLA$_2$ transforms oxidized phospholipids species into lysophosphatidylcholine (lysoPC); in turn, autotaxin transforms lysoPC into lysophosphatidic acid (lysoPA), which appears to play a role in the osteogenic reprogramming of VICs.[26,27]

Key regulators of osteogenesis, including *BMP2* and *RUNX2,* are under the control of *NOTCH1.* Expression of BMP2 and RUNX2 are increased in diseased aortic valves. Heritable forms of calcific aortic valve disease have been linked to *NOTCH1* mutations; more recently, a role for NOTCH1 in idiopathic forms of calcific aortic valve disease was discovered.[28,29] Hypomethylation of the promoter region of long noncoding RNA *H19* led to overexpression of *H19,* which was associated with mineralized aortic valves and upregulation of *BMP2* and *RUNX2.* This was shown to be mediated by repression of *NOTCH1* as a result of *H19* preventing recruitment of p53 to the *NOTCH1* promoter. Subsequent investigations showed that cadherin 11 (*CDH11*), which is enriched in diseased aortic valves and overexpressed in VICs from *Notch1+/-* mice, mediates *NOTCH1*-induced calcific aortic valve disease.[30] The roles of DNA methylation and noncoding RNAs in the pathophysiology of calcific aortic valve disease have been reviewed.[31] Despite progress in elucidating pathobiology, there is no medical therapy for calcific aortic valve disease, but several potentially promising therapeutic targets have been reviewed.[15,17,32]

Over time, progressive fibrocalcific remodeling of the aortic valve leaflets makes them less pliable and obstruction to flow out of the left ventricle develops and increases. This yields a chronic pressure overload state that leads to myocardial remodeling and dysfunction and accompanying changes in the pulmonary and systemic vasculature.

Left Ventricular Response: Structure and Function

Progressive valve obstruction imposes a chronic pressure overload state that leads to numerous changes in the structure and function of the left ventricle and accompanying changes in the pulmonary and systemic vasculature.[33-35]

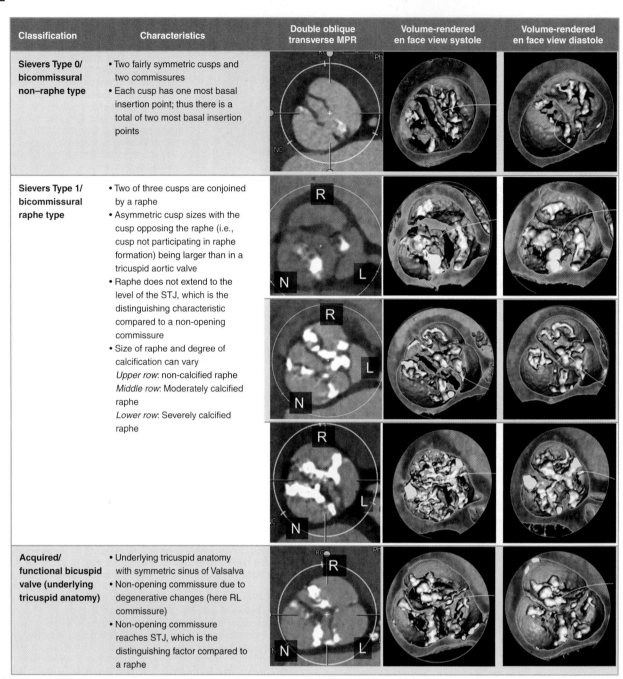

Classification	Characteristics	Double oblique transverse MPR	Volume-rendered en face view systole	Volume-rendered en face view diastole
Sievers Type 0/ bicommissural non–raphe type	• Two fairly symmetric cusps and two commissures • Each cusp has one most basal insertion point; thus there is a total of two most basal insertion points			
Sievers Type 1/ bicommissural raphe type	• Two of three cusps are conjoined by a raphe • Asymmetric cusp sizes with the cusp opposing the raphe (i.e., cusp not participating in raphe formation) being larger than in a tricuspid aortic valve • Raphe does not extend to the level of the STJ, which is the distinguishing characteristic compared to a non-opening commissure • Size of raphe and degree of calcification can vary *Upper row*: non-calcified raphe *Middle row*: Moderately calcified raphe *Lower row*: Severely calcified raphe			
Acquired/ functional bicuspid valve (underlying tricuspid anatomy)	• Underlying tricuspid anatomy with symmetric sinus of Valsalva • Non-opening commissure due to degenerative changes (here RL commissure) • Non-opening commissure reaches STJ, which is the distinguishing factor compared to a raphe			

FIGURE 72.3 Differing morphologies and calcification patterns of bicuspid aortic valves by cardiac CT. *STJ,* Sinotubular junction. (From Blanke P, et al. Computed tomography imaging in the context of transcatheter aortic valve implantation (TAVI)/transcatheter aortic valve replacement (TAVR). *JACC Cardiovasc Imaging.* 2019;12:1-24.)

provoke angina that may not be experienced at rest. Myocardial flow reserve is independently associated with aerobic exercise capacity and HF functional class in severe AS and appears to be influenced by the extent of LV hypertrophic remodeling and fibrosis, endothelial cell loss, and severity of valve obstruction.[51,52]

Left Ventricular Diastolic Function. Hypertrophic remodeling also impairs diastolic myocardial relaxation and increases stiffness, as modulated by cardiovascular and metabolic comorbidities.[53] Higher cardiomyocyte stiffness, increased myocardial fibrosis, advanced-glycation end products, and metabolic abnormalities each contribute to increased chamber stiffness and higher end-diastolic pressures.[43] Atrial contraction plays a particularly important role in filling of the left ventricle in AS because it increases LVEDP without causing a concomitant elevation of mean left atrial pressure. This "booster pump" function of the left atrium prevents the pulmonary venous and capillary pressures from rising to levels that would produce pulmonary congestion, while maintaining LVEDP at the elevated level necessary for effective contraction of the hypertrophied left ventricle. Loss of appropriately timed, vigorous

atrial contraction, as occurs in atrial fibrillation (AF) or atrioventricular (AV) dissociation, may result in rapid clinical deterioration in patients with severe AS. After relief of the pressure overload with AVR, diastolic dysfunction may revert toward normal with regression of hypertrophy, but some degree of long-term diastolic dysfunction typically persists.[53,54] Worse diastolic function before AVR and worse residual diastolic dysfunction after AVR have been associated with worse long-term outcomes.[53,54] The severity of diastolic dysfunction may also influence the clinical consequences of aortic regurgitation (AR) after TAVR.[55]

Left Ventricular Systolic Function. LV systolic function, as measured by the LVEF, generally remains preserved until late in the disease process in most patients with AS, but emerging data indicate that ejection fraction (EF) may begin to decline in patients before AS is considered severe.[1,56] What characterizes a "normal" or "preserved" EF in the setting of AS is not clear. Traditionally, it has been characterized as an EF 50% or greater, but accumulating evidence indicates that an EF <60% is associated with poor post-AVR outcomes, suggesting that the threshold indicative of impaired/

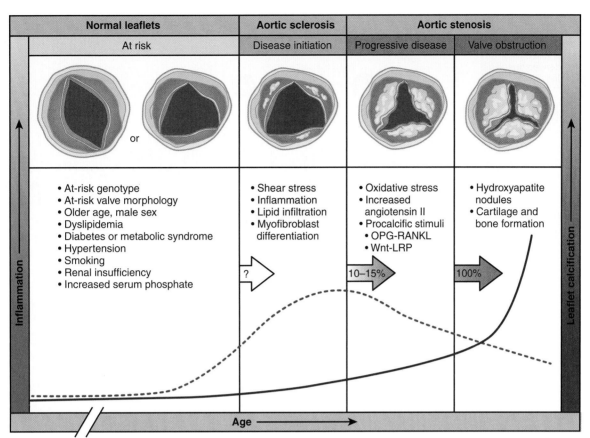

FIGURE 72.4 Disease mechanisms and time course of calcific aortic stenosis (AS): relationship among disease stage, valve anatomy, clinical risk factors, mechanisms of disease, and patient's age. Endothelial disruption with inflammation (*dashed line*) and lipid infiltration are key elements in the initiation of disease. There are few data on the prevalence of disease initiation in at-risk patients, and progressive disease develops in only a subgroup of these patients. Progressive leaflet disease, which is associated with several disease pathways, develops in approximately 10% to 15% of patients with AS. Once these disease mechanisms are activated, leaflet calcification results in severe AS in almost all patients. With end-stage disease, tissue calcification (*red line*) is the predominant tissue change, resulting in valve obstruction. Current imaging approaches are reliable only when substantial leaflet changes are present (in patients with progressive disease or valve obstruction), which limits clinical studies of interventions to prevent or slow the progression of early disease. *LRP,* Lipoprotein receptor–related protein complex; *OPG,* osteoprotegerin; *RANKL,* receptor activator of nuclear factor-κB ligand. (From Otto CM, Prendergast B. Aortic-valve stenosis: from patients at risk to severe valve obstruction. *N Engl J Med.* 2014;371:744-756.)

reduced EF in the setting of AS may need to be changed.[57-61] Before a reduction in EF occurs, more subtle systolic dysfunction can be detected as reduced longitudinal systolic strain, which is associated with worse outcomes in patients with severe AS[59,62] (see Chapter 16). The development and severity of systolic dysfunction results from a complex interplay of factors, including the severity of valve obstruction, metabolic abnormalities, vascular load, maladaptive hypertrophy (resulting in impaired contractility), ischemia, and fibrosis.[1,38,45] Eventually, a subset of patients develops overt systolic dysfunction manifested by a reduced LVEF. In these patients, systolic function usually improves after the ventricle is unloaded by AVR; the amount of recovery depends on many factors, including the degree to which systolic dysfunction was affected by afterload mismatch versus myocardial fibrosis and altered contractility.[63-65]

Pulmonary and Systemic Vasculature Response
The hypertrophied and pressure-overloaded left ventricle transmits increased pressure to the pulmonary vasculature, which leads to pulmonary hypertension in many patients with AS, becoming severe in 15% to 20%. Although patients may initially manifest pulmonary venous hypertension alone, some will go on to develop increased pulmonary vascular resistance, perhaps influenced by specific comorbidities and chronicity of pulmonary venous hypertension.[66-68] Among asymptomatic patients, exercise-induced pulmonary hypertension is associated with decreased event-free survival, and among patients undergoing TAVR or surgical AVR (SAVR), the presence and severity of pulmonary hypertension is associated with increased postoperative mortality.[67,68] Elevated pulmonary artery pressures decrease in some patients after AVR, but not all; residual pulmonary hypertension is associated with worse clinical outcomes.[69,70]

The systemic vasculature also makes an important contribution to total LV afterload.[33,66,71-73] Hemodynamic studies with agents that

dilate the systemic vasculature show an acute increase in LV stroke volume, underscoring that changes in vascular properties can unload the left ventricle despite no change in the valvular obstruction[66,74] (see also Classic References, Khot). Measures of increased vascular load, including arterial stiffness, global load (integrating both valvular and vascular load), and systolic blood pressure, have been associated with adverse LV remodeling, impaired LV function, and worse clinical outcomes.[72,75] In patients with AS, characterization of systemic vascular properties is conditioned by upstream obstruction; valve replacement unmasks and induces stiffer vascular behavior (Fig. 72.9).[71] Accordingly, in patients with AS, the load on the LV is a combined load at the valvular and vascular level; increased vascular load may identify patients who benefit less from AVR and may be a target for adjunctive medical therapy to optimize outcomes.

CLINICAL PRESENTATION

The diagnosis of AS is most often made on auscultation of a murmur suggestive of AS, followed by confirmation with echocardiography. When AS is not severe and symptoms are absent, patients are reevaluated clinically and with echocardiography based on the AS severity. Generally, repeat imaging is performed every 6 to 12 months for severe AS, every 1 to 2 years for moderate AS, and every 3 to 5 years for mild AS, unless a change in signs or symptoms prompts repeat imaging sooner.[57]

Symptoms
The cardinal manifestations of acquired AS are exertional dyspnea, angina, syncope, and ultimately HF.[1,14] Many patients are diagnosed

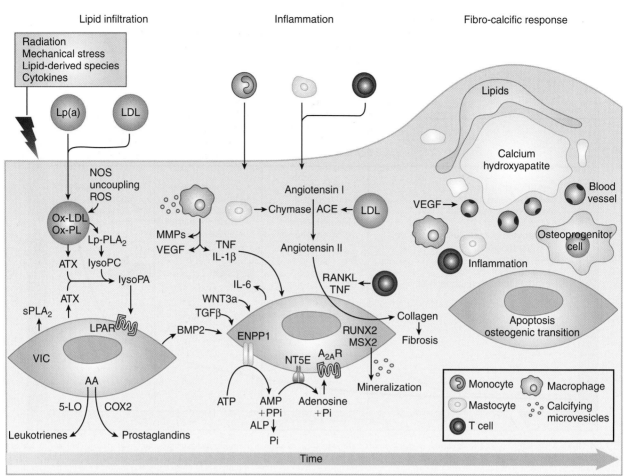

FIGURE 72.5 Pathogenesis of calcific aortic stenosis. Endothelial damage allows infiltration of lipids, specifically low-density lipoprotein (*LDL*) and lipoprotein(a) [*Lp(a)*], into the fibrosa and triggers the recruitment of inflammatory cells into the aortic valve. Endothelial injury can be triggered by several factors, including lipid-derived species, cytokines, mechanical stress, and radiation injury. The production of reactive oxygen species (*ROS*) is promoted by the uncoupling of nitric oxide synthase (*NOS*), which increases the oxidation of lipids and further intensifies the secretion of cytokines. Enzymes transported in the aortic valve by lipoproteins (i.e., LDL, Lp[a]) such as lipoprotein-associated phospholipase A$_2$ (*Lp-PLA$_2$*) and ectonucleotide pyrophosphatase/phosphodiesterase 2 (ENPP2), also known as autotoxin (*ATX*), produce lysophospholipid derivatives. ATX, which is also secreted by valve interstitial cells (*VICs*), transforms lysophosphatidylcholine (*lysoPC*) into lysophosphatidic acid (*lysoPA*). Several factors, including lysoPA, the receptor activator of nuclear factor-κB ligand (*RANKL;* also known as TNFSF11), and WNT3a, promote the osteogenic transition of VIC. Arachidonic acid (*AA*) generated by cytosolic PLA$_2$ promotes the production of eicosanoids such as prostaglandins and leukotrienes through prostaglandin G/H synthase 2 (PTGS2; also known as cyclooxygenase 2 [*COX2*]) and 5-lipoxygenase (*5-LO*) pathways, respectively. In turn, eicosanoids promote inflammation and mineralization. Chymase and angiotensin-converting enzyme (*ACE*) promote production of angiotensin II, which increases synthesis and secretion of collagen by VIC. Because of increased production of matrix metalloproteinases (*MMPs*) and decreased synthesis of tissue inhibitors of metalloproteinases (TIMPs), disorganized fibrous tissue accumulates within the aortic valve. Microcalcification begins early in the disease, driven by microvesicles secreted by VIC and macrophages. In addition, overexpression of ectonucleotidases—ENPP1, 5'-nucleotidase ecto (*NT5E*), and alkaline phosphatase (*ALP*)—promotes both apoptosis and osteogenic-mediated mineralization. Bone morphogenetic protein 2 (*BMP2*) leads to osteogenic transdifferentiation, which is associated with the expression of bone-related transcription factors (e.g., runt-related transcription factor 2 [*RUNX2*] and homeobox protein MSX2). Osteoblast-like cells subsequently coordinate calcification of the aortic valve as part of a highly regulated process analogous to skeletal bone formation. Deposition of mineralized matrix is accompanied by fibrosis and neovascularization, which is abetted by vascular endothelial growth factor (*VEGF*). In turn, neovascularization increases the recruitment of inflammatory cells and bone marrow–derived osteoprogenitor cells. *A$_{2A}$R,* Adenosine A$_{2A}$ receptor; *sPLA$_2$,* secreted phospholipase A$_2$; *LPAR,* lysophosphatidic acid receptor; *Ox-PL,* oxidized phospholipid; *Ox-LDL,* oxidized LDL; *TGFβ,* transforming growth factor beta; *TNF,* tumor necrosis factor. (From Lindman BR, et al. Calcific aortic stenosis. *Nat Rev Dis Primers.* 2016;2:16006.)

before symptom onset on the basis of the finding of a systolic murmur on physical examination, with confirmation of the diagnosis by echocardiography. Symptoms can develop at any age but typically begin at age 50 to 70 years with BAV stenosis and in those older than 70 with calcific stenosis of a trileaflet valve, although even in this age group approximately 40% of patients with AS have a congenital BAV (see Classic References, Roberts and Ko).

The most common clinical presentation in patients with a known diagnosis of AS who are followed prospectively is a gradual decrease in exercise tolerance, fatigue, or dyspnea on exertion. However, in some cases, symptom onset can be more abrupt and severe.[76] The mechanism of exertional dyspnea may be LV diastolic dysfunction, with an excessive rise in end-diastolic pressure leading to pulmonary congestion. Alternatively, exertional symptoms may be a result of the limited ability to increase cardiac output with exercise. More severe exertional dyspnea, with orthopnea, paroxysmal nocturnal dyspnea, and pulmonary edema are relatively late symptoms in patients with AS; in current practice, intervention typically is undertaken before this disease stage.

Angina is a frequent symptom of patients with severe AS, indicates myocardial ischemia, and usually resembles the angina observed in

patients with CAD in that it is usually precipitated by exertion and relieved by rest (see Chapters 35 and 40). In patients without CAD, angina results from the combination of the increased O$_2$ needs of hypertrophied myocardium and reduction of O$_2$ delivery due to decreased myocardial capillary density, endothelial cell loss, and increased LVEDP, which reduce the coronary perfusion pressure gradient and impair myocardial flow reserve. In patients with CAD, angina is caused by a combination of epicardial coronary artery obstruction and the O$_2$ imbalance characteristic of AS. Very rarely, angina results from calcific emboli to the coronary vascular bed.

Syncope most often is caused by the reduced cerebral perfusion that occurs during exertion when arterial pressure declines because of systemic vasodilation and an inadequate increase in cardiac output related to valvular stenosis. Syncope also has been attributed to malfunction of the baroreceptor mechanism in severe AS (see Chapter 102), as well as to a vasodepressor response to a greatly elevated LV systolic pressure during exercise. Premonitory symptoms of syncope are common. Exertional hypotension also may be manifested as "graying-out spells" or dizziness on effort. Syncope at rest may be caused by transient AF with loss of the atrial contribution to LV filling,

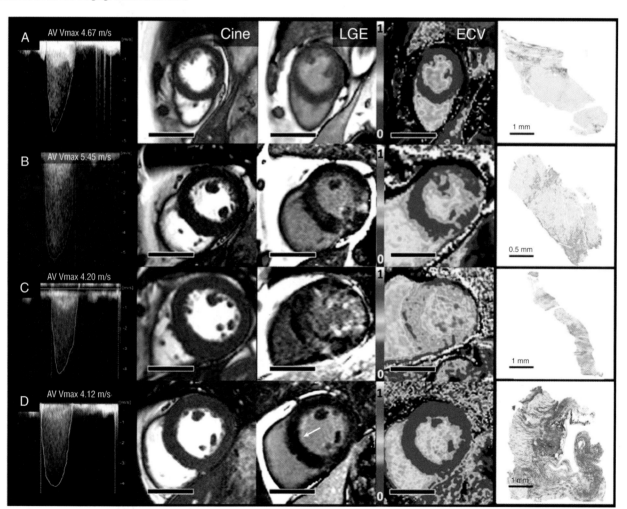

FIGURE 72.6 Hypertrophic remodeling in response to pressure overload from aortic stenosis. (From Bing R, et al. Imaging and impact of myocardial fibrosis in aortic stenosis. *JACC Cardiovasc Imaging.* 2019;12:283-296.)

FIGURE 72.7 Diffuse and replacement myocardial fibrosis in aortic stenosis. Aortic stenosis, myocardial hypertrophy, and fibrosis by imaging and biopsy. *Column 1,* Four exemplar patients showing continuous-wave Doppler (maximum velocities >4 m/sec). *Column 2 (Cine),* Short-axis cine stills demonstrating degrees of left ventricular hypertrophy. *Column 3 (LGE),* Matching late gadolinium enhancement images. *Column 4 (ECV),* Matching extracellular volume fraction. *Column 5,* Myocardial biopsy sample stained with picrosirius red (collagen volume fraction [CVF]). Patient **A** has minimal left ventricular hypertrophy [LVH], no LGE, an ECV of 28.4% and minimal biopsy subendocardial fibrosis (CVF 4.6%). Patient **B** has concentric LVH, patchy noninfarct LGE, an ECV of 29.9%, and moderate biopsy fibrosis (CVF 19.3%). Patient **C** has concentric LVH, widespread noninfarct LGE, an ECV of 36.5%, and severe biopsy fibrosis (CVF 24.5%). Patient **D** has mild concentric LVH, subtle subendocardial LGE (*arrow*), an ECV of 24.5%, thickened endocardium, and subendocardial scarring. Scale bars (columns 2–4) equal 5 cm. (From Treibel TA, et al. Reappraising myocardial fibrosis in severe aortic stenosis: an invasive and non-invasive study in 133 patients. *Eur Heart J.* 2018;39:699-709.)

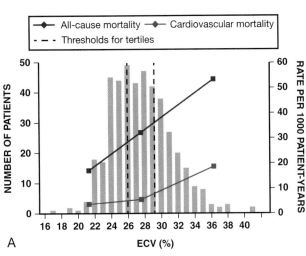

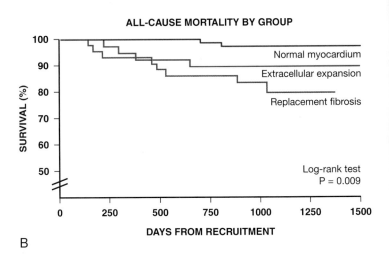

FIGURE 72.8 Myocardial fibrosis and mortality in aortic stenosis. A, Frequency distribution of magnitude of extracellular volume fraction (ECV, expressed as percent of left ventricular myocardium) in patients with aortic stenosis, and association of ECV with all-cause and cardiovascular mortality. **B,** Survival in subgroups of patients with AS defined by normal myocardium, extracellular expansion, and replacement fibrosis. (**A** from Everett RJ, et al. Extracellular myocardial volume in patients with aortic stenosis. *J Am Coll Cardiol.* 2020;75:304-316. **B** from Chin CWL, et al. Myocardial fibrosis and cardiac decompensation in aortic stenosis. *JACC Cardiovasc Imaging.* 2017;10:1320-1333.)

which causes a precipitous decline in cardiac output, or to transient AV block caused by extension of the calcification of the valve into the conduction system.

Gastrointestinal bleeding may develop in patients with severe AS, often associated with angiodysplasia (most frequently of the right colon) or other vascular malformations. This complication arises from shear stress–induced platelet aggregation with a reduction in high-molecular-weight multimers of von Willebrand factor and increases in proteolytic subunit fragments.[77] These abnormalities correlate with the severity of AS and are correctable by AVR.

An increased risk of infective endocarditis has been documented in patients with aortic valve disease, particularly in younger patients with a BAV (see Chapter 80). Cerebral emboli resulting in stroke or transient ischemic attacks may be caused by microthrombi on thickened BAVs. Calcific AS rarely may cause embolization of calcium to various organs, including the heart, kidneys, and brain.

Physical Examination

The key features of the physical examination in patients with AS are palpation of the carotid upstroke, evaluation of the systolic murmur, assessment of splitting of the second heart sound (S_2), and examination for signs of HF (see Chapters 13 and 49).

The carotid upstroke directly reflects the arterial pressure waveform. The expected finding with severe AS is a slow-rising, late-peaking, low-amplitude carotid pulse, the *parvus and tardus* carotid impulse. When present, this finding is specific for severe AS. However, many adults with AS have concurrent conditions, such as AR or systemic hypertension, that affect the arterial pressure curve and the carotid impulse. Thus, an apparently normal carotid impulse is not reliable for excluding the diagnosis of severe AS. In addition, with severe AS, radiation of the murmur to the carotid arteries may result in a palpable thrill or carotid shudder.

Auscultation

Overall, auscultation has relatively poor sensitivity and specificity for detecting AS, even among cardiologists.[78] The ejection systolic murmur of AS typically is late-peaking and heard best at the base of the heart, with radiation to the carotids. Cessation of the murmur before A_2 is helpful in differentiation from a pansystolic mitral murmur. In patients with calcified aortic valves, the systolic murmur is loudest at the base of the heart, but high-frequency components may radiate to the apex—the so-called *Gallavardin phenomenon*, in which the murmur may be

so prominent that it is mistaken for the murmur of mitral regurgitation (MR). In general, a louder and later-peaking murmur indicates more severe stenosis. However, although a systolic murmur of grade 3 intensity or greater is relatively specific for severe AS, this finding is insensitive, and many patients with severe AS have only a grade 2 murmur. When the left ventricle fails and stroke volume falls, the systolic murmur of AS becomes softer; rarely, it disappears altogether.

Splitting of S_2 is helpful in excluding the diagnosis of severe AS, because normal splitting implies the aortic valve leaflets are flexible enough to create an audible closing sound (A_2). With severe AS, S_2 may be single because (1) calcification and immobility of the aortic valve make A_2 inaudible, (2) closure of the pulmonic valve (P_2) is buried in the prolonged aortic ejection murmur, or (3) prolongation of LV systole makes A_2 coincide with P_2. The intensity of the systolic murmur varies from beat to beat when the duration of diastolic filling varies, as in AF or after a premature contraction. This characteristic is helpful in differentiating AS from MR, in which the murmur usually is unaffected. The murmur of valvular AS is augmented by squatting, which increases stroke volume. It is reduced in intensity during the strain of the Valsalva maneuver and on standing, both of which reduce transvalvular flow.

Diagnostic Testing

Echocardiography

Echocardiography is the standard approach for evaluating and following patients with AS and selecting them for valve replacement (see Chapter 16). Echocardiographic imaging allows for characterization of valve anatomy, including the cause of AS (see Fig. 16.40), a qualitative impression of valve calcification (see Fig. 16.42), and sometimes allows direct imaging of the orifice area using three-dimensional imaging.[78] Echocardiographic imaging is also invaluable for the evaluation of LVH and systolic function, with calculation of EF, measurement of aortic sinus dimensions, and detection of associated AR and mitral valve disease. Longitudinal systolic strain imaging has emerged as a more sensitive measure of LV function and predicts adverse clinical events, including mortality.[59,62]

Doppler echocardiography allows measurement of indices to determine the severity of AS, including peak transvalvular jet velocity (which is used to calculate the peak transvalvular pressure gradient with the modified Bernoulli equation), mean transvalvular pressure gradient, and aortic valve area (AVA) (calculated using the continuity equation) (Fig 72.10).[79,80] Both AVA and pressure gradient calculations from Doppler data have been well validated compared with invasive

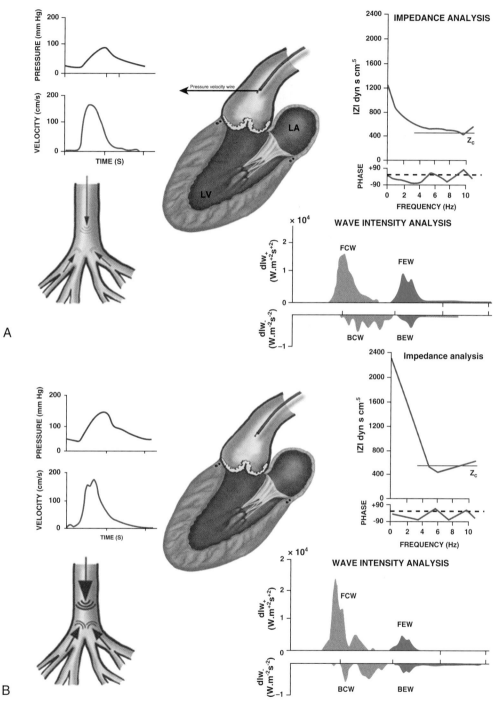

FIGURE 72.9 Aortic impedance and wave intensity analysis are shown in a patient before (A) and after (B) transcatheter aortic valve replacement (TAVR). Aortic systolic and pulse pressures increased after TAVR. Fourier decomposition of the simultaneous aortic pressure and velocity signals shows that SVR and the first three harmonic frequencies of the impedance spectrum (Z) increase after TAVR. Wave intensity analysis was used to separate total wave intensity into contributions from the forward (dIw+) and backward (dIw–) traveling waves. Compression waves (*gold*) increase pressure, and expansion waves (*green*) decrease aortic pressure. The forward compression wave (FCW) increases immediately after TAVR. *BCW,* Backward compression wave; *BEW,* backward expansion wave; *dIw,* wave intensity; *FEW,* forward expansion wave; *LA,* left atrium; *LV,* left ventricle; *SVR,* systemic vascular resistance. (From Yotti R, et al. Systemic vascular load in calcific degenerative aortic valve stenosis: insight from percutaneous valve replacement. *J Am Coll Cardiol.* 2015;65:423-433.)

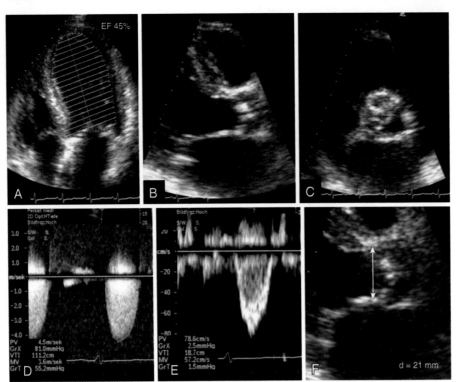

FIGURE 72.10 Assessment of aortic stenosis severity. A, The Simpson method is used to assess LV function by ejection fraction (EF). **B,** The long-axis view is used to assess the morphology, degree of calcification, and opening movement. **C,** The short axis further assesses morphology and the number of cusps. **D,** CW Doppler measures peak velocity, mean gradient, and the aortic velocity-time integral (VTI). **E,** Pulsed-wave Doppler is used to measure prestenotic velocity and the VTI in the LV outflow tract (LVOT). **F,** LVOT diameter (*d, double-headed arrow*) in zoom mode is used to calculate LVOT area. Images show a severely stenosed calcified tricuspid aortic valve with a mean gradient of 55 mm Hg, a calculated aortic valve area of 0.6 cm², and a reduced EF of 45%. (From Otto CM, ed. *The Practice of Clinical Echocardiography.* 6th ed. Philadelphia: Elsevier; 2022.)

hemodynamics and in terms of their ability to predict clinical outcome. However, the accuracy of these measures requires an experienced laboratory with meticulous attention to technical details. Evaluation of AS severity is affected by the presence of systemic hypertension, and reevaluation after blood pressure control may be necessary.[81] In patients with LV dysfunction and low cardiac output, assessing the severity of AS can be enhanced by assessing hemodynamic changes during dobutamine infusion (see later). In some patients, additional measures of AS severity may be necessary, such as correction for poststenotic pressure recovery or three-dimensional transesophageal echocardiography (TEE) of valve anatomy. The combination of pulsed, continuous-wave, and color flow Doppler echocardiography is helpful in detecting and determining the severity of AR (which coexists in approximately 75% of patients with predominant AS) and in estimating pulmonary artery pressure.

Exercise Stress Testing. Because patients may tailor their lifestyle to minimize symptoms or may ascribe fatigue and dyspnea to deconditioning or aging, they may not recognize early symptoms as important warning signals, although these symptoms often can be elicited by a careful history. Exercise testing may be helpful in apparently asymptomatic patients or when symptoms are vague (e.g., fatigue) to unmask symptoms or demonstrate limited exercise capacity or an abnormal blood pressure response.[57,82] Exercise stress testing should be attended by a physician and should be absolutely avoided in clearly symptomatic patients.

Cardiac Computed Tomography. The use and value of CT is rapidly expanding in patients with calcific aortic valve disease (see Chapter 20). CT is useful for evaluating aortic dilation in patients with evidence or suspicion of aortic root disease on echocardiography or chest radiography, particularly those with a bicuspid valve. Measurement of aortic dimensions at several levels, including the sinuses of Valsalva, sinotubular junction, and ascending aorta, is necessary for clinical decision making and surgical planning. CT is increasingly used to assess valve calcification to predict the rate of disease progression or, more often, when the severity of the stenosis is in doubt, particularly in those with low-flow, low-gradient AS

(Fig. 72.11).[83-85] It is complementary to echocardiography in assessing valve morphology (see Fig. 20.20B) and provides valuable information on the location and extent of calcification; this can guide treatment decisions regarding transcatheter versus surgical valve replacement and, if a transcatheter approach is selected, valve choice (see Fig. 72.3).[86-89] CT is also a routine part of the preprocedural evaluation of patients undergoing SAVR or TAVR (see Chapter 74), principally to look for a porcelain aorta, as well as determine appropriate valve sizing and assess aortic and peripheral arterial anatomy for a potential transcatheter approach (see Fig. 20.23).[86] Finally, as the quality and resolution of CT have rapidly improved, a gated CT coronary angiogram (with assessment of fractional flow reserve as warranted) may be used to evaluate for CAD instead of routine invasive angiography before AVR.[90,91]

Cardiac Catheterization. In almost all patients, the echocardiographic examination provides the important hemodynamic information required for patient management. Cardiac catheterization is now recommended only when noninvasive tests are inconclusive, when clinical and echocardiographic findings are discrepant, and for coronary angiography before AVR[57] (see Chapters 21 and 22).

Other Imaging Modalities
Cardiac Magnetic Resonance Imaging. Cardiac magnetic resonance (CMR) is useful for assessing LV volume, function, and mass, especially in settings in which this information cannot be obtained readily from echocardiography (see Chapter 19).[92] CMR is also excellent for assessing aortic dimensions in patients with a bicuspid valve, particularly to avoid radiation when serial imaging is needed over many years. Given the adverse prognosis associated with the presence and severity of myocardial fibrosis, CMR with T1 mapping and late gadolinium enhancement (LGE) may be used to risk-stratify patients with AS (see Figs. 72.6 through 72.8).[34,42-47] CMR is also sometimes used instead of CT to assess valve morphology, vascular anatomy, and annular dimensions in preparation for TAVR, although CMR is not recommended for assessment of stenosis severity because of underestimation of transvalvular velocities.[92]

Positron Emission Tomography. Active uptake of ¹⁸F-fluoride in the aortic valve on positron emission tomography (PET) identifies active tissue calcification and ¹⁸F-fluorodeoxyglucose uptake is a marker of valvular inflammation (see Chapter 18). These tracers are associated with disease progression and predict changes in severity of aortic valve calcification on serial CT studies (Fig. 72.12).[93-95] This may become a useful surrogate end point for trials testing therapies to slow the progression of calcific aortic valve disease, but further studies are needed.

Multimodality Imaging for Cardiac Amyloidosis. Transthyretin cardiac amyloidosis (ATTR-CA) is increasingly recognized as a coexistent disease process in individuals with AS, particularly those with low-flow or low-gradient AS.[96-98] Up to 16% of patients undergoing TAVR have been identified as having ATTR-CA, which is associated with more advanced cardiac structural and functional abnormalities. Multiple imaging modalities (see Chapters 16, 18, and 19) may be helpful in assessing for ATTR-CM, including echocardiographic strain, cardiac MRI, and technetium pyrophosphate (Fig. 72.13; see also Figs. 18.34, 18.35, and 19.13).[34] Even emerging methods to assess extracellular volume with CT may be useful.[99] Although ATTR-CA in a patient with severe AS may not make TAVR futile, it may be associated with worse outcomes, and emerging therapies for ATTR-CA should be considered.[98,100] This is an evolving area that requires additional research to determine the best method(s) for screening and treatment.

DISEASE COURSE AND STAGING

The disease course for a patient with AS is characterized by (1) progressive narrowing/obstruction of the valve with its attendant consequences for myocardial and vascular remodeling/dysfunction and (2)

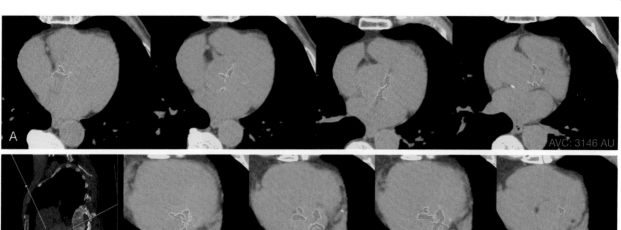

Aortic valve calcification (AVC)

FIGURE 72.11 Aortic valve calcification quantified by cardiac CT. Multiplanar reformat images in "native" axial **(A)** and "en face" **(B)** views showing aortic valve calcification (AVC) (*pink*). Note that, with the use of the "en face" reconstructed view, the calcification score is decreased by 37% and that aortic stenosis severity would be classified as nonsevere. Thus, "en face" view measurement of aortic valve calcification must not be used to assess AVC severity. (From Pawade T, et al. Why and how to measure aortic valve calcification in patients with aortic stenosis. *JACC Cardiovasc Imaging.* 2019;12:1835-1848.)

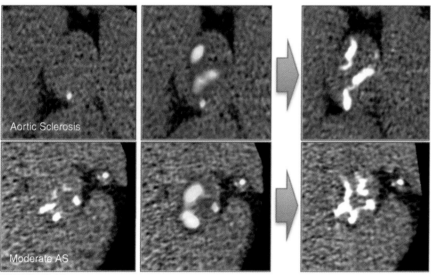

FIGURE 72.12 Valvular 18F-fluoride uptake predicts the progression of calcification in aortic stenosis. Two patients with calcific aortic valve disease. *Left,* Baseline CT images. *Middle,* Fused positron emission tomography (PET)/CT images showing increased 18F-fluoride valvular uptake (*red/yellow areas*). *Right,* Repeat CT scans after 2 years with new areas of macroscopic calcium (*white areas*) in a similar distribution to that of baseline PET uptake. (From Jenkins WS, et al. Valvular (18)F-fluoride and (18)F-fluorodeoxyglucose uptake predict disease progression and clinical outcome in patients with aortic stenosis. *J Am Coll Cardiol* 2015;66:1200-1201.)

Progressive Aortic Stenosis (Stage B; Mild to Moderate Valve Obstruction)

In adults with calcific AS, a significant burden of leaflet disease is present before obstruction to outflow develops. However, once even mild obstruction is present, hemodynamic progression occurs in almost all patients, with the interval from mild to severe obstruction ranging from less than 5 to more than 10 years. There is substantial patient-to-patient variability in the rate of progression; factors associated with more rapid hemodynamic progression include older age, more severe leaflet calcification, renal insufficiency, hypertension, obesity, metabolic syndrome, smoking, hyperlipidemia, and elevated circulating levels of Lp(a) and increased activity of Lp-PLA$_2$.[1,23,24,57] A greater initial increase in transvalvular gradient portends faster progression.[102] *Moderate* AS is characterized by an aortic jet velocity of 3.0 to 3.9 m/sec or mean transvalvular pressure gradient of 20 to 39 mm Hg, usually with an AVA of 1.0 to 1.5 cm². *Mild* AS is characterized by an aortic jet velocity of 2.0 to 2.9 m/sec or mean transvalvular pressure gradient less than 20 mm Hg, usually with aortic orifice of 1.5 to 2.0 cm² (see Table 72.2).[57,79]

ultimately the development of symptoms. These are reflected in the staging nomenclature of the American College of Cardiology/American Heart Association (ACC/AHA) Valvular Heart Disease Guidelines (Table 72.2).[57] Stage A includes those at risk for AS; stage B includes progressive AS (mild to moderate valve obstruction); stage C includes individuals with severe AS but no symptoms with LVEF ≥50% (C1) or with overt LV dysfunction (LVEF <50%) (C2); and stage D includes individuals with severe AS and symptoms broken down into three different subgroups (D1, D2, and D3) based on differing hemodynamics.[57]

The degree of stenosis associated with symptom onset varies among patients. Although stenosis is on average more severe in symptomatic than in asymptomatic patients, marked overlap is evident in all measures of severity between these two groups. Once AS is severe, only about 50% of patients report symptoms.[101] Markers of more rapid symptom onset include greater valve calcification, higher transvalvular gradient, more rapid increase in transvalvular gradient, and higher B-type natriuretic peptide, among others.[57]

Classification of Severe Aortic Stenosis

Criteria have been developed for characterizing severe AS; they are useful for categorizing patients, but it is important to recognize their limitations and imprecision. They should not be rigidly adhered to in isolation when determining clinical management. Clinical decisions are based on consideration of symptom status, severity of AS as determined by echocardiography, and LV systolic function. In some cases, additional measures of valve calcification by CT and hemodynamic stress with B-type natriuretic peptide (BNP) or N-terminal (NT)-pro hormone BNP (NT-proBNP) can provide important data regarding AS severity and its effect on the left ventricle. Additional factors, such as energy loss index, valvular impedance, or evaluation with changing

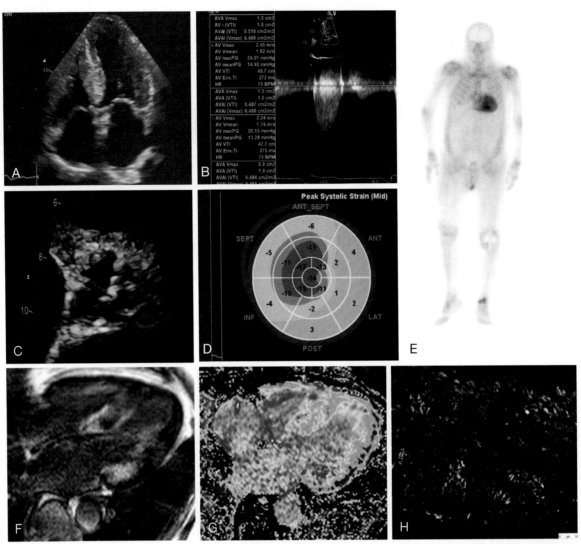

FIGURE 72.13 Multimodality imaging to detect cardiac amyloid in a patient with aortic stenosis. A, Although the echocardiogram showed left ventricular hypertrophy, this was attributed to the myocardial response to severe valve gradients **(B)** due to a heavily calcified tricuspid aortic valve **(C). D,** Strain imaging showed a characteristic apical sparing. **E,** Bone scintigraphy showed Perugini grade 2 cardiac uptake. Cardiac magnetic resonance showed transmural late gadolinium enhancement with higher signal from the myocardium than from the blood pool **(F),** and elevated native myocardial ECV **(G). H,** Diagnosis was confirmed as transthyretin amyloidosis on cardiac biopsy. (From Treibel TA, et al. Multimodality imaging markers of adverse myocardial remodeling in aortic stenosis. *JACC Cardiovasc Imaging.* 2019;12:1532-1548.)

loading conditions (e.g., dobutamine stress) or with exercise, are under investigation for evaluation of disease severity.[74,103]

The most specific definition for severe AS is a peak jet velocity of 4.0 m/sec or greater or mean gradient of 40 mm Hg or greater, usually accompanied by an AVA of 1.0 cm² or less (see Table 72.2 and Fig. 72.10).[57] When aortic velocity or gradient meets these criteria, severe AS is present and classified as stage C in asymptomatic patients and stage D1 in symptomatic patients. Classification of stenosis severity is more complex when AVA is 1.0 cm² or less, but mean pressure gradient is less than 40 mm Hg and peak jet velocity is less than 4.0 m/sec. This apparent discordance in indices of AS severity occurs because at a normal flow rate, an AVA of 1.0 corresponds to a mean gradient of 30.[104,105] This is a common clinical conundrum because over one third of patients with severe AS with an AVA of 1.0 cm² or less have a peak jet velocity less than 4.0 m/sec or mean gradient less than 40 mm Hg (stages D2 and D3 in Table 72.2).[104-106] Clinical judgment and expert imaging are the keys to differentiating patients with severe low-flow, low-gradient AS from those with moderate AS.

Asymptomatic Severe Aortic Stenosis (Stage C)

Stage C1 is defined as high-gradient severe AS with no symptoms and preserved systolic function (see Table 72.2). Prospective studies evaluating the rate of progression to symptomatic AS in initially asymptomatic patients are summarized in eTable 72.1. The strongest predictor

of progression to symptoms is the Doppler aortic jet velocity[106] (see also Classic References, Otto). Survival free of symptoms is 84% at 2 years when aortic velocity is less than 3 m/sec, compared with only 21% when velocity is greater than 4 m/sec (Fig. 72.14A). In adults with severe AS (Doppler velocity >4 m/sec), outcome can be further predicted by the magnitude of the Doppler velocity (Fig. 72.14B), as well as by the severity of aortic valve calcification.[84] In such studies, most events consisted of the development of symptoms prompting AVR and not sudden death in otherwise asymptomatic patients. However, retrospective studies have reported cases of sudden death in apparently asymptomatic adults with severe AS.[60]

Stage C2 is defined as high-gradient severe AS with no symptoms but overt LV systolic dysfunction with an LVEF <50%. However, several recent studies indicate that an LVEF of 50% to 60% is linked to a worse prognosis among patients with severe AS.[57-61] Accordingly, an LVEF of 60% is probably a better cutoff for indicating an LVEF below which abnormal function has developed in response to pressure overload from AS; expeditious AVR even in the absence of symptoms may be warranted below this higher LVEF threshold.

Symptomatic Severe Aortic Stenosis (Stage D)

Once even mild symptoms are present, survival is poor unless outflow obstruction is relieved. Expected survival for patients with severe symptomatic AS will differ somewhat based on the age, number of comorbidities,

TABLE 72.2 Stages of Valvular Aortic Stenosis (AS)

STAGE	DEFINITION	VALVE ANATOMY	VALVE HEMODYNAMICS	HEMODYNAMIC CONSEQUENCES	SYMPTOMS
A	At risk of AS	Bicuspid aortic valve (or other congenital valve anomaly) Aortic valve sclerosis	Aortic Vmax <2 m/sec with normal leaflet motion	None	None
B	Progressive AS	Mild to moderate leaflet calcification/fibrosis of a bicuspid or trileaflet valve with some reduction in systolic motion *or* Rheumatic valve changes with commissural fusion	**Mild AS:** Aortic Vmax 2.0-2.9 m/sec or mean ΔP <20 mm Hg **Moderate AS:** Aortic Vmax 3.0-3.9 m/sec or mean ΔP 20-39 mm Hg	Early LV diastolic dysfunction may be present Normal LVEF	None
C	Asymptomatic severe AS				
C1	Asymptomatic severe AS	Severe leaflet calcification/fibrosis or congenital stenosis with severely reduced leaflet opening	**Severe AS:** Aortic Vmax ≥4 m/sec or mean ΔP ≥40 mm Hg AVA typically is ≤1 cm² (or AVAi ≤0.6 cm²/m²) Very severe AS is an aortic Vmax ≥5 m/sec, or mean ΔP ≥ 60 mm Hg	LV diastolic dysfunction Mild LV hypertrophy Normal LVEF	None Exercise testing is reasonable to confirm symptom status
C2	Asymptomatic severe AS with LV systolic dysfunction	Severe leaflet calcification/fibrosis or congenital stenosis with severely reduced leaflet opening	Aortic Vmax ≥4 m/sec or mean ΔP ≥40 mm Hg AVA typically is ≤1 cm² (or AVAi ≤0.6 cm²/m²) but not required to define severe AS	LVEF <50%	None
D	Symptomatic severe AS				
D1	Symptomatic severe high-gradient AS	Severe leaflet calcification/fibrosis or congenital stenosis with severely reduced leaflet opening	**Severe AS:** Aortic Vmax ≥4 m/sec, or mean ΔP ≥40 mm Hg AVA typically is ≤1 cm² (or AVAi ≤0.6 cm²/m²), but may be larger with mixed AS/AR	LV diastolic dysfunction LV hypertrophy Pulmonary hypertension may be present	Exertional dyspnea or decreased exercise tolerance Exertional angina Exertional syncope or presyncope
D2	Symptomatic severe low-flow, low-gradient AS with reduced LVEF	Severe leaflet calcification/fibrosis with severely reduced leaflet motion	AVA ≤1 cm² with resting aortic Vmax <4 m/sec, or mean ΔP <40 mm Hg Dobutamine stress echo shows AVA ≤1 cm² with Vmax ≥4 m/sec at any flow rate	LV diastolic dysfunction LV hypertrophy LVEF <50%	HF Angina Syncope or presyncope
D3	Symptomatic severe low-gradient AS with normal LVEF or paradoxical low-flow severe AS	Severe leaflet calcification/fibrosis with severely reduced leaflet motion	AVA <1.0 cm² (AVAi <0.6 cm²/m²) with aortic Vmax <4 m/sec, or mean ΔP <40 mm Hg *and* stroke volume index <35 mL/m² Measured when patient is normotensive (systolic BP <140 mm Hg)	Increased LV relative wall thickness Small LV chamber with low stroke volume Restrictive diastolic filling LVEF ≥50%	HF Angina Syncope or presyncope

AVA, Aortic valve area; *AVAi, AVA* indexed to body surface area; *BP,* blood pressure; *HF,* heart failure; *LVEF,* left ventricular ejection fraction; *ΔP,* pressure gradient; *Vmax,* maximum aortic jet velocity.
From Otto CM, et al. 2020 AHA/ACC guideline for the management of patients with valvular heart disease: a report of the American College of Cardiology/American Heart Association Task Force on Practice Guidelines. *J Am Coll Cardiol.* 2021;77:e25-e197.

and severity of HF of the cohort examined, but average survival without AVR is only 1 to 3 years after symptom onset. Among symptomatic patients with severe AS, the outlook is poorest when the left ventricle has failed and the cardiac output and transvalvular gradient are both low. The risk of sudden death is high with symptomatic severe AS, so these patients should be promptly referred for AVR. In patients who do not undergo AVR, recurrent hospitalizations for angina and decompensated HF are common, associated with significant consumption of health care resources.[107]

Symptomatic Severe High-Gradient Aortic Stenosis (Stage D1)
Severe high-gradient AS is defined as peak jet velocity of 4.0 m/sec or greater or mean gradient of 40 mm Hg or greater, usually accompanied

by an AVA of 1.0 cm² or less (or indexed AVA of 0.6 cm²/m² or less) (see Table 72.2). Occasionally, AVA may be larger with mixed AS and AR. With alignment of all hemodynamic indices of AS severity, these patients have the clearest evidence of severe AS and warrant prompt referral for AVR.

Symptomatic Severe Low-Flow, Low-Gradient Aortic Stenosis with Reduced LVEF (Stage D2)
Classic low-flow, low-gradient AS (stage D2) is defined as AVA of 1.0 cm² or less with an aortic velocity less than 4.0 m/sec or mean gradient less than 40 mm Hg and LVEF less than 50% (see Table 72.2). Patients with HF symptoms and stage D2 AS often create a diagnostic dilemma for the clinician because their clinical presentation

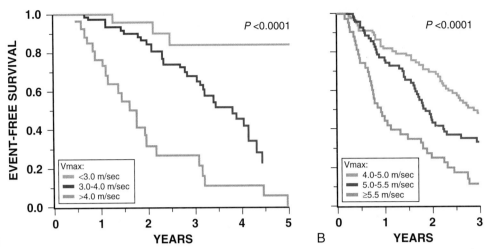

FIGURE 72.14 **Event-free survival based on initial peak aortic jet velocity. A,** Natural history as reflected by event-free survival in asymptomatic patients with aortic stenosis. Initial peak aortic jet velocity (Vmax) stratifies patients according to the likelihood that symptoms requiring valve replacement will develop over time. **B,** Outcomes with very severe aortic stenosis. Kaplan-Meier event-free survival rate for patients with Vmax of 4.0 m/sec or greater. In both **A** and **B,** most "events" consisted of the onset of symptoms warranting aortic valve replacement. (**A** from Otto CM, et al. A prospective study of asymptomatic valvular aortic stenosis: clinical, echocardiographic, and exercise predictors of outcome. *Circulation.* 1997;95:2262; **B** from Rosenhek R, et al. Natural history of very severe aortic stenosis. *Circulation.* 2010;121:151.)

and hemodynamic data may be indistinguishable from those of patients with dilated cardiomyopathy and a calcified valve that is not severely stenotic.[57,83] Severe AS can be distinguished from moderate AS with primary LV dysfunction based on the changes in valve hemodynamics during transient increases in flow, usually by increasing cardiac output with dobutamine[79,83] (see Chapter 16). Severe AS is present if there is an increase in aortic velocity to at least 4 m/sec at any flow rate, with AVA that remains less than 1.0 cm². Dobutamine echocardiography also provides evidence of myocardial contractile reserve (increase in stroke volume >20% from baseline), which historically has been an important predictor of operative risk and survival after SAVR in these patients.[83] However, even in patients who lack contractile reserve, SAVR is associated with better survival (approximately 50% at 5 years) than medical therapy, and more recent studies in patients undergoing TAVR have shown equivalent improvement in LVEF and survival in patients with and without contractile reserve.[65,108]

Symptomatic Severe Low-Flow, Low-Gradient Aortic Stenosis with Preserved LVEF (Stage D3)

Low-flow, low-gradient AS also can occur with a normal LVEF (≥50%) (see Table 72.2), typically in elderly patients with a small, hypertrophied left ventricle or those with concurrent hypertension. This is often referred to as "paradoxical" low-flow, low-gradient AS because despite a normal EF, transaortic flow is low (stroke volume index <35 mL/m²).[57,79,83] Distinguishing truly severe AS from moderate AS can be challenging. Measurement errors should be ruled out and small body size accounted for (an indexed AVA ≤0.6 cm²/m² is consistent with severe AS).[79] Dobutamine has been used to augment flow to distinguish truly severe AS from pseudosevere AS, but is less preferred in these patients with a small, hypertrophied ventricle and marked diastolic dysfunction.[109] Evaluation of valve hemodynamics after treatment of hypertension and, increasingly, CT assessment of valve calcification can be helpful in establishing the diagnosis of severe AS and is being used to identify patients with a severely calcified valve.[57,79,83]

TREATMENT

Medical Management
Medical therapy has thus far been shown to have no effect on disease progression in patients with AS.[1,14,32] Furthermore, both observational

studies and randomized clinical trials (RCTs) convincingly demonstrate that AVR is superior to medical therapy in patients with severe symptomatic AS. The risk of sudden death increases dramatically once symptoms are present, and patients should be advised to report promptly the development of any symptoms possibly related to AS. In asymptomatic patients with AS of any degree, evaluation and treatment for conventional cardiovascular risk factors is recommended in accordance with established guidelines (see Chapter 25).

Hypertension accompanies AS in many patients.[110] Because of traditional teaching that AS is a disease with fixed afterload, there often has been reluctance to treat hypertension because of concerns that vasodilation would not be offset by an increase in stroke volume. However, several studies have demonstrated that vasodilation is accompanied by increases in stroke volume, even in patients with severe AS[66] (see also Classic References, Khot). Hypertension imposes an additional load on the left ventricle and is associated with more adverse hypertrophic LV remodeling. Although treatment of hypertension may not reduce AS-related events, it should be treated because of the well-known adverse association between hypertension and vascular events and mortality.[111] Whether blood pressure targets should be the same (versus slightly higher) for patients with AS as the general population is unclear.[111] There is no one class of medicines established as the preferred treatment of hypertension in patients with AS, but because the renin-angiotensin system is upregulated in the valve and ventricle of patients with AS, angiotensin-converting-enzyme (ACE) inhibitors or angiotensin receptor blockers (ARBs) may be preferentially considered. Small studies have demonstrated their safety, and some suggest a clinical benefit, but larger-scale randomized studies are needed.

Concomitant CAD is common in middle-aged and elderly patients with AS. Primary and secondary prevention guidelines should be followed, and the decision of whether to prescribe a statin medication should not be influenced by the presence of AS. RCTs testing the use of statins in patients with mild AS to more advanced disease were adequately powered and showed no improvement in mortality, time to AVR, or rate of AS progression in the treatment versus placebo groups.[15]

AF or atrial flutter develop in up to one third of older patients with AS, perhaps exacerbated by left atrial enlargement related to diastolic dysfunction. When such an arrhythmia is observed in a patient with AS, the possibility of associated mitral valvular disease should be considered. When AF occurs, the rapid ventricular rate may precipitate symptoms, and the loss of atrial contribution to LV filling and a sudden fall in cardiac output may cause serious hypotension. If this occurs, AF should be treated promptly, usually with cardioversion. New-onset AF in a previously asymptomatic patient with severe AS may be a marker of impending symptom onset. For those with AF and native valve AS, as well as those treated with a bioprosthetic valve more than 3 months ago, anticoagulation with a non–vitamin K oral anticoagulant is an effective alternative to warfarin.[57]

In patients with HF and volume overload, AVR is indicated, but diuretics may reduce congestion and provide some symptomatic relief before intervention. Patients with decompensated HF may benefit from medical therapy as a bridge to definitive therapy with AVR. Nitroprusside has been used during hemodynamic monitoring in the intensive care unit to unload the left heart, reduce congestion, and improve forward flow (see Classic References, Khot). Similarly, phosphodiesterase type 5 inhibition has been shown to provide acute improvements in pulmonary and systemic hemodynamics resulting in biventricular unloading.[66] These medications may improve the patient's hemodynamic status, allowing the AVR procedure to be performed more safely.

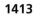

TABLE 72.3 Indications for Aortic Valve Replacement in Patients with Aortic Stenosis

COR	LOE	RECOMMENDATIONS
1	A	1. In adults with severe high-gradient AS (stage D1) and symptoms of exertional dyspnea, HF, angina, syncope, or presyncope by history or on exercise testing, AVR is indicated.
1	B-NR	2. In asymptomatic patients with severe AS and an LVEF <50% (stage C2). AVR is indicated.
1	B-NR	3. In asymptomatic patients with severe AS (stage C1) who are undergoing cardiac surgery for other indications, AVR is indicated.
1	B-NR	4. In symptomatic patients with low-flow, low-gradient severe AS with reduced LVEF (stage D2). AVR is recommended.
1	B-NR	5. In symptomatic patients with low-flow, low-gradient severe AS with normal LVEF (stage D3), AVR is recommended if AS is the most likely cause of symptoms.
2a	B-NR	6. In apparently asymptomatic patients with severe AS (stage C1) and low surgical risk, AVR is reasonable when an exercise test demonstrates decreased exercise tolerance (normalized for age and sex) or a fall in systolic blood pressure of ≥10 mm Hg from baseline to peak exercise.
2a	B-R	7. In asymptomatic patients with very severe AS (defined as an aortic velocity of ≥5 m/s) and low surgical risk, AVR is reasonable.
2a	B-NR	8. In apparently asymptomatic patients with severe AS (stage C1) and low surgical risk, AVR is reasonable when the serum B-type natriuretic peptide (BNP) level is greater than three times normal.
2a	B-NR	9. In asymptomatic patients with high-gradient severe AS (stage C1) and low surgical risk. AVR is reasonable when serial testing shows an increase in aortic velocity ≥0.3 m/s per year.
2b	B-NR	10. In asymptomatic patients with severe high-gradient AS (stage C1) and a progressive decrease in LVEF on at least three serial imaging studies to <60%, AVR may be considered.
2b	C-EO	11. In patients with moderate AS (stage B) who are undergoing cardiac surgery for other indications. AVR may be considered.

AS, Aortic stenosis; *AVR,* aortic valve replacement; *HF,* heart failure *LVEF,* left ventricular ejection fraction.
From Otto CM, et al. 2020 AHA/ACC guideline for the management of patients with valvular heart disease: a report of the American College of Cardiology/American Heart Association Task Force on Practice Guidelines. *J Am Coll Cardiol.* 2021;77:e25-e197.

Balloon Aortic Valvuloplasty

AVR is the procedure of choice for relief of outflow obstruction in adults with valvular AS. Balloon aortic valvuloplasty has only a modest hemodynamic effect in patients with calcific AS. It can provide short-term improvement in survival and quality of life, but these benefits are not sustained.[112] Accordingly, balloon aortic valvuloplasty is not recommended as an alternative to valve replacement for calcific AS. In selected cases, it might be reasonable as a bridge to definitive treatment with AVR in unstable patients or as a palliative procedure in patients who are not candidates for AVR.[57]

Aortic Valve Replacement

Recommendations regarding indications for and timing of AVR, type of valve used, and procedural approach require discussions within a multidisciplinary heart team and shared decision making with the patient and family.[57] Current recommendations for AVR in the 2020 revised ACC/AHA guidelines for management of valvular heart disease are shown in Table 72.3. AVR is recommended (Class I) for adults with symptomatic severe AS (stages D1, D2, and D3), even if symptoms are mild (Fig. 72.15).[57,113] AVR also is recommended (Class I) for severe AS with a LVEF less than 50% and for patients with severe asymptomatic AS who are undergoing coronary artery bypass grafting (CABG) or other forms of heart surgery. In addition, AVR is reasonable (Class IIa) for apparently asymptomatic patients with severe high-gradient AS when exercise testing provokes symptoms or a fall in blood pressure. AVR is also reasonable (Class IIa) in asymptomatic patients at low surgical risk when (1) AS is very severe (Vmax ≥5 m/sec), (2) there is rapid disease progression, or (3) BNP is greater than three times the upper limit of normal. AVR may be considered (Class IIb) when there is a progressive decrease in LVEF on at least three serial imaging studies to less than 60%.[57] Further studies are needed to determine whether other indexes of risk warrant earlier intervention in asymptomatic patients with severe AS. These include evidence of myocardial fibrosis, impaired longitudinal strain, pulmonary hypertension, and moderate or severe LVH, among others.[40,42,59,62]

The management of asymptomatic patients is the subject of ongoing study and debate.[114] A prospective observational study of initially asymptomatic Japanese patients with severe AS compared outcome in those who underwent early surgery versus a "watchful waiting" strategy.[115] With propensity matching to adjust for baseline differences between the two groups, the survival rate was significantly higher in the 291 patients with early surgery compared to the 291 initially followed conservatively. However, it is noteworthy that 31% of patients in the conservative group who developed symptoms did not undergo AVR, and this accounted for 17% of the deaths during "watchful waiting." Although this and other retrospective studies comparing prompt AVR versus medical therapy[116] are suggestive, propensity matching has its limitations. The nonperformance of AVR in many patients in the medical therapy group either initially or when criteria for AVR develop limit the value of these comparisons for informing optimal timing of AVR. Thus, the role of early AVR in asymptomatic patients can be determined only with appropriately designed RCTs.

Recently, a small trial randomized 145 asymptomatic patients with very severe AS (AVA ≤0.75 cm² or peak jet velocity ≥4.5 m/sec or higher or mean gradient ≥50 mm Hg or higher) to early SAVR (within 2 months of randomization) or conservative therapy with referral to SAVR when symptoms or overt LV dysfunction developed.[117] The primary end point of operative mortality or cardiovascular mortality occurred in 1% in the early surgery group and 15% in the conservative care group (HR 0.09, 95% CI 0.01 to 0.67); death from any cause occurred in 7% in the early surgery group and 21% in the conservative care group (HR 0.33, 95% CI 0.12 to 0.90). These randomized data are helpful in clarifying optimal timing of AVR in asymptomatic patients, but a couple of limitations should be considered: only younger, lower risk patients with very severe AS were included, and the small sample size with few events yielded wide confidence intervals. Several larger RCTs are under way testing the optimal timing of TAVR in asymptomatic patients; these include older, higher-risk patients and modestly less severe AS, albeit generally still high-gradient severe AS.[114] Additional RCTs are needed to

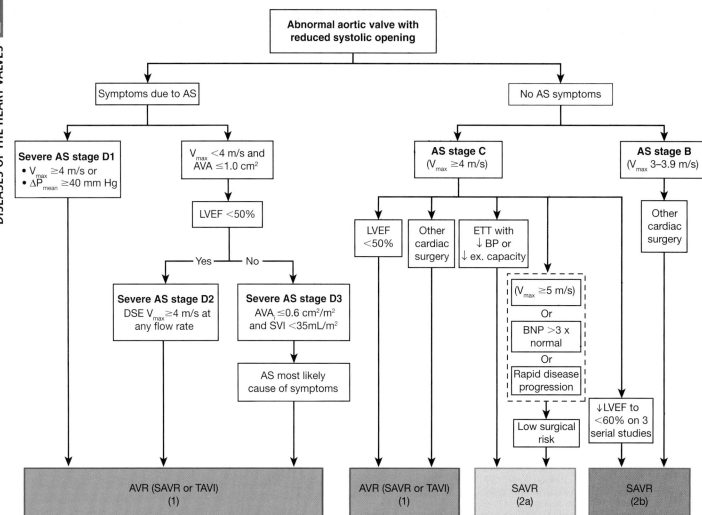

FIGURE 72.15 Recommendations for aortic valve replacement (*AVR*) in patients with aortic stenosis (*AS*). Colors correspond to Table 72.3. *Arrows* show the decision pathways that result in a recommendation for AVR. Periodic monitoring is indicated for all patients in whom AVR is not yet indicated, including those with asymptomatic (stage C) and symptomatic (stage D) AS and those with low-gradient AS (stage D2 or D3) who do not meet the criteria for intervention. See Fig 72.16 for choice of valve type (mechanical versus bioprosthetic [TAVI or SAVR]) when AVR is indicated. *AVA,* Aortic valve area; *AVA$_i$,* aortic valve area index; *BNP,* B-type natriuretic peptide; *BP,* blood pressure; *DSE,* dobutamine stress echocardiography; *ETT,* exercise treadmill test; *ex,* exercise; *LVEF,* left ventricular ejection fraction; *ΔP$_{mean}$,* mean systolic pressure gradient between LV and aorta; *SAVR,* surgical aortic valve replacement; *SVI,* stroke volume index; *TAVI,* transcatheter aortic valve implantation; *TAVR,* transcatheter aortic valve replacement; *V$_{max}$,* maximum velocity. (From Otto CM, et al. 2020 AHA/ACC guideline for the management of patients with valvular heart disease: a report of the American College of Cardiology/American Heart Association Task Force on Practice Guidelines. *J Am Coll Cardiol.* 2021;77:e25-197.)

clarify optimal timing of SAVR and TAVR in numerous subgroups of patients with moderate and severe AS.

In patients fulfilling current criteria for AVR, the next series of decisions revolves around a surgical or transcatheter approach. Current recommendations for SAVR or TAVR are shown in Table 72.4 and Fig. 72.16 (see also Fig. 72.15). For patients with life expectancy less than 1 year or anticipated poor quality of life not related to their AS, AVR is likely futile and palliative care is recommended.[57,118,119]

In general, AVR leads to an improvement in symptoms, quality of life, and functional capacity and lower rates of hospitalization and death. These clinical improvements are accompanied by reverse remodeling in the heart and improvements in LV function; however, cardiac recovery is variable and often incomplete with untoward consequences.[34,41,43,46,48,120]

Surgical Aortic Valve Replacement

The Society of Thoracic Surgeons (STS) 2020 update on outcomes (reporting data for the year 2018) cited an overall 30-day mortality rate of 1.9% in 25,274 patients undergoing isolated SAVR and 3.6% in 15,855 patients undergoing SAVR and CABG.[121] In patients younger than 70

with minimal comorbidities, the operative risk of mortality is less than 1% in many centers. Medicare data from the past decade indicate that the 30-day mortality after SAVR in patients aged 65 and older in the United States has decreased from 7.6% in 1999 to 4.2% in 2011, with the most marked decrease in patients aged 85 and older, in whom the 30-day mortality has decreased from 12.3% to 5.8%.[122] Therefore, advanced age should not be considered a contraindication to operation, although the majority of such patients are now treated with TAVR. Overall surgical volumes are declining as the volume of TAVR procedures steadily increases (63,361 in 2018).[121] This has the effect of also reducing SAVR mortality rates. The 30-day SAVR mortality rate also is significantly related to the number of AVR procedures performed at each hospital. Risk factors associated with a higher mortality rate include a high New York Heart Association functional class, impaired LV function, advanced age, the presence of associated CAD, and other comorbidities.

Transcatheter Aortic Valve Replacement

Over the last decade, TAVR has transformed the treatment of patients with calcific AS (see Chapter 74). Initial RCTs showed TAVR to be

TABLE 72.4 Recommendations for Choice of SAVR Versus TAVR for Patients for Whom a Bioprosthetic AVR Is Appropriate

COR	LOE	RECOMMENDATIONS
1	A	1. For symptomatic and asymptomatic patients with severe AS and any indication for AVR who are younger than 65 years of age or have a life expectancy >20 years. SAVR is recommended.
1	A	2. For symptomatic patients with severe AS who are 65 to 80 years of age and have no anatomic contraindication to transfemoral TAVI, either SAVR or transfemoral TAVI is recommended after shared decision making about the balance between expected patient longevity and valve durability.
1	A	3. For symptomatic patients with severe AS who are older than 80 years of age or for younger patients with a life expectancy <10 years and no anatomic contraindication to transfemoral TAVI, transfemoral TAVI is recommended in preference to SAVR.
1	B-NR	4. In asymptomatic patients with severe AS and an LVEF <50% who are 80 years of age or younger and have no anatomic contraindication to transfemoral TAVI, the decision between TAVI and SAVR should follow the same recommendations as for symptomatic patients in Recommendations 1, 2, and 3 above.
1	B-NR	5. For asymptomatic patients with severe AS and an abnormal exercise test, very severe AS, rapid progression, or an elevated BNP (COR 2a indications for AVR), SAVR is recommended in preference to TAVI.
1	A	6. For patients with an indication for AVR for whom a bioprosthetic valve is preferred but valve, vascular anatomy, or other factors are not suitable for transfemoral TAVI, SAVR is recommended.
1	A	7. For symptomatic patients of any age with severe AS and a high or prohibitive surgical risk, TAVI is recommended if predicted post-TAVI survival is >12 months with an acceptable quality of life.
1	C-EO	8. For symptomatic patients with severe AS for whom predicted post-TAVI or post-SAVR survival is <12 months or for whom minimal improvement in quality of life is expected, palliative care is recommended after shared decision making, including discussion of patient preferences and values.
2b	C-EO	9. In critically ill patients with severe AS, percutaneous aortic balloon dilation may be considered as a bridge to SAVR or TAVI.

AS, Aortic stenosis; *LVEF*, left ventricular ejection fraction; *SAVR*, surgical aortic valve replacement; *TAVI*, transcatheter aortic valve implantation.
From Otto CM, et al. 2020 AHA/ACC guideline for the management of patients with valvular heart disease: a report of the American College of Cardiology/American Heart Association Task Force on Practice Guidelines *J Am Coll Cardiol.* 2021;77:e25-e197.

superior to medical therapy (usually accompanied by balloon aortic valvuloplasty) in patients who were at prohibitive risk for surgery. Subsequently, in patients deemed high, intermediate, and low risk for surgery, TAVR was shown to be noninferior and, in some trials/subgroups, superior to SAVR.[123-127] Accordingly, TAVR is approved for the treatment of severe AS at all level of levels of risk. The most common approach to valve implantation is *transfemoral* (~95% of cases), particularly as sheath size progressively decreases. Although 5-year data on transcatheter valve durability are encouraging, longer-term data are needed particularly as we move toward treating younger, lower-risk patients.[128]

Patient Selection for TAVR or SAVR
The choice of SAVR versus TAVR should come after a decision that AVR is indicated (see Fig. 72.15). Recommendations for type of valve (mechanical versus bioprosthetic) and type of procedure (surgical versus transcatheter) are outlined in detail in Fig. 72.16. Given the complexity of issues to consider, it is recommended that these decisions occur in the environment of a multidisciplinary heart valve team of cardiac surgeons, interventional cardiologists, clinical and imaging experts in valve disease, and nurses, anesthetists, and geriatricians as needed.[57] Shared decision making with the patient and family is also essential, so that their values and preferences can be incorporated into any treatment decision.[57,129,130] As the field, experience, and technology have evolved, the choice between TAVR and SAVR has become less about patient/surgical risk (because of comorbidities) and more about age, anatomy, and accompanying coronary, valve, or aortic pathology (Table 72.5). TAVR is favored for individuals 80 years and older and those at high or extreme surgical risk, whereas SAVR is favored in those younger than 65 years of age (see Fig. 72.16). Beyond that, multiple factors should be considered to match a specific patient with the right therapy; in many cases, either TAVR or SAVR will be reasonable options. A significant area of uncertainty relates to younger patient age due to uncertainty regarding transcatheter valve durability, higher need for pacemakers after TAVR, and the anticipated need for multiple lifetime procedures if a bioprosthetic valve is implanted. Related to that is uncertainty regarding how to treat patients with BAV anatomy

because of uncertainties regarding TAVR efficacy in BAVs, which are encountered more frequently in young patients, and those with a BAV were routinely excluded from the randomized trials comparing TAVR to SAVR. However, TAVR has been performed in patients with a bicuspid valve with excellent results,[1,131-133] but patient age, valve anatomy, extent and location of calcification, and associated aortopathy all influence anticipated success with TAVR and degree of clinical equipoise between the two treatment options. Randomized trials are being considered to clarify optimal management of patients with bicuspid AS.

Postprocedural Issues
Even after treatment of AS with AVR, several issues remain important for clinical management to optimize patient outcomes. As is true after other cardiovascular events, participation in *cardiac rehabilitation* after heart valve surgery is associated with lower rates of death and rehospitalization over the first postprocedure year; however, only a minority participate.[134] In the case of *structural valve degeneration and valve thrombosis*, bioprosthetic valves, both surgical and transcatheter, are prone to develop valve thrombosis and/or degenerate (e.g., calcify, pannus, leaflet tearing) over time (see Chapter 79). The incidence, consequences, and treatment implications of valve thrombosis are still being examined.[135] In some cases, there will be a marked early increase in transvalvular gradient as a result of valve thrombosis that is often responsive to treatment with anticoagulation. Ongoing surveillance with echocardiography and, as indicated, four-dimensional CT is important to detect these issues early. Although AVR improves HF symptoms and quality of life on the whole, a sizeable minority has *residual HF* after AVR, resulting in rehospitalization and less or no improvement in quality of life.[119,136,137] Accordingly, rather than simply viewing AVR as the curative "fix" for AS, treatment of HF with a reduced or preserved EF with appropriate medical therapy is critical to optimize outcomes. Some studies suggest that blood pressure targets for patients treated with AVR for AS may need to be slightly higher than for the general population, although further studies are needed to clarify this issue.[72,138]

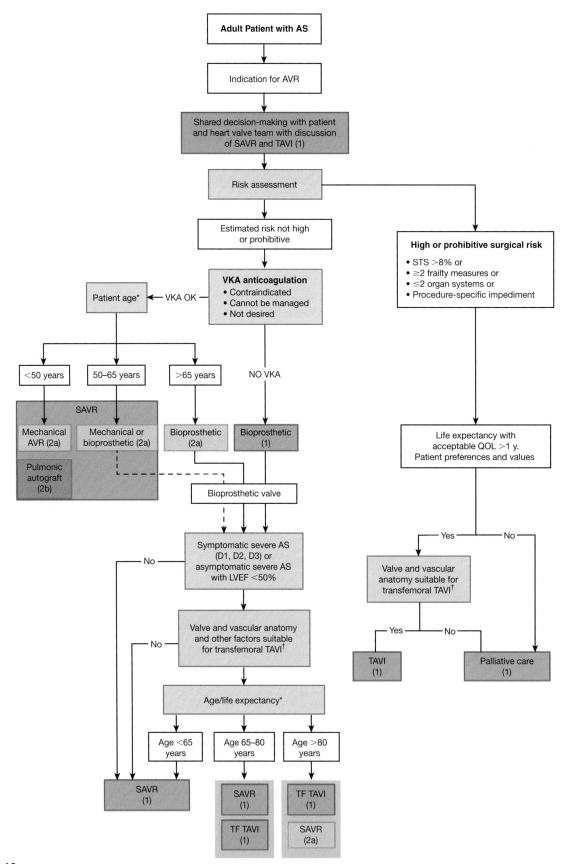

FIGURE 72.16 Selection of surgical versus transcatheter aortic valve replacement. Colors correspond to Table 72.3.*Approximate ages, based on U.S. Actuarial Life Expectancy tables, are provided for guidance. The balance between expected patient longevity and valve durability varies continuously across the age range, with more durable valves preferred for patients with a longer life expectancy. Bioprosthetic valve durability is finite (with shorter durability for younger patients), whereas mechanical valves are very durable but require lifelong anticoagulation. Long-term (20 years) data on outcomes with surgical bioprosthetic valves are available; robust data on transcatheter bioprosthetic valves extend to only 5 years, leading to uncertainty about longer-term outcomes. The decision about valve type should be individualized on the basis of patient-specific factors that might affect expected longevity. † Placement of a transcatheter valve requires vascular anatomy that allows transfemoral delivery and the absence of aortic root dilation that would require surgical replacement. Valvular anatomy must be suitable for placement of the specific prosthetic valve, including annulus size and shape, leaflet number and calcification, and coronary ostial height. *AS,* Aortic stenosis; *AVR,* aortic valve replacement; *LVEF,* left ventricular ejection fraction; *QOL,* quality of life; *SAVR,* surgical aortic valve replacement; *STS,* Society of Thoracic Surgeons; *TAVI,* transcatheter aortic valve implantation; *TF,* transfemoral; and *VKA,* vitamin K antagonist. (From Otto CM, et al. 2020 AHA/ACC guideline for the management of patients with valvular heart disease: a report of the American College of Cardiology/ American Heart Association Task Force on Practice Guidelines. *J Am Coll Cardiol.* 2021;77:e25-197.)

TABLE 72.5 Factors to Consider for Patient Selection for Transcatheter Versus Surgical Aortic Valve Replacement

Age
Bicuspid versus tricuspid valve
Valve calcification (amount, location)
Aortic size
Annulus size
Concomitant severe mitral or tricuspid valve disease
Extent, location, and complexity of coronary disease
Severity of left ventricular dysfunction
Transfemoral vascular access

CLASSIC REFERENCES

Grossman W, Jones D, McLaurin LP. Wall stress and patterns of hypertrophy in the human left ventricle. *J Clin Invest*. 1975;56:56–64.

Hill JA, Karimi M, Kutschke W, et al. Cardiac hypertrophy is not a required compensatory response to short-term pressure overload. *Circulation*. 2000;101:2863–2869.

Khot UN, Novaro GM, Popovic ZB, et al. Nitroprusside in critically ill patients with left ventricular dysfunction and aortic stenosis. *N Engl J Med*. 2003;348:1756–1763.

Otto CM, Burwash IG, Legget ME, et al. Prospective study of asymptomatic valvular aortic stenosis. Clinical, echocardiographic, and exercise predictors of outcome. *Circulation*. 1997;95:2262–2270.

Roberts WC, Ko JM. Frequency by decades of unicuspid, bicuspid, and tricuspid aortic valves in adults having isolated aortic valve replacement for aortic stenosis, with or without associated aortic regurgitation. *Circulation*. 2005;111:920–925.

REFERENCES

Epidemiology

1. Lindman BR, Clavel MA, Mathieu P, et al. Calcific aortic stenosis. *Nat Rev Dis Primers*. 2016;2:16006.
2. Osnabrugge RL, Mylotte D, Head SJ, et al. Aortic stenosis in the elderly: disease prevalence and number of candidates for transcatheter aortic valve replacement: a meta-analysis and modeling study. *J Am Coll Cardiol*. 2013;62:1002–1012.
3. d'Arcy JL, Coffey S, Loudon MA, et al. Large-scale community echocardiographic screening reveals a major burden of undiagnosed valvular heart disease in older people: the OxVALVE Population Cohort Study. *Eur Heart J*. 2016;37:3515–3522.
4. Coffey S, Cox B, Williams MJ. The prevalence, incidence, progression, and risks of aortic valve sclerosis: a systematic review and meta-analysis. *J Am Coll Cardiol*. 2014;63:2852–2861.
5. Yan AT, Koh M, Chan KK, et al. Association between cardiovascular risk factors and aortic stenosis: the CANHEART aortic stenosis study. *J Am Coll Cardiol*. 2017;69:1523–1532.
6. Lindman BR. Aortic stenosis: moving from treatment to prevention. *J Am Coll Cardiol*. 2017;69:1533–1535.
7. Prakash SK, Bosse Y, Muehlschlegel JD, et al. A roadmap to investigate the genetic basis of bicuspid aortic valve and its complications: insights from the International BAVCon (Bicuspid Aortic Valve Consortium). *J Am Coll Cardiol*. 2014;64:832–839.
8. Verma S, Siu SC. Aortic dilatation in patients with bicuspid aortic valve. *N Engl J Med*. 2014;370:1920–1929.
9. Michelena HI, Prakash SK, Della Corte A, et al. Bicuspid aortic valve: identifying knowledge gaps and rising to the challenge from the international Bicuspid Aortic Valve Consortium (BAVCon). *Circulation*. 2014;129:2691–2704.
10. Sherrah AG, Andvik S, van der Linde D, et al. Nonsyndromic thoracic aortic aneurysm and dissection outcomes with marfan syndrome versus bicuspid aortic valve aneurysm. *J Am Coll Cardiol*. 2016;67:618–626.
11. Masri A, Svensson LG, Griffin BP, et al. Contemporary natural history of bicuspid aortic valve disease: a systematic review. *Heart*. 2017;103:1323–1330.
12. Detaint D, Michelena HI, Nkomo VT, et al. Aortic dilatation patterns and rates in adults with bicuspid aortic valves: a comparative study with Marfan syndrome and degenerative aortopathy. *Heart*. 2014;100:126–134.
13. Braverman AC, Cheng A. The bicuspid aortic valve and associated aortic disease. In: Otto CM, Bonow RO, eds. *Valvular Heart Disease: A Companion to Braunwald's Heart Disease*. 5th ed. Philadelphia: Saunders; 2021:197–222.

Pathophysiology: Calcification and Obstruction

14. Otto C, Prendergast B. Aortic-valve stenosis–from patients at risk to severe valve obstruction. *N Engl J Med*. 2014;371:744–576.
15. Hutcheson JD, Aikawa E, Merryman WD. Potential drug targets for calcific aortic valve disease. *Nat Rev Cardiol*. 2014;11:218–231.
16. Zheng KH, Tzolos E, Dweck MR. Pathophysiology of aortic stenosis and future perspectives for medical therapy. *Cardiol Clin*. 2020;38:1–12.
17. Marquis-Gravel G, Redfors B, Leon MB, et al. Medical treatment of aortic stenosis. *Circulation*. 2016;134:1766–1784.
18. Thanassoulis G. Clinical and genetic risk factors for calcific valve disease. In: Otto CM, Bonow RO, eds. *Valvular Heart Disease: A Companion to Braunwald's Heart Disease*. 5th ed. Philadelphia: Saunders; 2021:66–78.
19. Thanassoulis G, Campbell CY, Owens DS, et al. Genetic associations with valvular calcification and aortic stenosis. *N Engl J Med*. 2013;368:503–512.
20. Kamstrup PR, Tybjærg-Hansen A, Nordestgaard BG. Elevated lipoprotein(a) and risk of aortic valve stenosis in the general population. *J Am Coll Cardiol*. 2014;63:470–477.
21. Cairns BJ, Coffey S, Travis RC, et al. A replicated, genome-wide significant association of aortic stenosis with a genetic variant for lipoprotein(a): meta-analysis of published and novel data. *Circulation*. 2017;135:1181–1183.
22. Perrot N, Theriault S, Dina C, et al. Genetic Variation in LPA, calcific aortic valve stenosis in patients undergoing cardiac surgery, and familial risk of aortic valve microcalcification. *JAMA Cardiol*. 2019;4:620–627.
23. Capoulade R, Chan KL, Yeang C, et al. Oxidized phospholipids, lipoprotein(a), and progression of calcific aortic valve stenosis. *J Am Coll Cardiol*. 2015;66:1236–4126.
24. Capoulade R, Mahmut A, Tastet L, et al. Impact of plasma Lp-PLA2 activity on the progression of aortic stenosis: the PROGRESSA study. *JACC Cardiovasc Imaging*. 2015;8:26–33.
25. Mahmut A, Boulanger MC, El Husseini D, et al. Elevated expression of lipoprotein-associated phospholipase A2 in calcific aortic valve disease: implications for valve mineralization. *J Am Coll Cardiol*. 2014;63:460–469.
26. Bouchareb R, Mahmut A, Nsaibia MJ, et al. Autotaxin derived from lipoprotein(a) and valve interstitial cells promotes inflammation and mineralization of the aortic valve. *Circulation*. 2015;132:677–690.
27. Rogers MA, Aikawa E. A Not-So-Little role for lipoprotein(a) in the development of calcific aortic valve disease. *Circulation*. 2015;132:621–362.
28. Hadji F, Boulanger MC, Guay SP, et al. Altered DNA methylation of long noncoding RNA H19 in calcific aortic valve disease promotes mineralization by silencing NOTCH1. *Circulation*. 2016;134:1848–1862.
29. Merryman WD, Clark CR. Lnc-ing NOTCH1 to idiopathic calcific aortic valve disease. *Circulation*. 2016;134:1863–1865.
30. Clark CR, Bowler MA, Snider JC, et al. Targeting cadherin-11 prevents notch1-mediated calcific aortic valve disease. *Circulation*. 2017;135:2448–2450.
31. Menon V, Lincoln J. The genetic regulation of aortic valve development and calcific disease. *Front Cardiovasc Med*. 2018;5:162.
32. Lindman BR, Merryman WD. Unloading the stenotic path to identifying medical therapy for calcific aortic valve disease: barriers and opportunities. *Circulation*. 2021;143:1455–1457.

Pathophysiology: Left Ventricular Response

33. Lindman BR. Left ventricular and vascular changes in valvular heart disease. In: Otto CM, Bonow RO, eds. *Valvular Heart Disease: A Companion to Braunwald's Heart Disease*. 5th ed. Philadelphia: Saunders; 2021:79–93.
34. Treibel TA, Badiani S, Lloyd G, et al. Multimodality imaging markers of adverse myocardial remodeling in aortic stenosis. *JACC Cardiovasc Imaging*. 2019;12:1532–1548.
35. Dweck MR, Boon NA, Newby DE. Calcific aortic stenosis: a disease of the valve and the myocardium. *J Am Coll Cardiol*. 2012;60:1854–1863.
36. Carabello BA. Is cardiac hypertrophy good or bad? The answer, of course, is yes. *JACC Cardiovasc Imaging*. 2014;7:1081–1083.
37. Petrov G, Dworatzek E, Schulze TM, et al. Maladaptive remodeling is associated with impaired survival in women but not in men after aortic valve replacement. *JACC Cardiovasc Imaging*. 2014;7:1073–1080.
38. Lindman BR, Arnold SV, Madrazo JA, et al. The adverse impact of diabetes mellitus on left ventricular remodeling and function in patients with severe aortic stenosis. *Circ Heart Fail*. 2011;4:286–292.
39. Beach JM, Mihaljevic T, Rajeswaran J, et al. Ventricular hypertrophy and left atrial dilatation persist and are associated with reduced survival after valve replacement for aortic stenosis. *J Thorac Cardiovasc Surg*. 2014;147:362–369.e8.
40. Gonzales H, Douglas PS, Pibarot P, et al. Left ventricular hypertrophy and clinical outcomes over 5 Years after TAVR: an analysis of the PARTNER trials and registries. *JACC Cardiovasc Interv*. 2020;13:1329–1339.
41. Chau KH, Douglas PS, Pibarot P, et al. Regression of left ventricular mass after transcatheter aortic valve replacement: the PARTNER trials and registries. *J Am Coll Cardiol*. 2020;75:2446–2458.
42. Everett RJ, Treibel TA, Fukui M, et al. Extracellular myocardial volume in patients with aortic stenosis. *J Am Coll Cardiol*. 2020;75:304–316.
43. Chin CWL, Everett RJ, Kwiecinski J, et al. Myocardial fibrosis and cardiac decompensation in aortic stenosis. *JACC Cardiovasc Imaging*. 2017;10:1320–1333.
44. Papanastasiou CA, Kokkinidis DG, Kampaktsis PN, et al. The prognostic role of late gadolinium enhancement in aortic stenosis: a systematic review and meta-analysis. *JACC Cardiovasc Imaging*. 2020;13:385–392.
45. Treibel TA, Lopez B, Gonzalez A, et al. Reappraising myocardial fibrosis in severe aortic stenosis: an invasive and non-invasive study in 133 patients. *Eur Heart J*. 2018;39:699–709.
46. Treibel TA, Kozor R, Schofield R, et al. Reverse myocardial remodeling following valve replacement in patients with aortic stenosis. *J Am Coll Cardiol*. 2018;71:860–871.
47. Bing R, Cavalcante JL, Everett RJ, et al. Imaging and impact of myocardial fibrosis in aortic stenosis. *JACC Cardiovasc Imaging*. 2019;12:283–296.
48. Weidemann F, Herrmann S, Stork S, et al. Impact of myocardial fibrosis in patients with symptomatic severe aortic stenosis. *Circulation*. 2009;120:577–584.
49. Naya M, Chiba S, Iwano H, et al. Myocardial oxidative metabolism is increased due to haemodynamic overload in patients with aortic valve stenosis: assessment using 11C-acetate positron emission tomography. *Eur J Nucl Med Mol Imaging*. 2010;37:2242–2248.
50. Ahn JH, Kim SM, Park SJ, et al. Coronary Microvascular dysfunction as a mechanism of angina in severe AS: prospective adenosine-stress CMR study. *J Am Coll Cardiol*. 2016;67:1412–1422.
51. Singh A, Jerosch-Herold M, Bekele S, et al. Determinants of exercise capacity and myocardial perfusion reserve in asymptomatic patients with aortic stenosis. *JACC Cardiovasc Imaging*. 2020;13:178–180.
52. Mahmod M, Chan K, Raman B, et al. Histological evidence for impaired myocardial perfusion reserve in severe aortic stenosis. *JACC Cardiovasc Imaging*. 2019;12:2276–2278.
53. Kampaktsis PN, Kokkinidis DG, Wong SC, et al. The role and clinical implications of diastolic dysfunction in aortic stenosis. *Heart*. 2017;103:1481–1487.
54. Ong G, Pibarot P, Redfors B, et al. Diastolic function and clinical outcomes after transcatheter aortic valve replacement: PARTNER 2 SAPIEN 3 registry. *J Am Coll Cardiol*. 2020;76:2940–2951.
55. Kampaktsis PN, Bang CN, Chiu Wong S, et al. Prognostic importance of diastolic dysfunction in relation to post procedural aortic insufficiency in patients undergoing transcatheter aortic valve replacement. *Catheter Cardiovasc Interv*. 2017;89:445–451.
56. Ito S, Miranda WR, Nkomo VT, et al. Reduced left ventricular ejection fraction in patients with aortic stenosis. *J Am Coll Cardiol*. 2018;71:1313–1321.
57. Otto CM, Nishimura RA, Bonow RO, et al. 2020 ACC/AHA guideline for the management of patients with valvular heart disease: a report of the American College of Cardiology/American Heart Association Joint Committee on Clinical Practice Guidelines. *J Am Coll Cardiol*. 2021;77:e25–e197.
58. Dahl JS, Eleid MF, Michelena HI, et al. Effect of left ventricular ejection fraction on postoperative outcome in patients with severe aortic stenosis undergoing aortic valve replacement. *Circ Cardiovasc Imaging*. 2015;8:e002917.
59. Dahl JS, Magne J, Pellikka PA, et al. Assessment of Subclinical left ventricular dysfunction in aortic stenosis. *JACC Cardiovasc Imaging*. 2019;12:163–171.
60. Lancellotti P, Magne J, Dulgheru R, et al. Outcomes of patients with asymptomatic aortic stenosis followed up in heart valve clinics. *JAMA Cardiol*. 2018;3:1060–1068.
61. Taniguchi T, Morimoto T, Shiomi H, et al. Prognostic impact of left ventricular ejection fraction in patients with severe aortic stenosis. *JACC Cardiovasc Interv*. 2018;11:145–157.
62. Magne J, Cosyns B, Popescu BA, et al. Distribution and Prognostic significance of left ventricular global longitudinal strain in asymptomatic significant aortic stenosis: an individual participant data meta-analysis. *JACC Cardiovasc Imaging*. 2019;12:84–92.
63. Elmariah S, Palacios IF, McAndrew T, et al. Outcomes of transcatheter and surgical aortic valve replacement in high-risk patients with aortic stenosis and left ventricular dysfunction: results from the Placement of Aortic Transcatheter Valves (PARTNER) trial (cohort A). *Circ Cardiovasc Interv*. 2013;6:604–614.
64. Dauerman HL, Reardon MJ, Popma JJ, et al. Early recovery of left ventricular systolic function after CoreValve transcatheter aortic valve replacement. *Circ Cardiovasc Interv*. 2016;9:e003425.

65. Maes F, Lerakis S, Barbosa Ribeiro H, et al. Outcomes from transcatheter aortic valve replacement in patients with low-flow, low-gradient aortic stenosis and left ventricular ejection fraction less than 30%: a Substudy from the TOPAS-TAVI registry. *JAMA Cardiol*. 2019;4:64–70.

Pathophysiology: Pulmonary and Systemic Vasculature Response

66. Lindman BR, Zajarias A, Madrazo JA, et al. Effects of phosphodiesterase type 5 inhibition on systemic and pulmonary hemodynamics and ventricular function in patients with severe symptomatic aortic stenosis. *Circulation*. 2012;125:2353–2362.
67. Lindman BR, Zajarias A, Maniar HS, et al. Risk stratification in patients with pulmonary hypertension undergoing transcatheter aortic valve replacement. *Heart*. 2015;101:1656–1664.
68. O'Sullivan CJ, Wenaweser P, Ceylan O, et al. Effect of pulmonary hypertension hemodynamic presentation on clinical outcomes in patients with severe symptomatic aortic valve stenosis undergoing transcatheter aortic valve implantation: insights from the new proposed pulmonary hypertension classification. *Circ Cardiovasc Interv*. 2015;8:e002358.
69. Testa L, Latib A, De Marco F, et al. Persistence of severe pulmonary hypertension after transcatheter aortic valve replacement: incidence and prognostic impact. *Circ Cardiovasc Interv*. 2016;9:e003563.
70. Masri A, Abdelkarim I, Sharbaugh MS, et al. Outcomes of persistent pulmonary hypertension following transcatheter aortic valve replacement. *Heart*. 2018;104:821–827.
71. Yotti R, Bermejo J, Gutierrez-Ibanes E, et al. Systemic vascular load in calcific degenerative aortic valve stenosis: insight from percutaneous valve replacement. *J Am Coll Cardiol*. 2015;65:423–433.
72. Lindman BR, Otto CM, Douglas PS, et al. Blood pressure and arterial load after transcatheter aortic valve replacement for aortic stenosis. *Circ Cardiovasc Imaging*. 2017;10:e006308.
73. Ben-Assa E, Brown J, Keshavarz-Motamed Z, et al. Ventricular stroke work and vascular impedance refine the characterization of patients with aortic stenosis. *Sci Transl Med*. 2019;11:eaaw0181.
74. Lloyd JW, Nishimura RA, Borlaug BA, et al. Hemodynamic response to nitroprusside in patients with low-gradient severe aortic stenosis and preserved ejection fraction. *J Am Coll Cardiol*. 2017;70:1339–1348.
75. Chirinos JA, Akers SR, Schelbert E, et al. Arterial properties as determinants of left ventricular mass and fibrosis in severe aortic stenosis: findings from ACRIN PA 4008. *J Am Heart Assoc*. 2019;8:e03742.

Clinical Presentation and Diagnostic Testing

76. Zilberszac R, Gabriel H, Schemper M, et al. Asymptomatic severe aortic stenosis in the elderly. *JACC Cardiovasc Imaging*. 2017;10:43–50.
77. Loscalzo J. From clinical observation to mechanism–Heyde's syndrome. *N Engl J Med*. 2012;367:1954–1956.
78. Thoenes M, Bramlage P, Zamorano P, et al. Patient screening for early detection of aortic stenosis (AS): review of current practice and future perspectives. *J Thorac Dis*. 2018;10:5584–5594.
79. Baumgartner H, Hung J, Bermejo J, et al. Recommendations on the echocardiographic assessment of aortic valve stenosis: a focused update from the European Association of Cardiovascular Imaging and the American Society of Echocardiography. *J Am Soc Echocardiogr*. 2017;30:372–392.
80. Hahn RT, Cavalcante JL. Imaging the aortic valve. In: Otto CM, Bonow RO, eds. *Valvular Heart Disease: A Companion to Braunwald's Heart Disease*. 5th ed. Philadelphia Saunders; 2013:124–155.
81. Eleid MF, Nishimura RA, Sorajja P, et al. Systemic hypertension in low-gradient severe aortic stenosis with preserved ejection fraction. *Circulation*. 2013;128:1349–1353.
82. Redfors B, Pibarot P, Gillam LD, et al. Stress testing in asymptomatic aortic stenosis. *Circulation*. 2017;135:1956–1976.
83. Clavel MA, Magne J, Pibarot P. Low-gradient aortic stenosis. *Eur Heart J*. 2016;37:2645–2657.
84. Pawade T, Clavel MA, Tribouilloy C, et al. Computed tomography aortic valve calcium scoring in patients with aortic stenosis. *Circ Cardiovasc Imaging*. 2018;11:e007146.
85. Pawade T, Sheth T, Guzzetti E, et al. Why and how to measure aortic valve calcification in patients with aortic stenosis. *JACC Cardiovasc Imaging*. 2019;12:1835–1848.
86. Blanke P, Weir-McCall JR, Achenbach S, et al. Computed tomography imaging in the context of Transcatheter Aortic Valve Implantation (TAVI)/Transcatheter Aortic Valve Replacement (TAVR): an expert consensus document of the society of cardiovascular computed tomography. *JACC Cardiovasc Imaging*. 2019;12:1–24.
87. Yoon SH, Lefevre T, Ahn JM, et al. Transcatheter aortic valve replacement with early- and New-Generation Devices in bicuspid aortic valve stenosis. *J Am Coll Cardiol*. 2016;68:1195–1205.
88. Yoon SH, Kim WK, Dhoble A, et al. Bicuspid aortic valve morphology and outcomes after transcatheter aortic valve replacement. *J Am Coll Cardiol*. 2020;76:1018–1030.
89. Okuno T, Asami M, Heg D, et al. Impact of left ventricular outflow tract calcification on procedural outcomes after transcatheter aortic valve replacement. *JACC Cardiovasc Interv*. 2020;13:1789–1799.
90. Michail M, Ihdayhid AR, Comella A, et al. Feasibility and Validity of computed tomography-derived fractional flow reserve in patients with severe aortic stenosis: the CAST-FFR study. *Circ Cardiovasc Interv*. 2021;14:e009586.
91. Strong C, Ferreira A, Teles RC, et al. Diagnostic accuracy of computed tomography angiography for the exclusion of coronary artery disease in candidates for transcatheter aortic valve implantation. *Sci Rep*. 2019;9:19942.
92. Cavalcante JL, Lalude OO, Schoenhagen P, et al. Cardiovascular magnetic resonance imaging for structural and valvular heart disease interventions. *JACC Cardiovasc Interv*. 2016;9:399–425.
93. Dweck MR, Jones C, Joshi NV, et al. Assessment of valvular calcification and inflammation by positron emission tomography in patients with aortic stenosis. *Circulation*. 2012;125:76–86.
94. Dweck MR, Jenkins WS, Vesey AT, et al. 18F-sodium fluoride uptake is a marker of active calcification and disease progression in patients with aortic stenosis. *Circ Cardiovasc Imaging*. 2014;7:371–378.
95. Jenkins WS, Vesey AT, Shah AS, et al. Valvular (18)F-fluoride and (18)F-fluorodeoxyglucose uptake predict disease progression and clinical outcome in patients with aortic stenosis. *J Am Coll Cardiol*. 2015;66:1200–1201.
96. Castano A, Narotsky DL, Hamid N, et al. Unveiling transthyretin cardiac amyloidosis and its predictors among elderly patients with severe aortic stenosis undergoing transcatheter aortic valve replacement. *Eur Heart J*. 2017;38:2879–2887.
97. Scully PR, Treibel TA, Fontana M, et al. Prevalence of cardiac amyloidosis in patients referred for transcatheter aortic valve replacement. *J Am Coll Cardiol*. 2018;71:463–464.
98. Cavalcante JL, Rijal S, Abdelkarim I, et al. Cardiac amyloidosis is prevalent in older patients with aortic stenosis and carries worse prognosis. *J Cardiovasc Magn Reson*. 2017;19:98.
99. Scully PR, Patel KP, Saberwal B, et al. Identifying cardiac amyloid in aortic stenosis: ECV quantification by CT in TAVR patients. *JACC Cardiovasc Imaging*. 2020;13:2177–2189.
100. Maurer MS, Schwartz JH, Gundapaneni B, et al. Tafamidis treatment for patients with transthyretin amyloid cardiomyopathy. *N Engl J Med*. 2018;379:1007–1016.

Disease Course and Staging

101. Genereux P, Stone GW, O'Gara PT, et al. Natural history, diagnostic approaches, and therapeutic strategies for patients with asymptomatic severe aortic stenosis. *J Am Coll Cardiol*. 2016;67:2263–2288.
102. Nayeri A, Xu M, Farber-Eger E, et al. Initial changes in peak aortic jet velocity and mean gradient predict progression to severe aortic stenosis. *Int J Cardiol Heart Vasc*. 2020;30:100592.
103. Bahlmann E, Gerdts E, Cramariuc D, et al. Prognostic value of energy loss index in asymptomatic aortic stenosis. *Circulation*. 2013;127:1149–1156.
104. Minners J, Allgeier M, Gohlke-Baerwolf C, et al. Inconsistent grading of aortic valve stenosis by current guidelines: haemodynamic studies in patients with apparently normal left ventricular function. *Heart*. 2010;96:1463–1468.
105. Berthelot-Richer M, Pibarot P, Capoulade R, et al. Discordant grading of aortic stenosis severity: echocardiographic predictors of survival benefit associated with aortic valve replacement. *JACC Cardiovasc Imaging*. 2016;9:797–805.
106. Linefsky JP, Otto CM. Aortic stenosis: clinical presentation, disease stages, and timing of intervention. In: Otto CM, Bonow RO, eds. *Valvular Heart Disease: A Companion to Braunwald's Heart Disease*. 5th ed. Philadelphia Saunders; 2013:124–155.
107. Clark MA, Arnold SV, Duhay FG, et al. Five-year clinical and economic outcomes among patients with medically managed severe aortic stenosis: results from a Medicare claims analysis. *Circ Cardiovasc Qual Outcomes*. 2012;5:697–704.
108. Ribeiro HB, Lerakis S, Gilard M, et al. Transcatheter aortic valve replacement in patients with low-flow, low-gradient aortic stenosis: the TOPAS-TAVI Registry. *J Am Coll Cardiol*. 2018;71:1297–1308.
109. Clavel MA, Ennezat PV, Marechaux S, et al. Stress echocardiography to assess stenosis severity and predict outcome in patients with paradoxical low-flow, low-gradient aortic stenosis and preserved LVEF. *JACC Cardiovasc Imaging*. 2013;6:175–183.

Treatment

110. Lindman BR, Otto CM. Time to treat hypertension in patients with aortic stenosis. *Circulation*. 2013;128:1281–1283.
111. Nielsen OW, Sajadieh A, Sabbah M, et al. Assessing optimal blood pressure in patients with asymptomatic aortic valve stenosis: the SEAS study. *Circulation*. 2016;134:455–468.
112. Kapadia S, Stewart WJ, Anderson WN, et al. Outcomes of inoperable symptomatic aortic stenosis patients not undergoing aortic valve replacement: insight into the impact of balloon aortic valvuloplasty from the PARTNER trial (Placement of AoRtic TraNscathetER Valve trial). *JACC Cardiovasc Interv*. 2015;8:324–333.
113. Baumgartner H, Falk V, Bax JJ, et al. 2017 ESC/EACTS Guidelines for the management of valvular heart disease. *Eur Heart J*. 2017;38:2739–2791.
114. Lindman BR, Dweck MR, Lancellotti P, et al. Management of asymptomatic severe aortic stenosis: evolving concepts in timing of valve replacement. *JACC Cardiovasc Imaging*. 2020;13:481–493.
115. Taniguchi T, Morimoto T, Shiomi H, et al. Initial surgical versus conservative strategies in patients with asymptomatic severe aortic stenosis. *J Am Coll Cardiol*. 2015;66:2827–2838.
116. Campo J, Tsoris A, Kruse J, et al. Prognosis of severe asymptomatic aortic stenosis with and without surgery. *Ann Thorac Surg*. 2019;108:74–80.
117. Kang DH, Park SJ, Lee SA, et al. Early surgery or conservative care for asymptomatic aortic stenosis. *N Engl J Med*. 2020;382:111–119.
118. Lindman BR, Alexander KP, O'Gara PT, et al. Futility, benefit, and transcatheter aortic valve replacement. *JACC Cardiovasc Interv*. 2014;7:707–716.
119. Arnold SV, Afilalo J, Spertus JA, et al. Prediction of poor outcome after transcatheter aortic valve replacement. *J Am Coll Cardiol*. 2016;68:1868–1877.
120. Kafa R, Kusunose K, Goodman AL, et al. Association of abnormal postoperative left ventricular global longitudinal strain with outcomes in severe aortic stenosis following aortic valve replacement. *JAMA Cardiol*. 2016;1:494–496.
121. Bowdish ME, D'Agostino RS, Thourani VH, et al. The society of thoracic surgeons adult cardiac surgery database: 2020 update on outcomes and research. *Ann Thorac Surg*. 2020;109:1646–1655.
122. Barreto-Filho JA, Wang Y, Dodson JA, et al. Trends in aortic valve replacement for elderly patients in the United States, 1999-2011. *J Am Med Assoc*. 2013;310:2078–2085.
123. Adams DH, Popma JJ, Reardon MJ, et al. Transcatheter aortic-valve replacement with a self-expanding prosthesis. *N Engl J Med*. 2014;370:1790–1798.
124. Leon MB, Smith CR, Mack MJ, et al. Transcatheter or surgical aortic-valve replacement in intermediate-risk patients. *N Engl J Med*. 2016;374:1609–1620.
125. Mack MJ, Leon MB, Thourani VH, et al. Transcatheter aortic-valve replacement with a balloon-expandable valve in low-risk patients. *N Engl J Med*. 2019;380:1695–1705.
126. Reardon MJ, Van Mieghem NM, Popma JJ, et al. Surgical or transcatheter aortic-valve replacement in intermediate-risk patients. *N Engl J Med*. 2017;376:1321–1331.
127. Popma JJ, Deeb GM, Yakubov SJ, et al. Transcatheter aortic-valve replacement with a self-expanding valve in low-risk patients. *N Engl J Med*. 2019;380:1706–1715.
128. Pibarot P, Ternacle J, Jaber WA, et al. Structural deterioration of transcatheter versus surgical aortic valve bioprostheses in the PARTNER-2 trial. *J Am Coll Cardiol*. 2020;76:1830–1843.
129. Coylewright M, O'Neill E, Sherman A, et al. The learning curve for shared decision-making in symptomatic aortic stenosis. *JAMA Cardiol*. 2020;5:442–448.
130. Lindman BR, Perpetua E. Incorporating the patient voice into shared decision-making for the treatment of aortic stenosis. *JAMA Cardiol*. 2020;5:380–381.
131. Makkar RR, Yoon SH, Leon MB, et al. Association between transcatheter aortic valve replacement for bicuspid vs tricuspid aortic stenosis and mortality or stroke. *J Am Med Assoc*. 2019;321:2193–2202.
132. Forrest JK, Kaple RK, Ramlawi B, et al. Transcatheter aortic valve replacement in bicuspid versus tricuspid aortic valves from the STS/ACC TVT Registry. *JACC Cardiovasc Interv*. 2020;13:1749–1759.
133. Halim SA, Edwards FH, Dai D, et al. Outcomes of transcatheter aortic valve replacement in patients with bicuspid aortic valve disease: a report from the Society of Thoracic Surgeons/American College of Cardiology transcatheter valve therapy Registry. *Circulation*. 2020;141:1071–1079.
134. Patel DK, Duncan MS, Shah AS, et al. Association of Cardiac Rehabilitation with decreased hospitalization and mortality risk after cardiac valve surgery. *JAMA Cardiol*. 2019;4:1250–1259.
135. Goel K, Lindman BR. Hypoattenuated leaflet thickening after transcatheter aortic valve replacement: expanding the evidence base but questions remain. *Circ Cardiovasc Imaging*. 2019;12:e010151.
136. Vemulapalli S, Dai D, Hammill BG, et al. Hospital resource utilization before and after transcatheter aortic valve replacement: the STS/ACC TVT Registry. *J Am Coll Cardiol*. 2019;73:1135–1146.
137. O'Leary JM, Clavel MA, Chen S, et al. Association of natriuretic peptide levels after transcatheter aortic valve replacement with subsequent clinical outcomes. *JAMA Cardiol*. 2020;5:1113–1123.
138. Lindman BR, Goel K, Bermejo J, et al. Lower blood pressure after transcatheter or surgical aortic valve replacement is associated with increased mortality. *J Am Heart Assoc*. 2019;8:e014020.

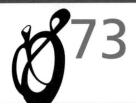# 73 Aortic Regurgitation

ROBERT O. BONOW AND RICK A. NISHIMURA

CAUSES AND PATHOLOGY

Aortic regurgitation (AR) can result from primary disease of the aortic valve leaflets and/or dilation of the aortic root and ascending aorta (Table 73.1).[1] Among patients with isolated AR who undergo aortic valve replacement (AVR), the percentage with primary disease of the aorta has been increasing steadily during the past few decades; it now represents the most common cause, accounting for more than 50% of all such patients in some series.

Valvular Disease

There are two predominant groups of patients who present with AR caused by a primary valve abnormality that is at least moderately severe. One group is comprised of young adults with noncalcified bicuspid aortic valves (BAVs) age 20 through 40 with AR caused by incomplete closure and/or prolapse of a valve leaflet. The other group consists or patients age 60 or older with calcific aortic valve disease. Although these latter patients usually have aortic stenosis (AS) as the primary valve disorder (see Chapter 72), among patients with significant calcific AS some degree (usually mild) of AR is often present. Other common causes of valve disorders leading to AR include infective endocarditis (see Chapter 80), in which the infection may destroy or cause perforation of a leaflet, or the vegetations may interfere with proper coaptation of the cusps; chest trauma resulting in valve disruption or a tear of the ascending aorta leading to valve prolapse; and rheumatic heart disease, particularly in low and middle income countries in which rheumatic fever is endemic (see Chapter 81). In rheumatic aortic valve disease, fusion of the commissures and fibrotic retraction of leaflet tissue lead to a fixed orifice with a central defect often producing combined AS and AR (see Fig. 72.1C). Associated mitral valve involvement is usually present (see Chapter 75). Progressive AR may also occur in patients with congenital heart disease (see Chapter 82), including those with a large ventricular septal defect, as well as in patients with membranous subaortic stenosis and as a complication of percutaneous balloon aortic valvuloplasty. Progressive AR also may occur in patients with myxomatous proliferation of the aortic valve. Increasingly common causes of valvular AR are structural deterioration of a bioprosthetic valve (see Chapter 79) and both central and paravalvular AR in patients who have undergone transcatheter aortic valve replacement (TAVR) (see Chapter 74).

Less common valvular causes of AR include various forms of congenital AR, such as unicommissural and quadricuspid valves,[2,3] or rupture of a congenitally fenestrated valve, particularly in the presence of hypertension. AR may also occur in association with systemic lupus erythematosus, rheumatoid arthritis, ankylosing spondylitis, Jaccoud arthropathy, Takayasu disease, Whipple disease, Crohn disease, and, in the past, the use of certain anorectic drugs.

Disease of the Aortic Root and Ascending Aorta

AR secondary to marked dilation of the ascending aorta (see Chapter 42) is now more common than primary valve disease in patients undergoing AVR for isolated AR. The conditions responsible for aortic root disease include age-related (degenerative) aortic dilation, systemic hypertension, aortic dilation related to BAVs,[4,5] cystic medial necrosis of the aorta (either isolated or associated with classic Marfan syndrome), aortic dissection, osteogenesis imperfecta, syphilitic aortitis, ankylosing spondylitis, Behçet syndrome, psoriatic arthritis (see Chapter 97), arthritis associated with ulcerative colitis, relapsing polychondritis, reactive arthritis, and giant cell arteritis, as well as exposure to some appetite-suppressant drugs.

When the aortic annulus becomes greatly dilated, the aortic leaflets separate and AR may ensue. Dissection of the diseased aortic wall may cause or aggravate the AR. Dilation of the aortic root also may have secondary effects on the aortic valve because dilation causes tension and bowing of the individual cusps, which may thicken and retract. This defect leads to intensification of the AR, further dilating the ascending aorta and leading to a vicious cycle in which, as is the case for mitral regurgitation (MR) (see Chapter 76), more regurgitation leads to more regurgitation.

CHRONIC AORTIC REGURGITATION

Pathophysiology

Left Ventricular Remodeling and Function. In contrast with MR, in which a fraction of the left ventricular (LV) stroke volume is ejected into the low-pressure left atrium, in AR the entire LV stroke volume is ejected into a high-pressure chamber (i.e., the aorta), although the low aortic diastolic pressure does facilitate ventricular emptying during early systole (Fig. 73.1). In MR, especially acute MR, the reduction of wall tension (i.e., reduced afterload) allows more complete systolic emptying; in AR, the increase in LV end-diastolic volume (i.e., increased preload) provides hemodynamic compensation.

Severe AR may occur with a normal effective forward stroke volume and a normal LV ejection fraction (EF) ([forward plus regurgitant stroke volume]/[end-diastolic volume]), together with an elevated LV end-diastolic volume, pressure, and stress[6] (Fig. 73.2). In accord with Laplace's law, which indicates that wall tension is related to the product of the intraventricular pressure and radius divided by wall thickness (see Chapter 46), LV dilation also increases the LV systolic tension required to develop any level of systolic pressure. Thus in AR, there is an increase in both preload and afterload. LV systolic function is maintained through the combination of chamber dilation and hypertrophy. This leads to eccentric hypertrophy, with replication of sarcomeres in series and elongation of myocytes and myocardial fibers (see Classic References, Grossman et al.). In compensated AR, sufficient wall thickening results in a normal ratio of LV wall thickness to cavity radius. Under these conditions, end-diastolic wall stress is maintained at or returns to normal levels. In AS, in contrast, changes include pressure overload (concentric) hypertrophy with replication of sarcomeres, largely in parallel, and an increased ratio of wall thickness to radius, but in both AR and AS, an increase in interstitial connective tissue develops (see Chapter 72). In AR, LV mass usually is greatly increased, often to levels even higher than in isolated AS. As AR persists and increases in severity over time, however, wall thickening fails to keep pace with the hemodynamic load, and end-systolic wall stress rises. At this point, the afterload mismatch results in a decline in systolic function, and the LVEF falls (see Fig. 73.2).

TABLE 73.1 Causes of Aortic Regurgitation

Leaflet Abnormalities

Rheumatic disease

Aortic valve sclerosis and calcification

Congenital abnormalities (bicuspid, unicuspid, and quadricuspid valves; aortic regurgitation associated with discrete subaortic stenosis and ventricular septal defect)

Infective endocarditis

Myxomatous valve disease

Complicating balloon valvuloplasty and transcatheter aortic valve implantation

Rare causes (drugs, leaflet fenestration, irradiation, nonbacterial endocarditis, trauma)

Aortic Root Abnormalities

Chronic hypertension

Marfan syndrome

Annulo-aortic ectasia

Aortic dissection

Ehlers-Danlos syndrome

Osteogenesis imperfecta

Atherosclerotic aneurysm

Syphilitic aortitis

Other systemic inflammatory disorders (giant cell aortitis, Takayasu disease, Reiter syndrome)

Combined Valve and Aortic Root Abnormalities

Bicuspid aortic valve

Ankylosing spondylitis

From Evangelista A, et al. Aortic regurgitation: clinical presentation, disease stages, and management. In Otto CM, Bonow RO, editors. Valvular Heart Disese. A Companion to Braunwald's Heart Disease. 5th ed. Philadelphia: Elsevier; 2021, pp. 179-196.

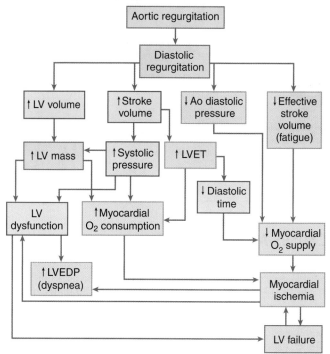

FIGURE 73.1 Pathophysiology of aortic regurgitation. Regurgitation results in an increased left ventricular (LV) volume, increased stroke volume, increased aortic (Ao) systolic pressure, and decreased effective stroke volume. Increased LV volume results in an increased LV mass, which may lead to LV dysfunction and failure. Increased LV stroke volume increases systolic pressure and prolongation of LV ejection time (LVET). Increased LV systolic pressure results in a decrease in diastolic time. Decreased diastolic time (myocardial perfusion time), diastolic aortic pressure, and effective stroke volume lead to reduced myocardial O_2 supply. Increased myocardial O_2 consumption and decreased myocardial O_2 supply produce myocardial ischemia, which further impairs LV function. *LVEDP,* Left ventricular end-diastolic pressure. (From Boudoulas H, Gravanis MB. Valvular heart disease. In Gravanis MB, editor. Cardiovascular Disorders: Pathogenesis and Pathophysiology. St Louis: Mosby; 1993, p. 64.)

Patients with severe chronic AR, left unchecked, can develop the largest LV end-diastolic volumes of any form of heart disease, resulting in so-called cor bovinum. However, end-diastolic pressure is not uniformly elevated (i.e., LV compliance often is increased; see Fig. 73.2). The adaptive response to gradually increasing, chronic AR permits the ventricle to function as an effective high-compliance pump, handling a large stroke volume, often with little increase in filling pressure. During exercise, peripheral vascular resistance declines and, with an increase in heart rate, diastole shortens and the regurgitation per beat decreases, facilitating an increment in effective (forward) cardiac output without substantial increases in end-diastolic volume and pressure. The EF and related ejection phase indices are often within normal limits, both at rest and during exercise, even though myocardial function, as reflected in the slope of the end-systolic pressure-volume relationship, is depressed.

As the left ventricle decompensates, interstitial fibrosis increases, compliance declines, and LV end-diastolic pressure and volume rise (see Fig. 73.2). In advanced stages of decompensation, left atrial, pulmonary artery wedge, pulmonary arterial, right ventricular (RV), and right atrial pressures rise and the effective (forward) cardiac output falls, at first during exercise and then at rest. The normal decline in LV end-systolic volume (ESV) or the rise in LVEF fails to occur during exercise. Symptoms of heart failure develop, particularly those secondary to pulmonary congestion.

Myocardial Ischemia

When acute AR is induced experimentally, myocardial oxygen requirements rise substantially, secondary to an increase in wall tension. In patients with chronic severe AR, total myocardial oxygen requirements also are augmented by the increase in LV mass (see Fig 73.1). Because the major portion of coronary blood flow occurs during diastole, when aortic pressure is lower than normal in AR, coronary perfusion pressure is reduced. Studies in experimentally induced AR have shown a reduction in coronary flow reserve, with a change in forward coronary flow from diastole to systole. The result, a combination of increased oxygen demands and reduced supply, sets the stage for the development of myocardial ischemia, especially during exercise. Thus patients with severe AR exhibit a reduction of coronary reserve, which may be responsible for myocardial ischemia and which may in turn play a role in the deterioration of LV function.

Clinical Presentation

The clinical stages of chronic AR are indicated in Table 73.2, demonstrating the progressive nature of the disease.[7]

Symptoms

In chronic severe AR, the left ventricle gradually enlarges while the patient remains asymptomatic.[1,7,8] Symptoms of reduced cardiac reserve or myocardial ischemia develop, most often in the fourth or fifth decade of life, and usually only after considerable cardiomegaly and myocardial dysfunction have occurred. The principal manifestations, including exertional dyspnea, orthopnea, and paroxysmal nocturnal dyspnea, usually develop gradually. Angina pectoris is prominent late in the course; nocturnal angina may be troublesome and often is accompanied by diaphoresis, which occurs when the heart rate slows and arterial diastolic pressure falls to extremely low levels. Patients with severe AR often complain of an uncomfortable awareness of the heartbeat, especially in supine position lying on left side, and thoracic discomfort caused by pounding of the heart against the chest wall. Tachycardia, occurring with emotional stress or exertion, may cause palpitations and head pounding. Premature ventricular contractions are particularly distressing because of the great heave of the volume-loaded left ventricle during the postextrasystolic beat. These complaints may be present for many years before symptoms of overt LV dysfunction develop.

Physical Examination

In patients with chronic, severe AR, the head may bob with each heartbeat (de Musset sign), and water hammer pulses, with abrupt distention and quick collapse (Corrigan pulse), are evident. The arterial pulse often is prominent and can be best appreciated by palpation of the radial artery with the patient's arm elevated (see Chapter 13). A bisferiens pulse may be present and is more readily recognized in the brachial and femoral arteries than in the carotid arteries. A variety of auscultatory

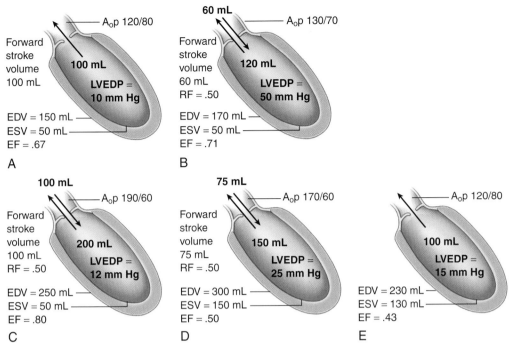

FIGURE 73.2 Hemodynamics of aortic regurgitation (AR). **A,** Normal conditions. **B,** The hemodynamic changes that occur in severe acute AR. Although total stroke volume is increased, forward stroke volume is reduced. Left ventricular end-diastolic pressure (LVEDP) rises dramatically. **C,** Hemodynamic changes occurring in chronic compensated AR. Eccentric hypertrophy produces increased end-diastolic volume (EDV), which permits an increase in total, as well as forward, stroke volume. The volume overload is accommodated, and LV filling pressure is normalized. Ventricular emptying and end-systolic volume (ESV) remain normal. **D,** In chronic decompensated AR, impaired LV emptying produces an increase in ESV and a fall in ejection fraction (EF), total stroke volume, and forward stroke volume. Further cardiac dilation and re-elevation of LV filling pressure occur. **E,** Immediately after valve replacement, preload estimated by EDV decreases, as does filling pressure. ESV also is decreased, but to a lesser extent. The result is an initial fall in EF. Despite these changes, elimination of AR leads to an increase in forward stroke volume, and with time, EF increases. *A$_o$p,* Aortic pressure; *RF,* regurgitant fraction. (From Carabello BA. Aortic regurgitation: hemodynamic determinants of prognosis. In Cohn LH, DiSesa VJ, editors. Aortic Regurgitation: Medical and Surgical Management. New York: Marcel Dekker; 1986, pp. 99-101.)

findings provide confirmation of a wide pulse pressure. The Traube sign (also known as pistol shot sounds) refers to booming systolic and diastolic sounds heard over the femoral artery, the Müller sign consists of systolic pulsations of the uvula, and the Duroziez sign consists of a systolic murmur heard over the femoral artery when it is compressed proximally and a diastolic murmur when it is compressed distally. Capillary pulsations (the Quincke sign) can be detected by transmitting a light through the patient's fingertips or exerting gentle pressure on the tip of a fingernail.

Systolic arterial pressure is elevated, and diastolic pressure is abnormally low. The reduction in diastolic pressure reflects severity of AR and has prognostic implications.[9,10] Korotkoff sounds often persist to zero even though the intra-arterial pressure rarely falls below 30 mm Hg. The point of change in Korotkoff sounds (i.e., the muffling of these sounds in phase IV) correlates with the diastolic pressure. As heart failure develops, peripheral vasoconstriction may occur and arterial diastolic pressure may rise, even though severe AR is present.[9]

The apical impulse is diffuse and hyperdynamic and is displaced laterally and inferiorly. A rapid ventricular filling wave often is palpable at the apex. The augmented stroke volume may create a systolic thrill at the base of the heart or suprasternal notch, and over the carotid arteries. In many patients, a carotid shudder is palpable.

Auscultation

The diastolic murmur, the principal physical finding in AR, is of high frequency and begins immediately after A$_2$. It may be distinguished from the murmur of pulmonic regurgitation by its earlier onset (i.e., immediately after A$_2$ rather than after P$_2$) and usually by the presence of a widened pulse pressure. The murmur is heard best with the diaphragm of the stethoscope when the patient is sitting up and leaning forward, with the breath held in deep exhalation. In severe AR, the murmur reaches an early peak and then shows a dominant decrescendo pattern throughout diastole.

The severity of AR correlates better with the duration than with the intensity of the murmur. In mild AR, the murmur may be limited to

early diastole and typically is high pitched and blowing. In severe AR, the murmur is holodiastolic and may have a rough quality. When the murmur is musical (cooing dove murmur), it usually signifies eversion or perforation of an aortic cusp. In patients with severe AR and LV decompensation, equilibration of aortic and LV pressures in late diastole abolishes the late diastolic component of the regurgitant murmur. When AR is caused by primary valvular disease, the diastolic murmur is heard best along the left sternal border in the third and fourth intercostal spaces. However, when it is caused mainly by dilation of the ascending aorta, the murmur often is more readily audible along the right sternal border.

Many patients with chronic AR have a harsh systolic outflow murmur caused by the increased total LV stroke volume and ejection rate, which often radiates to the carotid vessels. The systolic murmur often is more readily audible than the diastolic murmur. It may be higher pitched and less rasping than the murmur of AS but often is accompanied by a systolic thrill. Palpation of the carotid pulses will elucidate the cause of the systolic murmur and differentiate it from the murmur of AS.

A third heart sound (S$_3$) correlates with an increased LV end-diastolic volume. Its development may be a sign of impaired LV function, which is useful in identifying patients with severe AR who are candidates for surgical treatment. A mid-diastolic and late diastolic apical rumble, the *Austin Flint murmur*, is common in severe AR and may occur in the presence of a normal mitral valve. This murmur appears to be created by severe AR impinging on the anterior leaflet of the mitral valve or the free LV wall; convincing evidence for obstruction to mitral inflow in these patients is lacking.

Diagnostic Testing
Echocardiography

Echocardiography (see Chapter 16) is essential in evaluating cause (Fig. 73.3) and severity of AR as it impacts LV volume and function.[1,11] Anatomic findings such a BAV, thickening of the valve cusps, other congenital abnormalities, prolapse of the valve, a flail leaflet, or vegetation (see Fig. 80.4) are usually well delineated. In addition to leaflet anatomy and motion, the size and shape of the aortic root can be evaluated, although visualization of the ascending aorta is not always adequate, necessitating additional imaging tests in some cases. Transthoracic imaging usually is satisfactory, but transesophageal echocardiography (TEE) often provides more detail, particularly of the aortic root.

TEE is useful for the measurement of LV end-diastolic and end-systolic dimensions and volumes, EF, and mass.[11,12] Current recommendations for assessment of LV dilation emphasize measurement of LV volumes as well as linear dimensions, and criteria for normal dimensions and volumes as well as mild, moderate, and severe LV dilation have been published by the American Society of Echocardiography (ASE).[13] Three-dimensional (3D) and contrast echocardiography will enhance the accuracy of the volume measurements.[14] Recent studies have suggested that LVESV, indexed to body surface area, is a strong predictor of adverse clinical outcomes.[15,16] These measurements, when made serially, are of great value in selecting the optimal time for surgical intervention. When LV volumes are measured, meticulous attention

TABLE 73.2 Clinical Stages of Chronic Aortic Regurgitation (AR)

STAGE	DEFINITION	VALVE ANATOMY	VALVE HEMODYNAMICS	HEMODYNAMIC CONSEQUENCES	SYMPTOMS
A	At risk of AR	Bicuspid aortic valve (or other congenital valve anomaly) Aortic valve sclerosis Diseases of the aortic sinuses or ascending aorta History of rheumatic fever or known rheumatic heart disease IE	AR severity none or trace	None	None
B	Progressive AR	Mild to moderate calcification of a trileaflet valve or bicuspid aortic valve (or other congenital valve anomaly) Dilated aortic sinuses Rheumatic valve changes Previous IE	**Mild AR:** Jet width <25% of LVOT Vena contracta <0.3 cm RVol <30 mL/beat RF <30% ERO <0.10 cm² Angiography grade 1+ **Moderate AR:** Jet width 25%-64% of LVOT Vena contracta 0.3-0.6 cm RVol 30-59 mL/beat RF 30%-49% ERO 0.10-0.29 cm² Angiography grade 2+	Normal LV systolic function Normal LV volume or mild LV dilation	None
C	Asymptomatic severe AR	Calcific aortic valve disease Bicuspid valve (or other congenital abnormality) Dilated aortic sinuses or ascending aorta Rheumatic valve changes IE with abnormal leaflet closure or perforation	**Severe AR:** Jet width ≥65% of LVOT Vena contracta >0.6 cm Holodiastolic flow reversal in proximal abdominal aorta RVol ≥60 mL/beat RF ≥50% ERO ≥0.3 cm² Angiography grade 3+ to 4+ In addition, diagnosis of chronic severe AR requires evidence of LV dilation	C1: Normal LVEF (>55%) and mild to moderate LV dilation (LVESD ≤50 mm) C2: Abnormal LV systolic function with depressed LVEF (≤55%) or severe LV dilation (LVESD >50 mm or indexed LVESD >25 mm/m²)	None; exercise testing is reasonable to confirm symptom status
D	Symptomatic severe AR	Calcific valve disease Bicuspid valve (or other congenital abnormality) Dilated aortic sinuses or ascending aorta Rheumatic valve changes Previous IE with abnormal leaflet closure or perforation	**Severe AR:** Doppler jet width ≥65% of LVOT Vena contracta >0.6 cm Holodiastolic flow reversal in the proximal abdominal aorta RVol ≥60 mL/beat RF ≥50% ERO ≥0.3 cm² Angiography grade 3+ to 4+ In addition, diagnosis of chronic severe AR requires evidence of LV dilation	Symptomatic severe AR may occur with normal systolic function (LVEF >55%), mild to moderate LV dysfunction (LVEF 40% to 55%), or severe LV dysfunction (LVEF <40%). Moderate to severe LV dilation is present	Exertional dyspnea or angina, or more severe HF symptoms

AR, Aortic regurgitation; *ERO,* effective regurgitant orifice; *HF,* heart failure; *IE,* infective endocarditis; *LVEF,* left ventricular ejection fraction; *LVESD,* left ventricular end-systolic dimension; *LVOT,* left ventricular outflow tract; *RF,* regurgitant fraction; *RVol,* regurgitant volume.
From Otto CM, et al. 2020 AHA/ACC guideline for the management of patients with valvular heart disease: a report of the American College of Cardiology/American Heart Association Task Force on Practice Guidelines. J Am Coll Cardiol. 2021;77:e25-197.

to detail is needed, ensuring that the endocardium is well seen and the apex is not foreshortened, according to the ASE guidelines.

Doppler echocardiography and color flow Doppler imaging are the most sensitive and accurate noninvasive techniques for the diagnosis and evaluation of AR. They readily detect mild degrees of AR that may be inaudible on physical examination. As the severity of AR increases, there will be a larger area of turbulence in the LV outflow tract on color flow imaging, but this is only a semi-qualitative measure. There are indirect Doppler findings in severe AR including a high LV outflow velocity, reversal of flow in the descending aorta, and a short

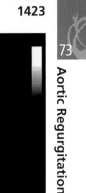

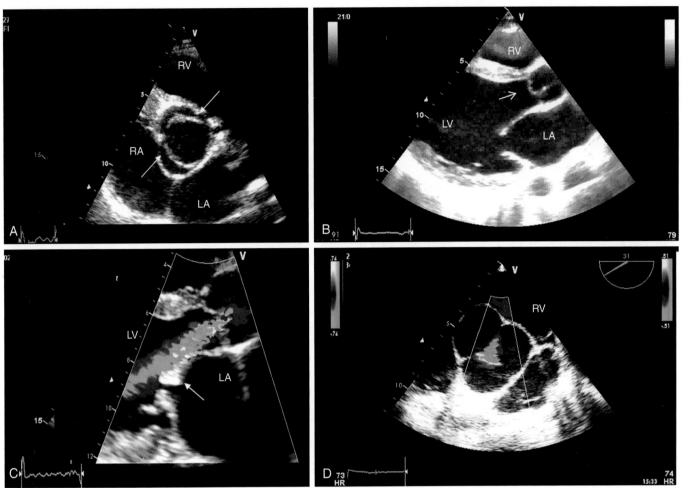

FIGURE 73.3 **A,** Transthoracic parasternal short-axis view shows a bicuspid aortic valve. **B,** Myxomatous aortic valve with prolapse of the right coronary cusp (*arrow*). **C,** Rheumatic valvular disease with mitral (*arrow*) and aortic involvement. **D,** Transesophageal echocardiography shows a central regurgitant orifice due to an annulo-aortic ectasia. *Ao,* Aorta; *LA,* left atrium; *LV,* left ventricle; *RV,* right ventricle. (From Evangelista A, et al. Aortic regurgitation: clinical presentation, disease stages, and management. In Otto CM, Bonow RO, editors. Valvular Heart Disease. A Companion to Braunwald's Heart Disease. 5th ed. Philadelphia: Elsevier; 2021, pp. 179-196.)

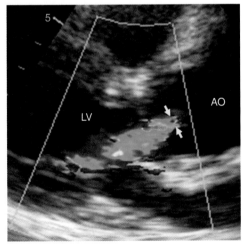

FIGURE 73.4 Parasternal long-axis view shows the vena contracta (*arrows*) of the regurgitant flow by Doppler in a patient with severe aortic regurgitation. *AO,* Aorta; *LV,* left ventricle. (From Evangelista A, et al. Aortic regurgitation: clinical presentation, disease stages, and management. In Otto CM, Bonow RO, editors. Valvular Heart Disease. A Companion to Braunwald's Heart Disease. 5th ed. Philadelphia: Elsevier; 2021, pp. 179-196.)

diastolic half-time of the AR continuous wave signal. Both the AR orifice size and AR flow can be estimated quantitatively[11] (Figs. 73.4 and 73.5; see also Fig 16.46), and such determinations are strongly recommended.[7,12] These quantitative data provide the basis for the definitions of mild, moderate, and severe AR in current guidelines (see

Table 73.2). Serial studies permit determination of the progression of AR and its effect on the left ventricle.

Cardiac Magnetic Resonance

Cardiac magnetic resonance (CMR) (see Chapter 19) is useful for assessing the degree of aortic dilation in patients with BAV and other diseases affecting the aortic root and ascending aorta, and it provides accurate measurements of regurgitant volumes and the regurgitant orifice to assess severity of AR on the basis of the antegrade and retrograde flow volumes in the ascending aorta (Fig. 73.6; see also Fig. 19.16). CMR is the most accurate noninvasive technique for assessing LVESV, end-diastolic volume, and mass,[11,14,17-19] and is recommended when echocardiographic evaluation of LV size and function or severity of regurgitation is suboptimal.[7,12]

Angiography

For angiographic assessment of AR, contrast material should be injected rapidly (i.e., at 55 to 60 mL at 20 mL/sec/sec) into the aortic root, and filming should be carried out in the right and left anterior oblique projections (see Chapter 22). Opacification may be improved by filming during a Valsalva maneuver.

Disease Course
Asymptomatic Patients

Patients with mild or moderate AR who are asymptomatic with normal or only minimally increased cardiac size require no therapy but should be followed clinically and by echocardiography every 12 or 24 months. Asymptomatic patients with chronic severe AR and normal LV systolic function should be examined at intervals of approximately 6 months. In

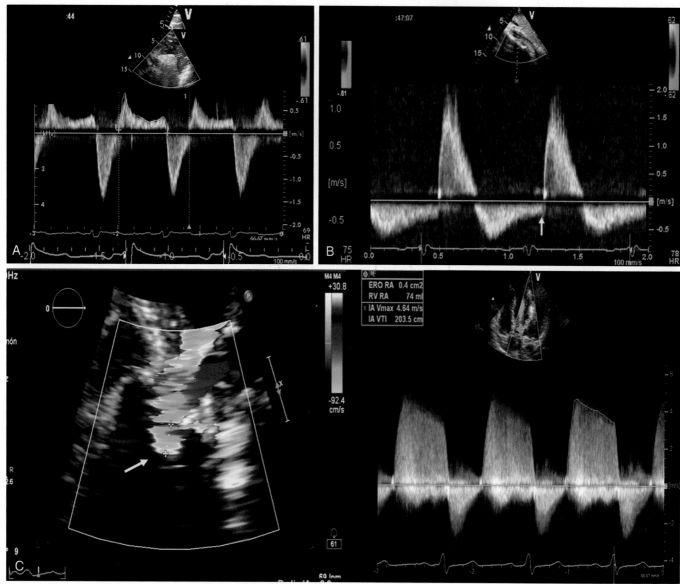

FIGURE 73.5 Assessment of severity of aortic regurgitation (AR). A, Diastolic flow reversal in the descending thoracic aorta by pulse-wave Doppler. The velocity-time integral is 22 cm, and end-diastolic velocity is greater than 20 cm/s. **B,** Holodiastolic flow reversal in the abdominal aorta *(arrow)* in a patient with severe AR. **C,** Quantitative assessment of AR severity using the proximal isovelocity surface area (PISA) method shows severe AR with effective regurgitant orifice area (EROA) of 0.40 cm² and regurgitant volume 74 mL/beat. (From Evangelista A, et al. Aortic regurgitation: clinical presentation, disease stages, and management. In Otto CM, Bonow RO, editors. Valvular Heart Disease. A Companion to Braunwald's Heart Disease. 5th ed. Philadelphia: Elsevier; 2021, pp. 179-196.)

addition to clinical examination, serial echocardiographic assessments of LV size and EF should be made. CMR usually is not necessary but may be useful in patients whose noninvasive test results are inconclusive or discordant with clinical findings or when further evaluation of aortic size is needed (see Fig. 73.6). Patients with mild to moderate AR and those with severe AR with a normal LVEF and only mild ventricular dilation may engage in aerobic forms of exercise. However, patients with AR who have limitations of cardiac reserve and/or evidence of declining LV function should not engage in competitive sports or strenuous activities.[20]

Moderately severe or even severe chronic AR often is associated with a generally favorable prognosis for many years. Quantitative measures of AR severity predict clinical outcome, and LV size and systolic function also are strong predictors of clinical outcome.[1,7,15,21-26] In a study of 251 asymptomatic patients (mean age, 61 years), the 10-year survival was 94% ± 4% in those with mild AR, compared with 69% ± 9% in those with severe AR (see Classic References, Detaint et al.) (Fig. 73.7). In contrast, in series involving younger asymptomatic patients (mean age, 39 years) with severe AR and a normal LVEF, the mortality rate was less than 1% per year,[7,8] and more than 45% of the patients remained asymptomatic with normal LV function at 10 years. The average rate of developing symptoms or LV systolic dysfunction in these latter series was less than 6% per year (see Classic References, Bonow et al.).

Gradual deterioration of LV function may occur even during the asymptomatic period, and some patients may incur significant impairment of systolic function before the onset of symptoms (see Table 73.2). Numerous surgical series over the past two decades have indicated that depressed LVEF is among the most important determinants of mortality after AVR, particularly as LV dysfunction may become irreversible and not improve after AVR.[7,8,22,23,25-27] LV dysfunction is more likely to be reversible if detected early, before EF becomes severely depressed, before the left ventricle becomes markedly dilated, and before significant symptoms develop. It is, therefore, important to intervene surgically before these changes have become irreversible.[1,7,8,23,27-29] Measures of LV systolic volume and systolic function are the most important predictors of clinical course in asymptomatic patients.[7,8,15] Biomarkers such as brain natriuretic peptide (BNP)[30] and assessment of myocardial strain[30-33] also may play a role in the future in identifying high-risk patients, based on small series published to date, but more work is necessary before these additional measures are recommended for routine management.

Symptomatic Patients

As is the case for AS (see Chapter 72) once the patient becomes symptomatic, the downhill course becomes rapidly progressive. Congestive heart failure, punctuated by episodes of acute pulmonary edema, and sudden

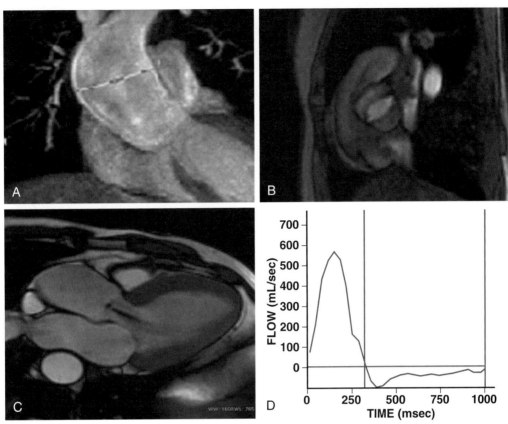

FIGURE 73.6 Cardiac magnetic resonance images showing a bicuspid aortic valve with aortic regurgitation and ascending aorta dilation. A, Fast single-shot steady-state free precession (SSFP) image in a coronal view. **B,** Retrospectively reconstructed magnitude image from a phase-contrast sequence showing a bicuspid aortic valve. **C,** Balanced SSFP image. Oblique axial left ventricle inflow-outflow view, showing grade 2 AR. **D,** Flow-versus-time plot for the ascending aorta. Antegrade flow was calculated at 140 mL/beat, retrograde flow at 40 mL/beat, and aortic regurgitant fraction of 33%. (From Tornos P, et al. Aortic regurgitation. In Otto CM, Bonow RO, editors. Valvular Heart Disease: A Companion to Braunwald's Heart Disease. 4th ed. Philadelphia: Saunders; 2013, pp. 163-178.)

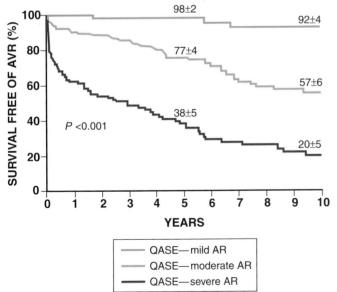

FIGURE 73.7 Composite endpoint of survival free of surgery for aortic regurgitation after diagnosis in asymptomatic patients. Patients are stratified according to quantitative criteria of the American Society of Echocardiography (QASE) for AR grading. The QASE–severe AR is defined as regurgitant volume (RV) greater than 60 mL/beat or effective regurgitant orifice (ERO) greater than 30 mm², the QASE–mild AR is defined as RV less than 30 mL/beat and ERO less than 10 mm², and the QASE–moderate AR is defined as greater than mild but not reaching QASE–severe criteria. The 5- and 10-year rates of the endpoint (± standard error) are indicated. Note the wide difference in outcomes according to QASE grading at baseline. *AVR,* Aortic valve replacement. (From Detaint D, et al. Quantitative echocardiographic determinants of clinical outcome in asymptomatic patients with aortic regurgitation: a prospective study. JACC Cardiovasc Imaging 2008;1:1-11.)

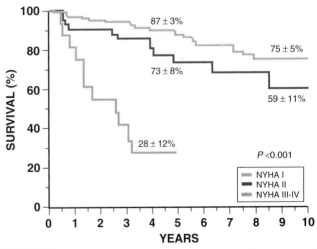

FIGURE 73.8 Survival without surgery in 242 patients with chronic aortic regurgitation, demonstrating the importance of symptoms in determining outcome. Patients with New York Heart Association (NYHA) class III or IV symptoms had a survival of only 28% at 4 years. In contrast, the 10-year survival in patients in NYHA class I was 75%, which was identical to that for an age-matched normal population. (From Dujardin KS, et al. Mortality and morbidity of aortic regurgitation in clinical practice: a long-term follow-up study. Circulation 1999;99:1851-1857.)

death may occur, usually in previously symptomatic patients who have considerable LV dilation. Data compiled in the presurgical era indicate that without surgical treatment, death usually occurred within 4 years after the development of angina pectoris and within 2 years after the onset of heart failure. Even in the current era, 4-year survival without surgery in patients with New York Heart Association (NYHA) class III or IV symptoms is only approximately 30% (see Classic References, Dujardin et al.) (Fig. 73.8).

TABLE 73.3 Indications for Aortic Valve Surgery in Patients with Aortic Regurgitation

COR	LOE	RECOMMENDATIONS
1	B-NR	1. In symptomatic patients with severe AR (stage D), aortic valve surgery is indicated regardless of LV systolic function
1	B-NR	2. In asymptomatic patients with chronic severe AR and LV systolic dysfunction (LVEF ≤55%) (stage C2), aortic valve surgery is indicated if no other cause for systolic dysfunction is identified
1	C-EO	3. In patients with severe AR (stage C or D) who are undergoing cardiac surgery for other indications, aortic valve surgery is indicated
2a	B-NR	4. In asymptomatic patients with severe AR and normal LV systolic function (LVEF >55%), aortic valve surgery is reasonable when the LV is severely enlarged (LVESD >50 mm or indexed LVESD >25 mm/m²) (stage C2)
2a	C-EO	5. In patients with moderate AR (stage B) who are undergoing cardiac or aortic surgery for other indications, aortic valve surgery is reasonable
2b	B-NR	6. In asymptomatic patients with severe AR and normal LV systolic function at rest (LVEF >55%; stage CI) and low surgical risk, aortic valve surgery may be considered when there is a progressive decline in LVEF on at least three serial studies to the low-normal range (LVEF 55% to 60%) or a progressive increase in LV dilation into the severe range (LVEDD >65 mm)
3: Harm	B-NR	7. In patients with isolated severe AR who have indications for SAVR and are candidates for surgery, TAVI should not be performed.

AR, Aortic regurgitation; *COR,* class of recommendation; *EO,* expert opinion; *LOE,* level of evidence; *LVEDD,* left ventricular end-diastolic dimension; *LVEF,* left ventricular ejection fraction; *LVESD,* left ventricular end-systolic dimension; *NR,* nonrandomized data; *SAVR,* surgical aortic valve replacement; *TAVI,* transcatheter aortic valve implantation.
From Otto CM, et al. 2020 AHA/ACC guideline for the management of patients with valvular heart disease: a report of the American College of Cardiology/American Heart Association Task Force on Practice Guidelines. J Am Coll Cardiol 2021;77:e25-197.

Treatment of Chronic Aortic Regurgitation

Medical Therapy

No specific therapy to prevent disease progression in chronic AR is currently available. Randomized clinical trials of dihydropyridine calcium channel antagonists and angiotensin-converting enzyme (ACE) inhibitors have not shown consistent clinical benefit in terms of blunting progression of LV dilation or delaying in need for AVR, and definitive recommendations regarding the indications for these drugs are not possible.[1,7]

Although there is no specific therapy to improve clinical outcomes in patients with chronic AR, it is recommended to treat hypertension (systolic blood pressure [SBP] >140 mm Hg), coronary artery disease (CAD), atrial arrhythmias, and any other cardiovascular comorbidities according to established guidelines.[7,23] For symptomatic patients. chronic medical therapy may be necessary for some patients who refuse surgery or are considered to have a prohibitive risk of surgery because of comorbid conditions. These patients should receive an aggressive evidence-based heart failure regimen (see Chapter 50) with ACE inhibitors (and perhaps other vasodilators), diuretics, and salt restriction; beta blockers may also be beneficial. Even though nitroglycerin and other nitrates are not as helpful in relieving anginal pain in patients with AR as they are in patients with CAD or AS, they are reasonable to try. In patients who are candidates for surgery but who have severely decompensated LV dysfunction, vasodilator therapy may be particularly helpful to stabilize patients prior to AVR.

Surgical Treatment

INDICATIONS FOR VALVE REPLACEMENT. Patients with chronic severe AR may be stable for years. However, long-standing volume overload will eventually result in irreversible LV dysfunction. In addition, the risk of isolated AVR has significantly decreased over the years, with an operative risk less than 3% when performed at experienced centers. Thus is it important to balance the immediate risks of AVR and continuing risks of an implanted prosthetic valve against the hazards of allowing a severe volume overload to irreversibly damage the left ventricle.

The current recommendations for AVR for patients with chronic severe AR in the 2020 American College of Cardiology (ACC)/American Heart Association (AHA) guidelines for the management of patients with valvular heart disease[7] are shown in Table 73.3, and the proposed management pathway is depicted in Fig. 73.9. Previous thresholds for depressed LVEF as an indication for surgery were set at 50%, but recent data indicate higher long-term postoperative risk in patients undergoing surgery with LVEF below 55% (in some series, 60%).[15,26,27] The 2020 revised guidelines have set the threshold for surgery at an LVEF of 55% or less.

SYMPTOMATIC PATIENTS. Because severe symptoms (NYHA class III or IV) are independent risk factors for poor postoperative survival, which has been confirmed in recent series,[22,25,26,27] surgery should be carried out in patients with even mild symptoms (NYHA class II) before severe LV dysfunction has developed.[1,7,8,23,34] Even after successful correction of AR, patients with severe LV dysfunction may have persistent cardiomegaly and depressed LV function. Such patients often exhibit persistent histologic changes in the left ventricle, including massive fiber hypertrophy and increased interstitial fibrous tissue. Therefore it is highly desirable to operate on patients before irreversible LV changes have occurred, and surgery is indicated for patients with severe chronic AR and any symptoms.

On the other hand, surgery should not be withheld in symptomatic patients with even moderate to severe LV systolic dysfunction, as outcomes are better with surgery than with medical therapy, and there is always the possibility of improvement in LV function following surgery with the addition of guideline-directed medical therapy.[35-37] Management with a multidisciplinary heart team and shared decision making with the patient and caregivers are essential in selecting high-risk patients for surgical intervention.[7,38]

ASYMPTOMATIC PATIENTS. In the absence of obvious contraindications or serious comorbidity, surgical treatment is advisable for asymptomatic patients with chronic severe AR with either an LVEF of 55% or less or a severe increase in LVESD (defined as end-systolic diameter [ESD] greater than 50 mm or indexed LVESD greater than 25 mm/m²),[7] as shown in Fig 73.9. Because of their excellent prognosis in the short and medium term, operative correction should be deferred in patients with chronic severe AR without these indications for surgery. This includes those who are asymptomatic, exhibit good exercise tolerance, and have an LVEF greater than 55% without severe LV dilation as defined previously or progressive LV dilation on serial echocardiograms. Between these two ends of the clinical-hemodynamic spectrum are many patients in whom it may be difficult to balance the immediate risks of AVR and the continuing risks of an implanted prosthetic valve against the hazards of allowing a severe volume overload to damage the left ventricle. Once again, a multidisciplinary heart team should be consulted when difficult decisions must be made.[38]

Because AR has complex effects on preload and afterload, the selection of appropriate indices of ventricular contractility to identify patients for operation is challenging. Serial changes in LV end-diastolic and ESVs or dimensions can be used to detect the relative deterioration of LV function. Although LV end-diastolic and ESVs and ejection phase indices (e.g., LVEF) are strongly influenced by loading conditions, they are nonetheless useful empirical predictors of postoperative function. Global longitudinal strain has the advantage of being a less

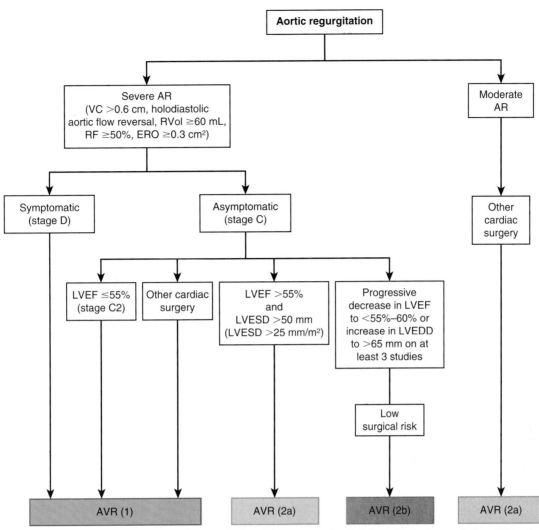

FIGURE 73.9 Management of patients with chronic aortic regurgitation. Colors correspond to Table 73.3. *AR,* Aortic regurgitation; *AVR,* aortic valve replacement; *EDD,* end-diastolic dimension; *EF,* ejection fraction; *ERO,* effective regurgitant orifice; *ESD,* end-systolic dimension; *LV,* left ventricular; *RF,* regurgitant fraction; *RVol,* regurgitant volume; *VC,* vena contracta. (From Otto CM, Nishimura, RA, Bonow RO, et al. 2020 AHA/ACC guideline for the management of patients with valvular heart disease: a report of the American College of Cardiology/American Heart Association Task Force on Practice Guidelines. J Am Coll Cardiol 2021;77:e25-197.)

load-dependent index of LV function,[30-33] but more data are needed before definitive recommendations can be made.

Serial echocardiographic measurements should be made with side-by-side comparison of previous serial studies. A consistent change in dimensions or volumes, greater than measurement variability, must be ensured before recommending AVR for asymptomatic patients on the basis of these numbers alone. This usually involves progressive changes over at least three sequential studies.

Although asymptomatic patients with chronic severe AR but normal LV function have an excellent prognosis over the short term, they need to be evaluated with frequent clinical evaluations and serial echocardiograms. LVESD is valuable in predicting outcome in asymptomatic patients. Patients with chronic severe AR and an ESD less than 40 mm almost invariably remain stable and can be followed without need for surgery in the near term (see Classic References, Bonow et al.). However, patients with an ESD of more than 50 mm have a 19% likelihood per year of developing symptoms of LV dysfunction, and those with an ESD more than 55 mm are at increased risk for development of irreversible LV dysfunction if they do not undergo AVR. Indexed LVESD or LVESV, which adjust for body size, may be more robust indicators for timing of surgical intervention than absolute dimensions and volumes.[7] Patients with an LVESD index of 2.5 cm/m² or LVESV index of 45 mL/m² or greater are at higher risk for adverse outcomes[15,16] (see also Classic References, Detaint et al.), and the LVESV index value of 45 mL/m² matches the ASE criteria for severe LV dilation.[13] Although the current guideline recommendations for surgical intervention are

based on an LVESD index threshold of 25 mm/m² (see Table 73.3 and Fig. 73.9),[7] recent studies have consistently suggested that lower thresholds of LVESD index should be considered to optimize long-term survival after AVR (Fig. 73.10).[22,25,26] In addition, observational studies in asymptomatic patients with chronic severe AR and normal LV systolic function have reported greater long-term postoperative survival rates in those undergoing early AVR compared with those followed conservatively with AVR based on guidelines recommendations.[27,28] These data have fueled discussions regarding earlier intervention to enhance long-term prognosis of patients with chronic severe AR,[29,39] a topic that warrants future clinical trials.

The indications for AVR for patients with chronic severe AR secondary to aortic sinus or ascending aortic disease are similar to those for patients with primary valvular disease. In addition, in patients undergoing AVR for severe AR, concomitant surgery to repair the aortic sinuses or replace the ascending aorta is indicated if the amount of aortic dilation is greater than 45 mm.[7,23,40] As is the case for patients with other valvular lesions, adult surgical candidates who may have underlying CAD, based on symptoms, age, sex, and risk factors, should undergo preoperative coronary angiography. Those with significant proximal coronary artery stenoses should undergo revascularization at the time of AVR.

OPERATIVE PROCEDURES. The standard surgical approach for chronic AR is AVR. Concurrent aortic root replacement is performed when aortic dilation is the cause of or accompanies valve dysfunction. However, experience is accumulating with surgical aortic valve repair, which is a viable option for selected younger patients in experienced

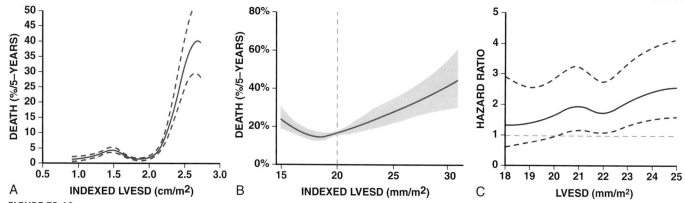

FIGURE 73.10 Association of preoperative left ventricular end-systolic dimension (LVESD) indexed to body surface area (BSA) and postoperative survival after aortic valve replacement. In all three series, postoperative risk rises as a continuous function above 20 mm/m^2 and thus lower than current recommendation for intervention of 25 mm/m^2. *Dashed lines* indicate confidence intervals. (**A** from Mentias A, et al. Long-term outcomes in patients with aortic regurgitation and preserved left ventricular ejection fraction. J Am Coll Cardiol 2016;68:2144-2153; **B** from Yang LT, et al. Outcomes in chronic hemodynamically significant aortic regurgitation and limitations of current guidelines. J Am Coll Cardiol 2019;73:1741-1752; and **C** from de Meester C, et al. Do guideline-based indications result in an outcome penalty for patients with severe aortic regurgitation? JACC Cardiovasc Imaging 2019;12:2126-2138.)

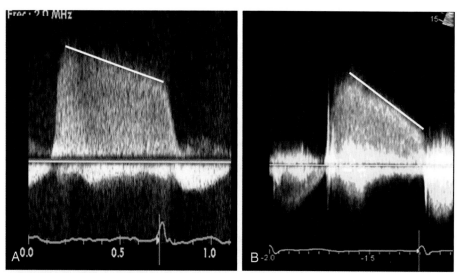

FIGURE 73.11 Diastolic Doppler signals. **A,** Chronic severe aortic regurgitation (AR). **B,** Acute severe AR. Notice the steeper deceleration slope in the acute phase, which is due to the equalization of LV and aortic diastolic pressures. (From Evangelista A, et al. Aortic regurgitation: clinical presentation, disease stages, and management. In Otto CM, Bonow RO, editors. Valvular Heart Disease. A Companion to Braunwald's Heart Disease. 5th ed. Philadelphia: Elsevier; 2021, pp. 179-196.)

centers, particularly those who are candidates for valve-sparing aortic root reconstruction.[41-44] However, unlike patients with chronic MR (see Chapter 76), the large majority of patients with pure AR will require AVR rather than repair. A Ross procedure is an option for selected young adults in centers of excellence skilled in this operation,[45-48] but the long-term results of the Ross procedure for AR are poorer than if performed for AS. TAVR for AR is under investigation but is not an established approach,[49,50] and it is not recommended in current guidelines (see Table 73.3).[7]

ACUTE AORTIC REGURGITATION

Pathophysiology and Clinical Presentation

Acute AR is caused most commonly by infective endocarditis, aortic dissection, or trauma (see Chapters 42 and 80). The characteristic features of acute AR are tachycardia and an increase in LV diastolic pressure. In contrast with the pathophysiologic events in chronic AR just described, in which the left ventricle can adapt over time to the increased hemodynamic load, in acute AR the regurgitant volume fills a ventricle of normal size that cannot accommodate the combined large regurgitant volume and inflow from the left atrium. Because the ability of total stroke volume to rise acutely is limited, forward stroke volume declines. The sudden increase in LV filling causes the LV diastolic pressure to rise rapidly above left atrial pressure during early diastole (see Fig. 73.2), causing the mitral valve to close prematurely

in diastole. The tachycardia may compensate for the reduced forward stroke volume, and the LV and aortic systolic pressures may exhibit little change. However, acute severe AR may cause profound hypotension and cardiogenic shock. In light of the limited ability of the left ventricle to tolerate acute severe AR, patients with this valvular lesion often develop clinical manifestations of sudden cardiovascular collapse, including weakness, severe dyspnea, and profound hypotension secondary to the reduced stroke volume and elevated left atrial pressure. In some patients, the aortic diastolic pressure equilibrates with the elevated LV diastolic pressure.

Physical Examination. Patients with acute severe AR characteristically appear gravely ill, with tachycardia, severe peripheral vasoconstriction, cyanosis, and sometimes pulmonary congestion and edema. Depending on the etiology of the acute AR, signs suggestive of endocarditis or aortic dissection may be present. The peripheral signs of AR are often not impressive and certainly not as dramatic as in patients with chronic AR. The normal or only slightly widened pulse pressure may lead to significant underestimation of the severity of the valvular lesion. The LV impulse is normal or almost normal, and the rocking motion of the chest characteristic of chronic AR is not apparent. S$_1$ may be soft or absent because of premature closure of the mitral valve, and the sound of mitral valve closure in mid- or late diastole occasionally is audible. Closure of the mitral valve may be incomplete, however, and diastolic MR may occur.

The early diastolic murmur of acute AR is lower pitched and of shorter duration compared with that of chronic AR, because as LV diastolic pressure rises, the (reverse) pressure gradient between the aorta and left ventricle is rapidly reduced. A systolic murmur is common, resulting in to-and-fro sounds. The Austin Flint murmur often is present but is of brief duration and ceases when LV pressure exceeds left atrial pressure in diastole. With premature diastolic closure of the mitral valve, the presystolic portion of the Austin Flint murmur is eliminated.

Echocardiography. In acute AR, the echocardiogram reveals a dense, diastolic Doppler signal (Fig. 73.11) with a short diastolic half time and an end-diastolic velocity approaching zero. There may also be premature closure of the mitral valve with diastolic MR on the Doppler traces due to the LV diastolic pressure exceeding the left atrial pressure at late diastole. LV size and EF are usually normal, although contractility may be enhanced and EF increased due to the compensatory adrenergic surge. These findings contrast with those in chronic AR, in which end-diastolic dimensions and wall motion are increased. TEE is often useful to clarify the underlying reason for the acute regurgitation, particularly to identify an ascending aortic dissection or endocarditis.

Electrocardiography. In acute AR, the electrocardiogram (ECG) will usually show sinus tachycardia. If endocarditis is a possible etiology, progressive severity of heart block on serial ECGs may indicate the presence and expansion of an accompanying aortic root abscess.

Radiography. In acute AR, radiographic examination often reveals evidence of marked pulmonary edema. The cardiac silhouette usually is remarkably normal, although left atrial enlargement may be present, and depending on the cause of the AR, enlargement of the ascending aorta may be seen.

Management of Acute Aortic Regurgitation

Because early death caused by LV failure is frequent in patients with acute severe AR, prompt surgical intervention is indicated. Even a normal ventricle cannot sustain the burden of acute, severe volume overload. Therefore the risk of acute AR is much greater than that of chronic AR. While the patient is being prepared for surgery, treatment with an intravenous positive inotropic agent (dopamine or dobutamine) and/or a vasodilator (nitroprusside) often is necessary. The agent and dosage should be selected on the basis of arterial pressure (see Chapter 49). Beta blockers and intra-aortic balloon counterpulsation are contraindicated, because either lowering the heart rate or augmenting peripheral resistance during diastole can lead to rapid hemodynamic decompensation. In hemodynamically stable patients with acute AR secondary to active infective endocarditis, operation may be deferred to allow 5 to 7 days of intensive antibiotic therapy (see Chapter 80). However, AVR should be undertaken at the earliest sign of hemodynamic instability or if there is any evidence of abscess formation. If an acute aortic dissection is the cause for the AR, the aorta will also need to be fixed during surgery.

CLASSIC REFERENCES

Bonow R, Lakatos E, Maron B, Epstein S. Serial long-term assessment of the natural history of asymptomatic patients with chronic aortic regurgitation and normal left ventricular systolic function. *Circulation*. 1991;84:1625–1635.

Detaint D, Messika-Zeitoun D, Maalouf J, et al. Quantitative echocardiographic determinants of clinical outcome in asymptomatic patients with aortic regurgitation: a prospective study. *JACC Cardiovasc Imaging*. 2008;1:1–11.

Dujardin KS, Enriquez-Sarano M, Schaff HV, et al. Mortality and morbidity of aortic regurgitation in clinical practice: a long-term follow-up study. *Circulation*. 1999;99:1851–1857.

Grossman W, Jones D, McLaurin LP. Wall stress and patterns of hypertrophy in the human left ventricle. *J Clin Invest*. 1975;56:56–64.

REFERENCES

Causes and Pathology

1. Evangelista A, Tornos P, Bonow RO. Aortic regurgitation: clinical presentation, disease stages, and management. In: Otto CM, Bonow RO, eds. *Valvular Heart Disease. A Companion to Braunwald's Heart Disease*. 5th ed. Philadelphia: Elsevier; 2021:179–196.
2. Slostad BD, Witt CM, O'Leary PW, et al. Unicuspid aortic valve: demographics, comorbidities, echocardiographic features, and long-term outcomes. *Circulation*. 2019;140:1853–1855.
3. Tsang MYC, Abudiab MM, Ammash NM, et al. Quadricuspid aortic valve: characteristics, associated structural cardiovascular abnormalities, and clinical outcomes. *Circulation*. 2016;133:312–319.
4. Braverman AC, Cheng A. The bicuspid aortic valve and associated aortic disease. In: Otto CM, Bonow RO, eds. *Valvular Heart Disease: A Companion to Braunwald's Heart Disease*. 5th ed. Philadelphia Saunders; 2013:197–222.
5. Verma S, Siu SC. Aortic dilatation in patients with bicuspid aortic valve. *N Engl J Med*. 2014;370:1920–1929.

Chronic AR – Pathophysiology and Clinical Presentation

6. Zilberszac R, Gabriel H, Schemper M, et al. Outcome of combined stenotic and regurgitant aortic valve disease. *J Am Coll Cardiol*. 2013;61:1489–1495.
7. Otto CM, Nishimura RA, Bonow RO, et al. 2020 ACC/AHA guideline for the management of patients with valvular heart disease: a report of the American College of Cardiology/American Heart Association joint committee on clinical practice guidelines. *J Am Coll Cardiol*. 2021;77:e25–e197.
8. Bonow RO. Chronic mitral regurgitation and aortic regurgitation: have indications for surgery changed? *J Am Coll Cardiol*. 2013;61:693–701.
9. Yang LT, Pellikka PA, Enriquez-Sarano M, et al. Diastolic blood pressure and heart rate are independently associated with mortality in chronic aortic regurgitation. *J Am Coll Cardiol*. 2020;75:29–39.
10. Chambers J. Aortic regurgitation: the value of clinical signs. *J Am Coll Cardiol*. 2020;75:40–41.

Chronic AR – Diagnostic Testing

11. Hahn RT, Cavalcante JL. Imaging the aortic valve. In: Otto CM, Bonow RO, eds. *Valvular Heart Disease: A Companion to Braunwald's Heart Disease*. 5th ed. Philadelphia Saunders; 2013:124–155.
12. Zoghbi WA, Adams D, Bonow RO, et al. Recommendations for non-invasive evaluation of native valvular regurgitation. A report from the American Society of Echocardiography developed in collaboration with the Society for Cardiovascular Magnetic Resonance. *J Am Soc Echocardiogr*. 2017;30:303–371.
13. Lang RM, Badano LP, Mor-Avi V, et al. Recommendations for cardiac chamber quantification by echocardiography in adults: an update from the American Society of Echocardiography and the European Association of Cardiovascular Imaging. *J Am Soc Echocardiogr*. 2015;28:1–39.
14. Ewe SH, Delgado V, van der Geest R, et al. Accuracy of three-dimensional versus two-dimensional echocardiography for quantification of aortic regurgitation and validation by three-dimensional three-directional velocity-encoded magnetic resonance imaging. *Am J Cardiol*. 2013;112:560–566.
15. Yang LT, Anand V, Zambito E, et al. Association of echocardiographic left ventricular end-systolic volume and volume-derived ejection fraction with outcome in asymptomatic chronic aortic regurgitation. *JAMA Cardiol*. 2021;6:189–198.
16. Bonow RO, O'Gara PT. Left ventricular end-systolic volume in chronic aortic regurgitation – finally, a step forward. *JAMA Cardiol*. 2021;6:189–199.
17. Cavalcante JL, Lalude OO, Schoenhagen P, Lerakis S. Cardiovascular magnetic resonance imaging for structural and valvular heart disease interventions. *JACC Cardiovasc Interv*. 2016;9:399–425.
18. Harris AW, Krieger EV, Kim M, et al. Cardiac magnetic resonance imaging versus transthoracic echocardiography for prediction of outcomes in chronic aortic or mitral regurgitation. *Am J Cardiol*. 2017;119:1074–1081.
19. Kammerlander AA, Wiesinger M, Duca F, et al. Diagnostic and prognostic utility of cardiac magnetic resonance imaging in aortic regurgitation. *JACC Cardiovasc Imaging*. 2019;12:1474–1483.

Chronic AR – Disease Course and Treatment

20. Bonow RO, Nishimura R, Thompson PD, Udelson JE. Eligibility and disqualification recommendations for competitive athletes with cardiovascular abnormalities. Task Force 5: valvular heart disease. A scientific statement from the American Heart Association and American College of Cardiology. *J Am Coll Cardiol*. 2015;66:2385–2392.
21. Kusunose K, Cremer PC, Tsutsui RS, et al. Regurgitant volume informs rate of progressive cardiac dysfunction in asymptomatic patients with chronic aortic or mitral regurgitation. *JACC Cardiovasc Imaging*. 2015;8:14–23.
22. Mentias A, Feng K, Alashi A, et al. Long-term outcomes in patients with aortic regurgitation and preserved left ventricular ejection fraction. *J Am Coll Cardiol*. 2016;68:2144–2153.
23. Baumgartner H, Falk V, Bax JJ, et al. 2017 ESC/ EACTS guidelines for the management of valvular heart disease. *Eur Heart J*. 2017;38:2739–2791.
24. Yang LT, Enriquez-Sarano M, Michelena HI, et al. Predictors of progression in patients with stage B aortic regurgitation. *J Am Coll Cardiol*. 2019;74:2480–2492.
25. Yang LT, Michelena HI, Scott CG, et al. Outcomes in chronic hemodynamically significant aortic regurgitation and limitations of current guidelines. *J Am Coll Cardiol*. 2019;73:1741–1752.
26. de Meester C, Gerber BL, Vancraeynest D, et al. Do guideline-based indications result in an outcome penalty for patients with severe aortic regurgitation? *J Am Coll Cardiol Imaging*. 2019;12:2126–2138.
27. Murashita T, Schaff HV, Suri RM, et al. Impact of left ventricular systolic function on outcome of correction of chronic severe aortic valve regurgitation: implications for timing of surgical intervention. *Ann Thorac Surg*. 2017;103:1222–1228.
28. Wang Y, Jiang W, Liu J, et al. Early surgery versus conventional treatment for asymptomatic severe aortic regurgitation with normal ejection fraction and left ventricular dilatation. *Eur J Cardio Thorac Surg*. 2017;52:118–124.
29. Desai MY, Svensson L. Chronic severe aortic regurgitation: should we lower operating thresholds? *Circulation*. 2019;140:1045–1047.
30. Lee JKT, Franzone A, Lanz J, et al. Early detection of subclinical myocardial damage in chronic aortic regurgitation and strategies for timely treatment of asymptomatic patients. *Circulation*. 2018;137:184–196.
31. Kusunose K, Agarwal S, Marwick TH, et al. Decision making in asymptomatic aortic regurgitation in the era of guidelines incremental values of resting and exercise cardiac dysfunction. *Circ Cardiovasc Imaging*. 2014;7:352–362.
32. Ewe SH, Haeck MLA, Ng ACT, et al. Detection of subtle left ventricular systolic dysfunction in patients with significant aortic regurgitation and preserved left ventricular ejection fraction: speckle tracking echocardiographic analysis. *Eur Heart J Cardiovasc Imaging*. 2015;16:992–999.
33. Alashi AA, Khullar T, Mentias A, et al. Long-term outcomes after aortic valve surgery in patients with asymptomatic chronic aortic regurgitation and preserved LVEF: impact of baseline and follow-up global longitudinal strain. *JACC Cardiovasc Imaging*. 2020;13:12–21.
34. Bonow RO, Leon MB, Doshi D, Moat N. Management strategies and future challenges for aortic valve disease. *Lancet*. 2016;387:1312–1323.
35. Kaneko T, Ejiofor JI, Neely RC, et al. Aortic regurgitation with markedly reduced left ventricular function is not a contraindication for aortic valve replacement. *Ann Thorac Surg*. 2016;102:41–47.
36. Fiedler AG, Bhambhani V, Laikhter E, et al. Aortic valve replacement associated with survival in severe regurgitation and low ejection fraction. *Heart*. 2018;104:835–840.
37. McConkey HZR, Rajani R, Prendergast BD. Improving outcomes in chronic aortic regurgitation: timely diagnosis, access to specialist assessment and earlier surgery. *Heart*. 2018;104:794–795.
38. Nishimura RA, O'Gara PT, Bavaria JE, et al. 2019 AATS/ACC/ASE/SCAI/STS expert consensus systems of care document: a proposal to optimize care for patients with valvular heart disease: a joint report of the American Association for Thoracic Surgery, American College of Cardiology, American Society of Echocardiography, Society for Cardiovascular Angiography and Interventions, and Society of Thoracic Surgeons. *J Am Coll Cardiol*. 2019;73:2609–2635.
39. O'Gara PT, Sun YP. Timing of valve interventions in patients with chronic aortic regurgitation: are we waiting too long? *J Am Coll Cardiol*. 2019;73:1753–1755.
40. Hiratzka LF, Creager MA, Isselbacher EM, et al. Surgery for aortic dilatation in patients with bicuspid aortic valves: a statement of clarification from the American College of Cardiology/American Heart Association Task Force on clinical practice guidelines. *J Am Coll Cardiol*. 2016;67:724–731.

Chronic AR – Aortic Valve Repair, Ross Procedure, TAVR

41. El Khoury G, de Kerchove L. Principles of aortic valve repair. *J Thorac Cardiovasc Surg*. 2013;145:S26–S29.
42. Ugur M, Schaff HV, Suri R, et al. Late outcome of noncoronary sinus replacement in patients with bicuspid aortic valves and aortopathy. *Ann Thorac Surg*. 2014;97:1242–1246.
43. Ouzounian M, Rao V, Manlhiot C, et al. Valve-sparing root replacement compared with composite valve graft procedures in patients with aortic root dilation. *J Am Coll Cardiol*. 2016;68:1838–1847.
44. Schneider U, Hofmann C, Schöpe J, et al. Long-term results of differentiated anatomic reconstruction of bicuspid aortic valves. *JAMA Cardiol*. 2020;5:1366–1373.
45. Mazine A, El-Hamamsy I, Verma S, et al. Primer on the Ross procedure in adults for cardiologists and cardiac surgeons. *J Am Coll Cardiol*. 2018;72: 2761–2177.
46. Martin E, Mohammadi S, Jacques F, et al. Clinical outcomes following the Ross procedure in adults: a 25-year longitudinal study. *J Am Coll Cardiol*. 2017;70:1890–1899.
47. Romeo JLR Papageorgiou G, da Costa FFD, et al. Long-term clinical and echocardiographic outcomes in young and middle-aged adults undergoing the Ross procedure. *JAMA Cardiol*. 2021;6(5):539–548. https://doi.org/10.1001/jamacardio.2020.7434.
48. Aboud A, Charitos EI, Fujita B, et al. Long-term outcomes of patients undergoing the Ross procedure. *J Am Coll Cardiol*. 2021;77:1412–1422.
49. Sawaya FJ, Deutsch MA, Seiffert M, et al. Safety and efficacy of transcatheter aortic valve replacement in the treatment of pure aortic regurgitation in native valves and failing surgical bioprostheses: results from an International registry study. *JACC Cardiovasc Interv*. 2017;10:1048–1056.
50. Jiang J, Liu X, He Y, et al. Transcatheter aortic valve replacement for pure native aortic valve regurgitation: a systematic review. *Cardiology*. 2018;141:132–140.

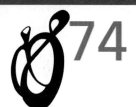

74 Transcatheter Aortic Valve Replacement

MARTIN B. LEON AND MICHAEL J. MACK

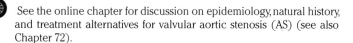

EPIDEMIOLOGY, NATURAL HISTORY, AND TREATMENT ALTERNATIVES FOR VALVULAR AORTIC STENOSIS

See the online chapter for discussion on epidemiology, natural history, and treatment alternatives for valvular aortic stenosis (AS) (see also Chapter 72).

HISTORY AND BACKGROUND OF TRANSCATHETER AORTIC VALVE REPLACEMENT (TAVR)

The combination of an aging population and accrued comorbidities rendered an enlarging segment of severe AS patients as poor candidates (real or perceived) for open surgical aortic valve replacement (AVR). Thus, a search for meaningful less-invasive catheter-based treatment options became a compelling clinical need.

Predicate Technologies Including Balloon Aortic Valvuloplasty

The first transcatheter approach embraced by interventional valve therapists for AS was balloon aortic valvuloplasty, introduced in 1986.[11] Early results from a U.S. registry of 492 patients demonstrated acute hemodynamic improvement, but mortality was 7.5% within 7 days and 34% within 1 year, and periprocedural complications were frequent.[12,13] The failure of balloon aortic valvuloplasty as a definitive therapy for AS was well documented in 165 patients with median follow-up of 3.9 years; freedom from either death, surgical AVR, or repeat balloon valvuloplasty at 1, 2, and 3 years was 40%, 19%, and 6%, respectively.[14] More recently, in the first PARTNER trial,[1] among the cohort of 102 patients randomized to standard therapy and receiving balloon aortic valvuloplasty within 30 days, despite acute hemodynamic improvement and few periprocedural complications, by 6 months and 1 year, mortality was 25.5% and 47.3% respectively.[15] Based upon these findings, balloon aortic valvuloplasty should not be considered as an alternative to surgical AVR for calcific AS and can only be recommended as a bridge to definitive AVR (surgical or transcatheter) in unstable patients or as short-term symptom palliation for patients who are not candidates for AVR.

The initial concept of an implantable bioprosthetic aortic valve mounted to a stent and delivered on a catheter was characterized in a closed-chested acute porcine model in 1992.[16] Excised porcine aortic valves, sewn to a homemade wire frame and crimped onto balloon catheters were delivered retrograde across the aortic valve and deployed at a transannular location after balloon inflation.[16] Several years later, a dedicated commercial program developed refined versions of this concept for durability testing, animal implants, human cadaver feasibility studies, and first-in-human cases. The early prototypes used three bovine pericardial leaflets, which were sewn to a tubular-slotted, balloon-expandable stainless-steel stent and crimped onto commercial noncompliant balloon valvuloplasty catheters. After accelerated pulse duplicator testing and 2 years of animal studies, the prototype devices were ready for compassionate-use human cases.

The Proof-of-Concept First-in-Human Case

See the online chapter.

THE EARLY YEARS OF TAVR

Outcomes in Patients Not Suitable for Surgery Using Early TAVR Technologies

The acronyms TAVI (transcatheter aortic valve implantation) and TAVR (transcatheter aortic valve replacement) have been used interchangeably; TAVI used more frequently in Europe and TAVR used more frequently in the United States and Asia. After the first-human use experiences, TAVR with first-generation balloon-expandable valves was applied sparingly in compassionate-use patients who were rejected for surgery. Additional discussion of early TAVR experiences is available in the online chapter.

These early TAVR clinical experiences were negatively impacted by first-generation technology, evolving procedural methods with inexperienced operators, and patient selection favoring the poorest candidates for surgery, which amplified the frequency and severity of post-treatment complications and adverse clinical events.

Patient Surgical Risk Profiles and Comorbidity Assessments

Initially, the expectations for TAVR were to provide an acceptable alternative for severe symptomatic AS patients who were not suitable for surgery. Implicit in the early case selection for TAVR was a stratification process for surgical risk. Multiple predictive risk scores have been developed and validated to help stratify a patient's risk for mortality

Additional content is available online at Elsevier eBooks for Practicing Clinicians

or morbidity after aortic valve surgery, either alone or combined with coronary revascularization. The most frequently used model in the United States is the STS predictive risk of operative mortality (PROM).[22] Common comorbidities contributing to increased surgical risk include chronic kidney disease, chronic lung disease (especially oxygen dependent), prior stroke, and vascular disease (coronary and peripheral). Risk stratification of AS patients, according to the most recent STS database, indicated a predicted mortality of 1.4% in low-risk (STS-PROM <4%, 80% of all patients), 5.1% in intermediate-risk (STS-PROM 4% to 8%), and 11.8% in high-risk (STS-PROM >8%) patients.[10] Additional discussion of frailty as a comorbidity is available online.

Introduction to the Heart Team

The use of multidisciplinary health care provider teams to manage complex medical problems has become a common theme in organ transplantation and oncology tumor boards. Likewise, the optimal management of severe AS in elderly patients with comorbid conditions has required a multidisciplinary "heart team" comprising the collective expertise of valve cardiologists, cardiac surgeons, interventional cardiologists trained in structural heart disease, imaging experts, gerontologists, other medical subspecialists, and advanced nursing practitioners. The roles of the heart team extend from the initial patient contact to valve clinic assessments, diagnostic decision making, inpatient procedural management, and subsequent follow-up care. The importance of the heart team was emphasized in the 2014 American College of Cardiology (ACC)/American Heart Association (AHA) guidelines for the management of valvular heart disease,[26] wherein the heart team was designated a class I recommendation for centers involved in TAVR care.

TAVR EVIDENCE-BASED CLINICAL RESEARCH

An Ecosystem for Aortic Valve Clinical Research

This material is presented in the online chapter.

Randomized Clinical Trials According to Surgical Risk Strata

Having created an ecosystem for aortic valve research, a series of landmark randomized clinical trials with both balloon-expandable and self-expanding TAVR systems were performed largely in the United States, which served to establish the evidence base for appropriate clinical indications. Based upon surgical risk stratification into de-escalating categories of prohibitive (or extreme), high, intermediate, and low risk for surgical valve replacement, available TAVR systems were randomized against standard therapies. Additional discussion of TAVR clinical trial methodology is available online.

Primary Clinical Endpoints

The first randomized TAVR trial in AS was the PARTNER trial in elderly patients who were considered unsuitable candidates for surgery due to coexisting conditions with a 50% or more predicted probability of either death by 30 days after surgery or a serious irreversible complication[1] (eTable 74.1). In 358 patients with severe symptomatic AS, the rate of death from any cause at 1 year (the primary endpoint) was 30.7% with balloon-expandable TAVR compared with 50.7% with nonsurgical standard therapies, consisting of medical treatment and balloon aortic valvuloplasty (hazard ratio 0.55 with TAVR; 95% confidence interval [CI], 0.40 to 0.74; $P < 0.001$) (eTables 74.2 and 74.3; Fig. 74.1A). After 5 years' follow-up,[30] the absolute 20% difference in all-cause mortality favoring TAVR was maintained, resulting in an increase in median survival from 11.7 months with standard therapy to 31.0 months after TAVR ($P < 0.0001$). Similar outcomes were observed in extreme-risk AS patients after TAVR using a self-expanding bioprosthesis.[31]

Concurrent with the extreme-risk trials and balloon-expandable and self-expanding TAVR was randomized versus surgery in high-risk AS patients[32,33] (eTable 74.1). The primary endpoint, death from any cause at 1 year, was noninferior for the comparison of TAVR versus surgery

(eTables 74.2 and 74.3; Fig. 74.1B and C), and the results were maintained after 5 years' follow-up.[34,35] Next, larger trials in intermediate-risk patients were performed with an expanded primary endpoint including all-cause death or disabling stroke after 2 years.[36,37] In the balloon-expandable TAVR intermediate-risk trial, 2032 patients were randomized to either TAVR or surgery and the rate of death or stroke at 2 years was similar in the TAVR (19.3%) and surgery (21.1%) groups ($P = 0.001$ for noninferiority)[36] (eTables 74.1–74.3 and eFig. 74.2A). After 5 years' follow-up,[38] the overall primary endpoint results were still similar between the groups. However, in those TAVR patients requiring transapical access (23.7% of the study cohort) due to unfavorable anatomic factors precluding the transfemoral approach, surgical AVR was superior to TAVR. In the self-expanding TAVR intermediate-risk trial, 1746 were randomized and the estimated rate of death or stroke at 2 years (Bayesian analysis) was 12.6% in the TAVR group and 14.0% in the surgery group (posterior probability of noninferiority >0.999)[37] (eTables 74.1–74.3 and eFig. 74.2B). Importantly, the high- and intermediate-risk AS patients treated in these trials were elderly ($\geq$ 80 years), with multiple comorbidities (STS scores ranged from 4% to 12%) and frequent frailty.

Given the favorable TAVR results in previous higher surgical risk trials, using current generation balloon-expandable and self-expanding TAVR systems and evolved procedural methods, trials were recently undertaken in younger, low-risk patients, which represents a high proportion of the patients currently being treated with severe AVR. Enrollment was confined to patients with tricuspid valve disease with transfemoral access and favorable anatomy for TAVR and surgery. The balloon-expandable low-risk PARTNER trial randomized 1000 patients with a mean age 73 years and mean STS score 1.9% to either transfemoral TAVR or surgery[39] (eTable 74.1). The primary composite endpoint of death, stroke, or cardiovascular rehospitalization within 1 year was significantly lower in the TAVR group than in the surgery group (8.5% versus 15.1%; $P = 0.001$ for superiority)[39] (eTables 74.2 and 74.3; Fig. 74.2A). The self-expanding TAVR low-risk trial randomized 1468 patients with a mean age 74 years and mean STS score 1.9%[40] (eTable 74.1). The primary endpoint of all-cause death or disabling stroke at 2 years was an estimated rate of 5.3% in the TAVR group and 6.7% in the surgery group (Bayesian methods, posterior probability of noninferiority > 0.999)[40] (eTables 74.2 and 74.3; Fig. 74.2B).

Based on these early-term results in selected patients who are similar to those randomized in the clinical trials, TAVR should be considered as an alternative therapy to surgery for severe symptomatic AS (see guideline recommendations).

Key Secondary Outcomes

In addition to the clinical outcomes comprising the primary endpoint of randomized TAVR trials, other important secondary endpoints that impact patient morbidity, hospital stay, or late mortality must be considered when comparing the safety and efficacy of new versus standard therapies. eTables 74.2 and 74.3 detail key secondary endpoints at 30 days and 1 year for TAVR and control therapies.[1,32,33,36,37,39,40] See the online chapter for additional discussion.

Echocardiographic Findings

Using echocardiography-derived measurements, reduction in aortic valve gradients and improvement in aortic valve areas have been similar with both transcatheter and surgical bioprosthetic valves, as determined by core laboratory assessments from the randomized trials.[32,33,36,37,39,40] In fact, many studies suggest greater hemodynamic improvements with transcatheter compared to surgical valves[40] (eFig. 74.3). Moreover, sustained improvement in antegrade hemodynamics for both transcatheter and surgical valves has been observed in studies with 5-year echocardiography follow-up[34,35,38] (eFig. 74.4A and B). Further discussion of echo findings after TAVR is available online. Other echo findings after relief of AS with both surgical and transcatheter replacement valves have been progressive regression of LV hypertrophy over time, reduction in functional mitral regurgitation, and improvement in LV ejection fraction, especially in patients with reduced baseline LV systolic function.

Paravalvular aortic regurgitation (PVR) after TAVR was commonly seen during the early registries and was increased compared with surgically implanted bioprostheses in the randomized trials[32,33,36,37,39,40]

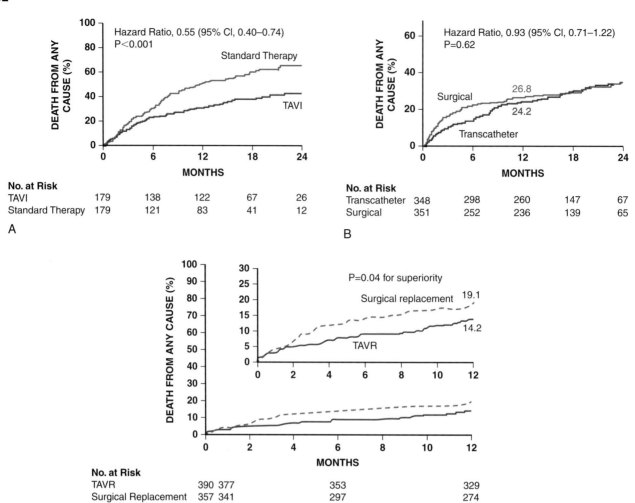

FIGURE 74.1 TAVR versus surgery randomized trials in extreme and high-risk patients; primary endpoint, all-cause death at 1 year. **A,** Extreme-risk patients with balloon-expandable TAVR. **B,** High-risk patients with balloon-expandable TAVR. **C,** High-risk patients with self-expanding TAVR. (From Leon MB, et al. Transcatheter aortic-valve implantation for aortic stenosis in patients who cannot undergo surgery. N Engl J Med 2010;363:1597-1607; Smith CR, et al. Transcatheter versus surgical aortic-valve replacement in high-risk patients. N Engl J Med 2011;364:2187-2198; Adams DH, et al. Transcatheter aortic-valve replacement with a self-expanding prosthesis. N Engl J Med 2014;370:1790-1798.)

(eFig. 74.5A). In most studies, moderate or severe (but not mild) PVR was associated with increased late mortality after TAVR[36] (eFig. 74.5B). Due to technology and procedural enhancements, recent TAVR systems have shown a reduction in moderate or severe PVR, which is now comparable to surgical valves, but there remains a significant difference favoring surgery in mild PVR[39] (eFig. 74.6).

Quality-of-Life Assessments

Beginning with the highest surgical risk patients, TAVR resulted in a dramatic improvement in cardiac symptoms and functional capacity, as determined by a significant decrease in the New York Heart Association (NYHA) functional class. At baseline, 75% to 95% of patients had functional class III or IV symptoms, which was reduced to 15% to 25% within one month after treatment (eFig. 74.7A). Additional discussion of quality-of-life assessments is available online.

In the low-risk balloon-expandable TAVR randomized trial, when expressed as ordinal categorical improvement variables, TAVR was associated with greater symptom benefit compared to surgery, both early and late[44] (eFig. 74.8).

National TAVR Registries

After regulatory approval in Europe of early TAVR systems in 2007, many countries (most notably France, Germany, Italy, and the United Kingdom) established national registries to capture representative data

from the emerging TAVR treatment experiences. Additional discussion of TAVR registries is available online.

Perhaps the most comprehensive and useful of the national registries has been the United States joint initiative of the Society of Thoracic Surgeons (STS) and the ACC with multiple other stakeholders (e.g., industry sponsors) to form the Transcatheter Valve Therapy (TVT) registry soon after the initial U.S. Food and Drug Administration (FDA) approval of the first balloon-expandable TAVR system in the United States in 2011.[45] (See the online chapter.)

The relationship of procedural volume and patient outcomes was described from the TVT registry.[47] An inverse volume–mortality association was observed for transfemoral TAVR procedures; mortality at 30 days was higher and more variable at hospitals with a low procedural volume than at hospitals with a high procedural volume.

The 2020 TVT registry comprehensive report included 276,316 TAVR patients representing 715 U.S. sites from 2011 through 2019, all three FDA-approved TAVR manufacturers, and all FDA-approved clinical indications.[48] During the TVT registry experience, TAVR volume has increased yearly from 14,000 to 73,000 cases per year, and the annual number of TAVR procedures exceeded the total number of surgical AVRs in 2018[48] (eFig. 74.9). Changes over time in patient demographics included a reduction in patient median age from 84 to 80 years, an increase in transfemoral access cases from 47% to 95%, and lower median STS scores from 6.9% to 4.4%, indicating a lower proportion of high-risk patients. Concurrently, clinical outcomes improved significantly over time; 30-day mortality decreased from 7.5% to 2.5%, 30-day

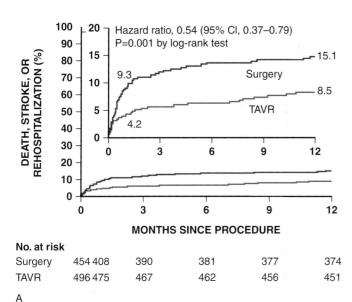

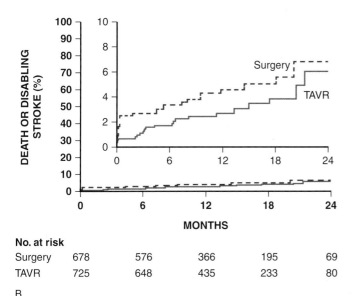

FIGURE 74.2 TAVR versus surgery randomized trials in low-risk patients. **A,** Primary endpoint, all-cause death or all stroke, or CV rehospitalization at 1 year; low-risk patients with balloon-expandable TAVR. **B,** Primary endpoint, all-cause death or disabling stroke at 2 years; low-risk patients with self-expanding TAVR. (From Mack MJ, et al. Transcatheter aortic-valve replacement with a balloon-expandable valve in low-risk patients. N Engl J Med 2019;380:1695-1705; Popma JJ, et al. Transcatheter aortic-valve replacement with a self-expanding valve in low-risk patients. N Engl J Med 2019;380:1706-1715.)

strokes from 2.8% to 2.3%, the need for new pacemakers diminished from 15.1% to 10.8%, length of hospital stay diminished from a median of 7 to 2 days, and patients discharged post-TAVR to home increased from 62% to 90%. Undoubtedly, a portion of the improved outcomes has been due to expanding treatment cohorts with reduced risk profiles, but the combination of procedural simplification, technology advances, and increased operator and site experience are likely also playing significant roles.

Society-Based Guidelines and Appropriate Use Criteria

In patients with severe AS and indications for AVR using a bioprosthetic valve, the choice of either surgery or TAVR has evolved with increasing clinical trial evidence. The ACC/AHA 2020 valvular heart disease guidelines[8] have expanded the recommended use of TAVR (either preferred or as an alternative to surgery) to four class 1 categories (Table 74.1). TAVR is the preferred recommendation for symptomatic patients (1) with high or prohibitive surgical risk (regardless

TABLE 74.1 Class 1 Recommendations for TAVR (ACC/AHA 2020 Guidelines)

COR	LOE	RECOMMENDATION
1	A	For symptomatic patients of any age with severe AS and a high or prohibitive surgical risk, TAVR is recommended if predicted post-TAVR survival is >12 months with an acceptable quality of life
1	A	For symptomatic patients with severe AS who are >80 years of age or for younger patients with a life expectancy <10 years and no anatomic contraindication to transfemoral access, TAVR is recommended
1	A	For symptomatic patients with severe AS who are 65 to 80 years of age and no anatomic contraindication to transfemoral access, after shared decision making, TAVR is an alternative to SAVR
1	B-NR	In asymptomatic patients with severe AS and an LVEF <50% who are ≤80 years of age and no anatomic contraindication to transfemoral access, TAVR is an alternative to SAVR (preference according to age)

COR, Class of recommendation; *LOE,* level of evidence; *LVEF,* left ventricular ejection fraction; *NR,* nonrandomized.
From Otto CM, et al. 2020 ACC/AHA Guideline for the management of patients with valvular heart disease: a report of the American College of Cardiology/American Heart Association Joint Committee on Clinical Practice Guidelines. J Am Coll Cardiol 2020.

of age) if predicted post-TAVR survival is >12 months with an acceptable quality of life and (2) >80 years of age (or younger with a life expectancy <10 years) without contraindications to transfemoral TAVR. After shared decision making, TAVR is an alternative to surgery for (1) symptomatic patients from 65 to 80 years of age without contraindications to transfemoral TAVR and (2) asymptomatic patients with an LV ejection fraction <50% (preference according to age). Clearly, the choice of surgery or TAVR is determined by four factors: (1) age and life expectancy, favoring TAVR in older patients with reduced life expectancy and surgery in younger patients with longer life expectancy, due to less well-understood bioprosthetic valve durability with TAVR; (2) clinical comorbidities, which favor the less-invasive TAVR procedure; (3) anatomic constraints challenging the safety of surgery (e.g., hostile chest wall deformities) or TAVR (e.g., suitability for transfemoral access); and (4) shared decision making in which a careful discussion with patients includes lifestyle preferences and explanations of known and unknown factors accounting for risks and benefits of each procedure. A flow diagram, which incorporates the current ACC/AHA guideline recommendations depicting the nodal points for choosing surgery versus TAVR in AVR-indicated patients, is provided (Fig. 74.3).

Not infrequently, the complexity of individual case scenarios cannot be captured easily within the confines of formal recommendation categories. Case-based decisions often require greater flexibility and should incorporate clinical experience and judgment. An additional guidance tool for TAVR practitioners is the development of appropriate use criteria for numerous AS case situations,[49] which details expert opinions on reasonable clinical management decisions.

TAVR TECHNOLOGY EVOLUTION

Anatomy (Components) of a TAVR System

Development of a transcatheter system for bioprosthetic AVR requires the integration of three basic foundational components: a bioprosthetic trileaflet valve, mounted on an expandable metallic frame or scaffold, which is attached to and incorporated with a catheter delivery system. Bioprosthetic valve materials generally consist of predetermined thickness bovine or porcine pericardium of prespecified geometry treated with glutaraldehyde fixation and anticalcification processes.

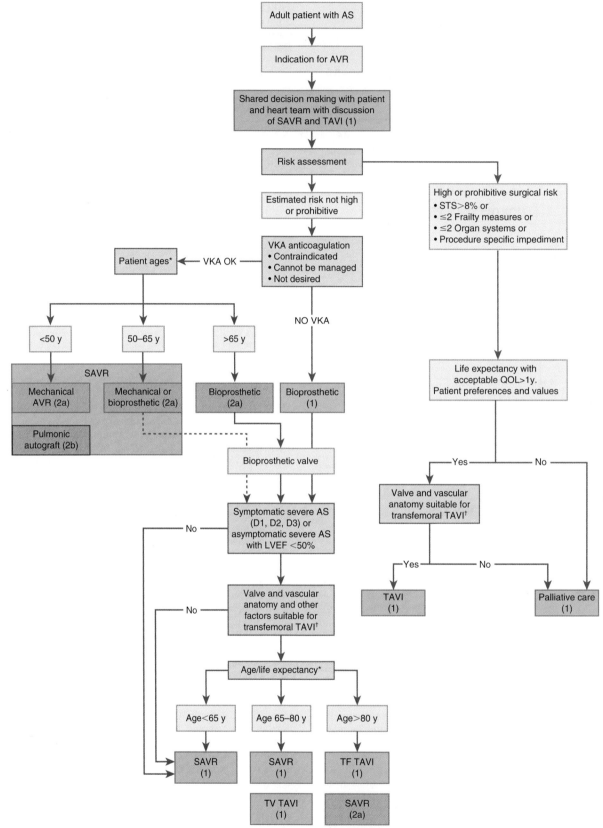

FIGURE 74.3 Choice of SAVR versus TAVI when AVR is indicated for valvular AS, based on the 2020 ACC/AHA valve guidelines recommendations. Green boxes denote class I recommendations. D1, Symptomatic severe high-gradient AS; D2, Symptomatic severe low-flow, low-gradient AS with reduced LVEF; D3, Symptomatic severe low-gradient AS with normal LVEF or paradoxical low-flow severe AS. *Approximate ages, based on US Actuarial Life Expectancy tables, are provided for guidance. The balance between expected patient longevity and valve durability varies continuously across the age range, with more durable valves preferred for patients with a longer life expectancy. †Placement of a transcatheter valve requires vascular anatomy that allows transfemoral delivery and the absence of aortic root dilation that would require surgical replacement. Valvular anatomy must be suitable for placement of the specific prosthetic valve, including annulus size and shape, leaflet number and calcification, and coronary ostial height. (From Otto CM, et al. 2020 ACC/AHA Guideline for the management of patients with valvular heart disease: a report of the American College of Cardiology/American Heart Association Joint Committee on Clinical Practice Guidelines. J Am Coll Cardiol 2020;77(4):e25-e197.)

The leaflets are sewn or attached to short, balloon-expandable metallic frames or to long, super-elastic nitinol self-expanding platforms. The valve-frame composite is compressed or crimped onto catheter delivery systems that facilitate frame expansion via either underlying noncompliant balloon inflation or overlying sheath retraction. After appropriate valve sizing (using CT-imaging formulas and accounting for 10% to 20% oversizing) and correct axial positioning within the aortic annulus, the valve-frame is deployed to the desired location with retention mediated by radial expansion of the frame against high-friction elements of the calcified native aortic valve complex. Various catheter-based delivery systems have been developed, some with directional steerability features, and all attempting to reduce overall system profiles to optimize use of the common femoral artery as the primary vascular access site. Other important features of TAVR systems include the implant location of the bioprosthetic valve, either intra-annular or supra-annular, the available valve sizes to match the range of annulus dimensions (from 18- through 30-mm mean diameter), and the frame length and geometry affecting catheter access to the coronary arteries.

Rapid Progression of TAVR Technologies to the Modern Era

Since the initial experiences with balloon-expandable and self-expanding TAVR systems,[11,20] there have been dramatic improvements in all TAVR components (Figs. 74.4 and 74.5). Additional discussion of TAVR technology evolution is available online.

Clearly, rapid technology evolution of both balloon-expandable and self-expanding TAVR systems have resulted in current generation devices that can treat almost all aortic annulus dimensions with user-friendly, low-profile delivery catheters for transfemoral access, repositionable features with predictable valve deployment, and reduced PVR.

Other TAVR Systems and Comparative Device versus Device Studies

Given the success of TAVR as a new therapy alternative for AS, there has been an explosion of novel technologies that have been developed and examined in clinical studies. New TAVR systems are shown in eFig. 74.10. Additional discussion of other new TAVR systems is available online.

Accessory Devices for TAVR

The use of off-the-shelf or purpose-driven accessory devices to either facilitate or reduce complications associated with TAVR has rapidly matured over the past decade. Presently, the routine TAVR procedure may be performed with dedicated preshaped 0.035" guidewires of different shapes, special large-diameter balloon catheters for pre- and especially post-dilation to optimize valve implantation, new temporary pacing catheters for valve deployment, expandable and in-line vascular sheaths to assist with low-profile transfemoral access, large-hole vascular closure devices to assist with arterial closure after sheath removal, and catheter-based cerebral embolic protection devices to reduce periprocedural neurologic events.

From the earliest TAVR studies, among the most concerning complications were vascular events due to high-profile sheaths and/or catheters straining the limits of iliofemoral anatomy[52] and embolic strokes due to device interactions with the ascending aorta and/or aortic valve.[53] Additional discussion of vascular closure devices is available online.

The risk of brain injury associated with embolic particulate debris liberated during TAVR procedures depends on the specific definitions applied and the intensity of diagnostic neuroimaging studies.[55] Temporary catheter-based intravascular filters and deflectors have been used in clinical trials to protect the brain from embolic neurologic events during TAVR. Additional discussion of cerebral embolic protection devices is available online.

Importantly, significant clinical stroke reduction after TAVR has not been confirmed, so the systematic use of cerebral protection devices is left up to the physician's judgment until ongoing large, randomized stroke studies are completed.

TAVR PROCEDURAL MATURATION

Computed Tomography Imaging for Procedural Planning

Computed tomography (CT) contrast imaging has become a fundamental diagnostic and procedure planning tool for all TAVR procedures. Most critically, CT is routinely used to optimally select the transcatheter valve size[57] and to assess anatomic features of the iliofemoral arteries to determine the suitability of transfemoral access for a given TAVR system. Additional discussion of CT-imaging for TAVR is available online.

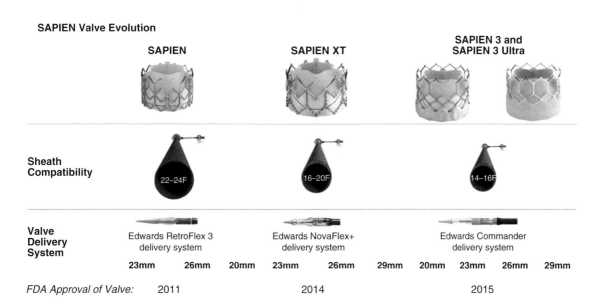

FIGURE 74.4 Evolution of balloon-expandable SAPIEN valves (Edwards Lifesciences), sheath compatibility, and valve delivery systems from initial FDA approval to the current generation.

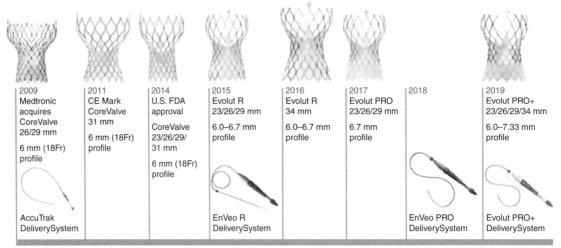

FIGURE 74.5 Evolution of self-expanding CoreValve-Evolut valves (Medtronic) and valve delivery systems from prior to initial FDA approval to the current generation.

Echocardiography for Diagnosis, Procedure-Planning and Follow-Up

The most useful and widely utilized imaging modality for evaluating aortic valve disease is transthoracic echocardiography (two- and three-dimensional). In the management of TAVR patients, echocardiography is used (1) pretreatment for diagnosis of stenosis severity and for procedure planning; (2) intra-procedure to determine the etiology of complications and to assess PVR; and (3) during follow-up as a clinical and research tool to assess long-term bioprosthetic valve function, especially in the setting of recurrent symptoms.[59] In addition, echocardiography provides critical quantitative and qualitative information to correctly stratify low-flow AS syndromes and to monitor LV mass regression, LV function (both systolic and diastolic), RV function, and concomitant mitral and tricuspid valve disease.[60] In post-TAVR patients, routine transthoracic echocardiograms are usually incorporated into follow-up clinical assessments, at 1- or 2-year intervals, or in response to symptom changes.

Minimalist Approach (Including Conscious Sedation Anesthesia)

Undoubtedly, among the most impactful advances in TAVR therapy has been the progressive evolution to a simplified or "minimalist" clinical care management strategy. The minimalist approach is meant to preserve patient safety while leveraging the less-invasive features of a transcatheter procedure to improve efficiencies, reduce costs, and create a more patient-friendly experience. An initially controversial but key aspect of the minimalist strategy was the elimination of routine general anesthesia with associated transesophageal echocardiography during the TAVR procedure, which was replaced by conscious sedation and transthoracic echocardiography. Additional discussion of the minimalist TAVR strategy is available online.

Importantly, although many components of the minimalist TAVR strategy can be used in most patients, thoughtful screening and triage is necessary. A minority of AS patients have high-risk clinical or anatomic factors, wherein the use of general anesthesia with transesophageal echocardiography guidance or other precautionary measures are advisable to optimize patient safety.

Alternative Vascular Access Strategies

Currently, transfemoral access for TAVR procedures is performed in >95% of all patients treated in the United States,[48] largely related to markedly smaller arterial sheath size requirements. There has been a corresponding decline in transthoracic access TAVR procedures (either transapical or direct aorta entry sites) due to evidence for increased complications with inferior early and late clinical outcomes.[36] For those remaining TAVR patients in whom transfemoral access is not possible, depending on operator experience and training, the most frequently used alternatives are transaxillary, transcarotid, and transcaval approaches.

TAVR-ASSOCIATED COMPLICATIONS

Intraprocedural Complications

Intraprocedural major complications during TAVR have declined over time and are currently uncommon. In the 2020 TVT registry report of >275,000 TAVR procedures overall and 73,000 in 2019, the incidence of acute structural complications (annulus rupture, chamber perforation, and valve embolization), need for cardiopulmonary bypass support, and conversion to open heart surgery were all <0.5%.[48] The very low incidence of intraprocedural complications has allowed more procedures to be safely performed in catherization laboratory settings with less formal surgical backup requirements in many centers.

Coronary Obstruction

Acute coronary obstruction during TAVR is rare due to careful preoperative CT-imaging for risk assessment. Important CT-measurements are the coronary orifice height above the aortic annulus and size of the sinuses of Valsalva relative to the annulus and the ascending aorta relative to the type and size of the planned valve. In patients deemed to be at high risk for coronary obstruction, coronary protection with preemptive wiring of the at-risk coronary ostia and eventual stent implantation in cases of coronary flow impairment is a potential strategy to prevent coronary obstruction. In a recent international registry, preemptive wiring was employed in 2.2% of TAVR cases deemed high risk for coronary obstruction followed by coronary stent deployment in 61% of these cases.[64]

Vascular Complications

The most frequent intraprocedural complication is related to transfemoral access with major vascular complications reported in 1.5% of patients.[48] The combination of preprocedure planning with CT-imaging, utilization of suture-based vascular closure devices for percutaneous common femoral artery repair, and the expanding use of ultrasound guidance to perform controlled common femoral artery access has reduced the frequency of minor and major vascular complications during TAVR. If vascular complications do occur, most can be successfully managed by an experienced operator using an endovascular approach, with the seldom need for surgical cutdown and open repair.

Postprocedural Complications
Neurologic Events

The 2% incidence of periprocedural stroke after TAVR has remained constant over the past 5 years.[48] A recent propensity-matched study compared strokes after transfemoral TAVR and surgical AVR in randomized trials (see the online chapter).[65]

Although cerebral embolic protection during TAVR is approved by the FDA,[56] the lack of definitive stroke prevention evidence has resulted in variable adoption with use in approximately 20% of cases in 2019.[48]

Conduction Disturbances

New atrioventricular conduction disturbances after TAVR remain an ongoing concern without complete resolution. The incidence of new permanent pacemaker (PPM) implantation due to high-degree atrioventricular block ranges from 6% to 7% with balloon-expandable valves to 17% to 18% with self-expanding valves, with an overall national rate of 11% for TAVR.[39,40,48] There has been a focus on procedural techniques to avoid oversizing the valve relative to the annulus and to minimize the depth of valve implantation to reduce trauma to the membranous septum, which have been shown to reduce the need for new PPM. Clinical management algorithms have been developed to guide optimal patient screening for advanced atrioventricular block after TAVR and the indications for PPM implantation.[66]

As younger patients with a longer life expectancy undergo TAVR, the importance of avoiding the need for permanent pacing increases. Another concern is an increase in the incidence of new left bundle branch block after TAVR, which has been demonstrated to be associated with decreased long-term survival.[67]

Paravalvular Regurgitation

The early TAVR randomized trials clearly indicated that PVR was more common after TAVR compared with surgery and was associated with increased late mortality.[68] The incidence of moderate-severe PVR post-TAVR has diminished significantly to approximately 1.5%, based on site reports in the most recent TVT registry.[48] There are a number of factors responsible for reduced PVR: (1) the routine use of CT-imaging to accurately assess annular dimensions for selection of the optimal valve size; (2) new generation transcatheter valve designs, which incorporate external wraps (polymers or biologic materials) to fill gaps and promote flush contact with the annulus; and (3) intraprocedure recognition of PVR and the use of post-dilation strategies which commonly resolves or greatly diminishes the severity of PVR. Placement of a second valve inside the initial valve (TAVR in TAVR) can help to resolve the PVR if initial placement location was imprecise. Finally, if moderate or severe PVR persists after the procedure, transcatheter device closure, most commonly using a vascular plug, can be performed and is usually successful.[69]

Prosthesis–Patient Mismatch

Prosthesis–patient mismatch is a condition where the effective orifice area (EOA) of a normally functioning prosthesis is too small in relation to the patient's body size and has been associated with worse outcomes after surgical AVR. Although TAVR prostheses generally have larger valve orifices, a recent analysis of the TVT registry demonstrated that severe and moderate prosthesis-patient mismatches were present following TAVR in 12% and 25% of patients, respectively.[70] Predictors of severe prosthesis-patient mismatch included small (≤23-mm diameter) valve prosthesis, valve-in-valve procedures, larger body surface area, female sex, younger age, non-white/Hispanic race, lower ejection fraction, atrial fibrillation (AF), and severe mitral or tricuspid regurgitation. Severe prosthesis-patient mismatch was associated with higher mortality and heart failure rehospitalization at 1 year. Recent studies have noted that Doppler echocardiography may overestimate the severity of prosthesis-patient mismatch post-TAVR due to pressure recovery considerations and assumptions made in calculating transvalvular gradients in a nonstenotic prosthetic valve. This has been demonstrated by a hemodynamic discordance, with systematically higher echocardiographic measurements of postprocedure transvalvular gradients compared with simultaneously measured invasive gradients.[71]

Other Complications

The incidence of other important complications after TAVR is low,[48] including major or life-threatening bleeding 4% to 5%, acute kidney injury ~1%, and endocarditis <1%. The frequency of endocarditis after TAVR is approximately the same as after surgical AVR.

TAVR AND CONCOMITANT CARDIAC DISEASES

See the online chapter for discussion on aortic stenosis (AS) and multivalve disease, AS and AF, AS and coronary artery disease (CAD), and TAVR in low-gradient AS.

TAVR IN SURGICAL BIOPROSTHETIC AORTIC VALVE FAILURE

The use of TAVR for the management of surgical bioprosthetic valve failure as an alternative to reoperative surgical AVR has become broadly adopted in clinical practice. The previously implanted surgical bioprosthesis serves as an ideal "landing zone" for TAVR implantation, and the risks of PVR and new PPMs are greatly reduced. The initial experience in the United States was reported in the TVT registry beginning in 2013 with 455 cases, and by 2019, there were almost 5000 valve-in-valve (ViV) cases performed.[48,85] The results of the PARTNER trial with ViV treatment in 365 high- and intermediate-risk patients using early generation balloon-expandable TAVR indicated a 1-year all-cause mortality of 12.4%, improved hemodynamics, and a dramatic improvement in quality-of-life measures.[86]

Current issues regarding aortic ViV procedures include the potential for coronary obstruction at the time of implant, prosthesis–patient mismatch, and unknown long-term valve durability. Patients who are at higher risk for coronary obstruction include those with surgical valves with externally mounted leaflets, low coronary artery orifices, and reduced space in the aortic sinuses around the surgical valve. The likelihood of coronary obstruction due to deflection of the surgical valve leaflet over the coronary ostia can be mitigated by splitting the leaflet of the surgical valve using a guidewire electrocautery technique, the so-called BASILICA procedure.[87] An ongoing clinical trial has demonstrated successful BASILICA pretreatment followed by uneventful ViV in patients at high risk for coronary obstruction. The presence or creation of prosthesis–patient mismatch especially with small surgical valves remains a limitation of the ViV procedure.[88] The use of supra-annular self-expanding TAVR systems is recommended in these challenging circumstances to achieve the lowest possible transvalvular gradients. Another approach is to fracture the surgical bioprosthesis with high-pressure noncompliant balloon inflations during ViV procedures, which further expands the surgical frame and results in improved hemodynamics after subsequent TAVR.[89] This technique has been used predominantly in patients with small surgical bioprostheses to enlarge the patient cohort for ViV therapy. Whether valve frame fracturing should be limited to smaller size surgical valves (19 and 21 mm) and in patients at risk for severe prosthesis-patient mismatch or should be performed routinely in all surgical valves to optimize the reduction in transvalvular gradients has been a point of controversy. A new surgical valve has also been developed, which is ideally suited to subsequent ViV, as the frame is designed to expand during subsequent ViV. The use of oral anticoagulants after ViV procedures due to possibly higher rates of valve thrombosis remains unknown. There is also increasing experience with placing TAVR valves within degenerated TAVR valves (TAV in TAV), a procedure likely to be more widely utilized in the coming years.[90]

GAPS IN TAVR KNOWLEDGE AND ONGOING CONTROVERSIES

Durability of TAVR Systems

Valve durability is now a critical issue as TAVR evolves to include younger, low-risk patients who are likely to survive for several decades after the procedure. The tissue from both surgical and transcatheter bioprostheses is prone to structural valve deterioration (SVD), which could lead to hemodynamic valve dysfunction. Durability is determined by numerous factors including tissue origin and thickness, anticalcification treatments, leaflet and valve design, and clinical factors such as patient age and metabolic abnormalities. In studies of surgical valves, SVD commonly begins 8 years after implantation, with marked acceleration after 10 years.[91] Follow-up surgical series indicate that the overall freedom from reintervention or death in patients with surgical aortic valves is approximately 95% at 5 years, 70% to 90% at 10 years, and 50% to 80% at 15 years.[92]

Long-term durability and freedom from SVD are largely unknown for TAVR, especially since the bulk of the early TAVR experiences were in elderly patients with limited life expectancy. Recent reports from Denmark (NOTION trial) and the United Kingdom (UK-TAVI registry) using early TAVR systems have provided some durability information for TAVR between 5 and 10 years.[93,94] In the randomized NOTION trial through 6 years, SVD was significantly greater for surgical aortic valve replacement (SAVR) than TAVR, and bioprosthetic valve failure was extremely low and similar for both groups. The UK-TAVI observational registry reported 91% of surviving patients remaining free of SVD between 5 and 10 years post-implantation, and the incidence of moderate or severe SVD was approximately 9% at a mean of 6 years. Although these data are reassuring, caution is still warranted in extending the indications for TAVR to young, low-risk patients.

Treatment of Bicuspid Aortic Valve Disease

Patients with known bicuspid aortic valve disease (BAVD) were excluded from the pivotal randomized trials of TAVR due to the uncertainty of TAVR prosthesis performance in complex bicuspid anatomies. Concerns regarding TAVR in BAVD relate to the more oval shape of the aortic annulus and the bulky eccentric calcification of the leaflets, raphe, and LV outflow tract. Indeed, these concerns were borne out in the early experience with TAVR using first-generation devices that led to a higher incidence of annular rupture, moderate-severe PVR, and the need for new PPMs.[95] However, with greater experience, especially in properly selected patients with less hostile anatomy using newer generation devices, the outcomes have been similar to TAVR in patients with tricuspid AS.[96] The role of TAVR in BAVD will be of greater importance as TAVR is used to treat younger patients who have a higher incidence of BAVD. Based on CT-imaging and clinical experience, it appears that TAVR may be suitable for some BAVD patients with a non- or minimally calcified raphe and those without bulky eccentric calcification of the valve leaflets and LV outflow tract. Likewise, there is consensus that younger patients with bulky, eccentric calcification at risk for annular rupture, marked annular ovality, and ascending aortic aneurysmal disease are best treated with surgery. Whether a randomized trial to clearly define the best management strategies in BAVD patients between these two extremes has been an ongoing controversy.

TAVR for Aortic Regurgitation

TAVR devices have been used mainly for the treatment of calcific AS due to the reliance on calcified native valve tissue for secure prosthesis anchoring. There has been early experience with currently approved devices in patients with pure aortic regurgitation (AR). A registry report of 331 patients with severe AR showed improvement in clinical outcomes with later generation balloon-expandable and self-expanding TAVR systems, emphasizing the need for device over-expansion and careful case selection.[97] Novel TAVR designs for the treatment of AR with features to secure the prosthetic valve to the underlying native leaflets (eFig. 74.10) are promising and are in various stages of clinical evaluation in the United States and elsewhere.

Managing the Young, Low-Risk Patient with AS

The management of young, low-risk patients with AS is in a state of rapid evolution and will be based on further evidence development. Clearly, valve durability is of greater importance in younger patients and there are scant TAVR durability data beyond 5 years, although there is no signal of premature SVD in transcatheter bioprostheses. Also, younger patients have a higher incidence of BAVD, and the additional burdens of increased anatomic complexity must

be considered. Based on current best available evidence, clinical management should apply an algorithm where the first decision is whether a tissue or mechanical valve is preferred. In general, patients <50 years are best treated with a mechanical valve if anticoagulation is acceptable, and in patients >60 to 65 years, a bioprosthetic valve is preferable. Shared decision making with patients in their 50s regarding the advantages and disadvantages of valve choice (anticoagulation versus durability) is appropriate. Once the decision for a tissue valve is made, the next decision is TAVR versus surgery, which also requires a careful shared decision-making process. Fewer than 10% of patients in the low-risk TAVR trials were <65 years, so long-term durability is unknown. The use of ViV TAVR after the first valve, be it a TAVR or surgery, may potentially lengthen the time to the next surgical intervention. Ongoing discussions are active among thought leaders regarding the lifetime management of young patients with AS, with a goal to generate evidence that can help to decide the most appropriate sequence for procedures (e.g., surgery or TAVR first).

Subclinical Leaflet Thrombosis

With the expanded use of CT-imaging, the detection of subclinical leaflet thrombosis on bioprosthetic valves has become readily available.[98] The sentinel imaging findings—hypoattenuated leaflet thickening (HALT) and reduced leaflet motion—were observed in approximately 20% of patients during the first year after TVR. To determine the frequency, natural history, and clinical relevance of these imaging findings, CT-surveillance substudies were imbedded in both low-risk randomized TAVR trials.[99,100] The PARTNER 3 CT-substudy[99] found that subclinical leaflet thrombosis was more frequent in transcatheter compared with surgical valves at 30 days but not at 1 year, a significant minority of patients had either resolution of 1-month HALT by 1 year or newly appearing HALT at 1 year, and the impact of HALT on thromboembolic complications and SVD was indeterminate and required long-term follow-up. Based on these studies, there is reasonable consensus that routine CT-evaluations or systematic anticoagulation therapy is not warranted after TAVR and should only be considered if thromboembolic complications are present (e.g., stroke or retinal artery embolus) or if there is an unexplained early increase in transvalvular aortic valve gradients.

Optimal Antithrombotic Therapies

Based on experience with coronary stents, dual antiplatelet therapy for 6 months became the early default antithrombotic management of patients after TAVR. However, multiple studies have demonstrated an increased incidence of bleeding complications with dual antiplatelet therapy compared with aspirin monotherapy without added benefit in reducing thromboembolic complications.[101] In a recent randomized trial, the direct factor Xa inhibitor rivaroxaban was associated with a higher incidence of death, thromboembolic complications, and bleeding compared with antiplatelet therapy. However, antithrombotic therapy was associated with a lower incidence of HALT in a substudy.[102,103] At the current time, aspirin monotherapy (or another single antiplatelet agent) is the preferred post-TAVR pharmacotherapy strategy in patients without recent coronary stents and without other indications for antithrombotic agents.

FUTURE TAVR DIRECTIONS

See the online chapter for discussion on future TAVR directions, including next-generation valve technology, expanded clinical indications, asymptomatic severe AS, moderate AS, and the modern era heart team.

REFERENCES

Background

1. Leon MB, Smith CR, Mack M, et al. Transcatheter aortic-valve implantation for aortic stenosis in patients who cannot undergo surgery. *N Engl J Med.* 2010;363:1597–1607.
2. Genereux P, Pibarot P, Redfors B, et al. Staging classification of aortic stenosis based on the extent of cardiac damage. *Eur Heart J.* 2017;38:3351–3358.
3. Roberts WC, Ko JM. Frequency by decades of unicuspid, bicuspid, and tricuspid aortic valves in adults having isolated aortic valve replacement for aortic stenosis, with or without associated aortic regurgitation. *Circulation.* 2005;111:920–925.
4. d'Arcy JL, Coffey S, Loudon MA, et al. Large-scale community echocardiographic screening reveals a major burden of undiagnosed valvular heart disease in older people: the OxVALVE Population Cohort Study. *Eur Heart J.* 2016;37:3515–3522.
5. Osnabrugge RL, Mylotte D, Head SJ, et al. Aortic stenosis in the elderly: disease prevalence and number of candidates for transcatheter aortic valve replacement: a meta-analysis and modeling study. *J Am Coll Cardiol.* 2013;62:1002–1012.
6. Baumgartner H, Falk V, Bax JJ, et al. 2017 ESC/EACTS Guidelines for the management of valvular heart disease. *Eur Heart J.* 2017;38:2739–2791.
7. Nishimura RA, Otto CM, Bonow RO, et al. 2017 AHA/ACC focused update of the 2014 AHA/ACC guideline for the management of patients with valvular heart disease: a report of the American College of Cardiology/American Heart Association Task Force on Clinical Practice Guidelines. *Circulation.* 2017;135:e1159–e1195.
8. Otto CM, Nishimura RA, Bonow RO, et al. 2020 ACC/AHA guideline for the management of patients with valvular heart disease: a report of the American College of Cardiology/American Heart Association Joint Committee on Clinical Practice Guidelines. *J Am Coll Cardiol.* 2020;77(4):e25–e197.
9. Bonow RO. Improving outlook for elderly patients with aortic stenosis. *J Am Med Assoc.* 2013;310:2045–2047.
10. Thourani VH, Suri RM, Gunter RL, et al. Contemporary real-world outcomes of surgical aortic valve replacement in 141,905 low-risk, intermediate-risk, and high-risk patients. *Ann Thorac Surg.* 2015;99:55–61.
11. Cribier A, Savin T, Saoudi N, et al. Percutaneous transluminal valvuloplasty of acquired aortic stenosis in elderly patients: an alternative to valve replacement? *Lancet.* 1986;1:63–67.
12. McKay RG. The Mansfield scientific aortic valvuloplasty registry: overview of acute hemodynamic results and procedural complications. *J Am Coll Cardiol.* 1991;17:485–491.
13. O'Neill W W. Predictors of long-term survival after percutaneous aortic valvuloplasty: report of the Mansfield scientific balloon aortic valvuloplasty registry. *J Am Coll Cardiol.* 1991;17:193–198.
14. Lieberman EB, Bashore TM, Hermiller JB, et al. Balloon aortic valvuloplasty in adults: failure of procedure to improve long-term survival. *J Am Coll Cardiol.* 1995;26:1522–1528.
15. Kapadia S, Stewart WJ, Anderson WN, et al. Outcomes of inoperable symptomatic aortic stenosis patients not undergoing aortic valve replacement: insight into the impact of balloon aortic valvuloplasty from the PARTNER trial (Placement of AoRTic TraNscathetER Valve trial). *JACC Cardiovasc Interv.* 2015;8:324–333.
16. Andersen HR, Knudsen LL, Hasenkam JM. Transluminal implantation of artificial heart valves. Description of a new expandable aortic valve and initial results with implantation by catheter technique in closed chest pigs. *Eur Heart J.* 1992;13:704–708.
17. Cribier A, Eltchaninoff H, Bash A, et al. Percutaneous transcatheter implantation of an aortic valve prosthesis for calcific aortic stenosis: first human case description. *Circulation.* 2002;106:3006–3008.
18. Cribier A, Eltchaninoff H, Tron C, et al. Treatment of calcific aortic stenosis with the percutaneous heart valve: mid-term follow-up from the initial feasibility studies: the French experience. *J Am Coll Cardiol.* 2006;47:1214–1223.
19. Kodali SK, O'Neill WW, Moses JW, et al. Early and late (one year) outcomes following transcatheter aortic valve implantation in patients with severe aortic stenosis (from the United States REVIVAL trial). *Am J Cardiol.* 2011;107:1058–1064.
20. Grube E, Laborde JC, Zickmann B, et al. First report on a human percutaneous transluminal implantation of a self-expanding valve prosthesis for interventional treatment of aortic valve stenosis. *Catheter Cardiovasc Interv.* 2005;66:465–469.

Evolution of TAVR

21. Grube E, Schuler G, Buellesfeld L, et al. Percutaneous aortic valve replacement for severe aortic stenosis in high-risk patients using the second- and current third-generation self-expanding CoreValve prosthesis: device success and 30-day clinical outcome. *J Am Coll Cardiol.* 2007;50:69–76.
22. Shahian DM, Jacobs JP, Badhwar V, et al. The society of thoracic surgeons 2018 adult cardiac surgery risk models: part 1-background, design considerations, and model development. *Ann Thorac Surg.* 2018;105:1411–1418.
23. Fried LP, Tangen CM, Walston J, et al. Frailty in older adults: evidence for a phenotype. *J Gerontol A Biol Sci Med Sci.* 2001;56:M146–M156.
24. Green P, Woglom AE, Genereux P, et al. The impact of frailty status on survival after transcatheter aortic valve replacement in older adults with severe aortic stenosis: a single-center experience. *JACC Cardiovasc Interv.* 2012;5:974–981.
25. Afilalo J, Lauck S, Kim DH, et al. Frailty in older adults undergoing aortic valve replacement: the FRAILTY-AVR study. *J Am Coll Cardiol.* 2017;70:689–700.
26. Nishimura RA, Otto CM, Bonow RO, et al. 2014 AHA/ACC guideline for the management of patients with valvular heart disease: a report of the American College of Cardiology/American Heart Association Task Force on Practice Guidelines. *J Am Coll Cardiol.* 2014;63:e57–e185.
27. Leon MB, Piazza N, Nikolsky E, et al. Standardized endpoint definitions for transcatheter aortic valve implantation clinical trials: a consensus report from the valve academic research consortium. *J Am Coll Cardiol.* 2011;57:253–269.
28. Kappetein AP, Head SJ, Genereux P, et al. Updated standardized endpoint definitions for transcatheter aortic valve implantation: the Valve Academic Research Consortium-2 consensus document. *J Am Coll Cardiol.* 2012;60:1438–1454.
29. Genereux P, Piazza N, Alu MC, et al. Valve Academic Research Consortium 3: updated endpoint definitions for aortic valve clinical research. *Eur Heart J.* 2020.
30. Kapadia SR, Leon MB, Makkar RR, et al. 5-year outcomes of transcatheter aortic valve replacement compared with standard treatment for patients with inoperable aortic stenosis (PARTNER 1): a randomised controlled trial. *Lancet.* 2015;385:2485–2491.
31. Popma JJ, Adams DH, Reardon MJ, et al. Transcatheter aortic valve replacement using a self-expanding bioprosthesis in patients with severe aortic stenosis at extreme risk for surgery. *J Am Coll Cardiol.* 2014;63:1972–1981.
32. Smith CR, Leon MB, Mack MJ, et al. Transcatheter versus surgical aortic-valve replacement in high-risk patients. *N Engl J Med.* 2011;364:2187–2198.
33. Adams DH, Popma JJ, Reardon MJ, et al. Transcatheter aortic-valve replacement with a self-expanding prosthesis. *N Engl J Med.* 2014;370:1790–1798.
34. Mack MJ, Leon MB, Smith CR, et al. 5-year outcomes of transcatheter aortic valve replacement or surgical aortic valve replacement for high surgical risk patients with aortic stenosis (PARTNER 1): a randomised controlled trial. *Lancet.* 2015;385:2477–2484.
35. Gleason TG, Reardon MJ, Popma JJ, et al. 5-Year outcomes of self-expanding transcatheter versus surgical aortic valve replacement in high-risk patients. *J Am Coll Cardiol.* 2018;72:2687–2696.

36. Leon MB, Smith CR, Mack MJ, et al. Transcatheter or surgical aortic-valve replacement in intermediate-risk patients. *N Engl J Med.* 2016;374:1609–1620.
37. Reardon MJ, Van Mieghem NM, Popma JJ, et al. Surgical or transcatheter aortic-valve replacement in intermediate-risk patients. *N Engl J Med.* 2017;376:1321–1331.
38. Makkar RR, Thourani VH, Mack MJ, et al. Five-year outcomes of transcatheter or surgical aortic-valve replacement. *N Engl J Med.* 2020;382:799–809.
39. Mack MJ, Leon MB, Thourani VH, et al. Transcatheter aortic-valve replacement with a balloon-expandable valve in low-risk patients. *N Engl J Med.* 2019;380:1695–1705.
40. Popma JJ, Deeb GM, Yakubov SJ, et al. Transcatheter aortic-valve replacement with a self-expanding valve in low-risk patients. *N Engl J Med.* 2019;380:1706–1715.
41. Reynolds MR, Magnuson EA, Wang K, et al. Health-related quality of life after transcatheter or surgical aortic valve replacement in high-risk patients with severe aortic stenosis: results from the PARTNER (Placement of AoRTic TraNscathetER Valve) Trial (Cohort A). *J Am Coll Cardiol.* 2012;60:548–5558.
42. Arnold SV, Reynolds MR, Wang K, et al. Health status after transcatheter or surgical aortic valve replacement in patients with severe aortic stenosis at increased surgical risk: results from the CoreValve US pivotal trial. *JACC Cardiovasc Interv.* 2015;8:1207–1217.
43. Baron SJ, Arnold SV, Wang K, et al. Health status benefits of transcatheter vs surgical aortic valve replacement in patients with severe aortic stenosis at intermediate surgical risk: results from the PARTNER 2 randomized clinical trial. *JAMA Cardiol.* 2017;2:837–845.
44. Baron SJ, Magnuson EA, Lu M, et al. Health status after transcatheter versus surgical aortic valve replacement in low-risk patients with aortic stenosis. *J Am Coll Cardiol.* 2019;74:2833–2842.
45. Carroll JD, Edwards FH, Marinac-Dabic D, et al. The STS-ACC transcatheter valve therapy national registry: a new partnership and infrastructure for the introduction and surveillance of medical devices and therapies. *J Am Coll Cardiol.* 2013;62:1026–1034.
46. Holmes Jr DR, Nishimura RA, Grover FL, et al. Annual outcomes with transcatheter valve therapy: from the STS/ACC TVT registry. *J Am Coll Cardiol.* 2015;66:2813–2823.
47. Vemulapalli S, Carroll JD, Mack MJ, et al. Procedural volume and outcomes for transcatheter aortic-valve replacement. *N Engl J Med.* 2019;380:2541–2550.
48. Carroll JD, Mack MJ, Vemulapalli S, et al. STS-ACC TVT registry of transcatheter aortic valve replacement. *J Am Coll Cardiol.* 2020;76:2492–2516.
49. Bonow RO, Brown AS, Gillam LD, et al. ACC/AATS/AHA/ASE/EACTS/HVS/SCA/SCAI/SCCT/SCMR/STS 2017 appropriate use criteria for the treatment of patients with severe aortic stenosis: a report of the American College of Cardiology Appropriate Use Criteria Task Force, American Association for Thoracic Surgery, American Heart Association, American Society of Echocardiography, European Association for Cardio-Thoracic Surgery, Heart Valve Society, Society of Cardiovascular Anesthesiologists, Society for Cardiovascular Angiography and Interventions, Society of Cardiovascular Computed Tomography, Society for Cardiovascular Magnetic Resonance, and Society of Thoracic Surgeons. *J Am Coll Cardiol.* 2017;70:2566–2598.
50. Feldman TE, Reardon MJ, Rajagopal V, et al. Effect of mechanically expanded vs self-expanding transcatheter aortic valve replacement on mortality and major adverse clinical events in high-risk patients with aortic stenosis: the REPRISE III randomized clinical trial. *J Am Med Assoc.* 2018;319:27–37.
51. Makkar RR, Cheng W, Waksman R, et al. Self-expanding intra-annular versus commercially available transcatheter heart valves in high and extreme risk patients with severe aortic stenosis (PORTICO IDE): a randomised, controlled, non-inferiority trial. *Lancet.* 2020;396:669–683.

Complications of TAVR

52. Genereux P, Webb JG, Svensson LG, et al. Vascular complications after transcatheter aortic valve replacement: insights from the PARTNER (Placement of AoRTic TraNscathetER Valve) trial. *J Am Coll Cardiol.* 2012;60:1043–1052.
53. Schaff HV. Transcatheter aortic-valve implantation-at what price? *N Engl J Med.* 2011;364:2256–2258.
54. Wood DA, Krajcer Z, Sathananthan J, et al. Pivotal clinical study to evaluate the safety and effectiveness of the MANTA percutaneous vascular closure device. *Circ Cardiovasc Interv.* 2019;12:e007258.
55. Lansky AJ, Messe SR, Brickman AM, et al. Proposed standardized neurological endpoints for cardiovascular clinical trials: an academic research consortium initiative. *J Am Coll Cardiol.* 2017;69:679–691.
56. Kapadia SR, Kodali S, Makkar R, et al. Protection against cerebral embolism during transcatheter aortic valve replacement. *J Am Coll Cardiol.* 2017;69:367–377.
57. Blanke P, Pibarot P, Hahn R, et al. Computed tomography-based oversizing degrees and incidence of paravalvular regurgitation of a new generation transcatheter heart valve. *JACC Cardiovasc Interv.* 2017;10:810–820.
58. Blanke P, Weir-McCall JR, Achenbach S, et al. Computed tomography imaging in the context of Transcatheter Aortic Valve Implantation (TAVI)/Transcatheter Aortic Valve Replacement (TAVR): an expert consensus document of the society of cardiovascular computed tomography. *JACC Cardiovasc Imaging.* 2019;12:1–24.
59. Douglas PS, Leon MB, Mack MJ, et al. Longitudinal hemodynamics of transcatheter and surgical aortic valves in the PARTNER trial. *JAMA Cardiol.* 2017;2:1197–1206.
60. Pibarot P, Salaun E, Dahou A, et al. Echocardiographic results of transcatheter versus surgical aortic valve replacement in low-risk patients: the PARTNER 3 trial. *Circulation.* 2020;141:1527–1537.
61. Babaliaros V, Devireddy C, Lerakis S, et al. Comparison of transfemoral transcatheter aortic valve replacement performed in the catheterization laboratory (minimalist approach) versus hybrid operating room (standard approach): outcomes and cost analysis. *JACC Cardiovasc Interv.* 2014;7:898–904.
62. Wood DA, Lauck SB, Cairns JA, et al. The Vancouver 3M (multidisciplinary, multimodality, but minimalist) clinical pathway facilitates safe next-day discharge home at low-, medium-, and high-volume transfemoral transcatheter aortic valve replacement centers: the 3M TAVR study. *JACC Cardiovasc Interv.* 2019;12:459–469.
63. Lederman RJ, Greenbaum AB, Rogers T, et al. Anatomic suitability for transcaval access based on computed tomography. *JACC Cardiovasc Interv.* 2017;10:1–10.
64. Palmerini T, Chakravarty T, Saia F, et al. Coronary protection to prevent coronary obstruction during TAVR: a multicenter international registry. *JACC Cardiovasc Interv.* 2020;13:739–747.
65. Kapadia SR, Huded CP, Kodali SK, et al. Stroke after surgical versus transfemoral transcatheter aortic valve replacement in the PARTNER trial. *J Am Coll Cardiol.* 2018;72:2415–2426.
66. Rodes-Cabau J, Ellenbogen KA, Krahn AD, et al. Management of conduction disturbances associated with transcatheter aortic valve replacement: JACC scientific expert panel. *J Am Coll Cardiol.* 2019;74:1086–1106.
67. Nazif TM, Chen S, George I, et al. New-onset left bundle branch block after transcatheter aortic valve replacement is associated with adverse long-term clinical outcomes in intermediate-risk patients: an analysis from the PARTNER II trial. *Eur Heart J.* 2019;40:2218–2227.
68. Kodali S, Pibarot P, Douglas PS, et al. Paravalvular regurgitation after transcatheter aortic valve replacement with the Edwards sapien valve in the PARTNER trial: characterizing patients and impact on outcomes. *Eur Heart J.* 2015;36:449–456.
69. Calvert PA, Northridge DB, Malik IS, et al. Percutaneous device closure of paravalvular leak: combined experience from the United Kingdom and Ireland. *Circulation.* 2016;134:934–944.
70. Herrmann HC, Daneshvar SA, Fonarow GC, et al. Prosthesis-patient mismatch in patients undergoing transcatheter aortic valve replacement: from the STS/ACC TVT registry. *J Am Coll Cardiol.* 2018;72:2701–2711.

75 Mitral Stenosis

Y.S. CHANDRASHEKHAR

Mitral stenosis (MS), known in the literature since at least the 1669 description by John Mayow and a major manifestation of rheumatic heart disease (RHD), remains an important problem worldwide. While the developed world has all but eliminated RHD, it continues to be a major cause of heart disease, morbidity, and mortality in the low and middle income countries (LMICs; 5.6 billion people or 80% of humanity) (see Chapter 81), especially affecting children and young adults in their most productive age.[1] It has, however, not disappeared entirely from the West—rheumatic MS (RMS) is occasionally seen in some under-resourced communities and among immigrants from areas with high prevalence of rheumatic fever; more importantly, nonrheumatic forms of MS are being increasingly seen—the degenerative MS (DMS) associated with mitral annular calcification (MAC), MS after radiation to the chest, and MS after surgical or percutaneous mitral valve interventions. Classic RMS can be prevented with good secondary prophylaxis for acute rheumatic fever (ARF) and can also be diagnosed as well as treated with relative ease. Nonrheumatic MS is more difficult to diagnose and may need specialized treatment options. It is, therefore, very important to recognize and understand multiple etiologic subsets of MS (eFig. 75.1) since they have very different natural history and strategies of prevention and treatment.

EPIDEMIOLOGY AND SECULAR TRENDS

Rheumatic Mitral Stenosis

There is, unfortunately, scarcity of good data on the prevalence of RHD and MS. A 2015 Global Burden of Disease modeling estimate puts the total prevalence of RHD at approximately 33.4 million cases (see Chapter 81),[1] and the mitral valve is involved most commonly in RHD. Subclinical disease, detectable by echocardiographic screening, is seven to eight times more common than clinically detectable disease[2] and would reveal an even larger prevalence of MS.

RMS is now largely concentrated among the LMICs that are endemic for group A Streptococcus (GAS) pharyngitis and ARF.[3] ARF-related carditis often occurs among children in the second decade and MS follows a couple of decades later. Classic RMS is more common in women, even though ARF is equally common in both sexes. Repeated episodes of untreated GAS pharyngeal infection accelerate its progression. The mechanism for valve damage is not clear but is thought to be autoimmune response to GAS moieties that mimic valve antigens and involves both humoral and cellular immune mechanisms.[4] There are some differences in how RMS behaves in endemic (South and East Asia, sub-Saharan Africa, and indigenous populations of Oceania) and nonendemic regions.[5] The former sees a more aggressive course: Patients are symptomatic at a younger age, often presenting in the second to fourth decade, approximately 75% of the patients don't recall an ARF episode, and the disease progresses more rapidly with higher mitral valve gradients that need earlier intervention.[3] Patients in the nonendemic regions seem to present with a more indolent course: They have slower progression and present much later (fifth to seventh decades), with suboptimal morphology for intervention, generally lower gradients and multiple other comorbidities (see Classic References, Shaw et al.).

Nonrheumatic Mitral Stenosis

DMS is most common in the Western world and is mainly MAC related,[6] although MS after mitral valve interventions[7] is increasingly seen in tertiary care centers (see eFig. 75.1). MAC-associated DMS has not been studied as extensively as RMS and its prevalence is not known, but it is thought to occur in about 1% to 2% of patients with MAC.[8] In a recent series, DMS due to MAC constituted 41% of patients with severe MS on echocardiography.[6] DMS is also being recognized increasingly (11% to 18%) in patients with aortic stenosis (AS) referred for transcatheter aortic valve replacement (TAVR). Other causes of MS are extremely rare and do not have good epidemiologic data.

DEFINITION OF DISEASE AND SEVERITY

Increased resistance at any level in the atrioventricular circuit (net AV resistance) can generate the MS physiology: obstruction to left atrial (LA) outflow and pressure gradient across the mitral valve, with consequent remodeling in the LA and pulmonary bed. Understanding this complexity is important since it may call for therapeutic approaches to DMS that differ from those applicable to patients with RMS.[9-11] The normal mitral valve area (MVA) is ≥4.0 cm². A gradient across the mitral valve starts to form with reduction in MVA to 2.0 cm², considered mild MS, and symptoms begin to appear, initially with exercise. Symptoms, more consistently develop at ≤1.5 cm² and are associated with a 5 to 10 mm Hg gradient. Significant hemodynamic changes (gradients in excess of 10 mm Hg) and resting symptoms are common at MVA ≤1.0 cm².[9] Guidelines consider "severe" MS based on when symptoms occur and where intervention can improve them, and ≤1.5 cm² is the recommended threshold for this.[9,10] However, some patients can develop significant symptoms with just moderate MS (MVA between 1.5 and 2.0 cm²) and can be selectively considered for intervention if other causes for their symptoms are excluded. Gradients depend on many hemodynamic variables including heart rate or flow and are not generally used to define severity. MAC-associated DMS currently uses the same definition as RMS, but the relation between MVA, gradients, and symptoms is much different than in RMS and might need an updated definition. MS due to a prosthetic valve is generally defined as resting mean valve gradient ≥5 mm Hg, peak mitral inflow velocity ≥1.9 msec, or effective orifice area ≤2 cm².

RHEUMATIC MITRAL STENOSIS

Pathology

Cardiac valve involvement in ARF starts with inflammation at the valve edges. It progresses to leaflet thickening and retraction along with variable degrees of calcification, all of which can lead to loss of flexibility. The main abnormality is fusion of the mitral leaflets in critical areas at their medial and lateral edges (commissural fusion), and the valve opening, narrowest at the valve tips, becomes a rigid structure that is oval or fish mouth shaped (Fig. 75.1; see also Fig. 16.32; see Videos 75.1, 75.2, and 75.3). The proximal and mid parts of the leaflets preserve some flexibility which results in the hockey stick appearance of the anterior leaflet in diastole. More severe disease extends into the subvalvular apparatus creating a dense mat of fused and shortened chordae that adds an additional level of resistance. Understanding pathology is crucial for clinical management.

Clinical Pathophysiology

The clinical consequences of MS depend on the degree of stenosis and consequent elevation in LA pressure (Fig. 75.2).[11] RMS is characterized by commissural fusion rather than just stiff valve leaflets and hence a relatively fixed orifice, and unlike AS, changes very little with varying hemodynamic conditions. An increased LA pressure is then needed to maintain left ventricular (LV) filling and preserve cardiac output.

Left Atrial Pressure

While MVA defines anatomic severity, it is the LA pressure that determines clinical symptoms[11] and improvement after definitive therapies like percutaneous balloon mitral valvuloplasty (BMV; see Fig. 78.1) or surgery.[11,12] LA pressure (measured indirectly as the gradient across the mitral valve), however, is highly variable (Fig. 75.3) depending on the time allowed for diastolic filling (heart rate) and flow (cardiac output). Tachycardia is one of the most important factors in increasing LA pressures since it significantly reduces diastolic filling time and compromises forward flow, which is immediately seen as high mitral valve gradients and worsening symptoms. Atrial contraction helps overcome the resistance at the mitral valve level and preserve forward

flow in MS—not surprisingly, the loss of atrial contraction and tachycardia during atrial fibrillation (AF) can precipitate clinical worsening even in patients previously asymptomatic. Since the gradient across the mitral valve increases as a square of the flow, small increases in the latter can have large effects on the gradient and its resulting symptoms, as seen in pregnancy, severe anemia, thyrotoxicosis, systemic infection, and other hyperdynamic states.

Chamber compliance (LA and to some extent, LV) also plays a role in development of symptoms, abnormal exercise hemodynamics, pulmonary hypertension (PAH), and degree of relief after relief of stenosis. A newly recognized subset termed low gradient MS (MVA <1.5 cm², mean gradient <10 mm Hg, and significant symptoms) is now being recognized in the developed world and may account for a significant proportion of patients coming to BMV in some centers. Some patients with these hemodynamic findings—constituting 11% of BMV patients in one series[12]—appear to have a physiology akin to heart failure with preserved ejection fraction superimposed on MS (see Chapter 51) and is characterized by older individuals with normal intrinsic LV contractility, decreased LV compliance, and high arterial afterload. They respond suboptimally to BMV, highlighting that reduced LV compliance may explain symptoms that do not respond to treatment of MS alone.[12]

Backward transmission of high LA pressures results in pulmonary venous hypertension and increased lung water; lung congestion explains exercise intolerance and dyspnea (and pulmonary edema in the most severe cases), and its relief, with diuretics or definitive MS treatment, is associated with immediate clinical benefit through reversing these changes. Signs of low cardiac output (due to severe flow restriction at the mitral valve and PAH) appear only at a much later stage.

Some compensatory mechanisms alter the relationship between LA pressure increase and symptoms. Chronically elevated LA pressure results in alveolar/interstitial thickening that limits alveolar edema, and increased lymphatic drainage helps redistribute alveolar fluid. This can improve symptoms for a short period before progressive MS overcomes these mechanisms. The development of PAH also ameliorates these symptoms but at the expense of right heart overload and possibly low cardiac output. Long-standing adverse changes in the lung and pulmonary vasculature can persist after relief of MS, explaining the lack of a direct relationship between hemodynamic improvement and changes in pulmonary function or exercise capacity. Prolonged elevation of LA pressure and LA remodeling can result in LA fibrosis that affects LA compliance. This may not be reversible after BMV, and low net AV compliance, which reflects the LA-LV as a unit, predicts both need for intervention and worse prognosis after BMV.

Left Atrial Function

The LA cannot empty readily in MS and remodels as a consequence of both increased pressure and volume. LA function is variably affected depending on severity of MS and degree of fibrosis and can be a form of atrial myopathy. LA volume is increased and LA emptying fraction is reduced. LA strain abnormalities are an early marker for LA dysfunction, can be seen in asymptomatic subjects with moderate MS, and are common in both RMS and DMS. Conduit strain is affected particularly in RMS and both reservoir strain (reflecting LA filling) and conduit strain (a marker for early diastolic emptying) are reduced, especially in patients with MAC. Abnormal peak atrial longitudinal strain (PALS) is associated with reduced

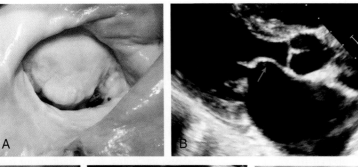
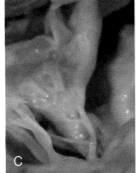
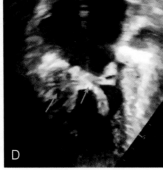
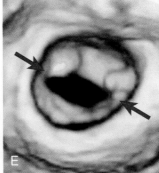

FIGURE 75.1 Pathology of mitral stenosis and imaging correlations. A, Fused commissures are the hallmark of rheumatic MS. Fusion starts along the valve tips and progresses to limit the opening from both ends. **B,** Some pliability of the rest of the leaflet causes a hockey stick appearance of the anterior leaflet on 2D echocardiography (*arrow*) (Video 75.1). **C,** Fibrosis and fusion extend to the sub-valvular apparatus resulting in matted and retracted chordae, which (**D**) can be seen on echocardiography (*arrows*) (see Video 75.2). **E,** Fusion of the commissures (*arrows*) creates a fish-mouth appearance as demonstrated on 3D echocardiography (see Video 75.3)

functional capacity, predicts future AF, and identifies adverse prognosis in asymptomatic subjects with moderate MS.

Left Ventricular Function

LV function is abnormal in some studies and is hypothesized to be due to multiple mechanisms (inflammatory process, tethering due to the rigid valve apparatus, altered LV compliance). However, it is not prominent in most patients with RMS but may be more prevalent in DMS due to coexisting comorbidities. LV deformation, a more sensitive parameter for LV function, however, is commonly abnormal in RMS and improves rapidly after BMV. Deformation parameters are normal when indexed to LV end-diastolic volume, suggesting this to be an effect of loading conditions rather than intrinsic myocardial dysfunction. Preliminary evidence suggests that impaired LV global longitudinal strain (GLS) might predict progression in milder forms of MS and outcomes after BMV over and above traditional measures. Post-BMV improvement in GLS is smaller in patients with suboptimal outcomes and often associated with an increase in LV end-diastolic pressure (LVEDP) after BMV, suggesting some degree of intrinsic diastolic dysfunction. Nevertheless, there is no immediately actionable clinical correlate for this subtle degree of LV dysfunction. LV diastolic dysfunction is difficult to diagnose in patients with MS and most indices including those with speckle tracking cannot accurately detect elevated LVEDP, an important marker of poor outcomes after BMV.

Right Ventricular Function

Overt RV dysfunction occurs late in the course of MS and is often a consequence of PAH. RV enlargement and elevated PA pressures track the severity of MS. These findings convey adverse prognosis even in patients treated with BMV or surgery. RV strain is emerging as a useful marker for subtle RV dysfunction even before onset of other signs, and it improves rapidly after BMV. Whether deformation imaging can be used to fine tune timing of intervention is not known at present.

Natural History

The stages of RMS as defined in the 2020 ACC/AHA guidelines for the management of patients with valvular heart disease[9] are shown in Table 75.1. Unlike rheumatic mitral regurgitation (MR) that starts proximate to the ARF episode, MS is a late presentation, is unlikely to regress, and progresses in severity in the majority of patients. Data on the natural history of untreated MS are very old[11] and have little relevance for patients seen today. In addition, the natural history of MS has diverged between LMICs (RMS) and the developed world (very little RMS and increasing DMS). A few things to take away from these studies include the following:

1. Valve area in RMS decreases approximately 0.09 cm^2 per year. Age, hemodynamic severity at diagnosis, and degree of valve deformity seem to predict progression. About a third show higher rate of progression, but this is not easily predictable from traditional clinical variables. Recurrent episodes of ARF mediate faster progression in LMICs but this evolution can occur even without repeated episodes suggesting some role for other factors like hemodynamic damage and scarring.
2. Symptoms are an important trigger for definitive therapy and have strong prognostic value. It takes approximately one to two decades to develop significant MS. About half of the

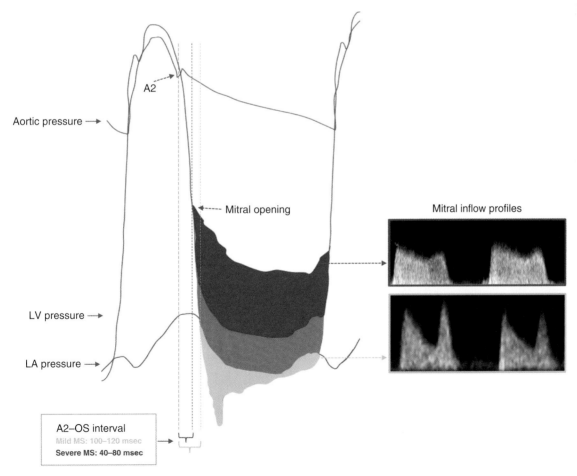

FIGURE 75.2 Hemodynamics of mitral stenosis. Severity of MS determines the magnitude of the diastolic pressure gradient between left atrium (LA) and left ventricle (LV). As MS progress from mild (*green*) to moderate (*blue*) to severe (*red*), the increasing pressure gradient causes the opening snap (OS) to occur earlier, thus shortening the time interval between aortic valve closure (A2) and OS. The corresponding Doppler inflow profiles show longer deceleration time and reduction in atrial augmentation as LA pressure increases.

asymptomatic patients with MS then develop symptoms over the next decade and most are symptomatic in two decades after onset of MS.

3. Symptomatic patients with severe MS do poorly without intervention, with a mortality that varies from 8% to 13% per year in the first 5 years. Severe symptoms denote worse prognosis—untreated, only 15% of patients in New York Heart Association (NYHA) functional Class IV and 60% in NYHA Class III survived for 5 years. Treating severe symptomatic MS with surgery in the pre-BMV era improved this otherwise dismal natural history.

4. Patients can first present with AF; almost 20% presented with an embolic episode in the past but early detection of AF in MS and aggressive use of oral anticoagulants (OACs) has markedly reduced this complication.

5. Latent RHD, diagnosed through screening echocardiography, identifies patients at risk for progression, especially without prophylaxis (see Chapter 81). Approximately 15% to 20% will progress especially if they have clear structural heart disease.

Diagnosis
Clinical Presentation

Clinical features of RMS, to some extent, depend on where patients live. There is no better description of signs and symptoms of classic MS than in the famous writings of Paul Wood (see Classic References, Wood) but that now apply mainly to subjects in locations with high endemic burden of ARF and suboptimal care. These patients are younger, have higher gradients, have lower MVA, and have low prevalence of AF and thus present with more typical signs and symptoms of MS. Patients from higher income countries[11-14] are often likely to be older, hypertensive, overweight and in AF; they can have comorbidities that can obscure the classic signs and symptoms of MS and present with lower gradients.

Dyspnea, initially on exertion and then at rest, is the usual presentation in MS. Paroxysmal nocturnal dyspnea and orthopnea are seen in severe symptomatic MS but may become less common with longer duration of untreated illness, as compensatory mechanisms in the lung and pulmonary circulation attenuate alveolar edema. Transition to the symptomatic phase is often precipitated by tachycardia or conditions generating increased flow across the valve—AF and pregnancy commonly bring asymptomatic patients to attention in LMICs. Clinical presentation is influenced by age, other comorbidities (like diastolic dysfunction), and presence of PAH. Onset of significant PAH, or aggressive use of diuretics and beta blockers, may reduce dyspnea but increase fatigue and symptoms of low cardiac output. Traditionally, a rise in LA pressure during exercise was thought to mediate exercise intolerance, but the correlation between MVA, gradient, and exercise capacity is imperfect. Newer data[15] suggest that exercise intolerance is mainly due to a combination of abnormalities comparable to those in patients with

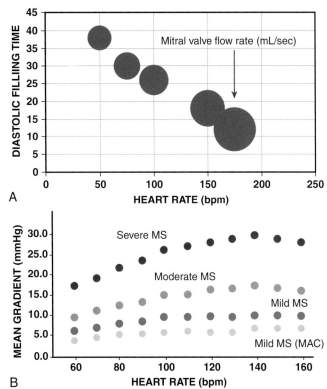

FIGURE 75.3 Relation between heart rate, diastolic filling time, and pressure gradient in mitral stenosis. **A,** Increasing heart rate causes sequential reduction in diastolic filling period. **B,** The reduced diastolic filling time at increasing heart rates is associated with exacerbation of the mitral pressure gradient, which is most marked with severe MS. Thus, higher heart rates are likely to precipitate symptoms.

TABLE 75.1 Stages of Mitral Stenosis (MS)

STAGE	DEFINITION	VALVE ANATOMY	VALVE HEMODYNAMICS*	HEMODYNAMIC CONSEQUENCES	SYMPTOMS
A	At risk for MS	Mild valve doming during diastole	Normal transmitral flow velocity	None	None
B	Progressive MS	Rheumatic valve changes with commissural fusion and diastolic doming of mitral valve leaflets Planimetered MVA >1.5 cm²	Increased transmitral flow velocities MVA >1.5 cm² Diastolic pressure half-time <150 msec	Mild to moderate LA enlargement Normal pulmonary pressure at rest	None
C	Asymptomatic severe MS	Rheumatic valve changes with commissural fusion and diastolic doming of mitral valve leaflets Planimetered MVA ≤1.5 cm²	MVA ≤1.5 cm² Diastolic pressure half-time ≥150 msec	Severe LA enlargement Elevated PASP >50 mm Hg	None
D	Symptomatic severe MS	Rheumatic valve changes with commissural fusion and diastolic doming of mitral valve leaflets Planimetered MVA ≤1.5 cm²	MVA ≤1.5 cm² Diastolic pressure half-time ≥150 msec	Severe LA enlargement Elevated PASP >50 mm Hg	Decreased exercise tolerance Exertional dyspnea

*The transmitral mean pressure gradient should be obtained to determine the full hemodynamic effect of the MS and usually is greater than 5 to 10 mm Hg in severe MS; however, because of the variability of the mean pressure gradient with heart rate and forward flow, it has not been included in the criteria for severity.
LA, Left atrial; MVA, mitral valve area; PASP, pulmonary artery systolic pressure.
From Otto CM, et al. 2020 AHA/ACC guideline for the management of patients with valvular heart disease: a report of the American College of Cardiology/American Heart Association Task Force on Practice Guidelines. J Am Coll Cardiol 2021;77:e25-197.

heart failure (chronotropic incompetence, abnormal stroke volume reserve, impaired ventilation, and low peak A–VO$_2$ difference). Palpitations, often a consequence of AF, are seen in the later stages of the disease and increase with age. Pulmonary edema is now seen rarely, except in LMICs, especially in pregnant patients with previously undetected disease. Severe PAH can result in angina or symptoms of right heart failure. The dilated LA (Ortner syndrome—hoarseness due to compression of the recurrent laryngeal nerve) or pulmonary artery can cause pressure effects. Stroke (especially in undetected AF) and hemoptysis (from pulmonary venous hypertension or ruptured bronchial veins) were not uncommon symptoms in the past but are now seen infrequently.

Physical Examination

Bedside physical signs of RMS can be divided into those arising from the pathologic mitral valve itself and those that are consequences of severe MS. The former includes a loud S$_1$ (and a tapping apex), the opening snap (OS), and mid-diastolic murmur with presystolic accentuation. The latter include the usual signs of AF, pulmonary venous and arterial hypertension, tricuspid regurgitation (TR), right heart failure, and, in late stages, systemic hypoperfusion.

The S$_1$ is often loud with a pliable mitral valve, but significant leaflet restriction (with fibrosis, calcification or subvalvular pathology) can decrease its intensity. The OS is a classic feature of RMS and arises at the peak of a rapid and forced opening of the restricted mitral leaflet by high LA pressure. It denotes two important things: (1) its presence along with a loud S$_1$ implies a pliable mitral valve that is likely to be a good candidate for BMV; (2) its timing helps in assessing severity of MS (see Fig. 75.2)—a higher LA pressure opens the mitral valve earlier, and, therefore, time between aortic closure sound and mitral OS (A2-OS interval) is inversely proportional to the severity of MS. As with a loud S$_1$, increasing calcification and rigidity of the body of the leaflets diminishes OS and might indicate unfavorable anatomy for percutaneous intervention.

The murmur in MS is difficult to hear and needs practice and a quiet room for best detection; tachycardia with mild exercise can bring out the findings. It is a low pitched diastolic rumble, best heard at the apex with the bell of the stethoscope while the patient is in the left lateral position. Its onset follows the OS, but may be heard just during presystolic accentuation in mild MS and gradually increases in length with increasing severity of stenosis. A presystolic accentuation (coinciding with atrial contraction) is prominent unless the patient is in AF. The RMS murmur is less discernable in patients with obesity, chronic obstructive pulmonary disease (COPD), or AF with a rapid ventricular response. The length of the murmur correlates with severity of MS but the intensity does not. Severe MS can occasionally have a thrill. S$_3$ (which occurs later in diastole, is softer and not generally confused with OS) and S$_4$ are not usually audible and their presence excludes severe MS. MR murmurs are not common in severe MS although a TR murmur (in the left lower sternal area that increases in inspiration) might be prominent in patients with significant PAH and RV enlargement. Some murmurs may mimic MS—those from high flow across the mitral valve (severe MR, some shunts like ventricular septal defect, or patent ductus arteriosus with high Qp/Qs or other high flow conditions) can be differentiated from MS by their clinical context, short murmurs, lack of an OS, and often the presence of an S$_3$. The Austin Flint murmur of aortic regurgitation (AR) usually does not have a loud S$_1$, OS, or presystolic accentuation and there are clear signs of significant AR (see Chapter 73). Tricuspid stenosis can accompany MS and has a diastolic murmur that increases with inspiration. Physical examination also helps to address two pertinent clinical questions at the bedside: how severe is the MS and how suitable is the valve for BMV. A short A2-OS interval followed by a long murmur starting earlier in diastole with prominent presystolic accentuation and signs of PAH or RV overload in a patient with limiting symptoms suggests severe MS. Loud S$_1$ and prominent OS indicates a pliable valve that could be suitable for BMV.

Echocardiography

Echocardiography is the mainstay of diagnosis in all forms of MS[11] (see Chapter 16)—it is the best modality to detect the presence and severity of LA outflow obstruction and evaluate its severity as well as hemodynamic consequences (Fig. 75.4; see also Fig. 16.34; see also Videos 75.4 and 75.5). It identifies the etiology of MS and is crucial for determining suitability of various interventions. Finally, it allows evaluation of other valve and myocardial disease that might affect the course of MS.

Each etiology has characteristic echo signatures but questions about severity of obstruction (MVA and gradients) are common to all conditions. MVA is best assessed with planimetry in all patients with RMS since it is the most accurate method if done correctly (tracing the inner edge at valve tips in mid-diastole of a completely seen, enface orifice of good image quality) and less subject to effect of changing loading conditions. However, two-dimensional (2D) echo may underestimate severity and is less optimal for understanding anatomy (e.g., commissural morphology pre and postintervention); 3D overcomes many of these limitations, is more reproducible, and should be used where possible (see Fig. 16.33).[16] Planimetry is not a good option for MVA in DMS and the continuity equation may work better. Pressure half time is useful to assess valve area in RMS but is not accurate in valves with prior intervention or in DMS since it is influenced by chamber compliance and multiple other factors. The proximal isovelocity surface area (PISA) method and continuity equation (see Fig. 16.35) can provide good measurements but are more complex and the latter is not useful if there is either AR or MR. MS following previous intervention like BMV poses special issues, and planimetry, especially with 3D, is the best option.

Gradients measured from Doppler tracings are reasonably accurate in reflecting the hemodynamic conditions at that given moment and are suitable for all kinds of MS, including DMS. It is important to recognize that gradients are heart rate and flow dependent and thus

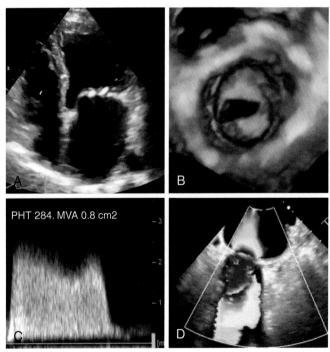

PHT 284. MVA 0.8 cm2

FIGURE 75.4 Echocardiography for diagnosing MS. 2D and 3D echocardiography is the best method to define morphology, assess severity (valve area and gradients), complications like left atrial thrombus and other valve pathology. **A,** Thickened mitral valve leaflets and large left atrium identified on four-chamber 2D echo view (see Video 75.4). **B,** Commissural fusion and fish mouth deformity seen on 3D echo (see Video 75.5). **C,** High inflow velocities, longer pressure half time, persisting gradient during diastasis and reduction in atrial contribution are characteristics of severe MS, **D,** Transesophageal echo showing clear flow convergence (PISA shell) with higher velocities.

could change appreciably between studies. All echo measurements should be interpreted in the correct clinical context, and discrepancies between MVA, gradients, and symptoms should be adjudicated thoughtfully by appropriately synthesizing multiple parameters. Transesophageal echocardiography (TEE), both 2D and 3D (see Chapter 16), provides greater details of valve anatomy and is very useful for excluding LA clot, although computed tomography (CT) can substitute for this. TEE is often used during BMV to guide the procedure as well as assess immediate results and complications.

An important role of echocardiography is to assess suitability for intervention, and at least four scoring systems for RMS are in use. Scoring systems have limitations including semiquantitative assessment and suboptimal reproducibility, and they do not reflect the contribution of each individual component of adverse outcome with equal accuracy. No single scoring method is preferable over another,[16] and ultimately, most centers use scores with which they are comfortable. The most often used score is the Wilkins score that combines leaflet mobility and calcification along with leaflet and subvalvular thickening into a numerical score (see Table 16.9 and Classic References, Wilkins et al.). It has good predictive accuracy for both short- and long-term outcome (see Fig. 78.2) but misses the effect of commissural calcification and the degree of preexisting MR and is not very effective in prognosticating the midrange of scores. Patients with suboptimal scores are not automatically destined for bad outcomes, and many centers successfully perform BMV in moderately suboptimal scores. Leaflet and commissural calcification and subvalvular pathology might have a disproportionate effect on outcomes and permit better triage of patients even with optimal Wilkins scores. A newer score, incorporating leaflet displacement and asymmetry in commissural remodeling,[17] was found to be better at predicting procedural outcome than Wilkins scores, and another one using 3D might be capable of identifying structural abnormalities better.

Additional Diagnostic Investigations
EKG and Chest X-Ray
Both EKG and chest x-ray can show consequences of MS in the form of LA enlargement (P mitrale) and RV pressure overload. In the later stages, the EKG can show AF and x-ray can show the presence and degree of pulmonary congestion.

Exercise Testing in MS
Exercise testing can be performed safely in most patients with MS and plays an important role in evaluating patients with severe MS who are asymptomatic or have equivocal symptoms and those who are symptomatic with moderate MS.[9,10] Stress echo can document exercise limitation and resolve discordance between symptoms and clinical or echocardiographic severity, and finding exercise-induced PAH can indicate need for BMV (see Chapter 16). In asymptomatic patients, exercise testing can also predict prognosis in multiple forms of MS including RMS, DMS, and prosthetic valve MS.[7] Dobutamine stress has been used in the past but is not currently a good option in most patients.

Other Diagnostic Tests
CT or cardiac magnetic resonance can provide information about valve anatomy and function but are rarely needed and are used when there is some other indication for them. Cardiac catheterization is rarely needed unless there are other specific clinical questions that it can best answer (e.g., coronary artery disease).

Associated Conditions
Atrial Fibrillation
AF is a dreaded complication of MS—it is common, increases with age and severity of MS, worsens hemodynamic as well as clinical status, is an important determinant of the high risk of stroke, and can limit survival in patients with RMS.[5,11,18] AF seems to be driven by both LA stretch and possibly inflammation, which together can cause structural and electrical remodeling (see Chapter 66). LA size

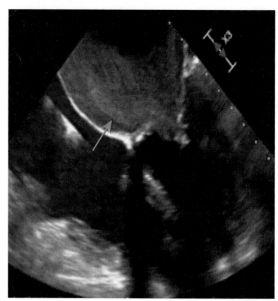

FIGURE 75.5 Severe MS promotes left atrial stasis. Blood stasis (*arrow*) promotes left atrial thrombosis and predisposes to embolic stroke (see Video 75.6).

and hemodynamic abnormalities relate to its occurrence and persistence. LA fibrosis is common, and subtle changes in LA function in the form of reduced PALS might precede onset of AF. AF worsens symptoms through a loss of atrial contribution to LV filling and cardiac output as well as the effect of fast heart rates. It facilitates stroke risk by further promoting stasis (Fig. 75.5; see also Video 75.6). Age has a strong influence on its occurrence. AF is uncommon (<5%) in young patients with RMS coming for BMV in the LMICs but is very prevalent (>60%) in the aging MS population in the West. The incidence of new AF in RMS is unclear but almost 20% developed AF over a median of 6-year follow-up in a recent study[19]; the average annual event rate was 3.5 % per year and increased to 6.0 % per year with even mildly increased LA size and pressure, with a correspondingly high event rate (embolism and death). Larger LA dimension and MVA of 1.5 cm^2 or less were good predictors for new-onset AF. The combination of MS and AF poses considerable risk for embolic events; patients with MS and AF are many times more likely to have embolic complications than MS without AF or AF without MS, and risk may be as high as patients with prosthetic valves—consequently, OACs (warfarin and not direct acting OACs) are strongly recommended in such patients irrespective of lesion severity or CHADS$_2$VASc scores.[9,10] Threshold to use OACs is lower than in other forms of valvular heart disease since AF can be intermittent, and even transient episodes (<30 sec) detected on ambulatory monitoring significantly increase risk of thromboembolic events. Moreover, patients with MS have been occasionally shown to have evidence of LA thrombus or may experience embolic events even when in sinus rhythm. The European guidelines even recommend considering OACs in patients with RMS in sinus rhythm if they have dense spontaneous LA echocardiographic contrast (see Fig. 75.5) and/or LA dilation.[10] Rate control is difficult to achieve in RMS but strategies are similar to those in the other patients with AF. Ivabradine has been used with some success. Restoring sinus rhythm is more likely in the presence of a small LA, short duration of AF, and less severe MS. Rhythm control improves quality of life and exercise tolerance, especially in those with small LA and durable results. Unless needed urgently, electrical cardioversion is best done after BMV. AF with MS has a high recurrence after cardioversion and antiarrhythmic drugs, especially amiodarone, are often needed for maintaining sinus rhythm. Pulmonary vein isolation is not as well studied in patients with RMS as in those with AF without MS, but there is some evidence of efficacy in these patients. Restoring sinus rhythm with a surgical maze procedure increases chances of remaining in sinus rhythm and reduces risk of embolism. AF does not appreciably affect success of BMV but adversely influences long-term event-free survival. AF is not consistently prevented with BMV, supporting efforts to reduce its occurrence in the first place; however, BMV in patients with AF is associated with less systemic embolism. Nonetheless, patients continue to have significant residual risk (approximately 20% embolic event rate in the next 5 years) and need adequate anticoagulation.

Pulmonary Hypertension

PAH is quite common in patients with symptomatic RMS, but prevalence depends on age, as well as duration and severity of MS. Some degree of PAH is seen in almost 80% of patients coming to BMV in various series and one-third have systolic PA pressure (PAP) greater than 50 mm Hg. The prevalence may be even higher for PAH during exercise or if the newest PAH definition is used (see Chapter 88). While primarily dependent on the severity of MS, mitral gradients correlate imperfectly with PAP, and net AV compliance might better reflect its genesis. PAH often is post capillary (mean PAP ≥25 mm Hg, mean pulmonary artery wedge pressure (PAWP) >15 mm Hg, low transpulmonary gradient, pulmonary vascular resistance (PVR) ≤3 WU) and is a consequence of pulmonary venous hypertension. However, chronically elevated PAP, especially in some hyperresponders, can mediate structural remodeling in the pulmonary arterial system, resulting in a combination of pre and postcapillary hypertension (mean PAP ≥25 mm Hg, mean PAWP >15 mm Hg, PVR >3 WU). Remodeling in PAH is mediated by mechanical stretch as well as inflammatory cytokine and growth factors and affects both arterioles and venules. PAH mediates RV dysfunction and TR, but the correlation with RV failure is not linear. PAH adversely affects long-term prognosis, even in patients treated with BMV or surgical mitral valve repair or replacement. However, patients with severe PAH have good immediate results with BMV in that PAH resolves in most patients quite rapidly and continues to improve further in the next few months unless there is suboptimal relief of MS, worsening MR, or valve restenosis. PAH may persist in a small proportion of patients despite optimal BMV results, and this might depend on whether the remodeling was reversible (mainly involving venules with vessel edema, or loose fibrosis) or irreversible (severe arteriolar hyperplasia and plexiform lesions), but these factors are difficult to identify a priori. Given its adverse influence, PAH is a class IIa trigger for therapeutic intervention in asymptomatic patients with PA systolic pressure >50 mm Hg in the both the U.S. and European guidelines.[9,10] While some drugs can influence PAH temporarily, relief of MS is the only proven treatment.

Pregnancy

Worldwide, MS is one of the most common valve conditions in pregnant women with structural heart disease.[20,21] In the European Registry of Pregnancy and Cardiac Disease (ROPAC), 10% of cases were MS, and MS was first detected during pregnancy in 25%.[20] This problem is magnified in those living in the world's poorest countries such as sub-Saharan Africa and the indigenous people of Oceania. Pregnancy poses a special burden in patients with MS given the unfavorable confluence of tachycardia and increased cardiac output. Cardiac output peaks in the second trimester (see Chapter 92), and patients with MS are often first detected at this time or present with worsening symptoms around 24 to 30 weeks of gestation. Delivery is the other dangerous time period; a third of pregnant patients developing heart failure due to MS become symptomatic around the time of delivery and in the first week postpartum, often in the first 72 hours, due to high LA pressures caused by increased venous return following relief of inferior vena cava (IVC) compression and autotransfusion of blood from the utero-placental circuit after delivery. Pregnant patients with mild MS usually tolerate the stress of pregnancy but need careful attention since 16% to 24% of patients can develop symptomatic heart failure.[20] Complications occur mainly in patients with symptomatic (NYHA II or greater) moderate to severe MS, of whom almost 40% to 50% require hospitalization, mainly for heart failure, compared to a quarter in those with asymptomatic moderate MS. Moderate or severe MS should, therefore, be detected and corrected if possible before pregnancy, as patients have four times fewer adverse events if intervention is

undertaken prior to conception.[20] The modified WHO risk stratification algorithm appropriately classifies untreated severe MS as a Class IV risk (pregnancy is contraindicated)

Diagnosis and Treatment

Diagnosis of MS remains largely the same as in the nonpregnant patient but with some nuances. Physiologic changes of pregnancy (peripheral vasodilation, hyperdynamic circulation, increased blood volume, tachycardia, anemia, elevated diaphragm, compression of IVC) can cause dyspnea, leg edema, loud S_1, and mitral murmurs (see Chapter 92)—these can mimic RMS but normal pregnancy is not accompanied by prominent diastolic murmurs or an OS; echocardiography remains diagnostic even though the gradient might be affected by hemodynamic conditions. Pressure half time is not as validated in this population and planimetry remains the reference standard as in the nonpregnant patient. There are few good prospective data but systematic reviews suggest that severe MS during pregnancy is adverse for both the mother and the child. Age, significant PAH, heart failure, and reduced ejection fraction are factors associated with poor maternal and fetal outcome. Maternal mortality is increased (3% range with severe MS and 0% to 2% with moderate MS), and is especially worse with PAH and in resource poor countries. There is an excess of stillbirth and neonatal death (2% to 4%) as well as preterm birth (up to 20%), related to compromised uteroplacental flow. Much of the morbidity can be minimized with adequate prepregnancy evaluation/counseling and early access to better care. Activity is allowed as tolerated but those with severe PAH might need some restriction.[21] Management of tachycardia and diuresis for dyspnea are the foundation of conservative treatment. AF is not uncommon in pregnant patients with severe MS (16%) and can precipitate symptoms, pulmonary edema, and rarely a cerebral vascular accident.[20] Drugs used to control rate, rhythm, and thrombotic risk have unique effects on the fetus. Beta blockers can cause fetal bradycardia, hypoglycemia, and a mild increase in premature births, but no major congenital abnormalities have been conclusively identified. Intrauterine growth restriction has been described especially for atenolol used in the second trimester. Calcium channel blockers can be used for rate control (FDA Category D) but amiodarone is contraindicated. Diuretics can affect uteroplacental perfusion and amniotic volume but have been used with few major adverse effects. Direct current cardioversion can be performed, if needed urgently. Anticoagulation needs thoughtful planning and use per guidelines.[9,22]

A significant portion of the excess mortality associated with severe MS occurs during delivery. Careful planning and proper medical supervision, however, results in good outcomes in the majority of patients. Vaginal delivery is the best option for patients with mild MS and mild symptoms (NYHA I-II) and asymptomatic moderate MS. Caesarean delivery is indicated in those with severe symptoms (NYHA III-IV) or moderate symptoms with significant PAH, and when BMV could not be undertaken previously.[10]

Percutaneous Balloon Mitral Valvuloplasty

BMV is safe and very effective for treating severe MS during pregnancy. Success rates are very high with minimal mortality (except in patients with florid heart failure), fluoroscopy times are under 10 minutes, and gradients fall immediately with excellent symptomatic improvement. Fetal development and growth and development of the child are unaffected. These results are far superior to those obtained with surgical intervention in pregnant patients. Not surprisingly, BMV is the treatment of choice for managing such patients but the success depends on the time of intervention. BMV before 20 weeks of gestation has poorer fetal outcomes and should be delayed as much as reasonable, optimally to after 24 weeks. Standard criteria for intrapregnancy BMV for MS include severe MS, NYHA Class III or IV symptoms while on optimal medical treatment, and suitable valve anatomy. Contraindications remain the same as in nonpregnant patients. Mitral valve surgery is used in refractory NYHA Class IV heart failure if BMV is not possible but has a high risk (9% of mothers and almost one-third of babies do not survive the procedure) and needs careful thought before proceeding.

Treatment

Patients with RMS should, whenever possible, be treated according to the current ACC/AHA and European guidelines.[9,10]

Medical Therapy

Severe symptomatic RMS is clearly a mechanical obstruction that needs structural intervention (either BMV or surgery). Medical therapy does not change the progression of the disease but can be a reasonable temporary measure before definitive therapy and is also useful in some mildly symptomatic patients who are not yet candidates for definitive therapy or as a palliative measure in those not suitable for any intervention. It mainly involves rate control, management of secondary conditions that could worsen MS (including AF, anemia, thyrotoxicosis, or infection), and judicious diuresis in patients who still continue to have exercise intolerance. At the same time, secondary prophylaxis for ARF and OACs to prevent embolic events should be meticulously offered per guideline recommendations. Patients with RMS with any incidence of AF and those in sinus rhythm with history of prior thromboembolism or LA thrombus should receive OACs. It is reasonable to consider OACs in patients with severely dilated LA or those with severe spontaneous contrast in the LA per European guidelines (no U.S. recommendation). Direct-acting OACs are not recommended. Rate control with any suitable drug is indicated in patients with AF and a rapid ventricular response and may help in patients in sinus rhythm who develop significant symptoms during exercise. Beta blockers decrease heart rates, thus creating longer diastolic filling time and reduced gradients but have not been consistently shown to improve exercise capacity.[15] Ivabradine might better control tachycardia during exercise than beta blockers. Digoxin is helpful only in patients with AF.

Transcatheter Interventional Therapy

Indications for intervention in RMS in the 2020 ACC/AHA guidelines are shown in Table 75.2 and Fig. 75.6. BMV and surgery (mostly open valve repair and rarely valve replacement) are effective but have particular indications. BMV is a very efficacious as well as cost effective treatment and is the preferred modality in most patients with valve area <1.5 cm² and suitable anatomy (see Chapter 78). It might be considered in those with valve area >1.5 cm² if symptoms can be clearly attributed to MS, especially if they develop high PAP. BMV might also be considered rather than offering surgery in patients with somewhat unfavorable anatomy, particularly those at high surgical risk, if performed at a comprehensive valve center.[9] Asymptomatic patients are not currently recommended intervention unless they have severe PAH (>50 mm Hg) or new-onset AF and have favorable anatomy. Additional factors that might be considered in asymptomatic patients include those with very high thromboembolic risk, are considering pregnancy, or scheduled to undergo major noncardiac surgery. Some preliminary observational studies support earlier performance of BMV in asymptomatic subjects with moderate stenosis and good valve morphology but there are no randomized trials to support this. Surgery is offered only in patients when BMV cannot be done safely due to adverse valve morphology or major contraindication, when the patient is having cardiac surgery for other reasons, or when the patient needs treatment for MS but there are other concomitant conditions that require surgical therapy like moderate to severe MR or TR, AS, or coronary artery disease (CAD).

The ideal patient is one with good valve morphology scores, MR <grade II, and few comorbidities. An LA thrombus is a contraindication for the procedure even though some experienced centers have safely performed BMV after 2 to 3 months of OAC. BMV has high success rates in patients with favorable morphology (>90%). Predictors of procedural success include extent of valve thickening, mobility and subvalvular involvement, uneven leaflet thickening, commissural asymmetry, and calcification (Fig. 75.7; see also Videos 75.2 and 75.7). Although none of the scores based on echocardiography are very good at predicting outcomes, a Wilkins score <8 in general predicts good outcomes (see Fig. 78.2), while those with a score >11 are best treated with surgery.[9] Patients with intermediate scores (between 9 and 11) can still have reasonable results and should be considered for BMV in experienced centers. The more recently designed scores[17,23,24] seemed to reclassify risk and predict long-term outcomes more robustly. The use of 3D echo is likely to improve triage to BMV.[16]

An MVA ≥1.5 cm² and MR ≤2/4 (without in-hospital major adverse cardiac and cerebrovascular events) are considered to be a good result after BMV.[23] Increase in MVA and reduction in gradient and PAP are durable over the long term in the majority of patients. The results are more durable in patients with favorable anatomy before BMV.[23] A post-procedure area of >1.8 cm² seems to predict good long-term outcomes. There has been a trend toward offering BMV in a larger pool of patients, especially in higher income countries.[13] Over the years, patients coming to BMV are older, have more AF and PAH, have a higher NYHA functional class, and have more suboptimal valve morphology (valvular and subvalvular calcification, MR and previous intervention).[14] As a result, while almost 90% of the patients in Western series had a good outcome after BMV in the past, more recent data show a success rate

---

TABLE 75.2 Recommendations for Intervention for Rheumatic Mitral Stenosis

COR	LOE	RECOMMENDATIONS
1	A	1. In symptomatic patients (NYHA Class II, III, or IV) with severe rheumatic MS (mitral valve area ≤1.5 cm², Stage D) and favorable valve morphology with less than moderate (2+) MR* in the absence of LA thrombus. PMBC is recommended if it can be performed at a comprehensive valve center.
1	B-NR	2. In severely symptomatic patients (NYHA Class III or IV) with severe rheumatic MS (mitral valve area ≤1.5 cm², Stage D) who (1) are not candidates for PMBC, (2) have failed a previous PMBC, (3) require other cardiac procedures, or (4) do not have access to PMBC, mitral valve surgery (repair, commissurotomy, or valve replacement) is indicated.
2a	B-NR	3. In asymptomatic patients with severe rheumatic MS (mitral valve area ≤1.5 cm², Stage C) and favorable valve morphology with less than 2 + MR in the absence of LA thrombus who have elevated pulmonary pressures (pulmonary artery systolic pressure >50 mm Hg), PMBC is reasonable if it can be performed at a comprehensive valve center.
2b	C-LD	4. In asymptomatic patients with severe rheumatic MS (mitral valve area ≤1.5 cm², Stage C) and favorable valve morphology with less than 2f/ MR* in the absence of LA thrombus who have new onset of AF, PMBC may be considered if it can be performed at a comprehensive valve center.
2b	C-LD	5. In symptomatic patients (NYHA Class II, III, or IV) with rheumatic MS and a mitral valve area >1.5 cm², if there is evidence of hemodynamically significant rheumatic MS on the basis of a pulmonary artery wedge pressure >25 mm Hg or a mean mitral valve gradient >15 mm Hg during exercise, PMBC may be considered if it can be performed at a comprehensive valve center.
2b	B-NR	6. In severely symptomatic patients (NYHA Class III or IV) with severe rheumatic MS (mitral valve area ≤1.5 cm², Stage D) who have a suboptimal valve anatomy and who are not candidates for surgery or are at high risk for surgery, PMBC may be considered if it can be performed at a comprehensive valve center.

*2+ on a 0 to 4+ scale according to Sellar's criteria or less than moderate by Doppler echocardiography.
PMBC, Percutaneous mitral balloon commissurotomy.
(From Otto CM, et al. 2020 AHA/ACC guideline for the management of patients with valvular heart disease: a report of the American College of Cardiology/American Heart Association Task Force on Practice Guidelines. J Am Coll Cardiol 2021;77:e25-197.)

of about 75%.[14] Cardiac complications (5%) including strokes (3%) are also slightly higher than in previous decades, as is the need for surgery (6%).[13] Success rates in LMICs continue to remain much higher (over 90%) and juvenile patients seem to have a particularly effective treatment with BMV.

Complications

Some degree of mild MR or worsening MR has been reported in 20% of patients in recent series.[24] It generally is tolerated well and remains stable or improves. MR arising from commissural splitting actually predicts a good outcome. Acute severe MR is one of the most feared complication of BMV but is rare (<1% to 2%). Severe MR due to tear of the anterior leaflet central scallop or damage to the subvalvular apparatus usually requires early surgery. Most other patients tolerate severe MR initially with only a minority needing emergency intervention. Significant MR, however, affects long-term outcomes adversely. A small interatrial shunt develops within 48 hours of BMV in 60% to 70% of patients, but this persists in less than 10% over the long term, especially if the MS is relieved.

Long-Term Results

Age and procedural success determine long-term outcomes.[14,17] Nearly 80% of patients undergoing BMV remain free of death, need for mitral surgery, or repeat BMV over the next 15 years[25] and about two-thirds remain so after 20 years. However, results also depend on the age of the patient and the era when BMV was performed. A study from France (patient age 49 ± 14) reported that the 20-year rate of good functional results (survival without cardiovascular death, severe symptoms [NYHA Class III-IV], mitral surgery, or repeat BMV) was only 30.2 ± 2.0%.[23] Greater age, higher NYHA class, and suboptimal relief of MS during the initial procedure were factors associated with outcome. Post-BMV restenosis, which is strongly related to suboptimal immediate results, affects long-term outcomes.[26] It develops over many years

and can be treated with repeat BMV with reasonable success if the mechanism is once again fusion of commissures. In patients with restenosis, results of repeat BMV are comparable to surgery but may be less successful if MS is due to valve leaflet rigidity and degeneration.

Surgical Intervention

Surgery is indicated in patients with contraindication for BMV, in those in whom BMV was unsuccessful, and in those with other conditions that would warrant surgery (TR, AS, or CAD).[9] A maze procedure and LA ligation can be performed concomitantly to reduce AF burden and related morbidity. Three types of surgery are offered for MS: closed mitral valvotomy (CMV), open mitral valvotomy (OMV), and mitral valve replacement (MVR). There is good long-term experience with all the three methods, and the results are durable with low rates of MR and reoperation. CMV is not practiced widely except in LMICs where it is economical and has reasonably good results in experienced centers; however, increases in MVA are less and outcomes suboptimal compared to OMV or BMV. Hence, BMV should be chosen over CMV, when both are available. OMV is the surgical procedure of choice, especially in the young. It has excellent results that are comparable to MVR but avoids many of the long-term issues with prosthetic valves. OMV is associated with mortality rates under 2%, excellent relief of symptoms, excellent long-term survival (96% at 10 years), and freedom from reoperation (98% at 9 years). Unless there are distinct indications for its use, MVR is the least preferred option due to higher risk, need for anticoagulation with mechanical valves, and high bioprosthesis failure rate in young patients. MVR has higher operative mortality (3% to 10%) and lower 10-year survival than OMV, but these statistics might reflect a more suboptimal patient substrate.

Comparison with BMV

Randomized clinical trials with limited-term follow-up show that results of BMV are as good or perhaps better than surgery. Robust long-term

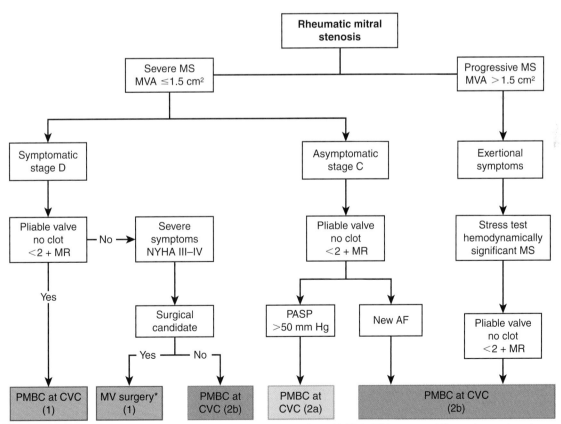

FIGURE 75.6 **Management strategy for rheumatic mitral stenosis.** Colors correspond to Table 75.2. *MV surgery could be repair, commissurotomy, or valve replacement. *AF,* Atrial fibrillation; *CVC,* comprehensive valve center; *MR,* mitral regurgitation; *MS,* mitral stenosis; *MV,* mitral valve; *MVA,* mitral valve area; *NYHA,* New York Heart Association; *PASP,* pulmonary artery systolic pressure; *PMBC,* percutaneous mitral balloon commissurotomy. (From Otto CM, et al. 2020 AHA/ACC guideline for the management of patients with valvular heart disease: a report of the American College of Cardiology/American Heart Association Task Force on Practice Guidelines. J Am Coll Cardiol 2021;77:e25-197.)

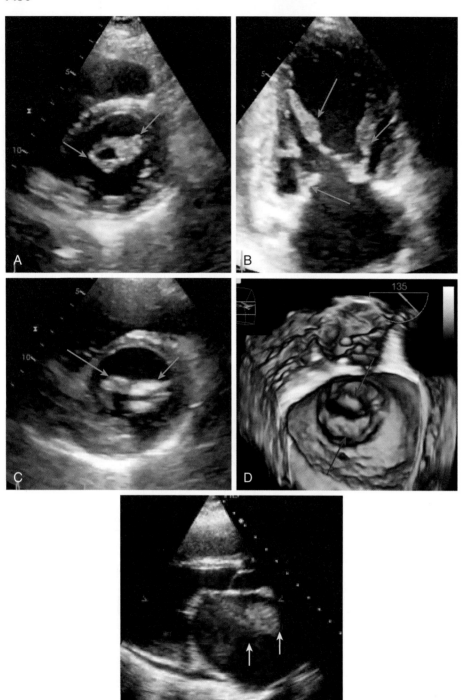

FIGURE 75.7 Echocardiographic features identifying poor suitability for percutaneous balloon mitral valvuloplasty (BMV). 2D and 3D echo is the best method to define less favorable morphology, risk of complications, and contraindications. **A,** Severe asymmetric commissural fusion could indicate that BMV may distribute force nonuniformly, thus increasing risk of suboptimal results and noncommissural tears (see Video 75.7). **B,** Severe fusion and matting of the subvalvular apparatus is a marker for increased risk of persistent gradient and complications after BMV (see Video 75.2). **C,** Asymmetric calcification of leaflets and commissures is a marker of risk of MR after BMV. **D,** Fibrotic leaflets with uneven leaflet thickening can influence results of BMV. **E,** Left atrial thrombus (arrows) is an absolute contraindication for BMV.

head-to-head comparisons with BMV are lacking, but intermediate outcomes of BMV and surgery are largely similar with higher procedural morbidity after surgery.[27] Long-term survival advantage of BMV over surgery has not been conclusively shown in the past and will be even more difficult to show in future, given that patients referred for surgery are usually those who are not favorable candidates for BMV. Surgery for restenosis carries a higher risk due to older age and other comorbidities, and BMV should be the first option whenever feasible.[26]

NONRHEUMATIC MITRAL STENOSIS

A number of conditions can cause nonrheumatic MS (see eFig. 75.1), and they each have many nuances of their own.

Degenerative MS Related to Mitral Annular Calcification

MAC is a chronic process that causes extensive calcification of the mitral valve annulus with extension into the base of both leaflets (see Fig. 17.6). It is now becoming an important cause of MS in the developed world. MAC increases as the population ages and, not surprisingly, MAC related MS is increasingly observed in aging societies. It has many atypical features, has pathophysiology that is somewhat different from RMS, is difficult to diagnose, and has limited treatment options.

The exact mechanism for MS is not clear but a number of factors including reduced diastolic annular expansion and stiff leaflets have been postulated. Both severity and pattern of distribution of MAC influence the degree of LA outflow obstruction. MAC in the anterior annulus, involvement of the anterior leaflet and in particular the A2 scallop, and extension into more than half of the leaflet length seem to predict development and severity of MS. Unlike RMS, there is no commissural fusion or subvalvular involvement (Fig. 75.8). The posterior leaflet is often very restricted due to significant calcification but the tips of both leaflets remain mobile. The mitral gradient due to MAC increases variably, roughly 0.8 ± 2.4 mm Hg/year and MVA decreases 0.05 cm^2/year, which is slower than in RMS.[11] PAH can be severe (>50 mm Hg), but only a small proportion (roughly 20%) of patients progress to systolic PAP >50 mm Hg.[6]

Diagnosis of hemodynamically significant DMS is difficult. The classic patients are older adults, often women, with multiple comorbidities including hypertension, heart failure with preserved ejection fraction (see Chapter 51), AF, COPD, and significant LV hypertrophy that make diagnosis difficult.[11] There may occasionally be a short diastolic rumble, but not the classical signs of RMS such as a loud S$_1$ or OS. Symptomatic patients with severe DMS have modest gradients and higher MVA (e.g., 8.0 ± 3.8 mm Hg and 1.26 ± 0.19 cm^2, respectively in the Mayo series[6]) than RMS. Defining severity of MS and proving it is the proximate cause for the patient's symptoms are quite challenging.[28] The main abnormality in DMS involves the base of the valve leaflets rather than the tips as in RMS and is unevenly distributed around the valve inflow. Early mitral filling is often preserved and late diastolic gradients can become minimal in beats with long RR intervals, unlike in RMS (Fig. 75.9). In addition, comorbidities reduce LA compliance and increase LV stiffness, both of which can lead to elevated LA pressure despite smaller Doppler gradients across the

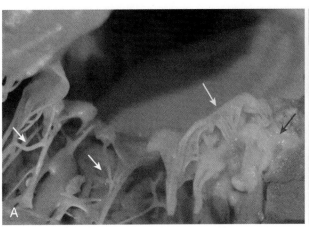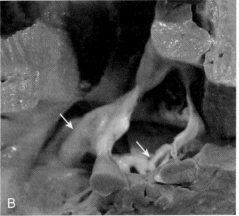

FIGURE 75.8 Pathologic distinction between degenerative and rheumatic MS. A, In this example of degenerative MS, the posterior annulus has severe mitral annular calcification (MAC; *red arrow*) that extends into the posterior mitral leaflet (PML; *yellow arrow*). The PML is thick and rigid, adding resistance to left atrial outflow. In severe cases, MAC extends into the anterior mitral leaflet, making MS more likely. The rest of the valve, including its tips, are spared and opens normally. The subvalvular apparatus is also unaffected (*white arrows*) and commissures are not fused. The narrowed valve orifice thus is at the base of the valve rather than at the leaflet tips, and BMV is not an option. **B,** In rheumatic MS, the annulus is unaffected and the pathology is in the valve edges, commissures and the subvalvular apparatus (*arrows*). The narrowed valve orifice is thus at the tips of the leaflets, and valve areas tend to be smaller than those of degenerative MS caused by MAC.

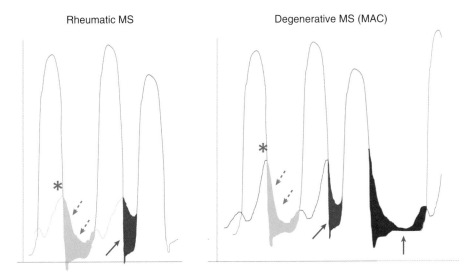

Rheumatic MS   Degenerative MS (MAC)

FIGURE 75.9 Pathophysiology of rheumatic MS versus degenerative MS caused but mitral annular calcification (MAC). Left, In rheumatic MS, the mitral valve area (MVA) is fixed and the early rapid filling phase is slow (*green arrows*) with significant gradient continuing during diastasis and atrial contraction. A premature beat (or tachycardia) will shorten diastole and increase the transmitral gradient (*red*). **Right,** In degenerative MS caused by MAC, the orifice is not as fixed and is comparatively larger than that in rheumatic MS. The left atrial (LA) and left ventricular end-diastolic pressure (LVEDP) are greater, but early rapid filling is better preserved (*green arrows*). The elevated LVEDP increases LA pressure above that due to mitral valve resistance alone. A premature beat has less of an impact on LA pressures. Long RR intervals allow more complete LA emptying, and significantly lower LA pressure, and the gradient is appreciably reduced during diastasis (*blue arrow*), something that is not usually seen in severe rheumatic MS. *Mitral valve opening.

discrepancy between echocardiographic MVA, gradients, and symptoms. The 3D planimetry lacks robust validation in DMS. Finally, mitral valve diastolic PISA is useful in calculating MVA in RMS, but this has not been well validated in DMS. In patients without significant MR or AR, a careful analysis using the continuity equation is probably the best way to diagnose severe DMS. Exercise testing might help clarify the hemodynamic effects of DMS (eFig. 75.2) in patients with symptoms but unclear severity of DMS.[7] CT is being used increasingly in studying MAC since it provides exquisite details about location, severity, circumferential extent and distribution of calcification into the mitral leaflets (see Fig. 75.10) that are far better than obtained from echocardiography. It may allow planimetry and calcium quantitation[30] that has clinical implications. Furthermore, it is a prerequisite for planning MAC related interventions.

Associated Aortic Stenosis

MAC is commonly seen in patients with AS (50% have MAC and 11% to 18% have MS, majority due to DMS) (see Chapter 72), and associated DMS, even if mild, affects short- and long-term outcomes, including stroke, with or without intervention for AS.[31,32] Recognizing MS is thus vital in patients with AS being considered for intervention, but the presence of both can make evaluation of MS difficult. AS can result in low flow-low gradient MS. Planimetry may not be accurate due to significant calcification, and pressure half time is unreliable. MS severity even with use of the continuity equation is commonly overestimated in patients with AS. Half of patients with concomitant AS and MS show increased MVAs after treatment of AS, suggesting low stroke volume before aortic intervention created a pseudo-MS. True DMS in the other half (predicted by preintervention MVA <1.5 cm², and a rigid annulus with calcification that extended into both leaflets) adversely influences outcome after AS intervention.[31]

Natural History

The natural history of MAC-related DMS is incompletely understood. DMS is associated with poor survival, mainly a consequence of the extensive comorbidities, with 1-year mortality in the 32% range. The majority of patients (60%) with severe DMS in a contemporary series[6] had symptoms, with dyspnea being the most common, while asymptomatic patients developed symptoms at the rate of 7% to 8% per year. Adverse events are fairly common (47% at 1 year, almost 75% over longer follow-up), and almost 50% of the patients died during the short follow-up of 2.8 ± 3.0 years.

mitral valve; it is sometimes difficult to be certain that MAC related mitral inflow obstruction rather than comorbidities is the dominant cause of symptoms. Not surprisingly, elevated LA and LV end-diastolic pressures often continue to be seen in some patients even after successful interventions.

Multiple techniques are often used to image and understand the etiology of symptoms (Fig. 75.10; see also Videos 75.8 and 75.9) in patients with MAC.[29] Planimetry, the reference standard for RMS, may not work well since MS is not a fixed obstruction at one level (e.g., at the leaflet tip in RMS) but is a result of increased resistance at the level of the leaflet base and annulus level as well as reduced opening angle of the calcified leaflet base. The difference in shape of the stenosed valve (dome shape in RMS and tubular funnel shape in DMS) can have differential effects on pressure loss and result in different effective MVAs or gradients. Extensive calcium can obscure the valve orifice outlines so planimetry is difficult. Pressure half time is affected by LV and LA compliance, which leads to an overestimate of the MVA, creating a

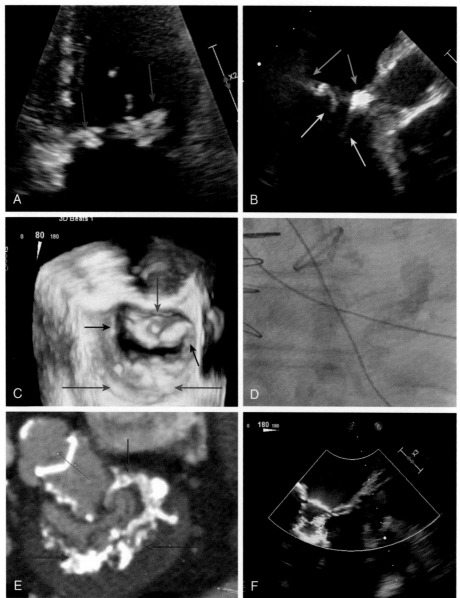

FIGURE 75.10 Imaging in degenerative MS due to mitral annular calcification (MAC). A, Extensive MAC (*arrows*) in a patient with MAC associated MS. **B,** The MAC starts from the annulus and extends for some length into the base of the leaflets (*orange arrows*), making them stiff. The rest of the leaflet is spared (*yellow arrows*). **C,** 3D echo shows extensive MAC (*red arrows*) (see Video 75.8). Unlike rheumatic MS there is no commissural fusion (*black arrows*). **D,** MAC is well visualized on x-ray (see Video 75.9). **E,** CT is the best modality for quantitation. **F,** Flow convergence shell is not impressive, suggesting lower gradient and relatively larger valve area despite severe symptoms.

associated with adverse outcomes including AV groove disruption. In addition, surgical risk is heightened by patient age and comorbidities. Complication rates, not surprisingly, tend to be high and rarely, procedures like mitral valve bypass (LA to LV conduit) might be needed. Many patients do report reduced symptoms if they survive surgery, but long-term survival studies are lacking. Transcatheter techniques are under development, and transcatheter mitral valve replacement (TMVR) and (ViMAC) with balloon-expandable transcatheter aortic valves have shown some promise. These are currently reserved for highly symptomatic patients with significant surgical risk. Early results from the TMVR in MAC Global Registry[33] in 116 severely symptomatic patients at extreme surgical risk indicate procedural success in 76.7% of patients but 15% needed a second valve due to suboptimal results (migration or severe MR). One year all-cause mortality was 54%, and the majority of the survivors (72%) were in NYHA functional Class I or II. The mean mitral gradient was reduced from 11.5 mm Hg to 5.8 mm Hg, the mean MVA increased from 1.3 cm² to 1.9 cm², and 75% of patients had no or trace MR. TMVR is feasible in patients with severe MAC but is associated with high 30-day and 1-year mortality, with LV outflow tract (LVOT) obstruction being the most dreaded complication (11.2%). Another multicenter study also confirmed suboptimal results in ViMAC compared to excellent outcomes for patients with transcatheter valve-in-valve for degenerated bioprostheses despite similar high surgical risk.[34] Early and midterm mortality after transcatheter ViMAC were high (35% and 63%, respectively). These early disappointing results may improve in the future with more optimal use of multimodality imaging for predicting LVOT obstruction and optimal valve sizing, dedicated MAC-related valve designs and more precise anticoagulation protocols.

Treatment

Therapeutic options in DMS are limited but evolving. A lack of good quality data prevents clear recommendations for treating DMS, unlike in RMS.[9-11] Medical therapy, in the form of diuretics and beta blockers to slow the heart rate, is commonly used in symptomatic DMS. However, mortality remains high with medical therapy.[6] Despite this dismal prognosis, MAC-related interventional procedures are performed only in a minority of patients, even in major medical centers. As an example, only 16% of such symptomatic patients underwent nonmedical therapies, of which 85% were surgical MVR.[6] BMV is not an option in DMS given that the abnormality does not involve commissural fusion. There are no effective methods to decalcify MAC and replacing the valve, either surgically or with transcatheter valve in MAC (ViMAC) using a transcatheter aortic valve device (see Chapter 78) are the only choices at this time. Surgical options have suboptimal results due to difficulty in suturing the new valve into heavily calcified segments, and extensive debriding of the annulus to adequately seat a valve is often

Radiotherapy-Induced MS

Valvular heart disease, including MS, is a time- and dose-dependent complication of chest radiation, particularly when using protocols that did not adequately shield nontarget structures. It takes decades to rise to clinical attention and can be a combination of MR and MS, the latter happening about two decades after exposure. Severe calcification of the cardiac fibrous skeleton, especially in the aortomitral curtain, the anterior annulus and anterior leaflet, is common but is not accompanied by subvalvular involvement or commissural fusion (Fig. 75.11; see also Videos 75.10 and 75.11). Radiation-associated MS is often accompanied by involvement of the aortic valve as well as restrictive myocardial disease. Treatment of radiation-associated MS is suboptimal but general principles remain the same as with other forms of MS.

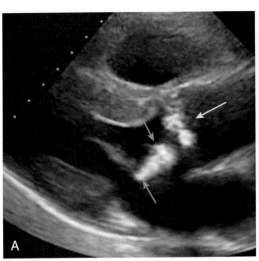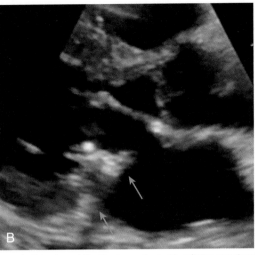

FIGURE 75.11 Nonrheumatic MS due to prior radiation therapy. A, Extensive calcification in a patient with radiation associated MS is predominantly in the "aortic-mitral curtain" (*orange arrows*), which is a classic sign of radiation induced valvular damage. In addition, the patient has calcific aortic stenosis (*yellow arrow*), which occurs before the onset of MS. Commissural fusion does not occur and hence balloon dilation is not an option (see Video 75.10). **B,** In contrast, degenerative MS related to mitral annular calcification most commonly involves the posterior annulus and then extends around the annulus and into the base of the leaflets. Aorto-mitral curtain calcification is not prominent (see Video 75.11).

MS Following Interventional and Surgical Therapies

A number of mitral valve interventions both surgical (prosthetic valves, Alfieri stitch, or mitral repair with annuloplasty) and percutaneous mitral valve clips (see Chapters 76 and 78) are becoming an important cause for MS in the Western world; indeed, MS related to prosthetic valve dysfunction was more common than even calcific DMS in the most recent experience at a major tertiary center.[7] Surgical series report MVA <1.5 cm² in approximately 20% of patients after surgical mitral valve repair for primary MR. These patients require a very nuanced evaluation since identifying prosthesis-related dysfunction as the main cause of LA outflow obstruction is difficult. However, it needs to be diagnosed correctly since it has specific therapeutic options, and intervention seems to improve mortality. Prosthetic valves can cause an MS-like syndrome either with disease affecting the operating valve orifice (thrombus, pannus, leaflet thickening and degeneration, or calcification and very rarely commissural fusion) or prosthesis-patient mismatch (PPM) (see Chapter 79). Both repeat surgical MVR and transcatheter mitral valve-in-valve replacement are options for treating MS due to degenerated mitral bioprostheses. These options seem to have largely similar outcomes in preliminary studies despite a 2 mm Hg higher gradient in the valve-in-valve group.[35] Data in 1529 high-risk patients (50% with MS) from the Society of Thoracic Surgeons/American College of Cardiology Transcatheter Valve Therapy Registry showed very high procedural success of transcatheter valve-in-valve (96.8%), good valve function that was maintained at 1 year, and low risks of valve thrombosis, LVOT obstruction (0.9%), and all-cause mortality (16.7% at 1 year).[36] The choice of therapy depends on the risk-benefit profile of the patient, expertise of the heart team, and need for other surgery (such as treatment of TR, which is seen in up to 50% of patients with prosthetic mitral valve stenosis). Smaller bioprosthetic valves (<23 mm) may perhaps be best treated with surgery to avoid higher gradients after transcatheter valve-in-valve. This transcatheter option was initially offered only to patients at high risk for repeat cardiac surgery but is now being used increasingly in patients who are somewhat lower risk (see Chapter 78). However, durability of the procedure and whether small residual valve gradients have future consequences need to be resolved.

PPM after MVR is fairly common, ranging between 30% and 85% by effective orifice area criteria (see Chapter 79). Unlike aortic valve PPM, there is conflicting data whether PPM after MVR significantly influences long-term prognosis. Clinically significant PPM is treated surgically but newer valve designs may provide other options in future.

Annuloplasty procedures during surgical repair of MR, especially when using a smaller-sized ring, can cause functional MS, which mediates PAH, new-onset AF, lower exercise capacity, and poorer quality of life even after abolishing the MR.[37] Treatment is often repeat surgery, but there is growing experience with transcatheter valve-in-ring procedures, which might be a reasonable option in some selected patients. About one-quarter to one-third of patients develop mitral valve gradients greater than 5 mm Hg (most in the 5 to 10 mm Hg range) after transcatheter edge-to-edge mitral clip procedures (see Chapter 78).[38] Preprocedure MVA <4 cm², preexisting gradients, significant leaflet calcification, and implanting >2 clips predict development of gradients of this magnitude. Clip-related MS, especially in patients with primary MR,[39] has poorer long-term outcomes including risk of death, AF, and reintervention. Residual MR has adverse outcomes but MS (>5 mm Hg) may be worse,[38] and both together are even more detrimental; there is thus a delicate balance between how aggressive one can be with clips to abolish MR and the risk of an unfavorable gradient. Diagnosing MS in the presence of a clip and two orifices is difficult. Measuring the hemodynamics of the larger orifice or averaging both has been suggested, but no single method has been well validated. Surgery provides definitive therapy; the valve can be repaired in 50% to 60% of cases but this becomes more difficult with an increasing number of clips. There is a 9% risk of early mortality, depending on urgency of surgery and the extent of patient comorbidities, and a 60% to 70% survival at 1 to 2 years.

CLASSIC REFERENCES

Shaw TR, Sutaria N, Prendergast B. Clinical and haemodynamic profiles of young, middle aged, and elderly patients with mitral stenosis undergoing mitral balloon valvotomy. *Heart.* 2003;89:1430–1436.

Wilkins GT, Weyman AE, Abascal VM, et al. Percutaneous balloon dilatation of the mitral valve: an analysis of echocardiographic variables related to outcome and the mechanism of dilatation. *Br Heart J.* 1988;60:299–308.

Wood P. An appreciation of mitral stenosis. I. Clinical features. *Br Med J.* 1954;1(4870):1051–1063.

REFERENCES

Epidemiology and Secular Trends

1. Watkins DA, Johnson CO, Colquhoun SM, et al. Global, regional, and national burden of rheumatic heart. Disease, 1990–2015. *New Engl J Med.* 2017;377:713–722.
2. Rothenbuhler M, O'Sullivan CJ, Stortecky S, et al. Active surveillance for rheumatic heart disease in endemic regions: a systematic review and meta-analysis of prevalence among children and adolescents. *Lancet Glob Health.* 2014;2:e717–e726.
3. Zuhlke L, Engel ME, Karthikeyan G, et al. Characteristics, complications, and gaps in evidence-based interventions in rheumatic heart disease: the Global Rheumatic Heart Disease Registry (the REMEDY study). *Eur Heart J.* 2015;36:1115–1122.
4. Tandon R, Sharma M, Chandrashekhar Y, et al. Revisiting the pathogenesis of rheumatic fever and carditis. *Nat Rev Cardiol.* 2013;10:171–177.
5. Zuhlke L, Karthikeyan G, Engel ME, et al. Clinical outcomes in 3343 children and adults with rheumatic heart disease from 14 low- and middle-income countries: two-year follow-up of the global Rheumatic Heart Disease Registry (the REMEDY study). *Circulation.* 2016;134:1456–1466.
6. Kato N, Padang R, Scott CG, et al. The natural history of severe calcific mitral stenosis. *J Am Coll Cardiol.* 2020;75:3048–3057.
7. Gentry JL, Parikh PK, Alashi A, et al. Characteristics and outcomes in a contemporary group of patients with susepcted significant mitral stenosis undergoing treadmill stress echocardiography. *Circ Cardiovasc Imaging.* 2019;12:e009062.
8. Nishimura RA, Vahanian A, Eleid MF, Mack MJ. Mitral valve disease—current management and future challenges. *Lancet.* 2016;387:1324–1334.
9. Otto CM, Nishimura RA, Bonow RO, et al. 2020 ACC/AHA guideline for the management of patients with valvular heart disease: executive summary: a report of the American College of Cardiology/American Heart Association joint committee on clinical practice guidelines. *J Am Coll Cardiol.* 2021;77:e25–197.
10. Baumgartner H, Falk V, Bax JJ, et al. 2017 ESC/EACTS Guidelines for the management of valvular heart disease. *Eur Heart J.* 2017;38:2739–2791.

Rheumatic Mitral Stenosis: Pathophysiology, Natural History, Diagnosis

11. Chandrashekhar Y, Westaby S, Narula J. Mitral stenosis. *Lancet*. 2009;374:1271–1283.
12. El Sabbagh A, Reddy YN, Barros-Gomes S, et al. Low-gradient severe mitral stenosis: hemodynamic profiles, clinical characteristics, and outcomes. *J Am Heart Assoc*. 2019;8:e010736.
13. Badheka AO, Shah N, Ghatak A, et al. Balloon mitral valvuloplasty in the United States: a 13-year perspective. *Am J Med*. 2014;127(1126).e1–12.
14. Desnos C, Iung B, Himbert D, et al. Temporal trends on percutaneous mitral commissurotomy: 30 years of experience. *J Am Heart Assoc*. 2019;8:e012031.
15. Laufer-Perl M, Gura Y, Shimiaie J, et al. Mechanisms of effort intolerance in patients with rheumatic mitral stenosis. *JACC Cardiovasc Imaging*. 2017;10:622–633.
16. Wunderlich NC, Beigel R, Siegel RJ. Management of mitral stenosis using 2D and 3D echo-Doppler imaging. *JACC Cardiovasc Imaging*. 2013;6:1191–1205.
17. Nunes MC, Tan TC, Elmariah S, et al. The echo score revisited: impact of incorporating commissural morphology and leaflet displacement to the prediction of outcome for patients undergoing percutaneous mitral valvuloplasty. *Circulation*. 2014;129:886–895.

Rheumatic Mitral Stenosis: Atrial Fibrillation, Pregnancy

18. Iung B, Leenhardt A, Extramiana F. Management of atrial fibrillation in patients with rheumatic mitral stenosis. *Heart*. 2018;104:1062–1068.
19. Kim H, Cho G, Kim Y, et al. Development of atrial fibrillation in patients with rheumatic mitral valve disease in sinus rhythm. *Int J Cardiovasc Imaging*. 2015;31:735–742.
20. van Hagen IM, Thorne SA, Taha N, et al. Pregnancy outcomes in women with rheumatic mitral valve disease: results from the registry of pregnancy and cardiac disease. *Circulation*. 2018;137:806–816.
21. Elkayam U, Goland S, Pieper PG, Silverside CK. High-risk cardiac disease in pregnancy: Part 1. *J Am Coll Cardiol*. 2016;68:396–410.
22. Regit-Azgrosek V, Roos-Hesselink JW, Bauersachs J, ESC Scientific Document Group, et al. 2018 ESC guidelines for the management of cardiovascular diseases during pregnancy. *Eur Heart J*. 2018;39:3165–3241.

Rheumatic Mitral Stenosis: Treatment

23. Bouleti C, Iung B, Laouenan C, et al. Late results of percutaneous mitral commissurotomy up to 20 years: development and validation of a risk score predicting late functional results from a series of 912 patients. *Circulation*. 2012;125:2119–2127.
24. Nunes MCP, Levine RA, Braulio R, et al. Mitral regurgitation after percutaneous mitral valvuloplasty: insights into mechanisms and impact on clinical outcomes. *JACC Cardiovasc Imaging*. 2020;13:2513–2526.
25. Meneguz-Moreno RA, Costa JR, Gomes NL, et al. Very long term follow-up after percutaneous balloon mitral valvuloplasty. *JACC Cardiovasc Interv*. 2018;11:1945–1952.
26. Bouleti C, Iung B, Himbert D, et al. Reinterventions after percutaneous mitral commissurotomy during long-term follow-up, up to 20 years: the role of repeat percutaneous mitral commissurotomy. *Eur Heart J*. 2013;34:1923–1930.
27. Singh AD, Mian A, Devasenapathy N, et al. Percutaneous mitral commissurotomy versus surgical commissurotomy for rheumatic mitral stenosis: a systematic review and meta-analysis of randomised controlled trials. *Heart*. 2020;106:1094–1101.

Degenerative Mitral Stenosis Due to Mitral Annular Calcification

28. Reddy YVN, Murgo JP, Nishimura RA. Complexity of defining severe "stenosis" from mitral annular calcification. *Circulation*. 2019;140:523–525.
29. Eleid MF, Foley TA, Said SM, et al. Severe mitral annular calcification: multimodality imaging for therapeutic strategies and interventions. *JACC Cardiovasc Imaging*. 2016;9:1318–1337.
30. Guerrero M, Wang DD, Pursnani A, et al. A cardiac computed tomography-based score to categorize mitral annular calcification severity and predict valve embolization. *JACC Cardiovasc Imaging*. 2020;13:1945–1957.
31. Kato N, Padang R, Pislaru C, et al. Hemodynamics and prognostic impact of concomitant mitral stenosis in patients undergoing surgical or transcatheter aortic valve replacement for aortic stenosis. *Circulation*. 2019;140:1251–1260.
32. Asami M, Windecker S, Praz F, et al. Transcatheter aortic valve replacement in patients with concomitant mitral stenosis. *Eur Heart J*. 2019;40:1342–1351.
33. Guerrero M, Urena M, Himbert D, et al. 1-Year outcomes of transcatheter mitral valve replacement in patients with severe mitral annular calcification. *J Am Coll Cardiol*. 2018;71:1841–1853.

Mitral Stenosis Following Surgical or Transcatheter Mitral Valve Procedures

34. Yoon SH, Whisenant BK, Bleiziffer S, et al. Outcomes of transcatheter mitral valve replacement for degenerated bioprostheses, failed annuloplasty rings, and mitral annular calcification. *Eur Heart J*. 2019;40:441–451.
35. Kamioka N, Babaliaros V, Morse MA, et al. Comparison of clinical and echocardiographic outcomes after surgical redo mitral valve replacement and transcatheter mitral valve-in-valve therapy. *JACC Cardiovasc Interv*. 2018;11:1131–1138.
36. Whisenant B, Kapadia SR, Eleid MF, et al. One-year outcomes of mitral valve-in-valve using the SAPIEN 3 transcatheter heart valve. *JAMA Cardiol*. 2020;5:1245–1252.
37. Kawamoto N, Fujita T, Fukushima S, et al. Functional mitral stenosis after mitral valve repair for type II dysfunction: determinants and impacts on long-term outcome. *Eur J Cardio Thorac Surg*. 2018;54:453–459.
38. Neuss M, Schau T, Isotani A, et al. Elevated mitral valve pressure gradient after MitraClip implantation deteriorates longterm outcome in patients with severe mitral regurgitation and severe heart failure. *JACC Cardiovasc Interv*. 2017;10:931–939.
39. Patzelt J, Zhang W, Sauter R, et al. Elevated mitral valve pressure gradient is predictive of long-term outcome after percutaneous edge-to-edge mitral valve repair in patients with degenerative Mitral Regurgitation (MR), but not in functional MR. *J Am Heart Assoc*. 2019;8:e011366.

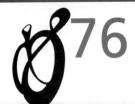

76 Mitral Regurgitation

REBECCA TUNG HAHN AND ROBERT O. BONOW

The prevalence of valvular heart disease increases with age, and population studies have shown mitral regurgitation (MR) of either primary or secondary cause is the most prevalent valvular disorder, occurring in 9% to 10% of elderly patients in United States (see Nkomo et al., Classic References). Prognosis and treatment, however, are distinctly different based on the cause of the MR,[1] and thus accurate diagnosis of valve morphology is an important first step in determining the appropriate treatment options.[2] The following chapter will review mitral valve (MV) anatomy, characterize morphologic and etiologic features and outcomes associated with primary and secondary disease, and then discuss current and investigational treatment options.

MITRAL VALVE ANATOMY

The MV is a complex three-dimensional structure involving multiple, anatomically distinct components (see Perloff and Roberts, Classic References). Coordinated interaction of the annulus, commissures, leaflets, chordae tendineae, papillary muscles, and left ventricle is crucial for MV functional integrity (Fig. 76.1). Abnormalities of any of these structures may cause MR.

Mitral Annulus

The mitral annulus is not a single, well-defined ring of connective tissue but is instead a multifaceted structure made up of the convergence of several components: the atrial and ventricular muscular walls, the hinge line of the mitral leaflets, the epicardial adipose tissue, a discontinuous semi-circle of fibrous tissue on its posterior aspect, and a band of connective tissue at its anterior aspect.[3] The annulus is often described as saddle-shaped on three-dimensional studies with anterior and posterior peaks and nadirs near the medial and lateral fibrous trigones (see Levine et al., Classic References). The anterior "horn" of the saddle is composed of the curved band of connective tissue that adjoins the annulus of the aorta at the level of the left and noncoronary cusps, referred to as the "aorto-mitral curtain" by surgeons and the 'intervalvular fibrosa' by imagers.[4] This band of tissue is continuous with the anterior MV leaflet, which hinges where the left atrial (LA) wall joins the leaflet. This hinge-point is more apical, usually below the fibrous trigones; thus, measurement of the annulus by multimodality imaging often demarcates the anterior annulus by cutting off the aorto-mitral curtain superior to the trigone-to-trigone line, making the annulus D-shaped: the straight component is conventionally named the anterior mitral annulus, and the curved component is the posterior mitral annulus.[5] The posterior annulus is less fibrotic and moves with myocardial contraction, allowing for systolic bending and apical displacement of the medial and lateral horns, increasing saddle height but reducing circumferential area. The mitral annulus is innervated

and supplies blood vessels to the leaflets.[6] Because it forms the convergence of the atrial and ventricular myocardium, the posterior annulus may dilate in the setting of either left ventricular (LV) or LA dilation and is also prone to age-related degenerative calcification.

Mitral Leaflets

Due to the oblique orientation of the mitral apparatus relative to the anatomic axes of the body, the anterior and posterior MV leaflets are oriented in a more anterosuperior and posteroinferior position.[7] The anterior leaflet is longer radially and thicker than the posterior leaflet, because it must withstand significantly higher tensile load. The posterior leaflet is longer circumferentially and more flexible. Two leaflet segmentation schemes have been proposed. The most commonly used classification scheme was proposed by Carpentier (Fig. 76.2A; see also Fig. 16.31) (see Carpentier, Classic References). Because the posterior leaflet typically has two well-defined indentations, there are three separate sections or "scallops" referred to as P1 (anterolateral), P2 (middle), and P3 (posteromedial). The anterior leaflet typically is devoid of indentations, so the anterior leaflet opposing P1 is designated as A1 (anterior segment), the segment opposite to P2 is A2 (middle segment), and the segment opposite to P3 is A3 (posterior segment). A modification of the Carpentier scheme (see Fig. 76.2B) divides the large middle segment into lateral (A2L and P2L) and medial (A2M and P2M) halves, which respects the separate chordal origins of the leaflets. The anterior and posterior leaflets come into direct continuity at the anterolateral and posteromedial commissures; commissural tissue may range from a few millimeters to distinct leaflets or scallops.

Mitral Valve Chordae and Papillary Muscles

The chordae tendineae are responsible for determining the position and tension on the leaflets at LV end-systole. The chordae are composed of collagen and elastin, are surrounded by a layer of endothelium, and originate from the heads of the papillary muscles or infrequently from the inferolateral ventricular wall. There are multiple chordal classification systems based on the origin (i.e., apical or basal portion of the papillary muscles), attachment site within the mitral complex (i.e., leaflet, interpapillary, myocardial wall), and insertion site on the mitral leaflets, to name a few.[8] The classification by leaflet insertion is the most often used with marginal or primary chordae inserting on the free margin of the mitral leaflets and secondary chordae inserting on the ventricular (rough zone) surface of the leaflets preventing billowing while reducing tension on the leaflet tissues. "Strut" chordae are thicker, secondary chordae and attach to the anterior MV leaflet with a broad, muscular base. These chordae have greater viscoelasticity than marginal chordae[9] and may play a role in determining dynamic ventricular shape and function due to their contribution to

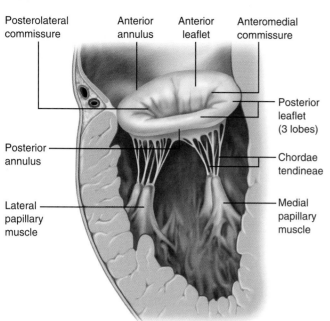

FIGURE 76.1 Continuity of the mitral apparatus and the left ventricular (LV) myocardium. Mitral regurgitation (MR) may be caused by any condition that affects the leaflets or the structure and function of the left ventricle. Similarly, a surgical procedure that disrupts the mitral apparatus in an attempt to correct MR will have adverse effects on LV geometry, volume, and function. (From Otto CM. Evaluation and management of chronic mitral regurgitation. *N Engl J Med.* 2001;345:740-746.)

A

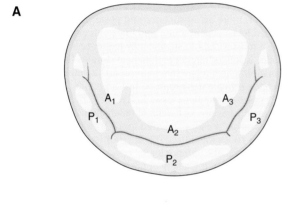

B

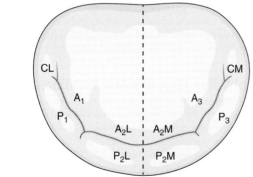

FIGURE 76.2 Classification of mitral valve segmentation, viewed from the atrial aspect of the valve. A, Segmentation model of Carpentier. **B,** Proposed adaptation by Shah. *CL,* lateral commissure; *CM,* medial commissure. (**A** modified from Carpentier A. Cardiac valve surgery: the "French correction." *J Thorac Cardiovasc Surg.* 1983;86:323-337; **B** modified from Shah PM. Current concepts in mitral valve prolapse: diagnosis and management. *J Cardiol.* 2010;56:125-133.)

ventricular-valve continuity. *Tertiary or basal chordae* insert on the posterior leaflet base and mitral annulus.

There are two papillary muscles; the anterolateral arises from the apicolateral third of the LV, and the posteromedial arises from the middle of the LV inferior wall. The anterolateral papillary muscle is

composed of an anterior and posterior head, and the posteromedial papillary muscle is usually composed of anterior, intermediate, and posterior heads. Because the papillary muscles connect directly to the LV, any geometric change in LV shape can change the axial relationship of the chordae and leaflets, resulting in poor leaflet coaptation. The posteromedial papillary muscle gives chordae to the medial half of both leaflets (i.e., posteromedial commissure, A3, P3, A2M, and P2M). Similarly, the anterolateral papillary muscle chordae attach to the lateral half of the MV leaflets (i.e., anterolateral commissure, A1, P1, A2L, and P2L). The midline of the valve is a relatively chordal-free zone.

MECHANISMS OF MITRAL REGURGITATION

Normal Mitral Valve Physiology

The MV complex described earlier must work in concert to close the annular orifice in systole without permitting regurgitation while maximizing forward flow during diastole under low pressure conditions. An appreciation of the dynamic nature of the MV is integral to the understanding of the morphologic abnormalities resulting in MR. In addition, the MV apparatus is thought to have the capacity to modify its structure in response to both genetic and biomechanical stresses.[10]

Three-dimensional imaging studies have shown that during the isovolumic contraction period in early systole, anteroposterior contraction occurs with accentuated folding across the fixed intercommissural diameter such that the annular saddle shape (with anteroposterior high points and mediolateral low points) is accentuated with resulting approximation of anterior and posterior leaflets. With LV contraction and longitudinal LV shortening, the annulus moves toward the apex while the papillary muscles contract to maintain the distance between the mitral annulus and papillary muscle tips. The papillary muscles that attach to the posterior half of the LV maintain leaflet closure in the posterior LV cavity away from the LV outflow tract (LVOT). At the same time, the mitral annulus and aortic annulus angle becomes more acute during systole to facilitate blood flow out the LVOT.

Mitral Regurgitation Morphologic Classifications

The 2020 American College of Cardiology/American Heart Association (ACC/AHA) guideline for the management of patients with valvular heart disease[1] and the 2020 focused update of the 2017 ACC expert consensus decision pathway on the management of MR[2] emphasize the importance of an initial assessment of its cause, mechanism, and severity. The major causes of MR include myxomatous degeneration (mitral valve prolapse [MVP] and ruptured mitral chordae), rheumatic heart disease, infective endocarditis, hypertrophic cardiomyopathy, annular calcification, dilated cardiomyopathy, and ischemic heart disease (Table 76.1). Less common causes of MR include collagen vascular diseases, trauma, the hypereosinophilic syndrome, carcinoid, and exposure to certain drugs. The morphologic classification for MR described by Carpentier (see Carpentier, Classic References) are based on the mobility of the MV leaflets (Fig. 76.3). A variety of causes are associated with each type of leaflet motion.

Type I MR involves normal mobility of leaflets with poor coaptation due to annular dilation or perforation or cleft/indentations of a leaflet. Etiologies associated with leaflet disruption are considered primary MR and include endocarditis and iatrogenic trauma. Congenital isolated cleft MV leaflets or deep indentations also may be associated with significant MR.[11] Atrial and annular dilation causing MR or atriogenic MR (Fig. 76.4, upper left), is a morphologic subtype of secondary MR and is usually associated with chronic atrial fibrillation (AF) or heart failure (HF) with preserved ejection fraction (EF), both resulting in progressive remodeling of the LA.[12-14] The LV dimensions, papillary muscles, chordae, and leaflets are typically intrinsically normal; however, in the setting of chronic AF or increased LA pressures, a number of anatomic derangements result in MR: LA dilation results in annular dilation and flattening, insufficient leaflet remodeling or leaflet thickening exceeds the increase in mitral annular area, and abnormal atrial-annular dynamics reduce normal leaflet coaptation mechanics.[14,15] Studies have suggested that maintenance of sinus rhythm may result in reduction of MR.[16] A possible subtype of atriogenic MR is atriogenic leaflet tethering.[17] This entity is still associated with LA and annular dilation, but because the posterior leaflet is attached to the junction of the LA and LV myocardium, progressive annular dilation may result in deviation of the leaflet attachment toward the outer wall of

TABLE 76.1 Causes of Acute and Chronic Mitral Regurgitation

Acute	Chronic
Mitral Annulus Disorders	**Inflammatory**
• Infective endocarditis (abscess formation)	• Rheumatic heart disease
• Trauma (valvular heart surgery)	• Systemic lupus erythematosus
• Paravalvular leak caused by suture interruption (surgical technical problems or infective endocarditis)	• Scleroderma
Mitral Leaflet Disorders	**Degenerative**
• Infective endocarditis (perforation or interfering with valve closure by vegetation)	• Myxomatous degeneration of mitral valve leaflets (Barlow click-murmur syndrome, prolapsing leaflet, mitral valve prolapse)
• Trauma (tear during percutaneous balloon mitral valvotomy or penetrating chest injury)	• Marfan syndrome
• Tumors (atrial myxoma)	• Ehlers-Danlos syndrome
• Myxomatous degeneration	• Pseudoxanthoma elasticum
• Systemic lupus erythematosus (Libman-Sacks lesion)	• Calcification of mitral valve annulus
Rupture of Chordae Tendineae	**Infective**
• Idiopathic (e.g., spontaneous)	• Infective endocarditis affecting normal, abnormal, or prosthetic mitral valves
• Myxomatous degeneration (mitral valve prolapse, Marfan syndrome, Ehlers-Danlos syndrome)	**Structural**
• Infective endocarditis	• Ruptured chordae tendineae (spontaneous or secondary to myocardial infarction, trauma, mitral valve prolapse, endocarditis)
• Acute rheumatic fever	• Rupture or dysfunction of papillary muscle (ischemia or myocardial infarction)
• Trauma (percutaneous balloon valvotomy, blunt chest trauma)	• Dilation of mitral valve annulus and left ventricular cavity (congestive cardiomyopathies, aneurysmal dilation of left ventricle)
Papillary Muscle Disorders	• Hypertrophic cardiomyopathy
• Coronary artery disease (causing dysfunction and rarely rupture)	• Paravalvular prosthetic leak
• Acute global left ventricular dysfunction	**Congenital**
• Infiltrative diseases (amyloidosis, sarcoidosis)	• Mitral valve clefts or fenestrations
• Trauma	• Parachute mitral valve abnormality in association with:
Primary Mitral Valve Prosthetic Disorders	• Endocardial cushion defects
• Porcine cusp perforation (endocarditis)	• Endocardial fibroelastosis
• Porcine cusp degeneration	• Transposition of great arteries
• Mechanical failure (strut fracture)	• Anomalous origin of left coronary artery
• Immobilized disc or ball of the mechanical prosthesis	

Data from Jutzy KR, Al-Zaibag M. Acute mitral and aortic valve regurgitation. In: Al-Zaibag M, Duran CMG, eds. *Valvular Heart Disease*. New York: Marcel Dekker; 1994:345-362; and Haffajee CI. Chronic mitral regurgitation. In: Dalen JE, Alpert JS, eds. *Valvular Heart Disease*. 2nd ed. Boston: Little, Brown; 1987;112

the LV myocardium and result in restriction of posterior leaflet motion in both systole and diastole with malcoaptation of the anterior leaflet and a posteriorly directed MR jet.

Type II MR involves excessive motion of the margin of a leaflet segment above the annular plane. This has been referred to as degenerative MR, also a morphologic subtype of primary MR. The two classic subtypes are MVP and leaflet flail with ruptured chordae. The two phenotypes related to these morphologic subtypes are fibroelastic deficiency and myxomatous degeneration. Fibroelastic deficiency is seen as a degenerative disease, and thus patients are older and the disease is typically localized to one or two segments and can involve ruptured chordae with leaflet redundancy and thickening primarily on the flail segment (typically posterior, especially P2). Although considered a "specific" sign of significant MR according to American Society of Echocardiography (ASE) guidelines,[18] a flail mitral leaflet is not synonymous with severe MR and can be associated with only mild or moderate MR.[19] In fibroelastic deficiency, leaflet area remains constant throughout the cardiac cycle with relatively normal annular dynamics and often holosystolic MR. Conversely, myxomatous disease is seen in younger patients with familial clustering and a variety of genetic abnormalities have been identified.[20] Myxomatous valves usually show generalized redundancy, cellular proliferation, and increased matrix production, resulting in thickening of both leaflets (Fig. 76.5), involving multiple segments and prolapse volume and height increases in late systole (see Fig. 76.4, upper right). In myxomatous disease, the mitral annulus is typically dilated and annular dynamics may be altered with the largest annular area in late systole, contributing to the presence of late-systolic MR.[21] In addition, there is loss of early-systolic area

contraction and saddle-shape deepening that may also contribute to leaflet malcoaptation. It is uncertain whether these diseases are variants along a single pathophysiologic spectrum; however, recent data showing distinct physiologic differences suggest that they are related but separate entities. A ruptured chordae and flail segment may occur with either phenotype.

Type III disease is associated with restricted mobility of leaflets, resulting in coaptation of leaflets in the ventricular level. This attenuated mobility can be diastolic and systolic (type IIIa) or just systolic (type IIIb). The first type (type IIIa) is the result of thickening and shortening of leaflets, chordae, or annulus secondary to inflammatory or congenital disease and is considered a form of primary MR. Classic etiologies associated with this mechanism are rheumatic heart disease (see Fig. 76.4, lower left), carcinoid, radiation induced, and mitral annular calcification–related MR. These entities share the same pathomorphologic changes: thickening, retraction, and rigidity of leaflets and attached chordae, which restricts both systolic and diastolic leaflet motion. In type IIIb the attenuated mobility is entirely systolic and is associated with LV enlargement, displacement of papillary muscles away from the mitral annulus, and systolic tethering of mitral leaflets transferred through the tensed chordae tendineae. This is the second morphologic subtype, considered secondary MR. A loss of annular folding across the intercommissural axis and the loss of saddle shape accentuation in early systole, play a role in early-systolic type IIIb MR just as it does in myxomatous MV disease.[22]

In general, types II and IIIa usually are caused by primary disorders of the MV leaflets, whereas types I and IIIb have relatively normal leaflets, which are distorted by LV and annular remodeling, resulting in secondary MR.

Dysfunction	Ventricular View	Atrial View	Etiologic Disorder
Type I Normal leaflet motion	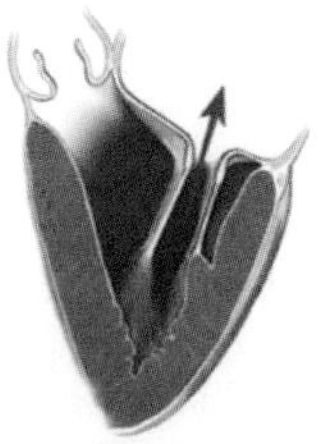	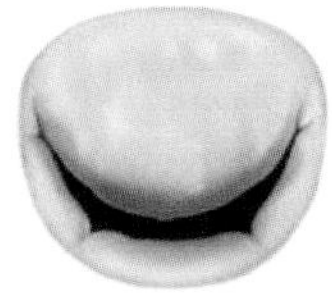	Ischemic cardiomyopathy Dilated cardiomyopathy Endocarditis Congenital

Type II
Increased leaflet motion
(leaflet prolapse)
	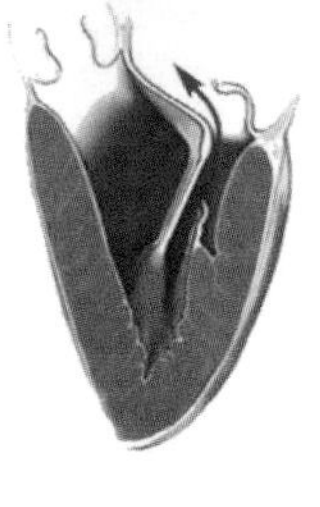	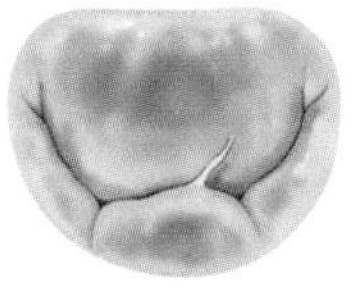	Degenerative disease
			  Fibroelastic deficiency
			  Marfan syndrome
			  Forme fruste Barlow
			  Barlow disease
			Endocarditis
			Rheumatic disease
			Trauma
			Ischemic cardiomyopathy
			Ehlers-Danlos syndrome

Type IIIA Restricted leaflet motion (restricted opening)	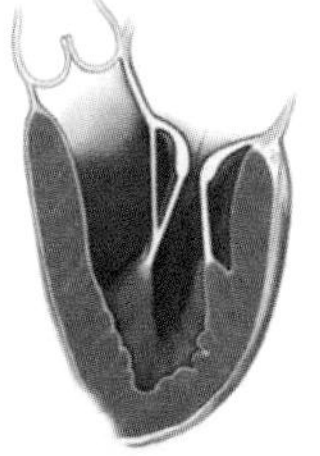	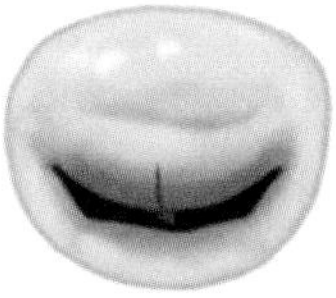	Rheumatic disease Carcinoid disease Radiation Lupus erythematosus Ergotamine use Hypereosinophilic syndrome Mucopolysaccharidosis
Type IIIB Restricted leaflet motion (restricted closure)	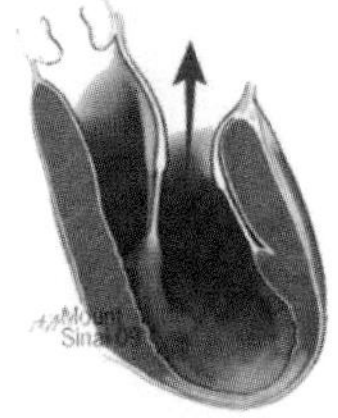	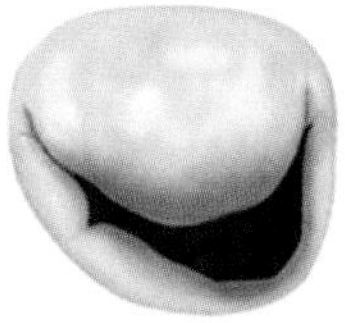	Ischemic cardiomyopathy Dilated cardiomyopathy

FIGURE 76.3 Pathophysiologic triad approach to mitral regurgitation (MR) and its multifactorial etiology. The mechanism of leaflet dysfunction defines the three types of MR. (From Castillo JG, Adams DH. Mitral valve repair and replacement. In: Otto CM, Bonow RO, eds. *Valvular Heart Disease: A Companion to Braunwald's Heart Disease.* Philadelphia: Saunders; 2013:327-340.)

PRIMARY MITRAL REGURGITATION

Clinical Presentation

The clinical stages of primary chronic degenerative MR are indicated in Table 76.2, demonstrating the progressive nature of the disease.

Symptoms

The nature and severity of symptoms in patients with chronic MR are functions of a combination of interrelated factors, including the severity of MR, rate of its progression, level of LA, pulmonary venous, and pulmonary arterial (PA) pressure, presence of episodic or chronic atrial tachyarrhythmias, and presence of associated valvular, myocardial, or coronary artery disease. In addition, there may be symptoms related to the underlying pathogenic cause of the MR (e.g., endocarditis, lupus, or Marfan syndrome). Many patients with severe MR remain completely asymptomatic, though close questioning of the patient or family may reveal subtle reductions in functional capacity (i.e., chronic weakness or fatigue). Symptoms may occur with preserved LV contractile function in patients with chronic MR who have severely elevated pulmonary venous pressures or AF. In other patients, symptoms herald LV decompensation.

Physical Examination (see Chapter 13)

Palpation of the arterial pulse is helpful in differentiating aortic stenosis (AS) from MR, both of which may produce a prominent systolic murmur at the base of the heart and apex (see Chapter 13). The carotid arterial upstroke is sharp in severe MR and delayed in AS; the volume of the pulse may be normal or reduced in the presence of HF. The cardiac impulse, like the arterial pulse, is brisk and hyperdynamic. It is displaced to the left, and a prominent LV filling wave is frequently palpable in thin patients.

Auscultation. S_1, produced by MV closure, is often diminished in patients with primary MR and defective valve leaflets. Wide splitting of S_2 is common and results from shortening of LV ejection and an earlier A_2 as a consequence of reduced resistance to LV ejection. In patients with severe pulmonary hypertension, P_2 is louder than A_2. The abnormal increase in the flow rate across the mitral orifice during the rapid filling phase is often associated with an S_3, which should not be interpreted as a feature of HF in these patients, and this may be accompanied by a brief diastolic rumble.

The systolic murmur is the most prominent physical finding; it must be differentiated from the systolic murmur of AS, tricuspid regurgitation, and ventricular septal defect. In most patients with severe MR, the systolic murmur commences immediately after the soft S_1 and continues beyond and may obscure A_2 because of the persisting pressure difference between the LV and LA after aortic valve closure. The holosystolic murmur of chronic MR is usually constant in intensity, blowing, high-pitched, and loudest at the apex, with frequent radiation to the left axilla and left infrascapular area, particularly with posteriorly directed jets. Radiation toward the sternum or aortic area, however, may occur with abnormalities of the posterior leaflet associated with an anteriorly directed regurgitant jet and is particularly common in patients with MVP and flail involving this leaflet (see Fig. 16.26). The murmur shows little change, even in the presence of large beat-to-beat variations of LV stroke volume, as in AF. This finding contrasts with that in most midsystolic (ejection) murmurs, such as in AS, which vary greatly in intensity with stroke volume and therefore with the duration of diastole. Little correlation has been found between the intensity of the systolic murmur and severity of MR.

The murmur of MR may be holosystolic, late systolic, or early systolic. When the murmur is confined to late systole, the regurgitation usually is secondary to MVP and may follow one or more mid-systolic clicks and typically is not severe. Such late systolic MR is often associated with a normal S_1 because initial closure of the MV cusps may be unimpaired. A midsystolic click preceding a mid- to late-systolic murmur, and the

response of that murmur to a number of maneuvers helps establish the diagnosis of MVP (discussed subsequently). Early systolic murmurs are typical of acute MR. When the LA v wave is markedly elevated in acute MR, the murmur may diminish or disappear in late systole as the reverse pressure gradient declines. As noted, a short, low-pitched diastolic murmur following S_3 may be audible in patients with severe MR, even without accompanying MS, due to increased early diastolic flow.

Dynamic Auscultation. Auscultation during positional changes or the Valsalva maneuver can be quite helpful in characterizing the MR murmur. When MR is holosystolic, it typically varies little during respiration. However, sudden standing usually diminishes the murmur, whereas squatting augments it. The late systolic murmur of MVP behaves in the opposite direction, decreasing in duration with squatting and increasing in duration with standing. Similarly, with the Valsalva maneuver, MVP clicks may occur earlier in systole with lengthening of the murmur. Holosystolic MR murmur is often softer during the strain of the Valsalva maneuver and shows a left-sided response (i.e., a transient overshoot that occurs six to eight beats after release of the strain). The murmur of MR usually is intensified by isometric exercise, differentiating it from the systolic murmurs of valvular AS and obstructive hypertrophic cardiomyopathy, both of which are reduced by this intervention.

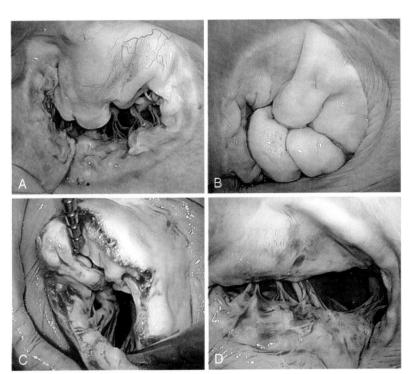

FIGURE 76.4 **Valve lesions in mitral regurgitation. A,** Severe annular dilation leading to type I dysfunction. **B,** Severe myxomatous changes with redundant, thick, and bulky segments in a patient with Barlow disease and type II dysfunction. **C,** Rheumatic mitral valve disease with classic "fish mouth" appearance and type IIIA dysfunction. **D,** Ischemic mitral valve disease caused by severe tethering of the P_3 scallop leading to type HIB dysfunction. (From Castillo JG, Adams DH. Mitral valve repair and replacement. In: Otto CM, Bonow RO, eds. *Valvular Heart Disease: A Companion to Braunwald's Heart Disease.* 5th ed. Philadelphia: Saunders; 2021:370-379.)

Echocardiography (see Chapter 16)

Echocardiography plays an integral role in the diagnosis of primary MR, in determining its cause and potential for repair, and in quantifying its severity (see Chapter 16). Assessment of MR severity by echocardiography can be divided into four general categories: structural, qualitative, semi-quantitative, and quantitative.[18] Structural assessment of patients with severe MR, includes not only the determination of valve morphology and mechanisms of MR (see Figs, 16.36, 16.37, and 80.5), but should also provide measures of LV systolic function, severity of dilation of the LV and LA, and right heart size and function. Quantification of mitral leaflet lengths, severity of tethering, and the severity of leaflet displacement into the atrium may be important for determining the success of surgical or transcatheter interventions.

All other assessments of MR severity rely on a number of Doppler echocardiographic modalities. Doppler echocardiography in MR characteristically reveals a high-velocity systolic jet in the LA during systole.[23] Qualitative assessment of MR severity uses color Doppler to assess the color jet area and flow convergence (vena contracta), and continuous wave Doppler to evaluate the density and shape of the regurgitant jet spectral profile (see eFig.16.26).

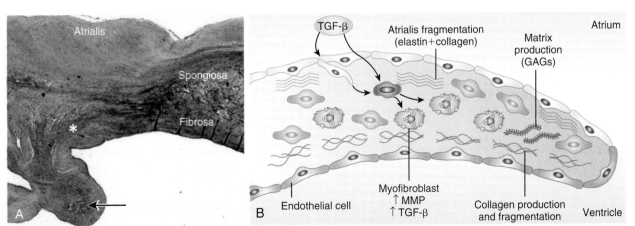

FIGURE 76.5 **Mechanisms of mitral valve prolapse (MVP). A,** Mitral valve stained with hematoxylin and eosin to define the lesion of MVP as disruption of the fibrosa by myxoid extracellular matrix (*), which also infiltrates the collagen core of the chordae tendineae, one of which was ruptured (*arrow*). The elastin lamina beneath the atrialis is also disrupted **B,** Schematic showing the mechanism of myxomatous degeneration, with activation of valve interstitial cells to myofibroblasts that increase matrix production and turnover, secrete MMPs that drive collagen and elastin fragmentation, and release transforming growth factor (TGF)-β, which in turn promotes further cell proliferation and myofibroblast differentiation. *GAGs,* Glycosaminoglycans; *MMP,* matrix metalloproteinase. (From Levine RA, et al. Mitral valve disease: morphology and mechanisms. *Nat Rev Cardiol.* 2015;12:689-710.)

TABLE 76.2 Stages of Chronic Primary Mitral Regurgitation

STAGE	DEFINITION	VALVE ANATOMY	VALVE HEMODYNAMICS*	HEMODYNAMIC CONSEQUENCES	SYMPTOMS
A	At risk for MR	Mild MVP with normal coaptation Mild valve thickening and leaflet restriction	No MR jet or small central jet area <20% LA on Doppler Small vena contracta <0.3 cm	None	None
B	Progressive MR	Moderate to severe MVP with normal coaptation Rheumatic valve changes with leaflet restriction and loss of central coaptation Previous IE	Central jet MR 20%-40% LA or late systolic eccentric jet MR Vena contracta <0.7 cm Rvol <60 mL RF <50% ERO <0.40 cm² Angiographic grade 1-2+	Mild LA enlargement No LV enlargement Normal pulmonary pressure	None
C	Asymptomatic severe MR	Severe MVP with loss of coaptation or flail leaflet Rheumatic valve changes with leaflet restriction and loss of central coaptation Previous IE Thickening of leaflets with radiation heart disease	Central jet MR >40% LA or holosystolic eccentric jet MR Vena contracta ≥0.7 cm Rvol ≥60 mL RF ≥50% ERO ≥0.40 cm² Angiographic grade 3-4+	Moderate or severe LA enlargement LV enlargement Pulmonary hypertension may be present at rest or with exercise. C1: LVEF >60% and LVESD <40 mm C2: LVEF ≤60% and LVESD ≥40 mm	None
D	Symptomatic severe MR	Severe MVP with loss of coaptation or flail leaflet Rheumatic valve changes with leaflet restriction and loss of central coaptation Previous IE Thickening of leaflets with radiation heart disease	Central jet MR >40% LA or holosystolic eccentric jet MR Vena contracta ≥0.7 cm Rvol ≥60 mL RF ≥50% ERO ≥0.40 cm² Angiographic grade 3-4+	Moderate or severe LA enlargement LV enlargement Pulmonary hypertension present	Decreased exercise tolerance Exertional dyspnea

ERO, Effective regurgitant orifice; *IE,* infective endocarditis; *LA,* left atrium; *LV,* left ventricle; *LVEF,* left ventricular ejection fraction; *LVESD,* left ventricular end-systolic dimension; *MR,* mitral regurgitation; *MVP,* mitral valve prolapse; *RF,* regurgitant fraction; *Rvol,* regurgitant volume.
*Several valve hemodynamic criteria are provided for assessment of MR severity, but not all criteria for each category will be present in each patient. Classification of MR severity as mild, moderate, or severe depends on data quality and integration of these parameters in conjunction with other clinical evidence.
From Otto CM, et al. 2020 AHA/ACC guideline for the management of patients with valvular heart disease: a report of the American College of Cardiology/American Heart Association Task Force on Practice Guidelines. *J Am Coll Cardiol.* 2021;77:e25-197.

Because color flow jet areas are significantly influenced by the driving pressure (LV-LA gradient) and momentum within the LA, hemodynamic factors (i.e., blood pressure, LA and LV compliance), jet eccentricity, as well as instrument factors (i.e., transmit power and frequency, receiver gain, Nyquist limit, and wall filter) limit the accuracy of this approach.[23] Importantly, though, the color Doppler jet duration and direction can give important clues as to the mechanism of the MR. In primary MR, the jet may be late systolic with a direction typically away from the most significant anatomic lesion, so posterior prolapse or flail typically produces an anterior jet and vice versa. With secondary MR, regurgitation is frequently bimodal, peaking in both early and late systole, with or without directionality depending on the presence of anterior leaflet override of a tethered posterior leaflet.

Semi-quantitative assessment of MR severity include measurements of components of the color Doppler regurgitant jet: flow convergence, jet width at the vena contracta, and jet area (see eFig. 16.26). Because these measurements are performed at a single point in the cardiac cycle and assume a symmetric regurgitant orifice, semi-quantitative methods become less accurate in the setting of temporal variability, nonplanar leaflet conformation and noncircular regurgitant orifices.

Quantification of MR Severity
Quantitative methods to measure regurgitant fraction, regurgitant volume (Rvol), and regurgitant orifice area have greater accuracy when done carefully (Fig. 76.6), and these methods are strongly recommended (see Table 76.2).[1,2,18] There are three methods for quantifying MR severity: proximal isovelocity surface area (PISA), volumetric Doppler, and three-dimensional direct planimetry of the vena contracta area.

The PISA method is perhaps the most practical quantitative method for daily use (see Chapter 16).[18,23] It exploits the predictable flow acceleration leading into the MV, which forms roughly hemispheric isovelocity shells that can be highlighted by shifting the aliasing velocity of the color display and identified where the color changes from blue to red (see Fig. 16.38). If the radial distance is r from the vena contracta to the contour with velocity v, then the flow rate Q will be given by

$$Q = 2\pi r^2 v$$

from which the effective regurgitant orifice area (EROA) can be obtained by dividing Q by the maximal velocity through the orifice obtained by continuous-wave (CW) Doppler (Vmax). A handy simplification that works in the majority of cases assumes approximately 100 mm Hg driving pressure across the regurgitant orifice (leading, via the Bernoulli equation, to a 5 m/sec maximal jet velocity). If the aliasing velocity is set to (approximately) 40 cm/sec, the math simplifies to EROA = r^2/2. An approximation to Rvol can be obtained by multiplying EROA by the velocity time integral of the regurgitant CW signal.

There are some important caveats to use of the PISA equation, the most critical of which involves nonholosystolic jets, such as those occurring with MVP in which the MR does not begin until the latter half of systole. In this case, the MR is much less severe than a single frame showing either the largest jet, vena contracta, or convergence zone would imply. Additional pitfalls include situations in which there are two or more regurgitant jets. Finally, the PISA method quantifies EROA with calculation of the Rvol. Regurgitant fraction requires a measure of total LV stroke volume and thus cannot be directly measured by this technique.

The volumetric Doppler method (see Fig 16.39) quantifies Rvol as the difference between the diastolic stroke volume across the MV and the forward stroke volume (typically using the LV outflow stroke volume). The expertise required to accurately measure these stroke volumes make this method less practical for general use. However, this method is not limited by MR temporal variability, multiple jets, or elliptical orifice. In addition, this method allows the quantitation of all three measures of MR severity important for making decisions about

intervention: regurgitant fraction, Rvol, and EROA. This is the preferred method in many comprehensive valve centers.

Finally, improvements in three-dimensional imaging permit acquisition of color Doppler volumes for direct planimetry of the vena contracta area. This method is more difficult for transthoracic compared with transesophageal echocardiography.

Supportive evidence for MR severity can be found in pulmonary venous flow (see eFig. 16.26). The normal pattern of systolic (S) wave greater than diastolic (D) wave generally indicates mild MR, frank systolic reversal indicates severe MR, but the common "blunted" pattern (S < D) may be seen in all degrees of MR. A transmitral E-wave >1.2 m/sec is supportive of severe MR, whereas a pattern with E < A virtually excludes severe MR. Doppler echocardiography also is an important tool to estimate the PA systolic pressure and to determine the presence and severity of associated aortic or tricuspid regurgitation.

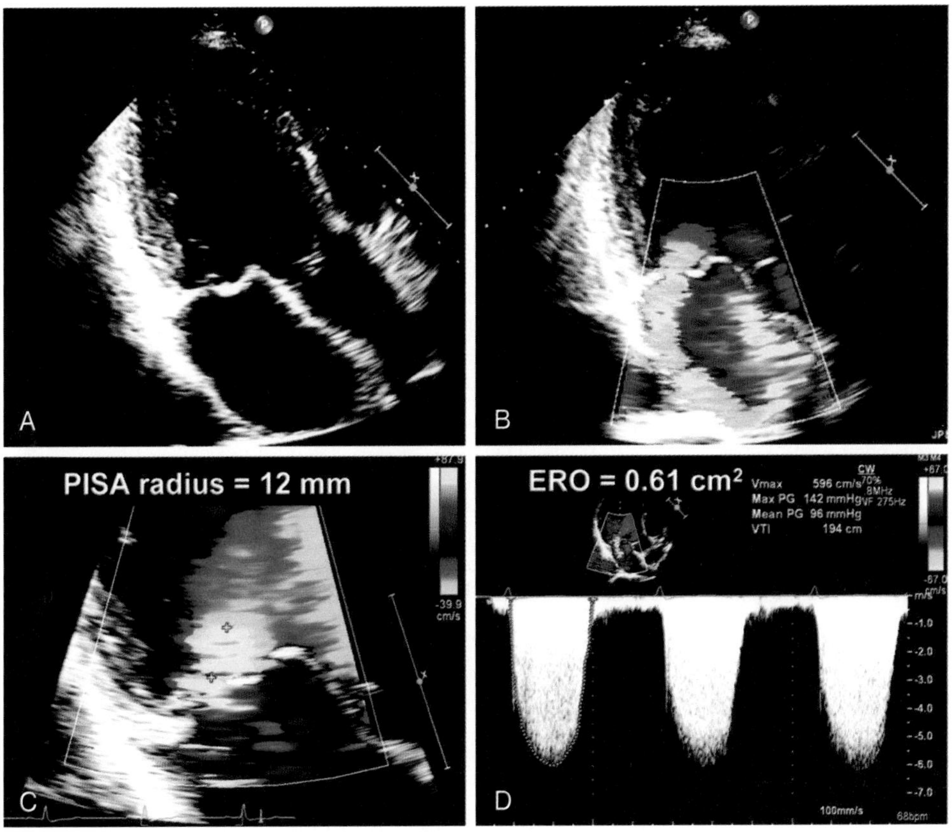

Transesophageal Echocardiography

Transesophageal echocardiography (TEE) may be needed in addition to transthoracic imaging for assessment of the detailed anatomy of the regurgitant MV, the mechanisms of MR, and the severity of MR in some patients (see Chapter 16). Because the MV is in the far-field of all transthoracic imaging planes, TEE has significant advantages for imaging the morphology of the valve and severity of MR, particularly when transthoracic imaging is limited or discordant with clinical presentation. TEE imaging is also recommended for patients in whom surgical or transcatheter intervention is contemplated to assess anatomic suitability.[1] Three-dimensional imaging and three-dimensional color Doppler[24] help elucidate the mechanism and severity of MR (Fig. 76.7; see also Fig. 16.36) but also becomes an essential tool to guide interventions.

Exercise Echocardiography

Assessment of LV function, MR severity, and PA systolic pressure can be extremely helpful in determining severity of MR and hemodynamic abnormalities (e.g., pulmonary hypertension) during exercise.[25] This is a useful objective means to evaluate symptomatic patients who appear to

FIGURE 76.6 **Severe mitral regurgitation (MR) caused by prolapse of the mitral valve with quantitative determination of effective regurgitant orifice area (ERO) on echocardiography. A** and **B,** Severe prolapse of the mitral valve with severe MR. **C** and **D,** ERO was calculated with the proximal isovelocity surface area (PISA) radius and peak velocity of the MR jet. (From Kang DH, et al. Comparison of early surgery versus conventional treatment in asymptomatic severe mitral regurgitation. *Circulation.* 2009;119:797-804.)

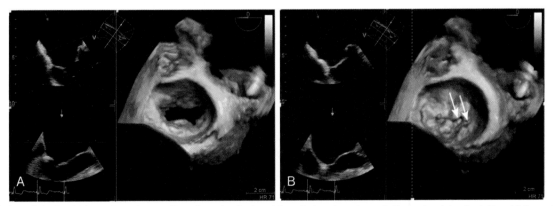

FIGURE 76.7 Three-dimensional echocardiography now allows direct visualization of the pathology, here demonstrating ruptured chordae to P_2 and P_3 (*arrows*). **A,** Ventricular diastole. **B,** Systole.

have less than severe MR at rest and, alternatively, to determine functional status and dynamic changes in hemodynamics in patients who otherwise appear stable and asymptomatic with severe MR (see section on Symptoms). Late-systolic MR may become more holosystolic with exercise, particularly if PA pressure rises significantly. Treadmill or bicycle exercise is appropriate in patients with MR. When ordering a treadmill exercise echo, one should provide guidance to the sonographer as to the priority for the various datasets to be obtained after exercise, because it is often impossible to obtain diagnostic mitral and tricuspid imaging and wall motion assessment while heart rate is still optimally high. If the focus is on the MV, rapid acquisition of mitral color and CW Doppler and tricuspid CW Doppler will usually be the priority. Semi-supine exercise testing on an appropriate tilted table allows continuous echocardiographic monitoring for quantifying changes in valvular regurgitation severity, LV function, and pulmonary pressure, offering significant advantages for the assessment of MR patients. Dobutamine echocardiography has little role in assessing organic MR but may be useful for ischemia or viability assessment in secondary MR (see section on Secondary Mitral Regurgitation).

OTHER DIAGNOSTIC EVALUATION MODALITIES (SEE PART III)
Electrocardiography
The principal electrocardiogram (ECG) findings are LA enlargement and AF. ECG evidence of LV enlargement occurs in approximately one third of patients with severe MR. Approximately 15% of patients exhibit ECG evidence of right ventricular (RV) hypertrophy, a change that reflects the presence of pulmonary hypertension of sufficient severity to counterbalance the hypertrophied LV in patients with MR.

Radiography
Cardiomegaly with LV enlargement, and particularly with LA enlargement, is a common finding in patients with chronic severe MR. Although the LA may be severely enlarged, little correlation has been found between LA size and pressure. Interstitial edema with Kerley B lines frequently is seen in patients with acute MR or with progressive LV failure.

Calcification of the mitral annulus, an important cause of MR in older adults, is most prominent in the posterior third of the cardiac silhouette. The lesion is best visualized on chest films exposed in the lateral or right anterior oblique projections (see Chapter 17), in which it appears as a dense, coarse, C-shaped opacity.

Cardiac Magnetic Resonance
Cardiac magnetic resonance (CMR) (see Chapter 19) provides accurate measurements of regurgitant flow that correlates well with quantitative Doppler imaging. It also is the most accurate noninvasive technique for measuring LV end-diastolic volume (EDV), end-systolic volume (ESV), and mass,[26] and is included in guidelines for imaging in valvular regurgitation.[18] Although detailed visualization of MV structure and function is obtained more reliably with echocardiography, particularly TEE, CMR offers a promising approach for accurate assessment of regurgitant severity and its impact on chamber size.[27]

CMR also has an evolving role for identifying the presence and severity of myocardial fibrosis for risk stratification of patients with MVP who have ventricular tachyarrhythmias and/or mitral annular disjunction (see section on Mitral Annular Disjunction).

Cardiac Computed Tomography
Cardiac CT imaging can provide useful structural information about the regurgitant MV (see Chapter 20),[28-30] with particular value in sizing the mitral annulus and quantifying the degree of annular calcification.[31] It appears to be particularly useful in planning for percutaneous MV replacement[32] and has been used in conjunction with three-dimensional printing to ensure an adequate fit of the proposed valve within the mitral apparatus.[33,34] Some have proposed CT imaging for quantification of the chamber volumes and regurgitant severity, specifically the planimetered size of the anatomic regurgitant orifice area, but this will likely remain adjunctive given the availability of echocardiography and CMR.

Left Ventricular Angiography
Given the availability of echocardiography and CMR, there is little reason to perform left ventriculography for the purpose of characterizing MR. The prompt appearance of contrast material in the LA after its injection into the LV indicates the presence of MR. The injection should be rapid enough to permit LV opacification but slow enough to avoid the development of premature ventricular contractions, which can induce spurious regurgitation (see Chapter 22). The Rvol can be estimated from the difference between the total LV stroke volume, estimated by angiocardiography, and the simultaneous measurement of the effective forward stroke volume by the Fick method.

Natural History

Although primary MR may be caused by Carpentier type I (perforation or cleft) and type IIIA (leaflet/chordal thickening) diseases, MVP is the most common cause of chronic primary MR in developed countries and is defined by an overriding of the annulus by a leaflet edge with displacement of the coaptation point into the atrium. Leaflet "flail" implies coaptation failure with eversion of the free edge of a leaflet into the LA, usually consequent to chordal rupture (see Fig. 76.7; see also Fig. 16.36). Echocardiography has been central to the diagnosis of MVP and flail (see Chapter 16). Because of the normal saddle shape of the annulus, diagnostic criteria for MVP were refined to include single-leaflet or bileaflet displacement >2 mm beyond the long-axis annular plane, with >5 mm leaflet thickening.[35,36] Using this more specific criteria, the prevalence of echocardiographically diagnosed MVP is ~2% to 3%. Multimodality imaging is useful to confirm the severity of regurgitation and assess myocardial fibrosis, which can accompany variants of this disease.[18,36,37]

Although screening of the general population indicates that many individuals with MVP have few clinical symptoms in large clinical populations, the disease is strongly associated with HF, need for valve surgery, development of AF, and increased mortality.[38] In a community-based study of 833 asymptomatic patients with MVP, 10-year all-cause mortality was 19% ± 2% and cardiovascular mortality was 9% ± 2% (see Avierinos et al., Classic References). In a retrospective analysis of patients presenting with moderate or severe MR, a primary etiology was identified in approximately one-third of patients, of whom >70% had MVP.[39] Compared with patients with secondary MR, patients with moderate or severe primary MR had larger Rvol, moderate cardiac remodeling, normal stroke volume index, and mildly elevated pulmonary pressure, yet had a 40% 5-year HF rate and increased risk of mortality (risk ratio, 1.83 [1.50 to 2.22]; $P < 0.0001$).[39] An increase in mortality with MVP is related to the quantitative severity of MR (adjusted hazard ratio [HR], 1.15; 95% confidence interval [CI], 1.10 to 1.20; $P < 0.0001$ per 10 mm^2).[40]

Left Ventricular Volumes and Systolic Function
In addition to severity of MR, outcomes are associated with LV size, with mortality risk increasing linearly with LV end-systolic dimension (ESD) >40 mm (HR, 1.15; 95% CI 1.04 to 1.27 per 1-mm increment) or LVESD index ≥22 mm/m^2 (adjusted HR 1.12; 95% CI, 1.01 to 1.23 per 1-mm/m^2 LVESD increment; $p = 0.01$).[41] Although surgery was associated with reduced mortality (adjusted HR, 0.62; 95% CI, 0.45 to 0.86; $p = 0.0035$), LVESD ≥40 mm was an independent predictor of reduced postsurgical survival.

In the setting of chronic severe MR, the LV end-diastolic volume (LVEDV) increases, which, by means of the Laplace principle, results in increased systolic LV wall stress, a stimulus for eccentric hypertrophy. Initially the reduced afterload is associated with increased ejection phase indices of myocardial contractility (i.e., LV ejection fraction [LVEF], fractional fiber shortening, and velocity of circumferential fiber shortening). However, prolonged hemodynamic overload ultimately leads to myocardial decompensation, an increase in LV end-diastolic pressure, and eventually a decrease in LV contractility despite only modest decreases in LVEF, which often remains in the normal or near-normal range. Long-term follow-up of 1875 patients with significant MR secondary to flail MV in the Mitral Regurgitation International Database (MIDA) registry,[42] patients with LVEF of 45% to 60% represented a large proportion of patients (23%), who rarely exhibited overt symptoms, and had higher mortality compared with EF >60%. An LVEF <60% was associated with an adjusted HR of 1.51 (1.22 to 1.87) and an EF <45% with an adjusted HR of 2.46 (1.67 to 3.61). The benefit of surgery was significant in the groups with EF <45% (adjusted HR, 0.28 [0.17 to

0.56]) and with EF of 45% to 60% (adjusted HR, 0.34 [0.21 to 0.64]).[42,43] A measure of longitudinal LV mechanics, global longitudinal strain (GLS) may be a more sensitive and accurate measurement of LV function than LVEF (see Chapter 16). In a study of 593 patients with severe primary MR (Barlow disease, fibroelastic deficiency, or forme fruste) who underwent MV surgery, LV-GLS ≥−20.6% (more impaired) showed significantlu worse survival than did patients with LV-GLS ≤−20.6% (p < 0.001) and GLS LV-GLS had incremental prognostic value over clinical risk factors for long-term survival.[44] The role of GLS in determining the timing of surgery remains unexplored.

Mitral Annular Disjunction

Mitral annular disjunction (MAD) has received growing awareness as a marker for risk of ventricular arrhythmias and sudden death in patients with MVP. This term describes abnormal spatial displacement of the point of insertion of the posterior MV leaflet, which results in a wide separation between the LA wall and MV junction and the LV attachment.[37,45] MAD has gained attention in recent years because of its association with frequent premature ventricular beats and nonsustained ventricular tachycardia, suggesting that it may be a marker of a "malignant" form of MVP. Although the incidence of sudden cardiac death is low among patients with MVP (estimated to be 0.2% to 0.4% per year),[46] this incidence is 3 times higher than that in the general population; thus, the prevalence of MVP of 2% to 3% suggests that the absolute number at risk is considerable. CMR imaging has shown late gadolinium enhancement indicative of myocardial fibrosis in patients with arrhythmias and MAD.[27,47,48] Additional risk findings include inverted or biphasic T waves, QT dispersion, QT prolongation, and premature ventricular contractions originating from the LVOT and papillary muscles, paradoxical systolic increase of the mitral annulus diameter, and increased tissue Doppler velocity of the mitral annulus.[37,46] In early studies, MAD was reported as a specific finding in patients with MVP, but more recent studies suggest that MAD associated with arrhythmias can occur in those without MVP and may be a separate morphologic entity.[47] Although arrhythmogenic MVP has been associated with increased MR severity,[47] recent data have shown no association with either MR severity or LV systolic dysfunction.[49]

Symptoms

The onset of symptoms in patients with severe chronic primary MR, regardless of LV function, is also associated with poor outcomes. Although "watchful waiting" often has been the treatment strategy for asymptomatic patients with severe organic MR, there is growing evidence that patients with severe primary MR who have no or minimal symptoms not only have lower operative mortality but would have improved long-term outcomes if surgery was performed before the onset of symptoms,[43,50] with societal recommendations to consider early surgery in patients who are candidates for MV repair.[1,2,51] Propensity score matching of early surgery and initial medical management groups in the MIDA registry confirmed higher survival after early surgery (HR, 0.52; 95% CI, 0.35 to 0.79; P= 0.002).[43] In the absence of symptoms, 10-year survival was also better with early surgery (84%; 95% CI, 78% to 90%) compared with initial medical management (78%; 95% CI, 72% to 85%; P=0.04). There was also an independent protective effect associated with early surgery upon late HF risk. Notably in this study, 93% of patients had MV repair performed. Similarly, in a study of 1234 patients with primary MR who underwent MV repair, long-term (median 13 years) survival was significantly associated with severity of symptoms, with highest survival rates among those who were asymptomatic before surgery (Fig. 76.8).[50] There is growing use of exercise testing to either elicit symptoms in asymptomatic patients with severe MR or confirm the cause of symptoms in patients with less than severe MR.[1,25]

A MIDA score has been proposed in which clinical parameters are used to assess mortality risk, which would be applicable to both medical and surgical treatment.[52] The several clinical parameters of the MIDA score and their point assignments (determined by Cox proportional hazard, competing risk, and competing risk with imputation models) are age ≥65 years (3 points), symptoms (3 points), RV systolic pressure >50 mm Hg (2 points), AF (1 point), LA diameter ≥55 mm (1 point), LV end-systolic diameter ≥40 mm (1 point), and LVEF ≤60% (1 point). MIDA score was associated with long-term risk of death under

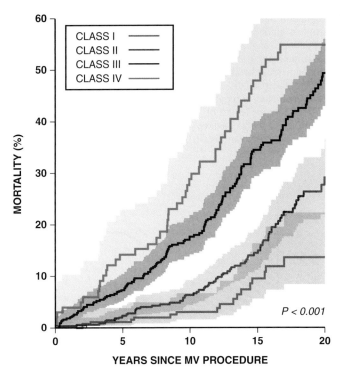

FIGURE 76.8 Survival over the course of 2 decades after mitral valve (MV) repair among 1234 patients with severe primary mitral regurgitation. Long-term postoperative survival was significantly associated with presence and severity of preoperative symptoms. (From David TE, et al. Long-term results of mitral valve repair for regurgitation due to leaflet prolapse. *J Am Coll Cardiol.* 2019;74:1044-1053.)

medical management (adjusted HR [95% CI] per unit 1.13 [1.01 to 1.22]; P < 0.001) (c = 0.81; standard deviation [SD] 0.03) and postsurgical outcome (adjusted HR [95% CI] per unit 1.35 [1.19 to 1.54]; P < 0.001). Although a simple risk score for both medical and surgical treatment (and that outperforms the standard surgical risk scores) will be of use to the clinician, the importance of integrating these and other comorbidities and weighing them against the expected benefit of surgical repair cannot be overemphasized. Both U.S. and European guidelines strongly support the involvement of the multidisciplinary heart team, for consensus decision making and with shared decision making with patient and family.[1,51]

Management of Primary Mitral Regurgitation

Medical Therapy for Primary Mitral Regurgitation

In the setting of a primary valvular disorder, medical management is limited and there are no specific recommendations for medical therapy of chronic primary MR. Treatment of hypertension is warranted according to standard guidelines for management of high blood pressure, and notably in doing so severity of MR will be reduced. However, vasodilator therapy is not indicated in normotensive patients with chronic primary MR and normal LVEF. Reduced preload and/or afterload may actually worsen MR in MVP. A meta-analysis of 19 studies evaluating the use of angiotensin-converting enzyme inhibitors and angiotensin receptor blockers (ARBs) showed only a modest change in regurgitant fraction (~8%)[53] and there is no strong evidence of benefit on clinical outcomes.[54] In the setting of reduced LVEF (<60%), however, standard guideline-directed medical therapy is indicated.

With acute, hemodynamically significant primary MR (i.e., flail), vasodilator therapy can increase forward flow but is often limited by systemic hypotension. In these instances, intra-aortic balloon counterpulsation can be helpful to treat acute severe MR.

Surgical Therapy for Primary Mitral Regurgitation

As noted previously, surgical intervention is warranted in patients with severe primary MR who are symptomatic or who have LV systolic

DISEASES OF THE HEART VALVES

dysfunction, defined as LVEF <60% or LVESD >40 mm.[1,51] Both U.S. and European guidelines recommendations are also concordant in stating that it is reasonable (Class IIa) to proceed with surgical MV repair in asymptomatic patients with severe primary MR and preserved LV function, with referral to centers that can provide durable repair at low operative risk (<1% mortality). Patients should be referred to centers experienced in repair, and patients with more complex forms of MR (e.g., anterior leaflet or bileaflet prolapse) should be referred to comprehensive valve centers.[1,2] Repair success increases with surgical volume and expertise (Fig. 76.9), which should be considered when referring a patient for surgery.[55-57] In addition, MV repair has superior outcomes to biological or mechanical MV replacement.[58] Unfortunately, national data persist in showing that many patients who are candidates for repair are treated with MV replacement, particularly at lower volume institutions.[59]

Indications for surgical intervention for chronic primary MR according to the revised ACC/AHA guidelines on management of patients with valvular heart disease[1] are listed in Table 76.3, along with a schema for patient management based on these guidelines recommendations (Fig. 76.10).

Transcatheter Therapy for Primary Mitral Regurgitation
Edge-to-Edge Repair

Transcatheter MV repair using an edge-to-edge clip between the anterior and posterior leaflets (see Fig. 78.3) is safe and effective in reducing severity of primary MR (see Chapter 78). Surgical MV repair is more effective at reducing or eliminating MR compared with the clip, but in randomized trials the clinical outcomes with the transcatheter repair were not inferior to outcomes with surgery.[60] In addition, anticipated progressive worsening after clip therapy has not been observed.

Studies of the MV clip have demonstrated improved symptoms and a reduction in MR by 2 to 3 grades leading to reverse remodeling of the LV. The revised 2020 ACC/AHA guidelines indicate that it is reasonable to perform transcatheter MV edge-to-edge repair (Class IIa) in severely symptomatic patients with primary MR who are considered at high or prohibitive surgical risk, if MV anatomy is favorable for the repair procedure and patient life expectancy is at least 1 year (see Table 76.3 and Fig. 76.10).

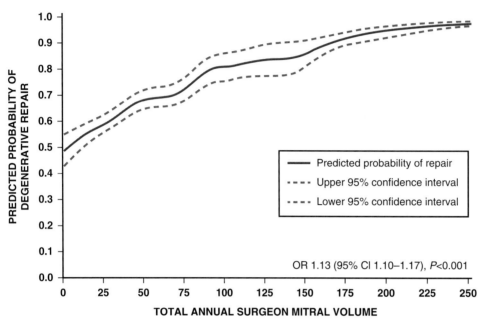

OR 1.13 (95% CI 1.10–1.17), P<0.001

FIGURE 76.9 Predicted probability of mitral repair for primary mitral regurgitation (MR) according to total annual surgeon mitral valve volume. After adjustment for preoperative risk factors, degenerative repair probability is significantly associated with total annual mitral valve surgeon volume. Data based on 5475 patients undergoing surgery by 313 surgeons in 41 hospitals in New York State. *CI,* Confidence interval; *OR,* odds ratio. (From Chikwe J, et al. Relation of mitral valve surgery volume to repair rate, durability, and survival. *J Am Coll Cardiol.* 2017;69:2397-2406.)

TABLE 76.3 Recommendations for Intervention for Chronic Primary Mitral Regurgitation.

COR	LOE	RECOMMENDATIONS
1	B-NR	1. In symptomatic patients with severe primary MR (stage D), mitral valve intervention is recommended irrespective of LV systolic function.
1	B-NR	2. In asymptomatic patients with severe primary MR and LV systolic dysfunction (LVEF ≤60%, LVESD ≥40 mm) (stage C2), mitral valve surgery is recommended.
1	B-NR	3. In patients with severe primary MR for whom surgery is indicated, mitral valve repair is recommended in preference to mitral valve replacement when the anatomic cause of MR is degenerative disease, if a successful and durable repair is possible.
2a	B-NR	4. In asymptomatic patients with severe primary MR and normal LV systolic function (LVEF ≥60% and LVESD ≤40 mm) (stage C1), mitral valve repair is reasonable when the likelihood of a successful and durable repair without residual MR is >95% with an expected mortality rate of <1%, when it can be performed at a primary or comprehensive valve center.
2b	C-LD	5. In asymptomatic patients with severe primary MR and normal LV systolic function (LVEF >60% and LVESD <40 mm) (stage C1) but with a progressive increase in LV size or decrease in EF on ≥3 serial imaging studies, mitral valve surgery may be considered irrespective of the probability of a successful and durable repair.
2a	B-NR	6. In severely symptomatic patients (NYHA Class III or IV) with primary severe MR and high or prohibitive surgical risk, transcatheter edge-to-edge repair (TEER) is reasonable if mitral valve anatomy is favorable for the repair procedure and patient life expectancy is at least 1 year.
2b	B-NR	7. In symptomatic patients with severe primary MR attributable to rheumatic valve disease, mitral valve repair may be considered at a comprehensive valve center by an experienced team when surgical treatment is indicated, if a durable and successful repair is likely.
3: Harm	B-NR	8. In patients with severe primary MR in which leaflet pathology is limited to less than half the posterior leaflet, mitral valve replacement should not be performed unless mitral valve repair has been attempted at a primary or comprehensive valve center and was unsuccessful.

EF, Ejection fraction; *LV,* left ventricle; *LVEF,* LV ejection fraction; *LVESD,* LV end-systolic dimension; *MR,* mitral regurgitation; *NYHA,* New York Heart Association.
From Otto CM, et al. 2020 AHA/ACC guideline for the management of patients with valvular heart disease: a report of the American College of Cardiology/American Heart Association Task Force on Practice Guidelines. *J Am Coll Cardiol.* 2021;77:e25-197.

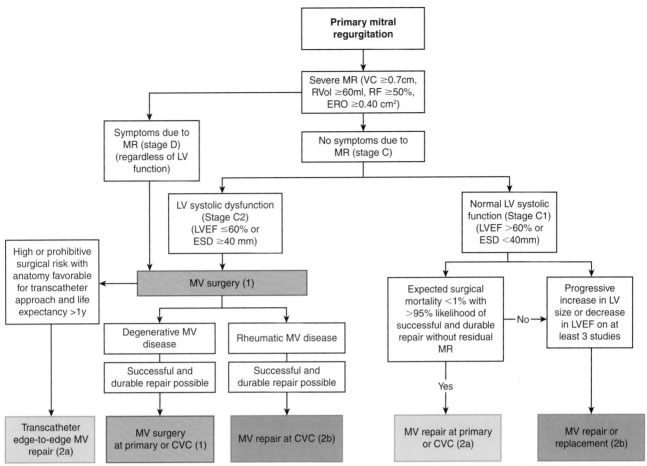

FIGURE 76.10 Management strategy for intervention for primary mitral regurgitation. Colors correspond to Table 76.3. *CVC,* Comprehensive valve center; *ERO,* effective regurgitant orifice; *ESD,* end-systolic dimension; *LVEF,* ejection fraction; *MR,* mitral regurgitation; *MV,* mitral valve; *MVR,* mitral valve replacement; *RF,* regurgitant fraction; *RVol,* regurgitant volume; *VC,* vena contracta. (From Otto CM, et al. 2020 AHA/ACC guideline for the management of patients with valvular heart disease: a report of the American College of Cardiology/American Heart Association Task Force on Practice Guidelines. *J Am Coll Cardiol.* 2021;77:e25-e197.)

A retrospective study of 100 low- to intermediate-risk elderly patients with primary MR treated with edge-to-edge repair compared with 206 patients with isolated surgical repair, showed that transcatheter repair resulted in lower acute postoperative complications and improved 1-year survival compared with surgery. However, the transcatheter approach was associated with greater MR recurrence and reduced survival beyond 1 year.[61] Another study that assigned patients to surgical versus transcatheter repair based on recommendations of a heart team[62] showed that such an individualized treatment strategy was effective. Low-risk patients with favorable anatomy were assigned to surgical repair, whereas high-risk patients with favorable anatomy for edge-to-edge repair underwent transcatheter therapy, and those with unfavorable anatomy were assigned to surgical replacement. Overall, surgical repair patients had higher 4-year survival (HR, 0.40; 95% CI, 0.26 to 0.63); $p < 0.001$) and fewer combined endpoints (HR, 0.51; 95% CI, 0.32 to 0.80; $p < 0.001$) compared with the other interventions, but the 4-year mortality for edge-to-edge repair for primary MR was low (~10%). Results of a meta-analysis of nine studies investigating the 1-year outcome of transcatheter edge-to-edge repair in patients with secondary versus primary MR ($n = 2615$) showed no significant differences in mortality rate (RR 1.26; 95% CI: 0.90 to 1.77; $p = 0.18$).[63]

The ideal anatomy for edge-to-edge repair for nonrheumatic primary MR come from the EVEREST trial and include involvement limited to the A2/P2 scallop, absence of calcium in the grasping zone, baseline MV area ≥4 cm², flail width <15 mm and flail gap <10 mm.[64] Several authors, however, have shown the feasibility of expanding these criteria.[65-67]

Investigational Devices

A number of other devices are under investigation for transcatheter repair of both primary and secondary MR. These include edge-to-edge devices, chordal repair therapies, and annuloplasty devices (see Fig. 78.6). In addition, trials of transcatheter approaches to MV replacement (TMVR) are in progress. These devices are discussed in detail in Chapter 78.

SECONDARY MITRAL REGURGITATION

Pathophysiology

The two main etiologies of secondary MR are annular dilation or atriogenic MR (Carpentier type I) and leaflet tethering from a ventricular disease (Carpentier IIIA) (see Fig 76.2). Atriogenic MR has gained increasing recognition as the etiology of MR in the setting of normal LV mechanics. Recent studies suggest the underlying mechanism is related to insufficient leaflet growth, LA dilation and annular dilation with altered annular dynamics.[15,17,68] In patients with HF and preserved EF (HFpEF), the Acute Decompensated Heart Failure Syndromes (ATTEND) registry found a significantly higher risk of reaching the clinical endpoint in patients with mild or moderate/severe secondary MR compared with patients without MR. Abe et al.[69] showed a prevalence of MR of ~8% in a HFpEF population, a significantly higher prevalence of adverse events (cardiac death, hospitalization from worsening HF, or mitral/tricuspid valve surgery) with a HR of 4.0; 95% CI, 2.3 to 7.0 per 1-grade increase. Although specific treatment of atriogenic MR in the setting of HFpEF has not been systematically studied, rhythm control may play a role. Atriogenic MR decreases in response to restoration of sinus rhythm after AF cardioversion and ablation.[16,70]

Secondary MR stemming from LV dilation and systolic dysfunction, often with concomitant mitral annular dilation, is a common consequence of ischemic and nonischemic cardiomyopathies (see Chapters 40 and 52).[71,72] The clinical stages of secondary MR are indicated in Table 76.4. In the setting of LV dysfunction and dilation, secondary MR results from displacement of the papillary muscles, tethering of the MV leaflets, and alteration of annular mechanics.[10,38] The etiology of LV dysfunction can be either ischemic or nonischemic (see Fig. 16.27B). A number of mechanisms may contribute to malcoaptation of the MV leaflets in secondary MR (Fig. 76.11; see also Fig. 16.37): (1) global and/or regional LV dilation/dysfunction that decreases the closing forces of the leaflets, (2) displacement of the papillary muscles with tethering of the leaflets into the ventricular cavity, which outweighs the closing forces, (3) dilation and dysfunction of the annulus, and (4) inadequate leaflet adaptation to ventricular or atrial enlargement.[10,73,74] The anatomic features associated with these mechanisms thus predict the severity of MR and recurrence after surgical repair: mitral leaflet tethering and restricted closure, asymmetric displacement and abnormal contraction of the LV wall underlying the papillary muscles, decreased shortening of the distance between the papillary muscles, and increased LV sphericity.[10]

Clinical Presentation

Symptoms

Patients with secondary MR related to LV dysfunction often present with HF symptoms, but many are asymptomatic (at least with regard to the MR), with MR detected incidentally on physical examination or echocardiography. AF is common.

Physical Examination. An apical S_3 is a common finding. Unlike primary MR, the systolic murmur of secondary MR related to LV dilation

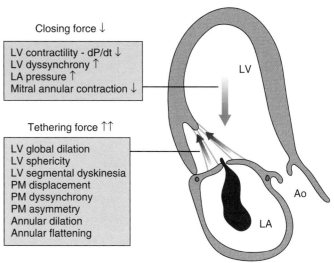

Closing force ↓

LV contractility - dP/dt ↓
LV dyssynchrony ↑
LA pressure ↑
Mitral annular contraction ↓

Tethering force ↑↑

LV global dilation
LV sphericity
LV segmental dyskinesia
PM displacement
PM dyssynchrony
PM asymmetry
Annular dilation
Annular flattening

FIGURE 76.11 Tethering and closing forces. The imbalance between tethering and closing forces result in secondary mitral regurgitation. (From Bertrand PB, et al. Exercise dynamics in secondary mitral regurgitation: pathophysiology and therapeutic implications. *Circulation.* 2017;135:297-314.)

TABLE 76.4 Stages of Chronic Secondary Mitral Regurgitation					
STAGE	DEFINITION	VALVE ANATOMY	VALVE HEMODYNAMICS*	ASSOCIATED CLINICAL FINDINGS	SYMPTOMS
A	At risk of MR	Normal valve leaflets, chords, and annulus in a patient with coronary disease or cardiomyopathy	No MR jet or small central jet area <20% LA on Doppler. Small vena contracta <0.30 cm	Normal or mildly dilated LV size with fixed (infarction) or inducible (ischemia) regional wall motion abnormalities. Primary myocardial disease with LV dilation and systolic dysfunction	Symptoms attributable to coronary ischemia or HF may be present that respond to revascularization and appropriate medical therapy
B	Progressive MR	Regional wall motion abnormalities with mild tethering of mitral leaflet. Annular dilation with mild loss of central coaptation of the mitral leaflets	ERO[†] <0.40 cm². Rvol <60 mL. RF <50%	Regional wall motion abnormalities with reduced LV systolic function. LV dilation and systolic dysfunction attributable to primary myocardial disease	Symptoms attributable to coronary ischemia or HF may be present that respond to revascularization and appropriate medical therapy
C	Asymptomatic severe MR	Regional wall motion abnormalities and/or LV dilation with severe tethering of mitral leaflet. Annular dilation with severe loss of central coaptation of the mitral leaflets	ERO[†] ≥0.40 cm². Rvol ≥60 mL. RF ≥50%	Regional wall motion abnormalities with reduced LV systolic function. LV dilation and systolic dysfunction attributable to primary myocardial disease	Symptoms attributable to coronary ischemia or HF may be present that respond to revascularization and appropriate medical therapy
D	Symptomatic severe MR	Regional wall motion abnormalities and/or LV dilation with severe tethering of mitral leaflet. Annular dilation with severe loss of central coaptation of mitral leaflets	ERO[†] ≥0.40 cm². Rvol ≥60 mL. RF ≥50%	Regional wall motion abnormalities with reduced LV systolic function. LV dilation and systolic dysfunction attributable to primary myocardial disease	HF symptoms attributable to MR persist even after revascularization and optimization of medical therapy. Decreased exercise tolerance. Exertional dyspnea

ERO, Effective regurgitant orifice; *HF,* heart failure; *LA,* left atrium; *LV,* left ventricular; *MR,* mitral regurgitation; *RF,* regurgitant fraction; *Rvol,* regurgitant volume.

*Several valve hemodynamic criteria are provided for assessment of MR severity, but not all criteria for each category will be present in each patient. Categorization of MR severity as mild, moderate, or severe depends on data quality and integration of these parameters in conjunction with other clinical evidence.

†The measurement of the proximal isovelocity surface area (PISA) by two-dimensional transthoracic echocardiography (TTE) in patients with secondary MR underestimates the true ERO because of the crescentic shape of the proximal convergence.

From Otto CM, et al. 2020 AHA/ACC guideline for the management of patients with valvular heart disease: a report of the American College of Cardiology/American Heart Association Task Force on Practice Guidelines. *J Am Coll Cardiol.* 2021;77:e25-197.

may be soft and barely audible, particularly in those patients with non-holosystolic MR that becomes minimal in midsystole. Thus, the physical examination can be misleading regarding the presence and severity of secondary MR. The murmur of papillary muscle dysfunction may occur in late systole and is highly variable, often accentuated or holosystolic during acute myocardial ischemia and absent when ischemia is relieved.

Echocardiography

Quantifying the severity of secondary MR by echocardiography has a number of limitations that resulted in the past in conflicting criteria in the American and European guidelines. Using the standard PISA method to assess MR severity, an EROA of 0.2 cm^2 has been associated with worse prognosis in secondary MR (Fig. 76.12) (see Grigioni et al., Classic References). Thus, European guidelines have used this cutoff to define "severe" disease.[51] However, underestimation of MR severity by this method may arise given the dynamic nature and crescent shape of the orifice in secondary MR.[75] Recognizing this issue, as well as needing to differentiate between prognostically severe and quantitatively severe secondary MR, both ASE and ACC/AHA guidelines grade severe secondary MR and primary MR the same using the cutoffs of EROA ≥0.4 cm^2, Rvol ≥60 mL and regurgitant fraction ≥50%.[1,2,18]

The various quantitative echocardiographic criteria may be discordant in secondary MR, making an assessment of severity more difficult (see Chapter 16). Rvol is dependent on loading conditions and chamber function and compliance. For instance, for the same regurgitant orifice, a higher LV systolic pressure may result in a larger Rvol and in the setting of LV dysfunction with reduced stroke volume, a low Rvol may be associated with a high regurgitant fraction. In a recent study of 423 patients with HF, Bartko et al. used the PISA method to measure EROA and Rvol, and the biplane Simpson LV volume to calculate regurgitant fraction.[76] Importantly, there was increased 5-year mortality associated with each of the measures of severity with HRs ranging from 1.37 to 1.50 ($P < 0.001$). Spline-curve analyses showed a linearly increasing risk enabling the ability to stratify patients into low-risk (EROA <20 mm^2 and Rvol <30 mL), intermediate-risk (EROA 20 to 29 mm^2 and Rvol 30 to 44 mL), and high-risk (EROA ≥30 mm^2 and Rvol ≥45 mL) groups. In the intermediate-risk group, a regurgitant fraction ≥50% was an indicator of hemodynamic severe secondary MR associated with poor outcome ($p = 0.017$). These cutoffs should be evaluated in larger patient populations and prospective trials.

Kamperidis et al.,[77] demonstrated that LV GLS is an early and more sensitive marker of LV systolic dysfunction than LVEF in patients with nonischemic dilated cardiomyopathy and significant secondary MR. In addition, Namazi and associates showed the incremental prognostic

value of LV GLS (in addition to LVEF) in secondary MR.[78] Patients with a more impaired LV GLS (> −7.0%) experienced higher mortality rates than those with a more preserved LV GLS (≤ −7.0%).

Cardiac Magnetic Resonance

CMR is useful in assessing severity of LV remodeling and contractile dysfunction as well as the pattern of myocardial fibrosis as it relates to regional dysfunction and papillary muscle dysfunction[18,79] (see Chapter 19, particularly Fig. 19.17).

Management of Secondary Mitral Regurgitation

Medical Therapy for Secondary Mitral Regurgitation

Patients with secondary MR stemming from LV dilation and dysfunction should undergo aggressive evidence-based medical management for LV systolic dysfunction[80] (see Chapter 50). In contrast to primary MR, a beneficial effect of medical therapy in patients with secondary MR, with respect to both valve function and clinical outcomes, is well established. However, this benefit is mainly attributed to a favorable impact of medical therapy on the underlying disease. Medical therapies have been shown to reduce MR in up to 40% of patients and are associated with improved outcomes.[81] Guideline-directed medical therapy (GDMT) including inhibitors of the renin-angiotensin-aldosterone system (RAAS) and beta-adrenergic blockers can significantly reduce secondary MR in 30% to 40% of patients with HF. In addition, HF guidelines have been updated to include the use of angiotensin receptor neprilysin inhibition (ARNI) in the treatment of symptomatic LV systolic dysfunction,[80] and treatment with sacubitril/valsartan has been associated with reduction in EROA related to reduction in LVEDV index ($p = 0.044$).[82] Significant reductions in secondary MR also occur with cardiac resynchronization therapy (CRT)[83] (see Chapters 50 and 58). Bartko et al.[84] showed that restoration of longitudinal papillary muscle synchronicity correlated with regression of secondary MR, which was associated with a better prognosis during the 8-year follow-up period compared with patients with no improvement in MR (adjusted HR, 0.41; 95% CI, 0.18 to 0.91; $p = 0.028$). Finally, guideline-directed management of significant coronary artery disease in the setting of ischemic MR should be instituted.[85,86]

Surgical Therapy for Secondary Mitral Regurgitation

In atriogenic secondary MR, small single-site case series[87] report good short-term outcomes after annuloplasty. However, the need for surgical intervention to treat atriogenic MR beyond rhythm control has been questioned.[16]

MV surgery is recommended at the time of coronary artery bypass surgery (CABG) in patients with LV dysfunction and severe ischemic MR. Whether concomitant MV repair should be performed during CABG in patients with moderate ischemic MR was addressed in the randomized trial conducted by the Cardiothoracic Surgical Trials Network (CTSN).[88] This trial randomized 301 patients with moderate MR (defined for this study as EROA between 0.2 and 0.4 cm^2) all requiring CABG to MV repair (with annuloplasty) versus CABG alone. Although there were significantly more patients with moderate or greater MR at 12 months in the no-repair group (31.0% versus 11.2%; $p < 0.001$), there was no difference between groups in the prespecified primary endpoint of postoperative LV end-systolic volume (ESV), nor was there any difference in mortality or major adverse cardiac events (Fig. 76.13).[88]

These results illustrate that in patients with secondary MR, the primary problem is disease of the LV myocardium, and prognosis is strongly influenced by the degree of LV dysfunction and residual ischemia. MV repair or replacement in these latter patients has a less beneficial effect on long-term outcome, particularly in those with ischemic MR, than in patients with primary MR. Thus, the indications for MV surgery are less clear for secondary MR than for primary MR, exemplified by there being no Class I or IIa indications for isolated surgery in secondary MR in the current ACC/AHA guidelines.[1] Moreover, unlike repair of primary MR caused by myxomatous disease or fibroelastic deficiency, in which an experienced surgeon can

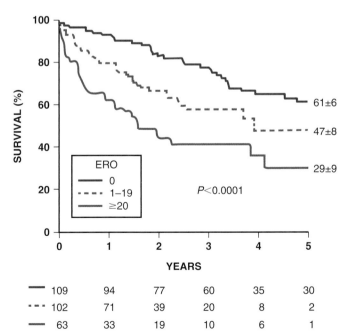

FIGURE 76.12 Survival in 303 patients with previous myocardial infarction and mean ejection fraction 34%, subgrouped by effective regurgitant orifice (ERO) according to presence and severity of ischemic mitral regurgitation (MR). Any degree of ischemic MR was associated with worse outcome than no MR. (From Grigioni F, et al. Ischemic mitral regurgitation: long-term outcome and prognostic implications with quantitative Doppler assessment. *Circulation.* 2001;103:1759-1764.)

DISEASES OF THE HEART VALVES

VIII

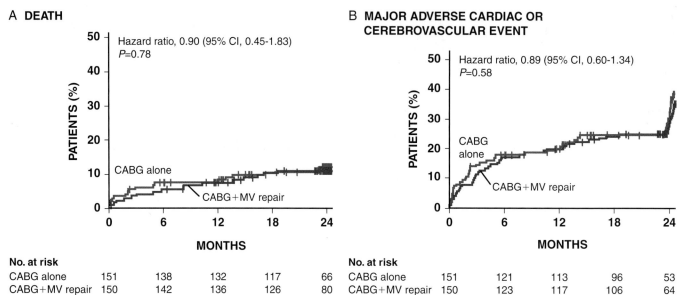

FIGURE 76.13 Two-year outcomes of patients with moderate mitral regurgitation undergoing coronary artery bypass graft (CABG) who were randomized to CABG alone versus CABG plus mitral valve (MV) repair. **A,** Death. **B,** Composite endpoint of major adverse cardiac or cerebrovascular events. (From Michler RE, et al. Two-year outcomes of surgical treatment of moderate ischemic mitral regurgitation. *N Engl J Med.* 2016;374:1932-1941.)

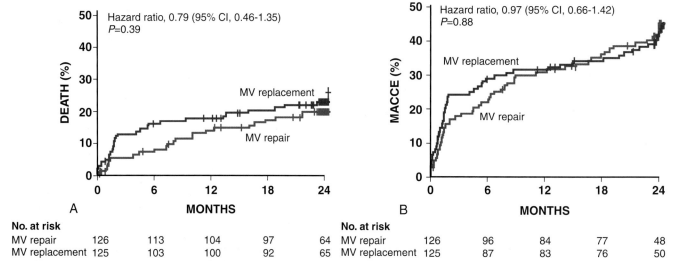

FIGURE 76.14 Postoperative outcomes of patients with ischemic mitral regurgitation randomly assigned to mitral valve (MV) repair versus replacement. **A,** Mortality. **B,** Composite endpoint of death, stroke, repeat MV surgery, hospitalization for heart failure, and increase in NYHA functional class by 1 or more. *MACCE,* major adverse cardiac or cerebrovascular events. (From Goldstein D, et al. Two-year outcomes of surgical treatment of severe ischemic mitral regurgitation. *N Engl J Med.* 2016;374:344–353.)

produce results that are durable for decades, MV repair of secondary MR is often not durable because of progression of the underlying LV myocardial disease. This has fueled suggestions that MV replacement might provide a more durable surgical solution to secondary MR with reduced recurrence rates. This hypothesis was addressed in a CTSN prospective randomized clinical trial of MV repair versus replacement in 251 patients with severe ischemic MR,[89] which demonstrated that MV replacement achieved equivalent degrees of reduction in LV volume compared with repair, with less recurrent MR during the follow-up period out to 2 years (Fig. 76.14). This result was driven by the 32.6% of repair patients who developed recurrent moderate or greater MR at 1 year, rising to 58.8% at 2 years. Among the patients with recurrent MR, LVESV index was significantly larger than in those without recurrence (62.6 ± 26.9 and 42.7 ± 26.4 mL, respectively; $p< 0.001$). These data have informed predictive models to identify patients most likely to fail a MV repair,[90] including those with larger EROA, outward tethering of the valve, and inferobasal aneurysms. In multivariate analysis, the ratio of LVESD to annuloplasty ring diameter was most predictive of recurrent MR.[91] Such patients appear to be better served by a chordal-sparing MV replacement.

Transcatheter Therapy for Secondary Mitral Regurgitation

One of the major new recommendations in the 2020 ACC/AHA guidelines is the indication for transcatheter edge-to-edge MV repair in patients with secondary MR.[1] The Cardiovascular Outcomes Assessment of the MitraClip Percutaneous Therapy for Heart Failure Patients with Functional Mitral Regurgitation (COAPT) trial,[92] which randomized patients with LV dysfunction and secondary MR to GDMT alone versus GDMT plus transcatheter edge-to-edge repair showed a significant reduction in the primary endpoint, rehospitalization for HF, and secondary endpoints of reduction in mortality, and combined endpoints of mortality and rehospitalization for HF (see Fig. 78.5). This seminal trial led the U.S. Food and Drug Administration to approve the edge-to-edge repair device for severe secondary MR as well as a Class IIa recommendation in the revised guidelines (Table 76.5 and Fig. 76.15). However, the Multicentre Study of Percutaneous Mitral Valve Repair MitraClip Device in Patients With Severe Secondary Mitral Regurgitation (MITRA-FR) trial,[93] which also randomized patients with LV dysfunction and secondary MR to GDMT alone versus GDMT plus transcatheter edge-to-edge repair, reported no significant benefit to edge-to-edge repair in the primary combined endpoint of survival or rehospitalization for HF (Fig. 76.16).

TABLE 76.5 Recommendations for Intervention for Chronic Secondary Mitral Regurgitation

COR	LOE	RECOMMENDATIONS
2a	B-R	1. In patients with chronic severe secondary MR related to LV systolic dysfunction (LVEF <50%) who have persistent symptoms (NYHA Class II, III, or IV) while on optimal GDMT for HF (stage D), TEER is reasonable in patients with appropriate anatomy as defined on TEE and with LVEF between 20% and 50%, LVESD ≤70 mm, and pulmonary artery systolic pressure ≤70 mm Hg.
2a	B-NR	2. In patients with severe secondary MR (stages C and D), mitral valve surgery is reasonable when CABG is undertaken for the treatment of myocardial ischemia.
2b	B-NR	3. In patients with chronic severe secondary MR from atrial annular dilation with preserved LV systolic function (LVEF ≥50%) who have severe persistent symptoms (NYHA Class III or IV) despite therapy for HF and therapy for associated AF or other comorbidities (stage D), mitral valve surgery may be considered.
2b	B-NR	4. In patients with chronic severe secondary MR related to LV systolic dysfunction (LVEF <50%) who have persistent severe symptoms (NYHA class III or IV) while on optimal GDMT for HF (stage D), mitral valve surgery may be considered.
2b	B-R	5. In patients with CAD and chronic severe secondary MR related to LV systolic dysfunction (LVEF <50%) (stage D) who are undergoing mitral valve surgery because of severe symptoms (NYHA class III or IV) that persist despite GDMT for HF, chordal-sparing mitral valve replacement may be reasonable to choose over downsized annuloplasty repair.

CABG, Coronary artery bypass graft; *CAD,* coronary artery disease; *GDMT,* guideline-directed medical therapy; *HF,* heart failure; *LVEF,* left ventricular ejection fraction; *LVESD,* left ventricular end-systolic dimension; *MR,* mitral regurgitation; *NYHA,* New York Heart Association; *TEE,* transesophageal echocardiography; *TEER,* transcatheter edge-to-edge repair.
From Otto CM, et al. 2020 AHA/ACC guideline for the management of patients with valvular heart disease: a report of the American College of Cardiology/American Heart Association Task Force on Practice Guidelines. *J Am Coll Cardiol.* 2021;77:e25-197.

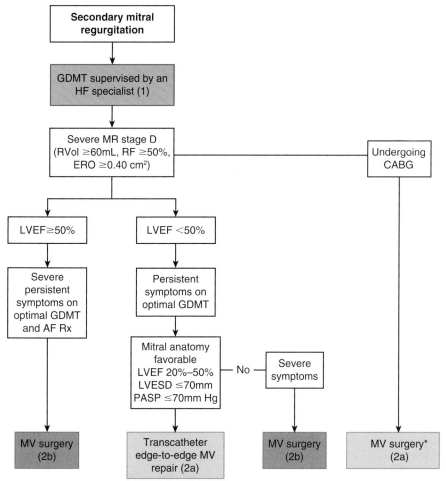

FIGURE 76.15 Management strategy for intervention for secondary mitral regurgitation. Colors correspond to Table 76.5. *AF,* Atrial fibrillation; *CABG, coronary* artery bypass graft; *ERO,* effective regurgitant orifice; *GDMT,* guideline-directed management and therapy; *HF,* heart failure; *LVEF,* left ventricular ejection fraction; *LVESD,* left ventricular end-systolic dimension; *MR,* mitral regurgitation; *MV,* mitral valve; *PASP,* pulmonary artery systolic pressure; *RF,* regurgitant fraction; *Rvol,* regurgitant volume; *Rx,* medication. (From Otto CM, et al. 2020 AHA/ACC guideline for the management of patients with valvular heart disease: a report of the American College of Cardiology/American Heart Association Task Force on Practice Guidelines. *J Am Coll Cardiol.* 2021;77:e25-197.)

These discordant results have led to extensive discussion and reevaluation of trial design, inclusion criteria, and patient populations that could explain the differences in results, as well as determine the appropriate patient populations for this therapy.

Differences in the COAPT and MITR-FR trial design and inclusion criteria may help explain the apparent discordance between the trials.[94] Randomization for COAPT occurred only after aggressive GDMT was achieved, including CRT as indicated, and stable for 3 months, and the primary efficacy outcome was rehospitalization for heart failure within 24 months; a relatively low percent of patients received ARB or ARNI therapy. Randomization for the MITRA-FR trial, however, occurred after identification of appropriate LVEF and MR criteria, and GDMT could continue to be fine-tuned during the course of the trial for both randomized cohorts; and a higher percentage of patients in both arms were treated with RAAS blockers. All-cause mortality rates at 1 year were similar for both treatment groups between the two trials. However, by 2 years the mortality rate for the GDMT arm in COAPT was worse (46% in COAPT versus 34% in MITRA-FR).[92,95]

Inclusion criteria for the trials was also different given the different thresholds for MR severity in the guidelines at the time of trial design. Because the EROA of the COAPT population was larger than that in MITRA-FR (~40 mm² compared with ~30 mm²) and the LVEDV index was smaller (~101 mL/m² versus ~135 mL/m²), the concept of proportionate and disproportionate secondary MR was proposed as a possible physiologic construct to understand the differences in the trials. To support this theory, Grayburn et al.[96] showed a linear relationship between MR severity (EROA) to LVEDV based on the Gorlin equation, using constant LVEF of 30% and regurgitant fraction of 50%. Using an EROA/EDV ratio of 0.14, the COAPT trial population had a disproportionately greater degree of MR relative to EDV, whereas the MITRA-FR patients had a proportionate degree of MR.[97] Thus, the argument was made that the COAPT patients were more likely to benefit from treatments to reduce MR severity than the MITRA-FR patients. In an opposing analysis, Gaasch et al.[98] used the Rvol/EDV ratio to argue that both trial populations had proportionate MR. Understandably, the physiologic relationship of MR severity to LV size depends not only on the etiology of the MR (ischemic versus

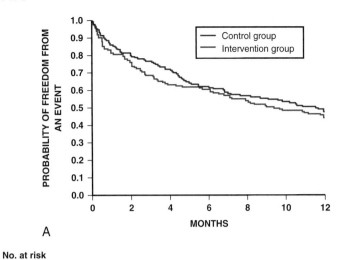

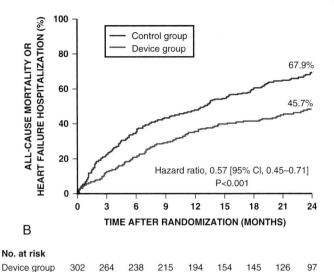

FIGURE 76.16 Outcomes of the MITRA-FR and COAPT trials. A, Freedom from death or hospitalization for heart failure in the MITRA-FR trial, the primary endpoint. **B,** Incidence of death or hospitalization for heart failure in the COAPT trial, a secondary endpoint. The primary endpoint in COAPT was hospitalization for heart failure. The secondary endpoint is shown here to compare outcomes to those with MITRA-FR using similar endpoints. (**A** from Obadia J-F, et al. Percutaneous repair or medical treatment for secondary mitral regurgitation. *N Engl J Med.* 2018;379:2297-2306; **B** from Stone GW, et al. Transcatheter mitral-valve repair in patients with heart failure. *N Engl J Med.* 2018;379:2307-2318.)

nonischemic) but also on hemodynamic load (preload and afterload), LV volume and function, and ventricular/atrial compliance, which may also be affected by disease duration, presence of AF, and underlying LV pathology.[99] More recent analyses of both trials,[100,101] including longer follow-up of the COAPT trial[102] and single site experience[103] suggest that severity of MR, LV remodeling, or their combination may not readily predict response to edge-to-edge repair in secondary MR.

Investigational Devices

A number of devices are under investigation for treatment of secondary MR (see Chapter 78), with focus on both transcatheter MV repair and TMVR.[104] As with surgery for secondary MR, TMVR has theoretical advantages compared with MV repair, because TMVR is applicable to a number of different anatomies and will virtually eliminate MR (see Fig. 78.7).

ACUTE MITRAL REGURGITATION

The causes of acute MR (see Table 76.1) are diverse and represent acute manifestations of disease processes that may, under other circumstances, cause chronic MR. Especially important causes of acute MR are spontaneous rupture of chordae tendineae (see Fig. 76.7), infective endocarditis with disruption of valve leaflets or chordal rupture (see Fig. 16.74A), ischemic dysfunction or rupture of a papillary muscle (see Fig. 16.21A), and malfunction of a prosthetic valve (see Fig. 79.5G).

Clinical Presentation

Acute severe MR causes a marked reduction in forward stroke volume, slight reduction in ESV, and increase in EDV. One major hemodynamic difference between acute and chronic MR derives from the differences in LA compliance. Patients who develop acute severe MR usually have a normal-size LA, with normal or reduced LA compliance. The LA pressure rises abruptly, which often leads to pulmonary edema, marked elevation of pulmonary vascular resistance, and right-sided heart failure.

Because the *v* wave is markedly elevated in patients with acute severe MR, the reverse pressure gradient between the LV and LA declines at the end of systole, and the murmur may be decrescendo rather than holosystolic, ending well before A_2. It usually is lower pitched and softer than the murmur of chronic MR. A left-sided S_4 frequently is found. Pulmonary hypertension, which is common in patients with acute MR, may increase the intensity of P_2, and the murmurs of pulmonary regurgitation and tricuspid regurgitation also may develop, along with a right-sided S_4. In patients with severe, acute MR, a *v* wave (late systolic pressure rise) in the pulmonary artery pressure pulse may rarely cause premature closure of the pulmonary valve, an early P_2, and paradoxical splitting of S_2. Acute MR, even if severe, often does not increase overall cardiac size, as seen on the chest radiograph, and may produce only mild LA enlargement despite marked elevation of LA pressure.

In addition, the echocardiogram may show little initial increase in the internal diameter of the LA or LV, but increased systolic motion of the LV is prominent. Characteristic features on Doppler echocardiography are the severe jet of MR and elevation of the pulmonary artery systolic pressure. Similar to the physical examination, the high atrial *v* wave can lead to early cessation of MR and a triangular CW Doppler profile instead of the usual parabolic shape. Careful interrogation of the valve by both transthoracic and transesophageal echo is essential to identify the mechanism and underlying etiology of the acute valve dysfunction (see Chapter 16).

In severe MR secondary to acute myocardial infarction, pulmonary edema, hypotension, and frank cardiogenic shock may develop. It is essential to determine the cause of the MR, which may be a ruptured papillary muscle, annular dilation from severe LV dilation, or papillary muscle displacement with leaflet tethering.[105]

Medical Management of Acute Mitral Regurgitation

Afterload reduction is particularly important in treating patients with acute MR. Intravenous nitroprusside may be lifesaving in patients with acute MR caused by rupture of the head of a papillary muscle complicating an acute myocardial infarction. It may permit stabilization of clinical status, thereby allowing coronary arteriography and surgery to be performed with the patient in optimal condition. In patients with acute MR who are hypotensive, an inotropic agent such as dobutamine should be administered with the nitroprusside. Intra-aortic balloon counterpulsation may be necessary to stabilize the patient while preparations for surgery are made.

Surgical Treatment of Acute Mitral Regurgitation

Emergency surgical treatment may be required for patients with acute LV failure caused by acute severe MR. Emergency surgery is associated with higher mortality rates than those for elective surgery for chronic MR.[106] However, unless patients with acute severe MR and heart failure are treated aggressively, a fatal outcome is almost certain.

Acute papillary muscle rupture requires emergency surgery with MV repair or replacement. In patients with papillary muscle dysfunction, initial treatment should consist of hemodynamic stabilization, usually with the aid of an intra-aortic balloon pump, and surgery should be considered for those patients who do not experience improvement with aggressive medical therapy. If patients with MR can be stabilized by medical treatment, it is preferable to defer operation until 4 to 6 weeks after the infarction if possible. Vasodilator treatment may be useful during this period. However, medical management should not be prolonged if multisystem (renal and/or pulmonary) failure develops.

Surgical mortality rates also are higher in patients with acute MR and refractory HF (NYHA Class IV), those with prosthetic valve dysfunction, and those with active infective endocarditis (of a native or prosthetic valve). Despite the higher surgical risks, the efficacy of early operation has been established in patients with infective endocarditis complicated by medically uncontrollable congestive heart failure and/or recurrent emboli.

Transcatheter Treatment of Acute Mitral Regurgitation

Experience is limited with percutaneous approaches to acute MR, although early reports support the selective use of the MitraClip in postinfarct MR[107] and even endocarditis, once the infection has been cleared.[108]

CLASSIC REFERENCES

Avierinos J-F, Gersh BJ, Melton LJ, et al. Natural history of asymptomatic mitral valve prolapse in the community. *Circulation*. 2002;106:1355–1361.

Carpentier A. Cardiac valve surgery–the "French correction". *J Thorac Cardiovasc Surg*. 1983;86:323–337.

Grigioni F, Enriquez-Sarano M, Zehr KJ, et al. Ischemic mitral regurgitation: long-term outcome and prognostic implications with quantitative doppler assessment. *Circulation*. 2001;103:1759–1764.

Levine RA, Handschumacher MD, Sanfilippo AJ, et al. Three-dimensional echocardiographic reconstruction of the mitral valve, with implications for the diagnosis of mitral valve prolapse. *Circulation*. 1989;80:589–598.

Nkomo VT, Gardin JM, Skelton TN, et al. Burden of valvular heart diseases: a population-based study. *Lancet*. 2006;368:1005–1011.

Perloff JK, Roberts WC. The mitral apparatus. Functional anatomy of mitral regurgitation. *Circulation*. 1972;46(2):227–239.

REFERENCES

1. Otto CM, Nishimura RA, Bonow RO, et al. 2020 AHA/ACC guideline for the management of patients with valvular heart disease: a report of the American College of Cardiology/American Heart Association task force on practice guidelines. *J Am Coll Cardiol*. 2021;77:e25–e197.
2. Bonow RO, O'Gara PT, Adams DH, et al. 2020 Focused update of the 2017 ACC expert consensus decision pathway on the management of mitral regurgitation. A report of the American College of Cardiology solution set oversight committee. *J Am Coll Cardiol*. 2020;75:2236–2270.

Mitral Valve Anatomy and Mechanisms of Regurgitation

3. Faletra FF, Leo LA, Paiocchi VL, et al. Anatomy of mitral annulus insights from non-invasive imaging techniques. *Eur Heart J Cardiovasc Imaging*. 2019;20:843–587.
4. Maréchaux S, Illman JE, Huynh J, et al. Functional anatomy and pathophysiologic principles in mitral regurgitation: non-invasive assessment. *Prog Cardiovasc Dis*. 2017;60:289–304.
5. Blanke P, Naoum C, Webb J, et al. Multimodality imaging in the context of transcatheter mitral valve replacement: establishing consensus among modalities and disciplines. *JACC Cardiovasc Imaging*. 2015;8:1191–1208.
6. Dal-Bianco JP, Levine RA. Anatomy of the mitral valve apparatus: role of 2D and 3D echocardiography. *Cardiol Clin*. 2013;31:151–164.
7. Theriault-Lauzier P, Andalib A, Martucci G, et al. Fluoroscopic anatomy of left-sided heart structures for transcatheter interventions: insight from multislice computed tomography. *JACC Cardiovasc Interv*. 2014;7:947–957.
8. Gunnal SA, Wabale RN, Farooqui MS. Morphological study of chordae tendinae in human cadaveric hearts. *Heart Views*. 2015;16:1–12.
9. Wilcox AG, Buchan KG, Espino DM. Frequency and diameter dependent viscoelastic properties of mitral valve chordae tendineae. *J Mech Behav Biomed Mater*. 2014;30:186–195.
10. Levine RA, Hagége AA, Judge DP, et al. Mitral valve disease—morphology and mechanisms. *Nat Rev Cardiol*. 2015;12:689–710.
11. Narang A, Addetia K, Weinert L, et al. Diagnosis of isolated cleft mitral valve using three-dimensional echocardiography. *J Am Soc Echocardiogr*. 2018;31:1161–1167.
12. Tang Z, Fan YT, Wang Y, et al. Mitral annular and left ventricular dynamics in atrial functional mitral regurgitation: a three-dimensional and speckle-tracking echocardiographic study. *J Am Soc Echocardiogr*. 2019;32:503–513.
13. Muraru D, Guta AC, Ochoa-Jimenez RC, et al. Functional regurgitation of atrioventricular valves and atrial fibrillation: an elusive pathophysiological link deserving further attention. *J Am Soc Echocardiogr*. 2020;33:42–53.
14. Kagiyama N, Mondillo S, Yoshida K, et al. Subtypes of atrial functional mitral regurgitation: imaging insights into their mechanisms and therapeutic implications. *JACC Cardiovasc Imaging*. 2020;13:820–835.
15. Deferm S, Bertrand PB, Verbrugge FH, et al. Atrial functional mitral regurgitation: JACC review topic of the week. *J Am Coll Cardiol*. 2019;73:2465–2476.
16. Gertz ZM, Raina A, Saghy L, et al. Evidence of atrial functional mitral regurgitation due to atrial fibrillation: reversal with arrhythmia control. *J Am Coll Cardiol*. 2011;58:1474–1481.
17. Silbiger JJ. Mechanistic insights into atrial functional mitral regurgitation: far more complicated than just left atrial remodeling. *Echocardiography*. 2019;36:164–169.
18. Zoghbi WA, Adams D, Bonow RO, et al. Recommendations for noninvasive evaluation of native valvular regurgitation: a report from the American Society of Echocardiography Developed in Collaboration with the Society for Cardiovascular Magnetic Resonance. *J Am Soc Echocardiogr*. 2017;30:303–371.
19. Kehl DW, Rader F, Siegel RJ. Echocardiographic features and clinical outcomes of flail mitral leaflet without severe mitral regurgitation. *J Am Soc Echocardiogr*. 2017;30:1162–1168.
20. Le Tourneau T, Mérot J, Rimbert A, et al. Genetics of syndromic and non-syndromic mitral valve prolapse. *Heart*. 2018;104:978–984.
21. Lee AP, Hsiung MC, Salgo IS, et al. Quantitative analysis of mitral valve morphology in mitral valve prolapse with real-time 3-dimensional echocardiography: importance of annular saddle shape in the pathogenesis of mitral regurgitation. *Circulation*. 2013;127:832–841.
22. Topilsky Y, Vaturi O, Watanabe N, et al. Real-time 3-dimensional dynamics of functional mitral regurgitation: a prospective quantitative and mechanistic study. *J Am Heart Assoc*. 2013;2:e000039.

Primary Mitral Regurgitation: Echocardiography and Other Diagnostic Modalities

23. Narang A, Puthumana J, Thomas JD. Diagnostic evaluation of mitral regurgitation. In: Otto CM, Bonow RO, eds. *Valvular Heart Disease: A Companion to Braunwald's Heart Disease*. 5th ed. Philadelphia: Saunders; 2021:289–310.
24. Tsang W, Freed BH, Lang RM. Three-dimensional anatomy of the aortic and mitral valves. In: Otto CM, Bonow RO, eds. *Valvular Heart Disease: A Companion to Braunwald's Heart Disease*. 5th ed. Philadelphia: Saunders; 2013:22–42.
25. Lancellotti P, Pellikka PA, Budts W, et al. The clinical use of stress echocardiography in non-ischaemic heart disease: recommendations from the European Association of Cardiovascular

Imaging and the American Society of Echocardiography. *Eur Heart J Cardiovasc Imaging*. 2016;17:1191–1229.
26. Kawel-Boehm N, Maceira A, Valsangiacomo-Buechel ER, et al. Normal values for cardiovascular magnetic resonance in adults and children. *J Cardiovasc Magn Reson*. 2015;17:29.
27. Uretsky S, Gillam L, Lang R, et al. Discordance between echocardiography and MRI in the assessment of mitral regurgitation severity: a prospective multicenter trial. *J Am Coll Cardiol*. 2015;65:1078–1088.
28. Naoum C, Blanke P, Cavalcante JL, et al. Cardiac computed tomography and magnetic resonance imaging in the evaluation of mitral and tricuspid valve disease: implications for transcatheter interventions. *Circ Cardiovasc Imaging*. 2017;10:pii: e005331. https://doi.org/10.1161/CIRCIMAGING.116.005331.
29. Koo HJ, Yang DH, Oh SY, et al. Demonstration of mitral valve prolapse with CT for planning of mitral valve repair. *Radiographics*. 2014;34:1537–1552.
30. van Rosendael PJ, Katsanos S, Kamperidis V, et al. New insights on Carpentier I mitral regurgitation from multidetector row computed tomography. *Am J Cardiol*. 2014;114:763–768.
31. Mak GJ, Blanke P, Ong K, et al. Three-dimensional echocardiography compared with computed tomography to determine mitral annulus size before transcatheter mitral valve implantation. *Circ Cardiovasc Imaging*. 2016;9:pii: e004176. https://doi.org/10.1161/CIRCIMAGING.115.004176.
32. Blanke P, Dvir D, Cheung A, et al. Mitral annular evaluation with CT in the context of transcatheter mitral valve replacement. *JACC Cardiovasc Imaging*. 2015;8:612–615.
33. Vukicevic M, Mosadegh B, Min JK, et al. Cardiac 3D printing and its future directions. *JACC Cardiovasc Imaging*. 2017;10:171–184.
34. Vukicevic M, Puperi DS, Grande-Allen KJ, et al. 3D Printed modeling of the mitral valve for catheter-based structural interventions. *Ann Biomed Eng*. 2017;45:508–519.

Primary Mitral Regurgitation: Natural History

35. Delling FN, Vasan RS. Epidemiology and pathophysiology of mitral valve prolapse. *Circulation*. 2014;129:2158–2170.
36. Parwani P, Avierinos JF, Levine RA, et al. Mitral valve prolapse: multimodality imaging and genetic insights. *Prog Cardiovasc Dis*. 2017;60:361–369.
37. Basso C, Iliceto S, Thiene G, et al. Mitral valve prolapse, ventricular arrhythmias, and sudden death. *Circulation*. 2019;140:952–964.
38. El Sabbagh A, Reddy YNV, Nishimura RA. Mitral valve regurgitation in the contemporary era: insights into diagnosis, management, and future directions. *JACC Cardiovascular Imaging*. 2018;11:628–643.
39. Dziadzko V, Dziadzko M, Medina-Inojosa JR, et al. Causes and mechanisms of isolated mitral regurgitation in the community: clinical context and outcome. *Eur Heart J*. 2019;40:2194–2202.
40. Antoine C, Benfari G, Michelena HI, et al. Clinical outcome of degenerative mitral regurgitation: critical importance of echocardiographic quantitative assessment in routine practice. *Circulation*. 2018;138:1317–1326.
41. Tribouilloy C, Grigioni F, Avierinos JF, et al. Survival implication of left ventricular end-systolic diameter in mitral regurgitation due to flail leaflets. A Long-Term Follow-Up Multicenter Study. *J Am Coll Cardiol*. 2009;54:1961–1968.
42. Tribouilloy C, Rusinaru D, Grigioni F, et al. Long-term mortality associated with left ventricular dysfunction in mitral regurgitation due to flail leaflets: a multicenter analysis. *Circ Cardiovasc Imaging*. 2014;7:363–370.
43. Suri RM, Vanoverschelde JL, Grigioni F, et al. Association between early surgical intervention vs watchful waiting and outcomes for mitral regurgitation due to flail mitral valve leaflets. *J Am Med Assoc*. 2013;310:609–616.
44. Hiemstra YL, Tomsic A, van Wijngaarden SE, et al. Prognostic value of global longitudinal strain and etiology after surgery for primary mitral regurgitation. *JACC: Cardiovasc Imaging*. 2020;13:577–585.
45. Enriquez-Sarano M. Mitral annular disjunction: the forgotten component of myxomatous mitral valve disease. *JACC Cardiovasc Imaging*. 2017;10:1434–1436.
46. Muthukumar L, Jahangir A, Jan MF, et al. Association between malignant mitral valve prolapse and sudden cardiac death: a review. *JAMA Cardiol*. 2020;5:1053–1061.
47. Dejgaard LA, Skjølsvik ET, Lie ØH, et al. The mitral annulus disjunction arrhythmic syndrome. *J Am Coll Cardiol*. 2018;72:1600–1609.
48. Perazzolo Marra M, Basso C, De Lazzari M, et al. Morphofunctional abnormalities of mitral annulus and arrhythmic mitral valve prolapse. *Circ Cardiovasc Imaging*. 2016;9:e005030.
49. Essayagh B, Sabbag A, Antoine C, et al. Presentation and outcome of arrhythmic mitral valve prolapse. *J Am Coll Cardiol*. 2020;76:637–649.
50. David TE, David CM, Tsang W, et al. Long-Term results of mitral valve repair for regurgitation due to leaflet prolapse. *J Am Coll Cardiol*. 2019;74:1044–1053.

Primary Mitral Regurgitation: Management

51. Baumgartner H, Falk V, Bax JJ, et al. 2017 ESC/EACTS guidelines for the management of valvular heart disease: the Task Force for the management of valvular heart disease of the European Society of Cardiology (ESC) and the European Association for Cardio-Thoracic Surgery (EACTS). *Eur Heart J*. 2017;38:2739–2791.
52. Grigioni F, Clavel MA, Vanoverschelde JL, et al. The MIDA Mortality Risk Score: development and external validation of a prognostic model for early and late death in degenerative mitral regurgitation. *Eur Heart J*. 2018;39:1281–1291.
53. Strauss CE, Duval S, Pastorius D, Harris KM. Pharmacotherapy in the treatment of mitral regurgitation: a systematic review. *J Heart Valve Dis*. 2012;21:275–285.
54. Katsi V, Georgiopoulos G, Magkas N, et al. The role of arterial hypertension in mitral valve regurgitation. *Curr Hypertens Rep*. 2019;21:20.
55. LaPar DJ, Ailawadi G, Isbell JM, et al. Mitral valve repair rates correlate with surgeon and institutional experience. *J Thorac Cardiovasc Surg*. 2014;148:995–1003.
56. Chikwe J, Toyoda N, Anyanwu AC, et al. Relation of mitral valve surgery volume to repair rate, durability, and survival. *J Am Coll Cardiol*. 2017;69:2397–2406.
57. Badhwar V, Vemulapalli S, Mack MA, et al. Volume-Outcome association of mitral valve surgery in the United States. *JAMA Cardiol*. 2020;5:1092–1101.
58. Lazam S, Vanoverschelde JL, Tribouilloy C, et al. Twenty-year outcome after mitral repair versus replacement for severe degenerative mitral regurgitation. *Circulation*. 2017;135:410–422.
59. Gammie JS, Chikwe J, Badhwar V, et al. Isolated mitral valve surgery: the society of thoracic surgeons adult cardiac surgery database analysis. *Ann Thorac Surg*. 2018;106:716–727.
60. Feldman T, Kar S, Elmariah S, et al. Randomized comparison of percutaneous repair and surgery for mitral regurgitation: 5-year results of EVEREST II. *J Am Coll Cardiol*. 2015;66:2844–2854.
61. Buzzatti N, Maisano F, Latib A, et al. Comparison of outcomes of percutaneous MitraClip versus surgical repair or replacement for degenerative mitral regurgitation in octogenarians. *Am J Cardiol*. 2015;115:487–492.
62. Külling M, Corti R, Noll G, et al. Heart team approach in treatment of mitral regurgitation: patient selection and outcome. *Open Heart*. 2020;7:e001280. https://doi.org/10.1136/openhrt-2020-001280.
63. Chiarito M, Pagnesi M, Martino EA, et al. Outcome after percutaneous edge-to-edge mitral repair for functional and degenerative mitral regurgitation: a systematic review and meta-analysis. *Heart*. 2018;104:306–312.
64. Feldman T, Foster E, Glower DD, et al. Percutaneous repair or surgery for mitral regurgitation. *N Engl J Med*. 2011;364:1395–1406.

65. Attizzani GF, Ohno Y, Capodanno D, et al. Extended use of percutaneous edge-to-edge mitral valve repair beyond EVEREST (Endovascular Valve Edge-To-Edge Repair) criteria: 30-day and 12-month clinical and echocardiographic outcomes from the GRASP (Getting Reduction of Mitral Insufficiency by Percutaneous Clip Implantation) registry. *JACC Cardiovasc Interv.* 2015;8:74–82.

66. Bottari VE, Tamborini G, Bartorelli AL, Alamanni F, Pepi M. MitraClip implantation in a previous surgical mitral valve edge-to-edge repair. *JACC Cardiovasc Interv.* 2015;8:111–113.

67. Hahn RT. Transcatheter valve replacement and valve repair: review of procedures and intraprocedural echocardiographic imaging. *Circ Res.* 2016;119:341–356.

Secondary Mitral Regurgitation: Pathophysiology

68. Machino-Ohtsuka T, Seo Y, Ishizu T, et al. Novel mechanistic insights into atrial functional mitral regurgitation: 3-dimensional echocardiographic study. *Circ J.* 2016;80:2240–2248.

69. Abe Y, Akamatsu K, Ito K, et al. Prevalence and prognostic significance of functional mitral and tricuspid regurgitation despite preserved left ventricular ejection fraction in atrial fibrillation patients. *Circ J.* 2018;82:1451–1458.

70. Reddy ST, Belden W, Doyle M, et al. Mitral regurgitation recovery and atrial reverse remodeling following pulmonary vein isolation procedure in patients with atrial fibrillation: a clinical observation proof-of-concept cardiac MRI study. *J Interv Card Electrophysiol.* 2013;37:307–315.

71. Grayburn PA. Secondary (functional) mitral regurgitation in ischemic and dilated cardiomyopathy. In: Otto CM, Bonow RO, eds. *Valvular Heart Disease: A Companion to Braunwald's Heart Disease.* 5th ed. Philadelphia: Saunders; 2013:354–369.

72. O'Gara PT, Mack MJ. Secondary mitral regurgitation. *N Engl J Med.* 2020;383:1458–1467.

73. Bertrand PB, Schwammenthal E, Levine RA, et al. Exercise dynamics in secondary mitral regurgitation: pathophysiology and therapeutic implications. *Circulation.* 2017;135:297–314.

74. Kimura T, Roger VL, Watanabe N, et al. The unique mechanism of functional mitral regurgitation in acute myocardial infarction: a prospective dynamic 4D quantitative echocardiographic study. *Eur Heart J Cardiovasc Imaging.* 2019;20:396–406.

Secondary Mitral Regurgitation: Echocardiography and Other Diagnostic Modalities

75. Grayburn PA, Carabello B, Hung J, et al. Defining "severe" secondary mitral regurgitation: emphasizing an integrated approach. *J Am Coll Cardiol.* 2014;64:2792–2801.

76. Bartko PE, Arfsten H, Heitzinger G, et al. A unifying concept for the quantitative assessment of secondary mitral regurgitation. *J Am Coll Cardiol.* 2019;73:2506–2517.

77. Kamperidis V, Marsan NA, Delgado V, et al. Left ventricular systolic function assessment in secondary mitral regurgitation: left ventricular ejection fraction vs. speckle tracking global longitudinal strain. *Eur Heart J.* 2016;37:811–681.

78. Namazi F, van der Bijl P, Hirasawa K, et al. Prognostic value of left ventricular global longitudinal strain in patients with secondary mitral regurgitation. *J Am Coll Cardiol.* 2020;75:750–758.

79. Chinitz JS, Chen D, Goyal P, et al. Mitral apparatus assessment by delayed enhancement CMR: relative impact of infarct distribution on mitral regurgitation. *JACC Cardiovasc Imaging.* 2013;6:220–234.

Secondary Mitral Regurgitation: Management

80. Yancy CW, Jessup M, Bozkurt B, et al. 2017 ACC/AHA/HFSA focused update of the 2013 ACCF/AHA guideline for the management of heart failure: a report of the American College of Cardiology/American Heart Association Task Force on Clinical Practice Guidelines and the Heart Failure Society of America. *Circulation.* 2017;136:e137–e161.

81. Nasser R, Van Assche L, Vorlat A, et al. Evolution of functional mitral regurgitation and prognosis in medically managed heart failure patients with reduced ejection fraction. *JACC Heart Fail.* 2017;5:652–659.

82. Kang DH, Park S-J, Shin SH, et al. Angiotensin receptor neprilysin inhibitor for functional mitral regurgitation. *Circulation.* 2019;139:1354–1365.

83. Levine RA, Nagata Y, Dal-Bianco JP. Left ventricular dyssynchrony and the mitral valve apparatus: an orchestra that needs to play in sync. *JACC Cardiovasc Imaging.* 2019;12:1738–1740.

84. Bartko PE, Arfsten H, Heitzinger G, et al. Papillary muscle dyssynchrony-mediated functional mitral regurgitation: mechanistic insights and modulation by cardiac resynchronization. *JACC Cardiovasc Imaging.* 2019;12:1728–1737.

85. Fihn SD, Blankenship JC, Alexander KP, et al. 2014 ACC/AHA/AATS/PCNA/SCAI/STS focused update of the guideline for the diagnosis and management of patients with stable ischemic heart disease: a report of the American College of Cardiology/American Heart Association Task Force on Practice Guidelines, and the American Association for Thoracic Surgery, Preventive Cardiovascular Nurses Association, Society for Cardiovascular Angiography and Interventions, and Society of Thoracic Surgeons. *J Am Coll Cardiol.* 2014;64:1929–4199.

86. Knuuti J, Wijns W, Saraste A, et al. 2019 ESC Guidelines for the diagnosis and management of chronic coronary syndromes: the task force for the diagnosis and management of chronic coronary syndromes of the European Society of Cardiology (ESC). *Eur Heart J.* 2019;41:407–747.

87. Takahashi Y, Abe Y, Sasaki Y, et al. Mitral valve repair for atrial functional mitral regurgitation in patients with chronic atrial fibrillation. *Interact Cardiovasc Thorac Surg.* 2015;21:163–168.

88. Michler RE, Smith PK, Parides MK, et al. Two-year outcomes of surgical treatment of moderate ischemic mitral regurgitation. *N Engl J Med.* 2016;374:1932–1941.

89. Goldstein D, Moskowitz AJ, Gelijns AC, et al. Two-year outcomes of surgical treatment of severe ischemic mitral regurgitation. *N Engl J Med.* 2016;374:344–353.

90. Kron IL, Hung J, Overbey JR, et al. Predicting recurrent mitral regurgitation after mitral valve repair for severe ischemic mitral regurgitation. *J Thorac Cardiovasc Surg.* 2015;149:752–761e1.

91. Capoulade R, Zeng X, Overbey JR, et al. Impact of left ventricular to mitral valve ring mismatch on recurrent ischemic mitral regurgitation after ring annuloplasty. *Circulation.* 2016;134:1247–1256.

92. Stone GW, Lindenfeld J, Abraham WT, et al. Transcatheter mitral-valve repair in patients with heart failure. *N Engl J Med.* 2018;379:2307–2318.

93. Obadia JF, Messika-Zeitoun D, Leurent G, et al. Percutaneous repair or medical treatment for secondary mitral regurgitation. *N Engl J Med.* 2018;379:2297–2306.

94. Nishimura RA, Bonow RO. Percutaneous repair of secondary mitral regurgitation: a tale of two trials. *N Engl J Med.* 2018;379:2374–2376.

95. Iung B, Armoiry X, Vahanian A, et al. Percutaneous repair or medical treatment for secondary mitral regurgitation: outcomes at 2 years. *Eur J Heart Fail.* 2019;21:1619–1627.

96. Grayburn PA, Carabello B, Hung J, et al. Defining "severe" secondary mitral regurgitation: emphasizing an integrated approach. *J Am Coll Cardiol.* 2014;64:2792–2801.

97. Packer M, Grayburn PA. New evidence supporting a novel conceptual framework for distinguishing proportionate and disproportionate functional mitral regurgitation. *JAMA Cardiol.* 2020;5:469–475.

98. Gaasch WG, Aurigemma GP, Meyer TE. An appraisal of the association of clinical outcomes with the severity of regurgitant volume relative to end-diastolic volume in patients with secondary mitral regurgitation. *JAMA Cardiol.* 2020;5:469–475.

99. Hahn RT. Disproportionate emphasis on proportionate mitral regurgitation: are there better measures of regurgitant severity? *JAMA Cardiol.* 2020;5:377–379.

100. Grayburn PA, Sannino A, Cohen DJ, et al. Predictors of clinical response to transcatheter reduction of secondary mitral regurgitation: the COAPT trial. *J Am Coll Cardiol.* 2020;76:1007–1014.

101. Messika-Zeitoun D, Iung B, Armoiry X, et al. Impact of mitral regurgitation severity and left ventricular remodeling on outcome after MitraClip implantation: results from the mitra-FR trial. *JACC Cardiovasc Imaging.* 2021;14:742–752.

102. Lindenfeld J, Abraham WT, Grayburn PA, et al. Association of effective regurgitation orifice area to left ventricular end-diastolic volume ratio with transcatheter mitral valve repair outcomes: a secondary analysis of the COAPT trial. *JAMA Cardiol.* 2021;6:427–436.

103. Adamo M, Cani DS, Gavazzoni M, et al. Impact of disproportionate secondary mitral regurgitation in patients undergoing edge-to-edge percutaneous mitral valve repair. *EuroIntervention.* 2020;16:413–420.

104. Mangieri A, Laricchia A, Giannini F, et al. Emerging technologies for percutaneous mitral valve repair. *Front Cardiovasc Med.* 2019;6:161.

Acute Mitral Regurgitation

105. Bajaj A, Sethi A, Rathor P, et al. Acute complications of myocardial infarction in the current era: diagnosis and management. *J Investig Med.* 2015;63:844–855.

106. Chatterjee S, Rankin JS, Gammie JS, et al. Isolated mitral valve surgery risk in 77,836 patients from the society of thoracic surgeons database. *Ann Thorac Surg.* 2013;96:1587–1595.

107. Adamo M, Curello S, Chiari E, et al. Percutaneous edge-to-edge mitral valve repair for the treatment of acute mitral regurgitation complicating myocardial infarction: a single centre experience. *Int J Cardiol.* 2017;234:53–57.

108. Chandrashekar P, Fender EA, Al-Hijji MA, et al. Novel use of MitraClip for severe mitral regurgitation due to infective endocarditis. *J Invasive Cardiol.* 2017;29:E21–E22.

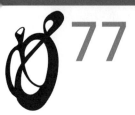

77 Tricuspid, Pulmonic, and Multivalvular Disease

PATRICIA A. PELLIKKA AND VUYISILE T. NKOMO

TRICUSPID STENOSIS

Causes and Pathology

Tricuspid stenosis (TS) is almost always rheumatic in origin, although rheumatic valve disease more commonly affects left-sided valves.[1] Other causes of obstruction to right atrial emptying are unusual and include congenital tricuspid atresia (see Chapter 82); right atrial tumors, which may produce a clinical picture suggesting rapidly progressive TS; and device leads, which more often are associated with tricuspid regurgitation (TR) but can become looped and fused to the tricuspid valve apparatus, and if multiple could cause obstruction. The carcinoid syndrome (see Chapter 52) and use of ergot-related drugs more frequently produce TR, which if severe, contributes to a gradient across the tricuspid valve (Video 77.1).[2] Dysfunction, including thrombosis, of a tricuspid mechanical or bioprosthetic valve can result in stenosis. Rarely, endomyocardial fibrosis, tricuspid valve vegetations, or extracardiac tumors cause obstruction to right ventricular (RV) inflow. Localized compression of the right atrium by a pericardial effusion may also lead to RV inflow obstruction and may be unrecognized if the effusion is mistaken for the right atrium (Fig. 77.1 and Video 77.2).

Most patients with rheumatic tricuspid valve disease have TR or a combination of TS and TR. Isolated rheumatic tricuspid valve disease is uncommon, and this lesion generally accompanies mitral valve disease, which dominates the presentation (see Chapters 75 and 76). In many patients with TS, the aortic valve also is involved (i.e., trivalvular stenosis is present). TS is found at autopsy in approximately 15% of patients with rheumatic heart disease but is of clinical significance in only approximately 5%. Organic tricuspid valve disease is more common in India, Pakistan, and other developing nations near the equator than in North America or Western Europe. The anatomic changes of rheumatic TS resemble those of mitral stenosis (MS), with fusion and shortening of the chordae tendineae and fusion of the leaflets at their edges, producing a diaphragm with a fixed central aperture, typically without calcification. Like MS, TS is more common in women. The right atrium often is greatly dilated in TS, and its walls are thickened. There may be evidence of severe passive congestion, with enlargement of the liver and spleen, and right atrial thrombus formation which may extend into the vena cava or cause pulmonary embolism.

Pathophysiology

A diastolic pressure gradient between the right atrium and ventricle—the hemodynamic expression of TS—is augmented when the transvalvular blood flow increases during inspiration or exercise and is reduced when the blood flow declines during expiration. A relatively modest diastolic pressure gradient (i.e., a mean gradient of only 5 mmHg) usually is sufficient to elevate the mean right atrial pressure to levels that result in systemic venous congestion and, unless sodium intake has been restricted or diuretics have been given, is associated ultimately with jugular venous distention, ascites, and edema. In patients with sinus rhythm, the right atrial *a* wave may be very tall. Resting cardiac output usually is markedly reduced and fails to rise during exercise. This accounts for the normal or only slightly elevated left atrial, pulmonary arterial, and RV systolic pressures, despite the frequent presence of accompanying mitral valvular disease.

A mean diastolic pressure gradient across the tricuspid valve as low as 2 mmHg and the typical echocardiographic appearance of leaflet restriction or doming is sufficient to establish the diagnosis of TS. Exercise, deep inspiration, and the rapid infusion of fluids or the administration of atropine may greatly enhance a borderline pressure gradient in a patient with TS. The diagnosis is generally made with transthoracic echocardiography; occasionally, transesophageal echocardiography (TEE) or other imaging such as cardiac magnetic resonance imaging (CMR) or computed tomography (CT) is necessary. Invasive assessment is rarely necessary.

Clinical Presentation

Symptoms. The low cardiac output in TS causes fatigue, and patients often experience discomfort from hepatomegaly, ascites, and anasarca (see Table 77.1). The severity of these symptoms, which are secondary to an elevated systemic venous pressure, is out of proportion to the degree of dyspnea. Some patients complain of a fluttering discomfort in the neck, caused by giant *a* waves in the jugular venous pulse. Occasionally, the symptoms of MS (severe dyspnea, orthopnea, and paroxysmal nocturnal dyspnea) may be masked by severe TS because the latter prevents surges of blood into the pulmonary circulation behind the stenotic mitral valve. The absence of symptoms of pulmonary congestion in a patient with obvious MS should suggest the possibility of TS.

Physical Examination (see Chapter 13). Because of the high frequency with which MS occurs in patients with TS, the similarity in the physical findings between the two valvular lesions, and the subtlety of physical findings in TS, echocardiography is essential to diagnose TS. The physical findings of TS may be attributed to MS, which is more common and associated with a louder murmur. Therefore a high index of clinical suspicion is required to detect TS. In the presence of sinus rhythm, the *a* wave in the jugular venous pulse is tall, and a presystolic hepatic pulsation often is palpable. The *y* descent is slow and barely appreciable. The lung fields are clear and, despite engorged neck veins

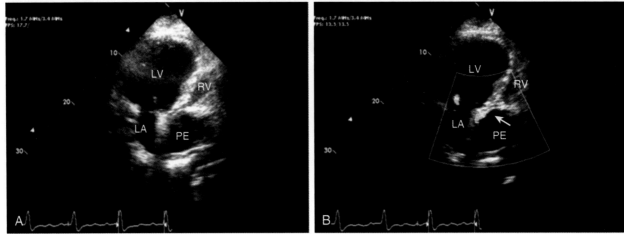

FIGURE 77.1 A, Apical four-chamber view showing localized pericardial effusion (PE) compressing the right atrium and assuming the shape of the right atrium. **B,** There is compression and significant narrowing of right ventricular inflow with a slit-like opening confirmed by color Doppler (*arrow*). Clinically the patient was in shock and underwent redo sternotomy and removal of a large hematoma around the diaphragmatic surface which was causing extrinsic compression of the right atrium. *LA,* Left atrium; *LV,* left ventricle; *RV,* right ventricle; *PE,* pericardial effusion.

TABLE 77.1 Clinical and Laboratory Features of Rheumatic Tricuspid Stenosis

History
• Progressive fatigue, edema, anorexia
• Minimal orthopnea, paroxysmal nocturnal dyspnea
• Rheumatic fever in two thirds of patients
• Female preponderance
• Pulmonary edema and hemoptysis rare

Physical Findings
• Signs of multivalvular involvement
• Diastolic rumble at lower left sternal border, increasing in intensity with inspiration
• Often confused with mitral stenosis
• Peripheral cyanosis
• Neck vein distention, with prominent *a* waves and slow *y* descent
• Absent right ventricular lift
• Associated murmurs of mitral and aortic valve disease
• Hepatic pulsation
• Ascites, peripheral edema

Imaging Findings
• ECG—tall right atrial P waves and no right ventricular hypertrophy
• Chest radiograph—dilated right atrium without enlarged pulmonary artery segment
• Echocardiogram—diastolic doming of tricuspid valve leaflets, thickening of valve, diastolic pressure gradient across tricuspid valve, right atrial enlargement

Modified from Ockene IS. Tricuspid valve disease. In Dalen JE, Alpert JS, eds. *Valvular Heart Disease.* 2nd ed. Boston: Little, Brown; 1987:356, 390.

and the presence of ascites and anasarca, the patient may be comfortable while lying flat. Thus, the diagnosis of TS may be suspected from inspection of the jugular venous pulse in a patient with MS but without clinical evidence of pulmonary hypertension. This suspicion is strengthened when a diastolic thrill is palpable at the lower left sternal border, particularly if the thrill appears or becomes more prominent during inspiration.

The auscultatory findings of the accompanying MS usually are prominent and often overshadow the more subtle signs of TS. A tricuspid opening snap (OS) may be audible but often is difficult to distinguish from a mitral OS. However, the tricuspid OS usually follows the mitral OS and is localized to the lower left sternal border, whereas the mitral

OS usually is most prominent at the apex and radiates more widely. The diastolic murmur of TS is also commonly heard best along the lower left parasternal border in the fourth intercostal space and usually is softer, higher-pitched, and shorter in duration than the murmur of MS. The presystolic component of the TS murmur has a scratchy quality and a crescendo-decrescendo configuration that diminishes before S_1. The diastolic murmur and OS of TS both are augmented by maneuvers that increase trans-tricuspid valve flow, including inspiration, the Mueller maneuver (forced inspiration against a closed glottis), assumption of the right lateral decubitus position, leg raising, inhalation of amyl nitrite, squatting, and isotonic exercise. They are reduced during expiration or the strain of the Valsalva maneuver and return to control levels immediately (i.e., within two or three beats) after the Valsalva release.

Echocardiography. The tricuspid valve should be carefully inspected at the time of echocardiography in any patient with known or suspected rheumatic heart disease or other valve disease known to affect multiple valves. The echocardiographic changes (see Chapter 16) of the tricuspid valve in rheumatic TS resemble those observed in the mitral valve in rheumatic MS (see Fig. 16.47). Two-dimensional echocardiography characteristically shows diastolic doming of the leaflets (Video 77.3), thickening and restricted motion of the other leaflets, reduced separation of the tips of the leaflets, and a reduction in diameter of the tricuspid orifice. The presence of commissural fusion and the anatomy of the valve and subvalvular apparatus should also be assessed, as these features may impact therapy. TEE allows added delineation of the details of valve structure. Doppler echocardiography can be helpful in assessment of the tricuspid valve even when 2-dimensional images are suboptimal. In TS, Doppler shows a prolonged slope of antegrade flow and compares well with cardiac catheterization in the quantification of TS and assessment of associated TR. Doppler evaluation of TS has largely replaced the need for catheterization to assess severity. Severe TS is characterized by a valve area of ≤1cm² as assessed by the continuity equation. The pressure half-time is generally greater than 190 msec, and the right atrium and inferior vena cava are dilated. The mean pressure gradient across the tricuspid valve varies with heart rate, but a mean gradient ≥5 mm Hg is consistent with significant TS.[3] Additional assessment of valve morphology may be provided by three-dimensional echocardiography, which allows en face views of the tricuspid valve from the atrial and ventricular aspects with simultaneous views of all three leaflets (Video 77.4).

Other Diagnostic Evaluation Modalities

Electrocardiography. In the absence of atrial fibrillation (AF) in a patient with valvular heart disease, TS is suggested by the presence of electrocardiographic evidence of right atrial enlargement (see Chapter 14). The P wave amplitude in leads II and V_1 exceeds 0.25 mV. Because most patients with TS have mitral valve disease, the electrocardiographic signs of biatrial enlargement commonly are seen. The amplitude of the QRS complex in lead V_1 may be reduced by the dilated right atrium.

Radiography. The key radiologic finding is marked cardiomegaly with conspicuous enlargement of the right atrium (i.e., prominence of the right heart border), which extends into a dilated superior vena cava and azygos vein, but without conspicuous dilation of the pulmonary artery. The vascular changes in the lungs characteristic of mitral valvular disease may be masked, with little or no interstitial edema or vascular redistribution, but left atrial enlargement may be present.

The stenotic tricuspid valve can also be visualized with CMR or computed tomographic imaging and right atrial and ventricular volumes quantified.

Cardiac Catheterization. Invasive hemodynamic assessment of TS is rarely needed but is appropriate in the symptomatic patient in whom the physical findings and noninvasive data are discordant. It may occasionally be undertaken in patients undergoing invasive hemodynamic assessment for another indication. Right atrial and RV pressures can be recorded simultaneously, using two catheters or a single catheter with a double lumen, with one lumen opening on either side of the tricuspid valve.

Management

Although the fundamental approach to the management of severe TS is surgical treatment, intensive sodium restriction and diuretic therapy may diminish those symptoms secondary to the accumulation of excess salt and water. If AF is present, ventricular rate control is needed to improve diastolic filling. A preparatory period of diuresis may diminish hepatic congestion, thereby improving hepatic function sufficiently to diminish the risks of subsequent operation.

Most patients with TS have coexisting valvular disease that requires surgery. Surgical treatment of TS should be carried out at the time of mitral valve repair or replacement in patients with TS in whom the mean diastolic pressure gradient exceeds 5 mm Hg and the tricuspid orifice is less than approximately 2.0 cm². The final decision concerning surgical treatment is sometimes made at the operating table.

Because TS almost always is accompanied by some TR, simple finger fracture valvotomy may not result in significant hemodynamic improvement but may merely substitute severe TR for TS. However, open valvotomy or commissurotomy in which the stenotic tricuspid valve is converted into a functionally bicuspid valve may result in improvement, but annuloplasty may also be necessary if annular dilatation is present.[4] The commissures between the anterior and septal leaflets and between the posterior and septal leaflets are opened. It is not advisable to open the commissure between the anterior and posterior leaflets for fear of producing severe TR. If open valvotomy does not restore reasonably normal valve function, the tricuspid valve may have to be replaced. A large bioprosthesis is preferred to a mechanical prosthesis in the tricuspid position because of the high risk of thrombosis of the latter and the longer durability of bioprostheses in the tricuspid than in the mitral or aortic positions. Tricuspid balloon valvuloplasty is feasible, but has limited efficacy as it may result in significant TR. It may be considered in the rare patient without TR, but because of lack of long-term outcome data, surgical therapy is preferred.

TRICUSPID REGURGITATION

Causes and Pathology

A trivial to mild degree of TR is commonly seen with echocardiography in patients with a normal right heart and structurally normal tricuspid valve. This is of no consequence and under normal conditions, does not increase in severity. However, various conditions can lead to greater degrees of TR. The most common cause of TR is not intrinsic involvement of the valve itself (i.e., primary TR) but rather dilation of the right ventricle and of the tricuspid annulus causing secondary (functional) TR (see Table 77.2).[5] Right heart dilatation may result from volume overload as seen with left-to-right shunts in atrial septal defects or anomalous pulmonary venous connections. Dilatation may be a complication of RV failure of any cause (see Fig. 16.48). It is observed in patients with RV hypertension secondary to any form of cardiac or pulmonary vascular disease. Thus, secondary TR may be seen in left-sided

valve disease, acute or chronic pulmonary thromboembolic disease, or chronic obstructive lung disease.[6,7] In general, a RV systolic pressure greater than 55 mm Hg will cause functional TR. TR can also occur secondary to RV infarction, congenital heart disease (e.g., pulmonic stenosis [PS] and pulmonary hypertension secondary to Eisenmenger syndrome; see Chapter 82), primary pulmonary hypertension (see Chapter 88) and cor pulmonale. In infants, TR may complicate RV failure secondary to neonatal pulmonary diseases and pulmonary hypertension with persistence of the fetal pulmonary circulation. In all these cases, TR reflects the presence of, and in turn aggravates, severe RV failure. Functional TR may diminish or disappear as the right ventricle decreases in size with the treatment of heart failure. TR can also occur as a consequence of dilation of the annulus in the Marfan syndrome, in which RV dilation secondary to pulmonary hypertension is not present. Acute or chronic AF can also lead to functional TR from tricuspid annulus dilatation, and AF is an important cause of isolated TR.[6,8]

A variety of disease processes can affect the tricuspid valve apparatus directly and lead to regurgitation (primary TR).[1,5] Organic TR may occur on a congenital basis (see Chapter 82), as part of Ebstein anomaly, defects involving the atrioventricular canal, when the tricuspid valve is involved in the formation of an aneurysm of the ventricular septum, or in corrected transposition of the great arteries, or it may occur as an isolated congenital lesion. Rheumatic fever may involve the tricuspid valve directly. When this occurs, it usually causes scarring of the valve leaflets and/or chordae tendineae, leading to limited leaflet mobility and either isolated TR or a combination of TR and TS. Rheumatic involvement of the mitral, and often aortic, valves coexist.

TR may result from prolapse of the tricuspid valve caused by myxomatous changes in the valve and chordae tendineae; prolapse of the

TABLE 77.2 Causes and Mechanisms of Pure Tricuspid Regurgitation

Causes

Anatomically Abnormal Valve

- Rheumatic

- Nonrheumatic
  Infective endocarditis
  Ebstein anomaly
  Floppy (prolapse)
  Congenital (non-Ebstein anomaly)
  Carcinoid
  Papillary muscle dysfunction
  Trauma
  Connective tissue disorders (Marfan syndrome)
  Rheumatoid arthritis
  Radiation injury

Anatomically Normal Valve (Functional, dilated annulus)

- Elevated right ventricular systolic pressure

- Chronic atrial fibrillation

- Restrictive cardiomyopathy

Mechanisms

CONDITION	LEAFLET AREA	ANNULAR CIRCUMFERENCE	LEAFLET INSERTION
Floppy	↑	↑	Normal
Ebstein anomaly	↑	↑	Abnormal
Pulmonary/right ventricular systolic hypertension	Normal	↑	Normal
Papillary muscle dysfunction	Normal	Normal	Normal
Carcinoid	↓/Normal	Normal	Normal
Rheumatic	↓/Normal	Normal	Normal
Infective endocarditis	↓/Normal	Normal	Normal

Modified from Waller BF. Rheumatic and nonrheumatic conditions producing valvular heart disease. In Frankl WS, Brest AN, eds. *Cardiovascular Clinics: Valvular Heart Disease: Comprehensive Evaluation and Management.* Philadelphia, FA: Davis; 1989:35, 95.

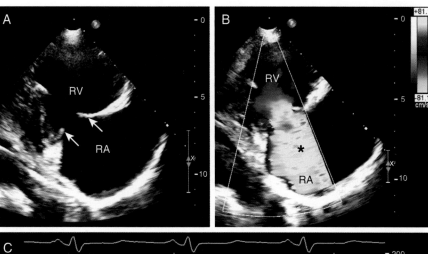

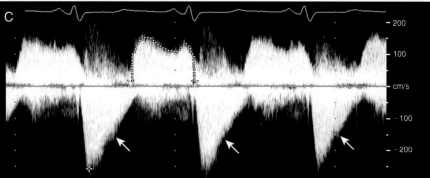

FIGURE 77.2 Transthoracic echocardiographic images of the tricuspid valve in a patient with carcinoid valvular heart disease. **A,** Two-dimensional parasternal long axis image of the tricuspid valve inflow view in mid-systole demonstrating a marked thickening and restriction of the tricuspid valve leaflets (*arrow*) resulting in failure of leaflet closure. **B,** Color Doppler imaging of the tricuspid valve in the parasternal long axis tricuspid valve inflow view in mid-systole demonstrating a broad regurgitant jet which occupies the entire right atrium consistent with severe tricuspid valve regurgitation (*asterisk*). **C,** Continuous wave Doppler imaging across the tricuspid valve demonstrating a dense, systolic, "dagger-shaped" tricuspid regurgitant jet consistent with severe tricuspid valve regurgitation (*arrows*). Less severe forms of tricuspid regurgitation are typically associated with parabolic shaped regurgitant jets. *RA,* Right atrium; *RV,* right ventricle. (From Luis SA, Pellikka PA. Carcinoid heart disease: diagnosis and management. *Best Pract Res Clin Endocrinol Metab.* 2016;30:149–158. https://doi.org/10.1016/j.beem.2015.09.005\.)

mitral valve is usually present in these patients as well. Prolapse of the tricuspid valve has been estimated to occur in 20% of all patients with mitral valve prolapse (MVP), but compared to MVP, diagnostic criteria are less well-defined. Tricuspid valve prolapse also may be associated with atrial septal defect.

Distortion of the tricuspid leaflets by transvenous pacemaker and defibrillator leads is an increasingly common cause of clinically significant TR.[9,10] Injury to the tricuspid valve or subvalvular apparatus may complicate endomyocardial biopsy.

TR or the combination of TR and TS is an important feature of the carcinoid syndrome (Fig. 77.2; see also Fig. 16.49), which leads to focal or diffuse deposits of fibrous tissue on the endocardium of the valvular cusps and cardiac chambers and on the intima of the great veins and coronary sinus (see Chapter 52). The white, fibrous carcinoid plaques are most extensive on the right side of the heart, where they usually are deposited on the ventricular surfaces of the tricuspid valve and cause the cusps to adhere to the underlying RV wall, thereby producing TR. A similar process may affect the tricuspid valve in patients who have used drugs that increase serotonin levels or simulate its effect on serotonin receptors (see Video 77.1). These include the anorectic drugs, fenfluramine and phentermine; ergot derivatives used for treating migraine headaches (ergotamine and methylsergide) or Parkinson disease (pergolide or cabergoline); or the synthetic stimulant and hallucinogen, 3,4-methylenedioxymethamphetamine (Ecstasy).

Other causes of TR include penetrating and nonpenetrating trauma,[11] dilated cardiomyopathy, and infective endocarditis (Video 77.5) (particularly staphylococcal endocarditis in intravenous drug users). Endomyocardial fibrosis with shortening of the tricuspid leaflets and chordae tendineae is an important cause of TR in tropical Africa, Asia, and South America. Less common causes of TR include cardiac tumors (particularly right atrial myxoma), endomyocardial fibrosis, methysergide-induced valvular disease, and systemic lupus erythematosus involving the tricuspid valve.

Clinical Presentation

The clinical stages of TR are depicted in Table 77.3.[3]

Symptoms. In the absence of pulmonary hypertension or RV failure, TR generally is well tolerated. When pulmonary hypertension and TR coexist, cardiac output declines and the manifestations of right-sided heart failure become intensified. Thus, the symptoms of TR result from a reduced cardiac output and from ascites, painful congestive hepatomegaly, and massive edema. Occasionally, patients exhibit throbbing pulsations in the neck, which intensify on effort and are caused by jugular venous distention, and systolic pulsations of the eyeballs also have been described. In the many patients with TR who have mitral valve disease, the symptoms of the latter usually predominate. Symptoms of pulmonary congestion may abate as TR develops but are replaced by weakness, fatigue, and other manifestations of a depressed cardiac output.

Physical Examination (see Chapter 13). In patients with severe TR, evidence of weight loss and cachexia, cyanosis, and jaundice are often present on inspection. AF is common. Jugular venous distention also is evident, the normal *x* and *x*′ descents disappear, and a prominent systolic wave—a *c-v* wave (or *s* wave)—is apparent. The descent of this wave, *y* descent, is sharp and becomes the most prominent feature of the venous pulse except with coexisting TS, in which case it is slowed. A venous systolic thrill and murmur in the neck may be present in patients with severe TR. The RV impulse is hyperdynamic and thrusting in quality. Initially, systolic pulsations of an enlarged tender liver are frequent. However, in patients with chronic TR and congestive cirrhosis, the liver may become firm and nontender. Ascites and edema are frequent.

On auscultation, the murmur of mild TR may be absent or very subtle and of short duration. When TR occurs in the absence of pulmonary hypertension (e.g., infective endocarditis [see Video 77.5] or after trauma), the murmur usually is of low intensity and limited to the first half of systole. With greater degrees of TR, auscultation usually reveals an S_3 originating from the right ventricle, which is accentuated by inspiration. When TR is associated with and secondary to pulmonary hypertension, P_2 is accentuated as well. When TR occurs in the presence of pulmonary hypertension, the systolic murmur usually is high-pitched, pansystolic, and loudest in the fourth intercostal space in the parasternal region but occasionally is loudest in the subxiphoid area. When the right ventricle is greatly dilated and occupies the anterior surface of the heart, the murmur may be prominent at the apex and difficult to distinguish from that produced by mitral regurgitation (MR).

TABLE 77.3 Stages of Tricuspid Regurgitation

STAGE	DEFINITION	VALVE HEMODYNAMICS	HEMODYNAMIC CONSEQUENCES	CLINICAL SYMPTOMS AND PRESENTATION
B	Progressive TR	Central jet ≤50% RA	None	None
		Vena contracta width ≤0.7 cm		
		ERO ≤0.4 cm²		
		R Vol ≤45 mL		
C	Asymptomatic severe TR	Central jet >50% RA	Dilated RV and RA	Elevated venous pressure
		Vena contracta width >0.7 cm	Elevated RA with cV wave	No symptoms
		ERO >0.4 cm²		
		R Vol >45 mL		
		Dense CW signal with dagger shape		
		Hepatic vein systolic flow reversal		
D1	Symptomatic severe TR	Central jet >50% RA	Dilated RV and RA	Elevated venous pressure
		Vena contracta width >0.7 cm	Elevated RA with cV wave	Dyspnea on exertion, fatigue, ascites, edema
		ERO >0.4 cm²		
		R Vol >45 mL		
		Dense CW signal with dagger shape		
		Hepatic vein systolic flow reversal		

CW, Continuous wave Doppler signal; *ERO*, effective regurgitant orifice; *RA*, right atrium; *RV*, right ventricle; *R Vol*, regurgitant volume; *TR*, tricuspid regurgitation.
From Otto, Nishimura, RA, Bonow RO, CM, et al. 2020 AHA/ACC guideline for the management of patients with valvular heart disease: a report of the American College of Cardiology/American Heart Association Task Force on Practice Guidelines. *J Am Coll Cardiol*. 2021. doi.org/10.1016/j.jacc.2020.11.018.

The response of the systolic murmur to respiration and other maneuvers is of considerable aid in establishing the diagnosis of TR. The murmur characteristically is augmented during inspiration (Carvallo sign) with inspiration being associated with an increase in RV size and tricuspid valve annulus dimension, as well as an increase in regurgitant orifice area.[12] However, when the failing ventricle can no longer increase its stroke volume with the patient in the recumbent or sitting position, the inspiratory augmentation may be elicited by standing. The murmur also increases during the Mueller maneuver (see earlier), exercise, leg raising, and hepatic compression. It demonstrates an immediate overshoot after release of the Valsalva strain but is reduced in intensity and duration in the standing position and during the strain of the Valsalva maneuver. Increased atrioventricular flow across the tricuspid orifice in diastole may cause a short early diastolic flow rumble in the left parasternal region following S_3. Tricuspid valve prolapse, like MVP, causes nonejection systolic clicks and late systolic murmurs. In tricuspid valve prolapse, however, these findings are more prominent at the lower left sternal border. With inspiration, the clicks occur later and the murmurs intensify and become shorter in duration.

Echocardiography. The goal of echocardiography is to estimate the severity of TR and assess pulmonary arterial pressure and RV function.[13,14] In patients with TR secondary to dilation of the tricuspid annulus, the right atrium, right ventricle, and tricuspid annulus all usually are greatly dilated on echocardiography.[15] Doppler of the hepatic vein in severe TR shows systolic flow reversals (Fig. 77.3). There is evidence of RV diastolic overload with paradoxical motion of the ventricular septum similar to that observed in atrial septal defect. Severity of TR can be assessed by measuring vena contracta (Fig. 77.4) and regurgitant volume and effective regurgitant area quantified by quantitative Doppler or proximal isovelocity surface area method. Exaggerated motion and delayed closure of the tricuspid valve are evident in patients with Ebstein anomaly. Prolapse of the tricuspid valve caused by myxomatous degeneration may be evident on echocardiography. Echocardiographic indications of tricuspid valve abnormalities, especially TR by Doppler examination, can be detected in the vast majority of patients with carcinoid heart disease (see Fig. 77.2). A similar appearance of the tricuspid valve may be seen in patients who have used drugs that increase serotonin levels or simulate its effect on serotonin receptors (see Video 77.1). In patients with TR caused by endocarditis, echocardiography may reveal vegetations on the valve or a flail valve (see Video 77.5). TEE enhances detection of TR, but the degree of TR may be reduced compared to transthoracic

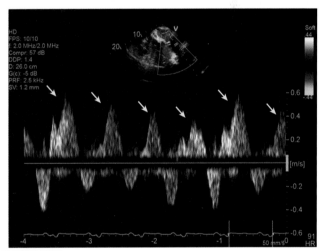

FIGURE 77.3 Pulsed-wave Doppler of the hepatic vein in a patient with severe tricuspid valve regurgitation showing significant hepatic vein systolic flow reversals (*arrows*).

echocardiography because of sedation given during TEE. Doppler echocardiography is a sensitive technique for visualizing the TR jet. The magnitude of TR can be quantified using techniques similar to those used to evaluate MR.[13,15]

Other Diagnostic Evaluation Modalities

Electrocardiography. ECG changes usually are nonspecific and characteristic of the lesion causing TR. Incomplete right bundle branch block, Q waves in lead V_1, and AF commonly are found.

Radiography. Marked cardiomegaly and a prominent right atrium are usually evident in patients with functional TR. Evidence of elevated right atrial pressure may include distention of the azygos vein and the presence of a pleural effusion. Ascites with upward displacement of the diaphragm may be present. Systolic pulsations of the right atrium may be present on fluoroscopy.

Cardiac Magnetic Resonance and Computed Tomography. CMR and CT are both useful for determining the three-dimensional geometric relationships between the right ventricle and the tricuspid annulus and leaflets in patients with functional TR.[16]

FIGURE 77.4 Transesophageal orthogonal views of the tricuspid valve showing severe tricuspid valve regurgitation with a large vena contracta of 1.68 cm in a patient with long-standing atrial fibrillation and functional tricuspid valve regurgitation from severe right atrial enlargement and tricuspid annulus dilation.

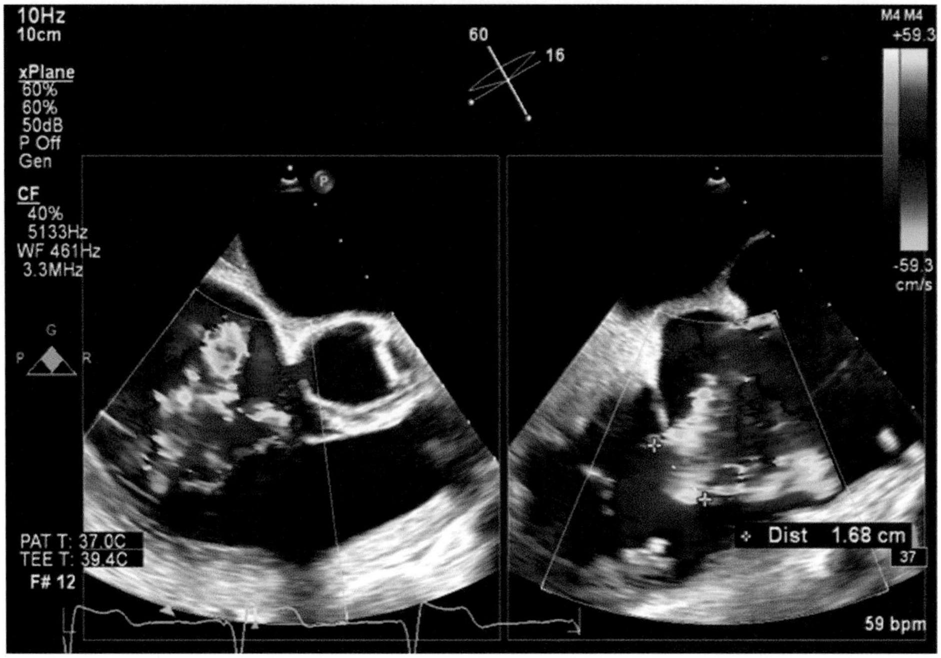

TABLE 77.4 ACC/AHA Guidelines for Intervention for Tricuspid Regurgitation

COR	LOE	INDICATION
1	B-NR	In patients with severe TR (Stages C and D) undergoing left-sided valve surgery, tricuspid valve surgery is recommended
2a	B-NR	In patients with progressive TR (Stage B) undergoing left-sided valve surgery, tricuspid valve surgery can be beneficial in the context of either (1) tricuspid annular dilation (tricuspid annulus end diastolic diameter >4.0 cm) or (2) prior signs and symptoms of right-sided HF
2a	B-NR	In patients with signs and symptoms of right-sided HF and severe primary TR (Stage D), isolated tricuspid valve surgery can be beneficial to reduce symptoms and recurrent hospitalizations
2a	B-NR	In patients with signs and symptoms of right-sided HF and severe isolated secondary TR attributable to annular dilation (in the absence of pulmonary hypertension or left-sided disease) who are poorly responsive to medical therapy (Stage D), isolated tricuspid valve surgery can be beneficial to reduce symptoms and recurrent hospitalizations.
2b	C-LD	In asymptomatic patients with severe primary TR (Stage C) and progressive RV dilation or systolic dysfunction, isolated tricuspid valve surgery may be considered
2b	B-NR	In patients with signs and symptoms of right-sided HF and severe TR (Stage D) who have undergone previous left-sided valve surgery, reoperation with isolated tricuspid valve surgery may be considered in the absence of severe pulmonary hypertension or severe RV systolic dysfunction

HF, heart failure; *LD*, limited data; *LOE*, level of evidence; *NR*, based on non-randomized studies; *RV*, right ventricular; *TR*, tricuspid regurgitation; *TS*, tricuspid stenosis.
From Otto CM, Nishimura, RA, Bonow RO, et al. 2020 AHA/ACC guideline for the management of patients with valvular heart disease: a report of the American College of Cardiology/American Heart Association Task Force on Practice Guidelines. *J Am Coll Cardiol*. 2021. doi.org/10.1016/j.jacc.2020.11.018.

Hemodynamic Findings. The right atrial and RV end-diastolic pressures often are elevated in TR, whether the condition is caused by organic disease of the tricuspid valve or is secondary to RV systolic overload. The right atrial pressure tracing usually reveals absence of the x descent and a prominent v or c-v wave (ventricularization of the atrial pressure). Absence of these findings essentially excludes moderate or severe TR. As the severity of TR increases, the contour of the right atrial pressure pulse increasingly resembles that of the RV pressure pulse. A rise or no change in right atrial pressure on deep inspiration, rather than the usual fall, is a characteristic finding.[17] Determination of the pulmonary arterial (or RV) systolic pressure may be helpful in deciding whether the TR is primary (caused by disease of the valve or its supporting structures) or functional (secondary to RV dilation). A pulmonary arterial or RV systolic pressure less than 40 mm Hg favors a primary cause, whereas a pressure greater than 55 mm Hg suggests that TR is secondary.

Management

TR in the absence of pulmonary hypertension is initially well tolerated. However, if TR is severe and sustained, eventually right heart failure will endure, which is associated with increased hospitalizations and excess mortality[18,19]; thus, appropriate consideration of and timing for surgery are indicated (see Table 77.4). Functional TR in the setting of pulmonary hypertension is associated with heart failure and poor survival.[20]

With the development of annuloplasty techniques, with or without an annuloplasty ring, surgical treatment of acquired TR secondary to annular dilation has greatly improved.[21,22] Repair rates have continued to increase significantly in the context of concomitant cardiac surgery; isolated tricuspid valve repair or replacement remains substantially underutilized.[23] At the time of mitral valve surgery in patients with TR secondary to pulmonary hypertension, the severity of the regurgitation should be assessed. It should be determined whether the TR is secondary to pulmonary hypertension, in which case the valve is normal, or whether it is secondary to other disease processes. Patients with mild TR without annular dilation usually do not require surgical treatment; pulmonary vascular pressures decline after successful mitral valve surgery, and the mild TR tends to disappear. However, even mild TR should be repaired if there is dilation of the tricuspid annulus, because the TR is likely to progress in severity if left untreated.[3,22] Excellent results have been reported in patients with mild to moderate TR using suture annuloplasty of the posterior (unsupported) portion of the annulus.[24] Patients with severe TR require ring annuloplasty.[25] Surgical mortality rates have continued to decrease over time. Contemporary data shows positive long-term outcomes associated with concomitant tricuspid valve repair at the time of left-heart valve surgery or coronary artery bypass surgery, irrespective of degree of TR,[26] although a doubling of risk of permanent pacemaker implantation was noted with use of tricuspid ring annuloplasty during mitral valve surgery.[26] Residual TR after tricuspid annuloplasty is determined principally by the degree of preoperative tricuspid leaflet tethering.[27] If these procedures do not provide a good functional result at the operating table, as assessed by TEE, valve replacement using a large bioprosthesis may be required. Transcatheter approaches to tricuspid valve repair and replacement using various methods and devices (see Chapter 78) are feasible and currently being studied in clinical trials.[28–30]

When organic disease of the tricuspid valve (Ebstein anomaly or carcinoid heart disease) causes TR severe enough to require surgery, valve replacement usually is needed. The risk of thrombosis of mechanical prostheses is greater in the tricuspid than in the mitral or aortic positions, presumably because pressure and flow rates are lower in the right side of the heart. For this reason, the artificial valve of choice for the tricuspid position in adults is a bioprosthesis. Graft durability of more than 10 years has been established. Postoperative vitamin K antagonist therapy is recommended after bioprosthetic tricuspid valve replacement in patients with carcinoid heart disease, because of a potential for thrombosis.[31]

In treating the difficult problem of tricuspid endocarditis (see Video 77.5) in intravenous drug users (see Chapter 80), total excision of the tricuspid valve without immediate replacement generally can be tolerated by these patients, who usually do not have associated pulmonary hypertension. However, management decisions should be made by a heart valve team, including cardiology, cardiac surgery, and infectious disease specialists. Diseased valvular tissue should be excised to eradicate the endocarditis (see Video 77.5), and antibiotic treatment can then be continued. RV dysfunction will eventually occur if the resultant severe TR is untreated. A bioprosthetic valve may therefore be inserted several months after valve excision and control of the infection.

PULMONIC STENOSIS

Causes and Pathology

Congenital PS is the most common etiology of PS with an estimated worldwide birth prevalence of 0.5 per 1000 live births, and a higher prevalence in Asia.[32] Noonan syndrome is associated with PS, and PS may be seen with tetralogy of Fallot, Williams syndrome, and with other congenital heart defects. The pulmonary valve may be bicuspid, unicommissural, acommissural, or dysplastic. Manifestations in children and adults are discussed in Chapter 82. Rheumatic inflammation of the pulmonic valve is very uncommon, is usually associated with involvement of other valves, and rarely leads to serious deformity. Carcinoid heart disease often involves the pulmonary valve, and plaques, similar to those involving the tricuspid valve, are often present in the outflow tract of the right ventricle of patients with malignant carcinoid. The plaques result in constriction of the pulmonary valve annulus, retraction, thickening and fusion of the valve cusps, and a combination of PS and pulmonic regurgitation (PR) (see Fig. 77.3).[2] Another cause of PS is extrinsic compression by cardiac tumors or by aneurysm of the sinus of Valsalva.

Clinical Presentation

It is not until PS is severe that symptoms develop. These symptoms include fatigue, dyspnea, exertional pre-syncope or syncope, and eventually, right heart failure.

Physical Examination

The systolic ejection murmur of PS is heard at the left base and increases with inspiration. With increasing severity of PS, the ejection click moves closer to the first heart sound; the click disappears in severe PS. With severe PS, the jugular venous pulse shows a prominent a wave. A RV lift becomes palpable.

Management

Management of congenital PS focuses on balloon dilation when PS is severe or the patient is symptomatic (see Chapter 82). For the mixed stenosis and regurgitation of carcinoid involvement of the pulmonic valve, patch annuloplasty at the time of pulmonic valve replacement is frequently advisable.[31] Transcatheter pulmonary valve replacement is increasingly being used for pulmonary stenosis, atresia, or regurgitation.[33] Long-term outcome after surgical treatment of PS is excellent.[34]

PULMONIC REGURGITATION

Causes and Pathology

PR can result from dilation of the valve ring secondary to pulmonary hypertension (of any cause) or from dilation of the pulmonary artery. Infective endocarditis can involve the pulmonic valve, resulting in valve regurgitation. As more patients with congenital heart disease survive to adulthood, there is an increasing population of young adults with residual PR after surgical treatment of tetralogy of Fallot (Fig. 77.5) or surgical or transcatheter treatment of congenital PS. PR also may result from various lesions that directly affect the pulmonic valve. These include congenital malformations, such as absent, malformed, fenestrated, or supernumerary leaflets. These anomalies may occur as isolated lesions but more often are associated with other congenital anomalies, particularly tetralogy of Fallot, ventricular septal defect, and pulmonic valvular stenosis. Less common causes include trauma, carcinoid syndrome, in which leaflet thickening and retraction results in mixed stenosis and regurgitation (Fig. 77.6; see also Fig. 16.49), rheumatic involvement, injury produced by a pulmonary artery flow-directed catheter, syphilis, and chest trauma.

Clinical Presentation

Like TR, isolated PR causes RV volume overload and may be tolerated for many years without difficulty unless it complicates, or is complicated by, pulmonary hypertension. In this case, PR usually is accompanied by and aggravates RV failure. Patients with PR caused by infective endocarditis who develop septic pulmonary emboli and pulmonary hypertension often exhibit severe RV failure. In most patients, the clinical manifestations of the primary disease are severe and usually overshadow the PR.

Physical Examination. The right ventricle is hyperdynamic and produces palpable systolic pulsations in the left parasternal area, and an enlarged pulmonary artery often produces systolic pulsations in the second left intercostal space. Sometimes systolic and diastolic thrills are felt in the same area. A tap reflecting pulmonic valve closure is usually palpable in the second intercostal space in patients with pulmonary hypertension and secondary PR.

Auscultation. P_2 is not audible in patients with congenital absence of the pulmonic valve; however, this sound is accentuated in patients with PR secondary to pulmonary hypertension. Wide splitting of S_2 caused by prolongation of RV ejection accompanying the augmented RV stroke volume may be noted. A nonvalvular systolic ejection click generated by the sudden expansion of the pulmonary artery by the augmented RV stroke volume frequently initiates a midsystolic ejection murmur, most prominent in the second left intercostal space. An S_3 and S_4 originating from the right ventricle are often audible in the fourth intercostal space at the left parasternal area, and are augmented by inspiration.

In the absence of pulmonary hypertension, the diastolic murmur of PR is low-pitched and usually is heard best at the third and fourth left intercostal spaces adjacent to the sternum. The regurgitant murmur reflects the diastolic pressure gradient between the pulmonary artery and the right ventricle; as these pressures are usually lower than left-sided pressures, the murmur of PR is less likely to be heard than that of a similar grade of aortic regurgitation (AR). The PR murmur commences when pressures in the pulmonary artery and right ventricle diverge, approximately 0.04 second after P_2. The murmur becomes louder during inspiration.

When systolic pulmonary arterial pressure exceeds approximately 55 mm Hg, dilation of the pulmonic annulus produces a high-velocity regurgitant jet resulting in the audible murmur of PR, or Graham Steell

DISEASES OF THE HEART VALVES

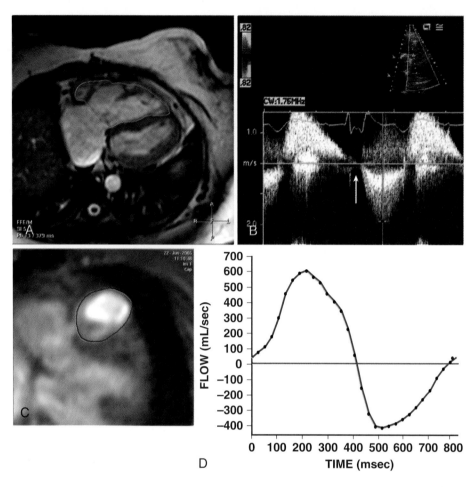

FIGURE 77.5 Cardiac magnetic resonance imaging (CMR) and Doppler echocardiographic evaluation in a 40-year-old woman who underwent repair of tetralogy of Fallot as a child. She was asymptomatic, but significant right ventricular (RV) enlargement was seen on echocardiography. **A,** RV dilation (*green circled area*) was confirmed in the CMR images, with a calculated RV end-diastolic volume of 444 mL. **B,** The Doppler tracing shows a dense signal in diastole with a steep deceleration slope that reaches the baseline before the end of diastole (*arrow*). **C,** Interrogation of pulmonary artery flow in the CMR phase-velocity images was performed by drawing a region of interest (*red circle*) around the pulmonary artery. **D,** Graph of the pulmonary artery flow within the region of interest indicated in **C** demonstrates both antegrade and retrograde flow. The total RV stroke volume was 245 mL, with antegrade flow of 98 mL, yielding a regurgitant fraction of 67%.

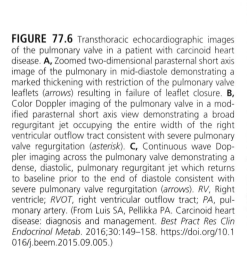

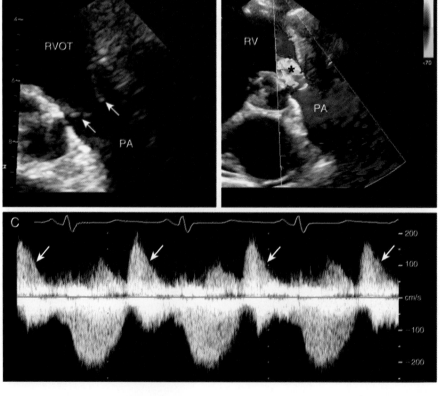

FIGURE 77.6 Transthoracic echocardiographic images of the pulmonary valve in a patient with carcinoid heart disease. **A,** Zoomed two-dimensional parasternal short axis image of the pulmonary in mid-diastole demonstrating a marked thickening with restriction of the pulmonary valve leaflets (*arrows*) resulting in failure of leaflet closure. **B,** Color Doppler imaging of the pulmonary valve in a modified parasternal short axis view demonstrating a broad regurgitant jet occupying the entire width of the right ventricular outflow tract consistent with severe pulmonary valve regurgitation (*asterisk*). **C,** Continuous wave Doppler imaging across the pulmonary valve demonstrating a dense, diastolic, pulmonary regurgitant jet which returns to baseline prior to the end of diastole consistent with severe pulmonary valve regurgitation (*arrows*). *RV,* Right ventricle; *RVOT,* right ventricular outflow tract; *PA,* pulmonary artery. (From Luis SA, Pellikka PA. Carcinoid heart disease: diagnosis and management. *Best Pract Res Clin Endocrinol Metab.* 2016;30:149–158. https://doi.org/10.1016/j.beem.2015.09.005.)

murmur. This murmur is high-pitched, blowing, and decrescendo, beginning immediately after P_2, and is most prominent in the left parasternal region in the second to fourth intercostal spaces. Thus, although it resembles the murmur of AR, it usually is accompanied by severe pulmonary hypertension—that is, an accentuated P_2 or fused S_2, an ejection sound, and a systolic murmur of TR, and not by a widened arterial pulse pressure. Sometimes, a low-frequency presystolic murmur is present, originating from increased diastolic flow across the tricuspid valve.

The murmur of PR secondary to pulmonary hypertension usually increases in intensity with inspiration, is diminished during the Valsalva strain, and returns to baseline intensity almost immediately after release of the Valsalva strain. This PR murmur resembles and may be confused with the diastolic blowing murmur of AR. However, a diastolic blowing murmur along the left sternal border in patients with rheumatic heart disease and pulmonary hypertension (even in the absence of peripheral signs of AR) usually is caused by AR rather than PR.

Echocardiography. A trivial or mild degree of PR can be detected by Doppler echocardiography in most normal patients. With more severe degrees, two-dimensional echocardiography shows RV dilation, and RV hypertrophy, in patients with pulmonary hypertension. RV function can be evaluated. Abnormal motion of the septum characteristic of volume overload of the right ventricle in diastole and/or septal flutter may be evident. The motion of the pulmonic valve may point to the cause of the PR. Absence of *a* waves and systolic notching of the posterior leaflet suggest pulmonary hypertension; large *a* waves indicate PS. Doppler echocardiography is extremely accurate in detecting PR and in helping estimate its severity (see Fig. 77.6; see also Fig. 16.50). Severe PR is associated with a reduced pressure half-time, indicating rapid equalization of pressure in the right ventricle and pulmonary artery. Additionally, the density of the Doppler profile of the jet is increased, and reversal of flow in the pulmonary artery by color flow imaging can be detected a distance from the valve. Abnormal Doppler signals in the RV outflow tract with velocity sustained throughout diastole are generally observed in patients in whom PR is caused by dilation of the valve ring secondary to pulmonary hypertension. When the velocity falls during diastole, the pulmonary artery pressure is usually normal, and the regurgitation is caused by an abnormality of the valve itself.

Other Diagnostic Evaluation Modalities

Electrocardiography. In the absence of pulmonary hypertension, PR is seen on an ECG as RV diastolic overload—an rSr (or rsR) configuration in the right precordial leads. PR secondary to pulmonary hypertension is usually associated with ECG evidence of RV hypertrophy.

Radiography. The pulmonary artery and right ventricle are usually enlarged, but these signs are nonspecific. Fluoroscopy may demonstrate pronounced pulsation of the main pulmonary artery.

CMR may be used to assess pulmonic valve anatomy, recognize any obstruction above or below the valve, measure pulmonary artery dilation, and quantify PR severity (see Fig. 77.5). CMR also is useful in evaluating RV dilation and systolic function.[35] Alternatively, cardiac CT may be used.[35]

Management

Except in patients with previous surgery for tetralogy of Fallot or similar RV outflow obstruction, or carcinoid heart disease, PR alone is seldom severe enough to require specific treatment. Treatment of the primary condition, such as infective endocarditis, or the lesion responsible for the pulmonary hypertension, such as surgery for mitral valvular disease, often ameliorates the PR. The timing of surgery for severe PR is based on the degree of RV dilation and evidence of systolic dysfunction.[3,36] In these patients, valve replacement may be carried out, preferably with a pulmonary allograft. There is growing experience with catheter-based approaches to pulmonic valve replacement in native pulmonic valve disease and in PR after surgical correction of congenital heart defects (see Chapter 82).[33]

MULTIVALVULAR DISEASE

Various clinical and hemodynamic syndromes can be produced by different combinations of valvular abnormalities. Multivalvular involvement has diverse causes (Table 77.5). It is frequently caused by rheumatic fever but is also seen in congenital heart disease, carcinoid

TABLE 77.5 Causes of Multivalvular Heart Disease

Acquired

Systemic diseases
- Infective endocarditis
- Carcinoid heart disease
- Systemic lupus erythematosus

Cardiac diseases
- Infective endocarditis
- Rheumatic heart disease

Degenerative
- Calcific diseases, increased with age, prior radiation, chronic kidney disease

Iatrogenic
- Adverse drug effects—ergot-related antagonists
- Radiation therapy

Functional (annulus dilatation)
- Due to ischemic heart disease, hypertensive heart disease, chronic arrhythmia, pulmonary hypertension, cardiomyopathy

Congenital

Connective tissue disorders
- Marfan syndrome, Ehlers-Danlos syndrome

Other
- Trisomy 18, 13, and 15
- Shone syndrome
- Ochronosis

Mixed

Multiple conditions may contribute to valve dysfunction
- Degenerative diseases may lead to associated functional disease
- Congenital heart disease may predispose to infective endocarditis or degenerative disease

heart disease, radiation heart disease, and connective tissue disorders. Degenerative calcific valve disease of the elderly is increasingly recognized to impact multiple valves. Myxomatous MR and prolapse may be associated with tricuspid valve prolapse and TR, or with pulmonary hypertension, tricuspid annulus dilation and TR. Marfan syndrome and other connective tissue disorders may cause multivalve prolapse and dilation, resulting in multivalvular regurgitation. Degenerative calcification of the aortic valve may be associated with degenerative mitral annular calcification, resulting in concomitant aortic stenosis (AS) and MR. Different pathologic conditions may affect two valves in the same patient (e.g., infective endocarditis on the aortic valve causing AR and ischemia causing MR).

In patients with multivalvular disease, the clinical manifestations depend on the relative severity of each lesion. When the valvular abnormalities are of approximately equal severity, clinical manifestations produced by the more proximal (upstream) of the two valvular lesions (i.e., the mitral valve in patients with combined mitral and aortic valvular disease and the tricuspid valve in patients with combined tricuspid and mitral valvular disease) are generally more prominent than those produced by the distal lesion. Thus, the proximal lesion tends to mask the distal lesion.

It is important to recognize multivalvular involvement preoperatively because failure to correct all significant valvular disease at the time of surgery increases mortality. Specific recommendations exist for concomitant valve surgery in patients undergoing surgery on another valve.[3,37] In patients with multivalvular disease, the relative severity of each lesion may be difficult to estimate by clinical examination because one lesion may mask the manifestations of the other. Therefore, patients suspected of having multivalvular involvement and who are being considered for surgical treatment should undergo careful clinical evaluation and full Doppler echocardiographic evaluation. Stress echocardiography is well suited to assess multivalvular disease and may be especially useful when the patient's symptoms are disproportionate to the resting hemodynamics. Mixed stenotic and regurgitant lesions can be assessed with a combination of two- or three-dimensional imaging, including planimetry of stenotic orifices, color flow imaging and Doppler. Multiple valves can be systematically assessed during exercise[38]; this is particularly helpful in assessing patients with exertional symptoms, especially when these seem disproportionate to findings on imaging at rest. Right and left cardiac catheterization may occasionally be necessary. If there is any question concerning the presence of significant AS in patients undergoing mitral valve surgery, the aortic valve should be inspected because overlooking this condition can lead to a high perioperative mortality. Similarly, it is useful to palpate the tricuspid valve at the time of mitral valve surgery. Intraoperative TEE is also important to assess the impact of repair of one valve lesion on another.

Mitral Stenosis and Aortic Valve Disease

Aortic valve involvement is present in approximately one third of patients with rheumatic MS. Rheumatic aortic valve disease may result in primary regurgitation, stenosis, or mixed stenosis and regurgitation. AR is evident on physical examination in approximately two thirds of patients with severe MS, but only approximately 10% of patients with MS have severe rheumatic AR. On physical examination, a proximal lesion may mask signs of a distal lesion. For example, significant AR may be missed in patients with severe MS because the widened pulse pressure may be absent. An accentuated S_1 and an OS in a patient with AR should suggest the possibility of mitral valvular disease. AS is evident on physical examination based on the typical murmur, even when MS is present; however, the cardiac output tends to be reduced more than that in patients with isolated AS. On physical examination, a S_4 (which is common in patients with pure AS) usually is not present. The midsystolic murmur characteristic of AS may be reduced in intensity and duration because the stroke volume is reduced by the MS.

Echocardiography is of decisive value in evaluating patients with rheumatic disease and allows accurate diagnosis of the presence and severity of multivalve involvement, taking into consideration the altered flow conditions with serial lesions. In the setting of severe AS, MS severity may be overestimated, especially when indexed stroke volume is reduced. True MS in patients with severe AS can be recognized by Doppler-derived mitral valve area ≤1.5 cm² and the extension of calcification to both anterior and posterior mitral leaflets and is associated with excess mortality.[39]

Because double-valve replacement is associated with increased short- and long-term risks, balloon mitral valvuloplasty (BMV) can be the first procedure if MS is the predominant lesion, with subsequent aortic valve replacement (AVR) when needed. If percutaneous BMV is not an option or concurrent AVR is needed, surgical valvotomy may be considered.

It is vital to recognize the presence of hemodynamically significant aortic valvular disease (i.e., AS and/or AR) preoperatively in patients who are to undergo BMV. This procedure may be hazardous because it can impose a sudden hemodynamic load on the left ventricle that had previously been protected by the MS and may lead to acute pulmonary edema.

Aortic Stenosis and Mitral Regurgitation

AS is often accompanied by MR caused by MVP, annular calcification, rheumatic disease, or functional MR. The increased left ventricular (LV) pressure secondary to LV outflow obstruction may augment the volume of MR flow, whereas the presence of MR may diminish the ventricular preload necessary to maintain the LV stroke volume in patients with AS. The result is a reduced forward cardiac output and marked left atrial and pulmonary venous hypertension. Significant MR is one explanation for low output AS (see Chapter 72).[40] The development of AF (caused by left atrial enlargement) has an adverse hemodynamic effect in the presence of AS. Physical findings may be confusing because it may be difficult to recognize two distinct systolic murmurs. However, on echocardiography, the cause and severity of AS and MR can be accurately diagnosed. In most cases, MR is mild to moderate and it is appropriate to treat AS alone. When MR is severe or there is significant structural mitral valve disease, concurrent mitral repair (whenever possible) or valve replacement at the time of AVR should be considered.

Aortic Regurgitation and Mitral Regurgitation

The relatively infrequent combination of AR and MR may be caused by rheumatic heart disease, prolapse of the aortic and mitral valves secondary to myxomatous degeneration, or dilation of both annuli in patients with connective tissue disorders, or IE. The clinical features of AR usually predominate, and it is sometimes difficult to determine whether the MR is caused by organic involvement of this valve or by dilation of the mitral valve ring secondary to LV enlargement. When both valvular leaks are

severe, this combination of lesions is poorly tolerated. The normal mitral valve ordinarily serves as a backup to the aortic valve, and premature (diastolic) closure of the mitral valve limits the volume of reflux that occurs in patients with acute AR. With severe combined regurgitant lesions, regardless of the cause of the mitral lesion, blood may reflux from the aorta through both chambers of the left side of the heart into the pulmonary veins. Physical and laboratory examinations usually show evidence of both lesions. An S_3 and a brisk arterial pulse frequently are present. The relative severity of each lesion can be assessed best by Doppler echocardiography, especially using proximal isovelocity surface area or vena contracta methods, three-dimensional imaging, or contrast angiography. This combination of lesions leads to severe LV dilation. MR that occurs in patients with AR secondary to LV dilation often regresses after AVR alone. If severe, the MR may be corrected by annuloplasty at the time of AVR. An intrinsically normal mitral valve that is regurgitant because of a dilated annulus should not be replaced.

Surgical Treatment of Multivalvular Disease

Timing and indication for surgery is typically driven by the more severe predominant valve lesion.[3,37,41] The long-term survival following multivalvular surgery depends strongly on the preoperative functional status. Patients operated on for combined AR and MR have poorer outcomes than patients undergoing double-valve replacement for any of the other combinations of lesions, presumably because both AR and MR may produce irreversible LV damage. Surgical or transcatheter mitral valve repair for MR or balloon mitral valvotomy for MS performed in combination with AVR may be preferable to double-valve replacement and should be considered. Moreover, most patients will experience some decrease in functional MR severity after AVR. In the setting of planned AVR, management of coexistent MR should take into consideration the severity of MR, its mechanism, operative risks and co-morbidities. Risk factors that reduce long-term survival after double-valve replacement include advanced age, less favorable functional status, decreased LV ejection fraction, greater LV enlargement, and accompanying ischemic heart disease requiring coronary artery bypass grafting.

In view of the higher risks, a higher threshold is required for multivalvular versus single-valve surgery. Thus, patients generally are advised not to undergo multivalvular surgery until they reach late New York Heart Association (NYHA) functional class II or class III, unless they exhibit evidence of declining LV function. Despite a detailed noninvasive and invasive workup, the decision to treat more than one valve often is made on the basis of findings on palpation or direct inspection at the operating table, or the findings on intraoperative TEE.

Triple- and Quadruple-Valve Disease

Hemodynamically significant disease involving the mitral, aortic, and tricuspid valves is uncommon and typically is caused by rheumatic heart disease. Carcinoid heart disease can sometimes involve three or four valves.[31] Patients with multivalvular disease may present in advanced heart failure with marked cardiomegaly, and surgical correction of all significant valvular lesions is imperative. However, triple- or quadruple-valve replacement is a long and complex operation. Early in the experience with this procedure, the mortality rate was 20% for patients in NYHA class III and 40% for patients in class IV. More recently, the mortality rate has declined but is still substantial and should be reserved for high-volume cardiac surgical centers.[42] In many patients with triple-valvular disease, it is possible to replace the aortic valve, repair the mitral valve, and perform a tricuspid annuloplasty or valvuloplasty.

Patients who survive triple- or quadruple-valve replacement surgery usually experience substantial clinical improvement during the early postoperative period, and postoperative catheterization studies show marked reductions in pulmonary arterial and capillary pressures. However, some patients die of arrhythmias or congestive heart failure in the late postoperative period despite normally functioning prostheses. The cause of cardiac failure in this situation is unknown, but may be related to intraoperative myocardial ischemia, microemboli from the multiple prostheses, or continued subclinical episodes of rheumatic myocarditis.

When multiple prosthetic valves must be inserted, it is logical to select two bioprostheses or two mechanical prostheses for the left side of the heart. If the patient is to be exposed to the hazards of anticoagulants for one mechanical prosthesis, it seems unreasonable to add the potential risks of early failure of a bioprosthesis. However, if two mechanical prostheses are selected for the left side of the heart, the use of a bioprosthesis in the tricuspid position is suggested. Repair instead of replacement of the mitral and tricuspid valves during triple valve surgery is associated with improved short-term outcomes.[43] Percutaneous therapies are a growing alternative to surgical intervention when valve lesions are amenable to percutaneous intervention and surgical risk is increased (see Chapters 74 and 78).[41]

REFERENCES

Tricuspid Stenosis

1. Rodes-Cabau J, Taramasso M, O'Gara PT. Diagnosis and treatment of tricuspid valve disease: current and future perspectives. *Lancet.* 2016;388:2431–2442.
2. Luis SA, Pellikka PA. Carcinoid heart disease: diagnosis and management. *Best Pract Res Clin Endocrinol Metab.* 2016;30:149–158.
3. Otto CM, Nishimura RA, Bonow RO, et al. 2020 AHA/ACC guideline for the management of patients with valvular heart disease: a report of the American College of Cardiology/American Heart Association Task Force on Practice guidelines. *J Am Coll Cardiol.* 2021. https://doi.org/10.1016/j.jacc.2020.11.018.
4. Cevasco M, Shekar PS. Surgical management of tricuspid stenosis. *Ann Cardiothorac Surg.* 2017;6:275–282.

Tricuspid Regurgitation—Pathophysiology and Clinical Presentation

5. Asmarats L, Taramasso M, Rodes-Cabau J. Tricuspid valve disease: diagnosis, prognosis and management of a rapidly evolving field. *Nat Rev Cardiol.* 2019;16:538–554.
6. Benfari G, Antoine C, Miller WL, et al. Excess mortality associated with functional tricuspid regurgitation complicating heart failure with reduced ejection fraction. *Circulation.* 2019;140:196–206.
7. Essayagh B, Antoine C, Benfari G, et al. Functional tricuspid regurgitation of degenerative mitral valve disease: a crucial determinant of survival. *Eur Heart J.* 2020;41:1918–1929.
8. Topilsky Y, Nkomo VT, Vatury O, et al. Clinical outcome of isolated tricuspid regurgitation. *JACC Cardiovasc Imaging.* 2014;7:1185–1194.
9. Hoke U, Auger D, Thijssen J, et al. Significant lead-induced tricuspid regurgitation is associated with poor prognosis at long-term follow-up. *Heart.* 2014;100:960–968.
10. Ebrille E, Chang JD, Zimetbaum PJ. Tricuspid valve dysfunction caused by right ventricular leads. *Card Electrophysiol Clin.* 2018;10:447–452.
11. Zhang Z, Yin K, Dong L, et al. Surgical management of traumatic tricuspid insufficiency. *J Card Surg.* 2017;32:342–346.
12. Topilsky Y, Tribouilloy C, Michelena HI, et al. Pathophysiology of tricuspid regurgitation: quantitative Doppler echocardiographic assessment of respiratory dependence. *Circulation.* 2010;122:1505–1513.
13. Topilsky Y, Michelena HI, Messika-Zeitoun D, Enriquez Sarano M. Doppler-echocardiographic assessment of tricuspid regurgitation. *Prog Cardiovasc Dis.* 2018;61:397–403.
14. Badano LP, Hahn R, Rodriguez-Zanella H, et al. Morphological assessment of the tricuspid apparatus and grading regurgitation severity in patients with functional tricuspid regurgitation: thinking outside the box. *JACC Cardiovasc Imaging.* 2019;12:652–664.
15. Hahn RT, Thomas JD, Khalique OK, et al. Imaging assessment of tricuspid regurgitation severity. *JACC Cardiovasc Imaging.* 2019;12:469–490.
16. Naoum C, Blanke P, Cavalcante JL, Leipsic J. Cardiac computed tomography and magnetic resonance imaging in the evaluation of mitral and tricuspid valve disease: implications for transcatheter interventions. *Circ Cardiovasc Imaging.* 2017;10. https://doi.org/10.1161/CIRCIMAGING.116.005331.
17. Syed FF, Schaff HV, Oh JK. Constrictive pericarditis–a curable diastolic heart failure. *Nat Rev Cardiol.* 2014;11:530–544.

Tricuspid Regurgitation—Management

18. Topilsky Y, Maltais S, Medina Inojosa J, et al. Burden of tricuspid regurgitation in patients diagnosed in the community setting. *JACC Cardiovasc Imaging.* 2019;12:433–442.
19. Fender EA, Petrescu I, Ionescu F, et al. Prognostic importance and predictors of survival in isolated tricuspid regurgitation: a growing problem. *Mayo Clin Proc.* 2019;94:2032–2039.
20. Chen L, Larsen CM, Le RJ, et al. The prognostic significance of tricuspid valve regurgitation in pulmonary arterial hypertension. *Clin Respir J.* 2018;12:1572–1580.
21. Hamandi M, Smith RL, Ryan WH, et al. Outcomes of isolated tricuspid valve surgery have improved in the modern era. *Ann Thorac Surg.* 2019;108:11–15.
22. Antunes MJ, Rodriguez-Palomares J, Prendergast B, et al. Management of tricuspid valve regurgitation: position statement of the European Society of Cardiology working groups of cardiovascular surgery and valvular heart disease. *Eur J Cardio Thorac Surg.* 2017;52:1022–1030.
23. Alqahtani F, Berzingi CO, Aljohani S, et al. Contemporary trends in the use and outcomes of surgical treatment of tricuspid regurgitation. *J Am Heart Assoc.* 2017;6. https://doi.org/10.1161/JAHA.117.007597.
24. Pagnesi M, Montalto C, Mangieri A, et al. Tricuspid annuloplasty versus a conservative approach in patients with functional tricuspid regurgitation undergoing left-sided heart valve surgery: a study-level meta-analysis. *Int J Cardiol.* 2017;240:138–144.
25. Parolari A, Barili F, Pilozzi A, Pacini D. Ring or suture annuloplasty for tricuspid regurgitation? A meta-analysis review. *Ann Thorac Surg.* 2014;98:2255–2263.
26. Badhwar V, Rankin JS, He M, et al. Performing concomitant tricuspid valve repair at the time of mitral valve operations is not associated with increased operative mortality. *Ann Thorac Surg.* 2017;103:587–593.
27. Yiu KH, Wong A, Pu L, et al. Prognostic value of preoperative right ventricular geometry and tricuspid valve tethering area in patients undergoing tricuspid annuloplasty. *Circulation.* 2014;129:87–92.
28. Taramasso M, Pozzoli A, Guidotti A, et al. Percutaneous tricuspid valve therapies: the new frontier. *Eur Heart J.* 2017;38:639–647.
29. Nickenig G, Weber M, Lurz P, et al. Transcatheter edge-to-edge repair for reduction of tricuspid regurgitation: 6-month outcomes of the TRILUMINATE single-arm study. *Lancet.* 2019;394:2002–2011.
30. Nickenig G, Weber M, Schueler R, et al. 6-Month outcomes of tricuspid valve reconstruction for patients with severe tricuspid regurgitation. *J Am Coll Cardiol.* 2019;73:1905–1915.
31. Connolly HM, Schaff HV, Abel MD, et al. Early and late outcomes of surgical treatment in carcinoid heart disease. *J Am Coll Cardiol.* 2015;66:2189–2196.

Pulmonic Stenosis and Pulmonic Regurgitation

32. van der Linde D, Konings EE, Slager MA, et al. Birth prevalence of congenital heart disease worldwide: a systematic review and meta-analysis. *J Am Coll Cardiol.* 2011;58:2241–2247.
33. Alkashkari W, Alsubei A, Hijazi ZM. Transcatheter pulmonary valve replacement: current state of art. *Curr Cardiol Rep.* 2018;20:27.
34. Cuypers JA, Menting ME, Opic P, et al. The unnatural history of pulmonary stenosis up to 40 years after surgical repair. *Heart.* 2017;103:273–279.
35. Chambers JB, Myerson SG, Rajani R, et al. Multimodality imaging in heart valve disease. *Open Heart.* 2016;3:e000330.
36. Cramer JW, Ginde S, Hill GD, et al. Tricuspid repair at pulmonary valve replacement does not alter outcomes in tetralogy of Fallot. *Ann Thorac Surg.* 2015;99:899–904.

Multivalvular Disease

37. Baumgartner H, Falk V, Bax JJ, et al. 2017 ESC/EACTS Guidelines for the management of valvular heart disease. *Eur Heart J.* 2017;38:2739–2791.
38. Lancellotti P, Pellikka PA, Budts W, et al. The clinical use of stress echocardiography in non-ischaemic heart disease: recommendations from the European Association of Cardiovascular Imaging and the American Society of Echocardiography. *Eur Heart J Cardiovasc Imaging.* 2016;17:1191–1229.
39. Kato N, Padang R, Pislaru C, et al. Hemodynamics and prognostic impact of concomitant mitral stenosis in patients undergoing surgical or transcatheter aortic valve replacement for aortic stenosis. *Circulation.* 2019;140:1251–1260.
40. Pislaru SV, Pellikka PA. The spectrum of low-output low-gradient aortic stenosis with normal ejection fraction. *Heart.* 2016;102:665–671.
41. Unger P, Pibarot P, Tribouilloy C, et al. Multiple and mixed valvular heart diseases. *Circ Cardiovasc Imaging.* 2018;11:e007862.
42. Pagni S, Ganzel BL, Singh R, et al. Clinical outcome after triple-valve operations in the modern era: are elderly patients at increased surgical risk? *Ann Thorac Surg.* 2014;97:569–576.
43. Suri RM, Thourani VH, Englum BR, et al. The expanding role of mitral valve repair in triple valve operations: contemporary North American outcomes in 8,021 patients. *Ann Thorac Surg.* 2014;97:1513–1519; discussion 1519.

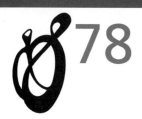

78 Transcatheter Therapies for Mitral and Tricuspid Valvular Heart Disease

HOWARD C. HERRMANN AND MICHAEL J. REARDON

The impetus for the development of transcatheter therapies for valvular heart disease (VHD) arises from two major factors. First, a transcatheter therapy can avoid the risks associated with more invasive surgical approaches, particularly those associated with cardiopulmonary bypass and median sternotomy, while preserving or enhancing outcomes. Second, the patient wants to avoid the invasiveness and prolonged recovery associated with major surgery. However, these factors must always be balanced with the efficacy of the transcatheter approach. In this regard, the patient will always prefer a transcatheter approach that is less invasive, provides a faster patient recovery, and has similar efficacy to a more invasive surgical approach. However, a less efficacious approach, even if safer and associated with faster recovery, will require more complex decision making that takes into account the patient's age, comorbidities, and goals of care.

Historically, the first and quite successful transcatheter therapy for VHD was balloon valvuloplasty for congenital pulmonic stenosis, developed by Dr. Jean Kan in 1982. That led to a decade of extension of balloon therapies to the treatment of mitral stenosis (MS) and aortic stenosis (AS), transcatheter aortic valve replacement (TAVR) for severe aortic stenosis, and opened the door to other transcatheter therapies for regurgitation lesions, such as MitraClip (Abbott Vascular, Santa Clara, California) repair for mitral regurgitation (MR) and new innovative approaches under development for tricuspid regurgitation (TR). The success of TAVR with both balloon-expandable and self-expanding prostheses for severe, symptomatic AS and MitraClip for MR has ushered in an entire medical specialty focused on transcatheter therapy of VHD. This chapter addresses the indications, techniques, and clinical and investigational therapies available for MS, MR, and TR.

MITRAL STENOSIS (SEE CHAPTER 75)

In the patient with severe and symptomatic MS, transthoracic echocardiography (TTE) is key to diagnose and confirm the functional severity of the stenosis (see Chapter 14).

Mitral Balloon Valvuloplasty

Determining the morphology of the mitral valve and subvalvular apparatus is important in preprocedural planning for mitral balloon valvuloplasty (MBV). The suitability of a valve for MBV can be determined using a morphologic score; the most widely used is the system of Wilkins (see Classic References), which assigns a score of 1 to 4 for leaflet mobility, valve thickening, calcification, and subvalvular thickening (see Table 14.9). Recently, the incorporation of additional echocardiographic measures including commissural calcification and

asymmetry and leaflet displacement have allowed refinement and improved accuracy for predicting outcome.[1] The severity of concomitant MR is also a key determining factor for MBV, both as it relates to the final result, which may increase up to one grade, and to confirm that the patient's symptoms are indeed caused by valvular obstruction and not concomitant regurgitation. In the latter case, surgical mitral valve replacement may be a better option for symptomatic relief. Transesophageal echocardiography (TEE) is a final step to assess further the severity of MR and valve morphology and to ensure the absence of left atrial (LA) thrombus before MBV. Some patients with severe calcification of the mitral annulus and leaflets, who are not candidates for balloon valvuloplasty, may be candidates for placement of a balloon-expandable transcatheter mitral valve replacement with a device initially approved for TAVR for AS. However, in a report of more than 100 such patients, the 30-day and 1-year mortality was high at 25% and 54%, respectively.[2] For other patients with less calcification and a suboptimal balloon morphology or mixed stenosis and regurgitation, a dedicated transcatheter mitral valve replacement may be another alternative.[3]

Indications

MBV is indicated in symptomatic MS patients who have at least moderate to severe MS, favorable valve morphology, absence of LA thrombus, and less than moderate to severe MR. In patients with rheumatic MS and calcified nonpliable valves who are at high risk or unsuitable for open surgery, MBV may be a reasonable alternative to provide palliative symptomatic relief. MBV may also be considered in asymptomatic patients with moderate to severe MS and new-onset atrial fibrillation after excluding LA thrombus (class IIb). In patients with symptoms and mild MS (mitral valve area [MVA] >1.5 cm^2), MBV can be considered if there is evidence of significant MS with exercise testing (class IIb).[4] The mechanism of benefit is separation of the fused commissures, which relieves the physical obstruction, thereby reducing the gradient and increasing MVA.

Procedure. The transvenous antegrade transseptal route is typically used to gain access to the left atrium to perform MBV. Inoue first used a self-positioning latex balloon wrapped with a nylon mesh to allow phased balloon expansion in 1982 and described the technique in 1984 (see Classic References). The double-balloon technique involves two peripheral arterial balloons tracked over separate guidewires placed in the left ventricle and simultaneously inflated.

The double-balloon technique was the first one used in the United States. Following transseptal catheterization and therapeutic anticoagulation, a balloon-tipped end-hole catheter is used to traverse the mitral valve via the transseptal puncture site. This catheter is navigated to the apex of the left ventricle, and once positioned, a 260-cm guidewire is

Additional content is available online at Elsevier eBooks for Practicing Clinicians

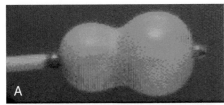
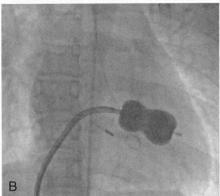

FIGURE 78.1 A, Inoue mitral balloon valvuloplasty catheter and three-stage balloon. **B,** Partially inflated Inoue balloon positioned across the mitral valve. Note an intracardiac echocardiographic catheter in the right ventricle and a pigtail catheter in the left ventricle.

the advantage of avoiding the endotracheal intubation and general anesthesia usually required for TEE.

MITRAL REGURGITATION

Unlike MS, which is caused primarily by rheumatic fever, MR is a more diverse disease that results from dysfunction of any of the portions of the complex mitral valve apparatus, including the leaflets, chords, annulus, and left ventricle. As discussed in Chapter 76, MR is often further classified into *primary* (organic or degenerative) disease, which affects the leaflets (e.g., fibromuscular dysplasia, mitral valve prolapse, and rheumatic disease), and *secondary* (ischemic or functional) disease, which spares the leaflets (e.g., diseases of atrium and ventricle, including ischemic dysfunction and dilated cardiomyopathy). Patients with severe MR have decreased survival, whether symptomatic or not, and surgery is often recommended.[6] In asymptomatic patients with primary MR and preserved LV function, a "watchful waiting" or "active surveillance" approach can be considered until the development of symptoms, LV dysfunction, pulmonary hypertension, or atrial fibrillation,[7] and current guidelines recommend surgery in patients who have reached these endpoints.[4] Surgery may also be considered for asymptomatic patients with normal LV function in whom there is a high likelihood of successful mitral valve repair.[4]

Rationale for Transcatheter Therapy

Surgery improves survival in observational studies but is associated with mortality rates of 1% to 5% and additional morbidity rates of 10% to 20%, including stroke, reoperation, renal failure, and prolonged ventilation.[8] The risks of surgery are particularly high in patients who are elderly or have LV dysfunction and secondary MR. In one study of more than 30,000 patients undergoing mitral valve replacement, mortality increased from 4.1% in those younger than 50 years to 17.0% in octogenarians,[9] although these outcomes improved in a more recent report.[10] The risks and morbidity of surgery coupled with patient preference have stimulated attempts to develop less invasive solutions.

When considering percutaneous or transcatheter approaches for mitral repair, it is useful to classify them according to the major structural abnormality that they address.[11] Unlike the extensive toolbox available to the mitral surgeon, transcatheter approaches are much more limited and often able to address only a single major element of the dysfunctional valve that contributes to MR.[12]

Table 78.1 lists some of the devices, their manufacturers, and current state of development.

Leaflet Repair with MitraClip Device

MitraClip (Abbott Vascular) was the first transcatheter mitral valve repair technology to receive CE (Conformité Européenne) Mark approval (European Union) and has now also received FDA approval for patients with primary (degenerative) MR and prohibitive surgical risk as well as for heart failure patients with left ventricular dysfunction (secondary MR) despite optimal medical therapy (Fig. 78.3). This system replicates the Alfieri stitch operation, in which the middle scallops of the posterior and anterior leaflets (P2 and A2, respectively) are sutured together to create a double-orifice mitral valve. The operation, although usually performed with adjunctive ring annuloplasty, has proved effective and durable in a wide variety of pathologies as well as in select patients without annuloplasty.[13]

Trials with MitraClip have confirmed its feasibility (e.g., Endovascular Valve Edge-to-Edge Repair Study [EVEREST] I), and its safety and efficacy were compared with those of surgical repair in a randomized trial (EVEREST II).[14] The procedure is performed with standard catheterization techniques using a transseptal approach from the right femoral vein.[15] The clip delivery system is introduced through a 24F sheath into the left atrium, where it can be guided by TEE using a series of turning knobs through the mitral valve into the left ventricle. A properly aligned and oriented clip can grasp the P2 and A2 segments of the leaflets from

then placed in the LV apex or looped across the aortic valve into the descending aorta. A second guidewire is placed using a similar technique or by using a dual-lumen catheter. Two 18- or 20-mm dilation balloons are tracked and positioned on the wires and inflated simultaneously to dilate the valve.

The Inoue technique has mostly replaced the double-balloon technique, in part because there is no risk of left ventricular (LV) perforation with the Inoue balloon (Fig. 78.1). The initial size of the Inoue balloon is based on patient's height. Once inserted over a guidewire into the left atrium, it can be steered across the mitral valve orifice with an internal stylet and then sequentially inflated multiple times over a 4-mm diameter range, with both hemodynamic and echocardiographic results assessed, to achieve the maximal dilation with the least increase in grade of MR. As such, it is important to evaluate carefully for severe commissural calcium preprocedurally. Calcium does not split with balloon inflation but does increase the potential for tearing the leaflets creating MR.

A reduction in mean mitral valve gradient by 50% or an increase in MVA greater than 1.5 cm² is considered a successful result and can be achieved in more than 80% of appropriately selected patients. An increase in MR by more than one grade after balloon inflation should signal an end to the procedure despite a residual gradient. Event-free survival after MBV is influenced by valve morphology. In a large study of 879 North American patients with a mean follow-up of 4.2 ± 3.7 years, there was a greater immediate increase in MVA after MBV and improved long-term survival (82% versus 57%; *P* < 0.0001) in patients with a Wilkins score of 8 or less (Fig. 78.2). Patients with higher echocardiographic scores have more events in the long term, including need for repeat MBV, need for mitral valve surgery, and death (Fig. 78.2B). In multivariate analysis, age, post-MBV MR grade of 3+ or higher, prior surgical commissurotomy, New York Heart Association (NYHA) Class IV symptoms, and elevated post-MBV pulmonary artery systolic pressure were all independently associated with worse outcome at follow-up.

The most common complication from MBV, severe MR, occurs in 2% to 10% of patients, with no significant difference between the Inoue and double-balloon techniques. Overall procedural mortality is approximately 1%. Other, less common procedural complications include pericardial tamponade, embolic events, vascular complications, arrhythmias, bleeding, stroke, myocardial infarction, residual atrial septal defect, and LV perforation.

Echocardiography is essential for many aspects of MBV, including the transseptal puncture and assessment of postprocedural results and complications (see Chapter 14). TEE is considered the gold standard, and 3D TEE has been shown to be superior to TTE in reducing fluoroscopy time and the interval from first transseptal puncture to first balloon inflation.[5] Intracardiac echocardiography can also be used, with

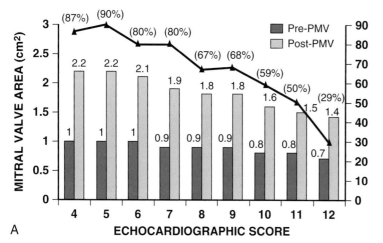

A

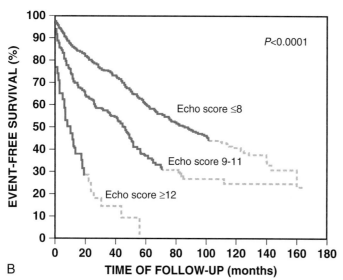

B

FIGURE 78.2 Results of mitral balloon valvuloplasty relative to preprocedural Wilkins score derived from echocardiography. A, *Bars* indicate mitral valve area before and after percutaneous mitral valvuloplasty (PMV) as a function of the echocardiographic score, and the connected *triangles* indicate procedural success rate. **B,** Association between echocardiographic score and postprocedural event-free survival. (From Palacios IF, et al. Which patients benefit from percutaneous mitral valvuloplasty? Prevalvuloplasty and postvalvuloplasty variables that predict long-term outcome. Circulation 2002;105:1465-1471. Copyright 2002 American Heart Association Inc.)

the ventricular side to create leaflet apposition. Once leaflet insertion is confirmed by echocardiography, the clip can be released. If a suboptimal grasp occurs, the leaflet can be released, allowing repositioning before a second grasp attempt. Additionally, a second or more clips can be placed as needed for optimal MR reduction.

In the randomized EVEREST II trial, 184 patients received MitraClip therapy and 95 underwent surgical repair or replacement.[16] These patients were almost a decade older (mean age, 67 years) than in usual surgical series and had more comorbidities. Major adverse events at 30 days were significantly less frequent with MitraClip therapy (9.6% versus 57% with surgery; $P < 0.0001$), although much of the difference could be attributed to the greater need for blood transfusions with surgery. The freedom from the combined outcome of death, mitral valve surgery, and MR severity greater than 2+ at 12 months was higher with surgery (73%) than with MitraClip therapy (55%; $P = 0.0007$). In patients with acute MitraClip therapy success, the result appears durable, with a very low rate of later mitral valve surgery.[17]

Subsequent analyses of this study and additional registries have demonstrated persistent reductions in MR grade, improvement in NYHA functional class, and reduction in LV dimensions with MitraClip therapy.[17] Other studies have shown a lack of MS, no effect of initial rhythm on results, and importantly, greater benefit than with surgery for higher-risk patients (Fig. 78.4). Although the EVEREST II trial failed to demonstrate efficacy equivalent to that of surgery for a diverse group

of patients with varied risk and etiology, the EVEREST High-Risk Registry and prohibitive-risk patient subset, combined with the experience outside the United States, indicate a more appropriate role in high-risk patients.

A new indication has recently emerged for MitraClip therapy in heart failure patients with secondary MR based on the results of the COAPT (Clinical Outcomes Assessment of the MitraClip Percutaneous Therapy for High Surgical Risk Patients) trial. This landmark trial compared the MitraClip device with medical therapy in patients with secondary MR in 614 patients after initial optimal medical therapy.[18] After 24 months of follow-up, there was a close to 50% reduction in the annualized rate of all hospitalizations for heart failure and an approximately 40% reduction in all-cause mortality with a very low rate of device-related complications (4%) (Fig. 78.5). In contrast, a similar French study failed to demonstrate a difference between heart failure patients treated with MitraClip and optimal medical management at 12 months of follow-up.[19] There are a number of reasons why these two similar trials had conflicting results, including different inclusion and exclusions, primary endpoints, operator experience, and procedural results.[20] An additional trial in this space (RESHAPE HF2) has not yet been reported and may add further clarity to who are the best candidates for MitraClip repair. Several other devices, designed to provide leaflet repair, including NeoChord, Mitra-Spacer, and MitraFlex, are in preclinical or phase I evaluation (see Table 78.1). The PASCAL edge-to-edge repair device has some similarities to MitraClip in that it is used to create a double orifice mitral valve, but has wider grasping elements and a central spacer.[21] In an initial report of 62 patients treated with this device, 98% and 86% had MR grade ≤2+ and ≤1+, respectively at 30 days.[21] A comparison of this device and MitraClip (The CLASP Study of Edwards PASCAL Transcatheter Mitral Valve Repair System Study; NCT03170349) is underway.

Indirect Annuloplasty

The venous anatomy of the heart is of particular interest for treating MR because of the ease of access (from the right internal jugular vein) and the location of the great cardiac vein in proximity to the posterior mitral annulus. Some of the first attempts to treat MR without surgery consisted of mimicking surgical ring annuloplasty through placement of devices in the coronary sinus, so-called indirect or percutaneous coronary sinus annuloplasty. The goal of this approach is to remodel the posterior annulus, cinching the great cardiac vein or pushing on the posterior annulus from the vein to improve leaflet coaptation.

The CARILLON XE2 Mitral Contour System (Cardiac Dimensions) has CE Mark and uses anchors placed in the coronary sinus that are pulled toward each other with a cinching device to reduce the mitral annular dimension by traction (Fig. 78.6). Early evaluation in the Amadeus study demonstrated feasibility, with implantation in 30 of 48 patients and modest improvement in quantitative measures of MR with a small risk of coronary compromise (15%) and death (one patient). More recently, a redesigned device was tested in the TITAN (Transcatheter Implantation of Carillon Mitral Annuloplasty Device) trial.[22] Among 65 patients with secondary MR (62% ischemic), the device was implanted successfully in 36 patients, with a mean age of 62 years, mean ejection fraction (EF) of 29%, predominantly NYHA Functional Class III symptoms, and 2+ (30%), 3+ (55%), or 4+ (15%) grade MR. Quantitative measures of MR were better at 6 and 12 months than in 17 patients who did not receive implants. In the most recent randomized, blinded, and sham-controlled evaluation of this device (REDUCE FMR, NCT02325830), a statistically significant modest difference in MR volume was observed at 1 year despite many missing echocardiograms.[23]

In general, indirect annuloplasty devices may be able to provide modest MR reduction in select patients, but likely less than that achievable surgically with a complete ring placed directly on the annulus. The limited efficacy is related to the location of the coronary sinus relative to the annulus (up to

TABLE 78.1 Devices for Transcatheter Mitral Valve Repair and Replacement

TYPE/INDICATION	BRAND NAME	MANUFACTURER	STATUS
Leaflet/chordal	MitraClip	Abbott Vascular, Abbott Park, Ill	CE Mark
			FDA approved
	NeoChord DS1000 System	NeoChord, Eden Prairie, Minn	CE Mark
			U.S. IDE trial
	Harpoon NeoChord	Edwards Lifesciences, Irvine, Calif	Phase 1 (OUS)
	Mitra-Spacer	Cardiosolutions, West Bridgewater, Mass	Phase 1 (OUS)
	MitraFlex	TransCardiac Therapeutics, Atlanta, Ga	Preclinical
	Middle Peak Medical	Middle Peak Medical, Palo Alto, Calif	Phase 1 (OUS)
Indirect annuloplasty	CARILLON XE2 Mitral Contour System	Cardiac Dimensions, Kirkland, Wis	CE Mark
	Kardium MR	Kardium, Richmond, British Columbia, Canada	Preclinical
	Cerclage annuloplasty	National Heart, Lung and Blood Institute, Bethesda, Md	Phase 1 (OUS)
Direct or left ventricular annuloplasty	Mitralign Percutaneous Annuloplasty System	Mitralign, Tewksbury, Mass	CE Mark
	GDS Accucinch System	Guided Delivery Systems, Santa Clara, Calif	Phase 1 (OUS)
	Boa RF Catheter	QuantumCor, Laguna Niguel, Calif	Preclinical
	Cardioband	Valtech Cardio, Or Yehuda, Israel	CE Mark
	Millipede System	Millipede, Santa Rosa, Calif	Phase 1 (OUS)
	Arto System	MVRx, Belmont, Calif	Phase 1 (OUS)
Hybrid surgical	Adjustable Annuloplasty Ring	Mitral Solutions, Fort Lauderdale, Fla	Phase 1 (OUS)
	enCor ring	MiCardia Corporation, Irvine, Calif	CE Mark
			Phase 1
Left ventricular remodeling	The Basal Annuloplasty of the Cardia Externally (BACE)	Mardil Medical, Minneapolis, Minnesota	Phase 1 (OUS)
	Tendyne Repair	Tendyne Holdings, Baltimore, Md	Preclinical
	MitraSpacer	Cardiosolutions, Stoughton, Mass	Phase 1 (OUS)
Replacement	CardiAQ-Edwards	Edwards Lifesciences, Irvine, Calif	Phase 1 (OUS)
			U.S. EFS
	Tendyne	Abbott Vascular, Chicago	Phase 1 (OUS)
			U.S. EFS
	Tiara	Neovasc, Richmond, British Columbia, Canada	Phase 1 (OUS)
			U.S. EFS
	Intrepid (Twelve)	Medtronic, Minneapolis, Minn	Phase 1 (OUS)
			U.S. EFS
	Caisson	Caisson Interventional, Maple Grove, Minn	U.S. EFS

CE, Conformité Européenne (European Union); EFS, early feasibility study; FDA, U.S. Food and Drug Administration; IDE, investigational device exemption; OUS, outside United States.

10 mm more cranial), great individual anatomic variability, and limited benefit of partial annular remodeling. Whether this level of efficacy will result in sufficient symptomatic improvement and LV remodeling to justify the procedure requires further study. Some "super-responders" may be identified on the basis of anatomic considerations before the procedure. The risks of this approach must also be considered. In addition to the risk for damage to the cardiac venous system, devices in this location can compress the left circumflex or diagonal coronary arteries, which traverse between the coronary sinus and the mitral annulus in most patients.[22,23]

In this regard, one novel indirect approach to reduce the septal-lateral dimension that deserves further consideration is the *cerclage annuloplasty* technique, which recently entered clinical evaluation. This approach attempts to create a more complete circumferential annuloplasty by placing a suture from the coronary sinus through a septal perforator vein into the right atrium or ventricle, where it is snared and tensioned with the proximal end from the right atrium to create a closed pursestring suture.[24] The procedure is guided by cardiac MRI and also uses a novel rigid protection device to avoid coronary compression.

Direct Annuloplasty and Left Ventricular Remodeling Techniques

Several devices have been developed to remodel more directly the mitral annulus, in part because of the limitations of indirect coronary

sinus annuloplasty described earlier (see Table 78.1). The Mitralign Percutaneous Annuloplasty System (Mitralign) was originally based on the surgical techniques of Paneth's posterior suture plication. In this procedure a transaortic catheter is advanced to the left ventricle and used to deliver pledgeted anchors through the posterior annulus that can be pulled together to shorten (plicate) the annulus up to 17 mm (with two implants) (Fig. 78.6B). In 50 of 71 patients successfully treated in a phase I trial, septal-lateral dimension was reduced about 2 mm, MR grade at 6 months was reduced by a mean of 1.3 grades in 50% of patients, and modest symptomatic improvement was observed.[25] The Accucinch (Guided Delivery Systems) device utilizes a catheter approach to place up to 12 anchors along the ventricular myocardium just below the valve plane (percutaneous ventriculoplasty). This approach may be able to reduce MR as well as improve LV function in patients with heart failure. In a preliminary report of 21 patients, reductions in LV end-systolic volume (28%), effective regurgitant orifice area (37%), and an increase in LV ejection fraction (33%) were observed at 6 months.[26]

More recently, the Cardioband annuloplasty system (Valtech Cardio, Or Yehuda, Israel) received CE Mark. This is an adjustable, catheter-delivered, sutureless device that is inserted transseptally and directly anchored on the atrial side of the annulus with subsequent adjustment (Fig. 78.6C). In a phase I European study, 31 high-risk patients with severe secondary MR received treatment.[27] Mean septal-lateral

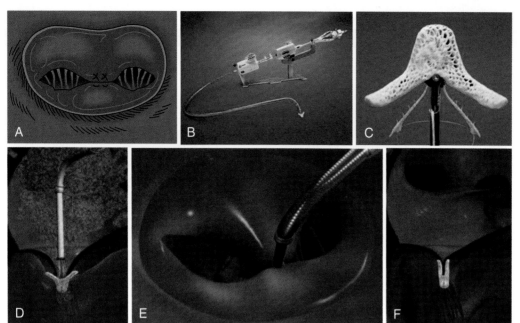

FIGURE 78.3 MitraClip leaflet coaptation system (Abbott Vascular) creates a bridge between the P2 and A2 segments of the mitral valve similar to the Alfieri stitch operation **(A)** utilizing a clip delivery system **(B)** and the MitraClip NT **(C)**. Drawings of side **(D)** and left atrial **(E)** views of the clip delivery system as it is advanced through the mitral valve in the open position prior to grasping of the leaflets. **F,** The final result is illustrated after the clip has been released and the delivery system removed. (Courtesy Abbott Vascular, Inc.)

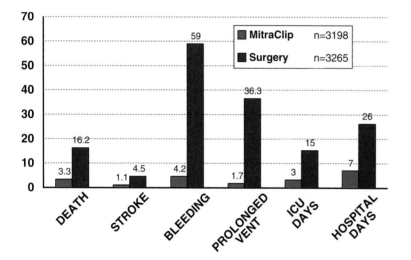

FIGURE 78.4 Meta-analysis of outcomes of the MitraClip compared with mitral valve surgery in high-risk patients. *ICU,* Intensive care unit; *Vent,* ventilation. (From Philip F, et al. MitraClip for severe symptomatic mitral regurgitation in patients at high surgical risk. Catheter Cardiovasc Interv 2014;84:581-590.)

to treat ischemic MR at the time of coronary artery bypass graft (CABG) surgery. In a preliminary report of 11 patients treated in India, MR grade was reduced acutely from grade 3.3 to 0.6. Preclinical work with a transcatheter approach to approximate the papillary muscles is also in development (Tendyne Repair).

Transcatheter Mitral Valve Replacement

The rationale for transcatheter mitral valve replacement (TMVR) is based on several lessons learned from surgical valve replacement[29,30] and results thus far with transcatheter mitral valve repair. With the current state of technologic development and clinical experience, transcatheter repairs do not appear to reduce MR to the same extent as surgical repairs. Moreover, in patients with secondary ischemic MR, mitral valve replacement (MVR) appears to provide more complete and durable elimination of MR than valve repair. In a surgical trial of 251 patients with severe ischemic MR randomized to mitral repair versus chordal-sparing MVR,[31] recurrent moderate or severe MR was higher at 12 months in the repair group (32.6%) than the replacement group (2.3%).

Early experience with valve-in-valve treatment using TAVR devices in previously implanted degenerating surgical mitral bioprostheses and annuloplasty rings has confirmed the feasibility of this approach. Balloon-expandable TAVR prostheses were initially implanted in degenerating bioprostheses and surgical annuloplasty rings via a transapical approach.[32] Subsequently, the feasibility of transseptal delivery and transatrial delivery has been demonstrated. Complications, including valve embolization, bleeding, and death, have been reported, but the early results have generally been favorable, with excellent reduction in MR grade and low residual transmitral gradients, resulting in the Sapien 3 device receiving FDA approval for this indication.[33]

Despite these initial demonstrations of the feasibility of transcatheter mitral valve-in-valve implantation, de novo placement of such devices in native valves, even those with mitral annular calcification, has proved more challenging.[34] Compared with TAVR, mitral devices need to be larger, and fixation to the diseased mitral apparatus is hampered by the greater valve complexity, lack of calcium, potential need for orientation, and noncircular annular shape.

Most current designs use a stent-based bioprosthesis that is self-expanding, anchors to attach to the annulus and/or leaflets, and a sealing skirt. Because the size of the mitral annulus requires a large prosthesis, initial experience has been with transapical delivery systems, although early experience with several transseptal and transatrial delivery approaches is underway. Novel devices that use a two-stage deployment with separate anchoring and valve portions are also being tested.[30]

At least five TMVR devices have entered early feasibility investigation clinically in the United States (Fig. 78.7; see also Table 78.1), and more than 30 are in early development. The initial experience with TMVR has been challenging, in part from inclusion of compassionately treated patients with multiple comorbidities and predominantly

dimension was reduced from 37 to 29 mm, with initial reduction in MR grade to "trace" or "mild" in 93% of patients and to moderate MR or less at 30 days in 88%.[27] In a subsequent report of 60 patients with a procedural success rate of 68%, moderate or less MR at 1 year was observed in 61% of patients and was associated with improvements in functional status and quality of life.[28] The basis for devices to treat MR by affecting the shape of the left ventricle arises from the pathophysiology of secondary ischemic or functional MR (see Chapter 76). Changes in the inferior and lateral left ventricle from infarction can lead to tethering or tenting of the posterior leaflet, allowing anterior leaflet override as the mechanism of MR. Similarly, failure of leaflet coaptation from global LV enlargement causing annular distention is the major mechanism for MR in dilated cardiomyopathy.[18] Although ring annuloplasty can often ameliorate MR caused by LV distortion, procedures that also address the underlying LV pathology may be more beneficial. The Basal Annuloplasty of the Cardia Externally (BACE) device (Mardil) is a surgically implanted external tension band placed around the heart externally

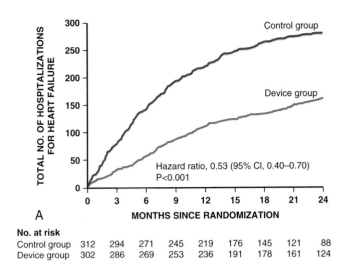

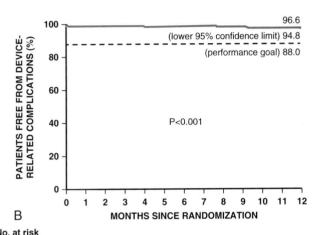

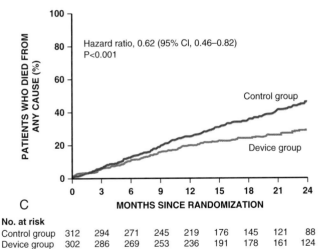

FIGURE 78.5 Primary effectiveness and safety end points and death in patients with secondary mitral regurgitation and heart failure from the COAPT trial. **A,** The cumulative incidence of the primary effectiveness end point of all hospitalizations for heart failure within 24 months of follow-up among patients who underwent transcatheter mitral-valve repair and received guideline-directed medical therapy (device group) and among those who received guideline-directed medical therapy alone (control group). The data shown here do not account for the competing risk of death, which was considered in the joint frailty model. A total of 160 hospitalizations for heart failure occurred in 92 patients in the device group, and a total of 283 hospitalizations for heart failure occurred in 151 patients in the control group. **B,** The rate of the primary safety endpoint of freedom from device-related complications at 12 months among the 293 patients in whom device implantation was attempted, as compared with an objective performance goal. **C,** Time-to-event curves for all-cause mortality in the device group and the control group. (From Stone GW, et al. Transcatheter mitral-valve repair in patients with heart failure. N Engl J Med 2018;379:2307-2318.)

treated with a relatively invasive transapical approach. Current trials are therefore targeting high-risk, but not inoperable, patients with both primary and secondary MR. Phase II study investigators will address that most patients with secondary MR do not have high short-term mortality and therefore are frequently medically managed. Overcoming procedural complications of TMVR will be essential to realize the symptomatic benefits compared with medical care. Patient comorbidities, cardiac and noncardiac, could hamper and confound comparative evaluations.

In the largest study of such a device to date, Sorajja and colleagues[35] treated 30 patients at high risk for surgery with a transcatheter transapical self-expanding nitinol prosthesis supporting a trileaflet porcine pericardial valve (Tendyne Mitral Valve System, Abbott Vascular, Roseville, Minnesota). The device was successfully implanted in 97 of 100 patients (97%) with no procedural deaths. The 30-day rates of mortality and stroke were 6% and 2%, respectively. At 1 year, MR was absent in 98% of patients and associated with significant improvements in symptoms and quality of life. Based on these results, this became the first TMVR device to attain CE Mark approval, and it is currently being evaluated in a pivotal US trial comparing it to MitraClip (SUMMIT trial, NCT03433274).

It is hoped that improvements in devices, operator and procedural experience, and patient selection will lead to better outcomes. The potential advantages of this approach include the avoidance of both the surgical incision and the effects of cardiopulmonary bypass. Such devices could be fully sparing of the subvalvular apparatus and provide MR reduction that is equivalent to that achieved with surgical valve replacement. However, the early high mortality, although in very-high-risk patients receiving the device as a compassionate approach, has tempered some of the early enthusiasm for TMVR.[36]

In this regard, it is useful to emphasize that TMVR is not a "mitral TAVR."[36,37] The mitral valve is more complex than the aortic valve, and MR has a vast array of etiologies. Unlike AS, MR is not as often a disease of elderly persons, and repair (not replacement) is the preferred surgical therapy, especially for patients with primary MR. Replacement may have less favorable effects on normal vortex flow and LV remodeling than successful repair.[38] Transcatheter prostheses in the mitral position will likely have lower durability, more risks associated with paravalvular leak,[39] and a greater risk of embolization, LV outflow tract obstruction, and thrombosis. Finally, the more frequent association with TR, which may need to be addressed, and the lower short-term mortality will be impediments to the design of rigorous clinical trials.[33,36]

TRICUSPID REGURGITATION

Tricuspid regurgitation (TR) is a common valve lesion that increases with age and affects about 1.6 million people in the United States and more than 70 million worldwide.[40,41] Focused analysis of the population of Olmsted County showed a prevalence of 0.55% for moderate or greater TR,[42] which would give an estimate of 160,000 to 240,000 cases of moderate or greater TR in the United States.[43] The majority of TR cases are functional and are associated with increased mortality.[42-45] Despite this high prevalence and association with increased mortality, <10,000 surgeries a year are performed in the United States for tricuspid valve disease, and in Olmsted County, only 2.6% of the patients with moderate or greater TR had surgery during the follow-up period.[42] Much of the apparent reticence to operate on isolated TR comes from the reported mortality in the surgical literature, which has ranged from 8% to 16%,[46-49] although mortality as low as 3.3% has been reported in a contemporary surgical series.[50] This reluctance to operate on patients with TR has led to the tricuspid valve being referred to as the "forgotten valve." In addition, the poor surgical outcomes in many series have fostered late referral for treatment. Many patients, by the time they are referred for potential intervention, have developed comorbidities, including liver failure, renal failure, coagulopathy, and end-stage heart failure, further increasing the risk of any intervention. The remodeling associated with TR results in increased annular and right ventricular size further increasing leaflet restriction and TR. Tricuspid regurgitation begets worsening tricuspid regurgitation. Understanding this has

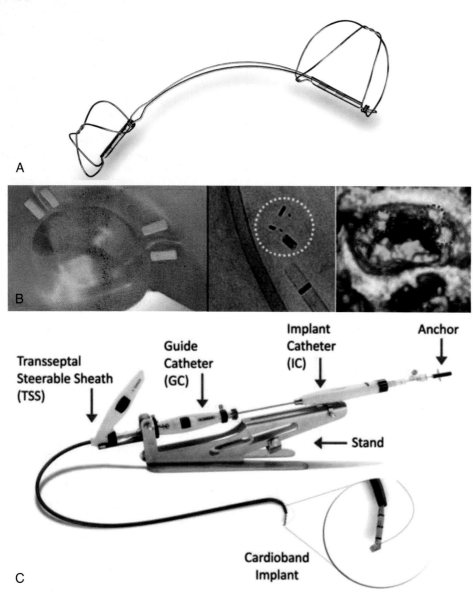

FIGURE 78.6 Evolving devices for mitral valve repair. A, Carillon XE2 Mitral Contour System (Cardiac Dimensions) **B,** Mitralign Percutaneous Annuloplasty System (Mitralign, Tewksbury, Mass). **C,** Cardioband annuloplasty system (Valtech Cardio, Or Yehuda, Israel). (From Nickenig G, et al. Treatment of functional mitral valve regurgitation with a percutaneous annuloplasty system. J Am Coll Cardiol 2016;67:2927-2936.)

Current evidence suggests that this is not correct and that TR that is moderate or greater is an independent risk for mortality (Fig. 78.8).[42,43,52,56] Even with this mortality risk, current guidelines only have a class I recommendation for TR surgery if left-sided valve surgery is being done.[57] When tricuspid valve repair is added to surgery for mitral valve repair in patients with moderate or greater TR, there is no increase in mortality but there is a significantly lower late rate of TR and better right ventricular recovery.[58] There is a clear undertreatment of significant TR, suggesting a large unmet need. Recognizing this unmet need has led clinicians to refocus on what has been often referred to as the forgotten valve. Transcatheter tricuspid valve intervention (TTVI) is emerging as a potential less invasive option to treat TR. It is hoped that this less invasive transcatheter approach, especially if it can prove safer, will lead to earlier intervention for TR to slow the progression of the associated heart failure. Most TTVI procedures mimic surgical procedures already in use. Isolated surgical tricuspid valve repair has a lower mortality than isolated surgical tricuspid valve replacement.[47,59] It is unknown if this difference will extend to transcatheter approaches as well, but this would seem likely as long as the repair is successful in decreasing the TR and durable. Transcatheter TR correction devices fall into several broad categories of annular remodeling, leaflet remodeling, spacers, and novel approaches such as caval valves or tricuspid valve replacement (Fig. 78.9). It is early in the development of TTVI procedures, and data are currently limited and the specific devices are likely to change with time, but the categories remain consistent. The tricuspid valve presents several physiologic and anatomic challenges for the interventionist. Anatomically, the tricuspid valve borders the right coronary artery and the atrioventricular node, placing both at risk for injury. Most TR is functional in nature and more related to right ventricular and TV annular enlargement than actual valve pathology. Surgical repair of functional atrioventricular valve pathology has not proven as consistent or durable as repair of primary lesions. At this time, it is also unknown if this applies to TTVI. Physiologically, TR is often associated with right heart failure and congestive liver failure and its consequences. An increased Model of End-Stage Liver Disease (MELD) score from liver congestion is associated with an increase in mortality for tricuspid valve interventions.[60] Choosing patients with right heart function that is likely to recover and allow the patient to survive and benefit from the procedure is crucial.

helped reignite interest in tricuspid valve intervention for TR, particularly with a less invasive transcatheter approach.[51]

Pathophysiology

The tricuspid valve is the largest and most caudal of the cardiac valves. Tricuspid regurgitation is primary in about 10% of cases, but less common in developed countries.[52] Primary TR can occur in congenital anomalies such as Ebstein anomaly, trauma, or carcinoid syndrome. Increasing causes of primary TR in developed countries are pacemaker and defibrillator leads across the valve and endocarditis, especially IV drug–related cases. Secondary or functional TR accounts for 90% of the cases. Secondary TR is the result of a negative remodeling of the right ventricle with normal valve leaflets. This leads to increased annular size and leaflet tethering producing TR.[53] Left-sided heart disease and pulmonary hypertension are common causes of negative remodeling and TR. Chronic atrial fibrillation can cause annular enlargement rather than right ventricular remodeling as a cause of TR.[54]

Treatment

In very early experience, TR was largely managed medically with the belief that it would improve with treatment of the underlying cause.[55]

Annuloplasty Devices

Surgeons have used annuloplasty bands and rings for mitral valve repair in both primary and secondary mitral regurgitation. Transcatheter annuloplasty devices attempt to replicate the annular remodeling achieved by surgical devices. Although transcatheter approaches, particularly with partial annuloplasty and bicuspidization techniques, may not be as efficacious as rigid surgical rings, the freedom from at least moderate TR at long-term follow-up was still achievable in the majority of patients[61] (Fig. 78.10).

The Cardioband transcatheter annuloplasty device fixes a partial annuloplasty band to the valve annulus with anchors using a transseptal approach that can then be tightened or cinched. The results with Cardioband were presented in the TRI-REPAIR (Tricuspid Regurgitation Repair With Cardioband Transcatheter System) study (NCT02981953).[62] This was a 30-patient prospective feasibility study with a primary performance endpoint of successful access, deployment, and positioning of the device with reduction of the septolateral annular diameter. The cases were carefully selected for anatomic and physiologic suitability and patients with pacemaker leads crossing the valve were excluded. Technical success was 100% with a 6.8% mortality at 30 days and 10% at 6 months. TR improved, but at 6 months, four patients still had torrential TR. Of note, three patients had a right coronary artery injury that was corrected with angioplasty in two of these patients and one was left untreated and led to the death of the patient. Other annuloplasty devices include the IRIS annuloplasty ring is a complete rigid ring anchored on the supravalvular annulus and then can be differentially cinched down to an appropriate annulus size and shape,[63,64] and the TriCinch device, which attempts to replicate the surgical Kay procedure, eliminating the posterior TV leaflet and converting the valve into a bileaflet valve.[63,64] This is a two-component device. The first part is a stainless-steel corkscrew implant, to be placed in the anterior annulus of the TV, in proximity to the anteroposterior commissure, which is connected to a self-expanding nitinol stent that is deployed below the hepatic region of the inferior vena cava. Once the corkscrew is deployed, the nitinol stent is pulled down into the inferior vena cava until the appropriate tension on the tricuspid valve annulus reduces the posterior leaflet to approximate a Kay repair. The stent is then deployed locking the system into place. The Percutaneous 4TECH TriCinch Coil Tricuspid Valve Repair System early feasibility study is ongoing (NCT03632967). The TriAlign system also attempts to replicate the Kay repair. The device is a transjugular suture-based tricuspid valve annuloplasty system that reduces tricuspid annular diameter by plication of the posterior leaflet.[65] The early results with this device were reported in the SCOUT

FIGURE 78.7 Transcatheter mitral valve replacement devices in early U.S. feasibility evaluation. *Top row,* CardiAQ-Edwards Transcatheter Mitral Valve (Edwards Lifesciences, Irvine, Calif) and Tendyne (Courtesy Abbott). *Bottom row,* Intrepid (Medtronic, Minneapolis, Minn), Tiara (Neovasc, Richmond, BC, Canada), and Caisson (Caisson Interventional, Maple Grove, Minn).

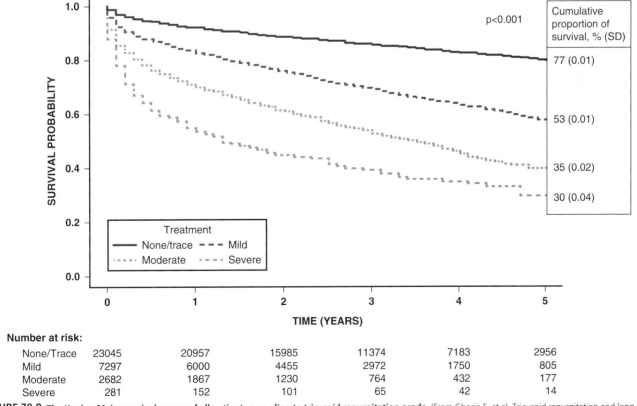

Number at risk:						
None/Trace	23045	20957	15985	11374	7183	2956
Mild	7297	6000	4455	2972	1750	805
Moderate	2682	1867	1230	764	432	177
Severe	281	152	101	65	42	14

FIGURE 78.8 The Kaplan-Meier survival curves of all patients according to tricuspid regurgitation grade. (From Chorin E, et al. Tricuspid regurgitation and long-term clinical outcomes. Eur Heart J Cardiovasc Imaging 2020;21:157-165.)

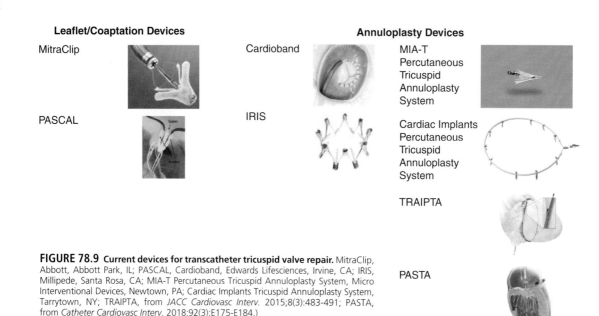

Leaflet/Coaptation Devices

MitraClip

PASCAL

Cardioband

IRIS

Annuloplasty Devices

MIA-T Percutaneous Tricuspid Annuloplasty System

Cardiac Implants Percutaneous Tricuspid Annuloplasty System

TRAIPTA

PASTA

FIGURE 78.9 Current devices for transcatheter tricuspid valve repair. MitraClip, Abbott, Abbott Park, IL; PASCAL, Cardioband, Edwards Lifesciences, Irvine, CA; IRIS, Millipede, Santa Rosa, CA; MIA-T Percutaneous Tricuspid Annuloplasty System, Micro Interventional Devices, Newtown, PA; Cardiac Implants Tricuspid Annuloplasty System, Tarrytown, NY; TRAIPTA, from *JACC Cardiovasc Interv.* 2015;8(3):483-491; PASTA, from *Catheter Cardiovasc Interv.* 2018;92(3):E175-E184.)

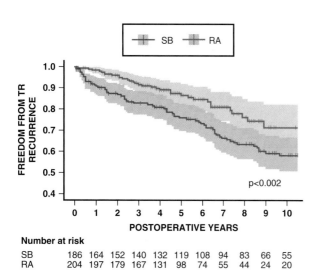

Number at risk

SB	186	164	152	140	132	119	108	94	83	66	55
RA	204	197	179	167	131	98	74	55	44	24	20

FIGURE 78.10 Freedom from TR recurrence (≥ moderate) with surgical ring annuloplasty (RA) versus suture bicuspidization (SB). (From Hirji S, et al. Outcomes after tricuspid valve repair with ring versus suture bicuspidization annuloplasty. Ann Thorac Surg 2020;110(3):821-828.)

(Percutaneous Tricuspid Valve Annuloplasty System for Symptomatic Chronic Functional Tricuspid Regurgitation) trial (NCT03225612).[66] Fifteen patients were treated with this device, with a technical success of 80% at 30 days.

Finally, a minimally invasive annuloplasty (MIA) device that utilizes proprietary anchors with a suture cinching approach is being studied in a OUS trial (STTAR, Study of Transcatheter Tricuspid Annuloplasty, Microinterventional Devices, Inc., Newtown, Penn). More than 30 patients have been treated with this device with reportedly good safety and efficacy, and a U.S. trial is planned.

Leaflet Clip Devices

Both the MitraClip and Pascal clip devices are being tested in the tricuspid position, usually clipping the anterior and septal leaflets.[63] The results for MitraClip from the TRIVALVE registry included 249 patients with a technical success rate of 96%.[67] The rate of TR of 3+ or more was decreased from 97% preprocedure to 23% at discharge. Preexisting pacemaker was present in 30% of these patients. This trial also excluded preexisting pacemakers. The hospital mortality was 2.8%. Mortality at 1 year was 20.3% and the 1-year combined endpoint of

mortality or rehospitalization occurred in 31% of patients. The TRILUMINATE trial (NCT03227757) is a prospective, single-arm, multicenter study at 21 sites in Europe and the United States using MitraClip in severe TR and is currently ongoing.

Valve Spacer Devices

The FORMA system consists of a spacer and a rail, which is anchored within the right ventricular apex under echocardiography guidance. The spacer will passively expand using holes within the shaft. The spacer gives the valve leaflets something to coapt against to reduce TR.[63,68,69] The device is being tested in the SPACER trial (NCVT02787408).

Caval Devices

Heterotopic implantation of valve(s) into the inferior vena cava alone or with the superior vena cava also has been done to protect the hepatic and renal venous circulation from the high pressures related to TR without actually eliminating the TR.[70,71] Two early trials, HOVER (NCT2339974) and TRICAVAL (NC02387696), are assessing this approach.

Tricuspid Valve Replacement Devices

Finally, valves for complete TV replacement are being developed and are early in their use. The NaviGate valve is an early stented, trileaflet valve fabricated from equine pericardium and a self-expanding tapered nitinol stent.[72] The valve is placed thru a small right anterior thoracotomy and early compassionate use in five patients has been reported with all patients having a successful implant.[73] The LUV_VALVE (Jenscare Biotechnology) and Trisol valve (Mor Research Applications) are two addition valve replacement platforms beginning early feasibility testing.[74] Finally, the Edwards EVOQUE mitral transcatheter valve and Medtronic's Intrepid device are also undergoing U.S. early feasibility evaluation for the treatment of TR.

SUMMARY

All of the transcatheter tricuspid valve device systems are early in their development and use. Preliminary results suggest safety and that TR does not need to be completely corrected to improve the patient's clinical status. Comparing transcatheter tricuspid intervention to medical therapy suggests that intervention provides better survival as well as less heart failure hospitalization (Fig. 78.11).[75] This will prompt continued work in this area.

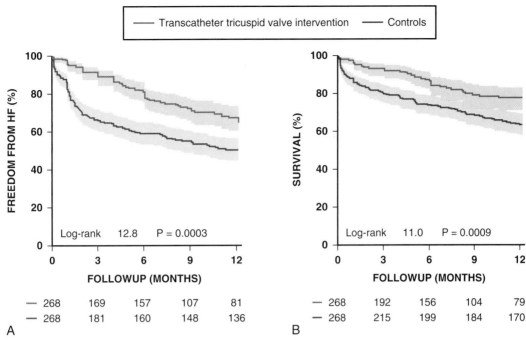

FIGURE 78.11 Transcatheter treatment of severe tricuspid regurgitation, primary and secondary endpoints: freedom from heart failure (**A**) and survival (**B**). (From Taramasso M, et al. Transcatheter versus medical treatment of patients with symptomatic severe tricuspid regurgitation. J Am Coll Cardiol 2019;74:2998-3000.)

CONCLUSION

Transcatheter therapy of VHD is an exciting, evolving, and growing area of cardiovascular medicine and surgery. The initial success of balloon valvuloplasty for stenotic lesions leading to the more recent growth of TAVR revolutionized the modern approach to AS. The complexity of the mitral valve apparatus and the myriad causes of mitral regurgitation led to slower growth and success of transcatheter mitral valve repair and replacement. However, fueled by the ever-growing prevalence of heart failure in the aging U.S. population[76]—most of these older patients with heart failure have significant MR—and aided by the ingenuity of physicians and engineers, we can anticipate that transcatheter mitral and tricuspid valve therapies will become an available option for many patients in the near future.

CLASSIC REFERENCES

Andersen HR, Knudsen LL, Hasemkam JM. Transluminal implantation of artificial heart valves: description of a new expandable aortic valve and initial results with implantation by catheter technique in closed chest pigs. *Eur Heart J.* 1992;13:704–708.

Cribier A, Eltchaninoff H, Bash A, et al. Percutaneous transcatheter implantation of an aortic valve prosthesis for calcific aortic stenosis: first human case description. *Circulation.* 2002;106:3006–3008.

Cribier A, Savin TSN, Rocha PBJ, Letac B. Percutaneous transluminal valvuloplasty of acquired aortic stenosis in elderly patients: an alternative to valve replacement? *Lancet.* 1986;1:63–67.

Harken DE, Scroff MS, Taylor MC. Partial and complete prostheses in aortic insufficiency. *J Thorac Cardiovasc Surg.* 1960;40:744–762.

Inoue K, Owaki T, Nakamura T, et al. Clinical application of transvenous mitral commissurotomy by a new balloon catheter. *J Thorac Cardiovasc Surg.* 1984;87:394–402.

National Heart, Lung and Blood Institute (NHLBI). Percutaneous balloon aortic valvuloplasty: acute and 30 day follow up results in 674 patients from the NHLBI Balloon Valvuplasty Registry. *Circulation.* 1991;84:2383–2397.

Wilkins GT, Weyman AE, Abascal VM, et al. Percutaneous balloon dilatation of the mitral valve: an analysis of echocardiographic variables related to outcome and the mechanism of dilatation. *Br Heart J.* 1988;60:299–308.

REFERENCES
Mitral Stenosis

1. Nunes MCP, Tan TC, Elmariah S, et al. The Echo score revisited. *Circulation.* 2014;129:886–895.
2. Guerrero M, Urena M, Himbert D, et al. 1-Year outcomes of transcatheter mitral valve replacement in patients with severe mitral annular calcification. *J Am Coll Cardiol.* 2018;71:1841–1853.
3. Fiorilli PN, Herrmann HC. Transcatheter mitral valve replacement: rationale and current status. *Annu Rev Med.* 2020;71:249–261.
4. Nishimura RA, Otto CM, Bonow RO, et al. 2014 AHA/ACC guideline for the management of patients with valvular heart disease: a report of the American College of Cardiology/American Heart Association task force on practice guidelines. *J Am Coll Cardiol.* 2014;63:e57–e185.
5. Eng MH, Salcedo EE, Kim M, et al. Implementation of real-time three-dimensional transesophageal echocardiography for mitral balloon valvuloplasty. *Catheter Cardiovasc Interv.* 2013;82:994–998.

Mitral Regurgitation

6. Glower DD. Surgical approaches to mitral regurgitation. *J Am Coll Cardiol.* 2012;60:1315–1322.
7. Rosenhek R, Rader F, Klaar U, et al. Outcome of watchful waiting in asymptomatic severe mitral regurgitation. *Circulation.* 2006;113:2238–2244.
8. Gammie JS, O'Brien SM, Griffith BP, et al. Influence of hospital procedural volume on care process and mortality for patients undergoing elective surgery for mitral regurgitation. *Circulation.* 2007;115:881–887.
9. Mehta RH, Eagle KA, Coombs LP, et al. Influence of age on outcomes in patients undergoing mitral valve replacement. *Ann Thorac Surg.* 2002;74:1459–1467.
10. Chatterjee S, Rankin JS, Gammie JS, et al. Isolated mitral valve surgery risk in 77,836 patients from the Society of Thoracic Surgeons database. *Ann Thorac Surg.* 2013;96:1587–1594.
11. Chaim PTL, Ruiz CE. Percutaneous mitral valve repair: a classification of the technology. *JACC Cardiovasc Interv.* 2011;4:1–13.
12. Herrmann HC, Maisano F. Transcatheter therapy of mitral regurgitation. *Circulation.* 2014;130:1712–1722.
13. Maisano F, Caldarola A, Blasio A, et al. Midterm results of edge-to-edge mitral valve repair without annuloplasty. *J Thorac Cardiovasc Surg.* 2003;126:1987–1997.
14. Feldman T, Foster E, Glower D, et al. Percutaneous repair or surgery for mitral regurgitation. *N Engl J Med.* 2011;364:1395–1406.
15. Silvestry FE, Rodriguez LL, Herrmann HC, et al. Echocardiographic guidance and assessment of percutaneous repair for mitral regurgitation with the Evalve MitraClip: lessons learned from EVEREST I. *J Am Soc Echocardiogr.* 2007;20:1131–1140.
16. Feldman T, Kar S, Elmariah S, et al. Randomized comparison of percutaneous repair and surgery for mitral regurgitation. *J Am Coll Cardiol.* 2015;66:2844–2854.
17. Philip F, Athappan G, Tuzcu EM, et al. MitraClip for severe symptomatic mitral regurgitation in patients at high surgical risk. *Catheter Cardiovasc Interv.* 2014;84:581–590.
18. Stone GW, Lindenfeld JA, Abraham WT, et al. Transcatheter mitral-valve repair in patients with heart failure. *N Engl J Med.* 2018;379:2307–2318.
19. Obadia JF, Messika-Zeitoun D, Iung LB, et al. Percutaneous repair or medical treatment for secondary mitral regurgitation. *N Engl J Med.* 2018;379:2297–2306.
20. Pibarot P, Delgado V, Bax JJ. MITRA-FR vs. COAPT: lessons from two trials with diametrically opposed results. *Eur Heart J Cardiovasc Imaging.* 2019;20:620–624.
21. Lim DS, Kar S, Spargias K, et al. Transcatheter valve repair for patients with mitral regurgitation. *JACC Cardiovasc Interv.* 2019;12:1369–1378.
22. Siminiak T, Wu JC, Haude M, et al. Treatment of functional mitral regurgitation by percutaneous annuloplasty: results of the TITAN Trial. *Eur J Heart Fail.* 2012;14:931–938.
23. Witte KK, Lipiecki J, Siminiak T, et al. The REDUCE FMR trial. *JACC Heart Fail.* 2019;7:945–955.
24. Kim JH, Kocaturk O, Ozturk C, et al. Mitral cerclage annuloplasty, a novel transcatheter treatment for secondary mitral valve regurgitation: initial results in swine. *J Am Coll Cardiol.* 2009;54:638–651.
25. Nickenig G, Schueler R, Dager A, et al. Treatment of functional mitral valve regurgitation with a percutaneous annuloplasty system. *J Am Coll Cardiol.* 2016;67:2927–2936.
26. Reisman M, Wudel J, Martin S, et al. TCT-88 6-month outcomes of an early feasibility study of the AccuCinch left ventricular repair system in patients with heart failure and functional mitral regurgitation. *J Am Coll Cardiol.* 2019;74(suppl 13):B88 (abstract).
27. Maisano F, Taramasso M, Nickenig G, et al. Cardioband, a transcatheter surgical-like direct mitral valve annuloplasty system: early results of the feasibility trial. *Eur Heart J.* 2016;37:817–825.
28. Messika-Zeitoun D, Nickenig G, Latib A, et al. Transcatheter mitral valve repair for functional mitral regurgitation using the Cardioband system: 1 year outcomes. *Eur Heart J.* 2019;40:466–472.
29. Herrmann HC. Transcatheter mitral valve implantation. *Cardiac Interv Today.* 2009:82–85.
30. Fiorilli PN, Herrmann HC. Transcatheter mitral valve replacement: rationale and current status. *Annu Rev Med.* 2020;71:249–261.
31. Acker MA, Parides MK, Perrault LP, et al. Mitral valve repair versus replacement for severe ischemic mitral regurgitation. *N Engl J Med.* 2014;370:23–32.
32. Cheung A, Webb JG, Barbanti M, et al. 5-Year experience with transcatheter transapical mitral valve-in-valve implantation for bioprosthetic valve dysfunction. *J Am Coll Cardiol.* 2013;61:1759–1766.
33. Grover FL, Vemulapalli S, Carroll JD, et al. 2016 annual report of the Society of Thoracic Surgeons/American College of Cardiology transcatheter valve therapy registry. *J Am Coll Cardiol.* 2017;69:1215–1230.
34. Guerrero M, Dvir D, Himbert D, et al. Transcatheter mitral valve replacement in native mitral valve disease with severe mitral annular calcification. *JACC Cardiovasc Interv.* 2016;9:1361–1371.
35. Sorajja P, Moat N, Badhwar V, et al. Initial feasibility study of a new transcatheter mitral prosthesis. *J Am Coll Cardiol.* 2019;73:1250–1260.
36. Herrmann HC, Chitwood WR. Transcatheter mitral valve replacement clears the first hurdle. *J Am Coll Cardiol.* 2017;69:392–394.

DISEASES OF THE HEART VALVES VIII

37. Anyanwu AC, Adams DH. Transcatheter mitral valve replacement. *J Am Coll Cardiol.* 2014;64:1820–1824.

38. Pedrizetti G, La Canna G, Alfieri O, et al. The vortex: an early predictor of cardiovascular outcome? *Nat Rev Cardiol.* 2014;11:545–553.

39. Taramasso M, Maisano F, Denti P, et al. Surgical treatment of paravalvular leak: long-term results in a single center experience (up to 14 years). *J Thorac Cardiovasc Surg.* 2015;149:1270–1275.

Tricuspid Regurgitation

40. Singh JP, Evans JC, Levy D, et al. Prevalence and clinical determinants of mitral, tricuspid, and aortic regurgitation (the Framingham Heart Study). *Am J Cardiol.* 1999;83:897–902.

41. Demir OM, Razzoli D, Mangieri A, et al. Transcatheter tricuspid valve replacement: principles and design. *Front Cardiovasc Med.* 2018;5:129.

42. Topilsky Y, Maltais S, Medina Inojosa J, et al. Burden of tricuspid regurgitation in patients diagnosed in the community setting. *JACC Cardiovasc Imaging.* 2019;12:433–442.

43. Enriquez-Sarano M, Messika-Zeitoun D, Topilsky Y, et al. Tricuspid regurgitation is a public health crisis. *Prog Cardiovasc Dis.* 2019;62:447–451.

44. Kazum SS, Sagie A, Shochat T, et al. Prevalence, echocardiographic correlations, and clinical outcome of tricuspid regurgitation in patients with significant left ventricular dysfunction. *Am J Med.* 2019;132:81–87.

45. Benfari G, Antoine C, Miller WL, et al. Excess mortality associated with functional tricuspid regurgitation complicating heart failure with reduced ejection fraction. *Circulation.* 2019;140:196–206.

46. Zack CJ, Fender EA, Chandrashekar P, et al. National trends and outcomes in isolated tricuspid valve surgery. *J Am Coll Cardiol.* 2017;70:2953–2960.

47. Alqahtani F, Berzingi CO, Aljohani S, et al. Contemporary trends in the use and outcomes of surgical treatment of tricuspid regurgitation. *J Am Heart Assoc.* 2017;6(12):e007597.

48. Axtell AL, Bhambhani V, Moonsamy P, et al. Surgery does not improve survival in patients with isolated severe tricuspid regurgitation. *J Am Coll Cardiol.* 2019;74:715–725.

49. Ejiofor JI, Neely RC, Yammine M, et al. Surgical outcomes of isolated tricuspid valve procedures: repair versus replacement. *Ann Cardiothorac Surg.* 2017;6:214–222.

50. Hamandi M, Smith RL, Ryan WH, et al. Outcomes of isolated tricuspid valve surgery have improved in the modern era. *Ann Thorac Surg.* 2019;108:11–15.

51. Taramasso M, Pozzoli A, Guidotti A, et al. Percutaneous tricuspid valve therapies: the new frontier. *Eur Heart J.* 2017;38:639–647.

52. Arsalan M, Walther T, Smith 2nd RL, Grayburn PA. Tricuspid regurgitation diagnosis and treatment. *Eur Heart J.* 2017;38:634–638.

53. Dreyfus GD, Martin RP, Chan KM, et al. Functional tricuspid regurgitation: a need to revise our understanding. *J Am Coll Cardiol.* 2015;65:2331–2336.

54. Topilsky Y, Khanna A, Le Tourneau T, et al. Clinical context and mechanism of functional tricuspid regurgitation in patients with and without pulmonary hypertension. *Circ Cardiovasc Imaging.* 2012;5:314–323.

55. Braunwald NS, Ross Jr J, Morrow AG. Conservative management of tricuspid regurgitation in patients undergoing mitral valve replacement. *Circulation.* 1967;35:I63–I69.

56. Chorin E, Rozenbaum Z, Topilsky Y, et al. Tricuspid regurgitation and long-term clinical outcomes. *Eur Heart J Cardiovasc Imaging.* 2020;21:157–165.

57. Nishimura RA, Otto CM, Bonow RO, et al. 2014 AHA/ACC guideline for the management of patients with valvular heart disease: executive summary: a report of the American College of Cardiology/American Heart Association task force on practice guidelines. *J Am Coll Cardiol.* 2014;63:2438–2488.

58. Chikwe J, Itagaki S, Anyanwu A, Adams DH. Impact of concomitant tricuspid annuloplasty on tricuspid regurgitation, right ventricular function, and pulmonary artery hypertension after repair of mitral valve prolapse. *J Am Coll Cardiol.* 2015;65:1931–1938.

59. Wong WK, Chen SW, Chou AH, et al. Late outcomes of valve repair versus replacement in isolated and concomitant tricuspid valve surgery: a Nationwide Cohort Study. *J Am Heart Assoc.* 2020:e015637.

60. Ailawadi G, Lapar DJ, Swenson BR, et al. Model for end-stage liver disease predicts mortality for tricuspid valve surgery. *Ann Thorac Surg.* 2009;87:1460–1467. discussion 1467-8.

61. Hirji S, Yazdchi F, Kiehm S, et al. Outcomes after tricuspid valve repair with ring versus suture bicuspidization annuloplasty. *Ann Thorac Surg.* 2020;110(3):821–828.

62. Nickenig G, Weber M, Schueler R, et al. 6-Month outcomes of tricuspid valve reconstruction for patients with severe tricuspid regurgitation. *J Am Coll Cardiol.* 2019;73:1905–1915.

63. Kolte D, Elmariah S. Current state of transcatheter tricuspid valve repair. *Cardiovasc Diagn Ther.* 2020;10:89–97.

64. Rogers JH, Boyd WD, Bolling SF. Tricuspid annuloplasty with the Millipede ring. *Prog Cardiovasc Dis.* 2019;62(6):486–487.

65. Besler C, Meduri CU, Lurz P. Transcatheter treatment of functional tricuspid regurgitation using the Trialign device. *Interv Cardiol.* 2018;13:8–13.

66. Hahn RT, Meduri CU, Davidson CJ, et al. Early feasibility study of a transcatheter tricuspid valve annuloplasty: SCOUT trial 30-day results. *J Am Coll Cardiol.* 2017;69:1795–1806.

67. Mehr M, Taramasso M, Besler C, et al. 1-Year outcomes after edge-to-edge valve repair for symptomatic tricuspid regurgitation: results from the TriValve Registry. *JACC Cardiovasc Interv.* 2019;12:1451–1461.

68. Puri R, Rodes-Cabau J. The FORMA repair system. *Interv Cardiol Clin.* 2018;7:47–55.

69. Asmarats L, Perlman G, Praz F, et al. Long-term outcomes of the FORMA transcatheter tricuspid valve repair system for the treatment of severe tricuspid regurgitation: insights from the first-in-human experience. *JACC Cardiovasc Interv.* 2019;12:1438–1447.

70. Lauten A, Dreger H, Schofer J, et al. Caval valve implantation for treatment of severe tricuspid regurgitation. *J Am Coll Cardiol.* 2018;71:1183–1184.

71. O'Neill BP. Caval valve implantation: are 2 valves better than 1? *Circ Cardiovasc Interv.* 2018;11:e006334.

72. Elgharably H, Harb SC, Kapadia S, et al. Transcatheter innovations in tricuspid regurgitation: navigate. *Prog Cardiovasc Dis.* 2019;62:493–495.

73. Hahn RT, George I, Kodali SK, et al. Early single-site experience with transcatheter tricuspid valve replacement. *JACC Cardiovasc Imaging.* 2019;12:416–429.

74. Asmarats L, Taramasso M, Rodes-Cabau J. Tricuspid valve disease: diagnosis, prognosis and management of a rapidly evolving field. *Nat Rev Cardiol.* 2019;16:538–554.

75. Taramasso M, Benfari G, van der Bijl P, et al. Transcatheter versus medical treatment of patients with symptomatic severe tricuspid regurgitation. *J Am Coll Cardiol.* 2019;74:2998–3008.

Conclusion

76. Benjamin EJ, Blaha MJ, Chiuve SE, et al. Heart disease and stroke statistics—2017 update. A report from the American Heart Association. *Circulation.* 2017;135:e146–e603.

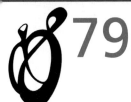

79 Prosthetic Heart Valves

PHILIPPE PIBAROT AND PATRICK T. O'GARA

The past six decades have witnessed extraordinary advancements in patient survival and functional outcomes following heart valve replacement surgery. Continued refinements in prosthetic valve design and performance, surgical and percutaneous techniques, myocardial preservation, systemic perfusion, cerebral protection, and anesthetic management have enabled the application of surgical and transcatheter valve therapy to an increasingly wider spectrum of patients. Minimally invasive surgical approaches and the use of primary valve repair for mitral or aortic valve pathology when anatomically appropriate are now the routine in the vast majority of comprehensive valve centers.[1] Heart valve teams provide multidisciplinary assessment and treatment of complex patients, including with the use of transcatheter interventions when appropriate. Over 57,000 aortic valve replacement (AVR) and over 19,000 mitral valve replacement (MVR) operations (with or without coronary artery bypass) were reported to the Society of Thoracic Surgeons (STS) National Adult Cardiac Database in calendar year 2019, whereas 72,991 transcatheter aortic valve replacement (TAVRs) and 1164 transcatheter mitral valve replacements (TMVRs, all within the confines of clinical trials) were reported to the STS/American College of Cardiology (ACC) Transcatheter Valve Therapy Registry in calendar year 2019.[2,3] The COVID-19 pandemic was associated with a significant decrease in the volume of valve replacement procedures reported to both registries in the calendar year 2020. Familiarity with the specific hemodynamic attributes, durability, thrombogenicity, and inherent limitations of currently available heart valve substitutes, as well as their potential for long-term complications, is critical for appropriate clinical decision making in patients in whom repair is not appropriate or feasible. The choice of valve prosthesis is inherently a trade-off between durability and risk of thromboembolism, with the associated hazards and lifestyle limitations of anticoagulation. The ideal heart valve substitute remains an elusive goal.

TYPES OF PROSTHETIC HEART VALVES

Mechanical Valves

There are three basic types of mechanical prosthetic valves: bileaflet, tilting disc, and ball-cage (Fig. 79.1). The St. Jude bileaflet valve is the most frequently implanted mechanical prosthesis worldwide. It consists of two pyrolytic semi-circular "leaflets" or discs with a slit-like central orifice between the two leaflets and two larger semi-circular orifices laterally. The opening angle of the leaflets relative to the annulus plane ranges from 75 to 90 degrees. The Carbomedics valve is a variation of the St. Jude prosthesis that can be rotated to prevent limitation of leaflet excursion by subvalvular tissue. For a given valve annulus size, the effective orifice areas (EOAs) are generally larger and transprosthetic pressure gradients are lower for the bileaflet mechanical valves compared with the tilting disc valves. Because the central orifice is smaller than the lateral orifices in bileaflet valves, the blood

flow velocity may be locally higher within the inflow aspect of the central orifice; this phenomenon may yield to overestimation of gradient and underestimation of EOA by transthoracic echocardiography (TTE) (see Chapter 16).[4,5] Bileaflet valves typically have a small amount of normal regurgitation ("washing jet") designed in part to decrease the risk of thrombus formation. A small central jet and two converging jets emanating from the hinge points of the disc can be visualized on color Doppler flow imaging.

Tilting disc or monoleaflet valves use a single circular disc that rotates within a rigid annulus to occlude or open the valve orifice. The disc is secured by lateral or central metal struts. The opening angle of the disc relative to the valve annulus ranges from 60 to 80 degrees, resulting in two orifices of different size. The nonperpendicular opening angle of the valve occluder tends to slightly increase the resistance to blood flow, particularly in the major orifices. Tilting disc valves also have a small amount of regurgitation, arising from small gaps at the perimeter of the valve.

The bulky Starr-Edwards ball-cage valve, the oldest commercially available prosthetic heart valve first used in 1965, is no longer implanted. The ball-cage valve is more thrombogenic and has less favorable hemodynamic performance characteristics than either bileaflet or tilting disc valves.

Currently available mechanical valves have excellent long-term durability, with up to 45 years for the Starr-Edwards valve and more than 35 years for the St. Jude valve. Structural deterioration, exemplified by some older generation Bjork-Shiley (strut fracture with disc embolization) and Starr-Edwards (ball variance) prostheses, is now extremely rare. Ten-year freedom from valve-related death exceeds 90% for both St. Jude and Carbomedics bileaflet valves. All patients with mechanical valves require lifelong anticoagulation with a vitamin K antagonist (VKA).[6] Long-term issues associated with mechanical valves include infective endocarditis, paravalvular leaks, hemolytic anemia, valve thrombosis/thromboembolism, pannus ingrowth, and hemorrhagic complications related to anticoagulation (Fig. 79.2).

Tissue Valves

Tissue or biological valves include stented and stentless bioprostheses (porcine, bovine), homografts (or allografts) from human cadaveric sources, and autografts of pericardial or pulmonic valve origin (see Fig. 79.1). They provide an alternative, less thrombogenic heart valve substitute for which long-term anticoagulation in the absence of additional risk factors for thromboembolism is not required.

Stented Bioprosthetic Valves

The traditional design of a heterograft valve consists of three biologic leaflets made from the porcine aortic valve or bovine pericardium treated with glutaraldehyde to reduce its antigenicity. The leaflets are

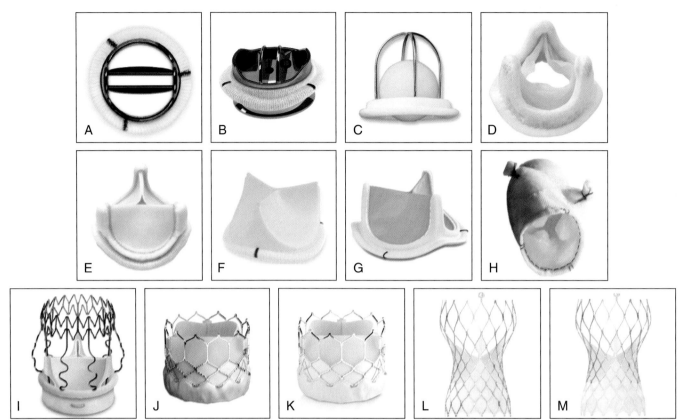

FIGURE 79.1 Different types and models of prosthetic valves. A, Bileaflet St. Jude mechanical valve. **B,** On-X heart valve (with permission of CryoLife). **C,** Caged ball Starr-Edwards mechanical valve. **D,** Stented porcine Medtronic Mosaic bioprosthetic valve. **E,** Stented bovine pericardial Edwards Magna bioprosthetic valve. **F,** Stented bovine pericardial Abbott Trifecta bioprosthetic valve. **G,** Stented bovine pericardial Edwards Inspiris bioprosthetic valve. **H,** Stentless porcine Medtronic Freestyle bioprosthetic valve. **I,** Sutureless Sorin Perceval bioprosthetic valve. **J,** Transcatheter balloon-expandable Edwards SAPIEN 3 bioprosthetic valve. **K,** Transcatheter balloon-expandable Edwards SAPIEN 3 Ultra bioprosthetic valve. **L,** Transcatheter self-expanding Medtronic CoreValve Evolut R bioprosthetic valve. **M,** Transcatheter self-expanding Medtronic CoreValve Evolut PRO bioprosthetic valve.

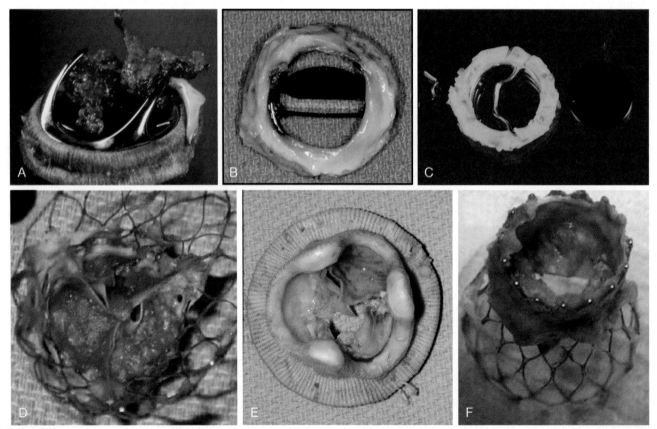

FIGURE 79.2 Prosthetic valve complications. A, Obstructive thrombosis of a Lillehei-Kaster tilting disc mechanical valve. **B,** Pannus ingrowth interacting with leaflet opening in a St. Jude Medical bileaflet mechanical valve. **C,** Rupture of the outlet strut and leaflet escape in a Björk-Shiley mechanical valve. **D,** Thrombosis in a self-expanding transcatheter aortic valve. **E,** Leaflet calcific degeneration and tear in a porcine bioprosthesis. **F,** Leaflet calcific degeneration and stenosis in a self-expanding transcatheter aortic valve. (Courtesy Dr. Siamak Mohammadi, Québec Heart & Lung Institute, Québec (**A** and **C**); Dr. Christian Couture, Québec Heart & Lung Institute, Québec (**B**); Dr. Gosta Petterson, Cleveland Clinic, Cleveland (**E**); **D** from Latib A, et al. Treatment and clinical outcomes of transcatheter heart valve thrombosis. Circ Cardiovasc Interv 2015;8:1-8; **F** from Seeburger J, et al. Structural valve deterioration of a CoreValve prosthesis 9 months after implantation. Eur Heart J 2013;34:1607.)

mounted on a metal or polymeric stented ring; they open to a circular orifice in systole, resembling the anatomy of the native aortic valve (see Fig. 79.1). The vast majority of bioprosthetic valves are treated with anti-calcifying agents or processes. The Inspiris Resilia Aortic Valve (Edwards LifeSciences, Irvine, CA) incorporates newer anti-calcification technology and an expandable sewing ring to accommodate future valve-in-valve implantation for symptomatic, severe structural valve deterioration (SVD).[7,8] The Perceval valve (LivaNova, London, UK) is a sutureless bioprosthetic valve designed to reduce intraoperative times.[8a,8b] The current generation of bovine pericardial valves offers improved hemodynamic performance compared with earlier generations.[9-14] A small degree of regurgitation can be detected by color Doppler flow imaging in 10% of normally functioning bioprostheses. One limitation of earlier generations of bioprosthetic valves was their limited durability due to SVD, typically beginning within 5 to 7 years after implantation but varying by position and age at implant, with tissue changes characterized by calcification, fibrosis, tears, and perforations. SVD occurs earlier for mitral than for aortic bioprosthetic valves, perhaps due to exposure of the mitral prosthesis to relatively higher left ventricular (LV) closing pressures. The process of SVD is accelerated in younger patients, in those with disordered calcium metabolism (end-stage renal disease), and, possibly, in pregnant women independent of younger age. With current generation bioprosthetic pericardial valves, durability is excellent, with SVD rates of 2% to 10% at 10 years, 10% to 20% at 15 years, and 40% at 20 years.[9,10] Premature SVD, however, was an issue with the certain models of the Sorin Mitroflow valve.[15]

Stentless Bioprosthetic Valves
The rigid sewing ring and stent-based construction of certain bioprostheses allow for easier implantation and maintenance of the three-dimensional relationships of the leaflets. However, these features also contribute to impaired hemodynamic performance. Stentless porcine valves (see Fig. 79.1) were developed in part to address these issues. Their use has been restricted to the aortic position. Implantation is technically more challenging, whether deployed in a subcoronary position or as part of a mini-root, and hence they are preferred by only a minority of surgeons. Early postoperative mean gradients can be <15 mm Hg with further improvement in valve performance over time due to aortic root remodeling, resulting in lower peak exercise transvalvular gradients and more rapid reduction in LV mass.[16]

Homografts
Aortic valve homografts are harvested from human cadavers within 24 hours of death and are treated with antibiotics and cryopreserved at –196°C. They are most commonly implanted in the form of a total root replacement with reimplantation of the coronary arteries. Homograft valves appear resistant to infection and are preferred by some surgeons for management of aortic valve and root endocarditis in the active phase (see Chapter 80). Neither immune suppression nor routine anticoagulation is required. Despite earlier expectations, long-term durability beyond 10 years is not superior to that for current generation pericardial valves[17] and reoperation may be technically more challenging due to calcification of the cylinder.

Autografts
In the Ross procedure, the patient's own pulmonic valve (or autograft) is harvested as a small tissue block containing the pulmonic valve, annulus, and proximal pulmonary artery and inserted in the aortic position usually as a complete root replacement with reimplantation of the coronary arteries.[17] The pulmonic valve and right ventricular outflow tract are then replaced with either an aortic or a pulmonic homograft. Thus, the procedure requires two separate valve operations, a longer time on cardiopulmonary bypass, and a steep learning curve. With appropriate selection of young patients by expert surgeons at experienced centers of excellence, operative mortality rates are <1% and 20-year survival rates as high as 95% and similar or slightly lower to the general population.[18,19] Advantages of the autograft include the ability to increase in size during childhood growth, excellent hemodynamic performance characteristics, lack of thrombogenicity, and resistance to infection. The hemodynamic performance characteristics of the pulmonary autograft are similar to those of a normal, native aortic valve. The procedure is usually reserved for children and young adults but should be avoided in patients with dilated aortic roots given the unacceptably high incidence of accelerated degeneration, pulmonary autograft dilation, and significant regurgitation.[20] The critical requirements of surgical skill and institutional experience cannot be overstated.[6]

Transcatheter Bioprosthetic Valves
TAVR is a valuable alternative to surgical AVR in patients across the surgical risk spectrum (see Chapters 72 and 74). Two main types of transcatheter aortic valves are currently used: balloon-expandable valves (BEV) and self-expanding valves (SEV) (see Fig. 79.1).

The Edwards LifeSciences (Irvine, CA) SAPIEN 3 and SAPIEN 3 Ultra BEVs consist of a three-leaflet pericardial bovine valve mounted in a cobalt chromium frame. These valves are available in several sizes. The Medtronic (Minneapolis, MN) EVOLUT-R and EVOLUT-Pro+ SEVs consist of three leaflets of porcine pericardium seated relatively higher in a nitinol frame to provide supra-annular placement and are also available in several sizes.

The vast majority of TAVR procedures are performed via a transfemoral approach, which is associated with lower mortality, fewer complications, and quicker recovery compared with alternative access site approaches (e.g., subclavian, carotid, transcaval, transaortic, apical). The choice of SEV versus BEV is highly operator dependent, though there are anatomic and echocardiographic considerations to be taken into account. Intermediate term durability appears similar, though the risk of permanent pacemaker implantation is higher with SEVs. Other risk factors for the development of high-grade AV block after TAVR have been identified.[21] Leaflet thrombosis can be recognized by the appearance of hypoattenuated leaflet thickening (HALT) on ECG-gated computed tomography (CT) and occurs in 10% to 20% of patients 30 days after TAVR, compared with approximately 5% to 15% after surgical AVR (SAVR).[22-24] Subclinical leaflet thrombosis, that is HALT in the absence of thromboembolic complications or a progressive increase in the transvalvular gradient, appears to be a dynamic phenomenon for which indications for treatment are uncertain.

For a given aortic annulus size, TAVR valves often have larger EOAs, lower gradients, and lower incidence of severe prosthesis-patient mismatch compared with SAVR valves.[25-28] Paravalvular leak (PVL) is, however, more frequent following TAVR and may result in adverse long-term consequences depending on its severity.[29] The risk of PVL has decreased over time with iterative improvements in valve design, preprocedural imaging, patient selection and intraprocedural techniques.[28,30] Some studies have suggested that SEVs have slightly larger EOAs and lower gradients but somewhat higher rates of PVL than BEVs.[31] The rate of SVD over short- to intermediate-term follow-up for the SAPIEN 3 valve is comparable to that of bioprosthetic SAVR valves.[32]

COMPARISON OF MECHANICAL AND TISSUE VALVES
Obvious differences between valve types relate to durability (i.e., theoretically indefinite for mechanical versus limited for tissue valves) and need for anticoagulation (i.e., obligatory use for mechanical versus none for tissue valves absent other risk factors for thromboembolism). Short- to intermediate-term hemodynamic performance characteristics with low-profile mechanical prostheses (e.g., St. Jude) are comparable to those with stented tissue valves of similar size. There are no important differences in rates of prosthetic valve endocarditis (PVE), though some series have suggested a higher incidence of early (<1 year) infection with mechanical valves versus bioprostheses.[33] In the Veterans Affairs randomized trial conducted between 1977 and 1982, patients undergoing AVR had a better 15-year survival with a mechanical valve than with a bioprosthetic valve, whereas there was no difference in survival with mechanical versus biological MVR (see Classic Reference, Hammermeister et al.). With AVR, the increased mortality among patients treated with a bioprosthesis was driven largely by the higher rate of SVD. There was an increased risk of bleeding with mechanical valve replacement, but no significant differences were observed for other valve-related complications such as thromboembolism or PVE. A smaller randomized trial of patients 55 to 70 years of age with aortic

valve disease also showed no difference in late survival between newer generation mechanical and bioprosthetic valves, with higher rates of SVD and reoperation in patients with bioprostheses but no other differences in secondary endpoints.[34] In an analysis of over 39,000 AVR patients aged 65 to 80 years reported to the STS Adult Cardiac Surgery Database and linked to Medicare, patients receiving a bioprosthesis had a similar adjusted risk for death, higher risks for reoperation and endocarditis, and lower risks for stroke and bleeding, compared with patients receiving a mechanical valve.[35] Two propensity-matched analyses from New York's Statewide Planning and Research Cooperative System (SPARCS) reported no survival differences for patients 50 to 69 years of age undergoing mechanical versus bioprosthetic, AVR, or MVR.[36,37] Rates of stroke and bleeding were higher, whereas rates of reoperation were lower, among mechanical valve recipients. A survival advantage among patients in this age group who underwent mechanical rather than bioprosthetic valve replacement was, however, reported from the Swedish system for the Enhancement and Development of Evidence-based care in Heart disease Evaluated According to Recommended Therapies (SWEDEHEART) register.[38] Stroke risk was similar between the groups, though bleeding rates were higher and need for reoperation lower after mechanical valve replacement. Overall survival and rates of reoperation, stroke, and bleeding after bioprosthetic versus mechanical valve replacement were examined in a 2017 report from the California Office of Statewide Health Planning and Development.[39] Among patients 45 to 54 years of age who underwent SAVR, receipt of a biological prosthesis was associated with a significantly higher 15-year mortality rate than receipt of a mechanical prosthesis. Among patients undergoing surgical MVR, use of a mechanical valve was associated with lower mortality up to age 69. There was significant decrease in the use of mechanical valves over the 17-year period examined (1996 to 2013). Rates of reoperation were lower but rates of bleeding and stroke were higher for those who received a mechanical valve.[39]

CHOICE OF VALVE REPLACEMENT PROCEDURE AND PROSTHESIS

Once the indication for valve intervention is established, the next step is to select the type of procedure (repair versus replacement) and the type of prosthetic valve to be used should replacement be necessary. The 2020 AHA/ACC guidelines for the management of patients with valvular heart disease advocate shared decision making regarding the choice of intervention (repair or replacement, transcatheter or surgical) as well as the type of prosthetic valve (mechanical valve or bioprosthesis).[6] This choice is based on consideration of several factors including patient age, expected longevity and comorbidities, valve durability, expected hemodynamics for a specific valve type and size, surgical or interventional risk, the potential need for and safety of long-term anticoagulation, and patient preferences.

CHOICE OF PROCEDURE

For patients meeting an indication for AVR, the choice of TAVR versus SAVR begins with assessment of surgical risk considering patient age and life expectancy (see Chapters 72 and 74). The ultimate choice also hinges on technical factors related to access (transfemoral versus alternative route), aortic valve and root anatomy, the extent and severity of calcification, the height of the coronary arteries, and the need for additional cardiac surgery (e.g., root or ascending aortic replacement, coronary artery bypass grafting). TAVR is preferred for prohibitive or high surgical risk patients provided life expectancy with reasonable quality exceeds 1 year. SAVR is preferred for low or intermediate surgical risk patients younger than 65 due to the paucity of data regarding TAVR valve durability beyond 5 years. For patients 65 to 80 years of age, the choice between TAVR and SAVR is largely driven by patient preference and the need for concomitant surgery. TAVR is generally preferred for patients over age 80.[6] Recommendations regarding TAVR apply primarily to patients with trileaflet aortic stenosis, although the use of TAVR for selected patients with bicuspid aortic valve stenosis has increased rapidly.

In patients with chronic severe primary mitral regurgitation (MR) who meet an indication for mitral valve surgery, mitral valve repair is recommended in preference to MVR when a successful and durable repair can be accomplished (see Chapter 76).[6] Transcatheter mitral valve repair using an edge-to-edge clip device is reserved for prohibitive surgical risk patients with primary MR. In patients with severe chronic secondary MR in the setting of ischemic cardiomyopathy referred for coronary artery bypass graft, concomitant MVR may be superior to mitral valve repair because it is associated with lower rates of recurrent moderate to severe regurgitation.[40] Transcatheter edge-to-edge repair (TEER) is reasonable

for selected patients with heart failure, reduced ejection fraction and moderately severe to severe MR (see Chapter 78).[6,41]

Tricuspid valve annuloplasty repair is frequently performed at the time of left-sided valve surgery when secondary tricuspid regurgitation (TR) is severe or when there is significant tricuspid annular dilation (>40 mm) despite only mild or moderate degrees of TR or a history of right-sided heart failure (see Chapter 77).[42] Tricuspid valve replacement is undertaken for severe primary tricuspid valve disease that cannot be repaired, such as with advanced rheumatic disease, carcinoid, or destructive endocarditis.[6] Surgical or transcatheter pulmonic valve replacement in the adult is rare.

CHOICE OF PROSTHETIC VALVE

A bioprosthesis is recommended in patients of any age for whom anticoagulant therapy is contraindicated, cannot be managed appropriately, or is not desired. A mechanical prosthesis is reasonable for SAVR in patients <50 years old who do not have a contraindication to antico-agulation, whereas a bioprosthesis is reasonable in SAVR patients >65 years old.[6] Either a bioprosthetic or mechanical valve is reasonable in SAVR patients between 50 and 65 years old. When MVR is necessary, a mechanical prosthesis is reasonable for patients <65 years old and a bioprosthesis is reasonable for patients ≥65 years old. For women contemplating pregnancy, a bioprosthesis is preferred to avoid the hazards of anticoagulation. The choice of prosthesis in patients with end-stage renal disease is challenging and should take into account life expectancy.

MEDICAL MANAGEMENT AND SURVEILLANCE AFTER VALVE REPLACEMENT

Antithrombotic Therapy

General Principles

Table 79.1 presents the antithrombotic regimens included in the 2020 AHA/ACC guideline for different types of procedures and prosthetic valves.[6] All patients with mechanical heart valves require lifelong anticoagulation with a VKA, the intensity of which varies as a function of valve type or thrombogenicity, valve position and number, and the presence of additional risk factors for thromboembolism, such as atrial fibrillation, LV systolic dysfunction, a history of thromboembolism, and hypercoagulable state (see Table 79.1). Anticoagulant therapy with non-vitamin K oral anticoagulants (NOACs) should not be used in patients with mechanical prostheses, although they can be used in patients with bioprosthetic valves or annuloplasty rings at a distance from surgery.[6] The addition of low-dose aspirin to VKA therapy can be considered in patients with mechanical valves when dictated by another indication. Although there is no clear consensus, a VKA may be used even in the absence of risk factors for thromboembolism for the first 3 to 6 months after bioprosthetic AVR or MVR.[6] Longer-term treatment of low thromboembolic risk bioprosthetic AVR and MVR patients consists of low-dose aspirin, although there are no randomized data to support this practice. In the absence of an indication for anticoagulation, single-agent antiplatelet therapy with low-dose aspirin is reasonable after TAVR.[6,43,44] For patients with an indication for anticoagulation, monotherapy with either a VKA or NOAC is reasonable after TAVR.[6] Treatment following TAVR with low-dose rivaroxaban (10 mg daily) plus aspirin (75 to 100 mg daily for the first 3 months) is contraindicated.[45]

Interruption of Antithrombotic Therapy

In the planned interruption of VKA therapy for noncardiac surgery, the following must be taken into account: the nature of the procedure; the magnitude of risk of thromboembolism based on valve type, position, and number; underlying patient risk factors; the length of time over which therapy is to be interrupted; and the competing risk of periprocedural hemorrhage.[6] Low-risk patients with low-profile bileaflet or tilting disc valves in the aortic position can usually stop VKA therapy 3 to 5 days before noncardiac surgery and then resume it postoperatively as soon as it is considered safe, without the need for a heparin "bridge." In all other patients, either low-molecular-weight heparin (LMWH) or intravenous unfractionated heparin

TABLE 79.1 Antithrombotic Therapy in Patients with Prosthetic Valves

COR**	LOE		VKA (TARGET INR)	ASPIRIN (75-100 MG)	CLOPIDOGREL (75 MG)
		Mechanical Valves			
I	B-NR	**AVR**–Bileaflet or current generation single tilting disc valves and no risk factors for thromboembolism*	Yes (INR: 2.5)	If indicated‡	
I	B-NR	**AVR**–Older-generation valves† and/or any risk factor for thromboembolism*	Yes (INR: 3.0)	If indicated‡	
I	B-NR	**MVR**–Mechanical valves	Yes (INR: 3.0)	If indicated‡	
IIb	B-NR	**AVR**–On-X valve and no risk factors for thromboembolism	Yes (INR: 1.5-2.0) §	Yes	
		Surgical Bioprosthetic Valves			
IIa	B-NR	AVR or MVR–Initial 3-6 months	Yes (2.5)		
IIa	B-NR	AVR or MVR–Lifelong		Yes	
		Transcatheter Aortic Valves			
IIb	B-NR	TAVR–Initial 3-6 months¶		Yes	Yes
IIb	B-NR	TAVR–Initial 3-6 months¶	Yes		
IIa	B-NR	TAVR–Lifelong		Yes	

AVR, Aortic valve replacement; *MVR,* mitral valve replacement; *INR,* international normalized ratio; *VKA,* vitamin K antagonist; *TAVR,* transcatheter aortic valve implantation.
*Risk factors for thromboembolism: Atrial fibrillation, LV dysfunction (LVEF ≤35%), LA dilation (LA diameter ≥50 mm), previous thromboembolism, and hypercoagulable condition.
†Ball-in-cage valves, older generation of single tilting-disc valves.
‡Addition of low-dose aspirin in low bleeding risk patients may be predicated on development of independent indication during follow-up, such as intra-coronary stent implantation.
§INR goal 2.5 for the first 3 months after On-X SAVR; INR goal 1.5-2.0 thereafter with lifelong continuation of low-dose aspirin.
¶If low risk of bleeding, one of the two antithrombotic therapies (aspirin + clopidogrel or VKA) but not both may be considered.
**COR refers to the AHA/ACC 2020 Valvular Heart Disease Class of Recommendation for each scenario. Class I indicates that the recommendation should be followed and the treatment given. Class IIa indicates that the recommendation is reasonable, and Class IIb indicates that the recommendation may be considered.
From Otto CM, et al. 2020 AHA/ACC guideline for the management of patients with valvular heart disease: a report of the American College of Cardiology/American Heart Association Task Force on Practice Guidelines. J Am Coll Cardiol 2021;77:e25-197.

(UFH) should be given on an individualized basis both before and after surgery, as directed by the surgeon. The use of LMWH avoids the need for preoperative hospitalization. For patients with a bioprosthetic valve or annuloplasty ring receiving an anticoagulant, it is reasonable to consider the need for bridging on the basis of the CHA_2DS_2-VASc score and the risk of bleeding. There is a paucity of randomized trial data and significant institutional and operator variability in the use of bridging strategies for noncardiac surgery in patients with prosthetic valves.

Pregnancy (see Chapter 92)

Pregnant patients with prosthetic valves should be followed carefully because of the increased hemodynamic burden that can cause or worsen heart failure if there is prosthetic valve dysfunction and also because of the hypercoagulable state related to pregnancy that increases the risk of valve thrombosis. All antithrombotic regimens carry an increased risk to the fetus, an increased risk of miscarriage, and an increased risk of hemorrhagic complications for the mother. Hence, patients require appropriate counseling, close monitoring, and adjustment of anticoagulation therapy. In pregnant patients with mechanical valves, warfarin is reasonable in the first trimester if the dose is ≤5 mg/day and is recommended to achieve a therapeutic international normalized ratio (INR) target in the second and third trimesters.[6] Discontinuation of warfarin with initiation of intravenous UFH is recommended before planned vaginal delivery in pregnant patients with a mechanical valve.

Infective Endocarditis Prophylaxis (see Chapter 80)

Patients with prosthetic valves are at increased risk for infective endocarditis because of the foreign valve surface and sewing ring (see Chapter 80). Antibiotic prophylaxis is indicated for patients with prosthetic valves who undergo dental procedures that involve manipulation of gingival tissue, the periapical region of teeth, or perforation of the oral mucosa, and it is not recommended for non-dental procedures such as transesophageal echocardiography, esophagogastroduodenoscopy, colonoscopy, or cystoscopy (unless there is active infection in these areas).[6,33]

Clinical Assessment

Postoperative visits should begin approximately 3 to 4 weeks after valve implantation. The first visit is focused on ensuring a smooth transition from hospital/rehabilitation facility to home, reconciling medications, and assessing neurocognitive function, wound healing, volume status, heart rhythm, and the auscultatory characteristics of prosthetic valve function. The history at subsequent visits is tailored to detect symptoms suggestive of heart failure or reduced functional capacity, arrhythmia, thromboembolism, or infection. Adherence to the recommended schedule of INR determinations and the relative time spent in the therapeutic range should be assessed in all VKA anticoagulated patients. Problems with bleeding should be identified. A focused cardiovascular examination is repeated at each visit. Instructions regarding antibiotic prophylaxis are repeated. After the 6-month mark, follow-up visits can be conducted annually unless interim problems arise.

A chest radiograph is obtained by the surgeon at the first visit to assess for residual pleural fluid, pneumothorax, lung aeration, and heart size. An electrocardiogram is routinely performed and should be reviewed for rhythm, conduction, and dynamic repolarization changes. Postoperative baseline values for hemoglobin, hematocrit, lactate dehydrogenase (LDH), and bilirubin should be established for patients with mechanical heart valves, allowing future comparisons should hemolysis be suspected. It is less useful to follow the serum haptoglobin. Other laboratory studies are performed as clinically relevant.

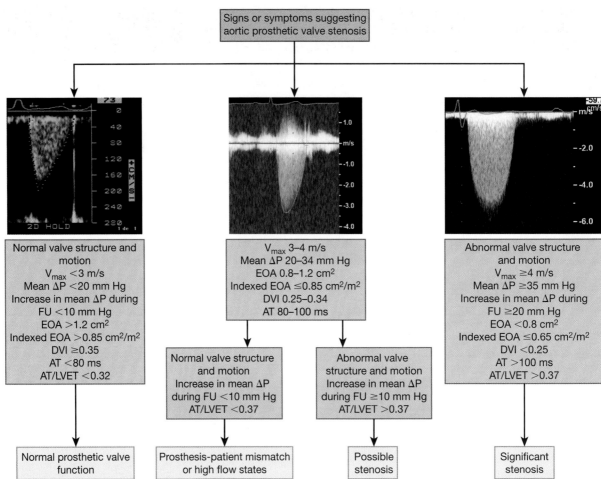

FIGURE 79.3 Evaluation of aortic prosthetic valve stenosis. A practical approach to evaluation of possible prosthetic aortic stenosis is to begin with standard measures of stenosis severity, including maximal velocity (V_{max}), mean pressure gradient (ΔP), effective orifice area (EOA), and Doppler velocity index (DVI: ratio of left ventricular outflow tract to aortic velocity). Normal values for each valve type and size should be referenced, but simple thresholds of 3 and 4 m/s for V_{max} and 20 and 35 mm Hg for mean ΔP are a quick first step. For patients with intermediate measures of stenosis severity, the assessment of valve structure and motion and of the changes in ΔP, EOA, and DVI during follow-up (FU) can be helpful to differentiate normal prosthetic valve function with concomitant prosthesis-patient mismatch or high flow states versus prosthetic valve stenosis. The shape of the transprosthetic flow velocity curve may also be helpful with a triangular shape (short acceleration time [AT], i.e., time to peak velocity relative to LV ejection time [LVET]) suggesting normal valve function and a rounded waveform (increased AT/LVET ratio) suggesting significant stenosis. Additional imaging including transesophageal echocardiography, cinefluoroscopy, or cardiac CT may be needed to assess valve leaflet structure and motion.

Echocardiography (see Chapter 16)

An initial TTE examination performed 6 weeks to 3 months after prosthetic valve implantation is recommended to assess the results of surgery and serve as a baseline for comparison should complications or deterioration occur later (see Figs. 16.51, 16.52, and 16.53).[6] Repeat TTE (as well as transesophageal echocardiography (TEE), fluoroscopy, or gated cardiac CT) is recommended if there is a change in clinical symptoms or signs suggesting valve dysfunction. In patients with a bioprosthetic surgical valve, routine TTE follow-up is recommended at 5 and 10 years and then annually thereafter. Presently, annual TTE studies are recommended for TAVR patients.[6] Studies estimate that 25% to 30% of patients with a bioprosthesis implanted for less than 10 years in the aortic position have some degree of valve degeneration/dysfunction.[10] In patients with mechanical valves, routine annual echocardiography is not indicated in the absence of a change in clinical status.

A complete echocardiogram includes two-dimensional imaging of the prosthetic valve; evaluation of the valve leaflet/occluder morphology and mobility; measurement of the transprosthetic velocity and gradients, valve EOA, and Doppler velocity index; estimation of the degree of regurgitation; evaluation of LV size and systolic function; and calculation of systolic pulmonary arterial pressure (see Chapter 16).[4,5,46,47] Paravalvular regurgitation is more common following TAVR than SAVR and the measurement of valve EOA is more challenging in transcatheter valves than in surgical valves due to the presence of the valve stent in the LV outflow tract.[6,48]

EVALUATION AND TREATMENT OF PROSTHETIC VALVE DYSFUNCTION AND COMPLICATIONS

The suspicion of prosthetic valve dysfunction may be heightened by the appreciation of a new murmur or symptom in a patient with a prosthetic valve or the incidental finding of abnormally high flow velocities and gradients detected during routine echocardiography. Doppler-echocardiography is the method of choice to evaluate prosthetic valve function, identify and quantitate prosthetic valve stenosis or regurgitation, and identify prosthesis-patient mismatch (PPM) (Figs. 79.3 and 79.4).[4,5,46] Cinefluoroscopy and ECG-gated cardiac CT may also be helpful to evaluate leaflet mobility in mechanical and bioprosthetic valves, respectively.[5] Prosthetic valve stenosis may be caused by thrombus formation, pannus ingrowth (or a combination of both) (see Figs. 16.55 and 20.21), leaflet calcification in the case of bioprosthetic valves, and vegetations. Prosthetic valve regurgitation may be related to thrombus formation (mechanical valves), leaflet tear (bioprostheses), vegetations, or PVL.

Prosthesis-Patient Mismatch

PPM occurs when the size of a normally functioning prosthetic valve is too small in relation to the patient's body size and thus to the patient's cardiac output requirements, resulting in abnormally high postoperative gradients. PPM is defined as an indexed EOA <0.85 cm² (severe:

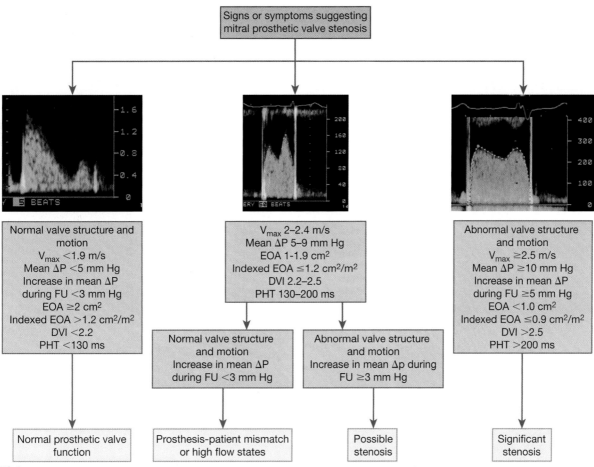

FIGURE 79.4 **Evaluation of mitral prosthetic valve stenosis.** The evaluation starts with standard measures of stenosis severity including maximal velocity (V_{max}), mean pressure gradient (mean ΔP), effective orifice area (EOA), and pressure half-time (PHT). Doppler velocity index (DVI) is the ratio of mitral to left ventricular outflow tract velocity, and therefore an elevated value is abnormal. Normal values for each valve type and size should be referenced, but the thresholds shown are a quick first step. In patients with intermediate measures of stenosis severity, the differential diagnosis includes significant stenosis, prosthesis-patient mismatch (PPM), and a high flow state. Additional imaging including transesophageal echocardiography, cinefluoroscopy, or cardiac CT may be needed to assess valve leaflet structure and motion. *FU,* Follow-up.

<0.65 cm²) for aortic prosthetic valves and EOA <1.2 cm² (severe: <0.9 cm²) for mitral prosthetic valves. The prevalence of moderate PPM ranges from 20% to 70% and that of severe PPM from 2% to 10% following AVR or MVR, respectively.[49] Patients with aortic PPM have higher functional class and worse exercise capacity, reduced regression of LV hypertrophy, more adverse cardiac events, and increased risk of both perioperative and late mortality after SAVR when compared with patients who do not have PPM.[49] Patients with mitral PPM have persisting pulmonary hypertension and increased incidence of congestive heart failure and death. A greater clinical impact of aortic PPM is also observed in specific groups of patients such as those with preexisting LV dysfunction or severe LV hypertrophy, and/or concomitant MR, as well as in those <65 to 70 years old. PPM is less frequent with TAVR compared with SAVR, particularly in the subset of patients with a small aortic annulus.[25,50] To reduce the incidence of postoperative PPM, aortic root enlargement is often performed to allow for implantation of a larger prosthesis. Figures 79.3 and 79.4 provide algorithms for differentiating between normal prosthetic valve function, PPM, and intrinsic valve dysfunction due to SVD, thrombus, or pannus.

Structural Valve Deterioration

Mechanical prostheses have an excellent durability, and SVD is extremely rare with contemporary valves. On the other hand, SVD due to leaflet calcification and/or collagen fiber disruption is the major cause of bioprosthetic valve failure. SVD may lead to leaflet stiffening and progressive stenosis or leaflet tear with transvalvular regurgitation[13,51] (Fig. 79.5; see also Fig. 16.56). Although SVD of bioprostheses has long been considered a purely passive degenerative process, more recent studies suggest that active and potentially modifiable processes may be involved including lipid infiltration,

inflammation, immune rejection, and active mineralization. Transcatheter valve-in-valve implantation offers a valuable alternative to surgery for patients with failed bioprosthetic valves who are at higher risk for reoperation (see Chapters 74 and 78). Nearly 4500 valve-in-valve implants were reported to the STS/ACC TVT Registry in 2019.[2]

Paravalvular Leak

PVL occurs external to the prosthetic valve at the interface between the valve ring and the native valve annulus (see Fig. 79.5). It can occur as a result of inadequate technique, suture dehiscence, compromised native tissue integrity (dense calcification, extensive myxomatous degeneration), infection, or chronic abrasion of the sewing ring against a calcified or rigid annulus. The magnitude of the regurgitant volume will depend on the size of the orifice. A small and hemodynamically inconsequential PVL is usually discovered incidentally during routine TTE with color Doppler flow imaging. No change in management would be indicated. Small PVLs may, however, be associated with significant intravascular hemolysis and anemia as red blood cells are forced through a narrow orifice at high velocities. Despite a high clinical index of suspicion in this circumstance, a new, regurgitant murmur may not be audible. TEE may be necessary to differentiate paravalvular versus transvalvular regurgitation and to visualize the defect appropriately, especially with mitral prostheses. Larger PVLs may result in significant volume overload and heart failure, to an extent that reoperation or catheter closure with an occluder device might be indicated. Significant PVL may develop during the late postoperative period and if such is the case, this is often the result of endocarditis. Management can prove quite challenging and a conservative approach with medical therapy may be chosen.

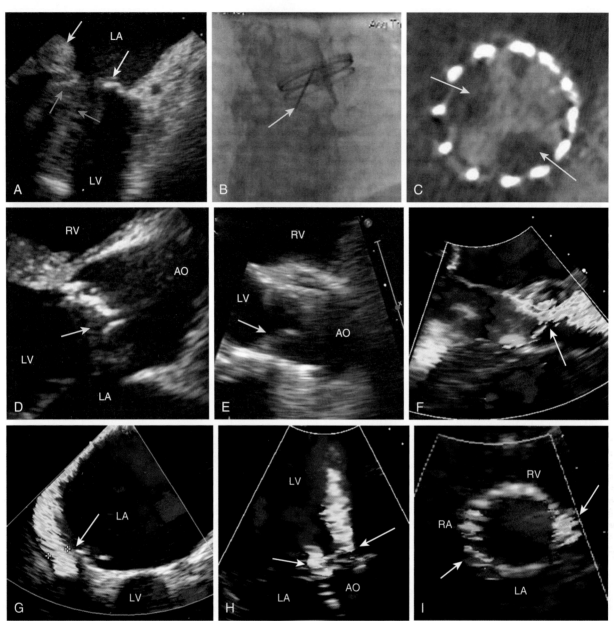

FIGURE 79.5 Imaging of prosthetic valve dysfunction. A, Transesophageal echocardiographic view of an obstructed mitral bileaflet mechanical valve. *Yellow arrow,* large-size thrombus; *white arrow,* pannus; *blue arrow,* mobile leaflet; *green arrow,* immobile leaflet (Video 79.1). **B,** Cinefluoroscopy of bileaflet mechanical valve showing an immobile leaflet (*yellow arrow*) (Video 79.2). **C,** Multi-detector computed tomography with contrast injection showing an area of hypoattenuation (*yellow arrows*) indicating thrombi on two of the leaflets of a balloon expandable transcatheter valve. **D,** Transthoracic echocardiographic view of a stented bioprosthetic valve with calcific degeneration, thickening, and reduced mobility of the leaflets (*yellow arrow*) (Video 79.3). **E** and **F,** Transthoracic echocardiographic views of an obstructive valve leaflet thrombus in a balloon-expandable transcatheter aortic valve. The leaflets are thickened (**E,** *yellow arrow*) and the width of the transprosthetic flow jet on color-Doppler is narrowed (**F,** *white arrow*) (Video 79.4); **G,** Transesophageal color Doppler echocardiographic view of a severe paravalvular leak (*white arrow*) in a mitral mechanical valve; **H** and **I,** Transthoracic color Doppler echocardiographic views (**H,** apical three-chamber; **I,** parasternal short-axis) of two paravalvular regurgitant jets (*white arrows*) in a transcatheter aortic valve (Video 79.5). (Courtesy Dr. Steven A. Goldstein, Washington Hospital Center **(A)**; Dr. John Chambers, Guy's and St. Thomas Hospitals, London, UK **(D)**; and Dr Arsène Basmadjian, Montreal Heart Institute, Montreal, Canada **(G)**.)

PVL is more frequent following TAVR compared with SAVR (see Chapter 74); its incidence is significantly lower with newer generation TAVR bioprostheses.[26,52,53] Because PVL jets after TAVR are often multiple, irregular, and eccentric, the imaging and grading of PVL can be challenging (see Fig. 79.5; see also Fig. 16.57). A multi-window, multi-parametric, integrative approach is essential to assess the severity of PVL by Doppler-echocardiography (see Chapter 16).[46-48] Other imaging modalities, such as cineangiography, cardiac CT, and cardiac magnetic resonance, as well as serum biomarkers, may also be useful to complement or corroborate the findings on TTE and TEE. The use of corrective procedures such as repeat balloon dilation, valve-in-valve implantation, and/or transcatheter leak closure may be considered depending on the severity of PVL and the risk of procedural complications.

Thromboembolism and Bleeding

Thromboembolisms are a major source of morbidity in patients with prosthetic heart valves. The incidence of clinically recognizable events ranges from 0.6% to 2.3% per patient-year,[6] an estimate that does not account for any subclinical episodes, which might be detected with sensitive imaging techniques.[54] Thromboembolic incidence rates are similar for nonanticoagulated patients with bioprostheses and appropriately anticoagulated patients with mechanical valves. Risk factors for thromboembolism include the inherent thrombogenicity of the prosthesis, valve position (mitral > aortic), valve number, time spent out of the therapeutic range of VKA anticoagulation, a history of thromboembolism, hypercoagulable state, atrial fibrillation, left atrial enlargement, and LV systolic dysfunction. The risk of bleeding, estimated at 1% per patient-year, increases with age and the intensity of anticoagulation. In patients with uncontrollable bleeding who require reversal of anticoagulation, administration of prothrombin complex concentrate is reasonable.[6] Antidotes to oral anti-Xa and antithrombin agents are also available.

Management of a thromboembolic event in patients with mechanical valves generally proceeds along one or more of the following lines: (1) For patients whose INR is subtherapeutic, the dose of the VKA is advanced to achieve the intended INR range; (2) for patients whose INR is in the therapeutic range, the dose of the VKA is advanced to achieve a higher INR range and/or low-dose aspirin is added if not already used; (3) the patient and family are informed about the increased risks of bleeding; (4) the potential for drug interactions is reviewed. Reoperation to implant a less thrombogenic valve is rarely undertaken for patients with recurrent thromboemboli despite aggressive antithrombotic therapy.

Prosthetic Valve Thrombosis (see Chapter 20)

The incidence of mechanical valve thrombosis is estimated at 0.3% to 1.3% per patient-year in high-income countries, but as high as 6% per patient-year in low- to middle-income countries.[6] Thrombosis of a mechanical heart valve can have devastating consequences (see Figs. 79.2 and 79.5; see also Fig. 16.54). Bioprosthetic (surgical or transcatheter) valve thrombosis is less common but does occur (see Figs. 20.21 and 20.24). A CT substudy of the PARTNER 3 trial observed a 30-day incidence of 13% among TAVR patients versus 5% for SAVR patients (see Chapter 74).[22] However, 56% of patients with HALT at 30 days showed resolution by 1 year, whereas 21% of patients without HALT at 30 days had evidence of leaflet thrombosis at 1 year. The 1-year prevalence of HALT was 28% for TAVR patients and 20% for SAVR patients.[22] The CT substudy of the EVOLUT Low Risk trial reported similar incidence of HALT in TAVR versus SAVR at 30 days (17.3% versus 16.5%) and 1 year (31% versus 27%).[24] Oral anticoagulation is reasonable for patients with bioprosthetic valve thrombosis and clinical symptoms (thromboembolism) or progressive prosthetic valve gradients with evidence of leaflet dysfunction; a VKA may be preferred.[6] The clinical significance and benefit of treatment for subclinical leaflet thrombosis is less clear (see Figs. 79.2 and 79.5).[22,23,55]

Clinical suspicion of mechanical prosthetic valve thrombosis should be raised by symptoms of heart failure, thromboembolism, and/or low cardiac output, coupled with a decrease in the intensity of the valve closure sounds new and pathologic murmurs and/or documentation of inadequate anticoagulation. Thrombosis is more common in the mitral and tricuspid positions than in the aortic position. Although differentiation from pannus formation can be difficult, the clinical context usually allows accurate diagnosis. Evaluation with TTE/TEE can help guide management decisions.[4,5] Confirmation of abnormal leaflet or disc excursion in the presence of an occluding thrombus can also be obtained with cinefluoroscopy or ECG-gated cardiac CT (see Fig. 79.5; see also Fig 20.20D).[5,22,24,56]

Emergency surgery is reasonable for patients with left-sided mechanical valve thrombosis and shock or New York Heart Association (NYHA) functional class III to IV symptoms and for patients with a large thrombus burden (≥0.8 cm² on TEE).[6] Slow infusion, low-dose fibrinolytic therapy is reasonable for patients with recent onset (<2 weeks) NYHA class I to II symptoms and small thrombus burden (<0.8 cm²) or for sicker patients with larger thrombi when surgery is either not available or inadvisable. Fibrinolytic therapy is generally recommended for patients with right-sided prosthetic valve thrombosis.[6] Some patients with no or minimal symptoms and small thrombi can often be managed with intravenous UFH alone and then converted to fibrinolytic therapy if unsuccessful. Any course of fibrinolytic therapy is followed at the appropriate interval by a continuous infusion of UFH during the transition to VKA therapy targeted to a higher INR with or without low-dose aspirin. Serial TTE studies are useful to assess the response to treatment.

Infective Endocarditis (see Chapter 80)

PVE is the most severe form of infective endocarditis and occurs in 1% to 6% of patients with valve prostheses accounting for 10% to 30% of all cases of infective endocarditis (see Chapter 80).[33,57] PVE is an extremely serious condition with high in-hospital mortality rates (20% to 50%). The diagnosis based on the Modified Duke Criteria relies predominantly on the combination of positive blood cultures and echocardiographic evidence of prosthetic valve infection, including vegetations, paravalvular abscess, or a new paravalvular regurgitation.[33] TEE is essential in patients with prosthetic valves because of its greater sensitivity in detecting these abnormalities (see Figs. 80.6 and 80.7). Increased uptake of ¹⁸Fluorodeoxyglucose measured by positron emission

tomography CT (PET-CT) may improve the early diagnosis of PVE (see Figs. 18.40 and 18.41).[58-60] Despite prompt and appropriate antibiotic treatment, many patients with PVE will eventually require surgery. Medical treatment alone is more likely to succeed in late PVE (occurring >6 months after surgery) and in nonstaphylococcal infections. Surgery should be considered in the following situations: heart failure; failure of antibiotic treatment; hemodynamically significant prosthetic valve regurgitation, especially if associated with deterioration of LV function; large vegetations (>10 mm in size); persistently positive blood cultures on therapy; recurrent emboli with persistent vegetations; and intracardiac fistula formation.[6] PVE after TAVR occurs predominantly within the first year after the procedure. Its incidence is low (0.5% to 1% per patient-year) but in-hospital (~35%) and 2-year (~67%) mortality rates are high,[61] likely reflective of patient age and comorbidities.

Hemolytic Anemia

The development of a non-immune hemolytic anemia after valve replacement or repair is usually attributable to PVL with intravascular red blood cell destruction. Diagnosis is based on a high index of suspicion, coupled with laboratory evidence of hemolysis, including the characteristic changes in red blood cells morphology (schistocytes), elevated indirect bilirubin and LDH, a high reticulocyte count, and depressed serum haptoglobin. Reoperative surgery or catheter closure of the defect is indicated when heart failure, a persistent transfusion requirement, or poor quality of life intervenes. Empiric medical measures include iron and folic acid replacement therapy and beta-adrenoreceptor blockers. It is important to exclude PVE as a cause.

CLASSIC REFERENCES
Hammermeister K, Sethi GK, Henderson WG, et al. Outcomes 15 years after valve replacement with a mechanical versus a bioprosthetic valve: final report of the veterans affairs randomized trial. J Am Coll Cardiol. 2000;36:1152–1158.

REFERENCES
1. Nishimura RA, O'Gara PT, Bavaria JE, et al. 2019 AATS/ACC/ASE/SCAI/STS expert consensus systems of care document: a proposal to optimize care for patients with valvular heart disease: a joint report of the American Association for Thoracic Surgery, American College of Cardiology, American Society of Echocardiography, Society for Cardiovascular Angiography and Interventions and Society of Thoracic Surgeons. J Am Coll Cardiol. 2019;73:2609–2635.
2. Carroll JD, Mack MJ, Vemulapalli S, et al. STS-ACC TVT registry of transcatheter aortic valve replacement. J Am Coll Cardiol. 2020;76:2492–2516.
3. Vemulapalli S, Dai D, Hammill BG, et al. Hospital resource utilization before and after transcatheter aortic valve replacement: the STS/ACC TVT registry. J Am Coll Cardiol. 2019;73:1135–1146.

Types of Prosthetic Heart Valves
4. Zoghbi WA, Chambers JB, Dumesnil JG, et al. Recommendations for evaluation of prosthetic valves with echocardiography and Doppler ultrasound: a report from the American Society of Echocardiography's guidelines and standards committee and the task force on prosthetic valves, developed in conjunction with the American College of Cardiology Cardiovascular Imaging Committee, Cardiac Imaging Committee of the American Heart Association, the European Association of Echocardiography, a registered branch of the European Society of Cardiology, the Japanese Society of Echocardiography and the Canadian Society of Echocardiography, endorsed by the American College of Cardiology Foundation, American Heart Association, European Association of Echocardiography, a registered branch of the European Society of Cardiology, the Japanese Society of Echocardiography, and Canadian Society of Echocardiography. J Am Soc Echocardiogr. 2009;22:975–1014.
5. Lancellotti P, Pibarot P, Chambers J, et al. Recommendations for the imaging assessment of prosthetic heart valves: a report from the European Association of Cardiovascular imaging endorsed by the Chinese Society of Echocardiography, the Interamerican Society of Echocardiography and the Brazilian Department of Cardiovascular Imaging. Eur Heart J Cardiovasc Imaging. 2016;17:589–590.
6. Otto CM, Nishimura RA, Bonow RO, et al. 2020 ACC/AHA guideline for the management of patients with valvular heart disease: executive summary: a report of the American College of Cardiology/American Heart Association joint committee on clinical practice guidelines. J Am Coll Cardiol. 2021;77:e25–e197.
7. Puskas JD, Bavaria JE, Svensson LG, et al. The COMMENCE trial: 2-year outcomes with an aortic bioprosthesis with RESILIA tissue. Eur J Cardio Thorac Surg. 2017;52:432–439.
8. Meuris B, Borger MA, Bourguignon T, et al. Durability of bioprosthetic aortic valves in patients under the age of 60 years - rationale and design of the international INDURE registry. J Cardiothorac Surg. 2020;15:119.
8a. Lorusso R, Folliguet T, Shrestha M, et al. Sutureless versus stented bioprostheses for aortic valve replacement: the randomized PERSIST-AVR study design. Thorac Cardiovasc Surg. 2020;68:114–123.
8b. Szecel D, Eurlings R, Rega F, et al. Perceval sutureless aortic valve implantation: mid-term outcomes. Ann Thorac Surg. 2021;111:1331–1337.
9. Johnston DR, Soltesz EG, Vakil N, et al. Long-term durability of bioprosthetic aortic valves: implications from 12,569 implants. Ann Thorac Surg. 2015;99:1239–1247.
10. Bourguignon T, Bouquiaux-Stablo AL, Candolfi P, et al. Very long-term outcomes of the Carpentier-Edwards Perimount valve in aortic position. Ann Thorac Surg. 2015;99:831–837.
11. Rodriguez-Gabella T, Voisine P, Dagenais F, et al. Long-term outcomes following surgical aortic bioprosthesis implantation. J Am Coll Cardiol. 2018;71:1401–1412.
12. Salaun E, Mahjoub H, Dahou A, et al. Hemodynamic deterioration of surgically implanted bioprosthetic aortic valves. J Am Coll Cardiol. 2018;72:241–251.
13. Salaun E, Clavel MA, Rodés-Cabau J, Pibarot P. Bioprosthetic aortic valve durability in the era of transcatheter aortic valve implantation. Heart. 2018;104:1323–1332.

1504

VIII DISEASES OF THE HEART VALVES

80 Infectious Endocarditis and Infections of Indwelling Devices

LARRY M. BADDOUR, NANDAN S. ANAVEKAR, JUAN A. CRESTANELLO, AND WALTER R. WILSON

Infections involving the heart valves (infectious endocarditis [IE]) and those that involve cardiovascular devices, including permanent pacemakers, implantable cardioverter-defibrillators (ICDs), coronary stents, and ventricular assist devices, are associated with substantial morbidity and mortality. As indications for devices continue to expand, infectious complications, including those that may require device removal, are becoming more commonplace. Because IE and other types of cardiovascular infections are often caused by multidrug-resistant (MDR) organisms acquired in the health care setting, there are fewer drugs are available for treating these infections and increased likelihood of drug-related toxicities. In addition, longer durations of therapy may be needed, which can increase the rate of drug-induced adverse events. These factors call for a multidisciplinary approach to cardiac infections.

INFECTIVE ENDOCARDITIS

IE has the proclivity to cause complications both at the cardiac valve site and at extracardiac locations that can predispose affected patients to serious morbidity and mortality. Management of IE therefore requires a team approach, which generally includes, at a minimum, specialists in infectious diseases, cardiovascular medicine, and cardiovascular surgery with particular expertise in IE. Thus every patient with IE should be managed in the inpatient setting of a medical center with experienced medical and surgical specialists to provide care, which often includes emergent diagnostic and surgical interventions. This "team" approach in IE management is warranted in medical centers that care for IE patients, and this approach of diagnosis and management has resulted in improved outcomes.

Epidemiology

The global burden of disease from IE is largely unknown. Much of the world's population lives in developing countries, where many people do not have routine access to advanced medical care, and usually no local or national infrastructure exists for disease reporting (see Chapter 2). Thus the clinical characterization of IE is biased, shaped by the collective experiences at large teaching facilities in countries where patient access is available and disease reporting is done. However, even in many developed countries, including the United States, IE is not included among the diagnoses requiring mandatory reporting to public health agencies that would define a statewide or national disease incidence or burden.

IE is a heterogeneous syndrome that is heavily influenced by the epidemiology of the infection. For example, in developing countries where rheumatic fever is still endemic, younger adults with longstanding rheumatic heart disease frequently present with a subacute clinical course spanning several weeks that involves left-sided native valve infection caused by viridans group streptococci (VGS). In contrast, in large, teaching, tertiary care centers in developed countries, patients with previous health care exposure frequently present with an acute illness that can be measured in days and is caused primarily by Staphylococcus aureus, with numerous anatomic sites of metastatic foci of infection and worse outcomes. Injection drug use (IDU) as a complication of the opioid epidemic currently active in the United States is another factor contributing to the escalating rate of IE due to S. aureus and has been prominent in rural settings. All types of care centers have provided care for these patients who are often seen in primary care settings initially with subsequent transfer to larger institutions with IE expertise.

The incidence of IE is influenced by multiple host factors that modify the risk of infection. Such factors include the underlying anatomic (usually valvular) cardiac conditions that result in turbulent blood flow and endothelial cell disruption (see later, Pathogenesis). In addition, aging of the population in developed countries has resulted in more patients with myxomatous degeneration of the mitral valve, with subsequent prolapse and insufficiency (see Chapter 76). At the same time, a dramatic fall in the incidence of rheumatic fever in developed countries has reduced the overall risk of IE in younger persons. Advances in medicine also alter the incidence of IE. For example, reduced use of tunneled catheters and increasing use of arteriovenous fistulas for chronic hemodialysis will reduce the risk of bloodstream infection and complicating IE. Improvement in oral health in developed countries also may affect the incidence of IE, but this notion remains to be proven.

Population-based studies[1,2] have been used to estimate both the incidence of IE and its clinical characterization, but complete case ascertainment is difficult to secure. For example, in the United States, patients may receive medical care in locations that are not in their place of residence. Thus large medical centers that have unique team expertise in IE management may be unable to obtain complete case ascertainment in a population because of changing referral patterns or second-party coverage. Data generated from a population-based investigation will have limited applicability (generalizability) if the cohort under study is not representative of other populations in demographic or clinical features.

Incidence studies of IE are limited in number and in geographic coverage of populations. Adjusted annual incidence rates reported among more recent surveys from Western Europe and Olmsted County, Minnesota, have varied and have ranged from approximately 3 to 14 cases per 100,000 persons annually.[3] Incidence trends have slowly increased in some countries with an expected increase due to increased IDU in the United States (see later). Historically, a sex predilection has been noted, with males more often affected by IE, and has been, in part, due to IDU, which more frequently is reported among men. This male predominance may be fading; an increasing prevalence of female IDU with IE has been noted in many rural areas in the United States in the current opioid epidemic.[4] In addition, the female incidence had increased with a high level of health care exposure cited as a predisposing condition for the development of IE in a recent analysis.[2] Health care exposure, including both nosocomial and non-nosocomial exposure, has been recognized only recently[2,5,6] as a major contributor to the development of IE. Not only do indwelling central venous catheters and hemodialysis predispose to bloodstream infection, but infection with antimicrobial resistant pathogens is more likely to occur as a consequence of health care–related exposure. The virulence of some of these pathogens, in particular methicillin-resistant S. aureus (MRSA), is notable and is associated with increased mortality in patients with IE.

As alluded to previously in this section, people who inject drugs (PWID) are a unique group at increased risk for IE and the current opioid epidemic has magnified the effect of IDU on IE in the United States. Surgery for drug use–associated IE increased 2.7-fold from 2011 to 2018, with higher rates observed in the East South Central and South Atlantic regions.[7] These patients tend to be young, male, and otherwise healthy, except for having hepatitis C virus infection, which is highly prevalent. The prevalence of human immunodeficiency virus (HIV) infection has been considerably less to date. The contact of these patients with the health care system often is limited to short stays in an emergency department (ED).

MICROBIOLOGY

A vast array of bacteria and fungi can cause IE,[8] as is evident in novel case reports and literature reviews of IE caused by unusual organisms. Although changes in the prevalence of pathogens causing IE have emerged in recent years because of critical changes in the epidemiology of IE in developed countries,[2,9] the overall distribution of infecting organisms has remained the same, with gram-positive cocci being predominant. These include streptococcal, staphylococcal, and enterococcal species. Important virulence factors unique to each genus group appear to be operative in infection pathogenesis (see later). It is therefore not surprising that the modified Duke criteria[10] listed only these three groups of pathogens as "typical microorganisms" in the designation of the major criterion of "blood culture positive" for IE (see later).

Streptococcal Species

Among streptococci, the VGS are the predominant organisms that cause IE. A "subacute" presentation is typical, with symptoms of infection present for weeks to a few months, with low-grade fever, night sweats, and fatigue being common. These organisms normally are found in the mouth of humans and tend to cause indolent infections. Sustained bacteremia due to this group of bacteria should prompt a consideration of the diagnosis of IE, as few other infection syndromes cause sustained bloodstream infection. The viridans group includes several evolving species of streptococci and currently includes *sanguis, oralis (mitis), salivarius, mutans, intermedius, anginosus,* and *constellatus.* The latter three species have been referred to the "*Streptococcus anginosus* or *S. milleri* group" and are unique in that they have a proclivity to produce abscess formation and metastatic infection foci, both within the heart and in extracardiac locations in IE patients.

The genera of *Gemella, Abiotrophia,* and *Granulicatella* have generally been included in discussions of VGS. For *Gemella,* one species designated as *morbillorum* was previously listed in the *Streptococcus* genus. These organisms can cause IE and exhibit metabolic characteristics similar to those previously referred to "nutritionally variant streptococci," and have been reassigned to *Abiotrophia* and *Granulicatella* genera. The recommended medical therapy for infections caused by these unique organisms is discussed later (see Antimicrobial Therapy).

The VGS constitute a predominant cause of native valve infection acquired in the community setting, in both developing and developed nations. A common substrate for infection from these organisms has been rheumatic valvular disease, but as mentioned, the incidence of acute rheumatic fever has fallen dramatically in developed countries.

Similar to other bacteria, VGS have developed resistance to some antibiotics. Fortunately, resistance to penicillin is seen in a small minority of IE isolates. Resistance is not based on beta-lactamase production, and the definitions used[8] to characterize strains as being "penicillin resistant" are not the same as the break points recommended by the Clinical and Laboratory Standards Institute (CLSI). This distinction can be confusing because selection of antibiotic therapy is based on in vitro susceptibility results.

In contrast to VGS, beta-hemolytic streptococci typically cause an acute presentation of IE. PWID and elderly persons are two at-risk groups. Complications are common and often involve valve destruction and extracardiac sites, frequently musculoskeletal, of infection. The prevalence of beta-hemolytic streptococci among cases of IE is less than 10%. Beta-hemolytic streptococci have remained uniquely susceptible to penicillin, with extremely rare exceptions. Nevertheless, it is prudent to obtain susceptibility testing on all IE-related isolates. Surgery is often required for management of severe valvular and perivalvular involvement (see later).

Streptococcus gallolyticus (formerly known as *S. bovis*) deserves particular attention. The organism usually is found in the gastrointestinal (GI) tract, and when recovered from blood culture, whether related to IE or not, an examination for an underlying GI lesion, including colon cancer, should be performed. Although it currently is the cause of less than 10% of cases of IE, the expectation is that it will become more prominent in aging populations and those with increasing restrictions on cancer prevention screening.

Historically, IE from *Streptococcus pneumoniae* has received considerable attention. Although it continues to be a common cause of community-acquired bloodstream infection that often is related to pneumonia, it is a rare cause of IE today. When *S. pneumoniae* does cause IE, the clinical presentation is usually acute and associated with valve destruction. It can be associated with meningitis as well as other intracranial complications. Invasive isolates of pneumococci tend to be penicillin susceptible, but susceptibility testing is required to confirm this notion. As with IE from beta-hemolytic streptococci, surgery often is required to address valve-related complications.

Staphylococcal Species

Staphylococci are gram-positive cocci that are well recognized as causes of IE. *S. aureus* is a common cause of both native and prosthetic valve endocarditis (PVE).[8,9] The presentation in cases caused by *S. aureus* is acute in onset and often associated with considerable systemic toxicity. In cases of left-sided heart infection, morbidity and mortality rates are high, despite appropriate therapy, including surgical intervention. Right-sided heart infection, predominantly of the tricuspid valve in PWID, has a much higher cure rate than that for left-sided heart infection, and mortality rates are low, unless bilateral infection is present. Unfortunately, the rate of IE from *S. aureus* is increasing, in part because of an increased exposure to health care and IDU. *S. aureus* predominates in both PWID and non–drug users with IE and accounted for 42.1% of IE related to drug use versus 24.3% of non–drug use IE cases who underwent valve surgery in one large series.[7] In addition, resistance to oxacillin and other antibiotics also has increased, which has made treatment more difficult.

Although coagulase-negative staphylococci are recognized as frequent pathogens of prosthetic valve infection, they also can infrequently cause native valve infection. Although these infections usually are subacute in presentation, the morbidity and mortality associated with IE caused by coagulase-negative staphylococci are considerable. Of the more than 30 species of coagulase-negative staphylococci, two deserve special attention. *Staphylococcus epidermidis* is the most commonly identified species to cause bacteremia and IE. *Staphylococcus lugdunensis* is another species that causes both native and PVE and tends to be more virulent than the other species of coagulase-negative staphylococci. Because this group of organisms is the most common cause of contaminated blood cultures, a delay in diagnosis can be due to misinterpretation of blood culture results. Multiple sets of blood culture specimens should therefore be collected to better distinguish contamination from bloodstream infection. Except for *S. lugdunensis*, which usually is penicillin susceptible, other species of coagulase-negative staphylococci are more drug resistant, and, accordingly, fewer treatment options exist.

Enterococcal Species

Age is strongly associated with the development of IE caused by enterococcal species, with the prevalence of these organisms in IE cases doubling among elderly persons compared with young adults.

The large majority of IE cases is by *Enterococcus faecalis* and is associated with genitourinary (GU) tract abnormalities. In the past, enterococcal IE was community acquired, and enterococci were well recognized as part of the normal gut flora in humans. More recently, enterococcal species associated with health care exposure and central venous catheter use have caused IE, and typically presents subacutely. MDR enterococcal species, in particular *Enterococcus faecium*, can cause IE that is difficult to cure; this includes infection caused by vancomycin-resistant strains collectively termed *vancomycin-resistant enterococci* (VRE).

HACEK Organisms

HACEK organisms are fastidious gram-negative bacilli comprising *Haemophilus* species (other than *H. influenzae*); *Aggregatibacter actinomycetemcomitans* (formerly *Actinobacillus actinomycetemcomitans*) and *Aggregatibacter aphrophilus* (formerly *Haemophilus aphrophilus*); *Cardiobacterium hominis; Eikenella corrodens;* and *Kingella kingae* and *Kingella denitrificans*. They colonize the oropharynx and upper respiratory tract, causing subacute IE presentation that is community acquired. Most of the organisms in blood cultures may require several days of incubation. Because of the indolent clinical course, diagnosis often is delayed, with the formation of large vegetations observed at echocardiography. As a result, embolism to the brain or other systemic sites occurs frequently.

Aerobic Gram-Negative Bacilli

In view of their universal causation of bloodstream infection, it is noteworthy that IE caused by aerobic gram-negative bacilli is rare. This observation attests to the particular virulence factors that characterize gram-positive cocci in IE pathogenesis and are not found in gram-negative bacilli. This group includes *Escherichia coli, Klebsiella* spp., *Enterobacter* spp., *Pseudomonas* spp., and others. In cases of IE caused by these organisms, presentations generally have been acute and sometimes associated with systemic toxicity, including sepsis and its complications. IE can be either community or health care associated. Outcomes of IE caused by aerobic gram-negative bacilli are characterized by increased morbidity and mortality rates.

Fungi

Fungi are extremely rare causes of IE. Identification of these organisms often is difficult because some do not grow in routine blood culture media. Even when selected culture media are used, fungal isolation may not be achieved. Thus fungi can cause either blood culture–positive or culture-negative IE.

The bulk of these infections are caused by *Candida* spp., although a broad array of fungi may cause IE. These infections usually are health care associated and involve prosthetic valves, often arising as a result of a central venous catheter infection. An indwelling right-heart catheter, such as a flotation catheter, can denude a valve and nonvalvular endothelial surface, predisposing the patient to fungal (or bacterial) right-sided IE. In addition, IDU is a well-recognized risk factor for fungal IE; in one multicenter investigation, fungal IE was twice as common in drug users (3.13%) as compared with that (1.5%) in non–drug users.[7]

Clinical presentations range in severity from acute to subacute. Complications are frequent, and surgical intervention is recommended as a routine intervention, particularly with infections caused by molds such as *Aspergillus* spp. Because relapsing IE is a concern and can be delayed in onset, many clinicians advocate the use of lifelong oral antifungal suppressive therapy, usually with an azole, after initial parenteral therapy is completed.

Culture-Negative Endocarditis

In most cases designated as blood culture–negative endocarditis, the pathogen is not recovered from blood cultures due to a patient's recent exposure to an antimicrobial that had suppressive or killing activity against the pathogen. In addition, with some uncommon causes of culture-negative endocarditis, the pathogen either will not grow in routine blood culture media or grows slowly in the media and is not detected in the time used for blood cultures. In the former scenario, nothing can be done. In the latter, blood cultures can be held for an extended period, at least 14 days, to determine if an isolate is recovered. Other techniques, such as special culture methods or serologic studies, also are used to isolate or identify infection. Organisms that should be included in this category include fungi, *Coxiella burnetii, Bartonella* spp., *Brucella* spp., *Tropheryma whippelii, Cutibacterium* (previously known as *Propionibacterium*) spp., and *Legionella* spp.

Pathogenesis

Two overarching aspects of endocarditis pathogenesis have been identified.[8] Already noted is a primary predilection for development of IE from an underlying valvular or nonvalvular cardiac structural abnormality that results in blood flow turbulence, endothelial disruption, and platelet and fibrin deposition. This lesion, termed *nonbacterial thrombotic endocarditis* (NBTE), serves as a nidus for subsequent adhesion by bacteria or fungi in the bloodstream. This pathway is thought to account for a majority of cases of IE, most often related to left-sided valvular stenosis or regurgitation. This picture of pathogenesis is mirrored, in many ways, in the animal model of endocarditis that has been used for decades to examine the pathogenesis, treatment, and prevention of IE. The microbiologic and histopathologic findings in infected animals reflect those seen in humans. A second factor is that infection may involve normal valves. Some reservations regarding this pathway of infection seem appropriate, because it is impossible to know if a valve is completely normal, including its endothelial surface, before onset of valve infection. In addition, animals do not develop experimental endocarditis after an intravascular challenge with a relatively large inoculum of virulent organisms, in particular *S. aureus*, in the absence of a previous disruption of the cardiac endothelial surface. Nevertheless, in vitro endothelial cell cultures studies have demonstrated uptake of organisms by endothelial cells.

The predominance of gram-positive cocci as causing IE deserves additional comment. Advances in molecular biologic techniques have resulted in the ability to define virulence factors that are unique to these organisms.[11] Infectivity studies that have compared "wild-type" parent strains to molecularly "engineered" strains using an experimental IE model have been of critical importance in defining virulence factors among strains of staphylococci, streptococci, and enterococci. Some of these factors serve as "adhesins" and are largely responsible for initial bacterial attachment to an NBTE nidus or to endothelial cells. They also are responsible for the attachment to medical devices, including prosthetic valves and cardiovascular implantable electronic device (CIED) leads. In this regard, biofilm formation occurs with some of these organisms and is important in both native tissue and prosthetic valve infections, in the context of factors responsible for the propagation of IE after initial bacterial attachment.

The findings from these investigations are expected to affect future treatment and prevention of IE. Novel vaccines containing bacterial proteins that function as adhesins and are good immunogens are being examined, for example, and already have proven to be efficacious in the prevention of experimental IE. In this case, the protein (FimA) is expressed by several VGS species in the pathogenesis of IE. In addition, it is conceivable that work focusing on treatment and prevention of dental caries by VGS could have some role in the management and prevention of IE.

Clinical Presentation
Predisposing Cardiac Conditions

Our understanding of predisposing conditions to IE has evolved over the decades since early clinical series were reported. More recently, the International Collaboration on Endocarditis–Prospective Cohort Study (ICE-PCS)[9] has detailed the clinical presentation in 2781 patients with definite IE. Native valve IE was predominant (72%), followed by PVE (21%) and permanent pacemaker or ICD IE (7%). Consistent with numerous earlier series, this international cohort study found that IE manifests with definite vegetations most frequently in the mitral valve position (41%), followed by the aortic valve position (38%), whereas the tricuspid (12%) and pulmonary (1%) valves were much less frequently involved.[9]

Preexisting valvular regurgitant lesions are much more prone to infection than stenotic lesions. It has been suggested that the incidence of IE is directly related to the impact of pressure on the closed valve, with shear stress disruption of the valvular endothelium in the vicinity of the egressing regurgitant jet. In the presence of the Venturi effect, circulating organisms are deposited within the high-velocity, lowered-pressure eddy zones of the regurgitant orifice of the receiving chamber, leading to the typical localization of vegetations on the upstream aspect of the infected valve.

Mitral regurgitation associated with degenerative mitral valve prolapse (MVP), particularly with advanced myxomatous leaflet thickening, is the most common predisposing condition for IE and is far more common than rheumatic mitral valve disease.[9] A recent population-based study demonstrated that an increased incidence of IE in patients with MVP was associated with either preexisting mitral regurgitation of at least moderate severity, or flail mitral leaflet.[12] Functional mitral regurgitation, associated with left ventricular (LV) remodeling causing malcoaptation of intrinsically normal mitral leaflets in a low-pressure, low-cardiac-output state (see Chapter 76), is quite uncommonly complicated by IE. The second most common native valve lesion predisposing to IE is aortic regurgitation. The risk of IE in patients with bicuspid aortic valve (BAV) is low (see Chapter 72), with an incidence of approximately 2% during follow-up periods ranging from 9 to 20 years.[13,14] BAV, however, is relatively common (16% to 43%) in case series of confirmed aortic valve IE,[15,16] is associated with a high incidence of periannular complications of IE (50% to 64%), and is a strong independent predictor of perivalvular extension of infection, where the infection extends beyond the valve annulus to involve adjacent cardiac structures.[15] In patients older than 65 years of age, non-rheumatic aortic stenosis is seen as the aortic valve lesion in IE at a rate almost three times that of younger patients (28% and 10%, respectively).[17] Structurally normal valves may also be affected in IE, with risk associations of advanced age, renal failure requiring hemodialysis, and infection caused by *S. aureus* or enterococci.[18]

Congenital heart disease (CHD) (see Chapter 82), other than BAV disease, is a predisposing condition to IE in approximately 5% to 12% of cases.[1,9,19] Unrepaired ventricular septal defects are the most frequent CHD lesions associated with IE, followed by ventricular outflow tract obstructive lesions, such as with tetralogy of Fallot.[20] Any highly turbulent shunt lesion can predispose affected patients to IE, as can the presence of prosthetic material used for palliative shunts, conduits, or shunt closures, particularly if a residual shunt is present after intervention. Low-velocity, low-turbulence shunt lesions, such as secundum atrial septal defect, are much less prone to endocardial disruption and are associated with a very low incidence of IE.[20]

Additional conditions contribute to the anatomic cardiac lesions in the predisposition to risk of IE. These include a history of previous IE, the presence of chronic intravenous (IV) access, IV drug abuse, and indwelling endocavitary devices. Predisposing general medical conditions include diabetes mellitus, underlying malignancy, renal failure requiring hemodialysis, and chronic immunosuppressive therapy.[9,19] A history of an invasive or dental procedure can be identified in approximately 25% of patients within 60 days of clinical presentation with IE.[9] A history of cardiac disease may be present in approximately 50% to 65% of patients.[21] Superimposed and of mounting concern is the increasing frequency of health care–associated IE. In a report from the ICE-PCS investigators,[22] 19% of the cases in a study cohort of 1622 patients with IE were considered to be nosocomial (defined as related to hospitalization for more than 2 days before presentation with IE). An additional 16% of cases were related to non-nosocomial health care (e.g., outpatient hemodialysis, IV chemotherapy, wound care, or residence in a long-term care facility) received within 30 days of onset of symptoms of IE.

A recent study demonstrated that a portal of pathogen entry responsible for IE could be identified in almost 75% of patients if a systematic search was pursued.[23] In this study, the most common entry site was cutaneous (40%), associated with health care delivery, such as vascular access or a surgical site, or sites used for IV drug abuse. The second most common (29%) portal of entry was oral/dental, with an active infection implicated much more frequently than a prior dental procedure. Thirdly, a GI source was detected in 23% of patients, in the majority with colonic neoplasm, or less commonly, ulcerative or inflammatory disease. Far less (<5%) frequently, a GU, otorhinolaryngottic, or respiratory portal of entry was detected.[23]

Symptoms

The presentation of IE encompasses a broad spectrum of symptoms and is influenced by multiple contributing factors (Figs. 80.1 and 80.2).

These factors would include (1) the virulence of the infecting organism and persistence of bacteremia, (2) extent of local tissue destruction of the involved valve(s) and hemodynamic sequelae, (3) perivalvular extension of infection, (4) septic embolization to any organ in the systemic arterial circulation or to the lungs, as in the case of right-sided IE, and (5) the consequences of circulating immune complexes and systemic immunopathologic factors.

The diverse potential symptoms associated with IE are listed in Table 80.1. The frequency of symptoms has been approximated from numerous clinical series in both the older and more contemporary literature. Fever (>38°C) is the most common presenting symptom, in up to 95% of patients, but may be absent in up to 20% of cases, particularly in elderly persons,[17] the immunocompromised, patients treated with previous empiric antibiotic therapy, or patients with CIED infections.[24,25] Fever defervescence usually occurs within 5 to 7 days of appropriate antibiotic therapy. Persistence of fever may indicate progressive infection with perivalvular extension such as abscess, septic embolization, an extracardiac site of infection (native or prosthetic), infected indwelling catheters or devices, inadequate antibiotic treatment of a resistant organism, or even an adverse reaction to the antibiotic therapy itself.

Other nonspecific constitutional symptoms of infection, such as chills, sweats, cough, headache, malaise, nausea, myalgias, and arthralgias, are less common accompanying symptoms and may be noted in approximately 20% to 40% of patients. In more protracted subacute cases of IE, symptoms and signs such as anorexia, weight loss, weakness, arthralgias, and abdominal pain may also occur in 5% to 30% of patients, misleading the clinician to pursue incorrect diagnoses such as malignancy, connective tissue disease, or other chronic infection or systemic inflammatory disorders.

Dyspnea is important to recognize because they may indicate a severe hemodynamic lesion, usually left-sided valvular regurgitation. Associated symptoms of orthopnea and paroxysmal nocturnal dyspnea herald the onset of heart failure (HF). Early recognition of HF symptoms is imperative because it is the most common complication of IE, has the greatest impact on prognosis, is the most frequent indication for surgical intervention, and is the most important predictor of poor outcome with surgical therapy for IE.[26] HF complicates the course of approximately 30% to 50% of patients with IE,[9,19,27,28] and even with early surgical intervention, still doubles in-hospital mortality to almost 25%.[28]

A variety of chest pain syndromes can accompany IE. Pleuritic chest pain may result from septic pulmonary embolization and infarction complicating tricuspid IE. Much less common is angina pectoris related to embolization of vegetation fragments into the coronary circulation, which complicates IE in approximately 1% of the cases. Musculoskeletal chest symptoms related to systemic infection or superimposed infectious pneumonitis also would be in the differential diagnosis.

Physical Examination (see Chapter 13)

Potential findings on physical examination are delineated in Table 80.2. These data are approximated from both older and more recently reported clinical series.[9,19,22,26–28] A definite murmur is audible in at least 80% of patients on presentation, particularly with left-sided IE. In the large ICE-PCS collaboration, the murmur was new in almost 50% of the patients.[9] The same cohort study found that worsening of a preexisting murmur occurred in 20% of cases. The presence of a new heart murmur also is noted more frequently in patients with IE complicated by HF,[26] and an S_3 gallop and pulmonary rales would further substantiate this diagnosis. Murmurs are detected in less than half of patients with IE complicating an implanted cardiac device[24] and are infrequently heard in patients with right-sided IE. Heart murmurs associated with acute IE complicated by extensive left-sided valvular destruction with acute, severe regurgitation may also be deceptively unimpressive because of rapid equalization of pressures between the chambers that diminishes the substrate for turbulent flow. Precipitous HF, pulmonary edema, and cardiogenic shock are most often associated with severe acute aortic regurgitation associated with IE, less so by severe acute mitral regurgitation. Severe tricuspid regurgitation, even as an acute complication of IE, is much better tolerated.

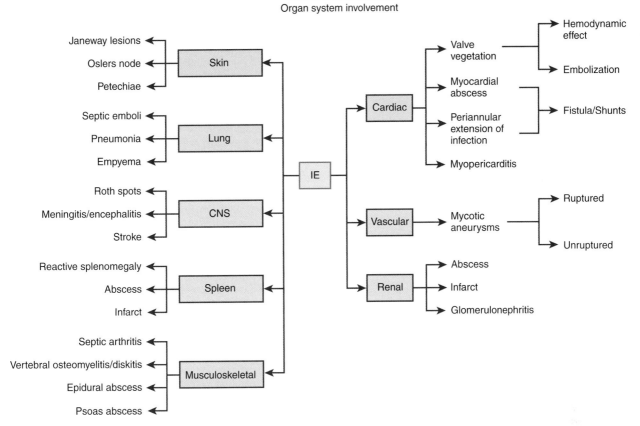

FIGURE 80.1 Clinical manifestations of organ system involvement due to infective endocarditis.

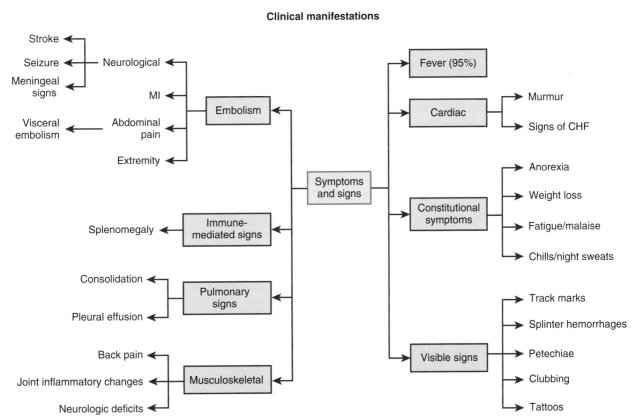

FIGURE 80.2 Signs and symptoms of infective endocarditis and its complications.

TABLE 80.1 Symptoms in Infective Endocarditis

SYMPTOM	PATIENTS AFFECTED (%)
Fever	80–95
Chills	40–70
Weakness	40–50
Malaise	20–40
Sweats	20–40
Anorexia	20–40
Headache	20–40
Dyspnea	20–40
Cough	20–30
Weight loss	20–30
Myalgia/arthralgia	10–30
Stroke	10–20
Confusion/delirium	10–20
Nausea/vomiting	10–20
Edema	5–15
Chest pain	5–15
Abdominal pain	5–15
Hemoptysis	5–10
Back pain	5–10

TABLE 80.2 Physical Findings in Infective Endocarditis

FINDING	PATIENTS AFFECTED (%)
Fever	80–90
Heart murmur	75–85
New murmur	10–50
Changing murmur	5–20
Central neurologic abnormality	20–40
Splenomegaly	10–40
Petechiae/conjunctival hemorrhage	10–40
Splinter hemorrhages	5–15
Janeway lesions	5–10
Osler nodes	3–10
Retinal lesion or Roth spot	2–10

A central neurologic abnormality can often be identified, and focal deficits consistent with stroke may be detected in 10% to 20% of patients (see Chapter 45).[9,26] In subacute, indolent IE, an acute stroke typically is the event that prompts the patient to seek medical attention. Most frequently, the stroke is cardioembolic in nature but may infrequently result from complications of intracranial cerebrovascular mycotic aneurysm, such as hemorrhagic rupture. Seizures, visual deficits, cranial nerve deficits, subarachnoid hemorrhage, and toxic encephalopathy are other potential neurologic complications of IE. The development of neurologic deterioration during the course of IE is associated with significantly increased mortality.

Abdominal examination may elicit nonspecific findings of tenderness and discomfort, particularly in the left upper quadrant, suggestive of splenic embolization and infarction, particularly if complicated by splenic abscess. The spleen is a common site of septic embolization. This most often is not identified by localized symptoms or findings but is discovered incidentally on computed tomography (CT) or using other imaging techniques. Splenomegaly usually is seen in subacute IE and is reported in approximately 10% of patients in more recent clinical series in which the diagnosis is established earlier in the course of the disease.[9,19,22]

As a result of advances leading to earlier diagnosis and therapy, the classic peripheral manifestations of IE are now infrequently observed. Petechiae are the most common, occurring on the conjunctivae, oral mucosa, or extremities. Janeway lesions are painless hemorrhagic macules with a predilection for the soles or palms and are sequelae of peripheral septic embolization, most often associated with staphylococcal IE. Splinter subungual hemorrhages also are painless, dark-red linear lesions in the proximal nailbed and may coalesce. Brown distal splinter lesions at the tips of the nails are quite common in patients who perform manual labor and are caused by trauma, not infection. *Osler nodes* are painful, erythematous, nodular lesions usually located in the pads of the fingers and toes and are the result of immune complex deposition and focal vasculitis. *Roth spots* are retinal hemorrhages with a pale center of coagulated fibrin and also are related to immune complex–mediated vasculitis secondary to IE. An immune complex–mediated diffuse glomerulonephritis rarely may be associated with these findings. Both Osler nodes and Roth spots can be observed with other disorders, such as systemic lupus erythematosus (SLE), leukemia, and nonbacterial endocarditis. Aside from petechiae and conjunctival hemorrhage, these peripheral findings were detected in less than 10% of patients in the recent ICE-PCS cohort.[9] A recent multicenter prospective cohort study of 1804 patients with IE confirmed similar results as pertains to the spectrum of clinical presentations and physical examination findings.[29]

Diagnosis

The protean clinical presentations and manifestations of IE encompass a broad differential diagnosis in the patient presenting with fever without a readily apparent cause. Other primary cardiac diagnoses that may potentially mimic IE include acute rheumatic fever, left atrial (LA) myxoma, antiphospholipid antibody syndrome, and nonbacterial thrombotic or marantic endocarditis. A number of connective tissue disorders, including SLE, reactive arthritis, polymyalgia rheumatica, and vasculitides, may be additional diagnostic considerations in select patients, as well as many other serious syndromes of infectious disease. The index of suspicion for IE incrementally increases in the presence of predisposing cardiac conditions, new or changing murmurs, bloodstream infection, clinical evidence of embolic phenomena, and evolving HF or certain other hemodynamic abnormalities.

In 1994, Durack and associates proposed diagnostic criteria, subsequently known as the Duke criteria, to establish the diagnosis of definite or possible IE, and also to reject the diagnosis of IE. These criteria incorporated direct histopathologic evidence of IE or major clinical criteria, namely, blood culture positivity and evidence of endocardial involvement, supplemented by minor clinical criteria, for the definite diagnosis of IE. Thereafter, multiple clinical series using the Duke criteria in the diagnosis of IE reported the sensitivity to be in the range of 80%, with both specificity and negative predictive value (NPV) exceeding 90%.[8,26] Recognizing the increasing impact of *S. aureus* IE, the potential for IE associated with *C. burnetii* infection, and the evolving role of transesophageal echocardiography (TEE) in the diagnosis of IE, Li and colleagues[10] proposed the modified Duke criteria (Table 80.3). *Major clinical criteria* include (1) blood culture positivity for bacteria typically associated with IE, or persistently positive cultures for organisms uncommonly associated with IE, or a blood culture or serology clearly positive for *C. burnetii* and (2) evidence of endocardial involvement by echocardiography demonstrating vegetation, significantly new valvular regurgitation, dehiscence of a prosthetic valve, or findings consistent with perivalvular extension of infection, such as abscess. *Minor clinical criteria* include (1) predisposing cardiac conditions or IV drug use; (2) persistent fever with temperatures greater than 38°C without an alternative explanation; (3) vascular phenomena such as systemic or pulmonary embolism, mycotic aneurysm, or intracranial or cutaneous hemorrhagic lesions; (4) immunologic phenomena such as Osler nodes, Roth spots, or glomerulonephritis; and (5) positive blood culture status not meeting major criteria or serologic evidence of active infection with an organism that could be associated with IE. By this diagnostic classification, a *definite* clinical diagnosis of IE is established in the presence of (a) two major criteria or (b) one

TABLE 80.3 Definition of Infective Endocarditis: Modified Duke Criteria

Definite Infective Endocarditis

Pathologic Criteria

- Microorganisms demonstrated by results of cultures or histologic examination of a vegetation, a vegetation that has embolized, or an intracardiac abscess specimen; or
- Pathologic lesions; vegetation, or intracardiac abscess confirmed by results of histologic examination showing active endocarditis

Clinical Criteria

- 2 major criteria, or
- 1 major criterion and 3 minor criteria, or
- 5 minor criteria

Possible Infective Endocarditis

- 1 major criterion and 1 minor criterion, or
- 3 minor criteria

Rejected Diagnosis of Infective Endocarditis

- Firm alternate diagnosis explaining evidence of suspected IE, or
- Resolution of IE syndrome with antibiotic therapy for ≤4 days, or
- No evidence of IE at surgery or autopsy, on antibiotic therapy for ≤4 days, or
- Does not meet criteria for possible IE

Definition of Terms Used in the Modified Duke Criteria for Diagnosis of Infective Endocarditis

Major Criteria

Blood culture findings positive for IE
  Typical microorganisms consistent with IE from two separate blood cultures:
  - *Viridans streptococci, Streptococcus gallolyticus* (formerly known as *S. bovis*), *Staphylococcus aureus,* HACEK group, or
  - Community-acquired enterococci, in the absence of a primary focus, or
  Microorganisms consistent with IE from persistently positive blood culture findings, defined as:
  - ≥2 positive culture findings of blood samples drawn >12 hr apart, or
  - 3 or most of ≥4 separate culture findings of blood (with first and last sample drawn ≥1 hr apart)
  - Single positive blood culture for *Coxiella burnetii* or anti–phase I IgG titer ≥1:800

Evidence of endocardial involvement
  Echocardiographic findings positive for IE (TEE recommended in patients with prosthetic valves, rated at least possible IE by clinical criteria or complicated IE [paravalvular abscess]; TTE as first test in other patients), defined as follows:
  - Oscillating intracardiac mass on valve or supporting structures, in the path of regurgitant jets, or on implanted material in the absence of an alternative anatomic explanation, or
  - Abscess, or
  - New partial dehiscence of prosthetic valve
  New valvular regurgitation; worsening or changing of preexisting murmur not sufficient

Minor Criteria

- Predisposition, predisposing heart condition, or intravenous drug use
- Fever—temperature >38°C
- Vascular phenomena, major arterial emboli, septic pulmonary infarcts, mycotic aneurysm, intracranial hemorrhage, conjunctival hemorrhages, and Janeway lesions
- Immunologic phenomena: glomerulonephritis, Osler nodes, Roth spots, and rheumatoid factor
- Microbiologic evidence: positive blood culture finding but does not meet a major criterion as noted above (excludes single positive culture findings for coagulase-negative staphylococci and organisms that do not cause endocarditis) or serologic evidence of active infection with organism consistent with IE

HACEK, Haemophilus spp., other than *H. influenzae; Aggregatibacter actinomycetemcomitans* [formerly *Actinobacillus actinomycetemcomitans*], *Aggregatibacter aphrophilus* [formerly *Haemophilus aphrophilus*]; *Cardiobacterium hominis; Eikenella corrodens; Kingella kingae* and *Kingella denitrificans; IE,* infective endocarditis; *TEE,* transesophageal echocardiography; *TTE,* transthoracic echocardiography.
Modified from Li JS, Sexton DJ, Mick N, et al. Proposed modifications to the Duke criteria for the diagnosis of infective endocarditis. *Clin Infect Dis.* 2000;30:633.

major and three minor criteria, or (c) five minor criteria. A *possible* clinical diagnosis of IE is appropriate in the presence of (a) one major and one minor criterion or (b) three minor criteria. The diagnosis of IE is *rejected* if clinical evaluation (a) does not meet criteria for possible IE or (b) reveals complete resolution of a suspected IE syndrome or absence of anatomic evidence for IE on a course of antibiotic therapy for 4 days or less, or if (c) an alternative diagnosis explaining the initial presentation is confirmed.

Since their publication in 2000, the modified Duke criteria have been validated in subsequent investigations of diagnostic accuracy (confirmed to be high) and also clinical and epidemiologic utility and have been endorsed by guideline documents pertinent to the evaluation and management of the patient with IE.[8,26] In view of the vast heterogeneity of clinical presentations of IE, the modified Duke criteria must always be used in combination with circumspect clinical judgment.

Diagnostic Testing

MICROBIOLOGY

The microbiology and epidemiology of pathogens that cause IE are detailed earlier in this chapter. As determined from data summarized from contemporary cohort series,[9,22,30–33] organisms identified in patients with IE in a variety of clinical settings are listed in Table 80.4. In community-acquired IE, VGS remain the most frequently isolated organism, followed closely by *S. aureus*, which is the predominant organism implicated in health care–associated IE, accounting for more than 40% of cases both in and out of the hospital environment. A defined portal of entry, such as an intravascular catheter or tissue disruption from a recent surgical or dental procedure, can be implicated in 25% to 67% of such cases.[19,22,30] MRSA IE is much more common in health care–associated than in community-acquired IE (47% versus 12%, respectively).[22] In IE associated with IV drug abuse, *S. aureus* accounts for almost 70% of cases.[9]

In patients with prosthetic valves (see Chapter 79), early PVE has been defined as occurring as early as 60 days or less[31] up to 1 year[26,32,33] after surgery. *S. aureus* also is the leading pathogen in early PVE, accounting for approximately 35% of cases, of which approximately one-fourth are MRSA,[31] followed closely by coagulase-negative staphylococci. Streptococcal early PVE is unusual. Late PVE is caused less often by staphylococci, which nevertheless are still the most common infecting organism, and a higher occurrence of infections with both VGS and *S. gallolyticus* (formerly *S. bovis*) has been documented. As with community-acquired native valve IE, enterococcal infections account for approximately 10% of cases of both early and late PVE.

Negative blood culture results are observed in approximately 5% to 15% of the cases for both native and prosthetic valve IE. In the large ICE-PCS, 62% of patients with culture-negative IE had received antibiotic therapy within 7 days of obtaining the initial blood culture.[9] Other reasons for blood culture negativity would include IE caused by fastidious organisms or unusual pathogens such as *Bartonella* or *Legionella* spp., *C. burnetii*, or fungi, as stated earlier Rapid detection of pathogens associated with IE by polymerase chain reaction (PCR) techniques may become a reliable alternative to standard blood culture techniques in such cases.[34]

OTHER BLOOD TESTING

The complete blood count often is abnormal in IE. In patients with subacute IE, a normochromic normocytic anemia of variable severity is detected in a majority of patients, often with low serum iron and total iron-binding capacity. Even with the systemic infection of IE, a leukocytosis with a left differential shift may be detected in only 50% to 60% of patients[32] and is more common with acute than with subacute IE. Leukopenia also may infrequently occur with subacute IE and usually is associated with splenomegaly. Thrombocytopenia may occur in approximately 10% of patients and has been found to be a predictor of early adverse outcome in IE. Sy and colleagues[35] reported a hazard ratio (HR) of approximately 1.13 for each 20×10^9/L decrement in the platelet count as a multivariate predictor of mortality from days 1 to 15 after presentation with IE.[35]

The erythrocyte sedimentation rate (ESR) usually is elevated in patients with IE, and in ICE-PCS, was elevated in 61% of patients. This large cohort study found that an elevated ESR was independently associated with a decreased risk of in-hospital death, presumably because of an association with subacute IE with a more indolent course.[9] The same study found that the C-reactive protein (CRP) also was elevated in approximately 60% of patients, whereas the rheumatoid factor concentration was abnormal in 5%[9]—the latter usually a feature of protracted subacute IE, not acute IE. Inclusion of ESR and CRP in the minor

modified Duke criteria for the diagnosis of IE has been proposed but is not endorsed by current guideline recommedations.[8]

Procalcitonin (PCT) is another protein that rises in response to a proinflammatory stimulus, particularly with severe bacterial infection. A meta-analysis of six studies, including 1006 patients with suspected IE, found PCT to be only 64% sensitive and 73% specific for the diagnosis of IE, and was less accurate than CRP.[36] PCT and other bacteremia-activated markers, such as cellular and vascular adhesion molecules, are currently not recommended as routine biomarkers for the diagnosis of IE.[37]

A new elevation in serum creatinine occurs in 10% to 30% of patients with IE[26] and may be related to multifactorial reasons including renal hypoperfusion from severe sepsis or HF, embolic renal infarction, immune complex–mediated glomerulonephritis, and toxicity from either antibiotic therapy or contrast agents used for imaging. Renal dysfunction developing within the first 8 days of presentation is independently predictive of early IE mortality, with HR of 1.13 per incremental increase in serum creatinine of 0.23 mg/dL,[35] and persistent serum creatinine elevation to greater than 2 mg/dL is predictive of 2-year mortality.[29] Urinalysis usually demonstrates hematuria and proteinuria. In cases of immune complex glomerulonephritis, red blood cell casts are evident, associated with depressed serum complement levels.

Limited studies conducted with small numbers of patients have assessed the prognostic value of cardiac biomarkers in IE. The cardiac troponins may be elevated from ventricular wall stress in HF, myocardial injury with myocardial abscess or embolic infarction, or septicemia alone. An increase in troponin I level to greater than 0.4 ng/mL significantly increases the risk of in-hospital mortality and need for early valve replacement.[38] A subset analysis of ICE-PCS demonstrated that in patients with IE, a troponin T level of 0.08 ng/mL or higher was associated with increased risk of cardiac abscess, central nervous system (CNS) events, and death IE.[39] An elevation of the B-type natriuretic peptide (BNP) level to 400 pg/mL or higher also has been associated with a fourfold risk of the same three complications of IE, even with exclusion of patients with LV dysfunction or severe left-sided valve regurgitation.[40] In another study, elevation of the NT-proBNP level to 1500 pg/mL or higher at hospital admission was an independent predictor of need for surgical intervention or death within 30 days.[41]

Electrocardiogram

The 12-lead electrocardiogram (ECG) usually demonstrates nonspecific findings in patients with uncomplicated IE (Fig. 80.3). Because of the close proximity of the atrioventricular node and proximal intraventricular conduction system to the aortic valve and root, perivalvular extension of infection from this location is the most common cause of new atrioventricular block (AVB) of any degree or bundle branch block (BBB). With perivalvular extension of infection, the incidence of AVB ranges from 10% to 20%, whereas new BBB occurs in approximately 3%.[22,32] The occurrence of a new conduction abnormality also is a multivariate risk predictor for death associated with IE.[22] In a

TABLE 80.4 **Microbiology of Infective Endocarditis**

ORGANISM	COMMUNITY-ACQUIRED IE (%) (n = 1201)[23,30]	NATIVE VALVE HEALTH CARE–ASSOCIATED IE (%) NOSOCOMIAL (%) (n = 370)[22,53]	NON-NOSOCOMIAL (%) (n = 254)[22]	INTRAVENOUS DRUG USERS WITH IE (%) (n = 237)[9]	PROSTHETIC VALVE EARLY IE (%) (n = 140)[31,33]	LATE IE (%) (n = 390)[31,33]
Staphylococcus aureus	21	45	42	68	34	19
Coagulase-negative staphylococci	6	12	15	3	28	20
Enterococcus species	10	14	16	5	10	13
Viridans group streptococci	26	10	6	10	1	11
Streptococcus gallolyticus*	10	3	3	1	1	7
HACEK	3	0	0	0	0	2
Fungi	0	2	2	1	6	3
Other	13	7	10	7	6	15
Negative blood culture	11	7	6	5	14	10

*Formerly *Streptococcus bovis*.

HACEK, *Haemophilus* spp., other than *H. influenzae*; *Aggregatibacter actinomycetemcomitans* [formerly *Actinobacillus actinomycetemcomitans*], *Aggregatibacter aphrophilus* [formerly *Haemophilus aphrophilus*]; *Cardiobacterium hominis*; *Eikenella corrodens*; *Kingella kingae* and *Kingella denitrificans*; *IE*, infective endocarditis.

minority of patients, perivalvular extension complicating aortic valve IE may compromise proximal coronary artery patency, or emboli from aortic valve vegetations may cause damage, resulting in ischemic ECG changes or even ST-segment elevation acute coronary syndromes.[26] Ischemic ECG changes may also manifest secondary to hemodynamic sequelae resulting in coronary arterial demand supply mismatch. Other atrial and ventricular arrhythmias may potentially complicate structural or hemodynamic complications of IE, especially in the context of underlying LV dysfunction. In a recent investigation that included 507 patients with left-sided native valve IE, new-onset atrial fibrillation was independently associated with HF and in-hospital mortality.[42]

Imaging
Imaging for Diagnosis of Infective Endocarditis
A major clinical criterion for the diagnosis of IE based on the modified Duke criteria is the demonstration of endocardial involvement with vegetations, perivalvular extension of infection, or evidence of disruption of the integrity of either native or prosthetic valves (see Table 80.3). Echocardiography has been and remains the cornerstone of diagnostic imaging in the context of infective endocarditis (see Chapter 16) (see Fig. 80.3). Using early-generation imaging systems, initial studies reported a sensitivity of transthoracic echocardiography (TTE) as 40% to 60% for the detection of native valvular vegetations, and substantially less for prosthetic valve vegetations.[43] With evolving advances in harmonic imaging and numerous other techniques to improve spatial image resolution, sensitivity of current TTE imaging techniques for detection of native valve IE recently has been 82% and as high as 89%

if high-quality TTE images are available (Fig. 80.4; see also Fig. 16.74A).[44] The specificity for TTE in the diagnosis of IE has been reported as 70% to 90%.[28,43–45] The absence of regurgitant lesions of the mitral or aortic valves makes endocarditic involvement of these valves less likely.

TEE circumvents multiple potential impediments to TTE imaging, such as body habitus, pulmonary disease, and other sources of acoustic interference between the chest wall and heart. Owing to much closer proximity of the transducer to the heart, TEE is performed with higher-frequency imaging, greatly enhancing spatial resolution (Fig. 80.5; see also Fig. 16.74B). With numerous imaging projections available, multi-plane two-dimensional and three-dimensional TEE can characterize vegetations with a resolution size of approaching 2 to 3 mm, with a sensitivity in the range of 90% to 100% and specificity exceeding 90%.[43–46] PVE, characterized by a lower incidence of valvular vegetations (60% to 70%) and higher incidence of periannular infection and associated complications (30% to 50%), is difficult to detect with TTE, generally with a sensitivity of less than 50%.[26] Valvular vegetations have been more frequently identified with IE involving transcatheter-implanted aortic bioprostheses (see Chapter 74), with perivalvular complications less common than for surgically implanted prostheses.[47,48] With sensitivity reported in the range of 80% to 95% and specificity greater than 90%,[28,49] TEE clearly is the imaging procedure of choice for the evaluation of suspected PVE (Figs. 80.6 and 80.7).

In general, TTE is more readily available, entirely noninvasive, and provides a complete cardiovascular hemodynamic profile. Furthermore, TTE may perform similarly to TEE in evaluating anterior structures of the heart, including the tricuspid valve and right ventricular

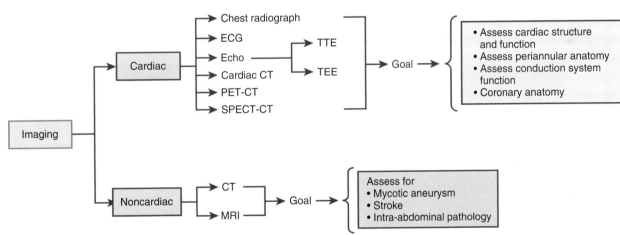

Investigations and diagnosis

FIGURE 80.3 Imaging techniques in the diagnosis and management of infective endocarditis and its complications.

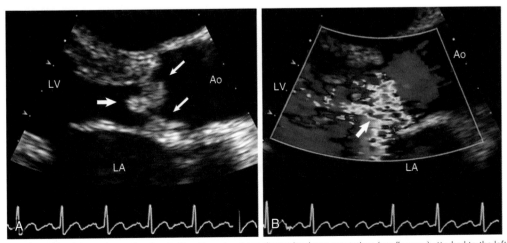

FIGURE 80.4 Infective endocarditis of the native aortic valve. **A,** Transthoracic echocardiography shows vegetations (*small arrows*) attached to the left ventricular aspects of the valve cusps and prolapsing into the left ventricular outflow tract (*large arrow*) during diastole. **B,** Severe aortic regurgitation (*arrow*) is shown by color Doppler. *Ao,* Ascending aorta; *LA,* left atrium; *LV,* left ventricle.

DISEASES OF THE HEART VALVES

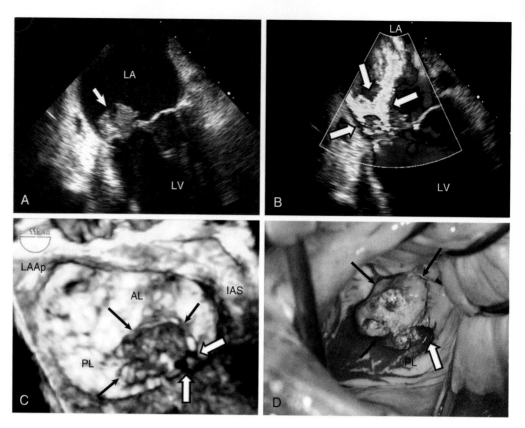

FIGURE 80.5 Infective endocarditis involving the mitral valve. **A,** Transesophageal echocardiography (TEE) image shows a large vegetation (*arrow*) attached to the atrial aspect of the posterior leaflet. **B,** Color Doppler image demonstrates a complex jet of mitral regurgitation (*arrows*) coursing through the body of the posterior mitral leaflet and vegetative mass, consistent with leaflet perforation. **C,** Three-dimensional TEE image of the mitral valve, as viewed from the left atrium (*LA*). Large vegetations (*black arrows*) are attached to the medial aspect of the posterior leaflet (*PL*), with perforation (*white arrows*) at the margin of the posteromedial commissure. **D,** Intraoperative visualization of the mitral valve as viewed from the left atriotomy. The large vegetative mass (*black arrows*) is attached to the posterior leaflet, and the posteromedial perforation (*white arrow*) is confirmed. *AL,* Anterior leaflet; *IAS,* interatrial septum; *LAAp,* left atrial appendage; *LV,* left ventricle.

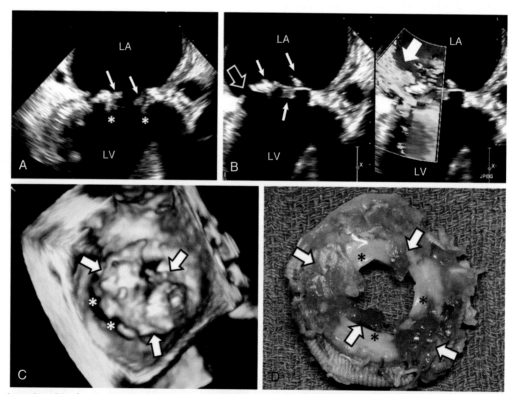

FIGURE 80.6 Infective endocarditis of a mitral bioprosthesis. **A,** On transesophageal echocardiography (TEE), multiple vegetations (*arrows*) can be seen within the inflow orifice of the bioprosthesis (*) during diastole. **B, Left,** During systole, a zone of inferolateral periannular prosthetic dehiscence (*large open arrow*) is evident with rocking motion of the prosthesis. Vegetations are present on the closed bioprosthetic leaflets and prosthetic annulus (*small arrows*). **Right,** Color Doppler image shows severe, eccentric periprosthetic mitral regurgitation (*large white arrow*) emanating from the zone of periannular dehiscence. *LA,* Left atrium; *LV,* left ventricle. **C,** Three-dimensional TEE view from the left atrium shows an extensive mass of vegetations encompassing the periannular margins (*arrows*), which was not fully appreciated by two-dimensional imaging. A large crescentic zone of periannular dehiscence (*) is well visualized. **D,** The surgically excised mitral bioprosthesis shows extensive vegetations (*arrows*) attached to the atrial aspects of the prosthesis. Pannus ingrowth (*) into the prosthetic orifice also is present.

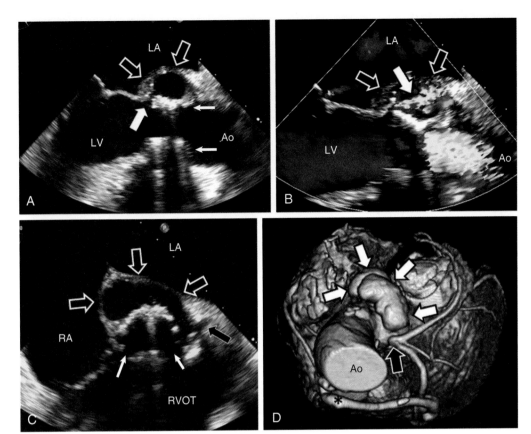

FIGURE 80.7 Periannular extension of infection complicating mechanical aortic prosthetic valve endocarditis. **A,** Transesophageal echocardiography (TEE) image shows a large, mycotic false aneurysm (*open arrows*) within the mitral-aortic intervalvular fibrosa adjacent to the prosthesis (*small arrows*). Communication with the left ventricular outflow tract is evident (*large white arrow*). **B,** Color Doppler image demonstrates flow communication (*arrow*) into the mycotic false aneurysm (*open arrows*) during systole, at which time the larger, color flow signal exits the aortic prosthesis into the ascending aorta (*Ao*). **C,** Short-axis TEE imaging of the mechanical aortic prosthesis (*small arrows*) indicates that the large mycotic false aneurysm (*large open arrows*) extends posteriorly adjacent to the left atrium (*LA*), bulges toward the right atrium (*RA*), and extends to the left main coronary artery (*black arrow*). **D,** Computed tomography with three-dimensional reconstruction, viewed from above and tilted anteriorly to show the posterior aortic root, shows the large posterolateral mycotic false aneurysm (*white arrows*) extending from the aortic root and encroaching upon the left main coronary artery (*black arrow*). A saphenous vein bypass graft (*) to the left anterior descending coronary artery also is seen. *LV,* Left ventricle; *RVOT,* right ventricular outflow tract.

outflow tract. In a study of IV drug users with suspected right-sided endocarditis, TTE performed as well as TEE in the detection of vegetations.[50] Because TTE and TEE provide complementary information, the most recent American Heart Association (AHA) guidelines[8] recommend both TTE and TEE be obtained in cases of suspected IE (Fig. 80.8). Variably mobile echodensities may be observed with echocardiography, particularly TEE. A differential diagnosis would include degenerative changes in a native valve, such as Lambl excrescences, endocardial fenestrations, ruptured or retracted chordae, and even acoustic artifacts reflected by calcified tissue. Valvular thickening, myxomatous changes, and sclerotic lesions move in concert with leaflet or cusp motion, without independent mobility of a vegetation, but may be difficult to discern from sessile vegetations. Filamentous valvular strands may be seen on both native and prosthetic valves. Thrombus associated with prosthetic valves may or may not be infected. Valvular neoplasms, such as papillary fibroelastoma or rarely myxomas, also are included in the differential. Vegetations of IE typically are located on the upstream, lower-pressure side of the regurgitant valve, have soft tissue echocardiographic density (particularly early in the course of infection) and often are multiple and lobulated, with motion independent of the valve structure. Hyperrefractile, discretely nodular, or filamentous echodensities located on the downstream side of the valve are much less likely to represent vegetations associated with IE.

In addition to confirming the diagnosis of IE, echocardiography provides important information regarding complications of IE that indicate the potential need for surgery (Table 80.5). In patients with suspect IE of a mechanical prosthetic valve, particularly in the mitral position, TEE is the diagnostic test of choice because of shadowing that could obscure standard TTE imaging. Cardiac CT can also be used to assess vegetations (see later) (see Fig. 80.3).

Imaging for Delineation of Complications of Endocarditis

LOCAL VALVULAR DESTRUCTION. Caused most frequently by left-sided valvular regurgitant lesions, HF may complicate the course of approximately 30% to 40% of patients with IE, is three times more common in native than in prosthetic valve IE, and is the primary

indication for early surgery in at least 50% to 60% of these patients.[26,28,50] New York Heart Association (NYHA) Functional Class III or IV HF complicating IE has the greatest impact on both medical and surgical prognosis, with reported in-hospital mortality rates in the range of 55% and 25%, respectively, in ICE-PCS.[50] HF most frequently is associated with aortic valve IE (30%), followed by mitral valve (20%) and tricuspid valve (<10%).[8]

New, moderate to severe valvular regurgitation may be detected by TEE in up to 70% of patients presenting with IE.[19] On imaging with TTE, and particularly with TEE, mechanisms contributing to valvular regurgitation include perforation, prolapse, and flail of the involved cusp or leaflet. Native valve perforations develop in 10% to 30% of patients with IE.[15,19,27,51] Even with TEE, which is much more sensitive than TTE (90% vs. 45%), perforations can be difficult to visualize using two-dimensional imaging alone. Three-dimensional TEE imaging can significantly enhance detection of valvular perforations complicating IE (see Fig. 80.5).[46] Color Doppler imaging can readily identify a perforation, with color flow convergence entraining into the perforation from the exiting chamber and a regurgitant jet traversing through the body of a cusp or leaflet. Saccular mycotic aneurysms, most often present on the atrial aspect of the mitral valve, may rupture, leaving a large defect in the leaflet. Extensive vegetations may also impede valvular coaptation, leading to regurgitation, or rarely may cause stenosis.

Infectious destruction of left-sided native valvular cusp or leaflet integrity and disruption of the valvular support apparatus can lead to acute severe valvular regurgitation complicated by precipitous HF, pulmonary edema, and hemodynamic instability (see Chapters 73 and 76). In addition to identifying the mechanism(s) of regurgitation, echocardiographic imaging typically demonstrates normal LV size and ejection fraction (EF). In acute severe aortic regurgitation, Doppler assessment will demonstrate evidence of rapid elevation of LV diastolic filling pressures with very short aortic regurgitant pressure half-times and a restrictive pattern of mitral inflow. Such hemodynamics are associated with premature closure of the mitral valve before the onset of systole. In acute severe mitral regurgitation, truncation of the usual parabolic continuous-wave Doppler regurgitant signal indicates

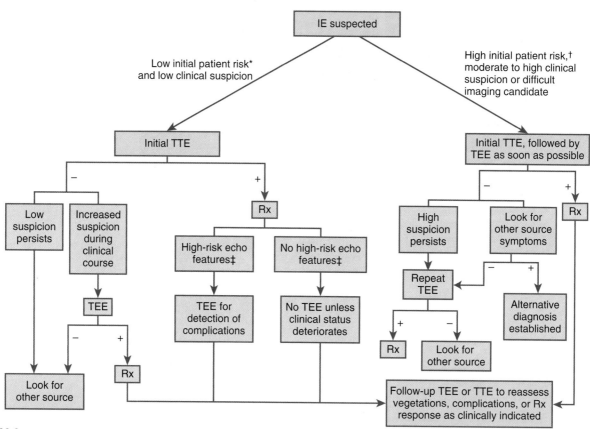

FIGURE 80.8 An approach to the diagnostic use of echocardiography (echo). *Rx*, Prescription; *TEE*, transesophageal echocardiography; *TTE*, transthoracic echocardiography. *For example, a patient with fever and a previously known heart murmur and no other stigmata of infective endocarditis (IE). †High initial patient risks include prosthetic heart valves, many congenital heart diseases, previous endocarditis, new murmur, heart failure, or other stigmata of endocarditis. ‡High-risk echocardiographic features include large or mobile vegetations, valvular insufficiency, suggestion of perivalvular extension, or secondary ventricular dysfunction (see text). (Modified from Baddour LM, Wilson WR, Bayer AS, et al. Infective endocarditis in adults: diagnosis, antimicrobial therapy, and management of complications. A scientific statement for healthcare professionals from the American Heart Association. *Circulation.* 2015;132:1435; and Habib G, et al. 2015 ESC guidelines for the management of infective endocarditis. The Task Force for the Management of Infective Endocarditis of the European Society of Cardiology. *Eur Heart J.* 2015;36:3075.)

TABLE 80.5 Echocardiographic Features That Suggest Potential Need for Surgical Intervention

Vegetation
Persistent vegetation after systemic embolization
Anterior mitral valve leaflet vegetation, particularly if it is highly mobile with size >10 mm*
One or more embolic events during the first 2 weeks of antimicrobial therapy*
Increase in vegetation size despite appropriate antimicrobial therapy*,†
Valvular Dysfunction
Acute aortic or mitral insufficiency with signs of ventricular failure†
Heart failure unresponsive to medical therapy†
Valve perforation or rupture†
Perivalvular Extension
Valvular dehiscence, rupture, or fistula†
New heart block†,‡
Large abscess or extension of abscess despite appropriate antimicrobial therapy†

*Surgery may be required because of risk of embolization.
†Surgery may be required because of heart failure or failure of medical therapy.
‡Echocardiography should not be the primary modality used to detect or monitor heart block.
See text for more complete discussion of indications for surgery based on vegetation characterizations.

late-systolic LV and LA pressure equilibration, consistent with a giant *v* wave noted on LA catheterization. Quantitative Doppler methods are quite useful to confirm the presence of acute severe regurgitation, because qualitative color flow jets may be complex, eccentric, or rapidly dissipating because of the loss of transvalvular pressure gradients.

PERIVALVULAR EXTENSION OF INFECTION. Perivalvular extension in IE includes the complications of periannular or intramyocardial abscess, mycotic false aneurysm, and fistula. The incidence of perivalvular extension ranges from 10% to almost 30% in native valve IE and at least 30% to 55% in PVE (see Figs. 80.6 and 80.7).[27,31] IE involving a transcatheter-implanted aortic bioprosthesis has been reported to have a lower incidence of complications from perivalvular extension of infection, such as abscess (15%), aortic mycotic pseudoaneurysm (4%), or aortoatrial fistula (4%).[47] Earlier series have reported the incidence of perivalvular extension of infection to approach 100% for aortic PVE.[8,26] Independent predictors of perivalvular extension are PVE, aortic valve involvement, and staphylococcal infection (from both coagulase-negative strains and *S. aureus*).[8,26] Periannular abscess has been reported in up to 50% of patients with native BAV IE (see Fig. 16.74C), versus 20% in those with a tricuspid aortic valve.[15] Persistent fever, ongoing bacteremia despite appropriate antibiotic therapy, chest pain, a new heart murmur, recurrent embolism, or HF all should alert the clinician to the possible presence of perivalvular extension. After HF, perivalvular extension of infection is the second most common indication for early surgical intervention for IE, and although surgery clearly confers an early survival benefit,[51] perivalvular extension remains an independent predictor of increased in-hospital and 1-year mortality.[9,26,27,50] In left-sided native valve *S. aureus* IE, the echocardiographic findings of perivalvular extension of infection, such as intracardiac abscess, and LVEF less than 40% have been strong independent predictors of in-hospital early mortality.[52]

It is recognized that the sensitivity of TTE for the diagnosis of perivalvular extension is at best 50%, and even less in PVE. TEE has a reported sensitivity of 80% to 90%, specificities of greater than 90%, with positive predictive value (PPV) and NPV of 85% to 90% for diagnosis of perivalvular extension.[8,45] Although TEE is quite sensitive for the diagnosis of aortic perivalvular extension, mitral annular calcification may obscure small regions of mitral perivalvular extension, particularly in the posterior aspects of the annulus.[53] On echocardiographic imaging, early perivalvular abscess usually appears as a nonhomogeneous, soft tissue, echodense thickening that distorts the margins of normal periannular anatomy.

With IE in the aortic valve position, a high predilection for perivalvular extension of infection to involve the *mitral-aortic intervalvular fibrosa* (MAIF) has been recognized. The MAIF is the fibrous zone of continuity between the noncoronary cusp of the aortic valve and insertion of the anterior mitral valve leaflet. Being one of the least vascular structures of the heart, the MAIF is more susceptible to infection and mycotic false aneurysm formation. On echocardiographic imaging of these false aneurysms, systolic expansion of an echolucent cavity can be appreciated within the infected MAIF (see Fig. 80.7), with color Doppler flow communication usually evident from the subvalvular LV outflow tract. Potential complications of MAIF mycotic false aneurysms include fistulous communications into the left atrium or aorta, extension around the aortic root, compression of the proximal left coronary arteries with resultant myocardial ischemia, systemic embolization, and rupture into the pericardial space.[53] Fistulas from aortic perivalvular extension of infection may track into any cardiac chamber and are best identified with TEE color flow Doppler techniques. Mitral valve IE complicated by perivalvular extension is less common, with much lower frequency of structural and conduction system sequelae. Prosthetic valve dehiscence is another manifestation of perivalvular extension of infection and usually is seen without impressive vegetations on the prosthesis itself (see Fig. 80.7). Imaging by TEE demonstrates crescentic defect adjacent to the sewing ring, variable rocking of the prosthesis, and periprosthetic regurgitation.

APPROACH TO ECHOCARDIOGRAPHIC IMAGING. Clinical risk assessment of the patient with suspected IE is the first step in deciding which echocardiographic imaging modality to use for evaluation (see Fig. 80.8 and Table 80.6). Patients with undifferentiated febrile syndromes, a chronic unchanged murmur, no physical examination findings suggestive of IE, and no high-risk cardiac anatomy (e.g., prosthetic valves or complex CHD) are characterized as being at initially low patient risk with a lower pretest likelihood of IE. High initial patient risk characteristics that present a high pretest probability of IE and likelihood of adverse outcome include clinical findings of a significant new heart murmur, peripheral stigmata of IE, new HF, *S. aureus* bacteremia, and high-risk cardiac anatomy, including the presence of a prosthetic valve or complex CHD.[2,8] Independent risk factors for IE (established in 10% to 15% of cases) in the presence of *S. aureus* bacteremia include community-acquired status, IV drug abuse, significant preexisting native valve disease, intracardiac prosthesis or CIED, prolonged (>72 hours) bacteremia, secondary foci of infection, and embolic event.[54-56]

As shown in Figure 80.8, patients at low initial risk should undergo TTE. In the absence of significant preexisting native valve disease or any prosthetic or implanted devices, adequate- or better-quality images detecting no vegetations exclude the diagnosis of IE, with NPV of 97% and sensitivity exceeding 90%.[54] With preexisting valve disease, the sensitivity approaches 60% but with a similar NPV if TTE image quality is adequate.[57] Even with *S. aureus* bacteremia, initial TTE imaging is reasonable in the absence of the previous risk factors.[8,56,58,59] If TTE images are limited or inadequate, TEE should be pursued. If TTE detects high-risk findings such as large (>10 mm in diameter) or highly mobile vegetations, suggests the presence of perivalvular extension of infection, or identifies new grade III to IV valvular regurgitation or new LV dysfunction, TEE should be promptly performed for further evaluation with the aim to definitively characterize the anatomic extent of infection and complications thereof. Patients at high risk (e.g., new-onset HF, significant new murmur, clinical stigmata of IE, prior IE, prosthetic heart valves/devices, complex CHD, *S. aureus* bacteremia) should undergo initial imaging with TEE (see Fig. 80.8), with supplemental TTE for complete semiquantitation of valvular regurgitation and delineation of left- and right-sided hemodynamics and ventricular function. If TEE is not immediately possible or available, TTE should be pursued first to avoid delay in imaging evaluation and diagnosis.

Provided that initial TTE images are of diagnostic quality and are negative for IE, if a low clinical suspicion for IE persists, other diagnoses

TABLE 80.6 Use of Echocardiography During Diagnosis and Treatment of Infective Endocarditis

Early
Echocardiography as soon as possible (<12 hr after initial evaluation)
TEE preferred; obtain TTE views of any abnormal findings for later comparison
TTE if TEE is not immediately available
TTE may be sufficient in small children
Repeat Echocardiography
TEE after positive TTE as soon as possible in patients at high risk for complications
TEE 7–10 days after initial TEE if suspicion exists without diagnosis of IE or with worrisome clinical course during early treatment of IE
Intraoperative
Prepump
Identification of vegetations, mechanism of regurgitation, abscesses, fistulas, and pseudoaneurysms
Postpump
Confirmation of successful repair of abnormal findings
Assessment of Residual Valve Dysfunction
Elevated afterload if necessary to avoid underestimating valve insufficiency or presence of residual abnormal flow
Completion of Therapy
Establish new baseline for valve function and morphology and ventricular size and function
TTE usually adequate; TEE or review of intraoperative TEE may be needed for complex anatomy to establish new baseline

IE, Infective endocarditis; *TEE,* transesophageal echocardiography; *TTE,* transthoracic echocardiography.

should be pursued (see Fig. 80.8). With increased clinical suspicion for IE throughout the patient's clinical course, an initially negative TTE should be followed up with TEE. If the initial TTE is positive for IE but high-risk findings as noted previously are lacking, TEE should not be mandatory, unless the patient is clinically unresponsive to antibiotic therapy or deteriorates during the clinical course. Any high-risk finding on TTE would warrant further evaluation with TEE.

As outlined in Figure 80.8, if the initial TEE is negative for IE and there is diminishing clinical suspicion of IE, other diagnoses should be evaluated. If IE remains high in the differential diagnosis, repeat TEE should be performed in 3 to 5 days, recognizing that NPV of two sequential TEE studies is 98%.[8] After an initial TEE is positive for IE, it should be repeated throughout the patient's course as clinically indicated, to assess response to antibiotic therapy or evaluate clinical or hemodynamic deterioration.

At the completion of antibiotic therapy, repeat echocardiography is indicated to establish a new post-treatment fingerprint of valvular morphology, residual vegetations, valvular regurgitation, and other hemodynamic factors and to assess ventricular function (see Table 80.6). Provided that images are of diagnostic quality, TTE should be adequate for this purpose. With complex anatomy, or if prosthetic valve function remains in question, TEE usually is indicated.

OTHER ADVANCED IMAGING. CT may be helpful in the evaluation of complications of endocarditis, including abscesses and pseudoaneurysms, and may be beneficial in surgical planning (see Fig. 80.3).[20] CT with angiography (multidetector computed tomographic angiography, or MDCTA) is a sensitive alternative imaging procedure for the evaluation of IE and perivalvular extension of infection (see Chapter 20). In a small group of patients with suspected IE, cardiac MDCTA was 96% sensitive for the detection of valvular vegetations, identical to that of multiplanar TEE, compared with intraoperative findings.[60] Both imaging techniques had specificity and PPV/NPV exceeding 95%. Excellent correlation was found between MDCTA and TEE in the determination of vegetation size and mobility; however, TEE was

DISEASES OF THE HEART VALVES

superior for the detection of small vegetations (≤4 mm) and valvular perforations. The sensitivity of MDCTA for the detection of perivalvular extension of infection confirmed at surgery was 100%, versus 89% for TEE, and it provided additional information regarding the extent of perivalvular extension that was not detected by TEE.[60] Similar findings have been reported in a series of patients with aortic PVE, with good accuracy of MDCTA in the detection of early perivalvular extension of infection (see Fig. 80.7), periannular abscess, false aneurysm, and prosthetic valve dehiscence compared with TEE and surgery.[61] The greatest advantage of cardiac CT in the setting of IE is its ability to couple the detection of complex cardiac anatomic abnormalities with coronary artery delineation, serving two important components of the diagnostic evaluation, particularly among patients who will require surgical intervention due to IE complications. In a study of 255 adults who underwent surgery for IE, TEE had statistically higher detection of vegetations (95.6% versus 70.0%, p < 0.0001) and leaflet perforations (81.3% versus 42.9%, p = 0.02) as compared with cardiac CTA; however, for detection of abscess/pseudoaneurysm, TEE had a similar sensitivity to cardiac CTA (90.5% versus 78.4%, p = 0.21).[52] There was no significant difference in perioperative outcomes whether coronary arteries were evaluated by CTA or ICA. Therefore there is a strong argument to consider cardiac CT as an alternate coronary artery imaging modality in IE patients with low to intermediate risk of disease but meet guideline recommendations for coronary artery imaging.

Recently, positron emission tomography (CT imaging with fluorine 18–fluorodeoxyglucose (^{18}F-FDG) has incrementally improved the diagnostic accuracy in evaluation of suspected PVE, particularly CIED IE, increasing the sensitivity from approximately 60% to 70% with the modified Duke criteria and TEE imaging alone to 87% to 97% with the addition of ^{18}F-FDG PET/CT (see Figs. 18.40 and 18.41).[62,63] This resulted primarily from enhanced identification of infection in the tissue spaces adjacent to the prosthetic valve or implanted device, and less from the identification of sites of secondary infection. This imaging technique has been proposed as an additional major Duke criterion for the diagnosis of prosthetic device IE,[62] but because of the current lack of large studies, routine use of ^{18}F-FDG PET/CT has not been endorsed by guideline-writing committees to date.[8,26] Moreover, ^{18}F-FDG PET/CT has not been of incremental value in the diagnosis of native valve IE.[64]

EMBOLISM. Embolic events are common early in the course of IE, particularly before the institution of appropriate antibiotic therapy. Over the past two decades, numerous studies have reported an overall incidence of embolic events that has ranged from 20% to 50%.[8,26] In more recent clinical series, the reported incidence of acute stroke complicating IE ranged from 10% to 23%,[9,17,19,22,27] with rates of 15% to 25% reported for other embolic events not causing stroke.[9,15,17] Both stroke and other embolic events complicating IE occur more frequently in patients younger than 65 years[17] and are adverse predictors of outcome and survival in IE.[8,26] In a multicenter study using admission-screening CT imaging in 384 patients presenting with IE, 26% had one site of embolism, and another 9% had multiple sites of embolism in the following distribution: CNS (38%), spleen (30%), renal (13%), lung (10%), peripheral artery (6%), mesenteric (2%), and coronary (1%). The embolic event was clinically silent in 15% of all patients. The incidence of cerebral embolic events probably is significantly underestimated by clinical assessment. In a study of 130 patients with definite or possible IE based on the modified Duke criteria, cerebral magnetic resonance imaging (MRI) detected acute ischemic lesions in 52% of patients and only 12% had acute neurologic symptoms.[65] In this study, MRI also demonstrated cerebral microhemorrhages in 57%, other hemorrhagic lesions in 8%, asymptomatic mycotic aneurysms in 8%, and abscesses in 6%. Screening cerebral MRI led to significant modification of the diagnosis or treatment plan in 28% of the entire study group.[65]

Peripheral embolization with or without metastatic infection also may be detected with PET/CT, and clinically unsuspected lesions of this nature were observed in 28% of patients in one small series.[66] Imaging with PET/CT also is useful in the detection of perivalvular extension of infection, particularly of the aortic root, and for identification of CIED infections.

Numerous studies have examined the ability of echocardiographic characterization of vegetations to predict risk of embolic events in

IE. More recent analyses have consistently shown that vegetations more than 10 mm in greatest dimension are independent predictors of embolism, with considerably higher risk with dimensions above 15 mm.[8,26,67–69] Before initiation of appropriate antibiotic therapy, large vegetations are associated with a greater than 40% risk of a clinically evident or silent embolic event. Pedunculated and highly mobile vegetations also are independently associated with embolic risk.[45] Both vegetation length of more than 10 mm and severe vegetation mobility are multivariate predictors of embolism, even after initiation of antibiotic therapy. Mitral valve vegetations, particularly on the anterior leaflet in native valve IE, are more likely to embolize than those in the aortic position; the embolic risk generally is equivalent in native and in prosthetic valve IE.[8,45,70]

The infecting organism also has an impact on embolic risk. S. aureus IE has been consistently implicated as an independent risk predictor for embolism; IE from S. gallolyticus and VGS is less implicated.[70] The presence of intracardiac perivalvular abscess is another independent risk for stroke associated with IE.[61]

Prediction of symptomatic embolism in IE has been proposed with the derivation and validation of a risk calculator using the variables of age, diabetes mellitus, atrial fibrillation, embolism before initiation of antibiotic therapy, vegetation length, and the presence of S. aureus infection. This calculator, known as the Embolic Risk French Calculator, is available online. Using this calculator, a 70-year-old patient with S. aureus IE, having all clinical risk variables present and vegetation size greater than 10 mm in length, would have an estimated 7-day embolic risk of 23%. The same-age patient with S. aureus IE but no clinical risk variables and vegetation size less than 10 mm would have an estimated 2% 7-day embolic risk.[71]

Over the past several decades, multiple clinical series have shown that the risk of embolism decreases dramatically, generally to less than 10% to 15%, within 1 week after initiation of appropriate antibiotic therapy.[8,26] The occurrence of stroke has been shown to fall to 3% after the first week of antibiotic therapy, with the overall incidence decreasing from 4.82 to 1.71 per 1000 patient-days during the second week of therapy.[70] With this documented response to antibiotic therapy, preemptive surgical intervention for potentially high-embolic-risk vegetations has not been previously advised unless there are recurrent embolic events despite ongoing appropriate antibiotic therapy.[8,26] This position has been challenged by a small study of patients with left-sided vegetations greater than 10 mm in diameter randomized to conventional management versus early surgery (within 48 hours).[72] On admission, almost 30% of each group had evidence of cerebral emboli and had no other indications for urgent surgical intervention. In patients randomized to conventional therapy, recurrent cerebral embolic events occurred in 13%, with an overall embolic event rate of 21% at 6 weeks, compared with a 0% over the same period for the early surgical patients; the in-hospital mortality was 3% for both groups.[72]

Recurrent embolic events or progressive increase in vegetation size despite appropriate antibiotic therapy, especially in the presence of significant perivalvular extension of infection or HF, would constitute clear indications for early surgical intervention.[8,26]

Thus far, no randomized controlled trials (RCTs) support the initiation of either antiplatelet or anticoagulant therapy to decrease embolic risk in IE. A retrospective analysis has suggested a lower occurrence of embolic events in patients who continue to receive antiplatelet therapy taken before the onset of IE.[73] In a larger prospective cohort analysis, established antiplatelet therapy did not reduce the incidence of cerebrovascular complications associated with IE but also did not increase the occurrence of hemorrhagic complications.[69] Therefore the initiation of aspirin or other antiplatelet agents as adjunctive therapy in IE is not currently recommended; however, the continuation of long-term antiplatelet therapy at the time of development of IE with no bleeding complications may be considered. Snygg-Martin et al.[59] reported that previously prescribed warfarin therapy, continued through the clinical course of left-sided native valve IE, was associated with a lower incidence of stroke, transient ischemic attack (TIA), and cerebral infections compared with those not receiving warfarin therapy (6% versus 26%, respectively), with the incidence of hemorrhagic complications being 2% in both groups.

ANTIMICROBIAL THERAPY

Not only is it important to diagnose IE, but it also is critical that an etiologic diagnosis be obtained to ensure that optimal antimicrobial therapy is provided for attempted cure.[8,75] Because of the rarity of presentation, diagnosis of IE often eludes nonspecialists, which results in the administration of empiric therapy for a variety of more common febrile illnesses. This empiricism can greatly reduce the sensitivity of subsequent blood cultures when the IE diagnosis is eventually considered. Thus initial empiricism results in a blood culture–negative presentation, which prompts administration of empiric antimicrobial therapy for IE. This scenario is a bane of infectious diseases specialists, who have traditionally cared for patients with IE. The antimicrobial regimen selected for therapy on the basis of the culture-negative state may not be curative. Moreover, the empiric regimen may include drugs, in particular aminoglycosides, that pose toxicity risks that might have been avoided had a pathogen been identified. Ultimately, this could result in a worst-case scenario in which a microbiologic cure is not achieved and irreversible toxicity occurs.

Some of the regimens employed in the treatment of IE are based on clinical trials with small numbers (dozens) of patients. Many of the regimens, however, are based on consensus opinion that is outlined in guidelines promulgated by societies or associations worldwide. Not surprisingly, these guidelines differ in their recommendations, which can be confusing for the practicing clinician.

Several tenets of medical management are important in defining an optimal antimicrobial regimen in each case of IE. First, consultation with a physician who is experienced in the care of patients with IE is mandatory; this usually involves a specialist trained in infectious diseases. Second, selection and dosing of antimicrobial therapy are based on both pharmacokinetic and pharmacodynamic characteristics of specific drugs and in vitro susceptibility testing results of an isolated pathogen in blood or tissue specimen culture-positive cases. Third, antimicrobial treatment should be prolonged (over weeks), high dose, parenteral, and "cidal" in its activity against a patient's isolate. Although important data were recently published regarding treatment regimens that include partial oral antibiotic dosing, more study is needed before regimens that include orally dosed antibiotics can be advocated for left-sided IE.[76] These aspects of medical therapy are necessary primarily because organisms in infected vegetations downregulate their metabolism once a relatively high concentration of organisms accumulate in vegetation tissue, which is an avascular structure.

Streptococci

Viridans Group Streptococci and *Streptococcus gallolyticus* (formerly *S. bovis*). Treatment regimens vary, depending on type of valve (native or prosthetic) and whether the streptococcal isolate is penicillin susceptible or not.[8] Regarding the latter issue, the definition of susceptibility to penicillin, as addressed previously, is based on minimum inhibitory concentrations (MICs) that are specific to treatment of the syndrome of IE; *highly penicillin-susceptible* status is defined as that of an isolate with an MIC of 0.12 µg/mL or less to penicillin. Therapy with either aqueous crystalline penicillin G sodium or ceftriaxone sodium should be microbiologically curative in 98% or more of patients with native valve IE who complete 4 weeks of treatment (Table 80.7). Because of the ease of administration of one dose per day of ceftriaxone parenterally, the bulk of therapy is with this agent rather than with intravenously administered aqueous crystalline penicillin G, which requires four to six doses per day. The once-a-day dosing of ceftriaxone sodium has been pivotal in some cases in allowing patients to avoid nursing home placement for multiple doses of antibiotic administration on a daily basis. The administration of one dose of ceftriaxone sodium each day is done in a variety of outpatient venues that routinely administer parenteral medications.

Vancomycin is recommended in patients who cannot tolerate penicillin or cephalosporin therapy because of a history of immunoglobulin E (IgE)-mediated allergic reactions (see Table 80.7). Before the preferred therapies of aqueous crystalline penicillin G or ceftriaxone are abandoned, consultation with an allergy specialist should be obtained, which may include oral amoxicillin challenge and/or skin testing to confirm that beta-lactam regimens are not a treatment option. Vancomycin should be administered intravenously for 4 weeks with serial, usually weekly, monitoring of serum trough levels, if the dose is stable and the renal status is not changing. The desired serum trough level is 10 to 15 µg/mL; serum peak vancomycin levels are not required for treatment.

TABLE 80.7 **Therapy of Native Valve Endocarditis Caused by Highly Penicillin-Susceptible Viridans Group Streptococci and *Streptococcus gallolyticus***

REGIMEN	DOSE* AND ROUTE	DURATION (WEEKS)	STRENGTH OF RECOMMENDATION	COMMENTS
Aqueous crystalline penicillin G sodium	12–18 million U/24 hr IV either continuously or in 4 or 6 equally divided doses	4	Class IIa, LOE: B	Preferred in most patients >65 years or patients with impairment of eighth cranial nerve function or renal function Ampicillin, 2 g IV every 4 hr, is reasonable alternative to penicillin if a penicillin shortage exists.
Or				
Ceftriaxone sodium	2 g/24 hr IV/IM in 1 dose	4	Class IIa, LOE: B	
Aqueous crystalline penicillin G sodium	12–18 million U/24 hr IV either continuously or in 6 equally divided doses	2	Class IIa, LOE: B	Two-week regimen not intended for patients with known cardiac or extracardiac abscess or for those with creatinine clearance of <20 mL/min, impaired eighth cranial nerve function, or *Abiotrophia, Granulicatella,* or *Gemella* spp. infection; gentamicin dose should be adjusted to achieve peak serum concentration of 3–4 µg/mL and trough serum concentration of <1 µg/mL when 3 divided doses are used; there are no optimal drug concentrations for single daily dosing.[†]
or				
Ceftriaxone sodium	2 g/24 hr IV or IM in 1 dose	2	Class IIa, LOE: B	
Plus				
Gentamicin sulfate[‡]	3 mg/kg/24 hr IV or IM in 1 dose	2		
Vancomycin hydrochloride[§]	30 mg/kg/24 hr IV in 2 equally divided doses	4	Class IIa, LOE: B	Vancomycin therapy is reasonable only for patients unable to tolerate penicillin or ceftriaxone; vancomycin dose should be adjusted to a trough concentration range of 10–15 µg/mL.

*Doses recommended are for patients with normal renal function.

[†]Data for once-daily dosing of aminoglycosides for children exist, but no data for treatment of infective endocarditis (IE) exist.

[‡]Other potentially nephrotoxic drugs (e.g., nonsteroidal antiinflammatory drugs) should be used with caution in patients receiving gentamicin therapy. Although it is preferred that gentamicin (3 mg/kg) be given as a single daily dose to adult patients with endocarditis caused by viridans group streptococci, as a second option, gentamicin can be administered daily in three equally divided doses.

[§]Vancomycin dosages should be infused during the course of at least 1 hour to reduce the risk of histamine-release "red man" syndrome.

Minimum inhibitory concentration (MIC) is ≤0.12 µg/mL. The subdivisions differ from Clinical and Laboratory Standards Institute–recommended break points that are used to define penicillin susceptibility.

IM, Intramuscularly; *IV,* intravenously; *LOE,* level of evidence.

From Baddour LM, Wilson WR, Bayer AS, et al. Infective endocarditis in adults: diagnosis, antimicrobial therapy, and management of complications. A scientific statement for healthcare professionals from the American Heart Association. *Circulation.* 2015;132:1435–1486.

For selected patients, a 2-week treatment regimen can be used, but this should be based on input from an infectious disease specialist. The combination regimen includes either aqueous crystalline penicillin G sodium or ceftriaxone sodium plus gentamicin sulfate (see Table 80.7). The 2-week regimen should be limited to cases of uncomplicated native valve IE caused by VGS or *S. gallolyticus* strains that are highly susceptible to penicillin. The regimen would not be appropriate in patients with underlying renal or eighth cranial nerve dysfunction. If the ceftriaxone-containing regimen is used, then the single daily dose of the drug should be administered immediately before or after gentamicin dosing. No recommended guidelines for monitoring serum gentamicin concentrations are currently available.

Penicillin resistance is divided into two categories for VGS and *S. gallolyticus* infection in patients with native valve IE. In one category, relative resistance to penicillin is defined as a penicillin MIC greater than 0.12 µg/mL to less than 0.5 µg/mL. In this group, 4 weeks of therapy is recommended with either aqueous crystalline penicillin G or ceftriaxone plus gentamicin once daily for the first 2 weeks of treatment (Table 80.8). Vancomycin can be used in patients who are not candidates for beta-lactam therapy. In the other category, penicillin resistance is defined as a penicillin MIC greater than 0.5 µg/mL. Fortunately, native valve IE due to these penicillin-resistant strains is rarely seen. In patients with these infections, a more aggressive course of therapy is recommended and is the same regimen as that used in the treatment of native valve IE caused by penicillin- and aminoglycoside-susceptible enterococci (see Table 80.7). Monotherapy with vancomycin should be administered in patients who are not candidates for the combination regimen.

Patients who have IE involving a prosthetic valve or prosthetic material (e.g., annuloplasty ring) due to VGS or *S. gallolyticus* should receive 6 weeks of antibiotic therapy (Table 80.9). In those infected with strains that are highly susceptible to penicillin (MIC <0.12 µg/mL), the addition of gentamicin for the first 2 weeks of either penicillin or ceftriaxone therapy is optional. In patients infected with streptococci that harbor any level of resistance to penicillin (MIC >0.12 µg/mL), combination therapy for 6 weeks is recommended. In patients who do not tolerate beta-lactam therapy, vancomycin as monotherapy should be administered for 6 weeks.

Bacteria Formerly Known as "Nutritionally Variant Streptococci." Because of their previous designation as "nutritionally variant streptococci," a discussion of organisms now included in nonstreptococcal categories is warranted, although the frequency of these organisms causing IE is low. *Abiotrophia defectiva* and *Granulicatella* spp. and *Gemella* spp. have unusual metabolic characteristics that can result in diminished activity of cell wall–active antibiotics to kill these organisms and thus decreased cure rates. Moreover, because of this characteristic, the ability to perform in vitro susceptibility testing is adversely affected, with potentially unreliable results.

Thus a regimen recommended for treatment of native valve IE is advocated (see Table 80.7).

Beta-Hemolytic Streptococci. Unlike IE caused by VGS and *S. gallolyticus*, IE caused by beta-hemolytic streptococci typically is characterized by an acute onset with rapid valve destruction and other complications that often require cardiovascular surgical intervention. Consultation with a specialist in infectious diseases and cardiology is recommended. Because IE is infrequently caused by these organisms, prospective clinical trial data for therapeutic decisions are lacking. Nevertheless, recommended therapy for IE caused by *Streptococcus pyogenes* (group A) includes either aqueous crystalline penicillin G or ceftriaxone or cefazolin, and treatment is for at least 4 weeks. For the other types (groups B, C, F, and G) of beta-hemolytic streptococcal infections, gentamicin is advocated by some clinicians for the first 2 weeks of treatment.

Staphylococci. As noted previously, staphylococci have become more prominent as causes of IE in developed countries. In addition, antibiotic resistance has dramatically increased over the years, and for many patients, therapeutic choices are limited, although use of these agents has been largely unexamined in prospective clinical trials.

Infections caused by oxacillin-susceptible staphylococci can be treated with either nafcillin or oxacillin that is administered intravenously over 6 weeks for left-sided native valve IE or complicated right-sided IE (Table 80.10). Although previously included as an optional agent to be given over the first 3 to 5 days of therapy,[8] gentamicin is no longer advocated because of nephrotoxicity risk.[76] Cefazolin is an option for patients with left-sided infection who are intolerant of penicillins but have not had an IgE-mediated allergic reaction to penicillins. Some experts advocate for the use of cefazolin over the antistaphylococcal penicillins.

For uncomplicated right-sided native valve IE caused by oxacillin-susceptible staphylococci, 2 weeks of antibiotic therapy with nafcillin or oxacillin is an option. For patients who are intolerant of beta-lactam therapy, vancomycin can be used, but many favor a longer treatment. Daptomycin, 6 mg/kg/day intravenously, is another treatment option in patients intolerant of beta-lactam therapy.

Defining an optimal treatment regimen for native valve IE, including left- and right-sided infection, caused by oxacillin-resistant staphylococci is a more difficult task. Currently, IV vancomycin is recommended, but cure rates are less than desired. Daptomycin and ceftaroline are treatment options in patients intolerant of or nonresponsive to vancomycin, but prospective trial data including large cohorts are lacking. In addition, combination therapy with daptomycin plus a variety of beta-lactams is undergoing evaluation.

Therapy for PVE caused by staphylococci involves more complex regimens because of the difficulty in curing infections involving prosthetic valve material. For oxacillin-susceptible strains, nafcillin or oxacillin is given for at least 6 weeks in combination with rifampin, which can be administered either intravenously or orally (Table 80.11). Cefazolin

TABLE 80.8 Therapy of Native Valve Endocarditis Caused by Strains of Viridans Group Streptococci and *Streptococcus gallolyticus* Relatively Resistant to Penicillin

REGIMEN	DOSE* AND ROUTE	DURATION (WEEKS)	STRENGTH OF RECOMMENDATION	COMMENTS
Aqueous crystalline penicillin G sodium	24 million U/24 hr IV either continuously or in 4–6 equally divided doses	4	Class IIa, LOE: B	It is reasonable to treat patients with IE caused penicillin-resistant (MIC ≥0.5 µg/mL) VGS strains with a combination of ampicillin or penicillin plus gentamicin as done for enterococcal IE with infectious diseases consultation. (Class IIa, LOE: C)
				Ampicillin, 2 g IV every 4 hr, is a reasonable alternative to penicillin if a penicillin shortage exists.
Plus				
Gentamicin sulfate†	3 mg/kg/24 hr IV or IM in 1 dose	2		Ceftriaxone may be a reasonable alternative treatment option for VGS isolates that are susceptible to ceftriaxone. (Class IIb, LOE: C)
Vancomycin hydrochloride‡	30 mg/kg/24 hr IV in 2 equally divided doses	4	Class IIa, LOE: C	Vancomycin therapy is reasonable only for patients unable to tolerate penicillin or ceftriaxone therapy.

*Doses recommended are for patients with normal renal function.
†See Table 80.7 for appropriate dose of gentamicin. Although it is preferred that gentamicin (3 mg/kg) be given as a single daily dose to adult patients with endocarditis caused by VGS, as a second option, gentamicin can be administered daily in three equally divided doses.
‡See Table 80.7 for appropriate dosage of vancomycin.
Minimum inhibitory concentration (MIC) is greater than 0.12 to less than 0.5 µg/mL for penicillin. The subdivisions differ from Clinical and Laboratory Standards Institute–recommended break points that are used to define penicillin susceptibility.
IE, Infective endocarditis; *IM,* intramuscularly; *IV,* intravenously *LOE,* level of evidence; *VGS,* Viridans Group Streptococci.
From Baddour LM, Wilson WR, Bayer AS, et al. Infective endocarditis in adults: diagnosis, antimicrobial therapy, and management of complications. A scientific statement for healthcare professionals from the American Heart Association. *Circulation.* 2015;132:1435–1486.

can be used if the patient is intolerant of penicillins and has not had an IgE-mediated allergic reaction. Gentamicin is recommended for the initial 2 weeks of treatment as well. In patients intolerant of gentamicin, or if the infecting isolate is resistant to gentamicin and other aminoglycosides, levofloxacin can be given, provided that the isolate is susceptible to this agent. For PVE caused by oxacillin-resistant strains, IV vancomycin should be given in combination with rifampin for at least 2 weeks and gentamicin for 2 weeks.

Enterococci. Enterococci are common causative organisms in IE, particularly in the elderly population and those with health care–associated infections, and treatment requires both penicillin or ampicillin and an aminoglycoside (usually gentamicin) for attempted cure of infection.

TABLE 80.9 Therapy for Endocarditis of Prosthetic Valves or Other Prosthetic Material Caused by Viridans Group Streptococci and *Streptococcus gallolyticus*

REGIMEN	DOSE* AND ROUTE	DURATION (WEEKS)	STRENGTH OF RECOMMENDATION	COMMENTS
Penicillin-Susceptible Strain (≤0.12 μg/mL)				
Aqueous crystalline penicillin G sodium	24 million U/24 hr IV either continuously or in 4–6 equally divided doses	6	Class IIa, LOE: B	Penicillin or ceftriaxone together with gentamicin has not demonstrated superior cure rates compared with monotherapy with penicillin or ceftriaxone for patients with highly susceptible strain.
Or				
Ceftriaxone	2 g/24 hr IV or IM in 1 dose	6	Class IIa, LOE: B	Ampicillin, 2 g IV every 4 hr, is reasonable alternative to penicillin if a penicillin shortage exists.
with or without				
Gentamicin sulfate†	3 mg/kg/24 hr IV or IM in 1 dose	2		Gentamicin therapy should not be administered to patients with creatinine clearance <30 mL/min.
Vancomycin hydrochloride‡	30 mg/kg/24 hr IV in 2 equally divided doses	6	Class IIa, LOE: B	Vancomycin is reasonable only for patients unable to tolerate penicillin or ceftriaxone.
Penicillin Relatively or Fully Resistant Strain (MIC >0.12 μg/mL)				
Aqueous crystalline penicillin sodium	24 million U/24 hr IV either continuously or in 4–6 equally divided doses	6	Class IIa, LOE: B	Ampicillin, 2 g IV every 4 hr, is a reasonable alternative to penicillin if a penicillin shortage exists.
Or				
Ceftriaxone	2 g/24 hr IV/IM in 1 dose	6	Class IIa, LOE: B	
Plus				
Gentamicin sulfate	3 mg/kg per 24 hr IV/IM in 1 dose	6		
Vancomycin hydrochloride	30 mg/kg/24 hr IV in 2 equally divided doses	6	Class IIa, LOE: B	Vancomycin is reasonable only for patients unable to tolerate penicillin or ceftriaxone.

*Doses recommended are for patients with normal renal function.
†See Table 80.7 for appropriate dose of gentamicin. Although it is preferred that gentamicin (3 mg/kg) be given as a single daily dose to adult patients with endocarditis resulting from VGS, as a second option, gentamicin can be administered daily in 3 equally divided doses.
‡See text and Table 80.7 for appropriate dose of vancomycin.
IM, Intramuscularly; *IV,* intravenously; *LOE,* level of evidence; *MIC,* minimum inhibitory concentration; *VGS,* Viridans Group Streptococci.
From Baddour LM, Wilson WR, Bayer AS, et al. Infective endocarditis in adults: diagnosis, antimicrobial therapy, and management of complications. A scientific statement for healthcare professionals from the American Heart Association. *Circulation.* 2015;132:1435–1486.

TABLE 80.10 Therapy for Endocarditis Caused by Staphylococci in the Absence of Prosthetic Materials

REGIMEN	DOSE* AND ROUTE	DURATION (WEEKS)	STRENGTH OF RECOMMENDATION	COMMENTS
Oxacillin-Susceptible Strains				
Nafcillin or oxacillin	12 g/24 hr IV in 4–6 equally divided doses	6	Class I, LOE: C	For complicated right-sided IE and for left-sided IE. For uncomplicated right-sided IE, 2 weeks (see text).
For penicillin-allergic (nonanaphylactoid-type) patients:				Consider skin testing for oxacillin-susceptible staphylococci and questionable history of immediate-type hypersensitivity to penicillin.
Cefazolin	6 g/24 hr IV in 3 equally divided doses	6	Class I, LOE: B	Cephalosporins should be avoided in patients with anaphylactoid-type hypersensitivity to beta-lactams; vancomycin should be used in these cases.
Oxacillin-Resistant Strains				
Vancomycin†	30 mg/kg/24 hr IV in 2 equally divided doses	6	Class I, LOE: C	Adjust vancomycin dose to achieve trough concentration of 10–20 μg/mL (see text for vancomycin alternatives).
Daptomycin	≥8 mg/kg/dose	6	Class IIb, LOE: B	Await additional study data to define optimal dosing.

*Doses recommended are for patients with normal renal function.
†For specific dosing adjustment and issues concerning vancomycin, see Table 80.7 footnotes.
IE, Infective endocarditis; *IV,* intravenously; *LOE,* level of evidence.
From Baddour LM, Wilson WR, Bayer AS, et al. Infective endocarditis in adults: diagnosis, antimicrobial therapy, and management of complications. A scientific statement for healthcare professionals from the American Heart Association. *Circulation.* 2015;132:1435–1486.

TABLE 80.11 Therapy for Endocarditis of Prosthetic Valves or Other Prosthetic Material Caused by Staphylococci

REGIMEN	DOSE* AND ROUTE	DURATION (WEEKS)	STRENGTH OF RECOMMENDATION	COMMENTS
Oxacillin-Susceptible Strains				
Nafcillin or oxacillin	12 g/24 hr IV in 6 equally divided doses	≥6	Class I, LOE: B	Vancomycin should be used in patients with immediate-type hypersensitivity reactions to beta-lactam antibiotics (see Table 80.7 for dosing guidelines).
plus				
Rifampin	900 mg/24 hr IV or orally in 3 equally divided doses	≥6		Cefazolin may be substituted for nafcillin or oxacillin in patients with non–immediate-type hypersensitivity reactions to penicillins.
plus				
Gentamicin†	3 mg/kg/24 hr IV or IM in 2 or 3 equally divided doses	2		
Oxacillin-Resistant Strains				
Vancomycin	30 mg/kg/24 hr in 2 equally divided doses	≥6	Class I, LOE: B	Adjust vancomycin to a trough concentration of 10–20 μg/mL.
Plus				
Rifampin	900 mg/24 hr IV/PO in 3 equally divided doses	≥6		
Plus				
Gentamicin	3 mg/kg/24 hr IV/IM in 2 or 3 equally divided doses	2		See text for gentamicin alternatives.

*Doses recommended are for patients with normal renal function.
†Gentamicin should be administered in close proximity to vancomycin, nafcillin, or oxacillin dosing. See Table 80.7 for appropriate dose of gentamicin.
IM, Intramuscularly; IV, intravenously; LOE, level of evidence; PO, orally.
From Baddour LM, Wilson WR, Bayer AS, et al. Infective endocarditis in adults: diagnosis, antimicrobial therapy, and management of complications. A scientific statement for healthcare professionals from the American Heart Association. *Circulation.* 2015;132:1435–1486.

E. faecalis accounts for the bulk (approximately 97%) of IE cases and are typically penicillin susceptible, while *E. faecium* and other enterococcal species are uncommon and may be resistant to penicillin and other agents. Because of the recommended 4 to 6 weeks of therapy, it often is difficult to complete the aminoglycoside-containing regimen in these older patients without the development of nephrotoxicity and/or ototoxicity. These adverse events are a greater concern in patients who are not candidates for penicillin therapy, usually because of previous allergic reaction, in whom vancomycin is combined with an aminoglycoside.

For native valve IE caused by strains that are susceptible to both penicillin and gentamicin, 4 weeks of antibiotic treatment is recommended in patients with symptoms for 3 months or less; 6 weeks is recommended for symptoms of IE longer than 3 months or for PVE (eTable 80.1). If an isolate is gentamicin resistant and streptomycin susceptible, streptomycin should be given with either ampicillin or penicillin (eTable 80.2).

When the isolate is *faecalis* species and resistant to all aminoglycosides or the patient is unable or unlikely to tolerate an aminoglycoside-containing regimen, a combination of "high-dose" ceftriaxone (4 g daily in two divided doses) with ampicillin has been successfully used,[77,78] but no head-to-head trials have been conducted to determine if the double–beta-lactam regimen is comparable in efficacy to the aminoglycoside-containing regimen. Nevertheless, historical data suggest comparable outcomes with the two regimens; thus double–beta-lactam therapy for IE caused by *E. faecalis* is a treatment option and has been included as a recommended regimen in the current AHA guidelines.[8,26] The beta-lactam combination should be administered for 6 weeks.

Some enterococcal isolates are penicillin resistant; most do not produce beta-lactamase as the mechanism of penicillin resistance and should be treated with a combination of vancomycin plus gentamicin. For the extremely rare isolate that produces beta-lactamase, ampicillin-sulbactam can be used with gentamicin (eTable 80.3). For enterococcal strains resistant to vancomycin (VRE) and penicillin, optimal treatment regimens are undefined, and therapy should be defined by a consulting infectious diseases expert. Often, daptomycin or linezolid is selected for use with other agents, depending on additional susceptibility results, which may require sending an isolate to a reference laboratory.

HACEK Organisms. The primary choice of therapy for IE caused by the HACEK group of organisms is ceftriaxone, given for 4 weeks for native valve infection and 6 weeks for PVE (eTable 80.4). Cefotaxime and ampicillin-sulbactam are acceptable alternative therapeutic agents, but their use has been limited because of the ease of dosing (once daily) with ceftriaxone, which is not shared by these other two treatment options. Fluoroquinolones should be efficacious as second-line agents, but clinical experience in IE treatment is limited.

Aerobic Gram-Negative Bacilli and Fungi. Although they rarely cause IE, coverage of both aerobic gram-negative bacilli and fungi is included here because many experts recommend a combined medical and surgical approach to management of IE caused by these pathogens.[26] Infectious diseases, cardiology, and cardiovascular surgery consultations should be sought in these cases. A lack of clinical trial data, reflecting in part the rarity of these syndromes, makes defining an optimal treatment regimen difficult.

Nevertheless, for IE caused by aerobic gram-negative bacilli, a combination of beta-lactam with an aminoglycoside is recommended, and the selection of these agents should be based on in vitro susceptibility testing results. A fluoroquinolone that is active against the isolated pathogen can be used instead of an aminoglycoside if the infecting isolate is aminoglycoside resistant or if the patient is intolerant of aminoglycosides.

Fungal IE primarily involves prosthetic valves and is characterized by poor outcomes. In some cases the infecting organism does not grow in routine blood cultures, and the infection can manifest as culture-negative endocarditis (discussed next). As noted previously, a majority of cases are caused by *Candida* spp., and many of the infections are health care associated. Because clinical trial data do not exist, defining an optimal treatment regimen is difficult, and drug therapy, which usually includes an amphotericin B–containing product, is associated with both infusion-related (rigors, fever, back pain, hypotension, bronchospasm, tachyarrhythmias) and delayed (nephrotoxicity, anemia, cation-wasting) adverse events that can be severe and limit use of these agents.[26] Moreover, relapse rates are high, even if valve surgery is done. The echinocandins (caspofungin, micafungin, and anidulafungin) have been useful in some patients who cannot tolerate an amphotericin B–containing regimen. Thus many experts advocate the use of long-term oral suppressive therapy once initial "induction" therapy is completed and an active oral agent is identified. Azole agents, including fluconazole and voriconazole, have been used most often. Unfortunately, none of the echinocandins is available for oral use. The complexity of antifungal selection warrants consultation with an expert in infectious diseases.

Culture-Negative Endocarditis. Empiricism begets empiricism. In most cases, when no pathogen is isolated in blood cultures or in other specimens (embolism, valve tissue), empiric antimicrobial therapy is started before specimen collection. Therefore selecting an optimal treatment regimen for these patients is difficult. Certainly, epidemiologic features of each case should be evaluated to assist in defining a treatment regimen (Table 80.12). In addition, the course of illness associated with the endocarditis presentation may offer clues to the cause of the infection and to the specific antibiotics already administered that might have

TABLE 80.12 Epidemiologic Clues in Etiologic Diagnosis of Culture-Negative Endocarditis

EPIDEMIOLOGIC FEATURE	COMMON MICROORGANISM
Injection drug use (IDU)	*Staphylococcus aureus*, including community-acquired oxacillin-resistant strains
	Coagulase-negative staphylococci
	Beta-hemolytic streptococci
	Fungi
	Aerobic gram-negative bacilli, including *Pseudomonas aeruginosa*
	Polymicrobial
Indwelling cardiovascular medical devices	*S. aureus*
	Coagulase-negative staphylococci
	Fungi
	Aerobic gram-negative bacilli
	Corynebacterium spp.
Genitourinary disorders, infection, and manipulation, including pregnancy, delivery, and abortion	*Enterococcus* spp.
	Group B streptococci (*S. agalactiae*)
	Listeria monocytogenes
	Aerobic gram-negative bacilli
	Neisseria gonorrhoeae
Chronic skin disorders, including recurrent infections	*S. aureus*
	Beta-hemolytic streptococci
Poor dental health, dental procedures	*Viridans group* streptococci (VGS)
	Nutritionally variant streptococci
	Abiotrophia defective
	Granulicatella spp.
	Gemella spp.
	HACEK organisms
Alcoholism, cirrhosis	*Bartonella* spp.
	Aeromonas spp.
	Listeria spp.
	Streptococcus pneumonia
	Beta-hemolytic streptococci
Burns	*S. aureus*
	Aerobic gram-negative bacilli, including *P. aeruginosa*
	Fungi
Diabetes mellitus	*S. aureus*
	Beta-hemolytic streptococci
	S. pneumoniae
Early (≤1 year) prosthetic valve placement	Coagulase-negative staphylococci
	S. aureus
	Aerobic gram-negative bacilli
	Fungi
	Corynebacterium spp.
	Legionella spp.
Late (>1 year) prosthetic valve placement	Coagulase-negative staphylococci
	S. aureus
	Viridans group streptococci
	Enterococcus spp.
	Fungi
	Corynebacterium spp.

TABLE 80.12 Epidemiologic Clues in Etiologic Diagnosis of Culture-Negative Endocarditis—cont'd

EPIDEMIOLOGIC FEATURE	COMMON MICROORGANISM
Dog or cat exposure	*Bartonella* spp.
	Pasteurella spp.
	Capnocytophaga spp.
Contact with contaminated milk or infected farm animals	*Brucella* spp.
	Coxiella burnetii
	Erysipelothrix spp.
Homeless, body lice	*Bartonella* spp.
HIV/AIDS	*Salmonella* spp.
	S. pneumonia
	S. aureus
Pneumonia, meningitis	*S. pneumoniae*
Solid-organ transplantation	*S. aureus*
	Aspergillus fumigatus
	Enterococcus spp.
	Candida spp.
Gastrointestinal lesions	*Streptococcus gallolyticus* (bovis)
	Enterococcus spp.
	Clostridium septicum

HACEK, Haemophilus spp., *Aggregatibacter* spp., *Cardiobacterium hominis, Eikenella corrodens,* and *Kingella* spp.; *HIV/AIDS,* human immunodeficiency virus infection and acquired immunodeficiency syndrome.
From Baddour LM, Wilson WR, Bayer AS, et al. Infective endocarditis in adults: diagnosis, antimicrobial therapy, and management of complications. A scientific statement for healthcare professionals from the American Heart Association. *Circulation.* 2015;132:1435–1486.

accounted for negative specimen (usually blood) cultures. In addition, an evaluation of blood and tissue should be done to determine if rare causes of endocarditis could account for a culture-negative presentation, particularly in patients who did not receive recent antimicrobial therapy. An evaluation of these rare causes of culture-negative endocarditis is outlined earlier.

Based on epidemiologic features and the most likely cadre of pathogens, a strategy for selection of antimicrobial therapy can be devised with input from an infectious diseases physician who has expertise in IE management. Considerations include the type of valve—native or prosthetic—and, with prosthetic valves, time since implantation of the valve. These regimens are necessarily broad to cover the most likely pathogens, which include the streptococci, staphylococci, enterococci, and HACEK organisms. Certain epidemiologic features may dictate broader coverage. The most troubling aspects of this approach are that the selected empiric therapy may not be adequate for a specific pathogen, and antimicrobials that would not be administered if the pathogen were identified will be given, with the potential for development of toxicity that may not be fully reversible.

Indications for and Timing of Surgery

The frequency with which surgery is used in the treatment of IE increased on average by 7% per decade between 1969 and 2000, with an attendant decrease in early mortality. In a recent study surgery for IE increased by 1.7-fold from 2011 to 2018 driven by drug use IE that increased 2.7-fold while non–drug use IE increased 1.4-fold (Geirsson et al).[7] In the current era, surgery is the mainstay of therapy for complicated IE. Current practice guidelines (largely based on observational series and expert opinion) advise that surgery should be considered in the presence of (1) HF, (2) features suggestive of a high risk of embolism, and (3) uncontrolled infection.[26,79] (See Tables 80G.3 and 80G.4 in the online chapter.) A review by Bannay and colleagues[80] demonstrated that early surgery led to significant improvements in survival after treatment for left-sided IE (adjusted HR for mortality, 0.55; 95% confidence interval [CI] 0.35 to 0.87;

P = 0.01). This benefit was further confirmed by a large, prospective, multinational study of the effect of early surgery on in-hospital mortality, accounting for treatment selection, survivorship, and hidden biases.[81] The investigators found that early surgery plus antimicrobial therapy (compared with medical management alone) was associated with a significant reduction in mortality in the overall cohort (12.1% versus 20.7%), as well as after propensity-based matching and adjustment for survivor bias (absolute risk reduction [ARR], −5.9%; *P* < 0.001). The results of these and other studies have led to management algorithms recommending the early consideration of surgical intervention after recognition of native valve IE.

Acute decompensated HF is the most frequently encountered reason for consideration of urgent surgical treatment. HF may be caused by severe regurgitation (aortic or mitral), intracardiac fistulas, or less often, vegetation-related valve obstruction. Emergent surgery for HF unresponsive to medical management is crucial, and swift intervention also is recommended, even if temporary stabilization of the patient can be achieved. Delayed surgery may be considered in the absence of HF after healing of acute endocarditic lesions, which in some circumstances may increase the likelihood of native valve repair.

Uncontrolled infection, the next most likely reason for surgical intervention, can be characterized broadly by increasing vegetation size, abscess formation, false aneurysms, or the creation of fistulas. Persistent fever frequently is associated with these anatomic findings. Early surgery is indicated in the setting of uncontrolled infection associated with persistent fever and positive blood cultures despite an appropriate antibiotic regimen, but surgery ideally should be delayed until after exclusion of extracardiac sources of infection. Perivalvular extension of infection is more common in aortic valve IE (10% to 40% in native valve IE and 56% to 100% in PVE). Some clinicians have noted that perivalvular abscesses most frequently occur in the posterior or lateral portions of the mitral annulus, whereas in aortic IE, extension can occur through the intervalvular fibrosa. The predictors of intervalvular fibrosa invasion include presence of a prosthetic valve (see Fig. 80.7), aortic location, and infection with coagulase-negative staphylococci. Pseudoaneurysms and fistula formation occur on average in 1.6% of cases and are more frequently related to *S. aureus* infection (46%). Other, less frequent manifestations of extension include ventricular septal defect, third-degree AVB, and acute coronary syndrome. Urgent surgery generally is recommended to treat perivalvular extension of infection (except in rare circumstances) and in cases of IE due to fungi, MDR organisms, and gram-negative bacteria. In general, perivalvular extension or infection with aggressive microorganisms warrants early surgery in the absence of severe comorbid disease that would otherwise be prognosis-limiting.

IE-related embolism is common (20% to 50% of cases) and can be fatal. Occult embolism may occur in approximately 20% of patients. A 2007 report indicated that the risk of embolism was highest in the first week after initiation of antibiotic therapy (4.8/1000 patient-days) and decreases thereafter (1.7/1000 patient-days).[82] Some experts therefore suggest that the greatest benefit to patient survival is the prevention of systemic embolization, which can best be realized during the first week of antibiotic therapy.

The exact timing of surgical intervention for embolism prevention should be based on the presence or absence of previous embolic events, other complications of IE, size and mobility of the vegetation, likelihood of conservative surgery (valve repair), and duration of antibiotic therapy.[80] Ultimately, extrapolation of surgical benefits also must consider factors of patient viability, comorbid conditions, potential consequences of conservative management, and patient preferences.

Surgery generally is recommended in the presence of large, mobile vegetations (>10 mm),[69] particularly after an embolic event occurring during treatment with appropriate antibiotics. Even if embolization has not occurred, the presence of HF, severe valvular dysfunction, persistent infection despite appropriate antibiotic therapy, or perivalvular abscess plus a large vegetation (>10 mm) constitutes an indication for earlier surgery. Only one small, randomized trial has evaluated the role of valve surgery in IE management.[69] Patients underwent valve surgery within 48 hours of randomization.

There were several exclusion criteria for enrollment, and patients had left-sided IE, severe valvular regurgitation without HF, and vegetations larger than 10 mm to be included in the study. Valve surgery patients had fewer embolic events in follow-up, but other outcome measures, including mortality and infection relapse rates, did not differ between the two groups (each with <40 patients).

When an indication for early surgical intervention is met, the next issue becomes the risk of surgery in the context of the illness and manifest complications, most importantly, neurologic complications. When an indication for surgical management is present, the timing of surgery is an important consideration. The European and U.S. guidelines on management of infective endocarditis differ on their definitions regarding surgical timing. In the European Society of Cardiology (ESC) guidelines, surgical timing is defined as either emergent (within 24 hours), urgent (within a few days) or elective (after 1 to 2 weeks of antibiotic therapy).[8,24] Despite these differences, both guidelines recommend avoiding a delay in surgical management of IE in the setting of progressive HF, uncontrolled infection, and prevention of embolism. Evidence for timing of surgical management of IE came from a randomized clinical trial from South Korea in which patients with left-sided, native valve endocarditis and severe valve disease with large vegetations were assigned to either early surgery (defined as within 48 hours of randomization) or conventional treatment.[69] The primary outcome was a composite of in-hospital death or embolic events within 6 weeks of randomization. Among the patients in the conventional treatment arm, 77% underwent surgery either at some point during the hospitalization or in follow up. Those who underwent early surgery had a significant reduction in the composite endpoint (HR 0.10; 95% CI, 0.01 to 0.82; *P* = 0.03). The benefit of early surgery was confirmed by other observational studies, one of which used propensity score matching to show that patients with native valve endocarditis who had surgery during index hospitalization had lower in-hospital mortality than those treated medically.[51]

A unique challenge is surgical timing in patients with prior stroke, especially hemorrhagic stroke, as postsurgical mortality in these patients is high in the first 4 weeks. In a retrospective analysis of a cohort of patients with left-sided endocarditis, patients with brain hemorrhage had a higher mortality when surgery was performed within 4 weeks as compared with delayed surgery.[83] The recommendation from the AHA guidelines states that it is reasonable to delay surgical intervention for at least 4 weeks in patients with major stroke or intracranial hemorrhage (ICH).[8]

Despite a progressive emphasis on earlier surgical intervention in distinct subgroups of patients with IE, a significant proportion still do not receive surgery even in the absence of stroke. In a prospective cohort of 863 patients with left-sided endocarditis and an indication for cardiac surgery, 24% did not undergo surgery with stroke being cited as the reason in nearly a quarter of cases.[84] Several risk score models are available to assist with the decision regarding surgical management,[85,86] and worse outcomes were present in older patients with multiple comorbidities including diabetes and renal disease.

Considerable debate surrounds the performance of surgical intervention with a history of recent neurologic embolization. Iung and coauthors[87] systematically performed cerebral and abdominal MRI in early IE and found neurologic lesions in 82% of cases (ischemic lesions in 25, microbleeds in 32, and silent aneurysms in 6), and abdominal lesions in 20 patients (34%). Of importance, these findings led to modifications of classification and/or therapy in 28% of patients. Rossi and colleagues[88] detailed a best-evidence summary of whether there is an ideal time for surgery in IE with cerebrovascular complications, including ICH, ruptured mycotic aneurysm, TIA, meningitis, encephalopathy, and brain abscess. The investigators recommended 1 to 2 weeks of antibiotic treatment before cardiac surgery is indicated. However, earlier surgery is indicated in HF (class I, level of evidence [LOE]: B) and uncontrolled infection (class I, LOE: B) and for prevention of embolic events (class I, LOE: B/C). After stroke, surgery should not be delayed in the absence of coma and once cerebral hemorrhage has been excluded by cranial CT (class IIa LOE: B). After a TIA or a silent cerebral embolism, surgery is recommended without delay (class I, LOE: B). After diagnosis of ICH, surgery should ideally be postponed for at least

1 month (class I, LOE: C). In the case of surgery for PVE, the general principles outlined for native valve IE should be followed. Every patient should have a repeated head CT scan immediately before the operation to rule out preoperative hemorrhagic transformation of a brain infarction. Presence of a hematoma warrants neurosurgical consultation and consideration of cerebral angiography to rule out a mycotic aneurysm.

Medical therapy in the setting of right-sided native valve IE is the mainstay of treatment, and surgical intervention most often can be deferred in the absence of (1) diuretic-resistant right-sided HF associated with severe tricuspid regurgitation, (2) fastidious organisms resistant to antimicrobial treatment (i.e., fungemia or persistent bacteremia for >7 days), or (3) vegetations larger than 20 mm in diameter associated with multiple pulmonary emboli and possible right-sided HF.

Surgical Intervention

Before surgical intervention, several considerations in addition to the confirmation of appropriate antibiotic therapy are important. First, coronary artery assessment using either cardiac catheterization or CT angiography is recommended, to ascertain whether concomitant coronary revascularization is necessary. Before the performance of cardiac surgery, identification of primary or secondary extracardiac sites of infection should be undertaken, and extirpation should be performed if practically possible.

The primary principles guiding surgical management of IE are (1) excision of infected material along with sterilization of remaining tissue and instruments, followed by (2) reconstruction of cardiac or valve structures to permit normal heart function. Valve repair almost always is a favored option in the treatment of valvular IE.[85] If the extent of débridement necessary to eradicate infection precludes valve reconstruction, prosthetic valve replacement may be necessary.

The specific techniques used are tailored to the anatomy encountered at operation. Perforations in a valve cusp or leaflet are reconstructed using pericardial patch or other matrix substances. In general, the use of prosthetic material should be minimized; however, in settings where valve replacement is required, consensus documents do not routinely recommend one particular valve substitute over another (i.e., mechanical vs. biologic).[89]

Reports have varied regarding frequency of mitral valve repair procedures. Data from one investigation suggest that mitral valve IE can be repaired in up to 80% of patients, particularly by experienced teams at referral centers.[90] Mitral valve repair in the United States was performed in only 25.8% of patients requiring valve surgery in one large, multicenter experience that included both IDU and non-IDU with IE.[7] A combination of traditional valvuloplasty techniques is utilized,[91] and results are assessed by intraoperative TEE (Table 80.13). Although theoretically appealing, mitral valve homografts and pulmonary autografts have failed to gain widespread acceptance.

In the setting of acute IE, mechanical or biologic (xenograft) aortic valve replacement may be required, with few early demonstrated differences between device types.[92,93] Homografts or stentless root xenograft conduits are selectively used to reconstruct severely affected aortic sinuses, repair abscess-related destruction, or correct aortoventricular discontinuity.[94]

Postsurgical outcomes depend on the etiologic microorganism, the extent of tissue destruction, the presence of systolic or diastolic HF, and comorbid conditions. Early operative mortality ranges between 5% and 15%.[95] A 2008 report suggested that surgery within the first week of antibiotic therapy is associated with in-hospital mortality rate of 15%, and the main predictor was periannular extension of disease; risk of recurrent IE was 12%.[96] With isolated infection of leaflets or cusps (particularly in the subacute/chronic phase), early mortality is lower and approaches that seen in normal valve repair and replacement surgery.

Postoperative complications in this high-risk patient population typically include profound intraoperative coagulopathy necessitating mediastinal reexploration, acute renal failure, stroke, low cardiac output, pneumonia, and AVB necessitating pacemaker implantation.[86,95,97]

Outpatient Management and Follow-Up Evaluation

Antimicrobial treatment of IE is done in the outpatient setting once microbiologic control of infection is obtained, and after surgical or other interventions, if required, are completed and clinical recovery is observed.[8] Parenteral therapy is delivered in a variety of settings, related in part to the individual patient's health care coverage; often, therapy is done in a patient's home by a family member who has received instruction regarding (usually) IV infusions. Serial laboratory monitoring for evidence of drug-related toxicity and serum concentrations of drugs, when applicable, is mandatory and can be accomplished in a variety of settings, including home health agencies, primary care offices, and infectious diseases clinics. Monitoring also includes serial visits with an experienced clinician to assess clinical status and evidence of drug tolerance and complications related to an indwelling venous catheter. As outlined earlier, beta-lactam antibiotics frequently are used in the treatment of IE caused by a variety of bacterial infections. These agents are well recognized to have various adverse effects, including diarrhea, which may or may not be caused by *Clostridioides difficile* infection, as well as rash, fever, neutropenia, and less often, hepatobiliary or renal toxicities.

Once parenteral antimicrobial therapy is completed (Table 80.14), the indwelling venous catheter should be removed because it can be a nidus of subsequent infection or of other, noninfectious complications, unless there is another need for the device. At completion of therapy, an echocardiogram should be obtained to serve as a baseline (see Table 80.6), because patients who have had an initial bout of IE, regardless of whether or not the valve was replaced, are at high risk for subsequent IE relapse or recurrence. Consultation with a cardiologist should determine whether TTE versus TEE is preferred. Daily dental hygiene and dental visits should be done to promote dental health.

Patients and their family members should be educated about aspects of IE,[8] in particular the importance of obtaining three sets of blood culture specimens if the patient develops fever any time in the future before taking any antibiotic. The critical aspect of securing multiple sets of blood cultures before initiating antibiotic therapy cannot be overemphasized. If a bloodstream infection is confirmed as the cause of the fever, an evaluation for relapsing or recurrent IE is necessary, which generally will include TEE in the evaluation for a source of the infection, in addition to initiating treatment for infection.

For PWID with IE, it is critical that addiction medicine consultation be obtained, preferably before hospital discharge, because these patients are at increased risk of recurrent IE with poorer outcomes, including mortality.[98]

TABLE 80.13 Frequency and Types of Operative Procedures in Patients with and Without Drug Use

VARIABLE	OVERALL (N = 34,905)	DRUG USE (N = 11,756)	NO DRUG USE (N = 23,149)	P-VALUE
First cardiovascular surgery	25,782 (73.9%)	9,654 (82.1%)	16,128 (69.7%)	<0.001
Aortic valve procedure	19,854 (56.9%)	5,253 (44.7%)	14,601 (63.1%)	<0.001
Mitral valve procedure	16,808 (48.2%)	4,636 (39.4%)	12,172 (52.6%)	<0.001
Tricuspid valve procedure	6,982 (20.0%)	4,624 (39.3%)	2,358 (10.2%)	<0.001
Pulmonary valve procedure	281 (0.8%)	138 (1.2%)	143 (0.6%)	<0.001
Multiple valve procedures	8,195 (23.5%)	2,621 (22.3%)	5,574 (24.1%)	

TABLE 80.14 Patient Care During and After Completion of Antimicrobial Treatment

Initiation Before or at Completion of Therapy
Echocardiography to establish new baseline
Drug rehabilitation referral for patients who use illicit injection drugs
Education on the signs of endocarditis and need for antibiotic prophylaxis for certain dental/surgical/invasive procedures
Thorough dental evaluation and treatment if not performed earlier in evaluation
Prompt removal of intravenous catheter at completion of antimicrobial therapy
Short-Term Follow-Up
At least three sets of blood cultures from separate sites for any febrile illness and before initiation of antibiotic therapy
Physical examination for evidence of heart failure
Evaluation for toxicity resulting from current/previous antimicrobial therapy
Long-Term Follow-Up
At least three sets of blood cultures from separate sites for any febrile illness and before initiation of antibiotic therapy
Evaluation of valvular and ventricular function (echocardiography)
Scrupulous oral hygiene and frequent dental professional office visits

From Baddour LM, Wilson WR, Bayer AS, et al. Infective endocarditis in adults: diagnosis, antimicrobial therapy, and management of complications. A scientific statement for healthcare professionals from the American Heart Association. *Circulation.* 2015;132:1435–1486.

CARDIOVASCULAR IMPLANTABLE ELECTRONIC DEVICE INFECTIONS

The number of patients with CIEDs has dramatically increased over the past two decades, and this trend will continue as the indications for their use expand (see Chapters 58 and 69) and the population continues to age. With this expansion of CIED placement, a concomitant increase in infections of these devices has been documented.[99–101] The accompanying morbidity, mortality, and financial burden from CIED infection have been substantial.

Epidemiology

Several database surveys suggest that the rate of CIED infection has increased more than the rate of device implantation.[101–103] Factors associated with increased CIED infection risk include device placement in older patients and those with more comorbidities (particularly renal failure), more leads placed per patient, increased need for device revision or replacement, and complications at the pocket site after device placement or revision, particularly hematoma formation and delayed or poor wound healing. Factors that reduce the likelihood of device infection include the administration of surgical site prophylaxis at the time of device placement or revision and a higher volume of devices implanted by the physician performing the procedure.

Clinical Syndromes

The most common presentation of CIED infections is that of erosion and/or inflammatory changes at the shoulder generator pocket site, with or without systemic manifestations of infection.[102] For others, systemic manifestations of infection prompt clinical evaluation with or without local findings of infection at the pocket site. Pulmonary manifestations, including pleuritic pain, lung infiltrates, and lung abscess, can develop. In addition, cardiac and peripheral stigmata of IE occur in patients with CIED infection, and there may be associated valve infection.

Microbiology

Staphylococcal species predominate as causes of CIED infection, accounting for 60% to 80% of infections in most series.[99–103] Both *S. aureus* and coagulase-negative staphylococci are common pathogens

and often are oxacillin resistant. Other gram-positive cocci, including streptococcal and enterococcal species, can cause CIED infection. Aerobic gram-negative bacilli and fungi are identified as pathogens in only a small minority of cases. Rarely, nontuberculous mycobacteria have been identified as causes of CIED infection.

Pathogenesis

Device infection pathogenesis involves the interactions of device, pathogen, and host.[103] Regarding the host, risk factors associated with infection have been outlined previously. For both the device and the pathogen, certain characteristics may not be unique to CIED infection but are considered operative in all types of device infections. Important among the pathogen-related mechanisms is biofilm formation. Bacteria and yeasts can attach and accumulate on the surface of a device, with eventual formation of a layer of organisms and amorphous material that harbors living organisms, able in this setting to evade normal host immune response and antimicrobial therapy. In addition to the mechanical barrier of the biofilm, organisms that accumulate in biofilms in this setting may alter their metabolic activities, protecting them from the static and cidal effects of certain antimicrobials.

On the basis of the proven efficacy of surgical site prophylaxis at CIED implantation, most CIED infections are believed to result from bacterial or fungal contamination of the device at placement. A less frequent mode of device contamination is lead infection occurring as a complication of bloodstream infection from an ectopic nidus such as an infected intravascular catheter.

Ongoing investigations are examining the surface components and physical and chemical aspects of a device and how those features interact with a pathogen's cell surface structures to either enhance or inhibit initial organism adherence to the device. Elucidation of mechanisms of initial pathogen adherence could lead to the development of devices that are more resistant to infection. Moreover, adjunctive therapies that could be administered at device placement or as vaccines before device placement may become available in the future to further reduce infection risks.

Diagnosis

The diagnosis of CIED infection is straightforward in cases where percutaneous device erosion has occurred or purulent drainage is present at a pocket site. Erythema, swelling, and pain at the pocket site also indicate infection. Distinguishing local findings due to early postoperative healing versus those due to infection can sometimes be challenging and may require serial patient examinations to determine the etiology of the local manifestations.

Blood cultures should be obtained in all cases of CIED infection, including those with clinical manifestations limited to the pocket site. The possibility of CIED infection should be considered in all patients with bloodstream infection. In patients with positive blood cultures, TEE should be performed. The sensitivity of TEE in detecting lead- and valve-related infection is superior to that of TTE.[99,100] A documented limitation of TEE, however, is that lead infection can occur with no abnormalities detected on the TEE image. Moreover, TEE identifies clots on leads in 5% to 10% of patients who have no infection. In select cases of CIED-IE, PET/CT may be helpful where pocket infection is not apparent and no alternative source of bloodstream infection is identified.

Ultimately, intraoperative findings and Gram staining and culture of deep pocket tissue and device samples obtained at complete device removal are useful in confirming CIED infection.

Management

A primary tenet of management of CIED infection includes complete device removal, if infection cure is the goal.[100,104] Despite the well-recognized risks of lead extraction,[104,105] it is essential to reduce the likelihood of relapsing infection. A management algorithm has been developed to assist in the care of patients with CIED infections (Figs. 80.9 and 80.10). Duration of antimicrobial therapy is based on the clinical syndrome of CIED infection and the identified pathogen. The recommended duration of antimicrobial therapy for the different infection syndromes is

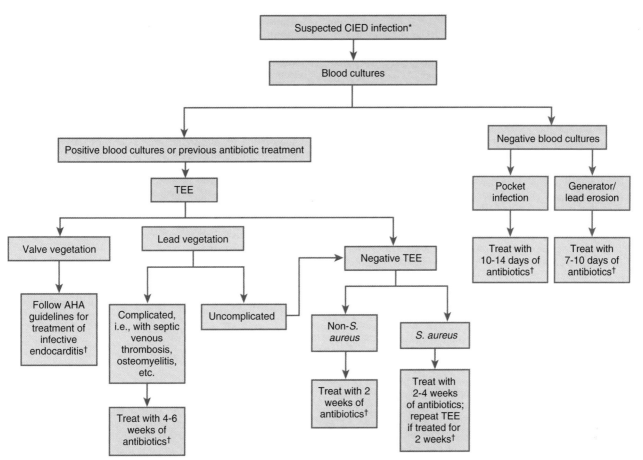

FIGURE 80.9 Approach to management of adults with cardiovascular implantable electronic device (CIED) infection. *A history, physical examination, chest radiograph, electrocardiogram, and echocardiographic device interrogation are standard baseline procedures before CIED removal. †Duration of antibiotics should be counted from the day of device explantation. Treatment can be extended to 4 or more weeks in the setting of metastatic septic complications (i.e., osteomyelitis, organ or deep abscess) or sustained bloodstream infection despite CIED removal. *AHA,* American Heart Association; *TEE,* transesophageal echocardiography. (Modified from Sohail MR, Uslan DZ, Khan AH, et al. Management and outcome of permanent pacemaker and implantable cardioverter-defibrillator infections. *J Am Coll Cardiol.* 2007;49:1851.)

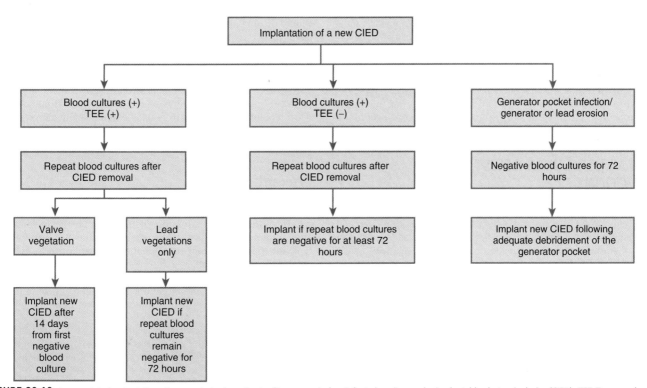

FIGURE 80.10 Approach to implantation of a new device in patients after removal of an infected cardiovascular implantable electronic device (CIED). *TEE,* Transesophageal echocardiography. (Modified from Sohail MR, Uslan DZ, Khan AH, et al. Management and outcome of permanent pacemaker and implantable cardioverter-defibrillator infections. *J Am Coll Cardiol.* 2007;49:1851.)

1528

not evidence based. Moreover, no evidence-based data are available to indicate the preferred route of therapy. In cases with complications such as valvular IE, duration of therapy can extend for 6 weeks or longer.

The optimal timing of new device placement is undefined. Each patient should undergo individualized assessment to determine the need for a new device. Some experts have advocated that a new device can be implanted 72 hours after removal of the infected device, provided that blood cultures are negative, no valvular IE is present, and control of infection at the pocket site is secured.[100,102]

Management of patients with bloodstream infection as the *sole* manifestation of an infection is more difficult.[100] In such patients a thorough evaluation, including TEE, identifies no nidus responsible for bloodstream infection. The obvious concern is that either the CIED is infected and serves as a source of bloodstream infection, or the bloodstream infection could secondarily infect the CIED. Decisions regarding device removal are complex. If the device is not removed, relapsing bloodstream infection is inevitable once antimicrobial therapy is completed, if the device is the source of bloodstream infection. Conversely, if the CIED is removed but was not infected, the patient was exposed to the risk and complications of device removal without benefit, as well as incurring considerable expense for the procedure.

Prophylaxis

Prospective, placebo-controlled, clinical trials and case-control and meta-analysis studies[106] consistently indicate that the preoperative administration of an antistaphylococcal antibiotic, usually cefazolin, given intravenously 30 to 60 minutes before device placement or revision, is effective in reducing the risk of CIED infection. If vancomycin is deemed a more appropriate choice, the IV administration should begin 2 hours before the procedure. Subsequent postoperative dosing is not recommended with either cefazolin or vancomycin.

Two "prevention" trials deserve particular comment. The PADIT examined a regimen that included preprocedural cefazolin *plus* vancomycin, intraoperative bacitracin pocket wash, and a 2-day postprocedural oral cephalexin course and demonstrated no benefit of this incremental treatment strategy in reducing CIED infections as compared with that of conventional single-dose, preprocedural cefazolin.[107] The WRAP-IT evaluated an antibacterial envelope that was placed at the time of generator implantation of CIED.[108] Major device infections were reduced as compared with that of standard prophylaxis measures and the envelope, which was absorbable, was well tolerated.

Antimicrobial prophylaxis is not recommended for patients with CIEDs who undergo invasive procedures, such as dental, GI, or GU procedures, because evidence-based data indicating that such procedures carry a risk of CIED infection are lacking. The predominance of staphylococci as the agents of CIED infection suggests that these invasive procedures probably are not responsible for device infection, and "secondary" prophylaxis is not warranted.

LEFT VENTRICULAR ASSIST DEVICE INFECTIONS

Major advances in the technologic aspects of LV assist devices (LVADs) have been pivotal in impacting patient survival,[109,110] and the demand for these devices continues to grow in the United States (see Chapter 59). Not surprisingly, device infection occurs in patients with LVADs and will continue to be a major complication of LVAD use as long as it remains a percutaneous device. The most dramatic change in infection risk among cardiac devices may be that associated with LVADs. Infection risks have fallen, largely because of improvements in device design, including reduction in size.

Characterizing the incidence, epidemiology, and risk factors associated with LVAD infections is difficult because of the striking design changes in these devices since their inception.[109,110] The first-generation, pulsatile-flow, volume-displacement devices, including Novacor, Heartmate XVE, and other Thoratec devices, have been associated with higher rates of infection than the more recently reported rates with the second-generation, continuous-flow devices, including Heartmate II, VentrAssist, and MicroMed DeBakey.

Three categories of LVAD infections have been identified based on the portion of the device that is infected. These designations are somewhat arbitrary, however, because infection can involve more than one portion of an LVAD. The most common presentation is that of driveline infection. Erythema and drainage at the driveline site, with or without systemic manifestations of infection, usually are present.

Pump pocket infection is a second infection presentation and can be a complication of driveline infection. Local pain or discomfort with systemic manifestations is present, and abnormal fluid collection is demonstrated on ultrasound examination or CT. Fluid aspiration or surgical drainage procedures yield purulent material.

LVAD-associated IE is the least often diagnosed of the three presentations, but some cases may go undiagnosed (or may be diagnosed only at autopsy) because diagnostic tools such as TEE lack sensitivity. This diagnosis should be considered in all patients with sustained bloodstream infection and no other cardiovascular device that could serve as a nidus for sustained bacteremia or fungemia.

Microbiology

Staphylococcal species are the predominant causes of LVAD infection,[109,110] and oxacillin resistance is common. Less often, a panoply of other bacteria, encompassing enterococci (including VRE) and *Pseudomonas* spp., and fungi (*Candida* spp.) are identified as pathogens. Treatment options, particularly as oral therapy, usually are limited because of the MDR profiles of these pathogens.

Management

The medical management of LVAD infections is difficult. Ideally, the device would be completely removed, but this approach requires surgical intervention and is associated with considerable morbidity and mortality. Therefore antimicrobial therapy is the mainstay of management and often is used for prolonged periods on a recurrent basis. In addition, antimicrobial selection is difficult because of the characteristic multidrug resistance of infecting pathogens and the underlying comorbidities that increase the likelihood of drug toxicity (e.g., chronic renal failure and colistin or aminoglycoside use for MDR *Pseudomonas aeruginosa* infection).

Regardless of site of device infection, blood culture specimens should be obtained in every case of LVAD infection. Positive blood cultures can occur in patients without systemic signs of infection and can indicate the presence of a more complicated infection (e.g., IE rather than only driveline infection) or infection of another cardiovascular device, such as a prosthetic valve or CIED.

A variety of surgical interventions are used in the management of LVAD infection. Such interventions range from local soft tissue débridement for driveline infection to heart transplantation with LVAD removal in an effort to control refractory LVAD endocarditis and its associated complications.

Prevention

Placebo-controlled trials indicating the efficacy of antibiotic prophylaxis at LVAD placement (surgical site prophylaxis) are lacking. Nevertheless, the adoption of this practice is universal,[109,110] and multiple (up to five) antimicrobials often are administered, typically including some combination of vancomycin, rifampin, cefepime, ciprofloxacin, and fluconazole. The duration of antimicrobial prophylaxis after LVAD implantation also has varied widely, with 24 hours as a minimal duration. In some centers, nasal mupirocin also is used for a variable duration both before and after LVAD implantation.

Meticulous daily care at the driveline exit site is advocated. Patient and family education and serial visits with specialized caregivers are critical in infection prevention and in securing an early diagnosis.

GUIDELINES

The Guidelines for Infective Endocarditis are in the online chapter.

REFERENCES

Epidemiology

1. Tleyjeh IM, Abdel-Latif A, Rahbi H, et al. A systematic review of population-based studies of infective endocarditis. *Chest*. 2007;132:1025–1035.
2. de Sa DDC, Tleyjeh IM, Anavekar NS, et al. Epidemiological trends of infective endocarditis: a population-based study in Olmsted County, Minnesota. *Mayo Clin Proc*. 2010;85:422–426.
3. Keller K, Hobohm L, Munzel T, Ostad MA. Incidence of infective endocarditis before and after the guideline modification regarding a more restrictive use of prophylactic antibiotics therapy in the USA and Europe. *Minerva Cardioangiol*. 2019;67:200–206.
4. Schranz AJ, Fleischauer A, Chu VH, et al. Trends in drug use-associated infective endocarditis and heart valve surgery, 2007 to 2017: a study of statewide discharge data. *Ann Intern Med*. 2019;170:31–40.
5. Siegman-Igra Y, Koifman B, Porat R, et al. Healthcare associated infective endocarditis: a distinct entity. *Scand J Infect Dis*. 2008;40:474–480.
6. Fedeli U, Schievano E, Buonfrate D, et al. Increasing incidence and mortality of infective endocarditis: a population-based study through a record-linkage system. *BMC Infect Dis*. 2011;11:48.
7. Geirsson A, Schranz A, Jawitz O, et al. The evolving burden of drug use associated infective endocarditis in the United States. *Ann Thorac Surg*. 2020;110(4):1185–1192.

Pathophysiology, Presentation, and Diagnosis

8. Baddour LM, Wilson WR, Bayer AS, et al. Infective endocarditis in adults: diagnosis, antimicrobial therapy, and management of complications: a scientific statement for healthcare professionals from the American Heart Association. *Circulation*. 2015;132:1435–1486.
9. Murdoch DR, Corey GR, Hoen B, et al. Clinical presentation, etiology, and outcome of infective endocarditis in the 21st century: the international collaboration on endocarditis–prospective cohort study. *Arch Int Med*. 2009;169:463–473.
10. Li JS, Sexton DJ, Mick N, et al. Proposed modifications to the Duke criteria for the diagnosis of infective endocarditis. *Clin Infect Dis*. 2000;30:633–638.
11. Holland TL, Baddour LM, Bayer AS, et al. Infective endocarditis. *Nat Rev Dis Primers*. 2016;2:16059.
12. Katan O, Michelena HI, Avierinos J-F, et al. Incidence and predictors of infective endocarditis in mitral valve prolapse: a population-based study. *Mayo Clin Proc*. 2016;91:336–342.
13. Tzemos N, Therrien J, Yip J, et al. Outcomes in adults with bicuspid aortic valves. *J Am Med Assoc*. 2008;300:1317–1325.
14. Michelena HI, Desjardins VA, Avierinos JF, et al. Natural history of asymptomatic patients with normally functioning or minimally dysfunctional bicuspid aortic valve in the community. *Circulation*. 2008;117:2776–2784.
15. Tribouilloy C, Rusinaru D, Sorel C, et al. Clinical characteristics and outcome of infective endocarditis in adults with bicuspid aortic valves: a multicentre observational study. *Heart*. 2010;96:1723–1729.
16. Kahveci G, Bayrak F, Pala S, et al. Impact of bicuspid aortic valve on complications and death in infective endocarditis of native aortic valves. *Tex Heart Inst J*. 2009;36:111–116.
17. Durante-Mangoni E, Bradley S, Selton-Suty C, et al. Current features of infective endocarditis in elderly patients: results of the international collaboration on endocarditis prospective cohort study. *Arch Intern Med*. 2008;168:2095–2103.
18. Sun BJ, Choi S-W, Park K-H, et al. Infective endocarditis involving apparently structurally normal valves in patients without previously recognized predisposing heart disease. *J Am Coll Cardiol*. 2015;65:307–309.
19. Lopez J, Revilla A, Vilacosta I, et al. Age-dependent profile of left-sided infective endocarditis: a 3-center experience. *Circulation*. 2010;121:892–897.
20. Knirsch W, Nadal D. Infective endocarditis in congenital heart disease. *Eur J Pediatr*. 2011;170:1111.
21. Duval X, Delahaye F, Alla F, et al. Temporal trends in infective endocarditis in the context of prophylaxis guideline modifications: three successive population-based surveys. *J Am Coll Cardiol*. 2012;59:1968–1976.
22. Benito N, Miró JM, de Lazzari E, et al. Health care–associated native valve endocarditis: importance of non-nosocomial acquisition. *Ann Intern Med*. 2009;150:586–594.
23. Delahaye F, M'Hammedi A, Guerpillon B, et al. Systematic search for present and potential portals of entry for infective endocarditis. *J Am Coll Cardiol*. 2016;67:151–158.
24. Sohail MR, Uslan DZ, Khan AH, et al. Infective endocarditis complicating permanent pacemaker and implantable cardioverter-defibrillator infection. *Mayo Clin Proc*. 2008;83:46–53.
25. Athan E, Chu VH, Tattevin P, et al. Clinical characteristics and outcome of infective endocarditis involving implantable cardiac devices. *J Am Med Assoc*. 2012;307:1727–1735.
26. Habib G, Lancellotti P, Antunes MJ, et al. 2015 ESC guidelines for the management of infective endocarditis: the task Force for the management of infective endocarditis of the European Society of Cardiology (ESC) endorsed by: European Association for Cardio-Thoracic Surgery (EACTS), The European Association of Nuclear Medicine (EANM). *Eur Heart J*. 2015;36:3075–3128.
27. López J, Fernández-Hidalgo N, Revilla A, et al. Internal and external validation of a model to predict adverse outcomes in patients with left-sided infective endocarditis. *Heart (British Cardiac Society)*. 2011;97:1138–1142.
28. Nadji G, Rusinaru D, Rémadi J-P, et al. Heart failure in left-sided native valve infective endocarditis: characteristics, prognosis, and results of surgical treatment. *Eur J Heart Fail*. 2009;11:668–675.
29. Muñoz P, Kestler M, De Alarcon A, et al. Current epidemiology and outcome of infective endocarditis: a multicenter, prospective, cohort study. *Medicine*. 2015;94:e1816.
30. Hill EE, Herijgers P, Claus P, et al. Infective endocarditis: changing epidemiology and predictors of 6-month mortality: a prospective cohort study. *Eur Heart J*. 2007;28:196–203.
31. Wang A, Athan E, Pappas PA, et al. Contemporary clinical profile and outcome of prosthetic valve endocarditis. *J Am Med Assoc*. 2007;297:1354–1361.
32. López J, Revilla A, Vilacosta I, et al. Definition, clinical profile, microbiological spectrum, and prognostic factors of early-onset prosthetic valve endocarditis. *Eur Heart J*. 2007;28:760–765.
33. Hill EE, Herregods M-C, Vanderschueren S, et al. Management of prosthetic valve infective endocarditis. *Am J Cardiol*. 2008;101:1174–1178.
34. Que Y-A, Moreillon P. Infective endocarditis. *Nat Rev Cardiol*. 2011;8:322–336.
35. Sy RW, Chawantanpipat C, Richmond DR, Kritharides L. Development and validation of a time-dependent risk model for predicting mortality in infective endocarditis. *Eur Heart J*. 2009;32:2016–2026.
36. Yu C-W, Juan L-I, Hsu S-C, et al. Role of procalcitonin in the diagnosis of infective endocarditis: a meta-analysis. *Am J Emerg Med*. 2013;31:935–941.
37. Snipsøyr MG, Ludvigsen M, Petersen E, et al. A systematic review of biomarkers in the diagnosis of infective endocarditis. *Int J Cardiol*. 2016;202:564–570.
38. Tsenovoy P, Aronow WS, Joseph J, Kopacz MS. Patients with infective endocarditis and increased cardiac troponin I levels have a higher incidence of in-hospital mortality and valve replacement than those with normal cardiac troponin I levels. *Cardiology*. 2009;112:202–204.
39. Stancoven AB, Shiue AB, Khera A, et al. Association of troponin T, detected with highly sensitive assay, and outcomes in infective endocarditis. *Am J Cardiol*. 2011;108:416–420.
40. Shiue AB, Stancoven AB, Purcell JB, et al. Relation of level of B-type natriuretic peptide with outcomes in patients with infective endocarditis. *Am J Cardiol*. 2010;106:1011–1015.
41. Kahveci G, Bayrak F, Mutlu B, et al. Prognostic value of N-terminal pro-B-type natriuretic peptide in patients with active infective endocarditis. *Am J Cardiol*. 2007;99:1429–1433.
42. Ferrera C, Vilacosta I, Fernández C, et al. Usefulness of new-onset atrial fibrillation, as a strong predictor of heart failure and death in patients with native left-sided infective endocarditis. *Am J Cardiol*. 2016;117:427–433.
43. Tornos P, Gonzalez-Alujas T, Thuny F, Habib G. Infective endocarditis: the European viewpoint. *Curr Prob Cardiol*. 2011;36:175–222.

Echocardiography

44. Casella F, Rana B, Casazza G, et al. The potential impact of contemporary transthoracic echocardiography on the management of patients with native valve endocarditis: a comparison with transesophageal echocardiography. *Echocardiography*. 2009;26:900–906.
45. Habib G, Badano L, Tribouilloy C, et al. Recommendations for the practice of echocardiography in infective endocarditis. *Eur J Echo*. 2010;11:202–219.
46. Hansalia S, Biswas M, Dutta R, et al. The value of live/real time three-dimensional transesophageal echocardiography in the assessment of valvular vegetations. *Echocardiography*. 2009;26:1264–1273.
47. Amat-Santos IJ, Messika-Zeitoun D, Eltchaninoff H, et al. Infective endocarditis after transcatheter aortic valve implantation. *Circulation*. 2015;131:1566–1574.
48. Latib A, Naim C, De Bonis M, et al. TAVR-associated prosthetic valve infective endocarditis: results of a large, multicenter registry. *J Am Coll Cardiol*. 2014;64:2176–2178.
49. Banchs J, Yusuf SW. Echocardiographic evaluation of cardiac infections. *Expert Rev Cardiovasc Ther*. 2012;10:1–4.
50. Román JS, Vilacosta I, Zamorano J, et al. Transesophageal echocardiography in right-sided endocarditis. *J Am Coll Cardiol*. 1993;21:1226–1230.
51. Kiefer T, Park L, Tribouilloy C, et al. Association between valvular surgery and mortality among patients with infective endocarditis complicated by heart failure. *J Am Med Assoc*. 2011;306:2239–2247.
52. Lauridsen TK, Park L, Tong SYC, et al. Echocardiographic findings predict in-hospital and 1-year mortality in left-sided native valve *Staphylococcus aureus* endocarditis. *Circ Cardiovasc Imag*. 2015;8:e003397.
53. Hill EE, Herijgers P, Claus P, et al. Abscess in infective endocarditis: the value of transesophageal echocardiography and outcome: a 5-year study. *Am Heart J*. 2007;154:923–928.
54. Showler A, Burry L, Bai AD, et al. Use of transthoracic echocardiography in the management of low-risk staphylococcus aureus bacteremia: results from a retrospective multicenter cohort study. *JACC Cardiovasc Imaging*. 2015;8:924–931.
55. Palraj BR, Baddour LM, Hess EP, et al. Predicting Risk of Endocarditis Using a Clinical Tool (PREDICT): scoring system to guide use of echocardiography in the management of Staphylococcus aureus bacteremia. *Clin Infect Dis*. 2015;61:18–28.
56. Tubiana S, Duval X, Alla F, et al. The VIRSTA score, a prediction score to estimate risk of infective endocarditis and determine priority for echocardiography in patients with Staphylococcus aureus bacteremia. *J Infect*. 2016;72:544–553.
57. Barton TL, Mottram PM, Stuart RL, et al. Transthoracic echocardiography is still useful in the initial evaluation of patients with suspected infective endocarditis: evaluation of a large cohort at a tertiary referral center. *Mayo Clin Proc*. 2014;89:799–805.

Complications

58. Snygg-Martin U, Rasmussen RV, Hassager C, et al. The relationship between cerebrovascular complications and previously established use of antiplatelet therapy in left-sided infective endocarditis. *Scand J Infect Dis*. 2011;43:899–904.
59. Snygg-Martin U, Rasmussen RV, Hassager C, et al. Warfarin therapy and incidence of cerebrovascular complications in left-sided native valve endocarditis. *Eur J Clin Microbiol Infect Dis*. 2011;30:151–157.
60. Sudhakar S, Sewani A, Agrawal M, Uretsky BF. Pseudoaneurysm of the Mitral-Aortic Intervalvular Fibrosa (MAIVF): a comprehensive review. *J Am Soc Echocardiogr*. 2010;23:1009–1018.
61. Feuchtner GM, Stolzmann P, Dichtl W, et al. Multislice computed tomography in infective endocarditis: comparison with transesophageal echocardiography and intraoperative findings. *J Am Coll Cardiol*. 2009;53:436–444.
62. Sims JR, Anavekar NS, Chandrasekaran K, et al. Utility of cardiac computed tomography scanning in the diagnosis and pre-operative evaluation of patients with infective endocarditis. *Int J Cardiovasc Imaging*. 2018;34:1155–1163.
63. Fagman E, Perrotta S, Bech-Hanssen O, et al. ECG-gated computed tomography: a new role for patients with suspected aortic prosthetic valve endocarditis. *Eur Radiol*. 2012;22:2407–2414.
64. Saby L, Laas O, Habib G, et al. Positron emission tomography/computed tomography for diagnosis of prosthetic valve endocarditis: increased valvular 18F-fluorodeoxyglucose uptake as a novel major criterion. *J Am Coll Cardiol*. 2013;61:2374–2382.
65. Pizzi MN, Roque A, Fernandez-Hidalgo N, et al. Improving the diagnosis of infective endocarditis in prosthetic valves and intracardiac devices with 18F-fluordeoxyglucose positron emission tomography/computed tomography angiography: initial results at an infective endocarditis referral center. *Circulation*. 2015;132:1113–1126.
66. Millar BC, Habib G, Moore JE. New diagnostic approaches in infective endocarditis. *Heart*. 2016;102:796–807.
67. Duval X, Iung B, Klein I, et al. Effect of early cerebral magnetic resonance imaging on clinical decisions in infective endocarditis: a prospective study. *Ann Intern Med*. 2010;152:497–504.

Management

68. Van Riet J, Hill EE, Gheysens O, et al. 18F-FDG PET/CT for early detection of embolism and metastatic infection in patients with infective endocarditis. *Eur J Nucl Med Molec Imaging*. 2010;37:1189–1197.
69. Kang D-H, Kim Y-J, Kim S-H, et al. Early surgery versus conventional treatment for infective endocarditis. *N Engl J Mede*. 2012;366:2466–2473.
70. Berdejo J, Shibayama K, Harada K, et al. Evaluation of vegetation size and its relationship with embolism in infective endocarditis. *Circ Cardiovasc Imaging*. 2014;7:149–154.
71. Pfister R, Betton Y, Freyhaus FT, et al. Three-dimensional compared to two-dimensional transesophageal echocardiography for diagnosis of infective endocarditis. *Infection*. 2016;44:725–731.
72. Dickerman SA, Abrutyn E, Barsic B, et al. The relationship between the initiation of antimicrobial therapy and the incidence of stroke in infective endocarditis: an analysis from the ICE Prospective Cohort Study (ICE-PCS). *Am Heart J*. 2007;154:1086–1094.
73. Hubert S, Thuny F, Resseguier N, et al. Prediction of symptomatic embolism in infective endocarditis: construction and validation of a risk calculator in a multicenter cohort. *J Am Coll Cardiol*. 2013;62:1384–1392.
74. Anavekar NS, Tleyjeh IM, Anavekar NS, et al. Impact of prior antiplatelet therapy on risk of embolism in infective endocarditis. *Clin Infect Dis*. 2007;44:1180–1186.
75. Thuny F, Grisoli D, Collart F, et al. Management of infective endocarditis: challenges and perspectives. *Lancet*. 2012;379:965–975.
76. Iversen K, Ihlemann N, Gill SU, et al. Partial oral versus intravenous antibiotic treatment of endocarditis. *New Engl J Med*. 2018;380:415–424.
77. Cosgrove SE, Vigliani GA, Fowler Jr VG, et al. Initial low-dose gentamicin for staphylococcus aureus bacteremia and endocarditis is nephrotoxic. *Clin Inf Dis*. 2009;48:713–721.
78. Gavaldà J, Len O, Miró JM, et al. Brief communication: treatment of enterococcus faecalis endocarditis with ampicillin plus ceftriaxone. *Ann Intern Med*. 2007;146:574–579.

79. Nishimura RA, Otto CM, Bonow RO, et al. 2014 AHA/ACC guideline for the management of patients with valvular heart disease: executive summary. *Circulation*. 2014;129:2440–2492.

80. Bannay A, Hoen B, Duval X, et al. The impact of valve surgery on short- and long-term mortality in left-sided infective endocarditis: do differences in methodological approaches explain previous conflicting results? *Eur Heart J*. 2009;32:2003–2015.

81. Lalani T, Cabell CH, Benjamin DK, et al. Analysis of the impact of early surgery on in-hospital mortality of native valve endocarditis. *Circulation*. 2010;121:1005–1013.

82. Thuny F, Beurtheret S, Mancini J, et al. The timing of surgery influences mortality and morbidity in adults with severe complicated infective endocarditis: a propensity analysis. *Eur Heart J*. 2009;32:2027–2033.

83. García-Cabrera E, Fernández-Hidalgo N, Almirante B, et al. Neurological complications of infective endocarditis. *Circulation*. 2013;127:2272–2284.

84. Chu VH, Park LP, Athan E, et al. Association between surgical indications, operative risk, and clinical outcome in infective endocarditis. *Circulation*. 2015;131:131–140.

85. Martínez-Sellés M, Muñoz P, Arnáiz A, et al. Valve surgery in active infective endocarditis: a simple score to predict in-hospital prognosis. *Int J Cardiol*. 2014;175:133–137.

86. Gaca JG, Sheng S, Daneshmand MA, et al. Outcomes for endocarditis surgery in North America: a simplified risk scoring system. *J Thorac Cardiovasc Surg*. 2011;141:98–106.e2.

87. Iung B, Klein I, Mourvillier B, et al. Respective effects of early cerebral and abdominal magnetic resonance imaging on clinical decisions in infective endocarditis. *Eur Heart J Cardiovasc Imaging*. 2012;13:703–710.

88. Rossi M, Gallo A, De Silva RJ, Sayeed R. What is the optimal timing for surgery in infective endocarditis with cerebrovascular complications? *Interact Cardiovasc Thorac Surg*. 2011;14:72–80.

89. Fernández-Hidalgo N, Almirante B, Gavaldà J, et al. Ampicillin plus ceftriaxone is as effective as ampicillin plus gentamicin for treating enterococcus faecalis infective endocarditis. *Clin Infect Dis*. 2013;56:1261–1268.

90. Prendergast BD, Tornos P. Surgery for infective endocarditis. *Circulation*. 2010;121:1141–1152.

91. Suri RM, Burkhart HM, Daly RC, et al. Robotic mitral valve repair for all prolapse subsets using techniques identical to open valvuloplasty: establishing the benchmark against which percutaneous interventions should be judged. *J Thorac Cardiovasc Surg*. 2011;142:970–979.

92. Minakata K, Schaff HV, Zehr KJ, et al. Is repair of aortic valve regurgitation a safe alternative to valve replacement? *J Thorac Cardiovasc Surg*. 2004;127:645–653.

93. Avierinos J-F, Thuny F, Chalvignac V, et al. Surgical treatment of active aortic endocarditis: homografts are not the cornerstone of outcome. *Ann Thorac Surg*. 2007;84:1935–1942.

94. Lopes S, Calvinho P, de Oliveira F, Antunes M. Allograft aortic root replacement in complex prosthetic endocarditis. *Eur J Cardio Thorac Surg*. 2007;32:126–132.

95. David TE, Gavra G, Feindel CM, et al. Surgical treatment of active infective endocarditis: a continued challenge. *J Thorac Cardiovasc Surg*. 2007;133:144–149.

96. Thuny F, Beurtheret S, Gariboldi V, et al. Outcome after surgical treatment performed within the first week of antimicrobial therapy during infective endocarditis: a prospective study. *Arch Cardiovasc Dis*. 2008;101:687–695.

97. de Kerchove L, Vanoverschelde J-L, Poncelet A, et al. Reconstructive surgery in active mitral valve endocarditis: feasibility, safety and durability. *Eur J Cardio Thorac Surg*. 2007;31:592–599.

98. Nguemeni Tiako MJ, Mori M, Bin Mahmood SU, et al. Recidivism is the leading cause of death among intravenous drug users who underwent cardiac surgery for infective endocarditis. *Semin Thorac Cardiovasc Surg*. 2019;31:40–45.

Implantable Device Infections

99. Baddour LM, Cha Y-M, Wilson WR. Infections of cardiovascular implantable electronic devices. *N Engl J Med*. 2012;367:842–849.

100. Baddour LM, Epstein AE, Erickson CC, et al. Update on cardiovascular implantable electronic device infections and their management. *Circulation*. 2010;121:458–477.

101. Greenspon AJ, Patel JD, Lau E, et al. 16-Year trends in the infection burden for pacemakers and implantable cardioverter-defibrillators in the United States: 1993 to 2008. *J Am Coll Cardiol*. 2011;58:1001–1006.

102. Sohail MR, Uslan DZ, Khan AH, et al. Management and outcome of permanent pacemaker and implantable cardioverter-defibrillator infections. *J Am Coll Cardiol*. 2007;49:1851–1859.

103. Nagpal A, Baddour LM, Sohail MR. Microbiology and pathogenesis of cardiovascular implantable electronic device infections. *Circ Arrhythm Electrophysiol*. 2012;5:433–441.

104. Wilkoff BL, Love CJ, Byrd CL, et al. Transvenous lead extraction: Heart Rhythm Society Expert consensus on facilities, training, indications, and patient management: this document was endorsed by the American Heart Association (AHA). *Heart Rhythm*. 2009;6:1085–1104.

105. Bracke F. Complications and lead extraction in cardiac pacing and defibrillation. *Neth Heart J*. 2008;16:S28–S31.

106. de Oliveira JC, Martinelli M, Nishioka SA, et al. Efficacy of antibiotic prophylaxis before the implantation of pacemakers and cardioverter-defibrillators: results of a large, prospective, randomized, double-blinded, placebo-controlled trial. *Circ Arrhythm Electrophysiol*. 2009;2:29–34.

107. Krahn AD, Longtin Y, Philippon F, et al. Prevention of arrhythmia device infection trial: the PADIT trial. *J Am Coll Cardiol*. 2018;72:3098–3109.

108. Tarakji KG, Mittal S, Kennergren C, et al. Antibacterial envelope to prevent cardiac implantable device infection. *N Engl J Med*. 2019;380:1895–1905.

109. Nienaber JJC, Kusne S, Riaz T, et al. Clinical manifestations and management of left ventricular assist device–associated infections. *Clin Infect Dis*. 2013;57:1438–1448.

110. O'Horo JC, Abu Saleh OM, Stulak JM, et al. Left ventricular assist device infections: a systematic review. *ASAIO J*. 2018;64:287–294.

Guidelines

111. Wilson WR, Gewitz M, Lockhart PB, et al; American Heart Association Young Hearts Rheumatic Fever, Endocarditis and Kawasaki Disease Committee of the Council on Lifelong Congenital Heart Disease and Heart Health in the Young; Council on Cardiovascular and Stroke Nursing; and the Council on Quality of Care and Outcomes Research. Prevention of Viridans Group Streptococcal Infective Endocarditis: A Scientific Statement From the American Heart Association. *Circulation*. 2021;143(20):e963-e978.

112. Otto CM, Nishimura RA, Bonow RO, et al. 2020 ACC/AHA Guideline for the Management of Patients With Valvular Heart Disease: Executive Summary: A Report of the American College of Cardiology/American Heart Association Joint Committee on Clinical Practice Guidelines. *J Am Coll Cardiol*. 2021;77(4) 450–500.

81 Rheumatic Fever

ANA OLGA MOCUMBI

Rheumatic fever (RF) is a leading cause of acquired heart disease in children and young adults worldwide. It is an illness preceded by a pharyngeal infection with group A beta-hemolytic streptococci (GAS), occurring most often between 5 and 15 years. The inflammatory process causes damage to collagen fibrils and connective tissue ground substance, resulting typically in combinations of arthritis, carditis, erythema marginatum, subcutaneous nodules, and chorea. The diagnosis is based on applying the modified Jones criteria to information gleaned from the history, examination, laboratory testing, individual risk, and, more recently, echocardiographic data (see "Diagnosis"). The treatment includes aspirin or other nonsteroid anti-inflammatory drugs, corticosteroids during severe carditis, and antimicrobials to eradicate residual streptococcal infection and prevent reinfection.

In allusion to the fleeting arthritis and damaging carditis that is characteristic of RF, the French physician Ernst-Charles Lasegue famously said, in 1884, that *"rheumatic fever licks the joints but bites the heart."* Indeed, it is the destructive effect on the heart that leads to the chronic sequelae of the RF—rheumatic heart disease (RHD)—a preventable cause of health failure, stroke, endocarditis, and premature deaths in highly endemic areas.

EPIDEMIOLOGY

The burden of RF remains uncertain due to the complexity of its diagnosis, which includes epidemiologic considerations, a high level of awareness, trained health professionals who can recognize subtle signs, and complementary tests that are not always readily available.

The burden of RF and RHD is most salient within marginalized communities in developed nations as well as in low- and middle-income regions.[1] Worldwide, incidence is 19/100,000 (range, 5 to 51/100,000), with lowest rates (<10/100,000) in North America and Western Europe and highest rates (>10/100,000) in Eastern Europe, the Middle East, Asia, Africa, Australia, and New Zealand.[2] The condition is more prevalent among young people, particularly between the ages of 5 to 30, and although its occurrence is similar between women and men, the inherent biological factors, the risk of illness during pregnancy, exposure to GAS through child rearing, and poor accessibility to resources make women approximately 1.8 times more susceptible to developing RHD.[3]

Four changing patterns for the burden of RF have been recognized over the past 150 years (Fig. 81.1). Curve A is typical of industrialized countries and represents the preantibiotic fall in RF incidence. This decrease preceding the introduction of antibiotics in the 1940s is almost certainly the result of improved socioeconomic standards, less overcrowded housing, and improved access to medical care; for example, in the United States, the incidence per 100,000 population was 100 at the start of the 20th century, was 45 to 65 between 1935 and 1960, and is currently estimated at less than 10 cases per 100,000.[4] Curve B shows persistently high incidence of RF in developing regions and among indigenous populations of some developed countries, such as Australia and New Zealand. The incidence of RF per 100,000/year among 5- to 14-year-old indigenous Australian children is as high as 162 in men and 228 in women.[5] This hyperendemic pattern is found in the majority of the population living in Africa, the Middle East, Asia, Eastern Europe, South America, and indigenous communities of Australasia. However, in Curve C, some developing countries—Cuba, Costa Rica, Martinique, Guadeloupe, and Tunisia—have experienced a fall in the incidence of RF after implementation of comprehensive public health programs of primary and secondary prevention of RF.[6] Finally, outbreaks of RF have been reported in affluent communities in the United States and Italy[7] (see also Veasy et al., Classic References). In Curve D, there is a sustained resurgence of RF and RHD in central Asia,[8] where the incidence of RF had fallen to the same levels as Japan in the 1970s but rose sharply in the post-Soviet period to levels associated with developing countries. This may reflect weakening of the primary care system and the economic crisis of the post-Soviet period (see Tulchinsky and Varavikova, Classic References).

The attack rate, defined as the percentage of patients with untreated GAS pharyngitis who develop acute RF (ARF), varies from <1.0% to 3.0%. Higher attack rates occur with certain streptococcal M protein serotypes and a stronger host immune response, likely resulting from undefined genetic predisposition[2] and factors such as the carrier state.[1,9]

Rheumatic arthritis was found in around 10% of family members of RHD cases undergoing cardiac surgery in Egypt,[10] and cardiac sequelae were detected in asymptomatic children during active community-based screening.[11] The strict application of the updated Jones criteria[12] still leads to underdiagnosis of RF in highly endemic regions[13]; the most effective predictors—arthritis, carditis, chorea, aortic regurgitation, significant mitral regurgitation, thick anterior mitral valve leaflets, elevated acute phase reactants, positive family history, and prolonged PR interval—show an overall prediction accuracy of 81.4%, with high sensitivity of 93% and specificity of 62%.[13]

PATHOGENESIS

RF is a multifactorial disease that follows GAS *(the agent)* pharyngitis in a susceptible individual *(the host)* who lives under deprived social conditions *(the environment)*. The theory of molecular mimicry holds

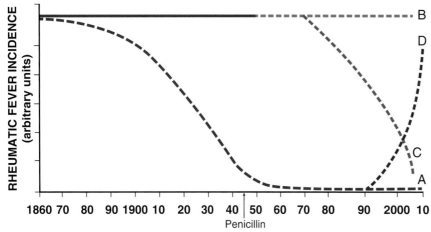

FIGURE 81.1 Incidence of rheumatic fever (RF): four patterns over the past 150 years. Curve A represents the preantibiotic fall in incidence of RF that is typical of industrialized countries. Curve B is typical of the persistent high incidence in regions of the world with no comprehensive program for prevention such as Africa and South Asia. Curve C shows the postantibiotic fall in the incidence of RF in countries that instituted comprehensive programs for primary and secondary prevention of RF, such as Cuba, Costa Rica, Martinique, and Guadeloupe. Curve D shows the fall and rise in the incidence of RF in the formerly Soviet republics of Central Asia. (Modified from Parry E, et al., editors. Principles of Medicine in Africa. 3rd ed. Cambridge: Cambridge University Press; 2004, p 861.)

that GAS pharyngitis triggers an autoimmune response in susceptible individuals by cross-reacting with similar epitopes in the heart, brain, joints, and skin, and that repeated episodes of RF lead to RHD.[1,14] In situations of untreated epidemic GAS pharyngitis, up to 3% of patients develop the disease.[15] The risk of RF is substantially reduced by effective antibiotic therapy.

The Agent
Epidemiologic data, immunologic observations, and the preventive effect of antibiotic treatment for pharyngitis demonstrated in clinical trials strongly support the causative role of untreated GAS pharyngitis in RF (see Dajani, Classic References). There is also growing evidence regarding the potential role of GAS skin infections in causing ARF, either alone or in combination with GAS pharyngitis.[16] Initial suggestions came from a report of RF following streptococcal wound infection (see Popat and Riding, Classic References). This may be particularly important in Africa, where excoriation of highly endemic scabies lesions can lead to secondary pyoderma infection, most commonly by *Staphylococcus aureus* and GAS.[17]

The hypothesis of molecular mimicry in the pathogenesis of RF[1] state that patients with RHD have cross-reactive autoantibodies that target the dominant GAS epitope of the group A carbohydrate, N-acetyl-beta-d-glucosamine (GlcNAc), and laminin and laminar basement membrane in heart valve endothelium. T cells in peripheral blood and heart valves of RHD patients cross-react with streptococcal M protein and cardiac myosin. Furthermore, autoantibodies against the GAS carbohydrate epitope GlcNAc and cardiac myosin appear during progression of RHD. In addition, autoantibodies against collagen that are cross-reactive may form because of the release of collagen from damaged valves.

The *two-hit hypothesis* for the initiation of disease proposes that antibody attack of valve endothelium facilitates the extravasation of T cells through activated epithelium into valve tissue, leading to the formation of granulomatous nodules called Aschoff bodies, characteristic of rheumatic myocarditis (Fig. 81.2). The area of central necrosis is surrounded by a ring of plump histiocytes, called Anitschkow cells. These nodules were discovered by Ludwig Aschoff and Paul Rudolf Geipel and thus are occasionally called Aschoff-Geipel bodies.

Human monoclonal antibodies (mAbs) derived from patients with disease target GlcNAc, gangliosides, and dopamine receptors on the surface of neuronal cells in the brain. Human mAbs and autoantibodies in Sydenham chorea activate calcium/calmodulin-dependent protein kinase II (CaMKii) in neuronal cells and recognize the intracellular protein biomarker tubulin.

The Host
Genetic predisposition to RF and RHD has been hypothesized by findings from familial studies, as well as observed associations between genes located in the human leukocyte antigens (HLA) on chromosome 6p21.3

and elsewhere in the genome. Currently, several lines of epidemiologic evidence support the role of hereditary factors in susceptibility to RF. First, the lifetime cumulative incidence of RF in populations exposed to rheumatogenic GAS infection is constant at 3% to 6% regardless of geography or ethnicity,[18] suggesting that the proportion of susceptible individuals is the same in all continental populations worldwide.[12] Second, the chance of an individual with a family history of RF acquiring the disease is nearly five times greater than that of an individual who has no such hereditary predisposition.[12] This familial aggregation of RHD has been supported by a study of children raised separately from parents with RHD, who had a relative risk of 2.93 for the development of RF compared with children whose parents did not have RHD.[12] The heritability of RF, at 60%, highlights the importance of heredity as a major susceptibility factor of the disease.

Studies conducted to search for specific genetic susceptibility factors in RF have targeted genes controlling the adaptive immune response (e.g., HLA class II alleles, cytotoxic T-cell lymphocyte antigen 4), the innate immune response (e.g., ficolin 2, mannose-binding lectin 2, receptor for Fc fragments of IgG, Toll-like receptor 2), cytokine genes (e.g., tumor necrosis factor-α, transforming growth factor-β, interleukin-1 receptor A, interleukin-10), and B-cell alloantigens. Significant associations have been found between genetic factors and RF, but studies either conflict or are not replicated.[12] Therefore, it is not possible at the present to predict the individuals who are at risk of developing RF following an episode of untreated GAS pharyngitis.

The Environment
RF is generally associated with low socioeconomic status. The incidence of RF has been falling consistently in industrialized countries since the mid-19th century, independently of the advent of penicillin, possible related to less crowding, improved housing and nutritional status, higher levels of parental employment, and better access to health care (see Fig. 81.1, Curve A). In endemic regions, the risk of RF is linked to high levels of deprivation based on household income, access to telephone and car, education level, and housing, as well as overcrowding and unemployment.

Pathogenesis of Acute Rheumatic Fever
The reason for the difference in complications resulting from GAS infections of the pharynx and of other areas of the body is not well understood. Pharyngeal infection with GAS leads to activation of the innate immune system. Neutrophils, macrophages, and dendritic cells phagocytose the bacteria and then present antigens to T cells; this leads to activation of humoral (antibodies) and cellular immune responses (CD4+ T-cell activation). The driving mechanism of ARF is the immune response becoming cross-reactive with human tissues: Carditis is caused by both cross-reactive antibodies and T cells, arthritis by immune complex deposition, chorea by antibody binding to neuronal cells and the skin, and subcutaneous manifestations by a delayed hypersensitivity reaction.[19]

Pathologic Features
The pathology of ARF varies by site with the joints, heart, skin, and central nervous system (CNS) being most often affected. Cardiac involvement manifests as carditis, typically affecting valves and endocardium, then myocardium, and finally pericardium. In ARF, Aschoff bodies (Fig. 81.2) often develop in the myocardium and other parts of the heart; the incidental finding of Aschoff nodules diagnoses acute rheumatic myocarditis.[20] Fibrinous nonspecific pericarditis, sometimes with effusion, occurs only in patients with endocardial inflammation and usually subsides without permanent damage.

Joint involvement manifests as nonspecific synovial inflammation; if biopsied, it sometimes shows small foci resembling Aschoff bodies (granulomatous collections of leukocytes, myocytes, and interstitial collagen). Unlike the cardiac findings, however, the abnormalities of the joints are not chronic and do not leave scarring or residual abnormalities.

Subcutaneous nodules appear indistinguishable from those of juvenile idiopathic arthritis (JIA), but biopsy shows features resembling Aschoff bodies. Erythema marginatum differs histologically from other skin lesions with similar macroscopic appearance (e.g., the rash of systemic JIA, Henoch-Schönlein purpura, erythema chronicum migrans, and erythema multiforme). Perivascular neutrophilic and mononuclear infiltrates of the dermis is usually found.

Sydenham chorea manifests as hyperperfusion and increased metabolism in the basal ganglia. Increased levels of antineuronal antibodies have also been shown.[21]

CLINICAL FEATURES

The typical attack of RF follows an episode of GAS infection—usually symptoms of GAS pharyngitis—after a latent period of 2 to 3 weeks, during which there are no clinical or laboratory evidence of active inflammation. However, as many as one-third of patients who develop RF do so after asymptomatic GAS, and in outbreaks up to 58% of patients have no symptoms of pharyngitis. Preceding symptomatic pharyngitis is recognized in only about two-thirds of patients with ARF in high-income countries, and even less in endemic regions.

A first episode of ARF can occur at any age but occurs most often between 4 and 15 years, ages that are also the peak years for streptococcal pharyngitis. However, in developing countries there are reports of RHD occurring at age 3 to 5 years. ARF typically involves some combination of the joints, heart, skin, and CNS. The most common major sign

is polyarthritis, which occurs in two-thirds to three-quarters of patients, followed by carditis and chorea. The illness usually begins with high fever, but in some patients the fever may be low-grade or absent.

Arthritis

Joint involvement is more common and more severe in young adults (100%) than in teenagers (82%) and children (66%). At the onset of the illness the joint involvement is asymmetric and usually affects the lower limbs initially before spreading to the upper limbs. *Migratory polyarthritis* is the most common manifestation of ARF, occurring in about 35% to 66% of children, often accompanied by fever. In some cases the joint involvement may be additive rather than migratory, with several joints affected simultaneously; thus in untreated patients the number of joints affected varies between 6 and 16. The affected joint may be inflamed for only a few days to 1 week before inflammation subsides. The polyarthritis is severe for approximately 1 week in two-thirds of the patients and may last for another 1 or 2 weeks in the remainder, before it resolves completely. If the joint swelling persists after 4 weeks, it becomes necessary to consider other conditions, such as JIA or systemic lupus erythematosus (SLE).

Monarthritis occurs in high-risk indigenous populations (e.g., in Australia, India, Fiji), as has been reported in 17% to 25% of patients. Joints become extremely painful and tender; these symptoms are often out of proportion to the modest warmth and swelling present on examination (this is in contrast to the arthritis of Lyme disease, in which the examination findings tend to be more severe than the symptoms). The large joints such as ankles, knees, elbows, and wrists are usually involved. Shoulders, hips, and small joints of the hands and feet may also be involved, but almost never alone. If vertebral joints are affected, another disorder should be suspected. Joint pain and fever usually subside within 2 weeks and seldom last more than 1 month.

The synovial fluid has characteristics of sterile inflammation. There may be reduction in complement components C1q, C3, and C4, suggesting their consumption by immune complexes. Radiographs may show features of a join effusion, but no other abnormality is noted.

Jaccoud arthritis or arthropathy (or chronic post-RF arthropathy) is a rare manifestation of RF characterized by deformities of the fingers and toes (Fig. 81.3). The condition may occur after repeated attacks of RF and results from recurrent inflammation of the fibrous articular capsule. There is ulnar deviation of the fingers, especially the fourth and fifth fingers, flexion of the metacarpophalangeal joints, and hyperextension of the proximal interphalangeal joints (i.e., swan neck deformity). The hand is usually painless, and there are no signs of inflammation. The deformities usually correctible but may become fixed in the later stages. There are no true erosions on radiography, and the rheumatoid factor is usually negative. A similar form of arthropathy is seen in patients with SLE.

Because the arthritis of RF responds promptly to nonsteroidal anti-inflammatory drugs (NSAIDs), the classic presentation of a migratory polyarthritis may be infrequent in regions where NSAID self-medication or prescription is common; this may explain the apparent fall in incidence of RF in some developing countries.[22]

Poststreptococcal reactive arthritis (PSRA) is diagnosed in patients who have arthritis that is not typical of RF but who have evidence of recent streptococcal infection. This condition occurs after a shorter latent period than RF, is less responsive to NSAIDs, may be associated with renal manifestations, and evidence of carditis is infrequent. The distinction between PSRA and RF is unclear, and many would recommend that a diagnosis of PSRA not be made in populations where RF is common. Even if the diagnosis is considered, it is appropriate to offer a period of secondary prophylaxis with penicillin, as for episodes of acute RF, in such populations.

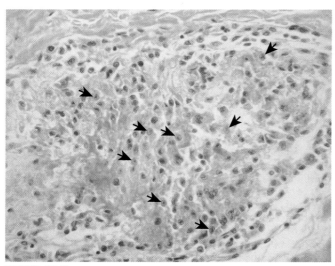

FIGURE 81.2 The Aschoff body of rheumatic fever. Photomicrography of an Aschoff nodule from the heart in a case of acute rheumatic fever. The nodule is composed of Anitschkow cells; these have clear nuclei with a central bar of chromatin, said to resemble a caterpillar. There is a central area of fibrin. This central necrosis is further surrounded by a mononuclear cell infiltrate. Myocardial fibers adjacent to the Aschoff body are undergoing destruction. (From Sebire NJ, et al., editors. Diagnostic Pediatric Surgical Pathology. London: Churchill Livingstone; 2010.)

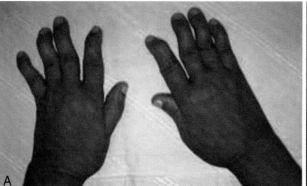
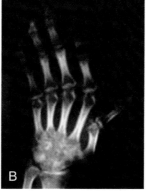

FIGURE 81.3 Post-rheumatic fever Jaccoud arthropathy. **A,** Swan neck deformity in Jaccoud arthropathy, with ulnar deviation and metacarpophalangeal subluxation. **B,** Plain radiograph of the left hand showing deformities but not erosions. (From Santiago MB. Jaccoud's arthropathy. Best Prac Res Rheumatol 2011;25:715.)

TABLE 81.1 World Heart Federation Minimum Criteria for the Diagnosis of Pathologic Valvular Regurgitation Caused by Rheumatic Carditis

ECHOCARDIOGRAPHIC FEATURES IN RHEUMATIC VALVULITIS			
DOPPLER FINDINGS		MORPHOLOGIC FINDINGS	
Pathologic mitral regurgitation*	Pathologic aortic regurgitation*	Acute mitral valve changes	Aortic valve changes in carditis or chronic RHD
Seen in at least two views	Seen in the least two views	Annular dilatation	Irregular or focal leaflet thickening
		Chordal elongation	
Jet length ≥2 cm in at least one view†	Jet length ≥1 cm in at least one view†	Chordal rupture resulting in flail leaflet with severe mitral regurgitation	Coaptation defect
Peak velocity > 3 m/sec	Peak velocity >3 m/sec	Anterior (or less commonly posterior leaflet tip prolapse)	Restricted leaflet motion
Pansystolic jet in the least one envelope	Pandiastolic jet in at least one envelope	Beading/nodularity of leaflet tips	Leaflet prolapse

*All four criteria must be met.
†A regurgitant jet length should be measured from the vena contracta to the last pixel of regurgitant color (blue or red) on the nonmagnified (nonzoomed) images.
The listed criteria provide a set of objective measures to distinguish physiologic valvular regurgitation from pathologic regurgitation but are not specific for rheumatic carditis. Morphologic abnormalities presented may or may not be present.
RHD, Rheumatic heart disease.
Adapted from Remenyi B, et al. World Heart Federation criteria for echocardiographic diagnosis of rheumatic heart disease: an evidence-based guideline. Nat Rev Cardiol 2012;9:297-309; Dougherty S, et al. Acute Rheumatic Fever and Rheumatic Heart Disease. 1st ed. Philadelphia: Elsevier; 2020.

Carditis

The incidence of carditis during the initial attack of RF varies from 40% to 91% depending on the selection of patients, the age of patient, and whether the diagnosis is made on clinical assessment alone or combined with echocardiography.[11] Carditis is the most serious manifestation of RF because it may lead to chronic RHD. It may be asymptomatic and detected during clinical examination of patients with arthritis or chorea. Heart failure results from a combination of carditis and valvular dysfunction and occurs in 5% to 10% of the initial episodes, more frequently during recurrences of RF. Patients may have high fever, chest pain, or both; tachycardia is common, especially during sleep. In about 50% of cases, cardiac damage (i.e., persistent valve dysfunction) occurs much later. The symptoms and signs depend on whether there is involvement of the pericardium, myocardium, or heart valves. Although considered to be a pancarditis, valvulitis is the most consistent feature of ARF, and if it is not present, the diagnosis should be reconsidered.

Valvulitis

The clinical diagnosis of valvulitis has classically been made by auscultation of murmurs, but subclinical cases detected by echocardiography may occur in up to 18% of cases of ARF. When heart murmurs are not heard at initial examination, repeated clinical examinations and echocardiography are recommended. The most common valvular lesion is mitral regurgitation; aortic regurgitation is less common. Stenotic lesions are uncommon in the early stages of RF, but a transient apical mid-diastolic murmur (Carey-Coombs) may occur in association with the murmur of mitral regurgitation. Murmurs often persist indefinitely; if no worsening occurs during the next 2 to 3 weeks, new manifestations of carditis seldom follow. In the presence of history of previous RHD, a change in the character of the murmurs or the appearance of a new murmur is indicative of acute rheumatic carditis.

Myocarditis

Inflammation of the myocardium is unlikely to be rheumatic in origin in the absence of valvulitis. Patients with myocarditis develop cardiomegaly or congestive heart failure, which may be severe and life threatening. Electrocardiographic abnormalities include varying degrees of heart block.

Pericarditis

Pericarditis occurs in approximately 10% of patients and may be manifested by anterior chest pain and a pericardial friction rub. The pericardial effusion may sometimes be large, but cardiac tamponade is rare and constrictive pericarditis does not occur.

Echocardiography is recommended for all patients with suspected or definite ARF, as it is more sensitive and specific than cardiac auscultation for detection of acute rheumatic carditis. (See Vasan et al., Classic References.) Table 81.1 outlines the World Heart Federation minimum echocardiographic criteria for pathologic regurgitation caused by rheumatic carditis.

Sydenham Chorea

The CNS is affected in up to 40% of children with RF,[23] predominating in females after puberty. The latent period between GAS pharyngitis and chorea is longer (6 to 8 weeks) than for arthritis and carditis; its onset is typically insidious and may be preceded by inappropriate laughing or crying. It can last for up to 2 years (usually 8 to 15 weeks); if it occurs in isolation, all inflammatory markers may be normal and the diagnosis may be overlooked as an indicator of ARF. It does not occur simultaneously with arthritis but may coexist with carditis.

Sydenham chorea, also referred to as St. Vitus dance, consists of rapid, involuntary, purposeless, and irregular jerking movements that may begin in the hands but often become generalized, involving the feet and face and interfering with voluntary activity; they disappear during sleep. The purposeless movements are associated with hypotonia, weakness (sometimes mistaken for paralysis), and loss of fine motor control.

Characteristic findings include fluctuating grip strength (milkmaid's grip), tongue fasciculations or tongue darting (patients intermittently involuntarily withdraw the tongue when attempting to protrude it for 30 seconds, the so-called jack-in-the-box tongue), facial grimacing, and explosive speech with or without tongue clucking. Emotional lability manifests in personality changes, with inappropriate behavior, restlessness, outburst of anger and crying, and learning difficulties; previously undiagnosed obsessive-compulsive behavior may be unmasked in many patients. The term pediatric autoimmune neuropsychiatric disorders associated with streptococcal infections (PANDAS) is used for children with tic or obsessive-compulsive disorders triggered by GAS infection, without cardiac valve damage. In populations at high risk of RF the suspicion of PANDAS should be considered as a manifestation of ARF and managed with secondary prophylaxis.

Cutaneous and Subcutaneous Features

Rarely, subcutaneous nodules and erythema marginatum develop in patients already having carditis, arthritis, or chorea; they almost never occur alone. The subcutaneous nodules of RF occur most frequently on the extensor surfaces of large joints. They may be detected over the occiput, elbows, knees, ankles, and Achilles tendons. Ordinarily, the

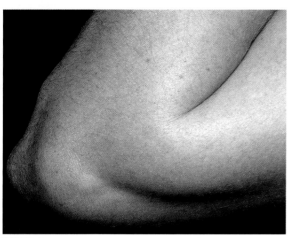

FIGURE 81.4 Subcutaneous nodules of rheumatic fever over the bony prominences of the elbow. (From Beeman LB, et al. Cardiology. In Zetelli BJ, et al., editors. Atlas of Pediatric Physical Diagnosis. 6th ed. Philadelphia: Saunders; 2012.)

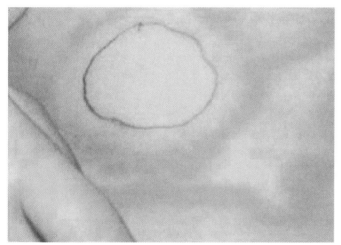

FIGURE 81.5 Erythema marginatum in acute rheumatic fever. The pen mark shows the location of the rash approximately 60 minutes previously. (From Cohen J, Powderly WG. Infectious Diseases. 2nd ed. St Louis: Mosby; 2004.)

nodules are firm, painless, and freely movable over the subcutaneous tissue; they vary in size from 0.5 to 2 cm and tend to occur in crops that may be related to the severity of the carditis (Fig. 81.4). They are transitory (seldom more than 1 month) and respond to treatment of joint or heart inflammation. Fewer than 10% of children with ARF have nodules.

Erythema Marginatum

Erythema marginatum occurs as a serpiginous, flat or slightly raised, nonscarring, and painless rash in fewer than 6% of children. The rash usually appears on the trunk and proximal extremities but not the face (Fig. 81.5), and is evanescent, pink, and nonpruritic. It extends centrifugally while the skin at the center returns to normal, always with an irregular serpiginous border. It sometimes lasts less than 1 day and may become more prominent after a shower. Its appearance is often delayed after the inciting streptococcal infection, with or after the other manifestations of rheumatic inflammation.

Other Manifestations

Fever (≥38.5°C), tachycardia during sleep, tachycardia out of proportion to fever, anorexia, and malaise can be prominent but are not specific. The temperature usually decreases within 1 week, rarely lasting more than 4 weeks. Abdominal pain and anorexia can occur because of the hepatic involvement in heart failure or because of concomitant mesenteric adenitis; rarely, the situation may resemble acute appendicitis.

DIAGNOSIS

No specific test exists to confirm conclusively a diagnosis of RF, which is based on the Jones criteria modified several times since T. Duckett Jones in 1944 first formulated them (see Bland and Jones, Classic References). The American Heart Association published the most recent revision in 2015[14] (Table 81.2). Diagnosis of a first episode of ARF is based on two major criteria, or one major and two minor criteria, each along with evidence of preceding GAS infection. Sydenham chorea alone (i.e., without minor criteria) fulfills diagnostic criteria if other causes of movement disorder are ruled out. Recent scarlet fever is highly suggestive.

Evidence of Preceding GAS Infection

Recent GAS infection is suggested by a recent history of pharyngitis and confirmed by one or more of the following: throat swab culture (positive in about 11% of patients with diagnosis of RF), an increased— or preferably rising—antistreptolysin O (ASO) titer, or a positive rapid antigen detection test (RADT) in a child with clinical manifestations suggestive of streptococcal pharyngitis. However, it is extremely difficult to distinguish patients with true GAS pharyngitis from carriers who have viral pharyngitis when throat swab culturing alone is used to diagnose GAS pharyngitis. Most studies assessing the incidence of GAS pharyngitis use throat swabbing and culture; while a RADT may be used, laboratory culture is still considered the most specific means of GAS confirmation.

Clinical symptoms are combined with RADT or culturing when diagnosing GAS pharyngitis. At present, serologic testing of antistreptolysin and anti-DNase B antibody titers in two blood samples taken 2 to 4 weeks apart with seroconversion is thought to distinguish true GAS pharyngitis from pharyngeal GAS carriers.[16] Throat cultures and RADT tests are often negative by the time ARF manifests, whereas ASO titers and anti-DNase B typically peak 3 to 6 weeks after GAS pharyngitis; about 80% of children with ARF have a significantly elevated ASO titer. As throat swab cultures have limited accuracy for ARF diagnosis (10% to 20%), polymerase chain reaction (PCR) based tests have been used with more than 90% specificity.

Revised Jones Criteria

The 2015 revised Jones criteria incorporate three main changes. First, subclinical valvulitis detected by echocardiography is accepted as a major criterion for the diagnosis of ARF in all patient populations. Second, there is recognition that the clinical utility of the Jones criteria is determined by the pretest probability and background disease prevalence in the population. To avoid over diagnosis in low-incidence populations (ARF incidence <2/100,000 school-aged children, usually 5 to 14 years old, per year, or all-age prevalence of RHD of >1/1000 population per year) and underdiagnosis in high-risk populations, variability in applying diagnostic criteria in low-risk versus high-risk populations has been introduced in line with the Australian guidelines.[12] Finally, in moderate- to high-risk communities, monoarthritis and polyarthralgia have been added to polyarthritis as major criteria, and a temperature of 38°C and monoarthralgia are the revised minor criteria (Table 81.2). The clinical entity "possible" RF is appropriate for clinical judgment in parts of the world where RF remains common and where it is not possible to fulfill the criteria due to lack of laboratory facilities to conduct all investigations to exclude RF.[12,19] Suspected RF in high-incidence setting warrants secondary prophylaxis for 12 months and reevaluation based on history, physical examination, and echocardiogram.

Other Tests

Electrocardiogram (ECG) reveals a prolonged PR interval in only 35% of children with ARF; higher-degree heart block may occur but is uncommon. Other ECG abnormalities may be due to pericarditis, enlargement of ventricles or atria, or arrhythmias.

Echocardiography can detect evidence of carditis even in patients without apparent murmurs. It is recommended for all patients with confirmed or suspected ARF to detect subclinical carditis in patients with apparently isolated Sydenham chorea and to monitor the status of patients with recurrences of carditis or chronic RHD. Not all echocardiographic abnormalities represent rheumatic carditis; isolated trivial

TABLE 81.2 2015 American Heart Association Revised Jones Criteria for Diagnosis of Acute Rheumatic Fever

A. FOR ALL PATIENT POPULATIONS WITH EVIDENCE OF PRECEDING GAS INFECTION	
Diagnosis: Initial ARF	Two major manifestations or one major plus two minor manifestations
Diagnosis: Recurrent ARF	Two major, or one major and two minor, or three minor manifestations
B. MAJOR CRITERIA	
Low-Risk Populations*	**Moderate and High-Risk Populations**
Carditis[†]	Carditis[†]
• Clinical and/or subclinical	• Clinical and/or subclinical
Arthritis	Arthritis
• Polyarthritis only	• Monoarthritis or polyarthritis
	• Polyarthralgia[‡]
Chorea	Chorea
Erythema marginatum	Erythema marginatum
Subcutaneous nodules	Subcutaneous nodules
C. MINOR CRITERIA	
Low-Risk Populations*	**Moderate and High-Risk Populations**
Polyarthralgia	Monoarthralgia
Fever ≥ 38.5°C	Fever ≥ 38°C
ESR ≥60 mm in the first hour and/or CRP ≥ mg/dL[§]	ESR ≥30 mm/hr and/or CRP ≥3.0 mg/dL[§]
Prolonged PR interval after accounting for age variability (unless carditis is a major criterion)	Prolonged PR interval after accounting for age variability (unless carditis is a major criterion)

From Dougherty S, et al. Acute Rheumatic Fever and Rheumatic Heart Disease. 1st ed. Elsevier; 2020.

*Annual acute rheumatic fever (ARF) incidence of <2/100,000 school-aged children or all-age rheumatic heart disease (RHD) prevalence of <1/1000 people per year.
[†]Defined as echocardiographic valvulitis (Table 81.1).
[‡]Polyarthralgia should only be considered as a major manifestation in moderate- and high-risk populations after exclusion of other causes.
[§]C-reactive protein (CRP) value must be greater than the normal laboratory upper limit. In addition, because the erythrocyte sedimentation rate (ESR) might evolve during the course of ARF, peak ESR values should be used.
Joint manifestations are only considered in either the major or the minor category, but not in both categories in the same patient.

valvar regurgitation or trivial pericardial effusion may be nonspecific. To maintain specificity, echocardiographic and Doppler results should meet the criteria for acute rheumatic carditis (Table 81.1).

Chest X-rays can detect cardiomegaly, a common manifestation of carditis in ARF.

Erythrocyte sedimentation rate (ESR) and serum C-reactive protein (CRP) are sensitive but not specific. The ESR is typically >60 mm/hr, while CRP is >30 mg/L and often >70 mg/L. Because it rises and falls faster than ESR, a normal CRP may confirm that inflammation is resolving in a patient with prolonged ESR elevation after acute symptoms have subsided. In the absence of carditis, ESR usually returns to normal within 3 months. Evidence of acute inflammation, including ESR, usually subsides within 5 months in uncomplicated carditis.

The *white blood cell (WBC)* count reaches 12,000 to 20,000/μL and may go higher with corticosteroid therapy. *Serum cardiac marker* levels may be obtained; normal cardiac troponin I levels exclude prominent myocardial damage.

Joint aspiration may be needed to exclude other causes of arthritis (e.g., infection). The joint fluid is usually cloudy and yellow, with an elevated WBC count composed primarily of neutrophils; culture is negative. Complement levels are usually normal or slightly decreased, compared with decreased levels in other inflammatory arthritis.

Biopsy of a subcutaneous nodule can aid in early diagnosis, especially when other major clinical manifestations are absent.

Differential Diagnosis

The differential diagnosis of ARF includes JIA (especially systemic and, less so, polyarticular), Lyme disease, reactive arthritis, arthropathy of sickle cell disease, leukemia or other cancer, SLE, embolic bacterial endocarditis, serum sickness, Kawasaki disease, drug reactions, and gonococcal arthritis. These are usually distinguished by history or specific laboratory tests. Absence of previous GAS infection, diurnal variation of the fever, evanescent rash, and prolonged symptomatic joint inflammation usually distinguish systemic JIA from ARF.

Recurrences

Recurrent episodes of ARF often mimic the initial attack; carditis tends to recur in patients who have had moderate to severe carditis in the past, and chorea without carditis recurs in patients who had chorea without carditis initially. The diagnosis of recurrent ARF requires two major, one major and two minor, or three minor criteria. While the Jones criteria were designed for the evaluation of ARF (rather than for a possible recurrence), if patients have a reliable history of ARF or RHD and GAS infection is documented, they may be used to establish the presence of a recurrence. Finally, in established RHD, a recurrence of ARF can be diagnosed by the presence of two minor criteria plus evidence of a preceding GAS infection.

NATURAL HISTORY

Patients who have had RF have about a 50% likelihood of having a recurrence if they have another episode of untreated GAS pharyngitis. In endemic areas for RHD it is usual to see patients with severe RHD and superimposed ARF, particularly carditis. Episodes of Sydenham chorea usually last several months and resolve completely in most patients, but about one-third of patients have recurrences. Joint inflammation may take one month to subside if not treated but does not lead to residual damage.

Prognosis following an episode of ARF depends mostly on how severely the heart is affected, and whether it is a recurrent episode of ARF. Murmurs eventually disappear in about half of patients whose acute episodes were manifested by mild carditis without major cardiac enlargement or decompensation; however, chronic valvular disease can occur, typically over years or decades, in patients who recovered from the acute episode with no evidence of valvular disease. Chronic RHD is the cause of 25% to 45% of all cardiovascular disease and a major cause of heart failure in developing countries.

MANAGEMENT

The primary goals of the treatment of a proven attack of ARF are to suppress the inflammatory response and minimize its effects on the heart and joints, to eradicate GAS from the pharynx, to provide relief of acute symptoms, and to initiate prophylaxis to prevent recurrent heart disease. The management of ARF is summarized in Table 81.3.

General Management

Patients should limit their activities if they have symptoms of arthritis, chorea, or heart failure. Strenuous exertion should be avoided, especially in patients with carditis. In asymptomatic carditis, strict bed rest has no proven value, despite its traditional usage. Bed rest appears to be appropriate to lessen joint pain, and its duration should be individually determined. Ambulation can usually be started once fever has subsided and acute-phase reactants are returning to normal.

Antibiotic Treatment

Although poststreptococcal inflammation is well developed by the time ARF is detected, and throat swabs are rarely positive for GAS, a 10-day course of oral penicillin or amoxicillin, or a single injection of intramuscular benzathine penicillin (or erythromycin if allergic to penicillin) is used to eradicate any lingering organisms; however, this conventional strategy is untested. Thereafter, secondary prophylaxis should be commenced as described later.

TABLE 81.3 Management Protocol for Acute Rheumatic Fever

Diagnosis
- Admission to hospital
- Investigation to confirm ARF and to exclude other pathologies
- Blood tests including acute-phase reactants and serology for the streptococcal organism
- Electrocardiogram
- Echocardiographic evaluation

Eradication of GAS
- Oral penicillin V* for 10 days OR single dose of intramuscular benzathine penicillin G
- Treatment of coexisting streptococcal impetigo

Arthritis/Arthralgia and Symptomatic Treatment
- Paracetamol until the diagnosis has been confirmed
- NSAIDs (naproxen is preferably used)
- Corticosteroids in cases where NSAIDs cannot be used

Carditis/Heart Failure
- Bed rest, fluid restriction, heart failure medications (furosemide, spironolactone, ACEI)
- Corticosteroids for severe heart failure if surgery is not indicated or unavailable
- Surgery for intractable heart failure associated with severe mitral or aortic regurgitation; preferable to defer surgery until acute rheumatic activity has resolved

Chorea
- Penicillin V* orally or intramuscular benzathine penicillin G
- Haloperidol or carbamazepine can be considered if the abnormal movements interfere with daily activities
- Valproic acid reserved for refractory cases
- Multidisciplinary input as required for significant motor or neuropsychiatric manifestations

Discharge Procedure
- Discharge once there is clinical improvement and reduction in ESR or CRP
- Notification to health authorities
- Patient and family education
- Secondary prophylaxis
- Outpatient follow-up

*Also known as phenoxymethylpenicillin or penicillin V potassium (PVK).
ACEI, Angiotensin-converting enzyme inhibitor; *CRP*, C-reactive protein; *ESR*, erythrocyte sedimentation rate; *GAS*, group A streptococcal; *NSAIDs*, nonsteroidal anti-inflammatory drugs.
From Dougherty S, et al. Acute Rheumatic Fever and Rheumatic Heart Disease. 1st ed. Elsevier; 2020:31-54.

Aspirin and Other Anti-Inflammatory Drugs

Anti-inflammatory agents used include salicylates, NSAIDs, and corticosteroids. Eight randomized clinical trials (RCTs), involving 996 people and conducted between 1950 and 2001, compared anti-inflammatory agents (e.g., aspirin, corticosteroids, immunoglobulins, pentoxifylline) with placebo or controls and anti-inflammatory agents with one another, in both adults and children with ARF (according to Jones or modified Jones criteria)[24]; several steroidal agents were compared to aspirin, placebo, or no treatment. Overall, there was no significant difference in the risk of cardiac disease at 1 year between the corticosteroid-treated and aspirin-treated groups. Thus, there is little evidence of benefit of using corticosteroids or IV immunoglobulins to reduce the risk of heart valve lesions in patients with ARF.[24] However, these trials assessed cardiac involvement on clinical grounds only, and thus observer error and interobserver variability of clinical methodology could invalidate the results. Moreover, the short duration of the

follow-up does not guarantee that important cardiac sequelae did not develop in the ensuing decades.

Aspirin controls fever and pain and should be given to all patients with arthritis and/or mild carditis. Although aspirin has been used for many decades, there are surprisingly few data from RCTs to define the optimal dosing schedule. Symptomatic ARF responds dramatically to aspirin and if no improvement is seen after 24 to 48 hours of high-dose aspirin therapy, the diagnosis of ARF should be reconsidered. Salicylate toxicity is the limiting factor to aspirin therapy and is manifested by tinnitus, headache, or hyperpnea; it may not appear until after 1 week of therapy. Salicylate levels are measured only to manage toxicity. Enteric-coated, buffered, or complex salicylate molecules provide no advantage.

Other NSAIDs have been reported to be effective in small trials; naproxen (7.5 to 10 mg/kg po bid) is the most studied. However, other NSAIDs have few advantages over aspirin, especially in the first week of therapy when salicylism is uncommon.

Prednisone is recommended instead of aspirin for patients with moderate to severe carditis, as judged by a combination of clinical findings, presence of cardiac enlargement, and possibly by severely abnormal echocardiography results. The appropriate dosage is 1 to 2 mg/kg/day oral (up to 60 mg/day) divided in two or three doses. If inflammation is not suppressed after 2 days or for cases of severe heart failure, an IV corticosteroid pulse of methylprednisolone succinate (30 mg/kg IV once/day, maximum 1 g/day for 3 successive days) may be given. Oral corticosteroids are typically given for 2 to 4 weeks and then tapered over another 2 to 3 weeks. Aspirin should be started during the corticosteroid taper and continued for 2 to 4 weeks after the corticosteroid has been stopped.

The duration of therapy depends on the severity of the attack, presence of carditis, and rate of response to treatment. Milder attacks with little or no carditis may be treated with salicylates for approximately 1 month or until inflammation (clinical and laboratory evidence) has subsided. More severe cases may require 2 to 3 months of corticosteroid therapy before this can be gradually weaned. Up to 5% of patients may still have rheumatic activity despite 6 months of therapy. Occasionally a "rebound" of inflammatory activity can occur when anti-inflammatory agents are reduced and may require salicylate treatment. Inflammatory markers such as ESR and CRP may be used to monitor disease activity and response to treatment. Recurrences of mild cardiac inflammation (indicated by fever or chest pain) may subside spontaneously; anti-inflammatory drugs should be resumed if recurrent symptoms last longer than a few days or if heart failure is uncontrolled by standard management.

Antibiotic Prophylaxis

Antistreptococcal prophylaxis (with penicillin) should be maintained continuously after the initial episode of ARF to prevent recurrences. See section titled Secondary Prevention.

PREVENTION
Primordial Prevention

Improvement of social conditions and increasing access to primary health care have been associated with dramatic fall in the incidence of RF even before the advent of antibiotics (see Fig. 81.1, Curve A). Therefore, primordial prevention requires improving the broad determinants of health in people at high risk, including environmental, economic, social, behavioral, and cultural.

Primary Prevention

Antibiotic treatment of proven or presumed GAS pharyngitis with intramuscular (IM) penicillin appears to reduce the attack rate by as much as 80%.[15] Eradication of GAS from the upper respiratory tract can usually be achieved with a single IM injection of benzathine penicillin or by a 10-day course of oral penicillin.[15] Although the use of IM penicillin is supported by clinical trials, few trials have tested the efficacy of oral

TABLE 81.4 Drug Regimens for Primary and Secondary Prevention of Rheumatic Fever

ANTIBIOTICS FOR GROUP A STREPTOCOCCAL PHARYNGITIS				
AGENT	**DOSE**	**ROUTE**	**DURATION**	**RATING**
Penicillins				
Penicillin V (phenoxymethyl penicillin)	**Children** (≤27 kg [≤60 lb]) 250 mg 2-3 times daily **Children** (>27 kg [>60 lb]) **Adolescents and adults:** 500 mg 2-3 times daily	Oral	10 days	IB
Amoxicillin	50 mg/kg once daily (maximum 1 g)	Oral	10 days	IB
Benzathine penicillin G	600,000 U for patients ≤27 kg (≤60 lb), 1,200,000 U for patients >27 kg (>60 lb)	Intramuscular	Once	IB
For Individuals Allergic to Penicillin				
Narrow-spectrum cephalosporin* (cephalexin, cefadroxil)	Variable	Oral	10 days	IB
Clindamycin	20 mg/kg per day divided in three doses (maximum 1.8 g/day)	Oral	10 days	IIaB
Azithromycin	12 mg/kg once daily (maximum 500 mg)	Oral	5 days	IIaB
Clarithromycin	15 mg/kg per day divided bid (maximum 250 mg bid)	Oral	10 days	IIaB
Recommendations for Secondary Prevention of Acute Rheumatic Fever				

- Secondary prophylaxis of acute rheumatic fever (ARF) and rheumatic heart disease (RHD) comprises long-term antibiotic therapy for an individual's diagnosis with ARF or RHD to prevent ARF recurrences triggered by recurrent group A streptococcal (GAS) infection and therefore prevent the development of RHD or worsening of existing RHD.
- International guidelines differ slightly on recommendations of antibiotic choice, duration, and patient groups in whom it is indicated.
- Key standard recommendations usually include use of parental (intramuscular) benzathine penicillin G (BPG) every 4 weeks in individuals diagnosed with ARF and/or RHD for minimum 5- to 10-year period after diagnosis of the most recent ARF episode, or to the age of 21, whichever comes later. In some countries, duration for severe cases is lifelong.

*To be avoided in those with immediate (type I) hypersensitivity to penicillin.
Rating indicates classification of recommendation and level of evidence (LOE) (e.g., IB indicates class I, LOE B); bid bis in die (twice per day).
Adapted from Dougherty S, et al. Acute Rheumatic Fever and Rheumatic Heart Disease. 1st ed. Elsevier; 2020:31-54.

penicillin for the primary prevention of RF. Table 81.4 presents drug regimens of choice for primary prevention.

A cluster-randomized RCT in Nepal tested the utility of echocardiographic screening and primary prevention as a public health strategy to prevent ARF,[11] and there has been successful application of primary prevention within a comprehensive public health program in Cuba, Costa Rica, and the French islands of Martinique and Guadeloupe (see Fig. 81.1, Curve C).[6] Finally, a study conducted in South Africa showed that a strategy of using a clinical decision rule to diagnose GAS pharyngitis without culturing, associated with provision of treatment with a single IM benzathine penicillin (BPG) injection, was cost-effective in a high-risk community,[25] where culturing for RF is prohibitively expensive. Evidence from the clinical trial on primary prevention[15] and this cost-effectiveness study[25] support the treatment of symptomatic cases of GAS pharyngitis diagnosed on clinical grounds as a cost-effective public health strategy for primary prevention of RF in the context of a comprehensive national prevention program. Potential barriers to the effectiveness of primary prevention of RF solely with antibiotic therapy of GAS pharyngitis include the fact that as many as one-third of patients who develop RF do not recall any symptoms of pharyngitis, and that in outbreaks, symptoms of pharyngitis are absent in up to 58% of those infected.

Secondary Prevention

RCTs strongly support the superiority of IM compared with oral penicillin for prevention of RF recurrences (see Manyemba and Mayosi, Classic References). Shorter intervals between injections are more effective. Evidence strongly supports injections every 2 weeks (with an almost 50% reduction in the risk of RF recurrence compared with injections every 4 weeks), while it is less strong for injections taken every 3 weeks.

Recommendations for the optimal duration of secondary prophylaxis are largely empiric and based on observational studies. The duration should be individualized, taking into account the socioeconomic conditions, the risk of exposure to GAS, and the previous history of

carditis with or without valve involvement. Children without carditis should receive prophylaxis for 5 years or until age 21, whichever is longer; those with carditis with mild mitral regurgitation or healed carditis should receive prophylaxis for 10 years or until age 25 (whichever is longer). Children with carditis and evidence of residual heart damage, or those who had valve surgery, should receive prophylaxis indefinitely or, alternatively, until age 40. Finally, prophylaxis should be lifelong in all patients with severe valvular disease who have close contact with young children because these have a high rate of GAS carriage.

FUTURE PERSPECTIVES

Comprehensive programs that include primary and secondary prevention interventions are effective in reducing the incidence of ARF and RHD in endemic countries[7] and thus are recommended by the World Health Organization.

However, the diagnosis of ARF is complex, and despite involving clinical, laboratory, and echocardiographic measurements, the Jones criteria are not very sensitive or specific in countries with a high incidence. An understanding of the molecular genetic mechanisms underlying host susceptibility to enhance the Jones criteria has been hampered by the relatively small number of candidate genes in RF/RHD. There is thus the need for large-scale multicenter studies with different populations to obtain reliable and reproducible findings.[26]

There is a clear case for development of vaccines against streptococci given the large disease burden, and there are multiple vaccine candidates in clinical and preclinical development.[27-29] Demonstration of vaccine efficacy against pharyngitis and skin infections constitutes a key near-term strategic goal, which will need investments and collaborative partnerships to diversify and advance vaccine candidates.

CLASSIC REFERENCES

Bland EF, Duckett Jones T. Rheumatic fever and rheumatic heart disease; a twenty year report on 1000 patients followed since childhood. *Circulation.* 1951;4:836–843.
Dajani AS. Current status of nonsuppurative complications of group A Streptococci. *Pediatr Infect Dis J.* 1991;10:S25–S27.

Manyemba J, Mayosi BM. Intramuscular penicillin is more effective than oral penicillin in secondary prevention of rheumatic fever: a systematic review. *S Afr Med J*. 2003;93:212–218.

Popat K, Riding W. Acute rheumatic fever following streptococcal wound infection. *Postgrad Med J*. 1976;52:165–170.

Tulchinsky TH, Varavikova EA. Addressing the epidemiologic transition in the former Soviet Union: strategies for health system and public health reform in Russia. *Am J Public Health*. 1996;86:313–320.

Vasan RS, Shrivastava S, Vijayakumar M, et al. Echocardiographic evaluation of patients with acute rheumatic fever and rheumatic carditis. *Circulation*. 1996;94:73–82.

Veasy LG, Wiedmeirer SE, Orsmond GS, et al. Resurgence of acute rheumatic fever in the intermountain area of the United States. *N Engl J Med*. 1987;316:421–427.

REFERENCES

Pathogenesis

1. Carapetis JR, McDonald M, Wilson NJ. Acute rheumatic fever. *Lancet*. 2005;366:155–168.
2. Watkins DA, Johnson CO, Colquhoun SM, et al. Global, regional, and national burden of rheumatic heart disease, 1990–2015. *N Engl J Med*. 2017;377:713–722.
3. Zühlke LJ, Beaton A, Engel ME, et al. Group A Streptococcus, acute rheumatic fever and rheumatic heart disease: epidemiology and clinical considerations. *Curr Treat Options Cardiovasc Med*. 2017;19:15.
4. Carapetis JR, Beaton A, Cunningham MW, et al. Acute rheumatic fever and rheumatic heart disease. *Nat Rev Dis Primers*. 2016;2:15084.
5. Lawrence JG, Carapetis JR, Griffiths K, et al. Acute rheumatic fever and rheumatic heart disease: incidence and progression in the Northern Territory of Australia, 1997 to 2010. *Circulation*. 2013;128:492–501.
6. Mayosi BM. Screening for rheumatic heart disease in eastern Nepal. *JAMA Cardiol*. 2016;1:96–97.
7. Pastore S, De Cunto A, Benettoni A, et al. The resurgence of rheumatic fever in develop country area: the role of echocardiography. *Rheumatology*. 2011;50:396–400.
8. Nulu S, Bukhman G, Kwan GF. Rheumatic heart disease: the unfinished global agenda. *Cardiol Clin*. 2017;35:165–180.
9. Yokchoo N, Patanarapeelert N, Patanarapeelert K. The effect of group A streptococcal carrier on the epidemic model of acute rheumatic fever. *Theor Biol Med Model*. 2019;16:14.
10. Ghamrawy A, Ibrahim NN, Abd El-Wahab EW. How accurate is the diagnosis of rheumatic fever in Egypt? Data from the national rheumatic heart disease prevention and control program (2006-2018). *PLoS Negl Trop Dis*. 2020;14(8):e0008558. https://doi.org/10.1371/journal.pntd.0008558.
11. Karki P, Uranw S, Bastola S, et al. Effectiveness of systematic echocardiographic screening for rheumatic heart disease in Nepalese school children: a cluster randomized comparison. *JAMA Cardiol*. 2021. https://doi.org/10.1001/jamacardio.2020.7050.
12. Gewitz MH, Baltimore RS, Tani LY, et al. Revision of the Jones Criteria for the diagnosis of acute rheumatic fever in the era of doppler echocardiography: a scientific statement from the American Heart Association. *Circulation*. 2015;131:1806–1818.
13. Aty-Marzouk PA, Hamza H, Mosaad N, et al. New guidelines for diagnosis of rheumatic fever: do they apply to all populations? *Turk J Pediatr*. 2020;62:411–423.

Pathogenesis

14. Bright PD, Mayosi BM, Martin WJ. An immunological perspective on rheumatic heart disease pathogenesis: more questions than answer. *Heart*. 2016;102:1527–1532.
15. Lennon D, Stewart J, Aderson P. Primary prevention of rheumatic fever. *Pediatr Infect Dis J*. 2016;35:820.
16. Bennett J, Moreland NJ, Oliver J, et al. Understanding group A streptococcal pharyngitis and skin infections as causes of rheumatic fever: protocol for a prospective disease incidence study. *BMC Infect Dis*. 2019;19:633.
17. Armitage EP, Senghore E, Darboe S, et al. High burden and seasonal variation of paediatric scabies and pyoderma prevalence in the Gambia: a cross-sectional study. *PLoS Negl Trop Dis*. 2019;13:e0007801. https://doi.org/10.1371/journal.pntd.0007801.
18. Woldu B, Bloomfield GS. Rheumatic heart disease in the twenty-first century. *Curr Cardiol Rep*. 2016;18:96.
19. Dougherty S, Nascmento B, Carapetis J. Clinical evaluation and diagnosis of acute rheumatic fever. In: Dougherty S, et al., ed. *Acute Rheumatic Fever and Rheumatic Heart Disease*. 1st ed. Elsevier; 2020:31–54.
20. Spina GS, Sampaio RO, Branco CE, et al. Incidental histological diagnosis of acute rheumatic myocarditis: case report and review of the literature. *Front Pediatr*. 2014;2:126.
21. Chain JL, Alvarez K, Mascaro-Blanco A, et al. Autoantibody biomarkers for basal Ganglia Encephalitis in Sydenham chorea and pediatric autoimmune neuropsychiatric disorder associated with streptococcal infections. *Front Psychiatry*. 2020;11:564.

Clinical Features, Diagnosis, Treatment, Prevention

22. Branco CE, Sampaio RO, Branco MM, et al. Rheumatic fever: neglected and underdiagnosed disease- new perspective on diagnosis and prevention. *Arq Bras Cardiol*. 2016;107:482–484.
23. Beier K, Pratt DP. Sydenham Chorea. 2020 Jul 21. In: *StatPearls [Internet]*. Treasure Island (FL): StatPearls Publishing; 2020 Jan–. PMID: 28613588.
24. Cilliers A, Manyemba J, Adler AJ, Saloojee H. Autoinflammatory treatment for carditis in acute rheumatic fever. *Cochrane Database Syst Rev*. 2012;(6):CD003176.
25. Irlam J Mayosi BM, Engel M, Gaziano T. Primary prevention of acute rheumatic fever and rheumatic heart disease with penicillin in South Africa children with pharyngitis: a cost-effectiveness analysis. *Circ Cardiovasc Qual Outcomes*. 2013;6:343–351.

Future Perspectives

26. Muhamed B, Shaboodien G, Engel ME. Genetic variants in rheumatic fever and rheumatic heart disease. *Am J Med Genet C Semin Med Genet*. 2020;184:159–177.
27. Steer AC, Carapetis JR, Dale JB, et al. Status of research and development of vaccines for streptococcus pyogenes. *Vaccine*. 2016;34:2953–2958.
28. Rivera-Hernandez T, Carnathan DG, Jones S, et al. An Experimental group A Streptococcus vaccine that reduces pharyngitis and Tonsillitis in a Nonhuman primate model. *mBio*. 2019;10(2):e00693-19. https://doi.org/10.1128/mBio.00693-19.
29. Vekemans J, Gouvea-Reis F, Kim JH, et al. The Path to group A Streptococcus vaccines: world health Organization research and development Technology Roadmap and Preferred Product characteristics. *Clin Infect Dis*. 2019;69:877–883.

82 Congenital Heart Disease in the Adolescent and Adult

ANNE MARIE VALENTE, ADAM L. DORFMAN, SONYA V. BABU-NARAYAN, AND ERIC V. KRIEGER

GENERAL CONSIDERATIONS

The number of adults living with congenital heart disease (CHD) is growing faster than the number of children with CHD, and now is estimated to be at least 1.4 million adults in the United States alone.[1,2] At least 20% of these adult congenital heart disease (ACHD) patients have complex cardiovascular anatomy and suffer from multi-system organ involvement. Lifelong follow-up in coordination with, or directly by, clinicians with expertise in ACHD is recommended. This chapter describes the long-term complications of living with CHD and highlights many of the potential comorbidities, discusses CHD nomenclature and cardiac development, and summarizes the more common CHD lesions that may be encountered in adulthood.

Access and Delivery of ACHD Care

In 2001, the 32nd Bethesda Conference addressed the changing profile of adults living with CHD by developing guidelines for delivery of care. In this document, congenital heart defects are grouped according to anatomic complexity. As the field has grown, there has been a recognition of the limitations of this system, which does not incorporate comorbidities or physiology into the levels of anatomic complexity. Therefore, in 2018, the American College of Cardiology (ACC) and the American Heart Association (AHA) released an updated set of ACHD guidelines which incorporates not only the anatomical classification (Table 82.1A) but also the physiological stage (Table 82.1B) of each patient.[3] This classification scheme is used throughout the guidelines to provide lesion-specific frequency of follow-up, testing, and general management.

Inherent in these guidelines is the expectation that any adult with CHD who has anything other than simple, unrepaired, isolated lesions or fully repaired shunt lesions should be managed in conjunction with an ACHD cardiologist. There is also emphasis that the most complex ACHD patients should receive the majority of their care at a center with dedicated ACHD expertise, as data confirms that ACHD patients cared for in specialized centers have lower mortality than those receiving care in centers lacking specific ACHD programs.[4] In 2020, revised guidelines for management of ACHD patients were released by the European Society of Cardiology.[5] This document includes sections on staffing requirements for ACHD expert centers, consideration of palliative care planning, expanded recommendations on arrhythmia and pulmonary hypertension (PH) management, and the emerging role of biomarkers and catheter-based interventions in ACHD patients.

Transition to ACHD Care

Due to advances in the management of CHD, a once life-threatening childhood illness is now often transformed into a chronic adult condition. With early surgical intervention, the majority of patients are repaired but not cured and require lifelong surveillance. Therefore, there is a critical need for successful transition and transfer of CHD patients from pediatric to adult CHD care. However, multiple barriers prevent effective transition. These barriers range from lack of a structured transition program to provider-patient/parent attachment, or unavailability of ACHD providers.[6] Pediatric cardiology programs should partner with an ACHD program to allow for successful transition and transfer of care. Transition discussions should begin at the age of 12 years, with the expectation of complete transfer to ACHD care

🌐 Additional content is available online at Elsevier eBooks for Practicing Clinicians

TABLE 82.1A Anatomic Classification of Congenital Heart Conditions

	CHD ANATOMY*		
	I: Simple	II: Moderate Complexity	III: Great Complexity (or Complex)
	Native disease • Isolated small ASD • Isolated small VSD • Mild isolated pulmonic stenosis **Repaired conditions** • Previously ligated or occluded ductus arteriosus • Repaired secundum ASD or sinus venosus defect without significant residual shunt or chamber enlargement • Repaired VSD without significant residual shunt or chamber enlargement	**Repaired or unrepaired conditions** • Aorto-left ventricular fistula • Anomalous pulmonary venous connection, partial or total • Anomalous coronary artery arising from the pulmonary artery • Anomalous aortic origin of a coronary artery from the opposite sinus • AVSD (partial or complete, including primum ASD) • Congenital aortic valve disease • Congenital mitral valve disease • Coarctation of the aorta • Ebstein anomaly (disease spectrum includes mild, moderate, and severe variations) • Infundibular right ventricular outflow obstruction • Ostium primum ASD • Moderate and large unrepaired secundum ASD • Moderate and large persistently patent ductus arteriosus • Pulmonary valve regurgitation (moderate or greater) • Pulmonary valve stenosis (moderate or greater) • Peripheral pulmonary stenosis • Sinus of Valsalva fistula/aneurysm • Sinus venosus defect • Subvalvar aortic stenosis (excluding HCM; HCM not addressed in these guidelines) • Supravalvar aortic stenosis • Straddling atrioventricular valve • Repaired tetralogy of Fallot • VSD with associated abnormality and/or moderate or greater shunt	• Cyanotic congenital heart defect (unrepaired or palliated, all forms) • Double-outlet ventricle • Fontan procedure • Interrupted aortic arch • Mitral atresia • Single ventricle (including double inlet left ventricle, tricuspid atresia, hypoplastic left heart, any other anatomic abnormality with a functionally single ventricle) • Pulmonary atresia (all forms) • TGA (classic or d-TGA; CCTGA or l-TGA) • Truncus arteriosus • Other abnormalities of atrioventricular and ventriculoarterial connection (i.e., crisscross heart, isomerism, heterotaxy syndromes, ventricular inversion)

*This list is not meant to be comprehensive; other conditions may be important in individual patients.
ACHD, Adult congenital heart disease; *AP,* anatomic and physiological; *ASD,* atrial septal defect; *AVSD,* atrioventricular septal defect; *CCTGA,* congenitally corrected transposition of the great arteries; *CHD,* congenital heart disease; *d- TGA,* dextro-transposition of the great arteries; *FC,* functional class; *HCM,* hypertrophic cardiomyopathy; *l-TGA,* levo-transposition of the great arteries; *NYHA,* New York Heart Association; *TGA,* transposition of the great arteries; *VSD,* ventricular septal defect.
Modified from Stout KK, Daniels CJ, Aboulhosn J, et al. 2018 AHA/ACC Guideline for the Management of Adults With Congenital Heart Disease: A report of the American College of Cardiology/American Heart Association Task Force on Clinical Practice Guidelines. *J Am Coll Cardiol.* 2019;73(12):1494–1563.

TABLE 82.1B Physiologic Stages of Adult Congenital Heart Disease Patient Classification

	A	B	C	D
Symptoms	NYHA FC I symptoms	NYHA FC II symptoms	NYHA FC III symptoms	NYHA IV symptoms
Valvular Disease		Mild	Significant	
Arrhythmias		Not requiring treatment	Controlled with treatment	Refractory to treatment
Hemodynamic Sequelae		Mild (mild aortic enlargement, mild ventricular enlargement, mild ventricular dysfunction)	Moderate or greater ventricular dysfunction (systemic, pulmonic, or both) Moderate aortic enlargement	Severe aortic enlargement
Exercise Capacity	Normal	Abnormal objective cardiac limitation to exercise		
Other	Normal renal, hepatic, and pulmonary function	Trivial or small shunt (not hemodynamically significant)	Venous or arterial stenosis Mild or moderate hypoxemia/cyanosis Hemodynamically significant shunt Pulmonary hypertension End-organ dysfunction responsive to therapy	Severe hypoxemia (almost always associated with cyanosis) Severe pulmonary hypertension Eisenmenger syndrome Refractory end-organ dysfunction

Modified from Stout KK, Daniels CJ, Aboulhosn JA, et al. 2018 AHA/ACC Guideline for the Management of Adults With Congenital Heart Disease: A report of the American College of Cardiology/American Heart Association Task Force on Clinical Practice Guidelines. *J Am Coll Cardiol.* 2019;73(12):1494–1563.

by 21 years of age. The probability of a successful transfer is directly related to documentation of the need for such in the medical record and formal educational interventions geared at understanding self-management skills.[7]

Clinical Evaluation

In caring for adults with CHD, it is helpful to understand some of the common terminology regarding congenital anatomy and prior procedures (Table 82.2). Many ACHD patients have had surgical interventions as children, and it is essential to understand the specific procedures and potential sequelae from these interventions. The physical examination of ACHD patients may also provide unique clues to prior procedures when the recorded history is unclear. Location of surgical scars will indicate whether a patient has had a lateral thoracotomy, such as with a patent ductus arteriosus (PDA) ligation or aortic coarctation repair. Additionally, absence of a radial pulse on the ipsilateral arm as a thoracotomy scar may suggest that the subclavian artery was sacrificed in the repair (such as a subclavian flap repair for coarctation of the aorta or a prior classic Blalock-Taussig-Thomas [BTT] shunt).

TABLE 82.2 Common Congenital Heart Disease Eponyms

ANATOMY EPONYMS	ANATOMIC DESCRIPTION
Bland-White-Garland syndrome	Anomalous left coronary artery from the pulmonary artery (ALCAPA)
Eisenmenger syndrome	Pulmonary hypertension with cyanosis due to right to left shunting
Gerbode defect	Septal defect resulting in direct left ventricle to right atrium shunt
Holmes Heart	Double inlet left ventricle with D-looped ventricles and normally related great vessels
Raghib defect	Coronary sinus septal defect in the presence of a left superior vena cava
Scimitar syndrome	Partial anomalous pulmonary venous connections of the right lower pulmonary vein to the IVC-RA junction, often accompanied by pulmonary artery hypoplasia and aortopulmonary collateral formation.
Shone syndrome	Series of left-sided obstructive lesions
Taussig-Bing Malformation	Form of double outlet right ventricle with D-malposed, side-by-side great vessels, sub-pulmonary VSD, hypoplastic aortic arch

SURGICAL EPONYMS	PROCEDURE DESCRIPTION
Baffes procedure	Early palliative procedure for transposition of the great arteries, with the inferior vena cava directed to the left atrium via homograft
Blalock-Taussig(-Thomas) shunt	"Classic"—direct end to end anastomosis of subclavian artery to pulmonary artery
	"Modified"—tube graft from subclavian artery to pulmonary artery
Brock Procedure	Closed infundibular resection for relief of pulmonary stenosis
Fontan or Fontan-Kreutzer	Atriopulmonary anastomosis for single ventricle heart disease
Fontan-Björk Modification	Includes the right ventricle into the pulmonary circulation, was the unique modification for tricuspid atresia
Glenn	"Classic"—end to end anastomosis of superior vena cava to right pulmonary artery
	"bidirectional"—end to side anastomosis of superior vena cava to right pulmonary artery
Kawashima	Bidirectional Glenn in context of interrupted inferior vena cava with azygos continuation to the superior vena cava
Lecompte Maneuver	Anterior translocation of the pulmonary arteries, so that both branch pulmonary arteries run anterior to the aorta. Most commonly used as part of the arterial switch operation
Mustard/Senning	Atrial switch operations for transposition of the great arteries, with atrial baffling using native atrial (Senning) or pericardial (Mustard) tissue to redirect systemic and pulmonary venous flow
Nikaidoh	In double outlet right ventricle, posterior translocation of the aortic root towards the left ventricle, with baffling of the left ventricle to the aorta in its new position
Norwood	Neonatal palliative procedure for hypoplastic left heart syndrome including aortic arch reconstruction with anastomosis of the native aorta to the pulmonary artery, which becomes the "neo-aorta," as well as atrial septectomy and a modified BT shunt
Potts shunt	Direct anastomosis of the left pulmonary artery to the descending aorta
Rastelli	Intra-cardiac routing of the left ventricle to the aorta, which arose from the right ventricle. Usually accompanied by a right ventricle to pulmonary artery conduit.
Takeuchi repair	Intrapulmonary baffle of the left coronary artery performed for anomalous left coronary artery from the pulmonary artery
Waterston shunt	Direct anastomosis of the right pulmonary artery to the ascending aorta

IVC, Inferior vena cava; *RA*, right atrium; *VSD*, ventricular septal defect.

The physical examination is also revealing in adult patients with newly discovered CHD, such as fixed splitting of the second heart sound in a patient with an unrepaired atrial septal defect (ASD), or diminished lower extremity pulses in a patient with an aortic coarctation. A classic physical examination finding in a patient with pulmonary stenosis is a systolic ejection click which decreases in intensity with inspiration.

The electrocardiogram (ECG) is an important tool in the assessment of CHD. The heart rhythm and rate, as well as the atrioventricular (AV) conduction, can be evaluated (see Chapter 14 and the ECG figures in the online chapter). Table 82.3 lists some of the common arrhythmias and ECG findings in various CHD conditions. The chest radiograph is an additional valuable tool in the assessment of the patient with CHD. Cardiac imaging plays an essential role in the management of ACHD patients. In 2020, Appropriate Use Criteria for multimodality imaging for follow-up care of CHD was released. This document presents 1035 unique scenarios to consider and rates various noninvasive imaging modalities into three categories: appropriate, may be appropriate, or rarely appropriate.[8]

The choice of when to obtain an echocardiogram, cardiac magnetic resonance (CMR), computed tomography (CT), nuclear scintigraphy, cardiac catheterization with x-ray angiography, or a combination of these modalities is dictated by the pertinent clinical question(s) and

by a host of patient- and modality-related factors. Echocardiography remains the cornerstone of cardiac imaging in the CHD patient (see also Chapter 16). However, as patients age, acoustic windows may be suboptimal, and the other imaging modalities such as CMR (see also Chapter 19) or cardiac CT (CCT, see also Chapter 20) are advantageous. Due to the need for serial imaging, cumulative exposure to ionizing radiation should be taken into account as ACHD patients have increased risk for malignancy, perhaps related to these procedures. Cardiopulmonary exercise testing and measurement of biomarkers play an important role in the serial follow-up and the timing of intervention and re-intervention. Cardiac catheterization (see also Chapter 21) is recommended in any ACHD patient with signs of elevated pulmonary artery (PA) pressure to determine pulmonary vascular resistance (PVR). There should be a low threshold for cardiac catheterization in any ACHD patient with new symptoms not explained with noninvasive testing, particularly in complex CHD patients.

Noncardiac Complications in the ACHD Patient

As ACHD patients age, extracardiac complications become increasingly prevalent and affect patients' long-term outcomes.[9] These

TABLE 82.3 Common Arrhythmias and Typical ECG Abnormalities Seen in Adults with Congenital Heart Disease

ACHD CONDITION	COMMON ARRHYTHMIAS	TYPICAL ECG ABNORMALITIES
D-loop TGA, status post atrial switch (Mustard or Senning)	• Sinus node dysfunction • IART • Sudden death	• Right axis deviation • Right ventricular hypertrophy with strain
L-loop TGA	• Complete heart block	• Q-waves in right precordial leads and absent septal Q waves in the left precordial leads • PR prolongation or AV block
Fontan circulation	• Sinus node dysfunction • IART • Atrial fibrillation	• Depends on intracardiac anatomy
Atrioventricular septal defects	• Complete heart block • IART	• Left axis deviation • Right bundle branch block
Ebstein anomaly	• Accessory pathways and pre-excitation • IART • Atrial fibrillation	• Right atrial enlargement • Right bundle branch block with QRS fragmentation • Low-amplitude QRS • First-degree AV block but PR interval can be short if accessory pathways present
Tetralogy of Fallot	• Ventricular tachycardia • IART • Sudden death	• Right atrial enlargement • Right axis deviation • Right bundle branch block with QRS fragmentation
Eisenmenger syndrome	• IART • Sudden death	• Right atrial enlargement • Right axis deviation • Right ventricular hypertrophy

ACHD, Adult congenital heart disease; *AV,* atrioventricular; *IART,* interatrial re-entrant tachycardia; *TGA,* transposition of the great arteries.

noncardiac complications may be present in ACHD patients, regardless of their level of complexity and may involve any organ system (Table 82.4). Many ACHD patients live with subclinical levels of organ dysfunction and small perturbations in their hemodynamics may result in dramatic decline in function. Abnormal lung function is common in ACHD patients, and up to 40% of ACHD patients have abnormal pulmonary function tests. There are multiple mechanisms for abnormal pulmonary mechanics in ACHD patients, such as restrictive lung disease in postoperative patients. Other patients may have diaphragmatic paralysis due to phrenic nerve injury, asymmetric pulmonary blood flow due to branch PA abnormalities or acquired conditions, such as sleep apnea. ACHD patients are more prone to develop pulmonary thrombosis and embolism, pulmonary hemorrhage, and pneumonia. Pneumonia is one of the leading causes of noncardiac death in ACHD patients.[10] There are specific pulmonary complications that may be seen in certain ACHD conditions, such as plastic bronchitis in patients living with Fontan physiology. Hemoptysis may occur in up to one-third of ACHD patients with Eisenmenger syndrome. PH is found in up to 10% of ACHD patients and is strongly associated with increased morbidity and mortality (see section on Pulmonary Hypertension and Eisenmenger Syndrome).

Renal dysfunction is common in ACHD patients and has been shown to be a primary driver of high-resource utilization for ACHD hospitalizations, accounting for up to one-third of hospital charges.[11] While cyanotic ACHD patients have the highest prevalence of impaired renal function, non-cyanotic ACHD patients also develop renal insufficiency with age, and renal impairment is directly associated with mortality in these patients. Therefore, it is prudent to assess renal function at regular intervals in aging ACHD patients. Cystatin C-based estimated glomerular filtration rate (eGFR) more accurately predicts clinical effects in ACHD patients than creatinine-based eGFR.[12]

The prevalence of liver disease among ACHD patients is poorly characterized and most likely underestimated. The majority of the evidence of hepatic dysfunction in ACHD patients has been focused on Fontan-associated liver disease (FALD).[13] The pathologic findings can range

from congestive hepatopathy to frank cirrhosis. Patients may have varying degrees of fibrosis with nodular regeneration. The etiology of hepatic dysfunction is most likely multifactorial, with systemic venous congestion and/or ischemia coupled with non-hemodynamic factors such as drug or viral-induced injury (see section on Fontan-Associated Liver Disease). Hepatitis C remains an important cause of liver disease in older ACHD patients, particularly those who received blood transfusions prior to 1992. Hematologic abnormalities in ACHD patients are common and include anemia, which is associated with increased mortality. Abnormalities of the coagulation system are observed in patients with Fontan physiology and are associated with bleeding and thrombotic complications. Cyanotic patients with erythrocytosis are at risk for hyperviscosity symptoms (see Eisenmenger section). Endocrinopathies and metabolic disorders are common in ACHD patients and may include thyroid disorders, obesity, diabetes, dyslipidemia, and disorders of calcium metabolism. Cancer is the second leading cause of non-cardiovascular death in ACHD patients,[10] with certain malignancies having an increased prevalence in specific CHD conditions, that is, hepatocellular carcinoma in adults with Fontan physiology. There is an increased risk of infectious and immunological complications in the ACHD population. The incidence of stroke is higher in ACHD patients than the general population.[14] Lastly, there is a growing body of evidence on the association of neurocognitive defects and CHD. At least one-third of ACHD patients report a mood or anxiety related disorder and many patients have deficits in executive function. These cognitive defects and psychosocial challenges have an impact on health status, education, employment, and quality of life.

CONGENITAL ANATOMY

Congenital Nomenclature

One of the challenges in caring for adults with CHD is the inconsistent terminology used to describe the anatomy and several classification systems have been proposed. Drs. Stella and Richard Van Praagh

TABLE 82.4 Noncardiac Complications in Adult Congenital Heart Disease

Neurologic	Increased incidence of occult or clinically evident strokes
	Decreased level of executive functioning skills
	Anxiety, post-traumatic stress disorder, depression
	Psychosocial disorders
	Neurodevelopmental deficits
Lungs	Restrictive lung disease
	Pulmonary vascular disease
	Pulmonary hypertension
	Pulmonary hemorrhage
	Plastic bronchitis
Immunology/ infectious disease	Protein-losing enteropathy
	Infective endocarditis
	Pneumonia
	Brain abscess
Renal	Decreased perfusion
	Chronic kidney disease
	Cardiorenal syndrome
Hepatic	Liver fibrosis
	Congestive hepatopathy
	Cardiac cirrhosis
	Fontan associated liver disease
Endocrine	Thyroid
	Calcium hemostasis/Bone health
	Obesity/Metabolic syndrome
	Diabetes
	Dyslipidemia
Vascular	Chronic venous insufficiency
	Cerebrovascular disease
	Aortopathy
	Endothelial dysfunction
	Hypertension
	Peripheral venous/arterial disease
Orthopedic	Scoliosis
	Kyphosis
Hematologic	Anemia
	Coagulopathies
	Secondary erythrocytosis/iron deficiency/ hyperuricemia (cyanotic CHD)
	Thromboembolism
Oncology	Low-dose ionizing radiation and malignancy
	Hepatocellular carcinoma
	Age-appropriate cancer screening

championed the segmental approach for description of congenital anatomy. In this approach, the heart is composed of several segments that are analyzed separately before formulating a comprehensive diagnosis. The principal segments are the atria, the ventricles, and the great arteries, which are joined together by the AV canal and the conus (infundibulum). In the normal heart, the right ventricle (RV) is right-sided and organized inflow-to-outflow from right to left, while the left ventricle (LV) is left-sided and organized inflow-to-outflow from left to right. It is important to determine the segmental alignments: that is, what drains into what. For example, in the normal heart the right atrium

(RA) is aligned with the RV and the RV is aligned with the PA. Similarly, in a normal heart the left atrium (LA) is aligned with the LV and the LV is aligned with the aorta. Finally, the segmental connections, the way in which adjacent segments are physically linked to each other, are described. For example, in the normal heart the RV is connected to the PA by a complete muscular conus (infundibulum), while the LV is connected to the aorta by aortic-mitral fibrous continuity (without a complete conus). Alignment and connection are distinct concepts and both are important, especially in complex defects.

Cardiac Development (Fig. 82.1)

The heart starts to form in the third week of gestation and is nearly fully formed by 8 weeks gestation. Mesodermal precardiac cells migrate to form the cardiac crescents (primary heart fields) in anterior lateral plate mesoderm, which are then brought together to form a primary linear heart tube by ventral closure of the embryo. Cells of the second heart field continue to proliferate outside the heart and are added to the heart tube over the course of embryogenesis, contributing to the atria, the RV, and outflow tract. Additionally, cardiac neural crest cells migrate into the developing heart in the 5th to 6th weeks and are essential for septation of the outflow, formation of the semilunar valves, and patterning of the aortic arches. Once formed, the heart tube grows and elongates by addition of cells from the second heart field. The ends of the heart tube are relatively fixed by the pericardial sac so that as it elongates it must loop (bend), and in the vast majority of hearts the loop falls to the right (D-loop). Further elongation pushes the mid-portion of the tube (future ventricles) inferior or caudal to the inflow, resulting in the normal relationship between the atria and ventricles. Further growth pushes the outflow medially and is associated with outflow rotation, both processes essential for normal alignment of the outflow. Finally, the proximal part of the outflow is incorporated in the RV, shortening the outflow in association with further rotation. While this remodeling is occurring, the outflow is undergoing septation under the influence of cardiac neural crest cells. Septation proceeds from distal to proximal, culminating in formation and muscularization of the infundibular, or muscular, outflow septum, which inserts onto the superior endocardial cushion at the rightward rim of the outflow foramen, walling the aorta into the LV via the outflow foramen and the PA directly into the RV (Video 82.1).

Genetic Considerations

CHD is the most commonly occurring birth defect and genetic etiologies are increasingly being recognized. Several hundred genes have been identified to either cause or contribute to CHD.[15] Epidemiological studies have suggested that a genetic or environmental cause can be identified in up to 30% of CHD cases. Single-gene disorders are found in 3% to 5%, gross chromosomal anomalies/aneuploidy in 8% to 10%, and pathogenic copy number variants in up to 25% of CHD cases. Environmental causes are identifiable in 2% of CHD cases. The remainder of CHD is presumed to be multifactorial.[16]

Sequence variants in CHD genes can cause both sporadic and inherited forms of CHD. Sequence variants in the same genes may be associated with different cardiac phenotypes, not only between families but also within families. Additionally, there is evolving evidence that some of the outcomes in patients with CHD may be influenced by the underlying genetic cause.[17]

Down syndrome is the most common aneuploidy and is usually caused by trisomy 21. It is also the most common chromosome abnormality associated with CHD. Fifty percent of children born with Down syndrome have CHD, most commonly defects in the AV canal. Table 82.5 lists certain genetic syndromes and associated congenital cardiac conditions.

LONG-TERM CONSIDERATIONS

Arrhythmias in Adult Congenital Heart Disease
Demographics and Prognosis

Arrhythmias are prevalent in ACHD patients. The frequency of arrhythmias increases with age and disease complexity. Arrhythmia causes

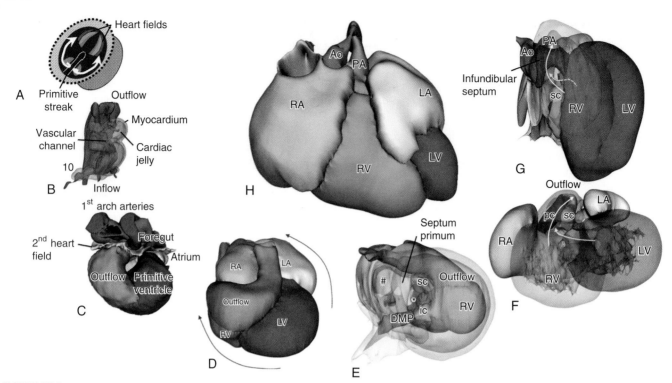

FIGURE 82.1 Developmental highlights. **A,** Carnegie stage (CS) 7-disc embryo during mid 3rd week illustrating gastrulation through the primitive streak to form the mesoderm and rostral migration of pre-cardiac mesoderm to form the 1st *(blue)* and 2nd *(yellow)* heart fields. **B,** CS 10 heart in the early 4th week showing the newly formed tubular heart. The vascular channel is seen through the semitransparent myocardium and cardiac jelly. **C,** CS 11 heart at mid 4th week. The heart tube is enlarged and lengthened by addition of cells from the proliferating 2nd heart field at both the outflow and inflow ends. As it lengthens in the confined pericardial space the heart tube bends or loops, usually to the right (**D** or dextral looping), leading to the final shape of the heart with ventricles caudal and atria rostral. **D,** CS 13 heart at the beginning of the 5th week showing chamber development by ballooning outgrowth of proliferating myocytes at specified points around the outer or greater curvature of the looped heart tube. Lengthening of the outflow pushes it centrally between the developing atria (*LA,* left atrium; *LV,* left ventricle; *RA,* right atrium; *RV,* right ventricular). **E,** CS 15 heart at the beginning of the 6th week. Looking through the semitransparent right posterior wall of the right atrium shows the septum primum (primary atrial septum) in yellow and the dorsal mesenchymal protrusion (DMP) in purple, the main components of the atrial septation complex. The DMP, a prong of cells originating from 2nd heart field, will continue to invade, filling the space between the superior *(sc)* and inferior *(ic)* endocardial cushions and closing ostium primum (*) completing atrial septation and contributing to division of the atrioventricular (AV) canal into left (mitral) and right (tricuspid) orifices. By this stage ostium secundum (#) or the foramen ovale has formed by breakdown of the septum primum at its origin from the posterior-superior atrial wall. The AV canal has begun to expand rightward so that it drains both atria into only the left ventricle (LV). **F,** CS 17 heart at the beginning of the 7th week viewed from the apex with the ventricles and outflow semitransparent showing the shortened and partially rotated outflow, resulting in spiraling of the parietal (pc) and septal (sc) outflow cushions or ridges about each other. The cushions have begun to fuse together distally under the influence of neural crest cells dividing the outflow into an anterior pulmonary *(white arrow)* and a posterior aortic *(yellow arrow)* pathway. Further anticlockwise rotation will bring the aortic pathway closer to the interventricular foramen, the eventual LV outflow. **G,** CS 19 heart at the end of the 7th week viewed from right and anterior with the RV semitransparent and the RA removed. Complete septation of the outflows is accomplished by formation and muscularization of the infundibular septum as the proximal parts of the outflow cushions fuse. The membranous septum forms where the developing infundibular septum joins the superior endocardial cushion *(sc)*. The LV pathway to the aorta *(yellow arrow)* through the interventricular foramen is on the far side of the infundibular septum and the pathway from RV to pulmonary artery *(white arrow)* is on the near side. **H,** CS 23 heart at the end of embryogenesis (end of 8th week) showing the completed but still immature fetal heart. Also see Video 82.1.

morbidity and mortality in adults with CHD and is the most frequent cause for hospital admission in adults with CHD. Patients with CHD with arrhythmia have a worse prognosis than those without.

New arrhythmias in a patient with CHD should prompt a careful evaluation to determine whether there is a hemodynamic cause for the arrhythmia. In many cases worsening ventricular dysfunction, valve dysfunction, or filling pressures can precipitate new rhythm disturbances. Echocardiography may yield information but in some catheterization is required.

The demographics and mechanisms of arrhythmia are very different in ACHD patients compared to adults with acquired heart disease: ACHD patients develop arrhythmia at a much younger age, frequently in their late teens or early 20s for patients with complex forms of CHD. Patients with ACHD are likely to have re-entrant arrhythmia related to surgical scars or around patches although diffuse fibrosis may predispose to arrhythmias as well. Patients with CHD are often intolerant of arrhythmia and in most instances restoration of sinus rhythm is preferred over rate control. In 2014 the Pediatric and Congenital Electrophysiology Society and the Heart Rhythm Society published a comprehensive consensus statement on the management of arrhythmias in adults with CHD.[18] Arrhythmias are discussed further in the sections on individual lesions.

Diagnostic Testing

Resting ECG is indicated in most patients with CHD. Common ECG abnormalities are shown in Table 82.3. Because rhythm disturbances

become more prevalent with increasing age, serial ECG monitoring is needed for patients at high risk for arrhythmia such as those with tetralogy of Fallot (TOF), Ebstein anomaly, Fontan circulation, transposition of the great arteries (TGA), and others.

Ambulatory ECG monitoring is useful to investigate palpitations and to screen for occult arrhythmia in asymptomatic patients. In patients with TOF asymptomatic nonsustained ventricular tachycardia (VT) recorded on Holter monitoring predicts clinical VT. In other CHD lesions, however, the clinical significance of asymptomatic arrhythmias seen on ambulatory ECG remains unknown. Exercise ECG monitoring is useful for patients with exercise-induced symptoms. Implantable loop recorders can be used for patients with infrequent but worrisome symptoms of arrhythmia.

The need for invasive electrophysiology (EP) study with programmed stimulation and electroanatomic mapping should be determined on a case-by-case basis. Inducible sustained VT is a risk factor for clinical VT and sudden death in patients with repaired TOF and is discussed in more detail in the section on Tetralogy of Fallot. The prognostic value of programmed electrical stimulation has not been determined in other forms of CHD and, in some conditions such as TGA, is not of prognostic value.[18]

Types of Arrhythmia

The type of arrhythmia encountered depends both on the native CHD lesion as well as the type of surgical repair (see Table 82.3).

TABLE 82.5 Genetic Syndromes and Congenital Heart Disease

SYNDROME	GENE(S)	CARDIAC DISEASE	% CONGENITAL HD	ASSOCIATED FINDINGS
Alagille	*JAG 1* *Notch2*	Pps, tof, pa	>90	Bile duct paucity, butterfly vertebrae, renal defects
CHARGE	*CHD7*	TOF, PDA, DORV, AVSD, VSD	75–85	Coloboma, choanal atresia, genital hypoplasia, ear anomalies, hearing loss, developmental delay, growth retardation, intellectual disability
22q11.2DS	*TBX1*	Conotruncal defects, VSD, IAA, ASD, VR	74–85	Cleft palate, bifid uvula, velopharyngeal insufficiency, microcephaly, hypocalcemia, immune deficit, psychiatric disorder, learning disability
Ellis-van Creveld	*EVC* *EVC2*	Common atrium	60	Skeletal dysplasia, short limbs, polydactyly, short ribs, dysplastic nails, respiratory insufficiency
Holt-Oram	*TBX5*	VSD, ASD, AVSD, conduction defects	50	Absent, hypoplastic, or triphalangeal thumbs; phocomelia; defects of radius; limb defects more prominent on left
Kabuki	*KMT2D* *KDM6A*	CoA, BAV, VSD, TOF, TGA, HLHS	50	Growth deficiency, wide palpebral fissures, large protuberant ears, fetal finger pads, intellectual disability, clinodactyly
Noonan	*PTPN11* *SOS1* *RAF1* *KRAS* *NRAS* *RIT1* *SHOC2* *SOS2* *BRAF*	Dysplastic PVS, ASD, TOF, AVSD, HCM, VSD, PDA	75	Short stature, hypertelorism, down-slanting palpebral fissures, ptosis, low posterior hairline, pectus deformity, bleeding disorder, chylothorax, cryptorchidism
VACTERAL association	Unknown	VSD, ASD, HLHS, PDA, TGA, TOF, TA	53–80	Vertebral anomalies, anal atresia, tracheoesophageal fistula, renal anomalies, radial dysplasia, thumb hypoplasia, single umbilical artery
Williams-Beuren	7q11/23 deletion (*ELN*)	SVAS, PAS, VSD, ASD	80	Unusual facies, thick lips, strabismus, stellate iris pattern, intellectual disability

ASD, Atrial septal defect; *AVSD*, atrioventricular septal defect; *BAV*, bicuspid aortic valve; *CoA*, coarctation of the aorta; *DORV*, double outlet right ventricle; *HCM*, hypertrophic cardiomyopathy; *HLHS*, hypoplastic left heart syndrome; *IAA*, interrupted aortic arch; *PA*, pulmonary atresia; *PAS*, pulmonary artery stenosis; *PDA*, patent ductus arteriosus; *PPS*, peripheral pulmonary stenosis; *PVS*, pulmonary valve stenosis; *TOF*, tetralogy of Fallot; *VR*, vascular ring; *VSD*, ventricular septal defect; *TGA*, transposition of the great arteries; *TA*, truncus arteriosus; *SVAS*, supravalvular aortic stenosis.
Modified from Pierpont ME, Brueckner M, Chung WK, et al. Genetic basis for congenital heart disease: revisited: a scientific statement from the American Heart Association. *Circulation*. 2018;138(21):e653–e711.

Bradyarrhythmia

Sinus Node Dysfunction

Sinus node dysfunction is most commonly related to surgical injury. Sinus node dysfunction is commonly encountered in patients with D-loop TGA who have undergone a Mustard or Senning operation and is also common following repair for ASD or sinus venosus defects. Patients with Glenn shunt or Fontan circulation may have sinus node dysfunction.

Atrial pacing is required for symptomatic sinus node dysfunction. Transvenous pacing is usually preferred but may be technically difficult in patients who have had surgical manipulation of the superior vena cava (SVC) (who are the same patients who are predisposed to sinus node dysfunction). Patients who have had a Fontan operation with an extracardiac conduit and those with open atrial shunts typically require epicardial pacing. Transvenous atrial pacing may be possible in patients with a lateral tunnel or atriopulmonary Fontan. Transvenous pacing is typically possible following the Mustard or Senning procedure or after repair of a superior sinus venosus defect but endocardial leads increase the risk of SVC stenosis or obstruction.

Heart Block

Heart block is common in patients with L-loop TGA as the AV node is superiorly and anteriorly displaced. The incidence of complete heart block in L-loop TGA is 2% per year. Patients with double-inlet LV also have a high incidence of heart block. Heart block is common in adults who had surgical repair of an atrioventricular septal defect (AVSD) as the AV node and His bundles are displaced posteriorly and

can be injured by ventricular septal defect (VSD) closure, although modern surgical techniques have decreased the likelihood of heart block in this population. Finally, complete heart block is a common post-surgical complication from patients who have had resection of a subaortic membrane or multiple operations on the left ventricular outflow tract (LVOT).

Pacemakers are used to treat heart block. Transvenous pacemakers are preferred when technically feasible. Biventricular pacing with cardiac resynchronization may be desirable for patients with underlying ventricular dysfunction or a systemic RV who require chronic ventricular pacing.

Tachyarrhythmias

Interatrial Re-Entrant Tachycardia

Interatrial re-entrant tachycardia (IART) is the most common tachyarrhythmia in CHD, accounting for 62% of atrial arrhythmias.[19] The cumulative incidence of IART approaches 50% by age 65 and occurs in a wide variety of CHD lesions.[20] IART can conduct around an anatomic obstacle such as an ASD patch or an atriotomy scar. While it may occur in children, frequency increases by young adulthood as progressive atrial fibrosis contributes to arrhythmogenesis. IART is exceedingly common in patients who have had a Mustard or Senning operation and for those with an atriopulmonary Fontan. In patients who have undergone the atrial switch operation, IART is a dangerous arrhythmia which may convert to polymorphic VT or pulseless electrical activity as the noncompliant interatrial baffles and systemic RV perform poorly at high heart rates. Patients with Fontan circulation also tolerate chronic

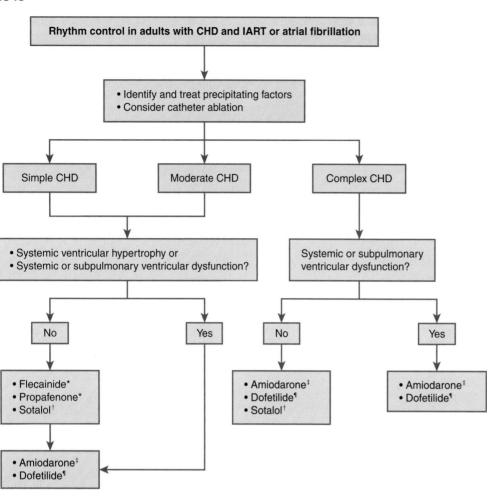

FIGURE 82.2 Rhythm control in adults with congenital heart disease (CHD) and intra-atrial reentrant tachycardia (IART) or atrial fibrillation. (From Khairy P, Van Hare GF, Balaji S, et al. PACES/HRS expert consensus statement on the recognition and management of arrhythmias in adult congenital heart disease. *Heart Rhythm.* 2014;11:e102–e665.)

patient's underlying congenital anatomy and consider risk factors for pro-arrhythmia such as ventricular dysfunction or QTc prolongation (Fig. 82.2). Sotalol and dofetilide are often preferred in patients with complex CHD. Amiodarone has considerable cumulative toxicity so is usually not a preferred first-line anti-arrhythmic in younger patients but is sometimes required for patients with ventricular dysfunction.

Which patients with atrial arrhythmia and CHD require long-term anticoagulation remains an area of active investigation. Risk models such as CHA_2DS_2-VASc are not validated in CHD and should not be relied upon because CHD patients have a much higher rate of thromboembolism than similarly aged patients with acquired heart disease, even in the absence of conventional risk factors.[22] Patients with Fontan circulation and IART should receive long-term anticoagulation. Patients with atrial arrhythmia and complex CHD should be considered for long-term anticoagulation as well. Both vitamin K antagonists and direct oral anticoagulants have been used successfully in adult patients with CHD.[23]

Atrial Fibrillation (see Chapter 66)
As patients with CHD age, atrial fibrillation becomes more common and is the most common atrial arrhythmia in adults with CHD older than age 50. Adults with CHD have a greater than 20-fold increased risk of developing atrial fibrillation compared to age matched controls; by age 42 greater than 8% of CHD patients have a diagnosis of atrial fibrillation.[19] Atrial fibrillation is most common in those with traditional risk factors such as obesity, tobacco use, and hypertension. Atrial fibrillation is common in patients with AV valve regurgitation, LVOT obstruction, Ebstein anomaly, Fontan circulation, ASDs, and AVSDs.

Compared with IART, atrial fibrillation is less reliably treated with catheter ablation. However, other principles related to rhythm control and anticoagulation, as discussed above, are broadly similar.

Ventricular Tachycardia and Sudden Death (see Chapters 67 and 70)
Sudden death is the second most common cause of cardiac death in adults with CHD following heart failure, and accounts for approximately 20% of death in patients with CHD, occurring at a rate of ~0.1% per patient year. Patients with TOF, TGA with a systemic RV, Fontan circulation, Eisenmenger syndrome, and complex forms of CHD are at the highest risk for ventricular arrhythmias and sudden cardiac death. Fortunately, the frequency of sudden death may be declining due to improved risk stratification, implantable cardioverter defibrillators (ICDs), and improvements in surgical technique (such as earlier definitive surgical repair and avoidance of ventriculotomies).[10,20] Ventricular arrhythmias are often macroreentrant scar-based arrhythmias. Discrete or diffuse replacement fibrosis also contributes to ventricular arrhythmia.

IART poorly and restoration of sinus rhythm is desirable. Patients with atrial arrhythmias have a 50% increased risk of mortality and double the morbidity compared to patients without atrial arrhythmia.[21] Acute termination of arrhythmia is usually performed with electrical cardioversion after atrial thrombus has been excluded with transesophageal echocardiography (TEE) or gated CCT. Pace termination or pharmacologic cardioversion can be performed in selected patients. Anticoagulation is required for at least 4 weeks following cardioversion.

Rhythm control is usually preferred over rate control for adults with CHD and IART. Catheter ablation is often effective and used as first-line therapy when IART is recurrent. Ablation should be performed by an electrophysiologist with experience in CHD as the mechanisms of reentry are due to surgical patches and unconventional anatomy not typically seen in acquired heart disease. Trans-baffle punctures are often required in patients with Mustard/Senning operations or Fontan circulation where the majority of patients have multiple IART circuits.

Medical therapy is a useful adjunct to catheter ablation or can be used when ablation is unsuccessful. AV nodal blockade with beta-blockers or calcium blockers is reasonable to prevent rapid ventricular response. Anti-arrhythmic drug choice must be tailored to the

Risk stratification to predict which patients are at risk for sudden death is challenging. Patients with a systemic LV and severe systolic dysfunction are thought to be high risk. A combination of clinical, ECG, and imaging parameters identify high-risk patients with repaired TOF and is discussed in detail in the section on Tetralogy of Fallot. Invasive EP studies further identify patients with repaired TOF but have not been shown to be predictive in other forms of CHD.

Secondary prevention ICDs are appropriate for patients with clinical sustained VT or aborted sudden cardiac death. Antiarrhythmic drugs may be adjunctive and catheter ablation can reduce the risk of ICD shocks. Results of catheter ablation for VT in repaired TOF are discussed separately.

Pacemakers and Implantable Defibrillators (see Chapter 69)

Pacemakers and ICDs are required in many patients with CHD. Indications for pacemakers are sinus node dysfunction and heart block. Indications for primary and secondary prevention ICDs are shown in Table 82.6.

Unfortunately, patients with CHD are at high risk for device complications such as lead fractures or device infections, which occur in up to 26% of adults with CHD. Both appropriate and inappropriate shocks are common in ACHD patients with ICDs. In a meta-analysis, appropriate shock rate was 22% at 3.3 years and inappropriate shock rate was 35% at 4.3 years follow-up, each higher than is seen in acquired heart disease.[24] Improvements in device algorithms and programming may reduce the risk of inappropriate shocks in contemporary cohorts.

Device implantation can be difficult in patients with surgically manipulated or variant venous anatomy (such as following Mustard/Senning procedures). Pacemakers should be epicardial in patients with intracardiac shunts, single ventricle, or ventricular leads in Fontan circulation. Cardiac resynchronization leads may be technically difficult due to variation in the location of the coronary sinus (CS) os. A proposed algorithm for cardiac resynchronization therapy (CRT) in CHD is shown in Fig. 82.3.

Because of the higher risk of device complications, both appropriate and inappropriate shocks, and the challenges with device implantation, the risk-benefit ratio of devices needs to be weighed carefully and in conjunction with ACHD providers and electrophysiologists experienced in CHD.

Heart Failure, Transplantation, and Mechanical Circulatory Support (see Part VI)

Epidemiology

Despite continued improvements in outcomes for those born with CHD, most adults with CHD, particularly for those with moderate or complex CHD, die from cardiac causes. Heart failure remains a major source of morbidity and the dominant cause of death for adults with CHD in the modern era, accounting for up to 40% of the ACHD mortality.[10]

The rate of heart failure hospitalizations among adults with CHD is increasing at a rapid rate. Hospitalizations for adults with CHD is associated with longer length of stay, high resource utilization, and poor in-hospital and long-term outcomes.[25] Heart failure is most common in patients with high anatomic or physiologic complexity including single ventricle anatomy, systemic RV, PH, and cyanosis. However, even patients with simple forms of CHD are at increased long-term risk of heart failure.[26]

Clinical Features

The clinical presentation of heart failure in patients with CHD is diverse. Typical symptoms such as pulmonary congestion, edema, and dyspnea on exertion may not be present. Often arrhythmia, hypoxemia, or exertional fatigue may be the presenting symptoms of heart failure in patients with CHD. Many patients with CHD have adapted to their lifelong cardiac condition and may under-report functional limitations. Cardiopulmonary exercise testing is useful to elicit sub-clinical deterioration, even in patients who report that they feel well. Patients with CHD and heart failure often have elevated biomarkers. Elevations in brain natriuretic peptide (BNP), troponin, and other biomarkers are associated with heart failure and poor outcomes in adults with CHD.[27]

TABLE 82.6 Indications for Implantable Defibrillators in Adults With Congenital Heart Disease

COR	LOE	RECOMMENDATION
SECONDARY PREVENTION		
I	B	ICD therapy is indicated in adults with CHD who are survivors of cardiac arrest due to ventricular fibrillation or hemodynamically unstable VT after evaluation to define the cause of the event and exclude any completely reversible etiology
I	B	ICD therapy is indicated in adults with CHD and spontaneous sustained VT who have undergone hemodynamic and electrophysiologic evaluation.
	C	Catheter ablation or surgery may offer a reasonable alternative or adjunct to ICD therapy in carefully selected patients
PRIMARY PREVENTION		
I	B	ICD therapy is indicated in adults with CHD and a systemic left ventricular ejection fraction ≤ 35%, biventricular physiology, and NYHA Class II or III symptoms
IIa	B	ICD therapy is reasonable in selected adults with tetralogy of Fallot and multiple risk factors for sudden cardiac death such as left ventricular systolic or diastolic dysfunction, nonsustained VT, QRS duration ≥180 ms, extensive right ventricular scarring, or inducible sustained VT at electrophysiologic study
IIb	C	ICD therapy may be reasonable in adults with a single or systemic right ventricular ejection fraction <35%, particularly in the presence of additional risk factors such as complex ventricular arrhythmias, unexplained syncope, NYHA functional Class II or III symptoms, QRS duration ≥140 msec, or severe systemic atrioventricular valve
		Regurgitation
IIb	B	ICD therapy may be considered in adults with CHD and syncope of unknown origin with hemodynamically significant sustained ventricular tachycardia or fibrillation inducible at electrophysiologic study
IIb	C	ICD therapy may be considered for adults with syncope and moderate or complex CHD in whom there is a high clinical suspicion of ventricular arrhythmia and in whom thorough invasive and noninvasive investigations have failed to define a cause
IIb	C	ICD therapy may be considered in adults with CHD and a systemic ventricular ejection fraction <35% in the absence of overt symptoms (NYHA class I) or other known risk factors

CHD, congenital heart disease; COR, class of recommendation; ICD, implantable cardioverter-defibrillator; LOE, level of evidence; NYHA, New York Heart Association; VT, ventricular tachycardia.
Adapted from Khairy P, Van Hare GF, Balaji S, et al. PACES/HRS expert consensus statement on the recognition and management of arrhythmias in adult congenital heart disease. *Heart Rhythm.* 2014;11(10):e102–e165.

Pathophysiology

The etiology and pathophysiology of heart failure in adults with CHD is often quite different from that of adults with acquired cardiovascular disease. The majority of heart failure in adults with acquired cardiovascular disease is secondary to left ventricular systolic or diastolic dysfunction; this is not true in adults with CHD. Adults with CHD are more likely to have a single ventricle, systemic RV, associated pulmonary vascular disease, residual shunt, or residual outflow obstruction as an underlying etiology of heart failure.

The pathophysiologic basis of heart failure differs depending on the underlying lesions. Volume loading from shunts and valvular regurgitation cause ventricular dilation and, if untreated, ventricular dysfunction. Residual outflow obstruction can result from sub-valvular or valvular stenosis as well as peripheral arterial narrowing, such as aortic

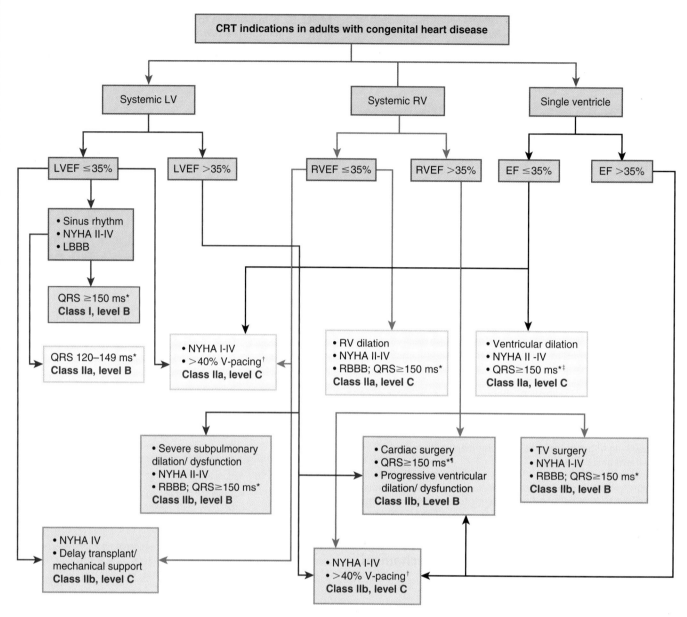

FIGURE 82.3 Recommendations for cardiac resynchronization therapy (CRT) in adults with congenital heart disease. (From Khairy P, Van Hare GF, Balaji S, et al. PACES/HRS expert consensus statement on the recognition and management of arrhythmias in adult congenital heart disease. *Heart Rhythm*. 2014;11:e102–e665.)

coarctation. Obstructive lesions can induce ventricular hypertrophy and dysfunction.

Patients with a systemic RV (such as those with D-loop TGA treated with an atrial switch procedure or those with L-loop TGA) are at high risk for ventricular dysfunction. The systemic RV is predisposed to systolic dysfunction due to unfavorable myocardial fiber orientation, nonconical shape, coronary supply-demand mismatch, and volume loading from tricuspid regurgitation.

Heart failure is exceedingly common in adults who have undergone the Fontan operation; transplant-free survival is less than 70% 25 years after the Fontan operation and most patients develop heart failure by age 40.[28] The mechanisms for heart failure after the Fontan operation are multifactorial and incompletely understood. Not all patients have overt ventricular or valvular dysfunction. Fontan failure is characterized by chronically elevated central venous pressure, low cardiac output, cyanosis due to collaterals, ascites, and cirrhosis.

Medical Therapy

Patients with CHD and heart failure should be managed at a specialty CHD center. The pathophysiologic basis of heart failure in CHD differs from that of acquired heart failure, therefore, it is often difficult to know which treatments are effective in CHD. Patients with CHD have been excluded from most heart failure trials and few studies have examined CHD patients specifically. Nonetheless, clinicians must make decisions about how to use medical therapy in patients with CHD, even in the absence of definitive data.

Prior to turning to medical therapy for heart failure, residual hemodynamic lesions such as shunts, valve dysfunction, and outflow obstruction should be sought out and treated. In many cases, trans-thoracic echocardiography (TTE) is insufficient and cross-sectional imaging or invasive hemodynamics are needed to define the cause of symptoms.

Standard guideline-directed medical therapy (GDMT) is likely effective when taken by CHD patients with a systemic LV who have heart failure due to left ventricular systolic dysfunction after residual hemodynamic lesions have been addressed. The efficacy of GDMT in other populations is less well established. Angiotensin blockade is commonly used in patients with a systemic RV and systolic dysfunction. However, the largest trial of Renin-Angiotensin-Aldosterone System (RAAS) blockade in patients with a systemic RV did not improve right ventricular ejection fraction. There is very little data to suggest that beta-blockers are beneficial for patients with a systemic RV. Pulmonary vasodilators, including PDE5-inhibitors and endothelin receptor antagonists, have been shown to improve functional class and exercise capacity in patients with Fontan circulation.[29] Newer heart failure medications such as sacubitril/valsartan, ivabradine, and dapagliflozin have not been prospectively studied in patients with CHD. Finally, modifiable risk factors such as hypertension, diabetes, obesity, and sleep apnea should be aggressively treated in CHD patients with heart failure.

Cardiac Resynchronization

CRT via multi-site pacing is appropriate for patients with a systemic LV, spontaneous or pacing-induced left bundle-branch block, and heart failure. The role of CRT in other forms of CHD is not as well established.[30]

Patients with a systemic RV (particularly those with L-loop TGA) have a high incidence of heart block as well as frequent need for ventricular pacing. Multiple observational studies suggest benefit of CRT in patients with a systemic RV, although the data are generally retrospective and uncontrolled. Placing CRT leads is technically more difficult in patients with a systemic RV due to variability in the location of the CS os, variant coronary vein anatomy, and the presence of surgical interatrial baffles. It is reasonable to consider placement of epicardial multi-site pacing leads in selected patients if they are going for cardiac surgery for other indications.

The benefit of CRT in patients with single ventricle anatomy following the Fontan operation is not well established. Additionally, multi-site pacing requires epicardial lead placement.

Transplantation

Patients with CHD and heart failure refractory to medical therapy should be considered for heart transplantation. Since 2000, the number of ACHD patients listed for transplantation and ultimately transplanted has doubled. Adult CHD patients account for more than 4% of adult heart transplantations done in the United States.

Compared to patients with acquired heart failure, CHD patients listed for heart transplantation are younger, more likely to have a prior sternotomy, less likely to have coronary artery disease, and less likely to have a left ventricular assist device. Alloimmunization secondary to prior transfusions or homograft implantation can prolong waitlist times, require desensitization, or make some patients ineligible for transplantation. Many patients with CHD have important comorbidities such as cirrhosis, chronic kidney disease, restrictive lung disease (as a consequence of prior chest surgery), or pulmonary vascular disease which may make them high-risk, or even ineligible for cardiac transplantation. For all these reasons, many patients with CHD and advanced heart failure are never listed for heart transplantation. Even those patients who are ultimately listed for transplantation are more likely to be delisted or

die without transplantation than patients with acquired cardiovascular disease.[31]

Due to the high complexity and prevalence of comorbidities in CHD patients with advanced heart failure, a multidisciplinary team consisting of ACHD specialists, advanced heart failure specialists, and cardiac surgeons with experience in both congenital and transplant surgery should evaluate all ACHD patients considered for transplantation. Necessarily, this process should take place at an ACHD specialty center.

Patients with CHD are listed at UNOS Status 4 in the allocation system adopted in 2018. They share status urgency with ambulatory patients with a left ventricular assist device, patients with cardiac amyloidosis, and those awaiting re-transplantation. Many of the criteria used to justify higher-urgency status, such as poor hemodynamics, inotropic support, or mechanical circulatory support may not be applicable to patients with ACHD. Therefore, patients with ACHD may require an exception to be listed at higher urgency in order to reflect their acuity and higher waitlist mortality.[32]

Patients with CHD have high operative risk which is reflected by increased in-hospital and 1-year mortality following transplantation. This early risk is mitigated by low late graft failure and mortality compared to those with acquired heart disease so that long-term survival is not lower for ACHD patients undergoing transplantation (Fig. 82.4).[33,34] For this reason, organ allocation to ACHD patients results in acceptable utility of donor hearts. Because of the high surgical risk and complexity of transplant in CHD, transplant should be performed at specialty ACHD centers.[35] When performed at high-volume ACHD transplant centers, outcomes are improved.

Mechanical Circulatory Support

ACHD patients with advanced heart failure have higher anatomic and physiologic complexity than those with acquired heart failure, therefore, mechanical circulatory support may not provide the same benefit. Left ventricular assist devices are appropriate for patients with advanced heart failure due to left ventricular systolic dysfunction who meet conventional indications for mechanical support. In carefully selected patients, ventricular assist devices can be used in patients with Fontan circulation, systemic RVs, or complex anatomy but this requires careful surgical planning and a multidisciplinary approach. ACHD patients have higher mortality after ventricular assist device placement than those with acquired heart disease.[36]

Palliative Care

It is important to acknowledge each patient's desires for care, as in ACHD patients nearing end-of-life the frequency of hospitalizations, intensive care admission, and increased length of hospital stay appear greater (despite younger age) than for adults with cancer. In a retrospective study of ACHD patients who died during a hospitalization, only a minority had engaged in end-of-life discussions with their providers. Data suggests that both adults with CHD, as well as their providers, would like to participate in advanced care planning and discussion of palliative care.[37]

Aortopathies in Congenital Heart Disease

Aortic dilation is common in adults with CHD, particularly in patients with bicuspid aortic valve (BAV) and conotruncal defects.[38] BAV is prevalent in 2% of the general population. The most common complications in BAV are stenosis or regurgitation of the valve, however, ascending aortic dilation occurs in at least 50% of patients (see Chapter 42). Aortopathy is a common finding in patients with conotruncal anomalies because the arterial walls are derived from cardiac neural crest and second heart field cells, either or both of which can be abnormal in these defects. For example, marked histologic abnormalities have been documented in the aortic root and ascending aorta present from infancy in patients with TOF. Aortic dilation is common in adults with repaired TOF, with up to 25% of adults with repaired TOF having an aortic

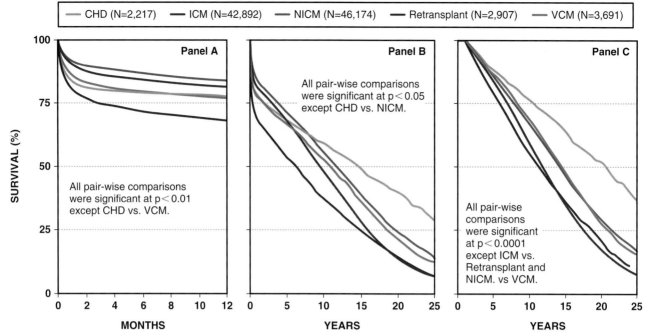

FIGURE 82.4 Kaplan-Meier curve demonstrating 1-year survival (**A**), long-term survival (**B**), and long-term survival conditional on survival to 1 year by diagnosis (**C**). January 1982–June 2014. *CHD*, Congenital heart disease; *ICM*, ischemic cardiomyopathy; *NICM*, non-ischemic cardiomyopathy; *VCM*, valvular cardiomyopathy. (From Lund LH. The Registry of the International Society for Heart and Lung Transplantation. Thirty-Third Adult Heart Transplantation Report—2016; Focus Theme: Primary Diagnostic Indications for Transplant. *J Heart Lung Transplant.* 2016;35[10]:1158–1169.)

root diameter larger than 4 cm; however, only 6.6% have *indexed* aortic values above the expected limits. Similarly, 50% of children with D-loop TGA have aortic root dilation 10 years after arterial switch operation; however, this dilation does not appear to be progressive. Despite the high prevalence of dilated ascending aorta in patients with conotruncal anomalies aortic dissection is exceedingly rare.

In following CHD patients serially over time, one must recognize that aortic measurements will vary depending on the specific imaging modality and measurement technique. Echocardiography labs may have various imaging protocols for aortic measurements that must be considered when comparing serial studies. The current multimodality imaging guidelines for the thoracic aorta in adults advocate obtaining aortic root measurements at end-diastole with a leading edge–to–leading edge technique, whereas imaging guidelines for pediatric echocardiograms, which are often used in echocardiography labs specializing in CHD, suggest obtaining aortic root measurements in mid-systole with an inner edge–to–inner edge technique.[39]

Subacute Bacterial Endocarditis

Patients with ACHD have an increased risk of developing subacute bacterial endocarditis (SBE), and this is associated with significant morbidity and mortality (see Chapter 80).[40] The most common pathogens responsible for SBE include *Streptococcus viridans, Staphylococcus* species, and *Enterococcus* species. Antibiotic prophylaxis is recommended prior to dental procedures for ACHD patients with high-risk characteristics, which include: (1) prior episodes of SBE, (2) prosthetic valves (including transcatheter), (3) valve repair using a prosthetic ring, (4) residual intracardiac shunts adjacent to prosthetic material, (5) cyanotic CHD, (6) any CHD repaired with prosthetic material up to 6 months after the procedure or lifelong if residual shunt or valvular regurgitation remains, and (7) for cardiac transplant recipients who develop cardiac valvulopathy. In a registry of over 14,000 ACHD patients, the incidence of SBE was 1.33 cases per 1000-person years. Valve-containing prosthetics were found to be an important independent risk factor for SBE, both short and long term after implantation, whereas non-valve-containing prosthetics (including valve repair) are associated with greater risk only in the short term (<6 months) after implantation (Fig. 82.5).[41] ACHD patients should be educated about symptoms of SBE and the importance of good oral hygiene and of obtaining blood cultures before starting antibiotic treatment in situations with concerning features for infection.

Pregnancy in Women With Congenital Heart Disease (see Chapter 92)

Profound hemodynamic changes occur during pregnancy, which are usually well tolerated by women with structurally normal hearts; however, these changes may not be tolerated as well in women with underlying CHD. Despite the fact that most women do not have cardiac complications during pregnancy, cardiovascular disease is the leading cause of indirect maternal mortality. All women with CHD should receive preconception counseling to determine maternal cardiac, obstetrical, and fetal risks, and potential long-term risks to the mother. Additionally, an individualized plan of care that addresses expectations and contingencies should be developed for and with women with CHD who are pregnant or who may become pregnant and shared with the patient and all caregivers (AHA/ACC Class I recommendation, level of evidence C-LD).

Men and women of childbearing age with CHD should be counseled on the risk of CHD recurrence in offspring and fetal echocardiography offered if either parent has CHD.

Several risk stratification scores have been developed for maternal cardiac conditions. The CARPREG 2 investigators reported the maternal outcomes of 1938 pregnancies in women with cardiac disease (63% CHD), and 16% of women experienced an adverse cardiac outcome, primarily heart failure and arrhythmias. The highest-weighted risk factors (weight of three points) include a prior history of cardiac events or arrhythmias, decreased functional status (New York Heart Association, NYHA, Class ≥III), and presence of a mechanical heart valve. Risk factors that account for two points include: ventricular dysfunction, high-risk left-sided valve disease/LVOT obstruction, PH, coronary artery disease, and high-risk aortopathy. One point was assigned for late pregnancy assessment or no prior cardiac intervention. The predicted risks for cardiac events stratified according to point score were ≤1 point (5%), 2 points (10%), 3 points (15%), 4 points (22%), and >4 points (41%).[42]

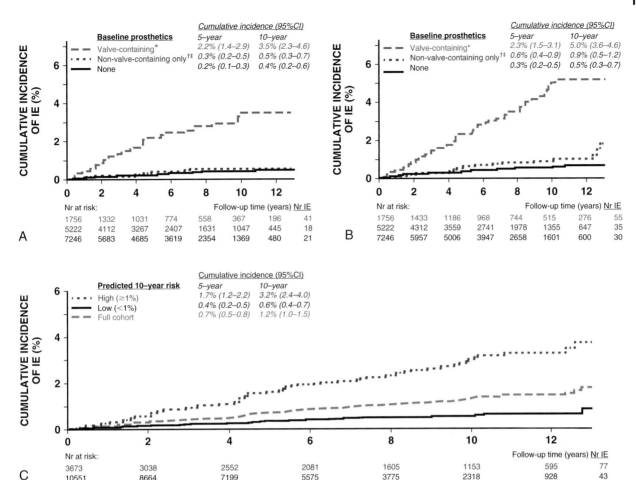

FIGURE 82.5 Cumulative incidence of infectious endocarditis (IE) in adults with congenital heart disease during follow-up by presence of prosthetic material at baseline (**A** and **B**) and predicted risj category (**C**). (From Kuijpers JM, Koolbergen DR, Groenink M, et al. Incidence, risk factors, and predictors of infective endocarditis in adult congenital heart disease: focus on the use of prosthetic material. *Eur Heart J.* 2017;38:2048–2056.)

The European Society of Cardiology published an extensive set of guidelines for management of cardiovascular diseases during pregnancy which includes the modified WHO risk classification, listed in Table 82.7. The recommended follow-up for women with WHO risk category II is every trimester; women with WHO risk category ≥III should be seen monthly or bimonthly.[43] Women with a high risk of maternal morbidity or mortality, including women with pulmonary arterial hypertension (PAH), Eisenmenger syndrome, severe systemic ventricular dysfunction, severe left-sided obstructive lesions, or in physiological stage D should be counselled against pregnancy and consider termination if they become pregnant.[44]

Exercise and Sports Participation (see Chapter 32)
Benefits of Physical Exercise
Virtually all patients with CHD should be encouraged to be physically active, exercise, and maintain physical fitness. Physical activity promotes cardiovascular and mental health; people who exercise regularly have an improved quality of life, better exercise capacity, and are less likely to suffer from obesity or type 2 diabetes. Even patients with complex CHD, such as Fontan circulation, derive benefits from regular physical exercise.[45]

Despite the benefits of exercise, physicians, parents, or patients may have concerns about the risk of sudden death with exercise and restrict physical activity or competitive sports. The risk of sudden death during exercise is very low for adults with CHD and observational studies do not suggest that exercise restriction reduces the risk of sudden death, perhaps because the majority of sudden death in patients with CHD occurs at rest, not with exercise.[46] At least in part due to these exercise restrictions, patients with CHD have lower levels of physical activity than patients without CHD and only 30%

of patients with CHD achieve the recommended levels of physical activity.[47]

Individualized Exercise Programs
Patients with CHD require individualized counseling regarding exercise recommendations or restrictions.[48] In general, patients with CHD have lower exercise capacity than patients without CHD and there is considerable heterogeneity across different diagnoses (Fig. 82.6).[49] Patients with moderate or complex anatomy or physiology may benefit from formal exercise testing to establish baseline exercise capacity and demonstrate safety of exercise. Patients with high-risk anatomy or physiology should be discouraged from participating in high-intensity sports and counseled toward lower-intensity physical activity (Table 82.8).

Low-risk patients can begin a training program at approximately 70% maximal predicted heart rate at least three times per week (totaling 150 minutes/week) and increase intensity or duration over time.

Competitive Sports
There are important differences between competitive sports and recreational exercise. In competitive sports, participants cannot reliably self-regulate effort and require high-intensity burst efforts imposed by coaches or playing conditions. For these reasons, competitive sports are thought to pose greater risk.

The AHA and ACC published a consensus statement on eligibility for participation in competitive sports in 2015.[50] Sports are graded in terms of their static and dynamic components and appropriateness for competition depends on the native anatomy and the presence of residual sequelae following repair. In many patients, pre-participation stress testing can provide useful information about the patient's exercise capacity, hemodynamics with exercise, and the presence of exercise-induced arrhythmias that can help guide decision making. Particularly

TABLE 82.7 Modified WHO Classification for Maternal Cardiac Risk

	mWHO I	mWHO II	mWHO II–III	mWHO III	mWHO IV
Diagnosis (if otherwise well and uncomplicated)	Small or mild • Pulmonary stenosis • Patent ductus arteriosus • Mitral valve prolapse • Successfully repaired simple lesions (atrial or ventricular septal defect, patent ductus arteriosus, anomalous pulmonary venous drainage) • Atrial or ventricular ectopic beats, isolated	Unoperated atrial or ventricular septal defect Repaired tetralogy of Fallot Most arrythmias (supraventricular arrhythmias) Turner syndrome without aortic dilatation	Mild left ventricular impairment (EF > 45%) Hypertrophic cardiomyopathy Native or tissue valve disease not considered WHO I or IV (mild mitral stenosis, moderate aortic stenosis) Marfan or other HTAD syndrome without aortic dilatation Aorta < 45 mm in bicuspid aortic valve pathology Repaired coarctation Atrioventricular septal defect	Moderate left ventricular impairment (EF 30%–45%) Previous peripartum cardiomyopathy without any residual left ventricular impairment Mechanical valve Systemic right ventricle with good or mildly decreased ventricular function Fontan circulation If otherwise the patient is well and the cardiac condition uncomplicated Unrepaired cyanotic heart disease Other complex heart disease Moderate mitral stenosis Severe asymptomatic aortic stenosis Moderate aortic dilatation (40–45 mm in Marfan syndrome or other HTAD; 45–50 mm in bicuspid aortic valve, Turner syndrome ASI 20–25 mm/m², tetralogy of Fallot <50 mm) Ventricular tachycardia	Pulmonary arterial hypertension Severe systemic ventricular dysfunction (EF < 30% or NYHA Class III–IV) Previous peripartum cardiomyopathy with any residual left ventricular impairment Severe mitral stenosis Severe symptomatic aortic stenosis Systemic right ventricle with moderate or severely decreased ventricular function Severe aortic dilatation (>45 mm in Marfan syndrome or other HTAD, > 50 mm in bicuspid aortic valve, Turner syndrome ASI > 25/mm/m², tetralogy of Fallot > 50 mm) Vascular Ehlers-Danlos Severe (re)coarctation Fontan with any complication
Risk	No detectable increased risk of maternal mortality and no/mild increased risk in morbidity	Small increased risk of maternal mortality or moderate increase in morbidity	Intermediate increased risk of maternal mortality or moderate to severe increase in morbidity	Significantly increased risk of maternal mortality or severe morbidity	Extremely high risk of maternal mortality or severe morbidity

Modified from Regitz-Zagrosek V, Roos-Hesselink JW, Bauersachs J, et al. 2018 ESC guidelines for the management of cardiovascular diseases during pregnancy. *Eur Heart J.* 2018;39:3165–3241.

for teenagers and adults shared decision making is often required following a detailed conversation about risks.

SPECIFIC DEFECTS

Left-to-Right Shunt Lesions

The physiology of a left-to-right shunt involves flow of pulmonary venous, or oxygenated, blood toward systemic venous, or deoxygenated, chambers or vessels. The degree of left-to-right shunting determines the amount of chamber dilation and is dictated by the size of the defect as well as the diastolic properties of the heart and the resistance in the great arteries. In general, shunt lesions proximal to the tricuspid valve (such as ASDs and anomalous pulmonary venous return) cause right heart dilation, those below the tricuspid valve (such as VSDs and PDAs) cause left heart dilation (Table 82.9). Small shunts may close spontaneously during childhood or remain small and hemodynamically insignificant. However, larger shunts that are not corrected early in life have the potential to cause elevations in PVR with reversal of the direction of flow from right-to-left leading to cyanosis and Eisenmenger syndrome (see section on Eisenmenger Syndrome).

The invasive evaluation of cardiac shunts should include the calculation of pulmonary and systemic vascular resistance (SVR). The ratio of pulmonary blood flow (Qp) to systemic blood flow (Qs) may be determined either noninvasively or by cardiac catheterization. Fig. 82.7 displays invasive hemodynamics in such a patient, with calculations of Qp/Qs and vascular resistance.

Atrial Septal Defects and Partial Anomalous Pulmonary Veins

Anatomic Description and Prevalence

There are multiple locations for interatrial communications, and a detailed understanding of the atrial septal anatomy is needed. Fig. 82.8 illustrates various locations of ASDs. The prevalence of ASD is 0.88 per 1000 adults. The most common type of ASD is a secundum ASD (Fig. 82.9), which is a true deficiency in the atrial septum, in the region of the fossa ovalis. This should be differentiated from a patent foramen ovale (PFO), which is persistence of patency of the flap valve of the fossa ovalis (not associated with right-sided cardiac dilation) and persists in up to 25% of adults. Primum ASDs may be considered in the spectrum of AVSDs (Fig. 82.10, Video 82.2A,B) and involve a deficiency in the region of the AV valves and are associated with a cleft in the mitral valve. Sinus venosus defects occur in the sinus venosus septum posterior to the true atrial septum and usually involve anomalous right-sided pulmonary venous return (Fig. 82.11). CS defects (also called unroofed CSs) are rare and involve direct communication of the CS and the LA due to complete or partial unroofing of the CS and are often accompanied by a persistent left-sided SVC.

Patients may also have anomalous pulmonary venous connections not associated with an ASD, known as partial anomalous pulmonary venous connection (PAPVC). PAPVC may be associated with either right- or left-sided pulmonary veins which can have several possible anomalous connections, with the most common being a left upper pulmonary vein to an ascending vertical vein into the brachiocephalic

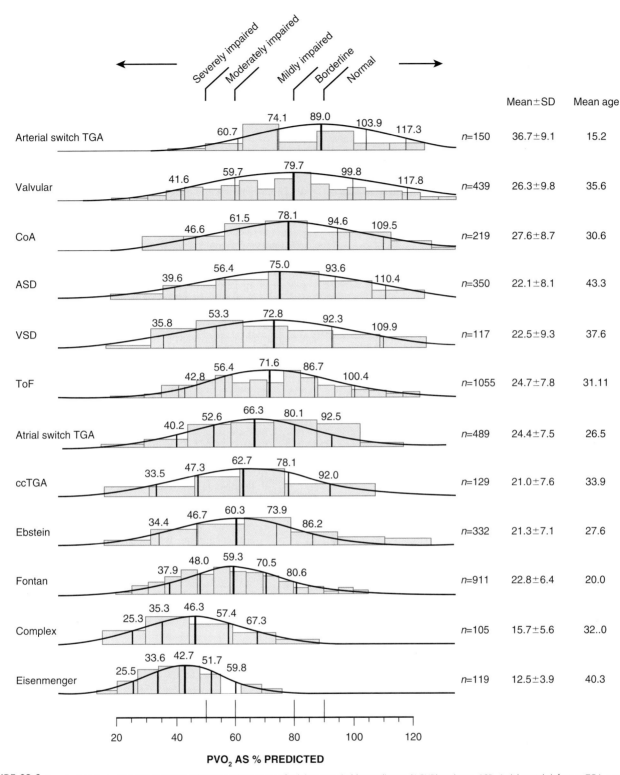

FIGURE 82.6 Range of peak oxygen consumption values in various types of adult congenital heart disease (ACHD) patients. *ASD,* Atrial septal defect; *ccTGA,* congenitally corrected transposition of the great arteries; *CoA,* coarctation of the aorta; *pVO₂,* peak oxygen consumption; *TGA,* transposition of the great arteries; *ToF,* tetralogy of Fallot; *VSD,* ventricular septal defect. (From Kempny A, Dimopoulos K, Uebing A, et al. Reference values for exercise limitations among adults with congenital heart disease. Relation to activities of daily life—single centre experience and review of published data. *Eur Heart J.* 2012;33:1386–396.)

vein or the right upper pulmonary vein draining to the SVC (Fig. 82.12). In the latter case, careful attention should be paid to ensure that there is not an associated sinus venosus defect. When the right-sided pulmonary veins connect to the inferior vena cava (IVC), this is called a scimitar vein. Isolated PAPVC involving a single pulmonary vein may cause mild degrees of right heart overload, but rarely require surgical correction.

Clinical Features

It is not uncommon for adults to have an ASD incidentally discovered at the time of imaging for unrelated issues. Symptoms, when they occur, most commonly include exercise intolerance, palpitations, or dyspnea with exertion. Supraventricular arrhythmias develop by 40 years of age in about 10% of patients and become increasingly prevalent with advancing age. The presence of cyanosis should alert one to the possibility of shunt reversal and Eisenmenger syndrome or, alternatively, to a prominent eustachian valve directing the inferior vena caval flow to the LA via a secundum ASD or sinus venosus defect of the inferior vena caval type. Pulse oximetry at rest and during exercise is recommended for evaluation of adults with unrepaired or repaired ASD with residual shunt to determine the direction and magnitude of the shunt.

The classic physical examination of an ASD is a wide, fixed splitting of the second heart sound, which is due to prolonged RV ejection and increased PA capacitance, which, in turn, delay pulmonary valve

TABLE 82.8 Congenital Conditions* in Which High-Intensity Exercise Should be Avoided

Cyanosis
High risk coronary anomalies
Hypoxemia
Severe aortic dilation
Severe outflow tract obstruction
Severe pulmonary hypertension
Severe ventricular dysfunction
Ventricular arrhythmias

*This list does not include non–adult congenital heart disease (ACHD) high-risk lesions such as hypertrophic cardiomyopathy, channelopathies, or arrhythmogenic cardiomyopathy. See Chapters 52, 54 and 63.

A. Cardiac Output

Systemic blood flow (L/min)

$$Qs = \dfrac{VO_2}{\dfrac{(13.6)(Hb)(Ao\ O^2\ sat - SVC\ O_2\ sat)}{100}}$$

Pulmonary blood flow (L/min)

$$Qp^* = \dfrac{VO_2}{\dfrac{(13.6)(Hb)(Ao\ O^2\ sat - SVC\ O_2\ sat)}{100}}$$

*Last, Qp can be inaccurate when there are multiple sources of pulmonary blood flow with differing oxygen contents and their relative contribution to flow is unknown.

B. Shunt Fraction

$$\dfrac{Qp}{Qs} = \dfrac{(Ao\ O_2\ sat - MVS\ O_2\ sat)}{(PV\ O_2\ sat - PA\ O_2\ sat)}$$

C. Vascular Resistance (mmHg/L/min)

$$Systemic\ Vascular\ Resistance\ (SVR) = \dfrac{Mean\ Aop - Mean\ RAp}{Qs}$$

$$Pulmonary\ Vascular\ Resistance\ (PVR) = \dfrac{Mean\ PAp - Mean\ LAp}{Qp}$$

FIGURE 82.7 Calculations of flow and resistance. **A,** Calculations of blood flow based on the Fick principle, oxygen consumption (VO₂) equals the delivered oxygen (cardiac output × arterial O₂ content) minus the returned oxygen (cardiac output × venous O₂ content). Rearranging this equation, the cardiac output (Qs) can be calculated. In room air, the contribution of dissolved oxygen is minimal, and left out of the equation. **B,** The shunt fraction (Qp/Qs) accounts for effective blood flow and provides the contribution of intracardiac shunts. The net shunt Qp:Qs summarizes the excess/deficit of flow across the pulmonary vascular bed relative to systemic, reflecting the totality of all unique sources of left-to-right, and right-to-left, intra- and extra-cardiac shunts. **C,** The vascular resistance across the systemic and pulmonary vascular beds and is calculated by the change in mean pressure divided by the flow through the circulatory bed. It is measured in Wood units (mm Hg/L/min), and is often indexed to body surface area (m²). *Ao,* Aorta; *Aop,* aortic pressure; *Hb,* hemoglobin; *LAp,* left atrial pressure; *MVS,* mixed venous saturation; *O₂ sat,* oxygen saturation; *PA,* pulmonary artery; *PAp,* pulmonary artery pressure; *PV,* pulmonary venous; *PVR,* pulmonary vascular resistance; *Qp,* pulmonary blood flow; *Qs,* systemic blood flow; *RAp,* right atrial pressure; *SVC,* superior vena cava; *SVR,* systemic vascular resistance; *VO₂,* oxygen consumption.

TABLE 82.9 Expected Chamber Enlargement With Cardiac Shunts

SHUNT	RA	RV	PA	LA	LV	AORTA
ASD	+	+	+			
VSD		±	+	+	+	
PDA			+	+	+	+

closure. Pulmonary flow murmurs are common. The ECG commonly displays a rightward QRS axis and an incomplete right bundle branch block (RBBB). The classic chest radiograph features are of cardiomegaly (from right atrial and right ventricular enlargement), and dilated central pulmonary arteries with pulmonary congestion. Cardiac imaging is essential in determining the anatomy of the atrial septum and pulmonary venous drainage. TTE is the initial imaging test, however, other imaging modalities, such as TEE, CMR, and CCT may be needed to confirm the anatomy. The 2020 Appropriate Use Criteria guidelines rate these modalities as always appropriate for the evaluation prior to planned surgical repair for sinus venous defects or for patients with a change in clinical status or new symptoms.

Repairs

When an ASD is discovered in an adult, if there is any degree of right heart dilation associated with symptoms, closure should be considered.[51] It is important to verify the direction of the shunt as left-to-right.

The next step is to verify that the PVR is less than ⅓ the SVR, the PA systolic pressure is less than 50% systemic, there is right heart enlargement, and the Qp/Qs is at least 1.5:1. The majority of secundum ASDs may be closed percutaneously (Fig. 82.13), however, surgical closure is required for sinus venosus defects, primum ASDs, or CS septal defects. It is reasonable to close an ASD in an asymptomatic patient with right heart enlargement (AHA/ACC Class IIa recommendation, level of evidence C-LD). If invasive hemodynamic assessment confirms significant elevations in PVR and/or pulmonary pressure, collaboration between ACHD and PH providers is important (see section on Eisenmenger syndrome).

Surgical closure is typically performed using a patch of autologous pericardium or synthetic material with an open sternotomy and cardiopulmonary bypass. The operative mortality is low, however, postoperative complications of post-pericardiotomy syndrome or atrial arrhythmias may occur. Special attention must be paid to those defects with partial anomalous pulmonary venous drainage, as redirecting the pulmonary venous flow may result in pulmonary vein stenosis. In patients with primum ASDs, care must be taken in closing the mitral valve cleft to avoid mitral stenosis or residual regurgitation.

Transcatheter closure is now widely accepted as an alternative to surgical repair for the majority of secundum ASDs. Several devices are available and range in size and configuration. Adequate rims of the defect must be demonstrated to ensure safe transcatheter closure. Post-procedural complications include atrial arrhythmias, heart block, thrombus formation on the device, and rarely device mobilization or erosion.

Long-Term Outcomes and Complications

Patients who undergo ASD repair prior to the age of 25 years have favorable outcomes. However, surgical repair does not provide proven benefit in reducing arrhythmia burden in older adults. Following closure, patients with significant residual shunt, valvular or ventricular dysfunction, arrhythmias, and/or PH should be followed at regular intervals with TTE. The imaging recommendations for patients following transcatheter ASD closure are dictated by the specific manufacturer, but in general, TTE is performed at 1 week, 1 month, and then annually for at least 5 years following closure. Any patient who has had a transcatheter ASD device placed who presents with chest pain

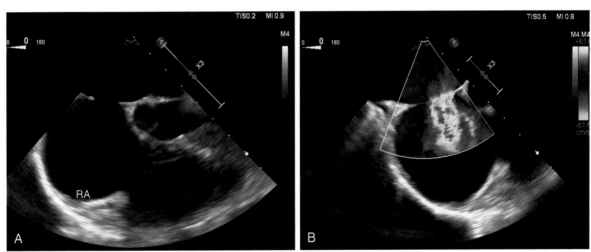

Confines of true atrial septum

Superior
sinus venosus defect

Atrioventricular
septal defect
(ostium primum)

Fossa ovalis
(ostium secundum)
defect

Inferior
sinus venosus defect

Coronary sinus defect

FIGURE 82.8 Various atrial level shunts. (From Webb GA, et al. Congenital heart disease in the adult and pediatric patient. In: Zipes P, et al., eds. *Braunwald's Heart Disease.* 11th ed. Philadelphia: Elsevier; 2019.)

should have an urgent evaluation to rule out device erosion, which occurs in 1 in 1000 cases.

Patients with ASD and elevated PVR require closely monitored management as PAH can progress even after ASD closure.

Atrioventricular Septal Defects
Anatomic Description and Prevalence

AVSDs are a spectrum of lesions that involve deficiencies of the AV septum, often accompanied by anomalies of the AV valves. AVSDs are the result of failed fusion of the endocardial cushions, and comprise up to 5% of CHD. These include primum ASDs, partial or complete AV canal defects (Fig. 82.14). Complete AVSDs are characterized by both an atrial and ventricular level defect with a common AV valve, usually comprised of five leaflets. A partial AVSD does not have a VSD component, and almost always has a cleft in the anterior mitral valve leaflet. A unique anatomic feature in patients with AVSD is elongation of the LVOT, due to the aortic valve being displaced anteriorly. This results in a scooped-out appearance of the ventricular septum and a shortened LV inlet, creating a "goose neck" appearance (Fig. 82.15). The severity of the defect is dictated by several factors including size of the shunt, extent of AV valve abnormalities, size discrepancy of the ventricle, and presence of additional anomalies, including LVOT obstruction.

Clinical Features

The great majority of patients with AVSD undergo repair in childhood. Older patients with large AVSDs which have not been repaired early in life usually develop irreversible pulmonary vascular disease and Eisenmenger syndrome, precluding complete repair. More commonly, adults with a history of AVSD repair in childhood present with symptoms from residual left AV valve regurgitation and stenosis, LVOT obstruction, or atrial arrhythmias.

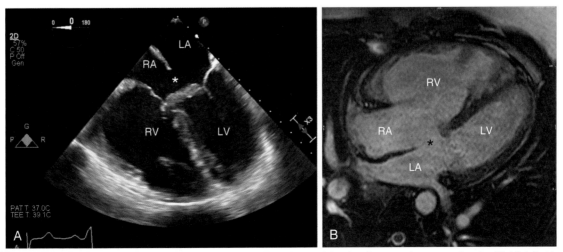

FIGURE 82.9 Transesophageal echocardiogram in the transverse plane. **A,** 2-D image of a secundum atrial septal defect (ASD). **B** Color Doppler showing flow through the ASD from the left atrium to the right atrium. *LA,* Left atrium; *RA,* right atrium.

FIGURE 82.10 Ostium primum atrial septal defect shown by transesophageal echocardiogram (**A**) and cardiac magnetic resonance imaging (**B**). *LA,* Left atrium; *LV,* left ventricular; *RA,* right atrium; *RV,* right ventricle; *asterisk,* atrial septal defect.

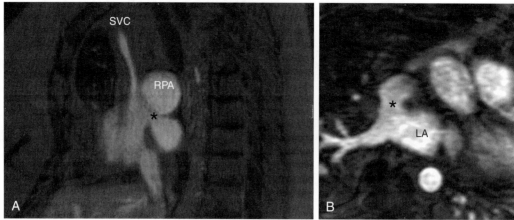

FIGURE 82.11 Gadolinium-enhanced 3-D MR angiogram of a superior-type sinus venosus defect **(A)**, sagittal oblique projection showing the superior vena cava (SVC) in its length and the defect superior to the true atrial septum *(asterisk)*. Note the dilated right pulmonary artery (RPA) in this patient with pulmonary hypertension and longstanding pulmonary overcirculation. **B,** Axial oblique image demonstrating the distal SVC with the defect at its posterior margin *(asterisk)* and communication with the left atrium (LA).

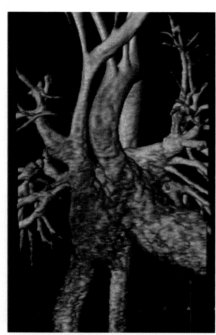

FIGURE 82.12 3-D reconstruction of gadolinium-enhanced MR angiogram in coronal view showing partial anomalous pulmonary venous connection of the right upper pulmonary vein to the superior vena cava.

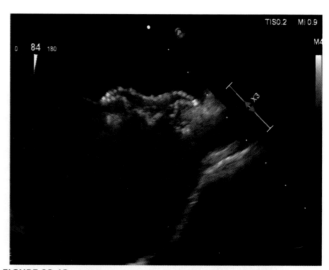

FIGURE 82.13 Transesophageal echo image in the near-vertical plane showing an Amplatzer septal occluder device positioned in a secundum ASD. The SVC is to the right of the image. *SVC,* Superior vena cava.

Surgical Repairs

Indications for surgical intervention of AVSD in adults are similar to those for ASD closure. These include a net left-to-right shunt (Qp:Qs ≥1.5:1), PA systolic pressure less than 50% systemic, and PVR less than one third systemic. Pre-operative cardiac catheterization may be required to assess for PH. For adults with prior repair, left AV valve regurgitation is the most common reason for later surgical reintervention.

Long-Term Outcomes and Complications

Survival after AVSD defects repair is good, yet reoperation for left AV valve disease and LVOT obstruction remains significant.[52] Other late complications include patch dehiscence or residual septal defects and development of complete heart block. Those adults with repaired AVSD and any degree of PH must be followed closely.

Ventricular Septal Defects

Anatomic Description and Prevalence

VSDs are the most common form of CHD, and the reported incidence of isolated VSDs varies widely, from 1.5 to 53 per 1000 live births. There are several classification schemes used to describe VSDs (Table 82.10). Fig. 82.16 demonstrates the locations of VSDs.

Clinical Features

Many isolated muscular and perimembranous VSDs are small and close spontaneously in childhood. However, there are several clinical presentations of VSDs in adults (Fig. 82.17, Video 82.3). Patients living with small, restrictive VSDs are usually asymptomatic with a harsh holosystolic murmur on exam. Continuous wave Doppler through these defects reveals a high velocity, often greater than 5 msec, which confirms the pressure-restrictive physiology. In this case, the left-to-right shunt is minimal, and there is usually not left ventricular dilation. Other adults may present with prior VSD surgical repair in childhood, some of whom have residual patch margin leaks. A small number of adults will present with moderate- or large-size VSDs which have not undergone closure. These patients must be assessed for elevated PVR and the presence of Eisenmenger syndrome.

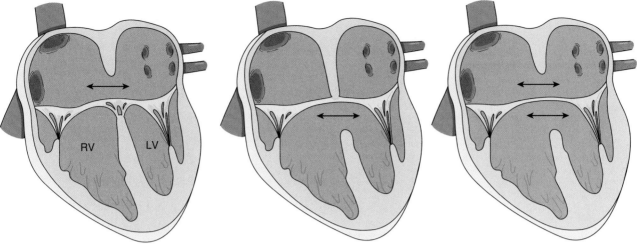

FIGURE 82.14 Various types of atrioventriucular canal (AVC) defects. The right diagram illustrates an exclusively atrial level communication, with the common atrioventricular (AV) valve densely attached to the ventricular septum. The type of AVC is termed a *primum atrial septal defect (ASD)*. The middle diagram has an exclusively ventricular communication. The common AV valve is fused with the inferior limbic band of septum secundum, and thus there is no primum ASD. The left diagram has both atrial and ventricular defects and is termed *complete common AVC defect*. *LV*, Left ventricle; *RV*, right ventricle. (Modified from Libby P. *Essential Atlas of Cardiovascular Disease*. New York: Springer; 2009.)

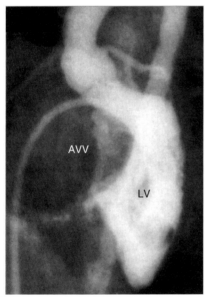

FIGURE 82.15 Angiogram of the left ventricular outflow tract demonstrating the classic "gooseneck" deformity in a patient with a primum atrial septal defect. This appearance is the result of the inlet dimension of the left ventricle being shorter than the outlet dimension. *AVV*, Atrioventricular valve; *LV*, left ventricle. (Modified from Libby P. *Essential Atlas of Cardiovascular Disease*. New York: Springer; 2009.)

TABLE 82.10 Ventricular Septal Defect Nomenclature

CHS	VAN PRAAGH	ANDERSON	OTHER
Perimembranous	Conoventricular*	Perimembranous outlet	Subaortic
Subarterial	Conal septal		Supracristal
Inlet	Atrioventricular canal	Juxta-arterial	Inlet
Muscular		Perimembranous	
	Muscular	Muscular	

*Not all conoventricular defects are in the perimembranous septum.

Repairs

Adults with a VSD and evidence of left ventricular volume overload and hemodynamically significant shunts (Qp:Qs ≥ 1.5:1) should undergo VSD closure if PA systolic pressure is less than 50% systemic and PVR is less than one third systemic (AHA/ACC Class I recommendation, level of evidence B-NR). It is reasonable to close conal septal VSDs in the presence of significant aortic regurgitation. The gold standard for VSD closure remains surgical direct suture closure or patch. However, transcatheter device occlusion of selected muscular and perimembranous defects is possible with favorable outcomes.[53]

Long-Term Outcomes and Complications

The prognosis for adults with surgically closed VSDs is generally favorable. However, studies have demonstrated these patients may have impaired ventricular contractility, compromised ventilatory response, reduced cardiac output during exercise, and lower functional capacity.[54]

Long-term surveillance is recommended for adults with prior VSD closure and any valvular dysfunction, ventricular dysfunction, arrhythmias, or PH.

Patent Ductus Arteriosus
Anatomic Description and Prevalence

The ductus arteriosus, derived from the distal left sixth primitive arch, connects the PA to the descending aorta in fetal life and normally closes within the first day of life. It may remain patent, particularly in premature infants. A PDA is found in about 0.3% to 0.8% of term infants.

Clinical Features

A PDA can range from a small hemodynamically insignificant lesion that is not heard on auscultation to one that is large enough to cause congestive heart failure and PH and Eisenmenger syndrome. Measurement of oxygen saturation should be performed in feet and both hands in adults with a PDA to assess for the presence of right-to-left shunting, as cyanosis is caused by right-to-left shunting in PDA predominantly downstream from the ductal insertion into the aorta. Adults with a hemodynamically significant PDA typically have a wide pulse pressure. On auscultation, a classic murmur is heard best just below the left clavicle and typically extends from systole past the second heart sound into diastole and peripheral pulses may be bounding.

Repairs

PDA closure in adults is recommended if left atrial or LV enlargement is present and attributable to PDA with net left-to-right shunt, PA systolic pressure is less than 50% systemic, and PVR less than one third systemic. Closure is usually feasible by transcatheter techniques.

Long-Term Outcomes and Complications

Patients with device occlusion or after surgical closure should be examined periodically for possible recanalization. Those patients with post-procedural left pulmonary artery (LPA) or aortic obstruction should be imaged at regular intervals. Endocarditis prophylaxis is recommended for 6 months following PDA device closure for life if any residual defect persists following device closure. Patients with a silent or small PDA do not require endocarditis prophylaxis.

---

for include low voltage QRS, peaked tall P waves (>2.5 mm) in leads II and VI due to right atrial enlargement or "Himalayan" p waves (>5 mm height), prolonged PR interval, or importantly a short PR interval and delta wave reflective of pre-excitation from an accessory pathway. Complete or incomplete RBBB is common in adults. An RSR pattern consistent with right ventricular conduction delay is typically seen in lead V1. Atrial flutter or fibrillation are common. The chest radiograph may show cardiomegaly, decreased pulmonary vascular markings, a small aorta and pulmonary trunk shadow, and may classically be described as showing a "boxed shaped" heart. Echocardiography (Fig. 82.19, Video 82.4A-C) must characterize the valve leaflets and subvalvar apparatus, the presence and flow direction in any PFO or ASD, and quantify tricuspid regurgitation. At TEE the tricuspid valve anterior leaflet and its distal tethering points are quite far from the probe and the combination of TTE and TEE or CMR may be necessary to fully evaluate valve morphology, function, and suitability for different surgical approaches. CMR is used to assess the degree of displacement and rotation of the tricuspid valve, quantify tricuspid regurgitation, RV volumes and RV systolic function, LV volumes which may be small, cardiac output which may be low, and Qp:Qs for measurement of cardiac shunt. CMR-derived RV and LV systolic dysfunction are associated with mortality and sustained VT.[55] Reduced or deteriorating exercise tolerance seen on cardiopulmonary exercise testing may prompt repair.

Long-term Outcomes and Complications
Unrepaired Ebstein Anomaly
Natural history outcomes for 72 adults with unoperated Ebstein anomaly demonstrated decreased survival due to biventricular failure or sudden death which were predicted by younger age at diagnosis, male gender, increased cardiothoracic ratio ≥0.65, and severity of valve displacement.[56] In a similar sized cohort major adverse cardiovascular events in adults with Ebstein anomaly were preceded by atrial tachycardia in the vast majority, which itself was often preceded by RV dilation and systolic dysfunction, and more anatomically severe Ebstein anomaly. LV or RV systolic dysfunction predicts adverse events. Atrial arrhythmia increases in prevalence with age. Atrioventricular reentrant tachycardia (AVRT) is the most common. In patients with symptomatic arrhythmias, or pre-excitation on the ECG, electrophysiologic testing followed by ablation is recommended. It is preferable to treat arrhythmia with ablation before surgery as following tricuspid valve surgery access to right-sided accessory pathways and the slow pathway in AV node re-entry tachycardia may be hindered.[5] Multiple accessory pathways in conjunction with atrial tachycardia and atrial fibrillation are associated with sudden death. Identification

of Ebstein patients at high risk for late life-threatening arrhythmias requires improvement.

Tricuspid Valve Repair and Replacement Surgery
The goal of surgery is to increase pulmonary blood flow, minimize tricuspid regurgitation, eliminate interatrial shunting, and improve RV function. Surgery is recommended for symptoms, heart failure attributed to tricuspid valve disease, exercise intolerance demonstrated by exercise testing, or progressive systolic dysfunction. It may also be considered for progressive RV enlargement, desaturation from right to left shunt, paroxysmal embolism, or atrial tachyarrhythmia. Timing of surgery is challenging especially for patients who are minimally symptomatic.

Tricuspid valve repair is preferred when feasible. The RV is usually plicated, shunts are closed, and adjunctive ablation may be performed. A large mobile anterior leaflet with a free leading edge and sufficient septal leaflet tissue is favorable for repair. The degree to which the inferior posterior chordae are shortened and tethered, of leaflet adherence, and rotation of the leaflets into the RVOT are determinants of whether the valve can be repaired or whether it must be replaced. Repair should be performed by a congenital surgeon with specific experience in Ebstein surgery.

There are many different types of valve repair described for Ebstein anomaly.

Tricuspid valve repair with the cone reconstruction was first proposed in 2004 and involves delamination of the anterior tricuspid valve leaflet from the RV endocardium, detaching and rotating it to bring the redundant leaflets to the level of the true tricuspid annulus to form a cone-shaped valve and longitudinal plication of the atrialized RV to restore RV geometry and function. A bidirectional Glenn procedure may be added as part of a "one and a half ventricle repair" when the RV is judged incapable to support the pulmonary circulation due to small size or poor function. Bidirectional Glenn may improve the chances of successful tricuspid valve repair by decreasing RV preload and increasing LV preload. In adults the creation of a Glenn shunt reduces the volume returning to the right heart by about one third. Reintervention may be required for recurrent tricuspid regurgitation post repair or failure of prosthetic tricuspid valves.

Transcatheter Atrial Septal Defect/Patent Foramen Ovale Closure
Device closure of ASD/PFO should be considered for paradoxical embolism but requires careful evaluation before intervention to exclude induction of RA pressure increase or fall in cardiac output. Intervention for cyanosis is considered in highly selected cases as it

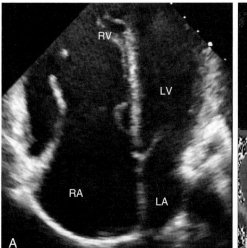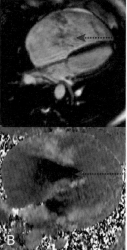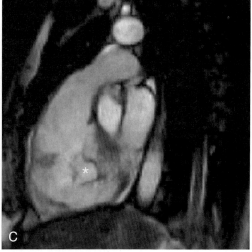

FIGURE 82.19 Ebstein malformation of the tricuspid valve. Four-chamber transthoracic echo showing mild apical displacement of the septal leaflet of the tricuspid valve compared to the origin of the mitral valve, with tricuspid annular dilatation and failure of coaptation of the tricuspid valve leaflets. The severe TR jet *(arrow)* is also seen on the four-chamber cardiac magnetic resonance cine (**B,** *top*) and by inplane velocity mapping (**B,** *bottom*). The valve leaflets are rotated toward the RV outflow tract (**C**) with an obvious coaptation gap *(asterisk)*. *LA,* Left atrium; *LV,* left ventricle; *RA,* right atrium; *RV,* right ventricle.

can result in further increase in right heart pressures and decrease in systemic cardiac output.

Ventricular Dysfunction, Heart Failure, and Transplantation

It is easy to overestimate RV contractility in Ebstein anomaly as systolic ejection of stroke volume is also to the low-pressure RA. When the left ventricle is underfilled or compressed it may be unable to generate a normal cardiac output despite preserved contractility. Cardiac transplantation is considered for patients with severe LV or severe biventricular dysfunction.

Pulmonary Stenosis

Anatomic Description and Prevalence

Isolated valvular pulmonary stenosis is one of the more common forms of CHD. The valve is typically formed abnormally; it may be bicuspid or monocuspid and may include dysplastic leaflets, incomplete opening of the commissures and systolic doming, or some combination of these. The severity of the lesion is defined by the echocardiography estimated peak instantaneous gradient, with mild stenosis less than or equal to 36 mm Hg (3 msec), moderate as 36 to 64 mm Hg (3 to 4 msec), and severe as greater than 64 mm Hg (4 msec). Severe pulmonary stenosis will typically be intervened upon during childhood. Mild and sometimes moderate disease may present in adulthood without prior intervention. The adult presenting with congenital valvular pulmonary stenosis may have some combination of pulmonary stenosis, pulmonary regurgitation, or both, depending on their original lesion and whether they underwent intervention during childhood.

Pulmonary valve disease can be seen in association with several genetic and chromosomal lesions. These can include Noonan syndrome or Williams syndrome.[57] While this lesion can be seen in association with some chromosomal non-disjunction syndromes, it would be quite rare for a patient with trisomy 13 or 18 to survive to adulthood.

Clinical Features and Diagnostic Testing

Patients are often asymptomatic. However, longstanding pulmonary stenosis will often lead to a hypertrophied and stiff RV, which may present with progressive exercise intolerance or signs and symptoms of heart failure. If there is an associated PFO or ASD, the noncompliant RV can lead to right-to-left shunting at the atrial level and cyanosis, particularly with exercise. Physical findings reflect pulmonary valve and RV disease. Cardiovascular exam will include a crescendo-decrescendo systolic ejection murmur of variable intensity and often a systolic ejection click. This click becomes softer with inspiration. The non-compliant RV will lead to a lift on palpation and a prominent jugular a wave. Hepatomegaly is uncommon except with advanced disease. Patients with significant pulmonary regurgitation will have a low-pitched diastolic decrescendo murmur, which can become higher pitched in the presence of PH. Mixed disease leads to a "to-and-fro" murmur of pulmonary stenosis and regurgitation.

Echocardiography is the mainstay of diagnosis for pulmonary stenosis (Fig. 82.20, Video 82.5). In patients with moderate stenosis or greater, TTE is appropriate to perform yearly.[3] Echo can assess for severity of stenosis and regurgitation, as well as for qualitative change in RV size and function. Signs of increased RV filling pressure include RA dilation, IVC dilation, and increased A wave reversal in the hepatic veins. End diastolic forward flow in the PA suggests impaired RV compliance.

CMR can quantify RV size and function. CMR is particularly useful for patients who have had intervention and developed pulmonary regurgitation as RV function and pulmonary regurgitation can both be assessed. Compared to patients with repaired TOF and severe pulmonary regurgitation, this patient population may have equal RV dilation but typically have more preserved RV systolic function.[58]

Cardiopulmonary exercise testing is recommended every 2 years for moderate valve disease. Serial decline in exercise capacity may prompt intervention.

Surgical Repairs

Repair of valvular pulmonary stenosis can be performed by transcatheter balloon valvuloplasty or with open surgical techniques. Balloon pulmonary valvuloplasty is usually preferred in the contemporary era, but many adults had surgical valvotomy in childhood. Less frequent is the Brock procedure, a blind surgical valvotomy performed through the infundibulum, which has fallen out of use. The result of any of these procedures is often pulmonary regurgitation; complete relief of stenosis is often accompanied by moderate or greater regurgitation, and some patients have no residual valve function whatsoever.

Long-Term Outcomes and Complications

Overall outcomes of valvar pulmonary stenosis as well as pulmonary regurgitation as a result of valve intervention are quite good. Patients with mild pulmonary stenosis rarely progress or require intervention. More significant valve dysfunction can lead to impairment of RV systolic and diastolic function, with complications related to the RV disease.

Indications for Intervention or Re-Intervention

The indications for primary intervention on pulmonary stenosis are straightforward. The 2018 ACC/AHA guidelines for the management of the adult with congenital heart disease recommend intervention as a class I indication for moderate or severe valvar pulmonary stenosis in the presence of symptoms including heart failure, exercise intolerance, or cyanosis. Primary intervention by balloon valvuloplasty is recommended, with surgical repair recommended for patients who have a contraindication to or have failed the transcatheter intervention. For asymptomatic patients with severe valvar pulmonary stenosis, intervention is considered reasonable, as a class IIa indication.

The indications for pulmonary valve replacement in the patient with mixed pulmonary stenosis and regurgitation are less clear. Pulmonary

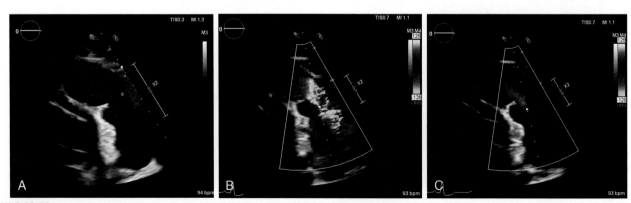

FIGURE 82.20 Transthoracic echocardiogram in the parasternal long axis view. **A**, 2-D image of the right ventricular outflow tract with the pulmonary valve open in systole. Note the thickened and mildly doming valve leaflet and dilated main pulmonary artery. **B**, Color Doppler image of antegrade flow through the stenotic pulmonary valve with turbulent and aliased flow. **C**, Color Doppler image in diastole of a narrow regurgitant jet through the pulmonary valve.

valve replacement is indicated for the patient with at least moderate regurgitation, RV dilation, and the presence of symptoms that can be attributed to the heart disease. In the absence of symptoms, there are not clear indications for valve replacement. Intervention may be reasonable in the patient with progressive changes in RV dilation or dysfunction, or with decreasing exercise capacity. Thresholds for intervention in TOF should not necessarily be extrapolated to patients with pulmonary stenosis.

Tetralogy of Fallot

Anatomic Description and Prevalence

TOF is the most common cyanotic congenital heart defect, comprising a "tetrad" of overriding aorta, VSD, pulmonary stenosis, and right ventricular hypertrophy (Fig. 82.21). Anterocephalad deviation of the outlet septum together with hypertrophy of the septoparietal trabeculations causes subpulmonary stenosis. The pulmonary valve, main and branch pulmonary arteries may also be narrow. Hypoplasia of the pulmonary arteries has been reported to be as frequent as 50%. Associated anomalies include right aortic arch, present in about 25% of patients, and anomalous course of the coronary arteries, the most common with a left anterior descending artery that originates from the right coronary artery and crosses the RVOT. This may be of surgical importance, sometimes necessitating the use of a RV-to-PA conduit. An ASD, a second muscular inlet VSD, or an AVSD—usually in the setting of Down syndrome—can coexist with TOF.

There are important anatomic variations of TOF. TOF with pulmonary atresia with major aortopulmonary collateral arteries (MAPCAs) is an extreme form of TOF present in approximately 15% of all cases. There is absence of any direct connection between the heart and the pulmonary arterial tree, a large VSD and two ventricles. Prior to repair blood reaches the pulmonary bed through the PDA and or MAPCAs. Repair is via unifocalization of MAPCAs, closure of the VSD, and RVOT reconstruction with a conduit.

Another anatomic variant is TOF with absent pulmonary valve, in which there is marked stenosis of the pulmonary valve annulus with poorly formed or absent valve leaflets and severely dilated or aneurysmal pulmonary arteries which may produce airway compression at birth.

Patients with repaired TOF constitute one of the largest groups of ACHD patients surviving into adulthood. Life expectancy depends on the precise underlying anatomy and nature and timing of previous interventions and is excellent for those with uncomplicated anatomy, early primary repair, and good biventricular function.

Clinical Features and Diagnostic Testing

Patients are followed lifelong at varying intervals depending on their clinical status. Symptoms include shortness of breath on exertion, palpitations, or syncope. The clinical examination will typically include normal oxygen saturations. A diastolic to-and-fro murmur in the pulmonary area signifies pulmonary regurgitation. An RV heave and a single second heart sound are present if pulmonary regurgitation is severe. Overt signs of right heart failure such as hepatomegaly, increased jugular venous pressure, and edema are uncommon. ECG will commonly show complete right bundle branch in older adults dependent on the reparative surgical technique. BNP is predictive of mortality.[59] Other diagnostic testing may include chest radiograph, echocardiography, CMR, and cardiopulmonary exercise testing. Ambulatory ECG monitoring, CCT, cardiac catheterization, and diagnostic electrophysiological studies are performed by clinical indication.

Knowledge of the patient's surgical history and most recent physiological status is critical for influencing appropriate frequency of diagnostic imaging and vital for decision-making related to indications for intervention for pulmonary regurgitation, RVOT obstruction, residual VSD, ascending aortic dilatation with aortic regurgitation, RV and LV dysfunction, arrhythmia, or endocarditis.

Echocardiography is routinely used for all patients including screening for significant pulmonary regurgitation and right heart dilatation and for assessing ventricular function. Severity of RVOT obstruction, tricuspid regurgitation, and diastolic dysfunction and presence of residual VSD are optimally assessed with echocardiography. Quantification of right atrial size is helpful as large right atrial area has been associated with sustained tachyarrhythmias in these patients.[60] Furthermore, Doppler can identify the presence of a restrictive RV with the presence

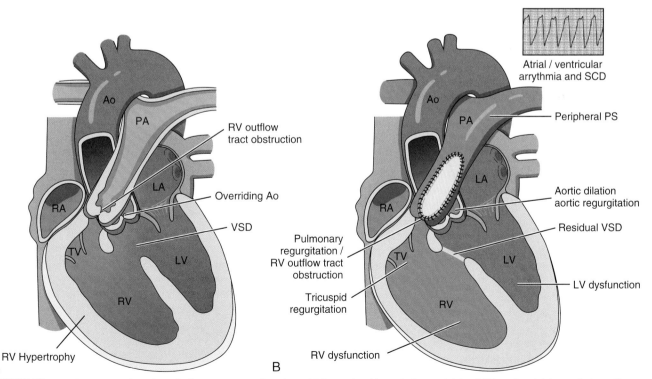

FIGURE 82.21 A, Native anatomy of tetralogy of Fallot. **B,** Anatomy of tetralogy of Fallot repair, with ventricular septal defect (VSD) patch and right ventricular outflow tract patch. Note the indication of various possible complications following surgery. *Ao,* Aorta; *LA,* left atrium; *LV,* left ventricle; *PA,* pulmonary artery; *PS,* pulmonary stenosis; *RA,* right atrium; *RV,* right ventricle; *SCD,* sudden cardiac death; *TV,* tricuspid valve. (From Baumgartner H, De Backer J. 2020 ESC guidelines for the management of adult congenital heart disease. *Eur Heart J.* 2020;42[6]:563–645.)

of an antegrade "a" wave (end-diastolic forward flow) in the RVOT on pulse wave Doppler throughout the respiratory cycle demonstrating a filled, non-compliant RV which is unable to distend further (Fig. 82.22).

CMR imaging is used for accurate assessment of right ventricular volume and function, severity of pulmonary regurgitation (Fig. 82.23), the entire RVOT including branch pulmonary arteries and the course of the proximal coronary arteries, size of both the aortic root and ascending aorta, quantification of tricuspid and aortic regurgitation, and if redo surgery is being planned shows the proximity of these structures to the sternum. RVOT regional wall motion abnormalities and aneurysms (Fig. 82.24, Video 82.6A,B) are common; the RVOT akinetic area length predicts the onset of sustained ventricular arrhythmia. RV volumes quantified by CMR in the context of moderate or severe pulmonary regurgitation are followed serially for progressive dilatation and to inform optimal timing for pulmonary valve replacement. Late gadolinium enhancement imaging correlates with adverse prognosis in adults with repaired TOF, hence may be useful in selected cases for decision-making. Cardiopulmonary exercise testing is crucial for objective measure of exercise capacity which is related to prognosis and facilitates decision-making regarding valve replacement. CCT is used primarily for coronary artery relationships to the RVOT, extent of calcification and RVOT and PA dimensions in the planning of transcatheter pulmonary valve implantation, and for coronary artery assessment preoperatively in older patients or delineation of MAPCAs in selected patients. Ambulatory ECG monitoring, event recorders, and diagnostic EP study are used in patients with arrhythmia symptoms or who are considered high risk or suspected high risk for arrhythmia. Inducible VT during EP study has prognostic value for future clinical VT and sudden cardiac death.

Cardiac catheterization for diagnostic purposes alone is rarely indicated for asymptomatic TOF patients. Preoperative assessment of TOF with pulmonary atresia with MAPCAs usually includes delineation of the arterial supply to both lungs by selective catheterization and angiography to show the course and segmental supply from the collateral arteries and central pulmonary arteries.

Surgical Repair

Those born in developed countries have usually undergone surgical repair with closure of the VSD and relief of pulmonary stenosis with resection of RV muscle bundles in the RVOT with or without more extensive right ventricular outflow reconstruction. Since surgical repair of TOF was introduced in the 1950s[61] survival rates of greater than 90% are expected beyond 40 years from repair. Therefore, repaired TOF constitutes one of the most common conditions seen in ACHD outpatient care.[62] The surgical strategy for repair has evolved with time: Previously

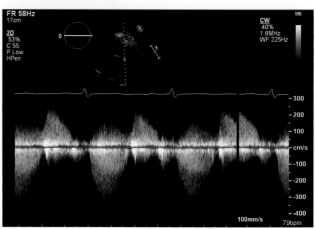

FIGURE 82.22 Spectral Doppler tracing of the main pulmonary artery in repaired tetralogy of Fallot; forward flow is seen in systole and retrograde flow of pulmonary regurgitation in diastole. Note the end diastolic forward flow in the main pulmonary artery corresponding to atrial systole, just before the QRS complex.

many infants received a BTT shunt prior to repair but now early primary repair is common. Due to recognition of the deleterious effects of pulmonary regurgitation, transannular patch is avoided where possible to preserve the integrity of the pulmonary valve. Patients with TOF with pulmonary atresia and those with anomalous left coronary artery from the right sinus may undergo a RV-to-PA artery conduit repair.

Long-Term Outcomes and Complications
Anatomic Sequalae

Table 82.11 lists the common sequelae of repaired TOF. Pulmonary regurgitation is a common sequela in repaired TOF patients particularly in patients who received a transannular patch repair. Patients with repaired TOF and pulmonary regurgitation are often asymptomatic for several decades; however, if untreated, severe pulmonary regurgitation results in RV dilatation and dysfunction, arrhythmia, heart failure, and even death.

In the past several decades, advancements have been made to determine the optimal timing of pulmonary valve replacement prior to symptoms and irreversible RV dysfunction. Symptomatic patients with significant pulmonary regurgitation should undergo valve replacement. The optimal threshold for elective pulmonary valve replacement for asymptomatic patients with significant pulmonary regurgitation is a subject of ongoing research. Pulmonary valve replacement is considered when RV end-systolic volume indexed to body surface area

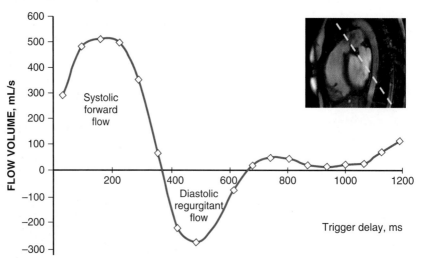

FIGURE 82.23 Cardiac magnetic resonance (CMR) quantification of pulmonary regurgitation after repair of tetralogy of Fallot. Pulmonary regurgitation is quantified by CMR in a cross section transecting the main pulmonary artery in the plane shown inset. The resultant through-plane phase contrast velocity mapping acquisition is used to plot forward flow to the lungs and to derive a pulmonary regurgitant fraction from integration of areas contained by forward and reversed flow curves. Typically, significant pulmonary regurgitation has a pulmonary regurgitant fraction ≥40%; this is greater with distal pulmonary obstruction or increased pulmonary artery compliance and less with subpulmonary stenosis or restrictive RV physiology. *ms*, milliseconds.

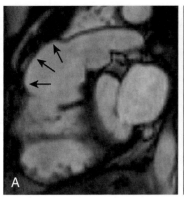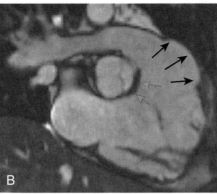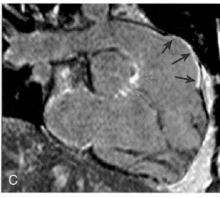

FIGURE 82.24 Right ventricular (RV) outflow tract aneurysmal or akinetic regions following tetralogy of Fallot repair. In older adults, RV outflow tract akinetic and or aneurysmal regions are common, are due to previous more generous resection of RV muscle bands with or without RV outflow tract or transannular patch augmentation, and contribute to worse RV ejection fraction. In the same patient this large akinetic RV outflow tract region is indicated by arrows in RV outflow tract **(A)** and RV in out **(B)** cine planes and its length was nearly 50 mm. **C,** Late gadolinium enhancement cardiac magnetic resonance (CMR) demonstrates fibrosis corresponding to the regional wall motion abnormality *(red arrows)* and there is fibrosis at the ventricular septal defect closure site *(blue arrows).*

TABLE 82.11 Common Long-Term Issues in Repaired Tetralogy of Fallot

RV volume overload
  Pulmonary regurgitation
  Tricuspid regurgitation
  Left-to-right shunt
    • VSD
    • Atrial septal defect
    • Systemic-to-pulmonary collaterals

RV pressure overload
  RVOT obstruction or pulmonary artery stenosis
  Pulmonary vascular disease
  Pulmonary venous hypertension secondary to LV diastolic dysfunction

RV systolic or diastolic dysfunction

LV systolic or diastolic dysfunction

Aortic regurgitation

Ventricular conduction delay and dyssynchrony

Arrhythmias
  Atrial flutter
  Atrial fibrillation
  Ventricular tachycardia

LV, Left ventricle; *RV,* right ventricle; *RVOT,* right ventricular outflow tract; *VSD,* ventricular septal defect.

reaches 80 mL/m² (or end-diastolic volume index reaches 160 mL/m²) as these RV volume thresholds predict normalization of RV volume following intervention. Right ventricular dysfunction is an indication for valve replacement.[3,63–65]

Transcatheter pulmonary valve implantation is an option when the anatomy of the RVOT and coronary arteries is favorable for available valves. Patients after previous surgical pulmonary valve replacement with a homograft or xenograft are usually suitable for transcatheter pulmonary valve implantation.

Symptomatic patients with severe RVOT obstruction require intervention. In those without symptoms intervention is indicated depending on objective exercise capacity, decreased or decreasing RV function, increasing tricuspid regurgitation, and presence of right-to-left shunting. Patients with discrete branch pulmonary stenosis, increased RV pressure, and reduced lung perfusion at CMR may benefit from branch PA dilatation and stenting.

Residual VSD may occur in up to 10% of repaired TOF patients and is often due to incomplete repair or VSD patch dehiscence.

Aortic dilatation not only at sinus level but of the ascending aorta is common after repaired TOF particularly after later repair, palliative shunt, with right aortic arch, and in men. Reassuringly progression

is slow and acute aortic dissection in the setting of repaired TOF is extremely rare.[66] Aortic dilatation may be associated with aortic regurgitation.

Ventricular Dilation and Dysfunction and Heart Failure

Heart failure is the most common cause of death in patients with repaired TOF.[10] Patients may have systolic or diastolic dysfunction of the LV or the RV. Pulmonary regurgitation can lead to RV dilatation and dysfunction. Tricuspid regurgitation may be a complication of previous surgical VSD closure or secondary to RV dilatation. LV dysfunction is present in greater than 20% of patients with repaired TOF and may result from ventricular-ventricular interaction, electromechanical dyssynchrony, or ischemia. LV dysfunction is more common in patients with previous palliative shunt, late repair, or aortic regurgitation and is associated with increased mortality.

Randomized controlled trials of medical therapies targeted at right ventricular dysfunction have been small, underpowered, and have not shown benefit.

Arrhythmia and Risk Stratification for Sudden Cardiac Death

Both atrial and ventricular arrhythmia increase in prevalence after around 35 years of age. The most common is IART related to the cavotricuspid isthmus, right atriotomy, and dilatation of the RA which is amenable to ablation. Atrial fibrillation from the LA can be difficult to treat. Monomorphic or polymorphic sustained VT may be fatal, the former typically associated with ventricular dysfunction.[67]

Ventricular arrhythmia is an important cause of sudden death, putative risk factors for which include prior LV systolic and diastolic dysfunction, sustained ventricular and atrial tachyarrhythmia, systolic RV dysfunction, excessive RV hypertrophy, QRS duration ≥180 milliseconds, QRS fragmentation, LV systolic or diastolic dysfunction, extensive fibrosis at CMR, and inducible VT at EP testing.[3,63,68] The latter invasive testing is performed in selected patients with multiple noninvasively derived risk factors. The INDICATOR study of 873 repaired TOF patients showed that CMR derived impaired RV and LV ejection fraction and increased RV mass/volume ratio together with history of sustained atrial arrhythmia predicted mortality and sustained VT during follow-up.[69]

Targeting anatomical isthmuses prophylactically by VT catheter ablation may be an effective way to obliterate the usual VT substrates but any role in patient-specific risk stratification requires further investigation. VT ablation may be a treatment of choice in patients with good RV and LV function in centers with appropriate expertise.[70] For patients surviving sustained VT or cardiac arrest an ICD is usually indicated for secondary prevention. Preoperative RV dysfunction and RV hypertrophy may confer ongoing risk of mortality and sustained VT even after pulmonary valve replacement.[71]

Robust algorithms to appropriately weight risk factors for individuals for indications for primary prevention ICD remain lacking. As in all cardiology these are likely to benefit selected patients with at least 3.5%/year mortality risk. Clinical practice is to consider automatic implantable cardioverter defibrillators (AICDs) in selected repaired TOF patients with multiple VT risk factors among LV dysfunction, non-sustained and symptomatic VT, QRS duration ≥180 milliseconds, extensive RV scarring on CMR, or inducible VT at programmed electrical stimulation and remains controversial.

Transposition of the Great Arteries
Anatomic Description and Prevalence
In D-loop TGA the aorta arises from the RV and the PA arises from the LV; that is ventriculo-arterial discordance. With this anatomy the pulmonary and systemic circulations are in parallel rather than in series; de-oxygenated blood recirculates through the systemic circulation while oxygenated blood recirculates through the pulmonary circulation (Fig. 82.25). Therefore, without mixing or correction, TGA is not survivable. TGA occurs in approximately 30/100,000 live births, accounting for approximately 6% of congenital heart defects making it the second most common cyanotic congenital heart defect, following TOF.

In the vast majority of patients with TGA, the atria are normally positioned and the AV connections are normal. Venous return is typically normal. The great arteries are transposed with the aortic valve anterior and rightward to the pulmonic valve (D-loop transposition). In some, the aortic valve is directly anterior to the pulmonic valve or the valves can be side-by-side.

TGA is frequently associated with other congenital malformations. Approximately 35% of patients have a concomitant VSD. The VSD is most typically malalignment, peri-membranous, or muscular. LVOT obstruction (native pulmonic or sub-pulmonic obstruction) is common. Mechanisms for LVOT obstruction include a discrete fibrous membrane in the LVOT, systolic anterior motion of the mitral valve, and valvular pulmonic stenosis.

Coronary artery anomalies are very common in TGA, and of clinical importance in those repaired with an arterial switch operation, discussed below. Approximately ⅔ of patients have a "typical" coronary artery pattern in which the left coronary arises from the left posterior sinus and the right coronary arises from the right posterior sinus. A single coronary artery is present in 10% and intra-arterial course is present in approximately 5%.

Unless repaired, TGA is lethal within the first year of life. Therefore, virtually all adults with TGA will have undergone a prior surgical repair.

Clinical Features
Unrepaired TGA in the adult is exceedingly rare. The physical exam will be dominated by profound cyanosis and erythrocytosis. The physical findings of the repaired patient depend entirely on the type of repair.

Surgical Repairs
Atrial Switch Operation
The atrial switch operation was the surgical repair for TGA from 1957 until the 1980s at which point it was replaced by the arterial switch operation (discussed below). The atrial switch procedure is often referred to by the eponyms Mustard procedure or Senning procedure. In the atrial switch, venous return is re-directed to create a circulation in series and resolve cyanosis. The SVC and IVC are re-routed leftward toward the mitral valve and the LV via inter-atrial baffles. The pulmonary veins are re-routed anteriorly and rightward, toward the tricuspid valve and the RV. Following the atrial switch operation, de-oxygenated blood flows from the SVC/IVC through the mitral valve, to the sub-pulmonic LV, where it is pumped to the PA and the lungs. Oxygenated blood returns via pulmonary veins, flows to the tricuspid valve and the systemic RV, and is pumped to the aorta. Therefore, following the atrial switch operation, the RV is the systemic ventricle, the tricuspid valve is the systemic AV valve, and the LV and mitral valve support the pulmonary circulation (Fig. 82.25B).

Arterial Switch Operation
In the contemporary era the arterial switch operation is the preferred treatment for TGA because it results in a systemic LV. In the arterial switch operation, the surgeon transects the great arteries above the sinuses and anastomoses them to the contralateral root. The coronary arteries must be removed from the native aortic root and re-anastomosed to the neo-aortic root, the most technically challenging portion of the operation and a source of operative morbidity in the early years of the arterial switch. Often draping the pulmonary arteries over the ascending aorta is required. Following the arterial switch operation, the LV supports the systemic circulation and the RV supports the pulmonary circulation (Fig. 82.25C).

Rastelli Operation
The Rastelli operation is a surgical option for infants with TGA, large VSD, and pulmonic stenosis. The surgeon over-sews the native pulmonic valve and places an angled VSD patch to direct oxygenated blood from the LV, across the VSD, and to the aortic valve. A RV-to-PA conduit provides for pulmonary blood flow (Fig. 82.25D).

Long-Term Outcomes and Complications Following the Atrial Switch Operation
While the atrial switch operation (Mustard or Senning) was revolutionary in that it allowed infants born with TGA to survive childhood, late complications are common in adults who have been treated with these operations (Table 82.12).

Ventricular Dysfunction
Following the atrial switch operation, the RV is the systemic ventricle. While systemic right ventricular systolic dysfunction is relatively uncommon in childhood, progressive deterioration is typical. By age 30 years, only a minority of patients are NYHA Functional Class I and up to a quarter have clinical heart failure.[72,73] There are multiple reasons why the RV is predisposed to systolic dysfunction when exposed to high afterload including unfavorable myocardial fiber orientation, non-conical ventricular geometry, and tricuspid (systemic AV valve) regurgitation imposing additional volume loading. Right ventricular dilation and dysfunction lead to annular enlargement and secondary tricuspid (systemic AV valve) regurgitation. The superimposed volume load on the systemic RV accelerates ventricular dysfunction and makes patients more likely to develop heart failure with reduced ejection fraction.

Systolic function of the systemic RV can be evaluated qualitatively by TTE. Quantitative assessment of systemic right ventricular systolic function is difficult by echocardiography: Parameters such as TAPSE, fractional area change, and tissue Doppler are not well validated in patients with a systemic RV. Cardiac MR remains the gold standard for quantification of RV systolic function.

Medical management of systemic right ventricular systolic dysfunction is discussed in more detail in the section on heart failure in CHD. There is no conclusive evidence that standard GDMT impacts ejection fraction, functional class, or clinical outcomes; however, ACE inhibitors and angiotensin receptor antagonists are commonly used in patients with a systemic RV and clinical heart failure with systolic dysfunction.

Baffle Complications
The interatrial baffles which divert pulmonary and systemic venous blood to the contralateral ventricle are predisposed to malfunction as well. The pathways can become narrowed, most commonly in the SVC limb (Fig. 82.26, Video 82.7A,B). Some patients may present with symptoms of SVC syndrome such as facial swelling or headache, although most are asymptomatic due to decompression down the azygous vein. Percutaneous stents usually effectively relieve symptomatic pathway obstruction so surgical baffle reconstruction is rarely required. Transvenous pacemaker or defibrillator leads are risk factors for SVC pathway obstruction and, when possible, are extracted prior to stent implantation to avoid jailing the lead between the SVC and the stent. Obstruction within the pulmonary venous pathway is less common and would present with symptoms of pulmonary edema. Pathway obstruction within the IVC limb is

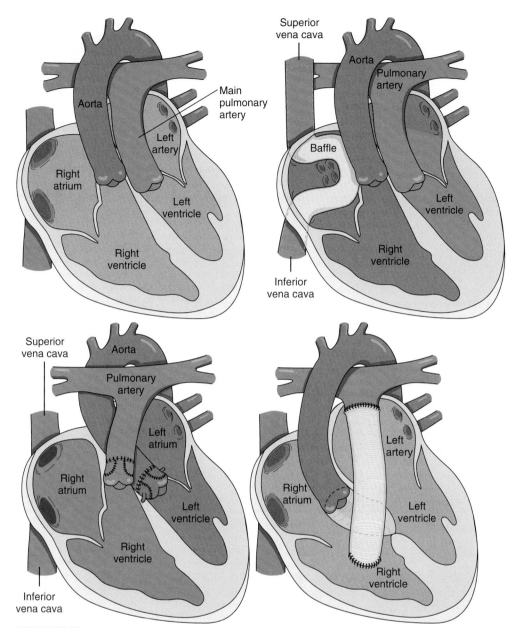

FIGURE 82.25 **A,** D-loop transposition of the great arteries, unrepaired with intact ventricular septum. The aorta is anterior and rightward of the pulmonary artery, and arising from the right ventricle. **B,** Following the atrial switch operation, the aorta continues to arise from the right ventricle; the systemic venous return has been baffled to the mitral valve and left ventricle, and the pulmonary venous return runs posterior to the systemic venous baffle to the tricuspid valve and right ventricle. **C,** Following the arterial switch operation, there is now ventriculo-arterial concordance, with the neo-aorta arising from the left ventricle. Note the suture lines above the coronary arteries on the neo-aorta and on the neo-pulmonary artery. **D,** Following Rastelli oper-ation, a patch has been placed to direct the left ventricle through a ventricular septal defect to the native aorta, which sits above the right ventricle. A conduit has been placed from the right ventricle to the pulmonary arteries.

antiarrhythmic drugs.[74] Over ⅓ of patients with an atrial switch proce-dure have sinus node dysfunction or other bradyarrhythmia requiring a pacemaker. Transvenous pacemaker leads are a risk factor for SVC path-way obstruction.

Long-Term Complications Following the Arterial Switch Operation

Late outcomes after the arterial switch are favorable compared to the atrial switch (see Table 82.12). Following the arterial switch the LV is the systemic ventricle and there are no interatrial baffles. Consequently, the risk of heart failure and arrhyth-mia is low after the arterial switch operation.

Coronary Artery Stenosis

The most technically difficult aspect of the arterial switch operation is the coronary transfer from the native aortic root to the neo-aortic root. The surgery is more challenging in patients with variant coronary artery patterns, single coronary arteries, or intramural coronary arteries, approx-imately ⅓ of patients with TGA. Cor-onary artery ostial stenosis typically presents within the first year after the arterial switch operation but can present in adolescence or adulthood with ventricular dysfunction, angina, ventricular arrhythmia, or sudden cardiac death. Patients with any of these symptoms should undergo coronary evaluation with invasive angiography, CT angiography, or stress testing. Percutaneous and surgical revascularization are both reason-able treatment options.

Aortic Dilation and Regurgitation

Following the arterial switch oper-ation, the neo-aortic valve and root (native pulmonic valve and root) are predisposed to dilation and secondary neo-aortic valve regurgi-tation. The rate of dissection is not known following the arterial switch

relatively rare but presents with lower extremity edema, ascites, or hepatic congestion.

A communication between the systemic venous pathway and the pulmonary venous pathway is called a baffle leak. Baffle leaks can lead to resting or exertional desaturation and can present with exer-cise intolerance, chamber dilation, or paradoxical embolism. Shunts are often bidirectional. Agitated saline injection on TTE show opacifi-cation of the systemic RV. Baffle leak is a risk for paradoxical embolism. Baffle leaks can be closed percutaneously, either with an ASD occluder device or a covered stent.

Atrial Arrhythmia

The extensive atrial suture lines used to create interatrial baffles pre-dispose patients to developing atrial arrhythmias. Interatrial re-entry tachycardia is common in adults who have undergone atrial switch procedure. Atrial tachyarrhythmias are associated with sudden car-diac death so should be treated aggressively, either with ablation or

operation, but there are very few reports of aortic dissection or rupture following the arterial switch operation. Indications for surgery on neo-aortic valve regurgitation mirror that for intervention for native aortic regurgitation and are based on symptoms, ventricular dilation, or the presence of ventricular dysfunction.

Supravalvar Pulmonic Stenosis

Supravalvar pulmonic stenosis can occur just above the pulmonic valve or in the branch pulmonary arteries. Proximal supravalvar pul-monic stenosis is well demonstrated by TTE but branch PA stenosis may be difficult to visualize by echocardiography; a high parasternal or suprasternal notch imaging can show the branch pulmonary arter-ies splayed over the mid-ascending aorta. MR angiography visualizes the degree of stenosis and using phase contrast MR in the branch pul-monary arteries provides quantitative flow data to each lung. When branch PA stenosis causes symptoms or right ventricular hypertension, percutaneous angioplasty with stenting is typically effective treatment.

TABLE 82.12 Common Complications Following Repair of Transposition of the Great Arteries

SURGICAL CORRECTION	COMPLICATION	TYPICAL SIGNS AND SYMPTOMS	DIAGNOSTIC EVALUATION	TYPICAL TREATMENT
Atrial switch operation (Mustard or Senning)	Baffle leak	Exercise intolerance, cyanosis, erythrocytosis, paradoxical embolism	TTE with agitated saline, TEE, gated cardiac CT, cardiac MR	Transcatheter closure with covered stent or ASD occlude device
	Pathway obstruction	Facial swelling, headaches, often asymptomatic	CT or MR angiography. Invasive angiography	If symptomatic, angioplasty with stenting; may require pacemaker lead extraction
	Interatrial re-entrant tachycardia	Palpitations, syncope	ECG, ambulatory monitoring, invasive EP study	Ablation, antiarrhythmic drugs
	Sinus node dysfunction	Exercise intolerance, syncope	ECG, ambulatory monitoring	Pacemaker
	Ventricular dysfunction	Exercise intolerance, congestive heart failure	TTE, cardiac MR	RAAS inhibition (although efficacy not well documented), diuretics, advanced HF pathway
Arterial switch operation	Ostial coronary artery stenosis	Angina, ventricular arrhythmias	Stress testing, CT, or invasive coronary angiography	Percutaneous or surgical revascularization
	Branch pulmonary artery stenosis	Exercise intolerance, chest discomfort; systolic murmur	TTE, CT, or MR angiography; quantitative nuclear lung perfusion scan	Balloon angioplasty with stenting; surgical pulmonary artery reconstruction
	Neo-aortic root dilation	None	TTE, CT, or MR angiography	Surgical neo-aortic root replacement for severe enlargement
	Neo-aortic valve regurgitation	Exercise intolerance; diastolic murmur	TTE, cardiac MR	Surgical neo-aortic valve replacement
Rastelli operation	Right ventricle to pulmonary artery conduit stenosis	Exercise intolerance, systolic murmur (often ≥ grade 3), right ventricular dysfunction	TTE	Transcatheter pulmonary valve implantation or surgical conduit replacement
	Right ventricle to pulmonary artery conduit regurgitation	Exercise intolerance, diastolic murmur, right ventricular dysfunction	TTE, cardiac MR	Transcatheter pulmonary valve implantation; occasionally surgical conduit revision

CT, Computed tomography; *EP,* electrophysiology; *HF,* heart failure; *MR:* Magnetic resonance; *RAAS:* Renin-angiotensin-aldosterone; *TEE,* Transesophageal echocardiography, *TTE,* transthoracic echocardiography.

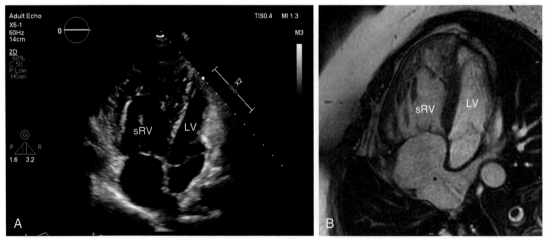

FIGURE 82.26 D-loop transposition of the great arteries s/p atrial switch operation. **A,** Transthoracic echocardiogram from apical view showing a hypertrophied and dilated systemic right ventricle and a thin-walled and pancaked left ventricle (LV). **B,** Steady state free precession cardiac MRI image in a similar plane showing the pulmonary venous pathway *(asterisk)* to the systemic, hypertrophied right ventricle.

Long-Term Complications Following the Rastelli Operation

Following the Rastelli operation, the LV is the systemic ventricle and the RV supplies the lungs via a RV-to-PA conduit. Children often require multiple conduit revisions during childhood as the conduit does not grow with the child. Late morbidity in adulthood is typically due to conduit stenosis, regurgitation, or mixed dysfunction (see Table 82.12).

Symptoms of conduit dysfunction include exercise intolerance and patients may show signs of right-sided heart failure. Conduit stenosis generates a systolic murmur (often grade III or higher) and conduit regurgitation generates a diastolic decrescendo murmur. Usually, echocardiography is useful to visualize the conduit and is particularly useful for quantifying obstruction. In some patients the conduit is obscured by the sternum. CMR with phase contrast and contrast enhanced angiography provide information on conduit anatomy and can be used to quantify regurgitation. In many patients with conduit dysfunction, transcatheter pulmonary valve implantation is effective for both stenosis and regurgitation. In some patients the conduit may be too small for percutaneous therapy. In others, conduit expansion results in coronary artery compression. In these patients surgical conduit replacement is required. Occasionally, following the Rastelli operation, patients may have residual VSD.

Congenitally Corrected Transposition of the Great Arteries

Anatomic Description and Prevalence

L-loop TGA, also called congenitally corrected TGA (ccTGA), is an uncommon congenital heart defect, accounting for less than 1% of CHD. L-loop TGA is characterized by AV discordance and ventriculo-arterial discordance; deoxygenated blood goes from the vena cavae to the RA, through the mitral valve to the LV, and then to the PA. Oxygenated blood returns via the pulmonary veins to the LA, through the tricuspid valve to the RV, and then is ejected to the aorta (Fig. 82.27). Therefore, L-loop TGA is a non-cyanotic congenital heart defect. Unoperated patients with L-loop TGA have a systemic RV. In the most common form of L-loop TGA the atria are normally situated, and there is ventricular inversion with the RV lying leftward and posterior. The great arteries are L-transposed with the aortic valve anterior and leftward of the pulmonic valve. Approximately 10% of patients with L-loop TGA have atrial situs inversus and mirror image dextrocardia; the physiology is unaltered by this variation.

The majority of patients with L-loop TGA have associated cardiovascular defects. More than half have a VSD. Subpulmonic or valvular pulmonic stenosis are common. The majority have a congenitally abnormal tricuspid (systemic AV) valve which shares features of Ebstein anomaly.

Clinical Features

Patients with L-loop TGA and no associated cardiac defects may remain asymptomatic and even go undiagnosed for decades. Those with ventricular dysfunction may have exercise intolerance or signs of heart failure. Because the AV node is displaced, patients with L-loop TGA have an abnormal conduction system which predisposes to complete heart block at a rate of 2% per year. The physical examination in L-loop TGA without associated lesions may be nearly normal with the exception of a single second heart sound (as the pulmonic closure sound is obscured by its posterior location). ECG shows absent septal Q-waves in the left precordial leads. AV block may be present. Chest radiograph typically shows a narrow and straight mediastinal silhouette. Patients with concomitant valve dysfunction will

have associated murmurs. Fig. 82.28 illustrates imaging examples of L-loop TGA (Video 82.8).

Surgical Repairs

Patients with L-loop TGA and no associated cardiac anomalies do not necessarily require surgery, although this will leave them with a systemic RV.

The double switch operation (Fig. 82.29) is a technically complex surgery which results in the LV in the sub-aortic position. In patients without a VSD, this consists of an atrial switch procedure (Mustard or Senning) and an arterial switch procedure. In patients with a VSD, the double switch can be achieved via an atrial switch and Rastelli operation.

Some patients with L-loop TGA and a pulmonic stenosis undergo a LV-to-PA conduit (and VSD closure, if indicated). This is a simpler surgery than the double-switch operation, but leaves the patient with a systemic RV and tricuspid valve.

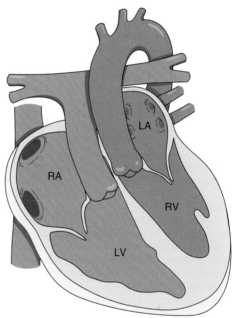

FIGURE 82.27 Diagram of L-loop transposition of the great arteries, demonstrating atrioventricular and ventriculoarterial discordance. Note the shading showing deoxygenated blood in the left ventricle and oxygenated blood in the right ventricle. *LA*, Left atrium; *LV*, Left ventricle, *RA*, right atrium; *RV*, right ventricle. (Modified from Libby P. *Essential Atlas of Cardiovascular Disease*. New York: Springer; 2009.)

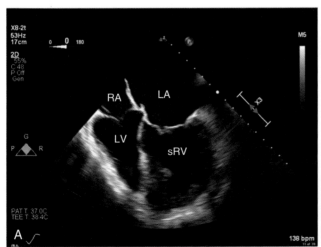 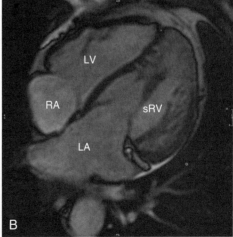

FIGURE 82.28 L-loop transposition of the great arteries. **A,** Transesophageal echocardiogram in transverse view showing atrioventricular discordance. **B,** Cardiac MRI steady state free precession cine imaging in a similar horizontal long axis plane. *LA*, Left atrium, *LV*, left ventricle, *RA*, right atrium, *sRV*, systemic right ventricle.

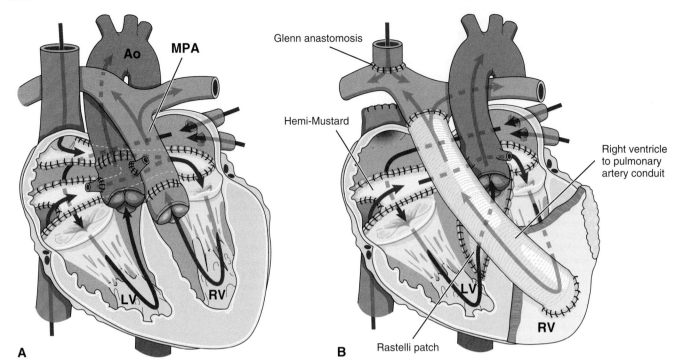

FIGURE 82.29 Diagram of two surgical options for L-loop transposition of the great arteries. **A,** Double switch operation, consisting of an atrial level switch and arterial switch. Note the superior vena cava (SVC) and inferior vena cava (IVC) blood baffled to the left-sided tricuspid valve and right ventricle (with *blue arrows*) and pulmonary venous blood flowing to the right-sided mitral valve and left ventricle (with *red arrows*). Suture lines are seen on the neo-aorta and neo-pulmonary artery following arterial switch. **B,** Hemi-Mustard and Rastelli operations. In this panel, the IVC blood is baffled to the left-sided tricuspid valve and right ventricle *(blue arrows)* and the SVC is directly anastomosed to the right pulmonary artery in end-to-side fashion (bidirectional Glenn). The right-sided left ventricle has been baffled through the native ventricular septal defect to the L-transposed aorta, forming a pathway for oxygenated blood. There is a conduit placed from the right ventricle to the pulmonary artery. *Ao,* Aorta; *LV,* left ventricle; *MPA,* main pulmonary artery; *RV,* right ventricle. (From Otto CM, ed. *The Practice of Clinical Echocardiography.* 5th ed. Philadelphia: Elsevier; 2017.)

Late Complications

Patients with L-loop TGA and no prior surgical repair are susceptible to regurgitation of the systemic tricuspid valve, systolic dysfunction of the systemic RV, and complete heart block. Tricuspid regurgitation is usually organic and results from a congenitally abnormal tricuspid valve with Ebstein-like features. Patients with symptomatic tricuspid regurgitation should be considered for valve replacement surgery as valve repair has poor long-term outcomes.[75,76] Because tricuspid regurgitation drives right ventricular systolic dysfunction, valve replacement should also be considered in the asymptomatic patient. Outcomes are better when valve replacement is performed in patients with preserved right ventricular systolic function, particularly with a right ventricular ejection fraction greater than 40%.

Medical management of systemic right ventricular systolic dysfunction is discussed in more detail in the section on heart failure in CHD.

Because of the abnormal location of the AV node and the conduction system in L-loop TGA, patients are predisposed to complete heart block. Serial monitoring with ECG and ambulatory monitors is warranted, as the incidence of complete heart block is as high as 2%/year and permanent pacemaker implantation may be required.

Patients who have undergone the double-switch procedure have a systemic LV, so they are less susceptible to ventricular dysfunction and less impacted by tricuspid regurgitation. However, they may develop any of the problems associated with the double switch such as baffle complications, coronary ostial stenosis, or conduit dysfunction. These complications, appropriate testing, and management are discussed in the section on D-loop TGA.

Double Outlet Right Ventricle
Anatomic Description and Prevalence

Double outlet RV (DORV) is a conotruncal anomaly in which both great arteries are completely or nearly completely aligned with the RV. DORV varies in complexity from a simple form that is physiologically

like a VSD to extremely complex defects associated with heterotaxy syndrome. The key anatomic features of DORV are the VSD, the infundibular septum, and the position of the arterial roots. The location of the VSD is almost always the same—between the limbs of the septal band. The commitment of the VSD to an arterial root is dependent on the orientation and size of the infundibular septum and the position of the arterial roots. Fig. 82.30 illustrates the relationship between the VSD and arterial roots in some common forms of DORV. Most often the VSD is aligned with the rightward aorta because the infundibular septum attaches to the muscular septum leftward and superior to the VSD, shielding the PA from the VSD. In 30% of cases the VSD is aligned with the PA because the infundibular septum extends anterior and rightward away from the muscular septum and under the aorta, shielding it from the VSD. If the infundibular septum is hypoplastic or absent, there is nothing to shield either arterial root from the VSD and it is doubly committed. In rare cases, the VSD is distant from the arterial roots and uncommitted to either. These are usually muscular or inlet defects.

The position of the great arteries is also important in determining the relationship between the VSD and the arterial roots. The aorta is usually posterior to or side by side with the PA if there is a subaortic VSD. However, in cases with a subpulmonic VSD, the aorta is usually side by side or anterior to the PA. In rare cases the aorta is to the left of the PA, so what would usually be a subpulmonary VSD becomes subaortic and vice versa.

There are four common physiologic variations of DORV that dictate the clinical presentation and approach to surgical repair:
1. VSD physiology: DORV with large subaortic VSD and no pulmonic stenosis
2. TOF physiology: DORV with subaortic VSD and pulmonic stenosis
3. TGA physiology: DORV with subpulmonary VSD with or without aortic obstruction
4. Single ventricle physiology: DORV with mitral atresia, severely unbalanced AV canal defect, or other cause of significant ventricular hypoplasia

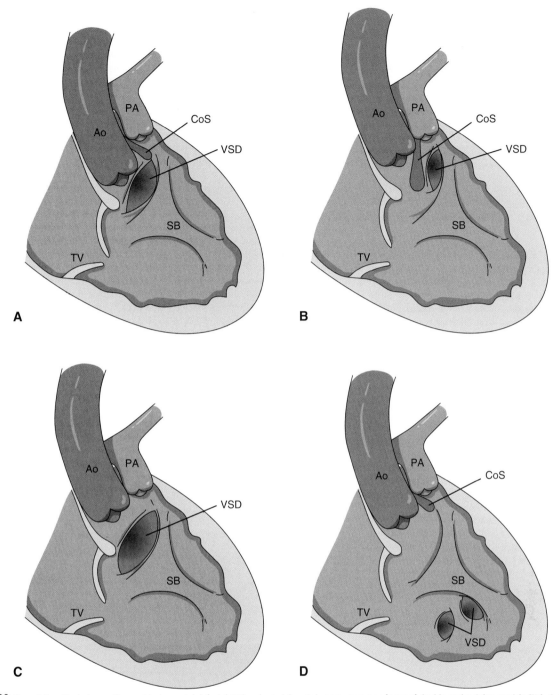

FIGURE 82.30 The relationship between the ventricular septal defect *(VSD)* and arterial roots in some common forms of double-outlet right ventricle (RV). **A,** Subaortic VSD. **B,** Subpulmonary VSD. **C,** Doubly committed VSD. **D,** Remote VSD. *Ao,* Aorta; *CoS,* conal septum; *PA,* pulmonary artery; *SB,* septal band; *TV,* tricuspid valve. (Modified from Lopez L. Double outlet ventricles. In: Lai WW, Mertens MM, Cohen MS, Geva T, eds. *Echocardiography in Pediatric and Congenital Heart Disease: From Fetus to Adult.* Wiley-Blackwell; 2009.)

A specific subset of DORV patients with subpulmonary VSD, bilateral conus, and side-by-side semilunar valves is known as "Taussig-Bing" anomaly. These patients often require frequent interventions in adult life to address residual obstruction in both outflow tracts.

Clinical Features

The clinical presentation of a child with DORV is dependent on the lesion with the most similar anatomy and physiology (TOF or TGA physiology).

Repairs

The surgical approach to DORV depends on the intracardiac anatomy. The position of the VSD and relationship to the great arteries is critical to the surgical approach. In the most common form (subaortic VSD), the surgical goals include establishing LV to aortic continuity by patching the VSD to tunnel the LV to the aorta. This pathway is often long and tortuous and, in some cases, the VSD must be enlarged to create this tunnel. Care must be taken to avoid creation of LVOT obstruction, which may result in the need for reoperation. If there is pulmonary stenosis (PS), relief of obstruction must be accomplished by either patch enlargement of the RVOT, valvotomy, or insertion of a conduit to establish RV-to-PA continuity.

For patients with DORV and a subpulmonary VSD, the surgical repair is similar to those with D-loop TGA with a baffle from the LV to the pulmonary valve and arterial switch operation. For patients with unfavorable anatomy for a biventricular repair, patients are staged to a Fontan palliation.

Long-Term Outcomes and Complications

There is limited data on long-term outcomes of patients with DORV. Reinterventions are most commonly done for LVOT obstruction. The mechanism of LVOT obstruction is believed to be related to subaortic membrane and muscle hypertrophy or restriction at the level of the VSD.[77]

Truncus Arteriosus

Anatomic Description and Prevalence

Truncus arteriosus is an uncommon type of congenital heart defect in which a single arterial trunk arises from the heart, giving origin to the coronary arteries, PAs, and systemic arteries, in that order. In most cases, a VSD and single semilunar valve are present. This semilunar valve is usually tricuspid but is quadricuspid in one-third of cases and usually overrides the ventricular septum through an outlet VSD.

Clinical Features

Without treatment, the mean age of death is 2.5 months, most often from heart failure. Unoperated children that do survive usually develop PH. Although rare, isolated cases of survival into adulthood with unrepaired truncus arteriosus have been reported, and these patients usually have Eisenmenger syndrome.

Repairs

Earlier surgical intervention is preferred. The surgical repair involves removing the PAs from the truncal root, patch closure of the VSD, and placement of a conduit between the RV and PAs. In cases in which the truncal valve is dysfunctional, repair or replacement with a homograft is performed.

Long-Term Outcomes and Complications

Important risk factors for perioperative death are severe truncal valve regurgitation, an interrupted aortic arch, coronary artery anomalies, and age at initial operation older than 100 days. Patients with only one PA are especially prone to early development of severe pulmonary vascular disease.

Postoperatively, patients are followed with serial imaging to monitor for RV-to-PA conduit dysfunction, branch PA obstruction, truncal valve dysfunction, and root dilation. Conduit dysfunction is common and replacement, or transcatheter pulmonary valve implantation, is required in most adults with repaired truncus arteriosus. Truncal (aortic) root dilation is common and can cause truncal valve regurgitation. Dissection is rare.

In adults with prior truncus arteriosus repair, decreased right ventricular ejection fraction and smaller ascending aorta on CMR were associated with adverse clinical events.[78]

Cor Triatriatum

Anatomic description and prevalence

Cor triatriatum is a rare lesion in which a membrane separates the LA *(sinister)* or the RA *(dexter)* into two compartments. The remainder of this section will consider the left atrial type. Anatomically, the membrane is proximal to the left atrial appendage, so that the pulmonary veins drain into the proximal chamber and the appendage and mitral valve are in the distal chamber. This landmark classically divides cor triatriatum from a supravalvar mitral ring, which is located distal to the left atrial appendage. The membrane may or may not be obstructive; a nonobstructive or mildly obstructive membrane may never require intervention.

Surgical repair of cor triatriatum consists of resection of the intraatrial membrane. It should be done with low levels of morbidity or complication. Repair is indicated for patients showing signs or symptoms of obstruction, which is physiologically analogous to pulmonary vein stenosis, leading to congestive heart failure, respiratory symptoms, lung pathology, and PH. Atrial flutter or fibrillation is not uncommon.[79] The membrane should also be resected in a patient presenting to the operating room for associated cardiac disease, such as ASD or VSD. Repair may also be considered for the asymptomatic patient with a high gradient across the membrane, which would commonly be considered in the 8 to 10 mm Hg range, although this is not based on strong published outcomes data.

Clinical Features and Diagnostic Testing

The ECG may show left atrial enlargement and depending on severity of disease could have findings consistent with PH. Echo is the mainstay of diagnosis (Fig. 82.31, Video 82.9A,B). Transthoracic echo can clearly demonstrate the obstructive membrane, often from parasternal long axis or short axis and apical 4-chamber views. Adding color Doppler shows where blood flow can pass through the membrane and assesses for obstruction, with gradients measured by spectral Doppler. If acoustic windows are insufficient for diagnosis, TEE is an excellent choice to show the posteriorly located membrane within the LA. Rarely, CMR or CT can be required to demonstrate the membrane and the anatomy of the pulmonary veins.

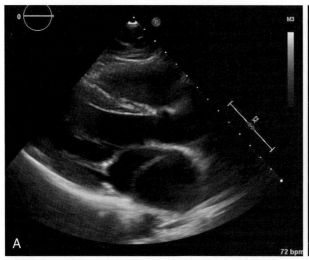
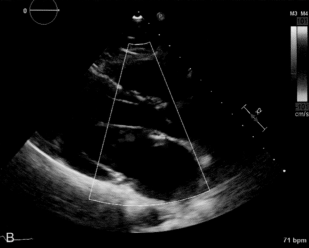

FIGURE 82.31 A, Transthoracic echocardiogram in the parasternal long axis view demonstrating cor triatriatum membrane within the left atrium. **B,** Color Doppler from the same window demonstrating a small flow jet around the obstructive membrane.

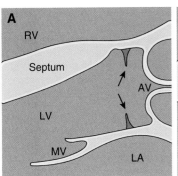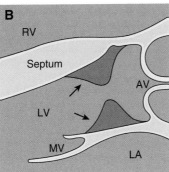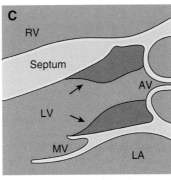

FIGURE 82.32 Types of subaortic stenosis. **A,** Discrete subaortic membrane *(arrows).* **B,** Thick fibromuscular ridge *(arrows).* **C,** Tunnel or tubular *(arrows). AV,* Aortic valve; *LA,* left atrium; *LV,* left ventricle; *MV,* mitral valve; *RV,* right ventricle. (From Devabhaktuni SR, Chakfeh E, Malik AO, et al. Subvalvular aortic stenosis: a review of current literature. *Clin Cardiol.* 2018;41[1]:131–136.)

Long-term Outcomes and Complications

Outcomes following repair of cor triatriatum are generally excellent. There is an incidence of pulmonary vein stenosis following repair, which should be investigated in any patient with recurrent symptoms.

Subvalvular Left Ventricular Outflow Tract Obstruction

Anatomic Description and Prevalence

LVOT obstruction proximal to the aortic valve can occur from a variety of different mechanisms including a discrete subaortic membrane, a fibromuscular ridge, or tunnel-like LVOT obstruction due to outflow tract hypoplasia (Fig. 82.32). LVOT obstruction due to hypertrophic cardiomyopathy is discussed separately (see Chapter 54.)

Subaortic obstruction due to a discrete subaortic membrane is a frequent cause of LVOT obstruction in children and is more common in males. It rarely occurs in infancy but may become manifest in early childhood or in adult years. It usually consists of a ridge of fibrous or fibromuscular tissue in the LVOT. The membrane is often circumferential extending both onto the septal surface anteriorly and the base of the anterior leaflet of the mitral valve posteriorly. The fibrous tissue may extend onto the aortic valve leaflets contributing to concomitant aortic regurgitation. Subaortic membranes or fibromuscular tunnels may exist with other left-sided obstructive lesions such as cor triatriatum sinister, supra-annular mitral ring, BAV, and aortic coarctation as part of Shone syndrome.

Subaortic obstruction can occur as a component of other forms of CHD as well. Patients with an AVSD may have LVOT obstruction due to elongation of the LVOT and chordal attachments of the left AV valve to the septum. Patients with a VSD may have prolapse of the tricuspid valve through the VSD or bowing of the membranous portion of the septum into the LVOT.

Clinical Features and Diagnostic Testing

Patients with isolated subaortic stenosis may present with dyspnea on exertion or with an asymptomatic harsh systolic ejection murmur. ECG may show left ventricular hypertrophy if the obstruction is severe. Untreated LVOT obstruction causes LV hypertrophy and, if severe, LV systolic and diastolic dysfunction.

The high-velocity jet from a subaortic membrane causes barotrauma to the aortic valve leaflets which induces leaflet thickening and fibrosis and predisposing to aortic regurgitation. Aortic regurgitation is present in the majority of patients with significant LVOT obstruction from a subaortic membrane and is usually mild. Aortic regurgitation is most common in patients with high outflow gradients. At the time of surgery in one large series, only 27% were free from aortic regurgitation.[80]

Echocardiography is the most useful test to determine the anatomy and severity of LVOT obstruction. A subaortic membrane typically appears as a linear membrane below the level of the aortic valve. It is seen from the parasternal long-axis view or the apical 3-chamber view on TTE. Color Doppler and pulsed-wave Doppler determines the level of obstruction. Continuous-wave Doppler echocardiography determines the severity of obstruction. Concomitant aortic regurgitation is common and color and spectral Doppler should be used to determine the aortic regurgitation severity. The aortic valve is typically tricommissural. However, eccentric flow from the LVOT obstruction can cause asymmetric opening, giving the impression of a BAV.

TEE is often helpful in distinguishing subaortic stenosis from valvular aortic stenosis, and determining whether the membrane encroaches onto the aortic valve leaflets (Fig. 82.33, Video 82.10A,B). CCT, cardiac MRI, and cardiac catheterization are rarely required for the evaluation of subaortic stenosis and are reserved for patients with inadequate echocardiographic windows. Cardiac MRI to evaluate LVOT obstruction due to hypertrophic cardiomyopathy is discussed elsewhere. Exercise testing can help determine the functional impact of LVOT obstruction in patients without overt symptoms.

Repairs

Symptomatic patients with severe LVOT obstruction (maximum gradient > 50 mm Hg, mean gradient > 30 mm Hg) should be referred for repair. Repair is also appropriate for patients with severe obstruction and reduced exertional capacity on exercise testing. Patients with subaortic stenosis and heart failure should also undergo repair,[3] even with moderate gradients (maximum gradient 30 to 50 mm Hg) because the low cardiac output from heart failure may lead to reduced gradients, even if obstruction is severe. Because high gradients are associated with progressive aortic regurgitation, asymptomatic patients with high gradients and aortic regurgitation can consider subaortic membrane resection in order to prevent progressive aortic regurgitation.

The treatment for LVOT obstruction is surgical. Surgery involves membrane resection with enucleation to the base of the membrane; some surgeons advocate for a concomitant limited myectomy. Occasionally LVOT enlargement with a Konno or Manougian procedure is needed. Patients with severe aortic regurgitation require valve replacement. Surgical mortality is low and immediate postoperative results are usually excellent.

Long-Term Outcomes and Complications

Late recurrence of LVOT obstruction and re-growth of a subaortic membrane is common. Following resection, the average rate of gradient increase is ~1.4 mm Hg/year and is more likely to recur in older patients and in females. Some (but not all) studies have suggested that combining myectomy with membrane resection results in less likelihood of recurrence and avoids the need for reoperation.[81] However, myectomy increases the risk of heart block (up to 4%) and iatrogenic VSD. Many patients require repeat surgery for recurrence of subaortic membrane years or decades after their initial intervention. It remains uncertain whether resection of the subaortic membrane prevents progression of aortic regurgitation.[82] For these reasons, long-term follow-up with serial echocardiography is needed for all patients who have undergone prior intervention for subaortic stenosis.

Supravalvar Aortic Stenosis

Anatomic Description and Prevalence

Supravalvar aortic stenosis (SVAS) refers to a narrowing in the ascending aorta. Morphologically it is most commonly an hourglass-shaped narrowing but can also occur from a fibrous ridge, or tubular hypoplasia of the proximal ascending aorta.

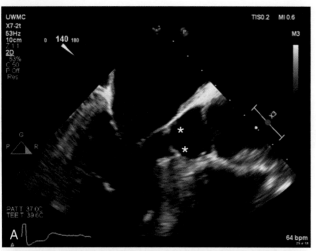

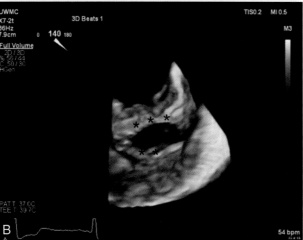

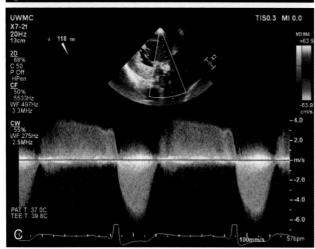

FIGURE 82.33 Transesophageal echocardiogram of a patient with a discrete sub-aortic membrane. **A,** Mid-esophageal window at 140 degrees showing the circumferential membrane on the septum and the base of the anterior leaflet of the mitral valve *(asterisk).* **B,** Three-dimensional view from the left ventricle looking out toward the aortic valve. **C,** Deep transgastric window with continuous wave Doppler across the left ventricular outflow tract showing severe left ventricular outflow tract obstruction (peak velocity 5.8 msec) and mild aortic regurgitation.

SVAS results as a consequence of mutations of ELN, the gene which encodes for the elastin protein, on chromosome 7q11.23. Most cases of SVAS result from new mutations but can also be transmitted in an autosomal dominant fashion. SVAS results from a combination of smooth muscle hyperplasia and deficient circumferential growth in the affected arteries.[83] In addition to causing supravalvar stenosis, ELN mutation frequently causes stenosis in other proximal arteries such as the brachiocephalic vessels, branch pulmonary arteries, and ostial coronary arteries.

The majority of ELN mutations are associated with Williams syndrome (OMIM 194050) but SVAS can also exist in a non-syndromic familial form. In addition to SVAS stenosis, Williams syndrome includes characteristic dysmorphic facial features (broad forehead, stellate irises, upturned nose, pointed chin; often described as "elfin" facies), hypercalcemia, hypothyroidism, diabetes mellitus, intellectual disability, and often an outgoing ("cocktail party") personality. SVAS affects up to 65% of patients with Williams syndrome. Other cardiovascular abnormalities include peripheral PA stenosis, ostial coronary artery stenosis, and hypertension.

Clinical Features and Diagnostic Testing

Physical examination findings may reveal hypertension. Four extremity blood pressures should be performed with the patient supine; if pressure is lower in the legs than the arms, hypoplasia of the descending aorta should be suspected. Patients with hypoplasia of the descending aorta may have an abdominal bruit and peripheral pulses may be diminished. SVAS results in a systolic ejection murmur. Patients with peripheral PA stenosis will have a murmur which radiates to the intrascapular regions. Facial and physical features of Williams syndrome may be present. There is a high incidence of sudden cardiac death in patients with Williams syndrome. Sudden death often occurs during noncardiac procedures and with induction of anesthesia. Careful periprocedural preparation is required. Patients who are at highest risk include young children, those with severe outflow tract obstruction, those with documented coronary artery involvement, or patients with prior history of arrhythmia or cardiovascular event.[84,85]

ECG reflects left ventricular pressure overload and may demonstrate LV hypertrophy. QTc prolongation is common in Williams syndrome.

Echocardiography is the primary imaging modality used to evaluate the morphology and severity of outflow tract obstruction in patients with SVAS. 2D imaging from the parasternal long axis view can usually define the anatomy and spectral Doppler is used to measure the degree of obstruction. Echocardiography is also appropriate to evaluate for LV hypertrophy in patients with SVAS or hypertension. Continuous wave Doppler from the high right parasternal window often yields the highest gradients. Right ventricular systolic pressures should also be calculated during echocardiography due to the high frequency of supravalvar PS and peripheral PA stenosis. CT or MR angiography is superior to echocardiography at imaging the branch pulmonary arteries and the head-and-neck vessels, particularly in adults.

Patients with ventricular dysfunction or symptoms of angina should be evaluated for coronary artery stenosis. Stenosis is often ostial but can also include diffuse stenosis or segments of ectasia and stenosis. Aortic valve leaflets may have unusual attachments to the ascending aorta which can also contribute to coronary artery obstruction. Coronary angiography remains the gold standard for the diagnosis of ostial coronary artery stenosis, but gated CCT scan can be diagnostic in many cases.

Repair

Surgery remains the mainstay of treatment. Patch arterioplasty is effective to treat most instances of SVAS and peripheral PA stenosis. Surgery usually provides more durable results than catheter intervention, which can be predisposed to in-stent restenosis.

Long-term Outcomes and Complications

Hypertension should be managed aggressively. Anatomic contributors, such as renal artery stenosis or diffuse hypoplasia of the descending thoracic aorta should be excluded. Medical therapy with calcium channel blockers or beta-blockers is appropriate. ACE inhibitors or angiotensin receptor blockers are appropriate for patients after renal artery stenosis has been excluded.

Due to the risk of sudden cardiac death with induction of anesthesia careful preparation is required. A cardiologist and anesthesia team familiar with Williams syndrome should evaluate the patient prior to procedures. Patients should maintain euvolemia whenever possible and agents which abruptly drop preload or afterload should be avoided whenever possible.

Coarctation of the Aorta
Anatomic Description and Prevalence

Coarctation of the aorta, first described by Morgagni in 1760, involves a localized or tubular narrowing in the aorta or aortic interruption. It is characterized by a generalized arteriopathy with decreased aortic compliance. Thus, systemic hypertension is common in adults even after excellent results from repair.[86]

Typically, coarctation is juxtaductal, located at the junction of the distal aortic arch and the descending aorta beyond the origin of the left subclavian artery. Rarely it occurs elsewhere in the aorta. Coarctation is formed by a localized shelf in the posterior and lateral aortic wall opposite or close to the ductus arteriosus. It can be tubular extending toward the origin of the subclavian artery and can involve the transverse aortic arch. Hypoplastic aortic arch is common and this or a "Gothic-shaped arch" is particularly associated with hypertension without residual obstruction at the coarctation site. Associated anomalies are common and include BAV (50% to 85%), VSD, mitral valve abnormalities, subaortic obstruction, anomalous origin of the right subclavian artery, and intracranial aneurysm (particularly Berry aneurysms in the Circle of Willis). Coarctation is common in certain syndromes, including Shone, Turners, Williams-Beuren, Noonan, hypoplastic left heart syndrome (HLHS), and other complex CHD. Shone syndrome is the association with coarctation of the aorta with mitral valve disease (parachute or supramitral ring) and multilevel left-sided outflow tract obstruction (subaortic or aortic valve stenosis).

Clinical Features and Diagnostic Testing

Coarctation of the aorta presents with a bimodal distribution. Severe coarctation may present as a neonate with shock and/or heart failure and a ductal-dependent circulation. Less severe forms of coarctation can present in adulthood discovered incidentally while screening for causes of systemic hypertension. Adults living with coarctation have impaired long-term survival and in particular there is morbidity related to hypertension, aortic valve disease, and post-repair complications at the site of the coarctation including aneurysmal dilatation, rupture, or dissection. Left heart failure, endocarditis, premature coronary artery and cerebral artery disease also occur as well as complications related to associated lesions.[86]

Symptoms in adults with coarctation when present include systemic hypertension, headache, and leg claudication. On physical examination, blood pressure measurements should be taken in the right arm as left arm blood pressure may be misleadingly low if the left subclavian artery was sacrificed in the repair. Lower extremity blood pressure measurement should also be made as a systolic blood pressure gradient between the right arm and lower limb ≥20 mm Hg indicates significant coarctation. Femoral pulses may be reduced and there may be brachial-femoral delay. If present, a murmur associated with discrete coarctation is systolic and best heard from the back. Continuous interscapular murmurs are suggestive of collateral arterial flow. Fundoscopy may show hypertensive retinopathy.

The 12-lead ECG should be assessed for features of left ventricular hypertrophy, left atrial enlargement, and ischemia. Chest radiograph may show erosion of the undersurface of the outer third of a posterior 2nd to 9th rib due to collaterals called rib notching. This may be present unilaterally if either the left or right subclavian artery arises distal to the coarctation. The "figure 3" sign of coarctation refers to the silhouette of aortic dilatation both before (pre-stenotic) and after (post-stenotic) the coarctation site (Fig. 82.34, Video 82.11). Ambulatory 24-hour right arm blood pressure measurement is useful for screening for hypertension during follow-up which is important even in those without important residual coarctation. Echocardiography is used to assess the aortic valve, aortic root, coarctation site, LV function, and mass. Evidence of increased velocity at the coarctation site can be sought with the use of continuous wave Doppler from suprasternal views (Fig. 82.35, Video 82.12). Doppler evidence of a diastolic tail in the descending thoracic aorta and continuous-flow pattern in the abdominal aorta suggests significant stenosis at the level of coarctation. CMR is routine in coarctation diagnosis, assessing suitability for transcatheter stenting or hybrid repair and follow-up, and is cost effective. CMR is used for quantification of LV mass, evaluating the entire aorta including for arch hypoplasia or Gothic angulation, severity of coarctation, and quantification of collateral flow. It also identifies complications post repair (e.g., aneurysms, false aneurysms, recoarctation, or residual stenosis), presence of aberrant subclavian arteries, and for the morphology and function of the aortic valve. All adults with coarctation should undergo cross-sectional imaging (usually CMR) at least once. Cardiac CT is more suited for assessing stent lumen and fracture, and coronary arteries. Exercise testing may reveal exercise-induced hypertension which is prognostically important in patients with repaired coarctation, as it has been linked to adverse ventricular remodeling (left ventricular hypertrophy). At cardiac catheterization, a peak-to-peak gradient across the coarctation site ≥20 mm Hg in the absence of well-developed collateral circulation is considered significant.

When an extensive collateral circulation is present increased systolic and diastolic gradient assessed by echocardiography or peak velocity at CMR are not reliable to detect severe coarctation nor is pressure gradient at cardiac catheterization.

Long-Term Outcomes and Complications

Lifelong expert surveillance for late complications is essential with cross-sectional imaging at intervals of at least 3 to 5 years.[87] Hypertension is a major determinant of late mortality after coarctation repair.[88] Hypertension prior to treatment of coarctation may resolve at first but recur or persist in over 50% of adults especially if intervention was at an older age. When there is new hypertension the coarctation should be reassessed to determine if there is a hemodynamic target for intervention. Hypertension is common without any residual coarctation as the aorta proximal to the coarctation site is abnormal with decreased compliance. Medical treatment choices for hypertension are

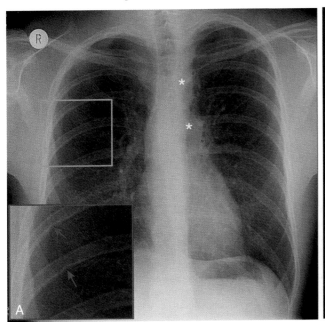
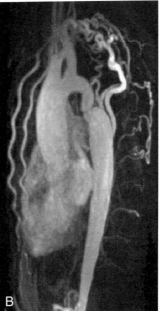

FIGURE 82.34 A, Chest radiograph reveals rib notching *(arrows)* in the 3rd to 5th ribs bilaterally as shown. The "figure 3" mediastinal silhouette *(blue)* is associated with coarctation and made by the distal aortic arch/dilated left subclavian artery and the post-stenotic dilatation of the descending aorta *(asterisks)*. **B,** CMR contrast enhanced angiography confirmed coarctation of the aorta with collaterals.

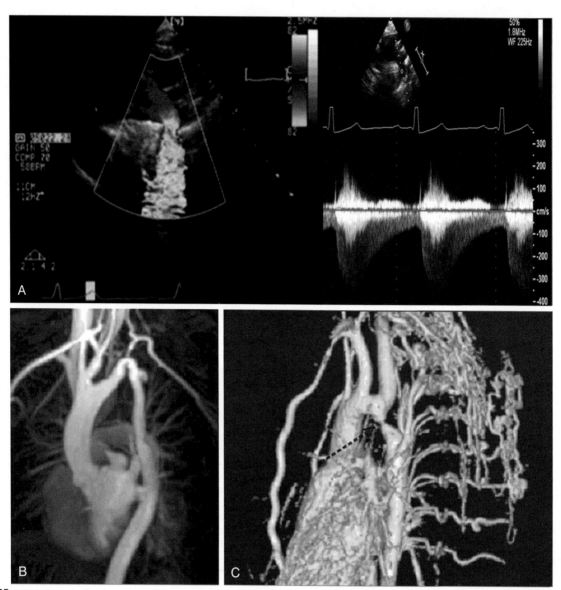

FIGURE 82.35 A, Turbulent color flow in the descending aorta with peak velocity above 3.5 msec. In the suprasternal continuous wave Doppler there is a double envelope reflecting both flow proximal to the aorta and high velocity flow across the coarctation site and there is a diastolic tail. **B,** Complex coarctation with hypoplastic arch, acute angulation, and tortuosity between the proximal arch and the descending aorta and a long (~8 cm) length segment of tubular hypoplasia. **C,** Severe coarctation with multiple large collaterals *(arrow)*.

as per standard guidelines. Proactive and aggressive control of blood pressure, and hyperlipidemia if present, is important given the need to prevent atherosclerotic heart disease and cerebral vascular disease.

The decision to intervene for coarctation or recoarctation of the aorta depends on blood pressure, gradient, and stenosis morphology. In adults, surgery is rarely needed and stenting is the treatment of choice when technically feasible. Repair (endovascular or surgical) of coarctation or recoarctation is indicated in hypertensive patients with an invasive peak-to-peak gradient ≥20 mm Hg. Coarctation stenting is also considered when feasible for hypertensive patients with a coarctation diameter ≤50% of the aortic diameter at the diaphragm regardless of peak-to-peak gradient and in normotensive coarctation with peak-to-peak gradient ≥20 mm Hg. Covered stents have been developed to prevent and treat acute wall injury associated with aortic coarctation.[89] Surgery to repair coarctation in adults may be indicated to treat more complex anatomy including interrupted aortic arch and long segment coarctation with options including an interposition graft and bypass grafts including ascending to descending aorta conduits.

Patients who have undergone balloon dilatation without stenting of coarctation at a younger age commonly need reintervention. Balloon dilatation can result in aneurysm formation at the site of coarctation or dissection. These complications are reduced by primary stenting

which is the usual first-line treatment for adults. Aneurysms at the site of the surgical coarctation repair also occur and this is particularly concerning for adults with a history of Dacron patch aortoplasty (Fig. 82.36, Video 82.13). The aortic wall opposite to the patch becomes aneurysmal and the false aneurysm at the suture line can also occur. Interposition grafts are at particular risk of false aneurysm. Associated ascending aortopathy with aneurysmal dilatation often related to a BAV and aortic valve disease itself may progress and require intervention.

Interrupted Aortic Arch

Interrupted aortic arch is a rare (<1.5% of all congenital heart defects) and severe CHD also associated with DiGeorge syndrome. Interrupted aortic arch occurs distal to the left subclavian artery (type A), between the left carotid artery and the left subclavian artery (type B) and uncommonly (<1%) between the brachiocephalic trunk and the left carotid artery (type C). It is associated with aberrant right subclavian artery which often arises distal to the interruption.

Adult survivors will usually have had previous childhood surgery with an interposition graft and possibly closure of VSD and subaortic stenosis resection. Associated intracardiac lesions typically include

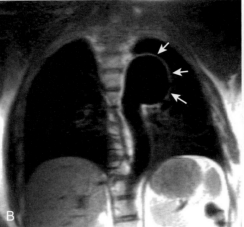
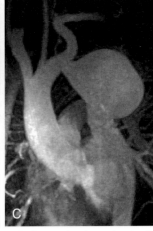

FIGURE 82.36 Dacron patch coarctation site aneurysm. **A,** Chest radiography done as routine surveillance after Dacron patch repair of coarctation shows alarming dilatation of the aorta *(arrows)* also revealed with the corresponding coronal plane MR image (**B,** *arrows*). **C,** The large, rounded aneurysm is just below the left subclavian artery branch, measures 53 × 55 × 64 mm, and is likely a contained false aneurysm. There is no residual coarctation.

VSD (80% to 90%), PDA, BAV, and complex congenital heart conditions, namely aortopulmonary window, double outlet RV, TGA, truncus arteriosus, single ventricle, or AVSD. Posterior deviation of the outlet septum in those with a VSD can result in LV outflow tract obstruction. During follow-up, reintervention for either LV outflow tract obstruction or recurrent aortic arch obstruction may be needed.

Vascular Rings
Anatomic Description and Prevalence
A vascular ring is an abnormality of aortic arch development which is defined as complete surrounding of the esophagus and trachea by vascular structures. This is distinct from an LPA sling, in which the LPA passes posterior to the trachea but anterior to the esophagus. The vessels comprising a vascular ring may all be patent or may include fibrous ligamenta, such as a ductal ligament or atretic arch.

A detailed discussion of the embryology of vascular ring formation is beyond the scope of this chapter. Briefly, there are six paired arches that form early in embryology; several of these arches fully or partially regress, while others form the aortic arch, its primary brachiocephalic branches, the proximal Pas, and ductus arteriosus. Errors in the pattern of regression can result in various forms of vascular ring.

The most common forms of vascular ring include double aortic arch and right aortic arch with aberrant left subclavian artery (Fig. 82.37). In the former, the right aortic arch is nearly always the dominant vessel, with a hypoplastic or atretic left aortic arch completing the ring. In the latter, there is a diverticulum of Kommerell at the origin of the aberrant subclavian vessel from the proximal descending aorta, which is a dilated proximal portion of the vessel due to the origin of the ductus arteriosus from that area and the high amount of ductal flow during fetal life. The presence of this diverticulum signifies that if the ductus is not patent, there is a ductal ligament arising from this region. There are several other rarer forms of vascular ring, but concepts for management are the same.

Vascular rings are rare lesions overall, although the true prevalence is probably not known due to a percentage of these lesions that never present clinically. Additionally, as repair is indicated for those lesions that present with symptoms, the vast majority of symptomatic rings are repaired in childhood. However, there is rare incidence of new symptoms first presenting in adulthood, as well as scattered cases that may have been symptomatic but eluded medical attention during childhood. There are also rare cases who may present with recurrent symptoms of respiratory changes or dysphagia in adulthood following correction in childhood.

Clinical Features and Diagnostic Testing
The most common symptomatic presentation for an adult with a vascular ring is dysphagia. Respiratory symptoms more commonly present

in childhood, but adults can present with wheezing or stridor, particularly with exertion, as well as dyspnea on exertion. Vascular rings can also present incidentally, such as with the discovery of a right aortic arch by chest x-ray leading to additional testing. Physical exam may include the aforementioned respiratory signs, but is otherwise typically not revealing.

The presence of a vascular ring is classically demonstrated by a barium swallow, with the finding of a posterior indentation of the esophagus. Most patients now receive further testing prior to considering surgery.

Echocardiography is often suggestive, but overall limited for this diagnosis, particularly in the presence of poor acoustic windows. Imaging at the suprasternal notch should demonstrate arch sidedness or a double aortic arch. An aberrant subclavian artery can be very difficult to visualize directly, but absence of normal bifurcation of the innominate artery is suggestive. In addition, the presence of a right aortic arch in an otherwise anatomically normal heart is highly suspicious for a vascular ring. Cross-sectional imaging by CT or MRI is diagnostic for a vascular ring and best characterizes the individual components of the anatomy; the presence of a ductal or arch ligament cannot be directly visualized except in the unusual case of extensive calcification, but can be inferred by the remainder of the anatomy. CT is superior for imaging the airway directly but MRI can also diagnose related airway compression.

Surgical Repairs
The classic surgical management of a vascular ring consists of releasing the ring by ligation and division of a patent vascular structure, or division of a ductal or aortic arch ligamentum. Opening the ring allows the vessels to release and affords greater space for the trachea and esophagus and is usually curative. This is performed via thoracotomy on whichever side the structure is found for division, usually the left.

There are some who advocate for more extensive surgery for vascular rings that include a diverticulum of Kommerell, such as a right aortic arch with aberrant left subclavian artery.[90] This typically includes translocation of the aberrant subclavian artery to the ipsilateral carotid artery, along with resection of the diverticulum of Kommerell. Note that this procedure has to include division of the ductal ligamentum, or the vascular ring has not been released and symptoms will not be relieved. It has been described via thoracotomy as a single procedure, or in two stages with a lower neck incision followed by thoracotomy.[90,91] This has also been described as hybrid repair, in which the subclavian artery is surgically translocated to the carotid artery, followed by endovascular exclusion of the diverticulum with embolization material and/or stent grafting of the descending aorta across the diverticulum. The argument in favor of the more extensive operation is that the diverticulum of Kommerell can compress the airway even after release of the vascular

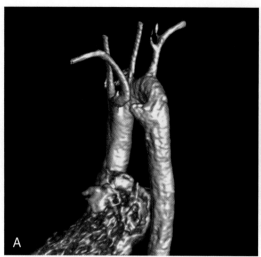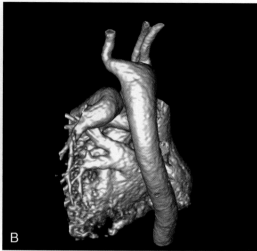

FIGURE 82.37 3-D reconstructions of gadolinium-enhanced MR angiograms. **A**, View from posterior and to the left of a double aortic arch with atresia of the distal left arch distal to the left subclavian artery. **B**, Posterior view of a right aortic arch with diverticulum of Kommerell and aberrant left subclavian artery; note the dilated diverticulum of Kommerell arising from the distal aortic arch.

ring, leading to recurrent symptoms, or can become aneurysmal and even rupture, causing a catastrophic event. The true incidence of diverticulum of Kommerell aneurysm and/or rupture is not known given the unclear incidence of vascular rings.

Diverticulum of Kommerell in the context of a left aortic arch with aberrant right subclavian artery almost always does not comprise a vascular ring but can cause dysphagia and can also become aneurysmal or rupture. There is a wealth of literature on the management of this condition, with serial imaging and sometimes surgical or endovascular repair, which remains somewhat controversial with a wide spectrum of approaches.[92] Surgical series in the literature are selected for more severe disease and the true incidence and therefore rate of complication remains unknown. However, it is crucial when assessing a patient with a diverticulum of Kommerell to discern whether there is the concomitant presence of a vascular ring (usually with a right aortic arch). If so, endovascular repair without surgical release of the ring will not relieve symptoms.

Long-Term Outcomes and Complications

Outcomes of vascular ring repair are excellent overall. However, as the vast majority of childhood repairs will have no further symptoms, those presenting to adult cardiology are selected for late or recurrent symptoms. After repair in adulthood, recurrent dysphagia has been reported in 14% of patients.[90] While this can have an anatomic basis, there may also be a functional component of esophageal dysmotility related to long-standing compression. As discussed, the rate of complications for a diverticulum of Kommerell is not known.

Anomalous Coronary Artery From the Pulmonary Artery

A coronary artery arising from the PA is an uncommon coronary anomaly. Anomalous left coronary artery from the pulmonary artery (ALCAPA) is more common than anomalous right coronary artery from the pulmonary artery (ARCAPA).

In patients with ALCAPA or ARCAPA, myocardial perfusion is via the coronary artery which arises normally from the aorta and is typically quite dilated. The anomalous coronary artery is supplied retrograde via collaterals and then drains into the PA. Because coronary artery pressure is higher than PA pressure, the anomalous coronary does not receive anterograde flow from the PA.

The degree of myocardial ischemia present in patients with ALCAPA or ARCAPA depends on the degree of collateralization and the coronary perfusion pressure. Most patients with ALCAPA present in infancy or early childhood with left ventricular systolic dysfunction, arrhythmias, or ischemic mitral regurgitation. Patients with ARCAPA typically

have a more favorable clinical course and may escape detection until adulthood.

Diagnosis should be suspected in infants or young children with ventricular dysfunction or secondary mitral regurgitation. Adults may show a dilated coronary artery or robust collaterals on echocardiography (Fig. 82.38, Video 82.14). Coronary angiography demonstrates a dilated coronary artery arising from the aorta which fills the anomalous artery via collaterals and drains into the PA (Fig. 82.39, Video 82.15). CT angiography is useful to delineate the coronary anatomy and facilitate surgical planning (Fig. 82.40, Video 82.16).

Surgery is indicated for patients with ALCAPA and patients with ARCAPA who have ventricular dysfunction, angina, or demonstrable ischemia. Options for surgical repair depend on the anatomy and the proximity of the anomalous coronary to the aorta. Direct reimplantation of the anomalous coronary artery into the aorta is preferred when technically feasible. Otherwise, the coronary artery can be supplied via an intrapulmonary tunnel to baffle the coronary to the aorta (Takeuchi repair). In some patients ligation and coronary artery bypass surgery is required. Operations in ALCAPA and ARCAPA should be performed by a congenital heart surgeon.

Single Ventricle
Anatomic Description and Prevalence

Single ventricle heart disease comprises several distinct anatomic lesions, which may represent a true anatomic single ventricle lesion, or a functional single ventricle lesion, in which a 2nd ventricle is present but is not adequate to supply the systemic or pulmonary circulation. Except in the rare case of congenital balance between the systemic and pulmonary circulations, these lesions require early palliative surgery for survival.

Tricuspid atresia is a functional single ventricle lesion, in which the tricuspid valve does not form. It is uncommon, with an incidence of approximately 1.2 per 10,000 live births.[93] This lesion is categorized by the relationship of the great vessels and the degree of pulmonary stenosis present at birth. There is typically a hypoplastic RV, and the great vessels can be in normal (S) position, D-transposed, or L-transposed. Decision making for neonatal surgery is dependent on the degree of obstruction to systemic or pulmonary outflow.

HLHS consists of a spectrum of left-sided obstructive lesions from mitral and aortic stenosis with a small LV to mitral and aortic atresia with a nearly absent left ventricular cavity. The incidence of this lesion is approximately 1.6 per 10,000 live births. HLHS typically includes severe hypoplasia of the aorta, requiring surgical reconstruction. Neonatal surgery includes aortic reconstruction with anastomosis to the

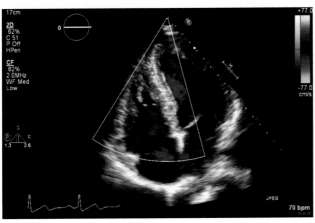

FIGURE 82.38 Transthoracic echocardiogram in apical 4-chamber view with color Doppler in a patient with anomalous right coronary artery from the pulmonary artery (ARCAPA). Note the extensive coronary collaterals seen by color Doppler. Also see Video 82.14.

native PA to create a systemic outflow from the RV, opening of the atrial septum, and providing pulmonary blood flow from one of several surgical shunt options.

Double inlet LV is an anatomic single ventricle lesion in which both AV valves are in continuity with the LV. The sinus of the RV does not form, though there remains an infundibular outflow tract connected by a bulboventricular foramen to the LV. The ventricles can be D- or L-looped, and the great vessels can be in normal (S), D-transposed, or L-transposed position, so that either the aorta or the PA can be related to the hypoplastic infundibular outflow. These relationships help determine decision making for initial palliative surgery. Double inlet/double outlet RV is a very rare example of true anatomic single ventricle disease, in which there is an embryonic RV associated with both AV valves and both systemic and pulmonary outlets, with no vestigial LV.

There are several other congenital defects that include two ventricles, but sometimes require single ventricle palliation, depending on details of the anatomy. Complete AV canal defect can be unbalanced; that is, the common valve can sit nearly entirely over one or the other ventricle, leaving a hypoplastic second ventricle and no option for a two-ventricle type of repair. Transposition of the great vessels can be complicated by other lesions such as VSDs and pulmonary outflow obstruction. A two-ventricle repair may not be achievable if the pulmonary valve is not usable as a "neo-aortic" valve and if a surgical pathway cannot be constructed from the LV through the VSD to the native aortic valve. Straddling of AV valves can also complicate a two-ventricle repair in this lesion. In these cases, an eventual Fontan palliation may be pursued.

Surgical Palliation

This section will not discuss patients who had single ventricle heart disease but have since received a heart transplant. Nearly all adult congenital patients with single ventricle heart disease will have received what is widely known as a Fontan palliation (Fig. 82.41), after the original surgical description by Drs. Fontan and Baudet in 1971.[94] This is generally reached in staged palliation, with the ultimate result of all systemic venous return bypassing the heart to flow passively directly to the pulmonary circulation, while the single functional ventricle acts as the systemic pump. There are several versions of the Fontan circulation, which will be discussed below.

The current surgical approach often includes neonatal surgery to achieve a stable systemic outflow and balance between systemic and pulmonary circulation to provide adequate oxygenation but protect the pulmonary circulation from pressure or volume overload, followed by a superior cavopulmonary anastomosis later in the first year of life, after which pulmonary circulation is provided by direct, passive flow of the superior systemic venous return to the lungs. This is ultimately followed by the Fontan procedure, which depending on version of procedure and individual center preference, is typically performed

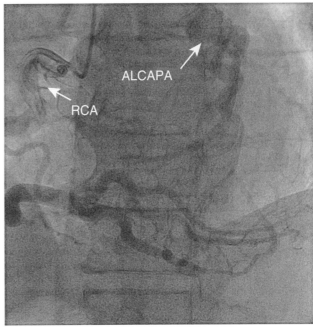

FIGURE 82.39 Coronary angiography in the right coronary artery (RCA) in a patient with anomalous left coronary artery from the pulmonary artery (ALCAPA). Note the dilated right coronary artery and left coronary artery which fills retrograde via collaterals and drains to the pulmonary artery. Also see Video 82.15.

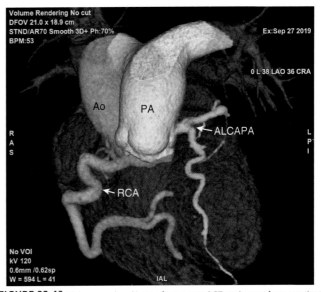

FIGURE 82.40 Volume rendered image from a gated CT angiogram from a patient with anomalous left coronary artery from the pulmonary artery (ALCAPA). Note the dilated right coronary artery (RCA) arising from the aorta (Ao) and the ALCAPA draining into the pulmonary artery (PA). Also see Video 82.16.

sometime between 18 months and 4 years of age. It is important to have some understanding of the stages of palliation, as some patients are unable to proceed down this pathway due to problems such as increased PVR, and rarely may present in adulthood with physiology of an aortopulmonary shunt or superior cavopulmonary anastomosis, typically with severe cyanosis.

The details of the Fontan palliation have gone through multiple iterations. The type of operation seen in an individual patient may have implications related to the likelihood of various complications in adulthood. The three most commonly seen versions of the Fontan circulation in adults include the extracardiac Fontan, the lateral tunnel Fontan, and direct right atrial to PA anastomosis, which is closer to the original described operation and has fallen out of favor. There

Classic Fontan

Atriopulmonary Fontan

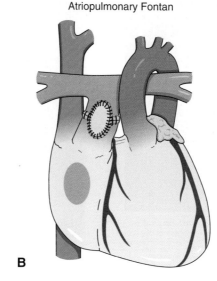

A

B

Lateral Tunnel Fontan

Extracardiac Fontan

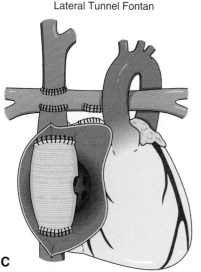

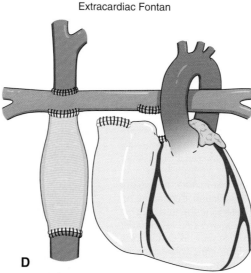

C

D

FIGURE 82.41 Diagrammatic representation of the various types of Fontan surgeries. **A,** The classic style Fontan, which consists of a conduit from the inferior vena cava to the left pulmonary artery and a classic right Glenn procedure (superior vena cava to the right pulmonary artery). **B,** The atriopulmonary connection has been largely abandoned due to dilation of the right atrium predisposing to thrombosis and atrial arrhythmias. **C,** Lateral tunnel is widely used in part due to the ease of creating a fenestration in this type. **D,** Extracardiac conduits are often used as it does not create extensive atrial sutures and may be performed off bypass. (Modified from Libby P. *Essential Atlas of Cardiovascular Disease.* New York: Springer; 2009.)

to the right atrial appendage. This often led to marked dilation of the RA due to exposure to chronic high pressure.

Clinical Features and Diagnostic Testing

The adult with a Fontan circulation may frequently present with dyspnea with activity, from exercise to basic activities of daily living. There is inherently less ability to augment stroke volume with demand in this circulation, and many patients may have chronotropic incompetence by adulthood as well. Palpitations are also a frequent complaint. Other symptoms may be related to end-organ damage from long-term impaired cardiac output.

There can be many findings on exam that are important to assess. Signs of chronic cyanosis such as clubbing of the digits may be present in patients with a Fontan, and are near-ubiquitous in adults with single ventricle disease who do not have a Fontan operation. Cardiac exam will show a single S1 and S2 on auscultation. Rhythm may reveal a rapid intra-atrial reentrant tachycardia or premature atrial or ventricular contractions. Any murmurs heard are typically pathologic, potentially related to AV or semilunar valve regurgitation or another inefficiency of the intracardiac circulation. A patient with an aortopulmonary shunt will have a continuous murmur. A small percentage of patients will have dextrocardia detected on exam. Hepatomegaly is frequently observed, and may be accompanied by ascites. Lower extremity edema is less common.

The routine care of the patient with a Fontan circulation includes considered use of cardiac-specific testing as well as monitoring for complications related to other organs. Routine history and physical exam should be performed at least yearly, more frequently for active problems.

Electrocardiography is routine with yearly clinic follow-up, as well as in the assessment for patients presenting with palpitations or other signs of arrhythmia.

Imaging assessment with either echocardiography or CMR is considered a Class I indication annually for this patient population, with CMR performed in lieu of echo typically every 2 to 3 years.[3] Echocardiography is useful for assessment of ventricular size and function, valve stenosis, and regurgitation, and the Fontan pathway and presence of a fenestration. Acoustic windows can limit the usefulness of echocardiography in this patient population. CMR also visualizes ventricular function and is a superior option for quantification of right ventricular size and function in particular (Fig. 82.42, Video 82.17A,B). Valve regurgitation can be quantified. CMR also provides superior visualization of the complete Fontan pathway and branch pulmonary arteries, including flow assessment for differential pulmonary blood flow and aorto-pulmonary or veno-venous collateralization. Placement of stainless-steel embolization coils in the past can severely limit CMR visualization due to magnetic susceptibility artifact. CT scanning overcomes artifacts related to coils and other implants and can also be used to provide excellent visualization of

are some other rarely seen versions of this circulation with variations in how the systemic venous blood is routed to the pulmonary circulation.

The extracardiac Fontan is currently in wide use. Surgically, this consists of a conduit placed outside of the heart, routing the IVC and hepatic veins directly to the pulmonary arteries. This is most typically preceded by a superior cavopulmonary anastomosis commonly known as a bidirectional Glenn operation, which is an end-to-side anastomosis of the SVC to the right pulmonary artery (RPA) (this can also be done on the left in the presence of a left SVC).

The lateral tunnel Fontan has become less prevalent but was the most common version of the Fontan operation and as such, is seen in many adults with single ventricle heart disease. In this operation the IVC and hepatic flow is tunneled through the RA, usually using the atrial wall as part of the tunnel, and anastomosed directly to the pulmonary arteries. This operation was often performed with a fenestration in the wall of the tunnel, enabling a small right-to-left shunt and mild systemic desaturation.

Direct right atrial to PA anastomosis was usually used specifically for patients with tricuspid atresia. In this version of the Fontan operation, the atrial septum was closed and the pulmonary arteries anastomosed

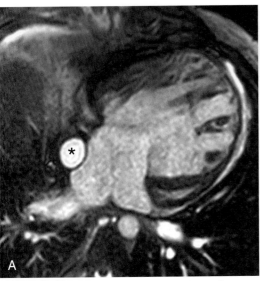 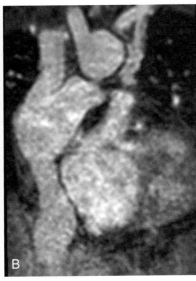

FIGURE 82.42 A, Still image from a cine steady state free precession MRI sequence in the horizontal long axis view; hypoplastic left heart syndrome s/p lateral tunnel Fontan. The right ventricle (RV) is dilated; the tricuspid valve is open at the beginning of diastole. There is a severely hypoplastic left ventricle seen. The Fontan pathway *(asterisk)* is at the rightward aspect of the right atrium; no fenestration is seen in this plane. **B,** 3-D steady state free precession image in the coronal oblique projection showing the Fontan pathway with inferior vena cava (IVC) and superior vena cava (SVC) draining into the lateral tunnel; the pulmonary arteries in this patient arise from the pathway to the left of the SVC after a previous hemi-Fontan procedure.

the Fontan pathway and pulmonary arteries, with less physiologic information compared to CMR.

Exercise testing is recommended every 1 to 3 years depending on severity of an individual patient's disease state.[3] This can comprise full cardiopulmonary exercise testing or a 6-minute walk test. Trends in exercise ability over time can be useful for medical management.

Cardiac catheterization provides the best assessment of intracardiac and Fontan pathway pressures and PVR. Patients undergoing Fontan revision surgery should have a pre-operative catheterization. For symptomatic patients, cardiac catheterization is considered a Class IIa indication if imaging does not provide adequate information.[3]

Basic metabolic profile testing, bNPPT/INR, total cholesterol, and complete blood count can be performed every 1 to 2 years and are considered a class IIa indication for Fontan patients. Testing provides greater information regarding liver and kidney function, as well as changes in hematocrit that can be related to chronic cyanosis or iron deficiency.

Liver ultrasound or MRI is indicated to assess the status of FALD. Expert consensus recommends hepatic imaging every 1 to 2 years.[95]

Long-Term Outcomes and Complications

Overall 20-year survival following the Fontan operation in two large series was 61% and 74%.[96,97] Survival has improved over time, and it is estimated that current 30-year survival for a child newly receiving a Fontan operation is approximately 85%. Complications are common and varied.

Ventricular Dilation, Dysfunction, and Heart Failure

The development of ventricular dilation in the Fontan patient is a marker for bad outcomes.[98] Dilation can result directly from pump failure and adaptation to decreased ejection fraction, but more commonly from lesions that volume-load the single ventricle. The single morphologic RV has been associated with decreased long-term survival, often with AV valve regurgitation as the precipitating and progressive lesion leading to single RV dilation and dysfunction.[28] Other volume loading lesions that can lead to progressive ventricular dilation, dysfunction, and failure include aortic or neo-aortic regurgitation and extensive aortopulmonary collateral vessels. CMR is an excellent imaging modality for the quantification of ventricular size and function, as well as for identifying potential etiologies for ventricular dilation.

Failure of the Fontan circulation can result from numerous hemodynamic insults. Primary pump failure may be a common final pathway

resulting from valve regurgitation, volume overload from collateral flow, or chronic myocardial damage which could be related to multiple operations on cardiopulmonary bypass during childhood, chronic hypoxia in some patients, or coronary artery insufficiency. In addition, the nature of the Fontan physiology is such that increasing pressure in the Fontan pathway can result from increased ventricular diastolic pressure, increased atrial pressure related to AV valve regurgitation, or increased PVR. Chronically high (>20 mm Hg) pressure in the Fontan pathway will eventually lead to other complications. There is interest in the use of pulmonary vasodilators in patients with a Fontan; there are some data suggesting this can improve exercise performance but no data suggesting changes in mortality or serious complications.[99]

Cardiac transplantation is ultimately indicated for failure of the Fontan circulation that is not amenable to medical or other interventional therapy. This can be related to pump failure, to high pressures in the Fontan circuit, or to other complications discussed below, such as FALD or protein-losing enteropathy (PLE). Importantly, transplantation of a Fontan patient is complex. The anatomy of systemic and pulmonary veins and arteries can vary widely, leading to challenging surgical situations for anastomosis of the donor heart to the recipient blood vessels. This requires a surgeon experienced in transplant of CHD patients. Physiology can also lead to complications, as Fontan patients for whom transplantation is indicated often have numerous comorbidities. These challenges lead to worse outcomes compared to standard transplantation. A recent analysis of national discharge data showed far higher in-hospital mortality for adult Fontan transplant patients compared to other adult transplants, 26.3% versus 5.3%.[100]

Arrhythmia

The development of atrial tachyarrhythmias in the Fontan patient is frequent. Notably, this has changed with time as newer surgical approaches to the Fontan have significantly altered the substrate for generating intra-atrial re-entrant tachycardia. The progression from atriopulmonary to lateral tunnel to extra-cardiac Fontan has brought benefit in a reduction in incidence of atrial arrhythmia, which was one of the driving factors in the development of these newer techniques. Still, periodic home Holter monitoring is routine for these patients. For patients with an atriopulmonary Fontan, the development of arrhythmia is nearly ubiquitous by the third decade of life.[101] IART is most common, but atrial fibrillation is also seen. The lateral tunnel Fontan improved substantially on this incidence, with a 15-year freedom from atrial tachyarrhythmia of 83%, and the extracardiac Fontan more so, with a 15-year freedom of 92%.[102] Need for pacemaker, usually for sinoatrial node dysfunction, is not infrequent. However, this too is more common in the atriopulmonary Fontan, with incidence of 21.5% at late follow-up, compared to 11% for lateral tunnel and 3.5% for extracardiac, meaning that the overall incidence will likely decrease as the newer forms of the operation progressively account for greater percentages of the adult Fontan population.[103]

Cyanosis

The Fontan circulation ideally includes complete separation of the pulmonary and systemic circulations. Therefore, cyanosis in the Fontan patient is a concerning finding. There are several anatomic factors that can lead to cyanosis. The lateral tunnel Fontan often includes a surgical fenestration to allow pulmonary to systemic shunting to relieve pressure on the pulmonary circulation. These fenestrations often close spontaneously, or may be closed with trans-catheter device placement. The adult with a patent fenestration, or other leak in a lateral tunnel Fontan baffle, will have a degree of cyanosis, depending on the size of the shunt. Increasing cyanosis with a stable fenestration or baffle leak could suggest an increase in PVR. This diagnosis can often be made by TTE. If acoustic windows are limiting, TEE can often be diagnostic.

Patients may present with cyanosis due to the development of systemic vein to pulmonary vein collateral vessels. These also form in part as a response to abnormal pressure within the systemic veins. These collateral vessels can become markedly dilated and tortuous. They can sometimes be diagnosed by echocardiography, but this can be difficult. MRI or CT can noninvasively diagnose veno-venous collaterals, and MRI has the added benefit of flow analysis to measure degree of shunting. If indicated, veno-venous collaterals can often be closed with embolization coils or other devices by catheterization.

Cyanosis in the Fontan patient can also be due to formation of pulmonary arteriovenous malformations (AVMs). These are most likely to occur when there is an imbalance of systemic venous blood to the lungs such that hepatic venous effluent goes only to one lung. The existence of a "hepatic factor" that inhibits AVM formation has been widely postulated, although not identified; the lung that does not receive flow of hepatic venous blood is at risk of AVM formation. Pulmonary AVMs can be diagnosed be echocardiography with agitated saline contrast. There is typically rapid return of contrast via the pulmonary veins to the LA, within 2 to 3 beats of the contrast arriving in the Fontan pathway. Localization of AVMs to the left or right lung can be accomplished in the catheterization lab, with direct injection of agitated saline into the LPA and RPA with simultaneous echo visualization of the heart. Treatment is challenging. A surgical revision of the Fontan pathway can help reroute hepatic venous blood to the affected lung.

Protein-Losing Enteropathy and Plastic Bronchitis

PLE is a severe complication of the Fontan, carrying high levels of morbidity and significant mortality, although the latter has improved over time. It is difficult to cure and is typically managed as a chronic disease with acute-on-chronic exacerbations. In PLE, protein is lost into the intestinal lumen, probably via abnormal lymphatic channels. This results in reduced serum oncotic pressure and systemic edema, as well as complications from the specific proteins lost, such as immune deficiency from loss of immunoglobulin. The etiology is not precisely known, but likely includes components of high systemic venous pressure, chronic inflammation, and chronic low cardiac output. There are no clear methods to predict which Fontan patients will develop this complication. This can be diagnosed clinically, with confirmation by stool alpha-1 antitrypsin levels. Treatment of exacerbations is largely symptomatic, consisting largely of albumin infusions combined with diuresis to repair fluid imbalance.[95] Other medications used include enteral corticosteroids for direct enteral anti-inflammatory properties, spironolactone, perhaps as another anti-inflammatory agent or as a diuretic. Unfractionated heparin is sometimes effective but not consistently so. More definitive treatment is invasive, with some effect of fenestration creation, although this leads to increased cyanosis, various direct interventions on the lymphatic system, or ultimately, heart transplantation.

Plastic bronchitis has a lower prevalence than PLE. This condition is similarly related to lymphatic abnormalities, leading to protein drainage into the airways and the formation of bronchial casts. These are often coughed up by the patient but can lead to acute airway decompensation. Treatment focuses on pulmonary toilet, including inhaled tissue plasminogen activator and percussive vests. Like PLE, the Fontan circulation is also assessed and invasive treatment to improve hemodynamics may be helpful, also including heart transplantation.

Abnormalities of the Aorta and Pulmonary Arteries

Many patients with a Fontan circulation had one or more interventions during childhood on their pulmonary arteries and/or their aorta. There may be residual or progressive lesions in those vessels as a result. Many single ventricle patients, particularly single RV, require aortic reconstruction as neonates. They may present as adults with aortic coarctation or aneurysm. Diagnosis is typically first made with echocardiography, but CT or MRI can be more definitive at times and

is particularly important for surgical planning. Treatment of recurrent coarctation is usually by balloon angioplasty and possible stenting in the catheterization laboratory. Aneurysm of the ascending aorta or transverse arch typically requires surgical repair, which can carry considerable morbidity and mortality. PA pathology often comprises discrete narrowings or diffuse hypoplasia. Patients who required aortic arch reconstruction are at higher risk for diffuse hypoplasia of the LPA. Echo imaging of the pulmonary arteries can be technically challenging due to limited acoustic windows. Most often, screening CT or MRI is used to make these diagnoses. MRI has the added benefit of calculating differential antegrade pulmonary blood flow. Discrete lesions can be addressed in the catheterization laboratory, usually with stenting. Diffusely hypoplastic vessels may not have a clear interventional option.

Fontan-Associated Liver Disease

Hepatic disease is eventually ubiquitous in Fontan patients. This is primarily related to a lifetime of elevated central venous pressure to the mid-teens and higher, leading to passive congestion and eventually cardiac cirrhosis. In adults who had surgery in the 1970s and 1980s, this may be compounded by chronic hepatitis C infection. Additionally, the Fontan patient often has impaired cardiac output and is in a chronic inflammatory state, all of which may lead to hepatic disease. Serum biomarkers are often not specifically diagnostic. Synthetic function is typically preserved until late stage of disease, and transaminases and gamma-glutamyl transferases (GGT) may often be mildly elevated. Regular imaging with ultrasound or MRI is indicated every 1 to 2 years. Hepatocellular carcinoma is a rare complication of FALD and can be suspected based on serum screening for alpha-fetoprotein and diagnosed with imaging. There is increasing experience with combined heart-liver transplantation, with small single center studies showing good survival.[104,105]

PULMONARY HYPERTENSION AND EISENMENGER SYNDROME

Demographics and Prognosis

More than 5% of ACHD patients have concurrent PH, as defined by a mean pulmonary arterial pressure of greater than 20 mm Hg.[106] ACHD patients with PH have more symptoms, worse exercise capacity, and are more likely to be hospitalized than ACHD patients without PH. Mortality is increased in ACHD patients who have PH. While PH can complicate almost any form of ACHD, it is most common in patients with shunt lesions, late repair, Down syndrome, and female gender.

Classification

Several distinct mechanisms contribute to PH in patients with CHD. It is critical to define the pathophysiology of PH in order to appropriately evaluate and treat the patient. The 6th World Symposium on Pulmonary Hypertension updated the classification of PH in patients with CHD (Table 82.13). In most cases, PH can be separated into pre-capillary and post-capillary etiologies, although mixed and complex forms exist. Pre-capillary PH (or PAH) is characterized by mPAP greater than 20 mm Hg, pulmonary capillary wedge pressure (PCWP) ≤ 15 mm Hg, and an elevated transpulmonary gradient (TPG) and PVR ≥ 3 Wood units (WU). PAH is most commonly seen in patients with shunt lesions and results from adverse pulmonary vascular remodeling characterized by vasoconstriction, smooth muscle hypertrophy, and intimal proliferation which is histopathologically indistinguishable from other forms of WHO Group 1 PAH (see Chapter 88). In its most severe form, pre-capillary PAH results in markedly elevated PVR, shunt reversal, and Eisenmenger syndrome (see below). Post-capillary PH is characterized by mPAP greater than 20 mm Hg with an elevated PCWP (>15 mm Hg) and a normal TPG and normal PVR less than 3 WU. Post-capillary PH is caused by left heart disease such as ventricular dysfunction, inflow or outflow obstruction, or severe regurgitant lesions. Often patients have overlapping etiologies of PH with combined pre- and post-capillary PH with elevations in PCWP, TPG, and PVR.

TABLE 82.13 Classification of Pulmonary Hypertension in Patients With Congenital Heart Disease

GROUPING ACCORDING TO SIXTH WORLD SYMPOSIUM ON PULMONARY HYPERTENSION	SUBGROUP
Group 1	(A) Eisenmenger syndrome
	(B) PAH associated with systemic-to-pulmonary shunt
	(C) PAH and coincidental/small defect
	(D) PAH following corrective surgery/defect closure
Group 2	Left heart disease (e.g., systemic ventricular dysfunction, valve disease)
	Pulmonary vein stenosis
	Isolated
	Associated (BPD, prematurity)
	Cor triatriatum
	Obstructed total anomalous pulmonary venous return
	Mitral/aortic stenosis (including supra-/subvalvular)
	Coarctation of the aorta
Group 3	BPD
	Lung disease (e.g., restrictive lung defect)
	OSA/nocturnal hypoventilation
Group 4	PH due to pulmonary artery obstructions
	Congenital
	Related to previous surgery
	Related to other conditions (e.g., sarcoidosis)
Group 5 (complex CHD)	Segmental PH
	Isolated pulmonary artery of ductal origin
	Absent pulmonary artery
	Pulmonary atresia with VSD and MAPCAs
	Hemitruncus
	Other
	Single ventricle
	Unoperated
	Operated
	Scimitar syndrome

BPD, Bronchopulmonary dysplasia; *CHD*, congenital heart disease; *MAPCA*, major aortopulmonary collateral artery; *PAH*, pulmonary arterial hypertension; *PH*, pulmonary hypertension; *VSD*, ventricular septal defect.
Based on the updated clinical classification of pulmonary hypertension from the *Proceedings of the 6th World Symposium on Pulmonary Hypertension*. Modified from Constantine A, Dimopoulos K, Opotowsky AR. Congenital heart disease and pulmonary hypertension. *Cardiol Clin.* 2020;38(3):445–456.

Patients with ACHD and suspected PH require invasive cardiac catheterization to define the severity and mechanism of the patient's PH. In patients with open shunt lesions, a "shunt run" is required and the systemic and pulmonary blood flood must be calculated separately in order to accurately calculate resistances. Using standard sampling techniques will lead to spurious results for PVR calculations. Patients with CHD and pre-capillary PH should be managed in conjunction with a PH specialist.

Eisenmenger Syndrome

Eisenmenger syndrome occurs when patients with a left-to-right shunt develop irreversible pulmonary vascular injury and severe PAH in response to pulmonary over-circulation. When PVR surpasses SVR

TABLE 82.14 Noncardiac Complications of Eisenmenger Syndrome

Hematologic	Erythrocytosis
	Iron deficiency
	Leukopenia
	Thrombocytopenia
	Hyperviscosity
Rheumatologic	Hyperuricemia
	Gout
	Arthritis
	Myalgias
Infectious	Endocarditis
	Pneumonia
	Intracranial abscesses
Pulmonary	Hemoptysis

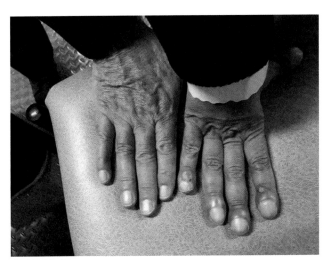

FIGURE 82.43 Cyanosis and digital clubbing in a patient with Eisenmenger syndrome *(right side of image)* compared to a healthy family member *(left side of image)*.

shunt direction reverses leading to cyanosis. Eisenmenger syndrome is most common in patients with large unrepaired post-tricuspid shunts such as AVSDs, VSD, or PDA in which cases Eisenmenger syndrome develops during the first few years of life. Eisenmenger syndrome can also exist in patients with complex intracardiac anatomy and is commonly seen in patients with truncus arteriosus, if unrepaired. A minority of patients (<10%) with unrepaired pre-tricuspid shunts, such as an ASD, also develop Eisenmenger syndrome. In these cases, Eisenmenger syndrome typically develops in adulthood. It is unknown why some patients with pre-tricuspid shunts develop Eisenmenger syndrome, but it is more common in women and other genetic or environmental factors may contribute. Due to improved diagnosis and treatment of CHD, Eisenmenger syndrome is rare in high-income nations but remains prevalent in regions where access to congenital heart surgery is limited.

Eisenmenger syndrome is a multi-organ systemic disease (Table 82.14). Chronic cyanosis induces a secondary erythrocytosis which leads to iron deficiency and hyperviscosity.[107] Hematologic dysregulation results in predisposition to both hemorrhage and thrombosis. Patients are therefore at risk for hemoptysis but also at risk for paradoxical embolism and cerebrovascular accidents.

Clinical Features

Patients with Eisenmenger syndrome demonstrate central cyanosis and digital clubbing (Fig. 82.43). Physical examination findings and laboratory abnormalities common in Eisenmenger syndrome can be found in Table 82.15.

TABLE 82.15 Physical and laboratory findings typical for Eisenmenger syndrome

Vital Signs	Hypoxemia
Physical Exam	Central cyanosis
	Hypertrophic osteoarthropathy (digital clubbing)
	Prominent jugular venous a-wave
	Right parasternal heave or lift
	Loud P2
	S3 or S4
	High-pitched diastolic murmur of pulmonary regurgitation
	Systolic murmurs may be faint or absent
Laboratory	Erythrocytosis
	Iron deficiency
	Thrombocytopenia
	Leukopenia
	Elevated BNP
	Hyperuricemia
Chest radiograph	Dilation of pulmonary arteries
	Peripheral pulmonary artery pruning
	Right atrial and right ventricular enlargement
ECG	Right atrial enlargement
	Right axis deviation
	Biventricular hypertrophy
	ST-T wave abnormalities
Transthoracic echocardiography	Right ventricular enlargement
	Right ventricular hypertrophy
	Pulmonary artery enlargement
	Pulmonary hypertension
	Large shunt defect with low-velocity flow; PDA can be difficult to visualize

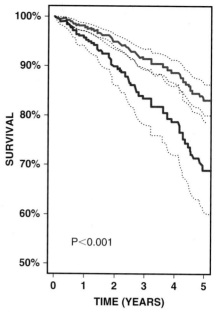

FIGURE 82.44 Survival by underlying shunt type in patients with Eisenmenger syndrome. Adjusted survival curves for patients with pre-tricuspid lesions *(red)* and post-tricuspid or complex shunts *(blue)* with 95% confidence intervals. (From Kempny A. Predictors of death in contemporary adult patients with Eisenmenger syndrome: a multicenter study. *Circulation.* 2017;135[15]:1432–1440.)

TABLE 82.16 Conditions to Avoid in Eisenmenger Syndrome

CONDITION TO AVOID	RATIONALE
Volume depletion	May worsen hyperviscosity
Excessive heat	May worsen hyperviscosity
Nonessential noncardiac surgery	High risk of operative morbidity or mortality. Anesthesia should be provided by cardiac anesthesiologist familiar with Eisenmenger syndrome.
Iron deficiency	May worsen hyperviscosity. Worsens symptoms. Patients should be tested for iron deficiency and iron should be replaced judiciously, with frequent monitoring.
Routine phlebotomy	Increases risk of stroke. Worsens iron deficiency. Phlebotomy should be reserved for symptomatic patients with adequate iron stores when symptoms are refractory to hydration.
Endocardial pacing	Increases risk of stroke
Pregnancy	High risk of maternal mortality (>30%). High risk of spontaneous abortion or miscarriage
Estrogen containing contraception	Increases risk of thrombotic complication.

Exercise capacity is markedly reduced in patients with Eisenmenger syndrome, worse than all other forms of ACHD. Symptoms may be nonspecific and include fatigue, dyspnea, arthralgias, chest pain, syncope, headache, hemoptysis, or stroke.

The prognosis of patients with Eisenmenger is variable, but better than other forms of severe PAH. Death during childhood is rare but becomes much more common during the 4th decade of life or later.[108] In a large multi-center study of patients with Eisenmenger syndrome including 1098 patients, on multivariable analysis, mortality was higher in patients with pre-tricuspid shunts, older age, lower resting oxygen saturations, non-sinus rhythm, and pericardial effusions (Fig. 82.44).[108] As with other forms of PAH, poor functional status and reduced 6-minute walk distance are also predictors of mortality. The most common causes of death include sudden death, congestive heart failure, and pulmonary hemorrhage. Patients are at risk from death during noncardiac surgery or infections, particularly brain abscesses. Antibiotic prophylaxis is required in all patients with Eisenmenger syndrome.

Management of Eisenmenger Syndrome

Patients with Eisenmenger syndrome should be managed at a comprehensive ACHD center with expertise in both CHD and PH. Patients should be seen at least annually with imaging and laboratory assessment. Much of the management of Eisenmenger syndrome is supportive. Patients should be counseled to avoid scenarios which are known to worsen outcomes in patients with Eisenmenger syndrome (Table 82.16). Specifically, patients should be counseled against volume depletion, extreme exercise, and extreme heat, as these can worsen hyperviscosity.

Pregnancy is absolutely contraindicated in Eisenmenger syndrome as it is associated with very high levels of maternal mortality (>30%) and fetal loss.[109] Effective non-estrogen containing contraception is required for women with Eisenmenger; options include intrauterine devices (IUDs), Depo-Provera injections, and progesterone eluting subcutaneous implantations (e.g., Nexplanon). Surgical sterilization is less commonly performed with the advent of less invasive contraception options. If pregnancy occurs, early termination should be encouraged.

Most patients with Eisenmenger syndrome develop a secondary erythrocytosis as an adaptive response to chronic cyanosis. The degree of erythrocytosis is proportional to the degree of cyanosis. Hematocrit greater than 60% is common, but in the compensated state rarely leads to hyperviscosity. Routine phlebotomy in asymptomatic patients is contraindicated as it increases the risk of stroke.

For patients who are experiencing symptoms suggestive of hyperviscosity (headache, lethargy, visual disturbances, paresthesia, myalgias) iron deficiency should first be excluded. Iron deficiency is common in patients with Eisenmenger syndrome and symptoms overlap with those of hyperviscosity. Volume depletion should also be excluded and corrected; this is usually effective at relieving the symptoms of hyperviscosity. In patients who are iron replete and volume replete but still have moderate or severe symptoms of hyperviscosity there is a limited role for therapeutic phlebotomy. Phlebotomy should be accompanied by simultaneous volume expansion with saline and frequent hemodynamic monitoring.

Pulmonary vasodilators should be considered in patients with Eisenmenger syndrome. The BREATH-5 randomized double-blind placebo-controlled trial demonstrated that bosentan improved exercise capacity and hemodynamics compared to placebo in patients with Eisenmenger syndrome to ASD, VSD, or PDA. However, the more recent MAESTRO trial did not show similar benefit with the use of macitentan[110] in a more heterogenous group of Eisenmenger patients. Epidemiologic data and smaller trials suggest benefit from sildenafil in Eisenmenger syndrome. Calcium channel blockers should not be used due to their negative inotropic effects.

Patients with Eisenmenger syndrome and advanced symptoms refractory to medical therapy can be considered for combined heart-lung transplantation or lung transplantation with repair of the cardiac defect. Outcomes in Eisenmenger syndrome are comparable to combined heart-lung transplantation in other conditions. A recent multinational study identified 63 patients who underwent heart-lung or lung transplantation for Eisenmenger syndrome. Early mortality was 11% and 15-year survival following transplantation was 41%.[111]

REFERENCES

General Considerations

1. Marelli AJ, Ionescu-Ittu R, Mackie AS, et al. Lifetime prevalence of congenital heart disease in the general population from 2000 to 2010. Circulation. 2014;130:749–756.
2. Gilboa SM, Devine OJ, Kucik JE, et al. Congenital heart defects in the United States: estimating the magnitude of the affected population in 2010. Circulation. 2016;134:101–109.
3. Stout KK, Daniels CJ, Aboulhosn JA, et al. 2018 AHA/ACC guideline for the management of adults with congenital heart disease: executive summary: a report of the American College of Cardiology/American heart association Task Force on clinical practice guidelines. J Am Coll Cardiol. 2018.
4. Mylotte D, Pilote L, Ionescu-Ittu R, et al. Specialized adult congenital heart disease care: the impact of policy on mortality. Circulation. 2014;129:1804–1812.
5. Baumgartner H, Bonhoeffer P, De Groot NM, et al. ESC Guidelines for the management of grown-up congenital heart disease (new version 2010). Eur Heart J. 2010;31:2915–2957.
6. Fernandes SM, Marelli A, Hile DM, Daniels CJ. Access and delivery of adult congenital heart disease care in the United States: quality-driven team-based care. Cardiol Clin. 2020;38:295–304.
7. Mackie AS, Rempel GR, Kovacs AH, et al. Transition intervention for adolescents with congenital heart disease. J Am Coll Cardiol. 2018;71:1768–1777.
8. Sachdeva R, Valente AM, Armstrong AK, et al. ACC/AHA/ASE/HRS/ISACHD/SCAI/SCCT/SCMR/SOPE 2020 appropriate use criteria for multimodality imaging during the follow-up care of patients with congenital heart disease: a report of the American College of Cardiology Solution Set Oversight Committee and Appropriate Use Criteria Task Force, American Heart Association, American Society of Echocardiography, Heart Rhythm Society, International Society for Adult Congenital Heart Disease, Society for Cardiovascular Angiography and Interventions, Society of Cardiovascular Computed Tomography, Society for Cardiovascular Magnetic Resonance, and Society of Pediatric Echocardiography. J Am Coll Cardiol. 2020;75:657–703.

Long-Term Considerations

9. Lui GK, Saidi A, Bhatt AB, et al. Diagnosis and management of noncardiac complications in adults with congenital heart disease: a scientific statement from the American heart association. Circulation. 2017;136:e348–e392.
10. Diller GP, Kempny A, Alonso-Gonzalez R, et al. Survival prospects and circumstances of death in contemporary adult congenital heart disease patients under follow-up at a large tertiary centre. Circulation. 2015;132:2118–2125.
11. Bhatt AB, Rajabali A, He W, Benavidez OJ. High resource use among adult congenital heart surgery admissions in adult hospitals: risk factors and association with death and comorbidities. Congenit Heart Dis. 2015;10:13–20.
12. Opotowsky AR, Carazo M, Singh MN, et al. Creatinine versus cystatin C to estimate glomerular filtration rate in adults with congenital heart disease: results of the Boston Adult Congenital Heart Disease Biobank. Am Heart J. 2019;214:142–155.
13. Wu FM, Kogon B, Earing MG, et al. Liver health in adults with Fontan circulation: a multicenter cross-sectional study. J Thorac Cardiovasc Surg. 2017;153:656–664.
14. Lanz J, Brophy JM, Therrien J, et al. Stroke in adults with congenital heart disease: incidence, cumulative risk, and predictors. Circulation. 2015;132:2385–2394.
15. Zaidi S, Brueckner M. Genetics and genomics of congenital heart disease. Circ Res. 2017;120:923–940.
16. Pierpont ME, Brueckner M, Chung WK, et al. Genetic basis for congenital heart disease: revisited: a scientific statement from the American heart association. Circulation. 2018;138:e653–e711.
17. Gelb BD. History of our understanding of the causes of congenital heart disease. Circ Cardiovasc Genet. 2015;8:529–536.
18. Khairy P, Van Hare GF, Balaji S, et al. PACES/HRS expert consensus statement on the recognition and management of arrhythmias in adult congenital heart disease: developed in partnership between the Pediatric and Congenital Electrophysiology Society (PACES) and the Heart Rhythm Society (HRS). Endorsed by the governing bodies of PACES, HRS, the American College of Cardiology (ACC), the American Heart Association (AHA), the European Heart Rhythm Association (EHRA), the Canadian Heart Rhythm Society (CHRS), and the International Society for Adult Congenital Heart Disease (ISACHD). Heart Rhythm. 2014;11:e102–e165.
19. Labombarda F, Hamilton R, Shohoudi A, et al. Increasing prevalence of atrial fibrillation and permanent atrial arrhythmias in congenital heart disease. J Am Coll Cardiol. 2017;70:857–865.
20. Moore JP, Khairy P. Adults with congenital heart disease and arrhythmia management. Cardiol Clin. 2020;38:417–434.
21. Bouchardy J, Therrien J, Pilote L, et al. Atrial arrhythmias in adults with congenital heart disease. Circulation. 2009;120:1679–1686.
22. Masuda K, Ishizu T, Niwa K, et al. Increased risk of thromboembolic events in adult congenital heart disease patients with atrial tachyarrhythmias. Int J Cardiol. 2017;234:69–75.
23. Yang H, Bouma BJ, Dimopoulos K, et al. Non-vitamin K antagonist oral anticoagulants (NOACs) for thromboembolic prevention, are they safe in congenital heart disease? Results of a worldwide study. Int J Cardiol. 2020;299:123–130.
24. Vehmeijer JT, Brouwer TF, Limpens J, et al. Implantable cardioverter-defibrillators in adults with congenital heart disease: a systematic review and meta-analysis. Eur Heart J. 2016;37:1439–1448.
25. Burchill LJ, Gao L, Kovacs AH, et al. Hospitalization trends and health resource use for adult congenital heart disease-related heart failure. J Am Heart Assoc. 2018;7:e008775.
26. Videbaek J, Laursen HB, Olsen M, et al. Long-term nationwide follow-up study of simple congenital heart disease diagnosed in otherwise healthy children. Circulation. 2016;133:474–483.
27. Baggen VJ, van den Bosch AE, Eindhoven JA, et al. Prognostic value of N-terminal pro-B-type natriuretic peptide, troponin-T, and growth-differentiation factor 15 in adult congenital heart disease. Circulation. 2017;135:264–279.
28. Moon J, Shen L, Likosky DS, Sood V, et al. Relationship of ventricular morphology and atrioventricular valve function to long-term outcomes following fontan procedures. J Am Coll Cardiol. 2020;76:419–431.
29. Hebert A, Mikkelsen UR, Thilen U, et al. Bosentan improves exercise capacity in adolescents and adults after fontan operation: the TEMPO (Treatment with Endothelin Receptor Antagonist in Fontan Patients, a Randomized, Placebo-Controlled, Double-Blind Study Measuring Peak Oxygen Consumption) study. Circulation. 2014;130:2021–2030.
30. Moore JP, Cho D, Lin JP, et al. Implantation techniques and outcomes after cardiac resynchronization therapy for congenitally corrected transposition of the great arteries. Heart Rhythm. 2018;15(12):1808–1815.
31. Alshawabkeh LI, Hu N, Carter KD, et al. Wait-list outcomes for adults with congenital heart disease listed for heart transplantation in the U.S. J Am Coll Cardiol. 2016;68:908–917.
32. OPTN/UNOS Thoracic Organ Transplantation Committee. Review Board (RB) Guidance for Adult Congenital Heart Disease (CHD) Exception Requests; 2017.
33. Menachem JN, Lindenfeld J, Schlendorf K, et al. Center volume and post-transplant survival among adults with congenital heart disease. J Heart Lung Transplant. 2018;37:1351–1360.
34. Lund LH, Edwards LB, Dipchand AI, et al. The registry of the International Society for heart and lung transplantation: thirty-third adult heart transplantation report-2016; focus Theme: primary diagnostic indications for transplant. J Heart Lung Transplant. 2016;35:1158–1169.
35. Nguyen VP, Dolgner SJ, Dardas TF, et al. Improved outcomes of heart transplantation in adults with congenital heart disease receiving regionalized care. J Am Coll Cardiol. 2019;74:2908–2918.
36. VanderPluym CJ, Cedars A, Eghtesady P, et al. Outcomes following implantation of mechanical circulatory support in adults with congenital heart disease: an analysis of the Interagency Registry for Mechanically Assisted Circulatory Support (INTERMACS). J Heart Lung Transplant. 2018;37:89–99.
37. Schwerzmann M, Goossens E, Gallego P, et al. Recommendations for advance care planning in adults with congenital heart disease: a position paper from the ESC Working group of adult congenital heart disease, the Association of Cardiovascular Nursing and Allied Professions (ACNAP), the European Association for Palliative Care (EAPC), and the International Society for Adult Congenital Heart Disease (ISACHD). Eur Heart J. 2020.
38. Kuijpers JM, Mulder BJ. Aortopathies in adult congenital heart disease and genetic aortopathy syndromes: management strategies and indications for surgery. Heart. 2017;103:952–966.
39. Lopez L, Colan SD, Frommelt PC, et al. Recommendations for quantification methods during the performance of a pediatric echocardiogram: a report from the pediatric measurements writing group of the American Society of echocardiography pediatric and congenital heart disease council. J Am Soc Echocardiogr. 2010;23:465–495; quiz 576-7.
40. Tutarel O, Alonso-Gonzalez R, Montanaro C, et al. Infective endocarditis in adults with congenital heart disease remains a lethal disease. Heart. 2018;104:161–165.
41. Kuijpers JM, Koolbergen DR, Groenink M, et al. Incidence, risk factors, and predictors of infective endocarditis in adult congenital heart disease: focus on the use of prosthetic material. Eur Heart J. 2017;38:2048–2056.
42. Silversides CK, Grewal J, Mason J, et al. Pregnancy outcomes in women with heart disease: the CARPREG II study. J Am Coll Cardiol. 2018;71:2419–2430.
43. Regitz-Zagrosek V, Roos-Hesselink JW, Bauersachs J, et al. 2018 ESC Guidelines for the management of cardiovascular diseases during pregnancy. Eur Heart J. 2018;39:3165–3241.
44. Stout KK, Daniels CJ, Aboulhosn JA, et al. 2018 AHA/ACC guideline for the management of adults with congenital heart disease: a report of the American College of cardiology/American heart association Task Force on clinical practice guidelines. J Am Coll Cardiol. 2019;73(12):1494–1563.
45. Holbein CE, Veldtman GR, Moons P, et al. Perceived health mediates effects of physical activity on quality of life in patients with a fontan circulation. Am J Cardiol. 2019;124:144–150.
46. Jortveit J, Eskedal L, Hirth A, et al. Sudden unexpected death in children with congenital heart defects. Eur Heart J. 2016;37:621–626.
47. Ko JM, White KS, Kovacs AH, et al. Physical activity-related drivers of perceived health status in adults with congenital heart disease. Am J Cardiol. 2018;122:1437–1442.
48. Buber J, Shafer K. Cardiopulmonary exercise testing and sports participation in adults with congenital heart disease. Heart. 2019;105:1670–1679.
49. Kempny A, Dimopoulos K, Uebing A, et al. Reference values for exercise limitations among adults with congenital heart disease. Relation to activities of daily life–single centre experience and review of published data. Eur Heart J. 2012;33:1386–1396.
50. Van Hare GF, Ackerman MJ, Evangelista JA, et al. Eligibility and disqualification recommendations for competitive athletes with cardiovascular abnormalities: task Force 4: congenital heart disease: a scientific statement from the American heart association and American College of cardiology. Circulation. 2015;132:e281–e291.

Specific Defects

51. Oster M, Bhatt AB, Zaragoza-Macias E, et al. Interventional therapy versus medical therapy for secundum atrial septal defect: a systematic review (Part 2) for the 2018 AHA/ACC guideline for the management of adults with congenital heart disease: a report of the American College of cardiology/American heart association Task Force on clinical practice guidelines. Circulation. 2019;139:e814–e830.
52. Mery CM, Zea-Vera R, Chacon-Portillo MA, et al. Contemporary results after repair of partial and transitional atrioventricular septal defects. J Thorac Cardiovasc Surg. 2019;157:1117–1127.e4.
53. Bergmann M, Germann CP, Nordmeyer J, et al. Short- and long-term outcome after interventional VSD closure: a single-center experience in pediatric and adult patients. Pediatr Cardiol. 2020.
54. Maagaard M, Eckerstrom F, Boutrup N, Hjortdal VE. Functional capacity past age 40 in patients with congenital ventricular septal defects. J Am Heart Assoc. 2020;9:e015956.
55. Rydman R, Shiina Y, Diller GP, et al. Major adverse events and atrial tachycardia in Ebstein's anomaly predicted by cardiovascular magnetic resonance. Heart. 2018;104:37–44.

56. Attie F, Rosas M, Rijlaarsdam M, et al. The adult patient with ebstein anomaly - outcome in 72 unoperated patients. *Medicine*. 2000;79:27–36.
57. De Backer J, Bondue A, Budts W, et al. Genetic counselling and testing in adults with congenital heart disease: a consensus document of the ESC Working group of grown-up congenital heart disease, the ESC working group on aorta and peripheral vascular disease and the European Society of Human genetics. *Eur J Prev Cardiol*. 2020;27:1423–1435.
58. Joynt MR, Yu S, Dorfman AL, et al. Differential impact of pulmonary regurgitation on patients with surgically repaired pulmonary stenosis versus tetralogy of Fallot. *Am J Cardiol*. 2016;117:289–294.
59. Heng EL, Bolger AP, Kempny A, et al. Neurohormonal activation and its relation to outcomes late after repair of tetralogy of Fallot. *Heart*. 2015;101:447–454.
60. Bonello B, Kempny A, Uebing A, et al. Right atrial area and right ventricular outflow tract akinetic length predict sustained tachyarrhythmia in repaired tetralogy of Fallot. *Int J Cardiol*. 2013;168:3280–3286.
61. Lillehei CW, Cohen M, Warden HE, Varco RL. The direct-vision intracardiac correction of congenital anomalies by controlled cross circulation; results in thirty-two patients with ventricular septal defects, tetralogy of Fallot, and atrioventricularis communis defects. *Surgery*. 1955;38:11–29.
62. Cuypers JA, Menting ME, Konings EE, et al. Unnatural history of tetralogy of Fallot: prospective follow-up of 40 years after surgical correction. *Circulation*. 2014;130:1944–1953.
63. Baumgartner H, De Backer J. 2020 ESC Guidelines for the management of adult congenital heart disease. *Eur Heart J*. 2020;42(6):563–645.
64. Bokma JP, Geva T, Sleeper LA, et al. A propensity score-adjusted analysis of clinical outcomes after pulmonary valve replacement in tetralogy of Fallot. *Heart*. 2018;104:738–744.
65. Heng EL, Gatzoulis MA, Uebing A, et al. Immediate and midterm cardiac remodeling after surgical pulmonary valve replacement in adults with repaired tetralogy of Fallot: a prospective cardiovascular magnetic resonance and clinical study. *Circulation*. 2017;136:1703–1713.
66. Bonello B, Shore DF, Uebing A, et al. Aortic dilatation in repaired tetralogy of Fallot. *JACC Cardiovasc Imaging*. 2018;11:150–152.
67. Gatzoulis MA, Balaji S, Webber SA, et al. Risk factors for arrhythmia and sudden cardiac death late after repair of tetralogy of Fallot: a multicentre study. *Lancet*. 2000;356:975–981.
68. Khairy P, Van Hare GF, Balaji S, et al. PACES/HRS expert consensus statement on the recognition and management of arrhythmias in adult congenital heart disease: developed in partnership between the Pediatric and Congenital Electrophysiology Society (PACES) and the Heart Rhythm Society (HRS). Endorsed by the governing bodies of PACES, HRS, the American College of Cardiology (ACC), the American Heart Association (AHA), the European Heart Rhythm Association (EHRA), the Canadian Heart Rhythm Society (CHRS), and the International Society for Adult Congenital Heart Disease (ISACHD). *Can J Cardiol*. 2014;30:e1–e63.
69. Valente AM, Gauvreau K, Assenza GE, et al. Contemporary predictors of death and sustained ventricular tachycardia in patients with repaired tetralogy of Fallot enrolled in the INDICATOR cohort. *Heart*. 2014;100:247–253.
70. Kapel GF, Reichlin T, Wijnmaalen AP, et al. Re-entry using anatomically determined isthmuses: a curable ventricular tachycardia in repaired congenital heart disease. *Circ Arrhythm Electrophysiol*. 2015;8:102–109.
71. Geva T, Mulder B, Gauvreau K, et al. Preoperative predictors of death and sustained ventricular tachycardia after pulmonary valve replacement in patients with repaired tetralogy of Fallot enrolled in the INDICATOR cohort. *Circulation*. 2018.
72. Couperus LE, Vliegen HW, Zandstra TE, et al. Long-term outcome after atrial correction for transposition of the great arteries. *Heart*. 2019;105:790–796.
73. Cuypers JA, Eindhoven JA, Slager MA, et al. The natural and unnatural history of the Mustard procedure: long-term outcome up to 40 years. *Eur Heart J*. 2014;35:1666–1674.
74. Khairy P, Harris L, Landzberg MJ, et al. Sudden death and defibrillators in transposition of the great arteries with intra-atrial baffles: a multicenter study. *Circ Arrhythm Electrophysiol*. 2008;1:250–257.
75. Koolbergen DR, Ahmed Y, Bouma BJ, et al. Follow-up after tricuspid valve surgery in adult patients with systemic right ventricles. *Eur J Cardio Thorac Surg*. 2016;50:456–463.
76. Deng L, Xu J, Tang Y, et al. Long-term outcomes of tricuspid valve surgery in patients with congenitally corrected transposition of the great arteries. *J Am Heart Assoc*. 2018;7.
77. Oladunjoye O, Piekarski B, Baird C, et al. Repair of double outlet right ventricle: midterm outcomes. *J Thorac Cardiovasc Surg*. 2019.
78. Robinson Vimala L, Hanneman K, et al. Characteristics of cardiovascular magnetic resonance imaging and outcomes in adults with repaired truncus arteriosus. *Am J Cardiol*. 2019;124:1636–1642.
79. Rudiene V, Hjortshoj CMS, Glaveckaite S, et al. Cor triatriatum sinistrum diagnosed in the adulthood: a systematic review. *Heart*. 2019;105:1197–1202.
80. van der Linde D, Roos-Hesselink JW, Rizopoulos D, et al. Surgical outcome of discrete subaortic stenosis in adults: a multicenter study. *Circulation*. 2013;127:1184–1191.e1-4.
81. Tefera E, Gedlu E, Bezabih A, et al. Outcome in children operated for membranous subaortic stenosis: membrane resection plus aggressive septal myectomy versus membrane resection alone. *World J Pediatr Congenit Heart Surg*. 2015;6:424–428.
82. Tal N, Golender J, Rechtman Y, et al. Long-term aortic valve function in patients with or without surgical treatment for discrete subaortic stenosis. *Pediatr Cardiol*. 2021;42(2):324–330.
83. Jiao Y, Li G, Korneva A, et al. Deficient circumferential growth is the primary determinant of aortic obstruction attributable to partial elastin deficiency. *Arterioscler Thromb Vasc Biol*. 2017;37:930–941.
84. Collins 2nd RT. Cardiovascular disease in Williams syndrome. *Curr Opin Pediatr*. 2018;30:609–615.
85. Latham GJ, Ross FJ, Eisses MJ, et al. Perioperative morbidity in children with elastin arteriopathy. *Paediatr Anaesth*. 2016;26:926–935.
86. Lee MGY, Babu-Narayan SV, Kempny A, et al. Long-term mortality and cardiovascular burden for adult survivors of coarctation of the aorta. *Heart*. 2019;105:1190–1196.
87. Choudhary P, Canniffe C, Jackson DJ, et al. Late outcomes in adults with coarctation of the aorta. *Heart*. 2015;101:1190–1195.
88. Rinnstrom D, Dellborg M, Thilen U, et al. Hypertension in adults with repaired coarctation of the aorta. *Am Heart J*. 2016;181:10–15.
89. Taggart NW, Minahan M, Cabalka AK, et al. Immediate outcomes of covered stent placement for treatment or prevention of aortic wall injury associated with coarctation of the aorta (COAST II). *JACC Cardiovasc Interv*. 2016;9:484–493.
90. Saran N, Dearani J, Said S, et al. Vascular rings in adults: outcome of surgical management. *Ann Thorac Surg*. 2019;108:1217–1227.
91. Luciano D, Mitchell J, Fraisse A, et al. Kommerell diverticulum should Be removed in children with vascular ring and aberrant left subclavian artery. *Ann Thorac Surg*. 2015;100:2293–2297.
92. Vinnakota A, Idrees JJ, Rosinski BF, et al. Outcomes of repair of Kommerell diverticulum. *Ann Thorac Surg*. 2019;108:1745–1750.
93. Hoffman JI, Kaplan S. The incidence of congenital heart disease. *J Am Coll Cardiol*. 2002;39:1890–1900.
94. Fontan F, Baudet E. Surgical repair of tricuspid atresia. *Thorax*. 1971;26:240–248.
95. Rychik J, Atz AM, Celermajer DS, et al. Evaluation and management of the child and adult with fontan circulation: a scientific statement from the American heart association. *Circulation*. 2019: CIR0000000000000696.
96. Pundi KN, Johnson JN, Dearani JA, et al. 40-Year follow-up after the fontan operation: long-term outcomes of 1,052 patients. *J Am Coll Cardiol*. 2015;66:1700–1710.
97. Downing TE, Allen KY, Glatz AC, et al. Long-term survival after the Fontan operation: twenty years of experience at a single center. *J Thorac Cardiovasc Surg*. 2017;154:243–253 e2.
98. Rathod RH, Prakash A, Kim YY, et al. Cardiac magnetic resonance parameters predict transplantation-free survival in patients with fontan circulation. *Circ Cardiovasc Imaging*. 2014;7:502–509.
99. Goldberg DJ, Zak V, Goldstein BH, et al. Results of the FUEL trial. *Circulation*. 2020;141:641–651.
100. Hernandez GA, Lemor A, Clark D, et al. Heart transplantation and in-hospital outcomes in adult congenital heart disease patients with Fontan: a decade nationwide analysis from 2004 to 2014. *J Card Surg*. 2020;35:603–608.
101. Quinton E, Nightingale P, Hudsmith L, et al. Prevalence of atrial tachyarrhythmia in adults after Fontan operation. *Heart*. 2015;101:1672–1677.
102. Ben Ali W, Bouhout I, Khairy P, et al. Extracardiac versus lateral tunnel fontan: a meta-analysis of long-term results. *Ann Thorac Surg*. 2019;107:837–843.
103. Dennis M, Zannino D, du Plessis K, et al. Clinical outcomes in adolescents and adults after the fontan procedure. *J Am Coll Cardiol*. 2018;71:1009–1017.
104. Vaikunth SS, Concepcion W, Daugherty T, et al. Short-term outcomes of en bloc combined heart and liver transplantation in the failing Fontan. *Clin Transplant*. 2019;33:e13540.
105. Reardon LC, DePasquale EC, Tarabay J, et al. Heart and heart-liver transplantation in adults with failing Fontan physiology. *Clin Transplant*. 2018;32:e13329.
106. Simonneau G, Montani D, Celermajer DS, et al. Haemodynamic definitions and updated clinical classification of pulmonary hypertension. *Eur Respir J*. 2019;53.

Eisenmenger Syndrome

107. Arvanitaki A, Giannakoulas G, Baumgartner H, Lammers AE. Eisenmenger syndrome: diagnosis, prognosis and clinical management. *Heart*. 2020;106:1638–1645.
108. Kempny A, Hjortshoj CS, Gu H, et al. Predictors of death in contemporary adult patients with eisenmenger syndrome: a multicenter study. *Circulation*. 2017;135:1432–1440.
109. Duan R, Xu X, Wang X, et al. Pregnancy outcome in women with Eisenmenger's syndrome: a case series from west China. *BMC Pregnancy Childbirth*. 2016;16:356.
110. Gatzoulis MA, Landzberg M, Beghetti M, et al. Evaluation of macitentan in patients with eisenmenger syndrome. *Circulation*. 2019;139:51–63.
111. Hjortshoj CS, Gilljam T, Dellgren G, et al. Outcome after heart-lung or lung transplantation in patients with Eisenmenger syndrome. *Heart*. 2020;106:127–132.

 # 83 Catheter-Based Treatment of Congenital Heart Disease in Adults

SHABANA SHAHANAVAZ, JOHN M. LASALA, AND DAVID T. BALZER

Advances in surgical and medical care have led to rapid growth in the number and state of adults living with congenital heart disease (see Chapter 82). Consequently there has been an increase in the volume and variety of transcatheter interventional procedures applicable to adult congenital heart disease (ACHD) patients. ACHDs span a wide spectrum with heterogeneous anomalies involving all aspects of cardiovascular physiology such that specialized training has become a necessity for anyone caring for such patients. Multiple professional societies including ACC, AHA, and SCAI have published recommendations regarding the delivery of ACHD interventional care. Current consensus explicitly states that interventional procedures should be performed at regional ACHD centers by qualified and experienced ACHD specialists, and in laboratories with appropriate staffing and experience to fulfill this task.[1,2] In addition, because of the complexity of disorders in these patients, any site undertaking the care of adults with congenital heart disease must have a well-established multidisciplinary team that includes congenital cardiothoracic surgeons, cardiac anesthesiologists, cardiac intensivists, and congenital cardiologists.[1,2] Pediatric interventional cardiologists are also key persons on the team, and partnerships between adult congenital interventionalists and pediatric interventional cardiologists are mandatory. As the capabilities of the congenital catheterization laboratory continue to evolve, the line between surgical and catheter-based interventions will become more and more blurred. Many interventions already take place in highly specialized hybrid operating suites whereby interventional cardiologists work alongside their cardiothoracic surgery colleagues. This combined model of intervention will continue to be adapted for adult congenital interventions, and it is this ongoing evolution that makes the field so exciting. Furthermore, as interventional approaches change, the indications for intervention become a "moving target." As a result, national guidelines outdate sooner than later; therefore, interventional cardiologists who treat adults must remain current about the ever-changing medical literature on this topic. In this chapter, we review major areas in which catheter-based interventions have become well established for adults with congenital heart disease. The topic of congenital heart disease in adults is reviewed in Chapter 82.

VALVULAR INTERVENTIONS

The first static pulmonary balloon valvuloplasty was performed in 1982; successful catheter-based interventions have since been performed on all types of cardiac valves.[3–5] Although valvuloplasty defined the early era of congenital interventional catheterization, valve replacement is defining the current era.

Pulmonary Valvuloplasty

Congenital valvular pulmonary stenosis accounts for 5% to 10% of all congenital heart disease.[6] In most cases, the stenosis is due to fusion of commissures with normal valve leaflets leading to "doming" of the valve leaflets, but rarely due to dysplastic leaflets. Static pulmonary valvuloplasty (aimed at separating the fused leaflets) was first performed in the early 1980s and has replaced surgical valvotomy as the initial intervention in cases of typical isolated valvar pulmonary stenosis.[5] Valvuloplasty for thick and/or dysplastic valves is less successful; moreover, balloon dilation will be unsuccessful in relieving any muscular subvalvar stenosis. Indications for pulmonary valvuloplasty in adults with congenital heart disease have been outlined elsewhere (see Chapter 82).[1] Before pulmonary valvuloplasty is performed, a complete right heart catheterization should be performed, followed by right ventricular (RV) angiography to profile the right ventricular outflow tract (RVOT). Angiographic measurements of the pulmonary annulus allows for the selection of the appropriately sized balloon, which is approximately 120% of the measured pulmonary annulus. Successful balloon valvuloplasty can usually be achieved with low pressure inflation of a compliant balloon. In patients with large annulus, double balloons can be used to achieve adequate dilation.[7] After dilation of the pulmonary valve, repeat angiography should be performed to rule out vascular injury. Pulmonary regurgitation is best assessed on post procedure echocardiography.

OUTCOMES AND COMPLICATIONS
Case selection is critical for optimizing outcomes. Patients with typical pulmonary valve stenosis will have relatively thin leaflets with partial fusion and will respond well to balloon valvuloplasty.[5] The most common complication of pulmonary valvuloplasty is pulmonary regurgitation (<10% with 2+ or greater pulmonary regurgitation), which is usually well tolerated. Major adverse events or unplanned surgeries were not reported for patients with typical valvar stenosis in the most recent report from the National Cardiovascular Data Registry (NCDR).[8]

Pulmonary Valve Replacement

Patients presenting for pulmonary valve replacement typically have a history of congenital heart disease and may have undergone multiple cardiac surgeries. The most common initial pathologies present in these patients are tetralogy of Fallot with associated pulmonary atresia, stenosis, or absence of the pulmonary valve, pulmonary valve dysfunction following a Ross procedure and truncus arteriosus.[9] The unifying component of the surgical repair in these patients is the frequent presence of a RV to pulmonary artery conduit, which is a prosthetic or tissue graft that is placed to bypass or reconstruct the

DISEASES OF THE MYOCARDIUM, PERICARDIUM, AND PULMONARY VASCULATURE BED

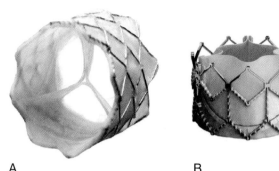

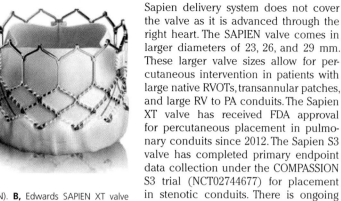

A   B   C

FIGURE 83.1 Transcatheter valves. **A,** Melody valve (Medtronic, Minneapolis, MN). **B,** Edwards SAPIEN XT valve (Edwards Lifesciences LLC, Irvine, CA). **C,** Edwards SAPIEN S3 valve (Edwards Lifesciences LLC, Irvine, CA).

RVOT. Over time, these conduits often develop progressive stenosis, regurgitation or a combination of these. Patients can present with symptoms of exercise intolerance, congestive heart failure and dysrhythmias heralding significant RV dysfunction. In an effort to avoid such dysfunction, relief of stenosis and placement of a competent valve are warranted. Determining the optimal timing for pulmonary valve replacement remains an issue; there are currently several indications in symptomatic[1] and asymptomatic[10] patients with pulmonary valve disease (see Chapter 82).

Pulmonary Valve Systems

There are currently two available valve systems approved by the Food and Drug Administration (FDA) for transcatheter pulmonary valve replacement (TPVR): Melody Transcatheter Pulmonary Valve (Medtronic, Inc., Minneapolis), and SAPIEN XT Pulmonic Valve (Edwards Lifesciences, Irvine, CA). Each has its own unique strengths and weaknesses.

Melody Valve

In 2000, Bonhoeffer and colleagues published the first successful percutaneous placement of his prototype stent-mounted valve in the pulmonary valve.[11] The rights to Bonhoeffer's valve design were acquired by Medtronic, Inc. (Minneapolis, MN) to develop the Melody valve (Fig. 83.1A). The Melody valve is composed of a valved segment of bovine internal jugular vein that is fixed with glutaraldehyde and then sutured to a platinum-iridium stent frame.[12] A percutaneous introducer, Ensemble Delivery sheath (Medtronic, Inc., Minneapolis, MN) covers the valve and is used to deliver the valve. Once in proper position, the sheath on the Ensemble system is pulled back to expose the valve, and via two sequential balloon dilations, the valve is deployed. RVOT stenting is routinely performed prior to valve deployment to prevent stent fractures of the Melody valve frame. There are currently two sizes of Melody valves available: 20 and 22 mm, with the delivery system available in three sizes: 18, 20, and 22 mm (Video 83.1).

SAPIEN Valve

The Edwards SAPIEN transcatheter heart valve (Irvine, CA) was originally designed for placement in the aortic position, but was found to have high success rates when placed in the pulmonary valve position, with the first successful pulmonary implantation in 2006.[13,14] This device is composed of bovine pericardium of three equal-sized leaflets that are hand-sewn to a cobalt chromium balloon-expandable stent with a polyethylene terephthalate fabric cuff (Fig. 83.1B). Additionally, the S3 has a new outer polyethylene terephthalate skirt which decreases the incidence of paravalvular leak. The Sapien XT and S3 system is crimped onto the Novaflex and Commander delivery system (Edwards Lifesciences, Irvine, CA), respectively (Fig. 83.1C). The delivery systems minimize profile by allowing the valve to be crimped onto the shaft of the balloon and then pushed onto the balloon *in vivo* once advanced through the introducer sheath. The

Sapien delivery system does not cover the valve as it is advanced through the right heart. The SAPIEN valve comes in larger diameters of 23, 26, and 29 mm. These larger valve sizes allow for percutaneous intervention in patients with large native RVOTs, transannular patches, and large RV to PA conduits. The Sapien XT valve has received FDA approval for percutaneous placement in pulmonary conduits since 2012. The Sapien S3 valve has completed primary endpoint data collection under the COMPASSION S3 trial (NCT02744677) for placement in stenotic conduits. There is ongoing enrollment for Sapien S3 placement in bioprosthetic valves (Video 83.2).

OUTCOMES AND COMPLICATIONS

The Melody valve received US Food and Drug Administration approval under a Humanitarian Device Exemption (HDE) in 2010 and Pre–Market Approval in 2015 for the treatment of conduit dysfunction. In 2016, it received approval for valve-in-valve placement to combat bioprosthetic valve dysfunction. Early and intermediate[15] outcome data have demonstrated excellent procedural success and freedom from RVOT reintervention at rates of 98% at 3 years and 91% at 5 years from intervention. SAPIEN valves have had similarly good early outcomes[16] and favorable comparisons with the Melody valve.[17] Valve selection is influenced by patient cohort (conduit versus transannular patch), ease of use of the delivery system (stiffness and lack of flexibility of the delivery system for the Sapien), and operator experience/preference. Important procedural complications include vascular injury, conduit disruption, pulmonary artery perforation, stent or valve embolization, coronary artery compression, ventricular arrhythmias, and tricuspid valve injury. Long-term complications include stent frame fracture (Melody valve), valve dysfunction, and endocarditis.[16–18]

ARTERIAL INTERVENTIONS

The pathologic "arterial" conditions encountered most frequently by congenital interventionalists are related to anatomic lesions in the pulmonary arterial tree, followed by coarctations of the aorta. As in other interventional areas, technologic advances have increased the breadth of catheter-based treatments for congenital heart disease, as well as the quality and durability of the outcomes. In adult patients, stenting has become a well-established companion to angioplasty and has improved acute and long-term outcomes.

Pulmonary Angioplasty

Pulmonary artery abnormalities can be isolated or in association with other cardiac defects, and occur in 2% to 3% of all patients with congenital heart disease. Depending on the obstruction site, these lesions can result in elevated RV pressure or significant flow discrepancies between lung segments, thereby causing isolated lung hypertension. Indications for pulmonary arterial intervention have been described elsewhere (see Chapter 82).[1] There are currently no stents approved by the FDA for use in pulmonary arteries; however, Palmaz Genesis stents (Cordis, Milpitas, CA) and the EV3 family of stents (Covidien/Medtronic, Minneapolis, MN) have been used and have shown good radial strength, low profiles, and achievable diameters. In children or in small or distal pulmonary arteries in adults, it is reasonable to use premounted stents.

OUTCOMES AND COMPLICATIONS

The heterogeneous nature of pulmonary arterial disease has resulted in a wide spectrum of clinical outcomes following catheter-based interventions.[19,20] Both the anatomic location of the stenosis and its

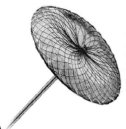 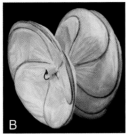 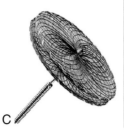 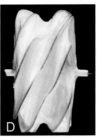

FIGURE 83.2 Various closure devices for atrial septal defects. **A,** Amplatzer Cribriform device (Abbott Inc., St. Paul, MN). **B,** GORE Cardioform Septal Occluder (W.L. GORE and Associates, Inc., Flagstaff, AZ). **C,** Amplatzer Septal Occluder (Abbott Inc., St. Paul, MN). **D,** Gore Cardioform ASD occlude (W.L. GORE and Associates, Inc., Flagstaff, AZ).

less than 10 mm Hg.[8] Complications include access injuries, vascular tears or dissections, stent embolization or malpositioning, restenosis, and aneurysm; and even death. For adults in the NCDR, 8.6% experienced an adverse event, but only one major adverse event occurred in 92 patients.[8] Long-term follow-up will continue to reveal the true risk of late aneurysm and restenosis in these patients. For children who are not fully grown, future dilations should be anticipated to keep pace with somatic growth.

circumstances of formation as a congenital or postoperative greatly contribute to the differences in clinical outcomes. Complications include vascular tears, stent embolization or malpositioning, pulmonary edema, and the need for unanticipated procedures or surgeries; some patients may not survive. A report from the NCDR revealed reasonable safety; in 245 procedures across all age-groups, adverse events were reported in 13.2% of cases and major adverse events in 1.2% of cases, and 2 patients died.[8]

Stenting for Coarctation of the Aorta

Coarctation is characterized by discrete narrowing of the thoracic aorta adjacent to where the ductus arteriosus was once inserted (see Chapter 82). Although it can present as an isolated lesion, it is also commonly found in genetic syndromes (Turner and Williams syndrome).[21] Hence, detailed investigation for the presence of coarctation should be made in these patients. The most common cardiovascular malformation associated with CoA is bicuspid aortic valve (BAV). Current guidelines recommend that patients with CoA undergo evaluation for intracranial aneurysms.[22] The increase in afterload imposed by the coarctation can result in left ventricular (LV) dysfunction and cardiogenic shock, which often develop in early infancy. More frequently, the body develops extensive collaterals through the chest wall, which minimize the increase in afterload and preserve systolic function. Over time, patients with coarctation will develop hypertension in varying degrees and, eventually, coronary artery disease and LV diastolic dysfunction. Transcatheter approach with stenting of the aorta is now considered a mainstay in the management of adults with native CoA and recoarctation. Coarctation stenting is typically performed by a retrograde approach via the femoral artery. After measuring the baseline gradient, angiography is performed and measurements of the distal aortic arch and thoracic aorta (at the level of the diaphragm) are recorded. The covered Cheatham pulmonary (CP) stent (NuMED, Inc., Hopkinton, NY) is approved by the FDA for use in coarctation, but other stents are often used off-label. The diameter of the implanted balloon should not be larger than that of the surrounding aorta or 3.5 times the narrowest dimension.[23] Stents are most frequently placed by balloon-in-balloon catheters because of their improved control. Once a stiff guidewire is positioned across the coarctation, a long sheath is positioned above the narrowed area and a mounted stent is advanced into position at the site of coarctation. The stent is uncovered and deployed with inflation of the balloon catheter. After successful placement of the stent, additional serial dilations of any residual waist may be considered. Follow-up angiography should be performed to rule out dissection or aneurysm before measuring the final pressure gradient. Indications for coarctation intervention are discussed elsewhere (see Chapter 82).[1] Comparisons between balloon angioplasty, aortic stenting, and surgical resection have been done, and catheter-based stenting has emerged as the preferred treatment modality for older children and adults (Video 83.3).

OUTCOMES AND COMPLICATIONS

Coarctation stenting is safe and compares favorably with surgery in regard to its ability to eliminate the pressure gradient.[8,23] The NCDR report noted more frequent stenting in older children and adults, with nearly 84% of stented patients achieving a postprocedural gradient of

SEPTAL INTERVENTIONS

Techniques for Closure of Atrial Septal Defects

Atrial septal defects (ASDs) are the third most common form of congenital heart disease. They occur in 56 to 100 live births per 100,000 infants.[6,24] Isolated ASDs will result in left-to-right shunting, with the magnitude of the shunt determined by ventricular compliance and atrioventricular valve stenosis. Significant left-to-right shunts result in RV dilation; if they are left unrepaired, they may ultimately result in pulmonary arterial muscularization and elevations in the pulmonary vascular resistance by the sixth decade of life. In an effort to avoid irreversible changes in pulmonary vascular resistance, early closure of significant ASDs has become standard practice. Transcatheter devices and techniques have evolved substantially since the first case was reported in 1976 by King and colleagues.[24] The currently available devices each have unique strengths and weaknesses (Fig. 83.2).[25] Indications for intervention have been previously outlined.[1]

Amplatzer Devices

Originally introduced in the mid-1990s, the Amplatzer Septal Occluder (ASO) (Abbott Inc., St. Paul, MN) has been used in thousands of cases worldwide. The ASO is made of woven nitinol wire that forms a self-centering device, with left and right atrial discs, and a central waist. The device is filled with interwoven Dacron polyester fibers to facilitate platelet aggregation and endothelialization. The device is secured to a delivery cable and introduced into the left atrium via the appropriately sized, proprietary TorqVue sheath. ASOs can treat ASDs of variable sizes as long as the atrial septal rim is substantial enough to allow for a secured placement of the. If the septal rim is deficient (<5 mm in contiguous zones), stable positioning will be more difficult to achieve and at times may not be possible. Numerous deployment techniques can be used if the septal rim is deficient, but are out of the scope of this chapter.[26–28] Shortly after the introduction of the ASO, Amplatzer developed the Cribriform device. In contrast to the ASO, the Cribriform device does not have a waist and is therefore not self-centering. Its primary benefit is that it can be placed in a small central defect and also covers numerous satellite defects. Its deployment is identical to that of the ASO, using the same TorqVue sheaths and delivery cables. The Amplatzer PFO occluder has been approved by the FDA for PFO closure in the context of cryptogenic stroke. It is made of two nitinol woven discs with integral Dacron patches and a fixed short waist (see Fig. 83.2). The Dacron patches are designed to stimulate endothelialization. The device comes in multiple sizes with the right atrial disc being larger than the left atrial disc. The Amplatzer Trevisio intravascular delivery system is a second generation delivery cable that has three sections with varying flexibility to decrease device distortion once positioned across the defect. The proximal portion is a stainless steel cable with moderate pushability. The middle part of the wire has a stainless steel cable with loosely wound stainless steel coil, and the distal part of the wire has a nitinol core with loosely wound stainless steel coil. The more flexible distal cable enables better assessment of final device position and is especially helpful in larger defects. Device sizing for the ASO should be based on the stop flow method of balloon sizing. In order to decrease the risk of device erosion, over inflation of the balloon should be avoided (not >1.5 × the static echocardiographic dimension). Device selection should be the same size (or at most 1 size larger) than the stop flow dimension. Defects with a deficient retroaortic rim (<5 mm) are considered higher risk for an erosion.

OUTCOMES AND COMPLICATIONS

The ASO demonstrated superior safety and similar closure rates when compared to surgery in the US Pivotal Trial. The postmarket approval study and multicenter community use trial have further solidified the ASO's position as a safe and effective device for transcatheter closure of an ASD or a patent foramen ovale (PFO).[29,30] Major adverse events reported include arrhythmias, device embolization, device erosion, device fracture, stroke, and left arterial thrombus. One of the most significant adverse events is device erosion. After the first reported case in 2002, AGA/St. Jude revised the ASO guidelines, but erosions continued to be reported to the Manufacturer and User Facility Device Experience (MAUDE) database. In response to ongoing erosion reports (<0.05% of worldwide sales, estimated to be approximately 0.1% of implants), the FDA and AGA/St. Jude made additional changes to the guidelines in an effort to minimize the erosion risk, and recommended closer follow-up with more frequent echocardiograms. In addition to erosion, several case reports in children and adults have demonstrated delayed endothelialization in the setting of endocarditis, and concerns have been raised regarding the optimal length of time for subacute bacterial endocarditis prophylaxis following device placement.[31] The RESPECT clinical trial (evaluating PFO closure with the Amplazter PFO Occluder) showed that among adults with a history of a cryptogenic ischemic stroke, closure of a PFO was associated with a lower rate of recurrent ischemic strokes than medical therapy alone during extended follow-up.[32]

GORE Devices

The GORE Helex device (no longer commercially available) was approved in 2006. It was not self-centering and therefore was relatively limited with regard to the sizes of defects it could effectively treat. GORE redesigned its septal occluder system which is now marketed as the GORE Cardioform Septal Occluder (GSO) (W.L. Gore and Associates, Flagstaff, AZ). The new device consists of a five-wire nitinol frame, which adds radial strength and improves structural integrity, and it is covered with the same expanded polytetrafluoroethylene (ePTFE) membrane as the original Helex device (see Fig. 83.2B). The redesigned delivery system is much more intuitive, and it maintains its novel retention cord mechanism. Owing to its non–self-centering design, the GSO can only close defects up to 18 mm in diameter. Similar to the GSO, the GORE Cardioform ASD occluder (GCA) is composed of a platinum–filled nitinol wire frame covered with ePTFE. The principal modification from the original GSO is its anatomically adaptable "intra–disc occluder" which expands to conform to the ASD size and shape, allowing different devices to treat a range of ASD diameters. The current device is locked by a nitinol pin running through the central eyelets, and has a retrieval cord attached to the right atrial eyelet. The available sizes are 27, 32, 37, 44, and 48 mm and are designed to treat defects ranging from 8 to 35 mm. These devices are not contraindicated in defects with deficient retroaortic rim since there is no erosion risk (Video 83.4).

OUTCOMES AND COMPLICATIONS

The GSO was approved by the FDA in 2012 and has demonstrated comparable safety and efficacy to the ASO in closure of PFO and ASD.[33] In contrast to the ASO, there is no report of device erosion following implantation of a GORE device. Overall, percutaneous device placement has emerged as the preferred intervention for ASDs because of its excellent outcomes and safety records. The Gore ASSURED clinical study was a prospective single arm registry that evaluated the safety and efficacy of the GCA device. The study showed excellent technical success with 100% closure rate and low adverse event rates.[34] The REDUCE study determined safety and efficacy of PFO closure with the GORE CARDIO-FORM Septal Occluder or GORE HELEX Septal Occluder plus antiplatelet medical management compared to antiplatelet medical management

alone in patients with a PFO and history of cryptogenic stroke.[35] The risk of subsequent ischemic stroke was lower among those assigned to PFO closure combined with antiplatelet therapy than those assigned to antiplatelet therapy alone. Current recommendations from the American Academy of Neurology states that clinicians can recommend closure following a discussion of potential benefits (absolute recurrent stroke risk reduction of 3.4% at 5 years) and risks (periprocedural complication rate of 3.9% and increased absolute rate of non-periprocedural atrial fibrillation of 0.33% per year) in patients <60 years of age with a PFO and embolic infarct and no other mechanism of stroke identified (level C).[36]

Techniques for Closure of Superior Sinus Venosus Atrial Septal Defects

The superior sinus venosus ASD is a congenital abnormality that is caused by a deficiency of the common wall between the superior vena cava (SVC) and the right sided pulmonary veins (see Chapter 82). This defect is frequently associated with an anomalous drainage of the right-sided pulmonary veins to the SVC. Traditionally, this defect is treated by surgical correction. However, advances in current covered stent technology has led to a transcatheter approach. This novel technique uses a covered stent deployed in the SVC-RA, closing the interatrial communication and redirecting pulmonary venous flow to the left atrium. In the presence of anomalous drainage of the right sided pulmonary veins higher in the SVC, surgical repair with reimplantation of the veins and patch closure of the sinus venosus ASD is recommended.[37]

Techniques for Closure of Ventricular Septal Defects

Ventricular septal defects (VSDs) are the most common congenital heart defects and can range in size from tiny pinholes to near absence of the septum (see also Chapter 82). VSDs can be an isolated finding or associated with other complex congenital heart diseases, primarily conotruncal defects (e.g., tetralogy of Fallot, double-outlet right ventricle, transposition of the great arteries). The ventricular septum has four primary regions: inlet, outlet, perimembranous area, and muscular area. Defects can occur in any location and extend to adjacent regions. The shunt through a VSD is predicated on ventricular outflow obstruction and downstream vascular resistance. The management of VSD is a complex topic beyond the scope of this chapter, and indications for intervention have been previously described (see Chapter 82).[1] Catheter-based device closure of muscular, traumatic, postoperative residual, and postinfarct VSDs has become a reasonable alternative to surgery. Perimembranous VSD remains controversial because of the associated risk of heart block. Inlet VSDs are not amenable to transcatheter techniques because there is no circumferential tissue for secured placement of device (Video 83.5).[38] Percutaneous closure of VSDs that are secondary to myocardial infarction has been attempted with a variety of devices (Amplatzer Septal Occluder and Amplater muscular VSD device). The Amplatzer Post Infarct muscular VSD device (Abbott Inc., St. Paul, MN) has larger disks and a longer waist (10 mm) than the Amplatzer muscular VSD device, in order to accommodate the thicker adult interventricular septum. This indication has received FDA approval. Details regarding timing of post infarct VSD intervention are outside the scope of this chapter.

OUTCOMES AND COMPLICATIONS

Complications specific to transcatheter device closure of VSDs include aortic regurgitation, tricuspid regurgitation, rhythm disturbances, and atrioventricular (AV block); death occurs rarely. In a review of the European registry of transcatheter VSD devices, Carminati and associates[39] found that VSDs in the perimembranous location were at increased risk for developing complete AV block. When similar devices were used, others found similar rates of AV block, ranging from 2% to 6%.[40–42] Interestingly, a lower risk of AV block has been seen in some cases

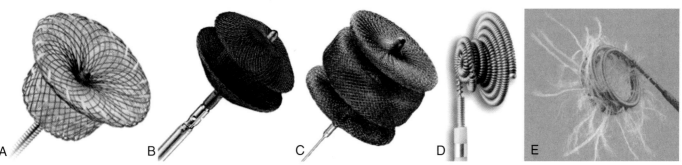

FIGURE 83.3 Various closure devices for patent ductus arteriosus. **A,** Amplatzer Ductal Occluder (St. Jude Medical, St. Paul, MN). **B,** Amplatzer Ductal Occluder II (St. Jude Medical, St. Paul, MN). **C,** Amplatzer Vascular Plug II (St. Jude Medical, St. Paul, MN). **D,** Nit-Occlud PDA Occluder (PFM Medical AG, Köln, Germany).

when the first-generation Amplatzer ductal occluders were used.[43] Review of outcomes for device closure of VSD's post myocardial infarction show that the mortality among overall surgical repair and percutaneous closure was significantly lower than medical management alone (P< 0.001 for all comparisons). The overall mortality with percutaneous closure was lower compared with late surgical closure (P < 0.0001).[44]

Treatment of Patent Ductus Arteriosus

Patent ductus arteriosus (PDA) is a frequent congenital heart defect that is most commonly detected in infancy through the associated murmur (see also Chapter 82). After birth, several important physiologic changes lead to early functional closure of the ductus followed by an anatomic closure in subsequent weeks to months. For patients in whom the ductus persists, the elevation in systemic vascular resistance and drop in pulmonary vascular resistance promotes a left-to-right shunt with resultant pulmonary overcirculation and left heart dilation. Left untreated, a large PDA can lead to significant heart failure, atrial arrhythmias (secondary to atrial hypertension), and pulmonary hypertension. PDA can be a site for infective endarteritis in rare cases.[45] Prior to catheter-based interventions, significant PDAs were ligated surgically via posterolateral thoracotomy. Indications for intervention have been outlined elsewhere.[1] From coils to vascular plugs to dedicated occlusion devices, the interventionalist has multiple options for PDA occlusion (Fig. 83.3). There is consensus regarding the indication for closure in large PDAs with associated left heart dilation despite a current controversy with respect to the need for closing "silent" PDAs.[46]

Amplatzer Duct Occluders (First- and Second-Generation)

The ADO-I device is made of a nitinol wire mesh packed with Dacron polyester fabric to facilitate platelet aggregation and endothelialization. The second-generation ADO-II has symmetric retention skirts, which allow it to be placed in an antegrade or a retrograde fashion. The ADO-II is not packed with polyester fibers because the nitinol wire weave is tighter than in ADO-I.

Amplatzer Vascular Plugs (Second- and Fourth-Generation)

In patients with long, tubular ducts, a vascular plug may be the optimal occlusion device. Vascular plugs have a conveniently low profile and work well in ducts with sufficient length to ensure that the left pulmonary artery and aorta are not obstructed. The AVP-II has a wide assortment of sizes (3 to 22 mm). The AVP-IV has fewer available sizes (4 to 8 mm) and is slightly longer than AVP-II, but it offers an even lower profile, to easily navigate tortuous anatomy.

Nit-Occlud Device

The Nit-Occlud device (PFM Medical, Carlsbad, CA) has a single nitinol wire coil, which can be wound in a funnel shape when it

is advanced from the catheter. The Nit-Occlud device can be delivered via a 4 Fr guide catheter with a controlled-release mechanism. The Nit-Occlud comes in multiple sizes with variable levels of wire stiffness.

Standard Coiling

After small ducts have been crossed, they can be reliably occluded with simple coils or detachable coils.

OUTCOMES AND COMPLICATIONS

Transcatheter closure of PDA has become a reliable procedure with excellent technical success and good efficacy.[6] Numerous articles have reviewed the outcomes of detachable coils and the Amplatzer devices, and found the overall closure rate to be approximately 94%.[8,47] Serious adverse events are extremely rare.[6] Minor complications (vascular injuries, device embolization, residual shunts, blood loss requiring transfusion, hemolysis, and aortic or pulmonary artery narrowing not requiring intervention) occur in the young, but rarely in adults.[6]

FUTURE PERSPECTIVES

The transcatheter management of structural congenital heart disease in adults has undergone rapid advances over the past decade. Pulmonary valve implants have become standard therapy for patients with pulmonic valve stenosis and/or regurgitation in circumferential conduits and within bioprosthetic valves. Currently approved therapies to manage circumferential RVOTs include surgically placed conduits, and TPVR with bioprosthetic valves. In addition to standard valve-in-valve therapy, intentional fracture of the surgical bioprosthetic valve frame using ultra-high-pressure balloons can be a means of facilitating further expansion of the valve in the aortic, pulmonary, and tricuspid positions.[48]

Unfortunately, most patients with dysfunctional RVOTs have large, compliant, non-circumferential outflow tracts previously modified by either surgical placement of a transannular patch or catheter-based balloon valvuloplasty. In recent years, several self-expanding, percutaneous valve devices have been designed and are in various stages of clinical testing for patients with these types of RVOT. The Harmony TPV is a porcine pericardial tissue valve mounted on a self-expanding nitinol frame (Fig. 83.4). The Harmony valve recently was studied as a part of an early feasibility trial where 20 patients underwent device implantation.[49] In contrast, the Alterra Adaptive Prestent (Edwards Lifesciences) is a valveless stent designed to be used as a docking adaptor for the 29 mm SAPIEN 3 THV within the RVOT. It is comprised of a covered self-expanding nitinol frame assembly that has 40-mm symmetrical inflow and outflow diameters and a 27-mm central section that serves as a landing zone for a 29 mm SAPIEN 3 valve (eFig. 83.1).[50] Both of these devices are promising catheter-based treatment plans of congenital heart disease in adults.

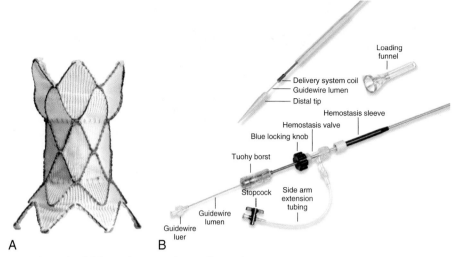

FIGURE 83.4 A, Harmony TPV porcine pericardial tissue valve mounted on a self expanding nitinol stent. **B,** The delivery system is a 25 Fr coil loading catheter with an integrated sheath.

REFERENCES

Valvular Interventions

1. Warnes CA, Williams GR, Bashore TM, et al. ACC/AHA 2008 guidelines for the management of adults with congenital heart disease: a report of the American College of Cardiology/American Heart Association task Force on Practice guidelines (Writing Committee to develop guidelines on the management of adults with congenital heart disease). Developed in Collaboration with the American Society of Echocardiography, heart rhythm society, International society for adult congenital heart disease, society for cardiovascular angiography and interventions, and society of thoracic surgeons. *J Am Coll Cardiol.* 2008;52(23):e143–e263.
2. Aboulhosn JA, Hijazi ZM, Kavinsky CJ, et al. SCAI position statement on adult congenital cardiac interventional training, competencies and organizational recommendations. *Catheter Cardiovasc Interv.* 2020;96(3):643–650.
3. Nishimura RA, Otto CM, Bonow RO, et al. 2014 AHA/ACC guideline for the management of patients with valvular heart disease: a report of the American College of Cardiology/American Heart Association task Force on Practice guidelines. *J Am Coll Cardiol.* 2014;63(22):e57–e185.
4. Kan JS, White RI, Mitchell SE, Gardner TJ. Percutaneous balloon valvuloplasty: a new method for treating congenital pulmonary valve stenosis. *N Engl J Med.* 1982;307:540–542.
5. Rao PS. Percutaneous balloon pulmonary valvuloplasty: state of the art. *Catheter Cardiovasc Interv.* 2007;69(5):747–763.
6. Hoffman JI, Kaplan S. The incidence of congenital heart disease. *J Am Coll Cardiol.* 2002;39(12):1890–1900. https://doi.org/10.1016.
7. Mullins CE, Nihill MR, Vick GWIII, et al. Double balloon technique for dilation of valvular or vessel stenosis in congenital and acquired heart disease. *J Am Coll Cardiol.* 1987;10:107–114.
8. Moore JW, Vincent RN, Beekman RH, et al. Procedural results and safety of common interventional procedures in congenital heart disease: initial report from the National Cardiovascular Data Registry. *J Am Coll Cardiol.* 2014;64(23):2439–2451.
9. Marelli AJ, Ionescu-Ittu R, Mackie AS, et al. Lifetime prevalence of congenital heart disease in the general population from 2000 to 2010. *Circulation.* 2014;130(9):749–756.
10. Geva T. Indications for pulmonary valve replacement in repaired tetralogy of Fallot: the quest continues. *Circulation.* 2013;128(17):1855–1857.
11. Bonhoeffer P, Boudjemline Y, Saliba Z, et al. Percutaneous replacement of pulmonary valve in a right-ventricle to pulmonary-artery prosthetic conduit with valve dysfunction. *Lancet.* 2000;356:1403–1405.
12. McElhinney DB, Hennesen JT. The Melody(R) valve and Ensemble(R) delivery system for transcatheter pulmonary valve replacement. *Ann N Y Acad Sci.* 2013;1291:77–85.
13. Leon MB, Smith CR, Mack M, et al. Transcatheter aortic-valve implantation for aortic stenosis in patients who cannot undergo surgery. *N Engl J Med.* 2010;363(17):1597–1607.
14. Garay F, Webb J, Hijazi ZM. Percutaneous replacement of pulmonary valve using the Edwards-Cribier percutaneous heart valve: first report in a human patient. *Catheter Cardiovasc Interv.* 2006;67:659–662.
15. Cheatham JP, Hellenbrand WE, Zahn EM, et al. Clinical and hemodynamic outcomes up to 7 years after transcatheter pulmonary valve replacement in the US Melody valve investigational device exemption trial. *Circulation.* 2015;131(22):1960–1970.
16. Holzer RJ, Hijazi ZM. Transcatheter pulmonary valve replacement: state of the art. *Catheter Cardiovasc Interv.* 2016;87(1):117–128.
17. McElhinney DB, Hellenbrand WE, Zahn M, et al. Short- and medium-term outcomes after transcatheter pulmonary valve placement in the expanded multicenter US Melody valve trial. *Circulation.* 2010;122(5):507–516.
18. McElhinney DB, Benson LN, Eicken A, et al. Infective endocarditis after transcatheter pulmonary valve replacement using the Melody valve: combined results of 3 prospective North American and European studies. *Circ Cardiovasc Interv.* 2013;6(3):292–300.
19. Bergersen L, Gauvreau K, Lock JE, Jenkins KJ, et al. Recent results of pulmonary arterial angioplasty: the differences between proximal and distal lesions. *Cardiol Young.* 2005;15(6):597–604.
20. Bergersen L, Gauvreau K, Justino H, et al. Randomized trial of cutting balloon compared with high-pressure angioplasty for the treatment of resistant pulmonary artery stenosis. *Circulation.* 2011;124(22):2388–2396.

Arterial Interventions

21. Lin AE, Craig TB, Elizabeth G, et al. Adults with genetic syndromes and cardiovascular abnormalities: clinical history and management. *Genet Med.* 2008;10(7):469–494.
22. Thompson BG, Brown Jr RD, Amin-Hanjani S, et al. Guidelines for the management of patients with unruptured intracranial aneurysms: a guideline for healthcare professionals from the American Heart Association/American Stroke Association. *Stroke.* 2015;46:2368–2400.
23. Salcher M, et al. Balloon dilatation and stenting for aortic coarctation: a systematic review and meta-analysis. *Circ Cardiovasc Interv.* 2016;9(6):e003153.

Septal Interventions

24. King TD, Thompson SL, Steiner C, et al. Secundum atrial septal defect. Nonoperative closure during cardiac catheterization. *J Am Med Assoc.* 1976;235:2506–2509.
25. Geva T, Martins JD, Wald RM. Atrial septal defects. *Lancet.* 2014;383(9932):1921–1932.
26. Dalvi B. Balloon assisted technique for closure of large atrial septal defects. *Images Paediatr Cardiol.* 2008;10(4):5–9.
27. Pinto R, Jain S, Dalvi B. Transcatheter closure of large atrial septal defects in children using the left atrial disc engagement-disengagement technique (LADEDT): technical considerations and short term results. *Catheter Cardiovasc Interv.* 2013;82(6):935–943.
28. Varma C, et al. Outcomes and alternative techniques for device closure of the large secundum atrial septal defect. *Catheter Cardiovasc Interv.* 2004;61(1):131–139.
29. Turner DR, et al. Closure of secundum atrial septal defects with the Amplatzer Septal Occluder: a prospective, multicenter, post-approval study. *Circ Cardiovasc Interv.* 2017;10:e004212.
30. Everett AD, et al. Community use of the Amplatzer atrial septal occluder: results of the multicenter MAGIC atrial septal defect study. *Pediatr Cardiol.* 2009;30(3):240–247.
31. Nguyen AK, et al. Endocarditis and incomplete endothelialization 12 years after Amplatzer septal occluder deployment. *Tex Heart Inst J.* 2016;43(3):227–231.
32. Saver JL, Carroll JD, Thaler DE, et al. Long-term outcomes of patent foramen ovale closure or medical therapy after stroke. *N Engl J Med.* 2017;377:1022–1032.
33. Grohmann J, et al. Transcatheter closure of atrial septal defects in children and adolescents: single-center experience with the GORE septal occluder. *Catheter Cardiovasc Interv.* 2014;84(6):E51–E57.
34. Sommer RJ, Love BA, Paolillo JA, et al. ASSURED clinical study: new GORE® CARDIOFORM ASD occluder for transcatheter closure of atrial septal defect [published online ahead of print, 2020 Jan 14]. *Catheter Cardiovasc Interv.* 2020;95(7):1285–1295.
35. Søndergaard L, Kasner SE, Rhodes JF, et al. Patent foramen ovale closure or antiplatelet therapy for cryptogenic stroke [published correction appears in N. Engl J Med. 2020;382(10):978.
36. Steven RM, Gary SG, David MK, et al. Kasner. Practice advisory update summary: patent foramen ovale and secondary stroke prevention. *Rep Guideline Subcommittee of the American Academy of Neurology.* First published April 29. 2020. https://doi.org/10.1212.
37. Hansen JH, Duong P, Jivanji SGM, et al. Transcatheter correction of superior sinus venosus atrial septal defects as an alternative to surgical treatment. *J Am Coll Cardiol.* 2020;75(11):1266–1278.
38. Yang L, Tai BC, Khin LA, et al. A systematic review on the efficacy and safety of transcatheter device closure of ventricular septal defects (VSD). *J Interv Cardiol.* 2014;27(3):260–272.
39. Carminati M, Butera G, Chessa M, et al. Transcatheter closure of congenital ventricular septal defects: results of the European Registry. *Eur Heart J.* 2007;28(19):2361–2368.
40. Fu Y-C, Bass J, Amin Z, et al. Transcatheter closure of perimembranous ventricular septal defects using the new Amplatzer membranous VSD occluder: results of the U.S. phase I trial. *J Am Coll Cardiol.* 2006;47(2):319–325.
41. Butera G, Carminati M, Chessa M, et al. Transcatheter closure of perimembranous ventricular septal defects: early and long-term results. *J Am Coll Cardiol.* 2007;50(12):1189–1195.
42. Butera G, Gaio G, Carminati M. Is steroid therapy enough to reverse complete atrioventricular block after percutaneous perimembranous ventricular septal defect closure? *J Cardiovasc Med (Hagerstown).* 2009;10(5):412–414.
43. Mahimarangaiah J, Subramanian A, Hemannasetty S, et al. Transcatheter closure of perimembranous ventricular septal defects with ductal occluders. *Cardiol Young.* 2015;25(5):918–926.
44. Omar S, Morgan GL, Panchal HB, et al. Management of post-myocardial infarction ventricular septal defects: a critical assessment. *J Interv Cardiol.* 2018;31(6):939–948. https://doi.org/10.1111.
45. Sabzi F, Faraji R. Adult patent ductus arteriosus complicated by endocarditis and hemolytic anemia. *Colomb Méd.* 2015;46(2):80–83.
46. Fortescue EB, Lock JE, Galvin T, et al. To close or not to close: the very small patent ductus arteriosus. *Congenit Heart Dis.* 2010;5(4):354–365.
47. Jin M, Liang Y-M, Wang X-F, et al. A retrospective study of 1,526 cases of transcatheter occlusion of patent ductus arteriosus. *Chin Med J.* 2015;128(17):2284–2289.

Future Perspectives

48. Shahanavaz S, Asnes JD, Grohmann J, et al. Intentional fracture of bioprosthetic valve frames in patients undergoing valve-in-valve transcatheter pulmonary valve replacement. *Circ Cardiovasc Interv.* 2018;11(8):e006453. https://doi.org/10.1161.
49. Bergersen L, Benson LN, Gillespie MJ, et al. Harmony feasibility trial: acute and short-term outcomes with a self-expanding transcatheter pulmonary valve. *JACC Cardiovasc Interv.* 2017;10(17):1763–1773.
50. Zahn EM, Chang JC, Armer D, Garg R. First human implant of the Alterra Adaptive PrestentTM: a new self-expanding device designed to remodel the right ventricular outflow tract. *Catheter Cardiovasc Interv.* 2018;91(6):1125–1129.

84 Cardiomyopathies Induced by Drugs or Toxins

ROBERT A. KLONER AND SHEREIF REZKALLA

Many natural and synthetic substances and environmental exposures may affect the heart adversely. Accordingly, it is important to understand the myriad ways in which these substances may influence the cardiovascular system. Many of these substances are used and abused by people throughout the world. With better understanding of the full extent of the pathophysiology of these toxins, we may be able to curb the problems associated with the use of these substances, as well as their associated economic burden. Chapter 56 discusses the toxicities of various chemotherapeutic agents.

ALCOHOL

History

Ancient Egyptians were one of the first civilizations to manufacture beer for both pleasure and religious rituals. In ancient China, rice wine was a tradition and consumed in moderation.[1] In the 16th century, distilled liquor was prepared and termed *alcohol*. The potential beneficial effects that alcohol could have on the heart were first described in medieval times. In the United States, the 21st amendment was added to the Constitution, which ended prohibition; since then, alcohol has become a widely available product.

For several decades, the deleterious effects of excessive alcohol intake on organ systems, including the cardiovascular system, have become widely recognized, and alcohol abuse is now considered a major cause of morbidity, mortality, and burden to the economics of society. The following section discusses the types of damage that excess alcohol causes to the heart and blood vessels.

Epidemiology

Alcohol is the most commonly used and abused substance across the globe. Approximately 40% of adults use alcohol worldwide. In the United States, approximately 70% of adults use alcohol. Eastern Europe and the former Soviet Union report the highest rates of alcohol consumption, at 10 L of pure alcohol per person per year, while the lowest areas of consumption are southeast Asia and the Middle East, at less than 2.5 L per person per year of pure alcohol.[2] Because of the heavy economic burden of alcohol abuse, the World Health Organization had a goal of decreasing alcohol consumption by 10%. Unfortunately, that goal was not achieved, and in fact, alcohol consumption is on the rise.

Although men consume significantly more alcohol compared with women, the latter are more sensitive to the drug, and the prevalence of alcoholic cardiomyopathy is equal between men and women. Moderate drinking is considered up to one drink per day in women and up to two drinks per day in men. Binge drinking (four drinks for women and five drinks for men in approximately 2 hours, resulting in blood alcohol concentration to 0.08 g/dL or greater) is becoming an increasing problem. Binge drinking in the elderly is on the rise, and it is estimated to occur in approximately 10% of adults older than 65 years of age.[3] Definitions of heavy drinking (Centers for Disease Control and Prevention [CDC]) include 15 drinks or more per week for men and 8 drinks or more per week for women. Both binge drinking and heavy drinking are associated with alcohol use disorder or alcoholism, the inability to control drinking related to both physical and emotional dependence upon alcohol consumption. There have been recent concerns that isolation during the COVID-19 pandemic crisis of 2020 may be associated with an increase in alcohol abuse.

Pharmacology and Pathophysiology

When ingested, ethanol is oxidized by the enzyme alcohol dehydrogenase into acetaldehyde. Acetaldehyde is then oxidized into acetic acid and acetate by the enzyme aldehyde dehydrogenase. These metabolites have an impact on cardiac myocytes, impairing mitochondrial function, enhancing oxidative stress, and increasing myocyte apoptosis,[4] ultimately leading to both systolic and diastolic cardiac dysfunction. The deleterious effects of alcohol drinking depend on the amount consumed and the duration of consumption. The degree of alcohol-induced cardiac effects varies by individual based on many genotypic and phenotypic variants. Although various manifestations of alcoholic heart disease are mainly associated with chronic heavy alcohol abuse, acute binge drinking may also cause myocardial injury, enhance inflammation, and result in cardiac arrhythmias. Other factors that contribute to the cardiac effects of alcohol include associated nutritional deficiencies as well as many additives that may be found in different alcoholic drinks.

Alcoholic Cardiomyopathy

Heavy alcohol drinking for prolonged periods of time affects systolic and diastolic heart function and may lead to overt heart failure (see Chapter 52).[5] The amount of alcohol drinking to be considered an alcoholic is generally more than 90 g/day of alcohol for 5 years or more. William MacKenzie first described the cardiac effects of alcohol in 1902, calling it alcoholic heart disease. As many as 30% of chronic alcoholics have evidence of left ventricular (LV) dysfunction by two-dimensional echocardiography. Alcoholic cardiomyopathy represents approximately 20% to 30% of cases of nonischemic dilated cardiomyopathy. The incidence is affected by both phenotypic and genotypic factors. Increased amounts of alcohol consumed per day and a long duration of alcohol use are associated with higher incidence of cardiomyopathy. Women are more susceptible to the development of the disease. The clinical picture of this disease ranges from asymptomatic cardiac abnormalities to clinically advanced congestive heart failure with symptoms of dyspnea, fatigue, and exercise intolerance; the clinical findings on physical examination include jugular venous congestion, rales in the lungs, and peripheral edema (see also Chapter 48). In history taking, the term *social drinking* does not capture the extent of alcohol use. The type, number of drinks per day, and the duration of drinking is essential in evaluating such patients. A 12-lead electrocardiogram (ECG) may show sinus tachycardia (particularly during acute intoxication), nonspecific ST and T wave abnormality, right and left bundle branch block, and various atrial and ventricular arrhythmias. Chest radiography shows cardiomegaly and pulmonary congestion when patients are in decompensated heart failure.[6] Echocardiography is an important non-invasive diagnostic modality. The earliest echocardiographic abnormality in heavy alcohol drinkers is diastolic dysfunction, present in at least one-third of asymptomatic patients. With progression of the disease, global systolic dysfunction ensues, and the echocardiogram may be indistinguishable from advanced idiopathic nonischemic cardiomyopathy. Atrial and ventricular thrombi may be detected in advanced cases, resulting in systemic embolization. Longitudinal, circumferential, and radial strain echocardiography can detect very early cases of alcoholic cardiomyopathy, which will aid in early detection and management of the disease.[7]

The histopathology of alcoholic cardiomyopathy is similar to dilated cardiomyopathy, except there is lower myocyte count in histologic sections in the former compared to the latter.[8] Guzzo-Merello et al.[9] followed 94 consecutive patients with alcoholic cardiomyopathy for a median follow-up of approximately 5 years. In that study, 5% of patients died from heart failure, 8.5% had sudden death, and 15% ended up with cardiac transplant. The remaining patients either remained clinically stable or improved after reducing alcohol intake. Atrial fibrillation, absence of beta blocker therapy, and QRS duration longer than 120 milliseconds were associated with poor prognosis.

Management of alcoholic cardiomyopathy parallels the treatment for heart failure with a reduced ejection fraction (see Chapter 50). Abstinence of alcohol drinking should be the first major component of treatment. Patients who stopped drinking or even decreased drinking to mild or moderate levels demonstrated improvement in LV ejection fraction upon follow-up. Patients who completely stop drinking alcohol may normalize their ejection fraction in 1 year. Factors that were associated with the best recovery of ejection fraction included narrow QRS, beta blocker therapy, and lack of use or need for diuretic therapy.[10]

Cardiac Arrhythmias

Frequent atrial and ventricular arrhythmias reported with alcohol drinking are secondary to the effect of alcohol on atrial muscle and ventricular myocytes as well as electrolyte abnormalities. The most common abnormality, and the one that needs more attention in the clinical setting, is atrial fibrillation.[11] Low levels of alcohol intake, with only one standard drink per day, is not associated with increased incidence of atrial fibrillation. Moderate drinking increases the incidence of atrial fibrillation in males only, whereas heavy drinking is associated with atrial arrhythmias in both sexes. The Framingham study showed an increase in the incidence of atrial fibrillation in 34% of patients who consumed more than three standard drinks per day. In a randomized study, 140 patients who consumed at least 10 drinks per week and had atrial fibrillation were randomized to either continuing drinking or no drinking. Those who stopped drinking had significantly lower incidence of atrial fibrillation.[12]

Several decades ago, "holiday heart" syndrome was described as cardiac arrhythmias that were mainly atrial flutter and atrial fibrillation.[13]

This syndrome describes patients who consume excessive alcohol on weekends and holidays, who then develop these arrhythmias a day or two later. It is more common in men than in women, occurs in patients with an apparently normal heart, and has a relatively benign prognosis.

Ventricular arrhythmias occur with heavy alcohol drinking and may be fatal. A V-shaped or J-shaped curve that characterizes the relationship between alcohol drinking and mortality has been described. Mild to moderate drinking is associated with lower cardiovascular mortality, whereas heavy drinking leads to increased mortality.[14] Alcohol drinking was followed in 33,593 healthy volunteers who drank alcohol for 26 years. Significant alcohol drinking was associated with higher mortality (Fig. 84.1).[15] Alcohol drinking in the presence of left bundle branch block and decreased ventricular function are determinants of malignant ventricular arrhythmias.[16]

Alcohol and Lipid Metabolism

Alcohol increases high-density lipoprotein (HDL) and may reduce low-density lipoprotein (LDL). It may even have some favorable effect on lipoprotein(a) (Fig. 84.2).[17] In addition, moderate intake of beer enhances the antioxidative properties of HDL; thus it prevents lipid deposition in blood vessel walls. Severe alcohol consumption may increase triglyceride levels, blunting the beneficial effect of moderate alcohol drinking.[18,19]

Alcohol and Coronary Artery Disease

In addition to a potential benefit on HDL levels, alcohol may have other protective effects that limit coronary atherosclerosis. Systemic inflammation is shown to promote atherosclerosis. Alcohol has antioxidant and antiinflammatory effects.[20] It is associated with a decrease in C-reactive protein as well as interleukin-6.[21] The beneficial effect is limited to low to moderate drinking,[22] and it appears to be more pronounced in men compared with women. In heavy drinkers, the opposite occurs. Heavy drinking and binge drinking are associated with an increase in inflammatory markers.[23] After mild to moderate alcohol drinking, there is a decrease in platelet aggregation. However, binge drinking may have the opposite effect, which may account for the increase in cardiac events following binge drinking. Some alcoholic beverages, specifically wine, contain resveratrol, which has an antioxidant effect that stimulates mitochondria biogenesis.[24] It is quite clear that low to moderate alcohol consumption is associated with a decreased risk of atherosclerotic burden.[25] Mild alcohol drinking, particularly wine, is associated with a decrease in cardiovascular risk. There is a favorable effect on mortality when mild alcohol

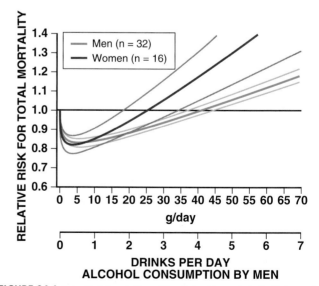

FIGURE 84.1 Risk of total mortality and its relationship to alcoholic drinks per day in both men and women. (From Di Castelnuovo A, Costanzo S, Bagnardi V, et al. Alcohol dosing and total mortality in men and women: an updated meta-analysis of 34 prospective studies. *Arch Intern Med.* 2006;166[22]:2437–2445.)

drinking is combined with other healthy lifestyle factors such as no smoking, a healthy diet, and moderate physical activity.[26] The American Heart Association (AHA) suggests that if a person already drinks, their intake be limited, with one or two drinks per day for men and only one drink for women. A "drink" is considered to be 12 ounces of beer, 5 ounces of wine, or a mixed drink containing 1.5 ounces of hard liquor. However, the AHA does not recommend that people start drinking to lower their cardiovascular risk.

Alcohol and Hypertension

Mild alcohol drinking does not affect blood pressure. However, heavy alcohol drinking, which initially may cause vasodilation, may later result in an increase in blood pressure. It is expected that controlling excessive alcohol drinking in people 40 to 60 years of age will result

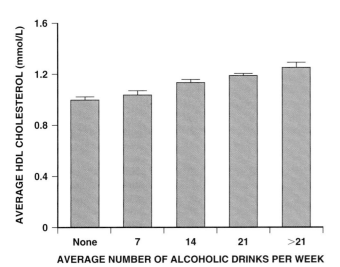

FIGURE 84.2 Relationship between average high-density lipoprotein (HDL) levels and average number of alcoholic drinks per week. (Modified from Suh I, Shaten BJ, Cutler JA, et al. Alcohol use and mortality from coronary heart disease: the role of high-density lipoprotein cholesterol. *Ann Intern Med.* 1992;116:881–887.)

in a decrease in hypertension, and that is expected in both men and women.[27] In a randomized study, 25 normotensive volunteers received either 375 mL of red wine or a nonalcoholic beverage. Blood pressure fell 4 hours after drinking alcohol but was significantly higher 24 hours later as compared with the control subjects. When drinking is combined with weight gain and smoking, the effect on blood pressure is accentuated. The deleterious and protective effects of alcohol on the cardiovascular system are summarized in Figure 84.3.

ELECTRONIC CIGARETTES

The Effect of Electronic Cigarettes/Vaping on the Cardiovascular System

It is well known that smoking tobacco cigarettes leads to a number of health problems including ischemic heart disease, lung cancer, other forms of cancer, chronic obstructive lung disease, and peripheral vascular disease. Tobacco smoking accelerates atherosclerosis and leads to myocardial infarction (MI), stroke, and peripheral arterial disease. Carbon monoxide in tobacco smoke reduces oxygen availability. The nicotine in tobacco smoke is known to stimulate the sympathetic nervous system, which results in an increase in heart rate, blood pressure, heart contractility, and coronary vasoconstriction. Nicotine lowers HDL cholesterol, increases triglyceride levels, and induces endothelial dysfunction. Tobacco smoke results in oxidant chemicals, particulates, and combustion products that cause inflammation, endothelial dysfunction, and activates clotting mechanisms.

There is a common perception that electronic (e-)cigarettes may be safer than tobacco cigarettes because they lack the tars that cause cancer and do not contain as many of the over 4000 chemical compounds that are created by a burning tobacco cigarette. It is also thought that they might help smokers quit tobacco smoking. E-cigarettes consist of a liquid cartridge that typically contains propylene glycol and vegetable glycerin and may contain nicotine at various doses (including very high doses). The e-liquid may also contain flavorings, some of which are fruit flavored and sweet and appeal to young people. The e-cigarette devices also include a sensor, a microprocessor, and a battery. The electronic cigarette is activated with inhalation by the sensor or by pushing a button; this triggers the heating of coils, which then vaporizes

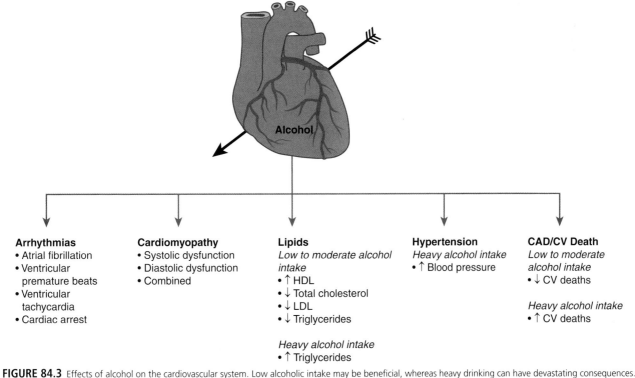

FIGURE 84.3 Effects of alcohol on the cardiovascular system. Low alcoholic intake may be beneficial, whereas heavy drinking can have devastating consequences.

DISEASES OF THE MYOCARDIUM, PERICARDIUM, AND PULMONARY VASCULATURE BED

the e-liquid within the cartridge. E-cigarette vapors reach the mouth or the air and condense into particles that form an aerosol. Some of the devices have a light that simulates the glow of a lit cigarette, which is turned on by the microprocessor. Although e-cigarettes do not contain tar or generate carbon monoxide as do tobacco cigarettes,[28] when the e-liquid is heated the results may include formation of formaldehyde, acetaldehyde, and acrolein, which result in reactive oxygen species and inflammation that can contribute to an acceleration of atherosclerosis and clotting. Electronic cigarettes are commonly used as a nicotine delivery device. Nicotine can result in the cardiovascular effects described earlier and is addictive. In addition, the high temperatures of e- cigarettes can result in the generation of very small particulate matter that can enter the lungs and possibly the vasculature to a greater extent than tobacco cigarettes and contribute to vascular damage. Metals and flavoring contained in e-cigarette vapor can contribute to adverse cardiovascular effects including inflammation.[29]

Electronic cigarettes have been around since approximately 2003, and they have become increasingly popular, even as overall tobacco smoking has declined. It is estimated that approximately 9 million adults in the United States vape on a regular basis. In 2019, approximately 28% of high school students reported using e-cigarettes, while only 5.8% reported smoking tobacco cigarettes. Approximately 10.5% of middle school students reported using e-cigarettes. E-cigarette use increased from 12% to 21% among high school students from 2017 to 2018.

Preclinical and clinical studies have examined the effects of e-cigarettes on the cardiovascular system. Variable effects on hemodynamics such as blood pressure and heart rate have been reported. One study showed that in people who smoked an e-cigarette with nicotine or standard cigarettes, both demonstrated an increase in blood pressure.[30] Blood pressure was elevated for a longer time (45 minutes) after using an e-cigarette with nicotine than with a standard cigarette (15 minutes). Those who smoked e-cigarettes without nicotine did not have an increase in blood pressure. Studies of heart rate variability have shown the use of e-cigarettes with nicotine was associated with a marked shift in cardiac sympathovagal balance towards sympathetic predominance, whereas this shift did not occur with e–cigarettes without nicotine. Some studies have suggested that e-cigarette vapor causes endothelial dysfunction with reduced flow–mediated vasodilation, increased vascular resistance, vascular stiffness, and reduced distal blood flow velocity. Although some studies suggested that nicotine was the cause, others suggested that the e-cigarette vapor itself was causing vascular abnormalities including abnormalities in endothelial cells. Other studies suggested that e-cigarettes increased low density lipoprotein oxidation and increased platelet activation. Flavoring, especially cinnamon flavoring, has been associated with abnormalities induced by e-cigarettes in an experimental model.[31] In these studies, e-cigarette flavoring caused decreased endothelial cell viability, increased reactive oxygen species levels, and increased inflammatory cytokine expression in human-induced pluripotent stem cell–derived endothelial cells. The long-term effects of e-cigarettes on the cardiovascular system are largely unknown.

One study suggested that e-cigarettes were more effective than standard, already approved nicotine replacement therapies for smoking cessation.[32] However, the AHA recommended using e-cigarettes for smoking cessation only as a last resort. They recommended behavioral support, nicotine patches, bupropion, or varenicline. In an observational study of over 69,000 participants from the National Health Interview Surveys, daily use of e-cigarettes was an independent factor associated with increased odds of suffering from a myocardial infarction (nearly double that of conventional tobacco smoking). There was a fivefold risk of having a myocardial infarction in individuals who used both standard cigarettes plus e-cigarettes compared with those who did not use either.[33] In a cross-sectional study of 400,000 participants from a 2016 behavioral risk factor surveillance study, the odds of having a stroke were 71% higher in e-cigarette users versus nonusers. In addition, the incidence of myocardial infarction was 59% greater in e-cigarette users than nonusers, and the incidence of angina pectoris was 40% higher in e-cigarette users than nonusers.[34] Thus, although e-cigarettes might help with smoking cessation, there may be consequences, including increased rates of myocardial infarction, stroke, endothelial dysfunction, increased platelet aggregation, and possible other cardiovascular effects.

E-Cigarette or Vaping Product Use Associated Lung Injury (see Chapter 28)

Beginning in July 2019, a new form of lung injury was described in people who vape and has now exploded into a true epidemic.[35] The condition is now known as E-cigarette or vaping product use associated lung injury (EVALI). As of January 14, 2020, there have now been over 2660 clinical cases of EVALI reported, with 60 deaths in the United States. Over 90% of victims have been hospitalized, and over 30% required respirators. Cases have been reported in nearly all states in the United States. The typical victim is a young male who has been using e-cigarettes (vaping) within days to weeks of the illness. The patients present with respiratory distress including shortness of breath, cough, chest pain, fever, fatigue, and gastrointestinal symptoms including nausea, vomiting, and diarrhea. The patients are often hypoxic. Chest radiography typically shows ground glass–appearing bilateral pulmonary infiltrates. Histology has shown pneumonitis, bronchiolitis, and diffuse alveolar damage. Some reports have described lipid-laden macrophages. The phenomenon has been observed in people using a wide variety of e-cigarette liquid brands, substances, and devices. The exact cause of EVALI remains to be determined. Of note, over 80% of cases included use of tetrahydrocannabinol (THC). One leading theory suggested by the CDC is that contaminants such as vitamin E acetate oil, which is often used to dilute THC, may be responsible for EVALI. However, although studies have shown that there is an association between the presence of vitamin E acetate in the lungs of victims and the presence of EVALI, these studies have not clearly demonstrated that vitamin E is responsible for the pulmonary problems that develop. Over 60% of the victims of EVALI also used e-liquid that contained nicotine. Although vitamin E acetate and nicotine may contribute to EVALI, additional studies will be necessary to determine the role of these agents. Other than stopping vaping, there is no specific treatment, as yet, for EVALI other than supportive measures and hospitalization if needed. Influenza testing should be considered, and other causes of pneumonia and respiratory distress (including COVID-19) should be ruled out and treated. Some patients have responded to corticosteroids.

COCAINE

History and Epidemiology

Cocaine is an active chemical found in the plant *Erythroxylon coca* and has been used since the Inca empire 5000 years ago. Alfred Neimann isolated cocaine in 1860, and the drug was initially used as a local anesthetic. Because of its special properties, including its stimulant effect, it was mixed with wine (Vin Mariani, 1865) and soft drinks (Coca-Cola, 1888). In 1914, it was legally classified as a narcotic substance, and its use was largely limited to addicts. In the early 1980s, a cheap, potent form of crystallized cocaine, referred to as crack cocaine (so named because of the crackling or popping sound it makes when heated) was introduced, which has led to an increase in cardiac events related to cocaine use.[36] Although cocaine use in the general population is trending downward, it is still one of the most commonly used illicit drugs in subjects seeking care in hospital emergency departments, and it is one of the most frequent causes of drug-related deaths reported by medical examiners in the United States. Importantly, cocaine use is rising among high school students, with a prevalence of approximately 5%.[37]

Pathophysiology

The onset and duration of cocaine's effects depend on its route of use, which consequently leads to varying cardiovascular and hemodynamic effects.[38] In general, the intravenous and inhaled (i.e., smoked) routes have a very rapid onset of action (seconds) and short-lived (30 minutes) duration when compared with the mucosally absorbed (e.g., oral, nasal [i.e., snorted], rectal, vaginal) routes. When applied locally, cocaine acts as an anesthetic by virtue of its inhibition of membrane permeability to sodium during depolarization, thereby blocking the initiation and transmission of electrical signals. When given systemically, it blocks the presynaptic reuptake of norepinephrine and dopamine, thereby producing an excess of these neurotransmitters at the site of the postsynaptic receptor (Fig. 84.4A). Experimental studies in dogs showed cocaine injection led to diffuse coronary artery spasm, reduced regional coronary blood flow, and a marked decrease in both systolic and diastolic cardiac function within minutes.[36] Cocaine induces vasoconstriction in normal coronary arteries but exerts a particularly marked vasoconstrictive effect in diseased segments (Fig. 84.4B). As a result, cocaine users with atherosclerotic coronary artery disease probably have an especially high risk for an ischemic event after cocaine use. Cocaine-induced coronary arterial vasoconstriction results primarily from the stimulation of coronary arterial alpha-adrenergic receptors because it is reversed by phentolamine (an alpha-adrenergic antagonist) and exacerbated by propranolol (a beta-adrenergic antagonist). Although it was suspected initially that the decrease in coronary blood flow was solely responsible for the myocardial dysfunction, rigorous time analysis studies suggested that cocaine has a direct negative effect on cardiac myocytes that can lead to cardiac dysfunction. Cocaine acts as a powerful sympathomimetic agent, with increases in circulating catecholamine levels leading to increases in blood pressure and heart rate, both of which increase oxygen demand.[36] The increase in oxygen demand combined with a decrease in blood supply due to coronary artery vasoconstriction explains various ischemic events temporally related to cocaine use. The effect of intranasal cocaine use in 42 smokers was studied in the catheterization laboratory. Cocaine resulted in an increase in the rate-pressure product, as well as a decrease in the diameter of the diseased segments of the coronary arteries. This combination of increased oxygen demand and decreased myocardial oxygen supply may explain the deleterious effects of cocaine on the human heart.[39] Additional studies suggested that cocaine enhances platelet aggregation, a mechanism that may contribute to the development of MI (Fig. 84.4B).

Clinical Presentation

Considering the deleterious effects that cocaine can have on disrupting the oxygen supply/demand balance in the heart, it is not surprising that chest pain is the chief complaint in cocaine abusers presenting to emergency departments. The risk of MI increases up to 24-fold in the first hour after cocaine abuse.[39] Chest pain may be related to cardiac involvement including acute MI, or alternatively, be noncardiac in nature. Two large-scale registries revealed that the incidence of MI among cocaine abusers who presented with chest pain was only 6%, suggesting that there are likely extracardiac cocaine-related causes of chest pain (e.g., pleuritic, musculoskeletal).

Based on the earlier observations, a stepped approach is recommended for the evaluation of patients presenting with cocaine-related chest pain, to reduce unnecessary hospitalizations and interventions. As shown in Figure 84.5, these patients should be first evaluated by history, physical examination, and vital signs, followed by an ECG and measurement of cardiac troponins. A recent review of 363,143 hospitalized patients with cocaine-induced chest pain revealed that only 0.69% suffered an acute MI. Moreover, the mortality rate in these patients was low (0.09%), suggesting that patients without ST-segment elevation can be safely observed in the emergency department.[40] The current American College of Cardiology (ACC)/AHA guidelines recommend that stable patients with cocaine-related chest pain should be observed for at least 12 hours (see Chapter 39).

Patients with ECG evidence of persistent ST-segment elevation that is nonresponsive to nitrates should be directly referred for coronary angiography, for consideration for possible angioplasty and stent implantation. Management of cocaine-induced MI is similar to non–drug-related MI (see Chapters 37, 38, and 39), with some exceptions. Immediate use of aspirin and clopidogrel is recommended because of the increased platelet aggregation and increased coronary thrombosis (see Fig. 84.4B). Although drug-eluting stents are occasionally used

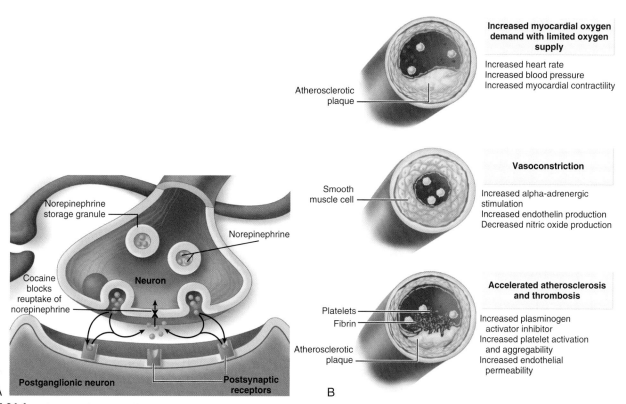

FIGURE 84.4 Mechanisms of cocaine toxicity. **A,** Mechanism by which cocaine alters sympathetic tone. Cocaine blocks the reuptake of norepinephrine by the preganglionic neuron (X), thereby resulting in excess amounts of this neurotransmitter at postganglionic receptor sites. **B,** Mechanisms by which cocaine may induce myocardial ischemia or infarction. Cocaine may induce myocardial ischemia or infarction by increasing the determinants of myocardial oxygen demand in the setting of limited oxygen supply *(top),* causing intense coronary arterial vasoconstriction *(middle)* or inducing accelerated atherosclerosis and thrombosis *(bottom).*

in the management of cocaine abusers, the majority of these patients usually receive bare-metal stents, and both the 2008 and 2012 ACC/AHA scientific statements recommend the use of bare-metal stents in cocaine users.[39] If immediate percutaneous intervention is not available, thrombolytic therapy should be initiated, unless otherwise contraindicated. If the patient's history suggests a low risk for cardiac events, the 12-lead ECG is normal, and the troponin level is within normal limits, then outpatient follow-up is adequate (see Fig. 84.5).

Nitrates, phentolamine (an alpha-receptor blocker), and verapamil (a calcium channel blocker) have been shown to reverse cocaine-induced coronary vasoconstriction in the controlled setting of the cardiac catheterization laboratory and are used to manage cocaine-induced chest pain. Although beta blockers represent an essential therapy in the mitigation of hyperadrenergic states and are known to reduce myocardial oxygen demand, the use of beta blockers in the setting of cocaine-induced vasoconstriction is still debated because of the concern that β_1/β_2-blockade might lead to unopposed alpha-stimulation, resulting in coronary artery vasoconstriction. ACC/AHA guidelines recommend against using beta-blockers in the setting of acute coronary syndromes with signs of acute cocaine intoxication (class III, Level of Evidence: C) unless patients are receiving a vasodilator. More recent studies examining beta blocker use in cocaine-exposed patients with acute coronary syndromes have shown that beta blockers are safe and potentially efficacious.[41] The 2012 AHA/ACC guidelines endorse the use of nonselective beta blockers in patients with persistent hypertensive or tachycardia after cocaine use, provided the patients are treated with a vasodilator (Class IIb, Level of Evidence: C). Although combined beta blocker and alpha blockers (e.g., labetalol and carvedilol) should theoretically be safer than nonselective beta blockers because they avoid unopposed alpha-stimulation, head-to-head comparisons of combined beta blocker and alpha blockers versus nonselective beta blockers have not been performed in patients with cocaine-induced chest pain.

Aortic Dissection

Because aortic dissection or rupture has been temporally related to cocaine use, it should be considered a possible cause of chest pain in cocaine users (see also Chapter 42). Cocaine has been implicated as a causative factor in 0.5% to 37% of cases of aortic dissection, with an average interval from cocaine use to the onset of symptoms of 12 hours (range, 0 to 24). Dissection probably results from a cocaine-induced increase in systemic arterial pressure. In addition to aortic rupture, cocaine-related rupture of mycotic and intracerebral aneurysms has been reported. Also, in patients with suspected MI, the possibility of aortic dissection should be considered before the use of thrombolytic therapy.

Myocardial Dysfunction

Long-term cocaine abuse has been associated with LV hypertrophy, as well as with LV diastolic and/or systolic dysfunction. The presence of LV dysfunction may be related to the occurrence of MI or repetitive episodes of myocardial ischemia. In addition, cocaine exerts a depressant effect on cardiac myocytes in animal studies, as well as in human myocytes. Cases of Takotsubo cardiomyopathy have been described following cocaine use (see Chapter 52).[42] Treatment of symptomatic heart failure arising after cocaine use follows the same guidelines for treating non-cocaine users with heart failure (see Chapter 50).[43] Stopping the use of cocaine may result in a significant improvement of LV function.

Cardiac Arrhythmias

Cardiac arrhythmias are a frequent finding in cocaine users presenting to the emergency department, including various atrial arrhythmias and ventricular arrhythmias such as ventricular extrasystoles, ventricular tachycardia, and ventricular fibrillation. Arrhythmias may be secondary to myocardial ischemia and MI as well as LV dysfunction. Cocaine may affect the generation and conduction of cardiac impulses by several mechanisms. First, its sympathomimetic properties may increase ventricular irritability and lower the threshold for fibrillation. Second, it inhibits action potential generation and conduction (i.e., it prolongs the QRS and QT intervals) as a result of its sodium channel–blocking effects. In so doing, it acts in a manner similar to that of a class I antiarrhythmic agent. Accordingly, Brugada-type electrocardiographic features and torsades de pointes have been observed following cocaine use. Third, cocaine increases the intracellular calcium concentration, which may result in afterdepolarizations and triggered ventricular arrhythmias. Fourth, it reduces vagal activity, thereby potentiating its sympathomimetic effects.

Acute cocaine use may result in ischemic strokes in young adults.[44] The enhanced sympathetic activity, prothrombotic effects, and cerebral vasoconstriction may be contributing factors. Another clinical manifestation of cocaine use is pulmonary hypertension. Similar to systemic hypertension, a retrospective study showed a fivefold increase in pulmonary hypertension in cocaine users compared with an age-sex-race–matched control group.[45]

COCAETHYLENE

In individuals who use cocaine in temporal proximity to the ingestion of ethanol, hepatic transesterification leads to the production of cocaethylene, a unique metabolic by-product of cocaine. Cocaethylene has a similar mechanism of action to cocaine, but it is more potent. Similar to cocaine, cocaethylene blocks reuptake of dopamine at the synaptic cleft, thereby possibly potentiating the systemic toxic

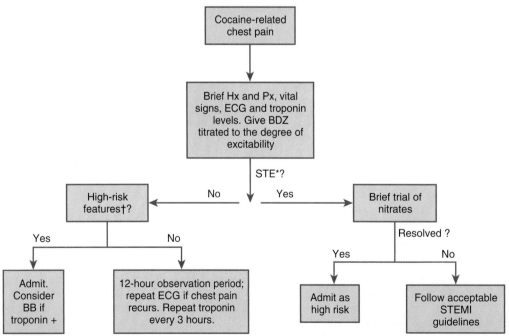

FIGURE 84.5 Algorithm for management of cocaine-induced chest pain in the emergency department. *STE is defined as ST-segment elevation of ≥2 mm. †High-risk features: hemodynamic instability, positive cardiac troponin, recurrent chest pain. *BB*, Beta blocker; *BDZ*, benzodiazepine; *ECG*, electrocardiogram; *STEMI*, ST elevation myocardial infarction. (From Havakuk O, Rezkalla SH, Kloner RA. The cardiovascular effects of cocaine. *J Am Coll Cardiol.* 2017;70:101–113.)

effects of cocaine. People who use cocaine and drink alcohol present with an exaggerated clinical presentation of cocaine use and have a higher mortality rate when compared with either drug alone.[46]

OTHER CARDIAC STIMULANTS

In addition to cocaine, there are a host of other stimulant drugs that can affect the heart.[47] Prescription drugs such as amphetamines and illicitly produced drugs such as methamphetamines and methylenedioxymethamphetamine (MDMA, ecstasy) are examples of some of these agents. These drugs are psychoactive stimulants that can result in sensations of euphoria, empathogenic-entactogenic (feelings of oneness, emotional communion, relatedness, empathy, sympathy), and hallucinations.

Amphetamines and Methamphetamines

The first amphetamines were marketed for nasal congestion, followed by the use amphetamines for narcolepsy and attention-deficit hyperactivity disorders. Some forms of amphetamines are sold illegally, for example, crystal methamphetamine or ice. These agents are central nervous system stimulants that release catecholamines, including norepinephrine, dopamine, and serotonin from presynaptic nerve terminals and prevent their reuptake, resulting in a hyperadrenergic state. These agents can increase heart rate and blood pressure and have been associated with a number of cardiac problems such as chest pain and acute coronary artery syndromes, including acute MI, vasospasm, cardiomyopathy, and acute pulmonary edema.

In a study of 230 patients with a history of acute amphetamine and methamphetamine abuse and positive urine tests (mainly young males), the most common electrocardiographic findings were sinus tachycardia, prolonged QT interval, and arrhythmia (supraventricular and ventricular). Additionally, there were elevations in creatine kinase-MB and troponin I levels. Most patients had normal echocardiograms, while a small number (7%) had LV systolic and/or diastolic dysfunction.[48] In a retrospective study from New Zealand, 30 patients with a history of amphetamine abuse admitted with heart failure and echocardiographic features of cardiomyopathy (LV ejection fraction 22 ± 8%) were identified. At presentation, four were in cardiogenic shock and five required ICU admission for inotropic support and mechanical ventilation. Most did not recover LV function despite optimal treatment, and five died from end stage heart failure.[49] In another study, investigators used the SphygmoCor system to assess the degree of arterial stiffening in users of recreational amphetamines such as "speed," "ecstasy," and "ice." Amphetamine users, both men and women, demonstrated evidence of accelerated cardiovascular aging, even when adjusting for other cardiovascular risk factors.[50] An analysis of 894 cases of methamphetamine-related deaths in Australia revealed a mean age of 38 years, with 79% being male. Of the deaths, 76% were associated with enlarged hearts, and LV hypertrophy was present in 19% of cases. Of all cases, 19% had severe coronary artery disease, and 20% had replacement fibrosis within the cardiac walls. Evidence of hypertension based on histologic findings was present in 33% of cases. The conclusion of this autopsy analysis was that cardiovascular disease was highly prevalent in these patients who used methamphetamine, despite their young age. In another study, young male methamphetamine users were found to have higher blood pressure, greater LV mass, and impaired diastolic ventricular function by echocardiographic measures, compared with age-matched male controls. Additionally, the methamphetamine abusers had evidence of reduced myocardial perfusion by myocardial contrast echocardiography.[51]

Methamphetamine use has also now been associated with a dissection of multiple coronary arteries, heart failure, and severe ischemic cardiomyopathy. Experimental studies showed that methamphetamine induces cardiac damage by increasing apoptosis (programmed cell death) in cardiomyocytes and reducing protein expression of melusin (a protein that is a mechanotransducer and is important in maintaining normal cardiac function).[52]

Pulmonary hypertension has also been associated with methamphetamine use (see Chapter 88).[53] In contrast to patients with idiopathic pulmonary hypertension, patients with methamphetamine-associated pulmonary hypertension were more likely to be males, have more severe symptoms of heart failure, have higher right atrial

pressure, and demonstrate lower stroke volume index. The patients with methamphetamine-related pulmonary hypertension had more than double the risk of deteriorating clinically and dying compared with patients with idiopathic pulmonary hypertension. The authors concluded that methamphetamine-associated pulmonary artery hypertension is an especially severe form of pulmonary hypertension that is progressive and has a poor outcome.

Khat and Cathinones

Khat is a flowering plant used for its neurostimulant effect. It has two active ingredients: cathine and cathinone. The plant is native to East Africa and the Arabian peninsula and is used in cultural and social situations. Khat is chewed like tobacco, can be made into tea or chewable paste, or can be smoked or added to food. Like other stimulants, it has sympathomimetic properties and is associated with increased heart rate and blood pressure. Khat has been linked to MIs, dilated cardiomyopathy, hypertension, and stroke. Synthetic cathinones, often marketed as "bath salts," have also been associated with cardiac disease, including sudden death and myocarditis.[54]

MARIJUANA

Marijuana is a psychoactive substance produced by drying the leaves and flowering tops of several species of the cannabis plant. It contains several endogenous cannabinoids, the most studied of which is trans-Δ^9-tetrahydrocannabinol (Δ–9–THC). THC is the active component of marijuana that is responsible for its psychoactive properties; it also has sympathomimetic effects that have been linked to cardiovascular side effects.[55] The cannabinoids in marijuana exert their effects by binding two cannabinoid receptors: cannabinoid receptor 1 (CB_1) and cannabinoid receptor 2 (CB_2). CB_1 and CB_2 both belong to a superfamily of metabotropic G protein–coupled receptors. CB_1 receptors are found predominantly in neurons of the brain, whereas CB_2 receptors are present in immune cells, vascular smooth muscle cells, and cardiac myocytes.

The effect of smoking marijuana on the cardiovascular system has been studied in healthy volunteers. Marijuana use resulted in an increase in pulse rate (thereby increasing myocardial oxygen demand) and various electrocardiographic changes, such as P wave abnormalities, as well as nonspecific ST and T wave abnormalities shortly after use. These effects were blocked by beta blockers.[55] The cardiovascular and many other side effects led the Surgeon General of the United States to issue a warning about the cardiac toxicity of marijuana use more than four decades ago. Despite that, and despite federal government laws declaring marijuana use illegal, many states in the United States have legalized marijuana use for recreational purposes. By early 2021, 16 states and the District of Columbia legalized the drug for such recreational purposes, and 36 states plus the District of Columbia legalized the use of medical marijuana. This section of the chapter focuses on various reported cardiovascular effects of marijuana use. It should be noted that the current medical literature is based on temporal associations between marijuana use and increased cardiovascular events, and the safety of marijuana has not been evaluated in controlled studies.

Atrial Arrhythmias

Various atrial arrhythmias have been reported following marijuana use.[56] Both tachycardias and sinus bradycardia have been reported after smoking the drug. The patients often were relatively young, without known risk factors, and the atrial arrhythmias were temporally related to the drug use. The most commonly reported atrial arrhythmia is atrial fibrillation, which was reported in 26% of published cases.[57]

Ventricular Arrhythmias

Ventricular arrhythmias, such as premature ventricular beats and ventricular tachycardia, have been reported to occur in people following marijuana use. The authors reported a case of syncope after marijuana use, associated with inducible ventricular tachycardia during electrophysiology study and no-reflow during coronary angiography. After the patient stopped using marijuana, no-reflow resolved and the ventricular tachycardia was no longer inducible.[58] There are no controlled studies determining the incidence of ventricular tachycardias in marijuana users.

Abouk et al.[59] studied the rate of death attributed to the cardiovascular system in the states that legalized marijuana. They compared death rates before and then after legalizing marijuana. There was a significant increase in death rate after legalizing marijuana, which was more pronounced in men. Whether this observation was secondary to ventricular arrhythmias, coronary artery disease, or other causes is not known. Other reports described unexpected sudden cardiac death following marijuana use, as well as synthetic cannabinoid use.[60]

Acute Coronary Syndromes

Marijuana inhalation results in increased myocardial oxygen demand in addition to creation of reactive oxygen radicals, endothelial dysfunction, and effects on human platelets. Most reports strongly suggest an increase in the incidence of acute coronary syndromes following marijuana use. Patients tend to be younger, with no other significant risk factors for the development of MI. Angiography during presentation of ST-segment elevation MI showed coronary thrombosis in normal coronary arteries or at sites in mildly atherosclerotic arteries. Some cases had normal appearing epicardial coronary arteries with coronary artery no-reflow.

Colorado was one of the earlier states to legalize marijuana use. Review of emergency department records in Colorado showed an increase in cardiovascular events following legalization of recreational use of marijuana.[61] In a report from France, there was an increase in patients who presented to the emergency department following marijuana use. When compared with nonusers who presented with similar cardiovascular complications, there was a 25% increase in mortality in those who were marijuana users. The increase in marijuana use in the United States, and indeed in many other countries across the world, and the emergence of more potent marijuana plants and synthetic cannabinoids clearly compound the problem. A study using hospital records from the national inpatient sample in the United States showed an increase in the number of marijuana users who were admitted with acute cardiovascular events. Figure 84.6 illustrates the cardiovascular complications of marijuana. Not all reports suggest a relation between marijuana use and cardiovascular events, however. A long-term follow-up of the CARDIA study followed young marijuana users for 25 years. Neither recent use nor cumulative lifetime marijuana use was associated with increased incidence of cardiovascular events.[62] However, this study may represent older preparations of marijuana and lower THC concentrations than are now present in contemporary marijuana preparations.

Neurologic Events

Marijuana use may result in cognitive dysfunction, behavioral problems, and memory attention disorders. Additionally, reports of ischemic strokes, and rarely hemorrhagic strokes, were reported. Transient ischemic attacks were reported as well. The mechanisms of such events are not well elucidated but are likely similar to that of cardiac ischemic events. Data from the Behavioral Risk Factor Surveillance System show that marijuana use for therapeutic and recreational purposes results in increased stroke incidence in young adults with recent use.[63] The odds of stroke occurrence increased in subjects who used the drug frequently compared with those who only occasionally used the drug.

Cannabidiol Oil

Cannabidiol (CBD) oil is a product derived from the plant cannabis sativa. CBD is another component of marijuana, but it lacks the psychoactive effect of THC. It has a favorable effect as a pain reliever, anti-inflammatory, and anxiety-relieving agent. No cardiac side effects were noticed during the use of CBD oils, and there are reports that it may reduce both resting and stress-induced hypertension.[64]

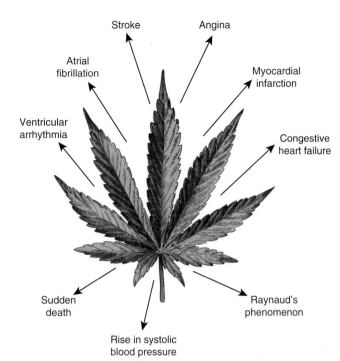

FIGURE 84.6 Cardiovascular complications of marijuana. (Modified from Rezkalla S, Kloner RA. Cardiovascular effects of marijuana. *Trends Cardiovasc Med.* 2019;29:403–407.)

ENERGY DRINKS AND CAFFEINE

Energy drinks have become increasingly popular as a dietary supplement among young people in the United States. They are often used to enhance physical performance, mental acuity, and concentration, to induce weight loss, to improve energy level, and to counteract the effects of alcohol. They contain a number of stimulants, primarily caffeine, which is usually present in much higher concentrations than in coffee or other beverages. For example, energy drinks may contain between 154 and 505 mg of caffeine in a 16- to 24-ounce can, whereas a 6.5-ounce cup of coffee contains 80 to 120 mg of caffeine, tea has 50 mg, and a 12-ounce can of cola has no more than 65 mg of caffeine.[65] Other stimulants found in energy drinks may include guarana, a plant from South America (also known as Brazilian cocoa) that is also high in caffeine content but is typically not included in the total estimate of caffeine in energy drinks. These beverages also contain taurine, sugars, ginseng (which can increase blood pressure), B vitamins, and other additives. Caffeine has sympathomimetic effects and increases cytosolic calcium concentration by inhibiting calcium reuptake in the sarcoplasmic reticulum. It can increase sinus rate, but in doses associated with moderate coffee drinking it does not stimulate atrial fibrillation, nor is it associated with ventricular arrhythmias at moderate doses. However, caffeine overdose is associated with tachycardia, arrhythmias, and hypertension. Energy drinks, especially when taken in excess, can be associated with cardiac arrhythmias, prolonged QT interval, MI, cardiac death, and aortic dissection.[66] Increases in heart rate, blood pressure, and stroke volume and contractility can occur with energy drink excess. Svatikova et al.[67] studied 25 healthy volunteers randomized to receive either placebo or a commercially available energy drink. In this study, the energy drink increased systolic, diastolic, and mean blood pressure and increased norepinephrine levels, but did not increase heart rate. Some reports of acute MI associated with energy drinks revealed patent coronary arteries at the time of catheterization, while one was associated with an intracoronary thrombus. Coronary vasospasm and/or increased platelet aggregation due to energy drinks have been considered possible mechanisms by which MI occurred. In one systematic study of platelet aggregation, volunteers were given water or energy drinks, and platelet function was measured before and 60 minutes after consumption. Energy drinks caused a significant increase in platelet aggregability to arachidonic acid–induced activation, but not with several other activating factors.[68] Practitioners and consumers should be made aware of the potential cardiac dangers of energy drinks.

OPIATES

Opioids are drugs used for pain relief, but their use is often abused, and in recent years this has resulted in increased use with deleterious consequences and the "opioid crisis" in the United States. Examples of opioids include opium, morphine, heroin, hydrocodone, oxycodone, and fentanyl. One of the leading side effects of opioids is respiratory depression that can lead to respiratory arrest. However, opioids have important adverse cardiovascular effects as well. Some of these drugs prolong the QT interval, a phenomenon that can result in the life-threatening ventricular arrhythmia, torsades de pointes, which can cause sudden cardiac death. Methadone is high risk for causing QT prolongation and ventricular arrhythmias, even at low doses. Tramadol, fentanyl, and oxycodone are intermediate in risk and may be more of a problem at higher doses. Morphine and buprenorphine are lower risk and do not usually cause QT prolongation or torsades de pointes at routine dosing levels. Other arrhythmias have been reported in opium consumers including supra-ventricular arrhythmias, atrial fibrillation, sinus bradycardia, and heart block, especially in those with underlying heart disease.[69] Opioids can also cause hypotension, bradycardia, and can reduce cardiac contractility. One study showed that opioids and sedatives represent independent risk factors for in-hospital cardiopulmonary arrest and resuscitation.[70] High doses of opioids should be used with caution, and periodic monitoring of the ECG and QT interval should be considered in high-risk users and patients participating in opioid maintenance treatment programs, where they are exposed to these drugs on a chronic basis. There has been concern that opioids might be associated with an increase in atherosclerotic diseases. In a large prospective cohort study of over 29,000 participants over 5 years, female prescription opioid users—but not male users—had a higher risk of coronary heart disease and cardiovascular death. There was no increase in stroke among opioid users.[71]

HEAVY METALS

Heavy metals have been implicated in heart disease, but many of the studies are older and may include exposures that are now outdated (e.g., cobalt in beer). A recent meta-analysis showed exposure to the heavy metals arsenic, lead, cadmium, and copper was associated with increased cardiovascular disease including coronary artery disease and stroke. However, mercury was not associated with an increase in cardiovascular disease.[72] Heavy metal exposure (including exposure to cadmium, lead, and mercury) has been implicated as contributing to metabolic syndrome. A recent analysis concluded that, although heavy metals may contribute to this syndrome, data were inconclusive and sometimes conflicting; the authors recommended a need for better prospective, standardized studies to determine the importance of heavy metals in the mechanism of metabolic syndrome.[73] People can be exposed to cadmium through food, cigarette smoke, air pollution, or occupational exposure. Cadmium increases reactive oxygen species and depletes natural antioxidants. Exposure to this heavy metal has been associated with endothelial and smooth muscle dysfunction, hypertension, atherosclerosis, and diabetes. Although chelation therapy is one approach to removing cadmium, recent studies suggest that the antioxidants curcumin and tetrahydrocurcumin may play a protective role in dealing with cadmium exposure.[74] A recent analysis showed that prenatal exposure to lead was a risk factor for congenital heart disease in the child (see Chapter 82).[75] Iron overload or hemochromatosis of the cardiovascular system is discussed in other sections of this book (see Chapter 52).

FUTURE DIRECTIONS

In this chapter, we discussed a variety of natural and synthetic drugs and toxins linked to significant deleterious cardiac events. Unfortunately, the precise mechanism of their effects is often unknown, and as a result, effective treatment is not established. This information is essential to avoid agents that interfere with specific molecular pathways that regulate cardiac function and to develop therapy that limits cardiotoxicity. Health care providers and the patients or subjects who use these drugs would benefit from a true understanding of their potential risks to the cardiovascular system. Finally, when new medications are approved for use, postmarketing studies should be required to identify any cardiotoxic effects that may occur infrequently and hence are not evident when the drug is studied in limited numbers of subjects, or only in the presence of concomitant conditions.

ACKNOWLEDGMENT

The authors gratefully acknowledge the editing and technical support of Marie Fleisner in the preparation of this chapter.

REFERENCES

Alcohol

1. Maisch B. Alcoholic cardiomyopathy. The result of dosage and individual predisposition. *Herz.* 2016;41:484–493.
2. Axley PD, Richardson CT, Singal AK. Epidemiology of alcohol consumption and societal burden of alcoholism and alcoholic liver disease. *Clin Liver Dis.* 2019;23:39–50.
3. Han BH, Moore AA, Ferris R, Palamar JJ. Binge drinking among older adults in the United States, 2015-2017. *J Am Geriatr Soc.* 2019;67:2139–2144.
4. Steiner JL, Lang CH. Etiology of alcoholic cardiomyopathy: mitochondria, oxidative stress and apoptosis. *Int J Biochem Cell Biol.* 2017;89:125–135.
5. Piano MR. Alcohol's effects on the cardiovascular system. *Alcohol Res.* 2017;38:219–241.
6. Mirijello A, Tarli C, Vassallo GA, et al. Alcoholic cardiomyopathy: What is known and what is not known. *Eur J Intern Med.* 2017;43:1–5.
7. Wang Y, Li G, Sun Y, et al. Left ventricular strain and rotation by 2-D speckle tracking echocardiography identify early alcoholic cardiomyopathy. *Ultrasound Med Biol.* 2016;42:1741–1749.
8. Li X, Nie Y, Lian H, Hu S. Histopathologic features of alcoholic cardiomyopathy compared with idiopathic dilated cardiomyopathy. *Medicine (Baltim).* 2018;97:e12259.
9. Guzzo-Merello G, Segovia J, Dominguez F, et al. Natural history and prognostic factors in alcoholic cardiomyopathy. *JACC Heart Fail.* 2015;3:78–86.
10. Amor-Salamanca A, Guzzo-Merello G, Gonzalez-Lopez E, et al. Prognostic impact and predictors of ejection fraction recovery in patients with alcoholic cardiomyopathy. *Rev Esp Cardiol.* 2018;71:612–619.
11. Gallagher C, Hendriks JM, Elliott AD, et al. Alcohol and incident atrial fibrillation—a systemic review and meta-analysis. *Int J Cardiol.* 2017;246:46–52.
12. Voskoboinik A, Kalman JM, De Siliva A, et al. Alcohol abstinence in drinkers with atrial fibrillation. *N Engl J Med.* 2020;382:20–28.
13. Brown KN, Yelamanchili VS, Goel A. Holiday heart syndrome. In: *StatPearls.* Treasure Island (FL): StatPearls Publishing; 2020.
14. Haseeb S, Alexander B, Baranchuk A. Wine and cardiovascular health: a comprehensive review. *Circulation.* 2017;136:1434–1448.
15. Whitfield JB, Heath AC, Madden PAF, et al. Effects of high alcohol intake, alcohol-related symptoms and smoking on mortality. *Addiction.* 2018;113:158–166.
16. Guzzo-Merello G, Dominguez F, Gonzalez-Lopez E, et al. Malignant ventricular arrhythmias in alcoholic cardiomyopathy. *Int J Cardiol.* 2015;199:99–105.
17. Vu KN, Ballantyne CM, Hoogeveen RC, et al. Causal role of alcohol consumption in an improved lipid profile: the Atherosclerosis Risk in Communities (ARIC) Study. *PloS One.* 2016;11:e0148765.
18. Padro T, Muñoz-García N, Vilahur G, et al. Moderate beer intake and cardiovascular health in overweight individuals. *Nutrients.* 2018;10:1237.
19. You M, Arteel GE. Effect of ethanol on lipid metabolism. *J Hepatol.* 2019;70:237–248.
20. Migliori M, Panichi V, de la Torre R, et al. Anti-inflammatory effect of white wine in CKD patients and healthy volunteers. *Blood Purif.* 2015;39:218–223.
21. Relja B, Menke J, Wagner N, et al. Effects of positive blood alcohol concentration on outcome and systemic interleukin-6 in major trauma patients. *Injury.* 2016;47:640–645.
22. Giacosa A, Barale R, Bavaresco L, et al. Mediterranean way of drinking and longevity. *Crit Rev Food Sci Nutr.* 2016;56:635–640.
23. Orio L, Anton M, Rodriguez-Rojo IC, et al. Young alcohol binge drinkers have elevated blood endotoxin, peripheral inflammation and low cortisol levels: neuropsychological correlations in women. *Addict Biol.* 2018;23:1130–1144.
24. Xia N, Daiber A, Forstermann U, Li H. Antioxidant effects of resveratrol in the cardiovascular system. *Br J Pharmacol.* 2017;174:1633–1646.
25. Golan R, Shai I, Gepner Y, et al. Effect of wine on carotid atherosclerosis in type 2 diabetes: a 2-year randomized controlled trial. *Eur J Clin Nutr.* 2018;72:871–878.
26. Li Y, Pan A, Wang DD, et al. Impact of healthy lifestyle factors on life expectancies in the US population. *Circulation.* 2018;138:345–355.
27. Rehm J, Gmel G, Sierra C, Gual A. Reduction of mortality following better detection of hypertension and alcohol problems in primary health care in Spain. *Adicciones.* 2018;30:9–18.

E-Cigarettes

28. MacDonald A, Middlekauff HR. Electronic cigarettes and cardiovascular health: what do we know so far? *Vasc Health Risk Manag.* 2019;15:159–174.
29. Buchanan ND, Grimmer JA, Tanwar V, et al. Cardiovascular risk of electronic cigarettes: a review of preclinical and clinical studies. *Cardiovasc Res.* 2020;116:14–50.
30. Franzen KF, Willig J, Cayo Talavera S, et al. E-Cigarettes and cigarettes worsen peripheral and central hemodynamics as well as arterial stiffness: a randomized, double-blinded pilot study. *Vasc Med.* 2018;23:419–425.

31. Lee WH, Ong S-G, Zhou Y, et al. Modeling cardiovascular risks of e-cigarettes with human-induced pluripotent stem cell-derived endothelial cells. *J Am Coll Cardiol*. 2019;73:2722–2737.

32. Hajek P, Phillips-Waller A, Przulj D, et al. A randomized trial of E-cigarettes versus nicotine-replacement therapy. *N Engl J Med*. 2019;380:626–637.

33. Alzahrani T, Pena I, Temesgen N, Glantz SA. Association between electronic cigarette use and myocardial infarction. *Am J Prev Med*. 2018;55:455–461.

34. Ndunda PM. Electronic cigarette use is associated with a higher risk of stroke. *Stroke*. 2019;50:A9.

35. Layden JE, Ghinai I, Pray I, et al. Pulmonary illness related to E-cigarette use in Illinois and Wisconsin—Final Report. *N Engl J Med*. 2020;382:903–916.

Cocaine

36. Stankowski RV, Kloner RA, Rezkalla SH. Cardiovascular consequences of cocaine use. *Trends Cardiovasc Med*. 2015;25:517–526.

37. Schneider KE, Krawczyk N, Xuan Z, Johnson RM. Past 15-year trends in lifetime cocaine use among US high school students. *Drug Alcohol Depend*. 2018;183:69–72.

38. Anderson JL, Adams CD, Antman EM, et al. 2012 ACCF/AHA focused update incorporated into the ACCF/AHA 2007 guidelines for the management of patients with unstable angina/non-ST-elevation myocardial infarction: a report of the American College of Cardiology Foundation/American Heart Association Task Force on Practice Guidelines. *J Am Coll Cardiol*. 2013;61:e179–e347.

39. Havakuk O, Rezkalla SH, Kloner RA. The cardiovascular effects of cocaine. *J Am Coll Cardiol*. 2017;70:101–113.

40. Singh V, Rodriguez AP, Thakkar B, et al. Hospital admissions for chest pain associated with cocaine use in the United States. *Am J Med*. 2017;130:688–698.

41. Pham D, Addison D, Kayani W, et al. Outcomes of beta blocker use in cocaine-associated chest pain: a meta-analysis. *Emerg Med J*. 2018;35:559–563.

42. Gill D, Sheikh N, Ruiz VG, Liu K. Case report: cocaine-induced takotsubu cardiomyopathy. *Hellenic J Cardiol*. 2018;59:129–132.

43. Nguyen P, Kamran H, Nasir S, et al. Comparison of frequency of cardiovascular events and mortality in patients with heart failure using versus not using cocaine. *Am J Cardiol*. 2017;119:2030–2034.

44. Cheng YC, Ryan KA, Qadwai SA, et al. Cocaine use and risk of ischemic stroke in young adults. *Stroke*. 2016;47:918–922.

45. Alzghoul BN, Abualsuod A, Alqam B, et al. Cocaine use and pulmonary hypertension. *Am J Cardiol*. 2020;125:282–288.

46. Jones AW. Forensic drug profile: cocaethylene. *J Anal Toxicol*. 2019;43:155–160.

Other Stimulants

47. Duflou J. Psychostimulant use disorder and the heart. *Addiction*. 2020;115:175–183.

48. Bazmi E, Mousavi F, Giahchin L, et al. Cardiovascular complications of acute amphetamine abuse. Cross-sectional study. *Sultan Qaboos Univ Med J*. 2017;17:e31–e37.

49. Kueh S-HA, Gabriel RS, Lund M, et al. Clinical characteristics and outcomes of patients with amphetamine-associated cardiomyopathy in South Aukland, New Zealand. *Heart Lung Circ*. 2016;25:1087–1093.

50. Reece AS, Norman A, Hulse GK. Acceleration of cardiovascular-biological age by amphetamine exposure is a power function of chronological age. *Heart Asia*. 2017;9:30–38.

51. Darke S, Duflou J, Kaye S. Prevalence and nature of cardiovascular disease in methamphetamine-related death: a national study. *Drug Alcohol Depend*. 2017;179:174–179.

52. Sun X, Wang Y, Xia B, et al. Methamphetamine produces cardiac damage and apoptosis by decreasing melusin. *Toxicol Appl Pharmacol*. 2019;378:114543.

53. Zamanian RT, Hedlin H, Greuenwald P, et al. Features and outcomes of methamphetamine-associated pulmonary arterial hypertension. *Am J Respir Crit Care Med*. 2018;197:788–800.

54. Zaami S, Giorgetti R, Pichini S, et al. Synthetic cathinones related fatalities: an update. *Eur Rev Med Pharmacol Sci*. 2018;22:268–274.

Marijuana

55. Rezkalla S, Kloner RA. Cardiovascular effects of marijuana. *Trends Cardiovasc Med*. 2019;29:403–407.

56. Kariyanna PT, Wengrofsky P, Jayarangaiah A, et al. Marijuana and cardiac arrhythmias: a scoping study. *Int J Clin Res Trials*. 2019;4:132.

57. Adegbala O, Adejumo AC, Olakanmi O, et al. Relation of cannabis use and atrial fibrillation among patients hospitalized for heart failure. *Am J Cardiol*. 2018;122:129–134.

58. Rezkalla S, Stankowski R, Kloner RA. Cardiovascular effects of marijuana. *J Cardiovasc Pharmacol Ther*. 2016;21:452–455.

59. Abouk R, Adams S. Examining the relationship between medical cannabis laws and cardiovascular deaths in the US. *Int J Drug Policy*. 2018;53:1–7.

60. Drummer OH, Gerostamoulos D, Woodford NW. Cannabis as a cause of death: a review. *Forensic Sci Int*. 2019;298:298–306.

61. Roberts BA. Legalized cannabis in Colorado emergency departments: a cautionary review of negative health and safety effects. *West J Emerg Med*. 2019;20:557–572.

62. Reis JP, Auer R, Bancks MP, et al. Cumulative lifetime marijuana use and incident cardiovascular disease in middle age: the Coronary Artery Risk Development in Young Adults (CARDIA) study. *Am J Public Health*. 2017;107:601–606.

63. Parekh T, Pemmasani S, Desai R. Marijuana use among young adults (18–44 Years of age) and risk of stroke: a behavioral risk factor surveillance system survey analysis. *Stroke*. 2020;51:308–310.

64. Sultan SR, O'Sullivan SE, England TJ. The effects of acute and sustained cannabidiol dosing for seven days on the haemodynamics in healthy men: a randomised controlled trial. *Br J Clin Pharmacol*. 2020;86:1125–1138.

Energy Drinks and Caffeine

65. Sifferlin A. What's in your energy drink? *Time Magazine*. Feb 04, 2013. https://healthland.toime.com/2013/02/04whats-in-your-energy-drink/.

66. Mangi MA, Rehman H, Rafique M, Illovsky M. Energy drinks and the risk of cardiovascular disease: a review of current literature. *Cureus*. 2017;9:e1322.

67. Svatikova A, Covassin N, Somers KR, et al. A randomized trial of cardiovascular responses to energy drink consumption in healthy adults. *J Am Med Assoc*. 2015;314:2079–2082.

68. Pommerening MJ, Cardenas JC, Radwan ZA, et al. Hypercoagulability after energy drink consumption. *J Surg Res*. 2015;199:635–640.

Opiates and Heavy Metals

69. Behzadi M, Joukar S, Beik A. Opioids and cardiac arrhythmia: a literature review. *Med Princ Pract*. 2018;27:401–414.

70. Overdyk FJ, Dowling O, Marino J, et al. Association of opioids and sedatives with increased risk of in-hospital cardiopulmonary arrest from an Administrative Database. *PloS One*. 2016;11:e0150214.

71. Khodneva Y, Muntner P, Kertesz S, et al. Prescription opioid use and risk of coronary heart disease, stroke, and cardiovascular death among adults from a prospective cohort (REGARDS study). *Pain Med*. 2016;17:444–455.

72. Chowdhury R, Ramond A, O'Keeffe LM, et al. Environmental toxic metal contaminants and risk of cardiovascular disease: systemic review and meta-analysis. *BMJ*. 2018;362:k3310.

73. Planchart A, Green A, Hoyo C, Mattingly CJ. Heavy metal exposure and metabolic syndrome: evidence from human and model system studies. *Curr Environ Health Rep*. 2018;5:110–124.

74. Kukongviriyapan U, Apakjit K, Kukongviriyapan V. Oxidative stress and cardiovascular dysfunction associated with cadmium exposure: beneficial effects of curcumin and tetrahydrocurcumin. *Tohuku J Exp Med*. 2016;239:25–38.

75. Ou Y, Bloom MS, Nie Z, et al. Associations between toxic and essential trace elements in maternal blood and fetal congenital heart defects. *Environ Int*. 2017;106:127–134.

85 Cardiovascular Abnormalities in HIV-Infected Individuals

PRISCILLA Y. HSUE AND DAVID D. WATERS

Approximately 37,900,000 people were living with human immunodeficiency virus (HIV) infection at the end of 2018, and 1,700,000 had become newly infected that year.[1] An estimated 23,300,000 people living with HIV were accessing antiretroviral therapy (ART), up from 7,700,000 in 2010.[1] The introduction of ART in 1996 and its increasingly widespread availability since then have dramatically reduced HIV-related mortality rates and has transformed HIV into a chronic disease for those receiving treatment. As a consequence, between 2010 and 2030 the proportion of people with HIV infection aged 50 years or older will increase from 28% to 73%, and the proportion with cardiovascular disease (CVD) from 19% to 78%.[2] Over the same period the proportion taking a cardiovascular (CV) drug is projected to increase from 9% to 50%.

The types of CVD associated with HIV have changed from the pre-ART to the ART eras, (Fig. 85.1) and will likely evolve further.[3] In the pre-ART era, people with acquired immunodeficiency syndrome (AIDS) often had pericardial effusions and dilated cardiomyopathy; these complications still occur in persons without access to ART. Following the introduction of protease inhibitors (PIs) in the late 1990s, manifestations of atherosclerosis, specifically myocardial infarction (MI) and stroke, became prominent, and heart failure (HF), atrial fibrillation (AF), and sudden cardiac death have emerged.

CARDIOVASCULAR RISK FACTORS IN PEOPLE LIVING WITH HIV

People living with HIV have elevated traditional coronary risk factors, particularly those receiving ART, compared with noninfected persons. Dyslipidemia, metabolic syndrome, hypertension, and cigarette smoking are all more prevalent among subjects with HIV, leading to higher calculated Framingham risk scores in this group than in noninfected individuals. In the North American AIDS Cohort Collaboration on Research and Design, smoking, hypercholesterolemia, and hypertension were calculated to account for 37%, 44%, and 42% of MIs, respectively.[4] These risk factors also contributed to cancers and end-stage renal disease. Thus CV risk factors should merit aggressive treatment in people with HIV.

Dyslipidemia

The onset of HIV infection associates with a decrease in total cholesterol, low-density lipoprotein cholesterol (LDL-C), and high-density lipoprotein cholesterol (HDL-C), and an increase in triglyceride levels.[5] The effect of ART on lipid levels varies among the classes of ART drugs and even varies among drugs within the same class. Two or three ART drugs are usually used in combination to block replication of the virus by more than one mechanism. As a consequence, the effect of single drugs can be difficult to ascertain. As a general rule, PIs, nonnucleoside reverse transcriptase inhibitors (NNRTIs), and nucleoside reverse transcriptase inhibitors (NRTIs) increase triglyceride levels and may increase LDL-C levels.[5] The probability that each ART drug will adversely affect lipid levels is classified as low, intermediate, or high (Table 85.1).

PIs increase triglyceride levels; in particular, ritonavir can cause extreme hypertriglyceridemia exceeding 1000 mg/dL. Ritonavir-saquinavir, ritonavir-lopinavir, and ritonavir-tipranavir combinations can also increase triglycerides. Atazanavir, either alone or in combination with ritonavir, associates less with an increase in triglycerides compared with these other PIs. Older PIs such as ritonavir also increase LDL-C, probably by increasing intestinal cholesterol absorption and not by increased synthesis. PIs have variable effects on HDL-C levels, which are often already low in persons with HIV due to smoking.

NNRTIs also increase LDL-C levels but do not depress HDL-C levels.[5] Among NNRTIs, efavirenz associates with slightly more subjects developing hypercholesterolemia and hypertriglyceridemia in one study compared with nevirapine. Efavirenz can associate with greater increases in LDL-C but not total to HDL-C ratio compared with atazanavir-ritonavir. The newer NNRTI rilpivirine generally associates with lower total, HDL-C, LDL-C, and triglyceride levels than efavirenz. The NRTI tenofovir alafenamide, a newer formulation of tenofovir disoproxil fumarate (TDF), is associated with higher levels of LDL-C and HDL-C but similar total cholesterol to HDLC ratios compared with TDF.[5]

The integrase strand transfer inhibitors (INSTIs), raltegravir, elvitegravir, and dolutegravir, and the C-C chemokine receptor type 5 coreceptor antagonist maraviroc have favorable effects on lipids, particularly compared with older forms of ART. Switching from a ritonavir-boosted PI regimen to darunavir/cobicistat can reduce triglyceride levels.[6]

1604

DISEASES OF THE MYOCARDIUM, PERICARDIUM, AND PULMONARY VASCULATURE BED

FIGURE 85.1 Overview of changes in HIV treatment and HIV-associated cardiovascular diseases. The types of cardiovascular complications associated with HIV infection have changed in the pre-antiretroviral therapy (ART) and ART eras and are likely to continue evolving in the future as new medications and treatment approaches emerge. In the pre-ART era, dilated cardiomyopathy and pericardial effusions were the most commonly reported cardiovascular issues in patients living with HIV. After the introduction of protease inhibitors in the late 1990s, atherosclerotic complications including myocardial infarction were described. More recently, reports of heart failure and rhythm abnormalities are now emerging in the setting of HIV infection. In the future, among individuals with access to ART, HIV infection will be a chronic disease state with increased risk of coronary artery disease. *CCR5,* CC-chemokine receptor 5; *NNRTI,* non-nucleoside reverse-transcriptase inhibitor; *NRTI,* nucleoside reverse-transcriptase inhibitor.

TABLE 85.1 Probability of Adverse Effects on Lipid Levels with HIV Drugs

LIPID EFFECTS	PI	NRTI	NNRTI	INSTI	OTHER CLASSES
Low	Atazanavir	Tenofovir	Nevirapine	Raltegravir	Maraviroc
	Atazanavir/Ritonavir	Abacavir	Etravirine	Elvitegravir	Enfuvirtide
		Lamivudine	Rilpivirine	Dolutegravir	Ibalizumab
		Emtricitabine	Doravirine	Bictegravir	
Intermediate	Saquinavir/Ritonavir	Zidovudine	Efavirenz		Cobicistat
	Darunavir/Ritonavir	Didanosine			
	Fosamprenavir/Ritonavir				
High	Lopinavir/Ritonavir	Stavudine			
	Tipranavir/Ritonavir				
	indinavir/ritonavir				

HIV, Human immunodeficiency virus; *INSTI,* integrase strand transfer inhibitors; *NNRTI,* non-nucleoside reverse transcriptase inhibitor; *NRTI,* nucleoside reverse transcriptase inhibitor; *PI,* protease inhibitor.

Most of the studies examining the effects of ART on lipid levels were of relatively short duration and were usually carried out in North American or European populations. However, ART is now initiated most often in people living in sub-Saharan Africa, where less data are available on the metabolic effects of treatment. In a recent meta-analysis of 14 trials of 21,023 individuals assessed between 2003 and 2014 from this region, ART associated with an increased risk of hypertriglyceridemia (RR 2.05, 95% CI, 1.51 to 2.77).[7] No consistent associations were seen between ART and raised blood pressure, glucose, hemoglobin A$_{1c}$, and other lipids across these studies.

The use of newer ART with fewer adverse lipid consequences might lead to a reduction in CV risk among patients living with HIV. However, although not affecting lipids, integrase inhibitors cause weight gain,[8] which may increase CV risk particularly after long-term use.

Lipodystrophy, the Metabolic Syndrome, and Obesity

Lipodystrophy is a syndrome characterized by fat accumulation in the dorsocervical region and an increase in or preservation of visceral fat, with subcutaneous and peripheral fat loss, resulting in relative central adiposity. Early PIs and the NRTIs stavudine and didanosine associated with lipodystrophy in at least 20% to 35% of persons taking these drugs long term, but newer PIs such as atazanavir do not appear to induce lipodystrophy.

Lipodystrophy in people with HIV commonly associates with features of the metabolic syndrome: insulin resistance, impaired glucose tolerance, hypertriglyceridemia, low HDL-C levels, and hypertension. The prevalence of the metabolic syndrome in subjects with HIV varies from 8.5% to 52% in published reports, with rates at the higher end of this range reported in Latin American countries and rates at the lower end in multicenter studies where patients had less exposure to ART.[9] Development of the metabolic syndrome was common in the first 3 years after initiation of an ART regimen that included stavudine or lopinavir/ritonavir, but is less common with newer drugs. Most studies indicate that the metabolic syndrome predicts for CVD and death in persons with HIV.[9]

A growing body of recent evidence suggests that INSTIs cause weight gain and an increased prevalence of obesity.[10] In some circumstances, weight gain might not be viewed as harmful; for example, someone with advanced HIV beginning treatment, where weight gain would be part of a return-to-health phenomenon, or weight gain after switching from a regimen that caused anorexia or nausea and vomiting. In a pooled analysis of weight gain in eight randomized, controlled trials of 5680 treatment-naïve subjects with HIV, INSTI use associated with more weight gain than were PIs or NNRTIs, with dolutegravir and bictegravir associated with more weight gain than elvitegravir/cobicistat.[11] Among NNRTIs, rilpivirine was linked to more weight gain than efavirenz. Among NRTIs, tenofovir alafenamide associated with more weight gain than TDF, abacavir, or zidovudine. Weight gain was more common in women, African Americans, and those with lower CD4 cell counts. The long-term implications of weight gain in the setting of integrase inhibitors and HIV on CVD have not been well studied at this time.

Diabetes

Whether HIV infection itself associates with an increased risk of diabetes or whether the increased risk relates only to specific ART drugs has been controversial. The PIs indinavir and lopinavir/ritonavir and the thymidine analogue stavudine can cause insulin resistance[9]; however, these drugs are no longer recommended for initial treatment of HIV owing to their toxicity. In a large cohort study from Denmark, the risk of diabetes among patients with HIV infection was nearly triple that of the general population in 1996–1999, but this excess was absent in 1999–2010. The difference in risk in the two periods is likely due to a decreased use of drugs with adverse metabolic consequences.

In a meta-analysis of 39 studies of CV risk factors in 13,698 people with HIV, the prevalence of diabetes was 7.24% but ranged from 0.5% to 39.1%.[12] Diabetes is more prevalent in persons with HIV compared with controls in some studies; for example, in an HIV cohort in Malawi where subjects had received ART for more than 10 years, the prevalence of diabetes was higher than in controls at all ages studied, and at age 60 or older was 13.2% in persons with HIV compared with 1.7% in controls.[13]

Among people with HIV, physical inactivity associates strongly with CV risk factors, including diabetes. In a study of 11,719 individuals with HIV, only 13% reported high levels of physical activity.[14] Compared with this group, those reporting very low levels of physical activity were more likely to have elevated triglycerides, obesity, hypertension, and diabetes. Other factors may play a role in the development of diabetes, including chronic inflammation, poor control of HIV disease, hepatitis C co-infection, along with demographic factors such as older age and male gender.

Hypertension and Chronic Kidney Disease

The prevalence of hypertension among persons with HIV averaged 19.8%, ranging from 4.8% to 63.3%, in the recent, large meta-analysis, mentioned earlier, where the prevalence of diabetes was 7.24%.[12] In studies comparing subjects living with HIV to uninfected controls, hypertension is not consistently higher in the HIV groups; however, both hypertension and prehypertension increase the risk of MI in the presence of HIV, just as in uninfected persons.[15]

In a meta-analysis comprising 61 studies and more than 200,000 subjects with HIV, with balanced geographic distribution, the prevalence of chronic kidney disease (CKD) varied from 6.4% with the MDRD equation, 4.8% with CKD-EPI, and 12.3% with Cockcroft-Gault.[16] CKD was more prevalent in Africa and less prevalent in Europe compared with other regions. CKD associated with hypertension and diabetes but not sex, hepatitis B or C co-infection, CD4 count, or ART status.

When CKD is defined as either albuminuria or a decreased glomerular filtration rate, it associates with an increased risk of CV events in people with HIV. Among 35,357 subjects with HIV in the D:A:D cohort, lower glomerular filtration rate associated strongly with a higher risk of CVD.[17] The development of CKD in persons with previously normal renal function has been reported with some forms of ART; specifically, TDF and the PIs atazanavir/ritonavir and lopinavir/ritonavir.[18]

Smoking

Smoking rates are two to three times higher in HIV cohorts compared with the general population, in the range of 40% to 70% in most studies, and with a high average number of pack-years.[19] Vaping is also prevalent among people with HIV but has as yet received little attention in the literature. Among 3251 subjects from the Danish HIV Cohort Study and 13,004 controls from the Copenhagen General Population Study, the population-attributable fraction of current or past smoking for MI was 72% (95% CI 55% to 82%) for HIV-infected individuals and 24% (95% CI, 3% to 40%) for controls.[19] If all current smokers stopped smoking, 42% (95% CI 21% to 57%) and 21% (95% CI 12% to 28%) of all MIs could potentially be avoided in the HIV and control populations.

In a previous study these investigators calculated that more life-years were lost from smoking than with HIV: 12.3 life-years (95% CI 8.1 to 16.4) compared with 5.1 life-years (95% CI 1.6 to 8.5). A 35-year-old living with HIV had a median life expectancy of 62.6 years if a smoker and 78.4 years if a non-smoker. These numbers illustrate the importance of stopping smoking in the context of HIV. Smoking cessation programs have the same modest success rates in people with HIV infection as in individuals without HIV. In a meta-analysis of eight trials including 1822 patients with HIV who were smokers, behavioral interventions increased abstinence rates by half.[20] Intensive group therapy can double the rate of quitting, to 13% compared with 6.6% in controls in one study of subjects with HIV, but the difference had dissipated by 6 months.[21] In another recent study of HIV subjects, the doubling of the quit rate persisted to 3 years, albeit at low levels, 10.3% versus 4.2% of controls.[22]

Potential drug-drug interactions between ART and smoking cessation drugs have not been well studied. Reports of varenicline, bupropion, and nicotine-replacement therapy in people with HIV infection have generally been small, short, and uncontrolled but have shown similar safety and success rates to reports in individuals without HIV infection.

Smoking may contribute to worsening of HIV-related damage in the heart, kidney, and brain. Neurocognitive defects are common among older people living with HIV and are more prevalent and severe in smokers than in non-smokers.[23] A quarter to half of persons living with HIV have deficits in multiple cognitive domains, including memory, verbal fluency, processing speed, and executive function, impairing their ability to accomplish many common tasks of daily living. Nicotine has antiinflammatory properties, and nicotine withdrawal may worsen neurocognitive defects.[23] The presence of neurocognitive defects predicts failure of smoking cessation. Smoking thus impairs quality of life, as well as markedly shortening the duration of life in subjects with HIV. Smoking cessation reduces CV events in subjects living with HIV.[3] The incidence of MI decreases within the first year and at 2 to 3 years was much reduced, although still double the rate of non-smokers with HIV. Thus, smoking cessation is a very desirable goal.

MECHANISMS OF HIV-RELATED ATHEROGENESIS

The pathogenesis of atherosclerosis in the setting of HIV infection is complicated and incompletely understood. Contributing mechanisms include the effects of the HIV proteins on immune and vascular cells, the immunodeficiency caused by the HIV infection, co-infection with cytomegalovirus (CMV), translocation of microbial products from the gut, chronic inflammation, and immune activation (Fig. 85.2).

In individuals receiving ART with undetectable levels of the virus, the HIV infection is not cured and low-level transcription of HIV genes persists. HIV-encoded proteins such as transactivator of transcription

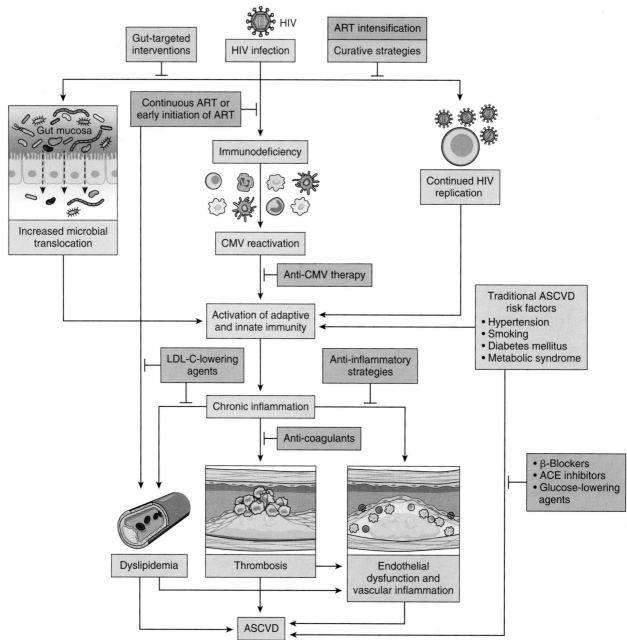

FIGURE 85.2 Pathophysiology and management of HIV-associated atherosclerotic cardiovascular disease. Schematic representation of the effects of HIV infection (*pink*) and the available strategies (*green*), as well as approaches under investigation (*purple*), for reducing the risk of atherosclerotic cardiovascular disease (ASCVD) and chronic inflammation in this patient population. In the setting of HIV infection, the increased microbial translocation from the gut, the continued HIV viral replication, and the HIV-induced immunodeficiency, along with traditional ASCVD risk factors, contribute to immune cell activation and chronic inflammation. HIV-specific interventions to reduce the risk of ASCVD include strategies targeted at co-infections (such as cytomegalovirus infection), use of newer antiretroviral therapies (ARTs) and intensification of ART. Strategies aimed at eradicating the HIV infection are under investigation. Treatments targeting traditional ASCVD risk factors, such as hypertension, diabetes mellitus, smoking and metabolic syndrome, are also critical for reducing the risk of ASCVD in patients living with HIV. Use of anticoagulants, beta blockers, angiotensin-converting enzyme (ACE) inhibitors and LDL cholesterol (LDL-C)-lowering agents (such as statins and PCSK9 inhibitors) reduce the risk of ASCVD in patients with cardiovascular disease without HIV infection and might, therefore, be useful in reducing the risk of HIV-associated ASCVD. Finally, strategies to lower inflammation, such as canakinumab, which has been reported to reduce cardiovascular events significantly in a non-HIV patient population, might also reduce the risk of HIV-associated ASCVD.

(Tat) and negative factor (Nef) induce inflammation and endothelial dysfunction.[24] In addition, the HIV envelope protein gp120 can stimulate endothelin-1 production.

CD4+ T cell depletion is the hallmark of HIV infection, and nadir CD4+ T cell count is a rough marker of the severity of immunodeficiency. Nadir CD4+ T cell count has been linked to increased carotid intima-media thickness (IMT), increased arterial stiffness, and incident MI.[3] The CD4:CD8 ratio, a marker of immunosenescence, predicts CV events in some but not in other studies. Thus, markers of immune system damage and viral detectability relate to CV events in HIV. Immune abnormalities persist in individuals with HIV infection even after successful treatment with ART. The mechanisms linking immune system damage to atherosclerosis have not been elucidated. Although

non–AIDS-related events, such as MI and stroke, are less common with complete viral suppression, such events still occur at rates higher than in an uninfected population.

Co-infection with CMV might play a part in HIV-associated atherosclerosis. Compared with uninfected individuals, subjects with HIV consistently have a higher proportion of CMV-specific CD8+ cells, with the highest levels seen in those receiving long-term ART with HIV suppression. CMV co-infection links strongly to HIV viral persistence and may also have a role in chronic immune activation and inflammation by expansion of the HIV reservoir. These CMV-specific T cell responses also correlate with markers of atherosclerosis, such as coronary artery calcification (CAC) and carotid IMT.[25] In the setting of HIV infection, high antibody titers to CMV, and to herpes simplex and varicella-zoster virus, associate with higher levels of biomarkers that accelerate inflammation and atherosclerosis.

Impairment of the gut barrier is an early feature of HIV infection, leading to microbial translocation, a process whereby microbial products leak through the intestinal barrier and cause immune activation.[3,26] Plasma levels of markers of microbial translocation such as soluble CD14 and lipopolysaccharide independently predict HIV disease progression and mortality in individuals not receiving ART. Whether these markers predict adverse outcomes in ART-treated individuals is unsettled; however, gut damage and microbial translocation persist even when HIV infection is suppressed by ART.[26] Plasma levels of the inflammatory markers interleukin-6 (IL-6) and tumor necrosis factor may be higher in individuals with higher levels of markers of microbial translocation. Although microbial translocation is thus another mechanism that might contribute to HIV-associated atherogenesis, interventions targeting this mechanism, specifically sevelamer, rifaximin, probiotics, and mesalamine, have not consistently lowered inflammatory markers or T cell activation.[3]

The three mechanisms discussed earlier, latent HIV infection, co-infection with other viruses, and microbial translocation, all stimulate atherogenesis by increasing inflammation. HIV infection associates with high plasma levels of inflammatory and coagulation markers, specifically C-reactive protein (CRP), IL-6, and D-dimer, and these biomarkers strongly predict CV events and all-cause mortality in individuals with HIV infection.[27] Subjects with HIV infection have higher arterial and lymph node inflammation as assessed by FDG-PET and CT imaging than uninfected individuals, and this marker of increased inflammation correlates with higher circulating levels of CRP, IL-6, and activated monocytes.[28]

Inflammation is a therapeutic target to reduce CV events in individuals with or without HIV infection (see Fig. 85.2). Statin therapy reduces inflammation, but the effects of statins on inflammatory markers seem to be attenuated in the presence of HIV infection.[29] Neither intensification of ART nor changing PI-based regimens to integrase inhibitors consistently reduces inflammatory markers. Short studies of aspirin treatment also had no effect on inflammatory markers in HIV infection.[30] Taken together, these findings suggest that strategies beyond ART and treatment of traditional CV risk factors are needed to reduce inflammation with the aim of lowering the risk of atherosclerosis in the setting of HIV infection.

Canakinumab, a monoclonal antibody targeting IL-1β, reduces CV events in patients with previous MI and a high-sensitivity CRP level of ≥2 mg/L.[31] In an on-treatment analysis, canakinumab-treated subjects who had a CRP reduction to <2 mg/L had significant reductions in CV endpoints, whereas no significant reduction in these outcomes was observed in patients who did not achieve a CRP reduction to this level.[32] Similar success was reported for individuals who achieved on-treatment IL-6 levels less than the study median value but not for those who did not.[33]

Would canakinumab reduce CV events in the setting of HIV? In a small study of subjects with HIV infection, canakinumab significantly reduced plasma IL-6 and CRP levels, with no effect on CD4, CD8, or RNA viral levels.[34] Inflammation in the bone marrow and arterial inflammation fell after canakinumab administration. By contrast, in the general population with stable atherosclerosis, methotrexate did not reduce inflammatory markers or improve clinical outcomes.[35] In a clinical trial in treated HIV, methotrexate lowered CD8 T cells and did not impact inflammation or endothelial function.[36] These small preliminary studies with inflammatory biomarkers as surrogate endpoints will hopefully lead to larger clinical trials of antiinflammatory therapies with CV endpoints in the population living with HIV.

Markers of inflammation and coagulation predict CV and other adverse events in individuals with HIV infection (Table 85.2).[37,38] The strong relationship between these markers and outcomes appears consistently across diverse HIV-infected populations including men, women, and different age groups. In combined data from three large cohorts of individuals with HIV infection, a 25% decrease in IL-6 or D-dimer levels in plasma associated independently with a 37% reduction in non-AIDS events or mortality.[39]

Biomarkers in HIV infection tend to group into clusters, with each cluster related to a cardiac phenotype.[40] The inflammatory phenotype is characterized by higher levels of CRP, IL-6, and D-dimer, whereas the cardiac cluster comprises higher levels of protein ST2 (also known as IL-1

receptor-like 1), N-terminal pro-B-type natriuretic peptide and growth/differentiation factor 15. Diastolic dysfunction is common with the inflammatory cluster of biomarkers, and pulmonary hypertension (PH) is more common in the cardiac cluster. Both groups associate with a three-fold increase in mortality over a 6.9-year follow-up after adjustment for other prognostic variables.[40] These biomarker clusters in patients with HIV might be helpful for selecting patients for appropriate therapy to prevent CV events.

The most obvious mechanism by which ART increases atherosclerosis is by worsening blood lipid levels. Interestingly, even after adjustment for blood lipid levels in the large D:A:D study, cumulative exposure to the NRTIs abacavir or didanosine or to the PIs lopinavir-ritonavir or indinavir associated with an increased risk of MI.

ART might also increase the risk of CV events through other mechanisms. Insulin resistance, lipodystrophy, and other patterns of fat distribution can contribute to atherogenesis. The NRTI abacavir has been linked to an increased risk of MI in some but not all studies. This increased risk has been attributed to increased platelet reactivity and to endothelial dysfunction. In the D:A:D study, a difference in the risk of MI was noted between two widely used PIs, with atazanavir being associated with a lower risk than darunavir. This reduced risk of MI may result from a protective effect of atazanavir because it increases bilirubin levels and elevated bilirubin levels independently predict lower incident CVD in HIV.[41] Overall, although current ART regimens appear to confer a much lower risk of CV events than older ART, longer-term data on newer regimens will be needed to ascertain this benefit.

Features of Atherosclerosis in People with HIV

Cardiac computed tomography (CCT) provides insight into the features of coronary disease in HIV patients.[42] The prevalence of CAC by CCT was not higher in HIV-infected individuals compared with controls across seven studies. However, CT angiographic studies reveal that noncalcified plaques are much more common in persons living with HIV than in uninfected controls.[43] In a meta-analysis of nine studies including 1229 HIV patients and 1029 controls, the prevalence of coronary stenosis greater than 30% or greater than 50%, or calcified plaques did not differ between HIV patients and controls.[44] However, noncalcified plaques were more than three times more likely to be present in HIV patients, 58% compared with 17%. Noncalcified plaques are more likely to be lipid-laden and inflammatory and exhibit imaging features associated with plaque rupture. HIV subjects with higher levels of arterial inflammation as assessed by FDG-PET imaging were more likely than those with lower levels of inflammation to have plaques with high-risk features.[45]

In non-HIV cohorts, carotid IMT associates with prevalent CVD and risk factors as well as increased risk of future stroke and MI. Many observational studies have compared carotid IMT in individuals with HIV and in controls.[42] Across these studies, carotid IMT averaged 0.04 mm thicker (95% CI 0.02 to 0.06 mm, p < 0.001) in subjects with HIV than in uninfected controls.[42] This conclusion should be viewed with caution due to differences among the studies in population characteristics, study designs, sample sizes, and ultrasound techniques. In some studies with serial measurements, carotid IMT progressed more rapidly in the HIV group than in controls. Carotid plaque also occurs more commonly in HIV patients compared with uninfected controls across six studies.[42] Carotid IMT independently predicts mortality in HIV.[46]

CORONARY DISEASE IN HIV SUBJECTS

Epidemiology

A recent systematic review that included 80 longitudinal studies with 793,635 individuals with HIV found a relative risk of CVD in persons living with HIV of 2.16 (95% CI 1.68 to 2.77) compared with uninfected individuals.[47] This risk resembles that of hypertension, diabetes, lipids, and smoking.[48] Over the past 26 years, the global population-attributable fraction of CVD due to HIV has tripled and now approaches 1%, with the greatest impact in sub-Saharan African and the Asia Pacific regions.[47] Thus the contribution of HIV to CVD is still small overall, but in an HIV-infected individual, HIV is as potent as any classical risk factor.

TABLE 85.2 Biomarkers of Inflammation and Coagulation Are Associated with Adverse Events in HIV Infection

STUDY (YEAR)	STUDY POPULATION	NUMBER OF PATIENTS	FOLLOW-UP	FINDINGS
SMART (2008)	Subjects with well-controlled HIV from 33 countries	5472	3700 person-years	IL-6 and D-dimer levels in plasma were strongly associated with all-cause mortality IL-6, CRP, and D-dimer levels in plasma were associated with increased risk of CVD
FRAM (2010)	Subjects with HIV	922	5 years	Fibrinogen and CRP levels were strong and independent predictors of mortality
ALLRT (2014)	Subjects with HIV and virologic suppression <1 yr after ART initiation	143	48–64 weeks after ART initiation	High IL-6, sTNFRI, sTNFRII, and D-dimer plasma levels and KT ratio at 1 year were associated with increased risk of non-AIDS events
VACS (2016)	Subjects with HIV and uninfected controls	2350	6.9 years	HIV infection was associated with elevated IL-6, sCD14, and D-dimer levels in plasma, which are associated with mortality
MACS (2016)	Subjects with well-controlled HIV	670	Up to 18 years	IL-6 and sCD14 levels in plasma were predictive of mortality
START (2017)	Subjects with HIV from 35 countries	4299	3.2 years	Baseline IL-6 and D-dimer levels in plasma were associated with the risk of AIDS, serious non-AIDS events or death

ART, Antiretroviral therapy; *CRP,* C-reactive protein; *CVD,* cardiovascular disease; *HIV,* human immunodeficiency virus; *IL-6,* interleukin-6; *KT,* kynurenine:tryptophan; *sCD14,* soluble CD14; *sTNFRI,* soluble tumor necrosis factor receptor type I; *sTNFRII,* soluble tumor necrosis factor receptor type II.

In addition to the elevated risk of an acute coronary syndrome (ACS), subjects with HIV have involvement of other vascular beds. The incidence of ischemia stroke increased by 25% in HIV-infected men compared with uninfected subjects in the Veterans Aging Cohort Study.[49] Peripheral arterial disease as assessed by ankle-brachial index was higher in subjects living with HIV compared with controls in a study from Copenhagen, and the difference persisted after adjustment for classic CV risk factors.[50]

Clinical Presentation

The clinical presentation of ACS differs in HIV-infected compared with uninfected individuals. HIV-infected individuals with ACS are on average more than a decade younger and are more likely to be men, to be current smokers, and to have low HDL-cholesterol levels. Their risk scores tend to be lower, and they are more likely to have single- rather than multiple-vessel coronary artery disease. In general, subjects with HIV hospitalized with ACS have excellent immediate outcomes.

In earlier studies, people with HIV had substantially higher rates of restenosis after percutaneous coronary interventions with bare metal stents, compared with uninfected individuals. More recent studies in which most patients received drug-eluting stents show similar medium-term outcomes between HIV subjects and matched controls.[51] A report from the Nationwide Inpatient Sample detected no increase in in-hospital mortality among 9771 HIV-infected individuals undergoing cardiac surgery, including coronary bypass, compared with matched, uninfected controls.[52] Long-term outcome studies after coronary bypass surgery have not been reported in large cohorts of persons living with HIV.

Some data indicate that HIV status of ACS patients influences the likelihood of receiving guideline-directed investigations and treatments. For example, in a U.S. Nationwide Impatient Sample from 2002 to 2011, comparing nearly 4000 HIV MI patients with more than 1.3 million uninfected MI patients, subjects with HIV were less likely to undergo invasive management (adjusted odds ratio [OR] 0.59, 95% CI 0.55 to 0.65), to undergo coronary bypass surgery (OR 0.66, 95% CI 0.57 to 0.76) or to receive drug-eluting stents (OR 0.83, 95% CI 0.76 to 0.92).[53] In a cohort of HIV subjects, 388 of 812 (48%) adjudicated MI were classified as type 2 MI (related to demand ischemia), a much higher rate than those reported in non-HIV populations.[54]

Treatment

The treatment of CHD in HIV-infected individuals should largely be guided by existing recommendations for uninfected patients in the absence of clinical trial data specific to HIV. However, two aspects specific to HIV deserve mention: (1) the potential contribution of ART to CVD, and (2) the treatment of lipid levels in HIV disease, for which separate guidelines have been devised.

Antiretroviral Therapy and Cardiovascular Disease

Since ART first became available in the 1990s, the indications for treatment and specific drug regimens have evolved rapidly. In earlier years, when the benefits of ART were more limited and treatment-related adverse effects were more common, the initiation of treatment was often delayed until subjects were at increased risk of immunosuppression. More recent studies suggest that the chronic immune stimulation and inflammation that accompanies early asymptomatic HIV infection can result in long-term morbidity. Thus, whereas treatment was initially restricted to those with low CD4 counts, it is now widely accepted that treatment should be started in all individuals with HIV infection with detectable viremia irrespective of CD4 cell count.[55] Initiation of ART is recommended as soon as possible in the setting of acute HIV infection because initiation prior to the development of HIV antibody positivity reduces the size of the latent HIV reservoir, reduces immune activation, and may protect against infection of central memory T cells. Early compared with deferred initiation of ART reduced AIDS-related and non–AIDS-related events in the START trial; this benefit did not reach statistical significance for CV outcomes, however.[56] Furthermore, early initiation of ART associated with increases in total and LDL-C but also decreased use of blood pressure medication.[57] The impact of early ART on CVD and CV risk in HIV remains unknown.

Planned discontinuation of early ART after a specific treatment duration is not recommended because the benefits do not persist and the subsequent viral rebound associates with increased clinical events and the potential for transmission.[55] Initiation of ART in elite controllers, defined as subjects with confirmed HIV infection and persistent undetectable HIV RNA without ART, remains controversial.[58] Of note, elite controllers are more likely to be hospitalized than individuals with controlled HIV, with CV hospitalizations being the most common.[59]

What combinations of drugs are recommended for initial therapy? The INSTIs have moved into a key role as first-line therapy because they are highly effective, with higher and more rapid rates of virologic suppression compared with PIs and NNRTIs, the previous mainstays of ART. INSTIs have the additional advantage of being extremely well tolerated. As discussed previously, weight gain is being increasingly recognized as a disquieting feature of modern ART combinations, with INSTIs being the main culprit.

TABLE 85.3 Metabolic Pathways of Statins and Interactions with ART

DRUG	METABOLISM	LIPOPHILIC	ART INTERACTIONS	COMMENT
Lovastatin	CYP3A4	Yes	PI, NNRTI	Limited potency
Simvastatin	CYP3A4	Yes	PI, NNRTI	Contraindicated
Pravastatin	Partial hepatic	No	PI	Limited potency
Fluvastatin	CYP2CY, CYP3A4	Yes		Limited potency
Atorvastatin	CYP3A4	Yes	PI	More potent
Rosuvastatin	CYP2C9 (<10%)	No	PI	More potent
Pitavastatin	Glucuronidation	Yes		Least D-D interaction; limited potency

ART, Antiretroviral therapy; *D-D,* drug-drug; *NNRTI,* non-nucleoside reverse transcriptase inhibitor; *PI,* protease inhibitor.

Guidelines recommend initial ART combinations.[55] Up to 96% of individuals who remain in care and receive ART have undetectable plasma HIV RNA levels. Several non–INSTI-containing regimens suppress HIV RNA in most subjects who adhere to therapy. These may be chosen based on individual clinical features, preferences, financial considerations, or unavailability of INSTIs.[55]

Pregnant women, those with hepatitis B or C co-infection, or those with opportunistic infections require modifications to ART.[55] Osteoporosis and fractures increase with HIV infection. During the first year or two after initiation of ART, patients may lose 2% to 6% of their bone mineral density. TDF-containing regimens associate with a greater initial decline in bone mineral density than TAF- or abacavir-containing regimens; thus, TDF is not recommended for patients with osteopenia or osteoporosis.[55]

Monitoring of kidney function with eGFR, urinalysis, and testing for glycosuria and albuminuria or proteinuria is recommended when ART is initiated or changed and every 6 months (along with HIV RNA) once HIV RNA is stable. TDF, especially with a boosted PI, increased the risk of CKD in cohort studies and thus is not recommended for subjects with an eGFR of less than 60 mL/min. Long-term data on TAF in subjects with preexisting renal disease are limited. TDF or TAF should be discontinued if renal function worsens, particularly if there is evidence of proximal tubular dysfunction.[55] Switching from TDF to TAF associates with an increase in lipids, mainly LDL-C and triglycerides.[60]

Improvements in ART have reduced the frequency of needing to switch drugs because of virologic failure and drug resistance. However, these improvements provide a rationale for switching therapy in some individuals who have virologic suppression with older regimens that are less convenient or that have more adverse effects. Reasons for considering switching therapy in such individuals include the development of adverse effects, the desire to reduce dosages or the number of pills taken, the occurrence of drug-drug interactions, or pregnancy. Some individuals may benefit from switching even if they are doing well on their current treatment. For instance, switching is reasonable for those taking regimens containing stavudine, didanosine, or zidovudine, because of long-term toxic effects, or older PIs that have higher pill burdens and greater metabolic toxicities than darunavir or atazanavir. Some drugs that are no longer recommended for initial use may be safely continued if well tolerated. For example, although nevirapine and efavirenz have substantial early toxic effects, they are safe and tolerable in the long term.[55]

Recommendations for laboratory monitoring include as close to the time of HIV diagnosis as possible and before beginning ART, measurement of: CD4 cell count; plasma HIV RNA level; serologic studies for hepatitis A, B, and C; serum chemistries, estimated creatinine clearance; complete blood cell count, and urine glucose and protein and genotyping for resistance to reverse transcriptase and PIs. Routine pretreatment screening for integrase resistance is not currently recommended. Screening for syphilis and mucosal nucleic acid amplification testing for chlamydia infection and gonorrhea should also be done at the time of HIV diagnosis, and a lipid profile should be obtained. Other laboratory assessments should be individualized, in keeping with current guidelines. If ART is initiated on the first visit, all laboratory specimens should be drawn before the first dose.

Treatment of Lipids in the Setting of HIV

Diet and lifestyle optimization should form the foundation for treatment of lipids in persons living with HIV.[5] As with all overweight individuals, caloric restriction and exercise should be used to attain ideal body weight. Reducing carbohydrate intake can improve triglyceride levels. In one report, fasting triglyceride levels and adipose tissue mass decreased, and muscle mass increased in HIV-infected men with hypertriglyceridemia after 16 weeks of resistance training. Nevertheless, diet and exercise by themselves rarely suffice to achieve adequate control.

A large number of controlled clinical trials have documented that LDL-C lowering, usually with statins, reduces the risk of CV events across a broad spectrum of patients without HIV infection. Similar data are not yet available for people living with HIV; however, the Randomized Trial to Prevent Vascular Events in HIV (REPRIEVE; clinicaltrials.gov NCT02344290) will address this issue. This trial has enrolled 7700 HIV-infected subjects without known CVD and randomized them to pitavastatin 4 mg/d or to placebo. The primary endpoint of REPRIEVE is a composite of CV events, and the trial is scheduled to be completed in early 2023.

Until recently, guidelines for cholesterol management have not specifically addressed individuals living with HIV. The 2016 European Society of Cardiology (ESC)/European Atherosclerosis Society (EAS) guidelines devote a short section to individuals with HIV infection and recommend dietary changes and exercise, as well as switching, when feasible, to a more lipid-friendly ART.[61] These guidelines also state that statin therapy should be considered to achieve the target LDL-C level of less than 2.6 mmol/L (100 mg/dL), the same target that is recommended for other patients at high risk of CVD.

The U.S. National Lipid Association recommended considering HIV infection as an independent risk factor for selecting drug therapy to lower LDL-C levels[62] but do not set specific LDL-C targets for subjects with HIV. Unfortunately, the 2013 American College of Cardiology/American Heart Association (ACC/AHA) guidelines based treatment recommendations on risk assessment tools that appear to be inaccurate in the setting of HIV. For example, in one recent study, high-risk coronary plaque morphology was seen on coronary CT angiography in 36% of 108 HIV patients, but the guidelines would recommend treatment for only 19% of them.[63] Similarly, in another study the guidelines failed to recommend therapy for two-thirds of individuals with HIV who had carotid plaque on ultrasound imaging.[64] The 2018 updated ACC/AHA guidelines state that HIV infection can be considered a CVD risk enhancer, which would favor starting moderate-intensity or high-intensity statin therapy.[65] These guidelines also recommend that a risk assessment, including fasting lipid profile, be done before and 4 to 12 weeks after starting ART.

Drug-drug interactions must be considered when using lipid-lowering drugs in persons living with HIV (Table 85.3). A systemic review of 18 clinical trials in HIV-infected subjects receiving ART confirmed that statin administration is safe when drug-drug interactions are taken into account.[66] Lovastatin and simvastatin are contraindicated with PIs because of the risk of rhabdomyolysis from high statin blood levels.[5] For the same reason, no more than 40 mg/day of atorvastatin should be used for individuals taking ritonavir-boosted PIs. Rosuvastatin blood levels increase when used with atazanavir/ritonavir and lopinavir/ritonavir, so limiting the rosuvastatin dose to 10 mg is advisable with these drugs. Pravastatin and fluvastatin are safe but do not lower LDL-C as much as atorvastatin or rosuvastatin. These weaker statins were widely used after the introduction of ART but are less popular now because of the growing realization, reflected in contemporary guidelines, that greater degrees of LDL-C lowering produce greater CV event reduction.[5] The proportion of subjects with HIV who had contraindicated statin use from PI has decreased from 2007 to 2015 but has increased in the setting of cobicistat-containing ART regimens,[54] which has similar interactions with statins to ritonavir.

Despite a lack of clinical trial outcomes data, pitavastatin is a good choice for individuals living with HIV because at higher doses its LDL-C–lowering effect is moderate, and because its metabolism is via glucuronidation, drug-drug interactions are avoided.[5] In a randomized, double-blind comparison study in 252 subjects with HIV, pitavastatin 4 mg/day reduced LDL-C by 31% and pravastatin 40 mg/day reduced LDL-C by 21%, with similar low rates of adverse events in the two treatment groups.[67]

As with other patients, statins should be the mainstay of lipid-lowering drug therapy for persons living with HIV. Several studies indicate that statins are underused in the setting of HIV even among eligible individuals.[68] In individuals with HIV who do not tolerate statins, ezetimibe is a safe option, albeit with limited LDL-C–lowering potency. Ezetimibe should be considered as add-on therapy for very-high-risk individuals with HIV who do not achieve sufficient LDL-C lowering with statins. Bile acid sequestrants are not recommended in the context of HIV because they increase triglyceride levels and their effects on the absorption of ART drugs have not been studied.[5] Add-on therapy can be problematic for individuals with HIV because they often already suffer from a high pill burden from ART and other medications.

Proprotein convertase subtilisin/kexin type 9 (PCSK9) inhibitors have not been widely studied in the setting of HIV but have several inherent advantages in this condition, including profound LDL-C lowering, a reduction in pill burden, avoidance of the drug-drug interactions of statins, and ease of use in patients with chronic liver disease, a common problem in this population. PCSK9 levels may be higher in persons with HIV compared with uninfected controls.[5] Switching ART to drugs that do not adversely affect lipid levels is a worthwhile strategy as long as viral suppression is maintained. Switching from older PIs to INSTIs can improve lipid levels but at the cost of an increased risk of virologic failure and thus is not recommended for individuals with a history of virologic failure.[5] Adding a statin might be preferable to switching for those not already taking a statin; in one study the addition of rosuvastatin 10 mg per day yielded better lipid results and was better tolerated compared with switching.[69]

Hypertriglyceridemia is a common finding in individuals with HIV and probably increases the risk of a CV event. Reducing alcohol and carbohydrate intake has a favorable effect in people with or without HIV infection. Consideration should be given to a change in ART to drugs that induce less hypertriglyceridemia. Fibrates reduce triglycerides, often at low doses, but have a drug-drug interaction with statins and some types of ART; for example, the lopinavir-ritonavir PI combination greatly reduces gemfibrozil absorption.[5] Monitoring of hepatic enzymes and creatine phosphokinase levels is advised for patients taking ART, a statin, and a fibrate. When triglycerides are greater than 1000 mg/dL, pancreatitis is a serious risk and urgent treatment is required.

Omega-3 fatty acids found in fish oil reduce triglyceride levels in persons with HIV and hypertriglyceridemia and has the advantage of no important drug-drug interactions; however, some fish oil preparations increase LDL-C levels modestly.[5] The Reduction of Cardiovascular Events with Icosapent Ethyl-Intervention Trial (REDUCE-IT) tested the effect of icosapent ethyl, a purified and quality-controlled pharmaceutical-grade eicosapentaenoic acid preparation, 2 g twice daily as add-on therapy with statins in 8179 patients with CVD or diabetes and other CV risk factors, and a fasting triglyceride level of 150 to 499 mg/dL.[70] After a median follow-up of 4.9 years, the primary endpoint, a composite of CV events, occurred in 17.2% of the icosapent ethyl patients compared with 22.0% of the placebo patients (HR 0.75, 95% CI 0.68 to 0.83). Although outcome data such as this are not available in the context of HIV, icosapent ethyl should now be considered as treatment for such persons with triglyceride levels in this range.

RISK ASSESSMENT AND SCREENING FOR CORONARY DISEASE

The tools used to calculate CV risk in the general population, (Framingham Risk Score, Systematic Coronary Risk Evaluation [SCORE] and the ACC/AHA pooled cohort equation), function poorly in HIV-infected cohorts.[71] A prediction model specific to HIV includes clinical variables, lipid levels, CD4 lymphocyte count, and ART history; a reduced model omits ART.[72] In the hands of its developers, the model performed better than the Framingham Risk Score, even after the Framingham score had been recalibrated to the HIV population. Studies comparing different models have reported that they yield quite different results with less overlap than would be expected. A recent AHA statement concluded that a clear best risk estimation model for HIV has not been identified.[73] Whatever risk assessment tool is use may underestimate true risk in the HIV population.

A 2019 AHA statement proposed a pragmatic approach to CV risk assessment in individuals with HIV (Fig. 85.3). The presence and extent of CAC as assessed by a CT scan strongly predict CV events in the general population and may be a useful risk assessment tool in subjects with HIV and intermediate risk.[73]

The 2019 AHA statement recommends consideration of selected CV risk enhancers identified in the 2018 ACC/AHA cholesterol clinical practice guidelines as likely atherosclerotic cardiovascular disease (ASCVD) risk enhancers in HIV (see Fig. 85.3).[73] These include early family history of MI or stroke (men, age <55 years; women, age <65 years), persistently elevated LDL-C ≥160 mg/dL, CKD, preeclampsia or premature menopause, subclinical atherosclerosis on imaging (including CAC), and high levels of selected biomarkers associated with elevated CV risk independently of traditional risk factors, specifically lipoprotein(a), CRP, and apolipoprotein B.

Cardiac screening for coronary disease may be cost-effective in intermediate risk subjects with HIV.[74] Of note, the ACC/AHA guidelines failed to recommend statin in more than two-thirds of HIV-infected individuals with evidence of carotid plaque >1.5 mm.[75] Depending on the clinical features of a patient, either screening for CAC, IMT, or a stress test would be an appropriate first step. An electrocardiogram should be done in all HIV-infected adults, and an echocardiogram is reasonable because of the high prevalence of left ventricular (LV) hypertrophy and LV dysfunction in this population (discussed later).

OTHER CARDIOVASCULAR CONDITIONS ASSOCIATED WITH HIV

Pulmonary Hypertension (see also Chapter 88)

The prevalence of idiopathic PH in the general population is estimated to be 1 to 2 persons per million, but in the setting of HIV the prevalence is several thousand times higher (0.5%). Studies where subjects with HIV were screened with Doppler echocardiography suggest that many more have asymptomatic mild PH and that the true prevalence considerably exceeds 0.5%. A revised definition of PH proposed in 2018 included a mean PA pressure greater than 20 mm Hg, a PA wedge pressure of 15 mm Hg or less, and a pulmonary vascular resistance of 3 Wood units or higher.[76] Implementation of this definition would increase the proportion of people with HIV who also have PH.

The pathology of PH associated with HIV infection is similar to that seen in PH patients without HIV. It includes intimal thickening of small pulmonary arteries with plexogenic lesions in the media, leading ultimately to obstruction of small pulmonary arteries. As with idiopathic PH, no single cause of HIV-associated PH has been identified, but many factors may contribute. Levels of inflammatory markers such as vascular endothelial growth factor-A, platelet-derived growth factor, and IL-1 and IL-6 increase in HIV-associated PH. Certain HIV proteins can activate endothelial cells indirectly, such as the envelope glycoprotein-120, which associate with higher levels of endothelin-1. Levels of endothelin-1 correlate with pulmonary artery systolic pressure among HIV-infected subjects with PH,[77] suggesting that this potent vasoconstrictor plays a central role in the pathogenesis of PH-HIV. Another potential mechanism is asymmetric dimethylarginine (ADMA)-induced endothelial

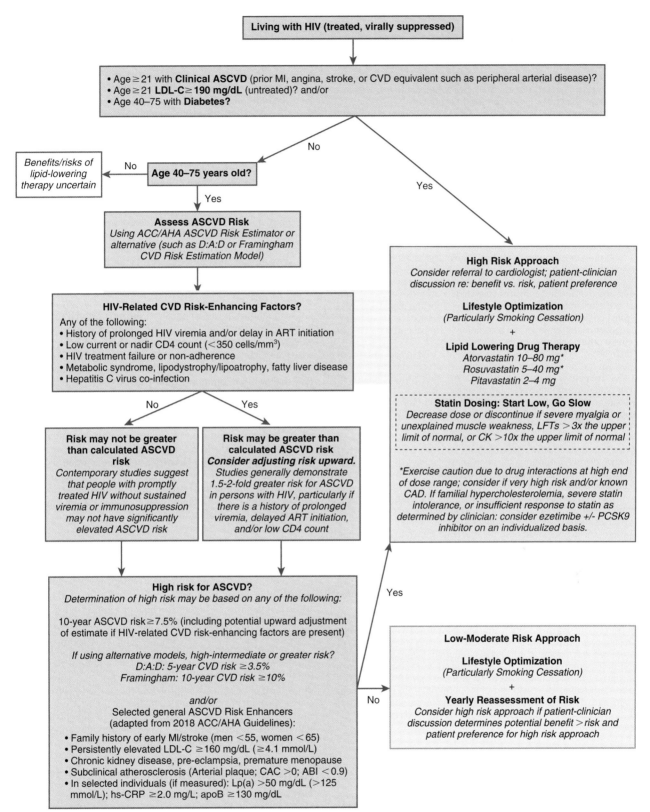

FIGURE 85.3 Pragmatic approach to atherosclerotic cardiovascular disease (ASCVD) risk assessment and prevention in treated HIV infection. This figure applies to people with treated HIV. For people with uncontrolled HIV, the first priority is appropriate HIV therapy to achieve viral suppression. Thresholds are based on findings of elevated CVD risk at current or nadir CD4 count less than 200, less than 350, and less than 500 cells/mm³. Hazard ratios and incidence rate ratios of 1.4–2.1 for myocardial infarction (MI) for people living with HIV (PLWH) versus uninfected people has been demonstrated in several studies. The hazard ratio of stroke for PLWH versus uninfected people was 1.40 in one study. *ABI,* Ankle-brachial index; *ACC/AHA,* American College of Cardiology/American Heart Association; *apoB,* apolipoprotein B; *ART,* antiretroviral therapy; *CAC,* coronary artery calcium; *CAD,* coronary artery disease; *CK,* creatine kinase; *CVD,* cardiovascular disease; *D:A:D,* Data Collection on Adverse Events of Anti-HIV Drugs; *hs-CRP,* high sensitivity C-reactive protein; *LFT,* liver function test; *LDL-C,* low-density lipoprotein cholesterol; *Lp(a),* lipoprotein A; *PCSK9,* proprotein convertase subtilisin-kexin type 9. (From Feinstein MJ, et al. Characteristics, prevention, and management of cardiovascular disease in people living with HIV: a scientific statement from the American Heart Association. *Circulation.* 2019;140:e98-e124, Fig 4.)

dysfunction, because elevated ADMA levels have been reported in HIV-associated PH.[78] Finally, a genetic predisposition to HIV-associated PH has been suggested, and some evidence indicates that autoimmunity may contribute.

Severe PH leads to worsening dyspnea, curtailed exercise capacity, right HF, and sudden cardiac death. PH may occur at any stage of HIV infection and does not appear to relate to CD4 count, ART, or other HIV-related factors. As the population with HIV ages, other conditions such as chronic pulmonary disease or HF may contribute to PH, mandating a thorough diagnostic evaluation for these patients.[79]

PH worsens outcomes in individuals with HIV, although asymptomatic subjects have a much better prognosis than do those with advanced dyspnea and reduced exercise tolerance. Death in PH-HIV is usually sudden or due to right HF and is rarely due to other HIV complications.[79] In one series of 77 PH-HIV subjects treated from 2000 to 2008, survival at 1, 3, and 5 years was 88%, 72%, and 63%, respectively. Predictors of survival were a cardiac index greater than 2.8 L/min/m^2 and a CD4 count of greater than 200 cells/μL. ART has not been shown to improve survival.[79]

Echocardiographic screening for PH is now recommended independent of symptoms for individuals with HIV and one of the following risk factors: female sex, intravenous drug or cocaine use, hepatitis C infection, high-prevalence country of origin, known Nef or Tat HIV proteins, and African-American patients.[80] Doppler estimates of PA systolic pressure are inaccurate both in the general population and in subjects with PH-HIV and thus are not sufficient to exclude a diagnosis of PH.[79] Right heart catheterization is the reference standard for the diagnosis of PH and must be performed before the initiation of PH-specific treatment.[79] Routine vasodilator testing is not recommended in patients with PH-HIV because a positive vasodilator test is rarely found.[79]

Treatment of PH-HIV is similar to treatment of PH in the absence of HIV, except for the issue of drug-drug interactions between PH therapy and ART. Pulmonary vasodilator testing reveals that a small minority of PH-HIV patients responds to calcium channel blockers.[81] The drug-drug interaction between calcium channel blockers and PIs means that the dose of the calcium channel blocker should be limited.

In case reports and small series, the phosphodiesterase type-5 inhibitors sildenafil, tadalafil, and vardenafil have been shown to improve dyspnea, functional class, exercise capacity, and mean pulmonary artery pressure in PH-HIV,[81] mirroring the improvements shown in clinical trials in PH without HIV. These drugs are metabolized by the 3A4 isoform of the cytochrome P450 system and interactions have been described with the PIs saquinavir, ritonavir, and indinavir. Thus, the dose of phosphodiesterase type-5 inhibitors in HIV-infected individuals who are concurrently on PIs should be carefully monitored.

The endothelin antagonist bosentan has been shown to improve pulmonary vascular resistance and exercise tolerance over 1 year of treatment, similar to the response expected in uninfected PH patients. The recommended dose of bosentan for individuals taking PIs is 62.5 mg/day or every other day instead of the usual dose of 125 mg twice daily. Studies of the selective endothelin receptor antagonists ambrisentan and sitaxsentan are limited to case reports in PH-HIV.

Several small series demonstrate that prostacyclin analogues induce hemodynamic benefit in PH-HIV.[82] Subcutaneous treprostinil and inhaled iloprost have improved functional capacity in the very small numbers of HIV-infected PH subjects that have been reported. Selexipag is a newer prostacyclin receptor agonist that was studied in 1156 patients in a randomized controlled trial; however, it included only 10 patients with PH-HIV.[83] In general, the treatment of PH in HIV-infected subjects does not appear to differ much from treatment in uninfected patients, except that specific clinical trial data are lacking in PH-HIV, and concomitant PI therapy introduces the problem of drug-drug interactions.

Heart Failure (see Part VI)

HF is a common accompaniment of HIV infection and portends a poor prognosis.[83] In the pre-ART era, HF generally resulted from HIV-associated cardiomyopathy and manifested as symptomatic systolic dysfunction with LV dilatation and a poor short-term outcome. This type of HF is still common with advanced HIV disease and AIDS in geographic areas where ART is not readily available.

In contrast, in the current era the diagnosis of HF includes many asymptomatic people living with HIV and often refers only to systolic or diastolic dysfunction detected by echocardiography. In a large cohort study of uninfected and HIV-infected U.S. veterans, where 2636

HF events occurred over 7.1 years of follow-up, HF with preserved ejection fraction (HFpEF) accounted for 34.6% of these, borderline HFpEF accounted for 15.5%, HF with reduced ejection fraction (HFrEF) for 37.1%, and HF of unknown type for 12.8%.[84] Compared with uninfected veterans, HIV-infected veterans had an increased risk of HFpEF (HR 1.21, 95% CI 1.03 to 1.41), borderline HFpEF (HR 1.37, 95% CI 1.09 to 1.72), and HFrEF (HR 1.61; 95% CI 1.40 to 1.86).

The pathophysiology of HIV-associated cardiomyopathy is multifactorial, with proposed causes including direct HIV infection with or without myocarditis, co-infection with other viruses such as Coxsackie virus B3 and CMV, opportunistic infections, and nutritional disorders.[83] HIV infection of the heart impairs systolic function. HIV gene products, such as tat, probably also contribute. Proinflammatory cytokines such as tumor necrosis factor and IL-1β also depress LV systolic function.

LV hypertrophy is more common in HIV-infected subjects than in controls. In a study from our group, HIV-infected participants had a mean 8 g/m^2 larger LV mass index compared with controls (p < 0.001). Higher LV mass index associated independently with lower nadir CD4 T cell count, suggesting that immunodeficiency might play a role in this process. Half of HIV subjects had diastolic dysfunction, and after adjusting for age and traditional risk factors, they were 2.4 times more likely to have diastolic dysfunction than controls. Both diastolic dysfunction and reduced ejection fraction predicted sudden cardiac death in our HIV cohort.[85]

The relationship of ART to HF in subjects with HIV is multifaceted. Some ART worsens glucose and lipid metabolism and associates with weight gain, factors that promote HF. ART has been blamed for otherwise unexplained LV hypertrophy in persons with HIV. On the other hand, ART prevents the cardiomyopathy and severe systolic dysfunction that was so common in the pre-ART era.[83] One ART, TDF, might reduce the risk of developing HF: in a large cohort of US veterans with HIV, HF risk was markedly lower in current TDF users (HR 0.68, 95% CI 0.53 to 0.86) compared with never users.[86] TDF might reduce the risk of HF by improving viral control and thus decreasing inflammation. The potential beneficial effect of TDF in HF requires confirmation.

In a cohort study from New York, with poorly controlled HIV and a high prevalence of drug use, PI-based regimens were associated with lower LV ejection fraction, higher pulmonary artery systolic pressure, and increased CV mortality as well as 30-day HF readmission among HIV-infected individuals with HF.[87]

Cardiac MRI provides insight into the subtle LV abnormalities that contribute to HF in the context of HIV. In one study, late gadolinium enhancement on cardiac MRI, a marker of cardiac fibrosis, was detected in 83% of 103 HIV subjects compared with only 16% of 92 controls.[88] The mean age of subjects in both groups was 45 years; ejection fraction was in the normal range but 6% lower in the HIV group, while LV mass was 7% higher. The high proportion of HIV subjects with myocardial fibrosis may not only contribute to incident HF but also the increased risk of sudden cardiac death in this group.

Treatment recommendations for HF in the setting of HIV are based upon trials done in uninfected HF patients and from guidelines based upon these trials (see also Chapters 48 to 51).[83] Thus, angiotensin-converting enzyme (ACE) inhibitors, beta blockers, aldosterone antagonists, digoxin, biventricular pacemakers, and AICDs should be used in persons with HIV as they are in uninfected patients with HF. Small numbers of HIV-infected subjects have undergone cardiac transplantation with excellent long-term survival.[89]

Arrhythmias and Sudden Cardiac Death (see Part VII)

HIV accentuates the risk of cardiac arrhythmias. The incidence of AF is rising as people with HIV age in the era of ART. In a large registry of U.S. veterans followed for a mean of 6.8 years from 1996 to 2011, 2.6% patients developed AF. Markers of HIV disease severity, specifically low CD4 count and high viral load, independently associate with the development of AF, along with expected clinical factors such as concomitant coronary disease, HF, alcoholism, renal dysfunction, and hypothyroidism. HIV infection associates with an increased risk for AF with an HR of 1.46, a magnitude of risk that is similar to established AF risk factors.[90]

As in the general population, management of AF aims to control the ventricular rate and to prevent embolic events. Scores to assess embolic risk do not appear to perform well in persons with AF and HIV.[91] Drugs used for rate control (diltiazem, verapamil) and newer anticoagulants (apixaban, rivaroxaban, ticagrelor) are metabolized by the CYP3A4 hepatic metabolism and thus interact with ART.[92] Although there are limited data available in HIV, dabigatran may have the least drug-drug interactions with ART.[93] Caution is therefore warranted in dose selection, and a dose adjustment may be indicated.

Subjects with HIV appear to be more susceptible to sudden cardiac death than uninfected persons. In a consecutive series of 2860 HIV patients followed for a mean of 3.7 years, the mean sudden cardiac death rate was 2.6 per 1000 person-years (95% CI 1.8 to 3.8), 4.5-fold higher than expected.[80] Sudden cardiac death patients had a higher prevalence of previous MI, cardiomyopathy, HF, and arrhythmias. LV systolic dysfunction and diastolic dysfunction, especially in the presence of detectable HIV RNA levels, predicted sudden cardiac death.[80] AICD implantation may be beneficial in subjects with HIV who meet criteria for a device. In one study comparing 59 HIV AICD subjects with 267 uninfected AICD controls, discharge rate over a mean follow-up of 19 months was higher in the HIV group (39% versus 20%, $P = 0.001$).[94]

Cerebrovascular Disease (see also Chapter 45)

As with ACS, the clinical features of ischemic stroke differ in HIV subjects compared with uninfected individuals. HIV stroke patients tend to be younger and male. Risk factors for ischemic stroke in the general population (i.e., hypertension, diabetes, smoking and dyslipidemia) are also risk factors for stroke in the setting of HIV. In the Veterans Aging Cohort Study the risk of ischemia stroke increased by 25% in HIV-infected men compared with uninfected subjects.[49] After adjustment, the risk of ischemic stroke was attenuated but still higher among HIV-infected men (HR 1.17, 95% CI 1.01 to 1.36, $P = 0.04$). HIV appears to increase the risk of ischemic stroke more in women than in men, with a risk that was almost doubled (HR 1.93, 95% CI 1.31 to 2.85) in one of the few studies of stroke incidence in HIV-infected women.[95] In a large series from the U.S. National Inpatient Sample, in-hospital mortality was higher in HIV-infected stroke than in uninfected stroke patients (7.6% versus 5.2%).[96]

The incidence of intracerebral hemorrhage is also higher in the setting of HIV, with an unadjusted incidence rate ratio of 1.85 (95% CI 1.37 to 2.47, p < 0.001).[97] In a multivariable model, HIV infection associated independently with a higher hazard of ICH, although its effect diminished with increasing age. A low CD4 count may associate with intracerebral hemorrhage.

More than one-third of strokes in persons with HIV are intracranial, as opposed to extracranial origin.[66] HIV crosses the blood-brain barrier early in the course of the infection and promotes inflammation of small vessels. During the first 6 months of ART in immunosuppressed individuals, the risk of stroke increases, perhaps due to small vessel thinning and erosion due to remodeling and neuroinflammation.[66] The relative contributions of atherosclerosis and inflammation to intracranial stroke in the context of HIV require further investigation.

The data linking ART to an increased risk of stroke are less compelling than the data for MI, possibly due to the lower incidence of stroke. A high viral load and a low CD4 count increase the risk of stroke. Yet even treated individuals with well-controlled infection show evidence of inflammation and immune activation and likely have increased risk for stroke.

The acute and long-term treatment of stroke in persons with HIV resembles that in uninfected individuals.[98] Primary and secondary prevention of stroke in subjects with HIV has great importance because of the increased risk in these individuals and because of their high prevalence of modifiable risk factors, notably smoking, dyslipidemia, and hypertension.

REFERENCES
General
1. Global HIV & AIDS Statistics—2019 Fact Sheet. https://www.unaids.org/en/resources/fact-sheet.
2. Smit M, Brinkman K, Geerlings S, et al. Future challenges for clinical care of an ageing population infected with HIV: a modelling study. *Lancet Infect Dis.* 2015;15:810–818.
3. Hsue PY, Waters DD. HIV infection and coronary heart disease: mechanisms and management. *Nat Rev Cardiol.* 2019;16:745–759.

Cardiovascular Risk Factors in People Living with HIV
4. Althoff KN, Gebo KA, Moore RD, et al. North American AIDS Cohort Collaboration on Research and Design. Contributions of traditional and HIV-related risk factors on non-AIDS-defining cancer, myocardial infarction, and end-stage liver and renal diseases in adults with HIV in the USA and Canada: a collaboration of cohort studies. *Lancet HIV.* 2019;6:e93–e104.
5. Waters DD, Hsue PY. Lipid abnormalities in persons living with HIV infection. *Can J Cardiol.* 2019;35:249–259.
6. Gori A, Antinori A, Vergori A, et al. Effectiveness of switching to darunavir/cobicistat in virologically-suppressed HIV-positive patients receiving ritonavir-boosted protease inhibitor-based regimen: the "STORE" study. *J Acquir Immune Defic Syndr.* 2020. (online ahead of print).
7. Ekoru K, Young EH, Dillon DG, et al. HIV treatment is associated with a two-fold higher probability of raised triglycerides: pooled analyses in 21023 individuals in sub-Saharan Africa. *Glob Health Epidemiol Genom.* 2018;3:e7.
8. Eckard AR, McComsey GA. Weight gain and integrase inhibitors. *Curr Opin Infect Dis.* 2020;33(1):10–19.
9. Nix LM, Tien PC. Metabolic syndrome, diabetes, and cardiovascular risk in HIV. *Curr HIV AIDS Rep.* 2014;11(3):271–278.
10. Hill A, Waters L, Pozniak A. Are new antiretroviral treatments increasing the risks of clinical obesity? *J Virus Erad.* 2019;5:41–43.
11. Sax PE, Erlandson KM, Lake JE, et al. Weight gain following initiation of antiretroviral therapy: risk factors in randomized comparative clinical trials. *CID.* 2019. (in press).
12. Grand M, Bia D, Diaz A. Cardiovascular risk assessment in people living with HIV: a systematic review and meta-analysis of real-life data. *Curr HIV Res.* 2020;18:5–18.
13. Mathabire Ru¨cker SC, Tayea A, Bitiliny J, et al. High rates of hypertension, diabetes, elevated low-density lipoprotein cholesterol, and cardiovascular disease risk factors in HIV- infected patients in Malawi. *AIDS.* 2018;32:253–260.
14. Willig AL, Webel AR, Westfall AO, et al. Physical activity trends and metabolic health outcomes in people living with HIV in the US, 2008-2015. *Prog Cardiovasc Dis.* 2020. https://doi.org/10.1016/j.pcad.2020.02.005. (on line ahead of print).
15. Armah KA, Chang CC, Baker JV, et al. Prehypertension, hypertension, and the risk of acute myocardial infarction in HIV-infected and -uninfected veterans. *Clin Infect Dis.* 2014;58(1):121–129.
16. Ekrikpo UE, Kengne AP, Bello AK, et al. Chronic kidney disease in the global adult HIV-infected population: a systematic review and meta-analysis. *PLoS One.* 2018;13(4):e0195443.
17. Ryom L, Lundgren JD, Ross M, et al. Renal impairment and cardiovascular disease in HIV- positive individuals: the D:A:D study. *J Infect Dis.* 2016;214:1212–1220.
18. Mocroft A, Lundgren JD, Ross M, et al. Current and cumulative exposure to potentially nephrotoxic antiretrovirals and development of chronic kidney disease in HIV-positive individuals with a normal baseline estimated glomerular filtration rate: a prospective international cohort study. *Lancet HIV.* 2016;3(1):e23–e32.
19. Rasmussen LD, Helleberg M, May MT, et al. Myocardial infarction among Danish HIV-infected individuals: population-attributable fractions associated with smoking. *Clin Infect Dis.* 2015;60(9):1415–1423.
20. Keith A, Dong Y, Shuter J, et al. Behavioral interventions for tobacco use in HIV-infected smokers: a meta-analysis. *J Acquir Immune Defic Syndr.* 2016;72:527–533.
21. Stanton CA, Kumar PN, Moadel AB, et al. A multicenter randomized controlled trial of intensive group therapy for tobacco treatment in HIV-infected cigarette smokers. *J Acquir Immune Defic Syndr.* 2020;83(4):405–414.
22. Shuter J, Kim RS, Durant S, Stanton CA. Long-term follow-up of smokers living with HIV after an intensive behavioral tobacco treatment intervention. *J Acquir Immune Defic Syndr.* 2020. (on line ahead of print).
23. Ghura S, Gross R, Jordan-Sciutto K, et al. Bidirectional associations among nicotine and tobacco smoke, neuroHIV, and anti-viral therapy. *J Neuroimmune Pharmacol.* 2019. https://doi.org/10.1007/s11481-019-09897-4. (on line ahead of print).

Mechanisms of HIV-Related Atherogenesis
24. Faust TB, Binning JM, Gross JD, Frankel AD. Making sense of multifunctional proteins: human immunodeficiency virus type 1 accessory and regulatory proteins and connections to transcription. *Annu Rev Virol.* 2017;4(1):241–260.
25. Knudsen A, Kristoffersen US, Panum I, et al. Coronary artery calcium and intima-media thickness are associated with level of cytomegalovirus immunoglobulin G in HIV-infected patients. *HIV Med.* 2018;20:60–62.
26. Tincati C, Douek DC, Marchetti G. Gut barrier structure, mucosal immunity and intestinal microbiota in the pathogenesis and treatment of HIV infection. *AIDS Res Ther.* 2016;13:19.
27. Borges AH, O'Connor JL, Phillips AN, et al. Interleukin 6 is a stronger predictor of clinical events than high-sensitivity C-reactive protein or D-dimer during HIV infection. *J Infect Dis.* 2016;214(3):408–416.
28. Tawakol A, Ishai A, Li D, et al. Association of arterial and lymph node inflammation with distinct inflammatory pathways in human immunodeficiency virus infection. *JAMA Cardiol.* 2017;2:163–171.
29. Toribio M, Fitch KV, Sanchez L, et al. Effects of pitavastatin and pravastatin on markers of immune activation and arterial inflammation in HIV. *AIDS.* 2017;31(6):797–806.
30. O'Brien MP, Hunt PW, Kitch PW, et al. A randomized placebo controlled trial of aspirin effects on immune activation in chronically human immunodeficiency virus-infected adults on virologically suppressive antiretroviral therapy. *Open Forum Infect Dis.* 2017;4(1):ofw278.
31. Ridker PM, Everett BM, Thuren T, et al. Antiinflammatory therapy with canakinumab for atherosclerotic disease. *N Engl J Med.* 2017;377:1119–1131.
32. Ridker PM, MacFadyen JG, Everett BM, et al. Relationship of C-reactive protein reduction to cardiovascular event reduction following treatment with canakinumab: a secondary analysis from the CANTOS randomised controlled trial. *Lancet.* 2018;391:319–328.
33. Ridker PM, Libby P, MacFadyen JG, et al. Modulation of the interleukin-6 signalling pathway and incidence rates of atherosclerotic events and all- cause mortality: analyses from the Canakinumab Anti-Inflammatory Thrombosis Outcomes Study (CANTOS). *Eur Heart J.* 2018;39:3499–3507.
34. Hsue PY, Li D, Ma Y, et al. IL-1beta inhibition reduces atherosclerotic inflammation in HIV infection. *J Am Coll Cardiol.* 2018;72:2809–2811.
35. Ridker PM, Everett BM, Pradhan A, et al. Low-dose methotrexate for the prevention of atherosclerotic events. *N Engl J Med.* 2019;380(8):752–762.
36. Hsue PY, Ribaudo HJ, Deeks SG, et al. Safety and impact of low-dose methotrexate on endothelial function and inflammation in individuals with treated human immunodeficiency virus: AIDS Clinical Trials Group Study A5314. *Clin Infect Dis.* 2019;68(11):1877–1886.
37. Borges AH, O'Connor JL, Phillips AN, et al. Interleukin 6 is a stronger predictor of clinical events than high-sensitivity C-reactive protein or D-dimer during HIV infection. *J Infect Dis.* 2016;214:408–416.
38. Nordell AD, McKenna M, Borges ÁH, et al. Severity of cardiovascular disease outcomes among patients with HIV is related to markers of inflammation and coagulation. *J Am Heart Assoc.* 2014;3:e000844.
39. Grund B, Baker JV, Deeks SG, et al. Relevance of interleukin-6 and D-dimer for serious non-AIDS morbidity and death among HIV-positive adults on suppressive antiretroviral therapy. *PLoS One.* 2016;11:e0155100.
40. Scherzer R, Shah SJ, Secemsky E, et al. Association of biomarker clusters with cardiac phenotypes and mortality in patients with HIV infection. *Circ Heart Fail.* 2018;11:e004312.

DISEASES OF THE MYOCARDIUM, PERICARDIUM, AND PULMONARY VASCULATURE BED

41. Marconi VC, Duncan MS, So-Armah K, et al. Bilirubin is inversely associated with cardiovascular disease among HIV-positive and HIV-negative individuals in VACS (Veterans Aging Cohort Study). *J Am Heart Assoc.* 2018;7(10):e007792.

Atherosclerosis in People with HIV/AIDS

42. Stein JH, Currier JS, Hsue PY. Arterial disease in patients with human immunodeficiency virus infection: what has imaging taught us? *JACC Cardiovasc Imaging.* 2014;7:515–525.
43. Post WS, Budoff M, Kingsley L, et al. Associations between HIV infection and subclinical coronary atherosclerosis: the Multicenter AIDS Cohort Study (MACS). *Ann Intern Med.* 2014;160:458–467.
44. D'Ascenzo F, Cerrato E, Calcagno A, et al. High prevalence at computed coronary tomography of non-calcified plaques in asymptomatic HIV patients treated with HAART: a meta-analysis. *Atherosclerosis.* 2015;240:197–2004.
45. Tawakol A, Lo J, Zanni MV, et al. Increased arterial inflammation relates to high-risk coronary plaque morphology in HIV-infected patients. *J Acquir Immune Defic Syndr.* 2014;66(2):164–171.
46. Hsu DC, Ma YF, Narwan A, et al. Plasma tissue factor and immune activation are associated with carotid intima-media thickness progression in treated HIV infection. *AIDS.* 2020;34(4):519–528.
47. Shah ASV, Stelzle D, Lee KK, et al. Global burden of atherosclerotic cardiovascular disease in people living with HIV: systematic review and meta-analysis. *Circulation.* 2018;138:1100–1112.
48. Hsue PY, Waters DD. Time to recognize HIV infection as a major cardiovascular risk factor. *Circulation.* 2018;138:1113–1115.
49. Sico JJ, Chang CC, So-Armah K, et al. HIV status and the risk of ischemic stroke among men. *Neurology.* 2015;84:1933–1940.
50. Knudsen AD, Gelpi M, Afzal S, et al. Brief report: prevalence of peripheral artery disease is higher in persons living with HIV compared with uninfected controls. *J Acquir Immune Defic Syndr.* 2018;79(3):381–385.
51. Badr S, Minha S, Kitabata H, et al. Safety and long-term outcomes after percutaneous coronary intervention in patients with human immunodeficiency virus. *Catheter Cardiovasc Interv.* 2015;85:192–198.
52. Robich MP, Schiltz N, Johnston DR, et al. Outcomes of patients with human immunodeficiency virus infection undergoing cardiovascular surgery in the United States. *J Thorac Cardiovasc Surg.* 2014;148:3066–3073.
53. Smilowitz NR, Gupta N, Guo Y, et al. Influence of human immunodeficiency virus seropositive status on the in-hospital management and outcomes of patients presenting with acute myocardial infarction. *J Invasive Cardiol.* 2016;28(10):403–409.
54. Rosenson RS, Colantonio LD, Burkholder GA, Chen L, Muntner P. Trends in utilization of statin therapy and contraindicated statin use in HIV-infected adults treated with antiretroviral therapy from 2007 through 2015. *J Am Heart Assoc.* 2018;7(24):e010345.
55. Günthard HF, Saag MS, Benson CA, et al. Antiretroviral drugs for treatment and prevention of HIV infection in adults. 2016 recommendations of the International Antiviral Society–USA Panel. *J Am Med Assoc.* 2016;316:191–210.
56. Lundgren JD, Babiker AG, Gordin F, et al. Initiation of antiretroviral therapy in early asymptomatic HIV infection. *N Engl J Med.* 2015;373(9):795–807.
57. Baker JV, Sharma S, Achhra AC, et al. Changes in cardiovascular disease risk factors with immediate versus deferred antiretroviral therapy initiation among HIV-positive participants in the START (Strategic Timing of Antiretroviral Treatment) Trial. *J Am Heart Assoc.* 2017;6(5):e004987.
58. Promer K, Karris MY. Current treatment options for HIV elite controllers: a review. *Curr Treat Options Infect Dis.* 2018;10(2):302–309.
59. Crowell TA, Gebo KA, Blankson JN, et al. Hospitalization rates and reasons among HIV elite controllers and persons with medically controlled HIV infection. *J Infect Dis.* 2015;211(11):1692–1702.
60. Milinkovic A, Berger F, Arenas-Pinto A, Mauss S. Reversible effect on lipids by switching from tenofovir disoproxil fumarate to tenofovir alafenamide and back. *AIDS.* 2019;33(15):2387–2391.
61. Landmesser U, Chapman MJ, Stock JK, et al. Update of ESC/EAS Task Force on practical clinical guidance for proprotein convertase subtilisin/kexin type 9 inhibition in patients with atherosclerotic cardiovascular disease or in familial hypercholesterolaemia. *Eur Heart J.* 2017;39:1131–1143. 2017.
62. Jacobson TA, Maki KC, Orringer CE, et al. National Lipid Association recommendations for patient-centered management of dyslipidemia: Part 2. *J Clin Lipidol.* 2015;9(suppl 6):S1–S122.
63. Zanni MV, Fitch KV, Feldpausch M, et al. 2013 American College of Cardiology/American Heart Association and 2004 Adult Treatment Panel III cholesterol guidelines applied to HIV-infected patients with/without subclinical high-risk coronary plaque. *AIDS.* 2014;28:2061–2070.
64. Phan BA, Weigel B, Ma Y, et al. Utility of 2013 American College of Cardiology/American Heart Association cholesterol guidelines in HIV-infected adults with carotid atherosclerosis. *Circ Cardiovasc Imaging.* 2017;10:e005995.
65. Grundy SM, Stone NJ, Bailey AL, et al. 2018 AHA/ACC/AACVPR/AAPA/ABC/ACPM/ADA/AGS/APhA/ASPC/NLA/PCNA guideline on the management of blood cholesterol: a report of the American College of Cardiology/American Heart Association task force on clinical practice guidelines. *Circulation.* 2019;139:e1082–e1143.
66. Feinstein MJ, Achenbach CJ, Stone NJ, et al. A systematic review of the usefulness of statin therapy in HIV-infected patients. *Am J Cardiol.* 2015;115:1760–1766.
67. Aberg JA, Sponseller CA, Ward DJ, et al. Pitavastatin versus pravastatin in adults with HIV-1 infection and dyslipidaemia (INTREPID): 12 week and 52 week results of a phase 4, multicentre, randomised, double-blind, superiority trial. *Lancet HIV.* 2017;4:e284–e294.

68. Clement ME, Park LP, Navar AM, et al. Statin utilization and recommendations among HIV- and HCV-infected veterans: a cohort study. *Clin Infect Dis.* 2016;63(3):407–413.
69. Lee FJ, Monteiro P, Baker D, et al. Rosuvastatin vs. protease inhibitor switching for hypercholesterolaemia: a randomized trial. *HIV Med.* 2016;17:605–614.
70. Bhatt DL, Steg G, Miller M, et al. Cardiovascular risk reduction with icosapent ethyl for hypertriglyceridemia. *N Engl J Med.* 2019;380:11–22.
71. Triant VA, Perez J, Regan S, et al. Cardiovascular risk prediction functions underestimate risk in HIV infection. *Circulation.* 2018;137:2203–2214.
72. Friis-Møller N, Ryom L, Smith C, et al. An updated prediction model of the global risk of cardiovascular disease in HIV-positive persons: the Data-collection on Adverse Effects of Anti-HIV Drugs (D:A:D) study. *Eur J Prev Cardiol.* 2016;23:214–223.
73. Feinstein MJ, Hsue PY, Benjamin LA, et al. Characteristics, prevention, and management of cardiovascular disease in people living with HIV: a scientific statement from the American Heart Association. *Circulation.* 2019;140:e98–e124.
74. Nolte JE, Neumann T, Manne JM, et al. Cost-effectiveness analysis of coronary artery disease screening in HIV-infected men. *Eur J Prev Cardiol.* 2014;21:972–729.
75. Phan BAP, Weigal B, Ma Y, et al. Utility of 2013 American College of Cardiology/American Heart Association cholesterol guidelines in HIV-infected adults with carotid atherosclerosis. *Circ Cardiovasc Imaging.* 2017;10(7):e005995.

Other Cardiovascular Conditions Associated with HIV

76. Simonneau G, Montani D, Celermajer DS, et al. Haemodynamic definitions and updated clinical classification of pulmonary hypertension. *Eur Respir J.* 2019;53(1).
77. Parikh RV, Ma Y, Scherzer R, et al. Endothelin-1 predicts hemodynamically assessed pulmonary artery hypertension in HIV infection. *PloS One.* 2016;11:e0146355.
78. Parikh RV, Scherzer R, Nitta EM, et al. Increased levels of asymmetric dimethylarginine are associated with pulmonary arterial hypertension in HIV infection. *AIDS.* 2014;28:511–519.
79. Basyal B, Jarrett H, Barnett CF. Pulmonary hypertension in HIV. *Can J Cardiol.* 2019;35:288–298.
80. Moyers BS, Secemsky EA, Vittinghoff E, et al. Effect of left ventricular dysfunction and viral load on risk of sudden cardiac death in patients with human immunodeficiency virus. *Am J Cardiol.* 2014;113(7):1260–1265.
81. Chinello P, Petrosillo N. Pharmacological treatment of HIV-associated pulmonary hypertension. *Expert Rev Clin Pharmacol.* 2016;9:715–725.
82. Sitbon O, Channick R, Chin KM, et al. Selexipag for the treatment of pulmonary arterial hypertension. *N Engl J Med.* 2015;373:2522–2533.
83. Hsue PY, Waters DD. Heart failure in persons living with HIV infection. *Curr Opin HIV AIDS.* 2017;12:534–539.
84. Freiberg MS, Chang CH, Skanderson M, et al. Association between HIV infection and the risk of heart failure with reduced ejection fraction and preserved ejection fraction in the antiretroviral therapy era: results from the veterans aging cohort study. *JAMA Cardiol.* 2017;2:536–546.
85. Moyers BS, Secemsky EA, Vittinghoff E, et al. Effect of left ventricular dysfunction and viral load on risk of sudden cardiac death in patients with human immunodeficiency virus. *Am J Cardiol.* 2014;113:1260–1265.
86. Chen R, Scherzer R, Hsue PY, et al. Association of tenofovir use with risk of incident heart failure in HIV-infected patients. *J Am Heart Assoc.* 2017;6:e005387.
87. Alvi RM, Neilan AM, Tariq N, et al. Protease inhibitors and cardiovascular outcomes in patients with HIV and heart failure. *J Am Coll Cardiol.* 2018;72(5):518–530.
88. Ntusi N, O'Dwyer E, Dorrell L, et al. HIV-1-related cardiovascular disease is associated with chronic inflammation, frequent pericardial effusions, and probable myocardial edema. *Circ Cardiovasc Imaging.* 2016;9:e004430.
89. Agüero F, Castel MA, Cocchi S, et al. An update on heart transplantation in human immunodeficiency virus-infected patients. *Am J Transplant.* 2016;16(1):21–28.
90. Sardana M, Hsue PY, Tseng ZH, et al. Human immunodeficiency virus infection and incident atrial fibrillation. *J Am Coll Cardiol.* 2019;74(11):1512–1514.
91. Chau KH, Scherzer R, Grunfeld C, et al. CHA2DS2-VASc score, warfarin use, and risk for thromboembolic events among HIV-infected persons with atrial fibrillation. *J Acquir Immune Defic Syndr.* 2017;76(1):90–97.
92. West TA, Perram J, Holloway CJ. Use of direct oral anticoagulants for treatment of atrial fibrillation in patients with HIV: a review. *Curr Opin HIV AIDS.* 2017;12(6):554–560.
93. Perram J, O'Dwyer E, Holloway C. Use of dabigatran with antiretrovirals. *HIV Med.* 2019;20(5):344–346.
94. Alvi RM, Neilan AM, Tariq N, et al. Incidence, predictors, and outcomes of implantable cardioverter-defibrillator discharge among people living with HIV. *J Am Heart Assoc.* 2018;7(18):e009857.
95. Chow FC, Regan S, Zanni MV, et al. Elevated ischemic stroke risk among women living with HIV infection. *AIDS.* 2018;32(1):59–67.
96. Sweeney EM, Thakur KT, Lyons JL, et al. Outcomes of intravenous tissue plasminogen activator for acute ischaemic stroke in HIV-infected adults. *Eur J Neurol.* 2014;21:1394–1399.
97. Chow FC, He W, Bachetti P, et al. Elevated rates of intracerebral hemorrhage in individuals from a US clinical care HIV cohort. *Neurology.* 2014;83(19):1705–1711.
98. Nguyen I, Kim AS, Chow FC. Prevention of stroke in people living with HIV. *Prog Cardiovasc Dis.* 2020; Jan 31;S0033-0620(20)30028_1.

 # 86 Pericardial Diseases

MARTIN M. LEWINTER, PAUL C. CREMER, AND ALLAN L. KLEIN

The pericardium is involved in a wide variety of diseases which result in some of the classic physical, imaging, and hemodynamic findings in cardiology. In this chapter we discuss the anatomy and physiology of the pericardium, acute and recurrent pericarditis, pericardial effusion and tamponade, constrictive and effusive-constrictive pericarditis (ECP), and selected specific etiologies.[1,2]

ANATOMY AND PHYSIOLOGY OF THE PERICARDIUM
The pericardium is composed of two layers,[3] the *visceral* pericardium, a monolayer of mesothelial cells and collagen and elastin fibers adherent to the epicardial surface of the heart, and the fibrous *parietal* pericardium, which is normally about 2 mm thick and surrounds most of the heart (Fig. 86.1). The parietal pericardium is largely acellular and contains collagen and elastin fibers. The visceral pericardium reflects back near the origins of the great vessels and is continuous with and forms the inner layer of the parietal pericardium. The pericardial space or sac is contained within these two layers, and normally contains up to 50 mL of serous fluid. The visceral-parietal reflection is a few centimeters proximal to the junctions of the cavae with the right atrium (RA); thus, portions of the caval vessels lie within the pericardial sac. Posterior to the left atrium (LA), the reflection occurs at the oblique sinus of the pericardium. The LA is largely extra-pericardial. The parietal pericardium has ligamentous attachments to the diaphragm, sternum, and other structures.

While its removal has no obvious negative consequences, the pericardium does function to maintain a relatively constant position of the heart in the thorax and provides a barrier to infection.[3] The pericardium is well-innervated with mechano- and chemoreceptors and phrenic afferent receptors which participate in reflexes arising from pericardium and/or epicardium (e.g., the Bezold-Jarisch reflex) and transmission of pericardial pain. The pericardium also secretes prostaglandins and related substances that may modulate neural traffic and coronary tone.

The best-characterized mechanical function of the pericardium is its *restraining* effect on cardiac volume.[3] This reflects the mechanical properties of the parietal pericardium. At low stresses the tissue is very elastic (eFig. 86.1, *top*). With further stretch, it abruptly becomes stiff and resistant to further stretch. The point on the stress-strain relation where this transition occurs is near the upper range of physiologic cardiac volumes. The *pressure-volume relation* of the pericardial sac reflects the properties of the tissue[3] (eFig. 86.1, *bottom, left curve*), that is, a flat, compliant segment transitioning relatively abruptly to a noncompliant segment around the upper limit of normal total cardiac volume. Thus, the sac has a relatively small reserve volume. When exceeded, the pressure within the sac operating on the surface of the heart increases rapidly and is transmitted into the cardiac chambers. The shape of the pericardial pressure-volume relation dictates that once a critical level of effusion is reached relatively small amounts of additional fluid will cause large increases in intra-pericardial pressure and markedly affect

cardiac function. Conversely, removal of small amounts of fluid can result in striking benefit. The shape of the pericardial pressure-volume relation also suggests that it *normally* restrains cardiac volume, that is, the force it exerts on the surface of the heart limits filling, with a component of *intra-cavitary* pressure reflecting the surface pressure. Studies with specially designed balloons[3] demonstrate a substantial surface pressure, especially when the upper limit of normal cardiac volume is exceeded.

Pericardial contact pressure has also been estimated by quantifying the shift in the right and left heart diastolic *pressure-volume relation* before and after pericardiectomy.[3] A decrease in pressure at a given volume is the *effective* pericardial pressure at that volume. Studies in normal canine hearts indicate negligible pressure at low normal filling volumes, with pressures in the 2 to 4 mm Hg range at the upper end of normal. At filling volumes above normal the pressure rapidly increases. Thus, at left-sided filling pressure approximately 25 mm Hg, contact pressure is approximately 10 mm Hg. Patients undergoing pericardiotomy during heart surgery develop mild postoperative increases in cardiac volume, consistent with relief of underlying, normal pericardial restraint to filling.

The normal pericardium also contributes to diastolic interaction,[3] defined here as transmission of intra-cavitary filling pressure to adjoining chambers. Thus, for example, a portion of right ventricular (RV) diastolic pressure is transmitted to the left ventricle (LV) across the interventricular septum and contributes to LV diastolic pressure. The overall effect of the pericardium is to more tightly couple right- and left-sided filling pressures. As cardiac volume increases the pericardium contributes increasingly to intra-cavitary filling pressures due to both external contact pressure and increased diastolic interaction. When the cardiac chambers dilate rapidly, the restraining effect of the pericardium and its contribution to diastolic interaction are augmented, resulting in a hemodynamic picture with features of both cardiac tamponade and constrictive pericarditis (CP), an example being RV myocardial infarction (MI).[3] Here, the right heart dilates rapidly such that total heart volume exceeds pericardial reserve volume. As a result, left- and right-sided filling pressures equilibrate at elevated levels and a paradoxical pulse and inspiratory increase in systemic venous pressure (Kussmaul's sign) may occur. Other conditions with similar effects include acute pulmonary embolus and sub-acute mitral regurgitation.[3]

Chronic cardiac dilatation, for example, dilated cardiomyopathy or regurgitant valvular disease, can result in total cardiac volume well in excess of the pericardial reserve volume yet exaggerated restraining effects are not observed. Thus, the pericardium adapts to accommodate chronic increases in cardiac volume. In experimental chronic volume overload, the pericardial pressure-volume relation shifts to the right and its slope decreases (eFig. 86.1, *bottom, right curve*), that is, it becomes more compliant, along with an increase in area and mass and a decreased effect on the diastolic pressure-volume relation.[3]

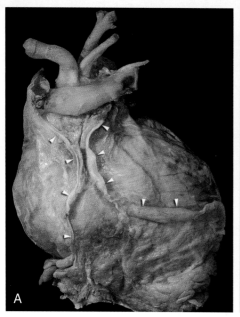 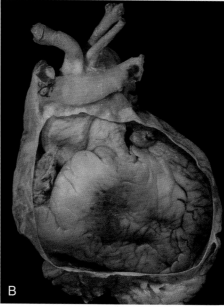

FIGURE 86.1 A, Anterior view of the intact parietal pericardial sac. The mediastinal pleura invest the lateral portion of the fibrous pericardium, with reflections indicated by the *arrowheads*. The space between the arrowheads corresponds to the attachment of the pericardium to the posterior surface of the sternum. Superiorly, the left innominate vein is seen merging with the superior vena cava. The branches of the aortic arch are just dorsal to the innominate vein. **B,** Anterior portion of the pericardial sac has been removed to show the heart and great vessels. The proximal segments of the great arteries are intrapericardial. (From Klein AL, Abbara S, Agler DA, et al. American Society of Echocardiography clinical recommendations for multimodality cardiovascular imaging of patients with pericardial disease: endorsed by the Society for Cardiovascular Magnetic Resonance and Society of Cardiovascular Computed Tomography. *J Am Soc Echocardiogr.* 2013;26(9):965–1012.e1015.)

ACUTE PERICARDITIS

Definition, Causes, Epidemiology, and Pathophysiology

Acute pericarditis is an inflammatory syndrome with or without pericardial effusion with a wide variety of causes (Table 86.1).[4–6] The prevalence of tuberculosis (TB) is a key element in the assessment of a suspected case of pericarditis. In developing regions where TB is endemic, it is the most common cause of pericarditis and effusion. TB is rare in developed countries and therefore is a far less important consideration.[4–6]

There are limited epidemiological data documenting the incidence and prevalence of acute pericarditis. At autopsy, the frequency is approximately 1%.[4,5] Pericarditis is common in the emergency department, accounting for up to 5% of patients with nonischemic chest pain.[5] A review of etiologies in published series is presented in Table 86.2. In developed countries, presumed viral and idiopathic etiologies are most common. We use *idiopathic* to denote acute pericarditis for which no specific cause is identified with routine diagnostic testing, as outlined below. Idiopathic cases are presumed to be viral. Testing for specific viruses is costly and has low yield and impact on management.[7,8] Such a term, although an admission of ignorance, is clinically meaningful if nonviral causes of pericarditis have been excluded, because treatment with antiinflammatory therapy is similar for all cases and prognosis is good.[9,10]

In a contemporary series from Northern Italy, the incidence of acute pericarditis was 27.7 cases/100,000 population/year with concomitant myocarditis in about 15%.[11] In hospitalized patients with acute pericarditis from Finland, the incidence rate of hospitalization was 3.32/100,000 population/year.[12] Men aged 16 to 65 years were at higher risk than women (RR 2.02). Acute pericarditis was the cause of 0.20% of all cardiovascular admissions. The proportion of admissions declined in younger patients. In-hospital mortality rate was 1.1% and increased with age and severe infections such as pneumonia or septicemia.

Most of the various causes of pericardial inflammation result in a response characterized by edema, thickening of the parietal layer, production of exudative pericardial fluid, and increased friction between the layers.[9] Acute pericarditis and myocarditis share common viral etiologies and, as noted, as many as 15% of pericarditis cases are associated with

myocarditis.[4,5,9,13] Coexistent myocarditis is usually manifested by modest release of cardiac biomarkers such as troponin (see Chapter 55). LV dysfunction is rare and the long-term prognosis of pericarditis complicated by myocarditis is excellent.[9,13] When ventricular function is normal the term "myopericarditis" is used. Cases with impaired function are labeled "perimyocarditis."

History and Differential Diagnosis

In greater than 90% of cases, the main symptom of acute pericarditis is chest pain, often quite severe.[4,5] It is usually retrosternal but may be localized to the left anterior chest and radiate to the neck, shoulders, and arms. Classically, the pain radiates to the trapezius ridge. Pericardial pain is pleuritic and worsened by lying down. Associated symptoms include dyspnea, cough, and occasionally hiccups. An antecedent history suggesting a viral illness is common. The history may provide clues to specific causative diagnoses. For example, a known malignancy or autoimmune disorder, high fevers with shaking chills, or weight loss suggest specific, nonidiopathic etiologies.

The differential diagnosis of chest pain is lengthy (see Chapters 35). Diagnoses most easily confused with pericarditis include myocardial ischemia/infarction, pneumonia with pleurisy, pulmonary embolism/infarction, costochondritis, and gastroesophageal reflux. Acute pericarditis is usually easily distinguished from myocardial ischemia, but further testing may be required. Other considerations include aortic dissection, intraabdominal processes, pneumothorax, and herpes zoster pain before skin lesions appear. Rarely, pericarditis can signal a preceding, silent MI.

Physical Examination

Patients with *uncomplicated* acute pericarditis often appear uncomfortable and anxious, with low-grade fever (<38°C) and sinus tachycardia. Arrhythmias are uncommon, although atrial fibrillation/flutter are reported in approximately 5% of cases.[14] The pathognomonic physical sign of acute pericarditis is the friction rub, reported in about one third of cases. Rubs are typically evanescent and may require repeated auscultation for detection.[5] The rub is ascribed to friction between pericardial layers. The classic rub consists of three components corresponding to ventricular systole, early diastole, and atrial contraction, and can be likened to the sound made when walking on crunchy snow. The rub is usually loudest at the lower left sternal border and best heard with the patient leaning forward. It is important to perform a thorough physical examination to look for clues to specific causative diagnoses as well as findings suggesting significant pericardial effusion.

Laboratory Testing

The electrocardiogram (ECG) is a key test for diagnosing acute pericarditis (see Chapter 14). The classic finding is "diffuse" ST-segment elevation (Fig. 86.2). The ST-segment vector points leftward, anterior, and inferior, with ST-segment elevation in all leads except aVR and often V_1. Usually, the ST segment is curved upward and resembles the current of injury of transmural ischemia. The distinction between acute pericarditis and transmural ischemia is usually not difficult because of more extensive lead involvement and lack of evolution to pathologic Q waves in pericarditis, and more prominent reciprocal ST depression in ischemia. However, ST elevation in pericarditis can at times involve a smaller number of leads and in some cases the ST segment more

TABLE 86.1 Categories of Diseases That Can Involve the Pericardium and Selected Specific Etiologies

Idiopathic*

Infectious

Viral* (echovirus, coxsackievirus, adenovirus, cytomegalovirus, hepatitis B, infectious mononucleosis, HIV/AIDS, SARS-CoV-2)

Bacterial* (*Mycobacterium tuberculosis, Mycobacterium avium-intracellulare*, pneumococcus, staphylococcus, streptococcus, mycoplasma, Lyme disease, *Haemophilus influenzae, Neisseria meningitides*, and many others)

HIV-associated*

Fungal (histoplasmosis, coccidioidomycosis, candida)

Protozoal

Inflammatory

Autoimmune diseases* (systemic lupus erythematosus, rheumatoid arthritis, scleroderma, dermatomyositis, Sjogren syndrome, inflammatory bowel disease, mixed)

Drug-induced autoimmune diseases* (procainamide, hydralazine, isoniazid, cyclosporine, etc.)

Arteritis (polyarteritis nodosa, temporal arteritis)

Post-cardiotomy/thoracotomy,* post-cardiac injury,* early and late post-myocardial infarction (Dressler syndrome*)

Autoinflammatory diseases* (tumor necrosis factor receptor-1 associated periodic syndrome, familial Mediterranean fever, others)

Miscellaneous: Sarcoidosis, Erdheim-Chester disease, Churg-Strauss disease, immunoglobulin G4 related diseases

Cancer

Primary: mesothelioma, fibrosarcoma, lipoma, etc.

Secondary*: breast and lung carcinoma, lymphomas, Kaposi sarcoma

Radiation-induced*

Early post-cardiac surgery and post-orthotopic heart transplantation

Hemopericardium

Trauma

Post-myocardial infarction free wall rupture

Endomyocardial biopsy

Dissecting aortic aneurysm

Device and procedure-related: percutaneous coronary procedures, implantable defibrillators and pacemakers, arrhythmia ablation, atrial septal defect closure, left atrial appendage isolation, percutaneous valve repair/replacement, laparoscopic hiatal hernia repair

Oral anticoagulants

Congenital

Cysts, diverticula, congenital absence

Miscellaneous

Stress cardiomyopathy

Cholesterol ("gold paint" pericarditis)

Chronic renal failure, dialysis-associated*

Chylopericardium

Hypo- and hyperthyroidism

Amyloidosis

Pneumopericardium

Polycystic kidney disease

Pulmonary arterial hypertension

*Etiologies that can present as the syndrome of acute pericarditis.

TABLE 86.2 Etiology of Pericarditis in Major Series

ETIOLOGY	REPORTED FREQUENCY (%)
Idiopathic	15% (Africa) to 80%–90% (Europe)
Infectious pericarditis	
Viral	Largely unknown
Bacterial:	
Tuberculosis	1%–4% developed countries, up to 70% (Africa)
Purulent	<1% developed countries, 2%–3% Africa
Other infectious causes	Rare, largely unknown
Noninfectious pericarditis	
Neoplastic	5%–9% to 35% (in tertiary referral centers)
Autoimmune	2%–24%
Other noninfectious causes	Rare (largely unknown)

PR-depression can occur without ST elevation and be the initial or sole ECG manifestation. Typical ECG evolution follows four stages: (1) PR depression and/or diffuse ST segment elevation, (2) normalization of ST segment, (3) T wave inversion with or without ST segment depression, and (4) normalization. The ECG often evolves without all four stages.

Although usually considered a hallmark of pericarditis, typical ECG changes reflect concomitant involvement of the myocardium, because the pericardium is electrically silent. For that reason, ECG changes are reported in no more than 60% of cases and are more common (>90%) with concomitant myocarditis.[13] Additional ECG changes that may constitute clues to the cause of pericarditis or associated findings include atrioventricular block in Lyme disease, pathologic Q waves signifying a previous, silent MI, and low-voltage or electrical alternans pointing toward significant effusion.

Many patients with acute pericarditis have a modestly elevated white blood cell count (WBC).[4,5] WBCs in excess of 13,000 to 14,000/mm[3] suggest a specific etiology. As noted earlier, as many as 15% of patients have coexistent myocarditis based on elevations in cardiac biomarkers such as troponin (see Chapter 55). Patients with myocarditis usually have ST-segment elevation.[13] Another concern in patients with elevated injury biomarkers is a prior silent MI followed by subsequent pericarditis. The latter usually occurs after large or late-presenting MIs with transmural ECG changes.[15]

Serum C-reactive protein (CRP) is elevated in approximately three-fourths of patients with acute pericarditis.[16] Normal values generally occur in patients seen very early or who have previously received anti-inflammatory drugs including corticosteroids. CRP usually normalizes within 1 week and in almost all cases by 4 weeks after initial evaluation. Failure to normalize CRP is independently associated with recurrent symptoms.[9] In addition to aiding in diagnosis, CRP can be used to monitor disease activity and individualize duration of therapy.[4,16] Although the utility of CRP for this purpose has not been prospectively validated, the association of elevated values with recurrences provides a rationale for measurement initially and when it is uncertain how long treatment should be maintained.

Chest radiograms are normal in uncomplicated acute pericarditis.[5] Occasionally, small pulmonary infiltrates or pleural effusions are present, presumably related to the underlying causative infection. Because small to moderate effusions may not cause an abnormal cardiac silhouette, even modest cardiac enlargement is of concern and generally associated with an effusion greater than 300 mL.

The echocardiographic-Doppler examination (see Chapter 16) is completely normal in approximately 40% of patients with acute pericarditis.[1,7] It is performed mainly to determine if an effusion is present and recommended in all patients with suspected pericarditis.[1,4] Pericardial effusion is reported in about 60% of cases of acute pericarditis and is usually small (<10 mm on semiquantitative echocardiographic assessment). Moderate (10 to 20 mm) or large effusions (>20 mm) are unusual and may signal a diagnosis other than *idiopathic* pericarditis. An effusion in a patient with a history consistent with acute pericarditis is confirmatory of the diagnosis.

closely resembles early repolarization. As with the rub, ECG changes can be dynamic. Frequent recordings can yield a diagnosis in patients who initially have neither rub nor ST elevation. PR-segment depression is also common and considered the earliest ECG sign of acute pericarditis, reflecting pericardial involvement overlying the atria (see Fig. 86.2).

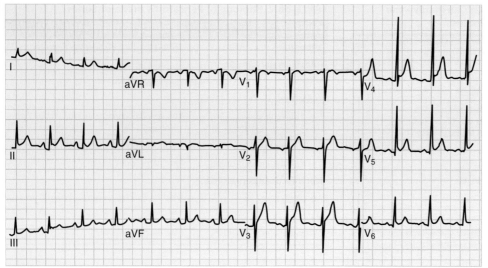

FIGURE 86.2 The electrocardiogram in acute pericarditis. Note both diffuse ST-segment elevation and PR-segment depression.

TABLE 86.3 Initial Approach to the Patient with Definite or Suspected Acute Pericarditis

1. If the diagnosis is suspected but not certain, listen often for pericardial rub and obtain ECGs frequently to check for diagnostic findings.

2. If the diagnosis is suspected or certain, obtain the following tests to help confirm the diagnosis (if necessary) and determine whether a specific causative diagnosis and/or significant associated conditions and/or complications are present:
   Hemogram
   hsCRP
   Troponin I
   Chest radiograph
   Echocardiogram
   Consider additional testing on the basis of clinical suspicion of a specific (non-idiopathic) etiology.

3. If the diagnosis is likely or certain, initiate therapy with an NSAID plus colchicine.

4. If diagnosis still uncertain consider CT scan or cardiac MRI to document pericardial inflammation.

CT, Computed tomography; *ECG,* electrocardiogram; *NSAID,* nonsteroidal antiinflammatory drugs.

Echocardiography is also useful in unusual cases where associated myocarditis is severe enough to alter ventricular function and to detect a previously silent MI. In uncomplicated acute pericarditis, it is rarely necessary to use imaging modalities other than echocardiography. However, in difficult cases computed tomography (CT) and/or cardiac magnetic resonance (CMR) imaging can help to detect pericardial thickening and/or active inflammation.[17,18]

Diagnosis, Natural History, and Management

ESC guidelines include the results of the first randomized clinical trials in pericarditis as well as more recent observational studies.[4] However, objective data to support recommendations for management of acute pericarditis and other pericardial diseases remain limited; most are based on expert opinion and consensus. According to the guidelines, the clinical diagnosis of acute pericarditis requires at least two of the following: (1) chest pain, (2) pericardial friction rub, (3) ECG changes consisting of typical ST elevation and/or PR depression, and (4) pericardial effusion.

In atypical presentations, additional imaging can be helpful in establishing the diagnosis. CT may show thickening or hyperattenuation of the pericardium. CMR may show pericardial edema based on fat-suppressed T2-weighted dark blood images, or delayed pericardial hyperenhancement indicative of ongoing inflammation.[17,18] Elevation

of biomarkers of inflammation (e.g., CRP) is supportive of the diagnosis, but not definitive.

Initial management is focused on confirming the diagnosis, screening for specific causes that would alter management, detection of effusion and other echocardiographic abnormalities, alleviation of symptoms, and directed treatment if a specific cause is discovered (Table 86.3). Certain features are associated with an increased risk of complications (mainly tamponade) (*inset*, Fig. 86.3). On this basis, triage of patients is possible after initial evaluation. We recommend the following routine testing: ECG, CBC, serum creatinine, CRP (or hsCRP), cardiac troponin, chest radiograph, and echocardiogram. Additional testing is guided by suspicion of a specific cause or complication. For example, if there are signs or symptoms concerning for systemic lupus erythematosus (SLE), an anti-nuclear antibody (ANA) titer is appropriate. However, low ANA titers are common in patients with *recurrent* idiopathic pericarditis without SLE criteria.[19] Thus, the significance of low ANA titers can be uncertain. Figure 86.3 and Table 86.3 summarize our recommendations for triage and initial management of patients with definite or suspected acute pericarditis.

Acute idiopathic pericarditis is a self-limited disease without significant complications or recurrence in 70% to 90% of patients.[5,9] If laboratory data do not contradict the diagnosis of *idiopathic* pericarditis, symptomatic treatment with nonsteroidal antiinflammatory drugs (NSAIDs) is recommended.[4,5,9] Restriction of physical activity until resolution of symptoms and normalization of CRP occurs is recommended. For athletes, return to sports is recommended after an arbitrary term of 3 months and only after symptoms have fully resolved and CRP, ECG, and echocardiogram have normalized.[4]

The choice of an antiinflammatory regimen is based on concomitant therapies (e.g., favoring aspirin [ASA] if antiplatelet therapy is required), patient preferences, and medical history (allergies, intolerances, etc.). Two alternative regimens with an excellent safety profile are recommended (Table 86.4): ibuprofen 600 to 800 mg orally three times daily, or ASA 750 to 1000 mg orally three times daily. Gastric protection in the form of a proton pump inhibitor should be provided. Many patients have satisfactory responses to the first few doses of an NSAID. A majority respond fully after 10 to 14 days and need no additional treatment. As noted, using normalization of CRP to guide duration of therapy is a reasonable alternative to a predetermined time course.[4,16] Once the patient is asymptomatic and CRP normalized, tapering rather than abrupt cessation of antiinflammatory drugs should be considered in an attempt to reduce recurrences (see Table 86.4).

Colchicine is recommended for 3 months as an adjunct to NSAIDs. When added to standard antiinflammatory therapy, colchicine reduces recurrences by approximately half[20] and speeds resolution of symptoms. Colchicine is thought to exert an antiinflammatory effect by blocking microtubule assembly in WBCs and inhibiting the inflammasome.[9] Weight-adjusted doses (0.5 to 0.6 mg orally every 12 hours or 0.5 to 0.6 mg once daily for patients <70 kg) are recommended.[4,20]

Patients with no more than small effusion and no high-risk features do not need to be admitted to hospital (see Fig. 86.3). Patients who do not respond well to initial treatment, have larger effusions, high-risk features, or a concerning etiology should be hospitalized for observation, further diagnostic testing, and treatment (see Fig. 86.3). In those who respond slowly to an NSAID and colchicine, analgesics allow time for a more complete response. Initial use of the IV route of administration for NSAIDs can be considered to more quickly alleviate symptoms.[4,21]

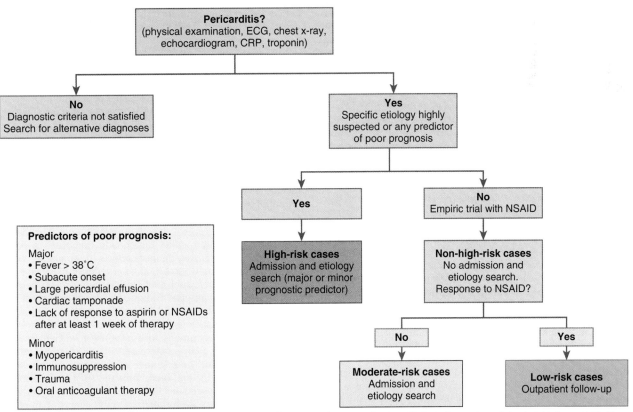

FIGURE 86.3 A proposed scheme for the triage and initial management of patients with suspected pericarditis, including markers of elevated risk (*box at left*). (From Adler Y, Charron P, Imazio M, et al. 2015 ESC Guidelines for the diagnosis and management of pericardial diseases: The Task Force for the Diagnosis and Management of Pericardial Diseases of the European Society of Cardiology (ESC)Endorsed by: The European Association for Cardio-Thoracic Surgery (EACTS). *Eur Heart J.* 2015;36[42]:2921–2964.)

TABLE 86.4 Empiric Antiinflammatory Therapy for Acute Idiopathic Pericarditis

DRUG	USUAL DOSING	INITIAL DURATION	TAPERING*
Aspirin	750–1000 mg every 8 hr	1–2 weeks	Decrease doses every week for 2–3 weeks, then discontinue
Ibuprofen	600–800 mg every 8 hr	1–2 weeks	Decrease doses every week for 2–3 weeks, then discontinue
Colchicine	0.5–0.6 mg once (<70 kg) or 0.5–0.6 mg twice daily (≥70 kg)	3 months	Optional, over 2–3 weeks

*Therapy duration is individualized and guided by symptoms and hsCRP. Maintain initial dose and taper only when asymptomatic and hsCRP is normalized.

Corticosteroid use should be minimized in patients with acute pericarditis because they may impair the clearance of infectious agents and short, high-dose courses may increase the risk of recurrence.[4,5,9] However, there are selected indications for their use: (1) contraindications to or failure of NSAID/colchicine, (2) underlying conditions (e.g., autoimmune diseases) whose primary treatment is corticosteroids, (3) concomitant diseases (e.g., renal failure), (4) pregnancy, and (5) concomitant therapies constituting relative contraindications to NSAIDs and/or colchicine (e.g., oral anticoagulants).[9,22] When used, relatively low doses of corticosteroids are recommended (e.g., prednisone 0.2 to 0.5 mg/kg daily) to minimize complications. Higher doses of corticosteroids are associated with major side effects in about one quarter of patients, leading to drug withdrawal, more hospitalizations, and more recurrences.[23] Tapering should be gradual, typically over 6 to 12 weeks, and guided by symptomatic response and CRP. Concurrent colchicine should be administrated during corticosteroid therapy.

Complications of acute pericarditis include effusion, tamponade, constriction, and recurrences. As noted earlier, small effusions are common. Relatively little is known about the incidence of more significant complications. In one study, over an average 31-month follow-up, tamponade developed in 3.1% and constriction in 1.5%.[24] Most complications occurred in patients with identified specific causes. In another study with longer follow-up, constriction developed in 1.8%. In the 83% of patients with idiopathic pericarditis, constriction developed in only 0.48%.[25] Thus, patients with idiopathic pericarditis can be reassured that development of constriction is exceedingly unlikely.

Recurrent Pericarditis

Recurrences occur in 15% to 30% of patients with idiopathic acute pericarditis.[5,9,26] Recurrences may seriously affect quality of life. They have not been associated with evolution to constriction.[25] A diagnosis of recurrent pericarditis requires new symptoms and signs of disease activity (friction rub, ECG changes, new or worsening pericardial effusion, elevation of CRP) after a symptom-free interval of at least 4 to 6 weeks.[4,5] It is not unusual for patients to have recurrent pain without objective evidence of disease activity. These patients may respond to repeated treatment but should not be classified as having a definite recurrence.

For recurrences, we recommend NSAID and colchicine in the same doses used for an initial episode. Therapy should be continued until complete resolution of symptoms and normalization of CRP, if elevated. At this point, the NSAID should be gradually tapered. If this therapy fails, corticosteroids may replace NSAID or may be added as "triple therapy." As for an initial episode, doses of 0.2 to 0.5 mg/kg/day of prednisone or equivalent are recommended for at least 2 to 4 weeks until resolution of symptoms and normalization of CRP, followed by gradual tapering every 2 to 4 weeks. Colchicine should be included for at least 6 months and up to 12 months for difficult cases.[9] For recurrence during corticosteroid tapering, we recommend maintaining the same dose if possible and controlling the recurrence by adding or increasing NSAID and/or starting colchicine if this has not been done. Some patients have recurrences which are mild and easily managed with re-institution of an NSAID for a brief period of time. These patients often do not have objective evidence of inflammation; an increase in corticosteroid dose or more intensive immunosuppressive therapy is not necessary.

For patients with colchicine-resistant and/or corticosteroid-dependent disease, additional therapies are available.[9,21] These patients are relatively rare, representing no more than 5% to 10% of recurrent pericarditis cases.[9,27] In this situation, CMR may help identify higher-risk patients and inform the expected clinical course and duration of treatment.[17,28–30] Potential alternative therapies include azathioprine (1 mg/kg/day with gradual dose increases and monitoring of WBC, transaminases, and amylase) and human intravenous immunoglobulin (400 to 500 mg/kg/day for 5 days with a possible repeat course after 1 month).[4,31] Interleukin-1 antagonists are a newer, very promising additional therapy for recurrent pericarditis.[21] Anakinra, a recombinant short-acting IL-1α and IL-1β cytokine receptor blocker, which is off-label, is one example (1 to 2 mg/kg/day up to 100 mg SC daily).[32] Optimal duration of therapy and whether tapering is required and if so how best to accomplish it have yet to be determined.[33] We generally treat patients with anakinra for 9 to 12 months followed by slow tapering. Recently, rilonacept (loading dose of 320 mg SC followed by 160 mg SC weekly), an IL-1α and IL-1β cytokine trap, has been shown to rapidly resolve acute episodes of recurrent pericarditis and markedly lower the risk of future recurrence by 96%.[33a,33b] Standard of care medications, including corticosteroids, were successfully discontinued as rilonacept was introduced. As a result, the drug received an indication for treatment of recurrent pericarditis from the FDA. The optimal duration of rilonacept is not known; however, the median duration in the RHAPSODY trial was 9 months (maximum 14 months), and tapering of rilonacept may not be required due to the gradual washout pharmacokinetics of the drug.[33c] The mechanisms of action of alternative antiinflammatory drugs for treatment of recurrent pericarditis are summarized in eFigure 86.2. For physicians who do not ordinarily prescribe these drugs, it is prudent to enlist the help of colleagues experienced in their use. In patients with pericarditis refractory to medical therapies, pericardiectomy may be considered.[34]

PERICARDIAL EFFUSION AND CARDIAC TAMPONADE

Etiology

Virtually any disease that involves the pericardium can cause an effusion (see Table 86.1).[3,4,7,35] In the developing world TB remains a major cause. In the developed world idiopathic pericarditis, malignancy, and percutaneous procedural complications are the most common causes of significant effusions.[4,35]

Effusions are common for several weeks to a few months following cardiac surgery and transplantation[4] but tamponade is unusual. Various miscellaneous, noninflammatory diseases can cause effusion (see Table 86.1), including transudates in patients with severe circulatory congestion. Bleeding into the pericardial sac occurs after blunt and penetrating trauma, following post-MI rupture of the LV free wall, and as a complication of various percutaneous cardiac procedures. Retrograde bleeding is a major cause of death due to aortic dissection (see Chapter 42). Effusions are also common in patients with pulmonary hypertension.[2] Asymptomatic pericardial effusions are sometimes discovered when a chest X-ray or echocardiogram is performed for unrelated indications, often in otherwise healthy individuals.[4]

Effusions with a high likelihood of progression to tamponade include bacterial, HIV-associated infections (see Chapter 80), bleeding, and neoplastic disease. Large effusions due to acute idiopathic pericarditis are infrequent, but account for significant numbers of tamponade cases because this diagnosis is so common. About 20% of large, symptomatic effusions without an obvious etiology following routine evaluation represent the initial presentation of a cancer.[4,36] Details of

pericardial effusion pertinent to selected, specific disease entities are discussed at the end of this chapter.

Pathophysiology and Hemodynamics

Formation of an effusion is usually a response to inflammatory, infectious, or neoplastic diseases involving the pericardium. Other diseases that can occasionally cause *noninflammatory* effusions include lymphomas with enlarged mediastinal lymph nodes,[3] circulatory congestion, and metabolic diseases including hypothyroidism and protein malnutrition.[3,4,7]

When an effusion accumulates, the pressure in the pericardial sac depends on the amount of fluid and the pericardial pressure-volume relation. The mechanical consequences of a high pressure acting on the surface of the heart mainly result from compression and collapse of right heart. Left heart underfilling then ensues from reduced right heart output. eFigure 86.3 depicts an experiment illustrating these principles. Clinically, cardiac tamponade comprises a continuum from an effusion causing minimal effects to circulatory collapse. A critical point occurs when an effusion reduces diastolic volume of the cardiac chambers such that cardiac output (CO) declines. The limited pericardial reserve volume dictates that modest amounts of rapidly accumulating fluid (150 to 200 mL) can impair cardiac function. In contrast, large, slowly accumulating effusions are often well-tolerated. The compensatory response to a hemodynamically significant effusion includes increased adrenergic tone and parasympathetic withdrawal. The resultant tachycardia and increased contractility[3] maintain CO and blood pressure (BP) for a period of time, but eventually they decline. Patients who cannot mount an adrenergic response are more susceptible to the effects of an effusion. In terminal tamponade, a depressor reflex with paradoxical bradycardia may supervene.

As fluid accumulates, left- and right-sided atrial and ventricular diastolic pressures rise and in severe tamponade equalize at a pressure similar to that in the pericardial sac, typically 20 to 25 mm Hg (Fig. 86.4). Equalization is closest during inspiration. Thus, *transmural* filling pressures are markedly reduced. Correspondingly, cardiac volumes progressively decline. The small end-diastolic ventricular volume (decreased preload) mainly accounts for reduced stroke volume (SV). Because of compensatory increases in contractility, end-systolic volume also decreases, but not enough to maintain SV.

In addition to elevated and equal intra-cavitary filling pressures, low transmural filling pressures, and small cardiac volumes, two other hemodynamic abnormalities are characteristic of tamponade.[3] One is loss of the y descent of the RA or systemic venous pressure wave (see Fig. 86.4). *x* and *y descents* correspond to periods when venous flow is increasing. Loss of the *y* descent has been explained based on the concept that total heart volume is fixed in severe tamponade.[3] Thus, blood can enter the heart only when blood is simultaneously leaving. The normal *y* descent begins when the tricuspid valve opens, that is, blood is not leaving. In tamponade inflow cannot increase and the descent is lost. The *x* descent occurs during ventricular ejection. Because blood is leaving the heart, inflow can increase and the *x* descent is retained. Loss of the *y* descent in systemic venous or RA pressure recordings is a useful clue to the presence of tamponade. An absent *y* descent and loss of diastolic venous inflow are considered classic.[3] However, in many cases in the modern era pulsed wave Doppler recordings reveal some degree of venous inflow into the right heart during ventricular diastole.[1,2] These patients may have ECP, with a mixed hemodynamic picture.

The second characteristic finding is the paradoxical pulse (Fig. 86.5), an abnormally large drop (>10 mm Hg) in systolic arterial pressure during inspiration. Other causes of *pulsus paradoxus* include CP, pulmonary embolus, and pulmonary disease with large variations in intra-thoracic pressure. The mechanism of the paradoxical pulse is multifactorial, but respiratory changes in systemic venous return are important.[3] In tamponade, in contrast to constriction, the normal inspiratory *increase* in systemic venous return is present and the normal inspiratory *decline* in systemic venous pressure is retained (Kussmaul's

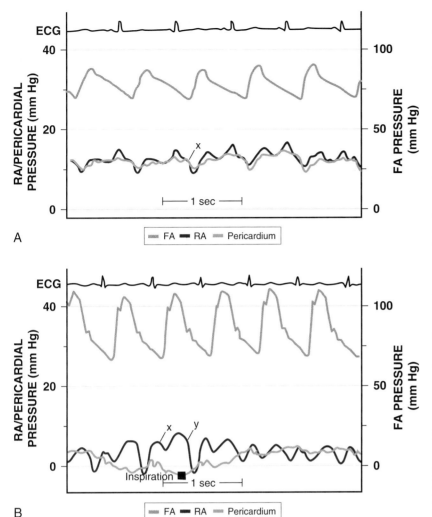

A

B

FIGURE 86.4 Femoral arterial (FA), right atrial (RA), and pericardial pressure before **(A)** and after **(B)** pericardiocentesis in a patient with cardiac tamponade. RA and pericardial pressure are about 15 mm Hg before pericardiocentesis. There is a minimal paradoxical pulse. RA x descent is present but y descent is absent before pericardiocentesis. Pericardiocentesis results in marked increase in FA pressure and decrease in RA pressure. During inspiration, pericardial pressure becomes negative, there is clear separation between RA and pericardial pressure, and y descent is now prominent, suggesting an effusive-constrictive picture. (From Baim DS, Grossman W, eds. *Grossman's Cardiac Catheterization, Angiography, and Intervention.* Philadelphia: Lippincott Williams & Wilkins, 2000:840.)

Although mean left- and right-sided filling pressures are typically 20 to 25 mm Hg, tamponade can occur at lower filling pressures, that is, low-pressure tamponade.[3,4,35] Low-pressure tamponade often occurs when there is a decrease in blood volume in the setting of a preexisting effusion which would not otherwise be significant. A modestly elevated pericardial pressure can lower transmural filling pressure to levels where SV is compromised. Because venous pressure is only modestly elevated or normal, the diagnosis may be missed. Low-pressure tamponade may be observed during hemodialysis, in patients with blood loss and volume depletion, and when diuretics are administered to patients with effusions. As many as 10% of patients undergoing closed pericardiocentesis may meet criteria for low-pressure tamponade. Compared with conventional tamponade, these patients are less often critically ill and signs of tamponade are less prominent.

Pericardial effusions can be loculated or localized, resulting in regional tamponade, most commonly after cardiac surgery.[3,4] Although reports are scarce, regional tamponade may cause atypical hemodynamic findings, for example, reduced CO with unilateral filling pressure elevation. Regional tamponade should be considered whenever there is hypotension in a setting where a loculated effusion is present. Rarely, large pleural effusions and pneumopericardium can compress the heart and cause tamponade.[3,4]

Clinical Presentation

A history pertinent to a specific disease etiology may be elicited. As noted earlier, asymptomatic effusions may be discovered in otherwise healthy individuals.[4] Specific etiologies are rarely found in these cases. Effusions per se do not cause symptoms without tamponade, although patients may have pain due to pericarditis. Patients with tamponade often complain of dyspnea (the mechanism is uncertain because there is no pulmonary congestion) and are more comfortable sitting forward. Other symptoms reflect the severity of CO and BP reduction.

The physical examination in pericardial effusion may provide clues to its etiology. In pericardial effusion without tamponade, the cardiovascular examination is normal except if the effusion is large, the cardiac impulse is difficult to palpate and heart sounds are muffled. A friction rub may of course be present. Tubular breath sounds may be heard in the left axilla or base due to bronchial compression. *Beck's triad,* hypotension, muffled heart sounds, and elevated jugular venous pressure, suggests severe tamponade. Patients with tamponade appear uncomfortable and display signs of reduced CO and shock, including tachypnea, diaphoresis, cool extremities, peripheral cyanosis, and depressed sensorium.[3,4,35] Hypotension is usually present, although in early stages compensatory mechanisms maintain BP. Some patients with subacute tamponade are initially *hypertensive.*[37] A paradoxical pulse is the rule, but it is important to be alert to situations where it may be absent. The paradox is quantified by cuff sphygmomanometry as the difference between the pressure at which Korotkoff sounds first appear and that at which they are present with each contraction. Tachycardia is also the rule unless heart rate lowering drugs have been administered, conduction system disease coexists, or a pre-terminal bradycardic reflex has supervened. The jugular venous pressure is markedly elevated except in low-pressure tamponade, and the y descent is usually absent. The normal decrease in venous pressure on inspiration is retained. Examination of the heart is simply consistent with effusion. Tamponade can be confused with anything that causes hypotension, shock, and elevated venous pressure, including decompensated heart failure, pulmonary embolus and other causes of pulmonary hypertension, and RV MI.

sign is *absent*). The increase in right heart filling pressure occurs, once again, under conditions where total heart volume is fixed and left heart volume markedly reduced. The interventricular septum shifts to the left in exaggerated fashion on inspiration, encroaching on the LV such that SV and pressure generation are further reduced (see Fig. 86.5). This is termed exaggerated ventricular interaction[1,7,35,36] (in distinction to the previous definition of ventricular interaction). Although the inspiratory increase in right heart volume (preload) increases RV SV, a few cardiac cycles are required to increase LV filling and SV and counteract the septal shift. Other factors that may contribute include increased afterload caused by transmission of negative intrathoracic pressure to the aorta and traction on the pericardium caused by descent of the diaphragm. Associated with these mechanisms, left and right heart pressure and SV variations are exaggerated and 180 degrees out of phase (see Figs. 86.4 and 86.5). Table 86.5 lists hemodynamic findings in tamponade compared with constriction. When there are preexisting elevations in diastolic pressures and/or volume, tamponade can occur without a paradoxical pulse.[3] Examples include chronic LV dysfunction, aortic regurgitation, and atrial septal defect. In patients with retrograde bleeding into the pericardial sac due to aortic dissection,[4] tamponade may occur without a paradoxical pulse because of aortic valve disruption and regurgitation.

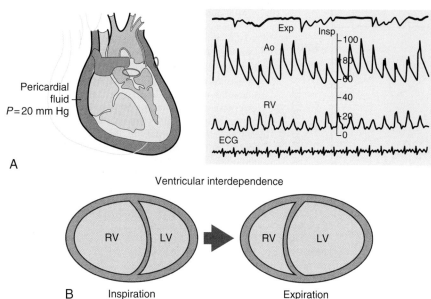

A

Ventricular interdependence

RV LV → RV LV

B Inspiration   Expiration

FIGURE 86.5 **A,** *Left,* illustration of leftward septal shift with encroachment of left ventricular (LV) volume during inspiration in cardiac tamponade. *Right,* respiration marker and aortic and right ventricular (RV) pressure tracings in cardiac tamponade. Note paradoxical pulse and 180 degrees out of phase respiratory variation in right and left-sided pressures. **B,** Exaggerated interventricular dependence in tamponade. On inspiration (*left*) there is a shift of the ventricular septum toward the LV, and on expiration (*right*) there is a shift of the ventricular septum toward the RV. (From Shabetai R. *The Pericardium.* New York: Grune & Stratton; 1981:266; and From Atherton JJ, Moore TD, Thomson HL, et al. *J Am Coll Cardiol.* 1998;31:413–418.)

TABLE 86.5 Hemodynamics in Cardiac Tamponade and Constrictive Pericarditis

	TAMPONADE	CONSTRICTION
Paradoxical pulse	Usually present	Present in approximately 1/3
Equal left/right filling	Present	Present pressures
Systemic venous wave morphology	Absent y descent	Prominent y descent (M or W shape)
Inspiratory change in systemic venous pressure	Decrease (normal)	Increase or no change (Kussmaul's sign)
"Square root" sign in ventricular pressure	Absent	Present

Laboratory Testing

ECG abnormalities include reduced voltage and electrical alternans (eFig. 86.4).[3,4] Reduced voltage is nonspecific and can be caused by emphysema, infiltrative myocardial disease, and pneumothorax. Electrical alternans is specific but relatively insensitive and caused by anterior-posterior swinging of the heart with each contraction. When pericarditis coexists, usual ECG findings may be present.

The chest radiograph reveals a normal cardiac silhouette until effusions are at least moderate in size. With larger effusions the antero-posterior cardiac silhouette assumes a rounded, flask-like appearance (eFig. 86.5). Lateral views may reveal the fat pad sign, a linear lucency at least 2 mm in width between chest wall and anterior surface of the heart caused by separation of epicardial from anterior mediastinal fat by the effusion. The lungs are oligemic.

M-mode and two-dimensional Doppler echocardiography are standard noninvasive methods for detection of effusion and tamponade (see also Chapter 16).[1,2,7,35,38] A significant effusion appears as a lucent separation between parietal and visceral pericardium for the entire cardiac cycle (Fig. 86.6 and Video 86.1). Small effusions are usually first evident over the posterobasal LV. With increasing effusions, the fluid spreads anteriorly, laterally, and behind the LA, where it is limited by the visceral pericardial reflection. Ultimately, the separation becomes

circumferential. Effusions are graded as trivial (only seen in systole), small (echo free space in diastole <10 mm), moderate (10 to 20 mm), large (>20 mm), and very large (>25 mm) (see Fig. 86.6).[7,35] Because speed of accumulation is critical, the hemodynamic significance of an effusion may not be correlated with its size. However, it is very unusual for tamponade to occur without a circumferential effusion. Frond-like or shaggy appearing structures in the pericardial space on echocardiography suggest clots, chronic inflammation, or neoplastic processes. CT and CMR are more accurate than transthoracic echocardiography for estimating pericardial thickness, although *transesophageal* echocardiography (TEE) is comparable.[1,2,7,35]

Several echocardiographic findings indicate that an effusion is large enough to cause hemodynamic compromise.[1,2,6,7] These include early diastolic collapse of RV, late diastolic indentation or collapse of RA, and exaggerated respiratory variation in RV and LV size and interventricular septal shifting during inspiration (septal bulge or "bounce"). Early diastolic RV collapse (Fig. 86.7, *right*; Video 86.1) and late diastolic RA collapse (see Fig. 86.7, *left*; Video 86.1) usually appear relatively early during tamponade,[1,2,7,35] when pericardial pressure transiently exceeds intra-cavitary pressure. Rarely, a large *pleural* effusion can cause right-sided chamber collapse.[7,35] Isolated *LV* and *LA* chamber collapse can occur with pericardial hematomas after cardiac surgery.[1,7,35] Cardiac chambers are small in tamponade and, as noted, the heart may swing antero-posteriorly (see Video 86.1). Distention of the inferior vena cava that does not diminish with inspiration is an important confirmatory finding. Doppler recordings demonstrate exaggerated respiratory variation in right- and left-sided venous and valvular flow, with inspiratory increases on the right and decreases on the left.[1,2,7,35] Caval inflow occurs largely during ventricular systole. These flow patterns are at least as sensitive for tamponade as M-mode and two-dimensional echocardiographic features.

With most effusions, transthoracic echocardiography provides sufficient diagnostic information for management decisions. TEE provides better quality images but is usually impractical in sick patients unless they are intubated. Fluoroscopy is useful in the cardiac catheterization laboratory for detection of procedure-related effusions that cause damping or abolition of cardiac pulsation. CT (see Chapter 20) and CMR (see Chapter 19) are useful adjuncts to echocardiography in characterizing effusion and tamponade,[39,40] but neither is ordinarily required and/or advisable in sick patients. They have a role when hemodynamics are atypical, other conditions complicate interpretation, the severity of tamponade is uncertain, or echocardiography is technically inadequate. Video 86.2 is a CMR cine image of a large, circumferential effusion and a small, under-filled LV. In this case, the RV was not compressed due to longstanding pulmonary hypertension, as evidenced by RV enlargement; thus, coexistent pulmonary hypertension modified echocardiographic signs of tamponade.

CT and MRI provide more detailed quantitation and regional localization of effusions than echocardiography and are useful with loculated and coexistent pleural effusions.[1,2,39,40] In Video 86.3, CMR demonstrates both large pericardial and pleural effusions in a patient with polyserositis. Pericardial thickness can be measured with both methods, allowing indirect assessment of the severity and chronicity of inflammation; MRI with gadolinium directly identifies inflammation. Clues to the nature of pericardial fluid can be gained from CT attenuation coefficients.[41] Attenuation similar to water suggests transudative effusion; attenuation denser than water suggests malignant, bloody or purulent fluid; and attenuation less dense than water, a chylous effusion. Malignant effusions are associated with a thicker pericardium than benign effusions. Finally, cine CT or CMR provides information similar to echocardiography for assessment of tamponade, for example, septal shifting, chamber collapse.

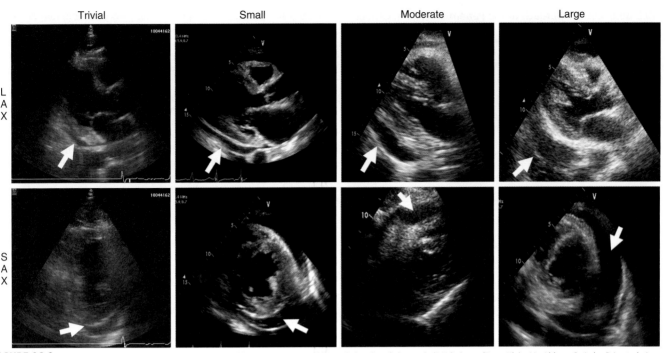

FIGURE 86.6 Trivial, small, moderate, and large pericardial effusions. Parasternal long axis (LAX) and short axis (SAX) views. (From Klein AL, Abbara S, Agler DA, et al. American Society of Echocardiography clinical recommendations for multimodality cardiovascular imaging of patients with pericardial disease: endorsed by the Society for Cardiovascular Magnetic Resonance and Society of Cardiovascular Computed Tomography. *J Am Soc Echocardiogr.* 2013;26:965–1012.e1015.)

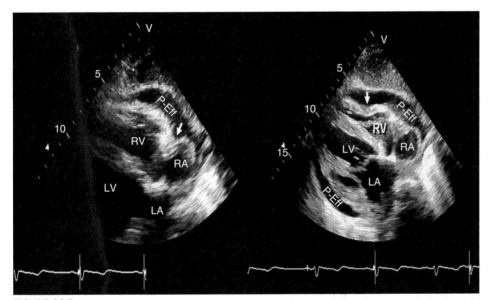

FIGURE 86.7 Two-dimensional echocardiographic subcostal view in a patient with cardiac tamponade showing right atrium (RA) *(left side)* and right ventricular (RV) *(right side)* indentation or "collapse" *(arrows)*. In RA and RV, indentation occurs during their respective relaxation when pressure is lowest, transiently falling below pericardial pressure. RA indentation occurs during early ventricular systole, whereas RV indentation occurs in early diastole. (From Klein AL, Abbara S, Agler DA, et al. American Society of Echocardiography clinical recommendations for multimodality cardiovascular imaging of patients with pericardial disease: endorsed by the Society for Cardiovascular Magnetic Resonance and Society of Cardiovascular Computed Tomography. *J Am Soc Echocardiogr.* 2013;26:965–1012.e1015.)

Management of Pericardial Effusion and Tamponade

Management is primarily dictated by whether tamponade is already present or has a high chance of developing (Table 86.6).[1,3,4,35] Situations where tamponade is a near-term threat include suspected bacterial pericarditis, hemopericardium, and any moderate to large effusion that is not thought to be chronic and/or is increasing in size. When tamponade is present or threatened, decision-making requires urgency and a low threshold for pericardiocentesis (see Table 86.6). *In the absence of actual or threatened tamponade,* management can be

more leisurely. This includes several categories of patients. Some have acute pericarditis with a small to moderate effusion detected as part of routine evaluation. Others do not have symptoms or signs of pericarditis or effusion but undergo echocardiography because of the presence of diseases known to involve the pericardium. The rest are asymptomatic and have effusions detected when tests are performed for reasons other than suspected pericardial disease, for example, screening, evaluation of an enlarged cardiac silhouette. Klein and colleagues[1] propose a three-step scoring system for pericardial effusion that awards points based on etiology, clinical presentation, and imaging to arrive at a cumulative score whose value dictates whether *urgent* drainage is warranted.

In many cases of effusion where tamponade is neither present nor threatened, an etiology will be evident or suggested based on the history and/or previous diagnostic tests. When the diagnosis is unclear, an assessment of specific etiologies should be undertaken, including diagnostic tests recommended for acute pericarditis and anything else dictated by the clinical picture, for example, neoplastic and autoimmune diseases, infections, and hypothyroidism.

In patients without actual or imminent tamponade, closed pericardiocentesis or, occasionally, surgical drainage (possibly with biopsy and/or creation of a window) may be undertaken for diagnostic purposes but is often not required. As discussed above, in many cases a diagnosis will either be obvious or become evident during initial investigations. Moreover, in this setting routine analysis of pericardial fluid has a low diagnostic yield.[4,35] In situations where pericardiocentesis is felt to be necessary for diagnosis, consideration should be given to open drainage with biopsy.

DISEASES OF THE MYOCARDIUM, PERICARDIUM, AND PULMONARY VASCULATURE BED

TABLE 86.6 Initial Approach to the Patient with a Pericardial Effusion

1. Determine if tamponade is present or threatened based on history, physical examination, echocardiogram.

2. If tamponade is not present or threatened:
   - if etiology not apparent, consider diagnostic tests as for acute pericarditis
   - if effusion is large, consider course of an NSAID + colchicine or corticosteroid and, if no response, consider closed pericardiocentesis

3. If tamponade is present or threatened:
   - urgent or emergent closed pericardiocentesis or careful monitoring if trial of medical treatment to reduce effusion is considered appropriate

Otherwise healthy patients with large, asymptomatic effusions and no evidence of tamponade or a specific etiology are a special category.[4,41] The effusions are by definition chronic and in general stable, but a minority (perhaps 20% to 30%) develop tamponade unpredictably. After closed pericardiocentesis the effusions may not reaccumulate. Thus, there is a rationale for pericardiocentesis following routine evaluation for specific etiologies as outlined above. Before undertaking pericardiocentesis a brief course of an NSAID or corticosteroid combined with colchicine may be considered. However, absent evidence of inflammation (increased CRP, gadolinium uptake on CMR), antiinflammatory regimens are not likely to be efficacious. Recurrence of this type of effusion after closed pericardiocentesis is considered an indication for a pericardial window or pericardiectomy.[4,41]

Patients with actual or threatened tamponade constitute medical emergencies. With the exception of those who do not wish prolongation of life (e.g., metastatic cancer), hospital admission and careful hemodynamic and echocardiographic monitoring is mandatory. The great majority require pericardiocentesis to treat or prevent tamponade, but there are some exceptions. Patients with acute, apparently idiopathic pericarditis with no more than mild tamponade can be treated for a brief period of time under careful monitoring with an NSAID and/or a corticosteroid combined with colchicine in an attempt to rapidly shrink the effusion. Patients with known inflammatory/autoimmune diseases can be treated similarly (there is no evidence that corticosteroids increase recurrences in these patients). Patients with *suspected* bacterial infections or hemopericardium *with small effusions (<10 mm)* should be considered to have threatened tamponade because of the etiology. These patients are appropriate for initial conservative management and careful monitoring because of the elevated risk of closed pericardiocentesis with smaller effusions.

Hemodynamic monitoring with a central venous or pulmonary artery catheter is often useful, especially in patients with threatened or mild tamponade in whom pericardiocentesis is deferred. Monitoring is also helpful *after* pericardiocentesis to assess reaccumulation and detect underlying constriction (see Fig. 86.4). Insertion of a catheter in the central circulation should not delay definitive therapy in critically ill patients.

For most patients in this category urgent or emergent pericardiocentesis is indicated. Once actual or threatened tamponade is diagnosed, intravenous hydration with normal saline should be instituted.[4,41] However, hydration as well as positive inotropes are temporizing measures that should not delay pericardiocentesis. In the vast majority of cases, echocardiographically guided *closed* pericardiocentesis is the method of choice. Before proceeding it is important to ensure that there is indeed an effusion large enough to cause tamponade that is amenable to a closed approach. Loculated effusions or effusions containing clots or fibrinous material increase the risk and difficulty of closed pericardiocentesis.

Whether to perform closed versus open pericardiocentesis in patients with *hemopericardium* is a difficult decision.[4,41] The danger of a closed approach is that lowering intra-pericardial pressure will allow more bleeding without affording an opportunity to correct its source. In cases of trauma or post-MI LV rupture, closed pericardiocentesis should usually be avoided. If bleeding is slower, closed pericardiocentesis is generally indicated because bleeding may stop spontaneously

and/or the procedure can provide temporary relief before definitive repair. Closed pericardiocentesis in patients with hemopericardium due to type A aortic dissection has been considered contraindicated. However, in one report closed pericardiocentesis using intermittent cycles of drainage dictated by systolic BP appeared safe and effective for stabilization.[42]

The usual approach to closed pericardiocentesis is para-apical needle insertion with echocardiographic guidance to minimize risks of myocardial puncture and assess completeness of fluid removal.[4] Occasionally, a sub-xyphoid site is preferred. Once the needle has entered the pericardial space, a modest amount of fluid is removed (perhaps 50 to 100 mL) in an effort to produce rapid improvement. A guidewire is then inserted and the needle replaced with a pigtail catheter, which is manipulated to maximize fluid removal. When possible, closed pericardiocentesis should be performed in an ICU procedure room or cardiac catheterization laboratory with experienced personnel available. Echocardiographically guided pericardiocentesis has a greater than 95% success rate and less than 2% serious complication rate.[43,44] Rarely, patients suffer "pericardial decompression syndrome" following closed or open drainage,[45] a poorly understood but life-threatening syndrome characterized by combinations of pulmonary edema and shock.

CT guidance is a valuable alternative to both echocardiographic guidance and open pericardiocentesis.[46] Its success rate and safety are comparable to echocardiographic guidance. It is particularly well suited for regional and/or loculated effusions and effusions where the usual needle insertion sites are felt to be unsafe.

If a pulmonary artery catheter has been inserted, RA and pulmonary capillary wedge pressure and CO should be monitored before, during, and after the procedure. Ideally, pericardial fluid pressure should also be measured. Hemodynamic monitoring is useful for several reasons. Initial measurements confirm and document severity of tamponade. Measurements after completion establish a baseline to assess reaccumulation. Some patients with tamponade have coexisting constriction (ECP), which is difficult to detect when an effusion dominates but becomes apparent after pericardiocentesis. Following pericardiocentesis, repeat echocardiography and in many cases continued hemodynamic monitoring should be used to assess reaccumulation. Intra-pericardial catheters should ideally be left in place for 2 to 3 days to allow continued drainage and minimize recurrence.[4,35,47]

Open pericardiocentesis is occasionally preferred for initial removal of fluid. Bleeding due to trauma and rupture of the LV free wall have been mentioned previously. Loculated effusions and/or effusions that are borderline in size are drained more safely in the operating room or using CT guidance. Recurring effusions, especially those causing tamponade, may initially be drained using a closed approach due to logistical considerations. However, open pericardiocentesis with possible biopsy and creation of a window are usually preferred for recurrences causing tamponade.[4,48]

Percutaneous balloon pericardiotomy and periocardioscopy have been used to drain fluid, create pericardial windows, and perform pericardial biopsy.[4,49] Balloon pericardiotomy is useful for malignant effusions and other situations where recurrence is common and a more definitive approach without surgery desirable. These methods appear safe and effective, but experience is confined to a few centers.

Pericardial Fluid Analysis

Normal pericardial fluid has the features of a plasma ultrafiltrate.[3] Lymphocytes are the predominant cell type. Although routine analysis does not have a very high yield for disease etiology, it is rewarding with bacterial infections and malignant effusions.[4,50] Measurements include WBC and differential, hematocrit glucose levels, and protein content. Although most effusions are exudates, detection of a transudate reduces diagnostic possibilities. Sanguineous appearing fluid is nonspecific and does not necessarily indicate active bleeding. Chylous effusions can occur after traumatic or surgical injury to the thoracic duct or obstruction by neoplasms. Cholesterol-rich ("gold paint") effusions occur in hypothyroidism. Pericardial fluid should be stained and cultured for bacteria and as much fluid as possible submitted for detection of malignant cells.

If TB pericarditis is suspected, several other tests are useful,[4,50,51] including unstimulated interferon-gamma (uIFN-γ), adenosine deaminase (ADA), lysozyme levels, and polymerase chain reaction (PCR). When TB is suspected at least one of these tests should be routine because of the time required for bacteriologic diagnosis.

Newer approaches for analysis of pericardial fluid have been investigated. There may be a role for measurement of tumor markers as a screen for malignant effusion.[4,52] Selected cytokine and related biomarkers measured in both pericardial fluid and serum[52] have shown promise in distinguishing various types of inflammatory effusions, but their roles are uncertain. In a small study, anti-myolemmal antibodies in pericardial fluid and serum were found to be predictive of recurrence in patients with chronic effusions.[53]

Pericardioscopy and Percutaneous Biopsy

Pericardioscopic-guided drainage of pericardial effusions was discussed earlier. When standard methods to evaluate the etiology of pericardial effusions are unsuccessful, extended pericardioscopically guided biopsies combined with immunological and molecular methods applied to both fluid and tissue (e.g., PCR)[49] have been advocated to improve diagnostic and management. This approach appears safe, but experience is limited.

CONSTRICTIVE PERICARDITIS

ETIOLOGY
CP is the end stage of an inflammatory process involving the pericardium. Many diseases listed in Table 86.1 can cause constriction. In the developed world common etiologies are idiopathic, post-surgical, and radiation injury.[3,4] TB was very common before the advent of effective therapy and remains important in developing countries.[54] Constriction can follow an initial insult by as little as several months and occasionally less, but typically takes years to develop. The end result is fibrosis, often calcification,

and adhesions of parietal and visceral pericardium. Figure 86.8 *(top)* illustrates the reciprocal relationship between the intense inflammation seen in acute and often in ECP (see below) and end-stage CP as inflammation diminishes and scarring and fibrosis gradually supervene. CMR images (see Fig. 86.8, *bottom*), discussed subsequently, demonstrate corresponding degrees of inflammation during this progression. Scarring is usually more or less symmetric and impedes filling of all heart chambers. Most patients have a thickened pericardium, but 18% are reported to have normal thickness on direct histopathologic examination and 28% on CT.[1,4,55] In a subset of patients with subacute inflammation constriction is transient and/or reversible by antiinflammatory drugs. This is observed early after cardiac surgery and in other patients with severe pericardial inflammation (discussed below).[3,9,17,28,56,57]

PATHOPHYSIOLOGY
The consequence of pericardial scarring and/or severe thickening is markedly restricted filling of the heart.[3,4] This results in elevated and equal filling pressures in all chambers and systemic and pulmonary veins. In early diastole the ventricles fill rapidly due to markedly elevated atrial pressures and accentuated ventricular suction related to small end-systolic volumes. During early to mid-diastole, filling abruptly ceases when cardiac volume reaches the limit set by the pericardium. Thus, almost all filling occurs early in diastole. Systemic venous congestion results in hepatic congestion, peripheral edema, ascites, anasarca, and cardiac cirrhosis. Reduced CO results from impaired filling and causes fatigue, muscle wasting, and weight loss. In "pure" constriction, ventricular contractile function is preserved, although ejection fraction (EF) can be reduced due to a small end-diastolic volume. In occasional patients, the myocardium is involved in inflammation and fibrosis, leading to contractile dysfunction that predicts a poor result after pericardiectomy.[4,58,59]

Failure of transmission of intrathoracic respiratory pressure changes to the cardiac chambers through the thickened pericardium is an important contributor to the pathophysiology of CP (Fig. 86.9, *top panel*). On inspiration the drop in intrathoracic pressure is transmitted to the pulmonary veins but not the left heart. Consequently, the small pulmonary venous to LA pressure gradient that normally drives left heart filling is reduced, resulting in decreased transmitral inflow. The inspiratory decrease in LV filling allows an increase in RV filling and a leftward

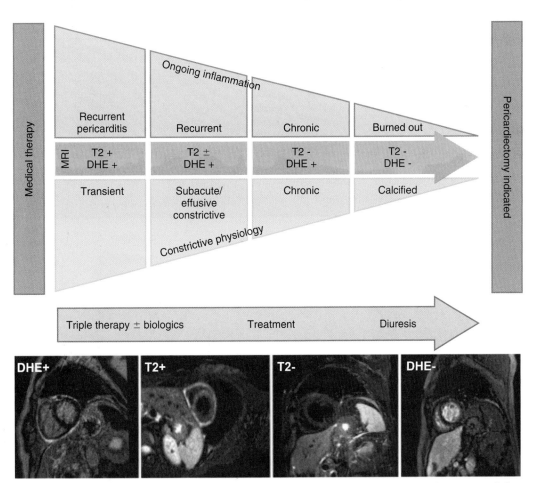

FIGURE 86.8 The spectrum of pericardial disease and its relation to inflammation (**top,** see text). Cardiac MRI **(bottom)** demonstrates the continuum of inflammatory disease starting with an acute phase and ending in burnt-out and/or calcific constrictive pericarditis. *DHE,* Delayed hyperenhancement. (From Chetrit M, et al. *J Am Coll Cardiol Imag.* 2020;13:1422–1437.)

interventricular septal shift. The opposite occurs with expiration (see Fig. 86.9, *middle and bottom panels*).[60–62] Similar to tamponade, these changes result in exaggerated respiratory variation in mitral and tricuspid inflow and LV and RV systolic and diastolic pressure and volumes (see Fig. 86.9, *bottom*). High systemic venous pressure and reduced CO induce renal retention of sodium and water. Inhibition of natriuretic peptides may exacerbate increased filling pressures.[63]

CLINICAL PRESENTATION

The usual presentation consists of signs and symptoms of right heart failure, lower extremity edema, vague abdominal complaints, and passive hepatic congestion, which can progress to ascites, anasarca, and jaundice due to cardiac cirrhosis. Signs and symptoms of left heart failure, dyspnea, cough, and orthopnea may also appear. Atrial fibrillation and tricuspid regurgitation, which further exacerbate venous pressure elevation, are common at this stage. At the end stage, effects of a chronically low CO are prominent, including fatigue, muscle wasting, and cachexia. Other findings include recurrent pleural effusions and syncope. CP can be mistaken for any cause of right heart failure, for example, RV systolic dysfunction, and end-stage liver disease.[60,61]

Physical Examination (see Chapter 13)

Physical findings include elevated jugular venous pressure with a prominent, rapidly collapsing *y*-descent. This, combined with a normal *x* descent, results in an M or W-shaped venous pressure contour. In patients with atrial fibrillation the *x* descent is lost, leaving only the prominent *y* descent. The latter is difficult to distinguish from tricuspid regurgitation which, as noted above, may also be present. *Kussmaul's sign*, an inspiratory increase in mean venous pressure, is usually present,[3] or pressure may simply fail to decrease on inspiration. Kussmaul's sign reflects loss of the normal increase in right heart venous return on inspiration, even though tricuspid flow increases. A paradoxical pulse occurs in perhaps one-third of patients, especially with an

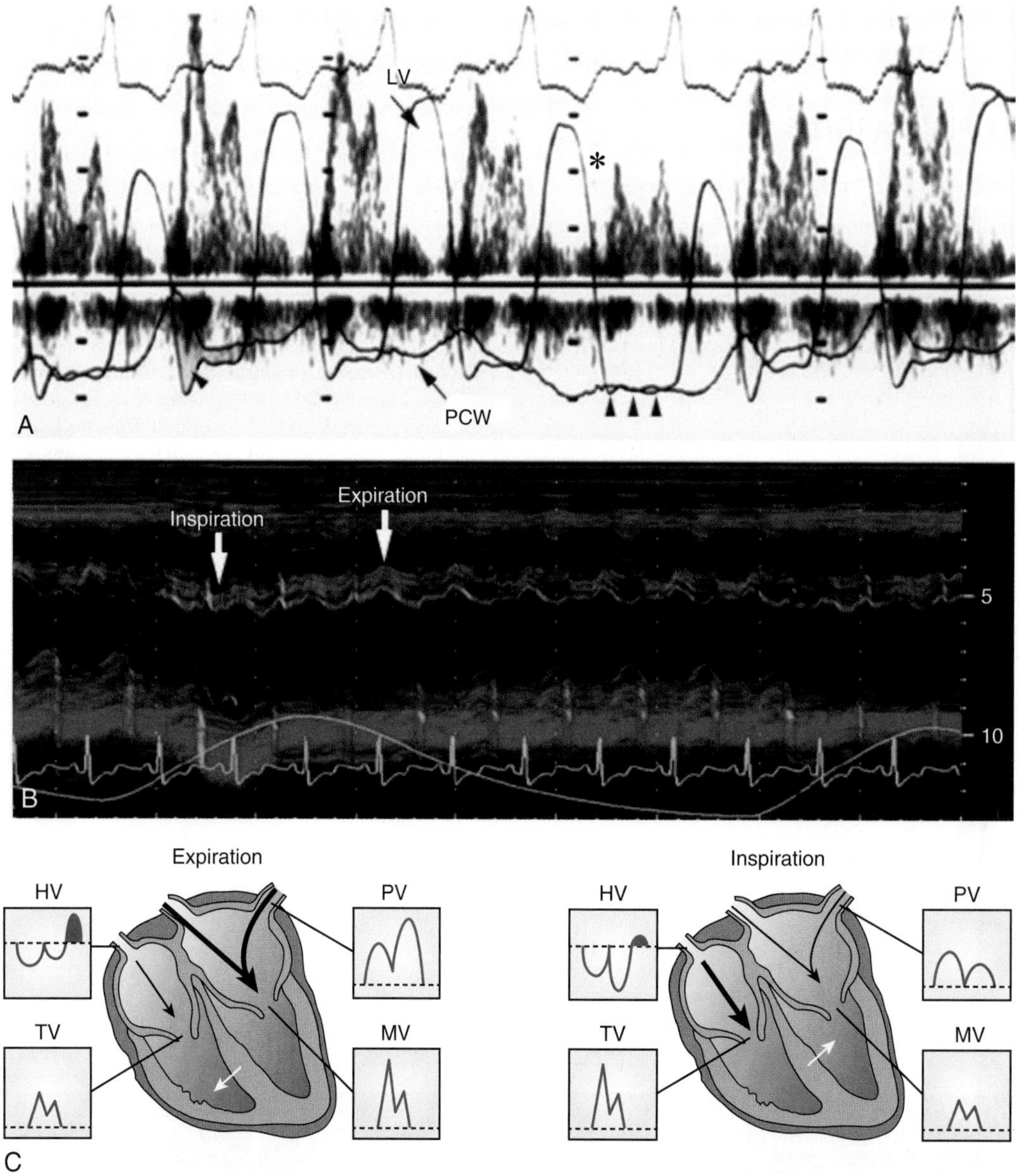

FIGURE 86.9 Ventricular interdependence and dissociation of intrathoracic and intracardiac pressure in patients with CP. **A,** LV and PCW pressures with simultaneous Doppler echocardiography of mitral inflow in a patient with constriction. Inspiration is associated with reduced left-sided filling gradient (*three arrowheads*) compared with the increased gradient with expiration (*yellow*) as the fall in intrathoracic pressure is transmitted to the pulmonary veins, but poorly to the LV. This is reflected by a fall in early mitral inflow velocity (*). **B,** Color M-mode echocardiogram with respirometer tracing showing septal bounce and ventricular interdependence in CP. Posterior displacement of the interventricular septum in early diastole is seen (*blue*). A posterior shift of the interventricular septum toward the LV during inspiration and toward the RV during expiration demonstrates ventricular interdependence. **C,** Typical changes of interventricular septal motion during respiration (*white arrows*) and blood velocities (*black arrows*). Insets show typical Doppler velocity versus time tracings across mitral (MV) and tricuspid (TV) valves and pulmonary (PV) and hepatic (HV) veins. (From Syed FF, et al. *Nat Rev Cardiol*. 2014;11:530–544.)

effusive-constrictive picture. It is probably best explained by the afore-mentioned lack of transmission of decreased intra-thoracic pressure to the left heart.[64] Table 86.5 reviews hemodynamic findings in tamponade versus constriction.

The most notable cardiac physical finding is the pericardial knock, an early diastolic sound best heard at the left sternal border and/or cardiac apex. It occurs slightly earlier and has a higher frequency content than a third heart sound and corresponds to early, abrupt cessation of ventricular filling. Widening of second sound splitting may also be present, as well as a tricuspid regurgitant murmur. Abdominal examination reveals hepatomegaly, often with palpable venous pulsations, and often ascites. Other signs of hepatic congestion/cirrhosis include jaundice, spider angiomata, and palmar erythema. Lower extremity edema is the rule. Muscle wasting, cachexia, and massive ascites and anasarca occur with end-stage constriction.

Laboratory Testing

There are no specific ECG findings. Nonspecific T wave abnormalities, reduced voltage, and left atrial enlargement may be present. Atrial fibrillation is common. On chest radiography, the cardiac silhouette can be enlarged due to a coexisting effusion. Pericardial calcification[65,66] is seen in a minority of patients and suggests TB (eFig. 86.6) but is not diagnostic of constrictive physiology. Pleural effusions are common and can be a presenting sign. If left heart filling pressures are markedly elevated pulmonary vascular congestion and redistribution may be present.

Echocardiography-Doppler Examination

M-mode and two-dimensional transthoracic and Doppler echo-cardiography and strain imaging are primary modalities for evaluating CP (see Chapter 16). Major findings include pericardial thickening and calcification (best appreciated with TEE), abrupt displacement of the interventricular septum during early diastole (septal "bounce") (see Fig. 86.9, middle; Video 86.4), and systemic venous congestion (dilated hepatic veins, inferior vena caval distention with blunted respiratory variation).[1,2,67] Premature pulmonic valve opening resulting from elevated RV early diastolic pressure and exaggerated septal shifting during respiration are common. As discussed above, LV EF is usually normal unless there is a marked decrease in end-diastolic volume or myocardial involvement. Mild to moderate biatrial enlargement is common.

Lack of transmission of intra-thoracic pressure to the cardiac chambers and resulting mitral/tricuspid inflow patterns have been discussed earlier. In accordance with these patterns, Doppler measurements usually reveal exaggerated respiratory variation in both mitral and tricuspid inflow velocity and tricuspid-mitral inflow velocity differences, with the latter 180 degrees out of phase (Fig. 86.9, bottom). Although there is some overlap with tamponade, these patterns have good sensitivity and specificity for diagnosing constriction and differentiating restrictive cardiomyopathy.[1,55,67,68] Typically, patients with CP demonstrate ≥ a 25% increase in mitral E velocity during expiration versus inspiration and increased diastolic flow reversal with expiration in the hepatic veins. Mitral E wave deceleration time is usually less than 160 milliseconds. Up to 20% of patients with CP do not exhibit typical respiratory changes, most likely because of markedly increased left atrial pressure and/or a mixed constrictive-restrictive pattern due to myocardial involvement. In patients without typical respiratory mitral-tricuspid flow findings, examination after maneuvers that decrease preload (head-up tilt, sitting) can unmask characteristic respiratory variations.

Respiratory mitral inflow variations similar to those in CP can be observed in chronic obstructive pulmonary disease (COPD), RV MI, pulmonary embolism, and pleural effusion.[1] These conditions have clinical and echocardiographic features that differentiate them from constriction. Superior vena caval flow velocities are helpful in distinguishing constriction from COPD. COPD patients display an increase in inspiratory superior vena caval systolic forward flow velocity not seen in constriction. As discussed earlier, TEE is superior to transthoracic

echocardiography for estimating pericardial thickness and correlates well with CT.[1,2,67]

Tissue Doppler and strain (deformation) imaging are useful adjuncts for diagnosing CP and distinguishing it from restrictive cardiomyopathy (see below).[1,2,67] Tissue Doppler reveals increased e' velocity of the medial mitral annulus and septal abnormalities corresponding to the "bounce." Lateral mitral annular e' is lower than medial annular e', termed "annulus reversus" (eFig. 86.7). In restrictive cardiomyopathy, the characteristic tall and narrow transmitral E is present, but e' is reduced. Regional variations in deformation and strain include reduced LV circumferential strain, torsion, and early diastolic untwisting, with preserved longitudinal strain. In contrast, in restriction circumferential strain and untwisting are preserved but reduced in the longitudinal direction. Regional longitudinal strain ratios of lateral LV wall/septum and RV free wall/septum indicative of pericardial-myocardial tethering are useful in differentiating constriction from constriction and improve after pericardiectomy (strain reversus).[69]

Cardiac Catheterization and Angiography (see Chapter 21)

Cardiac catheterization in patients with suspected CP provides documentation of hemodynamics and assists in distinguishing constriction from restrictive cardiomyopathy and in assessing myocardial involvement.[4,60] Coronary angiography is ordinarily performed in patients being considered for pericardiectomy. Rarely, external pinching or compression of a coronary artery by the pericardium is detected.

RA, RV diastolic, pulmonary capillary wedge, and pre-a wave LV diastolic pressures are elevated and equal, or nearly so, at around 20 to 25 mm Hg (Fig. 86.10). Differences of more than 3 to 5 mm Hg between left and right heart filling pressures are rare. The RA pressure tracing shows a preserved x descent, a prominent y descent, and roughly equal a and v wave heights, with resultant M or W configuration. RV and LV pressures reveal an early, marked diastolic dip and plateau ("square root" sign) (see Fig. 86.10).[60] Respiratory variation in LV and RV systolic and diastolic pressure is exaggerated. This has been quantified using the "systolic area index," the ratio of RV to LV systolic pressure × time[70] on inspiration versus expiration (see Fig. 86.10). A ratio greater than 1.1 strongly suggests constriction. Pulmonary artery and RV systolic pressures are often modestly elevated to 35 to 45 mm Hg. Greater elevation is not a feature of constriction. A ratio of RA pressure/ PCWP greater than 0.77 is an indicator of pericardial constraint that may distinguish pure constriction from constriction with myocardial involvement.[59,71] Hypovolemia, for example, due to diuretic therapy, can mask hemodynamic findings. Rapid infusion of 1 L of normal saline over 6 to 8 minutes may reveal typical features. SV is reduced but CO can be preserved because of tachycardia.

Computed Tomography and Cardiac Magnetic Resonance

ECG synchronized CT and EMR are important adjuncts to echocardiography-Doppler examinations in evaluating CP. CT (see Chapter 20) is helpful in detecting even minute amounts of pericardial calcification[1,17,55,66,67] (eFig. 86.7) and is the most accurate method for measuring thickness (normal <2 mm).[9] These features make CT well-suited for preoperative planning. CT may also obviate the need for invasive coronary angiography if vessels appear normal. Its major disadvantage is the frequent need for contrast medium to best display pericardial pathology. CMR (see Chapter 19) provides a detailed examination of the pericardium without the need for contrast or ionizing radiation. It is less sensitive for detecting calcification than CT and less accurate for measuring thickness. The "normal" pericardium visualized by CMR is up to 3 to 4 mm in thickness. This most likely reflects the entire pericardial "complex," with physiologic fluid representing a component of measured thickness. Cine acquisition MRI or CT are useful for detecting common findings of constriction (septal "bounce," ventricular interaction) when echocardiography is technically inadequate (see Video 86.4). Additional CT/CMR findings include distorted

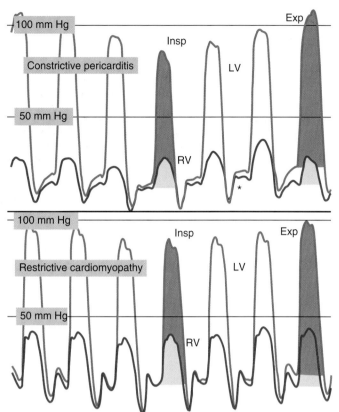

FIGURE 86.10 Top: LV (*blue*) and RV (*red*) pressure tracings in constrictive pericarditis. End-diastolic pressures are elevated and a "square root" sign (*) is present in both chambers. Enhanced ventricular interdependence is illustrated by visualization of the RV (*light gray*) and LV (*dark gray*) systolic areas under the curve for inspiration (*Insp*) and expiration (*Exp*). During inspiration the RV pressure curve area increases, whereas the LV pressure curve area decreases. **Bottom:** LV and RV pressures in restrictive cardiomyopathy. Although end-diastolic pressures are elevated and a "square root" sign (*) is present there is no evidence of enhanced ventricular interdependence; that is, changes in LV and RV pressure curve areas are parallel. (From Geske JB, Anavekar NS, Nishimura RA, et al. Differentiation of constriction and restriction: complex cardiovascular hemodynamics. *J Am Coll Cardiol.* 2016;68(21):2329–2347.)

ventricular contours, hepatic venous congestion, ascites, and pleural effusions.[17]

A thickened pericardium indicates acute and/or chronic pericarditis. Pericardial edema on T2 STIR and late gadolinium enhancement on CMR is more specific for active inflammation and may be useful in identifying patients who are candidates for management with antiinflammatory drugs (Fig. 86.11; see below).[3,9,17,28,56,57] Evidence of impaired diastolic filling and pericardial thickening, especially with calcification, is virtually diagnostic of constriction. Normal thickness argues against constriction but does not exclude it. Most patients with CP and normal thickness have calcification and distorted ventricular contours. The pericardium can be globally or focally thickened. Localized constriction caused by focal thickening is reported. In patients being considered for pericardiectomy, delineation of the location and severity of thickening and calcification by CT or CMR aids in risk stratification and surgical planning.

Differentiating Constrictive Pericarditis from Restrictive Cardiomyopathy

Because treatment differs, distinguishing CP from restrictive cardiomyopathy is important (Table 86.7).[60,72] Restrictive cardiomyopathy is increasingly recognized, in part due to the subgroup of patients with heart failure with preserved EF in whom transthyretin amyloidosis is diagnosed using technetium PYP scanning. The presentation and course of constriction and restriction overlap in many respects. A pericardial knock points to constriction. ECG and chest radiographic findings are mostly nonspecific. However, a calcified pericardium indicates constriction, whereas low QRS voltage

suggests amyloidosis. Echocardiographic distinctions are very helpful. Patients with restriction usually have thick-walled ventricles due to infiltrative processes or hypertrophy. Marked biatrial enlargement is typical of restriction but not constriction. In constriction, the most distinctive finding is the septal "bounce" and respirophasic shift.[68] As discussed above, the pericardium is usually but not invariably thickened in constriction.

Doppler flow measurements are also useful.[1,55,67] Enhanced respiratory variation in mitral inflow velocity (>25%) is seen in constriction but varies by less than 10% in restriction. In restriction, pulmonary venous systolic flow is blunted and diastolic flow is increased; this is not observed in constriction. Hepatic veins demonstrate enhanced expiratory flow reversal with constriction, in contrast to increased inspiratory flow reversal in restriction. Tissue Doppler and strain imaging can aid in differentiation.[1,55,67] Recently proposed criteria (respirophasic ventricular shift, preserved or increased medial mitral annulus e' velocity [>9 cm/sec], increased hepatic vein expiratory diastolic flow ratio [≥0.79]) distinguish constriction from restriction with sensitivity of 87% and specificity of 91%.[62,68]

Invasive hemodynamic differentiation between constriction and restrictive cardiomyopathy can be difficult. However, careful attention to the hemodynamic profile usually allows their distinction (see Table 86.6). In both, RV and LV diastolic pressures are markedly elevated. In restriction, LV diastolic pressure is usually higher than RV by at least 3 to 5 mm Hg, whereas in constriction LV and RV diastolic pressures track closely and rarely differ by more than 3 to 5 mm Hg. Severe pulmonary hypertension is sometimes observed in restriction but not in constriction. The absolute level of atrial or ventricular diastolic pressure is also useful, with extremely high pressures (>25 mm Hg) more common in restriction.[55,67,71] Finally, the systolic area index[70] is greater in constriction than restriction and reported to have high sensitivity and specificity for distinguishing between them.

CT or CMR, because of their ability to provide detailed assessment of pericardial thickness and calcification, are very useful in differentiating constriction from restriction,[2,67,71,73] although once again patients with constriction occasionally have normal thickness. PYP scanning has emerged as the primary means to diagnose cardiac. Brain natriuretic peptide (BNP) levels are elevated in restrictive cardiomyopathy but usually normal in constriction.[60]

Management

CP has a progressive but variable course. Radical surgical pericardiectomy is the definitive treatment in most patients. Pericardiectomy has been considered to have a relatively high perioperative mortality, ranging from 2 to nearly 20% in modern series.[74–76] However, this depends on the etiology of the constriction with a low mortality in idiopathic patients.

Risk factors for poor results include radiation-induced disease, comorbidities, especially COPD and renal insufficiency, coronary artery disease and prior cardiac surgery, reduced LV EF, cardiopulmonary bypass, and NYHA stage IV symptoms. Severely debilitated patients with stage IV symptoms in general have a prohibitively high risk. Relatively healthy older patients with mild constriction may be managed nonsurgically, with pericardiectomy held in reserve until the disease progresses. Otherwise, surgery should not be delayed once the diagnosis is made. Diuretics and salt restriction relieve volume overload, but patients ultimately become refractory. Because sinus tachycardia is compensatory, drugs that slow the heart rate should be avoided. In patients with atrial fibrillation and a rapid ventricular response, digoxin is recommended for rate control.

Pericardiectomy is performed through a median sternotomy, clamshell incision, or bilateral thoracotomy with or without cardiopulmonary bypass.[4,76] The visceral pericardium can be resected if involved. A more aggressive approach with complete removal of the pericardium has been advocated to facilitate access to the lateral, diaphragmatic, and posterior surfaces of the heart.[76] Ultrasonic or laser débridement[4] is an adjunct to conventional débridement or as the sole technique in patients with extensive, calcified adhesions. The "waffle" procedure,[77] in which multiple transverse and longitudinal incisions are made in

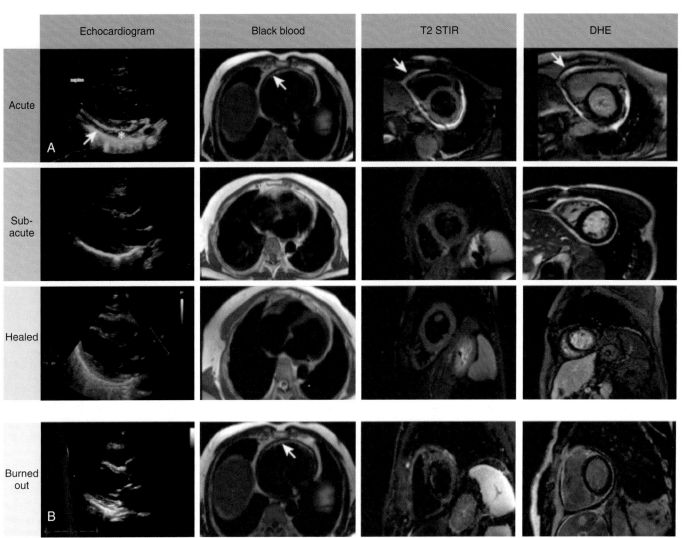

Echocardiogram	Black blood	T2 STIR	DHE

Acute

Sub-acute

Healed

Burned out

FIGURE 86.11 Changes in inflammation during the course of pericardial disease in a 27-year-old woman first seen after a recurrence of acute pericarditis. **A,** Initial (*acute*) stage echocardiogram shows a thickened pericardium (*) and a small effusion (*arrow*). Cardiac magnetic resonance shows acute inflammation with a thickened pericardium on black blood images (*arrow*), pericardial enhancement on T2 STIR and delayed images (DHE) (*arrow*). Triple therapy was intensified and anakinra introduced. Subsequent imaging showed a normal pericardial thickness, black blood sequences with interval resolution of T2 STIR enhancement but persistence of DHE signal suggesting a *subacute* stage of inflammation. After 8 months of treatment there was resolution of DHE with a normal-appearing pericardium on echocardiogram and black-blood sequences and normal T2 STIR suggesting a *healed* pericardium. **B,** Images from a 44-year-old man with idiopathic constrictive pericarditis. The echocardiogram appears normal, but black-blood sequences show a thickened pericardium (*arrow*). Furthermore, there is no signal on T2 STIR and DHE, which suggests "burned-out" disease. (From Chetrit M, et al. *J Am Coll Cardiol Imag.* 2020;13:1422–1437.)

the epicardial layer, is an alternative in patients with extensive epicardial involvement and can be done without cardiopulmonary bypass.

Hemodynamic and symptomatic improvement following pericardiectomy is achieved in some patients very soon after surgery. In others improvement may be delayed for weeks to months. Videos 86.5 and 86.6 are cine CMR images before and after successful pericardial stripping demonstrating relief of exaggerated respiratory variation in right and left heart volume. There have been several recent reports of long-term results of pericardiectomy for CP.[75,76] One-year survival ranges from 81% to 91%, five-year 64% to 85%, and 10-year 49% to 81%. Most survivors are free of adverse cardiovascular outcomes. Long-term results are worst in patients with radiation-induced disease, impaired renal function, reduced LV EF, moderate or severe tricuspid regurgitation, low serum sodium, and advanced age. LV diastolic function returns to normal in about 40% of patients early and 60% late after surgery. Poor responses to pericardiectomy have been attributed to myocardial atrophy or fibrosis, incomplete resection, and development of recurrent cardiac compression by mediastinal inflammation and fibrosis. Tricuspid regurgitation usually does not improve.

There have been several reports of transient or reversible CP.[3,9,17,28,56,57] Etiologies are diverse, but patients presenting early post-cardiac surgery appear to be common. Although features of constriction dominate, many patients have coexistent effusions and can be classified as ECP (see below). Because reported patients have been treated with various antiinflammatory regimens, it is possible the syndrome might disappear spontaneously. Reversible constriction typically resolves in 3 to 6 months or longer.[17] CMR gadolinium enhancement has been correlated with severity of inflammation in operative specimens.[17] Intensity of enhancement as well as pericardial thickness ≥3 mm on late enhancement images is predictive of a response to antiinflammatory drugs with resolution of constriction (see Figs. 86.8 and 86.11).[17] Responders also have higher hsCRP. It is not clear if patients with reversible constriction are as common as suggested in reported series,[17] which have been small and highly selected. Nonetheless, patients with intense late gadolinium enhancement on MRI, especially those with pericardial thickness greater than 3 mm, should be considered for a trial of antiinflammatory therapy, especially if they have had recent cardiac surgery, symptoms have appeared relatively rapidly, hsCRP is elevated, and there is not extensive calcification. NSAIDs, colchicine, and corticosteroids have been used separately and in various combinations with no clearly preferred regimen. As a practical matter, any antiinflammatory regimen should be administered for up to 6 months or longer if necessary to allow time for success but not so long that surgery is excessively delayed and/or significant side effects occur. Although there is no specific evidence to support it, we

TABLE 86.7 Hemodynamic and Echocardiographic Features of Constrictive Pericarditis Compared with Restrictive Cardiomyopathy

	CONSTRICTION	RESTRICTION
Prominent *y* descent in venous pressure	Present	Variable
Paradoxical pulse	Approximately 1/3 cases	Absent
Pericardial knock	Present	Absent
Equal right-left side filling pressures > right	Present	Left at least 3–5 mm Hg
Filling pressures >25 mm Hg	Rare	Common
Pulmonary artery systolic pressure >60 mm Hg	No	Common
"Square root" sign	Present	Variable
Respiratory variation in left-right pressures/flows	Exaggerated	Normal
Ventricular wall thickness	Normal	Usually increased
Pericardial thickness	Increased	Normal
Atrial size	Possible left atrium enlargement	Biatrial enlargement
Septal "bounce"	Present	Absent
Tissue Doppler E' velocity	Increased	Reduced
Speckle tracking	Normal longitudinal, decreased circumferential restoration	Decreased longitudinal, normal circumferential restoration

suggest "triple" therapy (NSAIDs, colchicine, and prednisone) in doses similar to those recommended for recurrent pericarditis. In the authors' experience, approximately 60% of these patients will not require surgery.

EFFUSIVE-CONSTRICTIVE PERICARDITIS

ECP combines elements of effusion/tamponade and constriction. Constrictive features usually are detected after pericardiocentesis.[4,78,79] Many cases of "transient" and/or medically treatable CP represent ECP. The course is quite variable, but usually subacute, from a few weeks to several months. An inflammatory effusion typically dominates early with constriction more prominent later, but there are many variations. The visceral pericardium is usually prominently involved. Figure 86.11 shows CMR images demonstrating varying effusion, pericardial thickening, and inflammation in a patient with a prolonged course of acute pericarditis leading to ECP (top three panels). For contrast, a patient with "burnt-out" CP is shown in the bottom of Figure 86.11. A proposed definition of underlying constriction is failure of RA pressure to decline by at least 50% to a level below 10 mm Hg when pericardial pressure is reduced to almost 0 mm Hg by pericardiocentesis and/or all detectable fluid is removed. A recent report revealed that echocardiographic-Doppler findings of constriction (respiratory variation in mitral inflow, hepatic vein expiratory diastolic flow reversal, respiratory septal shift) were most commonly seen before pericardiocentesis for effusion in those who *subsequently* developed effusion-constriction.[78,80,81] The reported incidence of ECP in patients with pericardial effusion varies from 1% to 15% in different series and may be especially high in TB.[78,79]

The most common causes of ECP are idiopathic, malignancy, radiation, post-pericardiotomy, and connective tissue diseases. TB is the leading cause in sub-Saharan Africa.[4,78,79] Physical, hemodynamic, and echocardiographic findings are mixtures of those associated with effusion and constriction and may vary with time as the syndrome progresses. Etiologic diagnosis occasionally requires acquisition of pericardial fluid and biopsy if the cause is not obvious and tamponade does not mandate pericardiocentesis. Management is tailored to the specific cause, if known. In idiopathic and post-pericardiotomy

cases, antiinflammatory treatment as described for noneffusive CP may provide a gratifying result with avoidance of pericardiectomy, but no guidance is available in regard to a specific approach. CMR with gadolinium uptake and measurement of hsCRP can be useful to identify patients with active inflammation who are more likely to respond to an antiinflammatory regimen. Pericardiectomy is ultimately required in many patients.

SPECIFIC ETIOLOGIES OF PERICARDIAL DISEASE
The pericardium is involved in numerous diseases (see Table 86.1), with selected etiologies discussed in the following sections.

Infectious Diseases
Viral Pericarditis. Viral pericarditis is presumed to be the most common infection in countries with low TB prevalence.[4] Numerous viruses have been implicated (see Table 86.1). Definitive diagnosis requires identification of viral particles or genomic material in pericardial fluid or tissue or antibody rises. This is impractical and/or unnecessary in almost all cases of acute pericarditis because management of immunocompetent patients is not affected by a specific viral diagnosis.

As of this writing, knowledge of pericardial involvement in COVID-19 is emerging. CT scans reveal pericardial effusions in a significant minority of patients; most are critically ill.[82,83] There is one published case report of pericardial effusion and tamponade, in association with myocarditis.[84] Others have been posted online. Reluctance to perform formal echocardiography (as opposed to point of care) has probably limited knowledge of natural history and clinical features of pericardial involvement. The mechanism of pericardial involvement is unclear.

Bacterial Pericarditis. In sub-Saharan Africa the most common bacterial cause of pericardial disease is TB. In the developed world TB and other forms of bacterial pericarditis are unusual in immunocompetent patients.

TB Pericarditis. TB pericarditis represents a secondary localization of a primary infection (usually pleural-pulmonary).[85] Specifics of the cytokine-mediated inflammatory response have been elucidated in recent years, with γ-interferon (IFN-γ) and IL-10 implicated.[85] Clinical presentations include acute pericarditis with effusion, isolated effusion, ECP, and CP. Acute pericarditis without effusion is very uncommon. Making the correct diagnosis is critical because mortality is 20% to 40% within 6 months of diagnosis absent effective treatment.

Diagnosis: A *definitive* diagnosis is based on detection of tubercle bacilli in pericardial fluid or tissue.[4,85] A *probable* diagnosis is based on evidence of disease elsewhere and/or a lymphocytic pericardial exudate with elevated IFN-γ, ADA or lysozyme levels. A presumptive diagnosis without evidence as outlined above is appropriate only in countries with high TB prevalence, followed by a positive response to therapy.[4,85]

Therapy: Rifampicin, isoniazid, pyrazinamide, and ethambutol for at least 2 months, followed by isoniazid and rifampicin for a total of 6 months is recommended. Treatment longer than 9 months gives no better results, increases costs, and risks poor compliance.[4,85,86]

Prognosis: In addition to its high untreated mortality, TB pericarditis has a 20% to 40% risk of evolving to constriction, often within 6 months.[4,85] Prompt antibiotic therapy is essential to prevent this. Additional treatments that may prevent constriction include intrapericardial urokinase[4] and adjunctive prednisolone for 6 weeks.[85,86] Corticosteroids should be avoided in HIV patients because they may increase HIV-associated malignancies. The role of colchicine is uncertain.[86] Even with optimal therapy the mortality of TB pericarditis remains high. Pericardiectomy is recommended if the patient's condition is not improving or is deteriorating after 4 to 8 weeks of therapy,[4] and in appropriately selected patients with more long-standing constriction.

Non-Tuberculous Bacterial Pericarditis. In developed countries, non-tuberculous bacterial pericarditis is rare, amounting to less than 1% cases. It is generally seen in the course of a critical febrile illness.[4] If bacterial pericarditis is suspected, urgent pericardiocentesis is mandatory for diagnosis, providing effusions are of sufficient size. Blood cultures should be obtained in any patient with pericarditis and fever greater than 38°C.[4]

Diagnosis: Pericardial fluid is usually purulent, with low glucose concentration and high WBC and neutrophil count. The diagnosis is made by microscopic detection of bacteria and/or positive cultures.[4]

Medical Therapy: IV antimicrobial therapy should be started empirically until bacteriological results are available. Prolonged drainage is crucial. Purulent effusions are often heavily loculated and likely to re-accumulate. Intrapericardial thrombolysis may help achieve adequate drainage before resorting to surgery. Subxiphoid pericardiostomy and rinsing of the pericardial sac should be considered.[4]

Prognosis: Bacterial pericarditis has a high mortality if untreated, and a high risk of evolving to constriction.[4]

Fungal Pericarditis. There has been a handful of case reports of fungal pericarditis. It is difficult to generalize about clinical features. Reported patients have presented with effusions and have had major comorbidities. Aspergillus and candida are among the organisms implicated.

Pericardial Disease and Human Immunodeficiency Virus

Various pericardial diseases have been reported in HIV patients (see Chapter 85). In the developed world, the epidemiology has been altered by highly active antiretroviral therapy (HAART). HAART has reduced all forms of cardiac involvement except for hypertensive heart disease and coronary artery disease, which are now the most common cardiac diseases in these patients.[87,88] Pericardial effusion, formerly the most common cardiovascular manifestation of HIV, is now rare. Patients receiving HAART have similar pericardial disease etiologies and prognosis as patients without HIV. In contrast, pericardial diseases are more complex and have a much poorer prognosis in untreated HIV and AIDS patients.[4,89] Small, asymptomatic effusions of uncertain etiology are common in untreated patients. TB remains the most common cause of larger effusions in African HIV-infected patients.[89] Less common forms of pericardial disease include various neoplasms, typical acute pericarditis, and myopericarditis. Constriction is rare.

Pericarditis in Patients with Renal Disease

Pericardial disease in patients with end-stage renal disease (ESRD) is less common in the era of widespread dialysis, but remains a significant problem and should be considered in patients with appropriate signs and symptoms.[4,90] Its pathophysiology is complex and probably multifactorial.[90] There are three main presentations[4,90]: (1) uremic pericarditis, often with moderate to large effusions, occurs before dialysis is initiated or within 8 weeks of initiation and is thought to be related to toxic metabolites; (2) "dialysis" pericarditis, occurring more than 8 weeks after dialysis initiation; and, rarely (3) CP. It is unclear if uremic and "dialysis" pericarditis truly differ from a pathophysiologic standpoint.

Some features of pericardial disease in patients with ESRD are distinctive. Chest pain is infrequent and one-third of patients are asymptomatic, and ECG changes are usually absent. Pericardial effusions are often bloody because of uremic coagulopathy. Tamponade is uncommon because effusions tend to develop gradually.

Intensive dialysis is effective in uremic pericarditis; in patients already receiving dialysis, intensification is less effective but remains a mainstay of treatment. Pericardiocentesis should be considered in patients unresponsive to dialysis and of course in those with tamponade. There are few data to guide use of antiinflammatory agents in ESRD.[4,90] Current guidelines[4] recommend NSAIDs, specifically 1 to 2 weeks of aspirin (750 to 1000 mg every 8 hours) or indomethacin (600 mg every 8 hours) as first-line therapy. NSAID bleeding complications are heightened in ESRD. Colchicine is relatively contraindicated but can be used on a short-term basis. Prednisone (0.2 to 0.5 mg/kg daily) may be prescribed to patients unresponsive or with contraindication/adverse effects to NSAIDs.

Pericardial Involvement in Autoimmune and Auto-inflammatory Diseases

Autoimmune diseases SLE, rheumatoid arthritis, scleroderma, sarcoidosis, inflammatory bowel disease) not infrequently cause pericarditis and/or effusion.[4,91,92] As many as 10% of patients with acute pericarditis may have an autoimmune disease. SLE accounts for the largest number; rarely, pericardial disease is its first manifestation. Pericardial involvement is usually related to activity of the underlying disease. Concomitant myocarditis may be present. CP is rare, but most common in rheumatoid arthritis.[4] Treatment of pericardial involvement is directed toward optimally treating the underlying disease and is best accomplished with close coordination between cardiologists, rheumatologists, and clinical immunologists.

Another group of patients, especially children, are affected by rare, auto-inflammatory periodic fevers (PFs).[4,93,94] PFs cause recurrent polyserositis, frequently including pericarditis. Most are caused by mutations resulting in dysregulation of inflammatory responses mediated by inflammasome IL-1β production, which is also implicated in recurrent idiopathic pericarditis. The most common PFs are familial Mediterranean fever (FMF) and tumor necrosis factor receptor–associated periodic syndrome. A positive family history for pericarditis or PFs, especially in a pediatric patient, a poor response to colchicine (in some PFs), and the need for corticosteroids or immunosuppressive agents such as anakinra are clues to these diseases. Genetic testing is required for diagnosis.

Various antiinflammatory regimens have been used for PFs.[93,94] Inflammasome-directed therapy, for example, anti-I-L1 α/β blockers (anakinra, rilonacept, canakinumab) or anti-TNF agents are highly effective for selected PFs.

Post-Cardiac Injury Syndromes. Post-cardiac injury syndromes (PCISs) include post-MI pericarditis, post-pericardiotomy syndrome (PPS), and posttraumatic pericarditis.[4,95–97] With the exception of *early* post-MI pericarditis, all are presumed to have an immune pathogenesis triggered by damage to pericardial tissue and/or blood in the pericardial sac associated with myocardial necrosis (*late* post-MI pericarditis), surgical trauma (PPS), or iatrogenic trauma (pericarditis after percutaneous procedures including coronary intervention [PCI], valve repair, arrhythmia ablation, device implantations, and left atrial isolation).

An immune-mediated pathogenesis is supported by a latent period, typically a few weeks, response to antiinflammatory drugs, and potential for recurrences. PCIS is an emerging cause of pericarditis because of an aging population and expansion of cardiac procedures.

Definition and Diagnostic Criteria: According to proposed criteria diagnosis of PCIS after cardiac injury requires at least two of the following[4,95]: (1) fever without an alternative cause, (2) pleuritic chest pain, (3) pericardial/pleural rubs, (4) pericardial effusion, (5) elevated CRP.

Specific considerations apply to post-MI pericarditis (see also Chapter 38). Two forms are recognized.[4] *Early* post-MI pericarditis occurs 1 to 3 days after MI. It is rare in the primary PCI era and is now seen after large, transmural MIs due to absent or late/failed reperfusion. *Late* post-MI pericarditis (*Dressler syndrome*) is also rare (<1% of MIs in the modern era) and also most common after large MIs.

Early post-MI pericarditis is usually asymptomatic and diagnosed by auscultation of a rub 1 to 3 days after the index event. Cardiac tamponade is rare. However, tamponade does occur with LV free wall rupture. Because of its association with large MIs, early post-MI pericarditis should alert the clinician to possible rupture, especially if an effusion is present. In the occasional symptomatic patient, pleuritic chest pain appears within the above time frame. It is important to distinguish pericardial from recurrent ischemic discomfort. Ordinarily, this is not difficult on clinical grounds. Typical ECG changes of acute pericarditis are uncommon. ECG changes usually involve subtle ST segment re-elevation in originally involved leads. Atypical T wave evolution (persistent upright T waves or early normalization of inverted T waves) appears to be sensitive for early post-MI pericarditis.[4] Late post-MI pericarditis occurs from 1 week to a few months after MI. Symptoms include fever and pleuritic chest pain. Physical examination may reveal pleural and/or pericardial rubs. The chest radiograph reveals pleural effusion and/or enlargement of the cardiac silhouette. The ECG often demonstrates typical acute pericarditis. Effusions are common but tamponade unusual.

Medical Therapy: Treatment guidelines recommend empiric antiinflammatory regimens as outlined for viral/idiopathic pericarditis.[4] Asymptomatic early post-MI pericarditis does not require treatment. Acetaminophen or aspirin are preferred for symptomatic patients.

Prognosis: The prognosis of PCIS is generally good. Long-term follow-up is warranted because CP has been reported in about 3% of cases.[25]

Pericardial Disease in Patients with Cancer

Most pericardial involvement in cancer occurs in the setting of metastatic disease, and may present as acute pericarditis, isolated effusion, ECP, or CP.[4,36,98] Malignant effusions are often moderate to large and frequently cause tamponade. They are usually caused by direct pericardial implants resulting from hematogenous spread and less commonly by lymphatic involvement. Virtually any metastatic cancers can involve the pericardium. Lung and breast carcinomas are most common. Lymphomas, leukemias, melanomas, and cancers of contiguous organs (e.g., esophagus) make up most of the rest. Cancer patients can also develop chemotherapy-related and radiation pericardial disease and are at risk for bacterial pericarditis.

The diagnosis of metastatic pericardial disease is based on confirmation of malignant infiltration of the pericardium by pericardial fluid cytology or biopsy.[4,36,98] A probable diagnosis is achieved by detection of tumor markers in pericardial fluid (CEA, GATA3, VEGF, and others).[4,52] None are accurate enough to definitively distinguish malignant from benign effusions. Evidence of malignant disease elsewhere with concomitant pericarditis and/or effusion is very suggestive. In almost two-thirds of patients with documented malignancy, pericardial effusion is due to nonmalignant causes, for example, radiation and other therapies or infections.[36,98]

Medical Therapy: Management of these patients requires a multidisciplinary approach including cardiologists, oncologists, and radiotherapists.[4,36,98,99]

General principles include the following:

1. Appropriate antineoplastic therapy.
2. Therapeutic and diagnostic pericardiocentesis for tamponade and as a diagnostic tool for moderate to large, suspicious effusions. Prolonged drainage is recommended to reduce the high recurrence rate (>40% to 50%). Additional interventions for recurrent effusions include surgical pericardial window and percutaneous balloon pericardiotomy.
3. Intrapericardial instillation of cytostatic/sclerosing agents is sometimes effective in preventing recurrences. The agent should be tailored to the type of cancer.
4. Radiation for controlling effusions in patients with radiosensitive cancers such as lymphomas and leukemias. Management is often palliative in patients with advanced disease and aimed at symptom relief rather than aggressive treatment of the underlying cancer.

Adverse pericardial effects of conventional cancer chemotherapeutic agents are rare and confined to case reports of acute pericarditis and/or effusion.[99] Several agents have been implicated including bleomycin and anthracyclines. Various adverse cardiovascular effects have been ascribed to kinase targeted drugs.[99] The main offender is dasatinib, used to treat leukemias. Dasatinib has been associated with pleural/pericardial effusions, including some cases of tamponade. Other kinase inhibitors appear to have less cardiovascular effects.

Pericardial disease has also been observed with several types of immunotherapy. IL-2, a T lymphocyte growth factor, is used to treat cancers such as renal cell carcinoma and melanoma. Myocarditis and pericarditis have been reported. More recently, immune checkpoint inhibitors (ICIs) have been used to treat various cancers. ICIs are antibodies directed against checkpoint or "brake" receptors on T-lymphocytes, important regulators of tumor growth. Resultant activation of the immune system has beneficial effects. About 1% of patients receiving ICIs have adverse cardiovascular effects, most commonly myocarditis and pericarditis with effusion and occasional tamponade.[99] Although the percentage of patients receiving ICIs who develop cardiovascular effects is small, this is an emerging problem because of the numbers of patients receiving these drugs and the seriousness of the effects. Pericardial tissue examination has revealed infiltration of lymphocytes and macrophages.

Pericarditis occurring as an adverse response to cancer treatment is treated with discontinuation of the offending agent and otherwise similarly to idiopathic pericarditis, that is, NSAIDs and colchicine, with corticosteroids used in poorly responsive patients. Patients with ICI-mediated pericarditis and severe myocarditis may require high-dose corticosteroids. Effusion and tamponade are treated as in other patients with malignant pericardial involvement.

Radiation-Induced Pericarditis

Chest radiation remains a significant cause of pericardial disease.[4,100,101] Radiation may also affect myocardium, valves, coronary arteries, and other mediastinal structures, promoting fibrosis.[100,101] Most cases occur in Hodgkin lymphoma, breast, or lung cancer patients. Modern treatment, including lower doses, better shielding, and dose calculation has reduced cardiovascular complications to about 2.5%.[4,100,101]

Radiation can induce early, transient, often sub-clinical acute or subacute pericarditis with or without effusion. CP is rare and may appear 2 to 20 years after treatment. Late constriction is dose-dependent and associated with an effusion late in the acute phase. Therapy for symptomatic pericarditis during the acute phase is similar to that for idiopathic pericarditis.[4] Concomitant myocardial damage contributes to poor outcomes after pericardiectomy for constriction.[4]

Thyroid-Associated Pericardial Disease

Pericardial effusions develop in 25% to 35% of patients with severe hypothyroidism (see Chapter 96).[4,102] These can be large but rarely cause tamponade. Hypothyroid effusions often have high concentrations of cholesterol. They gradually resolve with thyroid replacement. Rarely, effusion can occur in hyperthyroidism.

Pericardial Diseases in Pregnancy and Lactation

Insignificant pericardial effusions are observed in approximately 40% of healthy pregnant women (see Chapter 92).[102] Pregnancy does not influence the incidence, cause, or course of pericardial disease but it does impact management.[4,102] Acute pericarditis has a good prognosis with outcomes similar to the general population. NSAIDs may be prescribed during the first and early second trimester. After gestational week 20, all NSAIDs (except aspirin ≤100 mg/day) can cause constriction of the

ductus arteriosus and should either not be started or withdrawn. Relatively low-dose corticosteroids (e.g., prednisone 0.2 to 0.5 mg/kg/day) are an option that can be adopted for the entire duration of pregnancy. Absent a specific indication (e.g., FMF), colchicine is contraindicated during pregnancy.[4,102] Acetaminophen is allowed throughout pregnancy and breastfeeding as are proton pump inhibitors. During lactation, ibuprofen, indomethacin, naproxen, and prednisone are allowable. Colchicine is considered contraindicated, although in FMF patients no adverse effects on fertility, pregnancy, or fetal development have been reported.[4,102]

Pericardial Diseases in Children

Pericarditis is a significant cause of chest pain in children, accounting for about 5% of such patients in emergency departments.[4,103] The etiologic distribution differs from adults, with specific causes more common, including bacterial, auto-inflammatory diseases, and PCIS following surgical repair of congenital defects.[4,103] Children often have a more marked systemic inflammatory response, with a higher incidence of fever, pleuro-pulmonary involvement, and elevation of inflammatory markers.

There have been no randomized clinical trials in pediatric settings. Management follows the general scheme for adults, with appropriate dose adjustments.[4,103] Aspirin should generally be avoided because of the risk of Reye syndrome. Colchicine can be used, but corticosteroids should be restricted even more than in adults given particularly deleterious side effects (e.g., striae rubra, growth impairment). Biological agents such as anakinra and intravenous immunoglobulin have been advocated as alternatives.[104,105] Exercise restriction is difficult for children, especially in recurrent cases. Long-term prognosis is generally good, albeit related to the etiology of the underlying pericardial syndrome.

Stress Cardiomyopathy

Stress cardiomyopathy (Takotsubo syndrome) has been recognized for over two decades. Reversible ballooning of the apical LV was originally described, but variants are common. There are a number of case reports of pericarditis, effusion, and even cardiac tamponade.[106] The overall incidence of pericardial involvement is uncertain, but probably quite low. The mechanism is likely epicardial inflammation.

Hemopericardium

Any form of chest trauma can cause hemopericardium (see Chapter 71).[4] Post-MI free wall rupture occurs within several days of transmural MI (see Chapter 37). Hemopericardium due to retrograde bleeding into the pericardial sac is an important complication of type I aortic dissections (see Chapter 42). These patients may also have combined aortic regurgitation due to disruption of the aortic valve and tamponade without a paradoxical pulse. The role of pericardiocentesis has been discussed above.

Percutaneous cardiology procedures can be complicated by hemopericardium due to perforation of a cardiac chamber (with the exception of PCI).[4] Because these same procedures can cause PCIS, it is possible that blood in the pericardial sac can itself cause or worsen PCIS. Because of the proliferation of these procedures, they are now an important cause of hemopericardium. With experience the incidence of hemopericardium declines. Puncture of atrial or ventricular walls can occur during mitral valvuloplasty and during insertion of devices to correct mitral regurgitation.[4,107] Small pericardial effusions are observed rarely after device closure of atrial septal defects, most of which are asymptomatic.[108] Earlier reports of insertion of the Watchman left atrial appendage device and other left atrial isolation procedures indicated a relatively high incidence of perforation and effusions.[109] The Watchman has become the most commonly used device. Recent registry data indicate that rates of effusion have decreased, 0.2% for patients in atrial fibrillation and 1.5% for patients in sinus rhythm. Transcutaneous aortic valve implantation is complicated by about a 1% to 2% incidence of pericardial effusion/tamponade.[110]

Pericardial effusion and tamponade due to coronary perforation during PCI is now rare (see Chapter 41), with an incidence of 0.1% to 0.6%.[4,111] The clinical presentation is typically rapidly progressive cardiac decompensation, although occasionally it is delayed. The diagnosis is usually made by extravasation of dye from a coronary vessel. Loss of cardiac pulsation on fluoroscopy indicates a significant effusion. Management requires sealing the perforation, pericardiocentesis, and reversal of anticoagulation.[4,111] If a perforation cannot be managed percutaneously emergency surgery is indicated. Endomyocardial biopsy is occasionally complicated by perforation, but tamponade is unusual.[4]

Pericardial effusion and tamponade can occur as a complication of catheter-based arrhythmia procedures.[4,112,113] The incidence of effusion following atrial fibrillation ablation is on the order of 2% to 3%. Many patients can be managed conservatively and closed drainage is usually sufficient. Atrial flutter ablations have a 1% to 2% incidence of effusion; for supraventricular tachycardia ablations the incidence is 0.1% to 1.3%. Endocardial ventricular tachycardia ablations have a 1% to 3% risk of pericardial effusion. Epicardial ablations have a similar risk of effusion but a relatively high risk of tamponade.[113] RV perforation occasionally complicates pacemaker and implantable defibrillator lead insertion, but rarely causes tamponade.[114] Finally, tamponade is a rare complication of laparoscopic gastroesophageal surgery.[115] The incidence of *recurrent* pericarditis after percutaneous cardiac procedures is unknown. The authors believe this is an emerging problem.

Congenital Anomalies of the Pericardium

Pericardial cysts are rare, benign congenital malformations,[4,116] typically located at the right or left cardiophrenic angle. Cysts are typically round or elliptical and range from a few to greater than 20 cm. They are usually discovered as an incidental finding on imaging studies. They occasionally become symptomatic due to hemorrhage or infection, increasing in size and compressing adjacent structures.[116] On CT imaging, cysts appear as round or elliptical masses with the same density as water. Absent complications, cysts do not demonstrate contrast enhancement or delayed gadolinium uptake.

Surgery is not ordinarily recommended for pericardial cysts unless they become symptomatic. However, approximately 10% of apparent cysts actually represent pericardial diverticula with a persistent connection to the pericardial sac.[117] This may not be apparent on imaging studies and only identified at surgery. These lesions may cause atypical symptoms that are only relieved after surgery. Minimally invasive thoracoscopic resection or percutaneous aspiration are nonsurgical alternatives.

Congenital absence of the pericardium is very rare (see Chapter 82).[4,118] Usually part or all of the left parietal pericardium is absent, but partial absence of the right side is also reported. Partial absence of left pericardium is associated with atrial septal defect, bicuspid aortic valve, and pulmonary malformations. While usually asymptomatic, herniation of portions of the heart through the defect and/or torsion of great vessels can occur, with life-threatening consequences. Patients can have chest pain, syncope, or even sudden death. The ECG typically reveals incomplete right bundle branch block. Absence of all or most of the left pericardium results in a chest radiograph with a leftward shift of the cardiac silhouette and an elongated left heart border. Echocardiography reveals paradoxical septal motion and RV enlargement. CT or MRI establishes the diagnosis. Pericardiectomy ameliorates symptoms and prevents herniation.

Primary Pericardial Tumors

Various rare primary pericardial neoplasms have been reported, including mesotheliomas, fibrosarcomas, lymphangiomas, hemangiomas, teratomas, neurofibromas, and lipomas.[4] Many are locally invasive and/or compress cardiac structures or are detected because of an abnormal cardiac silhouette on chest radiograph. Mesotheliomas and fibrosarcomas are lethal, whereas others are benign. CT and CMR are helpful in delineating the anatomy of these tumors, but surgery is usually required for diagnosis and treatment.

REFERENCES

1. Klein AL, Abbara S, Agler DA, et al. American society of echocardiography clinical recommendations for multimodality cardiovascular imaging of patients with pericardial disease: endorsed by the society for cardiovascular magnetic resonance and society of cardiovascular computed tomography. *J Am Soc Echocardiogr.* 2013;26(9):965-1012.e1015.
2. Cosyns B, Plein S, Nihoyanopoulos P, et al. European Association of Cardiovascular Imaging (EACVI) position paper: multimodality imaging in pericardial disease. *Eur Heart J Cardiovasc Imaging.* 2015;16(1):12–31.
3. Shabetai R. *The Pericardium.* Norwell, MA: Kluwer Academic Publishers; 2003.
4. Adler Y, Charron P, Imazio M, et al. 2015 ESC guidelines for the diagnosis and management of pericardial diseases: the Task force for the diagnosis and management of pericardial diseases of the European Society of Cardiology (ESC) Endorsed by: The European Association for Cardio-Thoracic Surgery (EACTS). *Eur Heart J.* 2015;36(42):2921–2964.
5. Imazio M, Gaita F, LeWinter M. Evaluation and treatment of pericarditis: a systematic review. *J Am Med Assoc.* 2015;314(14):1498–1506.
6. Imazio M, Gaita F. Diagnosis and treatment of pericarditis. *Heart.* 2015;101(14):1159–1168.
7. Vakamudi S, Ho N, Cremer PC. Pericardial effusions: causes, diagnosis, and management. *Prog Cardiovasc Dis.* 2017;59(4):380–388.
8. Gouriet F, Levy PY, Casalta JP, et al. Etiology of pericarditis in a prospective cohort of 1162 cases. *Am J Med.* 2015;128(7). 784.e781-788.
9. Cremer PC, Kumar A, Kontzias A, et al. Complicated pericarditis: understanding risk factors and pathophysiology to inform imaging and treatment. *J Am Coll Cardiol.* 2016;68(21):2311–2328.
10. Brucato A, Imazio M, Cremer PC, et al. Recurrent pericarditis: still idiopathic? The pros and cons of a well-honoured term. *Intern Emerg Med.* 2018;13(6):839–844.
11. Imazio M, Cecchi E, Demichelis B, et al. Myopericarditis versus viral or idiopathic acute pericarditis. *Heart.* 2008;94(4):498–501.
12. Kytö V, Sipilä J, Rautava P. Clinical profile and influences on outcomes in patients hospitalized for acute pericarditis. *Circulation.* 2014;130(18):1601–1606.
13. Imazio M, Brucato A, Barbieri A, et al. Good prognosis for pericarditis with and without myocardial involvement: results from a multicenter, prospective cohort study. *Circulation.* 2013;128(1):42–49.
14. Imazio M, Lazaros G, Picardi E, et al. Incidence and prognostic significance of new onset atrial fibrillation/flutter in acute pericarditis. *Heart.* 2015;101(18):1463–1467.
15. Imazio M, Hoit BD. Post-cardiac injury syndromes. An emerging cause of pericardial diseases. *Int J Cardiol.* 2013;168(2):648–652.
16. Imazio M, Brucato A, Maestroni S, et al. Prevalence of C-reactive protein elevation and time course of normalization in acute pericarditis: implications for the diagnosis, therapy, and prognosis of pericarditis. *Circulation.* 2011;123(10):1092–1097.
17. Chetrit M, Xu B, Kwon DH, et al. Imaging-guided therapies for pericardial diseases. *JACC Cardiovasc Imaging.* 2019.
18. Chetrit M, Xu B, Verma BR, Klein AL. Multimodality imaging for the assessment of pericardial diseases. *Curr Cardiol Rep.* 2019;21(5):41.
19. Imazio M, Brucato A, Doria A, et al. Antinuclear antibodies in recurrent idiopathic pericarditis: prevalence and clinical significance. *Int J Cardiol.* 2009;136(3):289–293.
20. Imazio M, Brucato A, Cemin R, et al. A randomized trial of colchicine for acute pericarditis. *New Engl J Med.* 2013;369(16):1522–1528.
21. Xu B, Harb SC, Cremer PC. New insights into pericarditis: mechanisms of injury and therapeutic targets. *Curr Cardiol Rep.* 2017;19(7):60.
22. Rehman KA, Betancor J, Xu B, et al. Uremic pericarditis, pericardial effusion, and constrictive pericarditis in end-stage renal disease: insights and pathophysiology. *Clin Cardiol.* 2017;40(10):839–846.
23. Imazio M, Brucato A, Cumetti D, et al. Corticosteroids for recurrent pericarditis: high versus low doses: a nonrandomized observation. *Circulation.* 2008;118(6):667–671.
24. Imazio M, Cecchi E, Demichelis B, et al. Indicators of poor prognosis of acute pericarditis. *Circulation.* 2007;115(21):2739–2744.
25. Imazio M, Brucato A, Maestroni S, et al. Risk of constrictive pericarditis after acute pericarditis. *Circulation.* 2011;124(11):1270–1275.
26. Imazio M, Belli R, Brucato A, et al. Efficacy and safety of colchicine for treatment of multiple recurrences of pericarditis (CORP-2): a multicentre, double-blind, placebo-controlled, randomised trial. *Lancet.* 2014;383(9936):2232–2237.
27. Imazio M, Lazaros G, Brucato A, Gaita F. Recurrent pericarditis: new and emerging therapeutic options. *Nat Rev Cardiol.* 2016;13(2):99–105.
28. Cremer PC, Tariq MU, Karwa A, et al. Quantitative assessment of pericardial delayed hyperenhancement predicts clinical improvement in patients with constrictive pericarditis treated with anti-inflammatory therapy. *Circ Cardiovasc Imaging.* 2015;8(5):e003125.
29. Kumar A, Sato K, Yzeiraj E, et al. Quantitative pericardial delayed hyperenhancement informs clinical course in recurrent pericarditis. *JACC Cardiovasc Imaging.* 2017;10(11):1337–1346.
30. Kumar A, Sato K, Verma BR, et al. Quantitative assessment of pericardial delayed hyperenhancement helps identify patients with ongoing recurrences of pericarditis. *Open Heart.* 2018;5(2):e000944.
31. Imazio M, Lazaros G, Picardi E, et al. Intravenous human immunoglobulins for refractory recurrent pericarditis: a systematic review of all published cases. *J Cardiovasc Med.* 2016;17(4):263–269.
32. Brucato A, Imazio M, Gattorno M, et al. Effect of anakinra on recurrent pericarditis among patients with colchicine resistance and corticosteroid dependence: the AIRTRIP randomized clinical trial. *J Am Med Assoc.* 2016;316(18):1906–1912.
33. Imazio M, Andreis A, De Ferrari GM, et al. Anakinra for corticosteroid-dependent and colchicine-resistant pericarditis: the IRAP (International Registry of Anakinra for Pericarditis) study. *Eur J Prev Cardiol.* 2019.2047487319879534.
33a. Klein AL, Lin D, Cremer PC, et al. Efficacy and safety of rilonacept for recurrent pericarditis: results from a phase II clinical trial. *Heart.* 2021;107:488–496.
33b. Klein AL, Imazio M, Cremer P, et al. Phase 3 trial of tnterleukin-1 trap rilonacept in recurrent pericarditis. *N Engl J Med.* 2021;384:31–41.
33c. Klein AL, Imazio M, Paolini JF. Correspondence: Phase 3 trial of tnterleukin-1 trap rilonacept in recurrent pericarditis. *N Engl J Med.* 2021;384:1474–1476.
34. Khandaker MH, Schaff HV, Greason KL, et al. Pericardiectomy vs medical management in patients with relapsing pericarditis. *Mayo Clin Proc.* 2012;87(11):1062–1070.
35. Hoit BD. Pericardial effusion and cardiac tamponade in the new millennium. *Curr Cardiol Rep.* 2017;19(7):57.
36. Imazio M, Colopi M, De Ferrari GM. Pericardial diseases in patients with cancer: contemporary prevalence, management and outcomes. *Heart.* 2020;106(8):569–574.
37. Argulian E, Herzog E, Halpern DG, Messerli FH. Paradoxical hypertension with cardiac tamponade. *Am J Cardiol.* 2012;110(7):1066–1069.
38. Shabetai R, Oh JK. Pericardial effusion and compressive disorders of the heart: influence of new technology on unraveling its pathophysiology and hemodynamics. *New Braunwald_Cardiol Clin.* 2017;35(4):467–479.
39. O'Leary SM, Williams PL, Williams MP, et al. Imaging the pericardium: appearances on ECG-gated 64-detector row cardiac computed tomography. *Br J Radiol.* 2010;83(987):194–205.
40. Aldweib N, Farah V, Biederman RWW. Clinical utility of cardiac magnetic resonance imaging in pericardial diseases. *Curr Cardiol Rev.* 2018;14(3):200–212.
41. Imazio M, Adler Y. Management of pericardial effusion. *Eur Heart J.* 2013;34(16):1186–1197.
42. Hayashi T, Tsukube T, Yamashita T, et al. Impact of controlled pericardial drainage on critical cardiac tamponade with acute type A aortic dissection. *Circulation.* 2012;126(11 suppl 1):S97–S101.
43. Akyuz S, Zengin A, Arugaslan E, et al. Echo-guided pericardiocentesis in patients with clinically significant pericardial effusion. Outcomes over a 10-year period. *Braunwald_ Herz.* 2015;40(suppl 2):153–159.
44. Maggiolini S, Gentile G, Farina A, et al. Safety, efficacy, and complications of pericardiocentesis by real-time echo-monitored procedure. *Am J Cardiol.* 2016;117(8):1369–1374.
45. Pradhan R, Okabe T, Yoshida K, et al. Patient characteristics and predictors of mortality associated with pericardial decompression syndrome: a comprehensive analysis of published cases. *Eur Heart J Acute Cardiovasc Care.* 2015;4(2):113–120.
46. Vilela EM, Ruivo C, Guerreiro CE, et al. Computed tomography-guided pericardiocentesis: a systematic review concerning contemporary evidence and future perspectives. *Ther Adv Cardiovasc Dis.* 2018;12(11):299–307.
47. El Haddad D, Iliescu C, Yusuf SW, et al. Outcomes of cancer patients undergoing percutaneous pericardiocentesis for pericardial effusion. *J Am Coll Cardiol.* 2015;66(10):1119–1128.
48. Horr SE, Mentias A, Houghtaling PL, et al. Comparison of outcomes of pericardiocentesis versus surgical pericardial window in patients requiring drainage of pericardial effusions. *Am J Cardiol.* 2017;120(5):883–890.
49. Maisch B, Rupp H, Ristic A, Pankuweit S. Pericardioscopy and epi- and pericardial biopsy—a new window to the heart improving etiological diagnoses and permitting targeted intrapericardial therapy. *Heart Fail Rev.* 2013;18(3):317–328.
50. Azarbal A, LeWinter MM. Pericardial effusion. *Cardiol Clin.* 2017;35(4):515–524.
51. Abu Fanne R, Banai S, Chorin U, et al. Diagnostic yield of extensive infectious panel testing in acute pericarditis. *Cardiology.* 2011;119(3):134–139.

52. Karatolios K, Pankuweit S, Maisch B. Diagnostic value of biochemical biomarkers in malignant and non-malignant pericardial effusion. *Heart Fail Rev*. 2013;18(3):337–344.

53. Karatolios K, Pankuweit S, Richter A, et al. Anticardiac antibodies in patients with chronic pericardial effusion. *Dis Markers*. 2016;2016:9262741.

54. Uchi T, Hakuno D, Fukae T, et al. Armored heart because of tuberculous constrictive pericarditis. *Circ Cardiovasc Imaging*. 2019;12(3):e008726.

55. Cosyns B, Plein S, Nihoyanopoulos P, et al. European Association of Cardiovascular Imaging (EACVI) position paper: multimodality imaging in pericardial disease. *Eur Heart J Cardiovasc Imaging*. 2015;16(1):12–31.

56. Feng D, Glockner J, Kim K, et al. Cardiac magnetic resonance imaging pericardial late gadolinium enhancement and elevated inflammatory markers can predict the reversibility of constrictive pericarditis after antiinflammatory medical therapy: a pilot study. *Circulation*. 2011;124(17):1830–1837.

57. Gentry J, Klein AL, Jellis CL. Transient constrictive pericarditis: current diagnostic and therapeutic strategies. *Curr Cardiol Rep*. 2016;18(5):41.

58. Busch C, Penov K, Amorim PA, et al. Risk factors for mortality after pericardiectomy for chronic constrictive pericarditis in a large single-centre cohort. *Eur J Cardio Thorac Surg*. 2015;48(6):e110–e116.

59. Yang JH, Miranda WR, Borlaug BA, et al. Right atrial/pulmonary arterial wedge pressure ratio in primary and mixed constrictive pericarditis. *J Am Coll Cardiol*. 2019;73(25):3312–3321.

60. Geske JB, Anavekar NS, Nishimura RA, et al. Differentiation of constriction and restriction: complex cardiovascular hemodynamics. *J Am Coll Cardiol*. 2016;68(21):2329–2347.

61. Welch TD. Constrictive pericarditis: diagnosis, management and clinical outcomes. *Heart*. 2018;104(9):725–731.

62. Qamruddin S, Alkharabsheh SK, Sato K, et al. Differentiating constriction from restriction (from the mayo clinic echocardiographic criteria). *Am J Cardiol*. 2019;124(6):932–938.

63. Karaahmet T, Yilmaz F, Tigen K, et al. Diagnostic utility of plasma N-terminal pro-B-type natriuretic peptide and C-reactive protein levels in differential diagnosis of pericardial constriction and restrictive cardiomyopathy. *Congest Heart Fail*. 2009;15(6):265–270.

64. Miranda WR, Oh JK. Constrictive pericarditis: a practical clinical approach. *Prog Cardiovasc Dis*. 2017;59(4):369–379.

65. Bogaert J, Meyns B, Dymarkowski S, et al. Calcified constrictive pericarditis: prevalence, distribution patterns, and relationship to the myocardium. *JACC Cardiovasc Imaging*. 2016;9(8):1013–1014.

66. Senapati A, Isma'eel HA, Kumar A, et al. Disparity in spatial distribution of pericardial calcifications in constrictive pericarditis. *Open Heart*. 2018;5(2):e000835.

67. Alajaji W, Xu B, Sripariwuth A, et al. Noninvasive multimodality imaging for the diagnosis of constrictive pericarditis. *Circ Cardiovasc Imaging*. 2018;11(11):e007878.

68. Welch TD, Ling LH, Espinosa RE, et al. Echocardiographic diagnosis of constrictive pericarditis: mayo Clinic criteria. *Circ Cardiovasc Imaging*. 2014;7(3):526–534.

69. Kusunose K, Dahiya A, Popovic ZB, et al. Biventricular mechanics in constrictive pericarditis comparison with restrictive cardiomyopathy and impact of pericardiectomy. *Circ Cardiovasc Imaging*. 2013;6(3):399–406.

70. Talreja DR, Nishimura RA, Oh JK, Holmes DR. Constrictive pericarditis in the modern era: novel criteria for diagnosis in the cardiac catheterization laboratory. *J Am Coll Cardiol*. 2008;51(3):315–319.

71. Klein AL, Xu B. Constrictive pericarditis: differentiating the "purebred" from the "mixed bag". *J Am Coll Cardiol*. 2019;73(25):3322–3325.

72. Garcia MJ. Constrictive pericarditis versus restrictive cardiomyopathy? *J Am Coll Cardiol*. 2016;67(17):2061–2076.

73. Chetrit M, Natalie Szpakowski N, Desai MY. Multimodality imaging for the diagnosis and treatment of pericardial disease. *Expert Rev Cardiovasc Ther*. 2019:1–10.

74. Vistarini N, Chen C, Mazine A, et al. Pericardiectomy for constrictive pericarditis: 20 Years of experience at the montreal heart institute. *Ann Thorac Surg*. 2015;100(1):107–113.

75. Biçer M, Özdemir B, Kan İ., et al. Long-term outcomes of pericardiectomy for constrictive pericarditis. *J Cardiothorac Surg*. 2015;10. 177-177.

76. Gillaspie EA, Stulak JM, Daly RC, et al. A 20-year experience with isolated pericardiectomy: analysis of indications and outcomes. *J Thorac Cardiovasc Surg*. 2016;152(2):448–458.

77. Matsuura K, Mogi K, Takahara Y. Off-pump waffle procedure using an ultrasonic scalpel for constrictive pericarditis. *Eur J Cardio Thorac Surg*. 2015;47(5):e220–e222.

78. Kim KH, Miranda WR, Sinak LJ, et al. Effusive-constrictive pericarditis after pericardiocentesis: incidence, associated findings, and natural history. *JACC Cardiovasc Imaging*. 2018;11(4):534–541.

79. Klein AL, Cremer PC. Ephemeral effusive constrictive pathophysiology. *JACC Cardiovasc Imaging*. 2018;11(4):542–545.

80. Miranda WR, Newman DB, Oh JK. Effusive-constrictive pericarditis: doppler findings. *Curr Cardiol Rep*. 2019;21(11):144.

81. Miranda WR, Newman DB, Sinak LJ, et al. Pre- and post-pericardiocentesis echo-Doppler features of effusive-constrictive pericarditis compared with cardiac tamponade and constrictive pericarditis. *Eur Heart J Cardiovasc Imaging*. 2018.

82. Salehi S, Abedi A, Balakrishnan S, Gholamrezanezhad A. Coronavirus disease 2019 (COVID-19): a systematic review of imaging findings in 919 patients. *AJR Am J Roentgenol*. 2020:1–7.

83. Li K, Wu J, Wu F, et al. The clinical and chest CT features associated with severe and critical COVID-19 pneumonia. *Invest Radiol*. 2020;55(6):327–331.

84. Hua A, O'Gallagher K, Sado D, Byrne J. Life-threatening cardiac tamponade complicating myopericarditis in COVID-19. *New Braunwald_Eur Heart J*. 2020;41(22):2130.

85. Wiysonge CS, Ntsekhe M, Thabane L, et al. Interventions for treating tuberculous pericarditis. *Cochrane Database Syst Rev*. 2017;9(9):Cd000526.

86. Isiguzo G, Du Bruyn E, Howlett P, Ntsekhe M. Diagnosis and management of tuberculous pericarditis: what is new? *Curr Cardiol Rep*. 2020;22(1):2.

87. Manga P, McCutcheon K, Tsabedze N, et al. HIV and nonischemic heart disease. *J Am Coll Cardiol*. 2017;69(1):83–91.

88. Hsue PY. Mechanisms of cardiovascular disease in the setting of HIV infection. *Can J Cardiol*. 2019;35(3):238–248.

89. Noubiap JJ, Agbor VN, Ndoadoumgue AL, et al. Epidemiology of pericardial diseases in Africa: a systematic scoping review. *Heart*. 2019;105(3):180–188.

90. Rehman KA, Betancor J, Xu B, et al. Uremic pericarditis, pericardial effusion, and constrictive pericarditis in end-stage renal disease: insights and pathophysiology. *Clin Cardiol*. 2017;40(10):839–846.

91. Prasad M, Hermann J, Gabriel SE, et al. Cardiorheumatology: cardiac involvement in systemic rheumatic disease. *Nat Rev Cardiol*. 2015;12(3):168–176.

92. Lee KS, Kronbichler A, Eisenhut M, et al. Cardiovascular involvement in systemic rheumatic diseases: an integrated view for the treating physicians. *Autoimmun Rev*. 2018;17(3):201–214.

93. Rigante D, Cantarini L, Imazio M, et al. Autoinflammatory diseases and cardiovascular manifestations. *Ann Med*. 2011;43(5):341–346.

94. Krainer J, Siebenhandl S, Weinhausel A. Systemic autoinflammatory diseases. *J Autoimmun*. 2020;109:102421.

95. Tamarappoo BK, Klein AL. Post-pericardiotomy syndrome. *Curr Cardiol Rep*. 2016;18(11):116.

96. Verma BR, Banerjee K, Noll A, et al. Pericardial complications and postcardiac injury syndrome after cardiovascular implantable electronic device placement: a meta-analysis and systematic review. *Herz*. 2019.

97. Verma BR, Chetrit M, Gentry Iii JL, et al. Multimodality imaging in patients with post-cardiac injury syndrome. *Heart*. 2020;106(9):639–646.

98. Lestuzzi C, Berretta M, Tomkowski W. 2015 update on the diagnosis and management of neoplastic pericardial disease. *Expert Rev Cardiovasc Ther*. 2015;13(4):377–389.

99. Ala CK, Klein AL, Moslehi JJ. Cancer treatment-associated pericardial disease: epidemiology, clinical presentation, diagnosis, and management. *Curr Cardiol Rep*. 2019;21(12):156.

100. Szpakowski N, Desai MY. Radiation-associated pericardial disease. *Curr Cardiol Rep*. 2019;21(9):97.

101. Donnellan E, Jellis CL, Griffin BP. Radiation-associated cardiac disease: from molecular mechanisms to clinical management. *Curr Treat Options Cardiovasc Med*. 2019;21(5):22.

102. Chahine J, Ala CK, Gentry JL, et al. Pericardial diseases in patients with hypothyroidism. *Heart*. 2019;105(13):1027–1033.

103. Bergmann KR, Kharbanda A, Haveman L. Myocarditis and pericarditis in the pediatric patient: validated management strategies. *Pediatr Emerg Med Pract*. 2015;12(7):1–22. quiz 23.

104. Brucato A, Emmi G, Cantarini L, et al. Management of idiopathic recurrent pericarditis in adults and in children: a role for IL-1 receptor antagonism. *Intern Emerg Med*. 2018;13(4):475–489.

105. del Fresno MR, Peralta JE, Granados MA, et al. Intravenous immunoglobulin therapy for refractory recurrent pericarditis. *Pediatrics*. 2014;134(5):e1441–e1446.

106. Nagamori Y, Hamaoka T, Murai H, et al. Takotsubo cardiomyopathy complicated by cardiac tamponade due to non-hemorrhagic pericardial effusion: a case report. *BMC Cardiovasc Disord*. 2020;20(1):67.

107. Gheorghe L, Ielasi A, Rensing B, et al. Complications following percutaneous mitral valve repair. *Front Cardiovasc Med*. 2019;6:146.

108. Wang J, Patel M, Xiao M, et al. Incidence and predictors of asymptomatic pericardial effusion after transcatheter closure of atrial septal defect. *EuroIntervention*. 2016;12(2):e250–256.

109. Schmidt B, Betts TR, Sievert H, et al. Incidence of pericardial effusion after left atrial appendage closure: the impact of underlying heart rhythm-Data from the EWOLUTION study. *J Cardiovasc Electrophysiol*. 2018;29(7):973–978.

110. Hodson RW, Jin R, Ring ME, et al. Intrathoracic complications associated with trans-femoral transcatheter aortic valve replacement: implications for emergency surgical preparedness. *Catheter Cardiovasc Interv*. 2019.

111. Bauer T, Boeder N, Nef HM, et al. Fate of patients with coronary perforation complicating percutaneous coronary intervention (from the Euro heart survey percutaneous coronary intervention registry). *Am J Cardiol*. 2015;116(9):1363–1367.

112. Bhaskaran A, Chik W, Thomas S, et al. A review of the safety aspects of radio frequency ablation. *Int J Cardiol Heart Vasc*. 2015;8:147–153.

113. Liu XH, Chen CF, Gao XF, Xu YZ. Safety and efficacy of different catheter ablations for atrial fibrillation: a systematic review and meta-analysis. *Pacing Clin Electrophysiol*. 2016;39(8):883–899.

114. Ohlow MA, Lauer B, Brunelli M, Geller JC. Incidence and predictors of pericardial effusion after permanent heart rhythm device implantation: prospective evaluation of 968 consecutive patients. *Circ J*. 2013;77(4):975–981.

115. Sugumar H, Kearney LG, Srivastava PM. Pericardial tamponade: a life threatening complication of laparoscopic gastro-oesophageal surgery. *Heart Lung Circ*. 2012;21(4):237–239.

116. Khayata M, Alkharabsheh S, Shah NP, Klein AL. Pericardial cysts: a contemporary comprehensive review. *Curr Cardiol Rep*. 2019;21(7):64.

117. Money ME, Park C. Pericardial diverticula misdiagnosed as pericardial cysts. *J Thorac Cardiovasc Surg*. 2015;149(6):e103–e107.

118. Khayata M, Alkharabsheh S, Shah NP, et al. Case series, contemporary review and imaging guided diagnostic and management approach of congenital pericardial defects. *Open Heart*. 2020;7(1):e001103.

87 Pulmonary Embolism and Deep Vein Thrombosis

SAMUEL Z. GOLDHABER AND GREGORY PIAZZA

Venous thromboembolic disease (VTE), comprising both pulmonary embolism (PE) and deep vein thrombosis (DVT), contributes to substantial cardiovascular morbidity and mortality. PE causes more than 100,000 deaths annually in the United States, and the death rate is increasing (Fig. 87.1). Recently, there have been several advances in our understanding of these diseases and increasing recognition of the elevated VTE risk in certain groups, including patients with cancer and those in chronic care facilities, as well as greater understanding of risks and potential therapies in the pediatric population. There has also been increasing recognition of the role of inflammation in the pathogenesis of VTE, which shares pathophysiologic similarities with atherothrombosis.[1] This line of reasoning has uncovered a wide range of unconventional inflammation-related risk factors for PE, including sepsis, which is associated with a particularly high rate of VTE despite the use of thromboprophylaxis. Our knowledge of VTE genetics is also expanding rapidly, and recent large genetic studies have identified novel loci and led to development of polygenic risk scores for VTE.

Advances in diagnostic, therapeutic, and preventive strategies, coupled with novel perspectives on VTE pathophysiology, are emerging at an unprecedented pace. Clinical and electronic decision tools facilitate early VTE detection and improve prevention strategies. Novel oral anticoagulants (NOACs) such as dabigatran, rivaroxaban, apixaban, and edoxaban allow PE and DVT to be managed with fewer bleeding complications than with warfarin. Moreover, distinct advantages of NOAC therapy, including fixed dosing, the absence of drug-food interactions, the minimal number of drug-drug interactions, and the lack of need for testing blood coagulation levels simplify and enhance the safety of anticoagulation.

Finally, VTE and PE are being increasingly recognized as part of the syndrome associated with COVID-19, the disease caused by the SARS-CoV-2 virus and appear to be driven by the unique and thus far poorly understood inflammatory and thrombotic complications associated with the disease. Therapy for these patients has been particularly challenging and rapidly evolving.

EPIDEMIOLOGY

General Considerations

The incidence of VTE in North America and Europe is approximately 1.5 cases per 1000 person-years. About two-thirds of cases are DVT, and the rest are PE with or without DVT. Incidence increases with age and is similar in men and women. Approximately half of VTE occurs without antecedent trauma, surgery, immobilization, or cancer.

Death due to PE is increasing in the United States, particularly among young and middle-aged adults and has plateaued among those 65 years of age and older. In contrast, between 2000 and 2015 in Europe, age-standardized annual PE-related mortality rates decreased linearly from 12.8 to 6.5 deaths per 100,000.[2] These differences may reflect differences in patient demographics and comorbidities. In the United States, socioeconomically disadvantaged older adults hospitalized with PE have higher long-term mortality rates than their non-disadvantaged counterparts and are more likely to be readmitted within 30 and 90 days of discharge.[3] Most deaths in hospitalized patients with PE are sudden, characterized by pulseless electrical activity or resulting from multisystem organ failure caused by right heart dysfunction. Among

DISEASES OF THE MYOCARDIUM, PERICARDIUM, AND PULMONARY VASCULATURE BED

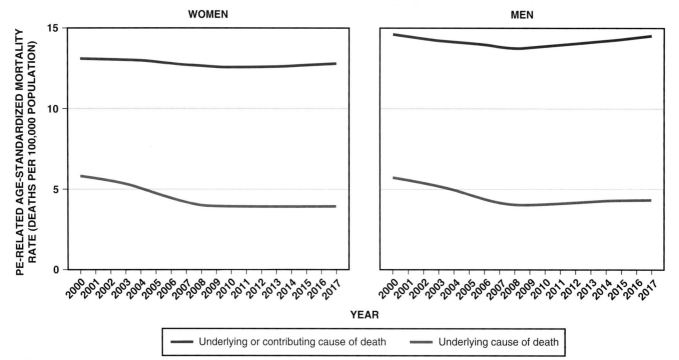

FIGURE 87.1 PE-related mortality in the United States, stratified by age and gender.

adults aged ≥65 years in the United States, the in-hospital case-fatality rate is approximately 4%, the 30-day readmission rate is 15%, and the 6-month mortality rate jumps to 20%.[4]

Clinical Risk Factors

Risk factors for VTE include advancing age, cancer, previous VTE, venous insufficiency, pregnancy, trauma, frailty, and immobility. Of those suffering VTE in the Worcester Venous Thromboembolism Study, 23% had undergone surgery, and 36% had been hospitalized within the preceding 3 months. Among those patients, less than 50% had received anticoagulant prophylaxis.[5]

Cardiovascular risk factors are associated with VTE. A meta-analysis of 63,552 patients with VTE and control subjects found that the relative risk for VTE was 2.3 for obesity, 1.5 for hypertension, 1.4 for diabetes mellitus, 1.2 for cigarette smoking, and 1.2 for hypercholesterolemia.[6] Heart failure (both reduced ejection fraction and preserved ejection fraction) triples the long-term risk of VTE.[7] Given the overlap between venous and arterial thrombosis risk factors, clinicians can counsel patients on steps to reduce VTE and coronary heart disease risk simultaneously.

Population-based cohort studies have shown that older age, smoking, and adiposity have been consistently linked to higher VTE risk.[8] In a study of more than 1 million women with a mean age of 56 years in the United Kingdom, VTE risk increased with increasing body mass index (BMI). Women with a BMI of 35 kg/m² or greater, for example, were three to four times more likely to develop VTE than women with a BMI between 22 and 25 kg/m².[9] A Spanish VTE registry called RIETE (Registro Informatizado de Enfermedad TromboEmbólica) included 18,023 patients with PE. Immobilized patients had a more than twofold increased risk of fatal PE. Of RIETE patients dying from PE, 43% had a history of recent immobilization for 4 days or longer.[10]

VTE is also a women's health issue. In the United States, PE accounts for 9% of all pregnancy-related deaths or approximately 1.5 deaths per 100,000 live births. Maternal deaths and maternal morbidity due to PE are more common among women who deliver by cesarean section.[11] Pregnancy, hormonal contraception, and postmenopausal hormonal therapy each contribute to increased risk. Use of progesterone-only birth control pills is not associated with increased VTE risk.

Long-haul air travel is a frequently discussed acquired risk factor, although the associated risk of fatal PE is less than 1/1 million air travelers. When death occurs, however, it is dramatic and especially tragic because the victim is often an otherwise healthy young person.

It has also been recognized that certain populations are at higher risk for VTE. Nursing home residency has been identified as an independent risk factor for VTE. Within Olmsted County, Minnesota, a Mayo Clinic study found that VTE incidence appears to be highest during the first week after admission to a nursing facility. The rate of VTE was 2.3%—nearly 30-fold higher than the incidence of VTE among all residents of Olmsted County. Nursing home residents with VTE had a twofold higher mortality rate compared with those who did not have VTE.[12] Unfortunately, appropriate guidelines for VTE prevention in nursing homes are lacking.

Cancer and Venous Thromboembolic

Some risk factors for VTE are not readily modifiable (Table 87.1). Cancer patients have a fourfold increased risk of VTE compared with the general population.[13] When unprovoked VTE occurs, there is about a 5% chance that occult cancer will be detected within the ensuing year.[14] For treatment of acute VTE in patients with established cancer, the National Comprehensive Cancer Network (NCCN) guidelines now recommend consideration of an NOAC rather than low molecular weight heparin (LMWH) monotherapy.[15]

As VTE patients with cancer survive longer due to advances in oncologic therapy, the frequency of VTE is increasing because cancer patients have a markedly increased incidence of VTE (see Chapter 57). Cancer-chemotherapy-associated VTE is common. Increased VTE risk is associated with solid tumors, especially adenocarcinomas of the pancreas, stomach, lung, esophagus, prostate, and colon. Less well known is that VTE risk also increases with "liquid tumors" such as myeloproliferative disorders, lymphoma, and leukemia.

Venous Thromboembolic in the Pediatric Population

Although the frequency of PE and DVT increases with age, VTE also afflicts infants, children, and teenagers.[16] VTE is increasingly diagnosed in pediatric patients, and anticoagulant use in this population has become common, despite the absence of US Food and Drug Administration (FDA) approval for this indication (see below). The increase in VTE diagnosis in children and adolescents

TABLE 87.1 Major Risk Factors for Venous Thromboembolism That Are Not Readily Modifiable

Advanced age
Arterial disease, including carotid and coronary disease
Personal or family history of venous thromboembolism
Recent surgery, trauma, or immobility, including stroke
Congestive heart failure
Chronic obstructive pulmonary disease
Acute infection
Blood transfusion
Erythropoietin-stimulating factor
Chronic inflammation (e.g., inflammatory bowel disease)
Chronic kidney disease
Air pollution
Long-haul air travel
Pregnancy, oral contraceptive pills, or postmenopausal hormone replacement therapy
Pacemaker, implantable cardioverter-defibrillator leads, or indwelling central venous catheter
Hypercoagulable states
Factor V Leiden resulting in activated protein C resistance
Prothrombin gene mutation 20210
Antithrombin deficiency
Protein C deficiency
Protein S deficiency
Antiphospholipid antibody syndrome (acquired, not inherited)

is probably due, in part, to increased awareness, improved imaging, and more frequent use of indwelling central venous catheters for chemotherapy and nutrition.

Hypercoagulable States

The two most common identified genetic causes of thrombophilia are factor V Leiden and the prothrombin gene mutation (see Chapter 95). Normally, a specified amount of activated protein C (aPC) can be added to plasma to prolong the activated partial thromboplastin time (aPTT). Patients with "aPC resistance" exhibit blunted aPTT prolongation and are predisposed to the development of PE and DVT. The phenotype of aPC resistance is associated with a single-point mutation, designated factor V Leiden, in the factor V gene. Factor V Leiden triples the risk of VTE and is associated with recurrent pregnancy loss, probably because of placental vein thrombosis. Use of oral estrogen-containing contraceptives by patients with factor V Leiden increases the VTE risk by at least 10-fold. A single-point mutation in the 3′untranslated region of the prothrombin gene (G-to-A transition at nucleotide position 20210) is associated with increased levels of prothrombin. The prothrombin gene mutation doubles the risk of VTE.

Antiphospholipid syndrome, the most common acquired thrombophilia, is a prothrombotic disorder that can cause venous or arterial thrombosis, thrombocytopenia, recurrent fetal loss, or acute ischemic encephalopathy. One of the following antiphospholipid antibodies must be present for at least 12 weeks to make the diagnosis: IgG or IgM anticardiolipin antibodies, anti-beta2-glycoprotein I, antiprothrombin, or lupus anticoagulant. The antiphospholipid syndrome heightens susceptibility to recurrent venous or arterial thrombosis if anticoagulation is discontinued. The antiphospholipid syndrome is often associated with other systemic autoimmune diseases such as systemic lupus erythematosus. However, primary antiphospholipid syndrome commonly occurs without other autoimmune manifestations.[17]

Obtaining a family history remains the fastest and most cost-effective method to identify a predisposition to venous thrombosis. Investigation with blood tests to detect known causes of hypercoagulability can be misleading. Consumption coagulopathy caused by venous thrombosis, for example, may be misdiagnosed as deficiency of antithrombin, protein C, or protein S. Heparin administration can depress antithrombin levels. Use of warfarin ordinarily causes a mild deficiency of protein C or protein S. Oral contraceptives and pregnancy also depress protein S levels.

Other Conditions Associated with Venous Thromboembolic

Chronic kidney disease is also associated with VTE,[18] probably because impaired kidney function heightens oxidative stress and inflammation. Other inflammation-based risk factors for VTE include Crohn disease, ulcerative colitis, rheumatoid arthritis, psoriasis, pneumonia, urinary tract infections, influenza, diabetes mellitus type 2, and inflammatory mediators such as transfused blood or erythropoietin stimulating factor.

Long-term Complications of Venous Thromboembolic and Risk of Subsequent Adverse Events

Major long-term complications of VTE include recurrent VTE, post-PE syndrome,[19] chronic thromboembolic pulmonary hypertension (CTEPH),[20] and postthrombotic syndrome (PTS, also called chronic venous insufficiency) of the legs.[21] PTS patients compared with controls report worse long-term physical health, mental health, and quality of life.[22] The most likely pathophysiological trigger for the development of CTEPH and PTS is thrombus persistence.[23]

The risk of subsequent arterial cardiovascular events doubles in VTE patients compared with controls.[24] Among 1023 Australian patients initially hospitalized with PE, the cumulative mortality rate was 32% over 5 years, with 40% of the deaths attributed to cardiovascular causes. Postdischarge mortality was 2.5 times higher than in an age- and gender-matched population.[25] In a Norwegian observational study of 29,506 participants with a median follow-up of 16 years, 1853 participants suffered myocardial infarction (MI), and 699 were diagnosed with VTE. MI was associated with a 72% increased risk of PE.[26] Heart failure[7] and chronic obstructive pulmonary disease (COPD) are also potent risk factors for in-hospital death among patients with VTE.

Pulmonary Embolism in COVID-19 Infection

VTE and PE are being increasingly recognized among patients diagnosed with COVID-19, the disease caused by the novel coronavirus SARS-CoV-2 (see Chapter 94). Patients triaged to the intensive care unit (ICU) have a high prevalence of PE as well as in situ pulmonary arterial thrombosis. In a multicenter prospective study of COVID-19 patients, the rate of VTE was 37% and was associated with an increased length of stay and a trend toward higher death rates due to PE.[27] Among 107 patients admitted to the Lille (France) University Hospital ICU with COVID-19 pneumonia, 21% suffered PE. The median time from ICU admission until a PE diagnosis was 6 days.[28] PE has also been reported in outpatients with COVID-19.[29] Proposed mechanisms for the development of macrovascular (Fig. 87.2A] and microvascular in situ thrombosis in the pulmonary vessels (Fig. 87.2B) include conventional risk factors such as immobility, pneumonia, fever, and obesity, as well as the inflammatory response (Fig. 87.2C), causing endothelial dysfunction and cytokine storm, which are known to occur in COVID-19 (**eFig. 87.1**).[30]

PATHOPHYSIOLOGY

ROLE OF COAGULATION AND PLATELETS IN VENOUS THROMBOEMBOLIC

VTE and atherothrombosis have intertwining risk factors and pathophysiology. The historical characterization of PE as a "red clot" disease, compared to atherothrombosis as a "white clot" disease, is no longer

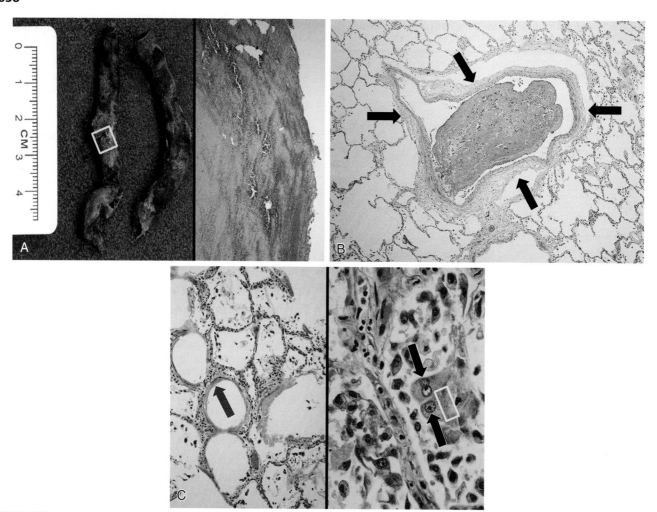

FIGURE 87.2 A, COVID-19 thrombosis: macroscopic thrombosis. *Left panel:* Right ventricular macroscopic thrombus originating in deep leg veins; yellow boxed area delineates a "chevron" with the imprint of venous valve markings. *Right panel:* Laminated microscopic thrombus. **B,** COVID-19 thrombosis: microscopic thrombosis. Microthrombus within a venule (*arrows*). **C,** COVID-19 thrombosis: acute respiratory distress syndrome triggers an inflammatory response that leads to arterial and venous thrombosis. *Left panel:* Arrow points to the hyaline membrane of an alveolus filled with transudative fluid. *Right panel:* Arrows point to two activated macrophages. Within the *yellow rectangle* there are multiple viral inclusion bodies. (Images kindly provided by Richard N. Mitchell, MD, PhD, and Robert F. Padera, MD, PhD.)

tenable. VTE is part of a pan-cardiovascular syndrome that includes coronary artery disease and cerebrovascular disease (Fig. 87.3). Virchow's triad of stasis, hypercoagulability, and endothelial injury often activates the pathophysiologic cascade leading to VTE. Inflammation is not included in Virchow's triad but is also a key precipitant. Infection and associated inflammation lead to the recruitment of platelets—one of the first steps necessary for thrombus initiation. Activated platelets release polyphosphates, procoagulant microparticles, and proinflammatory mediators. These activated platelets bind neutrophils and stimulate them to release nuclear material and form web-like extracellular networks containing DNA, histones, and neutrophil granule constituents. These networks are called *neutrophil extracellular traps* (NETs) and consist of DNA extruded from leukocytes to contain infections. These extracellular webs of chromatin, microbicidal proteins, and oxidant enzymes are prothrombotic and procoagulant. Histones stimulate platelet aggregation and promote platelet-dependent thrombin generation. As venous thrombi start to organize, neutrophils infiltrate the NETs. As thrombi mature, NETs provide the scaffold that binds red blood cells and promotes further platelet aggregation.[31] When not properly regulated, NETs have the potential to propagate inflammation and microvascular thrombosis, particularly in the lungs of patients with acute respiratory distress syndrome.[32]

Venous thrombi contain fibrin, red blood cells, platelets, and neutrophils (eFig 87.2). These thrombi flourish in an environment of stasis, low oxygen tension, oxidative stress, increased expression of proinflammatory gene products, and impaired endothelial cell regulatory capacity. Inflammation resulting from infection, transfusion, or erythropoietin-stimulating factor[33] activates a cascade of biochemical reactions in the vein endothelium that promotes thrombosis.[34]

The high recurrence rate of VTE in the absence of anticoagulation supports the hypothesis that venous thrombosis can persist as a subclinical and perhaps chronic inflammatory state that becomes clinically apparent intermittently, when activated platelets degranulate and release preformed proinflammatory mediators. In the JUPITER trial, an initially healthy cohort of 17,802 asymptomatic subjects with elevated baseline high-sensitivity C-reactive protein (hsCRP) levels was treated with rosuvastatin 20 mg daily and had a 43% reduction in symptomatic VTE.[35] The principal postulated mechanism of action was rosuvastatin's antiinflammatory effect, evidenced by its reduction of hsCRP levels.

MOLECULAR GENETICS AND VTE

The Million Veteran Program and the UK Biobank collaborated to perform a genome-wide association study on 26,066 cases and 624,053 controls. They identified 22 previously unknown loci and then developed a genome-wide polygenic risk score for VTE that identifies 5% of the population as at-risk carriers.[36] Common polymorphisms such as factor V Leiden and the prothrombin gene mutation account for an additional 5% of VTE heritability. Another research consortium identified 16 novel susceptibility loci for VTE, some of which were outside known coagulation pathways.[37] A polygenic risk score has been developed that identifies patients at greater than twofold increased risk for VTE.[38]

CARDIOPULMONARY DYNAMICS

PE can elicit a complex cardiopulmonary response that includes: (1) increased pulmonary vascular resistance due to vascular obstruction, hypoxemia, neurohumoral agents, and pulmonary artery baroreceptors; (2) impaired gas exchange caused by increased alveolar dead space

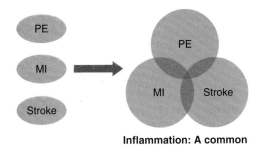

PE is a vascular medicine disease that overlaps with MI and stroke

PE

MI

Stroke

PE

MI   Stroke

Inflammation: A common underlying process

FIGURE 87.3 Pulmonary embolism (PE) is part of a pan-cardiovascular syndrome that includes myocardial infarction (MI) and stroke. Inflammation is a common underlying process.

from vascular obstruction and hypoxemia from alveolar hypoventilation and right-to-left shunting, as well as impaired carbon monoxide transfer caused by loss of gas exchange surface area; (3) alveolar hyperventilation caused by reflex stimulation of irritant receptors; (4) increased airway resistance due to bronchoconstriction; and (5) decreased pulmonary compliance due to edema, alveolar hemorrhage, and loss of surfactant.

The extent of pulmonary vascular obstruction, the presence of underlying cardiopulmonary disease, and the neurohumoral response determine whether and to what extent right ventricular dysfunction ensues. As pulmonary vascular resistance increases, pulmonary artery pressure rises. In response to pressure overload, the right ventricle (RV) releases cardiac biomarkers such as N-terminal prohormone-brain type natriuretic peptide (NT-proBNP), brain-type natriuretic peptide (BNP), and troponin, all of which portend an increased likelihood of adverse clinical outcomes.

The sudden rise in pulmonary artery pressure abruptly increases right ventricular afterload, with consequent elevation of right ventricular wall tension followed by right ventricular dilation and dysfunction (Fig. 87.4). As pressure in the RV increases further, the interventricular septum shifts toward the left, leading to underfilling and decreased left ventricular diastolic distensibility. With impaired filling of the left ventricle (LV), systemic cardiac output and systolic arterial pressure both decline, decreasing coronary perfusion and causing myocardial ischemia. Elevated right ventricular wall tension can reduce right coronary artery perfusion and increase right ventricular myocardial oxygen demand, causing ischemia. Perpetuation of this cycle can lead to right ventricular infarction, circulatory collapse, and death.

CLASSIFICATION OF PULMONARY EMBOLISM

Classification of acute PE (Table 87.2) can assist with prognostication and clinical management.[39] High-risk, also known as massive, PE accounts for 5% to 10% of cases. Catastrophic, or "super-massive," PE patients have refractory cardiogenic shock or require ongoing cardiopulmonary resuscitation. They may need mechanical circulatory support such as extracorporeal membrane oxygenation (ECMO) followed by surgical pulmonary embolectomy. Intermediate-risk or submassive PE is more common, occurring in approximately 20% to 25% of patients. Low-risk PE constitutes most PE cases—approximately 65% to 70%.

High-Risk Pulmonary Embolism

Patients with high-risk PE are susceptible to cardiogenic shock and multisystem organ failure. Renal insufficiency, hepatic dysfunction, and altered mentation are common findings. Their mortality rate approaches one-third.[40] PE is typically present bilaterally, sometimes as a "saddle" PE in the main pulmonary artery. Dyspnea is usually the most prominent symptom; chest pain and transient cyanosis occur less often; and systemic arterial hypotension requiring pressor support occurs frequently. Excessive fluid boluses may worsen right-sided heart

failure, rendering therapy more difficult. These patients may require heroic efforts to enable survival, such as venoarterial ECMO.[41]

Intermediate-Risk Pulmonary Embolism

Intermediate-risk PE patients present with normal systemic arterial pressure. The European Society of Cardiology (ESC) PE Guidelines subdivide intermediate-risk PE into intermediate-high- and intermediate-low-risk.[39] Patients with intermediate-high-risk PE present with both right ventricular hypokinesis and elevated cardiac biomarkers such as troponin, NT-proBNP, or BNP. Those with intermediate-low-risk PE present with right ventricular dysfunction, elevated cardiac biomarkers, or neither, but not both. Usually, one-third or more of the pulmonary artery vasculature is obstructed in intermediate-risk PE patients. Sudden onset of moderate pulmonary arterial hypertension (eFig. 87.3) and right ventricular enlargement is common. If patients have no previous history of cardiopulmonary disease, they may appear clinically well, but this initial impression may be misleading. They are at risk for recurrent PE, even with adequate anticoagulation. Most survive, but some will deteriorate clinically and require escalation of therapy with pressor support or advanced therapy.[42]

Low-Risk Pulmonary Embolism

Patients with low-risk PE do not exhibit markers of an adverse prognosis. They present with normal systemic arterial pressure and normal right ventricular function and do not have elevated cardiac biomarkers. They often have anatomically small PEs and appear clinically stable. Adequate anticoagulation usually results in an excellent clinical outcome. A subset with a reliable social network and clinical follow-up may be appropriate for home therapy.[43]

Pulmonary Infarction

Pulmonary infarction is characterized by pleuritic chest pain that may be unremitting or may wax and wane. The pleurisy is occasionally accompanied by hemoptysis. The embolus typically lodges in the peripheral pulmonary arterial tree, near the pleura (Fig. 87.5). Tissue infarction usually occurs 3 to 7 days after embolism. Signs and symptoms often include fever, leukocytosis, elevated erythrocyte sedimentation rate, and radiologic evidence of a wedge-shaped or pleural-based infiltrate.

Paradoxical Embolism

Paradoxical embolism may manifest with a sudden stroke, which may be misdiagnosed as "cryptogenic." The cause is a DVT that embolizes to the arterial system, usually through a patent foramen ovale or atrial septal defect. The DVT can be small and break away completely from a tiny leg vein, leaving no residual evidence of thrombosis that can be imaged on venous ultrasound examination.[44]

Nonthrombotic Pulmonary Embolism

Sources of embolism other than thrombus are uncommon. They include fat, tumor, air, and amniotic fluid. Fat embolism most often occurs after blunt trauma complicated by long bone fractures.[45] Air embolus can occur during placement or removal of a central venous catheter. Amniotic fluid embolism may be catastrophic and is characterized by respiratory failure, cardiogenic shock, and disseminated intravascular coagulation. Intravenous drug abusers sometimes self-inject contaminants such as hair, talc, and cotton; they are susceptible to septic PE.

Post-Pulmonary Embolism Syndrome

The post-PE syndrome is characterized by persistent symptoms, including chest pain and dyspnea, functional limitation, and exercise intolerance in the absence of pulmonary hypertension.[46] The impact of advanced therapies (i.e., systemic fibrinolysis or catheter-based intervention) on the frequency of post-PE syndrome remains unclear. However, in long-term follow-up from the PEITHO trial, systemic fibrinolysis did not decrease symptom burden or functional limitation in patients with intermediate-risk PE.[47]

Chronic Thromboembolic Pulmonary Hypertension (see Chapter 88)

CTEPH is characterized by persistent pulmonary arterial obstruction, pulmonary vasoconstriction, and a secondary small-vessel arteriopathy that results in chronic dyspnea, functional limitation, and progressive right ventricular failure.[48] CTEPH occurs in 2% to 4% of patients after PE. There are evolving therapeutic approaches for operable and inoperable disease.[49] Pulmonary thromboendarterectomy is the most effective and durable therapy. Pulmonary vasodilators, such as riociguat, can potentially improve symptoms and functional capacity in patients with inoperable disease or post-thromboendarterectomy pulmonary hypertension.[50] Balloon pulmonary angioplasty offers an additional option for patients who are not surgical candidates.[51] Because the evaluation and treatment are complex and evolving,

patients with CTEPH should be referred to specialized centers of excellence.

CLASSIFICATION OF DEEP VEIN THROMBOSIS

Lower-Extremity Deep Vein Thrombosis and the Relationship Between Deep Vein Thrombosis and Pulmonary Embolism

Patients present with DVT symptoms about twice as frequently as with PE symptoms. Leg DVT occurs approximately 10 times more often than upper-extremity DVT. The more proximal the thrombus is within the deep leg veins, the more likely it is to embolize and cause acute PE. When venous thrombi detach from their sites of formation, they travel through the venous system toward the vena cava. They pass through the right atrium and RV and then enter the pulmonary arterial circulation. An extremely large embolus may lodge at the bifurcation of the pulmonary artery, forming a saddle embolus (Fig. 87.6). In many patients with large PEs, ultrasonographic evidence of DVT is lacking, likely because the clot has already embolized to the lungs.

Isolated Calf Deep Vein Thrombosis

The clinical significance and treatment of isolated calf DVT have been the focus of ongoing investigation and debate. A randomized trial of injectable anticoagulation for 6 weeks in low-risk patients with isolated calf DVT did not reduce adverse outcomes, including extension of calf DVT, contralateral proximal DVT, and symptomatic PE at day 42 versus no treatment (3% vs. 5%; p=0.54), but did result in bleeding (4% vs. 0%; p=0.025).[52] In contrast, a meta-analysis found anticoagulation to be associated with a 50% reduction in recurrent VTE risk (6.5% vs. 12.0%; RR, 0.50; 95% CI, 0.31 to 0.79), without increasing the risk of major bleeding (0.4% vs. 0.7%; RR, 0.64; 95% CI, 0.15 to 2.73).[53] Anticoagulant therapy is typically prescribed in patients with symptomatic calf DVT.

Upper-Extremity Deep Vein Thrombosis

Upper-extremity DVT is an increasingly important clinical entity owing to more frequent placement of pacemakers and implantable cardioverter-defibrillators, as well as growing use of chronic indwelling catheters for chemotherapy and nutrition. The likelihood of upper-extremity DVT increases as the size and number of lumens of a peripherally inserted central catheter increase.[54] Catheter-based thrombosis is a major source of COVID-19-associated DVT.

A hospital initiative to use smaller-diameter catheters and to minimize the number of lumens can reduce the frequency of catheter-associated DVT.[55] Patients with upper-extremity DVT are at risk for PE, superior vena cava syndrome, loss of vascular access, and central venous stenosis of the subclavian or

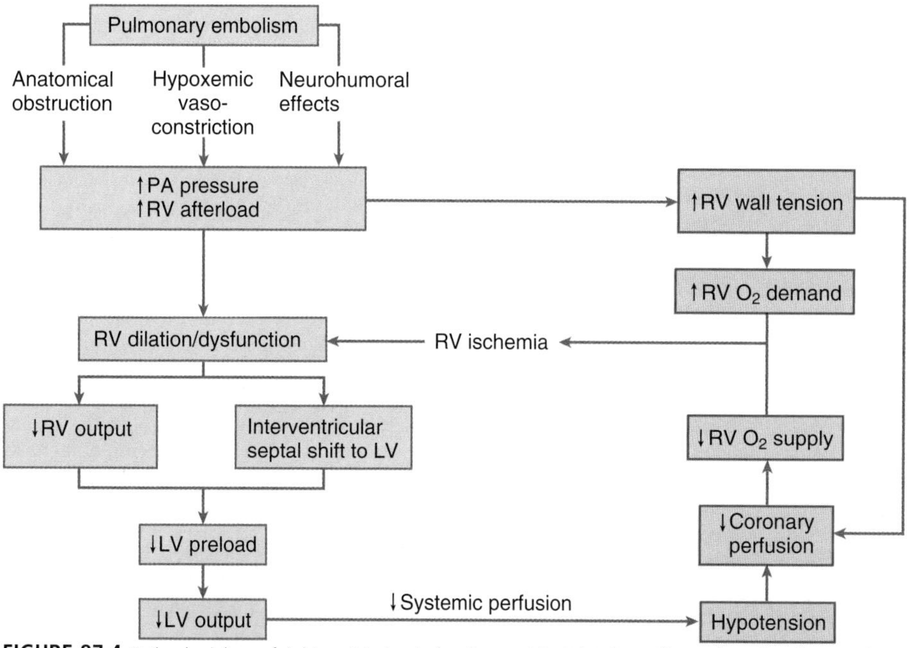

FIGURE 87.4 Pathophysiology of right ventricular dysfunction and its deleterious effects of causing decreased systemic arterial pressure, decreased coronary perfusion, and deteriorating ventricular function. *LV*, left ventricle/ventricular; *PA*, pulmonary artery; *RV*, right ventricle/ventricular.

TABLE 87.2 Classification of Acute Pulmonary Embolism

EUROPEAN SOCIETY OF CARDIOLOGY (ESC, 2019)	AMERICAN HEART ASSOCIATION (AHA, 2011)	HEMODYNAMIC STATUS	PE SEVERITY INDEX (PESI) (OR SIMPLIFIED PESI)	EVIDENCE OF DYSFUNCTION	TREATMENT
High risk	Massive	Unstable	High	Typically abnormal RV on imaging, elevated troponin, OR both	Anticoagulation and advanced therapy
Intermediate-high risk	Submassive	Stable	High	Abnormal RV on imaging, AND elevated troponin	Anticoagulation with advanced therapy if clinical deterioration
Intermediate-low risk			High	May have abnormal RV on imaging OR elevated troponin BUT not both	Anticoagulation
Low risk	Low risk	Stable	Low	None	Anticoagulation with home therapy in subset with reliable follow-up

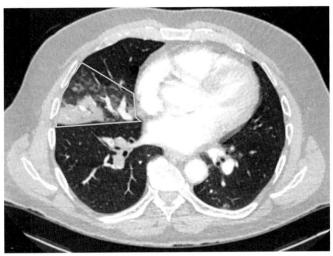

FIGURE 87.5 Chest computed tomography (CT) image showing a large, wedge-shaped (*outline*), right-sided pulmonary infarction.

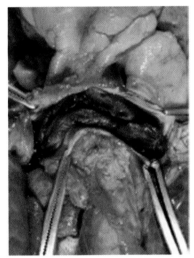

FIGURE 87.6 A 41-year-old woman with poorly controlled hypertension suffered an intracerebral hemorrhage, complicated 6 days later by acute pulmonary embolism. Emergency catheter embolectomy was unsuccessful, and she suffered cardiac arrest. At autopsy, a large saddle embolus extended from the root of the pulmonary artery into the left and right lungs.

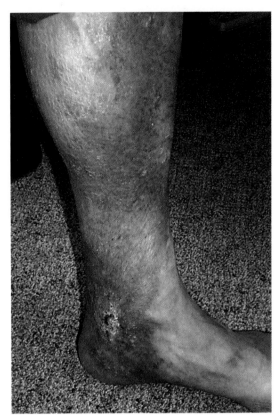

FIGURE 87.7 Left medial malleolus venous ulcer due to postthrombotic syndrome in a 57-year-old man with a history of left iliofemoral deep vein thrombosis (DVT) and extensive tobacco use. Note the extensive erythema of the skin of the left lower leg. (Courtesy Suresh Vedantham, MD.)

brachiocephalic veins. In a study of 3790 patients receiving peripherally inserted central catheters during hospitalization, central catheter use tripled the likelihood of upper-extremity DVT and increased the likelihood of leg DVT by about 50%.[56]

Postthrombotic Syndrome and Chronic Venous Insufficiency

Valve dysfunction in the deep venous system often results from damage due to DVT. Obstruction of the deep veins may further limit the outflow of blood, causing venous hypertension with leg muscle contraction. Abnormal hemodynamics in the large veins of the leg are transmitted into the microcirculation, causing venous microangiopathy. Patients with DVT who develop PTS have higher measured levels of inflammatory markers compared with those who do not.[57] Risk factors for PTS include iliofemoral DVT, recurrent ipsilateral DVT, persistent symptoms after 1 month of anticoagulation, increased BMI, advanced age, and suboptimal anticoagulation during the first 3 months after DVT diagnosis.[58] Physical findings may include varicose veins, abnormal pigmentation of the medial malleolus, and venous ulceration (Fig. 87.7). The economic impact of PTS is high[59] because of time lost from work and the expense of medical diagnosis and treatment. Chronic venous disease is associated with a reduced quality of life because of pain, decreased physical function, and decreased mobility. Vascular compression stockings (below-knee, 20 to 30 mm Hg or 30 to 40 mm Hg) do not prevent the development of PTS after

an acute proximal DVT.[60] However, for patients with venous insufficiency, vascular compression stockings are a mainstay of therapy, improving venous hemodynamics, reducing edema, alleviating calf discomfort, and minimizing skin discoloration. Supervised exercise training may have a role in treatment of PTS.[61]

Differentiating Lymphedema from Venous Insufficiency

Lymphedema may be misdiagnosed as chronic venous insufficiency. Leg discomfort due to lymphedema is usually caused by leg swelling or increased limb weight. In contrast, pain from venous insufficiency typically occurs during standing and is alleviated by leg elevation. Swelling from venous insufficiency tends to be symmetric in both legs and is often most marked in the calves. In contrast, lymphedema swelling affects the entire leg and foot but is rarely symmetric. Unlike venous insufficiency, swelling due to lymphedema does not decrease during the night. Some patients with lymphedema have a positive Kaposi-Stemmer sign—the skin on the dorsum of the base of the second toe cannot be pinched as a fold between the fingers.

Superficial Venous Thrombosis

Superficial venous thrombosis (thrombophlebitis) is associated with a small but finite risk of DVT and PE. In a large Danish population-based case-control study, the risk of VTE was 3.4% in the 3 months following diagnosis of superficial venous thrombosis. The risk of VTE remained at a fivefold increase for more than 5 years after the initial superficial venous thrombosis.[62] Treatment of superficial venous thrombosis has been studied in recent randomized trials (see below).

DIAGNOSIS

PE is notorious for masquerading as other illnesses, such as asthma, pneumonia, pleurisy, acute coronary syndrome, and congestive heart failure. PE often occurs concomitantly with other illnesses, especially pneumonia, asthma, and heart failure, thereby confounding the diagnostic workup. The most useful approach is a clinical assessment of likelihood, based on presenting symptoms and signs, in conjunction with judicious use of laboratory testing and diagnostic imaging.

Clinical Presentation

Symptoms and signs of PE are nonspecific. Hence, awareness of VTE risk factors and a clinical suspicion for PE are of paramount importance in guiding diagnostic testing. Dyspnea is the most frequent symptom, and tachypnea is the most frequent sign (Table 87.3). Severe dyspnea, syncope, or cyanosis portends a life-threatening PE. Severe pleuritic pain often signifies a PE located in the distal pulmonary arterial system, near the pleural lining.

Clues to a possible hemodynamically significant PE include: (1) acute cor pulmonale (acute right ventricular failure), with features such as distended neck veins, right-sided S_3 gallop, right ventricular heave, tachycardia, or tachypnea, especially if (2) there are echocardiographic findings of right ventricular dilation and hypokinesis or electrocardiographic evidence of acute cor pulmonale manifested by a new $S_1Q_3T_3$ pattern (Fig. 87.8), new right bundle branch block, or

TABLE 87.3 Most Common Symptoms and Signs of Pulmonary Embolism

Symptoms
Dyspnea
Chest pain, especially pleuritic or "positional"
Anxiety
Cough
Hemoptysis
Leg swelling and pain
Signs
Tachypnea
Tachycardia
Low-grade fever
Jugular venous distension
Tricuspid regurgitant murmur
Accentuated P_2
Leg edema, erythema, tenderness

right ventricular ischemia with inferior T wave inversion or with T wave inversion in leads V_1 through V_4. Clinical decision rules can stratify patients into groups with high clinical likelihood or non-high clinical likelihood of PE, using a set of seven bedside assessment questions known as the Wells criteria (Table 87.4).

Differential Diagnosis

The differential diagnosis of PE covers a wide spectrum, from life-threatening conditions—such as MI—to anxiety states (Table 87.5). Concomitant illnesses should be considered. For example, if pneumonia or heart failure does not respond to appropriate therapy, the possibility of coexisting PE should be considered. Idiopathic pulmonary arterial hypertension may manifest with sudden exacerbations that mimic acute PE.

Nonimaging Diagnostic Methods
Plasma D-Dimer Assay

The plasma D-dimer assay is a blood-screening test that relies on the following principle: most patients with PE have ongoing endogenous fibrinolysis that is not effective enough to prevent PE but that nevertheless breaks down some of the fibrin clot to D-dimers, cross-linked fragments of the fibrin protein that are present following fibrinolysis. Although elevated plasma concentrations of D-dimers are sensitive for the diagnosis of PE, they are not specific. Even in the absence of PE, levels are elevated for at least 1 week postoperatively and are abnormally high in patients with MI, sepsis, cancer, or almost any other systemic illness. This test is generally not useful for screening acutely ill hospitalized inpatients, because their D-dimer levels are usually elevated. However, the plasma D-dimer assay is ideally suited for screening outpatients or emergency department patients who have suspected PE but no coexisting acute systemic illness.

A normal plasma D-dimer enzyme-linked immunosorbent assay (ELISA) usually rules out PE in the absence of high clinical suspicion. These patients rarely warrant diagnostic imaging. However, when PE is strongly suspected or the patient has been hospitalized, a D-dimer ELISA should not be obtained, and one should proceed directly to chest computed tomography (CT) imaging.[63] Although the traditional upper limit of normal (ULN) for a D-dimer screening test is 500 ng/mL, the ULN should be increased for patients older than 50 years to 10 times the patient's age.[64] In addition to being a screening test for PE, an elevated D-dimer is an independent correlate of increased mortality and subsequent VTE across a broad variety of disease states.[65]

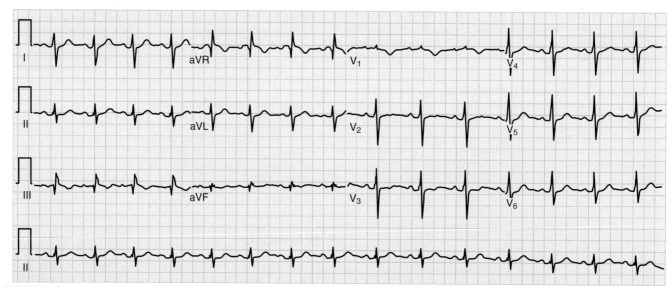

FIGURE 87.8 Electrocardiogram (ECG) from a 33-year-old man who presented with a left main pulmonary artery embolism on chest CT scan. He was hemodynamically stable, with normal right ventricular function on echocardiography. His troponin and brain-type natriuretic peptide (BNP) levels were normal. He was managed with anticoagulation alone. The initial ECG tracing shows an $S_1Q_3T_3$ (leads I and III) with an S wave in lead I, Q wave in lead III, and inverted T wave in lead III, and incomplete right bundle branch block, with inverted or flattened T waves in leads V_1 through V_4.

TABLE 87.4 Classic Wells Criteria to Assess Clinical Likelihood of Pulmonary Embolism

CRITERION	SCORING*
DVT symptoms or signs	3
An alternative diagnosis is less likely than PE	3
Heart rate >100 beats/min	1.5
Immobilization or surgery within 4 weeks	1.5
Previous DVT or PE	1.5
Hemoptysis	1
Cancer treated within 6 months or metastatic	1

DVT, Deep vein thrombosis; *PE*, pulmonary embolism.
*>4 score points = high probability; ≤4 score points = non–high probability.

TABLE 87.5 Differential Diagnosis of Pulmonary Embolism

Acute coronary syndromes

Chronic obstructive pulmonary disease exacerbation

Aortic dissection

Pneumonia

Acute bronchitis

Decompensated heart failure

Pulmonary hypertension

Pericardial disease

Intrathoracic malignancy

Musculoskeletal pain

Pneumothorax

Anxiety

Hepatobiliary or splenic pathology

Electrocardiogram

The electrocardiogram (ECG) helps exclude other conditions that may present similarly to acute PE, including acute MI and acute pericarditis. This test may lead the clinician toward a PE diagnosis in patients with electrocardiographic manifestations of right-sided heart strain. The most famous sign of right heart strain is the S1Q3T3 pattern, which consists of a deep S wave in lead I, a Q wave in lead III, and an inverted T wave in lead III, but the most common signs are sinus tachycardia and T wave inversion in leads V_1 to V_4 (see Fig. 87.8). Right-sided heart strain is not specific for PE and may be observed in patients with asthma, COPD, or idiopathic pulmonary hypertension. In patients with PE, the ECG may not be especially remarkable and may exhibit only sinus tachycardia, slight ST-segment and T wave abnormalities, or even an entirely normal appearance.

Imaging Methods
Chest Radiography

A near-normal radiographic appearance in the setting of severe respiratory compromise is highly suggestive of PE. Major chest radiographic abnormalities are uncommon. Focal oligemia (Westermark sign) indicates large central embolic occlusion. A peripheral wedge-shaped density above the diaphragm (Hampton hump) usually indicates pulmonary infarction (see Fig. 87.5). A subtle abnormality suggestive of PE is enlargement of the descending right pulmonary artery. The chest radiograph also can help identify patients with diseases that mimic PE, such as lobar pneumonia and pneumothorax, but patients with these illnesses also can have concomitant PE.

Lung Ultrasound

Point-of-care lung ultrasound has gained popularity in the evaluation of patients with dyspnea or chest pain in the emergency department and critical care settings.[66] PE may be suggested by

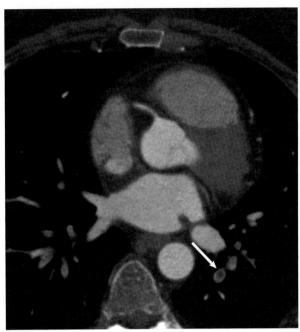

FIGURE 87.9 Small peripheral pulmonary embolism in the left lower lobe (*arrow*). (Courtesy U. Joseph Schoepf, MD.)

subpleural parenchymal consolidations visible on lung ultrasound when a pulmonary artery occlusion occurs.[67] Peripheral pulmonary consolidations identified on lung ultrasound can be observed in greater than 75% of patients having a PE.[67] While chest CT is still the best modality for PE diagnosis, point-of-care lung ultrasound may be a valuable alternative when clinical suspicion is high and the patient is not stable enough to travel safely to the CT scanner or CT is unavailable.[68] Lung ultrasound can also help distinguish PE from conditions such as heart failure, where B-lines will be present (see Chapter 16, echocardiography).

Chest Computed Tomography (see Chapter 20)

Chest CT has supplanted pulmonary radionuclide perfusion scintigraphy (see below) as the initial imaging test in most patients with suspected PE. Multidetector-row CT scanners can rapidly image the entire chest with submillimeter resolution. Three-dimensional images can be reconstructed, and color can be added electronically to enhance details of thrombus localization. The CT scan helps determine surgical or catheter accessibility to the thrombus in addition to alternative diagnoses that may require different therapy.[69] One cautionary note is that the CT scan may lead to overdiagnosis of PE due to breathing motion artifact or beam-hardening artifact.[70]

The latest generation of scanners can image thrombus in sixth-order vessels. These thrombi are so tiny that their clinical significance is uncertain (Fig. 87.9). The chest CT scan can also detect other pulmonary diseases that manifest in conjunction with PE or explain a clinical presentation that mimics PE. These diseases include pneumonia, atelectasis, pneumothorax, and pleural effusion, which may not be well-visualized on the chest radiograph.

For patients with suspected PE, the CT scan serves as a prognostic and diagnostic test. It shows a 4-chamber view of the heart and images the pulmonary arteries. Careful evaluation of the CT scan can detect signs of right ventricular dysfunction by analyzing (1) right ventricular-to-left ventricular end-diastolic diameter ratio (Fig. 87.10), (2) RV-to-LV volume ratio, (3) interventricular septal bowing toward the LV, and (4) reflux of contrast medium into the inferior vena cava (IVC).[71]

Right ventricular enlargement on CT correlates with right ventricular dysfunction and portends a complicated hospital course often marked by clinical deterioration. A RV-to-LV dimensional ratio of 0.9 or greater on a chest CT scan is abnormal and indicates right ventricular enlargement, correlating with right ventricular dysfunction on echocardiography.

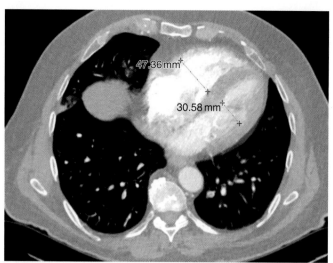

FIGURE 87.10 Enlarged right ventricle on chest CT in a patient with pulmonary embolism (PE). Normally, the ratio of the diameters of the right ventricle and the left ventricle is less than 0.9. This patient has an end-diastolic RV diameter of 47 mm and an end-diastolic LV diameter of 31 mm. The RV-to-LV diameter ratio of 1.5 is abnormally high and correlates with a poor prognosis. *LV,* Left ventricular; *RV,* right ventricular.

Echocardiography (see also Chapter 16)

Echocardiographic findings are normal in approximately half of unselected patients with acute PE, so echocardiography is not recommended as a routine diagnostic test for PE. Echocardiography is, however, a rapid, practical, and sensitive technique for detection of right ventricular overload among patients with established PE and helps identify patients who are at high risk for adverse events following PE. Moderate or severe right ventricular hypokinesis, persistent pulmonary hypertension, patent foramen ovale, and free-floating thrombus in the right atrium (Fig. 87.11A–E) or RV[72] are factors associated with high risk of death or recurrent thromboembolism. The presence of a specific pattern of regional right ventricular dysfunction, known as the "McConnell sign" and characterized by akinesis or dyskinesis of the mid right ventricular free wall with relative sparing of the base and apex, is highly specific for PE and often immediately recognizable by echocardiography (see also Chapter 16, Echocardiography). Echocardiography also can help identify illnesses that may mimic PE, such as MI and pericardial disease.

Venous Ultrasonography

The primary diagnostic criterion for DVT on ultrasound imaging is loss of vein compressibility (Fig. 87.12). Normally, the vein collapses completely when gentle pressure is applied to the overlying skin. Upper-extremity DVT can be more difficult to diagnose than leg DVT because the clavicle can hinder attempts to compress the subclavian vein. At least half of PE patients have no imaging evidence of DVT, probably because the entire DVT embolized to the pulmonary arteries. Therefore, if the level of clinical suspicion of PE is moderate or high, patients without evidence of DVT should undergo further investigation for PE.

Lung Scanning

Pulmonary radionuclide perfusion scintigraphy (lung scanning) uses radiolabeled aggregates of albumin or microspheres that lodge in the pulmonary microvasculature. Patients with large PE often have multiple perfusion defects. If ventilation scanning is performed on a patient with PE but no intrinsic lung disease, a normal ventilation study result is expected, yielding ventilation-perfusion mismatch that is interpreted as a high probability of PE. However, many patients with low-probability scans but with clinical findings strongly suggestive of PE do, in fact, have PE proven by invasive pulmonary angiography. Thus, clinical probability assessment helps to correctly interpret the scan results.

Most lung scans are nondiagnostic. An unequivocal normal or high-probability scan is the exception, not the rule. Interobserver variability is common, even among experts. Two principal indications for

obtaining a lung scan are renal insufficiency and an anaphylactic reaction to an intravenous contrast agent that cannot be suppressed with high-dose corticosteroids.

Magnetic Resonance Imaging

Gadolinium-enhanced magnetic resonance angiography (MRA) is far less sensitive than CT for the detection of PE, but unlike chest CT or catheter-based pulmonary angiography, MRA does not require ionizing radiation or injection of an iodinated contrast agent. Pulmonary MRA also can assess right ventricular size and function. Three-dimensional MRA can be performed during a single breath-hold and may provide high resolution from the main pulmonary artery through the segmental pulmonary artery branches. MRA has limited sensitivity for detection of distal PE and cannot be used as a stand-alone test to exclude PE.[73]

Pulmonary Angiography

Invasive pulmonary angiography formerly was the reference standard for the diagnosis of PE but is now rarely performed as a diagnostic test. However, use of this modality is routine when advanced interventions such as pharmacomechanical catheter-assisted therapy are planned. New thrombus usually has a concave edge. Chronic thrombus leads to bandlike defects called webs, in addition to intimal irregularities and abrupt narrowing or occlusion of lobar vessels.

Contrast Venography

Although contrast phlebography was once the reference standard for DVT diagnosis, venograms are rarely obtained now for diagnostic purposes. Venography is the first step, however, for evaluating patients with large femoral or iliofemoral DVT who will undergo invasive pharmacomechanical catheter-directed therapy.

Overall Strategy: An Integrated Diagnostic Approach

Suspected PE can be investigated with a wide array of diagnostic tests. The first step in an integrated diagnostic strategy (Fig. 87.13) is a directed history and physical examination to assess the clinical likelihood of acute PE. The finding of non-high clinical probability is followed by D-dimer testing; a normal D-dimer assay usually rules out PE. If the D-dimer is elevated, chest CT usually provides the definitive diagnosis or exclusion of PE. Electronic decision support at the time of ordering chest CT scans can reduce unwarranted imaging and increase the proportion of test results that are positive for PE.[74]

THERAPY

Risk Stratification (see Chapter 95)

PE manifests with a wide spectrum of acuity ranging from mild to severe. Therefore, rapid and accurate risk stratification is of paramount importance. Summoning the hospital's multidisciplinary PE response team (PERT) may be helpful in this regard.[75] Low-risk patients have an excellent prognosis with anticoagulation alone. High-risk patients may require intensive hemodynamic and respiratory support with pressors, mechanical ventilation, or ECMO.[76,77] In addition to anticoagulation, advanced management[78,79] options include systemic thrombolysis, pharmacomechanical catheter-assisted therapy, vena cava filter placement, or surgical embolectomy (Fig. 87.14).[80,81] The three key components for risk stratification are: (1) clinical evaluation, (2) assessment of right ventricular size and function, and (3) analysis of cardiac biomarkers to determine whether there is right ventricular microinfarction.

Clinical evaluation is straightforward if the PE patient looks and feels well and has no evidence of right ventricular dysfunction. The Pulmonary Embolism Severity Index (PESI) identifies 11 features from demographics, history, and clinical findings that can be weighted and scored to identify low-risk and high-risk patients (Table 87.6).[82] Clinicians should try to detect right ventricular dysfunction on physical examination by looking for distended jugular veins, a palpable

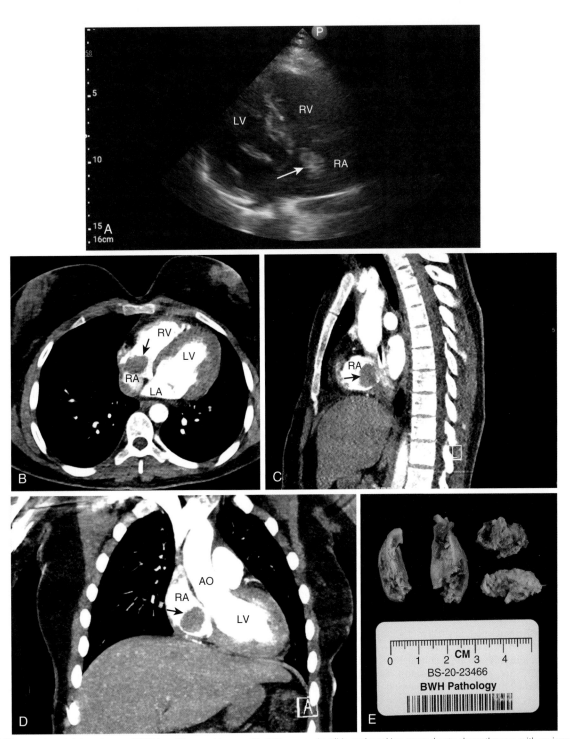

FIGURE 87.11 A, Right atrial thrombus on ECHO in a 60-year-old man with AML, myopericarditis, and cytokine storm due to chemotherapy, with an irregularly shaped 21 × 11 mm mobile mass in the right atrium. The mass intermittently prolapses partially through the tricuspid valve. There is no clear stalk or visible connection to the right atrial wall, interatrial septum, or tricuspid valve. **B** to **D,** Right atrial thrombus on chest CT of a 27-year-old woman with sickle cell disease who suffered three episodes of syncope heralded by lightheadedness and dizziness. Contrast-enhanced chest computed tomogram demonstrates clot-in-transit (black arrow) in a 27-year-old woman with sickle cell anemia. A large 26 × 18 mm filling defect in the right atrium is visualized in the axial (**B**), sagittal (**C**), and coronal views (**D**). *AO,* Aorta; *LA,* left atrium; *LV,* left ventricle; *RA,* right atrium; *RV,* right ventricle. The attending surgeon who excised the mass said, "I think her syncope was due to right ventricular inflow obstruction. The mass at surgery was bobbing in and out in front of the tricuspid valve, shutting down substantial flow into the right ventricle when in certain positions." **E,** Surgically excised right atrial thrombus seen on chest CT in **B** to **D.** It was *pink-red* and friable and measured 4.6 × 3.7 × 2.1 cm. The pathologist stated, "It does look mostly chronic with only a little bit of fresher thrombus." (Kindly provided by Robert F. Padera, MD, PhD, and Richard N. Mitchell, MD, PhD.)

left parasternal lift, a systolic murmur of tricuspid regurgitation, or an accentuated P_2. Clinical evaluation should integrate the results of electrocardiography that might show a right ventricular strain pattern (right bundle branch block, $S_1Q_3T_3$, negative T waves in leads V_1 through V_4), chest CT, echocardiography, and cardiac biomarkers of right ventricular microinfarction.

Parenteral Anticoagulation

Anticoagulation is the cornerstone of treatment for acute PE. Heparin, the most commonly used parenteral anticoagulant, acts primarily by binding to antithrombin, a protein that inhibits the coagulation factors thrombin (factor IIa) and factors Xa, IXa, XIa, and XIIa. Heparin subsequently promotes a conformational change

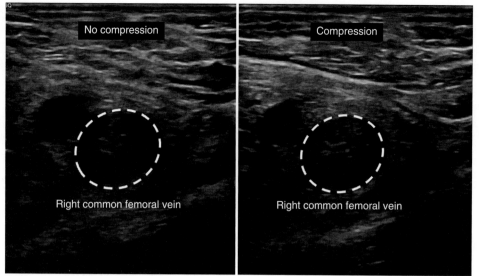

FIGURE 87.12 Acute right common femoral deep vein thrombosis (DVT) diagnosed by venous ultrasound examination of the leg. *Left:* Without compression. A cross-section of the right common femoral vein. The right common femoral vein is dilated. Thrombotic material can be visualized within the vein. The right common femoral artery is a smaller vessel, pulsating in real time, and is located at about 10 o'clock relative to the right common femoral vein. *Right:* With compression. Thrombotic material can be visualized within the vein. The dilated right common femoral vein fails to compress despite the technologist's firm pressure over the vein. Failure to compress the vein with manual pressure is the primary criterion for the diagnosis of DVT with venous ultrasound imaging. (Courtesy Gregory Piazza, MD, MS.)

in antithrombin that accelerates its activity approximately 100- to 1000-fold, thus preventing additional thrombus formation. Heparin does *not* directly dissolve thrombus. However, endogenous fibrinolytic mechanisms may lyse some of the previously formed thrombus. Beyond its anticoagulant activity, heparin also exerts pleiotropic effects, including antiinflammatory[83] and vasodilatory properties.[84]

Unfractionated Heparin

Unfractionated heparin (UFH) is a highly sulfated glycosaminoglycan that is partially purified, most often from pig intestinal mucosa. The intensity of continuous infusion intravenous UFH anticoagulation can be titrated by adjusting the infusion rate to reach a goal aPTT. The short half-life of UFH is advantageous for patients who may require subsequent insertion of an IVC filter, systemic thrombolysis, catheter-directed pharmacomechanical therapy, or surgical embolectomy.

For patients with average bleeding risk and normal hepatic function, UFH should be started with an intravenous bolus of 80 units/kg, followed by a continuous infusion at 18 units/kg/hr. The aPTT should be targeted between 1.5 and 2.5 times the control value. The therapeutic range commonly is 60 to 80 seconds. Monitoring continuous intravenous UFH infusions using anti-Xa assays (instead of aPTT) has some advantages, particularly in ill patients with multisystem organ failure, because this approach measures heparin's effect directly. It is especially useful for patients with a baseline elevated aPTT, such as those with lupus anticoagulant. The target level for therapeutic dosing is 0.3 to 0.7 units/mL.

Low-Molecular-Weight Heparin

LMWH consists of fragments of UFH that exhibit less binding to plasma proteins and endothelial cells. It therefore has greater bioavailability, with a more predictable dose response and a longer half-life compared with UFH. These features permit weight-based LMWH dosing without laboratory tests because no dose adjustment is needed in most cases. LMWH is gaining popularity for initial anticoagulation of intermediate-risk and high-risk PE because of the concern that administration of UFH does not rapidly and consistently achieve full therapeutic efficacy. The kidneys metabolize LMWH, and patients with renal impairment require downward adjustment of LMWH dosing. If a quantitative

assay is desired, an anti-Xa level can be obtained. Whether use of anti-Xa levels improves efficacy and safety remains controversial.

Fondaparinux

Fondaparinux is an anticoagulant pentasaccharide that specifically inhibits activated factor X. It can be thought of as an ultra-low-molecular-weight heparin. Fondaparinux's predictable and sustained pharmacokinetic properties allow a fixed-dose, once-daily subcutaneous injection, without the need for coagulation laboratory monitoring or dose adjustment. Fondaparinux has a 17-hour half-life, and its elimination is prolonged in patients with renal impairment. Fondaparinux is indicated for the initial treatment of acute PE and acute DVT. It is often used off-label for the management of suspected or proven heparin-induced thrombocytopenia (HIT) because it does not cross-react with heparin-induced antibodies.[85]

Heparin-Induced Thrombocytopenia

HIT is an immune-mediated complication of heparin.[86] It occurs more often with UFH than with LMWH. Immunoglobulin G antibodies bind to a heparin-platelet factor 4 complex to activate platelets, causing the release of prothrombotic microparticles. The microparticles promote excessive thrombin generation, which can result in paradoxical thrombosis despite thrombocytopenia. The thrombosis usually manifests as extensive and often bilateral DVT (sometimes affecting one upper extremity and one lower extremity) or PE, but presentations of MI, stroke, and unusual arterial thrombosis (such as mesenteric arterial thrombosis) also have been described.

The "4T Point Score" is a semiquantitative clinical screening test for HIT.[87] The four components are (1) **T**hrombocytopenia, (2) **T**iming of decrease in platelet count, (3) **T**hrombosis or other sequelae such as skin necrosis, and (4) absence of o**T**her explanation. HIT should be suspected when the platelet count decreases to less than 100,000 or to less than 50% of baseline. The thrombocytopenia is usually mild, in the range of 40,000 to 70,000. Typically, HIT occurs after 5 to 10 days of heparin exposure, most often in cardiac surgical ICUs. ELISA testing quantifies antiplatelet factor 4 (PF4)/heparin antibody levels, which are measured in optical density (OD) units. The higher the OD value, the more likely the diagnosis of HIT with thrombosis.[88] The serotonin release assay is the gold standard laboratory test for HIT.

When HIT is diagnosed, UFH or LMWH should be discontinued immediately, and patients should not receive platelet transfusions. Heparin "flushes" of intravenous lines should also be discontinued. For HIT with thrombosis, a parenteral direct thrombin inhibitor such as argatroban or bivalirudin should be used.

Warfarin Anticoagulation

Warfarin is a vitamin K antagonist, first approved for clinical use in 1954. It prevents gamma-carboxylation activation of coagulation factors II, VII, IX, and X. The full anticoagulant effect of warfarin becomes evident after 5 to 7 days, even if the prothrombin time, used to monitor warfarin's effect, becomes elevated more rapidly. For patients with VTE, the usual target INR range is between 2.0 and 3.0. Self-monitoring of INRs improves patient satisfaction and quality of life and may reduce the rate of bleeding and thromboembolic events.

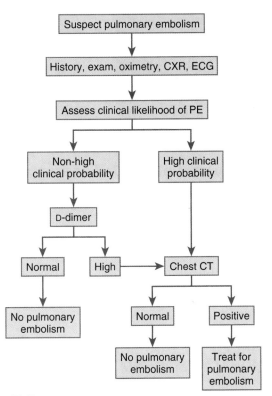

FIGURE 87.13 Integrated diagnostic approach for acute PE. *CXR,* Chest x-ray.

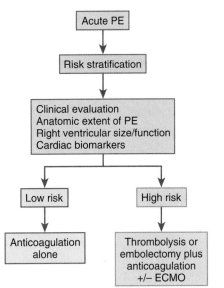

FIGURE 87.14 Management strategy for acute pulmonary embolism (PE), based on risk stratification. *ECMO,* Extracorporeal membrane oxygenation.

Warfarin Overlap with Heparin

Initiation of warfarin as monotherapy to treat acute VTE without UFH, LMWH, or fondaparinux may paradoxically exacerbate hypercoagulability, increasing the likelihood of recurrent thrombosis, by decreasing the levels of two endogenous anticoagulants, proteins C and S. Overlapping warfarin for at least 5 days with an immediately effective parenteral anticoagulant counteracts the procoagulant effect of unopposed warfarin.

Dosing and Monitoring of Warfarin

Dosing warfarin is both an art and a science. Warfarin traditionally is dosed using an "educated guess" coupled with trial and error. Many physicians begin with 5 mg daily. Debilitated or older adult patients require a reduced dose. High INRs from excessive warfarin predispose to bleeding complications. Warfarin-related major bleeding is the most common reason for adverse drug events and subsequent emergency hospitalization in older Americans. In contrast, subtherapeutic dosing makes patients vulnerable to recurrent VTE. All patients taking warfarin should wear a medical alert bracelet or necklace in case they require rapid reversal of warfarin. Warfarin also can have nonhemorrhagic side effects, such as alopecia and increased levels of arterial calcification.[89] In addition, warfarin may induce osteoporotic fractures.[90] Some patients complain of fatigue and "feeling cold".

Warfarin therapy is further plagued by multiple drug-drug and drug-food interactions. Centralized anticoagulation clinics, staffed by nurses or pharmacists, have eased the administrative burden of prescribing warfarin and have facilitated safer and more effective anticoagulation.

Warfarin "Bridging"

When patients undergo elective surgery or procedures such as colonoscopy, warfarin is temporarily discontinued. To ensure continued perioperative anticoagulation, "bridging" with LMWH used to be prescribed preoperatively while the warfarin activity washed out. However, the BRIDGE trial of atrial fibrillation patients showed that forgoing bridging was associated with a 59% reduction in major bleeding complications.[91] Subsequently, the practice of routine bridging has fallen out of favor.[92] Now, we forgo bridging with only a few exceptions, such as extreme thrombophilia or mechanical heart valves. For almost all patients, we instruct them to hold warfarin preoperatively (usually for 4 days) and on the day of surgery.

Novel Oral Anticoagulants

NOACs (see also Chapter 95) have a rapid onset of action and provide full anticoagulation within several hours of ingestion. They are prescribed in fixed doses without laboratory coagulation monitoring and have minimal drug-drug or drug-food interactions. These agents have a short half-life, so when they are stopped for an invasive diagnostic or surgical procedure, no bridging is needed. We usually instruct patients to hold NOACs for two days preoperatively and on the day of surgery. For VTE treatment, NOACs are noninferior to warfarin for efficacy and are superior to warfarin for safety.[93] In a meta-analysis of 24,455 patients with acute VTE, NOACs compared with warfarin had a 40% reduction in major bleeding, 61% reduction in nonfatal intracranial bleeding, and 64% reduction in fatal bleeding.[94]

Evolution of Oral Anticoagulants for Pulmonary Embolism and Deep Vein Thrombosis Treatment

Four NOACs are licensed for VTE treatment: dabigatran (an oral thrombin inhibitor),[95,96] and three factor Xa inhibitors[97]: rivaroxaban,[98,99] apixaban,[100] and edoxaban (Table 87.7).[101] For extended therapy after an initial 6-month course of anticoagulation, dabigatran was compared with warfarin and with placebo.[102] Rivaroxaban[98] and apixaban[103] were also compared against placebo in extended-therapy trials. These randomized trials showed that NOACs—in the doses tested—are safe and effective for extended-duration anticoagulation.

In children, the first major study of NOACs versus warfarin was undertaken with rivaroxaban. This global study included children from 107 pediatric hospitals in 28 countries. They all had documented acute VTE and had started heparin in the hospital. They were randomized to rivaroxaban versus warfarin in this 3-month, open-label trial. Rivaroxaban resulted in a similar low VTE recurrence risk and similar bleeding rate compared with standard warfarin anticoagulation.[104]

Managing Bleeding Complications from Anticoagulants

Protamine sulfate can be given for life-threatening bleeding caused by UFH or LMWH. Life-threatening bleeding caused by warfarin can be

TABLE 87.6 Pulmonary Embolism Severity Index and Simplified Pulmonary Embolism Severity Index: Predictors of Prognostic Risk

PESI Criteria*	
Age >80 years	Age in years
Male gender	+10
History of cancer	+30
History of heart failure	+10
History of chronic lung disease	+10
Heart rate ≥110 beats/min	+20
Systolic blood pressure <100 mm Hg	+30
Respiratory rate ≥30 breaths/min	+20
Temperature <36°C	+20
Altered mental status	+60
Arterial oxygen saturation <90%	+20
Simplified PESI† Criteria	
Age >80 years	+1
History of cancer	+1
History of heart failure or chronic lung disease	+1
Heart rate ≥110 beats/min	+1
Systolic blood pressure <100 mm Hg	+1
Arterial oxygen saturation <90%	+1

PE, Pulmonary embolism; *PESI*, Pulmonary Embolism Severity Index.
*Class 1 = ≤65; class 2 = 66 to 85; class 3 = 86 to 105; class 4 = 106 to 125; class 5 ≥126. In the PESI score, classes 1 and 2 are considered low risk, and classes 3 to 5 are considered high risk.
†Patients with a score of 0 are considered to be at low risk for PE; those with scores ≥1 are considered at high risk.

managed with prothrombin complex concentrates (PCC) to achieve immediate hemostasis.[105] For major bleeding, use idarucizumab to reverse dabigatran[106,107] and andexanet alfa to reverse rivaroxaban, apixaban, or edoxaban[108,109]

OPTIMAL DURATION OF ANTICOAGULATION AND SELECTION OF OPTIMAL ANTICOAGULANT

Risk of Recurrent Venous Thromboembolism after Discontinuation of Anticoagulation

VTE is associated with a high risk of recurrence after discontinuation of anticoagulation. Cardiovascular inflammation may explain the recurrent nature of VTE.[110] Accordingly, VTE is a chronic illness for many individuals, recurring in about 30% to 40% of patients who stop anticoagulation within 10 years after an initial event.[111–113] After discontinuing anticoagulation, men suffer recurrent VTE more often than women. In a meta-analysis of 7515 patients from 18 studies, men had a 41% recurrent VTE rate versus 29% for women at 10 years following the initial VTE.[114]

Persistent thrombus imaged on chest CT does not predict recurrent PE. Approximately half of patients with PE will have persistent thrombus on chest CT 6 months after the initial event. Abnormally elevated D-dimer levels after withdrawal of anticoagulation may signify ongoing hypercoagulability. However, the risk for recurrence in patients with a first unprovoked VTE who have a subsequent negative D-dimer result is not low enough to justify stopping anticoagulant therapy. In 319 patients with a negative D-dimer after completing 3 to 7 months of anticoagulation, the rate of recurrent VTE was 6.7% per patient-year.[115]

How to Determine the Optimal Duration of Anticoagulation

Until recently, most evidence-based clinical practice guidelines have dichotomized VTE into "provoked" and "unprovoked" silos. Such guidelines recommended extended treatment in patients with "unprovoked," or idiopathic, VTE. However, the definition of "provoked" VTE is challenging because triggers may be subtle, and recurrence risk can be high in those with clear provocation but enduring predisposing factors.[113,116] Accordingly, the 2019 ESC guidelines no longer endorse the terminology "provoked" and "unprovoked."[39] Instead, an individualized risk assessment is proposed in which only patients with an estimated recurrence risk of less than 3% per year should receive time-limited anticoagulant therapy. Attempts to refine prediction, including gender-specific models, have been proposed.[117,118]

Selection of an Optimal Oral Anticoagulant for Extended-Duration Anticoagulation

Apixaban, rivaroxaban, dabigatran, and warfarin have all been shown to safely and effectively reduce VTE recurrence in randomized trials of extended treatment (see Table 87.7). Low-intensity DOAC regimens offer enhanced safety while maintaining efficacy for long-term secondary prevention.[119,120] Low-dose aspirin has been investigated as an alternative for extended treatment but is only recommended for patients who refuse or are unable to tolerate anticoagulation.[39] Meta-analyses have confirmed the net clinical benefit of DOACs over warfarin, aspirin, or placebo.[121,122]

ADVANCED THERAPY FOR ACUTE PULMONARY EMBOLISM

Patients with high-risk PE or intermediate-high-risk PE that decompensates or fails to improve on anticoagulation generally warrant advanced therapy. Options include full-dose systemic fibrinolysis, half-dose systemic fibrinolysis, catheter-based therapy with or without fibrinolysis, surgical embolectomy, and IVC filter placement.

High-Risk Pulmonary Embolism

Multidisciplinary PERTs are being set up throughout the United States to immediately evaluate patients who present with high- or intermediate-high-risk PE. Team members have subspecialized cognitive and technical skills in PE, and the team approach promotes consensus and a unified, reasoned plan for the individual patient.[123,124]

Systemic Fibrinolysis Administered Through a Peripheral Vein. Fibrinolysis reverses right-sided heart failure by physical dissolution of anatomically obstructing pulmonary arterial thrombus. The hallmarks of successful therapy are reduction of right ventricular pressure overload and prevention of continued release of serotonin and other neurohumoral factors that exacerbate pulmonary hypertension.

When prescribing fibrinolysis, there are three dosing intensities: (1) full-dose systemic (licensed), (2) half-dose systemic (prescribed "off-label"), or (3) low-dose catheter-directed therapy.[78] The FDA has approved alteplase for high-risk PE, in a dose of 100 mg delivered through a peripheral vein as a continuous infusion over 2 hours, without concomitant heparin. Patients who receive fibrinolysis up to 14 days after onset of new symptoms or signs can derive benefit. Intracranial hemorrhage is the most feared and severe complication.

A meta-analysis examined patients randomized to fibrinolytic therapy versus anticoagulation alone, with most patients classified as intermediate-risk PE (1775 out of a total of 2115) because they had hemodynamic stability despite right ventricular dysfunction. Fibrinolysis resulted in a 47% reduction in all-cause mortality, a 60% decrease in recurrent PE, a 2.7-fold increased risk of major bleeding, and a 4.6-fold increased risk of intracranial hemorrhage.[125]

An alternative strategy has focused on half-dose systemic fibrinolysis. However, propensity-score-matched studies comparing outcomes in 3768 patients receiving 50 mg versus full-dose 100 mg of alteplase for PE demonstrated that half-dose fibrinolysis was associated with an increased requirement for treatment escalation (53.8% vs. 41.4%; p < 0.01), driven largely by rescue fibrinolysis (25.9% vs. 7.3%; p < 0.01) and catheter-directed therapy (14.2% vs. 3.8%; p< 0.01).[126] Furthermore, rates of hospital mortality (13% vs. 15%; p = 0.3), intracranial bleeding

Pulmonary Embolism and Deep Vein Thrombosis

TABLE 87.7 Novel Oral Anticoagulants for Venous Thromboembolism

DRUG/STUDY NAME	NOAC	WARFARIN
Dabigatran/ RE-COVER	(N = 1274)	(N = 1265)
	2.4% recurrence	2.1% recurrence
Dabigatran/ RE-MEDY	(N = 1430)	(N = 1426)
	1.8% recurrence	1.3% recurrence
Dabigatran/ RE-COVER II	(N = 1279)	(N = 1289)
	2.3% recurrence	2.2% recurrence
Rivaroxaban/ EINSTEIN Acute DVT	(N = 1731)	(N = 1718)
	2.1% recurrence	3.0% recurrence
Rivaroxaban/ EINSTEIN-PE	(N = 2420)	(N = 2413)
	2.1% recurrence;	1.8% recurrence;
	1.1% major bleeding	2.2% major bleeding
Apixaban AMPLIFY	(N = 2691)	(N = 2704)
	2.3% recurrence	2.7% recurrence
	0.6% major bleeding	1.8% major bleeding
Edoxaban/Hokusai—VTE	(N = 4143)	(N = 4149)
	3.2% recurrence	3.5% recurrence
	8.5% clinically relevant bleeding	10.3% clinically relevant bleeding
DRUG/STUDY NAME	**NOAC**	**PLACEBO**
Dabigatran/RE-SONATE	(N = 681)	(N = 662)
	0.4% recurrence	5.6% recurrence
Rivaroxaban/EINSTEIN DVT Continued Treatment	(N = 602)	(N = 594)
	1.3% recurrence	7.1% recurrence
Apixaban Extension VTE	(N = 829)	(N = 840)
	1.7% recurrence	8.8% recurrence
Einstein Choice	*Rivaroxaban 20 mg (N = 1107)*	*Aspirin 100 mg (N = 1131)*
	1.5%	4.4%
	Rivaroxaban 10 mg (N = 1127)	
	1.2%	

(0.5% vs. 0.4%; p = 0.67), gastrointestinal hemorrhage (1.6% vs. 1.6%; p = 0.99), and anemia (6.9% vs. 4.6%; p = 0.11) were similar.

Advances in Catheter-Based Therapy

The 1% to 3% rate of intracranial hemorrhage in patients with PE receiving systemic fibrinolysis has dampened enthusiasm for this potential life-saving therapy. Catheter-based reperfusion, however, holds the promise of efficacy, with lower rates of major bleeding owing to lower doses of a fibrinolytic agent or no need for fibrinolysis at all. Catheter-based therapy for acute PE includes pharmacomechanical therapy, catheter-directed fibrinolysis, and mechanical embolectomy. Catheter-based therapy that combines local fibrinolysis with mechanical thrombus "conditioning" may increase the efficacy of thrombus dissolution via higher local fibrinolytic drug concentrations and a greater exposed thrombus surface area. Because higher local drug concentration is achieved with a lower overall dose of fibrinolytic agent, catheter-based fibrinolysis may offer the advantage of decreased hemorrhagic complications.

Ultrasound-facilitated, catheter-directed fibrinolysis **(eFig. 87.4)** has been the most rigorously studied of these catheter-based techniques. In a European-based randomized controlled trial of 59 patients with intermediate-risk PE, ultrasound-facilitated, catheter-directed fibrinolysis with 20 mg of t-PA plus anticoagulation reduced a surrogate endpoint, RV-diameter-to-LV-diameter (RV-to-LV) ratio, from baseline to 24 hours to a greater extent than anticoagulation.[127] In the US-based, single-arm, multicenter SEATTLE II trial, the safety and efficacy of ultrasound-facilitated, catheter-directed fibrinolysis

(24 mg t-PA) was assessed in 150 patients with high- (N = 31) or intermediate-risk (N = 119) PE.[128] Mean RV-to-LV ratio decreased by 25%, mean pulmonary artery systolic pressure decreased by 30%, and mean modified Miller angiographic obstruction index diminished by 30% from pre-procedure to 48 hours post-procedure. Major bleeding occurred in 10% of patients with no intracranial hemorrhage. In 2014, the FDA cleared ultrasound-facilitated, catheter-directed fibrinolysis for PE treatment. In a subsequent dose-ranging trial, four accelerated-dosing regimens (8 mg/2 hours, 8 mg/4 hours, 12 mg/6 hours, and 24 mg/6 hours) for ultrasound-facilitated, catheter-directed fibrinolysis were evaluated in 101 patients with intermediate-risk PE.[129] All four regimens improved RV function comparable to 24 mg of t-PA administered over 12 to 24 hours, based on the CT-measured RV-to-LV ratio from baseline to 48 hours. A study utilizing a novel technique for three-dimensional reconstruction of the pulmonary vasculature from chest CT data obtained in the SEATTLE II trial showed that reduction in RV volume correlated with increased blood volume through the small peripheral, rather than large proximal, pulmonary arteries.[130] These data suggest that ultrasound-facilitated, catheter-directed fibrinolysis may relieve RV pressure overload via distal pulmonary artery reperfusion.

Purely mechanical catheter embolectomy techniques may have a niche in PE patients with contraindications to fibrinolytic therapy. The FlowTriever system (Inari Medical, Irvine, CA) is a large-bore device that mechanically engages thrombus via three self-expanding nitinol disks and then aspirates the thrombus. In a US-based single-arm, multicenter study of 106 patients with intermediate-risk PE, embolectomy with the FlowTriever system resulted in a 25% reduction

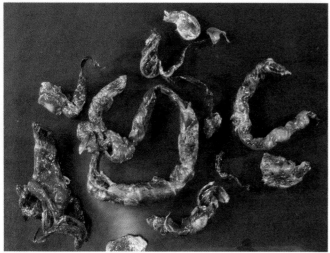

FIGURE 87.15 Surgical pulmonary embolectomy specimen in a 72-year-old woman who presented with presyncope, hypotension, and hypoxia. She was diagnosed with massive pulmonary embolism (PE) by chest CT scan and underwent successful emergency pulmonary embolectomy.

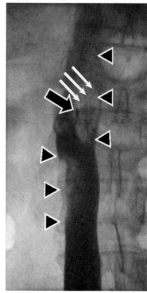

FIGURE 87.16 Large pulmonary embolism (PE)-in-transit, with thrombus (*arrowheads*) trapped below and visualized above the Bard Eclipse inferior vena cava filter. The force of the embolizing deep vein thrombosis (DVT) displaced one of the filter struts (*white arrows*). The "hook" to retrieve the filter is marked with the *black arrow.*

in CT-measured RV-to-LV ratio and 10% decrease in mean modified Miller index.[131] In the study, six major adverse events occurred within 48 hours of the procedure, including one major hemorrhage. The FlowTriever device received FDA clearance for treatment of PE in 2018. The Indigo Thrombectomy System (Penumbra, Inc, Alameda, CA) is a smaller-bore aspiration catheter that does not require fibrinolytic administration and was evaluated in a single-arm study of 119 patients with intermediate-risk PE (ClinicalTrials.gov identifier: NCT03218566). The Indigo System is intended for the removal of fresh, soft emboli and thrombi from vessels of the peripheral and venous systems using continuous aspiration. Treatment with the Indigo device resulted in a 27% reduction in the mean CT-measured RV-to-LV diameter ratio and was associated with three major adverse events.[132] It received FDA clearance in 2019.

Catheter-directed fibrinolysis without mechanical thrombus disruption has undergone limited prospective evaluation and may be a consideration for patients with high-risk or intermediate-high-risk PE,[133] although the data remain limited.[134] The 2019 ESC Guidelines offer catheter-based therapy as an alternative to surgical embolectomy for patients with high-risk PE in whom systemic fibrinolysis has failed or is contraindicated (Class IIa; Level of Evidence C) and as an alternative to systemic fibrinolysis in other PE patients who have experienced hemodynamic deterioration despite anticoagulation (Class IIa; Level of Evidence C).[39]

Surgical Embolectomy

Surgical embolectomy has reemerged for the management of patients with high-risk PE or intermediate-high-risk PE with severe right ventricular dysfunction and clinical deterioration despite anticoagulation, in whom contraindications preclude thrombolysis (Fig. 87.15). This procedure is also suitable for patients with acute PE who require surgical excision of a right atrial thrombus, closure of a patent foramen ovale, or excision of a clot-in-transit (Fig. 87.16). Surgical embolectomy can also be used as rescue therapy for patients whose PE is refractory to thrombolysis. Results are best when patients undergo surgery before they become pressor-dependent and before the onset of cardiogenic shock and multisystem organ failure.[135] Avoiding blind instrumentation of the fragile pulmonary arteries is imperative. Extraction is limited to directly visible clots. In experienced centers, surgical pulmonary embolectomy has been shown to be safe and effective.[136]

Inferior Vena Cava Filters

IVC filter insertion is considered in acute VTE patients (regardless of the size or clinical severity of the VTE) with contraindications to anticoagulation or with recurrent PE despite therapeutic anticoagulation.

Until recently, IVC filter insertion had also been considered on an individual basis for patients with intermediate- or high-risk PE who were tolerating therapeutic anticoagulation but in whom there was concern that a subsequent PE would likely be fatal. Such an indication was the focus of the PREPIC2 trial which randomly assigned 399 normotensive patients with acute PE, concomitant lower-extremity DVT, and at least 1 risk factor for adverse outcomes to retrievable IVC filter implantation plus anticoagulation versus anticoagulation alone.[137] Adjunctive insertion of a retrievable IVC filter, compared with anticoagulation alone, failed to reduce the risk of symptomatic recurrent PE or mortality at 3 or 6 months. In a meta-analysis of randomized controlled trials and prospective observational studies, IVC filters appear to reduce the short-term risk of subsequent PE, increase the long-term risk for DVT, and have no impact on overall mortality.[138]

Data demonstrate that retrievable IVC filters can be removed safely and easily, yet up to 50% remain permanently indwelling.[139] Device-related complications include strut fracture, filter migration, strut embolization, device tilt, IVC penetration, perforation of surrounding structures, PE, DVT, and IVC thrombosis. To avoid these complications, IVC filters should be retrieved as soon as no longer necessary and after anticoagulation has been safely started.

Deep Vein Thrombosis Interventions

Indications for catheter-directed DVT thrombolysis remain uncertain but usually include extensive iliofemoral and upper-extremity venous thrombosis. In Norway, the CaVenT study randomly assigned 209 patients with iliofemoral DVT to receive catheter-directed thrombolysis versus conventional therapy with LMWH bridging to warfarin. At 24 months, the frequency of PTS was 56% in the conventionally treated group, compared with 41% in the intervention group (p= 0.047). Iliofemoral patency was present in 66% of the intervention group, compared with 47% of the group receiving conventional anticoagulation.[140] The US-based ATTRACT trial randomly assigned 692 patients with acute iliofemoral or femoral DVT to receive either anticoagulation alone (LMWH or UFH) or anticoagulation and pharmacomechanical therapy.[141] Pharmacochemical therapy did not reduce the risk of PTS (47% in the intervention group vs. 48% in the anticoagulation alone group; RR, 0.96; 95% CI, 0.82 to 1.11), and resulted in a higher risk of major hemorrhage (1.7% vs. 0.3%; RR, 6.18; 95% CI, 0.78 to 49.2). Patients treated with catheter-directed thrombolysis had decreased rates of moderate-to-severe PTS, but quality of life did not differ. Based on these findings, pharmacomechanical therapy for acute lower-extremity DVT should be performed in experienced centers and reserved for highly selected patients with iliofemoral disease, severe symptoms or limb-threatening disease, and a low risk of bleeding.

Therapy in Patients with Cancer

LMWH has been traditionally prescribed as monotherapy without oral anticoagulation for cancer patients with VTE. In one randomized trial, dalteparin monotherapy reduced the recurrent VTE rate by about half compared with warfarin.[142] In a subsequent trial of tinzaparin monotherapy versus warfarin in cancer patients, tinzaparin-treated patients had an approximate 40% lower bleeding rate than those treated with warfarin.[143]

For cancer patients with acute VTE, NOACs are supplanting LMWH monotherapy, especially in patients who do not have gastrointestinal cancers. In the HOKUSAI-VTE Cancer trial of edoxaban versus dalteparin, edoxaban had less recurrent VTE than dalteparin but also had more major bleeding, primarily gastrointestinal.[144] Similarly, in the SELECT-D trial of rivaroxaban versus dalteparin, rivaroxaban had a lower rate of recurrent VTE but a higher rate of clinically relevant non-major bleeding than dalteparin.[145] The NCCN gave a top-tier recommendation to consider edoxaban or rivaroxaban when treating cancer patients with acute VTE and gave a limited recommendation to consider dabigatran or apixaban in situations where LMWH monotherapy was contraindicated or when patients declined LMWH injections.[20] Subsequently, the Caravaggio trial of apixaban versus dalteparin in 1155 cancer patients with acute VTE found that apixaban was noninferior to dalteparin both in preventing recurrent VTE and with respect to major bleeding.[146] There was a 5.6% recurrence rate with apixaban compared with a 7.9% recurrence rate with dalteparin (HR, 0.63; 95% CI, 0.37 to 1.07; p < 0.001 for noninferiority).

Treatment of Superficial Thrombophlebitis

Short-term use of fondaparinux (2.5 mg once daily for 45 days) is the best validated anticoagulation strategy.[147] In a randomized, open-label, noninferiority study of fondaparinux 2.5 mg daily versus rivaroxaban 10 mg daily for patients with superficial thrombophlebitis, rivaroxaban was found to be noninferior to fondaparinux and was not associated with more major bleeding.[148]

Therapy in Patients with Antiphospholipid Syndrome and Factor V Leiden

Antiphospholipid syndrome patients have an acquired, not a genetic, thrombophilia. They are susceptible to MI and stroke as well as to VTE. These patients are traditionally anticoagulated with warfarin rather than with NOACs. If anticoagulation is discontinued after a PE or DVT has occurred, these patients are at very high risk of suffering a recurrent event, with an incidence of at least 8% per year. In a randomized trial of rivaroxaban versus warfarin in patients with *severe* antiphospholipid syndrome, the trial was stopped early because rivaroxaban patients suffered more frequent thromboembolism than warfarin patients (12% vs. zero) and more major bleeding complications (7% vs. 3%).[149] However, with *mild* or *moderately severe* antiphospholipid syndrome, clinicians are prescribing NOACs rather than warfarin with increasing frequency.

Factor V Leiden is the most frequently diagnosed thrombophilia. It is genetic (autosomal dominant), not acquired. These patients are at higher-than-average risk of suffering a first-time acute PE or DVT. VTE is especially common if these individuals are taking estrogen-containing contraceptives. During pregnancy, they are susceptible to first-trimester miscarriage, presumed due to placental vein thrombosis, as well as to VTE. Two poorly understood observations about factor V Leiden are: (1) DVTs have a low embolization rate and if they do embolize, the PEs are typically smaller and less life-threatening than average; (2) the rate of recurrent VTE is not higher among Leiden patients compared with non-Leiden patients.

Therapy in Pediatric Populations

Guidelines for the use of anticoagulants in pediatrics are largely extrapolated from large randomized controlled trials in adults, smaller dose-finding and observational studies in children, and expert opinion. Randomized clinical trials of NOACs in pediatric VTE are ongoing.[150] More than 200 children participated in an open-label, single-arm, prospective cohort trial of dabigatran. Pharmacokinetics and pharmacodynamics of dabigatran were similar to those in adult VTE patients. Dabigatran showed a favorable safety profile for treating VTE in children aged ≥3 months to < 18 years.[151]

Emotional Support

PE impairs quality of life. In young adults diagnosed with VTE, the prescription of psychotropic drugs doubled compared with age- and gender-matched controls. Antidepressants were most frequently prescribed (53%), followed by sedatives (22%), anxiolytics (20%), and antipsychotics (5%).[152] VTE exacts a psychological toll on patients; many wonder if they will suffer a recurrent event and worry about the potential burden on their families, a diminished quality of life, and a shortened life span.[153]

Patients find PE to be emotionally draining, and they, along with their families, want to be reassured that they can expect good outcomes once the diagnosis has been established. Those affected by PE must confront issues such as genetic predisposition, potential long-term disability, changes in lifestyle related to anticoagulation, and the possibility of suffering a recurrent event. Clinicians can help allay this emotional burden by discussing the implications of PE with patients and their families, and PE support groups can help allay patient and family anxiety.

PREVENTION

Rationale for In-Hospital Venous Thromboembolism Prophylaxis

PE is the most preventable cause of in-hospital death. It may be difficult to detect, expensive and burdensome to treat, and potentially fatal. Fortunately, low fixed-dose anticoagulant prophylaxis is effective and safe during hospitalization (Table 87.8). Commonly used regimens include minidose UFH 5000 units three times daily, enoxaparin 40 mg daily, and dalteparin 5000 units daily. A multifaceted approach including electronic alerts, sharing comparative physician metrics, and continuing medical education can increase the frequency of appropriate VTE prophylaxis and reduce the incidence of 90-day symptomatic VTE.[154]

Rationale for Venous Thromboembolism Prophylaxis at Hospital Discharge

In the United States, about 7 million acutely ill medical patients at increased risk for VTE are hospitalized annually with conditions such as pneumonia, heart failure, and COPD. They account for more than 20% of the attributable risk for VTE. Thromboprophylaxis can halve their rate of VTE while hospitalized. However, venous stasis and immobilization tend to increase after hospital discharge because patients remain too weak and debilitated to walk at home. Prophylactic anticoagulation is discontinued at discharge, yet the peak incidence of acute VTE occurs within the first month after hospital stay.

To determine whether extended-duration administration of anticoagulation is superior to a standard course of prophylaxis with enoxaparin, the APEX trial compared the anti-Xa NOAC betrixaban, administered for 35 to 42 days, versus 6 to 14 days of enoxaparin, in 7513 hospitalized medically ill patients at risk for VTE. There was a 24% reduction in VTE among the extended-duration betrixaban patients compared with those assigned to enoxaparin. There was no difference in major bleeding between the two groups.[155] Ancillary APEX studies showed that betrixaban halved the rate of stroke compared with enoxaparin,[156] reduced the rate of cardiovascular mortality, MI, and stroke by 31%,[157] and halved the rate of rehospitalization.[158] Another ancillary APEX study showed that asymptomatic DVT is associated with an

DISEASES OF THE MYOCARDIUM, PERICARDIUM, AND PULMONARY VASCULATURE BED

TABLE 87.8 Regimens for Venous Thromboembolism Prevention

CONDITION	PROPHYLAXIS
Hospitalization with medical illness	Unfractionated heparin 5000 units SC bid or tid *or* Enoxaparin 40 mg SC qd *or* Dalteparin 2500 units or 5000 units SC qd *or* Fondaparinux 2.5 mg SC qd with normal renal function (in patients with a heparin allergy such as heparin-induced thrombocytopenia) *or* Rivaroxaban 10 mg qd started at hospital discharge and continued for 5 weeks
General surgery	Unfractionated heparin 5000 units SC bid or tid *or* Enoxaparin 40 mg SC qd *or* Dalteparin 2500 or 5000 units SC qd
Major orthopedic surgery	Warfarin (target INR 2.5) *or* Enoxaparin 30 mg SC bid *or* Enoxaparin 40 mg SC qd *or* Dalteparin 2500 or 5000 units SC qd *or* Fondaparinux 2.5 mg SC qd *or* Rivaroxaban 10 mg qd *or* Aspirin 81 mg BID *or* Rivaroxaban 10 mg qd for 5 days and then aspirin 81 mg daily thereafter Dabigatran 220 mg qd *or* Apixaban 2.5 mg twice daily

SC, Subcutaneous.

TABLE 87.9 Padua Prediction Score for Identification of Hospitalized Patients at Risk for Venous Thromboembolism

RISK FACTOR	SCORING
Cancer	3
Previous VTE	3
Immobility	3
Thrombophilia	3
Trauma/surgery	2
Age ≥70 years	1
Heart/respiratory failure	1
Acute MI or stroke	1
Infection/rheumatologic disorder	1
Obesity	1
Hormonal treatment	1

High risk for developing pulmonary embolism is defined as 4 score points or greater. *VTE,* Venous thromboembolic.

increased risk of death.[159] Betrixaban received FDA approval in 2017 for extended-duration VTE prophylaxis. However, the manufacturer withdrew it from the market for commercial reasons.

The MAGELLAN study of extended-duration VTE prophylaxis—rivaroxaban for 35 days versus enoxaparin for 10 days in medically ill patients being discharged from the hospital—showed that extended-duration rivaroxaban reduced the risk of VTE 23% more than enoxaparin. However, major bleeding complications were twice as frequent with rivaroxaban. Fatal bleeding occurred in 5 rivaroxaban patients compared with 1 enoxaparin patient.[160] Nevertheless, the benefit-risk profile of rivaroxaban became favorable when five groups at high bleeding risk were excluded: those with (1) active cancer, (2) dual antiplatelet therapy, (3) bronchiectasis/ pulmonary cavitation, (4) gastroduodenal ulcer, and (5) bleeding within 3 months of randomization.[161] In addition, rivaroxaban was compared against placebo in the MARINER trial of 12,024 medical patients being discharged from the hospital. The rivaroxaban group developed symptomatic VTE at half the rate of the placebo group. Major bleeding occurred more frequently in the rivaroxaban group but the difference with placebo was not statistically significant.[162] In 2019, the FDA approved rivaroxaban for extended-duration VTE prophylaxis at hospital discharge. In an ancillary MARINER study, rivaroxaban, like betrixaban, also reduced major adverse cardiovascular events by 28% compared with placebo.[163]

Whether extended-duration VTE prophylaxis is used in the United States remains to be seen. So far the uptake has been minimal. The absolute reduction in VTE is low, and cost-benefit analyses have not convinced clinicians or hospital administrators that the effort and expense to implement an extended-duration VTE prophylaxis program is worth the time and the money.[164]

In-Hospital Risk Factors for Venous Thromboembolism and Bleeding

The Padua Prediction Score is the most widely used risk assessment tool to aid clinicians in deciding whether to administer VTE prophylaxis to hospitalized medical patients. It has a point scoring system based on 11 variables (Table 87.9). A score of 4 or more points denotes a high risk for developing VTE. A simpler validated risk assessment model, developed at Intermountain Medical Center in Utah, predicts high risk if a patient has at least one of the following four risk factors: (1) previous VTE, (2) a medical indication for bed rest, (3) a peripherally inserted central venous catheter, or (4) cancer.[165] Pharmacologic thromboprophylaxis is

generally withheld if the bleeding risk is excessively high due to threatened, active, or recent major bleeding or thrombocytopenia.

Primary Prevention of Venous Thromboembolism in High-Risk Patients with Active Cancer

The double-blind, randomized AVERT trial with apixaban[166] and the CASSINI trial with rivaroxaban[167] compared NOACs with placebo to prevent VTE in high-risk patients with cancer. Both trials showed a substantial reduction in VTE, and both had low rates of major bleeding. It remains uncertain whether these trials will change clinical practice.[168]

Mechanical Prophylaxis in Medically Ill Patients

Unless there is an absolute contraindication to low-dose UFH or LMWH, hospitalized patients at high risk for developing VTE should receive pharmacological prophylaxis rather than mechanical prophylaxis. In a critical care unit trial of 2003 patients, all of whom were receiving thromboprophylaxis, the addition of adjunctive intermittent pneumatic compression did not lower the incidence of proximal leg DVT.[169]

Advances in Venous Thromboembolism Prophylaxis in Major Orthopedic Surgery

Extended prophylaxis after hospital discharge decreases the risk of PE and DVT among patients undergoing major orthopedic surgery, particularly total hip or knee replacement. There is evidence to support the use of almost any prophylactic measure in these patients.[170] Approved approaches include LMWH, warfarin, NOACs, and aspirin. The PEPPER Trial [NCT02810704] is randomizing about 20,000 patients undergoing total knee or hip replacement to warfarin (target INR 2.0) versus rivaroxaban 10 mg daily versus aspirin 81 mg twice daily for 30 days to determine whether any one of these three modalities has superior efficacy and safety.[171]

FUTURE PERSPECTIVES

PE is an illness we thought we understood well. However, new concepts are rapidly evolving regarding VTE pathophysiology in COVID-19, anticoagulation management, advanced therapy with thrombolysis, surgical embolectomy, and ECMO. Novel approaches to VTE prophylaxis are also being tested and challenged.

We used to celebrate the 50% decline of in-hospital PE mortality from 8% to 4%. Unfortunately, the overall US mortality rate, including the death rate from PE, is now increasing. The median age of death from PE has decreased from 73 years in 2000 to 68 years in 2017. Socioeconomically disadvantaged older adults hospitalized with PE have higher long-term mortality rates than their non-disadvantaged counterparts and are more likely to be readmitted within 30 days of hospital discharge.

Our understanding of VTE in patients with COVID-19 will continue to evolve. Moreover, as we begin to better understand the mechanisms underlying this disease, our treatment of thrombotic complications, including PE and VTE, will change.

With respect to the optimal duration of anticoagulation, the ESC PE Guidelines recommend that we no longer use the terms "provoked" and "unprovoked" when describing VTE and predicting the risk of recurrence. The guidelines also support a bold and novel directive: we should no longer provide a definitive "stop date" for anticoagulation, except for major trauma or major surgery. This is a major paradigm shift.

New anticoagulants are being developed that are expected to have a more favorable safety profile than currently available drugs. Two promising targets are inhibitors of factor XIa and factor XIIa. For those with congenital factor XIa deficiency, spontaneous bleeding is rare. Factor XIIa helps achieve thrombosis but has no role in hemostasis.[172] Major strides are being made in advanced therapies for high-risk PE as well. These include dose reduction of fibrinolytic agents and the deployment of novel catheters that either deliver drugs directly to the thrombus or remove large clots without the use of any fibrinolytic agent.

In prevention, implementation of in-hospital VTE prophylaxis is far-reaching. But now we must confront COVID-19, which causes PE despite thromboprophylaxis. The last frontier of VTE prevention is during the risky first 4 to 6 weeks after hospital discharge. While orthopedic and cancer surgeons have used postoperative extended-duration VTE prophylaxis for decades, this strategy is not endorsed by many healthcare providers who care for acute medically ill patients after hospital discharge.

We are privileged to witness such positive and rapid change in the field of PE and DVT. Clinicians, laboratory scientists, government agencies, business representatives, philanthropists, patients, and the public are working together to improve VTE awareness and to implement newly developed cutting-edge technologies, drugs, and best practices.

REFERENCES

1. Riva N, Donadini MP, Ageno W. Epidemiology and pathophysiology of venous thromboembolism: similarities with atherothrombosis and the role of inflammation. *Thromb Haemost.* 2015;113:1176–1183.

Epidemiology

2. Barco S, Mahmoudpour SH, Valerio L, et al. Trends in mortality related to pulmonary embolism in the European Region, 2000-15: analysis of vital registration data from the WHO Mortality Database. *Lancet Respir Med.* 2020;8:277–287.
3. Wadhera RK, Secemsky EA, Wang Y, et al. Association of socioeconomic disadvantage with mortality and readmissions among older adults hospitalized for pulmonary embolism in the United States. *J Am Heart Assoc.* 2021;10(13):e021117. https://doi.org/10.1161/JAHA.121.021117. Epub 2021 Jul 2.
4. Minges KE, Bikdeli B, Wang Y, et al. National trends in pulmonary embolism hospitalization rates and outcomes for adults aged >/=65 Years in the United States (1999 to 2010). *Am J Cardiol.* 2015;116:1436–1442.
5. Spencer FA, Lessard D, Emery C, et al. Venous thromboembolism in the outpatient setting. *Arch Intern Med.* 2007;167:1471–1475.
6. Ageno W, Becattini C, Brighton T, et al. Cardiovascular risk factors and venous thromboembolism: a meta-analysis. *Circulation.* 2008;117:93–102.
7. Fanola CL, Norby FL, Shah AM, et al. Incident heart failure and long-term risk for venous thromboembolism. *J Am Coll Cardiol.* 2020;75:148–158.
8. Gregson J, Kaptoge S, Bolton T, et al. Cardiovascular risk factors associated with venous thromboembolism. *JAMA Cardiol.* 2019;4:163–173.
9. Parkin L, Sweetland S, Balkwill A, et al. Body mass index, surgery, and risk of venous thromboembolism in middle-aged women: a cohort study. *Circulation.* 2012;125:1897–1904.
10. Nauffal D, Ballester M, Reyes RL, et al. Influence of recent immobilization and recent surgery on mortality in patients with pulmonary embolism. *J Thromb Haemost.* 2012;10:1752–1760.
11. Abe K, Kuklina EV, Hooper WC, Callaghan WM. Venous Thromboembolism as a cause of severe maternal morbidity and mortality in the United States. *Semin Perinatol.* 2019;43:200–204.
12. Petterson TM, Smith CY, Emerson JA, et al. Venous Thromboembolism (VTE) incidence and VTE-associated survival among olmsted county residents of local nursing homes. *Thromb Haemost.* 2018;118:1316–1328.
13. Hisada Y, Geddings JE, Ay C, Mackman N. Venous thrombosis and cancer: from mouse models to clinical trials. *J Thromb Haemost.* 2015;13:1372–1382.
14. van Es N, Le Gal G, Otten HM, et al. Screening for occult cancer in patients with unprovoked venous thromboembolism: a systematic review and meta-analysis of individual patient data. *Ann Intern Med.* 2017;167:410–417.
15. Streiff MB, Holmstrom B, Angelini D, et al. NCCN guidelines insights: cancer-associated venous thromboembolic disease, version 2.2018. *J Natl Compr Canc Netw.* 2018;16:1289–1303.
16. Sabapathy CA, Djouonang TN, Kahn SR, et al. Incidence trends and mortality from childhood venous thromboembolism: a population-based cohort study. *J Pediatr.* 2016;172:175–180.e171.
17. Garcia D, Erkan D. Diagnosis and management of the antiphospholipid syndrome. *N Engl J Med.* 2018;378:2010–2021.

18. Mahmoodi BK, Gansevoort RT, Naess IA, et al. Association of mild to moderate chronic kidney disease with venous thromboembolism: pooled analysis of five prospective general population cohorts. *Circulation.* 2012;126:1964–1971.
19. Dzikowska-Diduch O, Kostrubiec M, Kurnicka K, et al. The post-pulmonary syndrome—results of echocardiographic driven follow up after acute pulmonary embolism. *Thromb Res.* 2020;186:30–35.
20. Klok FA, Dzikowska-Diduch O, Kostrubiec M, et al. Derivation of a clinical prediction score for chronic thromboembolic pulmonary hypertension after acute pulmonary embolism. *J Thromb Haemost.* 2016;14:121–128.
21. Kahn SR, Comerota AJ, Cushman M, et al. The postthrombotic syndrome: evidence-based prevention, diagnosis, and treatment strategies: a scientific statement from the American Heart Association. *Circulation.* 2014;130:1636–1661.
22. Lubberts B, Paulino Pereira NR, et al. What is the effect of venous thromboembolism and related complications on patient reported health-related quality of life? A meta-analysis. *Thromb Haemost.* 2016;116.
23. Winter MP, Schernthaner GH, Lang IM. Chronic complications of venous thromboembolism. *J Thromb Haemost.* 2017;15:1531–1540.
24. Becattini C, Vedovati MC, Ageno W, et al. Incidence of arterial cardiovascular events after venous thromboembolism: a systematic review and a meta-analysis. *J Thromb Haemost.* 2010;8:891–897.
25. Ng AC, Chung T, Yong AS, et al. Long-term cardiovascular and noncardiovascular mortality of 1023 patients with confirmed acute pulmonary embolism. *Circ Cardiovasc Qual Outcomes.* 2011;4:122–128.
26. Rinde LB, Lind C, Smabrekke B, et al. Impact of incident myocardial infarction on the risk of venous thromboembolism: the Tromso Study. *J Thromb Haemost.* 2016;14:1183–1191.
27. Kaplan D, Casper TC, Elliott CG, et al. VTE incidence and risk factors in patients with severe sepsis and septic shock. *Chest.* 2015;148:1224–1230.
28. Poissy J, Goutay J, Caplan M, et al. Pulmonary embolism in COVID-19 patients: awareness of an increased prevalence. *Circulation.* 2020 Apr 24. https://doi.org/10.1161/CIRCULATIONAHA.120.047430.
29. Bompard F, Monnier H, Saab I, et al. Pulmonary embolism in patients with Covid-19 pneumonia. *Eur Respir J.* 2020:2001365. https://doi.org/10.1183/13993003.01365-2020.
30. Bikdeli B, Madhavan MV, Jimenez D, et al. COVID-19 and thrombotic or thromboembolic disease: implications for prevention, antithrombotic therapy, and follow-up. *J Am Coll Cardiol.* 2020.
31. Savchenko AS, Martinod K, Seidman MA, et al. Neutrophil extracellular traps form predominantly during the organizing stage of human venous thromboembolism development. *J Thromb Haemost.* 2014;12:860–870.
32. Zuo Y, Yalavarthi S, Shi H, et al. Neutrophil extracellular traps in COVID-19. *JCI Insight.* 2020;5(11):138999. https://doi.org/10.1172/jci.insight.138999.
33. Rogers MA, Levine DA, Blumberg N, et al. Triggers of hospitalization for venous thromboembolism. *Circulation.* 2012;125:2092–2099.
34. Tichelaar YI, Kluin-Nelemans HJ, Meijer K. Infections and inflammatory diseases as risk factors for venous thrombosis. A systematic review. *Thromb Haemost.* 2012;107:827–837.
35. Glynn RJ, Danielson E, Fonseca FA, et al. A randomized trial of rosuvastatin in the prevention of venous thromboembolism. *N Engl J Med.* 2009;360:1851–1861.
36. Klarin D, Busenkell E, Judy R, et al. Genome-wide association analysis of venous thromboembolism identifies new risk loci and genetic overlap with arterial vascular disease. *Nat Genet.* 2019;51:1574–1579.
37. Lindstrom S, Wang L, Smith EN, et al. Genomic and transcriptomic association studies identify 16 novel susceptibility loci for venous thromboembolism. *Blood.* 2019;134:1645–1657.
38. Marston NA, Gurmu Y, Melloni GEM, et al. The effect of PCSK9 (Proprotein Convertase Subtilisin/Kexin Type 9) inhibition on the risk of venous thromboembolism. *Circulation.* 2020;141:1600–1607.

Classification of Pulmonary Embolism

39. Konstantinides SV, Meyer G, Becattini C, et al. 2019 ESC Guidelines for the diagnosis and management of acute pulmonary embolism developed in collaboration with the European Respiratory Society (ERS). *Eur Heart J.* 2019.
40. Casazza F, Becattini C, Bongarzoni A, et al. Clinical features and short term outcomes of patients with acute pulmonary embolism. The Italian Pulmonary Embolism Registry (IPER). *Thromb Res.* 2012;130:847–852.
41. Yusuff HO, Zochios V, Vuylsteke A. Extracorporeal membrane oxygenation in acute massive pulmonary embolism: a systematic review. *Perfusion.* 2015;30:611–616.
42. Sista AK, Horowitz JM, Goldhaber SZ. Four key questions surrounding thrombolytic therapy for submassive pulmonary embolism. *Vasc Med.* 2016;21:47–52.
43. Hendriks SV, Klok FA, den Exter PL, et al. RV/LV ratio measurement seems to have no role in low risk patients with pulmonary embolism treated at home triaged by hestia criteria. *Am J Respir Crit Care Med.* 2020 Mar 23. https://doi.org/10.1164/rccm.202002-0267LE.
44. Windecker S, Stortecky S, Meier B. Paradoxical embolism. *J Am Coll Cardiol.* 2014;64:403–415.
45. Kosova E, Bergmark B, Piazza G. Fat embolism syndrome. *Circulation.* 2015;131:317–320.
46. Kahn SR, Akaberi A, Granton JT, et al. Quality of life, dyspnea, and functional exercise capacity following a first episode of pulmonary embolism: results of the ELOPE cohort study. *Am J Med.* 2017;130:990 e999-990 e921.
47. Konstantinides SV, Vicaut E, Danays T, et al. Impact of thrombolytic therapy on the long-term outcome of intermediate-risk pulmonary embolism. *J Am Coll Cardiol.* 2017;69:1536–1544.
48. Piazza G, Goldhaber SZ. Chronic thromboembolic pulmonary hypertension. *N Engl J Med.* 2011;364:351–360.
49. Mahmud E, Madani MM, Kim NH, et al. Chronic thromboembolic pulmonary hypertension: evolving therapeutic approaches for operable and inoperable disease. *J Am Coll Cardiol.* 2018;71:2468–2486.
50. Ghofrani HA, D'Armini AM, Grimminger F, et al. Riociguat for the treatment of chronic thromboembolic pulmonary hypertension. *N Engl J Med.* 2013;369:319–329.
51. Kataoka M, Inami T, Kawakami T, et al. Balloon pulmonary angioplasty (Percutaneous Transluminal Pulmonary Angioplasty) for chronic thromboembolic pulmonary hypertension: a Japanese perspective. *JACC Cardiovasc Interv.* 2019;12:1382–1388.
52. Righini M, Galanaud JP, Guenneguez H, et al. Anticoagulant therapy for symptomatic calf deep vein thrombosis (CACTUS): a randomised, double-blind, placebo-controlled trial. *Lancet Haematol.* 2016;3:e556–e562.
53. Franco L, Giustozzi M, Agnelli G, Becattini C. Anticoagulation in patients with isolated distal deep vein thrombosis: a meta-analysis. *J Thromb Haemost.* 2017;15:1142–1154.
54. Evans RS, Sharp JH, Linford LH, et al. Risk of symptomatic DVT associated with peripherally inserted central catheters. *Chest.* 2010;138:803–810.
55. Evans RS, Sharp JH, Linford LH, et al. Reduction of peripherally inserted central catheter-associated DVT. *Chest.* 2013;143:627–633.
56. Greene MT, Flanders SA, Woller SC, et al. The association between PICC use and venous thromboembolism in upper and lower extremities. *Am J Med.* 2015;128:986–993.e981.
57. Rabinovich A, Cohen JM, Cushman M, et al. Inflammation markers and their trajectories after deep vein thrombosis in relation to risk of post-thrombotic syndrome. *J Thromb Haemost.* 2015;13:398–408.
58. Galanaud JP, Righini M, Le Collen L, et al. Long-term risk of postthrombotic syndrome after symptomatic distal deep vein thrombosis: the CACTUS-PTS study. *J Thromb Haemost.* 2020;18:857–864.

59. Kachroo S, Boyd D, Bookhart BK, et al. Quality of life and economic costs associated with post-thrombotic syndrome. *Am J Health Syst Pharm*. 2012;69:567–572.
60. Kahn SR, Shapiro S, Wells PS, et al. Compression stockings to prevent post-thrombotic syndrome: a randomised placebo-controlled trial. *Lancet*. 2014;383:880–888.
61. Kahn SR, Shrier I, Shapiro S, et al. Six-month exercise training program to treat post-thrombotic syndrome: a randomized controlled two-centre trial. *CMAJ (Can Med Assoc J)*. 2011;183:37–44.
62. Cannegieter SC, Horvath-Puho E, Schmidt M, et al. Risk of venous and arterial thrombotic events in patients diagnosed with superficial vein thrombosis: a nationwide cohort study. *Blood*. 2015;125:229–235.

Diagnosis

63. Le Gal G, Righini M, Wells PS. D-dimer for pulmonary embolism. *J Am Med Assoc*. 2015;313:1668–1669.
64. Parpia S, Takach Lapner S, et al. Clinical pre-test probability adjusted versus age-adjusted D-dimer interpretation strategy for DVT diagnosis: a diagnostic individual patient data meta-analysis. *J Thromb Haemost*. 2020;18:669–675.
65. Halaby R, Popma CJ, Cohen A, et al. D-Dimer elevation and adverse outcomes. *J Thromb Thrombolysis*. 2015;39:55–59.
66. Picano E, Scali MC, Ciampi Q, Lichtenstein D. Lung ultrasound for the cardiologist. *JACC Cardiovasc Imaging*. 2018;11:1692–1705.
67. Squizzato A, Galli L, Gerdes VE. Point-of-care ultrasound in the diagnosis of pulmonary embolism. *Crit Ultrasound J*. 2015;7:7.
68. Bekgoz B, Kilicaslan I, Bildik F, et al. BLUE protocol ultrasonography in emergency department patients presenting with acute dyspnea. *Am J Emerg Med*. 2019;37:2020–2027.
69. Moore AJE, Wachsmann J, Chamarthy MR, et al. Imaging of acute pulmonary embolism: an update. *Cardiovasc Diagn Ther*. 2018;8:225–243.
70. Hutchinson BD, Navin P, Marom EM, et al. Overdiagnosis of pulmonary embolism by pulmonary CT angiography. *AJR Am J Roentgenol*. 2015;205:271–277.
71. Kang DK, Ramos-Duran L, Schoepf UJ, et al. Reproducibility of CT signs of right ventricular dysfunction in acute pulmonary embolism. *AJR Am J Roentgenol*. 2010;194:1500–1506.
72. Koc M, Kostrubiec M, Elikowski W, et al. Outcome of patients with right heart thrombi: the Right Heart Thrombi European Registry. *Eur Respir J*. 2016;47:869–875.
73. Li J, Feng L, Li J, Tang J. Diagnostic accuracy of magnetic resonance angiography for acute pulmonary embolism - a systematic review and meta-analysis. *Vasa*. 2016;45:149–154.
74. Raja AS, Ip IK, Prevedello LM, et al. Effect of computerized clinical decision support on the use and yield of CT pulmonary angiography in the emergency department. *Radiology*. 2012;262:468–474.

Anticoagulation Therapy

75. Carroll BJ, Beyer SE, Mehegan T, et al. Changes in care for acute pulmonary embolism with a multidisciplinary pulmonary embolism response team: PE response team. *Am J Med*. 2020; S0002-9343(20)30374-0. https://doi.org/10.1016/j.amjmed.2020.03.058.
76. Aso S, Matsui H, Fushimi K, Yasunaga H. In-hospital mortality and successful weaning from venoarterial extracorporeal membrane oxygenation: analysis of 5,263 patients using a National inpatient database in Japan. *Crit Care*. 2016;20:80. https://doi.org/10.1186/s13054-016-1261-1.
77. Meneveau N, Guillon B, Planquette B, et al. Outcomes after extracorporeal membrane oxygenation for the treatment of high-risk pulmonary embolism: a multicentre series of 52 cases. *Eur Heart J*. 2018;39:4196–4204.
78. Konstantinides SV, Warntges S. Acute phase treatment of venous thromboembolism: advanced therapy. Systemic fibrinolysis and pharmacomechanical therapy. *Thromb Haemost*. 2015;113:1202–1209.
79. Zhang R, Kobayashi T, Pugliese S, et al. Interventional therapies in acute pulmonary embolism. *Interv Cardiol Clin*. 2020;9:229–241.
80. Keeling WB, Bundt T, Leacche M, et al. Outcomes after surgical pulmonary embolectomy for acute pulmonary embolus: a multi-institutional study. *Ann Thorac Surg*. 2016;102(5):1498–1502.
81. Percy ED, Shah R, Hirji S, et al. National outcomes of surgical embolectomy for acute pulmonary embolism. *Ann Thorac Surg*. 2020;110(2):441–447.
82. Chan CM, Woods C, Shorr AF. The validation and reproducibility of the pulmonary embolism severity index. *J Thromb Haemost*. 2010;8:1509–1514.
83. Poterucha TJ, Libby P, Goldhaber SZ. More than an anticoagulant: do heparins have direct anti-inflammatory effects? *Thromb Haemost*. 2017;117(3):437–444.
84. Black SA, Cohen AT. Anticoagulation strategies for venous thromboembolism: moving towards a personalised approach. *Thromb Haemost*. 2015;114:660–669.
85. Kang M, Alahmadi M, Sawh S, et al. Fondaparinux for the treatment of suspected heparin-induced thrombocytopenia: a propensity score-matched study. *Blood*. 2015;125:924–929.
86. Salter BS, Weiner MM, Trinh MA, et al. Heparin-induced thrombocytopenia: a comprehensive clinical review. *J Am Coll Cardiol*. 2016;67:2519–2532.
87. Greinacher A. Clinical practice. heparin-induced thrombocytopenia. *N Engl J Med*. 2015;373:252–261.
88. Baroletti S, Hurwitz S, Conti NA, et al. Thrombosis in suspected heparin-induced thrombocytopenia occurs more often with high antibody levels. *Am J Med*. 2012;125:44–49.
89. Poterucha TJ, Goldhaber SZ. Warfarin and vascular calcification. *Am J Med*. 2016;129:635. e631–e634.
90. Binding C, Bjerring Olesen J, Abrahamsen B, et al. Osteoporotic fractures in patients with atrial fibrillation treated with conventional versus direct anticoagulants. *J Am Coll Cardiol*. 2019;74:2150–2158.
91. Douketis JD, Spyropoulos AC, Kaatz S, et al. Perioperative bridging anticoagulation in patients with atrial fibrillation. *N Engl J Med*. 2015;373:823–833.
92. Baumgartner C, de Kouchkovsky I, Whitaker E, Fang MC. Periprocedural bridging in patients with venous thromboembolism: a systematic review. *Am J Med*. 2019;132:722–732. e727.
93. Beyer-Westendorf J, Ageno W. Benefit-risk profile of non-vitamin K antagonist oral anticoagulants in the management of venous thromboembolism. *Thromb Haemost*. 2015;113:231–246.
94. van der Hulle T, Kooiman J, den Exter PL, et al. Effectiveness and safety of novel oral anticoagulants as compared with vitamin K antagonists in the treatment of acute symptomatic venous thromboembolism: a systematic review and meta-analysis. *J Thromb Haemost*. 2014;12:320–328.
95. Schulman S, Kearon C, Kakkar AK, et al. Dabigatran versus warfarin in the treatment of acute venous thromboembolism. *N Engl J Med*. 2009;361:2342–2352.
96. Schulman S, Kakkar AK, Goldhaber SZ, et al. Treatment of acute venous thromboembolism with dabigatran or warfarin and pooled analysis. *Circulation*. 2014;129:764–772.
97. Yeh CH, Gross PL, Weitz JI. Evolving use of new oral anticoagulants for treatment of venous thromboembolism. *Blood*. 2014;124:1020–1028.
98. Investigators E, Bauersachs R, Berkowitz SD, et al. Oral rivaroxaban for symptomatic venous thromboembolism. *N Engl J Med*. 2010;363:2499–2510.
99. Einstein-EP Investigators, Buller HR, Prins MH, et al. Oral rivaroxaban for the treatment of symptomatic pulmonary embolism. *N Engl J Med*. 2012;366:1287–1297.
100. Agnelli G, Buller HR, Cohen A, et al. Oral apixaban for the treatment of acute venous thromboembolism. *N Engl J Med*. 2013;369:799–808.
101. Hokusai VTEI, Buller HR, Decousus H, et al. Edoxaban versus warfarin for the treatment of symptomatic venous thromboembolism. *N Engl J Med*. 2013;369:1406–1415.
102. Schulman S, Kearon C, Kakkar AK, et al. Extended use of dabigatran, warfarin, or placebo in venous thromboembolism. *N Engl J Med*. 2013;368:709–718.
103. Agnelli G, Buller HR, Cohen A, et al. Apixaban for extended treatment of venous thromboembolism. *N Engl J Med*. 2013;368:699–708.
104. Male C, Lensing AWA, Palumbo JS, et al. Rivaroxaban compared with standard anticoagulants for the treatment of acute venous thromboembolism in children: a randomised, controlled, phase 3 trial. *Lancet Haematol*. 2020;7:e18–e27.
105. Hickey M, Gatien M, Taljaard M, et al. Outcomes of urgent warfarin reversal with frozen plasma versus prothrombin complex concentrate in the emergency department. *Circulation*. 2013;128:360–364.
106. Pollack Jr CV, Reilly PA, Eikelboom J, et al. Idarucizumab for dabigatran reversal. *N Engl J Med*. 2015;373:511–520.
107. Pollack Jr CV, Reilly PA, Weitz JI. Dabigatran reversal with idarucizumab. *N Engl J Med*. 2017;377:1691–1692.
108. Siegal DM, Curnutte JT, Connolly SJ, et al. Andexanet alfa for the reversal of factor Xa inhibitor activity. *N Engl J Med*. 2015;373:2413–2424.
109. Connolly SJ, Crowther M, Eikelboom JW, et al. Full study report of andexanet alfa for bleeding associated with factor Xa inhibitors. *N Engl J Med*. 2019;380:1326–1335.
110. Libby P, Hansson GK. From focal lipid storage to systemic inflammation: JACC review topic of the week. *J Am Coll Cardiol*. 2019;74:1594–1607.
111. Huang W, Goldberg RJ, Anderson FA, et al. Secular trends in occurrence of acute venous thromboembolism: the Worcester VTE study (1985-2009). *Am J Med*. 2014;127:829–839. e825.
112. Sogaard KK, Schmidt M, Pedersen L, et al. 30-year mortality after venous thromboembolism: a population-based cohort study. *Circulation*. 2014;130:829–836.
113. Albertsen IE, Nielsen PB, Sogaard M, et al. Risk of recurrent venous thromboembolism: a Danish Nationwide Cohort Study. *Am J Med*. 2018;131:1067–1074. e1064.
114. Khan F, Rahman A, Carrier M, et al. Long term risk of symptomatic recurrent venous thromboembolism after discontinuation of anticoagulant treatment for first unprovoked venous thromboembolism event: systematic review and meta-analysis. *BMJ*. 2019;366:l4363.
115. Kearon C, Spencer FA, O'Keeffe D, et al. D-dimer testing to select patients with a first unprovoked venous thromboembolism who can stop anticoagulant therapy: a cohort study. *Ann Intern Med*. 2015;162:27–34.
116. Kearon C, Ageno W, Cannegieter SC, et al. Categorization of patients as having provoked or unprovoked venous thromboembolism: guidance from the SSC of ISTH. *J Thromb Haemost*. 2016;14:1480–1483.
117. Rodger MA, Le Gal G, Anderson DR, et al. Validating the HERDOO2 rule to guide treatment duration for women with unprovoked venous thrombosis: multinational prospective cohort management study. *BMJ*. 2017;356:j1065.
118. Albertsen IE, Sogaard M, Goldhaber SZ, et al. Development of sex-stratified prediction models for recurrent venous thromboembolism: a Danish Nationwide Cohort Study. *Thromb Haemost*. 2020;120:805–814.
119. Agnelli G, Buller HR, Cohen A, et al. Apixaban for extended treatment of venous thromboembolism. *N Engl J Med*. 2013;368:699–708.
120. Weitz JI, Lensing AWA, Prins MH, et al. Rivaroxaban or aspirin for extended treatment of venous thromboembolism. *N Engl J Med*. 2017;376:1211–1222.
121. Vasanthamohan L, Boonyawat K, Chai-Adisaksopha C, Crowther M. Reduced-dose direct oral anticoagulants in the extended treatment of venous thromboembolism: a systematic review and meta-analysis. *J Thromb Haemost*. 2018;16:1288–1295.
122. Mai V, Guay CA, Perreault L, et al. Extended anticoagulation for VTE: a systematic review and meta-analysis. *Chest*. 2019;155:1199–1216.

Advanced Therapy

123. Dudzinski DM, Piazza G. Multidisciplinary pulmonary embolism response teams. *Circulation*. 2016;133:98–103.
124. Kolte D, Parikh SA, Piazza G, et al. Vascular teams in peripheral vascular disease. *J Am Coll Cardiol*. 2019;73:2477–2486.
125. Chatterjee S, Chakraborty A, Weinberg I, et al. Thrombolysis for pulmonary embolism and risk of all-cause mortality, major bleeding, and intracranial hemorrhage: a meta-analysis. *J Am Med Assoc*. 2014;311:2414–2421.
126. Kiser TH, Burnham EL, Clark B, et al. Half-dose versus full-dose alteplase for treatment of pulmonary embolism. *Crit Care Med*. 2018;46:1617–1625.
127. Kucher N, Boekstegers P, Muller OJ, et al. Randomized, controlled trial of ultrasound-assisted catheter-directed thrombolysis for acute intermediate-risk pulmonary embolism. *Circulation*. 2014;129:479–486.
128. Piazza G, Hohlfelder B, Jaff MR, et al. A prospective, single-arm, multicenter trial of ultrasound-facilitated, catheter-directed, low-dose fibrinolysis for acute massive and submassive pulmonary embolism: the SEATTLE II study. *JACC Cardiovasc Interv*. 2015;8:1382–1392.
129. Tapson VF, Sterling K, Jones N, et al. A randomized trial of the optimum duration of acoustic pulse thrombolysis procedure in acute intermediate-risk pulmonary embolism: the OPTALYSE PE trial. *JACC Cardiovasc Interv*. 2018;11:1401–1410.
130. Rahaghi FN, Estepar RSJ, Goldhaber SZ, et al. Quantification and significance of pulmonary vascular volume in predicting response to ultrasound-facilitated, catheter-directed fibrinolysis in acute pulmonary embolism (SEATTLE-3D). *Clin Cardiovasc Imaging*. 2019;12(12):e009903. https://doi.org/10.1161/CIRCIMAGING.119.009903. Epub 2019 Dec 17.
131. Tu T, Toma C, Tapson VF, et al. A prospective, single-arm, multicenter trial of catheter-directed mechanical thrombectomy for intermediate-risk acute pulmonary embolism: the FLARE study. *JACC Cardiovasc Interv*. 2019;12:859–869.
132. VIVA 2019: Penumbra Indigo Aspiration system IDE trial for acute PE meets primary safety and efficacy endpoints. [Electronic article]. *Vascular News*. 2019. *https://vascularnews.com/viva19-penumbra-indigo-aspiration-system-ide-trial-for-acute-pe-meets-primary-safety-and-efficacy-endpoints/*. Published 6 November 2019. Accessed 21 April 2020.
133. Kuo WT, Banerjee A, Kim PS, et al. Pulmonary Embolism Response to Fragmentation, Embolectomy, and Catheter Thrombolysis (PERFECT): initial results from a prospective multicenter registry. *Chest*. 2015;148:667–673.
134. Giri J, Sista AK, Weinberg I, et al. Interventional therapies for acute pulmonary embolism: current status and principles for the development of novel evidence: a scientific statement from the American Heart Association. *Circulation*. 2019;140:e774–e801.
135. Poterucha TJ, Bergmark B, Aranki S, et al. Surgical pulmonary embolectomy. *Circulation*. 2015;132:1146–1151.
136. Kolkailah AA, Hirji S, Piazza G, et al. Surgical pulmonary embolectomy and catheter-directed thrombolysis for treatment of submassive pulmonary embolism. *J Card Surg*. 2018;33:252–259.
137. Mismetti P, Laporte S, Pellerin O, et al. Effect of a retrievable inferior vena cava filter plus anticoagulation vs anticoagulation alone on risk of recurrent pulmonary embolism: a randomized clinical trial. *J Am Med Assoc*. 2015;313:1627–1635.
138. Bikdeli B, Chatterjee S, Desai NR, et al. Inferior vena cava filters to prevent pulmonary embolism: systematic review and meta-analysis. *J Am Coll Cardiol*. 2017;70:1587–1597.
139. Sutphin PD, Reis SP, McKune A, et al. Improving inferior vena cava filter retrieval rates with the define, measure, analyze, improve, control methodology. *J Vasc Interv Radiol*. 2015;26:491–498. e491.
140. Enden T, Haig Y, Klow NE, et al. Long-term outcome after additional catheter-directed thrombolysis versus standard treatment for acute iliofemoral deep vein thrombosis (the CaVenT study): a randomised controlled trial. *Lancet*. 2012;379:31–38.

141. Vedantham S, Goldhaber SZ, Julian JA, et al. Pharmacomechanical catheter-directed thrombolysis for deep-vein thrombosis. *N Engl J Med.* 2017;377:2240–2252.

142. Lee AY, Levine MN, Baker RI, et al. Low-molecular-weight heparin versus a coumarin for the prevention of recurrent venous thromboembolism in patients with cancer. *N Engl J Med.* 2003;349:146–153.

143. Lee AY, Kamphuisen PW, Meyer G, et al. Tinzaparin vs warfarin for treatment of acute venous thromboembolism in patients with active cancer: a randomized clinical trial. *J Am Med Assoc.* 2015;314:677–686.

144. Raskob GE, van Es N, Verhamme P, et al. Edoxaban for the treatment of cancer-associated venous thromboembolism. *N Engl J Med.* 2018;378:615–624.

145. Young AM, Marshall A, Thirlwall J, et al. Comparison of an oral factor Xa inhibitor with low molecular weight heparin in patients with cancer with venous thromboembolism: results of a randomized trial (SELECT-D). *J Clin Oncol.* 2018;36:2017–2023.

146. Agnelli G, Becattini C, Meyer G, et al. Apixaban for the treatment of venous thromboembolism associated with cancer. *N Engl J Med.* 2020;382:1599–1607.

147. Cosmi B. Management of superficial vein thrombosis. *J Thromb Haemost.* 2015;13:1175–1183.

148. Beyer-Westendorf J, Schellong SM, Gerlach H, et al. Prevention of thromboembolic complications in patients with superficial-vein thrombosis given rivaroxaban or fondaparinux: the open-label, randomised, non-inferiority SURPRISE phase 3b trial. *Lancet Haematol.* 2017;4:e105–e113.

149. Pengo V, Denas G, Zoppellaro G, et al. Rivaroxaban vs warfarin in high-risk patients with antiphospholipid syndrome. *Blood.* 2018;132:1365–1371.

150. Witmer C, Raffini L. Treatment of venous thromboembolism in pediatric patients. *Blood.* 2020;135:335–343.

151. Brandao LR, Albisetti M, Halton J, et al. Safety of dabigatran etexilate for the secondary prevention of venous thromboembolism in children. *Blood.* 2020;135:491–504.

152. Hojen AA, Gorst-Rasmussen A, Lip GY, et al. Use of psychotropic drugs following venous thromboembolism in youth. A nationwide cohort study. *Thromb Res.* 2015;135:643–647.

153. Hojen AA, Sorensen EE, Dreyer PS, et al. Long-term mental wellbeing of adolescents and young adults diagnosed with venous thromboembolism: results from a multistage mixed methods study. *J Thromb Haemost.* 2017;15:2333–2343.

Prevention

154. Woller SC, Stevens SM, Evans RS, et al. Electronic alerts, comparative practitioner metrics, and education improves thromboprophylaxis and reduces thrombosis. *Am J Med.* 2016;129:1124.e1117–e1126.

155. Cohen AT, Harrington RA, Goldhaber SZ, et al. Extended thromboprophylaxis with betrixaban in acutely ill medical patients. *N Engl J Med.* 2016;375:534–544.

156. Gibson CM, Chi G, Halaby R, et al. Extended-duration betrixaban reduces the risk of stroke versus standard-dose enoxaparin among hospitalized medically ill patients: an APEX trial substudy (Acute Medically Ill Venous Thromboembolism Prevention With Extended Duration Betrixaban). *Circulation.* 2017;135:648–655.

157. Nafee T, Gibson CM, Yee MK, et al. Reduction of cardiovascular mortality and ischemic events in acute medically ill patients. *Circulation.* 2019;139:1234–1236.

158. Chi G, Yee MK, Amin AN, et al. Extended-duration betrixaban reduces the risk of rehospitalization associated with venous thromboembolism among acutely ill hospitalized medical patients: findings from the APEX trial (Acute Medically Ill Venous Thromboembolism Prevention With Extended Duration Betrixaban Trial). *Circulation.* 2018;137:91–94.

159. Kalayci A, Gibson CM, Chi G, et al. Asymptomatic deep vein thrombosis is associated with an increased risk of death: insights from the APEX trial. *Thromb Haemost.* 2018;118:2046–2052.

160. Cohen AT, Spiro TE, Buller HR, et al. Rivaroxaban for thromboprophylaxis in acutely ill medical patients. *N Engl J Med.* 2013;368:513–523.

161. Spyropoulos AC, Lipardi C, Xu J, et al. Improved benefit risk profile of rivaroxaban in a subpopulation of the MAGELLAN study. *Clin Appl Thromb Hemost.* 2019;25:1076029619886022.

162. Spyropoulos AC, Ageno W, Albers GW, et al. Rivaroxaban for thromboprophylaxis after hospitalization for medical illness. *N Engl J Med.* 2018;379:1118–1127.

163. Spyropoulos AC. Post-discharge prophylaxis with rivaroxaban reduces fatal and major thromboembolic events in medically ill patients. *J Am Coll Cardiol.* 2020;75(25):3140–3147. https://doi.org/10.1016/j.jacc.2020.04.071. PMID: 32586587.

164. Goldhaber SZ. Thromboembolism prophylaxis for patients discharged from the hospital: easier said than done. *J Am Coll Cardiol.* 2020;75(25):3148–3150. https://doi.org/10.1016/j.jacc.2020.05.023. PMID: 32586588.

165. Woller SC, Stevens SM, Jones JP, et al. Derivation and validation of a simple model to identify venous thromboembolism risk in medical patients. *Am J Med.* 2011;124:947–954.e942.

166. Carrier M, Abou-Nassar K, Mallick R, et al. Apixaban to prevent venous thromboembolism in patients with cancer. *N Engl J Med.* 2019;380:711–719.

167. Khorana AA, Soff GA, Kakkar AK, et al. Rivaroxaban for thromboprophylaxis in high-risk ambulatory patients with cancer. *N Engl J Med.* 2019;380:720–728.

168. Agnelli G. Direct oral anticoagulants for thromboprophylaxis in ambulatory patients with cancer. *N Engl J Med.* 2019;380:781–783.

169. Arabi YM, Al-Hameed F, Burns KEA, et al. Adjunctive intermittent pneumatic compression for venous thromboprophylaxis. *N Engl J Med.* 2019;380:1305–1315.

170. Xu K, Chan NC, Ibrahim Q, et al. Reduction in mortality following elective major hip and knee surgery: a systematic review and meta-analysis. *Thromb Haemost.* 2019;119:668–674.

171. Pellegrini Jr VD, Eikelboom J, McCollister Evarts C, et al. Selection bias, orthopaedic style: knowing what we don't know about aspirin. *J Bone Joint Surg Am.* 2020;102:631–633.

172. Weitz JI, Chan NC. Novel antithrombotic strategies for treatment of venous thromboembolism. *Blood.* 2020;135:351–359.

88 Pulmonary Hypertension

BRADLEY A. MARON

Pulmonary hypertension (PH) is a specific although heterogeneous clinical disorder defined foremost by elevated pulmonary artery pressure. Pathogenic remodeling of medium and small pulmonary arterials increases pulmonary vascular resistance (PVR), which accompanies the hemodynamic pattern encountered in most PH patients clinically. Predominately, PH is caused by left heart disease or parenchymal lung disease. Pulmonary arterial hypertension (PAH), which was formerly termed *primary pulmonary hypertension*, is a distinct albeit uncommon subgroup of PH.[1] In PAH, interplay between genetic and molecular factors results in a classic plexogenic pulmonary arteriopathy occurring in the absence of other diseases that affect pulmonary artery pressure.

The pathophysiology of PH extends beyond the pulmonary circulation, and often includes right ventricular (RV) dysfunction, chronic kidney disease, overactivation of neurohumoral signaling pathways, and many other processes that impair global cardiovascular function and fitness.[2] This constellation of features forebodes disease burden, and informs treatment timing and escalation. Several recent advances have contemporized aspects central to PH epidemiology, diagnosis, prognosis, and patient management. For example, fresh insight on PH risk factors, the contribution of right ventricular-pulmonary arterial (RV-PA) uncoupling to right heart failure, and a widened cardiopulmonary hemodynamic risk spectrum have modernized the clinical profile of PH and caused a strategic shift emphasizing early diagnosis. Additionally, newly available medical and procedural therapies for PAH highlight continued progress toward improving quality of life and lifespan in patients affected by a disease once considered uniformly fatal. This chapter will begin by discussing the normal pulmonary circulation to provide an anatomic and physiological bases for understanding: (1) the classification of PH, (2) the pathology and pathobiology of PH, (3) the pathophysiology of PH, (4) and the clinical presentation, assessment, and treatment of patients with PH and PAH.

NORMAL PULMONARY CIRCULATION

The pulmonary vascular circuit originates from the main pulmonary artery, which measures approximately 2.7 to 2.9 cm in diameter, and divides into the right and left main pulmonary arteries. Iterative branching occurs proximal to distal along a course that tracks with each successive generation of bronchus. The main pulmonary arteries give rise to lobar arteries that branch into segmental, subsegmental, and intralobar arteries. Collectively, these aspects of the pulmonary circulatory tree comprise elastic arterials that are distensible at low transmural pressures, greater than 500 μm in diameter, and largely spared from adverse remodeling that underlies most pulmonary circulatory diseases.

By contrast, muscular pulmonary arteries and arterioles measure 100 to 500 μm and less than 100 μm in diameter, respectively, and are the principal structures affected in pulmonary circulatory diseases.[3] The wall of muscular arteries includes the single cell endothelial layer and muscular media, which is separated by the internal and external elastic laminae and densely populated with pulmonary artery smooth muscle cells. The adventitia is the outer most layer of muscular arteries and is comprised of fibroblasts, macrophage, progenitor cells, and vasovasorum. Pulmonary arterioles are pre-capillary structures that consist of a thin intima and single elastic lamina only. Alveolar capillaries measure 5 to 10μm in diameter and are lined with a continuous layer of endothelium enveloped by pericytes at focal connections, but do not include pulmonary artery smooth cells and, thus, are noncontractile.

Pulmonary Circulatory Physiology

The anatomy of the pulmonary vasculature is oriented in a parallel circuit, which permits high blood flow, low pressure, and low resistance (Fig. 88.1A). This is in contradistinction to the systemic vasculature that is organized as a circuit in series and designed to distribute cardiac output (CO) to regional beds. In the pulmonary circulation, multiplicative branching with successive smaller caliber vessels maximizes surface area to optimize gas exchange at the alveolar-capillary interface. Indeed, there are 280 billion capillaries, which outnumbers individual alveoli by a factor of 900-fold to cover 85% of all available alveolar surface area. The PVR reflects the ratio of change in pulmonary artery pressure (ΔP) to mean pulmonary blood flow (Q) (L/min); when this value is multiplied by 80, the result is expressed as mm Hg/L/min and referred to as a Wood unit (alternatively, resistance expressed as dyne*sec*cm⁻⁵ divided by 80 yields a Wood unit).[4] The calculated PVR may also be determined in clinical practice as: (mean pulmonary artery pressure [mPAP]-left atrial pressure)/CO. Because routine left atrial sampling is not practical, the pulmonary artery wedge pressure (PAWP) is used as a surrogate of this measurement.

Additional content is available online at Elsevier eBooks for Practicing Clinicians

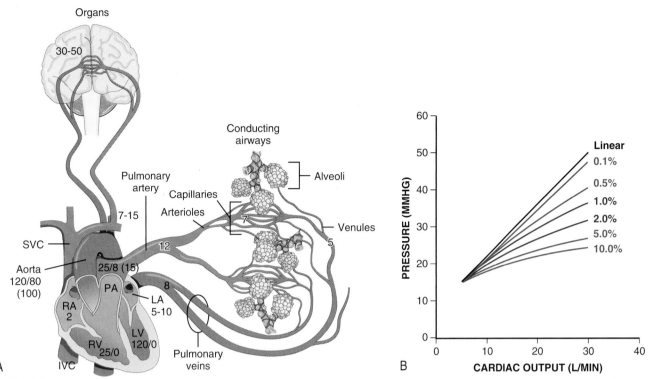

FIGURE 88.1 Pulmonary vascular anatomy and distensibility. **A,** Low pressure and low resistance characteristics of the pulmonary circulation permit optimal surface for gas exchange at the alveolar-capillary interface. Normal systolic and diastolic blood pressure values are presented in various compartments. *IVC*, Inferior vena cava; *LA*, left atrium; *LV*, left ventricle; *PA*, pulmonary artery; *RA*, right atrium; *RV*, right ventricle; *SVC*, superior vena cava. **B,** Modeled mean pulmonary arterial pressure–cardiac output relationships during dynamic exercise with progressively increased distensibility coefficients (α). The normal range of α values is 1% to 2%. (**A** adapted from Chamarthy MR et al. *Cardiovasc Diagn Ther* 2018 Jun;8(3):208–213; **B** from Lewis GD et al. *Circulation* 2013;128:1470–1479.)

Effect of Aging on the Pulmonary Circulation

Beyond the age of 35 years, there is a gradual decline in extensibility of the conduit pulmonary arteries, and an increase in muscularization of medium and small vessels. This is characterized by collagen deposition and deterioration of elastin, which, collectively causes mild fibrotic remodeling of the intima and vascular stiffening. The main pulmonary artery dilates slightly with age,[5] and the consequences of these age-related anatomical and histologic changes include a subtle rise in average mean mPAP and PVR, most evident in the seventh decade of life or greater.[6]

Pulmonary Venous System

A pulmonary venous network emerges from the alveolar-capillary interface with vessel diameter and branching ratios comparable to the arterial tree, totaling 15 enumerations.[7] Ultimately, three or four bronchial veins converge to a main pulmonary vein, in a pair per lung hilum. Overall, a total of four pulmonary veins articulate into the posterior left atrium. Small intra-pulmonary veins include a smooth muscle media, adventitia with vaso-vasorum, and elastin casing. Large pulmonary veins generally lack an elastic lamina and are muscular but are 60% less thick than pulmonary arteries with relatively more extracellular matrix. Sclerosis, fibrosis, and muscularization of pulmonary veins is recognized increasingly in the pathogenesis of left heart failure and other PH syndromes once considered to be exclusively due to arterial remodeling.[8]

Pulmonary Circulatory Physiology During Exercise

The average pulmonary blood flow at rest is 3.5 L/min/m², and at any moment 300 mL/m² of blood is in the pulmonary circulation of which approximately 25% occupies capillaries.[7] However, during exercise the cardiopulmonary apparatus must accommodate a fivefold or greater increase in CO. This dramatic shift affects mPAP via the direct effect of increased CO on intravascular blood volume and left atrial pressure.[9] It is important that the relationship between mPAP and CO is curvilinear in vivo (Fig. 88.1B). This allows the pulmonary circulatory unit to accommodate increased

blood volume without a proportional increase in pulmonary artery pressure, which would have a detrimental effect on RV afterload. The CO-mPAP relationship hinges on preserved distensibility, however, and pathological processes that impair normal pulmonary vascular compliance (even subtly) stand to disrupt cardiopulmonary physiology leading to a pathological state manifest by impaired exercise tolerance.[10]

CLASSIFICATION OF PULMONARY HYPERTENSION

In the 1950s, the British cardiologist Dr. Paul Wood assembled the first comprehensive data on PH patients. This classic work included observations from his own cohort at the National Heart and Brompton Hospitals, seminal descriptive publications on "primary pulmonary hypertension" by Castleman and Bland (1946), and pulmonary vascular pathology reports by Edwards (1950). Wood concluded upon six PH types: passive, hyperkinetic, obstructive, obliterative, vasoconstrictive, and polygenic (i.e., multifactorial). Given the rudimentary technology of that time compared to today, the sustained usefulness of this initial PH framework is quite remarkable. Indeed, the current PH classification overlaps with this scheme by Wood,[11] but now the cardiopulmonary hemodynamic profile is integrated directly with information on clinical disorders that predispose to pulmonary vascular disease. This collective, in turn, informs the pathophysiology (and presumed pathobiology) of an individual patient at point of care.

There are two broad, inter-related strategies by which to classify patients with PH.[12] First, the cardiopulmonary hemodynamic profile is used to assign patients into one of three categories: pre-capillary, isolated post-capillary, and combined pre- and post-capillary PH (Table 88.1). These designations aim to distinguish PH originating due to a pulmonary arterial lesion (pre-capillary) from disorders originating in the pulmonary venous bed or structures distal (post-capillary). Combined pre- and post-capillary PH refers to a post-capillary process that causes pulmonary arterial remodeling (indicated by increased PVR). Second, the comorbidity and demographic profile is used to assign individual patients into an

TABLE 88.1 Overlap Between Hemodynamic and Clinical Classification of Pulmonary Hypertension

DEFINITIONS	CHARACTERISTICS	PH CLINICAL GROUPS
Pre-capillary PH	mPAP >20 mm Hg	PAH
	PAWP ≤15 mm Hg	Lung disease
	PVR ≥3WU	Sleep-disordered breathing
		Miscellaneous causes
Isolated post-capillary PH (IpcPH)	mPAP >20 mm Hg	Left heart disease
	PAWP >15 mm Hg	Miscellaneous causes
	PVR <3 WU	
Combined pre- and post-capillary PH (CpcPH)	mPAP >20 mm Hg	Left heart disease
	PAWP >15 mm Hg	Miscellaneous causes
	PVR ≥3 WU	

mPAP, Mean pulmonary artery pressure; *PAH,* pulmonary arterial hypertension; *PAWP,* pulmonary artery wedge pressure; *PH,* pulmonary hypertension; *PVR,* pulmonary vascular resistance.
Adapted from Simonneau G, et al. *Eur Respir J.* 2019;53(1):180191.

TABLE 88.2 Revised Clinical Classification of Pulmonary Hypertension

1 PAH
　1.1 Idiopathic PAH
　1.2 Heritable PAH
　1.3 Drug- and toxin-induced PAH
　1.4 PAH associated with:
　　1.4.1 Connective tissue disease
　　1.4.2 HIV infection
　　1.4.3 Portal hypertension
　　1.4.4 Congenital heart disease
　　1.4.5 Schistosomiasis
　1.5 PAH long-term responders to calcium channel blockers
　1.6 PAH with overt features of venous/capillaries (PVOD/PCH) involvement
　1.7 Persistent PH of the newborn syndrome

2 PH due to left heart disease
　2.1 PH due to heart failure with preserved LVEF
　2.2 PH due to heart failure with reduced LVEF
　2.3 Valvular heart disease
　2.4 Congenital/acquired cardiovascular conditions leading to post-capillary PH

3 PH due to lung diseases and/or hypoxia
　3.1 Obstructive lung disease
　3.2 Restrictive lung disease
　3.3 Other lung disease with mixed restrictive/obstructive pattern
　3.4 Hypoxia without lung disease
　3.5 Developmental lung disorders

4 PH due to pulmonary artery obstructions
　4.1 Chronic thromboembolic PH
　4.2 Other pulmonary artery obstructions

5 PH with unclear and/or multifactorial mechanisms
　5.1 Hematological disorders
　5.2 Systemic and metabolic disorders
　5.3 Others
　5.4 Complex congenital heart disease

HIV, Human immunodeficiency virus; *LVEF,* left ventricular ejection fraction; *PAH,* pulmonary arterial hypertension; *PCH,* pulmonary capillary hemangiomatosis; *PH,* pulmonary hypertension; *PVOD,* pulmonary venoocclusive disease.
Adapted from Simonneau G, et al. *Eur Respir J.* 2019;53(1):801913.

appropriate clinical PH group (Table 88.2). It is important to note that certain clinical-hemodynamic combinations are not compatible; for example, PAH is exclusive of post-capillary PH.[1]

Hemodynamic Classifications

Elevated mPAP greater than 20 mm Hg diagnosed by invasive right heart catheterization (RHC) measured supine at rest is the sine qua non of PH. This is based on early-era normative data in 1,187 healthy research subjects showing that the median mPAP at rest was 14.0 ± 3.1 mm Hg. Using two times the SD, the upper limit of normal mPAP is 19 to 20 mm Hg.[13] These findings converge with results from large RHC databases suggesting that clinical risk emerges at mPAP approximately 19 mm Hg.[14] The relationship between mPAP and mortality is continuous, and patients referred for RHC with mPAP approximately 20 to 24 mm Hg and greater than 25 mm Hg have an all-cause adjusted mortality risk that is 1.23-fold and 2.16-fold greater, respectively, compared to mPAP less than 19 mm Hg. However, the association between mPAP and outcome is not homogenous throughout the mPAP continuum, as an increase by 1 mm Hg influences outcome risk to a greater extent between 20 and 25 mm Hg compared to levels indicative of severe disease (e.g., mPAP >40 mm Hg) (Fig. 88.2). It is also important to note that the normal mPAP increases slightly with age and may be as high as 22 mm Hg among those greater than 50 years. This should be considered when interpreting cardiopulmonary hemodynamics in symptomatic patients within this age range.[6,13]

A major branch point in the hemodynamic classification of PH patients is delineating pre-capillary PH from post-capillary PH. This is generally accomplished by turning to the PAWP, which transmits left ventricular end-diastolic pressure (LVEDP) in the absence of mitral valve disease or other mechanical obstruction between the pulmonary capillary network and LV. A PAWP greater than 15 mm Hg (or more conservatively >12 mm Hg) suggests pulmonary venous hypertension and post-capillary PH, whereas PAWP ≤15 mm Hg (or ≤12 mm Hg) indicates pre-capillary PH.[12] If a direct LVEDP measurement is performed, greater than 15 mm Hg is generally used to diagnose post-capillary PH (see section below on performing cardiac catheterization).

The most common form of PH that cardiologists will encounter in contemporary medical practice is in the setting of left heart disease. This includes patients with left ventricular systolic or diastolic dysfunction, mitral valvular disease of any type, stiff left atrial syndrome, and LV outflow tract or aortic valvular lesions, including obstructive hypertrophic cardiomyopathy. Virtually any left heart structural or functional abnormality from the ascending aorta to pulmonary venous bed may predispose patients to post-capillary PH. Thus, traditional risk factors for coronary artery disease, cardiomyopathy, left-sided structural heart disease, and mitral/aortic valvular heart disease are implicated directly or indirectly as PH risk factors as well. Notable examples include obstructive sleep apnea (OSA), tobacco use, connective tissue disease, and prior or active cardiotoxic chemotherapy. Processes that promote pathological remodeling of pulmonary arterials proximal to the lung capillary interface predispose patients to pre-capillary PH. Broadly, this encompasses patients with PAH, hypoxic lung or sleep disordered breathing conditions, and chronic thromboembolic pulmonary hypertension (CTEPH).

The prognostic implications of elevated mPAP have been affirmed in numerous studies involving patients with PH from almost all etiologies, particularly heart failure with reduced LV ejection fraction (HFrEF), mitral stenosis, idiopathic pulmonary fibrosis, chronic obstructive pulmonary disease (COPD), and sickle cell disease.[15,16] Nonetheless, physiological or easily reversible causes of mPAP greater than 20 mm Hg have been reported, such as anemia, pregnancy, and increased pulmonary blood flow states (e.g., highly conditioned athletes). To address this dilemma, PVR is used as a hemodynamic surrogate of pulmonary vascular disease, and the addition of PVR to mPAP increases the specificity of diagnosing PH compared to mPAP alone. A cut-off PVR equal to or greater than 3.0 Wood units (WU) distinguishes pulmonary vascular disease in PH patients; however, this demarcation is largely historical or based on observational studies in selected subgroups, such as those with idiopathic PAH, congenital heart defects with intracardiac shunt, and pulmonary fibrosis. Emergent data on the spectrum of PVR associated with adverse outcome suggests that greater than 2.2 WU may be sufficient to identify a pathogenic rise in mPAP, which differs in magnitude between pre- and post-capillary PH patients (**eFig. 88.1**).[17] Combined pre- and post-capillary PH is an overlapping pathophenotype that is characterized by pulmonary arterial remodeling due to chronic pulmonary venous hypertension, and in these patients mPAP

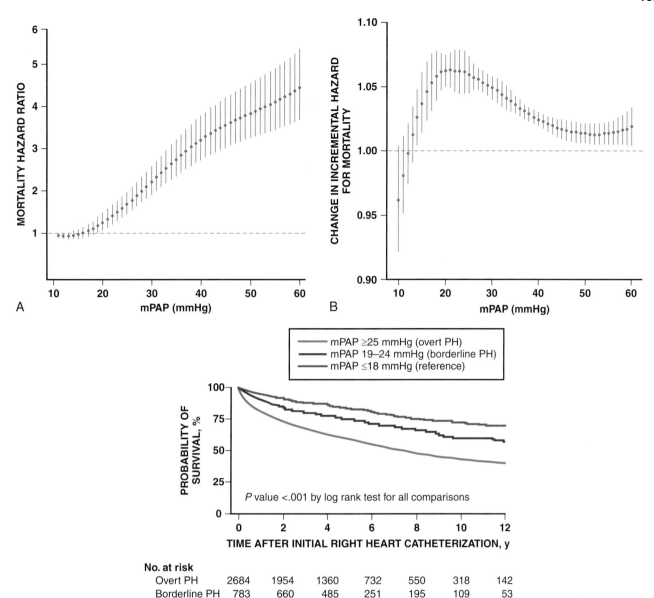

FIGURE 88.2 The association between pulmonary artery pressure and mortality. **A,** Data from a U.S. national cohort of patients referred for right heart catheterization were collected and the mean pulmonary artery pressure (mPAP) was modeled as a continuous variable. The association between all-cause mortality and mPAP emerges approximately 19 mm Hg and increases through approximately 60 mm Hg. **B,** Compared to mPAP levels at the high end of the continuum, an incremental increase by 1 mm Hg between approximately 20 and 25 mm Hg is associated with a greater change in clinical risk. **C,** The relationship between mildly elevated mPAP (>19 mm Hg) and adverse clinical outcome has been validated in several populations, demonstrated here by a Kaplan Meier analysis from patients referred for right heart catheterization (RHC) at Vanderbilt University. *PH,* Pulmonary hypertension. (**A** and **B** from Maron BA et al. *Circulation* 2016;133:1240–1248; **C** from Assad TR et al. *JAMA Cardiol* 2017;2:1361–1368.)

greater than 20 mm Hg, PAWP greater than 15 mm Hg, and PVR equal to or greater than 3.0 WU is used for diagnosis (see Table 88.1).[12]

Isolated Post-Capillary Pulmonary Hypertension Clinical Classifications
Heart Failure and Cardiomyopathy

The prevalence of PH in HFrEF populations is 30% to 50% when considering a pulmonary artery systolic pressure (PASP) cut-off greater than 45 mm Hg estimated echocardiographically.[18] This corresponds to a mPAP approximately 30 mm Hg, using the conversion method of Syyed: mPAP = 0.65 × PASP + 0.55 mm Hg. A stepwise increase in mortality risk of 6% to 8% is generally observed per 5 mm Hg rise in PASP. Catheter-based studies, which may be subject to referral bias, indicate that PH is present in 62% to 77% of HFrEF patients. Compared to idiopathic cardiomyopathy, patients with ischemic, infiltrative, hypertensive, or substance abuse cardiomyopathy tend to have higher mPAP at diagnosis. The adjusted mortality risk per 5 mm Hg

increase in mPAP is 85% in myocarditis compared to non-myocarditis patients.

In heart failure with preserved LV ejection fraction (HFpEF), the prevalence of PH is substantial and of greater clinical risk.[19] By some estimates, approximately 80% of HFpEF patients have PH (defined by an estimated PASP >35 mm Hg), which correlates with PAWP, and associates with a 30% mortality risk increase per 10 mm Hg PASP. Population studies in which RHC was used to directly measure cardiopulmonary hemodynamics suggest that more than half of patients have mPAP greater than 25 mm Hg, and compared to non-PH counterparts this group is at 33% higher risk for heart failure hospitalization rates. In obstructive hypertrophic cardiomyopathy, PH is observed in over half of patients referred for anterior septal myectomy.[20]

Valvular Heart Disease

The spectrum of PH severity reported in valvular heart disease is wide, which akin to data in cardiomyopathy patients is likely due to variable patient selection, method of assessment, and study enrollment criteria.[21,22] Across echocardiographic and RHC population studies, between 30% and 36% of asymptomatic aortic stenosis patients have at least mild PH, with severe PH observed in 20% of affected patients. In mitral stenosis, PH affects greater than 50% of patients, tracks strongly with symptoms, is a key determinant of management, and prognosticates outcome. Mitral stenosis patients with PASP greater than 60 mm Hg, for example, have a higher long-term rate of restenosis following mitral balloon valvuloplasty, and decreased 3-year survival following valvotomy compared to similar patients without severe PH. There is a positive association between mitral regurgitation grade and regurgitant orifice area with PASP. Moderate or severe PH is observed in greater than 50% of patients with severe primary mitral regurgitation, and is higher in subgroups with increased symptom burden. The average 5-year survival rate among primary mitral regurgitation patients is 25% less with PH compared to similar patients without PH. In secondary mitral valvular regurgitation, PH prevalence aligns with findings from HFrEF, in which approximately 40% of patients are affected. Stiff left atrial syndrome is probably underrecognized clinically, and certainly overlooked as a cause of PH even though impaired atrial compliance is a direct determinant of pulmonary venous congestion.[23]

Pre-Capillary Pulmonary Hypertension Clinical Classifications

Pulmonary Arterial Hypertension

Most PAH is idiopathic (iPAH) and prevalence depends somewhat on the methods for collecting population data. In studies from France, United Kingdom, Spain, Scotland, United States, and Ireland, the PAH prevalence is approximately 15 to 52 in 1 million population with an incidence of 2.4 to 7.1 cases per million per year.[24] The clinical profile of prevalent patients has evolved substantially since the initial NIH registry of PAH between 1981 and 1986. In that study, the mean age was 36 ± 15 years and the female to male ratio was 1.7.[1] Then, descriptions of PAH focused on women of childbearing age with connective tissue disease. However, modern registries suggest PAH affects patients across a broader age range: the Registry to Evaluate Early And Long-term PAH disease management (REVEAL),[25] inclusive of 54 U.S. centers, reported age at enrollment of 53 ± 15 years. Although the case distribution by gender remains stable compared with earlier reports, men tend to present with more severe disease burden compared with women, especially when diagnosis is made before age 45.[26,27] The female-predominant prevalence of PAH appears to be greater in black patients, although it remains unclear if this reflects a true racial trend or bias in access to care, or other factors.

Longitudinal outcome data from the NIH registry was in the era prior to pulmonary vasodilator therapies, and treatment was limited mainly to digoxin and diuretics. Accordingly, prognosis was dismal: the 1-, 3-, and 5-year survival rates were 68%, 48%, and 34%, respectively. Today, the 3-year survival approaches 84% in cross-sectional studies among patients treated with multiple drugs, although lifespan and quality of life remain greatly limited in most PAH patients.[28]

Hereditary Pulmonary Artery Hypertension

In 2001, Drs. John Newman and Jim Loyd and colleagues reported that a T354G variant in the *BMPR2* gene was common to 6 of 10 PAH patients across 5 subfamilies with affected members (reviewed in ref. 29). This large kindred genotype analysis gave rise to the field of hereditary PAH, which is a term that includes familial PAH (e.g., two or more affected family members) and simplex PAH (e.g., single occurrence in a family) when a pathogenic variant has been identified. Today, a BMRP2 variant is recognized as the most common genetic risk factor for PAH, identifiable in 70% of families with PAH and 10% of sporadic iPAH cases. However, a

TABLE 88.3 Key Genes Implicated in the Pathogenesis of Pulmonary Arterial Hypertension

GENES	NAME	BIOFUNCTIONALITY/PATHOGENICITY	CLINICAL PHENOTYPE
BMPR2	Bone Morphogenetic Protein Receptor Type 2	Pulmonary artery smooth muscle cell proliferation	Hereditary/familial PAH (germline)
		Endothelial dysfunction	PAH (de novo)
		Apoptosis-resistance	
		Dysregulated cellular metabolism	
ACVRL1	Activin A Receptor Like Type 1	Cell-surface receptor for the TGF-β superfamily of ligands	PAH associated with Hemorrhagic telangiectasia type 2
ENG	Endoglin	Regulates endothelial binding of TGF-β-1 and β-1 peptides	PAH associated with Hemorrhagic telangiectasia type 2
EIF2AK4	Eukaryotic Translation Initiation Factor 2 Alpha Kinase 4	Intimal fibrosis	Pulmonary venoocclusive disease
		Endothelial proliferation	Pulmonary capillary hemangiomatosis
GDF2	Growth differentiation factor 2	Regulates vascular quiescence	Hereditary/familial PAH
		Anti-apoptotic	
		Anti-proliferative	
		Inhibits vascular permeability	
TBX4	T-Box Transcription Factor 4	Developmental processes	Pediatric PAH
			Associated with small patella syndrome
ATP13A3	ATPase Family Homolog Up-Regulated In Senescence Cells 1	Cellular senescence	iPAH
SOX17	SRY-box 17	Erk an Wnt signaling	iPAH
		Immune response	
AQP1	Aquaporin 1	Pulmonary arterial smooth muscle cell migration and proliferation	Hereditary/familial PAH
		β-catenin signaling	
CAV1	Caveolin-1	Regulates physical colocalization of BMP receptors	Hereditary/familial PAH
		TGF-β signaling	
KCNK3	Potassium channel subfamily K member 3	Regulates membrane potential	Hereditary/familial PAH iPAH
		Vascular tone	

iPAH, Idiopathic pulmonary arterial hypertension; *TGF-β*, transforming growth factor-beta.

variant in any of 12 genes is considered pathogenic in PAH (Table 88.3), and evidence exists to implicate the involvement of 5 other potential genes.[29] Notable examples include variants in *ENG* and *ACVRL1* that code for endoglin and activin receptor-like kinase 1 (ALK-1), respectively, which are linked mechanistically to dysfunctional BMPR-2 and implicated in hereditary hemorrhagic telangiectasia-PAH. Most variants, including those affecting the BMPR-2 gene, are inherited in an autosomal dominant pattern, but exhibit reduced penetrance. Overall, fewer than 30% of PAH patients have single variants in causative genes.

Toxin-Induced Pulmonary Artery Hypertension

There is an established association between PAH and the anorexigens fenfluramine and dexfenfluramine, resulting in the discontinuation of these drugs for public use in 1997. Illicit methamphetamine use (in many cases leading to addiction), is a newly recognized worldwide epidemic affecting greater than 1% of the population aged 15 to 64 years in the United States, Australia, South Africa, and the United Kingdom among other countries (Fig. 88.3). Methamphetamines may account for up to 18% of non-idiopathic PAH, but data on the true prevalence of this population are lacking.[30] Pulmonary vascular remodeling from a mechanical injury induced by the drug packing material or as a result of molecular interactions with drug metabolites are proposed to cause PAH. Based on available data, the prognosis for methamphetamine PAH is concerning with a twofold risk of clinical worsening compared to iPAH and event-free survival at 5 years of 47%. The tyrosine kinase inhibitor dasatinib is associated with PAH, although this is unlikely a drug class effect.

Systemic Sclerosis with Pulmonary Artery Hypertension

Connective tissue disease-associated PAH accounts for approximately one in four cases of PAH overall, with systemic sclerosis (SSc) as the most common subtype. The overall prevalence of SSc-PAH is likely underestimated, but is at least 24 cases per million, which again is far greater than iPAH. Among SSc patients, the prevalence of PAH is 12% and up to 20% in patients with evidence of impaired lung diffusion capacity. However, PAH is the leading cause of death in SSc, and the mortality rate is fourfold greater than for iPAH.[31] The overall SSc syndrome includes immune dysfunction, inflammation, increased extracellular matrix remodeling, and fibrosis resulting in multiorgan injury, which provides a pathobiological basis for pulmonary vascular involvement. Although PAH may be observed in either the diffuse or limited cutaneous SSc subtypes, interstitial lung disease (pulmonary fibrosis) is particularly common in diffuse SSc. Therefore, it is important to determine if abnormal cardiopulmonary hemodynamics are in the setting of SSc-PAH or, conversely, due to PH from interstitial lung disease.

Infectious Pulmonary Artery Hypertension Subtypes

Schistosomiasis is a flatworm fluke parasite endemic to 52 countries, particularly Brazil and African nations, infecting between 200 and 300 million worldwide.[32] *Schistosomiasis mansoni* has a mandatory two-host life cycle that includes avian and snail. The cercariae are released by snail into fresh water, and gain access to humans via transdermal penetration. The result is an immune complex hypersensitivity reaction (i.e., Katayama fever) which self-resolves over 4 to 6 weeks. However, the worms mate in the portal circulation and the eggs themselves are transported to the pulmonary vasculature where granulomatous remodeling ensues resulting in a PAH clinical syndrome. The actual prevalence of Schistosomiasis-PAH is not known, but this is undoubtedly the most common cause of precapillary PH in developing countries. Pre-existing hepatosplenic disease increases PAH risk of infected hosts exponentially.

Pulmonary vascular dysfunction is a well-documented complication of human immunodeficiency virus (HIV), although uncertainty persists on the extent to which PAH, rather than elevated pulmonary artery pressure due to comorbid or iatrogenic causes, explain dyspnea or PH. From 7648 consecutive HIV-positive adults in France, 0.46% had PAH confirmed by RHC. Within HIV populations, the odds ratio of increased pulmonary artery pressure is 1.27 and 1.28 in patients with viral load greater than 500 copies/mL and CD4 cell count less than 200 cells/µL, respectively, which is associated with a risk-adjusted mortality increase of 78%.[33] Convincing evidence to suggest the virus directly infects pulmonary vascular cells is lacking, although vascular injury induced by viral proteins is plausible. Reports early in the COVID-19 pandemic suggest pulmonary vascular involvement in some patients, including key features consistent with end-stage disease such as frank right heart failure.[34] Understanding the longitudinal implications of COVID-19 on the development of PH, however, remain forthcoming.

Congenital Heart Disease

Pathogenic pulmonary vascular remodeling may develop in any patient with a large volume left-to-right intra- or extra-cardiac shunt, or an anatomic catastrophe that affects inflow or outflow (see Chapter 82). From a Dutch nationwide epidemiological study over a 15-year period, PH was reported in 63.7 per million children, which included 34% that had shunts amenable to immediate surgical correction. Among those patients with long-term PAH, 72% had a form of congenital heart disease.[35] As congenital heart disease patients

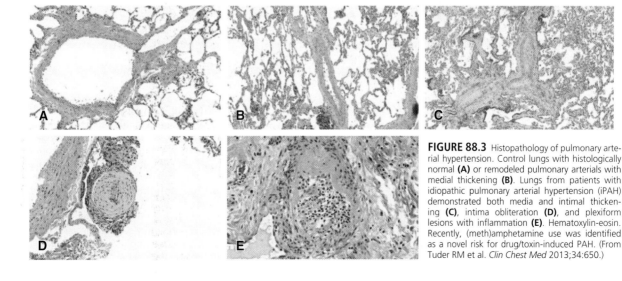

FIGURE 88.3 Histopathology of pulmonary arterial hypertension. Control lungs with histologically normal **(A)** or remodeled pulmonary arterials with medial thickening **(B)**. Lungs from patients with idiopathic pulmonary arterial hypertension (iPAH) demonstrated both media and intimal thickening **(C)**, intima obliteration **(D)**, and plexiform lesions with inflammation **(E)**. Hematoxylin-eosin. Recently, (meth)amphetamine use was identified as a novel risk for drug/toxin-induced PAH. (From Tuder RM et al. *Clin Chest Med* 2013;34:650.)

continue to live longer into adulthood, PAH will remain an important consideration for clinicians managing these patients. Indeed, cases discovered in the greater than or equal to seventh decade of life are well documented.

Lung Disease and Sleep Disordered Breathing

Approximately 90% of COPD patients have mPAP greater than 20 mm Hg, but only 5% have mPAP greater than 40 mm Hg.[36] Thus, severe PH in COPD is uncommon but when present is a risk factor for *cor pulmonale*. Similarly, PH is reported in 8% to 15% of mild idiopathic pulmonary fibrosis but may affect two-thirds of end-stage patients. Chronic PH is an uncommon manifestation of OSA, is almost always mild, and may be reversible with noninvasive ventilation (see Chapter 89). Nonetheless, given the expanding rate of obesity in the United States and other industrialized countries, OSA is an important and often overlooked PH risk factor.

Chronic Thromboembolic Pulmonary Hypertension

Thrombotic in situ pulmonary vascular remodeling resulting in PH occurs in approximately 3% of patients following luminal pulmonary embolism (see Chapter 87). Risk factors for developing CTEPH are not known, although elevated levels of factor VIII have been demonstrated in about 40% of patients. The clinical burden of CTEPH is mitigated fully in patients who are eligible and undergo successful surgical pulmonary thromboendarterectomy, which represents approximately two-thirds of patients. Surgical, medical, and percutaneous therapies for CTEPH are discussed below.

Pulmonary Venoocclusive Disease

Muscularization and sclerotic changes of pulmonary venules are the cornerstone findings of pulmonary venoocclusive disease (PVOD), which has an estimated annual incidence of 0.1 to 0.2 per million people.[37] Risk factors include auto-immune disorders, organic solvent exposure, medical therapy with alkylating agents (particularly mitomycin and cyclophosphamide), and certain genetic predispositions. No gender predominance has been established for the prevalence of PVOD.

Portopulmonary Hypertension

Portal hypertension with pre-capillary PH and PVR equal to or greater than 3.0 WU defines portopulmonary hypertension. Approximately 5% of cirrhotic patients have PH, although the prevalence is 16% in liver transplant referral populations. The detrimental effects of high CO and endotoxin release from liver dysfunction are proposed to underlie portopulmonary hypertension.[38] This is distinct from hepatopulmonary syndrome, for which hypoxemia from intrapulmonary vasodilation and impaired hypoxic vasoconstriction (without PH) is the hallmark feature.

Combined Pre- and Post-Capillary Pulmonary Hypertension
Left Heart Structural and Functional Disorders

Elevated PVR in patients with post-capillary PH is observed in many of the same circumstances associated with isolated post-capillary PH. Thus, there is overlap in the risk factors between these phenotypes, including diabetes mellitus; causes of LV dysfunction such as ischemic heart disease; valvular disease; and HFpEF. Although the genetic profile between these groups differs, it is not clear how genetic risk may protect or predispose to either clinical phenotype.[39] The combined pre-/post-capillary PH phenotype accounts for approximately 15% of all PH patients, although outcome is similar between this group and isolated post-capillary PH patients.[12,39]

PATHOLOGY

All forms of persistent PH are associated with pathogenic vascular remodeling, and most subtypes involve hypertrophic concentric muscularization, as well as fibrotic and (micro)thrombotic effacement of

distal pulmonary arterials. The main-, lobar-, and intra-lobar pulmonary arteries are usually phenotypically normal. Exceptions to this include congenital pulmonary stenosis, and proximal pulmonary arterial involvement in patients with CTEPH. In iPAH, certain forms of congenital heart disease, HIV-PAH, and Schistosomiasis-PAH there is a unique plexogenic vasculopathy (see Fig. 88.3). These focal but dense lesions are characterized by endothelial proliferation, the formation of microchannel networks, and irregular smooth muscle cell orientation in a glomeruloid pattern. The functional significance of these malformations is contested, but, nonetheless, their appearance is pathognomonic for PAH on autopsy.

Pulmonary venous remodeling is a classic feature of PVOD, which is a rare form of PH that overlaps histopathologically with pulmonary capillary hemangiomatosis (PCH). In both PVOD and PCH, arterial medial hypertrophy and/or intimal fibrosis, hemosiderosis, venulitis, and mild lymphocytic infiltrate are observed. In PVOD, obliteration of small pulmonary veins occurs due to sclerotic and fibrous thickening. A biallelic mutation in the *EIF2AK4* gene is associated with PVOD, and although chest radiation or other toxic exposures are related weakly to prevalence, definitive risk factors are lacking.[29] Autopsy specimens from patients with left heart failure show increased arterialization of pulmonary veins, including medial and intimal thickening that is largely concentric, and variable within the lung. These remodeling patterns correlate strongly with pulmonary artery pressure, providing a histopathological basis for the combined pre- and post-capillary PH hemodynamic pattern observed in some HFpEF and HFrEF patients.[8]

Unique pathology of CTEPH. Organized clot, defined by heavily fibrotic and obstructive lesions involving the intima and medial layers of distal pulmonary arterials, is a cornerstone feature of CTEPH. Strictures, webbing, dearborization, and collateralization with bronchial arterials is often also observed. It is important to note that vascular segments distal to the site of initial embolic injury are involved commonly, raising speculation that a propagative vasculopathy ultimately underlies the complete CTEPH pathophenotype.

PATHOBIOLOGY

The molecular basis of PAH is complex, and in blood vessels driven by interplay between signaling pathways that involve pulmonary artery endothelial cells, smooth muscle cells, pericytes, and adventitial fibroblasts (Fig. 88.4). Dysregulated cellular metabolism, specifically the preferential synthesis of lactic acid even under oxygen-rich circumstances (Warburg effect), apoptosis-resistance, post-transcriptional regulation of pro-fibrotic proteins, and epigenetic events underlie pathogenic changes to the ultrastructure of pulmonary arterioles.[40] A unifying, inciting trigger that perturbs vasoactive signaling pathways across patients is unlikely. Instead, susceptibility, in part genetic, to maladaptive responses following a stressor is more likely. Abnormalities in T cell (Treg cell)-dependent self-tolerance in PAH following an inflammatory insult leads to vascular infiltration of macrophages, mast cells, and B cells. This pathway may explain some forms of PAH, such as in HIV and SSc.

Activation of hypoxia signaling pathways (even in the absence of frank hypoxemia), nutritional (vitamin C) deficiencies, toxins, and other acquired risk factors stimulate pathogenetic events through alternative pathways. The accumulation of vascular reactive oxygen species is implicated in numerous maladaptive events that drive the PAH pathophenotype. For example, mitochondrial dysfunction perturbs the redox balance of pulmonary artery smooth muscle cells following hypoxia inducible factor (HIF)-1α stimulation, and increases cell survival through dynamin related protein-1/cyclin B1 signaling. Oxidative post-translational modification of a functionally essential cysteine in the SMAD3 docking region of NEDD9 results in pulmonary endothelial fibrillar collagen deposition and is identified recently as a potentially modifiable molecular mediator of PAH.[41] A predilection to metabolic dysfunction and overactivation of neurohumoral systems underlies the pathobiology of PAH (Fig. 88.5).

GENE-ENVIRONMENT INTERACTIONS

BMPR2 and other mutations
Impaired BMPR-II signaling
SNPs of: SERT, Kv1.5, and TRPC6
Epigenetic (DNMT, HDAC, MiRNA)
Sex hormone imbalance

Environmental triggers:
Anorexigens
Amphetamines
HIV
Schistosomiasis

PAH

BLOOD

Platelets
Th2
Treg
Macrophages
NK cells

↑ Platelet activation and serotonin release
ET-1/TxA2/NO+PGI$_2$
Adrenomedullin/BNP
Autoantibodies, growth factors
Cytokines (IL-6, MCP-1), NFkB

↑ **Vasoconstriction, inflammation, thrombosis**

INTIMA
ENDOTHELIUM

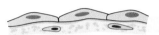

↓ VIP, NO+PGI$_2$, PPAR

↑ *Tissue factor, ADMA*
VIP receptors, PDGFR
PKM2

↑ Warburg metabolism
Thrombosis
Constrictors/dilatators
Proliferation/apoptosis

Endothelial dysfunction

MEDIA
SMOOTH MUSCLE CELLS

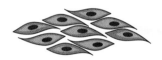

Kv1.5/2.1, PPAR, APoE
↓ Mitofusion2 (mitochondrial fusion)
MCUC function (mitochondrial Ca^{2+})
SOD2/PDH activity

↑ *Drp 1 (fission)*
HIF-1α, NFAT, and PDK
Survivin, 5-HHT, PDGF
Rho kinase, TRPC-6
Phosphodiesterase 5

↑ Warburg metabolism
Mitochondrial fission
Depolarized Ca^{2+} overloaded,
  Ca^{2+} sensitized proliferation/
  migration/apoptosis resistance

Vasoconstriction, vascular obstruction

ADVENTITIA
FIBROBLASTS

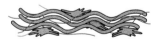

Collagen
Elastin

↑ *PKM2*
Elastase/MMP/tenascin
Inflammation (IL-6, MCP-1, NFkB)
Progenitor cells (+/–)
Proliferating fibroblasts
Adipocytokine: TNF-α, IL-6 ((APN)

↑ Warburg metabolism drives
  fibroblasts proliferation/
  migration and inflammatory
  cell influx
Elastin fragmentation

Fibrosis, vascular stiffening

RIGHT VENTRICLE

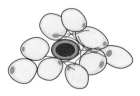

↓ Blood supply (ischemia/hibernation)
SERCA2A
Junctophilin 2

↑ *Mitochondrial fission*
Glycolysis
Adrenergic activation, fibrosis

↑ Warburg metabolism
T-tubule disarray
Fibrosis

↓ Contractility

RV-PA coupling
RV failure

FIGURE 88.4 FOR LEGEND SEE PAGE 1664.

FIGURE 88.4 Mechanisms implicated in pathogenesis of pulmonary arterial hypertension (PAH). PAH is a panvasculopathy, meaning that all layers of the vascular wall are involved. PAH is also reflective of gene environment interactions and has important genetic and epigenetic mechanisms. This figure shows abnormalities in the gene environment, blood, and each layer of the pulmonary artery, from intima (endothelial cells) to media (pulmonary arterial smooth muscle cells—PASMCs) to adventitia (fibroblasts). Because of the many reports that inform this composite figure, individual sources for the information are not referenced. The normal state is shown on the left side, the abnormalities that occur in PAH are highlighted in the middle section, and the consequences of these abnormalities are shown on the right. The net effect of these abnormalities is a state of vasoconstriction, inflammation, thrombosis with a hyperproliferative, apoptosis-resistant PASMC population, which promotes vasoconstriction and vascular obstruction, and excessive fibrosis, which reduces vascular compliance. These vascular changes ultimately increase RV afterload and impair RV-pulmonary artery coupling, leading to RV failure. *5-HHT*, 5 hydroxytryptamine; *ADMA*, asymmetric dimethylarginine; *APN*, adiponectin; *BMPR2*, bone morphogenetic protein receptor 2; *BNP*, brain natriuretic peptide; *Ca²⁺*, calcium; *DNAMT*, DNA methyltransferase; *Drp-1*, dynamin related protein 1; *ET-1*, endothelin-1; *HDAC*, histone deacetylases; *HIF*, hypoxia inducible factor; *IL*, interleukin; *MCP-1*, monocyte chemoattractant protein-1; *MCUC*, mitochondrial calcium uniporter complex; *miRNA*, micro RNA; *MMP*, matrix metalloproteinase; *NFAT*, nuclear factor of activated T cells; *NF-κB*, nuclear factor kappa light chain enhancer of activated B cells; *NK*, natural killer cells; *NO*, nitric oxide; *PDGFR*, platelet derived growth factor receptor; *PDGR*, platelet derived growth factor; *PDH*, pyruvate dehydrogenase; *PDK*, pyruvate dehydrogenase kinase; *PGI₂*, prostacyclin-I₂; *PKM-2*, pyruvate kinase M2; *PPAR*, peroxisome proliferator activated receptor; *SERCA*, sarco-endoplasmic reticulum Ca²⁺ ATPase; *SERT*, serotonin transporter; *SNP*, single nucleotide polymorphism; *SOD*, superoxide dismutase; *Th2*, T helper cells; *TNF*, tumor necrosis factor; *T-reg*, regulatory T cells; *TRPC*, transient receptor potential cation channel; *TxA2*, thromboxane A2; *VIP*, vasoactive intestinal peptide. (From Thenappan T et al. *BMJ* 2018;360:5492.)

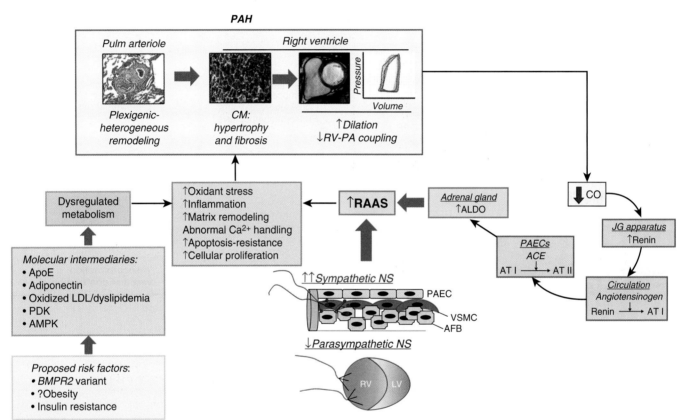

FIGURE 88.5 Dysregulated neurohumoral and metabolic signaling promote pulmonary arterial hypertension (PAH). Acquired and genetic risk factors predispose to dysregulated cellular metabolism involving pulmonary artery endothelial cells, pulmonary artery smooth muscle cells, and right ventricular (RV) cardiomyocytes. This induces various intermediate pathophenotypes involved in the progression of PAH (*red box*). Similarly, chronic elevation in RV afterload in PAH results in cavitary dilation and impaired efficiency, including decreased right ventricular–pulmonary arterial (RV–PA) coupling. A decrease in cardiac output up–regulates the renin–angiotensin–aldosterone system (RAAS), which is independently associated with cardiovascular remodeling and PAH progression. Abnormal sympathetic and parasympathetic nervous system (NS) increase pulmonary arterial tone and impair RV diastolic function, respectively, although the precise cellular targets modulating these effects remain incompletely characterized. *AFB*, Adventitial fibroblast; *ApoE*, apolipoprotein E; *Ang*, angiotensin; *BPMR2*, bone morphogenetic protein receptor–2; *CM*, cardiomyocyte; *CO*, cardiac output; *JG*, juxtaglomerular; *LV*, left ventricle; *PAEC*, pulmonary artery endothelial cell; *PDK*, pyruvate dehydrogenase kinase; *VSMC*, vascular smooth muscle cell. (From Maron BA et al. *Br J Pharmacol* 2020;177:1457–1471.)

ENDOTHELIN-1

Endothelin-1 (ET-1) is a 21-amino acid vasoactive peptide secreted from the endothelium and targets two G-protein coupled receptor isoforms. In pulmonary artery smooth muscle cells, simulation of the ET_A receptors by ET-1 leads to phospholipase C-β activation and subsequent increases in intracellular calcium (Ca^{2+}) bioavailability or, alternatively, influx of Ca^{2+} through plasma membrane channels. This mechanism induces an extremely potent vasoconstrictor as well as pro-mitogenic response. In pulmonary artery endothelial cells, stimulation of the ET_B-receptor activates endothelial nitric oxide synthase and subsequent nitric oxide (NO·) synthesis. Overall, these vasoconstrictor/pro-proliferative effects of ET_A-dependent signaling dominate ET-1 biofunctionality in pulmonary arterials. It is notable that increased ET-1 is not exclusive to PAH; in left heart failure there is a parabolic, positive association between ET-1 concentration and pulmonary artery pressure thereby implicating vascular congestion in the pulmonary release of ET-1.

PROSTAGLANDIN-I₂

Prostaglandin-I₂ (PGI₂) is a potential vasodilator, anti-platelet, and anti-inflammatory biochemical derivative of arachidonic acid, which under normal conditions is released from the endothelial membrane following phospholipid hydrolysis by phospholipase A2 in a reaction that requires cyclooxygenase. In PAH, endothelial dysfunction causes a depletion of bioactive PGI₂, which is associated with increased vascular tone and microthrombus. Additionally, 5-lipooxygenase, 5-hydroperoxyeicosatetraenoic acid, and leukotriene A₄ are lipoxygenase-dependent arachidonic acid metabolites that increase pulmonary vascular tone, induce pulmonary artery smooth muscle cells chemotaxis, and recruit mast cells.

NITRIC OXIDE

Activation of the heterodimeric protein soluble guanylyl cyclase in pulmonary artery smooth muscle cells by NO· results in the conversion of guanosine-5′-triphosphate (GTP) to the second messenger molecule cyclic guanosine monophosphate (cGMP). In turn, cGMP is either hydrolyzed to inactive 5′-GMP by the phosphodiesterase type-V (PDE-V) enzyme isoform, or stimulates protein kinase G-dependent blood vessel relaxation, platelet inhibition, and transcriptional changes that regulate ion channel conductance and cell survival favorably. In PAH and most other forms of PH, bioavailable NO· is decreased due to impaired endothelial nitric oxide synthase activity or via a scavenger effect by reactive oxygen species that converts NO· to peroxynitrite ($ONOO^-$) and other higher oxidative species.

SEROTONIN

This neurotransmitter is synthesized primarily by enterochromaffin cells of the gut from L-tryptophan, and is metabolized primarily by the liver (first pass) and lung.[42] However, expression of pulmonary endothelial tryptophan hydroxylase, which catalyzes the first step in serotonin synthesis, is increased in PAH and endothelial serotonin targets pulmonary artery smooth muscle cells via paracrine signaling to promote vasoconstriction, proliferation, mitogenesis, and inhibition of bone morphogenetic protein (BMP) signaling. Patients with PAH also have increased serotonin, and anorexigenic-PAH was described originally in the context of serotonergic weight-loss drugs (e.g., fenfluramine).

PATHOPHYSIOLOGY

The pulmonary vascular bed is a parallel circuit densely packed with blood vessels, evolved to maximize surface area for gas exchange at the alveolar interface, and is, therefore, a high-flow, low-resistance system. Pathogenic changes in the architecture of pulmonary arterials causes an early decline in pulmonary arterial compliance (RV stroke volume/pulmonary artery pulse pressure) prior to elevation in PVR, ultimately leading to increased pulmonary artery blood pressure.[43] It is important to recognize that pressure in the pulmonary circuit is determined, in part, by RV contractility. If RV failure is present, pulmonary artery pressure may be only mildly elevated despite severe pulmonary vascular remodeling (Fig. 88.6A). Alternatively, mildly elevated mPAP is observed in some physiological or immediately reversible states. Thus, staging PAH (and many forms of PH) is accomplished by considering PVR, which is related inversely to CO and may be viewed as an indirect hemodynamic surrogate of arterial remodeling severity.

Right Ventricular Dysfunction

The importance of RV performance in PH pathophysiology cannot be overemphasized, because diminished systolic function, decreased ejection fraction, cavitary dilation, and in some cases hypertrophy are prognostic for adverse outcome. In contrast to the LV, the RV is triangular, contracts in a predominately longitudinal plane, and is not governed by classical Frank-Starling mechanics. Furthermore, physiologic parameters familiar to anticipating load-dependent changes in LV contractility do not depict intrinsic RV function. Instead, understanding and predicting RV function hinges on the concept of efficient energy utilization. Specifically, the extent to which RV cardiac function and pulmonary vascular blood flow are matched is of central importance. Broadly, this is determined by the contribution of RV contractility that is dedicated to perfusing the lungs relative to RV work needed to maintain intravascular pulmonary arterial pressure. This relationship is referred to as RV-PA coupling (Fig. 88.6B).

Constructing the RV-PA coupling relationship requires direct measurement of the RV pressure-volume relationship, from which the end-systolic elastance (Ees) is determined by the slope of the end-systolic pressure versus the end-systolic volume.[44] Ventricular afterload is estimated from the pressure-volume relationship as arterial elastance (Ea), which is a measure of intrinsic (i.e., ventricular-independent) PVR. The Ees/Ea ratio quantifies RV-PA coupling. With increasing PVR, hypertrophic RV remodeling permits a matched increase in contractility. Ultimately, further hypertrophy is not possible or contra-productive. Cavitary dilation then ensues as a maladaptive response to defend stroke volume. In advanced-stage PH, the Ees/Ea ratio declines. Overall, the adult RV lacks pre-programmed molecular pathways that respond to pressure loading conditions in the same adaptive way that

is observed for the LV. It is important to recognize that RV dysfunction is observed as a consequence of pre-capillary, isolated post-capillary, and combined pre-/post-capillary PH.

Systemic Manifestations of Pulmonary Hypertension

The clinical phenotypic spectrum of PH, and, more specifically, PAH, has widened substantially in comparison to early reports focusing exclusively on pulmonary vascular remodeling. Regardless of the underlying cause, chronic RV dysfunction due to pulmonary vascular disease impacts nearly all organ systems.[2] In most cases, symptoms are secondary to end-organ damage from impaired CO that decreases perfusion in resistance (systemic) vascular beds. Examples include acute or exacerbation of chronic renal failure, leaky bowel syndrome, volitional muscle atrophy including diaphragmatic weakness, and cognitive impairment, or passive hepatic congestion due to elevated right atrial pressure. In PAH, neurohumoral overactivation, including increased circulating catecholamine levels and secondary hyperaldosteronism, associate with central cardiopulmonary hemodynamics and heart failure burden severity.[45] In turn, new onset depression, diabetes mellitus, and metabolic syndrome are common tertiary consequences of pulmonary vascular disease through impaired exercise tolerance or other life-limiting symptoms.

Beyond the secondary and tertiary manifestations of PH, it appears that some PAH subtypes involve primary but extra-pulmonary vascular mechanisms. Compared to iPAH, for example, patients with SSc-PAH demonstrate impaired RV-PA coupling at much lower RV afterload levels. This finding is linked to increased interstitial RV cardiac fibrosis and decreased maximal calcium-activated force, implying an intrinsic pathogenic feature of SSc-PAH that involves RV cardiomyocytes.[46] Other potential organs proposed in the primary PAH syndrome include (i) blood, by virtue of thrombocytopenia affecting 20% of PAH patients and microthrombosis observed at autopsy, and (ii) thyroid dysfunction, which is observed in up to approximately 25% of iPAH without a different explanation.[2]

PATIENT PRESENTATION AND CLINICAL ASSESSMENT

Patient Medical History

The presenting symptoms for PAH most often are shortness of breath, fatigue, abdominal distension, lower extremity edema, weakness, exercise limitation, or dyspnea with bending (bendopnea). Cardiac angina (due to either RV ischemia or left main coronary artery compression) and syncope (due to severely decreased CO) are high-risk presenting symptoms that are equivalent to a PAH emergency. Nevertheless, most PAH symptoms are nonspecific, which is a major barrier to timely diagnosis. In one-fifth of patients, the lag between initial presentation and diagnosis is greater than 2 years, particularly among those encountered before the age of 36 years. Pursuit of an explanation by which to account for symptoms in older patients may end after excluding more common cardiovascular diseases such as coronary artery disease, and PAH in often overlooked or misdiagnosed.

Physical Examination Findings

Although a "classic" physical examination for pulmonary hypertension (or PAH) does not exist, physicians should monitor for findings suggesting the presence or consequences of right-sided pressure and volume overload (see also Chapter 13). A loud or paradoxical P2 component of the second heart sound indicates accentuation of pulmonic closure. In severe PH, right-sided S3, RV lift, increased jugular venous pressure, and pulsatile liver may be observed. In cor pulmonale, decompensated right heart failure is the end-stage result of severe RV-PA uncoupling and should be considered in patients with systemic hypotension and cool lower extremities associated with severe functional limitation, heart failure symptoms at rest or with minimal activity, and/or mental status changes.

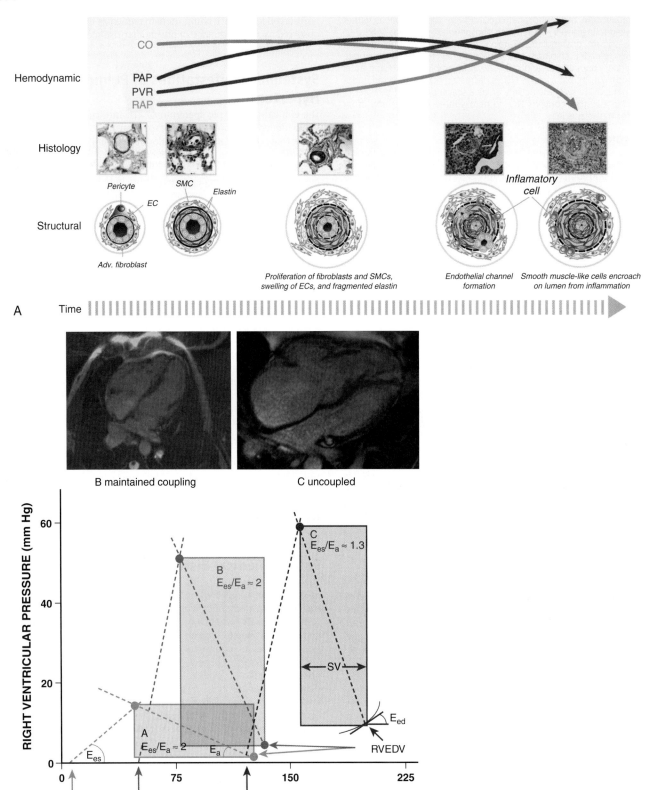

FIGURE 88.6 Hemodynamic and right ventricular pressure-volume relationship trajectory in pulmonary arterial hypertension. **A,** The trajectory of cardiopulmonary hemodynamics over time in patients with pulmonary arterial hypertension, overlaid with changes in the histology and structure of pulmonary arterials. (Adapted from Maron BA, et al. *Am J Respir Crit Care Med.* 2017;195:292–301.) **B** (*Top*), Right ventricular (RV) volumes at coupled stage and uncoupled stage in pulmonary hypertension (PH); (*Bottom*), Representative pressure-volume loops of control, PH with maintained coupling (early stage), and PH with increased RV volume. In regions *A* and *B*, E_{es}/E_a is within normal range, ventriculoarterial coupling is maintained, and wall stress is similar. In region *C*, volume is increased, E_{es}/E_a is decreased (uncoupling), and wall stress is increased. E_a, Measure of arterial load; E_{ed}, ventricular elastance at end-diastole; E_{es}, slope of the end-systolic pressure volume relation as a measure of RV contractility; *PVR*, pulmonary vascular resistance; *RVEDV*, right ventricular end-diastolic volume; *SV*, stroke volume; *Vd*, intercept with the volume axis. (From Vonk Noordegraaf A et al. *J Am Coll Cardiol* 2017;69:236–243.)

Approach to Diagnosis

The initial assessment of patients with suspected PH includes an electrocardiogram (ECG), chest roentgenogram, and echocardiogram (Fig. 88.7A–C).[38] In "real-world" practice, however, the possibility of PH is often deduced from results of these and other tests ordered for a different reason. Therefore, it is important to maintain a high clinical index of suspicion for PH when reviewing primary data and test results.

ECG. The pattern on ECG may indicate geometric changes in right heart structures such as right atrial enlargement or RV hypertrophy, which is suggested by an R/S ratio greater than 1 in lead V1 without other causes, or if the R wave amplitude in lead V1 is greater than 7 mm (see Chapter 14). An RV strain pattern (defined by RV hypertrophy with ST segment depression in V1 to V3) may be evident in advanced disease stages. In turn, LV hypertrophy and left atrial enlargement may point toward left heart disease PH rather than PAH.

Chest roentgenogram. The chest x-ray is abnormal in 90% of PAH patients, and findings include central pulmonary artery dilation, peripheral dearborization, right atrial and RV enlargement (see Chapter 17).[38] The presence of lung hyperinflation, pneumonia, or other features of primary lung disease, as well as features suggesting PE (e.g., Westermark sign, Hampton hump) may guide diagnosis.

Two-dimensional transthoracic echocardiography. Transthoracic echocardiography provides quantitative data noninvasively that is used to screen patients for PH, including PAH (see Chapter 16). However, this method *estimates* PASP by Doppler interrogation of a tricuspid regurgitant jet and does not determine right atrial pressure, PVR, or PAWP accurately, all of which are important for assessing PH clinically (Fig. 88.7D–G). In population studies, the Pearson correlation coefficient (r) for PASP estimated by echocardiography versus direct measurement using RHC (the gold standard diagnostic test, see below) ranges between 0.60 and 0.77 even when the two studies are performed in close temporal proximity. Wide chest anterior-posterior dimension, obstructive lung disease, and other factors that limit the acoustic windows may explain this finding. Furthermore, in one-third of patients with proven PH, a sufficient tricuspid jet is lacking and PASP is unmeasurable.[47] Thus, echocardiography alone is insufficient for diagnosing, classifying, and fully prognosticating patients.

Despite limitations associated with ultrasonographic assessment of hemodynamics, much key data on cardiac structure and function is acquired from echocardiography and useful in staging PH. For example, RV cavitary dilation, RV hypertrophy, hepatic vein dilation or blunted respirophasic dilation, and pericardial effusion inform right heart pathophysiology. Decreased pulmonary vascular distensibility results in the formation of a "notch" in the RV outflow tract Doppler envelope as well as decreased pulmonary artery acceleration time. When these are observed in the setting of a normal left atrial dimension, increased PVR greater than 3.0 WU may be present.

Because RV contraction occurs along a longitudinal rather than circumferential plane, calculating ejection fraction accurately from two-dimensional imaging is not possible. Instead, quantifying RV function can be accomplished by measuring "lunge" of the RV free wall at the level of the tricuspid valve. The tricuspid annular plane of systolic excursion (TAPSE) is generally measured in the apical 4-chamber view by aligning an M-mode cursor parallel to the RV free wall at the tricuspid annulus. The distance measured between end-diastole and end-systole is the TAPSE, and when ≤1.7 cm prognosticates adverse clinical outcome in PAH (Fig. 88.8H and I).[38] Other RV functional measures reported in PH assessment include longitudinal myocardial velocity (S'), fractional area change (FAC), Tei index speckle tracking, and ejection fraction by three-dimensional echocardiography (Table 88.4).

Left atrial diameter greater than 4.4 cm measured in the parasternal long axis view is often associated with left atrial hypertension, and this can be useful for calibrating the likelihood of PH from left heart disease. Agitated saline-enhanced echocardiography is warranted in patients with PH and structural cardiac abnormalities that predispose to intracardiac shunt or in whom unexplained hypoxemia is observed at rest or during exercise.

Pulmonary function tests and sleep study. Comorbid obstructive and restrictive lung disease is reported in up to 75% of cross-sectional populations enriched for prevalent cardiovascular diseases including heart failure, myocardial infarction, cardiac angina, and stroke. PH in patients with overlapping left heart and parenchymal lung disease is also common, and, therefore, it is important to consider diagnostic testing that characterizes lung structure and function in at-risk patients. Generally, pulmonary function test with spirometry and lung diffusion capacity of carbon monoxide (DLCO) is recommended in all patients suspected of PH. Patients with PAH may demonstrate modestly reduced lung volumes in the absence of marked obstructive, restrictive, or combined ventilatory defects that are more characteristic of parenchymal lung disease. Decreased DLCO is associated with pathogenic remodeling of the alveolar-capillary interface, and is therefore observed in PAH as well as many parenchymal lung diseases that do not include PH. Nonetheless, decreased DLCO is prognostic in PAH. OSA, which through hypoventilation predisposes to nocturnal

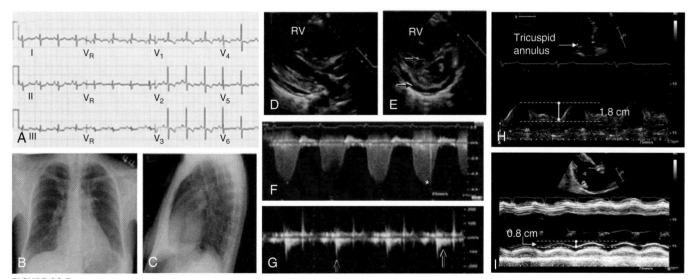

FIGURE 88.7 Representative findings from initial diagnostic tests in pulmonary arterial hypertension (PAH). Images obtained in a 43-year-old woman with idiopathic PAH. **A,** S1Q3T3 pattern noted consistent with right ventricle strain. T-wave inversion on anterior leads and ST depression is also suggestive of right ventricular hypertrophy (RVH) with strain (note early R wave predominance in V_1 to V_2 consistent with RVH). **B,** Chest roentgenography showing enlarged pulmonary artery and pruning of the distal pulmonary vasculature. **C,** Lateral chest roentgenography showing filling of the retrosternal space by an enlarged RV. **D,** Parasternal long axis echocardiography view showing dilated RV. **E,** Parasternal short axis echocardiography view showing fatted interventricular septum (*upper arrow*), severely dilated RV and pericardial effusion (*lower arrow*). **F,** Tricuspid regurgitation velocity (*asterisk*) is proportional to right ventricular systolic pressure and estimated by Bernoulli's equation. **G,** Measurement of pulmonary artery acceleration time (PAAT) (time from onset of flow to peak velocity) (*left arrow*) acquired from the RV outflow tract. Note the notching of the PA Doppler envelope, suggestive of pulmonary vascular hypertension (*right arrow*). **H,** The tricuspid plane of systolic excursion (TAPSE) that is normal (>1.7 cm). **I,** Abnormal in a patient with severe pulmonary hypertension. (**A-G** from Ryan JJ et al. *Pulm Circ* 2012;2:107–121; **H** and **I** courtesy Dr. Jayashri Aragam.)

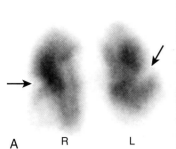
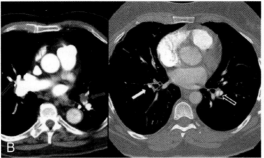
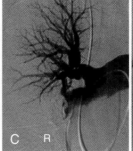
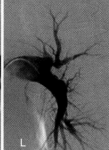

A   R   L   B   C   R   L

FIGURE 88.8 Imaging in chronic thromboembolic pulmonary hypertension (CTEPH). **A,** Nuclear ventilation/perfusion (V/Q) scintigraphy shows numerous mismatched perfusion defects (*arrows*). **B,** Computed tomographic pulmonary angiographic features of chronic thromboembolic disease. Left panel shows right middle lobe vessel narrowing (*open red arrow*) with lining thrombus versus intimal thickening involving the right descending pulmonary artery. Recanalized thrombus is seen in the left descending pulmonary artery (*solid red arrow*). Right panel shows marked vessel narrowing from organized clot in the right descending pulmonary artery (*solid white arrow*) and web in a proximal left lower lobe segmental vessel (*open white arrow*) **C,** Invasive pulmonary angiography demonstrates web and stricture filling defects, an occlusive arteriopathy in the central vasculature, as well as significant dearborization of distal pulmonary arterials bilaterally. (**B** and **C** from Mahmud E et al. *J Am Coll Cardiol* 2018;71:2468–2486.)

TABLE 88.4 Parameters Assessing Right Heart Structure and Function by Echocardiography Useful in Assessing Pulmonary Hypertension

ECHOCARDIOGRAPHIC RV PARAMETER	DESCRIPTION	DEFINITION	USE IN PH/PAH
Tricuspid annular plane systolic excursion (TAPSE)	Longitudinal movement of the RV free wall at the level of the tricuspid valve	Δ end-diastolic- end-systolic measurements acquired usually by M-mode in the apical 4-chamber view	<1.8 cm is prognostic for mortality in PAH
Longitudinal myocardial velocity	Peak velocity of RV longitudinal movement, indicating regional RV contractility	Doppler tissue imaging measures peak velocity (S′) of longitudinal movement of the tricuspid lateral annulus at systolic phase and representative of regional RV systolic function	<10 cm/sec is a marker of RV dysfunction
Right atrial area index	Right atrial size expressed as area, indexed to patient	Apical 4-chamber view at end-systole, corrected for height.	Prognosticates mortality and lung transplantation in PAH per ↑ 5 cm²
Myocardial performance (Tei) index	Measure of global RV performance	Sum of the isovolumic contraction and relaxation times divided by the ejection time.	>0.36 associates with PAH diagnosis; overall correlates with invasive hemodynamic measures, including mPAP and selected exercise parameters
RV fractional area change	Two-dimensional measure of global RV systolic function	(RV end-diastolic area – RV end-systolic area)/RV end-systolic area × 100	<35% suggests RV systolic dysfunction
RV strain and strain rate	Geometric changes to RV cavitary dimensions due to increased afterload	Angle-independent assessment of global and regional RV contractility	For < –12%: ↑ Clinical worsening ↑ 1- and 4-year mortality

mPAP, Mean pulmonary artery pressure; *PAH,* pulmonary arterial hypertension; *RV,* Right ventricle.

hypoxemia, and, thus, pulmonary vasoconstriction, should also be assessed by overnight oximetry or polysomnography in PAH patients or in those with otherwise unexplained PH.

Computed tomographic chest imaging and nuclear ventilation/perfusion (V/Q) scintigraphy. Noncontrast enhanced computed tomographic imaging of the lung is useful to delineate vascular from lung structural and parenchymal causes of PH, such as idiopathic pulmonary fibrosis. Mismatched perfusion defects on ventilation-perfusion (V/Q) scintigraphy is highly suggestive of CTEPH. When these imaging features are present, combining intermediate- and high-probability scan data results in a sensitivity and specificity of V/Q scan for CTPEH of approximately 100% and 86% to 90%, respectively (Fig. 88.8A).[48] In one study of 340 patients with severe PH, a proper V/Q scintigraphy was part of the diagnostic evaluation in only 16% of patients, emphasizing the need for clinicians to consider CTEPH in patients without a definitive cause of PH.[49] Staging CTEPH may require contrast-enhanced computed tomographic or digital subtraction pulmonary angiography, because operative candidacy hinges on anatomic distribution of *in situ* thrombosis that may not be fully evident by nuclear perfusion scanning alone (Fig. 88.8B,C).

Cardiac magnetic resonance (CMR) imaging. Quantitative assessment of RV ejection by CMR is useful for staging PH. This is a particularly important modality in patients for whom poor acoustic windows limit visualizing right heart structures by echocardiography. In PAH, the RV ejection fraction at baseline and in response to treatment prognosticates mortality, particularly when less than 35%. Similarly, there is an inverse association between RV ejection fraction and clinical outcome in patients with PH from left heart disease. Additionally, CMR integrates images across three dimensions, thereby providing optimal resolution for quantifying right atrial and RV chamber volume. Increased RV end-systolic and end-diastolic volumes are phenotypic patterns that correspond to uncoupled RV-PA pathophysiology but require CMR (or three-dimensional echocardiography) for assessing. Late gadolinium enhancement of the RV insertion points on T1 mapping, 4-dimensional quantitative pulmonary artery flow, and 3-dimensional magnetic resonance flow are next-generation imaging packages that show promise for optimizing right pathophenotype assessment in PH.

Positron emission tomography. Lung parenchymal uptake of fluorodeoxyglucose bound to 18-fluorine detected by positron emission tomography (¹⁸FDG-PET) is increased in iPAH patients compared to healthy controls. This supports mechanistic data on dysregulated cellular metabolism in pulmonary endothelial, pulmonary artery smooth muscle, and adventitial fibroblast cells from PAH patients (see Fig 88.4), suggesting that PET may ultimately offer an imaging correlate to stage the pathobiology of individual patients. Detection of the mannose receptor expressed on lung macrophages by PET has also been shown in pre-clinical models to detect early PAH,[50] but overall PET remains an investigational tool without defined clinical usefulness at present.

Exercise testing. Functional assessment using a 6-minute walk distance (6-MWD) or standard (noninvasive) cardiopulmonary exercise test (CPET) is critical to the management of patients with PH. In PAH particularly, symptom-limited functional capacity prognosticates key clinical events including need for therapy escalation, hospitalization, lung transplantation, and mortality. The 6-MWD should be performed according to American Thoracic Society guidelines (https://www.thoracic.org/statements/resources/pfet/sixminute.pdf) because performance is heavily influenceable under nonstandardized conditions. Performance on 6-MWD correlates with workload, heart rate, oxygen saturation, and dyspnea response (i.e., symptom burden), but is dependent on gait speed, age, weight, and muscle mass among other anthropometric variables.[51] In the Naughton-Balke treadmill protocol, incremental increases in workload by 1 metabolic equivalent at successive 2-minute stages is used to assess functional capacity.[51] In contrast to 6-MWD, performance on this test is less modifiable by external cues such as coaching or internal factors such as motivation.

> Exercise is a highly integrated process that beyond mechanical propulsion depends on O_2 uptake across the alveolar-capillary interface, normal O_2 delivery to target organs via CO, and preserved O_2 flux via diffusion across the skeletal muscle cell membrane. Peak volume of oxygen consumption (pVO_2) is a global determinant of cardiopulmonary and skeletal muscle fitness, and when measured using CPET correlates inversely with mortality in PAH and left heart failure patients.[52] In addition, CPET allows for assessment of the (assumed) anaerobic threshold, determined based on depletion of circulating bicarbonate that buffers excess protons (H^+) generated as a byproduct of lactic acid synthesis. This is identifiable by a succinct shift in the ratio of expired carbon dioxide to pVO_2, and when abnormal may suggest a pulmonary vascular limit to exercise. Additional CPET parameters that provide insight into pulmonary circulatory pathophysiology include an increase in the ratio of the peak minute ventilation to maximal voluntary ventilation (VE/MVV), widening of the difference between end-tidal partial pressure of oxygen (PETO_2), and end-tidal partial pressure of carbon dioxide (PETCO$_2$), and an increase in the ratio of minute ventilation to expired carbon dioxide ratio (VE/VCO_2), which suggest a pulmonary mechanical limit to exercise, intracardiac (or pulmonary) shunt, and poor aerobic fitness, respectively.

Cardiac catheterization. As time and financial pressures tilt emphasis to interventional opportunities, RHC seems to have been deemphasized in the current era (see Chapter 22). Nonetheless, perhaps no other widely available study in medicine provides as much integrated, real-time physiological data for use clinically, and a meticulous study is required to classify PH appropriately (see Table 88.1). Additional RHC indications include shock, guidance for pericardial disease, assessing constrictive versus restrictive cardiomyopathy, and quantifying shunt. A complete study includes the following three parts: oxyhemoglobin saturation (SaO_2) analysis in different vascular compartments, intravascular and intracardiac pressure measurement, CO assessment, and PAWP measurement (**e**Table 88.1). It is important to position the patient appropriately and "zero" the air-fluid interface in line with the phlebostatic axis (Fig. 88.9A–D).

Profiling the SaO_2 at different points within the superior vena cava (SVC), inferior vena cava (IVC), right atrium (RA), RV, and pulmonary artery (the latter referred to as the mixed venous SaO_2) is necessary to exclude intra- or extra-cardiac shunt. In turn, a "step-up" in SaO_2

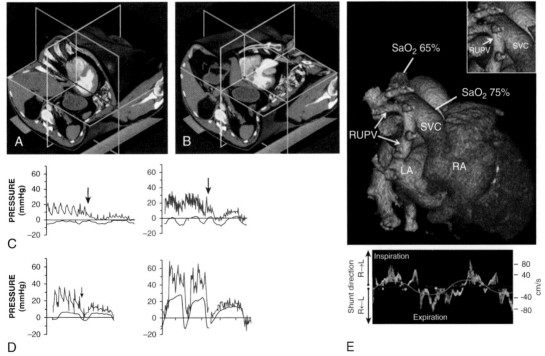

FIGURE 88.9 Anatomical and physiological considerations during right heart catheterization. **A,** Phlebostatic axis (*red line*): an axis running through the thorax at the junction of a transverse plane (*green*) passing through the fourth anterior intercostal space with a frontal plane (*blue*) passing midway between the posterior surface of the body and the base of the xiphoid process of the sternum. Suggested reference point (*red point*) defined by the intersection of the frontal plane (*blue*) at the midthoracic level, the transverse plane (*green*) at the level of fourth anterior intercostal space, and the midsagittal plane (*yellow*). In this patient, the reference point would be within the left atrium. **B,** Phlebostatic reference point (*red point*) defined by the intersection of the following planes: (1) midsagittal plane (*yellow*); (2) frontal plane (*blue*) anterior to the back 0.61 times the thickness of the chest; (3) transverse plane (*green*) caudal to the sternal notch 0.77 times the distance from the sternal notch to the tip of the xiphoid process. The reference point is within the right ventricle. **C,** Pulmonary artery pressure (*red line*) followed by pulmonary artery wedge pressure (*arrow*) in a normal subject at rest (*left*) and during exercise (*right*). Pleural pressure (*black line*) is on average negative with respiratory swings, which are amplified during exercise. **D,** Pulmonary artery pressure (*red line*) followed by pulmonary artery wedge pressure (*arrow*) in a patient with chronic obstructive pulmonary disease at rest (*left*) and during exercise (*right*). Pleural pressure (*black line*) shows respiratory swings, which appear transmitted to pulmonary vascular pressures. **E,** Multislice 3-dimensional reconstructive computed tomographic angiography performed in a 67-year-old man with newly diagnosed pulmonary hypertension due to a congenital anomalous pulmonary vein reveals an abnormal communication between the right upper pulmonary vein (RUPV) and superior vena cava (SVC) (provided at increased magnification in the *inset*) with normal insertion of the RUPV into the left atrium (LA). There is an oxyhemoglobin saturation "step-up" across the abnormal articulation point of the RUPV at the SVC. The Doppler signal demonstrates respirophasic bidirectional blood flow (i.e., shunt) through the RUPV. (**A,B** adapted from Kovacs G et al. *Am J Respir Crit Care Med* 2014;190:252–257; **C,D** from Naeije R, Boerrigter BG. *Eur Respir J* 2013;41:1002–1004; **E** adapted from Clarke JC et al. *Circ Cardiovasc Imaging* 2013;6(2):349–351.)

averaged across greater than 1 measurements between SVC-RA, RA-RV, or RV-PA of ≥7%, ≥5%, ≥5%, respectively, suggests the introduction of oxygenated blood to the right heart circulation through an anatomical shunt (Fig. 88.9E).[53] Characterizing shunt provides invaluable insight to PAH from Eisenmenger physiology (and subsequent right-to-left shunting), which in addition to specific congenital anatomic lesions is discussed in greater detail in Chapter 82.

In the absence of congenital pulmonic stenosis, a meaningful transpulmonary valvular gradient is not expected at rest. However, the compliance of the RV and pulmonary artery differs greatly, and, therefore, the diastolic measurements in these compartments are quite different normally. A RV end-diastolic pressure less than 10 mm Hg generally implies preserved RV function.

The CO is measured by direct pVO_2 analysis using a Douglas bag or metabolic cart; however this equipment is specialized and may be unavailable. More commonly, CO is measured indirectly using the estimated Fick (eFick) equation or thermodilutional (Td) method. The cardiac index corrects CO for body surface area and is often more useful clinically than CO alone for profiling the (dys)functional effects of cardiac performance. Accurate CO is critical, as these data bear on risk stratifying all forms of PH and guide the therapeutic approach to PAH in specific. Furthermore, the CO is used to calculate PVR, which itself is central to patient classification (see Table 88.1). Despite the importance of CO clinically there is only modest agreement between eFick and Td, and controversy exists regarding which is preferred in PH. One recent study using the national Veterans Affair catheterization database showed that Td or the average of eFick + Td was superior to eFick alone for predicting future mortality.[54]

The PAWP is a measure of LVEDP in the absence of mitral valve disease or pulmonary venous remodeling. Confirming optimal catheter placement in the wedge position may be challenging using the hemodynamic tracing alone but can be verified by measuring the wedge SaO_2 to confirm a venous sample.[55] Alternatively, a direct LVEDP measurement is recommended in cases where concordance between multiple PAWP measurements is lacking or the PAWP SaO_2 is less than 90%. It is essential to record the PAWP at end-expiration because wide undulation of the thorax (particularly in COPD) is associated with a transient decrease in PAWP levels. This, in turn, biases results toward over-diagnosing pre-capillary PH. Taken together, a diastolic transpulmonary gradient (calculated as the diastolic PAP – PAWP) ≥ 7 mm Hg and/or PVR ≥3 WU with PAWP or LVEDP ≥15 mm Hg suggests a contribution of left heart disease to PH.[55]

CARDIAC CATHETERIZATION DIAGNOSTIC MANEUVERS
Vasoreactivity Testing
Patients with idiopathic, hereditary, and drug/toxic-associated PAH should undergo vasoreactivity testing with inhaled NO•, intravenous prostacyclin, or intravenous adenosine. A positive test is defined by a decrease in mPAP ≥10 mm Hg to reach an mPAP ≤40 mm Hg with a decrease (or no change) in CO, and observed in approximately 5% of PAH patients.[1] However, identifying this patient subgroup has important implications on pharmacotherapeutic selection and outcome (see Approach to Treatment section below).

Confrontational Fluid Challenge
Differentiating PAH from PH-left heart disease may be challenging, especially in patients with borderline abnormal PAWP (13 to 15 mm Hg), risk factors for HFpEF, and/or on diuretic therapy. In these circumstances, monitoring a change in PAWP following the administration of 500 mL normal saline over 5 min may be useful for eliciting occult LV lusitropic impairment to uncover PH.[55] A rise in PAWP to greater than 18 mm Hg is suggestive of pulmonary PH-left heart disease, although universally accepted diagnostic criteria remain lacking.

Invasive Cardiopulmonary Exercise Testing
Supine or upright cycle ergometry with a pulmonary artery catheter, pneumotachograph, and radial artery catheter are the fundamental components of invasive cardiopulmonary exercise testing (iCPET), which is useful for interrogating the pathophysiological basis of unexplained dyspnea. In iCPET, continuous gas exchange data are integrated with serial invasive hemodynamic readings (including PAWP) as well as peripheral blood lactate, pH, and arterial content of oxygen among other variables. This approach aims to identify patients with the following potential disorders provoked by physical activity: pulmonary vascular disease with or without a component of left heart disease, peripheral oxygen extraction disorders (most often due to mitochondrial dysfunction), or neurovascular syndromes that may affect venous return to the RV (Table 88.5).[56] In 20% of patients referred for iCPET, a diagnosis of HFpEF is made demonstrating limitations to static cardiopulmonary hemodynamic assessment using only conventional RHC.

Risk Stratification
Standardized point-of-care risk assessment tools in PAH are available to guide clinical decision-making, including treatment escalation, and include the French Pulmonary Hypertension Network risk equation, REVEAL risk equation (v2.0), and the 2015 ESC/ERS Pulmonary Hypertension Guideline risk table (**eFig. 88.2**).[38,57] These scales generally integrate clinical, functional, echocardiographic, and biochemical data to generate a composite profile that corresponds to prognosis, but also provides a strategy to inform goal-directed therapy. The overarching goal of therapy is to achieve the lowest risk level possible, which generally means: 6-MWD greater than 440 m or pVO_2 greater than 15 mL/min/kg, right atrial area less than 18 cm², cardiac index greater than 2.5 L/min/m², and absent or low symptom burden with routine physical activity.[38]

TABLE 88.5 Hemodynamic Framework to Inform Exercise Intolerance Phenotypes

	AGE (Year)	PEAK MPAP (mm Hg)	PEAK PAWP (mm Hg)	PEAK PVR (WU)
PVD	≤50	>30	≤19	>1.34
	>50	>33	≤17	>2.10
LHD+PVD	≤50	—	>19	>1.34
	>50	—	>17	>2.10
LHD-noPVD	≤50		>19	≤1.34
	>50		>17	≤2.10

	pVO_2	PEAK CO	Ca-Vo₂/Hb	PEAK RAP (mm Hg)	PEAK PAWP (mm Hg)	PEAK MPAP (mm Hg)
Peripheral O₂ extraction disorder	<80% Predicted	≤80% Predicted	<0.80	—	—	—
Low ventricular filling	<80% Predicted	<80% Predicted	—	<9	<14	<30
Presumed normal	≥80% Predicted	≥80% Predicted	≥0.8	Per age-specific cutoffs in above table		

Exercise hemodynamic, peripheral blood metabolic, and peak VO₂ data criteria that are useful toward diagnosing exercise intolerance from otherwise unexplained dyspnea, although universally accepted diagnostic criteria for these patient subgroups remain lacking.
Ca-vo₂, Content of oxygen in arterial minus venous blood; *CO*, cardiac output; *Hb*, hemoglobin; *LHD*, left heart disease; *mPAP*, mean pulmonary artery pressure; *PAWP*, pulmonary artery wedge pressure; *Peak*, peak exercise; *PVD*, pulmonary vascular disease; *pVO₂*, peak volume of O₂ extraction; *PVR*, pulmonary vascular resistance; *RAP*, right atrial pressure.
From Oldham WM, et al. *Circ Res.* 2018;122(6):864–876.

INTEGRATED APPROACH TO DIAGNOSING PULMONARY HYPERTENSION

Patients with suspected PH based on symptoms should be evaluated further with ECG, chest roentgenography, and echocardiography (Fig. 88.10). Clinicians should focus on assessing comorbid lung and cardiovascular disease to explain findings suggesting PH; to this end, pursuing computed chest CT, pulmonary function testing with DLCO, and arterial blood gas analysis should be considered on an individualized basis. Exercise testing with 6-MWD or CPET is important to characterize symptom burden objectively, and doing so may also expand the profile of an individual patient by discovering helpful findings that are absent at rest, such as exertional hypoxemia or a pulmonary mechanical limit to exercise. Ultimately, diagnosing, classifying, and risk stratifying PH requires a complete RHC. Patients with otherwise unexplained dyspnea that do not meet a hemodynamic classification of PH may benefit from exercise RHC or iCPET to unmask HFpEF or other etiologies as a cause of symptoms. In such patients, increased left atrial size greater than 4.4 cm, obesity, atrial fibrillation, age greater than 60 years, treatment with ≥2 anti-hypertensive drugs, echocardiographic E/e′ ratio, or estimated PASP greater than 35 mm Hg may be sufficient to avoid invasive testing, as the presence of these features point toward HFpEF.[58]

It is incumbent on clinicians to integrate the totality of data from diagnostic testing, including RHC, for determining the most appropriate PH clinical classification. In the case of PAH, this is often informed by the absence of other cardiopulmonary diseases or known PH risk factors, and is suggested by a family history, drug/toxin exposure, or associated diseases such as SSc, HIV, or cirrhotic liver disease. Differentiating PAH from other PH phenotypes may be challenging in specific cases, including patients with left heart disease risk factors who present with severe PH, elevated PVR, and normal PAWP. Determining the contribution of standing diuretic therapy or other volume loading conditions on left heart disease can be determined by confrontational fluid challenge or exercise testing, as described above. In patients suspected of idiopathic, hereditary, or drug/toxin PAH, a positive hemodynamic response to testing with iNO is diagnostic for vasoreactive PAH (although a negative response does not *exclude* PAH). Compared to non-vasoreactive PAH patients, this subgroup is associated with a favorable prognosis including disease resolution in some patients when managed appropriately (Fig. 88.11).

Pulmonary Venoocclusive Disease

Diagnosing PVOD is a major challenge in clinical practice because the symptoms and hemodynamic pattern are often indistinguishable

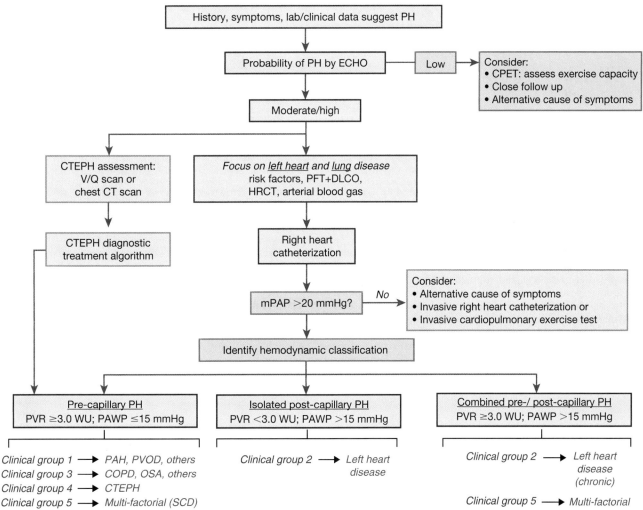

FIGURE 88.10 Integrated pathway for diagnosing pulmonary hypertension. In patients suspected of having pulmonary hypertension (PH) based on history, physical examination, and initial diagnostic testing (e.g., electrocardiogram, chest x-ray), a transthoracic echocardiogram (ECHO) is often used as the first quantitative test. In patients with moderate or high probability of PH based on echocardiography, assessment of left heart disease and pulmonary disease is warranted through various diagnostic tests, including pulmonary function testing with diffusion capacity for carbon monoxide (PFT+DLCO) and high-resolution computed tomography (HRCT). Patients should also be assessed for chronic thromboembolic pulmonary hypertension (CTEPH), initially by nuclear ventilation/perfusion (V/Q) scanning or contrast enhanced chest CT. The diagnosis of PH is made by right heart catheterization and requires a mean pulmonary artery pressure (mPAP) greater than 20 mm Hg. Patients are then classified by hemodynamic category (see Table 88.1 for details), which together with the clinical profile and other supporting data (e.g., serology, genetic testing) is used to determine the PH clinical group (see Table 88.2 for details). *COPD*, Chronic obstructive pulmonary disease; *CPET*, cardiopulmonary exercise test; *OSA*, obstructive sleep apnea; *PAH*, pulmonary arterial hypertension; *PAWP*, pulmonary artery wedge pressure; *PVOD*, pulmonary venoocclusive disease; *PVR*, pulmonary vascular resistance; *SCD*, sickle cell disease.

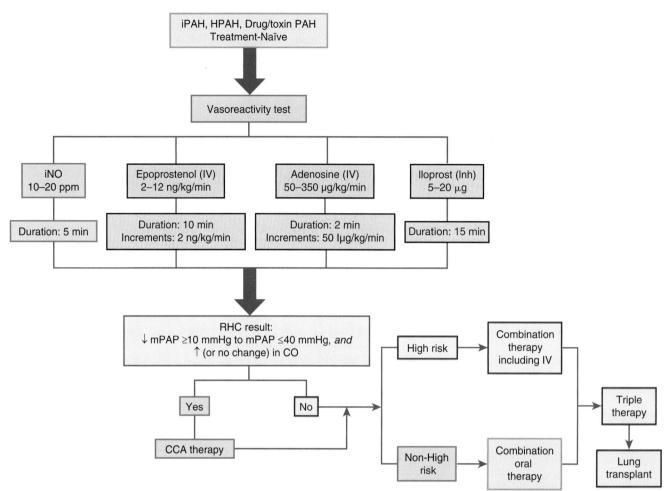

FIGURE 88.11 Vasoreactivity testing and overview of treatment in pulmonary arterial hypertension. Vasoreactivity is indicated in patients with idiopathic pulmonary arterial hypertension (iPAH), hereditary PAH (HPAH), and drug/toxin PAH. Inhaled nitric oxide (iNO) is the preferred agent for testing, although adenosine and prostacyclin analogues are suitable. In patients with a positive vasoreactivity test, high-dose calcium channel antagonist (CCA) therapy is first-line treatment in the absence of high-risk features. In patients without a positive vasoreactivity test, therapy selection is based on risk. Regardless of vasoreactivity results, chest pain, syncope, low cardiac index, and severe symptom burden are indications for intravenous (IV) prostacyclin therapy. Patients without both a positive vasoreactivity result and high-risk clinical features may be candidates for combination oral therapy. Suboptimal clinical response or clinical deterioration warrants consideration to triple therapy, and, if necessary lung transplantation. *CO*, cardiac output; *mPAP*, mean pulmonary artery pressure; *RHC*, right heart catheterization.

from PAH. Ultimately, the probability of PVOD hinges on a combination of factors, including clinical suspicion, genetic risk (e.g., biallelic *EIF2AK4* mutation), and subpleural thickened septal lines, centrilobular ground-glass opacities, and mediastinal lymphadenopathy on chest computed tomographic imaging (Table 88.6). Simultaneous measurement of LVEDP with multiple PAWP recordings from different pulmonary artery branches showing elevated PAWP:LVEDP ratio in some segments and normal ratio in other segments is suggestive, but not diagnostic of PVOD.[51] Lung biopsy remains the gold standard diagnostic test, but is generally avoided owing to the risk of major complication.[38] Unfortunately, PVOD may emerge as the operative diagnosis in patients that develop pulmonary edema following administration of pulmonary vasodilator therapy due to increased hydrostatic pressure proximal to fixed venous stenosis.

Chronic Thromboembolic Pulmonary Hypertension

A diagnosis of CTEPH must be suspected in any patient with prior PE and otherwise unexplained dyspnea or PH. The diagnostic approach to CTEPH is outlined in Figure 88.12, and integrates clinical data with imaging from V/Q, contrast enhanced chest CT, and pulmonary angiography. A subset of patients with symptoms (e.g., dyspnea and functional limitation) and evidence of pulmonary thromboembolic remodeling will present without PH. In this subgroup, chronic thromboembolic disease (CTED), ventilatory defects such as increased dead

space ventilation and (near) normal cardiopulmonary hemodynamics are reported.

TREATMENT

Pulmonary Arterial Hypertension

A multi-disciplinary care strategy is needed to optimize outcome in PAH, and patients should be evaluated prior to treatment at an expert referral center whenever possible. Supportive care with loop diuretics and supplemental oxygen attenuates pulmonary vascular congestion and hypoxic pulmonary vasoconstriction, which otherwise aggravate symptoms and worsen RV function. Approximately one-third of PAH patients in clinical trials are reported to use potassium-sparing diuretics (e.g., spironolactone, eplerenone), which may resolve hypokalemia and exert salutary clinical benefit by inhibiting aldosterone-mediated pulmonary vascular injury.[45] Digoxin may increase CO by as much as 10% in patients with RV failure due to PH, and attenuates the adverse effect of increased circulating norepinephrine on pulmonary vascular function. Vaccination against influenza and pneumococcal pneumonia is not evidenced-based, but is recommended owing to untoward complications from pneumonia in PAH patients. Routine anticoagulation is not recommended currently as part of the standard therapeutic approach.

Prescription exercise is a proven, albeit underused strategy for treating PAH. This may be due to delayed diagnosis, which is common and linked to advanced symptom burden at the time of presentation, or

TABLE 88.6 Comparison of Distinguishing Features Between Pulmonary Arterial Hypertension and Pulmonary Venoocclusive Disease

	PAH	PVOD
Genetics	Autosomal dominant (see Table 3)	Autosomal recessive (EIF2AK4)
Epidemiology	Approximately 15 cases/million	1–2 cases/million
		No gender predominance
	Female predominance (~2:1)	
Acquired risk factors	Anorexigens,	Chemotherapy (alkylating agents)
	Dasatinib	
	Interferon	
	Methamphetamines	
Associated conditions	Connective tissue disease, HIV infection, portal hypertension	Systemic sclerosis
Clinical Examination		
Hemoptysis	±	±
Pleural effusion	±	±
Right Heart Catheterization		
mPAP	↑	↑
PAWP	Normal	Normal
PVR	↑	↑
Pulmonary vasoreactivity	~5% in iPAH (predicts long-term CCA response)	~5% (not a predictor of CCA response)
Pulmonary Function Testing		
FEV₁, FVC, TLC	Normal	Normal
DLCO	Normal or mild ↓	↓↓↓
Resting PaO₂	Normal or mild ↓	↓↓↓
Exercise-desaturation	Often present	↓↓↓
Imaging		
Chest HRCT	Usually normal	Centrilobular ground-glass opacities, septal lines, mediastinal lymph node enlargement
V/Q scan	Usually normal	Usually normal
Treatment	Targeted PAH therapy is supported by RCTs	Risk of pulmonary edema; conflicting data on targeted PAH therapy, limited to small case series

DLCO, Diffusion capacity of carbon monoxide; *FEV₁*, forced expiratory volume in 1 second; *FVC*, forced vital capacity; *HIV*, human immunodeficiency virus; *HRCT*, high resolution computed tomography; *iPAH*, idiopathic pulmonary arterial hypertension; *mPAP*, mean pulmonary artery pressure; *PAH*, pulmonary arterial hypertension; *PaO₂*, partial pressure of oxygen; *PAWP*, pulmonary artery wedge pressure; *PVOD*, pulmonary venoocclusive disease; *PVR*, pulmonary vascular resistance; *RCTs*, randomized controlled trials; *TLC*, total lung capacity; *V/Q*, ventilation-perfusion. Adapted from Montani D, et al. *Eur Respir J.* 2016;47:1334–1335.

perhaps the misconception that moderated physical activity is dangerous. In one meta-analysis of 469 PAH patients, exercise improved 6-MWD by +53.3 m, pVO₂ by +1.8 mL/kg, and PASP by –3.7 mm Hg at week 15.[59] Inspiratory muscle training, too, is associated with an improvement in PAH endpoints.

At present, there are 14 U.S. Food and Drug Administration-approved PAH therapies that target NO· signaling, the endothelin receptor axis, or prostacyclin deficiency spanning oral, inhaled, subcutaneous (injectable and implantable), and intravenous delivery methods (Fig. 88.13A).[1] In patients without a positive vasoreactivity test, therapy selection is guided by clinical status: New York Heart Association Functional Class (NYHA FC) IV, cardiogenic shock by clinical or hemodynamic criteria (e.g., signs of impaired distal perfusion, cardiac index <2.1 l/min/m²), syncope, or chest pain (indicative of either RV ischemia or LMCA compression) are indications for continuous parenteral prostacyclin therapy.[38] For patients with a positive vasoreactivity test, high-dose calcium channel antagonist therapy is the initial treatment in the absence of high-risk findings.

Initial Management of Treatment-Naïve Pulmonary Arterial Hypertension Patients

An evidenced-based strategic shift in the approach to patients with newly diagnosed PAH (without an indication for immediate parenteral therapy) has emerged over the previous 5 years favoring the initiation of two oral PAH therapies. The Ambrisentan and Tadalafil in Patients with Pulmonary Arterial Hypertension (AMBITION) trial demonstrated a clear benefit in hard-clinical events among incident, treatment-naïve PAH patients administered combination ambrisentan (selective endothelin receptor-type A antagonist) plus tadalafil (PDE-V inhibitor) compared with monotherapy with either agent.[60] At a median of 517 days, an endpoint of death, hospitalization for PAH, disease progression, or unsatisfactory clinical response occurred in 18%, 34%, and 28% of patients randomized to combination therapy, ambrisentan monotherapy, and tadalafil monotherapy, respectively. The benefit of combination therapy corresponding to a 50% reduction in the hazard for achieving the composite endpoint (Fig. 88.13B–D). Data from observational cohort studies implies that the salutary benefit of combination therapy may not be exclusive to these drugs per se, and the evidence base is expanding in support of up-front treatment to triple therapy in highly selected patients. Conversely, monotherapy may be reasonable for patients that were initially administered one PAH drug and remain clinically stable or in whom prognosis is particularly favorable. Overall, personalizing a treatment plan for PAH should be done in collaboration with an expert referral center.

Therapeutic Escalation and End-Stage Disease

Generally, a low threshold to escalate therapy (e.g., dose uptitration or sequential addition of a new drug class) is warranted in PAH patients who demonstrate disease progression or, in turn, fail to demonstrate evidence of improvement. Hospitalization for heart failure and end-organ damage, particularly renal failure, are especially worrisome events that portend further decline and warrant adjustment to care. Indeed, referral for bilateral lung transplant evaluation should be considered in patients with suboptimal clinical response to the initial therapeutic approach. Although the 5-year post-transplant survival rate has improved in some series to 75% for PAH patients, availability of suitable donor lungs remains limited.[38] Temporizing (bridging) measures to transplantation in PAH include RV assist device or veno-arterial extracorporeal membrane oxygenation (V-A ECMO), although the precise indications and clinical profile that is best suited for these extreme measures is not clear. Balloon atrial septostomy, other interventional approaches that create a right-to-left shunt such as percutaneous Potts shunt, and salvage medical therapies may be considered to palliate symptoms in patients who are not candidates for lung transplant.

Genetic Counseling

Patients with idiopathic, familial, or anorexigen-associated PAH as well as PVOD/PCH should be considered for genetic counseling and testing. Generally, testing is focused first on the patient. Results are helpful if a pathogenetic variant is discovered in the patient, but not in unaffected family members. In this scenario, the risk of developing PAH in the unaffected family member is akin to the general population. Detecting the pathogenic variant harbored by a patient in a phenotype-negative family member is associated with an increased lifetime risk of developing PAH, although quantifying this risk with certainty is challenging due to the incomplete penetrant pattern of inheritance for most PAH variants. In the case of PVOD, identifying a biallelic EIF2AK4 mutation has direct implication on clinical management, as these patients tend to present at an earlier age and can be diagnosed and risk stratified for lung transplantation earlier by virtue of genetic testing results.

DISEASES OF THE MYOCARDIUM, PERICARDIUM, AND PULMONARY VASCULATURE BED

IX

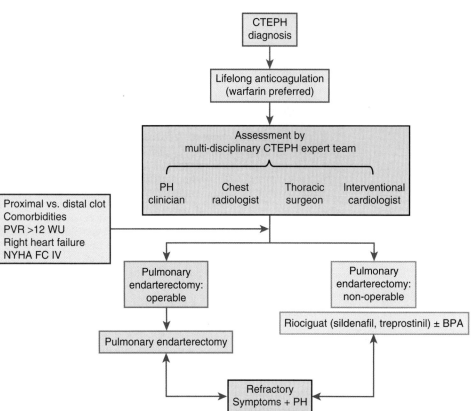

FIGURE 88.12 Chronic thromboembolic pulmonary hypertension (CTEPH) treatment algorithm. In patients diagnosed with CTEPH, lifelong anticoagulation with warfarin is generally indicated. Clinical decision-making requires a multidisciplinary expert team including a PH specialist, chest radiologist, (high pulmonary endarterectomy volume) thoracic surgeon, and interventional cardiologists (or interventional radiologist). Surgical pulmonary endarterectomy is the preferred treatment option, although operative candidacy may be mitigated by various high-risk features. In nonoperative patients, medical therapy and/or balloon pulmonary angioplasty (BPA) should be considered. *NHYA*, New York Heart Association; *PVR*, pulmonary vascular resistance.

Chronic Thromboembolic Pulmonary Hypertension (see Chapter 87)

Upon diagnosing CTEPH, all patients should be considered for surgical pulmonary thromboendarterectomy.[61] This is based on several lines of data indicating that surgery provides a distinct survival advantage and opportunity for complete or near complete resolution of symptoms. In one prospective study of 679 newly diagnosed CTEPH patients, the 3-year survival rate was 89% in operated patients compared to 70% in nonoperated patients.[62] Pulmonary thromboendarterectomy is performed through a median sternotomy and requires cardiopulmonary bypass as well as periods of hypothermic circulatory arrest to allow optimal visualization of clot. Technical success hinges on surgical accessibility and, importantly, the experience of the operator and surgical team. The probability of an optimal therapeutic response to surgery aligns with the relationship between the PH severity by cardiopulmonary hemodynamics and burden of thrombotic disease on imaging. Thus, distal disease, particularly subsegmental arterial involvement, raises anatomic concerns to the potential for therapeutic benefit. Other factors that may influence peri-operative risk include cardiovascular comorbidity burden, right heart failure, NYHA FC IV, and patients with very elevated PVR (>12 WU).[61]

In patients that are poor surgical candidates, have inoperable disease, or decline surgery, percutaneous balloon pulmonary angioplasty (BPA) at an expert referral center is a modern-day treatment option (Fig. 88.14). Matching data from digital subtraction pulmonary angiography with lung perfusion findings is used to assist in identifying target lesions, which otherwise may be difficult to discern owing to the complex and multifocal vasculopathy of CTEPH. Although angiographic evidence showing improvement in post-stenotic blood flow following BPA is often evident immediately, achieving significant clinical benefits from BPA requires multiple procedural attempts, generally requiring separate hospitalizations.[63] Additionally, peri-procedural complications

such as reperfusion injury, hemoptysis, or pulmonary artery perforation is reported in 15% of patients.[62] When these occur, pulmonary edema, hypoxemia, respiratory failure, and mortality are potential outcomes. In patients who are inoperable or in whom pulmonary thromboendarterectomy is associated with residual PH, therapy with the soluble guanylyl cyclase stimulator riociguat or the nonselective ERA macitentan can be useful for improving functional status and PVR.

Pulmonary Hypertension from Left Heart Disease

In PH from left heart disease (or any other specific cause), the principal goal of treatment is to optimize the underlying condition. This should include consideration to undiagnosed comorbid disease, such as COPD in patients with left heart disease, or vice-versa, including sleep apnea that is common to both. Conversely, PH drives decision-making in certain clinical scenarios, such as asymptomatic mitral valve regurgitation in which PASP greater than 50 mm Hg is a strong indication for valve repair or replacement. For management of PH due to conventional HFpEF or HFrEF, diuretic therapy remains the mainstay treatment (see Chapters 49 and 50). Implanting CardioMEMS heart failure system, which provides real-time pulmonary artery pressure monitoring, to guide diuretic dosing is an option for patients with a narrow therapeutic window (see Chapter 58). Efforts to repurpose pulmonary vasodilator therapy to either PH from cardiac or lung disease have been met mainly with negative or, at best, mixed data.[64] One exception is the minority of advanced heart failure patients post-left ventricular assist device implant with sustained PH. In this subgroup, PDE-V inhibitor therapy is effective for decreasing PVR as one strategy by which to delay, defer, or optimize candidacy for orthotropic heart transplantation.

There is a graded association between pre-operative PVR and peri-operative mortality following orthotopic heart transplantation that is particularly evident greater than 4 WU (and transpulmonary gradient greater than 15 mm Hg, calculated by the difference between mPAP and PAWP). In turn, PVR greater than 5 WU and transpulmonary gradient greater than 16 mm Hg is a relative contra-indication to heart transplantation. Acute vasodilator challenge should be performed if sPAP greater than 50 mm Hg, and either transpulmonary gradient ≥15 mm Hg (calculated by: mPAP – PAWP) or PVR greater than 3 WU and systemic systolic arterial pressure greater than 85 mm Hg.[55] However, consensus is lacking on the best vasodilator to use for testing in these circumstances, and data are variable on the relationship between PVR post-vasodilator challenge and outcome post-heart transplant. This scenario is complicated further by the fact that in many patients a reduction in PVR is accountable by increased PAWP.

SPECIAL CLINICAL CIRCUMSTANCES

High-Altitude Pulmonary Edema

At high altitude, particularly but not exclusively ≥2500 m, there are several environmental changes compared to sea level that bear directly on pulmonary vascular function, particularly hypobaric hypoxia. A fall in oxygen tension (measured as the partial pressure of O_2) detected at the

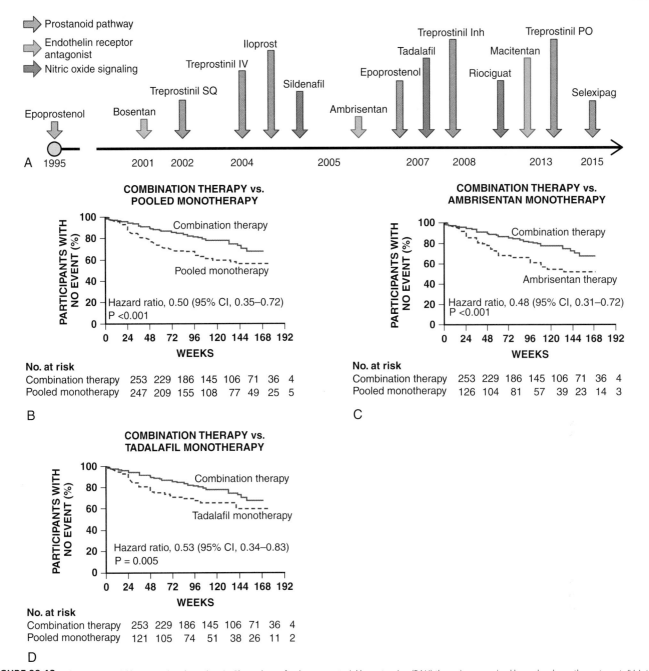

FIGURE 88.13 Pulmonary arterial hypertension therapies. **A,** Chronology of pulmonary arterial hypertension (PAH) therapies, organized by molecular pathway target. *IV,* Intravenous; *PO,* per oral; *SQ,* subcutaneous. Selexipag is a prostacyclin counterreceptor agonist, which differs from other same-class drugs that replace prostacyclin deficiency. **B-D,** Treatment-naïve PAH patients enrolled in the Ambrisentan and Tadalafil in Patients with Pulmonary Arterial Hypertension (AMBITION) trial were randomized to receive up-front monotherapy with the endothelin-type A receptor antagonist ambrisentan or the phosphodiesterase type-V inhibitor tadalafil, or the combination of both drugs. Kaplan-Meier curve for the primary endpoint, which was a time-to-event analysis of clinical failure, defined as death, hospitalization for worsening pulmonary arterial hypertension, disease progression, or unsatisfactory long-term clinical response. These data show comparisons in outcome for combination therapy vs. pooled monotherapy (**B**), ambrisentan monotherapy (**C**), and tadalafil monotherapy (**D**). (**B-D** from Galiè N et al. *N Engl J Med* 2015;373:834–844.)

level of the alveolar capillary is a major trigger of hypoxic pulmonary vasoconstriction. This occurs through membrane depolarization that propagates proximally, from capillary to arterials, leading to increased intrapulmonary artery smooth muscle cell Ca²⁺ levels. Teleologically, this appears necessary to shunt blood flow to lung regions that are "better" ventilated. There is a parabolic relationship between mPAP and altitude between 2000 and 4,500 m that ranges from 15 to 30 mm Hg, respectively.[65] Although this profile is compatible with normal living, the cardiopulmonary hemodynamic response to altitude varies substantially between individuals. Inhomogeneous hypoxic pulmonary vasoconstriction associated with rapid ascent causes high-altitude pulmonary edema (HAPE) arising from changes in capillary membrane permeability that lead to exudative effusion. The clinical syndrome includes shortness of breath and cough; treatment beyond prevention includes descent to a lower altitude, supplemental oxygen, and/or nifedipine.

The PH typical of high altitude is generally mild and tolerated clinically. In a population of Kyrgyz highlanders who dwell at approximately 3000 m above sea level, 14% have evidence of RV hypertrophy on ECG.[65] In patients with high-altitude PH, descent to lower altitude is important and may be lifesaving when the syndrome is complicated by heart failure. PDE-V inhibitor and acetazolamide therapies have also been reported effective at improving PH severity. The HAPE and high-altitude PH syndromes are distinct from acute or chronic mountain sickness, which are characterized by neurological symptoms in association with hypoventilation-induced overproduction of red blood cells and vasogenic cerebral edema.

DISEASES OF THE MYOCARDIUM, PERICARDIUM, AND PULMONARY VASCULATURE BED

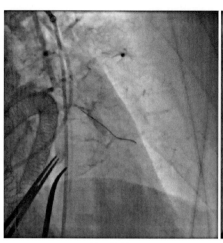
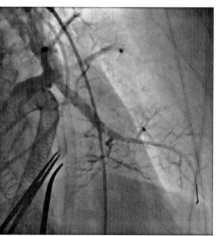

Pre-PBA

Post-PBA

FIGURE 88.14 Pulmonary balloon angioplasty (PBA) for chronic thromboembolic pulmonary hypertension (CTEPH). In inoperable CTEPH patients or in those with a suboptimal surgical result and residual symptoms, percutaneous pulmonary balloon angioplasty is a therapeutic option when performed at a PH center of excellence. Compared to pre-BPA, image of left pulmonary artery post-BPA demonstrates increased contrast flow to the lung periphery. (Adapted from Wiedenroth CB et al. *J Heart Lung Transpl* 2016;35:591–596.)

Sarcoidosis

Coalescing, non-necrotizing granulomas in clusters defines the pathology of sarcoidosis, which affects multiple organ systems including the lung parenchyma. The prevalence of PH in sarcoid patients varies widely and is biased by patient selection and method of assessment. Approximately 50% of sarcoid patients with exercise intolerance also have PH. Patients may present with either pre-capillary or post-capillary PH.[66] In the former, parenchymal fibrosis leading to arterial remodeling/destruction or direct granulomatous involvement of the vasculature underlies PH. In the latter, fibrosing mediastinitis, pulmonary venous involvement, or cardiac sarcoid including LV dysfunction should be considered. In one randomized clinical trial over 16 weeks, treatment with bosentan (nonselective endothelin receptor antagonist) did not improve 6-MWD or quality of life measures significantly.[66]

Sickle Cell Disease

Chronic hemolytic anemia is an important complication of sickle cell disease with direct ramifications on cardiopulmonary hemodynamics. The average basal CO for sickle cell disease patients approaches 11 liters/min, driven by low hemoglobin content (47 to 100 g/liter). It follows that PVR is low in sickle cell disease patients, which may be 50% of nonanemic healthy controls at baseline. Indeed, the upper limit of normal PVR in sickle cell disease is approximately 2.0 WU.[67] Red blood cell sickling itself is associated with increased release of intraerythrocytic hemoglobin that decreases NO· bioavailability and promotes the accumulation of vascular reactive oxygen species. This disruption in the redox balance of vascular cells underlies endothelial dysfunction, pulmonary artery smooth muscle cell proliferation, and in situ thrombosis. Indeed, pre-capillary PH is an established aspect of the sickle cell disease spectrum, affecting approximately 30% of patients. Long-standing high CO and plasma expansion from anemia also causes LV cavitary remodeling due to chronically elevated stroke volume. Over time, LV dysfunction may ensue, leading to pulmonary venous hypertension and post-capillary PH.

Overall, a stepwise increase in mPAP by 10 mm Hg is associated with a 1.7-fold increase in the mortality hazard. The pro-thrombotic potential in sickle cell disease elevates PVR (thus contributing to pre-capillary PH) and increases the risk of developing CTEPH. In fact, among sickle cell disease patients with PH, up to 25% are diagnosed with CTEPH. Therapy for sickle cell disease-PH should focus on correcting underlying anemia with hydroxyurea and blood transfusion. PDE-V inhibitor therapy may improve cardiopulmonary hemodynamics in this population but increases sickle cell vasoocclusive pain, and, therefore, should not be considered outside the advice and management of an expert referral center.[67]

Pregnancy (see Chapter 92)

Mortality or heart failure requiring lung transplantation is reported in 20% of pregnant women with PAH; therefore, it is recommended that patients avoid conception. Endothelin receptor antagonist therapy is teratogenic, and women of child-bearing age require counseling and a declaration of birth control prior to treatment. Pregnant PAH patients should be managed in a referral center with expertise in maternal-fetal medicine and pulmonary vascular disease.

Perioperative Management

Perioperative complication risk for noncardiac and nonobstetric surgeries is increased in PH; in one series of 114 PAH patients, major complications and mortality occurred in 6.1% and 3.5% of patients, respectively.[68] For PAH patients, general anesthesia should be avoided when possible. In patients requiring general anesthesia, an individualized care plan including cardiac anesthesia, intraoperative pulmonary artery catheter monitoring, and a plan to use inhaled therapies may prove useful.

FUTURE PERSPECTIVES

The PH field continues to evolve, including insight into the hemodynamic spectrum of clinical risk, a strategic shift in favor of aggressive early therapy in newly diagnosed PAH patients, and percutaneous interventions for selected patients affected by CTEPH. In particular, the mPAP threshold to diagnose PH is now greater than 20 mm Hg, placing emphasis on early diagnosis. Developing therapies specific to PH from left heart disease or lung disease remains a major goal. Overall, however, PH, including the PAH subtype, has emerged in the current era as a high-risk but manageable disease that should be considered in all patients with cardiopulmonary symptoms.

ACKNOWLEDGMENTS

Dr. Maron would like to acknowledge Dr. Stuart Rich, who authored an earlier version of this chapter which inspired many young physicians and students including Dr. Maron to pursue pulmonary hypertension in clinical and research endeavors.

Dr. Maron reports being a consultant for Actelion, and co-inventor on the following patents or patent application that are related to pulmonary hypertension (U.S. Patent #9,605,047; PCT/US2015/029672; Provisional ID: #62475955; Provisional ID: #24624; Provisional ID: #24622).

REFERENCES
Overview and Pulmonary Circulation
1. Maron BA, Galie N. Diagnosis, treatment, and clinical management of pulmonary arterial hypertension in the contemporary era: a review. *JAMA Cardiol.* 2016;1:1056–1065.
2. Rosenkranz S, Howard LS, Gomberg-Maitland M, Hoeper MM. Systemic consequences of pulmonary hypertension and right-sided heart failure. *Circulation.* 2020;141:678–693.
3. Tuder RM. Pulmonary vascular remodeling in pulmonary hypertension. *Cell Tissue Res.* 2017;367:643–649.
4. Rosenkranz S, Preston IR. Right heart catheterisation: best practice and pitfalls in pulmonary hypertension. *Eur Respir Rev.* 2015;24:642–652.
5. Raymond TE, Khabbaza JE, Yadav R, Tonelli AR. Significance of main pulmonary artery dilation on imaging studies. *Ann Am Thorac Soc.* 2014;11:1623–1632.
6. Kovacs G, Olschewski A, Berghold A, Olschewski H. Pulmonary vascular resistances during exercise in normal subjects: a systemic review. *Eur Respir J.* 2012;39:319–328.
7. Townsley MI. Structure and composition of pulmonary arteries, capillaries, and veins. *Compr Physiol.* 2012;2:675–709.
8. Fayyaz AU, Edwards WD, Maleszewski JJ, et al. Global pulmonary vascular remodeling in pulmonary hypertension associated with heart failure and preserved or reduced ejection fraction. *Circulation.* 2018;137:1796–1810.
9. Kovacs G, Herve P, Barbera JA, et al. An official European Respiratory Society statement: pulmonary haemodynamics during exercise. *Eur Respir J.* 2017;50:1700578.
10. Ho JE, Zern EK, Lau ES, et al. Exercise pulmonary hypertension predicts clinical outcomes in patients with dyspnea on effort. *J Am Coll Cardiol.* 2020;75:17–26.

Classification of Pulmonary Hypertension

11. Newman JH. Pulmonary hypertension by the method of Paul Wood. *Chest*. 2020;S0012-3692: 30428-1.
12. Simonneau G, Montani D, Celermajer DS, et al. Haemodynamic definitions and updated clinical classification of pulmonary hypertension. *Eur Respir J*. 2019;53:1801913.
13. Kovacs G, Douschan P, Maron BA, et al. Mildly increased pulmonary arterial pressure: a new disease entity or just a marker of poor prognosis? *Eur J Heart Fail*. 2019;21:1057–1061.
14. Maron BA, Hess E, Maddox TM, et al. Association of borderline pulmonary hypertension with mortality and hospitalization in a large patient cohort: insights from the Veterans Affairs Clinical Assessment, Reporting and Tracking program. *Circulation*. 2016;133:1240–1248.
15. Nishihara T, Yamamoto E, Tokitsu T, et al. New definition of pulmonary hypertension in patients with heart failure with preserved ejection fraction. *Am J Respir Crit Care Med*. 2019;200:386–388.
16. Nouraie M, Little JA, Hildesheim M, et al. Validation of a composite vascular high-risk profile for adult patients with sickle cell disease. *Am J Hematol*. 2019;94:E312–E314.
17. Maron BA, Brittain EL, Hess E, et al. The association between pulmonary vascular resistance and clinical outcomes in patients with pulmonary hypertension: a retrospective cohort study. *Lancet Respir Med*. 2020;S2213-2600(20)30317–9.
18. Guhaa A, Amione-Guerrab J, Park MH. Epidemiology of pulmonary hypertension in left heart disease. *Prog Cardiovasc Dis*. 2016;59:3–10.
19. Shah AM, Cikes M, Prasad N, et al. Echocardiographic features of patients with heart failure and preserved left ventricular ejection fraction. *J Am Coll Cardiol*. 2019;74:2858–2873.
20. Covella M, Rowin EJ, Hill NS, et al. Mechanism of progressive heart failure and significance of pulmonary hypertension in obstructive hypertrophic cardiomyopathy. *Circ Heart Fail*. 2017;10:e003689.
21. Magne J, Pibarot P, Sengupta PP, et al. Pulmonary hypertension in valvular disease: a comprehensive review on pathophysiology to therapy from the HAVEC Group. *JACC Cardiovasc Imaging*. 2015;8(1):83–99. https://doi.org/10.1016/j.jcmg.2014.12.003.
22. Nishimura RA, Otto CM, Bonow RO, et al. 2014. AHA/ACC guideline for the management of patients with valvular heart disease: executive summary: a report of the American College of Cardiology/American Heart Association Task Force on Practice Guidelines. *J Am Coll Cardiol*. 2014;63:2438–2488.
23. Caravita S, Mariani D, Blengino S, et al. Pulmonary hypertension due to a stiff left atrium: speckle tracking equivalents of large V-waves. *Echocardiography*. 2018;35:1464–1466.
24. Weatherald J, Reis A, Sitbon O, Humbert M, et al. Pulmonary arterial hypertension registries: past, present and into the future. *Eur Respir Rev*. 2019;28(154):190128.
25. Farber HW, Miller DP, Poms AD, et al. Five-Year outcomes of patients enrolled in the reveal registry. *Chest*. 2015;148:1043–1054.
26. Foderaro A, Ventetuolo CE. Pulmonary arterial hypertension and the sex hormone paradox. *Curr Hypertens Rep*. 2016;18:84.
27. Ventetuolo CE, Praestgaard A, Palevsky HI, et al. Sex and haemodynamics in pulmonary arterial hypertension. *Eur Respir J*. 2014;43:523–530.
28. Sitbon O, Sattlerr C, Bertoletti L, et al. Initial dual oral combination therapy in pulmonary arterial hypertension. *Eur Respir J*. 2016;47:1727–1736.
29. Morrell NW, Aldred MA, Chung WK, et al. Genetics and genomics of pulmonary arterial hypertension. *Eur Respir J*. 2019;53(1):1801899.
30. Zamanian RT, Hedlin H, Greuenwald P, et al. Features and outcomes of methamphetamine-associated pulmonary arterial hypertension. *Am J Respir Crit Care Med*. 2018;197:788–800.
31. Hassoun PM. The right ventricle in scleroderma (2013 Grover conference series). *Am J Respir Crit Care Med*. 2018;197:788–800.
32. Graham BB, Kumar R. Schistosomiasis and the pulmonary vasculature (2013 Grover Conference series). *Pulm Circ*. 2014;4:353–362.
33. Brittain EL, Duncan MS, Chang J, et al. Increased echocardiographic pulmonary pressure in HIV-infected and -uninfected individuals in the veterans aging cohort study. *Am J Respir Crit Care Med*. 2018;197:923–932.
34. Creel-Bulos C, Hockstein M, Amin N. Acute cor pulmonale in critically ill patients with Covid-19. *N Engl J Med*. 2020;382(21):e70.
35. van Loon RLE, Roofthooft MTR, Hillege HL, et al. Pediatric pulmonary hypertension in The Netherlands: epidemiology and characterization during the period 1991–2005. *Circulation*. 2011;124:1755–1764.
36. Nathan SD, Barbera JA, Gaine SP, et al. Pulmonary hypertension in chronic lung disease and hypoxia. *Eur Respir J*. 2019;53:1801914.
37. Montani D, Lau EEM, Dorfmuller P, et al. Pulmonary veno-occlusive disease. *Eur Respir J*. 2016;47:1518–1534.
38. Galiè N, Humbert M, Vachiery JL, et al. 2015 ESC/ERS Guidelines for the diagnosis and treatment of pulmonary hypertension. *Eur Respir J*. 2015:903–975.
39. Assad TR, Hemnes AR, Larkin EK, et al. Clinical and biological insights into combined post- and pre-capillary pulmonary hypertension. *J Am Coll Cardiol*. 2016;68(23):2525–2536.

Pathology, Pathobiology, and Pathophysiology

40. Archer SL. Acquired mitochondrial abnormalities, including epigenetic inhibition of superoxide dismutase 2, in pulmonary hypertension and cancer: therapeutic implications. *Adv Exp Med Biol*. 2016;903:29–53.
41. Samokhin AO, Stephens BA, Wertheim BM, et al. NEDD9 targets COL3A1 to promote endothelial fibrosis and pulmonary arterial hypertension. *Sci Transl Med*. 2018;10:445.
42. MacLean MR. The serotonin hypothesis in pulmonary hypertension revisited: targets for novel therapies (2017 Grover conference series). *Pulm Circ*. 2018;8: 2045894018759125.
43. Tedford RJ, Mudd JO, Girgis RE, et al. Right ventricular dysfunction in systemic sclerosis-associated pulmonary arterial hypertension. *Circ Heart Fail*. 2013;6:953–963.
44. Vonk Noordegraaf A, Westerhof BE, Westerhof N. The relationship between the right ventricle and its load in pulmonary hypertension. *J Am Coll Cardiol*. 2017;69:236–243.
45. Maron BA, Leopold JA. Emerging concepts in the molecular basis of pulmonary arterial hypertension: part ii: neurohormonal signaling contributes to the pulmonary vascular and right ventricular pathophenotype of pulmonary arterial hypertension. *Circulation*. 2015;131:2079–2091.
46. Hsu S, Kokkonen-Simon KM, Kirk JA, et al. Right ventricular myofilament functional differences in humans with systemic sclerosis-associated versus idiopathic pulmonary arterial hypertension. *Circulation*. 2018;137:2360–23670.

Integrated Approach to Diagnosis and Treatment

47. O'Leary JM, Assad TR, Xu M, et al. Lack of a tricuspid regurgitation Doppler signal and pulmonary hypertension by invasive measurement. *J Am Heart Assoc*. 2018;7:e009362.
48. Kim NH, Delcroix M, Jais X, et al. Chronic thromboembolic pulmonary hypertension. *Eur Respir J*. 2019;53:1801915.
49. Maron BA, Choudhary G, Khan UA, et al. Clinical profile and underdiagnosis of pulmonary hypertension in us veteran patients. *Circ Heart Fail*. 2013;6:906–912.
50. Park J-B, Suh M, Park J-Y, et al. Assessment of inflammation in pulmonary artery hypertension by 68 Ga-Mannosylated human serum albumin. *Am J Respir Crit Care Med*. 2020;201:95–106.
51. Rich JD, Rich S. Clinical diagnosis of pulmonary hypertension. *Circulation*. 2014;130:1820–1830.
52. Berry NC, Manyoo A, Oldham W, et al. Protocol for exercise hemodynamic assessment: performing an invasive cardiopulmonary exercise test in clinical practice. *Pulm Circ*. 2015;5:610–618.
53. Opotowsky AR. Clinical evaluation and management of pulmonary hypertension in the adult with congenital heart disease. *Circulation*. 2015;131:200–210.
54. Opotowsky AR, Hess E, Maron BA, et al. Thermodilution vs estimated fick cardiac output measurement in clinical practice: an analysis of mortality from the Veterans Affairs Clinical Assessment, Reporting, and Tracking (VA CART) program and Vanderbilt University. *JAMA Cardiol*. 2017;2:1090–1099.
55. Vachiéry JL, Tedford RJ, Rosenkranz S, et al. Pulmonary hypertension due to left heart disease. *Eur Respir J*. 2019;53:1801897.
56. Oldham WM, Oliveira RK, Wang RS, et al. Network analysis to risk stratify patients with exercise intolerance. *Circ Res*. 2018;122:864–876.
57. Benza RL, Gomberg-Maitland M, Elliott CG, et al. Predicting survival in patients with pulmonary arterial hypertension: the reveal risk score calculator 2.0 and comparison with ESC/ERS-based risk assessment strategies. *Chest*. 2019;156:323–337.
58. Reddy YNV, Carter RE, Obokata M, et al. A simple, evidence-based approach to help guide diagnosis of heart failure with preserved ejection fraction. *Circulation*. 2018;138:861–870.
59. Pandey A, Garg S, Khunger M, et al. Efficacy and safety of exercise training in chronic pulmonary hypertension. *Circ: Heart Fail*. 2015;8:1032–1043.
60. Galiè N, Barbera JA, Frost AE, et al. Initial use of ambrisentan plus tadalafil in pulmonary arterial hypertension. *N Engl J Med*. 2015;373:834–844.
61. Kim NH, Delcroix M, Jais X, et al. Chronic thromboembolic pulmonary hypertension. *Eur Respir J*. 2019;53:1801915.
62. Lang IM, Madani M. Update on chronic thromboembolic pulmonary hypertension. *Circulation*. 2014;130:508–518.
63. Auger WR. Surgical and percutaneous interventions for chronic thromboembolic pulmonary hypertension. *Cardiol Clin*. 2020;38:257–268.
64. Maron BA, Ryan JJ. A concerning trend for patients with pulmonary hypertension in the era of evidence-based medicine. *Circulation*. 2019;139(16):1861–1864.
65. Wilkins MR, Ghofrani H-A, Weissmann N, et al. Pathophysiology and treatment of high-altitude pulmonary vascular disease. *Circulation*. 2015;131:582–590.
66. Boucly A, Cottin V, Nunes H, et al. Management and long-term outcomes of sarcoidosis-associated pulmonary hypertension. *Eur Respir J*. 2017;50:1700465.
67. Gladwin MT. Cardiovascular complications and risk of death in sickle-cell disease. *Lancet*. 2016;387(10037):2565–2574.
68. Meyer S, McLaughlin VV, Seyfarth H-J, et al. Outcomes of noncardiac, nonobstetric surgery in patients with PAH: an international prospective survey. *Eur Respir J*. 2013;41:1302–1307.

89 Sleep-Disordered Breathing and Cardiac Disease

SUSAN REDLINE

Sleep-disordered breathing (SDB) is prevalent in patients with cardiac diseases, contributing to a reduced quality of life, a reduced functional capacity, and poor health. SDB causes acute and chronic physiologic stressors that can exacerbate cardiac ischemia, reduce systolic and diastolic function, cause cardiac structural and electrical remodeling, and increase the risk of cardiac arrhythmias and sudden death. Despite strong evidence linking SDB to cardiovascular disease (CVD), and the vulnerability of the cardiac patient to SDB-related stressors, SDB often goes unrecognized in cardiology practice, so there is potential for improved recognition and initiation of interventions. This chapter reviews aspects of SDB recognition, pathophysiology, and health outcomes relevant to cardiac disease.

DEFINITIONS

SDB refers to a spectrum of sleep-related breathing disorders that includes obstructive sleep apnea (OSA), central sleep apnea (CSA), Cheyne-Stokes respiration, and sleep-related hypoventilation. The mechanisms and risk factors for these disorders have overlapping as well as unique characteristics. Each is associated with impaired ventilation during sleep and sleep disruption, but differ with regard to degree of abnormalities in neuromuscular respiratory drive and airway collapsibility. The constellation of symptoms, the diagnostic criteria, and their associations with CVD are summarized in Table 89.1.

Typical symptoms of OSA include loud or disruptive snoring, snorting or gasping during sleep, poor sleep quality, unrefreshed sleep, and excessive daytime sleepiness. Diagnosis requires objective sleep testing using an in-laboratory polysomnograph or a home sleep apnea test, with demonstration of recurrent episodes of apneas and/or hypopneas. An apnea indicates a near absence of airflow during the period of upper airway obstruction for at least 10 seconds, while a hypopnea signifies a reduction in airflow relative to baseline accompanied by drop in oxygen saturation or a cortical arousal (Fig. 89.1).[1] Apneas and hypopneas are further classified as "obstructive" based on the occurrence of concurrent respiratory effort during periods of reduced or absent airflow, and otherwise as "central". Diagnostic criteria for OSA are: (1) symptoms of breathing disturbances during sleep (snoring, snorting, gasping, or breathing pauses) or daytime sleepiness or fatigue, despite sufficient opportunities to sleep and unexplained by other medical problems; and (2) five or more apneas or hypopneas per hour of sleep (apnea-hypopnea index [AHI]). OSA may be diagnosed in the absence of symptoms if the AHI is greater than 15). OSA severity is judged based on the frequency of breathing disturbances (AHI level), degree of hypoxemia and sleep disruption, and associated symptoms.

Excessive daytime sleepiness, in particular, marks severe disease that is associated with an increased risk of adverse CVD outcomes, as well as better adherence with OSA treatment. CSA often overlaps with OSA and is identified when more than 50% of respiratory disturbances are unaccompanied by respiratory effort.

The AHI and other indices of sleep are measured with multichannel overnight recordings. Polysomnography performed in the sleep laboratory records airflow, breathing effort and oxygen saturation, as well as data from the electroencephalogram, electrocardiogram, and leg muscles; providing the ability to identify apneas and hypopneas as well as stage sleep, quantify sleep fragmentation, and identify other sleep-related phenomena such as arrhythmias and periodic leg movements. Home-based sleep apnea tests collect data on breathing parameters, but do not typically record additional information. Although home sleep apnea tests are increasingly used due to their lower cost, in-laboratory polysomnography still serves to evaluate patients with complex comorbidities, such as heart failure (HF). When interpreting the results of home sleep apnea tests, it is important to note that they can underestimate the AHI by approximately 12%,[2] and larger misclassifications are likely in patients with poor sleep quality, such as those with HF, and in women, who typically have shorter respiratory events with less desaturation than men.

PATHOPHYSIOLOGY

Pathophysiology of Obstructive Sleep Apnea

The pharyngeal airway has no bony or cartilaginous support, and its size and shape change dynamically with each expiration and inspiration (when negative intraluminal pressure causes the airway to be "sucked" inward). Its patency therefore depends on the activation of pharyngeal dilator muscles, which decreases with sleep onset. Whether an apnea occurs depends on whether the level of neuromuscular activation of the upper airway muscles is adequate to overcome forces that promote airway collapse during sleep. The presence of an anatomically small airway (e.g., micrognathia, fat deposition in the lateral pharyngeal walls) and lying in the supine position (when gravitational and positional factors alter the position of the tongue and other soft tissues) increase the level of neuromuscular drive needed to maintain airway patency. Therefore, patients with small oropharyngeal airways due to craniofacial factors or excessive airway soft tissue have an increased risk for OSA. When a person is in the recumbent position, there can be a rostral redistribution of peripheral fluid from the lower extremities to the neck area, contributing to airway narrowing during sleep, and this factor can predispose patients

Additional content is available online at Elsevier eBooks for Practicing Clinicians

TABLE 89.1 Key Features of Obstructive Sleep Apnea and Central Sleep Apnea

	OBSTRUCTIVE SLEEP APNEA	CENTRAL SLEEP APNEA
Common presenting symptoms	Snoring, observed apneas, gasping or snorting during sleep, daytime sleepiness	Observed apneas, gasping or snorting during sleep, frequent awakenings, unrefreshed sleep, fatigue
Diagnosis	Home sleep apnea test or polysomnography showing AHI >5 with a predominance of obstructive apneas or hypopneas (>50%)	Polysomnography showing a predominance of central apneas or hypopneas (>50%) with a central apnea hypopnea index >5 Cheyne-Stokes respiration: ≥3 consecutive central apneas/central hypopneas separated by crescendo and decrescendo change in breathing amplitude with a cycle length ≥40 sec associated with central AHI >5
Associated risk factors	Obesity, male, middle-older age	Male, older age
Associated cardiovascular disease*	Resistant hypertension, stroke, heart failure (preserved and reduced ejection fraction), atrial fibrillation, coronary artery disease	Atrial fibrillation, heart failure (reduced or preserved ejection fraction), stroke, pulmonary hypertension, coronary artery disease

*Order shown indicating approximate relative strength of association.

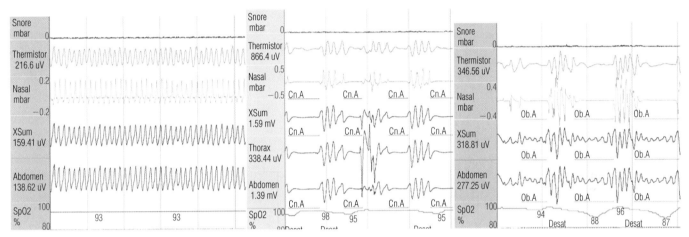

FIGURE 89.1 **Examples from an overnight sleep study, displaying respiratory channels.** The first panel shows normal breathing with stable oxygen saturation values. The second panel shows repetitive central apneas, characterized by 15- to 40-second periods of absent airflow (shown on the nasal and thermistor channels), with no associated respiratory effort of snoring, and oxyhemoglobin desaturation of 3% with each event. The third panel shows obstructive apneas, characterized by absent airflow with persistent effort on the thorax and abdominal channels, with deep desaturations (each panel is approximately 3 minutes long).

with HF and even mild peripheral edema or venous stasis to OSA.[3] Lung volume influences pharyngeal wall stiffness through tractional forces; therefore, reduced lung volumes, as may occur in obesity or with pulmonary congestion, can exacerbate propensity for OSA. Conversely, high lung volumes, as in chronic obstructive lung disease, may modestly protect against OSA. Increased nasal resistance (e.g., due to nasal septal deviation, polyps) promotes airway collapse by increasing the negative intraluminal suction pressure and is a risk factor for OSA in conditions such as pregnancy or allergy associated with nasal swelling.

Pharyngeal muscle activation depends both on the sensitivity of central and peripheral respiratory chemoreceptors and on neuromuscular responsiveness to CO_2 (Fig. 89.2).[4] During sleep, the blood CO_2 typically increases mildly, and this helps to activate respiratory muscles and stiffen airway dilators, protecting the upper airway (i.e., increasing critical closing pressure, P_{crit}). Depressed chemosensitivity and arousal response may prevent appropriate termination of apneas, prolonging the duration of the apnea and the severity of oxyhemoglobin desaturation. This ventilatory control problem can cause pathologic CO_2 retention and acidosis during sleep, a phenomenon common in obesity-hypoventilation and sleep-hypoventilation syndromes. Conversely, an overly sensitive response to CO_2 (i.e., reflecting high loop gain) can cause wide fluctuations in the ventilatory drive, resulting in central nervous system arousal and sleep fragmentation. Episodic hyperventilation can drive CO_2 levels to below the apneic threshold, precipitating cycles of apneas. This mechanism also occurs in CSA, and in its most extreme form is manifested as Cheyne-Stokes respiration.[5]

The severity of OSA can vary by sleep stage and position. During rapid eye movement (REM) sleep, the neuromuscular drive is low and fluctuating, sympathetic tone is high, and apneic events tend to

be longest and associated with the most severe oxyhemoglobin desaturation. "REM-dependent" OSA, characterized by a predominance of respiratory events in REM as compared to non-REM sleep, better predicts incident hypertension and mortality compared to the overall AHI level.[6] OSA also can worsen following acute ingestion of alcohol, which reduces neuromuscular activation, and when a person is in the supine position.

Pathophysiology of Central Sleep Apnea

In adults, CSA often occurs in association with cardiac or cerebrovascular disease. Its pathogenesis relates to a heightened sensitivity to CO_2 and a prolonged circulation delay between the pulmonary capillaries and carotid chemoreceptors, causing instability in breathing. Periods of hyperventilation cause CO_2 levels to fall below the apneic threshold, precipitating apneas and hypopneas. The occurrence of cycles of crescendo-decrescendo breathing is recognized as Cheyne-Stokes respiration; cycle lengths of 60 seconds are characteristic of patients with HF.

Risk Factors for and Recognition of Sleep-Disordered Breathing

OSA affects 34% of males and 17% of females between the ages of 30 to 70 years.[7] OSA and CVD commonly co-occur, reflecting both shared risk factors (e.g., central obesity) and causal relationships; therefore, the prevalence of OSA is as high as 40% to 80% in patients with hypertension, HF, or coronary heart disease (CHD).[5] Male sex, older age, and obesity are well-recognized OSA risk factors. OSA is two- to fourfold more prevalent in men than in women.[8] Factors that predispose men

DISEASES OF THE MYOCARDIUM, PERICARDIUM, AND PULMONARY VASCULATURE BED

IX

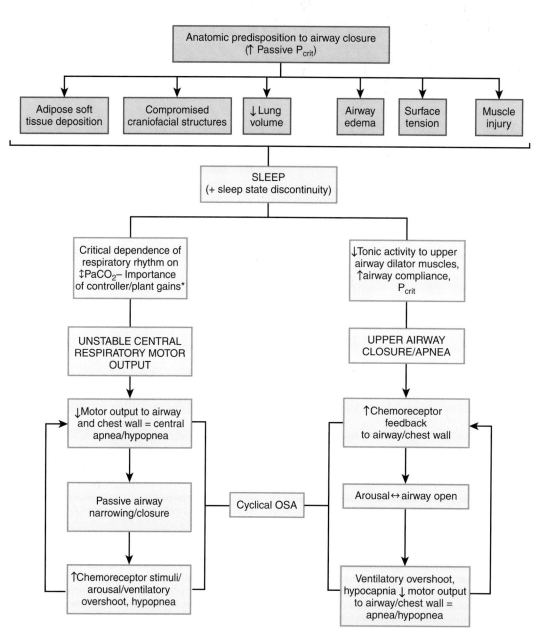

FIGURE 89.2 **Pathogenetic mechanisms leading to obstructive apneas.** *Controller/plant gains refer to the negative feedback loops that influence ventilation in response to a ventilatory disturbance (e.g., an apnea or change in pCO2). *Plant gain* refers to background drive to breathe; *controller gain* refers to the slope of changing ventilation in response to changes in pCO2 level. P_{crit}, critical closing pressure in the airway: the pressure at which the airway collapses. Passive P_{crit} is determined by the mechanical properties of the airway and surrounding tissues. A decrease in tonic activity to the airway dilator muscles refers to active P_{crit}. (From Dempsey JA, Veasey SC, Morgan BJ, O'Donnell CP. Pathophysiology of sleep apnea. *Physiol Rev.* 2010;90:47–112.)

to OSA include android patterns of adiposity (which predisposes to upper airway fat deposition) and relatively long pharyngeal length, which predisposes to collapsibility. OSA prevalence increases in women following menopause, and hormone replacement therapy is associated with reduced AHI levels, consistent with a role for sex hormones in modulating risk.[9] OSA severity increases not only in older women but also in older men, reflecting age-related comorbidities (e.g., cardiac diseases, neurologic diseases) and other age-related effects on airway stiffness and ventilation. OSA in elderly persons may differ from that in middle-aged individuals, with less prominent associations with snoring, obesity, autonomic system dysregulation, and CVD reported. It is not known whether differences in studies of middle-aged populations compared with older populations result from study biases or are true differences in OSA etiology and pathophysiology across the population.

Being overweight or obese accounts for approximately 40% to 60% of cases of OSA. Obese middle-aged individuals are fourfold or more likely to have OSA as compared with normal-weight individuals. Obesity contributes to OSA through effects on airway narrowing

caused by fat deposition in the tongue and parapharyngeal tissues and by reducing chest wall compliance and lung volumes. Obesity-associated cytokine levels also may influence ventilatory control and promote daytime sleepiness. Even a modest weight loss or weight gain can have an impact on the severity of OSA. For example, a 1% increase in the body mass index (BMI, kg/m²) is estimated to increase the AHI by 3%; this finding emphasizes the importance of weight management in OSA.[10] Approximately 20% of OSA patients are *not* obese, however, and the absence of obesity should not preclude an appropriate evaluation of patients with OSA symptoms. Other risk factors for OSA are craniofacial features that narrow the oropharyngeal airway, upper airway dilator muscle dysfunction, and abnormalities in ventilatory control.

A first-degree relative of a patient with OSA has an approximately twofold increased risk of OSA compared with someone without an affected relative.[11] Over 60% of the genetic variance explaining OSA is not associated with obesity, indicating the importance of multiple etiologic factors. Several genetic variants associated with OSA may also be associated with cardiac disease and abnormal lipid and glucose

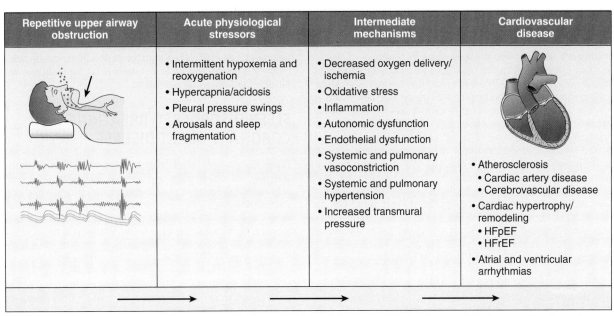

Repetitive upper airway obstruction	Acute physiological stressors	Intermediate mechanisms	Cardiovascular disease

	• Intermittent hypoxemia and reoxygenation
	• Hypercapnia/acidosis
	• Pleural pressure swings
	• Arousals and sleep fragmentation
		• Decreased oxygen delivery/ischemia
		• Oxidative stress
		• Inflammation
		• Autonomic dysfunction
		• Endothelial dysfunction
		• Systemic and pulmonary vasoconstriction
		• Systemic and pulmonary hypertension
		• Increased transmural pressure
			• Atherosclerosis
			  • Cardiac artery disease
			  • Cerebrovascular disease
			• Cardiac hypertrophy/remodeling
			  • HFpEF
			  • HFrEF
			• Atrial and ventricular arrhythmias

FIGURE 89.3 Mechanisms by which obstructive sleep apnea leads to physiological stressors, which then increase risk of atherosclerosis, cardiac remodeling, and arrhythmias.

levels, suggesting overlapping genetic mechanisms ("pleiotropy") for OSA and cardiac disease.[12] Sexual dimorphisms in genetic variants for OSA have been identified, similar to reports of sex-based differences in genetic variants for adiposity and cardiac disease.

Despite improved public awareness of OSA, it is estimated that more than 80% of individuals with moderate or severe OSA are undiagnosed.[13] Even among those diagnosed, more than 30% of patients report that the period between onset of symptoms and diagnosis exceeded 10 years.[14] Under-recognition is high among ethnic and minority groups and elderly individuals, particularly African Americans and older Asian Americans, groups also at risk for cardiometabolic diseases. Under-recognition in women may result from the preferential reporting of symptoms of fatigue rather than sleepiness, and the frequency of comorbid insomnia that can confound the diagnosis and reduce the sensitivity of screening questionnaires. Women often display REM-predominant OSA and may experience apneas that result in arousal without desaturation, findings that home sleep tests may miss.[15]

Risk factors for CSA are male sex, hypocapnia during wakefulness, and older age, as well as HF, CVD, and atrial fibrillation (AF).[16] Due to elevations in sympathetic drive, patients with CSA may not report sleepiness, and rather report symptoms of insomnia, such as difficulty falling asleep and frequent awakenings.

The role of routine screening for sleep apnea is not established. In 2017, The U.S. Preventive Services Task Force concluded that there was insufficient evidence to recommend routine screening for sleep apnea in primary care settings.[17] However, patients with diagnosed sleep apnea frequently report prolonged delays between the onset of symptoms and diagnosis and treatment, indicating a need to improve recognition. Screening questions (eFig. 89.1) or web-based algorithms that combine information on snoring frequency, age, BMI, and sex for calculating OSA risk[18] should be considered in cardiology practices, settings where sleep apnea prevalence is high, to improve identification and expedite treatment of this disorder.

Pathophysiologic Mechanisms That Link Sleep-Disordered Breathing to Cardiovascular Diseases

During healthy sleep, individuals experience a decrease in sympathetic nervous system activity and an increase in parasympathetic activity, with associated reductions in blood pressure (BP) and heart rate. Repetitive collapse of the upper airway that disrupts sleep continuity and causes arousal disturbs these patterns, resulting in surges in sympathetic activity and acute BP elevations.[19] Impaired gas exchange with intermittent hypoxia further affects the autonomic nervous system, as well as triggers the release of acute-phase proteins and reactive oxygen species. The release of these mediators may favor an augmented inflammatory and hypercoagulable state, exacerbating insulin resistance and lipolysis.[20] Hypoxia and autonomic nervous system alterations can contribute to electrical remodeling of the heart and myocyte injury. Oxyhemoglobin desaturation further compromises oxygenation of myocardial tissue. Inspiratory efforts against a closed glottis (with OSA) additionally cause wide swings in intrathoracic pressure, negatively affecting preload and afterload and left ventricular (LV) transmural pressure, increasing myocardial oxygen consumption, and impeding stroke volume. The pathophysiologic consequences of OSA are shown schematically in Figure 89.3, and summarized later in this chapter.

SLEEP-DISORDERED BREATHING AND HYPERTENSION

Approximately 30% of patients with essential hypertension (see also Chapter 26) and 80% of patients with resistant hypertension have OSA. Conversely, more than 50% of patients with OSA have hypertension.[21] Although the aggregation of hypertension and OSA partially reflects common risk factors, experimental animal and human data indicate that OSA is causally associated with hypertension.

OSA has both acute and chronic effects on BP. Acutely, BP and heart rate increase within 10 seconds of the termination of an apnea or hypopnea, corresponding to peak times of the arousal, ventilation, and oxygen saturation nadir. Frequent arousals trigger chemoreflexes and sympathetic output to the peripheral blood vessels, with consequent vasoconstriction, and altered renin-angiotensin-aldosterone system activity. Transient increases in BP can persist into the daytime. Chronic intermittent surges in BP also cause vascular remodeling.

OSA is associated with a non-dipping overnight BP pattern, increases in daytime BP to pre-hypertensive and hypertensive ranges, and an increased risk of poorly controlled and resistant hypertension. "Dose-response" associations are reported. Specifically, a 1-unit increase in the AHI is estimated to increase the odds of non-dipping systolic BP by 4%.[22] The Wisconsin Cohort Study, a prospective study of state employees, reported that the odds ratio, adjusted for obesity and other confounders, for the presence of hypertension after 4 years of follow-up was 2.9 for moderate or severe OSA.[23] The apneas and hypopneas occurring in REM sleep, rather than the AHI occurring across all sleep stages, appear to be most strongly associated with hypertension incidence.[6] During REM sleep, the sympathetic drive is highest, the muscular tone is lowest, and the respiratory events tend to last the longest and are associated with the most severe hypoxemia.

Over 30 randomized controlled trials have examined BP responses to positive airway pressure (PAP), the mainstay therapy for OSA.[24] Meta-analyses estimate that PAP treatment reduces the systolic and diastolic BP by an average of 2 to 3 mm Hg and 1.5 to 2 mm Hg, respectively. Generally, studies reported larger effects for nocturnal BP than daytime BP, and in individuals who have high PAP adherence or more severe OSA, or are younger, sleepier, or have resistant hypertension (with average BP improvements of 4 to 9 mm Hg). PAP also can improve non-dipping patterns, a well-established risk factor for all-cause mortality rates. The Heart Biomarker Evaluation in Apnea Treatment study compared PAP with supplemental oxygen therapy and usual care in patients with OSA at increased CVD risk, most of whom were under care of cardiologists and were using an average of 2.4 antihypertensive medications.[25] Relative to the usual care group, which included guideline-based management of CVD, the PAP group experienced significant lowering of mean 24-hour BP (by 2.4 mm Hg), with larger changes for the nocturnal BP (by 3.5 mm Hg). A meta-analysis that evaluated the influence of PAP on resistant hypertension estimated that PAP reduced ambulatory 24-hour systolic and diastolic BP by 7.2 and 5.0 mm Hg, respectively.[26] To address the role of PAP in reducing the incidence of hypertension, a multicenter trial conducted in Spain randomized 723 patients with moderate OSA but without significant sleepiness to PAP or usual care.[27] Over a median of 4 years of follow-up, an intention-to-treat analysis showed no reduction in the incidence of hypertension or CVD events with PAP. However, in an analysis of patients who used PAP for 4 hours or more per night, a 31% reduction in incident hypertension or CVD was observed and the magnitude of the 24-hour BP improvement was related directly to the hours of PAP use (each additional hour of PAP use resulted in a decrease in the average systolic BP of 1.3 mm Hg.)

The existing clinical trials highlight the importance of treatment adherence in achieving BP improvement. Other sources of variability in responses to OSA treatment include differences in residual apneic activity with treatment, severity of OSA, age, and cause of hypertension. The level of PAP adherence needed to obtain a significant BP reduction is unknown. Although a minimum threshold of 4 hours of CPAP use per night is commonly targeted, more than 6 hours of PAP use per night, including use during the late-night hours in REM sleep, is likely more effective. Suboptimal responses to PAP also may reflect delayed initiation of treatment; specifically, individuals with untreated OSA for years may undergo chronic remodeling of the vascular bed and changes in BP regulatory mechanisms that are not readily reversed with PAP. A variety of pathophysiologic processes contribute to hypertension, including insulin resistance, obesity, autonomic nervous system dysfunction, and variations in salt and fluid balance. OSA likely affects these mechanisms differently, and thus OSA treatment is expected to be more effective in certain subgroups. Biomarkers that reflect molecular mechanisms for CVD and/or sensitivity to hypoxia may play a future role for risk stratification. Such an approach is supported by an initial report that three microribonucleic acids associated with CVD predicted BP responses in patients with OSA and resistant hypertension.[28]

Alternative strategies, such as combined therapies (PAP, medications, and lifestyle) or physiologically targeted interventions, may prove to be superior to single therapies for some patients with both OSA and hypertension. The addition of PAP, when used for 4 hours or more per night, enhances the effects of pharmacotherapy in improving the BP.[29] Among obese patients with moderate OSA and elevations of C-reactive protein (CRP), a combination of weight loss plus PAP proved more effective in lowering the BP than PAP alone, suggesting the importance of concomitant lifestyle interventions in high-risk groups.[30] Early studies suggest that spironolactone[24] or renal denervation[24] may reduce both the severity of OSA and lower BP in patients with resistant hypertension.

Based on the existing evidence, the Seventh Report of the Joint National Committee on Prevention, Detection, Evaluation, and Treatment of High Blood Pressure (JNC 7) identified OSA as a treatable cause of hypertension.[31] Although average treatment effects are modest, long-term improvements of systolic BP by 2 to 3 mm Hg may reduce the risk of stroke and CHD by as much as 10%. Therefore, OSA treatment, especially when high levels of adherence are achieved and efficacy is greater, should have a beneficial population-level effect on adverse cardiovascular outcomes.

SLEEP-DISORDERED BREATHING AND CORONARY HEART DISEASE

There are multiple mechanisms by which SDB exacerbates atherosclerosis, including triggering sympathetic nervous system activity, augmenting the release of proinflammatory proteins and contributing to dyslipidemia, insulin resistance, and endothelial dysfunction. SDB-related episodes of recurrent hypoxemia activate leukocytes and endothelial cells, increase the expression of adhesion molecules, and lead to the release of oxygen free radicals, with levels that vary in proportion to the severity of SDB-related hypoxemia. Although the extent to which biomarker elevations are independent of obesity or other confounders is not clear, treatment of SDB, even for as short a time as 2 weeks, has been shown to reduce sympathetic activation, inflammation, oxidative stress, and endothelial dysfunction.[32]

OSA also may contribute to acute ischemia because of both decreased oxygen delivery (secondary to obstructed breathing) and increased oxygen consumption (due to elevated diastolic and transmural pressures and cardiac hypertrophy). Ischemic stressors may be most notable during the rebreathing phase of obstructive apneas, when large hemodynamic changes occur. The fractional flow reserve, a quantitative measurement of coronary artery stenosis, can dynamically vary with obstructive apneas because of fluctuations in the intrathoracic pressure that affect the venous and aortic pressures and coronary perfusion.[33] Patients with intermediate coronary lesions may experience intermittent myocardial ischemia as a result of cyclical changes in the coronary blood flow. Endothelial damage and compromised coronary vascular conductance may ensue due to surges in the BP and heart rate associated with sympathetic activation and reduced endothelial production of nitric oxide. Subclinical ischemia can be manifested on overnight electrocardiograms of patients with OSA, showing ST segment depression, which indicates nocturnal myocardial ischemia, and changes in QT dispersion, as well as paroxysms of ventricular tachycardia or AF that are associated temporally with the occurrence of apneas. Women with OSA have elevated levels of high-sensitivity troponin, a marker of subclinical myocardial injury; the level of troponin is one factor in the risk for HF or death in untreated OSA.[34]

Evidence for SDB as a CHD risk factor is found in large cohort studies that demonstrate that SDB is associated with an increased incidence of CHD and cardiovascular death. In over 5000 participants in the Multi-Ethnic Study of Atherosclerosis (MESA) who were free of known CVD at baseline and followed for 7.5 years, a physician-diagnosis of sleep apnea was associated with a 1.9 increased adjusted hazard ratio for incident cardiovascular events and a 2.4-fold higher mortality rate.[35] Several studies from Spain followed patients referred to sleep laboratories for periods of 5 to 10 years. Among men, untreated severe OSA was associated with a 2.9-fold increased risk of fatal cardiovascular events and a 3.2-fold increased risk of nonfatal cardiovascular events when compared with a control group. Among women followed for a median time of 72 months, the mortality rate was 3.5-fold higher in women with severe OSA than in female controls.[36] In the Sleep Heart Health Study cohort, moderate to severe SDB defined by an AHI ≥15 was associated with a 35% increased incidence of CHD over 8 years; among men younger than age 70 years, this risk was 70%.[37] In a prospective analysis of more than 10,000 individuals, patients with significant nocturnal hypoxemia had a nearly twofold increase in the risk of sudden cardiac death after potential confounders had been considered.[38] Use of quantitative metrics of hypoxia burden show particular promise for predicting those at risk for developing CHD-related death: individuals with the most severe degree of sleep-apnea hypoxic burden (in the highest quintile) had an approximately twofold increased risk of cardiovascular death compared to individuals with less hypoxia, even after adjusting for the AHI level and multiple other confounders.[39] Temporal support for a causal link between OSA and CHD comes from a study showing that individuals with OSA compared with those without OSA were more likely to experience a morning-peak onset of myocardial infarction[40] and die suddenly between midnight and 6:00 AM, the hours when apneas and hypopneas occur.[41]

Subclinical markers of atherosclerosis are also elevated in individuals with OSA compared to controls. In analyses adjusted for multiple confounders, coronary artery calcium burden (CAC Agatston score >400) was 40% more common in individuals with sleep apnea than in controls.[42] Furthermore, over 8 years, the CAC was more likely to progress in individuals with OSA compared to those without OSA.[43]

SDB appears to contribute to adverse outcomes among patients with CHD; patients with CHD who have OSA experience higher rates of major acute cardiovascular events than patients without OSA.[44,45] OSA is implicated in both plaque instability[47] and plaque vulnerability. Untreated OSA is associated with an increased need for a revascularization procedure as compared with rates in patients without OSA.[46] Infarct sizes are reported to be higher 3 months after myocardial infarction salvage procedures in patients with OSA than in patients without OSA.[47] In contrast, some research findings suggest that patients with SDB may develop collateral coronary blood flow from periods of intermittent hypoxemia, with resultant angiogenesis,[48] which may reduce the extent of myocardial injury immediately following an ischemic event.

Large observational studies demonstrate that patients with severe OSA treated with PAP have significantly reduced rates of fatal and nonfatal CVD compared to untreated patients. Patients with CHD treated with PAP are reported to have lower rates of nocturnal ischemia, acute coronary syndrome, need for coronary revascularization, and death from CVD compared to untreated patients with OSA. However, the data from several randomized controlled trials do not provide support for PAP in secondary prevention of CVD in patients with moderate to severe OSA. Interventions were PAP (or auto-titrating PAP) or conservative therapy. All studies excluded patients with significant sleepiness, and one also excluded those with severe overnight hypoxemia, reducing the generalizability of the results. Modest PAP adherence limited all studies, and the studies were underpowered to detect moderate improvements. The first study, following 725 patients without CVD for a median of 4 years, did not find a benefit for the PAP group. However, patients who used PAP for 4 hours or more per night experienced a significant improvement in the composite study outcome (incidence density ratio, 0.72; 95% confidence interval [CI], 0.52 to 0.98) compared with controls and nonadherent patients.[49] The Randomized Intervention with Continuous Positive Airway Pressure in Coronary Artery Disease and OSA (RICCADSA), randomized 244 non-sleepy patients with established CHD and moderate or severe OSA to PAP or usual care in a single European center.[50] At a median follow-up time of 57 months, the PAP group compared with the usual-care group had a 20% nonstatistically significant reduction in the primary composite endpoint. When restricted to patients using PAP for 4 hours or more per night, a significant 80% decrease in event rates was observed (HR, 0.29; 0.10 to 0.86). The multicenter international Sleep Apnea Cardiovascular Endpoints (SAVE) trial followed 2717 patients with a history of coronary artery or cerebrovascular disease for a mean of 3.7 years.[51] This study did not observe a difference in the primary composite CVD endpoint. A sub-analysis, however, showed that individuals adherent to PAP had a 40% significant reduction in cerebrovascular events compared with a propensity-matched subgroup from the usual-care group. The better effect for cerebrovascular disease than for the composite endpoint or CHD is in agreement with observational data showing stronger associations between OSA and cerebrovascular disease compared with CHD. Most recently, the Impact of Sleep Apnea Syndrome in the Evolution of Acute Coronary Syndrome (ISAACC) study randomized 1264 patients hospitalized with acute coronary syndrome with moderate to severe OSA to receive PAP therapy or usual care. Over a median follow-up of 3.4 years, the composite cardiovascular outcome did not significantly differ by intervention group (Hazard Ratio: 0.89 [95%CI, 0.68 to 1.17]).[52] The existing data suggest that PAP is unlikely to improve CVD outcomes unless it is used for at least 4 hours per night. However, the

SAVE study demonstrated that even suboptimal PAP use can improve quality of life and mood and result in fewer days of missed work, as well as possible cerebrovascular benefits, indicating positive effects in patients with CVD. The results of these studies emphasize the need to provide adherence support for patients prescribed PAP. In patients with CVD, adjunctive behavioral therapies (e.g., motivational education and problem solving) have demonstrated improvements of PAP use by an average of 90 minutes per night.

SLEEP-DISORDERED BREATHING, CARDIAC FUNCTION, AND HEART FAILURE

Both CSA and OSA are common in HF, present in up to 60% of HF patients.[53] CSA is the most common SDB variant associated with HF with a reduced ejection fraction (HFrEF), but OSA is predominant in HF with a preserved ejection fraction (HFpEF). Both OSA and CSA can occur in the same individual, underscoring the complex etiology and treatment of these disorders.

There is a bidirectional relationship between HF and SDB (Fig. 89.4). In patients with HF, pulmonary vascular congestion, elevated peripheral and central chemosensitivities, and a prolonged circulation time can cause hyperventilation, with instability in ventilation leading to apneas. Conversely, SDB may adversely affect cardiac function by contributing to systemic and pulmonary hypertension, non-dipping BP, atherosclerosis and ischemic injury, hypoxemia- and catecholamine-related myocyte injury, and cardiac remodeling. Hypoxia can trigger pulmonary vasoconstriction, which may increase the right ventricular afterload, cause right ventricular distention and leftward shift of the ventricular septum during diastole, impair LV filling, and reduce the stroke volume and cardiac output. SDB is increasingly recognized as a common cause of diastolic dysfunction, with effects attributable to chronic pressure overload, impaired coronary flow reserve, and inflammation leading to cardiac interstitial fibrosis.[54] Population studies show that the LV mass and LV mass-volume ratio (concentric remodeling) increase in proportion to the severity of SDB, with associations stronger in adults younger than 65 years of age.[55] Indices of diastolic dysfunction, including an increased E/A ratio, reduced mitral deceleration, and isovolumic relaxation, are higher in patients with SDB compared with controls.

Prospective studies demonstrate that SDB independently predicts new-onset HF. Middle-aged men with severe SDB (predominantly OSA) are estimated to have a 60% increased 8-year incidence of HF compared with men without SDB.[37] A 14-year prospective analysis of data from the Atherosclerosis Risk in Communities Study (ARIC) demonstrated that women with SDB have an approximately 30% increased incidence of HF or death compared with women without SDB, and also have an increased risk for developing LV hypertrophy.[34] In older men, the Outcomes of Sleep Disorders in Older Men Study demonstrated that the presence of SDB predicted a nearly twofold increased incidence of HF.[56] However, in this study, the risk was related to the presence of CSA or Cheyne-Stokes respiration rather than OSA. In patients with HF, SDB predicts HF exacerbations and progression, including an impaired quality of life, increased fatigue, a reduced functional status, more frequent hospitalizations, arrhythmias, and death.[57]

Current treatment strategies for OSA or CSA in patients with HF include optimization of cardiac function, with a focus on minimizing the fluid overload, and weight loss as appropriate. Exercise and elastic stockings can help prevent rostral redistribution of fluid. PAP treatment, by improving oxygenation, sympathetic activation, 24-hour BP profiles, subendocardial ischemia, preload and afterload, and inflammatory and oxidative stress, could improve cardiac function. Short-term studies demonstrate that PAP can reduce HF symptoms and improve quality of life and functional status. Small randomized controlled studies in HF also demonstrated that PAP improved the vascular and myocardial sympathetic nerve function, myocardial energetics, and diastolic dysfunction.[5] A meta-analysis estimated that PAP treatment in OSA and HF was associated with a 5.2% improvement in the LV ejection fraction.[58]

PAP therapies, however, have not been demonstrated to reduce mortality or the occurrence of cardiac events in rigorous clinical trials.

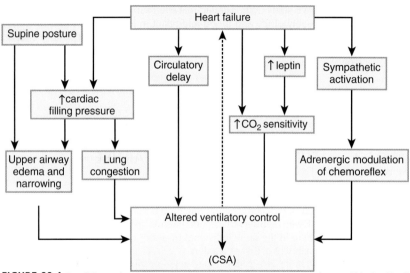

FIGURE 89.4 Possible mechanisms underlying development of CSA and the possible feedback from CSA resulting in exacerbation of heart failure. (From Somers VK, White DP, Amin R, et al. Sleep Apnea and Cardiovascular Disease: An American Heart Association/American College of Cardiology Foundation Scientific Statement From the American Heart Association Council for High Blood Pressure Research Professional Education Committee, Council on Clinical Cardiology, Stroke Council, and Council on Cardiovascular Nursing. *J Am Coll Cardiol*. 2008;52(8):686–717.)

Although a retrospective analysis of approximately 30,000 Medicare beneficiaries with newly diagnosed HF showed that treatment of SDB decreased rates of readmission, costs of health care, and mortality;[59] subsequent randomized controlled studies did not confirm these benefits. The first randomized controlled study—the Canadian Positive Airway Pressure (CANPAP) study—demonstrated that PAP improved several intermediate endpoints in patients with CSA and HFrEF (ejection fraction, catecholamines), but did not change mortality.[60] A potential explanation for this finding was that PAP did not adequately suppress central apneas, resulting in a suboptimal intervention. In support of this, a post hoc analysis suggested improved heart transplant-free survival in the subset of patients in whom CSA was suppressed.[61] Subsequently, two multinational studies were initiated to evaluate the role of a newer therapy—adaptive servoventilation (ASV)—a pressure device that delivers auto-adjusting pressure support on a breath-by-breath basis designed to suppress both obstructive and central apneas. The results of the first ASV trial, Treatment of Sleep-Disordered Breathing with Predominant Central Sleep Apnea by Adaptive Servo Ventilation in Patients with Heart Failure (SERVE-HF), conducted in 1345 patients with symptomatic HF and moderate to severe CSA, showed an unexpected 34% *increase* in CVD mortality rate with ASV as compared to usual care.[62] An advisory was subsequently issued against the use of ASV for treatment of patients with predominant CSA who have HFrEF with an ejection fraction of less than 45%. A second ongoing trial, Effect of ASV on Survival and Hospitalizations (ADVENT-HF), is testing an alternative ASV device in patients with OSA or CSA. Current consensus is that PAP can be used to treat symptoms of SDB such as sleepiness in patients with OSA or CSA who have HF, but that ASV should be avoided in patients with CSA with an ejection fraction less than 45%. This approach is reflected in the 2017 updated AHA/ACC Heart Failure Guidelines,[63] which highlighted (1) the importance of a formal sleep assessment to distinguish obstructive from CSA in patients with HF and symptoms of SDB or sleepiness; (2) use of PAP as a treatment strategy for improving sleep quality and daytime sleepiness; and (3) avoidance of ASV in patients with CSA and reduced ejection fraction.

The challenges of using pressure support therapies in patients with HF have stimulated investigations of alternative interventions. Nocturnal oxygen supplementation (NOS), which can stabilize breathing in patients with CSA and improve intermediate markers of cardiac function and quality of life, is under evaluation for use in patients with CSA and HFrEF in an ongoing multi-center trial (NCT03745898). Diaphragmatic stimulation, used to directly trigger or augment breathing efforts, is another approach potentially useful for treating CSA. An implantable unilateral transvenous phrenic nerve stimulator (PNS;

remede, Respicardia) was tested in 151 patients with CSA, 64% of whom had HF. The initial study results showed that more than half of a treatment group experienced more than a 50% reduction in the AHI at 6-months as well as experienced improved sleep quality and sleepiness, with effects stable for as long as 36 months.[64] Although small improvements in ejection fraction were observed, data on long term effects on survival are not available. The FDA granted pre-market approval for commercial use of the device in 2017 for treatment of moderate to severe CSA, with use restricted to centers with specific clinical expertise. Longer-term follow-up and assessment of the role of PNS across the spectrum of HF phenotypes are needed.

SLEEP-DISORDERED BREATHING AND CARDIAC ARRHYTHMIAS

Patients with SDB are predisposed to ventricular and atrial arrhythmias because of underlying cardiac risk factors and cardiac disease, as well as to the specific SDB-related stressors of intermittent hypoxemia, acidosis, sympathetic nervous system surges, and swings in intrathoracic pressures. Bradycardia and atrioventricular block may occur secondary to vagal stimulation accompanying apneas and hypoxemia. Susceptibility to atrial arrhythmias also reflects the vulnerability of the atrial walls to swings in intrathoracic pressure and mechanoreceptor activation, as well as sensitivity of the pulmonary vein ganglia to autonomic stimulation.[65] The degree of hypoxemia appears to be a potent stimulus for ventricular arrhythmias, sudden cardiac death, and recurrence of AF following cardioversion. Although the molecular mechanisms underlying these associations are not well understood, connexin remodeling, dysregulation of myocardial excitation/coupling, and phosphorylation of sodium channels are implicated in SDB-related atrial fibrosis and conduction and sinus node abnormalities.[66–68]

Abnormalities of P wave morphology and QT dispersion, indicative of underlying electrical conduction problems, have been observed in the overnight recordings of patients with SDB.[69] Moreover, apneas and hypopneas appear to be direct triggers of paroxysms of ventricular tachycardia and AF. Analysis of the temporal patterns of overnight arrhythmias demonstrated a 17-fold increased rate of arrhythmias occurring after an episode of apnea compared with a period of normal breathing.[70] Based on this analysis, a patient with moderate OSA (AHI 25) is estimated to experience one episode of a significant arrhythmia every 6 months attributable to apneic activity. In community studies, moderate or severe OSA was associated with a two- to fourfold increased risk of nocturnal arrhythmias; this finding suggested a basis for the observed increase in nocturnal sudden cardiac death in SDB.[71]

Of the arrhythmias, the link between OSA and AF has received the most study (see Chapter 66). OSA occurs in 21% to 74% of patients with AF[72] and is associated with increased hospitalization rates and symptom burden,[73] and recurrent AF after cardioversion.[74] Meta-analyses estimate that untreated OSA is associated with a 31% increased AF recurrence after catheter ablation.[75,76] A meta-analysis of observational studies estimated that PAP use in patients with OSA reduces the AF risk by 44%.[77] Observational studies also estimate that PAP can reduce risk of recurrent AF after cardioversion or catheter ablation to levels comparable to those in individuals without OSA and reduces the likelihood of progression to more permanent forms of AF.[74–76] A lower recurrence rate following ablation therapy in OSA patients treated with CPAP was reported to parallel PAP-related reductions in BP, atrial size, and ventricular mass,[78] supporting a physiological benefit of PAP. A consensus panel has identified OSA as an AF risk factor.[79] The high rate of AF recurrence in untreated patients has discouraged the use of ablation procedures until OSA is treated with PAP. However, it is important to note that there are no RCTs to support benefit: only one small RCT was conducted that was designed to address this question, which was negative,[80] and the SAVE trial provided no evidence for a benefit of PAP on an AF secondary outcome.[51]

FUTURE PERSPECTIVES

SDB is highly prevalent in patients with hypertension, coronary artery disease, HF (with or without a reduced ejection fraction), and atrial and ventricular arrhythmias. The profound nightly disturbances that occur with SDB cause a range of physiologic disturbances that adversely affect cardiac structure and function, and likely exacerbate the incidence and progression of these diseases. Treatment of OSA can improve the BP, ejection fraction, ventricular ectopy, and recurrence rate of AF, and can also improve the quality of life and mood in patients with CVD. The existing data indicate that patients with OSA who successfully use PAP have reduced rates of resistant hypertension and experience improved outcomes, including fewer cardiac and cerebrovascular events and lower mortality rates. Although the impact of directly treating CSA on cardiovascular outcomes remains uncertain, the presence of CSA predicts increased mortality rates as well as incident AF, and patients with CSA and HF may benefit from intensive HF therapy. Cardiologists may be increasingly involved in recognizing SDB and can use information on its pathophysiologic effects to tailor interventions and inform chronic disease management strategies.

REFERENCES

Epidemiology

1. Berry RB, Budhiraja R, Gottlieb DJ, et al. Rules for scoring respiratory events in sleep: update of the 2007 AASM manual for the scoring of sleep and associated events. Deliberations of the sleep apnea definitions task force of the American Academy of Sleep Medicine. *J Clin Sleep Med.* 2012;8(5):597–619.
2. Chai-Coetzer CL, Antic NA, Rowland LS, et al. A simplified model of screening questionnaire and home monitoring for obstructive sleep apnoea in primary care. *Thorax.* 2011;66(3):213–219.
3. White LH, Bradley TD. Role of nocturnal rostral fluid shift in the pathogenesis of obstructive and central sleep apnoea. *J Physiol (Lond).* 2013;591(5):1179–1193.
4. Dempsey JA, Veasey SC, Morgan BJ, O'Donnell CP. Pathophysiology of sleep apnea. *Physiol Rev.* 2010;90(1):47–112.
5. Javaheri S, Barbe F, Campos-Rodriguez F, et al. Sleep apnea: types, mechanisms, and clinical cardiovascular consequences. *J Am Coll Cardiol.* 2017;69(7):841–858.
6. Mokhlesi B, Finn LA, Hagen EW, et al. Obstructive sleep apnea during REM sleep and hypertension. Results of the Wisconsin Sleep Cohort. *Am J Respir Crit Care Med.* 2014;190(10):1158–1167.
7. Peppard PE, Young T, Barnet JH, et al. Increased prevalence of sleep-disordered breathing in adults. *Am J Epidemiol.* 2013;177(9):1006–1014.
8. Redline S, Strohl KP. Recognition and consequences of obstructive sleep apnea hypopnea syndrome. *Otolaryngol Clin North Am.* 1999;32(2):303–331.
9. Wimms A, Woehrle H, Ketheeswaran S, et al. Obstructive sleep apnea in women: specific issues and interventions. *BioMed Res Int.* 2016;2016:1764837.
10. Peppard PE, Young T, Palta M, et al. Longitudinal study of moderate weight change and sleep-disordered breathing. *J Am Med Assoc.* 2000;284(23):3015–3021.
11. Patel SR, Tishler PV. Familial and genetic factors. In: Kushida CA, ed. *Obstructive Sleep Apnea: Pathophysiology, Comorbidities, and Consequences.* New York: Informa Healthcare; 2007.
12. Chen H, Cade BE, Gleason KJ, et al. Multiethnic meta-analysis Identifies RAI1 as a possible obstructive sleep apnea-related quantitative trait locus in men. *Am J Respir Cell Mol Biol.* 2018;58(3):391–401.
13. Chen X, Wang R, Zee P, et al. Racial/ethnic differences in sleep disturbances: the Multi-Ethnic Study of Atherosclerosis (MESA). *Sleep.* 2015;38(6):877–888.
14. Redline S, Baker-Goodwin S, Bakker JP, et al. Patient partnerships transforming sleep medicine research and clinical care: perspectives from the sleep apnea patient-centered outcomes network. *J Clin Sleep Med.* 2016;12(7):1053–1058.
15. Won CHJ, Reid M, Sofer T, et al. Sex differences in obstructive sleep apnea phenotypes, the multi-ethnic study of atherosclerosis. *Sleep.* 2020;43(5).
16. Lyons OD, Bradley TD. Heart failure and sleep apnea. *Can J Cardiol.* 2015;31(7):898–908.
17. Jonas DE, Amick HR, Feltner C, et al. Screening for obstructive sleep apnea in adults: evidence report and systematic review for the US preventive services task force. *J Am Med Assoc.* 2017;317(4):415–433.
18. Shah N, Hanna DB, Teng Y, et al. Sex-specific prediction models for sleep apnea from the Hispanic community health study/study of Satinos. *Chest.* 2016;149(6):1409–1418.
19. Baltzis D, Bakker JP, Patel SR, Veves A. Obstructive sleep apnea and vascular diseases. *Compr Physiol.* 2016;6(3):1519–1528.
20. Orrù G, Storari M, Scano A, et al. Obstructive Sleep Apnea, oxidative stress, inflammation and endothelial dysfunction-An overview of predictive laboratory biomarkers. *Eur Rev Med Pharmacol Sci.* 2020;24(12):6939–6948.
21. Pedrosa RP, Drager LF, Gonzaga CC, et al. Obstructive sleep apnea: the most common secondary cause of hypertension associated with resistant hypertension. *Hypertension.* 2011;58(5):811–817.
22. Seif F, Patel SR, Walia HK, et al. Obstructive sleep apnea and diurnal nondipping hemodynamic indices in patients at increased cardiovascular risk. *J Hypertens.* 2014;32(2):267–275.
23. Peppard PE, Young T, Palta M, Skatrud J. Prospective study of the association between sleep-disordered breathing and hypertension. *N Engl J Med.* 2000;342(19):1378–1384.

Management

24. Liu L, Cao Q, Guo Z, Dai Q. Continuous positive airway pressure in patients with obstructive sleep apnea and resistant hypertension: a meta-analysis of randomized controlled trials. *J Clin Hypertens.* 2016;18(2):153–158.
25. Gottlieb DJ, Punjabi NM, Mehra R, et al. CPAP versus oxygen in obstructive sleep apnea. *N Engl J Med.* 2014;370(24):2276–2285.
26. Iftikhar IH, Valentine CW, Bittencourt LRA, et al. Effects of continuous positive airway pressure on blood pressure in patients with resistant hypertension and obstructive sleep apnea: a meta-analysis. *J Hypertens.* 2014;32(12):2341–2350; discussion 2350.
27. Martínez-García M-A, Capote F, Campos-Rodríguez F, et al. Effect of CPAP on blood pressure in patients with obstructive sleep apnea and resistant hypertension: the HIPARCO randomized clinical trial. *J Am Med Assoc.* 2013;310(22):2407–2415.
28. Sánchez-de-la-Torre M, Khalyfa A, Sánchez-de-la-Torre A, et al. Precision medicine in patients with resistant hypertension and obstructive sleep apnea: blood pressure response to continuous positive airway pressure treatment. *J Am Coll Cardiol.* 2015;66(9):1023–1032.
29. Thunström E, Manhem K, Rosengren A, Peker Y. Blood pressure response to losartan and continuous positive airway pressure in hypertension and obstructive sleep apnea. *Am J Respir Crit Care Med.* 2016;193(3):310–320.
30. Chirinos JA, Gurubhagavatula I, Teff K, et al. CPAP, weight loss, or both for obstructive sleep apnea. *N Engl J Med.* 2014;370(24):2265–2275.
31. National High Blood Pressure Education Program. *The Seventh Report of the Joint National Committee on Prevention, Detection, Evaluation, and Treatment of High Blood Pressure.* Bethesda (MD): National Heart, Lung, and Blood Institute (US); 2004.
32. Baessler A, Nadeem R, Harvey M, et al. Treatment for sleep apnea by continuous positive airway pressure improves levels of inflammatory markers - a meta-analysis. *J Inflamm.* 2013;10:13.
33. Mak GS, Kern MJ, Patel PM. Influence of obstructive sleep apnea and treatment with continuous positive airway pressure on fractional flow reserve measurements for coronary lesion assessment. *Catheter Cardiovasc Interv.* 2010;75(2):207–213.
34. Roca GQ, Redline S, Claggett B, et al. Sex-specific association of sleep apnea severity with subclinical myocardial injury, ventricular hypertrophy, and heart failure risk in a community-dwelling cohort: the atherosclerosis risk in communities-sleep heart health study. *Circulation.* 2015;132(14):1329–1337.
35. Yeboah J, Redline S, Johnson C, et al. Association between sleep apnea, snoring, incident cardiovascular events and all-cause mortality in an adult population: MESA. *Atherosclerosis.* 2011;219(2):963–968.
36. Campos-Rodriguez F, Martinez-Garcia MA, Reyes-Nuñez N, et al. Role of sleep apnea and continuous positive airway pressure therapy in the incidence of stroke or coronary heart disease in women. *Am J Respir Crit Care Med.* 2014;189(12):1544–1550.
37. Gottlieb DJ, Yenokyan G, Newman AB, et al. Prospective study of obstructive sleep apnea and incident coronary heart disease and heart failure: the sleep heart health study. *Circulation.* 2010;122(4):352–360.
38. Gami AS, Olson EJ, Shen WK, et al. Obstructive sleep apnea and the risk of sudden cardiac death: a longitudinal study of 10,701 adults. *J Am Coll Cardiol.* 2013;62(7):610–616.
39. Azarbarzin A, Sands SA, Stone KL, et al. The hypoxic burden of sleep apnoea predicts cardiovascular disease-related mortality: the Osteoporotic Fractures in Men Study and the Sleep Heart Health Study. *Eur Heart J.* 2019;40(14):1149–1157.
40. Nakashima H, Henmi T, Minami K, et al. Obstructive sleep apnoea increases the incidence of morning peak of onset in acute myocardial infarction. *Eur Heart J Acute Cardiovasc Care.* 2013;2(2):153–158.
41. Gami AS, Howard DE, Olson EJ, Somers VK. Day-night pattern of sudden death in obstructive sleep apnea. *N Engl J Med.* 2005;352(12):1206–1214.
42. Lutsey PL, McClelland RL, Duprez D, et al. Objectively measured sleep characteristics and prevalence of coronary artery calcification: the Multi-Ethnic Study of Atherosclerosis Sleep study. *Thorax.* 2015;70(9):880–887.
43. Kwon Y, Duprez DA, Jacobs DR, et al. Obstructive sleep apnea and progression of coronary artery calcium: the multi-ethnic study of atherosclerosis study. *J Am Heart Assoc.* 2014;3(5):e001241.
44. Mazaki T, Kasai T, Yokoi H, et al. Impact of sleep-disordered breathing on long-term outcomes in patients with acute coronary syndrome who have undergone primary percutaneous coronary intervention. *J Am Heart Assoc.* 2016;5(6).
45. Nakashima H, Kurobe M, Minami K, et al. Effects of moderate-to-severe obstructive sleep apnea on the clinical manifestations of plaque vulnerability and the progression of coronary atherosclerosis in patients with acute coronary syndrome. *Eur Heart J Acute Cardiovasc Care.* 2015;4(1):75–84.
46. Lee C-H, Sethi R, Li R, et al. Obstructive sleep apnea and cardiovascular events after percutaneous coronary intervention. *Circulation.* 2016;133(21):2008–2017.
47. Buchner S, Satzl A, Debl K, et al. Impact of sleep-disordered breathing on myocardial salvage and infarct size in patients with acute myocardial infarction. *Eur Heart J.* 2014;35(3):192–199.
48. Shah N, Redline S, Yaggi HK, et al. Obstructive sleep apnea and acute myocardial infarction severity: ischemic preconditioning? *Sleep Breath.* 2013;17(2):819–826.
49. Barbé F, Durán-Cantolla J, Sánchez-de-la-Torre M, et al. Effect of continuous positive airway pressure on the incidence of hypertension and cardiovascular events in nonsleepy patients with obstructive sleep apnea: a randomized controlled trial. *J Am Med Assoc.* 2012;307(20):2161–2168.
50. Peker Y, Glantz H, Eulenburg C, et al. Effect of positive airway pressure on cardiovascular outcomes in coronary artery disease patients with nonsleepy obstructive sleep apnea. The RICCADSA randomized controlled trial. *Am J Respir Crit Care Med.* 2016;194(5):613–620.
51. McEvoy RD, Antic NA, Heeley E, et al. CPAP for prevention of cardiovascular events in obstructive sleep apnea. *N Engl J Med.* 2016;375(10):919–931.
52. Sánchez-de-la-Torre M, Sánchez-de-la-Torre A, Bertran S, et al. Effect of obstructive sleep apnoea and its treatment with continuous positive airway pressure on the prevalence of cardiovascular events in patients with acute coronary syndrome (ISAACC study): a randomised controlled trial. *Lancet Respir Med.* 2020;8(4):359–367.

Heart Failure

53. Pearse SG, Cowie MR. Sleep-disordered breathing in heart failure. *Eur J Heart Fail.* 2016;18(4):353–361.
54. Bodez D, Damy T, Soulat-Dufour L, et al. Consequences of obstructive sleep apnoea syndrome on left ventricular geometry and diastolic function. *Arch Cardiovasc Dis.* 2016;109(8–9):494–503.
55. Javaheri S, Sharma RK, Wang R, et al. Association between obstructive sleep apnea and left ventricular structure by age and Gender: the multi-ethnic study of atherosclerosis. *Sleep.* 2016;39(3):523–529.
56. Javaheri S, Blackwell T, Ancoli-Israel S, et al. Sleep-disordered breathing and incident heart failure in older men. *Am J Respir Crit Care Med.* 2016;193(5):561–568.
57. Khayat R, Jarjoura D, Porter K, et al. Sleep disordered breathing and post-discharge mortality in patients with acute heart failure. *Eur Heart J.* 2015;36(23):1463–1469.
58. Sun H, Shi J, Li M, Chen X. Impact of continuous positive airway pressure treatment on left ventricular ejection fraction in patients with obstructive sleep apnea: a meta-analysis of randomized controlled trials. *PloS One.* 2013;8(5):e62298.
59. Javaheri S, Caref EB, Chen E, et al. Sleep apnea testing and outcomes in a large cohort of Medicare beneficiaries with newly diagnosed heart failure. *Am J Respir Crit Care Med.* 2011;183(4):539–546.
60. Bradley TD, Logan AG, Kimoff RJ, et al. Continuous positive airway pressure for central sleep apnea and heart failure. *N Engl J Med.* 2005;353(19):2025–2033.
61. Arzt M, Floras JS, Logan AG, et al. Suppression of central sleep apnea by continuous positive airway pressure and transplant-free survival in heart failure: a post hoc analysis of the Canadian Continuous Positive Airway Pressure for Patients with Central Sleep Apnea and Heart Failure Trial (CANPAP). *Circulation.* 2007;115(25):3173–3180.
62. Cowie MR, Woehrle H, Wegscheider K, et al. Adaptive servo-ventilation for central sleep apnea in systolic heart failure. *N Engl J Med.* 2015;373(12):1095–1105.

DISEASES OF THE MYOCARDIUM, PERICARDIUM, AND PULMONARY VASCULATURE BED

63. Yancy CW, Jessup M, Bozkurt B, et al. ACC/AHA/HFSA focused update of the 2013 ACCF/AHA guideline for the management of heart failure: a report of the American College of Cardiology/ American Heart Association task force on clinical practice guidelines and the heart failure Society of America. *J Am Coll Cardiol.* 2017;70(6):776–803. 2017.

64. Fox H, Oldenburg O, Javaheri S, et al. Long-term efficacy and safety of phrenic nerve stimulation for the treatment of central sleep apnea. *Sleep.* 2019;42(11).

65. Linz D, Woehrle H, Bitter T, et al. The importance of sleep-disordered breathing in cardiovascular disease. *Clin Res Cardiol.* 2015;104(9):705–718.

66. Dimitri H, Ng M, Brooks AG, et al. Atrial remodeling in obstructive sleep apnea: implications for atrial fibrillation. *Heart Rhythm.* 2012;9(3):321–327.

67. Bare DJ, Yan J, Ai X. Evidence of CaMKII-regulated late INa in atrial fibrillation patients with sleep apnea: one-Step closer to finding Plausible Therapeutic Targets for atrial fibrillation? *Circ Res.* 2020;126(5):616–618.

68. Lebek S, Pichler K, Reuthner K, et al. Enhanced CaMKII-dependent late INa induces atrial proarrhythmic activity in patients with sleep-disordered breathing. *Circ Res.* 2020;126(5):603–615.

69. Maeno K, Kasagi S, Ueda A, et al. Effects of obstructive sleep apnea and its treatment on signal-averaged P-wave duration in men. *Circ Arrhythm Electrophysiol.* 2013;6(2):287–293.

70. Monahan K, Storfer-Isser A, Mehra R, et al. Triggering of nocturnal arrhythmias by sleep-disordered breathing events. *J Am Coll Cardiol.* 2009;54(19):1797–1804.

71. Mehra R, Stone KL, Varosy PD, et al. Nocturnal Arrhythmias across a spectrum of obstructive and central sleep-disordered breathing in older men: outcomes of sleep disorders in older men (MrOS sleep) study. *Arch Intern Med.* 2009;169(12):1147–1155.

72. Linz D, McEvoy RD, Cowie MR, et al. Associations of obstructive sleep apnea with atrial fibrillation and continuous positive airway pressure treatment: a review. *JAMA Cardiol.* 2018;3(6):532–540.

73. Holmqvist F, Guan N, Zhu Z, et al. Impact of obstructive sleep apnea and continuous positive airway pressure therapy on outcomes in patients with atrial fibrillation-Results from the Outcomes Registry for Better Informed Treatment of Atrial Fibrillation (ORBIT-AF). *Am Heart J.* 2015;169(5):647–654.e2.

74. Kanagala R, Murali NS, Friedman PA, et al. Obstructive sleep apnea and the recurrence of atrial fibrillation. *Circulation.* 2003;107(20):2589–2594.

75. Li L, Wang Z, Li J, et al. Efficacy of catheter ablation of atrial fibrillation in patients with obstructive sleep apnoea with and without continuous positive airway pressure treatment: a meta-analysis of observational studies. *Europace.* 2014;16(9):1309–1314.

76. Ng CY, Liu T, Shehata M, et al. Meta-analysis of obstructive sleep apnea as predictor of atrial fibrillation recurrence after catheter ablation. *Am J Cardiol.* 2011;108(1):47–51.

77. Qureshi WT, Nasir UB, Alqalyoobi S, et al. Meta-analysis of continuous positive airway pressure as a therapy of atrial fibrillation in obstructive sleep apnea. *Am J Cardiol.* 2015;116(11):1767–1773.

78. Neilan TG, Farhad H, Dodson JA, et al. Effect of sleep apnea and continuous positive airway pressure on cardiac structure and recurrence of atrial fibrillation. *J Am Heart Assoc.* 2013;2(6):e000421.

79. Estes NAM, Sacco RL, Al-Khatib SM, et al. American Heart Association atrial fibrillation research summit: a conference report from the American Heart Association. *Circulation.* 2011;124(3):363–372.

80. Caples SM, Mansukhani MP, Friedman PA, Somers VK. The impact of continuous positive airway pressure treatment on the recurrence of atrial fibrillation post cardioversion: a randomized controlled trial. *Int J Cardiol.* 2019;278:133–136.

90 Cardiovascular Disease in Older Adults

DANIEL E. FORMAN, JEROME L. FLEG, NANETTE KASS WENGER, AND MICHAEL W. RICH

The population of older adults is expanding throughout the world. In the United States the population age ≥65 years, barely 3 million total in 1900, has climbed to about 46 million and is expected to reach almost 84 million by 2050.[1] The population age ≥85, only about 0.2% of the total in 1900, is anticipated to reach 5% to 6% by 2050. Across the European Union, 20% of the population is over age 65, and more than 29% of Japan's population is in this age group.[2] Extended lifespan increases exposure to mounting cardiovascular disease (CVD) risk factors and leads to injurious effects that are cumulative over time[3]; in addition, intrinsic age-related cellular and subcellular physiologic changes increase susceptibility to CVD incidence and progression.[4] Prevalence of almost every type of CVD increases with age, including many conditions that develop predominantly in older adults (e.g., degenerative aortic stenosis [AS], heart failure [HF] with preserved ejection fraction [HFpEF], sick sinus syndrome). Furthermore, CVD in older adults tends to be more complex than in younger populations, both in underlying pathophysiology and because it is more likely to occur in combination with multiple comorbidities. Approximately 70% of adults age ≥65 years in the United States have CVD, including 85% of those age ≥80 years,[5] with disproportionate hospitalizations, procedures, costs, and health care resource utilization. Adults age ≥75 years old comprise only about 6% of the current U.S. population but account for >50% of CVD deaths.

The biologic processes that predispose to CVD in old age also foster higher susceptibility to concomitant diseases and geriatric syndromes.[6] CVDs in older individuals thus occur in a context of comorbidities, frailty, sarcopenia, cognitive decline, and other non-CVDs that add to management complexity. In addition to increased morbidity and mortality, CVD in older adults is associated with higher vulnerability to functional decline and progressive disability, which in turn increase risk for CVD.[7]

WHAT IS AGING?

Although aging is customarily measured in chronologic years, more fundamental determinants of aging entail biologic stress over time (e.g., oxidative stress) in juxtaposition to diminishing homeostatic capacities contingent on telomeres, epigenetics, proteostasis, autophagy, and other subcellular factors.[8] Cellular senescence and the related phenomenon of inflammaging, or chronic low-grade inflammation, also increase with age[9] and catalyze development of CVD, comorbidities, and geriatric syndromes. Yet progression of subcellular aging phenomena and clinical manifestations are moderated by each person's lifelong health habits (e.g., nutrition, physical activity, sleep, alcohol), CVD risk factors, comorbidities, social structure (e.g., spouse, children), and intrinsic functional capacities (e.g., physical, cognitive). Although chronologic years are immutable, other aspects of aging can often be modified. Habitual exercise and/or caloric restriction, for example, reduce the trajectory of aging and susceptibility to age-related CVD.

AGE-ASSOCIATED CHANGES IN CARDIOVASCULAR STRUCTURE AND FUNCTION

Normal aging is associated with alterations in cellular function, molecular signaling, proteostasis, and other mechanistic variations that lead to progressive changes in cardiovascular (CV) structure and function. These changes induce localized and systemic neurohormonal responses, such as release of proinflammatory cytokines and upregulation of the renin-angiotensin-aldosterone system, that set the stage for age-related CVDs (Fig. 90.1).[4]

Vasculature

Prominent structural and functional changes affect the arterial system in older adults, even among those with no apparent CVD. The arterial wall media thickens due to smooth muscle cell hypertrophy, extracellular matrix accumulation, and calcium deposition. Intimal-medial thickness (IMT) increases almost threefold between ages 20 and 90 years in normotensive individuals.[8] The range of IMT also increases with age, suggesting a variable response to aging, likely due to different genetic and lifestyle factors.

Along with increased IMT, advancing age leads to fraying of elastic fibers as well as increases in collagen content and enzymatic cross-linking of extracellular matrix molecules in the arterial media that reduce distensibility and increase stiffness.[10] Irreversible non-enzymatic glycation-based crosslinking of collagen forms advanced glycation end products (AGEs) that exacerbate the stiffening.

Changes in both vasodilating nitric oxide (NO) and vasoconstricting angiotensin II also contribute to vascular aging. Age-dependent reductions in endothelium-dependent vasodilation have been attributed to reduced NO production.[10] Animal studies show both lower NO levels

CARDIOVASCULAR DISEASE IN SELECT POPULATIONS

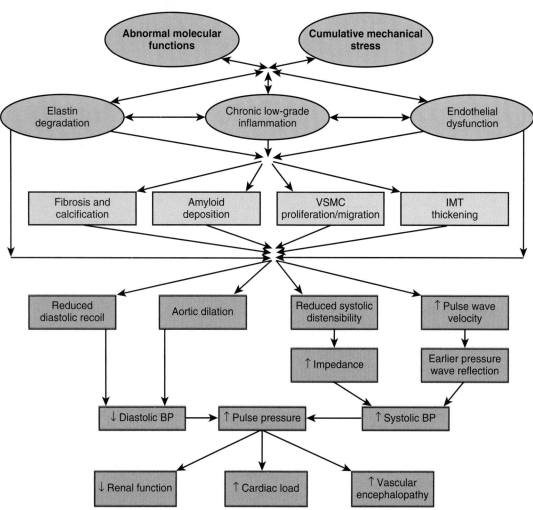

FIGURE 90.1 Conceptual model of arterial aging and its downstream effects. Age-associated molecular disorders and cumulative mechanical stress lead to a state of chronic inflammation, elastin degradation, and endothelial and vascular smooth muscle cell (VSMC) dysfunction. Downstream effects result in arterial wall calcification, fibrosis, amyloid deposition, VSMC proliferation, and intimal-medial thickening (IMT). These structural changes lead to functional alterations resulting in increased systolic blood pressure (BP) decreased diastolic BP, and widened pulse pressure. The increase in pulsatility leads to increased left ventricular load as well as elevated risks for chronic kidney disease and vascular dementia. (Adapted from Lakatta EG. So! What's aging? Is cardiovascular aging a disease? J Mol Cell Cardiol 2015;83:1-13.)

and reduced NO, consistent with reduced endothelial NO synthesis. Conversely, angiotensin II in the vessel wall increases 1000-fold with substantially increased angiotensin II signaling.

Both oxidative stress and chronic low-grade inflammation are key mediators of the structural and functional changes in the arterial wall with aging (see Chapter 24). Oxidative stress results from excessive generation of reactive oxygen species by enzymes such as NADPH oxidase, uncoupled NO synthase, and xanthine oxidase by the mitochondrial transport chain and from reduced antioxidant capacity. Increased reactive oxygen species and dysfunctional endothelial NO synthase contribute to age-associated decrements in endothelium-mediated vasodilation. Elevated oxidative stress also leads to enhanced protein oxidation, activation of inflammatory and endoplasmic reticulum stress responses, and apoptosis.

As a result of structural and functional changes in the arterial walls, stiffening of large- and medium-sized arteries occurs with aging, independent of disease. Systolic blood pressure (SBP) generally rises (see Chapter 26). In contrast, diastolic blood pressure (DBP) tends to rise until the sixth decade and declines thereafter due to reduced elastic recoil from the stiffer large arteries.[10] Pulse pressure, the difference between SBP and DBP, also increases with age, augmenting the pulsatile load on the heart and vasculature Pulse wave velocity (PWV), the speed with which an arterial pulse wave traverses the arterial tree, is another index of arterial stiffness. Aorto-femoral PWV increases two- to threefold across the adult lifespan in normotensive populations (see Chapter 43).

Left Ventricular (LV) Composition and Mass
With aging there is a decrease in the total number of cardiomyocytes, likely due to apoptosis, and an increase in their individual size (i.e.,

hypertrophy).[8] In both animal and human studies, apoptotic myocytes were more prevalent in the hearts of older men compared with women, paralleling an age-related decline of LV mass in men but not in women. Within the connective tissue, collagen content, fibrosis, and deposition of cardiac amyloid and lipofuscin all increase. The heart therefore becomes more fibrotic and stiffer with age.[11]

LV Wall Thickness, Cavity Size, and Shape
Despite the absence of an increase in cardiac mass with aging, there is a significant increase in myocardial thickness[11] due to increased cardiomyocyte size. Although concentric LV hypertrophy occurs, the interventricular septum increases in thickness more than the free wall, and there is a change in LV shape to a more spherical configuration. A more spherical ventricle is exposed to higher wall stress and is associated with higher incidence of LV dysfunction and HF (see Chapter 47). LV diastolic and systolic volumes decline with age and the LV mass/volume ratio increases in both sexes.[11]

Resting Cardiac Function
In healthy normotensive adults, resting LV shortening fraction and LV ejection fraction (LVEF), the two most commonly used measures of global LV systolic performance, are not affected by age.[11] Prolonged contractile activation of the thickened LV wall maintains a normal ejection time, and compensates for the late systolic augmentation of blood pressure (BP), preserving systolic LV pump function despite increased arterial stiffness. However, there is a modest decline in transmural global longitudinal strain and an increase in global circumferential strain with age. The increase in circumferential strain is likely a compensatory mechanism to maintain global LVEF.

TABLE 90.1 Relationship of Cardiovascular Aging in Healthy Humans to Cardiovascular Disease

AGE-ASSOCIATED CHANGES	PLAUSIBLE MECHANISMS	POSSIBLE RELATIONSHIP TO DISEASE
CV Structural Remodeling		
↑Vascular intimal thickness	↑ VSMC migration	Early stages of atherosclerosis matrix production
↑ Arterial stiffness	Elastin fragmentation and ↑ elastase activity	Systolic hypertension
	↑ Collagen production and cross-linking	
	Altered growth factor regulation and tissue repair	Atherosclerosis
↑ LV wall thickness	↑ LV myocyte size	↓ Early LV diastolic filling
	↓ Myocyte number and focal collagen deposition	↑ LV filling pressure/dyspnea
↑ Left atrial size	↑ Left atrial volume and pressure	↑ Risk of atrial fibrillation
Calcium deposits in valves and conduction system	Mechanical stress	Aortic stenosis
		Atrioventricular block
CV functional changes		
Altered vascular tone	↓ NO production/effects	Vascular stiffening and hypertension
	↓ βAR responses	
↓ CV reserve	↑Vascular load	Lower threshold for heart failure

βAR, Beta adrenergic receptor; CV, cardiovascular; LV, left ventricular, VSMC, vascular smooth muscle cell.

In contrast to systolic function, LV diastolic performance is prominently altered by aging. Whereas LV diastolic filling occurs primarily in early diastole in younger adults, transmitral early diastolic peak-filling rate declines by 30% to 50% between ages 20 and 80 years.[11] Conversely, there is an age-associated increase in peak A-wave velocity, which represents late LV filling facilitated by atrial contraction. The increase in late LV filling is mediated via a modest age-associated increase in left atrial size.[11] Tissue Doppler imaging in older adults shows lower E, e' and s', and greater E/e' compared with young individuals in both sedentary and trained persons.

Although age-related delays in early diastolic filling rate do not usually compromise end-diastolic volume and stroke volume at rest, stress-induced tachycardia (e.g., with exercise, fever, or other physiologic stress) is likely to exacerbate diastolic filling abnormalities. Tachycardia not only disproportionately shortens the time available for diastolic filling but also exacerbates impaired energy-dependent uptake of calcium into the sarcoplasmic reticulum. Therefore, fast heart rates are commonly associated with diastolic filling abnormalities, and the higher LV diastolic pressure is transmitted into the lungs despite normal resting LV systolic function. These findings are commonly manifested as HFpEF, especially when superimposed on other common age-associated comorbidities such as hypertension, diabetes, coronary heart disease (CHD), and atrial fibrillation (AF) (see Chapter 51).

The enlargement of the left atrium that occurs as a function of age and diastolic dysfunction occurs primarily after age 70 years[11] and increases susceptibility of older adults to AF. Whereas AF is often well tolerated in younger adults, it is more likely to provoke symptoms and clinical events among older individuals. Not only is AF commonly associated with poorly tolerated fast ventricular rates, but the AF-induced loss of the atrial boost to diastolic filling aggravates age-related diastolic filling impairment. Thus, older patients with AF are more likely than younger patients to incur reduced cardiac output and resultant dyspnea and fatigue (see Chapter 66).

Age-associated myocardial changes also predispose some older adults to myocardial ischemia and HF. A thicker LV predisposes to subendocardial ischemia by increasing the distance between the epicardial coronary arteries and the subendocardial myocytes. In addition, capillary growth and flow regulation in older hearts may not match the oxygen demands of the hypertrophied myocytes. These intramyocardial changes in capillary and flow-dynamics are compounded by peripheral arterial stiffening and accelerated PWV (i.e., faster reflected pressure waves in systole), such that subendocardial perfusion is no longer bolstered by augmented pressures in diastole,[10] leading to a decline in coronary perfusion pressure.

Amidst the aforementioned age-associated changes in the vasculature and heart (Table 90.1), especially when compounded by prolonged exposure to other CVD risk factors, CVD increases markedly in older adults. Intrinsic vulnerability to atherosclerosis in the vasculature predisposes to myocardial ischemia, MI, stroke, and peripheral arterial disease (PAD). Heart failure with reduced ejection fraction (HFrEF) may

TABLE 90.2 Common Age-Related Changes that Compound CVD Risks

Kidneys	↓ Glomerular filtration rate
	↓ Renal metabolism
Lungs	↓ Ventilatory capacity
	↑ Ventilation/perfusion mismatching
Musculoskeletal	↓ Skeletal muscle mass and function (sarcopenia)
	↓ Protein reserves
	↓ Bone mass
Immune function	↑ Susceptibility to infections
Hematopoietic	↑ Levels of coagulation factors
	↑ Platelet aggregability
	↑ Inhibitors of fibrinolysis
	↑ Anemia
Neurohormonal	↓ Cerebral autoregulatory
Liver	↓ Hepatic metabolism
Mood	↑ Depression
	↑ Anxiety
Sleep	↑ Obstructive sleep apnea

develop as the result of ischemic coronary events or prolonged hypertension, either of which can impair LV systolic function. However, HFpEF is more likely to develop in the setting of ventricular stiffening, especially in association with hypertension, AF, and diabetes, all of which increase with age. Furthermore, CV aging occurs in a context of other age-related changes that compound the effects of CVD (Table 90.2) (see Chapter 51). Risks associated with myocardial ischemia, HF and other CVD become significantly worsened in the presence of concomitant renal, metabolic, hematologic, pulmonary, and other noncardiac physiologic changes.

CV Response to Exercise

The ability to perform physical activity is highly relevant in clinical evaluation, especially in older adults. The CV response to aerobic exercise remains useful as a diagnostic and prognostic tool and is also strongly predictive of the ability of older individuals to withstand major procedures or aggressive therapies (see Chapter 32).

Aerobic Exercise Capacity. Cardiorespiratory fitness (defined by oxygen consumption [VO_2] max per kg weight at peak exercise) declines progressively with age. In cross-sectional studies, the decline is ~50% from the third to ninth decade. In longitudinal studies, a more

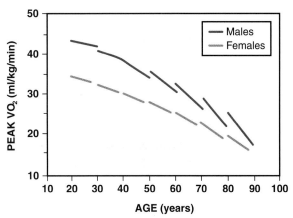

FIGURE 90.2 Longitudinal changes in peak oxygen (VO_2) consumption and maximal heart rate in healthy volunteers. Although the decrease in heart rate remained relatively constant over time at ~5% per decade, an accelerated age-associated decline occurs in peak VO_2 and oxygen pulse. (From Fleg JL, et al. Accelerated longitudinal decline of aerobic capacity in healthy older adults. Circulation. 2005 Aug 2;112(5):674-682.)

pronounced age-associated VO_2max decline is evident, regardless of habitual physical activity levels (Fig. 90.2).[11] The decline is only partially explained by changes in maximal heart rate and other CV parameters. Sarcopenia (i.e., atrophy and weakening of skeletal muscle) contributes significantly to age-associated decrease in VO_2 max. Age-related sarcopenia involves reduced number, size, and function of muscle fibers. By age 75 years, muscle mass typically represents ~15% of body weight compared with 30% in young adults. Fast twitch fibers atrophy to a greater extent than slow twitch fibers, which likely contributes to decrements in strength that are proportionally greater than the loss of muscle mass. Increased intramuscular fat and decreased mitochondrial bioenergetics contribute to reduced muscle function.[12] Furthermore, CVD has additional effect on skeletal muscle (most notably in HF) that compound impact of sarcopenia.[13]

The accelerated decline of aerobic capacity with age has important implications regarding functional independence and quality of life (QOL). Because many of the activities of daily living require fixed aerobic expenditures, they require a significantly larger percent of VO_2max in older than younger adults. When the energy required for an activity approaches or exceeds the aerobic capacity of an older individual, he or she will be less able and likely to perform it.[7]

Cardiac Function During Aerobic Exercise. In healthy adults, a ~50% decline in peak VO_2 between ages 20 and 80 years is accompanied by ~30% declines in cardiac output and ~20% declines in arteriovenous oxygen uptake. The decrease in cardiac index with age at maximal effort is due primarily to reduced heart rate.[11] Older individuals also have blunted capacity to reduce LV end-systolic volume (ESV) and to thereby augment LVEF with exercise to sustain higher capacity function (in part due to an age-related decline in adrenergic responsiveness). Some studies suggest this deficit may be offset by achieving a larger end-diastolic volume (EDV),[11] that is, the slower heart rate allows more time for LV filling, thereby providing a greater amount of blood in the heart at end-diastole. Nonetheless, maximum maximal LVEF often still diminishes with age due to insufficient diastolic expansion, reduced intrinsic myocardial contractility, increased arterial afterload, arterial-ventricular load mismatching, and blunted sympathetic modulation of LV contractility and arterial afterload.[10,11] The net effect of these changes is a marked reduction in CV reserve, such that even healthy older individuals free of CVD tend to become less able to maintain CV homeostasis in response to stress (e.g., major surgery or acute illness).

GERIATRIC DOMAINS PERTINENT TO CARDIOVASCULAR CARE

As described above, geriatric syndromes develop from the same biologic milieu as CVD in older adults. CVD in old age is likely to occur in combination with geriatric health care challenges that confound the standards of care that pertain primarily to younger and/or relatively more robust older populations (Table 90.3).

Multimorbidity

Multimorbidity or "multiple chronic conditions" denotes a situation in which two or more chronic conditions are active simultaneously. Multimorbidity shifts the therapeutic paradigm away from one that is oriented primarily to CVD-specific care to one that considers CVD in the context of competing conditions and priorities. For CVD therapies to achieve outcomes perceived as beneficial by a patient with multimorbidity, they must remain effective amidst conditions for which they were not intended or studied.[6]

Multimorbidity, prevalent in more than 70% of adults age ≥75 years[6] and in up to 90% of older HF patients, challenges the basic principles underlying conventional CV management. "Evidence-based" CVD guidelines typically rely on investigations that excluded study populations with significant comorbidities. Traditional therapy may be less applicable to patients with multiple diseases and concomitant medications. In a study of Medicare patients,[14] in those with HF, stroke, or AF, 50% had five or more comorbidities (Fig. 90.3). Moreover, the number of comorbidities correlates strongly with hospitalizations, cost of care, and mortality.

Management of CVD must be considered with added precautions as conventional therapies may provoke adverse effects; for example, antihypertensive medications are more likely to provoke falls in older patients with sarcopenia, Parkinson disease, or vision impairment. Furthermore, outcomes of older patients with CVD are often more likely to be affected by non-CVD comorbidities. For example, rehospitalization for HF may be caused by an infection or renal disease.

Frailty and Sarcopenia

Frailty denotes a state of vulnerability to stressors with limited reserves to stabilize declines across multiple physiologic systems.[15] Prevalence of frailty ranges from 10% to 70% in different CVD populations. Frail adults are prone to developing CVD and have worse outcomes and greater risks for harmful sequelae from standard therapies. With the advent of transcatheter aortic valve replacement (TAVR), interest in frailty accelerated among cardiology proceduralists as frailty often serves as a key selection criterion by which TAVR is considered (see Chapter 74). Subsequently, in the importance of frailty in informing personalized management has expanded to include care for acute coronary syndromes (ACS), CHD, and many other types of CVD.[15]

While the optimal assessment tool for frailty remains undefined, frailty is increasingly thought to be a biologic manifestation of inflammation[9]; circulating inflammatory biomarkers (high-sensitivity C-reactive protein and interleukin [IL]-6), as well as inflammatory cells (neutrophils and monocytes) are increased in frail individuals. Thus, CVD and frailty share inflammatory pathophysiology and tend to occur together. Older adults with CVD are more likely to be frail, and vice versa. Although geroscience insights implicate multiple subcellular mechanisms,[8] cellular senescence and associated inflammaging are significant components,[9,16] linking CVD, multimorbidity, frailty, and sarcopenia.

Sarcopenia is defined as a reduction in muscle strength and mass that is abnormally severe for an individual's age.[9] Whereas muscle atrophy is common with aging, sarcopenia entails muscle atrophy and weakening (dynapenia) that tends to be more common amid frailty and CVD. Inflammation is associated with reduced synthesis and activity of insulin-like growth factor 1 (IGF1), essential for muscle regeneration and maintenance of muscle integrity, and that also plays a role in mitigating plaque instability in atherosclerosis. In observational studies, high levels of IL-6 and low levels of IGF1 correlate with lower muscle strength and power, predicting frailty and associated risks of disability and death.

Two general approaches to identify frailty have evolved[17]: frailty conceptualized as an observable phenotype and frailty conceptualized as a numerical index. Fried advanced the premise of a "frailty phenotype" by identifying five specific physical characteristics that could be systematically assessed: weakness, low energy, slowed walking speed, decreased physical activity, and weight loss. Rockwood has championed an alternative approach in which frailty is conceptualized as an "index" of deficits of candidate variables, that is, a ratio of physical deficits as well as morbidities, disability, and other clinical variables that accumulate and progressively burden an individual. The magnitude and speed that deficits accumulate is applied as a gauge of vulnerability and risk. Variations on Fried's composite of physical phenotypic features include single-measure performance assessments including gait speed, handgrip strength, balance, or chair rise. Composite assessments such as the Timed Up and Go (TUG) and Sit to Stand tests[7] are also popular as they integrate multiple functional capabilities but usually entail more time and training to administer. A frailty tool app developed by Afilalo demonstrates their application (https://apps.apple.com/us/app/frailty-tool/id1330330931).

TABLE 90.3 Geriatric Syndromes and Clinical Implications

GERIATRIC SYNDROME	DIAGNOSIS/PREVALENCE	PROGNOSIS	DISEASE MANAGEMENT
Multimorbidity	Two or more chronic conditions (cardiac and noncardiac) that are active simultaneously Prevalence: 63% of those 65-74 years of age, 77% of those 75-84 years of age, and 83% of those ≥85 years of age	↑ Short and long-term prognostic risks due to CVD as well as non-CVD instability	Confounds customary CVD symptoms and signs Multiple diseases and providers often result in desynchronized or even contradictory aspects of care ↑ Likelihood that patients will experience high therapeutic burden
Frailty	State of vulnerability relating to diminished physiologic reserves across multiple physiologic systems Definition controversial: some define frailty as a phenotype, whereas others define frailty as an index of cumulative clinical deficits Prevalence: ranges from 10% to 60%, depending on the CVD burden, as well as the tool and cutoff chosen to define frailty.	↑ Risk from CVD as well as medical, device, percutaneous catheter, and surgical therapies used to treat CVD. ↑ Risks disability, falls, rehospitalization, poor quality of life, mortality	Guidelines-based therapy and procedures commonly overlook the impact of frailty on recommendations. Intensive care, bed rest, and functional decrements associated with many conventional therapies can exacerbate frailty and functional decline. Nutrition and exercise may help mitigate frailty and risks of frailty
Cognitive decline	Mild cognitive impairment (MCI)→ ↓ cognitive function without loss of function Prevalence estimates vary with the population and methods, but it rises with age, generally in the range of 2%-5% in those 60-55 to >20%-40% in those ≥90 years. Dementia → severe memory loss that interferes with daily life and loss of functional independence Prevalence increases with age, from ~5.0% of those aged 71-79 years to 35%-40% of those aged 90 and older.	↓ Independence ↓ Adherence ↓ Shared decision making ↓ QOL ↑ Hospitalization ↑ Mortality	Often confounds assessments of symptoms Often confounds accounts of present illness and PMHx Often confounds adherence Does not negate the potential value of therapeutic intervention, but it impacts the decision and implementation process
Delirium	Disturbance in cognition, attention, and consciousness or perception with fluctuating course Can manifest as agitated state or quiet and withdrawn High prevalence in older adults who are hospitalized, i.e., ~30%-60%.	↑ LOS ↑ Rehospitalization ↑ Functional decline ↑ Falls ↑ Long-term care ↑ Mortality	Predisposing risks include cognitive deficit, sensory limitations, and disorienting medications Treat by optimizing environment to increase orientation, avoid sedation, reduce meds, reduce pain
Polypharmacy	Multiple medications that have unintended interactive effects Polypharmacy usually considered four or more chronic medications 40% of older adults take ≥4 medications	↑ Adverse events (errors and drug interactions) ↑ Rehospitalizations ↑ Mortality	↑ Medication errors ↑ Drug–drug and drug–body interactions ↓ Adherence is common ↑ Under- and overtreatment both commonly occur Deprescribing is a relevant consideration
Disability	The inability to care for oneself or to manage one's own home	↑ Risk progressive functional and cognitive declines ↓ Self-reliance and self-efficacy ↑ Long-term care ↑ Mortality	Conventional care for CVD often contributes to a cycle of progressive disability, which highlights rationale for shared decision making for each aspect of therapy Suboptimal transitions are common contributors to disability, (e.g., hospital to home, and even hospital to postacute care)
Sensory loss	Vision and hearing deficits are common	↑ Risk progressive functional and cognitive declines ↓ Self-reliance and self-efficacy ↑ Long-term care ↑ Mortality	Conventional care for CVD often contributes to a cycle of progressive disability, which highlights rationale for shared decision making for each aspect of therapy Suboptimal transitions are common contributors to disability, (e.g., hospital to home, and even hospital to postacute care)
Incontinence	Urinary incontinence is common and often worsened by diuretics and other CVD meds		
Falls	Falls are common in older CVD patients as they can be provoked by environmental as well as syncopal etiologies and are often exacerbated by other geriatric syndromes such as polypharmacy, frailty, delirium, and visual deficits		

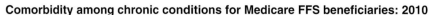

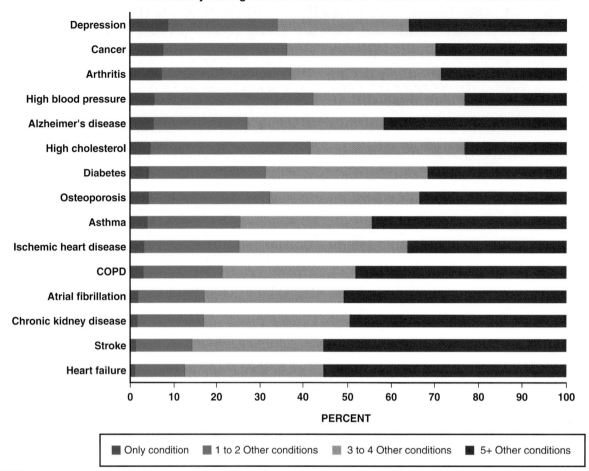

Comorbidity among chronic conditions for Medicare FFS beneficiaries: 2010

Legend: Only condition ■ 1 to 2 Other conditions ■ 3 to 4 Other conditions ■ 5+ Other conditions

FIGURE 90.3 Number of coexisting chronic conditions among Medicare fee-for-service (FFS) beneficiaries with common cardiovascular diagnoses. *COPD,* Chronic obstructive pulmonary disease. (From Centers for Medicare and Medicaid Services. Chronic Conditions Among Medicare Beneficiaries. Chartbook, 2012 Edition. Baltimore, 2012.)

Cognitive Impairment

Whereas dementia affects fewer than 5% of the population at 65 years, it affects more than 40% of those living past 85.[18] Prevalence is even higher in those with CVD, with causal relationships attributable to vascular disease, HF, AF, hypertension, hypotension, and frailty; relevant pathophysiology includes perfusion abnormalities, thrombosis, inflammation, mitochondrial dysfunction, and other factors.[19] For many older adults, cognitive decline may be insidious and subtle, often masked by a protective family and/or by a gradual withdrawal from activities and engagements that were previously routine. For those with overt dementia as well as those with subtle progressions of dementia, managing CVD often becomes disproportionately challenging. Clinical challenges relate to eliciting symptoms and past medical histories, making informed decisions, navigating diagnostic testing and procedures, and achieving reliable adherence and follow-up. Formalized testing of cognition may provide value, especially when cognition changes are subtle. Screening with the Montreal Cognitive Assessment (MoCA), Mini-Mental State Exam (MMSE), and miniCog are feasible options that can be integrated as part of CV care, with referral to a geriatrician or neurocognitive expert for further evaluation if indicated.

Delirium

Delirium is a disorder of disturbed attention that can manifest as agitated disruptive behavior or as quiet and withdrawn behavior that is less likely to elicit attention and corrective response. Delirium occurs in one-third of hospitalized patients ≥70 years, including 50% of those undergoing cardiac surgery and over 75% of those who require mechanical ventilation in an intensive care unit (ICU)[20] (see "Special Considerations" under "Noncardiac Surgery and Perioperative Management Considerations In Older Adults"). Baseline cognitive impairment significantly increases risks that delirium may occur. Mortality, morbidity, length of stay, cost, and discharge to a facility are all increased in those who become delirious. Multiple factors of hospitalization are likely to

trigger it, including the stress of a new environment, poor sleep, new medications, withdrawal from home medications, pain, dehydration, hypoxia, and metabolic shifts. Anticipatory screening by the Confusion Assessment Method (CAM) is a validated tool for screening in a hospital setting[21] and provides opportunity to mitigate precipitating factors.

Polypharmacy

Polypharmacy is common among older adults, with significant and sometimes dire consequences.[22] The Sloan survey showed that 44% of older men and 57% of older women received five or more prescription medications. In some cases polypharmacy relates to multimorbidity as multiple clinicians prescribe evidence-based medications oriented to different diseases. While disease guidelines are each supported by evidence, there is no guideline that addresses medications amidst multiple concurrent diseases and aggregate medical regimens.[23] Nonetheless, "quality indicators" used to assess the quality of care for individual diseases commonly reinforce tendencies for clinicians to prescribe guidelines-based medications irrespective of comorbidity and the total number of medications the patient is taking. Although most CVD guidelines acknowledge that clinical judgment is necessary to integrate evidence-based standards with each patient's circumstances, they do not provide a refined strategy to achieve such tailored care.

The safety risks associated with mounting numbers of medications in older adults are also affected by age-related changes in pharmacokinetics and pharmacodynamics[22] (see Chapter 9). The most significant age-related changes of pharmacokinetics pertain to renal metabolism. Glomerular filtration rate (GFR) decreases about 10% per decade in men and women. By age 80 years, GFR is typically one-half to two-thirds of that in younger adults. This reduction can be masked by overestimation of GFR using the Modified Diet in Renal Disease (MDRD) formula and the Chronic Kidney Disease Epidemiology Collaboration (CKD-EPI). The Cockroft-Gault is usually a preferred GFR equation; it accounts for age, sex, and weight, and characterizes a linear decrease of renal function. The dosage of many medications cleared by the kidney must be reduced in older patients with impaired renal function (e.g., digoxin, low-molecular-weight heparin [LMWH], glycoprotein IIb/IIIa inhibitors and, in some cases, direct-acting oral anticoagulants [DOACs]) (see Chapter 101).

Pharmacodynamic alterations are especially common amidst age-related changes in neuroautoregulation. Changes in thirst, temperature regulation, autonomic reflexes, sympathetic and cholinergic receptors, and cell signaling all impact the effects of medications, with greater susceptibility to orthostasis, syncope, falls, and other clinical sequelae.[24]

Drug–drug interactions are typical amidst polypharmacy, particularly when medications are metabolized by the same pathway.[25] Amiodarone, for example, inhibits CYP oxidative enzymes and increases drug levels of those medications that would normally be metabolized by this pathway (see Chapter 9). Adverse effects may also occur if clinical actions of medications are additive (e.g., administering aspirin, clopidogrel, and apixaban together will exacerbate bleeding risks) or competing (e.g., administering liraglutide and steroids together will decrease glucose control).

Drug–disease interactions occur as medications that benefit one chronic disease adversely affect another disease or syndrome. Beta blockers for cardiac ischemia may, for example, trigger bronchospasm in patients with concomitant chronic obstructive pulmonary disease (COPD). Calcium channel blockers can exacerbate chronic constipation, which is usually further compounded by sedentariness. Diuretics can aggravate incontinence and related social isolation and depression.

Disability
Disability refers to a physical or mental condition that limits a person's movements, senses, or activities. Whereas younger adults with CVD are usually able to rebound after a successful CVD hospitalization or therapy, an older adult has greater risks of new or worsening disability. Multimorbidity, frailty, sarcopenia, polypharmacy, and other geriatric syndromes predispose to disability in hospitalized older adults, especially in the context of deconditioning, cognitive impairment, malnutrition, and other burdens in older patients with CVD. The impact of hospital-related disability[26] is widespread and in some respects paradoxical, as older adults are especially vulnerable to morbid effects from the hospitalizations that are used to deliver care.

Notably, many CVD guideline-based therapies may inadvertently increase susceptibility to disability (e.g., increasing myalgias with statins and/or fatigue with beta blockers especially among adults. Recent CV trials reflect the growing recognition that the therapeutic priorities of many older patients differ from those who are young. In the ASPirin in Reducing Events in the Elderly (ASPREE)[27] trial, instead of focusing principally on thromboembolic events, bleeding and other disease metrics, the main endpoint was a "disability-free life," including freedom from dementia, for which there was no benefit of aspirin therapy.

PRECEPTS OF PATIENT-CENTERED CARE IN OLDER ADULTS

Although there is a tendency to refer to older adults as a distinct population with uniform health challenges, the variability between patients increases with age. Over a lifetime each individual encounters a diverse array of experiences, engages in a wide range of behaviors affecting health for better or worse, accumulates a highly variable list of health conditions of differing severity and impact, develops individualized attitudes about health care and preferences for care, and does all of these things in the context of uniquely personal psychosocial and family dynamics. As a result, people become progressively more heterogeneous with age. A fundamental challenge in caring for older patients with CVD is to integrate all of these factors, including prevalent geriatric syndromes, into a management plan that provides greatest weight to what is most important to the patient while maintaining sensitivity to competing non-CV comorbidities and social milieu that may greatly influence the patient's health care goals.

Diagnosis and Risk Assessment
Older adults are at increased risk for CVD due to age-related changes in CV physiology and the high prevalence of traditional CV risk factors at older age, especially hypertension, dyslipidemia, diabetes, obesity,

and sedentary lifestyle. However, older patients are also more likely to have ambiguous symptoms (i.e., symptoms with multiple often coexisting potential causes), atypical symptoms, or no symptoms despite advanced disease. Thus, a high index of suspicion for CVD is appropriate, and the clinician should be alert for subtle signs and symptoms that might suggest a new or worsening CV disorder. For example, a change in activity level or alterations in mood, cognition, or sleep and eating habits may reflect HF, severe CHD, or AF. Conversely, these same symptoms could be due to a host of other conditions, including depression, pulmonary or thyroid disease, or medication side effects. It is incumbent on the clinician to consider these possibilities before ordering a battery of diagnostic tests. Test selection, when indicated, should also include consideration of the clinical implications of test results. While this is true in patients of all ages, it is a consideration that becomes more germane in older adults. For example, an echocardiogram that is clearly warranted to assess LVEF to determine eligibility for an implantable cardioverter-defibrillator (ICD) in a middle-aged patient with HF becomes inappropriate for an 87-year-old woman who indicates that she does not want an ICD or in an older adult with limited life expectancy due to advanced comorbid illness.

Disease Management and Care Coordination
Given the likelihood of CVD occurring in a context of multimorbidity, most older patients have multiple providers, including physicians, advanced practice nurses, physician assistants, pharmacists, nutritionists, and therapists. While multiple providers offer complementary expertise, they predispose to fragmented care. The potential for mixed messaging, conflicting therapeutic plans, patient confusion, polypharmacy, and nonadherence is high. Although the primary care provider often assumes the role of medical "quarterback" to integrate care across multiple providers, decisions regarding medications, devices, procedures, and ongoing monitoring typically require CV expertise. Thus, CV clinicians must be skilled to work within such complex team relationships. Effective interpersonal skills and organization are increasingly requisite for effective CV care in older patients.

Application of Guidelines
Evidence-based practice CVD guidelines are based principally on randomized clinical trials in which older patients are underrepresented; those who are enrolled tend to be healthier with fewer comorbidities and geriatric syndromes than those encountered in clinical practice.[28] An additional limitation of guidelines is that recommendations are generally disease-specific and fail to adequately consider the impact of multimorbidity, cognitive impairment, or frailty. Other factors that may limit the relevance of guidelines to older patients include time-to-benefit versus time-to-harm, life expectancy, and patient burden. For many therapies, time-to-benefit is delayed, whereas adverse events may occur early during treatment. For example, ICD implantation is associated with an upfront procedural risk that is higher in patients ≥80 years, whereas the lifesaving benefit of an ICD may be delayed for years, if it occurs at all. Similarly, medication side effects often occur early after initiation, but benefit may not accrue for months to years. In the same way, patients with limited life expectancy due to very advanced age (i.e., ≥90 years) or competing illness may not survive long enough to derive benefit from some treatments. In addition, adherence to guideline recommendations often imposes burden on patients in the form of testing or additional medications that the patient, given the choice, would opt to forego. Importantly, in recent years many CV guidelines have acknowledged the above limitations and have advocated shared decision making in situations where applicability of recommendations is uncertain.

Shared Decision Making
Shared decision making (SDM) is a process by which an informed patient actively participates in decisions affecting the patient's health care.[29] The role of the clinician is to initially provide an unbiased

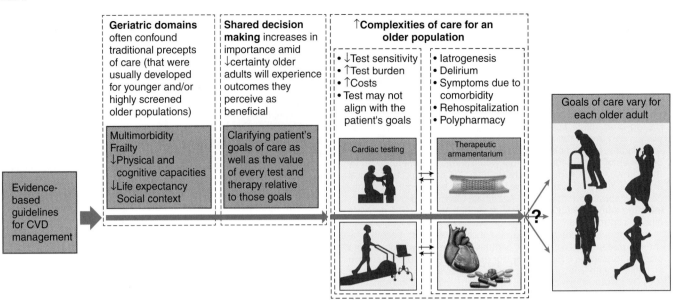

FIGURE 90.4 Among older adults with cardiovascular disease (CVD), clinical goals are more typically oriented to functional gains, independence, and quality of life (QOL), often with less priority ascribed to traditional CVD endpoints of major adverse cardiovascular events (MACE) that are emphasized in most major trials. Therapeutic risks are also relatively greater for older adults, particularly as geriatric syndromes compound the potential for harm. Given this ambiguous context, inclinations and oppositions for CVD therapy often vary from one patient to another, and shared decision-making becomes increasingly important. Nonetheless, shared decision-making is also challenged by common age-related limitations of health literacy and cognition.

summary of available options including advantages, disadvantages, and implications (in the case of testing). Following discussion with attention to patient concerns and questions, as well as incorporation of goals of care (e.g., QOL vs. length of life) and health care preferences (e.g., avoidance of risk and minimization of burden vs. willingness to accept risk and burden to achieve primary goal), a decision is made jointly by the patient (and family if appropriate) and the provider (Fig. 90.4). In most cases, decisions are not irrevocable and can be modified as circumstances, such as symptoms and comorbidities, evolve. In many cases, older patients, after being informed of the options and asking questions, will seek guidance from the clinician in reaching a decision. At this point, it is appropriate for the clinician to make a recommendation that is best aligned with the patient's goals and preferences.

Care Transitions, Skilled Nursing Facilities, and Long-Term Care

Care transition refers to any change in location of care delivery, for example, from hospital to postacute care or from skilled nursing facility to home. Older adults, especially those with multimorbidity, cognitive impairment, or frailty, are especially vulnerable to adverse outcomes during care transitions, including functional decline, medication errors, and delirium.[26] These perturbations often lead to rehospitalization and spiraling functional decline and progressive disability. To reduce the risk of adverse outcomes, effective care coordination is essential. In particular, meticulous medication reconciliation is required to ensure that the patient is taking all appropriately prescribed medications, but no medications that have been discontinued or which are no longer indicated. Minimizing polypharmacy and attention to potentially inappropriate medications in older adults, as defined by the Beers Criteria, is especially important.[30] A clinical pharmacist with experience in geriatric prescribing can play an invaluable role in ensuring safe and effective drug prescription and better medication adherence. Additional interventions that facilitate successful care transitions include frequent in-person or telephone follow-up and continuity of the care provider before, during, and after the transition.[31]

The role of postacute care for CVD patients is changing. In the past, older and sicker patients were routinely hospitalized for prolonged periods and were stable upon discharge to postacute care. As contemporary incentives encourage more rapid discharges from acute hospitalizations, increased numbers of older CVD patients are

being discharged to skilled nursing facilities (SNFs). Of the more than 1 million hospital discharges for HF each year in the United States, approximately 20% are discharged to SNFs. These patients often have residual volume overload, fluctuating renal function, and evolving medication regimens. Yet SNF staff often lack adequate training and are uncomfortable caring for moderately ill and potentially unstable CVD patients. In addition, systematized access to CVD clinicians may be limited. CMS has imposed mandatory quality metrics for SNFs to improve and standardize care, but apart from medication review, these metrics are not directly applicable to CV conditions.

CVD is highly prevalent in patients in long-term care facilities. This is a particularly vulnerable population with high prevalence of cognitive dysfunction, physical disability, frailty, and multiple coexisting medical conditions. However, data on optimal management of CVD in long-term care residents is sparse, as these patients have routinely been excluded from CV trials and few observational studies have focused on this group.

Palliative Care and End-of-Life Care

Palliative care focuses on alleviating symptoms, reducing physical and emotional suffering, and improving QOL; these are integral components of almost all medical care.[32] In addition to managing symptoms, palliative care addresses psychosocial and spiritual needs. It provides an extra layer of support, often in association with standard care. Palliative care improves QOL and may increase survival.[33] It is distinct from hospice care, which is oriented to patients with a prognosis of <6 months of expected survival, and who have agreed to forgo more aggressive treatment.

In some respects, geriatric cardiology and palliative care overlap. Many patients referred for palliative care are older and have CVD in the context of frailty, disability, and other care complexities that require a tailored approach to CV management. Although palliative care does not preclude standard care, including procedures such as percutaneous coronary intervention (PCI) or TAVR that may markedly improve QOL, most patients who choose to pursue palliative care have prioritized QOL and comfort over length of life. In other situations, geriatric cardiologists are at the crossroads of management and must facilitate decisions about which older, complex, frail patients may still benefit from prevention and intervention strategies that may forestall or reverse decline.

Among people ≥75 years, CVD is the leading cause of death, exceeding all other causes of death combined. As a result, CV providers and their patients often face end-of-life decisions, including decisions about resuscitation, thresholds of futility, and strategies to help families/surrogate caregivers if patients lose capacity to make their own decisions. In most instances it is effective to encourage and support older adults to develop an advance directive, clarifying what medical care they would or would not want in the event of a life-threatening or terminal illness, as well as designating durable power of attorney for health care. It is also useful when patients discuss these issues with their families or health care proxies so that there is clear understanding of their preferences. It is helpful for clinicians of older patients with CVD to initiate these discussions as part of routine care delivery (i.e., "normalize" the conversation). Studies have shown that most patients, especially those with advanced symptoms (e.g., New York Heart Association [NYHA] Class III–IV), prefer having these conversations with their trusted clinicians.

Deprescribing

Deprescribing is the process of reducing the dose or discontinuing medications that have become burdensome to the patient (e.g., due to side effects), are no longer aligned with the patient's goals of care, or are no longer likely to provide benefit or to have a favorable benefit-to-risk ratio.[34] Deprescribing is an integral component of good prescribing practice with the goals of reducing medication burden, decreasing risk of drug–drug and drug–disease interactions, and eliminating medications no longer likely to be beneficial or consistent with patients' goals and preferences. Older adults with declining life expectancy, high self-perceived medication burden, advanced dementia, or multiple competing comorbidities are good candidates for deprescribing, but even more vigorous adults can potentially benefit. Care transitions with comprehensive medication reconciliation offer an excellent opportunity for deprescribing, but all contacts with providers should include a medication review with consideration of medications that might be discontinued.

CORONARY HEART DISEASE

Epidemiology

Age-related vascular changes in conjunction with increasing prevalence and duration of traditional cardiac risk factors predispose to the development of CHD at older age, and age is the strongest risk factor for incident CHD (see Chapter 25). Similarly, the prevalence and mortality rates of CHD increase progressively with age. The Global Burden of Disease Study indicates that in men, approximately 50% of deaths attributable to CHD occur in those over age 70, whereas in women, almost 50% of CHD deaths occur among those over age 80.[35]

Presentation

Compared with younger individuals, older adults with stable CHD, especially those over age 80, are less likely to experience exertional angina and more likely to report shortness of breath, fatigue, or lack of energy as manifestations of myocardial ischemia. Similarly, dyspnea is the most common presenting symptom of acute MI in patients over age 80, and the prevalence of atypical symptoms, including indigestion, dizziness, and altered mentation increases with age. In addition, many older patients with CHD are asymptomatic, in part due to sedentary lifestyle, and the incidence of silent or clinically unrecognized MI increases with age (see Chapter 35). Older patients also tend to minimize symptoms or attribute them to age or other causes, especially when comorbid diseases complicate the experience.

Risk Stratification and Diagnosis

Neither the Pooled Cohorts Equations nor the Framingham Risk Score permit estimation of risk for CVD events in patients ≥80 years, but even in the absence of other risk factors or symptoms, patients in this age group are at increased risk. Similarly, the majority of men over age 65 and women over age 70 in the United States are in the intermediate risk category, as defined by current guidelines.[36] Further risk stratification

in older adults thus requires consideration of concomitant risk factors and symptoms.

The decision to pursue CHD evaluation in older adults is predicated on the pretest likelihood of disease, the probability that the test results will alter management, and patient preferences. In patients with relatively low pretest likelihood of severe CHD, mild to moderate symptoms that could potentially be controlled with medications, or clearly stated preference to avoid testing if possible, a conservative approach designed to control symptoms and risk factors is appropriate. For other patients, the decision-making process should start with a discussion of the advantages, disadvantages, and limitations of further testing in the context of the patient's goals of care. Results of two recent trials can be used to inform these discussions. In the PROMISE trial, 10,003 symptomatic patients with intermediate pretest likelihood of CHD were randomized to anatomical testing with coronary computed tomographic angiography (CCTA) or to functional testing (i.e., a stress test).[37] Over a median follow-up of 25 months, the primary outcome of death, MI, hospitalization for unstable angina, or major procedural complication occurred in 3.3% of the CCTA group and 3.0% of the stress test group, with no difference between groups and similar findings in patients younger or older than age 65. These findings indicate that the risk of a major adverse cardiac event during a 2-year follow-up period is quite low, and suggest that a conservative strategy, without testing, is reasonable for patients who prefer to avoid testing. The second study, the ISCHEMIA trial, randomized 5179 patients with moderate to severe ischemia on stress testing to an initial invasive strategy with coronary angiography and revascularization if indicated, or to an initial conservative strategy with intensive medical therapy.[38] Over a median follow-up of 3.2 years, there was no difference between groups in the primary outcome of CV death or MI, with similar findings across age groups. Patients randomized to the invasive strategy had better QOL, especially if they were more symptomatic at baseline. These results again provide rationale for conservative management, even in patients with moderate to severe symptoms, if the patient prefers to avoid testing and subsequent procedures.

In older patients who chose to proceed with further testing, the indications for stress testing, CCTA, and invasive angiography are similar to those in younger patients. If feasible, an exercise stress test is preferable to pharmacologic stress testing due to the important information derived on functional status, hemodynamic response to exercise, and occurrence of exercise-induced arrhythmias.[39] If appropriate, the exercise protocol should be modified to accommodate lower exercise capacity in older adults (i.e., starting at lower intensity and using smaller workload increments). Coronary CT angiography is less accurate in assessing lesion severity in older patients due to their high prevalence of coronary artery calcium (CAC).[39]

Management

Management of CHD (see Chapter 40) is similar in older and younger patients and includes control of risk factors, alleviation of symptoms, and prevention of complications (i.e., MI, death). Older patients are at increased risk for adverse effects from most medications, including bleeding with aspirin and other antithrombotic agents; bradycardia and hypotension with beta blockers; bradycardia, hypotension, pedal edema, constipation, and incontinence with calcium channel blockers (agent-specific); impaired renal function and hyperkalemia with ACE inhibitors (ACEI) and angiotensin receptor blockers (ARBs); and postural hypotension with nitrates. Statins in moderate- and high-intensities are recommended for adults >75 years, but risks of myalgias, fatigue, and reduced physical activity are increased.[40]

Invasive coronary angiography and revascularization are recommended for older adults with refractory symptoms, particularly those with significant ischemia on noninvasive diagnostic tests. In the Trial of Invasive versus Medical therapy in Elderly patients (TIME) study, symptom relief and exercise capacity during 4-year follow-up were better with revascularization than with optimized medical therapy alone in older patients with

CHD.[41] Similarly, the ISCHEMIA trial demonstrated improved QOL with revascularization in patients with high symptom burden.[39]

In older adults, PCI is associated with a modestly higher rate of procedural complications than in younger adults, including bleeding, stroke, and contrast-induced kidney injury. Dual antiplatelet therapy is associated with increased bleeding and transfusion risk in older patients. Bleeding risks can be minimized by using the radial artery approach and by weight- and renal dose-adjustments of anticoagulant and antiplatelet agents.

The choice of PCI versus coronary artery bypass grafting (CABG) involves consideration of the anatomy, comorbidities, functional capacity, frailty, and patient preferences. Although studies suggest that CABG is usually associated with less recurrence of symptoms and need for repeat revascularization, it also usually requires longer recovery and has a higher risk of stroke and procedure-related neurologic complications, including postoperative delirium.[41] Patients with diabetes or left main disease appear to have superior long-term outcomes with CABG. Although persistent cognitive decline following CABG has been reported, studies indicate this may primarily reflect unrecognized prior cognitive dysfunction.[42]

In assessing perioperative risk in older adults, physiologic status has greater import than chronologic age. The Euro SCORE and the Society of Thoracic Surgery (STS) risk score now include metrics of mobility and frailty (gait speed), respectively, in addition to surgical parameters and comorbidities, to help gauge short-term procedural risks and longer-term QOL outcomes. As discussed later (see "Cardiac Rehabilitation"), cardiac rehabilitation is also an integral component of CHD management.

Ischemia with Nonobstructive Coronary Arteries (INOCA)

INOCA is a multifactorial vascular syndrome in which an imbalance between oxygen supply and demand leads to ischemia in the absence of obstructive CHD.[43] Increasing age and age-related arterial stiffness are risk factors for INOCA, particularly in women, which in turn is associated with increased risk for CV events and impaired QOL. Many older adults have coronary microvascular dysfunction and diminished coronary flow reserve, as detected by positron emission tomography (PET), magnetic resonance imaging, or invasive coronary angiography. Treatment includes antiangina therapy and control of CV risk factors. A related syndrome, MI with nonobstructive coronary arteries (MINOCA), is more common in younger patients. However, in contrast to MINOCA, type 2 MI is more common in older adults. Type 2 MIs also result from supply–demand mismatch in the absence of obstructed coronary arteries when physiologic stresses (e.g., tachycardia, anemia, infections, hypertension) overwhelm limited CV flow reserves.

ACUTE CORONARY SYNDROMES (ACS) (SEE CHAPTERS 37 TO 39)

Epidemiology

In the United States, the average age at first acute MI is 65.6 years in men and 72.0 years in women.[44] In men, the incidence of MI peaks in the 65 to 74 year age group and declines at older ages, whereas the incidence in women increases progressively with age, surpassing that in men after age 85. The prevalence of MI in men increases from 2.8% at ages 40 to 59 to 11.5% at ages 60 to 79 and to 17.3% after age 80; comparable figures for women are 2.1%, 4.2%, and 12.7%. About 60% of hospitalizations for ACS are in patients ≥65 years, with approximately 85% of ACS mortality occurring in this age group; 32% to 43% of non-ST elevation (NSTE)-ACS admissions and 24% to 28% of ST-elevation MI (STEMI) admissions are in patients ≥75 years.[45] NSTE-ACS is far more prevalent than STEMI in the older population, as is type 2 MI.

Presentation

Older patients with ACS are less likely than younger patients to present with typical ischemic chest pain but more likely to experience dyspnea, diaphoresis, nausea and vomiting, presyncope or syncope, weakness, altered mental status, or confusion, even when chest discomfort is present. Chest pain is reported in only ~40% of those >85 years compared with almost 80% in those <65 years, often leading to delays in diagnosis and initiation of therapy. Heart failure, pulmonary edema, AF, bradyarrhythmias, hypotension, and shock all occur more frequently in older patients with ACS than in younger individuals, in part reflecting the marked reduction in CV reserve inherit to the aging process.

Diagnosis

Because older patients often present with atypical symptoms and NSTE-ACS, a heightened index of suspicion for ACS is required. The ECG may be nondiagnostic due to prior MI, conduction abnormalities, or paced rhythm, but ischemic ST-T changes carry the same implications as in younger patients. Older individuals tend to have higher baseline levels of troponin (cTn), such that 20% of community-dwelling adults >70 years have levels above the 99th percentile, and baseline levels tend to be higher in men than in women. These factors should be considered in evaluating the clinical significance of slight cTn elevations in older patients.[39] The emergence of high-sensitivity cTn (hs-cTn) could lead to over-diagnosis of ACS in older adults, with increased hospitalization and downstream testing, but additional data are needed.

Management

Older patients present complex challenges because of atypical symptomatology, high prevalence of cardiac and noncardiac comorbidities, age-related alterations in CV structure and physiology, and increased risk for adverse drug events and interactions due to polypharmacy. Although treatment standards for ACS do not differ with age, medication side effects, especially bleeding from antiplatelet and antithrombotic therapy, are more common in older patients.

Revascularization-STEMI

Timely reperfusion is the cornerstone of care for older patients with STEMI, with absolute benefits equal or greater than in younger patients given their higher mortality risks. However, older patients have more contraindications to reperfusion, and even if eligible are less likely to receive it. Primary PCI with stent placement is preferred over thrombolysis in older adults as it results in greater survival benefit, reduced reinfarction and need for repeat revascularization, and less intracranial hemorrhage. Fibrinolytic therapy has also been associated with an increased risk of myocardial rupture after age 75. If primary PCI cannot be performed within 120 minutes of symptom onset, fibrinolytic therapy is a reasonable option in carefully selected older patients with STEMI. In patients over age 75, streptokinase is associated with less intracranial bleeding than more fibrin-specific agents.

Revascularization-NSTE-ACS

Whereas randomized trials have shown benefit of an early invasive approach in high-risk ACS, including very old patients, management is frequently complicated by issues of multimorbidity, frailty, and geriatric domains that are coupled to MI pathophysiology.

Several trials have compared an invasive strategy to conservative management in older adults with NSTE-ACS with mixed results. In the After Eighty study, 457 patients ≥80 years were randomized to early catheterization and revascularization if indicated or to optimal medical therapy. During a median follow-up of 1.5 years, the invasive strategy was superior to the conservative strategy for the composite outcome of MI, need for urgent revascularization, stroke, or death.[46] The magnitude of benefit declined with age, and the small number of nonagenarians had no apparent benefit. There was no difference in bleeding complications, likely related to the predominant use of radial PCI access.[46]

Post-ACS Care and Discharge Planning

Older patients have longer lengths of stay following ACS, and frail individuals have even longer hospital stays and increased rates of discharge to institutional care. Older patients also have a high risk of rehospitalization and death, with a 50% increased mortality risk per 10-year increase in age starting at age 65. Utilization of recommended therapies mitigates these risks. Beta blockers have greater absolute benefit at older age in preventing subsequent MI and death than in younger groups. ACEIs and ARBs are beneficial in older patients, particularly those with HF or reduced LV systolic function. Statins are beneficial for secondary prevention in patients up to their early 80s but have not been adequately studied after age 80.[40] Dual antiplatelet therapy after PCI/stenting presents a challenge in older adults who also require anticoagulation for AF, deep vein thrombosis, mechanical heart valve, or other reasons. Recent studies and meta-analyses suggest that therapy with a P2Y12 inhibitor plus an oral anticoagulant, omitting aspirin, may be as effective as triple therapy in preventing MI, CV death, and ischemic stroke, with decreased bleeding.[47,48]

Comprehensive discharge planning includes the patient and family, and must address comorbidity, polypharmacy, and frailty, often in the context of impaired communication and cognition. Failure to understand and comply with the plan of care contributes to unreliable adherence, high rates of readmissions, and poor outcomes. The proportion of patients with ACS discharged to a postacute care facility or to home with home health services increases with age and with prevalent comorbidities, especially frailty and cognitive impairment. Cardiac rehabilitation (CR) has a Class IA recommendation following MI, PCI, or CABG, as well as in patients with stable CHD.[49] The benefits of CR extend to older adults and include reduced mortality, decreased hospitalizations, increased exercise tolerance, and improved QOL.

HEART FAILURE

Heart failure (see Part IV) epitomizes a convergence of CVD and geriatrics. The incidence and prevalence of HF rise exponentially with age, and entail the predisposing aspects of physiologic CV aging, mounting CVD risk factors over a lifetime, and geriatric syndromes. In addition, HF pathophysiology affects multiple systems (i.e., the heart as well as the vasculature, lungs, kidneys, and skeletal muscle).

Epidemiology

In the United States, HF is projected to increase from about 6.2 million currently to almost 8 million by 2030.[44] Prevalence more than doubles from 6% in those age 60 to 79 years to approximately 14% in those age ≥80 years; the mean age of patients with HF exceeds 70 years.[50] Whereas HF prevalence is higher in men than women through septuagenarian years, women predominate by age 80 and beyond. Incidence of HFpEF increases particularly rapidly among the very old[51]; underlying diastolic LV filling changes as well as high prevalence of hypertension, diabetes, AF, and other predisposing comorbid risks are all pervasive in older adults, intensifying susceptibility to HFpEF.[52] Hospital discharges for HF approximate 900,000 per year in the United States, comprising the most common reason for hospitalization in Medicare recipients, and progressively escalate as age increases. National Center for Health Statistics data show HF hospitalizations were 85.7/10,000 in adults age 65 to 74 years, 214.6/10,000 at age 75 to 84 years, and 430.7/10,000 for those age 85 years and older.[5]

Mortality rates from HF also increase with age, from <10/100,000 in adults age 45 to 49 years to 150/100,000 in octogenarians. Median survival was only 20 months for 825 patients ≥85 years versus 50 months for those <85 years in a study of 8507 hospitalized HF patients.[53] Atrial fibrillation, lower LVEF, and renal insufficiency were associated with greater long-term mortality. Risks for HF related to cumulative comorbid diseases are similar in older and younger adults, but the higher prevalence of comorbidity in older adults results in a higher attributable risk (i.e., prevalence times the relative risk) for developing HF despite a lower relative risk. Among Medicare beneficiaries, 65% of those with HF have five or more comorbidities, 25% have three to four comorbidities, and only 10% have two or fewer comorbidities.[14] High comorbidity burden is also associated with higher readmission rates and health care expenditures. The relationship between multimorbidity and HF is explained in part by the stresses induced by conditions superimposed upon age-related reduction in CV reserve. Inflammation associated with mounting comorbidity also exacerbates HF risks, particularly HFpEF.[52] Lifestyle factors (e.g., smoking, obesity, and low physical activity) add to HF risk in both older and younger populations.

Pathophysiology

Numerous population-based observational studies have demonstrated important age-related differences in the clinical profile and pathophysiology of HF[54] (see Chapter 47). More than half of older HF patients have a normal or near normal LVEF (i.e., HFpEF); in contrast, HF with reduced LVEF (HFrEF) represents the dominant form of HF in younger patients.

Diagnosis

Because HF affects multiple organ systems, no single test or procedure can definitively diagnose HF or exclude it (see Chapter 48). The specificity of one of the major Framingham diagnostic criteria for HF, orthopnea, or paroxysmal nocturnal dyspnea is low in older adults because these classic manifestations of HF can also be found in non-HF disorders such as pulmonary disease, deconditioning, and depression. Many older adults may attribute their HF symptoms to aging, thus delaying presentation until symptoms are more severe. Cognitive or sensory impairments may delay the diagnosis of HF in older adults.

Objective laboratory criteria are helpful in establishing the diagnosis of HF in older patients. A chest x-ray showing pulmonary venous hypertension and/or interstitial pulmonary edema is diagnostic. B-type natriuretic peptide (BNP) and N-terminal pro-BNP (NT-proBNP) levels increase with age, and higher cut points to diagnose HF are needed in older patients.[39] BNP levels are generally lower in HFpEF than HFrEF, making them less reliable as a diagnostic index for older adults, in whom HFpEF predominates.

Lifestyle HF Management

While lifestyle factors such as diet, physical activity, and patient/caregiver education retain an important role in older adults, rigid sodium and fluid restriction in older patients may reduce an already low caloric intake and exacerbate malnutrition and sarcopenia, both common in older HF patients and associated with adverse outcomes. In one trial, a sodium intake of 2.7 g/day reduced the rate of death or hospitalization by 25% compared with intake of 1.8 g/day.[55] Current guidelines suggest limiting sodium intake to <3 g/day in patients with stage C or D HF.[56]

Numerous trials have shown that exercise training in older patients with HFrEF improves functional capacity to a similar relative degree as in younger patients without increased safety concerns. The 2331 patient HF: A Controlled Trial Investigating Outcomes of Exercise Training (HF-ACTION) trial reported a similar modest improvement in a combined endpoint of all-cause mortality and hospitalizations as well as in combined CV mortality and HF hospitalizations in the 435 patients age ≥70 years compared with younger patients in a program of 36 supervised exercise sessions followed by home training for up to 4 years.[57] Based on the HF-ACTION results, Medicare approved outpatient supervised CR for stable HFrEF patients. Incorporating resistance exercises as well as flexibility and balance training is especially useful to counter age- and disease-associated deficits in these domains. In the absence of a formal training program, regular walking or other moderate intensity exercise is encouraged. Although an event-driven trial for exercise training in HFpEF is not available, many smaller trials suggest benefits, which may relate principally to improvements in peripheral mechanisms of disease (e.g., skeletal muscle and peripheral perfusion).

Because of the high hospitalization rates and their associated costs in older HF patients, much attention has been directed toward developing disease management programs to optimize HF patient care and improve outcomes. A meta-analysis of 47 trials including 10,869 older patients recently hospitalized for HF found that case management and multidisciplinary interventions probably reduced all-cause mortality, but clinic-based interventions had little or no effect on all-cause mortality. Case-management interventions, typically involving home visits and/or telephone follow-up, reduced HF readmissions at both 6 and 12 months' follow-up.[58] Multiple trials have also confirmed improved QOL from such programs. In older patients with NYHA Class III HF, an implanted pulmonary artery pressure sensor resulted in more medication changes and a 58% decrease in 30-day all-cause readmissions and 49% decrease in HF hospitalizations over 515 days mean follow-up.[59]

Pharmacotherapy for Chronic HFrEF (see Chapter 50)

Although ACEIs, ARBs, and beta blockers reduce CV events and improve survival in patients with HFrEF, this evidence base derives from RCTs that enrolled only modest numbers of patients age >75 years, and very few patients age ≥80. Benefits of each medication must be weighed against the risks associated with implicit polypharmacy of complex regimens in an older population prone to frailty, cognitive impairments, and other geriatric vulnerabilities. Frequent follow-up for adverse effects and need for medication adjustment is essential.

Diuretics. Diuretics remain the cornerstone for treatment of congestive signs and symptoms in chronic HFrEF despite the absence of RCT data that they reduce CV mortality. Observational studies suggest that chronic use may be associated with adverse outcomes, likely mediated by activation of neurohormones and electrolyte imbalances. Any of the three commonly used loop diuretics, furosemide, bumetanide, and torsemide may be considered for older adults, although absorption of bumetanide and torsemide is superior to furosemide. Doses are best started low and slowly uptitrated to achieve euvolemia; after which dose reduction can be tried. Serum electrolytes and renal function require more careful monitoring in older patients to reduce the risk for hypokalemia, hyponatremia, and prerenal azotemia. Concerns regarding incontinence and/or frequent voiding are also pertinent and may diminish an older patient's treatment experience and willingness to adhere to the medication.

ACEI OR ARB. Based on strong clinical trial evidence, older HFrEF patients who have no history of allergy or intolerance to an ACEI or ARB should be prescribed one of these drugs, starting at low doses. ARBs generally have fewer side effects. Close monitoring is required to avoid hypotension, hyperkalemia, or azotemia, especially in the first few weeks after initiating or up-titrating therapy. In RCTs, the average daily dose of ACEI or ARB was lower in older than younger patients.

Sacubitril-Valsartan Combination. The 2014 PARADIGM-HF study showed that the combination of the neprilysin inhibitor sacubitril and the ARB valsartan reduced total mortality by 16%, CV death by 20%, and HF hospitalization risk by 21% compared with the ACEI enalapril in 8442 patients with NYHA Class II to IV HFrEF. These benefits were similar in the 1563 patients >75 years as in younger groups.[60] Although hypotension, renal impairment, and hyperkalemia increased with age in both treatment arms, findings of more hypotension but less renal impairment or hyperkalemia with sacubitril-candesartan were consistent across age groups.

Beta Blockers. Unlike ACEI and ARB, a class effect is not evident for beta blockers in HFrEF. Clinical trial data supports only carvedilol, metoprolol succinate extended release, bisoprolol, nebivolol, and bucindolol, but the latter two drugs are not approved for HF in the United States. Although major RCTs of beta blockers included few patients ≥80 years, benefits appear similar across age. In hypertensive older patients with HFrEF, carvedilol may be a better beta blocker choice than metoprolol succinate or bisoprolol because of its vasodilating properties and tendency to lower BP more effectively. Side effects of beta blockers such as fatigue and/or chronotropic insufficiency are common in older patients, limiting maximal tolerated doses.

Aldosterone Antagonists. Despite powerful RCT evidence for efficacy of aldosterone antagonists in HFrEF, these drugs should be used with caution in older adults, with careful monitoring of renal function and serum potassium. While a high proportion of older participants participated in the Randomized Aldactone Evaluation Study (RALES), those enrolled were relatively healthy, and only about 20% of real-world very old HFrEF patients would have been eligible to enroll.[54] Generally, older patients with class III to IV HF should be started and maintained on spironolactone 12.5 mg daily or eplerenone 25 mg daily (or every other day if renal insufficiency is evident). Although hyperkalemia is a major limiting factor in older adults, the availability of the oral potassium-binding drug patiromer may enable more older individuals to benefit from aldosterone antagonists, but the risk of a prescribing cascade remains a concern.[22]

Digoxin. Even after two centuries of use, digitalis in HF patients is controversial. Despite its narrow therapeutic window and lack of life-prolonging benefits, the large DIG trial showed that digoxin reduced HF hospitalizations in HFrEF patients in sinus rhythm, including those ≥80 years. Because this trial antedated the widespread use of beta blockers and aldosterone antagonists, the benefit of digoxin in the current era is unclear. Recommended digoxin doses in older HFrEF patients are 0.125 mg/day or lower, which are likely to provide maximum clinical benefit with low risk of toxicity. While routine checking of serum digoxin concentration is not recommended, levels are indicated when symptoms or signs of digoxin toxicity are suspected.

Sodium Glucose Cotransport (SGLT)-2 Inhibitors. These drugs, originally developed as hypoglycemic agents, inhibit the reabsorption of both glucose and sodium from the distal renal tubule. Several recent studies have shown benefit of these drugs in HF patients with or without diabetes. In the DAPA-HF trial, dapagliflozin reduced the primary composite outcome of HF hospitalization, urgent HF visit, or CV death to a similar extent in age groups <55 years, 55 to 64, 65 to 74, and ≥75 years with HFrEF over an 18-month median follow-up without any age-related reduction in tolerability and safety compared with placebo.[61] Similar findings have been reported with empagliflozin.[62]

Other Pharmacologic Therapies. Although a RCT demonstrated a reduction of CV events with the combination of hydralazine and isosorbide dinitrate in younger (mean age 57 years) African Americans with HFrEF, adequate data in older patients is lacking. Intravenous inotropic agents, including dobutamine, milrinone, and levosimendan, have not been shown to improve clinical outcomes in patients with HF but may be considered as a palliative strategy in older patients with severe symptoms.

Nonmedicinal Options for Chronic HFrEF

Cardiac transplantation has been used successfully in highly selected patients in their 60s and early 70s with slightly higher surgical complications and mortality but fewer rejection episodes than in younger patients. Patients in their eighth decade and beyond are not generally cardiac transplant candidates. However, long-term or permanent LV assist devices (LVADs) have been shown to improve survival and QOL in such patients with end-stage HF. Risks of bleeding, infection, and thrombosis have been reduced with advent of continuous flow LVADs. An analysis of 1149 continuous flow LVAD recipients showed similar 1-year mortality in the 163 patients ≥70 years compared with younger patients, although gastrointestinal bleeding risk was higher in the older group.[63] Health-related QOL improved to a similar extent in 493 LVAD recipients age ≥70 years as in 977 younger recipients. Appropriate patient selection in experienced centers is critical for favorable outcomes.

Functionally active older HFrEF patients may benefit from cardiac surgical procedures. In one study, CABG improved survival in persons with reduced LVEF due to CHD, although the benefit was greater in younger individuals.[64] CABG may be considered for older HFrEF patients with multivessel CHD and evidence of ongoing myocardial ischemia with symptoms despite optimal medical therapy. Similarly, surgical or TAVR in older patients with HF due to severe AS is accompanied by markedly improved survival and functional status compared with medical therapy, although with higher bleeding and stroke risks and greater need for pacemaker implantation than in younger patients. Device therapy is discussed under "Cardiac Rhythm Abnormalities,"

Heart Failure with Preserved Ejection Fraction

More than half of older HF patients have HFpEF (see Chapter 51), and the prevalence is substantially higher in women than in men. The majority of patients with HFpEF have antecedent hypertension (60% to 80%). Multimorbidity is ubiquitous and often includes other CV disorders, such as CHD, AF, and valvular heart disease, as well as a wide range of non-CV conditions. Indeed, although HFpEF was once viewed as primarily a disorder of abnormal LV diastolic function, it is now considered to be a multifactorial systemic illness with complex pathogenesis involving aging, inflammation, multimorbidity, lifestyle, and genetic predisposition.[51] The prognosis for HFpEF is somewhat better than for HFrEF, but symptoms, QOL, and hospitalization rates are similar between the two forms of HF. However, despite multiple clinical trials investigating numerous agents, to date no pharmacologic or device-based interventions have demonstrated unequivocal efficacy in HFpEF. In the TOPCAT trial involving 3445 patients with HFpEF, spironolactone failed to reduce the primary composite endpoint of CV death, aborted cardiac arrest, or HF hospitalization but reduced HF hospitalization by a significant 17%.[65] In a posthoc subgroup analysis, spironolactone reduced the primary outcome by a significant 18% among patients enrolled in the Americas (United States, Canada, Brazil, Argentina), but not in those enrolled in Eastern Europe (Russia, Georgia), with similar results across the age spectrum, including patients age ≥75 years.[66] In the PARAGON-HF trial, 4822 patients with HFpEF (mean age 73 years, 53% women) were randomized to sacubitril-valsartan or to valsartan alone.[67] Although there was a 13% reduction in the composite primary outcome of CV mortality and total HF hospitalizations, the difference was not significant ($P = 0.06$). Prespecified subgroup analyses suggested that women and individuals with EF less than the median value of 57% benefitted from combined therapy.

Currently the management of HFpEF focuses on optimizing BP control, treating ischemia in patients with concomitant CHD, controlling heart rate in patients with AF, and avoiding excess dietary salt and fluid intake. In addition, aerobic exercise improves exercise tolerance in older adults with HFpEF, and weight loss with caloric restriction provides additional benefit in obese patients.[68] Diuretics are indicated to maintain euvolemia and minimize symptoms of shortness of breath and edema but must be used judiciously to avoid overdiuresis, which may lead to reduced organ perfusion and prerenal azotemia.

Cardiac Amyloidosis (see Chapter 53)

Transthyretin amyloid cardiomyopathy (ATTR) due to deposition of misfolded transthyretin protein in the myocardial interstitium, is an increasingly recognized cause of HFpEF in older adults.[69] Wild-type ATTR (ATTRwt) is an age-related disorder (formerly senile cardiac amyloid) that may contribute to 10% to 15% of HFpEF cases in older adults with a strong male predominance (>80% of cases). Hereditary ATTR (ATTRh) is related to specific genetic mutations, with the most common variant being present in 3% to 4% of African Americans. The cardiac manifestations of amyloid heart disease are similar to other forms of HFpEF, but noncardiac manifestations often include peripheral neuropathy, autonomic neuropathy (with orthostatic hypotension), bilateral carpal tunnel syndrome, and lumbar spinal stenosis. Low QRS voltage on electrocardiography is a classic feature of cardiac amyloid but is present in <50% of cases. Elevated cTn and NT-proBNP are common and correlate with prognosis but are nonspecific. Characteristic findings on echocardiography include increased LV wall thickness with normal or small LV cavity, markers of diastolic dysfunction, and abnormal global longitudinal strain with an "apical sparing" pattern. Recently bone-avid nuclear imaging has emerged as the noninvasive test of choice with high sensitivity and moderate specificity.[70] In patients in whom a light chain monoclonal gammopathy has been ruled out, a strongly positive bone-avid nuclear scan is diagnostic for ATTR, and biopsy is not required. In other cases, myocardial biopsy is needed to confirm the diagnosis.

Until recently there was no effective therapy for cardiac amyloid and the prognosis was poor, with a median survival of 2 to 4 years depending on type. However, tafamidis, a transthyretin-binding agent, was recently approved for treatment of ATTR amyloid based on the results of the ATTR-ACT trial.[71] In this study of 441 patients with ATTR cardiomyopathy (median age 75 years, 90% male, 81% white) tafamidis was associated with a 30% reduction in all-cause mortality, 32% reduction in CV-related hospitalizations, and better exercise tolerance and HF-related QOL over 30 months compared with placebo; tafamidis was generally well tolerated. Several other promising therapies for amyloidosis are currently under investigation.

Pulmonary Hypertension

Pulmonary hypertension (PH) (see Chapter 88) is increasingly recognized among older adults and is usually secondary to LV dysfunction. Differentiation of PH from HF or pulmonary disease is a key challenge, and specialized centers have evolved that focus on this differential.[72] HFpEF accompanied by pulmonary venous hypertension is associated with increased mortality as well as worse symptoms and diminished QOL.[73]

Pulmonary arterial hypertension (PAH) was once considered a disease that primarily affected young women, but it is increasingly recognized in the geriatric population. Recent Registry data show an increase in the proportion of older patients with PAH, particularly men. Given that <20% of patients who were enrolled in the clinical trials of the newer oral and parenteral therapies were older, extrapolation of the conclusions to older adults is uncertain.[74]

VALVULAR HEART DISEASE (SEE PART VIII)

Parallel to other age-associated changes in CV structure that may predispose to developing overt CVD, the cardiac valves undergo myxomatous degeneration and collagen infiltration, especially in the left heart. In the aortic valve, these processes manifest as valvular sclerosis, detected on physical exam by a short ejection murmur, and confirmed on echocardiography by leaflet thickening without calcification or orifice narrowing. Aortic sclerosis was observed in about half of individuals ≥85 years in the CHS. In ~2% of older adults, progressive calcification of the aortic leaflets results in valvular narrowing and AS. Aortic valvular regurgitation (AR), found in over a quarter of octogenarians, is usually due to annular dilation caused by chronic hypertension or leaflet calcification. In the mitral valve, myxomatous degeneration usually manifests as mitral regurgitation (MR) and is the primary mechanism for primary MR in older persons. Calcific deposits may also occur in the mitral valve leaflets, but more often in the mitral annulus, particularly in older women. Functional (i.e., secondary) MR is also common in seniors, usually due to ischemia-related papillary muscle dysfunction or to mitral annular dilation resulting from LV enlargement. Less common causes of mitral or aortic valvular regurgitation are endocarditis, rheumatic heart disease, mitral chordal rupture, aortic dissection, or trauma.

Aortic Stenosis

AS (see Chapter 72) is the prototypical valvular lesion in older adults, present in ~15% of those ≥65 years and is severe, as defined by a valve area <1 cm^2 or 0.6 cm^2/m^2 body surface area, in ~2%. In the majority, AS is secondary to calcification of a trileaflet AV; patients with congenital bicuspid valves generally present one to two decades earlier. Patients are usually asymptomatic on initial presentation with a harsh late-peaking systolic ejection murmur. In older sedentary individuals, the cardinal symptoms of angina, exercise intolerance, or syncope may not be reported because exertion sufficient to precipitate them occurs less frequently. The second heart sound is usually diminished and may be absent if calcification is extensive. In contrast to younger adults, the carotid artery upstroke is often not delayed because of large artery stiffening. The diagnosis is confirmed by Doppler echocardiography, which demonstrates the stenotic, calcified AV with a high transvalvular Doppler flow velocity, and a calculated AV area <1.0 cm^2. LV hypertrophy is generally present as well as reduced early diastolic LV filling rate. However, these latter findings are nonspecific because they are often present in older adults due to aging changes and hypertension.

The classic findings of severe AS on Doppler echocardiography are a stenotic, heavily calcified valve with restricted leaflet motion. A mean gradient across the AV ≥40 mm Hg and a peak flow velocity >4 m/sec with a LV stroke volume index ≥35 mL/m^2 signifies the most common hemodynamic pattern (high flow, high gradient). However, >40% of older patients have lower mean transvalvular gradients and/or peak velocities, that is, low gradient AS. About half of this latter group also have LV stroke volume indices of <35 mL/m^2, so called low flow, low gradient AS. This hemodynamic pattern is more common in women with small LV cavities and in patients with AF.[75] All-cause mortality over long-term follow-up is similar in medically treated patients with low flow, low gradient AS to that in the more typical high flow, high gradient pattern; both groups experience significant mortality reduction from AVR. However, the subset with high flow and low gradient does not generally have a mortality benefit from AVR.[75]

More robust older adults can generally undergo surgical AVR with acceptable morbidity and mortality. The 2020 ACC/AHA Guideline for the Management of Patients with Valvular Heart Disease[75a] recommends surgical AVR or transcatheter AVR after shared decision making among symptomatic patients ages 65 to 80 years. A tissue valve is generally preferred over a mechanical valve in older individuals to avoid the need for anticoagulation. Deterioration of bioprosthetic valves generally occurs more slowly in older than younger patients, increasing the likelihood that the prosthetic valve will not need to be replaced during the patient's remaining lifespan.

Transcatheter AVR (TAVR) has been transformative as an alternative for the sizable proportion of older patients with severe AS in a context of high surgical risks. In the initial PARTNER trial, 1-year mortality in otherwise inoperable patients with severe AS (mean age, 83 years; 54% women) randomized to TAVR was 30% compared with 50% in the medically treated group. Subsequent trials in patients at high and intermediate surgical risk showed similar 30-day and 1-year survival in patients randomized to TAVR vs. surgical AVR. In low risk patients (mean age, 73 years), the composite risk of death, stroke, or hospitalization at 1 year was significantly lower (8.5% vs. 15.1%) in patients randomized to TAVR compared to surgical AVR, as was hospital stay and risk of new-onset AF at 30 days.[76] Risks of stroke, vascular complications, permanent pacemaker implantation, and paravalvular leak are generally higher with TAVR, although strokes and vascular complication rates have decreased in recent trials.

In the Transcatheter Valve Therapy Registry, 30-day mortality after TAVR declined from 4% to 3% between 2013 and 2015 and 1-year mortality declined from 26% to 22%.[77] After TAVR, substantial improvement is seen in functional capacity, NYHA class, and QOL similar to surgical AVR. Excellent durability of TAVR, as defined by stability of the AV gradient and valve area, has been demonstrated to 5 years.

In the 2020 Guideline for the Management of Patients with Valvular Heart Disease,[75a] TAVR is recommended among symptomatic patients of any age with high or prohibitive surgical risk if predicted survival after intervention is >12 months with an acceptable quality of life. TAVR is also recommended for patients >80 years or any patient with life expectancy <10 years. As with other bioprosthetic valves, daily aspirin 75 to 100 mg is recommended as antithrombotic therapy.

Aortic Regurgitation

The prevalence of AR increases with age. Common causes of AR in older adults are valvular disease (degenerative or infectious) or aortic root dilation due to hypertension, connective tissue disease, aortic dissection, or trauma. Severe AR may be asymptomatic for many years; however, life expectancy without surgery is about 2 years in older individuals once HF develops. Left ventricular dilation, reduced EF, and moderate or greater PH predict higher mortality.

The classic diastolic high-pitched blowing murmur of AR is generally heard best at the lower left sternal border if due to valvular disease and at the upper right sternal border if due to aortic root dilation. Presence of a widened pulse pressure is not as helpful an ancillary sign of AR in older adults because they often have widened pulse pressure due to arterial stiffening. Definitive diagnosis of AR is made by quantifying the regurgitant jet on Doppler echocardiography. Chronic severe AR accompanied by a systolic LV dimension >4.5 cm or LVEF <50% is an indication for AVR even in the absence of symptoms.[78] Older patients are more likely to develop HF symptoms and LV dysfunction earlier in the disease course and have higher postoperative mortality than younger individuals. Operative mortality in older patients varies with LV function, increasing from <5% with normal function to 14% for LVEF <35%. Although moderate or severe AR has been a contraindication for TAVR to date, small series have shown successful treatment of AR by TAVR.[79] TAVR may become a reliable alternative to surgical AVR in high-risk older individuals with severe AR.

Mitral Stenosis

With the dramatic reduction in rheumatic heart disease in developed countries, mitral stenosis (MS) (see Chapter 75), the hallmark lesion of this disease, has become uncommon and is mostly confined to

foreign-born older adults, typically women, often with a prior mitral commissurotomy. Congestive symptoms generally indicate significant transmitral obstruction and a valve area <1.0 cm². Associated AF is more common in older patients with MS due to superimposed age-related left atrial enlargement and electrophysiologic changes. The resultant stasis of blood in the left atrium, especially the appendage, significantly increases risk for systemic thromboembolism, including stroke.

The pathognomonic low-pitched diastolic murmur of MS may be absent or of low intensity in older adults due to increased anteroposterior chest diameter or low stroke volume. In addition, the first heart sound may not be loud and the opening snap may be absent due to a fibrotic calcified mitral valve. Echocardiography is essential to confirm the diagnosis of MS, determine its severity, and characterize the extent of leaflet calcification and presence of associated MR.

In symptomatic older adults with severe MS, an intervention to increase mitral valve area is usually indicated. A percutaneous balloon valvulotomy may be suitable if the valve leaflets are not heavily calcified and their motion not severely restricted. However, success rates are below 50% in older patients and procedural complications and mortality are increased; cardiac tamponade occurs in ~5% and thromboembolism and death each in ~3%. Risks from mitral valve replacement (MVR) are also increased in older adults, with perioperative mortality ≥10%.

Mitral Annular Calcification

Mitral annular calcification (MAC) is an age-associated degenerative process that is more common in older women than men. It has been reported in about ~10% of community-dwelling adults age 45 to 84 years and much higher in those ≥85. The process parallels that in the AV, including the association with common atherosclerotic risk factors. Older patients with severe CKD have a particularly high rate of MAC. When MAC is extensive, it compromises the sphincter function of the mitral annulus and may stretch the mitral leaflets during systole, causing MR. Although MS may result from severe MAC that protrudes into the valve orifice, the MS is rarely severe. Calcific deposits from MAC may extend into the membranous ventricular septum, causing conduction disturbances. MAC increases the risk for endocarditis, especially perivalvular abscesses due to the avascularity of the annular tissue. Several studies have shown an increased risk of stroke or silent brain infarction in older patients with MAC. Although the net benefit of anticoagulation in patients with MAC is unclear, individuals with associated AF, MS, or severe MR are usually considered for such therapy.

Mitral Regurgitation

MR is common in older adults, with >10% of individuals age ≥75 years having at least moderate MR (see Chapter 76). Myxomatous degeneration is the most frequent structural etiology, with endocarditis, rheumatic heart disease, and papillary muscle rupture after MI less frequent causes. Functional MR is most often due to chronic LV and annular dilation or to ischemic papillary muscle dysfunction. Whereas myxomatous degeneration in younger populations typically presents as chest pain and mitral valve prolapse and is most common in women, in later life MR and congestive symptoms comprise the most common presentation, with similar prevalence in men and women. Chronic MR is often asymptomatic in older adults until it becomes severe. Presenting symptoms are initially exercise intolerance and fatigue, progressing to congestive symptoms as systolic LV function declines. Secondary PH is common in severe MR, and may result in right-sided HF.

Physical findings with significant MR are not generally altered by age; Doppler echocardiography quantifies the size of the regurgitant jet and provides insights regarding the etiology of MR based on leaflet and annular morphology and LV size and function. The prognosis of older patients with MR depends on its severity and etiology. Patients with acute MR secondary to papillary muscle rupture after an acute MI are an especially high-risk group due to the underlying myocardial insult and hemodynamic instability. Emergent surgical MVR with resection of the damaged papillary muscle and infarct zone is the treatment of choice. Patients with severe chronic MR and LV systolic dysfunction and/or dilation are also at high risk of adverse outcomes. Medical therapy for such patients should include ACEI/ARB and beta blockers, diuretics to relieve congestive symptoms, and rate or rhythm control of AF.

The 2020 ACC/AHA Guideline for the Management of Patients With Valvular Heart Disease recommends surgical repair in preference to valve replacement, provided that a successful and durable repair is technically feasible. In asymptomatic patients, surgery is recommended if LV ejection fraction (LVEF) ≤60% and/or LV end-systolic diameter ≥40 mm.[75a] Mitral valve repair is usually preferred over MVR for patients in their 70s and 80s, as results are similar to or better than MVR, including mortality ~5% or less and 70% to 80% 5-year survival. Functional status and

QOL are improved to a similar degree after MV repair or replacement. However, MVR is indicated when MV leaflets are fused, are extensively fibrotic or calcified, and have chordal shortening or fusion.

In parallel to the development of TAVR for treatment of severe AS, transcather mitral valve repair, now referred to as *transcatheter edge-to-edge repair* (TEER), provides a less invasive approach for severe MR. A MitraClip device "clips" the leaflets together, thereby reducing orifice size without affecting the annulus. In the Endovascular Valve Edge-to-Edge Repair Study (EVEREST) II, 351 older patients (mean age 76 years) with calculated surgical mortality risk ≥12% underwent MitraClip insertion. At 30 days, cardiac death occurred in 5%, MI in 1%, and stroke in 2.6%. At 12 months postprocedure, NYHA class and QOL had improved substantially, LV volumes were reduced, and MR severity was <2+ in 84% of patients.[80] A subsequent study of 564 patients of mean age 83 years reported 30-day mortality of 6%, strokes in 2%, and bleeding in 3%, with reduction of MR to grade <2 in 93%.[81] In older patients (mean age 72 years) with HF and moderate-to-severe or severe secondary MR who remained symptomatic despite maximal doses of guideline-directed medical therapy, transcatheter mitral-valve repair resulted in a lower rate of HF hospitalization and all-cause mortality over mean follow-up of 24 months compared with medical therapy alone.[82] Thus, TEER is an attractive option for a large proportion of high-risk older patients with severe MR. In the 2020 ACC/AHA Guideline for Management of Patients with Valvular Heart Disease, TEER is considered reasonable in patients with appropriate anatomy as defined on TEE and with LVEF between 20% and 50%, left ventricular end systolic diameter <70 mmHg, and pulmonary artery systolic pressure <70 mm Hg.[75a]

Endocarditis

Endocarditis (see Chapter 80) in older adults typically occurs as a result of indwelling vascular catheters, genitourinary or gastrointestinal instrumentation, pacemaker or ICD leads, prosthetic implants, or MAC. Diabetes and genitourinary and gastrointestinal cancer are major predisposing conditions. The most common pathogens in older adults are *Staphylococcus aureus*, often methicillin-resistant, *Streptococcus bovis*, and *Enterococci*. Morbidity and mortality from endocarditis are higher in older persons, due in part to comorbidities. In one large series, endocarditis incidence after TAVR was similar to that after surgical AVR and incurred a 36% in-hospital mortality.[83] Indications for endocarditis prophylaxis are similar regardless of age and include prosthetic valve implants, prior endocarditis, and cardiac transplantation.

CARDIAC RHYTHM ABNORMALITIES

Cardiac rhythm disorders (see Part VII) increase with age and become increasingly important contributors to morbidity and mortality.[84] Age-related changes in the heart and cardiac conduction system and the high prevalence of CVD provide substrates for arrhythmias. Fibrous, fatty, and calcific infiltration of the conduction system; calcification of the cardiac fibrous skeleton; reduction in the number of functioning sinus node pacemaker cells; impaired intracellular calcium handling; and blunted adrenergic responsiveness all increase the susceptibility to arrhythmias.[84] Cardiac amyloidosis is also increasingly recognized as etiologic for advanced AV block in older adults. Right and left bundle branch block increase with age.

Though the resting heart rate does not change with age, maximal heart rate decreases as a result of reduced sinus node responsivity to beta-adrenergic sympathetic stimulation[85]; beat-to-beat variability also decreases with age. Atrial ectopy occurs in about 10% of older individuals in the absence of known cardiac disease, with ventricular ectopy in 6% to 11% on resting ECG.

Supraventricular Arrhythmias
Atrial Fibrillation

Atrial fibrillation (see Chapter 66) occurs in about 12% of patients age ≥75 years and 18% of patients ≥85 years.[86] The high prevalence of AF relates to age-related changes in the atrial tissues, including fibrosis and conduction abnormalities that provide the substrate for electrical disarray. Hypertension and structural heart disease add to maladaptive atrial changes, which further predispose to AF.

The 2019 AHA/ACC/HRS Guideline for the Management of Patients with AF estimates that approximately one-third of patients with AF are ≥80 years.[87] Compared with younger adults, AF is more likely to occur in older adults in the absence of underlying heart disease. Common chronic comorbid conditions associated with AF include hypertension, CHD, obesity, sleep apnea, hyperlipidemia, and HF.

Symptoms of AF may include palpitations, light-headedness, chest discomfort, shortness of breath, fatigue, or decreased activity tolerance. Nonetheless, palpitations are less common than in younger patients and symptoms are frequently minimal or atypical. Acute pulmonary edema may occur with an abrupt loss of the atrial contribution to ventricular filling in a stiff LV. Less commonly, AF may be initially manifest as syncope, fall, or stroke.

The U.S. Preventive Services Task Force considers evidence insufficient for ECG screening for AF in old age, suggesting pulse palpation and confirmatory ECG.[88] The ESC guideline recommends AF screening at age ≥65 by pulse taking or an ECG rhythm strip (Class I); systematic ECG screening at age ≥75 is a Class IIb recommendation.[89] Wearable devices in the Apple Heart Study[90] suggest its utility to improve screening in older as well as younger adults.

Nonvalvular AF is associated with a fivefold increase in stroke. Strokes are often severe, and adverse outcomes are likely even after controlling for age and comorbidities. Increasing age is a potent risk factor for stroke, as highlighted in the CHA_2DS_2-VASc score, which assigns 1 point for age 65 to 74 years and 2 points for age ≥75 years. Thus, all persons age ≥75 years have a CHA_2DS_2-VASc score of ≥2 and are candidates for anticoagulation irrespective of whether the AF is paroxysmal, persistent, or permanent. In addition to the increased risk of stroke and HF, AF in older adults is associated with decreased physical performance and cognition,[91] shorter disability-free survival, and increased mortality.

Utility of anticoagulation is counterbalanced by increased risk of bleeding, particularly in older age. The HAS-BLED score reflects age-related bleeding risk, with "old age" defined as >65 years. The decision to initiate anticoagulation must integrate risks for stroke versus bleeding, as both increase with age. The frequent concomitant CHD may contribute to increased bleeding risk when dual antiplatelet agents are combined with anticoagulation. Multiple recent studies suggest the utility of using only a P2Y12 inhibitor (i.e., avoiding aspirin) in combination with warfarin[92] or a DOAC[93] with reduced bleeding events as compared with dual antiplatelet therapy.

Warfarin has been the traditional anticoagulant, with target international normalized ratio (INR) between and 2 and 2.5 recommended at older age. The estimated maintenance dose of warfarin is lower in senior adults, typically 2 to 5 mg daily, often initiated without a loading dose or with a loading dose of 5 mg. The requirements for regular INR surveillance as well as dietary limitations constitute significant challenges for older patients. Multiple drug interactions with warfarin pose added problems. Risk of osteoporosis also increases.[94] DOACs, dabigatran, rivaroxaban, apixaban, and edoxaban constitute favorable alternatives to warfarin without the need for dietary restriction or INR monitoring. Among patients ≥75 years, DOACs demonstrated similar or better stroke prevention efficacy with similar or less bleeding compared with warfarin.[95] Dose adjustment may be required based on age, body weight, and/or renal function. For older patients who are not candidates for anticoagulation, an alternative may be percutaneous left atrial appendage closure with the WATCHMAN device.[96]

Symptoms of AF may be managed by rate or rhythm control. Since rate control strategy is safer and usually as effective as pharmacologic rhythm control, it is the recommended first-line treatment in asymptomatic or mildly symptomatic patients of all ages. Class I options for achieving rate control include beta blockers and nondihydropyridine calcium channel blockers. Digoxin can aid in rate control in relatively sedentary individuals. Dronedarone is also useful. However, both nondihydropyridine calcium channel blockers and dronedarone are contraindicated in systolic HF. Given the vulnerability of older adults to medication-induced heart block, particularly with amiodarone and digitalis, the Rate Control Efficacy in Permanent Atrial Fibrillation (RACE) II trial assessed a more lenient rate control strategy. Therapy targeting heart rate <110 beats/min in older adults (Class IIb) without significant symptoms, CHD, or HF was comparable to strict rate control (<80 beats/min),[97] which may help to reduce need for cardiac pacing secondary to bradycardia.

Antiarrhythmic drugs have a higher incidence of adverse events in older adults due to the potential for drug interactions, unpredictable pharmacokinetics and pharmacodynamics, and variable renal function. A rhythm control strategy was associated with increased mortality in older adults in the Atrial Fibrillation Follow-up Investigation of Rhythm Management (AFFIRM) trial.[87] Since a rhythm control strategy does not obviate the need for anticoagulation, a rate control strategy is preferable in older adults. Nonetheless, maintenance of sinus rhythm has been associated with a better QOL and many clinicians still try to restore sinus rhythm in older adults at least once.

Atrioventricular node ablation to create complete heart block with pacemaker implantation has a Class IIa recommendation to achieve a regular rhythm in symptomatic patients in whom pharmacologic therapy has failed. Catheter or surgical AF ablation are also compelling considerations. Older adults commonly have large atria and chamber fibrosis that may reduce the likelihood of restoring and maintaining sinus rhythm. Nonetheless, the Catheter Ablation vs Antiarrhythmic Drug Therapy for Atrial Fibrillation (CABANA) trial suggests the potential of catheter ablation to improve QOL in older subgroups.[98] Radiofrequency ablation in patients with atrial flutter showed the success rate (86%) was comparable in patients ≥80 years to younger patients.[99]

Supraventricular Tachycardia (SVT). Episodes of supraventricular tachycardia (SVT; see Chapter 65) (short atrial runs, atrial tachycardia, atrioventricular nodal reentrant tachycardia [AVNRT] and atrioventricular reciprocating tachycardia [AVRT]) occur in up to 50% of the older population in 24-hour monitoring studies.[85] Management is similar to younger adults. Multifocal atrial tachycardia (MAT) is especially common in the setting of decompensated pulmonary disease; patients are often quite ill and symptomatic. Management of MAT is often constrained by poor tolerance of beta blockers and amiodarone and limitation of use of nondihydropyridine calcium channel blockers when there is LV dysfunction. The best outcome is achieved by control of the underlying pulmonary disease.

Bradyarrhythmias. Bradyarrhythmias (see Chapter 68) increase with age, primarily due to sinus node dysfunction and atrioventricular (AV) block. The number of sinus node pacemaker cells decreases to <10% functional cells by age 75.[85] Medications (e.g., donepezil for dementia) compound vulnerability to bradyarrhythmias. Similarly, bradyarrhythmia may be provoked by treatment for a tachyarrhythmia (e.g., tachy-brady variant of sick sinus syndrome). Hemodynamic effects may result from decreased cardiac output with dizziness, lightheadedness, falls, and syncope common sequelae, although symptoms may also include dyspnea, exercise intolerance, fatigue, or rarely chest pain. The ECG is the first diagnostic study, with a Holter monitor, event monitor, or implantable loop recorder also useful for detecting bradyarrhythmias. Assessment for chronotropic incompetence by exercise testing may be useful for patients with activity-related symptoms.

The initial management involves discontinuation of relevant medications (e.g., beta blockers, calcium channel blockers), if feasible. Presence of hypothyroidism and Lyme disease should also be considered. For persistent symptomatic bradycardia, permanent cardiac pacing is usually indicated (see Chapter 68). Greater than 75% of pacemaker implantations occur in patients age ≥65 years, with half >75 years. Pacemaker implantation has a Class I indication for sinus node dysfunction with documented symptomatic bradycardia or chronotropic incompetence, and Class II indication for symptoms at heart rate <40 beats/min.[100] Pacemaker implantation has a Class I indication for third-degree or advanced second-degree AV block with symptomatic bradycardia, an escape rhythm originating below the AV node or with a rate <40 beats/min, pauses ≥5 seconds, or after cardiac surgery without expectation for resolution.

Dual-chamber pacing improves QOL in older patents, likely because programmable pacing of both the atrial and ventricular rates improves diastolic flow and cardiac output, which are more dependent on the atrial contribution to ventricular filling in this population. Dual chamber pacing also reduces incidence of AF and decreases the rate of hospitalizations. Cardiac resynchronization therapy (CRT) has benefit for selected patients with symptomatic systolic HF (EF ≤35%) and a prolonged (≥150 msec) QRS as well as those with mild systolic dysfunction with an anticipated high pacing frequency (>40%). Class I indications for CRT are similar in older and younger patients.[100] Few patients age >75 years were enrolled in CRT trials; subgroup analyses from Cardiac Resynchronization-Heart Failure (CARE-HF), age <66 versus >66,[101] and Comparison of Medical Therapy, Pacing, and Defibrillation in Heart Failure (COMPANION), age ≤65 versus >65, suggest that older patients derive similar mortality benefit. In addition, CRT therapy improves gait speed, QOL, and frailty score in older HFrEF patients.

Ventricular Arrhythmias. Although the incidence of all ventricular arrhythmias (see Chapter 67) increases with age, sudden cardiac death (SCD) appears to decline after age 80 years, largely due to competing causes of death. No specific treatment is required for ventricular premature complexes (VPCs) in the absence of bothersome symptoms. Symptomatic VPCs often respond to low-dose beta blockade. Potentially life-threatening ventricular arrhythmias (i.e., sustained ventricular tachycardia and ventricular fibrillation) virtually always occur with structural heart disease such as ischemic or hypertensive cardiomyopathy.

Implantable Cardioverter Defibrillators and Cardiac Resynchronization Therapy: (See Chapter 69). The updated ACC/AHA/HRS 2008 Guidelines for device therapy of cardiac rhythm abnormalities do not address age-based indications and acknowledge that few clinical trials of device-based therapy have enrolled enough aged patients to reliably estimate the benefits. Relevance of comorbidities, limited life expectancy, and QOL issues are emphasized when considering ICDs for older adults.[100] In the Multicenter Automatic Defibrillator Implantation Trial (MADIT) II trial involving patients with a LVEF ≤30% and prior MI, ICD therapy improved survival in those age >70 years of age by more than 30% compared with conventional therapy. Nonetheless, the potential durability of ICD benefit is shorter and the risk of procedural complications higher in older patients. In a meta-analysis of the three major secondary prevention ICD trials (CASH, CIDS, AVID), patients ≥75 years old were more likely to die a nonarrhythmic death and there was no benefit from an ICD.[102]

The Guidelines address end-of-life issues and recommend that ICDs not be considered for patients with a life expectancy <1 year.[100] Implanting physicians are encouraged to discuss end-of-life issues before implantation and to encourage patients to complete advance directives and specifically address device management and deactivation if the patient becomes terminally ill.[103] Device deactivation in hospice care prevents multiple potentially painful shocks in terminally ill patients and may enable painless sudden death. While subcutaneous ICDs may have theoretical value for older patients, no trials of subcutaneous ICDs specifically address older adults.

VENOUS THROMBOEMBOLIC DISEASE

Epidemiology and Diagnosis

Deep vein thrombosis (DVT) and venous thromboembolism (VTE) (see Chapter 87), including pulmonary embolism (PE), increase exponentially with advancing age; increased blood thrombotic factors, limited mobility, and laxity of large venous valves contribute to risk. More than half of VTE follow surgery, injury, serious medical illness, or prolonged bed rest or occur with malignancy. A sharp increase in risk occurs after age 65, with a hazard ratio of 1.7 for every decade thereafter. Half of all patients with acute VTE are >70 years, and one-fourth are ≥80.[104] PE is more common than DVT in old age. There is increased hospital mortality with acute PE in older adults, with 1-year mortality of 39%, or 10% to 30% excess compared with younger individuals.[105]

In older adults, DVT has less typical symptoms such as lower extremity discomfort or difficulty with ambulation than at younger age, likely due to greater occurrence of proximal DVT without calf involvement. PE requires a high index of suspicion in any older patient admitted for shortness of breath. Pleuritic chest pain and hemoptysis are less common with PE than cough or syncope. Older adults with PE are more likely to have ECG abnormalities including tachycardia, $S_1Q_3T_3$, RBBB, AF, and anterior T wave abnormalities.[106]

Color flow imaging, in addition to duplex Doppler ultrasound, is highly accurate for diagnosis of DVT. D-dimer tests are highly sensitive for thrombus formation and can be used to exclude PE in patients with a low clinical probability. Application of age-adjusted cutoff values substantially increases the specificity without modifying the sensitivity.[107] In the age-adjusted D-dimer cutoff levels to rule out PE (ADJUST-PE) study, compared with a fixed D-dimer cutoff of 500 micrograms per liter, the combination of a pretest probability assessment with age-adjusted D-dimer cutoff, defined as age x 10, was associated with a larger number of patients in whom PE could be ruled out with a low likelihood of subsequent clinical VTE.[107]

Management

Aggressive VTE prophylaxis is the most important intervention, particularly early mobilization for hospitalized patients. Thromboprophylaxis with LMWH or low-dose unfractionated heparin is recommended, with extensive studies validating use in old age.[108] Fondaparinux is also effective. Intermittent pneumatic compression (IPC) and compression stockings are alternatives when anticoagulant bleeding risk is excessive, although IPC can cause skin injury, especially in frail older patients. Notably, routine use of compression stockings to prevent post-thrombotic syndrome in acute VTE is no longer recommended in the 2016 Guidelines.

The number of patients ≥75 years who require anticoagulation for DVT and VTE is rising. Management is challenging because both thrombosis and bleeding risks are high. Initial heparin therapy is requisite when starting warfarin. LMWH is preferable to unfractionated heparin because of simplicity of administration, less major bleeding risk, and lower mortality; LMWH also facilitates early hospital discharge and home management. Dose adjustment to body weight and renal function in older adults is essential. A meta-analysis of randomized trials confirmed that DOACs are associated with equal or greater efficacy than warfarin in older adults, with reduced bleeding and lower risk of VTE or VTE-related deaths.[109] Conventional anticoagulation for DVT lasts 3 months, but bleeding risks, particularly in patients >75 years and/or with concomitant cognitive impairments, falls, or other complexities often impact treatment duration. Unprovoked VTE is reasonably treated for longer duration when bleeding risk is acceptable.

Recently released American Society of Hematology guidelines recommend thromboprophylaxis in hospitalized medical patients with cancer, including LMWH or fondaparinux for surgical patients, LMWH or DOACs in ambulatory patients receiving systemic therapy at high risk of VTE, LMWH or DOAC for initial treatment of VTE, DOACs for the short-term treatment of VTE, and LMWH or DOACs for the long-term treatment of VTE.[109a]

Older adults are at high risk for PE and for adverse clinical outcomes and treatment-related complications. In an acutely ill PE patient with hypotension and hemodynamic instability, systemic thrombolysis, catheter-assisted thrombus removal or catheter-based thrombolysis are recommended.[110] For subsegmental PE and no proximal DVT, clinical surveillance is recommended rather than anticoagulation, with a low risk of recurrent VTE. However, anticoagulation is advised in patients with a high VTE risk.[108] Although the value of inferior vena cava filters (IVCFs) is controversial, an IVCF is recommended in patients with acute PE and contraindications to anticoagulation or active bleeding.

SYNCOPE

Background

Older adults are at increased risk for syncope (see Chapter 71) due to age-related changes in the CV system, including diminished baroreceptor responsiveness, impaired adrenergic responsiveness, and altered LV diastolic function, as well as increasing prevalence of CV and non-CV conditions and medications that predispose to syncope.[111] Prevalence of syncope exceeds 20% among adults aged ≥75 years; the annual incidence approaches 2% in those ≥80 years[112] and is substantially higher among nursing home residents. Prognosis of syncope worsens with age, with 2-year mortality rates of 25% to 30% in patients over 75 years. Syncope is also an important cause of injurious falls and associated disability in older adults.

Clinical Features and Etiology

The presentation of syncope is similar across the age spectrum, but older patients are less likely to recall preceding events. Amnesia for syncope is also common in older adults who fall, leading to misclassification of the etiology of falls and underdiagnosis of syncope.

Syncope in older adults is often multifactorial, reflecting the interplay between age-related CV changes, multimorbidity, and medications. Neurally-mediated syncope is the most frequent etiology in older adults, followed by orthostatic hypotension, dysautonomia, and CV etiologies. Neurally-mediated causes may be neurocardiogenic (vasovagal) or related to carotid sinus hypersensitivity (CSH), which is common in older adults although usually asymptomatic. Common causes of orthostatic hypotension and dysautonomia in older adults include diabetes, Parkinson disease, postprandial postural hypotension, dehydration, and prolonged bedrest (e.g., during hospitalization). Bradyarrhythmias due to sick sinus syndrome, conduction abnormalities, or medications are the most common cardiac causes of syncope in older adults. Supraventricular and ventricular tachyarrhythmias, as well as valvular heart disease (especially AS) and cardiomyopathies (hypertrophic cardiomyopathy, amyloid) are other important CV causes. The prognosis of cardiogenic syncope is worse than for other causes.

Evaluation

As in younger patients, a careful history is the cornerstone of the initial evaluation of syncope in older adults. However, the history in older patients may be less reliable due to impaired recall, cognitive impairment, anxiety, or medication side effects. A detailed assessment of medications is essential, including any recent changes in medications, adherence, and use of over-the-counter drugs and supplements. A complete physical examination should include measurement of heart rate and BP in the supine, sitting, and standing positions. Carotid sinus massage may be helpful if CSH is suspected.

Laboratory evaluation of syncope should be targeted to the most likely etiologies. If a cardiac cause is suspected, an echocardiogram and a period of ECG monitoring are usually appropriate. In patients with recurrent unexplained syncope, the implantable loop recorder has been associated with high diagnostic yield for an arrhythmic cause. Tilt-table testing may be helpful in evaluation of neurally-mediated syncope, but sensitivity and specificity are modest. Carotid duplex, head CT, EEG, brain MRI, and cardiac stress testing have very low diagnostic yield and should only be incorporated into the syncope evaluation in highly selected situations.[113]

Management

Management of syncope is oriented to the presumed etiology and is generally similar in younger and older patients. However, management of older patients is often complicated by age-related physiologic changes, comorbidities and geriatric syndromes, and polypharmacy. Optimal treatment of older adults requires consideration of each of these factors.

Syncope is a common cause of falls in older adults, and 35% of syncopal falls are associated with injury. Thus, a syncopal event should prompt a full evaluation of fall risk, including gait and balance testing, muscle strength, foot exam and assessment of footwear, review of predisposing medications (especially CV and psychoactive drugs) and neurologic exam to evaluate for neuropathy, Parkinson disease, and other neurologic deficits.

Numerous medications used to treat CV conditions may increase risk for syncope due to their effects on BP, heart rate, or heart rhythm. Medications that can prolong QTc, particularly when used in combination with other QTc-prolonging drugs, can induce syncope. Cholinesterase inhibitors used to treat Alzheimer disease (e.g., donepezil) may cause bradycardia, hypotension, and syncope, as can levodopa-carbidopa, a standard treatment for Parkinson disease. Alcohol, recreational drugs, and pain medications are additional potential causes of syncope. Deprescribing of potentially contributing medications, if clinically appropriate, should be considered.

Sarcopenia, frailty, malnutrition, cognitive impairment, and incontinence may contribute to syncope and should be treated as part of a holistic strategy to reduce risk of falls and syncope and improve function and QOL. Incontinence can contribute to syncope as a result of sudden standing in an attempt to get to the bathroom. Diuretics frequently exacerbate the problem, and dose adjustment is an important consideration. Referral to a geriatrician or urologist for further evaluation and management may be warranted.

PREVENTION

Efforts to prevent new or recurrent CV events in older adults center on control of modifiable factors known to facilitate development or progression of CV disease. Notably, most landmark clinical trials that established the treatment benefit included few if any individuals older than 70 to 75 years or only those without the comorbidities typically found in this age group. Competing risks for mortality from non-CV disorders may reduce the likelihood of demonstrating a survival benefit in older adults. However, benefits in respect to reducing CV events, preserving function, preserving cognition, reducing hospitalizations, and sustaining QOL are important rationales for prevention for many older adults.

Hypertension

Hypertension (see Chapter 26) is the most common CV risk factor among older men and women, with prevalence rates of ~70% in those aged 75 years and older.[10] Hypertension has the greatest population-attributable risk for CHD, cerebrovascular disease, and PAD among older adults. Over 70% of older adults with incident MI, stroke, acute aortic syndromes, and HF have preexisting hypertension. Hypertension is the most prevalent antecedent of HF, especially with preserved LVEF, and of chronic kidney disease.[5]

Before the 1980s, the age-associated elevation of SBP in older adults was generally considered a normal finding that did not warrant treatment. However, numerous observational studies have since documented that elevated SBP confers increased risk for CV morbidity and mortality.[114] After age 70 years, isolated systolic hypertension (ISH) accounts for >90% of all patients with hypertension.[10]

Multiple clinical trials in older cohorts have shown benefits of hypertension treatment.[115] Although only two trials showed significant reductions in total mortality, several showed substantial reductions in stroke and HF. The landmark HYpertension in the Very Elderly Trial (HYVET) demonstrated a 39% significant decrease in fatal stroke, 21% significant decrease in all-cause mortality, and 64% significant decrease in HF over 1.8 years mean follow-up in 3845 patients ≥80 years old with systolic BP ≥160 mm Hg treated with the thiazide-like diuretic indapamide to a target BP of 150/80 mm Hg versus placebo.[116] More recently, the Systolic Blood Pressure Intervention Trial (SPRINT) showed a 34% reduction in CV events and 33% reduction in mortality in 2636 patients aged ≥75 years with SBP >130 mm Hg randomized to a target of 120 mm Hg versus 140 mm Hg.[117] Based in part on these findings, the 2017 Update to the Hypertension Guidelines Committee recommended a target BP ≤130 mm Hg for persons in this age group.[114] In older patients with CHD, however, excessive lowering of DBP should be avoided to avert deleterious reductions in coronary blood flow. Some studies have found higher CHD rates when diastolic BP is reduced below 60 to 65 mm Hg.

Hypertension Management

Nonpharmacologic interventions are recommended as initial therapy to manage mild hypertension (see Chapter 26). Such an approach is especially useful in older adults to avoid or reduce the number and doses of antihypertensive drugs and their potential for adverse effects, biochemical changes, and high costs. For milder hypertension, lifestyle modifications may be the only treatment needed. These include aerobic exercise; reductions in excess body weight, mental stress, and intake of sodium and alcohol; smoking cessation; and adoption of the Dietary Approaches to Stop Hypertension (DASH) eating plan.[114]

Current guidelines recommend four major classes of antihypertensive drugs as first-line therapy: diuretics, ACEI, ARB, and calcium channel blockers. Two or more drugs will be required to achieve target BP levels in approximately two-thirds of seniors with hypertension. Combination therapy often allows lower individual drug dosages, minimizing dose-dependent side effects, and achieving longer duration of action and additive target organ protection,[114] although it also contributes to polypharmacy. The choice of specific agents is dictated by efficacy, tolerability, specific comorbidities, and cost. Given the age-related predisposition to orthostatic hypotension and changes in absorption, distribution, metabolism, and excretion of pharmacologic agents, therapy in older adults is best initiated at the lowest doses with gradual increments as tolerated. It is also important to assess resultant BP both seated and standing.

Dyslipidemia

Dyslipidemia (see Chapter 27) remains an important CV risk factor in older adults, although the relative risk imparted by lipid disorders may be attenuated compared with younger populations. Multiple cohort studies have shown that both total cholesterol and low density lipoprotein cholesterol (LDL-C) correlated significantly with fatal CHD in both sexes across a broad age range, including adults ≥65 years but with very few ≥80.[118] Despite the voluminous literature demonstrating reduction in CV events in both primary and secondary prevention populations receiving medications to lower LDL-C (primarily statins), the majority of patients in these trials were age <65 years old, with smaller enrollments in predominantly younger strata of older adults (Table 90.4).[40]

TABLE 90.4 Lipid Lowering Trials Supporting Secondary Prevention in Older Adults

TRIAL NAME	MEDICATION	N	AGE RANGE (YEAR)	% OLDER PATIENTS	FOLLOW-UP (YEARS)	OUTCOMES
4S	Simvastatin	4444	35-70	≥65 years (23%)	5.4	• 34% RRR in all-cause mortality • 34% RRR in MACE
HPS	Simvastatin	20,536	40-80	≥70 years (29%)	5	• 25% RRR in death or MI
CARE	Pravastatin	4159	21-75	≥65 years (31%)	5	• 24% RRR in death or MI
LIPID	Pravastatin	9014	31-75	≥65 years (36%)	6.1	• 24% RRR in all-cause mortality and cardiac mortality • 29% RRR in nonfatal MI • 20% RRR in coronary revascularization
PROSPER	Pravastatin	2565	70-82	≥70 years (100%)	3.2	• 20% RRR in CHD, nonfatal MI, and stroke*
TNT	Atorvastatin	10,001	35-75	≥65 years (38%)	4.9	• 19% RRR in composite endpoint of MACE, CHD-related death, nonfatal MI, or stroke
SAGE	Pravastatin vs. Atorvastatin	893	65-85	≥65 years (100%)	1	• 29% RRR in MACE and 67% RRR in death in atorvastatin group
ODYSSEY	Alirocumab	18,924	≥40	≥65 years (27%)	2.8	• 15% RRR in MACE with alirocumab
REDUCE-IT	Icosapent ethyl	8179	≥45	>65 years (46%)	4.9	• 25% RRR in MACE with icosapent ethyl

*Benefit was in the secondary prevention cohort with no benefit for the primary prevention cohort.
CHD, Coronary heart disease; *MACE,* major adverse cardiovascular events; *MI,* myocardial infarction; *RRR,* relative risk reduction.

Based on the available data, the 2018 ACC/AHA Prevention Guidelines continue to recommend statin therapy, designed to lower LDL-C by 30% to 49%, in patients older than 75 years with known CV disease and LDL-C of 70 to 189 mg/dL.[40] Recommendations are supported by data showing benefit in reducing major adverse CV events (MACE), including mortality, MI, strokes, and PAD for those expected to live sufficiently long to derive benefit. While recommendations differ from recommendations to initiate high-intensity statin therapy in adults 40 to 75 years old (with goals to lower LDL-C at least 50%), they do not recommend lowering doses when an older adult is already taking a high-dose statin and tolerating it well. High-intensity statin therapy is recommended for individuals with LDL-C ≥190 mg/dL regardless of age. In older individuals with CVD and LDL-C 70 to 189 mg/dL, the potential benefit of long-term statin therapy must be weighed against cost, inconvenience, and possible side effects. The Guidelines indicate that it may be reasonable to stop statin therapy when functional decline, multimorbidity, frailty, or reduced life expectancy limits the potential benefits of statin therapy.

The benefits of statins for primary prevention in older adults are less clear. In a meta-analysis of 28 statin trials involving over 186,000 patients, the proportional reduction in major vascular events was similar, irrespective of age, among patients with preexisting vascular disease, but appeared smaller among those older than among younger individuals not known to have vascular disease (P trend = 0.05).[119] A recent propensity-adjusted analysis in a study of over 300,000 veterans age ≥75 years (mean 81.1 years, 97% men) without known atherosclerotic cardiovascular disease (ASCVD) stands out by showing that statin use was associated with significant reductions in all-cause mortality (25%), CV mortality (20%), and composite ASCVD events (8%).[120] Findings were consistent across subgroups by age, including patients age ≥90 years. While the 2018 Guidelines currently provide only a Class IIb recommendation for statin therapy as primary prevention in older adults,[40] the Pragmatic Evaluation of Events and Benefits of Lipid-Lowering in Older Adults (PREVENTABLE) trial is expected to provide better data to guide management (NCT04262206).

The most common side effect observed with statins is myalgia, which occurs in about 5% of patients. Myopathy documented by elevated muscle enzyme levels is much less common, occurring in 0.01% to 0.05%. The most severe adverse effect, rhabdomyolysis, has an incidence of 3.4/100,000 person-years. Age is not an independent risk factor for these complications.

In older patients intolerant of statins or who cannot achieve their LDL-C goal on maximally tolerated statin doses, ezetimibe may be a useful adjunct. Ezetimibe reduces cholesterol absorption from the gut, generally reducing LDL-C 15% to 20%. Ezetimibe is generally well tolerated in older adults, though it reduced CV events by a modest 6% in the Improved Reduction of Outcomes: Vytorin Efficacy International Trial (IMPROVE-IT).[121]

Proprotein convertase subtilisin–kexin type 9 (PCSK9) inhibition represents another option to substantially lower LDL-C levels in patients who do not achieve guideline-recommended goals. In the Evaluation of Cardiovascular Outcomes After an Acute Coronary Syndrome During Treatment with Alirocumab (ODYSSEY OUTCOMES) trial, the PCSK9 inhibitor alirocumab added to high-intensity or maximum-tolerated statin treatment, reduced the primary composite endpoint of death from CHD, nonfatal MI, ischemic stroke, or unstable angina requiring hospitalization compared with placebo in 18,924 patients with a recent ACS. The 15% reduction in CV events was similar across age groups, including individuals ≥75 years old,[122] and adverse effects were not increased relative to placebo. Similar findings have been reported with evolocumab.[123] This newer drug class therefore represents an important advance in reducing CV events in older adults with CHD, although the current high cost is an impediment. Although fibrates are sometimes used to raise low HDL-C or to reduce elevated triglycerides, evidence supporting their benefit in reducing CVD events is sparse. The combination of gemfibrozil and statins is associated with an increased risk of rhabdomyolysis (0.12%) and should usually be avoided, especially in older adults. Niacin (nicotinic acid), the most effective drug available to raise HDL-C, also reduces elevated triglycerides but showed no benefit in reducing CV events in clinical trials. In the REDUCE-IT trial, icosapent ethyl, a highly purified eicosapentaenoic acid ethyl ester, lowered elevated triglyceride levels an average of 18% and reduced major CV events by 25%. However, the benefit was blunted in patients ≥65 years (HR = 0.87) compared with those <65 years (HR = 0.65), interaction P = 0.004.[124]

Diabetes

Advancing age is accompanied by reduced insulin sensitivity and secretion, contributing to greater glucose intolerance and higher rates of type 2 diabetes mellitus (see Chapter 31) in older adults. Approximately 15% of adults ≥65 years have been diagnosed diabetes, and in another 7% diabetes is undiagnosed.[118] An estimated 30% of older adults with diabetes have clinical CHD, double the prevalence in age-matched nondiabetics. Older adults with diabetes and CVD are at high risk for adverse macrovascular and microvascular outcomes as well as functional disability and geriatric syndromes (e.g., frailty and falls).

The primary treatment goals for older adults with diabetes include managing hyperglycemia and reducing risk of adverse clinical outcomes. Lifestyle modification is paramount. Weight loss can reduce insulin resistance and improve glycemic control. Dietary interventions that optimize macronutrient content as well as calorie count help improve glycemic control, independent of weight change. Regular aerobic and resistance exercise lower HbA$_{1c}$ by 0.5% to 1.0% in older adults, even without changes in body weight or fat mass.

Despite the benefits of lifestyle interventions, most older patients with diabetes require medications to achieve glycemic control. Because several large clinical trials have found either no effect or even increased mortality in older patients receiving intensive glycemic therapy, a less intensive target HbA$_{1c}$ of 7% to 7.9% is recommended for most older adults, especially those with longstanding diabetes and chronic comorbidities including CVD. Even higher targets may be considered for older patients with frailty or short life expectancy.[125]

Metformin has been favored as a first-line therapy due to its low risk for hypoglycemia and other adverse effects. Additional options include the short-acting sulfonylurea, glipizide, and the short-acting insulin secretagogue, repaglinide.[118] Two new agents worthy of consideration are the sodium-glucose cotransporter 2 inhibitors and the glucagon-like peptide-1 analogues, which reduced CV events in large RCTs. The reduced CV risk with empagliflozin was especially prominent in patients ≥65 years old.[126] If insulin therapy is needed, ultra-long-acting basal and very-short-acting prandial insulins are strongly preferred over intermediate-acting insulin formulations. Although tighter glycemic control in diabetes may help to avoid microvascular complications, greater CV risk reduction may be achieved from control of concurrent risk factors such as hypertension and dyslipidemia.[118]

Tobacco

Although only 8.4% of Americans ≥65 years were current smokers in 2018, 49.4% of men and 30.6% of women ≥65 years were former smokers.[5] Numerous studies have demonstrated that continued smoking increases the rate for recurrent coronary and vascular events in both younger and older patients; reduced CV event rates are seen among those who quit smoking. Over 12 years of follow-up, older men in the Oslo II study who quit smoking between screenings had 31% lower mortality than those who smoked at both screening visits.[127] A meta-analysis of 17 general population studies in over 1.2 million persons age ≥60 years from seven countries showed dose-dependent increased all-cause mortality rates in current smokers, with a mean relative mortality of 1.83 compared with never-smokers. Among former smokers, the mortality risk was attenuated to 1.34. Risk reduction from smoking cessation was seen even in persons age ≥80 years.[128] In a registry of patients with CHD, mortality rate was markedly lower in recent quitters than in persistent smokers. Smoking cessation also reduces the risk of new or recurrent stroke and improves claudication symptoms.

Physical Inactivity

Physical inactivity (see Chapter 25) is a well-established risk factor for multiple chronic diseases, including hypertension, type 2 diabetes, CHD, stroke, PAD, depression, osteoporosis, and certain cancers. Physical inactivity is also associated with increased CV mortality.[118] Because the biologic and clinical repercussions of a sedentary lifestyle exacerbate age-related pathophysiologic changes, the health consequences and societal costs of physical inactivity are especially relevant to older adults. Physical inactivity results in decreased functional capacity, increased risk of falling, worsened psychological status, and reduced cognitive function. In older adults, decreased physical activity constitutes the most common modifiable CV risk factor after hypertension. Only 18% of persons ≥75 years old report regular moderate or vigorous physical activity, and only 14% of men and 8% of women ≥65 years old report aerobic and muscle strengthening activities that meet the 2008 Federal physical activity guidelines. Patel et al. reported increased total mortality, especially CV mortality, over 14-year follow-up in men and women 50 to 74 years old who sat >6 hours/day compared with those sitting only 3 hours/day[129]; similar findings have been reported in other studies.[118]

Numerous observational studies and RCTs demonstrate that older adults benefit from initiating an exercise program; benefits include greater functional capacity, cognitive and psychological functioning, less mobility disability, better QOL, reduced recurrent CV events, and an increase in active life expectancy.[118] Consistently, regular physical activity mitigates CHD risk factors (including body weight, BP, serum lipids, and insulin sensitivity), improves bone density, and improves muscular strength, all key elements of health and well-being in older adults.[118] Even modest physical activity in older adults has been associated with lower CV risk.[130]

Physical Activity Prescription

The most important considerations when counseling regarding physical activity is to help shape a program that is pleasurable and achievable and that avoids injury or exacerbation of comorbid problems. Aerobics, strength, balance, and flexibility are all vital components. For adults willing to enter a formal exercise program, specific exercises can help improve tolerance of the physical demands of daily living and recreational activities. Generally, work intensities start lower than in younger patients, with smaller increments over time, especially in those with significant comorbidities that limit mobility (e.g., arthritis, pulmonary disease, and PAD). Increasing frequency and duration of exercise sessions should supersede increases in intensity to reduce the potential for overuse injuries. For adults who are disinclined to exercise in a program, increasing activity as part of daily living is also beneficial. Regular leisure activities such as walking, yoga, and gardening are all healthful.

Accumulating evidence suggests that activity benefits may increase in proportion to intensity. Reports in patients with established heart disease, including one study of patients with a mean age of 75 years, suggest that high intensity aerobic interval training can elicit greater improvement in exercise capacity than continuous exercise at a lower intensity.[118] Despite these encouraging data, such training is more complex than traditional training, necessitating more supervision for implementation and safety. Larger studies are needed to establish the efficacy and safety of high intensity interval training in older patients.

Cardiac Rehabilitation

Cardiac rehabilitation (CR; see Chapter 33) consists of structured exercise training combined with secondary prevention reinforcement, including individualized exercise prescription as well as close supervision and support.[118] It can be particularly helpful in catalyzing physical activity and wellness in adults who are sedentary amidst illness, deconditioning, and entrenched behavior patterns. Older adults with CHD who participated in supervised CR experienced 21% to 34% lower mortality than nonusers over the subsequent 5 years, independent of other risk factors.[131] Patients also benefit in increased physical capacity, independence, and self-efficacy after a hospitalization and/or CVD exacerbation, mitigating risks of posthospitalization disability.[49] Unfortunately, the vast majority of older patients do not participate in CR due to multiple factors, including lack of referral, logistical barriers, or socioeconomic barriers. Failure to refer, particularly for women, is a major contributor to the low participation of older adults. Participation in CR by Medicare eligible recipients is only ~12%.[118] Growing utilization of home-based CR may increase participation for some older adults, but geriatric complexities (e.g., frailty, cognitive impairments) may make home-based options more difficult for others.

Obesity (see Chapter 30)

An estimated two-thirds of seniors are overweight (body mass index [BMI] 25 to 30 kg/m^2) or obese (BMI ≥30 kg/m^2), closely paralleling rates in the general population. Data from NHANES suggest that 35% of noninstitutionalized women and 40% of men 65 to 74 years old are obese, as well as 27% of women and 26% of men ≥75 years.[5] Between 1988 and 1994 and from 2007 to 2008, obesity rates increased 30% to 40% in older women and 67% to 100% in older men.

Although overweight and obesity are associated with mildly increased mortality,[5] the risk ratio decreases as age advances. In obese patients with established CVD, multiple studies have demonstrated an obesity paradox; overweight and obese patients show greater survival than those of normal weight. Similar findings have been observed in older populations with CVD, but most of these studies have not differentiated between fat and lean mass, which likely plays an important role in health effects in old age. Sarcopenic obesity in an older adult does not confer mortality benefit.[132]

Diet (see Chapter 29)

Undernutrition is more common in older than younger individuals due to a combination of medical and socioeconomic factors: 5% to 10% of community dwelling persons aged >70 years are undernourished and prevalence increases to 30% to 65% in institutionalized older adults. Vitamin and mineral deficiencies are common in seniors due to inadequate intake, decreased absorption, and the effects of disease and medications. Vitamin D deficiency is particularly common in older adults due to low sunlight exposure and reduced synthesis by the skin and has been associated with increased CV mortality.[118] However, of the value of vitamin D supplementation remains unsubstantiated.[133]

It is useful for cardiologists and primary care providers to assess dietary intake of older patients, provide general dietary advice, and refer to a nutritionist if major dietary deficiencies or malnutrition are suspected. The Mediterranean diet (i.e., fruits, vegetables, whole grains, and nuts plus low intake of saturated fat) has been associated with beneficial effects on CV risk factors and outcomes in both older and younger adults. Some of these benefits may derive from flavonoids, which are abundant in fruits, vegetables, nuts, tea, and wine, and have anti-inflammatory and antioxidant effects. Higher flavonoid intake was associated with a lower risk of CV death in a population of 98,000 adults of initial mean age 70 years.[134]

NONCARDIAC SURGERY AND PERIOPERATIVE MANAGEMENT CONSIDERATIONS IN OLDER ADULTS

Background

As the population ages, the number of older adults undergoing surgical interventions has increased markedly and continues to expand. Physiologic age-related changes in all organ systems in conjunction with increasing comorbidity contribute to higher risk for perioperative complications and increase complexity of perioperative management in older patients. These factors should be considered in relation to the potential benefits of a surgical procedure and in the context of the older patient's overall goals of care. Patients should be encouraged to develop an advance directive and identify a health care proxy. Suspending a do-not-resuscitate designation is common during procedures, but management plans should be clarified in case there is a serious adverse event. Practice guidelines for optimal preoperative assessment and perioperative care of older adults undergoing surgery have been developed by the American College of Surgeons (ACS) in collaboration with the American Geriatrics Society (AGS).[135]

Risk Assessment

Several tools to evaluate risk of perioperative CV complications have been developed and validated. However, most of these instruments fail to consider geriatric conditions, including sarcopenia, frailty, functional limitations, multimorbidity, and cognitive impairment that heighten risk for adverse CV and non-CV outcomes following major surgery. Thus, the ACS/AGS Guideline for preoperative evaluation recommends that, in addition to CV risk assessment, older adults should be screened for history of falls, functional impairment, cognitive impairment, nutritional status, depression, and alcohol or substance abuse.[135]

Gait speed, as assessed by a timed walk over a measured distance (e.g., 5 meters), is a marker of frailty that has been shown to predict adverse surgical outcomes beyond standard assessments. Slow gait speed (<0.8 m/sec) adds significantly to conventional risk scores, such as the STS score,[15] and patients unable to perform the gait speed test are at highest surgical risk.

Perioperative Management

Age-related changes alter drug pharmacodynamics and pharmacokinetics, rendering older patients more vulnerable to anesthetic and analgesic complications. Although regional (epidural) anesthesia does not decrease mortality or risk of postoperative delirium or cognitive dysfunction, it is associated with better peripheral vascular circulation, less blood loss, improved pain control, reduced ileus, attenuation of thromboembolic complications, fewer respiratory complications, reduced postoperative narcotic requirements, and reduced surgical stress response.

Specific Complications

In addition to increased risk for cardiopulmonary complications following surgery, older adults are at risk for delirium, falls, functional and cognitive decline, urinary tract infections, acute kidney injury, poor nutrition, bowel disorders, pressure ulcers, hypothermia, and venous thromboembolism.[136]

Delirium, an acute decline in orientation and attention, occurs in up to 50% of older adults undergoing major surgery, and in over 80% of those who require mechanical ventilation in an ICU. Postoperative delirium is associated with increased length of stay and costs, falls, functional and cognitive decline, and mortality. An estimated 30% to 40% of delirium is avoidable through nonpharmacologic measures, including maintaining a normal sleep/wake cycle, presence of family, early mobilization, provision of hearing and vision aids, avoidance of restraints, and adequate hydration and pain management. It is essential to avoid deliriogenic medications, especially benzodiazepines and related drugs, antihistamines, and anticholinergics. The primary treatment for delirium involves correction of avoidable factors predisposing to its development. Short-term use of low-dose antipsychotic medication may be used to treat agitated or distressed patients who pose a risk of harm to themselves or others.

Postoperative cognitive dysfunction (POCD) entails deterioration in memory and executive function in the days to weeks after surgery, but confusion is not usually present. Incidence following major surgery has been reported to be >50%, but several studies suggest that POCD may reflect unrecognized baseline cognitive deficiencies,[42] highlighting the need for thorough preoperative assessments. POCD is associated with increased hospital stay and diminished QOL.

Decubitus ulcers are also common in older surgical patients. Risks include loss of subcutaneous tissue and decreased elasticity of the aged skin that predispose to damaged superficial tissues when skin is compressed for prolonged periods. There may be secondary infection, delayed recovery, and prolonged hospitalization, often with discharge to a transitional care facility. Preventive measures include routine postoperative skin examination, frequent repositioning, use of pressure redistributing support surfaces, pressure-relieving overlays in the operating room, and use of foam alternatives and heel protectors.

Older adults are susceptible to hypothermia due to impaired central and peripheral thermoregulatory function and the effects of anesthesia. It is particularly common among underweight or frail older adults and may contribute to electrolyte abnormalities, platelet dysfunction, increased risk for wound infection, and impaired drug metabolism. Warming to a core temperature of about 36°C is recommended with correction of electrolyte abnormalities.

Over 30% of hospitalized older adults experience functional decline during admission, and fewer than 50% return to their prior level of function within 1 year after discharge. Early mobilization is vital to minimize deconditioning, frailty, and sarcopenia. Early mobilization has also been associated with improved cardiac output and hemodynamics and reduced bone loss, hypocalcemia, joint contractures, constipation, incontinence, DVT, pressure ulcers, sensory deprivation, atelectasis, hypoxemia, pneumonia, depression, delirium, anxiety, and insomnia.

Postoperative aspiration pneumonia is also common, with risks compounded by cognitive decline, delirium, and sedation. Urinary tract infections and acute kidney injury can be minimized by avoiding nephrotoxins and urinary catheters and maintaining hydration.

Discharge Planning

Risk assessment at discharge must include consideration of hospitalization-associated disability, frailty, deconditioning, malnutrition, and altered cognition; all may provoke loss of independence and a cycle of functional decline. Postdischarge rehabilitation is critical whether delivered by home health or physical therapy and in an SNF or a rehabilitation facility.

PERIPHERAL ARTERIAL DISEASE, ABDOMINAL AORTIC ANEURYSM, AORTIC DISSECTION

This section is presented in the online chapter.

REFERENCES

General Considerations

1. Ortman JVV, Velkoff VA, Hogan H. The Older Population in the United States. http://www.census.gov/library/publications/2014/demo/p25-1140.html.
2. https://www.cia.gov/library/publications/the-world-factbook/fields/341.html.
3. Domanski MJ, Tian X, Wu CO, et al. Time course of LDL cholesterol exposure and cardiovascular disease event risk. *J Am Coll Cardiol.* 2020;76(13):1507–1516.
4. Lakatta EG. So! What's aging? Is cardiovascular aging a disease? *J Mol Cell Cardiol.* 2015;83:1–13.
5. Mozaffarian D, Benjamin EJ, Go AS, et al. Heart disease and stroke Statistics-2016 update: a report from the American heart association. *Circulation.* 2016;133(4):e38–360.
6. Forman DE, Maurer MS, Boyd C, et al. Multimorbidity in older adults with cardiovascular disease. *J Am Coll Cardiol.* 2018;71(19):2149–2161.
7. Forman DE, Arena R, Boxer R, et al. Prioritizing functional capacity as a principal end point for therapies oriented to older adults with cardiovascular disease: a scientific statement for Healthcare Professionals from the American heart association. *Circulation.* 2017;135(16):e894–e918.
8. Paneni F, Diaz Cañestro C, et al. The aging cardiovascular system: understanding it at the cellular and clinical levels. *J Am Coll Cardiol.* 2017;69(15):1952–1967.
9. Ferrucci L, Fabbri E. Inflammageing: chronic inflammation in ageing, cardiovascular disease, and frailty. *Nat Rev Cardiol.* 2018;15(9):505–522.
10. Aronow WS, Fleg JL, Pepine CJ, et al. ACCF/AHA 2011 expert consensus document on hypertension in the elderly: a report of the American College of cardiology Foundation Task Force on clinical expert consensus documents. *Circulation.* 2011;123(21):2434–2506.
11. Fleg JL, Strait J. Age-associated changes in cardiovascular structure and function: a fertile milieu for future disease. *Heart Fail Rev.* 2012;17(4–5):545–554.
12. Addison O, Marcus RL, Lastayo PC, Ryan AS. Intermuscular fat: a review of the consequences and causes. *Int J Endocrinol.* 2014;2014:309570.
13. Kitzman DW, Nicklas B, Kraus WE, et al. Skeletal muscle abnormalities and exercise intolerance in older patients with heart failure and preserved ejection fraction. *Am J Physiol Heart Circ Physiol.* 2014;306(9):H1364–H1370.
14. Arnett DK, Goodman RA, Halperin JL, et al. AHA/ACC/HHS strategies to enhance application of clinical practice guidelines in patients with cardiovascular disease and comorbid conditions: from the American Heart Association, American College of Cardiology, and U.S. Department of Health and Human Services. *J Am Coll Cardiol.* 2014;64(17):1851–1856.
15. Afilalo J, Alexander KP, Mack MJ, et al. Frailty assessment in the cardiovascular care of older adults. *J Am Coll Cardiol.* 2014;63(8):747–762.
16. Boccardi V, Mecocci P. The importance of cellular senescence in frailty and cardiovascular diseases. *Adv Exp Med Biol.* 2020;1216:79–86.
17. Forman DE, Alexander KP. Frailty: a vital sign for older adults with cardiovascular disease. *Can J Cardiol.* 2016;32(9):1082–1087.
18. Harada CN, Natelson Love MC, Triebel KL. Normal cognitive aging. *Clin Geriatr Med.* 2013;29(4):737–752.
19. Justin BN, Turek M, Hakim AM. Heart disease as a risk factor for dementia. *Clin Epidemiol.* 2013;5:135–145.
20. Marcantonio ER. Delirium in hospitalized older adults. *N Engl J Med.* 2017;377(15):1456–1466.
21. Damluji AA, Forman DE, van Diepen S, et al. Older adults in the cardiac intensive care unit: factoring geriatric syndromes in the management, prognosis, and process of care: a scientific statement from the American Heart Association. *Circulation.* 2020;141(2):e6–e32.

Medication Consideration

22. Schwartz JB, Schmader KE, Hanlon JT, et al. Pharmacotherapy in older adults with cardiovascular disease: report from an American College of cardiology, American geriatrics society, and National Institute on aging Workshop. *J Am Geriatr Soc.* 2019;67(2):371–380.
23. Allen LA, Fonarow GC, Liang L, et al. Medication initiation burden required to comply with heart failure guideline recommendations and hospital quality measures. *Circulation.* 2015;132(14):1347–1353.
24. Budnitz DS, Lovegrove MC, Shehab N, Richards CL. Emergency hospitalizations for adverse drug events in older Americans. *N Engl J Med.* 2011;365(21):2002–2012.
25. Rossello X, Pocock SJ, Julian DG. Long-term Use of cardiovascular drugs: challenges for Research and for patient care. *J Am Coll Cardiol.* 2015;66(11):1273–1285.
26. Krumholz HM. Post-hospital syndrome–an acquired, transient condition of generalized risk. *N Engl J Med.* 2013;368(2):100–102.
27. McNeil JJ, Woods RL, Nelson MR, et al. Effect of aspirin on disability-free survival in the healthy elderly. *N Engl J Med.* 2018;379(16):1499–1508.

Management Precepts

28. Rich MW, Chyun DA, Skolnick AH, et al. Knowledge Gaps in cardiovascular care of the older adult population: a scientific statement from the American heart association, American College of cardiology, and American geriatrics society. *Circulation*. 2016;133(21):2103–2122.
29. Boyd C, Smith CD, Masoudi FA, et al. Decision making for older adults with multiple chronic conditions: executive summary for the American geriatrics society guiding principles on the care of older adults with multimorbidity. *J Am Geriatr Soc*. 2019;67(4):665–673.
30. American geriatrics society 2019 updated AGS Beers Criteria® for potentially inappropriate medication use in older adults. *J Am Geriatr Soc*. 2019;67(4):674–694.
31. Tomlinson J, Cheong VL, Fylan B, et al. Successful care transitions for older people: a systematic review and meta-analysis of the effects of interventions that support medication continuity. *Age Ageing*. 2020;49(4):558–569.
32. Sullivan MF, Kirkpatrick JN. Palliative cardiovascular care: the right patient at the right time. *Clin Cardiol*. 2020;43(2):205–212.
33. Meyers DE, Goodlin SJ. End-of-Life decisions and palliative care in advanced heart failure. *Can J Cardiol*. 2016;32(9):1148–1156.

Ischemic Heart Disease

34. Krishnaswami A, Steinman MA, Goyal P, et al. Deprescribing in older adults with cardiovascular disease. *J Am Coll Cardiol*. 2019;73(20):2584–2595.
35. Moran AE, Forouzanfar MH, Roth GA, et al. Temporal trends in ischemic heart disease mortality in 21 world regions, 1980 to 2010: the Global Burden of Disease 2010 study. *Circulation*. 2014;129(14):1483–1492.
36. Mortensen MB, Fuster V, Muntendam P, et al. A simple disease-guided approach to personalize ACC/AHA-Recommended statin allocation in elderly people: the BioImage study. *J Am Coll Cardiol*. 2016;68(9):881–891.
37. Douglas PS, Hoffmann U. Outcomes of anatomical versus functional testing for coronary artery disease. *N Engl J Med*. 2015;372(1):1291–1300.
38. Maron DJ, Hochman JS, Reynolds HR, et al. Initial invasive or conservative strategy for stable coronary disease. *N Engl J Med*. 2020;382(15):1395–1407.
39. Forman DE, de Lemos JA, Shaw LJ, et al. Cardiovascular biomarkers and imaging in older adults: JACC Council Perspectives. *J Am Coll Cardiol*. 2020;76(13):1577–1594.
40. Grundy SM, Stone NJ, Bailey AL, et al. 2018 AHA/ACC/AACVPR/AAPA/ABC/ACPM/ADA/AGS/APhA/ASPC/NLA/PCNA guideline on the management of blood cholesterol: a report of the American College of cardiology/American heart association Task Force on clinical practice guidelines. *Circulation*. 2019;139(25):e1082–e1143.
41. Madhavan MV, Gersh BJ, Alexander KP, et al. Coronary artery disease in patients ≥80 Years of age. *J Am Coll Cardiol*. 2018;71(18):2015–2040.
42. Selnes OA, Gottesman RF, Grega MA, et al. Cognitive and neurologic outcomes after coronary-artery bypass surgery. *N Engl J Med*. 2012;366(3):250–257.
43. Bairey Merz CN, Pepine CJ, Walsh MN, Fleg JL. Ischemia and No obstructive coronary artery disease (INOCA): developing evidence-based therapies and Research Agenda for the Next decade. *Circulation*. 2017;135(11):1075–1092.
44. Virani SS, Alonso A, Benjamin EJ, et al. Heart disease and stroke statistics-2020 update: a report from the American Heart Association. *Circulation*. 2020;141(9):e139–e596.
45. Dai X, Busby-Whitehead J, Alexander KP. Acute coronary syndrome in the older adults. *J Geriatr Cardiol*. 2016;13(2):101–108.
46. Tegn N, Abdelnoor M, Aaberge L, et al. Invasive versus conservative strategy in patients aged 80 years or older with non-ST-elevation myocardial infarction or unstable angina pectoris (After Eighty study): an open-label randomised controlled trial. *Lancet*. 2016;387(10023):1057–1065.
47. Ravi V, Pulipati P, Vij A, Kodumuri V. Meta-analysis comparing double versus triple antithrombotic therapy in patients with atrial fibrillation and coronary artery disease. *Am J Cardiol*. 2020;125(1):19–28.
48. Lopes RD, Heizer G, Aronson R, et al. Antithrombotic therapy after acute coronary syndrome or PCI in atrial fibrillation. *N Engl J Med*. 2019;380(16):1509–1524.
49. Schopfer DW, Forman DE. Cardiac rehabilitation in older adults. *Can J Cardiol*. 2016;32(9):1088–1096.

Heart Failure

50. Gorodeski EZ, Goyal P, Hummel SL, et al. Domain management approach to heart failure in the geriatric patient: present and future. *J Am Coll Cardiol*. 2018;71(17):1921–1936.
51. Upadhya B, Kitzman DW. Heart failure with preserved ejection fraction: new approaches to diagnosis and management. *Clin Cardiol*. 2020;43(2):145–155.
52. Paulus WJ, Tschope C. A novel paradigm for heart failure with preserved ejection fraction: comorbidities drive myocardial dysfunction and remodeling through coronary microvascular endothelial inflammation. *J Am Coll Cardiol*. 2013;62(4):263–271.
53. Mogensen UM, Ersboll M, Andersen M, et al. Clinical characteristics and major comorbidities in heart failure patients more than 85 years of age compared with younger age groups. *Eur J Heart Fail*. 2011;13(11):1216–1223.
54. Pirmohamed A, Kitzman DW, Maurer MS. Heart failure in older adults: embracing complexity. *J Geriatr Cardiol*. 2016;13(1):8–14.
55. Paterna S, Gaspare P, Fasullo S, et al. Normal-sodium diet compared with low-sodium diet in compensated congestive heart failure: is sodium an old enemy or a new friend? *Clin Sci (Lond)*. 2008;114(3):221–230.
56. Yancy CW, Jessup M, Bozkurt B, et al. 2013 ACCF/AHA guideline for the management of heart failure: a report of the American College of cardiology Foundation/American heart association Task Force on practice guidelines. *J Am Coll Cardiol*. 2013;62(16):e147–239.
57. Forman DE, Sanderson BK, Josephson RA, et al. Heart failure as a newly approved diagnosis for cardiac rehabilitation: challenges and opportunities. *J Am Coll Cardiol*. 2015;65(24):2652–2659.
58. Takeda A, Martin N, Taylor RS, Taylor SJ. Disease management interventions for heart failure. *Cochrane Database Syst Rev*. 2019;1(1):Cd002752.
59. Adamson PB, Abraham WT, Stevenson LW, et al. Pulmonary artery pressure-guided heart failure management reduces 30-day readmissions. *Circ Heart Fail*. 2016;9(6).
60. Jhund PS, Fu M, Bayram E, et al. Efficacy and safety of LCZ696 (sacubitril-valsartan) according to age: insights from PARADIGM-HF. *Eur Heart J*. 2015;36(38):2576–2584.
61. Martinez FA, Serenelli M, Nicolau JC, et al. Efficacy and safety of dapagliflozin in heart failure with reduced ejection fraction according to age: insights from DAPA-HF. *Circulation*. 2020;141(2):100–111.
62. Packer M, Anker SD, Butler J, et al. Cardiovascular and renal outcomes with empagliflozin in heart failure. *N Engl J Med*. 2020.
63. Kim JH, Singh R, Pagani FD, et al. Ventricular assist device therapy in older patients with heart failure: characteristics and outcomes. *J Card Fail*. 2016;22(12):981–987.
64. Petrie MC, Jhund PS, She L, et al. Ten-year outcomes after coronary artery bypass grafting according to age in patients with heart failure and left ventricular systolic dysfunction: an analysis of the extended follow-up of the STICH trial (surgical treatment for ischemic heart failure). *Circulation*. 2016;134(18):1314–1324.
65. Pitt B, Pfeffer MA, Assmann SF, et al. Spironolactone for heart failure with preserved ejection fraction. *N Engl J Med*. 2014;370(15):1383–1392.
66. Pfeffer MA, Claggett B, Assmann SF, et al. Regional variation in patients and outcomes in the treatment of preserved cardiac function heart failure with an aldosterone antagonist (TOPCAT) trial. *Circulation*. 2015;131(1):34–42.
67. Solomon SD, McMurray JJV, Anand IS, et al. Angiotensin-neprilysin inhibition in heart failure with preserved ejection fraction. *N Engl J Med*. 2019;381(17):1609–1620.
68. Kitzman DW, Brubaker P, Morgan T, et al. Effect of caloric restriction or aerobic exercise training on peak oxygen consumption and quality of life in obese older patients with heart failure with preserved ejection fraction: a randomized clinical trial. *J Am Med Assoc*. 2016;315(1):36–46.
69. Ruberg FL, Grogan M, Hanna M, et al. Transthyretin amyloid cardiomyopathy: JACC state-of-the-art review. *J Am Coll Cardiol*. 2019;73(22):2872–2891.
70. Castano A, Haq M, Narotsky DL, et al. Multicenter study of planar Technetium 99m Pyrophosphate cardiac imaging: predicting survival for patients with ATTR cardiac amyloidosis. *JAMA Cardiol*. 2016;1(8):880–889.
71. Maurer MS, Schwartz JH, Gundapaneni B, et al. Tafamidis treatment for patients with transthyretin amyloid cardiomyopathy. *N Engl J Med*. 2018;379(11):1007–1016.
72. Berra G, Noble S, Soccal PM, et al. Pulmonary hypertension in the elderly: a different disease? *Breathe*. 2016;12(1):43–49.
73. Guazzi M, Gomberg-Maitland M, Arena R. Pulmonary hypertension in heart failure with preserved ejection fraction. *J Heart Lung Transplant*. 2015;34(3):273–281.
74. Campean IA, Lang IM. Treating pulmonary hypertension in the elderly. *Expert Opin Pharmacother*. 2020;21(10):1193–1200.
75. Bavishi C, Balasundaram K, Argulian E. Integration of flow-gradient patterns into clinical decision making for patients with suspected severe aortic stenosis and preserved LVEF: a systematic review of evidence and meta-analysis. *JACC Cardiovasc imaging*. 2016;9(11):1255–1263.

Valvular Heart Disease

75a. Otto CM, Nishimura RA, Bonow RO, et al. 2020 ACC/AHA Guideline for the Management of Patients With Valvular Heart Disease: Executive Summary: A Report of the American College of Cardiology/American Heart Association Joint Committee on Clinical Practice Guidelines. *J Am Coll Cardiol*. 2021;77(4):450–500.
76. Mack MJ, Leon MB, Thourani VH, et al. Transcatheter aortic-valve replacement with a balloon-Expandable valve in low-risk patients. *N Engl J Med*. 2019;380(18):1695–1705.
77. Grover FL, Vemulapalli S, Carroll JD, et al. 2016 annual report of the society of Thoracic Surgeons/American College of cardiology transcatheter valve therapy registry. *J Am Coll Cardiol*. 2016.
78. Nishimura RA, Otto CM, Bonow RO, et al. 2014 AHA/ACC guideline for the management of patients with valvular heart disease: executive summary: a report of the American College of Cardiology/American Heart Association Task Force on Practice Guidelines. *J Am Coll Cardiol*. 2014;63(22):2438–2488.
79. Franzone A, Piccolo R, Siontis GC, et al. Transcatheter aortic valve replacement for the treatment of pure native aortic valve regurgitation: a systematic review. *JACC Cardiovasc Interv*. 2016;9(22):2308–2317.
80. Glower DD, Kar S, Trento A, et al. Percutaneous mitral valve repair for mitral regurgitation in high-risk patients: results of the EVEREST II study. *J Am Coll Cardiol*. 2014;64(2):172–181.
81. Sorajja P, Mack M, Vemulapalli S, et al. Initial experience with commercial transcatheter mitral valve repair in the United States. *J Am Coll Cardiol*. 2016;67(10):1129–1140.
82. Stone GW, Lindenfeld J, Abraham WT, et al. Transcatheter mitral-valve repair in patients with heart failure. *N Engl J Med*. 2018;379(24):2307–2318.
83. Regueiro A, Linke A, Latib A, et al. Association between transcatheter aortic valve replacement and subsequent infective endocarditis and in-hospital death. *J Am Med Assoc*. 2016;316:1083–1092.

Arrhythmia

84. Curtis AB, Karki R, Hattoum A, Sharma UC. Arrhythmias in patients ≥80 Years of age: pathophysiology, management, and outcomes. *J Am Coll Cardiol*. 2018;71(18):2041–2057.
85. Chow GV, Marine JE, Fleg JL. Epidemiology of arrhythmias and conduction disorders in older adults. *Clin Geriatr Med*. 2012;28(4):539–553.
86. Hirsh DS, Wenger N. Atrial fibrillation in the elderly. *ESC CardioMed*. 2018:2221–2223.
87. January CT, Wann LS, Calkins H, et al. 2019 AHA/ACC/HRS focused update of the 2014 AHA/ACC/HRS guideline for the management of patients with atrial fibrillation: a report of the American College of cardiology/American heart association Task Force on clinical practice guidelines and the heart rhythm society in collaboration with the society of Thoracic Surgeons. *Circulation*. 2019;140(2):e125–e151.
88. Curry SJ, Krist AH, Owens DK, et al. Screening for atrial fibrillation with electrocardiography: US preventive services Task Force recommendation statement. *J Am Med Assoc*. 2018;320(5):478–484.
89. Kirchhof P, Benussi S, Kotecha D, et al. 2016 ESC Guidelines for the management of atrial fibrillation developed in collaboration with EACTS. *Eur Heart J*. 2016;37(38):2893–2962.
90. Perez MV, Mahaffey KW, Hedlin H, et al. Large-scale Assessment of a Smartwatch to identify atrial fibrillation. *N Engl J Med*. 2019;381(20):1909–1917.
91. Magnani JW, Wang N, Benjamin EJ, et al. Atrial fibrillation and declining physical performance in older adults: the health, aging, and body composition study. *Circ Arrhythm Electrophysiol*. 2016;9(5):e003525.
92. Khan SU, Osman M, Khan MU, et al. Dual versus triple therapy for atrial fibrillation after percutaneous coronary intervention: a systematic review and meta-analysis. *Ann Intern Med*. 2020;172(7):474–483.
93. Brunetti ND, Tricarico L, De Gennaro L, et al. Meta-analysis study on direct oral anticoagulants vs warfarin therapy in atrial fibrillation and PCI: dual or triple approach? *Int J Cardiol Heart Vasc*. 2020;29:100569.
94. Huang HK, Liu PP, Hsu JY, et al. Risk of osteoporosis in patients with atrial fibrillation using non-vitamin K antagonist oral anticoagulants or warfarin. *J Am Heart Assoc*. 2020;9(2):e013845.
95. Malik AH, Yandrapalli S, Aronow WS, et al. Meta-analysis of direct-acting oral anticoagulants compared with warfarin in patients >75 Years of age. *Am J Cardiol*. 2019;123(12):2051–2057.
96. Freeman JV, Varosy P, Price MJ, et al. The NCDR left atrial appendage occlusion registry. *J Am Coll Cardiol*. 2020;75(13):1503–1518.
97. Groenveld HF, Tijssen JG, Crijns HJ, et al. Rate control efficacy in permanent atrial fibrillation: successful and failed strict rate control against a background of lenient rate control: data from RACE II (Rate Control Efficacy in Permanent Atrial Fibrillation). *J Am Coll Cardiol*. 2013;61(7):741–748.
98. Packer DL, Mark DB, Robb RA, et al. Effect of catheter ablation vs antiarrhythmic drug therapy on mortality, stroke, bleeding, and cardiac arrest among patients with atrial fibrillation: the CABANA randomized clinical trial. *J Am Med Assoc*. 2019;321(13):1261–1274.
99. Brembilla-Perrot B, Olivier A, Sellal JM, et al. Influence of advancing age on clinical presentation, treatment efficacy and safety, and long-term outcome of pre-excitation syndromes: a retrospective cohort study of 961 patients included over a 25-year period. *BMJ Open*. 2016;6(5):e010520.
100. Epstein AE, DiMarco JP, Ellenbogen KA, et al. 2012 ACCF/AHA/HRS focused update incorporated into the ACCF/AHA/HRS 2008 guidelines for device-based therapy of cardiac rhythm abnormalities: a report of the American College of cardiology Foundation/American heart association Task Force on practice guidelines and the heart rhythm society. *Circulation*. 2013;127(3):e283–352.
101. Cleland JG, Freemantle N, Erdmann E, et al. Long-term mortality with cardiac resynchronization therapy in the Cardiac Resynchronization-Heart Failure (CARE-HF) trial. *Eur J Heart Fail*. 2012;14:628–634.
102. Vohra J. Implantable cardioverter defibrillators (ICDs) in octogenarians. *Heart Lung Circ*. 2014;23(3):213–216.

103. Hess PL, Matlock DD, Al-Khatib SM. Decision-making regarding primary prevention implantable cardioverter-defibrillators among older adults. *Clin Cardiol.* 2020;43(2):187–195.

Venous Thromboembolism

104. Boey JP, Gallus A. Drug treatment of venous thromboembolism in the elderly. *Drugs Aging.* 2016;33(7):475–490.
105. Lange N, Méan M, Stalder O, et al. Anticoagulation quality and clinical outcomes in multimorbid elderly patients with acute venous thromboembolism. *Thromb Res.* 2019;177:10–16.
106. Ali MS, Czarnecka-Kujawa K. Venous thromboembolism in the elderly. *Curr Geriatrics Rep.* 2016:132–139.
107. Righini M, Van Es J, Den Exter PL, et al. Age-adjusted D-dimer cutoff levels to rule out pulmonary embolism: the ADJUST-PE study. *J Am Med Assoc.* 2014;311(11):1117–1124.
108. Kearon C, Akl EA, Ornelas J, et al. Antithrombotic therapy for VTE disease: CHEST guideline and expert panel report. *Chest.* 2016;149(2):315–352.
109. Song ZK, Cao H, Wu H, et al. Current status of rivaroxaban in elderly patients with pulmonary embolism (Review). *Exp Ther Med.* 2020;19(4):2817–2825.
109a. Lyman GH, Carrier M, Ay C, et al. American Society of Hematology 2021 guidelines for management of venous thromboembolism: prevention and treatment in patients with cancer. *Blood Adv.* 2021;5(4):927–974.
110. Kim JS, Patel MHE, et al. Case series of elderly patients treated with catheter directed thrombolysis (CDT) for pulmonary embolism (PE) at large tertiary care center. *Am J Respir Crit Care Med.* 2020 (in press).
111. Goyal P, Maurer MS. Syncope in older adults. *J Geriatr Cardiol.* 2016;13(5):380–386.
112. O'Brien HAKR. Syncope in the elderly. *Eur Cardiol.* 2014;9(1):28–36.
113. Shen WK, Sheldon RS, Benditt DG, et al. 2017 ACC/AHA/HRS guideline for the evaluation and management of patients with syncope: a report of the American College of cardiology/American heart association Task Force on clinical practice guidelines and the heart rhythm society. *Circulation.* 2017;136(5):e60–e122.
114. Whelton PK, Carey RM, Aronow WS, et al. 2017 ACC/AHA/AAPA/ABC/ACPM/AGS/APhA/ASH/ASPC/NMA/PCNA guideline for the prevention, detection, evaluation, and management of high blood pressure in adults: executive summary: a report of the American College of cardiology/American heart association Task Force on clinical practice guidelines. *Circulation.* 2018;138(17):e426–e483.
115. Fleg JL, Aronow WS, Frishman WH. Cardiovascular drug therapy in the elderly: benefits and challenges. *Nat Rev Cardiol.* 2011;8(1):13–28.
116. Beckett NS, Peters R, Fletcher AE, et al. Treatment of hypertension in patients 80 years of age or older. *N Engl J Med.* 2008;358(18):1887–1898.
117. Williamson JD, Supiano MA, Applegate WB, et al. Intensive vs standard blood pressure control and cardiovascular disease outcomes in adults aged ≥75 Years: a randomized clinical trial. *J Am Med Assoc.* 2016;315(24):2673–2682.
118. Fleg JL, Forman DE, Berra K, et al. Secondary prevention of atherosclerotic cardiovascular disease in older adults: a scientific statement from the American Heart Association. *Circulation.* 2013;128(22):2422–2446.

119. Efficacy and safety of statin therapy in older people: a meta-analysis of individual participant data from 28 randomised controlled trials. *Lancet.* 2019;393(10170):407–415.
120. Orkaby AR, Driver JA, Ho YL, et al. Association of statin Use with all-cause and cardiovascular mortality in US Veterans 75 Years and older. *J Am Med Assoc.* 2020;324(1):68–78.
121. Cannon CP, Blazing MA, Giugliano RP, et al. Ezetimibe added to statin therapy after acute coronary syndromes. *N Engl J Med.* 2015;372(25):2387–2397.
122. Sinnaeve PR, Schwartz GG, Wojdyla DM, et al. Effect of alirocumab on cardiovascular outcomes after acute coronary syndromes according to age: an ODYSSEY OUTCOMES trial analysis. *Eur Heart J.* 2020;41(24):2248–2258.
123. Sever P, Gouni-Berthold I, Keech A, et al. LDL-cholesterol lowering with evolocumab, and outcomes according to age and sex in patients in the FOURIER Trial. *Eur J Prev Cardiol.* 2020. 2047487320902750.
124. Bhatt DL, Steg PG, Miller M, et al. Cardiovascular risk reduction with icosapent ethyl for hypertriglyceridemia. *N Engl J Med.* 2019;380(1):11–22.
125. Farrell B, Black C, Thompson W, et al. Deprescribing antihyperglycemic agents in older persons: evidence-based clinical practice guideline. *Can Fam Physician.* 2017;63(11):832–843.
126. Zinman B, Wanner C, Lachin JM, et al. Empagliflozin, cardiovascular outcomes, and mortality in type 2 diabetes. *N Engl J Med.* 2015;373(22):2117–2128.
127. Holme I, Anderssen SA. Increases in physical activity is as important as smoking cessation for reduction in total mortality in elderly men: 12 years of follow-up of the Oslo II study. *Br J Sports Med.* 2015;49(11):743–748.
128. Gellert C, Schottker B, Brenner H. Smoking and all-cause mortality in older people: systematic review and meta-analysis. *Arch Intern Med.* 2012;172(11):837–844.
129. Patel AV, Bernstein L, Deka A, et al. Leisure time spent sitting in relation to total mortality in a prospective cohort of US adults. *Am J Epidemiol.* 2010;172(4):419–429.
130. LaCroix AZ, Bellettiere J, Rillamas-Sun E, et al. Association of light physical activity measured by Accelerometry and incidence of coronary heart disease and cardiovascular disease in older women. *JAMA Netw Open.* 2019;2(3):e190419.
131. Suaya JA, Stason WB, Ades PA, et al. Cardiac rehabilitation and survival in older coronary patients. *J Am Coll Cardiol.* 2009;54(1):25–33.
132. Wannamethee SG, Atkins JL. Muscle loss and obesity: the health implications of sarcopenia and sarcopenic obesity. *Proc Nutr Soc.* 2015;74(4):405–412.
133. Manson JE, Cook NR, Lee IM, et al. Vitamin D supplements and prevention of cancer and cardiovascular disease. *N Engl J Med.* 2019;380(1):33–44.
134. McCullough ML, Peterson JJ, Patel R, et al. Flavonoid intake and cardiovascular disease mortality in a prospective cohort of US adults. *Am J Clin Nutr.* 2012;95(2):454–464.
135. Mohanty S, Rosenthal RA, Russell MM, et al. Optimal perioperative management of the geriatric patient: a best practices guideline from the American College of Surgeons NSQIP and the American geriatrics society. *J Am Coll Surg.* 2016;222(5):930–947.
136. Wolfe JD, Wolfe NK, Rich MW. Perioperative care of the geriatric patient for noncardiac surgery. *Clin Cardiol.* 2020;43(2):127–136.

91 Cardiovascular Disease in Women

MARTHA GULATI AND C. NOEL BAIREY MERZ

BACKGROUND

Cardiovascular disease (CVD) remains the leading cause of death among women, accounting for 420,184 deaths in women in 2018, and accounts for 1 in every 4 female deaths in the United States.[1] Approximately 60 million women are living with some form of CVD and the lifetime risk of developing CVD for a 40-year-old woman is estimated to be 1 in 2, with 1 in 3 at risk of developing coronary heart disease 1 in 5 developing heart failure (HF), and 1 in 5 having a stroke in their lifetime.[1] Since 2001, there had been a continuous decline in mortality from heart disease in women until 2010, where after mortality for CVD has risen in both sexes.[1] Nonetheless, the mortality rate from CVD in younger women (under the age of 55 years) has demonstrated no significant improvement in the last 2 decades, and these youngest women with CVD have the highest mortality rates.[2]

There are both sex (biological) and gender (sociocultural) differences in CVD and outcomes between women and men due to a number of variables including differences in the impact of traditional risk factors, sex-specific CVD risk factors, differences in treatment and management strategies for women for both primary and secondary prevention of CVD, and pathophysiological differences in CVD.

Prevention of CVD in women is influenced by awareness of the issue. Although more women have been dying from CVD than men in the United States, it was not until 1991 that the National Institutes of Health (NIH) established a policy that all NIH-funded trials must include both women and men in studies of conditions that affect both genders. In 2016 the NIH made it mandatory to include both sexes in cell and animal studies. While awareness of CVD as the leading cause of death in women has improved over time, it remains suboptimal, particularly in racial and ethnic minorities.[3] A nationally representative survey done by the Women's Health Alliance showed that even though 74% of women had one or more CVD risk factors, only 16% of women were informed that they were at risk for heart disease. Physician awareness, education, and assessment of women's CVD risk is also far from expected. This same survey showed that primary care physicians prioritized weight and breast health over concerns for CVD. Additionally, only 22% of primary care physicians and 42% of cardiologists felt well-equipped to assess CVD in women, and very few implemented the guidelines for CVD risk assessment in their practice in their women patients (16% of primary care physicians, 22% of cardiologists; p=NS).[3]

SEX, GENDER, AND GENETIC DIFFERENCES IN CARDIOVASCULAR DISEASE

The Institute of Medicine has defined *sex* as "the classification of living things, generally as male or female according to their reproductive organs and functions assigned by the chromosomal complement."[4] Sex differences result from true biological differences in the structure and function of the cardiovascular systems of men and women, in contrast with gender differences that stem from a person's self-representation resulting in psychosocial roles and behaviors imposed by society. Certainly, gender differences play a role in treatment of CVD and hence, impact outcomes but are very different from sex differences that arise from the genetic differences between men and women. Sex differences arise from the chromosomal differences between men (XY) and women (XX).

Genetic markers predictive of CVD remain undefined to date in women. The Multi-Ethnic Study of Atherosclerosis (MESA) is a study of subclinical CVD and risk factors that predict progression to clinically overt CVD and that predict progression of subclinical disease itself, in a diverse, population-based sample of 6814 men and women aged 45 to 84 unaffected with CVD. A genetic risk score (GRS) calculated using a literature-derived list of 46 SNPs predicted CHD in males but not women in MESA.[5] Currently there is no known genetic marker that can be used to improve risk assessment in women, beyond traditional methods.

CARDIOVASCULAR RISK FACTORS IN WOMEN (see Chapters 25 and 30)

TRADITIONAL CARDIOVASCULAR DISEASE RISK FACTORS AND THEIR IMPACT ON WOMEN

Age

Age powerfully predicts CVD, and specifically CHD. The prevalence of CVD increases with age in both men and women, but CHD events lag at least 10 years in women compared to men.[1] CHD increases in women after the age of 60, with 1 in 3 women having evidence of CHD after the age of 65 years, in contrast with 1 in 8 women aged 45 to 64. The atherosclerotic CVD (ASCVD) risk score increases with increasing age.[6] The highest sex difference in CHD mortality occurs in relatively young and middle-aged women, with relative stagnation in rates in contrast

Additional content is available online at Elsevier eBooks for Practicing Clinicians

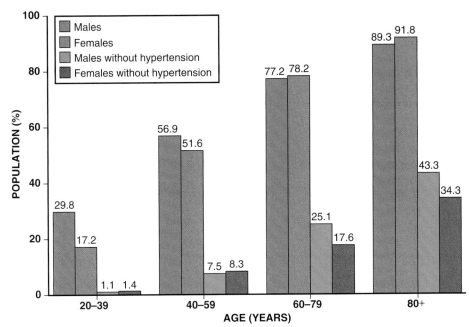

FIGURE 91.1 Prevalence of cardiovascular disease in US adults with and without hypertension (NHANES 2013–2016). (From Virani SS, et al. American Heart Association Council on Epidemiology and Prevention Statistics Committee and Stroke Statistics Subcommittee Heart Disease and Stroke Statistics-2020 Update: A Report from the American Heart Association. *Circulation.* 2020;141:e139–e596.)

with declines and no sex difference among older adult women and men.[7]

Family History
A history of CHD in a first-degree relative imparts risk on an individual. The 2018 American College of Cardiology/American Heart Association (ACC/AHA) guidelines on the treatment of blood cholesterol to reduce atherosclerotic cardiovascular risk in adults recommends consideration of a premature family history of CVD when assessing risk in asymptomatic adults.[8]

Hypertension (see also Chapter 26)
The definition of hypertension has changed, and as a result the prevalence of hypertension has increased with a lower threshold for the diagnosis of hypertension.[9] Based on the National Health and Nutrition Examination Survey (NHANES) 2017–2018, the overall prevalence of hypertension was similar among men (51.0%) and women (39.7%), which increases with age in both sexes. Women over the age of 60 have the same prevalence of hypertension compared with men (73.9% vs. 75.2%, respectively).[10] Women are more likely than men to have their hypertension controlled (53% vs. 46%), which does not change with age, in contrast with men where it worsens.[11] Hypertension rises two- to threefold in women taking second- and third-generation oral contraceptives, which raise blood pressure 7 to 8 mm Hg on average, however fourth-generation with drospirenone lower blood pressure.[12]

Hypertension has a greater adverse impact on CVD in women over the age of 60 when compared with men (Fig. 91.1).[1] Hypertension has an increased risk of the development of congestive HF, which is relatively greater in women. Women who present with strokes more likely have a history of hypertension than men. Indeed, the lifetime risk of stroke is greater in women compared with men, related to their greater life expectancy and the rise in stroke rates with age.

The effect of aging on blood pressure is not just a change due to menopause in women, as previously thought. Recent work has shown significant sex differences in blood pressure trajectories, where blood pressure actually increases more rapidly in women and begins early in life (Fig. 91.2).[13] The biological differences may explain the subsequent distinct pathophysiologic effects of hypertension, in addition to the variability in responsiveness to medications in women.

Diabetes (see also Chapter 31)
Diabetes increases the risk of CHD and confers greater risk for CHD in women than men, increasing a woman's risk of CHD by three-to sevenfold with only a two- to threefold increase in diabetic men. In addition,

the risk of fatal CHD in a diabetic woman increases 3.5 times versus nondiabetic woman, and higher than in diabetic men (relative risk of fatal CHD is 2.0 that of a nondiabetic man).[14] Importantly, even women with type 1 diabetes have twice the risk of fatal and nonfatal cardiovascular events, and a 40% greater risk of all-cause mortality compared with men.[15]

The American Diabetes Association suggests consideration of diabetes screening for women and men over the age of 45 years, and then every 3 years if the results are normal.[16] For women with a history of gestational diabetes, screening for diabetes should occur 6 to 12 weeks postpartum, with lifelong testing every 3 years. Additionally, the 2020 guidelines recommend screening women with polycystic ovarian syndrome (PCOS) if they are overweight or obese.[16]

Dyslipidemia (see also Chapter 27)
Dyslipidemia is common in women but steadily decreasing over time, based on the NHANES 2015–2018 data.[17] Elevated total cholesterol (>240 mg/dL) is present in 12.1% of adult women, compared with 10.5% of men. The only age group of women that had a lower total cholesterol than men are those under the age of 40. Overall, this may reflect undertreatment of dyslipidemia in women. There is evidence that women who are eligible for statin therapy are less likely to be treated with any statin or the recommended intensity of statin.[18] The reasons are both due to less prescribing of appropriate therapy and women declining or discontinuing treatment more frequently compared with men.

High-density lipoprotein (HDL) levels are higher in women,[17] and on average HDL-C levels in women are approximately 10 mg/dL higher than men throughout their lives. HDL is inversely associated with ASCVD events. Nonetheless, HDL as a target of therapy has to date not improved outcomes, and is not the target of the ASCVD risk assessment.

The ASCVD risk assessment focuses on low-density lipoprotein cholesterol (LDL-C) as the primary target of lipid-lowering therapy to reduce risk of CVD.[8] The use of nuclear magnetic resonance (NMR) spectroscopy lipoprofiles, apolipoproteins, particle size, and density are not endorsed by the current cholesterol guidelines in either men or women for cardiovascular risk assessment.[8]

Notably in women, adverse changes in the lipid profile accompany menopause and include increased levels of total cholesterol, LDL-C, and triglycerides and decreased levels of HDL-C, although it remains unclear how much risk factor worsening is related to aging as opposed to menopause-related hormonal changes.[19]

Cigarette Smoking
Cigarette smoking is the leading cause of preventable cardiovascular deaths. The use of cigarettes continues to decline in the United States, due to effective public health measures. Based on 2018 data, 16% of men and 12% of women reported tobacco use.[20] Although women smoke less than men, smoking cigarettes may be more detrimental in women than men. Female smokers die 14.5 years earlier than female nonsmokers and male smokers die 13.2 years earlier than male nonsmokers.[21] The use of oral contraceptives and cigarette use imparts an even greater risk of myocardial infarction than smoking alone, likely related to pro-thrombotic effects.

Cessation of smoking substantially reduces CVD risk in women; mortality risk among former smokers decreases nearly to that of never smokers.[22] It is important to recognize that smoking cessation works differently in women compared with men. Men have more nicotine receptors in their brain and nicotine replacement is more effective in men compared with women. Varenicline, on the other hand, has been shown to be more effective as a smoking cessation aid in women.[23]

Physical Activity/Physical Fitness (see also Chapters 32 and 33)
Physical activity benefits cardiovascular health but physical inactivity is common, with women more likely to report not meeting the physical activity guidelines than men (47% vs. 38%), which worsens with age.[24] Nonetheless, gender bias exists in physical activity measurement

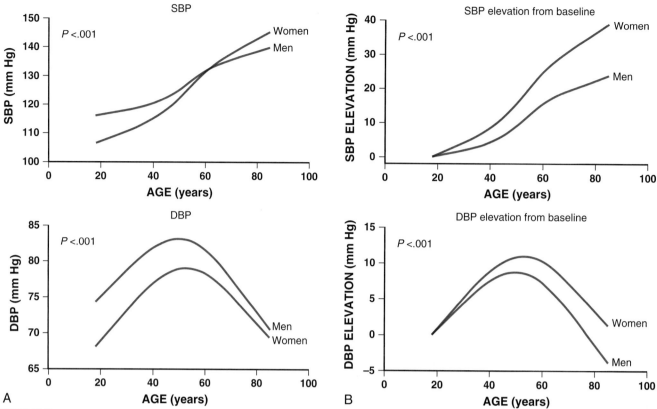

FIGURE 91.2 Sex-specific blood pressure changes over time in adults. (From Ji H, Kim A, Ebinger JE, et al. Sex differences in blood pressure trajectories over the life course. *JAMA Cardiol.* 2020;5[3]:19–26.)

instruments that do not collect domestic activities such as cooking, cleaning, and childcare, which may account for these observed differences. Using the 2008 U.S. federal physical activity guidelines, in every age group adult women reported performing less leisure-time physical activity than men in the 2017 National Health Interview Survey. Physical inactivity associates with higher blood pressure, worse cholesterol, poorer glucose metabolism, poorer mental health, and obesity. Physical inactivity, quantified by prolonged sitting time, has been shown to be an independent risk factor for CVD in women beyond leisure-time physical activity.[25]

Exercise capacity, also known as physical fitness, strongly and independently predicts all-cause mortality in asymptomatic women and can be quantified. In 4137 self-referred apparently healthy adults (2326 men, 1811 women; mean age: 42.8 ± 12.2 years) who underwent cardiopulmonary fitness testing, the low-fit women had a higher risk of dying from all-causes, CVD, and cancer during follow-up than those with moderate fitness and high fitness. At any point in time, low-fit women had a 28%, 34%, and 34% increased risk of dying from all-causes, CVD, and cancer compared with high-fit women (p < 0.01), respectively. In women, this relationship remained significant for all-cause and cancer mortality in the multivariable model (hazards ratio [HR] 1.63, p < 0.05 and HR 3.94, p < 0.01, respectively).[26]

Metabolic Syndrome (see also Chapters 30 and 31)
NHANES data from 2003 to 2014 indicate that 33.3% of women met the criteria for the metabolic syndrome, similar to that seen in men (35.3%, P < 0.01).[27] Those with the metabolic syndrome have an increased risk of developing CVD, and the association with the risk of MI has been demonstrated to be greater in women compared with men but no sex differences in the risk of stroke based on the presence of the metabolic syndrome.[28]

Obesity (see also Chapter 25)
Obesity, defined as a body mass index (BMI) of greater than 30 kg/m², is epidemic in the United States, with the 2017–2018 NHANES estimation of obesity in women at 41.8%, similar to that seen in men.[29] The rising incidence of diabetes associates closely with obesity. In the Nurses' Health Study, obesity was the most powerful predictor of diabetes, with women with a BMI ≥35 kg/m² having a relative risk for diabetes almost 40-fold greater than women with a BMI less than 23

kg/m². The pattern of obesity appears to be related to CVD, whereby elevated waist circumference above 35 inches, waist-to-hip ratio, and waist-to-height ratio, indicative of visceral obesity, is related to elevated CVD risk, whereas elevated BMI alone is not.[30]

Although obesity has also been associated with an increased mortality from CVD and shortened life expectancy from CVD, obesity is not an independent risk factor for CVD given that obesity is strongly associated with many of the traditional CHD risk factors. Notably, overweight, defined as a BMI of greater than 25 but less than 30 kg/m², is associated with lower mortality and CVD death compared to leaner counterparts. Obesity may simply be a marker for low physical activity and fitness levels. Prior work in women where both obesity and physical fitness were measured suggests that physically fit obese women are not at elevated risk, and conversely lean women who are not physically fit have elevated risk.[31]

High-Sensitivity C-Reactive Protein (see also Chapters 10 and 25)
Although high-sensitivity C-reactive protein (hsCRP) is not a causal risk factor for CVD, it may improve risk detection in women. Measuring hsCRP is not recommended in routine risk assessment of women, but rather as an option in those persons in the intermediate risk range based on the ASCVD risk score. An elevated hsCRP (>2.0 mg/L) is considered an ASCVD risk-enhancing factor.[6]

Sleep Apnea
Although sleep apnea is more prevalent in men compared with women, it is a very common issue in women and under-recognized in terms of its impact on CVD. In women, untreated obstructive sleep apnea is associated with an increased risk of hypertension, coronary artery disease (CAD), stroke, and atrial fibrillation.[32] Sleep apnea is believed to induce severe intermittent hypoxemia and CO_2 retention during sleep, with oxygen saturation sometimes dropping to ≤60%, disrupting the normal autonomic and hemodynamic responses to sleep.

Apnea often occurs repetitively through the night, and toward the end of an apneic episode, blood pressure rises and can reach levels as high as 240/130 mm Hg. This hemodynamic stress occurs simultaneously with severe hypoxemia, hypercapnia, and adrenergic activation, which in turn acts to promote CVD. Untreated sleep apnea in women is associated with 3.5 times greater risk of dying from CVD, yet this risk was reduced to the same as a woman without sleep apnea with appropriate treatment and continuous positive airway pressure.[32]

SEX-SPECIFIC RISK FACTORS
Age of Menarche
Age at onset of menarche is associated with ASCVD risk. Early menarche (occurring at or before the age of 12 years) and late onset menarche (>15 years) have both been shown to increase risk for adverse cardiovascular outcomes including myocardial infarction, stroke, and HF hospitalizations. In a 648-woman cohort from the WISE (Women's Ischemia Syndrome Evaluation) study, history of menarche at age ≤10 years and ≥15 years showed adverse cardiovascular events HR of 4.53 (95% CI 2.13 to 9.63) and 2.58 (95% CI 1.28 to 5.21), respectively, compared to women with menarche at age 12 years.[33]

Pregnancy-Associated Conditions:
Preterm Delivery. Preterm delivery, defined as births prior to 37 weeks gestation, complicates about 11% of deliveries worldwide. The underlying causes and mechanisms are not entirely clear but there is a strong association with preterm delivery and maternal risk of coronary heart disease and stroke, with the greatest risk associated with preterm deliveries before 32 weeks gestation.[34]

Eclampsia, Pre-eclampsia, and Pregnancy-Associated Hypertension (see also Chapter 92). Gestational hypertension of any sort associates with an increased risk of hypertension, chronic kidney disease, diabetes, stroke, and CVD (including HF, stroke, and myocardial infarction).[35] From the prospective UK Biobank cohort of over 220,000 women, those who reported hypertension during pregnancy were not just at greater risk of chronic hypertension, but also had a great risk of developing CAD, HF, aortic stenosis (AS), and mitral regurgitation over a median follow-up of 7 years (Fig. 91.3). From a causal standpoint, 64% of those with CAD and 49% of HF was driven by chronic hypertension, meaning treating hypertension in this group is of critical importance.[36]

Women with hypertensive disorders during pregnancy have a greater risk for stroke with the median age of a stroke in these women being ≤50 years, demonstrating an acceleration of CVD, despite premenopausal status and presumed low risk lessening emphasis on screening or treating of CVD risk factors.[37] Despite the association with elevated CVD events and labeling of pregnancy as a "stress test" for future CV events, some research suggests that the risk of CVD results from shared pre-pregnancy risk factors rather than any direct influence of the hypertensive disorder that occurred during pregnancy.[38] Hypertension during pregnancy is recognized as a risk-enhancing factor by the 2018 guidelines on the management of blood cholesterol.[8]

Gestational Diabetes (see also Chapter 92). Gestational diabetes increases the risk of future diabetes, but also increases the risk of CVD. A pooled analysis of nine studies that included over 5 million women demonstrated that women with gestational diabetes had a two-fold greater risk of cardiovascular events in the first 10 years postpartum, compared with women without gestational diabetes, even in those women who did not develop Type II diabetes.[39]

Small-for-Gestational-Age Infant. Small-for-gestational-age (SGA) delivery has been shown to be associated with an increased maternal risk of ASCVD. An SGA infant appears to be dose dependent, according to the severity of SGA as well as the number of SGA infants.[35]

Assisted Reproductive Therapies. Fertility hormonal therapies are estimated to be used in approximately 1% of births. The limited data available currently does not support an increased risk of ASCVD in women who undergo assisted reproductive therapy. In a systematic review of 41,910 women who received fertility therapy and 1,400,202 women who did not, there was no increased risk of a cardiac event (pooled HR: 0.91; 95% CI 0.67 to 1.25; I^2 = 36.6%) or diabetes mellitus (pooled HR 0.93, 95% CI 0.87 to 1.001; I^2 = 0%), however there was a trend toward higher risk of stroke (pooled HR 1.25, 95% CI 0.96 to 1.63; I^2 = 0%).[40] Although to date there has been no increase in subsequent ASCVD events in women who require reproductive therapies, there is a noted increase in hypertension while pregnant.

At this time, use of fertility therapy is not considered an independent risk factor for ASCVD. However, there is an early signal to suggest that women who have failed fertility therapy have an increased risk for future ASCVD events.[41] It is plausible that failed fertility therapy could be an indicator for future ASCVD risk as it poses a unique cardiometabolic stress test. This hypothesis warrants further investigation.

Polycystic Ovary Syndrome
Unique to women, PCOS associates with the development of many of the features of metabolic syndrome as well as insulin resistance, although first-degree male relatives also appear to have more insulin resistance. Women with PCOS have an increased prevalence of impaired glucose tolerance, the metabolic syndrome, and diabetes compared to women without PCOS.[42] Nonetheless, it remains unclear if PCOS is an independent risk factor for premature CVD in women. Based on the NHLBI-sponsored WISE (Women's Ischemia Syndrome Evaluation) study of postmenopausal women with PCOS and suspected myocardial ischemia, there was no greater risk of CVD or mortality over 10 years of follow-up.[42]

Functional Hypothalamic Amenorrhea (see also Chapter 96)
Up to 10% of premenopausal women have documented ovarian dysfunction with a larger proportion having subclinical hormonal dysfunction that may increase CVD risk. Functional hypothalamic amenorrhea (FHA) is a cause of a premenopausal ovarian dysfunction and occurs when gonadotropin-releasing hormone increases thereby increasing luteinizing hormone in a pulse frequency causing amenorrhea and hypoestrogenemia. Psychological stressors or metabolic insults such as caloric restriction or excessive exercise can induce FHA. Endothelial dysfunction, unfavorable lipid profiles, and premature CVD have been demonstrated in studies of young women with FHA.[43]

Premature Menopause and Premature Ovarian Insufficiency
The most common theory regarding the delayed onset of CAD in women compared with men is the role of circulating estrogen and its cardio-protective role. A meta-analysis concluded that women who had menopause at age younger than 45 years were more likely to have an incident coronary heart disease event (RR 1.50 [1.28 to 1.76]) compared to women undergoing menopause at ages ≥45 years.[44] The UK Biobank demonstrated that the earlier natural menopause occurs, the greater the risk of CHD and stroke.[45]

Premature ovarian insufficiency (POI) differs from premature menopause. It is defined as ovarian failure before the age of 40 years and results in a prolonged exposure of estrogen insufficiency. Reports have associated POI with an increased risk of CVD.[46] A meta-analysis from 10 observational studies with over 190,000 women demonstrated that POI was modestly associated with an increased incidence of coronary heart disease events (HR 1.69; $p = 0.0001$) but not with stroke.[47]

Premature menopause (before age 40 years) is a recognized risk-enhancing factor in the current ACC/AHA cholesterol guidelines.[8] Noting the presence of POI and the age of menopause should be part of any woman's ASCVD risk assessment.

Reproductive Hormones
Oral Contraceptive Therapy. For most women who are healthy and free of CVD and cardiovascular risk factors, the use of combination estrogen-progestin oral contraceptives associates with low relative and absolute risks of CVD. Women who are smokers over the age of 35, women with uncontrolled hypertension, a history of thromboembolic disease, or a history of ischemic heart disease (IHD) have an unacceptable level of CVD risk associated with oral contraceptives.[48]

Post-menopausal Hormone Therapy. A majority of CVD occurs after menopause in older women, in association with an increased burden of established CVD risk factors, hence the hypothesis that post-menopause hormone therapy reduces CVD risk, as supported by observational data. Nonetheless, randomized trials, such as Heart and Estrogen/Progestin Replacement Study (HERS) I, HERS II, Women's Health Initiative (WHI), and Raloxifene Use for The Heart (RUTH) did not find that hormone therapy or selective estrogen receptor modulators (SERMs) prevent either primary or secondary CVD events. Hormone replacement therapy and SERMS should not be used for the primary or secondary prevention of CVD.[49]

SEX-PREDOMINANT CARDIOVASCULAR DISEASE RISK FACTORS
Autoimmune Disease (see also Chapter 97)
Systemic inflammation in autoimmune disease, including rheumatoid arthritis (RA) and systemic erythematous lupus (SLE), may accelerate atherosclerosis and IHD and these diseases occur more frequently in women.[50] RA, SLE, and scleroderma associate with a significantly increased risk for CVD mortality.[50] Cardiovascular events often occur in younger women with SLE, with a risk for acute myocardial infarction 9- to 50-fold greater than the general population.[50] Traditional risk factors such as smoking, family history of premature CHD, hypertension, and elevated cholesterol do not completely account for the increased risk of CHD in patients with SLE. The 2018 ACC/AHA cholesterol guidelines include chronic inflammatory disorders as ASCVD risk enhancers which favor initiation of statin therapy for individuals with borderline ASCVD risk score.[8]

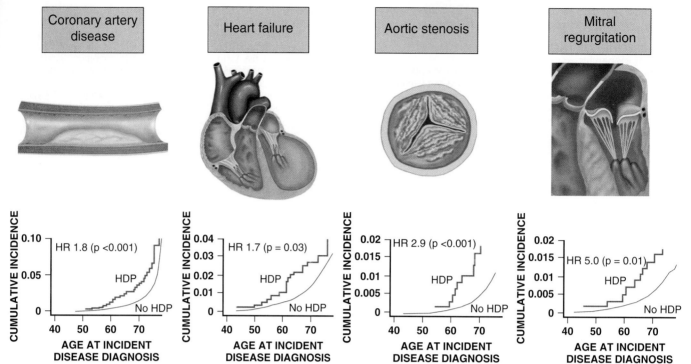

FIGURE 91.3 Hypertensive disorders in pregnancy and their relationship with cardiovascular disease. (From Honigberg MC, Zekavat SM, Aragam K, et al. Long-term cardiovascular risk in women with hypertension during pregnancy. *J Am Coll Cardiol.* 2019;74:2743–2754.)

Breast Cancer Therapy (see also Chapters 56 and 57)

Recent advancements in breast cancer treatment have led to improved survival but elevated risk of CVD.[51] The reasons for an increased risk of CVD appears to be the result of shared risk factors between breast cancer and CVD, in addition to the potential of direct cardiovascular injury that may accelerate atherosclerosis or HF.[52] Commonly used chemotherapeutic agents, such as anthracycline and trastuzumab, increase the risk of HF. In a large retrospective analysis of Medicare data of more than 45,000 older women who had early-stage breast cancer, the risk of developing HF was increased in women who received either trastuzumab (32.1/100 patients) or anthracycline plus trastuzumab (41.9/100 patients) compared with no adjuvant therapy (18.1/100 patients, p < 0.001). The addition of trastuzumab to anthracycline therapy added 12.1, 17.9, and 21.7 HF/cardiomyopathy events per 100 patients over 1, 2, and 3 years of follow-up, respectively. These rates are far higher than reported in early trials that established the use of trastuzumab.[52] Radiation therapy has an established association with the development of IHD. Exposure of the heart to ionizing radiation during radiotherapy for breast cancer increases the risk of IHD. The risk is directly proportional to the mean radiation dose to the heart, with an increase in CVD events of 7.4%/Gray (Gy) of radiation (95% CI, 2.9 to 14.5, p < 0.001). The risk of IHD begins within a few years after exposure and appears to continue for at least 20 years after the exposure. As expected, the risk for IHD is highest in women with pre-existing CVD risk factors.[52]

This period of breast cancer diagnosis and treatment is therefore an important window to provide ASCVD risk assessment, given that breast cancer is considered an ASCVD risk-enhancing factor.[8] Furthermore, a long-term post-treatment surveillance strategy needs to be implemented among these for monitoring late cardiotoxicity and/or non-therapy–related CVD event risk.

CARDIOVASCULAR DISEASE RISK ASSESSMENT (see also Chapter 25)

The role of ASCVD risk assessment is to identify those at highest risk of developing ASCVD, allowing guidance of appropriate intensity of screening and allocation of preventive therapy. Although there are a number of risk assessment tools available, the tool chosen should have been validated on the population on which it is being applied to. The risk estimator of choice in the United States remains the 2013 Pooled Cohort Equations (PCE), despite its acknowledged limitations in certain populations.[6] The 2018 ACC/AHA guidelines on the treatment of blood cholesterol to reduce ASCVD in adults relies on the PCE as the initial step in risk estimation, but incorporates nontraditional risk factors to refine the risk assessment.[8] The ASCVD risk estimator allows lifetime risk estimation for those aged 20 to 59 years, and 10-year risk estimation for those aged 40 to 75 years. Risk-enhancing factors allow individuals to be reclassified, and this includes the sex-specific and sex-predominant risk enhancers that impact women specifically.

ISCHEMIC HEART DISEASE IN WOMEN

Symptoms of Ischemia (see also Chapter 35)

Both sexes can experience the classic symptoms of myocardial ischemia. The perception that women may not experience chest pain or chest discomfort was based on retrospective data.[53,54] The National Registry of Myocardial Infarction demonstrated that women were more likely than men to present with a myocardial infarction without any chest pain at all (42 % vs. 31%, *P < 0.001*), particularly younger women who have the highest hospital mortality rates.[53] Nonetheless, more contemporary data has shown that symptoms of women and men are more alike than different. The Variation in Recovery: Role of Gender on Outcomes of Young AMI Patients (VIRGO) study reported presenting symptoms in women and men under the age of 55 years and found no differences in the report of chest pain by sex (87.2% women, 89.5% men) with AMI.[53] Young women were more likely to experience three or more associated symptoms, when compared with men. Similar findings were seen at all ages of AMI in the High-STEACS (High Sensitivity Troponin in the Evaluation of Patients with Acute Coronary Syndrome) trial. Those women diagnosed with AMI reported chest pain 92% of the time, comparable to the men at 91%.[55] Additionally, other "typical" symptoms were seen more in women compared with men (77% vs. 59%; *p = 0.007*) with AMI.

Certainly, for some women, the symptoms of ischemia may often be more nonspecific or less severe and can include shortness of breath; pain or discomfort in other body locations, such as that localized to the arm(s), shoulder, middle back, jaw, or epigastrium; indigestion; nausea or vomiting; diaphoresis; faintness or dizziness or syncope; fatigue; generalized weakness; or palpitations.[54] Nonetheless, most women do report chest pain or discomfort, along with additional symptoms. It is important to be aware of their risk and consider ischemia in the differential when women report such symptoms.

Delays in Care of Women

One barrier to the diagnosis of ischemia is delays in initiating care for women. This is a result of delays in women seeking care, in addition to delays in recognizing women being at risk by the healthcare team. The VIRGO study showed that young women also have delays in seeking care, and are more likely to present with AMI 6 or more hours after onset of symptoms, compared with men.[53] Additional delays occur upon presentation, with numerous studies documenting delays in care of women, particularly in initiating STEMI treatment and interventions, given public reporting of specific measures. Other work documents delays in reperfusion in women compared with men.[56] In-hospital and transfer times for percutaneous coronary intervention (PCI) were more likely to be exceeded in women compared with men (odds ratio [OR] 1.65, 95% CI 1.27 to 2.16), particularly when requiring transfer.

Diagnosis of Ischemia in Women

The classification of IHD risk in women refers to those females presenting for evaluation of suspected CAD who have chest discomfort or some ischemic equivalent including excessive dyspnea. Broadly characterized, pre-menopausal women with symptoms are typically low risk. Symptomatic women in their fifth decade of life should be considered at low-intermediate IHD risk, if they are capable of performing routine activities of daily living (ADL). If performance of routine ADL is compromised, a woman in her 50s should be elevated to the intermediate IHD risk category. Women in their 60s are also generally considered as intermediate IHD risk whereas women 70 and older are considered at high risk for CAD.[57] The low-intermediate or intermediate-risk woman is a candidate for an exercise ECG if they have a functional capacity estimate ≥5 METs (metabolic equivalent tests) using the Duke Activity Status Inventory (DASI). Intermediate-high IHD risk women with an abnormal 12 lead rest ECG should be referred for a CAD noninvasive imaging modality including pharmacologic stress myocardial perfusion imaging (MPI), Echo, or cardiovascular magnetic resonance (CMR) imaging or coronary computed tomography angiogram (CCTA). High-IHD–risk women with stable symptoms may be referred for a stress imaging modality for functional assessment of their ischemic burden and to guide post-test anti-ischemic therapies.[57]

These guidelines emphasize the usefulness of the traditional exercise stress test without imaging as the initial test of choice for women with a normal ECG and able to exercise. Although the ST segment depression with exercise may be less diagnostic of obstructive CAD in women, a negative exercise ECG stress test has significant diagnostic value. A markedly abnormal exercise ECG demonstrating 2 or more mm of ST segment changes, in particular when occurring at low workloads (<5 METs) or persisting for greater than 5 minutes into recovery, associates with a high likelihood of obstructive CAD for both women and men. It is important to note that the predictive value of stress testing is based on predicting obstructive CAD; an abnormal stress test in symptomatic women may still be consistent with IHD that is non-obstructive.

Although the IHD guidelines have not been recently updated, there are a number of trials that included women demonstrating the role of other imaging modalities. The Prospective Multicenter Imaging Study for Evaluation of Chest Pain (PROMISE) trial was a randomized trial that demonstrated that although coronary CTA (CCTA) was not superior to stress testing in low-to-intermediate–risk patients, it is an alternative test for evaluation of chest pain. In women, a positive CCTA (vs. negative CCTA) was more predictive of events (HR 5.9, 95% CI 3.3 to 10.4) than a positive stress test (vs. a negative stress test) (HR 2.3, 95% CI 1.2 to 4.3).[58] The role of CCTA is further enhanced by the randomized controlled SCOT-HEART (Scottish Computed Tomography of the Heart) trial, where CCTA imaging was associated with a significant reduction in nonfatal MI and deaths for coronary heart disease at 5 years, when compared with standard of care in those presenting with stable chest pain.[59]

With any imaging modality used in women, considerations must be made regarding the amount of radiation exposure. Many cardiac diagnostic procedures—including stress MPI, CCTA, and coronary angiography—expose women to varying doses of ionizing radiation. In those women for whom the benefit of IHD risk detection far exceeds the small projected cancer risk following exposure to ionizing radiation, radiation exposure should not be a consideration in physician decision-making.[60] For all other women, in particular low-risk pre-menopausal women, alternative tests without radiation exposure (i.e., exercise ECG) or a no-testing strategy should be applied. Applying appropriate use criteria can limit radiation exposure in women, lowering cancer risks due to imaging in the population. Emphasis on shared decision-making with patients on the impact of radiation exposure should be part of the process before testing is performed.

Interventions and Medical Therapy for Ischemic Heart Disease in Women

Optimal medical therapy for women with IHD does not differ from that for men. Nonetheless women often receive less intensive medical therapy and secondary preventive therapies, lifestyle counseling, or referral to cardiac rehabilitation, which ultimately influences outcomes.[61] SWEDEHEART (Swedish Web System for Enhancement and Development of Evidence–Based Care in Heart Disease Evaluated According to Recommended Therapies) included every hospital system in Sweden between 2003 and 2013 and demonstrated an excess mortality related to underuse of guideline-indicated therapies in those women with STEMI and NSTEMI, compared with men, after adjusting for age and comorbidities. Once adjusted for the sex disparities in medications, the excess mortality disappeared for NSTEMI at 1 year but persisted at 5 years (excess mortality risk ratio [EWMRR] 1.07, 95% CI 1.02 to 1.12) and for STEMI at 1 (EMRR 1.43, 95% CI 1.26 to 1.62) and 5 years (EMRR 1.31, 95% CI 1.19 to 1.43).[62] Gaps in outcomes could be reduced in women by using guideline-directed medical therapies in ACS.

In addition to the difference in medical therapy, there are sex differences in use of cardiac catheterization and revascularization use and timing (as discussed above), which associate with poorer outcomes in women with ACS. Based on the Acute Coronary Treatment and Intervention Outcomes Network Registry-Get with the Guidelines (ACTION Registry-GWTG) database for the treatment of STEMI and NSTEMI, there are sex and racial differences in not just medical therapy but also interventional therapies. In NSTEMI particularly, there were lower rates of invasive and interventional procedures, particularly pronounced in Black women.[63] In-hospital mortality after AMI remains higher in women compared with men in the ACTION-GWTG registry in those with obstructive CAD.[64] The Nationwide Inpatient Sample in a contemporary matched cohort found a significantly lower number of women underwent PTCA and other supportive procedures, which appears to be associated with significantly higher in-hospital mortality.[65] More recent analysis of the Nationwide Inpatient Sample looking at a more contemporary time from 2010 to 2016 demonstrated a persistence in disparities in reperfusion and revascularization therapies after STEMI in women, resulting in higher in-hospital mortality compared with men. Women had a higher overall in-hospital mortality than men (11% vs. 6.8%; OR 1.039, CI 1.003 to 1.007) which persisted with multi-variable adjustment. When stratified by age, this relationship persisted in the youngest (age 19 to 49 years) with a 25% elevated in-hospital mortality compared with men (adj OR 1.259, 95% CI 1.083 to 1.464).[66]

Furthermore, in randomized controlled PCI trials, women fare more poorly than men. In a pooled analysis of 10 randomized controlled PCI trials that included 2632 patients (22% women), women were older and had greater delays in reperfusion, but had better early post-MI left ventricular ejection fraction (LVEF) and similar infarct size to men.[67] Women still had higher adjusted 1-year rates of death or HF hospitalizations (HR 2.13, 95% CI 1.34 to 3.38), which were not explained by LVEF or infarct size.[67]

There is evidence that women do worse with incomplete revascularization compared with men after STEMI. A study of 589 consecutive STEMI patients followed for a median of 3.6 years demonstrated that women were equally likely to be incompletely revascularized (residual

SYNTAX score >8) compared with men, despite a lower burden of disease. These women who were incompletely revascularized were almost twice as likely as men to have repeat MI or die from cardiac causes, even after adjusting for risk (adjusted HR 1.77, 95% CI 1.13 to 2.77, p = 0.01).[68] This emphasizes the need for complete revascularization in women after STEMI.

Studies document increased bleeding risk in women undergoing PCI who receive glycoprotein IIb/IIIa inhibitors. The GLOBAL LEADERS randomized control trial that compared 1 month of dual antiplatelet therapy (DAPT) followed by 23 months of ticagrelor monotherapy with 12 months of DAPT following 21 months of aspirin found no difference in the efficacy or safety after 2 years with either antiplatelet regime.[69] Women experience an increased risk of bleeding and hemorrhagic stroke with either therapy, whereas men had lower risk of bleeding with ticagrelor monotherapy. Sex remains an independent predictor of bleeding post-PCI and has been demonstrated in the Nationwide Inpatient Sample of over 6.6 million patients with women having both an increased risk post PCI of in-hospital mortality (OR 1.20, 95% CI 1.16 to 1.23) and major bleeding (OR 1.81, 95% CI 1.77 to 1.86).[70]

A persistent pattern of higher mortality and poorer cardiovascular outcomes in women compared with men with IHD remains, mostly attributable to suboptimal use of guideline therapy in at-risk women, despite evidence that application of guideline therapy post-ACS reduces the mortality disparity in women, and that management of ACS and chronic angina with intensive medical therapy benefits both sexes equally.[71]

ISCHEMIC HEART DISEASE: BEYOND OBSTRUCTIVE CORONARY ARTERY DISEASE

Women have less anatomical obstructive CAD and relatively more preserved left ventricular function in the setting of both stable IHD and ACS.[72] Ischemia with no obstructive CAD is referred to as INOCA. Myocardial infarction with nonobstructive CAD is referred to as MINOCA. The traditional definition of obstructive CAD was any coronary stenosis greater than 70%,[73] but has been updated to include lesions of 50% to 70% where there is inducible ischemia or physiologic significant stenosis.

Ischemia with No Obstructive Coronary Artery Disease

INOCA is more frequently appreciated, with the recognition that obstructive lesions are not a prerequisite for ischemia. It can overlap with many features of MINOCA but exclusively refers to non-MI syndromes (Fig. 91.4).

Prevalence: In those who present with IHD and undergo angiography, approximately 50% have INOCA, with a higher prevalence in women compared with men (65% vs. 32%).[74] In a single-center study of all consecutive non-emergent cardiac angiograms, although women had a similar prevalence and extent of ischemia as men, women were more likely than men to have INOCA.[75] The odds of obstructive CAD in women undergoing coronary angiography is approximately half that compared with men, for an estimated prevalence of 2 to 3 million women with INOCA.

Pathophysiology: Studies have implicated adverse coronary reactivity, CMD, and plaque erosion/distal micro-embolization as contributory to INOCA pathophysiology. The prevalence may be increasing due to an increased recognition of these issues, in contrast with prior documentation of "false positive" ischemic imaging when no obstructive CAD was found. Additionally, more sensitive diagnostics, specifically advanced imaging techniques, are better able to detect IHD.

Prognosis: The lack of obstructive CAD does not imply a benign prognosis. Data from WISE has shown that symptomatic women with documented ischemia and nonobstructive CAD had a 10-year all-cause mortality and cardiac mortality of 17% and 11%, respectively.[76] In those women with normal coronary arteries but documented ischemia, the 10-year all-cause mortality and cardiac mortality was 10% and 6%, respectively.[76]

There are notable sex differences in outcomes in INOCA, with women having poorer outcomes when compared with men. Women with INOCA are four times more likely to be readmitted within 180 days for ACS when compared with men.[74] Coronary flow reserve (CFR) less than 2.5 is a significant incremental predictor of major adverse cardiac event (MACE) in both men and women, and by such stratification low CFR was a predictor of increased MACE rate (HR 1.06, 95% CI 1.01–1.12, p = 0.021), whereas low CBF was associated with increased risk of mortality (HR 1.12, 95% CI 1.01–1.24, p=0.038) and MACE in women undergoing invasive testing.[77]

Treatment: There is limited data regarding effectiveness of unique therapies for INOCA-related to outcomes. Nonetheless, treatment of stable IHD is necessary, but those with INOCA remain undertreated. When examining a number of studies, less than half of those with IHD are treated with guideline-recommended medical therapies for ischemia, including angiotensin-converting enzyme inhibitors

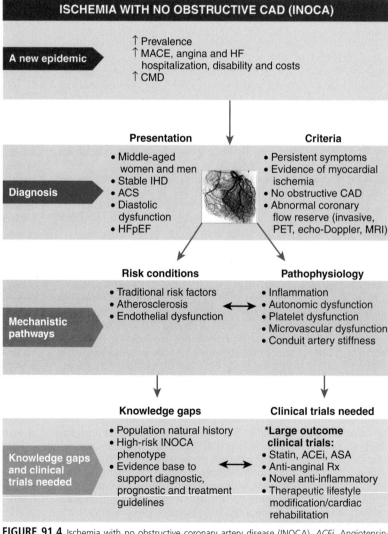

FIGURE 91.4 Ischemia with no obstructive coronary artery disease (INOCA). *ACEi,* Angiotensin-converting enzyme inhibitor; *ASA,* aspirin; *CAD,* coronary artery disease; *CMD,* coronary microvascular dysfunction; *HF,* heart failure; *HFpEF,* heart failure with preserved ejection fraction; *IHD,* ischemic heart disease; *MACE,* major adverse cardiac event; *MRI,* magnetic resonance imaging; *Rx,* prescription; *PET,* positron emission tomography. (From Bairey Merz CN, Pepine CJ, Walsh MN, Fleg JL. Ischemia and no obstructive coronary artery disease (INOCA): developing evidence-based therapies and research agenda for the next decade. *Circulation.* 2017;135(11):1075–1092.)

TABLE 91.1 Clinical Presentations with a Working Diagnosis of Myocardial Infarction with Nonobstructive Coronary Artery Disease

	UNDERLYING MECHANISM/ CLINICAL DISORDER	DIAGNOSTIC INVESTIGATIONS	TARGETED/EMPIRICAL THERAPIES
Noncoronary causes mimicking MINOCA	Supply-demand mismatch	History, identification of potential stressors	Treatment of underlying condition
	Takotsubo cardiomyopathy	Left ventricular angiogram, contrast MRI	GDMT for HF, ACE-I, beta blocker, mechanical circulatory support as needed
	Cardiomyopathies	Contrast cMRI	GDMT for HF, treatment of underlying cause
	Myocarditis	Contrast cMRI	GDMT for HF/myocarditis
Coronary causes of MINOCA	Plaque erosion/rupture	Angiogram review, consider IVUS/OCT	Aspirin, high-intensity statin, beta blocker, ACE-I, consider P2Y12 inhibitor
	Coronary vasospasm	Resolution with vasodilators, provocation testing, history of migraine medications or cocaine use	CCB, nitrates, cilostazol, consider statins
	Microvascular dysfunction	Invasive or noninvasive (PET) coronary blood flow and coronary flow reserve, cMRI	Lifestyle modification especially exercise, consider statin, ACE-I, beta blockers, L-arginine supplementation
	Coronary embolism/ thrombus	Angiogram review, consider IVUS/OCT, thrombophilia screen/workup	Consider anticoagulation, treatment of underlying thrombotic condition
	SCAD	Angiogram review, consider IVUS/OCT	Aspirin, beta-blocker, consider P2Y12 inhibitor

ACE-I, Angiotensin-converting enzyme inhibitor; *ARB,* angiotensin receptor blocker; *CCB,* calcium channel blocker; *cMRI,* cardiac magnetic resonance imaging; *GDMT,* guideline-directed medical therapy; *IVUS,* intravascular ultrasound; *MINOCA,* myocardial infarction in the absence of obstructive coronary artery disease; *OCT,* optical coherence tomography; *PET,* positron emission tomography; *SCAD,* spontaneous coronary artery dissection.
Adapted from Tamis-Holland JE, Jneid H, Reynolds HR, et al. Contemporary Diagnosis and Management of Patients With Myocardial Infarction in the Absence of Obstructive Coronary Artery Disease: A Scientific Statement From the American Heart Association. *Circulation.* 2019;139:e891–e908.

or angiotensin receptor blockers, beta blockers, calcium channel blockers, or statin therapies.[74] The under-treatment may be a result of diagnostic and therapeutic uncertainty, resulting in fewer secondary preventive therapies.

Myocardial Infarction with Nonobstructive Coronary Artery Disease

The increasing recognition of MI in those without obstructive CAD is now commonly referred to as MINOCA. MINOCA is not a single disease process and requires further evaluation to make a diagnosis and also exclude noncoronary etiologies of AMI (Table 91.1).[64]

Prevalence: MI in the absence of obstructive CAD occurs in 5% to 6% of all AMI, seen in both contemporary registries and prior ACS trials.[64] Women with ACS are twice as likely to have "normal" angiograms or demonstrate no obstructive CAD when compared with men, while the average of MINOCA is 58 years, compared with 61 years in those with AMI with obstructive CAD.[78] Given there are 1.4 million ACS events per year, 600,000 of which are women, this translates to 60,000 to 150,000 women with ACS and nonobstructive CAD.

Pathophysiology: MINOCA can be caused by both atherosclerotic and nonatherosclerotic causes (see Table 91.1).[79] Because it does not reflect only one disease process, not all MINOCA cases will have electrocardiographic changes and troponin elevations may be smaller than seen in obstructive AMI. Additionally, myocardial injury that is nonischemic (i.e., myocarditis, Takotsubo cardiomyopathy) can mimic myocardial infarction, and this distinction needs to be clarified by additional diagnostic testing because both injury and infarction will have elevations in troponin.[79]

Based on the Scientific Statement from the American Heart Association on Contemporary Diagnosis and Management of Patients with MINOCA, the underlying pathophysiology can be due to coronary vasospasm, CMD, coronary embolism or thrombosis, spontaneous coronary artery dissection (SCAD), and supply-demand mismatch.[79]

Prognosis: In the setting of an ACS, "normal" coronary arteries do not have a benign prognosis.[79] All-cause mortality appears to be lower in MINOCA compared with MI with obstructive CAD but is substantial (in-hospital mortality: 1.1 vs. 3.2%, *P = 0.001*; 12-month mortality: 6.7% vs. 3.5%, P = 0.003).[78]

Treatment: The current guidelines that exist for STEMI and NSTEMI do not differ by sex and no studies to date support the value of specific therapies of MINOCA, hence efforts to improve the application of guidelines in practice could improve MI and IHD outcomes in women. The management of MINOCA has a limited evidence-based literature and as described above, has multiple different possible pathophysiologies. To date, there are no prospective randomized, controlled trials for management of any of these. It is important to try to define the likely cause of MINOCA and assess for potential myocardial injury causes. Acute management should involve emergency supportive care, cardioprotective therapies irrespective of the cause of MINOCA, in addition to cause-targeted therapies. Secondary ASCVD preventive therapies should also be initiated.

Takotsubo Cardiomyopathy (see also Chapters 37 and 38)

Takotsubo cardiomyopathy accounts for 4% of those presenting with presumed ACS,[80] although the prevalence is higher in women, particularly post-menopausal women (5.9% to 7.5%), and female sex is one of the seven parameters of the diagnostic score. Takotsubo cardiomyopathy should be considered in women as part of the differential diagnosis of acute coronary syndrome.[80] Other names for this syndrome include "transient ventricular ballooning syndrome," "left ventricular apical ballooning syndrome," "stress-induced cardiomyopathy," "ampulla cardiomyopathy," and "broken heart syndrome." Women account for 90% of all Takotsubo cardiomyopathy cases.[80] The Fourth Universal Definition of MI does not consider Takotsubo cardiomyopathy an AMI and recognizes it as a separate syndrome, therefore it is not classified as a form of MINOCA.[81]

There are no randomized controlled trials assessing therapeutic options for Takotsubo cardiomyopathy. Beta blockers appear to provide no benefit for the index event or prevention of subsequent episodes.[82] There is some observational benefit of ACE-I with improved 1-year survival, but no guidance to duration of treatment necessary.[83] Although it is often thought that Takotsubo cardiomyopathy was benign because it was often reversible, in-hospital and long-term mortality is 4.1% and 5.6%, respectively based on the International Takotsubo Registry (InterTAK).[83] The Mayo Clinic Takotsubo registry demonstrated a 1-year survival of 94% but the leading cause of death was cancer, and cardiac deaths only accounted for 5% of all deaths. Although for Takotsubo cardiomyopathy is often reversible, it may recur in up to 5% to 10%.[80]

CARDIAC SURGERY

Coronary Artery Bypass Graft

Coronary artery bypass graft (CABG) surgery is a common procedure for the treatment of obstructive CAD for both men and women in the United States. Women undergo approximately 32% of CABG procedures annually.[1] For over 40 years, there has been a persistent sex disparity in outcomes with CABG, with women having higher perioperative morbidity and mortality after CABG than men.[84] When examining five US states from 2007 to 2014 which included 340,080 patients, women were 32% more likely to die compared with men, after adjusting for other factors including age, race, insurance, income, comorbidity index, surgical volumes, and year of procedure (adjusted OR 1.32, 95% CI 1.25 to 1.40). Women also had significantly greater risk of 30-day and 90-day readmissions. These sex differences noted have typically been explained by baseline differences in age, body size, coronary artery diameter, ASCVD risk factors, and other comorbidities. Nonetheless, risk assessment score includes sex as part of estimating risk of CABG, independent of other predictors. In an analysis of 72,824 patients women had significantly higher age–standardized mortality rate than men after CABG and combined CABG/mitral valve surgery. Men had lower rates of long-term mortality than women after isolated mitral valve repair, whereas women had lower rates of long-term mortality than men after isolated mitral valve replacement. There was a statistically significant association between female sex and long-term mortality after adjustment for key risk factors.[85] Data has been mixed in terms of outcomes based on sex, when off-pump CABG is performed. More contemporary cohorts have not shown a protective effect of off-pump CABG for women.

Valvular Heart Surgery

There are no sex-specific guidelines for valvular heart disease and valve surgery, although there are sex-specific outcome data after valve surgery. AS is the most common indication for valve replacement and women are older than men when presenting with symptomatic AS, have more exertional dyspnea, higher frailty scores, and more severe AS.[86] Smaller body size may also impact prosthetic valve size and affect outcomes, and as expected short-term survival is worse for women who undergo surgical replacement of the aortic valve.[86] Nonetheless, long-term outcomes suggest no gender differences in outcomes, and may even potentially favor women.

For mitral valve replacement surgery, regardless of type of valve replacement (mechanical or bioprosthetic), the evidence is inconsistent, with studies demonstrating women do worse than men, some with no difference in outcomes based on sex, and yet other studies demonstrating women have better long-term survival compared with men.[87] All risk calculators take sex into consideration and the risk scores are elevated for women compared with men.

Transcatheter Aortic Valve Intervention

Women referred for transcatheter aortic valve intervention (TAVI) have the same risk profile as women who are referred for surgical AVR. Female anatomy affects TAVI as well, including shorter distances from the coronary ostia to the annulus, increased calcification, and a more horizontal aorta, which can result in coronary obstruction necessitating conversion to open surgery.[88] On the other hand, small annuli in women results in less paravalvular regurgitation. Early TAVI trials limited transfemoral access in women due to lack of small sheath sizes but over time, the equipment has evolved.

In the early PARTNER trial of high-risk and inoperable patients with severe AS (1220 women and 1339 men), women had lower rates of renal disease, smoking, hyperlipidemia, and diabetes, yet higher STS mortality risk compared with men. Despite noting increased vascular and major bleeding complication in women, women had lower 1-year mortality rates with TAVI compared with men (19.0% vs. 25.6%, $P < 0.001$).[89] Women undergoing TAVI in a number of trials have demonstrated equal 30-day survival, but better long-term survival compared with men.[88–90]

Transcatheter Mitral Valve Repair

Recent data regarding transcatheter mitral valve repair (TMVR) with percutaneous edge-to-edge repair (MitraClip) has shown no difference by sex in terms of rehospitalization for HF but superior long-term survival in women compared with men.[91]

PERIPHERAL ARTERIAL DISEASE (see also Chapter 43)

Peripheral arterial disease (PAD) has a high prevalence in women in the United States, increasing with age and ranging from 2% at age 40 to as high as 25% in women 80 years or older, with more women with PAD over the age of 40 years compared with men. The incidence of PAD in women with chronic kidney disease has demonstrated significant sex differences, with women having a 1.53-fold greater adjusted PAD risk, compared to men in the Chronic Renal Insufficiency Cohort ($P < 0.001$).[92] Lower extremity PAD associates with equal morbidity and mortality and comparable health costs as IHD and ischemic stroke. PAD can be assessed using the ankle-brachial index (ABI), with the diagnosis of PAD when the ABI is less than 0.9.

There are sex differences in PAD symptoms. Women with PAD can lack the classical symptom of intermittent claudication and women are more likely to be asymptomatic than men. Like other CVD, there appears to be a long "latent phase" that can progress over time in women. In the K–VIS ELLA registry, a nationwide, multicenter, observational study that includes 3073 PAD patients undergoing endovascular therapy, women had higher rates of death, myocardial infarction, and major amputation than men and higher rates of complex lesions, procedural complications, and limb–specific adverse events.[93]

Women had lower amputation rates but still have persistent higher mortality than men.[94] Some studies have demonstrated that women with PAD that undergo endovascular therapy have poorer outcomes. Sex differences on survival after lower extremity PAD revascularization have been inconsistent but gender is often confounded by morbidity, age, and procedural factors that impact perioperative mortality. Women remain underrepresented in studies of PAD, contributing to the lack of sex-specific data or therapies.

Other forms of PAD also demonstrate sex differences. A single center in Canada has shown retrospectively that thoracic aortic aneurysms grow twice as fast in women, with aortic stiffness associated with the aneurysm growth in women but not in men.[95] Renal artery stenosis and abdominal aortic aneurysms are more common in men than women. Because abdominal aortic aneurysms are four times more likely in men, and less frequently associated with deaths in women, screening in asymptomatic women is not recommended, in contrast with men.[96]

HEART FAILURE (see also Chapters 47–52)

HF prevalence is increasing, and affects 3.2 million women in the United States, accounting for 54% of all people living with HF.[1] In 2016, there were 43,656 deaths in women due to HF, which accounted for more deaths in women compared with men (54.2% vs. 45.8%). Community surveillance data show that rates of hospitalization for HF are increasing over time, due to an increase in heart failure with preserved ejection fraction (HFpEF), which occurs more frequently in women.[97]

The risk factors associated with HF and its underlying pathophysiology differ by sex. Traditional risk factors, such as diabetes, obesity, hypertension, and tobacco use impact the risk of HF more in women than men. Additionally, psychological stress, a cause of Takotsubo cardiomyopathy, appears to have a greater impact on women than men. Women with HF have more hypertension, valvular heart disease, and thyroid disorders than men, but are less likely to have obstructive CAD. Even though obstructive CAD is less frequent in women, when it is present it is a stronger risk factor for the development of HF than hypertension. Risk factors selective for women include cardiac toxicity from chemotherapeutic drugs and radiation used for treatment of breast cancer and reproductive factors that can result in peripartum cardiomyopathy. Women who present with acute decompensated HF are twice as likely as men to have preserved left ventricular function or HFpEF[98] with obesity being a significant risk factor for women with HFpEF, particularly in African American women.[98] Even those women with an impaired LVEF will have a higher LVEF when compared with men. Notably, women with HF have a lower quality of life, lower functional capacity, more hospitalizations for HF, and more frequent depression. Nonetheless, overall survival is better for women compared with men with HF. This is not just a result of women having more HFpEF because mortality rates from HF do not relate to preserved or impaired ejection fraction in either sex, although those with ischemic cardiomyopathy have a worse prognosis.[99]

Peripartum Cardiomyopathy (see also Chapter 92)

Peripartum cardiomyopathy causes impaired LVEF that occurs in the last month of pregnancy or in the months after delivery (although the exact timing remains ill-defined) with no pre-existing cardiac disease and no identifiable cause.[100] Its incidence is estimated to be 1 in 4000 pregnancies and is associated with risk factors including advanced maternal age, African descent, high parity, twin pregnancy, usage of tocolytics, and poverty. After the diagnosis, about half recover their LVEF within 6 months, however 20% deteriorate and either die or require heart transplantation. Recovery appears to be related to a less severe decline in LVEF.[101] The risk of recurrence during subsequent pregnancy is greater in those with persistent left ventricular dysfunction (48% with significant deterioration, 16% died), although even those who recover have a high risk of recurrence (27% showed deterioration, no deaths).[102]

Heart Failure Diagnosis

There appear to be sex differences in the biomarker brain natriuretic peptide (BNP) used to diagnose HF and markers of cardiac stretch (natriuretic peptides) and fibrosis (galectin-3) are higher in women, whereas markers of cardiac injury (cardiac troponins) and inflammation (sST2) are higher in men.[103] Such differences may reflect sex-specific pathogenic processes associated with HF risk, but may also arise as a result of differences in sex hormone profiles and fat distribution. From a clinical perspective, sex-related differences in biomarker levels may affect the objectivity of biomarkers in HF management because what is considered to be "normal" in one sex may not be so in the other. Further studies are needed to delineate and understand the sex differences in HF biomarkers.

Heart Failure Treatment

Treatment for HF may benefit both sexes equally, however the under-representation of women in HF trials and the more prevalent HFpEF in women contributes to our lack of evidence regarding treatment of HF in women. The CHARM trials, along with others, showed women were more likely to have preserved left ventricular function (50%) than men (35%).[98] More recently, the PARAGON-HF trial demonstrated that angiotensin neprilysin inhibitor sacubitril/valsartan appeared to benefit women with HFpEF more than men.[104] Although the study did not show a difference overall in its primary outcomes of total HF hospitalization and CV deaths, it did show a significant 28% reduction in this endpoint in women, when compared to valsartan alone (rate ratio 0.73, 95% CI 0.59 to 0.90). Women with HFpEF are more symptomatic and have worse quality of life, but had lower mortality and fewer HF hospitalizations (Fig. 91.5).[105]

Device Use in Heart Failure

Implantable cardioverter-defibrillator (ICD) devices are underused in both sexes with HF, but particularly in women. None of the randomized trials for ICDs enrolled sufficient numbers of women to permit conclusions regarding sex differences and hence, have not demonstrated a mortality benefit in women. The differences may result in part from sex differences in body size and delayed presentation in women. Women are less likely to receive a defibrillator or CRT than men.[105] Examining ICD implantation for primary prevention in 11 countries in Europe between 2002 and 2014 finds fewer women received an ICD (19% of all ICD implantations). Nonetheless, women had a significantly lower mortality but also received fewer appropriate ICD shocks than men.[106]

CRT also shows benefit in both women and men with HF and wide QRS complex, but observational data from the National Cardiovascular Data Registry demonstrated that the mortality benefit is more pronounced in women, confirming earlier randomized trials that compared CRT to medical therapy alone.[107] Nonetheless, these devices are underused in women, as demonstrated in the Nationwide Inpatient Sample and Medicare/Medicaid Data.[108]

Mechanical Circulatory Support

Mechanical circulatory support (MCS) can bridge an HF patient to transplant or extend life. The commonest form of MCS is a left ventricular assist device (LVAD), and most LVADs are implanted into men (79%).[109] Looking at the Nationwide Inpatient Sample from 2004 to 2016, although LVADs are used more and have gotten smaller and more durable, women received these devices even less frequently, representing 26% of LVADs in 2004 and 22% by 2016.[110]

Cardiac Transplantation

Women are less likely to be listed for transplant and are less likely to receive a transplant, despite shorter waiting times for women. As of 2016, only 26% of all heart transplants in the United States occurred in women.[111] This, despite that fact that there appears to be no significant survival difference based on sex.[112] The survival difference is when waiting for transplantation. Women on LVAD support are less likely to be transplanted (62% vs. 76%, $P < 0.001$) and more likely to die or be removed from the transplant list as a result of worsening clinical status.[109] Female sex was a significant predictor of waitlist mortality (HR 1.51, $P < 0.001$).

Women who undergo heart transplantation have lower-risk features than men, with less IHD, diabetes, hypertension, smoking history, or prior cardiac surgery than men.[112] Women who eventually get a heart transplant do equally as well as men, despite the fact that women often get higher-risk transplanted hearts than men.[112]

ARRYTHMIA AND SUDDEN CARDIAC DEATH

Important sex differences in cardiac electrophysiology can impact arrhythmias and sudden cardiac death. Starting at puberty, women have higher resting heart rates compared to men. Women also have longer QT intervals, and a greater risk for drug-induced torsades de pointes. There are sex differences in the supraventricular tachycardias (SVTs). Atrioventricular (AV) nodal reentrant tachycardia (AVNRT) is twice as common in women as compared to men, compared to AV reentrant tachycardia as seen in the Wolff-Parkinson-White syndrome which is more common in men. Atrial and ventricular fibrillation also occur more frequently in men with Wolff-Parkinson-White syndrome. Globally, there continues to be an increase in the incidence and prevalence of atrial fibrillation for both men and women, but age-adjusted mortality due to atrial fibrillation has been shown to be comparable in women and men.[113] Compared to men, women with atrial fibrillation tend to be more symptomatic, have a higher risk of stroke and mortality, are less likely to receive anticoagulation and ablation procedures than men, and yet fare worse when treated with antiarrhythmic medications.[114] Women who experience sudden cardiac death are

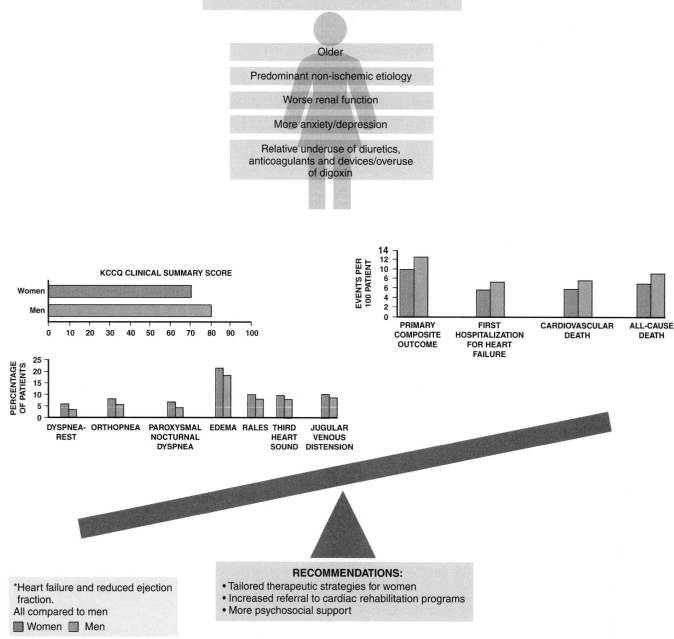

FIGURE 91.5 Women with heart failure with reduced ejection fraction. (From Dewan P, Rørth R, Jhund PS, et al. Differential impact of heart failure with reduced ejection fraction on men and women. *J Am Coll Cardiol.* 2019;73:29–40.)

older than men, and are less likely to have ischemic causes of sudden cardiac death.[115] Although women have an overall lower risk of sudden cardiac death, women with cardiac arrest who receive therapeutic hypothermia have significantly better outcomes than men, but are less likely than men to get recommended treatment after an out-of-hospital cardiac arrest.[116]

CARDIOVASCULAR DISEASE PREVENTION

Guidelines for CVD prevention in women were largely based on the "Effectiveness-Based Guidelines for the Prevention of Cardiovascular Disease in Women—2011 Update" but have been replaced by the 2018 ACC/AHA evidence-based guidelines on the treatment of blood cholesterol to reduce ASCVD in adults[8] and the 2019 ACC/AHA guidelines on the primary prevention of CVD.[7] These guidelines apply to both

women and men, with the focus on primary prevention of CVD. Secondary CVD prevention must be implemented once a diagnosis of CVD has been made.

An important component of secondary CVD prevention includes cardiac rehabilitation (see also Chapter 33). Cardiac rehabilitation improves functional capacity, decreases anginal symptoms, facilitates CVD risk reduction, and improves psychosocial well-being in both sexes. It also improves quality of life and medication compliance and reduces morbidity and mortality. Both sexes should be referred to cardiac rehabilitation after experiencing angina, any type of MI, postcoronary revascularization (either CABG or PCI), after valvular heart surgery, and those with chronic HF.[117] Nonetheless, cardiac rehabilitation is remarkably underused in the United States, with an estimated participation rate of only 10% to 20% of eligible patients, with women particularly under-referred and less likely to complete cardiac rehabilitation even if they enroll.[61]

ACKNOWLEDGMENTS

This work was supported by contracts from the National Heart, Lung and Blood Institutes, nos. N01-HV-68161, N01-HV-68162, N01-HV-68163, N01-HV-68164, grants U0164829, U01 HL649141, U01 HL649241, T32HL69751, 1R03AG032631 from the National Institute on Aging, GCRC grant MO1-RR00425 from the National Center for Research Resources and grants from the Gustavus and Louis Pfeiffer Research Foundation, Danville, NJ, The Women's Guild of Cedars-Sinai Medical Center, Los Angeles, CA, the Ladies Hospital Aid Society of Western Pennsylvania, Pittsburgh, PA, and QMED, Inc., Laurence Harbor, NJ, the Edythe L. Broad Women's Heart Research Fellowship, Cedars-Sinai Medical Center, Los Angeles, California, the Barbra Streisand Women's Cardiovascular Research and Education Program, Cedars-Sinai Medical Center, Los Angeles, The Society for Women's Health Research (SWHR), Washington, D.C. and the Linda Joy Pollin Women's Heart Health Program, and the Erika Glazer Women's Heart Health Project, Cedars-Sinai Medical Center, Los Angeles, California (CNBM).

REFERENCES

Epidemiology

1. Virani SS, et al. Heart disease and stroke statistics-2021 update: a report from the American Heart Association. *Circulation*; 2021:143(8):e254–e743.
2. Arora S, Stouffer GA, Kucharska-Newton AM, et al. Twenty year trends and sex differences in young adults hospitalized with acute myocardial infarction. *Circulation*. 2019;139:1047–1056.
3. Bairey Merz CN, Andersen H, Sprague E, et al. Knowledge, attitudes, and beliefs regarding cardiovascular disease in women: the women's heart alliance. *J Am Coll Cardiol*. 2017;70:123–132.
4. *Exploring the Biological Contributions to Human Health: Does Sex Matter?* The National Academies Press; 2001.
5. Hajek C, Guo X, Yao J, et al. Coronary heart disease genetic risk score predicts cardiovascular disease risk in men, not women. *Circ Genom Precis Med*. 2018;11:e002324.

Risk Factors

6. Arnett DK, Blumenthal RS, Albert MA, et al. 2019 ACC/AHA guideline on the primary prevention of cardiovascular disease: executive summary: a report of the American College of Cardiology/American heart association task force on clinical practice guidelines. *J Am Coll Cardiol*. 2019;74:1376–1414.
7. Wilmot KA, O'Flaherty M, Capewell S, et al. Coronary heart disease mortality declines in the United States from 1979 through 2011: evidence for stagnation in young adults, especially women. *Circulation*. 2015;132:997–1002.
8. Grundy SM, Stone NJ, Bailey AL, et al. 2018 AHA/ACC/AACVPR/AAPA/ABC/ACPM/ADA/AGS/APhA/ASPC/NLA/PCNA guideline on the management of blood cholesterol: a report of the American College of Cardiology/American heart association task force on clinical practice guidelines. *J Am Coll Cardiol*. 2019;73:e285–e350.
9. Whelton PK, Carey RM, Aronow WS, et al. 2017 ACC/AHA/AAPA/ABC/ACPM/AGS/APhA/ASH/ASPC/NMA/PCNA guideline for the prevention, detection, evaluation, and management of high blood pressure in adults: executive summary: a report of the American College of Cardiology/American heart association task force on clinical practice guidelines. *J Am Coll Cardiol*. 2018;71:2199–2269.
10. Ostchega Y, Fryar CD, Nwankwo T, Nguyen DT. *Hypertension Prevalence Among Adults Aged 18 and over: United States, 2017–2018*; 2020.
11. Fryar CD, Ostchega Y, Hales CM, et al. *Hypertension Prevalence and Control Among Adults: United States, 2015–2016*. NCHS Data Brief; 2017:1–8.
12. Giribela CR, Consolim-Colombo FM, Nisenbaum MG, et al. Effects of a combined oral contraceptive containing 20 mcg of ethinylestradiol and 3 mg of drospirenone on the blood pressure, renin-angiotensin-aldosterone system, insulin resistance, and androgenic profile of healthy young women. *Gynecol Endocrinol*. 2015;31:912–915.
13. Ji H, Kim A, Ebinger JE, et al. Sex differences in blood pressure trajectories over the life course. *JAMA Cardiol*. 2020.
14. Regensteiner JG, Golden S, Huebschmann AG, et al. Sex differences in the cardiovascular consequences of diabetes mellitus: a scientific statement from the American heart association. *Circulation*. 2015;132:2424–2447.
15. Huxley RR, Peters SA, Mishra GD, Woodward M. Risk of all-cause mortality and vascular events in women versus men with type 1 diabetes: a systematic review and meta-analysis. *Lancet Diabetes Endocrinol*. 2015;3:198–206.
16. Professional Practice Committee. Standards of medical care in diabetes-2020. *Diabetes Care*. 2020;43:S3.
17. Carroll MD, Fryar CD. *Total and High-Density Lipoprotein Cholesterol in Adults: United States, 2015–2018*; 2020.
18. Nanna MG, Wang TY, Xiang Q, et al. Sex differences in the use of statins in community practice. *Circ Cardiovasc Qual Outcomes*. 2019;12:e005562.
19. Polotsky HN, Polotsky AJ. Metabolic implications of menopause. *Semin Reprod Med*. 2010;28:426–434.
20. Creamer MR, Wang TW, Babb S, et al. Tobacco product use and cessation indicators among adults—United States, 2018. *MMWR Morb Mortal Wkly Rep*. 2019;68:1013–1019.
21. Palmer J, Lloyd A, Steele L, et al. Differential risk of ST-segment elevation myocardial infarction in male and female smokers. *J Am Coll Cardiol*. 2019;73:3259–3266.
22. Pirie K, Peto R, Reeves GK, et al. The 21st century hazards of smoking and benefits of stopping: a prospective study of one million women in the UK. *Lancet*. 2013;381:133–141.
23. McKee SA, Smith PH, Kaufman M, et al. Sex differences in varenicline efficacy for smoking cessation: a meta-analysis. *Nicotine Tob Res*. 2016;18:1002–1011.
24. Centers for Disease Control and Prevention. *Participation in Leisure-Time Aerobic and Muscle-Strengthening Activities that Meet the Federal 2008 Physical Activity Guidelines for Americans Among Adults Aged 18 and over, by Selected Characteristics: United States, Selected Years 1998–2017*; 2017:2020.
25. Chomistek AK, Cook NR, Rimm EB, et al. Physical activity and incident cardiovascular disease in women: is the relation modified by level of global cardiovascular risk? *J Am Heart Assoc*. 2018;7.
26. Imboden MT, Harber MP, Whaley MH, et al. Cardiorespiratory fitness and mortality in healthy men and women. *J Am Coll Cardiol*. 2018;72:2283–2292.
27. Shin D, Kongpakpaisarn K, Bohra C. Trends in the prevalence of metabolic syndrome and its components in the United States 2007–2014. *Int J Cardiol*. 2018;259:216–219.
28. Kazlauskiene L, Butnoriene J, Norkus A. Metabolic syndrome related to cardiovascular events in a 10-year prospective study. *Diabetol Metab Syndr*. 2015;7:102.
29. Hales CM, Carroll MD, Fryar CD, Ogden CL. *Prevalence of Obesity and Severe Obesity Among Adults: United States, 2017–2018*. NCHS Data Brief; 2020.
30. Manrique-Acevedo C, Chinnakotla B, Padilla J, et al. Obesity and cardiovascular disease in women. *Int J Obes (Lond)*. 2020;44:1210–1226.
31. Farrell SW, Barlow CE, Willis BL, et al. Cardiorespiratory fitness, different measures of adiposity, and cardiovascular disease mortality risk in women. *J Womens Health (Larchmt)*. 2020;29:319–326.
32. da Silva Paulitsch F, Zhang L. Continuous positive airway pressure for adults with obstructive sleep apnea and cardiovascular disease: a meta-analysis of randomized trials. *Sleep Med*. 2019;54:28–34.

Pregnancy and Endocrine Considerations

33. Lee JJ, Cook-Wiens G, Johnson BD, et al. Age at menarche and risk of cardiovascular disease outcomes: findings from the national heart Lung and blood institute-sponsored women's ischemia syndrome evaluation. *J Am Heart Assoc*. 2019;8:e012406.
34. Wu P, Gulati M, Kwok CS, et al. Preterm delivery and future risk of maternal cardiovascular disease: a systematic review and meta-analysis. *J Am Heart Assoc*. 2018;7.
35. Haas DM, Ehrenthal DB, Koch MA, et al. Pregnancy as a window to future cardiovascular health: design and implementation of the nuMoM2b heart health study. *Am J Epidemiol*. 2016;183:519–530.
36. Honigberg MC, Zekavat SM, Aragam K, et al. Long-term cardiovascular risk in women with hypertension during pregnancy. *J Am Coll Cardiol*. 2019;74:2743–2754.
37. Lo CCW, Lo ACQ, Leow SH, et al. Future cardiovascular disease risk for women with gestational hypertension: a systematic review and meta-analysis. *J Am Heart Assoc*. 2020:e013991.
38. Benschop L, Duvekot JJ, Roeters van Lennep JE. Future risk of cardiovascular disease risk factors and events in women after a hypertensive disorder of pregnancy. *Heart*. 2019;105:1273–1278.
39. Kramer CK, Campbell S, Retnakaran R. Gestational diabetes and the risk of cardiovascular disease in women: a systematic review and meta-analysis. *Diabetologia*. 2019;62:905–914.
40. Dayan N, Filion KB, Okano M, et al. Cardiovascular risk following fertility therapy: systematic review and meta-analysis. *J Am Coll Cardiol*. 2017;70:1203–1213.
41. Udell JA, Lu H, Redelmeier DA. Failure of fertility therapy and subsequent adverse cardiovascular events. *CMAJ*. 2017;189:E391–E397.
42. Merz CN, Shaw LJ, Azziz R, et al. Cardiovascular disease and 10-year mortality in postmenopausal women with clinical features of polycystic ovary syndrome. *J Womens Health (Larchmt)*. 2016;25:875–881.
43. Shufelt CL, Torbati T, Dutra E. Hypothalamic amenorrhea and the long-term health consequences. *Semin Reprod Med*. 2017;35:256–262.
44. Muka T, Oliver-Williams C, Kunutsor S, et al. Association of age at onset of menopause and time since onset of menopause with cardiovascular outcomes, intermediate vascular traits, and all-cause mortality: a systematic review and meta-analysis. *JAMA Cardiol*. 2016;1:767–776.
45. Peters SA, Woodward M. Women's reproductive factors and incident cardiovascular disease in the UK Biobank. *Heart*. 2018;104:1069–1075.
46. Christ J, Gunning M, Palla G, et al. Prolonged estrogen deprivation is associated with increased cardiovascular disease risk among women with primary ovarian insufficiency. *Fertil Steril*. 2017;108:e392.
47. Roeters van Lennep JE, Heida KY, Bots ML, et al. Cardiovascular disease risk in women with premature ovarian insufficiency: a systematic review and meta-analysis. *Eur J Prev Cardiol*. 2016;23:178–186.
48. Curtis KM, Jatlaoui TC, Tepper NK, et al. U.S. Selected practice recommendations for contraceptive use, 2016. *MMWR Recomm Rep (Morb Mortal Wkly Rep)*. 2016;65:1–66.
49. The 2017 hormone therapy position statement of the North American Menopause Society. *Menopause*. 2018;25:1362–1387.
50. Faccini A, Kaski JC, Camici PG. Coronary microvascular dysfunction in chronic inflammatory rheumatoid diseases. *Eur Heart J*. 2016;37:1799–1806.
51. Bradshaw PT, Stevens J, Khankari N, et al. Cardiovascular disease mortality among breast cancer survivors. *Epidemiology*. 2016;27:6–13.
52. Gulati M, Mulvagh SL. The connection between the breast and heart in a woman: breast cancer and cardiovascular disease. *Clin Cardiol*. 2018;41:253–257.
53. Lichtman JH, Leifheit EC, Safdar B, et al. Sex differences in the presentation and perception of symptoms among young patients with myocardial infarction: evidence from the VIRGO study (variation in recovery: role of gender on outcomes of young AMI patients). *Circulation*. 2018;137:781–790.
54. McSweeney JC, Rosenfeld AG, Abel WM, et al. Preventing and experiencing ischemic heart disease as a woman: state of the science: a scientific statement from the American Heart Association. *Circulation*. 2016;133:1302–1331.
55. Ferry AV, Anand A, Strachan FE, et al. Presenting symptoms in men and women diagnosed with myocardial infarction using sex-specific criteria. *J Am Heart Assoc*. 2019;8:e012307.
56. Bugiardini R, Ricci B, Cenko E, et al. Delayed care and mortality among women and men with myocardial infarction. *J Am Heart Assoc*. 2017;6.
57. Hendel RC, Jabbar AY, Mahata I. Initial diagnostic evaluation of stable coronary artery disease: the need for a patient-centered strategy. *J Am Heart Assoc*. 2017;6.
58. Hemal K, Pagidipati NJ, Coles A, et al. Sex differences in demographics, risk factors, presentation, and noninvasive testing in stable outpatients with suspected coronary artery disease: insights from the PROMISE trial. *JACC Cardiovasc Imaging*. 2016;9:337–346.

Ischemic Heart Disease

59. SCOT-Heart Investigators, Newby DE, Adamson PD, et al. Coronary CT angiography and 5-year risk of myocardial infarction. *N Engl J Med*. 2018;379:924–933.
60. Douglas PS, Hoffmann U, Patel MR, et al. Outcomes of anatomical versus functional testing for coronary artery disease. *N Engl J Med*. 2015;372:1291–1300.
61. Li S, Fonarow GC, Mukamal K, et al. Sex and racial disparities in cardiac rehabilitation referral at hospital discharge and Gaps in long-term mortality. *J Am Heart Assoc*. 2018;7.
62. Alabas OA, Gale CP, Hall M, et al. Sex differences in treatments, relative survival, and excess mortality following acute myocardial infarction: national cohort study using the SWEDEHEART registry. *J Am Heart Assoc*. 2017;6.
63. Anstey DE, Li S, Thomas L, et al. Race and sex differences in management and outcomes of patients after ST-elevation and non-ST-elevation myocardial infarct: results from the NCDR. *Clin Cardiol*. 2016;39:585–595.
64. Smilowitz NR, Mahajan AM, Roe MT, et al. Mortality of myocardial infarction by sex, age, and obstructive coronary artery disease status in the ACTION registry-GWTG (acute coronary treatment and intervention outcomes network registry-get with the guidelines). *Circ Cardiovasc Qual Outcomes*. 2017;10:e003443.
65. Malik JS, Jenner C, Ward PA. Maximising application of the aerosol box in protecting healthcare workers during the COVID-19 pandemic. *Anaesthesia*. 2020;75:974–975.
66. Liu J, Elbadawi A, Elgendy IY, et al. Age-stratified sex disparities in care and outcomes in patients with ST-elevation myocardial infarction. *Am J Med*. 2020.
67. Kosmidou I, Redfors B, Selker HP, et al. Infarct size, left ventricular function, and prognosis in women compared to men after primary percutaneous coronary intervention in ST-segment

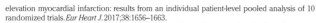

1722

CARDIOVASCULAR DISEASE IN SELECT POPULATIONS

X

elevation myocardial infarction: results from an individual patient-level pooled analysis of 10 randomized trials. *Eur Heart J*. 2017;38:1656–1663.

68. Burgess SN, Juergens CP, Nguyen TL, et al. Comparison of late cardiac death and myocardial infarction rates in women Vs. Men with ST-elevation myocardial infarction. *Am J Cardiol*. 2020;128:120–126.

69. Chichareon P, Modolo R, Kerkmeijer L, et al. Association of sex with outcomes in patients undergoing percutaneous coronary intervention: a subgroup Analysis of the GLOBAL LEADERS randomized clinical trial. *JAMA Cardiol*. 2019;1–10.

70. Potts J, Sirker A, Martinez SC, et al. Persistent sex disparities in clinical outcomes with percutaneous coronary intervention: Insights from 6.6 million PCI procedures in the United States. *PloS One*. 2018;13:e0203325.

71. Zhao M, Vaartjes I, Graham I, et al. Sex differences in risk factor management of coronary heart disease across three regions. *Heart*. 2017;103:1587–1594.

72. Tamis-Holland JE, Jneid H, Reynolds HR, et al. Contemporary diagnosis and management of patients with myocardial infarction in the absence of obstructive coronary artery disease: a scientific statement from the American heart association. *Circulation*. 2019;139:e891–e908.

73. Knuuti J, Wijns W, Aet al S. 2019 ESC Guidelines for the diagnosis and management of chronic coronary syndromes: the task force for the diagnosis and management of chronic coronary syndromes of the European Society of Cardiology (ESC). *Eur Heart J*. 2019;41:407–477.

74. Bairey Merz CN, Pepine CJ, Walsh MN, Fleg JL. Ischemia And No Obstructive Coronary Artery Disease (INOCA): developing evidence-based therapies and research agenda for the next decade. *Circulation*. 2017;135:1075–1092.

75. Ouellette ML, Loffler AI, Beller GA, et al. Clinical characteristics, sex differences, and outcomes in patients with normal or Near-normal coronary arteries, non-obstructive or obstructive coronary artery disease. *J Am Heart Assoc*. 2018;7.

76. Kenkre TS, Malhotra P, Johnson BD, et al. Ten-year mortality in the WISE study (Women's Ischemia Syndrome Evaluation). *Circ Cardiovasc Qual Outcomes*. 2017;10.

77. AlBadri A, Bairey Merz CN, Johnson BD, et al. Impact of abnormal coronary reactivity on long-term clinical outcomes in women. *J Am Coll Cardiol*. 2019;73:684–693.

78. Pasupathy S, Air T, Dreyer RP, et al. Systematic review of patients presenting with suspected myocardial infarction and nonobstructive coronary arteries. *Circulation*. 2015;131:861–870.

79. Tamis-Holland JE, Jneid H, Reynolds HR, et al. Contemporary diagnosis and management of patients with myocardial infarction in the absence of obstructive coronary artery disease: a scientific statement from the American Heart Association. *Circulation*. 2019;139:e891–e908.

80. El-Battrawy I, Santoro F, Stiermaier T, et al. Incidence and clinical impact of recurrent takotsubo syndrome: results from the GEIST registry. *J Am Heart Assoc*. 2019;8:e010753.

81. Thygesen K, Alpert JS, Jaffe AS, et al. Fourth universal definition of myocardial infarction (2018). *Circulation*. 2018;138:e618–e651.

82. Manginas A, Rigopoulos AG, Bigalke B, et al. Takotsubo syndrome—adding pieces to a complex puzzle. *BMC Cardiovasc Disord*. 2017;17:296.

83. Tornvall P, Collste O, Ehrenborg E, Jarnbert-Petterson H. A case-control study of risk markers and mortality in takotsubo stress cardiomyopathy. *J Am Coll Cardiol*. 2016;67:1931–1936.

84. Gupta S, Lui B, Ma X, et al. Sex differences in outcomes after coronary artery bypass grafting. *J Cardiothorac Vasc Anesth*. 2020.

85. Johnston A, Mesana TG, Lee DS, et al. Sex differences In long-term survival after major cardiac surgery: a population-based cohort study. *J Am Heart Assoc*. 2019;8:e013260.

Vascular Disease

86. Chaker Z, Badhwar V, Alqahtani F, et al. Sex differences in the utilization and outcomes of surgical aortic valve replacement for severe aortic stenosis. *J Am Heart Assoc*. 2017;6.

87. Mantovani A, Clavel MA, Michelena HI, et al. Enriquez-Sarano M. Comprehensive imaging in women with organic mitral regurgitation: implications for clinical outcome. *JACC Cardiovasc Imaging*. 2016;9:388–396.

88. Chandrasekhar J, Dangas G, Yu J, et al. Sex-based differences in outcomes with transcatheter aortic valve therapy: TVT registry from 2011 to 2014. *J Am Coll Cardiol*. 2016;68:2733–2744.

89. Kodali S, Williams MR, Doshi D, et al. Sex-specific differences at presentation and outcomes among patients undergoing transcatheter aortic valve replacement: a cohort study. *Ann Intern Med*. 2016;164:377–384.

90. Vlastra W, Chandrasekhar J, Garcia Del Blanco B, et al. Sex differences in transfemoral transcatheter aortic valve replacement. *J Am Coll Cardiol*. 2019;74:2758–2767.

91. Tigges E, Kalbacher D, Thomas C, et al. Transcatheter mitral valve repair in surgical high-risk patients: gender-specific acute and long-term outcomes. *BioMed Res Int*. 2016;2016:3934842.

Peripheral Arterial Disease

92. Wang GJ, Shaw PA, Townsend RR, et al. Sex differences in the incidence of peripheral artery disease in the chronic renal insufficiency cohort. *Circ Cardiovasc Qual Outcomes*. 2016;9:S86–S93.

93. Jackson EA, Munir K, Schreiber T, et al. Impact of sex on morbidity and mortality rates after lower extremity interventions for peripheral arterial disease: observations from the Blue Cross Blue Shield of Michigan Cardiovascular Consortium. *J Am Coll Cardiol*. 2014;63:2525–2530.

94. Schramm K, Rochon PJ. Gender differences in peripheral vascular disease. *Semin Intervent Radiol*. 2018;35:9–16.

95. Boczar KE, Cheung K, Boodhwani M, et al. Sex differences in thoracic aortic aneurysm growth. *Hypertension*. 2019;73:190–196.

96. Ali MU, Fitzpatrick-Lewis D, Miller J, et al. Screening for abdominal aortic aneurysm in asymptomatic adults. *J Vasc Surg*. 2016;64:1855–1868.

Heart Failure

97. Chang PP, Wruck LM, Shahar E, et al. Trends in hospitalizations and survival of acute decompensated heart failure in four US Communities (2005–2014): ARIC study community surveillance. *Circulation*. 2018;138:12–24.

98. Lam CSP, Arnott C, Beale AL, et al. Sex differences in heart failure. *Eur Heart J*. 2019;40:3859–3868c.

99. Beale AL, Nanayakkara S, Segan L, et al. Sex differences in heart failure with preserved ejection fraction pathophysiology: a detailed invasive hemodynamic and echocardiographic analysis. *JACC Heart Fail*. 2019;7:239–249.

100. Arany Z, Elkayam U. Peripartum cardiomyopathy. *Circulation*. 2016;133:1397–1409.

101. Davis MB, Arany Z, McNamara DM, et al. JACC state-of-the-art review. *J Am Coll Cardiol*. 2020;75:207–221.

102. McNamara DM, Elkayam U, Alharethi R, et al. Clinical outcomes for peripartum cardiomyopathy in North America: results of the IPAC study (investigations of pregnancy-associated cardiomyopathy). *J Am Coll Cardiol*. 2015;66:905–914.

103. Suthahar N, Meems LMG, Ho JE, de Boer RA. Sex-related differences in contemporary biomarkers for heart failure: a review. *Eur J Heart Fail*. 2020;22:775–788.

104. Solomon SD, McMurray JJV, Anand IS, et al. Angiotensin-neprilysin inhibition in heart failure with preserved ejection fraction. *N Engl J Med*. 2019;381:1609–1620.

105. Dewan P, Rorth R, Jhund PS, et al. Differential impact of heart failure with reduced ejection fraction on men and women. *J Am Coll Cardiol*. 2019;73:29–40.

106. Sticherling C, Arendacka B, Svendsen JH, et al. Sex differences in outcomes of primary prevention implantable cardioverter-defibrillator therapy: combined registry data from eleven European countries. *Europace*. 2018;20:963–970.

107. Zusterzeel R, Spatz ES, Curtis JP, et al. Cardiac resynchronization therapy in women versus men: observational comparative effectiveness study from the National Cardiovascular Data Registry. *Circ Cardiovasc Qual Outcomes*. 2015;8:S4–S11.

108. Randolph TC, Hellkamp AS, Zeitler EP, et al. Utilization of cardiac resynchronization therapy in eligible patients hospitalized for heart failure and its association with patient outcomes. *Am Heart J*. 2017;189:48–58.

109. DeFilippis EM, Truby LK, Garan AR, et al. Sex-related differences in use and outcomes of left ventricular assist devices as bridge to transplantation. *JACC Heart Fail*. 2019;7:250–257.

110. Joshi AA, Lerman JB, Sajja AP, et al. Sex-based differences in left ventricular assist device utilization: insights from the nationwide inpatient sample 2004 to 2016. *Circ Heart Fail*. 2019;12:e006082.

111. Colvin M, Smith JM, Hadley N, et al. OPTN/SRTR 2016 Annual data report: heart. *Am J Transplant*. 2018;18(suppl 1):291–362.

112. Moayedi Y, Fan CPS, Cherikh WS, et al. Survival outcomes after heart transplantation: does recipient sex matter? *Circ Heart Fail*. 2019;12:e006218.

113. Magnussen C, Niiranen TJ, Ojeda FM, et al. Sex differences and similarities in atrial fibrillation epidemiology, risk factors, and mortality in community cohorts: results from the biomarcare consortium (biomarker for cardiovascular risk assessment in Europe). *Circulation*. 2017;136:1588–1597.

114. Westerman S, Wenger N. Gender differences in atrial fibrillation: a review of epidemiology, management, and outcomes. *Curr Cardiol Rev*. 2019;15:136–144.

115. Haukilahti MAE, Holmstrom L, Vahatalo J, et al. Sudden cardiac death in women. *Circulation*. 2019;139:1012–1021.

116. Mumma BE, Umarov T. Sex differences in the prehospital management of out-of-hospital cardiac arrest. *Resuscitation*. 2016;105:161–164.

117. Thomas RJ, Balady G, Banka G, et al. 2018 ACC/AHA clinical performance and quality measures for cardiac rehabilitation: a report of the American College of Cardiology/American Heart Association task force on performance measures. *J Am Coll Cardiol*. 2018;71:1814–1837.

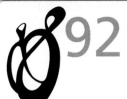

92 Pregnancy and Heart Disease

SAMUEL C. SIU AND CANDICE K. SILVERSIDES

Pregnancy results in hemodynamic and hormonal stress, which increases the risk of complications in women with heart disease. Over the past few decades, the number of pregnancies in women with cardiovascular disease has grown due to increases in the population of young women surviving with pediatric heart disease, older maternal age, and a higher prevalence of chronic medical conditions such as hypertension. Although many women are aware of their cardiovascular diagnosis prior to pregnancy, pregnancy can also unmask heart disease, and women can present with cardiovascular complications for the first time during pregnancy. Less commonly, pregnancy leads to de novo cardiac conditions, such as peripartum cardiomyopathy (PPCM) or coronary artery dissection. Along with increases in the population of pregnant women with cardiovascular disease, the field of cardio-obstetrics has grown, the medical community has a better understanding of pregnancy risks and treatment options, and standards of care have been established.[1-5] There is also increasing recognition that some pregnancy complications, such as preeclampsia, are associated with long-term maternal cardiovascular risks.[6]

The etiology of cardiac disease in women of childbearing age differs when compared with other cardiac cohorts. In high-income countries, congenital heart disease is the most common preexisting cardiac condition in pregnant women.[7,8] In contrast, rheumatic heart disease is much more common in low- and middle-income countries.[7] Arrhythmic disorders and cardiomyopathies are other commonly encountered cardiac conditions in cardio-obstetric clinics. Women may also have cardiovascular risk factors such has hypertension or diabetes, and these conditions are associated with adverse pregnancy outcomes.

During pregnancy, maternal morbidity and mortality are increased in women with heart disease.[8-10] Although maternal mortality secondary to cardiac disease is rare in high-income countries, when it occurs, it is frequently due to cardiovascular conditions such as cardiomyopathy, aortic dissection, or myocardial infarction (MI).[11,12] Maternal mortality is higher in low- and middle-income countries, and,[7] even in high-income countries, there are important racial differences.[13] In comparison, maternal cardiac morbidity is common and, depending on the population studied, occurs in 5% to 20% of pregnancies in women with heart disease.[7,8,14,15] The most common cardiac complications in women with heart disease are arrhythmias and heart failure. Timing of complications varies; arrhythmias typically occur in the second and third trimester, whereas heart failure occurs at the time of peak cardiac output, beginning at the end of second trimester and as well in the postpartum period (Fig. 92.1).[15] Some conditions, such as coarctation of the aorta, are associated with high rates of hypertensive disorders of pregnancy and preeclampsia. A significant proportion of maternal cardiovascular complications that occur in women with heart disease are preventable.[16,17]

Pregnancy complications may have late effects on maternal cardiovascular health. Pregnancy can lead to deterioration in ventricular or valve function, and, although these often return to normal after delivery, on occasion, deterioration can be permanent. For instance, pregnant women with atrial switch operations for complete transposition of the great arteries are at risk for permanent deterioration in subaortic right ventricular systolic function and worsening atrioventricular valve regurgitation.[18] Women with congenital heart disease who develop cardiac complications during pregnancy are at a higher risk of cardiovascular events later in life.[19] Similarly, women who develop complications related to placental dysfunction, such as preeclampsia and preterm birth, are at higher risk of maternal cardiovascular disease years after pregnancy compared with pregnant women who did not have complications.[6]

In addition to cardiac risks, pregnant women with cardiovascular disease are also at higher risk of obstetric and perinatal complications when compared with women without heart disease. For instance, women with Fontan operations or cyanotic heart disease and those using anticoagulants are at increased risk of postpartum hemorrhage.[20] Women with heart disease have higher rates of miscarriage, stillbirth, and neonatal death compared with women without heart disease.[8] Premature births and low birth weight babies are more common in women with heart disease, especially in women with complex congenital heart disease or pulmonary hypertension. In mothers and fathers with inherited cardiac conditions, transmission of heart disease to offspring can occur. The increased risk of obstetric and perinatal complications highlights the need for multidisciplinary care teams including maternal fetal medicine specialists, obstetric anesthetists, and neonatologists.

CARDIOVASCULAR CHANGES IN PREGNANCY

Pregnancy is associated with hemodynamic changes that are usually well tolerated in women with normal hearts. However, the hemodynamic changes of pregnancy can lead to cardiovascular complications, especially in women with preexisting heart disease. The hemodynamic changes of pregnancy begin as early as the sixth week of gestation, with increases in plasma volume (Table 92.1).[21] Early in pregnancy, the peripheral vascular resistance decreases and there is a corresponding small drop in blood pressure (BP) by 5 to 10 mm Hg below baseline until the third trimester, when the BP increases back to baseline. The heart rate increases by approximately

CARDIOVASCULAR DISEASE IN SELECT POPULATIONS X

10 beats/min above pre-pregnancy levels, and,[22] in combination with increases in stoke volume, there is a resultant increase in cardiac output by 30% to 50% (see Table 92.1). Twin pregnancies can increase the cardiac output by a further 10% to 15%. At the time of labor and delivery and immediately postpartum, cardiac output increases a further 60% to 80%. Catecholamines, release of inferior vena cava compression, autotransfusion from uterine contractions, and blood loss all contribute to further hemodynamic changes. Mobilization of fluid during the first week after delivery can result in heart failure in women with cardiomyopathy or severe outflow tract obstruction. Many of the hemodynamic changes resolve in the first 2 weeks after delivery, although complete resolution may take as long as 6 months. In addition to the hemodynamic changes, pregnancy results in increases in renal blood flow and glomerular filtration rate, cholesterol levels, insulin resistance, and clotting (see Table 92.1).

EVALUATION PRIOR TO PREGNANCY AND DURING PREGNANCY

Cardiac Findings During Normal Pregnancy

Fatigue, dyspnea, light-headedness, and palpitations are symptoms that can be associated with normal pregnancy.[23] Normal pregnancy results in cardiac examination findings including: (1) collapsing arterial pulses; (2) prominent jugular venous pulsations without elevation of jugular venous pressure; (3) laterally displaced apical impulse; (4) palpable right ventricle or pulmonary trunk; and (5) soft, short ejection systolic murmur best heard over the pulmonic area or left sternal border.[24] When it is difficult to differentiate between pregnancy-associated changes versus early cardiac decompensation, echocardiography, or B-type natriuretic peptide (BNP) level can be useful (a BNP value of 111 pg/mL has been proposed as having a positive likelihood ratio of 2.5 and a negative likelihood ratio of 0.1 for heart failure).[25] Pregnant women with heart disease have a higher BNP level than pregnant women without heart disease, and a BNP less than 100 pg/mL in the heart disease group had a 100% negative predictive value for cardiac complications.[26] Normal pregnancy is associated with electrocardiographic (sinus tachycardia, premature atrial or ventricular complexes, left QRS axis deviation, inferior Q waves, T wave flattening, ST depression, increased R/S ratio on right precordial leads) and chest radiographic (pleural effusion, straightening of left upper cardiac border, horizontal positioning of heart, increased lung vascular

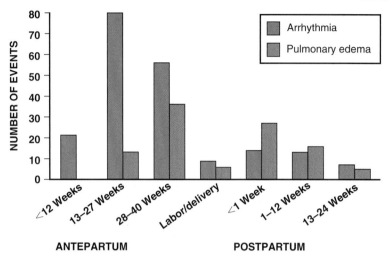

FIGURE 92.1 Timing of complications in women who develop arrhythmias or pulmonary edema during pregnancy. The y axis shows the total number of adverse events. The x axis shows the timing of presentation in women who develop pulmonary edema *(red bars)* or arrhythmias *(blue bars)*. (From Silversides CK, Grewal J, Mason J, et al. Pregnancy outcomes in women with heart disease: the CARPREG II study. *J Am Coll Cardiol.* 2018;71:2419–2430.)

TABLE 92.1 Normal Physiologic Changes in Pregnancy and Implications in Cardiovascular Conditions

ORGAN SYSTEM	NORMAL PHYSIOLOGIC CHANGES	IMPLICATIONS IN CARDIOVASCULAR CONDITIONS
Cardiovascular	During pregnancy: • ↑ Plasma flow (75%) ↑ cardiac output (CO) (30%–50%) ↓ systemic and pulmonary vascular resistance (SVR) and (PVR) During labor: • ↑ CO by 30% in active stage of labor • Increased circulating blood volume (300–500 mL) due to uterine contractions	• Cardiac complications in women with lesions that cannot tolerate volume loading (cardiomyopathy), decreases in SVR (Eisenmenger with intracardiac shunts) or with fixed obstruction (aortic or mitral stenosis) • Impaired hemodynamic adaptation • ↑ Mean arterial pressures (MAPs), SVR and ↓ CO in preeclampsia
Respiratory	• ↑ Metabolic rate and oxygen consumption • Mild compensated respiratory alkalosis	• Feeling of breathlessness during pregnancy • ↑ Minute ventilation in preeclampsia • Difficulty intubating in those who develop serious cardiac complications
Renal	• ↑ Plasma flow (75%) • ↑ Glomerular filtration rate (GFR) (40%–50%) • ↑ Proteinuria	• ↓ GFR ↓ uric acid clearance ↑ proteinuria in preeclampsia • Drug dosing may need to be adjusted based on GFR
Hematologic	• ↑ Plasma volume (50%) and red cell mass • ↑ Coagulation factors • ↓ Protein C • Compression of the inferior vena cava	• Physiologic anemia • ↑ Risk of thromboembolism in women with prosthetic heart valves, atrial fibrillation, Fontan circulation • ↓ Life span of platelets in and hemolysis in severe preeclampsia (HELLP syndrome)
Lipid metabolism	• ↑ Triglycerides, total cholesterol (50%) and in low-density lipoprotein cholesterol (LDL) (50%) and ↓ high-density lipoprotein cholesterol (HDL)	• ↑ Dyslipidemia with ↓ HDL ↑ free fatty acids in preeclampsia • Existing maternal dyslipidemia is associated with adverse pregnancy outcomes
Glucose metabolism	• ↑ Insulin resistance, mild diabetogenic state	• Gestational diabetes

From Sharma G, Ying Y, Silversides CK. The importance of cardiovascular risk assessment and pregnancy heart team in the management of cardiovascular disease in pregnancy. *Cardiol Clin.* 2020.

markings) findings that can mimic cardiac disease.[3,24] Similarly, one should be aware of the changes in echocardiographic data with normal pregnancy,[27] including: (1) increase in dimensions of all four cardiac chambers without changes in left ventricular ejection fraction; (2) increase in left ventricular wall thickness; (3) increasing degree of tricuspid regurgitation (TR) which usually does not exceed more than moderate in degree; and (4) changes in left ventricular mechanics (strain, twist, untwisting) and left atrial strain reflective of adaptive changes in LV volumes, mass, and loading conditions with advancing gestational age. Importantly the left ventricular diastolic dimension may exceed the normal limits reported in nonpregnant patients.[27]

Role of Cardiac Testing During Pregnancy

Transthoracic echocardiogram is the preferred imaging method in pregnancy, but imaging may be more technically challenging with cardiac displacement. When transesophageal echocardiography is performed in pregnancy to obtain data that cannot be obtained by transthoracic echocardiography, the imaging protocol should be abbreviated to minimize the potential risk of vomiting/aspiration due to delayed gastric emptying in pregnancy.[24] Exercise testing, with or without echocardiography, usually performed prior to pregnancy, should be limited to submaximal test if performed during pregnancy (peak heart rate not to exceed 70% to 80% of predicted maximum).[3,24] The use of dobutamine as a stress agent should be avoided.

The risk of fetal adverse outcome is highest with radiation exposure during the period of organogenesis during the first trimester.[28] A fetal exposure dose of less than 50 mGy is considered to be negligible risk. The fetal dose from chest radiography is less than 0.0001 mGy; however, maternal shielding should be used. Lung imaging with point of care ultrasound is an alternative when assessing for possible pulmonary edema or pulmonary pathology. Chest computed tomography (CT), if necessary for evaluation of pulmonary embolism or aortic pathology, should use low-radiation protocols (typically 0.01 to 0.66 mGy for CT pulmonary angiogram protocols). Cardiac magnetic resonance is an alternate to ionizing radiation imaging modalities, and gadolinium-based contrast should be avoided,[29] but may be less well tolerated due to greater time requirement for imaging. When cardiac catheterization is performed during pregnancy, radial approach is generally preferable (other than for suspected coronary artery dissection, see section on MI during pregnancy) and should be delayed until after period of organogenesis (>12 weeks gestational age)[3]; mean radiation exposure to the unshielded abdomen has been estimated to be 1.5 mGy with less than 20% reaching the fetus.[3] Electrophysiologic procedures for arrhythmias should best be deferred until after pregnancy or performed using a nonfluoroscopic system during pregnancy for refractory cases.[3,30]

Evaluation and Counseling Prior to and During Pregnancy

Pre-pregnancy counseling should be offered to females with heart disease who are of childbearing age, ideally during transition to adult cardiac care.[31] In those women who do not present until they are pregnant, counseling should be performed as early in pregnancy as possible.[16] Preconception counseling is universally recommended for all women with heart disease, preferably by a cardiac-obstetric or pregnancy heart team.[5] Physicians who provide this counseling should include, as a minimum, a cardiologist with expertise in management of pregnancy in women with heart disease, as well as an obstetrician with expertise in maternal fetal medicine.[8,31] The purposes of pre-pregnancy or pregnancy counseling are to provide risk assessment, risk reduction, and management planning to optimize risk or mitigate effects of complications.[2,16,31] Table 92.2 summarizes the general approach to evaluation and counseling. There is preliminary evidence that establishment of a cardio-obstetric clinic was associated with a reduction in the incidence of pulmonary edema.[15]

Risk Stratification

Heart failure and cardiac tachyarrhythmia comprised most of the nonfatal cardiac complications reported in large studies, with maternal mortality rate of 1% or less.[7,15,32,33] The rate of maternal cardiac complication is much higher in low- to middle-income countries or in populations with reduced access to health care.[8] Predictors of maternal cardiovascular complications (summarized in Table 92.3) can be obtained from cardiac history, maternal New York Heart Association (NYHA) functional class, oxygen saturation, and echocardiography. Comprehensive transthoracic echocardiography should be performed and interpreted by personnel experienced in the assessment of congenital and acquired heart disease. Of the various risk stratification approaches that incorporate individual predictors into an overall risk for maternal cardiac complications in women with spectrum of cardiac lesions, two are risk scores derived and validated from the prospective Canadian Cardiac Disease in Pregnancy Study (CARPREG).[8] The original CARPREG risk score incorporated four predictors, to classify pregnancies as being at low, intermediate, or high risk for maternal cardiovascular complications (Fig. 92.2, *left panel*). The CARPREG II risk score calculates the risk of maternal cardiovascular complications by functional, lesion specific, and process of care predictors (Fig. 92.2, *right panel*).[8] The third risk stratification tool, the modified

TABLE 92.2 Approach to Evaluation, Counseling, and Management: Before, During, and After Pregnancy

Preconception

Risk Assessment and Reduction
- Discuss maternal pregnancy risks (cardiac, obstetric, fetal)
- Discuss long-term maternal cardiac prognosis
- Discuss offspring risks including transmission of heart disease
- Referral to genetics when appropriate
- Modify medications as needed
- Smoking cessation and consideration of cardiac intervention prior to conception

Management Planning
- Referral to cardio-obstetric center
- Address assisted reproductive therapy safety in women with infertility
- Consider alternatives to pregnancy (surrogacy or adoption) in women with prohibitive pregnancy risks
- Discuss contraception options for women who want to avoid pregnancy
- Management during antepartum and peripartum period (see below)

Pregnancy and Delivery
- Referral to a cardio-obstetric center
- Consults with the pregnancy heart team including maternal fetal medicine and obstetric anesthesia
- Clinical surveillance throughout pregnancy with frequency of visits based on severity of disease
- Transthoracic echocardiographic surveillance during pregnancy
- Create and circulate a delivery plan including recommendations on the mode of delivery, induction, analgesia, safety of pushing, cardiac and postpartum monitoring
- Organize multidisciplinary conferences for complex or high-risk cases

Postpartum
- Ensure postpartum follow-up
- Medication modification for breastfeeding mothers
- Reestablish baseline in women with structural heart disease at 6 months postpartum
- Arrange postpartum cardiovascular risk assessment for women with pregnancy hypertension or maternal placental syndrome
- For women considering another pregnancy, reevaluate pregnancy risks
- Discuss contraception options

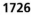

1726

CARDIOVASCULAR DISEASE IN SELECT POPULATIONS

X

TABLE 92.3 Predictors of Pregnancy Associated Complications in Women with Heart Disease

HOW PREDICTOR IS IDENTIFIED	MATERNAL CARDIAC COMPLICATIONS	FETAL AND NEONATAL COMPLICATIONS	GESTATIONAL HYPERTENSION	POSTPARTUM HEMORRHAGE
Baseline Clinical Assessment				
Cardiac events before pregnancy	Yes			
Cardiovascular medications before pregnancy	Yes	Yes		
NYHA functional class III or IV	Yes	Yes		
Anticoagulation		Yes		Yes
Cyanosis	Yes	Yes		Yes
Smoking during pregnancy	Yes	Yes		
Nulliparity			Yes	
Multiple gestation		Yes		
Cardiac Imaging (Primarily by Transthoracic Echocardiography) and Other Assessments				
Left heart obstruction	Yes	Yes		
Reduced systemic ventricular systolic dysfunction	Yes			
Pulmonary atrioventricular valve regurgitation (moderate/severe)	Yes			
Systemic atrioventricular valve regurgitation (moderate/severe)	Yes			
Pulmonary regurgitation or depressed subpulmonary ventricular function	Yes			
B-type natriuretic peptide level	Yes			
Cardiopulmonary test prior to pregnancy	Yes			
Maternal Cardiac Lesion				
Uncorrected or corrected cyanotic heart disease	Yes	Yes		
High-risk aortopathy	Yes			
Coronary artery disease	Yes			
Pulmonary hypertension	Yes	Yes		
Aortic coarctation			Yes	
Maternal systemic lupus erythematosus			Yes	
Aortic valve disease			Yes	
Mechanical prosthesis	Yes	Yes		
Modified World Health Organization Class	Yes			
Process of Care				
No prior cardiac interventions	Yes			
Late presentation for care	Yes			
Serial Assessments During Pregnancy				
Abnormal Uteroplacental Doppler		Yes		
Reduction in cardiac output between 1st and 3rd trimester		Yes		

NYHA, New York Heart Association.
From Grewal J, Windram J, Bottega et al; Canadian Cardiovascular Society: Clinical practice update on cardiovascular management of the pregnant patient. *Can J Cardiol.* 2021 Jul 1:S0828-282X(21)00356-1. https://doi.org/10.1016/j.cjca.2021.06.021; Silversides CK, Siu SC. Heart disease in pregnancy. In: Otto CH, ed. *The Practice of Clinical Echocardiography.* 6th ed. Philadelphia: Elsevier; 2020.

World Health Organization (mWHO) classification system, used an expert consensus approach to classify maternal cardiac lesions into five risk classes corresponding to increasing maternal cardiovascular risks (Table 92.4).[3] In a Canadian study, the CARPREG II risk score had superior predictive accuracy compared with the mWHO classification system.[34]

Risk scores and risk classification approaches should always be combined with clinical judgment. One approach is to identify pregnancies in women with cardiac lesions associated with high mortality risk or with devastating implications even if there is prompt intervention (Fig. 92.3).[8] Pregnancy should be discouraged in women with high-risk cardiac lesions (as listed on Fig. 92.3), and termination should be considered if pregnancy occurs. Pregnant women with high-risk lesions should receive their care by a maternal heart team and deliver at a referral center.

For pregnancies in women without the aforementioned high-risk lesions, a CARPREG II risk score could be used, with subsequent

modification after integrating patient (including exercise testing, compliance, comorbid conditions, socioeconomic status, anticoagulation) and lesion (i.e., type of cardiac lesions, type of operative repair, and late sequelae) specific information. For clinicians who prefer the mWHO risk-classification system, we recommend that general predictors of cardiovascular complications (e.g., prior history of heart failure and arrhythmias) be incorporated, which further stratify risk within each mWHO category (Fig. 92.4). Importantly, the cardiovascular complication rate can be as high as 5% in the low-risk group.[8] Assisted reproductive technologies (ARTs) confer additional risk to women with heart disease (see "Assisted Reproductive Technologies").[31]

Risk stratification should also include assessing the risk of noncardiac complications and long-term prognosis (see Table 92.3).[8] Maternal cardiovascular and fetal neonatal complications are related, likely reflecting the inability of the placenta to autoregulate blood flow. The likelihood of fetoneonatal complications

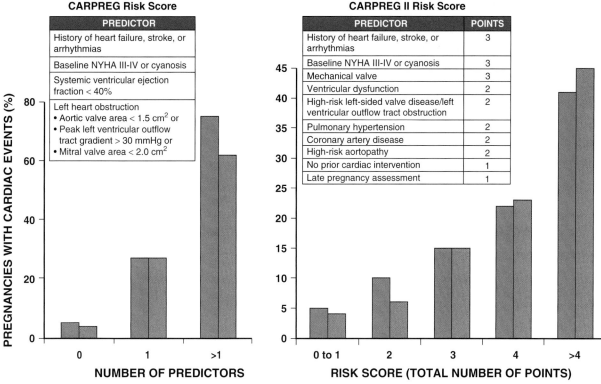

CARPREG Risk Score

PREDICTOR
History of heart failure, stroke, or arrhythmias
Baseline NYHA III-IV or cyanosis
Systemic ventricular ejection fraction < 40%
Left heart obstruction • Aortic valve area < 1.5 cm^2 or • Peak left ventricular outflow tract gradient > 30 mmHg or • Mitral valve area < 2.0 cm^2

CARPREG II Risk Score

PREDICTOR	POINTS
History of heart failure, stroke, or arrhythmias	3
Baseline NYHA III-IV or cyanosis	3
Mechanical valve	3
Ventricular dysfunction	2
High-risk left-sided valve disease/left ventricular outflow tract obstruction	2
Pulmonary hypertension	2
Coronary artery disease	2
High-risk aortopathy	2
No prior cardiac intervention	1
Late pregnancy assessment	1

FIGURE 92.2 Predicted and observed frequency of maternal cardiovascular event rates in the two Canadian Cardiac Disease in Pregnancy Study (CARPREG) risk scores.[15,31] **Left,** The original CARPREG risk score is based on four predictors, shown in the Predictor box. The predicted frequency of maternal cardiac events (in *blue*) is 5%, 27%, and 75%, corresponding to 0, 1, and greater than 1 predictor. The observed frequency of events in the validation group is shown in *red*. **Right,** The CARPREG II risk score is based on 10 variables, shown in the box. Each variable is assigned a weighted score (points). The sum of the points for all 10 variables represents the risk score. Risk scores are categorized into the five groups shown on the *x* axis: risk score of 0–1 points, score of 2 points, score of 3 points, score of 4 points, and score greater than 4 points, corresponding to predicted frequency of cardiac events (in *blue*) of 5%, 10%, 15%, 22%, and 41%, respectively. The observed frequency of cardiac events in the validation groups is in *red*. (From Silversides CK, Grewal J, Mason J, et al. Pregnancy outcomes in women with heart disease: the CARPREG II study. *J Am Coll Cardiol.* 2018;71:2419–2430; and Haberer K, Silversides CK. Congenital heart disease and women's health across the life span: focus on reproductive issues. *Can J Cardiol.* 2019;35:1652–1663.)

is increased when there are concurrent obstetric risk factors.[8] The obstetric and fetoneonatal risks emphasize the vital role of the multidisciplinary team in comprehensive risk assessment and counseling.[31] Pregnancy may accelerate subsequent progression to symptoms or cardiac decompensation in women with certain cardiac lesions.[8]

Management Planning

Preconception counseling provides opportunities to optimize risk by: (1) better defining the nature of the cardiac lesion and or functional capacity by exercise or cardiopulmonary testing, imaging, or cardiac catheterization; (2) stopping medications that are contraindicated in pregnancy (e.g., afterload reducing agents in heart failure treatment) for a trial period prior to pregnancy to ascertain clinical stability; (3) interventions such as smoking cessation or intervention for severe aortic/mitral stenosis (MS); and (4) genetic consultation if the women, her first-degree relative, or her partner has congenital a heart defect.[31,35] Regardless of when the counseling occurs, the following areas need to be discussed and management recommendations provided:

(A) Cardiovascular medications: Cardiovascular medications that are safe versus contraindicated during pregnancy (see general management section).[5,35]

(B) Site of pregnancy care/delivery: There are three possible options: (1) Exclusive care and delivery at referral center by maternal heart team (recommended for high-risk pregnancies); (2) Joint care by local cardiology or obstetric practitioners with delivery at local center, after initial evaluation by pregnancy heart team (non–high-risk pregnancies); or (3) Initial review by pregnancy heart team and local obstetric care (for low-risk pregnancies).[5,36]

(C) Fetal echocardiogram for same indications as for genetic counseling (see earlier).

(D) Management during labor and delivery (see also section on general management):
  (i) Vaginal delivery versus cardiac indications for cesarean delivery.[2]
  (ii) Spontaneous onset of labor versus induction
  (iii) Indications for invasive hemodynamic monitoring
  (iv) Continuous telemetry for patients with uncontrolled arrhythmias
  (v) Postpartum monitoring of the mother in coronary or intensive care units for women in high cardiac risk group, including women who required hemodynamic monitoring during labor and delivery.

For patients with pregnancy who are at high risk, a multidisciplinary meeting should be convened in the antepartum period to develop and document management plan during the peripartum and early postpartum periods.

ASSISTED REPRODUCTIVE TECHNOLOGIES

As with the general population, ARTs are being increasingly used for treatment of infertility and subfertility. In the cardiac population, some women, such as those with Fontan operations, cyanotic heart disease, or Turner syndrome, have higher rates of infertility.[20] Although ARTs improve the chances of pregnancy, they are associated with complications that may be dangerous for women with heart disease.

ARTs such as in vitro fertilization or intrauterine insemination usually follow medical treatment to stimulate ovulation, and this can result in ovarian hyperstimulation syndrome. Ovarian hyperstimulation syndrome, directly related to superovulation protocols, can be particularly problematic for women with heart disease as it leads to fluid shifts

TABLE 92.4 2018 Version of Modified World Health Organization Classification of Maternal Cardiovascular Risk

mWHO CLASS	CARDIAC LESIONS	MATERNAL CARDIAC RISK ASSIGNED BY 2018 GUIDELINES AUTHORS*	CLINICAL APPLICATION
Class I	• Small or mild pulmonary stenosis, patent ductus arteriosus, mitral valve prolapse • Successfully repaired simple lesions (atrial or ventricular septal defect, patent ductus arteriosus, anomalous pulmonary venous connection) • Atrial or ventricular ectopic beats, isolated	2.5%–5%	No detectable increased risk of maternal mortality and no/mild increase in morbidity
Class II	• Unoperated atrial or ventricular septal defect • Repaired tetralogy of Fallot • Most arrhythmias (supraventricular arrhythmias) • Turner syndrome without aortic dilation	5.7%–10.5%	Small increase in maternal risk mortality or moderate increase in morbidity
Class II or III	• Mild left ventricular impairment (EF > 45%) • Hypertrophic cardiomyopathy • Native or tissue valvular heart disease not considered WHO I or IV (mild mitral stenosis, moderate aortic stenosis) • Marfan or other HTAD syndrome without aortic dilatation • Aorta <45 mm in association with bicuspid aortic valve pathology • Repaired coarctation • Atrioventricular septal defect	10%–19%	Intermediate increased risk of maternal mortality or moderate to severe increase in morbidity
Class III	• Moderate left ventricular impairment (EF 30%–45%) • Previous peripartum cardiomyopathy without residual left ventricular impairment • Mechanical valve • Systemic right ventricle with good or mildly decreased ventricular function • Fontan circulation if otherwise well and the cardiac condition uncomplicated • Unrepaired cyanotic heart disease • Other complex congenital heart disease • Moderate mitral stenosis • Severe asymptomatic aortic stenosis • Moderate aortic dilation (40–45 mm in Marfan syndrome or other HTAD, 45–50 mm in bicuspid aortic valve, Turner syndrome ASI 20–25 mm/m², tetralogy of Fallot <50 mm) • Ventricular tachycardia	19%–27%	Significantly increased risk of maternal mortality or severe morbidity.
Class IV	• Pulmonary arterial hypertension • Severe systemic ventricular dysfunction (EF <30% or NYHA class III–IV) • Previous peripartum cardiomyopathy with any residual left ventricular impairment • Severe mitral stenosis • Severe symptomatic aortic stenosis • Systemic right ventricle with moderate or severely decreased ventricular function • Severe aortic dilatation (>45 mm in Marfan syndrome or other HTAD, >50 mm in bicuspid aortic valve, Turner syndrome ASI >25 mm/m², tetralogy of Fallot >50 mm) • Vascular Ehlers-Danlos • Severe (re)coarctation • Fontan with any complication	40%–100%	Extremely high risk of maternal mortality or severe morbidity

*Basis of risk estimates not provided.
ASI, Aortic size index; *EF,* ejection fraction; *HTAD,* heritable thoracic aortic disease; *mWHO,* modified World Health Organization; *NYHA,* New York Heart Association functional class.
From Regitz-Zagrosek V, Roos-Hesselink JW, Bauersachs J, et al. 2018 ESC Guidelines for the management of cardiovascular diseases during pregnancy. *Eur Heart J.* 2018;39:3165–3241.

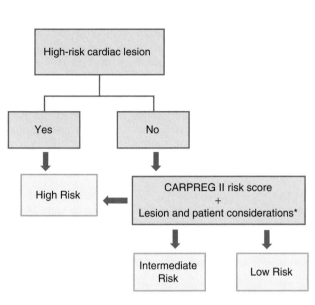

High-risk cardiac lesion
Eisenmenger syndrome or severe pulmonary hypertension
Prior peripartum cardiomyopathy with reduced left ventricular ejection fraction
Severe hereditary thoracic aortopathy • Marfan syndrome with aorta >45 mm or prior aortic replacement • Vascular Ehlers-Danlos syndrome • Turner syndrome with index aortic dimension >25 mm/m² or high risk features • Loeys-Dietz syndrome • Bicuspid aortopathy with aorta >50 mm
Symptomatic severe aortic or mitral stenosis
LV ejection fraction <30% or ventricular assist device
Fontan procedure with arrhythmia, ventricular systolic dysfunction, or other complications
Coronary artery dissection

FIGURE 92.3 A proposed approach for assessing risk of maternal cardiovascular complications in pregnant women with heart disease. *Denotes exercise testing, cardiac imaging data, compliance, comorbid conditions, and socioeconomic status, medications including anticoagulants. (From D'Souza RD, Silversides CK, Tomlinson GA, Siu SC. Assessing cardiac risk in pregnant women with heart disease: how risk scores are created and their role in clinical practice. *Can J Cardiol.* 2020;36:1011–1021.)

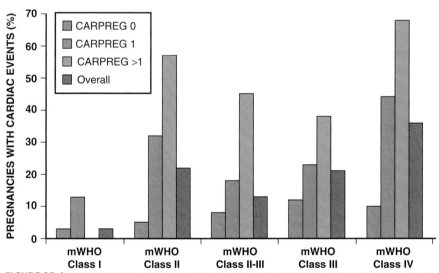

FIGURE 92.4 CARPREG Risk Score further stratifies risk within each mWHO Class. The *x* axis shows each modified World Health Organization (mWHO) class with the corresponding frequency of adverse primary maternal cardiovascular events (*y* axis). The overall maternal cardiac event rate during pregnancy for mWHO I, mWHO II, mWHO II to III, mWHO III, and mWHO IV was 3%, 22%, 13%, 21%, and 36%, respectively. There was a 12.5% event rate in pregnancies in which the mWHO class could not be determined. Each of the mWHO classes is further stratified according to CARPREG risk scores: 0, 1, and greater than 1. CARPREG denotes Cardiac Disease in Pregnancy Study. (From Silversides CK, Grewal J, Mason J, et al. Pregnancy outcomes in women with heart disease: the CARPREG II study. *J Am Coll Cardiol.* 2018;71:2419–2430.)

Multifetal gestations are more common in women receiving ARTs and are associated with increased hemodynamic stress when compared with singleton pregnancies. The additional hemodynamic stress may be poorly tolerated in women with severe forms of heart disease. In addition, twins and higher-order pregnancies are associated with higher rates of preeclampsia, preterm births, low birth weight babies, and neonatal mortality. One small study of fertility therapy in women with heart disease reported high rates of maternal and perinatal complications.[37] Although fertility therapy has not been shown to be associated with long-term cardiovascular risks, failed fertility therapy is associated with higher long-term cardiovascular events.[38]

Guidance is lacking on the optimal evaluation and treatment selection for women with heart disease. When making decisions about patient selection for ART, input from the cardiologist and the fertility specialist is crucial. Pregnancy is contraindicated in the presence of some serious cardiac conditions, and ARTs should be contraindicated in these same conditions.

GENERAL MANAGEMENT PRINCIPLES

Care of the pregnant women with heart disease requires a multidisciplinary team often referred to as the pregnancy heart team.[1,31] The pregnancy heart team includes cardiologists, maternal fetal medicine specialists, obstetric anesthetists, and nursing staff with expertise in pregnancy and heart disease. Other medical specialists (i.e., hematologists), geneticists, neonatologists, and social workers

into the extravascular space and thrombosis. Fluid shifts may be poorly tolerated in women with the Fontan operation and thrombosis poorly tolerated in women with mechanical valves. Therefore planning of superovulation protocols is important in women with heart disease and infertility. Women receiving in vitro fertilization are also at increased risk for pulmonary emboli, preeclampsia, and gestational hypertension.

are required for specific cases. The goal of the pregnancy heart team is to provide preconception counseling, coordinate pregnancy surveillance, treat complications, develop and disseminate delivery plans, and ensure appropriate postpartum follow-up (see Table 92.2).

The frequency of surveillance during pregnancy is based on the severity of the cardiac lesion and the maternal and fetal risk.[3,5] Women at low risk for cardiac complications are often seen once or twice during pregnancy with plans to deliver at a local obstetric center. Women at moderate or high risk for cardiac complications are followed more closely. In addition to clinic visits, pregnancy surveillance includes electrocardiograms, transthoracic echocardiograms, fetal ultrasounds, and, in some cases, placental ultrasounds or serial biomarkers such as BNP. Women with congenital heart disease should be offered a fetal echocardiogram at 18 to 22 weeks' gestation to assess for congenital cardiac malformation.

When using medications during pregnancy, consideration of the maternal benefit needs to be weighed against the potential for fetal toxicity. Most cardiac drugs cross the placental barrier and expose the fetus to the drug, and therefore the lowest possible dose should be used. Benefits and side effects of drugs should be discussed with all women receiving drugs during pregnancy. Teratogenic cardiac drugs should be stopped and switched to safer alternative drugs prior to pregnancy (Fig. 92.5). Drug safety during breastfeeding is based on the concentration of drug in the breast milk and may differ when compared with drug safety during pregnancy. The effectiveness of medications can be altered by the pregnancy associated changes in the volume of distribution, drug absorption, metabolism, and binding.[3,35] The doses of some medications, such as beta blockers, may need to be increased during pregnancy to achieve heart rate or BP control.

The safety profile of cardiovascular medications during pregnancy/lactation are summarized in Figure 92.5.[5,35] Medications that are contraindicated during pregnancy because of fetal toxicity or teratogenicity are: (1) atenolol; (2) angiotensin-converting enzyme inhibitors (ACE-Is) and angiotensin II receptor blockers (ARBs); (3) aldosterone antagonists; (4) statins; (5) direct oral anticoagulants; and (6) bosentan (endothelin receptor antagonists).[35] ACE-Is and ARBs cause second-trimester fetal nephrotoxicity, and ACE-Is are teratogenic. The recommendation to avoid atenolol, particularly in the first trimester, is based on concerns regarding higher rates of fetal growth restriction compared with other beta blockers. However, for women with heart disease, beta blockers usually do not have major effects on birth weight (mean weight reduction 191 g) when adjusted for other maternal risk factor for fetal growth restriction.[39] Recommendations to avoid statins in pregnancy may evolve with additional safety data in the future.[35]

For many of the newer cardiovascular medications, the fetal risk profile is not completely established and their use represent a balance between benefit versus fetal risk. Most drugs, except high-molecular-weight molecules such as heparin, cross the placenta and equilibrate in the fetal circulation over time. Importantly, some medications (ACE-Is) that are contraindicated during pregnancy can be used during lactation. The risk of some medications may be a related to gestational age. Warfarin is associated with an embryopathy when exposure occurs between 6 and 12 weeks' gestation and needs to be discontinued prior to 6 weeks' gestation. In the treatment of acute pericarditis during pregnancy during pregnancy, both aspirin (ASA) and nonsteroidal antiinflammatory drugs (NSAIDs) cross the placenta. Classic NSAIDs (ibuprofen, indomethacin, naproxen) or high-dose ASA can be used early in the pregnancy. After the 20th gestational week, all NSAIDs (except enteric coated ASA [ECASA] ≤100 mg daily) have the potential of causing constriction of the ductus arteriosus and impact fetal renal function and should be withdrawn by the 32nd gestational week.[40] Lowest effective doses of prednisone may be used during pregnancy. Ibuprofen, indomethacin, naproxen, and prednisone may be considered for lactating women. Colchicine is considered to be contraindicated during pregnancy and lactation, but data are incomplete.[40]

Drugs that are considered safe:

Arrhythmia
Adenosine, bisoprolol, digoxin*, lidocaine, metoprolol, nadolol, propranolol

Hypertension
Labetalol, methyl-dopa, metoprolol, nifedipine

Heart failure
Bumetanide, carvedilol, furosemide, metoprolol, dobutamine, dopamine, norepinephrine

Anticoagulation/antiplatelets/thrombolytics
Aspirin, low molecular weight heparin, unfractionated heparin

Drugs that are considered contraindicated:

Arrhythmia
Amiodarone**, atenolol, ivabradine

Hypertension/heart failure
ACE-inhibitors, aldosterone antagonists, ARBs, SGLT-2 inhibitors

Anticoagulation/antiplatelets/thrombolytics
Direct oral anticoagulants

Pulmonary hypertension/others
Bosentan and other endothelin receptor antagonists (ERA), statins

Data from observational studies is often conflicting regarding the safety of medication in pregnancy and lactation. Therefore the risks vs. benefits of treatment should be discussed with the patient on an individual basis. Potential adverse events should be anticipated and screened (e.g., growth restriction)

Drugs with limited/conflicting data/use with caution:

Arrhythmia
Diltiazem, flecainide, procainamide, propafenone, sotalol, verapamil

Hypertension/heart failure
Amlodipine, hydralazine, nitrates, nitroprusside, hydrochlorothiazide, metolazone, milrinone, torsemide

Anticoagulation/antiplatelets/thrombolytics
Clopidogrel, ticagrelor, warfarin argatroban, bivalirudin, fondaparinux, alteplase, streptokinase, tenecteplase

Pulmonary hypertension/others
Epoprostenol, iloprost, sildenafil, treprostinil

Drugs to avoid when breast feeding:
(again discuss the risks vs benefits of each agent)

Arrhythmia
Amiodarone, Ivabradine, sotalol

Hypertension/heart failure
ACE-inhibitors other than captopril, lisinopril or enalapril, aldosterone antagonists, ARBs, SGLT-2 inhibitors

Anticoagulation/antiplatelets/thrombolytics
Clopidogrel, direct oral anticoagulants

Pulmonary hypertension/others
Statins, bosentan & other ERAs

*Digoxin serum levels are unreliable during pregnancy. **May be used if other therapies have failed.

FIGURE 92.5 Safety profile of cardiovascular medications during pregnancy and lactation.[5,35] Summary of recent reviews of the use of cardiovascular medications during pregnancy and lactation.

When possible, a spontaneous vaginal delivery is preferred. Induction is usually reserved for logistical reasons (patient lives a long distance away from the hospital) or if a delivery is complex and a specific team is required to be present during delivery. Cesarean delivery is rarely required for cardiac indications except in women who do not have warfarin discontinued at least 2 weeks prior to delivery due to the risk of neonatal intracranial hemorrhage, those with severely dilated thoracic aortas, severe refractory heart failure, or hemodynamic instability. Vaginal deliveries can be conducted in the left lateral position to avoid compression of the inferior vena cava and optimize venous return. In women at high risk for complications, delivery planning should be made in conjunction with the pregnancy heart team and should take place at a cardiac and obstetric referral center. For some women, an assisted second stage of labor (i.e., with low forceps or vacuum extraction) may be helpful to prevent a long labor. Although routine endocarditis prophylaxis is no longer recommended for all pregnant women with heart disease, infective endocarditis prophylaxis is recommended at the time of labor and delivery in those at highest risk for endocarditis, such as women with prior endocarditis, mechanical valves, or cyanotic heart disease.

Most cardiac complications during pregnancy can be treated medically.[5] Heart failure should be treated with fluid and salt restriction and diuretics. It is important to identify and treat any precipitating factors such as tachyarrhythmias, infection, iatrogenic volume administration, and postpartum fluid shifts. Although ACE-Is and ARBs need to be stopped during pregnancy, afterload reduction with hydralazine and isosorbide dinitrate can be used.[36] Women who develop heart failure during pregnancy require close follow-up. Delivery needs to be planned carefully in women with antepartum complications, and treatment of heart failure prior to delivery is optimal. Hemodynamic monitoring with an arterial line should be considered for selected high-risk patients (severe left ventricular systolic dysfunction, severe aortic or MS, or pulmonary hypertension). Central venous and pulmonary artery catheters are rarely indicated and should be performed by an experienced operator after careful consideration of risk versus benefits.[3,24] Other than for obstetric and fetal indication, planned preterm delivery (<37 weeks' gestation) is seldom warranted for maternal cardiac reasons. Women with severe heart failure should be delivered at a center with availability of mechanical circulatory support as well as a transplant team.

Treatment of arrhythmias needs to be tailored to the individual and is based on the type of arrhythmia and the presence of underlying structural heart disease. Electrical cardioversion is safe during pregnancy, and women with tachyarrhythmias who are hemodynamically unstable require cardioversion. Bradycardias are less common during pregnancy. Pacemaker and implantable cardioverter defibrillators are safe during pregnancy and delivery. If cautery is used at the time of delivery, oversensing by the pacemaker is possible and therefore magnets should be available in the delivery room to use to eliminate oversensing.

Occasionally, women with refractory symptoms require a percutaneous or surgical intervention. Maternal abdominal lead shielding, radial approach, and procedural techniques can minimize radiation exposure to the fetus. Women with severe mitral, aortic, or pulmonary stenosis who have symptoms refractory to medical therapy may require a balloon valvuloplasty or, in very select cases, percutaneous valve insertion to relieve the outflow track obstruction. These procedures should be performed only at experienced centers because acute heart failure, arrhythmias, tamponade, and death have been reported. Obstetric back-up is required because precipitous labor can occur. Cardiac surgery during pregnancy should only be performed if no other options are available, because fetal mortality can occur in approximately 20% of cases. Urgent surgery, maternal comorbidities, and early gestational age are associated with the highest fetal risk.[3,41] Fetal risk can be mitigated by pulsatile perfusion, high pump flow, avoidance of hypothermic extracorporeal circulation, minimizing bypass times, and fetal monitoring.[3] Later in gestation, delivery followed by cardiac surgery is preferred

if there is adequate fetal maturity. In comparison, maternal surgical risks are similar to the nonpregnant population. A multidisciplinary pregnancy heart team with cardiology, cardiac surgery, anesthesia, obstetrics, and neonatology is necessary to optimize mother and offspring outcomes.

Cardiac arrest during pregnancy is managed similarly to the nonpregnant arrest, with the following modifications: (1) lateral uterine displacement during an arrest is required after 20 weeks' gestation; (2) intubation may be more difficult due to changes in airway mucosa; and (3) emergency cesarean delivery should be initiated if there has been no return of spontaneous circulation within 4 minutes of the onset of arrest in a pregnant women with a fundus height at or above the umbilicus.[42]

SPECIFIC CARDIOVASCULAR CONDITIONS

Hypertension (see Chapter 26)

Hypertensive disorders of pregnancy are one of the leading causes of maternal and perinatal mortality worldwide and responsible for 16% of maternal deaths in high-income countries.[2,43,44] They can be classified into four categories: preeclampsia/eclampsia, gestational hypertension, chronic hypertension, and chronic hypertension with superimposed preeclampsia (see eTable 92.1 for detailed diagnostic criteria). Although obstetric providers usually manage hypertensive disorders in pregnant women, cardiovascular practitioners should be aware of the overall management approach. Hypertension in pregnancy is defined as systolic blood pressure (SBP) of 140 mm Hg or greater or diastolic blood pressure (DBP) of 90 mm Hg or greater on two measurements at least 4 hours apart, with the proviso that the second measurement can be obtained within 15 minutes if the BP is severely elevated (SBP ≥160 mm Hg or DBP ≥110 mm Hg). The BP should be remeasured from the arm with the higher BP after an interval of at least 15 minutes if there is nonsevere elevation of BP.[2,43,44] Tobacco or caffeine use within 30 minutes prior to measurement can temporarily increases BP. Many women with first BP reading of 140/90 or greater will subsequently be found to have normal BP on repeated measurement.[45] Ambulatory BP monitoring can separate white coat versus chronic hypertension for women with persistent BP elevation of 140/90 mm Hg or less at less than 20 weeks' gestation. Patients with preexisting hypertension may have a falsely normal BP due to the reduced systemic vascular resistance that manifests by the 12th gestational week. Pregnant women with severe hypertension (BP ≥160/110 persistent for 15 minutes) should be triaged expeditiously and pharmacotherapy initiated to reduce risk of heart failure, stroke, or renal disease (Fig. 92.6).[44,45]

Preeclampsia is defined as: (1) hypertension (defined earlier) after 20 weeks' gestation in persons who were previously normotensive and (2) new-onset proteinuria **or** new-onset end-organ damage. In the presence of new-onset end-organ manifestations (see eTable 92.1), proteinuria is not needed to establish a diagnosis. One caveat is that gestational hypertension can manifest prior to 20 weeks, and previously undiagnosed chronic hypertension can present after 20 weeks, when the BP rises from its nadir in second trimester.[43,44] The current proposed mechanism for preeclampsia is uteroplacental ischemia resulting in imbalances in angiogenic and antiangiogenic factors.[44] Severe preeclampsia (see eTable 92.1) is an obstetrical emergency. The more severe form of preeclampsia, HELLP (hemolysis, elevated liver enzymes, and low platelet count) syndrome, usually presents in the third trimester and can present or progress in the postpartum period. Eclampsia, defined as new-onset seizures, the convulsive manifestation of preeclampsia, is a significant cause of maternal death, especially in low-resources settings. In a significant minority of cases, HELLP and eclampsia may not be preceded by hypertension or proteinuria.[44]

For those with less severe hypertension, pharmacotherapy can be initiated with any first-line agent (see Fig. 92.6). Current guidelines differ as to the threshold for initiation of pharmacotherapy in those women with less severe hypertension, as well as the optimal BP to be

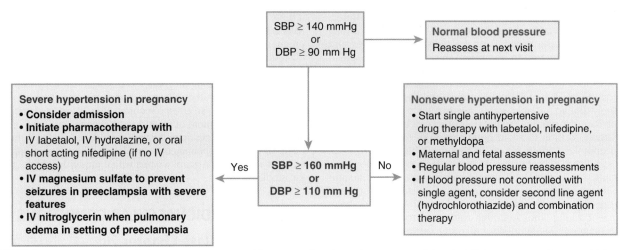

```
                    ┌──────────────────────┐
                    │  SBP ≥ 140 mmHg      │        ┌─────────────────────────┐
                    │         or           │───────▶│ Normal blood pressure   │
                    │  DBP ≥ 90 mm Hg      │        │ Reassess at next visit  │
                    └──────────────────────┘        └─────────────────────────┘
                               │
                               ▼
```

┌───┐   ┌──┐
│ **Severe hypertension in pregnancy**   │   │ **Nonsevere hypertension in pregnancy**   │
│ • **Consider admission**   │   │ • Start single antihypertensive   │
│ • **Initiate pharmacotherapy with**   │   ┌──────────────────┐   │   drug therapy with labetalol, nifedipine, │
│   IV labetalol, IV hydralazine, or oral   │ Yes │ SBP ≥ 160 mmHg   │ No │   or methyldopa   │
│   short acting nifedipine (if no IV   │◀─────│   or   │───▶│ • Maternal and fetal assessments   │
│   access)   │   │ DBP ≥ 110 mm Hg │   │ • Regular blood pressure reassessments   │
│ • **IV magnesium sulfate to prevent**   │   └──────────────────┘   │ • If blood pressure not controlled with   │
│   **seizures in preeclampsia with severe**│   │   single agent, consider second line agent │
│   **features**   │   │   (hydrochlorothiazide) and combination   │
│ • **IV nitroglycerin when pulmonary**   │   │   therapy   │
│   **edema in setting of preeclampsia**   │   │   │
└───┘   └──┘

FIGURE 92.6 Management algorithm for hypertension in pregnancy.[2,45] Summary of North American recommendations for initial management of women with hypertensive disorders of pregnancy.

achieved with treatment.[44–47] Tight control of BP (DBP <85 mm Hg) did not confer an improved maternal or perinatal outcome compared with less tight control of BP but did reduce the risk of developing severe hypertension.[45] Currently, the optimal goal for BP therapy varies between United States (range of 140 to 150/90 to 100 mm Hg), European (<140/90 mm Hg), and Canadian (<85 mm Hg diastolic BP) recommendations.[2,45,47] An important consideration is that hemoconcentration, rather than hypervolemia, is a frequent finding in patients with preeclampsia.

For prevention of preeclampsia, low-dose ASA should be initiated between 12 and 16 weeks' gestation (and ideally, no later than 20 weeks) and continued until at least 36 weeks' gestation in women in women with any high risk factors (chronic hypertension, prior preeclampsia , multifetal gestation, diabetes mellitus, renal disease, autoimmune disease, or preterm birth <34 weeks' gestation) or in women with more than 1 moderate risk factor (nulliparity, body mass index >30, family history of preeclampsia, age ≥35 years, socioeconomic status, or personal history factors).[2,44,48,49] In women with gestational hypertension or preeclampsia, the decision to deliver versus expectant treatment needs to consider the absence/presence of severe features of preeclampsia and gestational age.[44] Ambulatory follow-up and/or home BP monitoring should be continued in the postpartum period and therapy should be continued in those with postpartum hypertension (≥150/100 mm Hg).[2] Women with hypertension during pregnancy require longitudinal follow-up and risk factor modification because they are at elevated risk of developing hypertension or cardiovascular disease later in life.

CARDIOMYOPATHIES (SEE PART VI)

Common preexisting cardiopathies in women of childbearing age are dilated cardiomyopathy (DCM), hypertrophic cardiomyopathy (HCM), and cardiomyopathies related to congenital heart disease or valvular heart disease. Less common causes include: ischemic cardiomyopathy, tachycardiac-induced cardiomyopathy, arrhythmogenic right ventricular cardiomyopathy, noncompaction cardiomyopathy, restrictive cardiomyopathy, and Chagas disease in endemic areas. PPCM develops de novo during pregnancy. Pregnant women with cardiomyopathies are at risk for maternal and fetal complications and require careful preconception risk stratification and counseling.

DCM in women of childbearing age may be idiopathic or secondary to genetic defects (i.e., lamin A/C [*LMNA*], beta-myosin heavy chain [*MYH7*], or cardiac troponin T [*TNNT2*] mutation), prior myocarditis, or drug exposure (i.e., Adriamycin exposure) (eFig. 92.1).[50] Genetic counseling should be offered to women with DCM who have a family history of cardiomyopathy. Women with DCM are at risk of worsening left

ventricular systolic function, clinical heart failure, atrial or ventricular arrhythmia, thromboembolic complications, or, rarely, death.[3,51] Women with DCM who have good functional capacity and mild left ventricular systolic function often do well during pregnancy. Conversely, women with NYHA functional class III or IV and/or moderate or severe LV systolic dysfunction have high rates of cardiac complications including heart failure and arrhythmias.[51] Pregnancy is contraindicated in women with DCM and severe left ventricular systolic dysfunction.[3]

HCM is an inherited cardiomyopathy with autosomal dominant transmission, and transmission of HCM to offspring should be discussed at the time of the preconception visit because some women may wish to consider pre-implantation genetic screening. The HCM phenotype is variable and may have left ventricular outflow tract obstruction, diastolic or systolic dysfunction, or significant mitral regurgitation (MR). Atrial fibrillation (AF) and heart failure are the most common complications in pregnant women with HCM.[52] Maternal mortality, although rare, has been reported in women with high-risk features.[3] Most women with mild or moderate forms of HCM do not develop cardiac complications during pregnancy. Women with high-risk features such as severe left ventricular hypertrophy, syncope, prior ventricular tachycardia (VT), or severe left ventricular outflow tract obstruction can develop cardiac complications during pregnancy and require careful preconception assessment. In women with severe left ventricular outflow tract obstruction, epidural anesthesia should be used cautiously because it can result in hypotension and worsening of the outflow tract obstruction. Similarly, oxytocin may cause hypotension and tachycardia and should be given as a slow infusion. In women with obstructive HCM, avoidance of Valsalva and a facilitated second stage of labor is recommended at the time of labor and delivery.

PPCM is a cardiomyopathy that occurs de novo during pregnancy. Women typically present later in pregnancy or in the first few months postpartum with left ventricular systolic dysfunction (left ventricular ejection fraction [LVEF] <45%), heart failure, and embolic events. PPCM is a diagnosis of exclusion.[53] Older maternal age, Africa-American race, multigestation pregnancy, preeclampsia, and hypertension are risk factors for PPCM. The cause of PPCM is not known, but proposed mechanisms have included nutritional deficiencies, viral myocarditis, and autoimmune and vascular-hormonal processes. Treatment is similar to that for heart failure in general with diuresis, beta blockers, and afterload reduction. A mouse model for PPCM identified a 16-kDa prolactin fragment that resulted in vascular and myocardial dysfunction. Based on that finding and small human studies, bromocriptine, a suppressor of prolactin secretion, has been used as a therapy for PPCM.[53] Maternal recovery of left ventricular systolic function have been variable. In the North American Investigators of Pregnancy-Associated Cardiomyopathy (IPAC) study, approximately 70% of women had a left ventricular ejection fraction greater than

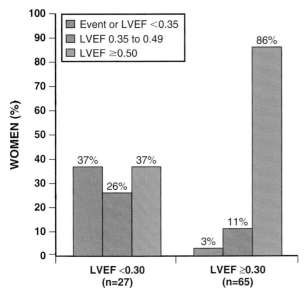

FIGURE 92.7 Recovery of left ventricular systolic function in women with peripartum cardiomyopathy. Comparison of left ventricular systolic function at 1 year post presentation based on the initial left ventricular ejection fraction. *Red column,* percentage of women with no recovery (event or final ejection fraction <0.35); *blue column,* percentage of women with partial recovery (final ejection fraction 0.35 to 0.49); *green column,* percentage of women with complete recovery (final ejection fraction ≥ 0.50). LVEF denotes left ventricular ejection fraction. (From McNamara DM, Elkayam U, Alharethi R, et al. Clinical outcomes for peripartum cardiomyopathy in North America: results of the IPAC study (investigations of pregnancy-associated cardiomyopathy). *J Am Coll Cardiol.* 2015;66:905–914.)

50% 1 year after their index presentation. Baseline left ventricular ejection fraction greater than 0.30 and left ventricular end diastolic dimensions less than 6.0 cm at presentation are prognostic markers associated with good recovery (Fig. 92.7).[54] One year after the index presentation in the IPAC study, 13% had experienced either a major cardiac event or had severe cardiomyopathy (LVEF <0.35). Higher mortality rates are reported in African Americans. Subsequent pregnancies carry risk, particularly in women in whom the left ventricular systolic function does not recover, and pregnancy is contraindicated in women with residual left ventricular systolic dysfunction because of the significant maternal mortality.[53]

Pregnancy after a heart transplant can be successful with careful planning. Pregnancy is not advised until at least 1 year after heart transplant and is contraindicated in women at high risk of rejection or with baseline graft dysfunction. All women should have preconception counseling so they can understand pregnancy risks and make medication modifications if necessary. A discussion about maternal life expectancy should be included as part of preconception counseling. Mycophenolate mofetil is teratogenic and should be stopped prior to conception. Alternatives to azathioprine should be used when possible. For those women who become pregnant, frequent surveillance of immunosuppressive medications is critical because changes in volume of distribution and metabolism may require dose adjustments during pregnancy and postpartum. Potential complications include rejection, graft dysfunction, and infection.[55] Hypertensive disorders of pregnancy occur in approximately 26% of pregnancies, and preeclampsia occurs in 18% of pregnancies.[55] Preterm deliveries occur in more than half of all pregnancies.[55] Immunosuppressive medications can impact the neonate, and therefore breastfeeding is not recommended.

MYOCARDIAL INFARCTION AND ISCHEMIC HEART DISEASE

Pregnancy is a risk factor for cardiac ischemic events,[2,56] relating to elevated pregnancy-associated increase in low-density lipoprotein (LDL) cholesterol levels, hypercoagulable state, inflammatory changes associated with preeclampsia/infection, hormonal weakening of the

arterial wall, increased vascular reactivity, or use of prostaglandin analog in postpartum hemorrhage.[57] Although ischemic heart disease was rarely encountered in the past, it is expected to increase in frequency with rising maternal age and increasing prevalence of atherosclerotic risk factors. The incidence of MI is estimated to be approximately 3 per 100,000 pregnancies, with a case fatality rate of approximately 5%.[58] Coronary atherosclerotic disease accounts for up to 40% of cases, spontaneous coronary artery dissection (SCAD) has been responsible for up to 43% of cases, and the remainder have been attributed to intracoronary thrombus (up to 17%) or coronary spasm (approximately 2%).[2,57] Majority of acute MI presented in the third trimester or postpartum period.[59] The diagnosis of MI during pregnancy is similar to that of nonpregnant patient[60] and may be misdiagnosed as dyspepsia or reflux.[57] ST elevation MI is more common than non–ST elevation MI, and up to two-thirds of MIs are anterior.

SCAD results in formation of an intramural hematoma which encroaches on the true coronary artery lumen.[57,61,62] Of the three types of SCAD, type 1 (typical appearance, multiple lumens, arterial wall stain) was encountered in less than one-third of cases. Confirming the diagnosis of type 2 (diffuse smooth stenosis, most common) and type 3 (mimic atherosclerosis; least common) SCAD usually requires intravascular ultrasound or optical coherence tomography.[61] Urgent angiography should be performed for suspected SCAD and for those presenting with ST elevation MI.[61] Because SCAD is a common cause of ST elevation MI in pregnant women, thrombolysis for acute ST-segment elevation myocardial infarction [STEMI] is not recommended. Thrombolytic agents do not cross the placenta but can cause maternal and placental bleeding. The risk of iatrogenic catheter-induced coronary artery dissection is higher (approximately 3%) than for standard coronary angiography, attributed to underlying vascular frailty in patients with SCAD. The risk of iatrogenic coronary dissection was higher with radial approach; thus the femoral approach may be preferred in the pregnant patient.[61] Technical recommendations have been proposed to reduce the risk of causing a new dissection or propagating an existing dissection.[63] Cardiac catheterization and coronary interventions in pregnant women should be performed by experienced operators at a referral center. It is reasonable to perform coronary angiography for a pregnant patient with non–ST elevation MI or acute coronary syndrome, but this need not be done emergently. A negative coronary CT angiography does not exclude SCAD.[61]

Although at least 70% of patients with SCAD will have angiographic healing on repeat angiography, these data are not based on consecutive sample or pregnant patients.[61] Medical therapy is the preferred strategy for SCAD, with inpatient monitoring for an extended period because up to 10% of conservatively managed patients may have extension of dissection within the first 7 days. Percutaneous coronary intervention (PCI) in patients with SCAD has consistently been reported to increase risk of complications and poor outcomes, likely related to increased coronary frailty. PCI or coronary artery bypass grafting (CABG) should be considered for those women with active or ongoing ischemia, hemodynamic instability, left main, or severe proximal two vessel dissection.[61] Meticulous angiographic and specific PCI techniques, designed to restore coronary flow without further propagating the dissection, have been proposed.[61] Patients with PCI should be on dual platelet therapy, and clopidogrel is viewed as the only "safe" inhibitor. Coronary artery surgery was not protective against recurrent SCAD, with the risk of graft occlusion from competitive flow from healing of the native coronary arteries.

Patients with MI should be on beta blockers and low-dose ASA. The indications for clopidogrel in patient who have not undergone PCI is less certain due to potential increase in bleeding risk. Nitrates and calcium channel blockers can be used for angina therapy. ACE-Is/ARBs and statins are not recommended during pregnancy. Nitrates, beta blockers, or low-molecular-weight or unfractionated heparin can be used for acute MI during pregnancy.[2,35,61] Doses of nitrates will need to be carefully titrated to avoid excessive maternal hypotension because the placenta cannot autoregulate BP. Pregnancy and delivery should be at a referral center with involvement of the maternal heart team. Current recommendation is for vaginal delivery with epidural anesthesia, with minimization of maternal efforts during vaginal delivery. Given that pregnancy is a risk factor for developing SCAD and the 3-year risk of major cardiac events for patients with SCAD in general is up to 30%,[61] future pregnancies should be discouraged.

Women with preexisting coronary artery disease or prior MI currently constitute a small proportion of pregnant women with heart disease.[15] However, a systematic review reported ischemic events occurred in 9% of pregnancies and the mortality rate was 2%; only 21% of pregnancies were uncomplicated (no maternal or fetal/neonatal complications).[56] Prior to pregnancy, women with coronary artery disease should undergo treatment of any correctable lesions that are associated with ischemia. For those women with significant coronary stenosis but further intervention is not possible, avoidance of pregnancy should be considered. Similar to patients with SCAD or MI during pregnancy, this high-risk group of patients should receive care by a pregnancy heart team and deliver at a center that can perform coronary revascularization and provide advanced cardiac therapies.[2] Low-dose ASA, beta₁ selective blockers, nitrates, and clopidogrel can be continued during pregnancy.[35] ACE-I can be reinitiated in the postpartum period, and some are safe for lactation (see general management section). Statins can be restarted in the postpartum period for women who are not lactating.[35]

NATIVE VALVULAR HEART DISEASE (SEE PART VIII)

Rheumatic MS is the most common type of valvular heart disease encountered in pregnant women globally.[64] Pregnancy-associated increase in stroke volume and heart rate results in elevation of the transmitral gradient and left atrial pressure, thereby increasing the likelihood of functional class deterioration, pulmonary edema, and atrial arrhythmia. The hypercoagulable state associated with pregnancy increases the risk of left atrial thrombus. The fetus is at increased rate of preterm birth, intrauterine growth restriction, and death, attributed to inability to augment cardiac

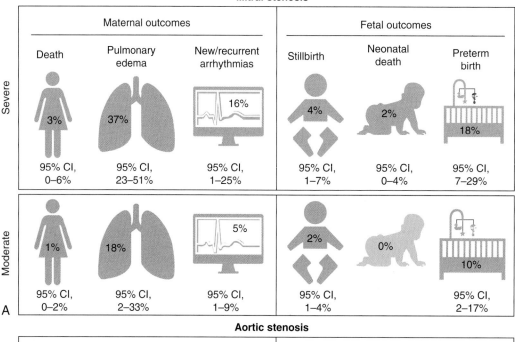

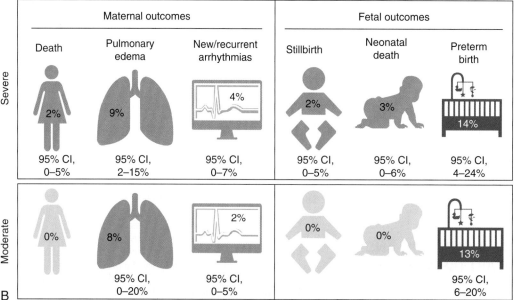

FIGURE 92.8 Maternal and fetal/neonatal outcomes by valve lesion and severity. Maternal and fetal complications in women with mitral (**A**) and aortic (**B**) stenosis as stratified by lesion severity. *CI,* Confidence interval. (From Ducas RA, Javier DA, D'Souza R, et al. Pregnancy outcomes in women with significant valve disease: a systematic review and meta-analysis. *Heart.* 2020;106:512–519.)

output and uteroplacental insufficiency. The frequency of complications generally corresponded to the severity of MS (Fig. 92.8A), and the risk within each class may be further elevated by symptoms, left ventricular systolic dysfunction, prior heart failure, or pulmonary artery hypertension.[65,66] Recent guidelines have reclassified mitral valve area of 1.5 cm^2 or less as severe or significant MS, which encompasses mitral valve area of 1.1 to 1.5 cm^2, which was formerly classified as moderate MS.[67] In countries with high prevalence of rheumatic heart disease and limited health care access, the mortality rate was 34%[68]; in contrast to the lower mortality reported in middle-high income countries (see Fig. 92.8A).[69]

Present guidelines have recommended percutaneous balloon valvuloplasty or mitral valve surgery prior to pregnancy for women with mitral valve area of 1.5 cm^2 or less,[3,67,70] to reduce the development of heart failure and AF (eTable 92.2). However, this strategy may not be applicable in women with access to specialty care and normal exercise tolerance, who are not at high thromboembolic risk and do not have pulmonary hypertension.[71] Pregnant women with MS should be followed serially during pregnancy, with a minimum frequency of at least once during the first trimester and again during the third trimester; those with severe MS will require more frequent follow-up. Mitral valve gradients will increase with increasing cardiac output during pregnancy, so assessment of MS severity should be by mitral valve area.[65] Beta$_1$ selective blockers are recommended,[67] especially in those with significant (moderate or severe) MS or symptoms. Deterioration in functional class may be an early warning sign of impending heart failure, and loop diuretics and increasing dose of beta blockers (or digoxin if intolerant to beta blockers) should be initiated along with restriction of activities. Exact heart rate goals with beta blockers have not been established. Atrial tachyarrhythmia is a frequent precipitant of maternal heart failure, especially in the third trimester.[5] Anticoagulation is recommended in those with AF, left atrial thrombus, or prior embolism. In those with significant MS and who are in sinus rhythm, anticoagulation is a consideration if there is spontaneous echocardiographic contrast in the left atrium, large left atrium (≥60 mL/m^2), or congestive heart failure.[3] Mitral valvuloplasty can be performed during pregnancy but is usually reserved for refractory symptoms or heart failure despite maximal medical therapy and hospitalization.

The risk of maternal and fetal mortality is lower in pregnancies in women with isolated MR.[66,69] However, moderate to severe MR is associated with heart failure in 23% of pregnancies in women with rheumatic heart disease and is an independent predictor of maternal cardiac complications regardless of etiology.[15,66] Therefore patients with moderate or severe MR should have serial follow-up in the antepartum period similar to patients with MS. Clinicians should also be aware that the reduced systemic vascular resistance during the antepartum may reduce the magnitude of MR during second to third trimester, leading to underestimation of its severity. We recommend that a single dose of intravenous loop diuretics be administered during the first several hours after delivery in patient with moderate or severe MR or MS, to reduce the likelihood of redistribution edema from autotransfusion following birth. For patients with predominant mitral valve disease, vaginal delivery with epidural anesthesia is the preferred mode of delivery, with cesarean delivery considered for patients with NYHA functional class III to IV or pulmonary hypertension, despite medical therapy. Mitral valve prolapse is considered to be a low-risk condition unless there is moderate or severe MR.

Aortic stenosis (AS) most commonly occurs as a result of bicuspid aortic valve (BAV) and limits the ability of the heart to increase cardiac output or adjust to changes in loading conditions during pregnancy,[23] increasing propensity for heart failure, ischemia, or hypotension.[23] Asymptomatic women with mild AS typically will tolerate pregnancy well. Women with moderate or severe AS are at risk for heart failure, arrhythmias, and angina, although the mortality risk in those with severe AS is low in the current era (Fig. 92.8B).[69] For subvalvular AS, a resting gradient greater than 30 mm Hg is considered to be hemodynamically significant.[15]

Current guidelines recommend exercise testing to risk stratify asymptomatic women with severe AS.[3,67] Aortic valve replacement is recommended in women with symptomatic AS or asymptomatic women with left ventricular ejection fraction less than 50% or abnormalities during exercise testing.[3,67] Although pre-pregnancy aortic valve replacement has been recommended in asymptomatic women with severe AS, this decision should be individualize based on left ventricular function and results of exercise testing.[3] Anatomic feasibility for a Ross procedure, with avoidance of long-term anticoagulation and potential for long-term valve longevity, would be an additional consideration.

Patients with AS require follow-up similar to mitral lesion, with diuretics treatment for heart failure (see eTable 92.2). How to deliver a woman with AS has not been established,[69] although cesarean is believed to reduce stress on the mother,[71] as well as facilitating logistics when there are plans for hemodynamic monitoring. Percutaneous valvuloplasty can be performed as a temporizing measure in those patients with refractory symptoms in the antepartum period. Valve replacement can be performed during pregnancy, or timed with a cesarean delivery, for life-threatening symptoms and where percutaneous approach is not possible.[4] Transcutaneous aortic valve replacement may be a potential option.

Aortic regurgitation is generally better tolerated than AS, and a small study reported that 29% of pregnancies in women with severe aortic regurgitation were complicated by pulmonary edema.[69] Functional deterioration will usually respond to loop diuretics.

Most women with significant valvular pulmonic stenosis would have been treated with percutaneous valvuloplasty in childhood. The small number of patients with severe pulmonic stenosis reported in studies have had generally good outcomes, with infrequent occurrence of right heart failure or deterioration in functional class.[71,18] Severe pulmonic regurgitation (PR) is also well tolerated, perhaps with the reduced pulmonary vascular resistance during pregnancy. Although there have been reports of right heart failure in patients with severe PR, many have been associated with right ventricular systolic dysfunction in patients with complex congenital lesions.[72] Isolated tricuspid stenosis is uncommonly encountered, and systematic outcome data are not available. With dilatation of tricuspid annulus with right ventricular enlargement during pregnancy, there can be an increase in TR,[27] and it is not unusual to see moderate TR during normal pregnancy. Women with isolated severe TR usually tolerate pregnancy well, when the right ventricle is not the systemic (subaortic) ventricle, although systematic data are absent. In patients with congenital cardiac lesions, moderate to severe TR was an independent predictor of cardiac complications,[72] but this finding has not been replicated by prospective studies.[15,73] Patients with right heart failure, or experiencing functional deterioration from right-sided valvular lesions, usually respond to loop diuretics; cardiac interventions can be deferred until after pregnancy.[71]

PROSTHETIC VALVES AND MANAGEMENT OF ANTICOAGULATION

Women with prosthetic valves are at risk for complications in pregnancy, and women should have preconception counseling for risk stratification and to discuss these risks. Compared with women with mechanical valves, those with bioprosthetic valves are at less risk for pregnancy-related complications as the valves are less thrombogenic and anticoagulation is not required.[74] Women with normal functioning bioprosthetic valves, good functional class, and normal left ventricular systolic function are at low risk for maternal cardiac complications. However, because valve degeneration occurs over time, some women with older valve implants may have abnormal valve function which increases pregnancy risk. Although pregnancy experience is limited, women with a Ross procedure (pulmonary valve autograft and bioprosthetic pulmonary valve) also have good pregnancy outcomes.[3]

Pregnancy in women with mechanical valves is associated with significant maternal and fetal risks. The most serious maternal complication is valve thrombosis, which can result in maternal mortality (Table 92.5).[75] The risk of valve thrombosis is related to a number of factors, including the type of anticoagulant used during pregnancy (warfarin less risk than heparin), the type of valve (newer generation valves less risk than older generation valves) and valve position (aortic position less risk than mitral position). There are three

TABLE 92.5 Maternal and Fetal Risk in Women with Mechanical Heart Valves

	PRIMARY MATERNAL AND FETAL OUTCOMES			
Anticoagulation Regimen	Maternal Mortality Estimate % (95% CI)	Thromboembolism Estimate % (95% CI)	Live Births Estimate % (95% CI)	Anticoagulant-Related Fetal and Neonatal Adverse Events Estimate % (95% CI)
Vitamin K antagonists (INR target 2.5–3.5)	0.9 (0.1, 1.6)	2.7 (1.4, 4.0)	64.5 (48.8, 80.2)*	2.0 (0.3, 3.7)*
Sequential treatment	2.0 (0.8, 3.1)	5.8 (3.8, 7.7)	79.9 (74.3, 85.6)	1.4 (0.3, 2.5)†
LMWH alone	2.9 (0.2, 5.7)	8.7 (3.9, 13.4)	92.0 (86.1, 98.0)	NA
UFH alone	3.4 (0, 7.7)	11.2 (2.8, 19.6)	69.5 (37.8, 100)	7.6 (0.1, 15.0)

*Of these, 7/407 (0.8% [0.0, 1.7]) represent embryopathy and 5/197 (2.1% [0.1, 4.1]) represent fetopathy.
†All cases represent fetopathy.
Estimates are presented as proportions per 100 affected pregnancies with 95% confidence intervals.
CI, Confidence intervals; INR, international normalized ratio; LMWH, low-molecular-weight heparin; NA, not applicable; UFH, unfractionated heparin.
From D'Souza R, Ostro J, Shah PS, Silversides CK, et al. Anticoagulation for pregnant women with mechanical heart valves: a systematic review and meta-analysis. Eur Heart J. 2017;38(19):1509-1516.

TABLE 92.6 International Recommendations for the Management of Anticoagulation in Pregnant Women with Mechanical Heart Valves[3,67,76]

	2018 EUROPEAN SOCIETY OF CARDIOLOGY GUIDELINES	2014 AMERICAN HEART ASSOCIATION/AMERICAN COLLEGE OF CARDIOLOGY GUIDELINES	2012 AMERICAN COLLEGE OF CHEST PHYSICIANS GUIDELINES
1st trimester	Warfarin dose <5 mg/day (or phenprocoumon <3 mg/day or acenocoumarol <2 mg/day) 1. VKA* 2. Adjusted-dose LMWH twice daily with monitoring of anti-Xa levels 4–6 hr post dose: Target anti-Xa level depends on valve site. Pre-dose target provided in recommendation footnotes 3. Adjusted-dose intravenous UFH (aPTT ≥2x control) Warfarin dose >5 mg/day 1. Adjusted-dose LMWH* twice daily with monitoring of anti-Xa levels 4–6 hr post dose: Target anti-Xa level depends on valve site. 2. Adjusted-dose intravenous UFH* (aPTT ≥ 2× control) 3. Continuation of VKA	Warfarin dose ≤5 mg/day 1. Warfarin* 2. Dose-adjusted LMWH ≥ two times daily (target anti-Xa level 0.8–1.2 U/mL 4–6 hr post dose) 3. Dose-adjusted continuous infusion UFH (aPTT at least 2 × control) Warfarin dose >5 mg/day 1. Dose-adjusted LMWH ≥ two times daily (target anti-Xa level 0.8-1.2 U/mL 4-6 hr post dose) * 2. Dose adjusted continuous infusion UFH (aPTT at least 2× control) *	Any of the following anticoagulant regimens are recommended: 1. Adjusted-dose bid LMWH throughout pregnancy, with doses adjusted to achieve the manufacturer's peak anti-Xa level 4 hr post dose 2. Adjusted-dose subcutaneous UFH throughout pregnancy administered every 12 hr in doses adjusted to keep the mid interval aPTT at least twice control or attain an anti-Xa heparin level of 0.35–0.70 units/mL 3. UFH or LMWH (as above) until the 13th week with substitution by VKA until close to delivery when UFH or LMWH is resumed. For women judged to be at very high risk of thromboembolism in whom concerns exist about the efficacy and safety of UFH or LMWH as dosed above (e.g., older-generation prosthesis in the mitral position or history of thromboembolism), VKA throughout pregnancy with replacement by UFH or LMWH (as above) close to delivery.
2nd and 3rd trimesters	1. VKA until 36 weeks' gestation†	1. Warfarin	
Addition of aspirin		Low-dose aspirin (75–100 mg daily) at the beginning of the 2nd trimester	Low-dose aspirin (75–100 mg daily)
Prior to delivery	1. Discontinue VKAs and start adjusted-dose intravenous UFH (aPTT ≥2× control) or adjusted-dose LMWH at 36 weeks' gestation 2. Replace LMWH with intravenous UFH (aPTT ≥ 2× control) at least 36 hr before planned delivery	1. Discontinue warfarin and dose-adjusted continuous infusion of UFH (aPTT at least 2× control)	1. UFH or LMWH is resumed close to delivery

*Option that received the highest grade of recommendation from among the competing options during that period of pregnancy.
†Option that received the highest grade of recommendation during the 2nd and 3rd trimesters, from among the competing options in the group with high dose of VKA.
aPTT, Activated partial thromboplastin time; INR, international normalized ratio; LMWH, low-molecular-weight heparin; UFH, unfractionated heparin; VKA, vitamin K antagonist (warfarin, phenprocoumon, or acenocoumarol).

anticoagulation options for pregnant women with mechanical valves: (a) warfarin or other vitamin K antagonists, (b) low-molecular-weight heparins, and (c) intravenous unfractionated heparin (Table 92.6). Direct oral anticoagulants are not safe for pregnant patients with mechanical valves. For pregnant women with mechanical valves, there is no perfect anticoagulant that is equally safe for both the mother and her child. Warfarin is associated with the lowest risk of valve thrombosis and maternal mortality for the mother but crosses the placenta and can cause warfarin embryopathy when used in

the first trimester and fetopathy when used later in pregnancy. Warfarin embryopathy appears to be dose dependent, with lower rates of embryopathy reported in women taking daily warfarin doses less than 5 mg.[72] Heparin does not cross the placenta and is therefore a safer alternative for the fetus but is less effective at preventing valve thrombosis and is associated with higher rates of maternal mortality.[75] One treatment strategy is to replace warfarin with low-molecular-weight heparin during embryogenesis (6 to 12 weeks' gestation) to prevent embryopathy. Use of low-molecular-weight heparin throughout pregnancy is an option for women who wish to avoid warfarin altogether, but this requires close follow-up throughout pregnancy because many of the reported cases of valve thrombosis were related to inadequate dosing and monitoring of anti-Xa levels. Peak anti-Xa levels should be measured frequently, with experts suggesting weekly to monthly anti-Xa monitoring during pregnancy.[3,67,76] In addition, some experts advocate measurement of trough levels to ensure consistently therapeutic anti-Xa levels and have developed a detailed treatment algorithm that considers valve position and type.[72] Anticoagulation surveillance during pregnancy in women with mechanical valves is often best done in conjunction with a hematologist with expertise in pregnancy. Unfractionated heparin is associated with high rates of valve thrombosis when given subcutaneously. Its use is recommended only when administered as a continuous intravenous infusion, in a hospital setting. At the time of delivery, women on anticoagulants are at risk for postpartum hemorrhage and should be monitored closely. Both heparin and warfarin are safe in the breastfeeding mother. Recommendations for anticoagulation in pregnant women with mechanical valves have been published by the American Heart Association/American College of Cardiology,[67] the American College of Chest Physicians,[76] and the European Society of Cardiology[3] (see Table 92.6). In view of the competing maternal and fetal risks, shared decision-making with women is required when choosing an anticoagulation regimen. All women should be followed in a tertiary care center by an experienced pregnancy heart team.

Mechanical valve thrombosis can be fatal and should be excluded in any pregnant women with new cardiac symptoms, heart failure, or significant increases in valve gradients on their echocardiogram. Diagnosis of a thrombosed valve is usually confirmed using transesophageal echocardiography or fluoroscopy. The choice of treatment options (heparin, thrombolytics, or surgery) is determined by the clinical stability of the patient, the size of the thrombus, and the availability of surgery.[72] An algorithm for treatment of left-sided mechanical valve thrombosis is shown on the on line eFigure 92.2.[77] Right-sided valve thrombosis is often treated with heparin or thrombolytics.

ARRHYTHMIAS (SEE PART VII)

Increases in plasma volume, hormonal-mediated changes in action potential, and autonomic changes are potential mechanisms contributing to an increased propensity to arrhythmias during pregnancy. Women who present with arrhythmias during pregnancy should have an echocardiogram to exclude structural heart disease and a Holter monitor to determine the burden of arrhythmias. The most frequently detected arrhythmias in pregnancy are atrial and ventricular premature beats, and generally these do not require therapy. Treatment of tachyarrhythmias needs to be tailored to the individual with consideration of the type of arrhythmia, the underlying heart disease, ventricular function, and the severity of symptoms.

Supraventricular tachycardia (SVT) is the most common arrhythmia in pregnant women and usually occurs in women with structurally normal hearts.[5] Women may present for the first time during pregnancy, or they may have a history of SVT. Women with a history of SVT and structural heart disease have approximately 50% recurrence rates during pregnancy.[78] Most women with SVT can be treated medically.[5,79] In women with acute SVT who are hemodynamically stable, vagal maneuvers and adenosine can used to terminate the arrhythmias. For women with a contraindication to adenosine or in whom adenosine is ineffective, intravenous beta blockers such as metoprolol or propranolol can be used (eFig. 92.3A,B). Experience with other antiarrhythmic agents is more limited and is usually reserved for those women who are highly symptomatic despite beta blockers or calcium channel blockers.

AF and atrial flutter (AFL) often occur in the setting of structural heart disease such as MS or congenital heart disease.[78,80] In general, in women who develop AF or AFL, rate control is preferred over rhythm control. Pregnant women with acute unstable AF or AFL require cardioversion (eFig. 92.4).[5] In pregnant women who are stable with rapid ventricular rates, beta blockers, or digoxin can be given to control the ventricular rate. As in the nonpregnant patient, pregnant women with AF/AFL for

more than 48 hours or of unknown duration require a transesophageal echocardiogram or 3 weeks of therapeutic anticoagulation prior to cardioversion. Pharmacologic cardioversion should be individualized, and the choice of antiarrhythmic should be based on the presence of structural heart disease and the left ventricular systolic function. Management of AF in patients with Wolff-Parkinson-White (WPW) requires special consideration as the rhythm can degenerate into an unstable preexcited rhythm if drugs such as beta blockers, calcium channel blockers, or digoxin are given as these drugs increase conduction over the accessory pathway. Therefore antiarrhythmic drugs that slow or block conduction over the pathway, such as flecainide, should be used to treat AF. Consideration of thromboembolism prophylaxis should be given to women who develop AF/AFL, especially those with structural heart disease or elevated $CHADS_2$ scores. Warfarin is associated with warfarin embryopathy when used between 6 and 12 weeks' gestation, and therefore low-molecular-weight heparin is often used during pregnancy. Direct oral anticoagulants are not recommended in pregnancy.

VT and ventricular fibrillation (VF) are rare during pregnancy. VT may be idiopathic, or it may occur in the setting of structural heart disease such as cardiomyopathies, valve disease, and congenital heart disease.[7,15] VT may be secondary to primary electrical diseases such as long QT syndrome (LQTS). Rarely, VT occurs in the setting of hypomagnesemia or hypertensive crises. Acute unstable VT or VF in pregnant women should be treated similarly to the nonpregnant patient with cardioversion or defibrillation (eFig. 92.5). Pharmacologic cardioversion with procainamide, amiodarone, or lidocaine may be appropriate in some cases of hemodynamically stable VT. Idiopathic VT is a monomorphic VT that typically originates from the right ventricular outflow tract. It is usually successfully treated with beta blockers or verapamil.[3] The risk of VT in women with LQTS, specifically LQT2 mutation, increases in the postpartum period.[81] Beta blockers are effective in preventing cardiac events in pregnant women with LQTS, and all women should be treated with beta blockers during pregnancy and postpartum.[81] VT in the setting of structural heart disease is more complex and requires and individualize approach to therapy. Amiodarone can affect fetal thyroid function and should be used only to treat recurrent VT and when other antiarrhythmic drugs are not suitable. In pregnant women with drug-refractory VT, catheter ablation may be considered and referral to a center that can offer radiofrequency catheter ablation without fluoroscopic guidance should be considered.

CONGENITAL HEART DISEASE (SEE CHAPTER 82)

The involvement of an adult congenital cardiologist, preferably as part of the pregnancy heart team, is recommended in the preconceptual counseling or care of pregnant women with congenital heart lesion. Review of prior clinical and procedural records will guide diagnostic tests and enable pregnancy management to be individualized.

Cardiac Shunts

Women with successful closure of isolated left-to-right shunts are at low risk for complications during pregnancy. In the absence of other risk factors such as cardiac arrhythmias, cardiac events after closure, systemic ventricular dysfunction, or pulmonary hypertension, women with repaired shunts can deliver at their local hospital. Women with unoperated atrial septal defect (ASD) usually tolerate pregnancy well. Overall frequency of arrhythmia, right heart failure, and thromboembolism is low.[3] In women of childbearing age, most unoperated ventricular septal defects (VSDs) or patent ductus arteriosus (PDA) are likely small (restrictive) as those with untreated significant shunts would have progressed to pulmonary hypertension in childhood. Women with small (restrictive) VSD or PDA, without other general risk factors, do not require additional cardiac precautions during the antepartum and peripartum period. For unrepaired ASD or VSD, repaired ASD or VSD with residual shunting, or patent foramen ovale, we recommend the use of air/particulate filters for indwelling IVs at time of labor and delivery, to reduce the chance of paradoxical right-to-left shunt.[23]

Cardiac shunts associated with pulmonary hypertension are discussed in the pulmonary hypertension section.

Left-Sided Obstruction

BAV is a common etiology of AS and aortic regurgitation (AR) in women in childbearing age. The management of AS and AR during pregnancy has been discussed earlier. An important association of BAV is ascending aorta dilatation and coarctation. Aortic dissection has been reported in women with BAV and aortopathy, although overall risk is lower than in women with aortopathy associated with Marfan syndrome.[23] The approach to the aortopathy associated with BAV is discussed in the aortopathy section.

Significant aortic coarctation impedes delivery of blood distally with adverse impact on the placental circulation, and increases the risk of intrauterine growth restriction and premature labor. Upper body hypertension and concomitant aortic valve disease pose additional risks. Maternal mortality has been reported, but this is rare in contemporary series.[23] Overtreatment of upper body hypertension during pregnancy could potentially result in hypotension distal to the coarctation site with adverse impact on fetal well-being. Even with successful coarctation repair, abnormal aortic compliance increases the risk of developing gestational hypertension.[23] An elevated descending aorta gradient may be a result of increase in flow, abnormal compliance, hypoplasia of the aorta, or true coarctation. Prolongation of the gradient into diastole (diastolic tail) as seen in the abdominal or descending aorta Doppler increases the certainty that true coarctation is present. Women with unrepaired coarctation or residual coarctation are at risk for aortic complication including dissection,[3] for which we offer empiric beta blockers therapy. Percutaneous intervention for residual or recurrent coarctation is best deferred until after pregnancy.[3]

Left-sided or systemic atrioventricular valvular regurgitation is treated similarly in those with acquired heart disease. Although isolated systemic atrioventricular valvular regurgitation may be well tolerated with heart failure/arrhythmia reported with low mortality, concomitant systemic ventricular systolic dysfunction will increase risk by impairing maternal adaptation to the regurgitant load during pregnancy. Those patients with moderate or severe regurgitation will need serial follow-up with consideration of postpartum intravenous loop diuretics to reduce the risk of redistribution pulmonary edema. Pulmonic and tricuspid valve disease has already been previously discussed in the section on native valvular disease.

Complex Congenital Lesions

The management considerations for selected complex congenital cardiac lesions are summarized on Table 92.7. Patients with complex congenital lesions represent a heterogeneous group, and their management during pregnancy has been extensively reviewed.[3,4,18,72] Women with complex congenital cardiac lesions should be followed by the pregnancy heart team, with the site of delivery determined by maternal risk, stability during pregnancy, and logistical considerations.

Unoperated Complex Congenital Lesions
Ebstein Anomaly

Acyanotic women with milder anatomic variations of Ebstein can expect to have an uncomplicated pregnancy, whereas women with severe Ebstein anomaly may be unable to tolerate the increased preload and cardiac output of pregnancy and are at risk for functional deterioration, right heart failure, and arrhythmia.[23] The overall frequency of cardiac complications during pregnancy is low (from 0% to ≤12%).[23,82] The associated lesions of preexcitation and interatrial shunting will increase cardiac risk during pregnancy. Those with the associated ASD or patent foramen ovale (PFO) may demonstrate reversal or increase in right-to-left shunting with pregnancy, leading to worsening cyanosis, with the risk of fetal loss, prematurity, or intrauterine growth restriction. Risk of preterm delivery and fetal mortality is increased.

Congenitally Corrected Transposition of Great Arteries

Systemic ventricular systolic dysfunction and significant systemic atrioventricular valvular regurgitation are common findings in adults with congenitally corrected transposition of the arteries. Importantly, significant systemic atrioventricular valvular regurgitation will mask systemic ventricular systolic dysfunction. Heart failure, endocarditis, stroke, or MI have been reported.[3,23] Pregnancy should be discouraged in patients with poor functional class, severe systemic ventricular systolic function, or severe systemic atrioventricular valvular regurgitation.[3]

Complex Congenital: Repaired
Repaired Tetralogy of Fallot

Pregnancy is usually well tolerated in women after repaired tetralogy, but risk is increased in the presence of left ventricular systolic dysfunction and/or severe PR with right ventricular dysfunction. Although right heart failure and arrhythmias have been reported in up to 12% of pregnancies, other series have reported lower complication rates.[3,23] Patients with VSD patch leak and residual right ventricular outflow tract obstruction usually tolerate pregnancy well as long as they are not cyanotic.[23,83]

Repaired Transposition of Great Arteries

Women born with repaired complete transposition of the great arteries would have undergone an atrial redirection operation (Mustard or Senning), an arterial switch operation (Jatene), or, less commonly, a Rastelli repair. Late complications after atrial redirection (baffle) operations include sinus node dysfunction, atrial arrhythmias, systemic ventricular dysfunction, and systemic atrioventricular valve regurgitation. Arrhythmias are the most common cardiac complication during pregnancy, and there is an increased risk of heart failure. Fetoneonatal complications are higher than in normal pregnancy. Pregnancy has been associated with progressive subaortic right ventricular dilation and deterioration in subaortic right ventricular function after pregnancy.[3,23] Baffle leak has been underrecognized (see Table 92.7). Pulmonary artery catheters should be discouraged due to potential problems with trapping of the catheter through the baffles. Reported experience during pregnancy in women treated with the arterial switch operation procedure remains limited,[3] but no maternal cardiovascular complications were observed in preliminary studies.[3,84] The main residua in those with Rastelli repair is right ventricular outflow tract conduit stenosis, which is usually well tolerated during pregnancy; those with severe conduit stenosis may experience functional deterioration, but right heart failure is uncommon.

Fontan

The ability of the heart to increase cardiac output during pregnancy is impaired following the Fontan operation, which directs systemic venous return to the pulmonary artery and bypasses the trabecular (or muscular) portion of the subpulmonary ventricle. Associated scarring and remodeling of the atria increase the risk of atrial arrhythmias while systemic venous stasis increases risk of atrial thrombi, particularly with atrial tachyarrhythmia. Importantly, adults with Fontan procedure may manifest reduced oxygen desaturation or cyanosis due to systemic to pulmonary collaterals or residual right to left shunt at the atrial level. Despite these concerns, low maternal mortality has been observed in pregnant women with Fontan procedure, likely reflecting patient selection as those with prior cardiac events, reduced systemic ventricular systolic function, or protein losing enteropathy were likely appropriately discouraged from pregnancy.[85] An overview reported SVT (9%) and heart failure (4%) with no maternal deaths.[20] Fetal and neonatal adverse outcomes remain common, with miscarriages complicating 45% of pregnancies and a high rate of antepartum bleeding (including abruptio placenta), prematurity, and cesarean delivery (11%, 59%, and 57%, respectively). Pregnant Fontan patients should deliver at a referral center and be cared for by a maternal heart team. Antiplatelet thromboprophylaxis should be considered (low-dose ECASA), with the use of low-molecular-weight heparin for those with prior history of embolism or atrial arrhythmias. Vaginal delivery is preferred.[3]

TABLE 92.7 Potential Complications and Management Recommendations for Pregnant Women with Complex Congenital Heart Lesions

CARDIAC LESION	CARDIAC COMPLICATIONS	MANAGEMENT RECOMMENDATIONS
Ebstein anomaly (unrepaired and repaired)	• Arrhythmias • Right heart failure • Paradoxical emboli • Oxygen desaturation from interatrial shunt	• Clinical and echocardiographic surveillance during pregnancy and postpartum including oxygen saturation • Echocardiographic monitoring of right ventricular systolic function • Air/particulate filters during labor and delivery for women with interatrial communications • Vaginal delivery preferred
Repaired tetralogy of Fallot	• Arrhythmias • Right heart failure	• Clinical and echocardiographic surveillance during pregnancy and postpartum • Echocardiographic monitoring of the right ventricular size, right ventricular systolic function, and pulmonary artery pressures • Autosomal dominant transmission of heart disease to offspring in women with 22q11.2 deletion syndrome • Vaginal delivery preferred
Arterial switch operation	• Arrhythmias • Aortic dilation or dissection • Heart failure in women with aortic regurgitation	• Clinical and echocardiographic surveillance during pregnancy and postpartum • Vaginal delivery preferred unless there is significant aortic dilation
Systemic right ventricle • Atrial switch operation (Mustard or Senning operation) • Congenitally corrected transposition of great arteries (unrepaired)	• Deterioration in ventricular function • Heart failure • Worsening systemic atrioventricular valve regurgitation • Arrhythmias • Heart failure	• Frequent clinical and echocardiographic surveillance during pregnancy and postpartum • Echocardiographic monitoring of the subaortic right ventricular size, systolic function, and atrioventricular valve regurgitation • Vaginal delivery with early epidural and a facilitated second stage of labor • Air/particulate filters during labor and delivery for women with atrial switch procedures • Avoid pulmonary catheters in women with atrial switch procedures • Postpartum monitoring for arrhythmias and heart failure
Fontan operation	• Arrhythmias • Heart failure • Thromboembolic complications • Bleeding complications	• Frequent clinical and echocardiographic surveillance during pregnancy and postpartum • Echocardiographic monitoring of subaortic ventricular function and atrioventricular valve regurgitation • Low-dose aspirin and consideration of anticoagulation for women at risk for thromboembolic complications • Prompt treatment of atrial arrhythmias • Prepare for preterm labor, which is common • Vaginal delivery with early epidural and a facilitated second stage of labor • Maintain adequate preload during delivery • Postpartum monitoring for arrhythmias and heart failure
Cyanotic congenital heart disease	• Mortality • Heart failure • Arrhythmias • Thromboembolism • Bleeding complications	• Frequent clinical and echocardiographic surveillance during pregnancy and postpartum including oxygen saturation • Supplemental oxygen and activity limitation • Air/particulate filters during labor and delivery • Consider thromboprophylaxis • Consider following brain natriuretic peptide • Preterm labor common • Vaginal delivery often possible • Postpartum monitoring for heart failure and arrhythmias

Cyanotic Congenital Heart Lesions

The cardiac causes of cyanosis in pregnant women without pulmonary artery hypertension are large shunts at atrial or ventricular levels, systemic venous to pulmonary venous collaterals, or reduced pulmonary blood flow. Maternal cardiovascular complications have been reported in approximately 30% of pregnancies and are related to maternal oxygen level. If the maternal oxygen saturation was 85% or less, the live birth rate was only 12%.[3] Supplemental oxygen and activity restriction are recommended. Thromboembolic prophylaxis has been proposed but must be balanced with the bleeding risk associated with cyanosis.[3]

Cyanosis is associated with abnormal thrombotic and bleeding tendency, and these patients are at risk for postpartum hemorrhage. Care by the pregnancy heart team and delivery at a referral center are recommended for pregnant women with cyanotic heart disease.

PULMONARY HYPERTENSION

Pulmonary arterial hypertension (PAH), from any cause, is associated with very high pregnancy risks. PAH is defined as a mean resting pulmonary arterial pressure greater than 25 mm Hg, and higher pulmonary arterial pressures are associated with higher risk. Maternal cardiac decompensation occurs because of the volume load on the right ventricle, the increased flow in the high-resistance pulmonary vascular bed, changes in intracardiac shunt flow with resulting desaturations, and thromboembolic events secondary to the prothrombotic effects of pregnancy. At delivery, adverse effects from anesthetic drugs and volume overload from intravenous fluids and volume shifts can further lead to cardiac decompensation. A review of pregnancy outcomes in women with PAH delivering between 1997 and 2007 reported a maternal mortality of 17%, 28%, and 33% in women with idiopathic PAH, congenital heart disease, and other causes, respectively.[86] Maternal mortality is the result of a number of causes, including right-sided heart failure, sudden death, pulmonary hypertensive crisis, and pulmonary embolism. Most maternal deaths occur within the first month after delivery. Although more favorable outcomes have been reported in women treated with pulmonary vasodilator therapy,[18,87-89] because of the high mortality risk, women with PAH should be advised against pregnancy and safe and reliable contraception should be provided. While women with idiopathic PAH or Eisenmenger syndrome are at the highest risk during pregnancy, pregnancy risks are high even when pulmonary hypertension is secondary to left heart disease.[90] Pregnant women with pulmonary hypertension are also at elevated risk of eclampsia, preterm delivery, and fetal death.[91]

For those women who become pregnant, termination often remains the safest option.[3] Those who choose to continue pregnancy require close antenatal follow-up with frequent clinic visits, transthoracic echocardiograms, and serum BNP levels.[18] Bosentan and other endothelin receptor antagonists are teratogenic and should be discontinued, ideally prior to pregnancy. Calcium channel blockers, phosphodiesterase-5 inhibitors, and prostacyclins have been used during pregnancy. During pregnancy and after delivery, fluid status should be followed closely to prevent right-sided heart failure. Joint care by the pregnancy heart and pulmonary hypertension team is important. All women should deliver at a tertiary care center with postpartum monitoring in the coronary/intensive care unit and careful diuresis. Women who are clinically stable can undergo vaginal delivery with early epidural anesthesia and an assisted second stage of delivery. Delivery is usually planned prior to 37 weeks' gestation.[18] Extended postpartum monitoring in hospital is recommended because many of the cardiac complications occur in the first postpartum week.

MARFAN SYNDROME AND INHERITED AORTOPATHIES

Increased cardiac output, hypervolemia, and the pregnancy-related changes in aorta media contribute to increased risk of aortic dilation and dissection.[18] Aortic dissection has been described in pregnant women with Marfan syndrome, Loeys-Dietz syndrome, vascular Ehlers-Danlos syndrome, Turner syndrome, and BAV.[92] The highest risk of dissection occurs in the third trimester or early postpartum.[18] The risk for complications varies according to the particular lesion.

In women with Marfan syndrome, the incidence of aortic dissection or rupture during pregnancy and postpartum period is eightfold higher than those who were not pregnant.[93] The overall risk of aortic dissection is approximately 3%, ranging from 1% in women with aortic diameters less than 40 mm, to approximately 10% in women with an aortic diameter greater than 40 mm, rapid dilatation, or previous ascending aortic dissection.[18] Aortic root replacement prior to pregnancy is not

protective from distal aortic dissection.[94,95] Similarly, it is possible for dissection to occur in an aorta that appears "normal" by imaging.

Loeys-Dietz syndrome is a high-risk lesion during pregnancy. Vascular dissection or rupture can occur in the presence of normal aorta dimensions and can occur despite aortic root replacement and optimal medical therapy. Pooled data reported a vascular dissection or rupture in 11% of pregnancies.[96] Uterine rupture has been reported. Vascular Ehlers-Danlos syndrome is extremely high risk, and like Loeys-Dietz syndrome (LDS), vascular rupture can occur despite normal aorta dimensions. Pregnant women with Turner syndrome are at significant risk of aortic dissection, preeclampsia, premature birth, low birth weight, and need for cesarean delivery.[97] Concurrent cardiac lesions (e.g., BAV or coarctation) increase the dissection risk.[18] Aorta measurements must be indexed to body surface area to adjust for the smaller stature in some patients with Turner syndrome. Aortic dissection has been described in women with Turner syndrome with prior root replacement as well as during ART-associated pregnancies.[3,97] Aortic dissection is much less common in women with BAV and aortopathy.[18] Early data on SMAD 3 mutation have reported favorable outcomes, but the patient numbers were small.[98]

All women with aortopathies considering pregnancy or already pregnant should be evaluated by and receive care by a maternal heart team at a referral center with echocardiographic assessment of the aorta, preferably supplemented by cardiac MR or CT before pregnancy. Pregnancy is contraindicated in Marfan and Loeys-Dietz syndrome with an ascending aorta greater than 45 mm, all patients with vascular Ehlers-Danlos syndrome, bicuspid associated aorta greater than 50 mm, and Turner syndrome with high-risk features (aortic size index [ASI] >2.5 cm/m^2 or history of aortic dissection).[3,72,97] Women with Marfan, Ehlers-Danlos, and Loeys-Dietz syndrome have a 50% chance of transmitting the syndrome to offspring. In addition, they are at increased risk for obstetric and fetoneonatal complications. Obstetric and neonatal complications (including preterm delivery from premature rupture of membranes and neonatal death) occur in approximately 40% of pregnancy in women with Marfan syndrome.[18]

For all aortopathies, serial echocardiographic evaluation of the aorta is recommended at least once during each trimester and increasing up to every 4 to 6 weeks in patients with aortic diameter greater than 40 mm, history of aortic surgery, or with progressive dilatation. TEE or cardiac magnetic resonance imaging (CMR) without gadolinium can be used for assessment if transthoracic echocardiogram is suboptimal.[18] Optimal hypertension control is crucial. Cesarean delivery is recommended in those with Marfan syndrome with aorta diameter greater than 40 mm (or progressive dilatation during pregnancy or prior aortic dissection repair), bicuspid aortopathy with aortic diameter greater than 45 mm, and Turner syndrome with ASI greater than 20 mm/m^2.[18] Plans for regional anesthesia should consider the high prevalence of dural ectasia in patients with Marfan syndrome. Prophylactic beta blockers (reducing heart rate by at least 20 beats/min) is recommended for pregnant patients with Marfan syndrome[18] and should be considered for Loey-Dietz, Turner syndrome, and in other aortopathies.[96,97] Beta blockers should also be considered when these patients undergo ARTs. A management algorithm for suspected aortic dissection during pregnancy is summarized in eFigure 92.6.[5]

CONTRACEPTION

There are multiple contraception formulations, including barrier method, estrogen-containing oral contraceptive pills, progestin-only contraceptives (oral and implantable), patches, subdermal implants, intrauterine devices, and sterilization procedures. Each of these contraceptive options has benefits, risks, and variable failure rates (eTable 92.3).[2] For women with heart disease, some forms of contraception can have important side effects and should be avoided. Barrier methods (male and female condoms, diaphragms, cervical caps) are safe for women with heart disease but have high failure rates and are therefore not suitable for women at high risk for complications who need reliable contraception. Estrogen-containing contraceptives, available as oral preparations, transdermal patches, and vaginal rings, have relatively low failure rates; however, the associated increased thromboembolic risks limit the use of these contraceptives in women with mechanical valves, Fontan circulation, severe left ventricular systolic dysfunction, coronary disease, or a history of thromboembolism. Progestin-only forms of contraception are not associated with thrombosis; however, progestin can lead to fluid retention, and progestin-only pills have higher failure rates than combined oral contraceptives and should not be used in women in whom pregnancy risks are prohibitive. Intrauterine devices have low failure rates and are effective for long periods of time, but implantation carries risk and can result in a profound vagal reaction which can be dangerous for women with pulmonary hypertension or Fontan circulation. For women with these high-risk conditions, intrauterine devices should be implanted in a monitored setting. In instances where pregnancy is contraindicated, permanent forms of contraception should be considered by the patient or her partner. Women with severe heart disease may have limited life expectancy, and it is important to consider that women may be outlived by their spouse, who may then want to father children in the future.

REFERENCES
Risk Assessment
1. Davis MB, Walsh MN. Cardio-obstetrics. *Circ Cardiovasc Qual Outcomes.* 2019;12:e005417.
2. Mehta LS, Warnes CA, Bradley E, et al. Cardiovascular considerations in caring for pregnant patients: a scientific statement from the American heart association. *Circulation.* 2020;141:e884–e903.
3. Regitz-Zagrosek V, Roos-Hesselink JW, Bauersachs J, et al. ESC Guidelines for the management of cardiovascular diseases during pregnancy. *Eur Heart J.* 2018;39:3165–3241. 2018.
4. Canobbio MM, Warnes CA, Aboulhosn J, et al. Management of pregnancy in patients with complex congenital heart disease: a scientific statement for healthcare professionals from the American heart association. *Circulation.* 2017;135:e50–e87.
5. Windram J, Grewal J, Bottega N, et al. Clinical practice update on cardiovascular management of the pregnant patient. *Can J Cardiol.* 2021 (in press).
6. Lane-Cordova AD, Khan SS, Grobman WA, et al. Long-term cardiovascular risks associated with adverse pregnancy outcomes: JACC review topic of the week. *J Am Coll Cardiol.* 2019;73:2106–2116.
7. Roos-Hesselink JW, Ruys TP, Stein JI, et al. Outcome of pregnancy in patients with structural or ischaemic heart disease: results of a registry of the European Society of Cardiology. *Eur Heart J.* 2013;34:657–665.
8. D'Souza RD, Silversides CK, Tomlinson GA, Siu SC. Assessing cardiac risk in pregnant women with heart disease: how risk scores are created and their role in clinical practice. *Can J Cardiol.* 2020;36:1011–1021.
9. Schlichting LE, Insaf TZ, Zaidi AN, et al. Maternal comorbidities and complications of delivery in pregnant women with congenital heart disease. *J Am Coll Cardiol.* 2019;73:2181–2191.
10. Ramage K, Grabowska K, Silversides C, et al. Association of adult congenital heart disease with pregnancy, maternal, and neonatal outcomes. *JAMA Netw Open.* 2019;2:e193667.
11. MBRRACE-UK. Saving lives, improving mothers' care: lessons learned to inform maternity care from the UK and Ireland confidential enquiries into maternal deaths and morbidity. 2015–17. 2019.
12. Main EK, McCain CL, Morton CH, et al. Pregnancy-related mortality in California: causes, characteristics, and improvement opportunities. *Obstet Gynecol.* 2015;125:938–947.
13. Petersen EE, Davis NL, Goodman D, et al. Racial/Ethnic disparities in pregnancy-related deaths—United States, 2007–2016. *MMWR Morb Mortal Wkly Rep.* 2019;68:762–765.
14. Drenthen W, Boersma E, Balci A, et al. Predictors of pregnancy complications in women with congenital heart disease. *Eur Heart J.* 2010;31:2124–2132.
15. Silversides CK, Grewal J, Mason J, et al. Pregnancy outcomes in women with heart disease: the CARPREG II study. *J Am Coll Cardiol.* 2018;71:2419–2430.
16. Pfaller B, Sathananthan G, Grewal J, et al. Preventing complications in pregnant women with cardiac disease. *J Am Coll Cardiol.* 2020;75:1443–1452.
17. Slomski A. Why do hundreds of us women die annually in childbirth? *J Am Med Assoc.* 2019;321:1239–1241.
18. Elkayam U, Goland S, Pieper PG, Silversides CK. High-risk cardiac disease in pregnancy: Part II. *J Am Coll Cardiol.* 2016;68:502–516.
19. Balint OH, Siu SC, Mason J, et al. Cardiac outcomes after pregnancy in women with congenital heart disease. *Heart.* 2010;96:1656–1661.
20. Garcia Ropero A, Baskar S, Roos Hesselink JW, et al. Pregnancy in women with a fontan circulation: a systematic review of the literature. *Circ Cardiovasc Qual Outcomes.* 2018;11:e004575.
21. Sharma G, Ying Y, Silversides CK. The importance of cardiovascular risk assessment and pregnancy heart team in the management of cardiovascular disease in pregnancy. *Cardiol Clin.* 2021;39:7–19.

Management
22. Green LJ, Mackillop LH, Salvi D, et al. Gestation-specific vital sign reference ranges in pregnancy. *Obstet Gynecol.* 2020;135:653–664.
23. Haberer K, Silversides CK, Colman JM, Siu SC. Pregnancy in young women with congenital heart disease. In: Allen HD, ed. *Moss & Adams' Heart Disease in Infants, Children, and Adolescents.* 10 ed. Baltimore: Lippincott Williams and Wildkins; 2021.
24. Elkayam U. Cardiovascular evaluation during pregnancy. In: Elkayam U, ed. *Cardiac Problems in Pregnancy.* 4th ed. Hoboken: Wiley Blackwell; 2018:19–31.
25. Malhame I, Hurlburt H, Larson L, et al. Sensitivity and specificity of B-type natriuretic peptide in diagnosing heart failure in pregnancy. *Obstet Gynecol.* 2019;134:440–449.
26. Tanous D, Siu SC, Mason J, et al. B-type natriuretic peptide in pregnant women with heart disease. *J Am Coll Cardiol.* 2010;56:1247–1253.
27. Silversides CK, Siu SC. Heart disease in pregnancy. In: Otto CM, ed. *The Practice of Clinical Echocardiography.* 6th ed. Phladelphia: Elsevier; 2020.
28. Colletti PM, Lee KH, Elkayam U. Cardiovascular imaging of the pregnant patient. *AJR Am J Roentgenol.* 2013;200:515–521.
29. Ray JG, Vermeulen MJ, Bharatha A, et al. Association between MRI exposure during pregnancy and fetal and childhood outcomes. *J Am Med Assoc.* 2016;316:952–961.
30. Brugada J, Katritsis DG, Arbelo E, et al. ESC Guidelines for the management of patients with supraventricular tachycardia the Task Force for the management of patients with supraventricular tachycardia of the European Society of Cardiology (ESC). *Eur Heart J.* 2020;41:655–720. 2019.
31. Haberer K, Silversides CK. Congenital heart disease and women's health across the life span: focus on reproductive issues. *Can J Cardiol.* 2019;35:1652–1663.

32. Lima FV, Yang J, Xu J, Stergiopoulos K. National trends and in-hospital outcomes in pregnant women with heart disease in the United States. *Am J Cardiol.* 2017;119:1694–1700.
33. van Hagen IM, Boersma E, Johnson MR, et al. Global cardiac risk assessment in the Registry of Pregnancy and Cardiac disease: results of a registry from the European Society of Cardiology. *Eur J Heart Fail.* 2016;18:523–533.
34. Siu SC, Evans KL, Foley MR. Risk assessment of the cardiac pregnant patient. *Clin Obstet Gynecol.* 2020;63:815–827.
35. Halpern DG, Weinberg CR, Pinnelas R, et al. Use of medication for cardiovascular disease during pregnancy: JACC state-of-the-art review. *J Am Coll Cardiol.* 2019;73:457–476.
36. Grewal J, Silversides CK, Colman JM. Pregnancy in women with heart disease: risk assessment and management of heart failure. *Heart Fail Clin.* 2014;10:117–129.
37. Dayan N, Laskin CA, Spitzer K, et al. Pregnancy complications in women with heart disease conceiving with fertility therapy. *J Am Coll Cardiol.* 2014;64:1862–1864.
38. Udell JA, Lu H, Redelmeier DA. Failure of fertility therapy and subsequent adverse cardiovascular events. *CMAJ (Can Med Assoc J).* 2017;189:E391–E397.
39. Grewal J, Siu SC, Lee T, et al. Impact of beta-blockers on birth weight in a high-risk cohort of pregnant women with CVD. *J Am Coll Cardiol.* 2020;75:2751–2752.
40. Adler Y, Charron P, Imazio M, et al. ESC guidelines for the diagnosis and management of pericardial diseases: the Task Force for the diagnosis and management of pericardial diseases of the European Society of Cardiology (ESC) Endorsed by: The European Association for Cardio-Thoracic Surgery (EACTS). *Eur Heart J.* 2015;36:2921–2964. 2015.
41. John AS, Gurley F, Schaff HV, et al. Cardiopulmonary bypass during pregnancy. *Ann Thorac Surg.* 2011;91:1191–1196.
42. Lavonas EJ, Drennan IR, Gabrielli A, et al. Part 10: special circumstances of resuscitation: 2015 American Heart Association guidelines update for cardiopulmonary resuscitation and emergency cardiovascular care. *Circulation.* 2015;132:S501–S518.
43. ACOG Practice Bulletin No. Chronic hypertension in pregnancy. *Obstet Gynecol.* 2019;133:e26–e50.203.
44. American College of Obstetricians and Gynecologists' Committee on Practice Bulletins-Obstetrics. Gestational hypertension and preeclampsia: ACOG practice Bulletin, number 222. *Obstet Gynecol.* 2020;135:e237–e260.
45. Butalia S, Audibert F, Cote AM, et al. Hypertension Canada's 2018 guidelines for the management of hypertension in pregnancy. *Can J Cardiol.* 2018;34:526–531.
46. Brown MA, Magee LA, Kenny LC, et al. The hypertensive disorders of pregnancy: ISSHP classification, diagnosis & management recommendations for international practice. *Pregnancy Hypertens.* 2018;13:291–310.
47. Williams B, Mancia G, Spiering W, et al. ESC/ESH Guidelines for the management of arterial hypertension. *Eur Heart J.* 2018;39:3021–3104. 2018.
48. D'Souza R, Kingdom J. Preeclampsia. *CMAJ.* 2016;188:1178.
49. Rolnik DL, Wright D, Poon LC, et al. Aspirin versus placebo in pregnancies at high risk for preterm preeclampsia. *N Engl J Med.* 2017;377:613–622.
50. Nolan M, Oikonomou EK, Silversides CK, et al. Impact of cancer therapy-related cardiac dysfunction on risk of heart failure in pregnancy. *JACC CardioOncol.* 2020;2:153–162.
51. Grewal J, Siu SC, Ross HJ, et al. Pregnancy outcomes in women with dilated cardiomyopathy. *J Am Coll Cardiol.* 2009;55:45–52.
52. Goland S, van Hagen IM, Elbaz-Greener G, et al. Pregnancy in women with hypertrophic cardiomyopathy: data from the European Society of Cardiology initiated Registry of Pregnancy and Cardiac disease (ROPAC). *Eur Heart J.* 2017;38:2683–2690.
53. Davis MB, Arany Z, McNamara DM, et al. Peripartum cardiomyopathy: JACC state-of-the-art review. *J Am Coll Cardiol.* 2020;75:207–221.
54. McNamara DM, Elkayam U, Alharethi R, et al. Clinical outcomes for peripartum cardiomyopathy in North America: results of the IPAC study (investigations of pregnancy-associated cardiomyopathy). *J Am Coll Cardiol.* 2015;66:905–914.
55. Acuna S, Zaffar N, Dong S, et al. Pregnancy outcomes in women with cardiothoracic transplants: a Systematic review and meta-analysis. *J Heart Lung Transplant.* 2020;39:93–102.
56. Lameijer H, Burchill LJ, Baris L, et al. Pregnancy in women with pre-existent ischaemic heart disease: a systematic review with individualised patient data. *Heart.* 2019;105:873–880.
57. Cauldwell M, Baris L, Roos-Hesselink JW, Johnson MR. Ischaemic heart disease and pregnancy. *Heart.* 2019;105:189–195.
58. Gibson P, Narous M, Firoz T, et al. Incidence of myocardial infarction in pregnancy: a systematic review and meta-analysis of population-based studies. *Eur Heart J Qual Care Clin Outcomes.* 2017;3:198–207.
59. Elkayam U, Jalnapurkar S, Barakkat MN, et al. Pregnancy-associated acute myocardial infarction: a review of contemporary experience in 150 cases between 2006 and 2011. *Circulation.* 2014;129:1695–1702.
60. Thygesen K, Alpert JS, Jaffe AS, et al. Fourth universal definition of myocardial infarction (2018). *Circulation.* 2018;138:e618–e651.
61. Hayes SN, Kim ESH, Saw J, et al. Spontaneous coronary artery dissection: current state of the science: a scientific statement from the American Heart Association. *Circulation.* 2018;137:e523–e557.
62. Tamis-Holland JE, Jneid H, Reynolds HR, et al. Contemporary diagnosis and management of patients with myocardial infarction in the absence of obstructive coronary artery disease: a scientific statement from the American Heart Association. *Circulation.* 2019;139:e891–e908.
63. Elkayam U, Havakuk O. Acute myocardial infarction and pregnancy. In: Elkayam U, ed. *Cardiac Problems in Pregnancy.* 4th ed. Hoboken: Wiley Blackwell; 2018:201–219.
64. French KA, Poppas A. Rheumatic heart disease in pregnancy: global challenges and clear opportunities. *Circulation.* 2018;137:817–819.
65. Silversides CK, Colman JM, Sermer M, Siu SC. Cardiac risk in pregnant women with rheumatic mitral stenosis. *Am J Cardiol.* 2003;91:1382–1385.
66. van Hagen IM, Thorne SA, Taha N, et al. Pregnancy outcomes in women with rheumatic mitral valve disease: results from the registry of pregnancy and cardiac disease. *Circulation.* 2018;137:806–816.
67. Nishimura RA, Otto CM, Bonow RO, et al. AHA/ACC guideline for the management of patients with valvular heart disease: a report of the American College of cardiology/American heart association Task Force on practice guidelines. *Circulation.* 2014;129:e521–e643. 2014.
68. Diao M, Kane A, Ndiaye MB, et al. Pregnancy in women with heart disease in sub-Saharan Africa. *Arch Cardiovasc Dis.* 2011;104:370–374.
69. Ducas RA, Javier DA, D'Souza R, et al. Pregnancy outcomes in women with significant valve disease: a systematic review and meta-analysis. *Heart.* 2020;106:512–519.
70. Baumgartner H, Falk V, Bax JJ, et al. ESC/EACTS Guidelines for the management of valvular heart disease. *Eur Heart J.* 2017;38:2739–2791. 2017.
71. Elkayam U. Native valvular heart disease and pregnancy. In: Elkayam U, ed. *Cardiac Problems in Pregnancy.* 4th ed. Hoboken: Wiley Blackwell; 2018:75–89.
72. Elkayam U, Goland S, Pieper PG, Silverside CK. High-risk cardiac disease in pregnancy: Part I. *J Am Coll Cardiol.* 2016;68:396–410.
73. Siu SC, Sermer M, Colman JM, et al. Prospective multicenter study of pregnancy outcomes in women with heart disease. *Circulation.* 2001;104:515–521.
74. North RA, Sadler L, Stewart AW, et al. Long-term survival and valve-related complications in young women with cardiac valve replacements. *Circulation.* 1999;99:2669–2676.
75. D'Souza R, Ostro J, Shah PS, et al. Anticoagulation for pregnant women with mechanical heart valves: a systematic review and meta-analysis. *Eur Heart J.* 2017;38(19):1509–1516.

76. Bates SM, Greer IA, Middeldorp S, et al. VTE, thrombophilia, antithrombotic therapy, and pregnancy: antithrombotic therapy and prevention of thrombosis, 9th ed: American college of chest physicians evidence-based clinical practice guidelines. *Chest.* 2012;141:e691S–e736S.

77. Bhagra CJ, D'Souza R, Silversides CK. Valvular heart disease and pregnancy part II: management of prosthetic valves. *Heart.* 2017;103:244–252.

78. Silversides CK, Harris L, Haberer K, et al. Recurrence rates of arrhythmias during pregnancy in women with previous tachyarrhythmia and impact on fetal and neonatal outcomes. *Am J Cardiol.* 2006;97:1206–1212.

79. Ghosh N, Luk A, Derzko C, et al. The acute treatment of maternal supraventricular tachycardias during pregnancy: a review of the literature. *J Obstet Gynaecol Can.* 2011;33:17–23.

80. Salam AM, Ertekin E, van Hagen IM, et al. Atrial fibrillation or flutter during pregnancy in patients with structural heart disease: data from the ROPAC (registry on pregnancy and cardiac disease). *JACC Clin Electrophysiol.* 2015;1:284–292.

81. Seth R, Moss AJ, McNitt S, et al. Long QT syndrome and pregnancy. *J Am Coll Cardiol.* 2007;49:1092–1098.

82. Lima FV, Koutrolou-Sotiropoulou P, Yen TY, Stergiopoulos K. Clinical characteristics and outcomes in pregnant women with Ebstein anomaly at the time of delivery in the USA: 2003–2012. *Arch Cardiovasc Dis.* 2016;109:390–398.

83. Egbe AC, El-Harasis M, Miranda WR, et al. Outcomes of pregnancy in patients with prior right ventricular outflow interventions. *J Am Heart Assoc.* 2019;8:e011730.

84. Stoll VM, Drury NE, Thorne S, et al. Pregnancy outcomes in women with transposition of the great arteries after an arterial switch operation. *JAMA Cardiol.* 2018;3:1119–1122.

85. Davis MB, Rogers IS. Pregnancy after fontan palliation: caution when details are lost in translation. *Circ Cardiovasc Qual Outcomes.* 2018;11:e004734.

86. Bedard E, Dimopoulos K, Gatzoulis MA. Has there been any progress made on pregnancy outcomes among women with pulmonary arterial hypertension? *Eur Heart J.* 2009;30:256–265.

87. Kiely DG, Condliffe R, Webster V, et al. Improved survival in pregnancy and pulmonary hypertension using a multiprofessional approach. *BJOG.* 2010;117:565–574.

88. Duarte AG, Thomas S, Safdar Z, et al. Management of pulmonary arterial hypertension during pregnancy: a retrospective, multicenter experience. *Chest.* 2013;143:1330–1336.

89. Jais X, Olsson KM, Barbera JA, et al. Pregnancy outcomes in pulmonary arterial hypertension in the modern management era. *Eur Respir J.* 2012;40:881–885.

90. Sliwa K, van Hagen IM, Budts W, et al. Pulmonary hypertension and pregnancy outcomes: data from the Registry of Pregnancy and Cardiac Disease (ROPAC) of the European Society of Cardiology. *Eur J Heart Fail.* 2016;18:1119–1128.

91. Thomas E, Yang J, Xu J, et al. Pulmonary hypertension and pregnancy outcomes: insights from the national inpatient sample. *J Am Heart Assoc.* 2017;6.

92. Kamel H, Roman MJ, Pitcher A, Devereux RB. Pregnancy and the risk of aortic dissection or rupture: a cohort-crossover analysis. *Circulation.* 2016;134:527–533.

93. Roman MJ, Pugh NL, Hendershot TP, et al. Aortic complications associated with pregnancy in Marfan syndrome: the NHLBI national registry of genetically triggered thoracic aortic aneurysms and cardiovascular conditions (GenTAC). *J Am Heart Assoc.* 2016;5.

94. Johnson MR, Roos Hesselink JW. Pregnancy, Marfan syndrome, and type-B aortic dissection. *BJOG.* 2018;125:494.

95. Sayama S, Takeda N, Iriyama T, et al. Peripartum type B aortic dissection in patients with Marfan syndrome who underwent aortic root replacement: a case series study. *BJOG.* 2018;125:487–493.

96. Frise CJ, Pitcher A, Mackillop L. Loeys-Dietz syndrome and pregnancy: the first ten years. *Int J Cardiol.* 2017;226:21–25.

97. Silberbach M, Roos-Hesselink JW, Andersen NH, et al. Cardiovascular health in turner syndrome: a scientific statement from the American Heart Association. *Circ Genom Precis Med.* 2018;11:e000048.

98. van Hagen IM, van der Linde D, van de Laar IM, et al. Pregnancy in women with SMAD3 mutation. *J Am Coll Cardiol.* 2017;69:1356–1358.

# 93 Heart Disease in Racially and Ethnically Diverse Populations

ALANNA A. MORRIS AND MICHELLE A. ALBERT

EPIDEMIOLOGY OF CARDIOVASCULAR DISEASE IN HETEROGENEOUS POPULATIONS

Cardiovascular Disease in Racial and Ethnic Groups

According to the 2017 National Center for Health Statistics (NHIS), the burden of coronary heart diseases (CHDs) varies by racial or ethnic group.[1] Although death rates from heart disease are declining for all race/ethnic groups, the rate of decline has been slower for race-ethnic minorities. In 2000, the age-adjusted death rate for heart disease was 326.5 per 100,000 people among non-Hispanic (NH) Blacks compared with 253.6 deaths per 100,000 among NH whites.[2] In 2017, the age-adjusted death rate had declined to 208.0 per 100,000 people among NH Blacks compared with 168.9 deaths per 100,000 among NH whites, thus preserving the higher rate of death for Blacks observed in 2000.[3] For Blacks and whites in the Atherosclerosis Risk In Communities (ARIC), Cardiovascular Health Study (CHS), and Reasons for Geographic And Racial Differences in Stroke (REGARDS) study, Black men were twice as likely to experience fatal CHD as white men (age-adjusted hazard ratio [HR], 2.09; 95% confidence interval [CI], 1.42 to 3.06), and Black women were more than twice as likely experience fatal CHD than white women (HR, 2.61; 95% CI, 1.57 to 4.34).[4] These differences in fatal CHD were largely attributable to social determinants of health and cardiovascular risk factors. Disparities in stroke prevalence and incidence are even greater.[1]

Hypertension (see also Chapter 26)

Blacks have higher rates of hypertension than other racial or ethnic groups.[5] Several proposed mechanisms may contribute to an increased incidence in Blacks (Fig. 93.1). Figure 93.2 presents the epidemiology of hypertension awareness, treatment, and control (see Fig. 93.3A-C) in the United States. Although rates of awareness in Blacks are higher (see Fig. 93.3A) than in other groups, and Blacks are more likely to be on treatment (see Fig. 93.3B) and use more medications to treat hypertension, Blacks have a lower rate of control than other racial or ethnic groups (see Fig. 93.3C).[6] American Indian/Alaska Natives (27.2%) also have higher rates of hypertension than Native Hawaiian or Other Pacific Islander (PI) (24.0%), Hispanic or LatinX (23.7%), white (24.8%), or Asian adults (21.9%).[1]

Among Hispanics/LatinXs, the hypertension prevalence varies considerably by subgroup. In the Hispanic Community Health Study/Study of LatinXs (HCHS/SOL), which measured blood pressure in 16,415 Hispanics/LatinXs (but does not include a comparison population of NHs), rates were highest among participants from Cuban, Puerto Rican, and Dominican ethnic backgrounds.[7] Hispanics/LatinXs are less likely to be aware of their hypertension and less likely to be treated than NH whites.[6,7]

National estimates of hypertension prevalence based on measured blood pressure in Asian Americans are lacking. Amongst the six largest Asian American populations (Asian Indian, Chinese, Filipino, Japanese, Korean, Vietnamese), Filipinos have particularly high rates of hypertension (53.2% to 59.9%), with poor awareness and control rates.[8] Filipino patients of older age, those with comorbid medical conditions, and those who did not smoke had improved hypertension treatment, and patients with health insurance had better blood pressure control. These findings suggest that better access to health care and an approach targeted toward multiple risk factors are needed to decrease the hypertension prevalence and risk among Filipinos.[9]

Type 2 Diabetes (see also Chapter 31)

The overall age-standardized prevalence of diabetes in the U.S. population is 14.6%, but Hispanics/LatinXs (16.6%), Blacks (18.3%), and Asians (16.4%) have a higher prevalence than NH whites (13.3%).[10]

The diabetes prevalence largely parallels the "epidemic" of obesity and physical inactivity, with evidence of disparities emerging even in childhood.[11,12] In the Hispanic/LatinX community, Dominicans, Puerto Ricans, and Mexicans (17% to 18%) seem to have a higher prevalence than South Americans and Cubans (10% to 13%).[13] Emerging research comparing the relative contributions of socioeconomic, environmental, and psychosocial factors, plus ancestry, to diabetes disparities has indicated that socioeconomic factors make up the largest group of mediating factors.[14]

Although the prevalence of diabetes generally parallels the obesity epidemic in most race/ethnic groups,[11] this has not been the case for Asian Americans. Asian Americans have on average a lower body mass index than other racial or ethnic groups but also display evidence of insulin resistance at lower values of body mass index which may be partly explained by differences in body fat distribution (see also Chapter 30).[11,15] PIs, South Asians, and Filipinos have prevalence of diabetes at least twofold to threefold higher than NH whites; prevalence of diabetes is also greater in Chinese, Japanese, Korean, and Southeast Asian adults compared with whites, although the magnitude of difference is less.[16] Filipinos and South/East Asians have higher rates of treatment than NH whites.

Cardiovascular Disease in Other Population Groups

Persons with psychological conditions and sexual minorities warrant increased attention because of their elevated risks of cardiovascular disease and its effects on health disparities. Psychological conditions including but not limited to anxiety, major depressive disorder, and bipolar disorder affected at least 46.6 million adults in 2017, with numerous others who are suffering but are undiagnosed and untreated.[17] This epidemic includes especially vulnerable populations, such as persons of lower socioeconomic status, the homeless, and military veterans.[18] An elevated cardiovascular risk is associated with adverse risk behaviors, isolation, limited contact with the health care system, and downward socioeconomic mobility; medications used to control some forms of mental illness can lead to weight gain and/or sedation, factors that contribute to decreases in motivation for physical activity (see also Chapter 99).[19]

Persons whose sexual orientation is lesbian, gay, bisexual, or transgender (LGBT) have not historically been considered "minorities," but they have emerged as sizeable social communities. Attention to the unique health needs in the LGBTQ population have traditionally focused on sexual health and less commonly on cardiovascular disease prevention and management. One exception that reflects the intersection between sexual and cardiovascular health relates to the shift of acquired immunodeficiency syndrome (AIDS) from an acute illness to a chronic illness, and its associated cardiovascular risks (see also Chapter 85). Although the burden of HIV/AIDS is not restricted to sexual minorities, the largest proportion of affected individuals are practicing male homosexuals and non-white minority women.[20] Medications used to manage HIV/AIDS have performed well in sparing associated wasting syndromes but as a result have yielded a higher burden of overweight and obesity and consequent metabolic disorders, including hypertension and diabetes.[21] HIV⁺ status (vs. HIV⁻ status) associates with reduced systolic heart function and an increased prevalence of left ventricular hypertrophy, even after adjustments have been made for metabolic factors. These cardiac changes may predispose individuals with HIV/AIDS to heart failure.[22,23]

Cardiovascular disease is a major cause of death among homeless adults, with mortality rates twofold to threefold higher than the general population.[24] Various factors contribute to the worse outcomes, including substance use, high burden of traditional and nontraditional cardiovascular risk factors, and limited access to health care.[25] Importantly, men (60%) and Black persons (39%) are overrepresented among homeless populations,[26] and 19% of persons who are transgender or gender-nonconforming have experienced homelessness at some point in their lives.[27]

CARDIOVASCULAR DISEASE MANAGEMENT

Lifestyle modification through behavioral intervention that focuses on weight loss, reduced sodium intake, increased physical activity, and reduced alcohol consumption remains the cornerstone of cardiovascular disease prevention and management.[28] When examining Life Simple 7 scores (an American Heart Association lifestyle metric) in National Health and Nutrition Examination Survey (NHANES) participants,

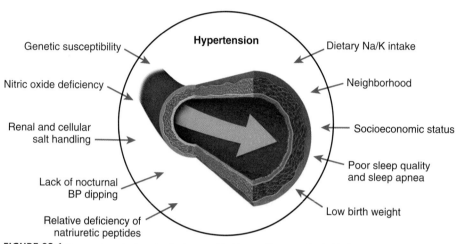

FIGURE 93.1 Proposed mechanisms for the increased incidence of hypertension in Blacks.

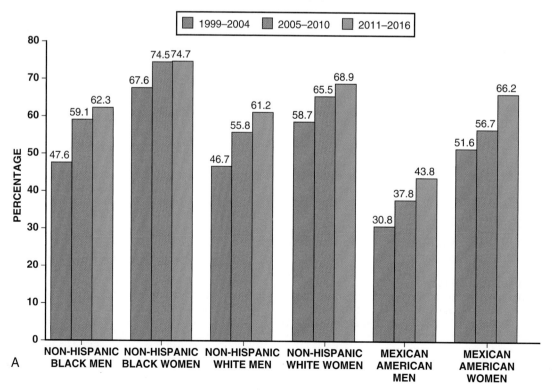

AGE-ADJUSTED AWARENESS OF HYPERTENSION AMONG US ADULTS WITH HYPERTENSION BY SEX AND RACE-ETHNICITY 1999–2016

A

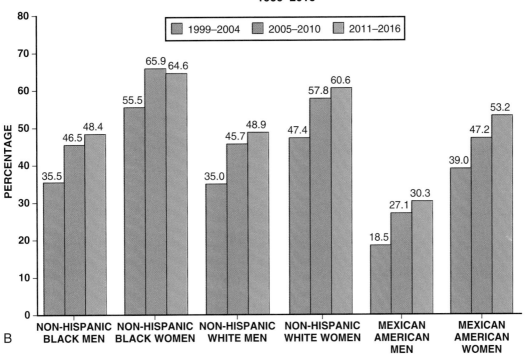

AGE-ADJUSTED TREATMENT OF HYPERTENSION AMONG US ADULTS WITH HYPERTENSION BY SEX AND RACE-ETHNICITY 1999–2016

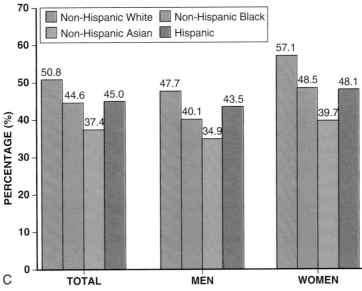

AGE-ADJUSTED PREVALENCE OF CONTROLLED HYPERTENSION AMONG US ADULTS AGED 18 AND OVER, BY SEX AND RACE AND HISPANIC ORIGIN: 2015–2016

FIGURE 93.2 Epidemiology of adults with hypertension by race/ethnicity, United States. (**A** and **B** based on American Heart Association Heart Disease and Stroke Statistics—2020 Update. *Circulation*. 2020;141:e139–e596. DOI: 10.1161/CIR.0000000000000757; **C**, adapted from Fryar CD, et al. Hypertension prevalence and control among adults, United States, 2015-2016, NCHS Data Brief 2017, no 289.)

Black and Mexican-American women scored significantly lower compared with white women, while differences between Black and white men were smaller and mostly nonsignificant.[29] Moreover, despite higher body mass index and/or atherosclerotic cardiovascular disease risk, Black women (adjusted odds ratio [OR] 0.8, 95% CI, 0.7 to 0.9) were less likely to attempt weight loss, and Hispanic women (adjusted OR 0.8, 95% CI 0.6 to 0.9) were less likely to report physical activity than white women. Black women (adjusted OR 0.6, 95% CI 0.5 to 0.7) were less likely than white women, and Hispanics (women adjusted OR 0.6, 95% CI 0.5 to 0.7; men adjusted OR 0.7, 95% CI 0.6 to 0.9) were less likely than whites to report a healthy diet.[30]

Social determinants of health, including housing instability, food insecurity, and access to safe facilities to engage in leisure time physical activity, can impact the ability for socioeconomically disadvantaged to engage in healthy lifestyle behaviors, and impede the efficacy of proven prevention recommendations.

Hypertension (see also Chapter 26)

The Systolic Blood Pressure Intervention Trial (SPRINT) studied antihypertensive drug therapy that focused on lowering the systolic blood pressure (SBP) to less than 120 mm Hg rather than to less than

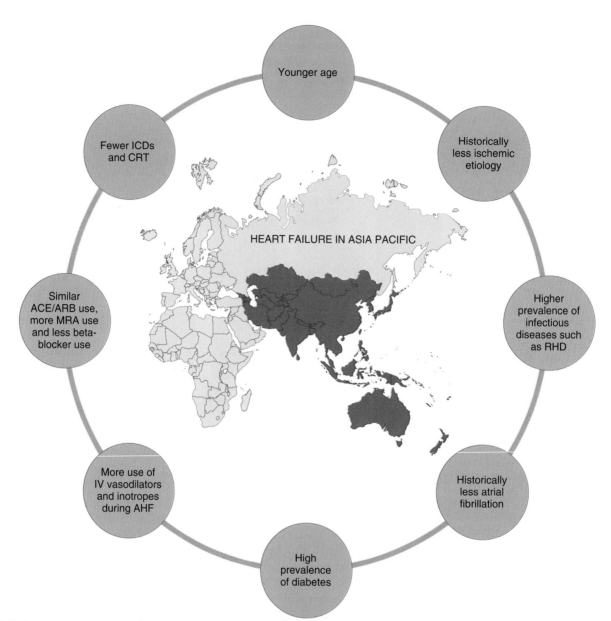

FIGURE 93.3 Heart failure phenotype in the Asian diaspora. (Adapted from Mentz RJ, Roessig L, Greenberg BH, et al. Heart failure clinical trials in East and Southeast Asia: understanding the importance and defining the next steps. *JACC Heart Fail*. 2016;4[6]:419–427.)

140 mm Hg in 9361 nondiabetic/stroke-free individuals whose SBP was 130 to 180 mm Hg and who had an increased cardiovascular disease risk (approximately 2%/year). The overall results showed that in the intensive therapy arm a 25% lower rate of combined outcomes for myocardial infarction (MI), acute coronary syndrome without MI, stroke, acute decompensated heart failure, or cardiovascular disease death, and a 27% reduced rate of all-cause mortality.[15] Stratified analyses revealed similar results in Blacks and non-Blacks, with a CI that included 1.0 among Blacks, and Blacks required an average of approximately 0.3 more antihypertensive medications.[31] Generalizability of the SPRINT population to the U.S. adult population 50 years old or older using NHANES data showed that 4% to 5% of Hispanics and Blacks compared with 9% of whites meet eligibility criteria for the study.[32] Nonetheless, only approximately 8.5% of Blacks and 14.2% of Hispanics with treated hypertension met the blood pressure targets identified in the SPRINT study, a finding that suggests there is substantial room for a hypertension-related cardiovascular disease risk reduction in these groups.

Pharmacotherapy informed by race or ethnicity for Black patients favors thiazide-type diuretics and calcium channel blocker drugs as first-line therapy in a majority of Blacks without contraindications (Table 93.1). A recent analysis of the NHANES suggests that Blacks were more likely to receive combination antihypertensive therapy (including diuretics and calcium channel blockers) compared with whites and Hispanics, and had the highest average number of antihypertensive medications (1.91, 95% CI, 1.84 to 1.97).[6] Despite this, only 31% of Blacks had their blood pressure controlled to recommended targets, as compared with 43% of whites. Hispanics were also less likely to have their blood pressure at recommended targets compared with whites but were less likely to be on antihypertensive therapy. Ongoing barriers to successful hypertension management in Black patients include lack of ambulatory self-monitoring of blood pressure, menthol cigarette smoking, lack of regular health care visits, and underinsurance.[33,34]

SPRINT included a substantial sample of race-ethnic minorities, and enrolled 984 (11%) Hispanics in the U.S. mainland and Puerto Rico.[35] Hispanics recruited into SPRINT were more likely to be uninsured and were on lower numbers of antihypertensive medications at baseline than NH subjects. Approximately 50% of Hispanic subjects in SPRINT had their blood pressure controlled to less than 140/90 mm Hg at baseline, similar to the NH subjects; better blood pressure control was more likely among those with a history of clinical cardiovascular disease. Many argue that because diabetes disproportionately affects the Hispanic population, use of a therapy targeted at the renin-angiotensin-aldosterone system may be more appropriate in Hispanics/LatinXs.[36]

TABLE 93.1 Hypertension Guidelines and Recommendations: Initial Drug Selection

GUIDELINE	EVIDENCE REVIEW METHODOLOGY	GENERAL ADULT POPULATION	GENERAL AFRICAN AMERICAN ADULT POPULATION	DIABETES MELLITUS	CHRONIC KIDNEY DISEASE
2017 Guideline for the Prevention, Detection, Evaluation, and Management of High Blood Pressure in Adults	Systematic review	ACE-I, ARB, CCB, thiazide	Thiazide, CCB	ACE-I, ARB, CCB, thiazide	ACE-I, ARB
International Society of Hypertension (2020)	Systematic review	ACE-I, ARB, CCB	ACE-I, ARB, CCB Thiazide-like diuretic	ACE-I, ARB, CCB, diuretics	ACE-I, ARB, CCB, diuretics
National Institute for Health and Care Excellence (2019)	Systematic review	≥55: CCB, ACE-I, ARB thiazide <55: ACE-I, ARB, CCB, thiazide	CCB, ACE-I, ARB, thiazide	ACE-I, ARB, CCB, thiazide	ACE-I, ARB
European Society of Hypertension and European Society of Cardiology (2018)	Consensus (graded)	ACE-I, ARB, CCB, diuretic, (consider BB if resistant)	Thiazide, CCB	ACE-I, ARB, CCB, diuretics	ACE-I, ARB, CCB, diuretics
Hypertension Canada Guidelines for Diagnosis, Risk Assessment, Prevention, and Treatment of Hypertension in Adults and Children (2018)	Consensus	ACE-I, ARB, CCB, thiazide	ACE-I are not recommended as first line	ACE-I, ARB, CCB, diuretic	ACE-I, ARB, diuretic
International Society on Hypertension in Blacks (2010)	Consensus	NA	Diuretic or CCB, RAS inhibitor plus CCB preferred over RAS inhibitor plus thiazide unless edema or high volume	ACE-I, ARB	ACE-I, ARB

ACE-I, Angiotensin-converting enzyme inhibitor; *ARB,* angiotensin-receptor blocker; *BB,* beta blocker; *CCB,* calcium channel blocker; *RAS,* renin-angiotensin system.
Adapted from Still CH, Ferdinand KC, Ogedegbe G, Wright JT Jr. Recognition and management of hypertension in older persons: focus on African Americans. *J Am Geriatr Soc.* 2015;63(10):2130–2138.

The general features of hypertension across the heterogeneous Asian diaspora appear similar. High salt intake, increased salt sensitivity, and more sustained 24-hour blood pressure elevations likely contribute to elevated risks of stroke compared with CHD among Asians.[37] The Japanese Society of Hypertension recommends the use of calcium channel blockers, angiotensin-converting enzyme inhibitors, and diuretics as first-line therapy for patients without other compelling indications.[13] Diuretics are recommended for salt-sensitive elderly Japanese patients. Like Blacks, South Asian patients develop hypertension at an earlier age and have accelerated end-organ damage compared with whites. Because morbidity and mortality data in South Asians are lacking, management principles resemble those of the general population, including early screening and use of combination therapy.[38]

Coronary Heart Disease

Almost 1 million percutaneous coronary interventions (PCIs) are performed annually in the United States for CHD. Blacks and Hispanics have longer wait times and are less likely to undergo PCI than whites, regardless of their insurance status.[39] Data from a large national improvement quality registry, ACTION Registry-GWTG of ST-segment elevation myocardial infarction (STEMI) and non-ST segment elevation myocardial infarction (NSTEMI) patients, showed that rates of catheterization were lower for NSTEMI and similar for STEMI in Blacks compared with whites.[40] Black patients were also less likely to have coronary artery bypass grafting (CABG). In general, Blacks and Hispanics have poorer revascularization outcomes, related to multidimensional influences, including individual, provider, hospital, and societal factors. For example, poorer CABG outcomes among Blacks and Hispanics relate in part to hospital quality and socioeconomic factors because poor and racial or ethnic minority patients receive care at lower-performing hospitals, according to standardized quality measures.[41,42] After enactment of the Massachusetts health care reform act in 2006, racial and ethnic disparities in those who received cardiovascular interventional care persisted.[43] However, counties in expansion states that participated in Medicaid expansion under the Affordable Care Act had fewer deaths per year from cardiovascular causes after Medicaid expansion compared with counties in nonexpansion states.[44]

Use of secondary prevention medications also varies by race and ethnicity. In the TReatment with ADP receptor iNhibitorS: Longitudinal Assessment of Treatment Patterns and Events after Acute Coronary Syndrome (TRANSLATE-ACS) study, race/ethnicity was not an independent predictor of medication nonadherence at 6 weeks post-MI. Financial hardship and depression associated with a higher risk of medication nonadherence, factors that may be more common in race/ethnic minorities. At 1 year post-MI, Black and Hispanic women seem to adhere least to medication regimens, suggesting that there is substantial room for improvement in post-MI care and understanding of treatment barriers in these patients.[45,46] Medication discontinuation is associated with side effects and physician discontinuation advice; higher rates of adherence are related to having private insurance, having assistance with paying for prescriptions, and having an outpatient follow-up appointment scheduled before hospital discharge.

In the context of dual antiplatelet therapy use after drug-eluting stent placement for acute coronary syndrome, there is limited specific data about racial and ethnic groups showing the effectiveness of the drugs and the adverse events that may occur, such as major bleeding. For example, the optimal duration of dual antiplatelet therapy after PCI may differ in East Asians compared with other groups, as there is some concern for higher bleeding risk in East Asians.[47] In addition, the efficacy of clopidogrel as an antiplatelet agent in Asians is of concern.[48]

Heart Failure

Blacks have a higher prevalence of heart failure, with an earlier onset and presentation than other racial and ethnic groups. Compared with whites, Blacks have almost a threefold increased risk for developing dilated cardiomyopathy, which is not fully explained by confounding variables such as hypertension or socioeconomic factors.[49] Emerging work suggests that there are complex relationships between heart failure with preserved ejection fraction (HFpEF) and race and ethnicity. Several key risk factors for HFpEF, including obesity, diabetes, and hypertension, are more common in Blacks. However, recent data suggest that amyloid deposition may be present in a substantial proportion of patients with clinical HFpEF, particularly with advanced age (see also Chapter 53).[50] The hereditary form of transthyretin (TTR)-related cardiac amyloidosis disproportionately affects Blacks, because the valine-to-isoleucine substitution at position 122 (V122I) mutation is carried by 3% to 5% of Black Americans.[51,52] Although the presence of the V122I variant associates strongly with the risk of heart failure, few Black patients are recognized as having a TTR-related cardiomyopathy or undergo genetic testing for TTR variants in routine clinical practice.[52,53]

Impaired vascular function caused by reduced endothelial nitric oxide synthesis and resultant endothelial dysfunction appears to contribute to the heart failure pathophysiology in Blacks.[54] The landmark African-American Heart Failure Trial (A-HeFT) study in 1052 Black patients with New York Heart Association Class III or IV heart failure showed a 43% reduction in deaths with fixed-dose isosorbide dinitrate and hydralazine treatment compared with placebo against a background of standard heart failure therapy.[55] In a subsequent Genetic Risk Assessment of Heart Failure (GRAHF) substudy of A-HeFT (n = 350 patients), a common GNB3 polymorphism, C825T associated with enhanced alpha$_2$-adrenergic receptor signaling, was associated with greater therapeutic effect of isosorbide dinitrate and hydralazine.[56]

Data regarding the prevalence of heart failure and effectiveness of therapeutic options in other race/ethnic groups are lacking despite their high prevalence of risk factors and structural heart disease. Among persons of Hispanic/LatinX background in the Echocardiographic Study of LatinXs (ECHO-SOL), left ventricular systolic and diastolic dysfunction were 3.6% and 50.3%, respectively, with more than 90% of the cardiac dysfunction categorized as subclinical or unrecognized.[57] Central Americans and Cuban Americans had a greater prevalence of diastolic dysfunction than Mexican Americans. Information about heart failure in Asians is sparse. Figure 93.3 illustrates the potential features of heart failure in Asia. In the United States, data from the GWTG-HF registry showed that Asians with heart failure were more likely to be younger males; to have hypertension, diabetes, and renal disease; and to be uninsured compared with whites.[58] Current Heart Failure Society of America/American Heart Association/American College of Cardiology (AHA/ACC) guidelines do not propose specific therapy for heart failure based on Hispanic ethnicity or Asian race.

Disparities in clinical heart failure outcomes exist based on race/ethnicity. Blacks have the highest risk of heart failure–related death.[59] The rate of heart failure hospitalization for Blacks is nearly 2.5-fold higher than the rate for whites, with costs that are significantly higher in the first year after an index hospitalization.[60,61] An analysis of the National Inpatient Sample showed the rate of heart failure hospitalization was 229% higher for Black males (P-for-trend = 0.141) and 240% higher for Black females (P-for-trend = 0.725) with reference to whites in 2013, with no significant change from 2002 to 2013.[60] Hispanic males had a 32% higher rate of heart failure hospitalization in 2002, and the difference narrowed to 4% (P-for-trend = 0.047) greater in 2013 relative to whites. For Hispanic females the rate was 55% greater in 2002 and narrowed to 8% greater (P-for-trend = 0.004) in 2013 relative to whites. Asian/PI males had a 27% lower rate in 2002 that improved to 43% (P-for-trend = 0.040) lower in 2013 relative to whites. For Asian/PI females the hospitalization rate was 24% lower in 2002 and improved to 43% (P-for-trend = 0.021) lower in 2013 relative to whites.

POTENTIAL FOR EMERGING SCIENTIFIC RESEARCH TO ADDRESS GROUP DISPARITIES IN CARDIOVASCULAR DISEASE

Despite what we have learned about the origin of disparities over the past few decades, disparities appear to be growing rather than shrinking. For areas with available clinical trial data for therapies that effectively treat cardiovascular disease in different racial and ethnic groups, comprehensive delivery and adherence present important challenges. Diversification of the workforce and increasing community outreach may also help, as prior research has shown that increasing the number of doctors who are race/ethnic minorities can improve adherence and the quality of communication experienced by patients.[62–64] Administering care in nontraditional settings in the community can also improve clinical outcomes. In a recent randomized controlled trial of Black male barbershop clients with uncontrolled hypertension, Black men randomized to a pharmacist-led intervention (in which barbers encouraged meetings in barbershops with specialty-trained pharmacists who prescribed drug therapy) achieved larger reductions

in blood pressure than Black men randomized to an active control approach where barbers encouraged lifestyle modification and doctor appointments.[64] Moreover, efforts to realize the potential of "precision" and "personalized" medicine should also target populations that experience the greatest burden of health disparities, lest unmet needs become more pronounced. In addition, longitudinal information is needed on recent immigrant populations, including those from Asia, where the cardiovascular risk varies markedly by country of origin, and those from Africa, where there is a burgeoning epidemic of cardiovascular disease associated with urbanization (see also Chapter 2. Specific issues in the near future include scaling, dissemination, and implementation of known effective strategies for prevention and treatment of cardiovascular disease in high-risk heterogeneous populations. Finally, the COVID-19 pandemic has unearthed the effect of CVD disparities contributing to the overwhelming impact of this pandemic in racial/ethnic minority and socioeconomically disadvantaged groups. The prevalence of certain conditions such as cardiomyopathy and CVD-related mortality will likely increase over time due to the impact of COVID-19 and thus research and interventions targeting the most affected populations is required.

ACKNOWLEDGMENTS

The authors thank Mercedes Carnethon, coauthor of this chapter from the previous edition of *Heart Disease*, for her contributions.

REFERENCES
Epidemiology
1. National Center for Health Statistics. *Summary Health Statistics Tables for US Adults.* National Health Interview Survey; 2018. http://ftp.cdc.gov/pub/Health_Statistics/NCHS/NHIS/SHS/2018_SHS_Table_A-1.pdf.
2. Miniño A, Arias E, Kochanek K, et al. Final Data for 2000. National Vital Statistics Reports. Vol 50 No 15. Hyattsville, Maryland: National Center for Health Statistics; 2002. https://www.cdc.gov/Nchs/data/nvsr/nvsr50/nvsr50_15.pdf.
3. National Center for Health Statistics Health, United States. *2017: With Special Feature on Mortality.* Hyattsville, MD: National Center for Health Statistics; 2018. https://www.cdc.gov/nchs/data/hus/hus17.pdf.
4. Colantonio LD, Gamboa CM, Richman JS, et al. Black-white differences in incident fatal, nonfatal, and total coronary heart disease. *Circulation.* 2017;136:152–166.
5. Prevalence of self-reported hypertension and antihypertensive medication use among adults—United States, 2017. *MMWR Morb Mortal Wkly Rep.* 2020;69:393–398. https://doi.org/10.15585/mmwr.mm6914a1. (Accessed May 1, 2020, 2020).

Hypertension
6. Gu A, Yue Y, Desai Raj P, Argulian E. Racial and ethnic differences in antihypertensive medication use and blood pressure control among US adults with hypertension. *Circ Cardiovasc Qual Outcomes.* 2017;10:e003166.
7. Sorlie PD, Allison MA, Avilés-Santa ML, et al. Prevalence of hypertension, awareness, treatment, and control in the hispanic community health study/study of LatinXs. *Am J Hypertens.* 2014;27:793–800.
8. Zhao B, Jose PO, Pu J, et al. Racial/ethnic differences in hypertension prevalence, treatment, and control for outpatients in Northern California 2010–2012. *Am J Hypertens.* 2014;28:631–639.
9. Ursua R, Aguilar D, Wyatt L, et al. Awareness, treatment and control of hypertension among Filipino immigrants. *J Gen Intern Med.* 2014;29:455–462.

Diabetes
10. Cheng YJ, Kanaya AM, Araneta MRG, et al. Prevalence of diabetes by race and ethnicity in the United States, 2011-2016. *J Am Med Assoc.* 2019;322:2389–2398.
11. Ogden CL, Carroll MD, Kit BK, Flegal KM. Prevalence of childhood and adult obesity in the United States, 2011-2012. *J Am Med Assoc.* 2014;311:806–814.
12. Dabelea D, Mayer-Davis EJ, Saydah S, et al. Prevalence of type 1 and type 2 diabetes among children and adolescents from 2001 to 2009. *J Am Med Assoc.* 2014;311:1778–1786.
13. Schneiderman N, Llabre M, Cowie CC, et al. Prevalence of diabetes among Hispanics/LatinXs from diverse backgrounds: the Hispanic community health study/study of LatinXs (HCHS/SOL). *Diabetes Care.* 2014;37:2233–2239.

Vulnerable Populations
14. Piccolo RS, Subramanian SV, Pearce N, et al. Relative contributions of socioeconomic, local environmental, psychosocial, lifestyle/behavioral, biophysiological, and ancestral factors to racial/ethnic disparities in type 2 diabetes. *Diabetes Care.* 2016;39:1208–1217.
15. Hsu WC, Araneta MR, Kanaya AM, et al. BMI cut points to identify at-risk Asian Americans for type 2 diabetes screening. *Diabetes Care.* 2015;38:150–158.
16. Gordon NP, Lin TY, Rau J, Lo JC. Aggregation of Asian-American subgroups masks meaningful differences in health and health risks among Asian ethnicities: an electronic health record based cohort study. *BMC Publ Health.* 2019;19:1551.
17. National Institute of Mental Health. Prevalence of Any Mental Illness. https://www.nimh.nih.gov/health/statistics/mental-illness.shtml#part_154785.
18. The 2019 Annual Homeless Assessment Report (AHAR) to Congress. https://files.hudexchange.info/resources/documents/2019-AHAR-Part-1.pdf.
19. Mental Health Medications. https://www.nimh.nih.gov/health/topics/mental-health-medications/index.shtml.
20. Centers for Disease Control and Prevention. *HIV Surveillance Report;* 2017:29. Published November 2018. http://www.cdc.gov/hiv/library/reports/hiv-surveillance.html.
21. Koethe JR, Jenkins CA, Lau B, et al. Rising obesity prevalence and weight gain among adults starting antiretroviral therapy in the United States and Canada. *AIDS Res Hum Retroviruses.* 2016;32:50–58.

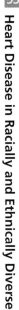
22. Freiberg MS, Chang C-CH, Skanderson M, et al. Association between HIV infection and the risk of heart failure with reduced ejection fraction and preserved ejection fraction in the antiretroviral therapy era: results from the veterans aging cohort study. *JAMA Cardiol.* 2017;2:536–546.

23. Womack JA, Chang CCH, So–Armah KA, et al. HIV infection and cardiovascular disease in women. *J Am Heart Assoc.* 2014;3:e001035.

24. Slockers MT, Nusselder WJ, Rietjens J, van Beeck EF. Unnatural death: a major but largely preventable cause-of-death among homeless people? *Eur J Public Health.* 2018;28:248–252.

25. Baggett TP, Liauw SS, Hwang SW. Cardiovascular disease and homelessness. *J Am Coll Cardiol.* 2018;71:2585.

26. Henry M, Watt R, Rosenthal L, et al. *The 2016 Annual Homeless Assessment Report (AHAR) to Congress: Part 1: Point-in-Time Estimates of Homelessness.* Washington DC: US Department of Housing and Urban Development; 2016.

27. *LGBTQ Homelessness. Published by the National Coalition for the Homeless*; 2017. https://nationalhomeless.org/wp-content/uploads/2017/06/LGBTQ-Homelessness.pdf.

Management Considerations

28. Arnett DK, Blumenthal RS, Albert MA, et al. 2019 ACC/AHA guideline on the primary prevention of cardiovascular disease: a report of the American College of Cardiology/American heart association task force on clinical practice guidelines. *Circulation.* 2019;140:e596–e646.

29. Pool LR, Ning H, Lloyd–Jones DM, Allen NB. Trends in racial/ethnic disparities in cardiovascular health among US adults from 1999–2012. *J Am Heart Assoc.* 2017;6:e006027.

30. Morris AA, Ko YA, Hutcheson SH, Quyyumi A. Race/ethnic and sex differences in the association of atherosclerotic cardiovascular disease risk and healthy lifestyle behaviors. *J Am Heart Assoc.* 2018;7:e008250.

31. Still CH, Rodriguez CJ, Wright Jr JT, et al. Clinical outcomes by race and ethnicity in the Systolic Blood Pressure Intervention Trial (SPRINT): a randomized clinical trial. *Am J Hypertens.* 2017;31:97–107.

32. Bress AP, Tanner RM, Hess R, et al. Generalizability of SPRINT results to the U.S. Adult population. *J Am Coll Cardiol.* 2016;67:463–472.

33. Still CH, Ferdinand KC, Ogedegbe G, Wright Jr JT. Recognition and management of hypertension in older persons: focus on African Americans. *J Am Geriatr Soc.* 2015;63:2130–2138.

34. Egan BM, Bland VJ, Brown AL, et al. Hypertension in African Americans aged 60 to 79 Years: statement from the international society of hypertension in blacks. *J Clin Hypertens.* 2015;17:252–259.

35. Rodriguez CJ, Still CH, Garcia KR, et al. Baseline blood pressure control in Hispanics: characteristics of Hispanics in the systolic blood pressure intervention trial. *J Clin Hypertens (Greenwich).* 2017;19:116–125.

36. Campbell PT, Krim SR, Lavie CJ, Ventura HO. Clinical characteristics, treatment patterns and outcomes of Hispanic hypertensive patients. *Prog Cardiovasc Dis.* 2014;57:244–252.

37. Kario K. Key points of the Japanese society of hypertension guidelines for the management of hypertension in 2014. *Pulse (Basel).* 2015;3:35–47.

38. Brewster LM, van Montfrans GA, Oehlers GP, Seedat YK. Systematic review: antihypertensive drug therapy in patients of African and South Asian ethnicity. *Intern Emerg Med.* 2016;11:355–374.

39. Graham G, Xiao Y-YK, Rappoport D, Siddiqi S. Population-level differences in revascularization treatment and outcomes among various United States subpopulations. *World J Cardiol.* 2016;8:24–40.

40. Anstey DE, Li S, Thomas L, et al. Race and Sex differences in management and outcomes of patients after ST-Elevation and non-ST-Elevation myocardial infarct: results from the NCDR. *Clin Cardiol.* 2016;39:585–595.

41. Rangrass G, Ghaferi AA, Dimick JB. Explaining racial disparities in outcomes after cardiac surgery: the role of hospital quality. *JAMA Surgery.* 2014;149:223–227.

42. Khera R, Vaughan-Sarrazin M, Rosenthal GE, Girotra S. Racial disparities in outcomes after cardiac surgery: the role of hospital quality. *Curr Cardiol Rep.* 2015;17:29.

43. Albert MA, Ayanian JZ, Silbaugh TS, et al. Early results of Massachusetts healthcare reform on racial, ethnic, and socioeconomic disparities in cardiovascular care. *Circulation.* 2014;129:2528–2538.

44. Khatana SAM, Bhatla A, Nathan AS, et al. Association of Medicaid expansion with cardiovascular mortality. *JAMA Cardiol.* 2019;4:671–679.

45. Lauffenburger JC, Robinson JG, Oramasionwu C, Fang G. Racial/Ethnic and gender gaps in the use of and adherence to evidence-based preventive therapies among elderly Medicare Part D beneficiaries after acute myocardial infarction. *Circulation.* 2014;129:754–763.

46. Albert MA. Not there yet. Medicare Part D and elimination of cardiovascular medication usage sociodemographic disparities after myocardial infarction. *Circulation.* 2014;129:723–724.

47. Ki Y-J, Kang J, Park J, et al. Efficacy and safety of long-term and short-term dual antiplatelet therapy: a meta-analysis of comparison between Asians and non-Asians. *J Clin Med.* 2020;9:652.

48. Brown SA, Pereira N. Pharmacogenomic impact of CYP2C19 variation on clopidogrel therapy in precision cardiovascular medicine. *J Pers Med.* 2018;8(1):8.

49. Bozkurt B, Colvin M, Cook J, et al. Current diagnostic and treatment strategies for specific dilated cardiomyopathies: a scientific statement from the American Heart Association. *Circulation.* 2016;134:e579–e646.

50. Mohammed SF, Mirzoyev SA, Edwards WD, et al. Left ventricular amyloid deposition in patients with heart failure and preserved ejection fraction. *JACC Heart Fail.* 2014;2:113–122.

51. Quarta CC, Buxbaum JN, Shah AM, et al. The amyloidogenic V122I transthyretin variant in elderly Black Americans. *N Eng J Med.* 2014;372:21–29.

52. Shah KB, Mankad AK, Castano A, et al. Transthyretin cardiac amyloidosis in Black Americans. *Circ Heart Fail.* 2016;9(6):e002558.

53. Damrauer SM, Chaudhary K, Cho JH, et al. Association of the V122I hereditary transthyretin amyloidosis genetic variant with heart failure among individuals of African or Hispanic/LatinX ancestry. *J Am Med Assoc.* 2019;322:2191–2202.

54. Ozkor MA, Rahman AM, Murrow JR, et al. Differences in vascular nitric oxide and endothelium-derived hyperpolarizing factor bioavailability in blacks and whites. *Arterioscler Thromb Vasc Biol.* 2014;34:1320–1327.

55. Taylor AL, Ziesche S, Yancy C, et al. Combination of isosorbide dinitrate and hydralazine in blacks with heart failure. *N Eng J Med.* 2004;351:2049–2057.

56. McNamara DM, Taylor AL, Tam SW, et al. G-protein beta-3 subunit genotype predicts enhanced benefit of fixed-dose isosorbide dinitrate and hydralazine: results of A-HeFT. *JACC Heart Fail.* 2014;2:551–557.

57. Mehta H, Armstrong A, Swett K, et al. Burden of systolic and diastolic left ventricular dysfunction among Hispanics in the United States: insights from the echocardiographic study of LatinXs. *Circ Heart Fail.* 2016;9:e002733-e.

58. Qian F, Fonarow GC, Krim SR, et al. Characteristics, quality of care, and in-hospital outcomes of Asian-American heart failure patients: findings from the American Heart Association get with the guidelines-heart failure program. *Int J Cardiol.* 2015;189:141–147.

59. Glynn P, Lloyd-Jones DM, Feinstein MJ, et al. Disparities in cardiovascular mortality related to heart failure in the United States. *J Am Coll Cardiol.* 2019;73:2354–2355.

60. Ziaeian B, Kominski GF, Ong MK, et al. National differences in trends for heart failure hospitalizations by Sex and race/ethnicity. *Circ Cardiovasc Qual Outcomes.* 2017;10:e003552.

61. Ziaeian B, Heidenreich PA, Xu H, et al. Medicare expenditures by race/ethnicity after hospitalization for heart failure with preserved ejection fraction. *JACC Heart Fail.* 2018;6:388.

62. Alsan M, Garrick O, Graziani G. Does diversity matter for health? Experimental evidence from Oakland. *Am Econ Rev.* 2019;109:4071–4111.

63. Shen MJ, Peterson EB, Costas-Muñiz R, et al. The effects of race and racial concordance on patient-physician communication: a systematic review of the literature. *J Racial Ethn Health Disparities.* 2018;5:117–140.

64. Victor RG, Lynch K, Li N, et al. A Cluster-randomized trial of blood-pressure reduction in Black barbershops. *N Eng J Med.* 2018;378:1291–1301.

94 Endemic and Pandemic Viral Illnesses and Cardiovascular Disease: Influenza and COVID-19

ORLY VARDENY, MOHAMMAD MADJID, AND SCOTT D. SOLOMON

INTRODUCTION

Over the past decade appreciation has grown that viral diseases can affect the cardiovascular system and contribute to cardiovascular disease (CVD). Influenza accounts for a substantial number of hospitalizations and deaths worldwide, and it has become increasingly evident that patients with CVD may have particular vulnerability to influenza-related complications and that influenza infection itself may contribute directly to CVD progression and events, including myocardial infarction (MI) and heart failure (HF). This association becomes even more evident when a large number of individuals in the population become infected, as has occurred several times in the past century in the setting of pandemics. In addition to influenza, other viruses, including respiratory syncytial virus (RSV), parainfluenza virus, adenovirus, human metapneumovirus, parvovirus, and enterovirus infections, have been implicated in CVD.

In late 2019, a novel coronavirus was found to be the cause of a cluster of cases of severe respiratory illness in Wuhan, China. This virus, SARS-CoV-2, and the disease it caused, COVID-19, quickly spread throughout the globe and was dubbed a global pandemic by the World Health Organization (WHO) on March 11, 2020. In addition to severe respiratory disease, often leading to a requirement for intensive care, mechanical ventilation, or death, this disease often affects the entire cardiovascular system, which may play a central role in the pathogenesis.

This chapter reviews the influence of endemic and pandemic viral infections, including influenza and COVID-19, on CVD. Several other viruses that directly affect the cardiovascular system, including parvovirus and coxsackie virus, are covered in other chapters (see Chapters 52 and 55). Due to the rapidly changing nature of our understanding of the pathophysiology and therapeutic options for COVID-19, this chapter focuses on established pathophysiology and treatment options at the time of writing (September 15, 2021) and will be updated online as more information becomes available.

INFLUENZA AND CARDIOVASCULAR RISK AND DISEASE

Influenza Virology

Influenza viruses are enveloped, negative-sense, single-stranded RNA viruses (~13.5-kb genome) that are characterized based on surface antigens and exist as A and B strains.[1] The hemagglutinin (HA) protein facilitates viral entry into the host cell and binds to the glycoprotein terminal sialic acid and glycolipid receptors. The neuraminidase protein (NA) facilitates viral release and affects viral evolution in concert with the HA protein. These two glycoproteins localize on the surface of the virus particle and are the main targets for protective antibodies generated from influenza virus infection or vaccination.

The segmental configuration of the influenza virus genome allows for reassortment, or interchange, of genetic RNA segments when two viruses of the same type infect the same cell. Thus influenza viruses undergo rapid antigenic *drifts* (defined as genetic variations in antigen structures stemming from point mutations in the HA and NA genes over time) and *shifts* (sudden genetic reassortment between two closely related influenza viral strains), which allow them to evade the host immune system. Although influenza B viruses primarily infect humans, the influenza A viruses (IAVs) are endemic in several species, including humans, birds, and pigs. Animal reservoirs offer a source of antigenically diverse HA and NA genes that can exchange between viral strains, creating virus variation, and occasionally forming novel influenza viruses that contain HA or NA segments from animals.[2] Reassortment of the influenza A pdm09 virus in which the HA H2 and polymerase PB1 genes of the avian H2N2 virus were replaced by two new avian H3 and PB1 genes led to a pandemic in 2009.[3] However, cases of swine- and avian-based zoonotic human transmission of influenza are rare, and are mainly confined to the avian H5N1 and H7N9 and the H3N2 variant viruses.

Pandemic influenza occurs every 20 to 50 years and stems from a viral strain that differs antigenically from previous strains. Because the human immune system is naive to the new virus, the overall lack of immunity in the population correlates with disease severity and excess mortality. Since 1918, the IAVs have caused four pandemics. The first and most severe pandemic in recent history, known as "Spanish influenza," occurred in 1918, was caused by an H1N1 IAV strain, and led to approximately 500 million infections and 50 to 100 million deaths worldwide. In 1957, the "Asian influenza" caused by an H2N2 IAV strain resulted in ~1.1 million deaths worldwide. In 1968, the "Hong Kong flu" caused by an A/H3N2 strain resulted in ~1 million deaths worldwide. The fourth pandemic in 2009, caused by the influenza A (H1N1) pdm09 virus, led to 151,700 to 575,400 deaths worldwide from 2009 to 2010. Since that time, this novel IAV has continued to spread as a seasonal influenza virus. Influenza B co-circulates with influenza A each year. Typically, outbreaks of influenza A and B in the northern and southern hemispheres can lead to as many as 5 million cases of severe influenza and up to 500,000 deaths worldwide in a single season.

The major societal burden from influenza is caused by influenza A and B through seasonal outbreaks, mostly during winter months

CARDIOVASCULAR DISEASE AND DISORDERS OF OTHER ORGANS

XI

when transmission conditions are more favorable due to low temperatures and humidity. Most infections occur in the pediatric population, although the most severe cases occur in younger children or in older adults. Children appear to be the main transmitters of influenza virus, evidenced by reduced incidence of severe influenza among older adults when children are vaccinated.[4]

Symptoms from influenza virus infection can vary from a mild upper respiratory disease limited to fever, sore throat, runny nose, cough, headache, muscle aches, and fatigue, to severe, in some cases leading to lethal influenza-induced pneumonia or due to a secondary bacterial infection. Influenza virus infection can also precipitate a wide range of nonrespiratory complications, including acute cardiovascular events.

Epidemiology of Influenza and Cardiovascular Disease

Several risk factors predispose patients to severe or lethal influenza infection. Due to lack of previous exposures, young children are more likely to develop worse symptoms and a higher fever and tend to shed larger amounts of virus for longer after being infected. Older adults are also at risk for more severe symptoms and infection-related complications, including hospitalizations, due to immunosenescence (reduced immune function with aging) and chronic conditions.[5] In addition to extremes of age, other groups at risk for severe disease, hospitalization, or death include those with concomitant pulmonary or cardiac conditions, neuromuscular disease, diabetes mellitus, and conditions that render patients immunocompromised. Obesity is associated with enhanced viral replication, and those with morbid obesity have increased risk for secondary bacterial infections and a reduced immune response to influenza vaccination. Pregnancy is also a risk factor for severe disease, possibly related to altered immune function coupled with increased cardiopulmonary demand; the risk appears to increase more with each trimester.[1]

Influenza and Acute Myocardial Infarction

Numerous observational studies utilizing case-control or case-only designs have reported associations between infection with influenza and other respiratory illnesses and acute MI, including a large self-controlled case series study including 115,112 individuals hospitalized for acute MI or stroke, which noted a fivefold increased risk for MI and a threefold increased risk for stroke within the first 3 days of an outpatient visit for various acute respiratory or urinary infections, including influenza.[6,7] Overall, influenza may account for between 3% and 6% of attributable risk for MI-related deaths. A patient-level study examining the relationship between laboratory-confirmed respiratory diagnosis and hospitalization for MI using insurance databases and public microbiology testing results found a 5-fold increased risk of acute MI within 7 days of influenza A and a 10-fold increased risk with influenza B. A significant time-dependent association was also detected with other respiratory viruses, including RSV, coronavirus, parainfluenza virus, adenovirus, human metapneumovirus, and enterovirus infections, adding to the evidence that various viral pathogens can precipitate atherothrombotic events.[8]

Influenza and Heart Failure

Influenza is also associated with increased risk for HF events. Increased overall hospitalization rates have been observed during influenza seasons compared with non-influenza seasons (adjusted hazard ratio [HR], 1.11; 95% confidence interval [CI], 1.03 to 1.20; P = 0.005).[9] In an analysis relating Centers for Disease Control and Prevention (CDC)-defined influenza-like illness (ILI) in four U.S. communities to rates of hospitalizations for HF or MI between 2010 and 2014, a 5% monthly absolute increase in influenza activity was associated with a 24% adjusted increase in hospitalizations for HF within the same month (incidence rate ratio (IRR), 1.24; 95% CI, 1.11 to 1.38; $P <$ 0.001) (Fig. 94.1).[10] Patients with HF also have increased risk for other adverse outcomes when hospitalized with influenza. In over 8 million HF patients from a national inpatient sample, those with influenza (0.67%) had an increased risk for in-hospital mortality (odds ratio [OR], 1.15; 95% CI, 1.03 to 1.30), acute respiratory failure (OR, 1.95; 95% CI 1.83 to 2.07), and requirement for mechanical ventilation (OR, 1.75; 95% CI, 1.62 to 1.89).[11]

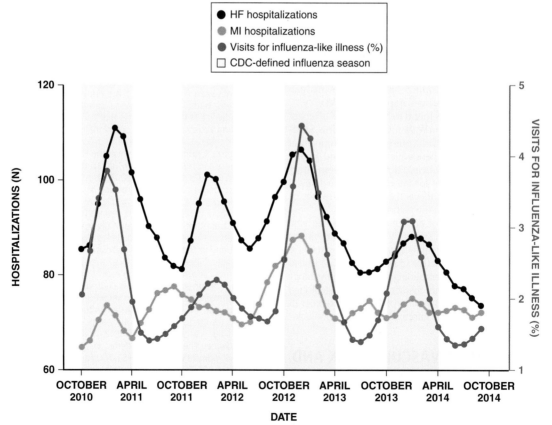

FIGURE 94.1 Association of timing of influenza season with hospitalizations for cardiovascular events. (From Kytömaa S, et al. Association of Influenza-like Illness Activity With Hospitalizations for Heart Failure: The Atherosclerosis Risk in Communities Study. JAMA Cardiol 2019;4(4):363-369.)

Influenza and Arrhythmia Risk

The incidence of cardiac arrest and sudden cardiac death (SCD) show seasonal variation, increasing during the winter in line with peak influenza season, and the likelihood of survival to hospital discharge after cardiac arrest was lowest during the winter.[12,13] A study of 481,516 out-of-hospital cardiac arrests in Japan reported a significant association between cardiac arrests and severe influenza epidemics (relative risk [RR], 1.25; 95% CI, 1.16, 1.34), with a more pronounced effect within 7 days of reported peaks in influenza activity, consistent with previous data on associations of influenza with acute MI. Ventricular tachyarrhythmias detected by implantable cardioverter-defibrillators (ICDs) have exhibited seasonal variation, with positive associations observed during the winter and during increased influenza activity.[14,15]

Because the risk of atrial fibrillation (AF) increases during winter months and colder temperatures,[16] a population case-control study in Taiwan related newly diagnosed AF to influenza infection during the previous year (adjusted OR, 1.18; 95% CI, 1.014 to 1.378; $P = 0.032$). Individuals who received influenza vaccination had a reduced risk for AF compared with unvaccinated people (adjusted OR, 0.881; 95% CI, 0.836 to 0.928; $P < 0.001$).[17]

Influenza and Myocarditis

Sporadic reports have linked myocarditis to influenza infection, varying from asymptomatic to fulminant myocarditis resulting in hemodynamic compromise, HF, or cardiogenic shock, requiring vasopressor or mechanical support. In cases of symptomatic myocarditis, patients typically present within 4 to 7 days of their illness with shortness of breath; pleuritic chest pain; and less frequently with hypotension, syncope, arrhythmia, or fulminant HF. Cases of fulminant myocarditis have been more common during pandemic influenza or during virulent years of seasonal influenza, as was the case during the 2009 H1N1 pandemic and during the particularly severe 2017/2018 influenza season. In case series, the majority of influenza-related myocarditis cases involved the A/H1N1 strain, followed by B-type and A/H3N2; HF was the most common complication (84% of cases), and over half of the cases required advanced cardiac support.[18]

Pathophysiology of Influenza and Cardiovascular Disease

Influenza affects the cardiovascular system through multiple mechanisms. Influenza virus has been localized to human coronary endothelial and smooth muscle cells.[19] Infection of mice with influenza A H3N2 virus led to severalfold increased expression of genes for monocyte chemoattractant protein-1 (MCP-1), interleukin-8 (IL-8), tissue factor (TF), plasminogen activator inhibitor 1 (PAI-1), vascular cell adhesion molecule 1 (VCAM-1), intercellular adhesion molecule (ICAM)-1, and E-selectin, whereas endothelial nitric oxide synthase (eNOS) expression decreased in endothelial cells.[19] In *Apo E*-deficient atherosclerotic mice, influenza virus A H3N2 can reside in the atherosclerotic plaques and myocardium, and the virus has been cultured from aorta and myocardium a week after infection in high titers, comparable to pulmonary tissue.[19] Infection also significantly increases plasma levels of proinflammatory cytokines and chemokines and can lead to an exaggerated cellular inflammatory response in atherosclerotic plaque, with a significant increase in plaque macrophage content.[19,20]

Viable virus could be detected in the myocardium of mice infected with influenza A within 12 days of infection, with evidence of oxidative stress-induced mitochondrial damage resulting in a low-energy state.[21] In addition, bacterial superinfection can complicate influenza infection, and likely contribute substantially to the risk in elderly individuals affected by influenza, and provide a rationale for administration of pneumococcal vaccine in this population.[22,23] The ability of influenza infection to directly infect arterial and myocardial tissues and to cause local arterial-level plus systemic proinflammatory effects, prothrombotic effects, and increases in pro-oxidative stress, in conjunction with nonspecific effects induced by demand ischemia, hypoxia, sympathetic stimulation, and myocardial depression, all contribute to an increased risk for multiple cardiovascular adverse outcomes (Fig. 94.2).[24-26]

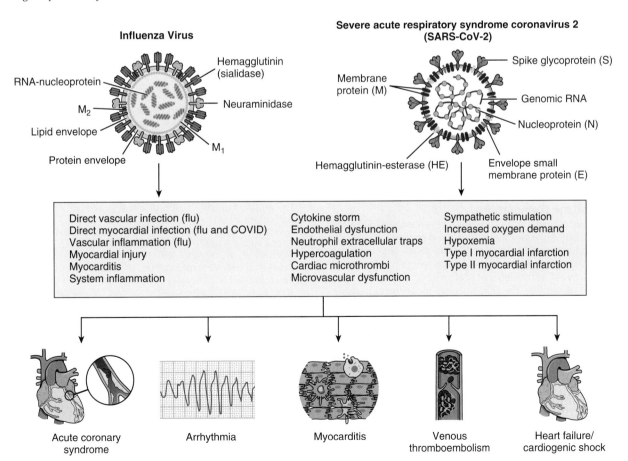

Cardiovascular manifestations

FIGURE 94.2 Mechanisms of acute viral infections on the cardiovascular system.

Influenza Prevention and Therapy

The association between influenza and CVD has stimulated growing interest in the role of influenza vaccination in the prevention of CVD. Several observational and small randomized, clinical trials (RCTs) have suggested that influenza vaccination can protect from adverse cardiovascular outcomes. To prevent influenza illness the CDC recommends annual influenza vaccination for individuals 6 months or older, unless contraindicated. Each year the WHO and the CDC Advisory Committee on Immunization Practices make recommendations for the influenza vaccine composition based on circulating strains in the Southern Hemisphere. Because antigenic mismatch can occur due to antigenic drifts or virus mutations during the period of production of vaccines, vaccine effectiveness (VE) can vary each year, with VE in recent years between 20% and 70%; nevertheless, vaccines confer some protection even during years with a poor antigenic match.

A large meta-analysis of six RCTs (four blinded, two open label) assessed the benefit of influenza vaccination on reducing major adverse cardiovascular events, including cardiovascular death or hospitalization for MI, unstable angina, stroke, HF, or urgent coronary revascularization in 6734 individuals, with numerically fewer deaths in the vaccinated group.[27] During a mean duration of follow-up of 7.9 months, the vaccine recipient group had fewer major adverse cardiovascular events compared with those who received placebo or no vaccination (RR, 0.64; 95% CI, 0.48, 0.86; $P = 0.003$), with an absolute risk difference of 1.74%. The effect was more pronounced in individuals with a recent acute coronary syndrome (ACS) compared with those without recent ACS.

In patients with HF, data on the effects of influenza vaccine on cardiac outcomes rely on observational studies due to the paucity of placebo-controlled trials. In a self-controlled case series from the United Kingdom between 1990 and 2013,[28] vaccinated individuals had a lower risk for hospitalization from cardiovascular (IRR, 0.73; 95% CI, 0.71, 0.76), respiratory infections (IRR 0.83, 95% CI 0.77, 0.90), or any cause (IRR, 0.96; 95% CI, 0.95, 0.98) relative to an adjacent vaccination-free year. Nevertheless, influenza vaccination in patients with HF remains low. In a post hoc analysis of the global PARADIGM-HF trial in over 8000 patients with HF with reduced ejection fraction (HFrEF), only 21% of patients with HF received influenza vaccination in the year of enrollment, with rates varying widely by country from less than 5% to 77%.[29] Vaccination was associated with an adjusted reduced risk for mortality (HR, 0.81; 95% CI, 0.67, 0.97; $P = 0.015$), but not all-cause hospitalizations, cardiovascular death, HF, or cardiopulmonary- or influenza-related hospitalizations. Similar reduction in HF-related outcomes were observed in a nation-wide observational cohort study from Denmark of greater than 130,000 individuals, with reductions in death and hospitalizations.[30] Observational data of influenza vaccination may indicate improved access to care, in addition to reflecting practice variation by region.

Influenza Vaccine Formulations

Influenza vaccine contains two strains from the A-lineage, A/H1N1 and A/H3N2, and either one or two strains from the B-lineage, B/Victoria or B/Yamagata, and are available in several formulations varying in their method of preparation (egg-based, cell culture, recombinant technology), in the amount of and number of vaccine antigens included, and in the presence of adjuvant. The CDC does not recommend preferentially one vaccine formulation over another, but it does emphasize the importance of annual vaccination. Immune responses to influenza vaccine are less robust among older individuals, which is a manifestation of immunosenescence. High-dose influenza vaccine that contains four times the amount of vaccine antigen as standard-dose influenza vaccine has been tested and approved in the United States and other regions for individuals age 65 or older. In a large, RCT of approximately 31,989 medically stable older adults, high-dose influenza vaccine reduced laboratory-confirmed symptomatic influenza by 24% compared with standard-dose vaccine,[31] with a suggestion of reduced risk in serious events caused by cardiac or pulmonary causes (rate ratio, 0.82; 95% CI, 0.73 to 0.93).[32]

The INVESTED trial compared high-dose vaccine with standard-dose vaccine in 5260 high-risk CVD participants; there was no reduction in cardiovascular or pulmonary hospitalizations.[33] Participants were randomized to high-dose trivalent inactivated influenza vaccine or standard-dose quadrivalent inactivated influenza vaccine and treated for up to three influenza seasons. The primary composite endpoint, death or cardiopulmonary hospitalization, did not differ between vaccine groups (HR, 1.06; 95% CI, 0.97, 1.17; $P = 0.21$), and results were consistent across secondary endpoints and within pre-specified subgroups, although high-dose vaccine was associated with more mild vaccine-related adverse events such as injection site pain, swelling, and myalgias. The low rates of hospitalizations ascribed to influenza or pneumonia were low overall, suggesting a modest attributable risk of these types of events to the overall risk for hospitalizations in this high-risk patient group.

Antiviral Therapies for Influenza

In addition to vaccination, antiviral agents may reduce the likelihood of influenza-related cardiovascular events, although available data are mostly observational. A large, propensity-matched, retrospective analysis of adults with a prior diagnosis of CVD suggested that treatment with oseltamivir in the first 48 hours after a diagnosis of influenza confers a significant reduction in the incidence of recurrent cardiovascular events (OR, 0.417; 95% CI, 0.349 to 0.498),[34] and at least one other retrospective study suggested potential benefit of oseltamivir in preventing stroke and transient ischemic attack (TIA) (HR, 0.56; 95% CI, 0.42 to 0.74).[35]

SARS-CoV-2 AND COVID-19

Coronavirus Virology and Epidemiology

Coronaviruses (Coronavirinae subfamily) fall into four groups of alpha, beta, gamma, and delta coronaviruses by phylogenetic clustering.[36] Alpha and beta coronaviruses cause infection in humans.[37] Coronaviruses contain four major structural proteins: the spike (S) protein, the nucleocapsid (N) protein, the membrane (M) protein, and the envelope (E) protein.[38] The spike protein, which resembles a crown in cross section and for which the viruses are named, mediates the attachment of the virus to the host cell receptor and subsequent fusion of the virus and cell membrane.

First discovered in the 1960s, the coronavirus family includes seven strains with the ability to infect humans (eFig. 94.1). Four viruses (i.e., HCoV-229E, HCoV-NL63, HCoV-OC43, and HCoV-HKU1) generally cause mild and self-resolving infections. Three other coronaviruses can cause severe and potentially fatal infections (Table 94.1): severe acute respiratory syndrome coronavirus (SARS-CoV), Middle East respiratory syndrome coronavirus (MERS-CoV), and severe acute respiratory syndrome coronavirus 2 (SARS-CoV-2).[39,40]

Severe Acute Respiratory Syndrome Coronavirus and Middle East Respiratory Syndrome. The SARS-CoV virus causing SARS infection

TABLE 94.1 Comparison of Coronaviruses with an Epidemic Potential

VIRUS	RECEPTOR	INCUBATION PERIOD	PREVALENCE OF UNDERLYING CARDIOVASCULAR DISEASE	AVERAGE CASE FATALITY RATE
SARS-CoV	ACE2	2-11 days	10%	10%
MERS-CoV	DPP4	2-13 days	30%	30%
SARS-CoV-2	ACE2	2-14 days	Up to 20% in hospitalized patients	2%-4% (Highly variable, based on multiple factors)

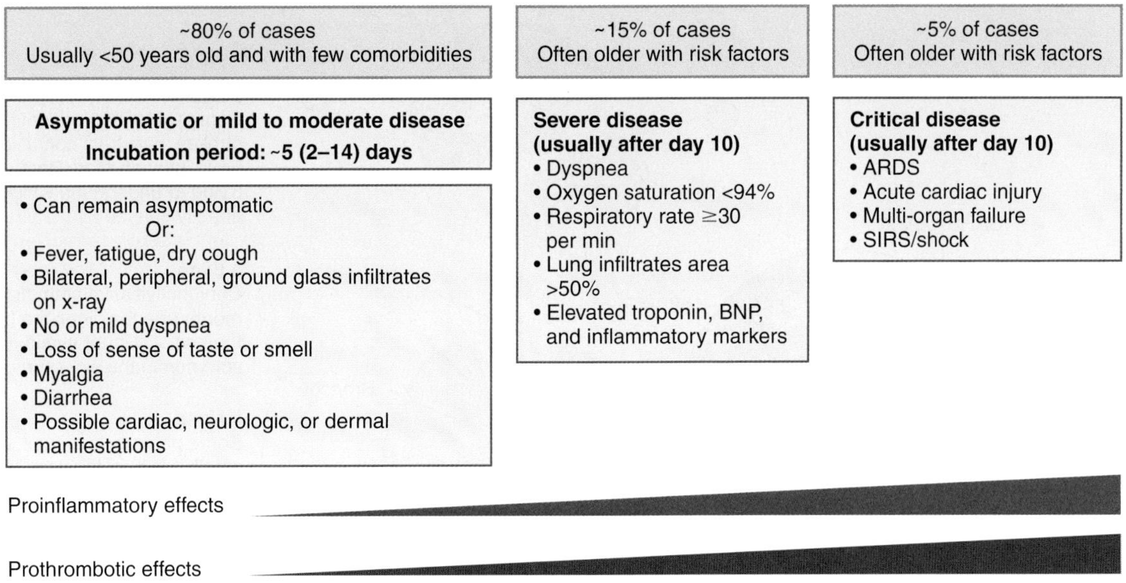

~80% of cases Usually <50 years old and with few comorbidities	~15% of cases Often older with risk factors	~5% of cases Often older with risk factors
Asymptomatic or mild to moderate disease **Incubation period: ~5 (2–14) days**	**Severe disease (usually after day 10)**	**Critical disease (usually after day 10)**
• Can remain asymptomatic Or: • Fever, fatigue, dry cough • Bilateral, peripheral, ground glass infiltrates on x-ray • No or mild dyspnea • Loss of sense of taste or smell • Myalgia • Diarrhea • Possible cardiac, neurologic, or dermal manifestations	• Dyspnea • Oxygen saturation <94% • Respiratory rate ≥30 per min • Lung infiltrates area >50% • Elevated troponin, BNP, and inflammatory markers	• ARDS • Acute cardiac injury • Multi-organ failure • SIRS/shock

Proinflammatory effects

Prothrombotic effects

FIGURE 94.3 Clinical course and manifestations of COVID-19.

first emerged in November 2002 in the Guangdong Province of China, likely related to a zoonotic transmission from the wild-animal markets. The virus most likely originated from bats with an intermediate host of civet cats.[41] SARS-CoV binds to and uses the angiotensin-converting enzyme 2 (ACE2) to enter host cells. ACE2 is abundantly expressed on the surfaces of endothelial cells of arteries, arterial smooth muscle, pericytes, and the epithelium of the respiratory tract and small intestine.[42] Primarily transmitted from symptomatic patients via respiratory droplets, SARS has an incubation period of 2 to 11 days after exposure,[43] and it affected 8096 people in 29 countries in 2003 with 774 cases of death reported worldwide (and 8 nonfatal cases in the United States). Cardiovascular complications reported with SARS in small case series included tachycardia, hypotension, bradycardia, ACS, MI, and thromboembolic events.[36,44-46]

The MERS-CoV outbreak emerged in Saudi Arabia (SA) in June 2012.[47] This virus also likely originated in bats with dromedary camels acting as the intermediate host for transmission to humans.[47] MERS-CoV enters the host cells through a serine peptidase, dipeptidyl peptidase 4 (DPP4),[42] and is transmitted from patients via respiratory secretions through close contact with an incubation period of 2 to 13 days.[43,48] MERS-CoV has been reported in about 2500 cases in 26 countries with a case fatality rate of 34.4%.[36,49] A systematic review of 637 patients with MERS-CoV showed a high prevalence of comorbidities among these patients including cardiac diseases (30%), hypertension (50%), diabetes (50%), and obesity (16%).[50]

Severe Acute Respiratory Syndrome CORONAVIRUS 2 and COVID-19

On December 31, 2019, a cluster of 27 cases of pneumonia of unknown etiology was reported in Wuhan, China. Patients had symptoms of viral pneumonia including fever, cough, chest discomfort, dyspnea, and bilateral lung infiltrates. The exact source of the initial infection remains unclear, although most of the initial cohort had an epidemiologic link to a wet market in Wuhan. The first genome sequence of the novel causative coronavirus was published on January 10, 2020, and the virus was later named SARS-CoV-2.[36] Human-to-human transmission was confirmed by January 20, 2020, and the disease reached epidemic peak in China by February 2020. On March 11, 2020, the WHO officially declared the global outbreak of COVID-19 as a pandemic.[51] By late March 2021, COVID-19 had affected 127 million and killed over 2.7 million individuals worldwide, and it has caused over 30 million infections and about 550,000 deaths in the United States.

SARS-CoV-2 belongs to the beta-CoVs group and shows about 89% nucleotide identity with bat virus and 79% with human SARS-CoV, and similarly uses ACE2 as the receptor to enter the host cell.[36] Transmission of SARS-CoV-2 occurs mainly by contact with an infected person or contaminated surface, exposure to virus-containing respiratory droplets, and exposure to virus-containing aerosols (<5 μm).[52] Fecal-oral transmission is also a rare route of transmission.[53]

The SARS-CoV-2 infection in adults can be either symptomatic or asymptomatic, and asymptomatic individuals still have the ability to transmit the disease. There are fewer symptomatic cases in children of 15 years old or younger. The primary symptoms of COVID-19 are fever, cough, and shortness of breath, although the full spectrum of symptoms is broad, and can include muscle pain, anorexia, malaise, sore throat, nasal congestion, anosmia, dyspnea, and headache. Symptoms may appear in as few as 2 days or as long as 14 days after exposure (Fig. 94.3).[36] The detected viral load is similar in asymptomatic and symptomatic COVID-19 patients, which explains the high potential for transmission of the virus from asymptomatic or minimally symptomatic patients to other persons.[54] COVID-19 is associated with multiple extrapulmonary manifestations (Fig. 94.4). Gastrointestinal symptoms such as diarrhea, abdominal pain, and vomiting occur in 2% to 10% of COVID-19 patients,[55] and SARS-CoV-2 patients' feces often contain viral RNA.[56]

As an RNA virus, SARS-CoV-2 is susceptible to mutation during replication. Mutations that persist after rounds of replication lead to the emergence of new *variants*[57,57a] and those with different phenotypic characteristics are termed *strains*. Three different nomenclature systems are used for naming and tracking SARS-CoV-2 variants. The World Health Organization (WHO) has introduced a simpler method of using Greek alphabet letters to identify variants of concern and variants of interest (eTable 94.1). Early in the pandemic, a novel variant, D614G, increased the efficacy of the virus to replicate and its ability to interact with the ACE2 receptor. Another variant, termed *alpha variant,* was initially identified in the United Kingdom and has additional mutations in the spike protein and is more easily transmissible with possibly higher mortality. The beta variant first identified in South Africa, also with mutations in the spike protein, shows high potential for transmissibility and is less likely to be effectively neutralized by convalescent serum, and might be less responsive to early vaccines based on the original circulating virus. The highly contagious delta variant, initially detected in India, has caused significant mortality, and first-generation vaccines may offer less protection against it.

Overall, the emergence of new variants is a cause for concern because they may have higher transmissibility, higher virulence, less susceptibility to treatments using monoclonal antibodies, and the potential ability to evade the body's innate or acquired immune responses, as well as the response to vaccines. Additional booster vaccine doses might become necessary to protect against them. It is yet not clear if new variants will have a different impact on the cardiovascular system.

Epidemiology of COVID-19 and Risk Factors
Comorbidities and COVID-19 Illness

Several comorbidities confer higher risk of requiring critical care from COVID-19, including advanced age, diabetes, hypertension, HF, and atherosclerotic CVD. Advanced age is associated with SARS-CoV-2 infection and worse disease severity, potentially related to immunosenescence, but also due to the presence of other comorbidities that portend a worse prognosis from COVID-19. Hypertension is the most prevalent comorbidity among patients with COVID-19 and affects approximately

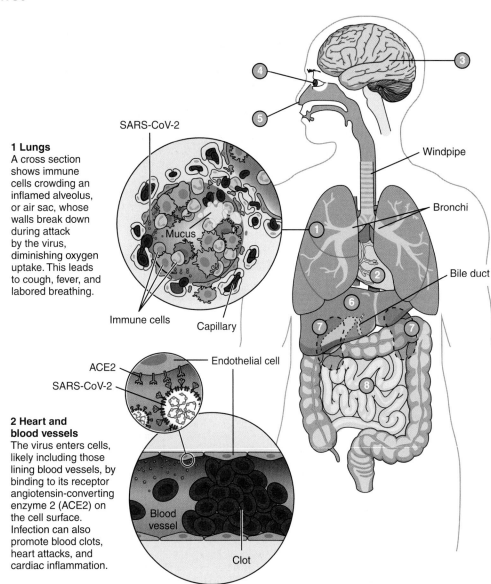

1 Lungs
A cross section shows immune cells crowding an inflamed alveolus, or air sac, whose walls break down during attack by the virus, diminishing oxygen uptake. This leads to cough, fever, and labored breathing.

2 Heart and blood vessels
The virus enters cells, likely including those lining blood vessels, by binding to its receptor angiotensin-converting enzyme 2 (ACE2) on the cell surface. Infection can also promote blood clots, heart attacks, and cardiac inflammation.

3 Brain
Some COVID-19 patients have strokes, seizures, confusion, and brain inflammation. Doctors are trying to understand which are directly caused by the virus.

4 Eyes
Conjunctivitis, inflammation of the membrane that lines the front of the eye and inner eyelid, is more common in the sickest patients.

5 Nose
Some patients lose their sense of smell. It is hypothesized that the virus may move up the nose's nerve endings and damage cells.

6 Liver
Up to half of hospitalized patients have enzyme levels that signal a struggling liver. An immune system in overdrive and drugs given to fight the virus may be causing the damage.

7 Kidneys
Kidney damage is common in severe cases and makes death more likely. The virus may attack the kidneys directly, or kidney failure may be a part of whole-body events such as plummeting blood pressure.

8 Intestines
Patient reports and biopsy data suggest the virus can infect the lower gastrointestinal tract, which is rich in ACE2. Some 20% or more of patients have diarrhea.

FIGURE 94.4 Extrapulmonary manifestations of COVID-19. (From Wadman M., et al. A rampage through the body. Science 2020;368(6489):356-360.)

30% of patients with severe COVID-19,[58] followed by diabetes mellitus, obesity, CVD, pulmonary disease, and cerebrovascular disease. Hypertension and CVD are associated with increased susceptibility to SARS-CoV-2 infection, and along with diabetes link to more severe COVID-19 and an increased mortality.

Individuals who meet criteria for obesity (body mass index [BMI] ≥30 kg/m²) also have increased risk for hospitalization for COVID-19, respiratory failure, and higher mortality even after adjustments for age, race, and comorbid conditions.[59] Obese individuals (WHO class I through III) are more likely to require mechanical ventilation or experience in-hospital death compared with nonobese patients (OR, 1.28 [95% CI 1.09 to 1.51], 1.57 [1.29 to 1.91], 1.80 [1.47 to 2.20], respectively). Obesity and age interact significantly, such that the association with obesity and adverse clinical outcomes was stronger for individuals younger than age 50 (p-interaction <0.05).

The mechanism by which increased BMI contributes to an adverse prognosis in COVID-19 is not entirely clear, but it may relate to increased inflammation from adipose tissue, which may stimulate production of inflammatory cytokines and increase the risk for cytokine storm (see later). Moreover, adipose tissue highly expresses ACE2,[60] which may contribute to the increased risk of more severe infection. In patients with more advanced disease, adverse respiratory mechanical factors, such as decreased pulmonary expiratory reserve volume, functional capacity, and respiratory system compliance, may also contribute to severity

of disease. Obesity is also often accompanied by other comorbidities known to increase risk for adverse clinical outcomes from COVID-19 illness such as hypertension, diabetes mellitus, and atherosclerotic CVD.

Racial and Ethnic Influences on COVID-19 Illness

Individuals from certain races and ethnic minority groups are at increased risk for COVID-19 and resultant hospitalizations, independent of age or other comorbid conditions.[61] Blacks were 3.6 more likely, Native Americans 3.4 times more likely, and Latinx individuals are 3.2 times more likely to die of COVID-19 when compared with whites, across all age groups, including younger adults who normally exhibit lower mortality rates.[62] Black Americans have a doubled risk of hospitalization from COVID-19 compared with white Americans, after adjustment for age, gender, residence, insurance plan, obesity and Charlson Comorbidity Index score.[63] Once hospitalized, Blacks and whites appear to have similar mortality rates.

Racial and ethnic disparities with COVID-19 infection and prognosis may arise from systemic structural disadvantages. Blacks are disproportionately represented in "essential worker" groups that were exempt from shelter-in-place efforts. Housing disadvantages with larger per household numbers are more common among Blacks and challenge social distancing initiatives, as is the use of public transportation. COVID-19 has exacerbated these disparities in the United States and across the globe.[64]

Clinical Cardiovascular Manifestations of COVID-19

Cardiovascular manifestations of COVID-19 vary, and acute infection links to a wide spectrum of cardiovascular complications, including ACS, stroke, acute-onset HF, arrhythmias, myocarditis, and cardiac arrest. Exactly how the disease leads to these complications remains unclear, although most likely it appears to be linked to the underlying inflammatory response that becomes unbridled in some patients, resulting in an immune-mediated thrombotic state (immunothrombosis).

Atherosclerotic Cardiovascular Syndromes: Acute Coronary Syndromes and Stroke in COVID-19 Patients

Respiratory infections are associated with ACSs, as noted previously for influenza.[26] SARS-CoV-2 can also trigger ACSs and strokes by producing profound proinflammatory and prothrombotic effects (see later). Early limited reports have suggested a higher thrombus burden in COVID-19 patients presenting with ST-elevation MI.[65] A Danish nationwide registry-based study of over 5000 patients with hospitalized COVID-19 revealed that the risk of acute MI and ischemic stroke were 5 and 10 times higher, respectively, during the first 14 days after COVID-19 infection compared with a period preceding known infection.[66]

Myocarditis due to COVID-19

Despite early reports of myocarditis in the setting of COVID-19, its actual incidence in the setting of COVID-19 infection appears quite low, with most evidence limited to case reports or small case series. Symptom presentation of cases thought to be myocarditis related to COVID-19 have varied from fatigue or dyspnea to chest pain or tightness on exertion. There have only been a few reports of fulminant myocarditis, evidenced by ventricular dysfunction and acute HF within a few weeks of confirmed SARS-CoV-2 infection. Although viral particles with the morphology and size of SARS-CoV-2 have been detected in myocardial interstitial macrophages, SARS-CoV-2 genomic material has not been detected in the cardiac myocytes (see later).[67]

COVID-19 and Heart Failure

COVID-19 is associated with increased risk for hospitalization and mortality in patients with prevalent HF and may also increase the risk of developing incident HF, particularly in at-risk individuals. Among 152 patients with a history of HF hospitalized with COVID-19 in a tertiary hospital in Spain, mortality rates were higher compared with those with COVID-19 and without HF ($n = 2928, 48.7\%$ vs. $19.0\%; P < 0.001$).[68] Of the 77 patients who developed acute HF, only 22.1% had a prior history of it, which supports the potential of the SARS-CoV-2 virus to result in myocardial damage. In a study of 132,312 patients with HF hospitalized between April and June 2020, using data from a large, multicenter, all-payer database inclusive of over 1000 health care entities and health systems in the United States, the in-hospital mortality rate for patients with HF hospitalized for COVID-19 was 24.2% compared with 2.6% in those hospitalized for acute HF and 4.6% in those who were hospitalized for other reasons during the same time frame.[69]

Arrhythmias in COVID-19

COVID-19 is associated with a wide array of arrhythmias. In general, acute infections can cause arrhythmias through multiple possible mechanisms, including direct infection of the myocardium, myocardial injury, myocarditis, hypoxia, ischemia, cytokine storm, and electrolyte disturbances.[70] Interruption of cardiac medications and iatrogenic effects of certain medications (i.e., chloroquine, hydroxychloroquine, azithromycin) used in COVID-19 may also contribute to the arrhythmogenic burden of COVID-19.

Overall, COVID-19-related arrhythmias are heterogeneous and include sinus tachycardia, AF, sinus bradycardia, complete heart block, ventricular tachycardia, ventricular fibrillation arrest, torsade de pointes, and pulseless electrical activity.[70,71] Although patients may develop sinus tachycardia during the infection period, the risk of other types of arrhythmias is lower and varies depending on the severity of the infection and the underlying condition of patients. Tachycardia

and palpitation are among common complaints in patients who have postacute sequelae SARS-CoV-2 (PASC, see later) infection. Limited reports from the Lombardy region in Italy and New York City described a temporal increase in out-of-hospital cardiac arrests during COVID-19 early peak activity, which could be ascribed to cardiac arrests or pulmonary embolism (PE).[72,73]

COVID-19 patients who are admitted to an intensive care unit (ICU) more commonly have severe and life-threatening arrhythmias. In a cohort of 700 patients (mean age 50 years, 45% men) with 11% in the ICU, 9 had cardiac arrest, all of which happened in ICU patients, and were due to pulseless electrical activity, asystole, or torsades de pointes, but not ventricular tachycardia or fibrillation.[74] Cardiac arrests, as expected, were associated with increased risk of in-hospital mortality; however, other arrhythmias (25 incident AF events, 9 significant bradyarrhythmias, and 10 nonsustained ventricular tachycardias [NSVTs]) were not.[74] In a large series of patients (3970 patients) admitted early in the pandemic to New York hospitals, new-onset atrial fibrillation/flutter was detected in 4% of COVID-19 patients, which was comparable to the same rate (4%) in a historic comparable cohort of patients hospitalized with influenza.[75] COVID-19 patients who developed atrial fibrillation/flutter were older and had higher levels of inflammatory biomarkers (i.e., C-reactive protein, IL-6), troponin, and D-dimer.[75]

Venous and Arterial Thromboembolism in COVID-19

Patients with COVID-19 exhibit increased rates of deep vein thrombosis (DVT) and PE (Fig. 94.5). A systematic review of 27 radiologic studies with 3342 patients showed high incidence rates of PE on computed tomography (CT) pulmonary angiography and DVT (17% and 15%, respectively).[76] PE was more frequent in patients admitted to the ICU (25%) compared with those not in the ICU (11%). Concomitant DVT was identified in 42% of patients with PE. The established guideline cutoffs for D-dimer used to exclude PE were applicable to patients with COVID-19.[76] Arterial thrombosis is less common in COVID-19 than venous thrombosis. In a retrospective study of 3334 hospitalized COVID-19 patients in New York (March to April 2020), 207 (6%) had venous thromboembolism (VTE) (3% PE and 4% DVT), whereas 11% had arterial thrombosis (2% ischemic stroke, 9% MI, and 1% systemic thromboembolism).[77] Patients with a thrombotic event had higher all-cause mortality than those without (43% vs. 21%; $P < 0.001$).

Multisystem Inflammatory Syndrome in Children

Initial experience with COVID-19 early during the pandemic suggested that children would not encounter the same degree of severity, complications, and sequelae from the SARS-CoV-2 virus. Albeit quite rare, a growing number of cases of an inflammatory shock syndrome in children prompted the CDC to define this manifestation as "multisystem inflammatory syndrome in children" (MIS-C).[78] MIS-C has several features akin to other known syndromes such as Kawasaki disease, Kawasaki shock syndrome, and toxic shock syndrome. It presents with prolonged fever, elevated inflammatory markers, and cardiovascular features such as arrhythmia, myocardial function depression, and valvular dysfunction. A survey that included 55 hospitals in Europe identified 286 cases that met a prespecified definition of persistent fever, inflammation, and cardiac involvement between February and June 2020.[79] Median age was 8.4 years, and 67% were male. Current or prior COVID-19 infection was confirmed in 65% of cases via polymerase chain reaction (PCR) or measurements of IgM or IgG antibodies. Only a minority of patients had preexisting congenital heart disease or autoimmune disorders. Among patients who had cardiac biomarkers checked, the majority had elevated troponin T or natriuretic peptides. Abnormal electrocardiogram (ECG) (primarily abnormal ST or T wave segment) occurred in 35% of cases and ejection fraction was impaired in 34% of cases, with 20% exhibiting sustained left ventricular systolic dysfunction at discharge. Although 30% of the cohort required inotropic support and 15% required mechanical ventilation, most patients had resolution of the acute manifestations and 93% of patients were discharged, suggesting a more benign course in children with MIS-C than adults with COVID-19, despite significant biomarker elevations and cardiovascular features.[80]

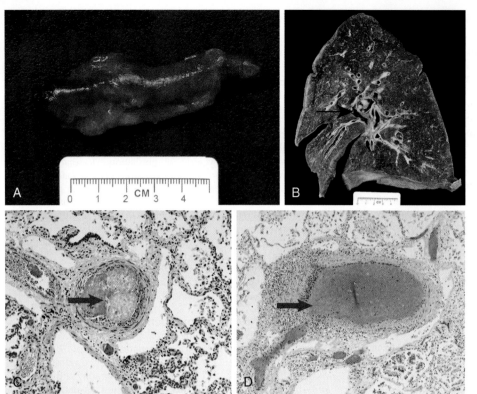

FIGURE 94.5 Gross and microscopic pathology of thromboembolism and vasculitis in COVID-19. A, Gross photograph of a deep vein thrombus removed from the femoral vein in a COVID-19 decedent. **B,** Gross photograph of a cross section of the right lung demonstrating extensive fatal thromboemboli *(arrow)* in a COVID-19 decedent. The background lung shows acute diffuse alveolar damage, characteristic of COVID-19 pneumonia. **C,** Photomicrograph of pulmonary thromboemboli *(arrow)* within small pulmonary arteries in the lung of a COVID-19 decedent. Microscopic thrombi/thromboemboli are common postmortem findings in the lungs, even in patients without known premortem clinical thromboembolic signs/symptoms. (Hematoxylin and eosin (H&E)-stained section, 400× original magnification.) **D,** Photomicrograph of vasculitis within a small pulmonary artery within the lung of a COVID-19 decedent. Vasculitis in the lungs is a rare finding in COVID-19 decedents. (H&E-stained section, 400× original magnification.) (Images courtesy Robert Padera, MD, Brigham and Women's Hospital.)

Biomarker Evidence of Myocardial Injury

Increased troponin levels indicate myocardial injury during the acute phase of infection, as defined as serum concentrations above a certain threshold (e.g., >0.03 ng/mL or levels above the 99th percentile upper reference limit), with or without accompanying electrocardiographic or echocardiographic evidence of acute ischemia.[81] Multiple mechanisms can elevate troponin including but not limited to ACSs,[82] type 1 or type 2 MI, myocarditis, cytokine storm, PE, or Takotsubo syndrome (stress-induced cardiomyopathy) with or without cardiogenic shock.[36,82-84] Chronic baseline conditions such as congestive HF or left ventricular hypertrophy can also raise troponin levels.[36,82] Biochemical evidence of myocardial injury portends worse clinical outcomes among hospitalized patients with COVID-19, and more commonly occurs in patients of older age and with comorbidities. Elevated troponin in COVID-19 has been associated with an increased risk for arrhythmias, respiratory failure, and mortality[85]; increased requirements for invasive and noninvasive mechanical ventilation; higher frequency of acute kidney injury, acute respiratory distress syndrome (ARDS), and coagulation disorders; and a greater than fourfold increased risk for death.[86] A multicenter study in 614 patients hospitalized with COVID-19 reported that elevated troponin occurred in 45.3% of patients and was associated with an increased in-hospital mortality (37% vs. 13%; HR, 1.71 [95% CI 1.13 to 2.59]; P = 0.01), independent of concomitant CVD.[87] Similarly, in a larger retrospective study of 2736 hospitalized patients, 36% had biochemical evidence of myocardial injury (any elevation of troponin I above the upper limits of normal), but less than a third had a history of CAD, and was associated with a 75% increased risk for in-hospital mortality.[81] Although evidence of the association of myocardial injury with adverse outcomes is consistent, it is unclear whether cardiac injury is a marker for disease severity or a direct contributor to COVID-19 morbidity and mortality.

Biomarkers Suggestive of Prothrombotic State

Patients with COVID-19 often have elevated levels of D-dimer, the degradation product of cross-linked fibrin monomers and a marker of coagulation and fibrinolysis. High D-dimer levels are associated with PE and VTE (see later). D-Dimer can be elevated in COVID-19 even in the absence of overt evidence of macrovascular thrombus, and elevated D-dimer levels are associated independently with mortality and a higher likelihood for requiring intubation.[88] High D-dimer levels are nonspecific and may indicate a hypercoagulable state, inflammation, pathologic fibrinolysis, microvascular angiopathy, and overall reflect COVID-19 illness severity.

Cardiac Imaging Findings in COVID-19

COVID-19 has been associated with abnormalities of cardiac structure and function in several studies, including echocardiographic evidence of left ventricular dysfunction, regional wall motion abnormalities, and mild reduction in right ventricular function.[89] Several cardiovascular magnetic resonance (CMR) imaging studies have noted myocardial abnormalities that persist after acute infection. In a study of 100 COVID-19 patients (33 of whom had been hospitalized), imaging was performed at a median of 71 days after diagnosis of COVID-19.[90] Pericardial effusion (>10 mm) was observed in 20% (20/100) of patients, and late gadolinium enhancement (LGE), reflecting scarring, was observed in 32% (32/100) (myocardial) and 22% (22/100) (pericardial) of the COVID-19 group. It was significantly more prevalent in COVID-19 patients than in healthy controls or risk factor-matched controls. In addition, other studies have noted high prevalence of myocardial edema post-COVID-19 infection. Whether abnormal CMR imaging findings observed after COVID-19 reflect permanent cardiac injury is unknown at this time due to the lack of long-term studies.

Effects of the COVID-19 Pandemic on Cardiovascular Health More Broadly

In addition to the effects of the disease on individuals infected with COVID-19, the pandemic has influenced cardiovascular health more broadly in the population. Early in the pandemic, a decrease in the incidence of hospitalization for acute MI, including both ST-segment elevation MI (STEMI) and non–ST-segment elevation MI (NSTEMI), by as much as 40% to 50% was noted compared with previous years (Fig. 94.6).[91-94] Northern Italy observed a 20% reduction in hospitalizations for MI during their peak surge of COVID-19 from February to May 2020 when compared with expected hospitalization rates based on historical data.[95] Unfortunately, this was paralleled with an increase in the number of out-of-hospital cardiac deaths.[95] The cause for the decline in acute MI in the overall population during COVID-19 peak surges likely arose for multiple reasons including patient avoidance of medical care due to fear of contracting COVID-19 in the emergency rooms or hospital settings and misdiagnosis or underappreciation of acute MI. Patients with COVID-19 also suffered longer door-to-CT, door-to-needle, and door-to-endovascular therapy times, with higher in-hospital mortality (OR, 4.34; 95% CI, 3.48 to 5.40).[96]

During peak COVID-19 surges, patients may ignore symptoms of myocardial ischemia, exacerbations of HF, or stroke, and delay seeking appropriate medical care. This delay may worsen outcomes and development of serious complications such as ischemic cardiomyopathy, increased risk of SCD, and development of rare but very high risk complications such as postinfarction myocardial rupture, ischemic ventricular septal defects, or ventricular aneurysms. Because of the potential hesitancy of patients to seek cardiovascular care in the setting of a pandemic, it is imperative to optimize safety measures in health care facilities to encourage patients to seek immediate care when facing early signs of heart attack and stroke. During high COVID-19 activity periods, patients should be screened and tested for coinfection and appropriate personal protective equipment should be utilized when performing emergency procedures on patients with unknown COVID-19 status.

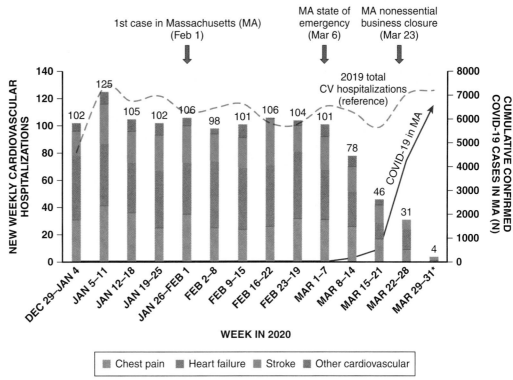

FIGURE 94.6 Decline in non–COVID-19-related cardiovascular hospitalizations during the SARS-CoV-2 pandemic. (From Bhatt AS, et al. Fewer hospitalizations for acute cardiovascular conditions during the COVID-19 pandemic. J Am Coll Cardiol 2020;76(3):280-288.)

MECHANISMS OF COVID-19 CARDIOVASCULAR DISEASE
Direct Effect on Cardiovascular Tissues
SARS-CoV-2 enters cells by binding to the ACE2 receptors in a process that is facilitated by transmembrane serine protease 2 (TMPRSS2). Both ACE2 and TMPRSS2 are present in multiple extrapulmonary tissues and are expressed in high concentrations in vascular tissues.[97] This may explain in part the high affinity of the virus for the circulatory system.[98] The presence of microthrombi in the myocardium parallels the finding of alveolar capillary microthrombi and widespread thrombosis with microangiopathy in pulmonary vessels of COVID-19 patients.[99] Multiple autopsy series have shown the presence of DVT and PE in these patients.[100,101] Major pulmonary and cardiac findings identified on autopsy are listed in Table 94.2. A systemic at review of 41 studies, including 316 autopsy cases, identified a variety of postmortem cardiac manifestations including cardiac dilatation (20%), acute ischemia (8%), intracardiac thrombi (2.5%), pericardial effusion (2.5%), and myocarditis in 1.5% of cases.[102] Direct infection of the myocardial cells with SARS-CoV-2 was extremely rare.

Histopathologic studies of cardiovascular tissues in COVID-19 have been mostly performed in a small series of deceased patients. They are subject to the inherent bias of studying the most severe cases, which likely decreases the findings' generalizability, yet they can provide critical information on the pathogenesis of the disease. SARS-CoV-2 RNA has been identified in a varying fraction of autopsied hearts, and true myocarditis (Fig. 94.7) has been generally rare.[101,103] In a small study of 15 hearts from COVID-19 victims, none revealed true myocarditis, and the virus was detected only in the myocytes of the left atrium of one case (with viral copies much less than lungs).[98] In another study of 104 endomyocardial biopsies performed during peak COID-19 activity in Germany, SARS-CoV-2 RNA was detected only in 5% of cases of clinically suspected myocarditis or new-onset HF.[104] A series of 39 serial autopsies in Germany identified SARS-CoV-2 RNA in 61.5% of cases and no myocarditis.[105] A high viral RNA load was detected in 16 (41%) cases and was associated with a proinflammatory cytokine response but was not associated with increased infiltration of mononuclear cells into the myocardium.[105] Indeed, a series of 40 autopsies in Italy revealed 14 patients with myocyte necrosis (of whom 3 had acute MI and 11 had focal myocyte necrosis).[106] Microthrombi rich in fibrin and terminal complement C5b-9 in myocardial capillaries, arterioles, and small muscular arteries were more common than large

TABLE 94.2 Important Pathology Findings in Autopsies of Subjects with COVID-19

Cardiac Pathology
Cardiomegaly
Cardiac dilation
Lymphocytic epicarditis/pericarditis
Lymphocytic myocarditis
Individual/focal myocyte necrosis
Acute ischemia
Intracardiac thrombi
Intramyocardial microthrombi in capillaries, arterioles, and small arteries
Pericardial effusion
Pulmonary Pathology
Severe endothelial injury
Acute pneumonitis
Interstitial pneumonitis
Interstitial lymphocytic pneumonitis
Incipient interstitial pneumonitis
Diffuse alveolar damage with perivascular T-cell infiltration
Bronchopneumonia with aspiration
Microthrombi in capillaries and small blood vessels
Microangiopathy and intussusceptive angiogenesis
Large pulmonary thromboemboli

epicardial coronary thrombi. This may explain presentations of STEMI in the absence of epicardial coronary obstruction.[107] In contrast with influenza, limited autopsy series have not shown infiltration of atherosclerotic plaques with inflammatory cells and/or plaque rupture after COVID-19.[101]

Cytokine Storm, Hyperinflammatory Response, and Endothelial Disease in COVID-19

Many patients with COVID-19 are asymptomatic or have mild to moderate disease. However, depending on age and comorbidities, up to 10% to 15% may develop severe disease requiring hospitalization, and up to 5% may need care in an ICU.[108] It is still unknown why some patients remain asymptomatic or have mild symptoms and why others progress to severe disease. Age, comorbidities, viral load, immune response, prior exposure (or lack of exposure) to coronaviruses, and inflammatory response play a role in this process.

Inflammation is an integral part of the innate immune response to infection. The inflammatory response begins after exposure to the pathogens and is expected to react proportionally to the pathogen burden and to return to baseline hemostasis after clearance of infectious burden. The balance between producing sufficient cytokines to clear the infection and avoiding hyperinflammation, which could damage the host cells, is pivotal for this process.[109]

SARS-CoV-2 infection triggers a robust systemic inflammatory response that can initiate a "cytokine storm" with a hyperinflammatory state, as evident by overproduction of a wide array of inflammatory mediators including circulating cytokines and chemokines, such as IL-1α, IL-1β, IL-2, IL-7, IL-6, IL-8, IL-10, tumor necrosis factor (TNF), interferon (IFN)-γ, granulocyte colony-stimulating factor (G-CSF), IFN-inducible protein-10 (IP-10), CCL2 (monocyte chemotactic protein [MCP]-1), CCL3 (macrophage inflammatory protein 1 alpha [MIP1α]), CXC-chemokine ligand 10 (CXCL10), C-reactive protein, ferritin, and D-dimers.[110-117] High serum levels of IL-6, IL-8, and TNF-α levels at the time of hospitalization powerfully predict patient survival ($P < 0.0001$, $P = 0.0205$, and $P = 0.0140$, respectively).[110] The cytokine storm likely contributes to the development of ARDS in COVID-19 patients, which has a mortality rate of up to 40% to 50%.[118] The hyperinflammation state of ARDS is characterized by increased proinflammatory cytokines, increased risk of shock, and poor clinical outcomes including multiorgan failure, and death.[116]

Although the term *cytokine storm* does not have an established definition,[118] it refers broadly to a hyperactive immune response characterized by the release of multiple proinflammatory mediators. However, these mediators are also part of our innate immune response and it is often challenging to distinguish a normal immune response from a dysregulated response leading to damage to host cells.[118] The cytokine response in COVID-19 is not universally exaggerated. In fact, a study of critically ill patients with COVID-19 with ARDS showed lower circulating cytokine levels when compared with patients with bacterial sepsis. The exact role of cytokines in the pathogenesis of COVID-19 remains undetermined and is subject of extensive research. At present, multiple clinical studies are under way to examine the potential benefit of targeting multiple inflammatory pathways in controlling COVID-19 and preventing its complications, noticeably ARDS (Fig. 94.8).[119-121]

Neutrophil extracellular trap (NET) formation may play an important role in the pathology of COVID-19. NETs are multimolecular, DNA-based, netlike structures made up of cytosolic and granule proteins and mitochondrial DNA originating from neutrophils in response to infections.[122] They may trap and limit dissemination of bacteria, fungi, and viruses. The inflammatory response in COVID-19 can activate NET formation.[116] Patients with COVID-19 have higher plasma levels of NET markers than healthy controls, and these markers correlate with

FIGURE 94.7 Lymphocytic myocarditis in COVID-19. A, Photomicrograph of lymphocytic myocarditis with myocyte necrosis in the myocardium of a profoundly immunosuppressed COVID-19 decedent. Hematoxylin and eosin-stained section, 400× original magnification. **B,** Photomicrograph of the same field as **(A)** of immunohistochemistry for the nucleocapsid protein of SARS-CoV-2 demonstrating positivity in the dying myocytes, but not in the associated endothelium or inflammatory infiltrate. 400× original magnification. (Images courtesy of Robert Padera, MD, Brigham and Women's Hospital.)

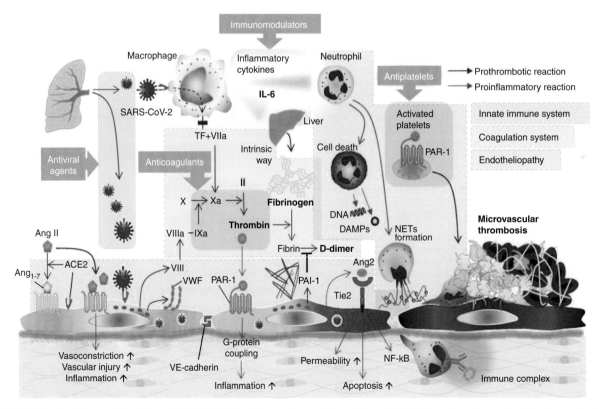

FIGURE 94.8 Pathophysiology of the effect of SARS-CoV-2. (From Connors JM, et al. Thrombosis and COVID-19: controversies and (tentative) conclusions. [published online ahead of print February 4, 2021]. *Clin Infect Dis.* https://doi.org/10.1093/cid/ciab096.)

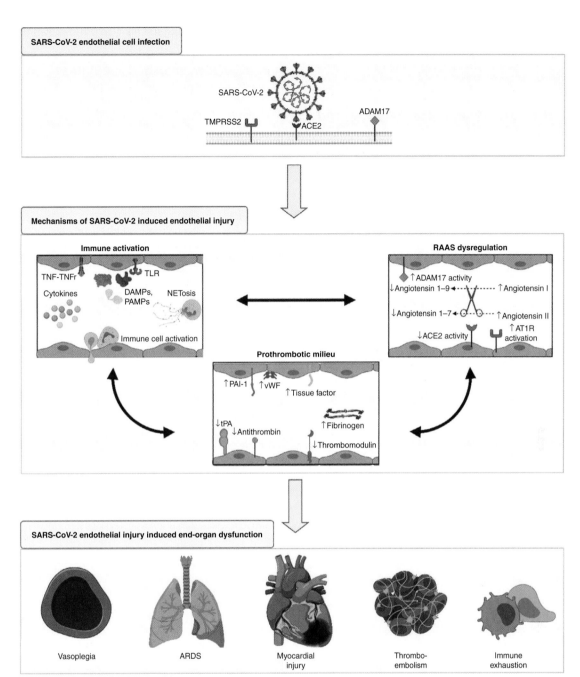

FIGURE 94.9 SARS-CoV-2-induced endothelial injury. Schematic of SARS-CoV-2 infection and proposed resulting endothelial injury, involving immune activation, prothrombotic milieu, and renin-angiotensin-aldosterone system (RAAS) dysregulation. These insults interact with each other to cause end-organ dysfunction that is manifest in many COVID-19 patients. *ADAM17,* A disintegrin and metalloproteinase 17; *ARDS,* acute respiratory distress syndrome; *AT1R,* angiotensin 1 receptor; *DAMPs,* damage-associated molecular patterns; *eNOS,* endothelial nitric oxide; *PAI-1,* plasminogen activator inhibitor-1; *PAMPs,* pathogen-associated molecular patterns; *TLR,* Toll-like receptor; *TMPRSS2,* transmembrane protease serine 2; *TNF,* tumor necrosis factor; *TNFr,* tumor necrosis factor receptor; *tPA,* tissue plasminogen activator; *vWF,* von Willebrand factor. (From Siddiqi HK, et al. COVID-19: a vascular disease. Trends Cardiovasc Med 2021;31:1-5.)

leukocyte numbers, neutrophils, inflammatory cytokines, and in vivo markers of coagulation, fibrinolysis, and endothelial damage. NET formation is associated with an increased risk of requiring respiratory support and worse short-term mortality.[123] A small case series of coronary thrombus samples aspirated during STEMI interventions detected NETs in all 5 patients with COVID-19, whereas it was detected in only 34 of 50 thrombi (68%) retrieved from noninfected controls.[124]

Another small in vitro study showed that neutrophils obtained from COVID-19 patients more readily release NETs compared with neutrophils from healthy individuals. NET production related directly with disease severity and was higher in intubated patients and in those who died later.[125] At autopsy, lungs show neutrophil-platelet accumulation in NET-containing microthrombi. In contrast, NET formation fell during convalescence after COVID-19.[125] SARS-CoV-2 induces a robust immunothrombotic process, which is part of the body's protective response to infections. However, NET formation induces a thrombogenic and cytotoxic environment that can damage epithelial and vascular

integrity and likely contributes to rapid pulmonary dysfunction and other complications.[116,126]

COVID-19 can provoke endothelial dysfunction (Fig. 94.9).[116] The normal endothelium has strong and unique anticoagulant, antithrombotic, vasodilatory, antioxidant, and pro-fibrinolytic properties.[116] (see Chapter 24). The release of proinflammatory cytokines during acute infections affect the endothelial cells and switch their homeostatic functions, leading to loss of many of their protective features.[84,116,127] Normally functioning endothelial cells effectively prevent platelet activation by producing nitric oxide, releasing prostacyclin, and expressing CD39 (an ecto-ADPase).[128] Endothelial dysfunction can cause cells to stop generating prostacyclin and produce thromboxane, which is a potent vasoconstrictor prostaglandin with prothrombotic effects. Endothelial injury can also disrupt the endothelial-dependent vasodilatation through impaired NOS expression and lead to production of endothelin-1, a potent vasoconstrictor.[129]

Moreover, the endothelial cells store von Willebrand factor (vWf) and P-selectin in a preformed state in intracellular granules called

Weibel-Palade bodies. Once activated, they can release vWf, which can facilitate platelet aggregates and thrombosis.[130] Additionally, the expression of TF after endothelial injury can activate the coagulation cascade leading to the well-known increased risk of thrombin generation and clot formation in COVID-19.[127]

Treatment of COVID-19 and COVID-19-Related Complications

The treatment of COVID-19 continues to evolve rapidly as more treatments complete testing in randomized trials.

Antiviral Therapy

Early-stage treatments include antivirals and anti-SARS-CoV-2 monoclonal antibodies. Remdesivir is a nucleoside analog that inhibits the RNA-dependent RNA polymerase, and the only U.S. Food and Drug Administration (FDA)-approved antiviral for the treatment of COVID-19. It is currently recommended for patients hospitalized with moderate COVID-19 who require supplemental oxygen, but benefit is not established in patients who require high-flow oxygen, noninvasive ventilation, or mechanical ventilation. Duration of treatment is 5 days, which may be extended to 10 days in the absence of clinical improvement.[131]

Anti-SARS-CoV-2 Monoclonal Antibodies

The FDA has issued emergency use authorizations (EUA) for several monoclonal antibodies. Bamlanivimab plus etesevimab (administered together) were authorized for the treatment of mild to moderate non-hospitalized COVID-19 in adults and pediatric patients (12 years of age or older weighing at least 40 kg).[132] In addition, the FDA has issued an EUA for casirivimab and imdevimab (administered together) for the treatment of mild to moderate non-hospitalized COVID-19 in adults and pediatric patients (12 years of age or older weighing at least 40 kg).[133] Other monoclonal antibodies are currently in development. Potential cardioprotective effects from anticytokine treatments are not yet determined due to inconsistency in clinical trial results.

Corticosteroid Therapy

Corticosteroids have shown benefit in the subset of patients with moderate COVID-19 who require supplemental oxygen. In the Randomized Evaluation of COVID-19 Therapy trial, dexamethasone (6 mg once daily for up to 10 days) reduced 28-day mortality, but patients who did not require oxygen did not benefit.[134] In the setting of more severe COVID-19, corticosteroids may negate the adverse inflammatory response that can lead to multiorgan failure. In a meta-analysis of 7 RCTs that enrolled 1703 critically ill patients (including those requiring mechanical ventilation) with COVID-19, use of systemic dexamethasone, hydrocortisone, or methylprednisolone resulted in a 34% reduced risk for all-cause mortality at 28 days.[135]

Other Management Considerations
Role of Anticoagulation in COVID-19

Many observational or smaller studies have investigated which patients with COVID-19 might benefit from anticoagulation or antiplatelet therapy at what dose and what stage of disease with varied results. While awaiting sufficiently powered, properly designed and executed blinded randomized trials, many institutions have adopted escalated-dose prophylaxis in all or specific groups of hospitalized patients with COVID-19. Consensus documents have generally recommended following the available evidence-based medicine recommendations to avoid a widespread usage of higher than prophylactic-dose anticoagulation unless used as part of a research study.[136]

In general, the risk of VTE in hospitalized patients peaked earlier in the pandemic but fell later with the adoption of prophylactic anticoagulation. A large study of nationwide population-based Danish registries suggested that the VTE risk in hospitalized COVID-19 patients is low to moderate and is not significantly higher than the VTE risk in hospitalized SARS-CoV-2-negative and influenza patients.[137] The risk of VTE in the postdischarge period and in outpatient COVID-19 cases may be mildly elevated but much less than the risk in acutely ill and hospitalized patients.

Anticoagulation Strategies in COVID-19

The potential benefit from anticoagulation needs to be balanced against the increased risk of bleeding and thrombocytopenia. There has been a clear paucity of high-quality data and a need for randomized clinical trials to assess the appropriate approach to anticoagulation in various COVID-19 patient populations. A few large studies have addressed these questions.

A large, open-label, adaptive, multiplatform, randomized clinical trial tested therapeutic-dose anticoagulation with heparin vs. usual-care pharmacologic thromboprophylaxis in more than 1000 *critically ill* patients with severe COVID-19. This multiplatform study incorporated data from the Randomized, Embedded, Multifactorial Adaptive Platform Trial for Community-Acquired Pneumonia (REMAP-CAP), the Accelerating COVID-19 Therapeutic Interventions and Vaccines-4 Antithrombotics Inpatient platform trial (ACTIV-4a), and the Antithrombotic Therapy to Ameliorate Complications of COVID-19 (ATTACC) trial.[138] In critically ill COVID-19 patients, an initial strategy of therapeutic dose anticoagulation with heparin did not result in a greater likelihood of survival to hospital discharge or a greater number of days free of intensive care unit (ICU)–level cardiovascular or respiratory organ support when compared to usual-care pharmacologic thromboprophylaxis. The usual-care thromboprophylaxis was determined by the local treating physicians and included either standard low-dose thromboprophylaxis or enhanced intermediate-dose thromboprophylaxis. This trial was stopped early due to meeting futility criteria. Major bleeding happened more often in patients assigned to therapeutic anticoagulation than those assigned to pharmacologic thromboprophylaxis. Major bleeding was infrequent.

Another multiplatform trial by the ATTACC, ACTIV-4a, and REMAP-CAP investigators studied the role of therapeutic anticoagulation in *non-critically ill* hospitalized COVID-19 patients.[139] In this open-label, adaptive, randomized controlled trial, more than 2000 non-critically ill patients hospitalized for COVID-19 were randomized to a pragmatic strategy of therapeutic-dose anticoagulation with heparin vs. usual-care pharmacological thromboprophylaxis (determined by the treating physicians per local protocols). An initial strategy of therapeutic-dose anticoagulation with heparin increased the probability of survival to hospital discharge and reduced the need for organ support. This study was stopped early when therapeutic-dose anticoagulation met the pre-specified criteria of superiority for patients on therapeutic-dose anticoagulation irrespective of baseline D-dimer. Major bleeding occurred infrequently.

The Intermediate vs. Standard-Dose Prophylactic Anticoagulation in Critically-Ill Patients With COVID-19: An Open Label Randomized Controlled Trial (INSPIRATION) was a multicenter trial that compared intermediate-dose (enoxaparin, 1 mg/kg daily) vs. standard-dose prophylactic anticoagulation (enoxaparin, 40 mg daily) in 600 adult patients admitted to the ICU with COVID-19.[140] On 30-day follow up, the primary efficacy outcome (a composite of venous or arterial thrombosis, treatment with extracorporeal membrane oxygenation, or mortality) showed no significant difference between the two groups.

Recommendations and living guidelines for prevention, diagnosis, and treatment of VTE are available (and continuously updated) on the websites of the American College of Cardiology (ACC), International Society on Thrombosis and Haemostasis (ISTH), American Society of Hematology (ASH), and American College of Chest Physicians (ACCP).

Angiotensin-Converting Enzyme Inhibitors and Angiotensin Receptor Blockers in the Setting of COVID-19

On discovery that SARS-CoV-2 uses ACE2 for host cell entry, concerns were raised regarding the potential for ACE inhibitors and ARBs to cause compensatory increases in expression of ACE2 and worsen prognosis among those with COVID-19. Observational studies evaluating outcomes associated with use of ACE inhibitors and ARBs among patients with confirmed COVID-19,[141,142] and RCTs comparing continuation or withdrawal of these agents among those hospitalized with COVID-19, showed no adverse effects on survival and other clinical outcomes.[143,144] Thus continuation of ACE inhibitors and ARBs during COVID-19 illness is recommended for patients treated with these medications.

Prevention of COVID-19: Vaccines

The discovery that neutralizing antibodies to SARS-CoV-2 primarily target the receptor binding domain of the S1 protein, also known as the spike protein, led to development of vaccine candidates within a year of release of the virus genome sequence. Several vaccines have been developed using nucleic acid platforms, non-replicating viral vectored platforms, inactivated virus, or recombinant subunit antigens. In the United States, the FDA has approved BNT162b2-mRNA (Pfizer-Bi-oNTech) mRNA COVID-19 vaccine for people 12 years or older (two injections, 21 days apart) and has issued emergency use authorization for mRNA-1273 (Moderna) vaccine for people 18 years or older (two injections, 28 days apart). The Ad26.COV2.S (Johnson & Johnson's Janssen) vaccine utilizes a viral vector platform with a replication-incompetent recombinant adenovirus type 26 (Ad26) vector and has received an EUA for single-dose administration for people 18 years or older. The AZD1222 (Oxford/AstraZeneca) vaccine is a single injection vaccine that utilizes a viral vector platform with modified adenovirus ChAdOx1 and is used extensively outside of the United States. Gam-COVID-Vac (Sputnik V) is a heterologous recombinant adenovirus (rAd)-based vaccine. It uses vectors rAd26 and rAd5 (both carrying the gene for SARS-CoV-2 glycoprotein S) and is given intramuscularly over a 21-day interval. Other promising and widely used vaccines include CoronaVac (by Sinovac Life Sciences), which contains inactivated SARS-CoV-2 virus, BBV152 (by Bharat Biotech International), which contains whole-virion inactivated SARS-CoV-2, and inactivated adjuvanted BBIBP-CorV (by Sinopharm/BBIBP) vaccines. Multiple other vaccines with various mechanisms of action are under development and investigation.

Vaccines have demonstrated efficacy in reducing COVID-19 morbidity and mortality in randomized clinical trials and in real world studies. Their widespread use has led to significant decrease in incident cases of COVID-19.

As of July 2021, the CDC Vaccine Adverse Event Reporting System (VAERS) received over 1100 reports of myocarditis or pericarditis and confirmed about 70% of these, after receipt of COVID-19 vaccination (primarily mRNA vaccines). The European Economic Area (EEA) has also reported myocarditis cases both with mRNA vaccines and with the AstraZeneca vaccine. Cases have been reported predominantly in young adults, more often in men, and usually after the second dose of the vaccine. Myocarditis, detectable by cardiac magnetic resonance, typically occurs within 3 to 5 days after vaccination and presents with chest discomfort, abnormal ECG, and troponin elevation. Although the exact mechanism is unknown, it is likely immune-mediated and eosinophilic myocarditis has been reported with prior vaccines. The possible incidence of asymptomatic cases, risk factors, management, and long-term effects have yet to be determined. Overall, myocarditis after COVID-19 immunization appears to be rare (~ 24 per million second doses), often mild, and likely self-resolving in the majority of cases. Treatment is primarily supportive.[145,146]

Rare cases of severe thrombosis with thrombocytopenia have been reported, primarily with the adenovirus-based vaccines, and have been termed *vaccine-induced immune thrombocytopenia and thrombosis* (VITT).[147,148] This syndrome is characterized by arterial or venous thrombosis, and has been reported in the cerebral sinuses (see Fig. 45.2) and splanchnic vessels, among others, in association with mild to severe thrombocytopenia. The mechanism appears to be similar to heparin-induced thrombocytopenia [HIT], and antibodies to platelet factor 4 (PF4)–polyanion have been identified by enzyme-linked immunosorbent assay (ELISA). Most cases have occurred in women under age 50 without recent exposure to heparin, with a peak time of symptom onset of 6 to 14 days after vaccination; and up to one third of initial cases resulted in death. Treatment is similar to that of HIT, including IVIG or non-heparin anticoagulation, although responses to these treatments is uncertain.

Postacute Sequelae SARS-CoV-2 Infection

Certain patients infected with SARS-CoV-2 continue to have symptoms for weeks to months after seeming recovery from the acute phase of the disease. Early reports suggest that up to 10% of COVID-19 patients may experience the "Long COVID syndrome" or PASC. The PASC symptoms are highly variable in variety, severity, and duration.

Preliminary studies suggest that up to 30% of patients may report symptoms as long as 9 months after acute infection.[149] Most common symptoms include but are not limited to fatigue, a decline in functional capacity and exercise tolerance, shortness of breath, sleeping issues, and palpitations. Some patients describe difficulty thinking clearly ("brain fog"), anxiety, and/or depression. The exact predictors, duration, extent of cardiac (or other organs) involvement, and the potential effects of various treatments for PASC require extensive research that has already started.

REFERENCES
Influenza and Cardiovascular Disease
1. Krammer F, Smith GJD, Fouchier RAM, et al. Influenza. Nat Rev Dis Primers. 2018;4(1):3.
2. Webster RG, Bean WJ, Gorman OT, et al. Evolution and ecology of influenza a viruses. Microbiol Rev. 1992;56(1):152–179.
3. Smith GJ, Vijaykrishna D, Bahl J, et al. Origins and evolutionary genomics of the 2009 swine-origin H1N1 influenza a epidemic. Nature. 2009;459(7250):1122–1125.
4. Cohen SA, Chui KK, Naumova EN. Influenza vaccination in young children reduces influenza-associated hospitalizations in older adults, 2002-2006. J Am Geriatr Soc. 2011;59(2):327–332.
5. Thompson WW, Shay DK, Weintraub E, et al. Influenza-associated hospitalizations in the United States. J Am Med Assoc. 2004;292(11):1333–1340.
6. Smeeth L, Thomas SL, Hall AJ, et al. Risk of myocardial infarction and stroke after acute infection or vaccination. New Engl J Med. 2004;351(25):2611–2618.
7. Warren-Gash C, Smeeth L, Hayward AC. Influenza as a trigger for acute myocardial infarction or death from cardiovascular disease: a systematic review. Lancet Infect Dis. 2009;9(10):601–610.
8. Kwong JC, Schwartz KL, Campitelli MA, et al. Acute myocardial infarction after laboratory-confirmed influenza infection. N Engl J Med. 2018;378(4):345–353.
9. Sandoval C, Walter SD, Krueger P, et al. Risk of hospitalization during influenza season among a cohort of patients with congestive heart failure. Epidemiol Infect. 2007;135(4):574–582.
10. Kytomaa S, Hegde S, Claggett B, et al. Association of influenza-like illness activity with hospitalizations for heart failure: the Atherosclerosis risk in communities study. JAMA Cardiol. 2019;4(4):363–369.
11. Panhwar MS, Kalra A, Gupta T, et al. Effect of influenza on outcomes in patients with heart failure. JACC Heart Fail. 2019;7(2):112–117.
12. Bagai A, McNally BF, Al-Khatib SM, et al. Temporal differences in out-of-hospital cardiac arrest incidence and survival. Circulation. 2013;128(24):2595–2602.
13. Herlitz J, Eek M, Holmberg M, Holmberg S. Diurnal, weekly and seasonal rhythm of out of hospital cardiac arrest in Sweden. Resuscitation. 2002;54(2):133–138.
14. Madjid M, Connolly AT, Nabutovsky Y, et al. Effect of high influenza activity on risk of ventricular arrhythmias requiring therapy in patients with implantable cardiac defibrillators and cardiac resynchronization therapy defibrillators. Am J Cardiol. 2019;124(1):44–50.
15. Muller D, Lampe F, Wegscheider K, et al. Annual distribution of ventricular tachycardias and ventricular fibrillation. Am Heart J. 2003;146(6):1061–1065.
16. Loomba RS. Seasonal variation in paroxysmal atrial fibrillation: a systematic review. J Atr Fibrillation. 2015;7(5):1201.
17. Chang TY, Chao TF, Liu CJ, et al. The association between influenza infection, vaccination, and atrial fibrillation: a nationwide case-control study. Heart Rhythm. 2016;13(6):1189–1194.
18. Sellers SA, Hagan RS, Hayden FG, Fischer 2nd WA. The hidden burden of influenza: a review of the extra-pulmonary complications of influenza infection. Influenza Other Respir Viruses. 2017;11(5):372–393.
19. Haidari M, Wyde PR, Litovsky S, et al. Influenza virus directly infects, inflames, and resides in the arteries of atherosclerotic and normal mice. Atherosclerosis. 2010;208(1):90–96.
20. Naghavi M, Wyde P, Litovsky S, et al. Influenza infection exerts prominent inflammatory and thrombotic effects on the atherosclerotic plaques of apolipoprotein E-deficient mice. Circulation. 2003;107(5):762–768.
21. Lin YH, Platt M, Gilley RP, et al. Influenza causes MLKL-driven cardiac proteome remodeling during convalescence. Circ Res. 2021.
22. Metersky ML, Masterton RG, Lode H, et al. Epidemiology, microbiology, and treatment considerations for bacterial pneumonia complicating influenza. Int J Infect Dis. 2012;16(5): e321–e331.
23. Musher DM, Rueda AM, Kaka AS, Mapara SM. The association between pneumococcal pneumonia and acute cardiac events. Clin Infect Dis. 2007;45(2):158–165.
24. Ng MP, Lee JC, Loke WM, et al. Does influenza a infection increase oxidative damage? Antioxid Redox Signal. 2014;21(7):1025–1031.
25. Madjid M, Aboshady I, Awan I, et al. Influenza and cardiovascular disease: is there a causal relationship? Tex Heart Inst J. 2004;31(1):4–13.

Influenza Prevention and Therapy
26. Corrales-Medina VF, Madjid M, Musher DM. Role of acute infection in triggering acute coronary syndromes. Lancet Infect Dis. 2010;10(2):83–92.
27. Udell JA, Zawi R, Bhatt DL, et al. Association between influenza vaccination and cardiovascular outcomes in high-risk patients: a meta-analysis. J Am Med Assoc. 2013;310(16):1711–1720.
28. Mohseni H, Kiran A, Khorshidi R, Rahimi K. Influenza vaccination and risk of hospitalization in patients with heart failure: a self-controlled case series study. Eur Heart J. 2017;38(5):326–333.
29. Vardeny O, Claggett B, Udell JA, et al. Influenza vaccination in patients with chronic heart failure: the PARADIGM-HF trial. JACC Heart Fail. 2016;4(2):152–158.
30. Modin D, Jorgensen ME, Gislason G, et al. Influenza vaccine in heart failure. Circulation. 2019;139(5):575–586.
31. DiazGranados CA, Dunning AJ, Kimmel M, et al. Efficacy of high-dose versus standard-dose influenza vaccine in older adults. New Engl J Med. 2014;371(7):635–645.
32. DiazGranados CA, Robertson CA, Talbot HK, et al. Prevention of serious events in adults 65 years of age or older: a comparison between high-dose and standard-dose inactivated influenza vaccines. Vaccine. 2015;33(38):4988–4993.
33. Vardeny O, Kim K, Udell JA, et al. Effect of high-dose trivalent vs standard-dose quadrivalent influenza vaccine on mortality or cardiopulmonary hospitalization in patients with high-risk cardiovascular disease: a randomized clinical trial. J Am Med Assoc. 2021;325(1):39–49.

34. Casscells SW, Granger E, Kress AM, et al. Use of oseltamivir after influenza infection is associated with reduced incidence of recurrent adverse cardiovascular outcomes among military health system beneficiaries with prior cardiovascular diseases. *Circ Cardiovasc Qual Outcomes*. 2009;2(2):108–115.
35. Madjid M, Curkendall S, Blumentals WA. The influence of oseltamivir treatment on the risk of stroke after influenza infection. *Cardiology*. 2009;113(2):98–107.

Corona viruses

36. Madjid M, Safavi-Naeini P, Solomon SD, Vardeny O. Potential effects of coronaviruses on the cardiovascular system: a review. *JAMA Cardiol*. 2020.
37. Zhang S-F, Tuo J-L, Huang X-B, et al. Epidemiology characteristics of human coronaviruses in patients with respiratory infection symptoms and phylogenetic analysis of HCoV-OC43 during 2010-2015 in Guangzhou. *PloS One*. 2018;13(1):e0191789-e.
38. Fehr AR, Perlman S. Coronaviruses: an overview of their replication and pathogenesis. *Methods Mol Biol*. 2015;1282:1–23.
39. Li W, Hulswit RJG, Kenney SP, et al. Broad receptor engagement of an emerging global coronavirus may potentiate its diverse cross-species transmissibility. *Proc Nat Acad Sci USA*. 2018;115(22):E5135–E5143.
40. Chen N, Zhou M, Dong X, et al. Epidemiological and clinical characteristics of 99 cases of 2019 novel coronavirus pneumonia in Wuhan, China: a descriptive study. *Lancet*. 2020.
41. Berry M, Gamieldien J, Fielding BC. Identification of new respiratory viruses in the new millennium. *Viruses*. 2015;7(3):996–1019.
42. Li F. Structure, function, and evolution of coronavirus spike proteins. *Ann Review Virol*. 2016;3(1):237–261.
43. Su S, Wong G, Shi W, et al. Epidemiology, genetic recombination, and pathogenesis of coronaviruses. *Trends Microbiol*. 2016;24(6):490–502.
44. Peiris JS, Chu CM, Cheng VC, et al. Clinical progression and viral load in a community outbreak of coronavirus-associated SARS pneumonia: a prospective study. *Lancet*. 2003;361(9371):1767–1772.
45. Chong PY, Chui P, Ling AE, et al. Analysis of deaths during the Severe Acute Respiratory Syndrome (SARS) epidemic in Singapore: challenges in determining a SARS diagnosis. *Arch Pathol Lab Med*. 2004;128(2):195–204.
46. Yu CM, Wong RS, Wu EB, et al. Cardiovascular complications of severe acute respiratory syndrome. *Postgrad Med J*. 2006;82(964):140–144.
47. Mohd HA, Al-Tawfiq JA, Memish ZA. Middle East Respiratory Syndrome Coronavirus (MERS-CoV) origin and animal reservoir. *Virol J*. 2016;13(1):87. https://doi.org/10.1186/s12985-016-0544-0.
48. Mackay IM, Arden KE. MERS coronavirus: diagnostics, epidemiology and transmission. *Virol J*. 2015;12(1):222. https://doi.org/10.1186/s12985-015-0439-5.
49. Oh MD, Park WB, Park SW, et al. Middle East respiratory syndrome: what we learned from the 2015 outbreak in the Republic of Korea. *Korean J Intern Med*. 2018;33(2):233–246.
50. Badawi A, Ryoo SG. Prevalence of comorbidities in the Middle East Respiratory Syndrome Coronavirus (MERS-CoV): a systematic review and meta-analysis. *Int J Infect Dis*. 2016;49:129–133.

SARS-CoV-2 and COVID-19

51. Hu B, Guo H, Zhou P, Shi ZL. Characteristics of SARS-CoV-2 and COVID-19. *Nat Rev Microbiol*. 2020.
52. The Lancet Respiratory M. COVID-19 transmission-up in the air. *Lancet Respir Med*. 2020;8(12):1159.
53. Hindson J. COVID-19: faecal-oral transmission? *Nat Rev Gastroenterol Hepatol*. 2020;17(5):259.
54. Zou L, Ruan F, Huang M, et al. SARS-CoV-2 viral load in upper respiratory specimens of infected patients. *N Engl J Med*. 2020.
55. Yeo C, Kaushal S, Yeo D. Enteric involvement of coronaviruses: is faecal–oral transmission of SARS-CoV-2 possible? *Lancet Gastroenterol Hepatol*. 2020;5(4):335–337.
56. Holshue ML, DeBolt C, Lindquist S, et al. First case of 2019 novel coronavirus in the United States. *N Engl J Med*. 2020. https://doi.org/10.1056/NEJMoa2001191.
57. Mascola JR, Graham BS, Fauci AS. SARS-CoV-2 viral variants-tackling a moving target. *J Am Med Assoc*. 2021.
57a. Konings F, Perkins MD, Kuhn JH, et al. SARS-CoV-2 variants of interest and concern naming scheme conducive for global discourse. *Nat Microbiol*. 2021;6:821–823.
58. Schiffrin EL, Flack JM, Ito S, et al. Hypertension and COVID-19. *Am J Hypertens*. 2020;33(5):373–374.
59. Hendren NS, de Lemos JA, Ayers C, et al. Association of body mass index and age with morbidity and mortality in patients hospitalized with COVID-19: results from the American Heart Association COVID-19 cardiovascular disease registry. *Circulation*. 2021;143(2):135–144.
60. Al-Benna S. Association of high level gene expression of ACE2 in adipose tissue with mortality of COVID-19 infection in obese patients. *Obes Med*. 2020;19:100283.
61. Rentsch CT, Kidwai-Khan F, Tate JP, et al. Patterns of COVID-19 testing and mortality by race and ethnicity among United States veterans: a nationwide cohort study. *PLoS Med*. 2020;17(9):e1003379.
62. Gross CP, Essien UR, Pasha S, et al. Racial and ethnic disparities in population-level Covid-19 mortality. *J Gen Intern Med*. 2020;35(10):3097–3099.
63. Price-Haywood EG, Burton J, Fort D, Seoane L. Hospitalization and mortality among Black patients and white patients with Covid-19. *New Engl J Med*. 2020;382(26):2534–2543.
64. Selden TM, Berdahl TA. COVID-19 and racial/ethnic disparities in health risk, employment, and household composition. *Health Aff*. 2020;39(9):1624–1632.

Cardiovascular Complications of COVID-19

65. Choudry FA, Hamshere SM, Rathod KS, et al. High thrombus burden in patients with COVID-19 presenting with ST-segment elevation myocardial infarction. *J Am Coll Cardiol*. 2020;76(10):1168–1176.
66. Modin D, Claggett B, Sindet-Pedersen C, et al. Acute COVID-19 and the incidence of ischemic stroke and acute myocardial infarction. *Circulation*. 2020;142(21):2080–2082.
67. Sala S, Peretto G, Gramegna M, et al. Acute myocarditis presenting as a reverse Tako-Tsubo syndrome in a patient with SARS-CoV-2 respiratory infection. *Eur Heart J*. 2020;41(19):1861–1862.
68. Rey JR, Caro-Codón J, Rosillo SO, et al. Heart failure in COVID-19 patients: prevalence, incidence and prognostic implications. *Eur J Heart Fail*. 2020;22(12):2205–2215.
69. Bhatt AS, Jering KS, Vaduganathan M, et al. Clinical outcomes in patients with heart failure hospitalized with COVID-19. *JACC Heart Fail*. 2021;9(1):65–73.
70. Dherange P, Lang J, Qian P, et al. Arrhythmias and COVID-19: a review. *JACC Clin Electrophysiol*. 2020;6(9):1193–1204.
71. Gopinathannair R, Merchant FM, Lakkireddy DR, et al. COVID-19 and cardiac arrhythmias: a global perspective on arrhythmia characteristics and management strategies. *J Interv Card Electrophysiol*. 2020;59(2):329–336.
72. Baldi E, Sechi GM, Mare C, et al. Out-of-Hospital cardiac arrest during the Covid-19 outbreak in Italy. *N Engl J Med*. 2020;383(5):496–498.
73. Goyal P, Choi JJ, Pinheiro LC, et al. Clinical characteristics of Covid-19 in New York city. *N Engl J Med*. 2020;382(24):2372–2374.
74. Bhatla A, Mayer MM, Adusumalli S, et al. COVID-19 and cardiac arrhythmias. *Heart Rhythm*. 2020;17(9):1439–1444.
75. Musikantow DR, Turagam MK, Sartori S, et al. Atrial fibrillation in patients hospitalized with COVID-19: incidence, predictors, outcomes and comparison to influenza. *JACC: Clinical Electrophysiology*. 2021.
76. Suh YJ, Hong H, Ohana M, Bompard F, et al. Pulmonary embolism and deep vein thrombosis in COVID-19: a systematic review and meta-analysis. *Radiology*. 2021;298(2):E70–E80.
77. Bilaloglu S, Aphinyanaphongs Y, Jones S, et al. Thrombosis in hospitalized patients with COVID-19 in a New York city health system. *J Am Med Assoc*. 2020;324(8):799–801.
78. Whittaker E, Bamford A, Kenny J, et al. Clinical characteristics of 58 children with a pediatric inflammatory multisystem syndrome temporally associated with SARS-CoV-2. *J Am Med Assoc*. 2020;324(3):259–269.
79. Valverde I, Singh Y, Sanchez-de-Toledo J, et al. Acute cardiovascular manifestations in 286 children with multisystem inflammatory syndrome associated with COVID-19 infection in Europe. *Circulation*. 2021;143(1):21–32.
80. Feldstein LR, Tenforde MW, Friedman KG, et al. Characteristics and outcomes of US children and adolescents with Multisystem Inflammatory Syndrome in Children (MIS-C) compared with severe acute COVID-19. *J Am Med Assoc*. 2021;325(11):1074–1087.
81. Lala A, Johnson KW, Januzzi JL, et al. Prevalence and impact of myocardial injury in patients hospitalized with COVID-19 infection. *J Am Coll Cardiol*. 2020;76(5):533–546.
82. Sandoval Y, Januzzi Jr JL, Jaffe AS. Cardiac troponin for the diagnosis and risk-stratification of myocardial injury in COVID-19: JACC review topic of the week. *J Am Coll Cardiol*. 2020. https://doi.org/10.1016/j.jacc.2020.06.068.
83. Kong N, Singh N, Mazzone S, et al. Takotsubo's syndrome presenting as cardiogenic shock in patients with COVID-19: a case-series and review of current literature. *Cardiovasc Revasc Med*. 2021.
84. Libby P. The heart in COVID-19: primary target or secondary bystander? *JACC Basic Transl Sci*. 2020;5(5):537–542.
85. Guo T, Fan Y, Chen M, et al. Cardiovascular implications of fatal outcomes of patients with Coronavirus Disease 2019 (COVID-19). *JAMA Cardiol*. 2020;5(7):811–818.
86. Shi S, Qin M, Shen B, et al. Association of cardiac injury with mortality in hospitalized patients with COVID-19 in Wuhan, China. *JAMA Cardiol*. 2020.
87. Lombardi CM, Carubelli V, Iorio A, et al. Association of troponin levels with mortality in Italian patients hospitalized with coronavirus disease 2019: results of a multicenter study. *JAMA Cardiol*. 2020;5(11):1274–1280.
88. Short SAP, Gupta S, Brenner SK, et al. D-dimer and death in critically ill patients with coronavirus disease 2019. *Crit Care Med*. 2021.
89. Szekely Y, Lichter Y, Taieb P, et al. Spectrum of cardiac manifestations in COVID-19: a systematic echocardiographic study. *Circulation*. 2020;142(4):342–353.
90. Puntmann VO, Carerj ML, Wieters I, et al. Outcomes of cardiovascular magnetic resonance imaging in patients recently recovered from Coronavirus Disease 2019 (COVID-19). *JAMA Cardiol*. 2020;5(11):1265–1273.
91. Garcia S, Albaghdadi MS, Meraj PM, et al. Reduction in ST-segment elevation cardiac catheterization laboratory activations in the United States during COVID-19 pandemic. *J Am Coll Cardiol*. 2020;75(22):2871–2872.
92. Solomon MD, McNulty EJ, Rana JS, et al. The Covid-19 pandemic and the incidence of acute myocardial infarction. *N Engl J Med*. 2020;383(7):691–693.
93. De Filippo O, D'Ascenzo F, Angelini F, et al. Reduced rate of hospital admissions for ACS during Covid-19 outbreak in northern Italy. *N Engl J Med*. 2020;383(1):88–89.
94. Mafham MM, Spata E, Goldacre R, et al. COVID-19 pandemic and admission rates for and management of acute coronary syndromes in England. *Lancet*. 2020;396(10248):381–389.
95. Campo G, Fortuna D, Berti E, et al. In- and out-of-hospital mortality for myocardial infarction during the first wave of the COVID-19 pandemic in Emilia-Romagna, Italy: a population-based observational study. *The Lancet Regional Health - Europe*. 221;3(100055).
96. Srivastava PK, Zhang S, Xian Y, et al. Acute ischemic stroke in patients with COVID-19: an analysis from get with the guidelines-stroke. *Stroke*. 2021;52(5):1826–1829.
97. Giustino G, Pinney SP, Lala A, et al. Coronavirus and cardiovascular disease, myocardial injury, and arrhythmia: JACC focus seminar. *J Am Coll Cardiol*. 2020;76(17):2011–2023.
98. Sakamoto A, Kawakami R, Kawai K, et al. ACE2 (Angiotensin-Converting Enzyme 2) and TMPRSS2 (Transmembrane Serine Protease 2) expression and localization of SARS-CoV-2 infection in the human heart. *Arterioscler Thromb Vasc Biol*. 2021;41(1):542–544.
99. Ackermann M, Verleden SE, Kuehnel M, et al. Pulmonary vascular endothelialitis, thrombosis, and angiogenesis in Covid-19. *N Engl J Med*. 2020;383(2):120–128.
100. Wichmann D, Sperhake JP, Lutgehetmann M, et al. Autopsy findings and venous thromboembolism in patients with COVID-19: a prospective cohort study. *Ann Intern Med*. 2020;173(4):268–277.
101. Buja LM, Wolf DA, Zhao B, et al. The emerging spectrum of cardiopulmonary pathology of the coronavirus disease 2019 (COVID-19): report of 3 autopsies from Houston, Texas, and review of autopsy findings from other United States cities. *Cardiovasc Pathol*. 2020;48:107233.
102. Roshdy A, Zaher S, Fayed H, Coghlan JG. COVID-19 and the heart: a systematic review of cardiac autopsies. *Front Cardiovasc Med*. 2021;7:626975.
103. Halushka MK, Vander Heide RS. Myocarditis is rare in COVID-19 autopsies: cardiovascular findings across 277 postmortem examinations. *Cardiovasc Pathol*. 2021;50:107300.
104. Escher F, Pietsch H, Aleshcheva G, et al. Detection of viral SARS-CoV-2 genomes and histopathological changes in endomyocardial biopsies. *ESC Heart Fail*. 2020;7(5):2440–2447.
105. Lindner D, Fitzek A, Bräuninger H, et al. Association of cardiac infection with SARS-CoV-2 in confirmed COVID-19 autopsy cases. *JAMA Cardiol*. 2020;5(11):1281–1285.
106. Pellegrini D, Kawakami R, Guagliumi G, et al. Microthrombi as a major cause of cardiac injury in COVID-19: a pathologic study. *Circulation*. 2021.
107. Guagliumi G, Sonzogni A, Pescetelli I, et al. Microthrombi and ST-segment-elevation myocardial infarction in COVID-19. *Circulation*. 2020;142(8):804–809.
108. Guan WJ, Ni ZY, Hu Y, et al. Clinical characteristics of coronavirus disease 2019 in China. *New Eng J Med*. 2020;58(4):711–712.
109. Fajgenbaum DC, June CH. Cytokine storm. *N Engl J Med*. 2020;383(23):2255–2273.
110. Del Valle DM, Kim-Schulze S, Huang HH, et al. An inflammatory cytokine signature predicts COVID-19 severity and survival. *Nat Med*. 2020;26(10):1636–1643.
111. Xu ZS, Shu T, Kang L, et al. Temporal profiling of plasma cytokines, chemokines and growth factors from mild, severe and fatal COVID-19 patients. *Signal Transduct Target Ther*. 2020;5(1):100.
112. Chen Y, Wang J, Liu C, et al. IP-10 and MCP-1 as biomarkers associated with disease severity of COVID-19. *Mol Med*. 2020;26(1):97.
113. Zizzo G, Cohen PL. Imperfect storm: is interleukin-33 the Achilles heel of COVID-19? *Lancet Rheumatol*. 2020;2(12):e779–e790.
114. Ye Q, Wang B, Mao J. The pathogenesis and treatment of the 'Cytokine Storm' in COVID-19. *J Infect*. 2020;80(6):607–613.
115. Hojyo S, Uchida M, Tanaka K, et al. How COVID-19 induces cytokine storm with high mortality. *Inflamm Regen*. 2020;40:37.
116. Libby P, Luscher T. COVID-19 is, in the end, an endothelial disease. *Eur Heart J*. 2020;41(32):3038–3044.
117. Mehta P, Porter JC, Manson JJ, et al. Therapeutic blockade of granulocyte macrophage colony-stimulating factor in COVID-19-associated hyperinflammation: challenges and opportunities. *Lancet Respir Med*. 2020;8(8):822–830.
118. Sinha P, Matthay MA, Calfee CS. Is a "cytokine storm" relevant to COVID-19? *JAMA Intern Med*. 2020;180(9):1152–1154.
119. Tang L, Yin Z, Hu Y, Mei H. Controlling cytokine storm is vital in COVID-19. *Front Immunol*. 2020;11:570993.
120. Quirch M, Lee J, Rehman S. Hazards of the cytokine storm and cytokine-targeted therapy in patients with COVID-19: review. *J Med Internet Res*. 2020;22(8):e20193.

121. Cron RQ, Schulert GS, Tattersall RS. Defining the scourge of COVID-19 hyperinflammatory syndrome. *Lancet Rheumatol*. 2020;2(12):e727–e729.
122. Brinkmann V, Reichard U, Goosmann C, et al. Neutrophil extracellular traps kill bacteria. *Science*. 2004;303(5663):1532–1535.
123. Ng H, Havervall S, Rosell A, et al. Circulating markers of neutrophil extracellular traps are of prognostic value in patients with COVID-19. *Arterioscler Thromb Vasc Biol*. 2020: ATVBAHA120315267.
124. Blasco A, Coronado M-J, Hernández-Terciado F, et al. Assessment of neutrophil extracellular traps in coronary thrombus of a case series of patients with COVID-19 and myocardial infarction. *JAMA Cardiol*. 2020;6(4):1–6.
125. Middleton EA, He X-Y, Denorme F, et al. Neutrophil extracellular traps contribute to immunothrombosis in COVID-19 acute respiratory distress syndrome. *Blood*. 2020;136(10):1169–1179.
126. Hidalgo A.A NET-thrombosis axis in COVID-19. *Blood*. 2020;136(10):1118–1119.
127. Folco EJ, Mawson TL, Vromman A, et al. Neutrophil extracellular traps induce endothelial cell activation and tissue factor production through interleukin-1alpha and cathepsin G. *Arterioscler Thromb Vasc Biol*. 2018;38(8):1901–1912.
128. Marcus AJ, Broekman MJ, Drosopoulos JH, et al. The endothelial cell ecto-ADPase responsible for inhibition of platelet function is CD39. *J Clin Invest*. 1997;99(6):1351–1360.
129. Gupta RM, Libby P, Barton M. Linking regulation of nitric oxide to endothelin-1: the Yin and Yang of vascular tone in the atherosclerotic plaque. *Atherosclerosis*. 2020;292:201–203.
130. Wagner DD. The Weibel-Palade body: the storage granule for von Willebrand factor and P-selectin. *Thromb Haemost*. 1993;70(1):105–110.

Management of COVID-19

131. Goldman JD, Lye DCB, Hui DS, et al. Remdesivir for 5 or 10 Days in patients with severe Covid-19. *New Engl J Med*. 2020;383(19):1827–1837.
132. Gottlieb RL, Nirula A, Chen P, et al. Effect of bamlanivimab as monotherapy or in combination with etesevimab on viral load in patients with mild to moderate COVID-19: a randomized clinical trial. *J Am Med Assoc*. 2021;325(7):632–644.
133. Weinreich DM, Sivapalasingam S, Norton T, et al. REGN-COV2, a neutralizing antibody cocktail, in outpatients with Covid-19. *New Engl J Med*. 2020;384(3):238–251.
134. RECOVERY Collaborative Group, Horby P, Lim WS, et al. Dexamethasone in hospitalized patients with Covid-19. *New Engl J Med*. 2021;384(8):693–704.
135. Sterne JAC, Diaz J, Villar J, et al. Corticosteroid therapy for critically ill patients with COVID-19: a structured summary of a study protocol for a prospective meta-analysis of randomized trials. *Trials*. 2020;21(1):734.
136. Moores LK, Tritschler T, Brosnahan S, et al. Prevention, diagnosis, and treatment of VTE in patients with coronavirus disease 2019: CHEST guideline and expert panel report. *Chest*. 2020;158(3):1143–1163.
137. Dalager-Pedersen M, Lund LC, Mariager T, et al. Venous thromboembolism and major bleeding in patients with COVID-19: a nationwide population-based cohort study. [published online ahead of print January 5, 2021]. *Clin Infect Dis*. https://doi.org/10.1093/cid/ciab003
138. The REMAP-CAP, ACTIV-4a, and ATTACC Investigators. Therapeutic anticoagulation with heparin in critically ill patients with Covid-19. *N Engl J Med*. https://doi.org/10.1056/NEJMoa2103417.
139. The ATTACC, ACTIV-4a, and REMAP-CAP Investigators. Therapeutic anticoagulation with heparin in noncritically ill patients with Covid-19. *N Engl J Med*. https://doi.org/10.1056/NEJMoa2105911.
140. INSPIRATION Investigators, Sadeghipour P, Talasaz AH, Rashidi F, et al. Effect of intermediate-dose vs standard-dose prophylactic anticoagulation on thrombotic events, extracorporeal membrane oxygenation treatment, or mortality among patients with COVID-19 admitted to the intensive care unit: The INSPIRATION randomized clinical trial. *JAMA*. 2021;325(16):1620–1630.
141. Reynolds HR, Adhikari S, Pulgarin C, et al. Renin-angiotensin-aldosterone system inhibitors and risk of Covid-19. *New Engl J Med*. 2020;382(25):2441–2448.
142. Mancia G, Rea F, Ludergnani M, et al. Renin-angiotensin-aldosterone system blockers and the risk of Covid-19. *New Engl J Med*. 2020;382(25):2431–2440.
143. Lopes RD, Macedo AVS, de Barros ESPGM, et al. Effect of discontinuing vs continuing angiotensin-converting enzyme inhibitors and angiotensin II receptor blockers on days alive and out of the hospital in patients admitted with COVID-19: a randomized clinical trial. *J Am Med Assoc*. 2021;325(3):254–264.
144. Cohen JB, Hanff TC, William P, et al. Continuation versus discontinuation of renin-angiotensin system inhibitors in patients admitted to hospital with COVID-19: a prospective, randomised, open-label trial. *Lancet Respir Med*. 2021;9(3):275–284.
145. Diaz GA, Parsons GT, Gering SK, et al. Myocarditis and pericarditis after vaccination for COVID-19. *JAMA*. 2021 Aug 4:e2113443.
146. Montgomery J, Ryan M, Engler R, et al. Myocarditis following immunization with mRNA COVID-19 vaccines in members of the US military. *JAMA Cardiol*. Published online June 29, 2021. https://doi.org/10.1001/jamacardio.2021.2833.
147. Pavord S, Scully M, Hunt BJ, et al. Clinical features of vaccine-induced immune thrombocytopenia and thrombosis. *N Engl J Med*. 2021. https://doi.org/10.1056/NEJMoa2109908. Epub ahead of print. PMID: 34379914.
148. Rizk JG, Gupta A, Sardar P, et al. Clinical characteristics and pharmacological management of COVID-19 vaccine-induced immune thrombotic thrombocytopenia with cerebral venous sinus thrombosis: a review. *JAMA Cardiol*. 2021. https://doi.org/10.1001/jamacardio.2021.3444. Epub ahead of print. PMID: 34374713.
149. Logue JK, Franko NM, McCulloch DJ, et al. Sequelae in adults at 6 months after COVID-19 infection. *JAMA Network Open*. 2021;4(2):e210830-e.

95 Hemostasis, Thrombosis, Fibrinolysis, and Cardiovascular Disease

JEFFREY I. WEITZ

Hemostasis preserves vascular integrity by balancing the physiologic processes that maintain blood fluidity under normal circumstances and prevent excessive bleeding after vascular injury. Preservation of blood fluidity depends on an intact vascular endothelium and a complex series of regulatory pathways that maintain platelets in a quiescent state and keep the coagulation system in check. In contrast, arrest of bleeding requires rapid formation of hemostatic plugs at sites of vascular injury to prevent exsanguination. Perturbation of hemostasis can lead to thrombosis, which can occur in arteries or veins and causes considerable morbidity and mortality. Arterial thrombosis is the most common cause of acute coronary syndrome, ischemic stroke, and limb gangrene, whereas thrombosis in the deep veins of the leg leads to postthrombotic syndrome and pulmonary embolism (see also Chapter 87).

Most arterial thrombi form on top of disrupted atherosclerotic plaques because plaque rupture exposes thrombogenic material in the core to blood (see also Chapters 24 and 37). This material then triggers platelet aggregation and fibrin formation, which results in the generation of a platelet-rich thrombus that temporarily or permanently occludes blood flow.[1] The consequent reduction in blood flow can cause acute coronary syndrome, transient ischemic attack, ischemic stroke, or acute limb ischemia.

In contrast to arterial thrombi, venous thrombi rarely form at sites of obvious vascular disruption.[2] Although venous thrombi can develop after surgical trauma to veins or arise due to indwelling venous catheters, they usually originate in valve cusps of the deep veins of the calf or in muscular sinuses, where there is stasis. Sluggish blood flow in these veins reduces oxygen supply to the avascular valve cusps. Hypoxemia induces endothelial cells lining the valve cusps to express adhesion molecules, which tether tissue factor–bearing leukocytes and microparticles onto their surface. The tissue factor then induces coagulation.[3] In addition, webs of chromatin released from activated neutrophils, called neutrophil extracellular traps (NETs), also contribute to thrombosis by providing a scaffold that binds platelets and promotes their activation and aggregation and by activating the contact system of coagulation.[4] Impaired blood flow exacerbates local thrombus formation by reducing clearance of activated clotting factors. Thrombi that extend into the proximal veins of the leg can dislodge and travel to the lungs to produce pulmonary embolism.

Arterial and venous thrombi contain platelets and fibrin, but the proportions differ. Arterial thrombi are rich in platelets because of high shear in the injured arteries.[1] In contrast, venous thrombi, which form under low-shear conditions, contain relatively few platelets and consist mostly of fibrin and trapped red cells.[2] Because of the predominance of platelets, arterial thrombi appear white, whereas venous thrombi appear red because of the trapped red cells.

The antithrombotic drugs used for prevention and treatment of thrombosis target components of thrombi and include antiplatelet drugs, which inhibit platelets; anticoagulants, which attenuate

coagulation; and fibrinolytic agents, which induce fibrin degradation (Fig. 95.1). With the predominance of platelets in arterial thrombi, strategies to inhibit or treat arterial thrombosis focus mainly on antiplatelet agents, although in the acute setting, anticoagulants and fibrinolytic agents may also be used. For occlusive arterial thrombi that require rapid restoration of blood flow, mechanical and/or pharmacologic methods enable thrombus extraction, compression, or degradation. Although rarely used for this indication, warfarin prevents recurrent ischemic events after acute myocardial infarction. The observations that the addition of low-dose rivaroxaban, an oral factor Xa inhibitor, to dual-antiplatelet therapy reduces recurrent ischemic events and stent thrombosis in patients with acute coronary syndrome, whereas its addition to aspirin reduces the risk of major adverse coronary and limb events in patients with stable coronary or peripheral artery disease, highlight the potential usefulness of anticoagulants on top of antiplatelet agents for secondary prevention (see also Chapters 40 and 43).[5,6]

Anticoagulants are the mainstay for prevention and treatment of venous thromboembolism (VTE), which includes deep vein thrombosis and pulmonary embolism.[2] Antiplatelet drugs are less effective than anticoagulants for prevention of venous thrombosis because of the limited platelet content of venous thrombi. Nonetheless, when given for secondary prevention, aspirin produces about a 30% reduction in risk for recurrent VTE,[7] a finding that highlights the overlap between venous and arterial thrombosis. Selected patients with VTE benefit from fibrinolytic therapy[2]; for example, patients with massive pulmonary embolism achieve more rapid restoration of pulmonary blood flow with systemic or catheter-directed fibrinolytic therapy than with anticoagulant therapy alone (see Chapter 87). Similarly, some patients with extensive iliac and/or femoral vein thrombosis may have a better outcome with catheter-directed fibrinolytic therapy and/or mechanical thrombus extraction in addition to anticoagulants.

This chapter reviews hemostasis and thrombosis and highlights the processes involved in platelet activation and aggregation, blood coagulation, and fibrinolysis. It reviews the major components of the hemostatic system: the vascular endothelium, platelets, and coagulation and fibrinolytic systems. The chapter then focuses on antiplatelet, anticoagulant, and fibrinolytic drugs in common use. It also provides a brief overview of new antithrombotic drugs in advanced stages of development.

HEMOSTATIC SYSTEM

Vascular Endothelium (see also Chapter 24)

A monolayer of endothelial cells lines the intimal surface of the circulatory tree and separates blood from the prothrombotic subendothelial components of the vessel wall. Accordingly, the vascular endothelium encompasses about 10^{13} cells and covers a vast surface area. Rather

Additional content is available online at Elsevier eBooks for Practicing Clinicians

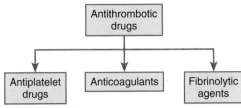

FIGURE 95.1 Classification of antithrombotic drugs.

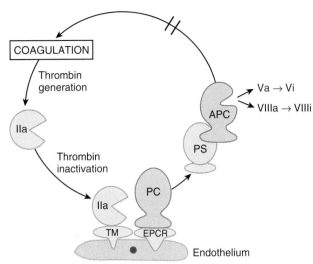

FIGURE 95.2 Protein C pathway. Activation of coagulation triggers thrombin (IIa) generation. Excess thrombin binds to thrombomodulin (TM) on the endothelial cell surface. Once bound, the substrate specificity of thrombin is altered such that it no longer acts as a procoagulant but becomes a potent activator of protein C (PC). The endothelial cell protein C receptor (EPCR) binds protein C and presents it to thrombomodulin-bound thrombin for activation. Activated protein C (APC), together with its cofactor protein S (PS), binds to the activated platelet surface and proteolytically degrades factors Va and VIIIa into inactive fragments (Vi and VIIIi). Degradation of these activated cofactors inhibits thrombin generation (double bar).

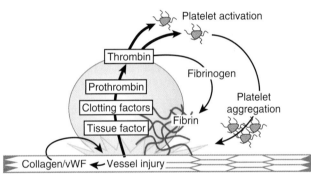

FIGURE 95.3 Central role of thrombin in thrombogenesis. Vascular injury simultaneously triggers platelet adhesion and activation, as well as activation of the coagulation system. Platelet activation is initiated by exposure of subendothelial collagen and von Willebrand factor (vWF), onto which platelets adhere. Adherent platelets become activated and release ADP and thromboxane A$_2$, platelet agonists that activate ambient platelets and recruit them to the site of injury. Coagulation, which is triggered by tissue factor exposed at the site of injury and enhanced by assembly of clotting factor complexes on the activated platelet surface, results in thrombin generation. Thrombin not only converts fibrinogen to fibrin but also serves as a potent platelet agonist. When platelets are activated, glycoprotein (GP) IIb/IIIa on their surfaces undergoes a conformational change that endows it with the capacity to ligate fibrinogen and mediate platelet aggregation. Fibrin strands then weave the platelet aggregates together to form a platelet/fibrin thrombus.

than serving as a static barrier, healthy vascular endothelium dynamically regulates hemostasis by inhibiting platelets, suppressing coagulation, and promoting fibrinolysis.

Platelet Inhibition

Endothelial cells synthesize prostacyclin and nitric oxide and release them into blood. These mediators not only serve to potently vasodilate but also inhibit platelet activation and subsequent aggregation by stimulating adenylate cyclase and increasing intracellular levels of cyclic adenosine monophosphate (cAMP). In addition, endothelial cells express the ecto-adenosine diphosphatase (ecto-ADPase) CD39 on their surface. This membrane-associated enzyme attenuates platelet activation by degrading ADP.[8]

Anticoagulant Activity

Intact endothelial cells actively regulate thrombin generation. Endothelial cells express heparan sulfate proteoglycans on their surface. Like medicinal heparin, heparan sulfate binds circulating antithrombin and enhances its activity. Heparan sulfate proteoglycans also bind tissue factor pathway inhibitor (TFPI), a naturally occurring inhibitor of coagulation.[9] Additional TFPI becomes tethered to the endothelial cell surface via glycosylphosphatidylinositol anchors. Administration of heparin or low-molecular-weight heparin (LMWH) displaces glycosaminoglycan-bound TFPI from the vascular endothelium, and the released TFPI may contribute to the antithrombotic activity of these drugs by inhibiting tissue factor–bound factor VIIa in a factor Xa–dependent manner.

Endothelial cells are central to the protein C anticoagulant pathway because they express thrombomodulin and endothelial cell protein C receptor (EPCR) on their surfaces.[10] The protein C pathway is initiated when thrombin binds to thrombomodulin. Once bound, the substrate specificity of thrombin is altered such that it no longer acts as a procoagulant but becomes a potent activator of protein C (Fig. 95.2). Activated protein C serves as an anticoagulant by degrading and inactivating activated factor V and factor VIII (factors Va and VIIIa, respectively), key cofactors involved in thrombin generation, in reactions enhanced by protein S. EPCR on the endothelial cell surface promotes this pathway about 20-fold by binding protein C and presenting it to the thrombin-thrombomodulin complex for activation. In addition to its role as an anticoagulant, activated protein C also regulates inflammation and preserves the barrier function of the endothelium.[10]

Fibrinolytic Activity

The vascular endothelium modulates fibrinolysis by synthesizing and releasing tissue and urokinase plasminogen activators (t-PA and u-PA, respectively), which initiate fibrinolysis by converting plasminogen to plasmin.[11] Whereas endothelial cells constitutively express t-PA, they produce u-PA in the settings of inflammation and wound repair. Endothelial cells also produce type 1 plasminogen activator inhibitor (PAI-1), the major regulator of both t-PA and u-PA. Therefore, net fibrinolytic activity depends on the dynamic balance between the release of plasminogen activators and PAI-1. Fibrinolysis localizes to the endothelial cell surface because these cells express annexin II, a coreceptor for plasminogen and t-PA that promotes their interaction. Hence, healthy vessels actively resist thrombosis and help maintain platelets in a quiescent state.[11]

Platelets

Platelets enter the circulation after the fragmentation of bone marrow megakaryocytes. Because they lack nuclei, platelets have a limited capacity to synthesize proteins. Thrombopoietin, a glycoprotein synthesized in the liver and kidneys, regulates megakaryocytic proliferation and maturation, as well as platelet production.[12] Once they enter the circulation, platelets have a life span of 7 to 10 days.

Damage to the intimal lining of the vessel exposes the underlying subendothelial matrix. Platelets home to sites of vascular disruption and adhere to the exposed matrix proteins.[13] Adherent platelets undergo activation and not only release substances that recruit additional platelets to the site of injury, but also promote thrombin generation and subsequent fibrin formation (Fig. 95.3). A potent platelet agonist, thrombin amplifies platelet recruitment and activation. Activated platelets then aggregate to form a plug that seals the leak in the vasculature. An understanding of the steps in these highly integrated processes helps pinpoint the sites of action of antiplatelet drugs and rationalizes the usefulness of anticoagulants for the treatment of arterial and venous thrombosis.

Adhesion

Platelets adhere to exposed collagen and von Willebrand factor (vWF) and form a monolayer that supports and promotes thrombin generation and subsequent fibrin formation.[13] These events depend on constitutively expressed receptors on the platelet surface, $\alpha_2\beta_1$ and glycoprotein VI (GP VI), which bind collagen, and GP Ibα and GP IIb/IIIa ($\alpha_{IIb}\beta_3$), which bind vWF. Receptors crowd the platelet surface, but those involved in adhesion are the most abundant. Each platelet has approximately 80,000 copies of GP IIb/IIIa and 25,000 copies of GP Ibα. Receptors cluster in cholesterol-enriched subdomains, which render them more mobile, thereby increasing the efficiency of platelet adhesion and subsequent activation.[1,2]

Under low-shear conditions, collagen can capture and activate platelets on its own. The captured platelets undergo cytoskeletal reorganization, which causes them to flatten out and adhere more closely to the damaged vessel wall. Under high-shear conditions, however, collagen and vWF must act in concert to support optimal platelet adhesion and activation. The vWF synthesized by endothelial cells and megakaryocytes assembles into multimers that range in size from 550 kDa to greater than 10,000 kDa.[1,14] Proteolytic processing of newly secreted vWF by the metalloproteinase ADAMTS13 (A Disintegrin-like And Metalloprotease with ThromboSpondin type 1 motif 13) reduces vWF multimer size, thereby preventing the accumulation of unusually large multimers. Deficiency of ADAMTS13 such as occurs with thrombotic thrombocytopenic purpura (TTP) results in microvascular thrombosis because these exceptionally large vWF multimers tether platelets to the endothelium.

When released from storage in the Weibel-Palade bodies of endothelial cells or the alpha-granules of platelets, most of the vWF enters the circulation, but the vWF released from the abluminal surface of endothelial cells accumulates in the subendothelial matrix, where it binds collagen via its A3 domain.[15] This surface-immobilized vWF can simultaneously bind platelets via its A1 domain. In contrast, circulating vWF does not react with unstimulated platelets. This difference in reactivity reflects the conformation of vWF; circulating vWF is in a coiled conformation, which prevents access of its platelet-binding domain to vWF receptors on the platelet surface, whereas immobilized vWF assumes an elongated shape, which exposes the platelet-binding A1 domain. In their extended conformation, large vWF multimers act as the molecular glue that tethers platelets to the damaged vessel wall with sufficient strength to withstand a higher shear force. Large vWF multimers provide additional binding sites for collagen and heighten platelet adhesion because platelets have more vWF receptors than collagen receptors.

Activation

Adhesion to collagen and vWF initiates signaling pathways that result in platelet activation. These pathways induce cyclooxygenase-1 (COX-1)-dependent synthesis and release of thromboxane A_2 and trigger the release of ADP from storage granules. Thromboxane A_2 is a potent vasoconstrictor and, like ADP, locally activates ambient platelets and recruits them to the site of injury, thereby expanding the platelet plug. To activate platelets, thromboxane A_2 and ADP must bind to their respective receptors on the platelet membrane. The thromboxane receptor (TP) is a G protein–coupled receptor that is found on platelets and the endothelium, which explains why thromboxane A_2 induces vasoconstriction as well as platelet activation.[16] ADP interacts with a family of G protein–coupled receptors on the platelet membrane. The most important of these is $P2Y_{12}$, which is the target of the thienopyridines (clopidogrel and prasugrel) and ticagrelor. $P2Y_1$ also contributes to ADP-induced platelet activation such that maximal ADP-induced platelet activation requires activation of both receptors and cangrelor. A third ADP receptor, $P2X_1$, is an adenosine triphosphate (ATP)-gated calcium channel. Platelet storage granules contain ATP, as well as ADP; the ATP released during the platelet activation process may contribute to the platelet recruitment process in a $P2X_1$-dependent fashion.

Although TP and the various ADP receptors signal through different pathways, they all trigger an increase in the intracellular concentration of calcium in platelets. The increase in calcium induces changes in platelet shape via cytoskeletal rearrangement, granule

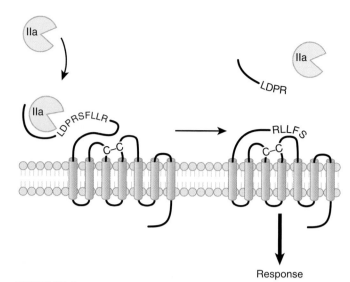

FIGURE 95.4 Activation of PAR-1 by thrombin. Thrombin (IIa) binds to the amino-terminal of the extracellular domain of PAR-1, where it cleaves a specific peptide bond. Cleavage of this bond generates a new amino-terminal sequence that acts as a tethered ligand and binds to the body of the receptor, thereby activating it. Thrombin then dissociates from the receptor. Analogues of the first five or six amino acids of the tethered ligand sequences, known as thrombin receptor agonist peptides, can independently activate PAR-1. *LDPRSFLLR*, Leu-Asp-Pro-Arg-Ser-Phe-Leu-Leu-Arg; *RLLFS*, Arg-Leu-Leu-Phe-Ser.

mobilization and release, and subsequent platelet aggregation. Activated platelets promote coagulation by expressing phosphatidylserine on their surface, an anionic phospholipid that supports the assembly of coagulation factor complexes. Once assembled, these clotting factor complexes trigger a burst of thrombin generation and subsequent fibrin formation. In addition to converting fibrinogen to fibrin, thrombin amplifies platelet recruitment and activation and promotes expansion of the platelet plug. Thrombin binds to protease-activated receptor types 1 and 4 (PAR-1 and PAR-4, respectively) on the platelet surface and cleaves their extended amino-terminal tails (Fig. 95.4), thereby generating new amino-termini that serve as tethered ligands that bind and activate the receptors.[17] Low concentrations of thrombin cleave PAR-1, whereas PAR-4 cleavage requires higher thrombin concentrations. Cleavage of either receptor triggers platelet activation.

In addition to providing a surface on which clotting factors assemble, activated platelets also promote fibrin formation and subsequent stabilization by enhancing the activation of factor V, factor VIII, factor XI, and factor XIII. Thus, a coordinated activation of platelets and coagulation, and formation of the fibrin network that results from the action of thrombin, help anchor the platelet aggregates at the site of injury. Activated platelets also release adhesive proteins, such as vWF, thrombospondin, and fibronectin, which may augment platelet adhesion at sites of injury, as well as growth factors such as platelet-derived growth factor (PDGF) and transforming growth factor-beta (TGF-β), which promote wound healing.

Platelet Aggregation

Aggregation serves as the final step in formation of the platelet plug by linking platelets to each other to form clumps. GP IIb/IIIa mediates these platelet-to-platelet linkages. On nonactivated platelets, GP IIb/IIIa exhibits minimal affinity for its ligands. Upon platelet activation, GP IIb/IIIa undergoes a conformational change that reflects transmission of inside-out signals from its cytoplasmic domain to its extracellular domain.[1,5] This transformation enhances the affinity of GP IIb/IIIa for its ligands, fibrinogen, and, under high-shear conditions, vWF. Arg-Gly-Asp (RGD) sequences located on fibrinogen and vWF, as well as a platelet-binding Lys-Gly-Asp (KGD) sequence on fibrinogen, mediate their interactions with GP IIb/IIIa. When subjected to high shear, circulating vWF elongates and exposes its platelet-binding domain, which enables its interaction with the conformationally activated GP IIb/IIIa.[18] Divalent fibrinogen and multivalent vWF molecules serve as bridges and bind adjacent platelets together. Once bound to GP IIb/IIIa, fibrinogen

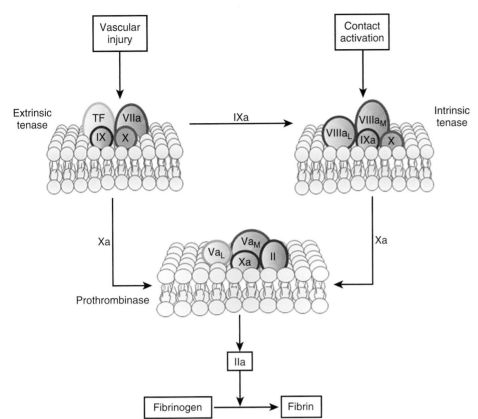

FIGURE 95.5 Coagulation system. Coagulation occurs through the action of discrete enzyme complexes composed of a vitamin K–dependent enzyme and a nonenzyme cofactor. These complexes assemble on anionic phospholipid membranes, such as the surface of activated platelets, in a calcium-dependent manner. Vascular injury exposes tissue factor (TF), which binds factor VIIa to form extrinsic tenase. Extrinsic tenase activates factors IX and X. Factor IXa binds to factor VIIIa to form intrinsic tenase, which activates factor X. Factor Xa binds to factor Va to form prothrombinase, which converts prothrombin (II) to thrombin (IIa). Thrombin then converts soluble fibrinogen to insoluble fibrin.

monocyte-derived microparticles (small membrane vesicles) also provide a source of tissue factor. When tissue factor–bearing monocytes or microparticles bind to platelets or other leukocytes and their plasma membranes fuse, transfer of tissue factor takes place. By binding to the adhesion molecules expressed on activated endothelial cells or to P-selectin on activated platelets, these tissue factor–bearing cells or microparticles can initiate or augment coagulation. This phenomenon probably explains how venous thrombi develop in the absence of obvious vessel wall injury.[2]

An integral membrane protein, tissue factor serves as a receptor for factor VII. Once bound, factor VII undergoes autoactivation, thereby forming the extrinsic tenase complex, which is a potent activator of factors IX and X or is activated by factor Xa. Upon activation, factors IXa and Xa serve as the enzyme components of intrinsic tenase and prothrombinase, respectively.

Intrinsic Tenase

Factor IXa binds to factor VIIIa on anionic cell surfaces to form the intrinsic tenase complex. Factor VIII circulates in blood in complex with vWF. Thrombin cleaves factor VIII and releases it from vWF, thereby converting it to its activated form. Activated platelets express binding sites for factor VIIIa. Once bound, factor VIIIa binds factor IXa in a calcium-dependent manner to form the intrinsic tenase complex, which then activates factor X. The change in catalytic efficiency of factor IXa–mediated activation of factor X that occurs with deletion of individual components of the intrinsic tenase complex highlights their importance. Absence of the membrane surface or factor VIIIa almost completely abolishes enzymatic activity, and the catalytic efficiency of the complete complex is 10^9-fold greater than that of factor IXa alone. Because intrinsic tenase activates factor X at a rate 50- to 100-fold faster than extrinsic tenase does, intrinsic tenase plays a critical role in the amplification of factor Xa and thrombin generation. The bleeding that occurs in patients with hemophilia A or B, which occurs with congenital or acquired deficiency of factor VIII or factor IX, respectively, highlights the importance of intrinsic tenase in hemostasis.

Prothrombinase

Factor Xa binds to factor Va, its activated cofactor, on anionic phospholipid membrane surfaces to form the prothrombinase complex. Activated platelets release factor V from their alpha granules, and this platelet-derived factor V may play a more important role in hemostasis than its plasma counterpart does. Although plasma factor V requires thrombin activation to exert its cofactor activity, the partially activated factor V released from platelets already exhibits substantial cofactor activity. Activated platelets express specific factor Va binding sites on their surface, and bound factor Va serves as a receptor for factor Xa. The catalytic efficiency of activation of prothrombin by factor Xa increases by 10^9-fold when factor Xa is incorporated into the prothrombinase complex. Prothrombin binds to the prothrombinase complex, where it undergoes conversion to thrombin in a reaction that releases prothrombin fragment 1.2 (F1.2). Plasma levels of F1.2 therefore provide a marker of prothrombin activation.

Fibrin Formation

Thrombin, the final effector in coagulation, converts soluble fibrinogen to insoluble fibrin. Fibrinogen is a dimeric molecule, each half

and vWF induce outside-inside signals that augment platelet activation and result in the activation of additional GP IIb/IIIa receptors, thus creating a positive feedback loop. Because GP IIb/IIIa serves as the final effector in platelet aggregation, it is a logical target for potent antiplatelet drugs. Fibrin, the ultimate product of the coagulation system, tethers the platelet aggregates together and anchors them to the site of injury.

Coagulation

Coagulation results in the generation of thrombin, which converts soluble fibrinogen to fibrin.[19] Coagulation occurs through the action of discrete enzyme complexes composed of a vitamin K–dependent enzyme and a nonenzyme cofactor that assemble on anionic phospholipid membranes in a calcium-dependent fashion. Each enzyme complex activates a vitamin K–dependent substrate that becomes the enzyme component of the subsequent complex (Fig. 95.5). Together, these complexes generate a small amount of thrombin that feeds back to amplify its own generation by activating the nonenzyme cofactors and platelets. The phosphatidylserine expressed on the surface of activated platelets provides an anionic surface on which the complexes assemble. The three enzyme complexes involved in thrombin generation are extrinsic tenase, intrinsic tenase, and prothrombinase. Although extrinsic tenase initiates the system under most circumstances, the contact system also plays a role in some situations.

Extrinsic Tenase

This complex forms on exposure of tissue factor–expressing cells to blood.[3] Tissue factor exposure occurs after atherosclerotic plaque rupture because the core of the plaque is rich in cells that express tissue factor. Denuding injury to the vessel wall also exposes the tissue factor constitutively expressed by subendothelial smooth muscle cells. In addition to cells in the vessel wall, cytokine activated monocytes and

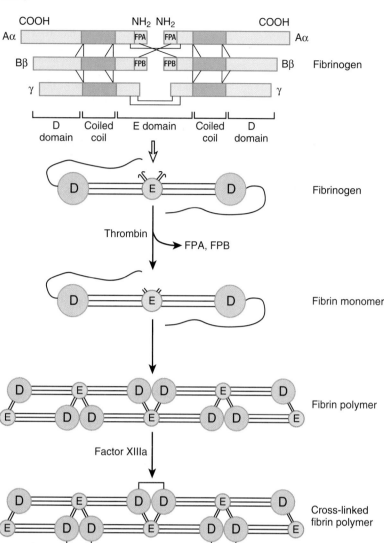

FIGURE 95.6 Fibrinogen structure and conversion of fibrinogen to fibrin. A dimer, each half of the fibrinogen molecule is composed of three polypeptide chains, the Aα, Bβ, and γ chains. Numerous disulfide bonds *(lines)* covalently link the chains together and join the two halves of the fibrinogen molecule to yield a trinodular structure with a central E domain linked via the coiled-coil regions to two lateral D domains. To convert fibrinogen to fibrin, thrombin cleaves specific peptide bonds at the amino (NH_2) terminals of the Aα and Bβ chains of fibrinogen to release fibrinopeptide A (FPA) and fibrinopeptide B (FPB), thereby generating fibrin monomer. Fibrin monomers polymerize to generate protofibrils arranged in a half-staggered overlapping manner. By covalently cross-linking the α and γ chains of adjacent fibrin monomers, factor XIIIa stabilizes the fibrin network and renders it resistant to degradation.

of which is composed of three polypeptide chains. the Aα, Bβ, and γ chains. Numerous disulfide bonds covalently link the chains together and join the two halves of the fibrinogen molecule (Fig. 95.6). Electron micrographic studies of fibrinogen reveal a trinodular structure with a central E domain flanked by two D domains. Crystal structures show symmetry of design with the central E domain, which contains the amino-terminals of the fibrinogen chains joined to the lateral D domains by coiled-coil regions.

Fibrinogen, the most abundant plasma protein involved in coagulation, circulates in an inactive form. Thrombin binds to the amino terminals of the Aα and Bβ chains of fibrinogen, where it cleaves specific peptide bonds to release fibrinopeptide A and fibrinopeptide B and generates fibrin monomers (see Fig. 95.6). Because they are products of the action of thrombin on fibrinogen, plasma levels provide an index of thrombin activity. Release of the fibrinopeptides creates new amino terminals that extend as knobs from the E domain of fibrinopeptides of one fibrin monomer and insert into preformed holes in the D domains of other fibrin monomers. This creates long strands known as protofibrils that consist of fibrin monomers noncovalently linked together in a half-staggered, overlapping manner.

Noncovalently linked fibrin protofibrils are unstable. By covalently cross-linking α- and γ-chains of adjacent fibrin monomers, factor XIIIa stabilizes the fibrin network in a calcium-dependent fashion and renders it relatively resistant to degradation. Factor XIII circulates in blood as a heterodimer consisting of two A and two B subunits. The active site and calcium binding sites of factor XIII are localized to the A subunit. Platelets contain large amounts of factor XIII in their cytoplasm, but platelet-derived factor XIII consists only of A subunits. Both plasma and platelet factor XIII are activated by thrombin.

Contact System

Current thinking views exposure of tissue factor as the sole pathway for activation of coagulation and regards the contact system—which includes factor XII, prekallikrein, and high-molecular-weight kininogen—as unimportant for hemostasis because patients deficient in these factors do not have bleeding problems. However, this concept is changing with emerging evidence that the contact system contributes to thrombosis. There are several mechanisms through which the contact system can be activated. First, blood-contacting medical devices such as stents or mechanical heart valves, and extracorporeal circuits such as those used for cardiopulmonary bypass or extracorporeal membrane oxygenation, trigger clotting by activating factor XII. Factor XIIa converts prekallikrein to kallikrein in a reaction accelerated by high-molecular-weight kininogen, and factor XIIa and kallikrein then feed back to activate additional factor XII. Factor XIIa propagates coagulation by activating factor XI (Fig. 95.7). Second, activated neutrophils extrude web-like structures known as neutrophil extracellular traps (NETs). Composed of nuclear DNA, histones, and proteases, NETs promote coagulation by binding and activating platelets, trapping red blood cells, and activating the contact pathway.[20] Third, polyphosphates released from the dense granules of activated platelets can activate factor XII and promote the inorganic activation of factor XI by thrombin.[21] Thus, surfaces and cells contribute to coagulation at numerous sites in the cascade.

Studies in animals and humans suggest that the contact system contributes to the growth of arterial and venous thrombi. Thus, mice deficient in factor XII or factor XI form small unstable thrombi at sites of arterial or venous damage.[20] Studies in humans undergoing knee arthroplasty have shown that lowering of factor XI levels with an antisense oligonucleotide or inhibiting factor XIa with an antibody reduces the risk of postoperative VTE to a greater extent than enoxaparin.[22,23] These findings identify factor XI and factor XII as potential targets for new anticoagulants.[24]

Fibrinolytic System

Fibrinolysis begins when plasminogen activators convert plasminogen to plasmin, which then degrades fibrin into soluble fragments (Fig. 95.8). Blood contains two immunologically and functionally distinct plasminogen activators, t-PA and u-PA. t-PA mediates intravascular fibrin degradation, whereas u-PA binds to a specific u-PA receptor (u-PAR) on the surface of cells, where it activates cell-bound plasminogen.[11] Consequently, pericellular proteolysis during cell migration and tissue remodeling and repair are the major functions of u-PA.

Regulation of fibrinolysis occurs at two levels. PAI-1 and, to a lesser extent, PAI-2 inhibit the plasminogen activators, whereas alpha$_2$-antiplasmin inhibits plasmin.[11] Endothelial cells synthesize PAI-1, which inhibits both t-PA and u-PA, whereas monocytes and the placenta synthesize PAI-2, which specifically inhibits u-PA. Thrombin-activated fibrinolysis inhibitor (TAFI) also attenuates fibrinolysis and provides a link between fibrinolysis and coagulation.[25] Impaired

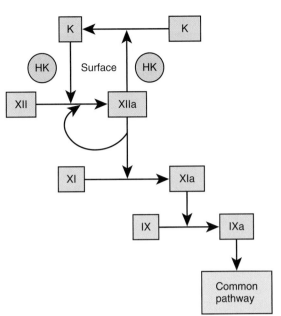

FIGURE 95.7 Contact system. Factor XII is activated by contact with negatively charged surfaces. Factor XIIa converts prekallikrein (PK) to kallikrein (K) and can feed back to activate more factor XII. Similarly, factor XIIa also can feed back to amplify its own generation. Approximately 75% of circulating PK is bound to high-molecular-weight kininogen (HK), which localizes it to anionic surfaces and promotes activation of PK. Factor XIIa propagates clotting by activating factor XI, which then activates factor IX, a process known as autoactivation. The resultant factor IXa assembles into the intrinsic tenase complex, which activates factor X to initiate the common pathway of coagulation.

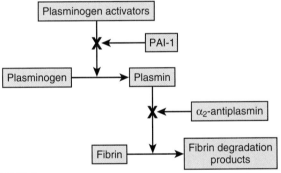

FIGURE 95.8 Fibrinolytic system and its regulation. Plasminogen activators convert plasminogen to plasmin. Plasmin then degrades fibrin into soluble fibrin degradation products. The system is regulated at two levels. Type 1 plasminogen activator inhibitor (PAI-1) inhibits the plasminogen activators, whereas alpha₂-antiplasmin serves as the major inhibitor of plasmin.

fibrinolysis promotes thrombus accumulation, whereas its excessive activation leads to bleeding.

Mechanism of Action of Tissue Plasminogen Activator

t-PA, a serine protease, contains five discrete domains: a fibronectin-like finger domain, an epidermal growth factor domain, two kringle domains, and a protease domain. Synthesized as a single-chain polypeptide, plasmin converts single-chain t-PA into a two-chain form. Both forms of t-PA convert plasminogen to plasmin. Native Glu-plasminogen is a single-chain polypeptide with a Glu residue at its amino-terminal. Plasmin cleavage near the amino-terminal generates Lys-plasminogen, a truncated form with a Lys residue at its new amino-terminal. t-PA cleaves a single peptide bond to convert single-chain Glu- or Lys-plasminogen into two-chain plasmin, which is composed of a heavy chain containing five kringle domains and a light chain containing the catalytic domain. Because its open conformation exposes the t-PA cleavage site, Lys-plasminogen is a better substrate for t-PA and u-PA than Glu-plasminogen is, which assumes a circular conformation that renders this bond less accessible.

t-PA has little enzymatic activity in the absence of fibrin, but its activity increases by at least three orders of magnitude when fibrin is present.[11] This increase in activity reflects the capacity of fibrin to serve as a template that binds t-PA and plasminogen and promotes their interaction. t-PA binds fibrin via its finger and second kringle domains, whereas plasminogen binds fibrin via its kringle domains. Kringle domains are loop-like structures that bind Lys residues on fibrin. Degradation of fibrin exposes more Lys residues, which provides additional binding sites for t-PA and plasminogen. Consequently, degrading fibrin stimulates activation of plasminogen by t-PA more than intact fibrin does.

Alpha₂-antiplasmin rapidly inhibits circulating plasmin by docking to its first kringle domain and then inhibiting the active site.[11] Because plasmin binds to fibrin via its kringle domains, plasmin generated on the fibrin surface resists inhibition by alpha₂-antiplasmin. This phenomenon endows fibrin-bound plasmin with the capacity to degrade fibrin. Factor XIIIa cross-links small amounts of alpha₂-antiplasmin onto fibrin, which prevents premature fibrinolysis.

Like fibrin, annexin II on endothelial cells binds t-PA and plasminogen and promotes the interaction of these proteins. Cell surface gangliosides and alpha-enolase may also bind plasminogen and promote its activation by altering its conformation into the more readily activated open form. Plasminogen binds to endothelial cells via its kringle domains. Lipoprotein(a), which also possesses kringle domains, impairs cell-based fibrinolysis by competing with plasminogen for cell surface binding (see also Chapter 27). This phenomenon may explain the association between elevated levels of lipoprotein(a) and atherosclerosis (see also Chapters 25 and 27).[26]

Mechanism of Action of Urokinase Plasminogen Activator

Synthesized as a single-chain polypeptide, single-chain u-PA (scu-PA) has minimal enzymatic activity. Plasmin readily converts scu-PA into an active two-chain form that can bind u-PAR on cell surfaces. Further cleavage at the amino-termini of two-chain u-PA yields a truncated, lower-molecular-weight form that lacks the u-PAR binding domain.[11]

Two-chain forms of u-PA readily convert plasminogen to plasmin in the absence or presence of fibrin. In contrast, scu-PA does not activate plasminogen in the absence of fibrin but can activate fibrin-bound plasminogen because plasminogen adopts a more open and readily activatable conformation when bound to fibrin. Like the higher-molecular-weight form of two-chain u-PA, scu-PA binds cell surface u-PAR, where plasmin can activate it. Many tumor cells elaborate u-PA and express u-PAR on their surface. Plasmin generated on these cells promotes their capacity to metastasize.[11] Inflammatory stimuli such as viruses and cardiovascular risk factors such as smoking and diabetes can trigger cleavage of membrane-bound u-PAR. Soluble u-PAR can cause acute kidney injury by inducing the formation of reactive oxygen species in the kidney tubules. The high levels of soluble u-PAR found in patients with COVID-19 may contribute to their predisposition to acute kidney injury.[27]

Mechanism of Action of Thrombin-Activatable Fibrinolysis Inhibitor

TAFI is synthesized in the liver and circulates in blood in a latent form, where thrombin bound to thrombomodulin can activate it. Unless bound to thrombomodulin, thrombin activates TAFI inefficiently.[25] Activated TAFI (TAFIa) attenuates fibrinolysis by cleaving Lys residues from the carboxy-termini of chains of degrading fibrin, thereby removing binding sites for plasminogen, plasmin, and t-PA. TAFI links fibrinolysis to coagulation in that the thrombin-thrombomodulin complex not only activates TAFI, which attenuates fibrinolysis, but also activates protein C, which mutes thrombin generation (see Fig. 95.2). TAFIa has a short half-life in plasma because the enzyme is unstable.[25] Genetic polymorphisms can result in the synthesis of more stable forms of TAFIa. Persistent attenuation of fibrinolysis by these variant forms of TAFIa may render patients susceptible to thrombosis.[25]

THROMBOSIS

A physiologic host defense mechanism, hemostasis focuses on arrest of bleeding by forming hemostatic plugs composed of platelets and fibrin at sites of vessel injury. In contrast, thrombosis reflects a pathologic process associated with intravascular thrombi that fill and occlude the lumens of arteries or veins.

Arterial Thrombosis (see also Chapter 24)

Most arterial thrombi occur on top of disrupted atherosclerotic plaques. Coronary plaques with a thin fibrous cap and a lipid-rich core are most prone to disruption.[1] Rupture of the fibrous cap exposes thrombogenic material in the lipid-rich core to blood and triggers platelet activation and thrombin generation. The extent of plaque disruption and the content of thrombogenic material in the plaque determine the consequences of the event, but host factors also contribute. Breakdown of the regulatory mechanisms that limit platelet activation and inhibit coagulation can augment thrombosis at sites of plaque disruption. Decreased production of nitric oxide and prostacyclin by diseased endothelial cells can trigger vasoconstriction and platelet activation.[28] Proinflammatory cytokines lower expression of thrombomodulin by endothelial cells, which promotes thrombin generation, and stimulate expression of PAI-1, which inhibits fibrinolysis.[29]

Products of blood coagulation contribute to atherogenesis, as well as to its complications. Microscopic erosions in the vessel wall trigger the formation of tiny platelet-rich thrombi. Activated platelets release PDGF and TGF-β, which promote a fibrotic response.[30] Thrombin generated at the site of injury not only activates platelets and converts fibrinogen to fibrin but also activates the thrombin receptor PAR-1 on smooth muscle cells and induces their proliferation, migration, and elaboration of extracellular matrix. Incorporation of microthrombi into plaque promotes their growth and decreased endothelial cell production of heparan sulfate—which normally limits smooth muscle proliferation—contributes to plaque expansion. The multiple links between atherosclerosis and thrombosis have prompted the term *atherothrombosis*.

Venous Thrombosis (see also Chapter 87)

Venous thrombosis may be caused by genetic or acquired hypercoagulable states or by such factors as advanced age, obesity, or cancer, which are usually acquired and are associated with immobility (Table 95.1). Inherited hypercoagulable states and these acquired risk factors combine to establish the intrinsic risk for thrombosis. Superimposed triggering factors, such as surgery, smoking, pregnancy, or hormonal therapy, modify this risk, and thrombosis occurs when the combination of genetic, acquired, and triggering forces exceeds a critical threshold (Fig. 95.9).

Some acquired or triggering factors entail a higher risk than do others. For example, major orthopedic surgery, neurosurgery, polytrauma, and metastatic cancer entail the highest risk, whereas prolonged bed rest, the presence of antiphospholipid antibodies, and the puerperium are associated with intermediate risk; pregnancy, obesity, long-distance travel, and the use of oral contraceptives or hormonal replacement therapy are mild risk factors. Up to half of patients with VTE before the age of 45 years have inherited hypercoagulable disorders (so-called thrombophilia), particularly those whose event occurred in the absence of risk factors or with minimal provocation, such as after minor trauma or a long-haul flight or with estrogen use. The following sections describe the inherited and acquired hypercoagulable states.

Inherited Hypercoagulable States

Inherited hypercoagulable states fall into two categories. Some are associated with gain-of-function mutations in procoagulant pathways, such as factor V Leiden, the prothrombin gene mutation, and increased levels of procoagulant proteins; others are associated with loss-of-function mutations of endogenous anticoagulant proteins, such as deficiencies of antithrombin, protein C, and protein S.[31] Although all of these inherited hypercoagulable disorders increase the risk for VTE, only increased levels of procoagulant proteins are clearly associated with an increased risk for arterial thrombosis.

TABLE 95.1 Classification of Hypercoagulable States

HEREDITARY	MIXED	ACQUIRED
Loss of Function		
Antithrombin deficiency	Hyperhomocysteinemia	Advanced age
Protein C deficiency		Previous venous thromboembolism
Protein S deficiency		Surgery
Gain of Function		Immobilization
Factor V Leiden		Obesity
Prothrombin gene mutation		Cancer
Elevated factor VIII, IX, or XI levels		Pregnancy, puerperium
		Drug-induced: L-asparaginase, hormonal therapy

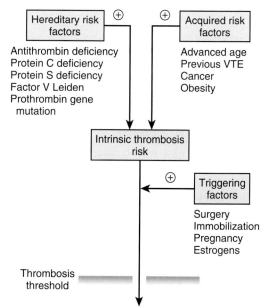

FIGURE 95.9 Thrombosis threshold. Hereditary and acquired risk factors combine to create an intrinsic risk for thrombosis. This risk is increased by extrinsic triggering factors. If the intrinsic and extrinsic forces exceed a critical threshold at which thrombin generation overwhelms protective mechanisms, thrombosis occurs. VTE, venous thromboembolism.

Factor V Leiden

The factor V Leiden mutation, present in about 5% of white individuals, is the most common inherited thrombophilia. Because of a founder effect, the mutation is less common in Hispanics and blacks and rare in Asians. Caused by a point mutation in the factor V gene, the defect results in the synthesis of a factor V molecule with a Gln residue in place of an Arg residue at position 506, one of three sites where activated protein C cleaves factor Va to inactivate it. Consequently, activated factor V Leiden resists rapid proteolysis and persists 10-fold longer in the presence of activated protein C than its wild-type counterpart does. The mutation is inherited in an autosomal dominant fashion. Individuals heterozygous for the factor V Leiden mutation have a fivefold increased risk for VTE; those homozygous for the mutation have a higher risk. However, the absolute risk for venous thrombosis is low with factor V Leiden, and with a yearly risk of 0.1% to 0.3%, patients with this disorder have a lifetime risk for thrombosis of only 5% to 10%.

An activated protein C resistance assay establishes the diagnosis of factor V Leiden in most cases. This assay involves calculation of the ratio of the activated partial thromboplastin time (APTT) measured after the addition of activated protein C divided by that determined before its addition. Use of factor V–deficient plasma increases the specificity of the test. When the clotting assay results are equivocal, genetic testing using a polymerase chain reaction (PCR)–based assay confirms the diagnosis.

Prothrombin Gene Mutation

The second most common thrombophilic disorder, the prothrombin gene mutation, reflects a G-to-A nucleotide transition at position 20210 in the 3′-untranslated region of the prothrombin gene. This mutation causes elevated levels of prothrombin, which enhance thrombin generation. The prevalence of the prothrombin gene mutation is about 3% in white persons and is lower in Asians and blacks. The mutation increases the risk for venous thrombosis to a similar extent as factor V Leiden does. Laboratory diagnosis depends on genetic screening after PCR amplification of the 3′-untranslated region of the prothrombin gene. Although persons heterozygous for this mutation have 30% higher levels of prothrombin than noncarriers do, the wide range of prothrombin levels in healthy individuals precludes the use of this phenotype for carrier identification.

Elevated Levels of Procoagulant Proteins

Elevated levels of factor VIII and other coagulation factors, including fibrinogen and factors IX and XI, appear to be independent risk factors for venous thrombosis. Increased levels of factor VIII are also associated with an up to threefold increase in the risk for myocardial infarction.[31] Although the molecular bases for the high levels of these coagulation factors have yet to be identified, genetic mechanisms probably contribute because these quantitative abnormalities have high heritability.

Antithrombin Deficiency

Synthesized in the liver, antithrombin regulates coagulation by forming a 1:1 covalent complex with thrombin, factor Xa, and other activated clotting factors. Heparan sulfate or heparin accelerates the rate of antithrombin interaction with its target proteases. Inherited antithrombin deficiency is rare; it occurs in approximately 1 in 2000 people and can be due to decreased synthesis of a normal protein or production of a dysfunctional protein. A parallel reduction in the levels of antithrombin antigen and activity identifies deficiencies caused by decreased synthesis, whereas decreased antithrombin activity in the presence of normal antigen levels identifies dysfunctional forms of antithrombin. Comparison of antithrombin activity with or without added heparin identifies variants with impaired heparin-binding capacity.

Acquired antithrombin deficiency results from decreased synthesis, increased consumption, or enhanced clearance. Decreased synthesis can occur in patients with severe hepatic disease, particularly cirrhosis, or in those given L-asparaginase. Increased activation of coagulation can result in antithrombin consumption in disorders such as extensive thrombosis, disseminated intravascular coagulation, severe sepsis, disseminated malignancy, or prolonged extracorporeal circulation. Heparin treatment can also reduce antithrombin levels up to 20% by enhancing the clearance of antithrombin. Severe antithrombin deficiency can develop in some patients with nephrotic syndrome because of loss of protein in urine.

Protein C Deficiency

Thrombin initiates the protein C pathway when it binds thrombomodulin on the endothelial cell surface (see Fig. 95.2). Thrombin bound to thrombomodulin activates protein C approximately 1000-fold more efficiently than free thrombin does.[10] EPCR augments this process 20-fold by binding protein C and presenting it to the thrombin-thrombomodulin complex for activation.[10] Activated protein C then becomes dissociated from the activation complex and decreases thrombin generation by inactivating factors Va and VIIIa on the activated platelet surface. For efficient inactivation of these factors, activated protein C must bind to protein S, its cofactor.

Protein C deficiency can be inherited or acquired. Approximately 1 in 200 adults has heterozygous protein C deficiency inherited in an autosomal dominant fashion, but most have no history of thrombosis. The variable phenotypic expression of hereditary protein C deficiency suggests the existence of other, yet unrecognized, modifying factors. In contrast to antithrombin deficiency, in which the homozygous state is associated with embryonic lethality, homozygous or doubly heterozygous protein C deficiency can occur. Newborns with these disorders often develop purpura fulminans characterized by widespread thrombosis.

Inherited protein C deficiency can result from decreased synthesis of normal protein or from synthesis of dysfunctional forms of protein C. Identification of the type of deficiency requires simultaneous measurement of protein C antigen and activity; reduced synthesis of a normal protein results in a parallel reduction in protein C antigen and activity, whereas synthesis of a dysfunctional protein results in normal antigen with reduced activity.

Acquired protein C deficiency can be due to decreased synthesis or increased consumption. Decreased synthesis can occur in patients with severe liver disease or in those given warfarin. Protein C consumption can occur with severe sepsis, with disseminated intravascular coagulation, and after surgery. Although antithrombin levels can be low in patients with nephrotic syndrome, protein C levels are normal or elevated in such patients.

Protein S Deficiency

Protein S serves as a cofactor for activated protein C (see Fig. 95.2). In addition, protein S may directly inhibit prothrombin activation because of its capacity to bind factors Va and Xa, components of the prothrombinase complex, in the presence of zinc. The importance of the direct anticoagulant activity of protein S is uncertain.

In the circulation, approximately 60% of total protein S is bound to C4b-binding protein, a complement component; only the remaining free 40% is functionally active. Diagnosis of protein S deficiency requires measurement of both the free and bound forms of protein S. Inherited protein S deficiency can result from reduced synthesis of the protein or synthesis of a dysfunctional protein. Acquired protein S deficiency can be due to decreased synthesis, increased consumption, loss, or shift of free protein S to the bound form. Decreased synthesis can occur in patients with severe liver disease or in those given warfarin or L-asparaginase. Increased consumption of protein S occurs in patients with acute thrombosis or disseminated intravascular coagulation. Patients with nephrotic syndrome can excrete free protein S in their urine, which causes decreased protein S activity. Total protein S levels in these patients are often normal because the levels of C4b-binding protein increase, thus shifting more protein S to the bound form. C4b-binding protein levels also increase in pregnancy and with the use of oral contraceptives. This shifts more protein S to the bound form and lowers the levels of free protein S and protein S activity. The consequences of this phenomenon are uncertain.

Other Hereditary Disorders

A polymorphism in the gene that encodes EPCR has been linked to venous thrombosis. Associated with EPCR shedding and high levels of soluble EPCR, this polymorphism reduces endothelial EPCR, and soluble EPCR competes with its endothelial cell counterpart for protein C binding.

A polymorphism in factor XIII that results in more rapid activation by thrombin is associated with a small reduction in the risk for VTE, myocardial infarction, and ischemic stroke in some but not all case-control studies.[32] The frequency of this polymorphism varies among different ethnic populations, and certain environmental factors, such as obesity and estrogen therapy, may augment its protective effect. More work is needed to determine the extent to which this polymorphism modulates the risk for thrombosis.

Acquired Hypercoagulable States (see also Chapter 87)

Acquired hypercoagulable states may develop during surgery and the period of immobilization following it; in persons of advanced age; in those who are obese, have cancer, are pregnant, or are taking estrogen therapy (oral contraceptive or hormone replacement therapy); or in those with a history of VTE, antiphospholipid syndrome, or hyperhomocysteinemia (see Table 95.1). These conditions can occur in isolation or in conjunction with hereditary hypercoagulable states.

Surgery and Immobilization

Surgery can directly damage veins, and immobilization after surgery leads to stasis in the deep veins of the leg. The risk for VTE in surgical patients depends on the patient's age, the type of surgery, and the presence of active cancer. Patients older than 65 years have a greater risk, and high-risk types of surgery include major orthopedic procedures, neurosurgery, and extensive abdominal or pelvic surgery, especially for cancer. Because the risk for VTE increases up to 20-fold in these patients, they require thromboprophylaxis until they gain full mobility. Hospitalization and nursing home confinement account for approximately 60% of cases of VTE, again reflecting the impact of immobilization. Hospitalization for medical illness accounts for a similar proportion of cases as hospitalization for surgery, thus highlighting the need for thromboprophylaxis in medical patients as well as in surgical patients. Extending thromboprophylaxis after hospital discharge may be beneficial in high-risk medical and surgical patients.[33,34]

Advanced Age

Predominantly a disease of older age, VTE in those younger than 50 years has an incidence of 1 per 10,000 and increases approximately 10-fold per decade thereafter. Men have an overall age-adjusted incidence rate approximately 1.2-fold higher than women. Although incidence rates are higher in women during the reproductive years, after 45 years of age, men have higher incidence rates. Many potential mechanisms may increase the incidence of VTE with advanced age, including decreased mobility, associated diseases, and vascular endothelium that is less resistant to thrombosis. Levels of procoagulant proteins also increase with age.

Obesity

The risk for VTE increases approximately 1.2-fold for every 10-kg/m^2 increase in body mass index, but the basis for the association between obesity and VTE is unclear. Obesity leads to immobility; in addition, adipose tissue, particularly visceral fat, expresses proinflammatory cytokines and adipokines, which may promote coagulation by increasing levels of procoagulant proteins or impair fibrinolysis by elevating levels of PAI-1.

Cancer

Approximately 20% of patients with VTE have cancer.[35] Cancer patients with VTE have reduced survival times compared with those without VTE. Patients with brain tumors, pancreatic cancer, or advanced ovarian or prostate cancer have particularly high rates of VTE. Treatment with chemotherapy, hormonal therapy, and biologic or gastric agents (such as erythropoietin, antiangiogenic drugs) further increases the risk, as do central venous catheters or surgery and immunotherapy for cancer. The pathogenesis of thrombosis in cancer patients is multifactorial and involves a complex interplay between the tumor, patient characteristics, and the hemostatic system. Many types of tumor cells express tissue factor or other procoagulants that can initiate coagulation. In addition to its role in coagulation, tissue factor also acts as a signaling molecule that promotes tumor proliferation and spread.[36] Patient characteristics that contribute to VTE include immobility and venous stasis secondary to extrinsic compression of major veins by tumor. Surgical procedures, central venous catheters, and chemotherapy can injure vessel walls. In addition, tamoxifen and selective estrogen receptor modulators (SERMs) induce an acquired hypercoagulable state by reducing levels of natural anticoagulant proteins.

A proportion of patients with unprovoked VTE have occult cancer. This observation has prompted some experts to recommend extensive screening for cancer in such patients, but the potential harms—including procedure-related morbidity, the psychological impact of false-positive test results, and the cost of screening—offsets any benefits of this approach. Studies comparing extensive cancer screening with

little or no screening in patients with unprovoked VTE have not demonstrated a reduction in cancer-related mortality rates with screening.[37] Therefore, unless symptoms suggestive of underlying cancer are present, only age-appropriate screening for breast, cervical, colon, and possibly prostate cancer is indicated because screening for these cancers may reduce mortality rates.

Pregnancy

Pregnant women have a fivefold to sixfold higher risk for VTE than do age-matched nonpregnant women. VTE occurs in approximately 1 in 1000 pregnancies, and in approximately 1 in 1000 women VTE develops in the postpartum period. VTE is the leading cause of maternal morbidity and mortality. Patient-related factors influence the risk for VTE in pregnancy and the puerperium, including age older than 35 years, body mass index higher than 29, cesarean delivery, thrombophilia, or a personal or family history of VTE. Ovarian hyperstimulation and multiparity also increase risk for thrombosis.

More than 90% of deep vein thrombi in pregnancy occur in the left leg, probably because the enlarged uterus compresses the left iliac vein. Hypercoagulability occurs in pregnancy because of the combination of venous stasis and changes in levels of blood proteins. Uterine enlargement reduces venous blood flow from the lower extremities. This is not the only contributor to venous stasis, however, because blood flow from the lower extremities begins to decrease by the end of the first trimester. Systemic factors also contribute to hypercoagulability. Thus, levels of procoagulant proteins, such as factor VIII, fibrinogen, and vWF increase in the third trimester of pregnancy. Coincidentally, suppression of the natural anticoagulant pathways takes place. These changes enhance thrombin generation, as evidenced by elevated levels of F1.2 and thrombin-antithrombin complexes.

About half the episodes of VTE in pregnancy occur in women with thrombophilia. The risk for VTE in women with thrombophilic defects depends on the type of abnormality and the presence of other risk factors. Risk appears highest in women with antithrombin, protein C, or protein S deficiency and lower in those with factor V Leiden or the prothrombin gene mutation. In general, these women have a higher daily risk for VTE in the postpartum period than during pregnancy. The risk during pregnancy is similar in all three trimesters. Therefore, women needing thromboprophylaxis require treatment throughout pregnancy and for at least 6 weeks postpartum.

Estrogen Therapy (see also Chapter 91)

Oral contraceptives, estrogen replacement therapy, and SERMs are all associated with an increased risk for VTE. The relatively high risk for VTE associated with first-generation oral contraceptives prompted the development of low-dose formulations. Currently available low-estrogen combination oral contraceptives contain 20 to 50 μg of ethinyl estradiol and one of several different progestins. Even use of these low-dose combination contraceptives is associated with a threefold to four-fold increased risk for VTE compared with nonusers. In absolute terms this translates to an incidence of 3 to 4 per 10,000 as compared with 5 to 10 per 100,000 in nonusers of reproductive age.

Although smoking increases the risk for myocardial infarction and stroke in women taking oral contraceptives, it is unclear whether smoking affects the risk for VTE. Obesity, however, increases the risk of both arterial and venous thrombosis. The risk for VTE is highest during the first year of oral contraceptive use and persists only for the duration of use. Case-control studies suggest a 20- to 30-fold higher risk for VTE in women with inherited thrombophilia who use oral contraceptives than in nonusers with thrombophilia or users without these defects. Despite the increased risk, routine screening for thrombophilia in young women considering oral contraceptive use is not recommended. Based on the incidence and case fatality rate of thrombotic events, estimates suggest that screening 400,000 women would detect 20,000 factor V Leiden carriers and that prevention of a single death would necessitate withholding oral contraceptives in all these women. Even larger numbers of women with less prevalent thrombophilic defects would require screening.

Hormonal replacement therapy with conjugated equine estrogen, with or without a progestin, is associated with a small increase in the risk for myocardial infarction, ischemic stroke, and VTE. SERMs, such as tamoxifen, are estrogen-like compounds that serve as an estrogen antagonist in the breast but as estrogen agonists in other tissues, such as bone and the uterus. Like estrogens, tamoxifen increases the risk for VTE by threefold to fourfold. The risk is higher in postmenopausal women, particularly those receiving systemic combination chemotherapy. Because of this risk, aromatase inhibitors, which antagonize estrogens by blocking their synthesis from androgens, are sometimes used in place of tamoxifen for the treatment of estrogen receptor–positive breast cancer. Aromatase inhibitors are associated with a lower risk for VTE than tamoxifen. Raloxifene, a SERM used to prevent osteoporosis, increases the risk for VTE threefold when compared with placebo, which contraindicates the use of raloxifene for prevention of osteoporosis in women with a history of VTE.

History of Previous Venous Thromboembolism
A history of previous VTE places patients at risk for recurrence. When anticoagulation treatment stops, patients with unprovoked VTE have a risk for recurrence of approximately 10% at 1 year and 30% at 5 years. This risk appears independent of whether an underlying thrombophilic defect is present, such as factor V Leiden or the prothrombin gene mutation. The risk for recurrent VTE is lower in patients whose incident event occurred in association with a transient major risk factor, such as surgery or trauma. These patients have a risk for recurrence of approximately 1% at 1 year and 5% at 5 years. Patients whose VTE occurred on the background of minor transient or persistent risk factors, such as a long-haul flight or chronic kidney disease, respectively, have an intermediate risk for recurrence. Patients at highest risk for recurrence are those with inherited deficiencies of antithrombin, protein C, or protein S; those with antiphospholipid syndrome; patients with advanced malignancy; or those homozygous for factor V Leiden or the prothrombin gene mutation. Their risk for recurrence likely ranges from 15% at 1 year to up to 50% at 5 years.

Antiphospholipid Syndrome
A heterogeneous group of autoantibodies directed against proteins that bind phospholipid to some antiphospholipid antibodies, known as lupus anticoagulants (LA), prolong phospholipid-dependent coagulation assays. Others, such as anticardiolipin (ACL) antibodies, target cardiolipin, and a subset of ACL antibodies recognizes other phospholipid-bound proteins, particularly beta$_2$-glycoprotein I. Patients with thrombosis in association with a persistent LA and/or ACL antibody have antiphospholipid syndrome. Primary antiphospholipid syndrome occurs in isolation, whereas secondary forms are associated with autoimmune disorders, such as systemic lupus erythematosus or other connective tissue diseases. Patients with antiphospholipid syndrome can have arterial, venous, or placental thrombosis. Arterial thrombosis can cause a transient ischemic attack, stroke, or myocardial infarction. Cerebral vein thrombosis can occur in addition to deep vein thrombosis and pulmonary embolism. Placental thrombosis probably causes pregnancy-related complications that characterize antiphospholipid syndrome. Such complications include fetal loss before 10 weeks of gestation and unexplained fetal death after 10 weeks of gestation, intrauterine growth restriction, preeclampsia, and eclampsia. Treatment with aspirin and/or LMWH during pregnancy may reduce the risk for these complications in women with antiphospholipid syndrome but not in those with other documented thrombophilic defects.

Laboratory diagnosis of antiphospholipid syndrome requires the presence of an LA or ACL antibody on tests taken at least 6 weeks apart. Diagnosis of an LA requires a battery of phospholipid-dependent clotting tests, whereas immunoassays detect ACL antibodies. Only ACL antibodies of medium to high titer and of the IgG or IgM subclass are associated with thrombosis. Approximately 3% to 10% of healthy individuals have ACL antibodies. Such antibodies also occur with certain infections, such as coronavirus disease (COVID-19), mycobacterial pneumonia, malaria, or parasitic disorders, and after exposure to some medications. Frequently, these antibodies are transient and of low titer. Approximately 30% to 50% of patients with systemic lupus erythematosus or other connective tissue disorders have ACL antibodies, and 10% to 20% have LA antibodies.

The mechanism by which antiphospholipid antibodies trigger thrombosis is unclear. These antibodies directly activate endothelial cells in culture and induce the expression of adhesion molecules that can tether tissue factor–bearing leukocytes or microparticles onto their surface. ACL antibodies also interfere with the protein C pathway, inhibit catalysis of antithrombin by endothelial heparan sulfate, and impair fibrinolysis. The relative importance of these mechanisms in humans remains unclear.

HYPERHOMOCYSTEINEMIA
Homocysteine serves as a methyl group donor during the metabolism of methionine, an essential amino acid derived from the diet. The interconversion of methionine and homocysteine depends on the availability of 5-methyltetrahydrofolate, a methyl group donor; vitamin B$_{12}$ and folate, cofactors in the interconversion; and the enzyme methionine synthase. Increased levels of homocysteine can result from increased production or reduced metabolism. Severe hyperhomocysteinemia and cystinuria, which are rare, usually result from deficiency of cystathionine beta-synthetase. The more common mild to moderate hyperhomocysteinemia often results from genetic mutations in methyltetrahydrofolate reductase (MTHFR) in association with nutritional deficiency of folate, vitamin B$_{12}$, or vitamin B$_6$. The common C677T and A1298C polymorphisms in MTHFR are associated with reduced enzymatic activity and increased thermolability, respectively, thereby increasing the requirement for nutritional cofactors. Hyperhomocysteinemia can also be associated with certain drugs, such as methotrexate, theophylline, cyclosporine, and most anticonvulsants, as well as with some chronic diseases, such as advanced renal disease, severe hepatic dysfunction, or hypothyroidism.

Although elevated levels of fasting serum homocysteine (>15 mmol/L) were once common, routine fortification of flour in North America with folic acid has lowered homocysteine levels in the general population. Elevated serum homocysteine may be associated with an increased risk for myocardial infarction, stroke, and peripheral artery disease, as well as VTE. Administration of folate along with vitamin B$_{12}$ and vitamin B$_6$ reduces levels of homocysteine. Nonetheless, randomized trials have shown that such therapy does not lower the risk for recurrent cardiovascular events in patients with coronary artery disease or stroke, nor does it lower the risk for recurrent VTE. Based on these negative trials and the declining incidence of hyperhomocysteinemia, enthusiasm for screening for hyperhomocysteinemia has declined.

TREATMENT OF THROMBOSIS
Antiplatelet Drugs
The commonly used antiplatelet drugs include aspirin, thienopyridines (ticlopidine, clopidogrel, and prasugrel), ticagrelor, cangrelor, dipyridamole, GPIIb/IIIa antagonists, and vorapaxar. Each agent has a distinct site of action (Fig. 95.10).

Aspirin
Aspirin is the most widely used antiplatelet agent worldwide. Because it is an inexpensive and effective drug, aspirin serves as the foundation of most antiplatelet strategies.

Mechanism of Action
Aspirin produces its antithrombotic effect by irreversibly acetylating and inhibiting platelet COX-1 (Fig. 95.10), a critical enzyme in the biosynthesis of thromboxane A$_2$. At high doses ($\approx$ 1 g/day), aspirin also inhibits COX-2, an inducible COX isoform found in endothelial cells and inflammatory cells.[38] In endothelial cells, COX-2 initiates the synthesis of prostacyclin, a potent vasodilator and inhibitor of platelet activation that antagonizes the effects of thromboxane A$_2$.

Indications
Aspirin is widely used for secondary prevention in patients with established coronary, cerebrovascular, or peripheral artery disease. In such patients, aspirin produces about a 20% reduction in the risk for cardiovascular death, myocardial infarction, or stroke.[38] Use of aspirin for

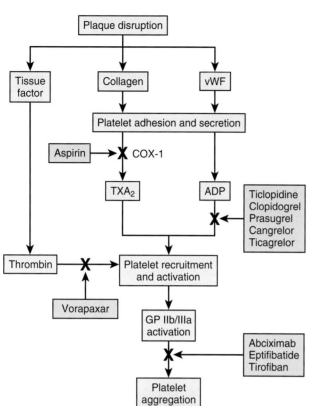

FIGURE 95.10 Sites of action of antiplatelet drugs. Aspirin inhibits the synthesis of thromboxane A_2 (TXA_2) by irreversibly acetylating cyclo-oxygenase 1 (COX-1). The reduced release of TXA_2 attenuates platelet activation and recruitment to the site of vascular injury. Ticlopidine, clopidogrel, and prasugrel irreversibly block $P2Y_{12}$, a key ADP receptor on the platelet surface; cangrelor and ticagrelor are reversible inhibitors of $P2Y_{12}$. Abciximab, eptifibatide, and tirofiban inhibit the final common pathway of platelet aggregation by blocking binding of fibrinogen and vWF to activated GP IIb/IIIa. Vorapaxar inhibits thrombin-mediated platelet activation by targeting protease-activated receptor-1 (PAR-1), the major thrombin receptor on platelets.

primary prevention is more controversial. Metaanalyses suggest that daily aspirin use produces a 20% to 25% reduction in the risk for a first cardiovascular event in patients at moderate to high risk for cardiovascular disease. Recent studies, however, have questioned whether the benefits of daily aspirin for primary cardiac protection outweigh its associated risks for gastrointestinal and intracerebral hemorrhage.[39,40] Consequently, aspirin is no longer recommended for primary cardiac prevention unless the baseline cardiovascular risk is at least 1% per year and 10% at 10 years (see also Chapter 25).[39]

Dosages
Usually administered at dosages of 75 to 325 mg once daily, there is no evidence that higher-dose aspirin is more effective than lower doses, and some meta-analyses suggest reduced efficacy with higher doses.[38] Because the side effects of aspirin, particularly gastrointestinal bleeding, depend on the dosage, daily aspirin dosages of 75 to 150 mg suffice for most indications. Rapid platelet inhibition requires an initial dose of non–enteric-coated aspirin of at least 160 mg.[38]

Side Effects
The most common side effects are gastrointestinal, and they range from dyspepsia to erosive gastritis or peptic ulcers with bleeding and perforation.[38] Use of enteric-coated or buffered aspirin in place of plain aspirin does not eliminate the risk for gastrointestinal side effects. The risk for major bleeding with aspirin is 1% to 3% per year. The concomitant use of aspirin and anticoagulants such as warfarin increases the risk for bleeding. When combined with warfarin or other oral anticoagulants, use of low-dose aspirin (75 to 100 mg daily) is best. Eradication of *Helicobacter pylori* infection and administration of proton pump inhibitors may reduce the risk for aspirin-induced upper gastrointestinal bleeding in patients with peptic ulcer disease.

Patients with a history of aspirin allergy characterized by bronchospasm should not receive aspirin. This problem occurs in approximately 0.3% of the general population but is more common in patients with chronic urticaria or asthma, particularly those with coexisting nasal polyps or chronic rhinitis.[41] Clopidogrel can be used in place of aspirin in such patients. Aspirin overdose is associated with hepatic and renal toxicity.

Aspirin Resistance
The term *aspirin resistance* is used to describe both clinical and laboratory phenomena.[42] A diagnosis of clinical aspirin resistance, defined as failure of aspirin to protect patients from ischemic vascular events, can be made only after such an event occurs. This retrospective diagnosis provides no opportunity to modify therapy. Furthermore, it is unrealistic to expect aspirin, which selectively blocks thromboxane A_2–induced platelet activation, to prevent all vascular events. The biochemical definition of aspirin resistance involves failure of the drug to inhibit thromboxane A_2 synthesis and/or arachidonic acid–induced platelet aggregation. Potential mechanisms for aspirin resistance include poor adherence, reduced or delayed absorption of aspirin due to its enteric coating,[43] thromboxane A_2 generation via pathways distinct from COX-1, increased activity of thromboxane A_2–independent pathways of platelet activation, use of concomitant medications that interfere with the action of aspirin, and pharmacogenetic factors. Tests used for the diagnosis of biochemical aspirin resistance include measurements of thromboxane B_2, the stable metabolite of thromboxane A_2, in serum or in urine, and assessment of arachidonic acid–induced platelet aggregation. These tests have not been standardized, however, and there is no evidence that they identify patients at risk for recurrent vascular events or that resistance can be reversed either by giving higher doses of aspirin or by adding other antiplatelet drugs. Until such information is available, testing for aspirin resistance remains a research tool.

Thienopyridines (see also Chapters 38 to 40)
The thienopyridines include ticlopidine, clopidogrel, and prasugrel, drugs that target $P2Y_{12}$, the key ADP receptor on platelet.

Mechanism of Action
The thienopyridines selectively inhibit ADP-induced platelet aggregation by irreversibly blocking $P2Y_{12}$ (see Fig. 95.10). These prodrugs require metabolic activation by the hepatic cytochrome P-450 (CYP) enzyme system. Therefore, when given in usual doses, ticlopidine and clopidogrel have a delayed onset of action. The metabolic activation of prasugrel is more efficient than that of clopidogrel. Consequently, prasugrel acts more rapidly and produces greater and more predictable inhibition of ADP-induced platelet aggregation than clopidogrel.[44] The active metabolites of the thienopyridines bind irreversibly to $P2Y_{12}$. Consequently, these drugs have prolonged action, which can present problems if patients require urgent surgery. To reduce the risk for bleeding, thienopyridine therapy must be stopped approximately 5 days before surgery.

Indications
When compared with aspirin in patients with recent ischemic stroke, myocardial infarction, or peripheral arterial disease, clopidogrel reduced the risk for cardiovascular death, myocardial infarction, and stroke by 8.7%. Therefore, clopidogrel is marginally more effective than aspirin, but it is more expensive, although the cost of clopidogrel has decreased now that generic forms are available. The combination of clopidogrel and aspirin capitalizes on the capacity of each drug to block complementary pathways of platelet activation. For example, this combination is recommended after stent implantation in coronary arteries. Chapter 41 discusses the use of antiplatelet agents after intervention.

The combination of clopidogrel and aspirin is also effective in patients with unstable angina (see also Chapter 39). In 12,562 such patients, the risk for cardiovascular death, myocardial infarction, or stroke was 9.3% in those randomly assigned to the combination of clopidogrel and aspirin and 11.4% in those given aspirin alone. This 20% relative risk reduction with combination therapy was highly statistically significant. However, combining clopidogrel with aspirin increases the risk for major bleeding to approximately 2% per year, a risk that persists even with a daily aspirin dose of 100 mg or less. Therefore, use of clopidogrel plus aspirin should be restricted to situations in which there is clear evidence of benefit. For example, this combination has not proved to be superior to clopidogrel alone in patients with acute ischemic stroke or to aspirin alone for primary prevention in those at risk for cardiovascular events.

Prasugrel was compared with clopidogrel in 13,608 patients with acute coronary syndromes scheduled to undergo percutaneous coronary intervention (PCI).[44] The incidence of the primary efficacy endpoint—a composite of cardiovascular death, myocardial infarction, and stroke—was significantly lower with prasugrel than with clopidogrel (9.9% and 12.1%, respectively), mainly because of a reduction in the incidence of nonfatal myocardial infarction. The incidence of stent thrombosis was also significantly lower with prasugrel than with clopidogrel (1.1% and 2.4%, respectively). These advantages, however, were at the expense of significantly higher rates of fatal bleeding (0.4% and 0.1%, respectively) and life-threatening bleeding (1.4% and 0.9%, respectively) with prasugrel. Because patients older than 75 years and those with a history of previous stroke or transient ischemic attack have a particularly high risk for bleeding, prasugrel should be avoided in older patients, and the drug is contraindicated in those with a history of cerebrovascular disease. Caution is required if prasugrel is used in patients weighing less than 60 kg or in those with renal impairment.

Dosages

Clopidogrel is given once daily at a dose of 75 mg.[38] Because its onset of action is delayed for several days, 300- to 600-mg loading doses of clopidogrel are given when rapid ADP receptor blockade is desired (see also Chapter 41). After a loading dose of 60 mg, prasugrel is given once daily at a dose of 10 mg.[38] Patients older than 75 years or weighing less than 60 kg should receive a daily prasugrel dose of 5 mg.

Clopidogrel Resistance

The capacity of clopidogrel to inhibit ADP-induced platelet aggregation varies among subjects.[45] This variability reflects, at least in part, genetic polymorphisms in the CYP isoenzymes involved in the metabolic activation of clopidogrel (see also Chapters 8, 38, and 39). The most important of these enzymes is CYP2C19. Clopidogrel-treated patients with the loss-of-function CYP2C19*2 allele exhibit reduced platelet inhibition in comparison with those with the wild-type CYP2C19*1 allele and experience a higher rate of cardiovascular events.[46] This is important because estimates suggest that up to 25% of whites, 30% of blacks, and 50% of Asians carry the loss-of-function allele, which may render them resistant to clopidogrel. Even patients with reduced-function CYP2C19*3, CYP2C19*4, or CYP2C19*5 alleles may derive less benefit from clopidogrel than do those with the full-function CYP2C19*1 allele. Patients with polymorphisms in ABCB1 may exhibit impaired clopidogrel absorption, and polymorphisms in CYP3A4 can contribute to reduced metabolic activation of clopidogrel. Polymorphisms in both these enzymes have been linked to adverse clinical outcomes. In contrast to their effect on the metabolic activation of clopidogrel, polymorphisms in CYP2C19 and CYP3A4 do not appear to influence activation of prasugrel, nor do they affect the response to ticagrelor.

Although concomitant administration of clopidogrel with proton pump inhibitors, which inhibit CYP2C19, reduces the effect of clopidogrel on ADP-induced platelet aggregation, this interaction has questionable clinical significance. Atorvastatin, a competitive inhibitor of CYP3A4, reduced the inhibitory effect of clopidogrel on ADP-induced platelet aggregation in one study, a finding unconfirmed in subsequent investigations.[47]

The influence of genetic polymorphisms on clinical outcomes with clopidogrel has raised the possibility that pharmacogenetic profiling and/or point-of-care platelet function testing could be used to identify clopidogrel-resistant patients so that they could be targeted for more intensive antiplatelet therapy.[48] Although up to 30% of clopidogrel-treated patients have evidence of reduced responsiveness to the drug, randomized clinical trials have failed to show that more intensive antiplatelet therapy improves the outcome in such patients.[49] Consequently, there is no indication for routine clopidogrel resistance testing at this time. Because their antiplatelet effects are more predictable, guidelines recommend prasugrel or ticagrelor instead of clopidogrel for high-risk patients.

Ticagrelor

As an orally active inhibitor of $P2Y_{12}$, ticagrelor differs from the thienopyridines in that it does not require metabolic activation and it produces reversible inhibition of the ADP receptor.

Mechanism of Action

Like the thienopyridines, ticagrelor inhibits $P2Y_{12}$. Because it does not require metabolic activation, ticagrelor has a more rapid onset and offset of action than clopidogrel does and it produces greater and more predictable inhibition of ADP-induced platelet aggregation.

Dosages

Ticagrelor is initiated with an oral loading dose of 180 mg followed by 90 mg twice daily. The dose does not need adjustment in patients with renal impairment, but caution is needed in patients with hepatic impairment or in those receiving potent inhibitors or inducers of CYP3A4 because ticagrelor is metabolized in the liver via CYP3A4. Ticagrelor is usually administered in conjunction with aspirin, and the daily aspirin dose should not exceed 100 mg. For secondary prevention at least 1 year after myocardial infarction, the dose of ticagrelor is reduced to 60 mg twice daily.

Side Effects

In addition to bleeding, a side effect of all $P2Y_{12}$ inhibitors, the most common side effects of ticagrelor are dyspnea, which can develop in up to 15% of patients, and bradyarrhythmias. The dyspnea, which tends to occur soon after initiating ticagrelor, is usually self-limited and mild in intensity but can be persistent and may necessitate drug discontinuation in some patients. Although the exact mechanism responsible for these side effects is unknown, they may be adenosine-mediated because ticagrelor inhibits its reuptake.

Although platelet transfusions may be useful to treat serious bleeding complications in patients taking clopidogrel or prasugrel, which bind irreversibly to $P2Y_{12}$, they are not effective for ticagrelor reversal because ticagrelor will bind to the transfused platelets. Bentracimab, an antibody fragment that binds ticagrelor and its metabolite with high affinity and rapidly reverses its inhibitory effects, is under development for ticagrelor reversal prior to urgent surgery or intervention or for patients with serious bleeding.[50]

Indications (see also Chapters 38 and 39)

When compared with clopidogrel in patients with acute coronary syndromes,[46] ticagrelor produced a greater reduction in the primary efficacy endpoint—a composite of cardiovascular death, myocardial infarction, and stroke at 1 year—than did clopidogrel (9.8% and 11.7%, respectively; $P = .001$). This difference reflected a significant reduction in both cardiovascular death (4.0% and 5.1%, respectively; $P = .001$) and myocardial infarction (5.8% and 6.9%, respectively; $P = .005$) with ticagrelor relative to clopidogrel. Rates of stroke were similar with ticagrelor and clopidogrel (1.5% and 1.3%, respectively), and there was no difference in rates of major bleeding. When minor bleeding was added to the major bleeding results, however, ticagrelor showed an increase relative to clopidogrel (16.1% and 14.6%, respectively; $P = .008$). Ticagrelor was also superior to clopidogrel in patients with acute coronary syndrome who underwent PCI or cardiac surgery. Based on these observations, guidelines give preference to ticagrelor over clopidogrel, particularly in higher-risk patients.

Cangrelor (see also Chapter 41)

Cangrelor is a rapidly acting reversible inhibitor of P2Y12 that is administered intravenously. It has an immediate onset of action, a half-life of 3 to 5 minutes, and an offset of action within an hour. Cangrelor is licensed for use in patients undergoing PCI and produces rapid ADP receptor blockade in those who have not received pretreatment with clopidogrel, prasugrel, or ticagrelor.[51]

Dipyridamole

A relatively weak antiplatelet agent on its own,[38] an extended-release formulation of dipyridamole combined with low-dose aspirin, a preparation marketed as Aggrenox, is used for prevention of stroke in patients with transient ischemic attacks.

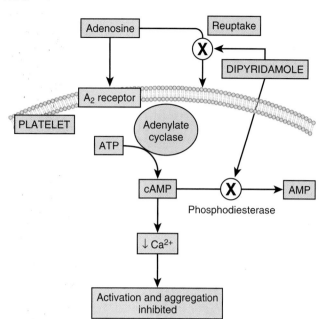

FIGURE 95.11 Mechanism of action of dipyridamole. Dipyridamole increases levels of cAMP in platelets by (1) blocking the reuptake of adenosine, thereby increasing the concentration of adenosine available to bind to the A$_2$ receptor, and (2) inhibiting phosphodiesterase-mediated cAMP degradation. By promoting calcium uptake, cAMP reduces intracellular levels of calcium. This, in turn, inhibits platelet activation and aggregation.

Mechanism of Action

By inhibiting phosphodiesterase, dipyridamole blocks the breakdown of cAMP. Increased levels of cAMP reduce intracellular calcium and inhibit platelet activation. Dipyridamole also blocks the uptake of adenosine by platelets and other cells. With more extracellular adenosine, there is a further increase in local cAMP levels because the platelet adenosine A$_2$ receptor and adenylate cyclase are coupled (Fig. 95.11).

Dosages

This fixed combination is given twice daily. Each capsule contains 200 mg of extended-release dipyridamole and 25 mg of aspirin.

Side Effects

Because dipyridamole has vasodilatory effects, caution is necessary in patients with coronary artery disease. Gastrointestinal complaints, headache, facial flushing, dizziness, and hypotension can also occur. These symptoms often subside with continued use of the drug.

Indications

Dipyridamole plus aspirin was compared with aspirin or dipyridamole alone and with placebo in patients with an ischemic stroke or a transient ischemic attack. The combination reduced the risk for stroke by 22.1% in comparison with aspirin and by 24.4% in comparison to dipyridamole.[52] A second trial compared dipyridamole plus aspirin with aspirin alone for secondary prevention in patients with ischemic stroke. Vascular death, stroke, or myocardial infarction occurred in 13% of patients given combination therapy and in 16% of those treated with aspirin alone. Although the combination of dipyridamole plus aspirin compares favorably with aspirin, the combination is not superior to clopidogrel. In a large, randomized trial that compared dipyridamole plus aspirin with clopidogrel for secondary prevention in patients with ischemic stroke, recurrent stroke event rates were similar (9.0% and 8.8%, respectively), as were rates of vascular death, stroke, and myocardial infarction (13.1% in both treatment arms). However, there was a trend toward more hemorrhagic strokes with dipyridamole plus aspirin than with clopidogrel (0.8% and 0.4%, respectively) and more major bleeding (4.1% and 3.8%, respectively).

Although dipyridamole/aspirin can replace aspirin for stroke prevention, because of the vasodilatory effects of dipyridamole and the

TABLE 95.2 Features of Glycoprotein IIb/IIIa Antagonists

FEATURE	ABCIXIMAB	EPTIFIBATIDE	TIROFIBAN
Description	Fab fragment of humanized mouse monoclonal antibody	Cyclical KGD-containing heptapeptide	Nonpeptidic RGD mimetic
Specific for GP IIb/IIIa	No	Yes	Yes
Plasma half-life	Short (min)	Long (2.5 hr)	Long (2.0 hr)
Platelet-bound half-life	Long (days)	Short (sec)	Short (sec)
Renal clearance	No	Yes	Yes

KGD, Lys-Gly-Asp sequence; *RGD*, Arg-Gly-Asp sequence.

paucity of data supporting the usefulness of this drug in patients with symptomatic coronary artery disease, dipyridamole/aspirin is contraindicated in such patients; clopidogrel is a better choice in patients with coronary artery disease.

Glycoprotein IIb/IIIa Receptor Antagonists (see also Chapters 38, 39, and 41)

As a class, parenteral GPIIb/IIIa receptor antagonists have a niche in patients with acute coronary syndromes. The three agents in this class are abciximab, eptifibatide, and tirofiban.

Mechanism of Action

A member of the integrin family of adhesion receptors, GPIIb/IIIa is expressed on the surface of platelets and megakaryocytes. With approximately 80,000 copies per platelet, GPIIb/IIIa is the most abundant receptor. GPIIb/IIIa is inactive on resting platelets. With platelet activation, however, inside-outside signal transduction pathways trigger conformational activation of the receptor. Once activated, GPIIb/IIIa binds fibrinogen and, under high-shear conditions, vWF. Once bound, fibrinogen and vWF bridge adjacent platelets together to induce platelet aggregation.

Although abciximab, eptifibatide, and tirofiban all target the GPIIb/IIIa receptor, they are structurally and pharmacologically distinct (Table 95.2).[45] Abciximab is a Fab fragment of a humanized murine monoclonal antibody directed against the activated form of GPIIb/IIIa. Abciximab binds to the activated receptor with high affinity and blocks the binding of adhesive molecules. In contrast to abciximab, eptifibatide and tirofiban are synthetic molecules. Eptifibatide is a cyclical heptapeptide that binds GPIIb/IIIa because it incorporates the KGD motif, whereas tirofiban is a nonpeptidic tyrosine derivative that acts as an RGD mimetic. With its long half-life, abciximab persists on the surface of platelets for up to 2 weeks. Eptifibatide and tirofiban have shorter half-lives.

In addition to targeting the GPIIb/IIIa receptor, abciximab (but not eptifibatide or tirofiban) also inhibits the closely related α$_{vβ3}$ receptor, which binds vitronectin, and α$_{Mβ2}$, a leukocyte integrin. Inhibition of α$_{vβ3}$ and α$_{Mβ2}$ may endow abciximab with antiinflammatory and/or antiproliferative properties that extend beyond platelet inhibition.

Dosages

All of the GPIIb/IIIa antagonists are given as an intravenous bolus followed by an infusion. Because of their renal clearance, eptifibatide and tirofiban doses require reduction in patients with renal insufficiency.

Side Effects

In addition to bleeding, thrombocytopenia is the most serious complication. Antibodies directed against neoantigens on GPIIb/IIIa that are exposed on antagonist binding cause thrombocytopenia, which is immune mediated. With abciximab, thrombocytopenia occurs in up to 5% of patients and is severe in approximately 1% of these individuals. Thrombocytopenia is less common with the other two agents and occurs in approximately 1% of patients.

Indications (see also Chapter 41)

Abciximab, eptifibatide, and tirofiban are used occasionally in patients undergoing PCI, particularly those with acute myocardial infarction, whereas tirofiban and eptifibatide are used in high-risk patients with unstable angina.

Vorapaxar

Unlike the other antiplatelet drugs, vorapaxar inhibits PAR-1, the major thrombin receptor on human platelets. Vorapaxar was compared with placebo for secondary prevention in 26,449 patients with previous myocardial infarction, ischemic stroke, or peripheral artery disease.[53] Overall, vorapaxar reduced the risk for cardiovascular death, myocardial infarction, or stroke by 13% but doubled the risk for intracranial bleeding. In the prespecified subgroup of 17,779 patients with previous myocardial infarction, however, vorapaxar reduced the risk for cardiovascular death, myocardial infarction, or stroke by 20% (from 9.7% to 8.1%). The rate of intracranial hemorrhage was higher with vorapaxar than with placebo (0.6% and 0.4%, respectively; P = .076), as was the rate of moderate or severe bleeding (3.4% and 2.1%, respectively; P < .001). Based on these data, the drug is now licensed for patients younger than 75 years with myocardial infarction who have no history of stroke, transient ischemic attack, or intracranial bleeding and who weigh more than 60 kg.

Anticoagulants

There are parenteral and oral anticoagulants. Currently available parenteral anticoagulants include heparin, LMWH, fondaparinux, a synthetic pentasaccharide, bivalirudin, and argatroban. Currently available oral anticoagulants include warfarin as well as dabigatran etexilate, which is an oral thrombin inhibitor, and rivaroxaban, apixaban, and edoxaban, which are oral factor Xa inhibitors.[54]

Parenteral Anticoagulants

Heparin

A sulfated polysaccharide, heparin is isolated from mammalian tissues rich in mast cells (Table 95.3). Most commercial heparin is derived from porcine intestinal mucosa and is a polymer of alternating D-glucuronic acid and N-acetyl-D-glucosamine residues.[55]

MECHANISM OF ACTION. Heparin acts as an anticoagulant by activating antithrombin (previously known as antithrombin III) and accelerating the rate at which it inhibits clotting enzymes, particularly thrombin and factor Xa. Antithrombin, the obligatory plasma cofactor for heparin, belongs to the serine protease inhibitor (serpin) superfamily. Synthesized in the liver and circulating in plasma at a concentration of 2.6 ± 0.4 µM, antithrombin acts as a suicide substrate for its target enzymes.

To activate antithrombin, heparin binds to the serpin via a unique pentasaccharide sequence found on a third of the chains of commercial heparin (Fig. 95.12). Heparin chains lacking this pentasaccharide sequence have little or no anticoagulant activity.[56] Once bound to antithrombin, heparin induces a conformational change in the reactive center loop of antithrombin that renders it more readily accessible to its target proteases. This conformational change enhances the rate at which antithrombin inhibits factor Xa by at least two orders of magnitude but has little effect on the rate of thrombin inhibition by antithrombin. To promote thrombin inhibition, heparin serves as a template that binds antithrombin and thrombin simultaneously. Formation of this ternary complex brings the enzyme in close apposition to the inhibitor, thereby promoting the formation of a stable covalent thrombin-antithrombin complex.

Only pentasaccharide-containing heparin chains composed of at least 18 saccharide units (which corresponds to a molecular weight of 5400) have sufficient length to bridge thrombin and antithrombin together.[56] With a mean molecular weight of 15,000 and a range of 5,000 to 30,000, almost all the chains of unfractionated heparin are long enough to provide this bridging function. Consequently, by definition, heparin has equal capacity to promote inhibition of thrombin and factor Xa by antithrombin and has an anti–factor Xa–to–anti–factor IIa (thrombin) ratio of 1:1. Heparin causes the release of TFPI from the

TABLE 95.3 Comparison of Features of Heparin, Low-Molecular-Weight Heparin, and Fondaparinux

FEATURES	HEPARIN	LMWH	FONDAPARINUX
Source	Biologic	Biologic	Synthetic
Molecular weight	15,000	5000	1500
Target	Xa and IIa	Xa and IIa	Xa
Bioavailability (%)	30	90	100
Half-life (hr)	1	4	17
Renal excretion	No	Yes	Yes
Antidote	Complete	Partial	No
Heparin-induced thrombocytopenia	<5%	<1%	Rare

LMWH, Low-molecular-weight heparin.

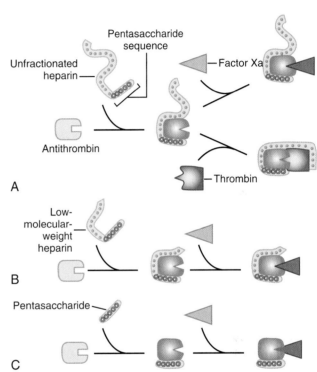

FIGURE 95.12 Mechanism of action of heparin, LMWH, and fondaparinux, a synthetic pentasaccharide. (A,) Heparin binds to antithrombin via its pentasaccharide sequence. This induces a conformational change in the reactive center loop of antithrombin that accelerates its interaction with factor Xa. To potentiate thrombin inhibition, heparin must simultaneously bind to antithrombin and thrombin. Only heparin chains composed of at least 18 saccharide units, which corresponds to a molecular weight of 5400, are of sufficient length to perform this bridging function. With a mean molecular weight of 15,000, all the heparin chains are long enough to do this. B, LMWH has greater capacity to potentiate factor Xa inhibition by antithrombin than thrombin does because with a mean molecular weight of 4500 to 6000, at least half of the LMWH chains are too short to bridge antithrombin to thrombin. C, Fondaparinux, a synthetic pentasaccharide, only accelerates inhibition of factor Xa by antithrombin because it is too short to bridge antithrombin to thrombin.

endothelium. A factor Xa–dependent inhibitor of tissue factor–bound factor VIIa,[9] TFPI may contribute to the antithrombotic activity of heparin. Longer heparin chains induce the release of more TFPI than shorter chains do.

PHARMACOLOGY OF HEPARIN. Heparin requires parenteral administration and is usually administered subcutaneously or by continuous intravenous infusion. If administered subcutaneously for the treatment of thrombosis, the dose must be high enough to overcome the limited bioavailability associated with this method of delivery. In the circulation, heparin binds to the endothelium and to plasma proteins other than antithrombin. Binding of heparin to endothelial cells explains its dose-dependent clearance. At low intravenous doses, the

CARDIOVASCULAR DISEASE AND DISORDERS OF OTHER ORGANS

XI

half-life of heparin is short because it rapidly binds to the endothelium. With higher intravenous doses of heparin, the half-life is longer because heparin clearance is slower once the endothelium is saturated. Clearance is mainly extrarenal; heparin binds to macrophages, which internalize and depolymerize the long heparin chains and secrete shorter chains back into the circulation. Because of its dose-dependent clearance mechanism, the plasma half-life of heparin ranges from 30 to 60 minutes with bolus intravenous doses of 25 and 100 units/kg, respectively.

Once heparin enters the circulation, it binds to plasma proteins other than antithrombin, a phenomenon that reduces the anticoagulant activity of heparin. Some of the heparin-binding proteins found in plasma are acute-phase reactants whose levels are elevated in ill patients. Activated platelets or endothelial cells release other proteins that can bind heparin, such as large multimers of vWF. Activated platelets also release platelet factor 4 (PF4), a highly cationic protein that binds heparin with high affinity. The large amounts of PF4 associated with platelet-rich arterial thrombi can neutralize the anticoagulant activity of heparin. This phenomenon may attenuate heparin's capacity to suppress thrombus growth.

Because levels of heparin binding–proteins in plasma vary from person to person, the anticoagulant response to fixed or weight-adjusted doses of heparin is unpredictable. Consequently, monitoring of coagulation is essential to ensure a therapeutic response, particularly when heparin is administered for the treatment of established thrombosis, because a subtherapeutic anticoagulant response may render patients at risk for recurrent thrombosis, whereas excessive anticoagulation increases the risk for bleeding.

MONITORING THE ANTICOAGULANT EFFECT OF HEPARIN. The APTT or anti-factor Xa level is used to monitor heparin.[57] Although the APTT is the test most often used for this purpose, there are problems with the assay: APTT reagents vary in their sensitivity to heparin, and the type of coagulometer used for testing can influence the results. Consequently, laboratories must establish a therapeutic APTT range with each reagent-coagulometer combination by measuring both the APTT and anti-factor Xa levels in plasma samples collected from heparin-treated patients. With most APTT reagents and coagulometers in current use, heparin levels are therapeutic with a twofold to three-fold prolongation of the APTT. Anti-factor Xa levels can also be used to monitor heparin therapy. With this test, therapeutic heparin levels range from 0.3 to 0.7 units/mL. Although this test is gaining in popularity, anti-factor Xa assays have yet to be standardized, and results can vary widely between laboratories.

Up to 25% of patients with VTE are heparin resistant; they require more than 35,000 units/day to achieve a therapeutic APTT. It is useful to measure anti-factor Xa levels in heparin-resistant patients because many will have a therapeutic anti-factor Xa level despite a subtherapeutic APTT. This dissociation in test results occurs because elevated plasma levels of fibrinogen and factor VIII, both acute-phase proteins, shorten the APTT but have no effect on anti-factor Xa levels.[57] Anti-factor Xa levels are better than the APTT for monitoring heparin in patients who exhibit this phenomenon. Patients with congenital or acquired antithrombin deficiency and those with elevated levels of heparin-binding proteins may also need high doses of heparin to achieve a therapeutic APTT or anti–factor Xa level. If there is good correlation between the APTT and the anti–factor Xa level, either test can be used for monitoring heparin therapy.

DOSAGES. For prophylaxis, heparin is usually given in fixed doses of 5000 units subcutaneously two or three times daily. With these low doses, monitoring of coagulation is unnecessary. In contrast, monitoring is essential when the drug is given in higher doses. Fixed-dose or weight-based heparin nomograms are used to standardize heparin regimens and to shorten the time required to achieve a therapeutic anticoagulant response. At least two heparin nomograms have been validated in patients with VTE, and both reduce the time required to achieve a therapeutic APTT. Weight-adjusted heparin nomograms have also been evaluated in patients with acute coronary syndromes. After an intravenous heparin bolus of 5000 units or 70 units/kg, a heparin infusion rate of 12 to 15 units/kg/hr is usually administered. In contrast, weight-adjusted heparin nomograms for patients with VTE use an

TABLE 95.4 Pharmacokinetic and Biophysical Limitations of Heparin

LIMITATIONS	MECHANISM
Poor bioavailability	Limited absorption of long heparin chains
Dose-dependent clearance	Binds to endothelial cells from subcutaneous injection sites
Variable anticoagulant response	Binds to plasma proteins; levels vary from patient to patient
Reduced activity in the vicinity of platelet-rich thrombi	Neutralized by platelet factor 4 released from activated platelets
Limited activity against factor Xa incorporated into the prothrombinase complex and thrombin bound to fibrin	Reduced capacity of heparin-antithrombin complex to inhibit factor Xa bound to activated platelets and thrombin bound to fibrin

initial bolus of 5000 units or 80 units/kg, followed by an infusion of 18 units/kg/hr. Thus achievement of a therapeutic APTT requires higher doses of heparin in patients with VTE than in those with acute coronary syndromes. This difference may reflect differences in thrombus burden. Heparin binds to fibrin, and the fibrin content of extensive deep vein thrombi is greater than that of coronary thrombi.

Traditionally, heparin manufacturers in North America measured heparin potency in USP units, with a unit defined as the concentration of heparin that prevents 1 mL of citrated sheep plasma from clotting for 1 hour after the addition of calcium. In contrast, manufacturers in Europe measured heparin potency with anti-Xa assays that use an international heparin standard for comparison. Because of problems with heparin contamination with oversulfated chondroitin sulfate,[55] which the USP assay system does not detect, North American heparin manufacturers now use the anti-Xa assay to measure heparin potency. Use of international units in place of USP units results in a 10% to 15% reduction in the heparin dose. This change is unlikely to affect patient care because dosing of heparin has been done this way in Europe for many years. Furthermore, heparin monitoring ensures a therapeutic anticoagulant response in high-risk situations, such as cardiopulmonary bypass surgery or PCI.

LIMITATIONS OF HEPARIN. Heparin has pharmacokinetic and biophysical limitations (Table 95.4). The pharmacokinetic limitations reflect heparin's propensity to bind in a pentasaccharide-independent fashion to cells and plasma proteins. Binding of heparin to endothelial cells explains its dose-dependent clearance, whereas binding to plasma proteins results in a variable anticoagulant response and can lead to heparin resistance.

The biophysical limitations of heparin reflect the inability of the heparin-antithrombin complex to inhibit factor Xa when it is incorporated into the prothrombinase complex, the complex that converts prothrombin to thrombin, and to inhibit thrombin bound to fibrin. Consequently, factor Xa bound to activated platelets within platelet-rich thrombi can generate thrombin, even in the presence of heparin. Thrombin bound to fibrin protects it from inhibition by the heparin-antithrombin complex. Clot-associated thrombin can then trigger growth of thrombi by locally activating platelets and amplifying its own generation through feedback activation of factors V, VIII, and XI. Neutralization of heparin by the high concentrations of PF4 released from activated platelets within the platelet-rich thrombus further compounds this problem.

SIDE EFFECTS. The most common side effect of heparin is bleeding. Other complications include thrombocytopenia, osteoporosis, and elevated levels of transaminases.

BLEEDING. The risk for heparin-induced bleeding increases with higher heparin doses. Concomitant administration of drugs that affect hemostasis, such as antiplatelet or fibrinolytic agents, increases the risk for bleeding, as does recent surgery or trauma.[58] Protamine sulfate will neutralize heparin in patients with serious bleeding. A mixture of basic polypeptides isolated from salmon sperm, protamine sulfate binds heparin with high affinity to form protamine-heparin complexes that undergo renal clearance. Typically, 1 mg of intravenous protamine

TABLE 95.5 Features of Heparin-Induced Thrombocytopenia

FEATURE	DETAILS
Thrombocytopenia	Platelet count of ≤100,000/µL or a decrease in platelet count of ≥50% from baseline
Timing	Platelet count falls 5 to 14 days after starting heparin
Type of heparin	More common with unfractionated heparin than with low-molecular-weight heparin
Type of patient	More common in surgical patients than in medical patients; more common in women than in men
Thrombosis	Venous thrombosis more common than arterial thrombosis

TABLE 95.6 Management of Heparin-Induced Thrombocytopenia

Stop all heparin.

Give an alternative anticoagulant, such as argatroban, bivalirudin, fondaparinux, rivaroxaban, or apixaban.

Do not give platelet transfusions.

Do not give warfarin until the platelet count returns to baseline levels; if warfarin was administered, give vitamin K to restore the international normalized ratio to normal.

Evaluate for thrombosis, particularly deep vein thrombosis.

TABLE 95.7 Advantages of Low-Molecular-Weight Heparin and Fondaparinux over Heparin

ADVANTAGE	CONSEQUENCE
Better bioavailability and longer half-life after subcutaneous injection	Can be given subcutaneously once or twice daily for both prophylaxis and treatment
Dose-independent clearance	Simplified dosing
Predictable anticoagulant response	Monitoring of coagulation is unnecessary in most patients
Lower risk for heparin-induced thrombocytopenia	Safer than heparin for short- or long-term administration
Lower risk for osteoporosis	Safer than heparin for long-term administration

sulfate neutralizes 100 units of heparin. Anaphylactoid reactions to protamine sulfate can occur, but administration by slow intravenous infusion reduces the risk for this problem.[59]

THROMBOCYTOPENIA. Heparin-induced thrombocytopenia (HIT) is an antibody-mediated process triggered by antibodies against neoantigens on PF4 that are exposed when heparin binds to this protein.[60] These antibodies, which are usually of the IgG subtype, bind simultaneously to the heparin-PF4 complex and to platelet Fc receptors. Such binding activates the platelets and generates platelet microparticles. Circulating microparticles are procoagulant because they express anionic phospholipids on their surface and can bind clotting factors, thereby promoting thrombin generation.

Typically, HIT occurs 5 to 14 days after the initiation of heparin therapy, but it may be manifested earlier if the patient has received heparin within the past 3 months (Table 95.5). Even a 50% decrease in the platelet count from the pretreatment value should raise suspicion of HIT in those receiving heparin. HIT is more common in surgical patients than in medical patients and, like many autoimmune disorders, occurs more frequently in females than in males.[60]

HIT is associated with either arterial or venous thrombosis. Venous thrombosis, which is manifested as deep vein thrombosis and/or pulmonary embolism, is more common than arterial thrombosis. Arterial thrombosis manifests as ischemic stroke or acute myocardial infarction. Rarely, platelet-rich thrombi in the distal aorta or iliac arteries can cause critical limb ischemia.

The diagnosis of HIT is established via enzyme-linked assays to detect antibodies against heparin-PF4 complexes or via platelet activation assays. Enzyme-linked assays are sensitive but are not specific and can be positive even in the absence of any clinical evidence of HIT.[61] The most specific diagnostic test is the serotonin release assay. This test involves quantification of serotonin release after exposure of washed platelets loaded with labeled serotonin to patient serum in the absence or presence of various concentrations of heparin. If the patient's serum contains HIT antibody, the addition of heparin induces platelet activation and subsequent serotonin release.

To manage HIT, heparin therapy should be stopped in patients with suspected or documented HIT, and an alternative anticoagulant should be administered to prevent or treat thrombosis (Table 95.6).[61] The agents most often used for this indication are parenteral direct thrombin inhibitors, such as argatroban or bivalirudin, or factor Xa inhibitors, such as fondaparinux, rivaroxaban or apixaban. Patients with HIT, particularly those with associated thrombosis, often have evidence of increased thrombin generation, which can lead to consumption of protein C. If these patients receive warfarin without a concomitant parenteral anticoagulant, the further decrease in protein C levels induced by the vitamin K antagonist can trigger skin necrosis. To avoid this problem, patients with HIT require treatment with a direct thrombin inhibitor, fondaparinux, rivaroxaban, or apixaban until the platelet count returns to normal levels. At this point, low-dose warfarin therapy can be introduced, and the thrombin inhibitor or fondaparinux can be discontinued when the anticoagulant response to warfarin has been therapeutic for at least 2 days.

OSTEOPOROSIS. Treatment with therapeutic doses of heparin for more than a month can cause a reduction in bone density. This occurs

in up to 30% of patients treated over the long term with heparin,[62] and symptomatic vertebral fractures occur in 2% to 3% of these individuals. Studies in vitro and in laboratory animals have provided insight into the pathogenesis of heparin-induced osteoporosis. These investigations suggest that heparin causes bone resorption by decreasing bone formation and enhancing bone resorption. Thus, heparin affects the activity of both osteoclasts and osteoblasts.

ELEVATED LEVELS OF TRANSAMINASES. Therapeutic doses of heparin frequently cause a modest elevation in serum levels of hepatic transaminases without a concomitant increase in the level of bilirubin. Levels of transaminases rapidly return to normal when use of the drug is stopped. The mechanism responsible for this phenomenon is unknown.

Low-Molecular-Weight Heparin

Consisting of smaller fragments of heparin, LMWH is prepared from unfractionated heparin by controlled enzymatic or chemical depolymerization. The mean molecular weight of LMWH is around 5000, one third the mean molecular weight of unfractionated heparin.[56] Because of its advantages over heparin (Table 95.7), LMWH has replaced heparin for most indications.

MECHANISM OF ACTION. Like heparin, LMWH exerts its anticoagulant activity by activating antithrombin. With a mean molecular weight of 5000, which corresponds to approximately 17 saccharide units, at least half of the pentasaccharide-containing chains of LMWH are too short to bridge thrombin to antithrombin (see Fig. 95.12). These chains retain the capacity to accelerate inhibition of factor Xa by antithrombin because this activity results largely from the conformational changes in antithrombin evoked by pentasaccharide binding. Consequently, LMWH catalyzes inhibition of factor Xa by antithrombin more than inhibition of thrombin.[63] Depending on their unique molecular weight distributions, LMWH preparations have anti–factor Xa to anti–factor IIa ratios ranging from 2:1 to 4:1 (see Table 95.3).

PHARMACOLOGY OF LOW-MOLECULAR-WEIGHT HEPARIN. Although usually given subcutaneously, LMWH can be administered intravenously if a rapid anticoagulant response is needed. LMWH has pharmacokinetic advantages over heparin. These advantages arise because the shorter heparin chains bind less avidly to endothelial cells, macrophages, and heparin-binding plasma proteins. Reduced binding to endothelial cells and macrophages eliminates the rapid, dose-dependent, and saturable mechanism of clearance that is a characteristic of unfractionated heparin. Instead, clearance of LMWH is not dose dependent and its plasma half-life is longer. Based on measurement of anti–factor Xa levels, LMWH has a plasma half-life of approximately 4 hours. Because of its renal clearance, LMWH can accumulate in patients with renal insufficiency.

LMWH exhibits approximately 90% bioavailability after subcutaneous injection.[63] Because LMWH binds less avidly to heparin-binding proteins in plasma than heparin does, LMWH produces a more predictable dose response, and resistance to LMWH is rare. With a longer half-life and more predictable anticoagulant response, LMWH can be given subcutaneously once or twice daily without monitoring coagulation, even when the drug is administered in treatment doses. These properties render LMWH more convenient than unfractionated heparin. Capitalizing on this feature, studies in patients with VTE have shown that home treatment with LMWH is as effective and safe as in-hospital treatment with continuous intravenous infusions of heparin.[63] Outpatient treatment with LMWH streamlines care, reduces health care costs, and increases patient satisfaction.

MONITORING OF LOW-MOLECULAR-WEIGHT HEPARIN. In most patients, LMWH does not require monitoring of coagulation. If monitoring is necessary, the anti–factor Xa level is measured because most LMWH preparations have little effect on the APTT. Therapeutic anti–factor Xa levels with LMWH range from 0.5 to 1.2 units/mL when measured 3 to 4 hours after drug administration. With prophylactic doses of LMWH, peak anti–factor Xa levels of 0.2 to 0.5 units/mL are desirable.[64]

Situations that may require LMWH monitoring include renal insufficiency and obesity. Monitoring of LMWH in patients with a creatinine clearance of 30 mL/min or less is advisable to ensure that no drug accumulation takes place. Although weight-adjusted LMWH dosages appear to produce therapeutic anti–factor Xa levels in overweight patients, this approach has not been well studied in those with morbid obesity. It may also be advisable to monitor the anticoagulant activity of LMWH during pregnancy because dose requirements can change, particularly in the third trimester. Monitoring should also be considered in high-risk settings, such as when patients with mechanical heart valves are given LMWH for prevention of valve thrombosis.

DOSAGES. The doses of LMWH recommended for prophylaxis or treatment vary depending on the preparation. For prophylaxis, once-daily subcutaneous doses of 4000 to 5000 units are often used, whereas doses of 2500 to 3000 units are given when the drug is administered twice daily. For treatment of VTE, a dose of 150 to 200 units/kg is given if the drug is administered once daily. If a twice-daily regimen is used, a dose of 100 units/kg is given. In patients with unstable angina, LMWH is administered subcutaneously twice daily at a dose of 100 to 120 units/kg. The dose is reduced in patients with renal impairment.

SIDE EFFECTS. The major complication of LMWH is bleeding. Meta-analyses suggest that the risk for major bleeding may be lower with LMWH than with unfractionated heparin. HIT and osteoporosis also are less common with LMWH than with unfractionated heparin.

BLEEDING. The risk for bleeding with LMWH increases when antiplatelet or fibrinolytic drugs are given concomitantly.[58] Recent surgery, trauma, or underlying hemostatic defects also increase the risk for bleeding with LMWH. Although protamine sulfate serves as an antidote for LMWH, it incompletely neutralizes the anticoagulant activity of LMWH because it binds only the longer chains.[56] Because longer chains contribute to thrombin inhibition by antithrombin, protamine sulfate completely reverses the anti–factor IIa activity of LMWH. In contrast, protamine sulfate only partially reverses the anti–factor Xa activity of LMWH because the shorter pentasaccharide-containing chains of LMWH do not bind protamine sulfate. Consequently, continuous intravenous unfractionated heparin may be a better choice than subcutaneous LMWH for patients at high risk for bleeding.

THROMBOCYTOPENIA. The risk for HIT is about fivefold lower with LMWH than with heparin.[55] LMWH binds less avidly to platelets and causes less release of PF4. Furthermore, with lower affinity for PF4 than for heparin, LMWH is less likely to induce the conformational changes in PF4 that trigger the formation of HIT antibodies.

LMWH should not be used to treat patients with HIT, because most HIT antibodies exhibit cross-reactivity with LMWH.[55] This in vitro cross-reactivity is not simply a laboratory phenomenon; thrombosis can occur in HIT patients treated with LMWH.

OSTEOPOROSIS. The risk for osteoporosis is lower with long-term LMWH than with heparin.[62] For extended treatment, therefore, LMWH is a better choice than heparin because of the lower risk for osteoporosis and HIT.

Fondaparinux

A synthetic analogue of the antithrombin-binding pentasaccharide sequence, fondaparinux differs from LMWH in several ways (see Table 95.3). Fondaparinux is licensed for thromboprophylaxis in medical, general surgical, and high-risk orthopedic patients and as an alternative to heparin or LMWH for the initial treatment of patients with established VTE. Although fondaparinux is licensed as an alternative to heparin or LMWH in patients with acute coronary syndrome in Europe and Canada, it is not approved for this indication in the United States.

MECHANISM OF ACTION. As a synthetic analogue of the antithrombin-binding pentasaccharide sequence found in heparin and LMWH, fondaparinux has a molecular weight of 1728. Fondaparinux binds only to antithrombin (see Fig. 95.12) and is too short to bridge thrombin to antithrombin. Consequently, fondaparinux catalyzes inhibition of factor Xa by antithrombin and does not enhance the rate of thrombin inhibition.[55]

PHARMACOLOGY OF FONDAPARINUX. (SEE ALSO CHAPTER 41). Fondaparinux exhibits complete bioavailability after subcutaneous injection. With no binding to endothelial cells or plasma proteins, clearance of fondaparinux does not depend on the dosage, and its plasma half-life is 17 hours. The drug is administered subcutaneously once daily. Because of its renal clearance, fondaparinux is contraindicated in patients with creatinine clearance lower than 30 mL/min, and it should be used with caution in those with a creatinine clearance lower than 50 mL/min.[64]

Fondaparinux produces a predictable anticoagulant response after administration in fixed doses because it does not bind to plasma proteins. The drug is given at a dosage of 2.5 mg once daily for prevention of VTE. For initial treatment of established VTE, fondaparinux is given at a dosage of 7.5 mg once daily. The dosage can be reduced to 5 mg once daily for those weighing less than 50 kg and increased to 10 mg for those heavier than 100 kg. When given in these doses, fondaparinux is as effective as heparin or LMWH for the initial treatment of patients with deep vein thrombosis or pulmonary embolism and produces similar rates of bleeding.[55]

Fondaparinux is used at a dosage of 2.5 mg once daily in patients with acute coronary syndromes. When this prophylactic dose of fondaparinux was compared with treatment doses of enoxaparin in patients with non–ST-segment elevation acute coronary syndrome, no difference in the rate of cardiovascular death, myocardial infarction, or stroke was seen at 9 days. The rate of major bleeding, however, was 50% lower with fondaparinux than with enoxaparin, which resulted in a 17% reduction in mortality rates at 1 month with fondaparinux. In patients with acute coronary syndromes who require PCI, there is a risk for catheter thrombosis with fondaparinux unless adjunctive heparin is given.

SIDE EFFECTS. Although fondaparinux can induce the formation of HIT antibodies, HIT rarely occurs.[61] This apparent paradox reflects the fact that induction of HIT requires heparin chains of sufficient length to bind multiple PF4 molecules. Fondaparinux is too short to do so. In contrast to LMWH, there is no cross-reactivity of fondaparinux with HIT antibodies. Consequently, fondaparinux appears to be effective for the treatment of HIT, although large clinical trials supporting its use are lacking.

The major side effect of fondaparinux is bleeding, and it has no antidote. Protamine sulfate has no effect on the anticoagulant activity of fondaparinux because it fails to bind to the drug. Recombinant activated factor VII has reversed the anticoagulant effects of fondaparinux in volunteers, but it is unknown whether this agent controls fondaparinux-induced bleeding.

TABLE 95.8 Comparison of the Properties of Hirudin, Bivalirudin, and Argatroban

PROPERTY	HIRUDIN	BIVALIRUDIN	ARGATROBAN
Molecular mass	7000	1980	527
Site or sites of interaction with thrombin	Active site and exosite 1	Active site and exosite 1	Active site
Renal clearance	Yes	No	No
Hepatic metabolism	No	No	Yes
Plasma half-life (minutes)	60	25	45

Parenteral Direct Thrombin Inhibitors

Heparin and LMWH indirectly inhibit thrombin because they require antithrombin to exert their anticoagulant activity. In contrast, direct thrombin inhibitors do not require a plasma cofactor; instead, they bind directly to thrombin and block its interaction with its substrates. Approved parenteral direct thrombin inhibitors include argatroban and bivalirudin; lepirudin, a recombinant form of hirudin, also falls within this class but is no longer available (Table 95.8). Argatroban is licensed for the treatment of HIT, whereas bivalirudin is approved as an alternative to heparin in patients undergoing PCI, including those with HIT.

Argatroban

Argatroban, a univalent inhibitor that targets the active site of thrombin, is metabolized in the liver.[65] Consequently, it must be used with caution in patients with hepatic insufficiency. Argatroban is administered by continuous intravenous infusion and has a plasma half-life of approximately 45 minutes. The APTT is used to monitor its anticoagulant effect, and the dosage is adjusted to achieve an APTT 1.5 to 3 times the baseline value, but not to exceed 100 seconds. Argatroban also prolongs the international normalized ratio (INR), a feature that can complicate transitioning of patients to warfarin. This problem can be circumvented by using levels of factor X in place of the INR to monitor warfarin. Alternatively, the argatroban infusion can be stopped for 2 to 3 hours before determination of the INR.

Bivalirudin (see also Chapter 41)

A synthetic 20–amino acid analogue of hirudin, bivalirudin is a divalent thrombin inhibitor.[65] Thus, the amino terminal portion of bivalirudin interacts with the active site of thrombin, whereas its carboxy terminal tail binds to exosite 1, the substrate-binding domain on thrombin. Bivalirudin has a plasma half-life of 25 minutes, the shortest half-life of all the parenteral direct thrombin inhibitors. It is degraded by peptidases and is partially excreted via the kidneys. When given in high doses in the cardiac catheterization laboratory, the anticoagulant activity of bivalirudin is monitored with the activated clotting time. With lower doses, its activity can be monitored using the APTT.

Studies comparing bivalirudin with heparin plus a GPIIb/IIIa antagonist suggest that bivalirudin produces less bleeding. This feature, plus its short half-life, renders bivalirudin a potential alternative to heparin in patients undergoing PCI. Bivalirudin has also been used successfully in patients with HIT who require PCI.[65]

Oral Anticoagulants

For over 60 years, the vitamin K antagonists, such as warfarin, were the only available oral anticoagulants. This situation changed with the introduction of the direct oral anticoagulants, which include dabigatran, rivaroxaban, apixaban, and edoxaban.

Warfarin

A water-soluble vitamin K antagonist initially developed as a rodenticide; warfarin is the coumarin derivative most often prescribed in North America. Like other vitamin K antagonists, warfarin interferes with the synthesis of vitamin K–dependent clotting proteins, which include prothrombin (factor II) and factors VII, IX, and X. Warfarin also impairs synthesis of the vitamin K–dependent anticoagulant proteins C and S.[66]

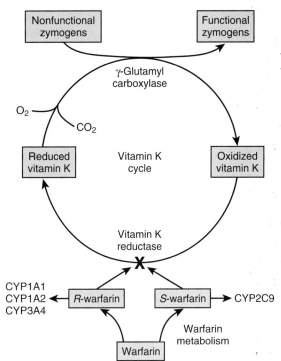

FIGURE 95.13 Mechanism of action of warfarin. A racemic mixture of *S*- and *R*-enantiomers, *S*-warfarin is most active. By blocking vitamin K epoxide reductase, warfarin inhibits the conversion of oxidized vitamin K into its reduced form. This inhibits vitamin K–dependent gamma-carboxylation of factors II, VII, IX, and X because reduced vitamin K serves as a cofactor for a gamma-glutamylcarboxylase, which catalyzes the gamma-carboxylation process, thereby converting prozymogens to zymogens capable of binding calcium and interacting with anionic phospholipid surfaces. *S*-warfarin is metabolized by CYP2C9. Common genetic polymorphisms in this enzyme can influence the metabolism of warfarin. Polymorphisms in the C1 subunit of vitamin K reductase (*VKORC1*) can also affect susceptibility of the enzyme to warfarin-induced inhibition, thereby influencing warfarin dosage requirements.

MECHANISM OF ACTION. All the vitamin K–dependent clotting factors possess glutamic acid residues at their N-terminals. A posttranslational modification adds a carboxyl group to the gamma carbon of these residues to generate gamma-carboxyglutamic acid. This modification is essential for expression of the activity of these clotting factors because it permits calcium-dependent binding of them to anionic phospholipid surfaces. A vitamin K–dependent carboxylase catalyzes the gamma-carboxylation. Thus, vitamin K from the diet undergoes reduction to vitamin K hydroquinone by vitamin K reductase (Fig. 95.13). Vitamin K hydroquinone serves as a cofactor for the carboxylase enzyme, which in the presence of carbon dioxide, replaces the hydrogen on the gamma carbon of glutamic acid residues with a carboxyl group. During this process, vitamin K hydroquinone is oxidized to vitamin K epoxide, which then undergoes reduction to vitamin K in a reaction catalyzed by vitamin K epoxide reductase.

Warfarin inhibits vitamin K epoxide reductase, thereby blocking the gamma-carboxylation process. This results in the synthesis of partially gamma-carboxylated clotting proteins with little or no biologic activity. Warfarin exerts its anticoagulant activity when the newly synthesized clotting factors with reduced activity gradually replace their fully active counterparts. The antithrombotic effect of warfarin requires a reduction in the functional levels of factor X and prothrombin, clotting factors with half-lives of 24 and 72 hours, respectively.[66] Because the antithrombotic effect of warfarin is delayed, patients with established thrombosis or at high risk for thrombosis require concomitant treatment with a rapidly acting parenteral anticoagulant, such as heparin, LMWH, or fondaparinux.[67]

PHARMACOLOGY. Warfarin is a racemic mixture of *R*- and *S*-isomers. It is rapidly and almost completely absorbed from the gastrointestinal tract. Levels of warfarin in blood peak approximately 90 minutes after administration. Racemic warfarin has a plasma half-life of 36 to 42 hours, and more than 97% of circulating warfarin is bound

TABLE 95.9 Frequencies of *CYP2C9* Genotypes and *VKORC1* Haplotypes in Different Populations and Their Effect on Warfarin Dose Requirements

GENOTYPE/ HAPLOTYPE	FREQUENCY (%)			DOSE REDUCTION COMPARED WITH WILD-TYPE (%)
	WHITES	BLACKS	ASIANS	
CYP2C9				
*1/*1	70	90	95	—
*1/*2	17	2	0	22
*1/*3	9	3	4	34
*2/*2	2	0	0	43
*2/*3	1	0	0	53
*3/*3	0	0	1	76
VKORC1				
Non-A/non-A	37	82	7	—
Non-A/A	45	12	30	26
A/A	18	6	63	50

to albumin. Only the small fraction of unbound warfarin is biologically active.[68]

Warfarin accumulates in the liver, where the two isomers are metabolized via distinct pathways. The more active *S*-enantiomer of warfarin is primarily metabolized by CYP2C9 (see Fig. 95.12). Two relatively common variants, *CYP2C9*2* and *CYP2C9*3*, encode an enzyme with reduced activity. Approximately 25% of whites have at least one variant allele of *CYP2C9*2* or *CYP2C9*3*; these variant alleles are less common in blacks and Asians (Table 95.9). Patients with one variant allele require 20% to 30% lower maintenance doses of warfarin, whereas those homozygous for these alleles require 50% to 70% lower doses than do those with the wild-type *CYP2C9*1* alleles. Consistent with the decreased warfarin dose requirement, patients with at least one *CYP2C9* variant allele are at increased risk for bleeding. Thus, when compared with individuals with no variant alleles, the relative risk for warfarin-associated bleeding in *CYP2C9*2* or *CYP2C9*3* carriers is 1.9 and 1.8, respectively.[68]

Warfarin interferes with the vitamin K cycle by inhibiting the C1 subunit of vitamin K epoxide reductase (VKORCI).[68] Polymorphisms in *VKORC1* can influence the anticoagulant response to warfarin. Several genetic variations of *VKORC1* are in strong linkage disequilibrium and have been designated as non-A haplotypes. *VKORC1* variants are more prevalent than variants of *CYP2C9*. Asians have the highest prevalence of *VKORC1* variants, followed by whites and blacks. Warfarin dose requirements for patients heterozygous or homozygous for the A haplotype are 25% and 50% lower, respectively, than the dose needed for patients with the non-A/non-A haplotype. Polymorphisms in *CYP2C9* and *VKORC1* explain up to 25% of the variability in warfarin dose requirements.[68] These findings prompted the U.S. Food and Drug Administration to amend the prescribing information for warfarin to recommend lower starting doses for patients with the *CYP2C9* and *VKORC1* genetic variants. In addition to genetic factors, fluctuations in the dietary intake of vitamin K, drugs, and various disease states influence the anticoagulant effect of warfarin. Consequently, computerized genotype-based warfarin-dosing algorithms also include pertinent patient characteristics, such as age, body weight, and concomitant medications.[68] Although these algorithms streamline warfarin dosing, randomized trials following time in therapeutic range with genotype-based warfarin dosing have yielded mixed results. It remains unclear whether better dose identification improves patient outcomes in terms of reducing hemorrhagic complications or recurrent thrombotic events.[68]

MONITORING. Warfarin therapy is most often monitored with the prothrombin time, a test sensitive to reductions in the levels of prothrombin, factor VII, and factor X.[69] The test involves the addition of thromboplastin, a reagent that contains tissue factor, phospholipid, and calcium, to citrated plasma and determination of the time until clot formation.

Thromboplastins vary in their sensitivity to reductions in the levels of vitamin K–dependent clotting factors. Consequently, less sensitive thromboplastins will trigger the administration of higher doses of warfarin to achieve a target prothrombin time. This issue can cause problems because higher doses of warfarin increase the risk for bleeding.

The INR was developed to circumvent many of the problems associated with the prothrombin time. To calculate the INR, the patient's prothrombin time is divided by the mean normal prothrombin time, and this ratio is then multiplied by the international sensitivity index (ISI), an index of the sensitivity of the thromboplastin used for determination of the prothrombin time to reductions in levels of the vitamin K–dependent clotting factors. Extremely sensitive thromboplastins have an ISI of 1.0. Most current thromboplastins have ISI values that range from 1.0 to 1.4.[69]

Although the INR has helped standardize anticoagulant practice, problems persist. The precision of INR determination varies depending on reagent-coagulometer combinations, which has led to variability in INR results. Unreliable reporting of the ISI by thromboplastin manufacturers also complicates determination of the INR. Furthermore, every laboratory must establish the mean normal prothrombin time with each new batch of thromboplastin reagent. To accomplish this, the prothrombin time must be measured in fresh plasma samples from at least 20 healthy volunteers via the same coagulometer that is used for patient samples.

For most indications, warfarin is administered at doses that produce a target INR of 2.0 to 3.0. An exception is patients with mechanical heart valves in the mitral position or in patients with a mechanical heart valve in other positions who have additional risk factors for stroke, such as atrial fibrillation, in whom a target INR of 2.5 to 3.5 is recommended. Studies in patients with atrial fibrillation demonstrate an increased risk for ischemic stroke when the INR falls below 1.7 and an increase in bleeding with INR values higher than 4.5. These findings highlight the narrow therapeutic window of vitamin K antagonists. In support of this concept, a study in patients receiving long-term warfarin therapy for unprovoked VTE demonstrated a higher rate of recurrent VTE with a target INR of 1.5 to 1.9 than with a target INR of 2.0 to 3.0.

DOSAGES. Warfarin is usually started at a dose of 5 to 10 mg. Lower doses are used for patients with *CYP2C9* or *VKORC1* polymorphisms that affect the pharmacodynamics or pharmacokinetics of warfarin and render patients more sensitive to the drug. The dose is then titrated to achieve the desired target INR. Because of its delayed onset of action, patients with established thrombosis or those at high risk for thrombosis are given concomitant treatment with a rapidly acting parenteral anticoagulant, such as heparin, LMWH, or fondaparinux. Initial prolongation of the INR reflects a reduction in the functional levels of factor VII. Consequently, concomitant treatment with the parenteral anticoagulant should be continued until the INR has been therapeutic for at least 2 consecutive days. A minimum 5-day course of parenteral anticoagulation is recommended to ensure that the levels of prothrombin have fallen into the therapeutic range with warfarin.

The narrow therapeutic window of warfarin renders frequent monitoring of coagulation necessary to ensure a therapeutic anticoagulant response. Even patients with stable warfarin dose requirements should have their INR determined every 3 to 4 weeks. Although some studies have raised the possibility that testing every 12 weeks may suffice in such patients, these results require confirmation in a larger number of patients.[70] More frequent INR monitoring is necessary with the introduction of new concomitant medications because many drugs enhance or reduce the anticoagulant effects of warfarin.

SIDE EFFECTS. Like all anticoagulants, the major side effect of warfarin is bleeding; a rare complication is skin necrosis. Warfarin crosses the placenta and can cause fetal abnormalities, so it should not be used during pregnancy.

BLEEDING. At least half of the bleeding complications with warfarin occur when the INR exceeds the therapeutic range. Bleeding complications may be mild, such as epistaxis or hematuria, or more severe, such as retroperitoneal or gastrointestinal bleeding. Life-threatening intracranial bleeding can also occur. To minimize the risk for bleeding, the INR should be maintained in the therapeutic range.

In asymptomatic patients whose INR is between 3.5 and 9, warfarin should be withheld until the INR returns to the therapeutic range. If the patient is at high risk for bleeding, sublingual or oral vitamin K can be administered. A vitamin K dose of 1 to 2.5 mg is usually adequate for patients with an INR between 4.9 and 9, whereas 2.5 to 5 mg can be used for those with an INR higher than 9. Higher doses of oral vitamin K (5 to 10 mg) produce more rapid reversal of the INR and may be helpful if the INR is excessively high.

Patients with serious bleeding need additional treatment. These patients require 10 mg of vitamin K by slow intravenous infusion with additional doses of vitamin K until the INR is in the normal range and four factor prothrombin complex concentrate to replace the vitamin K–dependent clotting proteins. Prothrombin complex concentrate is preferred over fresh frozen plasma for warfarin reversal because it normalizes the INR more rapidly and because the volume of administration is much smaller.[71]

Warfarin-treated patients who experience bleeding when their INR is in the therapeutic range require investigation of the cause of the bleeding. Those with gastrointestinal bleeding often have underlying peptic ulcer disease or a tumor. Similarly, investigation of hematuria or uterine bleeding in patients with a therapeutic INR may unmask a tumor of the genitourinary tract.

SKIN NECROSIS. A rare complication of warfarin, skin necrosis usually occurs 2 to 5 days after initiation of therapy. Well-demarcated erythematous lesions form on the thighs, buttocks, breasts, or toes. Typically, the center of the lesion becomes progressively necrotic. Examination of skin biopsy specimens taken from the borders of these lesions reveals thrombi in the microvasculature.

Warfarin-induced skin necrosis occurs in patients with congenital or acquired deficiencies of protein C or protein S or in patients with HIT whose heparin has been stopped but an alternate anticoagulant has not been given.[72,73] Initiation of warfarin therapy in these patients produces a precipitous fall in plasma levels of proteins C or S, thereby eliminating this important anticoagulant pathway before warfarin exerts an antithrombotic effect through lowering the functional levels of factor X and prothrombin. The resultant procoagulant state triggers thrombosis that is localized to the microvasculature of fatty tissues for unknown reasons.

Treatment of warfarin-induced skin necrosis involves discontinuation of warfarin and reversal with vitamin K, if needed. An alternative anticoagulant, such as heparin or LMWH, or fondaparinux or rivaroxaban in patients with HIT, should be given to patients with thrombosis. Protein C concentrates may accelerate healing of the skin lesions in protein C–deficient patients; fresh frozen plasma may be of value for those with protein S deficiency. Occasionally, skin grafting is necessary in those with extensive skin loss. Because of the potential for skin necrosis, patients with known protein C or protein S deficiency require overlapping treatment with a parenteral anticoagulant when initiating warfarin therapy. Warfarin should be started at low doses in these patients, and the parenteral anticoagulant should be continued until the INR is therapeutic for at least 2 to 3 consecutive days. Use of rivaroxaban or apixaban in place of warfarin can simplify management of such patients.

PREGNANCY. Warfarin crosses the placenta and can cause fetal abnormalities or bleeding. The fetal abnormalities include a characteristic embryopathy, which consists of nasal hypoplasia and stippled epiphyses. The risk for embryopathy is highest with warfarin administration in the first trimester of pregnancy. Central nervous system abnormalities can also occur with exposure to warfarin at any time during pregnancy. Finally, maternal administration of warfarin produces an anticoagulant effect in the fetus that can cause bleeding. This is of particular concern at delivery, when trauma to the head during passage through the birth canal can lead to intracranial bleeding. Because of these potential problems, warfarin is contraindicated in pregnancy, particularly in the first and third trimesters. Instead, heparin, LMWH, or fondaparinux can be given during pregnancy for prevention or treatment of thrombosis. Warfarin does not pass into breast milk and thus is safe for nursing mothers.

SPECIAL PROBLEMS. Patients with a lupus anticoagulant (LA) or those who need urgent or elective surgery present special challenges.

Although observational studies suggested that patients with thrombosis complicating antiphospholipid syndrome require higher-intensity warfarin regimens to prevent recurrent thromboembolic events, randomized trials indicated that usual-intensity warfarin treatment (INR of 2.0 to 3.0) is as effective as higher-intensity therapy and produces less bleeding.[74] Monitoring of warfarin can be problematic in patients with antiphospholipid syndrome if the LA prolongs the baseline INR; factor X levels can be used instead of the INR in such patients.

There is no need to stop warfarin treatment before procedures associated with a low risk for bleeding, including dental cleaning, simple dental extraction, cataract surgery, or skin biopsy.[75] In contrast, warfarin must be stopped 5 days before elective invasive procedures associated with a moderate or high risk for bleeding to allow the INR to return to normal levels. Only patients at high risk for thrombosis while not taking warfarin (such as those with mechanical heart valves in the mitral position or atrial fibrillation patients with a prior history of stroke) require bridging with once- or twice-daily subcutaneous injections of LMWH when the INR falls below 2.0. The last dose of LMWH should be given 12 to 24 hours before the procedure, depending on whether LMWH is administered twice or once daily, respectively. Once hemostasis is secure after the procedure, warfarin can be restarted. Thromboprophylaxis with LMWH can be given starting the day after major surgery and should be continued until the INR is therapeutic.

Direct Oral Anticoagulants (see also Chapters 38, 39, 66, and 87)

Direct oral anticoagulants that target thrombin or factor Xa are well established alternatives to warfarin. These drugs have a rapid onset of action and half-lives that permit once- or twice-daily administration. Designed to produce a predictable level of anticoagulation, direct oral anticoagulants are more convenient to administer than warfarin because they are given in fixed doses without the need for routine monitoring of coagulation. As a class, the direct oral anticoagulants are at least as effective as warfarin and produce less serious bleeding, particularly less intracranial hemorrhage.

MECHANISM OF ACTION. Direct oral anticoagulants are small molecules that bind reversibly to the active site of their target enzyme. Table 95.10 summarizes the pharmacologic features of these agents.

DOSAGES. For prevention of stroke in patients with nonvalvular atrial fibrillation, rivaroxaban is given at a dosage of 20 mg once daily, with a reduction to 15 mg once daily in patients with a creatinine clearance of 15 to 49 mL/min; dabigatran is given at a dosage of 150 mg twice daily, with a reduction to 75 mg twice daily in those with a creatinine clearance of 15 to 30 mL/min; apixaban is given at a dosage of 5 mg twice daily, with a reduction to 2.5 mg twice daily for patients with at least two of the "ABC" criteria (i.e., age over 80 years, body weight under 60 kg, and creatinine over 1.5 g/dL); and edoxaban is given at a dosage of 60 mg once daily for patients with a creatinine clearance of 50 to 95 mL/min and with a reduction to 30 mg once daily for patients with any one of the following criteria: creatinine clearance 15 to 50 mL/min,

TABLE 95.10 Comparison of the Features of the Direct Oral Anticoagulants

FEATURES	RIVAROX-ABAN	APIXABAN	EDOXABAN	DABIGATRAN
Target	Xa	Xa	Xa	IIa
Molecular weight	436	460	548	628
Prodrug	No	No	No	Yes
Bioavailability (%)	80	60	50	6
Time to peak (hr)	3	3	2	2
Half-life (hr)	7–11	12	9–14	12–17
Renal excretion (%)	33	25	50	80

body weight of 60 kg or less, or use of potent P-glycoprotein inhibitors, such as verapamil or quinidine.

Dabigatran, rivaroxaban, apixaban, and edoxaban are also licensed for treatment of patients with VTE. Dabigatran and edoxaban are started after patients have received at least a 5-day course of treatment with a parenteral anticoagulant such as LMWH; dabigatran is given at a dose of 150 mg twice daily provided the creatinine clearance is over 30 mL/min, and the dosage regimen for edoxaban is identical to that used in patients with atrial fibrillation. In contrast, rivaroxaban and apixaban can be given in all-oral regimens; rivaroxaban is started at a dose of 15 mg twice daily for 21 days and is then reduced to 20 mg once daily thereafter, whereas apixaban is started at a dose of 10 mg twice daily for 7 days and is then reduced to 5 mg twice daily thereafter.[54] For long-term secondary prevention, the dosage of apixaban can be lowered to 2.5 mg twice daily and the dose of rivaroxaban can be lowered to 10 mg once daily, doses that have safety profiles similar to those of placebo and aspirin, respectively.[54]

Dabigatran, rivaroxaban, and apixaban are licensed for thromboprophylaxis after elective hip or knee replacement surgery; edoxaban is not licensed for this indication except in Japan. Thromboprophylaxis is started after surgery and is often continued for 30 days in patients undergoing hip replacement and for 10 to 14 days in patients undergoing knee replacement. In lower-risk patients undergoing hip or knee replacement surgery, a 5-day course of rivaroxaban followed by a 30-day course of aspirin at a dose of 81 mg daily appears to be as effective and safe as extended thromboprophylaxis with rivaroxaban.[76] Dabigatran is given at a dose of 220 mg once daily, whereas rivaroxaban and apixaban are given at doses of 10 mg once daily and 2.5 mg twice daily, respectively. For secondary prevention of adverse cardiac or limb events in patients with coronary or peripheral artery disease, rivaroxaban is given at a dose of 2.5 mg twice daily on top of aspirin (81 or 100 mg once daily).

MONITORING. Although administered without routine monitoring, in some situations determination of the anticoagulant activity of the direct oral anticoagulants can be helpful,[77] including assessment of adherence, detection of accumulation or overdose, identification of bleeding mechanisms, and determination of activity before surgery or intervention. For qualitative assessment of anticoagulant activity, the prothrombin time can be used for factor Xa inhibitors and the APTT for dabigatran. Rivaroxaban and edoxaban prolong the prothrombin time more than apixaban does. In fact, because apixaban has such a limited effect on the prothrombin time, anti–factor Xa assays are needed to assess its activity.[77] The effect of the drugs on tests of coagulation varies depending on the reagents used to perform the tests, and variability increases with conversion of the prothrombin time to an INR. Chromogenic anti–factor Xa assays and the diluted thrombin clotting time or ecarin clotting or chromogenic assays with appropriate calibrators provide quantitative assays to measure plasma levels of the factor Xa inhibitors and dabigatran, respectively.[77]

SIDE EFFECTS. As with any anticoagulant, bleeding is the most common side effect of the direct oral anticoagulants. Although the direct oral anticoagulants are associated with less intracranial bleeding than warfarin is, the risk for gastrointestinal bleeding is higher with dabigatran (at the 150-mg, twice-daily dose), rivaroxaban, and edoxaban (at the 60-mg, once-daily dose) than with warfarin. Dyspepsia occurs in up to 10% of patients treated with dabigatran; this problem improves with time and can be minimized by taking the drug with food.

PERIPROCEDURAL MANAGEMENT. Like warfarin, the direct oral anticoagulants must be stopped before surgical procedures associated with a moderate or high risk for bleeding.[77,78] The drugs should be withheld for 1 to 2 days or longer if renal function is impaired. After surgery, patients should receive thromboprophylaxis with LMWH until hemostasis is restored, at which point the direct oral anticoagulants can be restarted.

Cardiac procedures such as atrial fibrillation ablation or pacemaker implantation can safely be performed without interruption of the direct oral anticoagulants. However, it may be prudent to hold the dose in the morning of the day of the procedure to avoid intervention at peak drug levels.

MANAGEMENT OF BLEEDING. With minor bleeding, withholding one or two doses of drug is usually sufficient.[79,80] With more serious bleeding, the approach is similar to that with warfarin, except that vitamin K administration is of no benefit; the anticoagulant and any antiplatelet drugs should be withheld, the patient should be resuscitated with fluids and blood products as necessary, and the bleeding site should be identified and managed. Coagulation testing will determine the extent of anticoagulation, and renal function should be assessed so that the half-life of the drug can be calculated.[79] Timing of the last dose of anticoagulant is important, and oral activated charcoal may help prevent absorption of drug administered in the past 4 hours particularly in cases of overdose. If bleeding continues or is life-threatening or if it occurs in a critical organ (e.g., the eye) or in a closed space (e.g., the pericardium or retroperitoneum), reversal of the anticoagulant should be considered.

Idarucizumab is licensed for dabigatran reversal in patients with serious bleeding or in those requiring urgent surgery or intervention.[81] A humanized antibody fragment, idarucizumab binds dabigatran with 350-fold higher affinity than that of dabigatran for thrombin to form an essentially irreversible complex that is cleared by the kidneys (Table 95.11). Idarucizumab is given intravenously as a 5-g bolus and is supplied in a box containing two 50-mL vials, each containing 2.5 g of idarucizumab.[81] Idarucizumab rapidly reverses the anticoagulant effects of dabigatran and normalizes the aPTT, diluted thrombin time, or ecarin clot time.[82]

Andexanet alfa is available for reversal of rivaroxaban, apixaban, and edoxaban. A recombinant variant of factor Xa without catalytic activity, andexanet serves as a decoy to sequester oral factor Xa inhibitors until they are cleared from the circulation.[81] Low- or high-dose intravenous andexanet regimens are used. The low-dose regimen starts with a bolus of 400 mg followed by an infusion of 4 mg/min for up to 120 minutes, whereas the high-dose regimen starts with a bolus of 800 mg followed by an infusion of 8 mg/min for up to 120 minutes.

TABLE 95.11 Reversal Agents for Direct Oral Anticoagulants

FEATURE	IDARUCIZUMAB	ANDEXANET ALFA	CIRAPARANTAG
Structure	Humanized antibody fragment	Recombinant human factor Xa variant	Synthetic, small cationic molecule
Mass (Da)	47,776	39,000	573
Mechanism of action	Binds dabigatran with high affinity	Competes with factors Xa for binding	Binds via hydrogen bonds
Target	Dabigatran	Rivaroxaban, apixaban, edoxaban and heparins	Dabigatran, rivaroxaban, apixaban, edoxaban and heparins
Administration	Intravenous bolus	Intravenous bolus followed by a 2-hour infusion	Intravenous bolus
Measurement of reversal	Activated partial thromboplastin time, diluted thrombin time, or ecarin clotting time or chromogenic assay	Calibrated anti-factor Xa assays	Whole-blood clotting time
Elimination	Renal (catabolism)	Not reported	Not reported
Cost	$3,500 per dose in the United States	$25,000 for low dose and double for high dose	Likely to be low

The low-dose regimen is used for reversal of doses of rivaroxaban or apixaban of 10 mg or 5 mg or less, respectively, or for any dose of rivaroxaban or apixaban if the last dose was taken more than 8 hours prior to presentation. The high-dose regimen is used to reverse rivaroxaban or apixaban doses over 10 and 5 mg, respectively, if the last dose was taken less than 8 hours since presentation, or for reversal if the dose of rivaroxaban or apixaban or the timing of the last dose is unknown (see Table 95.11). Andexanet alfa is expensive and is not available in all hospitals. Because of its cost, andexanet alfa is often reserved for reversal in patients with intracranial bleeds or for bleeds into a closed space such as retroperitoneal or pericardial bleeds. If andexanet is unavailable, the results of prospective cohort studies suggest that 4-factor prothrombin complex concentrate (25 to 50 units/kg) also is effective at restoring hemostasis.[81] If there is continued bleeding, activated prothrombin complex concentrate (50 units/kg) or recombinant factor VIIa (90 μg/kg) can be considered.[81]

Neither andexanet alfa nor 4-factor prothrombin complex concentrate has been evaluated for reversal in patients requiring urgent surgery or intervention. Furthermore, andexanet alfa not only reverses oral factor Xa inhibitors but also reverses heparin and LMWH. This could be problematic in patients who require cardiac surgery or vascular surgery, procedures where heparin is used routinely. To circumvent this problem, most surgical procedures and interventions can be done without reversal and 4-factor prothrombin complex concentrate can be given if necessary. For patients requiring surgery to stop bleeding such as those with a ruptured aortic aneurysm or with bleeding secondary to polytrauma, up front 4-factor prothrombin concentrate administration can be considered.

At an earlier stage of development than andexanet, ciraparantag is a synthetic, cationic small molecule that binds rivaroxaban, apixaban, and edoxaban, as well as dabigatran, heparin, LMWH, and fondaparinux. When given as an intravenous bolus to volunteers who took 60 mg of edoxaban, ciraparantag reduced the whole-blood clotting time in a concentration-dependent manner.[81] Because it binds citrate and other calcium chelators, routine tests of coagulation, such as the INR, APTT, or anti–factor Xa activity cannot be used to monitor ciraparantag reversal. Although the whole-blood clotting time may be useful for this purpose, the test is not widely available. Therefore, additional studies are needed before ciraparantag will be approved.

PREGNANCY. As small molecules, the direct oral anticoagulants can all pass through the placenta. Consequently, these agents are contraindicated in pregnancy, and when used by women of childbearing potential, appropriate contraception is important. Small amounts of rivaroxaban pass into breast milk, and it is unknown whether the other direct oral anticoagulants also do so. Therefore, direct oral anticoagulants should not be used in nursing mothers.

Novel Anticoagulants in Development
Although the direct oral anticoagulants represent a major advance over warfarin, the search for more effective and safer anticoagulants continues. Evidence that factor XII and factor XI, components of the contact system, are important for thrombus stabilization and growth has prompted development of anticoagulants that target these factors. Numerous phase 2 studies evaluating antisense oligonucleotides, inhibitory antibodies, and small molecule inhibitors are underway.[24]

Fibrinolytic Drugs (see also Chapter 38)
Used to degrade thrombi, fibrinolytic drugs are administered systemically or are delivered via catheters directly into the substance of the thrombus. Currently approved fibrinolytic agents include streptokinase; acylated plasminogen streptokinase activator complex (anistreplase); urokinase; recombinant t-PA (rt-PA), also known as alteplase or Activase; and two recombinant derivatives of rt-PA, tenecteplase and reteplase. Each of these agents acts by converting the proenzyme, plasminogen, to plasmin, the active enzyme.[11] There are two pools of plasminogen—circulating plasminogen and fibrin-bound plasminogen (Fig. 95.14). Plasminogen activators that preferentially activate fibrin-bound plasminogen are fibrin specific. In contrast, nonspecific plasminogen activators do not discriminate between fibrin-bound

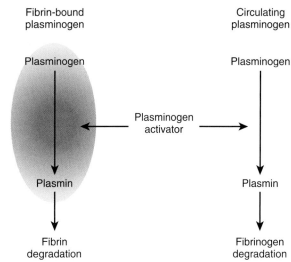

FIGURE 95.14 Consequences of activation of fibrin-bound or circulating plasminogen. The fibrin specificity of plasminogen activators reflects their capacity to distinguish between fibrin-bound and circulating plasminogen, which depends on their affinity for fibrin. Plasminogen activators with high affinity for fibrin preferentially activate fibrin-bound plasminogen. This results in the generation of plasmin on the fibrin surface. Fibrin-bound plasmin, which is protected from inactivation by alpha$_2$-antiplasmin, degrades fibrin to yield soluble fibrin degradation products. In contrast, plasminogen activators with little or no affinity for fibrin do not distinguish between fibrin-bound and circulating plasminogen. Activation of circulating plasminogen results in systemic plasminemia and subsequent degradation of fibrinogen and other clotting factors.

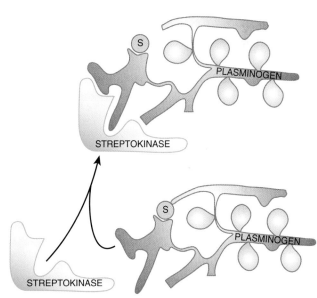

FIGURE 95.15 Mechanism of action of streptokinase. Streptokinase binds to plasminogen and induces a conformational change in plasminogen that exposes its active site. The streptokinase/plasmin(ogen) complex then serves as the activator of additional plasminogen molecules.

and circulating plasminogen.[83] Activation of circulating plasminogen results in the generation of unopposed plasmin, which can trigger the systemic lytic state. Alteplase and its derivatives are fibrin-specific plasminogen activators, whereas streptokinase, anistreplase, and urokinase are nonspecific agents.

Streptokinase
Unlike other plasminogen activators, streptokinase is not an enzyme and does not directly convert plasminogen to plasmin. Instead, it forms a 1:1 stoichiometric complex with plasminogen, thereby inducing a conformational change in plasminogen that exposes its active site (Fig. 95.15). This conformationally altered plasminogen then converts additional plasminogen molecules to plasmin.[84] Streptokinase

has no affinity for fibrin, and the streptokinase-plasminogen complex activates both free and fibrin-bound plasminogen. Activation of circulating plasminogen generates sufficient amounts of plasmin to overwhelm alpha$_2$-antiplasmin. Unopposed plasmin not only degrades fibrin in the occlusive thrombus but also induces a systemic lytic state.[83]

When given systemically to patients with acute myocardial infarction, streptokinase reduces mortality rates. For this indication the drug is usually administered as an intravenous infusion of 1.5 million units over a period of 30 to 60 minutes. Patients who receive streptokinase can form antibodies against it, as can patients with previous streptococcal infection. These antibodies can reduce the effectiveness of streptokinase. Allergic reactions occur in approximately 5% of patients treated with streptokinase. They may be manifested as a rash, fever, chills, and rigors; rarely, anaphylactic reactions can occur. Transient hypotension is common with streptokinase and probably reflects plasmin-mediated release of bradykinin. The hypotension usually responds to leg elevation and administration of intravenous fluids and low doses of vasopressors, such as dopamine or norepinephrine.

Anistreplase

To generate anistreplase, streptokinase is mixed with equimolar amounts of Lys-plasminogen, a plasmin-cleaved form of plasminogen with a Lys residue at its N-terminal. The active site of Lys-plasminogen exposed on combination with streptokinase is then blocked with an anisoyl group. After intravenous infusion, the anisoyl group is removed by deacylation, such that the complex has a half-life of approximately 100 minutes.[85] This allows drug administration via a single bolus infusion. Although it is more convenient to administer, anistreplase offers few mechanistic advantages over streptokinase. Like streptokinase, anistreplase does not distinguish between fibrin-bound and circulating plasminogen. Consequently, anistreplase produces a systemic lytic state. Similarly, allergic reactions and hypotension are just as frequent with anistreplase as they are with streptokinase. When anistreplase was compared with alteplase in patients with acute myocardial infarction, reperfusion was achieved more rapidly with alteplase than with anistreplase. Improved reperfusion was associated with a trend toward better clinical outcomes and reduced mortality rates with alteplase. The modest improvement in outcomes and the high cost of anistreplase have dampened enthusiasm for its use.

Urokinase

Originally isolated from cultured fetal kidney cells and later synthesized using recombinant DNA technology, urokinase is a two-chain serine protease with a molecular weight of 34,000.[11] Urokinase directly converts plasminogen to plasmin. Unlike streptokinase, urokinase is not immunogenic, and allergic reactions are rare. Urokinase produces a systemic lytic state because it does not discriminate between fibrin-bound and circulating plasminogen. Despite many years of use, systemic urokinase has never been evaluated for coronary fibrinolysis; instead, urokinase was mostly used for catheter-directed lysis of thrombi in the deep veins or in peripheral arteries. Because of production problems, urokinase is no longer available.

Alteplase

A recombinant form of single-chain t-PA, alteplase has a molecular weight of 68,000. Plasmin rapidly converts alteplase into its two-chain form. The interaction of alteplase with fibrin is mediated by the finger domain and, to a lesser extent, by the second kringle domain (Fig. 95.16).[11] Alteplase has a considerably higher affinity for fibrin than for fibrinogen. Consequently, the catalytic efficiency of plasminogen activation by alteplase is two to three orders of magnitude higher in the presence of fibrin than in the presence of fibrinogen.[83] Although alteplase preferentially activates plasminogen in the presence of fibrin, it is not as fibrin selective as first thought. Its fibrin specificity is limited because like fibrin, (DD)E, the major soluble degradation product of cross-linked fibrin, binds alteplase and plasminogen with high affinity. As a result, (DD)E is as potent as fibrin as a stimulator of plasminogen activation by alteplase. Plasmin generated on the

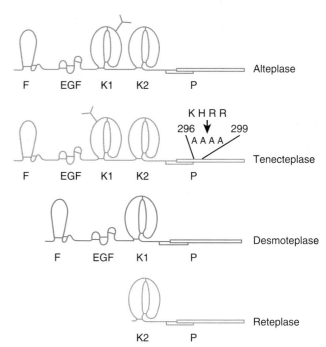

FIGURE 95.16 Domain structures of alteplase, tenecteplase, desmoteplase, and reteplase. The finger (F), epidermal growth factor (EGF), first and second kringles (K1 and K2, respectively), and protease (P) domains are illustrated. The glycosylation site (Y) on K1 has been repositioned in tenecteplase to endow it with a longer half-life. In addition, a tetra-alanine substitution in the protease domain renders tenecteplase resistant to PAI-1 inhibition. Desmoteplase differs from alteplase and tenecteplase in that it lacks a K2 domain. Reteplase is a truncated variant that lacks the F, EGF, and K1 domains.

fibrin surface results in thrombolysis, whereas plasmin generated on the surface of circulating (DD)E degrades fibrinogen. Fibrinogenolysis results in the accumulation of fragment X, a high-molecular-weight clottable fibrinogen degradation product. Incorporation of fragment X into hemostatic plugs formed at sites of vascular injury renders them susceptible to lysis.[86] This phenomenon may contribute to alteplase-induced bleeding.

A trial comparing alteplase with streptokinase for the treatment of patients with acute myocardial infarction demonstrated significantly lower mortality rates with alteplase than with streptokinase, although the absolute difference was small. Patients older than 75 years with anterior myocardial infarction presenting less than 6 hours after the onset of symptoms derived the greatest benefit from alteplase. Acute myocardial infarction or acute ischemic stroke is treated with an intravenous infusion of alteplase over a 60- to 90-minute period. The total dose of alteplase usually ranges from 90 to 100 mg. Allergic reactions and hypotension are rare, and alteplase is not immunogenic.

Tenecteplase

A genetically engineered variant of t-PA, tenecteplase was designed to have a longer half-life than t-PA and to be resistant to inactivation by PAI-1.[85] To prolong its half-life, a new glycosylation site was added to the first kringle domain (see Fig. 95.16). Because addition of this extra carbohydrate side chain reduced fibrin affinity, the existing glycosylation site on the first kringle domain was removed. To render the molecule resistant to inhibition by PAI-1, a tetra-alanine substitution was introduced at residues 296 to 299 in the protease domain, the region responsible for the interaction of t-PA with PAI-1.

Tenecteplase is more fibrin specific than t-PA. Although both agents bind to fibrin with similar affinity, the affinity of tenecteplase for (DD)E is significantly lower than that of t-PA. Consequently, (DD)E does not stimulate systemic plasminogen activation by tenecteplase to the same extent as t-PA does. As a result, tenecteplase produces less fibrinogenolysis than t-PA does.

For coronary fibrinolysis, tenecteplase is administered as a single intravenous bolus. In a large phase III trial that enrolled more than

16,000 patients, the 30-day mortality rate with single-bolus tenecteplase was like that with accelerated-dose t-PA. Although rates of intracranial hemorrhage were also similar with both treatments, patients given tenecteplase had less noncerebral bleeding and a reduced need for blood transfusions in comparison with those treated with t-PA. The improved safety profile of tenecteplase probably reflects its enhanced fibrin specificity.

Reteplase

A recombinant t-PA derivative, reteplase is a single-chain variant that lacks the finger, epidermal growth factor, and first kringle domains (see Fig. 95.16). This truncated derivative has a molecular weight of 39,000.[85] Reteplase binds fibrin with lower affinity than t-PA does because it lacks the finger domain. Because it is produced in *Escherichia coli*, reteplase is not glycosylated; this feature endows it with a plasma half-life longer than that of t-PA. Consequently, reteplase is given as two intravenous boluses separated by 30 minutes. Clinical trials in patients with acute myocardial infarction showed improved 30-day survival rates when reteplase was compared with streptokinase, but its noninferiority compared with alteplase.

Other Fibrinolytic Agents

Other fibrinolytic agents include desmoteplase (see Fig. 95.16), a recombinant form of the full-length plasminogen activator isolated from the saliva of the vampire bat, and alfimeprase, a truncated form of fibrolase, an enzyme isolated from the venom of the southern copperhead snake. Clinical studies with these agents have been disappointing. Desmoteplase, which is more fibrin specific than t-PA, was investigated for the treatment of acute ischemic stroke. Patients initially seen 3 to 9 hours after the onset of symptoms were randomly assigned to one or two doses of desmoteplase or to placebo. Overall response rates were low, and no differences from placebo were noted. Mortality rates were higher with desmoteplase.

Alfimeprase is a metalloproteinase that degrades fibrin and fibrinogen in a plasmin-independent fashion. In the circulation, alpha$_2$-macroglobulin inhibits alfimeprase, so alfimeprase must be delivered via a catheter directly into the thrombus. Despite promising phase II results, studies of alfimeprase for the treatment of peripheral arterial occlusion or for restoration of flow in blocked central venous catheters were stopped because of lack of efficacy. The disappointing results with desmoteplase and alfimeprase highlight the challenges of introducing new fibrinolytic drugs.

FUTURE PERSPECTIVES

Thrombosis in arteries or veins involves interplay among the vessel wall, platelets, the coagulation system, and fibrinolytic pathways. Activation of coagulation also triggers inflammatory pathways that may contribute to thrombosis. A better understanding of the biochemistry of platelet aggregation and blood coagulation and advances in structure-based drug design have identified new targets and prompted the development of novel antithrombotic drugs. Despite these advances, however, arterial and venous thromboembolic disorders remain a major cause of morbidity and death. The search for better targets and more potent, safer, or more convenient antiplatelet, anticoagulant, and fibrinolytic drugs continues.

REFERENCES

Hemostatic and Thrombotic Mechanisms

1. Bäck M, Yurdagul Jr A, Tabas I, et al. Inflammation and its resolution in atherosclerosis: mediators and therapeutic opportunities. *Nat Rev Cardiol*. 2019;16(7):389–406.
2. Chan NC, Weitz JI. Recent advances in understanding, diagnosing and treating venous thrombosis. *F1000Res*. 2020;9:F1000 Faculty Rev-1206.
3. Grover SP, Mackman N. Tissue factor: an essential mediator of hemostasis and trigger of thrombosis. *Arterioscl Thromb Vasc Biol*. 2018;38(4):709–725.
4. Thalin C, Hisada Y, Lundstrom S, et al. Neutrophil extracellular traps: Villains and targets in arterial, venous, and cancer-associated thrombosis. *Arterioscl Thromb Vasc Biol*. 2019;39(9):1724–1738.
5. Eikelboom JW, Connolly SJ, Bosch J, et al. Rivaroxaban with or without aspirin in stable cardiovascular disease. *N Engl J Med*. 2017;377(14):1319–1330.
6. Bonaca MP, Bauersachs RM, Anand SS, et al. Rivaroxaban in peripheral artery disease after revascularization. *N Engl J Med*. 2020;382(21):1994–2004.
7. Simes J, Becattini C, Agnelli G, et al. Aspirin for the prevention of recurrent venous thromboembolism: the inspire collaboration. *Circulation*. 2014;130(13):1062–1071.
8. Fuentes E, Palomo I. Extracellular ATP metabolism on vascular endothelial cells: a pathway with pro-thrombotic and anti-thrombotic molecules. *Vascul Pharmacol*. 2015;751–756.
9. Mast AE. Tissue factor pathway inhibitor: multiple anticoagulant activities for a single protein. *Arterioscl Thromb Vasc Biol*. 2016;36(1):9–14.
10. Griffin JH, Zlokovic BV, Mosnier LO. Activated protein c: Biased for translation. *Blood*. 2015;125(19):2898–2907.
11. Urano T, Castellino FJ, Suzuki Y. Regulation of plasminogen activation on cell surfaces and fibrin. *J Thromb Haemost*. 2018;16(8):1487–1497.
12. Baigger A, Blasczyk R, Figueiredo C. Towards the manufacture of megakaryocytes and platelets for clinical application. *Transfus Med Hemother*. 2017;44(3):165–173.
13. Becker RC, Sexton T, Smyth SS. Translational implications of platelets as vascular first responders. *Circ Res*. 2018;122(3):506–522.
14. Grover SP, Mackman N. Intrinsic pathway of coagulation and thrombosis. *Arterioscler Thromb Vasc Biol*. 2019;39(3):331–338.
15. Lenting PJ, Christophe OD, Denis CV. Von Willebrand factor biosynthesis, secretion, and clearance: connecting the far ends. *Blood*. 2015;125(13):2019–2028.
16. Gurbel PA, Kuliopulos A, Tantry US. G-protein-coupled receptors signaling pathways in new antiplatelet drug development. *Arterioscl Thromb Vasc Biol*. 2015;35(3):500–512.
17. Han X, Nieman MT. The domino effect triggered by the tethered ligand of the protease activated receptors. *Thromb Res*. 2020;19687–19698.
18. Jaffer IH, Weitz JI. The blood compatibility challenge. Part 1: Blood-contacting medical devices: the scope of the problem. *Acta Biomater*. 2019;942–10.
19. Ten Cate H, Hackeng TM, García de Frutos P. Coagulation factor and protease pathways in thrombosis and cardiovascular disease. *Thromb Haemost*. 2017;117(7):1265–1271.
20. Long AT, Kenne E, Jung R, et al. Contact system revisited: an interface between inflammation, coagulation, and innate immunity. *J Thrombosis Haemostasis*. 2016;14(3):427–437.
21. Baker C, Smith SA, Morrissey JH. Polyphosphate in thrombosis, hemostasis, and inflammation. *Res Pract Thromb Haemost*. 2019;3(1):18–25.
22. Buller HR, Bethune C, Bhanot S, et al. Factor XI antisense oligonucleotide for prevention of venous thrombosis. *N Engl J Med*. 2015;372(3):232–240.
23. Weitz JI, Bauersachs R, Becker B, et al. Effect of osocimab in preventing venous thromboembolism among patients undergoing knee arthroplasty: the foxtrot randomized clinical trial. *J Am Med Assoc*. 2020;323(2):130–139.
24. Fredenburgh JC, Weitz JI. New anticoagulants: moving beyond the direct oral anticoagulants. *J Thromb Haemost*. 2021;19(1):20–29.
25. Plug T, Meijers JC. Structure-function relationships in thrombin-activatable fibrinolysis inhibitor. *J Thromb Haemost*. 2016;14(4):633–644.
26. Bucci M, Tana C, Giamberardino MA, et al. Lp(a) and cardiovascular risk: investigating the hidden side of the moon. *Nutr Metab Cardiovasc Dis*. 2016;26(11):980–986.
27. Azam TU, Shadid HR, Blakely P, et al. Soluble urokinase receptor (supar) in covid-19-related aki. *J Am Soc Nephrol*. 2020;31(11):2725–2735.
28. Vanhoutte PM, Zhao Y, Xu A, et al. Thirty years of saying no: sources, fate, actions, and misfortunes of the endothelium-derived vasodilator mediator. *Circ Res*. 2016;119(2):375–396.
29. Loghmani H, Conway EM. Exploring traditional and nontraditional roles for thrombomodulin. *Blood*. 2018;132(2):148–158.
30. Leask A. Getting to the heart of the matter: new insights into cardiac fibrosis. *Circ Res*. 2015;116(7):1269–1276.
31. Martinelli I, De Stefano V, Mannucci PM. Inherited risk factors for venous thromboembolism. *Nat Rev Cardiol*. 2014;11(3):140–156.
32. Walton BL, Byrnes JR, Wolberg AS. Fibrinogen, red blood cells, and factor xiii in venous thrombosis. *J Thrombosis Haemostasis*. 2015;13 suppl 1S208-S15.
33. Cohen AT, Harrington RA, Goldhaber SZ, et al. Extended thromboprophylaxis with betrixaban in acutely ill medical patients. *N Engl J Med*. 2016;375(6):534–544.
34. Spyropoulos AC, Ageno W, Albers GW, et al. Rivaroxaban for thromboprophylaxis after hospitalization for medical illness. *N Engl J Med*. 2018;379(12):1118–1127.
35. Mahajan A, Brunson A, White R, et al. The epidemiology of cancer-associated venous thromboembolism: an update. *Semin Thromb Hemost*. 2019;45(4):321–325.
36. Hisada Y, Mackman N. Cancer-associated pathways and biomarkers of venous thrombosis. *Blood*. 2017;130(13):1499–1506.
37. Delluc A, Antic D, Lecumberri R, et al. Occult cancer screening in patients with venous thromboembolism: guidance from the SSC of the ISTH. *J Thromb Haemost*. 2017;15(10):2076–2079.

Treatment of Thrombosis

38. Yeung J, Li W, Holinstat M. Platelet signaling and disease: targeted therapy for thrombosis and other related diseases. *Pharmacol Rev*. 2018;70(3):526–548.
39. Dugani S, Ames JM, Manson JE, et al. Weighing the anti-ischemic benefits and bleeding risks from aspirin therapy: a rational approach. *Curr Atheroscler Rep*. 2018;20(3):15.
40. Raber I, McCarthy CP, Vaduganathan M, et al. The rise and fall of aspirin in the primary prevention of cardiovascular disease. *Lancet*. 2019;393(10186):2155–2167.
41. Wangberg H, White AA. Aspirin-exacerbated respiratory disease. *Curr Opin Immunol*. 2020.669-13.
42. Michelson AD, Bhatt DL. How I use laboratory monitoring of antiplatelet therapy. *Blood*. 2017;130(6):713–721.
43. Bhatt DL, Grosser T, Dong JF, et al. Enteric coating and aspirin nonresponsiveness in patients with type 2 diabetes mellitus. *J Am Coll Cardiol*. 2017;69(6):603–612.
44. Gurbel PA, Myat A, Kubica J, et al. State of the art: oral antiplatelet therapy. *JRSM Cardiovasc Dis*. 2016;520480004016652514.
45. Thomas MR, Storey RF. Clinical significance of residual platelet reactivity in patients treated with platelet p2y12 inhibitors. *Vascul Pharmacol*. 2016:8425–8427.
46. Sabatine MS, Mega JL. Pharmacogenomics of antiplatelet drugs. *Hematology Am Soc Hematol Educ Program*. 2014;(1):343–347.
47. Cuisset T, Quilici J. Cyp-mediated pharmacologic interference with optimal platelet inhibition. *J Cardiovasc Transl Res*. 2013;6(3):404–410.
48. Siller-Matula JM, Trenk D, Schror K, et al. How to improve the concept of individualised antiplatelet therapy with p2y12 receptor inhibitors–is an algorithm the answer? *Thromb Haemost*. 2015;113(1):37–52.
49. Pereira NL, Rihal CS, So DYF, et al. Clopidogrel pharmacogenetics. *Circ Cardiovasc Interv*. 2019;12(4):e007811.
50. Bhatt DL, Pollack CV, Weitz JI, et al. Antibody-based ticagrelor reversal agent in healthy volunteers. *N Engl J Med*. 2019;380(19):1825–1833.
51. Rollini F, Franchi F, Angiolillo DJ. Switching p2y12 receptor inhibiting therapies. *Interv Cardiol Clin*. 2017;6(1):67–89.
52. Kapil N, Datta YH, Alakbarova N, et al. Antiplatelet and anticoagulant therapies for prevention of ischemic stroke. *Clin Appl Thromb Hemost*. 2017;23(4):301–318.
53. Tantry US, Liu F, Chen G, et al. Vorapaxar in the secondary prevention of atherothrombosis. *Expert Rev Cardiovasc Ther*. 2015;13(12):1293–1305.
54. Chan NC, Weitz JI. Antithrombotic agents. *Circ Res*. 2019;124(3):426–436.
55. Mulloy B, Hogwood J, Gray E, et al. Pharmacology of heparin and related drugs. *Pharmacol Rev*. 2016;68(1):76–141.
56. Chandarajoti K, Liu J, Pawlinski R. The design and synthesis of new synthetic low-molecular-weight heparins. *J Thromb Haemost*. 2016;14(6):1135–1145.

1790

CARDIOVASCULAR DISEASE AND DISORDERS OF OTHER ORGANS

XI

57. Baluwala I, Favaloro EJ, Pasalic L. Therapeutic monitoring of unfractionated heparin - trials and tribulations. *Expert Rev Hematol.* 2017;10(7):595–605.
58. Piran S, Schulman S. Management of venous thromboembolism: an update. *Thromb J.* 2016;14(suppl 1):23.
59. Sokolowska E, Kalaska B, Miklosz J, et al. The toxicology of heparin reversal with protamine: past, present and future. *Expert Opin Drug Metab Toxicol.* 2016;12(8):897–909.
60. Greinacher A, Selleng K, Warkentin TE. Autoimmune heparin-induced thrombocytopenia. *J Thromb Haemost.* 2017;15(11):2099–2114.
61. Warkentin TE. Heparin-induced thrombocytopenia. *Curr Opin Crit Care.* 2015;21(6):576–585.
62. Signorelli SS, Scuto S, Marino E, et al. Anticoagulants and osteoporosis. *Int J Mol Sci.* 2019;20(21).
63. Spadarella G, Di Minno A, Donati MB, et al. From unfractionated heparin to pentasaccharide: Paradigm of rigorous science growing in the understanding of the in vivo thrombin generation. *Blood Rev.* 2020;39100613.
64. Babin JL, Traylor KL, Witt DM. Laboratory monitoring of low-molecular-weight heparin and fondaparinux. *Semin Thromb Hemost.* 2017;43(3):261–269.
65. van Es N, Bleker SM, Büller HR, et al. New developments in parenteral anticoagulation for arterial and venous thromboembolism. *Best Pract Res Clin Haematol.* 2013;26(2):203–213.
66. Mega JL, Simon T. Pharmacology of antithrombotic drugs: an assessment of oral antiplatelet and anticoagulant treatments. *Lancet.* 2015;386(9990):281–291.
67. Douketis JD. Navigating the anticoagulant landscape in 2017. *Cleveland Clin J Med.* 2017;84(10):768–778.
68. Fawzy AM, Lip GYH. Pharmacokinetics and pharmacodynamics of oral anticoagulants used in atrial fibrillation. *Expert Opin Drug Metab Toxicol.* 2019;15(5):381–398.
69. Dorgalaleh A, Favaloro EJ, Bahraini M, et al. Standardization of prothrombin time/international normalized ratio (PT/INR). *Int J Lab Hematol.* 2020.
70. Porter AL, Margolis AR, Staresinic CE, et al. Feasibility and safety of a 12-week inr follow-up protocol over 2 years in an anticoagulation clinic: a single-arm prospective cohort study. *J Thromb Thrombolysis.* 2019;47(2):200–208.
71. Milling TJ, Pollack CV. A review of guidelines on anticoagulation reversal across different clinical scenarios - is there a general consensus? *Am J Emerg Med.* 2020;38(9):1890–1903.
72. Dabiri G, Damstetter E, Chang Y, et al. Coagulation disorders and their cutaneous presentations: diagnostic work-up and treatment. *J Am Acad Dermatol.* 2016;74(5):795–804; quiz 805-6.
73. Warkentin TE, Greinacher A. Management of heparin-induced thrombocytopenia. *Curr Opin Hematol.* 2016;23(5):462–470.
74. Arachchillage DRJ, Laffan M. What is the appropriate anticoagulation strategy for thrombotic antiphospholipid syndrome? *Br J Haematol.* 2020;189(2):216–227.
75. Shaw JR, Kaplovitch E, Douketis J. Periprocedural management of oral anticoagulation. *Med Clin North Am.* 2020;104(4):709–726.
76. Anderson DR, Dunbar M, Murnaghan J, et al. Aspirin or rivaroxaban for vte prophylaxis after hip or knee arthroplasty. *N Engl J Med.* 2018;378(8):699–707.
77. Gosselin RC, Adcock DM. Douxfils J an update on laboratory assessment for direct oral anticoagulants (doacs). *Int J Lab Hematol.* 2019;41(S1):33–39.
78. Spyropoulos AC, Al-Badri A, Sherwood MW, et al. Periprocedural management of patients receiving a vitamin k antagonist or a direct oral anticoagulant requiring an elective procedure or surgery. *J Thromb Haemost.* 2016;14(5):875–885.
79. Siegal DM. Managing target-specific oral anticoagulant associated bleeding including an update on pharmacological reversal agents. *J Thromb Thrombolysis.* 2015;39(3):395–402.
80. Tomaselli GF, Mahaffey KW, Cuker A, et al. Acc expert consensus decision pathway on management of bleeding in patients on oral anticoagulants: a report of the American College of Cardiology Task Force on expert consensus decision pathways. *J Am Coll Cardiol.* 2017;70(24):3042–3067. 2017.
81. Shaw JR, Siegal DM. Pharmacological reversal of the direct oral anticoagulants-a comprehensive review of the literature. *Res Pract Thromb Haemost.* 2018;2(2):251–265.
82. Pollack Jr CV, Reilly PA, Eikelboom J, et al. Idarucizumab for dabigatran reversal. *N Engl J Med.* 2015;373(6):511–520.
83. Longstaff C, Kolev K. Basic mechanisms and regulation of fibrinolysis. *J Thrombosis Haemostasis.* 2015;13.suppl 1S98-105.
84. Verhamme IM, Panizzi PR, Bock PE. Pathogen activators of plasminogen. *J Thrombosis Haemostasis.* 2015;13 suppl 1S106-S14.
85. Khasa YP. The evolution of recombinant thrombolytics: current status and future directions. *Bioengineered.* 2017;8(4):331–358.
86. Matosevic B, Knoflach M, Werner P, et al. Fibrinogen degradation coagulopathy and bleeding complications after stroke thrombolysis. *Neurology.* 2013;80(13):1216–1224.

# 96 Endocrine Disorders and Cardiovascular Disease

BERNADETTE BIONDI

The endocrine system links tightly with many important cardiovascular diseases. As our understanding of the cellular and molecular effects of various hormones has evolved, we understand better the clinical manifestations that arise from excessive secretion of hormone and from glandular failure and subsequent hormone deficiency states.

This chapter reviews the spectrum of cardiac disease states that arise from changes in specific endocrine function. This approach allows us to explore the cellular mechanisms whereby various hormones can alter the cardiovascular system through actions on cardiac myocytes, vascular smooth muscle cells, and other target cells and tissues. In addition, this chapter discusses epidemiological studies and meta-analyses on cardiovascular morbidity and mortality associated with endocrine dysfunction to guide clinicians on the appropriate treatment of these patients.

PITUITARY HORMONES AND CARDIOVASCULAR DISEASE

The pituitary gland consists of two distinct anatomic portions. The anterior pituitary, or adenohypophysis, contains six different cell types; five of them produce polypeptide or glycoprotein hormones, and the sixth consists of nonsecretory chromophobic cells. The posterior pituitary, or neurohypophysis, is the anatomic location of the nerve terminals that secrete vasopressin (antidiuretic hormone) to control water balance or oxytocin, the milk letdown polypeptide.

Growth Hormone

The somatotropic cells secrete human growth hormone (hGH). Excessive secretion of hGH and insulin-like growth factor type 1 (IGF-1) by benign pituitary adenomas leads to the clinical syndrome of gigantism in youth before fusion of the bony epiphysis and to acromegaly in adults after maturation of the long bones.[1] hGH exerts its cellular effects through two major pathways. The first is by binding of the hormone to specific hGH receptors on target cells. Such receptors exist in the heart, skeletal muscle, fat, liver, and kidneys, as well as in many additional cell types throughout fetal development. The second growth-promoting effect of hGH results from stimulation of the synthesis of IGF-1. The liver produces the bulk of IGF-I, but other cell types can produce IGF-1 under the influence of hGH.[2] Shortly after identification

of the IGF family, this second messenger was thought to mediate most actions of hGH. The ability to promote glucose uptake and cellular protein synthesis gave rise to the term "insulin-like." IGF-1 binds to its cognate IGF-1 receptor, which localizes on almost all cell types. Genetic experiments have demonstrated that the presence of IGF-1 receptors on cell types links closely to the ability of these cells to divide. Studies in which the IGF-1 receptor was overexpressed in cardiac myocytes reportedly produced an increase in myocyte number and mitotic rate and enhanced the replication of post-differentiated myocytes.

Infusion of hGH or IGF-1 acutely changes cardiac function and hemodynamics. The acute increases in cardiac contractility and cardiac output may result, at least in part, from a decrease in systemic vascular resistance and left ventricular afterload.[3]

Cardiovascular Manifestations of Acromegaly

Acromegaly is a relatively uncommon condition with an annual incidence of 3 to 4 cases/million. Despite its rarity, this disorder is associated with markedly increased morbidity and mortality due to cardiovascular, respiratory, metabolic, and neoplastic complications, especially in undiagnosed and untreated patients.[4,5] The clinical disease activity of patients with an excess of hGH correlates better with serum levels of IGF-1 than with hGH concentrations.

About 60% of acromegalic patients develop cardiovascular disease. Hypertension, insulin resistance, diabetes mellitus, and hyperlipidemia represent the cardiovascular manifestations most frequently associated with acromegaly.[4,5] The Endocrine Society (ES) Clinical Practice Guidelines recommend that acromegalic patients undergo evaluation for associated comorbidities (hypertension, diabetes mellitus, cardiovascular disease, and sleep apnea).[6]

The cardiovascular and hemodynamic effects of acromegaly vary considerably depending on the patient's age and the disease's severity and duration. A specific acromegalic cardiomyopathy develops in patients with persistently increased secretion of hGH and IGF-1; this condition is characterized by a concentric biventricular hypertrophy, diastolic dysfunction, and mitral and aortic valve disease, and can occur even in the absence of cardiovascular risk factors.[3] The natural history of this specific cardiomyopathy has three phases.[3,7] The first phase typically develops in young patients with new onset acromegaly and involves a hyperkinetic syndrome with increased myocardial contractility and enhanced cardiac output. More evident hypertrophy usually develops during the second phase of cardiomyopathy which is associated with impaired diastolic filling and reduced cardiac performance during exercise. Impaired systolic function and low cardiac output progressively develop in the late phase of the disease in patients in whom acromegaly is undiagnosed or under-treated. Heart failure can complicate this late phase of the disease and portend a poor prognosis.[7] Hypertension, type 2 diabetes, and hyperlipidemia may further contribute to the impaired contractile function. Hypertension occurs with a mean prevalence of 33% to 46%, although the mechanism remains poorly understood. Administration of hGH promotes sodium retention and volume expansion while IGF-1 has a potent anti-natriuretic effect independent of any effect on aldosterone. Studies of the renin-angiotensin-aldosterone system have shown failure to inhibit release of renin optimally by volume expansion. Impaired glucose tolerance and diabetes mellitus are present in approximately 30% of acromegalic patients. Hyperlipidemia is principally characterized by hypertriglyceridemia and reduced high-density lipoprotein (HDL) cholesterol levels.

Acromegaly increases the prevalence of aortic and mitral valve disease. Patients with active acromegaly have a high prevalence of mitral and aortic abnormalities, which is higher in those with left ventricular hypertrophy. This condition can be considered one of the aspects of acromegalic cardiomyopathy because it is detectable even in young patients and in those with a short duration of the disease and can persist after treatment in cured patients. This persistence is likely to be correlated with the persistence of left ventricular hypertrophy and should be carefully monitored due to the risk of cardiac dysfunction. Progressive mitral regurgitation and increased left ventricular preload and afterload occur in patients with uncontrolled acromegaly. Patients with acromegaly can exhibit dilation of the aortic root, which is greater in men than in women. Left ventricular mass index is positively correlated with the diameter of the aorta, and patients with aortic ectasia usually have a greater left ventricular mass index than patients without this feature.

Although initial reports suggested that accelerated atherosclerosis impairs cardiac function in patients with longstanding acromegaly, a postmortem study revealed significant coronary artery disease in only 11% of patients dying of disease-related causes. Angiography showed normal or dilated coronary arteries in most cases. Fewer than 25% of the patients had positive nuclear stress tests, indicating that atherosclerosis and ischemic heart disease do not likely account for the marked degree of biventricular cardiac hypertrophy, cardiac failure, and cardiovascular mortality.

Abnormalities on the electrocardiogram (ECG), including left-axis deviation, septal Q waves, ST-T wave depression, abnormal QT dispersion, and conduction system defects, develop in up to 50% of patients with acromegaly. A variety of dysrhythmias can occur, including atrial and ventricular ectopic beats, sick sinus syndrome, and supraventricular and ventricular tachycardia.[8] Monitoring shows a fourfold increase in complex ventricular arrhythmias. Signal-averaged ECGs reveal a parallel rise late potential, a finding related to ventricular arrhythmia. Patients with active acromegaly more commonly show these electrophysiologic abnormalities than do treated patients. Patients with newly diagnosed, untreated acromegaly also manifest derangements in cardiac autonomic function, as measured by heart rate recovery and variability.

Acromegalic patients have an increased mortality compared to age- and gender-matched controls.[9] In uncontrolled acromegaly patients, the standardized mortality ratio (SMR) is significantly higher than the general population; however, mortality is strongly related to the disease control, which has normalized with the more frequent use of adjuvant therapy in the last decade.[9] In a 20-year follow-up study, the causes of death shifted from predominantly cardiovascular deaths (about 44%) during the first decade to predominantly cancer-related deaths in the next two decades.[10] Multiple studies have associated an increased risk of cancer of the gastrointestinal tract, colon, or lungs with this increased mortality.

Diagnosis

In 99% of the cases, acromegaly arises from benign adenomas of the anterior pituitary gland. At diagnosis most of these neoplasms are classified as macroadenomas (>10 mm), and patients have historical clinical evidence of having had the disease for longer than 10 years. The biochemical diagnosis of acromegaly depends on demonstrating elevated serum IGF-1 levels and lack of suppression of hGH to less than 1 μg/L following an oral glucose load.[6] Localization of the tumor occurs through magnetic resonance imaging (MRI) of the pituitary gland or computed tomographic (CT) scan when MRI is contraindicated or unavailable.

TREATMENT

Treatment aims to control tumor growth and normalize serum hGH and IGF-1 to reduce the risk of premature mortality and improve the quality of life.[11] Medical therapies include various options ranging from somatostatin analogs (SSAs) and somatostatin receptor ligands (SRLs) to GH, receptor antagonist pegvisomant, and dopamine agonists.[6,11] Pasireotide long-acting release (LAR), a long-acting somatostatin multireceptor ligand, can normalize IGF-1 in acromegalic patients who cannot be controlled with available SRLs; however, hyperglycemia develops in approximately half of the patients.[6,11]

Trans-sphenoidal surgery with resection of the adenoma cures about 50% to 70% of patients. Pre-operative medical therapy with SRLs is recommended to reduce surgical risk in patients with heart failure or severe comorbidities.[6,11]

The cardiovascular complications of acromegaly usually improve with disease modifying treatment and survival increases significantly in patients achieving disease remission, defined as the normalization of serum IGF-1 and serum hGH less than 1 μg/L.[6] hGH and/or IGF-1 levels that remain elevated after surgery mandate medical therapy.[6] Residual tumor mass following surgery may require radiotherapy if medical therapy is unavailable, unsuccessful, or not tolerated.[6] Cardiomyopathy, hypertension, valvular disease, and arrhythmias are the major causes of disease-associated morbidity and mortality. Surgery and medical treatment can all improve left ventricular hypertrophy and arrhythmias in patients who achieve biochemical control during treatment. Hyperglycemia, hypertension, and dyslipidemia should be treated promptly according to standard care. In the presence of a clinically relevant residual tumor that is unsuitable for resection, patients should be switched to pasireotide LAR or pegvisomant, in relation to the glycemia control.[6] Baseline fasting plasma glucose levels could help predict the onset of hyperglycemia during treatment with pegvisomant.

Growth Hormone Deficiency

hGH has an important role in the development of the normal heart and the maintenance of normal structure and function in the adult life. Children with untreated growth hormone deficiency (GHD) have an impaired cardiac structure, body composition, and cardiopulmonary functional capacity which can be restored after GH replacement therapy.[12] Even untreated adults with hGH deficiency have cardiac and endothelial dysfunction, insulin resistance, deranged lipid profile, increased carotid intima-media-thickness, elevated inflammatory markers, increased body fat with abdominal obesity, hypercoagulability, and decreased skeletal muscle mass and strength.[13] Early premature atherosclerosis can develop in hypopituitaric patients not receiving hGH therapy so that GH therapy should be continued after achieving adult height in patients with persistent growth hormone deficiency. Patients with untreated hypopituitarism have a doubled overall mortality, principally due to increased CV mortality.[14] Several reports have documented low IGF-1 levels as well as a blunted response to hypothalamic growth hormone-releasing hormone (GHRH) in patients with congestive heart failure (CHF) and severe LV dysfunction.[3,15] GH deficiency can be detected in about 30% of patients with CHF and is associated with an impaired LV remodeling.[3] A low IGF-1/GH ratio and high NT-proBNP levels were independent predictors of death in HF patients without cachexia, suggesting that low IGF-1 circulating levels in CHF can be linked to a progression of the disease, which GH replacement therapy is able to delay.[15] Treatment with recombinant human replacement therapy can have beneficial effects in patients with CHF (due to either ischemic or idiopathic dilated cardiomyopathy) with a coexisting GH deficiency.[16]

Prolactin Disease

The most common disorder of the anterior pituitary gland is small (<1.0 cm), prolactin-producing pituitary adenomas causing amenorrhea and galactorrhea. Prolactin plays a well-recognized stimulatory role in inflammation; prolactin receptors were localized in human coronary artery plaques, suggesting that prolactin might influence atherogenesis. Because hypothalamic dopamine normally inhibits prolactin secretion, dopamine agonists such as cabergoline and bromocriptine are first-line treatments. Patients with prolactinoma can have an unfavorable cardiovascular and metabolic risk profile. A decreased hypothalamic dopaminergic tone is involved in the pathogenesis of insulin resistance, while an increase in dopaminergic neurotransmission reduces food intake and induces energy expenditure. Moreover, suppression of dopaminergic tone is responsible for weight gain and metabolic abnormalities because the dopamine receptor type 2 is abundantly expressed on human pancreatic beta-cell and adipocytes, suggesting a regulatory role for peripheral dopamine in insulin and adipose functions. Exposure of pancreatic islet to prolactin (PRL) is known to stimulate insulin secretion and beta-cell proliferation. Medical treatment with dopamine-agonists (bromocriptine and cabergoline) can improve insulin resistance and metabolic abnormalities.[17] In a recent prospective study, a 5-mg/dL increment in prolactin was associated with increased odds of incidence of diabetes and hypertension.[18]

Treatment with low-dose cabergoline in hyperprolactinemia has been associated with an increased prevalence of tricuspid regurgitation in a recent meta-analysis.[19] Although the clinical significance of this finding has not been established, a complete echocardiographic evaluation could be indicated in patients treated with elevated doses of cabergoline, particularly for a long period.

ADRENAL HORMONES AND CARDIOVASCULAR DISEASE

Adrenocorticotropic Hormone and Cortisol

The adrenocorticotropic cells in the anterior pituitary synthesize a large protein (pro-opiomelanocortin), which is then processed within the corticotropic cell into a family of smaller proteins that include adrenocorticotrophic hormone (ACTH). The adrenal cortex zona glomerulosa produces aldosterone, and the zona fasciculata produces primarily cortisol and some androgenic steroids. The zona reticularis

produces cortisol and androgens as well. ACTH regulates the synthesis of cortisol in both the zona fasciculata and reticularis.

Cushing Disease and Cushing Syndrome

Cushing syndrome results from prolonged and inappropriately high exposure of tissues to glucocorticoids.[20] Excessive cortisol secretion and its attendant clinical disease state can arise from excessive release of ACTH by the pituitary (Cushing disease) or through the adenomatous or rarely malignant neoplastic process arising in the adrenal gland itself (Cushing syndrome).[21] Well-characterized conditions of adrenal glucocorticoid and mineralocorticoid excess appear to result from the excessively high levels of (ectopic) ACTH produced by small cell carcinoma of the lung, carcinoid tumors, pancreatic islet cell tumors, medullary thyroid cancer, and other adenocarcinomas and hematologic malignancies.[20] Clinical signs and symptoms of Cushing syndrome often develop in patients treated with exogenous steroids at doses equivalent to 20 mg of prednisone daily for more than 1 month. Cortisol, a member of the glucocorticoid family of steroid hormones, binds to receptors located within the cytoplasm of many cell types (Fig. 96.1). After binding cortisol these receptors translocate to the nucleus and function as transcription factors. Several cardiac genes contain glucocorticoid response elements in their promoter regions that confer transcriptional-level glucocorticoid responsiveness. Such genes include those that encode voltage-gated potassium channels, as well as protein kinases, which serve to phosphorylate and regulate the voltage-gated sodium channels. In addition, there are more rapidly acting, nontranscriptional pathways by which cortisol may regulate the activity of voltage-gated potassium channels.

Patients with Cushing disease can exhibit a variety of electrocardiographic changes. The duration of the PR interval appears to correlate inversely with adrenal cortisol production rates. The mechanism underlying this correlation may be related to the expression or regulation of the voltage-gated sodium channel (SCN5A). Changes in the ECG, specifically in the PR and QT intervals, may also arise from the direct (nongenomic) effects of glucocorticoids on the voltage-gated potassium channel (Kv1.5) in excitable tissues.

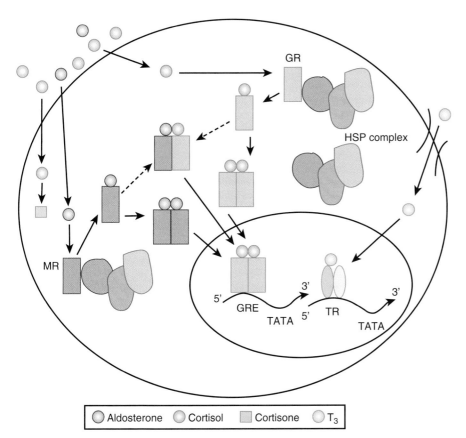

FIGURE 96.1 Generalized mechanism of action of the nuclear hormone receptor. The mineralocorticoid receptor (MR) has similar affinities for aldosterone and cortisol. Circulating levels of cortisol are 100 to 1000 times greater than those of aldosterone. In MR-responsive cells, the enzyme 11-beta-hydroxysteroid dehydrogenase metabolizes cortisol to cortisone, thereby allowing aldosterone to bind to the MR. The MR and glucocorticoid receptor (GR) are cytoplasmic receptors that after binding ligand, translocate to the nucleus and bind to glucocorticoid response elements (GREs) in the promoter regions of responsive genes. Triiodothyronine (T_3) is transported into the cell via specific membrane proteins and binds to thyroid hormone receptors (TRs), which are bound to thyroid hormone response elements in the promoter regions of T_3-responsive genes. *HSP*, heat shock protein; *TATA*, TATA box promoter region. (Courtesy Dr. S. Danzi.)

The cardiac effects of Cushing syndrome arise from the effects of glucocorticoids on the heart, liver, skeletal muscle, and fat tissue. The interaction between high cortisol levels and active mineralocorticoid receptor (MR) in cardiomyocytes induces cardiac remodeling and fibrosis, ventricular remodeling, and an impairment of relaxation.[21] It can also stimulate the expression of several pro-inflammatory and adhesion molecules, leading to increased myocardial stiffness and contractile dysfunction. Cortisol-mediated hypertension has multiple mechanisms in patients with Cushing[22]; cardiac structural and functional alterations are more severe in hypertensive patients, suggesting an interaction between the deleterious effects of hypertension and cortisol excess. Chronic cortisol hypersecretion can also cause central obesity, insulin resistance, dyslipidemia, a prothrombotic state, and metabolic syndrome. The prevalence of diabetes mellitus ranges between 18% and 30%.

A two- to fourfold increase in mortality has been reported in Cushing syndrome compared with the general population. This increased cardiovascular morbidity and mortality is largely due to cerebrovascular, peripheral vascular, and coronary artery disease, and CHF.[23–25] The cardiovascular risk may persist even after restoration of eucortisolaemia.[25] Recent evidence suggests an impaired cardiovascular profile even in patients with subclinical Cushing syndrome when compared with the general population; this condition is characterized by an incomplete post-dexamethasone cortisol suppression and adrenal incidentalomas.[26]

Diagnosis

The diagnosis of Cushing disease and Cushing syndrome requires the demonstration of increased cortisol production as reflected by an elevated 24-hour urinary free cortisol or nocturnal salivary cortisol level. ACTH measurement allows assessment of whether the disease is pituitary-, adrenal-, or ectopically based. An abnormal dexamethasone suppression test and a corticotropin-releasing hormone (CRH) test can help establish the cause of Cushing syndrome. Anatomic localization of the suspected lesions using MRI helps confirm laboratory findings.

TREATMENT

Treatment of excessive cortisol production depends on the underlying mechanisms.[27] Initial resection of primary lesion(s) is recommended for underlying Cushing disease (based in the pituitary) and also for Cushing disease related to ectopic and adrenal causes. Trans-sphenoidal selective adenomectomy with or without postoperative radiation therapy can partially or completely reverse the increased ACTH production by the anterior pituitary. Cushing syndrome requires surgical removal of one (adrenal adenoma, adrenal carcinoma) or both (multiple nodular) adrenal glands. Immediately after surgery, cortisol and mineralocorticoid (fludrocortisone [FST]) need to be replaced to prevent adrenal insufficiency.

Drug therapy before or after surgery can help control persistent cortisol production.[27] Pasireotide can decrease ACTH production from a pituitary tumor. The adrenal enzyme inhibitor ketoconazole may be used alone or in combination with metyrapone to enhance control of severe hypercortisolemia. Mitotane is used primarily to treat adrenal carcinoma. Mifepristone is approved in the United States for people with Cushing syndrome who have type 2 diabetes or glucose intolerance. This drug blocks the direct effect of cortisol on tissues and leads to an improvement in hypertension and/or diabetes in 40% to 60% of patients. Etomidate is useful where immediate parenteral action is required and in seriously ill patients who cannot take oral medications. The goal of therapy is the clinical normalization of cortisol levels.[27]

Primary Hyperaldosteronism

Primary hyperaldosteronism (PA) (see also Chapter 26) refers to a group of disorders in which aldosterone production is inappropriately high, relatively autonomous from the major regulators of secretion (angiotensin II and plasma potassium concentration), and non-suppressible by sodium loading.[28,29] It is the most common cause of secondary hypertension, with a prevalence of 20% in patients with resistant hypertension and 10% in those with severe hypertension.[30,31] Hypokalemia in the setting of hypertension should induce a prompt consideration of PA, although most patients with PA are not hypokalemic.[32] Common causes of PA include an adrenal adenoma, unilateral or bilateral adrenal hyperplasia, or, in rare cases, an adrenal carcinoma or an inherited condition: glucocorticoid-remediable aldosteronism (GRA).[28]

Aldosterone's mechanism of action on target tissues resembles that reported for glucocorticoids (see Fig. 96.1). Aldosterone enters cells and binds to the MR, which then translocates to the nucleus and promotes the expression of aldosterone-responsive genes. In addition to kidney cells, in which MRs control sodium transport, in vitro studies on rats have located these receptors in cardiac myocytes. MR is also expressed in vascular smooth muscle cells, endothelial cells, cells within brown adipose tissue, macrophages, and neurons in several brain regions.

In humans, primary aldosteronism causes cardiovascular damage; it can induce development of cardiac hypertrophy, myocardial fibrosis, diastolic dysfunction, and heart failure.[33,34] Stroke, nonfatal myocardial infarction, or atrial fibrillation are more frequent among patients with PA compared with patients with primary hypertension. Patients with PA also have an increased prevalence of metabolic syndrome and diabetes. Death resulting from cardiovascular causes is more common among patients with PA compared with matched control patients with primary hypertension. Fibrosis of the heart, adrenal glands, pancreas, and lungs has been found in autoptic studies in patients with PA.

In light of the cardiorenal and cerebrovascular implications stemming from an unrecognized and untreated PA, early diagnosis and screening are imperative. Primary aldosteronism should be investigated in patients with: (1) severe hypertension, systolic blood pressure ≥180, and diastolic blood pressure ≥110 mm Hg; (2) treatment-resistant hypertension (an office SBP/diastolic blood pressure ≥130/80 mm Hg and prescription of ≥3 antihypertensive medications at optimal doses, including a diuretic or an office SBP/diastolic blood pressure less than 130/80 mm Hg for a patient requiring ≥4 antihypertensive medications); (3) hypertension with spontaneous or diuretic-induced hypokalemia; (4) hypertension with incidentally discovered adrenal tumors; (5) hypertension and sleep apnea; (6) family history of early-onset hypertension or cerebrovascular accident at a young age (<40 years) (Table 96.1).[24,31]

Diagnosis

Plasma aldosterone/renin ratio detects possible PA.[28,31] Patients should have unrestricted dietary salt intake before testing and should be potassium replete. MR antagonists should be withdrawn for at least 4 weeks before testing, especially in patients with mild hypertension; for other drugs (beta-blockers, clonidine, methyldopa, non-steroidal anti-inflammatory drugs, ACE inhibitors, angiotensin receptor blockers, and dihydropyridine calcium blockers) a 2-week withdrawal should be sufficient. Correction of hypokalemia before testing is recommended. An aldosterone-to-renin ratio (ARR) greater than 20 is commonly used as the threshold for positive PA screening, with a sensitivity of 78% and a specificity of 83% in study participants with resistant hypertension.[28] Patients with an abnormal aldosterone/renin ratio undergo one or more confirmatory tests to definitively confirm or exclude the diagnosis.[28] The most commonly used suppression tests use saline loading (either by intravenous infusion or orally), FST, or a captopril challenge.

TABLE 96.1 Patients With a High Risk of Hyperaldosteronism[26,29]

- Severe hypertension: systolic blood pressure ≥180 and diastolic blood pressure ≥110 mm Hg
- Treatment-resistant hypertension
  - Office SBP/diastolic blood pressure ≥130/80 mm Hg and prescription of ≥3 antihypertensive medications at optimal doses, including a diuretic
  - Office SBP/diastolic blood pressure <130/80 mm Hg or prescription of ≥4 antihypertensive medications
- Hypertension with spontaneous or diuretic-induced hypokalemia
- Hypertension with adrenal incidentaloma
- Hypertension and sleep apnea
- Family history of early-onset hypertension or cerebrovascular accident at a young age (<40 years)

Caution should be used when performing confirmatory tests and hypokalemia, if present, should be corrected.

All patients with suspected disease should undergo adrenal CT to search for adrenocortical carcinoma,[28] although the value of CT scanning and MRI are debated because they cannot identify the source of aldosterone excess and micro-APAs (≤10 mm in diameter) are often undetectable by current imaging methods. Therefore, the available guidelines recommend performing adrenal venous sampling (AVS) before surgery to distinguish between unilateral and bilateral adrenal disease. Steroid profiling of adrenal vein and peripheral serum samples can distinguish between adenoma and hyperplasia; peripheral plasma 18-oxocortisol is higher in patients with adenoma than in those with bilateral hyperplasia, whereas cortisol, corticosterone, and dehydroepiandrosterone are lower.[35,36]

TREATMENT (See Also Chapters 26, 50, and 51)

Patients with PA and hypokalemia should receive slow-release potassium chloride supplementation to maintain plasma potassium.[28,31] The aldosterone antagonists, spironolactone or eplerenone (as a second choice) should be used to control hypertension, hypokalemia, and the deleterious CV effects of aldosterone hypersecretion.[28] Gynecomastia and sexual dysfunction can develop in 30% of cases in men; in these cases eplerenone can be used.[28] Close monitoring of electrolytes is essential when MR antagonists are used. Surgical treatment is practicable in young patients (<35 years) with spontaneous hypokalemia, marked aldosterone excess, and unilateral adrenal lesions with evidence of a cortical adenoma on adrenal CT.[28] Unilateral laparoscopic adrenalectomy can cure hypokalemia and improve or cure hypertension in such patients, lowering the risk of incidental CHF and all-cause mortality in a long-term follow-up.[37] Patients with a bilateral disease and those reluctant to undergo surgery should receive medical treatment with MR antagonists. In patients with GRA, low doses of glucocorticoid to lower ACTH and normalize BP and potassium levels represent the first-line treatment. In addition, if BP fails to normalize with glucocorticoid alone, an MR antagonist can be added.

Addison Disease

Primary adrenal insufficiency occurs when the adrenal cortex cannot produce sufficient glucocorticoids and/or mineralocorticoids.[38] Primary adrenal insufficiency arises most commonly from bilateral loss of adrenal function on an autoimmune basis; as a result of infection, hemorrhage, or metastatic malignancy; or in selected cases, from inborn errors of steroid hormone metabolism.[38] Addison disease can manifest itself at any age; it may be associated with other autoimmune disorders (e.g., Hashimoto thyroiditis, type 1 diabetes mellitus, autoimmune gastritis/pernicious anemia, and vitiligo). In contrast, secondary adrenal insufficiency, which results from pituitary-dependent loss of ACTH secretion, leads to a fall in glucocorticoid production, whereas mineralocorticoid production, including aldosterone, remains at relatively normal levels.

The non-cardiac symptoms—including increased pigmentation, abdominal pain with nausea and vomiting, hypoglycemia, and weight loss can be chronic, but tachycardia, hypotension, hyponatremia, hyperkalemia, loss of autonomic tone, cardiovascular collapse, and crisis may develop especially in acutely ill or untreated patients with Addison disease. Delayed treatment of more severe symptoms is likely to increase morbidity and mortality.

Laboratory findings (hyponatremia and hyperkalemia) indicate loss of aldosterone production (high renin levels).[39]

Hyperkalemia can alter findings on the ECG by producing low-amplitude P waves and peaked T waves. Blood pressure measurements uniformly show low diastolic pressure (<60 mm Hg) along with orthostatic changes that reflect loss of volume and acquired autonomic dysfunction. Patients with newly diagnosed, untreated Addison disease have reduced left ventricular end-systolic and end-diastolic dimensions in comparison to controls.

Diagnosis

Acute adrenal insufficiency characteristically occurs in the setting of acute stress, infection, or trauma in patients with chronic autoimmune adrenal insufficiency or in children with congenital abnormalities in cortisol metabolism. It can also develop as a result of bilateral adrenal hemorrhage in patients with severe systemic infection or diffuse intravascular coagulation. Secondary adrenal insufficiency can occur in the setting of hypopituitarism and is usually chronic, but acute changes caused by pituitary hemorrhage (apoplexy) or pituitary inflammation (lymphocytic hypophysitis) can also occur. Acute adrenal insufficiency can develop in patients treated with long-term suppressive doses of corticosteroids (>10 mg of prednisone for more than 1 month) if treatment is stopped precipitously or if an acute severe non–endocrine-related illness arises.

The diagnostic criteria include low cortisol levels (morning cortisol < 140 nmol/L [<5 μg/dL]) or when cortisol levels fail to rise above 500 nmol/L (20 μg /dL) 30 or 60 minutes after an intravenous injection of 250 μg of corticotropin.[39] The simultaneous measurement of plasma renin and aldosterone can help determine mineralocorticoid deficiency.

Treatment

Management of acute Addisonian crisis requires an adequate hydrocortisone replacement therapy (100 mg given as an initial IV bolus, then 100 mg every 8 to 12 hours for the first 24 hours, and tapering of the dose over the next 72 to 96 hours). Large volumes of normal saline with 5% dextrose can help address the intravascular fluid deficit. Potential underlying precipitating causes (including infection, acute cardiac or cerebral ischemia, or intra-abdominal emergency) require identification and treatment. Long-term treatment of adrenal insufficiency consists of oral corticosteroid therapy (hydrocortisone 20 mg) in two divided oral doses per day or prednisone (5 mg/day) administered orally once or twice daily.[39] A dual-release hydrocortisone preparation could be used, when possible, to mimic the cortisol circadian rhythm. Patients with confirmed aldosterone deficiency should receive mineralocorticoid replacement with fluorohydrocortisone (starting dose, 50 to 100 μg in adults). Diuretics and aldosterone antagonists such as spironolactone or eplerenone should be avoided.

PHEOCHROMOCYTOMA AND PARAGANGLIOMA

Pheochromocytomas (PCCs) and paragangliomas (PGLs), also named PPGLs, are tumors arising from neuroectodermal chromaffin cell in adrenal medulla or extra-adrenal paraganglia (see Chapter 26).[40,41] The 2017 WHO classification of adrenal tumors established anatomic criteria for PPGL classification and distinguished between PCCs originating from the adrenal medulla and PGLs originating from extra-adrenal paraganglia.[42] PGLs can be further divided according to clinical and biological behavior into: head and neck PGLs (HNPGLs) that originate from parasympathetic paraganglia and are characterized by a lack of catecholamine secretion, and sympathetic PGLs that originate from sympathetic paraganglia and are biochemically positive.[40–42] Head and neck PGLs are often multifocal, bilateral, sometimes recurrent, and rarely malignant (<5%). Sympathetic PGLs can be found everywhere from the skull base to the pelvic region, even though approximately 85% are located below the diaphragm. Metastatic disease is defined by the presence of PPGLs in nonchromaffin organs and occurs in about 5% to 20% of PCCs and 15% to 35% of sympathetic PGLs.[40]

Different familial autosomal dominant diseases have been identified: neurofibromatosis type 1 (NF1), multiple endocrine neoplasia type 2 (MEN2), von Hippel-Lindau (VHL) syndrome, and Carney triad (PGL, gastric stromal tumors, pulmonary chondromas).[43] When pheochromocytoma coexists with medullary thyroid carcinoma or occasionally with hyperparathyroidism, it is designated as MEN syndrome type 2A. In patients with MEN 2B, pheochromocytoma coexists with medullary thyroid cancer and with mucosal neuromas frequently seen on the lips and tongue. TMEM 127 encoding transmembrane protein 127 has been identified as a new susceptibility gene for PCC.[40,45] These patients have a malignancy rate less than 5% and adrenal catecholamine secreting PCC; bilateral PCCs can develop in a third of patients and rare cases of patients with extra-adrenal abdominal PGL and head and neck PGL have also been reported.[40] Myc-associated factor

X (MAX) adrenal tumors are bilateral in 67% of the cases and have malignant behavior in 25%.[40,45]

PPGLs are expected to have succinate dehydrogenase (SDHx) or fumarate hydratase (FH) mutations. About 22% to 70% PPGLs are caused by a single driver germ line mutation in SDHA, SDHB, SDHC, SDHD, and SDHAF2. SDHB-associated tumors can be malignant in more than 30% of the cases.[40] Succinate dehydrogenase gene A (SDHA) mutated paragangliomas PGL may be at high risk of metastases.[44] Next-generation sequencing (NGS) technology could be appropriate for carrying out genetic screening of these individuals.[46]

Clinical manifestations of pheochromocytoma include headache, palpitations, excessive sweating, tremulousness, chest pain, weight loss, and a variety of other constitutional complaints. Hypertension may be sustained or episodic but is usually constant and is paradoxically associated with orthostatic hypotension on arising in the morning. The paroxysmal attacks and classic symptoms result from episodic excessive catecholamine secretion. However, a small, but significant proportion of patients with pheochromocytoma are normotensive. Another rare sign can be the onset of diabetes in younger patients without typical risk factors for diabetes. Hypertensive crises can be induced after accidental tumor manipulation or during anesthesia. As a result of the release of norepinephrine and an increase in systemic vascular resistance, cardiac output is minimally (if at all) increased despite increases in the heart rate. The ECG can show left ventricular hypertrophy (LVH), as well as repolarization abnormalities, findings suggesting left ventricular strain. Although ventricular and atrial ectopy and episodes of supraventricular tachycardia can occur, little distinguishes the LVH from that of essential hypertension.

Patients with sympathetic PPGLs have a higher incidence of cardiovascular events before diagnosis. Impaired left ventricular function and cardiomyopathy can occur in patients with pheochromocytoma. The mechanism underlying this condition is complex and includes increased left ventricular work and LVH from associated hypertension; potential adverse effects of catecholamine excess on myocyte structure and contractility; and changes in coronary arteries, including thickening of the media, which presumably impairs blood flow to the myocardium. Patients with previously diagnosed or undiagnosed disease can show histologic evidence of myocarditis postmortem. The possibility of catecholamine-stimulated tachycardia in turn mediating left ventricular dysfunction should be addressed because treatments designed to slow the heart rate may improve the left ventricular function. Life-threatening cardiovascular manifestations of pheochromocytoma primarily result from hypertensive emergencies, abnormality of cardiac rhythm, and serious ventricular arrhythmias or conduction disturbances. Reversible dilated hypertrophic cardiomyopathy and Takotsubo cardiomyopathy are well established cardiac manifestations of pheochromocytoma. Rarely, pheochromocytoma can arise within the heart, presumably from chromaffin cells, which are part of the adrenergic autonomic paraganglia.

Diagnosis

An increase in norepinephrine, epinephrine, or its metabolites in serum or blood is essential for the diagnosis. Quantitative 24-hour urinary fractionated metanephrine levels are the most reliable screening indicators; they provide a sensitivity of 97% and a specificity of 91%.[43] There are at least four principal secretory profiles in PPGL: adrenergic, noradrenergic, dopaminergic, and silent. PCC and sympathetic PGL usually synthesize and secrete norepinephrine and/or epinephrine, while 23% of parasympathetic paraganglia-derived tumors secrete only dopamine.[40] Chromogranin A can be a useful biomarker in silent PPGLs and for monitoring the disease. Increased plasma levels of methoxytyramine (product of dopamine degradation) could discriminate patients with SDHx mutations and predict malignancy.[40] Interfering medications (anti-depressants, some anti-hypertensives, and other medications) and several foods which can cause false-positive elevations of these markers should be ruled out before testing patients with known or suspected PPGL. CT is the first-choice imaging modality because of its excellent spatial resolution for thorax, abdomen, and pelvis. MRI is recommended in patients with metastatic disease and

for detection of skull base and neck PGL.[131] I-metaiodobenzylguanidine can localize catecholamine-producing lesions.[123] MIBG SPECT/MRI has the highest sensitivity for adrenal PHEOs. 18F-fluorodeoxyglucose positron emission tomography scanning can visualize metastatic disease. FDOPA is extremely sensitive for patients with head/neck PGLs and particularly useful for patients with SDH mutations and/or biochemically silent PHEO/PGL. Promising results have been found with radiolabeled DOTA peptides (DOTATATE, DOTATOC, and DOTANOC), which target somatostatin receptors on the cell membrane; this tracer is superior to FDOPA PET/CT in the diagnosis of metastatic tumors.[47]

TREATMENT

Definitive treatment of pheochromocytoma requires removal of the lesion.[39] Accurate preoperative localization reduces operative mortality and eliminates the need for exploratory laparotomy. Endoscopic procedures are now standard for small tumors and open resection is indicated for large tumors (e.g., >6 cm) or invasive PCC.[41]

Preoperative pharmacologic treatment should be provided to prevent perioperative cardiovascular complications.[41] It includes 7 to 14 days of alpha-adrenergic blockade (usually with doxazosin, prazosin, or phenoxybenzamine) to normalize blood pressure. Beta-blocking drugs can normalize heart rate but should follow establishment of sufficient alpha blockade. Before surgical treatment, a high-sodium diet and fluid intake should be started to improve blood volume contraction and prevent severe hypotension after tumor removal. Operative intervention requires constant blood pressure monitoring, and intravenous phentolamine or sodium nitroprusside may be required to treat episodic hypertension intraoperatively.[41] Gauges of the success of surgery include effective blood pressure and symptom improvement, as well as measurement of urinary catecholamines 4 weeks after the procedure. Lifelong annual biochemical testing to assess for recurrent or metastatic disease is necessary.

PARATHYROID HORMONE AND CARDIOVASCULAR DISEASE

Diseases of the parathyroid glands can alter the cardiac function through two mechanisms. Parathyroid hormone (PTH), a protein hormone, can itself affect the heart, vascular smooth muscle cells, and endothelial cells. PTH-induced changes in serum calcium levels can also affect the cardiovascular system.[48]

PTH can bind to its receptor and alter the spontaneous beating rate of neonatal cardiac myocytes through an increase in intracellular cyclic adenosine monophosphate (cAMP). PTH can also alter calcium influx and cardiac contractility in adult cardiac myocytes and relaxation of vascular smooth muscle cells. Moreover, a variety of tissues, including cardiac myocytes produce the structurally related PTH-related peptide (PTHrP). PTHrP can bind to the PTH receptor on cardiac cells and stimulate accumulation of cAMP and contractile activity, as well as regulate L-type calcium currents. Long-term treatment with the recombinant human PTH may require monitoring for adverse cardiac effects.

Hyperparathyroidism

In primary hyperparathyroidism (PHPT) hypercalcemia (or high-normal serum calcium levels) occurs in presence of inappropriately normal or elevated PTH concentrations because of an overproduction of PTH. PHPT most often results from adenomatous enlargement of one of the four parathyroid glands.[48] Cardiovascular actions of hypercalcemia include increased cardiac contractility, shortening of the ventricular action potential duration (primarily through changes in phase 2), and blunting of the T wave and changes in the ST segment, occasionally suggesting cardiac ischemia. The QT interval shortens and occasionally the PR interval decreases. Treatment with digitalis glycosides appears to increase sensitivity of the heart to hypercalcemia. Increased PTH levels are associated with an increased risk of incident hypertension.[49] Patients with PHPT generally maintain normal left ventricular systolic function, but severe or chronic disease may impair diastolic function. Changes in left ventricular structure and function can improve after successful parathyroid surgery; higher preoperative PTH levels have been associated with greater improvements.[50] Even patients with normocalcemic PHPT have a higher risk of high blood pressure than subjects with normal PTH.[51]

Excess PTH (as seen in primary and secondary hyperparathyroidism) is associated with a higher incidence of hypertension, left ventricular hypertrophy, heart failure, cardiac arrhythmias, and valvular calcific disease, which may contribute to higher cardiac morbidity and mortality.[52,53] Several observational and population studies have discovered an association between elevated PTH and HF. This relationship may be attributed to the direct effects of PTH on cardiac myocytes, endothelial cells, and vascular smooth muscles. HF is an important predictor of cardiac morbidity and mortality, and there is increasing evidence that elevated PTH levels are an independent risk factor for incident HF.[52]

Hypercalcemia may lead to pathological changes in the heart, including the myocardial interstitium, and conducting systemic as well as calcific deposits in the valve cusps, annuli, and possibly coronary arteries. Although initially observed in fairly longstanding and severe hypercalcemia, so-called metastatic calcifications can also occur in secondary parathyroid disease arising from chronic renal failure, in which the serum calcium-phosphorus product constant is exceeded.

Diagnosis

A simultaneous increase in serum immunoreactive PTH (best represented by the intact PTH assay) with elevation of the serum calcium level establishes the diagnosis of PHPT. Other causes of hypercalcemia include malignancy with an increased level of PTHrP or hypercalcemia arising directly from bony metastases or neoplastic (lymphoma) or non-neoplastic disease (e.g., sarcoidosis) leading to an increase in the synthesis and release of 1,25-dihydroxyvitamin D_3.

TREATMENT
Treatment of hyperparathyroidism is the surgical removal of the parathyroid adenoma.[48] Calcimimetic medications (cinacalcet) can lower PTH concentrations and normalize serum calcium levels. Asymptomatic PHPT, routinely encountered in clinical endocrinology practice, may not require definitive treatment.

Hypocalcemia

Low serum levels of total and ionized calcium directly alter myocyte function. Hypocalcemia prolongs phase 2 of the action potential duration and the QT interval. Severe hypocalcemia can impair cardiac contractility and give rise to a diffuse musculoskeletal syndrome consisting of tetany and rhabdomyolysis. Primary hypoparathyroidism is rare and can develop after surgical removal of the parathyroid glands, as may occur after treatment of thyroid cancer, in the setting of polyglandular dysfunction syndromes, as a result of glandular agenesis (DiGeorge) syndrome, and in the rare heritable pseudohypoparathyroidism disorder. Recombinant human PTH offers a treatment option.[53]

Chronic renal failure is the most common cause of low serum calcium and high PTH levels. In patients suffering from such a condition, the effects of chronically high levels of PTH (secondary hyperparathyroidism) on the heart and cardiovascular system may be both causative and serve as a biomarker in assessing heart failure treatment strategies. In older adult patients with progression of aortic stenosis, a rise in serum PTH and bone remodeling occurs. The ability of PTH to stimulate G protein–coupled receptors may impair myocyte contractility and contribute to LVH. Cinacalcet can treat the secondary hyperparathyroidism associated with chronic renal failure.

Vitamin D

Most body tissues and cells express the vitamin D receptor. 1,25(OH)2D has a wide range of biological actions, including inhibiting cellular proliferation and inducing terminal differentiation, inhibiting angiogenesis, stimulating insulin production, and inhibiting renin production. Observational evidence suggests that lower levels of vitamin D are associated with an increased all-cause and cardiovascular morbidity. Vitamin D deficiency can contribute to coronary risk factors and cardiovascular disease; it predisposes to hypertension, diabetes mellitus and the metabolic syndrome, left ventricular hypertrophy, CHF, stroke, peripheral arterial disease, and chronic vascular inflammation.

THYROID HORMONE AND CARDIOVASCULAR DISEASE

The thyroid gland and the heart share a close relationship that arises in embryology. In ontogeny, the thyroid and heart migrate together. Changes in cardiovascular function across the entire spectrum of thyroid disease illustrate the close physiological relationship between the heart and thyroid.[54,55] Cardiovascular complications commonly occur in both subclinical and overt thyroid dysfunction.

Cellular Mechanisms of Thyroid Hormone Action on the Heart

Diagnosis and management of thyroid hormone–mediated cardiac disease states require understanding of the cellular mechanisms of thyroid hormone on the heart and vascular smooth muscle cells. Thyroid function is regulated by the hypothalamic-pituitary-thyroid (HPT) axis via a feedback mechanism. Secretion of thyroid stimulating hormone (TSH) by the pituitary gland is stimulated by hypothalamic TSH-releasing hormone (TRH), and TSH, in turn, stimulates the thyroid gland to release thyroxine (T_4) and triiodothyronine (T_3). TSH release is regulated directly by the negative feedback of thyroid hormone; this loop maintains the levels of circulating thyroid hormones and TSH in a physiological inverse relationship that defines the HPT axis set-point. This set-point is genetically determined although environmental factors, age, and systemic illness may induce changes in the HPT-axis.[56] The thyroid gland concentrates iodide and, through a series of enzymatic steps, synthesizes predominantly T_4 (about 80%) and a smaller percentage of triiodothyronine [T_3 about 20%]. Although T_4 is the main hormone produced by the thyroid gland, T_3 is the active hormone. Most circulating T_3 derives largely from T_4, thanks to the deiodinases activity in extrathyroidal peripheral tissues; 80% of the extrathyroidal T_3 is produced by deiodination of T_4.[57] Peripheral T_3 availability is regulated by three deiodinase isoforms, namely deiodinase type I (D1), type 2 (D2), and type 3 (D3).[57] The most important pathway of T_4 metabolism is its monodeiodination to active T_3 by D2 which catalyzes 5′ deiodination and converts T_4 to T_3. The deiodinase activity can change with aging and critical illness and D3 can arise in ischemic tissue.[58]

T_3 accounts for the vast majority of biological effects of TH. It increases myocardial oxygen consumption and tissue thermogenesis, regulates glucose and lipid metabolism, and acts on the heart and vascular smooth muscle cells (Fig. 96.2). Thyroid hormone regulates cardiac inotropy and chronotropy through direct and indirect mechanisms.[58,59] T_3 regulates the expression of genes that encode nuclear receptors and plasma membrane transport proteins within cardiac myocytes (eTable 96.1). Genomic effects of TH are mediated by TH nuclear receptors that are located in the intracellular compartment. T_3 is transported into the cytoplasm and several families of TH transporters have been identified; variations on binding protein levels can change the peripheral activity of THs.[54,59] The monocarboxylate transporters (MCTs) 8 and 10 are highly specific for iodothyronines and MCT10 has a greater capacity to transport T_3 than MCT8.[60,61] In humans, thyroid hormones bind intracellular DNA-binding proteins that combine as hormone receptor complexes to thyroid hormone response elements (TREs) in the regulatory regions of target genes. There are different subtypes of receptors—TRα1, TRα2, TRβ1, and TRβ2. TRα1 is mostly expressed in the trabecular myocardium. TRα2 does not bind T_3; however, it is able to bind TRE, thereby exerting a substantial negative effect on gene expression.[54,62] TRβ1 is only weakly expressed in the myocardium. After binding to the promoter regions, T_3 can activate or repress cardiac gene expression to regulate the synthesis of structural and regulatory cardiac proteins, cardiac membrane ion channels, and cell surface receptors, thus providing a molecular mechanism to explain many of the effects of thyroid hormone on the cardiovascular system (see eTable 96.1). Major T_3 targets include myosin heavy chain isoforms because T_3 up-regulates alpha-MHC, the fast myosin, and down-regulates β-MHC, the slow myosin. The human ventricle expresses principally beta-myosin, and limited alterations in isoform expression accompany thyroid disease states; however, changes in

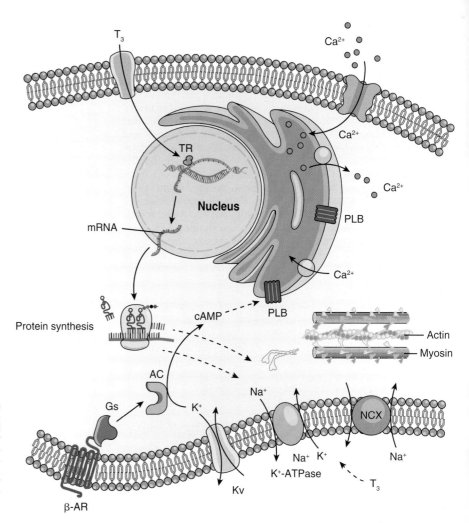

FIGURE 96.2 T_3 enters the cell via specific membrane transporters and binds to nuclear T_3 receptors. The complex binds to thyroid hormone response elements and regulates the transcription of specific genes. Non-nuclear T_3 actions on channels for Na^+, K^+, and Ca^{2+} ions are indicated. *AC*, adenylyl cyclase; *β-AR*, beta-adrenergic receptor; *Gs*, guanine nucleotide–binding protein subunit; *Kv*, voltage-gated potassium channel; *mRNA*, messenger RNA; *NCX*, sodium calcium exchanger; *PLB*, phospholamban; *TR*, T_3 receptor protein.

myosin heavy chain isoform expression can occur in the human atria in various diseases, including CHF and severe hypothyroidism, but are reversible with the appropriate therapy.[63,64] Sarcoplasmic reticulum Ca^{2+}-adenosine triphosphatase (ATPase) (SERCA2) is an important ion pump that determines the magnitude of myocyte calcium cycling (see Chapter 46). Reuptake of calcium into the sarcoendoplasmic reticulum, early in diastole, determines the rate at which the left ventricle relaxes (isovolumic relaxation time). SERCA2 is up-regulated and phospholamban is down-regulated by T_3 (PLB). This molecular mechanism can explain why diastolic function varies inversely across the entire spectrum of thyroid disease states, including even mild subclinical hypothyroidism (Fig. 96.3), contributing to the development of heart failure.[54] Changes in other myocyte genes include Na^+, K^+-ATPase, voltage-gated K^+ channels (Kv1.5 and Kv4.2), Na^+/Ca^{2+} exchanger, beta$_1$-adrenergic receptors, guanosine triphosphate–binding proteins, and the expression of cardiac-specific adenylyl cyclase catalytic subunit isoforms (V,VI).[54,62]

In addition to the well-characterized nuclear effects of thyroid hormone, some cardiac responses to thyroid hormone appear to result from non-transcriptional mechanisms,[65] as suggested by their relatively rapid onset of action, faster than attributable to changes in gene expression and protein synthesis, and non-susceptible to the effects of inhibitors of gene transcription. These indirect effects of TH largely occur at the plasma membrane, regulating ion transporter activity, and include ion channel activation (Na^+,K^+,Ca^{2+}) and regulation of specific signal transduction pathways.

T_3 decreases systemic vascular resistance through vascular smooth-muscle relaxation, which in turn decreases renal perfusion and leads to renin-angiotensin-aldosterone axis activation. T_3 also enhances the release of vasodilatory mediators by increasing metabolic and oxygen consumption. The activation of phosphatidylinositol 3-kinase (PI3K) and serine/threonine protein kinase (AKT) pathways cause

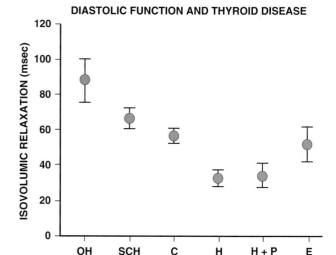

FIGURE 96.3 Diastolic function, as measured by the isovolumic relaxation time, varies over the entire range of thyroid disease, including overt hypothyroidism (OH), subclinical hypothyroidism (SCH), control (C), hyperthyroidism (H), hyperthyroidism after beta-adrenergic blockade (H + P), and hyperthyroidism after treatment to restore normal thyroid function (E).

the production of endothelial nitric oxide leading to a reduction in systemic vascular resistance through its effects on vascular smooth muscle cells.[66]

Diagnosis of Hyperthyroidism

The serum TSH level is the most widely used and sensitive marker for the diagnosis of thyroid dysfunction. Serum TSH levels decrease in hyperthyroidism due to the feedback of excessive T_4 and T_3 serum levels on thyrotropin pituitary synthesis and secretion. Overt hyperthyroidism is a severe clinical disorder induced by TH excess. Serum free thyroxine (FT_4) and or total (TT_3) or free triiodothyronine (FT_3) levels are above their respective reference ranges and serum TSH is suppressed in overt hyperthyroidism. In presence of abnormal TSH levels, measurement of FT_4 and TT_3 or FT_3 can help identify subclinical hyperthyroidism,[67,68] which is defined by subnormal serum TSH and normal serum FT_4 and/or total or FT_3 concentrations, although usually in the mid-to-high normal part of their reference ranges.[67,68] Subclinical hyperthyroidism can be classified into two categories: grade 1 subclinical hyperthyroidism, characterized by low detectable serum TSH levels (e.g., 0.1 to 0.4 mIU/L), and grade 2 subclinical hyperthyroidism in which serum TSH levels are completely undetectable (<0.1 mIU/L)[67,68]; 25% of patients with subclinical hyperthyroidism have grade 2 thyroid dysfunction. Patients with grade 2 subclinical hyperthyroidism are more likely to have an increased risk of progression to overt hyperthyroidism and negative CV adverse events.[67,68]

Overt and subclinical hyperthyroidism result most commonly from increased thyroid hormone synthesis related to Graves disease (GD), toxic adenoma (TA), or toxic multinodular goiter (TMNG). GD, an autoimmune form of hyperthyroidism, is the most common cause of overt and subclinical hyperthyroidism in iodine-replete countries.[67–69] TMNG and TA represent the main causes of thyroid hormone excess in areas with mild to moderate iodine deficiency.[67,68]

Cardiovascular Manifestations of Overt and Subclinical Hyperthyroidism

Changes in myocardial contractility and hemodynamics occur across the entire spectrum of thyroid disease (Table 96.2; see Fig. 96.3). Echocardiographic data indicate that, in humans, newly diagnosed thyrotoxicosis induces an improvement in left ventricular systolic function and an enhancement in left ventricular relaxation, diastolic flow velocities, and isovolumic relaxation time.[70] T_3 excess decreases systemic vascular resistance in arterioles of the peripheral circulation; this drop results in a smaller left ventricular end-systolic volume. A decrease in mean arterial pressure and activation of the

renin-angiotensin-aldosterone system increases serum angiotensin-converting enzyme activity and renal sodium reabsorption.[70] The enhanced plasma volume, coupled with increased erythropoietin synthesis expands blood volume; the improvement in diastolic relaxation of the heart contributes to increased left ventricular end-diastolic volume. Despite the marked reduction in systemic vascular resistance, the pulsatile arterial load undergoes a compensatory change and increased aortic input sustains the systolic arterial pressure.[70] Systolic arterial pressure almost invariably increases and diastolic arterial pressure decreases in subjects with overt hyperthyroidism, so that pulse pressure characteristically widens and mean arterial pressure only marginally decreases. Systolic hypertension may develop in up to 30% of hyperthyroid patients and is more pronounced in older patients. The net effect of an increased preload and a decreased afterload yields increased left ventricular stroke volume in hyperthyroidism.[70] In turn, the rise in heart rate and the increased stroke volume combine to cause a two- to threefold increase in cardiac output (see Table 96.2). Therefore, the hyperthyroid heart increases its performance through the modulation of hemodynamic loads; this positive effect on energy metabolism and oxygen consumption improves the left ventricle mechanical efficiency, optimizing its cardiac mechanical-energetic consumption.

Cardiovascular symptoms are an integral and often predominant clinical feature of patients with hyperthyroidism. Most patients experience palpitations resulting from increases in the rate and force of cardiac contractility. The increase in heart rate results from a decrease in parasympathetic stimulation and an increase in sympathetic tone. Heart rates higher than 90 beats/min at rest and during sleep commonly occur, the normal diurnal variation in heart rate is blunted, and the increase during exercise exaggerated.

Subclinical hyperthyroidism may increase heart rate, ventricular mass, arterial stiffness, and left atrial size, especially after long-term exposure to thyroid hormone excess.[67] It may exert unfavorable effects on cardiac morphology, inducing diastolic dysfunction and thereby impairing left ventricle performance (see Table 96.2).[67,68] Sinus tachycardia and atrial premature beats frequently occur in young patients; older patients (>60 years) usually do not have symptoms of adrenergic over-activity, but can develop atrial fibrillation.

Untreated hyperthyroidism is associated with increased CV morbidity and mortality.[67,68] Overt and subclinical hyperthyroidism have been associated with an increased risk of major CV events; this risk is mainly due to higher incidence of HF events.[71] Grade 2 subclinical hyperthyroidism has been associated with an increased risk of AF, HF, and coronary heart disease (CHD) in a meta-analysis assessing individual participant data (IPD) of euthyroid subjects and participants from high-quality prospective studies (see Table 96.2).[72]

Atrial Fibrillation in Overt and Subclinical Hyperthyroidism (see also Chapter 66)

Hyperthyroidism is linked to an increased supraventricular ectopic activity. Atrial fibrillation is a major cause for concern in patients with overt and subclinical hyperthyroidism[70,71] and may be the first symptom of thyroid hormone excess in older adults. T_3 increases systolic depolarization and diastolic repolarization and decreases the action potential duration and the refraction period of the atrial myocardium, as well as the atrial/ventricular nodal refraction period; the reduced inter-atrial action potential duration gives the substrate for atrial arrhythmias.[73]

There is unequivocal evidence that subclinical hyperthyroidism is also associated with an increased risk of atrial fibrillation. In an IPD meta-analysis from five prospective cohort studies, the overall hazard ratio (HR) for incident AF was significantly greater in participants with subclinical hyperthyroidism than in euthyroid controls during a mean follow-up of 8.8 years; grade 2 subclinical hyperthyroidism was associated with a higher risk of AF than grade 1 subclinical hyperthyroidism (see Table 96.2).[67,72] Absolute risks, but not relative risks, increase with aging. Additional analyses have explored whether there is a gradient of risk for developing AF even within the normal reference range of thyroid function tests. Data from the Rotterdam Study have shown that

TABLE 96.2 Effect of Thyroid Disease on Cardiovascular Function and Outcome

	OVERT HYPERTHYROIDISM AND GRADE 2 SUBCLINICAL HYPERTHYROIDISM (<0.1 mIU/L)	OVERT HYPOTHYROIDISM AND GRADE 2 SUBCLINICAL HYPOTHYROIDISM (TSH > 10 mIU/L)
Hypertension	Systolic hypertension Wide pulse pressure	Diastolic hypertension
Cardiac function	CO ↑ Systolic function ↑ Diastolic function ↑ Cardiac workload and LVM in long-term hyperthyroidism ↑ Cardiac preload ↑ Cardiac afterload ↓ Vascular reactivity ↑	CO ↓ Systolic function ↓ Diastolic function ↓ LVM → ↑ Arterial stiffness ↑ Cardiac preload ↓ Cardiac afterload ↑ Vascular reactivity ↓
Thrombogenicity	Coagulability ↑ Fibrinolysis ↑	Unclear
Cardiovascular outcome	Risk of atrial arrhythmias ↑ Risk of AF ↑ Risk of CHD ↑ Risk of HF ↑	Risk of CHD mortality with serum TSH > 7 mIU/L ↑ Risk of HF events with serum TSH > 7 mIU/L ↑

CHD, coronary heart disease; *LVM*, left ventricular mass; *TSH*, Thyroid stimulating hormone.

increasing FT_4 levels within the normal reference range are associated with an increased risk of AF.[74] In a meta-analysis in the Thyroid Studies Collaboration assessing IPD from 11 prospective studies, higher FT_4 levels at baseline in euthyroid individuals were associated with a significant increased risk of AF in age- and gender-adjusted analysis.[75]

Overt and subclinical hyperthyroidism have been associated with increased markers of thrombogenesis (fibrinogen and factor X levels). Hyperthyroid patients have higher von Willebrand antigen levels compared to euthyroid patients, leading to an enhanced platelet plug formation which subsequently decreases with treatment. Stroke is a potential complication of AF in overt hyperthyroidism leading to increased cerebrovascular events; on the contrary insufficient results have been reported in subclinical hyperthyroidism.[72,76]

The first-line treatment of atrial fibrillation and supraventricular tachycardia in patients with thyroid dysfunction should aim primarily to restore a euthyroid state.[68,77–79] Treatment of hyperthyroidism with antithyroid drugs should be the first-line therapy in patients with hyperthyroidism and atrial fibrillation to obtain conversion to sinus rhythm and to improve hemodynamics. A beta1-selective or nonselective agent may help to control the ventricular response. Beta blockers promptly improve the tachycardia-mediated component of ventricular dysfunction. Digitalis may help control the ventricular response in hyperthyroidism-associated atrial fibrillation, but because of the increased rate of digitalis clearance, the decreased sensitivity of drug action resulting from the high cellular levels of Na^+,K^+-ATPase, and the decreased parasympathetic tone, patients usually require higher doses. Anticoagulation, especially with the new non-vitamin K-dependent agents, in patients with hyperthyroidism and AF is controversial. The potential for systemic or cerebral embolization must be weighed against the risk for bleeding and complications. Pharmacological or electrical cardioversion should be considered in patients who do not recover normal rhythm spontaneously within 4 months of normalization of the thyroid function, after evaluation of the patient's age and underlying cardiac status. The ability to restore thyrotoxic patients to a euthyroid state and sinus rhythm justifies TSH testing in most patients with a recent onset of otherwise unexplained atrial fibrillation or other supraventricular arrhythmias.[77–79]

Heart Failure in Overt and Subclinical Hyperthyroidism

The cardiovascular alterations in hyperthyroidism include increased resting cardiac output and enhanced cardiac contractility (see Table 96.2). However, many hyperthyroid patients experience exercise intolerance and exertional dyspnea, caused in part by skeletal and respiratory muscle weakness.[70] The low vascular resistance and increased preload compromise cardiac functional reserve, which cannot rise further to accommodate the demands imposed by submaximal or maximal exercise. Despite the high cardiac output state, hyperthyroid patients have an impaired cardiopulmonary function during effort, which reflects their reduced CV and respiratory reserve during exercise. Nevertheless, a minority of patients have symptoms, including dyspnea on exertion, orthopnea, and paroxysmal nocturnal dyspnea, as well as signs demonstrating peripheral edema, elevated jugular venous pressure, or an S_3. This complex of findings, coupled with failure to increase the left ventricular ejection fraction with exercise, suggests a hyperthyroid cardiomyopathy. The term often used in this setting, *high-output failure*, is not appropriate because although resting cardiac output is as much as two to three times normal, the exercise intolerance does not appear to result from cardiac failure but rather from skeletal muscle weakness and perhaps associated pulmonary hypertension.[70,76] High-output states, however, can increase renal sodium reabsorption and expand plasma volume. Although systemic vascular resistance falls with hyperthyroidism, pulmonary vascular resistance does not, and because of the greater output to the pulmonary circulation, pulmonary arterial pressure increases. This leads to a rise in mean venous pressure, hepatic congestion, and peripheral edema of the type associated with primary pulmonary hypertension or right-sided heart failure. In patients with longstanding hyperthyroidism

and marked sinus tachycardia or atrial fibrillation, low cardiac output, impaired cardiac contractility with a low ejection fraction, and pulmonary congestion can develop—all consistent with heart failure.

A review of such cases suggests that the impairment in the left ventricular function results from the prolonged high heart rate and the development of a rate-related heart failure. When the left ventricle becomes dilated, mitral regurgitation may also develop (see Chapter 76). Recognition of this phenomenon is important as treatment aimed at slowing the heart rate or controlling the ventricular response in atrial fibrillation appears to improve left ventricular function, even before initiation of antithyroid therapy. Some patients with hyperthyroidism, similar to the overall CHF population, do not tolerate initiation of beta blockers in full doses. Patients critically ill who develop low cardiac output should be managed in an intensive care unit setting. Subclinical and overt hyperthyroidism are associated with 23% and 25% increased risk of major cardiovascular events (MACEs) respectively.[71] This risk is motivated by heart failure being about 15% to 20% higher respectively in subjects with subclinical hyperthyroidism and overt hyperthyroidism.[71] Pooled IPD data from six prospective cohort studies reported a significant risk of HF events in participants with grade 2 subclinical hyperthyroidism compared to grade 1.[72] Thyroid testing is highly recommended in patients with HF.[68]

CHD in Hyperthyroidism

A subset of thyrotoxic patients can experience angina-like chest pain. In older hyperthyroid patients with known or suspected coronary artery disease, the increase in cardiac work associated with the increase in cardiac output and cardiac contractility can produce myocardial ischemia, which can respond to beta blockers or lead to the restoration of a euthyroid state. Rarely patients, usually younger women, experience a syndrome of chest pain at rest associated with ischemic electrocardiographic changes. Cardiac catheterization has demonstrated that most of these patients have angiographically normal coronary arteries, but coronary vasospasm similar to that found in variant angina can occur (see also Chapters 40 and 91). Myocardial infarction rarely develops and these patients appear to respond to calcium channel–blocking agents or nitroglycerin.

A meta-analysis of IPD data from 10 prospective cohorts reported that grade 2 subclinical hyperthyroidism can increase the risk of CHD mortality (see Table 96.2).[72] The Rotterdam Study showed a higher risk of CVD events even in participants with high-normal FT_4 concentrations.[80]

Pulmonary Hypertension and Autoimmune Cardiovascular Involvement

Hyperthyroidism associates with a substantial degree of pulmonary hypertension (mean pulmonary artery systolic pressure >50 mm Hg).[76] Pulmonary hypertension in turn places a significant degree of stress and afterload on the right ventricle—thus implying that although systemic vascular resistance decreases with thyrotoxicosis, pulmonary vascular resistance does not. Correction of hyperthyroidism usually reduces pulmonary arterial pressure. Severe pulmonary hypertension may also reverse completely after successful treatment of hyperthyroidism. In addition to the reduction in pulmonary blood flow, a specific vasoactive effect of methimazole may explain the improvement in the pulmonary vasculature hemodynamics after treatment of hyperthyroidism.

Autoimmune hyperthyroidism occasionally links to autoimmune cardiovascular involvement. Pulmonary arterial hypertension, myxomatous cardiac valve disease, irreversible dilated cardiomyopathy, and peripartum cardiomyopathy have been reported in patients with GD.[76] Patients with autoimmune thyroid disease may have anticardiolipin antibodies and antiphospholipid syndrome.[76]

TREATMENT OF OVERT AND SUBCLINICAL HYPERTHYROIDISM

Graves disease tends to either resolve spontaneously or worsen with time. Methimazole is appropriate for younger adults with Graves disease, because this autoimmune condition may spontaneously remit

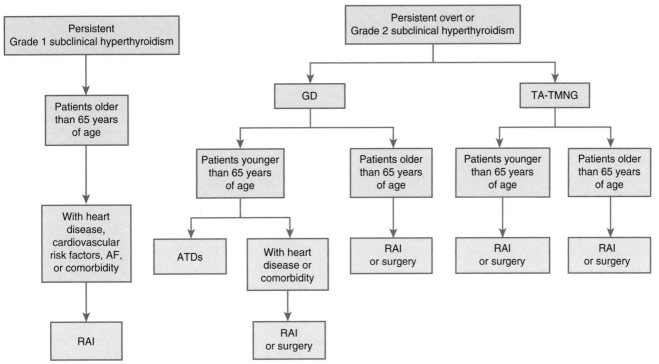

FIGURE 96.4 Treatment of overt and subclinical hyperthyroidism according to the etiology and degree of hyperthyroidism.

after a course of therapy; also patients with milder disease, that is, subclinical hyperthyroidism, are most likely to remit.[69] Radioiodine therapy is appropriate for older individuals with persistent Graves disease who have underlying comorbidities because definitive treatment is necessary to avoid the progression of cardiac disease (Fig. 96.4).[69,81]

Most patients with chronic subclinical hyperthyroidism have multinodular goiters or solitary nodules rather than autoimmune hyperthyroidism. Radioiodine would be the preferred treatment for individuals with overt or subclinical hyperthyroidism with a TMNG or a solitary autonomously functioning nodule.[67,69] Definitive therapy can then be safely performed with iodine-131 alone or in combination with an antithyroid drug (see Fig. 96.4).[67,68] Surgery would typically be reserved for patients with a large goiter and symptoms of compression, coexisting hyperparathyroidism, or suspicion of thyroid malignancy.[67,68] Treatment of subclinical hyperthyroidism is not recommended in asymptomatic younger persons or premenopausal women with milder degrees of lowering serum TSH (i.e., 0.1 to 0.4 mU/L) due to a lack of evidence of harm.[67,68]

Subclinical hyperthyroidism may develop during levothyroxine (L–T$_4$) therapy with doses that suppress serum TSH. Intentional TSH–suppressive doses of L–T$_4$ are only indicated in patients with a previous diagnosis of thyroid cancer with high risk of recurrences; the risk–benefit of TSH suppression should be considered in older patients.[82]

THYROID STORM

Patients with thyroid storm, the most severe form of hyperthyroidism, can display altered mental status, fever, gastrointestinal symptoms including pain, nausea, and rarely jaundice, exaggerated tachycardia, new onset supraventricular arrhythmias such as atrial fibrillation or hypotension, and cardiovascular collapse.[83] Takotsubo cardiomyopathy links to severe thyrotoxicosis and may be a manifestation of thyroid storm.

The mortality rate of thyroid storm can be as high as 50% and outcomes vary based on management of the cardiovascular manifestations. These patients require intensive care unit monitoring in addition to the use of antithyroid drugs, potassium iodide, and attention to other coexistent medical problems such as infection, trauma, or drugs such as amiodarone; they may tolerate intravenous administration of beta-adrenergic blocking drugs or calcium channel blockers poorly. The development of hypotensive cardiac arrest or worsening heart failure represents the untoward effects of such agents in patients with thyrotoxic heart disease. As noted above, intensive monitoring, judicious use of esmolol, and standard fluid and volume management with

simultaneous treatment to lower T$_4$ and T$_3$ can optimize the therapeutic response.[83]

Diagnosis of Overt and Subclinical Hypothyroidism

Overt hypothyroidism is a clinical condition in which TSH is increased and free thyroid hormones (especially FT$_4$) are low. The term myxedema is reserved for severe and/or complicated thyroid hormone deficiency in adults and is usually used to indicate a nonpitting edema caused by the accumulation of glycosaminoglycans in interstitial tissue. Subclinical hypothyroidism is diagnosed when serum TSH is above the upper limit of the normal reference range and free thyroid hormones are within their respective reference range. Patients may have a mild disease (TSH 4.5 to 9.9 mU/L) or a more severe dysfunction (TSH ≥ 10 mU/L).[84,85] Hashimoto thyroiditis represents the most common cause of acquired subclinical hypothyroidism in the adult. Thyroid surgery, radioiodine therapy, and, in some parts of the world, iodine deficiency are the most common causes of hypothyroidism.

Cardiovascular Effects of Overt and Subclinical Hypothyroidism

Hemodynamic changes occur in hypothyroidism (Fig. 96.5; see Table 96.2). Left ventricular function falls reversibly in hypothyroidism. Cardiac preload decreases due to the impaired diastolic function and decreased blood volume; left ventricular ejection fraction at rest and during exercise and cardiopulmonary exercise testing declines and tends to improve with restoration of euthyroidism.[86] Afterload increases in patients with hypothyroidism as a result of increased systemic vascular resistance, arterial stiffness, and endothelial dysfunction.[87] Systemic vascular resistance may increase as much as 30% and mean arterial pressure rise in up to 20% of patients with diastolic hypertension. Diastolic hypertension in patients with hypothyroidism is associated with a low renin level and a decrease in the hepatic synthesis of renin substrate. Cardiac output may decrease by as much as 30% to 40% in hypothyroidism. Despite the decrease in cardiac output and contractility of the hypothyroid myocardium, studies of myocardial metabolism have shown that the hypothyroid myocardium is energy-inefficient

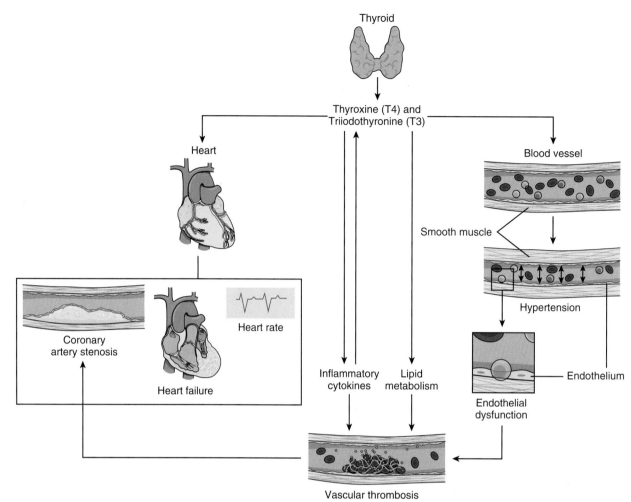

FIGURE 96.5 Effects of thyroid hormones (TH) on the risk of heart failure and coronary heart disease (effects on blood pressure, smooth muscle tone, endothelial function, lipid metabolism, and modulation of inflammatory pathways). (From Razvi S, Jabbar A, Pingitore A, et al. Thyroid hormones and cardiovascular function and diseases. *J Am Coll Cardiol.* 2018;71:1781.)

despite the low level of overall oxygen consumption. Indeed, increased afterload is one of the major factors determining myocardial oxygen consumption.

Pericardial effusions can occur in severe or long-standing hypothyroidism; occasionally, it can be large and cause the appearance of cardiomegaly on chest radiographs. Although rare, tamponade with hemodynamic compromise may occur. Echocardiography demonstrates small to moderate effusions in up to 30% of overtly hypothyroid patients; the effusions tend to resolve within weeks or months after initiation of thyroid hormone replacement therapy.

As a result of the changes in ion channel expression and parasympathetic tone, the ECG in hypothyroidism may show sinus bradycardia, low voltage, and prolongation of the action potential duration and QT interval. The QT prolongation predisposes patients to ventricular arrhythmias, and some patients have acquired torsades de pointes which can improve or completely resolve with thyroid hormone replacement.

Subclinical hypothyroidism can impair left ventricular filling and relaxation (see Fig. 96.3; Table 96.2).[84] It can also impair relaxation of vascular smooth muscle cells, inducing increases in systemic vascular resistance and arterial stiffness, as well as changes in endothelial function by reducing the availability of nitric oxide.[86–89]

Overt and subclinical hypothyroidism can progressively impair cardiac function leading to HF. A pooled analysis on a total of 2068 IPD data from six prospective studies reported an increased risk of HF events in patients with serum TSH greater than 7 to 10 mIU/L.[72,84] Some studies also demonstrate that subclinical hypothyroidism could potentially induce a worsening of the cardiac function in patients with preexisting HF leading to an increase in CV mortality.[90–92] Treatment of

hypothyroid patients with restoration of a euthyroid state resolves the CV changes in parallel with return of systemic vascular resistance to lower level (see Table 96.2).[93]

Coronary Heart Disease

Hypothyroidism also increases total and low-density lipoprotein (LDL) cholesterol in proportion to the rise in serum TSH levels.[94] Although thyroid hormone can alter cholesterol metabolism through multiple mechanisms, including a decrease in biliary excretion, the primary mechanism involves changes in the LDL metabolism caused by decreases in the numbers of the hepatic LDL receptor and reduced activity of cholesterol 7α-hydroxylase, an enzyme that lowers cholesterol levels. A recent study reported that the liver-selective thyroid hormone agonist eprotirome can lower cholesterol levels in statin-treated patients, in support of this concept.[95]

Increases in risk factors for atherosclerosis, including hypercholesterolemia, hypertension, endothelial dysfunction, and elevated levels of homocysteine, may elevate the risk for atherosclerosis and coronary and systemic vascular disease in patients with hypothyroidism (see Chapters 25 to 27) (see Fig. 96.5). Myocardial perfusion scans have demonstrated abnormalities suggestive of myocardial ischemia, but these defects appear to resolve with thyroid hormone treatment. A patient-level meta-analysis of several prospective cohort studies providing 542,494 person-years of follow-up has shown that subclinical hypothyroidism is associated with a higher risk of CV events and mortality in people with serum TSH greater than 7 mIU/L levels and even more in those with TSH levels greater than 10 mU/L irrespective of age.[84]

One of the major factors that affects CV risk in SCH populations is age and several observations have concluded that older individuals with grade 1 subclinical hypothyroidism may have a lower risk of CV disease than younger ones.[84] Treatment of mild disease is recommended in young patients with evidence of atherosclerotic cardiovascular disease, heart failure, or associated risk factors. Trials of L–T_4 in mild subclinical hypothyroidism using surrogate markers have shown improvements in the left ventricular function, vascular endothelial function, atherogenic lipid particles, or cardiac mitochondrial function.[84]

TSH screening is advisable in adults, particularly in patients with hypertension, hypercholesterolemia, hypertriglyceridemia, coronary or peripheral vascular disease, and unexplained pericardial or pleural effusions, as well as for various musculoskeletal syndromes or statin-associated myopathy.

TREATMENT OF HYPOTHYROIDISM

Replacement doses of purified preparations of L–T_4 (levothyroxine) are the treatment of choice in hypothyroid patients.[96,97] The optimal replacement dose of L–T_4 should take into account both the age of the patient and the cause of hypothyroidism. Indeed, the L–T_4 dosage should be lower in older adults and higher in patients with a more severe disease, particularly those who have undergone thyroidectomy or prior iodine treatment for GD. In all patients, thyroid hormone replacement should suffice to restore the serum TSH level to normal so that they are clinically and chemically euthyroid. The known effects of thyroid hormone on the heart and cardiovascular system do not support the concept that these patients benefit from maintenance of mild hypothyroidism.

Treatment of hypothyroidism yields predictable responses, especially from a cardiovascular perspective. Stepwise thyroid hormone replacement with L–T_4 incrementally decreases serum TSH, serum cholesterol, and serum creatine-kinase (CK) levels and improves left ventricular performance. Patients less than 50 years with no history of heart disease generally tolerate full replacement doses of L–T_4 (1.5 µg/kg/day) without concern for untoward cardiac effects. Patients greater than 50 years with known or suspected coronary artery disease have more complicated issues. Three major issues arise. Coronary artery bypass graft surgery (CABG) can be performed in patients with unstable angina, left main coronary artery disease, or three-vessel disease with impaired left ventricular function, even in the setting of overt hypothyroidism. Rarely a patient has sufficiently profound hypothyroidism to prolong bleeding times and partial thromboplastin times, which requires preoperative supplementation of clotting factors. Thyroid hormone replacement can be delayed until the postoperative period, when it can be administered in full doses parenterally or orally. Treatment of patients with known stable cardiac disease in whom cardiac revascularization is not clinically indicated should begin with low doses (12.5 µg) of L–T_4 and then stepwise increases (12.5 to 25 µg) every 6 to 8 weeks until the serum TSH level normalizes. Thyroid hormone replacement in this setting and its ability to lower systemic vascular resistance and decrease afterload, as well as improve myocardial efficiency, can actually decrease clinical signs of myocardial ischemia. In patients who, although potentially at risk for coronary artery disease, exhibit no clinical signs or symptoms, thyroid hormone replacement can start at low doses, generally in the range of 25 to 50 µg/day, and then increase by 25 µg every 6 to 8 weeks until the serum TSH level is normal. If signs or symptoms of ischemic heart disease develop, the same recommendations apply as for patients with known underlying heart diseases.

Despite the lack of definitive long-term studies on the outcome of mild-to-moderate hypothyroidism with and without replacement therapy, recommendations for treatment of patients with serum TSH ≥ 7 mIU/L have fallen on the side of replacement treatment with L–T_4.[84] Randomized controlled trials are needed to evaluate the clinical benefits and safety of treatment of SCH in reducing CV risk.

MYXEDEMA COMA

In the rare condition of myxedema coma, characterized by the development of hypothermia, altered mental status, hypotension, bradycardia, and hypoventilation, the need for thyroid hormone replacement is more of an emergency.[98] In patients with severe coma, treatment can be accomplished by intravenous administration of 200 µg of L–T_4 followed by 100 µg of L–T_4 per day to restore vital functions. L–T_3 may also be started simultaneously with L–T_4 in a starting dosage of 10 to 20 µg, followed by 10 µg every 6 hours for 1 or 2 days until the cerebral function of the patient improves. Patients with myxedema coma require intensive care unit monitoring with volume repletion, gentle warming, and ventilatory support in the presence of CO_2 retention. Administration of

hydrocortisone (50 to 100 mg three times daily) should be undertaken until the results of serum cortisol testing are obtained. When treated in this manner, hemodynamics, including systemic vascular resistance, cardiac output, and heart rate, improve within 24 to 48 hours. Severe hyponatremia should be corrected with the judicious administration of hypertonic saline solution (50 to 100 mL of 3% sodium chloride) followed by an IV bolus of 40 to 120 mg furosemide. This treatment should be used cautiously to avoid inadvertent correction of hyponatremia with its devastating consequences.

Amiodarone and Thyroid Function

Amiodarone is an iodine-rich antiarrhythmic agent used in the treatment of ventricular and atrial tachyarrhythmias; its 30% iodine content by weight and structural similarity to L–T_4 causes abnormalities in thyroid function test results in as many as 60% of the patients treated for short or long periods. The finding that dronedarone, a noniodinated benzofuran antiarrhythmic, does not alter thyroid function reinforces this concept.

Amiodarone inhibits entry of T_4 into cells and the intracellular conversion of T_4 to T_3 by inhibiting the 5′-monodeiodination of T_4 in the liver and pituitary. Inhibition of T_4 metabolism in the liver decreases serum T_3 and increases serum T_4 levels, whereas serum TSH levels initially remain normal. With more chronic treatment, T_4 synthesis and release from the thyroid gland can be inhibited, thereby producing an increase in TSH levels. Patients with autoimmune thyroid disease or enzymatic defects in thyroid hormone biosynthesis and even some patients without any risk factors can progress to overt chemical and clinical hypothyroidism.[99] The overall prevalence of hypothyroidism in amiodarone-treated patients is between 15% and 30%. Symptoms of hypothyroidism in this setting can be subtle and significant hypothyroidism can occur even in their absence. *Thyroid function should be measured every 3 months in all patients receiving amiodarone.* The effect on thyroid function does not depend on the dose and can occur at any time after initiating treatment; furthermore, because of the high lipid solubility and long half-life of amiodarone, this effect can persist up to 1 year after discontinuing therapy.

Less common but perhaps more challenging is the development of amiodarone-induced thyrotoxicosis (Table 96.3).[99] Although not initially observed in the iodine-replete American population, the experience from more iodine-deficient populations (such as Italy) suggests that it occurs with a prevalence as high as 10%. The onset was often sudden and could occur shortly after initiation of amiodarone therapy, during chronic treatment, or up to 1 year after stopping therapy. Clinical clues to the development of this condition include a new onset or recurrence of ventricular irritability (increased firing of an implantable cardioverter-defibrillator), decreased warfarin dose requirements, or return or worsening of the obstructive physiology of hypertrophic cardiomyopathy (see Chapter 54). Two forms of amiodarone-induced thyrotoxicosis can occur.[99] Type I occurs primarily in patients with preexisting thyroid disease and most commonly in iodine-deficient areas. These patients rarely have an increase in 24-hour radioiodine uptake and frequently some measures of thyroid autoimmunity, including antithyroid antibodies. In contrast, a variety of proinflammatory cytokines, including IL-6, presumably mediate type II thyroiditis. In this case, the toxic effect on the thyroid gland induces a release of preformed thyroid hormone through thyroiditis (type 2 amiodarone-induced thyrotoxicosis). This destructive process can continue for weeks or months and is usually associated with low to absent radioiodine uptake. Further experience has shown that these two types have substantial overlap in many of the distinguishing features. Amiodarone-induced thyrotoxicosis associates with a threefold increased risk for major adverse cardiovascular events, underscoring its clinical importance.[99] Table 96.3 proposes a scheme for thyroid function treatment in patients treated with amiodarone.

Because of the increased thyroidal and total-body iodine content, use of iodine-131 is almost always ineffective. Similarly, treatment with antithyroid drugs has marginal effectiveness. Corticosteroids (prednisone, 20 to 40 mg/day) provide benefit, perhaps with increased usefulness in patients with type II disease who have high serum levels of IL-6. However, corticosteroids can be instituted in all patients because when effective the response usually occurs within 2 to 4 weeks of initiating

TABLE 96.3 Treatment of Amiodarone-Associated Thyroid Dysfunction

Amiodarone-Induced Hypothyroidism (AIH)

- Amiodarone-induced thyrotoxicosis (AIT) can be diagnosed on the basis of classic signs and symptoms of hypothyroidism or hyperthyroidism or by routine (every 3–6 months) thyroid function testing
- Withdrawal of amiodarone is not necessary in patients with hypothyroidism
- L–T_4 treatment can be started at a low dose and progressively increased
- The target serum TSH level during levothyroxine therapy should be balanced with the risk of arrhythmias

Type 1 Amiodarone-Induced Thyrotoxicosis (AIT 1)

- Clinical hypothyroidism with a TSH level higher than 10 mIU/mL should be treated
- The treatment of choice is the use of antithyroid drugs
- Perchlorate at doses not exceeding 1 g/day can be useful in patients with resistant hyperthyroidism
- Total thyroidectomy should be performed in AIT 1 patients with a deterioration of the cardiovascular function or severe underlying cardiac disease and/or in patients with persistent hyperthyroidism unresponsive to medical therapies
- Hyperfunctioning thyroid gland can be definitely treated with thyroidectomy or radioiodine (RAI) treatment
- Euthyroidism should be restored before total thyroidectomy or RAI, when possible

Type 2 Amiodarone-Induced Thyrotoxicosis (AIT 2)

- Amiodarone can be continued only in patients with life-threatening arrhythmias and severe critical illness with poor prognosis
- The first-line treatment is the administration of oral glucocorticoids

Mixed/Indefinite Form of AIT

- Glucocorticoids should be added to thionamides

treatment. In patients unresponsive to glucocorticoids with evidence of hyperthyroidism—including weight loss, tachycardia, palpitations, worsening angina, ventricular tachycardia, or other untoward cardiac effects—treatment with antithyroid therapy (methimazole 10 to 30 mg/day) is variably effective and can cause considerable side effects. Total thyroidectomy can be performed safely and can rapidly reverse hyperthyroidism.[99] Preoperative treatment with beta blockers is indicated, and there have been no reported cases of resulting thyroid storm.

Whether amiodarone-mediated thyroid dysfunction should mandate discontinuation of therapy with the drug is an important issue. There is no evidence that stopping treatment with amiodarone hastens the resolution of chemical hyperthyroidism.

Changes in Thyroid Hormone Metabolism That Accompany Cardiac Disease

In addition to the changes in thyroid function that can result from classic thyroid disease, primary alterations in levels of serum total and free T_3 and occasionally in serum T_4 can accompany a variety of acute and chronic illnesses, including sepsis, starvation, and cardiac disease. In the absence of thyroid gland abnormality, changes in serum T_3 levels result from alterations in thyroid hormone metabolism. Some refer to such cases as nonthyroidal illness.[100] The mechanism for this decrease in serum T_3 levels is multifactorial and in part related to a decrease of 5'-monodeiodination in the liver. Up to 30% of patients with heart failure have a low serum T_3 level, a finding in patients treated with or without amiodarone. In patients with CHF, the fall in serum T_3 levels correlates with the severity of heart failure as assessed by the NYHA classification.[101] In addition, in patients with heart failure and preserved ejection fraction, the serum level of T_3 is inversely proportional to the level of pro-brain natriuretic peptide. The increased levels of inflammatory proteins (interleukins and cytokines such as IL-6, TNF-α, etc.) induce changes in thyroid hormone metabolism, type 2 deiodinase activity, and thyroid hormone receptors expression in patients with

heart failure, resulting in the development of tissue hypothyroidism in patients with severe heart failure. Changes occurring in the damaged myocardium and the reactivation of the fetal genotype in HF may suggest that the deleterious effects of hypothyroidism on the myocardium may benefit from T_3 replacement (eTable 96.2). In addition, TH treatment reduces interstitial fibrosis in animal models of ischemic and non-ischemic heart failure because of the inhibitory effect on metalloproteinases.

An antifibrotic effect of TH is also linked to the T_3-induced inhibition of the profibrotic pathways and supported by the association of low serum T_3 levels with the presence of cardiac fibrosis in patients with idiopathic dilated cardiomyopathy. A population-based study of patients with cardiac disease has shown how a low serum T_3 level strongly predicts all-cause and cardiovascular mortality. These observations led to studies examining the administration of L–T_4, L–T_3, or thyroid hormone analogs in patients with heart failure to potentially improve their prognosis. L–T_3 infusion in patients with chronic and stable dilated cardiomyopathy and low-T_3 syndrome improved cardiac performance and the neurohumoral milieu without a significant increase in myocardial O_2 consumption.[102] Larger multicenter trials for longer periods are needed to provide information on hard clinical outcomes such as mortality, arrhythmias, and hospitalizations before thyroid hormone therapy can be routinely prescribed in patients with heart failure as part of clinical practice.

Children and adults undergoing cardiac surgery with cardiopulmonary bypass demonstrate a predictable fall in serum T_3 levels in the perioperative period, which identifies patients at increased risk for morbidity and mortality. A prospective, randomized study has shown that especially in neonates, administration of T_3 in doses sufficient to restore serum T_3 levels to normal decreases the degree of therapeutic intervention and the need for postoperative inotropic agents.

THYROID HORMONES AND CARDIOPROTECTION

Following uncomplicated acute myocardial infarction (AMI), serum T_3 levels fall by about 20% and reach a nadir after approximately 96 hours. Experimental myocardial infarction in animals produces a similar decrease in serum T_3 levels, and replacement of T_3 levels to normal may increase left ventricular contractile function. Cardioprotection is an emerging target of therapeutic intervention in AMI to minimize irreversible ischemic damage and favor functional recovery of the ischemic-damaged myocardium. Low T_3 induces oxidative stress, increases the apoptotic rate, and is able to depress myocardial function, leading to worsened ventricular dysfunction (see eTable 96.2). There is some evidence in animal studies that thyroid hormones play a critical role in regeneration and repair during adult life. T_3 has a cardioprotective effect, owing to the activation of cytoprotective mechanisms, stimulation of cell growth and neo-angiogenesis, and regulation of mitochondrial dysfunction. Therefore, T_3 increases the post-ischemic recovery of myocardial function. The reduction in myocardial damage and the positive left ventricular remodeling induced by T_3 could delay or improve the evolution toward postischemic irreversible heart failure.

In a recent meta-analysis, patients with ischemic heart disease and concomitant Non-thyroidal illness syndrome (NTIS) or hypothyroidism had a higher risk of all-cause mortality and MACE.[103] However, despite these results, there is a need for future studies to clarify the causal relationship between these events and the association of NTIS or hypothyroidism in patients with ischemic heart disease. In a recent phase 2, randomized, controlled trial of oral T_3 in patients with STEMI and low serum free T_3 levels, the administration of T_3 in replacement doses for 6 months was proved to be safe and effective in reducing regional cardiac dysfunction and significantly increased stroke volume, as compared with no treatment.[104] Future randomized trials are necessary to demonstrate the safety and efficacy of thyroid hormone supplementation in patients with ischemic heart disease and NTIS or hypothyroidism before considering its routine use.

FUTURE PERSPECTIVES

Endocrine dysfunction can be responsible for hypertension, atrial fibrillation, coronary heart disease, and heart failure, increasing cardiovascular mortality. The identification of these disorders is important because appropriate treatment of the specific endocrine deficiency

TABLE 96.4 Clinical Features of Endocrine Dysfunctions: Diagnosis and Cardiovascular Outcome

CLINICAL FEATURES	POSSIBLE DIAGNOSIS	DIAGNOSTIC TESTS
Bradycardia	Hypothyroidism	TSH
Diastolic hypertension		FT$_3$
Fatigue		FT$_4$
Increased sensitivity to cold		ABTG
Constipation		ABTPO
Dry skin		Thyroid Doppler ultrasound
Weight gain		
Hoarseness		
Muscle weakness		
Elevated blood cholesterol levels		
Heart failure		
Coronary heart disease		
Systolic hypertension	Hyperthyroidism	TSH
Tachycardia		FT$_3$
Atrial arrhythmia		FT$_4$
Weight loss despite increased appetite		TG
Nervousness, anxiety, and irritability		ABTG
Tremor		ABTPO
Sweating		TSHR-Abs
Goiter		Thyroid Doppler ultrasound
Insomnia		Thyroid scan
Heart failure		
Coronary heart disease		
Young onset	Primary aldosteronism	Aldosterone/renin ratio
Sustained blood pressure		Confirmatory tests
Resistant hypertension with or without hypokalemia		Anatomic localization according to etiology
Diuretic-induced hypokalemia		Adrenal venous sampling
Muscle weakness		
Cramping		
Polyuria		
Incidental adrenal mass		
Young stroke		
Sleep apnea		
Family history of early-onset hypertension		
Myocardial fibrosis		
Paroxysmal hypertension	Pheochromocytoma	24-hr urinary fractionated metanephrines
Flushing		Plasma-free metanephrines
Headaches		Chromogranin A methoxytyramine
Sweating		Anatomic localization according to etiology
Palpitations		
Orthostatic hypotension		
Syncope		
Paradoxic blood pressure response to drugs, surgery, or anesthesia		
Incidentally discovered adrenal mass		
Family history of PPGL		
Previous PPGL		
Syndromic feature indicating a pheochromocytoma-related hereditary syndrome		

Continued

CARDIOVASCULAR DISEASE AND DISORDERS OF OTHER ORGANS

TABLE 96.4 Clinical Features of Endocrine Dysfunctions: Diagnosis and Cardiovascular Outcome—cont'd

CLINICAL FEATURES	POSSIBLE DIAGNOSIS	DIAGNOSTIC TESTS
Weight gain with central obesity and rounded face	Cushing syndrome	ACTH and cortisol levels
Pink or purple stretch marks on the skin of the abdomen, thighs, breasts, and arms		24-hr urinary cortisol
Fragile skin that bruises easily		Late-night salivary cortisol
Hypertension		Dexamethasone suppression test
Insulin resistance or type 2 diabetes		CRH test
Dyslipidemia		Anatomic localization according to etiology
Prothrombotic state		
Depression		
Increased pigmentation	Addison disease	ACTH and cortisol levels
Abdominal pain with nausea and vomiting		24-hr urinary cortisol
Hypotension		Intravenous injection of ACTH
Hypoglycemia		Anatomic evaluation according to etiology
Hyponatremia		
Hyperkalemia		
Loss of autonomic tone		
Enlarged hands and feet	Acromegaly	GH
Enlarged facial features		IGF1
Enlarged tongue		GH after oral glucose load
Hypertension		Localization of the tumor according to etiology
Insulin resistance		
Type 2 diabetes mellitus		
Hyperlipidemia		
Incidentally discovered pituitary tumors		
Sleep apnea		
Debilitating arthritis or carpal tunnel syndrome		
Cardiomegaly		
Concentric biventricular hypertrophy		
History of traumatic brain injury, subarachnoid hemorrhage, cranial irradiation, pituitary hemorrhage, or surgery	GH deficiency	GH
		IGF1
Central adiposity		IGF- Binding protein 3
Reduced lean muscle mass		GH-releasing hormone-arginine stimulation test
Impaired neuromuscular function		
Impaired lipid profile		
Depression, anxiety, social isolation		
Fatigue		
Impaired cardiac function		
Accelerated atherogenesis		
Increased risk of hypertension		
Prothrombotic state		
Decreased sweating and thermoregulation		
Changes in memory, processing speed, and attention		
Kidney stones	Primary hyperparathyroidism	Serum calcium level
Excessive urination		Urinary calcium
Abdominal pain		PTH
Bone and joint pain		1,25OH D3
Nausea, vomiting, or loss of appetite		Bone mineral density
Hypercalcemia or high-normal serum calcium levels		Technetium sestamibi scanning
Hypertension		

ACTH, Adrenocorticotrophic hormone; *IGF*, insulin-like growth factor; *PPGL*, pheochromocytoma and paraganglioma; *PTH*, parathyroid hormone *TSH*, thyroid stimulating hormone.

or excess can improve the cardiovascular outcome (Table 96.4). The fact that a variety of naturally occurring hormones have such profound effects on the heart and cardiovascular system also suggests that these actions can be harnessed to treat a variety of cardiovascular diseases. The ability of thyroid hormone to lower cholesterol levels, enhance cardiac contractility (especially diastolic function) via novel transcription-based mechanisms, and at the same time lower systemic vascular resistance provides a platform for developing novel therapies. In addition, the recognition that GH and serum T_3 levels alter in the setting of various forms of cardiac disease and heart failure can provide new biomarkers for assessing novel treatment strategies.

REFERENCES

For references to the older literature, please see the 11th edition of *Braunwald's Heart Disease*..

PITUITARY FUNCTION AND CARDIOVASCULAR DISEASE

Adrenal Function and Cardiovascular Disease

1. Melmed S. Pituitary-tumor endocrinopathies. *N Engl J Med.* 2020;382:937.
2. Higashi Y, Gautam S, Delafontaine P, Sukhanov S. IGF-1 and cardiovascular disease growth. *Horm IGF Res.* 2019;45(6).
3. Isgaard J, Arcopinto M, Karason K, Cittadini A. GH and the cardiovascular system: an update on a topic at heart. *Endocrine.* 2015;48:25.
4. Gadelha MR, Kasuki L, Lim DST, Fleseriu M. Systemic complications of acromegaly and the Impact of the current treatment Landscape: an update. *Endocr Rev.* 2019;40:268.
5. Ramos-Leví AM. Marazuela M Cardiovascular comorbidities in acromegaly: an update on their diagnosis and management. *Endocrine.* 2017;55:346.
6. Katznelson L, Laws Jr ER, Melmed S, et al. Acromegaly: an endocrine society clinical practice guideline. Endocrine Society. *J Clin Endocrinol Metab.* 2014;99:3933.
7. Sharma AN, Tan M, Amsterdam EA, Singh GD. Acromegalic cardiomyopathy: epidemiology, diagnosis, and management. *Clin Cardiol.* 2018;41:419.
8. Dural M, Kabakci G, Cinar N, et al. Assessment of cardiac autonomic functions by heart rate recovery, heart rate variability and QT dynamicity parameters in patients with acromegaly. *Pituitary.* 2014;17:163.
9. Bolfi F, Neves AF, Boguszewski CL. Nogueira N Mortality in acromegaly decreased in the last decade: a systematic review and meta-analysis. *Eur J Endocrinol.* 2018;179:59.
10. Ritvonen E, Loyttyniemi E, Jaatinen P, et al. Mortality in acromegaly: a 20-year follow-up study. *Endocr-Relat Cancer.* 2016;23:469.
11. Melmed S, Bronstein MD. Chanson P Consensus Statement on acromegaly therapeutic outcomes. *Nat Rev Endocrinol.* 2018;14:552.
12. Capalbo D, Barbieri F, Improda N, et al. Growth hormone improves cardiopulmonary capacity and body composition in children with growth hormone deficiency. *J Clin Endocrinol Metab.* 2017;102:4080.
13. Thomas JD, Dattani A, Zemrak F, et al. Characterisation of myocardial structure and function in adult-onset growth hormone deficiency using cardiac magnetic resonance. *Endocrine.* 2016;54(3):778e87.
14. Jasim S, Alahdab F, Ahmed AT, et al. Mortality in adults with hypopituitarism: a systematic review and meta-analysis. *Endocrine.* 2016;56:33.
15. Cittadini A, Marra AM, Arcopinto M, et al. Growth hormone replacement delays the progression of chronic heart failure combined with growth hormone deficiency: an extension of a randomized controlled single-blind study. *JACC Heart Fail1.* 2013;325.
16. Arcopinto M, Salzano A, Giallauria F, et al. Growth hormone deficiency is associated with worse cardiac function, physical performance, and outcome in chronic heart failure: insights from the T.O.S.CA. GHD study. *PloS One.* 2017;12(1):e0170058.
17. Lopez Vicchi F, Luque GM, Brie B, et al. Dopaminergic drugs in type 2 diabetes and glucose homeostasis. *Pharmacol Res.* 2016;109:74.
18. Kate E, Therkelsen BA, Tobin M, et al. Association between prolactin and incidence of cardiovascular risk factors in the framingham heart study. *J Am Heart Assoc.* 2016;5:e002640.
19. Stiles CE, Tetteh-Wayoe ET, Bestwick J, et al. A meta-analysis of the prevalence of cardiac valvulopathy in hyperprolactinemic patients treated with Cabergoline. *J Clin Endocrinol Metab.* 2018.

Adrenal Function and Cardiovascular Disease

20. Lacroix A, Feelders RA, Stratakis CA, Nieman LK. Cushing's syndrome. *Lancet.* 2015;386:913.
21. Kamenický P, Redheuil A, Roux C, et al. Cardiac structure and function in cushing's syndrome: a cardiac magnetic resonance imaging study. *J Clin Endocrinol Metab.* 2014;99:E2144.
22. Isidori AM, Graziadio C, Paragliola RM, et al. ABC Study Group. The hypertension of Cushing's syndrome: controversies in the pathophysiology and focus on cardiovascular complications. *J Hypertens.* 2015;33:44.
23. Javanmard P, Duan D, Geer EB. Mortality in patients with endogenous cushing's syndrome. *Endocrinol Metab Clin North Am.* 2018;47:313.
24. van Haalen FM, Broersen LH, Jorgensen JO, et al. Management of endocrine disease: mortality remains increased in Cushing's disease despite biochemical remission: a systematic review and meta-analysis. *Eur J Endocrinol.* 2015;172:R143.
25. Clayton RN, Jones PW, Reulen RC, et al. Mortality in patients with Cushing's disease more than 10 years after remission: a multicentre, multinational, retrospective cohort study. *Lancet Diabetes Endocrinol.* 2016;4:569.
26. Di Dalmazi G, Pasquali R. Adrenal adenomas, subclinical hypercortisolism, and cardiovascular outcomes. *Curr Opin Endocrinol Diabetes Obes.* 2015;22:163.
27. Nieman LK, Biller BM, Findling JW, et al. Treatment of cushing's syndrome: an endocrine society clinical practice guideline. *J Clin Endocrinol Metab.* 2015;100:2807.
28. Funder JW, Carey RM, Mantero F, et al. The management of primary aldosteronism: case detection, diagnosis, and treatment: an endocrine society clinical practice guideline. *J Clin Endocrinol Metab.* 2016;101:1889.
29. Vaidya A, Mulatero P, Baudrand R, Adler GL. The expanding spectrum of primary aldosteronism: implications for diagnosis, pathogenesis, and treatment. *Endocr Rev.* 2018;39:1057.
30. Monticone S, Burrello J, Tizzani D, et al. Prevalence and clinical manifestations of primary aldosteronism encountered in primary care practice. *J Am Coll Cardiol.* 2017;69:1811.
31. Byrd JB, Turcu AF, Auchus RJ. Primary aldosteronism. Practical approach to diagnosis and management. *Circulation.* 2018;138:823–835.
32. Rehan M, Raizman JE, Cavalier E, et al. Laboratory challenges in primary aldosteronism screening and diagnosis. *Clin Biochem.* 2015;48:377.
33. Monticone S, D'Ascenzo F, Moretti C, et al. Cardiovascular events and target organ damage in primary aldosteronism compared with essential hypertension: a systematic review and meta-analysis. *Lancet Diabetes Endocrinol.* 2018;6:41.
34. Huang WC, Chen YY, Lin YH, et al. TAIPAI study group incidental congestive heart failure in patients with aldosterone-producing adenomas. *J Am Heart Assoc.* 2019;8(24):e012410. 17.
35. Satoh F, Morimoto R, Ono Y, et al. Peripheral plasma 18-oxocortisol can discriminate unilateral adenoma from bilateral diseases in primary aldosteronism patients. *Hypertension.* 2015;65:1096.
36. Williams TA, Peitzsch M, Dietz AS, et al. Genotype-specific steroid profiles associated with aldosterone- producing adenomas. *Hypertension.* 2016;67:139.
37. Hundemer GL, Curhan GC, Yozamp N, et al. Cardiometabolic outcomes and mortality in medically treated primary aldosteronism: a retrospective cohort study. *Lancet Diabetes Endocrinol.* 2018;6:51.
38. Charmandari E, Nicolaides NC, Chrousos GP. Adrenal insufficiency. *Lancet.* 2014;383:2152.
39. Bornstein SR, Allolio B, Arlt W, et al. Diagnosis and treatment of primary adrenal insufficiency: an endocrine society clinical practice guideline. *J Clin Endocrinol Metab.* 2016;101:364.

Pheochromocytoma and Paraganglioma

40. Crona J, Taïeb D, Pacak K. New perspectives on pheochromocytoma and paraganglioma: toward a molecular classification. *Endocr Rev.* 2017;38:489.
41. Lenders JW, Duh QY, Eisenhofer G, et al. Pheochromocytoma and paraganglioma: an endocrine society clinical practice guideline. *J Clin Endocrinol Metab.* 2014;99:1915.
42. Lam AK. Update on adrenal tumours in 2017 World Health Organization (WHO) of endocrine tumours. *Endocr Pathol.* 2017.
43. Martucci VL, Pacak K. Pheochromocytoma and paraganglioma: diagnosis, genetics, management, and treatment. *Curr Probl Cancer.* 2014;38(7).
44. Tufton N, Ghelani R, Srirangalingam U, et al. SDHA mutated paragangliomas may be at high risk of metastasis. *Endocr Relat Cancer.* 2017;24:L43.
45. Bausch B, Schiavi F, Ni Y, et al. European-American-Asian Pheochromocytoma-Paraganglioma Registry Study Group. Clinical characterization of the pheochromocytoma and paraganglioma susceptibility genes SDHA, TMEM127, MAX, and SDHAF2 for gene-informed prevention. *JAMA Oncol.* 2017;3:1204.
46. Toledo RA, Burnichon N, Cascon A, et al. Consensus Statement on next-generation-sequencing-based diagnostic testing of hereditary phaeochromocytomas and paragangliomas. *Nat Rev Endocrinol.* 2017;3:233.
47. Janssen I, Chen CC, Millo CM, et al. PET/CT comparing (68)Ga-DOTATATE and other radiopharmaceuticals and in comparison with CT/MRI for the localization of sporadic metastatic pheochromocytoma and paraganglioma. *Eur J Nucl Med Mol Imaging.* 2016;43:1784.

Parathyroid Function, Calcium Metabolism, and Cardiovascular Disease

48. Bilezikian JP, Brandi ML, Eastell R, et al. Guidelines for the management of asymptomatic primary hyperparathyroidism: summary statement from the Fourth International Workshop. *J Clin Endocrinol Metab.* 2014;99:3561.
49. Yao L, Folsom AR, Pankow JS, et al. Parathyroid hormone and the risk of incident hypertension: the Atherosclerosis Risk in Communities study. *J Hypertens.* 2016;34:196.
50. McMahon D, Carrelli A, Palmeri N, et al. Effect of parathyroidectomy upon left ventricular mass in primary hyperparathyroidism: a meta-analysis. *J Clin Endocrinol Metab.* 2015;100:4399.
51. Chen G, Xue Y, Zhang Q, Wen, et al. Is normocalcemic primary hyperparathyroidism harmful or harmless? *J Clin Endocrinol Metab.* 2015;100:2420.
52. Pepe J, Cipriani C, Sonato C, et al. Cardiovascular manifestations of primary hyperparathyroidism: a narrative review. *Eur J Endocrinol.* 2017;77(6):R297–R308.
53. Bollerslev J, Rejnmark L, Marcocci C. European society of endocrinology clinical guideline: treatment of chronic hypoparathyroidism in adults. *Eur J Endocrinol.* 2015;173:G1–G20.

Thyroid Involvement in Cardiovascular Disease

54. Razvi S, Jabbar A, Pingitore A, et al. Thyroid hormones and cardiovascular function and diseases. *J Am Coll Cardiol.* 2018;71:1781.
55. Cappola AR, Desai AS, Medici M. Thyroid and cardiovascular disease research agenda for enhancing knowledge, prevention, and treatment. *Thyroid.* 2019;29:760.
56. Medici M, Visser WE, Visser TJ, Peeters RP. Genetic determination of the hypothalamic–pituitary–thyroid axis: where do we stand? *Endocr Rev.* 2015;36:214.
57. Bianco AC, Dumitrescu A, Gereben B, et al. Paradigms of dynamic control of thyroid hormone signaling. *Endocr Rev.* 2019;40:1000.
58. de Vries EM, Fliers E. Boelen A. The molecular basis of the non-thyroidal illness syndrome. *J Endocrinol.* 2015;225:R67–R81.
59. Danzi S, Klein I. Thyroid disease and the cardiovascular system. *Endocrinol Metab Clin North Am.* 2014;43:517.
60. Groeneweg S, van Geest FS, Peeters RP, et al. Thyroid hormone transporters. *Endocr Rev.* 2020;41(1).
61. Felmlee MA, Jones RS, Rodriguez-Cruz V, et al. Monocarboxylate transporters (SLC16): function, regulation, and role in health and disease. *Pharmacol Rev.* 2020;72(2):466.
62. Jabbar A, Pingitore A, Pearce SH, et al. Thyroid hormones and cardiovascular disease. *Nat Rev Cardiol.* 2017;14:39.
63. Wan W, Xu X, Zhao W, et al. Exercise training induced myosin heavy chain isoform alteration in the infarcted heart. *Appl Physiol Nutr Metab.* 2014;39(2):226.
64. Biondi B. The management of thyroid abnormalities in chronic heart failure. *Heart Fail Clin.* 2019;15:393.
65. Davis PJ, Goglia F, Leonard JL. Nongenomic actions of thyroid hormone. *Nat Rev Endocrinol.* 2016;12:111.
66. Gluvic ZM, Obradovic MM, Sudar-Milovanovicc EM, et al. Regulation of nitric oxide production in hypothyroidism. *Biomed Pharmacother.* 2020;124:109881.
67. Biondi B, Cooper DS. Subclinical hyperthyroidism. *N Engl J Med.* 2018;378:2411.
68. Biondi B, Bartalena L, Cooper DS, et al. The 2015 European thyroid association guidelines on diagnosis and treatment of endogenous subclinical hyperthyroidism. *Eur Thyroid J.* 2015;4:149.
69. Burch HB, Cooper DS. Management of Graves disease a review. *J Am Med Assoc.* 2015;314:2544.
70. Biondi B, Kahaly G. In: Luster M, Duntas L, Wartofsly L, eds. *Heart in Hyperthyroidism. The Thyroid and its Diseases. A Comprensive Guide for Clinicians.* Springer; 2019:367–375.
71. Selmer C, Olesen JB, Hansen ML, et al. Subclinical and overt thyroid dysfunction and risk of all-cause mortality and cardiovascular events: a large population study. *J Clin Endocrinol Metab.* 2014;99:2372.
72. Floriani C, Gencer B, Collet TH. Rodondi N Subclinical thyroid dysfunction and cardiovascular diseases: 2016 update. *Eur Heart J.* 2018;14:503.
73. Biondi B. Atrial fibrillation and hyperthyroidism. In: Lüscher TF, Camm AJ, Maurer G, Serruys PW, eds. *ESC Textbook of Cardiovascular Medicine.* 3rd ed. European Society of Cardiology.
74. Chaker L, Heeringa J, Dehghan A, et al. Normal thyroid function and the risk of atrial fibrillation: the Rotterdam Study. *J Clin Endocrinol Metab.* 2015;100:3718.
75. Baumgartner C, da Costa BR, Collet TH, et al. Thyroid studies collaboration. Thyroid function within the normal range, subclinical hypothyroidism, and the risk of atrial fibrillation. *Circulation. 8.* 2017;136(22):2100.
76. Biondi B. Impact of hyperthyroidism on the cardiovascular and musculoskeletal systems and management of subclinical Graves' disease. In Graves' disease: a comprehensive guide for clinicians. Editor R. Bahn Springer (New York). Editor R. Bahn Springer (New York) pages 133-146 ISBN 9781493925339.

77. Page RL, Joglar JA, Caldwell MA, et al. Evidence review committee chair 2015 ACC/AHA/HRS guideline for the management of adult patients with supraventricular tachycardia: a report of the American college of cardiology/American heart association task force onclinical practice guidelines and the heart rhythm society. *Circulation*. 2016;13(134):e232.

78. Al-Khatib SM, Arshad A, Balk EM, et al. Risk stratification for arrhythmic events in patients with asymptomatic pre-excitation: a systematic review for the 2015 ACC/AHA/HRS guideline for the management of adult patients with supraventricular tachycardia: a report of the American College of Cardiology/American Heart Association Task Force on clinical practice guidelines and the Heart Rhythm Society. *J Am Coll Cardiol*. 2016;67:1624–1638.

79. January CT, Wann LS, Alpert JS, et al. ACC/AHA task force member 2014. AHA/ACC/HRS guideline for the management of patients with atrial fibrillation: a report of the American college of cardiology/American heart association task force on practice guidelines and the heart rhythm society. *Circulation*. 2014;130.e199–267.

80. Bano A, Chaker L, Mattace-Raso FUS, et al. Thyroid function and the risk of atherosclerotic cardiovascular morbidity and mortality: the Rotterdam Study. *Circ Res*. 2017;121:1392.

81. De Leo S, Lee SY, Braverman LE. Hyperthyroidism. *Lancet*. 2016;388:906.

82. Biondi B, Cooper DS. Thyroid hormone suppression therapy. *Endocrinol Metab Clin North Am*. 2019;48(1):227.

83. Satoh T, Isozaki O, Suzuki A, et al. 2016 guidelines for the management of thyroid storm from the Japan thyroid association and Japan endocrine society (first edition). *Endocr J*. 2016;63:1025.

84. Biondi B, Cappola AR, Cooper DS. Subclinical hypothyroidism: a review. *J Am Med Assoc*. 2019;9(2):153.322.

85. Peeters RP. Subclinical hypothyroidism. *N Engl J Med*. 2017;376(26):2556.

86. Biondi B, Duntas. Heart in hypothyroidism. The thyroid and its diseases. In: Luster M, Duntas L, Wartofsly L, eds. *A Comprensive Guide for Clinicians*. Springer pp 255-263, 2019.

87. Klein I, Danzi S. Thyroid disease and the heart. *Curr Probl Cardiol*. 2016;41:65.

88. del Busto-Mesa A, Cabrera-Rego JO, Carrero-Fernández L, et al. Changes in arterial stiffness, carotid intima-media thickness, and epicardial fat after L-thyroxine replacement therapy in hypothyroidism. *Endocrinol Nutr*. 2015;62:270.

89. Aziz M, Kandimalla Y, Machavarapu A, et al. Effect of thyroxin treatment on carotid intima-media thickness (CIMT) reduction in patients with subclinical hypothyroidism (sch): a meta-analysis of clinical trials. *J Atheroscler Thromb*. 2017;24:643.

90. Chen S, Shauer A, Zwas DR, et al. The effect of thyroid function on clinical outcome in patients with heart failure. *Eur J Heart Fail*. 2014;16(2):217.

91. Ning N, Gao D, Triggiani V, et al. Prognostic role of hypothyroidism in heart failure a meta-analysis. *Medicine (Baltim)*. 2015;94(30):e1159.

92. Yang G, Wang Y, Ma A, Wang T. Subclinical thyroid dysfunction is associated with adverse prognosis in heart failure patients with reduced ejection fraction. *BMC Cardiovasc Disord*. 2019;19:83.

93. Kong LY, Gao X, Ding XY, et al. Left ventricular end-diastolic strain rate recovered in hypothyroidism following levothyroxine replacement therapy: a strain rate imaging study. *Echocardiography*. 2019;36:707.

94. Sinha RA, Singh BK, Yen PM. Direct effects of thyroid hormones on hepatic lipid metabolism. *Nat Rev Endocrinol*. 2018;14:259.

95. Olsson AG, Chester Ridgway E, Ladenson PW. Reductions in serum levels of LDL cholesterol, apolipoprotein B, triglycerides and lipoprotein(a) in hypercholesterolaemic patients treated with the liver-selective thyroid hormone receptor agonist eprotirome. *J Intern Med*. 2015;277:331.

96. Biondi B, Cooper DS. Thyroid hormone therapy for hypothyroidism. *Endocrine*. 2019;66(1):18.

97. Jonklaas J, Bianco AC, Bauer AJ, et al. American thyroid association task force on thyroid hormone replacement guidelines for the treatment of hypothyroidism: prepared by the American thyroid association task force on thyroid hormone replacement. *Thyroid*. 2014;24:1670.

98. Rizzo LFL, Mana DL, Bruno OD, Wartofsky L. Myxedema coma. *Medicina (B Aires)*. 2017;4(77):321.

99. Bartalena L, Bogazzi F, Chiovato L, et al. 2018 European Thyroid Association (ETA) guidelines for the management of amiodarone-associated thyroid dysfunction. *Eur Thyroid J*. 2018;7(55).

100. Fliers E, Bianco AC, Langouche L, Boelen A. Thyroid function in critically ill patients. *Lancet Diabetes Endocrinol*. 2015;3:816.

101. Rothberger GD, Gadhvi S, Michelakis N, Kumar A, et al. Usefulness of serum triiodothyronine (T3) to predict outcomes in patients hospitalized with acute heart failure. *Am J Cardiol*. 2017;119:599.

102. Vale C, Neves JS, von Hafe M, et al. The role of thyroid hormones in heart failure. *Cardiovasc Drugs Ther*. 2019;33:179–188.

103. Chang CY, Chien YJ, Lin PC, et al. Non-thyroidal illness syndrome and hypothyroidism in ischemic heart disease population: systematic review and meta-analysis. *J Clin Endocrinol Metab*. 2020.

104. Pingitore A, Mastorci F, Piaggi P, et al. Usefulness of triiodothyronine replacement therapy in patients with ST elevation myocardial infarction and borderline/reduced triiodothyronine levels (from the THIRST study). *Am J Cardiol*. 2019;123:905.

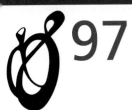

97 Rheumatic Diseases and the Cardiovascular System

JUSTIN C. MASON

The relationship between inflammatory rheumatic diseases and the cardiovascular system has long been recognized. As the treatment of these diseases has improved considerably over the last 30 years and increased survival, the importance and complexity of this interrelationship have achieved prominence. Indeed, we have entered an era in which established anti-rheumatic therapies are being trialed for the treatment of atherosclerosis.[1,2] Patients with multisystem rheumatic diseases may, on occasion, present initially to a cardiovascular physician or surgeon, and early recognition of the immune-mediated basis of the cardiovascular disease reduces morbidity and mortality. The vasculature may represent a primary target organ of the underlying rheumatic disease and can be affected at numerous sites and at micro- and macrovascular levels. Systemic sclerosis (SSc) impacts the microvessels and may be responsible for pulmonary arterial vasculopathy and pulmonary artery hypertension (PAH). Antineutrophil cytoplasmic antibody (ANCA)-associated systemic vasculitides (AASVs) affect arterioles preferentially, while the large-vessel vasculitides affect the aorta and its major branches. Antiphospholipid syndrome (APS) causes both venous and arterial thromboses. Cardiac complications influence morbidity and mortality and in systemic lupus erythematosus (SLE) include coronary arteritis, pericarditis, myocarditis, and valvular heart disease. Renal artery stenosis leading to uncontrolled hypertension is a feature of Takayasu arteritis (TA), and occlusive lesions in the subclavian, axillary, or iliac arteries may lead to limb claudication in patients with TA and giant cell arteritis (GCA). Inflammatory rheumatic diseases have equally important secondary effects on the cardiovascular system. Chronic systemic inflammation predisposes to endothelial dysfunction and increased arterial stiffness, thereby escalating the risk of cardiovascular events. Cardiovascular specialists increasingly recognize the significantly increased prevalence of cardiac dysrhythmias, premature myocardial infarction and stroke in patients suffering from rheumatoid arthritis (RA) and SLE.[3] Many outstanding clinical challenges remain; predominant among them are the development and rigorous evaluation of preventive strategies, early recognition, diagnosis and treatment of patients with rheumatic disease who have the highest risk for cardiovascular complications, alongside improved understanding of the underlying molecular mechanisms.

ATHEROSCLEROSIS AND THE RHEUMATIC DISEASES

Recognition of the role of inflammation in atherosclerosis has highlighted and stimulated study of the potential relationship between systemic inflammatory diseases and premature atherogenesis. This effort has substantially advanced our understanding of the epidemiology and underlying pathogenic mechanisms, revealing novel therapeutic targets. Current priorities include identification of patients most at risk and the development of preventive therapeutic strategies.[4,5] Evidence supporting an association between inflammatory diseases and premature cardiovascular events is best developed for RA and SLE. In addition, ankylosing spondylitis, psoriatic arthritis, AASV, TA, and APS may all associate with premature atherosclerosis. Cardiovascular specialists should consider an underlying inflammatory disease in young patients with otherwise unexplained angina, myocardial infarction, or stroke. Patients with a rheumatic disease who suffer a myocardial infarction have worse outcomes in terms of both heart failure and mortality than the age-matched general population.[3]

Endothelial Dysfunction and Vascular Injury

Homeostatic mechanisms promote a quiescent, antithrombotic, antiadhesive vascular endothelium and control vasodilation and permeability (see Chapters 24 and 36). Prolonged systemic inflammation such as that seen in RA and SLE may promote endothelial injury, increased endothelial apoptosis, and endothelial vasodilator dysfunction.

Traditional risk factors alone do not explain the increased burden of atherosclerosis, but inflammation may exacerbate the effects of classic risk factors.[6] When compared with the general population, patients with systemic inflammatory diseases more commonly exhibit endothelial dysfunction and increased aortic stiffness. Although the results of individual studies vary, effective treatment of the underlying inflammation may not always reverse the endothelial dysfunction or improve the aortic stiffness.[3,6,7] As plaque burden may not increase in rheumatologic diseases, systemic inflammatory environment may promote qualitative changes in plaques that predispose to plaque rupture, a conjecture supported by autopsy studies. Thus, both accelerated atherogenesis and higher-risk plaque may contribute to the observed increased incidence of premature cardiovascular events.[6,8]

Various molecular mechanisms mediate the increased risk for atherosclerotic disease and cardiovascular events. In addition to traditional cardiovascular risk factors, disease-related factors may include effects of the proinflammatory cytokines tumor necrosis factor-alpha (TNF-α), interleukin-1 (IL-1), interferon (IFN)-α, and IL-6 on endothelial activation, leukocyte adhesion, endothelial injury, and permeability. Chronic activation of toll-like receptor signaling, increased endothelial cell apoptosis and diminished capacity for repair may contribute. Autoantibodies (e.g., antiphospholipid antibodies), CD4+CD28- cytotoxic T cells, Th17/T$_{REG}$ imbalance, complement deficiency or excessive activation, genetic polymorphisms, and the deleterious effects of drugs, including corticosteroids and cyclosporine, are important.[3,6,8] The potential role for clonal hematopoiesis caused by somatic mutations in bone marrow stem cells also merits further investigation in autoimmune rheumatic disease (see also Chapter 24).[9]

Rheumatoid Arthritis

RA, an autoimmune, symmetric inflammatory polyarthritis with a female-to-male ratio of 3:1, affects up to 1% of the population in the Western world, with the onset of symptoms most commonly occurring between 30 and 50 years of age. Up to 80% of patients have a positive serum rheumatoid factor and/or anti–cyclic citrullinated peptide (CCP) antibodies. A systemic inflammatory response is evident, with low-grade fever, weight loss, raised erythrocyte sedimentation rate (ESR) and C-reactive protein (CRP), hypoalbuminemia, normochromic normocytic anemia, and thrombocytosis.

Atherosclerotic Disease in Rheumatoid Arthritis

A variety of studies have shown subclinical arterial disease with increased carotid intimal-media thickness (IMT) and early plaque development. Although RA independently raises the risk for atherosclerosis, the precise mechanistic relationship between RA and atherogenesis remains unknown. Similarly, the mechanisms and long-term outcomes of abnormalities in myocardial perfusion and coronary flow reserve in patients with RA and nonstenotic epicardial arteries remain to be established.[10] The initial abnormalities in vascular function may occur at or before the onset of RA symptoms.[11] The direct effect of chronic inflammation on vascular endothelium may itself promote atherogenesis, in addition to exacerbating the actions of traditional cardiovascular risk factors.[8,12] Moreover, the systemic inflammatory environment might contribute to the features of plaque and blood that promote cardiovascular events in patients with RA.[13]

Patients with RA have increased classic risk factors for atherosclerosis. Tobacco smoking associates with both cardiovascular risk and the development of RA. Similarly, insulin resistance and the metabolic syndrome are more common in RA. Patients with RA may have a dyslipidemia characterized by high triglyceride levels and low levels of high-density lipoprotein (HDL) and low-density lipoprotein (LDL) cholesterol.[14,15] The risk for myocardial infarction in patients with RA is considered similar to diabetes mellitus, and women with RA are twice as likely as age-matched controls in the general population to suffer myocardial infarction. Although death rates from both heart attack and stroke are comparable to that in the general population, events occur at an earlier age, with 50% of premature deaths in patients with RA being a direct consequence of cardiovascular disease. The excess mortality becomes apparent 7 to 10 years after diagnosis and associates with persistent disease activity and the presence of rheumatoid factor and anti-CCP antibodies. A recent review suggests that patients with RA who suffer a myocardial infarction have worse outcomes.[16] However, this situation is changing, reflecting improved recognition of excess risk.[17]

TREATMENT

Drug therapy for RA has evolved remarkably over the past 25 years, with the focus on biologic therapies and aggressive management of early disease. Clinical trials have demonstrated that this approach reduces symptoms and structural damage to joints. Increasing evidence suggests treatment to target to control synovitis also confers vascular protection.[3,18]

Methotrexate has become the most widely used disease-modifying antirheumatic drug (DMARD), and since its introduction, mortality from myocardial infarction in patients with RA has improved. Sulfasalazine and hydroxychloroquine may confer similar benefit. Patients who do not respond adequately to DMARD therapy should switch to biologic therapies. These include those targeting TNF-α (infliximab, adalimumab, etanercept, certolizumab, and golimumab), the IL-6 receptor (tocilizumab, sarilumab), CTLA4Ig (abatacept), and the B cell–depleting monoclonal antibody rituximab, alongside oral small molecules targeting the Janus kinases (JAK) (baricitinib, tofacitinib, upadacitinib, ruxolitinib).[19,20] An aggressive disease-modifying approach minimizes the use of nonsteroidal antiinflammatory drugs (NSAIDs) and the requirement for corticosteroid therapy. Glucocorticoids may worsen traditional risk factors including insulin resistance, hypertension, and lipid profiles and may hasten carotid plaque formation in RA.[12] Because NSAIDs and cyclo-oxygenase-2 (COX-2)-selective NSAIDs (coxibs), although effective, may elevate blood pressure and increase the frequency of thrombotic cardiovascular events, their use in patients with cardiovascular complications of inflammatory disease requires caution.[21] However, evidence suggests that NSAID use in patients with RA does not confer an increased risk for cardiovascular events, thus indicating that their anti-inflammatory effects predominate.

Definitive demonstration of the potential cardiovascular benefits of the biologic therapies requires the results of long-term prospective studies (see later). TNF-α promotes vascular endothelial activation and dysfunction and may lead to plaque destabilization, and hence blockade would appear to be an attractive therapeutic option. Infliximab therapy may improve endothelial function as measured by flow-mediated dilation 4 to 12 weeks after infusion, whereas etanercept has been reported to reduce aortic stiffness. Analysis of carotid IMT suggests that TNF-α antagonists reduce systemic inflammation and retard progression of IMT.[12] Tight therapeutic control of RA disease activity per se appears to have a beneficial effect on the risk for myocardial infarction.[18] Treatment of the arthritis must be combined with a careful review of classic risk factors, with appropriate steps taken to modify them. Despite this, too few patients are routinely assessed for cardiovascular risk.[22] Although we lack rigorous trials, most rheumatologists have a low threshold for addition of a statin.[23] Meanwhile, debate continues concerning the pros and cons of disease-specific cardiovascular risk calculators.[22] New guidelines have reviewed such issues.[14]

Systemic Lupus Erythematosus

SLE, a systemic autoimmune disease, predominates in women at a ratio of 9:1 and affects all racial groups but more commonly those of Afro-Caribbean, Asian, and Chinese extraction. Initial constitutional symptoms include night sweats, lethargy, malaise, and weight loss. Mucocutaneous features including the classic butterfly facial rash, oral ulcers, and alopecia are frequent. Serositis, myalgia, arthralgia, and Jaccoud nonerosive arthropathy also occur. Potentially life-threatening complications include glomerulonephritis with renal failure, central nervous system (CNS) involvement with cerebral vasculitis, pneumonitis, shrinking lung syndrome, and PAH. Hematologic involvement includes lymphopenia in most and frequently hemolytic anemia, neutropenia, and thrombocytopenia. Cardiac manifestations of SLE include pericarditis, myocarditis, endocarditis, aortitis, and coronary arteritis. Understanding of the pathogenesis of SLE continues to improve. A defect in apoptotic cell clearance results in the exposure of nuclear antigens to an immune system with hyperreactive B cells. Loss of immune tolerance results in the generation of autoantibodies and immune complexes. Deposition of immune complexes in target organs leads to the activation of complement and tissue injury.[24]

Most patients have high-titer antinuclear antibodies and antibodies against double-stranded DNA (dsDNA). The latter are more specific for the diagnosis of SLE, which is reinforced by the presence of antibodies against one or more nuclear antigens, including Sm, Ro, La, and ribonucleoprotein (RNP). Complement activation and consumption of C3 and C4 leading to reduced plasma levels characterize active disease. The ESR also rises in active disease, while CRP levels typically remain normal except in those with serositis or secondary infection.

Atherosclerotic Disease in Systemic Lupus Erythematosus

The increased risk for myocardial infarction and stroke in patients with SLE is somewhere between 2-fold and 10-fold and up to 50-fold greater than that in the general population. The young age of patients with SLE and cardiovascular disease (67% of female patients with SLE and a first cardiac event are less than 55 years of age) suggests that SLE accelerates arterial disease.[25,26] A study of 1874 cases (9485 person-years follow-up) revealed a 2.66-fold increase in the risk of myocardial infarction, stroke and coronary intervention when compared with the general population. Although the pattern and extent of coronary artery disease in SLE does not appear to differ (Fig. 97.1), the plaques may be more vulnerable to rupture. Patients with SLE have worse outcomes following myocardial infarction than the age-matched general population, with a higher risk for the development of cardiac failure and increased mortality.[8] This difference may result from late diagnosis of ischemic heart disease and a reluctance to treat aggressively.

Hypertension is common in SLE because of renal disease and the widespread use of glucocorticoids. Similarly, patients with SLE commonly have metabolic syndrome, which associates with renal impairment, higher corticosteroid doses, and Korean or Hispanic ethnicity. Patients with SLE also have lipid abnormalities, including high levels of very low-density lipoprotein (VLDL) and triglycerides, elevated or normal LDL cholesterol, reduced HDL cholesterol and impaired cholesterol efflux.[26]

TREATMENT

Mild SLE with rash and arthralgia can be treated with simple analgesics and NSAIDs, with hydroxychloroquine commonly added to minimize flares. Organ involvement, including mild renal impairment, hematologic abnormalities, myositis, arthritis, and cutaneous lesions, requires the addition of prednisone and typically an immunosuppressant such as mycophenolate mofetil (MMF), azathioprine, or methotrexate to aid in controlling the disease and to facilitate steroid sparing. Cyclophosphamide and corticosteroids remain the first-line treatment of life-threatening complications, including myocarditis, cerebritis, severe hematologic involvement, and glomerulonephritis. MMF often replaces cyclophosphamide for lupus nephritis because of its equivalent efficacy and concerns regarding the risk for permanent infertility seen in up to 50% of patients treated with cyclophosphamide.[27] Most rheumatologists and nephrologists consider rituximab an effective treatment of severe SLE, although clinical trials to date have proved disappointing. A variety of regimens have been used, including combinations of rituximab, prednisone, and cyclophosphamide.[28] Belimumab, a monoclonal antibody that binds to the soluble B lymphocyte stimulator and prevents its interaction with B cell surface receptors, has a modest disease-modifying effect in nonrenal SLE. Positive phase III trial data are emerging for belimumab in lupus nephritis, for IFN type 1 receptor antibody anifrolumab and calcineurin inhibitor voclosporin.[29]

Defining effective strategies for prevention of cardiovascular disease in patients with SLE will require long-term prospective trials with adjudicated cardiovascular endpoints. Undertreated and/or persistently active disease associates with accelerated atherogenesis. Therefore, adequate individualized immunosuppressive therapy should minimize cardiovascular complications. Hydroxychloroquine reduces LDL cholesterol and lowers mortality from cardiovascular disease in patients with SLE. Aggressive management of traditional risk factors is also advocated, including regular diligent monitoring and tight blood pressure control. Statins are widely used, particularly in patients with renal impairment. Caution and careful monitoring should be exercised in patients with active myositis, as statin therapy can exacerbate this complication. The clinical data available do not support significant protection against atherosclerosis by statins 2 to 3 years after initiation, although longer-term analysis is awaited.[26]

Atherosclerosis in Association With Other Rheumatic Diseases

The relationship between chronic inflammation and atherogenesis implies that many rheumatic diseases may be associated with premature and increased cardiovascular risk (Table 97.1). Because data in support of this hypothesis derive from relatively small studies, important current clinical challenges include the need to determine (1) which rheumatic diseases pose the greatest cardiovascular threat, (2) a means of identifying subsets of patients most at risk, and (3) evidence-based strategies to minimize cardiovascular events.

Ankylosing spondylitis, psoriatic arthritis, and gout all associate with atherosclerotic disease. Hyperuricemia independently predicts cardiovascular disease, and patients with gout often have hypertension, hyperlipidemia, obesity, and diabetes mellitus. Many drugs used for the treatment of cardiac disease, including diuretics, beta blockers, and low-dose aspirin, can increase serum uric acid levels. In contrast, losartan, angiotensin-converting enzyme (ACE) inhibitors, atorvastatin, and fenofibrate may reduce urate levels. Allopurinol may reduce the risk for congestive cardiac failure and cardiovascular-associated death, whereas an increased risk of cardiovascular death has been reported with febuxostat.[30] In addition to achieving a serum uric acid level lower than 0.36 mmol/L (6 mg/dL), patients with gout should receive dietary advice and aggressive management of cardiovascular risk factors.

Systematic review of articles on cardiovascular disease in psoriatic arthritis has revealed increased traditional risk factors, endothelial dysfunction, aortic stiffness, and subclinical atherosclerosis. The limited data available suggest that adequate suppression of inflammatory disease activity, which leads to improvement in endothelial dysfunction and carotid IMT, should be combined with regular assessment and

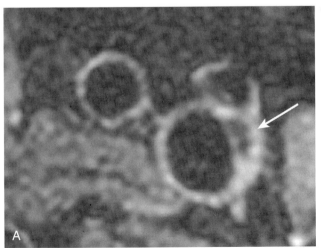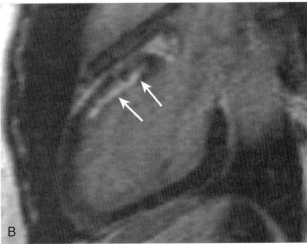

FIGURE 97.1 Atherosclerosis in systemic lupus erythematosus. **A,** Transaxial T2-weighted cardiac magnetic resonance (CMR) of the carotid bifurcation showing atherosclerotic plaque *(arrow)*. The lipid-filled core and fibrous cap can be seen along with evidence of calcification. **B,** CMR showing a two-chamber view in the late phase after gadolinium injection. Subendocardial late gadolinium enhancement is present in the anteroseptal left ventricle *(arrows)* and extends from the base of the heart to the midventricular region, consistent with a previous subendocardial myocardial infarction.

CARDIOVASCULAR DISEASE AND DISORDERS OF OTHER ORGANS

TABLE 97.1 Coronary Artery Involvement and the Rheumatic Diseases

Premature Atherosclerosis
Systemic lupus erythematosus
Rheumatoid arthritis
Ankylosing spondylitis
Psoriatic arthritis
Gout
Takayasu arteritis
Giant cell arteritis
Coronary Arteritis
Systemic lupus erythematosus
Takayasu arteritis
Kawasaki disease
Churg-Strauss syndrome
Polyarteritis nodosa
Granulomatous polyangiitis
Rheumatoid arthritis

control of traditional risk factors.[15,31] Patients with ankylosing spondylitis have also demonstrated impaired endothelial function, increased carotid IMT and pulse wave velocity, all of which indicate an increased risk for atherosclerosis.[31] The long-term impact of anti-TNF-α, and the pros and cons associated with increasing use of anti-IL-17 and anti-IL-12/23 therapies on the incidence of cardiovascular events in spondyloarthritides will emerge from international biologic registries.

VASCULITIDES (SEE CHAPTERS 42 AND 43)

The vasculitides, a heterogeneous group of diseases, represent a significant clinical challenge, both diagnostically and therapeutically. The primary systemic vasculitides are classified into large-, medium-, and small-vessel disease. This leaves a small group of unclassified conditions, including Behçet disease, relapsing polychondritis, primary CNS vasculitis, and Cogan syndrome.[32]

The histologic features of vasculitis include perivascular inflammatory infiltrates that may invade the arterial wall, fibrinoid necrosis, thrombosis, fibrosis, and scar formation. Fibrinoid necrosis, a specific feature of the medium- and small-vessel vasculitides, typically affects the tunica media. Complications include stenosis and occlusions resulting in organ ischemia, thrombosis, aneurysm formation, and hemorrhage. Although biopsy is optimal for making the diagnosis, suitable tissue may not always be accessible, or arterial biopsy may present unacceptable hazards, such as in patients with TA. Thus, diagnosis often depends on clinical findings, laboratory indices, and imaging.

The vasculitides have a complex, multifactorial, and poorly understood immunopathogenesis. The endothelium may be subject to complement-mediated injury as a consequence of immune complex deposition in polyarteritis nodosa (PAN) or rheumatoid vasculitis. In the medium- and small-vessel vasculitides, ANCAs may stimulate formation of neutrophil extracellular traps (NETs), which damage the endothelium. The proinflammatory cytokines TNF-α, IL-1, IL-6, and IFN-γ may activate the endothelium and induce the expression of adhesion molecules, including E-selectin, vascular cell adhesion molecule-1 (VCAM-1), and intercellular adhesion molecule-1 (ICAM-1), thereby facilitating leukocyte adhesion and recruitment into the vessel wall and surrounding tissue.

Cardiovascular disease in patients with vasculitis, although relatively rare, can be life-threatening. Aortitis, hypertension, coronary arteritis, valvular heart disease, pericarditis, myocarditis, conduction abnormalities, accelerated atherosclerosis, and cardiac failure can all occur. This section focuses on the vasculitides most likely to be encountered by cardiovascular disease specialists.

Large-Vessel Vasculitis
Giant Cell Arteritis
GCA affects large and medium-sized arteries. The disease affects those older than 50 years, with incidence increasing with age. GCA occurs most commonly in northern Europe, Scandinavia, and the United States in people of northern European ancestry. GCA typically affects extracranial branches of the aorta and, in addition to the temporal arteries, may involve the subclavian and axillary arteries, the thoracic aorta, and, on occasion, the vertebrobasilar circulation, and femoral and iliac arteries. Clinical features include fever, weight loss, malaise, headache, temporal artery thickening with loss of pulsation, scalp tenderness, and jaw claudication. The most feared complication, anterior ischemic optic neuropathy (AION), may be manifested as amaurosis fugax or sudden permanent visual loss. Up to 25% of patients present with systemic features without the classic sign of tenderness and temporal artery involvement. ^{18}F-fluorodeoxyglucose positron emission tomography (FDG-PET) has shown widespread FDG avidity throughout the aorta and subclavian and iliac arteries consistent with inflammation in more than 50% of patients.[33]

Pathogenesis
Histopathologic examination reveals localized fragmentation of the internal elastic lamina closely associated with an inflammatory infiltrate consisting predominantly of IFN-γ–producing CD4+ T lymphocytes, monocytes/macrophages, and occasional characteristic multinucleated giant cells. Activated CD83+ dendritic cells initiate the arterial wall inflammation and colocalize with activated T cells. Local synthesis of mediators such as platelet-derived growth factor leads to proliferation of smooth muscle cells and concentric stenosis of the arterial lumen (Fig. 97.2). Release of matrix metalloproteinases and generation of reactive oxygen species can result in arterial wall injury and aneurysm formation, typically involving the thoracic aorta.

Diagnosis
Biopsy is the definitive means of diagnosis and should be considered for all patients. However, the need for biopsy should not delay treatment. Temporal artery biopsy is positive in up to 80% of patients. Temporal artery ultrasound can reveal a characteristic halo sign with concentric homogeneous thickening of the arterial wall and evidence of flow disturbance and stenosis (see Fig. 97.2).[33]

Cardiovascular Complications
Although relatively rare, severe cardiovascular complications can occur and include aortic dissection and thoracic aortic aneurysms (Table 97.2).[33,34] Imaging and autopsy studies suggest that aortitis and aortic wall thickening are frequent in GCA, although their relationship with the development of aortic aneurysm remains unclear. Those with conventional cardiovascular risk factors including cigarette smoking, poorly controlled disease, and aortic regurgitation have a higher risk. Increased FDG uptake in the thoracic aorta can associate with an increased risk for aortic dilation. In the absence of guidelines, we recommend annual thoracic aortic screening for those with FDG-PET–positive thoracic aortic uptake or magnetic resonance angiography (MRA) or computed tomography angiography (CTA) evidence of aortic wall thickening and every 2 to 3 years in the remainder of patients. CTA and MRA are the optimal imaging techniques.[35] Pericarditis, coronary arteritis, limb ischemia, accelerated atherosclerosis, myocardial infarction, and cerebrovascular accidents all associate with GCA. Yet most outcome studies do not report increased mortality, so the impact of severe cardiovascular disease seems to be small.[36]

Takayasu Arteritis
TA, a granulomatous panarteritis, affects the aorta and its major branches, typically before the age of 40 years. The disease predominates in women, with a female-to-male ratio of up to 10:1. Because the diagnosis is often delayed, substantial arterial injury accrues.

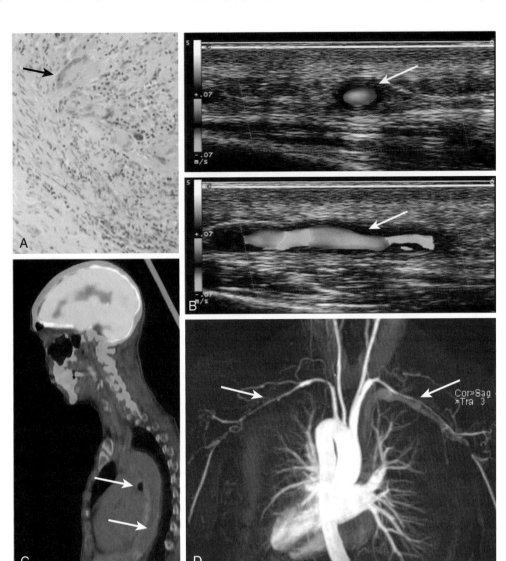

FIGURE 97.2 Giant cell arteritis (GCA). **A,** A temporal artery biopsy specimen stained with hematoxylin-eosin shows evidence of myofibroblast proliferation and vessel occlusion, a focal mononuclear cell inflammatory infiltrate, and the presence of multinucleated giant cells *(arrow).* **B,** Dark hypoechoic, circumferential wall thickening (halo sign) *(arrows)* is seen around the temporal artery lumen in active GCA in both transverse and longitudinal views. **C,** ^{18}FDG-PET-CT scan demonstrating uptake in the thoracic aorta, consistent with active arteritis. **D,** Magnetic resonance angiogram demonstrating bilateral stenosis of the left subclavian and axillary arteries *(arrows)* in a 60-year-old woman with upper limb ischemic symptoms. (**B** courtesy Dr. Wolfgang Schmidt, Medical Center for Rheumatology Berlin-Buch, Berlin, Germany.)

Presentation is typically nonspecific and associated with fever, night sweats, arthralgia, malaise, profound tiredness, and lethargy. TA may be accompanied by symptoms of upper limb claudication, and carotidynia occurs in up to 25% of patients. The aorta may be involved throughout its length, and even though any branches can be diseased, the most commonly affected are the subclavian and common carotid arteries. More than 90% of patients have stenotic/occlusive arterial lesions, whereas approximately 25% have aneurysms. The pulmonary arteries are involved in up to 50% of patients, and aortic valve regurgitation and coronary arteritis may occur (Fig. 97.3).[37]

TA has severe consequences, with 74% reporting compromised daily activities and 23% unable to work. In our cohort, survival at 15 years is higher than 95%; similarly, in the United States, 94% to 96% survival rates are reported, whereas in Korea the survival rate was 87% at 10 years. In Japan, 15-year survival rates have improved to 96.5%. However, the survival rate fell to 67% in a subset of patients with serious complications and/or a progressive disease course.

Pathogenesis
Arteritic lesions demonstrate adventitial thickening and focal leukocytic accumulation in the media with intimal hyperplasia. The leukocytes include activated dendritic cells, T and B lymphocytes, macrophages, and multinucleated giant cells (see Fig. 97.3). Growth factor–driven mesenchymal cell proliferation leads to intimal hyperplasia and fibrosis and subsequent arterial stenosis or occlusion. Local matrix metalloproteinase synthesis may predispose to aneurysmal dilation.

TABLE 97.2 Cardiovascular Disease in the Systemic Vasculitides

VASCULITIDES	CARDIOVASCULAR COMPLICATIONS
Large-Vessel Vasculitis	
Giant cell arteritis	Thoracic/abdominal artery aneurysm, limb ischemia, pericarditis, coronary arteritis, IHD, MI
Takayasu arteritis	Aortic regurgitation, limb ischemia, aortic stenosis, aortic aneurysm, stroke, hypertension, coronary arteritis and aneurysm, IHD, MI, myocarditis, cardiac failure
Kawasaki disease	Coronary artery aneurysm, MI, myocarditis, pericarditis, valvular dysfunction, cardiac failure
Medium-Vessel Vasculitis	
Eosinophilic granulomatosis with polyangiitis (Churg-Strauss syndrome)	Myocarditis, pericarditis, coronary arteritis, cardiomyopathy, cardiac fibrosis, valvular dysfunction, MI
Polyarteritis nodosa	Myocarditis, pericarditis, coronary arteritis, coronary aneurysm, hypertension, cardiac failure
Wegener granulomatosis (granulomatous polyangiitis)	Myocarditis, pericarditis, coronary arteritis, valvular heart disease, cardiac failure
Microscopic polyangiitis	Pericarditis, coronary microaneurysm, MI

IHD, Ischemic heart disease; *MI,* myocardial infarction.

Diagnosis

Diagnosis of TA depends principally on the physician including the disease in the differential diagnosis. The variable nature of the features of TA and the lack of constitutional symptoms in 30% to 50% of patients initially present a challenge to prompt diagnosis. In addition to improved physician awareness, a list of "red flags" that raise the possibility of TA is helpful (Table 97.3). One's index of suspicion must be high in young patients with an unexplained acute-phase response or hypertension. Similarly, common initial signs, including diminished or absent pulsation or arterial bruits, can suggest the diagnosis.

Laboratory abnormalities during active disease include raised ESR and CRP (in 75% of patients), often accompanied by normochromic normocytic anemia, thrombocytosis, hypergammaglobulinemia, and hypo-albuminemia. No specific autoantibodies or other serologic abnormalities exist. Noninvasive imaging is now the optimal means of diagnosis because tissue biopsy is rarely available. High-resolution ultrasound, cardiac magnetic resonance (CMR), MRA, CTA, and PET have all been studied.[35,38] Although the potential of these techniques is not in doubt, their specificity and sensitivity in the management of TA remain undetermined. ^{18}F-FDG-PET-CT may reveal evidence of active arteritis and lead to early detection of prestenotic disease. Demonstration of arterial wall enhancement, edema, or thickening on MRA and CTA may also facilitate the diagnosis of prestenotic disease, and stenoses and aneurysms can be readily identified and monitored (see Fig. 97.3). Color duplex ultrasound has particular use in assessing the common carotid and proximal subclavian arteries in TA. Homogeneous, bright concentric arterial wall thickening is a typical finding in affected common carotid arteries.

Cardiovascular Complications

In addition to the sequelae associated with cerebral, internal organ, and limb ischemia, aneurysms, PAH, or aortic rupture may develop. Cardiac complications include aortic valve insufficiency, accelerated atherosclerosis, cardiac ischemia, myocarditis, myocardial infarction, and heart failure. Coronary disease is often asymptomatic, as illustrated by the identification of silent myocardial injury in 27% of a cohort that we studied. Thallium stress scintigraphy revealed myocardial perfusion defects in 53%, whereas intra-arterial angiography has shown that up to 30% have coronary artery lesions typically affecting the ostia and proximal segments, with the left main coronary artery being most commonly affected. Ostial vasculitic coronary lesions are typically uncalcified, while more distal calcified lesions reflect secondary accelerated atherosclerosis. Neither MRA nor ^{18}F-FDG-PET-CT reliably identifies coronary arteritis, which is best identified by coronary CTA. Inflammation of the ascending aorta predisposes to coronary artery involvement, as well as to dilation of the aortic root with subsequent aortic valve regurgitation and the need for aortic valve replacement. Left ventricular dysfunction may affect up to 20% and may reflect myocarditis, ischemic heart disease, and hypertension. High blood pressure occurs commonly with renal artery stenosis often in association in TA.

Kawasaki Disease

Kawasaki disease (KD) predominantly affects children younger than 5 years with a peak incidence at 6 to 24 months of age. The vasculitis affects medium and small arteries, notably the coronary arteries. All racial groups may be affected, with the highest incidence is recorded in Asia (20 to 100 per 100,000 children <5 years of age). KD is an

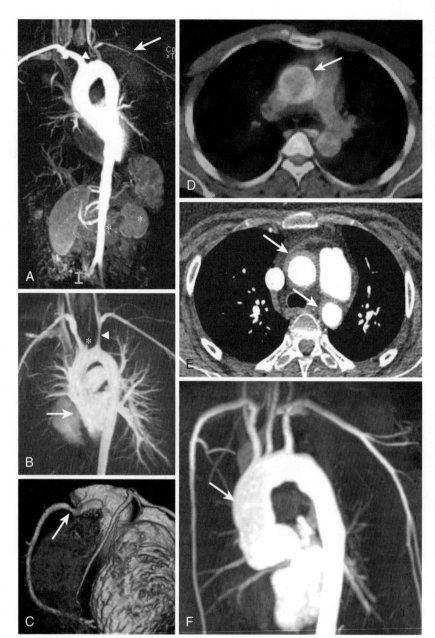

FIGURE 97.3 Takayasu arteritis. **A,** MRA demonstrating occlusion of the left common carotid artery (*arrowhead*), stenosis of the left subclavian artery with collateral formation (*arrow*), occlusion of the left renal artery and an atrophic left kidney (*asterisks*). **B,** MRA demonstrating severe stenosis of the right middle and lower lobe pulmonary arteries (*arrow*). The left common carotid artery is also occluded (*asterisk*) and there is stenosis of the left subclavian artery (*arrowhead*). **C,** Coronary CT angiogram demonstrating proximal ostial stenosis in the right coronary artery (*arrow*). **D,** [18]FDG-PET-CT scan demonstrating uptake in the aortic arch (*arrow*), consistent with active arteritis. **E,** CT angiography demonstrating thickening of the wall of the ascending and descending aorta (*arrows*). **F,** MRA revealing severe dilatation of the ascending aorta (*arrow*) requiring aortic valve replacement.

TABLE 97.3 "Red Flags" for Takayasu Arteritis

In patients younger than 40 years the following may indicative of TA:
Unexplained acute-phase response (raised ESR and/or CRP)
Carotidynia
Hypertension
Discrepant blood pressure between the arms (>10 mm Hg)
Absent/weak peripheral pulse or pulses
Limb claudication
Arterial bruit
Angina

CRP, C-reactive protein; *ESR,* erythrocyte sedimentation rate.

acute self-limited illness that typically resolves within 1 to 2 months, although mortality still remains 1% to 2%. Characteristic initial features include fever of 5 days' duration or longer, bilateral conjunctivitis, and mucocutaneous lesions, including red fissured lips and a strawberry tongue. Cervical lymphadenopathy may be prominent, with erythema affecting the palms and soles and a polymorphous exanthema.

Pathogenesis

The cause of KD is unknown, although occasional seasonal epidemics and increased incidence in siblings suggests infection may trigger the disease and lead to an uncontrolled immunologic response in a genetically susceptiblE host. Tissue specimens show endothelial injury, perhaps caused by proinflammatory cytokines and activated neutrophils. Infiltration of the arterial wall by neutrophils, T cells, and macrophages is associated with the development of arterial stenosis or, more commonly, aneurysms. Coronary artery aneurysms develop in up to 20% of patients during the first month of the illness, and 50% will regress in the following years. A variety of organisms have been implicated, including streptococci, staphylococci, and *Propionibacterium acnes*. Although no definitive evidence supports an infectious cause, the emergence of a Kawasaki-like syndrome in children affected by SARS-Cov-2 has reignited interest.[39]

Diagnosis

Neutrophilia, thrombocytosis, and a raised acute-phase response occur acutely. Echocardiography can detect coronary involvement from the second week of illness and can be used to monitor progress. Coronary angiography is not performed acutely because of the risk of precipitating myocardial infarction, but it can be used after 6 months to establish the degree of coronary artery involvement. The electrocardiogram (ECG) demonstrates abnormalities in up to 50% of patients, including tachycardia, T wave inversion, ST depression, atrioventricular block, and rarely, ventricular arrhythmia.

Cardiovascular Complications

Coronary artery aneurysms develop in up to 25% of untreated patients with KD. Sudden death can occur as a consequence of myocardial infarction following acute coronary thrombosis or rupture of a coronary artery aneurysm. Pericarditis, pericardial effusion, myocarditis, valvular dysfunction, and cardiac failure may all occur, whereas peripheral arterial involvement is less common but may affect the limb, renal, and visceral arteries.

Treatment

Intravenous immunoglobulin (IVIG) 2 g/kg over 10 to 12 hours should be prescribed as soon as diagnosis is made and within 10 days of presentation. Aspirin (30 to 100 mg/kg/day) is given concurrently until the patient is afebrile and then reduced to 3 to 5 mg/kg/day. This treatment combination reduces development of coronary artery aneurysm to 5%, with a significant impact on mortality. Ten to twenty percent of cases are resistant to IVIG. In this event a repeat course is recommended, and this can be combined with prednisone (2 mg/kg/day in divided doses). Alternative therapies for refractory disease, anti-TNF-α monoclonal infliximab (5 mg/kg IV over 2 hours) and the IL-1 receptor antagonist anakinra (100 to 200 mg/day SC), are both the subject of ongoing clinical trials.[40]

Most patients with KD have a good outcome. Yet in up to 20% of those with coronary artery aneurysms, coronary stenoses eventually develop, and these patients require long-term follow-up into adulthood by an experienced cardiologist. Although the risk for long-term complications, including myocardial infarction and sudden death, is greater in those with giant aneurysms, the risk for thrombosis and myocardial infarction still remains increased in those in whom aneurysms have regressed and throughout adult life.

Idiopathic Aortitis

Aortitis can complicate SLE, Cogan syndrome, Behçet disease, human leukocyte antigen (HLA) B27-positive spondyloarthropathy, KD, and GCA. Aortitis may also be idiopathic, although a number of such cases are now recognized to fall within the IgG4-related disease spectrum.[41] The clinical features are nonspecific and include malaise, lethargy, chest pain, fever, and weight loss, and the diagnosis is often missed, or made during incidental imaging or at the time of surgery. The ESR and CRP are typically raised, and the extent of the disease can be demonstrated by ^{18}F-FDG-CT-PET scanning and aortic MRA or CTA (Fig. 97.4). Dilation of the aortic root may require aortic valve and root replacement, whenever possible preceded by immunosuppressive therapy to control aortic wall inflammation. Treatment involves corticosteroids and a steroid-sparing immunosuppressant drug such as azathioprine, methotrexate, or MMF. The B-cell depleting antibody rituximab has proven particularly effective for IgG4-related disease.

Treatment of Large-Vessel Vasculitis

The evidence base for the treatment of large-vessel vasculitis is remarkably small. Although GCA and TA typically respond to steroids, gaining remission requires high doses and a considerable side effect burden. In GCA, the dependence on prednisone and conflicting evidence concerning the efficacy of steroid-sparing drugs, combined with concerns about AION, often result in overtreatment and considerable side effects. Indeed, 86% of patients experience glucocorticoid-related adverse events at 10-year follow-up. Both of these diseases have a high relapse rate when the dose of corticosteroid is tapered, suggesting persistent vasculitis. Potential mechanistic insight comes from the identification of two pathogenic pathways in GCA. Raised plasma IL-17 and Th17 cells in the arterial wall are rapidly reduced by prednisone therapy and remained suppressed as the dose is reduced. In contrast, the Th1-promoting cytokine IL-12 and IFN-γ-producing Th1 cells typically demonstrate corticosteroid resistance, which may account for the reemergence of disease.[33,42] Corticosteroid treatment of GCA should be tapered carefully to maintain remission and minimize side effects. Although the literature is somewhat conflicting, methotrexate may offer corticosteroid-sparing efficacy for those unable to reduce the dose of prednisone sufficiently.[43] Most patients with active TA require steroid-sparing immunosuppressive drugs. Methotrexate, MMF, and azathioprine are the most widely prescribed, and small open-label studies support their use.[37] In patients failing to respond or in those with life-threatening disease such as coronary arteritis or myocarditis, treatment with intravenous pulsed cyclophosphamide is recommended.

GiACTA, a double-blind, placebo-controlled study of the efficacy and safety of anti–IL-6 receptor monoclonal antibody tocilizumab in GCA reported that at 52 weeks, tocilizumab plus either a 26-week or 52-week prednisone taper demonstrated superiority in achieving sustained remission in GCA compared to the prednisone taper control arms alone.[44] While case reports also suggest that anti-TNF-α therapy can treat refractory GCA effectively, two small, randomized, placebo-controlled trials failed to demonstrate a significant clinically useful benefit. In patients with TA who fail to respond adequately to combination therapy with prednisone and steroid-sparing immunosuppressant drugs, including cyclophosphamide, current opinion is that both TNF-α and IL-6 blockade are effective, although clinical trial data is sparse.[45] A review of all published cases of TA treated with TNF-α antagonists found complete remission in 37%, partial remission in 53.5%, and no response in 9.5%. An initial placebo-controlled trial of tocilizumab in TA suggested a beneficial effect.[46] The suppression of both constitutional symptoms and CRP synthesis by tocilizumab complicates disease monitoring and may be falsely reassuring. Follow-up of patients with TA should therefore include angiographic monitoring, preferably with MRI because it avoids radiation exposure.[37]

Critical analysis of the published results suggests that percutaneous angioplasty or bypass surgery requires caution in patients with TA or GCA. Indications for surgical intervention include aneurysmal enlargement with risk for rupture, severe aortic regurgitation or coarctation, stenotic or occlusive lesions resulting in severe symptomatic coronary artery or cerebrovascular disease, uncontrolled hypertension as a consequence of renal artery stenosis, and stenoses leading to critical limb ischemia. Whenever possible, surgery should be delayed until immunosuppression has achieved clinical remission.[47]

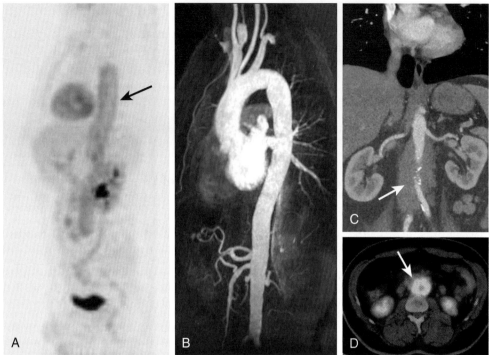

FIGURE 97.4 Idiopathic aortitis. **A,** ¹⁸F-FDG-PET scan demonstrating high-grade tracer uptake *(arrow)* in the aorta from below the level of the arch to just above the level of the aortic bifurcation, in keeping with aortitis. The activity is largely concentric around the aortic lumen. **B,** MRA showing aortic ectasia. **C,** IgG4-related disease with inflammatory peri-aortitis encasing the distal aorta below the renal arteries *(arrow)*. Calcification is seen within the aortic wall. **D,** ¹⁸F-FDG-PET scan reveals the inflammatory nature of the peri-aortitis with intense tracer uptake *(arrow)*.

Medium-Vessel Vasculitis

The medium-vessel vasculitides include Churg-Strauss syndrome (CSS, eosinophilic granulomatosis with polyangiitis, EGPA), granulomatosis with polyangiitis (GPA; Wegener granulomatosis), and microscopic polyangiitis (MPA). Although these diseases have overlapping features, they represent distinct clinical entities. GPA is most frequently associated with a cytoplasmic ANCA (cANCA) staining pattern that recognizes the antigen proteinase-3, whereas MPA most commonly associates with a perinuclear ANCA (pANCA) directed against myeloperoxidase.[48]

Eosinophilic Granulomatosis With Polyangiitis (Churg-Strauss Syndrome)

EGPA, a systemic small-vessel necrotizing vasculitis with a prevalence of 10 to 14 per million population, encompasses three disease phases. An initial prodrome characterized by allergic rhinitis, sinusitis, and asthma precedes peripheral blood eosinophilia and eosinophilic infiltrative lesions in the lung and myocardium. Some years later, a systemic phase follows with necrotizing vasculitis affecting the skin, peripheral nerves, gastrointestinal tract, and kidney (in 30%). Up to 40% of patients with EGPA are ANCA positive, most typically pANCA. ANCA-negative patients are more likely to suffer cardiopulmonary complications, whereas pANCA-positive patients seem to be more at risk for renal and peripheral nerve involvement. The diagnosis depends on the clinical features, imaging studies, ANCA, and whenever possible, biopsy results. Patients have a markedly raised peripheral eosinophil count and evidence of necrotizing vasculitis, including eosinophilic infiltration (Fig. 97.5).

The diagnosis of EGPA requires consideration of a number of alternatives, including GPA and MPA. A history of asthma, the presence of marked peripheral eosinophilia, and a dense eosinophilic infiltrate highly suggest EGPA. Viral infections, including cytomegalovirus and hepatitis B and C, must be excluded. In light of the eosinophilia, parasitic infestation, particularly by helminths, should be sought and excluded. Eosinophilia in the absence of demonstrable vasculitis may represent idiopathic hypereosinophilic syndrome or an underlying leukoproliferative disorder.

Cardiovascular Complications

Of all the vasculitides, EGPA most likely associates with severe and potentially fatal cardiac disease (see Table 97.2). Cardiac involvement complicates up to 60% of cases, and the disease spectrum includes pericarditis, myocarditis, coronary arteritis, myocardial infarction, cardiac fibrosis, arterial thrombosis, and valvular dysfunction. Cardiac disease is a prominent cause of death. Cardiomyopathy occurs as a result of ischemia secondary to arteritis affecting the intramyocardial arteries or, less frequently, the epicardial coronary arteries. Myocarditis associates with eosinophilic infiltration, fibrosis, and occasionally granuloma formation. Release of major basic protein and eosinophil-derived neurotoxin by infiltrating eosinophils can lead to direct tissue injury. Myocarditis may result in the development of restrictive, congestive, or dilated cardiomyopathy, or death.

Investigation

Cardiac involvement in EGPA requires urgent investigation, aggressive treatment, and initially, a 12-lead ECG and transthoracic echocardiography (see Fig. 97.5). Common findings include evidence of left ventricular dilation in 30% of patients, reduced shortening fraction, and increased cardiac wall echogenicity. Contrast-enhanced CMR provides the most sensitive means of detecting myocardial involvement.[49] If the diagnosis remains in doubt, endomyocardial biopsy may reveal eosinophilic infiltration with or without fibrosis, although vasculitis is rarely seen and the patchy nature of the disease renders diagnostic yield low.

Treatment

High-dose corticosteroid treatment typically results in a good response and associates with a 90% remission of disease. Relapses occur frequently on tapering steroid therapy, and prednisone-related side effects are common. In the presence of severe disease, including cardiac, gastrointestinal, CNS, and renal involvement, an immunosuppressant drug should be prescribed concomitantly. Although further clinical trials are required, the first choice of drug is pulsed intravenous cyclophosphamide. Once remission is achieved, generally by 3 to 6 months, cyclophosphamide can be replaced by azathioprine or methotrexate. In some patients with milder disease and evidence of steroid side effects, azathioprine or methotrexate should be added to

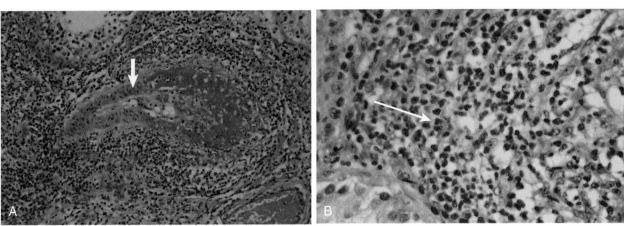

FIGURE 97.5 Churg-Strauss syndrome. **A,** Hematoxylin-eosin staining of a small artery *(arrow)* demonstrates fibrinoid necrosis and a dense perivascular mononuclear cell infiltrate. **B,** At higher magnification the inflammatory cells can be identified as predominantly eosinophils *(arrow)* with scattered macrophages.

aid in steroid tapering. In refractory disease, anecdotal case reports have suggested the effectiveness of IVIG or TNF-α blockade. The anti-IL-5 mAb mepolizumab has demonstrated efficacy in a randomized, placebo-controlled trial[50] and further results from the study of B cell depletion are awaited.[48]

Polyarteritis Nodosa

PAN is an increasingly rare disease characterized by a systemic necrotizing vasculitis of medium-sized arteries complicated by aneurysmal nodules. Viral infections, particularly with cytomegalovirus, human immunodeficiency virus, and hepatitis B and C virus, should be specifically sought and excluded. The classic type of PAN is an ANCA-negative vasculitis with the predominant clinical features including fever, malaise, arthralgia, weight loss, livedo reticularis, cutaneous nodules, and a vasculitic rash. Abdominal, cardiac, and testicular pain may occur, and some patients manifest mononeuritis multiplex. Hematuria, proteinuria, and/or hypertension indicates renal involvement.

The pathogenesis of PAN remains poorly understood. The initial vascular endothelial injury is followed by local release of IL-1 and TNF-α, which predispose to chronic inflammation and augmented leukocyte adhesion molecule expression. Recruitment of neutrophils is followed by monocyte infiltration, local endothelial disruption, thrombosis, and fibrinoid necrosis (Fig. 97.6). The associated arterial wall injury predisposes to aneurysm formation. The diagnosis of PAN is not straightforward. Although a biopsy can be definitive, yield is variable and dependent on an accessible lesion. A deep skin biopsy specimen from an involved nodular site is optimal. Combined sural nerve and muscle biopsy may also be helpful. Occasionally, nodules are detected on a medium-sized peripheral artery that can safely undergo biopsy. Renal biopsy should be approached with caution because of the risk for hemorrhage from microaneurysms. Despite increasing use of non-invasive imaging with CTA or MRA, mesenteric arteriography remains the most accurate way of identifying renal or hepatic microaneurysms.

Cardiovascular Complications

Cardiac involvement in PAN is often subclinical and clinically apparent in only 10% of patients. Congestive cardiac failure is most commonly seen and may reflect myocarditis or coronary arteritis. Alternatively, the underlying cause may be PAN-related renal disease complicated by hypertension. Five percent of patients develop pericarditis, as well as supraventricular tachycardia and valvular disease. Coronary angiography may reveal coronary artery microaneurysms, coronary arteritis, or coronary spasm. Coronary CTA may demonstrate coronary artery aneurysms.

Treatment

Glucocorticoids form the basis of treatment of PAN. In those with cardiac disease, significant proteinuria with or without renal impairment, CNS involvement, gastrointestinal disease, or mononeuritis multiplex, intravenous cyclophosphamide therapy is used initially. Some physicians prefer oral cyclophosphamide, and although side effects are more common, time until relapse may be longer. Six months of cyclophosphamide usually suffices to achieve disease remission, and treatment can be switched to oral azathioprine. In those with refractory disease, infliximab given in combination with methotrexate or azathioprine may provide benefit.

Granulomatosis With Polyangiitis (Wegener Granulomatosis)

GPA is a granulomatous necrotizing vasculitis that commonly affects the sinuses, upper airways, lungs, skin, joints, and kidneys. Diagnosis is based on clinical features, biopsy evidence, and typically a positive cANCA with antibodies against proteinase-3. The disease may be confined to the upper airways or be more generalized and include ocular inflammation, cutaneous vasculitis, arthralgia, cavitating lung lesions (Fig. 97.7), pulmonary hemorrhage, and acute renal failure. Clinical cardiac involvement is rare, although it has been reported in up to 30% of autopsy cases. The most frequently encountered problem is pericarditis, which can lead to hemodynamic compromise and tamponade. The presence of congestive cardiac failure is a poor prognostic sign and associated with 25% mortality in the first year. Underlying causes include coronary arteritis, myocarditis, and occasionally aortitis and valvular heart disease.

Microscopic Polyangiitis

MPA is most commonly associated with glomerulonephritis, renal impairment, and pulmonary hemorrhage. Cardiac disease is rarely clinically significant, but pericarditis occurs in 10% of patients, and congestive cardiac failure develops in up to 18%. Subclinical and occasionally symptomatic acute myocardial infarction can occur. Evidence from case reports and small series shows that this disease also features symptomatic aortitis and coronary artery microaneurysms.

Investigation

Cardiac involvement should initially be investigated noninvasively with modalities that include rest or stress echocardiography. Contrast-enhanced CMR can sensitively detect myocardial pathology, and coronary CTA can demonstrate coronary arteritis and microaneurysms. Echocardiography suggests valvular thickening is a common and typically asymptomatic finding in MPA. Aortic valve regurgitation may occur because of distortion and thickening of valve cusps or from aortic root dilation. On occasion, coronary arteriography may be required, and as for other vasculitides, it should be used cautiously in those suspected of having active coronary arteritis. When possible, steps should be taken to suppress disease activity with immunosuppressive therapy before angiography. Coronary arteritis can cause multiple small areas of myocardial infarction, which often remain clinically silent until the development of congestive cardiac failure. Occasionally, granulomas in conduction tissue precipitate cardiac dysrhythmia.

CARDIOVASCULAR DISEASE AND DISORDERS OF OTHER ORGANS

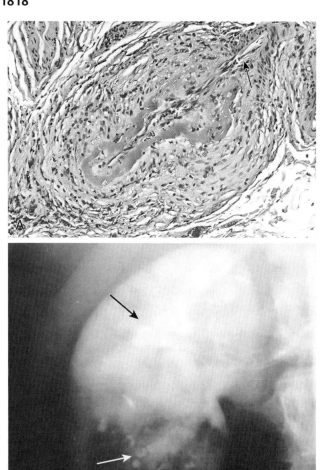

FIGURE 97.6 Polyarteritis nodosa (PAN). **A,** Photomicrograph of a hematoxylin–eosin–stained section of an artery biopsy specimen from a patient with PAN showing segmental fibrinoid necrosis, thrombotic occlusion of the lumen, and a small uninvolved remnant. **B,** Right renal angiogram showing multiple small aneurysms *(white arrow)* and a normal calyceal system *(black arrow)*. (From Mitchell RN. Blood Vessels. In: Kumar V, Abbas A, Aster JC, eds. *Robbins & Cotran Pathologic Basis of Disease.* 9th ed. Philadelphia: Elsevier Saunders; 2014.)

Treatment

For both GPA and MPA, high-dose prednisone (up to 1 mg/kg/day) is recommended at the onset and may be preceded by pulsed intravenous methylprednisolone if indicated. Patients with the most severe disease, including pulmonary hemorrhage, severe cardiac disease, or significant renal impairment, also receive pulsed intravenous cyclophosphamide to induce remission over the first 3 to 6 months, or alternatively B-cell depletion therapy with rituximab. In nonorgan threatening disease, remission can be achieved reliably with prednisolone in combination with methotrexate or MMF. Once remission is achieved, maintenance therapies may include azathioprine, methotrexate or rituximab, with continued prednisone tapering.[51] A range of novel therapies are under investigation including B-cell activating antagonist blisibimod, proteasome inhibitor bortezomib, abatacept targeting T-cell activation, and inhibition of the complement pathway with avacopan a C5a receptor antagonist.[48]

PERICARDITIS AND MYOCARDITIS

Pericarditis

Pericarditis commonly complicates the autoimmune connective tissue diseases, particularly SLE, SSc, and RA. Nonetheless, clinically

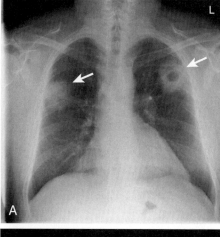
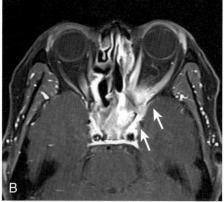
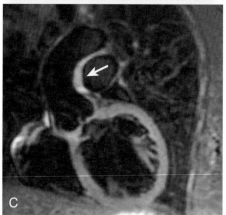

FIGURE 97.7 Granulomatosis with polyangiitis. **A,** Chest radiograph of a 36-year-old man showing pulmonary involvement with evidence of opacification and cavitation in the left upper lobe lesion *(arrows)*. **B,** CT scan of the orbits demonstrating confluent enhancing soft tissue at the left orbital apex as well as enhancing soft tissue opacifying the sinuses bilaterally (left > right) *(arrows)*. **C,** MRA demonstrating aortitis. The wall is thickened and enhancing around the root, extending to the left side of the ascending aorta.

significant pericarditis develops in fewer than 30% of patients. The reported prevalence ranges from 11% to 85%, depending on the type of study used to detect disease. Thus in necropsy studies, prevalence is high with pericardial involvement reported in 40% of individuals with RA, 40% to 80% of those with SLE, and up to 70% of those with SSc. Echocardiography detects pericardial thickening or small effusions in up to 50% of these patients. CMR can also define the extent of pericardial involvement.

Systemic Lupus Erythematosus

In SLE, pericarditis usually associates with disease flare and often with polyserositis. The symptoms are typically mild and consist of chest pain, which is worse on lying flat, and dyspnea, which may have a pleuritic component. Complicated pericarditis is rare, and in only 1% to 2%

is the effusion sufficiently large to cause cardiac tamponade. Constrictive pericarditis or infective pericarditis occur infrequently.

Rheumatoid Arthritis

Clinically significant pericarditis affects only 1% to 2% of patients with RA, more commonly male, seropositive patients. Constrictive pericarditis can develop over a period of months. Hemodynamically significant pericarditis, although reported, is extremely rare in patients being treated with antirheumatic therapy. Indeed, the more aggressive approach to management of RA and the increasing use of biologic therapies appear to have reduced the incidence of symptomatic pericarditis.

Systemic Sclerosis

The two most commonly encountered forms of scleroderma are diffuse cutaneous SSc (dSSc) and limited cutaneous SSc (lSSc). Following an initial vascular inflammatory phase, the predominant lesion is fibrosis, which affects multiple organs. In addition to the severe cutaneous manifestations, common clinical features include arthralgia, telangiectasia, pulmonary fibrosis, PAH, and esophageal dysmotility.[52] Renal crises are common and complicated by hypertension. Aggressive intervention is essential and includes the use of ACE inhibitors and calcium channel antagonists. This approach has transformed the prognosis.[53] Pericardial disease is common and more frequent in those with dSSc and a history of renal crisis. Echocardiography typically demonstrates small pericardial effusions, which are rarely hemodynamically significant. Rapidly accumulating large effusions may occur occasionally.

Pericardial Fluid Analysis

Analysis of pericardial fluid is rarely useful diagnostically unless infective pericarditis is suspected. Immune complexes, antinuclear and anti-dsDNA antibodies, complement consumption, and normal glucose levels have been reported in pericardial exudates from patients with SLE. In RA the pericardial fluid glucose concentration may be lower than that in plasma, and although rheumatoid factor activity is often detected, it is not considered diagnostic.

Treatment

In most cases a small pericardial effusion appears on a routine chest radiograph or echocardiogram and requires no specific treatment. Those with troublesome symptoms of pericarditis can receive a short course of an NSAID unless contraindicated. Colchicine is an important adjunctive therapeutic option in acute and chronic pericarditis. Likewise, low-dose oral prednisone may be required or used as an alternative.[54] Particularly recurrent cases require further optimization of the regular immunosuppressive therapy. Pericardial fluid accumulation may occasionally cause hemodynamic compromise requiring pericardiocentesis or, in recurrent cases, a pericardial window. For immunosuppressed patients, pericardial fluid should be analyzed for an infective cause. Advice should be sought from a microbiologist to ensure that the correct specimens are sent, including those required to exclude tuberculosis.

Myocarditis

Myocarditis is a rare but recognized cause of mortality in patients with autoimmune rheumatic diseases and is most commonly seen in patients with SLE, SSc, EGPA and polymyositis or dermatomyositis. Although most commonly present in those with an established rheumatic disease, myocarditis may be an initial feature requiring consideration of these conditions in the differential diagnosis of those with unexplained heart failure. The most common symptom of myocarditis is recent-onset exertional dyspnea with evidence of hypoxia. A patient rarely presents with severe heart failure at initial evaluation, and echocardiography usually reveals relatively modest changes in ventricular size and function. PAH must be excluded. In addition to standard blood tests, investigations should include: ESR, antinuclear antibody, antibodies against dsDNA and extractable nuclear antigens, rheumatoid factor, a myositis immunoblot screen, and complement factor C3 and C4 levels.

Systemic Lupus Erythematosus

Although the widespread use of more effective immunosuppressive regimens has reduced the prevalence of myocarditis in patients with SLE to fewer than 10%, much of which is subclinical, it remains an important and potentially life-threatening complication. Other potential causes of heart failure include hypertension, ischemic heart disease, valvular heart disease, and complications associated with renal failure.

The initial symptoms of myocarditis vary from low-grade fever, dyspnea, and palpitations to signs of severe heart failure. In addition to complement consumption, a raised ESR, and an increased titer of anti-dsDNA antibodies, the troponin I level may increase markedly. The ECG typically shows nonspecific findings such as sinus tachycardia, ST or T-wave changes. Supraventricular or ventricular tachycardias may also occur. Echocardiography aids in assessment (Fig. 97.8). Functional abnormalities may include segmental, regional, or global wall motion abnormalities; chamber dilation; and a reduced ejection fraction. In contrast, left ventricular hypertrophy in SLE more commonly associates with poorly controlled hypertension, whereas systolic and diastolic abnormalities in left ventricular function can associate with both hypertension and ischemic heart disease. CMR can detect myocarditis and myocardial fibrosis, and gadolinium or adenosine stress first-pass perfusion may demonstrate coronary microvascular dysfunction.[55] Indeed, CMR and PET identify coronary myocardial dysfunction and reduced coronary flow reserve in patients with SLE.

Opinion is divided on the use of endomyocardial biopsy. It will not permit a specific diagnosis of SLE per se. However, biopsy may identify an alternate cause or demonstrate an underlying inflammatory cause and features suggestive of SLE. Histopathologic analysis typically reveals small focal areas of fibrinoid necrosis with infiltration of lymphocytes and plasma cells, along with evidence of the deposition of immune complexes closely associated with myocyte bundles. Immunofluorescent studies may reveal granular staining and deposition of complement in and around myocardial blood vessels. Biopsy may also help exclude other potential causes of cardiomyopathy.

Systemic Sclerosis

Inflammatory myocarditis rarely results in symptomatic cardiomyopathy in patients with SSc; it affects mostly those with prominent skeletal muscle myositis. Echocardiography may demonstrate impaired diastolic and systolic function and a reduced ejection fraction, occasionally severe enough to cause cardiac failure. Endomyocardial biopsy most commonly reveals myocardial fibrosis. The fibrosis occurs focally and affects both ventricles. As with other lesions in SSc, microvascular disease is considered an important pathogenic factor.[52] Reduced coronary flow reserve occurs commonly, and subclinical myocardial ischemia probably contributes importantly to the ventricular dysfunction.

Myositis

Polymyositis and dermatomyositis affect the proximal skeletal muscles and can cause severe weakness. In dermatomyositis, additional characteristic cutaneous manifestations include a violaceous heliotrope rash, Gottron papules, and periungual erythema. In pediatric cases, subcutaneous calcification is common and vasculitis may lead to severe gut ischemia and hemorrhage. In adults, particularly those older than 60 years, dermatomyositis may be paraneoplastic. In severe cases, myositis involves the myocardium and pharyngeal or respiratory muscles and can be life-threatening. Creatine kinase levels rise markedly, and electromyography demonstrates fibrillation and polyphasic action potentials. MRI of the proximal limb muscles helps identify the muscles involved and those most amenable to biopsy. Histopathologic findings include muscle fiber necrosis and regeneration, a predominantly CD8+ T lymphocyte infiltrate, and HLA class I expression. Clinically significant myocarditis affects only 3%. Echocardiography may reveal ventricular dysfunction, whereas endomyocardial biopsy specimens demonstrate interstitial and perivascular lymphocytic infiltrates, contraction band necrosis, variable cardiomyocyte size, and degeneration and patchy fibrosis. Overt cardiac failure is rare; more common are rhythm and conduction abnormalities, including left anterior hemiblock and right bundle branch block.

Other Causes of Myocarditis

Even though postmortem studies have revealed evidence of myocarditis in patients with RA, it is seldom manifested clinically or causes heart failure. Although heart failure affects patients with RA more than it does age- and sex-matched controls, it predominantly reflects ischemia. Myocarditis also associates rarely with other rheumatic diseases, including ankylosing spondylitis, adult Still disease, GCA, and TA. In the latter it can be life-threatening.[56]

Treatment

Cardiac failure following myocarditis associated with autoimmune disease is treated with standard protocols and supportive interventions (see Chapter 50). Myocarditis in EGPA, TA, and SLE requires urgent corticosteroid treatment and, when severe, intravenous methylprednisolone, up to 1 g/day for 3 days, followed by oral prednisone, up to 1 mg/kg/day. These patients typically receive pulsed intravenous cyclophosphamide. For more modest disease, treatment can include the addition of, or increased dosages of, azathioprine or MMF. Some evidence suggests benefit of IVIG in resistant cases. Management of myocarditis complicating dermatomyositis or polymyositis uses a similar approach. Myocarditis in patients with SSc rarely requires aggressive treatment. Because high-dose corticosteroids increase the risk for renal crisis, early use of intravenous cyclophosphamide is favored.

VALVULAR HEART DISEASE

Clinically significant valvular disease can complicate many rheumatic diseases. Mechanisms may include direct damage to cardiac valve leaflets or aortic valve regurgitation as a consequence of aortitis affecting the ascending aorta.

Systemic Lupus Erythematosus

Valvular abnormalities occur commonly in patients with SLE, and necropsy studies have reported lesions in up to 75%. Verrucous endocarditis (Libman-Sacks endocarditis) and nonspecific valvular thickening occur most commonly. Valvulitis with rapid valvular dysfunction may also happen rarely. Transthoracic echocardiography detects verrucae in 2.5% to 12% and thickening in 4% to 38%, which increases to 30% and 43%, respectively, in those undergoing transesophageal echocardiography. Libman-Sacks lesions typically affect both valve surfaces, most commonly the mitral valve. Active valve lesions contain immunoglobulins, fibrin clumps, areas of focal necrosis, and a leukocytic infiltrate, whereas older healed lesions contain fibrous tissue predisposing to scarring and valve leaflet deformity. These abnormalities may cause valvular regurgitation. Libman-Sacks endocarditis occurs more commonly in SLE complicated by antiphospholipid antibodies and can accompany primary APS.

Libman-Sacks endocarditis is generally asymptomatic and may not cause a murmur. Assessment of SLE patients with a murmur may not be straightforward and requires exclusion of bacterial endocarditis. Echocardiography can help distinguish Libman-Sacks from infectious endocarditis, an important consideration in immunosuppressed patients. In contrast to the typically nonmobile vegetations of Libman-Sacks, bacterial vegetations usually localize at the valve leaflet closure line and demonstrate mobility that is independent of valve leaflet motion.

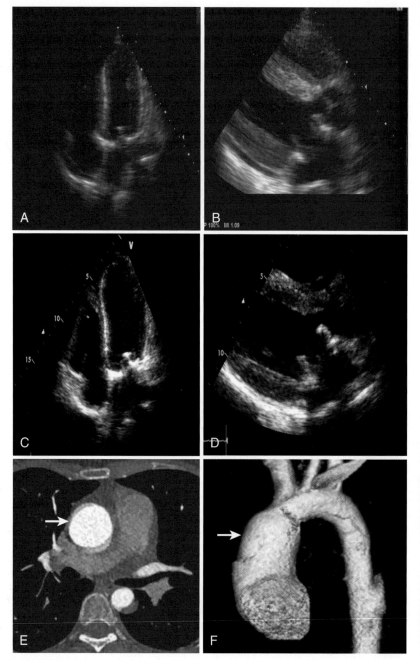

FIGURE 97.8 Myocarditis, aortitis and valvular heart disease. Myocarditis in systemic lupus erythematosus (SLE). **A** and **C,** Four-chamber view, **B** and **D,** Left ventricular view. In a 20-year-old patient with dyspnea and active SLE, the initial echocardiograms (**A** and **C**) showed mild impairment of ventricular function. Following symptomatic deterioration, the echocardiograms were repeated 6 days later (**B** and **D**) and demonstrated markedly increased thickening of the left ventricular wall with a bright signal suggestive of inflammatory infiltration. These findings were associated with substantial deterioration in left ventricular function. **E** and **F,** CTA of aorta in B27-positive ankylosing spondylitis complicated by aortitis and aortic root dilatation (*arrows*), resulting in aortic regurgitation requiring aortic valve and root replacement.

The presence of Libman-Sacks lesions increases the risk for secondary infective endocarditis, and prophylactic antibiotic prophylaxis should be considered to cover high-risk procedures such as invasive dental treatment (see Chapter 80). Complications of SLE-related valvular disease are rare, with hemodynamic effects seen in fewer than 5%. Valve replacement may be required for symptomatic regurgitation and occasionally for stenosis. The verrucous lesions may also embolize or rupture and lead to a cerebrovascular accident or peripheral embolism. Chordae tendineae rupture may also occur.

Treatment

Most patients require no specific treatment, although annual echocardiography can be used to monitor valve function. The introduction of corticosteroid therapy may have reduced the prevalence of Libman-Sacks endocarditis, and thus prednisone treatment may be considered in those with early active lesions. Patients with uncomplicated Libman-Sacks endocarditis with valve thickening on the echocardiogram are not routinely anticoagulated. However, in those with associated anti-phospholipid syndrome and no previous thrombosis, prophylactic low-dose aspirin is advised. Those with definitive vegetations, previous thrombosis or evidence of embolic phenomena should be considered for lifelong anticoagulation therapy.[57]

Seronegative Spondyloarthropathies

The seronegative spondyloarthropathies include ankylosing spondylitis, postinfectious reactive arthritis, inflammatory bowel disease-related arthritis, and psoriatic arthritis. HLA-B27 is associated with ankylosing spondylitis and reactive arthritis. The spondyloarthropathies share overlapping clinical features, including asymmetric, predominantly large-joint oligoarthritis, ocular inflammation, sacroiliitis, spinal disease, and enthesopathy. Ankylosing spondylitis and reactive arthritis commonly involve the aortic root and valve. Aortic valvulitis leads to aortic cusp thickening and retraction and subsequently to symptomatic aortic regurgitation, which may cause heart failure. Proximal aortitis affecting the ascending aorta leads to aortic root thickening and subsequently to dilation and aortic regurgitation (see Fig. 97.8), the prevalence of which relates to disease duration.

Treatment

Management of the spondyloarthropathies traditionally consisted of NSAIDs and, in more severe cases, the addition of DMARDs such as methotrexate, sulfasalazine, and leflunomide. Although these agents have some efficacy in the treatment of peripheral inflammatory arthritis, they have little effect on spinal inflammation. The use of TNF-α antagonists for ankylosing spondylitis and psoriatic arthropathy, and more recently agents targeting IL-17 and IL-12/23 pathways, is transforming control of these diseases, with beneficial effects on peripheral arthritis, spinal disease, and extra-articular complications, including uveitis.[58] Although evidence is currently limited, the initiation of biologic therapy in those with early signs and symptoms of aortitis may reduce the risk for cardiovascular complications, including aortic regurgitation.

Rheumatoid Arthritis

Valvular thickening commonly associates with RA in echocardiographic studies and at autopsy, but seldom causes clinical problems. Patients with seropositive RA and with prominent extra-articular nodular disease more frequently have valvular lesions. Echocardiography typically reveals mitral valve involvement, with valve thickening, asymptomatic mitral regurgitation, and prolapse being the predominant findings. Histopathologic examination of the valves demonstrates granulomatous nodular lesions. No specific treatment is indicated, although on occasion hemodynamically significant disease develops and requires mitral or aortic valve replacement.

Takayasu Arteritis

Cardiac valve dysfunction commonly complicates TA. In a series of 204 Korean patients, 23% had an abnormality in at least one valve, with regurgitation at the aortic valve found in 18% and at the mitral valve in 7.5%. Inflammation of the ascending aorta predisposes to dilation of the aortic root and aortic valve regurgitation. Approximately 15% of patients require aortic valve replacement with or without aortic root replacement with a graft. If possible, surgery should follow control of disease activity with immunosuppressive therapy.[47]

CARDIAC CONDUCTION DISTURBANCES

A variety of rheumatic diseases cause conduction abnormalities and cardiac rhythm disturbances, in part through a direct effect of systemic inflammation on cardiac electrophysiology.

Systemic Lupus Erythematosus and Sjögren Syndrome

Adult SLE seldom causes primary conduction abnormalities or rhythm disturbance, which may instead result from underlying ischemic heart disease or myocarditis. Female patients with SLE or Sjögren syndrome who test positive for antibodies against the Ro and/or La antigens carry the risk of bearing a child with congenital heart block, which may be complicated by myocarditis. These antibodies can cross the placenta and induce myocardial inflammation and may target the conduction system leading to fibrosis. The precise incidence is not established, but the usual figures quoted are 1 case in 20,000 live births with a range of 11,000 to 25,000. Patients with SLE, the overlap syndromes, and Sjögren syndrome should be screened for anti-Ro and anti-La before pregnancy and be counseled appropriately. The fetus of mothers known to be antibody positive should be screened in utero by echocardiography every 2 weeks from 16 weeks of gestation onward. Incomplete atrioventricular block can reverse, and myocarditis may respond to dexamethasone therapy. Complete atrioventricular block is irreversible and associated with up to 20% mortality, with 65% requiring insertion of a pacemaker.

Systemic Sclerosis

Conduction system disease affects up to 50% of SSc patients. The patchy myocardial fibrosis characteristically associated with SSc may account for the abnormalities seen with disruption of the conduction pathways. Supraventricular arrhythmias are usually benign and amenable to treatment. Ventricular conduction abnormalities also frequently occur in SSc. In these patients, ventricular ectopy is common and closely associated with sudden death.

Spondyloarthropathies

Conduction abnormalities frequently complicate the HLA-B27-related spondyloarthropathies. In ankylosing spondylitis, up to 30% of patients experience conduction system disease, predominantly caused by sub-aortic fibrosis extending into the septum and affecting the atrioventricular node. Atrioventricular conduction block occurs commonly and may become complete.

Polymyositis and Dermatomyositis

Conduction abnormalities are the most common cardiac manifestation of the myositis syndromes. Left anterior hemiblock and right bundle branch block occur most frequently and occasionally progress to complete heart block. The inflammation and fibrosis associated with polymyositis and dermatomyositis affect the conduction pathways, as demonstrated in 25% of autopsy cases.

Rheumatoid Arthritis

ECG screening studies in patients with RA have revealed arrhythmias or conducting system abnormalities in up to 50%, although they are usually clinically inapparent; RA patients have a twofold increase in sudden cardiac death compared to healthy controls.[59] Rheumatoid myocarditis and cardiac amyloid deposition can cause atrioventricular node conduction block. Similarly, rheumatoid nodules may disrupt the conduction system and cause all types of conduction abnormality.

PULMONARY ARTERIAL HYPERTENSION

PAH (see Chapter 88) is an important complication of the connective tissue diseases and is of concern to rheumatologists as a significant cause of premature mortality (Table 97.4). PAH often manifests late in disease evolution or remains undiagnosed. Furthermore, PAH frequently proves resistant to optimized treatment of the underlying connective tissue diseases. Notwithstanding, increased awareness, recognition of high-risk groups, improved screening and novel therapies point toward a better outlook.

CARDIOVASCULAR DISEASE AND DISORDERS OF OTHER ORGANS — XI

Systemic Sclerosis

SSc is the most resistant of the connective tissue diseases to treatment and has the highest mortality. PAH has very serious prognostic implications and is the most common single cause of SSc-related death. Novel therapeutic options offer renewed hope, and early data suggest improved survival.

Pathogenesis

Arterial remodeling is a central component in the pathogenesis of PAH and follows uncontrolled smooth muscle cell proliferation, deposition of extracellular matrix and subsequent fibrosis, vasoconstriction, and in situ thrombosis that together lead to increased pulmonary vascular resistance. Right ventricular dilation, dysfunction, and failure follow the development of PAH. Because PAH may develop very rapidly, effective screening strategies for patients with SSc are essential to detect PAH and allow early therapeutic intervention.

Screening

The prevalence of PAH in patients with SSc is up to 19%. PAH can occur as an early or late complication, and there is a lack of reliable predictive risk factors. Although more common with lSSc, PAH also frequently occurs in patients with dSSc. Pulmonary fibrosis can also complicate SSc and may exacerbate PAH (Fig. 97.9). Although debate continues regarding the frequency of screening, all patients must undergo an initial assessment, and annual screening is recommended thereafter to facilitate early diagnosis and improve survival. Annual screening should include echocardiography and pulmonary function testing.[60,61] In the latter, a low or falling carbon monoxide diffusing capacity may predict the development of PAH. In those with disease duration of more than 3 years and DLCO less than 60% the DETECT algorithm can be applied.[60,61] Echocardiographically assessed pulmonary artery pressure may miss early asymptomatic disease. The level of NT-pro-brain natriuretic protein (NT-proBNP) should be measured and relates to the degree of right ventricular dysfunction and the severity of PAH. Right-heart catheterization should follow positive screening results.[62]

Treatment and Outcome

The typical initial symptom of PAH is dyspnea. The diverse causes of this symptom often delay diagnosis until clinical evidence of hemodynamic impairment appears. The very poor 3-year survival rate of 47% to 56% also reflects delayed diagnosis, emphasizing the need for early diagnosis and treatment, which may improve outcome.[60] The aims of treatment include improvement in New York Heart Association (NYHA) functional class and quality of life, delay in clinical deterioration, and improved long-term outcome.[62] Although standard PAH outcome measures can assess response to treatment (Chapter 88), not all of them have been validated in patients with SSc and they may be complicated by coexistent conditions, including pulmonary fibrosis and musculoskeletal pain. Supported by clinical trials, treatment targets four main pathways with agents used alone and increasingly in combination.[60,63] Endothelin-1 receptor antagonists include bosentan, ambrisentan and macitentan. Epoprostenol, iloprost, treprostinil and selexipag target the prostacyclin pathway. The phosphodiesterase type 5 (PDE5) antagonists currently used are sildenafil and tadalafil. Riociguat, a soluble guanylate cyclase agonist has also been investigated in SSc PAH. Although efficacious, concerns remain about its safety in SSc.[63] Following clinical trial data, including that from AMBITION which demonstrated enhanced efficacy of ambrisentan and tadalafil in combination versus monotherapy,[63] the majority of specialist centers support the aggressive use of combination therapy in SSc patients considered at high risk of PAH.[60,63]

Systemic Lupus Erythematosus

The prevalence of PAH in patients with SLE varies between studies and was recently estimated to be between 0.5% and 17.5%. These patients are typically females of reproductive age, in whom PAH during pregnancy markedly increases the risk for mortality.

TABLE 97.4 Pulmonary Arterial Hypertension in Rheumatic Diseases

RHEUMATIC DISEASE	FEATURES OF PULMONARY ARTERIAL HYPERTENSION
Systemic sclerosis	Prevalence up to 19%. More common in lSSc. Annual screening recommended (echocardiography and pulmonary function). Disease >3 years and DLCO <60%, apply DETECT algorithm
PM/Scl overlap	Annual screening recommended. Survival rate at 3 years of 47%–56%
Systemic lupus erythematosus	Prevalence of 0.5%–17.5%. Survival rate at 3 years of 74%. Thrombotic arteriopathy is the most common underlying cause. 83% of patients have anticardiolipin antibodies. Patients with severe Raynaud phenomenon, anticardiolipin antibodies, and anti-U1RNP require screening
Rheumatoid arthritis	Prevalence data limited; reported to be up to 20%. Clinically significant disease rare, often secondary to COPD, chronic thromboembolic disease, or interstitial lung disease. Improved RA treatment may result in a reduced incidence
Sjögren syndrome	PAH a very rare complication of Sjögren syndrome. Usually occurs late in the course of disease. Prevalence unknown
Takayasu arteritis	Pulmonary arteritis present in up to 50% of patients. PAH prevalence of 12%. CMR or CTA and echocardiography required for screening.

CMR, Cardiac magnetic resonance; *COPD,* chronic obstructive pulmonary disease; *CTA,* computed tomography angiography; *lSSc,* limited cutaneous systemic sclerosis; *PAH,* pulmonary artery hypertension; *PM/Scl,* polymyositis/scleroderma; *RNP,* ribonucleoprotein.

Pathogenesis

In situ pulmonary thrombosis or chronic thromboembolic disease leading to thrombotic arteriopathy is the most common cause of PAH in patients with SLE, and 83% of such patients have anticardiolipin antibodies. Additional causes include pulmonary arteritis, underlying interstitial lung disease, and left-sided heart disease secondary to myocarditis, hypertension, or ischemic heart disease.

Clinical Findings and Diagnosis

Dyspnea, which may associate with fatigue, cough, and chest pain, is the typical initial symptom. The development of PAH does not necessarily reflect the duration of SLE or its severity. Limited data concerning predictive features indicate that patients with severe Raynaud phenomenon, anticardiolipin antibodies, and anti-U1RNP antibodies have more susceptibility to develop PAH. These patients should be screened annually with lung function, NT-proBNP levels, and echocardiography to estimate pulmonary artery pressure. Abnormality should be investigated further by right-heart catheterization.[64]

Treatment and Outcome

Management of PAH in patients with SLE uses a dual approach that combines optimized immunosuppression and vasodilator therapy,[65] although protocols vary between centers. Limited evidence supports therapeutic decisions in PAH associated with SLE. In contrast to SSc-related PAH, the response to increased corticosteroids and pulsed intravenous cyclophosphamide can be good, and once response is achieved, switching from cyclophosphamide to azathioprine or MMF can reduce toxicity. Stronger trial evidence is available for the use of the vasodilator therapies mentioned above. In those with anticardiolipin antibodies, life-long anticoagulation with warfarin is indicated. The 3-year survival rate of up to 89% is significantly higher than that in patients with SSc-related PAH.[64]

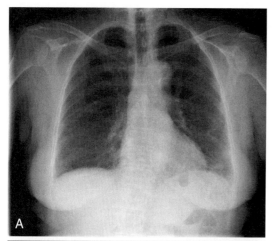

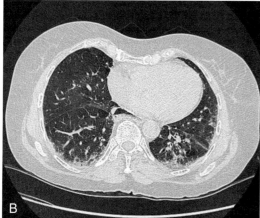

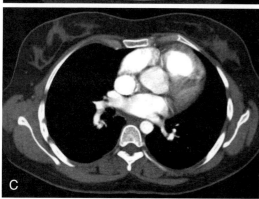

FIGURE 97.9 Systemic sclerosis. **A,** Chest radiograph of a patient with diffuse cutaneous systemic sclerosis showing interstitial shadowing, mainly in the lung bases, along with associated loss of volume, consistent with early pulmonary fibrosis. **B,** CT of the thorax demonstrating ground-glass opacity, subpleural honeycombing with thickening of the interlobular septa, and linear fibrotic bands, in keeping with pulmonary fibrosis. There is also evidence of associated mild traction bronchiectasis. **C,** Pulmonary CTA in a patient with limited cutaneous scleroderma and pulmonary hypertension. The right atrium and right ventricle are enlarged, and there is dilation of the pulmonary trunk.

Rheumatoid Arthritis

Pulmonary complications in RA include pleural effusions, pulmonary nodules, interstitial lung disease, bronchiolitis obliterans, and occasionally PAH. The prevalence of PAH in RA does not differ from that in the general population and does not warrant routine screening.[66] PAH in RA most commonly results from other underlying diseases, including chronic obstructive pulmonary disease, chronic pulmonary thromboembolism, hyperviscosity syndromes, lung surgery, or left-sided heart disease. PAH may also relate to extra-articular manifestations of RA, pulmonary fibrosis, or isolated pulmonary arteritis. Dyspnea is the most common initial symptom, and diagnosis is often delayed, not only

because dyspnea is initially attributed to other causes but because of limited exercise capacity in arthritic patients. Diagnosis of PAH by the measures outlined above should be followed by specific investigations such as high-resolution pulmonary CT, CTA, and pulmonary function tests to determine the underlying cause. No specific guidelines inform the treatment of PAH arising as a primary complication of RA. Active RA should be treated aggressively and preferably with biologic agents such as IL-6 receptor antagonists or rituximab. Specific treatment of PAH should also be considered as above.

Sjögren Syndrome

Clinically significant PAH very rarely complicates Sjögren syndrome and usually occurs late, most typically in patients with NYHA functional class III or IV, and the diagnosis is established as described for RA above.[67] Little evidence guides therapeutic decisions, and regimens vary considerably. Therapy with corticosteroids and immunosuppressive drugs, including azathioprine and cyclophosphamide, should be optimized to gain control of the underlying Sjögren syndrome activity. These measures may provide at least transient benefit in PAH, particularly in patients with evidence of active interstitial lung disease. Anecdotal evidence suggests beneficial effects of B cell depletion therapy with rituximab in patients with severe disease and may offer a future approach for those with PAH. In the majority enhanced immunosuppression is combined with standard PAH treatments described above.

Takayasu Arteritis

Pulmonary artery involvement in TA is often overlooked. Yet 50% of patients with TA have evidence of pulmonary arteritis in autopsy studies, and PAH develops in 12%. Even though pulmonary arteritis typically coexists with disease of the aorta, it can be isolated. Systemic hypertension and left ventricular dysfunction may cause secondary PAH. The pulmonary arterial lesions seen include stenoses, occlusions, and aneurysms. PAH may develop acutely early in the disease course or later and more insidiously following progressive pulmonary artery narrowing.[68] When present, symptoms may include dyspnea, chest pain, and peripheral edema. These symptoms are often ascribed to other causes, delaying diagnosis. Unless specifically sought, pulmonary artery involvement can be missed on initial radiologic studies. Dedicated CMR and contrast-enhanced CTA are the most sensitive detection modalities. Abnormalities should be pursued to exclude PAH with echocardiography and other studies as described above.

No available clinical trials guide therapeutic decisions. Aggressive treatment of the underlying arteritis with high-dose corticosteroids and a steroid-sparing drug such as methotrexate is recommended. Pulsed intravenous cyclophosphamide is typically reserved for nonresponders, and biologic therapies including antagonists of TNF-α or IL-6 receptor, should be considered early in refractory disease.[37] Warfarin is often used, particularly in those with evidence of thrombosis or pulmonary infarction. Case reports suggest antagonists of endothelin-1 and PDE5 may help in patients with more severe or resistance PAH. Open reconstructive surgery or percutaneous angioplasty may prove successful.

THROMBOSIS IN THE RHEUMATIC DISEASES (SEE ALSO CHAPTER 95)

Thrombosis is an important pathologic process in many rheumatic diseases and a cause of significant morbidity and mortality. Large-vessel thrombosis, both venous and arterial, can occur in Behçet disease and APS. Thrombosis in situ also occurs in small vessels, principally as the end result of chronic vessel wall hyperplasia or inflammation in diseases such as SSc, the vasculitides, and PAH. Chronic thromboembolic PAH can complicate SLE and SSc.

Activation of the coagulation cascade leading to thrombosis may be caused by abnormalities in the vessel wall, blood constituents, or blood flow (see Chapters 24 and 95). Abnormalities in endothelial function have particular relevance to rheumatic diseases. The prolonged systemic inflammation in patients with SLE, Behçet disease, and the vasculitides can cause endothelial apoptosis, a local inflammatory response, and endothelial activation. Cytokine-mediated endothelial activation disturbs anticoagulant and fibrinolytic mechanisms. Treatment of pro-thrombotic risk in these diseases requires consideration of approaches that include immunosuppression to control disease activity and minimize endothelial dysfunction, antiplatelet agents, anticoagulation, and the use of statins.

Antiphospholipid Syndrome (see Chapter 95)

APS associates with thrombosis (both arterial and venous) and with first-trimester fetal loss. Laboratory tests demonstrate antiphospholipid antibodies, most commonly anticardiolipin antibodies, anti-beta$_2$-glycoprotein-1 and/or a positive lupus anticoagulant test. Anticardiolipin antibodies, typically of the IgG or IgM isotype and present in medium to high titer, or the lupus anticoagulant should be demonstrated on at least two occasions 12 or more weeks apart. Antiphospholipid antibodies directed against beta$_2$-glycoprotein-1 may activate the endothelium, monocytes, and platelets. This leads to surface expression of cellular adhesion molecules and generation of tissue factor by both monocytes and the vascular endothelium. The increased tissue factor and thromboxane A$_2$ synthesis by platelets results in a procoagulant state. Thrombosis requires a second hit, such as that provided by activation of the complement cascade or intercurrent infection. Laboratory studies have demonstrated that antiphospholipid antibodies enhance leukocyte-endothelial cell interactions and induce thrombosis through inhibition of endothelial nitric oxide (eNOS) activation and nitric oxide biosynthesis. The mechanism involves binding of antibody to domain I of beta$_2$-glycoprotein-1 and impaired eNOS phosphorylation.[69] An important role for aPL-induced NET formation as a driver of thrombosis in APS has also emerged. Moreover, anti-NET antibodies in patients with primary APS may impair NET clearance and activate the complement cascade, novel data that may facilitate patient risk stratification and novel therapeutic approaches.[70]

Cardiovascular Disease

Valvular abnormalities are the most frequently reported cardiac abnormality in patients with APS. The most commonly detected lesions are verrucous (Libman-Sacks) endocarditis and nonspecific valvular thickening (see earlier) (Fig. 97.10). Although lesions are commonly found, clinically significant features are rare. Symptomatic disease is more frequent in those with high antibody titers. Congestive cardiac failure develops in up to 5% of patients, and 13% require cardiac valve replacement. Histologic analysis of the valves reveals deposition of antiphospholipid antibodies with complement activation. Occasionally, amaurosis fugax, transient ischemic attack, or stroke is seen as a consequence of arterial thromboembolism. Coronary thrombosis and myocardial infarction can complicate primary APS in 0.5% to 6% of patients, and intracardiac thrombi can also occur.[69,71] APS in patients with SLE may enhance their risk for myocardial infarction and stroke.

Treatment

Confirmed thrombosis in patients with APS requires anticoagulation. Most centers target an international normalized ratio (INR) of 2.5 to 3.5.[69,71] Some evidence supports the use of low-dose aspirin in patients with SLE complicated by antiphospholipid antibodies. In contrast, low-dose aspirin did not protect against deep venous thrombosis or pulmonary embolic disease in a study of men with primary APS. The role of direct oral anticoagulants (DOACs), including rivaroxaban, compared to vitamin K antagonists for the prevention of APS-related thrombosis remains the subject of on-going research. However, current clinical trial data and guidelines recommend against the use of DOACs in those with a high risk of thrombosis including triple positive patients (anticardiolipin Ab, anti-2-glycoprotein I Ab and lupus anticoagulant positive), while single or double positive patients established on DOACs may continue.[72]

Behçet Disease

Behçet disease occurs throughout the world but most commonly in Turkey, Iran, Japan, and Korea at 80 cases per 100,000 individuals, which

falls to 4 to 8 per 100,000 in the United States, France, Germany, and the United Kingdom. This multisystem disorder includes orogenital ulceration, acneiform skin lesions, and arthralgia. It may cause uveitis and blindness in the young. Arthralgia is common, and less frequently, patients suffer from meningoencephalitis, gastrointestinal ulceration, or vascular complications.

The vasculitis associated with Behçet disease predominantly affects the pulmonary arteries and veins, with thrombosis being a prominent clinical feature. Most thrombi are venous and cause superficial thrombophlebitis and deep venous thrombosis, including superior vena cava obstruction, cerebral vein thrombosis, and Budd-Chiari syndrome. In a small number of cases, pulmonary arterial vasculitis leads to in situ pulmonary arterial thrombosis. Although small studies have suggested that thrombosis is linked to the concurrent presence of a prothrombotic condition such as factor V Leiden or prothrombin mutations, this is not thought to be the cause in most. Indirect evidence suggests that the procoagulant state arises from an activated, adhesive, and prothrombotic endothelium due to chronic vascular inflammation. A clinical trial comparing treatment of thrombosis in Behçet disease with anticoagulation, immunosuppression, or a combination of both therapies supports this hypothesis. A higher proportion of patients treated with anticoagulation alone had recurrent thrombosis than did those prescribed immunosuppression.[73] Pulmonary arterial aneurysms are a rare life-threatening complication in Behçet disease (Fig. 97.11), and aneurysms may also occur in other arterial beds. Other cardiovascular complications occur in less than 10% and include pericarditis, myocarditis, intracardiac thrombosis, myocardial infarction, and myocardial aneurysm.

Treatment

The management of Behçet disease has advanced significantly in recent years.[74] The European League Against Rheumatism (EULAR) guidelines recommend immunosuppression for the treatment of thrombosis, an approach typically used in endemic areas. However, first-line treatment of these patients in emergency units in nonendemic areas is usually anticoagulation. This approach is appropriate because the cause of the thrombosis may not be immediately apparent, although patients with aneurysms have a substantial risk for bleeding. Patients should consult a specialist clinic for assessment of the need for long-term anticoagulation, immunosuppressive therapy, and noninvasive angiographic screening for aneurysms. Cardiovascular complications including arterial aneurysms are typically treated aggressively with cyclophosphamide, high-dose prednisone and anticoagulants to reduce inflammatory disease activity before surgical intervention, which may involve stenting via a percutaneous route or open surgical repair.[74] Because the lesions often recur, patients require regular screening. Second line treatments include anti-TNF-α therapy in those with recurrent aneurysms or those who fail to respond to cyclophosphamide (Fig. 97.11). For those with refractory disease, IFN-α has been used successfully, although side-effects are prominent. There is current interest in the use of other biologic agents including those targeting IL-1, IL-17, and IL-12/23.[74]

ANTIRHEUMATIC DRUGS AND CARDIOVASCULAR DISEASE

Drug therapy for the rheumatic diseases has undergone a dramatic transformation over the past 20 years and continues to do so. Contributory factors include advanced biologic insights, more accurate diagnostic tests and imaging data, improved understanding of the mechanistic actions of drugs, and the development of novel targeted therapies. This section emphasizes the beneficial and deleterious effects of antirheumatic drugs on the cardiovascular system.

Relationship Between Drug Treatment and Cardiovascular Disease

Although inflammation contributes to atherogenesis and patients with systemic inflammatory rheumatic diseases have a heightened risk for premature myocardial infarction and stroke, causality remains unproven.[8] The impact of antiinflammatory drugs on atherogenesis and the incidence of cardiovascular events has begun to provide insight in this regard.[4,75] Two recent trials demonstrate that the antiinflammatory effects associated with targeting the inflammasome reduces cardiovascular events.[1,2] Until recently, no clinical trial had convincingly demonstrated a beneficial effect of antiinflammatory drugs on cardiovascular outcomes. Indeed, the traditional NSAIDs or coxibs actually lead to a small but measurable increased risk for thrombosis. However, NSAID use in patients with inflammatory arthritis does not appear to confer increased cardiovascular risk, thus suggesting that their antiinflammatory role predominates.[76] Similarly, statins reduce serum CRP levels, and large clinical trials suggest that in part, statins provide vascular protection independent of their actions on LDL cholesterol, including immunomodulatory and antiinflammatory effects.

INTERLEUKIN-1 INHIBITION AND THE INFLAMMASOME
The CANTOS trial represented a step change in understanding the link between inflammation and atherothrombosis. The interleukin-1β monoclonal antibody canakinumab reduced cardiovascular events in patients with stable coronary artery disease and a baseline high-sensitivity-CRP >2 mg/L, if the hsCRP fell to <2 mg/L or the IL-6 level was reduced to less than the study median after 3 months' treatment (see Chapter 24).[1] Colchicine may act in part by targeting the inflammasome. COLCOT recruited participants to a randomized, double-blind trial of low dose colchicine (0.5 mg daily) within 30 days of myocardial infarction. The significant reduction in the composite primary endpoint of ischemic cardiovascular events in those receiving colchicine versus placebo predominantly reflected a reduction in stroke and in recurrent angina requiring coronary revascularization.[2]

TUMOR NECROSIS FACTOR-ALPHA ANTAGONISTS
TNF-α blockade affords an effective therapy for patients suffering from active RA, psoriatic arthritis, and ankylosing spondylitis. TNF-α can be targeted by monoclonal antibodies given intravenously or subcutaneously, or by subcutaneous injection of etanercept, a soluble TNF receptor fusion protein. The use of these agents is contraindicated in patients with established cardiovascular disease with evidence of NYHA class III and IV cardiac failure, and they should be used with caution in those with mild congestive cardiac failure.[4] In RA the combination of systemic inflammation and traditional risk factors is associated with rapid progression of carotid IMT. Treatment with methotrexate and TNF-α antagonists can reduce this progress,[12] with some evidence for a reduction in cardiovascular events.[77,78] Antiinflammatory treatments can reduce arterial ^{18}F-FDG avidity in patients with RA.[4,8,13,15]

INTERLEUKIN-6 INHIBITION
In light of the role of IL-6 signaling in atherogenesis, tocilizumab and sarilumab—inhibitors of IL-6R signaling—might be expected to have vasculoprotective effects and, at least in the short term, IL-6R inhibition may improve both endothelial function and aortic stiffness. However, these agents may also adversely affect lipid profiles and increase LDL cholesterol, thereby requiring the addition of a statin. Current data suggest that the rate of cardiovascular events in those receiving IL-6R inhibitors is equivalent to that in RA patients prescribed etanercept.[79]

INTERLEUKIN-17 INHIBITION
The role of IL-17A in atherothrombosis remains to be completely defined. Anti-IL-17 immunotherapy is increasingly used for the treatment of psoriasis and psoriatic arthritis. Clinical studies to date have not shown reduced cardiovascular risk.[80,81]

INTERLEUKIN-12 AND INTERLEUKIN-23 INHIBITION
Ustekinumab targets both IL-12 and IL-23 and is licensed for use in psoriasis and psoriatic arthritis. Preliminary clinical data derived from meta-analyses suggest that there might be an increased risk of major adverse cardiovascular events in those with pre-existing cardiovascular disease prescribed anti-IL12/23 antibodies.[4] As IL-23 selective monoclonal antibodies are now also entering clinical practice, cardiovascular risk data must be carefully sought.

B Cell Depletion
Rituximab targets CD20 and depletes B lymphocytes. Initially established as a treatment of B cell lymphoma, rituximab can control RA disease activity and reduce erosions. Similarly, rituximab exhibits efficacy equivalent to that of cyclophosphamide for the treatment of ANCA-associated vasculitis and may exert disease-modulating effects in SLE. Although long-term, adequately powered clinical trials with primary cardiovascular endpoints are required, evidence to date has not identified significant cardiovascular risk associated with rituximab therapy.[75,82] Conflicting results have been reported concerning its effect

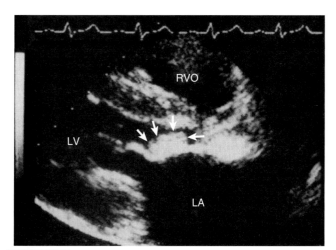

FIGURE 97.10 Parasternal long-axis view of the heart from a patient with SLE and high-titer antiphospholipid antibodies. A massive vegetation is seen on the ventricular surface of the anterior mitral leaflet *(arrows)*, but it is not interfering with valve mobility. *LA*, Left atrium; *LV*, left ventricle; *RVO*, right ventricular outflow; *SLE*, systemic lupus erythematosus. (Courtesy Professor Petros Nihoyannopoulos, National Heart and Lung Institute, Imperial College London.)

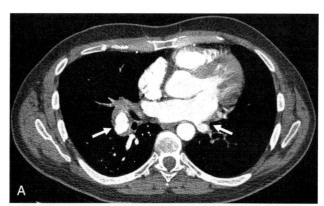
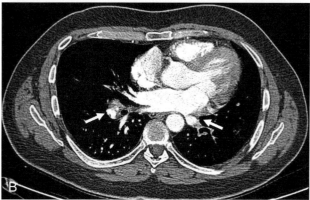

FIGURE 97.11 A, CT angiogram of a patient with Behçet disease showing bilateral pulmonary artery aneurysms *(arrows)*. **B,** Following 4 months of treatment with tumor necrosis factor-α antagonist infliximab, some reduction in the size of the pulmonary aneurysm on the right is seen. (Courtesy Professor Dorian Haskard, National Heart and Lung Institute, Imperial College London.)

on lipid profiles and these should be monitored. Following the reports of protective effects of B-cell depletion in mice with experimental atherosclerosis and myocardial infarction, a small phase I/II clinical trial of rituximab in patients suffering acute myocardial infarction showed reduced CRP and BNP (https://clinicaltrials.gov/ Identifier: NCT03072199).[4] Severe cardiovascular complications have occurred following rituximab infusions. Regulatory agency advice is that this treatment should be used with caution and the infusion rate reduced in those with preexisting cardiorespiratory disease and avoided in those with NYHA Class III and IV heart failure.

Methotrexate

Methotrexate in dosages up to 25 mg/wk has proven to be remarkably effective in treatment of RA and other inflammatory arthritides and is frequently used as a steroid-sparing drug in the vasculitides. The majority of clinical evidence suggests that methotrexate has a cardiovascular protective effect in patients with inflammatory arthritis, with those responding to methotrexate therapy demonstrating improvement in endothelial function. A recent consecutive meta-analysis confirmed early reports of a relative risk reduction in cardiovascular mortality in patients with RA and psoriatic arthritis prescribed methotrexate.[77] Novel additional mechanisms potentially underlying vascular protection include activation of an AMP-activated kinase and cyclic AMP response element-binding protein-dependent pathway[83] and beneficial effects on macrophage cholesterol handling.[84] These cardioprotective actions of methotrexate inspired the Cardiovascular Inflammation Reduction Trial (CIRT) in which patients with a previous myocardial infarction or multivessel coronary disease, as well as type 2 diabetes mellitus and/or the metabolic syndrome, were prescribed methotrexate (15 to 20 mg/wk) or placebo. No benefit from methotrexate was detected; this is likely because, and in contrast to CANTOS, CIRT participants had a median CRP of 1.5 mg/L at entry.[1,85] The different findings of CANTOS and CIRT imply that patient stratification and selection are essential for future studies.

Other Disease-Modifying Antirheumatic Drugs

The potential cardiovascular benefits of hydroxychloroquine, an antimalarial drug frequently used for the treatment of RA, SLE, and Sjögren syndrome, have become more widely recognized in recent years. Hydroxychloroquine lowers cholesterol and may improve both endothelial function and aortic stiffness. Clinical studies have demonstrated that hydroxychloroquine reduces the risk for cardiovascular events in patients with both RA and SLE. In contrast, concern regarding a prolonged QT interval, occasional association of high cumulative dosages with restrictive cardiomyopathy and with retinal damage require monitoring.

Cyclosporine continues to be used for the treatment of rheumatic disease on occasion, including polymyositis, Behçet diseases, SLE, and RA, as well as in many patients following organ transplantation. Clinical studies suggest that cyclosporine impairs flow-mediated vasodilation. At least in part, this effect reflects reduced eNOS activity and nitric oxide bioavailability. The adverse cardiovascular effects seen with cyclosporine may also reflect its propensity to induce hypertension and renal impairment. Alternative immunosuppressive drugs, used predominantly in the transplantation scenario, including tacrolimus and rapamycin (sirolimus), appear to have a more favorable vascular profile. JAK inhibitors (tofacitinib, baricitinib) are oral small inhibitors with disease-modifying efficacy in RA and psoriatic arthritis.[20] Data concerning effects of these agents on cardiovascular risk is sparse. A study of tofacitinib in RA reported an increase in cholesterol levels.[86]

Glucocorticoids

Glucocorticoids have undisputed efficacy in the treatment of systemic inflammatory diseases, including RA, SLE, and the vasculitides. Yet the substantial side effect burden concerns patients and physicians alike prompting the increased use of low-dose and rapid taper protocols. The influence of corticosteroid therapy on the progression of

atherosclerosis is complex and dependent on the context. Their impact on blood pressure and glucose and lipid metabolism may have a deleterious effect. In contrast, in SLE, evidence suggests that insufficient use of glucocorticoids risks persistently active and/or relapsing disease, thereby leading to an increased risk for accelerated atherogenesis. Thus combination therapy with a steroid-sparing drug such as azathioprine, MMF, methotrexate or biologic agents, which allows prednisone to be tapered to 7.5 mg/day or less, may be optimal.

Statins (see Chapters 25 and 27)

Large primary prevention trials indicate that statins can reduce cardiovascular morbidity and mortality, in part independently of changes in LDL cholesterol.[87] These actions have led to interest in statins as adjunctive therapy for rheumatic diseases, including RA and SLE, for which they have the potential to both reduce disease activity and lower cardiovascular risk.[88] Although meta-analyses indicate some antiinflammatory benefit,[89] clinical trial evidence supporting the routine use of statins in all patients with rheumatic diseases is relatively lacking. The recent Trial of Atorvastatin for the Primary Prevention of Cardiovascular Events in Patients with Rheumatoid Arthritis (TRACE RA) demonstrated the safety of atorvastatin 40 mg daily, a significant fall in the LDL cholesterol and a 34% cardiovascular events (CVE) risk reduction versus placebo, consistent with statin effects in other populations.[23] Although no guidelines exist, most rheumatologists currently consider the cardiovascular risk in patients with RA and SLE as equivalent to that in patients with diabetes mellitus. EULAR has suggested adding a 1.5× multiplier to standard cardiovascular risk calculations, while recent reports have recommended further expansion of the cardiovascular risk prediction score for RA.[75,90] Indications for a statin include an LDL cholesterol level of 190 mg/dL or higher, a long history of RA, a family history of hyperlipidemia, higher age at disease onset, and the presence of any other cardiovascular risk factors.[26]

Nonsteroidal Antiinflammatory Drugs

NSAIDs and coxibs are important and effective drugs for the treatment of pain and inflammation. Concerns regarding atherothrombotic complications have, however, raised reservations regarding their use. As a consequence, patients with rheumatic disease are often denied these medications inappropriately. Although current evidence suggests that both classes have a small, manageable, and dose-dependent risk for cardiovascular complications, establishing the degree of risk and the relative safety profiles between individual drugs is difficult because of clinical trial heterogeneity and a lack of randomized controlled trial data for older NSAIDs. Data overall suggest that no traditional NSAID or COX-2 inhibitor is entirely safe and that naproxen has the best cardiovascular profile as a result of its antiplatelet effects and that diclofenac may have the worst.[14,91] Despite these reservations, the absolute risk for a cardiovascular event is very low, and gastrointestinal bleeding and perforation likely represent the major long-term risk associated with NSAIDs (Table 97.5). Although coxibs are less likely to cause gastrointestinal problems, many guidelines recommend concomitant prescription of a proton pump inhibitor for patients taking either NSAIDs or coxibs for more than 10 to 14 days.

Current data concerning the use of NSAIDs and coxibs in rheumatic diseases are beginning to shift significantly. Data from studies comparing NSAIDs and coxibs in patients with arthritis do not support a class effect based on COX-2 selectivity. Moreover, longitudinal cohort analysis of NSAID use in RA and ankylosing spondylitis reveals only a small increase in cardiovascular events, which was lower than that recorded in the general population and with a low versus high intake of NSAIDs.[76] The difference may reflect the impact of these drugs on inflammation and minimization of an echo effect.[8,13] The study population is important, and few studies have looked in detail at patients with inflammatory arthritis. The Prospective Randomized Evaluation of Celecoxib Integrated Safety versus Ibuprofen or Naproxen (PRECISION) trial enrolled 24,081 RA or osteoarthritis patients with established or significant risk of cardiovascular disease.[21] Following

TABLE 97.5 Cardiovascular Versus Gastrointestinal Risk in Prescribing Nonsteroidal Antiinflammatory Drugs

Patients with CV risk who are taking aspirin should avoid tNSAIDs or coxibs if possible
If essential, consider naproxen plus a PPI if GI risk is low or a coxib in those with significant GI risk
Cardiovascular risk varies between individual tNSAIDs and coxibs
Risk for CV events appears lower in those with inflammatory rheumatic diseases.
Patients with cardiac failure or hypertension should avoid tNSAIDs and coxibs
Risk for a CV event with a tNSAID or coxib is <1% in those with <2 classic risk factors
Risk for a CV event may increase in older adults, men, and those with preexisting CV disease
Aspirin use increases the risk for GI events associated with tNSAIDs and coxibs
Coprescription of a PPI reduces the risk for GI events with tNSAIDs and coxibs
PPIs are more effective than H_2 antagonists or misoprostol for gastroprotection
Gastrointestinal risk varies between individual tNSAIDs
Use the lowest effective dose for the shortest period

coxibs, COX-2–selective antiinflammatory drugs; *CV*, cardiovascular; *GI*, gastrointestinal; *PPI*, proton pump inhibitor; *tNSAIDs*, traditional NSAIDs.

prescription of esomeprazole and randomization to moderate dose celecoxib, naproxen or ibuprofen, cardiovascular death, nonfatal stroke, and myocardial infarction were recorded. Although drug discontinuation rates were high, the trial revealed celecoxib to be noninferior to naproxen and ibuprofen with respect to cardiovascular safety and significantly safer than either comparator regarding gastrointestinal risk. These data provide important reassurance concerning the safety of moderate doses of celecoxib.

Wherever possible, NSAIDs and coxibs should be avoided in patients with known ischemic heart disease, previous thrombosis, poorly controlled hypertension, kidney disease, and cardiac failure. In patients in whom antiinflammatory drugs are being considered, an individualized assessment of both gastrointestinal and cardiovascular risk should be made. The patient should be encouraged to use these drugs when required and at the minimally effective dose rather than as a standing dose (see Table 97.5).

FUTURE PERSPECTIVES

The rapid development of novel biologics and small molecules targeting inflammatory pathways offers considerable promise for cardiovascular disease.[92] The current challenge is to design and perform adequately powered randomized clinical trials to investigate the efficacy of individual antiinflammatory drugs in preventing cardiovascular events. These drugs need to be affordable and sufficiently tractable for use in cardiovascular clinical practice. The data from the CANTOS and COLCOT clinical trials provide the impetus for further RCTs. The ultimate aim is to test the hypothesis that a relatively aggressive antiinflammatory approach, alongside conventional therapy, will confer additional benefit in those with known atherosclerotic coronary artery disease in the absence of an underlying rheumatic problem.

REFERENCES

Background

1. Ridker PM, Everett BM, Thuren T, et al. Antiinflammatory therapy with canakinumab for atherosclerotic disease. *N Engl J Med*. 2017;377:1119–1131.
2. Tardif JC, Kouz S, Waters DD, et al. Efficacy and safety of low-dose colchicine after myocardial infarction. *N Engl J Med*. 2019;381:2497–2505.
3. Prasad M, Hermann J, Gabriel SE, et al. Cardiorheumatology: cardiac involvement in systemic rheumatic disease. *Nat Rev Cardiol*. 2015;12:168–176.
4. Ait-Oufella H, Libby P, Tedgui A. Anticytokine immune therapy and atherothrombotic cardiovascular risk. *Arterioscler Thromb Vasc Biol*. 2019;39:1510–1519.
5. Libby P, Pasterkamp G, Crea F, Jang IK. Reassessing the mechanisms of acute coronary syndromes. *Circ Res*. 2019;124:150–160.
6. Skeoch S, Bruce IN. Atherosclerosis in rheumatoid arthritis: is it all about inflammation? *Nat Rev Rheumatol*. 2015;11:390–400.
7. Skeoch S, Williams H, Cristinacce P, et al. Evaluation of carotid plaque inflammation in patients with active rheumatoid arthritis using (18)F-fluorodeoxyglucose PET-CT and MRI: a pilot study. *Lancet*. 2015;385(suppl 1):S91.
8. Mason JC, Libby P. Cardiovascular disease in patients with chronic inflammation: mechanisms underlying premature cardiovascular events in rheumatologic conditions. *Eur Heart J*. 2015;36:482–489.
9. Jaiswal S, Libby P. Clonal haematopoiesis: connecting ageing and inflammation in cardiovascular disease. *Nat Rev Cardiol*. 2020;17:137–144.
10. Erre GL, Buscetta G, Paliogiannis P, et al. Coronary flow reserve in systemic rheumatic diseases: a systematic review and meta-analysis. *Rheumatol Int*. 2018;38:1179–1190.
11. Totoson P, Maguin-Gate K, Nappey M, et al. Microvascular abnormalities in adjuvant-induced arthritis: relationship to macrovascular endothelial function and markers of endothelial activation. *Arthritis Rheumatol*. 2015;67:1203–1213.
12. Del Rincon I, Polak JF, O'Leary DH, et al. Systemic inflammation and cardiovascular risk factors predict rapid progression of atherosclerosis in rheumatoid arthritis. *Ann Rheum Dis*. 2015;74:1118–1123.
13. Libby P, Nahrendorf M, Swirski FK. Leukocytes link local and systemic inflammation in ischemic cardiovascular disease: an expanded "cardiovascular continuum". *J Am Coll Cardiol*. 2016;67:1091–1103.
14. Agca R, Heslinga SC, Rollefstad S, et al. EULAR recommendations for cardiovascular disease risk management in patients with rheumatoid arthritis and other forms of inflammatory joint disorders: 2015/2016 update. *Ann Rheum Dis*. 2017;76:17–28.
15. Ferguson LD, Siebert S, McInnes IB, Sattar N. Cardiometabolic comorbidities in RA and PsA: lessons learned and future directions. *Nat Rev Rheumatol*. 2019;15:461–474.
16. Skielta M, Soderstrom L, Rantapaa-Dahlqvist S, et al. Trends in mortality, co-morbidity and treatment after acute myocardial infarction in patients with rheumatoid arthritis 1998-2013. *Eur Heart J Acute Cardiovasc Care*. 2020;9:931–938.
17. Elbadawi A, Ahmed HH, Elgendy IY, et al. Outcomes of acute myocardial infarction in patients with rheumatoid arthritis. *Am J Med*. 2020.
18. Solomon DH, Reed GW, Kremer JM, et al. Disease activity in rheumatoid arthritis and the risk of cardiovascular events. *Arthritis Rheumatol*. 2015;67:1449–1455.
19. Aletaha D. Precision medicine and management of rheumatoid arthritis. *J Autoimmun*. 2020;110:102405.
20. You H, Xu D, Zhao J, et al. JAK inhibitors: prospects in connective tissue diseases. *Clin Rev Allergy Immunol*. 2020.
21. Nissen SE, Yeomans ND, Solomon DH, et al. Cardiovascular safety of celecoxib, naproxen, or ibuprofen for arthritis. *N Engl J Med*. 2016;375:2519–2529.
22. Semb AG, Ikdahl E, Wibetoe G, Crowson C, Rollefstad S. Atherosclerotic cardiovascular disease prevention in rheumatoid arthritis. *Nat Rev Rheumatol*. 2020;16:361–379.
23. Kitas GD, Nightingale P, Armitage J, et al. A multicenter, randomized, placebo-controlled trial of atorvastatin for the primary prevention of cardiovascular events in patients with rheumatoid arthritis. *Arthritis Rheumatol*. 2019;71:1437–1449.
24. Catalina MD, Owen KA, Labonte AC, et al. The pathogenesis of systemic lupus erythematosus: harnessing big data to understand the molecular basis of lupus. *J Autoimmun*. 2019:102359.
25. Giannelou M, Mavragani CP. Cardiovascular disease in systemic lupus erythematosus: a comprehensive update. *J Autoimmun*. 2017;82:1–12.
26. Liu Y, Kaplan MJ. Cardiovascular disease in systemic lupus erythematosus: an update. *Curr Opin Rheumatol*. 2018;30:441–448.
27. Gatto M, Zen M, Iaccarino L, Doria A. New therapeutic strategies in systemic lupus erythematosus management. *Nat Rev Rheumatol*. 2019;15:30–48.
28. Murphy G, Isenberg DA. New therapies for systemic lupus erythematosus - past imperfect, future tense. *Nat Rev Rheumatol*. 2019;15:403–412.
29. van Vollenhoven R. String of successful trials in SLE: have we cracked the code? *Lupus Sci Med*. 2020;7:e000380.
30. Stamp LK, Dalbeth N. Prevention and treatment of gout. *Nat Rev Rheumatol*. 2019;15:68–70.

Vasculitides

31. Liew JW, Ramiro S, Gensler LS. Cardiovascular morbidity and mortality in ankylosing spondylitis and psoriatic arthritis. *Best Pract Res Clin Rheumatol*. 2018;32:369–389.
32. Watts RA, Robson J. Introduction, epidemiology and classification of vasculitis. *Best Pract Res Clin Rheumatol*. 2018;32:3–20.
33. Dejaco C, Brouwer E, Mason JC, et al. Giant cell arteritis and polymyalgia rheumatica: current challenges and opportunities. *Nat Rev Rheumatol*. 2017;13:578–592.
34. Berti A, Dejaco C. Update on the epidemiology, risk factors, and outcomes of systemic vasculitides. *Best Pract Res Clin Rheumatol*. 2018;32:271–294.
35. Dejaco C, Ramiro S, Duftner C, et al. EULAR recommendations for the use of imaging in large vessel vasculitis in clinical practice. *Ann Rheum Dis*. 2018;77:636–643.
36. Udayakumar PD, Chandran AK, Crowson CS, et al. Cardiovascular risk and acute coronary syndrome in giant cell arteritis: a population-based retrospective cohort study. *Arthritis Care Res (Hoboken)*. 2015;67:396–402.
37. Tombetti E, Mason JC. Takayasu arteritis: advanced understanding is leading to new horizons. *Rheumatology (Oxford)*. 2019;58:206–219.
38. Tombetti E, Mason JC. Application of imaging techniques for Takayasu arteritis. *Presse Med*. 2017;46:e215–e223.
39. Whittaker E, Bamford A, Kenny J, et al. Clinical characteristics of 58 children with a pediatric inflammatory multisystem syndrome temporally associated with SARS-CoV-2. *J Am Med Assoc*. 2020.
40. Soni PR, Noval Rivas M, Arditi M. A comprehensive update on Kawasaki disease vasculitis and myocarditis. *Curr Rheumatol Rep*. 2020;22:6.
41. Perugino CA, Wallace ZS, Meyersohn N, et al. Large vessel involvement by IgG4-related disease. *Medicine (Baltim)*. 2016;95:e3344.
42. Watanabe R, Goronzy JJ, Berry G, et al. Giant cell arteritis: from pathogenesis to therapeutic management. *Curr Treatm Opt Rheumatol*. 2016;2:126–137.
43. Mackie SL, Dejaco C, Appenzeller S, et al. British Society for Rheumatology guideline on diagnosis and treatment of giant cell arteritis. *Rheumatology (Oxford)*. 2020;59:e1–e23.
44. Stone JH, Tuckwell K, Dimonaco S, et al. Trial of tocilizumab in giant-cell arteritis. *N Engl J Med*. 2017;377:317–328.
45. Hellmich B, Agueda A, Monti S, et al. 2018 Update of the EULAR recommendations for the management of large vessel vasculitis. *Ann Rheum Dis*. 2020;79:19–30.
46. Nakaoka Y, Isobe M, Takei S, et al. Efficacy and safety of tocilizumab in patients with refractory Takayasu arteritis: results from a randomised, double-blind, placebo-controlled, phase 3 trial in Japan (the TAKT study). *Ann Rheum Dis*. 2018;77:348–354.

47. Mason JC. Surgical intervention and its role in Takayasu arteritis. *Best Pract Res Clin Rheumatol.* 2018;32:112–124.

48. Nakazawa D, Masuda S, Tomaru U, Ishizu A. Pathogenesis and therapeutic interventions for ANCA-associated vasculitis. *Nat Rev Rheumatol.* 2019;15:91–101.

49. Yune S, Choi DC, Lee BJ, et al. Detecting cardiac involvement with magnetic resonance in patients with active eosinophilic granulomatosis with polyangiitis. *Int J Cardiovasc Imaging.* 2016;32(suppl 1):155–162.

50. Wechsler ME, Akuthota P, Jayne D, et al. Mepolizumab or placebo for eosinophilic granulomatosis with polyangiitis. *N Engl J Med.* 2017;376:1921–1932.

51. Yates M, Watts RA, Bajema IM, et al. EULAR/ERA-EDTA recommendations for the management of ANCA-associated vasculitis. *Ann Rheum Dis.* 2016;75:1583–1594.

52. Denton CP, Khanna D. Systemic sclerosis. *Lancet.* 2017;390:1685–1699.

53. Volkmann ER, Varga J. Emerging targets of disease-modifying therapy for systemic sclerosis. *Nat Rev Rheumatol.* 2019;15:208–224.

54. Adler Y, Charron P, Imazio M, et al. 2015 ESC guidelines for the diagnosis and management of pericardial diseases: the task force for the diagnosis and management of pericardial diseases of the European Society of Cardiology (ESC) endorsed by: the European Association for Cardio-Thoracic Surgery (EACTS). *Eur Heart J.* 2015;36:2921–2964.

55. Mavrogeni S, Koutsogeorgopoulou L, Markousis-Mavrogenis G, et al. Cardiovascular magnetic resonance detects silent heart disease missed by echocardiography in systemic lupus erythematosus. *Lupus.* 2018;27:564–571.

56. Bechman K, Gopalan D, Nihoyannopoulos P, Mason JC. A cohort study reveals myocarditis to be a rare and life-threatening presentation of large vessel vasculitis. *Semin Arthritis Rheum.* 2017;47:241–246.

57. Kolitz T, Shiber S, Sharabi I, et al. Cardiac manifestations of antiphospholipid syndrome with focus on its primary form. *Front Immunol.* 2019;10:941.

58. Sieper J, Poddubnyy D, Miossec P. The IL-23-IL-17 pathway as a therapeutic target in axial spondyloarthritis. *Nat Rev Rheumatol.* 2019;15:747–757.

59. Lazzerini PE, Capecchi PL, Laghi-Pasini F. Systemic inflammation and arrhythmic risk: lessons from rheumatoid arthritis. *Eur Heart J.* 2017;38:1717–1727.

Pulmonary Hypertension

60. Denton CP, Wells AU, Coghlan JG. Major lung complications of systemic sclerosis. *Nat Rev Rheumatol.* 2018;14:511–527.

61. Saygin D, Domsic RT. Pulmonary arterial hypertension in systemic sclerosis: challenges in diagnosis, screening and treatment. *Open Access Rheumatol.* 2019;11:323–333.

62. Galie N, Humbert M, Vachiery JL, et al. 2015 ESC/ERS guidelines for the diagnosis and treatment of pulmonary hypertension: the joint task force for the diagnosis and treatment of pulmonary hypertension of the European Society of Cardiology (ESC) and the European Respiratory Society (ERS): endorsed by: association for European Paediatric and Congenital Cardiology (AEPC), International Society for Heart and Lung Transplantation (ISHLT). *Eur Heart J.* 2016;37:67–119.

63. Lee MH, Bull TM. The role of pulmonary arterial hypertension-targeted therapy in systemic sclerosis. *F1000Res.* 2019;8.

64. Hannah JR, D'Cruz DP. Pulmonary complications of systemic lupus erythematosus. *Semin Respir Crit Care Med.* 2019;40:227–234.

65. Kommireddy S, Bhyravavajhala S, Kurimeti K, et al. Pulmonary arterial hypertension in systemic lupus erythematosus may benefit by addition of immunosuppression to vasodilator therapy: an observational study. *Rheumatology (Oxford).* 2015;54:1673–1679.

66. Montani D, Henry J, O'Connell C, et al. Association between rheumatoid arthritis and pulmonary hypertension: data from the French pulmonary hypertension registry. *Respiration.* 2018;95:244–250.

67. Flament T, Bigot A, Chaigne B, et al. Pulmonary manifestations of Sjogren's syndrome. *Eur Respir Rev.* 2016;25:110–123.

68. He Y, Lv N, Dang A, Cheng N. Pulmonary artery involvement in patients with Takayasu arteritis. *J Rheumatol.* 2020;47:264–272.

Management Strategies

69. Petri M. Antiphospholipid syndrome. *Transl Res.* 2020.

70. Zuo Y, Yalavarthi S, Gockman K, et al. Anti-NET antibodies and impaired NET degradation in antiphospholipid syndrome. *Arthritis Rheumatol.* 2020.

71. Oliveira DC, Correia A, Oliveira C. The issue of the antiphospholipid antibody syndrome. *J Clin Med Res.* 2020;12:286–292.

72. Wahl D, Dufrost V. Direct oral anticoagulants in antiphospholipid syndrome: too early or too late? *Ann Intern Med.* 2019;171:765–766.

73. Emmi G, Bettiol A, Silvestri E, et al. Vascular Behcet's syndrome: an update. *Intern Emerg Med.* 2019;14:645–652.

74. Bettiol A, Hatemi G, Vannozzi L, et al. Treating the different phenotypes of behcet's syndrome. *Front Immunol.* 2019;10:2830.

75. Halacoglu J, Shea LA. Cardiovascular risk assessment and therapeutic implications in rheumatoid arthritis. *J Cardiovasc Transl Res.* 2020.

76. Braun J, Baraliakos X, Westhoff T. Nonsteroidal anti-inflammatory drugs and cardiovascular risk - a matter of indication. *Semin Arthritis Rheum.* 2020;50:285–288.

77. Roubille C, Richer V, Starnino T, et al. The effects of tumour necrosis factor inhibitors, methotrexate, non-steroidal anti-inflammatory drugs and corticosteroids on cardiovascular events in rheumatoid arthritis, psoriasis and psoriatic arthritis: a systematic review and meta-analysis. *Ann Rheum Dis.* 2015;74:480–489.

78. Low AS, Symmons DP, Lunt M, et al. Relationship between exposure to tumour necrosis factor inhibitor therapy and incidence and severity of myocardial infarction in patients with rheumatoid arthritis. *Ann Rheum Dis.* 2017;76:654–660.

79. Choy EH, De Benedetti F, Takeuchi T, et al. Translating IL-6 biology into effective treatments. *Nat Rev Rheumatol.* 2020;16:335–345.

80. Baeten D, Sieper J, Braun J, et al. Secukinumab, an interleukin-17A inhibitor, in ankylosing spondylitis. *N Engl J Med.* 2015;373:2534–2548.

81. Mease PJ, McInnes IB, Kirkham B, et al. Secukinumab inhibition of interleukin-17A in patients with psoriatic arthritis. *N Engl J Med.* 2015;373:1329–1339.

82. Cohen MD, Keystone E. Rituximab for rheumatoid arthritis. *Rheumatol Ther.* 2015;2:99–111.

83. Thornton CC, Al-Rashed F, Calay D, et al. Methotrexate-mediated activation of an AMPK-CREB-dependent pathway: a novel mechanism for vascular protection in chronic systemic inflammation. *Ann Rheum Dis.* 2016;75:439–448.

84. Ronda N, Greco D, Adorni MP, et al. Newly identified antiatherosclerotic activity of methotrexate and adalimumab: complementary effects on lipoprotein function and macrophage cholesterol metabolism. *Arthritis Rheumatol.* 2015;67:1155–1164.

85. Ridker PM, Everett BM, Pradhan A, et al. Low-dose methotrexate for the prevention of atherosclerotic events. *N Engl J Med.* 2019;380:752–762.

86. Charles-Schoeman C, Fleischmann R, Davignon J, et al. Potential mechanisms leading to the abnormal lipid profile in patients with rheumatoid arthritis versus healthy volunteers and reversal by tofacitinib. *Arthritis Rheumatol.* 2015;67:616–625.

87. Satoh M, Takahashi Y, Tabuchi T, et al. Cellular and molecular mechanisms of statins: an update on pleiotropic effects. *Clin Sci (Lond).* 2015;129:93–105.

88. Xing B, Yin YF, Zhao LD, et al. Effect of 3-hydroxy-3-methylglutaryl-coenzyme a reductase inhibitor on disease activity in patients with rheumatoid arthritis: a meta-analysis. *Medicine (Baltim).* 2015;94:e572.

89. Li GM, Zhao J, Li B, et al. The anti-inflammatory effects of statins on patients with rheumatoid arthritis: a systemic review and meta-analysis of 15 randomized controlled trials. *Autoimmun Rev.* 2018;17:215–225.

90. Solomon DH, Greenberg J, Curtis JR, et al. Derivation and internal validation of an expanded cardiovascular risk prediction score for rheumatoid arthritis: a Consortium of Rheumatology Researchers of North America Registry Study. *Arthritis Rheumatol.* 2015;67:1995–2003.

91. Schjerning AM, McGettigan P, Gislason G. Cardiovascular effects and safety of (non-aspirin) NSAIDs. *Nat Rev Cardiol.* 2020.

92. Ridker PM. Anticytokine agents: targeting interleukin signaling pathways for the treatment of atherothrombosis. *Circ Res.* 2019;124:437–450.

98 Tumors Affecting the Cardiovascular System

DANIEL J. LENIHAN, MICHAEL J. REARDON, AND W. GREGORY HUNDLEY

Cardiac masses frequently present significant diagnostic and therapeutic clinical challenges. In many cases, a cardiac mass is detected as an incidental finding and the resultant evaluation may culminate in the confirmation of a cardiac tumor; however, this is generally an uncommon event since other cardiac masses, including normal structures (particularly within the right atrium), thrombi, or valvular vegetations are more common.[1,2] This chapter describes the initial symptoms and signs that may indicate a cardiac tumor, followed by an explanation that often includes cardiovascular imaging. Once a cardiac tumor is suspected, the ultimate diagnosis is usually confirmed by a biopsy or surgery as histologic diagnosis has a direct bearing on further treatment planning. The remainder of the chapter focuses on the delineation and potential management of cardiac tumors as well as the overall anticipated outcomes. In many cases, the final pathologic diagnosis is typically confirmed by surgical removal after many difficult decisions regarding investigations and treatment are made in relation to the urgency of the clinical situation and initial presentation.

CLINICAL MANIFESTATION OF CARDIAC TUMORS

Initial Clinical Decision Making Regarding Cardiac Masses

Patients with cardiac tumors may present with no symptoms or physical findings and receive notification of an abnormality on an imaging examination performed for an unrelated indication. Alternatively, patients may experience nonspecific or detailed symptoms or signs that should alert practitioners to the possibility of a cardiac tumor (Table 98.1). The most important consideration in confirming the presence of a cardiac tumor is a high index of suspicion and the integration of symptoms, physical findings, and imaging characteristics in a logical manner to establish a clinically reasonable plan of action. The initial diagnostic test for a patient with concerning symptoms often involves an imaging test (Table 98.2), such as two-dimensional (2D) echocardiography (2D-echo) (see Chapter 16)[3] or cardiac magnetic resonance imaging (cMRI) (see Chapter 19).[4] Depending on the characteristics of this mass and the known comorbidities of the patient, additional imaging may be undertaken.[5] These including three-dimensional (3D) echo with or without contrast (see Chapter 16),[6] cMRI with gadolinium[7] (see Chapter 19), coronary angiography (to define the presence of coronary artery disease) (see Chapter 21),[8] positron emission testing (PET) to provide staging for cancer (see Chapter 18),[8] or computed tomography (CT) (see Chapter 20), including a CT angiogram (CTA) to

clarify intrathoracic structures.[9,10] Transesophageal echocardiography (TEE) can also provide very specific anatomical information that is critical to treatment planning (see Chapter 16).[8]

Clinical Scenarios When Evaluating a Cardiac Mass

In assessing a cardiac mass as the initial evaluation for a cardiac tumor, the clinical context in which the image was obtained is critical for making a diagnosis. A differential diagnosis of a cardiac mass is broad and includes tumors, thrombi, infection, and artifacts (Table 98.3). The most important characteristic would be evidence of perfusion into the mass as an indicator of a benign or malignant tumor.[5] When considering typically encountered clinical scenarios, a patient with new-onset heart failure and severe left ventricular (LV) dysfunction, who has a 2D-echo image that shows an apical mass, a cardiac tumor is quite unlikely. This suspicion would be firmly established if there was a severe wall motion abnormality in that region, the mass appeared distinct from the myocardial wall and was lobulated (Fig. 98.1). An LV mass with these characteristics is much more likely to be a thrombus as opposed to a tumor. Additionally, patients treated for cancer with indwelling catheters may experience development of abnormal masses, which may be observed during routine screening for cardiac dysfunction. As shown in Figure 98.2, this right atrial mass seen during transthoracic echocardiogram and then characterized more completely with cardiovascular MRI is consistent with a thrombus.

Another scenario involves a patient with a history of melanoma that is metastatic to other organs, who has routine cardiac imaging and a solid mass is seen in an unusual location. Since there is no wall motion abnormality and no significant valvular disease or clinical signs suggestive of infective endocarditis, a mobile mass on the tricuspid valve is very likely to be a metastatic lesion to the heart (Fig. 98.3). Another imaging characteristic that provides insight indicating a tumor is present is the behavior of the mass during cardiac motion. If a tumor is infiltrating the myocardium, it is unlikely to contract in a normal fashion. An LV myocardial apical mass contracting similarly to the surrounding tissue is likely to be either focal hypertrophy (Fig. 98.4) or LV noncompaction (Fig. 98.5)[11,12] as opposed to a cardiac tumor. Furthermore, progression of an image over time also may indicate the pathologic process. If a cardiac mass changes in size during serial imaging, suspicion of a cardiac tumor is much higher (eFig. 98.1). However, an LV apical mass that is stable for months or years is unlikely to be a malignant cardiac tumor as noted in Figures 98.4 and 98.5.

The exact nature and location of a mass is critical in the determination of the likelihood that it is a tumor. A classic example of this principle is lipomatous hypertrophy of the intraatrial septum (Fig. 98.6). The initial suspicion might be that this is a myxoma or other tumor, but an MRI with specific characteristics that are a hallmark for lipomatous hypertrophy will confirm the diagnosis.[13] Additionally, ridges of tissue including the crista terminalis or the eustachian valve remnant can also mimic cardiac masses (eFig. 98.2).

TABLE 98.1 Range of Clinical Findings That May Indicate a Cardiac Tumor

- Completely asymptomatic but an incidental abnormality on imaging
- Low-grade fevers
- Transient ischemic attack or cerebral vascular event
- Positional dyspnea
- Weight loss
- Peripheral embolic events
- Chest discomfort
- Congestive heart failure
- Upper extremity/neck swelling
- Lower extremity venous thrombosis
- Palpitations
- Arrhythmias
- Pericardial effusion/tamponade

TABLE 98.2 Common Testing That May Indicate the Possibility of a Cardiac Tumor

- Two or three dimensional echocardiography
- Chest x-ray
- Computed tomography (CT)
- CT angiography
- Magnetic resonance imaging
- Transesophageal echocardiography
- Positron emission tomography
- Nuclear scintigraphy

TABLE 98.3 Differential Diagnosis of Cardiac Masses

- Intracardiac thrombus
- Focal myocardial hypertrophy
- Left ventricular noncompaction
- Infectious (abscess)
- Primary cardiac tumor
- Secondary cardiac tumor (metastasis)
- Lipomatous hypertrophy of the septum
- Cyst
- Imaging artifact

Classification of Cardiac Tumors

Cardiac tumors are divided into primary and secondary tumors. Primary cardiac tumors are very rare, with an autopsy incidence of 1:2000.[14] These tumors include benign or malignant neoplasms that may arise from any tissue of the heart. In terms of primary tumors, approximately 80% are benign and these can be grouped as simple or complex, considering the treatment that is typically required. The approximately 20% of primary cardiac tumors remaining are malignant and usually are pathologically described as sarcomas.[15-17] Table 98.4 summarizes some of the pathologic descriptions of cardiac tumors that have been reported, albeit not an exhaustive list, since there have been many very specific pathologic descriptions and it can be difficult to adequately categorize them. Thus, general categories will be discussed in the remainder of this chapter. Figure 98.7 illustrates the types of tumor that may affect different chambers of the heart and pericardium. Secondary or metastatic cardiac tumors are 30 times more common than a primary neoplasm with an autopsy incidence of 1.7% to 14%[18] or 1:100.[14]

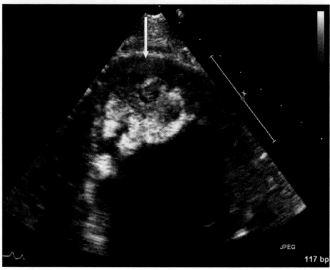

FIGURE 98.1 A large irregular mass noted in the left ventricular apex (*arrow*) in the context of a patient with severe left ventricular dysfunction. The edges are distinct from the myocardium classic for a thrombus.

BENIGN (NONMALIGNANT) PRIMARY CARDIAC TUMORS

The majority (>80%) of the primary cardiac tumors are nonmalignant; however, because of their location these frequently require surgical treatment.[19,20] Myxoma constitutes about 50% of all benign cardiac tumors in adults, but only a small percentage of such tumors in children.[21] Rhabdomyomas are the most common benign tumor in children and account for 40% to 60% of the pediatric cases.[20] Other benign cardiac tumors that have been described include fibromas, lipomas, hemangiomas, papillary fibroelastomas, cystic tumors of the AV node, and paragangliomas.

Simple Benign Tumors
Myxomas

Most myxomas (>80%) are most commonly found in the left atrium and in decreasing frequencies in the right atrium, right ventricle, and left ventricle (Fig. 98.8).[16,22] The incidence of cardiac myxoma peaks at 40 to 60 years of age, with a female to male ratio of approximately 3:1. Most myxomas occur sporadically but may be familial and occasionally these have been described in relation to a particular syndrome called Carney's complex, an autosomal-dominant condition associated with cardiac myxomas, myxomas in other regions (cutaneous or mammary), hyperpigmented skin lesions, hyperactivity of the adrenal or testicular glands, and pituitary tumors. Carney's complex occurs at a younger age and should be considered when cardiac myxomas are discovered in atypical locations in the heart.[15]

Etiology and Pathophysiology

The exact origin of myxoma cells remains uncertain, but they are thought to arise from remnants of subendocardial cells or multipotential mesenchymal cells in the region of the fossa ovalis, which can differentiate along a variety of cell lines. The hypothesis is that cardiac myxoma originates from a pluripotential stem cell, and myxoma cells express a variety of antigens and other endothelial markers. Myxomas typically form a pedunculated mass with a short broad base (85% of myxomas), but sessile forms can also occur.[19] Classically, myxomas appear yellowish, appear white or brownish, and are frequently friable. The tumor size can range from 1 cm to more than 10 cm, and the surface is smooth in the majority of the cases. A villous or papillary form of myxoma has been reported and contains a surface that consists of multiple fine or very fine villous, gelatinous, and fragile extensions that have a tendency to fragment spontaneously and are associated with embolic phenomena.[23] Histologically, myxomas are composed of

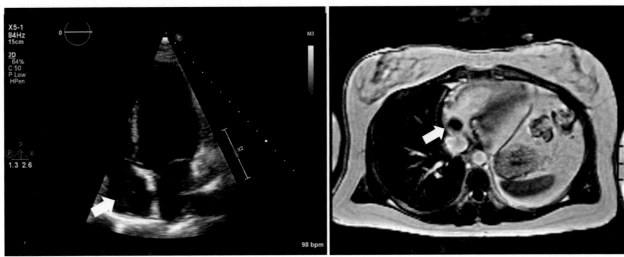

FIGURE 98.2 **Differentiation of tumor versus thrombus formation in 48-year-old woman treated for breast cancer. Left,** Four-chamber echocardiogram with new right atrial mass (*arrow*) that developed after the third round of anthracycline-based chemotherapy administered via an indwelling catheter. **Right,** Late gadolinium enhanced cardiac MRI demonstrating absence of contrast uptake within the mass consistent with a thrombus (*arrow*). The etiology of the thrombus in this case is related to the indwelling catheter (not shown) resting against the wall of the right atrium and serving as a nidus for thrombus formation.

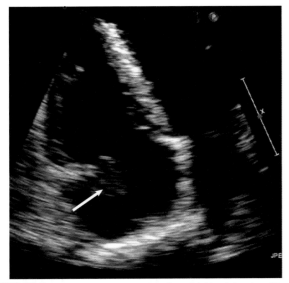

FIGURE 98.3 An irregular mass is noted on the atrial side of the tricuspid valve (*arrow*) in a patient with metastatic melanoma.

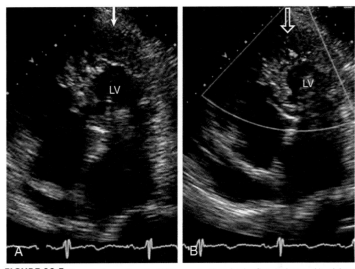

FIGURE 98.5 An apical mass is not solid (*arrow* in **A**) and color flow is detected in "lakes" within the apical mass (*arrow* in **B**). This is typical of noncompaction cardiomyopathy and this area does appear to contract.

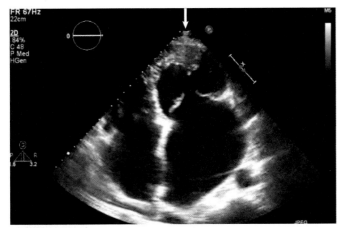

FIGURE 98.4 A four-chamber echo image showing focal apical hypertrophy (*arrow*) that resulted in severe diastolic heart failure. The apical mass contracted and was stable in appearance for years.

spindle and stellate shaped cells with myxoid stroma that may also contain endothelial cells, smooth muscle cells, and other elements surrounded within an acid mucopolysaccharide substance. Calcifications may also be seen in some cases.[19]

Clinical Manifestations

Patients commonly are asymptomatic and the tumor is found as an incidental finding on 2D-echo. When symptoms are present, dyspnea, especially dyspnea that is worse while lying on the left side, should alert the astute clinician to the possibility of a myxoma. Most clinical presentations related to myxoma result from mitral valve obstruction (syncope, dyspnea, and pulmonary edema) followed by embolic manifestations.[16,23] Patients may present with nonspecific symptoms such as fatigue, cough, low-grade fever, arthralgia, myalgia, weight loss, erythematous rash, and laboratory findings of anemia and increased erythrocyte sedimentation rate (ESR), C-reactive protein, and gamma globulin levels. Less commonly they may have thrombocytopenia, clubbing, cyanosis, or Raynaud's phenomenon. Physical exam findings can reveal a systolic murmur or a diastolic murmur suggestive of mitral stenosis. A tumor plop may potentially be heard (a low-pitched diastolic sound heard as the tumor prolapses into the left ventricle).[16,23] In one study, a cardiac auscultation abnormality was detected in 64% of patients,[24] and the most common auscultation

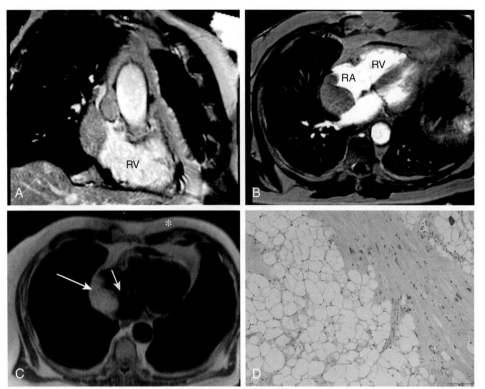

FIGURE 98.6 A and **B,** A large intraatrial mass (lipomatous septal hypertrophy) obstructing the inflow into the right atrium. **C,** MRI showing a large intraatrial mass with high intensity signal (*white arrow*) and sparing the region of fossa ovalis (*yellow arrow*). Also noted is the signal intensity is similar to the subcutaneous chest wall fat consistent with lipomatous hypertrophy of the intraatrial septum (*). **D,** There is an admixture of adipocytes, fibrosis, and entrapped hypertrophic cardiomyocytes. The adipocytes have variable size of cytoplasmic vacuolation, demonstrating a "hibernoma" or "brown fat" morphology. *RA,* Right atrium; *RV,* right ventricle.

TABLE 98.4 Pathologic Description of Cardiac Tumors

Benign
• Myxoma
• Paraganglioma
• Rhabdomyoma
• Fibroma
• Lipoma
• Hemangioma
• Papillary fibroelastoma
• Cystic tumor of the AV node
Malignant
• Sarcoma
• Lymphoma
Metastatic
• Renal cell carcinoma
• Melanoma
• Breast cancer
• Lung cancer
• Sarcoma
• Lymphoma
• Leukemia
• Cervical cancer

findings are a systolic murmur (in 50% of cases) followed by loud first heart sound (32%), an opening snap (26%), and a diastolic murmur (15%).[23] The reason for the systolic murmur may be caused by damage to the valves, failure of the leaflets to coapt, or narrowing of the outflow tract by the tumor. A diastolic murmur is present due to obstruction of the

mitral valve from the tumor. Tumor plop may be confused with a mitral opening snap or a third heart sound and can be detected in up to 15% of cases.[24] Chest examination may reveal fine crepitations consistent with pulmonary edema while there may be peripheral signs of embolic phenomenon. The physical evidence of embolic phenomenon will vary depending on the vascular territory involved. Involvement of cerebral vessels results in neurologic signs; involvement of coronary arteries may result in an acute coronary syndrome; intestinal arterial obstruction may result in ischemic bowel; and peripheral arterial obstruction can result in limb-threatening ischemia.

Laboratory Testing
Laboratory test abnormalities may include anemia, elevated serum gamma globulin, elevated ESR, and elevated serum C-reactive protein, which is present in approximately 75% of the patients.[23] There are no specific electrocardiogram (ECG) findings in myxoma. Chest x-ray findings are also nonspecific and include signs of congestive heart failure, cardiomegaly, and left atrial enlargement. In some cases, the tumor itself may be visible due to calcification.[24] A 2D echo usually should demonstrate a mass in the atrium, with the stalk attached to the interatrial septum but myxomas have been reported in all chambers of the heart.[22] A TEE provides specific delineation of the tumor including the size and origin. CT and MRI scans provide better delineation of the intracardiac mass, the extent of tumor in relation to extracardiac structures, and provide anatomical definition for preoperative planning (Table 98.5).

Treatment
The only definitive treatment of cardiac myxoma is surgical removal. Generally, the myxoma is surgically excised using cardiopulmonary bypass and cardioplegic arrest. The tumor is removed by either right or left atriotomy or combined atriotomy, depending on the site and extent of the tumor. The choice of technique also depends on associated conditions that need surgical intervention, such as valve repair or replacement, and coronary disease if present. Lifelong follow-up is needed, as myxomas have some tendency to recur. The recurrence rate of myxoma has varied but one large experience suggests that is quite low and may be below 1%.[23,25]

Fibroelastoma
Valvular structures may have a papillary fibroelastoma attached, which is often found incidentally. These are small in size, typically less than 2 cm, and most commonly occur on the aortic valve followed by the mitral valve. Rarely these may be found anywhere in the endocardial surface and the majority of fibroelastomas that have been reported are solitary, although multiple ones have been rarely reported.[26] Fibroelastomas may result in embolic phenomena, and when situated on the aortic valve or the left ventricle, can cause coronary ostial occlusion (Fig. 98.9).[27] Grossly, they have a characteristic frond like appearance, resembling a sea anemone, and histologically the tumor has an inner central core of collagen surrounded by a layer of acid mucopolysaccharides and covered by endothelial cells[26] (eFig. 98.3). For the most part, complete surgical resection is recommended for left-sided papillary fibroelastoma primarily because of the high likelihood of systemic embolism, which

can lead to stroke, myocardial infarction, peripheral embolism, and even sudden death. The decision for surgery in right-sided disease is more difficult as the number of asymptomatic right heart fibroelastomas is unknown and recommendation for surgery depends on the exact location, size, and potential risk to the patient. On imaging, especially echocardiographic imaging, there is a characteristic small, mobile, pedunculated, and very echo dense core that enables it to be differentiated from a vegetation or thrombi. Typically the structure of the valve can be preserved once the tumor is removed (see eFig. 98.3). The chance of recurrence appears low and there is no compelling data to continue anticoagulation long term unless there are other indications to do so.[28]

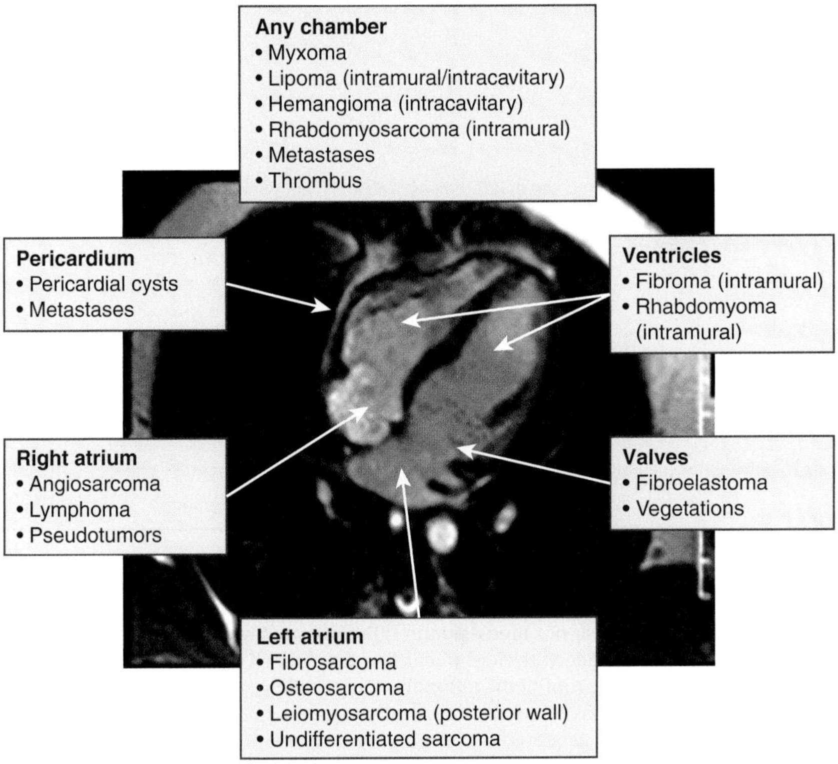

Rhabdomyomas

Rhabdomyomas are usually found in the ventricle and are the most common benign cardiac tumor found in children.[20,21] The majority of these patients have signs of or a family history of tuberous sclerosis.[20] In one study of patients with tuberous sclerosis complex, cardiac tumor was found in 48% of the patients, with an incidence of 66% in patients less than 2 years old.[29] Frequently, these patients are asymptomatic although some patients with rhabdomyoma may present clinically with arrhythmias and heart failure.[20,29] It is possible these tumors may regress with age but can sometimes grow or appear during puberty.[29] As a result of these uncertain outcomes, long-term clinical and echocardiographic follow-up is needed in patients with tuberous sclerosis. Most often, surgery can be avoided, although if arrhythmias become a symptomatic problem, antiarrhythmics and ultimately surgery may have to be considered.[20]

Lipomas

A lipoma is a rare benign cardiac tumor comprising only 3% of all benign tumors.[30] These tend to occur in the left ventricle or the right atrium but may be found anywhere in the heart as well as the pericardium. Although frequently asymptomatic, they may grow large enough to cause obstructive symptoms and require surgical intervention (see Fig. 98.6). Obstruction and compression of the superior vena cava may occur in patients with lipomas involving the right atrium.

Cystic Tumor of the AV Node (Previously Called Mesothelioma)

Because of their location near the atrioventricular node, these cystic tumors can present with varying degree of heart block or even sudden death.[31] Cardiac MRI is particularly useful in the diagnosis of this tumor.[32]

Other Very Rare Benign Cardiac Tumors

There are few very rare reports of hemangioma,[33,34] neurofibroma, teratomas,[35] leiomyoma, and lymphangioma; however, there are not enough data to summarize

Any chamber
• Myxoma
• Lipoma (intramural/intracavitary)
• Hemangioma (intracavitary)
• Rhabdomyosarcoma (intramural)
• Metastases
• Thrombus

Pericardium
• Pericardial cysts
• Metastases

Right atrium
• Angiosarcoma
• Lymphoma
• Pseudotumors

Left atrium
• Fibrosarcoma
• Osteosarcoma
• Leiomyosarcoma (posterior wall)
• Undifferentiated sarcoma

Ventricles
• Fibroma (intramural)
• Rhabdomyoma (intramural)

Valves
• Fibroelastoma
• Vegetations

FIGURE 98.7 Illustration of tumors or masses in the various chambers and structures of the heart.

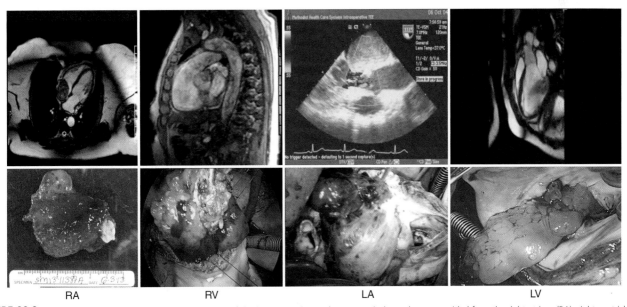

RA   RV   LA   LV

FIGURE 98.8 Myxomas have been reported in every chamber of the heart. Imaging and gross surgical samples are provided from the right atrium (RA), right ventricle (RV), left atrium (LA), and the left ventricle (LV). On all of the gross pictures from each chamber, the outward appearance is generally yellow to gray and can appear soft and villous or perhaps smooth and more solid. Note the lack of thrombus on the surface of each tumor.

TABLE 98.5 Imaging Characteristics of Tumors with Echo, CT, and cMRI

CARDIAC TUMOR	ECHOCARDIOGRAPHY (ECHO)	COMPUTED TOMOGRAPHY (CT)	MAGNETIC RESONANCE IMAGING (cMRI)
Myxoma	Mobile tumor	Narrow base of attachment	Mottled gadolinium contrast enhancement
	Frequently attached fossa ovalis	Heterogeneous with low attenuation	Mobile on cine imaging
	Heterogeneous echogenicity	Possible calcification	Varying (mixture of values on T1 mapping)
Papillary Fibroelastoma	Mobile valve leaflet mass	Mass seen on valve leaflets	Mobile mass on valve leaflets
			Variable gadolinium contrast enhancement
Lipoma	General thickening of interatrial septum	Low attenuation due to fat	High T1 signal
			Fat saturated images with low signal
Rhabdomyoma	Small lobulated hyperechoic intramuscular masses		Multiple masses with homogeneous signal intensity
			Uniform T1 and T2 values
Fibroma	Large intramural mass	Homogeneous with low attenuation	Uniform T1 and T2 values
		Calcification may be present	Isointense on T1-weighted images
		Large intramural mass	Large intramural mass
Hemangioma	Increased echogenicity	Heterogeneous with marked enhancement	Gadolinium enhancement present
Angiosarcoma	Invades across tissue boundaries	Invasive across tissue boundaries; low attenuation	Invasive across tissue boundaries
			Varying or heterogeneous gadolinium enhancement
	Pericardial effusion		Varying or heterogeneous T1 and T2 values
Lymphoma	Low echogenicity masses	Low attenuation masses	Enhancement with gadolinium that may be heterogeneous
	Pericardial effusion		
Metastases	Often multiple masses	Often multiple lesions	Often multiple lesions
	May have pericardial effusion		Gadolinium enhancement

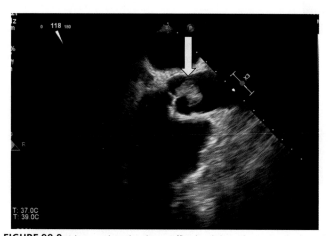

FIGURE 98.9 A large pedunculated mass affixed and above the aortic valve (*arrow*) was a papillary fibroelastoma confirmed at surgery. The valve was repaired successfully without replacement.

expected findings. Typically these tumors will be diagnosed after resection. Complete resection of the tumor is possible in most of the benign primary tumors, compared with malignant tumors, with a perioperative death of 1.4%.[36] Hemangiomas are characteristically vascular and maybe endocardial or epicardial (Fig. 98.10 and eFig. 98.4).[37]

Complex Benign Tumors
Paragangliomas
Cardiac paragangliomas are chromaffin-producing tumors arising from the neural crest cells of the sympathetic and parasympathetic

chains. Only 1% to 2% occur in the chest and most of these are in the posterior mediastinum.[25] The tumor may be located in the pericardial space with no intracardiac extension[38] but are often located around the roof of the left atrium and aortic root involving the cardiac structures[39] and can occur anywhere in the heart. When paraganglioma is suspected, a coronary CT angiogram or cardiac catheterization is necessary looking for large feeding vessels (Fig. 98.11). If present, this is almost pathognomonic for paraganglioma and diagnostic biopsy should be avoided due to the high risk of bleeding. Paragangliomas are a highly vascular tumor and may present with hypertension and chest pain.[38,40] The tumors originating from the roof of left atrium are often very large and require extensive surgery, including cardiac auto transplantation,[39] and should generally be confined to specialized centers. A coronary angiogram in these patients shows a characteristic "tumor blush" (Fig. 98.11C).[38,40] These tumors are further classified as hormonally active or inactive. Histology cannot reliably determine if the tumor is benign and about 10% will recur with metastatic disease. These tumors were originally referred to as malignant paraganglioma but the term "metastatic paraganglioma" is currently favored. Although large surgical cohorts are lacking, the author's (MR) current experience (Methodist Hospital, Houston, Texas) includes a total of 20 resections in 19 patients with two deaths and one recurrence as metastatic paraganglioma.[41]

Fibromas
These tumors are histologically composed primarily of fibroblasts or collagen. Typically these occur in childhood, although it can also occur in adults.[16,19,42] Most often a fibroma is located in the ventricle and interventricular septum, and patients may present with chest pain, pericardial effusion, heart failure, arrhythmias, and sudden death. Cardiomegaly is frequently seen on chest x-ray, which may also show the calcification within the tumor mass.[42] Frequently these tumors are associated with arrhythmias and might require multimodality treatment with medications, electrophysiologic procedures,

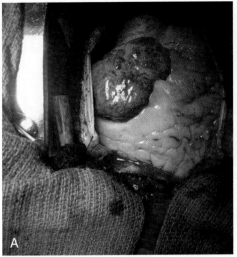
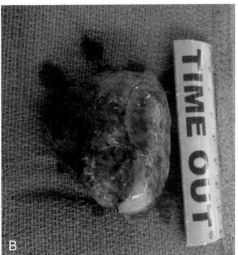
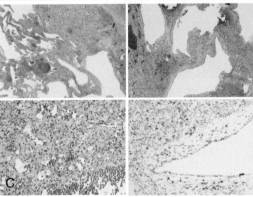
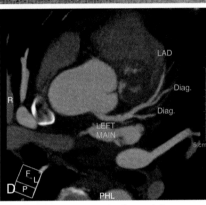

MALIGNANT PRIMARY CARDIAC TUMORS

Sarcomas

Primary cardiac tumors, both benign and malignant, are rare with a meta-analysis covering 22 studies showing an autopsy incidence of approximately 0.02% while primary cardiac sarcomas make up over 75% of these malignant tumors.[46] Primary cardiac sarcoma constitutes only about 1% of all soft tissue sarcomas.[47] The age of presentation for cardiac sarcomas ranges from 1 to 76 years, with a mean age around 40 years.[17,47] Studies using large U.S. national databases have confirmed the extreme rarity of primary cardiac sarcoma as well is its usual dismal outlook.[48,49] Angiosarcomas and unclassified sarcomas account for approximately 76% of all cardiac sarcomas, of which angiosarcomas are the most common.[50] Rhabdomyosarcoma is the most common form of cardiac sarcoma in children. Leiomyosarcoma, synovial sarcoma, osteosarcoma, fibrosarcoma, myxoid sarcoma, liposarcoma, mesenchymal sarcoma, neurofibrosarcoma, and malignant fibrous histiocytoma are other cardiac sarcomas observed.[15,17,50] Angiosarcomas are predominantly found on the right side while osteosarcomas and unclassified sarcomas are predominantly found on the left side of the heart.[50] Pericardial angiosarcomas are extremely rare.[51] Most published reports are from institutional series and generally have included 30 or fewer surgical cases.[17,52-54] The national French Sarcoma Group found 124 cases of primary cardiac sarcoma over 33 years

FIGURE 98.10 Primary cardiac hemangioma arising from the right coronary artery at the base of the aorta and right atrium. A, Complete resection was possible with uneventful postoperative course. **B,** The resected specimen was easily dissected free from adjacent structures and was supplied by the right coronary artery. **C,** Histologic and immunohistochemical features of the tumor. **Top left,** Low-power view showing large vascular spaces and more solid areas with small capillaries. There is a portion of residual cardiac muscle in the upper right corner (2× magnification). **Top right,** Medium-power view showing that the vascular spaces are lined by an attenuated endothelial lining with cells with small nuclei. Many of the spaces contain blood and fibrin and the intervening areas of capillary proliferation have blood and scattered chronic inflammatory cells (4×magnification). **Bottom left,** High-power view of the capillary rich area showing plump cells lining the vascular spaces (20× magnification). **Bottom right,** CD 31 immunohistochemistry showing strong brown staining of the lining cells of the large spaces and also of the plump cells in the capillary rich areas (20× magnification). **D,** CT angiography showing the mass adjacent to the right coronary artery.

and/or surgery. If surgical resection is performed, fibromas tend not to recur. A distinguishing feature of fibromas, contrasted to rhabdomyoma, is that there is classically calcification within the tumor.[19] Although these tumors can be extremely large when they involve the left ventricle, they tend to push the myocardium away, rather than replace it, allowing for resection of large tumors with preservation of ventricular function.[43]

Treatment

Most tumors, particularly benign masses, are relatively limited in size and do not have extensive adjacent cardiac involvement. The surgical approach, whether via median sternotomy or right thoracotomy, allows complete removal and repair of most resulting defects. However, there is a small group of tumors with complex cardiac involvement. These tumors may invade and obstruct pulmonary veins or the mitral annulus, which renders complete removal impossible with conventional surgical approaches. Pioneered by Reardon and colleagues in Houston, the complete removal of the heart with back table resection and reconstruction of the pulmonary veins and atria offers a potential cure or significant palliation in selected patients. The approach is similar to heart transplant cardiectomy allowing for exposure of the pulmonary veins and complete resection of atrial and even ventricular masses.[44] In their select series there was 100% 1-year survival among patients with benign tumors and 50% survival in patients with malignant tumors (primarily sarcoma).[45]

in France with 81 patients receiving surgical resection.[55] The largest single institution report found 131 primary cardiac sarcoma (PCS) cases over 25 years with 95 patients receiving surgical resection.[56] Three recent large national database studies in the United States have reinforced this rarity. The Surveillance, Epidemiology and End Results (SEER) database had 442 patients with PCS identified over 42 years (1973 to 2015) with only 218 (49.8%) having surgery.[48] The National Cancer Database (NCDB) was queried for 2004 to 2015 finding 617 patients with PSC over this 21-year period and 372 (60.3%) having surgery.[49] An additional study using the NCDB from 2004 to 2016 found 100,317 primary cardiac tumors, of which 826 (0.8%) were malignant and of these, 731 (88.5%) were sarcoma.[57] In this study, surgery was done on 442 (59.2%) of the primary malignant tumors and 225 (50.9%) had multimodality treatment in addition to their surgery.

As a result of this rarity, only a few institutions and even fewer individual physicians have an appreciable experience with treating this disease.[58] It is generally agreed that complete surgical resection is the mainstay of therapy. If surgery cannot be done, the 1-year survival is less than 10%.[59] Knowing when complete resection is possible and who would be an appropriate candidate can be difficult but is important for the clinician to understand. Additionally, the role of neoadjuvant and adjuvant chemotherapy and radiation therapy are poorly defined as most studies have been small, although recent evidence seems to be favoring both.[48,49,60-62] A clinically practical way to consider primary

CARDIOVASCULAR DISEASE AND DISORDERS OF OTHER ORGANS

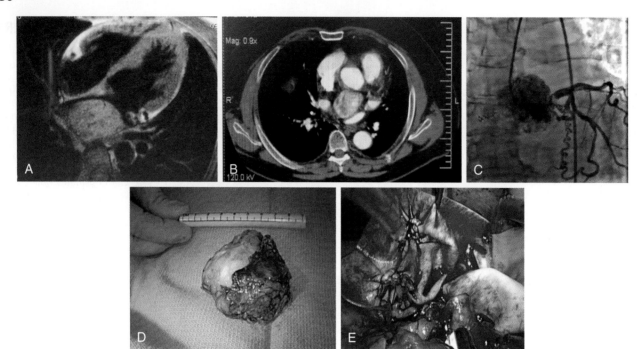

FIGURE 98.11 Imaging and pathology of the presentation for a paraganglioma. A, CMR image with a large hypervascular tumor of the left atrium. **B,** CT imaging demonstrates the tumor extends superiorly behind the aorta and pulmonary artery. **C,** Cardiac catheterization image that demonstrates giant vessels feeding the paraganglioma. **D,** Gross specimen, which shows the diffuse nature of the tumor. The smooth portion is part of the left atrial wall that had to be resected. There is no tissue plane between the tumor and the atrial wall. **E,** Posterior left atrial repair with bovine pericardium. (**C** from Chan EY, et al. Management of primary cardiac paraganglioma. J Thorac Cardiovasc Surg 2020;S0022-5223(20):32704-32705.)

cardiac sarcoma is by tumor location since this often determines the clinical presentation, urgency of treatment, and surgical options: (1) right heart, (2) left heart, or (3) pulmonary artery.

Clinical Manifestations

Cardiac tumors commonly cause symptoms by three separate mechanisms: obstruction, embolization, and arrhythmias. Rarely pericardial invasion and tamponade may be the first manifestation of the disease. Both atrial and ventricular tumors, when large enough, may result in obstructive symptoms and cause syncope, chest pain, dyspnea, or heart failure. The most common presenting symptoms include dyspnea, followed by chest pain, cough, syncope, hemoptysis, sudden death, fever, embolic events, and cardiac arrhythmias.[17] Large tumors on the right side, besides causing venous congestion, may also limit cardiac filling with sudden decreases in intravascular volume and potentially precipitating syncope in these patients. Left-sided cardiac tumors, if large enough, can also impair ventricular filling leading to syncope or heart failure (Fig. 98.12). Unfortunately, about 29% of cardiac sarcomas have metastatic disease at the time of presentation, typically in the lung.[17,51] Sarcomas, especially left-sided, are commonly associated with cardiac embolic events[15] and arrhythmia may be an important problem as well. A finding of a cardiac mass with pericardial effusion should raise the suspicion of a malignant cardiac tumor.[51] Commonly, pericardial effusion is due to associated pericardial involvement; however, a malignant effusion is not always proven.

Laboratory Investigations

Regardless of the imaging modalities used, malignant tumors of the heart often involve invasion of the tumor across tissue boundaries or planes including the pericardium, epicardium, endocardium, and valve planes. This feature often distinguishes these tumors from nonmalignant and other normal structures. Due to increasing use of CT scan and better modalities of cardiac imaging, the primary cardiac tumors may be identified at an earlier stage. ECG changes are usually nonspecific; however, heart block, ventricular hypertrophy, bundle branch blocks, atrial flutter, and atrial tachycardia may be present in some cases. Cardiomegaly is a common but nonspecific radiologic finding of cardiac sarcomas.[15] Echo is commonly used in the initial diagnosis of primary

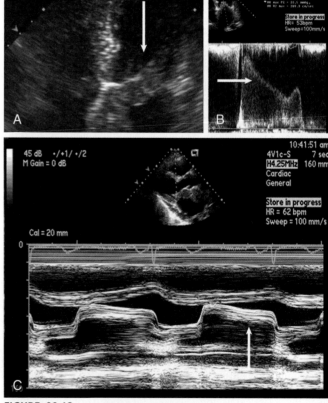

FIGURE 98.12 Echo Doppler images from a patient with sarcoma who presented with heart failure and mitral stenosis. A, Four-chamber image with mitral valve thickening (*arrow*). **B,** Increased velocity across the mitral valve showing stenosis (*arrow*). **C,** M-mode showing a classic mitral stenosis pattern.

cardiac tumors with transthoracic 2D, 3D, and contrast imaging being appropriate techniques. However, transthoracic echo has several well-known limitations: operator experience, lung interference due to pulmonary disease, narrow rib spaces, or unfavorable body habitus. TEE can provide more specific and detailed imaging than 2D echo especially structures that are more posterior such as the left atrium. Cross sectional imaging methods, such as CT and MRI, have an important role in the evaluation and further assessment of malignant cardiac tumors, especially in evaluation of myocardial invasion (Fig. 98.13), involvement of mediastinal structures, tissue characterization (Fig. 98.14), and vascularity (Table 98.5).[5,63]

Treatment

A complete resection is the optimal goal for surgical treatment.[15,17,64] Once surgical treatment is completed, adjuvant chemotherapy seems prudent although not widely studied but has shown to improve survival over surgery alone in a SEER database analysis.[48,64] It is possible that neoadjuvant therapy may be useful and has been shown to improve survival with some sarcomas, but this is speculative.[65] The most common chemotherapeutic regimen used for cardiac sarcomas is combined doxorubicin and ifosfamide.[51] A combination of docetaxel and gemcitabine also showed some response in various sarcomas and can be used as an alternative chemotherapeutic regimen.[51] Other treatment options include ifosfamide-epirubicin (doxorubicin)

and cyclophosphamide, vincristine, doxorubicin, and dacarbazine (CyVADIC).[47] Unlike other sarcomas, cardiac sarcomas overall have a very poor prognosis with a median survival rate of 6 months to 25 months after diagnosis.[16,19,50] The presence of tumor necrosis and metastases is associated with a poor prognosis[50] as is the presence of a right-sided cardiac sarcoma.[66] Sarcomas other than angiosarcomas, sarcomas on the left side of the heart, and completely resected sarcomas seem to have a better prognosis.[17] At the time of surgical resection, patients with negative surgical margins have a better survival.[66] Low-grade cardiac sarcoma on histologic grading may appear to have a better survival, although in one study there was no significant correlation between the histologic grade and survival.[17,50,67] For additional information regarding right heart, left heart, and pulmonary artery sarcomas, please see the online supplement for this chapter, "Treatment of Sarcomas."

Heart Tumor Team
Malignant primary cardiac tumors are rare, are exceedingly complex, and have a dismal survival without treatment. The treatment of primary cardiac tumors requires a multidisciplinary cardiac tumor team including cardio-oncologists, sarcoma oncologists, specialized cardiac surgeons, and imaging experts.[58] The author's (MR) current single institution published experience with primary cardiac sarcoma surgical resection includes 95 patients.[56] The mean survival for the entire group was 20 months. Most deaths are due to metastatic disease suggesting that better biologic treatment is the key to significantly improving survival.

SECONDARY CARDIAC TUMORS

The autopsy incidence of secondary cardiac tumors ranges from 1.7% to 14% (average 7.1%) in cancer patients and 0.7% to 3.5% (average 2.3%) in the general population.[18] In comparison to older series, there is a significant increase in the incidence of cardiac metastases in cancer patients after 1970, predominately due to improvement in imaging modalities (Figs. 98.15 and 98.16). Cardiac metastases can occur either by direct extension, via blood stream, by lymphatics, or by intracavitary diffusion through the inferior vena cava (IVC). Pericardial metastasis (69%) is the most common location followed by epicardial (34%), myocardial (32%), and endocardial metastases (5%).[68] The pericardium is most often involved due to direct invasion by the thoracic cancers, including breast and lung cancer. Abdominal and pelvic tumors may reach the right atrium through the IVC. The most common tumor exhibiting this tendency is renal cell carcinoma.[51] A recent review suggests that lung cancer is the most common cause of cardiac metastasis followed by esophageal cancer and hematologic malignancy.[16] The symptoms of cardiac metastases are extremely variable, depending on

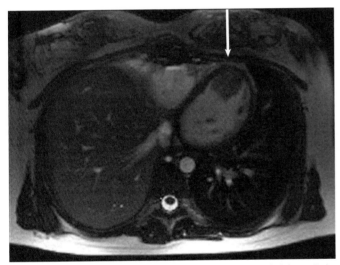

FIGURE 98.13 T_1-weighted cardiac magnetic resonance image of a left ventricular apical tumor of metastatic alveolar cell sarcoma. Note the indistinct nature of the tumor infiltrating the myocardium (*arrow*). This is in contrast to the distinct line that classically separates thrombus from myocardium.

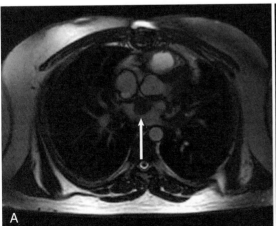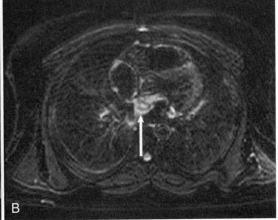

FIGURE 98.14 A, T_2-weighted image of a cardiac magnetic resonance image demonstrating a large left atrial mass near the anterior leaflet of the mitral valve. **B,** Contrast enhancement of the mass confirms a high degree of blood flow strongly suggesting an angiosarcoma.

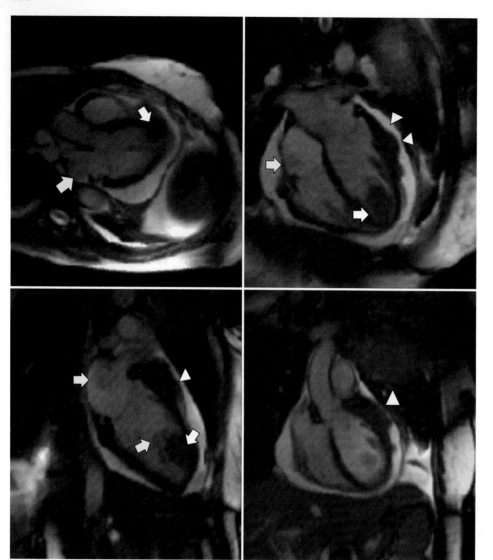

FIGURE 98.15 **A 39-nine-year-old with prior history of breast cancer presents with 2-day history of dyspnea and was referred for cardiac MRI after mass seen in LV apex on echocardiography. Top left,** Three-chamber view. **Top right,** Four-chamber view. **Bottom left,** Two-chamber view. **Bottom right,** Coronal view of the left ventricle. White arrows demonstrate cavitary masses of different texture (*solid white arrows and cystic yellow arrows*). Also, there are pericardial masses (*white triangles*) and a moderate-sized circumferential pericardial effusion. These findings are consistent with metastatic breast cancer.

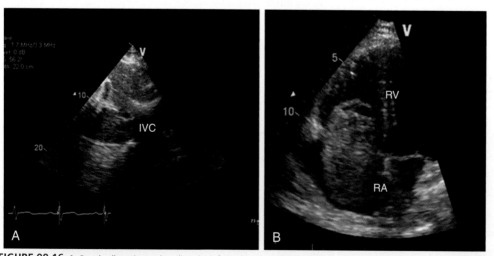

FIGURE 98.16 A, Renal cell carcinoma invading the inferior vena cava (IVC). **B,** Renal cell carcinoma invading the right atrium (RA) and prolapsing into the right ventricle (RV).

the location of the tumor. Dyspnea, palpitations, syncope, chest pain, and peripheral edema are common clinical presentations.[51,68] Heart failure, cardiac arrhythmias, heart blocks, acute myocardial infarction, myocardial rupture, systemic embolization, and superior vena cava syndrome (eFig. 98.5) are other manifestations of cardiac metastases. Multiple tumor metastases contributing to both pulmonary and systemic emboli can be observed as shown in Figure 98.15 in a woman with breast cancer. A new heart murmur or any new ECG finding without clear symptoms in a cancer patient should raise the suspicion of cardiac metastases. Typical ECG findings encountered patients with cardiac metastases are ST-T wave changes (mimicking myocardial ischemia or injury), new atrial fibrillation or flutter, and low voltages with electrical alternans indicating a significant pericardial effusion. The ECG findings of myocardial injury may indicate an invasion of the coronary vessels by tumor.[69]

Treatment

Treatment of metastatic cardiac tumors is usually palliative, as overall prognosis is poor, with >50% of patients dying within one year.[51] Palliative radiotherapy and chemotherapy in chemo-sensitive tumors are recommended.[18] In these patients, end-of-life care should be discussed and all efforts should be made to improve the quality of life (see Chapter 50). In highly selected cases, extraordinary surgical approaches can be attempted, such as auto transplantation, but this is an unusual option. The management of a malignant pericardial effusion is typically individualized to a local center experience and close collaboration between oncology and cardiology is necessary to ensure an optimal treatment plan. Recent data indicate that infusion of selected chemotherapy may be useful in patients who have a malignant effusion,[70] but this is not widely practiced.[71]

DIRECT AND INDIRECT COMPLICATIONS OF NEOPLASIA

Patients with cardiac and noncardiac neoplasia can develop direct and indirect complications that affect the pericardium and the superior vena cava. These topics are discussed briefly in the following section.

Pericardial Effusion

The differential diagnosis of a pericardial effusion in a patient with a known malignancy includes malignant effusion, radiation-induced or drug-induced pericarditis, idiopathic pericarditis, infectious (including tuberculosis, fungal, or bacterial), or iatrogenic, secondary to procedures (see Chapters 56 and 57). It is estimated that approximately 40% of patients with cancer and a pericardial effusion were found to have either radiation-induced or idiopathic and only a minority actually have malignant effusion.[53] Drug-induced pericarditis is typically seen after high-dose anthracycline or cyclophosphamide therapy (see Chapter 57). The management of patients with pericardial effusions secondary to metastatic disease and radiation is discussed in Chapter 86.

Cardiac Tamponade

The diagnosis and management of cardiac tamponade secondary to metastatic disease and radiation is discussed in Chapter 86.

Constrictive Pericarditis

Constrictive or effusive-constrictive pericarditis is a late complication of chest irradiation that may be becoming more common because of the longer survival of patients with breast cancer and Hodgkin disease who typically receive chest irradiation. This topic is covered in detail in Chapter 86.

Superior Vena Cava Syndrome

The superior vena cava (SVC) syndrome refers to clinical signs and symptoms that result from either partial or complete obstruction of blood flow through the SVC. This obstruction most commonly results from tumor infiltration of the vessel wall or from thrombotic occlusion. For additional information please refer to the online supplement for this chapter, "The Superior Vena Cava Syndrome in Cancer Patients."

FUTURE PERSPECTIVES

The clinical outcomes of patients who have a primary cardiac tumor heavily depend on early detection and prompt, appropriate treatment. It is a frequent phenomenon that cardiac tumors are only discovered after a patient experiences a period of confusing constellation of symptoms that are ultimately connected to an abnormal image that suggests a cardiac tumor. As a result, there is commonly an advanced stage of disease already at the time of diagnosis. Once a primary cardiac tumor is diagnosed, all patients should be managed by a multidisciplinary team including medical oncologists, radiation oncologists, cardiologists, and cardiac surgeons. Over the last few years, increasing use of imaging modalities (e.g., echo, MRI, and CT) has led to an increasing number of incidental findings of primary cardiac tumor. However, current imaging techniques may accurately differentiate tumors from other causes of masses seen on imaging slightly more than 50% of the time. With improvements in echocardiographic and CT/MRI imaging techniques, identification of all cardiac tumors will be done with a higher degree of certainty. No noninvasive technique can identify whether the tumor is benign or malignant and a pathologic sample is needed in all cases. Improvement in surgical technique has led to minimally invasive approaches, but this still entails general anesthesia, a surgical incision, and is a major stress for a patient. Continued refinement in the surgical tools and approaches will lead to less morbidity and mortality. Currently, there are no blood tests available that would point to metastasis, and this gap represents a large unmet clinical need.

REFERENCES
Clinical Manifestations
1. Zaragoza-Macias E, Chen MA, Gill EA. Real time three-dimensional echocardiography evaluation of intracardiac masses. *Echocardiography*. 2012;29:207–219.
2. Mankad R, Herrmann J. Cardiac tumors: echo assessment. *Echo Res Pract*. 2016;3:R65–R77.
3. Auger D, Pressacco J, Marcotte F, et al. Cardiac masses: an integrative approach using echocardiography and other imaging modalities. *Heart*. 2011;97:1101–1109.
4. O'Donnell DH, Abbara S, Chaithiraphan V, et al. Cardiac tumors: optimal cardiac MR sequences and spectrum of imaging appearances. *AJR Am J Roentgenol*. 2009;193:377–387.
5. Kassi M, Polsani V, Schutt RC, et al. Differentiating benign from malignant cardiac tumors with cardiac magnetic resonance imaging. *J Thorac Cardiovasc Surg*. 2019;157:1912–1922.e2.
6. Plana JC. Added value of real-time three-dimensional echocardiography in assessing cardiac masses. *Curr Cardiol Rep*. 2009;11:205–209.
7. Buckley O, Madan R, Kwong R, et al. Cardiac masses, part 1: imaging strategies and technical considerations. *AJR Am J Roentgenol*. 2011;197:W837–W841.
8. Buckley O, Madan R, Kwong R, et al. Cardiac masses, part 2: key imaging features for diagnosis and surgical planning. *AJR Am J Roentgenol*. 2011;197:W842–W851.
9. van Beek EJ, Stolpen AH, Khanna G, Thompson BH. CT and MRI of pericardial and cardiac neoplastic disease. *Canc Imag*. 2007;7:19–26.
10. Yuan SM, Shinfeld A, Lavee J, et al. Imaging morphology of cardiac tumours. *Cardiol J*. 2009;16:26–35.
11. Kohli SK, Pantazis AA, Shah JS, et al. Diagnosis of left-ventricular non-compaction in patients with left-ventricular systolic dysfunction: time for a reappraisal of diagnostic criteria? *Eur Heart J*. 2008;29:89–95.
12. Jacquier A, Thuny F, Jop B, et al. Measurement of trabeculated left ventricular mass using cardiac magnetic resonance imaging in the diagnosis of left ventricular non-compaction. *Eur Heart J*. 2010;31:1098–1104.
13. Xanthos T, Giannakopoulos N, Papadimitriou L. Lipomatous hypertrophy of the interatrial septum: a pathological and clinical approach. *Int J Cardiol*. 2007;121:4–8.
14. Basso C, Rizzo S, Valente M, Thiene G. Cardiac masses and tumours. *Heart*. 2016;102:1230–1245.
15. Neragi-Miandoab S, Kim J, Vlahakes GJ. Malignant tumours of the heart: a review of tumour type, diagnosis and therapy. *Clin Oncol (R Coll Radiol)*. 2007;19:748–756.
16. Ekmektzoglou KA, Samelis GF, Xanthos T. Heart and tumors: location, metastasis, clinical manifestations, diagnostic approaches and therapeutic considerations. *J Cardiovasc Med (Hagerstown)*. 2008;9:769–777.
17. Simpson L, Kumar SK, Okuno SH, et al. Malignant primary cardiac tumors: review of a single institution experience. *Cancer*. 2008;112:2440–2446.
18. Al-Mamgani A, Baartman L, Baaijens M, et al. Cardiac metastases. *Int J Clin Oncol*. 2008;13:369–372.
19. McManus B. Primary tumors of the heart. In: *Braunwald's Heart Disease*. 9th ed. Elsevier; 2011:1638–1650.

Benign Primary Cardiac Tumors
20. Burke A, Virmani R. Pediatric heart tumors. *Cardiovasc Pathol*. 2008;17:193–198.
21. Thomas-de-Montpreville V, Nottin R, Dulmet E, Serraf A. Heart tumors in children and adults: clinicopathological study of 59 patients from a surgical center. *Cardiovasc Pathol*. 2007;16:22–18.
22. Bakaeen FG, Reardon MJ, Coselli JS, et al. Surgical outcome in 85 patients with primary cardiac tumors. *Am J Surg*. 2003;186:641–647; discussion 647.
23. Acebo E, Val-Bernal JF, Gomez-Roman JJ, Revuelta JM. Clinicopathologic study and DNA analysis of 37 cardiac myxomas: a 28-year experience. *Chest*. 2003;123:1379–1385.
24. Pinede L, Duhaut P, Loire R. Clinical presentation of left atrial cardiac myxoma. A series of 112 consecutive cases. *Medicine*. 2001;80:159–172.
25. Yanagawa B, Chan EY, Cusimano RJ, Reardon MJ. Approach to surgery for cardiac tumors: primary simple, primary complex, and secondary. *Cardiol Clin*. 2019;37:525–531.
26. Sydow K, Willems S, Reichenspurner H, Meinertz T. Papillary fibroelastomas of the heart. *Thorac Cardiovasc Surgeon*. 2008;56:9–13.
27. Walkes JC, Bavare C, Blackmon S, Reardon MJ. Transaortic resection of an apical left ventricular fibroelastoma facilitated by a thoracoscope. *J Thorac Cardiovasc Surg*. 2007;134:793–794.
28. Abu Saleh WK, Al Jabbari O, Ramlawi B, Reardon MJ. Cardiac papillary fibroelastoma: single-institution experience with 14 surgical patients. *Tex Heart Inst J*. 2016;43:148–151.
29. Jozwiak S, Kotulska K, Kasprzyk-Obara J, et al. Clinical and genotype studies of cardiac tumors in 154 patients with tuberous sclerosis complex. *Pediatrics*. 2006;118:e1146–e1151.
30. Yu K, Liu Y, Wang H, et al. Epidemiological and pathological characteristics of cardiac tumors: a clinical study of 242 cases. *Interact Cardiovasc Thoracic Surg*. 2007;6:636–639.
31. Evans CA, Suvarna SK. Cystic atrioventricular node tumour: not a mesothelioma. *J Clin Pathol*. 2005;58:1232.
32. Tran TT, Starnes V, Wang X, et al. Cardiovascular magnetics resonance diagnosis of cystic tumor of the atrioventricular node. *J Cardiovasc Magn Res*. 2009;11:13.
33. Eftychiou C, Antoniades L. Cardiac hemangioma in the left ventricle and brief review of the literature. *J Cardiovasc Med (Hagerstown)*. 2009;10:565–567.
34. Wu G, Jones J, Sequeira IB, Pepelassis D. Congenital pericardial hemangioma responding to high-dose corticosteroid therapy. *Can J Cardiol*. 2009;25:e139–140.
35. Cohen R, Mirrer B, Loarte P, Navarro V. Intrapericardial mature cystic teratoma in an adult: case presentation. *Clin Cardiol*. 2013;36:6–9.
36. Centofanti P, Di Rosa E, Deorsola L, et al. Primary cardiac tumors: early and late results of surgical treatment in 91 patients. *Ann Thorac Surg*. 1999;68:1236–1241.
37. Abu Saleh WK, Al Jabbari O, Ramlawi B, et al. Case report: cardiac tumor resection and repair with porcine Xenograft. *Methodist Debakey Cardiovasc J*. 2016;12:116–118.
38. Rana O, Gonda P, Addis B, Greaves K. Image in cardiovascular medicine. Intrapericardial paraganglioma presenting as chest pain. *Circulation*. 2009;119:e373–375.
39. Ramlawi B, David EA, Kim MP, et al. Contemporary surgical management of cardiac paragangliomas. *Ann Thorac Surg*. 2012;93:1972–1976.
40. Khalid TJ, Zuberi O, Zuberi L, Khalid I. A rare case of cardiac paraganglioma presenting as anginal pain: a case report. *Cases J*. 2009;2:72.
41. Chan EY, Ali A, Umana JP, et al. Management of primary cardiac paraganglioma. *J Thorac Cardiovasc Surg*. 2020;S0022–S5223(20):32704–5. https://doi.org/10.1016/j.jtcvs.2020.09.100. Epub ahead of print. PMID: 33148444.
42. Burke AP, Rosado-de-Christenson M, Templeton PA, Virmani R. Cardiac fibroma: clinicopathologic correlates and surgical treatment. *J Thorac Cardiovasc Surg*. 1994;108:862–870.
43. Leja MJ, Perryman L, Reardon MJ. Resection of left ventricular fibroma with subacute papillary muscle rupture. *Tex Heart Inst J*. 2011;38:279–281.
44. Reardon MJ, DeFelice CA, Sheinbaum R, Baldwin JC. Cardiac autotransplant for surgical treatment of a malignant neoplasm. *Ann Thorac Surg*. 1999;67:1793–1795.
45. Ramlawi B, Al-Jabbari O, Blau LN, et al. Autotransplantation for the resection of complex left heart tumors. *Ann Thorac Surg*. 2014;98:863–868.

Malignant Primary Tumors
46. Reynen K. Frequency of primary tumors of the heart. *Am J Cardiol*. 1996;77:107.
47. Gupta A. Primary cardiac sarcomas. *Expert Rev Cardiovasc Ther*. 2008;6:1295–1297.
48. Yin K, Luo R, Wei Y, et al. Survival outcomes in patients with primary cardiac sarcoma in the United States. *J Thorac Cardiovasc Surg*. 2021;162(1):107–115.e2.
49. Hendriksen BS, Stahl KA, Hollenbeak CS, et al. Postoperative chemotherapy and radiation improve survival following cardiac sarcoma resection. *J Thorac Cardiovasc Surg*. 2019.
50. Kim CH, Dancer JY, Coffey D, et al. Clinicopathologic study of 24 patients with primary cardiac sarcomas: a 10-year single institution experience. *Human Pathol*. 2008;39:933–938.
51. Yusuf SW, Bathina JD, Qureshi S, et al. Cardiac tumors in a tertiary care cancer hospital: clinical features, echocardiographic findings, treatment and outcomes. *Heart Int*. 2012;7:e4.
52. Randhawa JS, Budd GT, Randhawa M, et al. Primary cardiac sarcoma: 25-year cleveland clinic experience. *Am J Clin Oncol*. 2016;39:593–599.

53. Li H, Xu D, Chen Z, et al. Prognostic analysis for survival after resections of localized primary cardiac sarcomas: a single-institution experience. *Ann Thorac Surg.* 2014;97:1379–1385.
54. Agaimy A, Rosch J, Weyand M, Strecker T. Primary and metastatic cardiac sarcomas: a 12-year experience at a German heart center. *Int J Clin Exp Pathol.* 2012;5:928–938.
55. Isambert N, Ray-Coquard I, Italiano A, et al. Primary cardiac sarcomas: a retrospective study of the French Sarcoma Group. *Eur J Cancer.* 2014;50:128–136.
56. Ramlawi B, Leja MJ, Abu Saleh WK, et al. Surgical treatment of primary cardiac sarcomas: review of a single-institution experience. *Ann Thorac Surg.* 2016;101:698–702.
57. Sultan I, Bianco V, Habertheuer A, et al. Long-term outcomes of primary cardiac malignancies: multi institutional results from the national cancer database. *J Am Coll Cardiol.* 2020;75(18):2338–2347.
58. Lestuzzi C, Reardon MJ. Primary cardiac malignancies: the need for a multidisciplinary approach and the role of the cardio-oncologist. *J Am Coll Cardiol.* 2020;75:2348–2351.
59. Leja MJ, Shah DJ, Reardon MJ. Primary cardiac tumors. *Tex Heart Inst J.* 2011;38:261–262.
60. Abu Saleh WK, Ramlawi B, Shapira OM, et al. Improved outcomes with the evolution of a neoadjuvant chemotherapy approach to right heart sarcoma. *Ann Thorac Surg.* 2017;104:90–96.
61. Wu Y, Million L, Moding EJ, et al. The impact of postoperative therapy on primary cardiac sarcoma. *J Thorac Cardiovasc Surg.* 2018;156:2194–2203.
62. Ravi V, Reardon MJ. Commentary: primary cardiac sarcoma-Systemic disease requires systemic therapy. *J Thorac Cardiovasc Surg.* 2019;S0022–5223(19):32391–32398.
63. Salanitri J, Lisle D, Rigsby C, et al. Benign cardiac tumours: cardiac CT and MRI imaging appearances. *J Med Imaging Radiat Oncol.* 2008;52:550–558.
64. Blackmon SH, Patel AR, Bruckner BA, et al. Cardiac autotransplantation for malignant or complex primary left-heart tumors. *Tex Heart Inst J.* 2008;35:296–300.
65. Pigott C, Welker M, Khosla P, Higgins RS. Improved outcome with multimodality therapy in primary cardiac angiosarcoma. *Nat Clin Pract Oncol.* 2008;5:112–115.
66. Kim MP, Correa AM, Blackmon S, et al. Outcomes after right-side heart sarcoma resection. *Ann Thorac Surg.* 2011;91:770–776.
67. Zhang PJ, Brooks JS, Goldblum JR, et al. Primary cardiac sarcomas: a clinicopathologic analysis of a series with follow-up information in 17 patients and emphasis on long-term survival. *Hum Pathol.* 2008;39:1385–1395.

Secondary Cardiac Tumors and Direct and Indirect Complications of Neoplasia

68. Bussani R, De-Giorgio F, Abbate A, Silvestri F. Cardiac metastases. *J Clin Pathol.* 2007;60:27–34.
69. Yusuf SW, Durand JB, Lenihan DJ. Wrap beats. *Am J Med.* 2007;120:417–419.
70. Maisch B, Ristic A, Pankuweit S. Evaluation and management of pericardial effusion in patients with neoplastic disease. *Prog Cardiovasc Dis.* 2010;53:157–163.
71. El Haddad D, Iliescu C, Yusuf SW, et al. Outcomes of cancer patients undergoing percutaneous pericardiocentesis for pericardial effusion. *J Am Coll Cardiol.* 2015;66:1119–1128.

99 Psychiatric and Psychosocial Aspects of Cardiovascular Disease

KENNETH E. FREEDLAND, ROBERT M. CARNEY, ERIC J. LENZE, AND MICHAEL W. RICH

Psychological stress and certain psychiatric disorders can have clinically significant cardiovascular (CV) effects. The CV consequences of acute psychological stress have been examined in naturalistic studies of responses to disasters and personal losses, as well as in controlled laboratory studies. Various forms of chronic stress and adversity, such as unemployment and financial difficulties, have been shown to increase the risk of developing coronary heart disease (CHD) and to exacerbate established CHD. Similarly, multiple psychiatric disorders including anxiety, posttraumatic stress disorder (PTSD), depression, and others have been found to increase the risk of developing CHD and other CV conditions and are associated with increased morbidity and mortality in patients with established CV disease (CVD).

This chapter provides an overview of the CV consequences of stress and psychiatric disorders and discusses the biobehavioral mechanisms that might explain these effects. It also discusses approaches to the evaluation and management of psychiatric comorbidities in cardiac patients, including psychotherapeutic interventions, medications, noninvasive procedures including electroconvulsive therapy (ECT) and transcranial magnetic stimulation (TMS), and other nonpharmacological interventions.

ACUTE STRESS AND EMOTIONAL AROUSAL

Stress and Emotional Triggers of Acute Cardiovascular Events

Cardiac event rates often surge in populations that are exposed *en masse* to extremely stressful events.[1] Acute myocardial infarctions (MIs) increased 35% in Los Angeles after the 1994 Northridge earthquake, and sudden cardiac deaths increased from 4.6 per day during the previous week to 24 on the day of the earthquake. The 1995 Great Hanshin (Kobe) earthquake produced a 3.5-fold increase in acute MIs and a significant increase in fatal MIs. In contrast, the 1989 Loma Prieta earthquake did not affect the rate of acute MIs. Whether a disaster triggers cardiac events may depend on the time of day that it strikes—whereas the Northridge earthquake hit at 4:30 AM, the Loma Prieta earthquake hit at 5:00 PM. Superimposition of an extremely stressful event on the stress of sudden early morning awakening may be especially dangerous for individuals who are at risk for an acute MI.

Cardiac event rates may also increase during wars and terrorist attacks. For example, CV mortality increased 58% on the first day of Iraqi missile attacks on Israel during the 1991 Persian Gulf War, primarily in the targeted cities. In contrast, CV mortality did not increase in New York City on September 11, 2001. Cardiac event rate changes may depend in part on whether the stressful situation is inescapable. Individuals who were in close proximity to the 9/11 attacks were at higher risk for stress-related disorders than were those who were farther away at the time.

Private stressors can also trigger CV events. In a Danish study, the death of a child increased the risk of a first MI by 31% and of a fatal MI by 58%. In the Determinants of MI Onset Study, the risk of MI increased 21-fold after the death of a loved one.[2] A U.K. study of older primary care patients found elevated 30-day rates of MI (rate ratio 2.14) and stroke (rate ratio 2.40) in bereaved compared to matched non-bereaved patients.[3]

Takotsubo cardiomyopathy mostly affects women and is usually associated with transient left ventricular dysfunction (see also Chapters 37, 38, and 50). The onset is preceded by a stressful event in about four out of five cases.[4] The cardiomyopathy frequently resolves within weeks but recurrences are common and patients (especially older ones) who have had this syndrome are at increased risk for mortality.[4]

Emotional triggers have been studied retrospectively in survivors of cardiac events. The trauma of having a cardiac event can affect a patient's recall of antecedent emotions, and recall bias can affect the validity of this type of research. Case-crossover designs, in which patients serve as their own controls, can reduce recall bias. The Determinants of MI Onset Study used this design and found a 2.43-fold increase in the incidence of acute MI within two hours after angry outbursts. A meta-analysis of case-crossover studies found that the risk of MI or acute coronary syndrome (ACS) was 4.74 times higher in the 2 hours after an angry outburst than at other times.[5]

Cardiovascular Responses to Everyday Stressors and Emotions

Ambulatory monitoring studies have documented a variety of CV responses to everyday stressors and negative emotions. For example, in patients with implantable cardioverter-defibrillators (ICDs), anger precedes about 15% of shocks compared to only 3% of control periods. Everyday stressors and negative emotions such as anger, tension, frustration, and sadness can reduce heart rate variability and trigger episodes of myocardial ischemia and ventricular ectopy in patients with CHD.

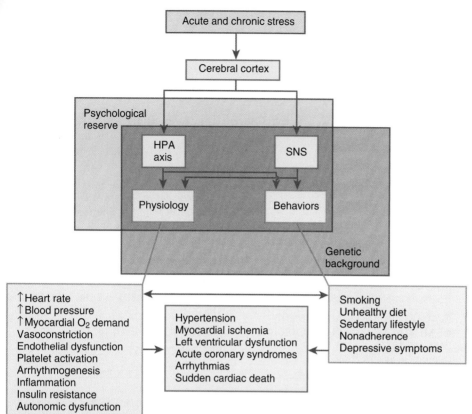

FIGURE 99.1 Potential mechanisms underlying the link between psychological factors and cardiovascular disease. *HPA,* Hypothalamic-pituitary-adrenal axis; *SNS,* sympathetic nervous system. (From Vaccarino V, Bremner JD. *Braunwald's Heart Disease: A Textbook of Cardiovascular Medicine.* 11th ed. Philadelphia, Elsevier, 2019.)

Mechanisms Underlying Acute Stress Effects

Several interrelated biobehavioral mechanisms have been implicated in the CV effects of acute stress. Mental stress-induced myocardial ischemia (MSMI) is accompanied by hemodynamic, neurohormonal, and vascular responses[6] and activation of brain areas involved in stress reactivity and depression (Fig. 99.1).[7] Among 196 patients with coronary disease in the Psychophysiological Investigations of Myocardial Ischemia (PIMI), 58% developed MSMI during mental stress testing. MSMI was accompanied by increases in heart rate, blood pressure, cardiac output, and systemic vascular resistance, a decrease in left ventricular ejection fraction, and wall motion abnormalities. In the more recent Mental Stress Ischemia Prognosis Study (MIPS) of 660 patients with coronary disease, mental stress testing increased the rate-pressure product, arterial stiffness, microvascular constriction, and plasma epinephrine,[8] as well as the inflammatory biomarkers IL-6, MCP-1, and MMP-9.[9] The 106 (16%) patients who developed MSMI had greater hemodynamic and vasoconstrictive responses to mental stress compared to MSMI-negative patients.[8] Normal epicardial coronary arteries and coronary microvessels dilate in response to acute mental stress. Diseased vessels paradoxically constrict in response to mental stress, and resistance vessel dilation is impaired. The coronary microvascular response to mental stress is endothelium-dependent and mediated by nitric oxide.[10]

CARDIOVASCULAR CONSEQUENCES OF CHRONIC STRESS (SEE ALSO CHAPTER 93)

Several sources of chronic stress have been identified as CV risk factors. These include childhood adversity, low socioeconomic status (SES), work stress, discrimination, stigmatization, and caregiving.

Childhood Adversity

Adverse childhood experiences (ACEs) include physical, sexual, and emotional abuse, as well as neglect, economic disadvantage, homelessness, exposure to violent crime, bullying, and other forms of victimization. Over 50% of the U.S. population has had at least one ACE. An American Heart Association scientific statement concluded that there is substantial evidence linking ACEs to cardiometabolic diseases later in life, including heart disease, diabetes, and stroke.[11] A recent analysis of Behavioral Risk Factor Surveillance System (BRFSS) data found dose-response relationships between ACE exposure and the incidence of CVD, as well as asthma, arthritis, chronic obstructive pulmonary disease (COPD), and depression. The associations with CVD and COPD were explained in part by smoking, heavy drinking, and obesity.[12] A separate analysis of BRFSS data also found that high exposure to ACEs was associated with CVD, but only in respondents with a history of depression.[13]

Socioeconomic Status

There has been extensive research on the health effects of low SES, also known as socioeconomic position. Most studies of the long-term effects of SES in childhood are based on parental or household income, education, or occupation. There is growing evidence that low childhood SES increases the risk of CVD in adulthood. For example, a longitudinal population-based cohort study in Finland found that growing up in a family with low SES predicts increased left ventricular mass and impaired diastolic function in middle age.[14]

Most studies associating adult SES with health outcomes use education, income, wealth, occupation, or employment status as indicators.[15] Early studies established that adult SES is related to CVD risk,[16] and more recent studies have strengthened the evidence. For example, a recent report from the Atherosclerosis Risk in Communities Study found that over a 24-year follow-up, the lowest SES group had a 1.92-fold higher risk of developing heart failure compared with the highest SES group after adjusting for income, education, deprivation, CV risk factors, and health care access.[17] A recent Medicare Expenditure Panel Survey report found that the lowest income group had the highest prevalence of cardiac risk factors including obesity, diabetes, hypertension, and physical inactivity. The trend in physical inactivity was particularly concerning, with a 71% increase in the lowest income group over a decade.[18] A study from the Swedish National Diabetes Register reported CV mortality hazard ratios (HRs) of 1.87 for the lowest versus highest income quintiles and 0.84 for individuals with college degrees versus those with less than 10 years of education.[19] SES effects have also been found in recent clinical follow-up studies. For example, low SES was associated with a high risk of all-cause mortality over 4.5 years in a retrospective study of 4503 patients who had been hospitalized with atrial fibrillation.[20]

Occupational Stress and Unemployment

A large body of research has linked various forms of occupational or work-related stress to CVD.[21] The job strain or demand-control model has dominated the research on occupational stress. It hypothesizes that demanding jobs in which the worker has little control are highly stressful, especially in socially unsupportive work environments. There is considerable evidence that job strain is a CV risk factor, at least among men. In an individual-level meta-analysis with 47,045 participants, individuals with job strain were more likely to have elevated Framingham Risk Scores (odds ratio, 1.13). A cumulative meta-analysis of 26 prospective cohort studies reported a HR for incident CHD of 1.34 for the presence versus absence of job strain.

The effort-reward imbalance model identifies another source of occupational stress. The rewards of some highly demanding jobs are insufficient in terms of compensation, job security, prospects for advancement, and/or prestige. The evidence for effort-reward imbalance as a CV risk factor in men is more limited than it is for job strain, and little is known about its effects in women. However, it predicted CV and all-cause mortality in men in the Kuopio Ischemic Heart Disease Risk Factor Study and CV mortality over 25 years in a prospective Finnish cohort study. Job strain predicted and effort-reward imbalance marginally predicted incident CHD in the Whitehall II study of male civil servants in London, but only among employees who were frequently subjected to unfair criticism or other forms of occupational injustice. Occupational injustice itself was an independent predictor of incident CHD, even after adjusting for job strain and effort-reward imbalance.

Job insecurity and unemployment have also been identified as contributors to poor CV health. An individual-level meta-analysis of 13 cohort studies found an adjusted relative risk of high versus low job security of 1.32 for incident CHD, with no differences between men and women or younger and older individuals. The CV risks of job insecurity were partly explained by lower SES and higher prevalence of CHD risk factors among job-insecure individuals.[22] An analysis of nationally representative prospective data on adults aged 51 to 75 years in the Health and Retirement Study showed that the risk of having an acute MI was significantly higher among unemployed than consistently employed workers (HR 1.35), and that there was a dose-response relationship with MI risk and the cumulative number of job losses. The first year of unemployment was an especially high-risk period.

Social Discrimination and Stigmatization

There is inconsistent evidence as to whether various forms of social discrimination and stigmatization, including discrimination based on race, age, sex, or sexual orientation, increase the risk of CVD. Some studies have yielded null or paradoxical results, such as findings from the Jackson Heart Study that racial discrimination among African Americans is associated with a lower risk of all-cause mortality[23] and from the Coronary Artery Risk Development in Young Adults (CARDIA) study that racial discrimination is inversely associated with coronary artery calcification. However, other studies do suggest that chronic exposure to discrimination or stigmatization can have adverse CV consequences.[24] For example, when participants in the National Epidemiological Survey on Alcohol and Related Conditions were grouped by state-level indicators of structural racism, there was a significantly greater past-year prevalence of acute MI among blacks living in states with high levels of structural racism compared to those living in low-structural racism states. Conversely, whites were less likely to have had an acute MI if they lived in a high- rather than a low-structural racism state.[25] Among participants in the Multi-Ethnic Study of Atherosclerosis who were initially free of clinical CVD, those who reported high lifetime levels of racial discrimination had a higher 10-year risk of incident CV events (adjusted HR, 1.36).[26] African American participants in the Jackson Heart Study without hypertension at baseline who experienced medium (HR, 1.49) or high (HR, 1.34) levels of racial discrimination were at increased risk for incident hypertension.[27] Thus, there is growing evidence that racial discrimination increases CVD risks in African Americans.

Caregiving

There has been limited research on the CV effects of chronic stress associated with caregiving for a family member with a debilitating chronic illness such as Alzheimer disease, and much of this work has focused on surrogate outcomes. Nevertheless, there is evidence that stressful caregiving over relatively long periods may promote CVD. In the Reasons for Geographic and Racial Differences in Stroke (REGARDS) study, Framingham Stroke Risk scores averaged 23% higher in participants who reported high caregiver strain compared to those with low or no caregiver strain. The risk was especially high in African American men. Caregiver strain did not affect Framingham CHD Risk scores in this study. Other studies have shown that caregiver stress can contribute to endothelial dysfunction, impairment of the cardiovagal baroreflex,[28] the development or worsening of cardiometabolic syndrome, and the development of carotid plaque.

Combinations of Chronic and Acute Stress

Acute stress is often superimposed on a background of chronic stress and other psychological (e.g., depression) and pathophysiological (e.g., unstable plaque) vulnerabilities. The "perfect storm" model proposes that when mental stress triggers an ACS, it does so in concert with these other factors.[29] Few studies have examined whether the CV effects of acute mental stress differ depending on the background level of chronic stress. However, a recent analysis of MIPS data showed that in patients with stable coronary disease, a high level of chronic psychosocial distress is associated with a blunted hemodynamic response to acute mental stress.[30] In prior studies, blunted CV reactivity to mental stress has been associated with obesity, smoking, and other health risk behaviors.[31]

MENTAL HEALTH AND PSYCHIATRIC DISORDERS

The Diagnostic and Statistical Manual of Mental Disorders (DSM-5)[32] provides a compendium of psychiatric disorders, along with the corresponding ICD-10 codes. Some of these disorders are prevalent in the general adult population, and even more prevalent in populations with chronic medical illness.[33] Conversely, certain medical conditions such as diabetes and CHD are highly prevalent among populations with serious mental illnesses.[34] A small number of psychiatric disorders, including PTSD and several mood and anxiety disorders, are of particular interest in the context of CVD because they have been identified as risk factors for the development of CVD or as predictors of adverse outcomes and poor health-related quality of life in patients with established CVD.

Mechanisms

The search for pathways that link psychiatric disorders to incident cardiac disease and subsequent cardiac events is ongoing, and many candidate mechanisms have been identified. The links between depression and cardiac outcomes have received the most study. Depression is associated with dysregulation of the autonomic nervous system (ANS) and the hypothalamic–pituitary–adrenal (HPA) axis, including higher levels of plasma and urinary catecholamines and cortisol, higher resting and mean 24-hour heart rates, and lower heart rate variability (see Fig. 99.1). Other studies have found elevated proinflammatory cytokines, acute-phase proteins, chemokines, and adhesion molecules, including increased levels of C-reactive protein (CRP), interleukin-6 (IL-6), and tumor necrosis factor (TNF). There is also evidence that depressed patients with CHD have elevated markers of coagulation and platelet activity, especially β-thromboglobulin and platelet factor 4. However, none of these abnormalities is present in every depressed patient,[35] and the proportion of the effect of depression on incident CHD or cardiac events (including mortality) explained by these factors is modest. This suggests that several pathways may be involved and that they differ across individuals.[36]

In addition to the physiological mechanisms, there are behavioral characteristics of depressed patients that likely contribute to the increased risk for CVD and adverse cardiac outcomes. Depressed patients are more likely to be sedentary, to smoke, and to engage in other unhealthy behaviors (e.g., poor diet, higher alcohol consumption) (see Fig. 99.1). Furthermore, depression predicts poor adherence to medication regimens, risk factor modification interventions including dietary regimens and smoking cessation programs, and cardiac rehabilitation.[36]

Shared Features Across Mental Disorders

As discussed below, there is now compelling evidence that a wide range of negative emotional states and psychiatric disorders increase the risk for incident CVD and for cardiac events in patients with established CVD. These observations have led to growing interest in elucidating common elements that might explain the risks. One such effort has been the attempt to identify underlying personality dimensions and temperaments associated with these psychiatric disorders and with the susceptibility to the effects of acute and chronic stress that might explain their CV effects. Type D (distressed) personality, which consists of a combination of neuroticism and social inhibition, is an example. Neuroticism is a personality trait that in itself has been associated with depression and anxiety disorders. The hypothesis that a single underlying personality type explains much of the effect of different negative affective states on CVD is intuitively appealing. It might also be more efficient to study a single unifying disorder than the growing number of negative affective states and disorders (e.g., distress, anger, hostility, depression, general anxiety, panic disorder, phobias, PTSD, vital exhaustion) that have been identified as risk factors for CVD. These disorders are often comorbid, and they share many of the same symptoms and many of the same putative mechanisms that may explain their effect on CVD (e.g., ANS dysfunction, increased inflammatory activity, poor diet, insufficient exercise, smoking). Furthermore, many drugs considered to be primarily antidepressants, and many forms of psychotherapy including cognitive behavior therapy (CBT), are used to treat depression, anxiety disorders, PTSD, and psychosocial distress associated with stressful situations. Thus, there is both mechanistic and therapeutic overlap between these ostensibly distinct psychiatric disorders, suggesting that an integrative approach to their evaluation and management may be warranted. Nonetheless, most research continues to study these affective states and psychiatric disorders individually as separate albeit related entities.

Anxiety

The 12-month prevalence of anxiety disorders in the United States is about 18%, and the lifetime prevalence is about 30% in women and 19% in men. There is evidence that anxiety is a risk factor for incident CHD, as well as atrial and ventricular arrhythmias. However, most studies of anxiety as a risk factor for cardiac morbidity and mortality have used self-report anxiety symptom questionnaires. There have been fewer studies of clinically diagnosed anxiety disorders.

A meta-analysis of 20 studies with nearly 250,000 individuals and a mean follow-up of 11.2 years found that anxious persons had a 26% increased risk for incident CHD (HR = 1.26; CI 1.15–1.38) and a nearly 50% increased risk of cardiac death (HR = 1.48; CI 1.14–1.92), independent of biological and demographic risk factors and health behaviors.[37] A more recent meta-analysis reported a 40% increased risk of developing CHD among anxious persons, but found significant heterogeneity of effect sizes across the studies.[38]

There is also evidence that anxiety is a risk factor for cardiac events in patients with established CHD.[39] However, anxiety is highly comorbid with depression,[40] making it difficult to separate the risks of incident CHD or subsequent cardiac events associated with anxiety from those of depression. Adding to this difficulty, patients with both anxiety and major depressive disorder are likely to be more severely depressed and impaired than depressed patients with little anxiety.[36] Thus, it has been difficult to demonstrate an effect of anxiety independent from depression in many studies.

Some anxiety disorders are associated with a daily experience of mild to moderate anxiety throughout the day. Individuals with specific phobias may be relatively free of anxiety at most times, but they experience anxiety or panic in certain situations such as when exposed to heights or to certain animals. Individuals with agoraphobia have an extreme fear of being away from home or in open spaces, crowds, or places from which it would be difficult to escape in an emergency. Individuals with panic disorder, with or without agoraphobia, experience episodes of extreme anxiety accompanied by highly elevated sympathetic nervous system activity. There is some evidence that these anxiety disorders may differ with respect to their risk for cardiac events and mortality, but not all studies have supported this conclusion. Nearly every review of this literature has concluded that larger, better quality studies are needed to address this question.

A few studies have found that some forms of anxiety may be beneficial in cardiac patients, at least at moderate levels. In one study, patients with a lifetime diagnosis of generalized anxiety disorder tended to have better CV outcomes than those without an anxiety diagnosis. A potential explanation for this finding is that a moderate level of anxiety, while perhaps unpleasant, may motivate patients to follow medical advice and engage in self-care after a diagnosis of heart disease. This may also explain why anxiety symptom questionnaires do not always predict worse outcomes in CHD patients. Much like depression, anxiety has been associated with poor sleep, lower activity level, poor diet, and increased smoking.[36] These factors may help explain poorer prognosis associated with anxiety.

In summary, there is moderate evidence that anxiety is a risk factor for incident CHD and cardiac events in patients with established CHD. However, there are fewer studies of anxiety than of depression as predictors of cardiac outcomes, and not all studies have found anxiety to be a significant independent predictor of incident CHD or cardiac events. Nevertheless, the consensus among most experts is that anxiety is likely to be a risk factor for incident CHD. More research is needed to determine whether this risk differs by type of anxiety disorder and the extent to which the effects of anxiety are independent from those of depression.

Posttraumatic Stress Disorder

PTSD may be triggered by a single traumatic, life-threatening event or by recurrent events. A diagnosis of PTSD requires exposure to a traumatic event, such as a natural disaster, injurious accident, combat, or a life-threatening medical event such as ACS, accompanied by intense fear or panic. This is followed by persistent painful and intrusive memories, nightmares and flashbacks, avoidance behavior, and hyperarousal. The lifetime prevalence of PTSD in the U.S. population is estimated to be as high as 8%, whereas approximately 18% of combat veterans have or will develop this disorder during their lifetime. PTSD is independently associated with an increased risk for incident CHD[41,42] and for recurrent cardiac events following an ACS. There is also evidence that PTSD is associated with increased risk for atrial fibrillation, heart failure, and CV mortality. Along with anxiety and depression, PTSD has been widely reported in patients with an implantable cardioverter defibrillator (ICD). PTSD also increases the long-term risk of mortality in patients with an ICD, independent of cardiac disease severity.

Although there are medications for PTSD, psychotherapeutic interventions may be more effective. The best-established approaches include prolonged exposure therapy and cognitive processing therapy. Prolonged exposure therapy involves repeated exposure to the traumatic event(s), through either guided imagination or stimuli such as photographs or videos. Cognitive processing therapy involves examination of thoughts and beliefs about the trauma and its meaning and consequences. Although these approaches can produce dramatic results in many cases, the response rate is only around 50% and the full remission rate is even lower. Thus, more work is needed to improve PTSD treatment outcomes and to determine whether effective treatment of this disorder reduces the risk for both incident CHD and cardiac events in patients with established CHD.

Depression

Of the psychosocial problems and psychiatric disorders that may be risk factors for incident CHD or for cardiac events in patients with established CHD, depression is by far the best studied. There have been over 100 studies of depression as a risk factor for incident CVD. Many different self-report questionnaires and diagnostic interviews have been used to define depression in these studies. Some studies have focused on older adults, on women or men only, or on patients with cardiac risk factors such as hypertension. Despite the heterogeneity of the methods for assessing and defining depression and of the populations examined, at least six meta-analyses have been performed. Five of them found a 60% to 80% increased risk of incident CHD associated with depression. One reported a more modest level of risk (30%), but all found that depression is a significant risk factor for developing CHD.[36]

Most studies have found that the risks associated with depression remain significant after adjustment for a variety of medical and demographic confounders. For example, Gan and colleagues[43] found that adjustment for established cardiac risk factors including smoking, body mass index (BMI), hypertension, diabetes, physical inactivity, and low SES did not substantially change the risk estimates for depression in their meta-analysis.

A recent cohort study conducted in 21 countries with 145,862 participants found the incidence of MI and CVD mortality to be about 20% higher in those with four or more symptoms of depression (11% of the total sample) compared to non-depressed participants.[44] This represents a lower estimate of risk than those reported in recent meta-analyses. Unlike the meta-analyses, however, these data were collected from many different countries with different standards of living, socioeconomic levels, and medical care. The effect of depression on MI and cardiac mortality was twice as high in urban compared to rural areas, regardless of economic level.

Depression has also been studied as a predictor of cardiac events and mortality in patients with established CHD. The point prevalence of major depression in the adult population is estimated to be about 5%. By contrast, 15% to 20% of patients with medically stable CHD have major depression, and up to 30% have significant depressive symptoms.[36] Over 300 studies have evaluated depression as a risk factor for medical morbidity and mortality in patients with established CHD and at least five meta-analyses have been published.[36]

One of the largest and most recent meta-analyses included 29 studies and found that depression was associated with a 2.7-fold increased risk for cardiac-related mortality, a 2.3-fold increased risk for all-cause mortality, and a 1.6-fold increased risk for CV events.[45] In one of the largest studies of depression and CV mortality in CHD, after extensive adjustment for major cardiac risk factors, including age, sex, smoking, systolic blood pressure, BMI, diabetes, social class, heavy alcohol use, and antidepressant medications, a 2.7-fold increased risk of cardiac death in patients with depression over a median follow-up period of 8 years was reported.

Thus, the preponderance of evidence indicates that depression is an independent risk factor for incident CHD and for cardiac events in persons with known heart disease. However, many established risk factors for CHD have been shown to be associated with depression, such as smoking and sedentary lifestyle.[36] Although residual confounding must be considered as a possible explanation for at least part of the association, after a careful review of the literature, a scientific panel convened by the American Heart Association issued a statement identifying depression as a major risk factor for cardiac morbidity and mortality after an ACS.[46] Correspondingly, the current ACC/AHA Practice Guidelines for the Management of Patients with ST-elevation MI recommend screening for depression, as well as anxiety and sleep disorders, in the post-MI period (Fig. 99.2).[47]

OTHER PSYCHIATRIC DISORDERS

Other psychiatric disorders may also be risk factors for the development of CHD or subsequent cardiac events, as well as early mortality. A study of over 47,000 community-dwelling adults from 17 countries with over 2 million person-years[48] reported the relationships between 16 DSM-IV psychiatric disorders and the risk of onset of 10 physical disorders including heart disease. After adjusting for age, sex, country, education, and smoking, they found significant associations between most of the 16 psychiatric disorders and the subsequent onset of most of the 10 physical conditions, including CVD. They concluded that the "piecemeal" perspective of evaluating a single mental disorder and medical disorder obscures the "broader message" that mental disorders of all types are associated with a wide range of chronic physical conditions, including CVDs. Although the investigators administered a standardized psychiatric diagnostic interview to all participants, they relied on the participants' self-report of the physical conditions, which the investigators acknowledged as a limitation of the study. Nevertheless, the study provides intriguing, suggestive evidence that many psychiatric disorders may be risk factors for a wide range of medical conditions including CVD.

Similarly, Vance and colleagues found that multiple psychiatric illnesses, including psychotic disorders, were associated with an increased risk of adverse cardiac outcomes in over 1.5 million men and 94,000 women military veterans who were receiving care in the Department of Veterans Affairs health system.[49] In addition, they reported that more severe psychiatric disorders had the largest effect sizes, even after controlling for standard CVD risk factors and psychotropic medication use. Weye and colleagues reported on the relationship between specific mental disorders and life expectancy in a population-based cohort study from Denmark that included nearly 7 million participants.[50] They found that the diagnosis of a mental disorder was associated with life expectancies shortened by 11.2 years in males and 7.9 years in females compared to those without mental disorders. The effects were most dramatic for alcohol use, but depression and anxiety disorders also predicted shorter life spans, in many cases in patients with CVD. In a recent study of 108,610 Canadian patients with acute MI, patients with comorbid schizophrenia (N = 1145, 1.1%) had an increased risk for all-cause, 1-year mortality (adjusted HR = 1.55; CI 1.37–1.77).[51] The association of schizophrenia with mortality was attenuated after adjusting for revascularization. Thus, there is ample evidence that many psychiatric disorders are risk markers for CVD, cardiac events, and early mortality.

Cognitive Impairment

The prevalence of cognitive impairment increases with age and with CVD. In addition, many mental disorders, such as depression, are also associated with cognitive impairment. As a result, individuals with comorbid CVD and mental disorders are at substantially increased risk for cognitive impairment. The presence of cognitive impairment complicates management of CV disease, as cognitively impaired individuals have difficulty remembering and following through on treatment plans, adhering to medication regimens, or accurately reporting symptoms. Even mildly cognitively impaired patients can have difficulty with adherence to their medication regimen, and they may need support with medication adherence, getting to appointments, following medical instructions, and making lifestyle changes such as exercising. Thus, it is essential to involve family or other caregivers in medical discussions with cognitively impaired patients. Cognitive impairment also necessitates screening for reversible causes of the impairment, in particular medications. Atropine (for bradyarrhythmias) and tertiary amine tricyclics such as amitriptyline, imipramine, or doxepin (most often for pain or sleep) can cause cognitive impairment and delirium due to their centrally acting antimuscarinic effects. In addition, benzodiazepines can cause cognitive impairment and delirium.

Older patients and patients with mental disorders should be screened for cognitive impairment. Effective approaches to screening include: (i) conducting brief tests of cognitive performance and (ii) asking a corroborative source whether the patient is having difficulties with memory or thinking. A simple screening test for cognitive impairment that takes only 1 to 2 minutes includes questions on orientation ("what is today's date?" "what floor are we on?"), memory (remember three objects, or a name and address; assess recall after 5 minutes), attention and information processing speed ("say the months of the year backwards, starting with December"), and executive function and visuospatial abilities ("please draw a clock face" then "draw the hands to show 10 after 11"). Corroborative sources should be individuals who know the patient well, have frequent contact with them, and can answer questions such as "how much difficulty do they have remembering new information?" and "how much trouble do they have understanding or doing complex things such as finances or shopping?" Family members may either downplay or over-report a patient's cognitive problems and often may note that their remote memory is intact. (This is common in mild to moderate Alzheimer dementia, in which recent but not remote recall is impaired.)

While there is increasing evidence that cognitive impairment can be prevented by CVD risk reduction,[52] once cognitive impairment occurs there are few therapies and they are only modestly effective. Two classes of cognitive enhancing medications, acetylcholinesterase inhibitors and stimulants, are commonly associated with CV effects. Acetylcholinesterase inhibitors include donepezil, rivastigmine, and galantamine. These medications are indicated for patients with dementia. They are also frequently prescribed off-label for patients with mild neurocognitive disorder (a milder level of cognitive impairment that

XI

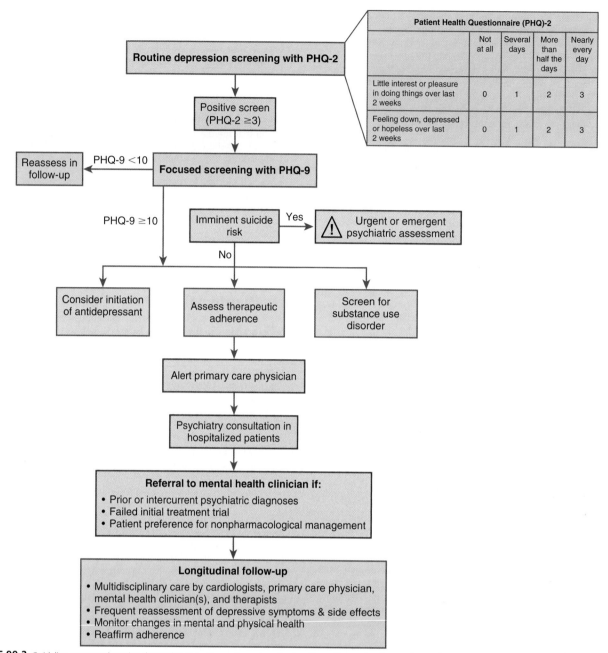

FIGURE 99.2 Guideline-supported routine depression screening pathway in patients with cardiovascular disease. (From Jha MK, Qamar A, Vaduganathan M, et al. Screening and management of depression in patients with cardiovascular disease: JACC state-of-the-art review. *J Am Coll Cardiol.* 2019;73[14]:1827–1845.)

often transitions to dementia) or even for cognitively normal older adults with subjective cognitive complaints. The cholinesterase inhibitors produce modest improvements in memory and other aspects of cognitive function. Their main cardiac effect is bradycardia through increasing cholinergic transmission. They can also increase the PR interval and cause, or be relatively contraindicated in, heart block.[53] As well, these drugs are sometimes poorly tolerated due to side effects of nausea, diarrhea, or depression. Memantine is not a cholinesterase inhibitor but is thought to act via glutamatergic N-methyl-D-aspartate (NMDA) antagonism and is unlikely to produce CV effects.

Stimulants include methylphenidate and amphetamine. They are typically used for attention deficit disorder in children, but many middle-aged and older adult patients take them for longstanding attention deficits or new-onset problems with concentration. They are also used for disorders of excessive somnolence and binge eating, and are sometimes used in stroke (e.g., for apathy) and depression. All of these conditions are more common in patients with CV disorders than in the general adult population; as a result, stimulant use in the CV population is not rare. In children, stimulants are widely regarded as safe, but in adults—particularly older adults—they have been associated

with CV complications, including MI, cerebrovascular events, ventricular arrhythmias, and sudden death. Causes of these complications may include increased blood pressure and heart rate and induced vasospasm via increased levels of catecholamines (norepinephrine and dopamine), vasculitis, and prolongation of the QTc interval.[54]

The decision to use cholinesterase inhibitors or stimulants in patients with CVD is often a complex one that requires balancing perceived benefits against the potential safety risks. Ideally, this can be best achieved through a multidisciplinary shared decision-making process involving the cardiologist, psychiatrist and/or geriatrician, and the patient and patient surrogate.

EVALUATION AND MANAGEMENT OF MENTAL HEALTH IN THE CARDIAC PATIENT

Current Guidelines

Although several psychiatric comorbidities are prevalent in patients with CVD and predict adverse outcomes, current cardiology and primary care practice guidelines address only some of them. Several organizations have provided guidance on screening, assessment, and/ or treatment of depression and anxiety in patient populations with or at risk for CVD.

The American Academy of Family Physicians recommends that patients with a recent ACS should be screened for depression, and strongly recommends that patients with clinically significant depression should be treated with antidepressant medications and/or CBT. The screening guidance is based on low-quality evidence, but treatment recommendations are based on moderate-quality evidence.[55] The United States Preventive Services Task Force (USPSTF) found convincing evidence to support depression screening for all adults and older adults in clinical practice settings.[56] The 2016 European Guidelines on Cardiovascular Disease Prevention in Clinical Practice recommend screening and evaluation of patients for depression, anxiety, and other psychiatric conditions (level of evidence B, Class IIa recommendation).[57] The European Society of Cardiology recommends assessment of depression and anxiety in patients after implantation of an ICD(level of evidence C, Class I recommendation).[58] The American College of Cardiology (ACC) and the American Heart Association (AHA) recommend recognition of depression as a risk factor for adverse medical outcomes in patients with an ACS[59] and screening for depression in patients with CHD.[60] In patients with an ST-elevation MI, the ACC and AHA also recommend screening for depression, anxiety, and sleep disorders (level of evidence C, Class I recommendation).[47] When indicated, depressed patients should be treated with CBT or selective serotonin reuptake inhibitors (SSRIs; level of evidence A, Class IIa recommendation), and anxiolytic agents should be used for the short-term treatment of anxiety (level of evidence C, Class IIa recommendation).[47]

Psychotherapy

Psychotherapies such as CBT or interpersonal psychotherapy are as effective as antidepressants for moderate to severe depression in medically well depressed patients. Anxiety disorders also respond well to CBT. CBT for depression is the best studied psychotherapy in patients with heart disease.[61] CBT helps patients identify dysfunctional thoughts, attitudes, and behaviors that may cause or prolong depressed mood and related symptoms. The patient learns to replace their dysfunctional cognitions and behaviors with more adaptive ones. These cognitive and behavioral changes improve the patient's mood. In addition, CBT promotes effective coping and problem-solving strategies, and it encourages patients to use behavioral activation, i.e., increased engagement in pleasant and productive activities, to further improve their mood. Antidepressant medications are often used to augment CBT or other psychotherapeutic interventions for patients who do not have a sufficient response after a month or two of therapy. This stepped-care approach to treating depression has been shown to be more effective than the usual care provided in typical clinical settings.[62]

Patients who are already taking multiple medications for their cardiac and other medical conditions often express a preference for psychotherapy over antidepressants or anxiolytics. In addition, many patients want to discuss problems related to their illness, as well as family, personal, and work-related concerns. Learning more effective ways of coping with their illness may also help improve their quality of life. CBT is an appropriate option for patients who are not only seeking relief from the symptoms of depression or anxiety, but who also want to address the distressing problems, stressors, or losses they are experiencing. If a patient with CVD is motivated to work on his or her problems and is cognitively intact, evidenced-based psychotherapies, such as CBT or interpersonal psychotherapy, are likely to be helpful in improving their depression and anxiety.[61] However, these psychotherapies may not be available in some communities, and psychotherapy is not always covered by medical insurance in the United States. Antidepressant or anxiolytic medications may be the best alternatives for patients who lack access to effective psychotherapeutic services.

Antidepressant Medications

Antidepressant medications are the most common type of treatment for depression and other mental disorders associated with an increased risk for CVD, including PTSD. Antidepressants appear to be more effective (compared to placebo) in patients with moderate or severe depression than in patients with mild depression. This suggests that patients with mild depression are about as likely to improve with watchful waiting

as with an antidepressant. Therefore, prior to initiating antidepressant treatment, providers should ensure that patients have sufficiently severe and persistent symptomatology to warrant starting a medication. Such evidence includes: mood is low (or anxious) most of the day, nearly every day; persistent negative thoughts about ones' self (i.e., guilt, worthlessness, hopelessness); symptoms cause persistent distress or functional impairment; and/or symptoms include recurrent thoughts about death (e.g., life is not worth living, it may be better to be dead than alive). Absent such severity markers, antidepressant medications are unlikely to be effective, and psychotherapy or watchful waiting is preferred.

One exception to this precept is for patients already taking an antidepressant, in whom "mild" depression or anxiety may indicate residual symptoms of an inadequately treated illness and should prompt a consideration of whether the antidepressant dose should be increased. As discussed below, antidepressants useful in patients with CVD include SSRIs (paroxetine, fluoxetine, sertraline, and others), mirtazapine, bupropion, venlafaxine, desvenlafaxine, and duloxetine).

Antidepressants act on the brain's monoaminergic neurotransmitter systems: serotonin, norepinephrine, and/or dopamine. Almost all antidepressants bind to and inhibit transporter proteins that are responsible for the reuptake of neurotransmitter into the neuron after it has been released into the synapse, thereby causing an increase in neurotransmitter within the synapse. Most antidepressant drugs block the serotonin transporter (serotonin reuptake inhibitors), the norepinephrine transporter (norepinephrine reuptake inhibitors [NRIs]), or a combination of the two (serotonin-norepinephrine reuptake inhibitors [SNRIs]). The process by which this molecular action reduces depression or other mental disorders remains unknown. Of note, these SNRIs effects are not confined to the brain and the synaptic cleft; for example, serotonin transporters are found in platelets, bone (osteoblasts, osteoclasts), and intestinal absorptive cells. The clinical significance of peripheral SSRI effects is not well understood, although there is substantial evidence for increased bleeding risks due to effects on platelets.

Many antidepressants also have other non-monoaminergic effects on the cholinergic, histaminergic, or alpha-adrenergic systems, which are sometimes called "off-target" effects because they are thought to be unrelated to the drug's therapeutic effects. The original tricyclic antidepressants tended to have widespread effects on these receptors, which were responsible for many of their side effects. For many of the newer antidepressants, the non-monoaminergic effects are minimal or have unknown clinical relevance, and some of these actions, such as sigma-1 receptor agonism, have been the subject of research for possible cardioprotective effects. Table 99.1 summarizes medications commonly used for the treatment of depression in patients with CVD, and general principles for prescribing antidepressant medications are shown in Table 99.2.

Tricyclic Antidepressants

Tricyclics were developed specifically for treating depression and were the first class of medications proven to be effective in patients with depression. They are also used for treating anxiety disorders, including panic disorder, and clomipramine is used for obsessive-compulsive disorder. With the development of newer agents, they are usually reserved for treatment-resistant cases. Tricyclics are frequently used at lower doses for non-psychiatric conditions such as chronic pain, migraine headaches, and insomnia. The mechanism of action is to increase norepinephrine and serotonin levels in the synapse. Representative agents include imipramine, doxepin, desipramine, clomipramine, nortriptyline, and amitriptyline.

The two most salient concerns regarding tricyclics for patients with CVD are their side effects and their potential for inducing QTc prolongation. Tricyclics have anticholinergic effects, which may cause dry mouth, constipation, memory problems, confusion, blurred vision, sexual dysfunction, and decreased urination. They also cause alpha-1 adrenergic blockade, which may lead to orthostatic hypotension, and anti-histaminergic effects, including sedation, increased appetite, and confusion. Generally, the tertiary amine tricyclics—amitriptyline, imipramine, doxepin, and clomipramine—have more significant effects at these receptors and hence more side effects compared to the secondary amine tricyclics nortriptyline and desipramine. For this reason, tertiary amine tricyclics are not recommended for older adults, who are more susceptible to the memory impairment and orthostatic hypotension associated with these medications.

TABLE 99.1 Commonly Used Antidepressant Medications

ANTIDEPRESSANT	TYPICAL DAILY STARTING DOSE	EFFECTIVE DAILY DOSE RANGE	COMMENTS
Selective Serotonin Reuptake Inhibitors (SSRIs)			
Escitalopram	5–10 mg	10–20 mg	Good first-line medications because of safety, tolerability, and ease of use
Sertraline	25–50 mg	50–200 mg	
Citalopram	10–20 mg	20–40 mg	QTc prolongation (avg 13 msec) at doses >20 mg in older adults Has mild antihistamine effects at higher doses.
Fluoxetine	10–20 mg	20–40 mg	Reduces metabolism of other drugs through CYP2D6 and CYP2B6 (moderate inhibitor)
Paroxetine	10–20 mg	20–40 mg	Reduces metabolism of other drugs through CYP2D6 and CYP2B6 (strong inhibitor)
Fluvoxamine	50 mg	100–300 mg	Reduces metabolism of other drugs through multiple CYP enzymes, particularly CYP2C19 and CYP1A2 (strong interaction)
Serotonin-Norepinephrine Reuptake Inhibitors (SNRIs)			Usually safe but can cause hypertension or orthostatic hypotension
Venlafaxine extended release	37.5–75 mg	150–300 mg	
Desvenlafaxine	50 mg	50–100 mg	
Duloxetine	30–60 mg	60–120 mg	Reduces metabolism of other drugs through CYP2D6 and CYP2B6 (moderate interaction)
Milnacipran	12.5–25 mg	50 mg twice daily	Under patent protection, expensive
Other Antidepressant Medications and Strategies			
Bupropion XL	150 mg	300–450 mg	Reduces metabolism of other drugs through CYP2D6 (strong interaction). Metabolized chiefly by CYP2B6 and can cause ataxia, falls, and rarely seizures at excessively high concentrations
Mirtazapine	7.5–15 mg	30–45 mg	Has strong antihistamine properties so can cause sedation and weight gain, even at low doses (15 mg or less)
Tricyclics	25–50 mg	Based on blood concentration	Pro-arrhythmic effects in ischemic heart disease. Can prolong QTc interval. Nortriptyline and desipramine are better tolerated
Vortioxetine	5 mg	5–20 mg	Well-tolerated alternative to SSRIs but under patent protection, expensive
Vilazodone	10 mg	40 mg	Under patent protection, expensive
Aripiprazole augmentation	2 mg	2–15 mg	Avoid in patients with or at risk for parkinsonism, can cause akathisia or rarely tardive dyskinesia Sometimes causes weight gain; recommend following lipids and glucose
Quetiapine augmentation	25 mg	50–300 mg	Can cause sedation and (often) weight gain, recommend monitoring lipids and glucose
Brexpiprazole augmentation	1 mg	2–4 mg	Avoid in patients with or at risk for parkinsonism, can cause akathisia or rarely tardive dyskinesia. Sometimes causes weight gain; recommend monitoring lipids and glucose

TABLE 99.2 General Principles for Prescribing Antidepressant Medications

1. Start low but use full dose range as needed and as tolerated.
2. Avoid drug-drug interactions when possible but do not stop an antidepressant medication that is helpful.
3. For patients who do not respond, switch to another class of agent. For those who respond partially, consider augmentation treatment.
4. After 1–2 failed trials, refer to psychiatry.
5. Psychotherapy works well in combination with antidepressants.

All tricyclics have quinidine-like properties, leading to an increase in the PR interval, prolongation of the QRS duration and QT interval, and flattening of the T wave on the electrocardiogram (ECG) (see also Chapter 14). These effects are usually only seen at the higher "antidepressant" doses. Tricyclics should be avoided in patients with preexisting cardiac conduction defects, a prolonged QT interval, heart failure, or ischemic heart disease including a recent MI. Additionally, if tricyclics are used for the treatment of depression (as opposed to low doses for migraine, for example), therapeutic drug level monitoring and ECG monitoring are recommended. Importantly, tricyclic medications

have been associated with an increased risk of malignant ventricular arrhythmias and sudden cardiac death (see also Chapters 9, 62, and 70). For patients who suffer a cardiac event while being treated with a tricyclic, there is a theoretical concern that abrupt withdrawal from the medication can also be associated with an increased risk of arrhythmias. A practical way to address these competing concerns is to taper the tricyclic medication slowly over two weeks, but more quickly if the patient has ongoing arrhythmias. Similarly, tricyclics should be tapered and stopped if prolongation of the QT interval or significant hypotension becomes problematic; if appropriate, the patient should be treated with an alternative medication such as an SSRI, venlafaxine, or bupropion (see below). These latter medications are preferred in patients who develop new onset depression after an acute MI.

Selective Serotonin Reuptake Inhibitors

The SSRIs include fluoxetine, paroxetine, fluvoxamine, citalopram, escitalopram, and sertraline. As the name implies, SSRIs block reuptake of serotonin into the neuron at the synapse. SSRIs have not been shown to have greater efficacy in the treatment of depression than the older tricyclics, but they have a more favorable side effect profile. Specifically, the SSRIs have no anticholinergic effects (except paroxetine) and no cardiac effects (except citalopram, which increases the QTc interval).

For these reasons, the SSRIs are good first-line antidepressant choices for the cardiac patient population.

Side effects of SSRIs include nausea, diarrhea, headache, insomnia (or sometimes somnolence), agitation, and sexual dysfunction, which may include loss of libido, delayed ejaculation, and erectile dysfunction. Most of these side effects are usually transient, with the exception of sexual dysfunction. Alternative antidepressants that do not cause sexual dysfunction include bupropion or mirtazapine, which are not in the SSRI class. SSRIs, especially fluoxetine, are associated with an increase in risk of bleeding. For cardiac patients taking aspirin or other antiplatelet or anticoagulant medication, this can be a significant concern. Abrupt cessation of an SSRI can result in a discontinuation syndrome, which, while not dangerous, can cause unpleasant symptoms including agitation, nervousness, and physical sensations like electrical shocks. Rarely SSRIs can cause akathisia and other extrapyramidal side effects, as can the antipsychotics. Akathisia includes feelings of restlessness, pacing, and internal stiffness, which are often very uncomfortable. All antidepressant medications carry the warning of an increased risk of suicidal thoughts in children and young adults under the age of 25, although this risk should not preclude their use in such populations.[63]

Based on several short-term trials, SSRIs are generally considered safe and effective in cardiac patients. Although treatment of depression has not been shown to improve cardiac outcomes, in several trials treatment responders appeared to have better cardiac outcomes than nonresponders, suggesting that antidepressant treatment, when effective for depression, improves cardiac outcomes. Conversely, several observational studies have shown an increased risk of cardiac death with longer-term use of SSRIs. A Danish nationwide study, for example, found a significant association between SSRI (as well as tricyclic antidepressant) use and out-of-hospital cardiac arrest, especially for citalopram and nortriptyline, whereas no association was found for other drug classes, such as the NRIs and the serotonin-norepinephrine dual reuptake inhibitors.[64] A prior analysis of the Nurses' Health Study also found that antidepressant use was associated with a threefold increase in the risk of sudden cardiac death, even after adjusting for the severity of depression and risk factors for CHD. In this study, the risk was similar for SSRIs and other antidepressants outside of the SSRI class. These observational data are difficult to interpret given the likelihood of confounding by indication[65]; i.e., the patients for whom antidepressants were prescribed may have had an inherently higher risk for cardiac arrest. Therefore, while it is not possible to make pragmatic recommendations based on these observational studies, it should be recognized that the risk of sudden cardiac death associated with antidepressant use is very low, and that the potential benefits of treating depression outweigh the risks.

Norepinephrine Reuptake Inhibitors

The NRIs block reuptake of norepinephrine into the neuron. Medications in this group include most of the tricyclics, such as nortriptyline and desipramine, as well as reboxetine. These drugs have a relatively favorable side effect profile and may be useful in individuals who do not respond to, or cannot tolerate, SSRIs.

Serotonin and Norepinephrine Dual Reuptake Inhibitors

Several antidepressants have dual reuptake inhibition for SNRIs, including venlafaxine, desvenlafaxine, milnacipran, and duloxetine. There is speculation that by affecting both neurotransmitters, these drugs provide a better treatment response for depression than SSRIs. In an analysis combining multiple studies, the response rate with venlafaxine, defined as at least a 50% reduction in symptoms of depression, was 74%, which was significantly better than SSRIs, with a 61% response rate, and tricyclics, with a 58% response. SNRIs are therefore often used as second-line agents in individuals who do not adequately respond to SSRIs.

Common side effects with SNRIs, including venlafaxine and duloxetine, include dizziness, constipation, dry mouth, headache, and changes in sleep. Rarely a serotonin syndrome may occur, with restlessness, shivering, and sweating. Venlafaxine has also been associated with a dose-dependent increase in blood pressure, which may be problematic for patients with comorbid hypertension or CVD. A recent study found that approximately 10% of previously-normotensive patients developed hypertension with high-dose venlafaxine, and orthostatic hypotension was also common.[66]

Monoamine Oxidase Inhibitors

Drugs that block the monoamine oxidase inhibitor enzyme (MAOI drugs), and therefore boost the monoamines (serotonin, norepinephrine), include selegiline/deprenyl, phenelzine, and tranylcypromine. They have a more favorable CV profile than the tricyclics, with little or no effect on cardiac conduction, although they can be associated with orthostatic hypotension (because of alpha-adrenergic blockade) and anticholinergic and antihistaminergic effects. The older MAOI drugs phenelzine and tranylcypromine in particular can cause potentially life-threatening elevations of blood pressure if taken with foods that are high in tyramine content, including wine, cheese, chocolate, and beer. This risk is much less for selegiline/deprenyl, especially at lower doses where it acts as a more selective MAOI. Drugs that can precipitate hypertensive reactions in a patient taking an MAOI include those with sympathomimetic effects (e.g., amphetamines, ephedrine, cocaine). MAOIs should not be taken with meperidine. Due to the risk of hypertensive crisis, the MAOIs are not recommended for use in cardiac patients, and indeed they are no longer commonly prescribed in general.

Antidepressants with Other Mechanisms of Action

Some drugs act on other neurotransmitter systems or their mechanism of action is poorly understood. Two commonly used drugs are bupropion and mirtazapine. Bupropion primarily acts on dopamine and norepinephrine systems and is used for both depression and smoking cessation. Side effects include weight loss and restlessness, as well as possible increases in blood pressure; in relatively rare cases, high doses can cause seizures or, in older adults, falls. Mirtazapine is a quadracyclic antidepressant that has actions on several different receptor systems. It blocks presynaptic noradrenergic alpha-2 receptors with resultant enhancement of norepinephrine release. Mirtazapine also increases serotonin release. Side effects include sweating and shivering, tiredness, strange dreams, dyslipidemia, weight gain, anxiety, and agitation. It can be associated with antihistaminergic effects and mild orthostatic hypotension. Short-term randomized trials in cardiac patients have not shown an increase in mortality or cardiovascular events associated with these medications.

Other drugs with mixed actions include trazodone and maprotiline. These drugs are rarely used for the treatment of depression, although trazodone is frequently prescribed as a hypnotic because of its sedative effect. The profile of these medications appears safe in terms of anticholinergic side effects and effects on the heart and blood pressure. Trazodone can cause priapism (extended painful erection that requires emergency treatment) in rare cases. It is a safe and often effective medication for induction of sleep that is not habit-forming. It is sometimes preferred to zolpidem and related insomnia medications, for example, when patients have alcohol or substance use disorders or side effects such as sleepwalking or hallucinations from zolpidem or similar drugs.

ANTIDEPRESSANTS AND CARDIAC QTc PROLONGATION. As noted above, tricyclic antidepressants prolong the QTc interval when used at doses sufficient to produce an antidepressant effect. Most of the newer SSRI and SNRI drugs have been studied with respect to QTc prolongation. Citalopram prolongs the QTc interval in a dose-dependent fashion, such that the FDA included a warning in its package insert stating that the drug should not be used at doses greater than 20 mg in older adults because of this risk. There is a similar concern with escitalopram, although at its usual dosing range of 10 to 20 mg it is not considered to produce sufficient QTc prolongation to advise against its use. Other SSRI/SNRI drugs appear to have less or no effect on the QTc interval. For example, a recent study of venlafaxine found no QTc prolongation even at high therapeutic doses.[67] CV clinicians may wish to advise against the use of citalopram when QTc prolongation is a concern (e.g., in older adults), and against escitalopram as an alternative in patients with citalopram-induced QTc prolongation. One exception is if the antidepressant is highly effective for the patient's depression, in which case the medication should be continued with monitoring of the QTc interval.

ANTIDEPRESSANTS AND DRUG-DRUG INTERACTIONS. The above sections described pharmacodynamic (i.e., receptor) effects of antidepressants, but many antidepressants also have relevant pharmacokinetic effects by reducing the metabolism of other drugs through inhibition of hepatic cytochrome P450 (CYP) enzymes (see also Chapter 9).

CARDIOVASCULAR DISEASE AND DISORDERS OF OTHER ORGANS

Thus, cardiac patients may have additional risks related to concomitant drugs whose metabolism is affected by these antidepressants. Drugs prone to cause these interactions include paroxetine and bupropion (strong inhibitors of CYP 2D6, which metabolizes many drugs including beta-blockers and several antiarrhythmic agents), fluoxetine and duloxetine (moderate inhibitors of CYP 2D6), and fluvoxamine (strong inhibitor of CYP 1A2, which metabolizes caffeine and theophylline, and CYP 2C19, which metabolizes clopidogrel). In contrast, escitalopram, sertraline, and venlafaxine have no significant effects on CYP enzymes. The practical implications of these drug-drug interactions remain controversial, in part because many drugs are metabolized by multiple enzymes (e.g., propranolol is metabolized by CYPs 2D6, 2C19, and 1A2) and blocking one enzyme may not have significant effects. However, many pharmacologists believe that these interactions are important, particularly in older adults. They can be avoided by prioritizing drugs without these effects as first-line treatments.

Electroconvulsive Therapy

ECT is used for the treatment of severe depression in patients who have had multiple failed trials of psychotherapy and medication. ECT has an 80% response rate, which is better than for medications, works quickly (within 2 to 3 weeks), and is a safe procedure for most individuals. Cardiologists may be asked to assess patient safety for ECT, as it may cause brief but profound hemodynamic changes, including bradycardia (up to frank asystole, which may last for a few seconds), followed by tachycardia and hypertension. These effects usually resolve within 20 minutes. Rare complications include persistent hypertension, arrhythmias, asystole lasting more than 5 seconds, ischemia, and heart failure. Older age and preexisting CVD, including hypertension, coronary artery disease, heart failure, aortic stenosis, atrial fibrillation, and implanted cardiac devices are associated with increased complication rates. Patients undergoing ECT should be monitored throughout the procedure and until stable after the procedure. With appropriate monitoring and management of medications, almost all patients can safely complete treatment.

While there are no absolute contraindications to ECT, the procedure should be delayed in patients who are hemodynamically unstable or who have new-onset or uncontrolled arrhythmias or hypertension. In patients with stable CHD and controlled hypertension, medications may be continued through the morning of the procedure. For patients with sustained post-ECT hypertension, antihypertensive therapy should be given after ECT and premedication used on the morning of subsequent ECT sessions; medications shown to be effective for this indication include labetalol, nicardipine, and clonidine.

In patients with an implanted pacemaker, the pacemaker should be tested before and after ECT; a magnet should be placed at the patient's bedside in the event that electrical interference leads to pacemaker inhibition and bradycardia. ECT appears safe in patients with an ICD. The detection mode of the ICD should be turned off during ECT, and continuous electrocardiographic monitoring should be maintained, with resuscitative equipment by the patient bedside in the event that external defibrillation is necessary.

Transcranial Magnetic Stimulation

TMS is a noninvasive therapy approved for treatment-resistant depression. It involves exposing the brain to a magnetic field, usually in the prefrontal cortex. It does not require sedation or the induction of a seizure and typically does not have any cardiac effects. It is increasingly being used as it has become more available and as shorter TMS sequences have been shown to be effective.[68]

Anxiolytic Medications

Benzodiazepines

In the 1960s benzodiazepines displaced barbiturates as the most commonly used medications for insomnia, and they were frequently prescribed for patients with anxiety and depression as well. Originally marketed as having less potential for dependence and abuse, this has not subsequently been borne out. Benzodiazepines act on the gamma-aminobutyric acid (GABA)-benzodiazepine receptor complex in the central nervous system, where they have a discrete binding site. This is the same complex that alcohol and the inhibitory transmitter GABA bind to. The most commonly prescribed benzodiazepines today include alprazolam, which is used primarily for anxiety attacks and panic disorder; clonazepam, which is used for epilepsy; and temazepam, which is used for insomnia. Other benzodiazepines include oxazepam, lorazepam, chlordiazepoxide, clorazepate, and diazepam, among others. Benzodiazepines are also used for treating in-patients with alcohol withdrawal, a not uncommon condition in patients hospitalized with CVD. Differences between benzodiazepines are related to the time of onset of action and duration of effect. Benzodiazepines increase sleep time by an average of about 1 hour per night. Side effects from benzodiazepines include daytime drowsiness, dizziness, light-headedness, falls, and memory problems. In addition, use of benzodiazepines is associated with a 60% increase in traffic accidents. This risk is further increased with concurrent alcohol usage and in older adults. In patients with cardiac disease and comorbid chronic pulmonary disease, benzodiazepines should be used with caution due to the potential for respiratory depression. This is of particular concern in obstructive sleep apnea because benzodiazepine-induced reductions in upper airway muscle tone and central nervous system response to hypoxia could result in an increased number and duration of apneic and hypopneic events.[69]

Benzodiazepines are habit-forming. As a result, patients can become resistant to stopping them, and in some cases their use can lead to abuse and addiction. Furthermore, abrupt cessation of benzodiazepines is often associated with a withdrawal syndrome that may include serious adverse events, including seizures and death. Therefore, discontinuation of long-term benzodiazepines should be gradual (e.g., 25% reduction every 2 weeks). The challenges associated with stopping benzodiazepines may lead to their inappropriate chronic use and potential risks from that use, which should be considered when initiating a new prescription.

Non-Benzodiazepine "Z-Drug" Medications

The so-call "Z drugs"—zaleplon, zolpidem, eszopiclone, and zopiclone—act on specific subsets of the GABA receptor and are mainly used for insomnia. Although they are commonly called "non-benzodiazepine" medications, they have not been shown to be more effective or safe than benzodiazepines. As with benzodiazepines, these medications can cause memory impairment, drowsiness, dizziness, and falls; they can also cause hallucinations and parasomnias such as sleepwalking. Zaleplon has a shorter half-life (1 hour) than zolpidem (2.5 hours) or eszopiclone (6 hours), and is better for promoting sleep onset as opposed to sleep maintenance. As with benzodiazepines, abrupt discontinuation of these medications may be associated with withdrawal symptoms, including serious and even life-threatening adverse events, especially if the drug is taken chronically at high dose.

Medications with Other Mechanisms of Action

Buspirone is effective in treating generalized anxiety disorder and is sometimes used as an augmenting agent in depression. It is an agonist of the serotonin 1A receptor and relatively free of next-day drowsiness and memory impairment, or the potential for dependence or abuse. Buspirone is preferable to the benzodiazepines for the treatment of anxiety in cardiac patients because it lacks respiratory suppressive effects and there are no known adverse cardiac effects. Other side effects are minimal, and include nausea, headache, and lightheadedness.

Alternative Medicines and Supplements

Several natural remedies, including St. John's wort and omega-3 fatty acids, have been used for the treatment of depression and anxiety. However, data from high-quality large controlled studies evaluating the safety and efficacy of these agents are limited. See the online supplement, Alternative Medicines and Supplements for Depression and Anxiety.

Mindfulness

Mindfulness is nonjudgmental awareness of one's own present thoughts, emotions, and behaviors. Mindfulness interventions combine elements of traditional meditation and CBT with a goal of learning to moderate emotional responses to day-to-day experiences. Controlled trials have shown reductions in distress and increases in feelings of general well-being in mindfulness groups compared to usual care. There is some evidence that mindfulness may augment the efficacy of antidepressants,[70] and it may help improve lifestyle risk factors, including smoking, diet, weight, and physical activity.[71] However, there is little evidence that mindfulness techniques improve CV outcomes, owing to the paucity of rigorous clinical trials in this area.

Tai chi and yoga are mindfulness techniques with multiple components thought to be helpful for CV health: physical exercise, stress reduction, emotional regulation, improved breathing efficiency, and social support. CV benefits with tai chi include improved blood pressure control, whereas yoga improves multiple CV risk factors including blood pressure, triglycerides, and insulin resistance.[72] Given the widespread availability and popularity of programs that include tai chi or yoga, they can play an important role in enhancing both CV and mental health.

Exercise

Multiple studies over the past 25 years have shown that various types of exercise are associated with salutary effects on depression (see also Chapter 32). Meta-analyses have consistently reported favorable effects of exercise, noting clinically significant benefits in medically well depressed patients. Similarly, a recent meta-analysis revealed that exercise-based cardiac rehabilitation alleviates symptoms of depression and anxiety among patients with recent MI or coronary artery bypass surgery.[73]

Current public health guidelines recommend 30 minutes of moderate intensity aerobic exercise at least 5 days per week, and this also appears to be an effective exercise "dose" to improve the mood of people with mild to moderate depression. Exercise may also be a useful adjunct to antidepressant medication in depressed patients who do not have a complete response to drug therapy.

Collaborative Care

Although depression and anxiety disorders are associated with worse prognosis and quality of life in patients with CVDs, they are infrequently recognized or treated by cardiology providers. Many primary care physicians, cardiologists, and other specialists are now using a collaborative care model to assist in the identification and treatment of psychiatric disorders in their practices. In this model, treatment for depression or anxiety is managed by the primary care physician or specialist, in consultation with a psychiatrist and/or other mental health professional, using a measurement-guided care plan based on evidence-based practice guidelines.[74] Studies in cardiology settings have generally found superior outcomes in patients receiving collaborative versus standard care, although this approach has had less of an impact in settings in which depression screening was already being practiced.[75]

SUMMARY AND FUTURE DIRECTIONS

To date, treatment of depression and anxiety have not been definitively shown to improve CV outcomes. However, recognition and management of these conditions, especially if they are severe or persistent, is essential for promoting patient wellness, enhancing quality of life, and improving patients' ability to adhere to treatments and lifestyle recommendations. In many cases the CV clinician can address the problem without an immediate referral to a mental health professional. Self-reported "anxiety" may reflect concern about their cardiac condition. Educating the patient about their heart disorder, listening to their concerns, and allowing the patient to express their worries often has a therapeutic effect and helps alleviate distress. It is important to determine if the patient is having thoughts of taking his or her own life or is having such severe impairment in functioning that referral to a psychiatrist, psychologist, or social worker is indicated; this depends both on the

severity of the condition and the type of treatment that might be appropriate (medications versus psychotherapy or counseling).

Antidepressants useful in patients with CVD include SSRIs (paroxetine, fluoxetine, sertraline, and others), mirtazapine, bupropion, venlafaxine, desvenlafaxine, and duloxetine, with careful monitoring of blood pressure for the latter 3 SNRI drugs. ECT and TMS are alternative non-pharmacological treatment options in selected cases. A healthy lifestyle, including physical activity tailored to patients' functional capabilities, should be recommended to reduce depression, improve well-being, and lower CV risk. Community resources include therapists, counselors, and social workers who can teach stress reduction and mindfulness techniques, either individually or in classes, as well as exercise, tai chi, and yoga classes. There are also many self-help books that patients can purchase to teach themselves these stress reduction techniques.

Numerous stressors, psychosocial factors, and psychiatric disorders have been found to increase the risk of incident CVD and to predict adverse outcomes in established CVD. Although these factors differ in many ways, some of their features overlap and they often co-occur in various combinations. In addition, the clinical presentations of some of these problems are highly heterogeneous. Further research is needed to characterize the highest-risk phenotypes and to identify factors that contribute to their development and persistence. Identification of these phenotypes will facilitate research on the biobehavioral mechanisms that link mental stress, psychosocial distress, and psychiatric disorders to adverse outcomes in CVD. It will also facilitate treatment research and make it possible to identify patients with mental health disorders who are at high risk for adverse cardiac outcomes.

ACKNOWLEDGMENT

The authors gratefully acknowledge Drs. Viola Vaccarino and J. Douglas Bremner, whose chapter on this topic in the prior edition of *Braunwald's Heart Disease: A Textbook of Cardiovascular Medicine* served as the basis for the current chapter.

REFERENCES

Acute Stress, Emotional Arousal, Cardiovascular Consequences of Chronic Stress
1. Zarifeh J, Mulder R. Natural disasters and the risk of cardiovascular disease. In: Alvarenga ME, Byrne D, eds. *Handbook of Psychocardiology*. New York, NY: Springer Berlin Heidelberg; 2016.
2. Mostofsky E, Maclure M, Sherwood JB, et al. Risk of acute myocardial infarction after the death of a significant person in one's life: the determinants of myocardial infarction onset study. *Circulation*. 2012;125(3):491–496.
3. Carey IM, Shah SM, DeWilde S, et al. Increased risk of acute cardiovascular events after partner bereavement: a matched cohort study. *JAMA Intern Med*. 2014;174(4):598–605.
4. Pelliccia F, Pasceri V, Patti G, et al. Long-term prognosis and outcome predictors in takotsubo syndrome: a systematic review and meta-regression study. *JACC Heart Fail*. 2019;7(2):143–154.
5. Mostofsky E, Penner EA, Mittleman MA. Outbursts of anger as a trigger of acute cardiovascular events: a systematic review and meta-analysis. *Eur Heart J*. 2014;35(21):1404–1410.
6. Hammadah M, Alkhoder A, Al Mheid I, et al. Hemodynamic, catecholamine, vasomotor and vascular responses: determinants of myocardial ischemia during mental stress. *Int J Cardiol*. 2017;243:47–53.
7. Bremner JD, Campanella C, Khan Z, et al. Brain mechanisms of stress and depression in coronary artery disease. *J Psychiatr Res*. 2019;109:76–88.
8. Hammadah M, Kim JH, Al Mheid I, et al. Coronary and peripheral vasomotor responses to mental stress. *J Am Heart Assoc*. 2018;7(10):e008532.
9. Hammadah M, Sullivan S, Pearce B, et al. Inflammatory response to mental stress and mental stress induced myocardial ischemia. *Brain Behav Immun*. 2018;68:90–97.
10. Khan SG, Melikian N, Shabeeh H, et al. The human coronary vasodilatory response to acute mental stress is mediated by neuronal nitric oxide synthase. *Am J Physiol Heart Circ Physiol*. 2017;313(3):H578–h583.
11. Suglia SF, Koenen KC, Boynton-Jarrett R, et al. Childhood and adolescent adversity and cardiometabolic outcomes: a scientific statement from the American heart association. *Circulation*. 2018;137(5):e15–e28.
12. Waehrer GM, Miller TR, Silverio Marques SC, et al. Disease burden of adverse childhood experiences across 14 states. *PloS One*. 2020;15(1):e0226134.
13. Salas J, van den Berk-Clark C, Skiöld-Hanlin S, et al. Adverse childhood experiences, depression, and cardiometabolic disease in a nationally representative sample. *J Psychosom Res*. 2019;127:109842.
14. Laitinen TT, Puolakka E, Ruohonen S, et al. Association of socioeconomic status in childhood with left ventricular structure and diastolic function in adulthood: the cardiovascular risk in young finns study. *JAMA Pediatr*. 2017;171(8):781–787.
15. Havranek EP, Mujahid MS, Barr DA, et al. Social determinants of risk and outcomes for cardiovascular disease: a scientific statement from the American Heart Association. *Circulation*. 2015;132(9):873–898.
16. Schultz WM, Kelli HM, Lisko JC, et al. Socioeconomic status and cardiovascular outcomes: challenges and interventions. *Circulation*. 2018;137(20):2166–2178.
17. Vart P, Matsushita K, Rawlings AM, et al. SES, heart failure, and N-terminal pro-b-type natriuretic peptide: the atherosclerosis risk in communities study. *Am J Prev Med*. 2018;54(2):229–236.
18. Valero-Elizondo J, Hong JC, Spatz ES, et al. Persistent socioeconomic disparities in cardiovascular risk factors and health in the United States: medical expenditure Panel Survey 2002-2013. *Atherosclerosis*. 2018;269:301–305.

19. Rawshani A, Svensson AM, Zethelius B, et al. Association between socioeconomic status and mortality, cardiovascular disease, and cancer in patients with type 2 diabetes. *JAMA Intern Med.* 2016;176(8):1146–1154.
20. Kargoli F, Shulman E, Aagaard P, et al. Socioeconomic status as a predictor of mortality in patients admitted with atrial fibrillation. *Am J Cardiol.* 2017;119(9):1378–1381.
21. Sara JD, Prasad M, Eleid MF, et al. Association between work-related stress and coronary heart disease: a review of prospective studies through the job strain, effort-reward balance, and organizational justice models. *J Am Heart Assoc.* 2018;7(9).
22. Virtanen M, Nyberg ST, Batty GD, et al. Perceived job insecurity as a risk factor for incident coronary heart disease: systematic review and meta-analysis. *BMJ (Clinical Research ed).* 2013;347:f4746.
23. Dunlay SM, Lippmann SJ, Greiner MA, et al. Perceived discrimination and cardiovascular outcomes in Older African Americans: insights from the Jackson heart study. *Mayo Clin Proc.* 2017;92(5):699–709.
24. Panza GA, Puhl RM, Taylor BA, et al. Links between discrimination and cardiovascular health among socially stigmatized groups: a systematic review. *PloS One.* 2019;14(6):e0217623.
25. Lukachko A, Hatzenbuehler ML, Keyes KM. Structural racism and myocardial infarction in the United States. *Soc Sci Med.* 2014;103:42–50.
26. Everson-Rose SA, Lutsey PL, Roetker NS, et al. Perceived discrimination and incident cardiovascular events: the multi-ethnic study of atherosclerosis. *Am J Epidemiol.* 2015;182(3):225–234.
27. Forde AT, Sims M, Muntner P, et al. Discrimination and hypertension risk among African Americans in the Jackson heart study. *Hypertension.* 2020. HYPERTENSIONAHA11914492.
28. Wu KK, Bos T, Mausbach BT, et al. Long-term caregiving is associated with impaired cardiovagal baroreflex. *J Psychosom Res.* 2017;103:29–33.
29. Burg MM, Edmondson D, Shimbo D, et al. The "perfect storm" and acute coronary syndrome onset: do psychosocial factors play a role? *Prog Cardiovasc Dis.* 2013;55(6):601–610.
30. Pimple P, Hammadah M, Wilmot K, et al. The relation of psychosocial distress with myocardial perfusion and stress-induced myocardial ischemia. *Psychosom Med.* 2019;81(4):363–371.
31. Phillips AC, Ginty AT, Hughes BM. The other side of the coin: blunted cardiovascular and cortisol reactivity are associated with negative health outcomes. *Int J Psychophysiol.* 2013;90(1):1–7.

Mental Health and Psychiatric Disorders, Evaluation

32. American Psychiatric Association. *DSM-5 Task Force. Diagnostic and Statistical Manual of Mental Disorders: DSM-5.* 5th ed. Washington, DC: American Psychiatric Association; 2013.
33. Thom R, Silbersweig DA, Boland RJ. Major depressive disorder in medical illness: a review of assessment, prevalence, and treatment options. *Psychosom Med.* 2019;81(3):246–255.
34. Janssen EM, McGinty EE, Azrin ST, et al. Review of the evidence: prevalence of medical conditions in the United States population with serious mental illness. *Gen Hosp Psychiatry.* 2015;37(3):199–222.
35. Stewart JC. One effect size does not fit all—is the depression-inflammation link missing in racial/ethnic minority individuals? *JAMA Psychiatry.* 2016;73(3):301–302.
36. Carney RM, Freedland KE. Depression and coronary heart disease. *Nat Rev Cardiol.* 2017;14(3):145–155.
37. Roest AM, Martens EJ, de Jonge P, Denollet J. Anxiety and risk of incident coronary heart disease: a meta-analysis. *J Am Coll Cardiol.* 2010;56(1):38–46.
38. Emdin CA, Odutayo A, Wong CX, et al. Meta-analysis of anxiety as a risk factor for cardiovascular disease. *Am J Cardiol.* 2016;118(4):511–519.
39. Allgulander C. Anxiety as a risk factor in cardiovascular disease. *Curr Opin Psychiatry.* 2016;29(1):13–17.
40. Tully PJ, Cosh SM, Baumeister H. The anxious heart in whose mind? A systematic review and meta-regression of factors associated with anxiety disorder diagnosis, treatment and morbidity risk in coronary heart disease. *J Psychosom Res.* 2014;77(6):439–448.
41. Ahmadi N, Hajsadeghi F, Mirshkarlo HB, et al. Post-traumatic stress disorder, coronary atherosclerosis, and mortality. *Am J Cardiol.* 2011;108(1):29–33.
42. Edmondson D, Kronish IM, Shaffer JA, et al. Posttraumatic stress disorder and risk for coronary heart disease: a meta-analytic review. *Am Heart J.* 2013;166(5):806–814.
43. Gan Y, Gong Y, Tong X, et al. Depression and the risk of coronary heart disease: a meta-analysis of prospective cohort studies. *BMC Psychiatr.* 2014;14:371.
44. Rajan S, McKee M, Rangarajan S, et al. Association of symptoms of depression with cardiovascular disease and mortality in low-, middle-, and high-income countries. *JAMA Psychiatry.* 2020;77(10):1052–1063.
45. Meijer A, Conradi HJ, Bos EH, et al. Adjusted prognostic association of depression following myocardial infarction with mortality and cardiovascular events: individual patient data meta-analysis. *Br J Psychiatry.* 2013;203(2):90–102.
46. Lichtman JH, Froelicher ES, Blumenthal JA, et al. Depression as a risk factor for poor prognosis among patients with acute coronary syndrome: systematic review and recommendations: a scientific statement from the American Heart Association. *Circulation.* 2014;129(12):1350–1369.
47. Antman EM, Anbe DT, Armstrong PW, et al. ACC/AHA guidelines for the management of patients with ST-elevation myocardial infarction—executive summary: a report of the American college of cardiology/American heart association task force on practice guidelines (writing committee to revise the 1999 guidelines for the management of patients with acute myocardial infarction). *Circulation.* 2004;110(5):588–636.
48. Scott KM, Lim C, Al-Hamzawi A, et al. Association of mental disorders with subsequent chronic physical conditions: world mental health surveys from 17 countries. *JAMA Psychiatry.* 2016;73(2):150–158.
49. Vance MC, Wiitala WL, Sussman JB, et al. Increased cardiovascular disease risk in veterans with mental illness. *Circ Cardiovasc Qual Outcomes.* 2019;12(10):e005563.
50. Weye N, Momen NC, Christensen MK, et al. Association of specific mental disorders with premature mortality in the Danish population using alternative measurement methods. *JAMA Netw Open.* 2020;3(6):e206646.
51. Hauck TS, Liu N, Wijeysundera HC, Kurdyak P. Mortality and revascularization among myocardial infarction patients with schizophrenia: a population-based cohort study. *Can J Psychiatry.* 2020;65(7):454–462.
52. Wolters FJ, Chibnik LB, Waziry R, et al. Twenty-seven-year time trends in dementia incidence in Europe and the United States: the alzheimer cohorts consortium. *Neurology.* 2020;95(5):e519–e531.
53. Isik AT, Soysal P, Stubbs B, et al. Cardiovascular outcomes of cholinesterase inhibitors in individuals with dementia: a meta-analysis and systematic review. *J Am Geriatr Soc.* 2018;66(9):1805–1811.
54. Westover AN, Halm EA. Do prescription stimulants increase the risk of adverse cardiovascular events?: a systematic review. *BMC Cardiovasc Disord.* 2012;12:41.

Evaluation and Management of Mental Health in the Cardiac Patient

55. Frost JL, Rich Jr RL, Robbins CW, et al. Depression following acute coronary syndrome events: screening and treatment guidelines from the AAFP. *Am Fam Physician.* 2019;99(12). Online.
56. Siu AL, Bibbins-Domingo K, Grossman DC, et al. Screening for depression in adults: US preventive services task force recommendation statement. *J Am Med Assoc.* 2016;315(4):380–387.
57. Piepoli MF, Hoes AW, Agewall S, et al. European guidelines on cardiovascular disease prevention in clinical practice: the sixth joint task force of the European society of cardiology and other societies on cardiovascular disease prevention in clinical practice (constituted by representatives of 10 societies and by invited experts)developed with the special contribution of the European Association for Cardiovascular Prevention & Rehabilitation (EACPR). *Eur Heart J.* 2016;37(29):2315–2381. 2016.
58. Priori SG, Blomström-Lundqvist C, Mazzanti A, et al. ESC guidelines for the management of patients with ventricular arrhythmias and the prevention of sudden cardiac death: the Task Force for the management of patients with ventricular arrhythmias and the prevention of sudden cardiac death of the European Society of Cardiology (ESC). endorsed by: association for European Paediatric and Congenital Cardiology (AEPC). *Eur Heart J.* 2015;36(41):2793–2867. 2015.
59. Lichtman JH, Froelicher ES, Blumenthal JA, et al. Depression as a risk factor for poor prognosis among patients with acute coronary syndrome: systematic review and recommendations: a scientific statement from the American Heart Association. *Circulation.* 2014;129(12):1350–1369.
60. Lichtman JH, Bigger Jr JT, Blumenthal JA, et al. Depression and coronary heart disease: recommendations for screening, referral, and treatment: a science advisory from the American heart association prevention committee of the council on cardiovascular nursing, council on clinical cardiology, council on epidemiology and prevention, and interdisciplinary council on quality of care and outcomes research: endorsed by the American psychiatric association. *Circulation.* 2008;118(17):1768–1775.
61. Freedland KE, Carney R,M, Rich MW, et al. Cognitive behavior therapy for depression and self-care in heart failure patients: a randomized clinical trial. *JAMA Intern Med.* 2015;175(11):1773–1782.
62. Davidson KW, Bigger JT, Burg MM, et al. Centralized, stepped, patient preference-based treatment for patients with post-acute coronary syndrome depression: CODIACS vanguard randomized controlled trial. *JAMA Intern Med.* 2013;173(11):997–1004.
63. Friedman RA. Antidepressants' black-box warning—10 years later. *N Engl J Med.* 2014;371(18):1666–1668.
64. Weeke P, Jensen A, FF, et al. Antidepressant use and risk of out-of-hospital cardiac arrest: a nationwide case-time-control study. *Clin Pharmacol Ther.* 2012;92(1):72–79.
65. Dragioti E, Solmi M, Favaro A, et al. Association of antidepressant use with adverse health outcomes: a systematic umbrella review. *JAMA Psychiatry.* 2019;76(12):1241–1255.
66. Wathra R, Mulsant BH, Thomson L, et al. Hypertension and orthostatic hypotension with venlafaxine treatment in depressed older adults. *J Psychopharmacol.* 2020;34(10):1112–1118.
67. Behlke LM, Lenze EJ, Pham B, et al. The effect of venlafaxine on ECG intervals during treatment for depression in older adults. *J Clin Psychopharmacol.* 2020;40(6):553–559.
68. Janicak PG, Dokucu ME. Transcranial magnetic stimulation for the treatment of major depression. *Neuropsychiatr Dis Treat.* 2015;11:1549–1560.
69. Heck T, Zolezzi M. Obstructive sleep apnea: management considerations in psychiatric patients. *Neuropsychiatr Dis Treat.* 2015;11:2691–2698.
70. Segal ZV, Dimidjian S, Beck A, et al. Outcomes of online mindfulness-based cognitive therapy for patients with residual depressive symptoms: a randomized clinical trial. *JAMA Psychiatry.* 2020;77(6):563–573.
71. Gotink RA, Younge JO, Wery MF, et al. Online mindfulness as a promising method to improve exercise capacity in heart disease: 12-month follow-up of a randomized controlled trial. *PloS One.* 2017;12(5):e0175923.
72. Cramer H, Lauche R, Haller H, et al. Effects of yoga on cardiovascular disease risk factors: a systematic review and meta-analysis. *Int J Cardiol.* 2014;173(2):170–183.
73. Zheng X, Zheng Y, Ma J, et al. Effect of exercise-based cardiac rehabilitation on anxiety and depression in patients with myocardial infarction: a systematic review and meta-analysis. *Heart Lung.* 2019;48(1):1–7.
74. Archer J, Bower P, Gilbody S, et al. Collaborative care for depression and anxiety problems. *Cochrane Database Syst Rev.* 2012;10:Cd006525.
75. Huffman JC, Mastromauro CA, Beach SR, et al. Collaborative care for depression and anxiety disorders in patients with recent cardiac events: the Management of Sadness and Anxiety in Cardiology (MOSAIC) randomized clinical trial. *JAMA Intern Med.* 2014;174(6):927–935.

100 Neuromuscular Disorders and Cardiovascular Disease

WILLIAM J. GROH, ELIZABETH M. MCNALLY, AND GORDON F. TOMASELLI

Neurologic diseases often affect the heart and vascular system, and in many cases, cardiovascular disease limits life expectancy and reduces quality of life in these patients. As such, cardiologists are an integral part of the medical team evaluating and treating patients with primary neurologic disorders. In several disorders, the cardiovascular manifestations are responsible for a greater risk than that attributable to the neurologic manifestations. This chapter reviews those neurologic disorders associated with important cardiovascular manifestations or sequelae.

NEUROMUSCULAR DISEASES

The neuromuscular diseases may be classified based on clinical features, molecular genetics, or pathophysiological consequences. This group includes disorders of muscle proteins dystrophin and sarcoglycans; membrane and filament proteins lamin A/C, emerin, and desmin; nucleotide repeat disorders such as myotonic dystrophy, Friedreich ataxia (FRDA), and spinobulbar muscular atrophy; and mitochondrial and metabolic disorders (eFig. 100.1).

MUSCULAR DYSTROPHIES

Muscular dystrophies are a group of inherited skeletal muscle diseases. Skeletal muscle and the heart are both striated muscles, and many muscular dystrophies have direct effects on cardiac muscle, with manifestations including heart failure, conduction disease and heart block, atrial and ventricular arrhythmias, and sudden death. With improved multidisciplinary care and, more recently, targeted treatment, patients are living longer and an increasing proportion manifest cardiac disease.[1] This section will review the genetics, pathogenesis, clinical presentation, cardiovascular manifestations, evaluation, prognosis, and treatment of muscular dystrophies with major cardiac involvement. These include:
- Duchenne and Becker muscular dystrophies
- Myotonic dystrophies
- Emery-Dreifuss muscular dystrophies and associated disorders
- Limb-girdle muscular dystrophies
- Facioscapulohumeral muscular dystrophy

Duchenne and Becker Muscular Dystrophy
Genetics and Pathogenesis
Duchenne muscular dystrophy (DMD) and Becker muscular dystrophy (BMD) are X-linked recessive disorders caused by mutations in one of the largest genes in the human genome, dystrophin (see also Chapters 7, 52, and 63). *Dystrophin* is located on the short arm of the X chromosome with 79 exons, spanning 2.4 Mb producing a 14 kb mRNA. Variable promoters produce different full-length and shorter versions of dystrophin expressed in muscle and brain, and the short 71 kDa isoform is ubiquitously expressed. Alternative splicing produces other isoforms expressed in the retina, kidney, brain, and peripheral nerves. About 60% of DMD cases are due to deletions of one or more exons; more rarely, duplications, small insertions/deletions, or point mutations produce disease (eFig.100.2). In DMD, mutations usually disrupt the reading frame or introduce a premature stop codon, leading to the absence of dystrophin. Mutations that maintain the reading frame produce internally truncated, relatively functional proteins, resulting in a milder form of the disease, BMD. Although the skeletal muscle symptoms are less severe, the majority of BMD patients also develop a cardiomyopathy, and it is the leading cause of death in patients with BMD.

The dystrophin protein and its associated glycoproteins provide a structural link between the myocyte cytoskeleton and extracellular matrix linking contractile proteins to the cell membrane (Fig. 100.1B). Absence of dystrophin leads to membrane fragility resulting in myofiber or cardiomyocyte necrosis and eventual loss of cells with fibrotic replacement. Mutations in the genes encoding dystrophin-associated glycoproteins also present with degeneration of cardiac and skeletal muscle. Cardiac myocytes lacking dystrophin are susceptible to mechanical damage.[2] Cardiac involvement is seen in both DMD and BMD and the severity is not correlated with the severity of skeletal muscle involvement. Mutations in specific domains of the dystrophin gene are associated with a higher risk for cardiomyopathy.[3] X-linked dilated cardiomyopathy arises from mutations that primarily affect cardiac dystrophin production which manifests as cardiac involvement without skeletal muscle dysfunction.

Clinical Presentation
DMD is the most common inherited neuromuscular disease, with an incidence of 1 case in 3600 to 6000 live male births.[4] Patients typically present with skeletal muscle weakness before the age of 5 years, which progresses if untreated such that boys become wheelchair-bound by their early teens (Fig. 100.2). Without support, death occurs by age 25 years, primarily from a combination of respiratory dysfunction and heart failure. A multidisciplinary treatment approach, including glucocorticoid steroids, ventilatory support, and cardiac therapy has improved survival rates.[1] BMD is less common than DMD, is associated with a highly variable presentation of skeletal muscle weakness compared to Duchenne (see Fig. 100.2), and carries a better prognosis, with most patients surviving to the age of 40 to 50 years or longer. In both Duchenne and Becker muscular dystrophies,

CARDIOVASCULAR DISEASE AND DISORDERS OF OTHER ORGANS

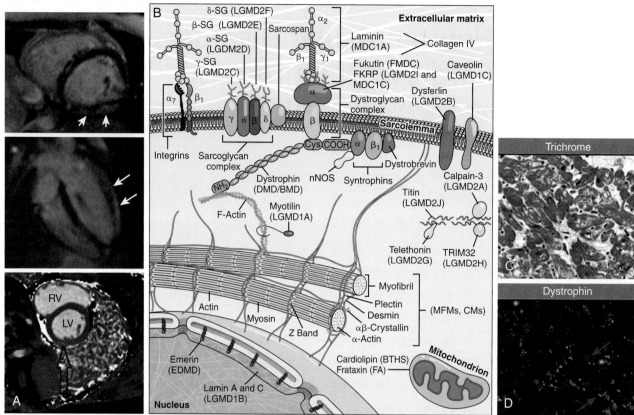

FIGURE 100.1 Cardiac involvement in Duchenne muscular dystrophy. **A** *(top, middle),* Late gadolinium enhancement (LGE) in MR images of a patient with Duchenne muscular dystrophy *(arrows* indicate areas of positive LGE, primarily in the inferior-lateral left ventricle). *Bottom,* T1 mapping shows variation *(orange)* in the LV wall consistent with fibrosis. **B,** Constitution of a cardiomyocyte cell membrane, demonstrating connection between the intramembranous sarcoglycan complex (α, β, γ, δ), dystroglycan complex (α and β), and dystrophin, which is linked to the intracellular actin cytoskeleton. The dystroglycan complex connects to the basal lamina on the extracellular side via laminin and to syntrophins and nitric oxide synthase (nNOS) via dystrobrevin (encoded by the *DTNA* gene). **C,** Trichrome staining of an endomyocardial biopsy sample taken from the patient in **A** showing irregular-sized cardiomyocytes in the presence of diffuse interstitial fibrosis *(red arrows).* **D,** Dystrophin staining: A few cardiomyocytes show discontinuous expression of dystrophin in the cell membrane *(red arrows),* whereas most cardiomyocytes have no dystrophin at all in their membranes. *BMD,* Becker muscular dystrophy; *DMD,* Duchenne muscular dystrophy; *LGMD,* limb-girdle muscular dystrophy. (**A** from Power LC, O'Grady GL, Hornung TS, et al. Imaging the heart to detect cardiomyopathy in Duchenne muscular dystrophy: a review. *Neuromuscul Disord.* 2018;28:717–730; Rochitte CE, Liberato G, Silva MC. Comprehensive assessment of cardiac involvement in muscular dystrophies by cardiac MR imaging. *Magn Reson Imaging Clin N Am.* 2019;27:521–531; **B** modified from Feingold B, Mahle WT, Auerbach S, et al. Management of cardiac involvement associated with neuromuscular diseases: a scientific statement from the American Heart Association. *Circulation.* 2017;136:e200–e231; **C** and **D** from Yilmaz A, Gdynia H-J, Ludolph AC, et al. Images in cardiovascular medicine: cardiomyopathy in a Duchenne muscular dystrophy carrier and her diseased son: similar pattern revealed by cardiovascular MRI. *Circulation.* 2010;121:e237.)

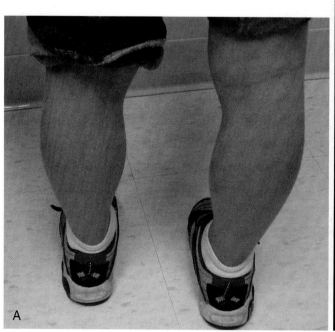
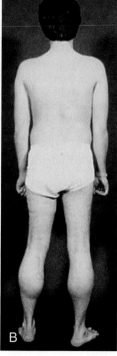

FIGURE 100.2 A, Calf pseudohypertrophy (related to an increase in fat, fibrous tissue, and diseased, poorly functioning muscle) in an 8-year-old boy with Duchenne muscular dystrophy. **B,** Becker muscular dystrophy in a 24-year-old man. Dystrophy of the shoulder girdle and calf pseudohypertrophy are evident. (**A** courtesy Dr. Laurence E. Walsh; **B** courtesy Dr. Robert M. Pascuzzi.)

elevated serum creatine kinase activity is observed, at levels more than 10 and 5 times normal values, respectively. Cardiac troponin T is elevated in up to one-half of patients likely related to immunoreactivity of the assay with diseased skeletal muscle. Cardiac troponin I remains normal in the majority of patients but has been observed to elevate in Duchenne patients with clinical features indicative of cardiomyopathy progression.[5]

Cardiovascular Manifestations

Most patients with DMD develop cardiomyopathy, but symptoms can be masked by activity limits due to skeletal muscle weakness. Sinus tachycardia is the earliest finding in the Duchenne heart, with the onset of clinically apparent cardiomyopathy common after the age of 10. Cardiac involvement can be diagnosed earlier by cardiac magnetic resonance imaging (MRI).[5-7] The majority of patients with DMD 18 years of age or older develop cardiomyopathy with reduced ejection fraction. Early involvement is observed in the inferobasal and lateral left ventricle (LV) (see Fig. 100.1A). As with the skeletal muscle weakness, cardiac involvement in Becker muscular dystrophy is more variable than in DMD, ranging from none or subclinical disease to severe cardiomyopathy requiring transplant. More than one-half of patients with subclinical or benign skeletal muscle disease were noted to have cardiac involvement if carefully evaluated. Progression in the severity of cardiac involvement is common. Cardiomyopathy can initially involve solely the right ventricle. The severity of cardiac involvement in both Duchenne and Becker muscular dystrophy can be independent of skeletal muscle involvement.

Thoracic deformities and a high diaphragm can alter the cardiovascular examination in patients with DMD. A reduction in the anterior-posterior chest dimension is commonly responsible for a systolic impulse displaced to the left sternal border, a grade 1 to 3/6 short midsystolic murmur in the second left interspace, and a loud pulmonary component of the second heart sound. In both Duchenne and Becker types of muscular dystrophy, mitral regurgitation is observed. The presence of mitral regurgitation is related to posterior papillary muscle dysfunction in DMD and to mitral annular dilation in BMD. Female carriers of Duchenne and Becker muscular dystrophy are at increased risk for dilated cardiomyopathy[8,9] and is consistent with increased susceptibility to cardiac injury in DMD carrier mice.[10]

Electrocardiography

In a majority of patients with DMD, the electrocardiogram (ECG) is abnormal (see Chapter 14). The classically described electrocardiographic pattern shows distinctive tall R waves and increased R/S amplitude in V_1 and deep narrow Q waves in the left precordial leads possibly related to the posterolateral left ventricular involvement (Fig. 100.3). Other common findings include a short PR interval and right ventricular hypertrophy. No association between the presence of a dilated cardiomyopathy and electrocardiographic abnormalities has been established. In BMD, electrocardiographic abnormalities are present in up to 75% of the patients. The electrocardiographic abnormalities observed include tall R waves and an increased R/S amplitude in V_1, akin to that seen in DMD. In patients with dilated cardiomyopathy, a left bundle branch block is also common.

Imaging

Clinical care guidelines recommend using screening echocardiography at diagnosis or by the age of 6 years; subsequently every 2 years until the age of 10; and annually thereafter in boys with DMD (this and other cardiac imaging modalities are described more fully in Chapters 16 to 20).[11] Cardiac MRI, especially with gadolinium contrast, is more sensitive in detecting subclinical ventricular involvement and fibrosis. The presence of fibrosis as indicated by late gadolinium enhancement on MRI predicted a subsequent decrement in left ventricular function.[7] Regional abnormalities in the posterobasal and lateral wall typically occur earlier than in other areas (see Fig. 100.1A). A process akin to left ventricular noncompaction can be observed, possibly resulting from compensatory mechanisms in response to the failing dystrophic myocardium. Mitral regurgitation can result from dystrophic changes in the posterior leaflet papillary muscles.

Arrhythmias

In DMD, persistent or labile sinus tachycardia is the most common arrhythmia recognized (see Chapter 65). Atrial arrhythmias, including atrial fibrillation and atrial flutter (see Chapter 66), occur in the setting of respiratory dysfunction and cor pulmonale or are associated with progression of dilated cardiomyopathy. Abnormalities in atrioventricular conduction have been observed, with both short and prolonged PR intervals recognized. Ventricular arrhythmias occur on monitoring in 30% of patients, primarily ventricular premature beats. Complex ventricular arrhythmias have been reported, more commonly in patients with advanced DMD. Sudden death occurs in DMD, typically in patients with end-stage muscular disease, and may occur due to arrhythmias or events like fat emboli.[12] Several follow-up studies have shown a correlation between sudden death and the presence of complex ventricular arrhythmias. The presence of ventricular arrhythmias was not a predictor for all-cause mortality. Arrhythmia manifestations in BMD are typically related to the severity of the associated structural cardiomyopathy. Distal conduction system disease with complete heart block and bundle branch reentry ventricular tachycardia has been observed (see Chapter 67).

Treatment and Prognosis

DMD is a progressive skeletal and cardiac muscle disorder. Glucocorticoid steroids and steroid derivatives are effective in delaying skeletal muscle disease progression and appear to decrease the progression to a dilated cardiomyopathy.[13] They constitute the mainstay of treatment for DMD and are part of the Care Considerations. Deflazacort is an FDA approved glucocorticoid for DMD, although prednisone is still commonly used. A retrospective analysis supports steroid benefit to the heart. The adverse side effects from long-term glucocorticoid treatment include obesity, osteoporosis, and metabolic syndrome. A novel dissociative steroid, vamolorone, is being investigated with initial promising results. Steroid treatment is not routinely recommended in BMD.

A cardiac cause for morbidity and mortality is playing an increasingly significant role in DMD because of improved multidisciplinary support for respiratory issues. There is an equal distribution of cardiac death from heart failure and sudden death. With evidence of reduced left ventricular function, even mildly reduced function, it is reasonable to offer guideline-directed heart failure management. Angiotensin-converting enzyme (ACE) inhibitors and beta blockers can improve left ventricular function in patients treated early. Angiotensin receptor blockers can be used if the patient cannot tolerate ACE inhibitors. The aldosterone antagonist, eplerenone, showed benefit in maintaining cardiac magnetic resonance left ventricular circumferential strain in boys already receiving ACE inhibitors or angiotensin receptor blockers.[14,15] Dosing, age, or clinical status at which pharmacotherapy should be initiated is unclear (see Chapters 49 and 50). Other advanced types of therapy such as implantable cardioverter-defibrillators (ICDs) play an uncertain role but should be considered individually based on clinical presentation using a shared decision-making approach (see Chapter 69). The use of left ventricular mechanical assist devices has been described. Whether heart failure therapies improve long-term outcomes is unclear. However, the age at death has increased, with the majority of patients surviving into their 30s, and recognition and treatment of the associated cardiomyopathy likely plays a role in that success. In patients with Becker muscular dystrophy, an improvement in left ventricular function also is observed after treatment with ACE inhibitors and beta blockers. Screening with left ventricular imaging is recommended as in DMD. Advanced heart failure therapy, including primary prevention ICDs, is appropriate in patients with cardiomyopathy. Patients with Becker muscular dystrophy with advanced heart failure can undergo cardiac transplantation, with expected outcomes similar to those for non–muscular dystrophy cohorts of age-matched patients with dilated cardiomyopathy.[16] Female carriers of Duchenne and BMD do not develop a cardiomyopathy during childhood, and screening can be delayed until later in adolescence. Cardiac transplantation also has been reported in carriers.

CARDIOVASCULAR DISEASE AND DISORDERS OF OTHER ORGANS

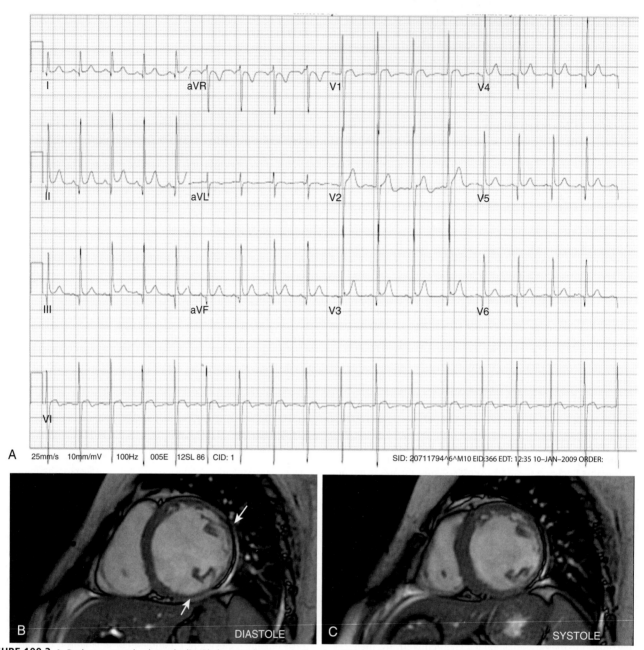

FIGURE 100.3 **A,** Duchenne muscular dystrophy (DMD) electrocardiogram reveals a short PR interval, an increase in the R/S ratio in the right precordial leads and narrow Q wave in the inferolateral leads. **B** and **C,** Cine sequences in the short axis view in diastole and systole showing dilation and thinning of the left ventricle wall particularly prominent in the inferior and lateral regions. (From Rochitte CE, Liberato G, Silva MC. Comprehensive assessment of cardiac involvement in muscular dystrophies by cardiac MR imaging. *Magn Reson Imaging Clin N Am.* 2019;27:521–531.)

Mutation-targeted treatment for Duchenne includes three forms of antisense mediated exon skipping that have been FDA approved, eteplirsen, golodirsen, and casimersen, and these agents treat different primary gene mutations (see eFig. 100.1). Adeno-associated viral gene therapy is in later stages of clinical investigation using micro-dystrophin, which is designed to convert Duchenne into Becker muscular dystrophy. On the horizon, CRISPR-Cas9-mediated gene editing is being designed to mediate more permanent exon skipping.[17,18]

Myotonic Dystrophies
Genetics and Pathogenesis

The myotonic dystrophies are autosomal dominant disorders characterized by myotonia, which is a delayed muscle relaxation after contraction, weakness, and atrophy of skeletal muscles, and systemic manifestations, including endocrine abnormalities, cataracts, cognitive impairment, and cardiac involvement (Fig. 100.4). Two distinct mutations are responsible for the myotonic dystrophies. In myotonic

dystrophy type 1 (Steinert disease), the mutation is an amplified trinucleotide cytosine-thymine-guanine (CTG) repeat on chromosome 19 in the 3′ untranslated region of dystrophia myotonica protein kinase *(DMPK)*. Normal individuals have 5 to 37 copies of the repeat, whereas patients with myotonic dystrophy have 50 to several thousand repeats. A direct correlation exists between an increasing number of CTG repeats and earlier age at onset and increasing severity of neuromuscular involvement (Table 100.1). Cardiac involvement including conduction disease, arrhythmias, and age at cardiovascular death also correlate with the length of repeat expansion (Fig. 100.5). It is typical for the CTG repeat to expand as it is passed from parents to offspring, resulting in the characteristic worsening clinical manifestations in subsequent generations, termed *anticipation*. Myotonic dystrophy type 2, also called proximal myotonic myopathy (PROMM), has generally less severe skeletal muscle and cardiac manifestations than type 1. Both congenital presentation and cognitive impairment are lacking in myotonic dystrophy type 2—typically, the most severely involved subsets of the type 1 patients. The genetic

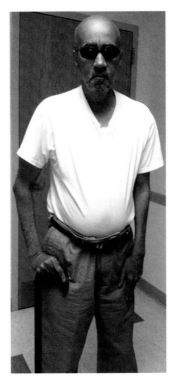

FIGURE 100.4 The patient is a 54-year-old man with myotonic dystrophy type 1. Typical characteristics of balding, thin face, and distal muscle atrophy are evident.

TABLE 100.1 Clinical Manifestation of Myotonic Dystrophy Type I

PHENOTYPE	CLINICAL	CTG LENGTH	ONSET
Congenital	Infantile hypotonia	>1000 (maternal)	Birth
	Respiratory failure		
	Learning disability		
	CV complications		
Childhood onset	Facial weakness	50–1000	1–10 yr
	Myotonia		
	Low IQ		
	Conduction defects		
"Classic DM1"	Myotonia	50–1000	10–30 yr
	Weakness (distal)		
	Conduction defects		
	Insulin resistance		
	Cataracts		
Late onset	Mild myotonia	50–100	20–70 yr
	Cataracts		

mutation responsible for myotonic dystrophy type 2 is a tetranucleotide repeat expansion, cytosine-cytosine-thymine-guanine (CCTG), found on chromosome 3 in intron 1 of the cellular nucleic acid binding protein (*CNBP* aka *ZNF9*). Intergenerational repeat contraction and expansion has been reported, and there is no apparent relationship between the degree of expansion and clinical severity. The prominent molecular mechanism by which both myotonic dystrophies exert their similar phenotypic presentations is by a toxic RNA gain-of-function effect. Large RNA expansions sequester and alter the function of nuclear RNA–binding proteins, resulting in aberrant mRNA splicing and polyadenylation. Cardiac involvement is related to the resultant dysregulation of multiple cardiac proteins that underlie contraction, calcium handling, excitability, and cell connectivity (Fig. 100.6).[19]

Clinical Presentation

The myotonic dystrophies are the most common inherited neuromuscular disorders in patients presenting as adults. Type 1 is more commonly diagnosed than type 2, except in certain areas of northern Europe. The global incidence of myotonic dystrophy type 1 has been estimated to be 1 in 8000 but higher in certain populations, such as French Canadians. The age at onset of symptoms and diagnosis averages 20 to 25 years. A congenital presentation is seen in severely affected patients with myotonic dystrophy type 1. Common early manifestations are related to weakness in the muscles of the face, neck, and distal extremities. Muscle weakness is progressive. On examination, myotonia can be demonstrated in the grip, thenar muscle group, and tongue (Fig. 100.7). A diagnosis can be made in asymptomatic patients using electromyography and genetic testing. Subcapsular ("Christmas tree") cataracts and early male-pattern baldness are common. Hyperinsulinemia, hyperglycemia, insulin resistance, diabetes, testicular failure, and adrenocortical dysregulation are seen in myotonic dystrophy type 1. Cardiac symptoms typically appear after the onset of skeletal muscle weakness but can be the initial manifestation. Patients with myotonic dystrophy type 2 exhibit muscle weakness, myotonia, cataracts, and endocrine abnormalities, as in type 1; however, age at symptom onset is typically older.

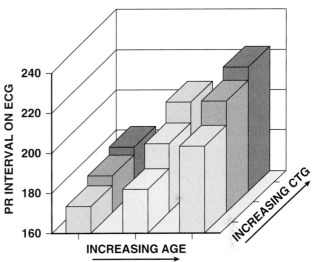

FIGURE 100.5 The relationship between the PR interval on the electrocardiogram and age and cytosine-thymine-guanine (CTG) repeat sequence expansion in 342 patients with myotonic dystrophy type 1. There is a direct relationship between age and CTG repeat sequence expansion and the severity of cardiac conduction disease, as quantified by the PR interval. The relationship suggests that cardiac involvement in myotonic dystrophy type 1 is a time-dependent degenerative process, with the rate of progression modulated by the extent of CTG repeat expansion. (From Groh WJ, Lowe MR, Zipes DP. Severity of cardiac conduction involvement and arrhythmias in myotonic dystrophy type 1 correlates with age and CTG repeat length. *J Cardiovasc Electrophysiol.* 2002;13:444.)

Cardiovascular Manifestations

Histopathology in the myotonic dystrophies shows cardiac myocyte hypertrophy and degeneration with fibrosis and fatty infiltration preferentially targeting the specialized conduction tissue, including the sinus node, atrioventricular node, and His-Purkinje system (Fig. 100.8). Degenerative changes are observed in working atrial and ventricular tissue but only rarely progress to a symptomatic dilated cardiomyopathy. It is not clear if there are differences in the cardiac pathology observed between myotonic dystrophy type 1 and 2. Patients with type 2 myotonic dystrophy typically demonstrate cardiac involvement later in life or not at all. The primary cardiac manifestations of the myotonic dystrophies are arrhythmias.

XI

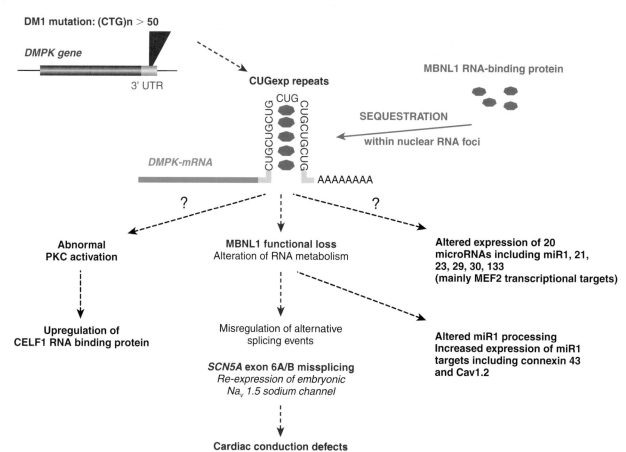

FIGURE 100.6 Multiple molecular mechanisms of cardiac involvement in type 1 myotonic dystrophy. Triplet nucleotide repeats in the 3′UTR of dystrophia myotonica protein kinase (DMPK) disrupt chromatin, can sequester muscle blind 1 (MBNL1), altering mRNA metabolism. Disruption of mRNA splicing and increased expression of microRNAs can cause dysregulation of target genes including sodium, calcium, chloride and gap junction channels, calcium handling proteins, troponins and the insulin receptor. *CELF1,* CUG binding protein Elav-like family member 1; *MEF2,* myocyte enhancer factor; *PKC,* protein kinase C; *UTR,* untranslated region.

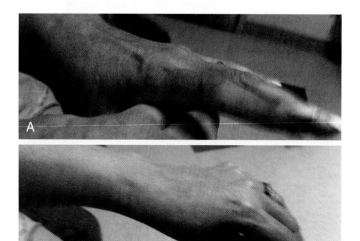

FIGURE 100.7 Grip myotonia in myotonic dystrophy. After exerting a grip **(A)** the patient is unable to fully open the hand **(B).**

Electrocardiography

A majority of adult patients with myotonic dystrophy type 1 exhibit electrocardiographic abnormalities. In a general middle-aged US myotonic population, abnormal electrocardiographic patterns were seen in 65% of the patients. Abnormalities included first-degree atrioventricular block in 42%, right bundle branch block in 3%, left bundle branch block in 4%, and nonspecific intraventricular conduction delay in 12%. Q-waves not associated with a known myocardial infarction are common. Electrocardiographic abnormalities are less common in younger patients. Conduction disease worsens with advancing age (Fig. 100.9).

Electrocardiographic abnormalities are less common in myotonic dystrophy type 2, occurring in approximately 20% of middle-aged patients.

Imaging and Heart Failure

Left ventricular systolic and diastolic dysfunction, left ventricular hypertrophy, mitral valve prolapse, regional wall motion abnormalities, and left atrial dilatation have been reported in patients with myotonic dystrophy type 1 at moderate prevalence rates. Clinical heart failure is observed but is less common than are arrhythmias. Left ventricular hypertrophy and ventricular dilation have been reported in myotonic dystrophy type 2. Cardiac MRI is more sensitive than echocardiography for detection of early cardiac involvement. Myocardial fibrosis is often observed in myotonic dystrophy and is associated with regional abnormalities in LV function. The association of global LV function and conduction abnormalities is more variable.[20-22]

Arrhythmias

A cardiac etiology is second only to respiratory failure as a cause of death in patients with myotonic dystrophy type 1. The major goal of management is evaluation of the risk for serious arrhythmias and sudden death (eFig. 100.3). Patients with myotonic dystrophy type 1 demonstrate a wide range of arrhythmias. At cardiac electrophysiologic study, the most common abnormality found is a prolonged His-ventricular (H-V) interval (Chapter 68). Conduction system disease can progress to symptomatic atrioventricular block and necessitate pacemaker implantation. The prevalence of permanent cardiac pacing in patients with myotonic dystrophy type 1 varies widely between studies based on referral patterns and the indications used for implant. Updated practice guidelines have recognized that asymptomatic conduction abnormalities in neuromuscular diseases such as myotonic dystrophy may warrant special consideration for pacing (Chapter 69).[23] Atrial arrhythmias, primarily atrial fibrillation and atrial flutter (Chapter 66), are the most common arrhythmias observed. Ventricular

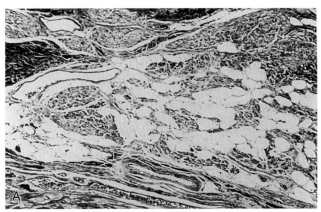

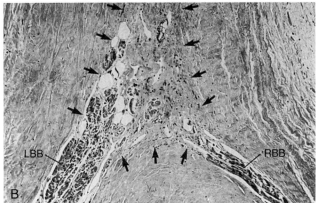

FIGURE 100.8 Histopathologic features of the atrioventricular bundle in myotonic dystrophy. **A,** Fatty infiltration in a specimen from a 57-year-old man (Masson trichrome stain, ×90). **B,** Focal replacement fibrosis and atrophy in a specimen from a 48-year-old woman. *Arrows* demarcate expected size and shape of the branching atrioventricular bundle (hematoxylin-eosin stain, ×90.) *LBB,* left bundle branch; *RBB,* right bundle branch. (From Nguyen HH, Wolfe JT 3rd, Holmes DR Jr, et al. Pathology of the cardiac conduction system in myotonic dystrophy: a study of 12 cases. *J Am Coll Cardiol.* 1988;11:662.)

tachycardia can occur. Patients with myotonic dystrophy type 1 are at risk for ventricular tachycardia occurring as a consequence of reentry in the diseased distal conduction system, as characterized by bundle branch reentry and interfascicular reentry tachycardia (Fig. 100.10). Therapy with right bundle branch or fascicular radiofrequency ablation can be curative (Chapter 67). Sudden death is responsible for 18% to 33% of deaths in myotonic dystrophy type 1; presumably, most are due to arrhythmias. Annual rates of sudden death in population studies vary between 0.25% and 2%. The mechanisms leading to sudden death are not clear. Distal conduction disease producing atrioventricular block can result in the lack of an appropriate escape rhythm and asystole or bradycardia-mediated ventricular fibrillation. Sudden death can occur in myotonic dystrophy type 1 despite pacing, implicating ventricular arrhythmias. Non-arrhythmic causes of sudden death, probably acute respiratory issues, play some role. Arrhythmias and sudden death have been reported in myotonic dystrophy type 2 but seem to be rarer than in type 1.

Treatment and Prognosis
Cardiac manifestations occur in both myotonic dystrophy types 1 and 2, and therefore diagnostic evaluation is essential in both.[24] Cardiac disease is observed at a younger age in myotonic dystrophy type 1 compared with type 2. Annual ECGs are recommended even in patients without symptoms or conduction disease. Echocardiography or other imaging modalities can determine if structural abnormalities are present. Cardiac imaging in adults should be done at diagnosis or with new symptoms. In the absence of significant abnormalities and symptoms, repeat evaluation every 3 to 5 years is appropriate. In the patient with reduced left ventricular function, standard therapy including ACE inhibitors and beta blockers has improved symptoms. There are no data on the role of ACE inhibitors or beta blockers in preventing the development of

a cardiomyopathy in myotonic dystrophy. Patients presenting with symptoms indicative of arrhythmias such as syncope and palpitations should undergo an evaluation, often including a cardiac electrophysiologic study, to determine an underlying causative disorder. The role and interval for ambulatory ECG (Holter) monitoring are not clear although periodic surveillance even in the absence of conduction system disease is prudent (Chapter 61). The presence of significant or progressive electrocardiographic abnormalities despite a lack of symptoms is an indication for consideration of prophylactic pacing.[23] The presence of severe electrocardiographic conduction abnormalities and atrial arrhythmias were independent risk factors for sudden death.[25] The strategy of pacing when the H-V interval is 70 milliseconds or more decreased sudden death in a large observational trial using propensity analysis for risk stratification. Patients with significant conduction defects who are candidates for pacemaker implantation should be evaluated for their risk of ventricular arrhythmias. If cardiac MRI reveals fibrosis or if LV dysfunction is present, programmed stimulation of the ventricle may be appropriate. If a ventricular tachyarrhythmia is inducible with a non-aggressive protocol, an ICD may be the preferred cardiac rhythm management device. In patients presenting with wide complex tachycardia, cardiac electrophysiologic study with particular evaluation for bundle branch reentry tachycardia should be done (Chapter 67). The use of cardiac resynchronization therapy may be appropriate in patients requiring ventricular pacing.

Treatment of myotonia, weakness, and muscle pain with sodium channel blocking drugs (mexiletine) in patients with myotonic dystrophy may be required. In the setting of a normal resting ECG and no evidence for cardiac involvement, mexiletine can be used without further evaluation. If the ECG demonstrates any conduction system disease, pacing may be required to safely use sodium channel blocking drugs. In situations in which pacing is not possible or desired, instituting drug therapy with electrocardiographic monitoring may be considered recognizing the risk of progressive conduction system disease. Similarly, the use of Na channel blocking drugs for the treatment of atrial fibrillation is contraindicated in patients with conduction system disease in the absence of a pacemaker.

Anesthesia in patients with myotonic dystrophy increases the risks of decreased gastrointestinal motility, respiratory failure, and arrhythmias. Patients may have unpredictable responses to neuromuscular blocking agents and careful monitoring during the perioperative period is mandatory. Monitored anesthesia during cardiac device implants should be done under an anesthesiologist's care.[24]

The course and prognosis of neuromuscular abnormalities in the myotonic dystrophies is variable (eTable 100.1).[26] Respiratory failure from progressive muscle dysfunction is the most common cause of death. Some patients, however, are only minimally limited by weakness up to the age of 60 to 70 years. Sudden death can reduce survival rates in patients with myotonic dystrophies, including those minimally symptomatic neuromuscular involvement. Decisions regarding primary prevention cardiac devices need to be made with full consideration of all aspects for the care of the myotonic patient.

Emery-Dreifuss Muscular Dystrophy and Associated Disorders
Genetics and Cardiac Pathology
Emery-Dreifuss muscular dystrophy (EDMD) is a spectrum of rare inherited disorders in which skeletal muscle symptoms are often mild but with cardiac involvement that is both common and serious. The disease (EDMD1) is classically inherited in an X-linked recessive fashion and the gene responsible, *STA*, encodes a nuclear membrane protein termed emerin (Table 100.2). EDMD is also inherited in an autosomal manner, the result of mutations in the *LMNA* gene that encodes the nuclear membrane proteins, lamins A and C. *LMNA* mutations also cause a spectrum of other diseases, including dilated cardiomyopathy and conduction system disease without skeletal muscle involvement and lipodystrophy (Chapter 52).[27] Nuclear membrane proteins such as emerin and lamins A and C provide structural support for the nucleus and interact with the cell's cytoskeletal proteins. The most common pattern of inheritance of LMNA mutations is autosomal dominant with variable expressivity and penetrance. Mutations throughout the *LMNA* gene have been documented in EDMD.

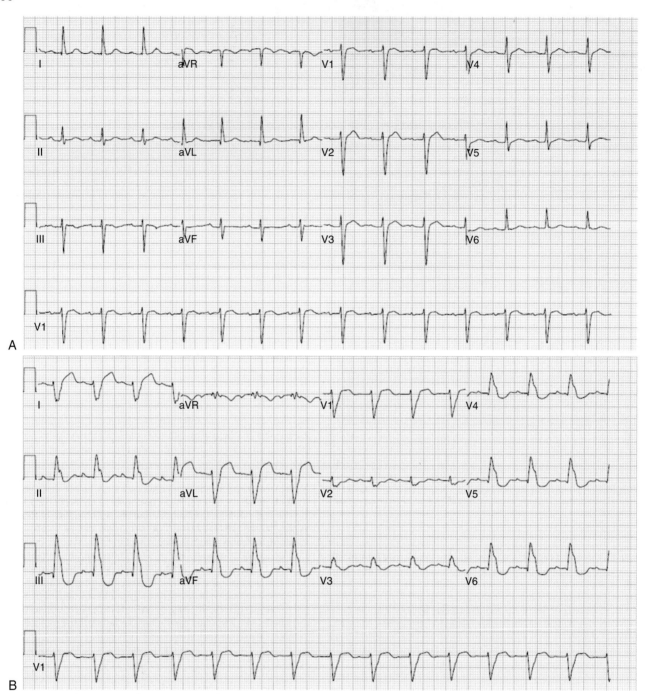

FIGURE 100.9 A and **B,** Electrocardiograms recorded 2 years apart in a 36-year-old woman with myotonic dystrophy (the *top tracings* are older). There is a dramatic increase in the QRS duration, ventricular axis shift, and increase in the PR interval consistent with progressive and severe conduction disease.

Clinical Presentation

EDMD is characterized by a triad of early contractures of the elbow, Achilles tendon, and posterior cervical muscles; slowly progressing muscle weakness and atrophy, primarily in humeroperoneal muscles; and cardiac involvement (Fig. 100.11). The disorder has been labeled "benign X-linked muscular dystrophy" to differentiate the slowly progressive muscular weakness from that of DMD. In the autosomal dominant and recessive inheritance of EDMD, a more variable phenotypic expression and penetrance are typically observed. Mutations in the lamin A/C gene are also responsible for an autosomal dominant familial partial lipodystrophy characterized by marked loss of subcutaneous fat, diabetes, hypertriglyceridemia, and cardiac abnormalities.

Cardiovascular Manifestations

In most patients with EDMD, the cardiac manifestations are the cause of mortality. Arrhythmias and dilated cardiomyopathy are the major

manifestations of cardiac disease in EDMD and its associated disorders (see eFig. 100.1). In X-linked recessive EDMD, abnormalities in impulse generation and conduction are common. Electrocardiographic abnormalities are usually apparent by age 20 to 30 years, commonly showing first-degree atrioventricular block. The atria appear to be involved earlier than the ventricles, with atrial fibrillation and atrial flutter, or more classically, permanent atrial standstill and junctional bradycardia. Abnormalities in impulse generation or conduction are present in virtually all patients by age 35 to 40 years, and requirement for pacing is typical. Ventricular arrhythmias occur, including sustained ventricular tachycardia and ventricular fibrillation. Sudden death, presumably due to cardiac disorders, before age 50 is observed and has informed the use of primary prevention ICDs.[12,28] Female carriers of X-linked recessive EDMD due to emerin mutations do not exhibit skeletal muscle disease but exhibit late cardiac disease, including conduction abnormalities, and more rarely sudden death. Although arrhythmias are the

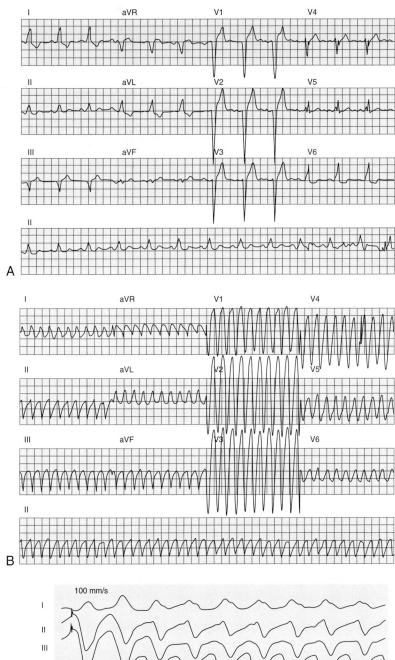

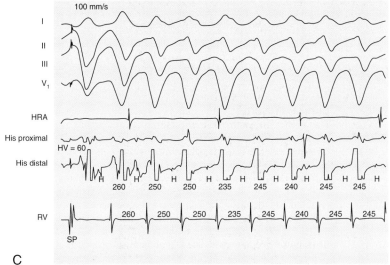

FIGURE 100.10 Bundle branch reentry tachycardia in a 34-year-old woman with myotonic dystrophy type 1 presenting with a symptomatic (recurrent syncope) wide-complex tachycardia. **A,** Electrocardiogram (ECG) showing sinus rhythm and a QRS complex with left bundle branch block. **B,** ECG showing a rapid monomorphic tachycardia easily inducible on electrophysiologic study, with left bundle morphology. **C,** Recordings during electrophysiologic study, including the surface ECG (leads I, II, III, V₁) and intracardiac ECGs (high right atrium, HRA, His proximal, His distal, and right ventricle, RV). A monomorphic ventricular tachycardia is induced with atrial-ventricular (A-V) dissociation and His association, consistent with bundle branch reentry tachycardia. Note, the H-H interval drives the subsequent V-V interval.

most common presentation of cardiac involvement in X-linked recessive EDMD, a dilated cardiomyopathy does occur. The dilated cardiomyopathy is more common in patients in whom the survival time has been improved with cardiac device implantation. Both autopsy and endomyocardial biopsy specimens have shown cardiac fibrosis.

Patients with disorders caused by lamin A and C mutations typically present at 20 to 40 years of age with cardiac conduction disease, atrial fibrillation, and dilated cardiomyopathy. Skeletal muscle disease typically is subclinical or absent. Progressive cardiomyopathy severe enough to require heart transplantation has been reported. Sudden death in those patients with dilated cardiomyopathy occurs. Pacing often is required for symptomatic heart block. ICDs are the appropriate cardiac device for a majority of these patients.

Treatment and Prognosis

Patients should be monitored for development of electrocardiographic conduction abnormalities and arrhythmias. Annual evaluation including an ECG is appropriate (eFig. 100.4). Sinus node dysfunction and atrial standstill are associated with AF often before the development of bradyarrhythmias. AF is associated with a relatively high frequency of embolic stroke, even in the absence of ventricular dysfunction; therefore, anticoagulation should be considered in patients with EDMD with atrial standstill or AF.[29] Sudden death even in patients with pacemakers has been observed. Primary prevention ICD is recommended in patients with EDMD and its associated disorders if significant electrocardiographic conduction disease is present and pacing is being considered.[12,28] The use of biventricular pacing should be considered in patients that require ventricular pacing. Whether ICDs should be considered only in certain subgroups of patients or in all patients with significant conduction disease or cardiomyopathy is not clear. In a large observational European series, risk factors for sudden death and appropriate ICD therapy included nonsustained ventricular tachycardia, left ventricular ejection fraction less than 45% at presentation, male sex, and lamin A or C non–missense mutations.[12] Routine imaging for evaluation of left ventricular function is appropriate in all patients with EDMD and the associated disorders. Although data are limited in this cohort, patients with LV dysfunction should be managed with guideline-recommended medical therapies, including ACEIs or ARBs, neprilysin inhibitors, beta blockers, and diuretics. Advanced HF treatment, including mechanical cardiac support (ventricular assist devices) and heart transplantation should be considered in appropriate patients. Female carriers of X-linked recessive EDMD develop conduction disease, and electrocardiographic monitoring on a routine basis is appropriate. Atrioventricular block can occur with anesthesia.

Limb-Girdle Muscular Dystrophies
Genetics and Pathophysiology

The limb-girdle muscular dystrophies are a group of over 25 muscle disorders with a limb-shoulder and pelvic girdle distribution of weakness, but with otherwise heterogeneous inheritance and genetic causes.[30,31] The naming convention is based on the mode of inheritance, with limb-girdle muscular dystrophy (LGMD)1 being transmitted as an autosomal dominant trait and LGMD2 as autosomal recessive. Within each class, there are subclasses of LGMDs identified by a letter designation. Autosomal recessive (subtypes 2A to 2Z), dominant (subtypes 1A to 1H), and sporadic patterns of inheritance have been observed. Genes involved include those encoding dystrophin-associated glycoproteins,

CARDIOVASCULAR DISEASE AND DISORDERS OF OTHER ORGANS

TABLE 100.2 Inheritance, Gene Locus, Disease Protein, and Cardiac Manifestations of Neuromuscular Disorders

DISEASE	OMIM	HERITANCE	GENE LOCUS	DISEASE PROTEIN	CARDIAC MANIFESTATIONS			
					Cardiomyopathy	Conduction abnormalities	Ventricular arrhythmia	Atrial arrhythmia
Duchenne MD	#310200	X-linked	Xp21	Dystrophin	+++	+	++	+
Becker MD	#300376	X-linked	Xp21	Dystrophin	+++	+	++	+
Limb-girdle MD, types 2C-G, I, J, N,Q	multiple	Autosomal recessive	Various	Sarcoglycans and others	+++	+	++	++
Myotonic dystrophy 1	#160900	Autosomal dominant	19q13	DMPK	+	+++	+	++
Myotonic dystrophy 2	#602668	AD	3q21	ZF9	Rare	+	+	+
Emery-Dreifuss MD, type 1	#310300	XL	Xq28	Emerin	++	+++	+++	++
Limb-girdle MD, type 1B	#150330	AD	1q11-21	Lamin A/C	+	++	+++	++
Fascioscapulohumeral MD	#158900	AD	4q35 D4Z4	DUX4	Rare	Rare	Rare	Rare
Friedreich ataxia	#229300	AR	9q21.11	Frataxin	+++ (HCM)	+++	+++	+
Kearns-Sayre syndrome	#530000	AD	mtDNA	Various	+	+++	+	++

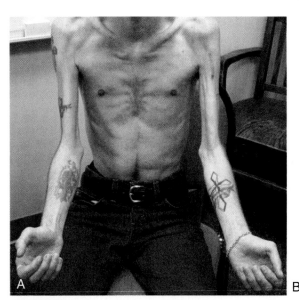

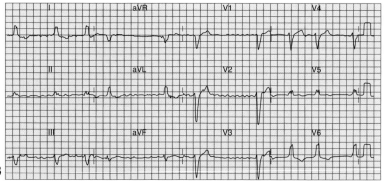

FIGURE 100.11 Emery-Dreifuss muscular dystrophy in a 28-year-old man presenting with syncope. **A,** Contractures of the elbow and atrophy in the humeroperoneal muscles. **B,** Electrocardiogram obtained at initial presentation showed atrial fibrillation with slow ventricular rate and a QRS complex with left bundle branch block. (Courtesy Dr. Robert M. Pascuzzi.)

sarcomeric proteins, sarcolemmal proteins, nuclear membrane proteins, and cellular enzymes. An autosomal dominant LGMD (subtype 1B) with a high prevalence of arrhythmias and a late dilated cardiomyopathy is caused by mutations encoding lamin A/C, as in EDMD. An autosomal recessive or sporadic LGMD associated with a progressive dilated cardiomyopathy is caused by mutations affecting the function of the dystrophin-glycoprotein complex, including sarcoglycan and fukutin-related proteins (subtypes 2C to 2F and 2I, respectively). The sarcoglycans interact with dystrophin-associated glycoproteins to counteract mechanical stress associated with contraction. Fukutin-related proteins affect glycosylation of a dystrophin-associated glycoprotein. An autosomal recessive LGMD associated with a variable onset of a dilated cardiomyopathy is caused by a mutation in a sarcolemmal repair protein termed dysferlin (subtype 2B) (see Fig. 100.1). Other more recently discovered and rarer subtypes of LGMD are variably associated with cardiac abnormalities in limited reports. A new nomenclature has been recommended.[32]

Clinical Presentation

The onset of proximal muscle weakness is variable but usually occurs before age 30. The recessive disorders tend to cause earlier and produce more severe weakness than the dominant disorders. Sarcoglycan-associated LGMDs more prominently affect flexor muscle groups and exhibit a rapidly progressive course, often with wheelchair confinement within a decade. Creatine kinase levels may be moderately to severely elevated. Patients commonly present with complaints of difficulty with walking or running secondary to pelvic girdle involvement. As the disease progresses, involvement of the shoulder muscles and then more distal muscles occurs, with sparing of facial involvement. Independent of the onset of skeletal muscle disease, effects on the heart are usually apparent by the second or third decade of life (eFig 100.5).

Cardiovascular Manifestations

As with many of the features of the limb-girdle muscular dystrophies, heterogeneity in the presence and degree of cardiac involvement is usual. Importantly, the severity of cardiac involvement may not be correlated with the degree of skeletal muscle impairment. The limb-girdle muscular dystrophies types 2C to 2F, termed *sarcoglycanopathies*, exhibit a dilated cardiomyopathy. Cardiac abnormalities are detected in a majority of patients typically a decade after skeletal muscle symptoms occur. Cardiomyopathy is less common in the subtype 2D than present in the other sarcoglycanopathies. ECGs show similar abnormalities as in Duchenne and Becker muscular dystrophy, including an increased R wave in V_1 and lateral Q waves. Imaging can show a progressive dilated cardiomyopathy. A severe cardiomyopathy, including presentation with heart failure in childhood, can occur. Sudden death associated with the cardiomyopathy has been reported.

LGMD type 2I, caused by mutations in fukutin-related proteins, is associated with a dilated cardiomyopathy. The mutation is also responsible for a form of congenital muscular dystrophy. The age at disease onset and severity of skeletal muscle involvement are variable, with symptoms emerging in some patients during childhood but more typically developing after the age of 20 years. Approximately one-half of patients with LGMD type 2I exhibit cardiac involvement (Fig. 100.12) more commonly reported in males. Cardiac findings include regional wall motion abnormalities or a dilated cardiomyopathy and heart failure. Conduction disease generally does not occur independent of structural cardiac involvement. LGMD type 2A due to calpain 3 mutations and type 2B, due to dysferlin gene mutations, have little cardiac involvement, although abnormalities can be detected on cardiac imaging.

The autosomal dominant LGMD type 1B is caused by mutations in the gene encoding lamins A and C with a clinical phenotype similar to EDMD. Skeletal muscle involvement is mild, with frequent and severe cardiac involvement. Atrioventricular block develops by early middle age, often necessitating pacing. Sudden death is observed even in patients with pacemakers. A progressive dilated cardiomyopathy can occur, typically after the development of conduction disease.

Treatment and Prognosis

Because of the heterogeneous nature of LGMD, specific recommendations for routine cardiac evaluation and therapy are based on the disease type. The frequency and severity of cardiac involvement in LGMD and in particular the laminopathies, mandates an aggressive approach to evaluation and management. This is particularly relevant in view of the often milder skeletal muscle disease in these patients. In addition to a thorough cardiovascular history and physical examination, the recommended evaluation includes resting and ambulatory ECGs, echocardiography, and cardiac MRI with contrast (in cases in which there is any suggestion of cardiac involvement).

Treatment of LV dysfunction even in the absence of clinical HF is appropriate and should include ACEIs or ARBs and beta blockers in the absence of contraindications. Patients with dilated cardiomyopathies respond to standard heart failure therapy. Heart transplantation has been reported. Prophylactic placement of an ICD instead of a pacemaker has been recommended in patients with lamin A and C mutation after conduction disease is observed akin to that in EDMD. In a large observational European series, risk factors for sudden death and appropriate ICD therapy included nonsustained ventricular tachycardia, left ventricular ejection fraction less than 45% at presentation, male sex, and lamin A or C non–missense mutations.[12]

Facioscapulohumeral Muscular Dystrophy
Genetics and Pathophysiology

Facioscapulohumeral muscular dystrophy is the third most common muscular dystrophy after the Duchenne and myotonic types.[33] Underreporting of disease prevalence is likely due to mild subclinical forms. It is an autosomal dominant disorder in which the primary genetic mutation occurs at chromosomal locus 4q35, with a contraction of a D4Z4 repeat sequence that leads to derepression of a retrogene, *DUX4* encoding a transcriptional regulator whose target genes are toxic to skeletal muscle (Table 100.2). *DUX4* derepression may result from repeat contraction induced chromatin hypomethylation (FSHD1, most common form) or as a consequence of a second mutation in SMCHD1, a gene involved in chromatin methylation of the D4Z4 region (FSHD2) (eFig. 100.6).

Clinical Presentation

The onset and rates of progression of muscle weakness are highly variable, with a distinct regional pattern starting in the face and periscapular region, then progressing caudally and distally in the upper body, then to the pelvic musculature. Muscle weakness in FSHD tends to be more asymmetric than other muscular dystrophies, except in advanced disease. Respiratory involvement is rare; however, some patients develop restrictive lung disease. In patients with large deletions in the D4Z4 region, high frequency hearing loss and retinal vascular disease with exudative retinopathy (Coats Disease) has been described.[34]

Cardiovascular Manifestations

Cardiac involvement in facioscapulohumeral muscular dystrophy is reported but does not constitute as significant a problem in prevalence or severity as in other muscular dystrophies. Cardiomyopathy, ventricular arrhythmias and symptomatic conduction disease are generally not observed. There are reports of supraventricular tachycardia (SVT) and asymptomatic right bundle branch block.

Treatment and Prognosis

Because significant clinical cardiac involvement is rare in facioscapulohumeral muscular dystrophy, specific monitoring or treatment recommendations are not well defined. Annual ECGs have been recommended.

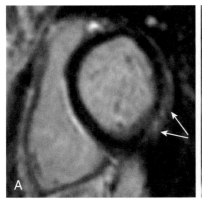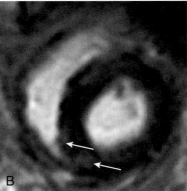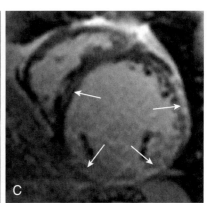

FIGURE 100.12 Cardiac magnetic resonance imaging findings in limb-girdle muscular dystrophy. Late gadolinium enhancement (*arrows*) in limb-girdle muscular dystrophy patients demonstrating focal epicardial (**A**) or midwall (**B**) enhancement. **C,** Patient with limb-girdle muscular dystrophy 2I and advanced dilated cardiomyopathy had extensive myocardial injury/fibrosis. (From Rosales XQ, Moser SJ, Tran T, et al. Cardiovascular magnetic resonance of cardiomyopathy in limb girdle muscular dystrophy 2B and 2I. *J Cardiovasc Magn Reson.* 2011;13:39.)

XI

Friedreich Ataxia

Genetics and Pathophysiology

Friedreich ataxia (FRDA) is an autosomal recessive, multisystem disease characterized by spinocerebellar degeneration. The clinical presentation includes ataxia of the limbs and trunk, dysarthria, loss of deep tendon reflexes, sensory abnormalities, skeletal deformities, diabetes mellitus, and cardiac involvement. The primary genetic abnormality is an unstable trinucleotide repeat expansion (guanine-adenine-adenine, GAA), in the first intron of frataxin gene *(FXN)* that inhibits its transcription. Frataxin is a 210–amino acid mitochondrial protein associated with iron homeostasis. Deficiency of the protein leads to mitochondrial iron aggregation increasing cell susceptibility to oxidative stress (eFig. 100.7). Messenger RNA for frataxin is highly expressed in the heart. Endomyocardial biopsy samples have shown deficient function in mitochondrial respiratory complex subunits and in aconitase, an iron-sulfur protein involved in iron homeostasis. Impaired mitochondrial lipid metabolism also may play a role in the cardiomyopathy in FRDA. Histopathologic examination has revealed myocyte hypertrophy due to proliferation of mitochondria, myocyte degeneration, interstitial fibrosis, active muscle necrosis, bizarre pleomorphic nuclei, and periodic acid–Schiff–(PAS) positive deposition in both large and small coronary arteries. Degeneration and fibrosis in cardiac nerves and ganglia and the conduction system also have been observed. An earlier age at symptom onset, increasing severity of neurologic symptoms, and worsening left ventricular hypertrophy are observed in patients in whom genetic testing shows a larger GAA repeat expansion.

Clinical Presentation

FRDA is one of the most common inherited ataxias. The development of neurologic symptoms before age 25 and typically around puberty is characteristic. Progressive, debilitating ataxia and loss of neuromuscular function, with the patient wheelchair-bound 10 to 20 years after symptom onset, is the usual course. Neurologic symptoms precede cardiac symptoms in most but not all cases.

Cardiovascular Manifestations

FRDA is associated with left ventricular hypertrophy (Fig. 100.13). Asymmetric septal hypertrophy is uncommon and a left ventricular outflow gradient is rare but has been observed. The prevalence of hypertrophy increases, particularly with a younger age at diagnosis and with increasing GAA trinucleotide expansion. ECG abnormalities are present in over 90% of patients with FRDA. Left ventricular hypertrophy is not always present on ECGs despite echocardiographic evidence. Widespread ST deviation and T wave inversions are common as is right axis deviation (Fig. 100.14). Patients with left ventricular hypertrophy without systolic dysfunction typically have no cardiac symptoms. About 10% of patients develop left ventricular systolic dysfunction with an ejection fraction of less than 50%.[35,36] Presentation with a dilated cardiomyopathy has been reported (Fig. 100.15). The dilated cardiomyopathy occurs as a transition from the hypertrophic cardiomyopathy. Atrial arrhythmias including atrial fibrillation and flutter are associated with the progression to a dilated cardiomyopathy. Similarly, ventricular tachycardias are generally coincident with the development of dilated cardiomyopathy. The hypertrophic cardiomyopathy of FRDA is not associated with serious ventricular arrhythmias, as observed in the other types of heritable hypertrophic cardiomyopathies. Myocardial fiber disarray is not commonly observed in the hypertrophic cardiomyopathy of FRDA. Sudden death likely due to ventricular arrhythmias has been reported, but a mechanism has not been well characterized.[12,36]

Treatment and Prognosis

Idebenone, a free radical scavenger, has modest but variable effectiveness for decreasing left ventricular hypertrophy in FRDA. Idebenone does not improve left ventricular systolic function. It is unclear whether the modest improvement in cardiac imaging parameters leads to an alteration in the clinical cardiovascular course. Idebenone and other antioxidants (vitamin E and coenzyme Q10) have been studied and do not improve neurologic outcomes. In a majority of patients with FRDA, neurologic dysfunction is progressive. Heart failure is the most common cause of death.[37] Arrhythmias complicate heart failure deaths in one third of patients. Respiratory dysfunction is the second most common cause of death. Death from heart failure occurs earlier than respiratory death, typically before the age of 30 years. The role of pharmacologic or defibrillator therapy in FRDA and dilated cardiomyopathy has not been evaluated, but such conventional therapy should be considered. Small case series describe cardiac transplantation in FRDA patients with mild neurological disease.[38]

LESS COMMON NEUROMUSCULAR DISEASES ASSOCIATED WITH CARDIAC MANIFESTATIONS

The Periodic Paralyses

Genetics and Clinical Presentation

The primary periodic paralyses are rare, non-dystrophic disorders of autosomal dominant inheritance associated with mutations in ion channel genes.[39] They can be classified into hypokalemic and hyperkalemic periodic paralyses and Andersen-Tawil syndrome (see Chapter 63). In addition, acquired hypokalemic periodic paralysis may complicate thyrotoxicosis, especially in Asian men. All patients present with episodic attacks of flaccid paralysis precipitated by variable environmental stimuli including cold and exercise, or with rest after exercise. The periodic paralyses may be complicated by a late-onset permanent skeletal myopathy. Hypokalemic periodic paralysis is characterized by episodic attacks of weakness exacerbated by carbohydrate load or occurring during rest after exercise and is associated with decreased serum potassium levels at onset. Penetrance is nearly complete in male patients and 50% in female patients. It is caused by point mutations in the dihydropyridine-sensitive calcium channel *(CACNA1S)* or in skeletal muscle sodium channel *(SCN4A)*. Approximately 20% of cases are of uncertain genetic cause. One third of the cases of thyrotoxic hypokalemic periodic paralysis are caused by mutations in an inward rectifier potassium channel, Kir2.6, which is regulated by thyroid hormone. Hyperkalemic periodic paralysis also manifests with episodic weakness but with symptoms worsening with potassium supplementation and decreasing with carbohydrate load. Potassium levels usually are high but may be normal during an attack. Hyperkalemic periodic paralysis is due primarily to mutations in *SCN4A*, but other loci also have been identified. Multiple different mutations

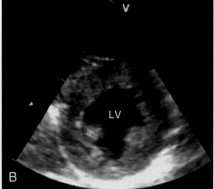

FIGURE 100.13 Hypertrophic cardiomyopathy in Friedreich ataxia. Echocardiographic apical 4-chamber (**A**) and short-axis (**B**) views from a Friedreich ataxia patient with left ventricular hypertrophy (LV wall thickness 15 mm). *LA*, left atrium; *LV*, left ventricle; *RA*, right atrium; *RV*, right ventricle. (From Weidemann F, Störk S, Liu D, et al. Cardiomyopathy of Friedreich ataxia. *J Neurochem*. 2013;126[suppl 1]:88.)

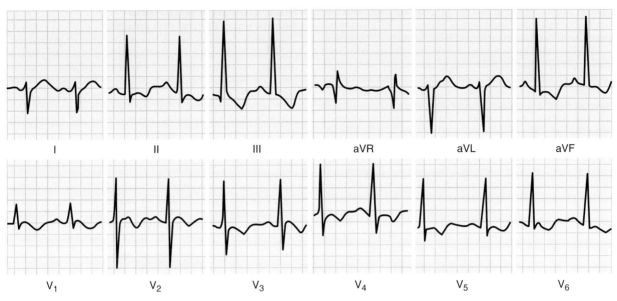

I   II   III   aVR   aVL   aVF

V₁   V₂   V₃   V₄   V₅   V₆

FIGURE 100.14 Electrocardiogram from a 34-year-old man with Friedreich ataxia. Widespread ST and T changes are evident. (Courtesy Dr. Charles Fisch, Indiana University School of Medicine, Indianapolis.)

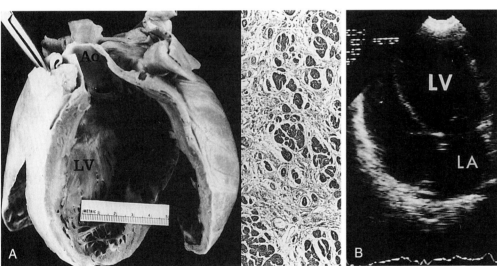

FIGURE 100.15 A, Gross and histologic specimens from a 17-year-old boy with Friedreich ataxia whose electrocardiogram progressed from a normal appearance at age 13 years to a minimally dilated, hypocontractile left ventricle (LV) 3 to 4 years later. The gross specimen *(left)* shows a mildly dilated LV with normal wall thickness. The microscopic section from the left ventricular free wall *(right)* shows marked connective tissue replacement. Although specifically sought, small-vessel coronary artery disease was not identified. **B,** Two-dimensional echocardiogram (apical window) showing the mildly dilated, thin-walled LV. *Ao,* aorta; *LA,* left atrium. (From Child JS, Perloff JK, Bach PM, et al. Cardiac involvement in Friedreich ataxia. *J Am Coll Cardiol.* 1986;7:1370.)

KCNJ2-mediated disease. The loss of function of IK1 is responsible for the large and prolonged U-wave.

Cardiovascular Manifestations

The periodic paralyses are associated with ventricular arrhythmias. Most arrhythmias occur in Andersen-Tawil syndrome and less often in hyperkalemic periodic paralysis. Bidirectional ventricular tachycardia (see Fig 100.16) has been observed without digitalis intoxication (Chapters 14 and 63). The episodes of bidirectional ventricular tachycardia are independent of attacks of muscle weakness, do not correlate with serum potassium levels, and can convert to sinus rhythm with exercise. The tachycardia typically is less than 150 beats/min and well tolerated. Andersen-Tawil syndrome is associated with modest prolongation in the QT interval but more specifically a prolonged and prominent U wave. Cardiac conduction

in this gene have been reported that result in a potassium-sensitive failure of inactivation (gain-of-function) in the sodium channel.

Andersen-Tawil syndrome (also designated as long QT syndrome 7) is a distinct periodic paralysis associated with dysmorphic physical features of short stature, low-set ears, micrognathia, hypertelorism, and clinodactyly; abnormalities on the ECG include an abnormal QT-U wave pattern and ventricular arrhythmias (Fig. 100.16).[39] Weakness can be triggered by low, normal, or high potassium levels. It can be inherited in an autosomal dominant fashion or can be sporadic. Phenotypic variability and incomplete penetrance can complicate the diagnosis for a given family. Mutations in the *KCNJ2* gene encoding the inward rectifier potassium channel subunit (Kir2.1), and inward rectifier current (IK1, responsible for maintaining the resting membrane potential) accounts for 60% of cases. The genetic cause(s) in the other 40% of patients is unknown but seemingly involve other proteins contributing to IK1 because the phenotype is indistinguishable from

abnormalities, atypical of long QT syndromes, have been observed in Andersen-Tawil syndrome. Torsades de pointes is observed in Andersen-Tawil syndrome but is less common than in the other long QT syndromes. Syncope, cardiac arrest, and sudden death have been reported in the periodic paralyses, most prominently in the Andersen-Tawil syndrome. The factors that portend an increased risk of life-threatening arrhythmias are not clear. The frequency of ventricular ectopy or non-sustained ventricular tachycardia on ambulatory monitoring did not differentiate Andersen-Tawil syndrome patients with and without syncope.[40]

Treatment and Prognosis

The episodes of weakness typically respond to measures that normalize potassium levels. Weakness in hyperkalemic periodic paralysis can respond to mexiletine. Weakness in hypokalemic periodic paralysis may respond to acetazolamide. Treatment targeting electrolyte abnormalities usually does not ameliorate arrhythmias or, if it does, affords only transient benefit. Improvement in symptomatic non-sustained ventricular tachycardia associated with a prolonged QT interval has been reported with beta-blocker therapy. Class 1A antiarrhythmic drugs can worsen muscle weakness and exacerbate arrhythmias associated with a prolonged QT interval. Bidirectional ventricular tachycardia, not associated with a prolonged QT interval, may not respond to beta-blocker therapy. Flecainide decreases the frequency of ventricular arrhythmias assessed by ambulatory monitoring and is associated with a good clinical outcome over 2 years in Andersen-Tawil syndrome.[40] Amiodarone and imipramine have also been shown to have efficacy in small series and case reports. The use of ICDs has been reported in Andersen-Tawil syndrome, primarily in those with symptomatic and drug-refractory sustained ventricular arrhythmias. Programming of defibrillators to avoid inappropriate discharges is problematic because ventricular tachycardia is often self-terminating. Prognosis in the Andersen-Tawil syndrome is reasonably good despite frequent episodes of ventricular ectopy.

Mitochondrial Disorders
Genetics and Clinical Presentation

The mitochondrial disorders, also termed mitochondrial myopathies, encephalomyopathies, or respiratory chain disorders, are a heterogeneous group of diseases resulting from abnormalities in mitochondrial function.[41] The list of distinct disorders is extensive (eTable 100.2) and includes deficiencies in electron transport chain proteins, mutations in mitochondrial DNA and tRNA, coenzyme Q10 deficiency, 3-methylglucatonic acidurias and abnormal iron handling. Mitochondrial DNA is inherited maternally, and some of these disorders are thus transmitted from mother to children of both sexes. Many other disorders result from abnormalities in nuclear DNA involved in mitochondrial form and function and are inherited in an autosomal or X-linked fashion. Sporadic cases can occur. Disease severity can vary among family members because both mutant and normal mitochondrial DNA can be present in tissue in variable proportions, a phenomenon termed *heteroplasmy*. Consistent with the energy-generating

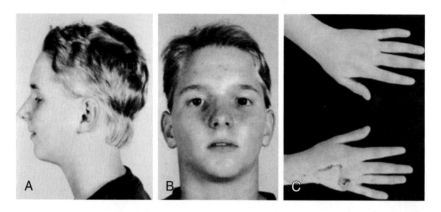

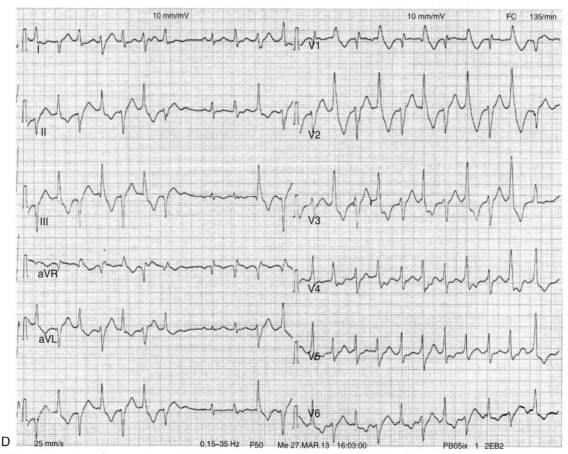

FIGURE 100.16 Andersen-Tawil syndrome. **A** and **B**, An affected patient exhibits characteristic low-set ears, hypertelorism, micrognathia, and clinodactyly of the fifth digits **(C)**. ECG from a patient with Andersen-Tawil syndrome before **(D)** and after flecainide **(E)**. (**D** and **E** from Maffe S, Paffoni P, Bergamasco L, et al. Therapeutic management of ventricular arrhythmias in Andersen-Tawil syndrome. *J Electrocardiol.* Jan–Feb 2020;58:37–42)

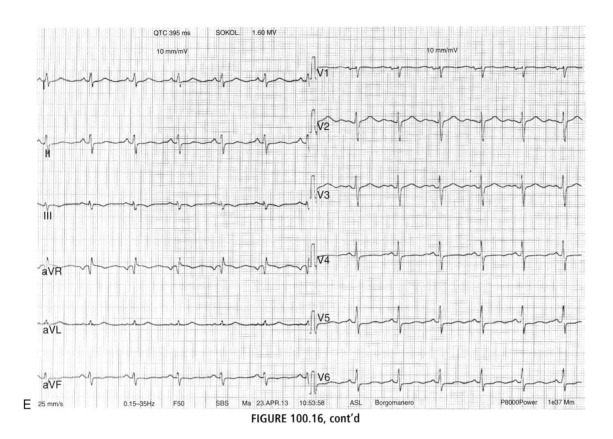

FIGURE 100.16, cont'd

role of mitochondria in all cells, these disorders have systemic manifestations. Tissue with a high respiratory workload such as brain and skeletal muscle, especially extraocular, retinal, and cardiac muscle, are primarily affected. Mitochondrial disorders that have cardiac manifestations may appear as part of several clinical phenotypes. *Chronic progressive external ophthalmoplegia* is characterized by involvement of the extraocular muscles and can also involve oropharyngeal muscles. It is primarily a sporadic disease. *Kearns-Sayre syndrome,* a subtype of chronic progressive external ophthalmoplegia, is characterized by ocular myopathy, pigmentary retinopathy, and age at onset before 20 years. Diabetes, deafness, and ataxia can also be associated. *Myoclonus epilepsy with red ragged fibers* (MERRF) is characterized by myoclonus, seizures, ataxia, dementia, and skeletal muscle weakness. *Mitochondrial myopathy with encephalopathy, lactic acidosis, and strokelike episodes* (MELAS) is the most common of the maternally inherited mitochondrial disorders and is characterized by encephalopathy, subacute stroke-like events, migraine-like headaches, recurrent emesis, extremity weakness, and short stature. *Leber hereditary optic neuropathy* causes subacute blindness, primarily in young men. Other, mitochondrial point mutation disorders, including neuropathy, ataxia, and retinitis pigmentosa *(NARP)* and *Leigh syndrome* (subacute necrotizing encephalomyelopathy) cause neurodegenerative disorders primarily in children. *Barth syndrome* is an X-linked mitochondrial disease manifested by hypotonia, growth retardation, cyclic neutropenia, and 3-methylglutaconic aciduria in children. It is caused by mutations in exons of the nuclear gene encoding tafazzin.

Cardiovascular Manifestations

Patients with mitochondrial myopathy can present with chest pain or, more typically, dyspnea with exertion. In chronic progressive external ophthalmoplegia, most commonly in the Kearns-Sayre syndrome variant, cardiac involvement manifests primarily as conduction abnormalities. In the Kearns-Sayre syndrome, atrioventricular block is observed, usually manifesting after eye involvement. The H-V interval is prolonged, consistent with distal conduction disease. Permanent pacing often is required by early- to mid-adulthood. An increased prevalence of ventricular preexcitation has also been

reported. Cardiac MRI demonstrates nonischemic, late gadolinium enhancement in approximately one third of patients and in some cases dilated cardiomyopathy.[41] Mutations in mitochondrial tRNA such as *MERRF* and *MELAS,* are typically associated with hypertrophic (symmetric or asymmetric) cardiomyopathy but dilated cardiomyopathy and rarely arrhythmogenic histiocytoid cardiomyopathy have been observed. Other disorders caused by mitochondrial point mutations can manifest with a similar cardiac phenotype of hypertrophic or dilated cardiomyopathy, often in children. Whether the dilated cardiomyopathy represents a progression from the hypertrophic cardiomyopathy or a separate syndrome is not clear. The dilated cardiomyopathy can result in heart failure and death. More than one half of patients with MELAS had non-ischemic, late gadolinium enhancement on cardiac MRI. Leber hereditary optic neuropathy can be associated with a hypertrophic cardiomyopathy and a short PR interval or preexcitation syndromes (Chapter 65). Barth syndrome is associated with left ventricular non-compaction and endocardial fibroelastosis or a hypertrophic or dilated cardiomyopathy. Heart failure and ventricular arrhythmias occur, often in young children.[42]

Treatment and Prognosis

There are currently no effective treatments for most mitochondrial disorders. There are strategies for managing some of the cardiac manifestations. In Kearns-Sayre syndrome, the implantation of a pacemaker has been advocated when significant or progressive conduction disease is present including in asymptomatic patients. The degree of conduction disease that warrants prophylactic pacing is not clear. ICDs are recommended in patients with both conduction disease and a dilated cardiomyopathy.[42] In the other mitochondrial disorders, an understanding of the potential and specific presentations for cardiac involvement is necessary. Cardiac evaluation, electrocardiography, echocardiography, and other imaging modalities are recommended. Prophylactic or symptomatic heart failure pharmacotherapy, although not studied in these rare diseases, would seem warranted. Improved survival rates in children with Barth syndrome receiving aggressive treatment for cardiomyopathy and neutropenia has been observed.[43]

Spinal Muscular Atrophy

Genetics and Clinical Presentation

Spinal muscular atrophy (SMA) is a lower motor neuron disorder manifesting as progressive, symmetric proximal muscular weakness.[44] It is the leading inherited cause of infant death. SMA is classified clinically by the age at symptom onset and disease severity into type I (Werdnig-Hoffman disease), type II (intermediate form), type III (Kugelberg-Welander disease), and type IV (adult-onset spinal muscular atrophy). SMA is inherited in autosomal recessive fashion or is sporadic. Mutations or deletions in the telomeric survival of motor neuron (*SMN*) gene are observed in most patients. The loss of functional SMN protein results in premature neuronal cell death.

Cardiovascular Manifestations

The SMN protein has primarily a motor neuron role. However, cardiac abnormalities can be present including sinus tachycardia.[44] Additionally, the profound respiratory muscle weakness that occurs in SMA can impact cardiac function.

Treatment and Prognosis

SMA type 1 is now treated with adeno-associated gene therapy as a one-time intravenous infusion. Onasemnogene abeparvovec is an FDA approved gene therapy for the treatment of SMA type 1 patients under the age of 2. Additionally, nusinersen is an antisense oligonucleotide-based exon skipping therapy also approved for the treatment of SMA, as is the oral small molecule splicing modulator risdiplam. Older symptomatic SMA patients can also receive treatment with nusinersen or risdiplam. Nusinersen is delivered intrathecally and requires repeated dosing, often three times a year. A prolonged lifespan for SMA type 1 patients is now being seen, and whether these treatments will uncover any cardiac defects remains to be seen.[45]

Myofibrillar Myopathies

Genetics and Clinical Presentation

The myofibrillar myopathies arise from mutations in genes encoding proteins of myofibrils. This includes mutations in *DES, CYRAB, MYOT, ZASP, BAG3, DNAJB6, TTN* and *FLNC*. The inheritance patterns can vary and the age of onset is from child to adult, with both familial and sporadic forms. *DES* encodes desmin, an abundant intermediate filament protein, expressed in cardiomyocytes.[46,47] Desmin has multiple functions in the heart and interacts with well over a dozen other proteins involved in contraction, maintenance of cell-cell contacts, apoptosis, and energetics. Acquired disruption of the intermediate filament network is a common pathological consequence in structural heart disease. DES mutation can lead to myopathic process that affects both heart and skeletal muscle.[46] The disorder is inherited primarily in autosomal dominant fashion, but autosomal recessive inheritance, and sporadic mutations have been reported. Typically, symptomatic skeletal muscle abnormalities, manifesting as respiratory dysfunction, will be observed prior to cardiac involvement. For any of the myofibrillar myopathies, muscle biopsy can be diagnostic. Variability in the phenotype is recognized and a cardiomyopathy can develop without obvious skeletal muscle abnormalities. Creatine kinase is mildly elevated in some patients.

FLNC encodes filamin C, a structural protein found at the Z disk and also at the sarcolemma. A distal skeletal myopathy is typically observed. Some variants have little or no skeletal muscle involvement but with serious cardiac issues. FLNC truncations have increased arrhythmia risks.

Cardiovascular Manifestations

The cardiac involvement observed in desmin myopathy typically consists of conduction system disease and, more rarely, ventricular arrhythmias, before the onset of a dilated or restrictive cardiomyopathy. An arrhythmogenic right ventricular cardiomyopathy–like phenotype has been reported.[48] Both sudden death and heart failure–related deaths can occur. Sudden death can occur despite pacemaker implantation.[12]

Similarly, filamin C-associated disease can present with different forms of cardiomyopathy including hypertrophic, restrictive, and dilated. Involvement of the right ventricle can lead to a clinical picture mimicking arrhythmogenic right ventricular cardiomyopathy. The majority of patients have frequent ventricular ectopy on monitoring and are at risk of ventricular arrhythmias and sudden death.

Treatment and Prognosis

The desmin and filamin-C associated myopathies should be considered in the differential diagnosis in individuals or families presenting with a skeletal or cardiac myopathy, including those with an arrhythmogenic right ventricular cardiomyopathy. Monitoring for the development of cardiac conduction and structural heart disease is necessary in affected families. Asymptomatic conduction disease on the ECG predicts future adverse cardiac events in desmin associated myopathies.[12] Primary prevention pacemakers or ICDs should be considered in those patients with significant conduction disease. It is not clear if the presence of conduction disease predicts future adverse cardiac events in filamin-C associated myopathies. Guideline based heart failure pharmacotherapy is recommended in these patients.

Guillain-Barré Syndrome

Clinical Presentation

The Guillain-Barré syndrome is an acute inflammatory demyelinating neuropathy characterized by peripheral, cranial, and autonomic nerve dysfunction (Chapter 102).[49] It is the most common acquired demyelinating neuropathy. Men are more commonly affected than women. In two thirds of affected patients, an acute viral or bacterial illness, or respiratory or gastrointestinal manifestations precede the onset of neurologic symptoms within 6 weeks. The disorder is typically associated with pain, paresthesias, and symmetric limb weakness that progresses proximally and can involve cranial and respiratory muscles. One fourth of affected patients require assisted ventilation.

Cardiovascular Manifestations

Non-ambulant patients are at increased risk for deep vein thrombosis and pulmonary emboli. Cardiac involvement related to accompanying autonomic nervous system dysfunction is seen in one-half of patients. Autonomic dysfunction, characterized by alternating sympathetic and parasympathetic hyperactivity poses a significant risk in Guillain-Barré syndrome patients and increases mortality rates. Moreover, there is no clear association between the severity of motor weakness and the degree and lability of autonomic dysfunction.[50] Cardiovascular manifestations include hypertension, orthostatic hypotension, resting sinus tachycardia, loss of heart rate variability, electrocardiographic ST abnormalities, and both bradycardia and tachycardias. Microneurographic recordings have shown increased sympathetic outflow during the acute illness, which normalizes with recovery. Extreme presentations of autonomic dysfunction have been associated with Takotsubo cardiomyopathy.[51] Life-threatening arrhythmias occur in Guillain-Barré syndrome, primarily in patients requiring assisted ventilation. Arrhythmias observed include asystole, symptomatic bradycardia, rapid atrial fibrillation, and ventricular tachycardia or fibrillation. Asystole commonly was associated with tracheal suctioning. Death may occur as a consequence of an arrhythmia.[52]

Treatment and Prognosis

Supportive care should include deep vein thrombosis prophylaxis in non-ambulant patients. Early plasmapheresis or intravenous immunoglobulin can improve recovery. In severely affected patients, especially those requiring assisted ventilation, cardiac rhythm monitoring is mandatory. It is reasonable to monitor the rhythm via telemetry in all those admitted with Guillain-Barré syndrome. If serious bradycardia or asystole is observed, temporary or permanent pacing can improve survival. Atropine or isoproterenol during tracheal suctioning can be of benefit. Takotsubo cardiomyopathy should be treated with beta blockers and routine treatment for left ventricular dysfunction and cardiac congestion (Chapters 48 and 50). The mortality rate in patients hospitalized with Guillain-Barré syndrome is as high as 15%. In patients who recover from Guillain-Barré syndrome, autonomic function also normalizes, and an increase in the long-term arrhythmia risk has not been observed.

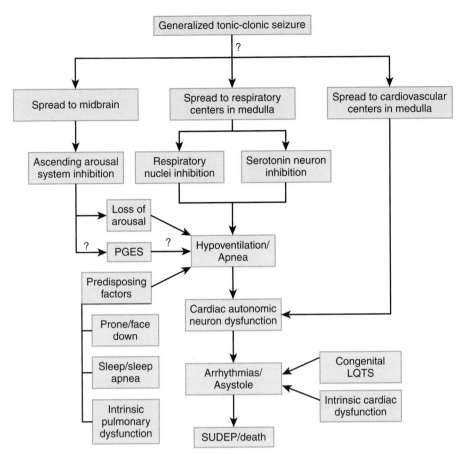

FIGURE 100.17 Pathophysiologic mechanisms underlying sudden unexpected death in epilepsy (SUDEP). SUDEP often results from a generalized tonic-clonic seizure, which leads to inhibition of specific midbrain- and medulla-mediated effects via an unknown pathway. Other factors shown may predispose these patients to SUDEP. *LQTS,* long QT syndrome; *PGES,* postictal generalized EEG suppression. (From Dlouhy BJ, Gehlbach BK, Richerson GB. Sudden unexpected death in epilepsy: basic mechanisms and clinical implications for prevention. *J Neurol Neurosurg Psychiatry.* 2016;87:402.)

Myasthenia Gravis
Clinical Presentation
Myasthenia gravis is a disorder of neuromuscular transmission resulting from production of antibody targeted to the nicotinic acetylcholine receptor or muscle-specific receptor tyrosine kinase.[53] The primary symptom, fluctuating weakness, usually begins with the eye and facial muscles and later can involve the large muscles of the limbs. Patients can present at any age, typically at a younger age in women and at an older age in men. Myasthenia gravis is commonly associated with hyperplasia or a benign or malignant tumor (thymoma) of the thymus gland. Multiple autoimmune diseases can complicate myasthenia gravis. With the development of immune check point inhibitors used in cancer treatment, myasthenia gravis has been associated with immune-related cardiotoxicity with cardiomyopathy and life-threatening ventricular arrhythmias.[54]

Cardiovascular Manifestations
Myocarditis can occur in patients with myasthenia gravis, especially in those with a thymoma (Chapters 55 and 94). The mechanism in myocarditis is a humoral immune response against proteins in striated muscle, including titin, the ryanodine receptor, and a potassium-channel protein (Kv1.4).[53] Up to 16% of patients with myasthenia gravis have cardiac manifestations not explained by another etiologic disorder. Presentation with arrhythmias, which can include atrial fibrillation, atrioventricular block, asystole, ventricular tachycardia, sudden death, or heart failure, is typical. Myasthenic crisis has been associated with stress cardiomyopathy.[55] Autopsy findings are consistent with myocarditis, often giant cell myocarditis. A polymyositis affecting both skeletal and cardiac muscle is seen. In some cases autonomic nervous system dysfunction may be associated with myasthenia gravis.[56]

Treatment and Prognosis
Myasthenia gravis is treated with anticholinesterases and immunosuppressive agents. Thymectomy is often indicated. Anticholinesterase agents may slow the sinus rate and cause heart block and hypotension. Pacing can be necessary. Whether immunosuppressive agents or thymectomy improve associated cardiac disease is unknown. Case reports have described the development of rapidly progressive and fatal heart failure within weeks after thymoma resection in patients in whom histologic examination showed giant cell myocarditis.

Myoglobinopathy
Myoglobinopathy is a recently described adult-onset autosomal dominant progressive centrifugal skeletal myopathy. The skeletal myopathy is variably associated with cardiomyopathy and HF. Myoglobin is highly expressed in the heart, and disease associated mutations have been suggested to accelerate oxygen dissociation from heme and alter the redox state of skeletal and cardiac tissues, increasing superoxide levels.[57] Sarcoplasmic inclusion bodies in both skeletal and cardiac muscle are the hallmark of the disease. The onset of skeletal muscle symptoms is the 5th decade of life with progression with patients becoming non-ambulant over a decade or two. The cause of death in these patients is both respiratory and cardiac failure.

ABCC9-Related Intellectual Disability Myopathy Syndrome
KATP channels (IK-ATP) are heterooctomers of an inwardly rectifying potassium channel, Kir6.x and regulatory sulfonylurea receptor, SURx (Chapter 62). In the pancreas and nerve, K-ATP channels are composed of Kir6.2 *(KCNJ8)* and SUR1 *(ABCC8).* In skeletal and cardiac muscle the channel is formed by the combination of Kir6.2 and SUR2A *(ABCC9).* Mutations in the channel subunits are associated with congenital forms of diabetes and hyperinsulinism as well as Cantu Sydrome.[58] Loss-of-function mutations in *ABCC9* have been described in a syndrome that includes mild intellectual disability, skeletal myopathy characterized by lordosis, facial dysmorphism, reddish-purple skin discoloration (cutis marmorata), abnormal dentition and dilated cardiomyopathy. KATP channel subunits are expressed broadly but the mechanism of production of the manifestations of disease is uncertain. The loss-of-function phenotype suggests that KATP channel activators may be useful in symptom control.

Epilepsy
Cardiovascular Manifestations
Epilepsy is a complex brain disorder characterized by recurrent unprovoked seizures.[59] Patients with epilepsy are at increased risk for sudden death of unknown cause, which has been termed *sudden unexpected death in epilepsy* (SUDEP) (Chapter 70). It is the leading cause of premature death in patients with epilepsy, with an incidence ranging from 0.6 to 9 per 1000 patient-years, depending on the population studied. It accounts for up to 18% of all deaths in people with epilepsy and a lifetime cumulative risk as high as 35% in patients with refractory epilepsy.[60] The mechanisms leading to sudden death in epilepsy are not clear and probably vary. Central or obstructive postictal apnea, mechanical suffocation possibly exacerbated by prone positioning, excessive respiratory secretions, acute pulmonary edema, and arrhythmias all may be involved (Fig. 100.17). A number of drugs affecting the brain prolong the QT interval and may contribute (Chapters 9 and 64).

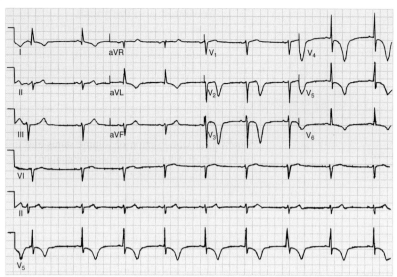

FIGURE 100.18 Electrocardiogram from a patient with cerebral hemorrhage. Deep and symmetric T wave inversions are evident. (Courtesy Dr. Charles Fisch, Indiana University School of Medicine, Indianapolis.)

The role of genetics is an area of active investigation[60] and early repolarization with seizure induced remodeling of cardiac electrophysiology has been suggested.[61–63] A majority of witnessed sudden deaths occur at or in proximity to the time of a seizure. Severe bradycardia with sinus arrest has been documented in monitored patients during seizures, including studies with an implantable loop recorder. Periictal bradycardia is more common in patients with temporal lobe seizures. Whether bradycardia has a role in epileptic patients who experience sudden death is not clear. Ventricular arrhythmia disorders such as long-QT syndrome or right ventricular dysplasia can manifest with symptoms suggestive of epilepsy and could be responsible for a small proportion of sudden deaths. The role of preexisting structural heart disease in SUDEP is uncertain, but the presence of heart disease will increase the arrhythmic risk of seizures. Observational studies have assessed risk factors for SUDEP. These include male sex, onset of epilepsy at a young age, a long duration of epilepsy, high seizure frequency especially of generalized tonic-clonic seizures, and the need for polytherapy to control seizures.

Treatment and Prognosis

A primary rhythm disorder needs to be considered in the differential diagnosis of epilepsy. Patients with poorly controlled epilepsy should be aggressively evaluated and treated at tertiary epilepsy centers. Medications to control seizures may increase the risk of life-threatening cardiac arrhythmias.[61] Particularly in refractory cases, epilepsy surgery should be strongly considered. Patients with ictal bradycardia can require pacemaker implantation. Nighttime supervision of the epileptic patient and supine sleeping positions should be considered although data are limited in support of efficacy of such maneuvers.[64]

Acute Cerebrovascular Disease
Cardiovascular Manifestations

Acute cerebrovascular diseases, including subarachnoid hemorrhage, other stroke syndromes, and head injury, can be associated with severe cardiac manifestations, which represent a major challenge in the management of these patients (Chapter 45). For example, severe adverse cardiac events including acute coronary syndrome, heart failure, and cardiac arrhythmia occur in approximately 20% of patients with ischemic stroke, occurring predominantly within the first 3 days after the event (eFig. 100.8).[65] The patient's age and burden of cardiovascular disease or risk correlate with the individual susceptibility to develop severe cardiovascular complications of stroke (eFig. 100.9). In addition, factors promoting electrical instability such as electrolyte abnormalities and drugs that prolong QT interval, as well as comorbidities that promote autonomic failure (e.g., diabetes) increase the risk of cardiac manifestations of brain injury.

The mechanism by which cardiac abnormalities occur with brain injury is related to autonomic nervous system dysfunction, with both increased sympathetic and parasympathetic output (Chapter 102). Excessive myocardial catecholamine release is primarily responsible for the observed cardiac pathology. Hypothalamic stimulation can reproduce the electrocardiographic changes observed in acute cerebrovascular disease. Electrocardiographic changes associated with hypothalamic stimulation or blood in the subarachnoid space can be diminished with spinal cord transection, stellate ganglion blockade, vagolytics, and adrenergic blockers. Electrocardiographic abnormalities are observed in approximately 70% of patients with subarachnoid hemorrhage. Abnormalities including ST elevation and depression, T-wave inversion, and pathologic Q-waves are observed. Peaked inverted T-waves and a prolonged QT interval can occur in a significant proportion of patients with electrocardiographic abnormalities associated with cerebrovascular disease (Fig. 100.18). Hypokalemia often seen in patients with subarachnoid hemorrhage can increase the likelihood of QT interval prolongation. Other stroke syndromes often are associated with abnormalities on the ECG, but whether these are related to the stroke syndrome or to underlying intrinsic cardiac disease often is difficult to discern. Prolongation of QT interval is more common in subarachnoid hemorrhage than in other stroke syndromes. Closed head trauma can cause electrocardiographic abnormalities similar to those in subarachnoid hemorrhage, including a prolonged QT interval. Myocardial damage with liberation of enzymes and subendocardial hemorrhage or fibrosis at autopsy can occur in the setting of acute cerebral disease. The term *neurogenic stunned myocardium* is used to describe the reversible syndrome. The process can manifest with selective apical involvement, a Takotsubo cardiomyopathy. Cardiac troponin elevation and echocardiographic evidence of left ventricular dysfunction are present in a significant proportion of patients with subarachnoid hemorrhage. Patients with a poorer neurologic status at admission are more likely to have higher peak troponin levels. Women are at higher risk for myocardial necrosis. Pulmonary edema can accompany the acute neurologic insult. The edema can have both a cardiogenic component, related to systemic hypertension and left ventricular dysfunction, and a neurogenic (pulmonary capillary leak) component. Life-threatening arrhythmias can occur in the setting of acute cerebrovascular disease. Ventricular tachycardia or fibrillation has been observed in patients with subarachnoid hemorrhage and head trauma. Torsades de pointes–type ventricular tachycardia can occur (Fig. 100.19) (Chapter 67), often in the setting of a prolonged QT interval and hypokalemia. Stroke syndromes other than subarachnoid hemorrhage appear to be only rarely associated with serious ventricular tachycardias. Atrial arrhythmias, including atrial fibrillation and regular supraventricular tachycardia, have been observed. Atrial fibrillation is most common in patients presenting with acute thromboembolic stroke. Separating an effect from the cause can be difficult. Bradycardias, including sinoatrial block, sinus arrest, and atrioventricular block, occur in up to 10% of patients with subarachnoid hemorrhage.

Treatment and Prognosis

Beta blockers are effective in decreasing myocardial damage and in controlling both supraventricular and ventricular arrhythmias associated with subarachnoid hemorrhage and head trauma. Beta blockers increase the likelihood of bradycardia and cannot be used in patients with hypotension requiring vasopressors. Life-threatening arrhythmias occur primarily in the first day after a neurologic event. Continuous electrocardiographic monitoring during this period is indicated. Careful monitoring of potassium levels, especially in patients with subarachnoid hemorrhage, is warranted. Refractory ventricular arrhythmias have been controlled effectively with stellate ganglion blockade. Electrocardiographic abnormalities reflect unfavorable intracranial factors but do not appear to portend a poor cardiovascular outcome. The magnitude of peak troponin elevation is predictive for adverse

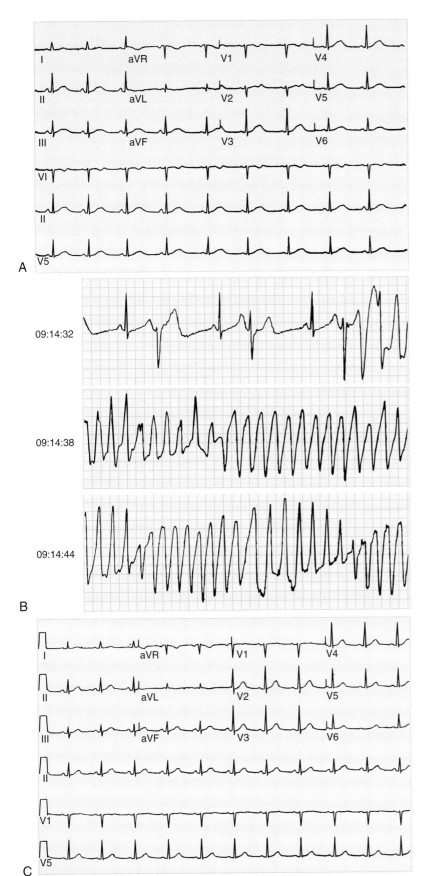

FIGURE 100.19 Cardiac manifestations with cerebral hemorrhage in a 49-year-old patient. **A,** ECG recorded within 3 hours of admission and 4 hours after onset of symptoms. QT interval prolongation is evident. **B,** Electrocardiographic monitoring 6 hours after admission. Ventricular bigeminy precedes the onset of polymorphic ventricular tachycardia. Cardioversion was required. The patient subsequently was treated with a beta-adrenergic blocker without further ventricular tachycardia. **C,** On an ECG obtained 2 weeks after hospital admission, the QT interval has normalized.

patient outcomes, including severe disability at hospital discharge and death.[65] Head injury (blunt trauma or gunshot wound) and cerebrovascular accidents are the leading causes of brain death in patients being considered as heart donors. These donors can manifest electrocardiographic abnormalities, hemodynamic instability, and myocardial dysfunction related primarily to adrenergic storm and not to intrinsic cardiac disease. Experimental studies on whether contractile performance recovers with transplantation are still controversial. Optimization of volume status and inotropic support with careful echocardiographic evaluation and possibly left-heart catheterization can allow the use of some donor hearts that would have otherwise been rejected.

CONCLUSIONS/FUTURE PERSPECTIVES

Neurologic diseases often affect the heart and vascular system, and in many cases, cardiovascular disease limits life expectancy and reduces quality of life in these patients. As such, cardiologists are an integral part in the medical evaluation and treatment of patients with primary neurologic disorders. In several disorders, the cardiovascular manifestations are responsible for a greater risk than that attributable to the neurologic manifestations. An area of ongoing investigation is understanding the mechanisms of cardiac disease produced by neurological and neuromuscular disorders. This work will identify precision diagnostics and therapeutics and has helped to inform biological and gene therapeutic treatment of these disorders.

REFERENCES
Muscular Dystrophies
1. Nikhanj A, Yogasundaram H, Miskew Nichols B, et al. Cardiac intervention improves heart disease and clinical outcomes in patients with muscular dystrophy in a multidisciplinary care setting. *J Am Heart Assoc.* 2020;9:e014004.
2. Kamdar F, Garry DJ. Dystrophin-deficient cardiomyopathy. *J Am Coll Cardiol.* 2016;67:2533–2546.
3. McNally EM, Kaltman JR, Benson DW, et al. Contemporary cardiac issues in Duchenne muscular dystrophy. Working group of the National Heart, Lung, and Blood Institute in collaboration with parent project muscular dystrophy. *Circulation.* 2015;131:1590–1598.
4. Mercuri E, Bonnemann CG, Muntoni F. Muscular dystrophies. *Lancet.* 2019;394:2025–2038.
5. Hor KN, Mah ML, Johnston P, et al. Advances in the diagnosis and management of cardiomyopathy in duchenne muscular dystrophy. *Neuromuscul Disord.* 2018;28:711–716.
6. Power LC, O'Grady GL, Hornung TS, et al. Imaging the heart to detect cardiomyopathy in Duchenne muscular dystrophy: a review. *Neuromuscul Disord.* 2018;28:717–730.
7. Rochitte CE, Liberato G, Silva MC. Comprehensive assessment of cardiac involvement in muscular dystrophies by cardiac MR imaging. *Magn Reson Imaging Clin N Am.* 2019;27:521–531.
8. Adachi K, Hashiguchi S, Saito M, et al. Detection and management of cardiomyopathy in female dystrophinopathy carriers. *J Neurol Sci.* 2018;386:74–80.
9. Ishizaki M, Kobayashi M, Adachi K, et al. Female dystrophinopathy: review of current literature. *Neuromuscul Disord.* 2018;28:572–581.
10. Meyers TA, Heitzman JA, Townsend D. DMD carrier model with mosaic dystrophin expression in the heart reveals complex vulnerability to myocardial injury. *Hum Mol Genet.* 2020;29:944–954.
11. Feingold B, Mahle WT, Auerbach S, et al. Management of cardiac involvement associated with neuromuscular diseases: a scientific statement from the American Heart Association. *Circulation.* 2017;136:e200–e231.
12. Finsterer J, Stollberger C, Maeztu C. Sudden cardiac death in neuromuscular disorders. *Int J Cardiol.* 2016;203:508–515.
13. Birnkrant DJ, Bushby K, Bann CM, et al. Diagnosis and management of Duchenne muscular dystrophy, part 2: respiratory, cardiac, bone health, and orthopaedic management. *Lancet Neurol.* 2018;17:347–361.
14. Bourke JP, Bueser T, Quinlivan R. Interventions for preventing and treating cardiac complications in Duchenne and Becker muscular dystrophy and x-linked dilated cardiomyopathy. *Cochrane Database Syst Rev.* 2018;10:CD009068.
15. Raman SV, Hor KN, Mazur W, et al. Stabilization of early Duchenne cardiomyopathy with aldosterone inhibition: results of the multicenter aidmd trial. *J Am Heart Assoc.* 2019;8:e013501.
16. Wells D, Rizwan R, Jefferies JL, et al. Heart transplantation in muscular dystrophy patients: is it a viable option? *Circ Heart Fail.* 2020;13:e005447.

17. Min YL, Bassel-Duby R, Olson EN. Crispr correction of duchenne muscular dystrophy. *Annu Rev Med*. 2019;70:239–255.
18. Verhaart IEC, Aartsma-Rus A. Therapeutic developments for duchenne muscular dystrophy. *Nat Rev Neurol*. 2019;15:373–386.
19. Wahbi K, Furling D. Cardiovascular manifestations of myotonic dystrophy. *Trends Cardiovasc Med*. 2020;30:232–238.
20. Luetkens JA, von Landenberg C, Isaak A, et al. Comprehensive cardiac magnetic resonance for assessment of cardiac involvement in myotonic muscular dystrophy type 1 and 2 without known cardiovascular disease. *Circ Cardiovasc Imaging*. 2019;12:e009100.
21. Cardona A, Arnold WD, Kissel JT, et al. Myocardial fibrosis by late gadolinium enhancement cardiovascular magnetic resonance in myotonic muscular dystrophy type 1: highly prevalent but not associated with surface conduction abnormality. *J Cardiovasc Magn Reson*. 2019;21:26.
22. Tanawuttiwat T, Wagner KR, Tomaselli G, et al. Left ventricular dysfunction and conduction disturbances in patients with myotonic muscular dystrophy type i and ii. *JAMA Cardiol*. 2017;2:225–228.
23. Kusumoto FM, Schoenfeld MH, Barrett C, et al. 2018 acc/aha/hrs guideline on the evaluation and management of patients with bradycardia and cardiac conduction delay: a report of the American college of cardiology/American heart association task force on clinical practice guidelines and the heart rhythm society. *J Am Coll Cardiol*. 2019;74:e51–e156.
24. McNally EM, Mann DL, Pinto Y, et al. Clinical care recommendations for cardiologists treating adults with myotonic dystrophy. *J Am Heart Assoc*. 2020;9:e014006.
25. Wahbi K, Babuty D, Probst V, et al. Incidence and predictors of sudden death, major conduction defects and sustained ventricular tachyarrhythmias in 1388 patients with myotonic dystrophy type 1. *Eur Heart J*. 2017;38:751–758.
26. Wahbi K, Porcher R, Laforet P, et al. Development and validation of a new scoring system to predict survival in patients with myotonic dystrophy type 1. *JAMA Neurol*. 2018;75:573–581.
27. Muchir A, Worman HJ. Emery-Dreifuss muscular dystrophy: focal point nuclear envelope. *Curr Opin Neurol*. 2019;32:728–734.
28. Wang S, Peng D. Cardiac involvement in Emery-Dreifuss muscular dystrophy and related management strategies. *Int Heart J*. 2019;60:12–18.
29. Limipitikul W, Ong CS, Tomaselli GF. Neuromuscular disease: cardiac manifestations and sudden death risk. *Card Electrophysiol Clin*. 2017;9:731–747.
30. Taghizadeh E, Rezaee M, Barreto GE, et al. Prevalence, pathological mechanisms, and genetic basis of limb-girdle muscular dystrophies: a review. *J Cell Physiol*. 2019;234:7874–7884.
31. Thompson R, Straub V. Limb-girdle muscular dystrophies - international collaborations for translational research. *Nat Rev Neurol*. 2016;12:294–309.
32. Straub V, Murphy A, Udd B, et al. 229th ENMC international workshop: limb girdle muscular dystrophies – Nomenclature and reformed classification Naarden, The Netherlands, 17–19 March 2017. *Neuromuscul Disord*. 2018;28(8):702–710.
33. Hamel J, Tawil R. Facioscapulohumeral muscular dystrophy: update on pathogenesis and future treatments. *Neurotherapeutics*. 2018;15:863–871.
34. Tawil R. Facioscapulohumeral muscular dystrophy. *Handb Clin Neurol*. 2018;148:541–548.
35. Sommerville RB, Vincenti MG, Winborn K, et al. Diagnosis and management of adult hereditary cardio-neuromuscular disorders: a model for the multidisciplinary care of complex genetic disorders. *Trends Cardiovasc Med*. 2017;27:51–58.
36. Arbustini E, Di Toro A, Giuliani L, et al. Cardiac phenotypes in hereditary muscle disorders: JACC state-of-the-art review. *J Am Coll Cardiol*. 2018;72:2485–2506.
37. Kearney M, Orrell RW, Fahey M, et al. Pharmacological treatments for Friedreich ataxia. *Cochrane Database Syst Rev*. 2016:CD007791.
38. McCormick A, Shinnick J, Schadt K, et al. Cardiac transplantation in Friedreich ataxia: extended follow-up. *J Neurol Sci*. 2017;375:471–473.
39. Statland JM, Fontaine B, Hanna MG, et al. Review of the diagnosis and treatment of periodic paralysis. *Muscle Nerve*. 2018;57:522–530.
40. Maffe S, Paffoni P, Bergamasco L, et al. Therapeutic management of ventricular arrhythmias in Andersen-Tawil syndrome. *J Electrocardiol*. 2020;58:37–42.

Other Neuromuscular Diseases

41. El-Hattab AW, Scaglia F. Mitochondrial cardiomyopathies. *Front Cardiovasc Med*. 2016;3:25.
42. Towbin JA, Jefferies JL. Cardiomyopathies due to left ventricular noncompaction, mitochondrial and storage diseases, and inborn errors of metabolism. *Circ Res*. 2017;121:838–854.
43. Kang SL, Forsey J, Dudley D, et al. Clinical characteristics and outcomes of cardiomyopathy in Barth syndrome: the UK experience. *Pediatr Cardiol*. 2016;37:167–176.
44. Nash LA, Burns JK, Chardon JW, et al. Spinal muscular atrophy: more than a disease of motor neurons? *Curr Mol Med*. 2016;16:779–792.
45. Levin AA. Treating disease at the rna level with oligonucleotides. *N Engl J Med*. 2019;380:57–70.
46. Tsikitis M, Galata Z, Mavroidis M, et al. Intermediate filaments in cardiomyopathy. *Biophys Rev*. 2018;10:1007–1031.
47. Brodehl A, Gaertner-Rommel A, Milting H. Molecular insights into cardiomyopathies associated with desmin (des) mutations. *Biophys Rev*. 2018;10:983–1006.
48. Finsterer J, Stollberger C. Arrhythmogenic right ventricular dysplasia in neuromuscular disorders. *Clin Med Insights Cardiol*. 2016;10:173–180.
49. Hilz MJ, Liu M, Roy S, et al. Cardiac involvement in peripheral neuropathies. *J Clin Neuromuscul Dis*. 2016;17:120–128.
50. Hilz MJ, Liu M, Roy S, et al. Autonomic dysfunction in the neurological intensive care unit. *Clin Auton Res*. 2019;29:301–311.
51. Jones T, Umaskanth N, De Boisanger J, et al. Guillain-barre syndrome complicated by Takotsubo cardiomyopathy: an under-recognised association. *BMJ Case Rep*. 2020;13.
52. Gupta S, Verma R, Sethi R, et al. Cardiovascular complications and its relationship with functional outcomes in Guillain-Barre syndrome. *QJM*. 2020;113:93–99.
53. Gilhus NE. Myasthenia gravis. *N Engl J Med*. 2016;375:2570–2581.
54. Hu JR, Florido R, Lipson EJ, et al. Cardiovascular toxicities associated with immune checkpoint inhibitors. *Cardiovasc Res*. 2019;115:854–868.
55. Desai R, Abbas SA, Fong HK, et al. Burden and impact of takotsubo syndrome in myasthenic crisis: a national inpatient perspective on the under-recognized but potentially fatal association. *Int J Cardiol*. 2020;299:63–66.
56. Kocabas ZU, Kizilay F, Basarici I, et al. Evaluation of cardiac autonomic functions in myasthenia gravis. *Neurol Res*. 2018;40:405–412.
57. Olive M, Engvall M, Ravenscroft G, et al. Myoglobinopathy is an adult-onset autosomal dominant myopathy with characteristic sarcoplasmic inclusions. *Nat Commun*. 2019;10:1396.
58. Smeland MF, McClenaghan C, Roessler HI, et al. ABCC9-related intellectual disability myopathy syndrome is a KATP channelopathy with loss-of-function mutations in ABCC9. *Nat Commun*. 2019;10:4457.
59. Krishnamurthy KB. Epilepsy. *Ann Intern Med*. 2016;164. ITC17-32.
60. Chahal CAA, Salloum MN, Alahdab F, et al. Systematic review of the genetics of sudden unexpected death in epilepsy: potential overlap with sudden cardiac death and arrhythmia-related genes. *J Am Heart Assoc*. 2020;9:e012264.
61. Li MCH, O'Brien TJ, Todaro M, et al. Acquired cardiac channelopathies in epilepsy: evidence, mechanisms, and clinical significance. *Epilepsia*. 2019;60:1753–1767.
62. Hayashi K, Kohno R, Akamatsu N, et al. Abnormal repolarization: a common electrocardiographic finding in patients with epilepsy. *J Cardiovasc Electrophysiol*. 2019;30:109–115.
63. Ufongene C, El Atrache R, Loddenkemper T, et al. Electrocardiographic changes associated with epilepsy beyond heart rate and their utilization in future seizure detection and forecasting methods. *Clin Neurophysiol*. 2020;131:866–879.
64. Maguire MJ, Jackson CF, Marson AG, et al. Treatments for the prevention of sudden unexpected death in epilepsy (SUDEP). *Cochrane Database Syst Rev*. 2020;4:CD011792.
65. Scheitz JF, Nolte CH, Doehner W, et al. Stroke-heart syndrome: clinical presentation and underlying mechanisms. *Lancet Neurol*. 2018;17:1109–1120.

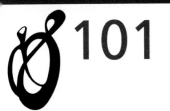 **101** Interface Between Renal Disease and Cardiovascular Illness

PETER A. MCCULLOUGH

Kidney disease confers increased risks for atherosclerotic cardiovascular disease (CVD), myocardial disease and heart failure (HF), arrhythmias, and valvular disease. Obesity, type 2 diabetes mellitus, hypertension (HTN), and increased longevity contribute to an expanding prevalence pool of patients with chronic kidney disease (CKD). Recognition of the stage of CKD is important in cardiology as it influences the approach to the screening, diagnosis, prognosis, and management of many cardiovascular problems as well as the use of many drugs. Both pharmacologic and interventional management of patients with heart disease can be designed to minimize risk to the kidneys and in some scenarios simultaneously improve the risk of major adverse renal and cardiovascular events.

THE CARDIORENAL INTERSECTION

The heart and kidney are inextricably linked in terms of hemodynamic and regulatory functions. In a normal 70-kg human, each kidney weighs about 130 to 170 g and receives blood flow of 400 mL/min per 100 g, which is approximately 20% to 25% of the cardiac output, allowing the needed flow to maintain glomerular filtration by approximately 1 million nephrons (Fig. 101.1). This flow is several times greater per unit weight than most other organs due to lower vascular resistance. Although the oxygen extraction is low, the kidneys account for about 8% of the total oxygen consumption of the body. The kidney has a central role in electrolyte balance, protein metabolism, and blood pressure regulation. Communication between these two organs occurs at multiple levels, including the sympathetic nervous system (SNS), the renin-angiotensin-aldosterone system (RAAS), vasopressin, endothelin, and the natriuretic peptides.

The obesity pandemic is spawning secondary epidemics of type 2 diabetes mellitus (DM) and HTN often leading to CKD and CVD.[1] Among those with DM for 25 years or more, the prevalence of diabetic nephropathy as a result of microvascular disease in type 1 and type 2 DM is about 50%.[2] Approximately half of all cases of end-stage renal disease (ESRD) result from diabetic nephropathy. All forms of kidney disease have a more rapid progression when there are maladaptive mutations in apoprotein L1 (bound to high-density lipoprotein particles and expressed in the podocytes, proximal tubules, and vascular endothelium). Mutant apoprotein L1 protects against African trypanosomiasis but is associated with both kidney and coronary heart disease (Fig. 101.2).[3] With the aging of the general population and cardiovascular care shifting toward the elderly, age-related decreased renal function comprises a major adverse prognostic factor after CVD events. CKD accelerates the progression of atherosclerosis, myocardial disease, valvular disease, and promotes an array of cardiac arrhythmias leading to sudden death.[4]

CHRONIC KIDNEY DISEASE AND CARDIOVASCULAR RISK

A range of estimated glomerular filtration rate (eGFR) values derived from equations defines CKD.[5] A common definition for CKD stipulates an eGFR of less than 60 mL/min/1.73 m^2 or the presence of kidney damage. With aging (age 20 to 80), the eGFR declines from about 130 to 60 mL/min/1.73 m^2, and a variety of pathobiological processes emerge when the eGFR drops below 60 mL/min/1.73 m^2 or stage 3 CKD (approximately a serum creatinine [Cr] of 1.2 mg/dL in a woman and 1.5 mg/dL in a man). Because Cr is a crude indicator of renal function and often underestimates renal dysfunction in women and the elderly, eGFR or creatinine clearance (CrCl) calculated by the CKD-EPI (Chronic Kidney Disease Epidemiology Collaboration) and Cockcroft-Gault equation, improve the assessment of renal function. CrCl is used most often for drug dosing since it incorporates body weight. For classification of disease, and prognosis, the CKD-EPI equation is preferred because it does not rely on body weight and associates best with adverse outcomes including death. The equation is: eGFR = $141 \times \min (Cr/\kappa, 1)\alpha \times \max(Cr/\kappa, 1) - 1.209 \times 0.993 \times$ age (yr) $\times 1.018$ [if female] $\times 1.159$ [if Black]; where: Cr is serum creatinine in mg/dL, κ is 0.7 for females and 0.9 for males, α is –0.329 for females and –0.411 for males, min indicates the minimum of Cr/κ or 1, and max indicates the maximum of Cr/κ or 1.

Another approved blood test reflecting renal filtration function and used in eGFR equations is Cystatin-C.[6] Cystatin C is a 13 kDa protein produced by all nucleated cells. Its low molecular mass and its high isoelectric point allow it to be freely filtered by the glomerulus and 100% reabsorbed by the proximal tubule. The serum concentration of cystatin C correlates with eGFR and, in combination with a stable production rate, provides a sensitive marker of renal filtration function. Serum levels of cystatin C do not depend on weight and height, muscle mass, age or sex, making it less variable than Cr. Furthermore,

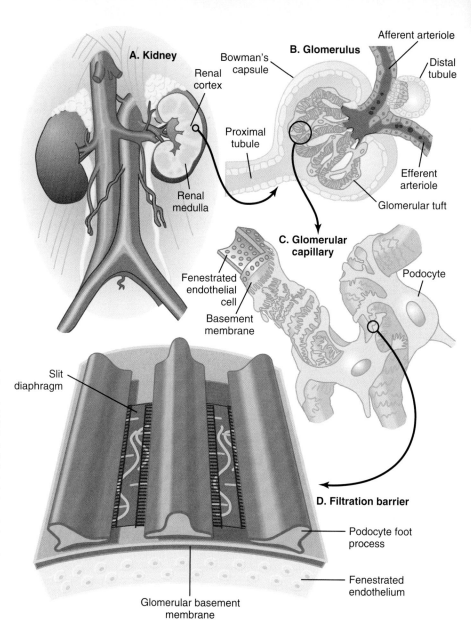

FIGURE 101.1 Normal structure of the glomerular vasculature. Each kidney contains about 1 million glomeruli in the renal cortex (*Part A, Kidney*). *Part B, Glomerulus,* shows an afferent arteriole entering Bowman's capsule and branching into several capillaries that form the glomerular tuft; the walls of the capillaries constitute the actual filter. The plasma filtrate (primary urine) is directed to the proximal tubule, whereas the unfiltered blood returns to the circulation through the efferent arteriole. The filtration barrier of the capillary wall contains an innermost fenestrated endothelium, the glomerular basement membrane, and a layer of interdigitating podocyte foot processes (*Part C, Glomerular capillary*). In *Part D, Filtration barrier,* a cross section through the glomerular capillary depicts the fenestrated endothelial layer and the glomerular basement membrane with overlying podocyte foot processes. An ultrathin slit diaphragm spans the filtration slit between the foot processes, slightly above the basement membrane. To show the slit diaphragm, the foot processes are drawn smaller than actual scale. (Adapted from Tryggvason K, Patrakka J, Wartiovaara J. Hereditary proteinuria syndromes and mechanisms of proteinuria. *N Engl J Med.* 2006;354[13]:1387–1401.)

measurements can be made and interpreted from a single random sample with reference intervals in women and men being 0.54 to 1.21 mg/L (median 0.85 mg/L, range 0.42 to 1.39 mg/L).

In addition, microalbuminuria at any level of eGFR indicates CKD and occurs as the result of endothelial dysfunction or damage in glomerular capillaries secondary to the metabolic syndrome, DM, and HTN. The most widely accepted definition of microalbuminuria is a random urine albumin/Cr ratio (ACR) of 30 to 300 mg/g. An ACR greater than 300 mg/g is considered gross proteinuria. The random, spot ACR is the office test for microalbuminuria recommended as part of the cardiovascular and renal risk assessment done by cardiologists and other specialists. Microalbuminuria independently predicts CVD risk for those with and without DM. The amount of albumin and protein in the urine is the most important prognostic factor for the rapid progression of CKD to ESRD.[7] In addition both the eGFR and degree of albuminuria contribute independently to the risks of future acute kidney injury (AKI), myocardial infarction (MI), stroke, HF, and death (Fig. 101.3).[8]

IMPLICATIONS OF ANEMIA DUE TO CHRONIC KIDNEY DISEASE

Blood hemoglobin (Hb) concentration is associated with CKD, and CVD. The World Health Organization defines anemia as a Hb level less than 13 g/dL in men and less than 12 g/dL in women:

approximately 9% of the general adult population meets this definition. Some 20% of patients with stable coronary disease and 30% to 60% of patients with HF have anemia due to CKD. Hence, anemia is a common and easily identifiable potential cause of constitutional symptoms as well as a potential diagnostic and therapeutic target, particularly in the setting of iron deficiency or reduced availability of vitamin B_{12} or folic acid.

Anemia is associated with multiple adverse outcomes, and decreases tissue oxygen delivery and utilization.[13] The cause of anemia in patients with CKD can be multifactorial due to impairment in iron transport and a relative deficiency of erythropoietin-α (EPO), an erythrocyte stimulating protein (ESP), which is normally produced by renal parenchymal cells in response to blood partial pressure of oxygen under the control of gene regulator hypoxia-inducible factor (HIF). Patients with CKD and HF resist the effects of EPO. In addition, increased circulating levels of hepcidin-25, an inhibitor of the ferroportin receptor, impair iron absorption and utilization throughout the body including the bone marrow. As Hb drops over the course of CKD, HF hospitalizations and death increase. Conversely, those patients who have had a spontaneous rise in Hb whether it be due to improved nutrition, reduced neurohormonal factors, or other unknown reasons, enjoy a significant reduction in endpoints over the next several years. This improvement is associated with a significant reduction in left ventricular mass index, suggesting a favorable change in left ventricular remodeling.

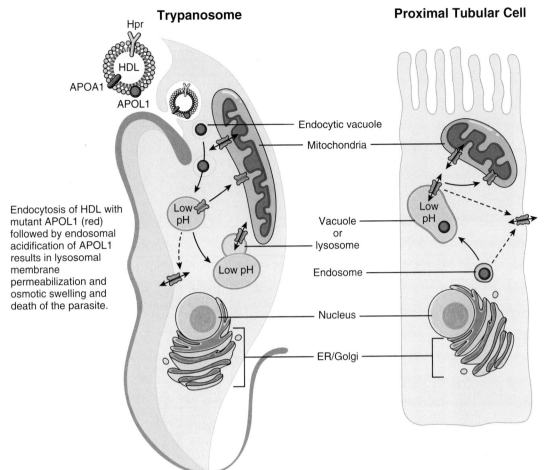

Trypanosome

Hpr
HDL
APOA1
APOL1

Endocytosis of HDL with mutant APOL1 (red) followed by endosomal acidification of APOL1 results in lysosomal membrane permeabilization and osmotic swelling and death of the parasite.

Proximal Tubular Cell

Endocytic vacuole
Mitochondria
Low pH
Vacuole or lysosome
Low pH
Endosome
Nucleus
ER/Golgi

Mutant APOL1 is produced by normal biosynthetic pathways within the cell. APOL1 caused an increase in endocytic activity and reduced organelle acidification, mitochondrial dysfunction, cell hypertrophy and death. APOL1 may insert into plasma membranes (dashed lines) of both trypanosomes and human kidney cells.

FIGURE 101.2 APOL1 killing mechanisms applied to trypanosomes and normal human kidney cells by intracellular, membrane-associated and intracellular APOL1. (Adapted from Bruggeman LA, O'Toole JF, Sedor JR. Identifying the Intracellular Function of APOL1. *J Am Soc Nephrol.* 2017;28[4]:1008–1011.)

Treatment of anemia with exogenous ESPs (EPO and darbepoetin-α) increasing the Hb level from below 10 g/dL to 12 g/dL has been linked to favorable changes in left ventricular remodeling, improved ejection fraction, improved functional classification, and higher levels of peak oxygen consumption with exercise testing. However, treatment with EPO and supplemental iron which is needed in approximately 70% of cases of ESRD, is associated with three problems: (1) increased platelet activity, thrombin generation, and resultant increased risk of thrombosis; (2) elevated endothelin and asymmetric dimethylarginine which theoretically reduces nitric oxide availability, and can raise blood pressure; and (3) worsened measures of oxidative stress. Randomized trials of ESAs targeting higher levels of Hb in CKD have shown higher rates of CVD events and no improvement in mortality, progression of CKD, or health-related quality of life.[9–11] The Reduction of Events With Darbepoetin Alfa in Heart Failure Trial Failure (RED-HF) randomized, 2278 patients with systolic HF and mild-to-moderate anemia (Hb = 9.0 to 12.0 g/dL) to receive darbepoetin alfa approximately 60 to 600 μg SQ q 2 to 4 weeks (target Hb = 13 g/dL) or placebo and found no reductions in HF hospitalizations or death, but a 35% excess risk of thromboembolic complications with the ESA.[12] When the dose exposure of ESA is taken into account, it appears that cardiovascular drug toxicity and not the Hb accounts for the adverse outcomes reported in ESA trials.[13] As a result of these trials, the current strategy is to use ESA sparingly to maintain a Hb concentration to avoid symptoms and the need for transfusion.

High-dose oral or intravenous iron may overcome the iron-reutilization defect in CKD anemia.[14] In a meta-analysis of 64 trials (including five studies of HF patients) comprising 9004 patients, iron associated with elevations in Hb and reductions in the need for transfusion.[15] Analysis of the five trials of HF patients with iron deficiency (509 patients received iron therapy and 342 controls) showed that intravenous iron is associated with reductions in HF hospitalizations

and cardiovascular death (OR 0.39, 95% CI 0.24 to 0.63, P = 0.0001) and improvements in multiple measures of functional status.[16] While these results need confirmation in large-scale clinical trials, they support consideration of iron repletion in patients with CKD, anemia, and HF when there is evidence of iron deficiency (iron saturation <20% and ferritin <200 ng/mL).

HIF is short-lived due to a prolylhydroxylase that breaks down this regulator of EPO expression. There are oral HIF prolyl hydroxylase inhibitors that stabilize HIF and allow greater endogenous production of EPO, improved iron transport, and elevated Hb concentrations.[17] Phase III trials have demonstrated efficacy in maintaining Hb along with cardiovascular safety in pre-dialysis CKD and ESRD.[18,19]

CONTRAST-INDUCED ACUTE KIDNEY INJURY (SEE ALSO CHAPTER 21 AND FIG. 21.2)

Iodinated contrast-induced acute kidney injury (CI-AKI) is most commonly defined by the Kidney Disease International Global Outcomes criteria of a ≥0.3 (mg/dL) rise in serum Cr from baseline within 48 hours of intravascular administration or a ≥50% elevation from baseline over the course of hospitalization.[20] The National Cardiovascular Data Registry Cath-PCI (n = 985,737 who underwent elective and urgent percutaneous coronary intervention [PCI]) reported 69,658 (7.1%) cases of CI-AKI (Cr rise ≥0.3 mg/dL) and 3005 (0.3%) cases of AKI requiring dialysis.[21] Transient rises in Cr are associated with longer hospital ward and intensive care unit stays, MI, stroke, HF, rehospitalization, and death after coronary angiography, PCI, and angiography followed by cardiac surgery (Fig. 101.4).[22]

Post angiography-AKI has three potential pathophysiologic mechanisms: (1) direct toxicity of iodinated contrast material to nephrons,

ALL-CAUSE MORTALITY

	ACR <10	ACR 10–29	ACR 30–299	ACR ≥300
eGFR >105	1.1	1.5	2.2	5.0
eGFR 90-105	Ref	1.4	1.5	3.1
eGFR 75-90	1.0	1.3	1.7	2.3
eGFR 60-75	1.0	1.4	1.8	2.7
eGFR 45-60	1.3	1.7	2.2	3.6
eGFR 30-45	1.9	2.3	3.3	4.9
eGFR 15-30	5.3	3.6	4.7	6.6

CARDIOVASCULAR MORTALITY

	ACR <10	ACR 10–29	ACR 30–299	ACR ≥300
eGFR >105	0.9	1.3	2.3	2.1
eGFR 90-105	Ref	1.5	1.7	3.7
eGFR 75-90	1.0	1.3	1.6	3.7
eGFR 60-75	1.0	1.4	2.0	4.1
eGFR 45-60	1.5	2.2	2.8	4.3
eGFR 30-45	2.2	2.7	3.4	5.2
eGFR 15-30	14	7.9	4.8	8.1

KIDNEY FAILURE (ESRD)

	ACR <10	ACR 10–29	ACR 30–299	ACR ≥300
eGFR >105	Ref	Ref	7.8	18
eGFR 90-105	Ref	Ref	11	20
eGFR 75-90	Ref	Ref	3.8	48
eGFR 60-75	Ref	Ref	7.4	67
eGFR 45-60	5.2	22	40	147
eGFR 30-45	56	74	294	763
eGFR 15-30	433	1044	1056	2286

AKI

	ACR <10	ACR 10–29	ACR 30–299	ACR ≥300
eGFR >105	Ref	Ref	2.7	8.4
eGFR 90-105	Ref	Ref	2.4	5.8
eGFR 75-90	Ref	Ref	2.5	4.1
eGFR 60-75	Ref	Ref	3.3	6.4
eGFR 45-60	2.2	4.9	6.4	5.9
eGFR 30-45	7.3	10	12	20
eGFR 15-30	17	17	21	29

PROGRESSIVE CKD

	ACR <10	ACR 10–29	ACR 30–299	ACR ≥300
eGFR >105	Ref	Ref	0.4	3.0
eGFR 90-105	Ref	Ref	0.9	3.3
eGFR 75-90	Ref	Ref	1.9	5.0
eGFR 60-75	Ref	Ref	3.2	8.1
eGFR 45-60	3.1	4.0	9.4	57
eGFR 30-45	3.0	19	15	22
eGFR 15-30	4.0	12	21	7.7

FIGURE 101.3 Relative risks of heart and kidney outcomes in cohorts where eGFR and ACR where measured. *ACR,* Albumin/Cr ratio; *AKI,* Acute kidney injury; *CKD,* chronic kidney disease; *eGFR,* estimated glomerular filtration rate; *ESRD,* end-stage renal disease. (Adapted from Chronic Kidney Disease Prognosis Consortium, Matsushita K, van der Velde M, et al. Association of estimated glomerular filtration rate and albuminuria with all-cause and cardiovascular mortality in general population cohorts: a collaborative meta-analysis. *Lancet.* 2010;375[9731]:2073–2081.)

(2) microshowers of atheroemboli to the kidneys (due to catheter and wire exchanges above the renal arteries), and (3) contrast material- and atheroemboli-induced intrarenal vasoconstriction. Direct toxicity to nephrons with iodinated contrast media appears related to the ionicity and osmolality of the contrast media given in the milieu of CKD.[22] Microshowers of cholesterol emboli may occur in about 50% of percutaneous interventions using an aortic approach; most episodes are clinically silent.[23] However, in approximately 1% of high-risk cases, an acute cholesterol emboli syndrome can develop, manifested by acute renal failure, mesenteric ischemia, decreased microcirculation to the extremities, and, in some cases, embolic stroke. Because there is less trans-aortic movement of wires and catheters, trans-radial coronary intervention is associated with approximately 22% to 50% lower rates of CI-AKI.[24,25] Intrarenal vasoconstriction as a pathological vascular response to contrast media in CKD and perhaps as an organ reaction to superimposed cholesterol microemboli also injure the kidney. Hypoxia triggers activation of the renal SNS and further reduces renal blood flow (Fig. 101.5). The most important predictor of CI-AKI is eGFR less than 60 mL/min/1.73 m², a proxy for a reduced number of functioning nephrons that must take on the filtration load with increased oxygen demands in the face of reduced delivery, and hence a greater susceptibility to cytotoxic, ischemic, and oxidative injury.[22]

PREVENTION OF CONTRAST-INDUCED ACUTE KIDNEY INJURY

Patients with preexisting CKD (baseline eGFR <60 mL/min/1.73 m²), and in particular, those with CKD and DM merit a mitigation strategy for CI-AKI. The presence of CKD, DM, and other risk factors including hemodynamic instability, use of intra-aortic balloon counterpulsation,

HF, older age, and anemia in the same patient entail a risk of CI-AKI over 50%.[26] The informed consent process of a high-risk patient before the use of intravascular iodinated contrast should include discussion of CI-AKI. CI-AKI prevention involves consideration of four issues: (1) intravascular volume expansion, (2) choice and quantity of contrast material, (3) trans-radial or femoral approach, and (4) postprocedural monitoring and expectant care.

Because iodinated contrast is water soluble, it is amenable to prevention strategies that expand intravascular volume, increase renal filtration and tubular flow of urine into collecting ducts, and then into the ureters and bladder. CI-AKI responds to intravascular administration of isotonic crystalloid solutions to enhance renal elimination of contrast via the urine. Numerous randomized trials have compared isotonic bicarbonate solutions to intravenous saline. The largest and highest quality trials have shown no differences in the rates of renal outcomes.[27,28] Patient factors should guide the use of either isotonic crystalloid solution. The POSEIDON (Prevention of Contrast Renal Injury with Different Hydration Strategies) trial randomized 396 patients with eGFR less than 60 mL/min/1.73 m² and one additional risk factor to a strategy of measurement of left ventricular end-diastolic pressure (LVEDP) and expanding plasma volume versus usual care. Each group had standard of care of normal saline 3 mL/kg for 1 hour before cardiac catheterization. The LVEDP guided approach with more intensive fluid administration during and after the procedure resulted in a 69% relative risk reduction in CI-AKI, p = 0.005. Thus, it is reasonable to consider a 250 mL intravenous administration of normal saline before the procedure and achieve a urine output of approximately 150 mL/hr throughout and after the procedure.

Randomized trials of iodinated contrast agents have demonstrated the lowest rates of CI-AKI with nonionic, iso-osmolar iodixanol. A meta-analysis restricted to 25 head-to-head, prospective, double-blind,

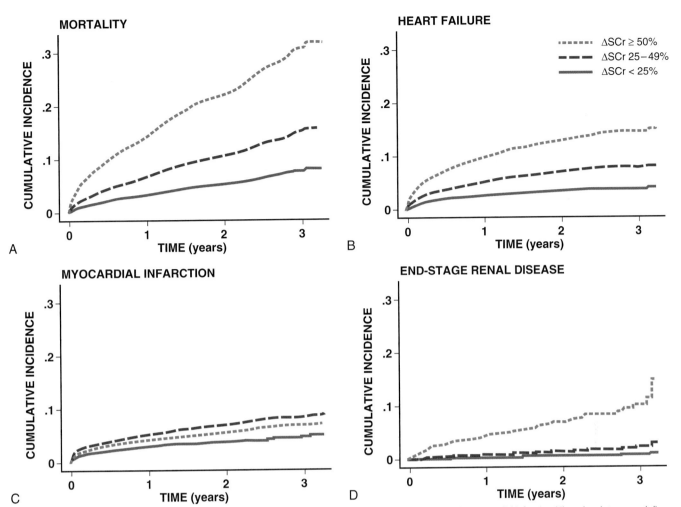

FIGURE 101.4 Cumulative incidence of all-cause mortality (**A**), hospitalization for heart failure (**B**), hospitalization for myocardial infarction (**C**), and end-stage renal disease following coronary angiography (**D**), according to severity of acute kidney injury as reflected by magnitude of change in serum creatinine (ΔScr) concentration after coronary angiography. Coronary angiography alone = 4219, with PCI = 8205, with cardiac surgery = 2412. *PCI,* Percutaneous coronary intervention. (Adapted from James MT, Ghali WA, Knudtson ML, et al. Associations between acute kidney injury and cardiovascular and renal outcomes after coronary angiography. *Circulation.* 2011;123[4]:409–416.)

randomized, controlled trials that compared iodixanol with low-osmolar contrast media (LOCM) in adult patients undergoing angiographic examinations with serum Cr values at baseline and following CM administration.[29] The relative risk of CI-AKI (Cr rise ≥0.5 mg/dL) occurring for iodixanol was 0.46, p= 0.004, compared to LOCM as summarized in Figure 101.6. These data indicate that iodixanol (290 mOsm/kg) is less nephrotoxic than LOCM agents with osmolalities ranging from 600 to 800 mOsm/kg when given intra-arterially. However, there appears to be no significant difference in rates of CI-AKI between iodixanol and LOCM when contrast is administered in lower-risk patients or intravenously.[29]

Although it is desirable to limit contrast to the smallest volume possible in any setting, there is disagreement about a "safe" contrast limit. The lower the eGFR, the less contrast material may cause CI-AKI. In general, it is desirable to limit the contrast medium to less than 30 mL for a diagnostic procedure and less than 100 mL for an interventional procedure. If staged procedures are planned, it is advantageous to have more than 10 days between the first and second contrast exposures if CI-AKI has occurred with the first procedure. As mentioned above, the trans-radial approach is associated with significantly lower risk of CI-AKI when controlling for all other factors.[30]

Most trials of preventive strategies for CI-AKI have been small, underpowered, and inconclusive. After many small, suggestive studies, a large (*n* = 2308) randomized trial of N-acetylcysteine 1200 mg p.o. bid the day before and after the procedure showed no differences in the rates of CI-AKI (12.7% for both groups), ESRD, or other outcomes.[31] This result received support from a larger trial (*n* = 5177) of diagnostic angiography and PCI demonstrating no impact of N-acetylcysteine or sodium

bicarbonate.[32] As a result, neither N-acetylcysteine nor any other drug or intravenous solution is approved for the prevention of CI-AKI.

A suggested algorithm for risk stratification and prevention of CI-AKI is shown in Figure 101.7. An eGFR less than 60 mL/min/1.73 m² mandates preprocedural volume expansion, use of trans-radial access if possible, iodixanol or LOCM as the contrast agent, and minimization of contrast volume. Postprocedural monitoring is critical in the current era of short stays and outpatient procedures. In general, high-risk patients in the hospital should have hydration started 1 to 3 hours before the procedure and continued at least 3 hours afterward. Serum Cr should be measured 24 hours after the procedure. Outpatients, particularly those with eGFR less than 60 mL/min/1.73 m², should have either an overnight stay or discharge to home with 48-hour follow-up and serum Cr measurement. If severe CI-AKI is going to develop, patients usually have a rise of Cr greater than 0.5 mg/dL in the first 24 hours after the procedure. Thus, for those who do not have this degree of serum Cr elevation and are otherwise uncomplicated, discharge to home may be considered. Those patients with eGFR less than 30 mL/min/1.73 m², should have a discussion of the possibility of dialysis and nephrology consultation for possible pre- and post-procedure hemofiltration and dialysis management.

CARDIAC SURGERY ASSOCIATED ACUTE KIDNEY INJURY

AKI occurs in approximately 15% of patients after forms of cardiac surgery with or without use of cardiopulmonary bypass. Rates of AKI are

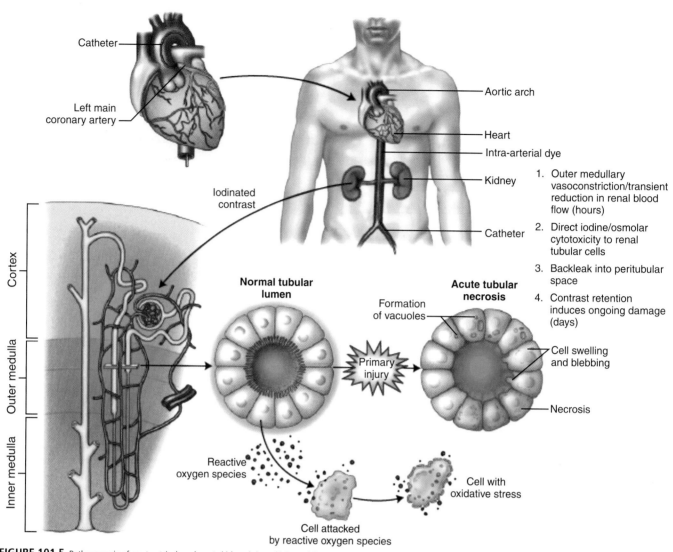

1. Outer medullary vasoconstriction/transient reduction in renal blood flow (hours)
2. Direct iodine/osmolar cytotoxicity to renal tubular cells
3. Backleak into peritubular space
4. Contrast retention induces ongoing damage (days)

FIGURE 101.5 Pathogenesis of contrast-induced acute kidney injury. (Adapted from Brown JR, McCullough PA. *Contrast Nephropathy and Kidney Injury Textbook of Cardiovascular Intervention.* Springer; 2011.)

Meta-analysis, year	Administration	CI-AKI definition	IOCM	LOCM	RR (95% CI)	*P* value	RR and 95% CI
McCullough, 2011	IV	≥0.5 mg/dL	158	157	0.968 (0.19–4.97)	0.968	
From, 2010	IV/IA	mixed	3192	3046	0.77 (0.56–1.06)	0.11	
Reed, 2009	IV/IA	mixed	1291	1289	0.79 (0.56–1.12)	0.189	
Heinrich, 2009	IV/IA	≥0.5 mg/dL	1303	1238	0.75 (0.44–1.26)	0.27	
McCullough, 2011	IA	≥0.5 mg/dL	2396	2373	0.46 (0.27–0.79)	0.004	

0.01 0.1 1 10 100

Favors IOCM
Iso-osmolar
iodixanol

Favors LOCM
Iomeprol
Iopamidol
Iopromide
Ioversol
others

FIGURE 101.6 Compilation of pooled odds ratios from head-to-head trials for IA, IV, and mixed IA and IV meta-analyses of the incidence of CI-AKI (defined as ≥0.5 mg/dL increase in sCr from baseline) demonstrating a leftward shift in pooled estimates moving from IV, to mixed IV/IA, and IA trials favoring the use of iodixanol. *CI-AKI*, Contrast-induced acute kidney injury. (Adapted from McCullough PA, Brown JR. Effects of intra-arterial and intravenous iso-osmolar contrast medium (iodixanol) on the risk of contrast-induced acute kidney injury: a meta-analysis. *Cardiorenal Med.* 2011;1[4]:220–234.)

higher when coronary angiography is done on the same day or less than 5 days between the angiogram and the surgery.[33] Cardiac surgery exposes patients to many factors including endogenous/exogenous toxins (free heme, catalytic iron), metabolic factors, ischemia and reperfusion, neurohormonal activation, inflammation, and oxidative stress, all of which may contribute to renal tubular injury heralded by reduced urine output and a rise in serum Cr after cardiac surgery.[34] KDIGO (Kidney Disease Global Outcomes) criteria can be used to identify AKI in this patient group (Fig. 101.8).[20] Various blood and urine markers may predict post-operative AKI.[34] Off-pump cardiac surgery

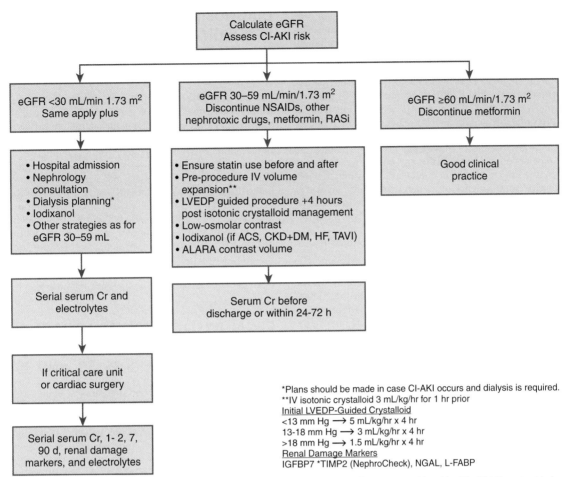

FIGURE 101.7 Algorithm for management of patients receiving iodinated contrast media. *ALARA,* As low as reasonably achievable; *CI-AKI,* contrast-induced acute kidney injury; *CKD,* chronic kidney disease; *Cr,* creatinine; *eGFR,* estimated glomerular filtration rate; *NSAIDs,* nonsteroidal anti-inflammatory agents. (Adapted from McCullough PA, Choi JP, Feghali GA, et al. Contrast-induced acute kidney injury. *J Am Coll Cardiol.* 2016;68[13]:1465–1473.)

Stage	Serum creatinine	Urine output
1	1.5–1.9 × baseline or ≥0.3 mg/dl (≥26.5 mmol/L) increase	<0.5 mL/kg/h for 6–12 h
2	2.0–2.9 × baseline	<0.5 mL/kg/h for >12 h
3	3.0 × baseline, or increase in serum creatinine ≥4.0 mg/dL (≥353.6 mmol/L), or initiation of RRT, or decrease in eGFR <35 mL/min/1.73 m² for patients <18 years	<0.3 mL/kg/h for ≥24 h or anuria for ≥12 h

FIGURE 101.8 Stages of acute kidney injury according to the KDIGO classification. *eGFR,* Estimated glomerular filtration rate; *KDIGO,* kidney disease: Improving global outcomes; *RRT,* renal replacement therapy. (Adapted from KDIGO AKI Work Group. KDIGO clinical practice guideline for acute kidney injury. *Kidney Int Suppl.* 2012;17:1–138.)

does not seem to lower rates of AKI. Trials of natriuretic peptides, corticosteroids, alpha melanocytic stimulating hormone agonists, complement inhibitors, and remote ischemic preconditioning have failed to prevent AKI. Thus, there are no accepted forms of prophylaxis or treatment for cardiac surgery associated with AKI at this time.

ACCELERATION OF VASCULAR CALCIFICATION

When the eGFR falls below 60 mL/min/1.73 m², filtration and elimination of phosphorus falls. In addition, a lower production of 1,25 dihydroxyvitamin D leads to a relative hypocalcemia. Thus, subtle degrees of hyperphosphatemia and hypocalcemia trigger increased release of parathyroid hormone (PTH) causing liberation of calcium and phosphorus from bone. The bone, in turn, produces greater amounts of fibroblast growth factor-23, which directs the kidneys to increase the clearance of phosphorus but also promotes left ventricular hypertrophy (LVH). As a result of this abnormal bone and mineral metabolism,

patients with ESRD have markedly increased absolute values and rates of accumulation of arterial calcification as well as LVH. A variety of in vitro stimuli can induce vascular smooth muscle cells to assume osteoblast-like functions, including handling of phosphorus, oxidized low-density lipoprotein cholesterol (LDL-C), vascular calcification factor, PTH, and PTH-related peptide.

No specific strategy to manipulate calcium-phosphorus balance or to treat secondary hyperparathyroidism changes the annual rate of increase in coronary artery calcium score or cardiovascular events.[35–37]

RENAL DISEASE AND HYPERTENSION (SEE ALSO CHAPTER 26)

The kidney is a central regulator of blood pressure and controls intraglomerular pressure through autoregulation. Sodium retention stimulates increases in systemic and renal arteriolar pressure in an attempt to force greater degrees of filtration in the glomerulus. Glomerular injury activates a variety of pathways that further increase systemic blood pressure. This effect sets up a vicious circle of more glomerular and tubulointerstitial injury and worsened HTN. A cornerstone of management of combined CKD and CVD is strict blood pressure control. In most patients with CKD and proteinuria, three or more antihypertensive agents are needed to achieve a goal blood pressure of less than 130/80 mm Hg.[38] The Systolic Blood Pressure Intervention Trial (SPRINT) randomized 9361 patients without DM having a mean eGFR of 71 mL/min/1.72 m² and found that a systolic blood pressure target of 120 mm Hg is associated with reduced rates of first occurrence of MI, acute coronary syndrome (ACS), stroke, HF, or death from cardiovascular causes. However, there were no differences in the rates of progression to CKD, ESRD, or any other renal outcome. When a significant (≥20%) reduction in eGFR was seen within the first 6 months of intensive combination antihypertensive therapy, there was a 33% reduction in cardiovascular events and no difference in mortality suggesting the blood pressure reduction should not be compromised for excess concern over Cr.[39] The key lifestyle issues for management of CKD and HTN include dietary changes with sodium restriction, weight reduction of ≥15% to a target body mass index less than 25 kg/m², and exercise for 60 min/day most days of the week. Pharmacological therapy aims for strict blood pressure control with an agent that antagonizes the RAAS often in combined action with a thiazide-type diuretic. Dihydropyridine calcium channel blockers alone because of relative afferent arteriolar dilation increase intraglomerular pressure and worsen glomerular injury, and thus should be avoided as singular agents for blood pressure control. Combinations of multiple RAAS-blocking drugs (angiotensin converting enzyme inhibitors [ACEI], angiotensin II receptor blockers [ARB], direct renin inhibitor) provide no additional benefit but cause more complications. Clinical clues such as poorly controlled blood pressure on more than three agents, abdominal bruits, smoking history, peripheral arterial disease, and a marked change in serum Cr with administration of ACEI/ARB should raise the possibility of bilateral renal artery stenosis.[40] Although renal artery stenosis accounts for less than 3% of ESRD cases, it represents a potentially treatable condition (see Chapters 26 and 44). Catheter-based renal sympathetic denervation improves blood pressure in patients with resistant HTN, and additional trials are addressing lesser degrees of HTN and clinical outcomes including major cardiovascular events including HF.[41]

DIAGNOSIS OF ACUTE CORONARY SYNDROMES IN PATIENTS WITH CHRONIC KIDNEY DISEASE (SEE ALSO CHAPTERS 38 AND 39)

Patients with CKD have higher rates of silent ischemia, which cluster with serious arrhythmias, HF, and other cardiac events. About half of stable outpatients with CKD will have a high-sensitivity cardiac troponin I (cTnI) or cTnT above the 99th percentile of normal.[42] The degree of elevation of cTn is associated with left ventricular mass, coronary disease, severity of renal disease, and all-cause mortality.[43] Thus with the use of high-sensitivity assays, in general, cTnI is more advantageous in the diagnostic evaluation of CKD or ESRD patients with acute chest discomfort, while chronic elevations of cTnT are more common and more prognostic in stable patients. The diagnosis of MI in patients with CKD or ESRD can be confirmed with serial troponin measurements demonstrating approximately fivefold rise above the first value since so many are above the 99th percentile of normal at baseline.[44] The skeletal myopathy of CKD can elevate creatine kinase, myoglobin, and some older generation cTnI/cTnT assays, making these tests less desirable.

RENAL DYSFUNCTION AS A PROGNOSTIC FACTOR IN ACUTE CORONARY SYNDROMES (SEE ALSO CHAPTERS 35, 38, AND 39)

Advances in the diagnosis and treatment of acute ACS include early paramedic response and defibrillation, coronary care units, and pharmacotherapy including antiplatelet agents, antithrombotics, beta receptor–blocking agents, RAAS blockade, lipid-lowering therapy, intravenous thrombolytic agents, and percutaneous intervention (Tables 101.1–101.3). CKD patients represent 30.5% of ST segment elevation MI (STEMI) and 42.9% of NSTEMI cases (Fig. 101.9) and have higher rates of in-hospital mortality in a graded fashion with worsened renal function (Fig. 101.10).[45] The degree of CKD is independently associated with 30-day and 1-year mortality after ACS. Reduced baseline

TABLE 101.1 Acute and Chronic Treatments for Coronary Artery Disease in Patients with Chronic Kidney Disease

MEDICATION	USE	CKD POPULATION	PHARMACOLOGY
Antiplatelet Agents			
Aspirin	Acute MI: 160–325 mg by mouth as soon as possible	No specific dosing adjustments in patients with CKD	Metabolism: liver, microsomal enzyme system
	MI prophylaxis: 81–162 mg by mouth once daily	Meta-analysis involving patients on dialysis demonstrated a benefit of aspirin therapy on cardiovascular outcomes	Renal clearance: 80%–100% 24–72 hr
	PCI: 325 mg by mouth 2 hr pre-surgery, then 160–325 mg by mouth maintenance		Excretion: principally in urine (80%–100%), sweat, saliva, feces
	UA: 75–162 mg by mouth once daily		
Clopidogrel	UA/NSTEMI: 300–600 mg initial loading dose, followed by 75 mg by mouth once daily with aspirin	No specific dosing adjustments in patients with CKD	Metabolism: CYP3A4, CYP2C19 (predominantly) and others to generate active metabolite; also by esterase to an inactive metabolite
	STEMI: 75 mg by mouth once daily with aspirin 75–162 mg per day		
	Recent MI: 75 mg by mouth once daily		Excretion: urine and feces
Prasugrel	ACS:	No specific dose adjustments in patients with CKD	Metabolism: liver; CYP450, CYP2B6, CYP2C9/CYP2C19 (minor), CYP3A4 substrate; CYP2B6 (weak) inhibitor
	Loading dose: 60 mg by mouth once		
	Maintenance dose: 10 mg by mouth once daily with aspirin 81–325 mg per day; bleeding risk may increase if weight <60 kg, consider 5 mg by mouth once daily (efficacy/safety not established)		Excretion: urine (68%) and feces (27%)
Ticagrelor	ACS with PCI and stent:	No specific dose adjustments in patients with CKD	Metabolism: hepatic CYP450
	Starting dose: 180 mg by mouth once		Excretion: bile primarily, urine <1%
	Maintenance dose: 90 mg by mouth twice daily		
	To be given for 1 year with aspirin as an alternative option for dual antiplatelet therapy		

Continued

TABLE 101.1 Acute and Chronic Treatments for Coronary Artery Disease in Patients with Chronic Kidney Disease—cont'd

MEDICATION	USE	CKD POPULATION	PHARMACOLOGY
Angiotensin Converting Enzyme Inhibitors			
For example, Captopril, zofenopril, enalapril, ramipril, quinapril, perindopril, lisinopril, benazepril, imidapril, trandolapril, fosinopril	Indicated for the treatment of hypertension, prevention of cardiovascular events including heart failure in those at risk, reduction in the progression of type 1 diabetic nephropathy, and reduction in cardiovascular events in patients post MI with left ventricular dysfunction or heart failure Also indicated for the treatment of heart failure	The dosing schedules may need to be individualized for each dialysis session in order to avoid intradialytic hypotension In general, reduce dose by 50%–75% in ESRD	Elimination: mainly renal with an elimination half-life of 12.6 hr in healthy individuals In patients with impaired renal function (CrCl ≤30 mL/min) a longer half-life and accumulation have been observed without clinical consequences
Angiotensin II Receptor Antagonists			
For example, Losartan, irbesartan, olmesartan, candesartan, valsartan, telmisartan	Indicated for treatment of hypertension, to reduce the progression of type 2 diabetic nephropathy, and reduce cardiovascular events in patients post-MI with left ventricular dysfunction or heart failure Indicated for heart failure in those intolerant to ACE inhibitors	As first-line treatment in the majority of patients with CKD, recommend the use of ACE inhibitors or ARBs; both have been shown to reduce LVH in patients on hemodialysis Levels of ARBs do not change significantly during hemodialysis	Losartan has 88% hepatic and 12% renal clearance
Calcium Channel Blockers			
Dihydropyridines: e.g., Amlodipine, felodipine, nicardipine, nifedipine, nimodipine, nitrendipine Nondihydropyridines: e.g., Diltiazem, verapamil	In UA/NSTEMI, if β-blockers are contraindicated, a non-dihydropyridine CCB should be chosen in the absence of clinically significant left ventricular dysfunction or other contraindications[44]	No specific dose adjustments for patients with CKD The management of chronic CAD in patients on dialysis should follow that of the general population and use of CCBs as indicated The hemodynamic and electrophysiologic effects of CCBs are markedly different from each other and should be evaluated when selecting a suitable therapy	Amlodipine has renal elimination as the major route of excretion with about 60% cleared in the urine Diltiazem undergoes primary liver metabolism
Nitrates			
Nitroglycerin	2% ointment Angina: 0.5–2 inches applied in morning and 6 hr later to truncal skin Heart failure: 1.5 inches, increase by 0.5–1 inch up to 4 inches, every 4 hr Sublingual: 0.4 mg for relief of chest pain in ACS Sublingual: 0.3-0.6 mg every 5 min Maximum: 3 doses within 15 min	No specific dose adjustments for patients with CKD Care must be used to avoid hypotension in low volume states such as dialysis sessions	Metabolism: mainly in liver, extrahepatic sites such as vascular wall, red blood cells Excretion: urine
Antianginal			
Ranolazine	500–1000 mg by mouth twice daily Max: 2000 mg/day	No specific dose adjustments for patients with CKD Prolongs QTc interval Recommend close monitoring	Excretion: urine 73%–75%, feces 25%

ACE, Angiotensin-converting enzyme; *ACS,* acute coronary syndromes; *ARB,* angiotensin-receptor blocker; *CAD,* coronary artery disease; *CCB,* calcium-channel blocker; *CKD,* chronic kidney disease; *CrCl,* creatinine clearance; *ESRD,* end-stage renal disease; *LVH,* left ventricular hypertrophy; *MI,* myocardial infarction; *NSTEMI,* non-ST-elevation myocardial infarction; *PCI,* percutaneous coronary intervention; *STEMI,* ST-elevation myocardial infarction; *UA,* unstable angina.

eGFR also predicts higher rates of AKI, bleeding, the development of HF, recurrent MI, rehospitalization, and stroke in the setting of ACS. Patients with ESRD have the highest mortality after MI of any large, chronic disease population.

REASONS FOR POOR OUTCOMES AFTER ACUTE CORONARY SYNDROMES IN PATIENTS WITH RENAL DYSFUNCTION

Patients with renal dysfunction may have poor cardiovascular outcomes after ACS for four reasons: (1) excess comorbidities associated with CKD and ESRD, in particular DM and left ventricular dysfunction, (2) therapeutic nihilism, (3) toxicity of therapies, and (4) special biological and pathophysiological factors in renal dysfunction that cause worsened outcomes.[46]

The primary defects that promote thrombosis attributable to uremia are cytokine elevation, excess thrombin generation, and decreased platelet aggregation. Hence, patients with CKD and ESRD can have increased rates of coronary thrombotic events and increased bleeding risks at the same time. In patients with renal dysfunction, the risks of bleeding increase with aspirin, unfractionated heparin, low-molecular-weight heparin, direct thrombin inhibitors, anti-factor Xa agents, thrombolytics, glycoprotein IIb/IIIa antagonists, and thienopyridine antiplatelet agents (Tables 101.4 and 101.5). Uremia causes platelet dysfunction by independent mechanisms that add to pharmacologic anti-platelet agents.[47]

Renal dysfunction creates a pro-inflammatory oxidative stress state, and is associated with higher rates of plaque rupture and incident

TABLE 101.2 β-Adrenergic Receptor Blockers in Patients with Chronic Kidney Disease*

MEDICATION	USE	CKD POPULATION	PHARMACOLOGY
Metoprolol	Acute MI	No specific dose adjustments for patients with CKD	Dialyzable: Yes.
	Metoprolol tartrate: 2.5–5 mg rapid IV every 2–5 min, up to 15 mg over 10–15 min, then 15 min after last IV and receiving 15 mg IV or 50 mg by mouth every 6 hr for 48 hr, then 50–100 mg by mouth twice daily	Recommend close monitoring for adverse effects	Metabolism: hepatic CYP2D6
	Angina		Metabolites: inactive
	Metoprolol tartrate: initially 50 mg by mouth twice daily then titrated to 200 mg by mouth twice daily		Excretion: urine 95%
	Heart failure		
	Metoprolol succinate: 25–100 mg by mouth once daily, target dose 200 mg/day		
Esmolol	Immediate control	No specific dose adjustments for patients with CKD	Metabolism: extensively metabolized by esterase in cytosol of red blood cells
	For intraoperative treatment give an 80 mg (approximately 1 mg/kg) bolus dose over 30 s followed by a 150 µg/kg/min infusion, if needed		Metabolites: major acid metabolite (ASL-8123), methanol (inactive)
	Maximum infusion rate: 300 µg/kg/min		Excretion: urine <1%–2%
	Gradual control		
	For postoperative treatment, give loading dosage infusion of 500 µg/kg/min over 1 min followed by a 4 min infusion of 50 µg/kg/min		
	If no effect within 5 min, repeat loading dose and follow with infusion increased to 100 µg/kg/min		
Carvedilol	Hypertension, HF, and post-MI protection:	No specific dose adjustments for patients with CKD	Elimination: mainly biliary
	6.25–25 mg by mouth twice daily	In a small study of patients on dialysis with dilated cardiomyopathies, carvedilol improved left ventricular function and decreased hospitalization, cardiovascular deaths and total mortality	Excretion: primarily via feces
	Start at 6.25 mg by mouth twice daily, then increase every 3–14 days to 12.5 mg by mouth twice daily, then 25 mg by mouth twice daily, then 50 mg twice daily for weight >85 kg		

*Hemodialysis reduces blood levels of atenolol, acebutolol, and nadolol; by contrast, levels of carvedilol and labetalol do not change significantly.
ACS, Acute coronary syndromes; *CKD*, chronic kidney disease; *HF*, heart failure; *IV*, intravenous; *MI*, myocardial infarction.

thrombotic CVD events. Patients with CKD have more proximal and extensive coronary artery disease (CAD) than the general population; thus, they have larger areas of myocardium at risk for ischemia and dysfunction. Finally, acute on chronic hyperactivation of neurohormonal systems including the RAAS, SNS, endothelin, vasopressin, without adequate counter-regulation by natriuretic peptides, nitric oxide, and other systems may promote worsened ischemia, myocardial dysfunction, and HF.

TREATMENT OF MYOCARDIAL INFARCTION IN PATIENTS WITH RENAL DYSFUNCTION (SEE CHAPTERS 38 AND 39)

Therapies that benefit the general population often yield enhanced benefit in patients with CKD and ESRD include aspirin, beta blockers, ACEI, ARB, aldosterone receptor antagonists.[48] Therapies that require dose adjustment on the basis of CrCl include low-molecular-weight heparins, bivalirudin, and glycoprotein IIb/IIIa antagonists. Given that the major inputs for bleeding risks include older age, low body weight, and renal dysfunction, Tables 101.4 and 101.5 also list agents that are approved in a weight-adjusted dose form and gives the currently recommended dose adjustments for commonly used antiplatelet and antithrombotic agents.[47] Greater utilization of such therapies, despite the heightened risk for complications, might attenuate the excess mortality reported in CKD and ESRD populations. There have been no randomized trials of PCI in patients with CKD or ESRD. However, in the large Swedish Web-system for Enhancement and Development of Evidence-based care in Heart disease Evaluated According to Recommended Therapies (SWEDEHEART) has observed an apparent benefit to revascularization in ACS in CKD groups with eGFR ≥15 mL/min/1.73 m² (Fig. 101.11).[49] Patients with more severe degrees of renal impairment and those on dialysis, although infrequently offered PCI, appeared to have no improvement in survival with interventional management.

CARDIORENAL SYNDROMES (SEE PART VI)

The term cardiorenal syndrome (CRS) refers to disorders of the heart and kidneys whereby acute or chronic dysfunction in one organ may induce acute or chronic dysfunction in the other. Patients with CKD, and in particular ESRD, have three key mechanical contributors to HF: pressure overload (related to HTN), volume overload, and cardiomyopathy (Fig. 101.12). Approximately 20% of patients approaching hemodialysis have a diagnosis of pre-existing HF. It is unclear how much of this diagnosis results purely from chronic volume overload from renal failure and how much is due to impaired systolic or diastolic function. CKD influences the blood levels of B-type natriuretic peptide (BNP) and to a greater extent with NT-proBNP.[50] In general, when the eGFR is less than 60 mL/min/1.73 m², higher cut points of 200 pg/mL and 1200 pg/mL should be used in the diagnosis of HF with BNP and NT-proBNP, respectively.

Once acute heart failure is recognized on clinical grounds, approximately 25% of patients will develop a CRS during the hospitalization characterized by a rise in serum Cr ≥0.3 mg/dL and a reduction in urine output (Fig. 101.13). These findings are not associated with markers of acute tubular injury suggesting that they reflect a transient renal hemodynamic problem.[51] Of those, approximately one third return to baseline, one third are left with worsened eGFR, and the final third have progressive cardiorenal disease resulting in either death or the need for renal replacement therapy.[52] Multiple studies have shown

TABLE 101.3 Lipid-Lowering Therapy for Primary and Secondary Prevention in Patients with Chronic Kidney Disease

MEDICATION	USE	CKD POPULATION	PHARMACOLOGY
Rosuvastatin	Cardiovascular event protection 10–40 mg by mouth once daily	Efficacy in LDL-C reduction in CKD demonstrated at doses as low as 2.5 mg daily	Metabolism: liver, CYP450 CYP2C9 Excretion: bile primarily, urine <2%
Simvastatin	Cardiovascular event protection: 20–40 mg by mouth once daily combined with ezetimibe 10 mg by mouth once daily Maximum dose: 40 mg by mouth given at hour of sleep	Consider starting dose at 5 mg in the evening in patients with CKD In SHARP, lipid lowering with statin + ezetimibe was beneficial in patients with CKD In HPS, simvastatin reduced the renal decline in patients with CKD	Metabolism: liver, CYP450 CYP3A4 Excretion: bile primarily, urine <2%
Atorvastatin	Cardiovascular event protection: 10–80 mg by mouth once daily	No specific dose adjustments for patients with CKD Atorvastatin 10 mg in patients with CKD revealed a significantly lower risk of the primary end point (nonfatal MI or cardiac death) when compared with placebo[110] With the TNT and GREACE studies, atorvastatin showed improvement in renal function in patients with CKD	Metabolism: liver, CYP450 CYP3A4 Excretion: bile primarily, urine <2%
Fluvastatin	Cardiovascular event protection: 40 mg by mouth twice daily Extended release: 80 mg by mouth once daily	No specific dose adjustments for patients with CKD Caution for increased risk of rhabdomyolysis A multicenter, randomized, double blind, placebo-controlled trial of fluvastatin was conducted in kidney transplant recipients. Fluvastatin reduced LDL cholesterol levels by 32%. Although the primary end point did not achieve statistical significance, secondary analysis showed that the fluvastatin group experienced fewer cardiac deaths and nonfatal MI than did the placebo group. Coronary intervention procedures were not significantly different between the two groups	Metabolism: liver, CYP450 CYP2C9 isozyme system (75%), and to a lesser extent by CYP3A4 (approximately 20%) and CYP2C8 (approximately 5%) Excretion: bile primarily 90%, urine 5%
Pravastatin	Cardiovascular event protection: Start: 40 mg by mouth once daily, may adjust dose every 4 weeks Maximum dose: 80 mg by mouth once daily	Start at 10 mg by mouth once daily in patients with CKD A randomized trial of pravastatin versus placebo in patients with previous MI and CKD in a secondary analysis showed coronary death or nonfatal MI was lower in patients receiving pravastatin, suggesting that pravastatin is effective for secondary prevention of cardiovascular events in patients with CKD	Metabolism: glucuronidation Excretion: bile primarily 70%, urine 20%
Pitavastatin	Lowering LDL-C and total cholesterol: Start: 1 mg by mouth once daily may adjust every 4 weeks Maximum dose: 4 mg by mouth once daily	Start at 1 mg po qd in patients with CKD	Metabolism: glucuronidation Excretion: bile primarily 79%, urine 15%
Ezetimibe	Lowering LDL-C and total cholesterol: Start 10 mg po qd	Start at 10 mg po qd with no renal dose adjustment, tested in ESRD	Metabolism: glucuronidation Excretion: Bile/feces 78%, urine 11%
Colesevelam hydrochloride	Lowering LDL-C and total cholesterol, improving glycemic control type 2 diabetes: Start 625 mg tabs, 3 tabs po bid	Start at 3 tabs po bid with no renal dose adjustment	Metabolism: no systemic absorption Excretion: feces
Evolocumab Humanized monoclonal IgG2 directed against PCSK9	Cardiovascular event protection: Start 140 mg SQ q 2 weeks or 420 mg SQ q 4 weeks	Start 140 mg SQ q 2 weeks or 420 mg SQ q 4 weeks with no renal dose adjustment	Metabolism: saturable target binding and proteolysis Excretion: none
Alirocumab Humanized monoclonal IgG1 directed against PCSK9	Cardiovascular event protection: Start 75 or 150 mg SQ q 2 weeks or 300 mg SQ q 4 weeks	Start 75 or 150 mg SQ q 2 weeks or 300 mg SQ q 4 weeks with no renal dose adjustment	Metabolism: saturable target binding and proteolysis Excretion: none

ACS, Acute coronary syndromes; *CKD,* chronic kidney disease; *ESRD,* end-stage renal disease; *LDL-C,* low-density lipoprotein cholesterol; *MI,* myocardial infarction.

that the predictors of CRS (type 1) include baseline eGFR, older age, female sex, increased baseline blood pressure, higher initial natriuretic peptide levels, and increased central venous pressure. Because CRS Type 1 in patients with HF rarely occurs in the prehospital phase and more commonly develops after treatment is started in-hospital, initial diuresis followed by inadequate plasma refill from the extravascular tissues has been implicated. Continued administration of loop diuretics, probably by further activating the RAAS and possibly worsening intra-renal hemodynamics, probably contribute to CRS Type 1 when diuresis is not maintained.

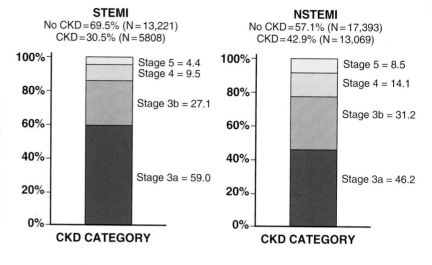

FIGURE 101.9 Prevalence of chronic kidney disease (CKD) and stages 3a, 3b, 4, and 5 (no dialysis) and dialysis presenting with ST segment elevation myocardial infarction (STEMI) and NSTEMI. Stage 3b as estimated glomerular filtration rate (eGFR) 30 to 44 mL/min/1.73 m²; Stage 4 CKD as eGFR between 15 and 29 mL/min/1.73 m², and Stage 5 CKD as an eGFR less than 15 mL/min/1.73 m² or dialysis therapy. (Adapted from Fox CS, Muntner P, Chen AY, et al. Acute Coronary Treatment and Intervention Outcomes Network registry. Use of evidence-based therapies in short-term outcomes of ST-segment elevation myocardial infarction and non-ST-segment elevation myocardial infarction in patients with chronic kidney disease: a report from the National Cardiovascular Data Acute Coronary Treatment and Intervention Outcomes Network registry. *Circulation.* 2010;121[3]:357–365.)

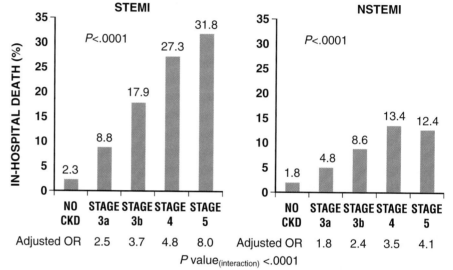

FIGURE 101.10 Crude rates and adjusted odds ratios for death by CKD stages among those presenting with STEMI and NSTEMI, with *P-trend and P-interaction* for STEMI versus NSTEMI by CKD stages. Stage 3a CKD was defined as an eGFR between 45 and 59 mL/min/1.73 m²; Stage 3b as eGFR 30 to 44 mL/min/1.73 m²; Stage 4 CKD as eGFR between 15 and 29 mL/min/1.73 m²; and Stage 5 CKD as an eGFR less than 15 mL/min/1.73 m² or dialysis therapy. *CKD,* Chronic kidney disease; *eGFR,* estimated glomerular filtration rate; *STEMI,* ST segment elevation myocardial infarction. (Adapted from Fox CS, Muntner P, Chen AY, et al. Use of evidence-based therapies in short-term outcomes of ST-segment elevation myocardial infarction and non-ST-segment elevation myocardial infarction in patients with chronic kidney disease: a report from the National Cardiovascular Data Acute Coronary Treatment and Intervention Outcomes Network registry. *Circulation.* 2010;121[3]:357–365.)

TABLE 101.4 Intravenous Glycoprotein IIb/IIIa Inhibitors for Unstable Angina/NSTEMI, STEMI, PCI

MEDICATION	USE	CKD POPULATION*	PHARMACOLOGY
Abciximab	Adjunct to PCI: 0.25 mg/kg IV bolus over at least 1 min, 10–60 min before start of PCI, then 0.125 µg/kg/min (not to exceed 10 µg/min) continuous IV infusion for 12 hr Unstable angina with PCI planned within 24 hr: 0.25 mg/kg IV bolus over at least 1 min, then 0.125 µg/kg/min (not to exceed 10 µg/min) IV infusion for 18–24 hr concluding 1 hr after PCI	No specific dose adjustments for patients with CKD Abciximab should also be considered as adjunctive therapy in patients with ACS on dialysis In CKD, safety of abciximab has been shown for creatinine levels >152.5 µmol/L Although increased bleeding with abciximab in patients with CKD has been reported, other studies have shown no increase in bleeding for CKD versus no CKD for abciximab in PCI	Metabolism: unknown, but likely by the reticuloendothelial system CYP450: unknown involvement Excretion: urine
Eptifibatide	ACS: 180 µg/kg IV bolus, then 2 µg/kg/min IV for up to 72 hr PCI: 180 µg/kg IV, then a continuous infusion at 2 µg/kg/min with another 180 µg/kg IV bolus 10 min after first bolus Continue infusion for at least 12 hr	Creatinine clearance <50 mL/min and ACS: 180 µg/kg IV, then continuous infusion 1 µg/kg/min Safety and use during hemodialysis is not established	Metabolism: other, minimal CYP450: unknown involvement Excretion: urine 50%
Tirofiban	In patients undergoing PCI, tirofiban is not recommended as an alternative to abciximab[43] ACS: 0.4 µg/kg/min IV for 30 min, then 0.1 µg/kg/min IV for 48–108 hr PCI: Continue 0.1 µg/kg/min IV through procedure and for 12–24 hr after	Creatinine clearance <30 mL/min and ACS: reduce dose to 50% of normal rate Safety and use during hemodialysis not established	Excretion: urine 65% (primarily unchanged), feces 25% (primarily unchanged)

ACS, Acute coronary syndromes; *CKD,* chronic kidney disease; *IV,* intravenous; *NSTEMI,* non-ST-elevation myocardial infarction; *PCI,* percutaneous coronary intervention; *STEMI,* ST-elevation myocardial infarction.

*When a glycoprotein IIb/IIIa antagonist is used, abciximab and tirofiban should be considered preferred agents as no dosing changes are required for abciximab, and dialysis-specific dosing recommendations are available for tirofiban. Increased bleeding but reduced in-hospital mortality in CKD patients with ACS treated with glycoprotein IIb/IIIa antagonists has also been shown.[49]

TABLE 101.5 Antithrombotic Agents for Acute Coronary Syndromes and Other Thrombotic Indications in Patients with Chronic Kidney Disease

MEDICATION	USE	CKD POPULATION	PHARMACOLOGY
Indirect Factor Xa Inhibitors			
Unfractionated heparin	Recommended dosage and desired aPTT values as per institutional protocol PCI: 60–100 units/kg IV given once Target ACT 250–350 sec In patients receiving glycoprotein IIb/IIIa inhibitor, give 50–70 units/kg IV to target ACT 200 sec STEMI, adjunct treatment, streptokinase use: 800 units/hr when <80 kg body weight or 1000 units/hr when >80 kg body weight Start: 5000 units IV, adjust dose to target aPTT 50–75 sec NSTEMI: 12-15 units/kg/hr IV Start: 60–70 units/kg IV; Max 5000 units bolus, max rate 1000 units/hr Adjust dose to target aPTT 50–75 sec	In patients with CKD, suggested starting dose of heparin is 50 IU/kg bolus, then 18 IU/kg/hr Monitor aPTT level and adjust accordingly as per institutional protocol	Metabolism: liver (partial) Metabolites: none Excretion: urine
Low-molecular-weight heparin (e.g., enoxaparin)	Unstable angina, non-Q-wave myocardial infarction: 1 mg/kg subcutaneously twice daily STEMI, aged <75 years: 30 mg IV bolus plus 1 mg/kg subcutaneously, then 1 mg/kg subcutaneously every 12 hr PCI: additional 0.3 mg/kg IV bolus if last subcutaneous administration given >8 hr before balloon inflation STEMI, aged >75 years: 0.75 mg/kg subcutaneously every 12 hr (no IV bolus)	CrCl <30 mL/min STEMI, aged <75 years: 30 mg IV bolus plus 1 mg/kg subcutaneously, then 1 mg/kg subcutaneously once a day STEMI, aged >75 years: 1 mg/kg subcutaneously once a day	Excretion: urine 40%
Direct Factor Xa Inhibitor			
Fondaparinux	Unstable angina/NSTEMI Conservative strategy: 2.5 mg subcutaneously once daily During PCI: add unfractionated heparin 50–60 units/kg IV bolus for prophylaxis of catheter thrombosis[49]	CrCl 30–50 mL/min: use with caution CrCl <30 mL/min: not indicated	Excretion: urine (primarily unchanged)
Direct Thrombin Inhibitors			
Bivalirudin	Intended for use with aspirin 300–325 mg/day 0.75 mg/kg IV bolus initially, followed by continuous infusion at rate of 1.75 mg/kg/hr for duration of procedure Perform ACT 5 min after bolus dose Administer additional 0.3 mg/kg bolus if necessary May continue infusion following PCI beyond 4 hr (optional post-PCI, at discretion of treating healthcare provider) initiated at rate of 0.2 mg/kg/hr for up to 20 hr as needed	CrCl 10–29 mL/min: usual bolus dose, then initial infusion of 1 mg/kg/hr IV up to 4 hr Hemodialysis: usual bolus dose, then initial infusion of 0.25 mg/kg/hr IV up to 4 hr Bivalirudin is a direct thrombin inhibitor with specific dosing adjustments for patients on dialysis and should be preferentially considered	Dialysable: with 25% reduction in levels Excretion: urine
Dabigatran	Indicated for prevention of stroke and thromboembolism associated with nonvalvular atrial fibrillation CrCl >30 mL/min: 150 mg by mouth twice daily	CrCl 15–30 mL/min: 75 mg by mouth twice daily CrCl <15 mL/min or hemodialysis: not indicated For patients currently taking dabigatran, wait 12 hr (CrCl ≥30 mL/min) or 24 hr (CrCl <30 mL/min) after the last dose of dabigatran before initiating treatment with a parenteral anticoagulant If possible, discontinue dabigatran 1–2 days (CrCl ≥50 mL/min) or 3–5 days (CrCl <50 mL/min) before invasive or surgical procedures because of increased risk of bleeding	Metabolism liver esterases and microsomal carboxylesterases Excretion: feces 7%, urine 86%

Continued

CARDIOVASCULAR DISEASE AND DISORDERS OF OTHER ORGANS

XI

TABLE 101.5 Antithrombotic Agents for Acute Coronary Syndromes and Other Thrombotic Indications in Patients with Chronic Kidney Disease—cont'd

MEDICATION	USE	CKD POPULATION	PHARMACOLOGY
Rivaroxaban	Indicated for prevention of stroke and thromboembolism associated with nonvalvular atrial fibrillation, venous thromboembolism (VTE) CrCl >50 mL/min: 15 mg by mouth bid for 3 weeks (acute anticoagulation for VTE) CrCl >50 mL/min: 20 mg by mouth at hour of sleep (chronic anticoagulation)	CrCl 15–50 mL/min: 15 mg by mouth at hour of sleep CrCl <15 mL/min: not indicated	Metabolism: liver CYP450 Excretion: feces 28%, urine 66% Half-life: 5–9 hr or 11–13 hr in elderly
Apixaban	Indicated for prevention of stroke and thromboembolism associated with nonvalvular atrial fibrillation, venous thromboembolism (VTE) 2.5 mg by mouth twice daily (VTE prophylaxis) 5 mg by mouth twice daily (chronic anticoagulation)	age ≥80 years, body weight ≤60 kg, or serum creatinine ≥1.5 mg/dL, the recommended dose is 2.5 mg orally twice daily	Metabolism: liver CYP450 CYP3A4/5 while CYP1A2, 2C8, 2C9, 2C19, and 2J2 are minor Excretion: feces 83%, urine 27%
Edoxaban	Indicated for prevention of stroke and thromboembolism associated with nonvalvular atrial fibrillation, venous thromboembolism (VTE) 60 mg by mouth once daily (VTE prophylaxis) 60 mg by mouth once daily (chronic anticoagulation)	CrCl >95 mL/min: Do not use; increased ischemic stroke compared with warfarin CrCl >50–95 mL/min 60 mg orally once daily CrCl 15–50 mL/min or <60 kg: 30 mg orally once daily	Metabolism: minimal Excretion: urine

ACS, Acute coronary syndromes; *ACT,* activated clotting time; *aPTT,* activated partial thromboplastin time; *CKD,* chronic kidney disease; *CrCl,* creatinine clearance; *IV,* intravenous; *NSTEMI,* non-ST-elevation myocardial infarction; *PCI,* percutaneous coronary intervention; *STEMI,* ST-elevation myocardial infarction.

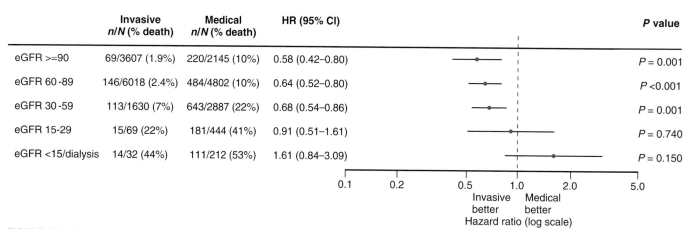

	Invasive *n/N* (% death)	Medical *n/N* (% death)	HR (95% CI)		P value
eGFR >=90	69/3607 (1.9%)	220/2145 (10%)	0.58 (0.42–0.80)		P = 0.001
eGFR 60-89	146/6018 (2.4%)	484/4802 (10%)	0.64 (0.52–0.80)		P <0.001
eGFR 30-59	113/1630 (7%)	643/2887 (22%)	0.68 (0.54–0.86)		P = 0.001
eGFR 15-29	15/69 (22%)	181/444 (41%)	0.91 (0.51–1.61)		P = 0.740
eGFR <15/dialysis	14/32 (44%)	111/212 (53%)	1.61 (0.84–3.09)		P = 0.150

FIGURE 101.11 Estimated hazard ratio for mortality at 1 year for patients treated either medically or with early revascularization. (Adapted from Szummer K, Lundman P, Jacobson SH, et al. Influence of renal function on the effects of early revascularization in non-ST-elevation myocardial infarction: data from the Swedish Web-System for Enhancement and Development of Evidence-Based Care in Heart Disease Evaluated According to Recommended Therapies (SWEDEHEART). *Circulation.* 2009;120[10]:851–858.)

There are no proven therapeutic strategies for CRS Type 1. Withdrawal of RAAS inhibition with the aim of improving azotemia is associated with increased risk of rehospitalization and mortality.[53] Hence, provided blood pressure is adequate and hyperkalemia is manageable, ACEI/ARB including MRA should be continued despite the development of azotemia.[54] Failed approaches include use of continuous furosemide infusions, low-dose dopamine, nesiritide, and programmatic use of inotropic agents. In the setting of poor arterial perfusion, dobutamine or milrinone are commonly used during hospitalizations to support the patient while ACE/ARB or sacubitril/valsartan, beta-blockers, and diuretics are optimized. Neither agent alone reduces mortality, but they do increase the risk of arrhythmias, and milrinone must be dose adjusted when the eGFR is below 45 mL/min/1.73 m² (Table 101.6). Patients with advanced HF have reduced renal blood flow, decreased glomerular filtration rate, enhanced proximal reabsorption of water, increased absorption of sodium along the loop of Henle, and an overall reduced capacity of the nephron to excrete water. Furthermore, reduced effective arterial blood volume stimulates vasopressin release, which plays a dominant role in worsening water retention. Hyponatremia and excess body water can be improved with the use of oral tolvaptan without worsening azotemia.[55]

Treatment efforts should be aimed at reducing congestion within a narrow management window (see Chapters 50 and 51) and improving left ventricular systolic function, often in the hospitalized setting, with the oral and intravenous therapies including diuretics mentioned previously. Observational studies and small trials utilizing continuous veno-venous ultrafiltration have shown mixed results in symptoms, reductions in fluid weight, length of stay, rehospitalization, and death.[56] Until larger trials help define the indicated population, optimal timing and mode of ultrafiltration, and demonstrate longer-term reductions in hospitalization and mortality, ultrafiltration can be considered a last-line approach for the patient with refractory CRS.

The management of the patient who is already receiving dialysis and has HF requires particular care. In general, proven HF therapies, provided they are tolerated, should be employed along with regular and ad hoc dialysis as needed to control volume overload. Clinicians should keep in mind that ACEI are dialyzed but angiotensin receptor blockers are not. Both agents are associated with reductions in mortality in ESRD patients in observational studies. Studies of frequent dialysis performed in the home at lower rates of ultrafiltration have consistently demonstrated lower rates of HF hospitalization and death.[57]

In ambulatory patients with HF with reduced ejection fraction and CKD, administration of sodium glucose cotransporter-2 inhibitors

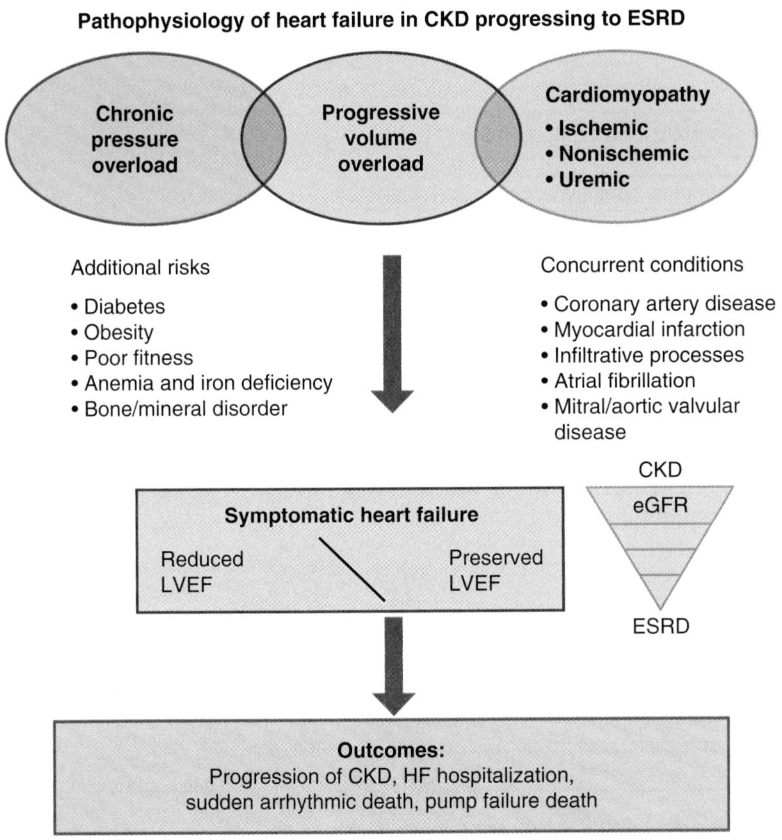

Pathophysiology of heart failure in CKD progressing to ESRD

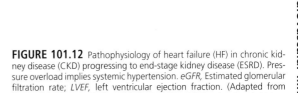

FIGURE 101.12 Pathophysiology of heart failure (HF) in chronic kidney disease (CKD) progressing to end-stage kidney disease (ESRD). Pressure overload implies systemic hypertension. *eGFR,* Estimated glomerular filtration rate; *LVEF,* left ventricular ejection fraction. (Adapted from House AA, Wanner C, Sarnak MJ, et al. Heart failure in chronic kidney disease: conclusions from a Kidney Disease: Improving Global Outcomes (KDIGO) Controversies Conference. *Kidney Int.* 2019;95[6]:1304–1317.)

(SGLT2i) offers considerable benefit for both HF and renal function.[58] These oral agents approved for use in type 2 diabetes, HF, and diabetic nephropathy induce glycosuria, urinary sodium loss, and a spectrum of secondary metabolic effects in the body. Across multiple trials there are consistent greater than 25% relative risk reductions in HF hospitalization, progression of CKD, ESRD, and cardiovascular death associated with these agents.[59,60]

In summary, CKD and HF present a particularly challenging scenario for clinicians and patients. Among patients with CKD, beta blockers, ACEI/ARB, sacubitril/valsartan, and SGLT2i are associated with both cardiac and renal benefits. Frequent outpatient monitoring and avoidance of overly aggressive diuresis are advised. Dialysis patients, despite having volume reduction with mechanical fluid removal, should have medical therapy with ACEIs or ARBs, beta blockers, and additional agents for blood pressure control if needed. Ideally, ESRD patients with HF would undergo frequent (daily) hemodialysis at home provided self- and partner-care can be delivered without difficulties.

CHRONIC KIDNEY DISEASE AND VALVULAR HEART DISEASE (SEE PART VIII)

CKD mineral and bone disorder (phosphate retention, relative hypocalcemia, increased PTH) are associated with valvular thickening and calcific deposits of the aortic and mitral valves occurs in patients with ESRD.[61] Approximately 80% of patients with ESRD have the murmur of aortic sclerosis and 40% have mitral annular calcification.[62] Patients with CKD and ESRD have rates of valve failure greater than in the general population.[63]

Bacterial endocarditis may develop in patients with ESRD who have temporary dialysis access catheters (see also Chapter 80.)[64] Endocarditis with common pathogens including *Staphylococcus, Streptococcus,* and *Enterococcus* in the mitral, aortic, or tricuspid valves, are associated with a risk of cerebral embolism of 40% and a mortality rate of 50% in ESRD.[64] It becomes very difficult to treat given the continued need for dialysis access and the delay in surgical placement of permanent arteriovenous shunts or fistulas. Unfortunately, surgical mortality

associated with valve replacement in ESRD related to endocarditis is very high. In the setting of ESRD, when valve surgery is carried out for endocarditis or other causes of valve failure, there has been no difference in survival among those who received tissue or mechanical valve prostheses. Thus, tissue valves are a reasonable choice given the complicating issue of chronic anticoagulation and bleeding with repeated dialysis vascular access.[65]

RENAL FUNCTION AND ARRHYTHMIAS (SEE PART VII)

Uremia, hyperkalemia, acidosis, and disorders of calcium-phosphorous balance all link to higher rates of atrial and ventricular arrhythmias. Given a concurrent substrate of LVH, left ventricular dilation, HF, and valvular disease, it is not surprising that higher rates of virtually all arrhythmias have been reported in CKD, including bradyarrhythmias and heart block. Hypokalemia after hemodialysis can be observed for 6 to 8 hours as the plasma potassium concentration equilibrates from approximately 2.0 mEq/liter to the normal range of 3.5 to 5.5 mEq/liter. During this time, there is an increased risk of sudden cardiac death.[66] There is a general trend to increase the potassium concentration of the dialysis fluid to reduce the large shifts in potassium in ESRD patients. Chronic hyperkalemia between dialysis sessions can be controlled with daily oral potassium binders (patiromer, sodium zirconium cyclosilicate).[67] Caveats for practical management include dose adjustment for many antiarrhythmic medications including dofetilide and sotalol (Table 101.7). One randomized trial failed to find a benefit with prophylactic implantable cardioverter-defibrillator (ICD) insertion in dialysis patients with LVEF ≥35%.[68] Observational studies suggest that ESRD patients who survive a sudden death event have a favorable benefit to risk ratio favoring ICD implantation; however, rates of infection are higher and when they occur are associated with in-hospital mortality of approximately 14%.[69] Of concern, CKD, and ESRD in particular, may cause elevated defibrillation thresholds and failure of ICDs and are associated with high rates of shock and antitachycardia pacing therapy than patients with normal renal function.[70] Until this association

XI

CARDIOVASCULAR DISEASE AND DISORDERS OF OTHER ORGANS

CKD-Associated Myocardial Changes
Myocyte hypertrophy
Myocyte dysfunction
↑↑Interstitial fibrosis
↓Capillary density
↑↑LV mass
Elevated serum troponin levels

CKD-Associated Vascular Changes
Accelerated atherosclerosis
↑Vascular stiffness
↓Smooth muscle density
Osteoblastic VSMC metaplasia
Intra- and extracellular calcification

Acute on Chronic Cardiac Disease

Chronic neurohormonal
↑SNS, RAS, aldosterone
↓Vitamin D
↑PTH
↑PO$_4$
Hypotestosteronism
↓EPO
↓Fe utilization
↓Na$^+$,K$^+$-ATPase

Inciting Events
↓Medical compliance
↑Sodium intake
Ischemia
Arrhythmias (AF)
OSA

Added insults
NSAID, TZD

Systolic or Diastolic Dysfunction or Both

Altered intrarenal hemodynamics

Decreased Perfusion — Increased venous pressure — Renal congestion

Precipitators
Diuretics
Vasodilators
Procedures

Toxicity
Vasoconstriction

Acute-on-Chronic Kidney Injury

DM+HTN + other CKD
Renal hypoperfusion
Decreased GFR
Resistance to diuretics
Resistance to ANP/BNP
Na + H$_2$O retention
Necrosis / apoptosis
Fibrosis

Acute Neurohormonal Activation
SNS + RAS + Aldosterone + Endothelin + ADH + renal vasoconstriction (adenosine) + prostaglandin dysregulation

Biomarkers
↑BNP/NT-proBNP
↑NGAL
↑KIM-1
↑IL-18
Catalytic iron
↑Cystatin C
↑Creatinine
Urine albumin
Many others

LV failure mechanisms
• Pressure overload
• Volume overload
• Cardiomyopathy

Humoral signaling

ANP/BNP — Natriuretic peptides — Blocked natriuresis

Anemia/relative ↓Epo/Fe transport blocked

IL-1, TNF-alpha

Monocyte activation

Endothelial dysfunction

Cytokine secretion

↓Tubuloglomerular function

↑Adhesion Molecules, ↑Enzymatic Activation, ↑Oxidative Stress

FIGURE 101.13 Pathophysiology of type 1 cardiorenal syndrome or worsening renal function after hospitalization for acutely decompensated heart failure. (Adapted from Herzog CA, Asinger RW, Berger AK, et al. Cardiovascular disease in chronic kidney disease. A clinical update from Kidney Disease: Improving Global Outcomes (KDIGO). *Kidney Int.* 2011;80[6]:572–586.)

is better understood, patients receiving ICDs should have frequent surveillance and consideration for noninvasive programmed stimulation for appropriate antitachycardia and defibrillation therapy.

CONSULTATIVE APPROACH TO SEVERE KIDNEY DISEASE AND HEMODIALYSIS PATIENTS

The prevalence of angiographically significant CAD ranges from 25% in young, non-diabetic hemodialysis patients, to 85% in older ESRD patients with long-standing DM.[71] Of those initiating dialysis, 87% have some structural abnormality on echocardiography including LVH, reduced LVEF, right ventricular hypertrophy or dysfunction, pulmonary HTN, or valvular disease.[72] Thus, many years of CKD must be associated with these progressive changes and we cannot attribute them solely to the dialysis procedure in most patients who are in the first few months of treatment. Cardiac death in dialysis patients younger than age 45 may be 100 times greater than that the general population. Medicare beneficiaries with CKD prior to initiation of dialysis are 60% more likely to have a billing claim submitted for the diagnosis of CVD and 70% more likely to have a claim submitted for "atherosclerotic heart disease." Of those claims incident to dialysis, a substantial proportion, perhaps the majority, have established CAD. In diabetic renal transplant candidates 30% will have one or more lesions with greater than 75% stenosis.[73] When comparing patients who undergo evaluation for CAD,

those with ESRD have substantially more numerous, proximal, and severe coronary artery lesions, as well as more severe left ventricular dysfunction. The patient with incipient ESRD on dialysis can be considered the highest cardiovascular risk patient in medicine with expected rates of CHD death that exceed many-fold than that expected for a non-ESRD patient, even those with a burden of several cardiovascular risk factors.

Despite the use of multiple medications, most published series of ESRD patients from either clinical trials or registries indicate the mean systolic blood pressure is approximately 155 mm Hg. Indeed 80% of ESRD patients have HTN, which is adequately controlled in only 30%. Peritoneal dialysis, more frequent in-center, and home hemodialysis are all associated with much better blood pressure control than thrice-weekly hemodialysis.[74] Home hemodialysis for 5 or more days in the week is associated with approximately 45% relative risk reduction in HF but at approximately 25% excess risk of more frequent access site and endovascular infections.[75] Arteriovenous fistulas used for dialysis access cause recirculation of blood in one of the extremities (usually with upper arm), and depending on size and proximity, can account for as much as approximately 25% shunting, resulting in right ventricular volume overload and development of HF.[76] Long-term cardiorenal protection involves two important concepts; blood pressure control, and use of an agent that blocks the RAAS such as an ACEI or ARB as the base of therapy. The RAAS appears to have considerable redundancy and is able to maintain is function, if not increase its overall level of activity, without participation by the kidneys. Hence this hyperactivation of the RAAS is a target for therapy even in anephric patients

TABLE 101.6 Selected Therapies for Heart Failure in Patients with Chronic Kidney Disease

MEDICATION	USE	CKD POPULATION	PHARMACOLOGY
Dobutamine	Acutely decompensated heart failure with low cardiac output. Continuous infusion: 5.0–15 µg/kg/min IV Initial rate 5.0 µg/kg/min IV titrate 5–20 µg/kg/min; no more than 40 µg/kg/min	No specific dose adjustments for patients with CKD Recommend close monitoring for adverse effects including arrhythmias Doses <5.0 µg/kg/min may produce hypotension	Metabolism: methylation of the catechol and hepatic conjugation. May increase renal clearance of other drugs in low cardiac output states
Milrinone	Acutely decompensated heart failure with low cardiac output. Loading dose of 50 µg/kg IV over 10 min, then start maintenance: 0.375–0.75 µg/kg/min	Recommended infusion rates (µg/kg/min) CrCl – mL/min/1.73 m² [CrCl >50]: No change [50]: 0.43 µg/kg/min [40]: 0.38 µg/kg/min [30]: 0.33 µg/kg/min [20]: 0.28 µg/kg/min [10]: 0.23 µg/kg/min [5]: 0.2 µg/kg/min	Excreted unchanged in the urine
Nesiritide	Acutely decompensated heart failure with pulmonary congestion. 2 µg/kg IV bolus over 1 min, then 0.01 µg/kg/min IV infusion. If hypotension, discontinue until stabilized, then restart at 30% lower dose	No specific dose adjustments for patients with CKD Recommend close monitoring for adverse effects including hypotension	Cleared by: (1) binding to cell surface clearance receptors with subsequent cellular internalization and lysosomal proteolysis; (2) proteolytic cleavage of the peptide by endopeptidases, such as neutral endopeptidase, which are present on the vascular luminal surface; and (3) renal filtration.
Nitroprusside	Acutely decompensated heart failure with vasoconstriction 0.25–0.8 mg/kg/min IV	No specific dose adjustments for patients with CKD Recommend close monitoring for adverse effects including hypotension and thiocyanate accumulation	Intraerythrocytic reaction but hepatic and renal function impacts thiocyanate accumulation
Valsartan/Sacubitril	Chronic HF with reduced LVEF sacubitril/valsartan 24/26, 49/51, 97/103 mg orally twice daily	No specific dose adjustments for patients with CKD, monitor Cr, BUN, K⁺, greater preservation of renal function compared to enalapril over time in HF	Metabolism: Sacubitril converted to LBQ657 by esterases, urine 52%–68%, feces 37%–48% Valsartan urine approximately 13%, feces 86%.
Dapagliflozin	Chronic HF with LVEF ≤40% with or without type 2 diabetes	Start 10 mg po qd with eGFR >30 mL/min/1.73 m² and continue to ESRD, no dose adjustments based on renal function	Metabolism: glucuronidation in liver, 75% eliminated in urine, 21% in feces
Ivabradine	Chronic HF with LVEF <35% and heart rate >70 start 5 mg orally twice daily and may reduce to 2.5 mg or increase to 7.5 mg twice daily depending on heart rate and tolerability	No specific dose adjustments for patients with CKD	Metabolism: liver CYP450 CYP3A4 Excretion: feces 96%, urine 4%
Hydralazine	Acute and chronic HF, intolerant to RAAS blockers, 25–50 mg by mouth t.i.d. or q.i.d.	Dose q8–16 hr with CrCl <10 mL/min	Hepatic clearance, 25%–40% removed with dialysis
Digoxin	Chronic systolic and diastolic heart failure, atrial fibrillation with rapid ventricular rate 0.25 mg by mouth qd	0.125 mg po qd or q.o.d.	50%–70% excreted unchanged in the urine. The half-life in anuric patients is prolonged to 3.5–5 days. Digoxin is not effectively removed from the body by dialysis
Patiromer	Reduction of potassium and control of hyperkalemia	8.4 g po qd, advance up to 25.2 g po daily, in general take 3 hr away from other medications, can be used in HF, CKD, ESRD	Metabolism: none Elimination: fecal
Sodium Zirconium Cyclosilicate	Reduction of potassium and control of hyperkalemia	5 or 10 g po qd, in general take 2 hr away from other medications, can be used in HF, CKD, ESRD	Metabolism: none Elimination: fecal

CKD, Chronic kidney disease; *CrCl*, creatinine clearance; *eGFR*, estimated glomerular filtration rate; *ESRD*, end-stage renal disease; *HF*, heart failure; *IV*, intravenous; *LVEF*, left ventricular ejection fraction; *RAAS*, renin-angiotensin-aldosterone system.

TABLE 101.7 Selected Anti-Arrhythmics in Patients with Chronic Kidney Disease

MEDICATION	USE	CKD POPULATION	PHARMACOLOGY
Amiodarone	Acute ventricular and acute and chronic atrial arrhythmias, First Rapid: 150 mg over 10 min (15 mg/min) Followed by Slow: 360 mg over 6 hr (1 mg/min) Maintenance infusion: 540 mg over the remaining 18 hr (0.5 mg/min) Oral 800–1600 mg/day in divided doses until a total of 10 g has been given; then 200–400 mg/day	No specific dose adjustments for patients with CKD	Eliminated primarily by hepatic metabolism and biliary excretion; negligible renal excretion
Dronedarone	Atrial fibrillation/atrial flutter 400 mg orally twice a day with morning and evening meals	No specific dose adjustments for patients with CKD	Dronedarone is extensively metabolized by the liver
Dofetilide	Atrial fibrillation/atrial flutter 500 μg p.o. bid initially. QTc interval should be measured 2–3 hr after the initial dose. If the QTc >15% of baseline, or if the QTc is >500 msec (550 msec in patients with ventricular conduction abnormalities), dofetilide should be adjusted. Continued monitoring for doses 2–5: QTc interval must be determined 2–3 hr after each subsequent dose of dofetilide for in-hospital doses 2–5. If the measured QTc is >500 msec (550 msec in patients with ventricular conduction abnormalities) dofetilide should be stopped.	[CrCl >60 mL/min]: 500 μg bid [40–60 mL/min]: 250 μg twice daily. [20–39 mL/min]: 125 μg twice daily. [<20 mL/min]: Contraindicated	Hepatic metabolism accounts for 20%–30%, 70%–80% renal elimination
Sotalol	Atrial fibrillation/atrial flutter 80–160 mg orally twice a day	CrCl 30–59 mL/min: The dosage interval should be increased to 24 hr. CrCl 10–29 mL/min: The dosage interval should be increased to 36–48 hr. CrCl less than 10 mL/min: Dose should be individualized.	Excreted unchanged in the kidney. Removed with dialysis

CKD, Chronic kidney disease; *CrCl,* creatinine clearance.

since ACEI/ARB can reduce LVH and possibly improve survival. A small trial demonstrated that ramipril can preserve residual urine output in those receiving peritoneal dialysis, which is a consistently favorable finding in ESRD.[77] A case-matched study of ESRD patients found that those who were taking ACEI or ARB had improved survival and this benefit appeared to get larger for longer durations of use.[78] ACEI/ARB therapy may worsen hyperkalemia in patients with ESRD. As tolerated, the clinician should consider adjusting the dialysis regimen to improve potassium removal and/or daily use of oral potassium binders.[79]

With an ACEI/ARB as a base of therapy, the antihypertensive regimen can be further modified according to blood pressure–lowering efficacy and CAD event reduction. Beta-blockers can be used as both an anti-hypertensive and anti-ischemic agents. In those with HF, beta-blockers improve left ventricular ejection fraction, and reduce rates of hospitalization, sudden death, and all-cause mortality. Patients with ESRD who receive beta-blockers after CAD events may have large relative risk reductions in all-cause mortality.

Additional choices of anti-hypertensive or cardioprotective agents should be based on ease of management and compliance, and lack of adverse effects. Guidelines for non-ESRD patients state the optimal office systolic blood pressure should be less than 130 mm Hg. The difficult task in the ESRD patient is to achieve these goals without having hypotension during dialysis sessions. Given the high rates of severe CAD in ESRD, hypotension during dialysis can worsen clinical and subclinical ischemia recognized as chest discomfort, shortness of breath, ST-segment depression on electrocardiography, and elevations of cTn on blood testing.

The goal of LDL-C reduction, in most cases with a statin and ezetimibe, in patients with ESRD is supported by a 17% reduction in major atherosclerotic events shown in the Study of Heart and Renal Protection in patients with predialysis CKD and ESRD.[80] Monoclonal antibodies against proprotein convertase subtilisin kexin 9 (PCSK9) can be used in CKD and ESRD to lower LDL-C in addition to maximally tolerated lipid-lowering therapy.[81] These agents additionally lower lipoprotein (a), which is commonly elevated in ESRD.[82] Colesevelam, a bile-acid sequestrant, also can aid in lowering serum phosphorus. Because of competing risk and reduced survival in CKD and ESRD, there are no trials demonstrating a mortality benefit with lipid-lowering therapy.

In ESRD with DM, blood glucose control to a target glycohemoglobin less than 7% can be expected to reduce rates of microvascular complications (retinopathy) and to a lesser extent, clinically important atherosclerotic disease elsewhere (MI, stroke, CVD death).[89] Patients with ESRD should stop smoking. The use of antiplatelet or antithrombotic agents for the prevention of CVD risk in ESRD requires caution.

In the setting of stable symptomatic CAD, an analysis from the Clinical Outcomes Utilizing Revascularization and Aggressive Drug Evaluation (COURAGE) trial suggested that PCI had no benefit over optimal medical therapy in patients with predialysis CKD.[83] The ISCHEMIA-CKD trial randomized 777 patients with moderate coronary ischemia and CKD (eGFR = 23 mL/min/1.73 m²) or on dialysis (51%) to an initial invasive strategy consisting of coronary angiography and revascularization (if appropriate) versus medical therapy alone and angiography reserved for those in whom medical therapy had failed.[84] While the rates of MI or cardiovascular death at 2.2 years were high (approximately 36.5%) in both groups, there was no benefit observed with the invasive approach. After symptomatic failure of optimal medical therapy in a patient with ESRD and CAD, the next step is coronary angiography and consideration of revascularization. In the common scenario of multivessel disease, multiple studies have shown that coronary artery bypass graft (CABG) surgery is associated with superior outcomes over PCI with drug-eluting stents probably due to more complete revascularization and protection from recurrent MI.[85] Patients with ESRD undergoing coronary revascularization procedures have increased risk for adverse events including death. Dialysis-dependent patients undergoing CABG face a 4.4-fold increased risk of in-hospital death, a 3.1 times greater risk of mediastinitis, and a 2.6-fold increased risk of stroke compared to those patients undergoing CABG who were not on dialysis.[48]

In summary, patients with ESRD have greater coronary heart disease risk than those with equivalent risk factor status without ESRD. An aggressive approach with medical management for CAD is warranted, even in the case of subclinical CAD. The threshold for diagnostic testing should be low in ESRD patients. When significant multivessel CAD is found, ESRD patients appear to benefit from revascularization with CABG compared to PCI, and if clinically reasonable, should be given that opportunity for improved survival and reduction in future cardiac events.

Considerations

Avoid AKI (e.g., radiocontrast, NSAIDs, aminoglycosides, vancomycin, lithium)
Treat iron-deficiency anemia
Treat vitamin B and thiamine deficiencies
Optimize CKD-MBD measures
Coronary revascularization
ICD/CRT as feasible and appropriate

Kidney transplantation
Nocturnal home hemodialysis
Peritoneal dialysis
In-center 3x/week dialysis

Digoxin
AF control

H-ISDN
• If RAASi/ARNI intolerant
• African American

Ivabradine
• On maximum tolerated β-blocker
Normal sinus rhythm heart rate >70

Mineralocorticoid antagonist
• If potassium is acceptable or manageable with K-binders

β-Adrenergic blocker
Carvedilol/metoprolol succinate/bisoprolol

ACEi or ARB if ACEi-intolerant or ARNi SGLT2i

Acute CRRT
IV thiazides
IV loop diuretics
Oral metolazone
Oral loop diuretics
Oral thiazides

FIGURE 101.14 Pharmacotherapy for the prevention and treatment of heart failure with reduced ejection fraction in chronic kidney disease (CKD) progressing to end-stage kidney disease. *ACEi*, Angiotensin-converting enzyme inhibitor; *AF*, atrial fibrillation; *AKI*, acute kidney injury; *ARB*, angiotensin II receptor blocker; *ARNi*, angiotensin receptor neprilysin inhibitor; *CKD-MBD*, chronic kidney disease–mineral bone disorder; *CRT*, cardiac resynchronization therapy; *CRRT*, continuous renal replacement therapy; *H-ISDN*, hydralazine-isosorbide dinitrate; *ICD*, implantable cardioverter-defibrillator; *NSAID*, nonsteroidal anti-inflammatory drug; *RAASi*, renin-angiotensin-aldosterone system inhibitor; *SGLT2i*, sodium glucose cotransporter 2 inhibitor. (Adapted from House AA, Wanner C, Sarnak MJ, et al. Heart failure in chronic kidney disease: conclusions from a Kidney Disease: Improving Global Outcomes (KDIGO) Controversies Conference. *Kidney Int.* 2019;95[6]:1304–1317.)

EVALUATION AND MANAGEMENT OF THE RENAL TRANSPLANT RECIPIENT

Cardiovascular screening is recommended in high-risk CKD patients before renal transplantation.[86] These include persons with DM, men over age 45 years, women over 55 years, previous history of ischemic heart disease, an abnormal electrocardiogram, left ventricular dysfunction, smoking history, and duration of dialysis more than 2 years. Controversies exist regarding the ideal screening test for CAD in ESRD patients. The choice of exercise versus pharmacologic stress and echocardiographic versus nuclear scintigraphic imaging requires individualization. Coronary cardiac computed tomographic angiography may be considered as another screening tool especially in the young with the understanding that it can exclude significant coronary disease and identify very-low-risk patients who may move on to renal transplantation.[87] However, substantial coronary artery calcification can render the interpretation of the computed tomographic angiogram difficult (see Chapter 20.) Coronary angiography and revascularization can be performed with very little loss of renal function in very low eGFR groups if done carefully with staged intervals between the diagnostic procedure and PCI or CABG.[88] After renal transplantation, treatment with lipid-lowering therapy (low potency statins, i.e., fluvastatin, pravastatin), is generally associated with a favorable benefit-to-risk ratio.[89] A meta-analysis of 22 studies (3465 participants) has supported the use of statins in renal transplant recipients for the reduction of cardiovascular events.[90] Finally, renal transplantation confers a relative freedom from the development of HF and associated complications and can be considered as a therapy in the overall schema of managing patients with combined heart and kidney failure (Fig. 101.14).[91]

SUMMARY

Recognition has increased over the last several decades that patients with CKD have a high risk for CVD. Frequent clinical scenarios in which renal function influences care include PCI, cardiac surgery, ACS, HF, valvular disease, and arrhythmias. Further study of the adverse metabolic milieu of CKD is likely to lead to generalizable diagnostic and therapeutic targets for the future management of renal patients with cardiovascular illness.

REFERENCES

Chronic Kidney Disease and Cardiovascular Risk

1. Szczech LA, Stewart RC, Su HL, et al. Primary care detection of chronic kidney disease in adults with type-2 diabetes: the ADD-CKD Study (awareness, detection and drug therapy in type 2 diabetes and chronic kidney disease). *PloS One.* 2014;9(11):e110535.
2. Ritz E, Zeng X-X, Rychlík I. Clinical manifestation and natural history of diabetic nephropathy. *Contrib Nephrol.* 2011;170:19–27.
3. Kruzel-Davila E, Wasser WG, Aviram S, Skorecki K. APOL1 nephropathy: from gene to mechanisms of kidney injury. *Nephrol Dial Transplant.* 2016;31(3):349–358.
4. Herzog CA, Asinger RW, Berger AK, et al. Cardiovascular disease in chronic kidney disease. a clinical update from kidney disease: improving Global Outcomes (KDIGO). *Kidney Int.* 2011;80(6):572–586.
5. Levey AS, Inker LA, Coresh J. GFR estimation: from physiology to public health. *Am J Kidney Dis.* 2014;63(5):820–834.
6. Ferguson TW, Komenda P, Tangri N. Cystatin C as a biomarker for estimating glomerular filtration rate. *Curr Opin Nephrol Hypertens.* 2015;24(3):295–300.
7. Amin AP, Whaley-Connell AT, Li S, et al. The synergistic relationship between estimated GFR and microalbuminuria in predicting long-term progression to ESRD or death in patients with diabetes: results from the Kidney Early Evaluation Program (KEEP). *Am J Kidney Dis.* 2013;61(4 suppl 2):S12–S23.
8. Matsushita K, Coresh J, Sang Y, et al. Estimated glomerular filtration rate and albuminuria for prediction of cardiovascular outcomes: a collaborative meta-analysis of individual participant data. *Lancet Diabetes Endocrinol.* 2015;3(7):514–525.
9. Palmer SC, Navaneethan SD, Craig JC, et al. Meta-analysis: erythropoiesis-stimulating agents in patients with chronic kidney disease. *Ann Intern Med.* 2010;153(1):23–33.
10. Covic A, Nistor I, Donciu MD, et al. Erythropoiesis-stimulating agents (ESA) for preventing the progression of chronic kidney disease: a meta-analysis of 19 studies. *Am J Nephrol.* 2014;40(3):263–279.
11. Collister D, Komenda P, Hiebert B, et al. The effect of erythropoietin-stimulating agents on health-related quality of life in anemia of chronic kidney disease: a systematic review and meta-analysis. *Ann Intern Med.* 2016;164(7):472–478.
12. Swedberg K, Young JB, Anand IS, et al. Treatment of anemia with darbepoetin alfa in systolic heart failure. *N Engl J Med.* 2013;368(13):1210–1219.
13. McCullough PA, Barnhart HX, Inrig JK, et al. Cardiovascular toxicity of epoetin-alfa in patients with chronic kidney disease. *Am J Nephrol.* 2013;37(6):549–558.
14. McCullough PA, Uhlig K, Neylan JF, et al. Usefulness of oral ferric citrate in patients with iron-deficiency anemia and chronic kidney disease with or without heart failure. *Am J Cardiol.* 2018;122(4):683–688.
15. Clevenger B, Gurusamy K, Klein AA, et al. Systematic review and meta-analysis of iron therapy in anaemic adults without chronic kidney disease: updated and abridged Cochrane review. *Eur J Heart Fail.* 2016.
16. Jankowska EA, Tkaczyszyn M, Suchocki T, et al. Effects of intravenous iron therapy in iron-deficient patients with systolic heart failure: a meta-analysis of randomized controlled trials. *Eur J Heart Fail.* 2016.
17. Maxwell PH, Eckardt KU. HIF prolyl hydroxylase inhibitors for the treatment of renal anaemia and beyond. *Nat Rev Nephrol.* 2016;12(3):157–168.
18. Chen N, Hao C, Liu BC, et al. Roxadustat treatment for anemia in patients undergoing long-term dialysis. *N Engl J Med.* 2019;381(11):1011–1022.
19. Liu J, Zhang A, Hayden JC, et al. Roxadustat (FG-4592) treatment for anemia in dialysis-dependent (DD) and not dialysis-dependent (NDD) chronic kidney disease patients: a systematic review and meta-analysis. *Pharmacol Res.* 2020;155:104747.

Contrast-Induced and Intervention-Associated Acute Kidney Injury

20. KDIGO AKI Work Group. KDIGO clinical practice guideline for acute kidney injury. *Kidney Int Suppl.* 2012;17:1–138.

21. Tsai TT, Patel UD, Chang TI, et al. Contemporary incidence, predictors, and outcomes of acute kidney injury in patients undergoing percutaneous coronary interventions: insights from the NCDR cath-PCI registry. *JACC Cardiovasc Interv*. 2014;7(1):1–9.

22. McCullough PA, Choi JP, Feghali GA, et al. Contrast-induced acute kidney injury. *J Am Coll Cardiol*. 2016;68(13):1465–1473.

23. Keeley EC, Grines CL. Scraping of aortic debris by coronary guiding catheters: a prospective evaluation of 1,000 cases. *J Am Coll Cardiol*. 1998;32(7):1861–1865.

24. Kooiman J, Seth M, Dixon S, et al. Risk of acute kidney injury after percutaneous coronary interventions using radial versus femoral vascular access: insights from the Blue Cross Blue Shield of Michigan Cardiovascular Consortium. *Circ Cardiovasc Interv*. 2014;7(2):190–198.

25. Cortese B, Sciahbasi A, Sebik R, et al. Comparison of risk of acute kidney injury after primary percutaneous coronary interventions with the transradial approach versus the transfemoral approach (from the PRIPITENA urban registry). *Am J Cardiol*. 2014;114(6):820–825.

26. Mehran R, Aymong ED, Nikolsky E, et al. A simple risk score for prediction of contrast-induced nephropathy after percutaneous coronary intervention: development and initial validation. *J Am Coll Cardiol*. 2004;44(7):1393–1399.

27. Solomon R, Gordon P, Manoukian SV, et al. Randomized trial of bicarbonate or saline study for the prevention of contrast-induced nephropathy in patients with CKD. *Clin J Am Soc Nephrol*. 2015;10(9):1519–1524.

28. Brar SS, Shen AY, Jorgensen MB, et al. Sodium bicarbonate vs sodium chloride for the prevention of contrast medium-induced nephropathy in patients undergoing coronary angiography: a randomized trial. *J Am Med Assoc*. 2008;300(9):1038–1046.

29. McCullough PA, Brown JR. Effects of intra-arterial and intravenous iso-osmolar contrast medium (iodixanol) on the risk of contrast-induced acute kidney injury: a meta-analysis. *Cardiorenal Med*. 2011;1(4):220–234.

30. Andò G, Gragnano F, Calabrò P, Valgimigli M. Radial vs femoral access for the prevention of acute kidney injury (AKI) after coronary angiography or intervention: a systematic review and meta-analysis. *Catheter Cardiovasc Interv*. 2018;92(7):E518-E526.

31. ACT Investigators. Acetylcysteine for prevention of renal outcomes in patients undergoing coronary and peripheral vascular angiography: main results from the randomized Acetylcysteine for Contrast-induced nephropathy Trial (ACT). *Circulation*. 2011;124(11):1250–1259.

32. Weisbord SD, Gallagher M, Jneid H, et al. Outcomes after angiography with sodium bicarbonate and acetylcysteine. *N Engl J Med*. 2018;378(7):603–614.

33. Tecson KM, Brown D, Choi JW, et al. Major adverse renal and cardiac events after coronary angiography and cardiac surgery. *Ann Thorac Surg*. 2018;105(6):1724–1730.

34. O'Neal JB, Shaw AD, Billings 4th FT. Acute kidney injury following cardiac surgery: current understanding and future directions. *Crit Care*. 2016;20(1):187.

Acceleration of Vascular Calcification

35. Raggi P, Chertow GM, Torres PU, et al. The ADVANCE study: a randomized study to evaluate the effects of cinacalcet plus low-dose vitamin D on vascular calcification in patients on hemodialysis. *Nephrol Dial Transplant*. 2011;26(4):1327–1339.

36. EVOLVE Trial Investigators, Chertow GM, Block GA, et al. Effect of cinacalcet on cardiovascular disease in patients undergoing dialysis. *N Engl J Med*. 2012;367(26):2482–2494.

37. Charytan DM, Fishbane S, Malyszko J, et al. Cardiorenal syndrome and the role of the bone-mineral axis and anemia. *Am J Kidney Dis*. 2015;66(2):196–205.

Renal Disease and Hypertension

38. Khouri Y, Steigerwalt SP, Alsamara M, McCullough PA. What is the ideal blood pressure goal for patients with stage III or higher chronic kidney disease?. *Curr Cardiol Rep*. 2011;13(6):492–501.

39. Beddhu S, Shen J, Cheung AK, et al. Implications of early decline in eGFR due to intensive BP control for cardiovascular outcomes in SPRINT. *J Am Soc Nephrol*. 2019;30(8):1523–1533.

40. Cohen MG, Pascua JA, Garcia-Ben M, et al. A simple prediction rule for significant renal artery stenosis in patients undergoing cardiac catheterization. *Am Heart J*. 2005;150(6):1204–1211.

41. Akinseye OA, Ralston WF, Johnson KC, et al. Renal sympathetic denervation: a comprehensive review [published online ahead of print, 2020 may 3]. *Curr Probl Cardiol*. 2020:100598.

Acute Coronary Syndromes in Patients with Chronic Kidney Disease

42. Twerenbold R, Wildi K, Jaeger C, et al. Optimal cutoff levels of more sensitive cardiac troponin assays for the early diagnosis of myocardial infarction in patients with renal dysfunction. *Circulation*. 2015;131(23):2041–2050.

43. deFilippi C, Seliger SL, Kelley W, et al. Interpreting cardiac troponin results from high-sensitivity assays in chronic kidney disease without acute coronary syndrome. *Clin Chem*. 2012;58(9):1342–1351.

44. Vasudevan A, Singer AJ, DeFilippi C, et al. Renal function and scaled troponin in patients presenting to the emergency department with symptoms of myocardial infarction. *Am J Nephrol*. 2017;45(4):304–309.

45. Fox CS, Muntner P, Chen AY, et al. Acute Coronary Treatment and Intervention Outcomes Network registry. Use of evidence-based therapies in short-term outcomes of ST-segment elevation myocardial infarction and non-ST-segment elevation myocardial infarction in patients with chronic kidney disease: a report from the National Cardiovascular Data Acute Coronary Treatment and Intervention Outcomes Network registry. *Circulation*. 2010;121(3):357–365.

46. McCullough PA. Why is chronic kidney disease the "spoiler" for cardiovascular outcomes?. *J Am Coll Cardiol*. 2003;41(5):725–728.

47. Sica D. The implications of renal impairment among patients undergoing percutaneous coronary intervention. *J Invasive Cardiol*. 2002;14(suppl B):30B-37B.

48. Roberts JK, McCullough PA. The management of acute coronary syndromes in patients with chronic kidney disease. *Adv Chronic Kidney Dis*. 2014;21(6):472–479.

49. Szummer K, Lundman P, Jacobson SH, et al. Influence of renal function on the effects of early revascularization in non-ST-elevation myocardial infarction: data from the Swedish web-system for enhancement and development of evidence-based care in heart disease evaluated according to recommended therapies (SWEDEHEART). *Circulation*. 2009;120(10):851–858.

Cardiorenal Syndromes

50. McCullough PA, Kluger AY. Interpreting the wide range of NT-proBNP concentrations in clinical decision making. *J Am Coll Cardiol*. 2018;71(11):1201–1203.

51. Rangaswami J, Bhalla V, Blair JEA, et al. American heart association council on the kidney in cardiovascular disease and council on clinical cardiology. Cardiorenal syndrome: classification, Pathophysiology, diagnosis, and treatment strategies: a scientific statement from the American heart association. *Circulation*. 2019;139(16):e840–e878.

52. Haase M, Müller C, Damman K, et al. Pathogenesis of cardiorenal syndrome type 1 in acute decompensated heart failure: workgroup statements from the eleventh consensus conference of the Acute Dialysis Quality Initiative (ADQI). *Contrib Nephrol*. 2013;182:99–116.

53. Oliveros E, Oni ET, Shahzad A, et al. Benefits and risks of continuing angiotensin-converting enzyme inhibitors, angiotensin II receptor antagonists, and mineralocorticoid receptor antagonists during hospitalizations for acute heart failure. *Cardiorenal Med*. 2020;10(2):69–84.

54. Singhania G, Ejaz AA, McCullough PA, et al. Continuation of chronic heart failure therapies during heart failure hospitalization - a review. *Rev Cardiovasc Med*. 2019;20(3):111–120.

55. Gunderson EG, Lillyblad MP, Fine M, et al. Tolvaptan for volume management in heart failure. *Pharmacotherapy*. 2019;39(4):473–485.

56. Costanzo MR, Ronco C, Abraham WT, et al. Extracorporeal ultrafiltration for fluid overload in heart failure: current status and prospects for further research. *J Am Coll Cardiol*. 2017;69(19):2428–2445.

57. Weinhandl ED, Gilbertson DT, Collins AJ. Mortality, hospitalization, and technique failure in daily home hemodialysis and matched peritoneal dialysis patients: a matched cohort study. *Am J Kidney Dis*. 2016;67(1):98–110.

58. Kluger AY, Tecson KM, Barbin CM, et al. Cardiorenal outcomes in the canvas, DECLARE-TIMI 58, and EMPA-REG outcome trials: a systematic review. *Rev Cardiovasc Med*. 2018;19(2):41–49.

59. Kluger AY, Tecson KM, et al. Class effects of SGLT2 inhibitors on cardiorenal outcomes. *Cardiovasc Diabetol*. 2019;18(1):99.

60. Lo KB, Gul F, Ram P, et al. The effects of SGLT2 inhibitors on cardiovascular and renal outcomes in diabetic patients: a systematic review and meta-analysis. *Cardiorenal Med*. 2020;10(1):1–10.

61. Roberts WC, Taylor MA, Shirani J. Cardiac findings at necropsy in patients with chronic kidney disease maintained on chronic hemodialysis. *Medicine (Baltim)*. 2012;91(3):165–178.

62. Roberts WC, Taylor MA, Shirani J. Cardiac findings at necropsy in patients with chronic kidney disease maintained on chronic hemodialysis. *Medicine (Baltim)*. 2012;91(3):165–178.

Chronic Kidney Disease and Valvular Heart Disease

63. Kim D, Shim CY, Hong GR, et al. Effect of end-stage renal disease on rate of progression of aortic stenosis. *Am J Cardiol*. 2016;117(12):1972–1977.

64. Kamalakannan D, Pai RM, Johnson LB, et al. Epidemiology and clinical outcomes of infective endocarditis in hemodialysis patients. *Ann Thorac Surg*. 2007;83(6):2081–2086.

65. Altarabsheh SE, Deo SV, Dunlay SM, et al. Tissue valves are preferable for patients with end-stage renal disease: an aggregate meta-analysis. *J Card Surg*. 2016.

Renal Function and Arrhythmias

66. Pun PH, Lehrich RW, Honeycutt EF, et al. Modifiable risk factors associated with sudden cardiac arrest within hemodialysis clinics. *Kidney Int*. 2011;79(2):218–227.

67. Palmer BF. Potassium binders for hyperkalemia in chronic kidney disease-diet, renin-angiotensin-aldosterone system inhibitor therapy, and hemodialysis. *Mayo Clin Proc*. 2020;95(2):339–354.

68. Jukema JW, Timal RJ, Rotmans JI, et al. Prophylactic use of implantable cardioverter-defibrillators in the prevention of sudden cardiac death in dialysis patients. *Circulation*. 2019;139(23):2628–2638.

69. Opelami O, Sakhuja A, Liu X, et al. Outcomes of infected cardiovascular implantable devices in dialysis patients. *Am J Nephrol*. 2014;40(3):280–287.

70. Hage FG, Aljaroudi W, Aggarwal H, et al. Outcomes of patients with chronic kidney disease and implantable cardiac defibrillator: primary versus secondary prevention. *Int J Cardiol*. 2013;165(1):113–116.

Consultative Approach to the Hemodialysis Patient

71. De Vriese AS, Vandecasteele SJ, Van den Bergh B, De Geeter FW. Should we screen for coronary artery disease in asymptomatic chronic dialysis patients?. *Kidney Int*. 2012;81(2):143–151.

72. McCullough PA, Roberts WC. Influence of chronic renal failure on cardiac structure. *J Am Coll Cardiol*. 2016;67(10):1183–1185.

73. De Lima JJ, Gowdak LH, de Paula FJ, et al. Coronary artery disease assessment and intervention in renal transplant patients: analysis from the KiHeart cohort. *Transplantation*. 2016;100(7):1580–1587.

74. Kotanko P, Garg AX, Depner T, et al. Effects of frequent hemodialysis on blood pressure: results from the randomized frequent hemodialysis network trials. *Hemodial Int*. 2015;19(3):386–401.

75. McCullough PA, Chan CT, Weinhandl ED, et al. Intensive hemodialysis, left ventricular hypertrophy, and cardiovascular disease. *Am J Kidney Dis*. 2016;68(5S1):S5-S14.

76. Rao NN, Dundon BK, Worthley MI, Faull RJ. The impact of arteriovenous fistulae for hemodialysis on the cardiovascular system. *Semin Dial*. 2016;29(3):214–221.

77. Li PK, Chow KM, Wong TY, et al. Effects of an angiotensin-converting enzyme inhibitor on residual renal function in patients receiving peritoneal dialysis. A randomized, controlled study. *Ann Intern Med*. 2003;139(2):105–112. PubMed PMID: 12859160.

78. Wu CK, Yang YH, Juang JM, et al. Effects of angiotensin converting enzyme inhibition or angiotensin receptor blockade in dialysis patients: a nationwide data survey and propensity analysis. *Medicine (Baltim)*. 2015;94(3):e424.

79. McCullough PA, Costanzo MR, Silver M, et al. Novel agents for the prevention and management of hyperkalemia. *Rev Cardiovasc Med*. 2015;16(2):140–155. Review. PubMed PMID: 26198561.

80. Baigent C, Landray MJ, Reith C, et al. The effects of lowering LDL cholesterol with simvastatin plus ezetimibe in patients with chronic kidney disease (Study of Heart and Renal Protection): a randomised placebo-controlled trial. *Lancet*. 2011;377(9784):2181–2192.

81. Charytan DM, Sabatine MS, Pedersen TR, et al. Efficacy and safety of evolocumab in chronic kidney disease in the FOURIER trial. *J Am Coll Cardiol*. 2019;73(23):2961–2970.

82. Watts GF, Chan DC, Pang J, et al. PCSK9 Inhibition with alirocumab increases the catabolism of lipoprotein(a) particles in statin-treated patients with elevated lipoprotein(a). *Metabolism*. 2020;107:154221.

83. Sedlis SP, Jurkovitz CT, Hartigan PM, et al. Optimal medical therapy with or without percutaneous coronary intervention for patients with stable coronary artery disease and chronic kidney disease. *Am J Cardiol*. 2009;104(12):1647–1653.

84. Bangalore S, Maron DJ, O'Brien SM, et al. Management of coronary disease in patients with advanced kidney disease. *N Engl J Med*. 2020;382(17):1608–1618.

85. Ashrith G, Lee VV, Elayda MA, et al. Short- and long-term outcomes of coronary artery bypass grafting or drug-eluting stent implantation for multivessel coronary artery disease in patients with chronic kidney disease. *Am J Cardiol*. 2010;106(3):348–353.

86. Lentine KL, Costa SP, Weir MR, et al. American heart association council on the kidney in cardiovascular disease and council on peripheral vascular disease. cardiac disease evaluation and management among kidney and liver transplantation candidates: a scientific statement from the American heart association and the American college of cardiology foundation. *J Am Coll Cardiol*. 2012;60(5):434–480.

87. Winther S, Svensson M, Jørgensen HS, et al. Diagnostic performance of coronary CT angiography and myocardial perfusion imaging in kidney transplantation candidates. *JACC Cardiovasc Imaging*. 2015;8(5):553–562.

88. Kumar N, Dahri L, Brown W, et al. Effect of elective coronary angiography on glomerular filtration rate in patients with advanced chronic kidney disease. *Clin J Am Soc Nephrol*. 2009;4(12):1907–1913.

89. Riella LV, Gabardi S, Chandraker A. Dyslipidemia and its therapeutic challenges in renal transplantation. *Am J Transplant*. 2012;12(8):1975–1982.

90. Palmer SC, Navaneethan SD, Craig JC, et al. HMG CoA reductase inhibitors (statins) for kidney transplant recipients. *Cochrane Database Syst Rev*. 2014;(1):CD005019.

91. House AA, Wanner C, Sarnak MJ, et al. Heart failure in chronic kidney disease: conclusions from a kidney disease: Improving Global Outcomes (KDIGO) Controversies conference. *Kidney Int*. 2019;95(6):1304–1317.

102 Cardiovascular Manifestations of Autonomic Disorders

JASON S. BRADFIELD AND KALYANAM SHIVKUMAR

The critical role of a balanced autonomic nervous system for appropriate function and responsiveness of the cardiovascular system is often overlooked. The interrelationship of these two systems is often thought of predominantly through the lens of abnormalities in blood pressure and heart rate in response to internal and external stimuli in patients with structurally "normal hearts" or secondary to primary neurologic abnormalities. However, the cardiovascular manifestations of autonomic dysfunction are much more complex. Autonomic dysfunction/dysregulation can be caused by direct cardiac insults, leading to abnormal afferent signaling and local remodeling subsequent progression to cardiac disorders from heart failure to atrial and ventricular arrhythmias and sudden cardiac death.

This chapter reviews cardiovascular autonomic anatomy and physiology in health and disease with further discussion of primary and secondary cardiovascular autonomic dysfunction and how this dysfunction can lead to benign as well as life-threatening disorders.

OVERVIEW OF ANATOMY AND PHYSIOLOGY OF THE AUTONOMIC NERVOUS SYSTEM

The autonomic nervous system regulates heart rate, cardiac contractility, and blood pressure and responds on a beat-to-beat basis to physiologic stress. This real-time response allows individuals to adjust to the external environment as well as to physiologic changes in multiple organ systems. Therefore, the "environment" that the autonomic nervous system is responding to is both internal and external encompassing a broad spectrum of stimuli including cardiovascular afferents, pressure, and volume sensors, as well as postural and visual stimuli.

Sympathetic, Parasympathetic, and Intrinsic Neuronal Control

The anatomy and physiology of the cardiovascular autonomic nervous system is a complex interplay of sympathetic, parasympathetic, and intrinsic neurons in addition to a number of well-established reflexes (Fig. 102.1). In addition to direct afferent and efferent connections between the brain and central nervous system and the heart and vascular system that control all aspects of cardiac physiologic function, visceral integration and reflexes maintain and optimize blood pressure. The sympathetic and parasympathetic systems are often thought of as opposing forces; however the intricate feedback between these

systems, the intrinsic cardiac nervous system, and numerous reflex arcs allows for highly refined regulation of cardiac electrical and mechanical function.

Cardiac autonomic nerves can anatomically be broken down into central, intrathoracic, and intrinsic cardiac components.[1,2] The cardiac intrinsic components are located in the epicardial fat pads and cardiac ganglia. These ganglionated plexi include afferent, efferent, and interconnecting neurons. The ganglia (located in the region of the posterior left atrium, aortopulmonary window, anterior/posterior right atrium, and junction of the inferior vena cava and inferior right atrium) give input to the sinus and atrioventricular nodes (Fig. 102.2). The left and right cardiac nerves are a combination of sympathetic and parasympathetic nerves entering and leaving the heart.

From the heart, afferent sensory neurons provide real-time information on cardiac status via parasympathetic (vagal trunk/nodose ganglia) and sympathetic (dorsal root ganglia) tracts to the higher centers. Efferent motor neurons travel from the central system to the epicardial cardiac structures. Sympathetic efferents travel from the intermediolateral spinal cord to the superior, middle, and cervicothoracic (stellate) ganglia. The pre-ganglionic neurons secrete acetylcholine that binds to nicotinic receptors. The post-ganglionic nerves then project from the stellate ganglia (C8-T1) plus T2-T4 to the epicardium of the atria and ventricles where the postganglionic neurons release norepinephrine, which binds to alpha- and beta-adrenergic receptors. Parasympathetic efferents originate in the nucleus ambiguous and medulla oblongata and travel through the vagus nerve to the cardiac ganglia. Approximately 80% of fibers in the vagus nerve are thought to be afferent, however. Parasympathetic pre-ganglionic neurons release acetylcholine to activate nicotinic and muscarinic cholinergic receptors. Post-ganglionic neurons secrete acetylcholine to activate muscarinic receptors in the myocardium and vasculature.

The sympathetic and parasympathetic nervous systems are generally thought of as parallel and separate systems, though there is some crossover between sympathetic and parasympathetic systems as well as afferent and efferent pathways. Identification of neuron types is often only possible by assessment of specific neurotransmitters (which is beyond the scope of this chapter). The antagonization that does occur happens at both pre- and postsynaptic levels. Norepinephrine and acetylcholine impair the release of the other and afferent signals are processed at multiple levels of the system. Further, the cotransmitter neuropeptide Y released from sympathetic nerves can also inhibit acetylcholine.[3] Cardiac electrophysiologic effects of sympathetic and parasympathetic systems are summarized in Table 102.1.[4]

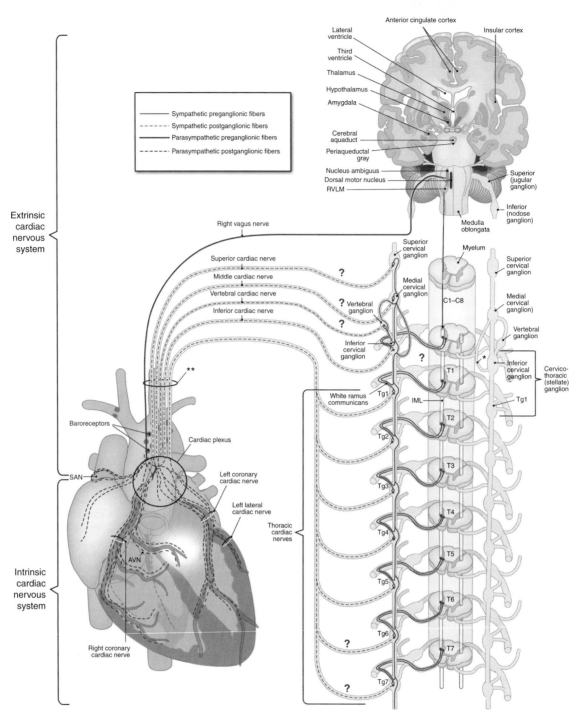

FIGURE 102.1 Overview of cardiac innervation. Schematic drawing of the cardiac autonomic nervous system. Preganglionic cardiac parasympathetic axons arise from neurons in either the nucleus ambiguus or dorsal motor nucleus of the vagus nerve; they run in cardiac branches of the vagus nerve (*solid blue lines*) to synapse in cardiac plexuses and ganglia from where postganglionic fibers (*dashed blue lines*) innervate the sinoatrial node (SAN), atrioventricular node (AVN), coronary arteries, and ventricular myocytes. Preganglionic cardiac sympathetic axons (*solid red lines*) arise from neurons in the intermediolateral cell columns (IMLs) of the upper four or five (possibly six or seven) thoracic spinal segments, that receive modulating input from several forebrain centers (e.g., the insular cortex, anterior cingulate cortex, central nuclei of the amygdala, and several hypothalamic nuclei interneurons); they leave the spinal cord through anterior (ventral) roots, enter the anterior (ventral) rami of spinal nerves and pass to the sympathetic chains through white rami communicantes to synapse in the upper thoracic (Tg) or cervical ganglia; postganglionic fibers (*dashed red lines*) from these ganglia form the sympathetic cardiac nerves. At the heart parasympathetic and sympathetic nerves converge to form the cardiac plexus from which atrial and ventricular autonomic innervation is arranged. The red question marks (*?*) indicate anatomical structures for which existence and/or involvement in cardiac sympathetic innervation are debated. *Ansa subclavia. **Vagal and sympathetic nerves intermingle before reaching the cardiac plexus and projecting on the heart. *RVLM*, rostral ventrolateral medulla. (From Wink J, et al. Human adult cardiac autonomic innervation: controversies in anatomical knowledge and relevance for cardiac neuromodulation. Auton Neurosci 2020;227:102674.)

Baroreflex

Autonomic innervation of arteries, veins, and capillaries control vascular tone and diameter. Afferent neurons respond to chemical and mechanical stimuli in regions such as the aortic arch and carotid sinus to regulate blood flow, blood pressure, and heart rate via baroreflexes with the ultimate goal of protecting cerebral perfusion.[5] Baroreceptors existing in the walls of major blood vessels (mechanoreceptors in the aortic arch, carotid sinus, origin of the right subclavian artery in addition to low pressure sensors in the atria and pulmonary artery) are activated by stretch related to blood pressure/volume and activate the brain stem predominantly via the vagus nerve. These mechanoreceptors are stretch-dependent, leading to an increased frequency of discharge in the glossopharyngeal nerve and the aortic nerve, which coalesce with the vagus nerve. The low-pressure cardiopulmonary baroreceptors

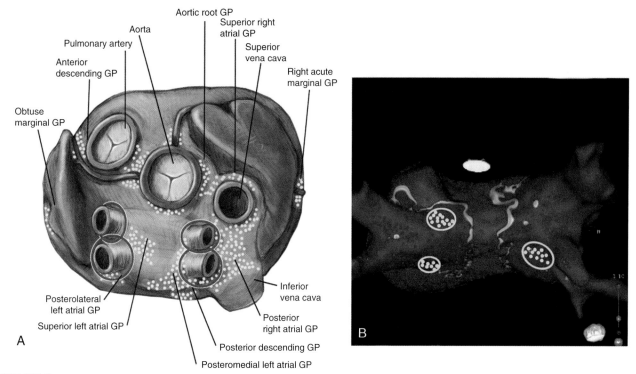

FIGURE 102.2 **Intrinsic cardiac nervous system. A,** Dense network of intrinsic cardiac ganglionated plexi (GP) (*yellow dots*) correlates anatomically with major cardiac vessels. These GP also crudely match ablation sites targeted by most pulmonary vein isolation (PVI) techniques (*red circles*) for atrial fibrillation. **B,** Electroanatomic map of PV after atrial fibrillation ablation, showing correlation of ablation sites with approximated sites of intrinsic cardiac GP (*encircled gray dots*). *Red,* low voltage tissue after pulmonary vein isolation (ablation); *Purple,* normal tissue (not ablated). (From Zhu C, et al. Neuromodulation for ventricular tachycardia and atrial fibrillation: a clinical scenario-based review. JACC Clin Electrophysiol 2019;5:881-896.)

TABLE 102.1 Sympathetic versus Parasympathetic Effects on Heart

CARDIAC PARAMETER	SYMPATHETIC ACTIVATION	PARASYMPATHETIC ACTIVATION	POTENTIAL MECHANISMS
Chronotropy (heart rate)	↑	↓	SNS: Increased SA node phase 4 slope due to increased L-type Ca and I_f currents. PSNS: Less steep phase 4 slope from increased magnitude of ligand-gated K current.
Ventricular action potential duration and refractory period	↓	↑	SNS leads to release of NE and beta-adrenergic receptors. Role of cotransmitters unknown. PNS releases ACh, which inhibits NE release and may also increase APD by muscarinic receptor activation.
Automaticity	↑	↓	SNS-mediated release of NE and beta-adrenergic receptor activation. Role of cotransmitters unknown. PNS releases ACh, which inhibits NE release and may also increase APD by muscarinic receptor activation.
Dispersion of repolarization	↑	↓	SNS: Causes heterogeneity in repolarization in infarcted hearts PNS: Reduces DOR by reducing dispersion in border zone of infarcts
Afterdepolarizations (EADs and DADs)	↑	↓	SNS: Causes calcium overload PNS: Reduces calcium entry

Ach, Acetylcholine; *APD,* action potential duration; *DAD,* delayed after depolarization; *DOR,* dispersion of repolarization; *EAD,* early after depolarization; *NE,* norepinephrine; *PNS,* parasympathetic nervous system activation; *SNS,* sympathetic nervous system activation.
From Wu P, Vaseghi M. The autonomic nervous system and ventricular arrhythmias in myocardial infarction and heart failure. *Pacing Clin Electrophysiol* 2020;43:172-180.

respond to volume, and when volume increases there is a vasodilatory response and drop in blood pressure in addition to a decrease in vasopressin, which leads to an increase in salt and water excretion.

Critical adjustment for postural changes is predominantly controlled through baroreflexes (Fig. 102.3). As vascular pressures change, the relative sympathetic to parasympathetic activity is modified to allow for increased vascular tone, cardiac contractility, and heart rate. Abruptly elevated blood pressure leads to increased stretch of baroreceptors and increased firing, causing decreased sympathetic and increased parasympathetic activity. This change in activity leads to reduced arteriolar resistance and decreased venous tone, as well as decreased heart rate and cardiac contractility.

With standing, less pressure is sensed by the baroreceptors, which leads to vasoconstriction and increased heart rate to prevent drop in blood pressure and associated symptoms. At rest, the baroreflex allows the parasympathetic input to predominate and inhibits sympathetic

output. This critical reflex is not consistently present for patients with orthostatic hypotension and vasovagal syncope discussed later. One must recall that the "intrinsic heart rate" of the sinus node is approximately 100 beats per minute (bpm), and what we consider normal resting heart rate (50 to 70 bpm) is the result of elevated parasympathetic input relative to sympathetic. Therefore, heart rate can be raised with decreased parasympathetic stimulation.

Chemoreflex

Chemoreceptors respond to hypoxia and hypercapnia. When activated they lead to vasoconstriction and hyperventilation. There are peripheral (carotid body) and central (brainstem) chemoreceptors. In obstructive sleep apnea, for example, chemoreflexes respond to the recurrent apnea/hypoxia with a sympathetic vasoconstriction and a

Baroreflex Measures

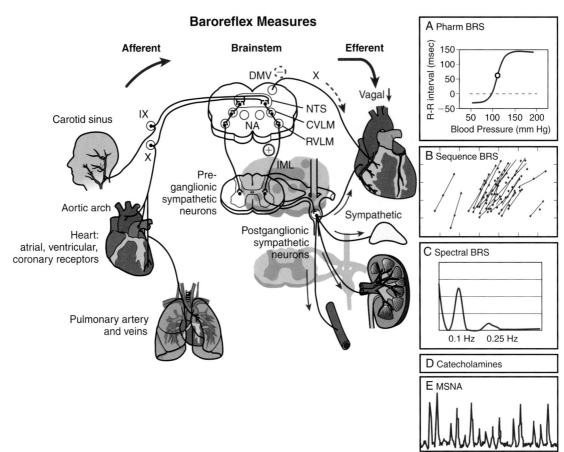

FIGURE 102.3 Diagram of the baroreflex in humans with methods of assessment. A to E, Five methods of assessing baroreflex sensitivity (BRS). **A,** Baroreflex properties can be assessed by pharmacologic probing with graduated doses of BP-elevating and/or BP-lowering drugs such as phenylephrine and nitroprusside. Changes in slope of the regression line between R-R interval changes and BP changes is referred to as *baroreflex sensitivity*. **B,** The same can be done by using spontaneous fluctuations of BP and R-R intervals, where sequences of heartbeats with increasing or decreasing BP and R-R prolongation are identified and analyzed. **C,** Spectral analysis of HR and BP variability allows assessment of sympathetic and vagal modulation of HR and BP. Cross-spectral transfer function analysis can be used to study the interactions and determine baroreflex sensitivity. **D,** Plasma catecholamine levels are essential markers for sympathetic activity. **E,** Recording of muscle sympathetic nerve activity (MSNA). MSNA is an instantaneous signal of current sympathetic activation, and it allows the estimation of sympathetic baroreflex sensitivity. *CVLM,* Caudal ventrolateral medulla; *DMV,* dorsal motor nucleus of vagus; *IML,* intermediolateral column of spinal cord; *NA,* nucleus ambiguous (vagus); *NTS,* nucleus tractus solitarius; *RVLM,* rostral ventrolateral medulla. (From Robertson D, Robertson RM. Cardiovascular Manifestations of Autonomic Disorders. In Zipes DP, et al., editors. Braunwald's Heart Disease: A Textbook Cardiovascular Medicine. 11th ed. Elsevier; 2019.)

bradycardic response, which is adaptive initially but ultimately can have pathologic consequences.

Diving Reflex

The diving reflex is a powerful reflex in response to diving under water in mammals to allow for prolonged submersion. There is a simultaneous increase in parasympathetic and sympathetic drive. Crucial organ oxygenation is protected including a dramatic bradycardia to decrease myocardial oxygen demand.

PATHOPHYSIOLOGY

Autonomic Dysfunction in the Setting of a Structurally Normal Heart

Autonomic dysregulation can lead to neurally mediated syncope from orthostatic hypotension/vasovagal syncope or carotid sinus syndrome.[6] These are disorders of autonomic reflexes. Other disorders such as postural tachycardia syndrome (POTS) and inappropriate sinus tachycardia (IST) are thought to be in part due to elevated sympathetic activity. These syndromes, which are more common in young women, can have significant overlap. Though not life-threatening, these disorders can significantly impair quality of life.

Vasovagal syncope occurs after upright posture or after painful stimuli or emotional stress. Prodromal symptoms of diaphoresis, a "warm sensation" and nausea, often occur. Vasovagal syncope is reported to occur in over 40% of women and 30% of men by the age of 60 due to

lack of effective reflex response to posture and venous pooling or in response to external stimuli. Decreased cardiac output and a potential paradoxical vasodilation with hypotension and possible bradycardia can lead to syncope. Treatment for vasovagal syncope, when episodes are frequent, include lifestyle modification, hydration, lower extremity compression stockings, beta blockers, and fludrocortisone/midodrine. While most vasovagal syncope involves a combination of hypotension and bradycardia (mixed), in some cases patients may have a primary "cardio-inhibitory" response with pronounced bradycardia that responds to pacemaker implantation.

POTS patients have symptoms (lightheadedness, palpitations, etc.) with standing that are associated with a rise in heart rate of ≥30 bpm without an associated drop in systolic blood pressure. POTS is much more prevalent in women (~75%) in the age range of 15 to 25 years, but overall prevalence is low at around 0.2%.[7] A full understanding of mechanism is not clear but has been postulated to involve components of autonomic denervation, hypovolemia, possible autoimmunity, hypervigilance, and deconditioning. In fact, a structured exercise program starting with recumbent exercises can be used as a treatment prior to considering pharmacologic therapies such as beta blockers. IST is a resting heart rate over 100 bpm, or over 90 bpm on average Holter monitor recordings, without reversible cause and associated with symptoms. IST occurs in less than 1.5% of the population. Similar to POTS, the cause is not completely understood. Medical therapy with beta blockers or Ivabradine (an I*f* current blocker) can be utilized to decrease heart rate in some cases.

Neural pathology can secondarily occur in a number of disorders including but not limited to diabetes, Parkinson disease, and multisystem atrophy. Neurologic injury including spinal cord disorders, severe head injury, subarachnoid hemorrhage, and stroke can manifest with distinct cardiac electrophysiologic abnormalities including brady- and tachyarrhythmias.[8,9] In some instances the resulting autonomic dysfunction is transient and can resolve with resolution of the primary pathology, such as in subarachnoid hemorrhage. In more chronic disease states, such as Parkinson or multisystem atrophy, the autonomic manifestations can be chronic and progressive.

Autonomic Dysfunction in the Setting of Intrinsic Cardiac Disease

Autonomic dysfunction can occur due to, and further exacerbate, primary cardiac pathology including myocardial infarction as well as ischemic and nonischemic cardiomyopathy and associated heart failure. These disorders can directly damage cardiac nerves. Subsequent increase in sympathetic (including increased cardiac norepinephrine spillover and increased activation of the renin-angiotensin-aldosterone system in the kidneys) and decrease in parasympathetic output may occur to maintain homeostasis; however, the persistent afferent pathologic signaling can lead to a cycle of worsening cardiac dysfunction and proarrhythmia.[10]

Persistently elevated sympathetic stimulation in heart failure can cause tachycardia, increased afterload, and ventricular remodeling. Subsequent changes can lead to downregulation of beta-1 receptors at the plasma membrane. Cardiac injury can lead to sympathetic nerve death, which is followed by heterogenous nerve sprouting at scar border zones and supersensitivity of denervated regions within the myocardium. The altered myocardium becomes prone to ventricular arrhythmias in the acute and chronic phases of disease. Interestingly, changes are not limited to the heart itself, with evidence that cardiac injury can lead to changes within the stellate ganglia.[11] When parasympathetic dysfunction is present, manifestations include abnormal heart rate response with tachycardia and decreased heart rate variability, which is a marker for increased mortality.[12]

PROARRHYTHMIA

Atrial Fibrillation

Mechanisms of atrial fibrillation (AF) are complex and incompletely understood. Pulmonary vein triggers are well established as the primary target of electrophysiologic intervention and increased ectopy can be triggered by sympathetic stimulation. However, numerous other factors including atrial stretch, fibrosis, altered calcium handling, and autonomic pathology are thought to be involved to varying degrees.

The posterior left atrium is highly innervated by ganglionated plexi with parasympathetic nerves predominating. The data for the relative contribution of vagal stimulation and the ganglionated plexi to the initiation and maintenance of AF is mixed. Vagal nerve stimulation can induce AF, and there are data that injection of botulinum toxin into the fat pads where ganglionated plexi reside can decrease AF episodes. Although relative contributions of the sympathetic and parasympathetic nervous system still need to be fully elucidated, the role of the autonomic nervous system in general is clear, exemplified by the fact that in orthotopic heart transplant patients (complete cardiac denervation), AF is rare, except for patients with active graft rejection.

Ventricular Tachycardia/Ventricular Fibrillation

Parasympathetic dysfunction is associated with sudden death, and reduced heart rate variability and baroreceptor sensitivity are measurable markers of said dysfunction. However, specific data for parasympathetic dysfunction and ventricular tachycardia/ventricular fibrillation (VT/VF) are limited, whereas data for the sympathetic nervous system contributing to ventricular arrhythmias are better

defined. Elevated sympathetic afferent and efferent signaling in heart disease leads to elevated norepinephrine and neuropeptide Y release, which is associated with vasoconstriction and cardiac remodeling as well as shortening of action potential and refractory period durations.[13,14] Both right and left stellate stimulation can cause early and late afterdepolarizations, even in normal hearts.[15] Nerve death, nerve sprouting at scar border zones, and supersensitivity, as noted above, can predispose to ventricular ectopy as well as creating a substrate for reentrant arrhythmias.

INVESTIGATIONS AND DIAGNOSIS

Testing to determine autonomic function/dysfunction during health and disease is challenging. While numerous testing measures have been assessed, the sensitivity and specificity of these tests is limited and the tests are not easily incorporated into clinical practice.[16] Heart rate variability, heart rate turbulence, baroreceptor sensitivity, and heart rate recovery have been used with variable success to assess cardiac autonomic dysfunction, but they are beyond the scope of this chapter (see Chapter 61). However, certain clinical assessments can be utilized with limited additional expertise.

Orthostatic Blood Pressure

Change from a supine to standing position can lead to ½ to 1 liter of blood to pool in the lower extremities and splanchnic venous system. This pooling leads to decreased venous return and associated decreased cardiac output. Decreased return and cardiac stroke volume/output leads to decreased afferent baroreceptor activity. The subsequent decrease in parasympathetic and increase in sympathetic tone causes vasoconstriction, increased cardiac contractility, and increased heart rate, which optimizes blood pressure and most importantly protects cerebral profusion. Appropriate orthostatic blood pressure can be easily tested at the bedside. It is important to ensure the patient has been lying flat for 10 minutes before the baseline blood pressure and heart rate are established. On standing, repeat measurements should be obtained at 1, 3, and 5 minutes and correlated with any symptoms (Fig. 102.4).

Tilt table testing can be utilized to assess orthostatic tolerance and the responses are potentially increased given that lower extremity muscle tone is not utilized with tilt table testing (Fig. 102.5). The four phases of vasovagal response seen during a tilt table test are well described by Jardine and colleagues and include early stabilization in response to upright posture, circulatory instability (early presyncope), terminal hypotension, and recovery with resumption of supine posture.[17] Tilt table testing, with prolonged passive postural stress, can be assessed in isolation or with the addition of pharmacologic agents such as isoproterenol or nitrates, though these medications reduce specificity. A "positive" tilt test doesn't define the cause of a patient's syncope but simply shows that the patient has a propensity for this abnormal reflex, which as noted above effects a large percentage of the population over time.

Valsalva Maneuver

The Valsalva maneuver can also be done at the bedside with electrocardiogram, blood pressure, and ideally expiratory pressure monitoring. After baseline measurements are obtained, the patient blows into a closed system to 40 mm Hg for 12 seconds. There is an initial increase in blood pressure due to the expiratory pressure being transmitted to the intrathoracic vessels. Subsequently, there is a fall in systolic blood pressure as the venous return is diminished, as is stroke volume. The fall in blood pressure is sensed and sympathetic simulation and parasympathetic withdrawal brings the blood pressure back up toward baseline and the heart rate elevates. Ultimately, venous return is restored and blood is pumped by a sympathetically activated heart and because the circulation is vasoconstricted, leading to an elevated blood pressure, which then stimulates the baroreceptors and causes sympathetic withdrawal and slowing of the heart rate.[18]

Cold Pressor Test

The cold pressor test involves placing a supine patient's hand in ice water for 3 to 5 minutes after obtaining baseline steady state heart rate and blood pressure. Rise in heart rate and blood pressure due to vasoconstriction in skeletal muscle can be monitored and may be abnormal if autonomic dysfunction is present.

Plasma Catecholamines

Plasma catecholamines including norepinephrine, epinephrine, and dopamine can be easily measured in plasma. However, in currently available assays the utility is limited for the assessment and treatment of most autonomic disorders. Approximately 80% to 90% of norepinephrine undergoes reuptake into neurons with 10% to 20% "spillover" that can be measured. These measurements can however be useful for evaluating for neuroendocrine tumors.

NEUROMODULATORY THERAPIES

Autonomic interventions predominantly target the overactivity of the sympathetic nervous system relative to the parasympathetic.[19] Blockade of the sympathetic nervous system via pharmacologic or interventional/surgical techniques (so-called neuraxial modulation) can reduce the risk of atrial and ventricular arrhythmias and the risk of sudden death. Parasympathetic modulation is also under evaluation to treat the component of dysregulation that contributes to heart failure (see Chapter 47) and atrial (see Chapters 65 and 66) and ventricular arrhythmias (see Chapter 67).

Pharmacologic Therapy

Therapy with beta blockers, angiotensin-converting enzyme inhibitors (ACE-I), angiotensin receptor blockers (ARB), and mineralocorticoid receptor antagonists have significant beneficial autonomic effects. Beta blockers inhibit the effect of norepinephrine on beta receptors and

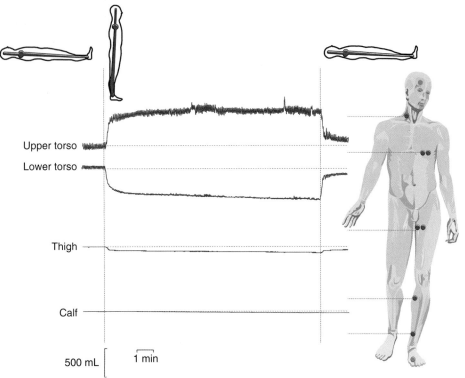

FIGURE 102.4 Orthostatic fluid shifts estimated by impedance. Change in impedance within segments of the human body during upright posture, reflecting shifts in fluid volume from the upper torso to the lower torso and to a lesser degree to the thighs. The increase in fluid in the splanchnic circulation forms the basis for considering studies of an abdominal binder to improve orthostatic tolerance in patients with orthostatic hypotension and orthostatic tachycardia. (From Robertson D, Robertson RM. Cardiovascular Manifestations of Autonomic Disorders. In Zipes DP, et al., editors. Braunwald's Heart Disease: A Textbook Cardiovascular Medicine. 11th ed. Elsevier; 2019.)

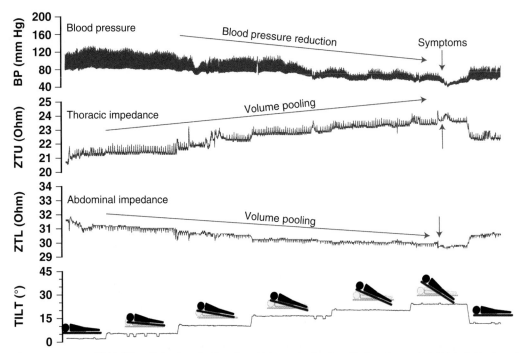

FIGURE 102.5 Impedance assessment of fluid shifts with head-up tilt. Note that with increasing head-up tilt, there is a gradual shift in fluid volume from the chest to the abdomen, reflecting pooling in the splanchnic/mesenteric circulation. Recovery of pooling begins immediately with the assumption of the supine posture. ZTU, ZTL (ohm), measure of impedance inversely related to fluid volume in the body segment referred to. (From Robertson D, Robertson RM. Cardiovascular Manifestations of Autonomic Disorders. In Zipes DP, et al., editors. Braunwald's Heart Disease: A Textbook Cardiovascular Medicine. 11th ed. Elsevier; 2019.)

help return the downregulated beta receptors to equilibrium. Additionally, they can inhibit intrinsic pacemaker currents and further reduce heart rate. Blockade of angiotensin II type I receptors inhibit norepinephrine levels, and therefore ACE-I and ARBs have benefit in treating autonomic dysregulation of heart failure when the renin-angiotensin-aldosterone system is upregulated. More extensive discussion of pharmacotherapy for heart failure and arrhythmia management are discussed elsewhere (see Chapters 50 and 64).

Sympathetic Modulation

Data for interventional and surgical autonomic modulation have predominantly been studied for arrhythmia management with limited data for heart failure (Fig. 102.6). Data are strongest for sympathetic denervation with more variable data for parasympathetic modulation to date (Table 102.2).

Thoracic Epidural Anesthesia/Percutaneous Stellate Block

Thoracic epidural anesthesia (TEA) blocks both afferent and efferent communication with the spinal cord. TEA is performed by delivering anesthetic (bupivacaine or ropivacaine) as 1 mL boluses and subsequent continuous infusion via an epidural needle to the T1-T2 or T2-T3 interspaces.

TEA has been shown to prolong myocardial refractory periods and has been utilized for the acute management of refractory ventricular arrhythmias. The largest series was reported by Do and colleagues. This was a multicenter retrospective series of 11 patients that underwent TEA for VT storm. In this series, response rate was modest, with 45% of patients demonstrating complete control of VT/VF and 9% having partial clinical benefit.[20] Clinical markers of success are limited in available data, as patients undergoing TEA did not have significant changes in blood pressure or heart rate that could be monitored for effect. However, patients that had a relative response (decreased arrhythmia burden) to general anesthesia were more likely to have further decrease in arrhythmia burden with TEA. Use of TEA may allow patients to avoid intubation/sedation or be woken from sedation to allow participation in their plan of care.

TEA cannot be utilized in the setting of anticoagulation or use of antiplatelets medications such as clopidogrel. An alternative to TEA that can be considered when anticoagulation or antiplatelets are mandatory is percutaneous stellate ganglion blockade. Stellate block can inhibit both afferent and efferent signaling at the level of the stellate ganglia. A systematic review of 38 cases demonstrated a reduction in ventricular arrhythmias and associated implantable cardioverter-defibrillator (ICD) therapies.[21] Similar to TEA, this procedure can be performed at the bedside. It is performed by injecting lidocaine or bupivacaine, using ultrasound guidance (to avoid the carotid artery or jugular vein) to target the stellate ganglia via a needle inserted in the supraclavicular region at the C6 transverse process.[22]

Renal Denervation

Renal artery denervation (RDN) of afferent and efferent nerves decreases sympathetic output to the heart and has been shown to decrease norepinephrine spillover.[23] Animal data show increased VF threshold and decreased ventricular arrhythmia burden.[24] RDN in its current clinical form (outside of studies of new technology) is performed with a standard open-irrigated cardiac ablation catheter delivering short circumferential ablation lesions within the renal arteries. More RDN-specific catheters and techniques are being evaluated.

RDN has shown promise for the management of atrial and ventricular arrhythmias as well as heart failure. The largest case series utilizing RDN for refractory ventricular arrhythmias was presented by Ukena and colleagues, who showed a significant decrease in ventricular arrhythmia burden at 1 and 3 months in 13 patients from 5 international centers.[25] RDN has also been shown to be adjunctive

to cardiac sympathetic denervation (CSD), discussed below.[26] In a series of 10 patients that had failed ablation and CSD, 6 (60%) had clinical benefit from RDN, suggesting that RDN has additional benefits even when other autonomic interventions such as CSD are unsuccessful.

RDN has been utilized to treat AF in greater numbers than for VT and has even been studied in a randomized trial (ERADICATE AF). ERADICATE AF compared ablation alone (n = 148) to ablation and RDN (n = 154) with a significant improvement in freedom from AF in the combined ablation and RDN group (72.1% versus 56.5%) at 12 months' follow-up.[27] Data from a meta-analysis further supports the benefit of RDN for the treatment of AF.[28]

Cardiac Sympathetic Denervation

Cardiac sympathetic denervation (CSD) has been shown to decrease VT/VF in various animal models and clinical series since the 1960s. CSD has been utilized for a variety of disorders including medication-refractory angina, long QT syndrome, and catecholaminergic VT, in addition to more recent data on patients with structural heart disease. CSD is performed by surgical removal of the lower one-third to half of the stellate ganglia and the T2-T4 ganglia and is most commonly performed with video-assisted thoracoscopic techniques.

CSD reduces VT inducibility and increases ventricular ARIs in a porcine model.[29] Further evidence in a canine model demonstrates reduced cardiac norepinephrine levels during ischemia and a significant reduction in VF when the heart is decentralized from the stellate ganglia and spinal cord.[30] CSD has been shown to decrease VT/VF refractory to antiarrhythmic drugs and catheter ablation in patients with structural heart disease. Vaseghi and colleagues followed initial data with intermediate and long-term results of 41 patients that underwent CSD.[31] Of the patients that underwent a bilateral approach, 48% were free of VT/VF at a mean follow-up of 367 days, but 90% had a significant overall reduction in ICD therapies. A subsequent multicenter series assessed 121 patients with a 1-year freedom from sustained ventricular arrhythmias or ICD shocks of 58%. Lower success was seen in patients with more advanced heart failure and slower VT rates.[32]

Augmentation of Parasympathetic Drive

Studies of parasympathetic stimulation for the treatment of heart failure and arrhythmia management have been mixed, and data is stronger for AF than for VT/VF. This may be due to variability in the frequencies, pulse widths, and intensities utilized in available studies that limit interpretation.[33]

Vagal Nerve Stimulation

Vagal nerve stimulation (VNS) has been shown in a porcine infarct model to stabilize electrical heterogeneity and reduce ventricular arrhythmia inducibility.[34] Low level VNS may have benefit for AF as well, with a randomized trial of low level stimulation in 54 patients that underwent cardiac surgery demonstrating a significant reduction in postoperative AF (12% versus 36%) as well as a reduction in inflammatory markers.[35] VNS trials in heart failure have shown mixed results. The ANTHEM Heart Failure trial showed improvements in ejection fraction, symptoms, and quality of life, but other studies have been negative.[36]

Tragal stimulation, via stimulation of the auricular branch of the vagus nerve, is a percutaneous method of increasing vagal tone and has shown benefit for management of AF. Low level stimulation over a 6-month period was associated with a decrease in AF burden compared with a sham control group in 52 patients with paroxysmal AF.[37]

Spinal Cord Stimulation

Spinal cord stimulation (SCS), performed by inserting electrodes in the epidural space, typically at the T2 to T4 level, can increase vagal tone and decrease sympathetic activity. SCS has shown promising

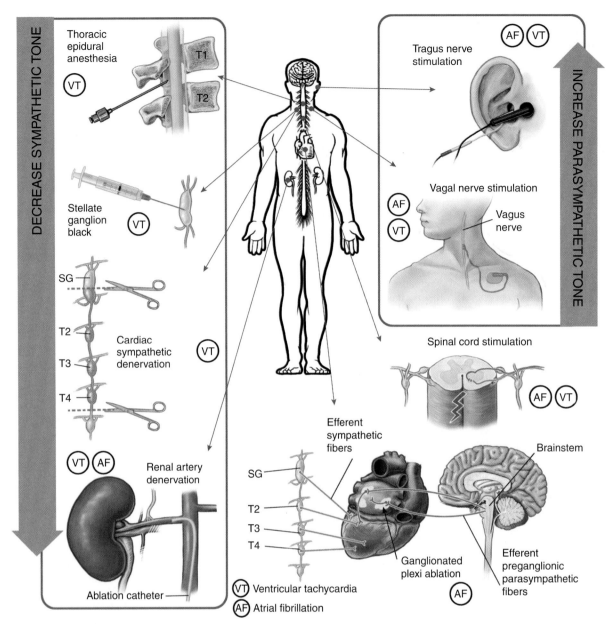

FIGURE 102.6 Schematic demonstrating options for autonomic modulation of arrhythmias. *AF,* Atrial fibrillation; *SG,* stellate ganglia; *T,* thoracic; *VT,* ventricular tachycardia. (From Zhu C, et al. Neuromodulation for ventricular tachycardia and atrial fibrillation: a clinical scenario-based review. JACC Clin Electrophysiol 2019;5:881-896.)

results in animal models with suggestion of improved myocardial function and reduced ventricular arrhythmias with prolonged ventricular refractory periods and decreased left stellate ganglia activity.[38,39] However, clinical studies such as the DEFEAT-HF study did not show significant differences in arrhythmia burden. A canine model of pacing-induced AF suggests SCS may reduce the incidence and burden of AF, but that benefit was only seen early in the disease process.[40]

Baroreceptor Stimulation

Targeting the carotid sinus baroreceptors via the placement of electrodes adjacent to the carotid bodies can increase parasympathetic afferent activity with a goal of augmenting vagal tone.[41] The Baroreflex Activation Therapy for Heart Failure (BEAT-HF) study, which utilized an implanted electrode, led to improvements in functional capacity and quality of life for patients with mild-moderate heart failure without an indication for cardiac resynchronization therapy.[42] No significant data exist to date for this method in the management of atrial or ventricular arrhythmias.

FUTURE PERSPECTIVES

Neurocardiology in general, and specifically assessing the autonomic influences during health and disease, is a growing area of basic, translational, and clinical research with a goal of clinical intervention. However, while our understanding of this complex system is progressing rapidly, there is still a remarkable amount of progress that needs to be made.

A number of autonomic disorders, including vasovagal syncope and IST, have very few efficacious treatments for a symptomatic patient population. Recent data suggest the potential benefit of ganglionated plexi ablation for neutrally mediated syncope.[43,44] Sun and colleagues assessed 57 patients who underwent cardioneural ablation and found that during 36-month follow-up, 91% remained syncope-free.

Novel concepts involving interventions on the autonomic nervous system to treat bradyarrhythmias are also gaining interest. Treatment of bradyarrhythmias (sinus node dysfunction, AV block) has largely been limited to pacemaker implantation, as these disorders were thought

TABLE 102.2 Studies of Autonomic Modulation Targeting the Sympathetic Nervous System

MODALITY	YEAR	CITATION	STUDY TYPE	N	ETIOLOGY OF CMY	TYPE OF VT	FOLLOW-UP	MAIN FINDINGS
Thoracic Epidural Anesthesia								
TEA	2017	Do et al.	Retrospective, multicenter	11	NiCMY (45%), iCMY (27%), other (28%)	VT storm: PMVT (27%), MMVT (73%)	Acute	45% complete response*, 9% partial response*, 45% no response
TEA	2010	Bourke et al.	Retrospective, multicenter	8	iCMY (50%), NiCMY (25%), other (25%)	VT storm: PMVT (37.5%), MMVT (62.5%)	6.2 ± 4.6 mo	≥80% reduction in arrhythmia burden in 6 of 8 patients
Percutaneous Sympathetic Ganglion Block								
SGB (89% Left)	2017	Meng et al.	Retrospective review	38	NiCMY (18%), iCMY (45%), unspecified (29%)	Mixed VT/VF (39%), PMVT (32%), MMVT (11%), VF (18%)	Hospital d/c (6-28 days)	83%-95% relative reduction in VA burden, 80.6% survived to hospital discharge
SGB (50% Bilateral, 50% Left)	2019	Tian et al.	Single-center case series	30	iCMY (57%), NiCMY (33%), idiopathic (7%), LQT (3%)	VT storm (40%), VT+VF storm (50%), VF storm (10%)	72 hr + f/u of 22 ± 16 mo	50% complete response^, 20% partial response^ at 72 hours post TEA. Overall 92% reduction in VA episodes (in patients with ICD)
Surgical Cardiac Sympathetic Denervation in Structural Heart Disease								
LCSD	2010	Bourke et al.	Retrospective, multicenter	9	NiCMY (22%), iCMY (22%), Sarcoid (22%), HCM (22%), ARVC (11%)	VT storm: PMVT (22%), MMVT (78%)	6.2 ± 4.6 mo	33% complete response+, 22% partial response+, 44% no response
BCSD (66%), LCSD (34%)	2014	Vaseghi et al.	Retrospective, single center	41	NiCMY (54%), iCMY (22%), HCM (7%), sarcoid (5%), other (12%)	Refractory VT or VT storm: MMVT (80%), PMVT/VF (20%)	367 ± 251 days	48% had 1-yr survival free of ICD shock after BCSD (30% after LCSD); 90% had reduction in ICD therapies
BCSD	2016	Saenz et al.	Retrospective, multicenter	75	Chagasic cardiomyopathy	MMVT	7 mo (IQR1-46)	Decrease in ICD shocks from median of 4 (range 2-30) before to 0 (range 0-2) after BCSD
BCSD (81%) LCSD (19%)	2017	Vaseghi et al.	Retrospective, multicenter	121	NiCMY (71%), iCMY (27%), mixed CMY (2%)	Recurrent VT or VT storm	1.5 ± 1.4 years	Reduction in ICD shocks from mean of 18 ± 30 in the year before to 2.0 ± 4.3 after CSD
BCSD	2019	Assis et al.	Retrospective, single center	8	ARVC	Refractory VT	1.9 ± 0.9 years	Reduction in ICD shocks/ sustained VT (12.6 ± 18.2 to 0.9 ± 1.4)
BCSD (80%) RCSD (20%)	2019	Okada et al.	Retrospective, single center	5	Cardiac sarcoidosis	Refractory VT	26 mo (IQR 5-29)	Reduction in ICD shocks from median of 5 (in the 6 months preceding CSD) to 0
Renal Sympathetic Denervation								
RDN	2014	Remo et al.	Retrospective, single center	4	iCMY (50%), NiCMY (50%)	Recurrent VT	8.8 mo (IQR 5-11)	Decrease in VT episodes from 11.0 ± 4.2 during the month pre-RDN to 0.3 ± 0.1/month post-RDN
RDN	2015	Armaganijan et al.	Prospective single center	10	Chagas CMY (60%), NiCMY (20%), iCMY (20%)	Refractory VA	6 mo (IQR 18 days, 6 mo)	Reduction in VT/VF episodes from 28.5 to 1, reduction in ICD shocks from 8 to 0
RDN	2016	Ukena et al.	Retrospective, multicenter	13	iCMY (54%), NiCMY (46%)	Refractory VAs: VF (62%), MMVT (54%), PMVT (46%)	12 mo	Reduction in VT/VF episodes from median of 21 in the month pre-RDN to 2 and 0 at 1 and 3 months post-RDN
RDN	2016	Evranos et al.	Propensity score-matched cohort	32	iCMY (62%), NiCMY (38%)	Refractory VA	15 mo (IQR 6-20)	Reduction in VT/VF/ICD therapies in RDN + ablation vs. ablation only group
RDN	2018	Jiang et al.	Prospective case series	8	DCM (63%), iCMY (25%), iCMY (12%)	VT storm or VA episodes on ICD interrogation	15 mo (IQR 6-30)	Reduction in VA episodes from 3.2 to 0.1 per mo
RDN (10% Left-sided only)	2019	Bradfield et al.	Retrospective, single center	10	NiCMY (90%), iCMY (10%)	Recurrent VT/VT storm: MMVT (70%), PMVT (30%)	23 mo	Reduction in ICD therapies (from 29.5 ± 25.2 to 7.1 ± 10.1) 6 mo pre-to 23 mo post-RDN

Continued

CARDIOVASCULAR DISEASE AND DISORDERS OF OTHER ORGANS

XI

TABLE 102.2

Follow-up is given as mean ± standard deviation or median (IQR); months, months of follow-up. *complete response, complete suppression of VT episodes (48 hours after TEA), *partial response (80% to 99% reduction in VT episodes); ^partial response not defined; +complete response = no VA within 1 week of procedure, +partial response = recurrence of VAs that did not fulfill definition of VT storm. ARVC, Arrhythmogenic right ventricular cardiomyopathy; ATP, anti-tachycardia pacing; BCSD/LCSD/RCSD, bilateral/left/right cardiac sympathetic denervation; CMY, cardiomyopathy; CPVT, catecholaminergic polymorphic ventricular tachycardia; DCM, dilated cardiomyopathy; HCM, hypertrophic cardiomyopathy; ICD, implantable cardioverter defibrillator; iCMY, ischemic cardiomyopathy; LQTS, long QT syndrome; MMVT, monomorphic ventricular tachycardia; NiCMY, nonischemic cardiomyopathy; PMVT, polymorphic ventricular tachycardia; RDN, renal sympathetic denervation; SGB, stellate ganglion blockade; TEA, thoracic epidural anesthesia; VF, ventricular fibrillation; VT, ventricular tachycardia.
From Nguyen LH, Vaseghi M. Sympathetic denervation for treatment of ventricular arrhythmias. J Atr Fibrillation 2020;13:2404.

---

to be secondary to irreversible conduction system fibrosis associated with normal aging, previous cardiac surgery (valve replacement, etc.), or other cardiac pathology (myocardial infarction, infiltrative/inflammatory cardiomyopathies). However, recent clinical evidence suggests that in at least a subset of this population cardioneural ablation, targeting specific cardiac ganglia, may increase the sinus rate and/or improve atrioventricular nodal conduction properties.[45]

With regard to primary cardiac disorders that lead to autonomic dysregulation such as myocardial infarction and/or ischemic or nonischemic cardiomyopathy, novel interventions have been developed for the treatment of cardiomyopathy and atrial and ventricular arrhythmias. As these techniques develop and as our understanding of the pathophysiology improves, many of these interventions, which are currently surgical such as CSD, will become catheter-based or even noninvasive. Additionally, while many of these procedures have shown promising results, substantial opportunity exists to optimize the techniques and to further delineate the best targets with comprehensive translational research.

REFERENCES

Overview

1. Hanna P, Rajendran PS, Ajijola OA, et al. Cardiac neuroanatomy - imaging nerves to define functional control. Auton Neurosci. 2017;207:48–58.
2. Ardell JL, Armour JA. Neurocardiology: structure-based function. Compr Physiol. 2016;6:1635–1653.
3. Dusi V, Zhu C, Ajijola OA. Neuromodulation approaches for cardiac arrhythmias: recent advances. Curr Cardiol Rep. 2019;21:32.
4. Wu P, Vaseghi M. The autonomic nervous system and ventricular arrhythmias in myocardial infarction and heart failure. Pacing Clin Electrophysiol. 2020;43:172–180.
5. Kaufmann H, Norcliffe-Kaufmann L, Palma JA. Baroreflex dysfunction. N Engl J Med. 2020;382:163–178.
6. Feigofsky S, Fedorowski A. Defining cardiac dysautonomia - different types, overlap syndromes; case-based presentations. J Atr Fibrillation. 2020;13:2403.

Pathophysiology

7. Sheldon RS, Grubb 2nd BP, Olshansky B, et al. 2015 heart rhythm society expert consensus statement on the diagnosis and treatment of postural tachycardia syndrome, inappropriate sinus tachycardia, and vasovagal syncope. Heart Rhythm. 2015;12:e41–e63.
8. Chen Z, Venkat P, Seyfried D, et al. Brain-heart interaction: cardiac complications after stroke. Circ Res. 2017;121:451–468.
9. Silvani A, Calandra-Buonaura G, Dampney RA, et al. Brain-heart interactions: physiology and clinical implications. Philos Trans A Math Phys Eng Sci. 2016;374.
10. Shivkumar K, Ajijola OA, Anand I, et al. Clinical neurocardiology defining the value of neuroscience-based cardiovascular therapeutics. J Physiol. 2016;594:3911–3954.
11. Nakamura K, Ajijola OA, Aliotta E, et al. Pathological effects of chronic myocardial infarction on peripheral neurons mediating cardiac neurotransmission. Auton Neurosci. 2016;197:34–40.
12. Sobowale CO, Hori Y, Ajijola OA. Neuromodulation therapy in heart failure: combined use of drugs and devices. J Innov Card Rhythm Manag. 2020;11:4151–4159.
13. Ajijola OA, Chatterjee NA, Gonzales MJ, et al. Coronary sinus neuropeptide Y levels and adverse outcomes in patients with stable chronic heart failure. JAMA Cardiol. 2020;5:318–325.
14. Herring N, Tapoulal N, Kalla M, et al. Oxford Acute Myocardial Infarction S. Neuropeptide-Y causes coronary microvascular constriction and is associated with reduced ejection fraction following ST-elevation myocardial infarction. Eur Heart J. 2019;40:1920–1929.
15. Yagishita D, Chui RW, Yamakawa K, et al. Sympathetic nerve stimulation, not circulating norepinephrine, modulates T-peak to T-end interval by increasing global dispersion of repolarization. Circ Arrhythm Electrophysiol. 2015;8:174–185.
16. Goldberger JJ, Arora R, Buckley U, et al. Autonomic nervous system dysfunction: JACC Focus Seminar. J Am Coll Cardiol. 2019;73:1189–1206.
17. Jardine DL, Wieling W, Brignole M, et al. The pathophysiology of the vasovagal response. Heart Rhythm. 2018;15:921–929.
18. Braunwald's Heart Disease: A Textbook of Cardiovascular Medicine. 11th ed: Elsevier.
19. Hanna P, Shivkumar K, Ardell JL. Calming the nervous heart: autonomic therapies in heart failure. Card Fail Rev. 2018;4:92–98.

Arrhythmia

20. Do DH, Bradfield J, Ajijola OA, et al. Thoracic epidural anesthesia can Be effective for the short-term management of ventricular tachycardia storm. J Am Heart Assoc. 2017;6.
21. Fudim M, Boortz-Marx R, Ganesh A, et al. Stellate ganglion blockade for the treatment of refractory ventricular arrhythmias: a systematic review and meta-analysis. J Cardiovasc Electrophysiol. 2017;28:1460–1467.
22. Fudim M, Boortz-Marx R, Patel CB, et al. Autonomic modulation for the treatment of ventricular arrhythmias: therapeutic use of percutaneous stellate ganglion blocks. J Cardiovasc Electrophysiol. 2017;28:446–449.
23. Bradfield JS, Vaseghi M, Shivkumar K. Renal denervation for refractory ventricular arrhythmias. Trends Cardiovasc Med. 2014;24:206–213.
24. Zhang WH, Zhou QN, Lu YM, et al. Renal denervation reduced ventricular arrhythmia after myocardial infarction by inhibiting sympathetic activity and remodeling. J Am Heart Assoc. 2018;7:e009938.
25. Ukena C, Mahfoud F, Ewen S, et al. Renal denervation for treatment of ventricular arrhythmias: data from an International Multicenter Registry. Clin Res Cardiol. 2016;105:873–879.
26. Bradfield JS, Hayase J, Liu K, et al. Renal denervation as adjunctive therapy to cardiac sympathetic denervation for ablation refractory ventricular tachycardia. Heart Rhythm. 2020;17:220–227.
27. Steinberg JS, Shabanov V, Ponomarev D, et al. Effect of renal denervation and catheter ablation vs catheter ablation alone on atrial fibrillation recurrence among patients with paroxysmal atrial fibrillation and hypertension: the ERADICATE-AF randomized clinical trial. J Am Med Assoc. 2020;323:248–255.
28. Atti V, Turagam MK, Garg J, et al. Renal sympathetic denervation improves clinical outcomes in patients undergoing catheter ablation for atrial fibrillation and history of hypertension: a meta-analysis. J Cardiovasc Electrophysiol. 2019;30:702–708.
29. Irie T, Yamakawa K, Hamon D, et al. Cardiac sympathetic innervation via middle cervical and stellate ganglia and antiarrhythmic mechanism of bilateral stellectomy. Am J Physiol Heart Circ Physiol. 2017;312:H392–H405.
30. Ardell JL, Foreman RD, Armour JA, et al. Cardiac sympathectomy and spinal cord stimulation attenuate reflex-mediated norepinephrine release during ischemia preventing ventricular fibrillation. JCI Insight. 2019;4.
31. Vaseghi M, Gima J, Kanaan C, et al. Cardiac sympathetic denervation in patients with refractory ventricular arrhythmias or electrical storm: intermediate and long-term follow-up. Heart Rhythm. 2014;11:360–366.
32. Vaseghi M, Barwad P, Malavassi Corrales FJ, et al. Cardiac sympathetic denervation for refractory ventricular arrhythmias. J Am Coll Cardiol. 2017;69:3070–3080.
33. Ardell JL, Nier H, Hammer M, et al. Defining the neural fulcrum for chronic vagus nerve stimulation: implications for integrated cardiac control. J Physiol. 2017;595:6887–6903.
34. Vaseghi M, Salavatian S, Rajendran PS, et al. Parasympathetic dysfunction and antiarrhythmic effect of vagal nerve stimulation following myocardial infarction. JCI Insight. 2017;2.
35. Stavrakis S, Humphrey MB, Scherlag B, et al. Low-level vagus nerve stimulation suppresses postoperative atrial fibrillation and inflammation: a randomized study. JACC Clin Electrophysiol. 2017;3:929–938.
36. Premchand RK, Sharma K, Mittal S, et al. Autonomic regulation therapy via left or right cervical vagus nerve stimulation in patients with chronic heart failure: results of the ANTHEM-HF trial. J Card Fail. 2014;20:808–816.
37. Stavrakis S, Humphrey MB, Scherlag BJ, et al. Low-level transcutaneous electrical vagus nerve stimulation suppresses atrial fibrillation. J Am Coll Cardiol. 2015;65:867–875.
38. Wang S, Zhou X, Huang B, et al. Spinal cord stimulation protects against ventricular arrhythmias by suppressing left stellate ganglion neural activity in an acute myocardial infarction canine model. Heart Rhythm. 2015;12:1628–1635.
39. Howard-Quijano K, Takamiya T, Dale EA, et al. Spinal cord stimulation reduces ventricular arrhythmias during acute ischemia by attenuation of regional myocardial excitability. Am J Physiol Heart Circ Physiol. 2017;313:H421–H431.
40. Ardell JL, Cardinal R, Beaumont E, et al. Chronic spinal cord stimulation modifies intrinsic cardiac synaptic efficacy in the suppression of atrial fibrillation. Auton Neurosci. 2014;186:38–44.
41. Wang Y, Dai M, Cao Q, et al. Carotid baroreceptor stimulation suppresses ventricular fibrillation in canines with chronic heart failure. Basic Res Cardiol. 2019;114:41.

Newer Modulating Therapies

42. Zile MR, Lindenfeld J, Weaver FA, et al. Baroreflex activation therapy in patients with heart failure with reduced ejection fraction. J Am Coll Cardiol. 2020;76:1–13.
43. Aksu T, Guler TE, Mutluer FO, et al. Electroanatomic-mapping-guided cardioneuroablation versus combined approach for vasovagal syncope: a cross-sectional observational study. J Interv Card Electrophysiol. 2019;54:177–188.
44. Sun W, Zheng L, Qiao Y, et al. Catheter ablation as a treatment for vasovagal syncope: long-term Outcome of Endocardial autonomic modification of the left atrium. J Am Heart Assoc. 2016;5:e003471.
45. Rivarola E, Hardy C, Sosa E, et al. Selective atrial vagal denervation guided by spectral mapping to treat advanced atrioventricular block. Europace. 2016;18:445–449.

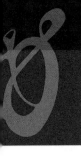

Disclosure Index

The following contributors have indicated that they have a relationship or affiliation that, in the context of their participation in the writing of a chapter for the twelfth edition of *Braunwald's Heart Disease,* could be perceived as a real or apparent conflict of interest, but they do not consider that it has influenced the writing of their chapter.

Codes for the disclosure information (institution[s] and nature of relationship[s]) are provided below.

RELATIONSHIP CODES

A—Stock options or bond holdings in a for-profit corporation or self-directed pension plan

B—Research grants

C—Employment (full or part-time)

D—Ownership or partnership

E—Consulting fees or other remuneration received by the contributor or immediate family

F—Nonremunerative positions, such as board member, trustee, unremunerated consultant, or public spokesperson

G—Receipt of royalties

H—Speakers bureau or CME lectures

INSTITUTION AND COMPANY CODES

001	4D Molecular Therapeutics
002	89Bio
003	ABBIVE
004	Abbott
005	Abbott Laboratories
006	Abbott Lantheus Medical Imaging
007	Abbott Medical
008	Abbott Vascular
009	ABBVIE
010	Abiomed
011	Acasti Pharma
012	ACC & ABIM
013	Acist
014	Acist Medical
015	Actelion Pharmaceuticals
016	Acutus Medical
017	Aetna
018	Afimmune
019	Agepha
020	Agile
021	Alexion Pharmaceuticals
022	AliveCor
023	Alkem Metabolics
024	Allegiant
025	Allergan
026	Alleviant
027	Alnylam
028	Althera
029	AM Pharma
030	Amarin
031	America's Test Kitchen
032	American Board of Internal Medicine
033	American Board of Vascular Medicine
034	American College of Cardiology
035	American College of Cardiology Foundation
036	American Heart Association
037	American Medical Association
038	American Regent

039	American Society of Nuclear Cardiology
040	Amgen
041	Ancora
042	Anthos Therapeutics
043	Anumana
044	Apnimed Inc
045	Apple
046	Applied Therapeutics
047	ARCA Biopharma
048	Arena
049	Arena Pharmaceuticals
050	Aria
051	ARIA CV
052	Arnold and Porter Law Firm
053	AstraZeneca, Inc.
054	AstraZeneca/Bristol Myers Squibb Alliance
055	Atricure
056	Attralus
057	Audentes
058	Avidity
059	AXON Therapies
060	Baim Institute
061	Barnes-Jewish Hospital Foundation
062	Bausch Health
063	Bayer Healthcare
064	Belvoir Publications
065	Beren Therapeutics
066	Beth Israel Deaconess
067	Biosense Webster
068	Biosensors
069	Biosig, Inc
070	Biotronik
071	BMS, Inc
072	Boehringer Ingelheim
073	Boston Biomedical Innovation Center
074	Boston Scientific Corporation
075	Boston Scientific Inc.

076	Boston Pharmaceuticals
077	Bracco
078	Brightseed
079	Bristol Meyers Squibb, Co.
080	BTG EKOS
081	Bunge
082	Calibrate
083	California Institute for Regenerative Medicine (CIRM)
084	Canadian Cardiovascular Society
085	Canadian Institutes of Health Research (CIHR)
086	Cantargia, Inc
087	Cardax
088	Cardiac Booster
089	Cardiac Dimensions
090	Cardiac Dimensions, Inc
091	Cardiac Phoenix
092	CardiaWave
093	Cardiol
094	Cardiology Today
095	Cardior Pharmaceuticals
096	Cardiora
097	Cardurion
098	Cardurion Pharmaceuticals
099	Caristo Diagnostics
100	Cartesian Therapeutics
101	Celladon
102	CellAegis
103	Cellprothera
104	CeloNova
105	Centre for Chronic Disease Control (New Delhi India)
106	Centre intégré universitaire de santé et de services sociaux de la Capitale-Nationale
107	CERC
108	Chiesi
109	Cine-Med Research
110	Civibiopharm

CONTRIBUTORS

Ackerman, Michael J.: E-005, G-022, G-043, G-075, E-126, E-205, E-224, E-236, G-355

Ades, Philip A.: B-251

Albert, Christine M.: B-005, B-301, E-301, B-327

Albert, Michelle: B-036, C-352

Attia, Zachi: A-022, A-148, A-260, F-186

Bairey Merz, C. Noel: B-299, E-207

Bakris, George L.: E-053, E-063, E-027, E-206, E-238, E-259, E-367, E-216

Balzer, David T.: E-005, E-145, E-236

Beckman, Joshua A.: C-040, C-063, B-079, C-211, C-210, C-258

Bers, Donald M.: E-249

Bhatnagar, Armin: B-256

Bhatt, Deepak L.: B-002, B-008, B-018, B-030, B-040, B-053, B-063, B-072, B-074, B-079, B-087, B-103, B-108, B-122, B-147, B-150, B-158, B-161, B-168, B-170, B-188, B-194, B-195, B-208, B-209, B-211, B-221, B-231, B-236, B-238, B-258, B-249, B-259, B-269, B-275, B-280, B-296, B-306, B-308, B-330, E-034, E-052, E-060, E-064, E-084, E-112, E-140, E-152, E-184, E-189, E-281, E-293, E-311, E-376, F-034, G-151,

Blankstein, Ron: B-040, E-040, G-355

Bohula, Erin A.: B-005, B-040, B-053, B-126, B-147, B-204, B-232, B-238, B-258, B-274, B-296, B-301, B-231, E-040, E-219, E-233, E-259, E-315

Bonaca, Mark P.: B-040, B-053, B-063, B-211, B-221, B-259, B-047, E-040, E-053, E-057, E-063, E-117, E-211, E-221, E-238, E-259, E-274, E-296, E-305, E-381

Bonow, Robert O.: C-257, E-037

Borlaug, Barry A.: E-213, E-050, E-238, E-258, E-150, E-259, B-256, B-234, B-118, B-053, B-240, B-333, B-179

Braunwald, Eugene: B-053, B-126, B-238, B-258, E-040, E-072, E-249, E-259, E-097, E-364

Braverman, Alan C.: F-226, G-355

Brush, John Elliot: C-313, F-143, F-032, F-034, G-131

Calkins, Hugh: E-236, E-067, B-075, E-075, E-055, E-032, E-355, E-007

Canty, John M.: B-256, B-358, E-220, E-289

Carney, Robert M.: A-274, B-251

Chandrashekhar, Y. S.: E-034

Chen, Peng-Shen: E-186

Chung, Mina K.: B-256, B-036, F-186, E-032, G-355, E-171, E-115, E-215, E-036, G-151, C-112

Cooper, Leslie T.: F-093, E-071, E-086, F-247

Creager, Mark A.: B-036, G-378, G-151, C-129, F-380

Cremer, Paul: B-258, B-217, C-322, C-217

Crestanello, Juan A.: C-228, E-236

Curtis, Anne B.: E-008, E-211, E-236, E-244, E-308, E-383

Dangas, George D.: B-008, B-074, B-276

Daubert, James P. B-005, E-005, E-067, E-070, E-074, C-140, E-383, E-373, E-160, E-243, E-277

de Lemos, James A.: B-005, E-035, E-036, E-040, E-296, B-301, E-267, E-320, C-166

Després, Jean-Pierre: C-350, C-106, B-085

Devries, Stephen: C-172

Di Carli, Marcelo F.: B-178, B-325

Dorbala, Sharmila: B-274, B-174, B-056, B-256, B-036, E-274, E-174, E-256, F-040

Duncker, Dirk J.: B-070, B-288, B-369, B-088

Ellenbogen, Kenneth A.: E-012, B-236, E-236, H-236, B-074, E-074, H-074, G-151, H-070, B-067, E-067, F-067

Everett IV, Thomas H.: B-256, C-201

Felker, G. Michael: E-005, B-036, E-048, B-063, E-072, E-079, B-040, E-040, B-125, E-125, B-238, E-236, B-249, B-251, E-258

Fleg, Jerome L.: C-251

Freedland, Kenneth E.: B-251, C-375, E-324

Friedman, Paul: G-228

Gaziano, J. Michael: B-258, E-063

Gaziano, Thomas A.: B-258, C-231, C-040, C-127, C-134, C-379

Genest, Jacques: B-085, B-165, E-238, E-258, E-294, F-084, H-040, H-306

Gillam, Linda: E-276, E-077, E-145, E-036, E-034

Giudicessi, John R.: A-182, A-274

Giugliano, Robert P.: B-040, E-040, B-042, B-126, E-126, E-239, E-030, E-034, E-053, E-072, E-079, E-121, E-124, E-150, E-157, E-178, E-182, E-211, E-221, E-274, E-303, E-304, E-314

Goldberger, Ary L.: B-151, C-066, G-321, B-251

Goldberger, Jeffrey J.: C-270, E-236

Goldhaber, Samuel Z.: B-063, B-072, B-079, B-080, B-126, B-211, B-251, E-072

Gulati, Martha: C-351

Hahn, Rebecca T.: H-008, H-145, H-276, E-008, E-074, H-145, H-276

Hasenfuss, Gerd: F-118, E-315, E-199, E-258, E-053, E-063, E-072

Herrmann, Howard C.: B-005, B-041, B-063, B-074, B-145, B-235, B-318, B-377, E-005, E-145, E-235, D-242

Herrmann, Joerg: G-151, B-250, B-228

Hershberger, Ray E.: G-355, B-251, B-252, C-261

Ho, Carolyn Y.: B-249, E-249, B-079, E-079, E-334

Hsue, Priscilla Y.: D-178, D-238

Hundley, Gregory: B-036, C-374, E-353, D-272, B-250, B-251, E-094

Inzucchi, Silvio E.: E-072, E-053, E-259, E-221, E-157, E-005, E-371, C-151, G-355, G-229

Joynt Maddox, Karen E: B-251, B-256, C-347

Kalman, Jonathan M.: B-067, B-005, B-236, H-067

Kapa, Suraj: A-069, A-346, B-005, B-075, B-211, A-148, A-332

Kern, Morton J.: H-008, H-075, H-276, H-014, H-264

Kinlay, Scott: C-358, R-132, R-256, E-114, F-033

Klein, Allan L.: B-217, E-322, E-274

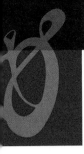

Index

Note: Page numbers followed by "f" indicate figures, "t" indicate tables, "b" indicate boxes.

A

a wave, 127–128
AAI pacing mode, 1327, 1327f
Abacavir, cardiovascular disease and, in HIV patients, 1605
ABCC9-related intellectual disability myopathy syndrome, 1869
Abciximab
  in myocardial infarction, renal dysfunction and, 1884t
  in percutaneous coronary intervention, 800.e1
  in thrombosis, 1778
Abdomen, examination of, 126
Abdominal pain, in rheumatic fever, 1535
Abdominojugular reflux, 128
Abetalipoproteinemia, 510b
Ablation, cryoballoon catheter, 1281, 1281f–1282f
Absolute benefit, 57–58
Absolute flow reserve, 620, 620f, 620.e1f
Absolute risk reduction, 58
Acarbose, in diabetes mellitus, 562t–563t, 569
Accelerated arteriosclerosis, after transplantation, 438–439, 439f–440f
Accelerated idioventricular rhythm, 1210t, 1292
  electrocardiography in, 1292, 1293f
  electrotherapy in, 1227b
  management of, 1292
Accentuated antagonism, 1178
Accessory pathways
  anatomic considerations, 1264b
  anterograde, 1217b–1218b
  arrhythmias associated with, 1266–1267
  atriofascicular, 1231b–1232b, 1268b–1270b, 1269f
  concealed *vs.* manifest, 1264b
  epidemiology of, 1264, 1264f
  localization, 1266b
  location of, 1231–1232, 1231f
  multiple, 1241f
  radiofrequency catheter ablation of, 1231–1232
  retrograde, 1217b–1218b, 1223b–1224b
  septal, 1231b–1232b
  tachycardias due to, 1264–1270
  unusual forms of, 1268.e1f, 1268b–1270b, 1269f
  WPW ECG, 1264–1266, 1264f–1266f
Accuracy, in biomarkers, 106
ACE inhibitors. *See* Angiotensin-converting enzyme (ACE) inhibitors
Acebutolol, in angina pectoris, 758t
Acetylcholine, of sinoatrial node, 1175.e1b
Acetylsalicylic acid. *See* Aspirin
Acidosis, coronary vascular resistance and, 616b–617b
Acoustic shadowing, in echocardiography, 215b–216b
Acquired atrioventricular block, 1162.e1, 1162.e3t
Acquired immunodeficiency syndrome (AIDS). *See* Human immunodeficiency virus (HIV) infection
Acromegaly, 487
  cardiovascular manifestations of, 1791–1793
  diagnosis of, 1792–1793
  treatment of, 1792b
ACTA2, 812
Actin, 892f, 893, 894f
Action potential. *See* Cardiac action potential
Action potential duration (APD)
  functional reentry and, 1187.e1f, 1185
  in heart failure, 924–925, 925.e1f
Action to Control Cardiovascular Risk in Diabetes (ACCORD) trial, 492
Active fixation leads, 1322b–1323b
Acupuncture, 593b–594b
  in hypertension, 595
Acute Addisonian crisis, 1795b

Acute aortic regurgitation, 1428–1429
  clinical presentation of, 1428–1429, 1428f, 1428b–1429b
  management of, 1428b–1429b
  pathophysiology of, 1428–1429, 1428f, 1428b–1429b
Acute aortic syndromes, 818, 818f
Acute cerebrovascular disease, 1870–1871, 1870f
Acute chest pain. *See* Chest pain
Acute coronary syndrome (ACS). *See also* Myocardial infarction
  acute heart failure and, 956b
  acute stress and, 1841
  in chronic kidney disease, 1880, 1880t–1881t
  in COVID-19 patients, 1757
  in diabetes mellitus, 571–573
  in elderly, 1696–1697
  evaluation of, 124t, 138
  magnetic resonance imaging in, 322b, 323f–324f
  marijuana use and, 1600, 1600b
  myocardial infarction, 636, 638f, 639
  non-ST elevation, 714–738, 715f
    amphetamine use and, 735
    biomarkers in, 717–718, 717f–718f, 718t–720t
    cardiac syndrome X and, 735
    chronic kidney disease and, 733b–734b
    clinical assessment of, 715–718
    cocaine use and, 735
    diabetes mellitus and, 733–734
    early risk stratification in, 735.e1
    electrocardiography in, 716–717
    epidemiology of, 714
    future perspectives in, 735, 735t
    glucose intolerance and, 733–734
    heart failure and, 734
    history of, 715
    invasive imaging of, 719
    management of, 721–732
      anticoagulant therapy in, 726–727, 735.e3
      anti-inflammatory therapies, 728
      anti-ischemic therapy in, 721–723, 723t, 735.e2
      antithrombotic therapy in, 723–726, 723f, 724t, 735.e2, 735.e4t
      bleeding and, 728
      coronary revascularization in, 735.e2
      discharge and posthospital care for, 732
      early hospital care for, 735.e1, 735.e2t
      evidence gaps in, 735.e3
      general measures in, 721
      guidelines on, 735.e1, 735.e1t
      hospital discharge in, 735.e2
      initial evaluation in, 735.e1, 735.e3f
      invasive *vs.* conservative, 728–731, 730f
      ischemia-guided strategy for, 731, 735.e2, 735.e5f
      lipid-lowering therapy in, 731–732, 732f
      performance measures and registries in, 735.e7t
      posthospital care in, 732
      risk factor modification, 735.e3
      timing of invasive approach, 731
    noninvasive testing for, 718–719, 721t
    in older adults, 732–733
    pathophysiology of, 714–715, 716f–717f, 716t
    physical examination in, 716
    Prinzmetal variant angina and, 734
    risk assessment of, 720, 722f
    risk criteria in, 735.e6t
    vasospastic angina, 734–735
    in women, 733
  OCT in, 381–382, 381f–382f
  percutaneous coronary interventions in, 787–793
  reasons for poor outcomes after, 1881–1882, 1884t–1886t

Acute coronary syndrome (ACS) *(Continued)*
  renal dysfunction as prognostic factor in, 1880–1881, 1880t–1883t, 1884f
  suspected, 293–294
  transcatheter aortic valve replacement and, 1436
  in women, 1717
Acute ischemia, electrophysiologic effects of, 1366b
Acute ischemic stroke
  management of, 879–886, 880t
    anticoagulation therapy for, 883–886, 885f
    endovascular therapy for, 881–883, 883f–884f, 884t
    intravenous recombinant tissue plasminogen activator, 880–881, 881f–883f, 881b, 882t
    other modalities for treatment of, 885b–886b
Acute kidney injury
  cardiac surgery associated, 1877–1879, 1879f
  contrast-induced, 1875–1876, 1877f–1878f
Acute limb ischemia (ALI), 854–855, 859
  clinical categories of, 854.e1t
  diagnostic tests in, 854, 854.e2t
  incidence of, 837–838
  pathogenesis of, 854, 854f
  prognosis of, 854, 854.e1f, 854.e1t
  treatment of, 854–855, 855f
Acute myocardial infarction
  cardiovascular disease and, 6–7, 6f
  influenza and, 1752
  pacemakers in
    asystole, 703
    permanent pacing in, 703
    temporary pacing in, 703
  secondary prevention after, 707–710
    anticoagulants as, 709–710, 709.e1f
    antiplatelet agents as, 708
    beta-adrenergic blocking agents as, 709
    calcium channel antagonists as, 710
    cardiac rehabilitation, 707
    depression, 707–708
    hormone therapy as, 710
    lifestyle modification, 707
    modification of lipid profile, 708
    nitrates as, 709
    nonsteroidal antiinflammatory drugs as, 710
    renin-angiotensin-aldosterone system as, 708–709
Acute pericarditis, 1616–1620
  causes of, 1616
  definition of, 1616, 1617t
  diagnosis of, 1618–1619
  differential diagnosis of, 1616
  electrocardiography in, 1616–1617, 1618f
  epidemiology of, 1616
  etiology of, 1617t
  history of, 1616
  laboratory testing in, 1616–1618
  management of, 1618–1619, 1618t–1619t, 1619f
  natural history of, 1618–1619
  physical examination in, 1616
  recurrent, 1619–1620, 1620.e1f
Acute vasospasm, 1100
Adams-Stokes attacks, 1318–1319
Adaptive design, 49–50
Adaptive immunity, in atherosclerosis, 432, 433f
Addison disease, 1795b
Adenoma
  of adrenal gland, 1794b
  of pituitary gland, 1792
Adenosine, 1211.e1t, 1208t–1210t, 1212t, 1214t, 1225, 1225b
  coronary vascular resistance and, 616b–617b
  pregnancy and, 1730f
Adenosine A₁ receptor antagonists, for acute heart failure, 971b–972b

Adenosine A$_2$ receptor agonists, as coronary vasodilators, 614b
Adenosine diphosphate receptor antagonists, in percutaneous coronary intervention, 799–800, 800.e1t
Adenovirus infection, 1080b–1081b
Adenylyl cyclase, 901–902
ADI pacing mode, reducing right ventricular pacing, 1328b, 1329f
Adipokines, in heart failure, 920.e1f, 920b–921b
Adiponectin, in heart failure, 920b–921b
Adipose tissue
  in heart failure with preserved and mildly reduced ejection, 1011b–1017b
  obesity and, 548
  visceral, as endocrine organ, 549, 550f–551f
Adiposity, causal inference for, 80
Adjunctive pharmacotherapy, in percutaneous coronary intervention, 787.e1, 787.e3t
Ado-trastuzumab Emtansine (T-DM1), 1095
ADRA2C, 1194
ADRB1, 1194
ADRB1 gene, 95t, 98
ADRB2 gene, 95t
Adrenal insufficiency, 1795b
Adrenergic inhibitors. *See* Beta adrenoceptor-blocking agents (beta blockers)
Adrenergic signaling systems, 899–903, 900t
Adrenocorticotropic hormone, 1793
Adrenomedullin, in heart failure, 920b–921b
Advanced heart failure, statins in, 517
Adventitia, 428, 428f
  in intravascular imaging, 379
AED. *See* Automated external defibrillator
Aerobic exercise
  capacity, age-associated changes in, 1687b–1690b, 1690f
  in hypertension, 595
African Americans
  heart failure in, 1001
  hypertension in, 1747t
Afterdepolarizations, 1180, 1181f
  delayed, 1180–1181, 1182f
    generation of, role of intracellular Ca^{2+}-handling abnormalities in, 1183.e1f, 1181–1183
  early, 1180, 1183
    drugs and, 1183
Afterload, 906
  abrupt increase in, 906–907
Age/aging. *See also* Older adults
  abdominal aortic aneurysm, 1709.e1
  acute coronary syndromes and, 1696–1697
  acute heart failure and, 946–947
  aortic dissection, 1709.e2
  cardiac rhythm abnormalities and, 1701–1702
  cardiovascular structure and function, associated changes in, 1687–1690, 1688f
    to exercise, 1687b–1690b, 1690f
    left ventricular, 1687b–1690b
    resting cardiac function, 1687b–1690b, 1689t
    vasculature, 1687b–1690b
  central sleep apnea and, 1679–1680
  coronary heart disease and, 1695–1696
  definition of, 1687
  epidemiology of, 25–26
  heart failure and, 933, 1697–1699
  lower extremity peripheral arterial disease and, 1709.e1
  obstructive sleep apnea and, 1679–1680
  STEMI-related mortality and, 636, 636.e1f
  sudden cardiac death and, 1352–1354, 1353f
  syncope and, 1703
  valvular heart disease and, 1699–1701
  venous thromboembolic disease and, 1702–1703, 1774
  visceral obesity and, 550
Air pollution, cardiovascular disease and, 31–37, 32f, 39.e1t
  cardiovascular effects of, 34–36, 35f
    approaches to communicate risk, 37
    arrhythmia, 36
    chronic kidney disease, 36
    diabetes, 36
    heart failure, 36
    hypertension, 35–36
    ischemic heart disease, 35
    mechanistic insights into, 36–37, 36f
    societal and personal strategies, 37
    venous thromboembolism, 36

Air pollution, cardiovascular disease and *(Continued)*
  cardiovascular mortality and, 34
  composition of, 31–34, 33t
    gaseous pollutants, 33
    household *vs.* ambient air pollution, 34
    particulate matter, 33–34
Airway, in cardiopulmonary resuscitation, 1372
Ajmaline, 1211.e1t, 1208t–1209t, 1212t, 1216, 1216b
Albiglutide, in diabetes mellitus, 562t–563t, 567
Alcohol, 535, 540t. *See also* Ethanol
Alcohol consumption, cardiovascular disease and, 459–461, 460f
Alcohol septal ablation, in hypertrophic cardiomyopathy, 1071–1072, 1075f
Alcoholic cardiomyopathy, 1041, 1593–1594
Aldosterone, 1025, 1793f, 1795b
  heart failure and, 983, 993–994
  hypertension and, 475–476
Aldosterone antagonists
  in chronic HFrEF, 1698b
  hyperkalemia due to, 988
  pregnancy and, 1730f
Aldosterone/renin ratio, 1794–1795
Alfimeprase, 1789b
Aliskiren, in heart failure, 996–997
Alkylating agents, cardiotoxic effects of, 1092t, 1094.e1
Alkylating-like agents, cardiotoxic effects of, 1092t, 1094.e1
Alleles, 73
Allen test, 386
Allergic reactions, after coronary angiography, 364b–366b
Allergy, to aspirin, 1776
Aloglipitin, in diabetes mellitus, 562t–563t, 566
Alpha adrenoceptor-blocking activity, 759.e1
Alpha-adrenergic receptor subtypes, 901
Alpha-galactosidase A deficiency, 1046
  echocardiography in, 222
Alteplase, 1788, 1788f
Alternans patterns, 171b–172b, 172f
Alternative payment models (APMs), cardiovascular disease and, 65–66
Ambrisentan, in pulmonary arterial hypertension, 1675f
Ambulatory blood pressure monitoring (ABPM), 482–483
Ambulatory electrocardiographic (Holter) recording, 1151–1153, 1154f–1155f, 1162.e2t, 1162.e3t
Ambulatory monitoring, in sudden cardiac death, 1378b–1379b
Amenorrhea, functional hypothalamic, 1710b–1714b
Amiloride, in heart failure, 983t, 984
Amiodarone, 1211.e1t, 1208t–1209t, 1212t, 1214t, 1220–1222, 1221t
  in atrial fibrillation, 1278
    in heart failure, 1002
  in chronic kidney disease, 1890t
  in pregnancy, 1730f
  thyroid function and, 1803–1804, 1804t
Amiodarone-induced thyrotoxicosis (AIT), 1803, 1804t
AMIOVERT trial, 1336t
Amlodipine, in angina pectoris, 760, 761t
Amniotic fluid embolism, sudden cardiac death and, 1363b–1365b
Amphetamines
  cardiovascular complications of, 1599, 1599b
  in non-ST elevation acute coronary syndromes, 735
Amphotericin B, in infective endocarditis, 1519b–1523b
Ampicillin-sulbactam, in infective endocarditis, 1519b–1523b
Amplatz catheters, 367, 368f
Amplatzer ASD closure device, echocardiography in, 257, 259f
Amplatzer devices, in atrial septal defects, 1589–1590, 1589f, 1590b
Amplatzer duct occluders, in congenital heart disease, 1591, 1591f
Amplatzer vascular plugs, in congenital heart disease, 1591, 1591f
Amylin mimetics, in diabetes mellitus, 562t–563t
Amyloid A, serum, in chest pain evaluation, 603b
Amyloidosis
  advanced circulatory support in, 1058b
  amyloidogenic light chain, 1052, 1058–1059
  amyloidogenic transthyretin, 1052–1053, 1059–1060, 1059t
    TTR silencers, 1060
    TTR stabilizers, 1059–1060

Amyloidosis *(Continued)*
  arrhythmia, management of, 1058b
  cardiac, 1044, 1052–1061, 1053t
    biomarkers of, 1056b
    biopsy in, 1056b
    clinical features of, 1054
    clinical management of, 1058–1060
    diagnosis of, 1055–1056, 1055f, 1057t
    epidemiology of, 1052–1053
    genotyping in, 1056b
    imaging in, 1056b, 1057f
    magnetic resonance imaging in, 326, 326f–327f
    pathophysiology of, 1053–1054
    prognosis of, 1054
  disease-targeted therapeutics for, 1058–1060
  echocardiography in, 220f, 222
  heart failure, management of, 1058b
  imaging, 284b
  organ transplantation and, 1058b
  radionuclide imaging in, 303–304, 304f–305f
  supportive non-disease-modifying therapies, 1058
Analgesics, for STEMI, 665–666
Analyses, alternative methods of, 46b–47b
Anastrozole, cardiotoxic effects of, 1092t
Andersen-Tawil syndrome (ATS), 1199, 1865, 1866f–1867f
  clinical description and manifestations of, 1199, 1200f
  electrocardiography in, 1199
  genetic basis of, 1192f, 1199b
  KCNJ2-Mediated, phenotypic correlates of, 1199
Andexanet alfa, 1786–1787, 1786t
Androgen deprivation therapy, 1092t, 1096
Anemia
  in chronic kidney disease, 1874–1875
  heart failure and, 977.e1f, 976–977
  prevalence of, 977b–978b
Anesthesia, for noncardiac surgery, 417–418, 417b–418b
  epidural, 418
  monitored anesthesia care in, 418
  regional, 418
  spinal, 418
Aneurysmal disease, atherosclerosis and, 439–440
Aneurysmectomy, left ventricular, 780.e1
Aneurysms
  aortic. *See* Aortic aneurysm(s)
  coronary artery, 749.e1
  left ventricular, 218b–219b
  sinus of Valsalva, echocardiography in, 244, 248f
Aneurysms-osteoarthritis syndrome, 811, 811t
Angina pectoris. *See also* Chest pain; Stable ischemic heart disease
  evaluation of, 123–124
  pain, mechanism of, 740.e1
  stable, 739–742
    assessment of, 740
    characteristics of, 739–740, 740.e1f
    classification of, 740
    clinical manifestations of, 739–740
    enhanced external counterpulsation for, 764.e1
    importance of pathophysiologic considerations, 742
    increased myocardial oxygen requirements and, 741–742
    nonpharmacologic treatment approaches to, 764
    pain in, 740–741
    pathophysiology of, 741–742, 741f
    percutaneous coronary intervention in, 786–787
    pharmacologic management of, 757–758, 757t
      beta adrenoceptor-blocking agents for, 757–758, 757f, 757t–758t, 760t
      calcium antagonists for, 758–760
      choice of initial therapy of, 763
      combination therapy in, 764
      integrated approach to, 764
      nitrates for, 760–762, 760.e1f, 762t
      selection of, 763–764
    physical examination in, 741
    relief of, 772
    risk models of, 749
    risk stratification in, 749
    spinal cord stimulation for, 764.e1
    transiently decreased oxygen supply and, 742
    treatment of associated diseases, 749
Angiogenesis, 628
  in plaques, 434–435, 434f
Angiographic stroke volume, 402

INDEX

I-21

Index

Femoral artery
    access complications of, 799.e1
    percutaneous technique, for cardiac catheterization, 386–388, 387f–389f
    for vascular access, 798–799
Femoral-popliteal artery disease, endovascular treatment of, 864–865, 864.e3f, 864f–865f
Fetus
    effects of warfarin on, 1785
    undernutrition effects on, 26
Fever, in STEMI, 654
18F-FDG metabolic imaging protocols, 286–288
18F-FDG PET/CT
    versus 99mTc-SPECT MPI, 311.e1f
    imaging in large-vessel vasculitis, 309f
    metabolic imaging protocols, 286–288
    to therapy in aortitis, 310f
Fiber
    dietary, 537f
    in dyslipidemia, 596b
Fibrates, 518
Fibric acid derivatives (fibrates), 518
    for coronary heart disease, 559
Fibrin, formation of, 1769–1770, 1770f
Fibrinogen, 1769–1770, 1770f
    in peripheral artery disease, 838
    serum, in STEMI, 652b
Fibrinolysis, 1766–1790
    anticoagulation with, 677
    antiplatelet therapy with, 678
    prehospital, in STEMI, 663–664
    STEMI and, 668–669
Fibrinolytic activity, vascular endothelium and, 1767
Fibrinolytic drugs, 1787–1789, 1787f
    alteplase as, 1788, 1788f
    anistreplase as, 1788
    reteplase as, 1788–1789
    streptokinase as, 1787–1789, 1787f
    tenecteplase as, 1788–1789
    urokinase as, 1788
Fibrinolytic system, 1770–1771, 1771f
Fibrinolytic therapy, effect of, 669–671, 669f–670f
    comparison of, 670, 670t, 670.e1f
    complications of, 670–671, 671f
    intracoronary fibrinolysis, 671
    late therapy, 671
    on left ventricular function, 670
Fibrinopeptide A, in STEMI, 652b
Fibroblasts, in heart failure, 928.e1f, 927f, 927b–929b
Fibroelastoma, papillary, 1832–1833, 1832.e1f
Fibromas, 1834–1835, 1834f
    echocardiography in, 253b, 253.e1f
Fibromuscular dysplasia (FMD), 488, 853, 853f, 853t
    in renal artery stenosis, 867
Fibrosis, endomyocardial, 1049
Fick method, for cardiac output measurements, 393–394, 395f
Fight-or-flight response, 899–900, 900f, 900t
Filipinos, hypertension in, 1743
Fine particles, 31–32
Finger cuffs, 483
Fingers, examination of, 126
First-degree atrioventricular (AV) block, 1315
    electrocardiography for, 1315, 1315f
Fish, 533f, 534, 540t
Fish eye disease, 513
Fish oils, 519–520
Fixed coupling, in premature ventricular complexes, 1288
Flamm's formula, 404
Flecainide, 1121.e1t, 1209t, 1212t, 1214t, 1217–1218, 1217b–1218b
    in atrial fibrillation, 1280
    in pregnancy, 1730f
Fluconazole, for infective endocarditis, 1519b–1523b
Fludrocortisone suppression test, for primary hyperaldosteronism, 485
Fluid retention, management of, in heart failure, 981–989, 982f
Fluid status, device-based therapies for management of, 989, 989b
Fluid-filled pressure systems, in pressure measurements, 392, 392.e1t
Fluoroquinolones, for infective endocarditis, from HACEK organisms, 1519b–1523b
Fluoroscopy, in pericardial effusion and cardiac tamponade, 1622

5-Fluorouracil, cardiotoxic effects of, 1092t, 1094.e1
Flutamide, cardiotoxic effects of, 1092t
Fluvastatin, in chronic kidney disease, 1883t
Focal atrial tachycardia, 1234f–1235f, 1234b–1235b, 1247–1251, 1248f–1249f
    acute management of, 1251b
    atomic distribution of, 1250–1251, 1251f
    chronic management, 1251b, 1252f
    clinical features of, 1248b
    diagnosis of, 1248–1251
    differential diagnosis of, 1248–1251
    epidemiology of, 1248b
    macroreentrant atrial tachycardia vs., 1248b–1249b
    management of, 1251b
    multifocal atrial tachycardia vs., 1248b–1249b, 1250f
Focal discharge, in atrial fibrillation, 1187
Focal fibromuscular dysplasia, 853
Focal ventricular fibrillation, 1241f
Fondaparinux, 1779t, 1782
    in chronic kidney disease, 1885t–1886t
    mechanism of action of, 1779f, 1782
    in NSTE-ACS, 727b
    in percutaneous coronary intervention, 787.e3t, 801
    pharmacology of, 1782
    in pulmonary embolism, 1646
    side effects of, 1782
Fontaine classification, of peripheral artery disease, 841, 841t
Fontan procedure, pregnancy and, 1738, 1739t
Fontan-associated liver disease, 1582
Food processing, 540–543
Foods, 532–535
Foramen ovale, patent. See Patent foramen ovale
Fosinopril, in heart failure, 991t
FOURIER (Further Cardiovascular Outcomes Research with PCSK9 Inhibition in Subjects with Elevated Risk) trial, 874b–877b
Fractional flow reserve, 619f, 621–622, 621f, 621.e1f, 621.e2f, 624f, 627f
    in percutaneous coronary intervention, 795
    in stable ischemic heart disease, 747, 765, 769f
Frailty, 1431.e1
    in elderly, 1690b–1693b
    extreme, aortic stenosis and, 1431.e1
    in physical examination, 125, 125t
Framing effects, information and, 59
Framingham Risk Score, 28, 1610
Frank-Starling effect, 895, 906
Friction rubs, in STEMI, 655
Friedreich ataxia, 1864, 1864f–1865f, 1864.e1f
Fruits, 532, 533f, 540t
Functional assessment, of pulmonary arterial hypertension, 1669
Functional reentry, 1187.e1f, 1185–1186, 1188f
Funduscopic examination, 126
Fungi, causing infective endocarditis, 1506b–1507b, 1512t
    antimicrobial therapy for, 1519b–1523b
Furosemide
    in heart failure, 982, 983t
    in pregnancy, 1730f
Fusiform aneurysm, 806–807
FXYD proteins, 1171b–1173b

G

G protein, 901, 902f
    inhibitory, 901b
    stimulatory, 901b
    third, 901b
Gadolinium-enhanced magnetic resonance angiography, for pulmonary embolism, 1644
Gallbladder disease, chest pain in, 600t
Ganglionated plexuses, 1179b
Gap junction channels, 1173–1175, 1175f
    alterations in, arrhythmias and, 1174b–1175b
    biochemical coupling and, 1173
    connexins of, 1174b–1175b
Gaseous pollutants, 33
Gastroepiploic artery, cannulation for, 367b–368b, 369f
Gastrointestinal conditions, chest pain in, 601
Gastrointestinal tract, aspirin effects on, 1775–1776
Gated blood pool scans, 284b
Gaucher disease, 1047–1048
Gender
    in acute heart failure, 946–947
    body mass index and, 24, 25f

Gender (Continued)
    hypertension and, 22–23, 22f
    obesity and, 23–24
    tobacco use and, 20–21, 21f
    total cholesterol and, 23, 24f
Gene therapy, for lipoprotein disorders, 522
General appearance, in patient evaluation, 125, 125t
Genetic architecture, 72
Genetic lipoprotein disorders, 509–510, 509t
Genetic susceptibility factors, in rheumatic fever, 1532b–1533b
Genetics
    in abdominal aortic aneurysms, 808
    in Andersen-Tawil syndrome, 1192f, 1199b
    in arrhythmogenic right ventricular cardiomyopathy, 1039b–1040b
    in atrial fibrillation, 1274
    in Brugada syndrome, 1192f, 1201b, 1202f
    in cardiac arrhythmias, 1191–1207
    of cardiovascular disease, 8
    cardiovascular medicine to
        applications of, 71–86
        translating, 72t
    in catecholaminergic polymorphic ventricular tachycardia, 1203f, 1203b
    central dogma, 71
    in dilated cardiomyopathy, 1035, 1035f–1036f
    disease risk prediction, 80–81
    DNA in, 71
    in early repolarization syndrome, 1204b
    epidemiologic associations, causal inference of, 77–80
    in familial atrial fibrillation, 1204b–1205b
    in familial hypercholesterolemia, 83
    future perspectives for, 85
    gene discovery, 75–77
        case-control studies, 75–77
        family-based studies, 75
        population-based studies of, 75–77
    genetic architecture, 72
    genetic variation in, 72–73, 72f–73f
        characterizing, 73–75, 73b–75b
    genome-wide association study for
        coronary artery disease, 77, 78f
        lipids, 76–77, 77f
    in heart failure, 921.e1f
    heritability in, 72
    human genetic variation, characterizing, 73–75, 73b–75b
    in hypertrophic cardiomyopathy, 1063, 1065t, 1066–1067, 1066f–1067f
    in idiopathic ventricular fibrillation, 1205.e1f, 1205b
    in long QT syndrome, 1191b–1193b, 1192f
    mendelian randomization principles and applications, 79–80
    next-generation technologies and therapeutics, 83–85
    on-target therapeutic side effect prediction, 82
    pathogenicity assessments and monogenic risk, 80–81, 80t
    population-based discovery of rare protein-coding variants associated
        with coronary artery disease, 77
    precision medicine, 82–83
    principles of, 71–75
    in progressive cardiac conduction disease, 1205b–1206b
    in restrictive cardiomyopathy, 1043–1044
    in short QT syndrome, 1192f, 1197b
    in sick sinus syndrome, 1206b
    in sudden cardiac death, 1354t, 1355f, 1356, 1377t
    therapeutic response prediction, 81–83
    in Timothy syndrome, 1192f, 1196b–1197b
    visceral obesity and, 550
Genome
    conceptual relationship of, 88f
    therapeutically targeting, 84–85
Genome-wide association study (GWAS), 93b–96b
Genomics, of cardiovascular disease, 8
Genotype, 71
Gentamicin, in infective endocarditis, from streptococcal species, 1519b–1523b, 1520t–1521t
Geriatric domains, pertinent to cardiovascular care, 1690–1693, 1691t
    cognitive impairment in, 1690b–1693b
    delirium in, 1690b–1693b
    disability in, 1690b–1693b

Volume 1 pp. 1-888 • **Volume 2** pp. 889-1902

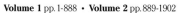